EMERY
AND
RIMOIN'S

Volume 1

Principles and Practice of

MEDICAL
GENETICS

FOURTH EDITION

Senior Advisory Editor
Alan E.H. Emery MD PhD DSc FRCPE FLS FRS(E)
Professor and Chief Medical Advisor
European Neuromuscular Centre
Department of Neurology
Royal Devon and Exeter Hospital
Exeter
UK

EMERY AND RIMOIN'S

Principles and Practice of

MEDICAL GENETICS

Volume 1

FOURTH EDITION

Edited by

DAVID L. RIMOIN MD PhD
Steven Spielberg Chairman of Pediatrics
Director, Medical Genetics Birth Defects Center
Cedars-Sinai Health System;
Professor of Pediatrics and Medicine
UCLA School of Medicine
Los Angeles, CA, USA

J. MICHAEL CONNOR MD DSc FRCP
Professor of Medical Genetics
Director, West of Scotland Regional Genetics Service
Institute of Medical Genetics
University of Glasgow Medical School
Yorkhill Hospitals
Glasgow, UK

REED E. PYERITZ MD PhD
Professor of Medicine and Genetics
Director, Division of Medical Genetics
University of Pennsylvania School of Medicine
Philadelphia, PA, USA

BRUCE R. KORF MD PhD
Medical Director, Harvard-Partners Center for Genetics and Genomics
Associate Professor of Neurology, Harvard Medical School,
Boston, MA, USA

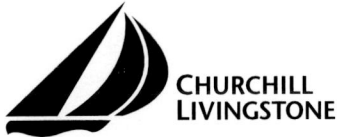

CHURCHILL LIVINGSTONE

London Edinburgh New York Philadelphia St Louis Sydney Toronto 2002

CHURCHILL LIVINGSTONE
An imprint of Harcourt Publishers Limited

First Edition © Longman Group UK Limited 1983
Second Edition © Longman Group UK Limited 1990
Third Edition © Pearson Professional Limited 1997

Fourth Edition published 2002

ISBN 0443064342

British Library Cataloguing in Publication Data
A catalogue record for this book is available from the British Library

Library of Congress Cataloging in Publication Data
A catalog record for this book is available from the Library of Congress

Note
Medical knowledge is constantly changing. As new information becomes
available, changes in treatment, procedures, equipment and the use of drugs
become necessary. The editors/authors/contributors and the publishers have
taken care to ensure that the information given in this text is accurate and
up to date. However, readers are strongly advised to confirm that the
information, especially with regard to drug usage, complies with the latest
legislation and standards of practice.

Existing UK nomenclature is changing to the system of Recommended
International Nonproprietary Names (rINNs). Until the UK names are no
longer in use, these more familiar names are used in this book in preference to
rINNs, details of which may be obtained from the
British National Formulary.

The
publisher's
policy is to use
**paper manufactured
from sustainable forests**

Printed in China by the RDC Group

Commissioning Editor: Michael J. Houston
Project Development Manager: Sheila Black
Project Manager: Cheryl Brant
Designer: Sarah Russell
Illustrations Manager: Mick Ruddy
Illustrator: Robin Dean

Contents

Contents

Contents

Contributors

David Aitken BSc MIBiol PhD FRCPath
Head of Biochemical Genetics, Institute of Medical Genetics, University of Glasgow Medical School, Yorkhill, Glasgow,UK

Judith Allanson MB ChB FRCP FRCP(C) FCCME FABMG
Professor of Pediatrics, University of Ottawa; Head, Clinical Section, Genetics Patient Service Unit, Children's Hospital of Eastern Ontatio, Ottawa, Canada

Chester Alper MD
Professor of Pediatrics, Harvard Medical School, The Center for Blood Research, Boston, MA, USA

Joanna Amberger BA
Data Curator, McKusick-Nathans Insitiue of Genetic Medicine, The John Hopkins University School of Medicine, Baltimore, MD, USA

Niall Anderson BSc PhD
Lecturer in Statistical Genetics, Department of Medicine and Therapeutics, University of Glasgow, Western Infirmary, Glasgow, UK

Karl Anderson MD
Professor, Department of Preventive Medicine and Community Health, Internal Medicine, Pharmacology and Toxicology, University of Texas Medical Branch, Galveston, TX, USA

Ingrun Anton-Lamprecht DSc
Professor and Former Director, Ultrastructure Research of the Skin, Department of Dermatology, Faculty of Medicine, Ruprecht-Karls University Heidelberg, Germany

Stylianos Antonarakis MD DSc
Professor and Director of Medical Genetics, Medical Genetics Division, University of Geneva Medical School and University Hospitals, Geneva, Switzerland

Reynir Arngrimsson MD CMCh PhD
Associate Professor of Clinical Genetics, Unit of Medical Genetics, University of Iceland; Chief Scientific Officer, Iceland Genomics Corporation, Reykjavik, Iceland

Veronique Arnould-Devuyst MD
Department of Opthalmology, Clinique Europe – St Michel, Brussels, Belgium

Kenneth Astrin PhD
Associate Professor of Human Genetics, Department of Human Genetics, Mount Sinai School of Medicine of NYU, New York, NY, USA

David Avram MD
Resident of Dermatology, Harvard Medical School, Massachusetts General Hospital, Wang Ambulatory Center, Boston, MA, USA

Felicia Axelrod MD
Carl Seaman Professor of Dysautonomia Treatment and Research, Department of Pediatrics; Professor of Neurology, New York University School of Medicine, New York, NY, USA

Howard P Baden MD
Professor of Dermatology, Harvard Medical School; Dermatologist, Massachusetts General Hospital; Senior Associate for Academic Affairs, Cutaneous Biology Research Centre, Charleston, MA, USA

Gregory S Barsh MD PhD
Associate Professor of Pediatrics and of Genetics, Department of Pediatrics, Stanford University, Stanford, CA, USA

Peter G. Barth MD PhD
Professor, Department of Pediatric Neurology, Emma Children's Hospital - AMC, University of Amsterdam, Amsterdam, The Netherlands

J B Bateman MD
Chair and Professor, Department of Opahthalmology, University of Colorado School of Medicine, Denver, CO, USA

David MW Beeson MA PhD
MRC Senior Non-Clinical Fellow, Neurosciences Group, Department of Clinical Neurology , Weatherall Insitute of Molecular Medicine, University of Oxford, Oxford, UK

Peter Beighton MD PhD, FRCP, FRCPCH, FRSSA
Emeritus Professor of Human Genetics, Faculty of Health Sciences, University of Cape Town, Cape Town, South Africa

Phillip Bennett BSc PhD MD FRCOG
Professor of Obstetrics & Gynaecology, Institute of Reproductive and Developmental, Biology, Imperial College School of Medicine, London, UK

Merrill Benson BA MS MD
Professor of Pathology and Laboratory Medicine, Professor of Medicine, Donald Merritt Professor of Medicial Genetics, Professor of Medical and Molecular Genetics, Neuropathology Division, Department of Pathology and Laboratory Medicine, Indiana University School of Medicine, Indianapolis, IN, USA

Katherine L Bergwerk MD
Attending, Cedars-Sinai Medical Centre, Los Angeles, Clinical Faculty, Jules Stein Eye Institute, UCLA School of Medicine, Los Angeles, CA, USA

Wade Berrettini MD PhD
The Karl E Rickels Professor of Psychiatry; Director, Centre for Neurology and Behavioral Sciences, University of Pennsylvania, Philadelphia, PA, USA

Wilma B Bias PhD
Professor Emerita, Department of Medicine, Division of Medical Genetics, Johns Hopkins School of Medicine and Department of Epidemiology, Johns Hopkins University School of Hygiene and Public Health, Baltimore, MD, USA

Donald M Black PhD BSc
Research Group Leader, Department of Cancer and Molecular Genetics, Beatson Institute for Cancer Research, Wolfson Laboratory for Molecular Pathology, Bearsden, Glasgow, UK

Eugene R Bleecker MD
Professor, Director of Centre for Human Genetics, Wake Forest University, Winston-Salem, NC, USA

Cornelius Boerkoel III MD PhD
Assistant Professor, Department of Molecular and Human Genetics, Baylor College of Medicine, Houston, TX, USA

Richard Boland MD
Professor of Medicine, Chief, Division of Gastroenterology, Department of Medicine, University of California School of Medicine, San Diego, La Jolla, CA, USA

Christopher L Bowlus MD
Assistant Professor of Internal Medicine, Division of Gastroenterology, Department of Internal Medicine, University of California Davis Medical Center, Sacramento, CA, USA

Michael Brown PhD
Assistant Professor, Department of Genetics and Molecular Medicine, Emory University of Medicine, Atlanta, GA, USA

Matthew Brown MD FRACP
Head of Spondyloarthritis and Bone Disease, Arthritis Research Campaign Senior Fellow, Wellcome Trust Centre for Human Genetics, Oxford, UK

John Burn MD FRCP FRCPCH FRCOGFMedSci
Professor of Clinical Genetics, Institute of Human Genetics, University of Newcastle upon Tyne, Newcastle upon Tyne, UK

Kate Bushby MB CHB MSc MD FRCP
Professor of Neuromuscular Genetics; Consultant Clinical Geneticist, Institute of Human Genetics, International Centre for Life, Newcastle upon Tyne, UK

Peter Byers MD
Professor, Department of Pathology and Division of Medical Genetics, Department of Medicine, University of Washington School of Medicine, Seattle, WA, USA

Janet Carter MRCPsych PhD
MRC Clinician Scientist Fellow, Honorary Senior Lecturer in Neuroscience and Consultant in Old Age Psychiatry, The Maudsley Hospital Trust and Institue of Psychiatry, Kings College, London, UK

Angela Carter BSc PhD
University Research Fellow, Academic Unit of Molecular Vascular Medicine, Research School of Medicine, Leeds General Infirmary, Leeds, UK

Lawrence W Castellani PhD
Associate Researcher, Department of Medicine - Cardiology, University of California Los Angeles, Los Angeles, CA, USA

Stephen Cederbaum MD
Professor, Departments of Psychiatry and Pediatrics/
Genetics; Chief, Division of Genetics, Department of
Pediatrics, University of California, Los Angeles;
Consultant in Metabolic Disorders, Southern California
Kaiser-Permanente, Los Angeles, CA, USA

Barton Childs MD
Professor Emeritus, Department of Pediatrics, The Johns
Hopkins University School of Medicine, Baltimore, MD,
USA

Mahesh Choolani MB BS MRCOG
Research Fellow, Maternal & Fetal Medicine Department,
Imperial College School of Medicine, Queens Charlotte's
Hospital Campus, London, UK

Namita Chowdhury PhD
Professor of Medicine and Molecular Genetics, Marion Bessin
Liver Center, Albert Einstein College of Medicine, NY, USA

Jayanta Chowdhury MD MRCP
Professor of Medicine and Molecular Genetics; Director,
Gastroenterology and Liver Diseases, Jack and Pearl
Resnick Campus; Director, Genetic Engineering Core
Laboratory, Marion Bessin, Liver Research, Marion Bessin
Liver Center, Albert Einstein College of Medicine, New
York, NY, USA

Thomas Chu MD PhD
Associate Director, Pharmacogenomics, Genset Corporation,
La Jolla; Assistant Clinical Professor of Pediatrics (voluntary),
University of California, San Diego, CA, USA

Robin D Clark MD
Head of Cancer Genetics Unit, Associate Professor of
Pediatrics, USC School of Medicine, Norris Cancer
Hospital, University of Southern California, Los Angeles,
CA, USA

Angus Clarke DM FRCP FRCPCH
Professor and HonoraryConsultant Clinical, Geneticist,
Department of Medical Genetics, University of Wales
College of Medicine, Cardiff, UK

Jill Clayton-Smith MBChB MRCP MD
Consultant Clinical Geneticist, Department of Medical
Genetics, St Mary's Hospital, Manchester, UK

**M Cohen BA, DMD, MSD, MCRCD (C), Cert IH,
MPH, PhD, FCCMG**
Professor of Oral & Maxillofacial Pathology, Pediatrics,
Community Health & Epidemology, Health Services
Administration, and Sociology & Social Anthropology,
Department of Oral and Maxillofacial Pathology, Dalhousie
University, Nova Scotia, Canada

David Cole MD PhD FCCMG FRCPC FACMG
Professor, Departments of Laboratory Medicine &
Pathology, Medicine and Pediatrics (Genetics), University
of Toronto; Director, Toronto General Hospital Genetic
Repository, University Health Network, Toronto, Canada

Michael Connor MD DSc FRCP
Professor of Medical Genetics, Director, West of Scotland
Regional Genetics Service, Institute of Medical Genetics,
University of Glasgow Medical School, Yorkhill Hospitals,
Glasgow, UK

Jackie Cook BA MB BS FRCP
Consultant Clinical Geneticist, North Trent Clinical
Genetics Service, Department of Clinical Genetics,
Sheffield Children's Hospital, Sheffield, UK

David N Cooper BSc PhD
Professor of Human Molecular Genetics, Institute of
Medical Genetics, University of Wales College of Medicine,
Cardiff, UK

Pierre Corvol MD
Professor of Medicine, Collège de France, Laboratoires
de Médecine Expérimentale, INSERM, Unité 36, Paris,
France

Edward Cotlier MD MSc (Hon. Yale)
Research Scientist, New York State Institute for
Developmental Disabilities, Staten Island, New York;
Former Chief of Division, Ophthalmic Genetics, Yale
University, New Haven, CT, USA

Donnell Creel PhD
Director, Electrophysiology Service, Department of
Opthalmology, University of Utah School of Medicine, Salt
Lake City, UT, USA

Jennifer A Crossley BSc PhD
Principal Scientist, Institute of Medical Genetics, University
of Glasgow Medical School, Yorkhill, Glasgow, UK

Garry Cutting MD
Professor, Pediatrics and Medicine, Institute for Genetic Medicine, Johns Hopkins University, School of Medicine, Baltimore, MD, USA

Stephen Daiger PhD
Professor of Medical Genetics, Human Genetics Center, School of Public Health, Houston, TX, USA

Alvin E Davis III MD
Senior Investigator, The Center for Blood Research, Harvard School of Medicine, Boston, MA, USA

Samir Deeb PhD
Research Professor of Medicine and Genetics, Genetics Department, University of Washington School of Medicine, Seattle, WA, USA

J Depaulo MD
Professor of Psychiatry, Department of Psychiatry, Johns Hopkins University School of Medicine, Baltimore, MD, USA

Robert Desnick MD PhD
Professor and Chairman, Department of Human Genetics, Mount Sinai School of Medicine of New York University, New York, NY, USA

Martin Dichgans PD, Dr.Med.
Neurologische Klinik, Klinikum Grosshadern, Ludwig Maximilians University, Munich, Germany

Sandra Disse-Nicodème PhD
Graduate Student, INSERM Unit 36, Collège de France, Paris, France

Anna Dominiczak MD FRCP FMedSci
BHF Professor of Cardiovascular Medicine, Department of Medicine and Therapeutics, Gardiner Institute, University of Glasgow, Glasgow, UK

Dian Donnai MB BS FRCP FRCOG
Professor, Department of Medical Genetics, St Mary's Hospital, Manchester, UK

Patricia Donohoue MD
Associate Professor, Division of Pediatrics, Endocrinology & Diabetes, University of Iowa Hospital & Clinics, Iowa City, IA, USA

Alysa Doyle PhD
Director of Neuropsychology, Clinical & Research Program in Pediatric Psychopharmacology, Massachusetts General Hospital; Instructor in Psychiatry, Harvard Medical School, Boston, MA, USA

Victor Dubowitz MD PhD FRCP FRCPCH
Emeritus Professor of Paediatrics, Dubowitz Neuromuscular Centre, Department of Paediatrics, Imperial College School of Medicine, Hammersmith Campus, London, UK

Sherman Elias MD
Professor and Head of Obstetrics and Gynecology, Professor of Molecular Genetics, Department of Obstetrics and Gynecology, University of Illinois at Chicago, Chicago, IL, USA

Frances Elmslie MB ChB MD MRCP
Consultant Clinical Geneticist, Department of Clinical Genetics, Guy's and St Thomas' NHS Trust, London, UK

Beverly Emanuel PhD
The Charles EH Upham Professor of Pediatrics, University of Pennsylvania School of Medicine, Chief, Division of Human Genetics and Molecular Biology, The Children's Hospital of Philadelphia, Philadelphia, PA, USA

Alan Emery MD, PhD, DSc, FRCP, FRCPE, FLS, FRSE
Professor & Chief Scientific Advisor, European Neuro-Muscular Centre, Department of Neurology, Royal Devon & Exeter Hospital, Exeter, UK

Charles J Epstein MD
Professor, Department of Pediatrics, University of California School of Medicine, San Francisco, CA, USA

Richard W Erbe MD
Chief, Division of Genetics, The Children's Hospital of Buffalo, Professor of Pediatrics and Medicine, School of Medicine and and Biomedical Sciences, State University of New York at Buffalo, NY, USA

Henry Erlich PhD
Director, Department of Human Genetics and Vice President, Discovery Research, Roche Molecular Systems Inc, Alameda CA, USA

Rena E Falk MD
Professor, Department of Pediatrics, University of California Los Angeles School of Medicine; Director, Prenatal Diagnosis Center, Associate Director Cytogenetics Laboratory, Medical Genetics Birth Defects Centre, Cedars-Sinai Medical Center, Los Angeles, CA, USA

Stephen V Faraone PhD
Associate Professor, Department of Psychiatry, Harvard Medical School, Boston, MD, USA

Malcolm Ferguson-Smith MB, ChB, FRCPath, FRCP(Glas), FMedSci, FRSE, FRS
Emeritus Professor of Pathology, Department of Clinical Veterinary Medicine, Centre for Veterinary Science, Cambridge, UK

Robert E Ferrell PhD
Professor, Department of Human Genetics, University of Pittsburgh Graduate School of Public Health, Pittsburgh, PA, USA

John K Fink MD
Associate Professor, Department of Neurology, University of Michigan, Ann Arbor, Director, Neurogenetic Disorders Clinic, MI, USA

Nathan Fischel-Ghodsian MD
Professor of Pediatrics, Department of Pediatrics, University of California, Cedars-Sinai Medical Center, Los Angeles, CA, USA

Delbert A Fisher MD
Professor Emeritus, Department of Pediatrics and Medicine, UCLA School of Medicine; Vice President, BP Science and Innovation, Quest Diagnostics Inc., San Juan Capistrano, CA, USA

Tatiana Foroud PhD
Assistant Professor, Department of Medical and Molecular Genetics, and Psychiatry, Indiana University School of Medicine, Indianapolis, IN, USA

Ragini Fredrich MD
Pediatrics and Nephrology Department of Pediatrics, University of Nevada School of Medicine, Las Vegas, NV, USA

Jan M Friedman MD PhD
Professor of Medical Genetics, Department of Medical Genetics, University of British Columbia, Vancouver, British Columbia, Canada

Mark R Gardiner MD FRCP
Professor of Paediatrics, Department of Paediatrics and Child Health, Royal Free and University College Medical, School, University College of London, London, UK

Jozef Gecz PhD
Senior Medical Scientist, Department of Cytogenetics and Molecular, Genetics, Women's and Children's Hospital, Senior Lecturer, Department of Paediatrics, University of Adelaide, Adelaide, South Australia, Australia

Tobias Gedde-Dahl Jr MD
Professor, Institute of Forensic Medicine, University of Oslo, Rikshospitalet, Oslo, Norway

Jeffrey W Gilger PhD
Director, Human Biology Program, University of Kansas, Lawrence, KA, USA

Anne-Paul Gimenez-Roqueplo MD PhD
Assistant Hospitalo-Universitaire, Département de Génétique, Hôpital Européen Georges Pompidou, Paris, France

David Ginsburg MD
Warner-Lambert/Parke-Davis Professor of Medicine; Investigator, Howard Hughes Medical Institute, Department of Internal Medicine and Human Genetics, University of Michigan Medical Center, Ann Arbor, MI, USA

Bertil Glader MD PhD
Professor of Pediatrics (Hematology / Oncology), Associate Dean for Continuing Medical Education, Stanford University School of Medicine, Stanford, CA, USA

Lowell Goldsmith MD
Professor of Dermatology, Dean Emeritus, Dermatology Department, Rochester University, Rochester, NY, USA

Stephen I Goodman MD
Professor, Department of Pediatrics, University of Colorado School of Medicine, Denver, CO, USA

Judith Goodship BSc, MBChB, MRCP(UK). MD. FRCP(UK)
Institute of Human Genetics, University of Newcastle upon Tyne, Newcastle-Upon-Tyne, UK

Ora Karp Gordon MD MS
Fellow in Medical Genetics, Cedars-Sinai Medical Center, Los Angeles, CA, USA

Gail E Graham MD, MSc, FRCPC, FCCMG
Assistant Professor of Medical Genetics, University of Calgary; Clinical Geneticist, Alberta Children's Hospital, Calgary, Alberta, Canada

John Graham MD ScD
Professor of Pediatrics, UCLA School of Medicine; Director of Clinical Genetics and Dysmorphology, Department of Pediatrics, Cedars-Sinai Medical Center, Los Angeles, CA, USA

Peter J Grant MD FRCP
Professor of Molecular Vascular Medicine, Honorary Consulant Physician, Academic Unit of Molecular and Vascular Medicine, Leeds General Infirmary, Leeds, UK

Wayne Grody MD PhD
Professor, Division of Medical Genetics and Molecular Pathology; Director, Diagnostic Molecular Pathology Laboratory, Departments of Pathology & Laboratory Medicine and Pediatrics, UCLA School of Medicine, Los Angeles, CA, USA

Jeffrey R Gruen MD
Associate Professor, Department of Pediatrics, Yale Child Health Research Center, Yale University School of Medicine, New Haven, CT, USA

Daniel J Gruskin MD
Medical Genetics Birth Defects Center, Cedars-Sinai Medical Center, Los Angeles, CA, USA

Gunnar Gundmundsson MD PhD
Staff Physician, Landspitali University Hospital, Department of Biochemistry and Molecular Biology, University of Iceland, Faculty of Medicine, Reykjavik, Iceland

Bevra H Hahn MD
Professor and Chief, Department of Medicine, Division of Rheumatology, University of California Los Angeles School of Medicine, Los Angeles, CA, USA

Judith Hall OC MD FRCP(C) FAAP FCCMG FABMG
Professor and Head, Department of Pediatrics, University of British Columbia, British Columbia Children's Hospital, Vancouver, British Columbia, Canada

James W Hanson MD
Senior Advisor for Medical Genetics and Acting Chief, Clinical and Genetic Epidemiology Research Branch, Division of Cancer Control and Population Sciences, National Cancer Institute, National Institutes of Health, Bethesda, MD, USA

Peter S Harper MD FRCP
Professor of Medical Genetics, University of Wales College of Medicine, Consultant Physician and Clinical Geneticist, University Hospital of Wales, Cardiff, UK

Michael Hayden MB ChB PhD FRCP(c) FRSC
Director and Senior Scientist, Center for Molecular Medicine and Therapeutics; Professor, Department of Medical Genetics, University of British Columbia, Vancouver, British Columbia, Canada

Vincent J Hearing PhD
Chief, Pigment Cell Biology Section, Laboratory of Cell Biology, National Institutes of Health, Bethesda, MD, USA

John Heckenlively MD
Underwood Professor of Ophthamology, Jules Stein Institute, UCLA, Los Angeles, CA, USA

Geoffrey N Hendy BSc PhD
Assistant Director, Calcium Research Laboratory, Royal Victoria Hospital; Professor of Medicine, McGill University Faculty of Medicine, Montreal, Quebec, Canada

Afif Hentati MD
Fellow, Department of Neurology, Northwestern University Medical School, Chicago, IL, USA

Hugo SA Heymans MD PhD
Professor of Pediatrics, Chair, Emma Children's Hospital/Academic Medical Centre, Amsterdam, The Netherlands

Harry R Hill MD
Professor of Pathology Pediatrics and Medicine; Head, Division of Clinical Pathology, University of Utah Medical Center, Salt Lake City, UT, USA

Richard Hillman MD
Professor of Child Health and of Biochemistry, Director of Metabolic Genetics, University of Missouri-Columbia, Columbia, MO, USA

Kurt Hirschhorn MD
Professor of Pediatrics, Human Genetics and Medicine, Mount Sinai School of Medicine, New York, USA

Rochelle Hirschhorn MD
Professor of Medicine, Department of Medicine, New York University School of Medicine, NY, USA

Susan Hodge DSc
Professor, Psychiatry and Biostatistics, Columbia University, New York, NY, USA

William Horton MD
Professor of Molecular & Medical Genetics, Oregon Health Sciences University; Director of Research, Shriners Hospital, Portland, OR, USA

Gary Hunninghake MD
Sterba Professor Medicine; Director, Division of Pumonary, Critical Care and Occupational Medicine, Department of Internal Medicine, University of Iowa College of Medicine and Veterans Administration Medical Center, Iowa City, IA, USA

Susan M Huson MD FRCP
Consultant Clinical Geneticist, Oxford Radcliffe Hospitals; Honorary Senior Clinical Lecturer, Nuffield Department of Medicine, University of Oxford, Oxford, UK

Sherwin Isenberg MD
Professor of Pediatrics and Ophthalmology; Vice-chairman, Jules Stein Eye Institute, UCLA School of Medicine, Los Angeles, CA, USA

Boris Ivandic MD
Professor of Medicine, Department of Medicine II, University of Luebeck, Luebeck, Germany

Ethylin Wang Jabs MD
Dr Frank V. Sutland Professor of Pediatric Genetics, Professor of Pediatrics, Medicine, and Plastic, Surgery, Johns Hopkins University, Baltimore, MD, USA

Hannu Jalanko MD PhD
Head, Department of Pediatric Nephrology and Transplantation, Hospital for Children and Adolescents, University of Helsinki, Helsinki, Finland

Henry Jampel MD MHS
Associate Professor, Department of Opthalmology, Johns Hopkins University School of Medicine, Baltimore, MD, USA

Xavier Jeunemaitre MD PhD
Professor of Genetics, Departement de Génétique, Hôpital Européen Georges Pompidou, Paris, France

Kenneth Jones MD
Professor of Pediatrics, Department of Pediatrics, University of California, San Diego, CA, USA

Marilyn C Jones MD
Adjunct Professor, Department of Pediatrics, University of California San Diego, Director, Dysmorphology and Genetics, Children's Hospital, San Diego, CA, USA

Stanley C Jordan MD
Professor of Pediatrics, Medical Director, Renal Transplantation and Transplant Immunology; Director, Pediatric Nephrology, UCLA School of Medicine, Los Angeles, CA, USA

Lucia F Jorge-Nebert BPharm PhD
Professor, Faculty of Pharmacy; Associate Director, DNA and Human Genomics Institute, University of Panama, Panama, Republic of Panama

Anne Joutel MD PhD
Chargée de Recherche, INSERM EPI 99 21 , Faculté de Médecine Lariboisière, Paris, France

Helena Kaariainen MD PhD
Director, Department of Medical Genetics, The Family Federation of Finland, Helsinki, Finland

Michael Kaback MD
Professor of Pediatrics and Reproductive Medicine, University of California San Diego School of Medicine, San Diego, CA, USA

Ajith Kadakol MD
Research Associate, Marion Bessin Liver Centre, Albert Einstein College of Medicine, New York, NY, USA

Elaine S Kamil MD
Associate Director Pediatric Nephrology, Professor of Pediatrics, Department of Pediatrics, Cedars-Sinai Medical Center, Los Angeles, CA, USA

Hooshang Kangarloo MD
Professor of Radiology & Pediatrics, University of California at Los Angeles, Los Angeles, CA, USA

Bronya JB Keats PhD
Professor and Acting Head, Department of Biometry and Genetics, Director, Center for Molecular and Human Genetics, Louisiana State University Health Sciences Center, New Orleans, LA, USA

Richard A King MD PhD
Professor of Medicine, Department of Medicine and Institute of Human Genetics, University of Minnesota, Minneapolis, MN, USA

Helen M Kingston MD FRCP DCH
Consultant Clinical Geneticist, Regional Genetic Service, St Mary's Hospital, UK

Dennis K Kinney PhD
Director, Genetic Laboratory, McLean Hospital, Belmont, MA; Assistant Professor of Psychology, Department of Psychiatry, Harvard Medical School, Boston, MA, USA

Yuri N Kobzev MD PhD
Fellow, Section of Haematology/Oncology, Department of Medicine, University of Chicago Medical Center, Chicago, IL, USA

Julie R Korenberg PhD MD
Vice Chair of Pediatrics for Research, Cedars-Sinai Medical Center; Geri & Richard Brawerman Chair of Molecular Genetics, Medical Genetics Birth Defects Center; Professor of Pediatrics and Human Genetics, University of California at Los Angeles, Los Angeles, CA, USA

Bruce R Korf MD PhD
Medical Director, Harvard-Partners Center for Human Genetics and Genomics; Associate Professor of Neurology, Harvard Medical School, Boston, MA, USA

Deborah Krakow MD,
Department of Obstetrics & Gynecology, Medical Genetics Birth Defects Center, Cedars-Sinai Medical Center, Los Angeles, CA, USA

Michael Krawczak PhD
Professor of Mathematical Genetics, Institute of Medical Genetics, University of Wales College of Medicine, Cardiff, UK

Berry Kremer MD PhD
Professor of Clinical Neurology, Department of Neurology, UMC Nijmegen, Netherlands

Ralph S Lachman MD
Professor of Radiology and Pediatrics, UCLA School of Medicine Los Angeles; Co-Director, International Skeletal Dysplasia Registry, Los Angeles, CA , USA

Wayne W K Lam MBChB MRCP
Consultant in Clinical Genetics, Clinical Genetics Department, Western General Hospital, Edinburgh, UK

Lawrence C Layman MD
Chief, Section of Reproductive Endocrinology, Infertility & Genetics, Department of Obstetrics and Gynecology, Developmental Biology Program, The Institute of Molecular Medicine and Genetics, The Medical College of Georgia, Augusta, GA, USA

Anna-Elina Lehesjoki MD PhD
Senior Fellow, Folkhalsan Institute of Genetics and Deparment of Medical Genetics, Academy of Finland, Helsinki, Finland

Frank Lehmann-Horn MD
Professor and Chair, Department of Applied Physiology, University of Ulm, Ulm, Germany

Jules G Leroy MD PhD
Emeritus Professor of Pediatrics & Medical Genetics, Ghent University Medical School, Ghent, Belgium

Michael A Levine MD
Professor of Pediatrics, Medicine and Pathology; Director, Division of Pediatric Endocrinology, Department of Pediatrics, Johns Hopkins University School of Medicine, Baltimore, MD, USA

Harvey L Levy MD
Senior Associate in Medicine/Genetics, The Children's Hospital, Boston; Associate Professor of Pediatrics, Harvard Medical School, Boston, MA, USA

Amy Feldman Lewanda MD
Medical Geneticist, Inova Fairfax Hospital for Children; Clinical Associate Professor of Pediatrics, University of Virginia, Clinical Assistant Professor of Pediatrics, George Washington University, Washington, DC, USA

Inge Liebaers MD PhD
Chairman & Professor, Centre for Medical Genetics, University Hospital, Dutch-Speaking Brussels Free University, Brussels, Belgium

Willy Lissens PhD
Head of Molecular Genetics Laboratory, Centre for Medical Genetics, University Hospital, Dutch Speaking Brussels Free University, Brussels, Belgium

Marie T Lott MA
Research Specialist Supervisor, Center for Molecular Medicine, Emory University School of Medicine, Atlanta, GA, USA

James R Lupski MD PhD FAAP FACMG FAAAS
Cullen Professor of Molecular and Human Genetics, Professor of Pediatrics and Director, Medical Scientist Training Program, Department of Molecular and Human Genetics, Baylor College of Medicine, Houston, TX, USA

Aldon J Lusis PhD
Professor, Department of Medicine, Department of Microbiology and Molecular Genetics and Department of Human Genetics, University of California Los Angeles, Los Angeles, CA, USA

Rhona M MacKie MD DSc FRS(E) FRCP FRCPath
Professor and Head of Department, Department of Dermatology, University of Glasgow, Glasgow, UK

Eamonn Maher BSc MB ChB MA MD FRCP
Professor of Medical Genetics, Section of Medical and Molecular Genetics, University of Birmingham, Edgbaston, Birmingham, UK

George M Martin MD
Professor of Pathology; Adjunct Professor of Genetics; Associate Director, Alzheimer's Disease Research Center, Department of Pathology, University of Washington, Seattle, WA, USA

Stephen Marx MD
Chief of Metabolic Diseases Branch and Chief of Genetics and Endocrinology Section, NIDDK / National Institutes of Health, Bethesda, MD, USA

Dietrich Matern MD
Assistant Professor, Department of Laboratory Medicine and Pathology, Co-director, Biochemical Genetics Laboratory, Division of Laboratory Genetics, Mayo Clinic and Foundation, Rochester, MN, USA

Irene Maumenee MD
Ort Professor of Opthalmology & Professor of Pediatrics, Center for Hereditary Eye Diseases, The Wilmer Eye Institute, Baltimore, MD, USA

Matthew J McGinniss PhD
Group Leader, Assay Design and Diagnostics, Sequenom Inc., San Diego; Adjunct Assistant Professor of Pediatrics, University of California San Diego, San Diego, CA, USA

Matthew McGue PhD
Professor and Chair, Department of Psychology, University of Minnesota, Minneapolis, MN, USA

Melvin G McInnis MD
Associate Professor, Department of Psychiatry and Behavioral, Sciences, Johns Hopkins University School of Medicine, Baltimore, MD, USA

William McKenna BA MD DSc FRCP FESC FACC
British Heart Foundation Professor of Molecular, Cardiovascular Sciences, Department of Cardiological Sciences, St George's Hospital Medical School, London, UK

Rona M MacKie CBE MD DSc FRCP FRCPath FRSE
Professor and Head of Department, Department of Dermatology, University of Glasgow, Glasgow, UK

Victor McKusick MD
University Professor of Medical Genetics, McKusick-Nathans Institute of Genetic Medicine, Johns Hopkins University School of Medicine, Baltimore, MD, USA

Stephen J Melzer MD
Professor of Medicine, Division of Gastroenterology, Department of Medicine, University of Maryland School of Medicine, Baltimore Veterans' Affairs Hospital, Baltimore, MD, USA

Eugenio Mercuri MD PhD
Lecturer in Paediatric Neurology, Dubowitz Neuromuscular Unit, Department of Paediatrics and Neonatal Medicine, London, UK

Deborah A Meyers PhD
Associate Professor , Centre For Human Genetics, Wake Forest University, Winston-Salem, NC, USA

Jeffrey E Ming MD PhD
Assistant Professor of Pediatrics, The Children's Hospital of Philadelphia, Department of Pediatrics, University of Pennsylvania School of Medicine, Philadelphia, PA, USA

Ganeshwar Mochida MD
Research Fellow, Neurology Department, Beth Israel Deaconess Medical Center, Boston, MA, USA

T K Mohandas PhD
Professor, Department of Pathology, Dartmouth Medical School; Director, Cytogenetics Laboratory, Dartmouth-Hitchcock Medical Center, Lebanon, NH, USA

Chanda T Moseley PhD
Postdoctoral Research Fellow, Division of Medical Genetics, Vanderbilt University School of Medicine, Nashville, TN, USA

Arno Motulsky MD
Professor Emeritus of Medicine and Genetics, Division of Medical Genetics, Department of Medicine, University of Washington, Seattle, WA, USA

Asha Moudgil MD
Associate Professor of Pediatrics, The George Washington University Department of Nephrology, Children's National Medical Center, Washington DC, USA

Robert Mueller MB BS BSc FRCP
Professor of Clinical Genetics, Department of Clinical Genetics, St James' University Hospital, Leeds, UK

Maximilian Muenke MD
Chief, Medical Genetics Branch, National Human Genome Research Institute, National Instiitues of Health, Bethesda, MD, USA

John Mulley BSc MScAgr PhD
Affiliate Associate Professor, Department of Molecular Biosciences and Genetics, University of Adelaide; Chief Geneticist, Department of Cytogenetics and Molecular Genetics, Centre of Medical Genetics, Adelaide, South Australia, Australia

A Linn Murphree MD
Director, The Retinoblastoma Center, Children's Hospital, Los Angeles, CA, USA

Edmond Murphy MD ScD
Professor Emeritus of Medicine, Johns Hopkins University, Baltimore, MD, USA

Michael F Murray MD
Fellow in Medical Genetics, Department of Medicine, Harvard Institutes of Medicine, Boston, MA, USA

Daniel Nebert MD
Professor of Environmental Health; Professor of Pediatrics & Developmental Biology, Division of Human Genetics, University of Cincinnati Medical Center, Cincinnati, OH, USA

Gerald T Nepom MD PhD
Director, Virginia Mason Research Center, Benaroya Research Institute, Seattle, WA, USA

Maria I New MD
Chairman & Professor of Pediatrics; Chief, Pediatric Endocrinology; Harold & Percy Uris Professor of Pediatric Endocrinology and Metabolism, New York Presbyterian Hospital, Weill Medical College of Cornell University, New York, NY, USA

Won G Ng PhD
Professor, Department of Pediatrics, University of Southern California School of Medicine, Division of Medical Genetics, Children's Hospital Los Angeles, Los Angeles, CA, USA

Robert Nickells PhD
Assistant Professor, Department of Ophthalmology and Visual Sciences, University of Wisconsin Medical School, Madison, WI, USA

Reijo Norio MD
Director Emeritus, Department of Medical Genetics, The Family Federation of Finland, Helsinki, Finland

William S Oetting PhD
Associate Professor, Department of Medicine, Institute of Human Genetics, University of Minnesota, Minneapolis, MN, USA

John Old BSc PhD FRCPath
Clinical Scientist and Reader in Haematology, Oxford University, Globinopathy Reference Laboratory, John Radcliffe Hospital, Oxford, UK

Puneet Opal MD PhD
Assistant Professor of Neurology, Baylor College of Medicine, Houston, TX, USA

Jonathon C Packham MRCP
Consultant Rheumatologist, Department of Rheumatology, University Hospital Trust, Birmingham, UK

Seymour Packman MD
Professor of Pediatrics and Director, Biochemical Genetics Service, Division of Medical Genetics, Department of Pediatrics, University of California San Francisco, San Francisco, CA, USA

Theodore M Page MD
Associate Research Neuroscientist, Department of Neurosciences, University of California San Diego, School of Medicine, La Jolla, CA, USA

Eberhard Passarge MD
Professor and Chairman, Department of Human Genetics, University of Essen, Essen, Germany

Leena Peltonen MD PhD
Professor and Chair, Department of Human Genetics, University of California Los Angeles, Los Angeles, CA, USA

Bruce F Pennington PhD
John Evans Professor, Department of Psychology, University of Denver, Denver, CO, USA

Alan K Percy MD
William Bew White Jr Professor of Pediatrics, Director, Division of Pediatric Neurology, University of Alabama at Birmingham, Birmingham, AL, USA

Margaret Pericak-Vance PhD
Professor and Chief, Section of Medical Genetics, Duke University Medical Center, Durham, NC, USA

John Phillips III MD FAAP FACMG
Professor of Pediatrics and Biochemistry; David T. Karzon Chair in Pediatrics; Director, Division of Medical Genetics, Department of Pediatrics, Vanderbilt University of Medicine, Nashville, TN, USA

Joanne Philpot BA MBBS MRCP
Consultant Paediatrician, Frimley Park Hospital, Surrey, UK

Leena Pulkkinen PhD
Research Associate Professor, Department of Dermatology and Cutaneous Biology, Jefferson Medical College, Philadelphia, PA, USA

Stefan M Pulst MD
Director and Carmen & Louis Warschaw Chair, Division of Neurology, Cedars-Sinai Medical Center; Professor of Medicine, University of California Los Angeles School of Medicine, Los Angeles, CA, USA

Reed E Pyeritz MD PhD FACP FACMG
Professor of Medicine and Genetics, Director, Division of Medical Genetics, University of Pennsylvania School of Medicine, Philadelphia, PA , USA

Yaron Rabinowitz MD
Associate Clinical Professor, Department of, Ophthalmology and Pediatrics, UCLA; Director of Ocular Genetics Research Program, Burns and Allen Research Institute, Cedars-Sinai Medical Center, Los Angeles, CA, USA

Leslie J Raffel MD
Associate Director, Common Diseases Genetics Program, Associate Professor of Pediatrics, UCLA, Cedars-Sinai Medical Center, Los Angeles, CA, USA

Gerald V Raymond MD
Assistant Professor in Neurology, John Hopkins University, Baltimore; Neurologist, Kennedy-Krieger Institute, Baltimore, MD, USA

Philip R Reilly MD JD
President and Chief Executive Officer, Shriver Center for Mental Retardation Inc., Waltham, MA, USA

David L Rimoin MD PhD
Steven Spielberg Chairman of Pediatrics; Director, Medical Genetics Birth Defects Center, Cedars-Sinai Health System, Professor of Pediatrics and Medicine, UCLA School of Medicine, Los Angeles, CA, USA

Piero Rinaldo MD PhD
Professor, Department of Laboratory Medicine and Pathology; Co-director, Biochemical Genetics Laboratory, Division of Laboratory Genetics, Mayo Clinic and Foundation, Rochester, MN, USA

Neil Risch PhD
Professor, Department of Genetics, Stanford University School of Medicine, Stanford, CA, USA

Asad Rizvi MD FRCPC
Cardiology Fellow, Hartford Hospital/University of Connecticut Health Center, Hartford, CT, USA

Charles H Roedeck MD BS BSc DSc FRCOG FRCPath FmedSci
Professor and Head, Department of Obstetrics and Gynaecology, University College of London, Director, Fetal Medicine Unit, University College London Hospitals, London, UK

Thomas F Roe MD
Professor, Department of Pediatrics, University of Southern California School of Medicine Los Angeles, Division of Endocrinology and Metabolism, Children's Hospital Los Angeles, Los Angeles, CA, USA

Fred S Rosen MD
James L Gamble Professor of Pediatrics, Harvard Medical School, Boston; President, The Centre for Blood Research, Boston, MA, USA

Allen D Roses MD
Senior Vice-President, Genetics Research, GlaxoSmithKline, Triangle Park, NC, USA

Jerome I Rotter MD
Director, Division of Medical Genetics, Professor of Medicine, Pediatrics and Human Genetics; Board of Governors' Chair in Medical Genetics, Burns and Allen Cedars-Sinai Research Institute, University of California Los Angeles School of Medicine, Los Angeles, CA, USA

Janet Rowley MD
Blum-Reise Distinguished Service Professor of Medicine, Molecular Genetics and Cell Biology, and of Human Genetics; Interim Deputy Dean for Science, Department of Medicine, Section of Hematology/Oncology, University of Chicago, Chicago, IL, USA

Reinhardt Rüdel PhD
Professor and Head, Department of General Physiology, University of Ulm, Ulm, Germany

Sabine Rudnik-Schöneborn MD
Consultant in Medical Genetics, Institute of Human Genetics, Technical University, Aachen, Germany

Michael Rutter MD FRCP FRCPsych FRS
Professor of Developmental Psychopathology, Social Genetics & Development Psychiatry Research Centre, Institute of Psychiatry, London, UK

Mohamed Sabry MBBCh DHCG MSc MD
Research Fellow, Division of Neurogenetics, Neurology Department, Harvard Medical School, Boston, MA, USA

Dessa Sadovnik PhD
Professor, Medical Genetics and Medicine (Neurology), Department of Medical Genetics, University of British Columbia, Vancouver, British Columbia, Canada

Ann M Saunders PhD
Associate Research Professor, Division of Neurology, Duke University Medical Center, Durham, NC, USA

Lori B Schaen MD
Resident in Dermatology, Department of Dermatology, University of Rochester, Rochester, NY, USA

Maren T Scheuner MD MPH
Director, GenRISK Program, Cedars-Sinai Medical Center, Los Angeles , Assistant Professor of Medicine, University of California Los Angeles School of Medicine, Los Angeles, CA, USA

Rhona R Schreck PhD
Professor of Pediatrics, UCLA School of Medicine, Director of Cytogenetics, Medical Genetics-Birth Defects Center, Cedars-Sinai Medical Center, Los Angeles, CA, USA

Edward H Schuchman PhD
Professor of Human Genetics; Member, Institute for Gene Therapy and Molecular Medicine, Mount Sinai School of Medicine, New York, NY, USA

Ulrike Schwarze MD
Acting Assistant Professor, Department of Pathology, University of Washington, Seattle, WA, USA

Danial S Scoles PhD
Associate Professor, Division of Neurology, Department of Medicine, University of California, UCLA School of Medicine; Research Scientist, Division of Neurology, Cedars-Sinai Medical Center, Los Angeles, CA, USA

J Edwin Seegmiller MD
Research Professor of Medicine, Department of Medicine, University of California San Diego, School of Medicine, La Jolla, CA, USA

David Seligson MD
Postgraduate Researcher, Departments of Human Genetics and Pathology & Laboratory Medicine, UCLA School of Medicine, Los Angeles, CA, USA

Stephanie Sherman PhD
Professor, Department of Genetics, Emory University School of Medicine, Atlanta, GA, USA

Lee P Shulman MD
Professor of Obstetrics and Gynecology and Molecular Genetics; Director, Division of Reproductive Genetics Deputy Head, Department of Obstetrics and Gynecology, University of Illinois at Chicago, Chicago, IL, USA

Teepu Siddique MD
Professor, Department of Neurology and Cell and Molecular Biology, Northwestern University Medical School, Chicago, IL, USA

David Sillence MB BS, MD (Melb), FRACP, FRCPA, FAFPHM, MACMG
Professor of Medical Genetics, Academic Department of Medical Genetics, The Children's Hospital, Westmead, New South Wales, Australia

Edwin Silverman MD PhD
Assistant Professor of Medicine, Channing Laboratory/ Pulmonary and Critical Care Medicine, Brigham and Women's Hospital, Boston, MA, USA

Neil S Silverman MD
Medical Director, Inpatient Obstetrics, Cedars-Sinai Medical Center, Los Angeles; Associate Professor, Obstetrics and Gynecology, UCLA School of Medicine, Los Angeles, CA, USA

Emily A Simonoff MD BA MRCPsych
Professor, Department of Child and Adolescent Psychiatry, Guy's, King's and St Thomas' Medical School and Institute of Psychiatry, London, UK

Joe Leigh Simpson MD
Ernst W Bertner Chairman and Professor, Department of Obstetrics and Gynecology; Professor, Department of Molecular and Human Genetics, Baylor College of Medicine, Houston, TX, USA

Kim Smith BA MRCPath
Head, Cytogenetics, Medical Genetics Laboratories, Addenbrooke's NHS Trust, Cambridge, UK

Shelley D Smith PhD FACMG
Professor of Pediatrics; Assistant Director, Center for Human Molecular Genetics, Munroe Meyer Institute, University of Nebraska Medical Center, Omaha, NB, USA

M Anne Spence PhD
Professor of Genetics, Department of Pediatrics, University of California, Irvine, CA, USA

Kevin Spencer BSc MSc CBiol CChem EurClin Chem, MIBiol, FRSC, FRCPath
Consultant Biochemist, Endocrine Unit, Clinical Biochemistry Department, Harold Wood Hospital, Romford, UK

Nancy Spinner PhD
Associate Professor of Pediatrics and Genetics, University of Pennsylvania School of Medicine; Director of Clinical Cytogenetics, Department of Pathology and Laboratory Medicine, Abramson Research Center, Philadelphia, PA, USA

Jürgen Spranger MD
Professor of Pediatrics, Children's Hospital, Johannes Gutenberg-Universität Mainz, Mainz, Germany

C Michael Steel FRCPE FRSE
Professor in Medical Science, University of St Andrews; Honorary Consultant Geneticist, Lothian Health and Tayside Health Board, Scotland, UK

Elizabeth Streeten MD
Assistant Professor, University of Maryland Hospital, Baltimore, MD, USA

Joel Sugar MD
Professor, Department of Ophthalmology, UIC Eye Center, University of Illinois Eye & Ear Infirmary, Chicago, IL, USA

C Gail Summers MD
Professor, Departments of Ophthalmology and Pediatrics, University of Minnesota, Minneapolis, MN, USA

Grant R Sutherland PhD DSc FAA FRS
Director, Department of Cytogenetics and Molecular Genetics, Women's and Children's Hospital, Adelaide, Adelaide, South Australia, Australia

Kent D Taylor PhD
Assistant Professor of Pediatrics, Departments of Medicine and Pediatrics, Burns and Allen Cedars-Sinai Research Institute, Los Angeles, CA, USA

Milhan Telatar PhD
Research Assistant, Department of Pathology and Laboratory Medicine, University of California Los Angeles, Los Angeles, CA, USA

Paul Thompson MD
Director, Preventative Cardiology, Hartford Hospital; Professor of Medicine, University of Connecticut, Hartford Hospital, Hartford, CT, USA

Edward Tobias PhD MRCP
GlaxoSmithKline Research Fellow, Department of Medical Genetics, University of Glasgow and Beatson Institute for Cancer Research, Glasgow; Honorary Consultant, Duncan Guthrie Institute of Medical Genetics, Yorkhill NHS Trust, Glasgow, UK

John Tolmie MB ChB FRCP(Glasg)
Consultant Clinical Geneticist, Duncan Guthrie Insitute of Medical Genetics, University of Glasgow Medical School, Yorkhill Hospitals NHS Trust, Glasgow, UK

Jeffrey A Towbin MD
Professor of Pediatrics (Cardiology) and Molecular & Human Genetics, Pediatric Cardiology, Texas Children's Hospital, Baylor College of Medicine, Houston, TX, USA

Massimo Trucco MD
Professor of Pediatrics, University of Pittsburgh, Children's Hospital of Pittsburgh, Pittsburgh, PA, USA

Betty P Tsao PhD
Associate Professor, Division of Rheumatology, Department of Medicine, University of California Los Angeles, Los Angeles, CA, USA

Dolly B Tyan PhD
Director, Histocompatibility and Immunogentics; Associate Director of Pediatrics, Medical Genetics – Birth Defects Center, Cedars Sinai Medical Center, Los Angeles, CA, USA

Jouni Uitto MD PhD
Professor and Chair, Department of Dermatology and Cutaneous Biology; Director, Jefferson Insitute of Molecular Medicine, Jefferson Medical College, Philadelphia, PA, USA

Sheila Unger MD, FRCPC, FAMBG, FCCMG
Staff Clinical Geneticist, Department of Genetics, The Hospital for Sick Children, Assistant Professor, Department of Pediatrics, University of Toronto, Toronto, Ontario, Canada

Andre Van Steirteghem MD PhD
Professor of Embryology and Reproductive Medicine, Centre for Reproductive Medicine, Academisch Ziekenhuis, Brussels, Belgium

James Versalovic MD PhD FCAP
Assistant Professor of Pathology, Harvard Medical School, Director of Molecular Diagnostics, Massachusetts General Hospital, Boston, MA, USA

Hans-Peter Vosberg MD
Group Leader, Department of Experimental Cardiology, Max Planck Institute for Physiological and Clinical Research, Bad Nauheim, Germany

Ann Walker MA CEG
Professor of Pediatrics, Division of Human Genetics, Department of Pediatrics, College of Medicine, University of California Irvine Medical Center, Orange, CA, USA

Douglas C Wallace PhD
Robert W Woodruff Professor of Medical Genetics, Professor and Director, Center for Molecular Medicine, Emory University School of Medicine, Atlanta, GA, USA

Carina Wallgren-Pettersson MD, PhD
Consultant in Medical Genetics, The Folkhalsan Department of Medical Genetics, University of Helsinki, Helsinki, Finland

Christopher Walsh MD PhD
Bullard Professor of Neurology, Harvard Medical School, Department of Neurology, Beth Israel Deaconess Medical Center, Boston, MA, USA

Ronald Wanders PhD
Professor of Clinical Enzymology and Inherited Disease, Departments of Clinical Chemistry and Pediatrics, University of Amsterdam, Academic Medical Centre, Amsterdam, The Netherlands

William R Wilcox MD PhD
Assistant Professor, Division of Medical Genetics, Department of Pediatrics, Cedars-Sinai Medical Center and University of California Los Angeles School of Medicine, Los Angeles, CA, USA

Nicholas Willcox MB Phd BChir
Professor of Neurosciences, Department of Clinical Neurology, Weatherall Institute of Molecular Medicine, University of Oxford, Oxford, UK

Robert C Wilson PhD
Associate Professor of Biochemistry, Department of Pediatrics, The New York Presbyterian Hospital/Weill Medical College of Cornell University, New York, NY, USA

Paul Wordsworth MA MB BS FRCP
Professor of Rheumatology, Nuffield Orthopaedic Centre, Headington, Oxford, UK

Huiying Yang MD PhD
Associate Director, Genetic Epidemiology; Asscociate Professor of Pediatrics, Departments of Medicine and Pedatrics, Burns and Allen Cedars-Sinai Research Institute and the University of California Los Angeles School of Medicine, Los Angeles, CA, USA

Kuender Yang MD PhD
Professor of Pediatrics and Deputy Director of Chang Gung Children's Hospital at Kaosiung, Kaohsiung, Taiwan

Ian Young MSc MD FRCP
Visiting Professor, Department of Clinical Genetics, Leicester Royal Infirmary, Leicester, UK

Donald Zack MD PhD
Professor, Departments of Ophthalmology, Molecular Biology & Genetics and Neuroscience, Johns Hopkins University School of Medicine, Baltimore, MD, USA

Klaus Zerres MD
Professor of Medicine; Chair Department of Human Genetics, Institut für Humangenetik, Aachen, Germany

Huda Zoghbi MD
Professor, Department of Pediatrics, Neurology, Neuroscience, and Molecular and Human Genetics, Baylor College of Medicine, Houston, TX, USA

Jonathan Zonana MD, Professor of Molecular and Medical Genetics and of Pediatrics, Oregon Health Science University, Portland, OR, USA

Foreword

In the Foreword for the first edition of *Principles and Practice of Medical Genetics*, dated 1983, I compared the book to William Osler's *Principles and Practice of Medicine* (1st Ed., 1892). I believed that there was an obvious parallelism between the two works not only in title, but also in breadth of scope, intended audience (both practitioners and students), and potential impact.

In the Foreword for the second edition, dated 1990, I commented on the advent of map-based gene discovery ("reverse genomics," later renamed "positional cloning"), the expansion in somatic cell genetics particularly in relation to cancer, and the extent to which molecular diagnostic methods had come into routine use in the practice of clinical genetics.

In the Foreword for the third edition, dated 1996, I looked back over the previous 5 or 6 years and marveled at the accelerating pace of discovery in the scientific basis of clinical genetics and at the expanding diagnostic armamentarium that was becoming available as a result. These advances included:

- The Human Genome Project, formally initiated on October 1, 1990, after the publication of the second edition of this textbook, had passed its fifth birthday and appeared to be ahead of schedule (and under budget) in its dual goal of locating all the genes and sequencing the entire genome. The benefits that were predicted were beginning to be realized.

- Mutations causing genetic disorders were being defined at the DNA level at a phenomenal rate. One or more disease-causing mutations had been identified at about 425 loci. At some loci, the separate mutations causing the same or similar phenotype were very numerous (e.g., over 400 different mutations in the CFTR gene causing cystic fibrosis). The success of mutation detection amplified greatly the power of DNA diagnosis and the dissection of phenotype-genotype relationships. The new mutation explosion was not solely quantitative; in addition, new types of mutations had been uncovered (e.g., expanded trinucleotide repeats that had been found to be the cause of many neurologic disorders, and mutations in mismatch repair genes ["mutator genes"] involved particularly in cancer).

- The precise mutational basis of some leading genetic disorders had been defined, including Marfan syndrome, achondroplasia, polycystic kidney disease, von Recklinghausen neurofibromatosis, and many more. In fact, before 1990 the mutant gene had been identified by positional cloning in only four disorders: chronic granulomatous disease, Duchenne muscular dystrophy, retinoblastoma, and cystic fibrosis. By the third edition, about 50 disorders had been characterized by this approach. For an even greater number of disorders, the mutant gene had been identified by the positional candidate gene approach (e.g., several forms of familial cardiomyopathy, hereditary hemorrhagic telangiectasia, two forms of Hirschsprung disease, several forms of Charcot-Marie-Tooth disease, two forms of hereditary nonpolyposis colon cancer, X-linked disorders, SCID, and many others).

- Congenital malformations had also yielded to elucidation by molecular genetic methods. Some of the best examples were provided by the craniosynostosis syndromes such as Crouzon syndrome, that are caused by mutations in fibroblast growth factor receptor genes. It turned out that mutations in the same gene can cause either neoplasia (in which case the gene is called an oncogene) or congenital anomaly (in which case the gene might be called a teratogene). Mutations in the *KIT* gene may cause piebaldism or mast cell leukemia; those in the *RET* gene, Hirschsprung disease or multiple endocrine neoplasia; and those in *PAX3*, Waardenburg syndrome or alveolar rhabdomyosarcoma.

- A particularly remarkable development of the previous six years was the extent to which common disorders ("complex traits"), with genetics traditionally described as multifactorial, had yielded to genetic analysis even at the molecular level. Colorectal cancer and Alzheimer disease were two of the leading examples. Colorectal disease proves to be indeed multifactorial in terms of polygenic/environmental causation. Alzheimer disease appeared to be an example of genetic heterogeneity with any one of a number of loci being capable of a major role in causation.

- The expanded knowledge of the mutational basis of genetic disease was opening up new opportunities for detection and prediction that go all the way from single-cell preimplantation diagnosis to population screening. Portended was a changing role for the clinical geneticist in overseeing and interpreting DNA testing, and in designing and supervising health and reproductive programs based on the findings.

- In the United States, professionalization of medical genetics had been signalled in the previous five years by the evolution of certifying boards (American Board of Medical Genetics, American Board of Genetic Counseling), and by the creation of the American College of Medical Genetics. Comparable developments had occurred in some other developed countries.

As I write this Foreword for the fourth edition, I am impressed that the five-year interval since the last edition has seen much greater advances in the scientific base of medical genetics than in either of the two previous inter-publication periods. In large part because of the human genome sequencing initiative, major new trends in human genetics research (representing paradigm shifts in some instances) have occurred:

- Structural genomics → functional genomics
- Genomics → proteomics
- Map-based gene discovery → sequence-based gene discovery
- Gene action → gene regulation
- Analysis of one gene → analysis of multiple genes in gene families, pathways or systems
- Etiology (specific mutation) → pathogenesis (mechanism)
- Monogenic disorders → multifactorial ("complex") disorders
- Specific DNA diagnosis → detection of susceptibility
- Study of one species → study of several species

Database searching (research *in silico* or cybergenetics) has become a primary method of genetics research. Also since the last edition, microarray ("chip") technology for profiling of the function of many genes or for screening for multiple genetic abnormalities has been fully developed.

By the time of the next edition of *Emery & Rimoin's Principles and Practice of Medical Genetics*, I predict that the impact of the scientific advances of the last five years will be fully evident in the clinical practice of medical genetics.

Victor A. McKusick, MD
University Professor of Medical Genetics
Johns Hopkins University School of Medicine
Baltimore, MD
USA

Preface

In the nearly twenty years that have elapsed since the first edition of this book was published, the field of medical genetics has experienced a period of explosive growth. The rate of change in the science and application of medical genetics that occurred in the period spanning the first through the third editions of this book has markedly accelerated. Genetics was viewed by most practitioners as an important but obscure corner of medicine. Now it is widely recognized that virtually all human disorders have a genetic component, and genetics is viewed as the key basic science in uncovering the mysteries of disease pathogenesis. The tools of molecular genetics have matured remarkably over these past two decades, to the point where the mutations that underlie most single-gene disorders are being reported week by week. This has resulted in insights into disease mechanisms that have solved medical puzzles that have existed for centuries. These advances are also providing new clinical approaches that vastly improve the ability to accurately diagnose these disorders, and in many instances offer new hope for treatment and prevention. Of even greater importance for the medical community and the public is the increasing ability to dissect the genetic contributions to common disorders. These remain dauntingly complex, but powerful molecular genetic and statistical tools are now being applied to the problem. The promise of new approaches to prevention and treatment represents a new paradigm that will transform the practice of medicine.

The recent announcement of a "working draft" of the human genome has captured public attention and raised both hopes and concerns. It remains to be seen how quickly and to what extent the genetic approach will be incorporated into the day-to-day practice of medicine. The complexity of translating scientific developments in genetics to clinical application is being increasingly recognized, particularly with respect to legal, ethical, psychological, and social implications. The need to inform colleagues throughout medicine about advances in genetics and the principles of their clinical application has never been greater.

The continued excitement and progress in our field is reflected in further expansion of this book with over 20 new chapters, necessitating three volumes. The number of genetic disorders understood at the molecular level has increased dramatically since the previous edition and common disorders not traditionally viewed as "genetic" are now included as genetic contributions are coming to light. We continue to be grateful for comments on previous editions provided by our colleagues. This edition is better for their input, and we accept full responsibility for the deficiencies that remain.

We warmly acknowledge, besides our contributing authors, the assistance of staff at Churchill Livingstone/ Elsevier Health Sciences in Edinburgh and London, and our personal assistant Sue Lief in Los Angeles. Once again, we thank Professor Victor A. McKusick, in many ways the father of present-day medical genetics, for writing the Foreword to this new edition and contributing to the chapter on the history of our field and as recent a compilation of the human gene map as our publishing process would permit. Finally, we appreciate the continued moral, scholarly, and spiritual support of Professor Alan E.H. Emery, one of the originators of this book.

David L. Rimoin, MD PhD
J. Michael Connor, MD DSc FRCP
Reed E. Pyeritz, MD PhD
Bruce R. Korf, MD PhD

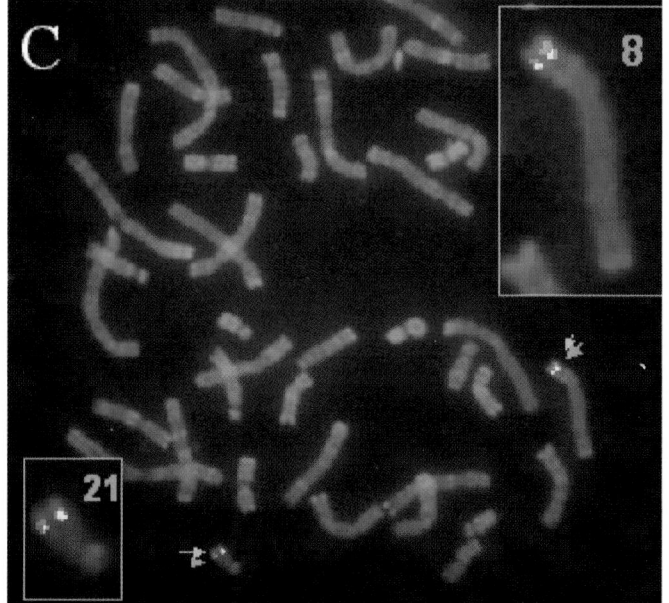

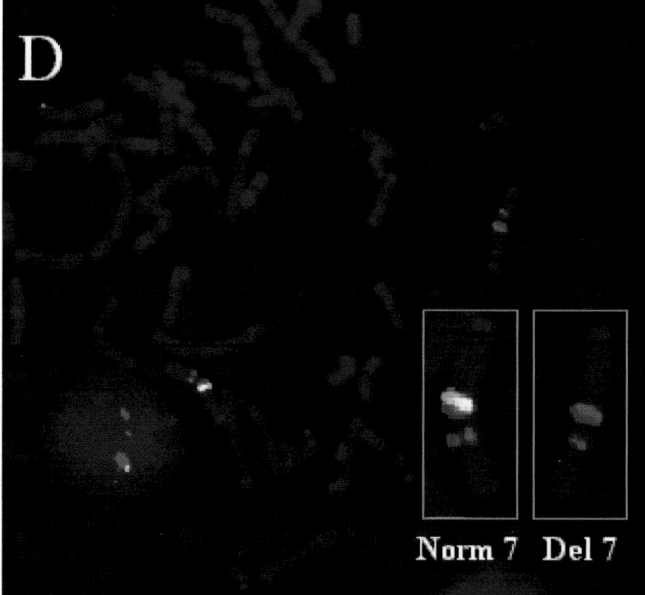

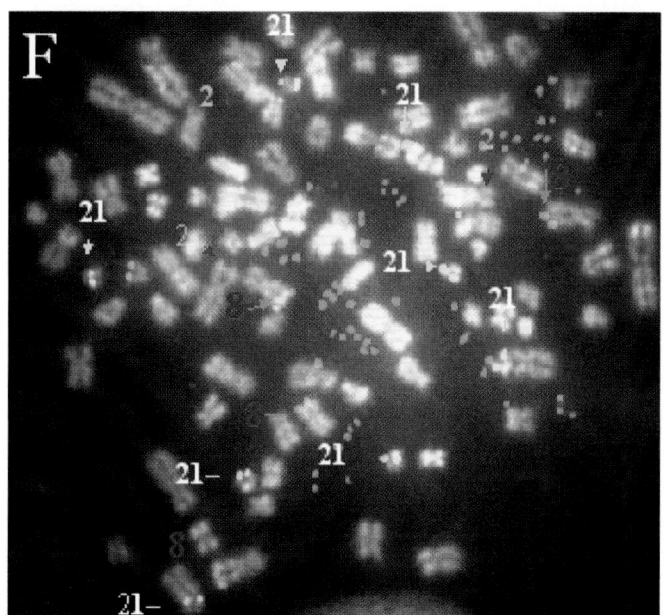

Plate 9.9. Fluorescence in situ hybridization

C. A subtle chromosomal rearrangement translocates the terminal band of chromosome 21 to the short arm of chromosome 8 is shown by two color FISH with two single copy BAC probes linked to DNA sequences on chromosome 21.

D. A deletion of chromosome band 7q11.2 in Williams syndrome is shown on one homolog using BAC DNAs containing the gene for elastin (in green) and for a flanking duplicated region (pink).

F. Gene amplification of the myc oncogene on dm (double minute) chromosome fragments (green) is shown in a highly aneuploid lymphoma specimen by using FISH with a BAC carrying myc. Chromosome numbers are noted.

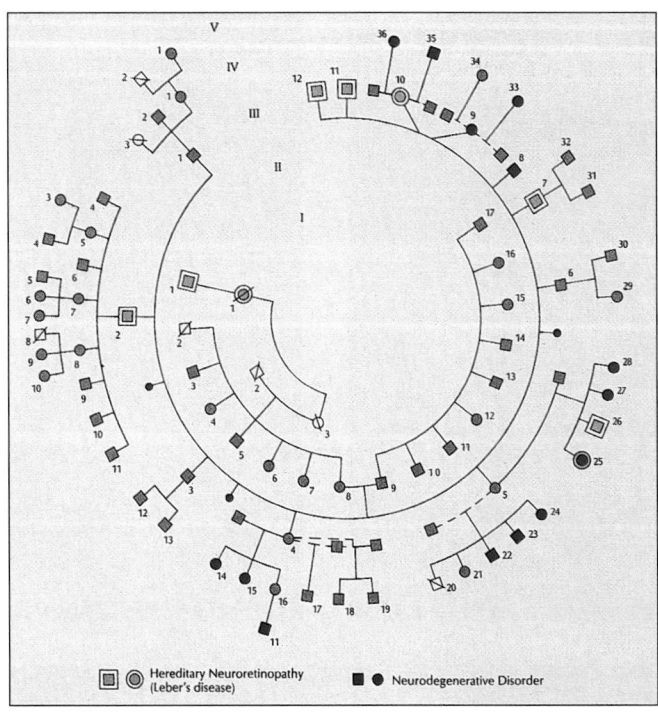

Plate 11.7. Hispanic family with maternally inherited LHON and/or dystonia due to the heteroplasmic mtDNA mutation at MTND6*LDYT14459A. Individuals with LHON experience acute onset optic atrophy and central vision loss, generally as young adults. Individuals with neurodegenerative disease have a much earlier age on onset and experience gait disturbance, rigidity, pseudobulbar syndrome, impaired intelligence, short stature, and frequently infantile bilateral striatal necrosis (IBSN). (Reproduced Novotny et al., 1986.)

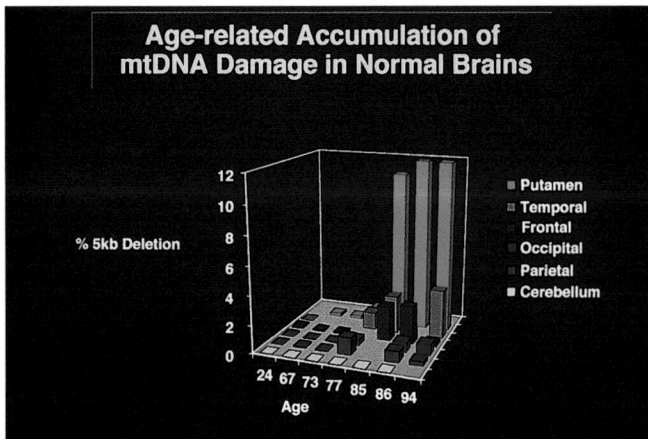

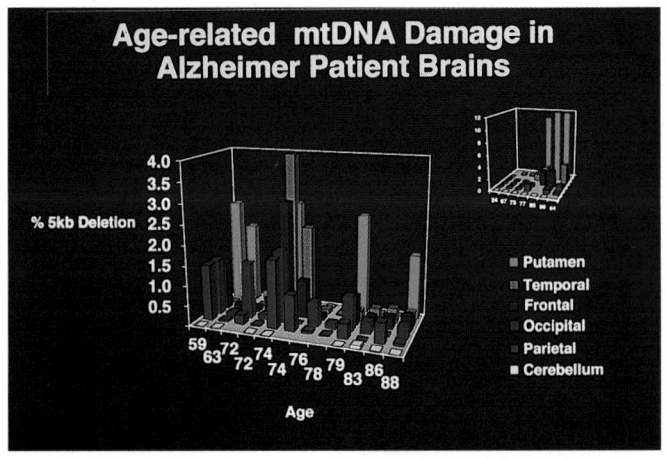

Plate 11.12. Levels of the common 5-kb deletion in different regions of the brains of normal controls and Alzheimer's disease patients Normal individuals (left-hand panel) experience an exponential increase in mtDNA deletions in the cortex and putamen after age 75 years. AD patients (right-hand panel). have high levels of deletion in the cortex prior to age 75 which are subsequently lost after age 75 years, possibly due to apoptosis (Reproduced from Corral-Debrinski et al., 1992a, 1994).)

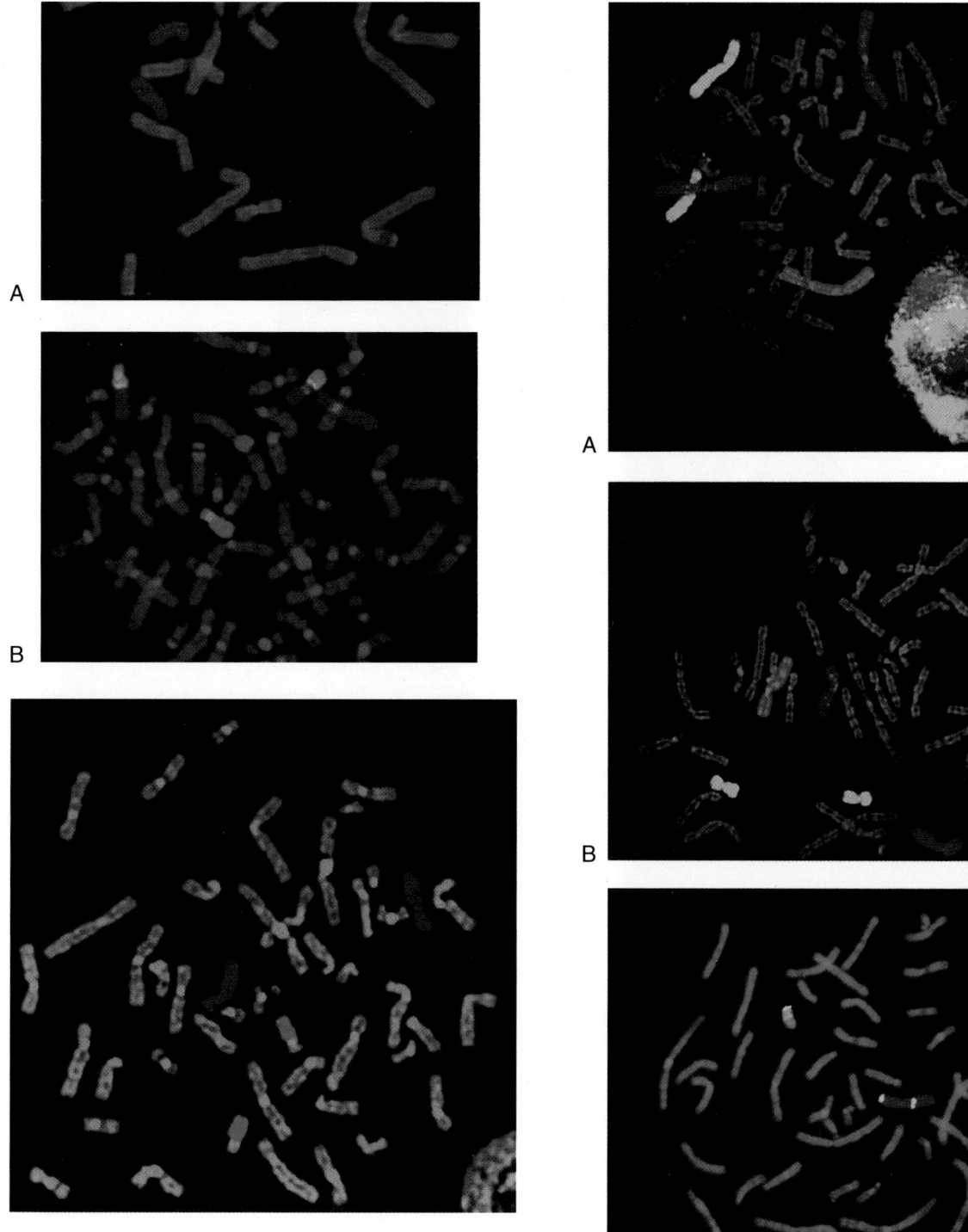

Plate 25.6. Forward chromosome painting revealing (A) an insertional translocation of 18q12.3–18q21.2 (red) into 4p15.2, (B) a 46,XX, t(8;18)(q11.2;q12.2) reciprocal translocation, and (C) a small marker chromosome identified as a ring 8 chromosome in a preparation hybridized with chromosome-specific paint probes (CAMBIO) for chromosome 8 (red) and chromosome 18 (green).

Plate 25.13. Chromosome painting using chromosome specific probes (CAMBIO Ltd., Cambridge, England) from flow sorted chromosomes (DAPI counterstain). (A) Chromosome 1 (red), chromosome 2 (green), and chromosome 6 (yellow). Interphase nucleus reveals chromosome domains within nucleus. (B) Chromosome 7 (green), chromosome 11(red), and chromosome 20 (yellow). (C) X chromosome (red), Y chromosome (green). Note Y signal (yellow) on XY homologous regions of Xp (tip) and Xq (proximaal third) and X signal (yellow) on XY homologous region of Yp (tip).

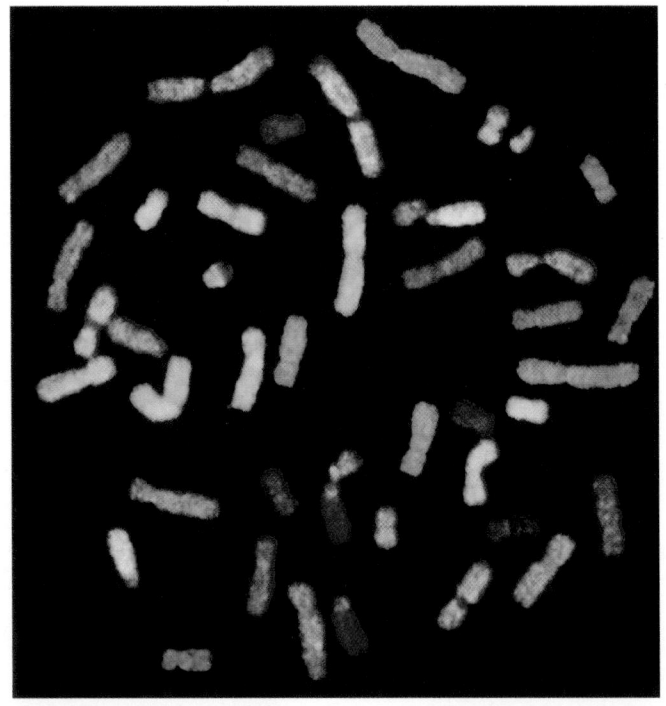

A

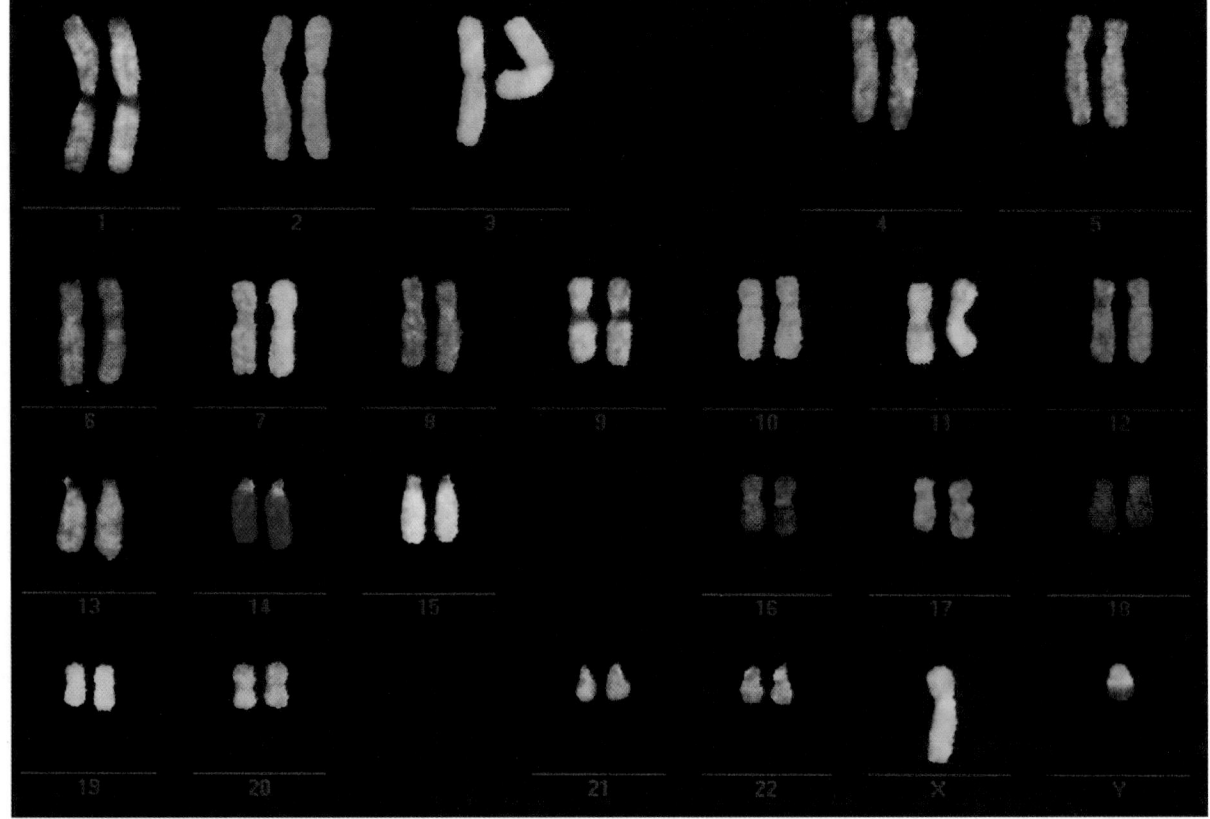

B

Plate 25.14. Multicolor FISH analysis of a normal human male metaphase using combinatorial chromosome-specific painting probes produced with five fluorescent dyes. (A) Raw image of metaphase in pseudocolor, (B) Karyotype of raw image. (C) M-FISH karyotype after chromosome identification by computer.

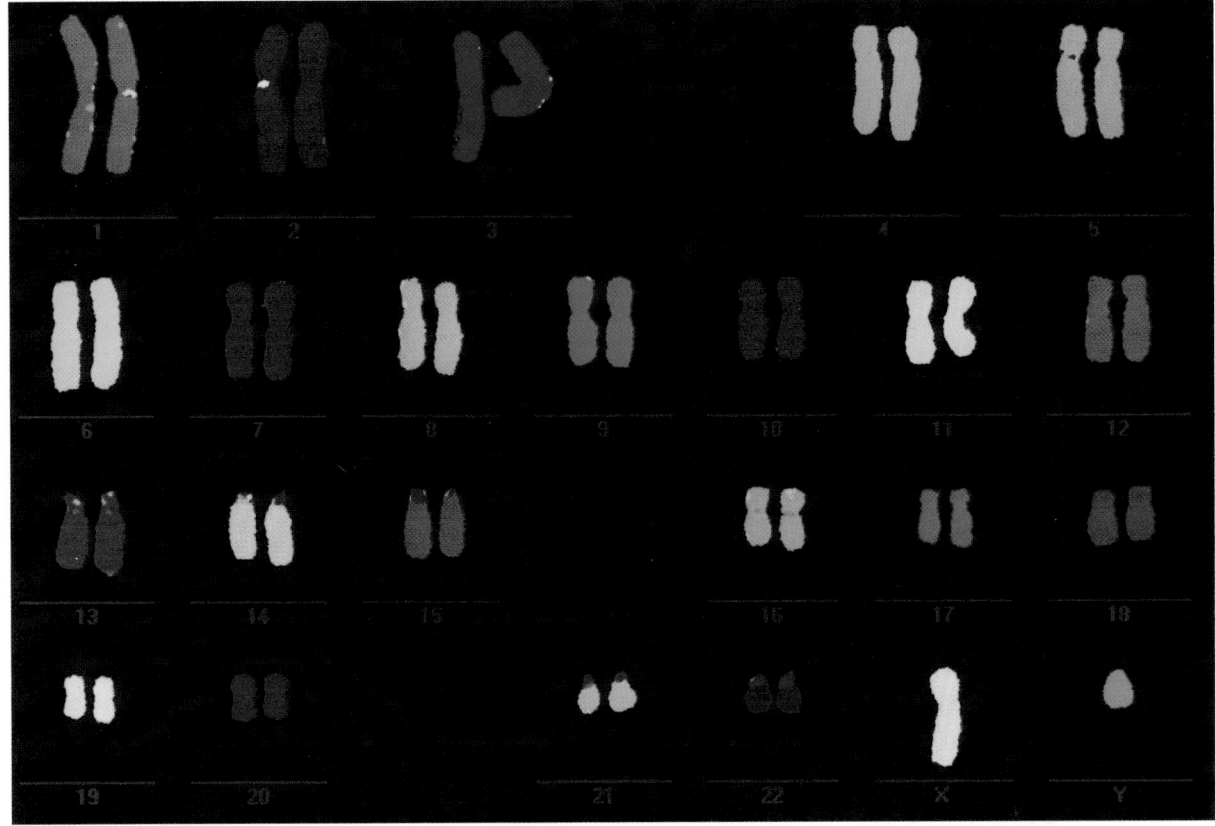

Plate 25.14. (C) .

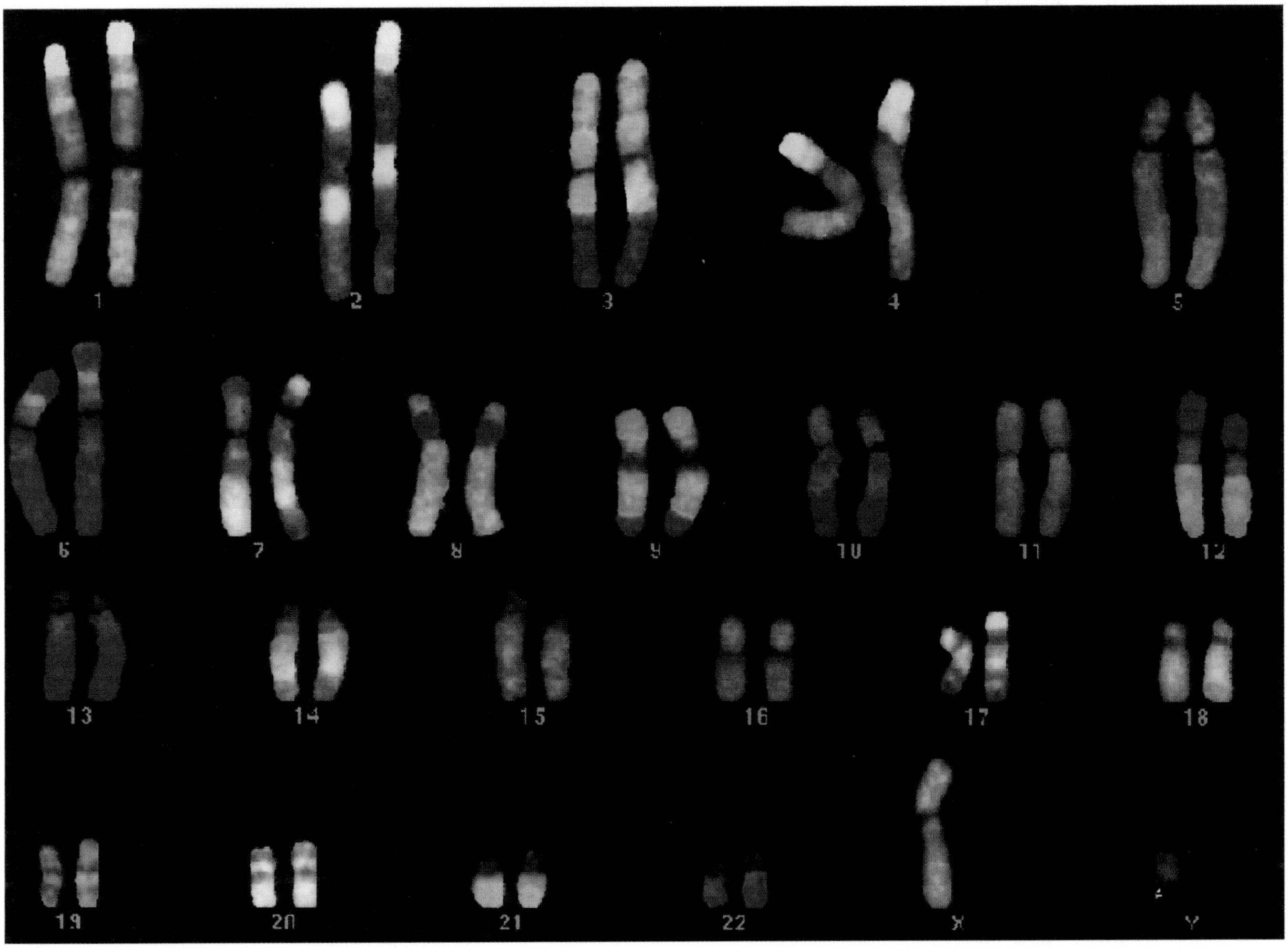

Plate 25.15. Color banding of human male metaphase using chromosome-specific gibbon painting probes. Color bands reflect interchromosomal rearrangements arising during divergence of human and gibbon. Note large pericentric inversion of right homologue of chromosome 7.

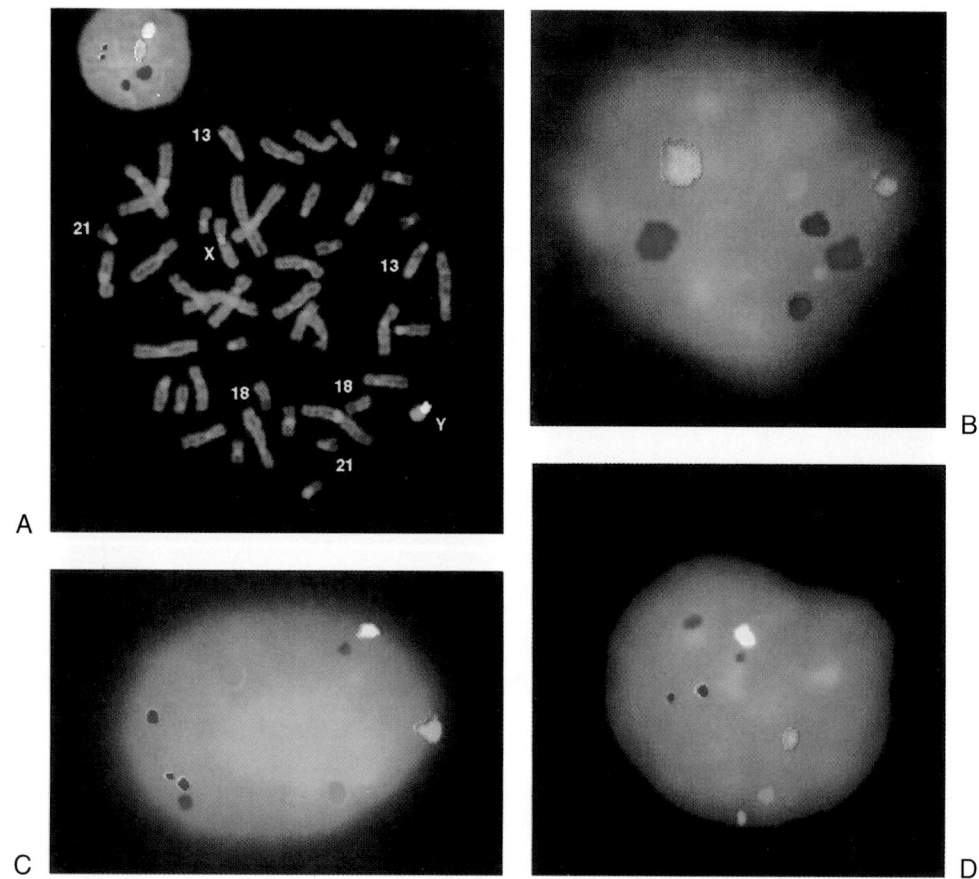

Plate 25.16. FISH probes useful for determining chromosome copy number in interphase nuclei. (A) Lymphocyte metaphase showing centromeric probes for X chromosome (lilac), Y chromosome (yellow), and chromosome 18 (blue); a YAC clone marks chromosome 13 (green) and acontig of two overlapping cosmids marks chromosome 21 (red). (B) Uncultured amniotic fluid cell nucleus from a female fetus hybridized with the above probes revealing normal copy number of each chromosome. (C) As above, rom male fetus with trisomy 21 (Down syndrome). (D) As above, from normal male fetus. (From Divane A et al., 1994, with permission.)

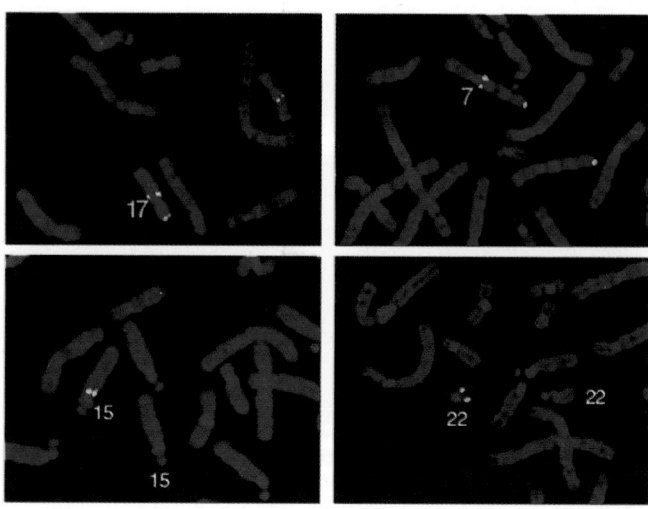

Plate 25.17. The diagnosis of microdeletion syndromes using labeled cosmid clones (ONCOR, Gaithersburg, USA) that map into the region involved in the deletion. (A) Miller-Dieker syndrome. Chromosome 17 identified by cosmid clone in 17q. Note loss of signal at 17q13 in one homologue (*right*). (B) Williams syndrome. Chromosome 7 identified by cosmid clone at distal end of 7q. Note loss of signal at the elastin locus on 7q11.23 in one homologue (*lower*). (C) Prader-Willi syndrome. One homologue of chromosome 15 shows loss of signal at 15q12. (D) DiGeorge syndrome. One homologue of chromosome 22 shows loss of signal at 22q11.

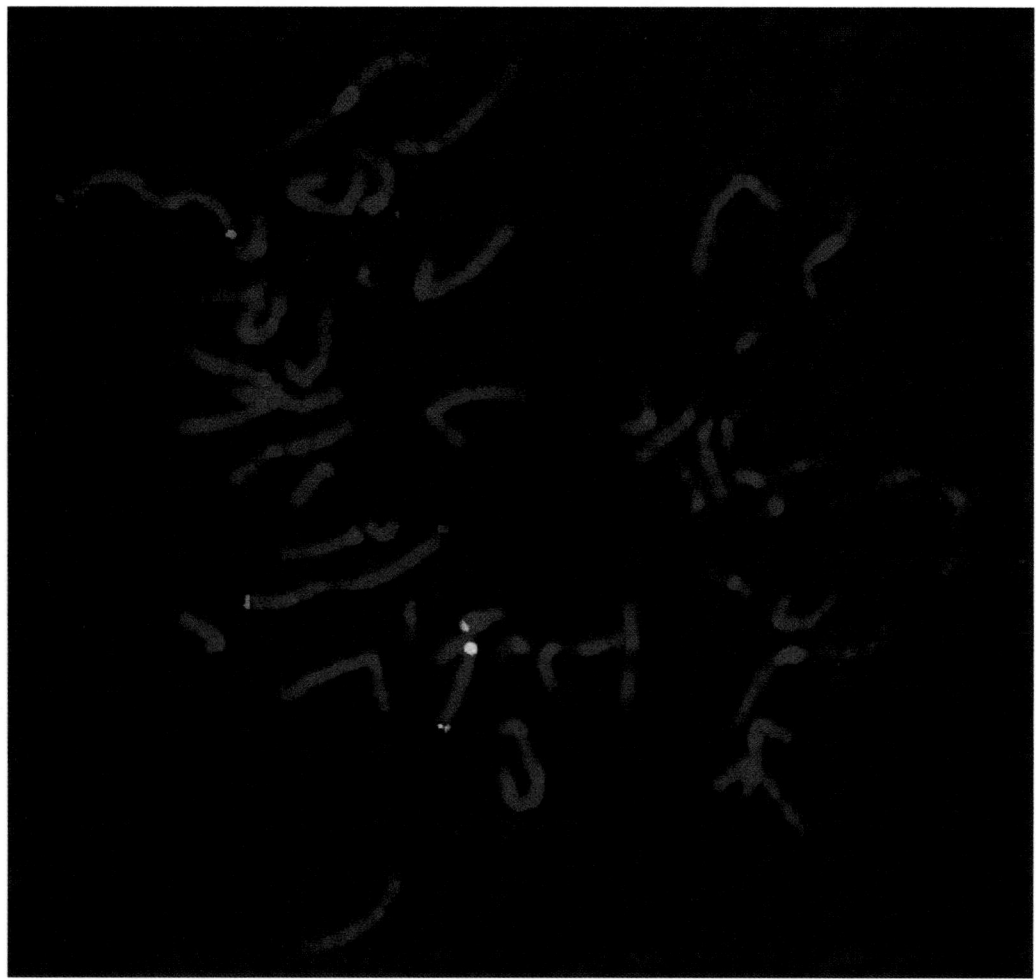

Plate 25.18. Human metaphase showing telomeric probes for chromosome 2p (Spectrum Green), 2q (Spectrum Orange) and pairing regions of Xq and Yq (Spectrum Green + Spectrum Orange). X alpha cenFromeric probe (Spectrum Aqua) identifies the X centromere.

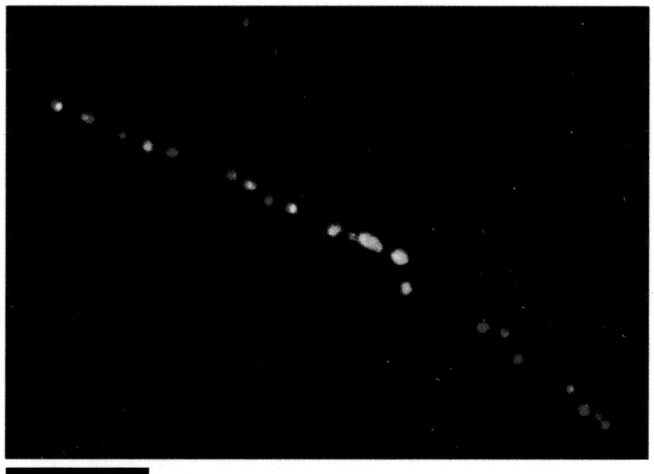

10μm

Plate 25.19. Fiber-FISH. Decondensation of chromatin by alkali treatment of fixed nuclei and hybridation of close;ly linked labeled cosmid clones. Three cosmids from the HLA region labeled with FITC, Texas Red, and a 50:50 mixture of FITC and Texas Red, respectively. Each cosmid measures 35 kb and there is a 5 to 10 Kb gap between the red and green cosmids.

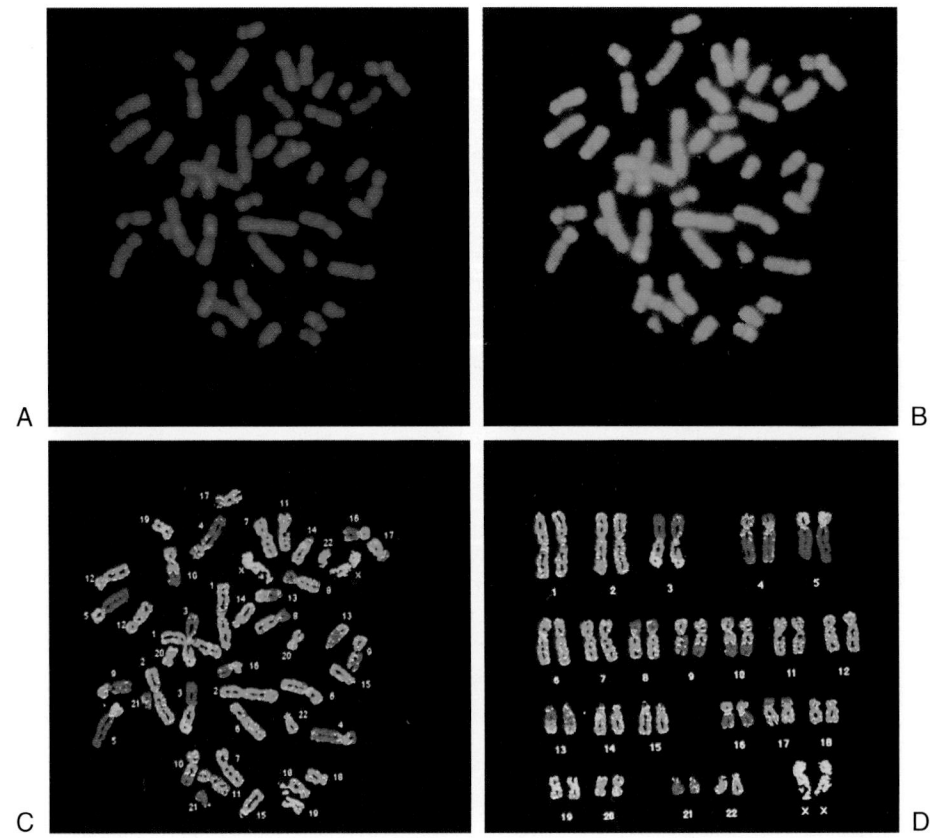

A B C D

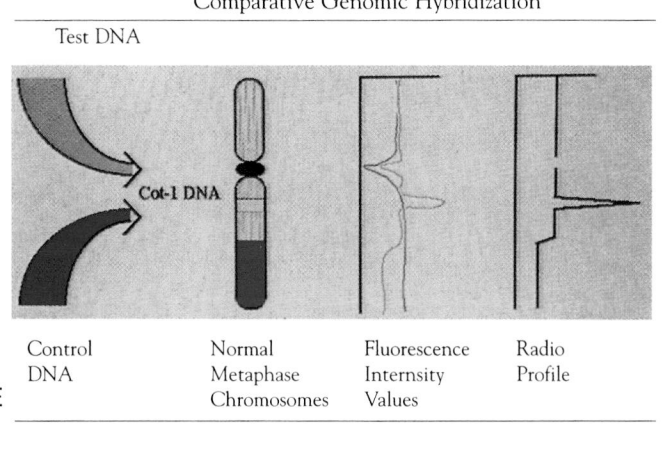

Comparative Genomic Hybridization

Test DNA

Cot-1 DNA

Control   Normal   Fluorescence   Radio
DNA   Metaphase   Internsity   Profile
                Chromosomes   Values

E

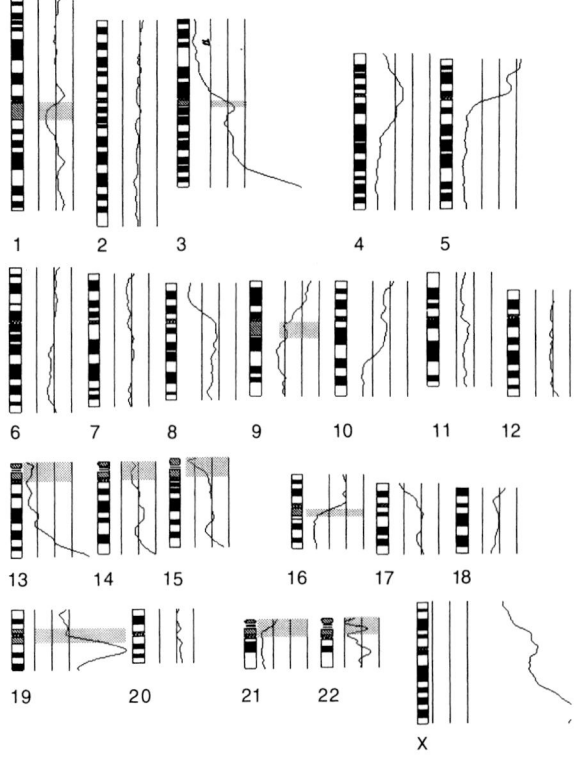

1 2 3 4 5

6 7 8 9 10 11 12

13 14 15 16 17 18

19 20 21 22 X

F

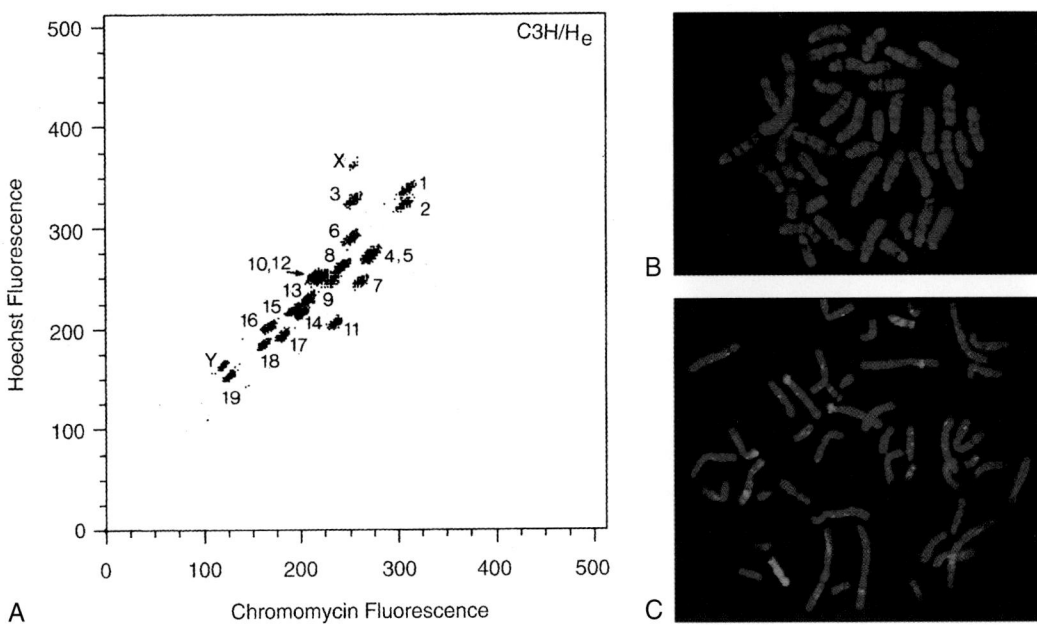

Plate 25.21. Cross species chromosome painting. (A) Flow karyotype of male C3H/He mouse showing separation of most of the autosomes and the sex chromosomes. (B) Mouse chromosome specific paint probe (CAMBIO Ltd., Cambridge, England) from chromosome 11 and hybridized to male mouse metaphase. (C) Mouse chromosome 11 paint hybridized to male human metaphse showing cross-species homology of conserved DNA sequences on chromosomes 17, 2p, distal 5q, 7q, and 22q.

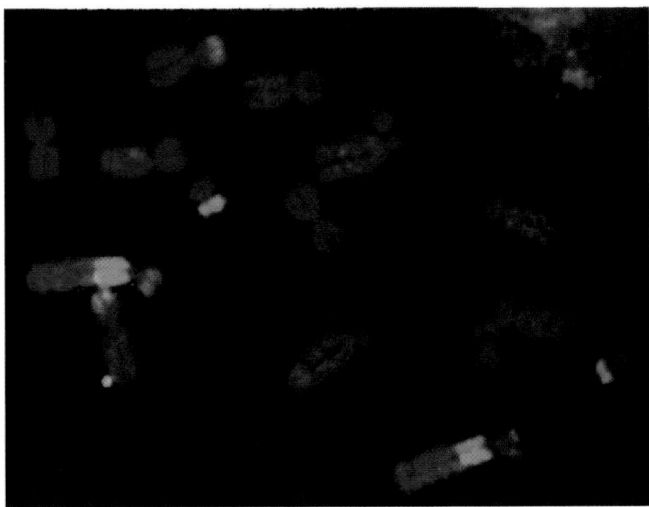

Plate 25.20. Comparative genomic hybridization (CGH) analysis of a small cell lung carcinoma (SCLC). (A) Hybridization of control DNA labeled with digoxigenin and visualized with TRITC (red) to a normal male metaphase. (B) The same metaphase hybridized with tumor DNA labeled with biotin and visualized with FITC (green). The images in (A) and (B) are merged in (C) and given false colors by image analysis to reveal areas of gain (green) and loss (red) of tumor DNA when the ratios of tumor DNA:control DNA are more than 1.5 and less than 0.5, respectively. Ratios between 0.5 and 1.5 are indicated in blue. (D) is the karyotype of this metaphase showing that the homologues of each chromosome have a consistent pattern. Fluorescence ratio along each chromosome are generated as illustrated in (E). In (F) ratio profiles for each chromosome have been determined derived from five metaphases of the same SCLC. The three vertical lines to the right of each chromosome idogram represent fluorescence ratios of 0.5, 1, and 1.5 (*from left to right*) between tumor and control DNA. The ratio profile (curve) represents the mean value of the five metaphases. The gray-shaded boxes represent chromosomal regions rich in heterochromatin that could not be interpreted due to abundance of repetitive DNA. All changes visible in (C) are confirmed by mean ration profile measurements. Note especially the loss of 3p, 5q, 10q, 13q, and 17p and the amplification of 3q, 5p, and 19q that are commonly observed in SCLC. (From Ried T et al., 1994, with permission. Courtesy of Dr Thomas Reid.)

Plate 25.22. Cross-species chromosome painting. Chromosomes 4 (red), 7 (green), and 9 (yellow) from the brush-tailed possum hybridized to chromosomes 1, 3, and 7 of the tammar wallaby. (From Rens et al., 1999, with permission.)

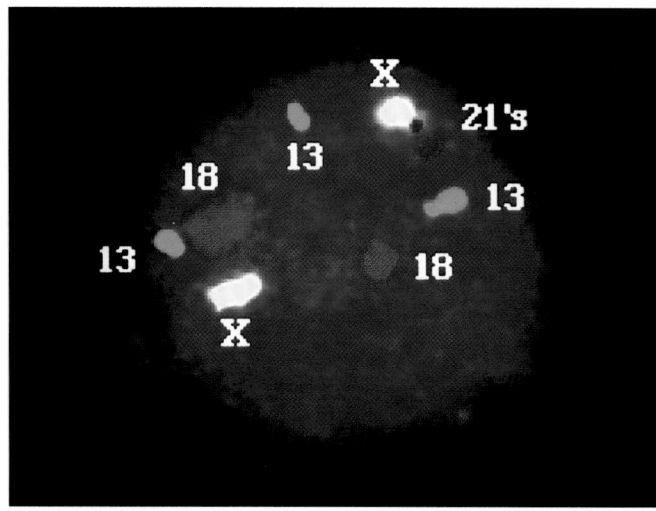

Plate 29.8. Five color FISH analysis of fetal cell obtained from maternal circulation. Fetus with 47,XX,+13 complement.

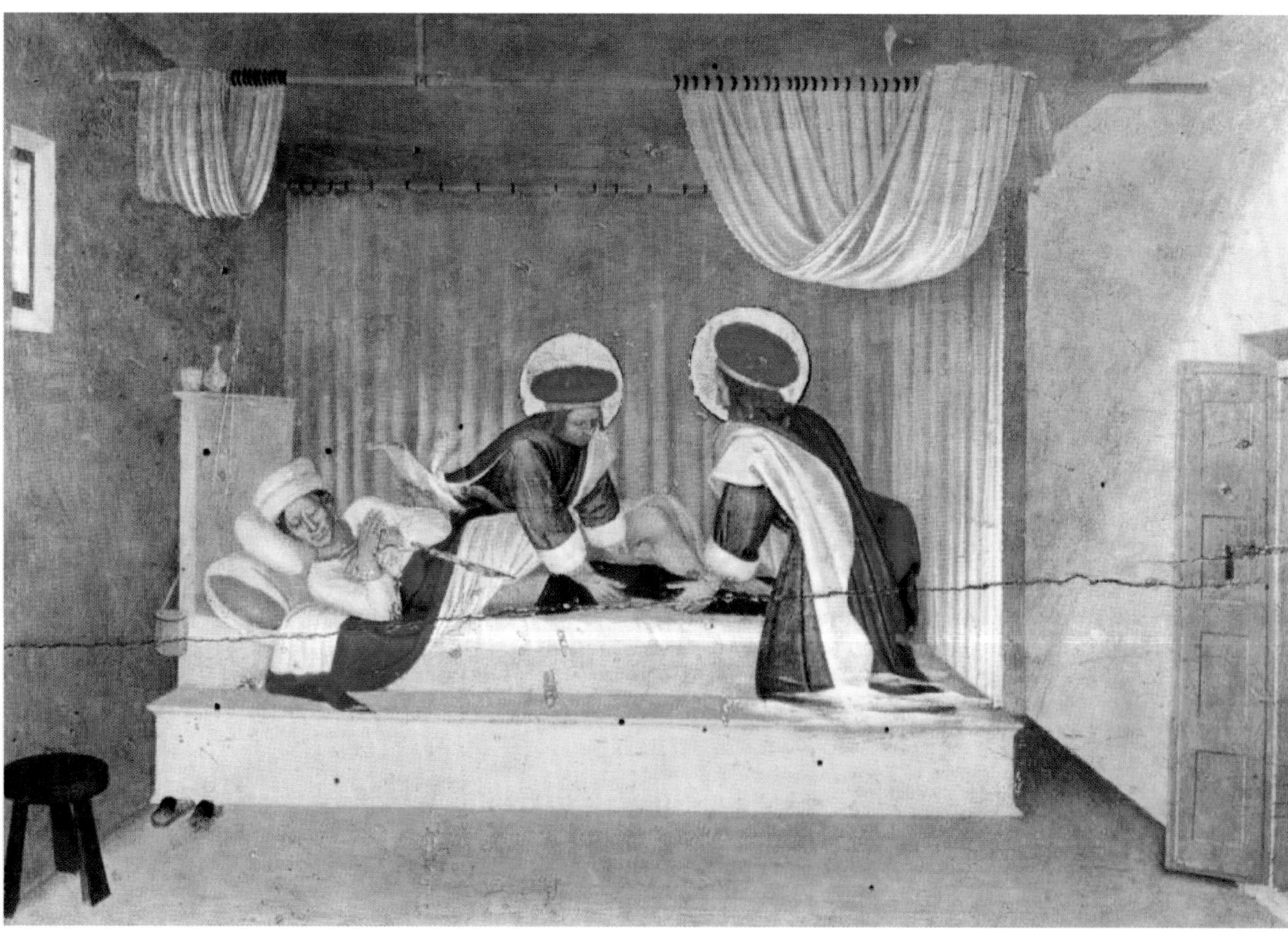

Plate 43.1. The miracle of Cosmas and Damian as portrayed by Fra Angelico in his painting conserved in the museum of San Marco Church in Florence, Italy.

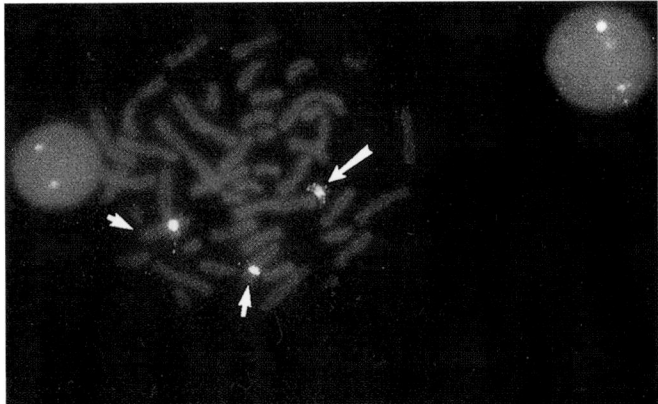

Plate 46.27. (B) Pohotomicrograph of a metaphase after fluorescence in situ hybridization using a biotin-labeled α-satellite probe for the pericentrometric region of chromosome 8. *Large arrow* indicates the brightly fluorescent marker chromosome. The two normal 8s (*smaller arrows*) also give a positive signal. (From Spinner NB, Rehberg-Grace K, Owens NL et al. (1995) Mosaicism for a chromosome 8 derived marker chromosome in a patient with manifestations of trisomy 8 mosaicism. Am J Med Genet 56:22–24, with permission.)

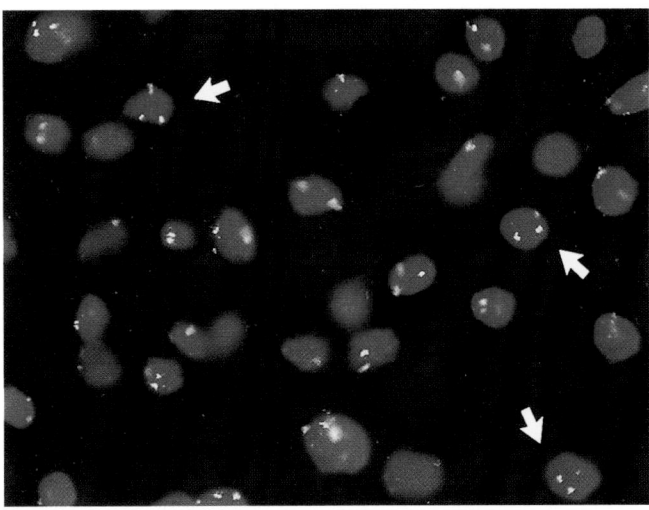

Plate 46.37. Photomicrograph of interphase cells from the buccal mucosa of a patient with Pallister-Killian syndrome after fluorescent in situ hybridization, using an α-satellite probe from the pericentromeric region of chromosome 12. Note that some cells in the field (*arrows*) have three signals, consistent with the presence of the isochromosome 12p.

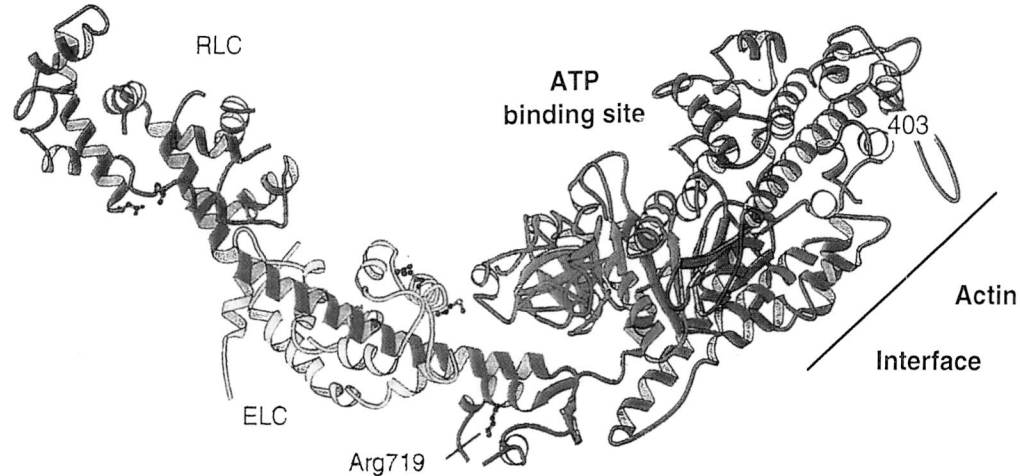

Plate 49.21. Three-dimensional representation of the myosin S1 structure. This scheme is based on the X-ray analysis of the chicken-fast skeletal muscle myosin (Rayment et al., 1993a). Due to the high degree of evolutionary conservation of myosins across species it applies with minor modifications to human cardiac myosin also. The ATP binding site (a cleft in the S1 head) and the actin binding interface are indicated. The two light chains, ELC (yellow) and RLC (purple) that bind to the α-helical neck are shown. The colors refer to the tryptic fragments of myosin: red 50 kDa, green 25 kDa and blue 20 kDa. The positions of two missense mutations, which are both associated with a severe course of HCM, are indicated: 403[Arg-Gln] and 719[Arg-Gln].

BASIC PRINCIPLES

History of medical genetics

Victor A. McKusick

Introduction

Medical genetics is the science of human biologic variation as it relates to health and disease. Clinical genetics is that part of medical genetics concerned with the health of individual humans and their families. Alternatively, clinical genetics can be defined as the science and practice of diagnosis, prevention, and management of genetic disorders.

Within recent years, medical genetics has become established as a clinical specialty, as the culmination of developments that began in 1956 with the description of the correct chromosome number of the human. With the discovery of specific microscopically visible chromosomal changes associated with clinical disorders, beginning with Down syndrome in January 1959, medical genetics acquired an anatomic base. Medical geneticists now had their specific organ—the genome—just as cardiologists had the heart and neurologists had the nervous system.

The anatomic base of medical genetics was greatly extended with the mapping of genes to chromosomes and specific chromosomal regions, at an ever-accelerating pace, over the past 30 years. Gene mapping has not only enlarged the base for medical genetics but, indeed, as pointed out to me by Charles Scriver (personal communication, 1980), has also provided a neo-Vesalian basis for all of medicine (McKusick, 1981). Medical historians tell us that the anatomy of Vesalius published in 1543 was of pivotal importance in the development of modern medicine. It was the basis of the physiology of William Harvey (1628) and the morbid anatomy of Morgagni (1761). Similarly, human gene mapping constitutes an approach to the study of abnormal gene function in all diseases; the gene-mapping approach has been adopted by researchers in almost all branches of medicine in the study of their most puzzling disorders. Through mapping, they have sought the basic defect in these disorders, and their clinical colleagues have used mapping information for diagnosis and carrier detection. The ultimate anatomic basis for medical genetics, the DNA sequence, is provided by the Human Genome Project.

In this brief history of medical genetics, I trace the foundations of the field that were laid between 1865, when Mendel published his work, and 1956, when the correct chromosome number was reported. I then discuss the events of the past 45 years that have seen the main evolution of the discipline. Finally, I attempt some projections for the future.

Foundations of medical genetics before 1956

Medical genetics in many developed countries is now a recognized specialty. In the United States, for example, an American Board of Medical Genetics certifies practitioners in the field, including PhD medical geneticists; the Board of Medical Genetics was the twenty-fourth to join the family of certifying American specialty boards, in 1991. Medical genetics is a rather unusual branch of clinical medicine; indeed, it may be nearly unique in that it originated out of a basic science. Most specialties started as crafts (or out of a technologic advance such as radiography) and only subsequently acquired basic science foundations.

The basic science that developed before 1956 and served as the foundation for the developments of the last 45 years included mendelism, cytogenetics, biochemical genetics, immunogenetics, and statistical, formal, and population genetics.

MENDELISM

The demonstration of the particulate nature of inheritance was the contribution of Gregor Mendel (1822–1884), a monk and later abbot in an Augustinian monastery (Fig. 1.1) in Brünn (now Brno), Moravia (now the Czech Republic). The terms *dominant* and *recessive* were his. The delay in recognition of his work has been attributed to various factors, but the most likely is poor timing; in 1865, when Mendel reported his findings and conclusions, the chromosomes had not yet been discovered. Because its physical basis, meiosis, had not yet been described, mendelism had no plausible basis to qualify it over other possible mechanisms of inheritance such as blending inheritance, which was favored by Francis Galton (1822–1911) and others of Mendel's contemporaries.

R A Fisher (1890–1962) (1936) raised a question as to whether Mendel's results were "too good," that is, that the data agreed too closely with the conclusions (see the discussion of this matter by Novitski, 1995). (Mendel's "Round" [R] versus "wrinkled" [r] trait in the garden pea has been shown to be due to a transposon insertion in the R gene for starch branching enzyme. The wrinkled state is due to lack of an osmotic effect present when the normally functioning enzyme is present. The first demonstration of mutation in the human due to insertion of a transposon was provided by the Kazazian group [Dombroski et al., 1991]: a movable element from chromosome 22 was inserted into the factor VIII gene causing hemophilia A.)

Human chromosomes, visualized in tumor cells in mitosis, were pictured in a paper by Walther Flemming (Fig. 1.2A),

professor of anatomy in Kiel, in 1882 (Fig. 1.2B). The term *chromosome* was introduced by Waldeyer in 1888. Mitosis and meiosis were described in the last quarter of the nine-

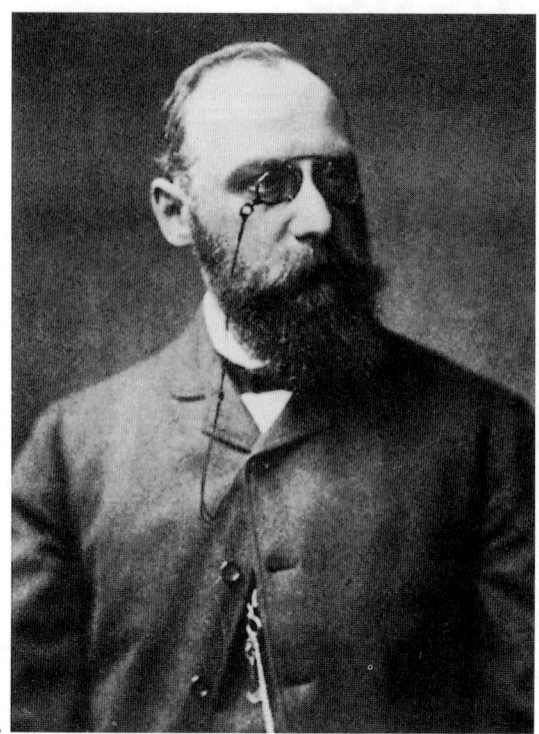

A

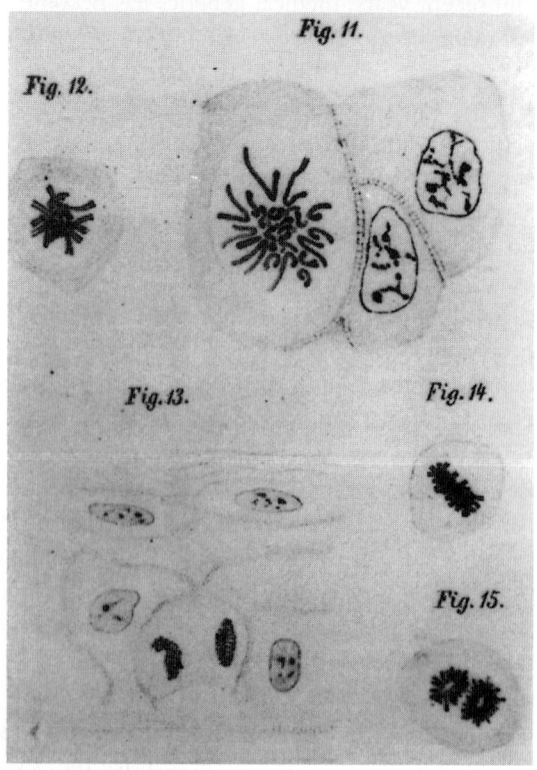

B

Fig. 1.2. (A) Walther Flemming (1843–1905), discoverer of chromosomes. (B) First illustration of human chromosomes, by Flemming (1882).

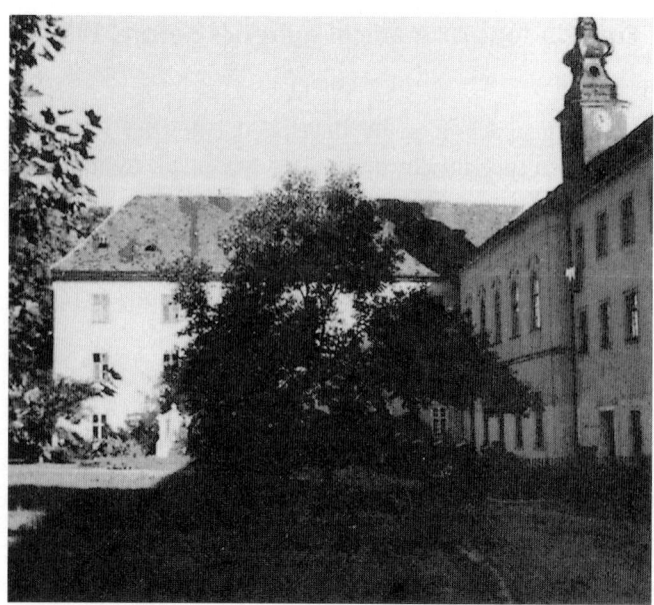

Fig. 1.1. Mendel's monastery as it appeared in 1971.

teenth century. (The term *meiosis* was introduced in 1905 by Farmer and Moore; the process had been previously referred to as the reduction divisions. The word *miosis*, usually taken to mean "reduction in size of the pupil," is from the same root. It is fortunate that the words are spelled differently in the two usages. In fact, Farmer and Moore spelled it *maiosis*. They wrote as follows: "We propose to apply the terms Maiosis or Maiotic phase to cover the whole series of nuclear changes included in the two divisions that were designated as Heterotype and Homotype by Flemming.")

During the 1880s, Roux, deVries, and Weismann developed the theory that the chromosomes carry determinants of heredity and development. The state of cytogenetics before the discovery of Mendel's work was reviewed by E B Wilson (Fig. 1.3) in his classic text (Wilson, 1896). In a discussion of the Roux-deVries-Weismann theory (pp. 182–185), Wilson (1896) wrote that

> the chromatin is a congeries or colony of invisible self-propagating vital units …, each of which has the power of determining the development of a particular quality. Weismann conceives these units … [to be] associated in linear groups to form the … chromosomes.

In 1900 mendelism was rediscovered independently by Hugo deVries (1848–1935) in Amsterdam, Carl F J E Correns (1864–1933) in Tübingen, Germany, and Erich von Tschermak (1871–1962) in Vienna, Austria. The chromosome theory of mendelism was put forward about 1903 by Walter S Sutton (1877–1916) (Fig. 1.4), then a graduate student at Columbia under E B Wilson (McKusick, 1960); and by Theodor Boveri (1862–1915) of Würzburg, Germany, a leading cytologist to whom Wilson dedicated his landmark book (1896). Sutton, a Kansas farm boy, had studied meiosis in the Kansas grasshopper at Kansas University under C E McClung. He was in New York in 1902, when William Bateson, the leading English champion for mendelism, lectured there on the subject. Sutton promptly recognized the behavior of Mendel's so-called factors in transmission from one generation to the next as exactly what one would expect if they were located on the chromosomes. The segregation of alleles and assortment of non-alleles were precisely what one would anticipate given the observed behavior of the chromosomes in meiosis.

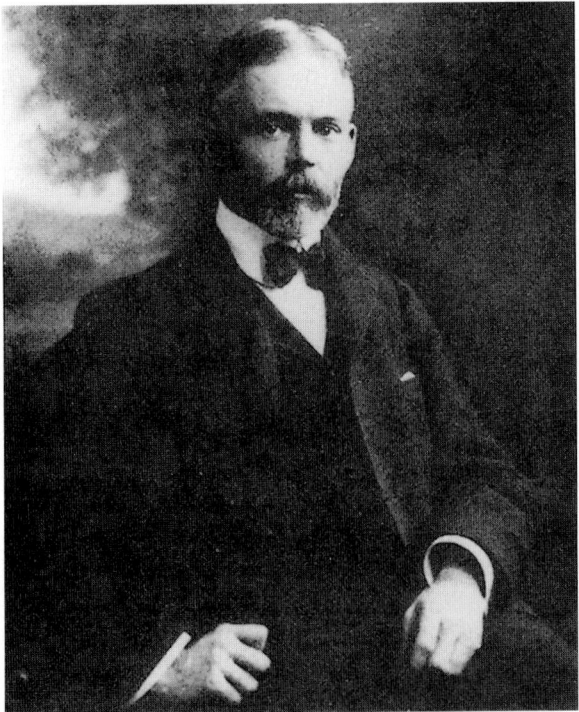

Fig. 1.3. E B Wilson (1856–1939), noted cytologist and author of *The Cell in Development and Inheritance* (1896).

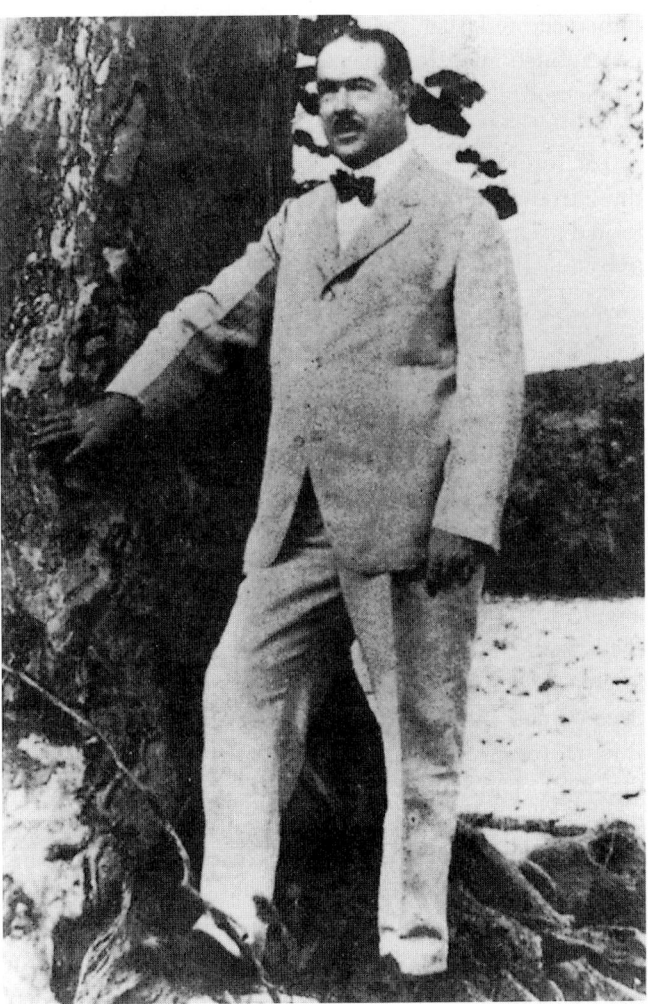

Fig. 1.4. Walter S Sutton (1877–1916), co-developer of the chromosome theory of mendelism.

William Bateson (1861–1926) had a difficult time converting biometricians to the mendelian view of heredity. These were the disciples of Francis Galton, including Karl Pearson (1856–1936), who favored blending inheritance. They were led to this view through experiences with the study of quantitative traits that we would call multifactorial. Their recalcitrance is evident in the following statement (Pearson et al, 1911):

> As we have seen in the course of this work albinism is a graded character, and we have every reason to believe that both in man and dogs separate grades are hereditary ... Mendelism is at present the mode—no other conception of heredity can even obtain a hearing. Yet one of the present writers at least believes that a reaction will shortly set in, and that the views of Galton will again come by their own.

The views of the biometricians and mendelists were reconciled by R A Fisher in a classic paper published in 1918. Fisher showed that the mendelian behavior of multiple genes functioning together can explain the findings of the biometricians in regard to quantitative traits. (In his 1918 paper, Fisher introduced the term *variance*.)

Bateson made many contributions to genetics, including the introduction of the term. In a letter written in 1905, related to a projected new professorship at Oxford University (which he did not receive), Bateson wrote as follows:

> If the Quick Fund were used for the foundation of a Professorship relating to Heredity and Variation the best title would, I think, be "The Quick Professorship of the Study of Heredity." No single word in common use quite gives this meaning. Such a word is badly wanted and if it were desirable to coin one "Genetics" might do. Either expression clearly includes Variation and the cognate phenomena.

Another of Bateson's accomplishments was the discovery (with Punnett) of linkage in the domestic fowl. They misinterpreted the phenomenon and assigned terms that have been perpetuated, however: coupling and repulsion signify whether the two mutant genes of particular interest are on the same chromosome or on opposite chromosomes, respectively. The true significance of linkage and the application of linkage and crossingover to chromosome mapping were contributions of Thomas Hunt Morgan (1866–1945) and his colleagues working in the famous "fly room" at Columbia (Fig. 1.5). Alfred Sturtevant was then a college undergraduate; Calvin Bridges and Hermann Muller were junior associates of Morgan. The unit of genetic map distance, the centimorgan (cM), was named for Morgan. An

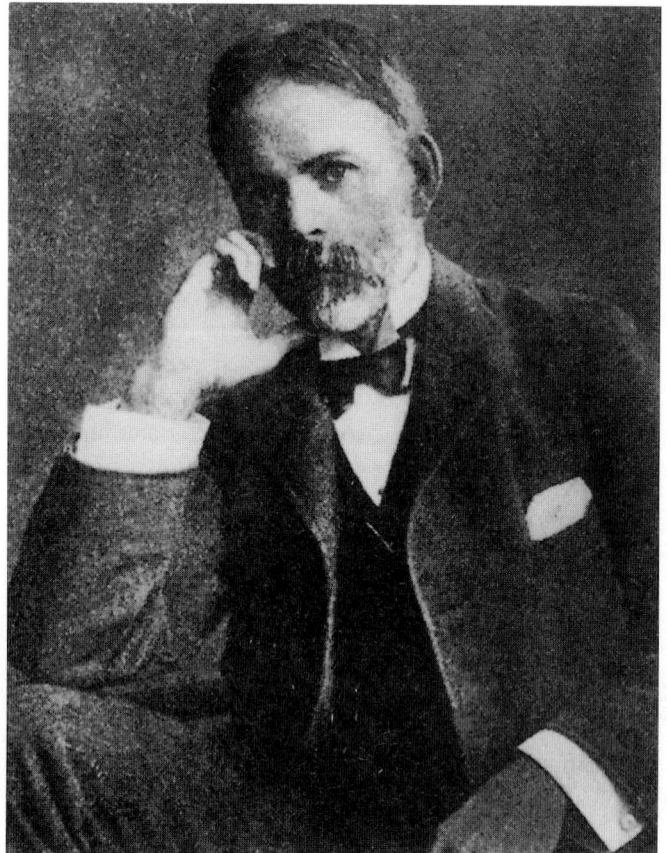

Fig. 1.5. Thomas Hunt Morgan (1866–1945), student of linkage and first American-born Nobel laureate in Medicine or Physiology. Photo c. 1910.

1892 PhD from Johns Hopkins University, he was the first native-born American to be awarded the Nobel prize in physiology or medicine (1933), given for his contributions to the concept of the gene.

In 1927, Hermann J Muller (1890–1967) demonstrated that X-irradiation produces an increase in the rate of mutation in *Drosophila*. For this work, he received the Nobel prize in 1946.

CYTOGENETICS

During the 50 years after Flemming's first picturing of human chromosomes in 1882, several attempts were made to determine the chromosome number in the human and to determine the human sex chromosome constitution. A particularly definitive paper appeared to be that of T S Painter (1923), in which the diploid number of 48 was arrived at from study of meiotic chromosomes in testicular material from a hanged criminal in Texas. (There is probably no basis for the favorite suggestion of graduate students that the man may have had the XYY syndrome and therefore appeared to have 24, rather than 23, bivalents.) Painter commented that in some of his best preparations, the diploid number appeared to be 46. As an important contribution of the paper, Painter established the human XY sex chromosome mechanism.

In 1949, Murray Barr, working with Bertram in London, Ontario, discovered the sex chromatin, otherwise known as the Barr body, or X chromatin. The distinctive body was visualized in the nucleus of neural cells of the cat. A neuroanatomist, Barr was studying changes in neural cells with repetitive stimulation of the nerves. Fortunately, he had sufficiently good records that he could establish that the unusual body in the interphase nuclei occurred only in female cats. Ten years later, when the XXY Klinefelter syndrome and the XO Turner syndrome, as well as other sex chromosome aneuploidies, were described, the correlation of the number of Barr bodies with the number of X chromosomes in excess of one was established. The correlation with X-inactivation and the Lyon hypothesis were likewise elaborated. Twenty years after the paper of Barr and Bertram (1949), the fluorescent (F) body, or Y chromatin, was discovered in interphase nuclei by Zech and Caspersson and colleagues (Caspersson et al. 1970a,b, 1971).

Three new techniques developed in the 1950s and early 1960s facilitated the burgeoning of human cytogenetics, including clinical cytogenetics. During the early 1950s, T C Hsu (sometimes known to his colleagues and friends as "tissue culture Hsu") was working in Galveston, when he accidentally discovered, through an error in the preparation of solutions, that hypotonicity causes nuclei to swell with dispersion of the mitotic chromosomes, improving visibility. In his paper, Hsu acknowledged that Hughes at Cambridge University had independently made the same discovery. This technical "trick" was used by J H Tjio and Albert Levan (1956) (Fig. 1.6A and B) in studies of the chromosomes of fetal lung cells in mitosis and by Charles Ford (Fig. 1.7A) and John Hamerton (Fig. 1.7B) in studies of meiotic testicular cells (1956) to determine that the correct chromosome number of the human is 2N = 46.

In the early days of clinical cytogenetics it was the practice to do bone marrow aspiration in order to get an adequate number of dividing cells for analysis. This requirement was avoided by the introduction of phytohemagglutinin by Peter Nowell (Nowell, 1960; Nowell and Hungerford, 1960a; 1960b). As its name implies, phytohemagglutinin is of plant origin and causes the agglutination of red cells. Its use was introduced by Edwin E Osgood (1899–1970) of Portland, Oregon, for the purpose of separating white blood cells from red blood cells. It was Nowell's observation that circulating lymphocytes exposed to phytohemagglutinin were stimulated to divide. Thus, it was possible to obtain from a sample of peripheral blood adequate numbers of dividing cells for chromosome studies.

The third technique of particular value to cytogenetics was the use of colchicine to arrest cell division in mitosis. Combined with phytohemagglutinin, it further helped

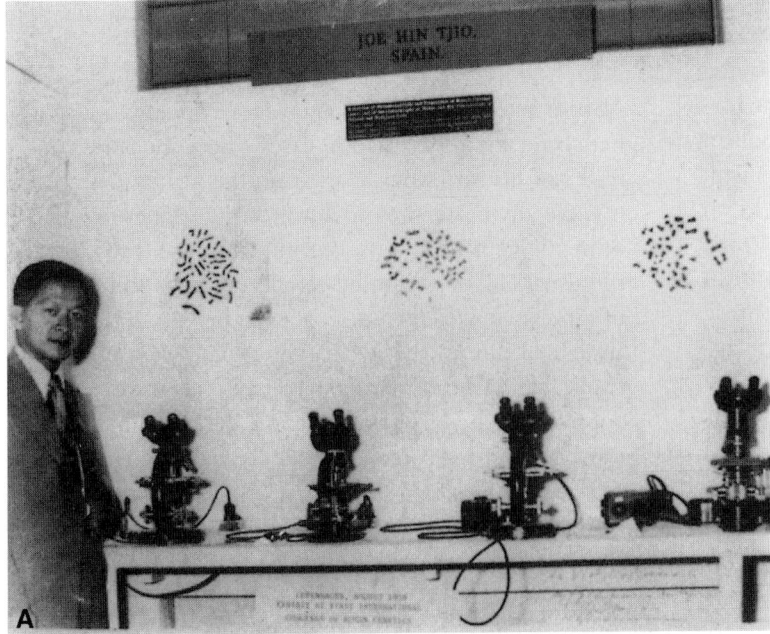
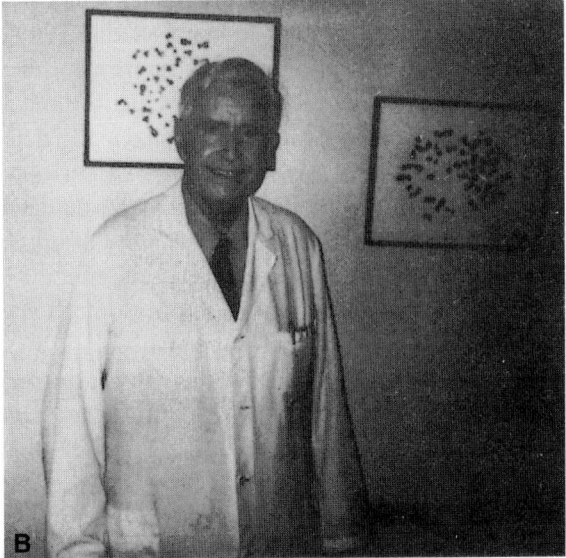

Fig. 1.6. (A) Exhibit by J H Tjio at first World Congress of Human Genetics in Copenhagen (1956). Demonstration of 2N = 46 in mitotic cells. (B) Albert Levan in Lund, Sweden, in 1989. Collaborator of Tjio in work published in 1956.

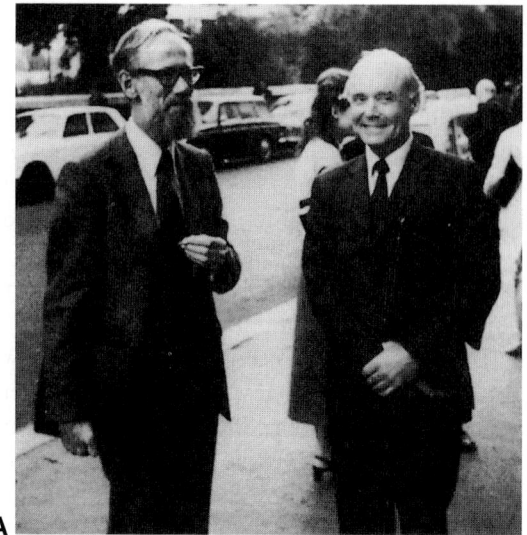
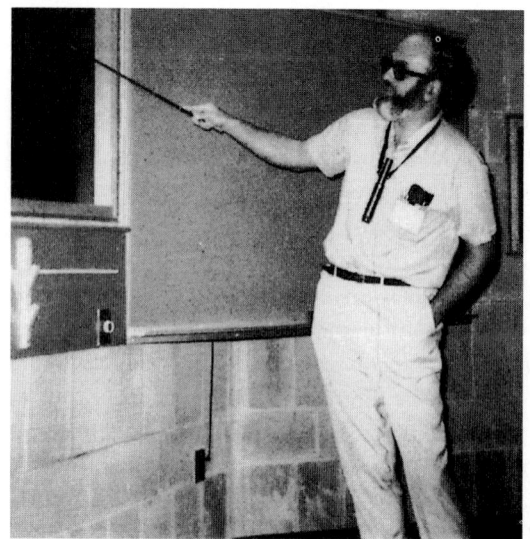

Fig. 1.7. Charles Ford (A), (at right) and John Hamerton (B) confirmed the 2N = 46 in meiotic cells in 1956. Photographs in 1971 and 1974, respectively.

ensure adequate numbers of cells at a stage of division optimal for chromosome identification and enumeration.

BIOCHEMICAL GENETICS

The acknowledged father of biochemical genetics is Archibald Garrod (1858–1936), who introduced the concept of *inborn errors of metabolism*, as well as the term (Bearn, 1993). Alkaptonuria was the first of the disorders he investigated. In his paper on this condition in 1902, after coaching by Bateson, he recognized that its inheritance was probably mendelian recessive because of the occurrence in both males and females with normal parents who were often consanguineous. In his famous Croonian lectures (delivered in 1908 and published in 1909), he formally unveiled the concept of inborn errors of metabolism and discussed three other conditions: pentosuria, albinism, and cystinuria. The nature of the enzymatic defect in all four of these disorders is now known. La Du et al. (1958) confirmed Garrod's prediction of an enzyme deficiency in alkaptonuria by demonstrating deficiency of homogentisic acid oxidase in a liver sample. The gene mutant in alkaptonuria has been mapped to chromosome 3 by linkage studies; the gene encoding homogentisic acid oxidase has been cloned and a number of disease-causing mutations identified therein (see OMIM 203500). The enzyme deficiency of tyrosinase in classic oculocutaneous albinism has been characterized all the way to the DNA level, and the enzymatic and genetic defects in other forms of albinism have been defined. On the basis of classic biochemistry, the enzyme defect in pentosuria is known to involve xylitol dehydrogenase (L-xylulose reductase); the gene has not been mapped. Cystinuria is not, strictly speaking, a Garrodian inborn error of metabolism, but a defect in renal (and intestinal) transport of dibasic amino acids. It is caused by mutation in an amino acid transporter gene located on chromosome 2.

Bateson, Garrod's contemporary and advisor in matters genetical, is credited with the useful piece of advice: "Treasure your exceptions!" He was referring to findings in experimental genetics and perhaps was emphasizing also the value of investigating rare mutants. The same message was conveyed by Archibald Garrod (1928). He quoted a letter written by William Harvey a few months before his death in 1657:

> Nature is nowhere accustomed more openly to display her secret mysteries than in cases where she shows traces of her workings apart from the beaten path; nor is there any better way to advance the proper practice of medicine than to give our minds to the discovery of the usual law of nature by careful investigation of cases of rarer forms of disease. For it has been found, in almost all things, that what they contain of useful or applicable nature is hardly perceived unless we are deprived of them, or they become deranged in some way.

Garrod was William Osler's immediate successor as Regius Professor of Medicine at Oxford University. He seems to have been sensitive to the prevailing view that the disorders he studied were unimportant because they were rare, especially in contrast to the infections and nutritional diseases rampant at that time. It was after his retirement from the Regius chair in 1927 that Garrod (1931) wrote *The Inborn Factors in Disease*, expanding his earlier *Inborn Errors of Metabolism* (1909) to the full-blown theory of biochemical individuality. Indeed, as pointed out by Barton Childs (1995), there was prophetic symbolism in the succession from Osler, who emphasized the disease that affected the patient, to Garrod, who focused on the patient affected by the disease.

Alkaptonuria was not the first inborn error of metabolism in which a specific enzyme deficiency was demonstrated. The first was hepatic glucose-6-phosphatase (G6P) deficiency demonstrated in glycogen storage disease type 1 by Carl and Gerty Cori (1952). (Diaphorase deficiency in methemoglobinemia was demonstrated by Gibson in 1948, but perhaps this cannot be considered a Garrodian inborn error of intermediary metabolism.) Deficiency of phenylalanine hydroxylase in phenylketonuria (PKU) was demonstrated soon after by Jervis (1953). Asbjørn Følling in Norway had described PKU in 1934. The molecular nature of a mutation of the gene encoding phenylalanine hydroxylase (*PAH*; MIM 261600) in PKU was first described by Savio Woo and colleagues in 1986 (DiLella et al., 1986).

Linus Pauling (1901–1994) introduced his concept of molecular disease during the late 1940s. It was an outgrowth of his focus on protein structure and specifically his work on sickle cell anemia (with Itano) (Pauling et al., 1949) demonstrating by electrophoresis that the hemoglobin molecule had an abnormal structure. By 1956, Vernon Ingram had narrowed the abnormality of the sickle hemoglobin molecule to a single peptide, and by 1957 to a single amino acid difference.

By 1956 also, Oliver Smithies was writing about starch gel electrophoresis, opening up the study of human variation at the protein level. With this and similar methods, Harry Harris (1919–1994) at the Galton Laboratory extended the Garrodian concept of biochemical individuality (Fig. 1.8).

As studies of the heredity of biochemical differences were going on, investigations of the chemistry of heredity were under way that would be the basis of what we now call molecular genetics. DNA had been discovered in fish sperm by Miescher in the nineteenth century. At the Rockefeller Institute for Medical Research in 1944, O T Avery, C M McLeod, and M McCarty demonstrated that the transforming factor, which changed the *Pneumococcus* from a rough form to a smooth form, is DNA. In 1953, Watson and Crick suggested a model for the structure of DNA consistent with its X-ray crystallography and with its biologic properties, including the capacity for replication.

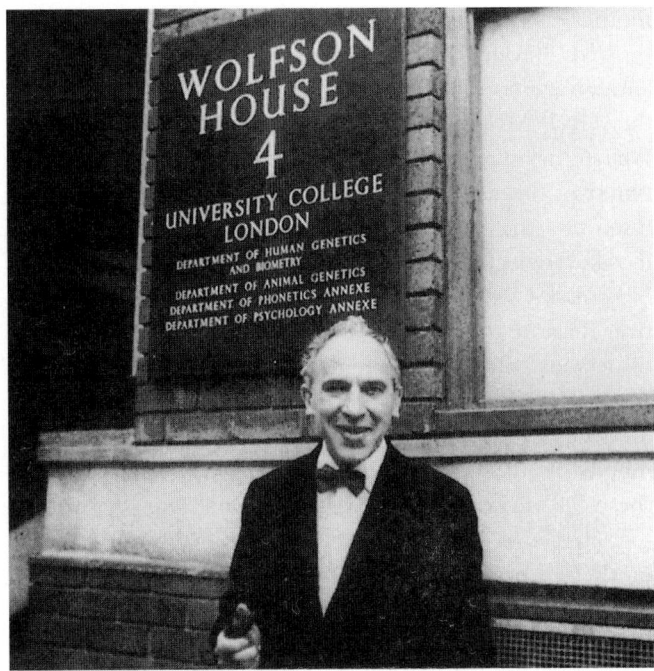

Fig. 1.8. Harry Harris (c. 1974).

IMMUNOGENETICS

Immunogenetics can be said to have had its start with the discovery of the ABO blood groups. These were demonstrated through the existence of "natural" antibodies (isoantibodies) by K Landsteiner in 1901. From the distribution of ABO blood types in populations, Felix Bernstein, in the early 1920s derived support for the multiple allele, one-locus explanation, rather than the alternative two-locus (A, non-A; and B, non-B) hypothesis. F Yamamoto et al. (1990) defined the molecular differences between the genes for blood groups O and A and between those for A and B.

The next-to-be-discovered blood group was MN, found by Landsteiner and Levine (1927). These workers injected rabbits with different samples of human red cells and absorbed the resulting rabbit immune serum with other red cell samples, until they found antibodies that distinguished human bloods of the same ABO type.

Yet other blood group systems were discovered on the basis of antibodies ("antisera") from mothers immunized to red cell antigens the fetus inherited from the father and antibodies from recipients of mismatched blood transfusions. The Rh blood group system is an example. As recounted by Race and Sanger (1975), Levine and Stetson (1939), in a brief but historic paper, described how the mother of a stillborn fetus suffered a severe hemolytic reaction to the transfusion of blood from her husband. The mother's serum agglutinated the cells of her husband and those of 80 out of 104 other ABO compatible donors. The antigen responsible was shown to be independent of the ABO, MN, and P groups. In 1940, Landsteiner and Weiner, having immunized rabbits and guinea pigs with the blood of the monkey *Macacus rhesus*, made the surprising discovery that the antibodies agglutinated not only the monkey red cells, but also the red cells of about 85% of New York City white people, who were said to be Rh positive. Because the anti-Rh antibody was found in the blood of persons who had suffered reaction to the transfusion of ABO-matched blood, and the antibody of Levine and Stetson (1939) was apparently identical to that raised in rabbits by injection of rhesus blood, the system was called rhesus (Rh). Levine et al. (1941) showed that erythroblastosis fetalis is the result of Rh incompatibility between mother and child. Years later it became known that rabbit anti-rhesus and human anti-Rh antibodies are in fact not the same, but it was too late to change the name. Instead, the rabbit anti-rhesus antibody was called anti-LW, in honor of Landsteiner and Weiner. The LW antigen was later shown to be encoded by a gene on chromosome 19 that is quite distinct from the *RH* gene on chromosome 1.

Before 1956, blood groups provided some of the clearest examples of the role of mendelism in the human, as well as some of the most important examples of the application of genetic principles in human health and disease, particularly blood transfusion and maternofetal Rh incompatibility.

STATISTICAL, FORMAL, AND POPULATION GENETICS

A cornerstone of population genetics is the *Hardy-Weinberg principle*, named for Godfrey Harold Hardy (1877–1947), distinguished mathematician of Cambridge University, and Wilhelm Weinberg (1862–1937), physician of Stuttgart, Germany, publishing independently in 1908. Hardy (1908) was stimulated to write a short paper to explain why a dominant gene would not, with the passage of generations, become inevitably and progressively more frequent. He published the paper in the American journal, *Science*, perhaps because he considered it a trivial contribution and would be embarrassed to publish it in a British journal.

R A Fisher, J B S Haldane (1892–1964), and Sewall Wright (1889–1988) were the great triumvirate of population genetics. Sewall Wright is noted for the concept and term *random genetic drift*. J B S Haldane (Fig. 1.9) made many contributions, including, with Julia Bell (Bell and Haldane, 1937), the first attempt at quantitation of linkage of two human traits, colorblindness and hemophilia. Fisher

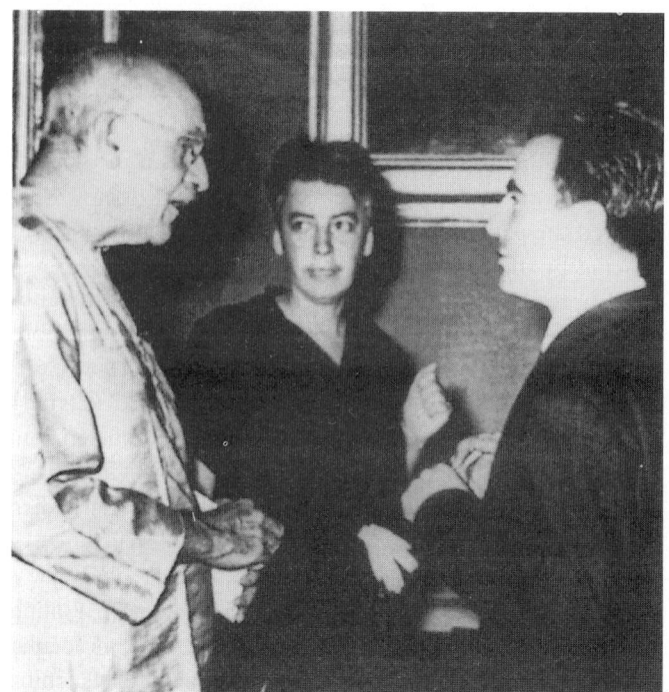

Fig. 1.9. J B S Haldane with Helen Spurway and Marcello Siniscalco at Second World Congress of Human Genetics, Rome, 1961.

proposed a multilocus, closely linked hypothesis for Rh blood groups and worked on methods for correcting for the bias of ascertainment affecting segregation analysis of autosomal recessive traits.

To test the recessive hypothesis for mode of inheritance in a given disorder in humans, the results of different types of matings must be observed as they are found, rather than being set up by design. In those families in which both parents are heterozygous carriers of a rare recessive trait, the presence of the recessive gene is often not recognizable unless a homozygote is included among the offspring. Thus, the ascertained families are a truncated sample of the whole. Furthermore, under the usual social circumstances, families with both parents heterozygous may be more likely to be ascertained if two, three, or four children are affected than they are if only one child is affected. Corrections for these so-called biases of ascertainment were devised by Weinberg of the Hardy-Weinberg law, Bernstein, of ABO fame, and Fritz Lenz and Lancelot Hogben, whose names are combined in the Lenz-Hogben correction, as well as by Fisher, Norman Bailey, and Newton E Morton. With the development of methods for identifying the presence of the recessive gene biochemically and ultimately by analysis of the DNA itself, such corrections became less often necessary.

Pre-1956 studies of genetic linkage in the human for the purpose of chromosome mapping are discussed later as part of a review of the history of that aspect of human genetics.

Growth and development of medical genetics: 1956 to the present

During the past 45 years, medical genetics has developed through a convergence of mendelism, cytogenetics, biochemical genetics, immunogenetics, and statistical, formal, and population genetics. The development in each of these areas is traced in the preceding part of this chapter. Since 1956, medical genetics, in building on these foundations, has been blessed with three methodologies more or less specific to the field. These are "chromosomology" (beginning about 1956), somatic cell genetics (beginning about 1966), and molecular genetics (beginning about 1976). As will be indicated later, transgenic mice and all methods for transfer of genes into cultured cells or whole organisms, beginning about 1986, constitute a fourth methodologic approach. The gene transfer methods, in combination with directed mutation and gene "knock-out," have already proved particularly useful in the analysis of the function of genes, normal and abnormal.

Two further major methodologic advances were database searching (research *in silico*, or cybergenomics) as a primary method of genetic and genomic research, and microarray technology for profiling of gene function. These began in the mid or late 1990s.

CHROMOSOMOLOGY

Following the lead of Margery Shaw (personal communication, 1971), I divide the history of human cytogenetics into five ages: (1) 1882–1956 (gestation), the period from the first publication on human chromosomes to the reports of the correct chromosome number; (2) 1956–1966 (a golden age of human clinical cytogenetics); (3) 1966–1969 (resting phase), a period when the field seemed to be "in the doldrums," with little progress; (4) 1969–1977 (the banding era); and (5) 1977 to the present (the era of molecular cytogenetics).

Jerome Lejeune (1926–1994) (Fig. 1.10) opened up the field of clinical cytogenetics with his report in January 1959 of the extra small chromosome in mongoloid idiocy, as Down syndrome was then called. (A letter in *The Lancet* in 1961, containing a list of 19 signatories resembling a short Who's Who in Human Genetics [Allen et al., 1961], established the eponymic designation as the preferred one. This is a prime example of the triumph of an eponym.)

The quinacrine fluorescence method was the first of the banding methods developed by Torbjørn Caspersson and colleagues (1970a,b 1971) and exploited by Peter Pearson and others. This was followed by the various methods of

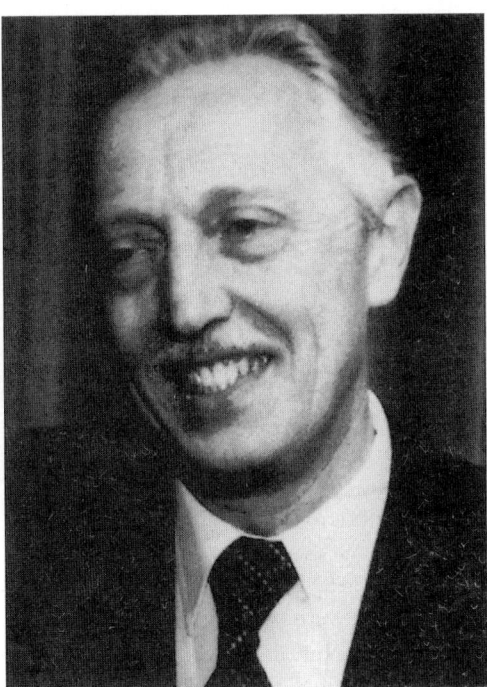

Fig. 1.10. Jerome Lejeune in Baltimore, 1984.

Giemsa staining following alkali and other treatments for so-called G-banding, and by the method called reverse banding, or R-banding, because the Giemsa-light bands were stained.

The banding techniques permitted the unique identification of each human chromosome. This was immensely useful in experimental situations such as the study of rodent/human somatic cell hybrids (see later under Somatic Cell Genetics) and in the precise characterization of chromosomal aberrations. An early result was the demonstration that the smallest autosome is not number 22, but rather number 21, the autosome trisomic in Down syndrome. Jerome Lejeune had thought that Down syndrome is trisomy of the next to the smallest autosome, not the smallest. Furthermore, it was demonstrated by Janet Rowley (1973) (Fig. 1.11) that the Philadelphia (Ph) chromosome involves the non-Down syndrome chromosome, number 22, and that it represents a reciprocal translocation (with chromosome 9), not a deletion. The precise delineation of deletions and other aberrations permitted deletion mapping and mapping by dosage effects. An early, perhaps the first, example was the assignment of the locus for red cell acid phosphatase (MIM 171500) to 2p25 by Ferguson-Smith et al. (1973). The refined cytogenetic delineation of aberrations in the chromosomes also permitted the recognition of "new" chromosomal syndromes. Since one could be reasonably certain of having a "pure culture" series of cases with the same anomaly, it was possible to establish karyotype-phenotype correlations. The trisomy 8 syndrome,

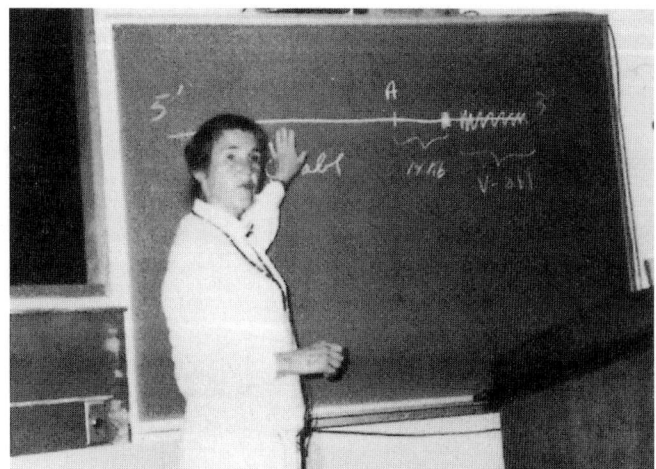

Fig. 1.11. Janet Rowley at Bar Harbor Course, 1983.

the 5q- syndrome, the Pallister-Killian syndrome, and the Jacobson syndrome were examples.

By 1977, high-resolution cytogenetics involving the banding of extended chromosome in cells arrested in prophase or prometaphase had been introduced independently by Jorge Yunis (1976), Uta Francke (Francke and Oliver, 1978), and the Manilovs. This improved further the identification of microdeletions in solid tumors such as Wilms tumor and retinoblastoma, in 11p13 and 13q14, respectively. It revealed specific chromosomal abnormalities in congenital disorders of previously obscure etiology, including Langer-Giedion syndrome, Prader-Willi syndrome, DiGeorge syndrome, and Beckwith-Wiedemann syndrome. It provided the basis for the concept of contiguous gene syndromes put forward by Roy Schmickel (1986).

The era of molecular cytogenetics, which persists to this day, began about 1977. With improved methods for studying DNA, the biochemical basis of banding was elucidated. The G+C-rich nature of the giemsa-light bands was demonstrated and this information was correlated with evidence that these bands are also gene rich. Chromosomal in situ hybridization with radiolabeled DNA probes was first made to work reliably for single copy genes in 1981, through the work of Mary Harper and Grady Saunders, Cynthia Morton, Malcolm A Ferguson-Smith (Fig. 1.12), and others. Because of high background noise and perhaps other factors, erroneous results had been previously obtained in experiments that attempted to map single-copy genes. Harper used dextran to create a "wad" of the isotopically labeled probe, thereby achieving a signal at the site of the particular gene that was well above the background level. In the initial paper by Harper et al. (1981), the method was used to map the insulin gene to the tip of the short arm of chromosome 11. Fluorescent in situ hybridization (FISH), a

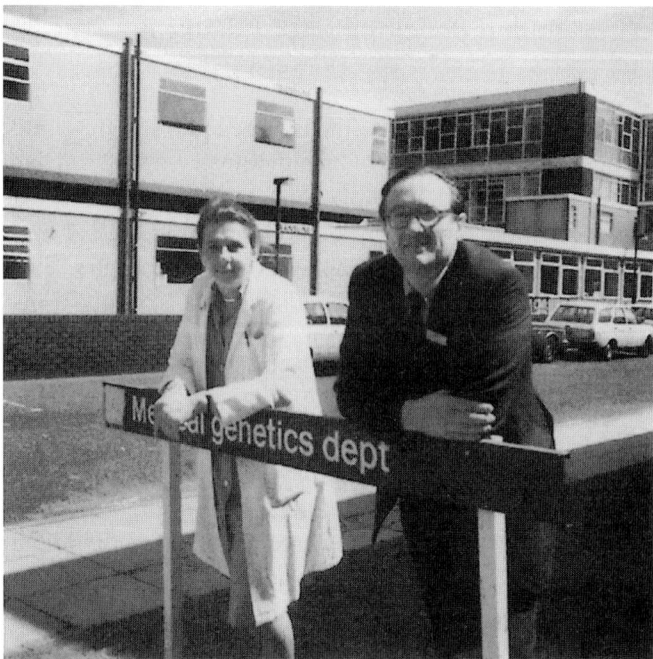

Fig. 1.12. Malcolm A Ferguson-Smith with Marie G Ferguson-Smith in Glasgow, 1981.

nonisotopic method, was developed by Ward et al., Landegent et al., and others in about 1985.

The combination of molecular techniques with cytogenetic techniques permitted chromosome mapping of oncogenes and identification of their role in hematologic malignancies associated with translocations. The *MYC* oncogene on chromosome 8 in Burkitt lymphoma was an early example elucidated by Carlo Croce, Philip Leder (Fig. 1.13), and others; the *ABL* oncogene on 9q, involved in chronic myeloid leukemia was worked out by Rowley, Heisterkamp, Grosveld (de Klein et al., 1982), and others. Chromosome sorting with fluorescence-activated devices, followed by

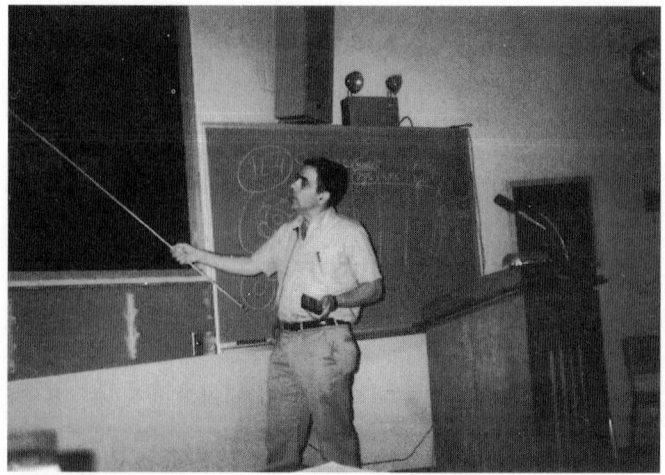

Fig. 1.13. Philip Leder at Bar Harbor Course, 1988.

analysis of gene content by molecular genetic methods, was developed; for example, Roger Lebo and colleagues (1984) used this method specifically for gene mapping.

Deletions were also found in association with neoplasms, usually solid tumors. The classic example is retinoblastoma. Lionel Penrose and colleagues (Lele et al, 1963) were the first to find a deletion in any neoplasm, a deletion in chromosome 13 in retinoblastoma. (Deletions in retinoblastoma played a role in proof of the Knudson hypothesis [Knudson et al, 1975] and in positional cloning of the *RB1* gene.)

Chromosome microdissection, another method of physical mapping, was developed for collection of DNA from specific regions that could then be subjected to molecular genetic studies. For example, the approach was used by the Horsthemke group (Lüdecke et al, 1989) to study the gene content of the region of 8q involved in Langer-Giedion syndrome, a contiguous gene syndrome (Schmickel, 1986).

SOMATIC CELL GENETICS

The second large methodologic advance in the era of human genetics since 1956 was somatic cell genetics. This has been contributory in several ways. In formal genetic analysis, it permitted the mapping of genes to specific human chromosomes or chromosome regions by the study of interspecies hybrids, between the human and the mouse, for example. It permitted the differentiation of allelism and nonallelism disorders on the basis of noncomplementation or complementation, respectively, when cells from different patients with a given disorder (e.g., xeroderma pigmentosum) were mixed. In a third place, it permitted the study of the biochemical essence of many inborn errors of metabolism in cultured cells, usually skin fibroblasts. In a fourth and perhaps its most important application, somatic cell genetics provided an effective approach to the investigation of that vast category of somatic cell genetic disease, neoplasia.

Somatic cell genetics can be said to have gotten its start in the mid-1960s. The techniques that had been developed for culturing cells during the previous decades and the findings of studies of cultured cells were a useful background. No cell line has been subjected to more extensive study than has the HeLa cell. This cell line was isolated from the cervical carcinoma of a patient named Henrietta Lacks (Fig. 1.14), who presented to the Johns Hopkins Hospital in early 1951 at the age of 31. Hers was one of some two dozen cervical carcinomas in which George O Gey (1899–1970) attempted to establish a cell line and the only one yielding a successful result. The fact that it was an unusual cancer, indeed an adenosquamous carcinoma rather than the usual squamous cervical carcinoma, was found on review of the histology by

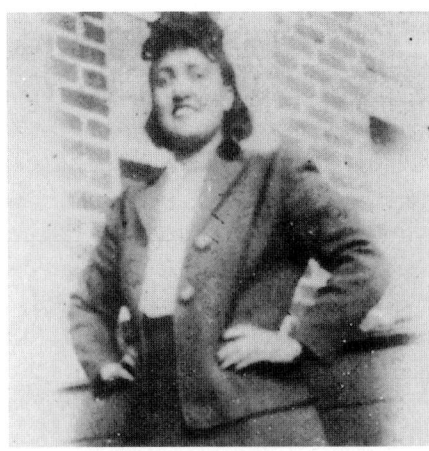

Fig. 1.14. Henrietta Lacks, whose cervical carcinoma was the source of the clonal HeLa cell line.

Howard W Jones and colleagues (1971). It had an unusual fungating appearance suggesting a venereal lesion and prompting a dark field analysis for spirochetes (which were not found). Although there was no evidence of invasion or metastasis at the time she was first seen and despite radium therapy, Mrs Lacks was dead in eight months. The genetic characteristics of the HeLa cell line, including HLA types, were determined by Susan Hsu et al. (1976) and compared with the findings in surviving members of her family. That Mrs Lacks was a heterozygote for glucose-6-phosphate dehydrogenase (G6PD) deficiency (G6PD A/B) was established by the fact that she had both G6PD-deficient and G6PD-normal sons. The Hela cell line is G6PD-deficient (G6PD-A), indicating its monoclonal origin; this fact was established by Philip Fialkow (1977) in studies of the monoclonality of cancers. The vigor of the HeLa cell line is attested to by the extent to which it has contaminated other cell lines in laboratories around the world (Jones et al., 1971).

Based on the information acquired from studies of cultured cells, the HeLa cell being the prototypic human cell line, cell culture achieved wide use in studies of inborn errors of metabolism in the 1960s. Among the first of such studies, based on the wide enzymatic repertoire of the fibroblast, was that of galactosemia by Bias and Kalckar and by Robert Krooth in the late 1950s and early 1960s. Later in the 1960s, when Seegmiller with Rosenbloom and Kelley was defining the deficiency of HPRT in the Lesch-Nyhan syndrome (Seegmiller et al, 1967), he would refer to making morning rounds on his tissue cultures. He alluded to the fact that cultured skin fibroblasts captured the essence of the patients' inborn errors of metabolism for study. Another notable example of the use of cultured cells in genetic studies was the Goldstein and Brown characterization, in the 1970s, of the low-density lipoprotein (LDL) receptor and its role in normal cholesterol metabolism and familial hyper-cholesterolemia.

The development of prenatal diagnosis by amniocentesis was dependent on the fortunate circumstance that the amniocyte for the most part demonstrates the same enzymatic activities (or deficiencies) in cell culture as do other cells and tissues of the patient. Exceptions, however, include conditions such as type 1 glycogen storage disease (von Gierke disease) in which deficiency of G6P had been demonstrated by the Coris. Phenylketonuria (PKU) proved to be another exception.

An important application of somatic cell genetics to formal genetics was the clonal proof of the Lyon hypothesis. Ronald Davidson, Harold Nitowsky, and Barton Childs (1963) provided the most compelling evidence in the human. These investigators cloned two classes of cells from cultures of females heterozygous for the A/B electrophoretic variant of G6PD, one class of cells being type A and the other type B.

All cancer is genetic disease, somatic cell genetic disease. The chromosome theory of cancer was first clearly enunciated by Theodor Boveri in his monograph of 1914 (see McKusick, 1985, for biographic details).

Somatic cell genetics has played a big role in the proof and clarification of the genetic basis of cancer. It provided the methods by which the clonal nature of cancers was proved. Much of the molecular genetics of cancer such as the demonstration of oncogenes has been discovered through somatic cell genetics. The triad of methodologies that have been successively employed beginning in 1956—chromosomology, somatic cell genetics, and molecular genetics—have all played a role.

A particularly substantial contribution of somatic cell genetics has been to gene mapping (see later), specifically physical mapping, that is, the assignment of genes to specific chromosomes and chromosomal regions, as opposed to genetic mapping, the determination of the interval between gene loci on the basis of amount of crossingover during meiosis. The method substituted interspecies (e.g., mouse and human) differences for interallelic differences used in meiosis-based linkage mapping. Somatic cell hybridization was what Haldane (Fig. 1.9) called a substitute for sex and Pontecorvo (Fig. 1.15) termed a parasexual method.

Somatic cell hybridization was made practical by the discovery of fusigens: first a virus, Sendai, by Y Okada (1958) and later a chemical, propylene glycol, by Guido Pontecorvo (1975) (Fig. 1.15). Both damage the plasma membrane of the co-cultivated rodent and human cells, encouraging fusion. In the second place, the development of selection media allowed the isolation of hybrid cells from among the numeri-

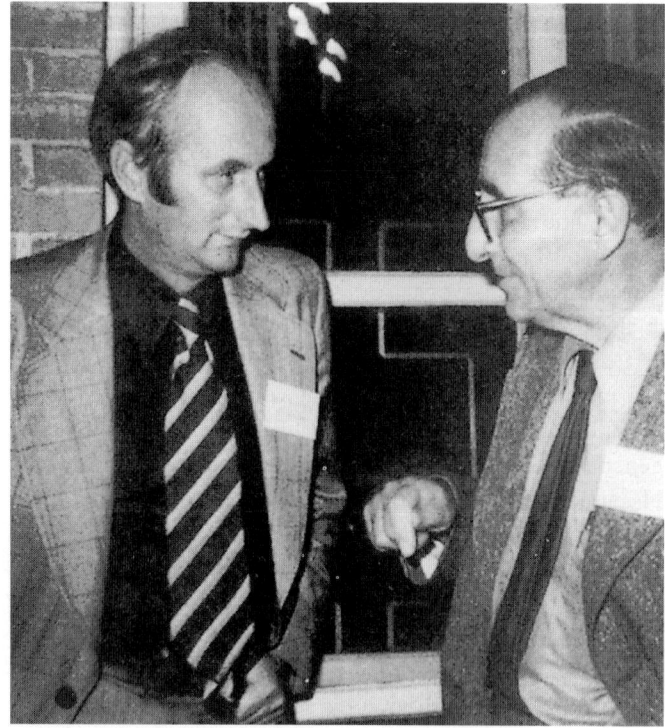

Fig. 1.15. Guido Pontecorvo (*right*) with Dirk Bootsma at Third Human Gene Mapping Workshop, Baltimore, 1975.

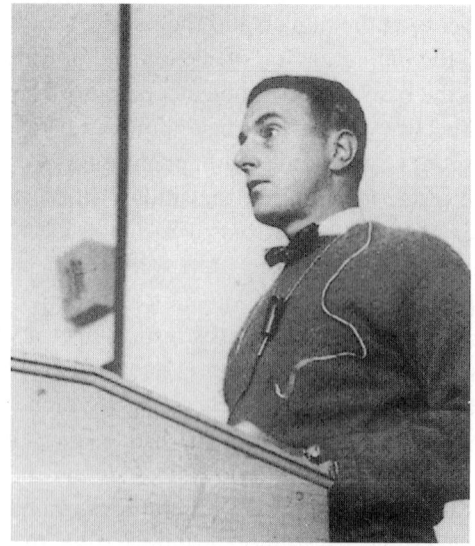

Fig. 1.16. John Littlefield at Bar Harbor Course, 1964.

cally overwhelming parental cells. The first of the selection media was hypoxanthine-aminopterin-thymidine (HAT), adapted to this use by John Littlefield (1964) (Fig. 1.16). The first human gene to be mapped by the method of somatic cell hybridization was that which encodes the cytosolic isozyme of thymidine kinase (TK1; MIM 188300). Mary Weiss and Howard Green (1967), who mapped TK1 to a specific chromosome, recognized the power of somatic cell hybridization for chromosome mapping. Barbara Migeon and C S Miller (1968) identified the TK1-bearing chromosome as belonging to group E and after the advent of chromosome banding, O J Miller et al. (1971) identified the chromosome as number 17. Through the work of Frank Ruddle (Fig. 1.17), Walter Bodmer (Fig. 1.18), and many others, the application of somatic cell genetics to chromosome mapping was exploited to the fullest. During the 1970s, the somatic hybrid cell method accounted for the largest part of the progress in gene mapping that was collated in the regular Human Gene Mapping Workshops begun in 1973 (McKusick and Ruddle, 1977).

MOLECULAR GENETICS

The foundations of molecular genetics were laid in the pre-1956 era by the discovery of DNA, called nuclein, by Miescher in 1867; the demonstration that the pneumococcal transforming factor is DNA by Oswald Avery, Colin MacLeod, and Maclyn McCarty (1944); and the solution of the structure of DNA by Watson and Crick (1953) (Fig. 1.19). Working out the three-letter code of DNA was begun by Marshall Nirenberg and Heinrich Matthei, who in 1961 observed the synthesis of a polypeptide composed solely of phenylalanine residues, when they used artificially synthesized RNA consisting only of uracil. Thereafter, the code was "cracked," one trinucleotide at a time, with the complete Rosetta stone of molecular genetics becoming available by 1966.

Restriction enzymes that cut DNA at the site of specific sequences were discovered by Werner Arber and Hamilton O Smith in about 1970, and Daniel Nathans showed that one can use the enzymes for mapping DNA, the so-called restriction map, first developed for SV40 viral DNA. The Southern blot method for displaying fragments of DNA

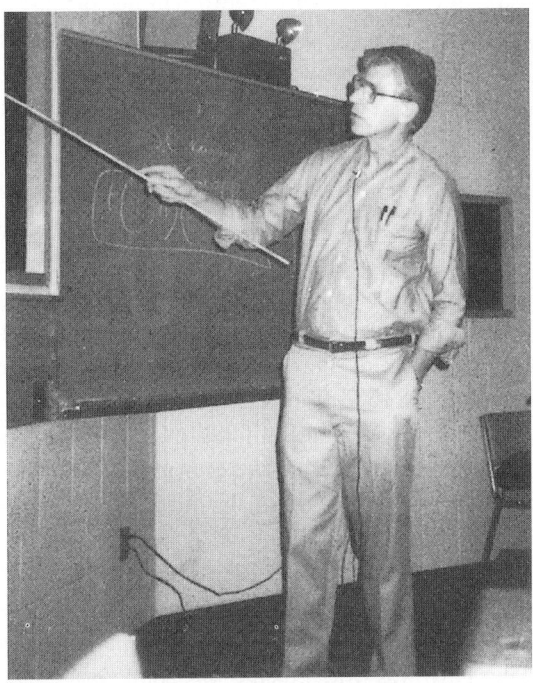

Fig. 1.17. Frank Ruddle at Bar Harbor Course, 1987.

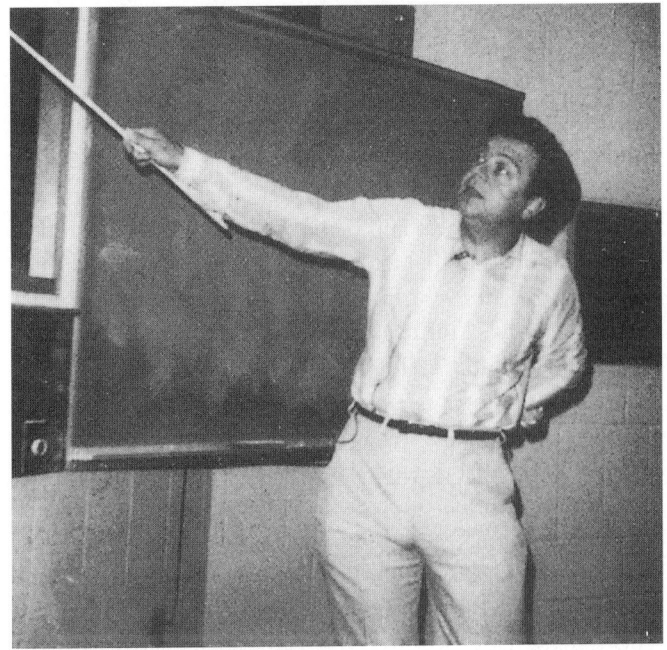

Fig. 1.18. Walter Bodmer at Bar Harbor Course, 1979.

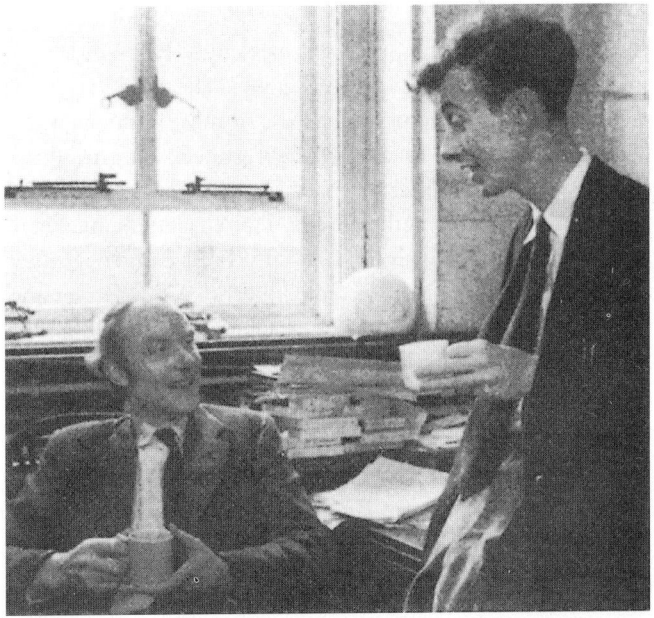

Fig. 1.19. Francis Crick (left) and James Watson at Cavendish Laboratory, University of Cambridge, 1953. (From Photo Researchers, with permission.)

created by dissection with restriction enzymes was developed by Edwin M Southern in 1975 (Southern, 1975).

The discovery of specific restriction endonucleases made possible the isolation of discrete molecular fragments of naturally occurring DNA for the first time. This capability was fundamental to the development of molecular cloning (Cohen et al, 1973), which opened up the era of recombinant DNA. The combination of molecular cloning and endonuclease restriction allowed the synthesis and isolation of any naturally occurring DNA that could be cloned into a useful vector and on the basis of flanking restriction sites, excised from it. The availability of a large variety of restriction enzymes significantly expanded the value of these methods.

The polymerase chain reaction (PCR) was a major addition to the molecular genetics armamentarium. PCR was formally unveiled in full technical detail by K Mullis et al. (1986) at the same historic Cold Spring Harbor Symposium on Quantitative Biology, Molecular Biology of *Homo sapiens*, at which the Human Genome Project was discussed in a historic rump session. Combined with specific restriction enzyme cleavage at the mutation site, the method had been used in the diagnosis of sickle cell anemia by J Saiki et al. (1985).

The first human gene to be cloned was chorionic sommatomammotropin, by Shine et al. (1977). About the same time, Tom Maniatis cloned two of the smallest human genes, those for the α- and β-chains of hemoglobin. Most genes are at least 20 times bigger, and a few are as much as 1000 times bigger, containing much noncoding DNA (i.e., introns). After the discovery of reverse transcriptase, it was possible to take a shortcut and clone only the coding part of the gene complementary to the processed messenger RNA (mRNA), so-called complementary DNA (cDNA). The cloning of large segments of DNA (up to a megabase or more) came in 1987 with the invention of YAC (yeast artificial chromosome) cloning by David Burke, Maynard Olson, and others (1987).

Two advanced methods for DNA sequencing were reported simultaneously in 1977, by Fred Sanger (Sanger et al., 1977) and by Maxam and Gilbert (1977). Sanger and Gilbert shared the Nobel Prize in Chemistry in 1980. The Sanger dideoxy method for DNA sequencing remained the basic technology upon which the genetics revolution of the last vintage of the twentieth century was based, albeit major advances in automation and other modifications were made.

CHROMOSOME MAPPING

The first assignment of a specific gene to a specific human chromosome can be credited to E B Wilson (Fig. 1.3),

Columbia University professor and colleague of Thomas Hunt Morgan (Fig. 1.5). Wilson (1911) wrote as follows:

> In the case of color blindness, for example, all the facts seem to follow under this assumption if the male be digametic (as Guyer's observations show to be the case in man). For in fertilization this character will pass with the affected X chromosome from the male into the female, and from the female into half her offspring of both sexes. Color blindness, being a recessive character, should therefore appear in neither daughters nor granddaughters, but in half the grandsons, as seems to be actually the case.

John Dalton (1766–1844), whose name is memorialized in the unit of molecular mass, had described his own colorblindness in the 1790s; Swiss ophthalmologist Horner had described the pedigree patterns we now recognize as typical of X-linked recessive inheritance. (Even earlier, as indicated by Rushton in 1994, Pliny Earle, a pioneer Philadelphia psychiatrist, in 1845 delineated the inheritance pattern of colorblindness on the basis of his own family.) The sex chromosome constitution of the human had been assumed to be either XY or XO in the male and XX in the female, as a result of studies by Wilson's colleague N M Stevens.

In a famous paper in 1915, J B S Haldane (1892–1964), with his sister Naomi and fellow student A D Sprunt, reported the first example of autosomal genetic linkage in a mammal. This was the linkage of "pink eye" (*p*) with albinism (*c*). The authors did not use the term linkage; the title of their paper was "Reduplication in mice." It was published in the early stages of the "War of 1914" (World War I), and in the first paragraph the authors stated: "Owing to the war it has been necessary to publish prematurely, as unfortunately one of us (ADS) has already been killed in France."

The first human genetic map interval to be estimated was that for colorblindness and hemophilia. The transmission of hemophilia in the characteristic X-linked pedigree pattern was described in New England families early in the nineteenth century (McKusick, 1962a). J B S Haldane with Julia Bell (Bell and Haldane, 1937) in 1937 attempted an estimate of the interval on the basis of published pedigrees, and Haldane with C A B Smith revised the estimate in 1947. They placed the interval in the vicinity of 10 cM; the fact that there are two forms of X-linked hemophilia (A, or classic hemophilia, and B, or Christmas disease) was not found until 1952, when in the Christmas issue of the *British Medical Journal*, Biggs and colleagues in Oxford, England, reported the case of a five-year-old boy named Christmas with hemophilia of a distinctive type. It was distinguishable from classic hemophilia by the fact that serum from Master Christmas corrected the clotting defect in the blood of patients with classic hemophilia. Subsequent studies of the linkage between hemophilia A and colorblindness showed very tight linkage and a reanalysis of the published hemophilia/cb data used originally by Haldane and colleagues led C A B Smith to conclude that the series was a mixture of two forms of hemophilia, one very tightly linked to colorblindness and one loosely linked or not linked at all. We now know that hemophilia B maps to the long arm of the X chromosome, but at a distance proximal to hemophilia A and colorblindness, which are at the very tip of the long arm.

During the 1930s and 1940s, considerable thought was given to what approaches might be used to identify genetic linkage, recognizing that it is necessary in the human to use matings as they are found; one cannot, of course, create the matings that are most informative as one can in mouse and fruit fly. Lionel Penrose (1898–1972) (Fig. 1.20) elaborated a sib-pair method in the 1930s (Penrose, 1935). The first autosomal linkage in the human was not identified until the early 1950s, when Jan Mohr (Fig. 1.21) demonstrated linkage of the Lutheran blood group and secretor factor loci as part of his doctoral thesis in the institute headed up by Tage Kemp (Fig. 1.21) in Copenhagen. Mohr was subsequently the director of that institute, and it was in his department that the first-to-be-discovered autosomal linkage group (Lutheran and secretor) was determined to be located on chromosome 19 (Eiberg et al., 1983).

The method logarithm of the odds (lods) was developed by C A B Smith in the 1950s and elaborated by Newton Morton. Using these methods, Morton (1956) demonstrated linkage of the elliptocytosis and Rh blood group loci (including the demonstration of genetic heterogeneity,

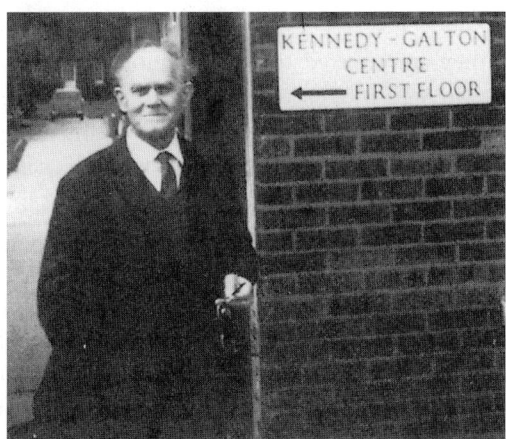

Fig. 1.20. Lionel Penrose, 1973.

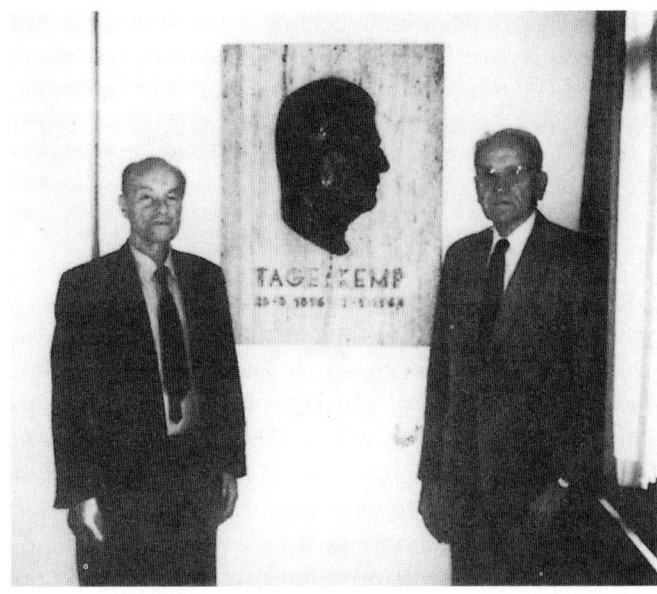

Fig. 1.21. Jan Mohr (left) and Victor McKusick with plaque honoring Tage Kemp (1896–1964), Copenhagen, 1979. Mohr was Kemp's successor as director of the Institute of Human Genetics in Copenhagen. Kemp was the convener of the First World Congress of Human Genetics (1956).

since some families did not show linkage). Renwick and others showed linkage of the ABO blood group to the nail-patella syndrome. All three of the early examples of autosomal linkage were established with blood groups (or, in the case of secretor factor, an "honorary" blood group), illustrating the pathetically limited repertoire of markers, a major handicap to gene mapping in that era. By 1951, when the first autosomal linkage was discovered in the human, at least eight autosomal linkage groups had been identified in the mouse. On the other hand, it was about the same time in the early 1950s that the first X-linked locus was identified in the mouse, whereas three dozen or more loci were known to be on the human X chromosome because of X-linked pedigree patterns.

The first gene to be assigned to a specific autosome was the Duffy blood group locus, which was localized to chromosome 1 by Donahue et al. (1968). At that time, R P Donahue was a candidate for the doctoral degree in human genetics at Johns Hopkins. As every graduate student in human genetics should probably do, he determined his own karyotype, although his thesis research was not on a cytogenetic problem. He identified a heteromorphism of the chromosome 1 pair. One chromosome 1 showed what looked like an uncoiled region (this was in the prebanding era) in the proximal portion of the long arm. Donahue had both the wit and the gumption to do a linkage study: the wit to sense that this might be a mendelizing character in his family, and the gumption to collect blood samples from widely scattered relatives, to determine marker traits, and to analyze the data. The analysis suggested linkage of the Duffy blood group locus to the "uncoiler" trait. Although the lod score was far below the value of 3.0 usually accepted as evidence for linkage, confirmation of the assignment came quickly from other workers.

After 1971, abundant information was collected on chromosome mapping by the method of somatic cell hybridization. Radiation by hybrid mapping (see p.18) made use of hybridization with rodent cells to "rescue" human cells in which random fragmentation of chromosomes had been produced by radiation. *In situ* hybridization of DNA probes to chromosomes, first with radioactively labeled probes and later with fluorescent probes, was a mapping method first made to work reliaby for single copy genes 1981.

About 1980, molecular genetics entered the chromosome mapping field. It contributed to the field in three ways: (1) it permitted direct identification of the human gene in somatic cell hybrids, so that it was possible to go directly for the gene, rather than requiring expression of the human gene in the hybrid cell; (2) it provided probes for chromosomal in situ hybridization, which was made to work for the first time in a reliable way for single copy genes in 1981; and (3) it provided DNA polymorphisms as markers for family linkage study, thereby providing a virtually limitless repertoire.

In a seminal paper (Botstein et al., 1980), David Botstein (Fig. 1.22), Ray White (Fig. 1.23), Michael Skolnick, and Ron Davis formally outlined the value of what they called restriction fragment length polymorphisms (RFLPs or "riflips") as linkage markers in family studies. In fact, the first RFLP had been discovered by Y-W Kan and A M Dozy (1978), an *Hpa*I variant 3′ to the β-globin locus, and Ellen Solomon and Walter Bodmer (1979) had suggested the value of such DNA variants as linkage markers:

> Given the range of available restriction enzymes, one can envisage finding enough markers to cover systematically the whole human genome. Thus, only 200–300 suitably selected probes might be needed to provide a genetic marker for, say, every 10% recombination. Such a set of genetic markers could revolutionise our ability to study the genetic determination of complex attributes and to follow the inheritance of traits.

The late Allan C Wilson (1934–1991) decried the use of the term restriction fragment *length* polymorphism, arguing that length mutations are one large class of mutations, the other being point mutations, and that it would be better to refer to these simply as restriction fragment polymorphisms.

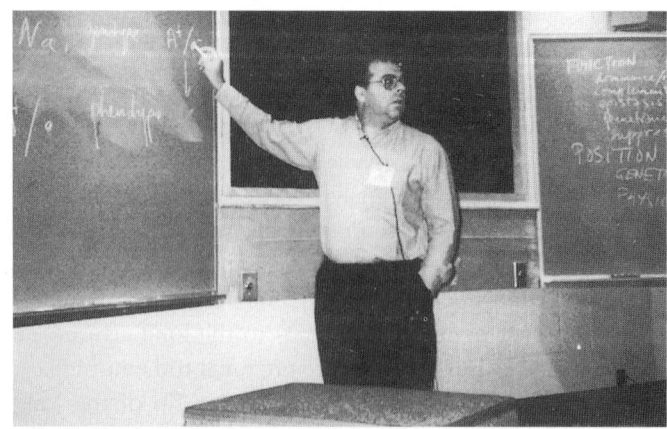

Fig. 1.22. David Botstein at Bar Harbor Course, 1987.

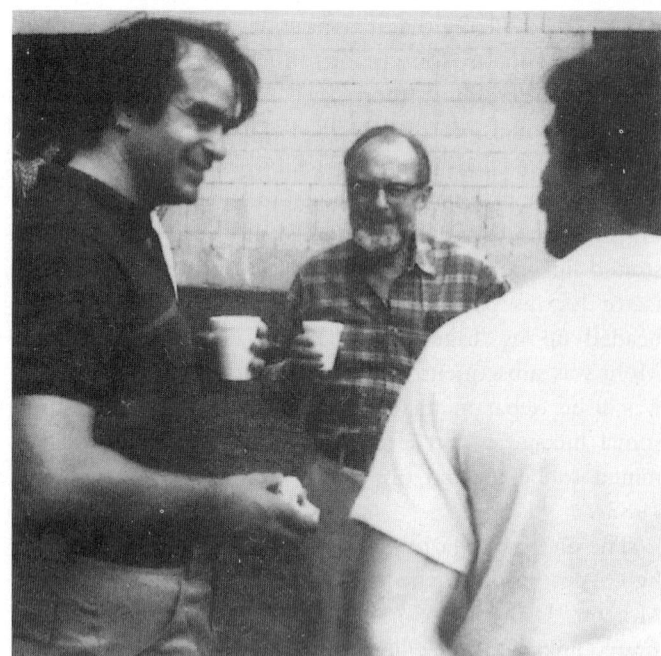

Fig. 1.23. Ray White (left), James Neel (middle) a Jospeh Nadeau at Bar Harbor, 1983.

In mice they are referred to as restriction fragment length variants (RFLVs). Indeed this is what they are, differences between inbred strains and not polymorphisms in the strict sense as defined by E B Ford of Oxford University as the occurrence together in the same habitat of two or more distinct forms of a species in such proportions that the rarest of them cannot be maintained by recurrent mutation. Indeed, RFLPs in the human, when first discovered in a small number of samples, could not be known to be polymorphisms in the terms of this definition; 1% is usually taken as the minimal frequency of the rarer allele. However, it turns out that most DNA variants are indeed highly variable and qualify as polymorphisms within the Ford definition.

A second form of DNA variation to be discovered was variable number of tandem repeats (VNTRs), introduced as hypervariable DNA markers for linkage studies, as well as for use in forensic science by Jeffreys et al. (1985) and by Nakamura, White and their colleagues (1987). The third major, and still more variable, type of DNA polymorphism is represented by the dinucleotide repeats, for example (CA)n, the so-called microsatellites. These were discovered and developed by James Weber at the Marshfield Clinic in Marshfield, Wisconsin, and by Michael Litt in Portland, Oregon; they are extensively exploited by many, particularly Jean Weissenbach in Paris, for the creation of genetic maps and the mapping of disease genes.

The first major successful application of RFLPs in linkage study was the mapping of the Huntington disease locus (HD) to the tip of chromosome 4 through linkage to the so-called GS8 RFLP; this marker at a locus designated D4S10 in the human gene mapping nomenclature was, in turn, mapped to that region of chromosome 4 by in situ hybridization. The initial demonstration of linkage was achieved by James Gusella et al. (1983) on samples assembled by Nancy Wexler (Fig. 1.24) from an extraordinarily large and extensively affected kindred with Huntington disease in the Lake Maracaibo region of Venezuela.

Haplotyping is the determination of markers close to, and on the same chromosome as, the mutation of interest. The term *haplotype* was first used in connection with the major histocompatibility types, HLA types. Haplotyping was developed particularly extensively by Haig Kazazian

(Fig. 1.25) and Stylianos Antonarakis (Fig. 1.26) at Johns Hopkins University in collaboration with Stuart Orkin in Boston and others, for identifying the presence of the gene

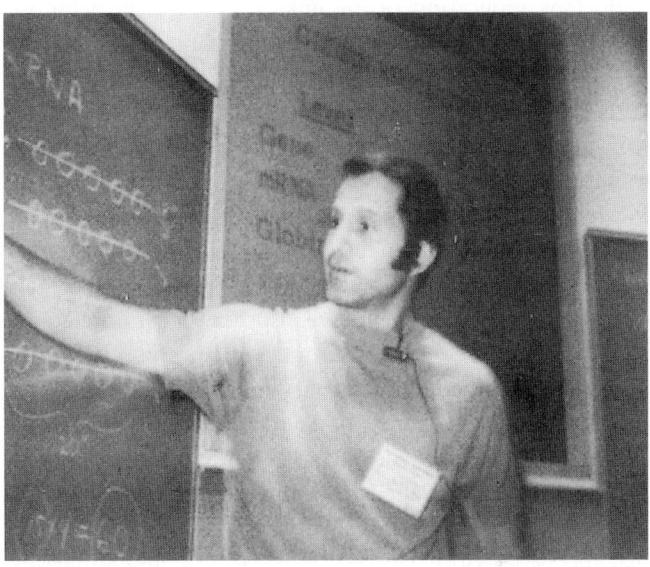

Fig. 1.25. Haig Kazazian at Bar Harbor, 1976.

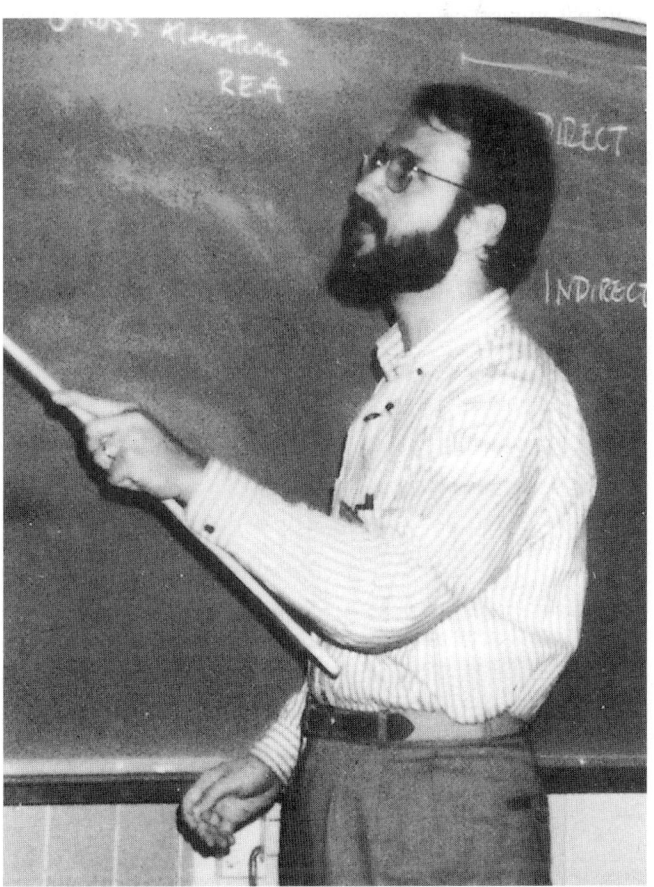

Fig. 1.26. Stylianos Antonarakis at Bar Harbor, 1988.

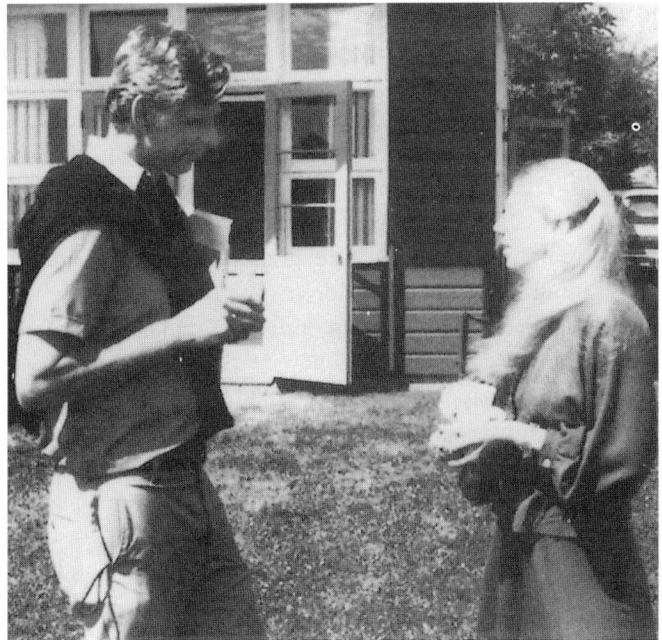

Fig. 1.24. Frank Ruddle (left) and Nancy Wexler at Bar Harbor, 1983.

for thalassemia in particular individuals. Since haplotypes represent closely linked markers, it is not unexpected that in families and even in population groups, common forms of thalassemia are associated with the same haplotype. This important application of the linkage principle in diagnosis and in population genetics (for tracing the multiple origins, e.g., of the sickle hemoglobin gene) was extended from the hemoglobinopathies to many inborn errors of metabolism, particularly cystic fibrosis. Because of the many different mutations capable of causing cystic fibrosis and because of the relatively high frequency of the "cystic fibrosis" gene, tracing it in families through the haplotype has been useful.

In some populations, such as the Finns and the Old Order Amish, many usually rare disorders occur in relatively high frequency because of a founder effect. In such populations, most individuals affected with a recessive disorder that is rare in the general population are homozygous for a particular haplotype. Indeed, as was theorized by C A B Smith in 1953 and elaborated more recently by Lander and Botstein (1987) (Fig. 1.27), patients with any rare autosomal recessive disorder, if the parents are consanguineous, will be expected to be homozygous for closely linked markers, that is, homozygous for a particular haplotype. This has indeed been shown to be the case in several disorders, including Bloom syndrome, diastrophic dysplasia, and alkaptonuria (Pollack et al., 1993). Of course, in founder populations, a specific haplotype is likely to be shared in common by persons affected with an autosomal dominant or X-linked recessive as well.

Linkage analysis by the study of PCR-amplified DNA from individual sperm was introduced by Norman Arnheim in 1988 (see Boehnke et al, 1989). Essentially, one could fill

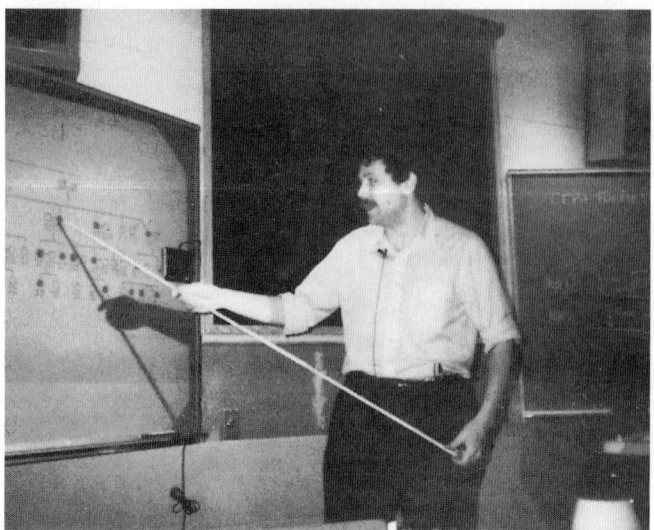

Fig. 1.27. Eric Lander at Bar Harbor, 1989.

in the sort of information contained in stick diagrams used to explain linkage in textbooks of genetics. With this approach, it was not necessary to have observations on diploid offspring to identify recombinants among the gametes produced by the parent.

Comparative mapping, most extensively pursued between mouse and humans, has been exploited as a clue to the likely location of genes in the human. A great deal of syntenic homology has been found between these two extensively studied species. The X chromosome in the human and in all other placental mammals has essentially the same genetic content, as was pointed out during the 1960s by Ohno (1967), who also pointed out that the X chromosome is about the same size in all these organisms. The extensive syntenic homology, in the case of the autosomes, between the human and the mouse came as a surprise to many. What I have chosen to call the Oxford grid (for example, see p.ccclxi of *Mendelian Inheritance in Man*, 12th edn., 1998) was developed by John H Edwards, professor of genetics at Oxford University, and collaborators, particularly A G Searle, at nearby Harwell.

The term *synteny*, meaning "on the same chromosome," was introduced by James H Renwick (1926–1994) (Fig. 1.28) in about 1970. It proved to be a useful term of distinction from linkage; two loci may be syntenic but not linked in the strict genetic sense because they are so far apart on the same chromosome that they assort independently through crossing over.

Renwick was also responsible for developing an early program for computer-assisted linkage analysis. Jurg Ott (1985) also developed programs, as have others. These facilitated widespread analysis of linkage data.

A development of great importance for advancement of genetic mapping was the creation of the Centre d'Études du Polymorphisme Humain (CEPH) in Paris by Jean Dausset in 1983. CEPH created and maintains a reference panel of family DNAs for mapping by linkage. The three-generation family units consist of the four grandparents, two parents, and a minimum of eight children. The data on markers, as they are determined in these reference families in many laboratories, are collated, and new markers and genetic disorders can be mapped against the reference panel.

Radiation hybrid mapping was first devised by Goss and Harris (1975) as a modification of mapping with somatic cell hybrids. It involved fragmentation of the human chromosomes by irradiation of cultured cells and the "rescue" of these cells by fusion with mouse cells. The method was revived and revamped about 1990 by Peter Goodfellow of Cambridge University (Goodfellow et al., 1990) and David Cox of Stanford University (Cox et al., 1990). Both created

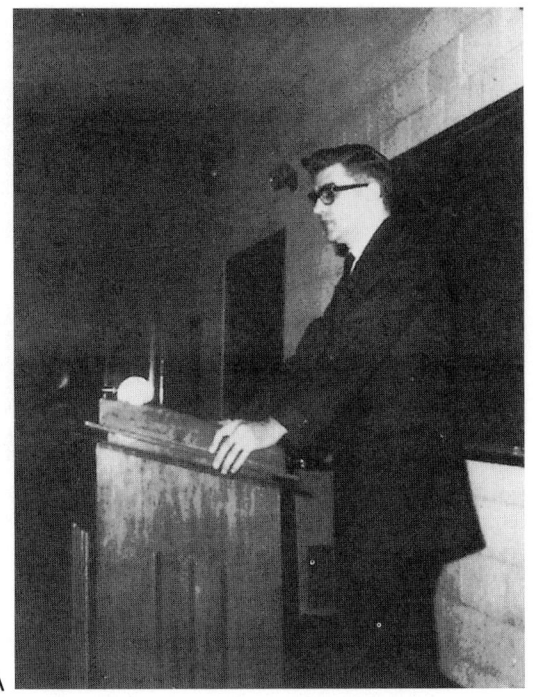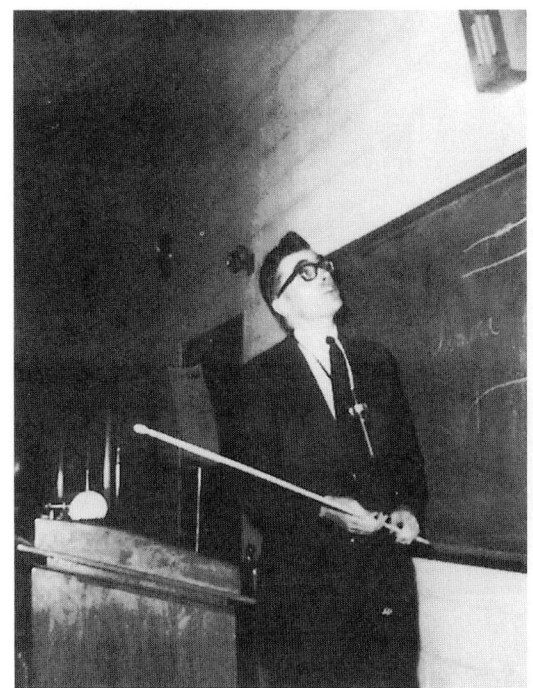

A   B

Fig. 1.28. (A and B) James Renwick at Bar Harbor, 1972.

DNA panels from cells with various human chromosomal content.

The creation of clone libraries, e.g., YACs, whose map location was known from radiation hybrid mapping or other methods made it possible to map a newly found sequence by hybridization or by linkage to a marker such as a sequence tagged site (STS) or gene known to be on the same clone fragment. STSs were proposed by Maynard Olson et al. (1989) as useful markers in mapping (Green and Olson, 1990).

THE HUMAN GENOME PROJECT AND GENOMICS

The goal of the Human Genome Project (HGP) is to locate all the 60,000 to 70,000 genes and sequence the entire 3 billion or more nucleotides of the haploid genome. It is primarily a mapping project; even sequencing is determining the ultimate map. In its initial form, however, it was not formally conceived as a mapping project. When proposed by Robert Sinsheimer, Walter Gilbert, Renato Dulbecco, and others in 1985–1986, the HGP was viewed as a project for complete *sequencing* of the genome. Previous progress in gene mapping and the value of the results were apparently unfamiliar to the leading promulgators, who were molecular geneticists. In part, objections to the Project raised between 1985, when it was first proposed, and 1990, its official start

date, resulted from the impression that it was an enterprise of mindless sequencing without much biology. (A factor also contributing to the unhappiness of many scientists with the Project was the price tag. The National Research Council/ National Academy of Sciences [NRC/NAS] committee on mapping and sequencing the human genome, commissioned in late 1986, and reporting out in February 1988, estimated that the "job" could be done in 15 years for $200 million a year. Journalists in particular advertised the HGP as a $3.0 billion project, which biologists coping with funding problems found disturbing. Of course, the *annual* budget of the National Institutes of Health [NIH] is approximately 50 times that figure [in 1988 dollars]!)

At a birth defects congress in the Hague in 1969, complete mapping of the genes on the human chromosomes had been proposed as an effective approach to solution of problems of congenital malformations and genetic disorders in general (McKusick, 1970) (Fig. 1.29). The proposal came close on the heels of the first manned moon landing in July 1969; complete genome mapping was seen as the next moon shot. The potential benefit of complete mapping was frequently emphasized thereafter. For example, it was advanced as an achievable goal for the last "vintage" of the twentieth century (McKusick, 1980). Human Gene Mapping Workshops, initiated by Frank Ruddle in New Haven, Connecticut, in 1973, continued in the same form until 1991, for collation of the world's

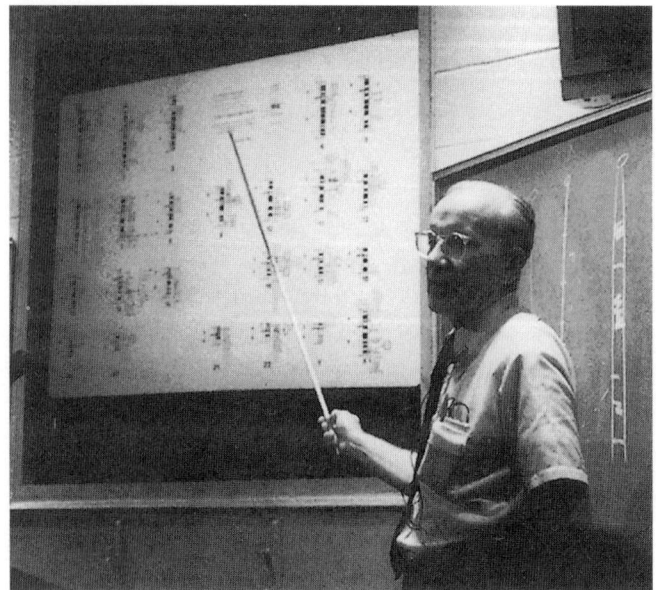

Fig. 1.29. Victor McKusick and the human gene map, Bar Harbor Course, 1981.

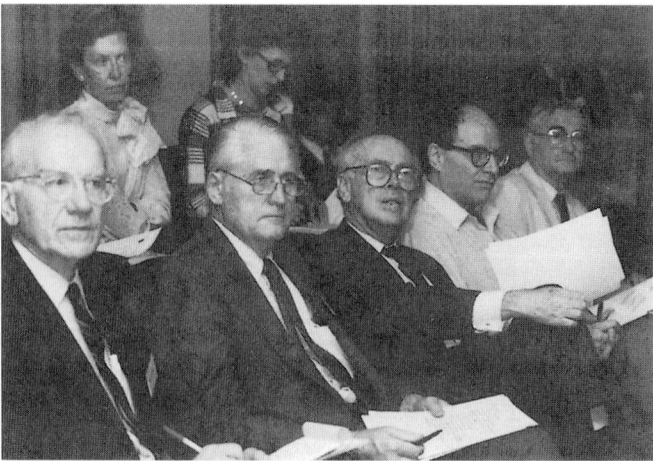

Fig. 1.30. At Howard Hughes Medical Institute-sponsored NIH conference on the proposed human genome project, July 1986. Left to right: Victor McKusick, L. H. ("Holly") Smith, James Watson, Walter Gilbert, Robert Sinsheimer.

experience in gene mapping. The function of these workshops was taken over by HUGO (see later).

It is true that the 1969 proposal had little apparent impact even though it was repeatedly restated over the next 15 years (McKusick, 1980; 1981). In 1969, the methodology that would make the HGP possible was not yet at hand. As outlined elsewhere, recombinant DNA technology and methods of efficient DNA sequencing came in the 1970s; improved methods for both genetic and physical mapping came in the 1980s. As pointed out by R Cook-Deegan (1994, p. 10) in his history of the HGP, whatever revisionist history might be written, the facts are that the HGP was conceived and promoted, not by medical geneticists, but by molecular biologists such as Robert Sinsheimer, Walter Gilbert (Fig. 1.30), and Renato Dulbecco, who worked predominantly on organisms other than the human. And it was conceived and promoted apparently in ignorance, for the most part, of what had been accomplished and proposed in the area of gene mapping. It is true that in the 1986 Cold Spring Harbor Symposium devoted to the human genome, a long review was given of the status of the human gene map (McKusick, 1986). This and the accompanying chromosome-by-chromosome lists of genes then mapped was an eye-opener to the molecular geneticists present. Also at that meeting, a rump session led by Gilbert and Paul Berg discussed the pros and cons of the proposed genome project (see Cook-Deegan, 1994, for photographs of Gilbert, Berg, and Botstein at that crucial meeting and for a summary of the discussion).

If 1985–1990 was a gestational period for the HGP, the NRC/NAS committee (1988) was the midwife. The offi-

cial birth date for the project in the United States was October 1, 1990, with federal funding jointly through the Department of Energy (DOE) (about one-third) and the NIH (about two-thirds). (The DOE through its national laboratories has long had a mandate to study the biologic effects of radiation. With the leadership of Charles DeLisi, then with the DOE, and the legislative initiative of Senator Nick Domenici of New Mexico, DOE became involved both intramurally [in its national laboratories] and extramurally in the HGP.)

James G Watson (Fig. 1.30) of Watson-Crick fame led the NIH program for its first three years, bringing to it both his prestige and his wisdom. At the same time he directed the newly created National Center for Human Genome Research (NCHGR), which functioned in much the same way as the individual institutes, he continued to direct the Cold Spring Harbor Laboratory on Long Island, New York. In 1993, Francis Collins (Fig. 1.31) became the director of the NCHGR and proceeded to develop an intramural program in medical genetics. This reflects his conviction that the HGP is primarily a gene-finding enterprise and is linked to clinical medicine as both an efficient way to find genes and an effective way to realize potential benefits in diagnosis, prevention, and management of genetic disorders. The "Center" became an institute, the National Human Genome Research Institute (NHGRI) January 1, 1995.

In parallel with the HGP in the United States, genome programs were developing in many other countries, particularly the United Kingdom, France, and Japan. In September 1988, a group of 32 scientists from 14 countries met in Montreux, Switzerland, to found the Human Genome Organisation (HUGO) (Fig. 1.32). As one member of the

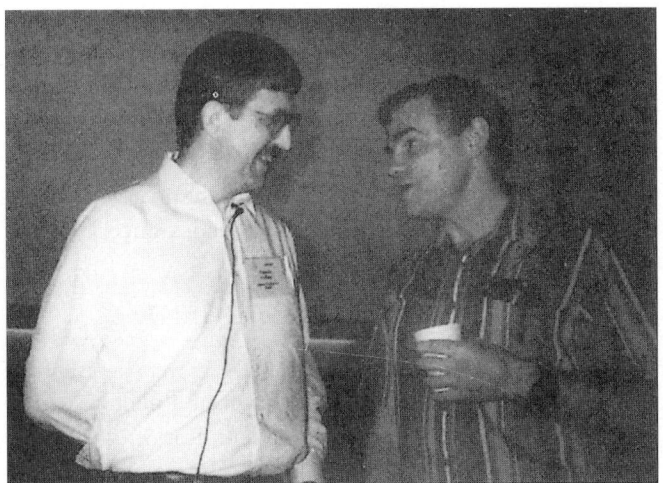

Fig. 1.31. Francis Collins (left) with Leroy Hood, Cold Spring Harbor, 1993.

organizing group, Norton Zinder, put it, "HUGO is a UN for the human genome." It is a coordinating organization. Its founder president Victor McKusick was succeeded by Walter Bodmer in 1990, by Thomas Caskey in 1993, by Grant Sutherland in 1996, and thereafter by Gert-Jan van Ommen followed by Lap-Chee Tsui.

The HGP progressed even faster than predicted, mainly because of new methods: PCR, YACs, STSs (Olson et al., 1989), microsatellite linkage markers, and others. The official start date for the HGP in the United States was October 1, 1990. The completion date predicted by the

15-year estimate made by the NRC/NAS Committee on Mapping and Sequencing the Human Genome (1988), was September 30, 2005. At the five-year mark, Francis Collins (1995) could report that the HGP was "ahead of schedule and under budget".

A phenomenal speeding up occurred in the last part of the 1990s, with announcement of a "first draft" of the complete sequence in June 2000. The acceleration can be credited to the development of improved high-thoughtput sequencers that used capillaries for the dideoxy method developed by Sanger in 1977; and particularly to the application to the human of "shot-gun" sequencing which had been successful in the first complete sequencing of a free-living organism, *H. influenzae*, by Hamilton Smith, Craig Venter and colleagues (Fleischmann et al., 1995). Previously the approach of the publicly funded HGP had been the creation of successive maps: a genetic linkage map of many genetic markers (e.g., Dib et al, 1996), a physical map of overlapping DNA segments, e.g., YACs (Chumakov et al, 1995), and finally the ultimate map, the DNA sequence. As opposed to this top-down approach, a bottom-up strategy, sequencing random fragments with assembly thereafter, was used by Venter and his colleagues in the private genome project of Celera to get the complete genome sequence of microorganisms and subsequently of *Drosophila* (Adams et al., 2000) and the human.

The Human Mitochondrial Genome Project (HMGP), although never called that, had been completed long before. The HMGP had been done in an order opposite to

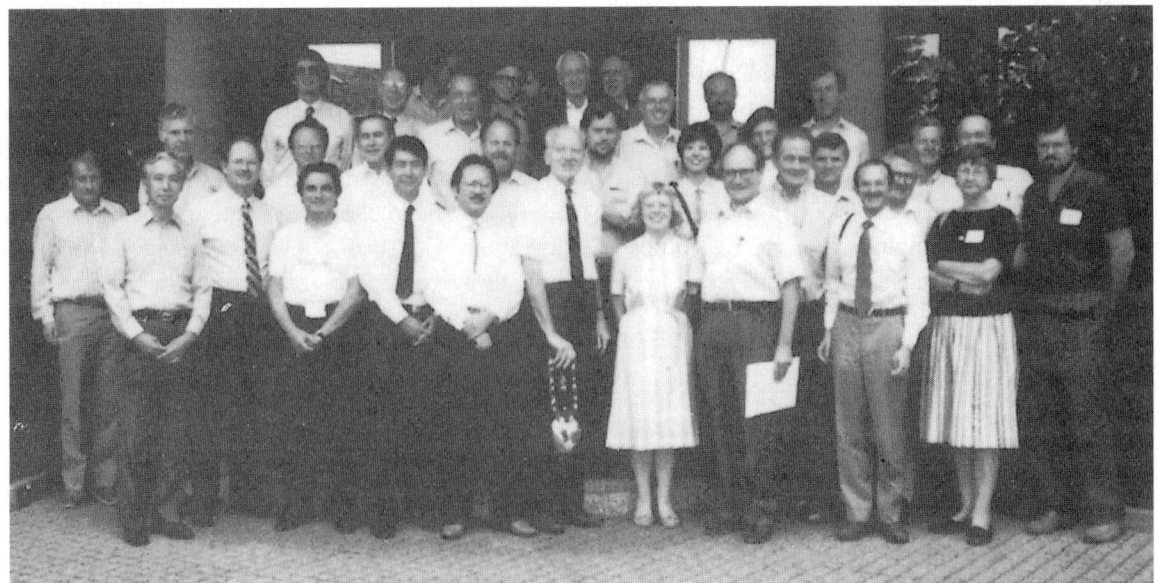

Fig. 1.32. Founding council for the Human Genome Organisation (HUGO) at Montreux, Switzerland, September, 1988 (11 members were absent). First row (left to right): Matsubara, Shows, Tocchini-Valentini, Honjo, Shimizu, McKusick (with Swiss cowbell), Lyon, Gilbert, Cantor, Robson, Karpov (observer). Second row: Hirt, Ruddle, Collins, Zinder, Sutherland, Cavanee, Hinton (staff), Strayer (staff), Tooze, Hood, Frézal, Cahill, Ferguson-Smith. Third row: Pearson, Dulbecco, Philipson, Jacob, Mirzabekov, Goodfellow (observer), Dausset, Watson, Worton, Southern, Grzeschik.

the way the HGP was conducted. The complete sequencing was done first, by the group of Fred Sanger at Cambridge University (Anderson et al., 1981). Then all the genes were identified, and finally disorders related to mutations in those genes were characterized.

The term *genome* appears to have been first used by Winkler in 1920 and to have been created by the elision of GENes and chromosOMEs to signify the set of chromosomes and the genes they contain (McKusick and Ruddle, 1987). Thus, it is an irregular hybrid from two Greek roots. The term *genomics* is of more recent mintage having been proposed in July, 1986 by Thomas H Roderick, of The Jackson Laboratory to designate the field of gene mapping and sequencing and specifically a new journal. The journal's inaugural editorial (McKusick and Ruddle, 1987) was entitled "A new discipline, a new name, a new journal." The next 10 years showed a remarkable growth of the field and widespread use of the term genomics, so that in 1996 an editorial was entitled "An established discipline, a commonly used name, a mature journal" (McKusick et al., 1996).

Goodfellow (1997) stated that he "would define genetics as the study of inheritance and genomics as the study of genomes". Adjectives added to the word genomics have indicated specific aspects or applications of genomics. Mapping and sequencing constitute *structural genomics*. "*Functional genomics*", continuing with Goodfellow's definitions, "is the attachment of information about function to knowledge of DNA sequence." *Pharmacogenomics* (Roses, 2000), *toxicogenomics*, *comparative genomics* and *physiologic* are some of the derivative terms for subfields of *genomics* (McKusick, 1997).

Leading approaches for functional genomics are transgenic methods, which involve manipulation of the particular sequence in transgenic animals. Another is database searching for similar sequences in other organisms where function is already known or can be determined more readily than is possible in the human. The latter is comparative genomics. Database searching has been referred to as research *in silico* or cybergenomics.

Already before the Human Genome Project was completed, intense attention was directed to the function of the genome in a global sense as reflected by the protein gene products. *Proteomics* was a term invented about 1995 by Mark Russell who used two-dimensional display methods for peptides (Pandey and Mann, 2000). *Physiomics*, a further derivation, is also called *systems analysis* or *systems biology* and refers further to function.

Functional genomics has also involved the study of gene expression as reflected by messenger RNA (mRNA). Description of coordinated gene expression in various tissues, at various stages of development and in various physiologic states, became possible with the development of microassay methods ("chip technology") and other methods such as SAGE (serial analysis of gene expression) in the latter part of the 1990s. These methods for profiling gene expression represent the sixth of the major methodologies that have advanced medical genetics since 1956.

CLINICAL APPLICATIONS OF GENE MAPPING

Gene mapping, defined as the location of a gene to a specific chromosome site and/or the identification of markers that are close neighbors, has clinical value in diagnosis by the linkage principle and usefulness in identifying the nature of the basic defect either through positional cloning or through the candidate gene approach. J B S Haldane (Fig. 1.9) suggested in the 1920s that diagnosis by the linkage principle would be both possible and useful. In 1956, after Fuchs had suggested amniocentesis as a method of diagnosis of fetal sex based on the presence or absence of a Barr body in amniocytes, John H Edwards (1956) suggested that with amniocentesis one could do prenatal diagnosis by the linkage principle. The idea was further developed by McKusick (1969), and McCurdy (1971) demonstrated its practicability in connection with the hemophilia A carrier status, using the very closely linked G6PD marker. Schrott and colleagues applied the approach in connection with the closely linked myotonic dystrophy and secretor loci, the secretor status of the fetus being determinable in amniotic fluid (Schrott et al., 1973; Schrott and Omenn, 1975). But the full strength of the linkage approach was not realized until the 1980s, when abundant DNA markers became available. As indicated earlier, haplotypes (i.e., clustered markers around the disease locus) were useful in the thalassemias and in some inborn errors of metabolism. Usually, however, linkage is an arduous, and not always practicable, approach because it requires the availability of multiple family members and heterozygosity of the marker traits in key individuals. Furthermore, even under ideal circumstances, the available markers may be a distance from the disease locus, creating the possibility of a small, but finite chance of recombination, yielding false results. Thus, it is preferable to go for DNA diagnosis, that is, diagnosis based on the precise gene lesion.

In those disorders in which an enzyme deficiency or other protein abnormality has been identified, the wild-type gene can be cloned and defects in the gene identified. In the case of many Mendelian disorders, however, the nature of the biochemical defect was a mystery until the introduction of the mapping approach to identifying the basic derangement. The first of the mystery diseases to be mapped by linkage to DNA markers was Huntington disease (Gusella et al., 1983). It was, however, almost exactly 10 years to the week before the nature of the gene defect was reported (Huntington's Disease Collaborative Research Group, 1993).

Map-based gene discovery involves positional cloning and the candidate gene approach. Positional cloning was referred to initially as reverse genetics (e.g., Orkin, 1986). Starting with the phenotype, mapping it and then going to the gene is, however, the approach of classic genetics; true reverse genetics will be increasingly practiced as fragments of DNA with transcriptional and other characteristics of a gene are investigated to determine their role in the phenotype, by methods such as transgenic, or "knock-out," mice. For this reason, Francis Collins (1992) (Fig. 1.31) suggested that the approach be called positional cloning, not reverse genetics (Ruddle, 1984; Orkin, 1986). Table 1.1 lists, in chronologic order of discovery, the disease-producing genes identified by

positional cloning (that is, "walking in" on the gene from flanking markers), up until January, 1994.

Whereas positional cloning and the candidate gene approach are map-based cloning, functional cloning starts with the functional gene product and uses reverse transcriptase to create a cDNA corresponding to the mRNA encoded by the particular gene. The candidate gene approach involves mapping the disease phenotype to a particular chromosomal location and then scrutinizing that chromosomal region for genes encoding enzymes or other proteins that might plausibly be implicated in the disease in question. Support for the involvement of the candidate gene in the disease is provided by the demonstration of absolute linkage of a RFLP or microsatellite marker within the gene with the disease in question, and the proof is clinched by the demonstration of a specific point mutation or other intragenic lesion. Elucidation of the defect in one form of hypertrophic cardiomyopathy by Seidman and colleagues (Jarcho et al., 1989; Geisterfer-Lowrance et al., 1990) is an early example.

Table 1.1. Map-Based Gene Discovery: Positional Cloning (selected examples)[a].

Disorder	Gene	Location	MIM No.	Year
Chronic granulomatous disease, X-linked	CYBB	Xp21.1	306400	1986
Duchenne muscular dystrophy	DMD	Xp21.2	310200	1986
Retinoblastoma	RB1	13q14.1–q14.2	180200	1986
Cystic fibrosis	CFTR	7q31.2	219700	1989
Wilms tumor	WT1	11p13	194070	1989
Neurofibromatosis type 1	NF1	17q11.2	162200	1990
Gonadal dysgenesis, XY female type	TDF, SRY	Yp11.3	480000	1990
Choroideremia	CHM	Xq21.2	303100	1990
Fragile X syndrome	FMR1	Xq27.3	309550	1991
Myotonic dystrophy	DM	19q13.2–q13.3	160900	1992
X-linked agammaglobulinemia	AGMX2	Xp22	300310	1993
Neurofibromatosis type 2	NF2	22q12.2	101000	1993
Huntington disease	HD	4p16.3	143100	1993
Multiple endocrine neoplastic type 2	RET	10q11.2	171400	1993
Breast cancer, familial, type 1	BRCA1	17q21	113705	1994
Polycystic kidney disease-1	PKD1	16p13.3	173900	1994
Tuberous sclerosis-2	TSC2	16p13	191092	1994
Breast cancer, familial, type 2	BRCA2	13q	600185	1995
Werner syndrome	WRN	8p	277700	1996
Multiple endocrine neoplasia, type 1	MEN1	11q	131100	1997
Peutz-Jeghers syndrome	STK11	19p	175200	1998
Rett syndrome	RTT	Xq	312750	1999
Ellis-van Creveld syndrome	EVC	4p	225500	2000
Cartilage-hair hypoplasia	RMRP	9p	250250	2001

Abbreviations: *MIM, Mendelian Inheritance in man (McKusick, 1998).* [a] *In addition to these mendelian disorders, many genes with somatic mutations involved in neoplasia have also been identified by positional cloning, starting, for example, from translocation breakpoints.*

Many methods for identification of intragenic lesions have been identified over the past 10 years. By late 1994, disease-producing point mutations had been identified in almost 350 genes, and in many of these (e.g., *CFTR*, *HBB*) they numbered in the hundreds.

EVOLUTION OF CLINICAL GENETICS

Knut Faber (1930) attributed to Mendel a major role in shaping our thinking about nosology, particularly the classification of disease and the delineation of distinct disease entities. The advent of the bacteriologic era in the decades immediately after Mendel also had a powerful effect on nosology. Both developments sharpened focus on etiology: the role of specific microorganisms or the role of specific mutant genes. Until little more than a century ago, jaundice, dropsy, anemia, and other disorders were treated like disease entities in medical textbooks and in medical thinking and practice. Although mendelian thinking contributed importantly to the general concepts in medicine, genetics did not become involved significantly in clinical medicine until after the acquisition of an anatomic base, beginning in the late 1950s.

One can point to several examples of pre-mendelian "pedigree genetics." Patterns characteristic of autosomal dominant and autosomal recessive inheritance were commented on by Maupertuis in the 1750s, by Adams in 1814 (Motulsky, 1959), and by Sedgwick in the 1860s. The X-linked recessive pattern of hemophilia was noted in a newspaper account in the 1790s and in medical reports by Otto in 1803 and Hay in 1813 of early New England families (McKusick, 1962a, b). Similarly, the X-linked recessive pedigree pattern of colorblindness was described clearly by Swiss ophthalmologist Horner in Zurich in 1876, and even earlier by Earle (1845) in Philadelphia.

The relationship of consanguinity to an increased frequency of genetic defects was demonstrated by Bemiss in 1857 in studies of congenital deafness.

Early post-mendelian examples of pedigree genetics include a report of albinism as a recessive by William E Castle at Harvard in 1902. Farabee, a graduate student with Castle, described brachydactyly as a mendelian dominant trait, basing his thesis research on a family in his home town of Old Concord, Pennsylvania. The family was subsequently updated by Haws and McKusick (1963). Harvey Cushing, the neurosurgeon and biographer of William Osler, published a large kindred with *symphalangism* (his term for anchylosis of the phalanges) in a paper with accompanying fold-out pedigree in the first issue of *Genetics* in 1916, which also contained the famous paper by Calvin Bridges on non-disjunction.

The three main principles of clinical genetics (perhaps they should be called the three main phenomena of significance to clinical genetics) are pleiotropism, genetic heterogeneity, and variability. The history of our understanding of each can be traced.

Pleiotropism refers to multiple phenotypic (i.e., clinical) effects of a single mutant gene. This phenomenon is important to clinical medicine because often an external feature that is part of the pleiotropism and that may be in itself benign and insignificant may point to the presence of serious internal disease and/or to the fact that the person is a carrier of the mutant gene. The term was introduced by Plate in 1910. Hadorn developed the concept in considerable detail on the basis of studies in *Drosophila*. In his *Animal Genetics and Medicine* (1947), Hans Grüneberg gave numerous examples, particularly from the mouse, and presented what he called "pedigrees of causes" relating all features of the syndrome back to a unitary defect. Analysis of pleiotropism, with the demonstration of plausible pedigrees of causes, was an important aspect of *Heritable Disorders of Connective Tissue* (McKusick, 1956). The evidence for a unitary basic defect was fundamental to research in Marfan syndrome and other disorders. It took more than 35 years for the prediction of a unitary connective tissue defect in Marfan syndrome to be substantiated and particularized (Dietz et al., 1991; McKusick, 1991).

Genetic heterogeneity means that any one of several genetic mechanisms can lead to the same or similar phenotype. The idea was implicit in the work of Johannsen of Copenhagen, who in the first decade of this century distinguished phenotype and genotype. It was he who introduced the two terms (as well as the word *gene*) and put forward the concept that the phenotype is no necessary indication of the genotype. Genetic heterogeneity is obviously of practical importance in clinical medicine, since the prognosis, appropriate genetic counseling, and effective treatment may vary among the several genetic forms of a given disorder. Many examples of genetic heterogeneity have been uncovered during the past 45 years, especially through the application of biochemical and molecular methods. A striking example was homocystinuria, which simulates Marfan syndrome closely because of dislocated lenses and skeletal features such as increased height, scoliosis, and deformity of the anterior chest, but homocystinuria has recessive, not dominant, inheritance; has thrombotic, not aortic, complications in the cardiovascular system; and, of course, has a biochemical marker in the form of homocystine in the urine.

Baur, Lenz, and Fischer, in their textbook in the 1930s, recognized genetic heterogeneity. William Allen, who is honored by the William Allen Award of the American Society of Human Genetics, wrote about genetic heterogeneity when he pointed out that some disorders, such as Charcot-Marie-Tooth disease, occur in autosomal dominant, autosomal recessive, and X-linked forms. Allen pointed out that as a generalization the autosomal recessive form is most severe, the autosomal dominant form mildest (and most variable), and the X-linked recessive form intermediate in severity. This generalization is sometimes called Lenz's law, after Fritz Lenz of the Baur, Lenz, and Fischer textbook (and father of Widukind Lenz, medical geneticist of Münster, Germany).

Harry Harris (1953) (Fig. 1.8) of London, emphasized

the heterogeneity of apparently simple "characters": One of the problems central to all studies in human genetics arises from the difficulty of knowing whether a particular difference has been characterized in, as it were, a "chemically pure" form. What appears at first sight to be a homogeneous entity readily identifiable by a particular technique, and presumably having a unitary genetical causation, turns out, with the application of newer techniques to the problem, to consist of more than one quite distinct phenomenon … The condition known as "cystinuria" provides a simple illustration of this point.

As one aspect of the "darker side" of heredity counseling, F Clarke Fraser (1956) pointed to genetic heterogeneity of clinical entities. He wrote: "A lot of difficulty comes from the fact that for many diseases two clinically similar cases may be genetically different, and thus have different genetic prognoses."

Newton E Morton (1956) demonstrated genetic heterogeneity in elliptocytosis when he found that the disorder is linked to the Rh blood group locus in some families and not in others.

Variation in the clinical picture is a characteristic of disease of all etiologies, both genetic and nongenetic. If the clinical picture resulting from a particular etiologic factor were invariant, clinical medicine would be child's play. Learning clinical medicine is, to large extent, learning how to cope with variation. As well as pointing out the significance of pleiotropism, Hans Grüneberg (1947) emphasized that variability can depend on the genetic background of the particular mutation. A frequently cited example from the mouse was provided by the work of L C Dunn (1893–1974), who found that the *Brachyury* mutation, usually manifested by a short tail, was accompanied by an almost normal tail in some genetic stocks.

Penetrance and expressivity are aspects of variation. The terms and the concepts they signify were introduced by Vogt in 1926 (Stern, 1960) and were used by Timofeeff-Ressovsky soon thereafter while he was working in Berlin with Vogt. (Timofeeff-Ressovsky, still in Berlin at the time the Russians captured the city in 1944, was sent to a gulag, where he was a fellow prisoner of Solzhenitzyn; see Solzhenitzyn's *Gulag Archipelago* for references to the evening intellectual interactions by which they helped maintain each other's sanity. Timofeeff-Ressovsky was partially "rehabilitated" toward the end of his life and attended the World Congress of Genetics in Moscow in 1978.)

Penetrance is an all-or-none phenomenon. Expressivity is variation in severity of a genetic disorder or trait. When expressivity is so low that the disorder cannot be recognized, the gene is said to be nonpenetrant. Obviously, nonpenetrance is to some extent related to the power of the methods for studying the phenotype. The more penetrating the method, the lower the frequency of nonpenetrance!

CLINICAL ARMAMENTARIUM OF MEDICAL GENETICS

Part of the reason for the creation of the American Board of Medical Genetics and comparable agencies in some other countries is the fact that since 1956 there is so much more that clinical geneticists can do. Thus, a mechanism is needed for oversight of the training and certification of practitioners.

Bradford Hill, the British biostatistician, suggested that the practice of medicine consists of seeking answers to three questions: What is wrong? The answer is diagnosis. What is going to happen? The answer is prognosis. What can be done about it? The answer is treatment. (David Danks of Melbourne suggested to me that the health professional should always keep a fourth question in mind: Why did it happen? The answer is etiology and pathogenesis, on which prevention and treatment can be based.)

Advances in diagnosis have come from both the clinic and the laboratory. Because the individual genetic disorders, of which there are many, are rare, clinical geneticists play a key role in diagnosis. For many of these disorders, there are not yet specific biochemical or other tests. Syndromology and dysmorphology are important aspects of the clinical geneticist's work. Cytogenetic diagnosis is his specific responsibility, at least for nonmalignant disorders. The oncologist makes heavy use of cytogenetic diagnosis, particularly in relation to hematologic malignancies.

Prognosis in clinical genetics has somewhat different implications than prognosis in other parts of clinical medicine. The question—What is going to happen?—relates not only to the person at hand, but also to other members of the family, particularly an unborn child. Testing for the carrier status in a condition such as Duchenne muscular dystrophy or hemophilia or for a disease in its presymptomatic stages as in Huntington disease, is obviously of great importance to prognostication.

Neonatal screening and population-based screening for specific genetic diseases, and prenatal screening for Down syndrome in mothers over 35 years of age, do not fit neatly into the Bradford Hill paradigm of clinical medicine. Although they do address the question—what is going to happen?—the question—what is wrong?—has not been asked. The question is not even—Is something wrong?—since all genetic disorders are not tested for.

These procedures are at the interface between clinical medicine and public health, or at least between clinical medicine and preventive medicine. I would not wish to suggest that I recognize a distinction between preventive medicine and clinical medicine; preventive medicine is an integral and exceedingly important aspect of clinical medicine.

Treatment is generally viewed as the "short suit" of clinical genetics. However, more can be accomplished than is realized, and I would emphasize that *management* is a better designation for the medical geneticist's role than is *treatment*, which implies a repertoire of measures almost exclusively pharmaceutical or surgical.

With this overview as a preamble, let me outline the development of the medical geneticist's clinical armamentarium over the past 45 years.

An important item in the armamentarium of the clinical geneticist is command of syndromology and dysmorphology. Genetic diseases include a large number of individually rare disorders many of which have little basis of diagnosis other than their particular clinical features. Syndromology is the art and science of recognizing distinct genetic entities by characteristic combinations of clinical manifestations. Robert Gorlin of Minneapolis and John Opitz of Madison, Wisconsin (later of Helena, Montana, and Salt Lake City), are two American syndromologists from among the many capable ones. Dysmorphology is the term introduced by David W Smith (1926–1981) of Seattle, Washington, as an improvement on clinical teratology. It implies syndromology and as well encompasses considerations of etiology and pathogenesis; for example, the mechanisms by which the several features of malformation syndrome occur together were part of David Smith's focus and his delineation of the fetal alcohol syndrome illustrated his attention not only to distinctive clinical features but also to causation. *Smith's Recognizable Patterns of Malformation Syndromes* (Jones, 1988) is a classic.

Many malformation syndromes and genetic disorders carry the name of a person, not always the first, who described the condition as a distinct entity. These eponyms have advantages when the basic nature of the disorder is unknown and thus a specific label based thereon is not possible. Usefully, eponyms remind medical geneticists of the roots of their field (Beighton, 1986). Place names (toponyms) likewise link the disorder to the geographic or ethnic setting of the first (or early) description of the disorder or protein (e.g., hemoglobin) variant. Tangier disease and familial Mediterranean fever are examples.

Neither syndromology nor dysmorphology is limited to genetic disorders, but congenital anomalies of all etiologies are the responsibility of clinical geneticists. They must keep in mind all causation, both genetic and nongenetic and an interaction of the two. It was no accident that the teratogenic action of thalidomide was detected by a medical geneticist Widukind Lenz, in the early 1960s. It was easy for a nongeneticist to consider phocomelia a genetic disorder; a geneticist would be more likely to recognize that the distribution of cases in time, place, and families was not consistent with a genetic basis.

Annual conferences entitled the Clinical Delineation of Birth Defects were initiated in 1968 at Johns Hopkins University with financial support of the March of Dimes. During their heyday, from 1968 to about 1978, these gatherings of the aficionados illustrated the attention given by clinical geneticists to the development of the field of syndromology/dysmorphology. The annual David W. Smith conferences continue in the same tradition.

Several computerized databases have been developed during the past 10 to 15 years as an aid to the syndromologist: the London Dysmorphology Database of Robin Winter; GenDiag of Ségolène Amye, Paris; and POSSUM of Agnes Bankier and David Danks of Melbourne.

A SYNTHESIS: 1956–2001

Interestingly, 1956 was not only the year that human chromosomology got off to a firm start but also the date of the first world congress of human genetics, in Copenhagen under the presidency of Tage Kemp. The tenth and most recent of these quinquennial congresses was held in 2001. The first congress was a splendid survey of the status of human genetics at the time. The subsequent congresses were milestones measuring progress since 1956 (McKusick, 1992).

At the first congress in 1956, Tjio and Levan (Fig. 1.6A and B) and Ford and Hamerton (Fig. 1.7A and B) were getting the chromosome number right. Newton Morton was writing on linkage analysis. Oliver Smithies was beginning to write on starch gel electrophoresis. Vernon Ingram was narrowing down the molecular defect in sickle hemoglobin to a single peptide, and the first edition of my *Heritable Disorders of Connective Tissue* (McKusick, 1956) was published.

Behold what happened between the first congress and the eighth held in Washington in 1991. From the anatomy of the chromosomes at the most elementary level of enumeration, we had gone to their dissection by both mechanical and molecular methods. Genetic linkage had enjoyed a phenomenal renaissance, and linkage was by then analyzed on populations of sperm studied individually by direct molecular methods. Rather than studying variation in proteins by electrophoresis, we were examining variation in the DNA itself. From the one example of sickle hemoglobin, the known mutational repertoire of the β-globin gene had expanded to more than 400, for example. At least one disease-related point mutation had been defined in more than 170 different genes, a count that had passed the 1000 mark by the end of 2000 (Antonarakis and Mc Kusick, 2000).

Among the heritable disorders of connective tissue, clinical delineation had been refined by molecular definition. For example, in the mucopolysaccharidoses, lumped under the Hurler syndrome in 1956, at least 10 enzymatically distinct entities had been defined and, in the disorders of the fibrous elements of connective tissue, precise intragenic lesions had been described in osteogenesis imperfecta, in some of the Ehlers-Danlos syndromes and skeletal dysplasias, and in the Marfan syndrome.

By the 1961 congress in Rome, chaired by Luigi Gedda, clinical chromosomology had arrived. From the findings in Turner syndrome and Klinefelter syndrome, the role of the Y chromosome in sex determination was realized; the existence of testis-determining factor (TDF) was deduced. The hypothesis of the single active X chromosome, advanced by Mary Lyon (Lyon, 1961, 1962) (Fig. 1.33), was the intellectually provocative new concept. Electrophoretic polymorphisms of serum proteins and red cell enzymes were being described. The "Philadelphia chromosome" was found in chronic myelogenous leukemia, one of the first pieces of evidence in humans supporting the chromosome theory of cancer (Nowell and Hungerford 1960 B).

By 1991, imprinting had taken the place of lyonization. TDF had been cloned and characterized under the label "sex-determining region of Y" (*SRY*). The fundamental basis of specific forms of cancer had been traced to specific genes—sometimes multiple, sequentially collaborating genes—and to specific mutations within genes.

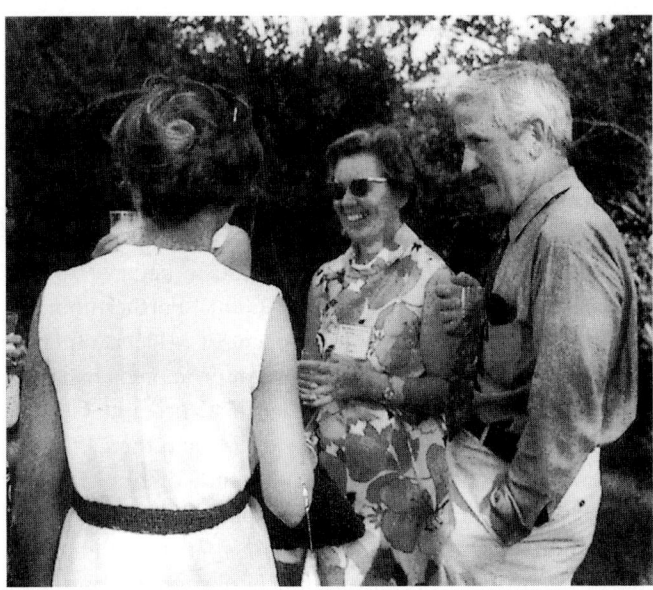

Fig. 1.33. Mary Lyon (center) with Wesley Whitten at Bar Harbor, 1971.

The Chicago congress in 1966 was under the presidency of Lionel S Penrose of London (Fig. 1.20). The genetic code had been completely deciphered that year. Somatic cell genetics had entered the scene for the study of inborn errors of metabolism. For example, it provided the strongest proof of the Lyon hypothesis and, through the study of cultured amniotic cells, opened the way for prenatal diagnosis by amniocentesis. The concept of lysosomal diseases had emerged, and the first edition of *Mendelian Inheritance in Man* (MIM) (McKusick, 1966), already computer based, was published earlier that year.

Review of the growth of successive editions of MIM provides an opportunity to engage in some scientometrics. As indicated by the original subtitle "Catalogs of Autosomal Dominant, Autosomal Recessive, and X-linked Phenotypes," MIM was an encyclopedia of phenotypes—genetic traits and disorders. But early on it was the intent that there should be one entry per gene locus, based largely on the philosophy that, if two genetic diseases or traits result from mutation at different loci, they are fundamentally distinct, however similar in phenotype they may be. Genetics is finding genes—gene hunting. The number of entries in successive editions of MIM can serve as one basis of quantifying progress in our field in the last 35 years. There were about 1500 entries in the first edition. In the 1960s, the only way we had to identify separate entries (read "gene loci") was by mendelizing phenotypes, sometimes aided by biochemical or immunologic characteristics or by genetic features such as linkage. In the 1970s, the rate of accession was accelerated by a parasexual method for gene identification and mapping, namely, somatic cell hybridization. By the 1980s, cloning of human genes was practiced. Accordingly, entries in MIM were created for genes when they were cloned, sequenced, and mapped, even though no mendelian phenotype had been associated. By the twelfth edition (McKusick, 1998), entries in MIM numbered 8587, an impressive figure but still a long way from the 60,000 to 70,000 expressed genes the human was then thought to have (Fields et al., 1994). (By the Fall of 2000, the number in the continuously updated online version, OMIM, was approaching 12,000.) Furthermore, by the 1990s, the evolution of the content of MIM as outlined above had lead to a self-redefinition that prompted change of the subtitle to "A Catalog of Human Genes and Genetic Disorders" in the eleventh edition (1994) and thereafter.

By the Paris congress in 1971, the study of inborn errors of metabolism in cultured cells had paid off. For example, elucidation of the defect in Lesch-Nyhan syndrome and the differentiation of various mucopolysaccharidoses had been accomplished through the study of cultured cells. Chromosome banding had been introduced and the first genes were being assigned to specific autosomes by linkage to chromosomal heteromorphisms and rearrangements and by interspecies somatic cell hybridization. There were four autosomal gene assignments by 1971.

Plotting the growth of the human gene map since 1971 is another exercise in scientometrics. By June 1976, just before the fifth Congress in Mexico City, at least one gene had been assigned to every chromosome. This was largely through the application of somatic cell hybridization. By the 1981 congress in Jerusalem, molecular genetic methods for gene mapping had entered the scene and were responsible for further acceleration of mapping in the 1980s. Molecular genetics provided probes for identification of human genes in rodent/human somatic cell hybrids. It provided probes for in situ hybridization to chromosomes and, importantly, it provided DNA markers (e.g., RFLPs, VNTRs) for family linkage studies, for mapping mendelian disorders of unknown biochemical basis. By the time of the 1991 congress, a total of at least 2300 genes had been mapped to specific chromosomes and, for most, to specific chromosomal regions.

By the fifth Congress in Mexico City in 1976, other advances of note included the concept of receptor diseases—disorders such as familial hypercholesterolemia (Goldstein and Brown, 1979) and androgen insensitivity—and Knudson et al, hypothesis of hereditary/sporadic tumors (Knudson, 1971; Knudson et al., 1975). The Philadelphia chromosome had been reinterpreted as a reciprocal translocation rather than a deletion.

By the 1981 Congress in Jerusalem, under the presidency of James V Neel (Fig. 1.34), in addition to the advances in the methods and results of gene mapping,

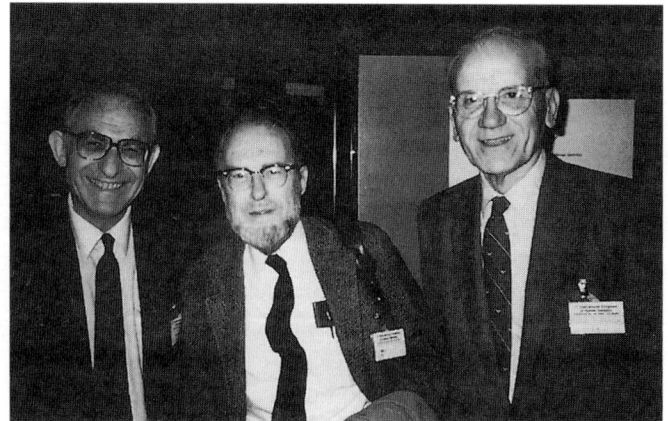

Fig. 1.34. Three presidents of the World Congress of Human Genetics: (left to right) Arno Motulsky (Berlin, 1986), James V Neel (Jerusalem, 1981), Victor McKusick (Washington, 1991). Photo from 1991. Neel died in 2000 at the age of 85.

human genes were being cloned, the genetic basis of antibody diversity was well on the way to elucidation, human variation was being studied with monoclonal antibodies, and one human chromosome had been completely sequenced—the mitochondrial chromosome.

By 1986 and the congress in Berlin, presided over by Arno Motulsky (Fig. 1.34), Huntington disease had been mapped using RFLPs—the first disorder of unknown biochemical basis mapped by this approach. VNTRs were a new class of markers. The previous spring, PCR had been unveiled at the Cold Spring Harbor Symposium, which had been devoted to the human genome. PFGE, DGGE, and CVS were introduced as acronyms for other new techniques or diagnostic methods. Contiguous gene syndromes were conceptualized and the deletions underlying them used for gene mapping and gene isolation. The approach, then called "reverse genetics," had succeeded in isolation of the gene for chronic granulomatous disease and at the very time of the congress was well on the way to characterization of the large gene that is mutant in Duchenne muscular dystrophy. Transgenic mice expressing human genes had been created. By molecular methods, the Knudson hypothesis had been proved for retinoblastoma; and the specific oncogenic molecular changes in the Philadelphia chromosome of chronic myeloid leukemia had been worked out, as well as those in the translocations underlying Burkitt lymphoma.

By the time of the eighth congress in 1991 (chaired by Victor McKusick; Fig. 1.34), the HGP had been launched. The HGP had been in a stage of debate and planning in 1986. The fruitfulness of positional cloning (alias reverse genetics) had been established for Duchenne muscular dystrophy, cystic fibrosis, neurofibromatoses, polyposis coli, and others. The candidate gene approach had also paid off for retinitis pigmentosa, hypertrophic cardiomyopathy, Marfan syndrome, and malignant hyperthermia. The genetics of common cancers such as colon cancer had been greatly clarified. *TDF* had been cloned. Specific mutations in the mitochondrial chromosome had been related to specific diseases. Imprinting and uniparental disomy were challenging concepts.

Between the eighth congress and the ninth (1996), in Rio de Janeiro, Brazil, with Newton Morton as president, ESTs (expressed sequence tags) were introduced (Adams et al., 1991) as a short-cut to the expressed part of the genome, the first free-living organism (H. *influenzae*) was completely sequenced (1995), a detailed linkage reference map using DNA markers was completed, a physical map of YAC contigs was published, radiation hybrid mapping came into wide use, the role of folic acid in birth defects was accepted as established and folic acid supplementation of food products introduced into practice. Preimplantation diagnosis at a 4- or 8-cell stage was added to in vitro fertilization (IVF), as a method for selection of non-mutant concepti.

Between the ninth congress in Rio de Janeiro and the tenth in Vienna in 2001 (G Utermann, President), database "mining" (research *in silico*, or cybergenomics) came in as a primary method of genomic research. As a result of positional cloning and related approaches to disease gene discovery well over 1000 genes had been found to have one or more disease-related mutations (Antonarakis and McKusick, 2000). Microassay methods ("chip technology") had been introduced for profiling gene expression and for gene diagnosis (Lockhart and Winzeler, 2000). Yeast became the first eukaryote to be completely sequenced (in the spring of 1996 shortly before the Rio Congress). *Caenorhabditis elegans*, a nematode, was the first metazoan completely sequenced (in 1999), followed by *Drosophila* (in 2000). On June 26, 2000, completion of a first draft of the complete human sequence was announced jointly by Venter and Collins, for the private and public projects, respectively, in a historic ceremony in the East Room of the White House, with connection by satellite to 10 Downing Street in London where Prime Minister Blair echoed President Clinton in emphasizing the significance of the event.

During the 1996–2001 interval, rapid progress toward the goal of the Human Genome Project was accompanied by the following paradigm shifts:

- from structural genomics to functional genomics;
- from map-based gene discovery to sequence-based gene discovery;
- from genetic disease diagnosis to detection of genetic predisposition of common disorders;
- from etiology (specific causation) to pathogenesis (mechanism);
- from a one-gene-at-a-time approach to study of systems, pathways and families of genes;
- from genomics to proteomics.

Another paradigm shift was from medical genetics to genetic medicine. This was not merely a change of name of institutions, although that did occur as in the program at Johns Hopkins which began in 1957 as the Division of Medical Genetics in the department of internal medicine, became in 1989 a multi-departmental Center for Medical Genetics, and in 1999 was transformed into an institute of genetic medicine. Beyond a change in name, this shift is a broadening of perspective. *Medical genetics* tends to imply an exclusive focus on rare mendelian disorders and chromosomal aberrations; *genetic medicine* reflects the fact that genetics pervades all parts of clinical medicine, that genetic factors are involved in all disease, and that genetic predisposition in the etiology of common disorders ("complex traits") is an important part of the science and practice of medical genetics.

Since 1956, human genetics has become *medicalized*, to use Motulsky's term, to an enormous extent. It has become *subspecialized*. Medical genetics has become *professionalized* through the development of clinical colleges and certifying organizations. During the past decade, human genetics has also become intensely *molecularized*. Molecular genetics pervades all aspects of human and medical genetics. Human genetics has become *commercialized* to an extent we might not have predicted. The field has also become *democratized* and *universalized*; its implications are felt in all aspects of society. It has become *consumerized*; consumerism is evident in the role of genetic support groups and foundations for funding of research on single genetic diseases.

FORTY YEARS IN THE HISTORY OF MEDICAL GENETICS

Mendelian Inheritance in Man (MIM) has recorded in detail the advances in medical genetics in the period since it was first initiated in 1960, as a catalog of X-linked traits (McKusick, 1962b). The catalog of recessives was undertaken in late 1962 in connection with studies of an inbred group, the Old Order Amish. The dominant catalog was created in 1963. The catalogs went on the computer in 1964. The first print edition of all three catalogs (a pioneer in computer-based publication) appeared in 1966, the twelfth in 1998. The 12 editions represent serial cross-sections of the field of medical genetics over four decades.

MIM was made publicly available online (under the designation OMIM) in 1987. OMIM (http://www.ncbi.nih.gov/omim) has the virtue of timeliness (it is updated almost daily) and easy searchability. The print version has usefulness in a non-electronic setting and as an archive.

The evolution of medical genetics since the early 1960s is illustrated in many ways by MIM (and OMIM). The subtitle at the beginning was "Catalogs of Autosomal Dominant, Autosomal Recessive, and X-linked Phenotypes". Although the gene behind the phenotype was always in mind (e.g., the X-linked catalog was created as an indication of the genetic constitution of the X chromosome), almost the only way to identify a gene was through a mendelizing phenotype, at the beginning. With molecular genetic advances, the subtitle in later print editions became "A Catalog of Human Genes and Genetic Disorders".

The future

Since the late 1980s, thought and discussion have been devoted to the future of human genetics to an unprecedented extent—largely growing out of the debate over the HGP and the planning for it. Rarely, if ever, has the future of a scientific field and its implications for society been given such wide and intense attention. An unusual and important feature of the federally funded Human Genome Project in the United States was support of research projects in the ethical, legal and societal implications (ELSI) of genome mapping and sequencing.

ELSI was a proactive effort to avoid misuse and abuse of new found genomic information. The history of eugenics and its misguided, unethical and immoral practices based on primitive knowledge of human genetics in the first half of the 20th century was a warning signal. The atrocities in Nazi Germany (Müller-Hill, 1985) were only the most flagrant, inhuman and abominable examples. Furthermore, it was anticipated that the power of information on the full genome of individuals and population groups would raise novel issues for society, medicine, and the law.

Completion of the human genome project provides a source book of the human that will be the basis for study in human biology and medicine for a long time to come. When all the genes have been found, we certainly still will not know, for most of them, their function even in solo, let alone in concert with the rest of the genome. True reverse genetics, in the New Genetics according to Walter Gilbert, David Botstein, and others, will involve working from specific DNA sequences of unknown function to the phenotype. Having in the past 35 years worked progressively from the phenotype to DNA, we will in the next 35 years be returning from DNA to the phenotype by determining the function of specific DNA sequences. Just as the function of much of the DNA remains to be determined even though the full sequence is known, the worldwide variation in that DNA is largely unknown, and long study will be required of the relationship between DNA variation and variation in function, critical to the understanding of evolution and the genetics of disease susceptibility and performance.

Study of the source book provided by the HGP should be particularly useful in the two great frontiers of human biology: how the mind works and how development is programmed. In the area of health and medicine, great benefit can be expected from the better understanding of genetic factors in multifactorial disorders which tend to be the common conditions such as hypertension and major mental illness. The source book will surely be very useful to the understanding of somatic cell genetic disease. Gene mapping and related studies have been primarily responsible for appreciation that in addition to the three classical categories of genetic disease—single gene disorders, multifactorial disorders, and chromosomal aberrations—somatic cell genetic disease is a large fourth category. This has been most extensively and definitively established through the definition of mutation as the basis of cancer. (Facetiously, it is suggested that medical genetics is taking over oncology.) Somatic cell mutations are likely to occupy us increasingly as the basis of congenital malformations, autoimmune processes and even aging. (McFarlane Burnett suggested about 1960 that somatic cell mutation is the basis of autoimmune processes and a somatic mutation theory of aging has been entertained for a long time.) The connection between oncogenesis and teratogenesis—between oncogenes and teratogens, if you will—is already adumbrated by the examples of Wilms tumor and Greig cephalosyndactyly syndrome, to mention two. It is to be assumed that somatic cell gene therapy not only for inherited diseases but perhaps also for some of these acquired somatic cell genetic diseases, especially neoplasia, will become available during the next decade.

Two scientific and technologic revolutions, the biologic revolution and the information revolution, converged in the human genome initiative. Information is power. Risks can accompany both the political and the scientific changes. Appropriately, ethical, legal, and societal implications of the human genome initiative are being examined in many parts of the world.

The methods developed by the HGP will allow the rapid and economical generation of information on the genomes of individuals. In the medical area, this information will widen the gap between what we know how to diagnose and what we know how to treat, between what we can diagnose in the presymptomatic state and what we can prevent. We have had that problem, for example, in the case of Huntington disease. The complete map and sequence is also likely to increase the gap between what we *think* we know and what we *really* know. But by this second gap, I refer in part to the likelihood that weak associations will be found between particular genomic constitutions and certain presumed characteristics such as criminality or alcoholism or elements of intelligence or performance. Some of these associations are likely to be spurious. Other weak associations may be found to be statistically valid but will be blown out of all proper proportion to the detriment of individuals and of groups. As geneticists, we have a responsibility to avoid unfounded conclusions and overblown interpretations and to inculcate the profound respect for the genetic variability that is the strength of the species and indeed of the individual—referring to the differences in the two genomes each of us has, one from the father and one from the mother.

The mere existence of the complete reference gene map and DNA sequence down to the last nucleotide may lead to the absurdity of reductionism, the misconception that we then know everything it means to be human, or to the absurdity of genetic determinism, that what we are is a direct and inevitable consequence of what our genome is. Our phenotypes are not "hard-wired" to our genotypes. Risk figures that state the chance of given common disorder in an individual based on a genome screen are probabilities, not certainties. They are more analogous to weather report than to a road map.

Thus, information on the reference gene map and sequence of the human may represent per se a hazard, if it distorts the way we think about ourselves and our fellow human beings. The ability to analyze the genomes of individuals is accompanied by risks of information misuse and abuse. We must be alert to the need to protect the privacy and confidentiality of the information that the human genome project will allow to be collected on the genetic constitution of individuals. We must make every effort to avoid the misuse or abuse of such information by third parties, and our governments may need to take measures to assure these protections under law.

Near the end of his terms of office, President Eisenhower warned against the dangers of the military industrial complex. It is appropriate to warn of a potential hazard of the genetic-commercial complex. The increasing availability of tests for presumed genetic quality or disqualify could lead the commercial sector and the Madison Avenue publicist to bring subtle or not so subtle pressure on couples to make value judgments in the choice of their gametes for reproduction. Autonomy in reproductive choice is a cornerstone of the ethics of genetic counseling. That reproductive choice would not be autonomous if subjected to the Madison Avenue type of pressure. Especially, trivialization of reproductive choices should be avoided.

As human geneticists, we are privileged to work in a scientifically important field and a field of intellectual challenge. Human genetics is a field that holds particular fascination because it involves the most fundamental and pervasive aspects of our own species, an added fascination that the physical sciences or pure mathematics, for example, cannot share. To have combined with this intellectual and anthropocentric fascination, the opportunity to contribute to human welfare and to be of service to families and individuals through medical genetics and clinical genetics is a privilege. The privilege carries with it responsibilities to which I have already referred.

REFERENCES

Adams MD and 12 others including Venter JC (1991) Complementary DNA sequencing: Expressed sequence tags and human genome project. Science 252:1651–1656

Adams MD and 194 others including Smith HO, Gibbs RA, Myers EW, Rubin GM, Venter JC (2000) The genome sequence of Drosophila melanogaster. Science 287:2185–95

Allen G, Benda CE, Böök JA, Carter CO and 15 others (1961) "Mongolism," letter. Lancet 1:775; also Am J Hum Genet 13:426

Anderson S, Bankier AT, Barrell BG et al. (1981) Sequence and organization of the human mitochondrial genome. Nature 290:457–465

Antonarakis SE, McKusick VA (2000) OMIM passes the 1,000-disease-gene mark. Nature Genet 25:11

Avery OT, MacLeod CM, McCarty M (1944) Studies on the chemical nature of the substance inducing transformation of pneumococcal types. Induction of transformation by a deoxyribonucleic acid fraction from *Pneumococcus* Type III. J Exp Med 79:137–158

Barr ML, Bertram LF (1949) A morphological distinction between neurones of the male and the female and the behavior of the nucleolar satellite during accelerated nucleoprotein synthesis. Nature 163:676–677

Bearn AG (1993) Archibald Garrod and the Individuality of Man. Clarendon Press, Oxford

Beighton P (1986) The Man Behind the Syndrome. Springer Verlag. N Y

Bell J, Haldane JBS (1937) The linkage between the genes for colour-blindness and haemophilia in man. Proc R Soc Lond Ser B 123:119–150

Biggs R, Douglas AS, Macfarlane RG et al. (1952) Christmas disease: A condition previously mistaken for haemophilia. BMJ 2:1378–1382

Boehnke M, Arnheim N, Li H, Collins FS (1989) Fine-structure genetic mapping of human chromosomes using the polymerase chain reaction on single sperm. Am J Hum Genet 45:21–32

Botstein D, White RL, Skolnick M, Davis RW (1980) Construction of a genetic linkage map in man using restriction fragment length polymorphisms. Am J Hum Genet 32:314–331

Burke DT, Carle GF, Olson MV (1987) Cloning of large segments of exogenous DNA into yeast by means of artificial chromosome vectors. Science 236:806

Caspersson T, Zech L, Johansson C (1970a) Differential banding of alkylating fluorochromes in human chromosomes. Exp Cell Res 60:315–319

Caspersson T, Zech L, Johansson C, Modest EJ (1970b) Quinocrine mustard fluorescent banding. Chromosoma 30:215–227

Caspersson T, Lomakka C, Zech L (1971) Fluorescent banding. Hereditas 67:89–102

Childs B (1995) The logic of disease. In Scriver CR, Beaudet AL, Sly WS, Valle D (eds): The Metabolic and Molecular Bases of Inherited Disease. McGraw-Hill, N Y p. 230.

Chumakov IM, and others including Cohen DA (1995) YAC contig map of the human genome. Nature 377:(suppl.) 175–297

Cohen S, Chang A, Boyer H, Helling R (1973) Construction of biologically functional bacterial plasmids in vitro. Proc Natl Acad Sci USA 70:3240–3244

Collins FS (1992) Positional cloning: Let's not call it reverse anymore. Nature Genet 1:3–6

Collins FS (1995) Ahead of schedule and under budget: The Genome Project passes its fifth birthday. Proc Natl Acad Sci USA 92:10821–10823

Cook-Deegan R (1994) The Gene Wars. Norton, N Y

Cori GT, Cori CF (1952) Glucose-6-phosphatase of the liver in glycogen storage disease. J Biol Chem 199:661–667

Cox DR, Burmeister M, Price ER, Kim S, Myers RM (1990) Radiation hybrid mapping: A somatic cell genetic method for constructing high-resolution maps of mammalian chromosomes. Science 250:245–250

Davidson RG, Nitowsky HM, Childs B (1963) Demonstration of two populations of cells in the human female heterozygous for glucose-6-phosphate dehydrogenase variants. Proc Natl Acad Sci USA 50:481–485

de Klein A, Geurts van Kessel A, Grosveld G et al. (1982) A cellular oncogene is translocated to the Philadelphia chromosome in chronic myelocytic leukaemia. Nature 300:765–767

Dib C and 13 others including Weissenbach J (1996) A comprehensive genetic map of the human genome based on 5,264 microsatellites. Nature 380:152–154

Dietz HC, Cutting GR, Pyeritz RE et al. (1991) Marfan syndrome caused by a recurrent de novo missense mutation in the fibrillin gene. Nature 353:337–339

DiLella AG, Marvit J, Lidsky AS et al. (1986) Tight linkage between a splicing mutation and a specific DNA haplotype in phenylketonuria. Nature 322:799–803

Dombroski BA, Mathias SL, Nanthakumar E et al. (1991) Isolation of an active human transposable element. Science 254:1805–1808

Donahue RP, Bias WB, Renwick JH, McKusick VA (1968) Probable assignment of the Duffy blood group locus to chromosome 1 in man. Proc Natl Acad Sci USA 61:949–955

Earle P (1845) On the inability to distinguish colors. Am J Med Sci 9:346–354

Edwards JH (1956) Antenatal detection of hereditary disorders, letter. Lancet 1:579

Eiberg H, Mohr J, Nielsen LS, Simonsen N (1983) Genetics and linkage relationships of the C3 polymorphism: discovery of C3-Se linkage and assignment of LES-C3-DM-Se-PEPD-Lu synteny to chromosome 19. Clin Genet 24:159–170

Faber K (1930) Nosography, 2nd edn. Hoeber, N Y

Farmer JB, Moore JES (1905) On the maiotic phase (reduction divisions) in animals and plants. Q J Microsc Sci 48:489

Ferguson-Smith MA, Newman BF, Ellis PM et al. (1973) Assignment by deletion of human red cell acid phosphatase gene locus to the short arm of chromosome 2. Nature 243:271–273

Fialkow PJ (1977) Clonal origin and stem cell evolution of human tumors. In Mulvihill JJ, Miller RW, Fraumeni JF Jr (eds): Genetics of Human Cancer. Raven, N Y, p. 439.

Fields C, Adams MD, White O, Venter JC (1994) How many genes in the human genome. Nature Genet 7:345–346

Fisher RA (1918) Correlation between relatives on the supposition of mendelian inheritance. Trans R Soc, Edinb 52:399–433

Fisher RA (1936) Has Mendel's work been rediscovered? Ann Sci 1:115–137

Fleischmann RD, Adams MD and 30 others including Smith HO and Venter JC (1995) Whole-genome random sequencing and assembly of Haemophilus influenzae Rd. Science 269:496–512

Flemming W (1882) Zellsubstanz. Kern & Zelltheilung. FCW Vogel, Leipzig

Ford CE, Hamerton JC (1956) The chromosomes of man. Nature 178:1020–1023

Francke U, Oliver N (1978) Quantitative analysis of high-resulution trypsin-Giemsa bands on human prometaphase chromosomes. Hum Genet 45:137–165

Fraser FC (1956) Heredity counseling: the darker side. Eugen Q 3:45

Garrod A (1909) Inborn Errors of Metabolism. Frowde, London

Garrod A (1928) The lessons of rare diseases. Lancet 1:1055–1060

Garrod A (1931) The Inborn Factors in Disease: An Essay. Clarendon Press, Oxford

Geisterfer-Lowrance AAT, Kass S, Tanigawa G et al. (1990) A molecular basis for familial hypertrophic cardiomyopathy: a beta cardiac myosin heavy chain gene missense mutation. Cell 62:999–1006

Goldstein JL, Brown MS (1979) The LDL receptor locus and the genetics of familial hypercholesterolemia. Annu Rev Genet 13:259–289

Goodfellow PJ, Povey S, Nevanlinna HA, Goodfellow PN (1990) Generation of a panel of somatic cell hybrids containing unselected fragments of human chromosome 10 by x-ray irradiation and cell fusion: Application to isolating the MEN2A region in hybrid cells. Somat Cell Molec Genet 16:163–171

Goss S, Harris H (1975) A new method for mapping genes in human chromosomes. Nature 255:680–684

Green ED, Olson MV (1990) Chromosomal region of the cystic fibrosis gene in yeast artificial chromosomes: a model for human genome mapping. Science 94:8

Grüneberg H (1947) Animal Genetics and Medicine. Hoeber, N Y

Gusella JF, Wexler NS, Conneally PM et al. (1983) A polymorphic DNA marker genetically linked to Huntington's disease. Nature 306:234–238

Haldane JBS, Smith CAB (1947) A new estimate of the linkage between the genes for colour-blindness and haemophilia in man. Ann Eugen 14:10–31

Haldane JBS, Sprunt AD, Haldane NM (1915) Reduplication in mice. J Genet 5:133–135

Hardy GH (1908) Mendelian proportions in a mixed population. Science 28:49–50

Harper ME, Ullrich A, Saunders GF (1981) Localization of the human insulin gene to the distal end of the short arm of chromosome 11. Proc Nat Acad Sci USA 78:4458–4460

Harris H (1953) An Introduction to Human Biochemical Genetics. Cambridge University Press, Cambridge, England, p. 19

Haws DV, McKusick VA (1963) Farabee's brachydactylous kindred revisited. Bull Johns Hopkins Hosp 113:20–30

Hsu SH, Schacter BZ, Delaney NL et al. (1976) Genetic characteristics of the HeLa cell. Science 191:392–394

Huntington's Disease Collaborative Research Group (1993) A novel gene containing a trinucleotide repeat that is expanded and unstable on Huntington's disease chromosomes. Cell 72:971–983

Jarcho JA, McKenna W, Pare JAP et al. (1989) Mapping a gene for familial hypertrophic cardiomyopathy to chromosome 14q1. N Engl J Med 321:1372–1378

Jeffreys A, Wilson V, Thein S (1985) Hypervariable "minisatellite" regions in human DNA. Science 314:67–73

Jervis GA (1953) Phenylpyruvic oligophrenia deficiency of phenylalanine-oxidizing system. Proc Soc Exp Biol Med 82:514–515

Jones HW Jr, McKusick VA, Harper PS, Wuu KD (1971) George O. Gey (1899–1970): The HeLa cell and a reappraisal of its origin. Obstet Gynecol 38:945–949

Jones KL (1988) Smith's Recognizable Patterns of Human Malformation, 4th edn. WB Saunders, Philadelphia

Kan YW, Dozy AM (1978) Polymorphism of DNA sequence adjacent to human beta-globin structural gene: Relationship to sickle mutation. Proc Nat Acad Sci USA 75:5631–5635

Knudson AG Jr (1971) Mutation and cancer: Statistical study of retinoblastoma. Proc Natl Acad Sci USA 68:820–823

Knudson AG Jr, Hethcote HW, Brown BW (1975) Mutation and childhood cancer: A probabilistic model for the incidence of retinoblastoma. Proc Natl Acad Sci USA 72:5116–5120

La Du BN, Zannoni VG, Laster L, Seegmiller JE (1958) The nature of the defect in tyrosine metabolism in alcaptonuria. J Biol Chem 230:251

Lander ES, Botstein D (1987) Homozygosity mapping: A way to map human recessive traits with the DNA of inbred children. Science 236:1567–1570

Landsteiner K, Levine P (1927) A new agglutinable factor differentiating individual human bloods. Proc Soc Exp Biol Med 24:600–602

Landsteiner K, Weiner AS (1940) An agglutinable factor in human blood recognized by immune sera for rhesus blood. Proc Soc Exp Biol Med 43:223

Lebo RV, Gorin F, Fletterick RJ et al. (1984) High-resolution chromosome sorting and DNA spot-blot analysis assign McArdle's syndrome to chromosome 11. Science 225:57–59

Lele KP, Penrose LS, Stallard HB (1963) Chromosome deletion in a case of retinoblastoma. Ann Hum Genet 27:171–174

Levine P, Stetson RE (1939) An unusual case of intragroup agglutination. JAMA 113:126–127

Levine P, Katzin EM, Burnham L (1941) Isoimmunization in pregnancy, its possible bearing on the etiology of erythroblastosis fetalis. JAMA 116:825–827

Littlefield JW (1964) Selection of hybrids from matings of fibroblasts in vitro and their presumed recombinants. Science 145:709–710

Lockhart DJ, Winzeler EA (2000) Genomics, gene expression and DNA arrays. Nature 405:827–836

Lüdecke HJ, Senger G, Claussen U, Horsthemke B (1989) Cloning defined regions of the human genome by microdissection of banded chromosomes and enzymatic amplification. Nature 338:348–350

Lyon MF (1961) Gene action in the X-chromosome of the mouse (*Mus musculus*) Nature 190:372–373

Lyon MF (1962) Sex chromatin and gene action in the mammalian X-chromosome. Am J Hum Genet 14:135–148

McCurdy PR (1971) Use of genetic linkage for the detection of female carriers of hemophilia. N Engl J Med 285:218–219

McKusick VA (1956) Heritable Disorders of Connective Tissue. CV Mosby, St. Louis

McKusick VA (1960) Walter S. Sutton and the physical basis of mendelism. Bull Hist Med 34:487

McKusick VA (1962a) Hemophilia in early New England: A follow-up of four kindreds in which hemophilia occurred in the pre-Revolutionary period. J Hist Med 17:342–364

McKusick VA (1962b) On the X chromosome of man. Quart Rev Biol 37:69–175

McKusick VA (1966) Mendelian Inheritance in Man, 1st edn. Johns Hopkins University Press, Baltimore (12th edn. 1998; OMIM—online version, URL http://www.ncbi.nih.nlm.gov/omim)

McKusick VA (1969) On lumpers and splitters, or the nosology of genetic disease. Perspect Biol Med 12:298–312

McKusick VA (1970) Prospects for progress, In Fraser FC, McKusick VA (eds): Congenital Malformations. Vol. 3. Third International Conference, The Hague, 1969. Excerpta Medica, Amsterdam, p. 407.

McKusick VA (1980) The anatomy of the human genome. Am J Med 69:267–276

McKusick VA (1981) The human genome through the eyes of Mercator and Vesalius. Trans Am Clin Climatol Assoc 42:66–90

McKusick VA (1985) Marcella O'Grady Boveri (1865–1950) and the chromosome theory of cancer. J Med Genet 22:431–440

McKusick VA (1986) The gene map of *Homo sapiens:* Status and prospectus. The molecular biology of *Homo sapiens.* Cold Spring Harbor Symp 51:15–27

McKusick VA (1991) The defect in Marfan syndrome. Nature 352:279–281

McKusick VA (1992) Human genetics: The last 35 years, the present, and the future. Am J Hum Genet 50:663–670

McKusick VA (1996) Genomics: An established discipline, a commonly used name, a mature journal. Genomics 31:1–2

McKusick VA (1997) Genomics: Structural and functional studies of genomes. Genomics 45:244–249

McKusick VA (1998) Mendelian Inheritance in Man, 12th edn. Johns Hopkins University Press, Baltimore

McKusick VA, Ruddle FH (1977) The status of the gene map of the human chromosomes. Science 396:390–405

McKusick VA, Ruddle FH (1987) A new discipline, a new name, a new journal. Genomics 1:1–2

Maxam AM, Gilbert W (1977) A new method for sequencing DNA. Proc Nat Acad Sci USA 74:1258–1262

Migeon BR, Miller CS (1968) Human-mouse somatic cell hybrids with single human chromosome (group E): Link with thymidine kinase activity. Science 162:1005–1006

Miller OJ, Allderdice PW, Miller DA (1971) Human thymidine kinase gene locus: Assignment to chromosome 17 in a hybrid of man and mouse cells. Science 173:244–245

Morton NE (1956) The detection and estimation of linkage between the genes for elliptocytosis and the Rh blood type. Am J Hum Genet 8:80–96

Motulsky AG (1959) Joseph Adams (1756–1818), a forgotten founder of medical genetics. Arch Intern Med 104:490–496

Müller-Hill B (1998) In Murderous Science, translated by Fraser GR. Oxford University Press, Oxford

Mullis K, Faloona F, Scharf S (1986) Specific enzymatic amplification of DNA in vitro: The polymerase chain reaction. Cold Spring Harbor Symp Quant Biol 51:263–273

Nakamura Y, Leppert M, O'Connell P et al. (1987) Variable number of tandem repeat (VNTR) markers for human gene mapping. Science 235:1616–1622

National Research Council/National Academy of Sciences Committee (1988) Mapping and Sequencing the Human Genome. National Academy of Sciences Press, Washington, DC

Novitski CE (1995) Another look at some of Mendel's results. J Hered 86:62–66

Nowell PC (1960) Phytohaemagglutinin: An initiator of mitosis in cultures of normal human leukocytes. Cancer Res 20:462–466

Nowell PC, Hungerford DA (1960a) A minute chromosome in human chronic granulocytic leukemia. Science 132:1497

Nowell PC, Hungerford DA (1960b) Chromosome studies on normal and leukemic human leukocytes. J Natl Cancer Inst 25:85–109

Ohno S (1967) Sex Chromosomes and Sex-linked Genes. Springer-Verlag, Berlin.

Okada Y (1958) The fusion of Ehrlich's tumor cells caused by H.V.J. virus in vitro. Bikens J 1:103–110

Olson M, Hood L, Cantor C, Botstein D (1989) A common language for physical mapping of the human genome. Science 245:1434–1435

Orkin SH (1986) Reverse genetics and human disease. Cell 47:845–850

Ott J (1985) Analysis of Human Genetic Linkage. Johns Hopkins University Press, Baltimore

Painter TS (1923) Studies in mammalian spermatogenesis. II. The spermatogenesis of man. J Exp Zool 37:291–336

Pandey A, Mann M (2000) Proteomics to study genes and genomes. Nature 405:837–846

Pauling LC, Itano HA, Singer SJ, Wells IC (1949) Sickle cell anemia, a molecular disease. Science 110:543–548

Pearson K, Nettleship E, Usher CH (1911) A Monograph on Albinism in Man. DuLau, London

Penrose LS (1935) The detection of autosomal linkage in data which consist of pairs of brothers and sisters of unspecified parentage. Ann Eugen 6:133–138

Pollack MR, Chou, Y-HW, Cerda JJ (1993) Homozygosity mapping of the gene for alkaptonuria to chromosome 3q2. Nature Genet 5: 201–204

Pontecorvo G (1975) Production of mammalian somatic cell hybrids by means of polyethylene glycol treatment. Somat Cell Mol Genet 4:397–400

Race RR, Sanger R (1975) Blood Groups in Man, 6th edn. FA Davis, Philadelphia, p 178

Roses AD (2000) Pharmacogenomics and the practice of medicine. Nature 405:857–865

Rowley JD (1973) A new consistent abnormality in chronic myelogenous leukemia identified by quinacrine fluorescence and Giemsa staining. Nature 243:290–293

Ruddle FH (1984) Reverse genetics and beyond. Am J Hum Genet 36:944–953

Rushton AR (1994) Genetics and Medicine in the United States 1800 to 1922. Johns Hopkins University Press, Baltimore

Saiki RK, Scharf S, Falsona F et al. (1985) Enzymatic amplification of beta-globin genomic sequences and restriction site analysis for diagnosis of sickle cell anemia. Science 230:1350–1354

Sanger F, Nicklen S, Coulson AR (1977) DNA sequencing with chain-terminating inhibitors. Proc Natl Acad Sci USA 74:5463–5467

Schmickel RD (1986) Contiguous gene syndromes: a component of recognizable syndromes. J Pediatr 109:231–241

Schrott HG, Karp L, Omenn GS (1973) Prenatal prediction in myotonic dystrophy: Guidelines for genetic counseling. Clin Genet 4:38–45

Schrott HG, Omenn GS (1975) Myotonic dystrophy: Opportunities for prenatal prediction. Neurology 25:789–791

Seegmiller JE, Rosenbloom FM, Kelley WN (1967) Enzyme defect associated with a sex-linked human neurological disorder and excessive purine synthesis. Science 155:1682–1684

Shine J, Seeburg PH, Martial JA et al. (1977) Construction and analysis of recombinant DNA for human chorionic somatomammotropin. Nature 270:494–499

Solomon E, Bodmer WF (1979) Evolution of sickle variant gene, letter. Lancet 1:923

Southern EM (1975) Detection of specific sequences among DNA fragments separated by gel electrophoresis. J Mol Biol 98:503–517

Stern C (1960) O. Vogt and the terms "penetrance" and "expressivity." Am J Hum Genet 12:141

Sutton WS (1903) The chromosomes in heredity. Biol Bull 4:231

Tjio JH, Levan A (1956) The chromosome number in man. Hereditas 42:1–6

Watson JD, Crick FHC (1953) Molecular structure of nucleic acids. A structure for deoxyribose nucleic acid. Nature 171:737–738

Weiss M, Green H (1967) Human-mouse hybrid cell lines containing partial complements of human chromosomes and functioning human genes. Proc Natl Acad Sci USA 58:1104–1111

Wilson EB (1896) The Cell in Development and Heredity, 1st edn. Macmillan, N Y

Wilson EB (1911) The sex chromosomes. Arch Mikrosk Anat Entwicklungsmech 77:249–271

Yamamoto F, Clausen H, White T et al. (1990) Molecular genetic basis of the histo-blood group ABO system. Nature 345:229–233

Yunis JJ (1976) High resolution of human chromosomes. Science 191:1268–1270

SUGGESTED READINGS

Bishop JE, Waldholz M (1990) Genome: The Story of the Most Astonishing Scientific Adventure of Our time—the Attempt to Map All the Genes of the Human Body. Simon and Schuster, N Y

Dunn LC (1965) A Short History of Genetics. McGraw-Hill, N Y

Guethlein LA (1990) The Bar Harbor course: A 30-year veteran in the teaching of human genetics. Am J Hum Genet 46:192–206

Hsu TC (1979) Human and Mammalian Cytogenetics: An Historic Perspective. Springer-Verlag, N Y

Judson HF (1979) The Eighth Day of Creation: The Makers of the Revolution in Biology. Simon & Schuster, N Y

Kevles DL (1985) In the Name of Eugenics: Genetics and the Uses of Human Heredity. Alfred A Knopf, N Y

Ludmerer LM (1972) Genetics and American Society: A Historical Approach. Johns Hopkins University Press, Baltimore

McKusick VA (1975) The growth and development of human genetics as a clinical discipline. Am J Human Genet 27:261–273

McKusick VA (1989) Forty years of medical genetics. JAMA 261:3155–3158

McKusick VA (1993) Medical genetics: A 40-year perspective on the evolution of a medical speciality from a basic science. JAMA 270:2351–2356

Portugal FH, Cohen JS (1977) A Century of DNA. A History of the Discovery of the Structure and Function of the Genetic Substance. MIT Press, Cambridge, MA

Ridley M (1999) Genome: The Autobiography of a Species in 23 Chapters. Fourth Estate, London

Schull WJ, Chakraborty R (eds) (1979) Human Genetics: A Selection of Insights. Dowden, Hutchinson and Ross, Stroudsburg, PA (Anthology of human genetics papers, reprinted in facsimile with comments. Part of Benchmark Papers in Genetics series)

Watson JD, Tooze J (1981) The DNA Story: A Documentary History of Gene Cloning. WA Freeman, San Francisco

Medicine in a genetic context

Barton Childs

Introduction

The history of science through the recently ended millennium is characterized by an exponential rate of expansion (De Solla Price, 1963). No aspect escaped, but biology, which is relatively new, has by all accounts exploded. Naturally these changes are reflected in new principles, new thinking, new ways of handling new information. Among the problems created is that of making these novelties available to practitioners of science of all kinds.

Among the ways suitable to medicine are massive volumes that contain detailed summaries of diseases, usually of one class, as endocrine, gastroenterological, or, as in the case of *Principles and Practice of Medical Genetics* (*PPMG*), inherited. And of course the pace of change requires revisions, always characterized by increases that reflect the rate of accumulation. Fission adds volumes whose pages, chapters, contributors and diseases all do their best to obey the exponential imperative. Each chapter represents one topic more or less, an expansible topic capable of embracing new disorders with each new edition, so the number of chapters is no guide to the number of diseases. In addition to new diseases, new paths of basic science are added, a characteristic of books that mirror progress in reductionist investigation. But where is reductionist biology taking us? Clearly, one direction is toward fragmentation; more and more is learned about increasingly restricted fields so that even specialities bifurcate and medicine becomes ever more splintered. But despite such assaults, whatever it is we call medicine has at bottom some integrity, some consistency, common grounds that are clearly revealed in *PPMG* as well as in its sister enterprise, *The Metabolic and Molecular Basis of Inherited Disease* (*MMBID*) (Scriver, 1995). One such

common ground is genetics. And since there is included in both of these books disorders of such a striking variety of cellular structures and metabolic mechanisms engaging every organ and organ system, it is easy to imagine that genetic variation is at the basis of all diseases. This idea is far from new, having been suggested even in the eighteenth and nineteenth centuries, when it took the form of diathesis and idiosyncrasy (Rosenberg, 1995). Then, in this century, it appears in the shape of a continuity between clear cut segregating monogenic diseases and varying degrees of familial aggregation of cases that suggest the outcomes of the actions of more than one gene acting in environments favorable for the onset of a disease. But now, with the advent of genomics which makes possible the study of the genetics of diseases of complex origin in families of patients who have affected relatives, as well as in those who do not, we are learning that genetic variation underlies the latter no less than the former, so the continuity of segregating to non-segregating familial aggregation, is extended to include cases where there is neither segregation nor aggregation (Lander, 1996). Perhaps we should require a disease to be shown *not* to be associated with any genetic variation, before saying it has no genetic basis.

All professions undergoing rapid change and increasing specialism face the same dilemma. The generalists who, as generalists, must keep up, find the density of new information daunting, even impossible to sort out and retain. So, books like *PPMG* are intended to present that information in an orderly way and in relation to specific diseases. But the job is no sooner done than even newer information arrives to change how the various disorders are perceived, and, of course, treated. Furthermore new diseases have been described and must be included. Hence another edition must appear. And that's not all. The various sciences that

37

contribute to our understanding are all changing too, providing new insights that challenge conventional thinking. Editors respond to this intense pressure by including articles that present not only new information but new insights, new ways of thinking about groups of diseases or perhaps all, and these usually appear at the beginning, hinting strongly that the reader of any later chapters would do well to read these preliminary ones.

It would seem that the editors of *PPMG* suppose that, for example, the principles of chromosomal organization or of genomics or of the investigations of diseases of complex origin would help the reader better to understand the chapters on developmental anomalies or the origins of high blood pressure, or inborn errors. And that may happen, given the effort. But each reader who makes this synthesis for himself or herself is likely to do it in the context of some specific disorder rather than to generalize the principles to all diseases. Indeed we lack a clearly articulated set of principles of disease as opposed to diseases. That is not to say that medicine lacks principles; the idea of the body as a machine that breaks and needs fixing is one, and the medical history, diagnosis, pathogenesis, treatment, prognosis and prevention all have a conceptual basis, as do the basic sciences related to medicine. But disease as a concept seems to be taken for granted. Textbooks of medicine, pediatrics, and pathology often begin with generalities, but not about disease. Medical texts sometimes begin by defining the practice of medicine, the meaning of signs and symptoms, the doctor–patient relationships and medical ethics, while pediatric texts include growth and development, relations with parents, and the special quality of the medicine of infants and children. Perhaps it is an expression of medicine's pragmatism. Why try to define something you know cannot be deciphered at a satisfactory level even though you know that level must be molecular? This is the view of the editors of Cecil's 21st edition published in 2000 (Goldman, 2000). The editors say "true understanding of disease processes depends upon levels of scientific knowledge that are just being discovered." Pathology probably comes nearest to touching on the principles of Disease in generalizing on cell injury, inflammation, cell death and tissue repair. But no book suggests that a student of medicine (and we are all students throughout the length of our careers) might take profit in an account of Disease as opposed to diseases, including: why we have it, who is likely to be affected and how, and when in the lifetime and what forms can it take as well as what are its constraints? That is, what are the explanatory generalizations that comprise a context within which to fit all diseases?

Similarly, definitions of Disease have fallen by the wayside. It is true that many such definitions have been offered; there is a sizable literature on the subject (Cohen, 1960; Temkin, 1963; King, 1982; Childs, 1999b). Perhaps today's reluctance stems from physicians' perception that we have not had the wherewithal for any but descriptions based on signs and symptoms rather than anything at its core. But today we are satisfied with a definition of a disease when pathogenesis is explained by reference to abnormality of some metabolic or homeostatic system, and we can describe the qualities of the proteins that compose the system. Now, if that is so, why may we not define Disease as a consequence of incongruence of a metabolic or homeostatic system with conditions of life? And since all such systems are composed of proteins capable of reflecting the variations of their genetic origins, is it not appropriate to agree with Vogel and Motulsky who, in the 3rd edition of their book, *Human Genetics*, proclaimed genetics as the principal "basic science for medicine" (Vogel and Motulsky, 1998)?

If genetics is the basic science for medicine it should be possible to construct a set of principles that characterize disease in a genetic context. That is, a set of generalizations shared by all diseases and framed in genetic terms. And there should be hierarchies of principles, inclusive and of increasing generality and forming a matrix embracing them all. What follows is one such matrix.

The principles of disease

A foundation for developing principles of disease exists in the ideas of Ernst Mayr (Mayr, 1961). Mayr perceives biology as divided into two areas differing in concept and method. One, functional biology, is concerned with the operation and interaction of molecules, systems and organisms. Causes are proximate, the viewpoint is inward and questions are commonly preceded by how; how does the organism function? The other biology, Mayr calls evolutionary. It is concerned with the history of functional biology, its causes are called ultimate, and its questions are prefaced by why; why in the sense of, what is the history of organisms, what are the conditions of the past that have made it possible to ask for answers to the how questions. The two biologies meet, or overlap, at the level of the DNA, so that the functional deals with everything after transcription, while the evolutionary centers on the history of the DNA as well as, presumably, with the evolution of the conditions of the environment within which organisms have attained their present state.

Mayr did not include disease in his description of the two biologies, but disease is no less biological than the ideal state, so there should be no difficulty in applying his principles to biological abnormality. So in relation to disease, the proximate causes are a) the products of the variant genes, and b) the experiences of the environment with which they are incongruent. Ultimate, or remote causes are a) the mechanisms of mutation and the causes of fluctuations through time of the elements of the gene pool, including selection, mating systems, founder effects and drift, and b) the means whereby cultures and social organization evolve. In disease, the variant gene products and the experiences of the environment with which they are incongruent, account for characteristic signs and symptoms, but in making available the particular proximate causes assembled by chance in particular patients, it is the remote causes that impart the stamp of individuality to the case.

So the model relates disease to causes, to the gene pool and ultimately to biological evolution as well as to the evolution of cultures, and to individuality, the latter a consequence of the specificities of both causes. And there are here elements for constructing a *context* of principles of disease, always remembering that the word context derives from the Latin word *contexere*, meaning to weave. That is, the principles must be seen to be related and interdependent so as to form a network of ideas within which to compose one's thoughts about each specific example of each disease.

There is a further feature of Mayr's views on biology, also crucial in its application to disease (Mayr 1982). It is the state of mind in which to observe patients. In medicine we tend to think of patients in relation to their disease; that is, as a class of people characterized by the name of the disease. This is what Mayr calls topological thinking. Although patients do differ somewhat one from another, they all share an essence: the disease. In contrast, Mayr proposes population thinking, in recognition that populations consist not of types but of unique individuals. So, in this context, disease has no essence, its variety is imparted by that of the unique individuals who experience it, each in their own private version, and the name of the disease is a convenience, an acknowledgment of the necessity to group patients for logistical purposes. The reader will surely agree that the fruits of the Human Genome Project (HGP) can be accommodated only in such a populational vein.

Why do we need such principles? Physicians are pragmatic; their way is determined by what they see before them, and students and especially residents, are intolerant of anything they can label "philosophical." But the principles are there, explaining the qualities and behaviors of diseases and they await exposition.

But haven't we already discovered them? Medicine is at a peak of success in diagnosis and treatment and moving rapidly to ever new heights of achievement. But all of the

changes may not be equally evident. For example, the analysis of pathogenesis, traditionally a top-down process, is beginning to give way to a bottom-up approach in which discovery of variant genes leads to variant protein products and thence to the same molecular analysis of pathogenesis. And the genetic heterogeneity and individuality of disease are not easily accommodated in traditional thinking. So we are changing how we look at disease, how we define it and classify it, and the language we use in describing it. For example, genomics and proteomics are new words that embody new ways (Lander, 1996; Lander and Weinberg, 2000; Burley et al, 1999). And these developments are changing our relationships to biology and to society. Biologists are expressing interest in the fates of the molecules they discover and the public is becoming aware of what molecular biology and genetics mean to them, as risk factors, for example (Andrews et al, 1994; Motulsky, 1999). So, since this same molecular genetics gives us new insights into the principles that govern – and have always governed – disease, should we not articulate those principles and weave them into our thinking?

Reasons for doing so lie in the need for coherence in medicine; coherence in the face of reductionist dispersion, coherence in bringing new developments to the whole of the medical enterprise and to the public, and coherence in medical education and the thinking that goes into it. No one can possibly know all the information there is, but we all need a context that can supply both a substrate upon which to apply the new, and a receptacle within which to encompass our own field. The principles of disease bear a relationship to those of diseases that resembles the relationship of military strategy to tactics, or of historiography to the practice of history, or of grammar to precision in learning and speaking a language. Once such principles have sunk into the unconscious, they remain there as a context and a basis from which the conscious thinking about the subject takes off. They are no longer "philosophy" but the basis for daily thought.

Defining disease

If we are to define disease it must be as loss of adaptation; the open system has had difficulty in maintaining homeostasis. So our question is, how is this failure of adaptation attained. The straightforward answer is to say that a variation in a homeostatic system was incongruent with its environment, whether within the cell or outside, and the mechanisms for compensation were inadequate, momentarily or permanently, to restore congruence. As a result, other systems were affected, and then still others. But this only tells us that the machine broke down. If we would define disease, we must know what variations can lead to what levels of incongruence. We must know the weaknesses in the evolution of organisms, or if not weaknesses, degrees of flexibility. That is, the origins of human disease lie in both human evolution and in that of the environment with which the human species has evolved to be congruent. And since both biological and cultural evolution are continuous, though at markedly different rates, congruence must be relative and changing.

Such questions have always been germane to the definition of disease, however infrequently posed, but they assume a new relevance now because of the frequent assertion that one need only know the molecular form of the incongruence to devise an appropriate treatment. That is, all of our problems could be solved at the molecular level. If this were true, we do not need to define disease except molecularly, and that is the vision we pursue. But before committing wholly to such a concept it is as well to probe further into the question, what is disease?

It may seem odd to ask such a question; surely it has been answered again and again. And so it has, and many times, but always within the descriptive limits of the period. Descriptions and definitions of disease have in history proceeded from the top down and from outside in. That is from a history of the illness only, to history plus inspection, then on to physical examination in life and at autopsy, to increasingly intimate inspections by radiological and newer visual means, as well as biochemical examination, and now molecular analysis. And now that we can proceed from the bottom up, beginning with genes identified by genomics to their protein products and to the homeostatic systems into which they are integrated, the definition of disease should be reconsidered.

History reveals two opposing definitions. One, called essentialist, proposes that diseases exist somehow and in some way as entities that attack their victims. The other, called nominalist, is represented as a change within, an altered state, or a deviation, in response to some stimulus. In the essentialist view the patient was healthy and was brought low by the disease, whereas in the nominalist, the disease is an expression of the particularity of the individual response to a stimulus. This modern-sounding construction was popular in the nineteenth century in the form of "diathesis", in which there was suggested some element of heredity as well as individual vulnerability (Scriver, 1989; Rosenberg, 1995). It was swept aside by the essentialist version, which emerged, in the latter part of the nineteenth and early twentieth centuries when microorganisms were discovered. Then the nominalist began to regain favor as, first biochemistry, then genetics, then molecular biology, flourished. Today,

although we still experience microbial scourges, the nominalist view prevails, perhaps because we can so easily see that the responses to diseases, even to microbial assaults, are a product of the individuality of the systems of homeostasis, and because we are more perceptive of the interrelationships of proximate and remote causes. But there is a lingering residuum of essentialism in molecular diagnosis, so often proclaimed to be a preliminary to some "designer" treatment, usually to be concocted by pharmaceutical companies who have made the word pharmacogenetics their own. Such a diagnosis in unobjectionable as far as it goes but it has implications. That is, it is an essentialist view insofar as: a) it emphasizes the disease without differentiating the patient, b) it includes only proximate causes; the gene and its product are perceived as no less essentialist than the microbe that attacks, and c) it is typological. Even though allelic heterogeneity may be acknowledged, the variation is around the expressions of the "classical case". There is no recognition that each patient will respond to the effects of the products of each gene individually, to say nothing of each designer drug. For many years the monogenic diseases were regarded in an essentialist, typological vein, but we have become more nominalist, more prone to population thinking and more ready to recognize the significant effects of variability of both the genetic and the environmental settings in which the principal gene effect is measured (Scriver, 1999). So, in defining disease we must take into account not just the gene that seems most relevant to the phenotype – after which the phenotype may be neglected in the interest of molecular treatment – but also keep alive the relationships of genes (or better, of their products) and phenotypes, the better to grasp the individuality of each, so as to tailor the particularity of the molecular treatment to the biological individuality of a very particular patient. Then, having that principle in mind, the necessity to group patients for treatment can be managed rationally.

So, in the end, how shall we define disease? The elements of Mayr's model must be satisfied. That is, the definition must include remote causes as well as proximate, and the relationship of both to the DNA. And it must be populational in concept, rather than typological, which is to say, it must be nominalist. So, one way of expressing it is: disease is a consequence of incongruence between genetically variable homeostatic systems and the kinds, intensities and durations of exposures to elements of the environments to which they are called upon to adapt.

No doubt objections will be raised. Is cyanide poisoning a disease? No human variation is needed. Nor is there variation in susceptibility to scurvy, although it is unquestionably a disease. But although cyanide will extinguish all life, scurvy is a disease of species; only we and the guinea pig among mammals are vulnerable. Still, it is fair to say that human homeostasis is uniformly incongruent with the presence of cyanide and the absence of ascorbic acid and so both quality for this definition. Others see poisoning and trauma as something other than disease and call them by other names – accidents for one. But again the human constitution is incongruent with bullets and car crashes and so is vulnerable. How about infections? We have genetically determined mechanisms, both well developed and efficient in coping with microbial invaders. Here the variability includes individual vulnerability in the many immunodeficiencies, as well as individual invulnerability, both relative and absolute, in individuals who are proof against infections with many organisms including one malaria parasite, the tubercle bacillus and the polio virus (Hill, 1999).

And if there are those that are proof against, who can doubt that there are individualities susceptible to particular organisms? In general microorganisms attack at cellular sites we define as strengths but which they have defined for their purposes as our weaknesses; for example, cell surface molecules designed for high efficiency as elements of metabolism, but which the organisms have adapted themselves to use as means of access. The point is that it is usually variation in the microbial, rather than the human, cell that brings particularity to the encounter, although there may be both. So, since variation in either human victim and microbial attacker or both, determine the nature of the encounter, infections fulfill the nominalist definition, even while, as entities, they are compatible with, were even the prototype of, the essentialist definition. Which suggests that both definitions are of historical interest only, suitable for levels of description of disease we have left behind. But they are still of value in showing how the more intimate we become with the human body, organ, and molecule, the more our concepts change, the more we need to shed old ideas and their locutions and adapt to what the new is telling us. But still we should observe that much of what is new was foreshadowed in the old. A leisurely reading of the chapter, "The inborn factors in infective diseases", in Archibald Garrod's book, *Inborn Factors in Disease*, published in 1931, underlines the validity of that observation (Scriver and Childs, 1989).

The how questions

In the Mayr model it is by way of the DNA that remote causes leave their imprint on the proximate, and it is the protein gene products that are the effectors of both. Once

we spoke of gene–environment interactions, but now we know that the actual contact between these sources of variation is by way of those proteins. Indeed, one way of perceiving the DNA is as a molecule that is helpless without proteins that carry out all its ends, including transcription and translation too (Fox-Keller, 1995). So the proteins carry on the life of the cell as elements in integrated systems, responding to influences from adjacent cells, distant organs and the outside, to maintain the open system in its uncertain relationships in life. They are, therefore, *unit steps of homeostasis*, and as such are pivotal in concepts of life, development, aging, health and disease.

Such a list of attainments is banal without explanation and illustration. In the following section are several ways in which the unit steps of homeostasis fulfill the purposes of the cell. They are called unit steps to convey their elemental state as units of pathways, and cascades, structural elements, protein machines, transducers in signaling systems, and transporters or receptors of molecules that are going somewhere. The phrase further implies units of integration into systems intended to maintain the organism's steady state; they are the node between nature and nurture and the phrase has the virtue of being indifferent to whether or not the specific protein fulfills a useful purpose or is disruptive. And finally, the unit steps have an important historical meaning, representing the central idea of Garrod's inborn error, Beadle and Tatum's one gene–one peptide, and Pauling's molecular disease (Garrod, 1902; Beadle, 1956; Pauling, 1949).

SOME QUALITIES OF THE UNIT STEP OF HOMEOSTASIS

As a unit of history

Clearly the DNA is an instrument of memory, a memory that in preserving the past, gives guidance for the future. That is, the future must always reflect the past, and the means whereby this Janus vision is attained is the protein gene product which repeats its phylogenetic history in its present composition and function, and predicts its future in its reincarnation through subsequent generations as itself or in the form of variants. Some of the variants have no future and their incongruence is noted by natural selection. Others are contingent, favorable for some conditions, inappropriate for others. And then there are those proteins, that are hardly changed from microbial ancestry and which represent core functions. In human society, political and religious systems have similar capacities for endurance, revealing fundamental, unchanged dogma associated with adaptation in ways that promote the cause with little change in the fundamentals. So the proteins that constitute our proteomes descend to us not only from our parents and other human antecedents, but, with variable conservation, from both the ancient and recent past.

As effectors of gene intention

We often speak of a gene or genes as being "for" something, by which we indicate some sort of direct relationship to a phenotype. That is, we seem to be saying that the gene's influence is determining. And so it is, if by determining we mean the sequences of bases in mRNA and of amino acids in a protein product. In this sense the gene is indeed "for" something. But each gene product has in addition, an emergent career of its own, not predicted at all, or only indirectly, by its gene. It assumes a position in the homeostatic device to which it belongs, and can now be said to be "for" that system, as the factor VIII gene is "for" both the factor VIII protein and "for" clotting. But it is far from determining of clotting; all the other elements are needed too, or, as we all well know, life-threatening bleeding occurs. And we know that in physiology, system is integrated with system in hierarchical relationships, so that the farther away from the steps of translation and first integration, the more dilute the gene's determining power becomes. No doubt the genes are involved wherever their products are to be found, but indirectly, and any one may have little power to shape the ultimate phenotype. In another sense the genes appear to be hardly involved at all beyond transcription because it is the quality of the protein product that determines its role in the economy of the cell, a role that is determined by how the protein folds and takes shape, a shape that must accommodate to the shapes of the products of other genes and they with still others. No doubt the protein's folding and shape reflect the information residing in its parent gene, but its gene has no control over the shapes of those other proteins with which it fits, to say nothing of how multiprotein machines work (Alberts, 1998). Here is a question not of genes but of how proteins interact. It is a matter of physiology. Indeed it is possible that as the fruits of the HGP and the proteomists filter into medicine we will hear a good deal less about genes and more about proteins (Gelbert, 1998). This could be less than ideal were the proteins not perceived to be as closely identified with the concept of variation as the genes. Let us see to it that they are.

As a unit of development

T.H. Morgan adopted drosophila as an organism suitable for the study of development (Kohler, 1994). But it didn't work out that way and his students led the way to the operational definition of the gene. So it is ironic that modern technology has made the fruit fly ideal for the very study that defied Morgan's efforts (Capecchi, 1997; Kornberg and Krosnaw, 2000).

In development the genes fulfill their intentions in the ways just described. Their products are the units of developmental change, assuming positions in systems appropriate for their conformation so as to give each organism a matrix, embodying a trajectory of change that is a product of how the embryo, fetus and baby meet and respond to experiences of intra-uterine and external environments. That is, development is a historical process; what the organism is today is built upon what it was yesterday and leads to what it will be tomorrow (Stent, 1981). And since the genes see to the continuity of their products throughout the changes of a lifetime, it is hardly likely that the influences of the past, however distant, would fail to influence the present. So if we would understand the origins and expressions of disease, it must be in the context of three time scales, all at once; that of phylogeny, that of development maturation and aging and that of the present (Waddington, 1957). To know what we begin with is to know potential incongruence, to know where development is taking, or has taken, us is to clothe the potential with the probable, one way or the other, and to know where we are at the moment is to know the strengths and weaknesses with which we face tomorrow. There is an increasing interest in the idea that some diseases of middle life have precursors, manifestations dating to early, even intrauterine, life. These expressions may not appear to relate to the disease they are said to characterize. Rather they may represent subtle changes in trajectories which, if pursued, emerge finally as disease (Marmot, 1997). How else could birth weight be related to Type II diabetes or heart attack?

As a unit of individuality

In medicine patients are seen one at a time. Each one is biologically unique, has different experiences and tells a different story. These expressions, together with the help of the laboratory and observations over time, are compared with those of the classical case to reach a diagnosis, and, allowing something for variation, treatment or management is devised. This thinking is typological, individuality is usually ignored and the doctor is in thrall to nosology. The method works well enough, but heterogeneity of proximate cause may be overlooked, and patients are likely to be aware when they are being perceived as representative of a class rather than as their unique selves. Now, molecular biology has given us the wherewithal to observe molecular individuality, that is, the capacity to make comparisons between individuals of variations in base pairs in the DNA and differences in amino acid sequences in proteins. The unit of individuality is the unit step of homeostasis and the expression of uniqueness lies in how the variant proteins affect each its own system, and the integrations of the latter with others, as well as how the systems respond to non-genetic proximate causes. Genomic analysis of single nucleotide polymorphisms (SNPs) suggests that the number of polymorphic loci expressed in amino acid substitution in proteins will turn out to be somewhat greater than the 30% we are accustomed to (Cargillet et al, 1999; Halushka et al, 1999). This is the substrate of variability within which additional "private" variants as well as clearly bad mutants express their effects, and all of this variation is made manifest in how the integrated homeostatic devices are fulfilling their duties. So, if each human being is unique by virtue of the variant proteins in his/her whole physiological apparatus, why should not each such human being express an experience with disease as variously as a career of health.

Variation contributed by variant proteins is far from all. Such variability is compounded by the individuality of the developmental and maturational trajectory characteristic of each person, a path determined no less strongly by the kinds, intensities and durations of experiences than by the protein gene products with which they interact. But the final arbiter of individuality is the remote causes, which determine the specificity of both genes and experiences. The variation in the parental gene pool is a sample of what is available to the species but it is necessarily limited, characterized by ethnicity and made local by founder effect, migration and mating customs. These are all influences that determine the particularity of an individual's genetic endowment. But if genetic individuality is both determined and constrained by the genetic raw material inherited at conception, so is the variety of experiences made possible and limited by the mores of the social and cultural milieux, itself often inherited, which shape our likes and dislikes, our indulgences and restraints, in short, the qualities and quantities of the experiences we encounter. So, in the end, it is the remote causes that confer the specificity of individuality, but the unit steps of homeostasis that supply the substrate. Of course the idea of variant proteins as units of individuality is not a new one, having been proposed by Archibald Garrod as "chemical individuality", as early as 1902 (Garrod, 1902).

The unit steps as effectors of disease

If the gene product is the implement of homeostasis, it follows that it is the effector of disease; certain of its variants are in some degree incongruent with the environment, inside the cell or out. That is, wherever the origins and mechanisms of pathogenesis have been laid bare, there are proteins at the root if it. How could it be otherwise, given that both structures and motivators of the functions of cells are proteins, and disease is a consequence of homeostatic incongruence. A critic might suggest infections as exceptions, but it is the congruence of the microorganism's structures with our unit steps of homeostasis that allows them to attach themselves to cell surfaces and then to release toxin or to gain access to the cell's interior and there to reproduce. It is they who define our strengths as weaknesses, our congruence as incongruence. And they do so by using the human gene products, the human unit steps of homeostasis.

The history of the realization of this role of the unit step in disease is of interest; it paralleled the successive descriptions and definitions of both genes and proteins (Childs, 1999b). We all know that Archibald Garrod was the first to call attention to alcaptonuria as a hereditary alternative form of metabolism due to failure of an enzymatically catalyzed step (Garrod, 1902). He called this, and other such metabolic aberrations, inborn errors to distinguish them from diseases. This was an insight of extraordinary penetration in which he recognized that the differences in protein composition that distinguished species must also differentiate individuals within species (Bearn, 1993). But even by 1909 when his first book, *Inborn Errors of Metabolism*, was published he could go no farther (Scriver 1989; Bearn, 1993). Little was known about protein structure, and nothing of sequence of amino acids, and it was not even established yet, to everyone's satisfaction, that enzymes were proteins (Fruton, 1972).

As for the gene in 1909, it was still defined statistically, and although phenotype and genotype were differentiated in that year, the gene was an unknown entity, perceived by Johannsen as, "an accounting or calculating unit". But by 1915 the gene had been defined operationally, so by then Garrod could have proposed the inborn errors as products of mutants of single genes. But he never did. Even in his 1931 book, *Inborn Factors in Disease*, he did not use the word gene despite a general recognition that genes were involved somehow in some diseases (Scriver and Childs, 1989; Bearn, 1993). For example, in 1927 Barker reported that, "No less than 223 heritable anomalies have been described in man already" (Barker, 1927). And others, not in medicine, recognized a biochemical relationship between genes and phenotypes: Wright in coat colors of guinea pigs and Wheldale in flower pigments (Wright, 1917; Scott-Moncrieff, 1981). Then in the late thirties and early forties the studies of Ephrussi, Beadle and Tatum, first in

Drosophila, then in *Neurospora*, provided a functional definition of the gene that brought gene and protein unequivocally together to clarify Garrod's observations, and capitalizing on rapid advances in biochemistry, to begin in the fifties an era of biochemical genetics (Beadle, 1956). Biochemical genetics was an ecumenical enterprise. If Garrod was its icon and Harry Harris its chief expositor, there were also contributions of non-geneticists, including Pauling's concept of molecular disease and the elaboration of the enzyme deficiencies in (Type I) glycogen storage disease, galactosemia and other disorders, all classical inborn errors, described by biochemists with no primary interest in genetics and who made no reference to Garrod or to Beadle-Tatum (Pauling et al, 1949; Cori and Cori, 1952; Isselbacher et al, 1956). But whatever the influence, the list of inborn errors expanded rapidly, soon attaining an exponential rate of increase that has never slackened.

It is worth noting that biochemical genetics flourished before the impact of the discovery of the double helix could be felt. But the latter developments led first to Yanofsky's definition of the structural gene with its correspondence to sequences in amino acids in proteins (Yanofsky, 1965) and later to the definition of the gene that includes both transcribed and nontranscribed DNA. And this led, in turn, to the development of genomics as an analytical method. Thus biochemical genetics whose analysis proceeds from the phenotype to the protein and its gene, met genomics whose analysis proceeds from the gene toward the phenotype by way of its protein product (Lander and Schork, 1994). And in time, the glamor passed from biochemical genetics to genomics, perhaps principally because the former had no way to tackle the genetics of complex disorders. Actually both are needed since phenotypes are not necessarily explained upon discovery of the gene or genes whose products are acting as proximate causes.

As the focal point in pathogenesis, the protein gene product provides an economical answer to the question of the origins of monogenic diseases. But the question of the moment is how to explain those called complex. The approach includes genomics, by which salient genes can be found and characterized (Lander and Weinberg, 2000). Further steps involve discovery of their proteins and the homeostatic devices to which they belong, after which the pathophysiology may be elucidated. Additional participation by genetically inclined thinkers lies in sorting out the heterogeneity by means of appropriate family studies, work that must be done before, or together with, efforts to tie treatments to the consequences of particular protein variants.

Today we scoff at such diagnostic "entities" as dropsy and consumption, having begun long since to resolve their heterogeneity. But the HGP will provide the means to show how much more we have to go to characterize distinctive versions of, say, heart attack and stroke. So numerous are the genetic contributors likely to be that a case might be made for everyone having his/her own version of heart attack, stroke, or other multigenic, multifactorial disorder. So family studies are vital for deciding which genes play important roles in which versions of the disease. The results will resemble those in the study of monogenic disorders; the heterogeneity will be of both loci and alleles, and the sets thereof will vary from family to family and individual to individual (Scriver, 1999). This kind of genetic thinking, not yet routine in medicine, is crucial to our understanding and represents an important principle of disease.

The protein product as a unit of selection

Neodarwinism is the outcome of a debate in which geneticists agreed that the object of selection must be phenotype, not genes, while evolutionary biologists, to whom the phenotype had been that object all along, agreed that both phenotypes, and their variation, originated in the genes (Mayr and Provine, 1980). If so, while the phenotype remains the unit of selection, it is the variable unit step or steps that cause it to qualify for that fate. In medicine we are not much concerned with the selection by which species attain their characteristics, but with what evolutionary biologists call "purifying" selection, that which removes "undesirable" genes prior to reproduction. So here again the protein product of the gene occupies a central position between two aspects of human biology. And here is yet another example of the cleavage between biology and medicine. The irony in the word purifying is not lost on the physician to whom the protection of life is uppermost, while to biology, with no stake in the individual, the question is purely one of understanding the rise and decline of species. But, in fact, variations in unit steps of homeostasis are no less the stuff of positive selection than negative.

As a hedge against genetic determinism

Institutions change and renew themselves but always they retain residual signs of their origins. No one would deny that all of the genetics of today stems from the concepts elaborated in the fly room at Columbia, or that we continue to use both concepts and language appropriate to the drosophilists' definition of the gene (Fox-Keller, 1995). Theirs was an operational definition in which authority for both heredity and cellular function was accorded to the gene. In his book, *What is Life*, Schroedinger spoke of the gene as, "law code and executive power" as well as "architect's plan and builder's craft in one" (Schroedinger, 1967). So the language of drosophila genetics included such locutions as: genes "for," gene-environment interaction, modifiers, penetrance and pleiotropy, all of which are perceived as properties of the gene, although we know now that they refer to events mediated by the protein unit steps of homeostasis. There is no question of the latter's specification by the genes, but in folding and assuming an appropriate position in a relevant homeostatic device, they become a part of mechanisms that regulate both themselves and the DNA. Thus it is not the genes that are penetrant, pleiotropic, or that interact with the environment, it is the proteins that do these actions that are removed from the genes' control.

It might be correct to speak of a "gene for", say an enzyme, or even for its pathway; for example, there is a "gene for" phenylalanine hydroxylase and "for" phenylalanine degradation. But in their further integration, proteins lose their identity in those of integrated functions, for which any single gene can no longer be perceived to have any authority.

There is another way in which the locution "gene for" is used. When we observe that a disease segregates, we say there is a "gene for" that disease, that one or more mutants act as proximate cause. That is exactly what the drosophilists did for their mutants, unconcerned with their ignorance of how a gene could shorten bristles or deform wings. We continue to use their discourse, even though we know that the protein product is the actual agent of function (Fox-Keller, 1995). But "genes for" is a tricky phrase. When we use it unthinkingly, as in genes for high blood pressure, say, we obscure our own inner view of the reality, whereas when we speak of variant proteins, there spring immediately to mind, pathways, cascades, receptors, transducers and feedback loops. There comes to mind as a further example, the article that appeared in the 1999 volume of the *Annual Review of Biochemistry* in which no less than 61 proteins were cited, all engaged in all sorts of ways in the maintenance of blood pressure (Garbers and Dubois, 1999). Incidentally, it is amusing to imagine that had Archibald Garrod come to alcaptonuria thinking like a geneticist of the time, he would probably have perceived it only as a recessive character, not an inborn error. But he came to it as a biochemist and saw it for what it was: a metabolic alternative due to the absence of an enzyme. He used the genetic evidence expressed in consanguinity to support the idea of heredity, not as evidence of a gene. So, rather than to perceive his lack of interest in genetics as a shortcoming, we should be glad of it because the idea of a "gene for" alkaptonuria could have stood in the way of his biochemical insights. But equally, had he pondered the work of the drosophilists emerging in print

from 1905 to 1920, and which included their operational definition of the gene, the second edition of his *Inborn Errors of Metabolism* published in 1926 must surely have anticipated the Beadle–Tatum one gene–one enzyme principle (Garrod, 1926).

So, if we human geneticists of today revert occasionally to the drosophiline mentality how likely are patients, their families and the public to escape? How are they to know that the words "gene for", say I.Q., artistic ability or criminal behavior, obscure the unfathomable complexity of the identity and actions of gene products integrated in hierarchies to compose cells, organs, and whole organisms, all in touch with one another and with the outside. The extremes to which "genes for" can go are summarized in a book called *The DNA Mystique: The Gene as a Cultural Icon* by Nelkin and Lindee (Nelkin and Linder, 1995). But fortunately we have our mental image of the products of the genes, the unit steps of homeostasis, with their multifarious behaviors as a bulwark against loose thinking.

As the goal of HGP

One road to the discovery of new principles of disease is the Human Genome Project (Collins, 1999). Lander has suggested that this bears the same relationship to biology as the Periodic Table bears to Chemistry (Lander and Weinberg, 2000). So it compels our attention. Further, it is the ultimate identifier of those homeostatic units that lie at the basis of pathogenesis.

Tens of thousands of genes and their products will be identified, and sooner or later, the products' roles in homeostasis will follow, with obvious benefits for investigation of pathogenesis, treatment and prevention. In addition, definitive samples of gene products, useful in defining disease, will be available for characterizing human biological properties hitherto unknown. A few examples of questions that will be asked, follow:

a) How variable is the human genome? Is it more, or less, than the estimates of Harris and Lewontin? Studies of SNPs suggest more (Cargill et al, 1999; Halushka et al, 1999). Nothing could be more useful than this answer since it is the common genes that so often act as modifiers and furnish the wherewithal for complex diseases. A roster of variant polymorphisms with their associations to disease, if any, would be immensely useful.

b) Is there an inborn error for every locus? And are all classes of proteins equally involved in diseases? In a comparison between 348 mutant proteins associated with inborn errors listed in *MMBID*, 7th edition, and a list of

3000 "core" proteins shared by yeast and *Caenorhabditis elegans*, the distribution of protein types in the two samples was remarkably similar (Jiminez-Sanchez et al, 2000). Although indirect, the suggestion is there that all protein types are involved in inborn errors, but we cannot yet say that there is an inborn error for every locus, however plausible the idea may be.

c) Are diseases characterized by the qualities of the proteins that are their proximate causes? For example, do enzyme deficiencies differ in some systematic way from disorders associated with receptors, transcription factors or structural proteins?

d) Are conserved genes over- or under-represented in disease? One might expect them to be over-represented on the assumption that they fulfill critical functions, or under-represented because their mutants might be so often lethal.

e) What is the role, if any, of developmental constraints in fostering or suppressing disease? These are limitations on the evolution of phenotypic variation expressed in developmental blind alleys. Kirschner and Gerhart have examined ways such constraints are loosened to allow new mutation and evolutionary progress. But would some of the latter be disease (Kirschner and Gerhart, 1998)? And Rutherford showed how, in drosophila, such constraint was exerted by a heat shock protein (Rutherford and Lindquist, 1998). When altered by mutation, the constraining force was lifted, and the effects of mutants suppressed by the wild type protein were observed. Some of these effects were developmental anomalies.

f) Are diseases characterized by the evolutionary age of the proteins that lie at their root? That is, we might suppose that inborn errors of housekeeping genes shared by remotely related species were the oldest. Do they differ in any particular from diseases of the most recent mammalian or human genes?

g) What are the implications for aging? Are some proteins more frequently the object of aging processes; or is it random? A recent paper in Science reported an increasing rate, with age, of errors in the mitotic machinery that led to multiple abnormalities of regulation of dozens of enzymes (Ly et al, 2000). So, will aging, which has been perceived by some as dishomeostasis, turn out to have the same molecular basis as disease?

Many other questions will be asked, many no doubt not now askable because the contexts in which they are relevant are unknown. The HGP will also change other aspects of our thinking. As more and more diseases are given molecu-

lar definition we will surely classify them differently, departing from the present anatomical, organ system, age-related rubrics, moving to more molecular designations. As heterogeneity is laid bare, old classes will go and new ones will come, reflecting a sharp revision in how we will see disease itself. In addition, our language will change. It is likely that we will refer less to genes and more to proteins so our residual drosophiline language is likely to go too. Of what use are words like modifier, epistasis, penetrance, pleiotropy and the like when visualizing the reality as actions and interactions of proteins, in, say, multiunit machines, or even in whole systems (Lander and Weinberg, 2000)? Which suggests also that we in medicine will be thinking less in units and more in multi-unit devices. Linear thinking may be out as complexity moves in. But maybe the most significant change in our thinking will be compelled by the definitive evidence of human variation and individuality. Typological thinking will give way to population thinking. No doubt there will always be use for the former at one level; that of the value of means and the classical case, but only as a preliminary to the population thinking that perceives the extent and impact of variation on human individuality.

Social impact

The unit step of homeostasis is attaining increasing prominence as a risk factor and signal for preventive action, and medicine has been adapting not only to their potential use, but to their impact on their possessors' lives. These concerns are well known to readers of *PPMG*; they have been the subject of many papers, books and committee reports and they touch on counseling, ethics, legal matters, and psychological impact (Anon, 1975; Holtzman, 1989; Holtzman and Watson, 1998; Andrews et al, 1994; Motulsky, 1999). They are mentioned here because of the potential uses of such risk factors in prevention. If the HGP fulfills its promise, there is the possibility to know the protein products of all genes known to participate in pathogenesis. Many scenarios as to the use of these markers have been offered. Only time will tell which, if any, is practical but we would be wise to continue our study and preparation. How to use information, available at birth, about many variant genes, perhaps dozens in single individuals, and known to be associated with diseases all across the life span, is something entirely new in medicine. Is it consonant with good medicine? Is it acceptable to the public? How do we prepare the public to make rational decisions about it? How do we prepare individuals to accept and use constructively, such emotionally loaded information? These questions can be answered only in colloquy with the public.

As a source of coherence

In concentrating on the specificities of the pathogenesis of each disease, reductionist investigation emphasizes the separateness of diseases. It exerts a centrifugal effect that adds to that of our conventional nosology, which divides medicine into specialties across which we interact collaboratively, when at all. But the concept of the unit step of homeostasis as the central focus of all pathogenesis provides a principle of disease that exerts a contrary, centripetal force that unifies the thinking about both disease and diseases. It is the difference between analysis and synthesis. Medical thinking, until recently, was in the main synthetic. It dealt with the body as a whole, no doubt because of ignorance of its parts. In contrast, in the thinking of today, the emphasis is on analysis; our attention is directed more to micro unitary parts, with less attention to the whole. But in acting as units of the mechanisms whereby an open system maintains its adaptation to an indifferent environment, the protein gene product is the effective link between those proximate and remote causes portrayed in the Mayr model. And that link is no less evident when unit step and environment are incongruent than when congruent. In the Mayr model the proximate causes are consequent upon the DNA and pose questions prefaced by how while the remote causes lead up to the DNA and pose questions prefaced by why. In this summary of the role of the protein gene product we have dealt with how questions. In the next section we examine the why questions and the principles they illustrate.

The why questions

Just as the questions preceded by how are answered by reference to proximate causes, so are the why questions answered by reference to remote causes. And the answers to the why questions contribute no less to the specificity of identity than the proximate. Indeed, they are the enablers, the ultimate arbiters of that specificity. So we are what we are by virtue of endowment, experience, development, maturation and aging, but the bounds of what we can be and the precise description of what we are, are determined by how the remote causes came to be what they are and how they were sampled in the making of the individual. So the answers to the why questions are likely to probe more widely and deeply than those preceeded by how. In fact they begin with the latter to give them specificity. And yet we spend most of our energies and money on seeking prox-

imate causes. The imperatives of treatment and prevention require it, yet it should be observed that it is the why questions that are most often asked by the public, particularly by those affected by disease. Medical education would do well to include them.

Why do we have disease?

Why is it that after all these eons of evolution, species have not evolved to perfect attunement with the environment? First, it must be said that we *are* remarkably well adapted. Increasing longevity suggests that in the developed world we are moving toward the ideal rectangular survival curve (Fries and Crapo, 1981). That is, we are moving in the direction, at least, of some probably unattainable minimal amount of disease compatible with some necessary degree of genetic diversity. In addition, the environment changes requiring new adaptation, and then observation suggests that nature never reaches for perfection but for some compromise that ensures perpetuation of species usually at the expense of individuals. For example, the fecundity of our own species is presumed to be of the order of only 25%, and not all of that makes it to maturity (Jacobs, 1990). But that a principal hazard to the global ecology is a surplus of human beings, is testimony to nature's way of doing business.

Since evolution proceeds by the intervention of natural selection, there must be something to select, and again, although there are mechanisms of astonishing precision to ensure the accuracy of replication of the DNA, they are not perfect either, and so, after the removal of individuals unlikely ever to survive or reproduce, we are still left with sufficient variation among individuals to adapt to the randomness of change in the environment. This includes genes that are either neutral under all conditions, or contingent; that is, adaptive under some conditions, but nonadaptive and conducive to incongruence and disease under others. So disease must be presumed to be a by-product of the necessity to have enough variability for all conditions.

Why this disease?

Patients often ask this question. Why, they ask, should I have diabetes or cancer, or why should my baby have this bizarre disease I've never even heard of? The media have spread the news of genetics so their question may be, "Is it in my genes, and if so where in the world did such genes come from?" So the questions are directed to both proximate and remote causes. First to the proximate which include the genetic endowment received by the patient at conception and which, together with the kinds, duration and intensities of experiences of the environment, created a developmental and maturational matrix that is an expression of individual potential from day to day. Then, the parental contribution to this matrix reflects the specificity of their genes, themselves representative of one or more gene pools, each with its own variable composition and history. The contributions of experiences are representative of qualities of the society the patient inhabits, qualities that vary with cultural history. And finally, the contribution of development and maturation, is that of a trajectory whose specificity is derived from both endowment and experiences as they create and characterize the evolving matrix within which the incongruence and disease are engendered. So the answer to the question of why this disease, requires us to acknowledge that while the disease is a consequence of incongruence between proximate causes, it was remote causes that account for the existence, availability and particularity of those proximate factors.

Why this person?

If patients are baffled by the disease they experience, they are angered by its apparent choice of themselves. "Why me?", is their injured cry. Of course the reasons reside in the origins and specificities of genes, experiences and development given in answer to the previous question, but "why me?" is a profoundly different question because, no matter how specific the genes, the experiences and the development, so long as it is only the disease itself that commands our attention, there is the possibility that we miss the full impact of the individuality of the patient, its multifariousness, its history, its uniqueness. There is always a healthy side to a sick patient with its own proximate and remote causes and its diversity. And it is in noting those qualities that some clinicians are distinguished from others to whom the particularity of the patient lies only in his or her variant molecules. In fact, it is in appealing to the particularity of the whole patient, molecules included, that the physician is able to help the patient to discover and to mobilize resources that may make the difference between a timely or a delayed recovery, or even between life and death.

Why at this time?

Perhaps the least understood by its victims is disease's apparent caprice in choosing when it strikes: the infant, blooming and full of promise, who wilts and dies, the robust, active college student who dies in one or two days of meningococcal meningitis; the busy, tireless 50 year old who is felled by cancer. No doubt in old age disease and death are less anomalous, more expected, and yet we must ask why one person is privileged to die at 90 while others have died untimely. But we know that there are reasons for ages at onset of diseases and that they are accommodated within the nominalist definition of disease. These reasons are embodied in human mortality curves which, in the developed world, are U shaped; declining sharply after birth, reaching a nadir at adolescence and beginning to rise again in young adult life. If we were to include life before birth, the post-natal decline would be seen to be the end of a steep drop through intra-uterine life.

Table 2.1 lists and contrasts qualities of the diseases experienced on the two sides of the U. How do we explain the differences? Again, appeal to remote causes gives the answers. All of the differences are those expected if the heritability of disease were to fall throughout life. The table tells us that indeed it does decline, the incidence of monogenic disease drops sharply before the nadir of the U, which suggest strong selection against disorders that imperil reproduction, leaving post-pubertal disease to be associated mainly with the kind of genetic variation that is contingent, implicated in disease only in the presence of non-genetic proximate cause, and representative of the kind of variation successful species exhibit. But, although the distribution of mortalities is U shaped, the principle of continuity is not defied; monogenic disease continues to occur even in late life, and diseases of complex origin are known in childhood, even in utero (Fig. 2.1).

Another way of perceiving in more detail the decline in prominence of the genetic impulse in disease, is to express it as a decline in a gradient of selective effect. The gradient

Table 2.1. Differences in Pre- and Postpubertal Diseases

	Prepubertal	Postpubertal
Mode of inheritance	Monogenic	Multifactorial
Age at onset	Early	Late
Frequency	Rare	Frequent
Latency	Short	Long
Affected relatives	Numerous	Few
Diagnostic specificity	High	Low
Number of diseases	Very many	Fewer
Burden	Great	Less
Sex differences	Occasional	Frequent
Influence of migration	No	Yes
Secular change	No	Yes
Effects of SES	Some	More
Success in treatment	Some	More
Heritability	High	Low
Predictability	High	Low

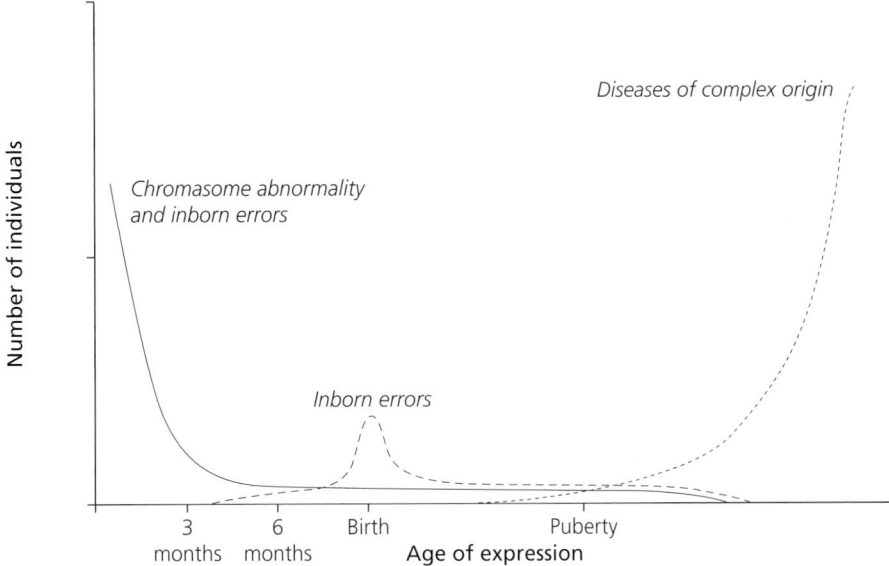

Fig. 2.1. Continuity of disease across the lifetime.

is not of genes, but of phenotypes and the weight of selection is heaviest in utero and least in old age. Burden is measured in risk to life, curtailment of reproduction and permanent disability. These are biological burdens such that loss of life in utero, even before implantation, is more burdensome than the death of a bread-winning parent at age 40 with all its social upheaval. The apparent discrepancy in these burdens is a consequence of a natural ambiguity in human life in which we have two selves, one biological, the other social. It is as if we live two lives, one in obedience to the biological imperative to survive to reproduce, the other to exploit endowment and opportunity to have a fulfilling social life. Obviously these lives are intertwined, but when in opposition, there is a schism that may lead to disease.

The gradient is at its peak in utero where for reasons we can only guess, the majority of conceptuses are found wanting and die. Because intrauterine life is protected from the outside, most of this mayhem is likely to be genetic; for example, known early losses are most frequently associated with chromosomal anomalies (Jacobs, 1990). But there must be inborn errors as well, involving among others, proteins specific to development. Then there are many known inborn errors with onset early in postnatal life and constituting a significant proportion of disease in newborns. In keeping with the biological desirability of a population of reproducers unencumbered by such mutants, 90% of single gene diseases will have been disclosed by puberty, 99% by the end of reproduction (Costa et al, 1985). As teenage passes into early adult life and that into mid-life, the residual monogenic disease consists mainly of the cases of earli-

est onset of complex diseases, the most severe, life threatening and resistant to treatment, while those with later onset, milder, more responsive to treatment are of complex origin, often irregularly familial or sporadic, a continuity commensurate with a high degree of heterogeneity of proximate cause. At the lowest end of the gradient are degrees of health expressed in resistance, completing the continuity that began with the mayhem in utero. Resistance to disease is little noticed in medicine where appeals to the doctor are only made when the patient is sick, but it is well known in infections.

In keeping with the concept of declining heritability we expect an increasing contribution of non-genetic variation. Most cancer takes its origin from mutation but it is mainly somatic and so may be counted as of environmental origin, perhaps as an aspect of aging. Aging is perceived as dishomeostasis, a product of cell loss and dysfunction due to denaturation of proteins. So while gerontologists, no doubt correctly, decline to see aging as disease, its expressions are associated with failure of the same gene products we associate with disease.

The decline in heritability is not monotonic but rises and falls according to developmental phase (Fig. 2.1) (Costa et al, 1985). For example, the genetically determined intrauterine disease has an early onset while fetal disease late in pregnancy is more likely to be of maternal origin; prematurity, placenta previa, hypertension, premature placental detachment and the like. Then there is a fresh spate of genetic disease in infancy, with deaths in childhood being more likely to be due to poisons, infections, accidents, and in some places, homicide. In adult life early onset cases of complex disorders are strongly conditioned by genetic variation, while late onset cases are likely to be non-familial (Childs and Scriver, 1986).

Reasons for this phenomenon are conjectural, but it makes sense if the effects of new sets of genes are exposed to selection at the beginning of each developmental phase. It is an observation that needs study. Another kind of continuity exhibited by the gradient of selective effect is the overlap of disorders characteristic of different developmental phases (Fig. 2.1). For example, most chromosomal anomalies are lethal in utero, but for some there is a backwash of liveborn babies. But not all malformations are due to chromosomal aberration, some are of complex origin, some are harmless and may be recognized only at autopsy or emerge only under conditions of unusual stress, as urinary tract infection in a patient with a single kidney, perhaps in adult life. Prepubertal life is characterized by monogenic disease, but Type I diabetes, asthma, inflammatory bowel disease and other disorders of complex origin sometimes have onset then too. When a disease has onset over a broad range of ages we must always wonder whether all the victims to whose disorder we give the same name, actually have the same disease. So in complex disorders the problem of naming will be with us until we are able to sort out the heterogeneity. In the end it seems likely that the number of diseases of adult life will be no less than those of the prepubertal years. No doubt genomics will identify the genes and the issue of names will be resolved.

One reason why this description of the decline in heritability, with its stops and starts and overlaps has been given prominence here is to illustrate the principle of the continuity of life, a continuity often ignored in both concept and organization. Hospitals, medical schools and medical education are arranged around age and organ system for perfectly good reasons, and the system has proved its worth. But molecular genetics provides a continuity that brings the specialities together in taking a longitudinal view of human life.

Prevention and treatment

One might suppose a priori that the Mayr model could not accommodate prevention and treatment of human disease. Biology is concerned with what is, and does not accommodate intervention; the minute one intervenes, what is, no longer is. And what could be more unnatural than government agencies that regulate how we deal with nature, or surgical transplantation of organs as a treatment, to say nothing of the idea of designer drugs for molecular defects. But we cannot escape our biological heritage, nor do we wish to, so perhaps the model is apposite after all.

All organisms are capable of adapting to, or otherwise defending themselves against, uncongenial environments. Some call upon homeostatic flexibility when under stress, others move to evade it; evolution has seen to these self-protective capabilities. For example, many organisms have molecular mechanisms to withstand stress; heat shock proteins are one (Hoffman and Parsons, 1991). Others are enzymes that detoxify foreign substances, and a third is up and down regulation of metabolic systems. Some organisms remove themselves from threats. In addition, animals that can, choose surroundings appropriate for their physiology and improve them too (Lewontin, 1983). So, in the sense that they know what experiences to avoid, animals practice prevention, and when attacked by disease or hurt in the course of the day's work, they fall back upon natural mechanisms by way of treatment. The difference between them and us is that we consciously intervene in both. But in the degree to which we seek out proximate causes intending to alter them by prevention or treatment, and in the degree to which we try consciously to influence social and cultural conditions with an eye to changing remote causes, we do fulfill the expectation of the model.

PREVENTION

Constituted separately from medicine and described as improvement in diet, housing and other living conditions, prevention has saved more lives than treatment (McKeown, 1976). And when microorganisms were identified as proximate causes, they became the target of prevention by quarantine and immunization; the latter remains a staple of medical care. These preventive measures were and are in the hands mainly of local government, while progress in fostering the ideas and promoting education in preventive medicine were and are the work of university-based schools of Public Health and Hygiene. After the fifties when antibiotics reduced the mortality of infections, other diseases like diabetes, cancer and kidney disorders came into focus. Then the ideas of preventive medicine and epidemiology which had been restricted to the control of infectious diseases in populations began to include prevention of non-infectious disease in individuals, leading to the establishment of organizations that included patients, their families and the public, and which were devoted to education and counseling of patients and relatives as well as the general public with the intention to prevent and to learn enough to treat these common disorders. The American Cancer Society, the American Diabetes Society and The March of Dimes come readily to mind. In the sixties and seventies as more and more inborn errors were described, this principle was applied also to the generation of a multitude of disease-related societies, each dedicated to education, treatment and prevention of one disease, the latter in the form of reproductive counseling, antenatal diagnosis and sometimes abortion. Then, as the molecular basis of these disorders was discovered, newborn screening for inborn errors was offered by many state health departments and intensive studies were undertaken of every aspect of this form of preventive medicine including screening, counseling and issues both ethical and legal (Bergsma, 1974; Anon, 1975; Lubs and de la Cruz, 1977; Hsia et al, 1979). The question then arose of testing relatives of patients with inborn errors, with an eye to reproductive advice, and the triumph of Tay-Sachs testing is one result (Anon, 1975; Andrews et al, 1994). And now that rapid progress is being made in unraveling the genomics and proteomics of complex disease, time will give us more risk factors in the way of variant genes and proteins. These developments are reviewed here in this detail to call attention to the movement of the focus of prevention away from populations to individuals, and now to the molecular emphasis in both prevention and treatment. Just as the discovery of genes associated with disease suggests the possibility of cure, so does it suggest prevention by testing of relatives and populations. Indeed the logic of prevention is even more powerful than that of cure. That is, unlike treatment which is always after-the-fact, and is occasionally as threatening as the disease it is designed to combat, prevention spares the organism such rigors even while far less disruptive of social and economic life. On the other hand, in keeping with the principle of continuity, the two are sometimes indistinguishable.

So, may we expect miracles of prevention now that we can identify proximate causes? Readers of *PPMG* know that we may not (Andrews et al, 1994; Holtzman, 1989; Holtzman and Watson, 1998; Motulsky, 1989). It is a matter of the continuity of the gradient of selective effect. At one end, the virtual elimination of Tay-Sachs disease among Jews and the prevention of a few other inborn errors by the same means represent successes of the high technology promoted by Lewis Thomas (Thomas, 1974). At the other end are healthy centenarians who attribute their robust health to some idiosyncratic behavior. But in between are those genes and their variant products whose virtues are a sometime thing, depending upon, on the one hand, the specificities of experiences over the lifetime, or,

on the other, their support, or reinforcement in failure, by the variant products of other genes. So the same variant gene product may be adequate in one person and fail in another, even in the same family. Or it may be within the same person adequate under one circumstance and insufficient under another. Thus, as a predictor, a gene may be of only limited use to an individual even while accepted as a significant risk in a population. This is a frequent problem of epidemiologically designated risk factors; it is not always clear to whom among their possessors the trait is actually risky—to say nothing of gradations in risk. It is the problem also of evidence-based medicine, which, however valuable in increasing the rigor of diagnosis and treatment, provides recommendations suitable for populations, not individuals (Sweeney et al, 1998; Tonelli, 1998; Mant, 1999). It is a matter of typological, as opposed to population, thinking. Of course the Human Genome Project will add greatly to the list of our genes and their proteins so that the exact identity of all of the units in pathways, and other homeostatic devices will be known, improving thereby the predictive value of various combinations of variants (Van Omenn et al, 1999). And, assuming increasing identification of exterior proximate causes, the accuracy and usefulness of preventive predictions may improve remarkably. The necessity for the advancement of knowledge of non-genetic proximate causes cannot be exaggerated. We need a project of similar scope and ambition to that of the HGP. In the meantime we should do what we can where we can, and for the rest, fall back upon an aspect of medicine that may have become unfashionable in modern times but which is perhaps more than ever needed; helping patients to live with uncertainty.

A far less likely, but more effective, means of health promotion is the control of remote causes. The virtue of such an approach is clearly indicated in the Mayr model wherein the relationship of the two kinds of causes and two kinds of biology is so lucidly stated. To influence by law the distributions of genes is both unconstitutional and in strong opposition to "liberty and the pursuit of happiness", but to influence the organization of society and culture for the betterment of health is not only possible but is already the aim of numerous government agencies, the even more numerous private disease-related societies, as well as physicians who have advised their patients to practice healthy ways. But what has not been emphasized, at least in the USA is the power of corporate action, of putting the weight of the whole medical profession socially and politically on the side of health promotion. Today in the USA this is impossible, and some will say it is undesirable, but the point to be made here is the logic of the position. On one side is the power of remote causes in the origin of disease (let us think here of the evolution, growth, organization, penetration and political powers of the tobacco industry) and on the other is the power of societies to organize themselves to influence those remote causes. In the USA it was public opinion followed by legal action that began the descent of the authority of tobacco. There are other social conditions likely to retard the advance of prevention. One of these is the combination in the public mind of a superficial grasp of progress in biology and genetics, and an unreasoning belief in the limitless potential of that progress. But for a recipient to respond realistically to the offer of prevention requires the ability to, a) differentiate between personal and populational probabilities, b) to grasp its potential for success or failure, and c) to participate constructively with a knowledgeable and sympathetic physician in greeting either success or failure. We don't often think of the evolution of education, or of the public grasp and acceptance of advances in medicine as remote causes of success or failure, but we should.

TREATMENT

The essence of Lewis Thomas' concept of high technology in treatment lay in the discovery of the exact point or points in the machine that were broken, and which could be repaired by a single, simple, straightforward maneuver (Thomas, 1974). One of his examples of such a treatment was the use of steroid in the adrenogenital syndrome. And after the fifties amid the rapid accumulation of newly described inborn errors there was optimism that such diseases would be brought under control (Scriver, 1967). But results so far have been something less. In the eighties Hayes tabulated successes and failures in 65 inborn errors, a part of a larger randomized sample of monogenic diseases taken from MIM 5 (Hayes et al, 1985). Table 2.2 shows that for 12% treatments were successful in rendering the patient normal or essentially so, while in 40% there was some improvement, often not very impressive, while about 48% showed no success at all. A further examination of success or failure in treatment of the same 65 diseases 10 years later was reported by Treacy with results shown in

Table 2.2 (Treacy et al, 1995). There was no increase in the number of very successful treatments, but some of the previously resistant disorders now yielded in some degree, often to such rigorous therapies as tissue and organ transplantation. These, Thomas saw as middle technologies, sometimes effective, but expensive and perhaps hard on the patient. A third look in 1999, this time including 517 inborn errors listed in the 7th edition of MMBID, gave much the same results (Table 2.2) (Treacy et al, 2000).

Given the qualities of the inborn errors that were the object of treatments the record is perhaps not surprising. Most are at or near the top of the gradient of selective effect, some are lethal, some are permanently crippling. And all are heterogeneous, some as to loci, all as to alleles. And we now know that we must expect equal heterogeneity among those shadowy modifiers we presume to exist (Scriver, 1999). So these disorders are simply the most intractable. But farther down the gradient, the diseases are more amenable, not necessarily to cure, but certainly to management. This seems to be telling us that there is a relationship between heritability and success in therapy. When the heritability is high in a population we expect less of treatment than when it is low; i.e. fewer patients are likely to respond satisfactorily. The history of treatment of rickets with vitamin D is exemplary. When, after the mid-forties rickets almost disappeared, nearly all that was left were several different kinds of monogenic vitamin D resistant rickets (Scriver and Childs, 1989). This experience seems to furnish medicine, especially preventive medicine, an aim, even a motto. We work to drive the heritability of disease toward 1.0. And we fervently hope that the gene therapists will confound the motto by inventing high technology treatments that subdue even the most "genetic" and even the most refractory of those disorders that continue to resist every effort to contain them. As for the complex disorders, they are resistant too, but in a different way. If every individual has his/her own set of proximate causes, the complexity is of a high degree. The problem is one of discovery of the non-genetic causes and trying to eliminate them, as well as discovering which sets of genetic causes pose vulnerability to the threats of those non-genetic influences, both in general and in each affected individual. No easy job, but we are up against a wily opponent. Many years ago Max Delbruck observed that, "any living cell carries with it the experiences of a billion years of experimentation by its ancestors. You cannot expect to explain so wise an old bird in a few simple words" (Delbruck, 1966). We are definitely embarked upon an effort to expose that wisdom. The next two or three editions of *PPMG* should show how wise the old bird is.

Table 2.2. Effectiveness of Treatment of Inborn Errors			
	1983 *Hayes*	*1993* *Treacy*	*2000* *Treacy*
Fully Beneficial	12*	12	12
Partially Beneficial	40	57	54
No Benefit	48	31	34

*Percent of total

Conclusion

The explanatory principles of disease begin with the capacity of the species for genetic variability, a capacity that is required for survival of species and that is experienced randomly resulting in genes whose products have, through time, conferred upon their recipients a status of congruence with equally variable environments. But sometimes the result is incongruence which can lead to disease. It is in the gene products, the protein unit steps of homeostasis that this species variability is expressed in congruence or incongruence: in health or disease. This expression occurs within a biochemical and molecular cellular matrix conditioned by interaction between such protein products and experiences of the environment through development, maturation and aging. Accordingly, analysis of pathogenesis must be pursued in three time scales all at once: that of phylogeny whence the genes and their products were derived, that of ontogeny, maturation and aging which condition the ever changing matrix, and that of the moment representing the impact of today's events. This principle, embracing the three time scales, incorporates also two kinds of causes, proximate and remote, which are expressed in the uniqueness of individuals. The incongruent proximate causes: variable protein unit steps of homeostasis and varying kinds, amounts and durations of experiences of the environment, account for the expressions of disease phenotypes that are subject to selection and incur the social stigmas that complicate the lives of their victims. Remote causes are constituted of the evolution and dynamics of both biological and social milieux that account for the nature and local availability of proximate causes, their unique assembly as genotypes and availability as experiences, to form combinations favorable for disease. And it is that particularity that determines who gets which disease at what time in life. The qualities of diseases are expressions of unique and variable human genomes arranged in a gradient of selective effect, a representation of the removal in early life of those unlikely to reproduce, and in post-reproductive life, a less intense test of survival in a variable environment. It is in the latter part of the range of the gradient that both prevention and treatment are likely to be most effective; prevention because changes in environment can be effective in avoiding disease, and treatment because the homeostasis can be characterized as inefficient and in need of a boost, rather than broken. The logic of prevention is more powerful than that of treatment, but we need both a more comprehensive knowledge of non-genetic proximate causes, and in time to learn, understand and adjust to the social dislocations any sudden spate of preventions could bring. But it is in part in the grasp of the possibility and plausibilities of both prevention and treatment, and in part in understanding the meaning in medicine of individuality and the virtues of population thinking in relation to it, that we may be able at once to pursue the reductionist path we have so successfully traversed, and return to embrace the integration, the humanity, of patients who appeal to us for relief of both the consequences of their molecular incongruities and the injury of the disease to that integrated humanity.

REFERENCES

Alberts B (1998) The cell as a collection of protein machines: Preparing the next generation of molecular biologists. Cell 92:291–294

Andrews LB, Fullarton JE, Holtzman NA, Motulsky AG (1994) Assessing Genetic Risks. National Academy Press, Washington DC

Anon, Genetic Screening (1975) Nat Acad Sci, Washington DC

Barker LF (1927) Heredity in the clinic. Am Jour Med Sci 173:597–605

Beadle GW (1956) Genes and chemical reactions in neurospora. Science 129:1715–1719

Bearn AG (1993) Archibald Garrod and the Individuality of Man. OUP, Oxford

Bergsma D (1974) Ethical, social and legal dimensions of screening for human genetic disease. Birth Defects Original Article Series 10 No 6

Burley SK, Almo SC, Bonnano JB et al. (1999) Structural genomics: Beyond the Human Genome Project. Nat Genet 23:151–157

Burnham JC (1982) America and medicine's golden age. What happened to it? Science 215:1474–1479

Capecchi MR (1997) Hox genes and mammalian development. Cold Spring Harbor Symp Quant Biol 62:273–278

Cargill M, Altshuler D, Ireland J et al. (1999) Characterization of single-nucleotide polymorphisms in coding regions of human genes. Nat Genet 22:231–238

Childs B, Scriver CR (1986) Age at onset and causes of disease. Persp Biol Med 29:437–460

Childs B (1999) Genetic medicine. Johns Hopkins Press, pp 35–43

Childs B (1999) The entry of genetics into medicine. Jour Urban Health 76:497–508

Cohen H (1960) The evolution of the concept of disease. In Lush B (ed): Concepts of Medicine, OUP, Oxford

Collins FS (1999) Shattuck lecture: Medical and societal consequences of the human genome project. New Eng Jour Med 341:28–37

Cori GT, Cori CF (1952) Glucose-6-phosphate of the liver in glycogen storage disease. J Biol Chem 199:661–667

Costa T, Scriver CR, Childs B (1985) The effect of Mendelian disease on human health: A measurement. Am Jour Med Genet 21:231–242

Delbruck M (1966) A physicist looks at biology. In Cairns J, Stent GS, Watson JD (eds): Phage and the Origins of Molecular Biology. Cold Spring Harbor Press, Cold Spring Harbor, NY, pp 9–22

De Solla Price DJ (1963) Little Science Big Science. Columbia U. Press, NY

Fox-Keller E (1995) Language and science: Genetics, embryology and the discourse of gene action. In Fox-Keller E (ed.): Refiguring Life. Columbia U. Press, NY

Fries JF, Crapo LM (1981) Vitality and Aging. WH Freeman, NY

Fruton JS (1972) Molecules and Life. Wiley-Interscience, NY

Garbers DL, Dubois SK (1999) The molecular basis of hypertension. Ann Rev Biochem 68:127–155

Garrod AE (1902) The incidence of alkaptonuria: A study in chemical individuality. Lancet 2:1616–1620

Garrod AE (1909) Inborn Errors of Metabolism, Oxford Press

Garrod AE (1926) Inborn Errors of Metabolism. 2nd edn, OUP, Oxford

Gelbert WM (1998) Databases in genomic research. Science 282:659–661

Goldman L, Bennett JC (2000) Cecil Textbook of Medicine, 21st edn. Saunders, NY

Halushka MK, Fan JB, Bentley K et al. (1999) Patterns of single-nucleotide polymorphisms in candidate genes for blood pressure homeostasis. Nat Genet 22:239–247

Hayes A, Costa T, Scriver CR, Childs B (1985) The effect of mendelian disease on human health. II: Response to treatments. Am Jour Med Genet 21:243–255

Hill AVS (1999) Genetics and genomics of infectious disease susceptibility. Brit Med Bull 55:401–413

Hoffmann AA, Parsons PA (1991) Evolutionary Genetics and Environmental Stress. OUP, NY

Holtzman NA (1989) Proceed with Caution. The Johns Hopkins Press, Baltimore

Holtzman NA, Watson MS (1998) Promoting Safe and Effective Genetic Testing in the United States. Johns Hopkins University Press, Baltimore

Hsia YE, Hirshhorn K, Silverberg RL, Godmillow L (1979) Counseling in Genetics. AL Liss, NY

Isselbacher KJ, Anderson EP, Kurahashi K, Kalckar HM (1956) Science, 123:635–636

Jacobs PA (1990) The role of chromosome abnormalities in reproductive failure. Reprod Nutr Dev supp 63s–74s

Jiminez-Sanchez G, Childs B, Valle D (2000) The effect of mendelian disease on human health. In Scriver CR, Beaudet AL, Sly WS, Valle D (eds): The Metabolic and Molecular Basis of Inherited Disease, 8th edn. McGraw-Hill, NY, pp 167–174

King L (1982) Medical Thinking. Princeton Press, Princeton

Kirschner M, Gerhart J (1998) Evolvability. Proc Nat Acad Sci 95:8420–8427

Knoppers BM, Labarge CM (1990) Genetic Screening: From newborns to DNA typing. Exerpta Medica, Amsterdam

Kohler RE (1994) Lords of the Fly. Univ. of Chicago Press, Chicago

Kornberg TB, Krosnow MA (2000) The drosophila genome sequence: Implications for biology and medicine. Science 287:2218–2220

Lander E, (1996) The new genomics: Global views of biology. Science 274:536–539

Lander ES, Schork NJ (1994) Genetic dissection of complex traits. Science 265:2037–2048

Lander ES, Weinberg RA (2000) Genomics: Journey to the center of biology. Science 287:1777–1782

Lewontin RC (1983) Gene, organism and environment. In Bendell DS (ed.): Evolution from Molecules to Men. CU Press, NY, pp 273–286

Lubs HA, de la Cruz F (1977) Genetic Counseling. Raven Press, NY

Ly DH, Lockhart DJ, Lerner RA, Shultz PG (2000) Mitotic misregulation and human aging. Science 287:2486–2492

Marmot MG (1997) Early life and adult disorder. Brit Med Bull 53:3–9

Mant D (1999) Can randomized trials inform clinical decisions about individual patients? Lancet 353:743–746

Maynard Smith J, Burian R, Kauffman S et al. (1985) Developmental constraints and evolution. Quart Rev Biol 60:265–287

Mayr E (1961) Cause and Effect in biology. Science 134:1501–1506

Mayr E (1982) The Growth of Biological Thought. Harvard Univ Press, Boston, pp 45–47

Mayr E, Provine WB (1980) The Evolutionary Synthesis. Harvard Univ. Press, Cambridge

Motulsky AG (1999) If I had a gene test, what would I have and who would I tell? Lancet 354: SI 35–SI37

McKeown J (1976) The Role of Medicine. Nuffield Trust, London

Nelkin D, Lindee MS (1995) The DNA Mystique. WH Freeman, NY

Pauling L, Itano HA, Singer SJ, Wells IC (1949) Sickle cell anemia, a molecular disease. Science 110:543–548

Rosenberg CE (1995) Banishing risk: or the more things change the more they remain the same. Persp Biol Med 39:28–42

Rosenberg CR (1979) Toward an ecology of knowledge. In The Organization of Knowledge in Modern America. The Johns Hopkins Press, Baltimore, pp 440–455

Rutherford S, Lindquist S (1998) Hsp 90 as a capacitor for morphological evolution. Nature 396: 336–346

Schroedinger E (1967) What is Life? Cambridge Univ. Press, p23

Scott-Moncrieff R (1981–1983) The classical period in chemical genetics. Notes and Records, Roy Soc London 36–37:125–154

Scriver CR (1967) Treatment in medical genetics. Proc. 3rd Int. Cong. Genetics. Johns Hopkins Press, Baltimore Crow JF, Neel JV (eds): p45

Scriver CR (1989) Changing heritability of nutritional disease: Another explanation for clustering. In Simopoulos A, Childs B (eds): Genetic Variation and Nutrition. Karger, New York, pp 60–71

Scriver CR (1999) Monogenic traits are not simple. Trends in Genetics 15:3–8

Scriver CR, Childs B (1989) Garrod's Inborn Factors in Disease. Oxford Press, New York

Scriver CR, Beaudet AL, Sly WS, Valle D (1995) The Metabolic and Molecular Basis of Metabolic Disease, 7th edn. McGraw-Hill, NY

Stent GS (1981) Strengths and weaknesses of the genetic approach to the development of the nervous system. In Cowan WM (ed): Studies in Developmental Neurobiology. Oxford Univ. Press, NY

Sweeney KG, MacAuley D, Gray DP (1998) Personal significance: The third dimension. Lancet 351:134–137

Temkin O (1963) The scientific approach to disease: Specific entity and individual sickness. In Crombie AC (ed): Historical Studies in Intellectual, Social and Technical Conditions for Scientific Discovery. Basic Books, NY, pp 629–647

Thomas L (1974) The future impact of science and technology on medicine. Bioscience 24:99

Tonelli MR (1998) The philosophical limits of evidence based medicine. Acad Med 73:1234–1240

Treacy E, Childs B, Scriver CR (1995) Response to treatment in hereditary metabolic disease: 1993 survey and 10 years comparison. Am Jour Hum Genet 56:359–367

Treacy EP, Valle D, Scriver CR (2000) Treatment of genetic disease. In Scriver CR, Beaudet AL, Sly WS, Valle D (eds): The Metabolic and Molecular Basis of Inherited Disease, 8th edn. McGraw-Hill, NY

Van Omenn GJB, Bakker E, den Dunnen JT (1999) The Human Genome Product and the future of diagnostics, treatment and prevention. Lancet 354: supp. si5–si10

Vogel F, Motulsky AG (1998) Human Genetics. Preface, 3rd edn. Springer-Verlag, NY

Yanofsky C (1965–1966) Gene structure and protein structure. Harvey Lectures 61:145–167

Waddington CH (1957) The Strategy of the Genes. Allen and Unwin, London

Wright S (1917) Color inheritance in mammals. Jour Hered 8:224–235

Nature and frequency of genetic disease

3

David L. Rimoin
J. Michael Connor
Reed E. Pyeritz
Bruce R. Korf

Genes are major determinants of human variation. It is estimated that any two copies of a randomly selected gene will differ at a single nucleotide base every 1–2 thousand bases. This implies that any person is heterozygous for as many as 40,000 amino acid substitutions (Cargill et al., 1999). The impact of genetically determined characteristics spans a continuum and may be nil at one extreme or lethal at the other. In determining a trait, one or two alleles may be all important, but more commonly genes interact with one another and with one or more environmental factors. This interaction between genetic and environmental factors is now apparent for numerous diseases and includes many conditions previously believed to have a purely environmental etiology. For example, genetically determined susceptibility has now been identified for several infections (see Ch. 42), for many drug-induced idiosyncrasies (see Ch. 21), and for several carcinogens (e.g., bladder cancer in aniline dye workers who are slow acetylators). We suspect that such interactions are commonplace and that relatively few conditions are solely environmental in causation. However, for definitions of the types and frequency of genetic disorders, we use the currently available information, with the proviso that these are all the minimum frequencies and based on imperfect categorization. For example, short stature as a manifestation of an inherited skeletal dysplasia would be considered a genetic disease, whereas extremes of normal variation of height due to interaction of several genes (as yet undefined) and environmental factors generally would not.

Furthermore, the interpretation will depend on the situation (e.g., red-green colorblindness may be a serious disability to the hunter-gatherer) or on the public perception (e.g., persons with albinism are considered blessed in some populations). Hence the distinction between normal variation and disease is blurred and, as variable criteria have been used in different surveys of genetic disease, this must be considered in their interpretation. With these points in mind, Table 3.1 presents a classification of types of genetic disease together with their frequencies.

Table 3.1. Types and frequencies of genetic diseases

Type	Frequency by age 25 yr	Frequency after 25 yr	Lifetime frequency
Chromosomal disorders	1.8/1000	2/1000	3.8/1000[a]
Single gene disorders	3.6/1000	16.4/1000	20/1000[b]
Multifactorial (part-genetic) disorders	46.4/1000	600/1000	646.4/1000[c]
Somatic cell (cumulative) genetic disorders	—	240/1000	240/1000[d]

[a] Excludes asymptomatic carriers of balanced structural rearrangements but includes numerical sex chromosomal disorders, many of which will be undiagnosed.
[b] Excludes carriers of premutations and of other mutations with few or no symptoms but includes mitochondrial gene mutations.
[c] For congenital malformations, only the proven part-genetic contribution is included, but for chronic disorders of adulthood the figure is an overall frequency estimate.
[d] Assumes that all cancers represent cumulative genetic mutations and excludes the inherited single gene cancer syndromes.

Frequency of genetic disease

Each type of genetic disease has a large number of subtypes; determination of individual and collective frequencies would require comprehensive investigation of a large sample of a specific population. This is clearly not practical. The situation is further complicated by the continued delineation of new subtypes of genetic disease, by difficulties in defining a boundary between a genetic disease of medical significance and a mild inherited trait (e.g., many mutations for von Willebrand disease), and by population variations in the frequencies of different genetic diseases. Thus, most of the available data pertain to specific conditions either in a sample of the general population or in specific populations (e.g., learning disabled). Extrapolation of such data to the overall population is difficult. One very useful attempt to circumvent these difficulties in estimating the frequency of genetic disease has been the creation and maintenance of the British Columbia Health Surveillance Registry (Baird et al., 1988). This Registry, established in 1952, uses multiple sources of ascertainment in a consecutive series of more than one million livebirths. Analysis of these data shows that before 25 years of age, at least 53 of 1000 liveborn individuals can be expected to have disease with an important genetic component. This figure of 53 of 1000 comprises 3.6 single gene disorders per 1000 (1.4 autosomal dominant, 1.7 autosomal recessive, and 0.5 X-linked recessive), 1.8 chromosomal disorders per 1000, 46.4 multifactorial, or part-genetic disorders per 1000, and 1.2 genetic type uncertain disorders per 1000. In this analysis, congenital abnormalities were included only if a multifactorial or part-genetic etiology had been established, but if all congenital abnormalities were included, the cumulative figure rose to more than 79 per 1000 livebirths. Although multiple sources of ascertainment were employed, systematic screening of the entire population for each disorder was not performed; hence, these figures are minimum estimates. They also include neither mild conditions that are unlikely to come to medical attention nor the contribution of genetic conditions to pregnancy loss, stillbirths, and diseases of middle and old age (see below).

CHROMOSOMAL DISORDERS

By definition, a chromosomal disorder is present if there is a visible alteration in the number or structure of the chromosomes. Using routine light microscopy, multiple newborn cytogenetic surveys reveal a frequency in liveborn children of 6 in 1000; of these, two-thirds are disabled either mentally or physically as a result (Tolmie, 1995). A proportion of the remainder will, in adult life, be at increased risk of either miscarriage or having a disabled child. These chromsomally abnormal liveborn infants comprise only a small proportion of all chromosomally abnormal conceptions. It is estimated that the rate of chromosomal abnormality in embryonic and fetal deaths is within the range 32% to 42%; the proportion of all recognized conceptuses that are chromosomally abnormal is thus 5% to 7% (Hook, 1992). In spontaneous abortions and liveborn infants, different types of chromosomal abnormality predominate; for example, trisomy 16 is the commonest autosomal trisomy in abortions, whereas trisomies for chromosome 21, 18, and 13 are the only autosomal trisomies occurring at appreciable frequencies in liveborns. Monosomy for the X chromosome (45,X) occurs in about 1% of all conceptions, but 98% of those affected do not reach term. Triploidy is also frequent in abortions, but is exceptional in newborns. The high frequency of chromosomally abnormal conceptions is mirrored by results of chromosome analysis in gametes, which reveal an approximate abnormality rate of 10% in sperm and 25% in oocytes (Pellestor, 1991). Since the great majority of chromosomal abnormalities are lethal in early gestation, the abnormality rate in stillbirths is considerably lower, at about 5% to 7%. The frequency is also higher than the liverborn frequency in selected populations. For example, Klinefelter syndrome is found in 10% of azoospermic infertile men, compared with a male birth incidence of 1 in 1000.

Routine light microscopy cannot resolve small amounts of missing or additional material (less than 4 Mb of DNA), and such microdeletions or microduplications would be missed by conventional microscopy. These can be detected with specific molecular probes coupled with fluorescent in situ hybridization (FISH); multiple microdeletion disorders have been defined in recent years and undoubtedly more await discovery (see Chs. 9 and 46). Such microdeletions, which epistemologically link "chromosomal disorders" with single gene disorders, account for a proportion of currently unexplained learning disability and multiple malformation syndromes (Flint et al., 1995).

SINGLE GENE DISORDERS

By definition, single gene disorders arise as a result of mutations in one or both alleles of a gene on an autosome or sex chromosome or in a mitochondrial gene. There have been many investigations into the overall frequency of single gene disorders. Many early estimates were misleadingly low due to underascertainment, especially of late-onset disorders (e.g., familial hypercholesterolemia, adult polycystic kidney disease, and Huntington disease). Carter (1977) reviewed the earlier literature and estimated an overall incidence of autosomal dominant traits of 7.0 in 1000 livebirths, of autosomal recessive traits of 2.5 in 1000 livebirths, and of X-linked disorders of 0.5 in 1000 livebirths. This gave a combined frequency of 10 in 1000 livebirths (1%). At that time, approximately 2500 single gene disorders had been delineated. The number of recognized mendelian phenotypes has since more than quadrupled (OMIM, 2000), and these new entities include several particularly common conditions (e.g., familial breast cancer syndromes, with a combined estimated frequency of 5 in 1000; hereditary nonpolyposis colon cancer syndromes, with a combined frequency of 5 in 1000). In addition, new technologies for DNA analysis have revealed a higher-than-expected frequency of generally asymptomatic people with one or two mutant alleles at a locus. For example, up to 1% of the population have a mutant allele for von Willebrand factor, but many of these people have few or no symptoms, so again there is the problem of the imprecise and variable boundary between a harmless variant and a clinically important one. Furthermore, DNA analysis has shown that for several important disorders, including myotonic dystrophy and fragile X syndrome, relatives of an affected individual may harbor a premutation that, although not detrimental to the carrier, has the potential for expansion to a full deleterious mutation in their offspring. The prevalence of such premutation carriers may be as high as 1 in 250 to 500 females for fragile X syndrome (see Ch. 103).

The frequencies of many single-gene disorders show population variation. This is readily understood for selected populations; for example, fragile X syndrome is found in 7% of developmentally delayed males, as compared with a general male population frequency of 1 in 4000. Geographic variation is also observed and may be explained by selection or by founder effects or attributed to random genetic drift. For example, selection has resulted in a carrier frequency of 1 in 3 for sickle cell anemia in parts of equatorial Africa, and the Afrikaners of South Africa have a high frequency of variegate porphyria and familial hypercholesterolaemia due to a founder effect. The carrier frequency for HFE, one of the genes responsible for hemochromatosis, is 1 in 10 in individuals of Celtic ancestry. Undoubtedly, more single-gene disorders are going to be delineated. In theory, at least one per locus will eventually be recognized (about 30,000) minus those with no or a mild phenotype and minus those incompatible with establishment/continuance of a pregnancy. Hence the overall estimates of frequencies shown in Table 3.1 are again minimum figures. There is already

overlap with the multifactorial or part-genetic category. For example, many patients with acute intermittent porphyria are asymptomatic in the absence of an environmental trigger, and epistatic involvement of other genes is believed to contribute to intrafamilial phenotypic variation for patients with the same mutation. As more gene-environment and gene-gene interactions are identified, the boundary between single gene disorders and multifactorial disorders will become further blurred.

MULTIFACTORIAL (OR PART-GENETIC) DISORDERS

Multifactorial disorders result from an interaction of one or more genes with one or more environmental factors. Thus, in effect the genetic contribution predisposes the individual to the actions of environmental agents. Such an interaction is suspected when conditions show an increased recurrence risk within families, which does not reach the level of risk or pattern seen for single gene disorders and when identical twin concordance exceeds that for nonidentical twins but is less than 100% (see Ch. 18). For most multifactorial disorders, however, the nature of the environmental agent(s) and the genetic predisposition are currently unclear and are the subject of intensive research efforts. The use of single nucleotide polymorphisms for linkage and association studies promises to accelerate progress in this area.

These multifactorial disorders are believed to account for approximately one-half of all congenital malformations and to be relevant to many common chronic disorders of adulthood, including hypertension, rheumatoid arthritis, psychoses, and senile dementia (complex common disorders). The former group had an estimated frequency of 46.4 in 1000 in the British Columbia survey (Baird et al., 1988) and the latter may be as high as 600 in 1000 (UNSEAR, 1986). In addition, a multifactorial etiology is suspected for many common psychological disorders of childhood, including dyslexia (5% to 10% of the population), specific language impairment (5% of children), and attention deficit-hyperactivity disorder (4% to 10% of children) (see Ch. 105). Hence the multifactorial disorder category represents the commonest type of genetic disease in both children and adults.

Multifactorial disorders also show considerable ethnic and geographic variation. For example, talipes equinovarus is some six times more common among Maoris than among Europeans, and neural tube defects were once 10 times more frequent in Ireland than in North America.

Often ignored, both intellectually and in research, are genotypes that *reduce* susceptibility to potentially harmful environmental factors. An understanding of alleles that provide protection from disease will yield insight into pathogenesis as well as novel approaches to therapy and prevention.

SOMATIC CELL (OR CUMULATIVE) GENETIC DISORDERS

In somatic cell (or cumulative) genetic disorders, the condition is caused by the additive effects of several mutations of different genes. This has been observed for numerous cancers (see Ch. 19); most of the mutations are usually confined to the tumor (i.e., to a group of somatic cells). The first step in the cascade of mutations may be inherited (i.e., involving germ cells and all somatic cells); these single gene disorders are included in the single gene disorder frequency in Table 3.1. Carcinogens are important causes of noninherited mutations, and genetic susceptibility is suspected to account for individual variation in risk on exposure. Somatic cell genetic disorders might also be involved in other clinical conditions such as autoimmune disorders and the aging process.

Morbidity and mortality due to genetic disease

The same general difficulties that pertain to the frequency estimates for genetic disorders (see above), also apply to estimates of the contribution of the various types of genetic disorder to morbidity and mortality during pregnancy, in childhood, and in adulthood. Hence these figures should be taken as minimum estimates.

CONCEPTION AND PREGNANCY

One in 15 recognized pregnancies spontaneously miscarries, and a higher percentage (up to 50%) of conceptions is lost before recognition of the pregnancy. The majority of these losses is caused by numerical chromosomal abnormalities.

CHILDHOOD

Since the turn of the century in many Western countries, advances in medicine and public health have resulted in a gradual decline in the contribution of environmental factors to childhood morbidity and mortality. The result of these changes has been to throw genetic disorders into greater prominence. These changes are well illustrated in data from surveys of the causes of childhood deaths in various U.K. hospitals (Table 3.2). Over the past half-century, the relative importance of genetic illness in childhood mortality has tripled, accounting for one-half of all deaths by 1976. By contrast, in developing countries, nongenetic causes of childhood mortality continue to predominate. For example, in Madras in 1976, more than 95% of childhood deaths in hospitals were due to nongenetic causes, in most cases, infectious diseases, and less than 5% were due to genetic causes (Emery AE, unpublished observations).

An idea of the contribution of genetic disease to morbidity can be judged from the prevalence of such diseases among pediatric inpatients. In reviewing 4115 in patients. Hall et al. (1978) found multifactorial disease in 22.1%, a single-gene disorder in 3.9% and a chromosomal disorder in 0.6%. Thus, more than 1 in 4 pediatric inpatients has a genetic disorder, as compared with the general population frequency estimate of 1 in 20 by 25 years of age (Table 3.1). This does not include the morbidity that did not lead to inpatient admission. In recent surveys of the learning disabled, the basis is genetic in more than one-half, which would give a population frequency of genetic disease associated with learning disability of 18 in 1000 school-age children (see Ch. 104).

ADULTHOOD

In Western countries, the commonest causes of death are cancer and cardiovascular disorders. All cancers are now known to have a cumulative genetic basis, and there is evidence for a major genetic contribution to cardiovascular

Table 3.2. Proportions of childhood deaths attributable to nongenetic and genetic causes

	London 1914[a] (%)	London 1954[a] (%)	Newcastle 1966[b] (%)	Edinburgh 1976[c] (%)
Nongenetic	83.5	62.5	58	50
Genetic				
Single gene disorder	2	12	8.5	8.9
Chromosomal disorder	—	—	2.5	2.9
Part-genetic disorder	14.5	25.5	31	38.2

[a] Carter (1956).
[b] Roberts et al. (1970).
[c] Emery, AE (unpublished observations).

disease. Single gene disorders causing diabetes or high blood pressure are relatively uncommon, but multifactorial inheritance accounts for a large proportion of patients with premature vascular disease and systemic hypertension (see Chs. 53 and 51). Similarly, there is a growing recognition of the importance of multifactorial inheritance for many other common disorders of adulthood responsible for both morbidity and mortality.

REFERENCES

Baird PA, Anderson TW, Newcombe HB, Lowry RB (1988) Genetic disorders in children and young adults: A population study. Am J Hum Genet 42:677–693

Cargill M, Altshuler D, Ireland J et al. (1999) Characterization of single-nucleotide polymorphisms in coding regions of human genes. Nature Genet 22:231–238

Carter CO (1956) Changing patterns in the causes of death at the Hospital for Sick Children. Great Ormond Street J 11:65–68

Carter CO (1977) Monogenic disorders. J Med Genet 14:316–320

Flint J, Wilkie AOM, Buckle VJ et al. (1995) The detection of subtelomeric chromosomal rearrangements in idiopathic mental retardation. Nature Genet 9:132–139

Hall JG, Powers EK, McIlvaine RT, Ean VH (1978) The frequency and familial burden of genetic disease in a paediatric hospital. Am J Med Genet 1:416–436

Hook EB (1992) Prevalence, risks and recurrence. trs. In Brock DJH, Rodeck CH, Ferguson-Smith MA (eds): Prenatal Diagnosis and Screening. Churchill-Livingstone, Edinburgh, p. 351.

Online Mendelian Inheritance in Man, OMIM ™. McKusick-Nathans Institute for Genetic Medicine, Johns Hopkins University (Baltimore, MD) and National Center for Biotechnology Information, National Library of Medicine (Bethesda, MD), 2000. World Wide Web URL: http://www.ncbi.nlm.nih.gov/omim

Pellestor F (1991) Frequency and distribution of aneuploidy in human female garnetes. Hum Genet 86:283–288

Roberts DF, Chavez J, Court SDM (1970) The genetic component in child mortality. Arch Dis Child 45:33–38

Tolmie JL (1995) Chromosome disorders. In Whittle MJ, Connor JM (eds): Prenatal Diagnosis in Obstetric Practice. Blackwell Scientific, Oxford, p. 34.

UNSEAR (1986) United Nations Scientific Committee on the Effects of Atomic Radiation. Report on the Genetic and Somatic Effects of Ionising Radiation. United Nations, NY

Genome structure and gene expression

Gregory Barsh

Charles J. Epstein

Leena Peltonen

Introduction

The chemical structure of genetic material as well as the storage, processing and transfer of genetic information from one generation to the next are basically the same in all living organisms. However, the recently published sequence of the human genome has revealed many interesting details, having some degree of specificity to man. The complexity of the human phenotype—when compared to that of other sequenced species—is not explained by the significantly higher number of genes. Instead of predicted 50,000–150,000 genes, only some 35,000 can be verified in the sequence. Multiple single nucleotide polymorphisms (SNPs), tissue-specific splice variations, complex posttranslational modifications and more complex use of protein domains create diversity in the gene products. In fact, not only one but several different polypeptides are synthesized based on the information coded by one gene. Only 7% of human genes appear to be vertebrate-specific, and interestingly those genes encode proteins associated with defense and immunity functions and proteins in the nervous system.

For the first time in human history we are in the position to define the exact structure of the human genome. We can identify the essential features of its structure, and determine how the message in the genome is translated to the complex functions of human cells and tissues. The Director of the Human Genome Project, Dr Francis Collins, has described the human genome as the story of man with three volumes: A history book, describing the details of the evolution of our species; a manual, with detailed building instructions for human cells and organs; and a new textbook of medicine, providing novel insights to our disease processes.

DOUBLE HELIX STRUCTURE, DNA REPLICATION, TRANSCRIPTION, AND RECOMBINATION

The function of the human genome is reliably to transfer information from one generation to the next. This is carried out in a semiconservative way: one of two parental DNA strands of the double helix remains intact in every cell division. Watson and Crick proposed that two DNA strands form a double helix by hydrogen bonding between the nitrogenous bases: guanine (G) pairs with cytosine(C) and adenine (A) pairs with thymine (T, or its analogue, uracil, in RNA) (Fig. 4.1) The hydrogen bonds formed between these pyrimidine-purine pairs (guanine and adenine are purines; cytosine, thymine, and uracil are pyrimidines)

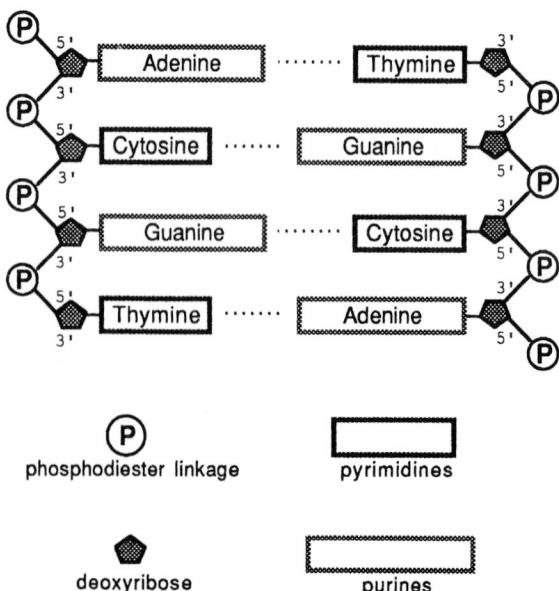

Fig. 4.1. Complementary structure of double-stranded DNA.

stabilize the double helix and glue the two *complementary* strands together. Two DNA-strands run in opposite directions (antiparallel). One strand runs in a 5′ to 3′ direction, the other in a 3′ to 5′ direction.

Replication

Genetic information is preserved by DNA replication, a process that produces identical copies of DNA molecules during each cell division into two daughter cells. During this process, the two parental strands separate, and each serves as a template for the synthesis of a new complementary strand by an enzyme, DNA polymerase (Fig. 4.2). Each daughter cell inherits one strand of the parental duplex. Every DNA-molecule thus contains a "young" strand that was synthesized in the parental cell and an "old" strand that was synthesized in the grandparent cell during DNA-replication when the cell prepares to divide. This guarantees intact information from one cell generation to

the next. The genome copies itself throughout millions of cell divisions during an individual's life with amazing precision, due to the semiconservative character of replication.

Transcription

The genome can copy itself with almost error-free efficiency; it can also produce multiple copies of meaningful (transcript producing) parts of the genome. The genes *are transcribed from* DNA into *messenger RNA* (mRNA) (Fig. 4.3). A single gene can give rise to multiple transcripts by means of alternative splicing and alternative transcription initiation and termination sites. During transcription, the DNA duplex unwinds, and one of the strands serves as the template for synthesis of a complementary RNA strand. RNA is distinguished from DNA by the presence of uracil instead of thymine, ribose instead of deoxyribose, and a different three-dimensional folding pattern. The mRNA molecules, opposite to DNA-molecules, are single stranded and function as the vehicle for *translating* nucleic acid into protein sequence.

In eukaryotes, three different RNA polymerases (I, II, and III, respectively) transcribe genes coding for mRNAs which will eventually be translated to proteins, as well as ribosomal RNAs (rRNA) and transfer RNAs (tRNA). Initiation of gene transcription requires additional proteins besides RNA polymerase; multiple *transcription factors* form the initiation complex. This complex gets attached to

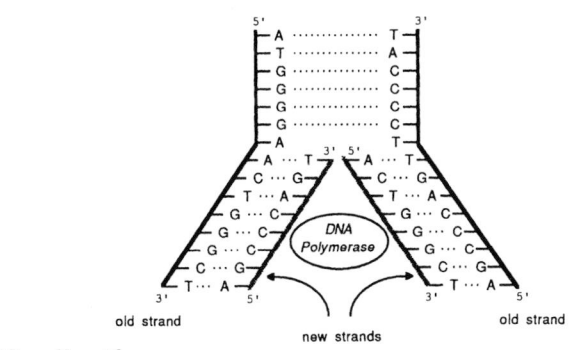

Replication

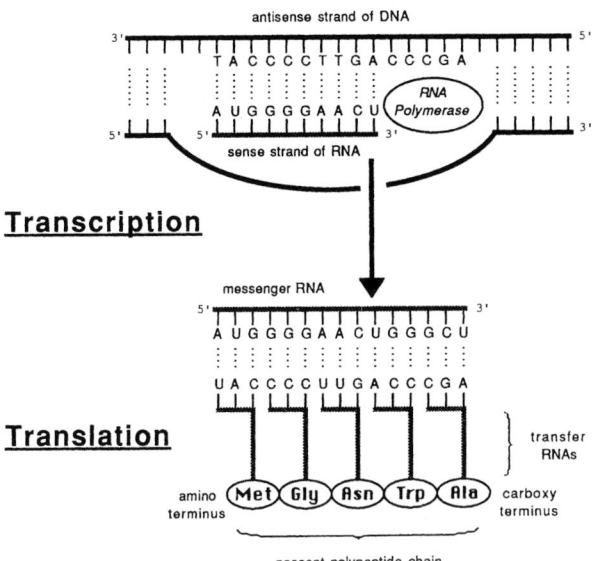

Transcription

Translation

Fig. 4.2. Flow of genetic information.

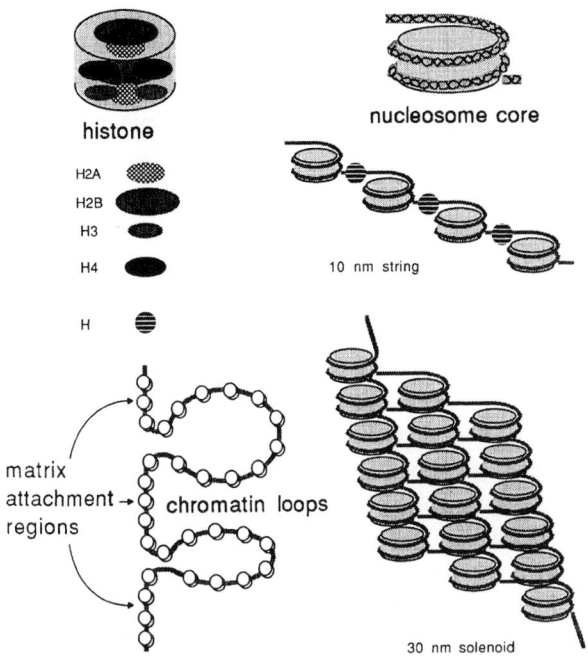

Fig. 4.3. Packaging of DNA into chromatin.

the initiation site of the transcription in the 5′ end of the gene and determines which genes are transcribed in different cell types or during different developmental stages of specific tissues. The transcription factors (including enhancers and inhibitors) also determine the level of gene expression. The enhancers and inhibitors can bind not only to the 5′ end of each gene but also to other regions; a typical binding site is the first intron in many mammalian genes.

Most typically only one of the two DNA-strands gets transcribed, and the consensus on the nomenclature annotating the DNA strand, which is similar to the transcribed mRNA sequence (however, with thymine instead of uracil), is to refer to it as a *sense* strand. The DNA sequence that serves as the transcriptional template is referred to as an *antisense* strand.

Recombination

Recombination is a physical exchange of chromosomal DNA between the parental chromosomes. During the "four strand stage" of meiosis, two duplex DNA molecules (from both parents) form a hybrid, and a single strand of one duplex (maternal) is paired with its complement from the other duplex (paternal). Single stranded DNA is exchanged between the homologous chromosomes and the process involves DNA strand breakage and resealing resulting in the precise recombination and exchange of DNA sequences between two homologous chromosomes. Recombinations are visible in the crossing over, and take place during both spermatogenesis and oogenesis. The frequency of recombinations is proportional to the distance between two gene loci in the chromosomal DNA strand, and this provides the basis for the determination of the genetic distance between two genetic loci. The proximity of two loci is measured by the percent recombination between them; a map distance of 1 centiMorgan indicates a 1% recombination frequency between two loci. On average one cM equals 1 million nucleotides, but there is wide variation in this ratio in different chromosomal regions. Average recombination rate increases as the length of the chromosomal arm decreases and the recombination rate tends to be suppressed near the centromeres.

The draft genome sequence has for the first time made it possible to compare the genetic and physical distances, and to analyze variations in recombination frequency in different chromosomal regions. On average one million base pairs (1 Mb) correspond to 1 cM (1% recombination frequency). However, there is tremendous local variation in individual chromosomes and the average recombination rate is higher in short chromosomal arms (2 Mb per cM). Further, the recombination rate is suppressed near the centromeres and higher in distal parts of the chromosomal arms. There is also significant variation in the recombination rates between the sexes. Some regions show higher recombination frequency in males, some in females.

Direction of the DNA and RNA-synthesis

Each chromosome in the human cell consists of a single double-helical DNA strand; an average chromosome contains some 4–5 cm of DNA-strand. The polarity of a single-stranded nucleic acid is defined by the position of phosphodiester bonds, which connect the 3′ hydroxyl group of one nucleoside to the 5′ hydroxyl group of the next (Fig. 4.1). A nucleoside is the combination of a purine or pyrimidine base with ribose (in RNA) or deoxyribose (in DNA), and a nucleotide is the combination of a nucleoside with one or more phosphate groups. The phosphate groups in a single nucleotide triphosphate are attached to the ribose or deoxyribose moiety via the 5′ hydroxyl residue, and two of the three phosphates are removed during incorporation of each nucleotide triphosphate into DNA or RNA. When the new DNA-strand is synthesized during replication or copied during transcription, the polymerase enzymes add new nucleotides to the 3′ hydroxyl group of a growing polynucleotide chain. The newly synthesized strand of RNA or DNA is said to begin at the 5′ terminus and to end at the 3′ terminus, thus the parental or template DNA-strand is "read" in the 3′ to 5′ direction, while the new strand is synthesized in the 5′ to 3′ direction. If two proteins are encoded by adjacent genes which lie on different strands, these genes are said to have opposite transcriptional orientations.

Organization of genomic DNA

The 3 billion base pair long genomic DNA of the human genome is packaged into 22 pairs of autosomes and X and Y sex chromosomes. The chromosomal DNA can be divided into regions of heterochromatin and euchromatin: heterochromatin representing the tightly packed regions of chromosomal DNA strands and euchromatin representing the "loose," actively transcribed DNA regions. Using cytogenetic staining methods, differently packed chromosomal regions can be viewed as G (Giemsa) bands, the banding pattern being characteristic to individual chromosomes and providing the basis for the cytogenetic identification of 23 different human chromosomes. From early on, the dark G-bands have been considered to reflect the "gene poor and GC-poor" regions, and the sequence information on the human genome has proven this concept to be true. Additionally, the sequence information has revealed tremendous differences in the GC content in different chromosomal regions. GC content may vary from 36% to 47% when about 50 Mb stretches in different chromosomal regions are analyzed.

Each of the 46 human chromosomes contains a single DNA duplex extending between the two telomeres. Were the length of DNA in an average-size human chromosome (130,000,000 bp) stretched end to end, it would be more than 100,000 times longer than a metaphase chromosome. This hundred-thousand fold redundancy of DNA packing is achieved by coiling and folding the double helix into a series of progressively shorter and thicker structures (Fig. 4.3). Proteins that bind to DNA help direct and organize this folding; the complex of DNA and protein is referred to as *chromatin*.

NUCLEOSOMES AND HIGHER-ORDER CHROMATIN STRUCTURE

The simplest level of chromatin structure is the organization of DNA and histones into *nucleosomes*. Each nucleo-

some is a 146-bp-long segment of DNA tightly wrapped almost two times around a histone core. This octamer core contains two molecules each of H2A, H2B, H3, and H4. Nucleosomes are a fundamental feature of all eukaryotic DNA; the octamer core histones are well conserved among even distantly related species. A fifth histone, H1, binds to the DNA just outside each nucleosome and is less well conserved. A region of linker DNA up to 80 bp in length usually separates adjacent nucleosomes, so that nucleosomes are spaced an average of 200 bp apart.

Nucleosomes represent the first level in the packaging of naked DNA into chromatin and appear in the electron microscope as a string of 10-nm "beads." The next level in packaging (Fig. 4.4) is the coiling of nucleosomes into a solenoid that contains six nucleosomes per turn, measures 30 nm in diameter, and is stabilized by interactions between H1 molecules bound to adjacent nucleosomes. Additional levels of folding can compress DNA into 300-nm fibers and a nearly 1000-nm metaphase chromatid, but the molecular basis of these packaging steps is not well understood.

EUCHROMATIN AND HETEROCHROMATIN

During metaphase, the entire chromosome is highly condensed, but at other times, most chromatin is organized into fibers of intermediate diameter, 30 to 300 nm, designated

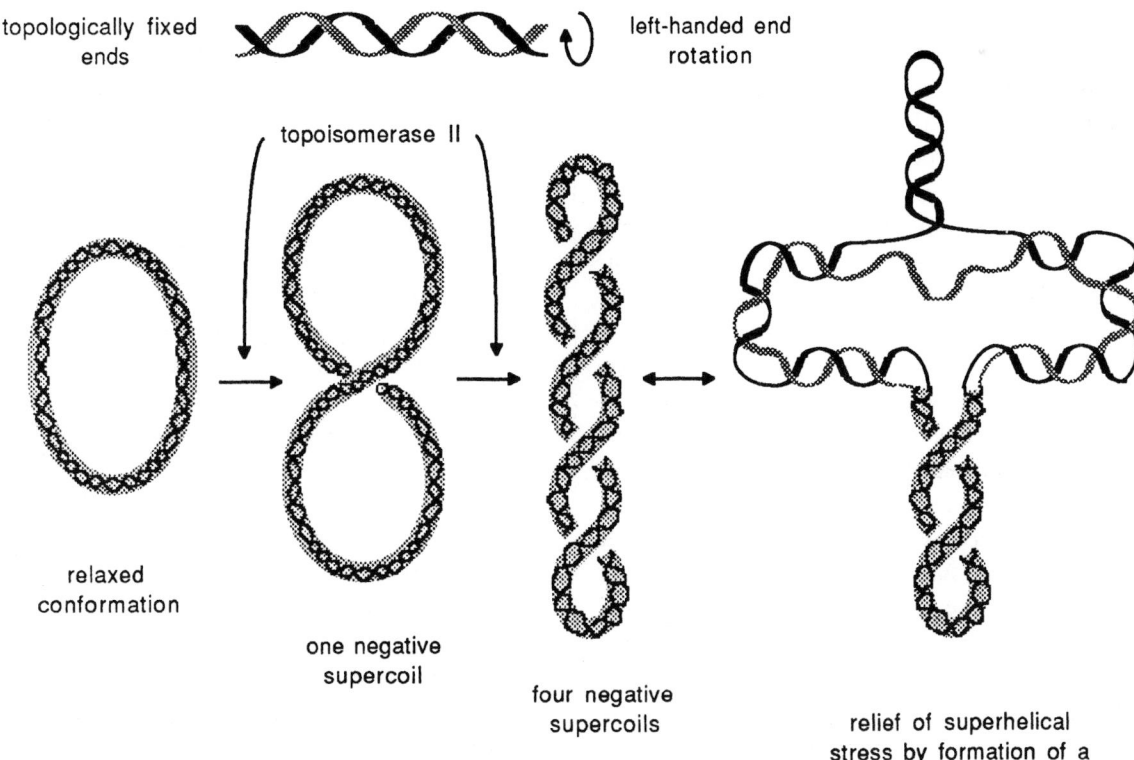

topologically fixed ends

left-handed end rotation

topoisomerase II

relaxed conformation

one negative supercoil

four negative supercoils

relief of superhelical stress by formation of a cruciform structure

Fig. 4.4. Superhelical turns in DNA.

euchromatin. However, some portions of the genome remain highly condensed throughout the entire cell cycle, replicate late during S phase, and are described as *heterochromatin*. Many areas of heterochromatin are located close to chromosome centromeres and to telomeres of acrocentric chromosomes, contain highly repetitive or simple-sequence DNA instead of genes, and may play a structural role in chromosome organization. A special form of heterochromatin is found in the inactive X chromosome in female cells, which contains genes but does not express them. This is partially due to a high degree of chromatin condensation that does not allow access of the DNA to gene regulatory proteins and transcriptional machinery. Inactive X heterochromatin remains highly condensed during the lifetime of somatic cells, but in germ cells it becomes active and euchromatic by the time of entrance into meiosis during oogenesis.

Formation of heterochromatin involves proteins that help direct condensation and packaging assembly of these proteins and DNA into heterochromatin. The molecular mechanisms behind heterochromatin formation have been exposed by studies of inactivation of the other X chromosome in female cells. Heterochromatin spreading is also thought to be involved in the initiation of X chromosome inactivation that occurs in all female cells, since condensation begins from a specific site on the X chromosome, the *X inactivation center, which in human is located on X q13*. At this center, the *XIST* gene encodes a 15 kb functional RNA product, which operates as an inactivator of many X chromosonal genes. *XIST* gets transcribed only from the inactive X chromosome and is thus an example of a gene that is subject to monoallelic expression. During early embryonic development, the X inactivation appears to happen randomly, the X inactivation being independent of the parental origin. However, when female somatic cells replicate their DNA and divide, the inactive X chromosome always gives rise to inactive daughter X chromosomes, even though the active X chromosome in the parent cell may have nearly the same DNA sequence as the inactive X.

XIST is essential for the initiation of X chromosomal inactivation but does not seem to be required for the maintenance of X inactivation. The effect of *XIST* RNA covers a very long genetic distance; *XIST* RNA inactivates genes at a significant interval from *XIST*. Although *XIST* is essential for the X inactivation center, other genes are also required. An X controlling element and a gene called *TSIX* are also required for the maintenance of X inactivation. Detailed analyses of the function of these genes have clarified some general details concerning the heterochromatin formation and gene inactivation.

CENTROMERES AND TELOMERES

Special features of the DNA molecule that comprises each human chromosome are required at the centromere and the telomere. Located close to most centromeres are many copies of a 171-bp sequence—alphoid repeats—that are highly condensed and form heterochromatin. Although the precise DNA sequences required for centromere function in mammals have not yet been determined, they are likely to lie close to alphoid repeat DNA and to bind structural proteins that serve as a site for kinetochore formation and spindle attachment during metaphase. Certain alphoid repeats are found close to the centromeres of all chromosomes, while others are specific for one or a small number of chromosomes. The proteins and DNA sequences that make up the centromere must also ensure that the two daughter chromatids are partitioned to different cells during cytokinesis.

Because template-directed replication of DNA can only be performed in a 5′-to-3′ direction, one strand of each duplex cannot be fully replicated at its 3′ terminus by DNA polymerase. Therefore, the telomeres of each human chromosome contain many copies of a short repeat, 5′-GGGTT-3′, that can be replicated using the enzyme telomerase. This enzyme has an RNA component that itself serves as a template and can elongate the 5′-GGGTT-3′ repeat in a manner that does not depend on the DNA strand.

Repeat content of the human genome

Less than 5% of the human genome sequence encodes proteins, whereas repeat sequences account for at least 50% of the sequence. The repeats fall into five categories: 1) Transposon-derived repeats, often referred as interspersed repeats; 2) inactive retroposed copies of cellular genes (referred as processed pseudogenes); 3) segmental duplications, consisting of blocks of around 10–300 kb which have been copied from one region of the genome into another; 4) blocks of tandemly repeated sequences such as centromeres and ribosomal gene clusters; and 5) simple sequence repeats, consisting of direct repeats of short sequences (like $(CA)_n$ or $(CGG)_n$ which have been extremely important for human genetic studies, since they have been used as genetic markers (see inter-individual variations in the human genome)

Transposable elements in humans, like in all mammals, fall into four types (Table 4.1): Long interspersed elements or LINEs; short interspersed elements or SINEs (including Alu-sequences); LTR retrotransposons; and DNA transposons. Both the number and age of transposable elements

Table 4.1. Number and nature of repeats in eukaryotic genomes

	Percentage of bases		
	Human	**Fly**	**Worm**
LINE/SINE	33.40	0.70	0.40
LTR	8.10	1.50	0.00
DNA	2.80	0.70	5.30
TOTAL	44.40	3.10	6.50

in the human genome is strikingly different from those in other species. The density of transposable elements is much higher in humans than in other species, and the human genome is filled with ancient transposons versus transposons of recent origin in other species. It thus appears that these repeats have prevailed due to significant evolutionary advantage, although their precise function is not well understood. Some chromosomes are extremely crowded with repeat elements, e.g., a 500 kb region in Xp has an overall transposable element density of 89%, whereas some chromosomal regions are nearly devoid of repeats, e.g., the homeobox gene clusters.

Pseudogenes are regions of DNA with many sequence elements of a potential transcriptional unit (e.g., promoter, protein coding region, splice junctions) that do not code for a functional product. They can originate after gene duplication if the duplicated sequence acquires a mutation that prevents its expression. For example, a member of the α globin gene family, $\Psi\zeta$, has all the sequence characteristics of a functional globin gene, but the protein-coding region contains a single point mutation which prevents expression of a full-length globin. A second way that pseudogenes originate is by the pathway of reverse transcription and integration. If the mRNA of a cellular gene is accidentally converted into cDNA by reverse transcriptase, a duplex DNA molecule can be formed that lacks introns and contains a polyA tract. Regions of DNA with this pattern are commonly found in genomic DNA, showing that cellular mRNAs are occasional substrates for reverse transcriptase and that the DNA products can integrate back into the genome.

Large segmental duplications are especially enriched into pericentromeric and to some extent subtelomeric regions of chromosomes. These interchromosomal duplications are sequences from elsewhere in the genome, sized at 1–200 kb and are much more common in humans than in yeast, fly or worm, suggesting a relatively recent origin for these duplications. This clustering of segmental duplications especially in pericentromeric regions may represent a damage-control mechanism; chromosomal breakage products are preferentially inserted into pericentromeric regions.

Interindividual variations in the human genome

Sequencing of the human genome has exposed multiple inter-individual variations. These variants include both simple sequence repeat polymorphisms and single nucleotide polymorphisms. Repeat polymorphisms can represent di-(mostly CA), tri- or tetranucleotide repeats, and they form the basis of the genetic map of the human genome. These repeat markers are multiallelic; the alleles differ in the length of the repeats and thus they can be used to identify the maternal and paternal alleles of individuals as well as to define recombinants between marker loci. The high degree of length polymorphism in the repeat number within the human population is due to frequent slippage by DNA-polymerase during replication. These simple sequence repeats comprise about 3% of the human genome and there is approximately one such repeat per 2 kb of genomic sequence. The repeats are more common in the regions that do not code for polypeptides; however, they can exist in the introns, and some repeats also affect the produced polypeptide that is part of the coding sequence. Well over 5000 repeat markers have been characterized, mapped, and ordered along chromosomal DNA strands. This facilitates PCR-based detection and electrophoretic size-separation of the alleles of each repeat polymorphism. Using this genetic map of the human genome, over 100 disease genes have already been mapped and isolated solely based on their chromosomal position.

Specific triple nucleotides can be unstable, expand and contract in meioses, and are hardly ever inherited in the same length to the next generation. If the repeat becomes excessively long, it can cause diseases like Huntington disease or spinocerebellar ataxia, which are both caused by the expanded repeat CAG in the coding region of a gene that results in a polyglutamine tract within the gene product. Some expanded repeats occur in 5′ and 3′ nontranslated regions and also result in a disease due to their effect on gene transcription.

Single nucleotide polymorphisms or SNPs are also nonrandomly distributed in the human genome. Over 2 million SNPs are identified in the genome sequence but only a small fraction, less than 1%, are predicted to impact the protein sequence. Based on the information provided by the Human Genome Sequencing Project, only some thousands, not millions, of genetic variations contribute to the structural diversity of human polypeptides. The single nucleotide diversity of autosomes is about 9×10^{-4}, and for the X chromosome the diversity is slightly less.

Gene structure and the molecular pathway of gene expression

STRUCTURE OF TRANSCRIPTIONAL UNITS–EXONS AND MRNA

Sequences coding for a single eukaryotic mRNA molecule are often separated by non-coding sequences into non-contiguous pieces along the chromosomal DNA strand (Fig. 4.5). The pieces that code for mature mRNA are referred to as *exons*. During transcription, the exons are spliced together from a larger precursor RNA that contains, in addition to the exons, interspersed noncoding pieces referred to as *introns*. The number of exons coding for a single mRNA molecule depends on the gene and the organism, but varies from one to more than one hundred. Human genes tend to have small exons, encoding an average of only 50 codons. These exons are separated by large introns, often exceeding 10 kb. The size distribution of exons and introns of human genes based on the analyzed sequence information and the comparison to worm and fly sequence is provided in Fig. 4.6 and Table 4.2.

Individual exons often correspond to structural and/or functional domains of the proteins for which they code, such as signal peptide of secretory polypeptides or heme binding domain of globin. For some complex proteins, domains encoded by single exons often appear in apparently

Table 4.2. Characteristics of human genes

	Median	*Mean*
Internal exon	122 bp	145 bp
Exon number	7	8.8
Introns	1,023 bp	3,365 bp
3'UTR	400 bp	770 bp
5'UTR	230 bp	300 bp
Coding sequence	1,100 bp	1,340 bp
Polypeptide	367 aa	447 aa
Genomic extent	14 kb	27 kb

unrelated proteins, suggesting that the evolution of these proteins may have been facilitated by the ability to bring together different protein subdomains by exon shuffling. The origin of intron/exon structure is thought to be extremely ancient and to predate the divergence of eukaryotes and prokaryotes. However, prokaryotes and small eukaryotes (e.g., yeast) have lost their introns during evolution, perhaps because of the strong selective pressure in these organisms to retain a small genome size.

Gene expression

The expression of individual genes can be regulated at multiple levels. Before a gene sequence gets translated into

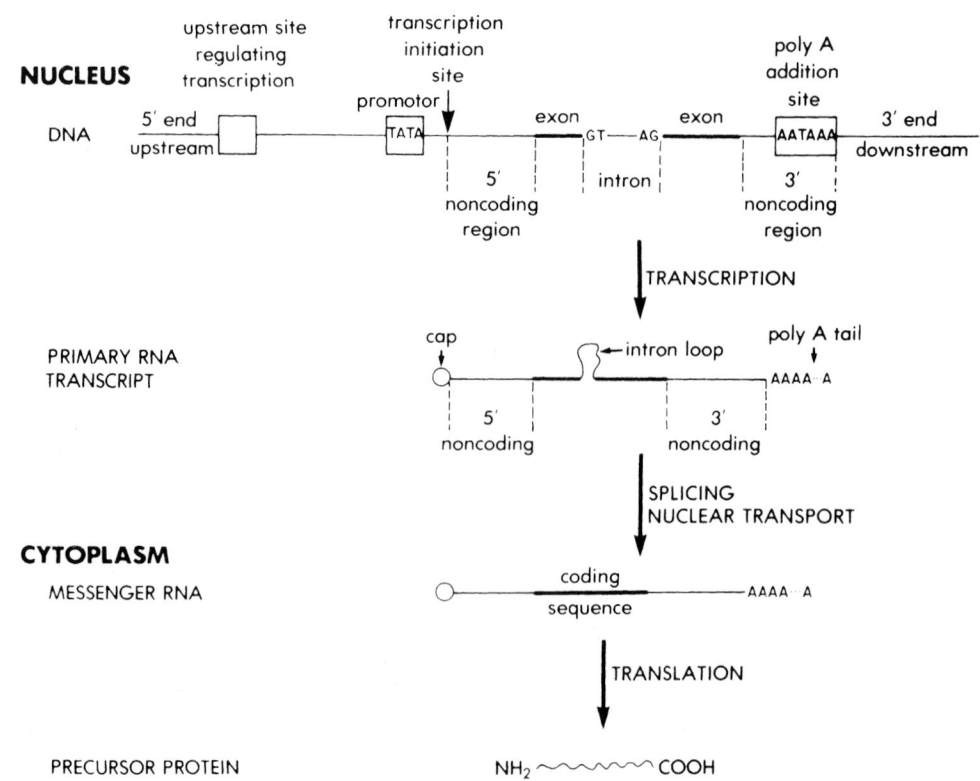

Fig. 4.5. Eukaryotic gene structure and the pathway of gene expression.

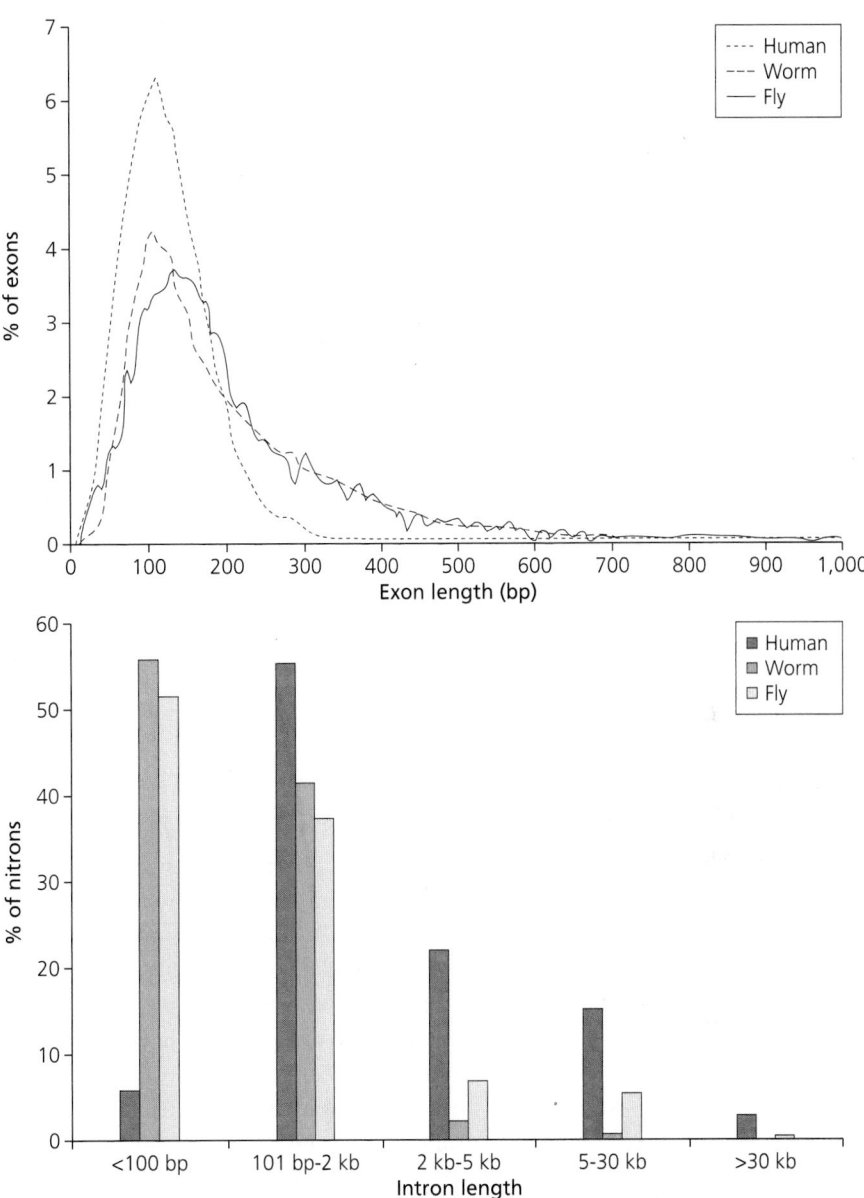

Fig. 4.6. Size distributions of exons and introns in human, worm and fly.

a polypeptide sequence, multiple events take place: Activation of the local DNA structure, followed by initiation and completion of transcription, processing of the primary transcript, transport of the modified transcript to the cytoplasm and translation of the mature mRNA. All these steps can be the target of regulation and potential control points of the gene expression. Some genes are needed in all cell and tissue types since they encode a crucial gene product. Such genes are often referred to as housekeeping genes. However, numerous human and mammalian genes show a highly restricted cell- or tissue-specific expression pattern, and this spatial or temporal restriction of gene expression can also occur at multiple levels.

Transcription

Initiation of transcription happens when the compact DNA structure is loosened and short sequence elements in the 5′ end of the gene guide and activate the DNA polymerase (Figure 4.7). A group of such sequences is often clustered upstream of the transcription initiation site and form the promoter. The *promoter* is a region of DNA in the 5′ end of the genes, that binds RNA polymerase.

There are different types of promoters for RNA polymerase I, II, and III. RNA polymerase I and III are dedicated to transcribe genes coding for RNA molecules (ribosomal RNA, transfer RNA), which assist in the translation of the polypeptide encoding genes. All RNA polymerases are large

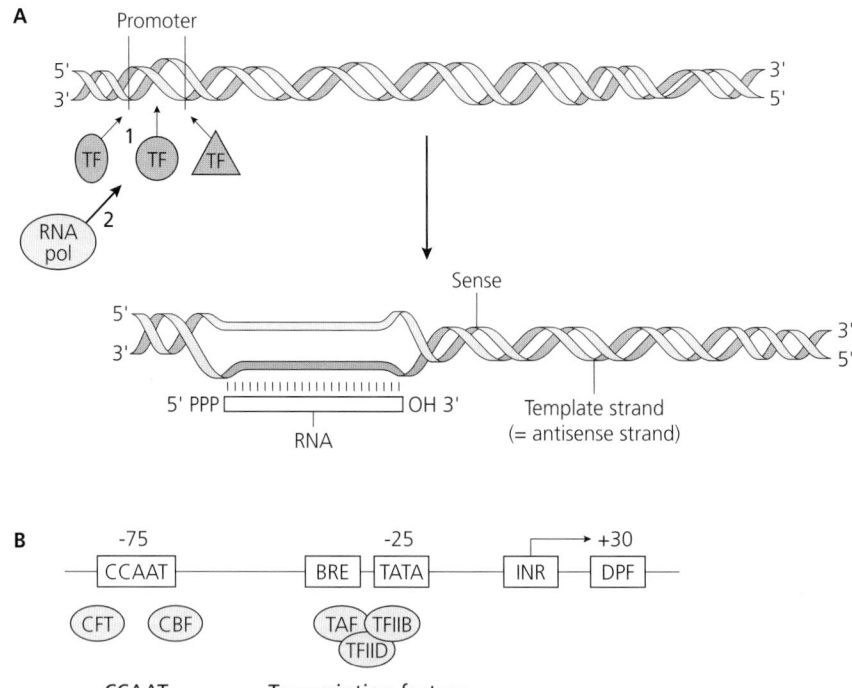

Fig. 4.7. Transcription of eukaryotic genes (A); basic promoter elements in eukaryotes (B).

proteins and appear as aggregates consisting of 8–14 subunits. Significant amounts of information exist on promoter sequences specific for these polymerases. The so-called basal apparatus, the generic minimal promoter sequence which is sufficient to initiate transcription of any protein coding gene, contains a polymerase II recognition signal as well as general transcription factors needed for the binding of the polymerase. This minimal promoter contains a consensus sequence 5′-TATA-3′ some 25 bp upstream of the site at which transcription begins, surrounded by GC-rich sequences, as well as the BRE sequence (transcription factor recognition element), the Inr (initiator) sequence at the start site of transcription and the DPE (downstream promoter element) some 30 bp 3′ from the transcription initiation site. Further, some 50–200 bps upstream is the CAAT box, to which several transcription factors bind. The minimal promoter binds a series of general transcription factors, which are relatively abundant proteins used to initiate the transcription of nearly all mRNAs. The usual nomenclature of the numerous transcription factors is TF followed by a Roman number to indicate the associated RNA polymerase. The general transcription factors like TFIIB, TFIID, TFIIE, TFIIF, and TFIIH facilitate the binding and activation of RNA polymerase II into an activated transcriptional complex.

Genes are constitutively expressed at some basal minimum rate determined by the core promoter. However, the transcription can be increased or totally switched off by additional positive or negative elements (enhancers or silencers), which regulate the efficiency and specificity with which a promoter is recognized by the transcriptional apparatus. These cis-acting regulatory elements are typically short sequences located some 200 bp upstream from the promoter sequence. Finally, gene expression can be regulated by the response elements to external stimuli. These response elements are often less than 1000 bp upstream from the transcription start site. The genes under common control share similar response elements, recognized by regulatory transcription factors. Some response elements are extremely well characterized, such as heat shock response elements or glucocorticoid response elements.

Promoters do not necessarily have to lie upstream of the transcriptional initiation site. In fact, transcription of the small 5S RNA gene by RNA polymerase III uses a promoter that lies 47 bp downstream of the transcription start site in the center of the coding sequence for 5S RNA. This promoter binds the general transcription factor TFIIIA, a large protein with several zinc fingers, which then, along with the factors TFIIIB and TFIIIC, binds RNA polymerase III in a manner such that the polymerase is positioned at the exact spot that transcription begins. Although the mechanism of TFIIIA binding appears to be a common one, promoters that lie in exon sequences may be limited to the special situations in which multicopy genes such as 5S RNA or tRNA are subject to coordinate regulation.

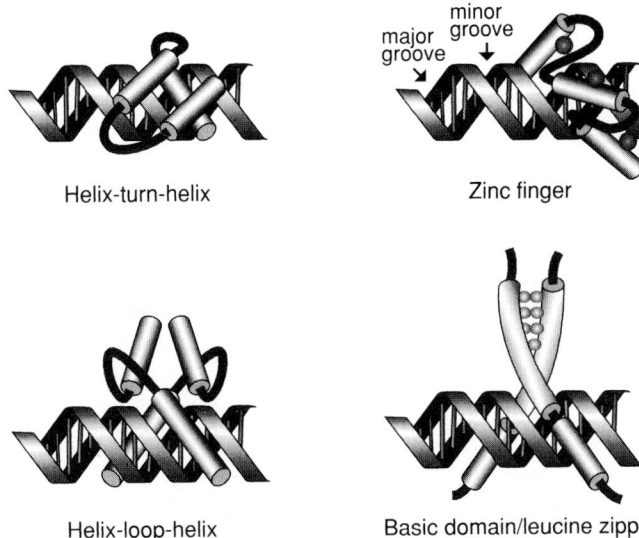

Fig. 4.8. Three-dimensional structure of DNA helix bound to transcription factors.

Comparison of many transcription factors has exposed some structural domains characteristic of the DNA binding character of these proteins (Fig. 4.8). These include zinc finger motifs, helix-turn-helix motifs, helix-loop-helix motifs and leucine zippers. The zinc finger motif involves binding a zinc-ion by four conservative amino acids to form a finger-like loop. The typical loop is 23 amino acids long and the finger structure is often tandemly repeated. The helix-turn-helix motif is a common element of homeobox proteins. It consists of two short alpha helices separated by a short stretch (turn) of amino acids. The helix-loop-helix motif consists of two alpha helices separated by a flexible loop that is flexible enough to allow two helices to pack against each other. The contact of the helix-loop-helix motif with DNA is considered to be looser than other transcription factors. The leucine zipper motif is a helical stretch of amino acids, leucine being every seventh amino acid and occuring once every two turns of the helix. Characteristic to all the transcription factors is that they recognize and bind a short nucleotide sequence and that their binding surface has extensive complementarity to the surface of the DNA double helix. Typically the eukaryotic transcription factors have two functional domains: an activation domain that interacts with other transcription factors (proteins) and a DNA binding domain that binds to the DNA of the target gene.

Enhancers and cis-acting regulatory elements

Enhancers were described originally as cis-acting sequences that increased transcriptional initiation but, unlike pro-moters, were not dependent on their orientation or their distance from the transcriptional start site. It now is apparent that enhancers are generally short (less than 20- to 30-bp) sequences that bind specific transcription factors, which in turn facilitate the assembly of an activated transcriptional complex at the promoter. Most enhancers function whether on the coding or noncoding strand of the DNA (i.e., in either orientation), can act up to several thousand base pairs distant from their promoter target, and are a more general form of cis-acting regulatory elements. Although some upstream regulatory elements can function in most cellular environments, most are active only in specific cell types and therefore play a central role in regulating tissue specificity of gene expression.

Silencers are regulatory elements that reduce transcription levels. They are less characterized than enhancers and some of them are position-dependent while others seem to be position-independent. They can bind transcription factors that act in transcriptional initiation, and many genes contain a combination of both positive and negative upstream regulatory elements which then act in concert on a single promoter. This allows gene expression to be controlled very precisely with regard to cell type, developmental stage, and environmental conditions. For example, upstream regulatory elements direct expression of the erythropoietin gene in a specific subset of renal cells at a certain time in development, and allow modulation of expression in response to changes in oxygenation. Boundary elements are insulators, some 0.5–3.0 kilobases long, which block or isolate the spreading of the effect of enhancers or silencers.

Mutations of gene promoters or enhancers can alter the pattern of expression but not the structure of a particular gene product. Some of the best-known examples are point mutations and partial deletions of the β-globin gene cluster that affect upstream regulatory sequences and lead to reduced expression of adult β-chains in β-thalassemia and/or increased expression of fetal γ-chains in hereditary persistence of fetal hemoglobin (HPFH).

PARTS OF A GENE THAT ARE TRANSCRIBED BUT NOT TRANSLATED

Introns and splice junctions

The number of introns in a simple transcriptional unit will be one less than the number of exons. More complicated arrangements exist in which an upstream exon can be spliced to any of several different downstream exons, or in which a complete transcriptional unit is nested inside the intron of a second transcriptional unit. In these situations, the same DNA sequence can be used both as exon and as intron, depending on the transcriptional unit. Regardless of how the transcriptional unit is organized, the borders between potential exons and introns always share common features thought to be involved in the splicing process itself. Beginning from the upstream or 5′ exon, these *splice junctions* have the sequence

... A<u>G</u>[<u>GT</u> ... A ... PyPyPyPyPyPyPyPyPy<u>N</u><u>AG</u>] ...

where the brackets contain intron sequences, the underlined sequences are characteristics of every splice junction, and the non-underlined sequences are characteristic of the consensus splice junctions. The conserved intron sequences serve a critical role in the splicing process, and many inherited diseases are caused by mutations of the GT or AG intron sequences that flank the splice junctions and result in the abnormal splicing and an abnormal polypeptide chain.

A transcribed precursor RNA molecule must have its introns spliced out and its ends modified before export to the cytoplasm as mature mRNA. Abnormalities in this process are likely to underlie the pathogenesis of mental retardation in the fragile X syndrome, since the mutated gene in that condition encodes a protein that binds to and facilitates the processing of hnRNA. The physical form of hnRNA is a ribonucleoprotein particle in which the hnRNA is bound to core proteins and organized as a series of beads. Small nuclear ribonucleoproteins (snRNPs) have a critical role in the splicing of hnRNA. They consist of 50 to 200 nucleotide long RNA molecules tightly associated with a group of about 10 different proteins. There are a limited number of RNA molecules in snRNPs (described as U1, U2, U3, etc.) and these are among the highly conserved sequences in different eukaryotes. The U1 to U6 snRNPs are integral components of spliceosomes, multienzyme complexes that stabilize intermediates in the splicing reaction. An initial intermediate of the splicing reaction is formed when the 5′ guanylate end of an intron is joined to an adenylate residue near the 3′ end of the intron through a 2′–5′ phosphodiester linkage (Fig. 4.9). After the completion of exon-exon fusion, the excised intron is released as a "lariat structure" with the adenine residue serving as the branch point of the lariat.

The genes encoding rRNA and tRNA also contain exons and introns, but are spliced by different mechanisms than those required for mRNA splicing. Self-splicing of RNA without any protein factors is known to happen in prokaryotes, which suggests that introns have an extremely ancient evolutionary origin, predating not only the eukaryote/prokaryote divergence, but perhaps the origin of proteins as well.

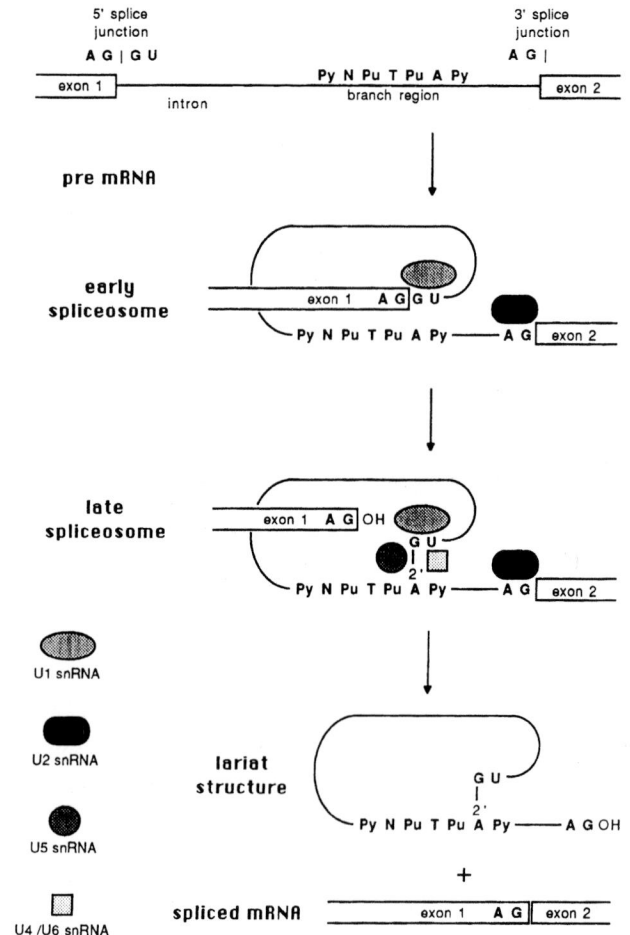

Fig. 4.9. Splicing of mRNA.

5′ untranslated sequences

During the processing of precursor RNA in the nucleus, 3′ termini as well as introns are removed. However, precursor RNA always begins with an exon, so the initial sequences in mRNA are also the first to be synthesized in the precursor RNA. Shortly after initiation of mRNA transcription, a methylguanylate residue is added to the 5′ end of the primary transcript (Fig. 4.5). This 5′ "cap" is a characteristic of every mRNA molecule, and the transcriptional start or initiation site is also referred to as the *capping site*. The 5′ *untranslated region* extends from the capping site to the beginning of protein-coding sequence and can be up to several hundred base pairs in length. The 5′-untranslated regions of most mRNAs contain a consensus sequence of 5′-CCAGCCAUG-3′ involved in the initiation of protein synthesis. In addition, some 5′-untranslated regions contain "upstream AUGs" that may affect the initiation of protein synthesis and thus could serve to control expression of selected genes at the translational level.

3′ untranslated sequences and transcriptional termination

The 3′ end of a mature mRNA molecule is created by cleavage of the primary precursor RNA and the addition of a several hundred nucleotide-long polyadenylic acid tail (Fig. 4.5). The site for cleavage is marked by the sequence 5′-AAUAAA-3′ 15 to 20 nucleotides upstream and by additional uncharacterized sequences 10 to 30 nucleotides downstream (in histone mRNAs, which do not have polyA tails, cleavage of the primary transcript is specified only by downstream sequence elements). The actual length of the primary transcript before cleavage is determined by *transcriptional termination* signals located another 500 to 2000 bp farther downstream of the polyA addition site.

Some complex transcriptional units contain several potential polyadenylation and/or transcription termination sites. It is often difficult to distinguish the latter from the former, since the product available for analysis (mRNA) has lost the portion of the 3′ terminus transcribed by RNA polymerase. Alternative polyadenylation (or termination) sites can determine final protein structure if the longer precursor RNA contains an exon not found in the shorter precursor RNA. In a simple case, two proteins with different C-terminal lengths are formed. But if alternative exon splice sites are made available in the longer precursor RNA, proteins with entirely different sequences can be produced.

The region from the last protein codon to the polyA addition site may contain up to several hundred nucleotides of a *3′ untranslated region*, which includes signals that affect mRNA processing and stability. Many mRNAs that are known to have a very short half-life contain a 50-nucleotide AU-rich sequence in the 3′ untranslated region. Removal or alteration of this sequence prolongs the half-life of mRNA, suggesting that the presence of AU-rich sequences in the 3′ untranslated region may be a general feature of genes that rapidly alter the level of their expression.

TRANSLATION OF RNA INTO PROTEIN

Genetic code

After intron sequences are spliced out of the primary RNA transcript and the 3′ terminus is generated (in most cases, by the addition of a polyA tail), the mature mRNA is transported from the nucleus to the cytoplasm, where it is translated into a polypeptide chain. In the cytoplasm, tRNA molecules provide a bridge between mRNA and free amino acids (Fig. 4.2). Adjacent groups of three nucleotides in mRNA (*codons*) each bind to complementary three nucleotide sequences in tRNA (*anticodons*). Unlike most other nucleic acids, tRNA molecules have a rigid tertiary structure. All tRNAs are L-shaped, with the anticodon located at one end and the amino acid-binding site at the other end. Modified nucleotides, such as methylguanosine (mG) and pseudouridine (ψ), are common in tRNA and help determine the specific three-dimensional characteristics of tRNA molecules. Aminoacyl tRNA synthetases specifically recognize different tRNAs and attach each tRNA to the correct amino acid. The last base in each codon is followed by the first base in the next, and thus the first codon in an mRNA molecule determines the *reading frame* for all subsequent codons.

The relationship between codon and amino acid sequence is referred to as the genetic code (Fig. 4.10). The different tertiary structures of each tRNA are specifically recognized by the proper tRNA synthetase, ensuring the accuracy of the code. Because the anticodon sequence itself does not determine tRNA tertiary structure, each amino acid may have several possible codons recognized by tRNAs with different anticodons but similar tertiary structure; that is, they are recognized by the same tRNA synthetase. For example, 5′-AAA-3′ $tRNA^{Phe}$ (the tRNA coding for phenylalanine with the anticodon 5′-AAA-3′) has the same tertiary structure and is charged by the same tRNA synthetase as 5′-GAA-3′ $tRNA^{Phe}$. Thus, codons 5′-UUU-3′ and 5′-UUC-3′ both code for phenylalanine using different tRNAs but the same tRNA synthetase. Additional redundancy in the genetic code arises because the third base pair in each codon-anticodon duplex (first base pair from the 5′ end of the anticodon) is often an exception to the "rules" of Watson-Crick base pairing. In particular, G:U or U:G base pairs are often found in the third position of a codon-anticodon duplex, and the guanine analogue, inosine, found only in tRNA, can pair or *wobble* with A, C, or U in the

UUU, UUC – Phe UUA, UUG – Leu	UCU, UCC, UCA, UCG – Ser	UAU, UAC – Tyr UAA – stop UAG – stop	UGU, UGC – Cys UGA – stop UGG – Trp
CUU, CUC, CUA, CUG – Leu	CCU, CCC, CCA, CCG – Pro	CAU, CAC – His CAA, CAG – Gln	CGU, CGC, CGA, CGG – Arg
AUU, AUC, AUA – Ile AUG – Met	ACU, ACC, ACA, ACG – Thr	AAU, AAC – Asn AAA, AAG – Lys	AGU, AGC – Ser AGA, AGG – Arg
GUU, GUC, GUA, GUG – Val	GCU, GCC, GCA, GCG – Ala	GAU, GAC – Asp GAA, GAG – Glu	GGU, GGC, GGA, GGG – Gly

Fig. 4.10. Genetic code.

codon. Despite the redundancy of the genetic code, synonymous codons are not used with equal frequency, and the pattern of codon usage (*codon bias*) may vary tremendously among different species and between nuclear and mitochondrial mRNAs.

The AUG codon, which codes for methionine, always begins the protein-coding portion of every mRNA molecule. Therefore, every newly synthesized peptide begins with a methionine. The tRNA^{Met} for this initiator AUG codon has a different tertiary structure from all other tRNAs, including the tRNA^{Met} that functions in elongation. Translation of most mRNAs begins with the first AUG from the 5′ end, which determines the reading frame for the rest of the mRNA molecule. The UAA, UAG, and UGA codons have no cognate tRNAs, and one of these codons ends or terminates the protein-coding portion of every mRNA molecule.

Mutations that change one codon into another that codes for a different amino acid produce a protein with an amino acid substitution and are described as *missense* mutations. However, the UAA, UAG, and UGA codons do not code for an amino acid but instead serve as a signal to terminate protein synthesis (see below). Mutations that produce one of these codons in the middle of a normal reading frame cause truncation of the newly synthesized protein during protein synthesis and are referred to as *nonsense* mutations.

Protein synthesis

The biochemistry of protein synthesis (Fig. 4.11) can be divided into the stages of initiation, elongation, and termination. All three processes occur on ribosomes, cytoplasmic particles of protein and RNA (rRNA) that align the different substrates of each reaction. Active ribosomes are grouped together as strings of up to 50 ribosomes per mRNA molecule (*polysomes*), but inactive ribosomes can be separated into pools of two subunits, described by their size or sedimentation coefficient (S value). The small 40S ribosomal subunit contains 18S rRNA and 33 different proteins, and the large 60S subunit contains 28S rRNA, 5.8S rRNA, 5S rRNA, and 50 different proteins. Translation begins with the formation of a preinitiation complex that contains the 40S ribosomal subunit, initiator tRNA^{Met}, GTP, and several protein initiation factors. One of these factors, eukaryotic initiation factor 2 (eIF-2), may be a rate-limiting component under certain conditions and thus serves as a target for the control of translational initiation. An mRNA molecule initially binds to the preinitiation complex in conjunction with several initiation factors that interact with the 5′ cap structure, after which the mRNA is "scanned" in a 3′ direction until the consensus sequence 5′-CCACC*AUG*G-3′ (*AUG* is the start codon) is reached. Binding of the 60S ribosomal subunit and dissociation of several initiation factors including eIF2 form a complex of proteins and subcellular particles poised to begin synthesis of the first peptide bond.

A ribosome contains room for two tRNAs and their respective amino acids (Fig. 4.11). One tRNA at the peptidyl or P site is connected to the amino acid that has just been incorporated into a nascent peptide chain, and another tRNA at the aminoacyl or A site is connected to a single amino acid ready to participate in protein synthesis. During elongation, a peptide bond is formed between the two adjacent amino acids, the ribosome moves to the next codon in mRNA, the tRNA at the P site dissociates from the nascent peptide chain, and the tRNA at the A site is translocated to the P site. This series of reactions is dependent on elongation factor 1 (EF1), which binds to free charged tRNAs in much the same way that eIF2 binds to the initiator tRNA^{Met}, and EF2, which facilitates translocation from the A site to the P site.

When a codon signifying termination of protein synthesis is reached (UAA, UAG, or UGA), the completed polypeptide separates from the tRNA at the P site, and the ribosome dissociates into inactive subunits. In bacteria and in yeast, a unique group of *suppressor* tRNA mutations is caused by changes in an anticodon that permit cognate binding of a particular tRNA to a termination codon. Point mutations in mRNA that would normally lead to premature termination of protein synthesis (e.g., by changing a UUA codon into a UAA codon), are then partially suppressed by the mutant tRNA. Suppressor tRNA mutations have not yet been identified in mammalian cells.

Protein localization

Gene products function in particular cellular compartments. Histones, tubulin, glycosyl transferases, peptide hormone receptors, and collagen are specifically localized to the nucleus, cytosol, Golgi, cell membrane, and extracellular space, respectively. Although many membranes contain pores large enough to accommodate a linear polypeptide chain, completely folded proteins are generally too large to fit through these pores. Besides the problem of translocating soluble proteins across membranes, proteins that remain attached to the membrane must be placed and oriented in specific ways. These problems—protein sorting, translocation, and membrane orientation—are solved by related biochemical mechanisms that depend on short

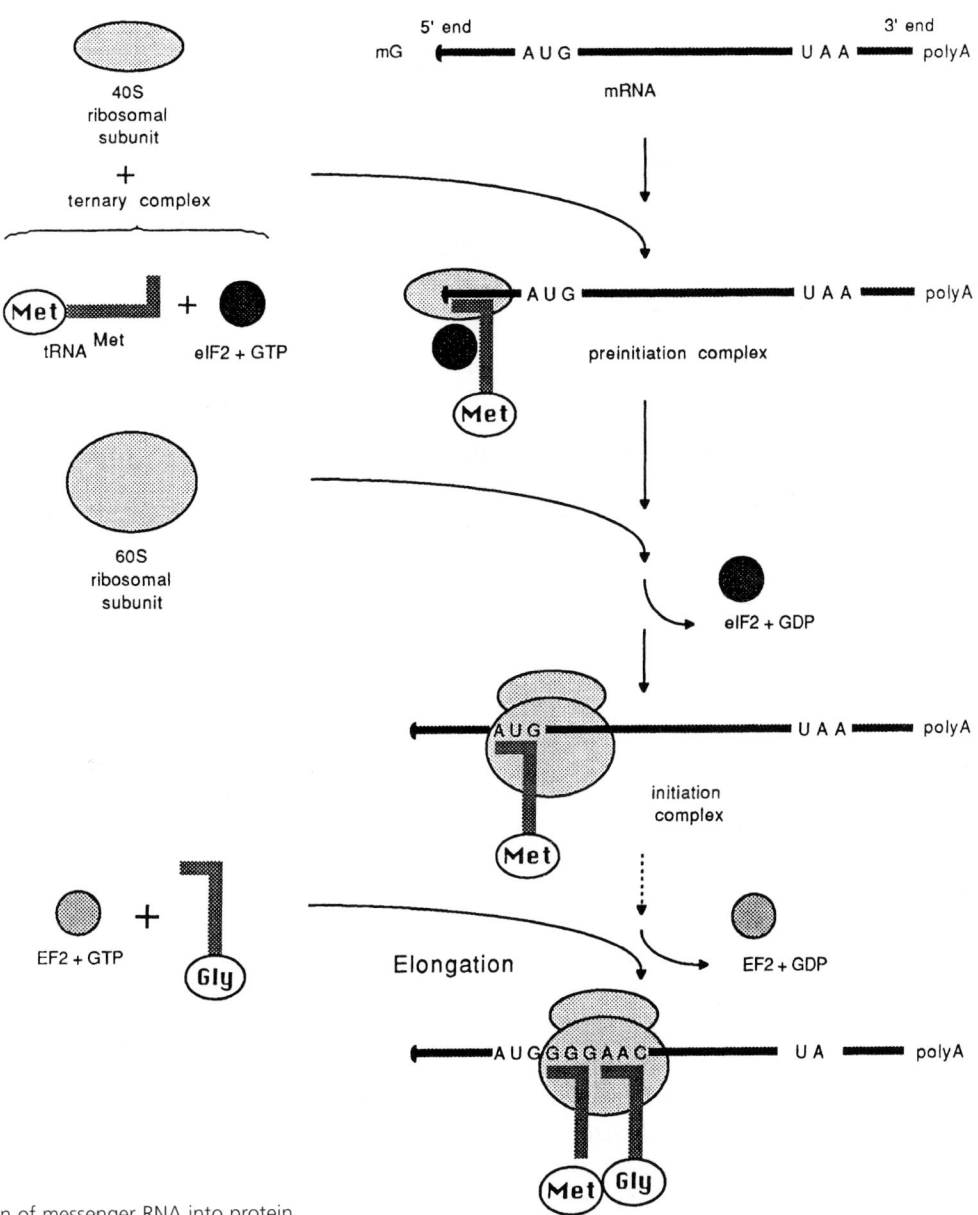

Fig. 4.11. Translation of messenger RNA into protein.

peptide sequences in each protein. One of the most well understood pathways is the initial sorting of gene products into those that will remain inside the cytosol or nucleus and those that pass across the endoplasmic reticulum which are then available for secretion into the extracellular space. This initial sorting is determined early in the translation of proteins destined to cross the endoplasmic reticulum by the presence of a specialized *signal sequence* of 20 to 30 amino acids usually located at the N-terminus (Fig. 4.12).

The signal sequence of a growing polypeptide chain is first "visible" when the polypeptide is approximately 70 amino acids long (about 35 amino acids are "hidden" by the ribosome) and binds to the protein/RNA complex, called the signal recognition particle (SRP). SRP stops further translation until bound to its receptor docking protein, located on the rough endoplasmic reticulum (ER) and associated with a hydrophilic membrane pore. The signal peptide passes through the pore, translation recommences, and the growing polypeptide crosses the membrane. After the completed protein has passed into the lumenal ER, signal peptidase, a protein on the lumenal surface of the ER, cleaves the signal peptide to complete the initial phase of protein sorting.

Extrusion of proteins from the RER pass through the Golgi into secretory vesicles; eventually, the extracellular space does not require specialized mechanisms other than

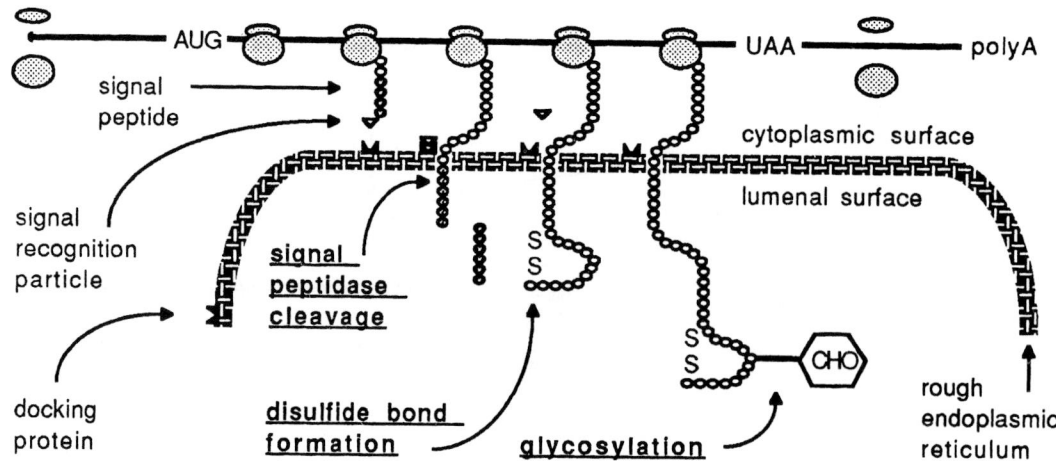

Fig. 4.12. Translocation of newly synthesized proteins across the endoplasmic reticulum.

the presence of a signal sequence and is sometimes described as a default pathway. Insertion and orientation of proteins into the cell membrane, however, requires additional sequences that function either to stop transfer across the membrane (stop transfer sequences), or to initiate transfer of an internal loop of the nascent polypeptide chain (start transfer sequences). Start transfer sequences are recognized by SRP-like N-terminal signal sequences but are not cleaved away from the protein after translocation. The number, order, and orientation of start transfer and stop transfer sequences determine the conformation of complex integral membrane proteins that span the membrane multiple times, such as rhodopsin. Some soluble proteins that contain the short peptide sequence Lys-Asp-Glu-Leu (KDEL) remain in the lumen of the RER, such as binding protein (BiP) and protein disulfide isomerase (PDI). Both BiP and PDI facilitate the folding of newly synthesized proteins in the RER. PDI catalyzes the rearrangement of Cys-Cys disulfide bonds; BiP is a so-called *chaperone* that binds temporarily to portions of other proteins normally not exposed to the surface and, in doing so, prevents partially folded proteins from aggregating. Soluble proteins destined for specialized compartments inside the cell such as lysosomes or peroxisomes use a signal sequence to gain access to the ER lumen but require additional mechanisms for localization. Lysosomal sorting depends on amino acid sequences that specify post-translational addition of a mannose-6-phosphate residue. Proteins containing this modification are selectively transferred from the Golgi to the lysosomal interior. Failure to modify proteins destined for the lysosome in this way is responsible for the inherited disease mucolipidosis II (I cell disease).

Transport of proteins into mitochondria also depends on a signal sequence usually located at the amino terminus,

albeit a different one from that used to facilitate the transport of proteins across the RER. Unlike RER proteins, for which translation and translocation are co-dependent, mitochondrial proteins are first translated completely, released into the cytosol, and then translocated into the mitochondrial matrix or the intermembrane space. The potential problem of translocating a completely folded protein across a membrane pore is solved for mitochondria by chaperone proteins of the hsp70 family, which bind to proteins destined for the mitochondria and prevent them from folding until after they have passed across the mitochondrial membrane.

Post-translational modification

Alterations to protein structure that occur after translation include the formation of disulfide bonds, hydroxylation, glycosylation, proteolytic cleavage, and phosphorylation. Phosphorylation of serine, tyrosine, and threonine residues is a common reversible modification that alters protein-protein interactions or controls enzymatic activity, mostly of intracellular proteins. The formation of disulfide bonds, hydroxylation, glycosylation, and proteolytic cleavage are generally not reversible and are confined mostly to extracellular proteins.

Intramolecular disulfide bond formation usually begins contranslationally as the growing polypeptide chain enters the lumen of the ER. Some proteins, such as immunoglobulin light chains, have a sequential pattern of intrachain disulfide bonds (e.g., between the first and second cysteines, third and fourth cysteines). Other proteins, such as proinsulin, have a more complicated pattern. Protein folding and establishment of the correct arrangement of disulfide bonds are the critical steps in proceeding from a one-dimensional DNA sequence to a three-dimensional protein structure, and in some cases, facilitate one another. Glycosylation of newly synthesized proteins may be O-linked via serine, threonine, or hydroxylysine residues, or N-linked via asparagine residues. O-linked glycosylation is catalyzed by glycosyl transferases, located on the lumenal surface of the Golgi apparatus. N-linked glycosylation begins with transfer of a 14-residue oligosaccharide from a lipid molecule, dolichol, embedded in the RER membrane to the asparagine residue of a growing polypeptide chain. At some sites, the oligosaccharide is highly modified by removal and addition of other carbohydrates to form a complex glycoprotein modification. Other sites are less modified and contain the original high-mannose composition of the dolichol intermediate. Many glycoprotein modifications help determine the specificity of extracellular protein-protein interactions, such as antigen-antibody binding or attachment of cells to the extracellular matrix.

Proteoglycans are a specialized class of extensively glycosylated proteins that contain a protein core with long disaccharide chains branching off at regular intervals and can contain as much as 95% carbohydrate by weight. Proteoglycans are extremely hydrophilic and form hydrated gels that provide structural integrity to the extracellular space. During growth and development, extracellular remodeling is accompanied by endocytosis and degradation of proteoglycans by lysosomal enzymes specific for different disaccharide chains; absence of these lysosomal enzymes produces the mucopolysaccharidoses such as Hunter syndrome or Hurler syndrome.

EXPRESSION OF HOUSEKEEPING AND TISSUE-SPECIFIC GENES

Many proteins that are operating in basic metabolic functions such as energy generation or nutrient transport are found in all cells, and the genes that encode these proteins are described as *housekeeping* genes. They are characteristically expressed at the relatively constant level in all cells. More specialized genes that are not housekeeping are used only at specific times and places during development. The sequence of the human genome has revealed that the most common genes in our genome are those encoding transcription factors and nucleic acid enzymes, which make up 13% out of those some 27,000 genes with known or putative function. Other highly represented genes encode receptors, kinases, and hydrolases. These and other housekeeping genes usually account for 90% or more of the transcripts expressed in any particular cell type. The functional distribution of encoded human proteins based on the current understanding of the genome sequence is given in Figure 4.13.

Analysis of sequence data has revealed that short tracts of DNA with a relatively large proportion of 5'-CG-3'

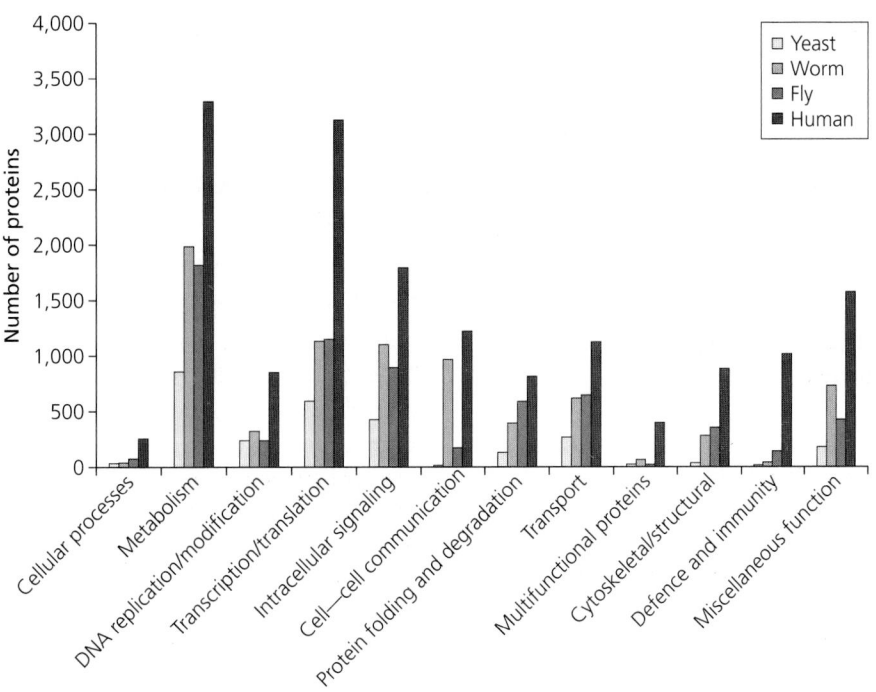

Fig. 4.13. Functional distribution of human gene products based on the genome sequence

dinucleotide pairs and a very high GC content are frequently located near the 5′ end of all housekeeping and also many specialized genes. The genome sequence analysis of almost 30,000 CpG islands has shown that they are characteristically short, more than 89% of them being less than 1800 bp long. The density of CpG islands substantially varies among chromosomal regions. Typically there are 5–15 CpG island per Mb, but the Y chromosome has an unusually low and chromosome 19 an unusually high content of them. The relative density of CpG islands seems to correlate reasonably well with the estimates of relative gene density based on the analyses of ESTs.

Gene families

Gene families consist of structurally (and usually functionally) related genes with a common evolutionary origin. Multiple levels of hierarchical subfamily structure are common. Examples include the immunoglobulin variable region (κ and λ), collagen (interstitial and basement membrane), and globin (α and β) gene families. Some gene family members, such as collagens, are dispersed among different chromosomal locations, but many others, such as the κ or λ variable region genes, are physically linked. Among gene families that exhibit linkage, members are usually oriented in the same direction. In some cases, linkage is thought to be an evolutionary "footprint" without functional significance, suggesting that evolutionary divergence of a gene family occurs through successive rounds of duplication in tandem arrays. However, in certain gene families, such as the immunoglobulins, linkage has been conserved during evolution because it provides a mechanism for co-ordinated or regulated control of expression. Members of gene families are often under similar control mechanisms of gene expression sharing, e.g., carrying similar response elements in their 5′ end.

Modification of DNA in chromosomes during development and reproduction

With the notable exception of the immune system, all cells of a single individual are identical in DNA content and sequence. However, structural modifications of DNA that differ among cell types play a critical role in the control of gene expression during development, differentiation, and reproduction. The two major ways in which DNA is modified—methylation of specific cytosine residues and alterations in chromatin structure—often occur in concert, and help explain alterations in gene expression that are stably inherited in daughter cells. For example, a basal keratinocyte and a hepatocyte have identical DNA sequences but have entirely different patterns of gene expression and cellular phenotypes that are stably inherited during cell division. Heritable phenotypic differences that are not mediated by a change in DNA sequence are described as *epigenetic*. Cellular differentiation, X chromosome inactivation, and parental imprinting (see below) are all examples of epigenetic changes.

GENOMIC MODIFICATION BY METHYLATION

The major site of DNA methylation in mammals is at the 5′ residue of cytosine in the dinucleotide sequence, 5′-CG-3′. Methylcytosine is easily mutable to thymine; the frequency of 5′-CG-3′ dinucleotide pairs in mammalian DNA is therefore quite low relative to other dinucleotides. About one-half of all 5′-CG-3′ sequences in every mammalian cell are methylated, but the CpG islands frequently located near housekeeping genes are usually not methylated. In many cases, methylation of 5′-CG-3′ sites in tissue-specific genes correlates with gene inactivation. For example, certain 5′-CG-3′ residues in the globin genes are methylated in non-erythroid cells but demethylated in reticulocytes. Because maintenance methylases act on hemimethylated duplex DNA, $[Il30]=\&^{5'\text{-mCG-}3'}_{3'\text{-GC-}5'}$, to produce a fully methylated duplex, $=\&^{5'\text{-mCG-}3'}_{3'\text{-GmC-}5'}$, methylation patterns are inherited in a semiconservative fashion during DNA replication and cell division, and provide one possible explanation for patterns of gene expression inherited in an epigenetic fashion.

GENOMIC MODIFICATION BY CHANGES IN CHROMATIN STRUCTURE

Another type of DNA modification that accompanies stable inheritance of a cellular phenotype is the degree of condensation and protein binding reflected in chromatin structure. In general, actively transcribed genes within euchromatin are relatively decondensed and lie on thin loops that may each contain 10 to 200 kb of DNA. Groups of actively transcribed genes are often located on the same loop, or *chromatin domain*. For example, the β-globin gene cluster contains five genes in nearly 100 kb and lies on chromatin that is relatively unfolded in erythroid cells but tightly folded in nonerythroid cells. A small portion of DNA several kilobases long, the locus control region, is located at one end of the β-globin cluster and acts in cis to initiate chromatin unfolding and gene expression over the entire cluster.

X CHROMOSOME INACTIVATION

X chromosome inactivation provides a mechanism for compensating the difference in gene dosage between females, whose somatic cells have two X chromosomes, and males, whose somatic cells have one X chromosome. Therefore, unlike autosomal genes, most of which are expressed in two functional copies per diploid cell, only one allele of most X-linked genes is expressed in female cells (because one of the two X chromosomes is inactivated) and in male cells (because only one X chromosome is present). X inactivation occurs early in development when the human embryo contains several hundred to several thousand cells and, except for placental tissues, occurs at random. During inactivation, a choice is made to inactivate either the paternally derived or the maternally derived X; this chromosome then remains inactive through all subsequent cell divisions. An important exception to X chromosome inactivation involves the distal tip of Xp, which is homologous to a portion of the Y chromosome. This so-called *pseudoautosomal region* contains approximately 2500 kb, is not inactivated, and undergoes recombination with the homologous region on the Y chromosome. In addition, a few genes on the rest of the X chromosome are never inactivated and are therefore always present in two functional copies per cell. Finally, two active X chromosomes are required for normal development of female germ cells, and the inactive X chromosome in germ cell precursors is reactivated during oogenesis.

PARENTAL IMPRINTING

A small number of autosomal genes have been identified in which only one of the two alleles remains active in somatic cells and in which the allele chosen for inactivation depends on parental origin. For example, the gene for an insulin-like growth factor 2 (*IGF-2*) lies on chromosome 11 but is only expressed on the paternally derived homologue. By contrast, the gene mutated in Angelman syndrome lies on chromosome 15 but is apparently expressed only from the maternally derived homologue. Studies in mice suggest that genes subject to parental imprinting undergo a structural modification during gametogenesis that is stably inherited and that later determines whether they are expressed. For example, specific 5′-CG-3′ sites close to the *Igf-2* gene are methylated differently in oogenesis than in spermatogenesis, and these differences in methylation patterns persist in somatic cells of the embryo after fertilization. Like X inactivation, the precise biochemical mechanisms responsible for parental imprinting are not completely understood.

The pathophysiology of certain genetic diseases depends on normal parental imprinting. For example, Prader-Willi syndrome, which commonly results from a microdeletion on chromosome 15, appears to be caused by a gene(s) expressed only on the paternally derived homolog because microdeletions of a maternally derived chromosome 15 do not produce Prader-Willi syndrome, while rare individuals who inherit both copies of chromosome 15 (uniparental disomy) from the mother do have Prader-Willi syndrome. Conversely, Angelman syndrome can result either from microdeletions of a maternally derived chromosome 15 or uniparental disomy for the paternal chromosome 15. As with *IGF2* and *H19*, the gene(s) for Prader-Willi and Angelman syndrome are distinct, yet closely linked and are apparently imprinted in opposite ways.

GENOMIC MODIFICATION BY REARRANGEMENT OF DNA—IMMUNOGLOBULIN GENES

A specialized form of genomic modification is the irreversible rearrangement of DNA that results in the production of antibody and T-cell receptor diversity. This special type of genomic modification has evolved to endow the immune system with tremendous flexibility in confronting foreign antigens. The germline encodes approximately 10^6 types of antibodies, but recombination during development of pre-B cells has the potential to produce more than 10^{15} types of antibodies. This special type of site-specific recombination occurs at short 10 to 20 nucleotide segments and combines regions that are very far apart in the germline and in nonimmune cells into a single gene. Recombination brings together two regions, V and J, to produce a functional light chain gene, while three regions—V, D, and J—are brought together to produce a functional heavy chain gene or T-cell receptor chain. These rearrangements are facilitated by a specialized set of proteins that catalyze site-specific recombination, and absence of recombination produces one form of severe combined immunodeficiency disease. In addition to V-D-J joining, heavy chain genes undergo a second type of DNA rearrangement known as immunoglobulin class switching, which allows a specific antigen-binding site to combine with different C-termini during an immune response. In the initial phases of an immune response, an antigen binding site, encoded by variable regions of heavy and light chains, is connected to the cell surface via the C-terminus of the heavy chain molecule as IgM or IgD. Later in the immune response, DNA recombination connects the same heavy chain variable region with a different C-terminus to produce IgG or IgA (Fig. 4.14).

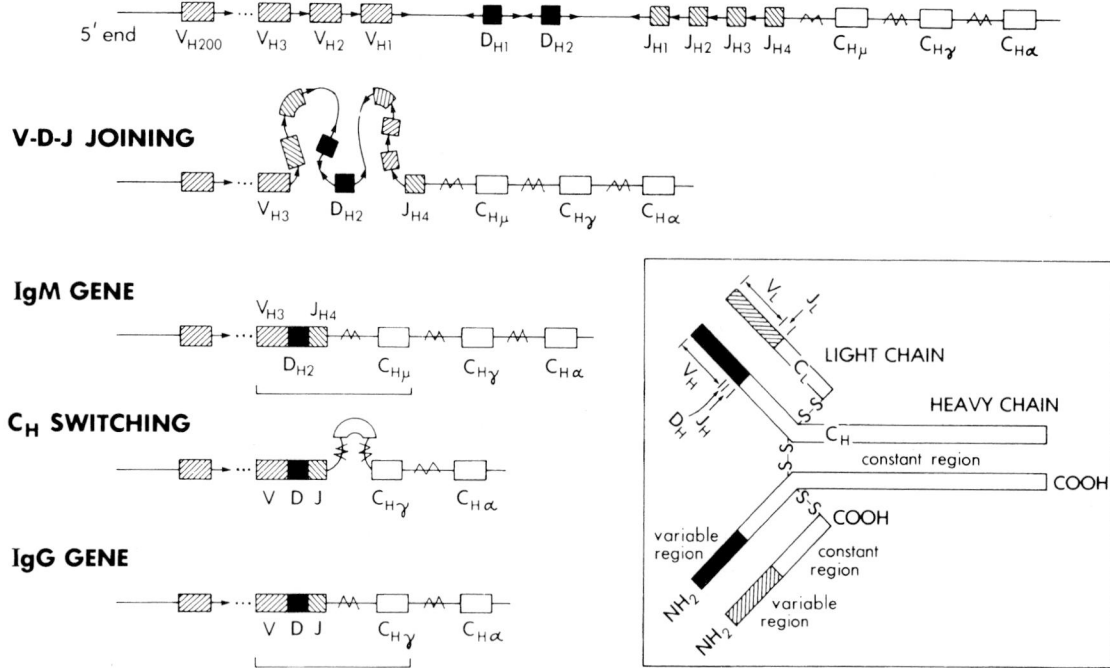

Fig. 4.14 Model of the DNA rearrangements associated with the expression of immunoglobulin heavy chain genes. *Arrows*, blocks of conserved sequences that can pair to facilitate V-D-J joining. The inset is a diagram of a completed immunoglobulin molecule, consisting of both light and heavy chains, with their respective variable and constant regions.

Glossary

Anticodon   The sequence in tRNA or in the noncoding strand of DNA that is complementary to the codon.

Antisense   The nucleic acid sequence complementary to that found in mRNA. Antisense nucleic acid-DNA or RNA-produced as a single strand can potentially bind to and interfere with the processing or translation of a particular mRNA molecule. A few anti sense RNA molecules are made normally that regulate gene expression, and many attempts are under way to use artificial antisense nucleic acids as therapeutic reagents.

Basic Domain/Leucine Zipper   A structural motif that both binds DNA (the basic region) and mediates protein dimerization (the leucine zipper) observed in many gene regulatory proteins including fos, jun, and C/EBPs.

Capping Site   The site in a gene at which transcription of RNA begins. Shortly after transcription, a methylguanylate residue is added or "capped" to the 5' end of mRNA molecules.

cDNA   Refers to DNA complementary to an mRNA molecule. A cDNA copy of a gene does not contain introns and may contain a segment of polyT complementary to the polyA tail of most mRNAs. cDNAs are made using reverse tran scriptase artificially in molecular cloning experiments and naturally during the life cycle of retroviruses and retrotransposons. A single-stranded cDNA synthesized from an RNA template by reverse transcriptase can be converted into a double-stranded cDNA by DNA polymerase.

Chaperone   A protein that aids in the folding and localization of other proteins by binding to hydrophobic regions of nascent or partially folded proteins that are normally not exposed in the mature protein.

Chromatin   The complex of DNA and intimately associated proteins that represents the normal state of genes in the nucleus.

Chromatin Domain   A region of chromatin that contains a group of actively transcribed genes and is often more unfolded and extended than are adjacent chromatin regions.

Codon   The three-nucleotide sequence in mRNA or DNA that encodes a single amino acid.

Codon Bias   For amino acids with degenerate codons, the frequency of codon usage usually is not equally distributed among all possibilities. For example, codons GGA, GGC, GGG, and GGU all code for glycine, but GGC and GGG are used less frequently than GGA or GGU.

Complementary   Two single-stranded nucleic acid molecules—DNA or RNA—are complementary when they form a succession of perfectly matched A:T and G:C base pairs in antiparallel orientation. Note that the sequence 5′-ATGC-3′ is complementary to 5′-GCAT-3′, and not to 5′-TACG-3′. Complementary sequences are produced during replication of DNA and transcription into RNA.

Consensus   Used in the context of molecular biology, a consensus DNA sequence describes a majority of different DNA sequences that bind the same gene regulatory protein.

CpG Island   A region of DNA often found close to the 5′ end of housekeeping genes that is relatively rich in 5′-CG-3′ dinucleotide sequences, where the C is often not methylated.

Cross-Strand Exchange   The four-stranded structure that forms the joint between two duplex DNA molecules during recombination.

Enhancer   The region or regions of a gene that bind specific gene regulatory proteins and thereby help determine the level and the cell type of gene expression.

Epigenetic   Any change in the phenotype of a cell or individual that is heritable but that does not involve a change in DNA sequence is described as epigenetic.

Euchromatin   The majority of nuclear DNA that remains relatively unfolded during most of the cell cycle and is therefore accessible to transcriptional machinery.

Exon   The portions of a duplex DNA molecule that encodes mature RNA.

Gene Conversion   One potential outcome of a cross-strand exchange whereby two homologous portions of paired duplex DNA molecules become identical in sequence. Gene conversion results in a unidirectional flow rather than an exchange of genetic information.

Helix-Loop-Helix   A structural motif that mediates dimerization of many gene regulatory proteins including those that regulate muscle development, such as MyoD and myogenin. These proteins bind to DNA using a basic region similar to that found in the bZIP motif and are often referred to as bHLH proteins. Some gene regulatory proteins such as MYC have both HLH and bZIP motifs.

Helix-Turn-Helix   A structural motif that binds DNA, observed in many gene regulatory proteins, including those that contain homeodomains.

Heterochromatin   Chromosomal regions that remain tightly folded during the entire cell cycle, replicate late during S phase, and do not contain actively transcribed genes. Some heterochromatin is purely structural, contains highly repetitive DNA, and is found close to centromeres, to telomeres of acrocentric chromosomes, and on the long arm of the Y chromosome. In addition, the X chromosome that has been inactivated in female cells folds into heterochromatin.

HnRNA   The immediate product of transcription in the nucleus, which consists of newly transcribed and partially processed RNA molecules of many different sizes.

Homeodomain   A structural motif that binds DNA and includes a helix-turn-helix section. A small subset (about 20) of genes encoding homeodomains play important roles in axial patterning and are referred to as HOX genes.

Housekeeping Gene   A gene required for general cellular metabolism and that is therefore transcribed in nearly every cell of the body.

Intron   The portions of a duplex DNA molecule that intervene between exons and are removed during RNA processing.

Locus Control Region   First defined for the β-globin cluster, the locus control region is a portion of DNA several kilobases in length required for high-level tissue-specific expression of every gene in the β-globin cluster.

Messenger RNA   The type of RNA that encodes protein. mRNA is transcribed by RNA polymerase II and a different set of general transcription factors than those used for other RNAs. Most but not all mRNAs (e.g., histone mRNAs) are polyadenylated at their 3′ termini.

Middle Repetitive DNA   An intermediate class of repetitive DNA with repeat lengths of approximately 100 to 10,000 bp that is generally distributed widely in euchromatin.

Missense   Base pair substitutions that alter the amino acid specified by a particular codon are described as missense mutations, to distinguish them from substitutions that produce a termination codon (nonsense mutations) or those that produce a degenerate codon (silent mutations). For example, an A-to-T mutation that changes the codon GGA to

GGU codon is silent because both codons specify glycine.

Nonsense   A base pair substitution that produces a termination codon (UGA, UAA, or UAG) and therefore results in a protein that is truncated prematurely.

Nucleosome   The smallest unit of chromatin that contains four pairs of histones and 146 bp of DNA folded into a compact bead-like structure.

Polysome   Translational machinery allows the coincident synthesis of multiple proteins from a single mRNA molecule. Ribosomes near the 5′ end of an mRNA molecule are associated with a short nascent polypeptide, while ribosomes near the 3′ end of an mRNA molecule are associated with a polypeptide that is nearly complete. A polysome is the subcellular complex containing one mRNA molecule bound to many ribosomes and their nascent polypeptide chains.

Promoter   The region of a gene that determines where RNA polymerase binds and initiates transcription. Most promoters are located within 100 nucleotides or so of the actual transcriptional start site.

Provirus   The double-stranded DNA copy of a retroviral genome found in the nucleus of a host cell.

Pseudoautosomal Region   The chromosome region on the distal tip of Xp and Yp that contains homologous genes and undergoes recombination during meiosis.

Reading Frame   In an mRNA molecule, the exact nucleotide at which translation begins determines which one of three possible reading frames will be used during translation, since adjacent groups of three nucleotides are "parsed" by the translational machinery. Insertions or deletions of nucleotides that are not multiples of three shift the reading frame of mRNA to encode an entirely different protein.

Recombination   The process whereby two homologous duplex DNA molecules exchange information by crossing over.

Retrotransposon   A DNA molecule that can copy or transpose itself from one site in the genome to another by first being transcribed into RNA, then generating a cDNA copy, and finally via recombination into genomic DNA. Retrotransposons have a life cycle similar to retroviruses but do not exist outside the cell.

RNA Editing   The process whereby the sequence of a mature RNA is altered so that is no longer corresponds to its DNA template.

Satellite DNA   Highly repetitive DNA (generally repeat lengths of less than 5 to 10 bp), often found in heterochromatin, that can be separated from the majority of genomic DNA by density-gradient centrifugation.

Sense   The nucleic acid sequence corresponding to mRNA and used, by convention, in the genetic code. Thus, the mRNA sequence 5′-AUG-3′ is the codon for the amino acid methionine, pairs with the anticodon 5′-CAU-3′ in a tRNA molecule, and is transcribed from a complementary template strand 5′-CAT-3′ in the parent DNA duplex. The terms *sense* and *coding* are often used interchangeably, as are the terms antisense and noncoding. Note that in the parent DNA duplex, the "coding" strand is complementary to the strand that serves as the template for producing mRNA.

Signal Sequence   A region of 15 to 40 amino acids that lies usually at the amino terminus of proteins destined for secretion, membrane insertion, or localization to the endoplasmic reticulum or Golgi apparatus.

Single-Copy DNA   The approximately 70% of DNA in the human genome that is not repeated and thus present in one copy per set of haploid chromosomes.

Spice Junction   The regions that span exon/intron boundaries, and that bind components of the splicing machinery.

Supercoil   The ability of a duplex DNA molecule to form loops or coils. Loops can be oriented in either the same or the opposite direction of the DNA double helix and are described, respectively, as positive or negative.

Transcription   The synthesis of RNA (messenger, ribosomal, or transfer) from DNA by RNA polymerase. Transcription occurs in the nucleus and is the major point at which gene expression is regulated.

Transcription factors   A set of proteins required for RNA synthesis. General transcription factors are required for all RNAs transcribed by a particular polymerase. Specific transcription factors, a subset of gene regulatory proteins, are required for particular genes or groups of genes and play a major role in determining the pattern of genes transcribed in each cell type.

Transcriptional termination   The process whereby RNA polymerase ceases to transcribe a particular gene. The site of transcriptional termination is almost always hundreds or thousands of nucletotides away from the end of mRNA molecules, whose 3′ ends are determined by polyadenylation.

Transfer RNA   tRNA molecules are short adapters that help convert mRNA sequence into amino acid sequence. Each tRNA folds into a unique three-dimensional configuration recognized by a specific tRNA synthetase that "charges" the tRNA with the correct amino acid. Thus, correct interpretation of the genetic code requires not only correct pairing between codon and anticodon, but also correct charging of each tRNA.

Translation The process whereby protein is synthesized from an mRNA sequence. Translation occurs in the cytoplasm and relies on a complex biochemical machinery that includes ribosomes and tRNA molecules.

Untranslated Region The portions of a gene that are tran scribed into mRNA but that are not translated into protein. By definition, untranslated regions are found in exons.

Wobble Base pairing between the codon of an mRNA molecule and an anticodon of a tRNA molecule is said to occasionally wobble at the third residue of the codon. Wobble base pairing is one of the factors that contributes to degeneracy of the genetic code whereby multiple codons specify the same amino acid.

X-Inactivation Center The site on the X chromosome from which inactivation and folding into heterochromatin commences.

Zinc Finger A structural motif that binds DNA and is observed in many gene regulatory proteins including TFIIIA, required for the transcription of small RNAs.

SUGGESTED READINGS

GENERAL

Alberts B, Bray D, Lewis J et al. (1994) Molecular Biology of the Cell, 3rd edn. Garland, NY

Darnell J, Lodish H, Baltimore D (1990) Molecular Cell Biology, 2nd edn. WH Freeman, NY

International Human Genome Sequencing Consortium (2001) Initial sequencing and analysis of the human genome. Nature 409:860–920

Lewin B (1994) Genes. Vol. V. Oxford University Press, New York

Venter JC, Adams MD, Myers EW et al. (2001) The sequence of human genome. Science 291:1304–1350

DNA STRUCTURE, REPLICATION, AND RECOMBINATION

Clark AJ, Sandler SJ (1994) Homologous genetic recombination: The pieces begin to fall into place. Crit Rev Microbiol 20:125–142

Hagerman PJ (1990) Sequence-directed curvature of DNA. Annu Rev Biochem 59:755–781

Kornberg A, Baker T (1992) DNA Replication. WH Freeman, NY

Schleif R (1992) DNA looping. Annu Rev Biochem 61:199–223

Trifonov EN (1991) DNA in profile. Trends Biochem Sci 16:467–470

DNA TRANSCRIPTION AND GENE REGULATORY PROTEINS

Gehring WJ, Muller M, Affolter M et al. (1990) The structure of the homeodomain and its functional implications. Trends Genet 6:323–329

Harrison SC, Aggarwal AK (1990) DNA recognition by proteins with the helix-turn-helix motif. Annu Rev Biochem 59:933–969

McKnight SL (1991) Molecular zippers in gene regulation. Sci Am 264:54–64

Pabo CO, Sauer RT (1992) Transcription factors: structural families and principles of DNA recognition. Annu Rev Biochem 61:1053–1095

Rhodes D, Klug A (1993) Zinc fingers. Sci Am 268:56–65

Schwabe JW, Rhodes D (1991) Beyond zinc fingers: steroid hormone receptors have a novel structural motif for DNA recognition. Trends Biochem Sci 16:291–296

White RJ, Jackson SP (1992) The TATA-binding protein: A central role in transcription by RNA polymerases I, II and III. Trends Genet 8:284–288

RNA PROCESSING

Atwater JA, Wisdom R, Verma IM (1990) Regulated mRNA stability. Annu Rev Genet 24:519–541

Hodges P, Scott J (1992) Apolipoprotein B mRNA editing: A new tier for the control of gene expression. Trends Biochem Sci 17:77–81

Ruby SW, Abelson J (1991) Pre-mRNA splicing in yeast. Trends Genet 7:79–85

PROTEIN SYNTHESIS

Altmann M, Trachsel H (1993) Regulation of translation initiation and modulation of cellular physiology. Trends Biochem Sci 18:429–432

Hershey JW (1991) Translational control in mammalian cells. Annu Rev Biochem 60:717–755

Maden T (1993) The translational apparatus, from Berlin. Trends Biochem Sci 18:155–157

CHROMATIN AND CHROMOSOME STRUCTURE

Blackburn EH (1992) Telomerases. Annu Rev Biochem 61:113–129

Grunstein M (1990) Nucleosomes: Regulators of transcription. Trends Genet 6:395–400

Hansen JC, Ausio J (1992) Chromatin dynamics and the modulation of genetic activity. Trends Biochem Sci 17:187–191

Morse RH (1992) Transcribed chromatin. Trends Biochem Sci 17:23–26

Moyzis RK (1991) The human telomere. Sci Am 265:48–55

Svaren J, Chalkley R (1990) The structure and assembly of active chromatin. Trends Genet 6:52–56

Willard HF (1990) Centromeres of mammalian chromosomes. Trends Genet 6:410–416

EPIGENETIC CONTROL: DNA METHYLATION, X-INACTIVATION, AND PARENTAL IMPRINTING

Landman OE (1991) The inheritance of acquired characteristics. Annu Rev Genet 25:1–20

Lyon MF (1993) Epigenetic inheritance in mammals. Trends Genet 9:123–128

Migeon BR (1994) X-chromosome inactivation: Molecular mechanisms and genetic consequences. Trends Genet 10:230–235

Moore T, Haig D (1991) Genomic imprinting in mammalian development: a parental tug-of-war. Trends Genet 7:45–49

Sapienza C (1990) Parental imprinting of genes. Sci Am 263:52–60

Varmuza S, Mann M (1994) Genomic imprinting—defusing the ovarian time bomb. Trends Genet 10:118–123

IMMUNE SYSTEM

Gellert M (1992) Molecular analysis of V(D)J recombination. Annu Rev Genet 26:425–446

Harriman W, Volk H, Defranoux N, Wabl M (1993) Immunoglobulin class switch recombination. Annu Rev Immunol 11:361–384

Schatz DG, Oettinger MA, Schlissel MS (1992) V(D)J recombination: molecular biology and regulation. Annu Rev Immunol 10:359–383

Mutations in human disease: nature and consequences

5

Stylianos E. Antonarakis
Michael Krawczak
David N. Cooper

Introduction

Recent advances have made possible the localization and isolation of numerous disease-related genes and the direct detection of the underlying pathological lesions. Single base-pair substitutions and micro-deletions are the commonest mutations in the human genome, the remainder comprising an assortment of insertions, duplications, inversions, expansions and complex rearrangements. Characterized mutations occur not only in coding sequences but also in promoter regions, splice junctions, within introns and untranslated regions. Mutations may interfere with any stage in the pathway of expression from gene to protein product. This chapter attempts to provide an overview of the nature of mutations causing human genetic disease and then considers their consequences for the clinical phenotype. Further detailed discussion on this topic can be found in Cooper et al. (1995) and in the monograph by Cooper and Krawczak (1993). The interested reader is also referred to Vogel (1990) for a detailed discussion of mutation rates and factors influencing the generation of mutations. Finally, there are two online databases that contain disease-related mutations: the first is the "Online Mendelian Inheritance in Man" (OMIM) and the second is the "Human Gene Mutation Database" (HGMD).

Neutral variation/DNA polymorphisms

There is enormous variation manifest in the DNA sequences of any two randomly chosen human haploid genomes.

Clearly, not all variations within a gene cause abnormal expression of abnormal protein products. Indeed, single nucleotide substitutions/polymorphisms (SNP) occur in 1/ 1000 nucleotides in intervening sequences and flanking DNA (Antonarakis et al., 1985; Cooper et al., 1985; Nickerson et al. 1998; Wang et al., 1998). These substitutions represent one form of DNA polymorphism that can be used as markers for specific regions of the genome. Similarly, some single nucleotide substitutions in the coding regions of genes may also be normal polymorphic variants even if they alter the polypeptide product (Orkin et al., 1982). For example, there are three common alternative sequences of the β-globin (*HBB*) gene on chromosome 11p. These forms differ at five nucleotides, one of which is within the first exon of the gene.

Another form of normal variation in our genome is the presence of variable numbers of tandem repeats (VNTR). The repeat unit can be 10 to 60 nucleotides in length and many different alleles may exist at a given locus (Wyman and White, 1980; Jeffreys et al., 1985). The combination of a VNTR and single nucleotide substitutions within the repeat unit results in an extremely high level of polymorphic variability that can be used as a bar code for the identification of different individuals (Jeffreys et al., 1990). The introduction of the polymerase chain reaction (PCR) (Saiki et al, 1985) permitted the rapid detection and analysis of variation in short sequence repeats (SSR), for example $(GT)_n$ repeats (Weber and May, 1989; Litt and Luty, 1989). These are common polymorphisms that occur on average one in 50 kilobases (kb) of DNA. The SSRs also display many alleles and the repeat unit can be two, three, four, five or more nucleotides. Poly (A) tracts may also be polymorphic, exhibiting variation in the number of A residues (Economou et al., 1990); many of these polymorphisms are localized at the ends of *Alu* repetitive elements. Another kind of poly-morphism in the human genome is the presence or absence of retrotransposons (i.e., *Alu* or LINE repetitive elements or pseudogenes) at specific locations (Anagnou et al., 1984; Cooper 1999). Finally, duplicational polymorphisms have been reported for some human genes, e.g. *HBA1, PRB1–4, HBZ, CYP21/C4A/C4B* (Cooper, 1999).

DNA polymorphisms have proven extremely useful in developing linkage maps for the human genome, for mapping monogenic and polygenic complex disorders, for determining the origin of aneuploidies and chromosomal abnormalities, for distinguishing normal from mutant chro-mosomes in genetic diagnoses, for performing forensic, paternity, and transplantation studies, for studying the evo-lution of the genome, the loss of heterozygosity in certain malignancies, the instability of the genome in certain tumors and recombination within the genome. However, in studying the role of a candidate gene in a given disorder, it is imperative to distinguish between mutations that cause a clinical phenotype and the polymorphic variability of the normal genome.

Disease-causing mutations

THE NATURE OF MUTATION

Figure 5.1A depicts the frequencies of the various mutation types responsible for molecularly characterized human genetic disorders, as recorded in the "Human Gene Mutation Database" (HGMD) (Krawczak et al., 2000a). HGMD records each mutation *once* regardless of the number of independent occurrences of that lesion. Figure 5.1B shows the frequency of the first mutation per disease recorded in "Mendelian Inheritance in Man" (MIM) and Antonarakis and McKusick, 2000. On 14 September 2000, HGMD contained some 23,800 different mutations in 1084 human genes, whereas MIM contained examples of allelic variants in 1070 human genes.

Nucleotide substitutions

Single nucleotide substitutions are the most frequent muta-tions in the genome (Fig. 5.1). Most of these alterations occur during DNA replication, which is an accurate, yet error-prone multistep process. The accuracy of DNA repli-cation depends on the fidelity of the replicative step and the efficiency of the subsequent error correction mechanisms (Loeb and Kunkel, 1982). Analysis of more than 7000

nucleotide substitutions associated with human disorders shows that the most common substitution for T (thymine) is to C (cytosine), for C it is to T, for A (adenine) it is to G (guanine) and for G it is to A (Krawczak et al., 1998). Transitions are therefore much more common than trans-versions. Roughly, 63% of substitutions are transitions (T to C, C to T, A to G, G to A) and 37% are transversions (T to A or G, A to T or C, G to C or T, C to G or A).

Among single nucleotide substitutions, there is one that predominates and it is the most common type of mutational lesion: CpG dinucleotides mutate to TpG at a frequency that is about 5 times higher than mutations in all other di-nucleotides (Youssoufian et al., 1986 1988; Cooper et al., 1995; Krawczak et al., 1998). This substitution, which when it occurs on one DNA strand generates TG, and on the other, CA (CG to TG or CA rule), represents a major cause of human genetic disease. This phenomenon was first observed in the factor VIII (*F8C*) gene in cases of hemo-philia A (Youssoufian et al., 1986), but it was soon noted in studies of many other genes (Cooper and Youssoufian, 1988). In deed, in hemophilia A, CG to TG or CA muta-tions account for 46% of point mutations in unrelated patients (Antonarakis et al., 1995). In the "Human Gene Mutation Database" (HGMD) (Krawczak et al., 2000a) such mutations account for ~23% of the total (Krawczak et al, 1998). Among CpG dinucleotide mutations, transi-tions to TG or CA account for ~90% of substitutions. The mechanism of this common type of mutation appears to be methylation-mediated deamination of 5-methylcytosine. In eukaryotic genomes, 5-methylcytosine (5 mC) occurs pre-dominantly in CpG dinucleotides, most of which appear to be methylated (see Cooper, 1983, for review). The 5 mC then undergoes spontaneous non-enzymatic deamination to form thymine (Fig. 5.2). There is a bias in terms of the origin of CpG to TpG mutations: most occur in male germ cells (M/F ratio is 7 to 1). One reason for this may be that sperm DNA is heavily methylated, whereas oocyte DNA is comparatively undermethylated (Driscoll and Migeon, 1990). Another reason may be the considerably higher number of germ-line cell divisions in males as compared to females (Hurst and Ellegren, 1998).

Deletions or insertions of a few nucleotides

Deletions or insertions of a few nucleotides are also fairly common in the human genome. Most of these are less than 20 base-pairs (bp) in length. Indeed, the majority of micro-deletions involve <5 nucleotides. In HGMD, deletion of 1 base-pair accounts for 40% of small deletions whilst an addi-tional 30% involve two or three nucleotides. The majority

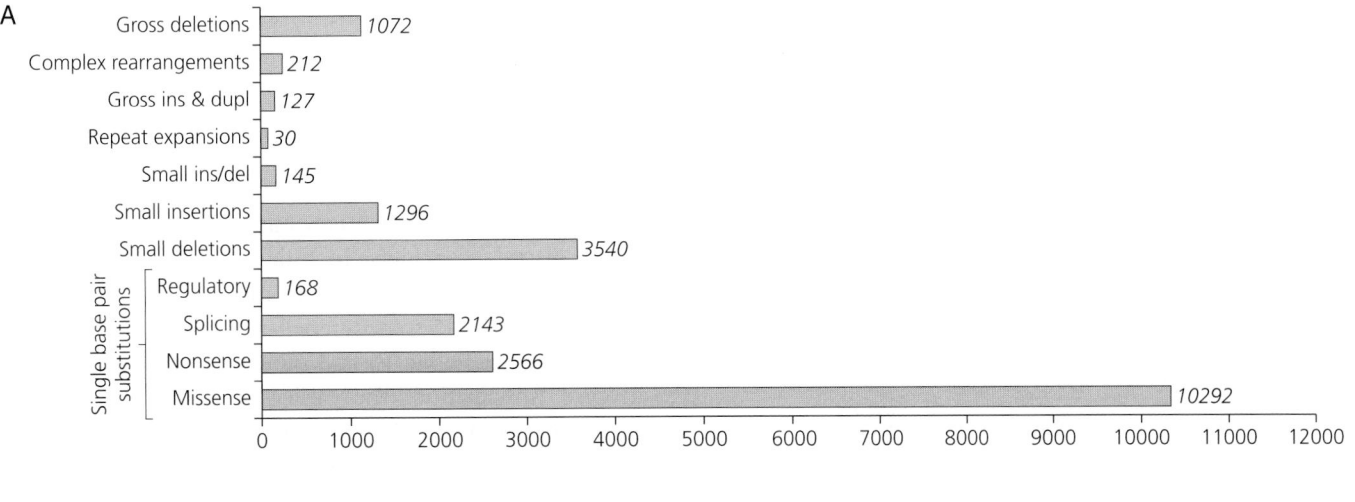

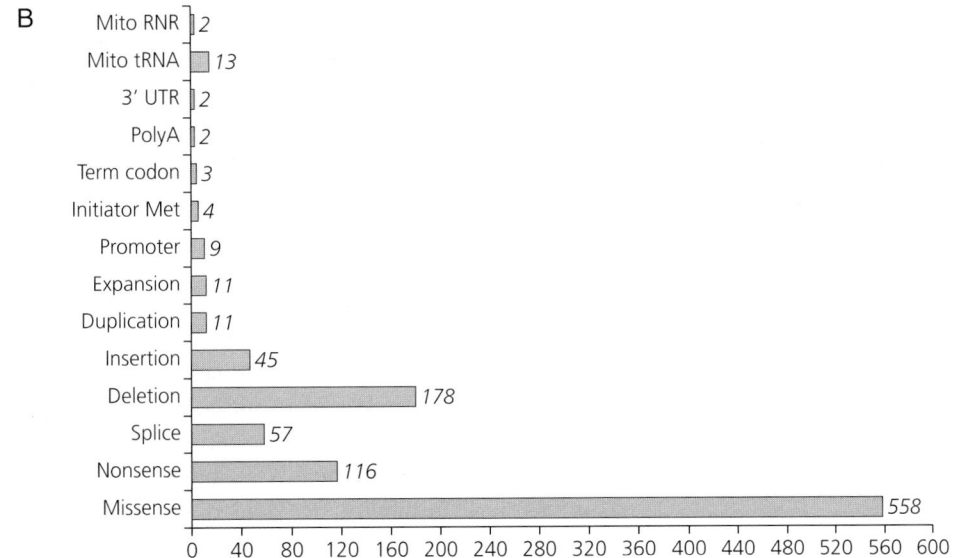

Fig. 5.1. (A) Spectrum of different types of human gene mutation logged in the Human Gene Mutation Database as of May 2000. (B) Spectrum of different types of human gene mutation logged as the first reported mutation per disease in Mendelian Inheritance in Man (data as of March 15, 2000).

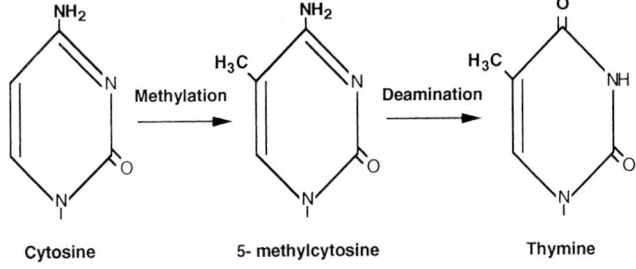

Fig. 5.2. Schematic representation of cytosine, 5'-methylcytosine and thymine, and the chemical events involved in the transformation of cytosine to thymine.

of small deletions recorded (78%) result in an alteration of the reading frame. Most micro-deletions occur in regions that contain direct repeats of 2 bp or more. The most common length of direct repeat is 3 bp (48% of direct repeats associated with short deletions) (Cooper et al., 1995). The most plausible mechanism for small deletions mediated by the presence of direct repeats is the slipped mispairing model of Efstratiadis, et al.. (1980) (Fig. 5.3). In addition, deletions of one or a few nucleotides frequently occur in runs of the same nucleotide, for example a poly (T) region (Kunkel, 1985). Finally, inverted repeats and «symmetric elements» are also frequently found in the immediate vicinity of micro-deletions (Cooper and Krawczak, 1993; Schmucker and Krawczak, 1997).

Micro-insertions (again up to 20 nucleotides) are rarer than micro-deletions; thus in HGMD there are three times more micro-deletions than micro-insertions recorded (Fig. 5.1A). Nearly half of these involve the insertion of

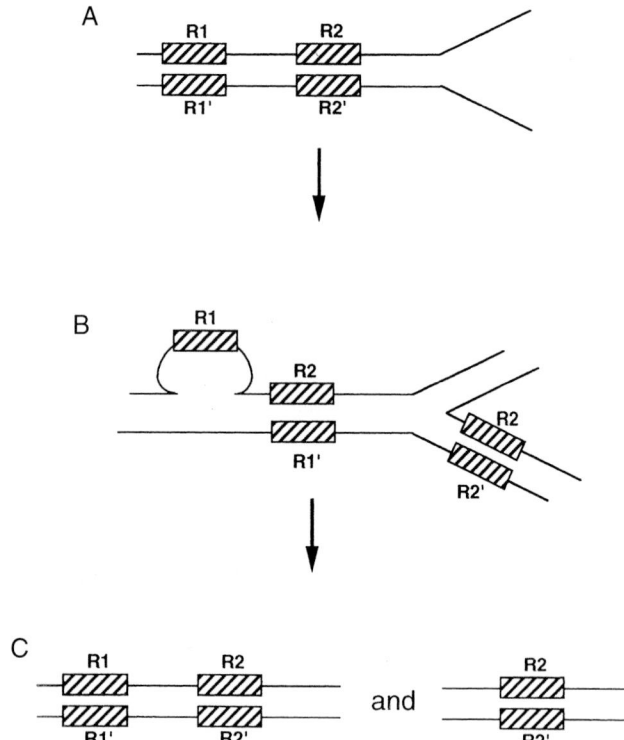

Fig. 5.3. Schematic representation of the slipped mispairing model of mutagenesis during DNA replication. (A) Double-stranded DNA containing R1 and R2 direct repeats. (B) Double-stranded DNA becoming single-stranded at the replication fork and repeat R2 base-pairs with R1' producing a single-stranded loop. (C) The loop is excised yielding two kinds of new double-stranded molecules: one contains a single repeat and lacks sequences between the repeats, the other has the parental configuration. From Cooper et al. (1995) The nature and mechanisms of human gene mutation. In Scriver et al. (eds) *Molecular Bases of Inherited Disease*, 7th edit. © 1995, McGraw-Hill.

only 1 nucleotide. As is the case with micro-deletions, most micro-insertions lead to alterations of the reading frame and are located in regions containing direct or inverted repeats or runs of the same nucleotide. Details of mechanisms of generation during replication can be found in Cooper and Krawczak (1991). There are insufficient data available to estimate the frequency ratio of micro-insertions or deletions in male or female germ cells. In the case of such lesions in the Factor VIII Mutation database, 56% of small deletions/insertions occur in DNA regions harbouring direct repeats or runs of the same nucleotide (Antonarakis et al., 1995).

Expansion of trinucleotide (and other) repeat sequences

Another mechanism of human gene mutation causing hereditary disease is the instability of certain trinucleotide repeats and their expansion in affected genes (Caskey et al.,

1992; Rousseau et al., 1992; Mandel, 1993). A growing number of disorders (a total of 30 recorded in HGMD), the majority of which involve neuromuscular tissues, have been found to be due to the expansion of trinucleotide repeats. The first such disease was fragile X, a common cause of male mental handicap, that mapped to chromosome Xq27.3. Table 5.1 lists some of the characteristics of these disorders which include Huntington disease, myotonic dystrophy, spinobulbar muscular atrophy, spinocerebellar ataxia 1, spinocerebellar ataxia 3 or Machado-Joseph disease, fragile E, and dentatorubral pallidoluysian atrophy. Anticipation (the earlier onset and more severe phenotype in successive generations) is a common phenomenon in these disorders (Harper et al., 1992). The trinucleotide involved is usually either CAG or CGG but occasionally CTG, GCG or GAA. It can be located in the 5′ untranslated region (UTR) as in the case of the *FMR1* gene underlying fragile X, in the coding region (as in Huntington disease, SCA1, SCA3 and Kennedy disease) coding for poly(Gln), in an intron as in Friedreich ataxia, or in the 3′ UTR as in myotonic dystrophy (Table 5.1). The expansion of the triplet repeat either silences the gene (abolishes its expression) or results in a dominant gain-of-function mutation mediated by the longer poly(Gln) peptide (Housman, 1995). The trinucleotide repeats are usually polymorphic in human populations. Rarely, however, the number of trinucleotide repeats lie within a high risk category that is termed premutation. In such a case, the premutation exhibits a high probability of further expansion (instability) to yield disease-related alleles (full mutation). In fragile X, for example, the normal polymorphic alleles of the CGG repeat contain between 10 and 50 triplets, the premutation between 50 and 200, and the full mutation more than 200 triplets (Fu et al., 1991). Expansion of premutations to full mutations only occurs during female meiotic transmission. The probability of repeat expansion correlates with repeat copy number in the premutated allele. Since the premutation must precede the appearance of a full mutation, all mothers of affected children carry either a full mutation or a premutation (Fu et al, 1991).

The precise mechanism of repeat expansion is unclear although it is known that DNA polymerase progression is blocked by CTG and CGG repeats and the resultant idling of the polymerase could serve to catalyse slippage leading to repeat expansion (Kang et al., 1995). In the case of spinocerebellar ataxia 1 (SCA1), interruption of the CAG repeat with a CAT unit is associated with a more stable trinucleotide repeat (Chung et al., 1993). More details about these dynamic mutations can be found in the appropriate chapters

Table 5.1 Various examples of disorders of trinucleotide and other repeat expansions

Disorder	Inheritance	Gene	Chr	OMIM#	Repeat	Normal	Mutant	Repeat location	Mutation type	Parental gender bias
1 Fragile X syndrome	XLD	FMR1	Xq27.3	309550	CGG	6-52	60-200 premutation 230-1000 full maturation	5'UTR	LOF, FraX	Paternal
2 Fragile E mental retardation	XLD	FMR2	Xq28	309548	GCC	7-35	130-150 premutation 230-750 full maturation	5'UTR	LOF, FraX	ND
3 Myotonic dystrophy	AD	DMPK	19q13	160900	CTG	5-37	50-3000	3'UTR	?Dom negative	Maternal
4 Spinobulbar muscular atrophy	XLD	AR	Xq13-21	313700	CAG	11-33	38-66	Coding	GOF, LOF	ND
5 Huntington disease	AD	HD	4p16.3	143100	CAG	6-39	36-121	Coding	GOF	Paternal
6 Dentatorubro-pallidoluysian atrophy	AD	DRPLA	12p13.31	125370	CAG	6-35	51-88	Coding	GOF	Paternal
7 Spinocerebellar ataxia 1	AD	SCA1/ATX1	6p23	601556	CAG	6-39	41-81	Coding	GOF	Paternal
8 Spinocerebellar ataxia 2	AD	SCA2/ATX2	12q24.1	601517	CAG	14-31	35-64	Coding	GOF	Paternal
9 Spinocerebellar ataxia 3	AD	SCA3/MJD1	14q32.1	109150	CAG	12-41	40-84	Coding	GOF	Paternal
10 Spinocerebellar ataxia 6/ Episodic ataxia type 2	AD	CACNA1A	19p13	601011	CAG	7-18	20-23 EA2 21-27 SCA6	Coding	ND	ND
11 Spinocerebellar ataxia 7	AD	SCA7	3p12-13	164500	CAG	7-17	38-130	Coding	GOF	Paternal
12 Friedreich ataxia	AR	FRDA1	9q13-21.2	229300	GAA	6-34	80 premutation 112-1700 full mutation	Intron 1	LOF, FraX	Maternal
13 Progressive myoclonus epilepsy 1	AR	CSTB	21q22.3	601145	CCCCGCCCCGCG	2-3	35-80	5' flanking	LOF	Paternal
14 Synpolydactyly	AD	HOXD13	2q31-q32	142989	(GCG)n(GCT)n(GCA)n	15	22-29	Coding	ND	?
15 Oculopharangeal muscular dystropy	AD	PABP2	14q11.2-q13	602279	GCG	6	7-13	Coding	ND	?

covering individual disorders, and in Wells and Warren, (1998).

A repeat expansion of 12 nucleotides (CCCGCCC-CGCG) in the 5′ flanking region of the *CSTB* gene causes one form of progressive myoclonus epilepsy (EPM1) (Lalioti et al., 1997). This indicates that repeat sequences other than trinucleotides could be expanded and cause human disorders.

Large deletions

Large deletions are common causes of certain disorders and rare in others. In most of the X-linked disorders, for example, large deletions account for about 5% of molecular defects. In other disorders, however, such as steroid sulfatase deficiency (STS), large deletions account for 84% of patients (Ballabio et al., 1989). The same is true for disorders like Duchenne muscular dystrophy, growth hormone deficiency and α-thalassemia (Den Dunnen et al., 1987; Vnencak-Jones and Phillips, 1990; Nicholls et al., 1987).

A considerable number of large deletions are probably generated by mispairing of homologous sequences and unequal recombination (Fig. 5.4). One of the best examples of homologous unequal recombination is the case of α-globin genes on chromosome 16p. As a result of a recent evolutionary duplication of the α-globin genes, extensive regions of sequence homology exist between the two closely linked α-genes. Unequal crossover results in either deletion of one α-gene or the creation of a fusion hybrid gene (Embury et al., 1980). The reciprocal product chromosomes carry three α-genes and are not associated with a clinical phenotype (Goossens et al., 1980). Another example of a fusion gene resulting from an unequal crossover is the case of Lepore characterized by a hybrid gene between the δ- and β-globin genes on chromosome 11p (Baglioni, 1962). In the case of steroid sulfatase deficiency, the deletion can be as large as one megabase (Shapiro et al., 1989). In Kallmann syndrome, translocation can occur as a result of unequal mispairing of X and Y homologous sequences (Guioli et al., 1992).

Several common genetic disorders are due to large deletions (or duplications) caused by unequal crossing-over of homologous sequences. Figure 5.5 depicts various examples that include a 1.5 Mb deletion of 17p12 in hereditary neuropathy with liability to pressure palsies (HNPP) (Reiter et al., 1998), deletion of 1.5 Mb of 17q11.2 in neurofibromatosis type 1 (Dorschner et al., 2000), deletion of 1.6 Mb of 7q11.23 in Williams syndrome (Francke, 1999), deletion of 5 Mb of 17p11.2 in Smith-Magenis syndrome (Juyal et al, 1996), deletion of either 3 Mb or more rarely 1.5 Mb of 22q11 in DiGeorge and velo-cardio-facial syndrome (Edelmann et al., 1999; Shaikh et al., 2000), and deletions of 4 Mb of 15q in Prader-Willi and Angelman syndromes (Christian et al., 1999). For a review of chromosomal duplicons mediating deletions or duplications, see Ji et al., 2000.

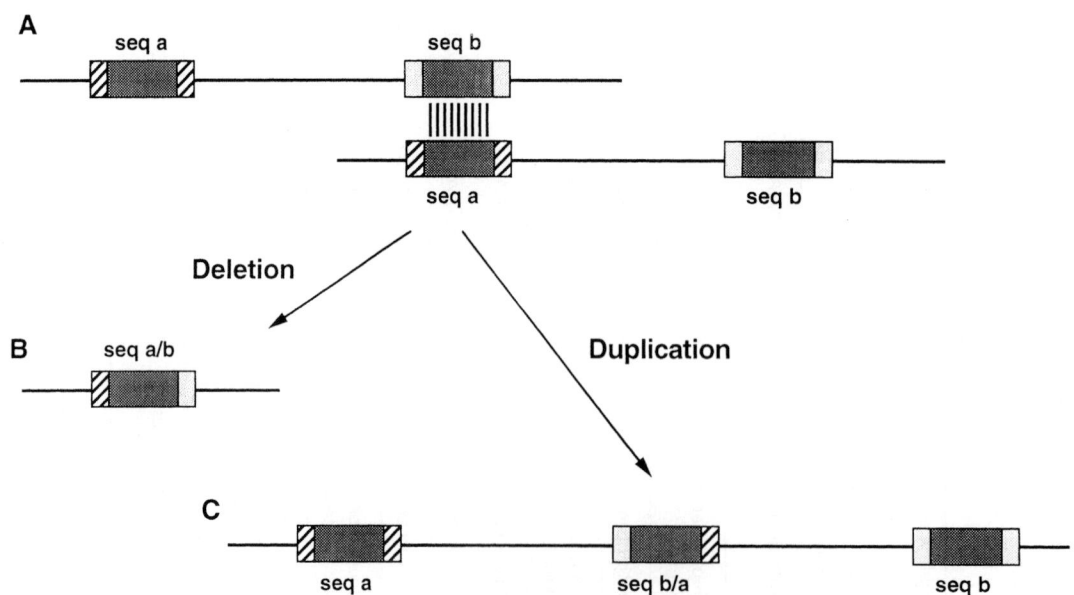

Fig. 5.4. (A) Homologous unequal recombination between similar regions of sequences a and b (seq a, seq b). The recombination events cause either (B) deletions or (C) duplications. In the case of a deletion, a hybrid sequence is generated with the first part from seq a and second from seq b. The middle sequence in (C) is also a hybrid sequence; the first part is from seq b and the second part is from seq a.

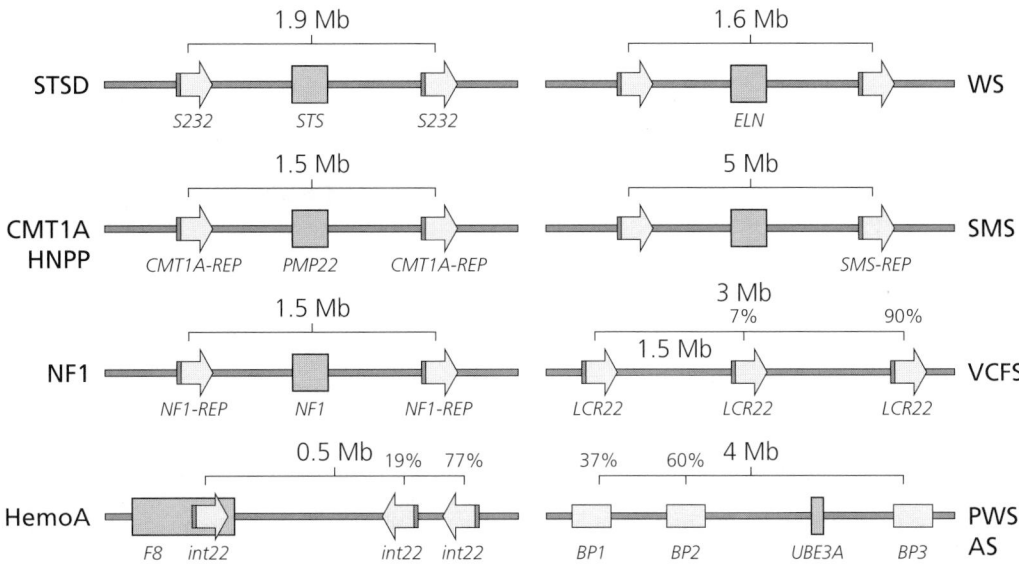

Fig. 5.5. Genes, duplicons and diseases. Unequal crossover between homologous sequences (duplicons) produce either deletions or duplications of the DNA between the duplicons. The duplicons are shown by arrows or clear boxes. Genes included in the duplications/deletions are shown as filled boxes. STSD, steroid sulfatase deficiency; CMTA1, Charcot-Marie-Tooth type A1; HNPP, hereditary neuropathy with liability to pressure palsies; NF1, neurofibromatosis 1; HemoA, hemophilia A; WS, Williams syndrome; SMS, Smith-Magenis syndrome; VCFS, Velo-cardio-facial syndrome; PWS, Prader-Willi syndrome; AS, Angelman syndrome.

In many cases of large deletion, homologous unequal crossover occurs between repetitive elements such as *Alu* sequences. The *Alu* repeat is the most abundant repetitive element with about 10^6 copies in the human genome (Deininger, 1989). The element is about 300 bp in length and consists of two similar regions separated by a short A-rich region. Unequal crossover can occur between *Alu* sequences oriented in either the opposite or the same direction; in addition, unequal crossings over have been noted between an *Alu* element and a non-repetitive DNA sequence without homology to *Alus*. The best examples of *Alu-Alu* recombination occur in the genes encoding the low-density lipoprotein receptor (*LDLR*) which underlies familial hypercholesterolemia, and complement component 1 inhibitor (*C1I*) (Lehrmann et al., 1987; Stoppa-Lyonnet et al., 1991). All but one of the breakpoints associated with *LDLR* gene deletions occur within *Alu* repeats. By contrast, deletions in other *Alu*-rich genes (e.g. *GLA1*) do not involve *Alu* repetitive elements (Kornreich et al., 1990).

Nonhomologous (illegitimate) recombination occurs between two DNA sites that share minimal sequence homology of a few base-pairs. This type of recombination during meiosis or alternatively, slipped mispairing during DNA replication mediated by short (two to eight) nucleotide direct repeats flanking the deletions is a common finding in many instances of large gene deletions (Roth and Wilson, 1986). Such deletions have been studied, for example, in hemophilia A;. a compilation of 46 junctions from large deletions revealed that about 50% shared 2- to 6-bp homology at the breakpoint junction, as compared with only 17% in which the deletion was due to *Alu-Alu* recombination (Woods-Samuels et al., 1991). Similar results have been reported from the intron 7 deletion hotspot in the Duchenne muscular dystrophy (*DMD*) gene; 8/9 deletion breakpoints examined were found to be flanked by DNA sequences with minimal homology (McNaughton et al., 1998).

Large insertions (via retrotransposition)

A less common but nevertheless still fascinating mechanism of human gene mutation is the de novo insertion of repetitive elements via retrotransposition. The phenomenon was first observed in humans in the factor VIII (*F8C*) gene in two unrelated de novo cases of severe hemophilia A (Kazazian et al., 1988). Truncated LINE (long interspersed) repetitive elements were introduced into exon 14 of the factor VIII (*F8C*) gene where they caused disruption of the reading frame. The inserted elements contained a poly(A) tract and caused a target site duplication of more than 12 nucleotides. Further analysis of these insertions revealed that, in one case, the inserted element was an exact but truncated copy of a full-length LINE element with open reading frames found at chromosome 22q11 (Dombroski et al., 1991). The master gene produces an mRNA that is probably reverse transcribed (possibly via a reverse transcriptase encoded by itself) and the double stranded nucleic acid is then reinserted into an A-rich

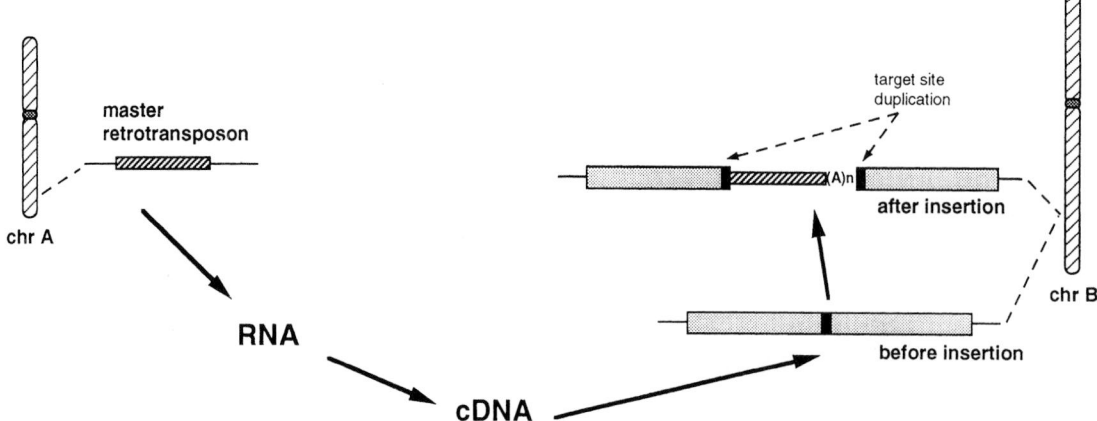

Fig. 5.6. Schematic representation of retrotransposition. A master retrotransposon from chromosome A is transcribed to RNA; then reverse transcribed to double-stranded DNA and inserted into an adenine-rich region of chromosome B. The transposon has a poly(A) tail and produces a target site duplication. From Cooper et al. (1995) The nature and mechanisms of human gene mutation. In Scriver et al. (eds) *The Metabolic and Molecular Bases of Inherited Disease*, 7th edit. © 1995, McGraw-Hill.

region of the genome (Fig. 5.6). More such insertions have been reported to date (Kazazian et al., 1998). It is noteworthy that insertions of these elements in introns of genes or flanking regions are probably not associated with disease, but instead represent rare, private polymorphisms (Woods-Samuels et al., 1989).

Similar retrotranspositions that involve members of the *Alu* family have also been reported in several genes (examples include *Alu* insertions into the *NF1* gene causing type 1 neurofibromatosis, into the factor IX gene [*F9*] causing hemophilia B, and into the cholinesterase (*BCHE*) gene in a case of acholinesterasemia Muratani et al., 1991; Wallace et al., 1991; Vidaud et al., 1993). Further study of these additional de novo insertions may eventually uncover the master *Alu* sequences that are transcribed and have a particular function.

Large insertion of repetitive elements

Insertion of non-retrotransposons, namely beta-satellite repeats has been recently observed in the human genome. An insertion of 18 copies of the 68 bp monomer of the beta-satellite repeat in exon 11 of the *TMPRSS3* gene on chromosome 21 caused one form of recessive non-syndromic deafness DFNB10 (Scott et al., 2001). This may be mediated by invasion of the genomic DNA by the small polydisperse circular DNA (spcDNA).

Inversions

The most common inversion found to date is that associated with the factor VIII (*F8C*) gene, which occurs via intra-chromosomal recombination mediated by a 9.5-kb sequence that is repeated three times in the last megabase of Xqter; once in intron 22 of the factor VIII (*F8C*) gene and twice about 400 kb telomeric to the first (Lakich et al., 1993; Naylor et al., 1993) (Fig. 5.7). Most inversions, which are high frequency independent recurring events, involve the distal sequence. Rossiter et al. (1994) have shown that the vast majority of inversions occur in male germ cells, perhaps because intrachromosomal recombination is inhibited by the presence of homologous X chromosomes (male to female ratio was estimated to be about 300 to 1). Almost all mothers of inversion hemophilia A cases are carriers of the abnormality. DNA diagnosis of the molecular lesion in severe hemophilia A has been greatly facilitated by the occurrence of this common inversion of the *F8C* gene. The frequency of de novo inversion has been estimated to be 7.2×10^{-6} per gamete per generation. Another example of inversion has been described in the *IDS* gene (also on Xq) in about 13% of cases of Hunter syndrome (Bondeson et al., 1995). Inversions of DNA sequences have also been reported in the β-globin gene cluster on 11p and in the *APOA1–APOC3–APOA4* gene cluster on 11q (Jennings et al., 1985; Karathanasis et al., 1987).

Duplications

Duplications of whole genes or exons have contributed very significantly to the evolution of the mammalian genome (Cooper, 1999). Most gene clusters (e.g., β-globin or Hox) owe their origin to duplications that have occurred during evolution. Furthermore, the presence of similar domains in proteins (e.g., immunoglobulin-like domains in many trans-

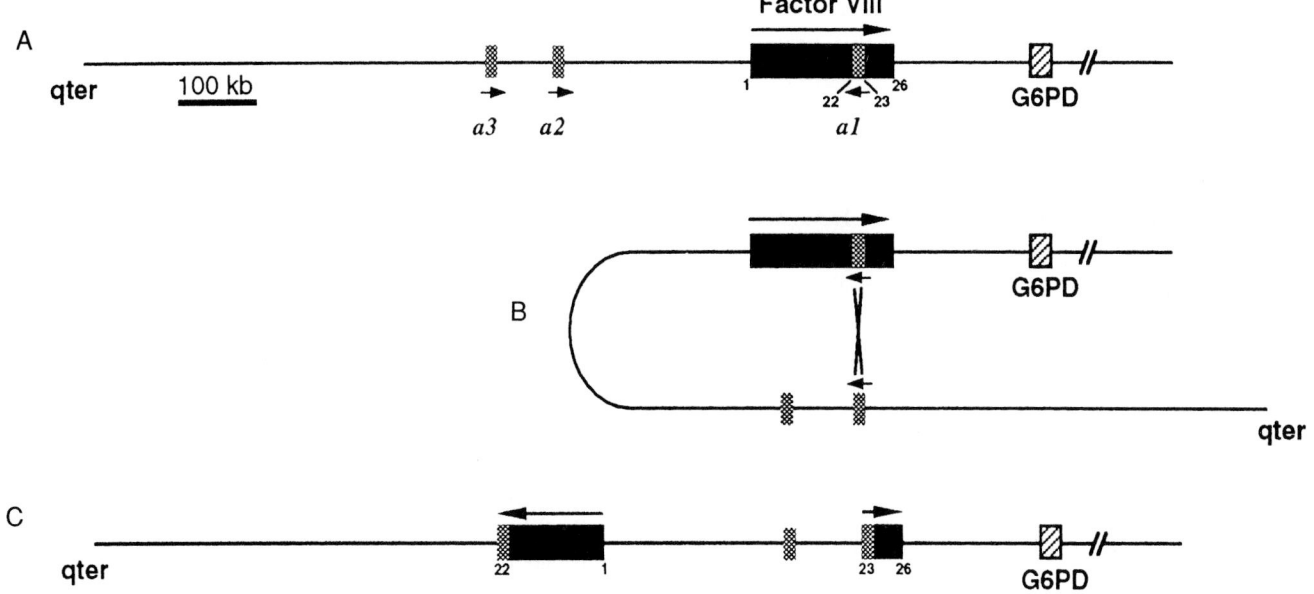

Fig. 5.7. Common inversion of factor VIII (*F8C*) gene in severe hemophilia A. (A) Schematic representation of the most distal 1 Mb of Xq. Regions α₁, α₂ and α₃ are 9.5 kb highly homologous DNA elements. The orientations of these sequences are shown by arrows. (B) Intrachromosomal recombination between elements α₁ and α₃. (C) The crossover results in the inversion of exons 1 to 22 of the *F8C* gene.

membrane proteins) are due to duplications of certain exons. Occasionally, however, duplications are also the cause of genetic disorders. The most frequent mechanism of duplication is homologous unequal crossover as described for large deletions. In fact, most large duplications are generated as the reciprocal product of a deletion resulting from homologous unequal crossover. Duplications are less common, however, than their theoretically reciprocal deletions (e.g., see Hu et al., 1990, for the *DMD* gene). This may be due to the non-pathogenicity of a duplication (e.g., α-globin genes), elimination of duplications as is the case for the *HPRT1* gene, or to the fact that not all mechanisms that lead to deletions also produce duplications. A large and common duplication has been identified in cases of Charcot-Marie-Tooth disease type 1A (Pentao et al., 1992). This duplication involves 1.5 Mb of DNA on chromosome 17 p containing the peripheral myelin protein 22 (*PMP22*) gene. It results from homologous unequal crossover events between 24 kb repeats that flank the duplicated region. The reciprocal deletion product of this recombination event is responsible for a completely different clinical phenotype: hereditary neuropathy with liability to pressure palsies (Fig. 5.5).

Gene conversion

Gene conversion is the modification of one of two alleles by the other. It involves the non-reciprocal correction of an acceptor gene or DNA sequence by a donor sequence which itself remains physically unchanged. In most known instances of gene conversion as a cause of human genetic disease, the functional gene has been wholly or partially converted to the sequence of a highly homologous and closely linked pseudogene which therefore acts as the donor sequence. Probable examples include the genes for steroid 21-hydroxylase (*CYP21*) (Tusié-Luna and White, 1995), polycystic kidney disease (*PKD1*) (Watnick et al., 1998), neutrophil cytosolic factor p47-*phox* (*NCF1*) (Görlach et al., 1997), immunoglobulin λ-like polypeptide 1 (*IGLL1*) (Minegishi et al., 1998), glucocerebrosidase (*GBA*) (Eyal et al., 1990), von Willebrand factor (*VWF*) (Eikenboom et al., 1994) and phosphomannomutase (*PMM2*) (Schollen et al., 1998). These gene/pseudogene pairs are all closely linked with the exception of the *VWF* gene (12p13) and its pseudogene (22q11–q13), and the *PMM2* gene (16p13) and its pseudogene (18p). Together, these two exceptions would seem to establish a precedent for the occurrence of gene conversion between unlinked loci in the human genome.

Insertion-deletions (Indels)

Indels are combined micro-insertions/micro-deletions, e.g., the 9 deleted base-pairs encoding codons 39–41 of the α2-globin (*HBA2*) gene were replaced by eight inserted bases that served to duplicate the adjacent downstream sequence (Oron-Karni et al., 1997). Indels constitute a fairly infrequent type of lesion causing human genetic disease; some 0.67% of lesions in HGMD fall into this category.

Other complex defects

Complex mutational events that involve combined gross duplications, deletions, and/or insertions of DNA sequence have also been observed and together constitute ~1% of entries in HGMD. One example of this type of gene defect is a 10.9 kb deletion coupled with a 95 bp inversion in the factor IX (*F9*) gene causing hemophilia B (Ketterling et al., 1993). The molecular characterization of this type of lesion is often extremely complicated and in most cases the underlying mutational mechanisms cannot be readily inferred.

Frequency of disease-producing mutations

The frequency of different molecular defects is not the same for every gene and every disorder. It depends largely on the DNA sequence characteristics of the gene in question (e.g., the presence of repeat units or homologous sequences), and the function of its encoded protein. For some genes, deletions predominate; for others, one special type of lesion such as inversion may be particularly common. Some genes exhibit mainly frameshifts and stop codons associated with a specific disorder whereas others manifest mainly missense mutations for a given phenotype, or perhaps expansions of trinucleotide repeats.

CONSEQUENCES OF MUTATIONS

Mutations affecting the amino acid sequence of the predicted protein, but not gene expression

Many missense mutations (i.e., nucleotide substitutions that result in an amino acid substitution) cause hereditary disease in humans. Missense mutations are of importance in understanding the structure or function of a protein since they usually occur in amino acid residues of structural or functional significance. It is sometimes difficult to establish a causative link between a missense mutation and a disease phenotype. The absence of the mutation in a large sample (usually 200 individuals) from the same ethnic group as the patient serves to exclude the possibility of a common polymorphism. Amino acid substitutions in evolutionarily conserved residues can also be good candidates for true pathogenicity. If the function of the protein is known, assessment of the effect of the missense mutation can be performed by in vitro mutagenesis and functional assay. Finally, the introduction of the mutation into an entire

organism (for example, in transgenic mice) and the study of its systemic effects provides one of the best means of assessing its contribution to a particular clinical phenotype. Amino acid substitutions can be shown to reduce or abolish the physiological function of a protein; for example, missense mutations have been identified in factor VIII that abolish thrombin cleavage which is necessary for its activation (Arai et al., 1989), interfere with binding to other proteins such as von Willebrand factor (Higuchi et al., 1990) or create or abolish N-glycosylation sites (Aly et al., 1992). In other proteins, mutations have been identified, for example in DNA binding domains, catalytic domains, transmembrane domains, ATP-binding regions, receptor-ligand contact sites, phosphorylation or other chemical modification sites. Missense mutations may also affect protein folding causing a dramatic change in secondary and tertiary structure such that the protein can no longer fulfill its physiological function.

Missense mutations can result in disease by (1) elimination or reduction of the physiological activity/role of the protein; (2) gain-of function by which the amino acid substitution creates new functional capabilities of the protein in biochemical and developmental processes in which the protein either does not participate or has a different role; (3) change of the target function of another protein as in the case of the mutation in the protein C cleavage site at Arg 506 of coagulation factor V, which is associated with thrombophilia (Bertina et al., 1994) or in the case of a mutation in the thrombin cleavage site of factor VIII that eliminates normal activation of factor VIII (Arai et al., 1989); and (4) participation of the mutant polypeptide in protein complexes, which renders the entire complex abnormal or nonfunctional, as in the case of the triple helical structure of certain collagens in which incorporation of one abnormal collagen chain results in protein suicide or abnormal structure that degrades rapidly (Byers, 1995).

Mutations affecting gene expression

Mutations that do not result in amino acid substitution invariably affect gene expression, i.e., transcription, RNA processing and maturation, translation or protein stability. Total or partial gene deletions, insertions, inversions, and other gross rearrangements obviously result in the loss of gene expression. These types of mutation are usually less frequent unless the genomic sequence environment of specific genes (e.g., presence of repeats) predisposes to such lesions. Disorders with high frequencies of gross rearrangements include α-thalassemia, Duchenne muscular dystrophy, steroid sulfatase deficiency and hemophilia A. Some partial gene deletions that eliminate one or a few exons in-frame result in milder clinical phenotypes because gene expression is not totally eliminated; the resulting protein may lack an amino acid domain that is not critical for its function (Youssoufian et al., 1987).

Transcription mutants

Mutations in known promoter motifs usually lead to reduced (or occasionally increased) mRNA levels. Such mutations have been studied in the TATA box of the β-globin (*HBB*) gene (Antonarakis et al., 1984). Other nucleotide substitutions in DNA motifs that bind transcription factors include those located in the CACCC motif of the β-globin (*HBB*) gene for transcription factor EKLF binding (Orkin et al., 1984; Perkins et al., 1995), several motifs in the γ-globin (*HBG*) genes (Collins et al., 1984), the CCAAT motif of the *F9* gene for C/EBP binding (Crossley and Brownlee, 1990), the SP1 motif of the human *LDLR* gene promoter (Koivisto et al., 1994) and the binding site for the transcription factor Oct-1 in the lipoprotein lipase (*LPL*) gene (Yang et al., 1995). These few examples are only representative of a total of >150 known promoter mutations causing human genetic disease (Krawczak et al., 2000b). The importance of these mutants lies in the specific DNA sequences thereby implicated in binding to transcription factors. Whilst most of the known mutations reduce the levels of mRNA production, some substitutions actually increase it; examples of the latter include various lesions in the promoters of the Gγ and Aγ globin genes that cause hereditary persistence of fetal hemoglobin due to inappropriate continuation of γ-globin gene expression in adult life (Weatherall et al., 1995). An increase in the distance of pro-moter elements from the transcriptional start site may also result in gene silencing. Such an example has been found in the promoter elements of the *CSTB* gene in progressive myoclonus epilepsy type 1 (EPM1) (Lalioti et al., 1999). Mutations that serve to alter the transcriptional regulation of gene expression have been reviewed by Semenza (1994).

Krawczak et al. (2000b) have demonstrated that the concomitant change in local DNA sequence complexity surrounding a substituted nucleotide is directly related to the likelihood of a regulatory mutation coming to clinical attention. This finding is consistent with the view that DNA sequence complexity is a critical determinant of gene regulatory function.

Polymorphisms in the promoter region that are associated with differential levels of gene expression may predispose to common disorders. For example, a G->A single nucleotide polymorphism (SNP) at nucleotide −6 relative to the transcriptional initiation site of the angiotensin (*AGT*) gene influences the basal level of transcription and may predispose to essential hypertension (Inoue et al., 1997). Some 1% of entries in HGMD are of this type.

mRNA splicing mutants

There are a wide variety of mutations in introns that affect normal RNA splicing (see Krawczak et al., 1992, for review). The most commonly found mutations occur in the invariant dinucleotides GT and AG found at the beginning and end of the donor (5′) and acceptor (3′) consensus splice sequences (see Fig. 5.8 for the consensus splice elements and Fig. 5.9 for the different kinds of RNA splicing abnormalities). Almost all of these mutations cause either exon skipping or cryptic splice site utilization resulting in the severe reduction or absence of

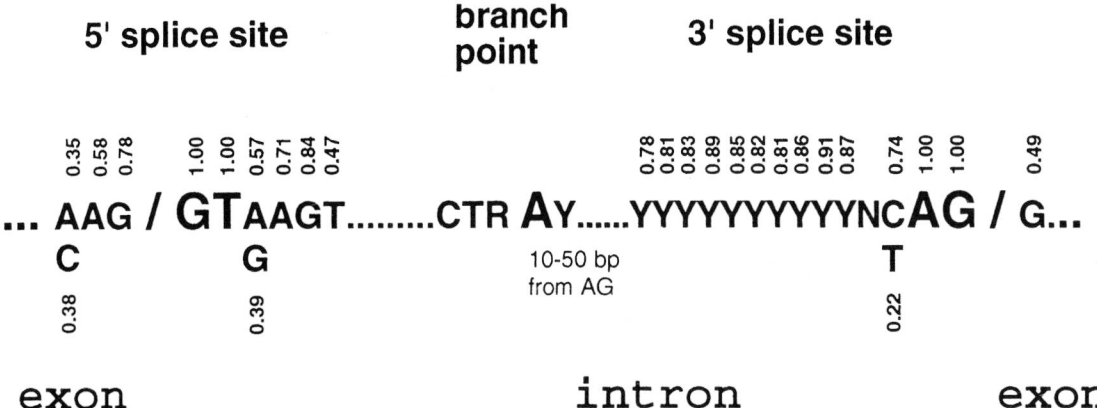

Fig. 5.8. Consensus sequences for the donor (5′ splice) and acceptor (3′ splice) sites and the branch-point. Numbers above or below the nucleotides correspond to frequencies of a given nucleotide in a large number of mammalian splice site sequences. Note that the dinucleotides GT and AG at the beginning and end of the intron are invariant.

Normal splicing

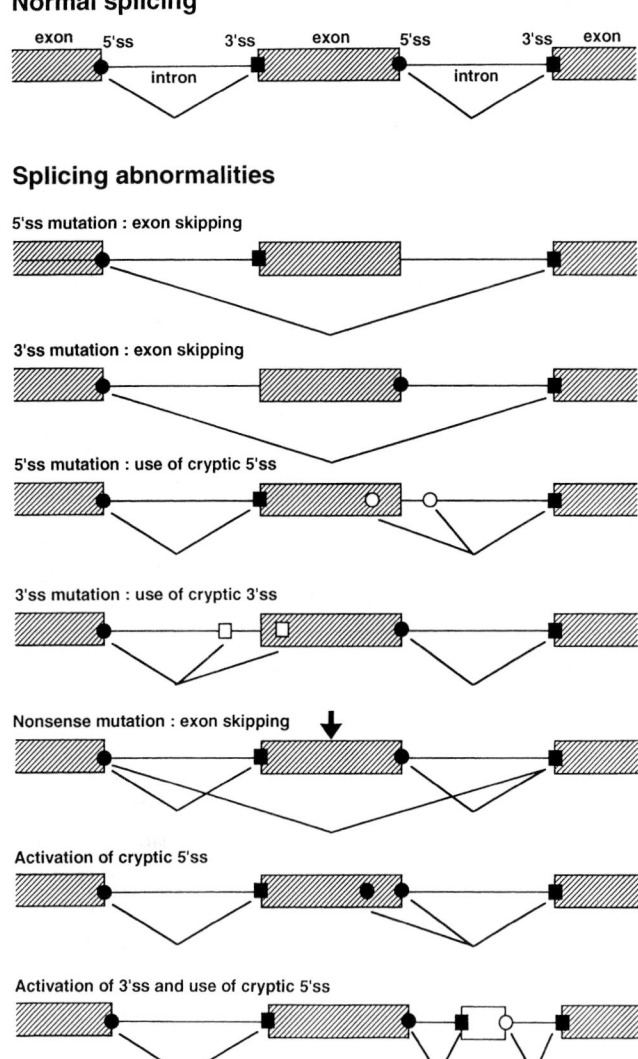

Splicing abnormalities

5'ss mutation : exon skipping

3'ss mutation : exon skipping

5'ss mutation : use of cryptic 5'ss

3'ss mutation : use of cryptic 3'ss

Nonsense mutation : exon skipping

Activation of cryptic 5'ss

Activation of 3'ss and use of cryptic 5'ss

Fig. 5.9. Examples of splicing abnormalities in introns of human genes. Exons are shown as striped boxes; introns as lines between exons. A black square denotes the normal 3' splice site; a black circle represents the normal 5' splice site. White squares and circles denote cryptic 3' and 5' splice sites, respectively. The arrow represents a nonsense mutation. In the example at the bottom of the panel, a new abnormal "exon" is shown in the second intron.

normally spliced mRNA. In addition, mutations in nucleotides +3, +4, +5, +6 and −1 of the consensus donor splice site have been observed, with variable severity of the RNA splicing defect. Similarly, mutations in positions −3 and the polypyrimidine tract of the consensus acceptor splice site have been noted. In the majority of these cases, some normal splicing occurs and the defect is not severe. Utilization of cryptic splice sites leads to the production of abnormal mature mRNA with premature stop codons or to the inclusion of additional amino acids after translation (see Cooper et al., 1995, for examples and references cited therein).

Other kinds of mutation in introns include those that cause the activation of cryptic splice sites (by altering a sequence so as to make it more similar to an authentic consensus splice site) or by creation of new splice sites (Treistman et al., 1983). In both instances, new intron splice patterns occur with consequent introduction of stop codons or abnormal peptides after translation. These mutations do not completely abolish normal splicing and are therefore not associated with the absence of normal mature mRNA. A mutation in a lariat structure branchpoint (Sharp, 1987) has been found in the *L1CAM* gene in a patient with X-linked hydrocephalus (Rosenthal et al., 1992). By contrast, another mutation in intron 5 of the type 2 neurofibromatosis (*NF2*) gene created a consensus branchpoint sequence and led to the activation of a cryptic exon (De Klein et al., 1998). Single base-pair substitutions within splicing enhancer sequences may also perturb splicing by promoting exon skipping; examples include a mutation in intron 3 of the growth hormone (*GH1*) gene causing short stature (Cogan et al., 1997) and a mutation in exon 5 of the adenosine deaminase (*ADA*) gene causing ADA deficiency (Santisteban et al., 1995).

Splice-mediated insertional inactivation involving an *Alu* repeat was first reported by Mitchell et al. (1991). Analysis of the ornithine δ-aminotransferase (*OAT*) mRNA of a patient with gyrate atrophy revealed a 142 nucleotide insertion at the junction of exons 3 and 4. An *Alu* sequence is normally present in intron 3 of the *OAT* gene 150 bp downstream of exon 3. The *Alu* sequence found in the cDNA was identical to this one, except that the patient was homozygous for a C→G transversion in the right arm of the *Alu* repeat which served to create a new 5' splice site. This activated an upstream cryptic 3' splice site [the poly(T) complement of the *Alu* poly(A) tail followed by an AG dinucleotide] and a new exon, containing the majority of the right arm of the *Alu* sequence, was recognized by the splicing apparatus and incorporated into the mRNA. The splice-mediated insertion of an *Alu* sequence in reverse orientation has also been reported in the *COL4A3* gene causing Alport syndrome (Knebelmann et al., 1995).

RNA cleavage-polyadenylation mutants

Few examples of RNA cleavage-polyadenylation mutations have been described. Those reported occur in the sequence AAUAAA, which is 10 to 30 nucleotides upstream of the polyadenylation site and is important for the endonucleolytic cleavage and polyadenylation of the mRNA. Mutation in this sequence of the beta-globin (*HBB*) gene results in mild thalassemia (Orkin et al., 1982). In these cases, normal polyadenylation and cleavage occurs at a level about 10% of normal. Alternative AAUAAA sites downstream of the mutated one are used, resulting in larger mRNAs which are highly unstable. Other mutations near the poly(A) cleavage sequence may result in mRNA destabilization; one such mutation has been described 12 bp upstream of the AAUAAA sequence of the β-globin (*HBB*) gene in a patient with β-thalassemia (Cai et al., 1992).

Cap site mutations

Transcription of the mRNA is initiated at the so-called cap site, which is protected from exonucleolytic degradation by the addition of α-methylguanine. A mutation of A to C at the cap site of the β-globin (*HBB*) gene was found in a patient with β-thalassemia (Wong et al., 1987). It is not, however, clear if this mutation causes reduced transcription or abnormal initiation of transcription since C is found in 6% of transcription start sites (Kozak, 1984) (the most common nucleotide (76%) at position +1 is A).

Mutations in untranslated regions

Sequence motifs in the 5′ UTRs of genes are thought to play a role in controlling the translation of the encoding mRNA. Thus mutations in the iron response element (IRE) in the 5′ UTR of the ferritin (*FTH1*) gene interfere with the post-transcriptional regulation of ferritin synthesis by decreasing the affinity of IRE for IRE-binding protein (Girelli et al., 1995). By contrast, decreases in the steady state level of β-globin (*HBB*) mRNA were noted in association with a single base deletion at position +10 (Athanassiadou et al., 1994) and a C→G transversion at position +33 (Ho et al., 1996) in the *HBB* 5′ UTR.

Sequences in the 3′ UTRs of genes are known to be involved in controlling mRNA cleavage/polyadenylation and determining mRNA stability, export, intracellular localization and translational efficiency. A G→A transition 69 nucleotides downstream of the polyadenylation site of the δ-globin (*HBD*) gene has been reported as a cause of δ-thalassemia (Moi et al., 1992); the mutation occurs within a GATA motif and serves to increase the binding affinity of the sequence for erythroid-specific DNA binding protein. Another important 3′ UTR mutation is the G20210A transition in the prothrombin (*F2*) gene; this lesion is associated with elevated plasma levels of prothrombin and an increased risk of venous thrombosis (Poort et al., 1996).

The phenotypic effects of lesions in untranslated regions and their clinical consequences have been reviewed recently by Cazzola and Skoda (2000).

Translation mutants

Initiation codon mutations

Mutations in the ATG translation initiation codon have been reported in several disorders (e.g., Pirastu et al., 1984). Instances of substitutions in all three nucleotides have been observed in β-thalassemia, Norrie disease, albinism, phenylketonuria, McArdle disease, and Albright osteodystrophy among others. Almost invariably, the mutation leads to severe reduction of steady-state mRNA levels similar to that associated with nonsense mutations. The mutant mRNA is presumably not translated. The first AUG codon occurs in the context of the so-called Kozak consensus sequence GCCA/GCCAUGG, which is thought to be recognized by the 40S ribosomal subunit (Kozak, 1991). Mutations at the initiator methionine ATG may completely abolish translation; however, the possibility exists of utilization of the mutant ATG with much reduced efficiency or translational initiation at the next available ATG codon.

Termination codon mutations

The classic example of a termination codon mutant is the case of the α_2-globin Constant Spring, with a mutation in the normal stop codon; this substitution leads to incorporation of an additional 31 amino acid residues in the α_2-globin polypeptide chain (Clegg et al., 1971). The resulting protein is unstable and does not interact properly with the β-globin chains of hemoglobin.

Frameshift mutations

A large number of frameshift mutations have been described in numerous disease-related genes. All lead to altered translation termination with abnormal polypeptide chain after the frameshifts; severe phenotypes are usually seen. Frameshifts occur with short deletions or insertions and exon skipping. The mechanism of these mutations was discussed earlier in this chapter.

Nonsense mutations

Nonsense mutations obviously cause premature termination of translation and truncated polypeptides. Almost 50% of nonsense mutations are to codon TGA and roughly 30% to TAA and 20% to TAG. About one-half of the new TGA codons are due to the CG to TG rule described earlier. Many such mutations have been described in a large number of disease-related genes. Nonsense mutations are usually associated with reduction in the steady state level of cytoplasmic mRNA (Benz et al., 1978), but this observation is not universal. One or more parameters could be affected: the transcription rate, the efficiency of mRNA processing or transport to the cytoplasm, or mRNA stability. In practical terms, the observation of greatly reduced or absent cytoplasmic mRNA associated with nonsense mutations has important implications for mutation screening. Thus attempts to obtain mRNA for RT–PCR and mutation detection may result in amplification of nucleic acid from only the non-nonsense mutation-bearing allele. Nonsense mutations in the factor VIII (*F8C*) gene (hemophilia A) and fibrillin (*FBN1*) gene (Marfan syndrome) have been associated with the skipping of exons containing these mutations (Dietz et al., 1993; Naylor et al., 1993). This observation has now been extended to other genes; exon skipping is either complete or partial. The mechanism underlying this phenomenon is unknown although a number of intriguing models have been proposed (Frischmeyer and Dietz, 1999).

Unstable protein mutants

Missense mutations can cause abnormal protein folding and are therefore associated with reduced expression owing to instability of the protein. Reviews of mutations that affect protein stability can be found in Alber (1989) and Pakula and Sauer (1989). For proteins that circulate in body fluids, most mutations are associated with CRM negative status in which the amount of protein correlates with the amount of activity or CRM reduced status in which the amount of activity is still lower than the amount of protein produced. Many such mutations have been seen in factor VIII causing mild/moderate hemophilia A (Antonarakis et al., 1994).

Wacey et al. (1999) have explored the nature of the biophysical properties of amino acid substitutions that increase their likelihood of coming to clinical attention; these include solvent inaccessibility, the number of adverse steric interactions introduced and a reduction in H-bond number.

Mutations in remote promoter elements/locus control regions

In the β-globin gene cluster, a regulatory region about 10 kb upstream of the epsilon globin (*HBE*) gene has been identified that is capable of directing a high level of position-independent β-globin gene expression (Grosveld et al., 1989). This region, termed the Locus Control Region (LCR), is thought to organize the entire 60 kb β-globin gene cluster into an active chromatin domain and to enhance the transcription of individual globin genes (Stamatoyannopoulos, 1991). A similar LCR is also present in the α-globin gene cluster and other gene clusters (Vyas et al., 1992). Deletions of the LCR in the β-globin gene cluster result in silencing of the β-globin and other genes of the cluster, even though the genes themselves are intact (Weatherall et al., 1995). A particular 25 kb deletion, known as Hispanic γδβ-thalassemia, which deletes sequences 9.5 to 39 kb upstream of the ε-globin gene including the LCR renders the β-globin gene 60 kb downstream of the deletion nonfunctional (Driscoll et al., 1989). This extraordinary effect of the deletion of the LCR is thought to be due to an altered (DNase I resistant) state of chromatin associated with nonfunctional genes. Several other examples of similar deletions in the LCR of the α-globin gene cluster have been reported (Liebhaber et al., 1990).

Gene inactivation by expansion of a trinucleotide repeat

Trinucleotide repeat expansion has been discussed earlier. When the trinucleotide repeat lies within the coding region, its expansion may result in an abnormal protein with gain-of-function due to the introduction of additional amino acids in the poly(Gln) region (Housman, 1995). In the case of fragile X, however, the $(CGG)_n$ repeat is located in the 5′ UTR of the *FMR1* gene, and its expansion to full mutation results in hypermethylation of the promoter region, loss of transcription and therefore silencing of the gene (Warren, 1994). By contrast, expansion of the CTG repeat in the 3′ UTR of the *DMPK* gene causing myotonic dystrophy does not abolish transcription but rather causes nuclear retention of transcripts (Davis et al., 1997). Gene inactivation can also be caused by altering the spacing of promoter elements from the transcriptional start site as in the case of the 12mer repeat expansion in the *CSTB* gene (Lalioti et al., 1999).

Mutations producing inappropriate gene expression

Hereditary persistence of fetal hemoglobin (HPFH) and hereditary persistence of α-fetoprotein (HPAFP) are two clinical conditions that are prototypes for the inappropriate expression of γ-globin and α-fetoprotein genes, respectively. Normally the levels of fetal hemoglobin (HbF; α2γ2) in adult life are very low, as there is a switch from fetal to adult hemoglobin during the perinatal period. Similarly, AFP is produced at high level in fetal liver but declines rapidly after birth. In HPFH and HPAFP, however, the levels of HbF and AFP, respectively, are inappropriately high in adult life. This is often due to single nucleotide substitutions in the promoter regions of Gγ (*HBG2*) or Aγ (*HBG1*) or *AFP* genes. A considerable number of mutations that occur in the region −114 to −202 of the γ-globin genes have been characterized and presumably cause persistent expression of their corresponding genes (Weatherall et al., 1995). A similar situation has been observed with a −119 mutation in the *AFP* gene (McVey et al., 1993). These mutations occur within DNA binding motifs for transcriptional regulators.

Abnormal proteins due to fusion of two different genes

The translation of fusion genes results in novel proteins with different or abnormal properties from their parent polypeptides. Fusion genes are either the result of (1) homologous unequal crossing-over, or (2) junction sequences at breakpoints of chromosomal translocations. Hemoglobin Lepore, a fusion of δ- and β-globin genes is the prime example of the first mechanism. Other examples of abnormal fusion genes due to unequal crossover include the case of glucocorticoid-suppressible hyperaldosteronism (GSH), an autosomal dominant form of hypertension, caused by over-secretion of aldosterone (Pascoe et al., 1992); some GSH patients have hybrid genes between *CYP11B1* and *CYP11B2*, two highly homologous cytochrome P450 genes in 8q22. The hybrid gene contains the regulatory elements of *CYP11B1*, expressed in the adrenal gland, and the 3′ coding region of *CYP11B2*, which is essential for aldosterone synthesis. Another example is the case of abnormalities of color vision resulting from fusion of the green and red colour pigment (*RCP*, *GCP*) genes (Nathans et al., 1986). Recombination between the Kallmann gene on Xp22.3 (*KALX*) and its homologue (*KALY*) at Yp11.21 results in a fusion gene that is transcriptionally inactive and is associated with Kallmann syndrome secondary to an X;Y translocation.

A growing number of hematologic malignancies are associated with abnormal fusion proteins, the genes of which are found at the breakpoints of chromosomal translocations. One of the first reported examples was the case of fusion of the *BCR* and *ABL* genes in the t(9; 22) known as Philadelphia (Ph) chromosome in chronic myelogenous leukemia. The *BCR* gene is on chromosome 22 and the *ABL* gene is on chromosome 9; after the translocation junction, a fusion gene is created with the promoter elements of the *ABL* gene and the 3′ half of the *BCR* gene (Bartram et al., 1983). A new abnormal protein is detected in the leukemia cells, the abnormal function of which prob-

ably contributes to the malignant phenotype. Another example is the case of Ewing sarcoma (a solid tumor of bone) in which an 11;22 translocation results in a fusion of the *FLI1* gene on 11q24 with the *EWS* gene on 22q12 (Delattre et al., 1992). This type of rearrangement has been reviewed by Rabbits (1994). Fusion genes can be readily identified by PCR and can serve either as diagnostic indicators for relapse in the disorders concerned or as indicators of the need for an alternative therapeutic regimen.

Mutations in genes involved in mismatch repair associated with genomic instability

Mutations that lead to abnormal or abolished function of genes encoding proteins involved in DNA mismatch repair are of particular importance because they lead to accumulation of mutations throughout the genome. For example, some forms of hereditary nonpolyposis colon cancer, which may account for up to 10% of colon carcinoma, are due to mutations in genes such as *MSH2* or *MLH1* that encode mismatch repair proteins (Fishel et al., 1993; Leach et al., 1993; Papadopoulos et al., 1993). In families with mutations in these genes, the DNA of tumor tissue shows considerable instability as detected by the generation of new alleles for numerous DNA polymorphic markers (Ionov et al., 1993). One of the genes affected by the genomic instability is the type II transforming growth factor-β (TGF-β) receptor, (*TGFB2R*) which has a run of 10 adenines in its coding region. This run of As is altered, resulting in a frameshift and absence of the receptor, which in turn releases the cell from TGF-β inhibitory effects and contributes to malignancy (Markowitz et al., 1995). The discovery and further study of genes of the mutation repair system will enhance our understanding of germline and somatic mutations.

General principles of genotype-phenotype correlations

Several general principles have emerged as a result of the intense study of causative mutations in genetic disorders. The following discussion highlights some of these principles. The reader is encouraged to use the on-line "Mendelian Inheritance in Man" (MIM) for further information or for specific genes and clinical phenotypes. The review of Wolf (1995) provides an excellent guide to the complex issues inherent in the study of the relationship between mutant genotype and clinical phenotype.

Mutations in the *same gene may be responsible for more than one disorder*. There are many examples to illustrate the principle that mutations in a single gene can cause different and distinct clinical phenotypes (allelic heterogeneity). Historically, the first example is that of the beta-globin (*HBB*) gene on 11pter. Mutations of this gene cause β-thalassemia, sickle cell disease and methemoglobinemia. The *L1CAM* gene on Xq28 has been shown to be mutated in hydrocephalus and stenosis of aqueduct of Sylvius, MASA syndrome (*m*ental retardation, *a*phasia, *s*huffling gait, *a*dducted thumbs), and spastic paraplegia 1. The *COL1A2* gene on 7q21–q22 is involved in four different clinical forms of osteogenesis imperfecta (types II, III, IV, and atypical) as well as Ehlers-Danlos syndrome type VII B. The fibroblast growth factor receptor 2 (*FGFR2*) gene is mutated in three different cranio-synostosis syndromes, namely Pfeiffer, Crouzon and Jackson-Weiss. The *COL2A1* gene is implicated in Stickler syndrome type 1, SED congenita, Kneist dysplasia, achondrogenesis-hypochondrogenesis type 2, precocious osteoarthritis, Wagner syndrome type 2, and SMED Strudwick type. In a recent survey of 1014 genes causing disorders in OMIM, 165 genes were associated with two disorders, 52 genes with three disorders, 24 genes with four disorders and 19 genes with five or more disorders (Antonarakis and McKusick, 2000).

One disorder may be caused by mutations in more than one gene. There is a plethora of similar clinical phenotypes due to mutations in different genes. This observation, also known as nonallelic or locus heterogeneity, is well understood thanks to linkage analyses for genetic disorders and the search for mutations in different genes. Thus tuberous sclerosis, a relatively common autosomal dominant disorder, is caused by lesions in at least two different loci: *TSC1* on 9q34 and *TSC2* on 16p13.3. Approximately 60% of TSC families show linkage to the *TSC2* locus and 40% to the *TSC1* locus. Hereditary nonpolyposis colon cancer has been associated with mutations in five different genes. *MLH1* on 3p, *MSH2* on 2p16, *PMS1* on 2q31–q33, *PMS2* on 7p22 and *MSH6* on 2p16. A recent survey of 804 disorders in OMIM for nonallelic heterogeneity revealed 26 disorders associated with two genes, 11 disorders with three genes, and four disorders with five genes. Retinitis pigmentosa has been associated with a total of 14 different genes and the list is still growing. We expect that disorders of complex or polygenic phenotypes, such as hypertension, atherosclerosis, diabetes, schizophrenia, and manic-depressive illness, will be associated with a considerable number of genes scattered throughout the genome.

One and the same mutation may be associated with different clinical phenotypes (polypheny). The clinical phenotype does not only depend on the one mutation in the responsi-

ble gene; it can be modified by the action of any of the other 30,000 to 40,000 genes in the genome (Wolf, 1997). The environment can also play an important role in the full development of the clinical phenotype. The classic sickle cell disease mutation in the β-globin (*HBB*) gene (Glu6Val) may be associated with severe or mild sickle cell disease. The amelioration of the severe clinical phenotype in this case can be attributed to the increased expression of γ-globin genes and the presence of high levels of HbF. The genomic environment of the β-globin gene cluster may therefore modify the severity of sickle cell disease as may genetic variation originating from other loci, e.g., the α-globin genes (Cooper and Krawczak, 1993). Another example of this phenomenon has recently been provided by studies of certain craniosynostoses. Both Pfeiffer and Crouzon syndromes can be associated with the same C342Y or C342R mutations in the *FGFR2* gene.

One of the best examples of the contribution of the environment to the phenotype of single gene disorders is that of phenylketonuria due to phenylalanine hydroxylase (PAH) deficiency. Individuals homozygous for mutations in the *PAH* gene develop severe mental handicap if fed a normal diet. However, the cognitive status remains normal if these individuals are fed with a special, phenylalanine-free diet.

Mutations in more than one gene may be required to express a given clinical phenotype (digenic inheritance). Digenic inheritance refers to clinical phenotypes caused by the co-inheritance of mutations in two unlinked genes. Thus one form of retinitis pigmentosa is due to the co-inheritance of mutations in the *RDS* gene on 6p *and* the *ROM* gene on 11q (Kajiwara et al., 1994). Individuals with either one or the other mutation, do not suffer from the disease. In similar vein, digenic inheritance of mutations in the *MITF* and *TYR* genes has been reported as a cause of Waardenburg syndrome type 2 in conjunction with ocular albism (Morell et al., 1997). This phenomenon may be common in polygenic disorders and in disorders with «low penetrance».

Different mutations in the same gene may give rise to distinct dominant and recessive forms of the same disease. Von Willebrand factor (vWF) deficiency is a relatively common monogenic disease of blood coagulation. Many mutations have been studied in the *VWF* gene on chromosome 12p. A fraction of mutations (usually deletions, nonsense codons, or frameshift mutations) cause vWF deficiency with a recessive mode of inheritance; other mutations however (mostly missense substitutions) are associated with a dominant mode of inheritance of the vWF deficiency (Nichols and Gunsburg, 1997).

Whereas the majority of hitherto characterized growth hormone (*GH1*) gene lesions (including gross deletions and missense/nonsense mutations) that underlie familial short stature are inherited in autosomal recessive fashion, there is a group of intron 3 splicing mutations that are characterized by a dominant mode of inheritance (Cogan et al., 1997). These lesions result in the in-frame skipping of exon 3 encoding 40 amino acids including a Cys residue. The dominant negative nature of this mutation is thought to be explicable in terms of the participation of the resulting free unpaired cysteine residue in an illegitimate intermolecular disulphide linkage leading to dimerization of the mutant molecule with a normal GH molecule and inhibition of GH secretion.

For a discussion of pathologic alterations of the normal imprinting mechanisms the reader is referred to the Chapter 14. For mutations in the mitochondrial genome see Chapter 11.

Why study mutation?

The sequencing of the human genome is now almost complete and its annotation well underway. Full exploitation of the emerging data, specifically in relation to understanding the etiology of inherited disease and disease predispositions, is however likely to be hampered by our ignorance of the basic processes underlying inter-individual, inter-population and inter-species genetic diversity. At the population level, such an understanding is seen as essential for any meaningful interpretation of the prevalence/incidence patterns observed for diseases with a genetic basis. Within families, it is a prerequisite for being able to explain how inter-individual variation arises and how variable phenotypic expression can be associated with identical gene lesions. Thus, for sequence data emerging from the Human Genome Project to be useful in the context of molecular medicine, they must eventually be related to the genetic variation underlying human inherited disease. To this end, the meta-analysis of pathological germline mutations in human genes should facilitate

(i)   the assessment of the spectrum of known genetic variation underlying human inherited disease,

(ii) the identification of factors determining the propensity of DNA sequences to undergo germline mutation,

(iii) the optimization of mutational screening strategies,

(iv) the identification of disease states that exhibit incomplete mutational spectra, prompting the search for, and detection of, novel gene lesions associated with different clinical phenotypes,

(v)   extrapolation toward the genetic basis of other, more complex traits and diseases,

(vi) our understanding of the biological function of a given protein,

(vii) meaningful comparison between the different mechanisms of mutagenesis underlying inherited and somatic disease,

(ix) studies of human genetic diseases in their evolutionary context.

ACKNOWLEDGMENTS

SEA wishes to thank the members of his laboratory for discussions, ideas and debates over the past 20 years; the Swiss National Science Foundation for grants 31–33965.92, 31–40500.94, 31–57149.99 and the Cantonal Hospital and University of Geneva Medical School for financial support. This chapter is dedicated to the memory of E S Antonarakis, who introduced SEA to critical and analytical thinking. DNC and MK are most grateful to Celera Genomics, the Deutsche Forschungsgemeinschaft, SmithKline-Beecham, the Genome Database, Pfizer and Pharmacia Corporation for their financial support.

REFERENCES

Alber T (1989) Mutational effects on protein stability. Annu Rev Biochem 58:765–798

Aly AM, Higuchi M, Kasper CK et al. (1992) Hemophilia A due to mutations that create new N-glycosylation sites. Proc Natl Acad Sci USA 89:4933–4937

Anagnou NP, O'Brien SJ, Shimada T et al. (1984) Chromosomal organization of the human DHFR genes: Dispersion, selective amplification, and a novel form of polymorphism. Proc Natl Acad Sci USA 81:5170–5174

Antonarakis SE, McKusick VA (2000) OMIM passes the 1,000-disease-gene mark. Nature Genet 25:11

Antonarakis SE, Kazazian HH Jr, Orkin SH (1985) DNA polymorphism and molecular pathology of the human globin gene clusters. Hum Genet 69:1–14

Antonarakis SE, Kazazian HH Jr, Tuddenham EGD (1995) Molecular etiology of factor VIII deficiency in hemophilia A. Hum Mutat 5:1–22

Antonarakis SE, Orkin SH, Cheng TC et al. (1984) β-Thalassemia in American Blacks: Novel mutations in the TATA box and IVS-2 acceptor splice site. Proc Natl Acad Sci USA 81:1154–1158

Arai M, Inaba H, Higuchi M et al. (1989) Direct characterization of factor VIII in plasma: Detection of a mutation altering a thrombin cleavage site (Arg 372, Arg 372-to-His). Proc Natl Acad Sci USA 86:4277–4281

Athanassiadou A, Papachatzopoulou A, Zoumbos N, Maniatis GM (1994) A novel β-thalassaemia mutation in the 5′ untranslated region of the β-globin gene. Br J Haematol 88:307–310

Baglioni C (1962) The fusion of two peptide chains in hemoglobin Lepore and its interpretation as a genetic deletion. Proc Natl Acad Sci USA 48:1880–1884

Ballabio A, Carrozzo R, Parenti G et al. (1989) Molecular heterogeneity of steroid sulfatase deficiency: A multicenter study of 57 unrelated patients at DNA and protein levels. Genomics 4:36–40

Bartram CR, de Klein A, Hogemeijer A et al. (1983) Translation of c-abl oncogene correlates with the presence of a Philadelphia chromosome in CMC. Nature 306:277–280

Benz EJ, Forget BG, Hillman DG et al. (1978) Variability in the amount of β-globin mRNA in β°-thalassaemia. Cell 14:299–312

Bertina RM, Koeleman BRC, Koster T et al. (1994) Mutation in blood coagulation factor V associated with resistance to activated protein C. Nature 369:64–67

Bondeson ML, Dahl N, Malmgren H et al. (1995) Inversion of the *IDS* gene resulting from recombination within IDS-related sequences is a common cause of the Hunter syndrome. Hum Mol Genet 4:615–621

Byers PH (1995) Disorders of collagen biosynthesis and structure. In Scriver CR, Beaudet AL, Sly WS, Valle D (eds): The Metabolic and Molecular Bases of Inherited Disease, p. 7029 7th edn. McGraw-Hill, N Y

Cai S-P, Eng B, Francombe WH et al. (1992) Two novel β-thalassemia mutations in the 5′ and 3′ noncoding regions of the β-globin gene. Blood 79:1342–1346

Caskey CT, Pizzuti A, Fu Y-H et al. (1992) Triplet repeat mutations in human diseases. Science 256:784–788

Cazzola M, Skoda RC (2000) Translational pathophysiology: A novel molecular mechanism of human disease. Blood 95:3280–3288

Christian SL, Fantes JA, Mewborn SK et al. (1999) Large genomic duplicons map to sites of instability in the Prader-Willi/Angelman syndrome chromosome region (15q11–q13). Hum Mol Genet 8:1025–37

Chung M, Ranum LPW, Duvick LA et al. (1993) Evidence for a mechanism predisposing to intergenerational CAG repeat instability in spinocerebellar ataxia type 1. Nature Genet 5:254–258

Clegg JB, Weatherall DJ, Milner PG (1971) Haemoglobin Constant Spring—a chain termination mutant? Nature 234:337–339

Cogan JD, Prince MA, Lekhakula S et al. (1997) A novel mechanism of aberrant pre-mRNA splicing in humans. Hum Mol Genet 6: 909–912

Collins FS, Stoeckert CJ, Serjeant GR et al. (1984) Gγβ+ hereditary persistence of fetal hemoglobin: Cosmid cloning and identification of a specific mutation 5′ to the Gγ gene. Proc Natal Acad Sci USA 81:4894–4898

Cooper DN (1983) Eukaryotic DNA methylation. Hum Genet 64:315–333

Cooper DN (1999) Human Gene Evolution. BIOS Scientific, Oxford.

Cooper DN, Krawczak M (1991) Mechanisms of insertional mutagenesis in human genes causing genetic disease. Hum Genet 87:409–415

Cooper DN, Krawczak M (1993) Human Gene Mutation. BIOS Scientific, Oxford

Cooper DN, Youssoufian H (1988) The CpG dinucleotide and human genetic disease. Hum Genet 78:151–155

Cooper DN, Smith BA, Cooke HJ et al. (1985) An estimate of unique DNA sequence heterozygosity in the human genome. Hum Genet 69:201–205

Cooper DN, Krawczak M, Antonarakis SE (1995) The nature and mechanisms of human gene mutation. In Scriver CR, Beaudet AL, Sly WS, Valle D (eds): The Metabolic and Molecular Bases of Inherited Disease, 7th edn. McGraw-Hill, N Y, p. 259

Crossley M, Brownlee GG (1990) Disruption of a C/EBP binding site in the factor IX promoter is associated with haemophilia B. Nature 345:444–446

Davis BM, McCurrach ME, Taneja KL et al. (1997) Expansion of a CUG trinucleotide repeat in the 3′ untranslated region of myotonic dystrophy protein kinase transcripts results in nuclear retention of transcripts. Proc Natl Acad Sci USA 94:7388–7393

De Klein A, Riegman PHJ, Bijlsma EK et al. (1998) A G→A transition creates a branchpoint sequence and activation of a cryptic exon, resulting in the hereditary disorder neurofibromatosis 2. Hum Mol Genet 7:393–398

Deininger PL (1989) SINEs: Short interspersed repetitive DNA elements in higher eukaryotes. In Berg DE, Howe MM (eds): Mobile DNA. American Society of Microbiology, Washington, DC, p. 619

Delattre O, Zuoman J, Plougastel B et al. (1992) Gene fusion with an ETS DNA-binding domain caused by chromosome translocation in human tumors. Nature 359:162–165

Den Dunnen JT, Bakker E, Klein Breteler EG et al. (1987) Direct detection of more than 50% of the Duchenne muscular dystrophy mutations by field inversion gels. Nature 329: 640–642

Dietz HC, Valle D, Francomano CA et al. (1993) The skipping of consecutive exons *in vivo* induced by nonsense mutations. Science 259:680–683

Dombroski BA, Mathias SL, Nanthakumar E et al. (1991) Isolation of an active human transposable element. Science 254:1805–1807

Dorschner MO, Sybert VP, Weaver M, Pletcher BA, Stephens K (2000) NF1 microdeletion breakpoints are clustered at flanking repetitive sequences. Hum Mol Genet 9:35–46

Driscoll DJ, Migeon BR (1990) Sex differences in methylation of single copy genes in human meiotic germ cells; implications for X-inactivation, parental imprinting, and origin of CpG mutations. Somat Cell Mol Genet 16:267–282

Driscoll MC, Dobkin CS, Alter BP (1989) γδβ-thalassaemia due to a *de novo* mutation deleting the 5′ β-globin gene activation-region hypersensitive sites. Proc Natl Acad Sci USA 86:7470–7474

Economou EP, Bergen A, Warren AC, Antonarakis SE (1990) The poly(A) tail of *Alu* repetitive elements is polymorphic in the human genome (AluVpA). Proc Natl Acad Sci USA 87:2951–2954

Edelmann L, Pandita RK, Morrow BE (1999) Low-copy repeats mediate the common 3-Mb deletion in patients with velo-cardio-facial syndrome. Am J Hum Genet. 64:1076–86

Efstratiadis A, Posakony JW, Maniatis T et al. (1980) The structure and evolution of the human β-globin gene family. Cell 21:653–668

Eikenboom JC, Vink T, Briët E et al. (1994) Multiple substitutions in the von Willebrand factor gene that mimic the pseudogene sequence. Proc Natl Acad Sci USA 91: 2221–2224

Embury SH, Miller JA, Dozy AM et al. (1980) Two different molecular organizations account for the single α-globin gene of the α-thalassaemia-2 genotype. J Clin Invest 66:1319–1324

Eyal N, Wilder S, Horowitz M (1990) Prevalent and rare mutations among Gaucher patients. Gene 96:277–283

Fishel R, Lescoe MK, Rao MR et al. (1993) The human mutator gene homolog MSH2 and its association with hereditary nonpolyposis colon cancer. Science 263:1625–1629

Francke U (1999) Williams-Beuren syndrome: Genes and mechanisms. Hum Mol Genet 8: 1947–54

Frischmeyer PA, Dietz HC (1999) Nonsense-mediated mRNA decay in health and disease. Hum Mol Genet 8:1893–1900

Fu Y-H, Kuhl DPA, Pizzuti A et al. (1991) Variation of the CGG repeat at the fragile X site results in genetic instability: Resolution of Sherman paradox. Cell 67: 1047–1058

Girelli D, Corrocher R, Bisceglia L et al. (1995) Molecular basis for the recently described hereditary hyperferritinemia-cataract syndrome: A mutation in the iron-responsive element of ferritin L-subunit gene (the Verona mutation). Blood 86:4050–4053

Görlach A, Lee PL, Roesler J et al. (1997) A p47-*phox* pseudogene carries the most common mutation causing p47-*phox*-deficient chronic granulomatous disease. J Clin Invest 100:1907–1918

Goossens M, Dozy AM, Embury SH et al. (1980) Triplicated α-globin loci in humans. Proc Natl Acad Sci USA 77:518–521

Grosveld F, van Assendelft GB, Greaves DR, Kollias G (1989) Position-independent high-level expression of the human β-globin gene in transgenic mice. Cell 51:975–985

Guioli S, Incerti B, Zanaria E et al. (1992) Kallmann syndrome due to a translocation resulting in an X/Y fusion gene. Nature Genet 1:337–340

Harper PS, Harley HG, Reardon W, Shaw DJ (1992) Anticipation in myotonic dystrophy: New light on an old problem. Am J Hum Genet 51:10–16

Higuchi M, Wong C, Kochhan L et al. (1990) Characterization of mutations in the factor VIII gene by direct sequencing of amplified genomic DNA. Genomics 6:65–71

Ho PJ, Rochette J, Fisher CA et al. (1996) Moderate reduction of β-globin gene transcript by a novel mutation in the 5′ untranslated region: A study of its interaction with other genotypes in two families. Blood 87:1170–1178

Housman D (1995) Gain of glutamines, gain of function? Nature Genet 10:3–4

Hu X, Ray PN, Murphy EG et al. (1990) Duplicational mutation at the Duchenne muscular dystrophy locus: Its frequency, distribution, origin and phenotype/genotype correlation. Am J Hum Genet 46:682–695

"Human Gene Mutation Database"
http://www.wwcm.ac.uk/uwcm/mg/hgmdo.html

Hurst LD, Ellegren H (1998) Sex biases in the mutation rates. Trends Genet 14:446–452

Inoue I, Nakajima T, Williams CS et al. (1997) A nucleotide substitution in the promoter of human angiotensinogen is associated with essential hypertension and affects basal transcription *in vitro*. J Clin Invest 99:1786–1797

Ionov Y, Pernado MA, Malkosyan S et al. (1993) Ubiquitous somatic mutations in simple repeated sequences reveal a new mechanism for colonic carcinogenesis. Nature 363: 558–561

Jeffreys AJ, Wilson V, Thein SL (1985) Hypervariable minisatellite regions in human DNA. Nature 314:67–73

Jeffreys AA, Neumann R, Wilson V (1990) Repeat unit sequence variation in minisatellites: A novel source of DNA polymorphism for studying variation and mutation by single molecular analysis. Cell 601:473–485

Jennings MW, Jones RW, Wood WG, Weatherall DJ (1985) Analysis of an inversion within the human β-globin gene cluster. Nucleic Acids Res 13:2897–2906

Ji Y, Eichler EE, Schwartz S, Nicholls RD (2000) Structure of chromosomal duplicons and their role in mediating human genomic disorders. Genome Res 10:597–610

Juyal RC, Figuera LE, Hauge X et al. (1996) Molecular analyses of 17p11.2 deletions in 62 Smith-Magenis syndrome patients. Am J Hum Genet 58:998–1007

Kajiwara K, Berson EL, Dryja TP (1994) Digeneic retinitis pigmentosa due to mutations at the unlinked peripherin/*RDS* and *ROM1* loci. Science 264:1604–1608

Kang S, Ohshima K, Simizu M et al. (1995) Pausing of DNA synthesis *in vitro* at specific loci in CTG and CGG triplet repeats from human hereditary disease genes. J Biol Chem 270:27014–27021

Karathanasis SK, Ferris E, Haddad IA (1987) DNA inversion within the apolipoproteins AI/CIII/AIV-encoding gene cluster of certain patients with premature atherosclerosis. Proc Natl Acad Sci USA 84:7198–7202

Kazazian HH Jr (1998) Mobile elements and disease. Curr Opin Genet Dev 8:343–50

Kazazian HH, Wong C, Youssoufian H et al. (1988) Haemophilia A resulting from *de novo* insertion of L1 sequences represents a novel mechanism for mutation in man. Nature 332:164–166

Ketterling RP, Ricke DO, Wurster MW, Sommer SS (1993) Deletions with inversions: Report of a mutation and review of the literature. Hum Mutat 2:53–57

Knebelmann B, Forestier L, Drouot L et al. (1995) Splice-mediated insertion of an *Alu* sequence in the *COL4A3* mRNA causing autosomal recessive Alport syndrome. Hum Mol Genet 4:675–679

Koivisto UM, Palvimo JJ, Janne OA, Kontula K (1994) A single base substitution in the proximal Sp1 site of the human *LDLR* promoter as a cause of familial hypercholesterolemia. Proc Natl Acad Sci USA 91:10526–10530

Kornreich R, Bishop DF, Desnick RJ (1990) α-Galactosidase A gene rearrangements causing Fabry disease. J Biol Chem 265:9319–9326

Kozak M (1984) Compilation and analysis of sequences upstream from the translational start site in eukaryotic mRNAs. Nucleic Acids Res 12:857–872

Kozak M (1991) Structural features in eukaryotic mRNAs that modulate the initiation of translation. J Biol Chem 266:19867–19870

Krawczak M, Reiss J, Cooper DN (1992) The mutational spectrum of single base-pair substitutions in mRNA splice junctions of human genes: Causes and consequences. Hum Genet 90:41–54

Krawczak M, Ball EV, Cooper DN (1998) Neighboring-nucleotide effects on the rates of germ-line single-base-pair substitution in human genes. Am J Hum Genet 63:474–488

Krawczak M, Ball EV, Fenton I et al. (2000a) Human Gene Mutation Database—a biomedical information and research resource. Hum Mutat 15:45–51

Krawczak M, Chuzhanova NA, Stenson PD et al. (2000b) Changes in primary DNA sequence complexity influence the phenotypic consequences of mutations in human gene regulatory regions. Hum Genet 107:362–365.

Kunkel TA (1985) The mutational specificity of DNA polymerases α and γ during *in vitro* DNA synthesis. J Biol Chem 260:12866–12874

Lakich D, Kazazian HH, Antonarakis SE, Gitschier J (1993) Inversions of the factor VIII gene as a common cause of severe hemophilia A. Nature Genet 5:236–241

Lalioti MD, Scott HS, Buresi C et al. (1997) Dodecamer repeat expansion in cystatin B gene in progressive myoclonus epilepsy. Nature 386:847–51

Lalioti MD, Scott HS, Antonarakis SE (1999) Altered spacing of promoter elements due to the dodecamer repeat expansion contributes to reduced expression of the cystatin B gene in EPM1. Hum Mol Genet 8:1791–1798

Leach FS, Nicolaides NC, Papadopoulos N et al. (1993) Mutations of a mut S homolog in hereditary non polyposis colon cancer. Cell 75:1215–1226

Lehrman MA, Goldstein JL, Russell DW, Brown MS (1987) Duplication of seven exons in LDL receptor gene caused by *Alu-Alu* recombination in a subject with familial hypercholesterolemia. Cell 48:827–835

Liebhaber SA, Grise E-U, Weiss I et al. (1990) Inactivation of human α-globin gene expression by a *de novo* deletion located upstream of the α-globin gene cluster. Proc Natl Acad Sci USA 87:9431–9431

Litt M, Luty JA (1989) A hypervariable microsatellite revealed by *in vitro* amplification of a dinucleotide repeat within the cardiac muscle gene. Am J Hum Genet 44:397–401

Loeb LA, Kunkel TA (1982) Fidelity of DNA synthesis. Annu Rev Biochem 52:429–457

McNaughton JC, Cockburn DJ, Hughes G et al. (1998) Is gene deletion in eukaryotes sequence-dependent? A study of nine deletion junctions and nineteen other deletion breakpoints in intron 7 of the human dystrophin gene. Gene 222:41–51

McVey JH, Michaelides K, Hansen LP et al. (1993) A G to A substitution in an HNF 1 binding site in the human *AFP* gene is associated with hereditary persistence of α-fetoprotein Hum Mol Genet 2:379–384

Mandel J-L (1993) Questions of expansion. Nature Genet 4:8–10

Markowitz S, Wang J, Myeroff L et al. (1995) Inactivation of the type II TGF-β receptor in colon cancer cells with microsatellite instability. Science 268: 1336–1338

Minegishi Y, Coustan-Smith E, Wang YH et al. (1998) Mutations in the human λ5/14.1 gene results in B cell deficiency and agammaglobulinemia. J Exp Med 187:71–77

Mitchell GA, Labuda D, Fontaine G et al. (1991) Splice-mediated insertion of an *Alu* sequence inactivates ornithine δ-aminotransferase: A role for *Alu* elements in human mutation. Proc Natl Acad Sci USA 88:815–819

Moi P, Loudainos G, Lavinha J et al. (1992) Delta-thalassemia due to a mutation in an erythroid-specific binding protein sequence 3′ to the delta-globin gene. Blood 79:512–516

Morell R, Spritz RA, Ho L et al. (1997) Apparent digenic inheritance of Waardenburg syndrome type 2 (WS2) and autosomal recessive ocular albinism (AROA). Hum Mol Genet 6:659–664

Muratani K, Hada T, Yamamoto Y et al. (1991) Inactivation of the cholinesterase gene by *Alu* insertion: possible mechanism for human gene transposition. Proc Natl Acad Sci USA 88:11315–11319

Nathans J, Piantanida TP, Eddy RL et al. (1986) Molecular genetics of inherited variation in human color vision. Science 232:203–210

Naylor JA, Green PM, Rizza CR, Giannelli F (1993) Analysis of factor VIII m RNA reveals defects in everyone of 28 hemophilia patients. Hum Mol Genet 2:11–17

Nicholls RD, Fischel-Ghodsian N, Higgs DR (1987) Recombination at the human α-globin gene cluster: Sequence features and topological constraints. Cell 49:369–378

Nickerson DA, Taylor SL, Weiss KM et al. (1998) DNA sequence diversity in a 9.7-kb region of the human lipoprotein lipase gene. Nature Genet 19:233–240

Nichols WC, Ginsburg D (1997) von Willebrand disease. Medicine 76:1–20

"Online Mendelian Inheritance in Man" (OMIM) *http://www. ncbi.nlm.nih.gov/omim*

Orkin SH, Kazazian HH, Antonarakis SE et al. (1982) Linkage of β-thalassemia mutations and β-globin gene polymorphisms with DNA polymorphisms in the human β-globin gene cluster. Nature 296:627–631

Orkin SH, Antonarakis SE, Kazazian HH Jr (1984) Base substitution at position –88 in a β-thalassemia globin gene: Further evidence for the role of distal promoter element ACACCC. J Biol Chem 259:8679–8681

Orkin SH, Cheng T-C, Antonarakis SE, Kazazian HH (1985) Thalassemia due to a mutation in the cleavage-polyadenylation signal of the human β-globin gene. EMBO J 4:453–456

Oron-Karni V, Filon D, Rund D, Oppenheim A (1997) A novel mechanism generating short deletion/insertions following slippage is suggested by a mutation in the human α2-globin gene. Hum Mol Genet 6:881–885

Pakula AA, Sauer RT (1989) Genetic analysis of protein stability and function. Annu Rev Genet 23:289–310

Papadopoulos N, Nicolaides NC, Wei YF et al. (1993) Mutations of a mut L homolog in hereditary colon cancer. Science 263:1625–1629

Pascoe L, Curnow KM, Slutsker L et al. (1992) Glucocorticoid-suppressible hyperaldosteronism results from hybrid genes created by unequal crossovers between *CYP11B1* and *CYP11B2*. Proc Natl Acad Sci USA 89:8327–8331

Pentao L, Wise CA, Chinault AC et al. (1992) Charcot-Marie-Tooth type 1A duplication appears to arise from recombination at repeat sequences flanking the 1.5 Mb monomer unit. Nature Genet 2:292–300

Perkins AC, Sharpe AH, Orkin SH (1995) Lethal β-thalassemia in mice lacking the erythroid CACCC-transcription factor EKLF. Nature 375:318–322

Pirastu M, Saglio G, Chang JC et al. (1984) Initiation codon mutation as a cause of α-thalassemia. J Biol Chem 259:12315–12317

Poort SR, Rosendaal FR, Reitsma PH, Bertina RM (1996) A common genetic variation in the 3′-untranslated region of the prothrombin gene is associated with elevated plasma prothrombin levels and an increase in venous thrombosis. Blood 88:3698–3703

Rabbits TH (1994) Chromosomal translocations in human cancer. Nature 372:143–149

Reiter LT, Hastings PJ, Nelis E et al. (1998) Human meiotic recombination products revealed by sequencing a hotspot for homologous strand exchange in multiple HNPP deletion patients. Am J Hum Genet. 62:1023–33

Rosenthal A, Jouet M, Kenwrick S (1992) Aberrant splicing of neural cell adhesion molecule L1 mRNA in a family with X-linked hydrocephalus. Nature Genet 2:107–112

Rossiter JP, Young M, Kimberland M et al. (1994) Factor VIII gene inversions causing severe hemophilia A originate almost exclusively in male germ cells Hum Mol Genet 7: 1038–1039

Roth DB, Wilson JH (1986) Nonhomologous recombination in mammalian cells: Role for short sequence homologies in the joining reaction. Mol Cell Biol 6:4295–4304

Rousseau F, Heitz D, Mandel J-L (1992) The unstable and methylatable mutations causing the fragile X syndrome. Hum Mutat 1:91–96

Saiki RK, Scharf S, Faloona F et al. (1985) Enzymatic amplification of β-globin genomic sequences and restriction site analysis for the diagnosis of sickle cell anemia. Science 230:1350–1354

Santisteban I, Arredondo-Vega FX, Kelly S et al. (1995) Three new adenosine deaminase mutations that define a splicing enhancer and cause severe and prtial phenotypes: Implications for evolution of a CpG hotspot anhd expression of a transduced ADA cDNA. Hum Mol Genet 4:2081–2087

Schmucker B, Krawczak M (1997) Meiotic microdeletion breakpoints in the BRCA1 gene are significantly associated with symmetric DNA-sequence elements. Am J Hum Genet 61: 1454–1456

Schollen E, Pardon E, Heykants L et al. (1998) Comparative analysis of the phosphomannomutase genes PMM1, PMM2 and PMM2psi: The sequence variation in the processed pseudogene is a reflection of the mutations found in the functional gene. Hum Mol Genet 7:157–164

Semenza G (1994) Transcriptional regulation of gene expression: Mechanisms and pathophysiology. Hum Mutat 3:180–199

Scott HS, Kudoh J, Wattenhofer M et al. (2001) Insertion of beta-satellite repeats identifies a transmembrane protease causing both congenital and childhood onset autosomal recessive deafness (DFNB8/10). Nature Genet 27:59–63.

Shaikh TH, Kurahashi H, Saitta SC (2000) Chromosome 22-specific low copy repeats and the 22q11.2 deletion syndrome: Genomic organization and deletion endpoint analysis. Hum Mol Genet. 9:489–501

Shapiro LJ, Yen P, Pomerantz D et al. (1989) Molecular studies of deletions at the human steroid sulphatase locus. Proc Natl Acad Sci USA 86:8477–8481

Sharp P (1987) Splicing of messenger RNA precursors. Science 235:767–771

Stamatoyannopoulos G (1991) Human hemoglobin switching. Science 252:383–384

Stoppa-Lyonnet D, Duponchel C, Meo T et al. (1991) Recombination biases in the rearranged C1-inhibitor genes of hereditary angioedema patients. Am J Hum Genet 49:1055–1062

Treistman R, Orkin SH, Maniatis T (1983) Specific transcription and RNA splicing defects in five cloned in β-thalassemia genes. Nature 302:591–596

Tusie-Luna M-T, White PC (1995) Gene conversions and unequal crossovers between *CYP21* (steroid 21-hydroxylase gene) and *CYP21P* involve different mechanisms. Proc Natl Acad Sci USA 92:10796–10800

Vidaud D, Vidaud M, Bahnak BR et al. (1993) Hemophilia B due to a *de novo* insertion of a human-specific *Alu* subfamily member within the coding region of the factor IX gene. Eur J Hum Genet 1:30–36

Vnencak-Jones CL, Phillips JA (1990) Hot spots for growth hormone gene deletions in homologous regions outside of *Alu* repeats. Science 250:1745–1748

Vogel F (1990) Mutation in man. In Emery AEH, Rimoin DL: (eds): Principles and Practice of Medical Genetics, 2nd edn. Churchill Livingstone, Edinburgh, p. 53

Vyas P, Vickers MA, Simmons DL et al. (1992) *Cis*-acting sequences regulating expression of the human α-globin cluster lie within constitutively open chromatin. Cell 69:781–793

Wacey AI, Cooper DN, Liney D et al. (1999) Disentangling the perturbational effects of amino acid substitutions in the DNA-binding domain of p53. Hum Genet 104:15–22

Wallace MR, Andersen LB, Saulino AM et al. (1991) A *de novo Alu* insertion results in neurofibromatosis type 1. Nature 353:864–866

Wang DG, Fan J-B, Siao C-J et al. (1998) Large scale identification, mapping, and genotyping of single-nucleotide polymorphisms in the human genome. Science 280:1077–1082

Warren ST, Nelson DL (1994) Advances in molecular analysis of fragile X syndrome JAMA 271:536–542

Watnick TJ, Gandolph MA, Weber H et al. (1988) Gene conversion is a likely cause of mutation in *PKD1*. Hum Mol Genet 7:1239–1243

Weatherall DJ, Clegg JB, Higgs DR, Wood WG (1995) The hemoglobinopathies. In Scriver CR, Beaudet AL, Sly WS, Valle D (eds): The Metabolic and Molecular Bases of Inherited Disease, 7th edn. McGraw-Hill, N Y, p. 3454

Weber JL, May PE (1989) Abundant class of human DNA polymorphisms which can be typed using the polymerase chain reaction. Am J Hum Genet 44:388–396

Wells RD, Warren ST (eds) (1998) Genetic Instabilities and Hereditary Neurological Diseases. Academic Press, San Diego

Wolf U (1995) The genetic contribution to the phenotype. Hum Genet 95:127–148

Wolf U (1997) Identical mutations and phenotypic variation. Hum Genet 100:305–321

Wong C, Dowling CE, Saiki RK et al. (1987) Characterization of β-thalassemia mutations using direct genomic sequencing of amplified single copy DNA. Nature 330:384–386

Woods-Samuels P, Kazazian HH, Antonarakis SE (1991) Nonhomologous recombination on the human genome: Deletions in the human factor VIII gene. Genomics 10:94–101

Woods-Samuels P, Wong C, Mathias SL et al. (1989) Characterization of a non-deleterious L1 insertion in an intron of the human factor VIII gene and evidence for open reading frame in functional L1 elements. Genomics 4:290–296

Wyman AR, White R (1980) A highly polymorphic locus in human DNA. Proc Natl Acad Sci USA 77:6754–6758

Yang WS, Nerin DN, Peng R et al. (1995) A mutation in the protomer of the *LPL* gene in a patient with familial combined hyperlipidemia and low LPL activity. Proc Natl Acad Sci USA 92:4462–4466

Youssoufian H, Kazazian HH, Phillips DG et al. (1986) Recurrent mutations in hemophilia A give evidence for CpG mutation hotspots. Nature 324:280–282

Youssoufian H, Antonarakis SE, Phillips DG et al. (1987) The molecular genetics of hemophilia A: Five different partial deletions of factor VIII:C gene. Proc Natl Acad Sci USA 84:3772–3776

Youssoufian H, Antonarakis SE, Bell W et al. (1988) Nonsense and missense mutations in hemophilia A: Estimate of the relative mutation rate at CG dinucleotides. Am J Hum Genet 42:718–725

Mendelian inheritance

6

Jackie Cook
Wayne Lam
Robert F. Mueller

Introduction

Unifactorial inheritance refers to those disorders that are due to the inheritance of a single mutant gene. The first descriptions of unifactorial inheritance were made by Mendel in 1865, when he published the results of his experiments on the garden pea in his paper "Versuche uber Pflanzen Hybriden" (Experiments on Plant Hybrids). His work was largely ignored until it was republished by Bateson in 1901, from which time the term mendelian inheritance became synonymous with unifactorial inheritance.

From the ratios that Mendel described in his experiments on the garden pea, and the work of subsequent researchers, including Bateson, four main conclusions were drawn (Peters, 1959):

1. Genes come in pairs (Mendel termed them factors), one inherited from each parent.
2. Individual genes can have different alleles, some of which (dominant traits) exert their effects over others (recessive traits)—the principle of dominance. In Mendel's own words "those characters which are transmitted entire, or almost unchanged in the hybridisation, and therefore in themselves constitute the characters of the hybrid, are termed the dominant, and those which become latent in the process recessive."
3. At meiosis alleles segregate from each other with each gamete receiving only one allele – the principle of segregation, or Mendel's first law.
4. The segregation of different pairs of alleles is independent – the principle of independent assortment, or Mendel's second law.

With time, these principles have had to be modified. For example, although most genes come in pairs, for genes on the sex chromosomes males only have one allele, that is, they are termed hemizygous. Also, although alleles of a gene on different chromosomes show independent assortment, genes that are physically close together on the same chromosome do not – a phenomenon that has allowed mapping of genes in the human genome through linkage studies. These principles, however, still form a useful set of rules designed to explain the inheritance of many inherited characteristics and disorders.

Diseases inherited in a mendelian fashion are categorized according to whether the gene is on an autosome or a sex chromosome and whether the trait is dominant or recessive.

Dominance and recessiveness

DEFINITION OF DOMINANCE

Fundamental to the understanding of mendelian inheritance are the concepts of dominance and recessiveness. Dominance is not a property intrinsic to a particular allele but describes the relationship between it and the corresponding allele on the homologous chromosome. If the phenotypes associated with the genotypes AA and AB are the same but differ from the phenotype of BB, allele A is dominant to allele B and, conversely, allele B is recessive to allele A. Therefore, A manifests in the heterozygous state. An example of a dominant disease allele is that for Huntington disease with most persons affected with the disease being heterozygous for a mutant allele. However, individuals have been identified from a large inbred

Venezuelan family who have been shown by molecular techniques to be homozygous for the mutant allele by virtue of both parents being affected with Huntington disease. Such individuals do not appear different phenotypically from heterozygotes for the disorder (Wexler et al., 1987).

If the phenotype of the heterozygous state, AB, is intermediate between the phenotypes of AA and BB, allele A is said to be incompletely dominant or semi-dominant to allele B. Although the skeletal dysplasia achondroplasia, associated with rhizomelic shortening of the limbs, characteristic facies with mid-face hypoplasia, exaggerated lumbar lordosis, limitation of hip and elbow extension, genu varum, and trident hand, was conventionally thought to be due to a dominant allele, homozygotes for the mutant gene have a much more severe skeletal dysplasia, resulting in early death from respiratory embarrassment due to a small thoracic cage and neurologic deficit due to hydrocephalus (Hall et al., 1969), clearly an example of incomplete or semidominance. Homozygotes for most dominant mutant alleles causing human genetic diseases occur so rarely that it is not known whether they exhibit complete or incomplete dominance.

If the phenotype of AB displays the phenotypic features of both the homozygotic states then alleles A and B are said to be co-dominant. The human ABO blood group system exhibits co-dominance as individuals with the genotype AB have the phenotypic characteristics of both genotypes AA and BB.

MECHANISMS OF DOMINANCE

Most mutations result in an allele that is recessive to the wild-type allele; the phenotype is therefore only expressed in the homozygous state. This is because most mutations result in an inactive gene product, but the reduced level of activity due to the remaining wild-type allele is sufficient to achieve the effects of that gene product, often because it involves an enzyme that is only required in small amounts as a catalyst in a metabolic pathway. Although in some recessive inborn errors of metabolism, it is possible to identify heterozygotes, more often than not, the only way to identify carriers is by direct mutation analysis, using molecular genetic techniques.

There are several mechanisms by which a mutation can lead to a dominant mutant allele whose phenotype is expressed in the heterozygous state (Wilkie, 1994).

Loss-of-function mutations

For most mutant alleles, loss of function will usually exhibit recessive behavior. Where a reduction in amount or reduced activity of the gene product results in the phenotypic features, this is termed haploinsufficiency (e.g., in a critical rate-limiting step of a metabolic pathway). Any reduction in the amount of gene product will result in that pathway not being able to function at full activity. The same appears to apply to regulatory genes that could have a threshold level of activity. *PAX3* is a gene coding for a DNA binding protein and point mutations in the gene result in Waardenburg syndrome characterized by deafness and pigmentary disturbances. Certain mutations in *PAX3* have been shown to abolish all protein function of that allele; therefore, the phenotype must be due to a dosage effect as it manifests in the heterozygous state (Tassabehji et al., 1993).

Another example in which the quantitative amount of a gene product is important are genes that produce proteins in large quantities (e.g., C1 esterase inhibitor), mutations of which cause the disorder hereditary angioneurotic edema. C1 esterase inhibitor is removed rapidly from the circulation at a rate independent of its concentration. Therefore, although heterozygotes produce 50% of the normal amount, they have only 15 to 20% of the normal amount in the circulation, leading to the clinical manifestations of the disorder (Lachmann and Rosen, 1984).

Gain-of-function mutations

Increased gene dosage

This mechanism involves an excess of gene product leading to a disease phenotype. Although gene dosage of critical regions or genes has been invoked as the cause for the phenotypic features associated with the autosomal trisomies, there are few examples involving single gene disorders. One example involves the *PMP22* gene, which codes for the peripheral myelin protein 22. Duplication of the DNA sequence of one allele is associated with hereditary sensory and motor neuropathy type 1 (Patel et al., 1992).

Ectopic or temporally altered mRNA expression

Ectopic or temporally altered mRNA is expressed when a mutation occurs that affects the time or place of gene expression and usually involves a regulatory part of the gene. For example, during development in erythroid precursor cells, there is a switch from the production of γ-globin to the production of the δ and β globin. This switch is controlled, at least in part, by the binding of transcription factors to the γ-globin promoter. Point mutations in the globin promoter region prevent the normal switch, resulting in the disorder of hereditary persistence of fetal hemoglobin (Martin et al., 1989).

Increased protein activity

Mutations can lead to proteins with a prolonged half-life or proteins that have lost their normal constitutive inhibitory regulatory activity. If a mutation occurs in a part of a gene that codes for the protein sequence acting as the recognition site for proteolytic degradation, this will not take place, with the protein remaining active. Many proteins possess domains that allow their activity to be reversibly inhibited. For example, skeletal muscle sodium channels undergo voltage-sensitive regulation, and mutations in the gene *SCN4A* that codes for the α-subunit of the sodium channels result in the disorder hyperkalemic periodic paralysis characterized by muscle myotonia and paralysis due to loss of regulatory inactivation of the sodium channel (Ptacek et al., 1991).

Dominant negative mutations

If a mutant allele interferes with the wild-type allele this is termed a dominant negative mutation. This could occur in a multimeric protein in which a mutant subunit has an intact binding domain but altered catalytic activity, affecting the function of the entire multimer. If a protein is a dimer, one mutant and one wild-type allele would result in only 25% normal dimers, with up to a 75% reduction in activity.

Many structural proteins are multimers (e.g., the various types of collagen proteins). Each of the collagen subunit genes has a central portion coding for repeating tripeptide units that are essential for the assembly of the collagen molecule. The disease osteogenesis imperfecta is caused by point mutations in the central portion of the collagen subunit genes leading to a structural deformation which will cause disruption of the whole collagen protein (Byers et al., 1991).

Toxic protein alterations

Toxic protein alterations are mutations that cause structural alterations in proteins that disrupt normal function, leading to toxic products that poison the cell, for example, the hereditary amyloidoses in which mutations in the transthyretin gene lead to resistance to proteolysis, hence to increased stability of the protein. The protein then undergoes multimerization and accumulates in the cell as fibrils causing disruption of the cell (Benson, 1991).

New protein functions

Some mutations have been found to confer a new function on a gene product. For example, a fatal bleeding disorder was found to be caused by a missense mutation in the α_1-antitrypsin gene, in which methionine was replaced by arginine at position 358, the effect of which was to convert α_1-antitrypsin, normally an inhibitor of elastase, into an inhibitor of thrombin. This thrombin inhibitory activity was not compensated for by an increase in endogenous coagulant production, resulting in a severe bleeding disorder (Owen et al., 1983).

Recessive mutations with dominant effects

The mechanisms described so far show how mutations can cause dominant effects at a cellular level by the effects on the proteins produced. It is possible to have mutations that show a dominant pattern of inheritance in families, yet are recessive at the cellular or molecular level; that is, the gene is inactivated but has no other effect. The classic example of this is the retinoblastoma gene *RB-1*, inactivation of which can lead to the formation of the developmental eye tumor, retinoblastoma. Families can show a dominant mode of inheritance for this disorder, yet cells heterozygous for the mutation are completely normal, the mutation itself being recessive.

The dominant pattern of inheritance of familial retinoblastoma results through transmission of a first mutation with a second somatic mutation occurring in the normal allele of at least one retinal cell during a critical period of development leading to the formation of a retinoblastoma, the so-called "two-hit hypothesis" (Knudson, 1971). There are several ways in which the normal allele in somatic cells can be inactivated. These include point mutations, deletions, translocations, and mitotic nondisjunction, resulting in loss of a whole chromosome. It is now known that the "two-hit" hypothesis applies to most of the dominantly inherited familial cancer syndromes in which the germline mutation in a tumor suppressor gene is recessive and a mutation in a somatic cell in the corresponding allele leads to the development of a tumor.

Autosomal dominant inheritance

DEFINITION

Autosomal dominant inheritance refers to disorders caused by genes located on the autosomes, thereby affecting both

Table 6.1 Characteristics of an Autosomal Dominant Inherited Disorder

Successive or multiple generations in a family are affected
Males and females are both affected in approximately equal proportions
Males and females can both be responsible for transmission
There is at least one instance of male-to-male transmission

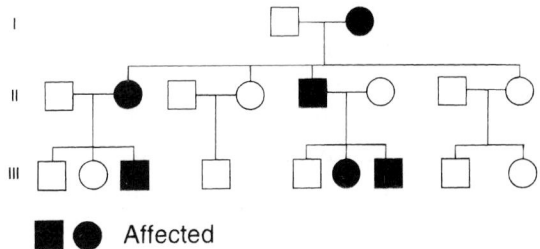

■ ● Affected

Fig. 6.1. Pedigree consistent with autosomal dominant inheritance.

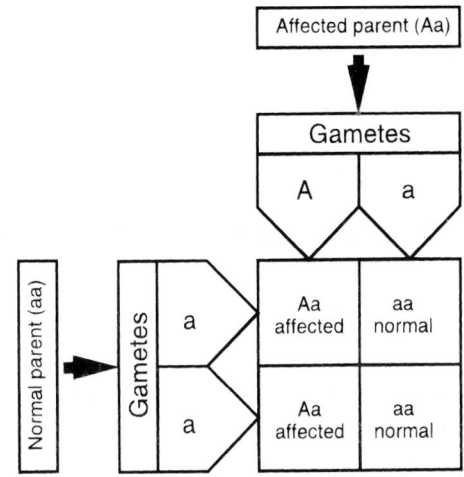

Fig. 6.2. Punnett's square of gametes and offspring in autosomal dominant inheritance.

males and females. The disease or mutant alleles are dominant to the wild-type alleles; therefore, the disorder is manifest in the heterozygote (i.e., individuals who possess both the wild-type and mutant allele). The necessary characteristics to be certain a disorder is inherited in an autosomal dominant manner are listed in Table 6.1 and depicted in Figure 6.1.

RECURRENCE RISKS

Since individuals with autosomal dominant disorders are heterozygous for a mutant and a normal allele, there is a 1 in 2 (50%) chance a gamete will carry the normal allele and a 1 in 2 (50%) chance a gamete will carry the mutant allele. Assuming that the individual's partner will contribute a normal allele, there is a 1 in 2 (50%) chance that the offspring will inherit the disorder with each pregnancy (Fig. 6.2).

PENETRANCE

There can be marked variability in the clinical manifestations of autosomal dominant disorders, with them often showing what is known as reduced penetrance (i.e., not every person with the mutant allele showing features of the disorder). The penetrance of a disorder is an index of the proportion of individuals with an allele who have manifestations of it. An allele is said to be nonpenetrant if an individual known to be heterozygous for the allele, either by pedigree analysis or by molecular investigation, shows no signs of the disorder when subjected to appropriate clinical investigation. The penetrance of some genes is dependent

on the age of the individual, as in Huntington disease, in which the penetrance is age dependent or is said to show delayed penetrance.

EXPRESSIVITY

The expressivity of a gene is the degree to which a phenotype is expressed in an individual. Many autosomal dominant diseases show variable expressivity such that individuals in the same family who carry an identical mutation can vary considerably in the severity of their disorder. For example, in autosomal dominant retinitis pigmentosa, individuals within the same family can show marked variation in the extent of their visual impairment.

ANTICIPATION

A disorder is said to demonstrate anticipation if the manifestations of the mutant allele increase in severity as it is passed down the generations. An example of a disorder that demonstrates anticipation is myotonic dystrophy. In a typical three generation family with myotonic dystrophy, the grandparent may have only cataracts without any muscle problems; in the next generation, affected individuals have muscle weakness and myotonia, while in the third generation, the family can present after a child is born with the congenital form of the disease with profound muscle hypotonia and life-threatening respiratory problems.

SEX INFLUENCE

Sex influence involves the expression of an autosomal allele that occurs more frequently in one sex than the other. An example in humans is gout, with males affected more frequently than females until after the menopause, an effect probably mediated by hormonal differences.

SEX LIMITATION

Some traits are manifested only in individuals of one sex, an extreme situation known as sex limitation. This can occur when a gene affects an organ only possessed by one of the sexes (e.g., unicornuate uterus).

PLEIOTROPY

Pleiotropy refers to the phenomenon in which a single gene is responsible for a number of distinct and seemingly unrelated phenotypic effects. For example, the allele causing neurofibromatosis type 1 can produce abnormalities of skin pigmentation, neurofibromas of the peripheral nerves, short stature, macrocephaly, skeletal abnormalities, and fits. Each one of the pleiotropic effects of an allele can show reduced or nonpenetrance and variable expressivity.

MECHANISMS OF REDUCED PENETRANCE AND VARIABLE EXPRESSIVITY

Some of the underlying mechanisms accounting for reduced penetrance and variable expressivity have been known for some time, while others are only now becoming apparent with the advent of modern molecular biologic techniques.

Environmental factors

Environmental influences can affect the expression of genes. This can involve factors in the internal environment, such as hormones, or in the external environment, such as the effect of certain drugs (e.g. barbiturates) in acute intermittent porphyria. This disorder is characterized by attacks of abdominal pain, constipation, and psychiatric disturbances and is due to a mutation in a gene coding for an enzyme involved in heme biosynthesis. Attacks can be precipitated by certain drugs including phenobarbital and the sulfonamides. Avoidance of these precipitating factors will result in the nonpenetrance of the disorder. Similarly, diet could affect the manifestation of familial hypercholesterolemia, such that the lower the intake of dietary cholesterol, the lower the serum cholesterol and the less severe or the later the manifestations of complications associated with the disorder.

Somatic mutations

Retinoblastoma has already been mentioned as an example of one of the familial cancer genes in which a "second-hit" somatic mutation needs to occur in order for the disorder to manifest.

Unstable DNA triplet repeat sequences

It is now known that there are a group of dominant genetic disorders in which the mutation is an unstable DNA triplet repeat sequence that expands in successive meioses and whose size correlates with the severity of the disorder. This accounts for the anticipation seen in such disorders as myotonic dystrophy and Huntington disease. Unstable DNA is discussed in greater detail later in this chapter.

Genetic background

Information from studies of inbred animals suggests that it is likely that the genetic background of an individual (i.e., the nature of particular alleles at other loci that interact with a mutant allele) will influence the expression of a disorder. Analysis of the effect of this type of interaction is complex and is poorly understood at present.

New dominant mutations

While nonpenetrance can be a possible cause of a dominant disorder arising in the offspring of completely normal parents, an alternative explanation is, however, that a mutation has arisen during transmission of the gene, that is, it represents a new mutation. This appears to be more common for certain disorders than others, such as in achondroplasia, in which in 80% of families the parents are of normal stature, reflecting the reduced reproductive fitness of adults with achondroplasia. The observation that achondroplasia occurred more frequently in last-born children of a sibship (Weinberg, 1912) was suggested by Penrose as attributable to increased paternal age associated with new mutations, on the basis that "older germ-cells, possessed by older parents, might be more likely to show deterioration, in the form of genetical changes" (Penrose, 1955).

Some dominant mutations are universally lethal before the affected individual reaches the reproductive age and therefore are always seen as new lethal dominant mutations. Several lethal disorders that were previously considered to be recessive are now known in many instances to be due to new dominant mutations, such as the perinatal lethal form (type II) of osteogenesis imperfecta (Byers et al., 1988a).

New dominant mutations that occur during gametogenesis are associated with a negligible recurrence risk for future siblings. However, if the disorder is compatible with survival to the reproductive age and the possibility of reproduction, the recurrence risks for the offspring of the affected individual is 50%.

Gonadal mosaicism

In the case of certain new dominant mutations, there is a small but significant risk that a second child will be affected despite both parents being clinically normal. The recent ability to determine the molecular basis of many of these disorders has shown that this finding can be explained by the phenomenon of gonadal mosaicism. This is the presence of two genetically different types of germ cell in an individual.

The mutational event occurs post-fertilization with the degree of mosaicism being dependent upon the time that it occurred. There is evidence that this usually occurs early in development as commitment of primordial cells to the germline occurs before tissue allocation (Soriano and Jaenisch, 1986) and in studies of individuals with gonadal mosaicism, up to 50% also have the mutation in a somatic cell line (Zlotogora, 1993).

The frequency of gonadal mosaicism differs between disorders. At present it is unclear why it is a frequent finding in some disorders such as fascioscapulohumeral dystrophy and osteogenesis imperfecta where mosaicism is found in approximately 19% and 15% of all cases (Kohler et al., 1996; Byers et al., 1988b) while in others such as achondroplasia there have only been a few rare case reports. This is an important point to remember when providing recurrence risk advice in genetic counselling.

Autosomal recessive inheritance

DEFINITION

Autosomal recessive inheritance refers to disorders due to genes located on the autosomes, but in which the disease alleles are recessive to the wild-type alleles and are therefore not evident in the heterozygous state, only being manifest in the homozygous state. The necessary characteristics to be certain that a disorder is inherited in an autosomal recessive manner are listed in Table 6.2 and depicted in Figure 6.3.

The parents of an individual with an autosomal recessive disorder are heterozygous for the disease allele and are usually referred to as being carriers for the disorder.

Table 6.2 Characteristics of an autosomal recessive inherited disorder

Both males and females are affected
The disorder normally occurs in only one generation, usually within a single sibship
The parents can be consanguinous

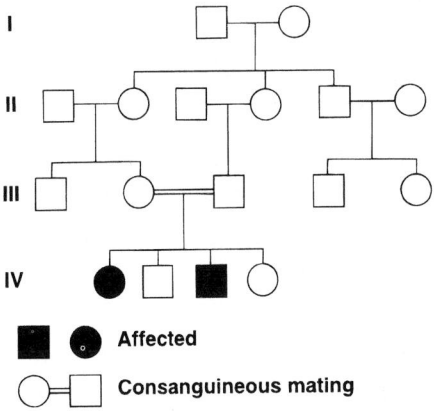

Fig. 6.3. Pedigree consistent with autosomal recessive inheritance.

CONSANGUINITY

If a couple are consanguineous they have at least one ancestor in common in the preceding few generations. This means that they are more likely to carry identical alleles inherited from this common ancestor and could both transmit an identical allele to their offspring, who would then be homozygous for that allele. A consanguineous couple has an increased risk that their offspring will be affected with a recessive disorder. The rarer a particular disease is in a population, the more likely the parents are to be consanguineous. For example, cystic fibrosis is the commonest autosomal recessive disorder in Caucasians in Western Europe, with an incidence of approximately 1 in 2,000. The incidence of consanguinity in the parents of children with cystic fibrosis is not appreciably greater than that in the general population. By contrast, with very rare autosomal recessive disorders such as alkaptonuria, 8 of the first 19 families originally described by Garrod were consanguineous (Garrod, 1902).

RECURRENCE RISKS

When two parents carrying the same disease allele reproduce, there is an equal chance that gametes contain the disease or the wild-type allele. There are four possible combinations of these gametes, resulting in a 1 in 4 (25%) chance of having a homozygous affected offspring, a 1 in 2

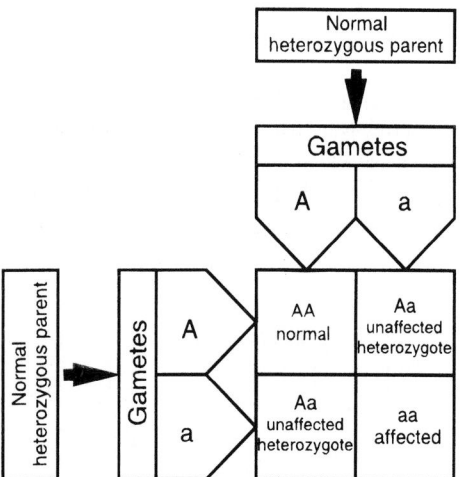

Fig. 6.4. Punnett's square of gametes and offspring for autosomal recessive inheritance.

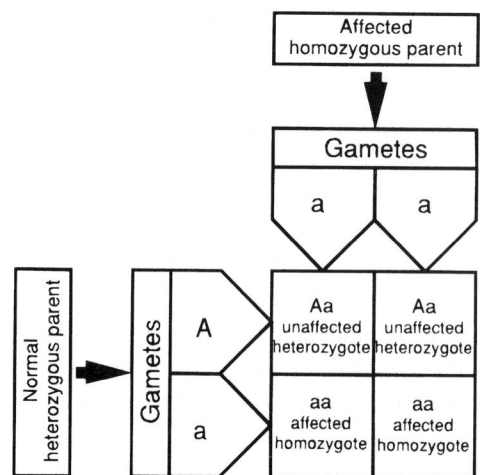

Fig. 6.6. Punnett's square for gametes and offspring of individuals with an autosomal recessive disorder and a partner heterozygous for the same disorder.

(50%) chance of having a heterozygous unaffected carrier offspring, and a 1 in 4 (25%) chance of having a homozygous unaffected offspring (Fig. 6.4).

When an individual with an autosomal recessive disorder has children, they will only produce gametes containing the disease allele. Since it is most likely that their partner will be homozygous for the wild-type allele, they will always contribute a normal allele and therefore all the children will be heterozygous carriers and unaffected (Fig. 6.5). If, however, an affected individual has children with a partner who happens to be heterozygous for the disease allele, there will be a 50% chance of transmitting the disorder, depending on whether the partner contributes a disease or a wild-type allele (Fig. 6.6). Such a pedigree is said to exhibit pseudodominance (Fig. 6.7).

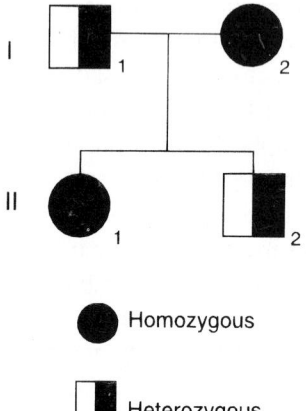

Fig. 6.7. Pedigree of an autosomal recessive disorder showing pseudodominance.

GENETIC HETEROGENEITY

It is not unusual in some recessive disorders, such as sensorineural deafness, for two affected individuals to have children. Assortative mating occurs in such instances because of social circumstances in which individuals with the same disability, such as deafness or visual impairment, are often educated together or share the same social facilities. If their disorder were due to a mutation in the same autosomal recessive gene, all their offspring would be affected. In a number of such studies involving the offspring of parents with inherited sensorineural deafness, however, a significant proportion of such matings lead to offspring with normal hearing (Chung and Brown, 1970). Although in some instances this could be due to other causes (e.g., acquired causes being mistaken for inherited

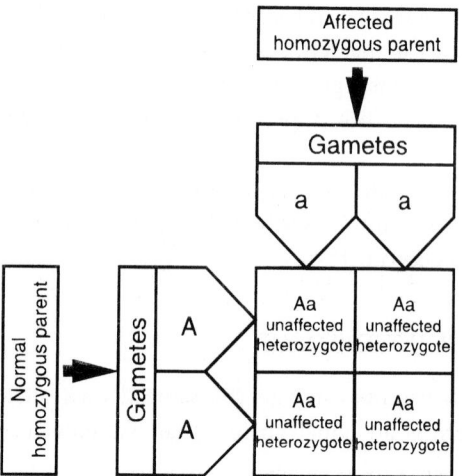

Fig. 6.5. Punnett's square for gametes and offspring of individuals with an autosomal recessive disorder and a normal partner.

deafness), in most instances the gene causing the deafness in the two parents is different, a phenomenon known as genetic heterogeneity. Each parent will transmit one mutant allele, but a wild-type allele of the gene causing their partner's deafness, therefore, the child is heterozygous for the two mutant alleles or what is known as a double heterozygote. The results of segregation analyses suggested that there are a number of different genes causing clinically indistinguishable autosomal recessive sensorineural deafness and this has now been confirmed with 28 loci identified to date. This type of genetic heterogeneity involving different genes is known as locus heterogeneity.

Heterogeneity can also exist at the same locus; thus, an individual affected with a recessively inherited disorder, often called a compound heterozygote, does not have the same two mutant alleles at the locus involved, unless a specific mutation is especially prevalent in a particular population or the affected individual is the offspring of a consanguineous relationship, in which case the allele is likely to be identical by descent. This is known as allelic or mutational heterogeneity. The specific mutations that an affected individual possesses can, in fact, determine the severity of the disorder, as in cystic fibrosis, in which individuals who are homozygous for the most common mutation in the cystic fibrosis gene, Δ-F508, have a higher incidence of pancreatic insufficiency (Kerem et al., 1990).

UNIPARENTAL DISOMY

Uniparental disomy, a mode of inheritance that was previously unexpected, has recently been recognized as responsible for unusual modes of inheritance. This involves both homologues of a chromosome pair being derived from the same parent. Uniparental disomy has been reported as a rare cause of the autosomal recessive disorder cystic fibrosis in the offspring of a couple where only one parent was a heterozygote carrier for the mutant allele, the affected offspring receiving both chromosome 7 homologues with the mutant allele from that parent (Voss et al., 1989). Uniparental disomy is covered in greater detail in a subsequent section of this chapter.

Sex-linked inheritance

Strictly speaking, sex-linked inheritance refers to the inheritance patterns shown by genes on the sex chromosomes. If the gene is on the X chromosome, it is said to show X-linked inheritance and, if on the Y chromosome, Y-linked or holandric inheritance.

X-LINKED RECESSIVE INHERITANCE

Definition

This form of inheritance is conventionally referred to as sex-linked inheritance. It refers to disorders due to recessive genes on the X chromosome. Males have a single X-chromosome and are therefore hemizygous for most of the alleles on the X chromosome, so that if they have a mutant allele, they will manifest the disorder. Females, on the other hand, will usually only manifest the disorder if they are homozygous for the disease allele and if heterozygous will usually be unaffected. Since it is rare for females to be homozygous for a mutant allele, X-linked recessive disorders usually only affect males.

The necessary characteristics to be certain a disorder is inherited in an X-linked recessive manner are listed in Table 6.3 and portrayed in Figure 6.8.

Recurrence risks

If a male affected with an X-linked recessive disorder survives to reproduce, he will always transmit his X chromosome with the mutant allele to his daughters, who will be obligate carriers. An affected male will always transmit his Y chromosome to a son and therefore none of his sons will be affected (Fig. 6.9). A carrier female has one X chromosome

Table 6.3 Characteristics of an X-linked recessive inherited disorder

Males are affected almost exclusively
Transmission occurs through unaffected or carrier females to their sons
Male-to-male transmission is not observed
Affected males are at risk of transmitting the disorder to their grandsons through their obligate carrier daughters

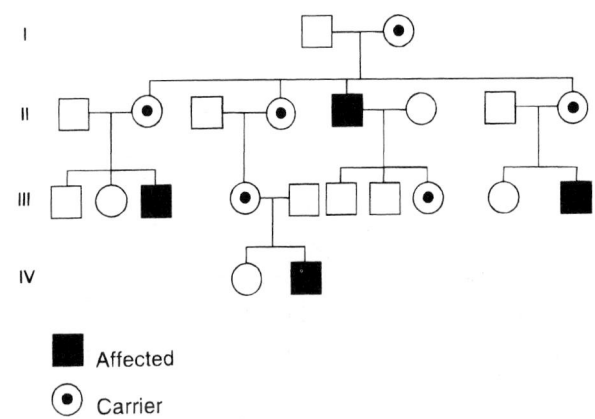

Fig. 6.8. Pedigree consistent with X-linked recessive inheritance.

■ Affected
⊙ Carrier

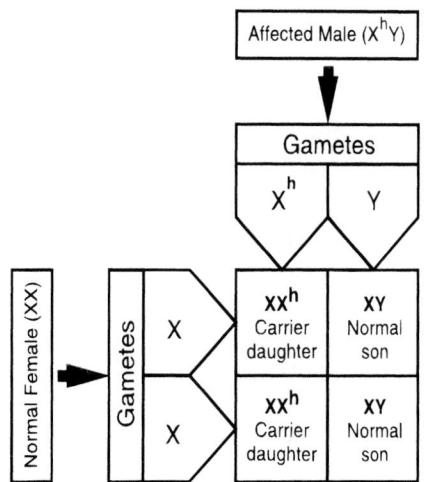

Fig. 6.9. Punnett's square for gametes and offspring of a male with an X-linked recessive disorder.

with the wild-type allele and one X chromosome with the disease allele; therefore, her sons have a 1 in 2 (50%) chance of being affected, while her daughters have a 1 in 2 (50%) chance of being carriers (Fig. 6.10).

For a female to be affected with an X-linked recessive disorder her mother would have to be a carrier and her father affected with the disorder. Obviously this situation is encountered only very rarely. Another possibility is that her mother is a carrier and the X chromosome transmitted by her father undergoes a new mutation. A female can also be affected by an X-linked recessive disorder if she has a single X chromosome (i.e., Turner syndrome), in which case she will be hemizygous for alleles on the X chromosome like a male.

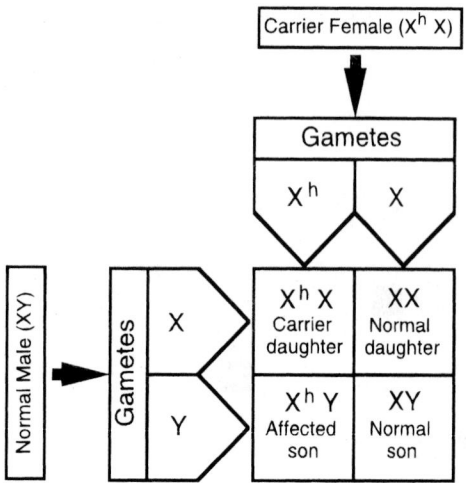

Fig. 6.10. Punnett's square for gametes and offspring of a carrier female of an X-linked disorder.

X inactivation

Early in the embryonic development one of the X chromosomes in females is inactivated in each cell with the result that the female, like the male, has a single functional X chromosome. In individuals with X chromosome aneuploidies, all but one of the X chromosomes are inactivated in each cell. The process of X inactivation is controlled by a region of the X chromosome, the X inactivation center, situated on the proximal portion of the long arm. X inactivation usually occurs as a random process, such that in approximately 50% of cells in a female, the maternally derived X chromosome is active and in the other 50% the paternally derived X chromosome is active. In females who are carriers of an X-linked recessive mutation, one-half of the cells will actively express the disease allele. Occasionally, this can be demonstrated clinically; for example, in X-linked retinitis pigmentosa, careful fundoscopic examination of the retina of a female carrier can show a mosaic pattern of pigmentation (Gieser et al., 1980).

Manifesting female carriers of X-linked recessive disorders

Although female carriers of X-linked recessive disorders are usually asymptomatic, they can manifest signs of the disorder. They are usually much less severely affected than males, however. There are a number of different mechanisms by which a female heterozygote can manifest signs of an X-linked recessive disorder but the underlying cause for each one is nonrandom or skewed X inactivation. In this situation, there is a departure from the normal random process of X inactivation, with a greater proportion of one X chromosome inactivated than the other. If in most cells the active X chromosome is the one with the mutant allele, a female can manifest the disorder.

Mechanisms of nonrandom X inactivation

A number of mechanisms can lead to nonrandom X inactivation:

1. *Chance*: Skewed X inactivation can occur by chance.
2. *Monozygotic twinning*: There have been several reports of monozygotic female twins, both heterozygous for a dystrophin gene deletion, one of whom was a manifesting carrier for Duchenne muscular dystrophy and the other an unaffected carrier (Richards et al., 1990). It was demonstrated that in lymphocytes and fibroblasts of the affected twin, the majority of active X chromosomes had the deletion, while in the unaffected

twin most active X chromosomes possessed the intact gene. It has been postulated that the twinning process could have been a consequence of cell surface differences as a result of X chromosome inactivation, leading to the separation of the two cell masses.

3. *Cytogenetic abnormalities*: In females with an X-autosome translocation, the normal X chromosome will be preferentially inactivated, maintaining the diploid state for the autosome involved in the translocation. If the translocation disrupts or interferes with the expression of a gene on the X chromosome, or the X chromosome involved in the translocation carries a disease allele, that female will manifest the disorder. The finding of X-autosome translocations in manifesting female carriers of Duchenne muscular dystrophy was instrumental in the mapping and cloning of the dystrophin gene (Bodrug et al., 1987).

4. *Elimination of cells expressing the mutant allele*: If a gene on the X chromosome is required for cell survival, the normal gene will always be found on the active X chromosome and the defective gene on the inactive X chromosome in the mature cell population, even though X inactivation occurred as a random process. This has been demonstrated in a number of disorders, including X-linked severe combined immunodeficiency, and can be used in the determination of carrier status for females at risk (Goodship et al., 1988).

Gonadal mosaicism

As with autosomal dominant disorders, gonadal mosaicism is an important phenomenon in X-linked recessive disorders, occurring particularly frequently in Duchenne muscular dystrophy, where it has been shown to occur in both male and female gametogenesis. It is important to take this into account when advising mothers of apparently sporadically affected males with Duchenne muscular dystrophy of recurrence risks (van Essen et al., 1992).

X-LINKED DOMINANT INHERITANCE

Definition

X-linked dominant inheritance is an uncommon form of inheritance and is caused by dominant disease alleles on the X chromosome. The disorder will manifest in both hemizygous males and heterozygous females. Random X inactivation would mean that females are less likely to be severely affected than hemizygous males, unless they are homozy-

Table 6.4 Characteristics of an X-Linked Dominant Inherited Disorder

Daughters of affected males always inherit the disorder
Sons of affected males never inherit the disorder
Affected females can transmit the disorder to offspring of both sexes
An excess of affected females exists in pedigrees for the disorder

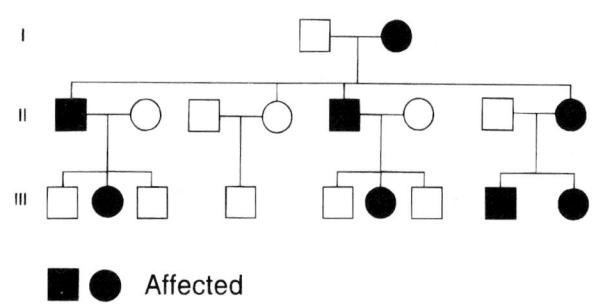

■ ● Affected

Fig. 6.11. Pedigree consistent with X-linked dominant inheritance.

gous for the disease allele. The characteristics of an X-linked dominant inherited disorder are listed in Table 6.4 and depicted in Figure 6.11.

Recurrence risks

Offspring of either sex have a 1 in 2 (50%) chance of inheriting the disorder from affected females (Fig. 6.12). The situation is different for males affected by X-linked dominant disorders whose daughters will always inherit the gene and whose sons cannot inherit the gene (Fig. 6.13). An example of an X-linked dominant disorder is vitamin D-

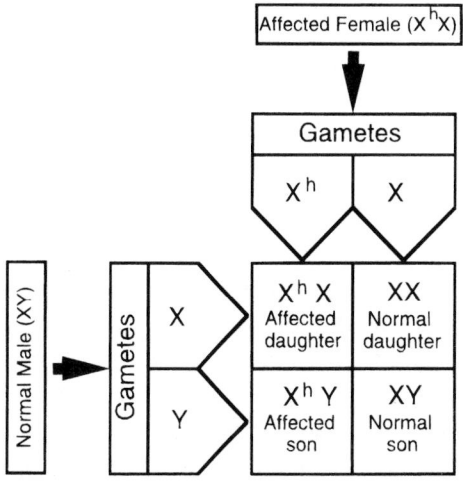

Fig. 6.12. Punnett's square for gametes and offspring of a female affected with an X-linked dominant disorder.

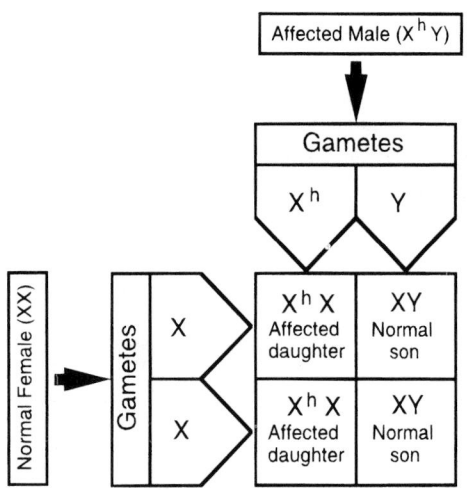

Fig. 6.13. Punnett's square for gametes and offspring of a male affected with an X-linked dominant disorder.

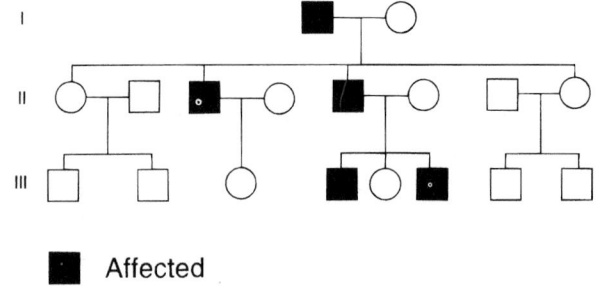

■ Affected

Fig. 6.14. Pedigree consistent with Y-linked inheritance.

resistant rickets. X inactivation results in females with this disorder having less severe skeletal changes than occur in affected males.

X-linked dominant lethal alleles

In some disorders due to mutant alleles of genes on the X chromosome, affected males are never or very rarely seen (e.g., incontinentia pigmenti and Goltz syndrome). This is thought to be due to a lethal effect of the mutant disease allele in the hemizygous male, resulting in nonviability of the conceptus during early embryonic development. As a consequence, if an affected female were to have children, one would expect a sex ratio of 2:1, female to male, in the offspring and that one-half of the females would be affected, while none of the male offspring would be affected. The majority of the mothers of females with these X-linked dominant lethal disorders are generally unaffected and the disease alleles are therefore thought to arise as new mutations.

Y-LINKED (HOLANDRIC) INHERITANCE

Y-linked, or holandric, inheritance refers to genes carried on the Y chromosome. They therefore will be present only in males, and the disorder would be passed on to all their sons only (Fig. 6.14). Although a number of traits, such as hairy ears, have been postulated to be inherited in this manner, there is no good evidence for this type of inheritance being associated with disease in humans. Genes involved in spermatogenesis have been mapped to the Y chromosome (Ma et al., 1993), but a male with a mutation

in a Y-linked gene involved in spermatogenesis would probably be infertile or hypofertile making it difficult to demonstrate Y-linked inheritance. This situation may well change with the use of techniques such as intracytoplasmic sperm injection (ICSI) to treat male infertility which will result in the transmission of the infertility to male offspring.

Partial sex linkage

A small region of sequence identity exists between the X and Y chromosomes located at the tips of the long and short arms, known as the pseudoautosomal regions of the sex chromosomes (Rappold, 1993). A high rate of recombination at the telomeres of the short arms is thought to be obligatory for normal meiosis of these chromosomes. The genes within these regions, known as pseudoautosomal genes, escape X inactivation in the female (Schiebel et al., 1993); therefore, both sexes have two active alleles at these loci. A pseudoautosomal gene *SHOX* has been postulated to account for some of the features seen in the numerical sex chromosome disorder Turner syndrome (Kosho et al., 1999).

There is no definite evidence, as yet, for a human genetic disorder caused by a pseudoautosomal gene but, given the high rate of recombination between the X and the Y, this type of inheritance could provide an explanation for disorders which appear to be X-linked in some families and Y-linked in others.

Nontraditional inheritance

Disorders have been known for many years that do not follow the rules of classic mendelian inheritance. Recent advances in molecular biology are now providing the explanations for these observations and will no doubt continue to provide new ones in the future.

UNSTABLE DNA TRIPLET REPEAT SEQUENCES

Definition

One assumption of mendelian genetics is that mutant alleles are transmitted from parent to offspring unchanged. An ever increasing number of disorders are now being described in which the underlying mutation is an expansion of a triplet nucleotide repeat sequence that is unstable and can change in size on transmission from parent to offspring. Triplet repeats occur throughout the human genome and are normally stably transmitted. Their normal function is unknown.

Premutations/full mutations

The size of the triplet repeat sequences involved in the various disorders recognized in humans is polymorphic in the general population, occurring with differing numbers of repeats. The disease state appears to occur when the size of the repeat sequence is greater than that normally seen in the general population. There is no absolute cut-off between the normal range of repeat numbers and those associated with the disease state, but triplet repeat numbers outside the normal range have been divided into premutations and full mutations. Premutations are expansions beyond the normal range but which are associated with a normal phenotype. They are, however, unstable in transmission and are more likely to mutate into a full mutation associated with the disease phenotype.

Instability and anticipation

In triplet repeat disorders there is a tendency for the size of the triplet repeat to increase as it is transmitted. In addition, it appears that the longer a repeat is, the more likely it is to expand further on transmission to the next generation. The size of the repeat shows a rough correlation with the severity and age of onset of the disorder in an individual. This has now been demonstrated to be the molecular explanation of the phenomenon of anticipation seen in many of the dominant triplet repeat diseases. The cause of the instability and propensity for expansion is unknown although there are many theories. One possible mechanism is slippage at DNA replication (Richards and Sutherland, 1994). The longer a repeat, the more likely two single stranded breaks are to occur within the repeat. Since the fragment is not anchored by a unique sequence, it is able to slip and repair could result in the introduction of more repeat copies than were present in the original sequence. Another possible mechanism for

the expansions is that the simple triplet-repeat tracts form alternative DNA structures such as hairpins, which interfere with accurate replication (Sinden, 1999). Triplet repeats of perfect sequence (i.e., CTGCTGCTG …) are much more unstable than imperfect repeats (i.e., CTGCTTCTG …), a fact that might support either mechanism. Such mechanisms would be postulated to lead to decreases in triplet-repeat size as well. It is not understood why increases in triplet-repeat size appears so much more frequently than decreases in size.

Another observation that is still not fully understood is that the size of the expansion can be influenced by the sex of the transmitting parent. For example, in myotonic dystrophy expansions are on average larger when transmitted by females. This could account for the observation that the vast majority of children with the congenital form of myotonic dystrophy, which is usually associated with a very large expansion, inherit the gene from their mother (Mulley et al., 1993).

Similarly, in fragile X mental retardation expansions of premutations to full mutations only occur in transmission through females. Analysis of sperm from males with a full mutation for fragile X mental retardation only shows the premutations (Reyniers et al., 1993). Rather than needing an explanation for why large expansions occur during female transmission, it could be more relevant to inquire why large expansions are not transmitted by the male. Conversely, in Huntington disease, there is a tendency for larger mutations to be transmitted by males. The juvenile form of Huntington disease, which is again associated with large expansions of the triplet repeat sequence, is almost always transmitted by the father (Andrew et al., 1993).

There is still much dispute as to whether the expansion of the trinucleotide repeat sequence occurs during meiosis, or as a result of mitotic instability during mitosis as a post-fertilization event, or both (Nelson and Warren, 1993). Sampling of different tissues in persons with fragile X mental retardation often shows a wide range of repeat sizes. As in meiotic transmission, the larger the expansion of the triplet repeat, the more unstable it becomes in somatic cells.

Effects of triplet repeat expansion

The triplet repeat disorders can be divided into two distinct groups. Type I disorders involve the expansion of CAG repeats, which encode an expanded polyglutamine tract, inserted into the open reading frame of a gene. Type II disorders involve repeat expansions in noncoding regions of genes. The commonest examples of the two types of disorders are shown in Table 6.5.

6   Basic principles

Table 6.5 Examples of Triplet Repeats in Human Genetic Disease

Disease	Repeat	Location
Type I Diseases		
Huntington Disease	CAG	Translated region coding for polyglutamine
Spinocerebellar Ataxia 1	CAG	Translated region coding for polyglutamine
Spinocerebellar Ataxia 2	CAG	Translated region coding for polyglutamine
Spinocerebellar Ataxia 3	CAG	Translated region coding for polyglutamine
Spinocerebellar Ataxia 6	CAG	Translated region coding for polyglutamine
Spinocerebellar Ataxia 7	CAG	Translated region coding for polyglutamine
Type II Diseases		
Fragile X Syndrome	CGG	5′ untranslated region
Myotonic Dystrophy	CTG	3′ untranslated region
Friedreich Ataxia	GAA	Intronic

Type I polyglutamine expansions

These have now been recognized as a major cause of inherited neurodegenerative disease. The basis of these diseases is a dominant toxic gain of function that occurs at the protein level and that increases with longer glutamine repeats. The novel toxic property seems to be due to misfolding of the polyglutamine domain. This may lead to both aggregation of protein and impaired proteolysis and many of these diseases show aggregations of mutant protein within the nucleus. Despite widespread expression of the various disease proteins, certain populations of neurons are particularly susceptible to degeneration, and the basis of this vulnerability remains a crucial question (Paulson, 1999).

Type II repeat diseases

There are probably several mechanisms involved in the pathology of type II repeat diseases where the repeat expansion occurs in a noncoding region of the gene.

1. *DNA methylation* In fragile X mental retardation, the trinucleotide repeat sequence occurs in the 5′ untranslated region of the *FMR1* gene and the full mutation interferes with the transcription of the gene. The full mutation is associated with methylation of an adjacent CpG island, a likely promoter region for the *FMR1* gene. It is not known, however, whether this methylation is a cause or consequence of the inactivity of the *FMR1* gene (Richards and Sutherland, 1992).

2. *RNA effects* Myotonic dystrophy is due to a CTG repeat in the 3′ untranslated region of the gene. One theory is that it exerts its effect at the RNA level. Untranslated RNA containing large numbers of CUG repeats may affect cell physiology by sequestering or activating specific proteins in the cell (Timchenko, 1999).

3. *Inhibition of transcription* Friedreich ataxia is different from the other triplet repeat diseases in that it is caused by a GAA repeat in the first intron and is inherited as a recessive. The expansion results in marked decreases in mRNA levels, thought to result from the formation of an unusual non-β DNA structure inhibiting transcription (Sinden, 1999).

FRAGILE X MENTAL RETARDATION— THE SHERMAN PARADOX

Until the discovery of unstable triplet repeats, the inheritance pattern of fragile X mental retardation was puzzling. Although initially presumed to be due to an X-linked recessive gene there were a number of observations that did not conform to classical X-linked recessive inheritance:

1. Thirty per cent of carrier females showed some degree of mental impairment, a proportion greater than one would expect with carrier females.

2. Males who were phenotypically normal (normal transmitting males) could pass a mutant allele to their daughters who were also phenotypically normal but who were at risk of having affected sons.

The risk of mental impairment in fragile X mental retardation pedigrees was noted to be contingent on the position of the individuals within a pedigree. The likelihood of mental impairment was higher in the offspring of intellectually normal daughters of transmitting males than in the offspring of intellectually normal mothers of transmitting males (Sherman paradox) (Sherman et al., 1984, 1985).

The finding that fragile X mental retardation is due to an unstable CGG trinucleotide repeat in the 5′ untranslated region of the *FMR1* gene provides an explanation for the Sherman paradox. The size of the repeat in the normal population varies from 6 to 50 repeats. The mothers of normal transmitting males have a premutation in the 60 to 69 triplet repeat range. This can be transmitted as a premutation to a normal transmitting male son or expand to a full mutation of greater than 200 repeats leading to an affected son (8.5% risk). Normal transmitting males pass the premutation on to their daughters who have slightly larger premutations, usually in the 70 to 89 repeat range, associated

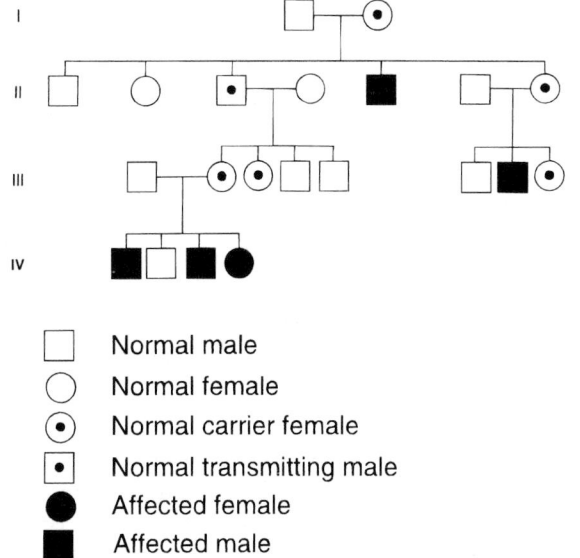

Normal male
Normal female
Normal carrier female
Normal transmitting male
Affected female
Affected male

Fig. 6.15. Pedigree of a family with fragile-X mental retardation.

with an increased risk of expansion upon transmission due to the larger repeat size. Once the triplet repeat size reaches 90 or more repeats, the risk of expansion approaches 100%, and the consequent risk of having an affected boy becomes 50%. Full mutations can result in mental impairment in females (Fu et al., 1991) (Fig. 6.15).

GENOMIC IMPRINTING

Definition

From our knowledge of mendelian inheritance it is assumed that genes from both parents play an equal role in early development. However, pronuclear transfer experiments have clearly demonstrated that the paternal and maternal genomes, despite their identical genetic contributions, are not functionally equivalent and both are essential for normal development. This phenomenon is attributed to differential epigenetic modifications of the germline leading to parental dependent silencing of some regions of the chromosome during development. This process is known as genomic imprinting and leads to the functional hemizygosity of a small number of genes, as only the paternal or maternal allele is expressed.

A gene is said to be maternally imprinted if the maternally derived allele is inactivated, and paternally imprinted if the paternally derived allele is inactivated. To date there has been much speculation on the purpose and origin of such a process; however, a true understanding has still to be elucidated.

Mechanism of imprinting

The mechanism of imprinting in the gametes is poorly understood but must satisfy four requirements (Tycko, 1994):

1. Imprinting must occur before fertilization.
2. Imprinting must be able to confer transcriptional silencing.
3. Imprinting must be stably transmitted through mitosis in somatic cells.
4. Imprinting must be reversible on passage through the opposite parental germline (i.e., if an allele is maternally imprinted, this must be removed in the gametes of a male offspring).

One approach towards elucidation of mechanisms has been to examine epigenetic properties that distinguish the maternal and paternal alleles. This process is most advanced for DNA methylation. Evidence for its involvement is that all imprinted genes show differences in methylation pattern, what are known as differential methylation regions (DMR), between maternal and paternal alleles (Neumann and Barlow, 1996). Methylation of genes in promoter regions can lead to transcriptional silencing which can be stably transmitted through mitosis by the action of DNA methyltransferase (Bird, 1992). DNA in sperm has been shown to have a different pattern of methylation than that of DNA from ova (Rubin et al., 1994). There is extensive reprogramming of the methylation pattern of the genome during preimplantation development of the zygote; however, at some imprinted sequences, the differences in methylation inherited from the gametes appear to survive reprogramming and as such may well coincide with putative imprinting signals for differentiation of alleles (Neumann and Barlow, 1996).

Another factor thought to play a part in imprinting, whether independently or in conjunction with DNA methylation, is chromatin structure. Chromatin structure can be studied by looking at sensitivity to DNA nucleases. Such studies have shown different chromatin organization on the methylated and unmethylated alleles of several imprinted genes (Khosla et al., 1999). It has been suggested that alternative chromatin organization may have a role in preventing the differential methylation regions from becoming methylated during development (Feil and Khosla, 1999).

Evidence for the role of genomic imprinting in human disease

There are several lines of evidence suggesting that genomic imprinting is involved in human genetic disease.

Pedigree analysis

A few diseases occur with equal frequencies in males and females but are transmitted exclusively or preferentially from one type of parent. An example is the disorder of familial glomus tumors. These benign chemodectomas usually present as an enlarging cervical mass or with a cranial nerve palsy. Although the tumors are seen in several generations in a family and occur both in males and in females, they are inherited almost exclusively via the paternal line and maternal transmission does not occur (Fig. 6.16). However, unaffected males with affected mothers or grandmothers can have affected children (van der Mey et al., 1989). This pattern of inheritance could be explained if an autosomal dominant gene is maternally imprinted such that it is inactivated during oogenesis and is reactivated during male spermatogenesis.

Uniparental disomy (UPD)

Uniparental disomy refers to the presence of both homologues of a chromosome pair or chromosomal region in a diploid offspring being derived from a single parent. If the two homologues are identical due to an error in meiosis II, this is known as uniparental isodisomy, while if the two homologues are different but still from the same parent due to a meiosis I error, this is known as uniparental heterodisomy.

Although the initial observation of UPD in humans was first reported in autosomal recessive disorders (Spence et al., 1988), it is now most well known because of the consequences of disrupting genomic imprinting. The proposed mechanism by which the abnormal phenotype manifests is the loss of the normal biparental contribution in a region where an imprinted gene resides. This results in either that individual having no actively expressed allele or having biallelic expression of that allele, dependent on the imprinting status and parent of origin of the UPD.

Potential mechanisms of uniparental disomy

1. *Trisomic rescue*: Meiotic nondisjunction in one gamete would result in an embryo trisomic for a chromosome. Loss of the chromosome from the parent contributing the single homologue would result in either uniparental heterodisomy or isodisomy depending on whether the error occurred in meiosis I or meiosis II (Hall, 1990; Kalousek et al., 1993) (Fig. 6.17A, B).
2. *Gamete complementation*: Meiotic nondisjunction could occur in one gamete fertilized by a gamete nullisomic for that chromosome (Wang et al., 1991). This may give rise to either heterodisomy or isodisomy (Fig. 6.17 C,D).
3. *Monosomy duplication*: A monosomic gamete could fertilize a nullisomic gamete which through chromosome duplication produces uniparental isodisomy (Spence et al., 1988) (Fig. 6.17E).
4. *Compensatory duplication*: Postzygotic duplication of one chromosome following the loss of the other homologous chromosome which was abnormal, giving rise to uniparental isodisomy (Petersen et al., 1992) (Fig. 6.17F).
5. *Heterochromatid exchange*: Postzygotic balanced heterochromatid cross-over leading to segmental uniparental isodisomy (Henry et al., 1993; Slatter et al., 1994) (Fig. 6.17G).

Syndromes associated with disruption of genomic imprinting

There are now several well recognized syndromes where abnormalities of imprinting are thought to be the cause, Prader–Willi and Angelman syndrome on chromosome 15 involving the region 15q11–13 and Beckwith–Wiedemann syndrome on chromosome 11 at 11p15.5.

Prader–Willi/Angelman syndrome

The Prader–Willi syndrome (PWS) is a disorder characterized by short stature, obesity, and mild to moderate learning difficulties. The Angelman syndrome (AS) is characterized by gait disturbance, epilepsy and severe learning difficulties. Over the last 15 years several findings have pointed to a parent of origin effect and it is now clear that PWS is caused by a deficiency of paternal gene expression within the

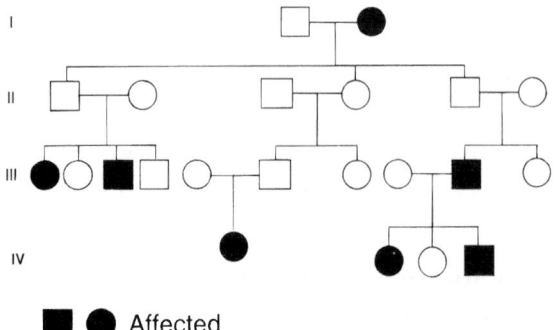

■ ● Affected

Fig. 6.16. Pedigree of a family with hereditary glomus tumors consistent with maternal imprinting.

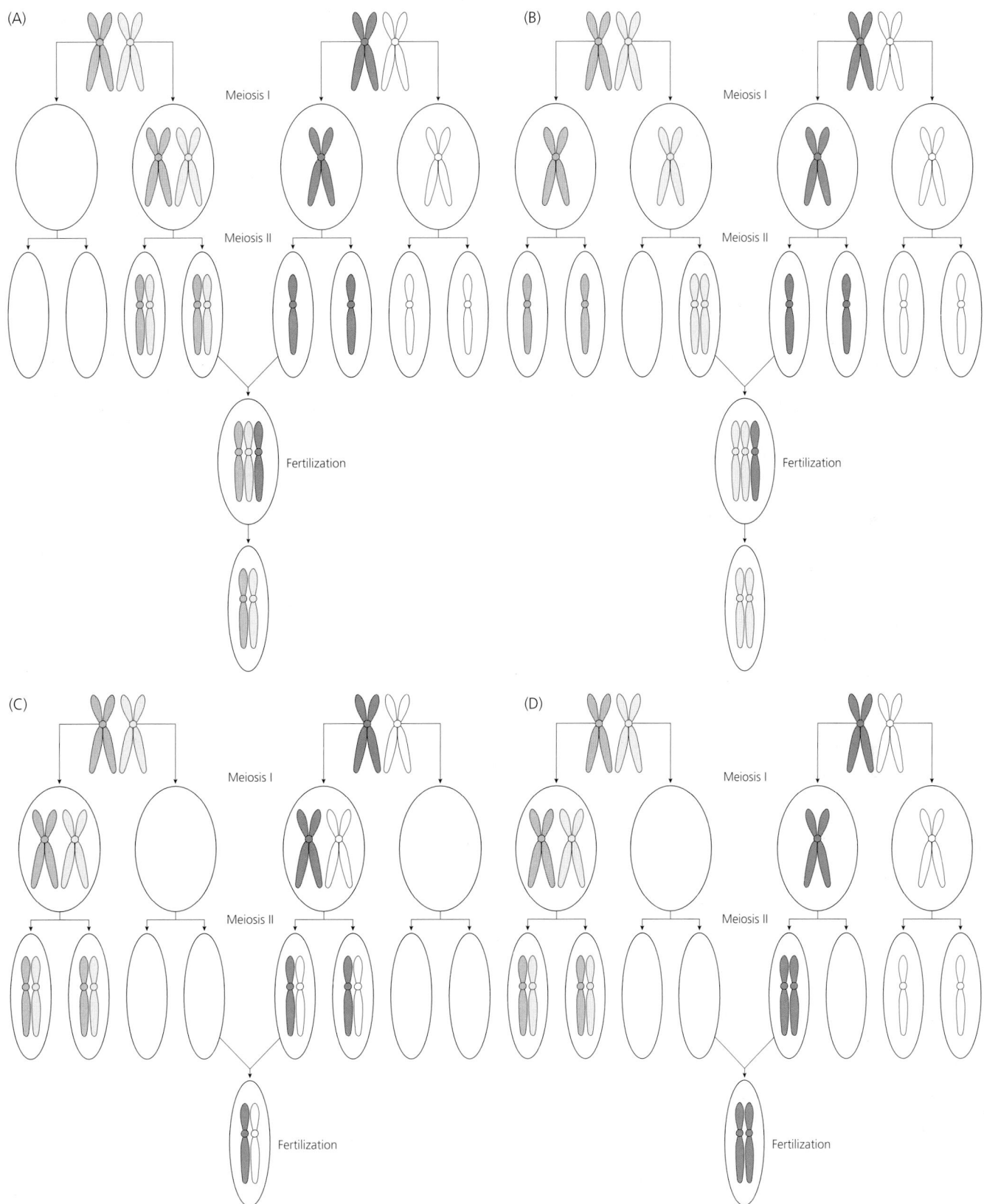

Fig. 6.17. Mechanisms of uniparental disomy. Trisomic rescue causing heterodisomy due to a meiosis I error (A). Trisomic rescue causing isodisomy due to a meiosis II error (B). Gamete complementation causing heterodisomy due to a meiosis I error (C). Gamete complementation causing isodisomy due to a meiosis II error (D).

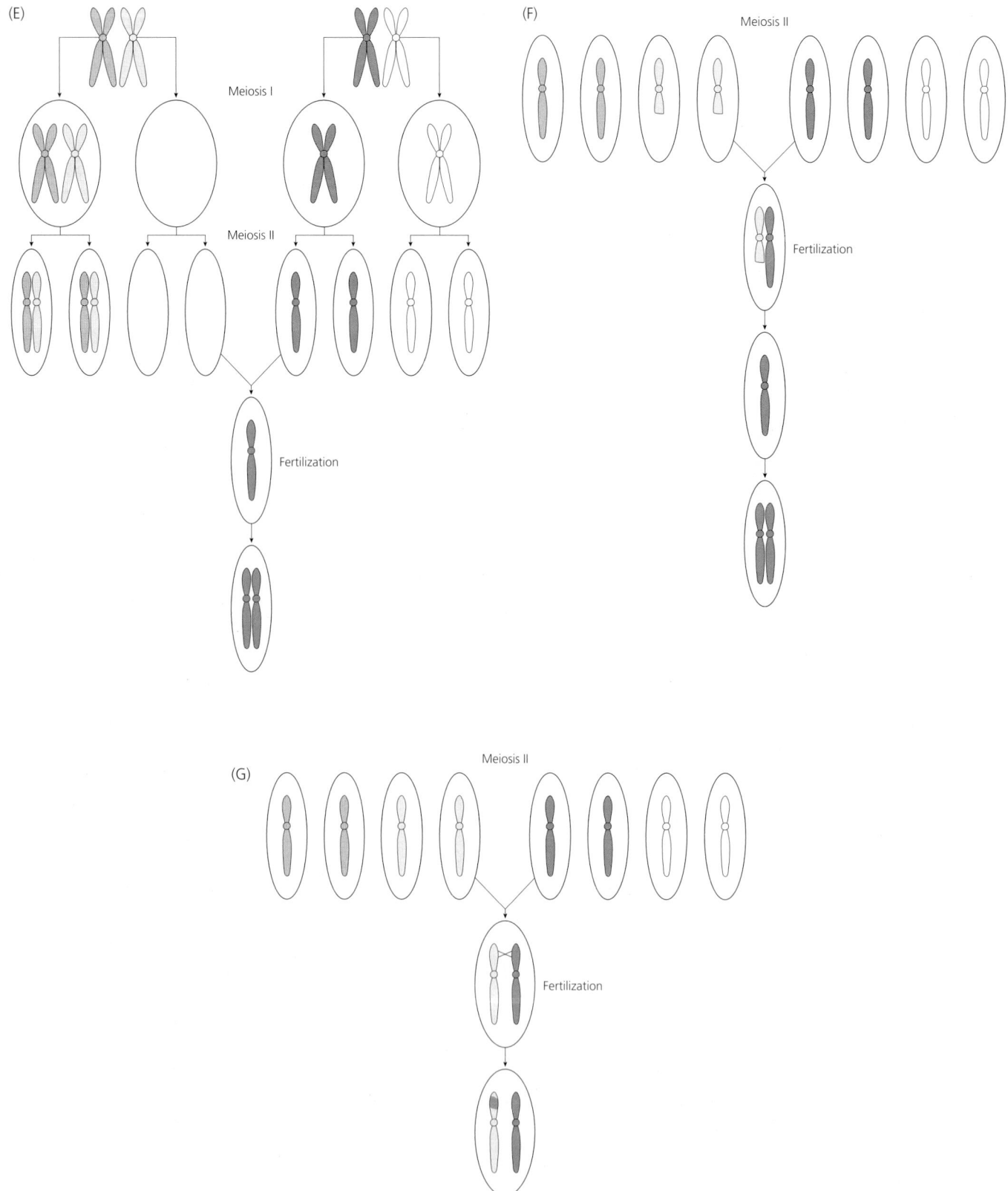

Fig. 6.17. Mechanisms of uniparental disomy. Monosomy duplication (E). Compensatory duplication due to loss of an abnormal chromosome (F). Heterochromatid exchange (G).

chromosome region 15q11–13, whereas AS is caused by a deficiency of maternal gene expression within the same region. The following mechanisms have been observed to cause the two disorders.

1. *Deletions*: Deletions of chromosome 15q11–13 are the major cause in both syndromes. In PWS this accounts for up to 70% of cases with deletions occurring on the paternally derived chromosome. Maternal deletions of the same region give rise to AS and accounts for around 60% of cases.
2. *Uniparental disomy*: Uniparental disomy is the next commonest cause with maternal UPD accounting for up to 30% of PWS cases. However only 2–3% of AS cases are due to paternal UPD.
3. *Abnormalities of imprinting*: In 2–3% of PWS the paternal allele has developed a maternal pattern of methylation, while in AS the maternal allele has developed a paternal pattern of methylation in 7–9% of cases. In both instances there is a normal biparental contribution of chromosomes and the abnormality is due to a putative imprinting centre mutation.

Within the critical region for PWS the possible candidate genes responsible for the disorder are the small ribonucleo-protein associated polypeptide N (*SNRPN*), necdin (*NDN*), zinc finger protein 127 (*ZNF127*) and a gene designated as imprinted in Prader–Willi (*IPW*) which has an intron/exon structure but does not have an identifiable coding capacity. All are preferentially expressed on the paternal allele (Christian et al., 1998; Jiang et al., 1998). In 1997 mutations were identified in the E6–AP ubiquitin-protein ligase (UBE3A) gene of patients with AS. UBE3A has a tissue specific pattern of imprinting and is preferentially expressed from the maternal allele in the human brain (Vu and Hoffman, 1997).

Beckwith–Wiedemann syndrome

Beckwith–Wiedemann syndrome (BWS) is a fetal overgrowth syndrome characterized by exomphalos, macroglossia, visceromegaly, hemihypertrophy, and gigantism (Beckwith, 1969). Affected individuals are at risk of developing an associated group of embryonal tumors including Wilms' tumor, adrenocortical carcinoma, hepatoblastoma and embryonal rhabdomyosarcoma.

The genetics of BWS are complex and a variety of mechanisms have been demonstrated to be involved in its pathogenesis; however, in each case imprinted genes from chromosome 11p15.5 have been implicated. These are either preferentially expressed from the maternal allele (e.g., *H19*,

the gene giving rise to the long QT syndrome *KCNQ1* and the putative tumour supressor gene *CDKN1C*) or from the paternal allele (e.g., insulin-like growth factor 2, *IGF2*). A number of features of Beckwith–Weidemann syndrome have indicated a role for genomic imprinting:

1. 2 to 3% of patients with BWS have cytogenetic abnormalities involving chromosome 11p15, which include paternally derived duplications of this region and maternally derived inversions and balanced translocations of this region (Weksberg et al., 1993a).
2. In 15% of cases, there is a family history of BWS with linkage to 11p15.5. In these cases, the phenotype only occurs with maternal transmission (Viljoen and Ramesar, 1992).
3. In 20% of sporadic cases of BWS, there is paternal uniparental isodisomy of chromosome 11. This arises as a post-zygotic mitotic event, so that affected individuals are mosaic for normal and disomic cell lines. There is a strong association between paternal uniparental disomy and hemihypertrophy, suggesting a localized overgrowth effect (Henry et al., 1993).
4. About 5–10% of sporadic BWS cases have an abnormal methylation pattern of the *IGF2/H19* domain resulting from conversion of the normal maternal allele specific methylation patterns of *IGF2* and *H19* to the paternal configuration. This is associated with absent *H19* expression and activation of *IGF2* expression from the maternal allele (Reik et al., 1995). By analogy, with the Angelman and Prader–Willi syndromes, these patients were proposed to have an imprinting centre mutation (Reik et al., 1995).

Loss of imprinting (LOI) of *IGF2* with expression from both alleles was found in up to 80% of sporadic BWS patients (Weksberg et al., 1993b, Joyce et al., 1997). The precise mechanism of LOI of *IGF2* is not known; however, the maternally expressed H19 gene has been implicated in some cases (Leighton et al., 1995), although LOI of IGF2 has been shown to also occur in an H19-independent manner (Brown et al., 1996; Joyce et al., 1997). Germline mutations in the *CDKN1C* gene occur in about 40% of familial cases and about 4% of sporadic patients (Lam et al., 1999). It is unclear at present how *IGF2* LOI and mutations in *CDKN1C* give rise to the BWS phenotype but recent evidence suggests that they act on a common growth control pathway (Caspary et al., 1999). In many BWS patients with chromosomal rearrangements, the breakpoint has been found to occur in the *KCNQ1* gene (Lee et al., 1997).

DIGENIC INHERITANCE

Genetic or locus heterogeneity by which different genes can cause clinically identical disorders has been discussed previously in this chapter. However, these cases are considered to be monogenic in that in any one family only one locus is thought to be defective. Reports of families with retinitis pigmentosa in which affected individuals are heterozygous for mutations in two different recessive genes (i.e., double heterozygotes) suggest the possibility of a previously undescribed mode of inheritance, known as digenic inheritance (Kajiwara et al., 1994).

Although the families they describe were initially thought to be compatible with autosomal dominant retinitis pigmentosa with reduced penetrance, the families showed a number of unusual features:

1. In each family, the disease originated in the offspring of unaffected individuals.
2. Affected individuals transmitted the disorder to statistically significantly fewer than 50% of their offspring.

On molecular testing, they found that both affected and unaffected individuals carried a mutation in the *peripherin/ RDS* gene. Affected individuals were also heterozygous for a mutation in the *ROM1* gene. These genes encode two of the polypeptide subunits of an oligomeric transmembrane protein complex present at the photoreceptor outer segment disc rims. Mutant *peripherin/RDS* protein can assemble with wild type *ROM1* to form structurally normal complexes but cannot assemble with mutant *ROM1* protein. Therefore only the combination of the two heterozygous mutations is pathogenic (Goldberg and Molday, 1996).

Digenic inheritance has also been demonstrated in inherited sensorineural deafness where mutations in different deafness genes have been shown to interact in a synergistic manner where each gene alone results in a mild and sometimes undiagnosed phenotype, but both together result in a more severe phenotype (Balciuniene et al., 1998).

MITOCHONDRIAL INHERITANCE

The nuclear chromosomes are not the only source of coding DNA sequences within the cell. Mitochondria possess their own DNA, which, as well as coding for mitochondrial tRNA and rRNA, also carries the genes for 12 structural proteins that are all mitochondrial enzyme subunits. Mutations within these genes have been shown to cause disease (e.g., Leber's hereditary optic neuropathy). The inheritance pattern of mitochondrial DNA is, however, very different from nuclear DNA. Mitochondria are exclusively maternally inherited. Therefore, mitochondrial mutations can only be transmitted through females although they can affect both sexes equally. Mitochondrial inheritance is discussed in more detail in Chapter 12.

REFERENCES

Andrew S, Goldberg P, Kremer B et al. (1993) The relationship between trinucleotide (CAG) repeat length and clinical features of Huntington's disease. Nat Genet 4:398–403

Balciuniene J, Dahl N, Borg E, Samuelsson E et al. (1998) Evidence for digenic inheritance of nonsyndromic hereditary hearing loss in a Swedish family. Am J Hum Genet 63(3):786–793

Beckwith JB (1969) Macroglossia, omphalocele, adrenal cytomegaly, gigantism and hyperplastic visceromegaly. Birth Defects Orig Art Ser V(2):188–196

Benson M (1991) Inherited amyloidosis. J Med Genet 28:73–78

Bird A (1992) The essentials of DNA methylation. Cell 70:5–8

Bodrug S, Ray P, Gonzalez I et al. (1987) Molecular analysis of a constitutional X-autosome translocation in a female with muscular dystrophy. Science 237:1620–1624

Brown KW, Villar AJ, Bickmore W et al. (1996) Imprinting mutation in the Beckwith–Weidemann syndrome leads to biallelic IGF2 expression through an H19 independent pathway. Hum Mol Genet 6:2027–2032

Byers P, Starman B, Cohn D, Horwitz A (1988a) A novel mutation causes a perinatal lethal form of osteogenesis imperfecta: An insertion in one alpha-1(I) collagen allele (COL1A1). J Biol Chem 263:7855–7861

Byers PH, Tsipouras P, Bonadio F et al. (1988b) Perinatal lethal osteogenesis imperfecta (OI type II): A biochemically heterogeneous disorder usually due to new mutations in the genes for type 1 collagen. Am J Hum Genet 42:237–248

Byers P, Wallis G, Willing M (1991) Osteogenesis imperfecta: translation of mutation to phenotype. J Med Genet 28:433–442

Caspary T, Cleary MA, Perlman EJ et al. (1999) Oppositely imprinted genes p57(Kip2) and IGF2 interact in a mouse model for Beckwith–Weidemann syndrome. Genes Dev 13:3115–3124

Christian SL, Bhatt NK, Martin SA et al. (1998) Integrated YAC contig map of the Prader-Willi/Angelman region on chromosome 15q11–q13 with average STS spacing of 35kb. Genome Res 8:146–157

Chung CS, Brown KS (1970) Family studies of early childhood deafness ascertained through the Clarke school for the deaf. Am J Hum Genet 22:630–644

Feil R and Khosla S (1999) Genomic imprinting in mammals—an interplay between chromatin and DNA methylation? Trends Genet 15:431–435

Fu YH, Kuhl DP, Pizzuti A et al. (1991) Variation of the CGG repeat at the fragile X site results in genetic instability: Resolution of the Sherman paradox. Cell 67:1047–1058

Garrod AE (1902) The incidence of alkaptonuria: A study in chemical individuality. Lancet 2:1616–1620

Gieser D, Fishman G, Cunha-Vaz J (1980) X-linked recessive retinitis pigmentosa and vitreous fluorophotometry. A study of female heterozygotes. Arch Ophthalmol 98:307–310

Goldberg AF, Molday RS (1996) Defective subunit assembly underlies a digenic form of retinitis pigmentosa linked to mutations in peripherin/rds and rom-1. Proc Natl Acad Sci USA 26;93(24):13726–13730

Goodship J, Malcolm S, Lau Y et al. (1988) Use of chromosome inactivation analysis to establish carrier status for X-linked severe combined immunodeficiency. Lancet 2:729–732

Hall JG, Dorst JP, Taybi H et al. (1969) Two probable cases of homozygosity for the achondroplasia gene. Birth Defects 4:24–34

Hall JG (1990) Genomic imprinting: Review and relevance to human disease. Am J Hum Genet 46:857–873

Henry I, Puesch A, Riesewijk A et al. (1993) Somatic mosaicism for partial paternal isodisomy in Wiedemann–Beckwith syndrome: a post fertilisation event. Eur J Hum Genet 1:19–29

Jiang Y, Tsai TF, Bressler J et al. (1998) Imprinting in Angelman and Prader–Willi syndromes. Curr Opin Genet Dev 8:334–342

Joyce JA, Lam WWK, Catchpoole DJ et al. (1997) Imprinting of IGF2 and H19: Lack of reciprocity in sporadic Beckwith–Weidemann syndrome. Hum Mol Genet 6:1543–1548

Kajiwara K, Berson E, Dryja T (1994) Digenic retinitis pigmentosa due to mutations at the unlinked peripherin/RDS and ROMI loci. Science 264:1604–1607

Kalousek DK, Langlois S, Barrett I et al. (1993) Uniparental disomy for chromosome 16 in humans. Am J Hum Genet 52:8–16

Kerem E, Corey M, Kerem B et al. (1990) The relation between genotype and phenotype in cystic fibrosis—analysis of the most common mutation (delta F508). N Engl J med 323:1517–1522

Khosla S, Aitchison A, Gregory R et al. (1999) Parental allele-specific chromatin configuration in a boundary-imprinting-control element upstream of the mouse H19 gene. Mol Cell Biology 19:2556–2566

Knudson A (1971) Mutation and cancer: statistical study of retinoblastoma. Proc Natl Acad Sci USA 68:820–823

Kohler J, Rupilius B, Otto M et al. (1996) Germline mosaicism in 4q35 fascioscapulohumeral muscular dystrophy (FSHD1A) occurring predominantly in oogenesis. Hum Genet 98:485–490

Kosho T, Muroya K, Nagai T et al. (1999) Skeletal features and growth patterns in 14 patients with haploinsufficiency of SHOX: implications for the development of Turner syndrome. J Clin Endocrinol Metab 84:4613–4621

Lachmann PJ, Rosen FS (1984) The catabolism of C1 inhibitor and the pathogenesis of hereditary angio-oedema. APMIS, section C, suppl 284. 92:35–39

Lam WWK, Hatada I, Ohishi S et al. (1999) Analysis of germline CDKNIC (p57^{KIP2}) mutations in familial and sporadic Beckwith–Weidemann syndrome (BWS) provides a novel genotype-phenotype correlation. J Med Genet 36:518–523

Lee MP, Hu RJ, Johnson LA et al. (1997) Human KVLQT1 gene shows tissue specific imprinting and encompasses Beckwith–Weidemann syndrome chromosomal rearrangements. Nat Genet 15:181–185

Leighton PA, Ingram RS, Eggenschwiler J et al. (1995) Disruption of imprinting caused by deletion of the H19 gene region in mice. Nature 375:34–39

Ma K, Inglis JD, Sharkey A et al. (1993) A Y chromosome gene family with RNA-binding homology: Candidates for the azoospermia factor AZF controlling human spermatogenesis. Cell 5:1287–1295

Martin DIK, Tsai SF, Orkin SH (1989) Increased gamma-globin expression in a non-deletion HPFH mediated by an erythroid-specific DNA-binding factor. Nature 338:435–438

Mulley J, Staples A, Donnelly A et al. (1993) Explanation for exclusive maternal origin for congenital form of myotonic dystrophy. Lancet 341:236–237

Nelson D, Warren S (1993) Trinucleotide repeat instability: When and where? Nat Genet 4:107–108

Neumann B, Barlow DP (1996) Multiple roles for DNA methylation in gametic imprinting. Curr Opin Genet Dev 6:733–740

Owen M, Brennan S, Lewis J, Carrell R (1983) Mutation of antitrypsin to antithrombin. N Engl J Med 309:694–698

Patel PI, Roa BB, Welcher AA et al. (1992) The gene for the peripheral myelin protein PMP-22 is a candidate for Charcot-Marie-Tooth disease type 1a. Nature Genet 1:159–165

Paulson H (1999) Protein fate in neurodegenerative proteinopathies: Polyglutamine diseases join the (mis)fold. Am J Hum Genet 64:339–345

Penrose L (1955) Parental age and mutation. Lancet 2:312–313

Peters J (1959) Classic Papers in Genetics. Prentice-Hall, London

Petersen MB, Bartsch O, Adelsberger PA et al. (1992) Uniparental isodisomy due to a duplication of chromosome 21 occurring in somatic cells monosomic for chromosome 21. Genomics 13:269–274

Ptacek LJ, George AL, Griggs RS et al. (1991) Identification of a mutation in the gene causing hyperkalaemic periodic paralysis. Cell 67:1021–1027

Rappold G (1993) The pseudoautosomal regions of the human sex chromosomes. Hum Genet 92:315–324

Reik W, Brown K, Schneid H et al. (1995) Imprinting mutations in the Beckwith–Weidemann syndrome suggested by an altered imprinting pattern in the IGF2-H19 domain. Hum Mol Genet 4:2379–2385

Reyniers E, Vits L, De Boulle K et al. (1993) The full mutation in the FMR-1 gene of male fragile-X patients is absent in their sperm. Nature Genet 4:143–146

Richards C, Watkins S, Hoffman E et al. (1990) Skewed X-inactivation in a female MZ twin results in Duchenne muscular dystrophy. Am J Hum Genet 46:672–681

Richards R, Sutherland G (1992) Heritable unstable DNA sequences. Nature Genet 1:7–9

Richards R, Sutherland G (1994) Simple repeat DNA is not replicated simply. Nature Genet 6:114–116

Rubin CM, van de Voort CA, Teplitz RL et al. (1994) Alu repeated DNAs are differentially methylated in primate germ cells. Nucleic Acids Res 22:5121–5127

Schiebel K, Weiss B, Wohrle D, Rappold G (1993) A human pseudoautosomal gene, ADP/ATP translocase, escapes X-inactivation whereas a homologue on Xq is subject to X-inactivation. Nature Genet 3:82–87

Sherman S, Morton N, Jacobs P, Turner G (1984) The marker (X) syndrome: a cytogenetic and genetic analysis. Ann Hum Genet 48:21–37

Sherman S, Jacobs P, Morton N et al. (1985) Further segregation analysis of the fragile X syndrome with special reference to transmitting males. Hum Genet 69:289–299

Sinden R (1999) Biological implications of the DNA structures associated with disease-causing triplet repeats. Am J Hum Genet. 64:346–353

Slatter RE, Elliott M, Welham K et al. (1994) Mosaic uniparental disomy in Beckwith–Weidemann syndrome. J Med Genet 31:749–753

Soriano P, Jaenisch R (1986) Retroviruses as probes for mammalian development: Allocation of cells to the somatic and germ cell lineages. Cell 46:19–29

Spence JE, Perciaccante G, Greig GM et al. (1988) Uniparental disomy as a mechanism for human genetic disease. Am J Hum Genet 42:217–226

Tassabehji M, Read A, Newton V et al. (1993) Mutations in the PAX3 gene causing Waardenburg syndrome type 1 and type 2. Nature Genet 3:26–30

Timchenko (1999) Myotonic dystrophy: The role of RNA CUG triplet repeats. Am J Hum Genet 64:360–364

Tycko B (1994) Genomic imprinting: Mechanism and role in human pathology. Am J Pathol 144:431–443

van der Mey A, Maaswinkel-Mooy P, Cornelisse C et al. (1989) Genomic imprinting in hereditary glomus tumours: Evidence for new genetic theory. Lancet 2:1291–1294 van Essen AJ et al. (1992) Parental origin and germline mosaicism of deletions and duplications of the dystrophin gene: A European study. Hum Genet 88:249–257

Viljoen D, Ramesar R (1992) Evidence for paternal imprinting in familial Beckwith–Wiedemann syndrome. J Med Genet 29:221–225

Voss R, Ben-Simon E, Avital A et al. (1989) isodisomy of chromosome 7 in a patient with cystic fibrosis: Could uniparental disomy be common in humans? Am J Hum Genet 45:373–380

Vu TH, Hoffman AR (1997) Imprinting of the Angelman syndrome gene, UBE3A, is restricted to brain. Nat Genet 17:12–13

Wang J-CC, Passage MB, Yen PH et al. (1991) Uniparental heterodisomy for chromosome 14 in a phenotypically abnormal familial balanced 13/14 translocation carrier. Am J Hum Genet 48:1069–1074

Weinberg W (1912) Zur Vererbung des Zwergwuches. Arch Rass Ges Biol 9:710–717

Weksberg R, Teshima I, Williams B et al. (1993a) Molecular characterisation of cytogenetic alterations associated with the Beckwith–Wiedemann syndrome phenotype refines the localisation and suggests the gene for BWS is imprinted. Hum Mol Genet 2:549–556

Weksberg R, Shen DR, Fei YL et al. (1993b) Disruption of insulin-like growth factor 2 imprinting in Beckwith–Weidemann syndrome. Nat Genet 5:143–150

Wexler NS, Young AB, Tanzi RE et al. (1987) Homozygotes for Huntington's disease. Nature 326:194–197

Wilkie A (1994) The molecular basis of genetic dominance. J Med Genet 31:89–98

Zlotogora J (1993) Mutations in von Recklinghausen neurofibromatosis. Am J Med Genet 46:182–184

Segregation analysis

M. Anne Spence
Susan E. Hodge

7

Introduction

Gregor Mendel defined the science of genetics when he proposed two simple laws governing the behavior of inheritance factors. These concepts are so basic that they are taken for granted in this age of mapping and cloning genes, yet much of our current knowledge depends heavily on the application of Mendel's two laws. His first law states that alleles, or alternative gene forms at a single locus, segregate, and, moreover, do so with equal probabilities. This principle forms the basis for this chapter. His second law states that alleles at different loci assort independently of each other. Violation of this principle constitutes linkage and provides the essential tool for the development of genetic maps (see Ch. 8). For complex and/or common disorders such as depression or epilepsy, techniques are being developed that use both principles simultaneously. We discuss these newest approaches later in the chapter but begin with the description of segregation analysis.

In experimental organisms, the segregation of alleles can be observed directly in constructed matings, by counting the phenotypes and numbers of offspring produced. These observations are simplified by a theoretical construct: We assume that the conveyance of hereditary information is particulate by nature and that each parent has two possible alternatives transmitted at random to the next generation. One simple ratio arises from the mating Aa × aa, where the heterozygote parent segregates the two alleles, A and a, in equal frequency. Here the expected ratio is equal numbers of Aa and aa offspring. It is easy to derive the ratio for the Aa × Aa mating type and confirm that the expected offspring proportions are one-fourth AA, one-half Aa, and one-fourth aa.

We use observed segregation ratios in three important ways in human genetics. First, they act as a criterion for a gene, since a trait under genetic control will segregate in families, and the frequencies of phenotypes should be consistent with mendelian ratios such as those above. Second, segregation ratios can provide a test for genetic heterogeneity. For example, the clinically similar phenotypes of retinitis pigmentosa result from three different patterns of segregation in families: autosomal dominant, autosomal recessive, and X-linked recessive (McKusick, 1994). The implications of heterogeneity are so important both for genetic counseling and for studies of the pathophysiology that sometimes we overlook the method by which the knowledge has been obtained. Finally, segregation patterns, defining the mode of inheritance for a trait, play an important role in genetic linkage studies.

Definitions and basic principles

For the segregation of alleles to be observed in families, the trait must exist in different forms (phenotypes) in the population; within any family at least one parent must possess two different alleles and produce children; and finally, we must have some method of locating the families which are segregating the trait so that the ratios may be determined in an unbiased and accurate fashion. The first two requirements for segregation analysis cannot be controlled by the genetic investigator, but the last point can and must be detailed by the scientist.

The simplest example is the segregation pattern for an autosomal dominant trait like Huntington disease or Marfan syndrome (McKusick, 1994). Because it is determined by a locus on an autosomal chromosome, the trait may be passed by either parent to offspring of either sex. The sex ratio among affected individuals is therefore 1:1. The dominant nature of the trait ensures that the heterozygotes express the phenotype, and a vertical transmission of the trait through multiple generations in families is a striking feature.

The segregation ratio for an autosomal dominant trait can be calculated directly from the family data. If the trait of interest is relatively common, such as brown eyes or freckling, individuals can be selected by a variety of techniques, including a random sample drawn from drivers' license files, voting registration files, or lists of those attending a university class. The individuals identified with the dominant trait are designated probands. (The term index case usually refers to the first proband in a family but is used by different investigators to denote any of several selection criteria and should not be equated with the term proband; see Marazita, 1995.)

Human geneticists are often interested in diseases that occur with relatively low frequencies. For rare diseases, the usual sampling scheme is to check hospital records, specialty clinics such as genetic counseling centers, schools for the blind or deaf, or other relevant institutions in order to identify affected individuals. For dominant diseases, the ascertainment of affected individuals does not alter the calculation of the segregation ratio, as long as this ratio is then determined by enumerating the proband's children. Every set of offspring must be included in the count, whether none, some, or all of the children are affected with the disease.

Autosomal dominant and X-linked inheritance

Once a ratio is obtained from the data, the question of interest may be addressed: Is the trait segregating in a genetic fashion? In order to test the hypothesis that the trait is genetic, the investigator must state the expected mendelian ratio, given the type of families ascertained. We begin with autosomal dominant inheritance. If the trait is thought to be autosomal dominant on the basis of vertical transmission in families and an equal sex ratio, we expect to ascertain families with only one affected parent (assuming a rare trait) who is heterozygous. The ratio obtained from the data may be compared directly with the expected 1:1 affected to normal ratio by a chi-square test or other appropriate statistic (Matthews and Farewell, 1985).

Failure to reject the hypothesis of the expected mendelian ratio means that the data appear compatible with the hypothesized mode of inheritance. This information may provide strong evidence for the genetic basis of the disease, but the investigator should keep the following considerations in mind when interpreting the test results. First, even if the actual ratio is the expected mendelian one, the sample may simply not be large enough to have sufficient power to reject the hypothesis. Second, other factors such as the environment may have produced the segregation pattern. The existence of a pattern is not conclusive evidence for a gene, although it is nearly conclusive for traits such as Huntington disease, because the pattern observed in the data is exactly that expected under the autosomal dominant model and the observation occurred in a large number of families from a variety of ethnic groups (McKusick, 1994). Recent mapping and cloning of the Huntington disease gene confirms the genetic hypothesis (Huntington's Disease Collaborative Research Group, 1993). By contrast, the suggestion using segregation data that the neurologic disorder Kuru was autosomal dominant proved incorrect, as it has been shown to be caused by a slow virus (Gajdusek et al., 1969). McGuffin and Huckle (1990) provide an amusing example of how a segregation analysis can provide strong evidence of genetic transmission for a trait (i.e., attending medical school) that is presumably not genetic.

On the other hand, a trait may show deviations from the expected ratio yet actually be dominant. It is important to examine the magnitude and type of deviation before rejecting the genetic hypothesis. Complications such as delayed age of onset (e.g., Huntington disease), variable expression (e.g., Marfan syndrome), and reduced penetrance (e.g., neurofibromatosis) produce deviations from the expected ratio. These complications can be recognized by the application of either genetic or clinical criteria. Genetic criteria define reduced penetrance when an unaffected parent transmits the disease to two or more children. Clinical criteria are required for diseases with pleiotropy, defined as the phenomenon whereby a single gene is responsible for a number of distinct and seemingly unrelated phenotypic effects (King and Stansfield, 1990), such as Marfan syndrome, in which the observation of patients with differing combinations of the phenotypes leads to the syndrome definition independent of the genetic analyses. A genetic etiology for the trait is tested by segregation analysis, using the expanded definition of the syndrome for the phenotype.

Although segregation analysis may not be definitive in the presence of complicating factors, the importance of a genetic etiology is often suggested by the analysis. Segregation analysis results are further substantiated by examination of larger pedigrees, studies of twins, population data, biochemical analyses, and, finally, gene linkage studies (see Ch. 8).

Families display a different segregation pattern when the trait is inherited in an X-linked fashion. The mendelian ratio now depends on the sex of the segregating parent, as well as the sex of the offspring. X-linked inheritance, whether recessive or dominant, produces such distinctive patterns in families that these diseases are more quickly identified and mapped than autosomal disorders. Estimated ratios can be calculated by the direct method for dominant traits and corrected for ascertainment with recessive traits as detailed below for autosomal conditions. The most critical observation for the X-linked recessive case is the absence of male-to-male transmission and for the X-linked dominant case is that all daughters of affected males are affected. The same complications that exist for autosomal dominant traits may affect the analyses of X-linked traits, namely reduced penetrance or variable expression. To complicate matters further, some phenotypes are sex-limited in their expression, for physiologic or anatomic reasons, even though their mode of inheritance is autosomal. These traits are distinguished by their segregation patterns if they are rare in the population.

Recessive inheritance and ascertainment issues

Recessive diseases introduce the additional complication that we need to allow for ascertainment. Recessive inheritance produces yet another distinctive segregation pattern as well. We still wish to calculate a segregation ratio and compare it with the mendelian expectation; however, in this case, ascertaining probands to examine the segregation ratio in their offspring breaks down completely, as affected individuals will most likely marry normal homozygotes and produce unaffected children. Thus, ascertaining through affected parents would be extremely inefficient.

How do we obtain data that will lead to a meaningful test of our hypothesis? When the trait is rare, the mating type producing most of the affected children consists of two heterozygous unaffected parents. The solution is to identify affected children of normal parents as probands and to examine the distribution of disease in their sibs, since sibs have one chance in four of being affected. This is called ascertainment through the children, and now the specific method of ascertaining probands becomes of major importance in segregation analysis. We will ascertain those families where the heterozygous parents produce at least one affected child. Failure to ascertain families with no affected children distorts the sample, and without ascertainment

correction, the number of affected will appear to be greater than expected, and the recessive mode of inheritance may be mistakenly rejected.

The effect of the distortion in the data due to ascertainment is clearly illustrated in Figure 7.1. The first column demonstrates a sample of families of size 3, segregating an autosomal recessive trait from heterozygous parents. The number of families of each type is predicted by the binomial expansion, so this sample in fact shows exactly what is expected. For example, sibships with all three sibs affected occur with the frequency of one-fourth × one-fourth × one-fourth, or 1/64. So one family in the sample of 64 families is shown as having all three sibs affected. Note that many of the families in the sample have no affected children and hence would not be ascertained. Thus, a sample ascertained through affected individuals will appear to contain too many affected individuals, although in fact there are too few unaffected individuals, in the sense that we are missing a large segment of the sample.

The degree of distortion in the data and a method to correct the ascertainment bias both depend on the investigator's choice of ascertainment scheme when planning the study. This decision defines who may be a proband, and this definition must be rigorously adhered to throughout the study. Variable ascertainment criteria create a situation where no one correction method is appropriate, and analysis may lead to false rejection or acceptance of the hypothesis (Greenberg, 1986). The examples in the next two sections will serve to illustrate two extremes of the selection choices, before we describe a more general approach in the third section.

TRUNCATE ASCERTAINMENT

When the search for probands is carried out for an extended period, and with many sources of ascertainment, all affected individuals within the study area will be identified. Under this truncate ascertainment scheme, every affected individual in the sample is independently ascertained, that is, found through an independent study source, as opposed to being identified by interview of family members. The probability that a family is included in the study is then independent of the number of affected individuals in the family, since every family with at least one affected child is sure to be ascertained. For a genetic trait, the distribution of affected members in the family is exactly that described by the mendelian ratio, with the exception that there are no families with all normal children. This is shown in the middle column of Figure 7.1, where the only change from the original, "perfect" sample is that the box containing families with all unaffected children is

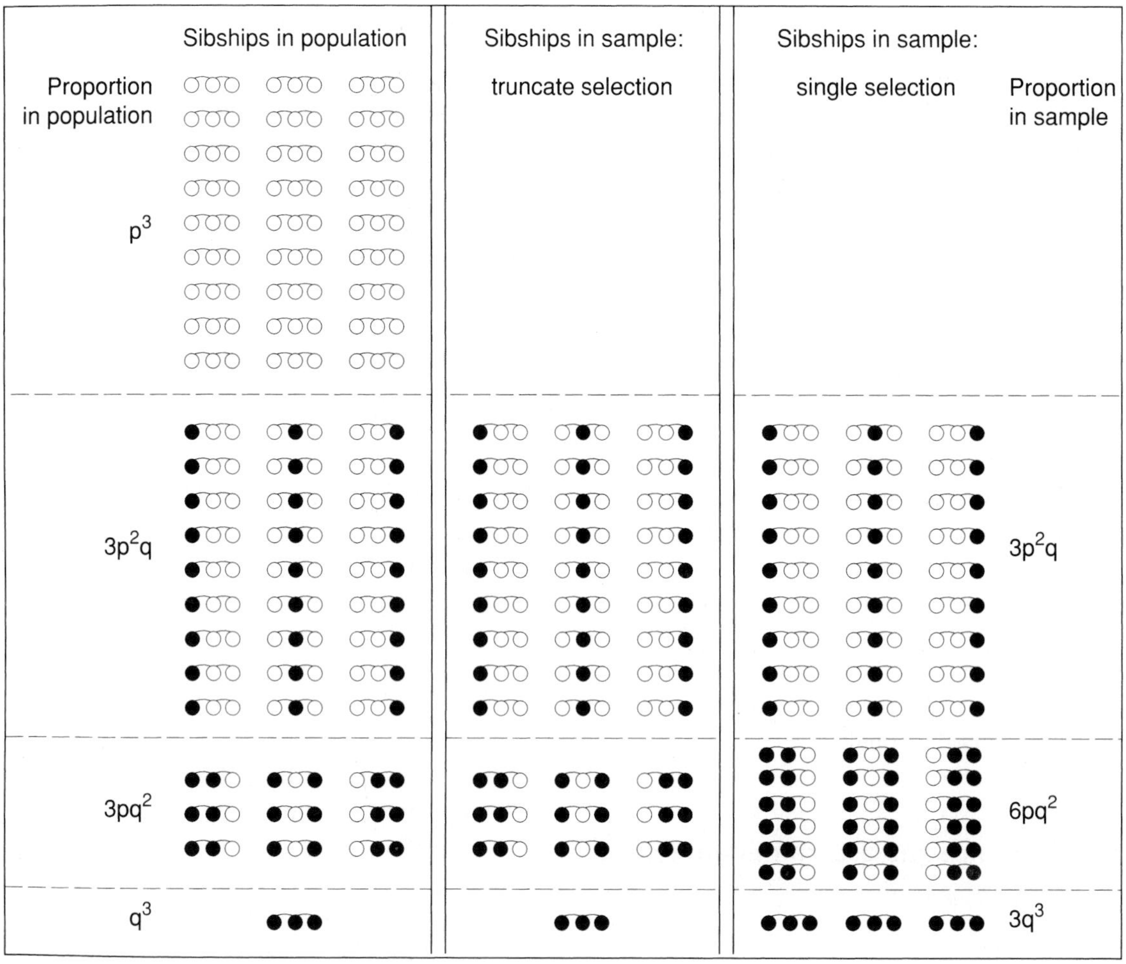

Fig. 7.1. Sibships of size three in the proportions in which they occur: (1) in the general population; (2) in truncate selection; (3) in single selection. Only sibships that are offspring of two heterozygous parents are considered. Thus, p = probability of unaffected offspring = 3/4, q = probability of affected offspring = 1/4. Solid circles indicate affected; open circles unaffected offspring. (Adapted from Sutton, 1988, with permission.)

now empty. Weinberg (1928) described the ascertainment bias and proposed the proband method for correcting for this bias (Tables 7.1 and 7.2). The principle is simple: one discards a proband and counts the number of remaining affected and unaffected sibs, repeating the step for each proband. These two tables reveal the serious distortion in the ratio before the correction, contrast this with the exact 3:1 ratio after the correction, and summarize the correction procedure. For example, count the sample in the middle column of Figure 7.1, using this procedure, and determine for yourself that in the corrected sample the proportion of affected siblings is 25%. What is the proportion in the uncorrected data?

SINGLE ASCERTAINMENT

A common alternative to truncate ascertainment is to choose one narrowly defined group for sampling. For example, one might define deaf children as probands, then

test all second-grade school children for hearing deficits. Under single ascertainment, almost every family sampled has only one proband – the probability that a family has more than one proband is very small. (The occasional exception could arise from, for example, twins.) The resulting sample will still contain only families with at least one affected member, just as under truncate ascertainment, but now the chance that a family is represented in the sample is proportional to the number of affected children, since a family with several deaf children has a better chance of having one of them in the second grade than a family with only one deaf child. This results in a greater proportion of the families in the sample having multiple affected children and leads to the differences observed in the right-hand column of Figure 7.1. Count the proportion of affected siblings in the single selection sample (right-hand column of Fig. 7.1) and note how it differs from the proportion in the truncate sample (middle column). This difference is also

Table 7.1. Estimation of Segregation Ratio Among Truncate Ascertainment Families With Normal Parents and Three Offspring—Expected Distributions of Families and Offspring

| Family Type | | Expected Frequency of Family Type | | Example: Ideal Sample of 37 Families | | | | |
| | | | | Observed No. | | | Corrected No. | |
Index (i)	Description	In Population	In an Ascertained Sample	NF(i) = No. of Families	SNU(i) = No. Unaff.	SNA(i) = No. Affected	CNU(i) = No. Unaff.	CNA(i) = No. Affected
0	3 unaff.	27/64	0	0	0	0	0	0
1	2 unaff. 1 aff.	27/64	27/37	27	54	27	54	0
2	1 unaff. 2 aff.	9/64	9/37	9	9	18	18	18
3	3 aff.	1/64	1/37	1	0	3	0	6
	Total	1	1	37	63	48	72	24

Table 7.2. Estimation of Segregation Ratio Among Truncate Ascertainment Families With Normal Parents and Three Offspring—Calculation of the Corrected Segregation Ratio

Uncorrected segregation ratio
SNU(T):SNA(T) = 63:48 = 21:16 = 1.3:1

Corrected segregation ratio
CNU(T):CNA(T) = 72:24 = 3:1

where

$$CNA(T) = \sum_{i=1}^{3} CNA(i)$$

$$CNU(T) = \sum_{i=1}^{3} CNU(i)$$

$$CNU(i) = i \times SNU(i)$$

$$CNA(i) = [SNA(i) - NF(i)] \times i$$

illustrated by comparing the idealized sample in Table 7.3 with that in Table 7.1. The Weinberg proband method will still correct the data if, and only if, the definition of proband is strictly applied and each family is included in the corrected sample only once, irrespective of the number of affected children. This is an exercise left to the reader to confirm.

Another type of methodology is illustrated in Table 7.4, one in which the expected mendelian ratio, rather than the data, is altered to account for the ascertainment. Since we know the ascertainment scheme and its impact ahead of time, the technique is one of the a priori methods. In principle, for single selection we predict that the proband in each family plus one quarter of the other sibs will be affected. In Table 7.4 the altered ratio is 1:1, as is the ratio in the observed data. For a real analysis, one would have families of different sizes and the corrected ratio would have to be calculated for each sibship size. The reader should calculate several ratios to demonstrate that the ratio approaches one-fourth as sibships become larger and that small families produce the greatest distortion.

MULTIPLE ASCERTAINMENT

The two methods illustrated above emphasize the importance of correcting for ascertainment bias and the need to apply the appropriate correction. However, real-life

Table 7.3. Estimation of Segregation Ratio Among Single Ascertainment Families With Normal Parents and Three Offspring—Expected Distributions of Families and Offspring

| Family Type | Expected Frequency of Family Type | | Example: Ideal Sample of 48 Families | | |
	In Population	In an Ascertained Sample	No. of Families	No. Unaffected	No. Affected
3 unaff.	27/64	0	0	0	0
2 unaff. 1 aff.	27/64	27/48	27	54	27
1 unaff. 2 aff.	9/64	18/48	18	18	36
3 aff.	1/64	3/48	3	0	9
Total:	1	1	48	72	72

Table 7.4. Estimation of Segregation Ratio Among Single Ascertainment Families With Normal Parents and Three Offspring—Calculation of the Corrected Segregation Ratio

$$\text{Expected segregation ratio} = \frac{\text{Number of affected offspring}}{\text{total offspring}} = \frac{1}{4}$$

$$\text{Corrected segregation ratio} = \frac{1 + (s - 1)\frac{1}{4}}{s}$$

where 1 refers to the (one) proband, and s is the sibship size

Example:

For families of size 3: $\dfrac{1 + (3 - 1)\frac{1}{4}}{3} = \dfrac{1 + \frac{1}{2}}{3} = \dfrac{1}{2}$

Corrected ratio = 1:1

Observed ratio = 72:72 = 1:1

ascertainment schemes rarely conform exactly to either the single or truncate paradigms; rather the data collected usually contain more than one proband per family, or contain affected individuals who are not probands. This sampling scheme, called multiple ascertainment (or multiple incomplete selection by Morton, 1959), falls between truncate and single ascertainment and requires its own method of correction. (There are also other ascertainment schemes that do not fall between single and truncate ascertainment; see Ewens and Shute, 1986b for details.)

The method of choice for multiple ascertainment is to use maximum likelihood techniques, where equations are fitted to the data by simultaneously estimating the segregation ratio, denoted ρ, and the ascertainment probability, denoted by π. The ascertainment probability is defined as the probability that an affected individual in the population will be ascertained as a proband. Under truncate ascertainment, π equals unity whereas under single ascertainment, π becomes very small, approaching zero (although π cannot equal zero, if a sample exists). Morton (1959, 1962) first described the methods, which are sufficiently complex numerically to require computer solution. The basic equation for multiple ascertainment is

$$P\,(r \mid \text{family ascertained}; s, p, \pi) =$$

$$\frac{\left[\binom{s}{r} p^{r}(1 - p)^{s - r}\right]\left[1 - (1 - \pi)^{r}\right]}{1 - (1 - p\pi)^{s}}$$

where the first term in brackets in the numerator gives the binomial probability of r affected among s sibs, the second tern in brackets represents the correction for the ascertainment and the denominator gives the total probability of the sample corrected for ascertainment.

A special application of multiple ascertainment arises where we require at least two probands in each family

(rather than requiring at least one proband, as above). The following equation describes the distribution of r affected individuals in sibships of size s ascertained through at least two probands:

$$P(r \mid \text{at least two probands}; s, p, \pi) =$$

$$\frac{\left[\binom{s}{r} p^{r}(1 - p)^{s - r}\right]\left[1 - \pi)^{r} - r\pi(1 - \pi)^{r - 1}\right]}{1 - (1 - p\pi)^{s} - sp\pi(1 - p\pi)^{s - 1}}$$

This sampling scheme is useful for traits where sporadic cases are suspected, as with autism (Ritvo et al., 1985) or diaphragmatic hernia (Bocian et al., 1986). Elandt-Johnson (1971) expanded the method to include equations for two-locus models.

The key to the technique is the simultaneous estimation of the ascertainment probability π and the segregation ratio p. This ensures the appropriate level of correction, assuming independent ascertainment for each proband. Several methods are available for estimating the ascertainment probability; for examples, see Morton (1962) or Gladstien et al., (1978). If the sample size is small, there will not be sufficient information for a simultaneous solution of the necessary equations, and the investigator will be forced to resort to a modification of the Weinberg method or some similar technique (e.g., Li and Mantel, 1968). The power of the maximum likelihood approach is that the equations may be expanded to include other features, such as an estimation of the proportion of sporadic cases. These analyses are best undertaken in consultation with a genetic epidemiologist, although computer programs for the analyses are generally available.

Complex segregation analysis

The application to human disease of the concepts of polygenic or multifactorial inheritance in the 1960s, and genetic heterogeneity in the 1970s, led to a greater awareness of the complexity of inheritance patterns for diseases. This awareness, coupled with improved computer technology, led to the development of complex segregation analysis models. Although the multifactorial inheritance model can be tested directly (Gladstien et al., 1978; see also Ch. 15), it is more appropriate statistically to test that hypothesis simultaneously with the alternative single-gene hypotheses. Morton and MacLean (1974) proposed the mixed model as a way to formulate complex segregation analysis for these simultaneous tests. The mixed model also depends on the distribution of affected individuals in families, but the etiology is partitioned among a major gene (single mendelian locus), polygenic or multifactorial inheritance, and the environment. The presence or absence of contributions from each component is tested statistically. The formulation of this mixed model is substantially more complex than that of the single-gene models, although the underlying maximum-likelihood approach is not unlike that used in the multiple ascertainment equations, as we have seen. Ascertainment is specified for each family, allowing the pooling of samples from different studies. Several reviews detail the mathematical formulation of these models and the complications in their application (Elston and Rao, 1978; Elston, 1980). Because of the number of parameters that must be estimated, these analyses may require even larger data sets – often hundreds of families – in order to achieve definitive results. An example of the application of these techniques is the study of nonsyndromic cleft lip with or without cleft palate, in which the analyses rejected the multifactorial threshold hypothesis (previously thought to be the mode of inheritance for birth defects), while confirming that a small proportion of the families segregated in an autosomal recessive fashion (Marazita et al., 1984; Chung et al., 1986).

In a parallel development to the mixed model, Elston and Stewart (1971) specified the basic algorithm for pedigree analysis. Their equations are evaluated over large pedigrees individually, and the segregation pattern is tested for conformity to expected mendelian patterns. Sufficiently large pedigrees can provide adequate information for testing the hypotheses, as illustrated by an analysis of hypercholesterolemia (Elston et al., 1975).

Complex segregation analysis for the mixed model was initially confined to nuclear families because of the computational complexities. Now it has been expanded to pedigrees through the addition of pointers (Lalouel and Morton, 1981) or the use of appropriate approximations (Hasstedt, 1982a, 1982b). Lalouel et al., (1983) also presented a unified model, which synthesized features of the Morton and Elston approaches described above. These methodologic efforts have culminated in a technique that permits the pooling of nuclear families and pedigrees, ascertained over a variety of sampling schemes, for testing hypotheses of single gene versus multifactorial transmission, and environmental contributions. The essence of major gene analysis still revolves around testing the transmission probabilities, that is, the expected mendelian segregation patterns.

Several investigators have advocated a new form of joint segregation-linkage analysis. The investigator calculates lod scores (as in linkage analysis; see Ch. 8), then maximizes the lod scores over specified mode of transmission, in order to determine which mode of transmission yields the highest maximum lod score. Prima facie this procedure seems illegitimate, because lod scores are calculated conditional on the mode of transmission, and one cannot in general maximize over what is being conditioned on. However, under certain conditions the procedure can be valid. The lod scores maximized over genetic models are called mod scores by Clerget-Darpoux et al., (1986) and Clerget-Darpoux and Bonaïti-Pellié (1992), and MMLS by Greenberg (1989); the approach was first suggested by Risch (1984). A major advantage of this approach is that one need not know how the data were ascertained; a major limitation is that one must have a marker linked reasonably tightly to one's disease of interest, in order for mod scores to yield any information. Hodge and Elston (1994) summarize properties of mod scores and practical guidelines for their use. This is a promising approach, and one that is still being studied, but it has not yet eliminated the need for classical segregation analysis.

Summary

Two areas in which work is continuing in segregation analysis are regression models for quantitative traits and new approaches to ascertainment. In an attempt to improve the power to detect loci influencing quantitative traits, Almasy and Blangero (1998) have developed a bivariate mixed discrete–continuous trait variance component approach. This permits the investigator to test for genetic and environmental effects on phenotypically correlated traits. An example of this approach is an analysis estimating the proportion of genetic variance of alcoholism attributed to common genetic effects with each of three personality traits (Czerwinski et al., 2000). The variance component approach has also been applied to linkage analysis while simultaneously estimating the major gene and random polygenic effects (Amos, 1994). These approaches appear promising, especially with quantitative traits where environmental factors are measured, but they also require an extensive amount of computation. Concerning ascertainment, it has long been recognized that the concept of a "proband" is not always applicable in real-life situations. Stene (1978), Greenberg (1986), Ewens and Shute (1986a, b), Ginsburg and Axenovich (1992), Vieland and Hodge (1995), and Hodge and Vieland (1996) are among those who have explored alternative approaches to ascertainment, but the details of these are beyond the scope of this chapter.

REFERENCES

Amos CL (1994) Robust variance-components approach for assessing genetic linkage in pedigrees. Am J Hum Genet 54:535–543

Almasy L, Blangero J (1998) Multipoint quantitative trait linkage analysis in general pedigrees. Am J Hum Genet 62:1198–1211

Bocian M, Spence MA, Marazita ML et al. (1986) Familial diaphragmatic defects: Early prenatal diagnosis and evidence for major gene inheritance. Am J Med Genet, Suppl. 2:163–176

Chung CS, Bixler D, Watanabe T et al. (1986) Segregation analysis of cleft lip with or without cleft palate: A comparison of Danish and Japanese data. Am J Hum Genet 39:603–611

Clerget-Darpoux F, Bonaïti-Pellié C (1992) Strategies on marker information for the study of human diseases. Ann Hum Genet 46:145–153

Clerget-Darpoux F, Bonaïti-Pellié C, Hochez J (1986) Effects of misspecifying genetic parameters in lod score analysis. Biometrics 42:393–399

Czerwinski SA, Mahaney MC, Williams JT, Almasy L, Blangero J (2000) Genetic analysis of personality traits and alcoholism using a mixed discrete-continuous trait variance component model. Genetic Epidemiology, in press

Elandt-Johnson RC (1971) Probability Models and Statistical Methods in Genetics. John Wiley & Sons, NY

Elston RC (1980) Segregation analysis In Mielke JH, Crawford MH (eds): Current Developments in Anthropological Genetics. Plenum, New York, p. 327

Elston RC, Rao DC (1978) Statistical modeling and analysis in human genetics. Ann Rev Biophys Bioeng 7:253–286

Elston RC, Stewart J (1971) A general model for the genetic analysis of pedigree data. Hum Hered 21:523–542

Elston RC, Namboodiri KK, Glueck CJ et al. (1975) Study of the genetic transmission of hypercholesterolemia and hypertriglyceridemia in a 195 member kindred. Ann Hum Genet 39:67–87

Ewens WJ, Shute NCE (1986a) A resolution of the ascertainment sampling problem. I. Theory. Theor Pop Biol 30:388–412

Ewens WJ, Shute NCE (1986b) The limits of ascertainment. Ann Hum Genet 50:399–402

Gajdusek DC, Rogers NG, Basnight CJ, Alpers M (1969) Transmission experiments with Kuru chimpanzees and the isolation of latent viruses from the explant tissues of affected animals. Ann NY Acad Sci 162: 529–550

Ginsburg EK, Axenovich TI (1992) A cooperative binomial ascertainment model. Am J Hum Genet 51:1156–1160

Gladstien K, Lange K, Spence MA (1978) A goodness-of-fit test for the polygenic threshold model: Application to pyloric stenosis. Am J Med Genet 2:7–13

Greenberg DA (1986) The effect of proband designation on segregation analysis. Am J Hum Genet 39:329–339

Greenberg DA (1989) Inferring mode of inheritance by comparison of lod scores. Am J Med Genet 35:480–486

Hasstedt SJ (1982a) A mixed-model likelihood approximation on large pedigrees. Comput Biomed Res 15:295–307

Hasstedt SJ (1982b) Linkage analysis using the mixed, major gene with general penetrance or three locus model. Cytogenet Cell Genet 6:284

Hodge SE, Elston RC (1994) Lods, wrods, and mods: the interpretation of lod scores calculated under different models. Genet Epidemiol 11: 329–342

Hodge SE, Vieland VJ (1996) The essence of single ascertainment. Genetics 144:1215–1223

Huntington's Disease Collaborative Research Group (1993) A novel gene containing a trinucleotide repeat that is expanded and unstable on Huntington's disease chromosomes. Cell 72:971–983

King RC, Stansfield WD (1990) A Dictionary of Genetics, 4th edn. Oxford, NY

Lalouel JM, Morton NE (1981) Complex segregation analysis with pointers. Hum Hered 31:312–321

Lalouel JM, Rao DC, Morton NE, Elston RC (1983) A unified model for complex segregation analysis. Am J Hum Genet 20:61–68

Li CC, Mantel N (1968) A simple method of estimating the segregation ratio under complete ascertainment. Am J Hum Genet 20:61–68

McGuffin P, Huckle P (1990) Simulation of Mendelism revisited: The recessive gene for attending medical school. Am J Hum Genet 46:994–999

McKusick VA (1994) Mendelian Inheritance in Man: Catalog of Autosomal Dominant, Autosomal Recessive, and X-Linked Phenotypes, 11th edn. Johns Hopkins University Press, Baltimore

Marazita M (1995) Defining "proband." Am J Hum Genet 57:981–982

Marazita ML, Spence MA, Melnick M (1984) Genetic analysis of cleft lip with or without cleft palate in Danish kindreds. Am J Med Genet 19: 9–18

Matthews DE, Farewell VT (1985) Using and Understanding Medical Statistics. S Karger, Basel

Morton NE (1959) Genetic tests under incomplete ascertainment. Am J Hum Genet 11:1–16

Morton NE (1962) Segregation and linkage. In Burdette J (ed): Methodology in Human Genetics. Holden-Day, San Francisco, p. 17

Morton NE, MacLean CJ (1974) Analysis of family resemblance. III. Complex segregation analysis of quantitative traits. Am J Hum Genet 26:489–503

Risch N (1984) Segregation analysis incorporating linkage markers. I. Single-locus models with application to type 1 diabetes. Am J Hum Genet 36:363–386

Ritvo ER, Spence MA, Freeman BJ, Mason-Brothers A et al. (1985) Evidence for autosomal recessive inheritance in 46 families with multiple incidences of autism. Am J Psychiatry 142:187–192

Stene J (1978) Choice of ascertainment model I. Discrimination between single-proband models by means of birth order data. Ann Hum Genet 42:219–229

Sutton NE (1988) An Introduction to Human Genetics. Harcourt, Brace & Jovanovitch, p. 41

Vieland VJ, Hodge SE (1995) Inherent intractability of the ascertainment problem for pedigree data: A general likelihood framework. Am J Hum Genet 56:33–43

Weinberg W (1928) Mathematische Grundlagen der Probandenmethode. Z Indukt Abstammungs Vererbungslehre 48:179–228

Analysis of genetic linkage

Niall H. Anderson

8

Introduction

Homologous chromosomes pair at meiosis and experience reciprocal exchanges by recombination; in consequence, each gametic chromosome is a patchwork of the two homologous chromosomes inherited from each parent. The probability that an exchange, or crossing-over, has occurred in the interval defined by any two loci is a function of the distance that separates them. Recombination events cannot be observed directly; rather, one can estimate their frequency by comparing the chromosomes of offspring to those of the parents, provided distinct alleles define inheritance at each locus.

Linkage analysis relies on genetic recombination to infer distance between loci by exploiting naturally occurring genetic variation to define genetic markers, using structured human families as an alternative to the experimental crosses practiced in laboratory animals. Conclusions are reached through statistical inference.

Through linkage analysis, genetic markers can be assembled into genetic maps of human chromosomes, and the familial segregation of inherited disorders can be followed through the phenotypes they define. Whenever a gene exerts a significant effect in the occurrence of a disease, linkage can be established between the disease phenotype and genetic markers, thereby defining the chromosomal region harboring the gene in which a deleterious mutation leads to expression of the disease. Such linked markers may be of diagnostic value; they also pave the way for the eventual isolation of the mutant gene.

Recombination and genetic distance

Recombination results from crossing-over between chromatids of paired chromosomes at the first division of meiosis. As illustrated in Figure 8.1, for recombination to be observed between two loci the following conditions must be satisfied: (1) distinct alleles are present on the two parental chromosomes at both loci; (2) the gamete recovered is derived from a recombinant chromatid; (3) the recombinant chromatid has experienced an *odd* number of crossings-over. Our present understanding of the mechanism of recombination has been derived from the analysis of meiosis under controlled crosses in experimental organisms, particularly in Ascomycetes such as *Neurospora* where all meiotic products are recovered in an ordered fashion (reviewed in White and Lalouel, 1987).

The probability that recombination will occur between two loci is in part a function of the physical distance separating them. That relationship, however, is not simple for several reasons: (1) as noted above, recombination results from an odd number of crossings-over, which are not

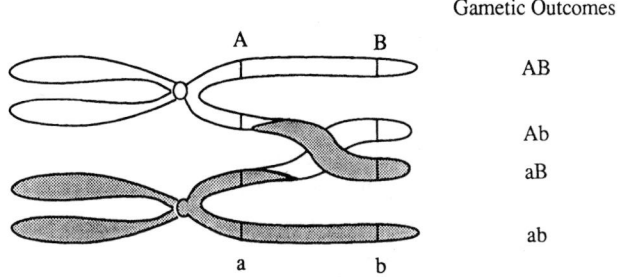

Fig. 8.1. Four-strand model of homologous recombination at the first division of meiosis.

directly observed; (2) the density of crossing-over appears to be variable along chromosomes; (3) multiple crossings-over do not appear to occur independently; rather, a crossing-over event tends to inhibit the occurrence of another in its vicinity, a phenomenon called positive interference. Therefore, the distance inferred between loci from genetic recombination is a functional measure only loosely related to physical separation. It is expressed in terms of crossing-over density in units of Morgans (M), 1 Morgan corresponding to that distance over which there occurs, on average, one crossing-over per chromatid.

The functional relationship between frequency of recombination and genetic distance depends on assumptions regarding interference. When no interference is assumed, crossings-over occur independently, following a Poisson process. As shown by Haldane (1919), recombination, r, and genetic distance, d, satisfy the relations

$$d = \frac{-\log_e (1 - 2r)}{2}$$

and

$$r = \frac{1 - e^{-2d}}{2}$$

Other functions that have been proposed to incorporate various degrees of interference have been reviewed elsewhere (White and Lalouel, 1987).

From published observations on chiasma counts in spermatogenesis, Renwick (1968) estimated the total genetic length of the human autosomal genome as 30 M. Given the estimate of 3 billion nucleotides derived for the human haploid genome (Kornberg, 1980), the common assumption is that, on average, 1 centiMorgan (cM) corresponds to 1 million nucleotides.

Genetic markers

Until it became possible to investigate sequence polymorphisms in arbitrary segments of human DNA, genetic markers for the human genome were limited to polymorphisms in plasma proteins that were recognized either by immunologic reactions or by electrophoretic assays. While all such markers are fully penetrant, some systems can only be defined phenotypically because of dominance relationships between alleles, as is the case for the ABO blood group system. Cotterman (1969) introduced a convenient factor-union algebra for expressing alleles and phenotypes in terms of the elementary factors that are identified experi-

Table 8.1. Factor-Union Algebra

Alleles	Factors		
	A_1	A_2	B
A_1	1	1	0
A_2	0	1	0
B	0	0	1
O	0	0	0

Phenotypes	Genotypes	Binary Codes
[A_1]	A_1A_1 or A_1A_2 or A_1O	110
[A_2]	A_2A_2 or A_2O	010
[A_1B]	A_1B	111
[O]	O	000

Genetic systems can be described through simple algebraic rules relating factors detected (antigens, DNA fragments etc.) to alleles, alleles to genotypes and phenotypes to genotypes. This is an example of the application of this Boolean algebra to the ABO blood group system (upper table), with four phenotypes given as an illustration (lower table).

mentally; this concept is illustrated in Table 8.1. Although more than 30 such systems were available for early linkage studies, the small number of those classical markers, their usually low heterozygosity, and the variety of experimental techniques required to characterize them, drastically limited their domain of application.

The exploitation of variation in DNA sequence to generate restriction fragment length polymorphisms (RFLPs) (Botstein et al., 1980) removed those restrictions. Cloned DNA sequences can reveal polymorphic loci after digestion of genomic DNA with appropriate restriction enzymes, by a procedure known as Southern blotting (Southern, 1975). Genomic DNA digested by a restriction enzyme is electrophoresed in an agarose gel, denatured, and transferred by capillary action to a paper or nylon support. Hybridization with a radiolabeled cloned DNA segment, or *probe*, followed by autoradiography, reveals DNA segments homologous to the probe. DNA sequence polymorphisms affecting such restriction sites yield variation in the length of the fragments revealed by this process.

Several types of genetic polymorphism can be recognized by this approach. The most common type of RFLP results from a mutation that destroys or creates a restriction site. In the majority of cases a single site exhibits polymorphism, leading to a diallelic system. It is not uncommon, however, for a probe to reveal polymorphism at several sites within the region with which it shares homology, particularly with large cloned segments or with probes derived from cDNA sequences. In such cases, a one-to-one relationship no longer exists between status of restriction sites and observed DNA fragments; what can be observed, however, is the presence or absence of bands of defined length. The factor-union system of Cotterman applies to all such systems and therefore provides a uniform coding scheme for all genetic markers. Or, a given probe may reveal polymorphisms with more than one restriction enzyme. In such instances, several genetic systems can be defined in the chromosomal region spanned by the probe, and these systems can be combined into haplotypes to define the multiallelic systems. However, the extent of polymorphism that can be defined by haplotypes may be limited by the occurrence of linkage disequilibrium over such limited genomic regions: certain combinations of alleles at distinct loci may tend to be observed more often on the same chromosome than is expected by chance.

Insertions or deletions within the interval defined by two invariant restriction sites may generate variation in the length of hybridizing fragments in the absence of restriction site polymorphism. This underlying mechanism is suspected when a similar size difference is noted between alleles defined with different restriction enzymes.

Loci containing a variable number of tandem repeats (VNTRs) of a short sequence of nucleotides represent a form of insertion/deletion polymorphism that is particularly useful for linkage analysis. The first locus of this kind was discovered by chance in a library of cloned DNA segments (Wyman and White, 1980). Subsequently, VNTRs were found associated with insulin, the first locus in which the tandem-repeat structure was defined (Bell et al., 1981, 1982), the *HRASL* locus (Goldfarb et al., 1982), the myoglobin locus (Jeffreys et al., 1985), and the ζ-globin locus (Proudfoot et al., 1982). The cloned sequence at the myoglobin locus, used as a probe of genomic DNA digested with an arbitrary enzyme, revealed a large number of distinct bands on Southern blots under hybridization conditions of low stringency. This indicated partial homology between the probe and a wide array of loci, dispersed throughout the human genome, that share a core oligomeric sequence. Using this core sequence, as well as several others since discovered, to screen cosmid libraries of human genomic DNA has resulted in the isolation of a large number of locus-specific probes. Because these probes reveal variation in a tandem array of repeats flanked by unique DNA sequences, allelic interpretation is straightforward. Examples of VNTR polymorphisms are presented in Figure 8.2. The loci identified by such probes usually display multiallelic series and a high degree of heterozygosity. The extent of polymorphism revealed in this way depends on the power of resolution afforded by the enzyme chosen and on the experimental conditions used for Southern blotting.

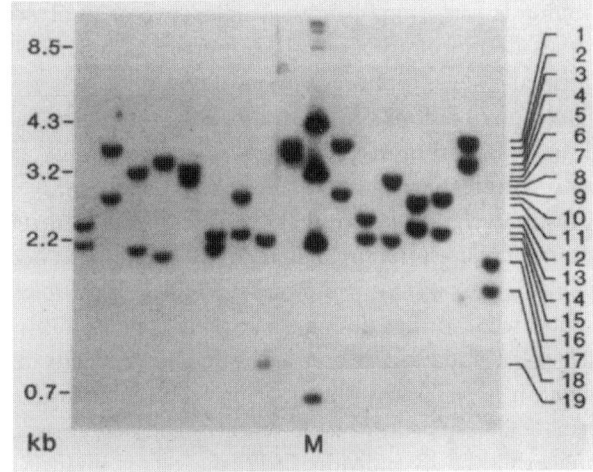

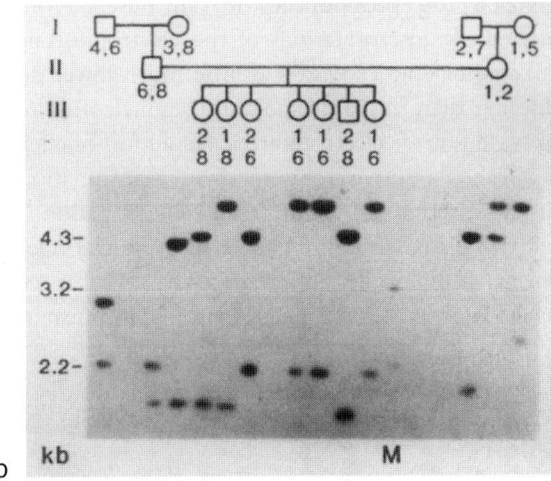

Fig. 8.2. Allelic variation revealed by the probe pYNH24 in 16 unrelated subjects *a*. and in a nuclear pedigree *b*. (Reprinted with permission from Nakamura et al., 1987, Science 235: 1616–1622. Copyright 1987, American Association for the Advancement of Science.)

A new series of polymorphisms (Litt and Luty, 1989; Weber and May, 1989), based on the variation in the number of copies of tandem repeats of simple sequence motifs (short tandem repeats – STR) involving one to four nucleotides, has further expanded the scope and power of marker studies for several reasons. The motifs are widely dispersed at high density throughout the genome: it is estimated that dinucleotide repeats occur, on average, every 80 kb. The degree of polymorphism they exhibit is usually high, with heterozygosity often in excess of 80%. Finally, the markers can be characterized by the polymerase chain reaction, and the polymorphisms are analysed under conditions that lend themselves to significant laboratory automation. DNA segments encompassing the repeats are enzymatically amplified by using oligonucleotide primers derived from unique sequences flanking a tandem repeat.

Detection is performed by either radioactive or fluorescent methods after labeling of one the primers. Size separation is performed by electrophoresis on polyacrylamide gels under denaturing conditions similar to those of sequencing gels.

Two polymorphisms based on single nucleotide and tetranucleotide repeats are presented in Figures 8.3 and 8.4, respectively. Alleles are characterized by the occurrence of bands of major intensity, but additional bands also occur, which differ in size from the major bands by multiples of the repeated motif. Although the precise mechanism by which this "laddering" effect arises has not been formally clarified, it is believed to be an artifact associated with the enzymatic amplification of the repeats. The degree of laddering exhibited by individual STR markers is highly variable. When too pronounced, it can obscure or even preclude allelic interpretations of the electrophoretic patterns. Tetranucleotides usually exhibit much lower degrees of laddering than single nucleotide or dinucleotide repeats and provide greater electrophoretic resolution of alleles.

However, the drive to even greater automation and higher throughput has prompted a reinvestigation of the feasibility of using large numbers of single nucleotide polymorphisms (commonly abbreviated to SNP) as genetic markers (Kruglyak, 1997). The lower polymorphism rate of

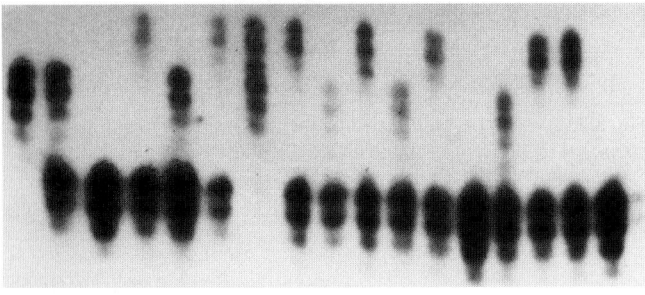

Fig. 8.3. Electrophoretic patterns revealed by marker UT5219, a single nucleotide repeat of adenine.

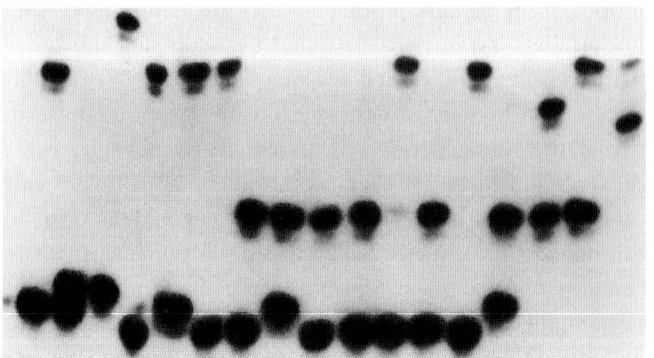

Fig. 8.4. Electrophoretic patterns revealed by marker UT453, a tetranucleotide repeat of the simple sequence AAAG.

the SNPs would be compensated by their greater availability (estimated at 1 per 1000 base pairs), and the speed and efficiency of automated genotyping procedures would be increased by only having to perform a plus/minus assay. Kruglyak (1997) suggested that a dense map of SNPs at 1 cM intervals would provide an efficient tool for initial genome screens in linkage studies, with areas of interest being followed up with markers of any available type (SNP, STR, VNTR, etc.).

With these new marker technologies, the density of markers available on human chromosomes has become very impressive. Individual contributions of multiple independent investigators and large-scale mapping efforts exemplified by the Genethon project (Dib et al., 1996) have yielded thousands of new markers. The Cooperative Human Linkage Center (CHLC) has attempted to provide reference maps integrating data from multiple sources, including markers based on dinucleotide repeats (Murray et al., 1994). A high-density map of the human genome, based on over a thousand tetranucleotide repeat markers, was developed in parallel (Utah Marker Development Group, 1995). Much of these data were combined by Broman et al (1998) into a comprehensive genetic map of over 8000 STR polymorphisms. Libraries of SNPs are growing rapidly: see, for example, Buetow et al. (1999) and HGBASE (2000).

Families

Families constitute the second essential resource for linkage analysis in humans. In experimental species, controlled crosses can be designed to investigate recombination optimally. For two diallelic series *A,a* and *B,b*, homozygous parental strains can be constructed and crossed, *AB/AB* X *ab/ab*, yielding a first generation (F1) of *AB/ab* individuals where the alleles inherited from each parent are located on distinct chromosomes. F1 individuals can be crossed to any parental line, say *AB/ab* X *AB/AB* (backcross), or they can be crossed among themselves, *AB/ab* X *AB/ab* (intercross). Because the chromosomal origin of each allele is unambiguous, recombination events can be directly identified in the offspring. Consequently, estimation of recombination involves very simple statistics.

Under the nonexperimental conditions that prevail in humans, a situation analogous to a backcross consists of a nuclear family where the observed parental genotypes are *AaBb* X *aabb*. Note, however, that the chromosomal distribution, or phase, of the alleles is unknown in the double het-

Table 8.2. Detection of Linkage in a Double Backcross, *AaBb* × *aabb*

Phase of First Parent		Prior Probability
Coupling	*AB/ab*	1/2
Repulsion	*Ab/aB*	1/2

Conditional Probabilities of Gametes Produced by First Parent

Phase	AB	Ab	aB	ab	Total
Coupling	$(1-r)/2$	$r/2$	$r/2$	$(1-r)/2$	1
Repulsion	$r/2$	$(1-r)/2$	$(1-r)/2$	$r/2$	1

r represents the recombination fraction between the A, a and B, b loci. The 4 possible progeny genotypes are AB/ab, Ab/ab, aB/ab, ab/ab, each with probability 1/4.

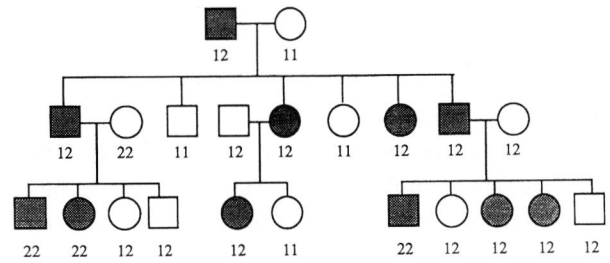

Fig. 8.6. Linkage analysis in a pedigree segregating a rare autosomal dominant disorder with complete penetrance. It yields a lod score of 3.31 at $r = 0$. When resolved into its four component nuclear families, the combined lod score is only 2.4.

erozygote: that parent may be either *AB/ab* or *Ab/aB*. For historical reasons, these two possible phases are usually called *coupling* and *repulsion*. As can be seen in Table 8.2, the interpretation of the genotypes observed in the offspring is different under each phase. It follows that, in such instances, recombination cannot be identified directly; rather, it is inferred by statistical methods (reviewed later in this chapter).

A more favorable situation can be created if one adds the grandparents to this nuclear family, a structure we will call a nuclear pedigree. When a parent is a double heterozygote, the genotype of the corresponding grandparents may elucidate the parental phase (Fig. 8.5). Note, however, that sometimes the parental phase may remain unresolved, with a probability inversely related to the heterozygosity of each marker.

Mendelian disorders are often investigated in yet more extended familial structures, or pedigrees, whether they are

recessive conditions in isolated populations or dominant disorders where inheritances can be followed along extended lineages. For a rare condition, such an ascertainment scheme may be the only way for a substantial number of affected individuals to be obtained for genetic analysis. Although the simple methods of linkage analysis applicable to nuclear families could be used for disease studies after resolution of extended pedigrees into their component nuclear families, information on phase provided by other relatives would be lost, as shown in Figure 8.6. In consequence, the analysis of whole pedigrees is usually performed with the assistance of computer programs such as LIPED (Ott, 1974) for pairs of loci or VITESSE (O'Connell and Weeks, 1995) for two or more loci.

Simple structures still contain some information about linkage. As pointed out by Smith (1953), affected sib pairs or single inbred recessive patients can be informative. The sib-pair approach has less power than conventional linkage analysis based on familial segregation: however, it may be well suited to common diseases with undefined, complex modes of inheritance, as it requires minimal genetic assumptions (see Ch. 12). While inbred recessive homozygotes may be of greater value than was previously anticipated, given the markers and genetic maps now available (Lander and Botstein, 1987), complex inbred populations and the fact that identical alleles are not necessarily identical by descent may impose practical limitations. The emphasis here is on classical linkage analysis as applied to simple mendelian disorders.

Statistical methods

MAXIMUM LIKELIHOOD

In most practical applications of linkage analysis in humans, phase is unknown in at least some individuals, and

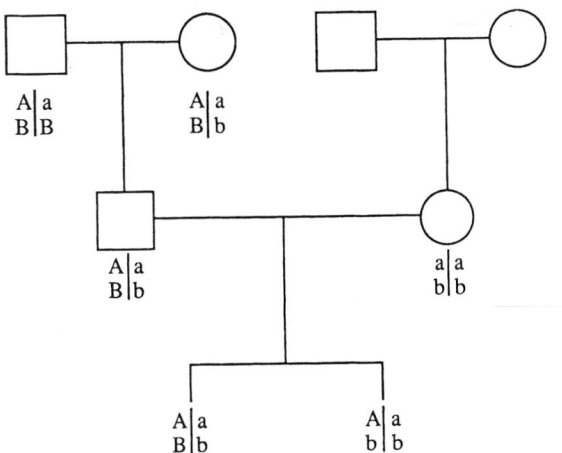

Fig. 8.5. Determination of phase in a nuclear pedigree. When the grandparents are not available for genotyping, the double heterozygote of the second generation may be of either phase *AB/ab* or *Ab/aB*.

therefore the recombination events are not directly reflected by the observations. Rather, recombination frequencies are estimated by statistical methods from the available observations.

Linkage between two loci is not an event, but a hypothesis that can be submitted to a statistical test. In linkage analysis, statistical inference is performed by the method of maximum likelihood, a general approach that estimates parameters specifying probability distributions and evaluates the relative merit of competing hypotheses (Edwards, 1984). A probability distribution is assumed, which involves one or more parameters that specify the distribution. For two loci, the simplest situation of linkage analysis, this distribution depends on the particular family structures sampled, and it is expressed as a function of the recombination frequency, r. A hypothesis is contemplated, namely, that the two loci are linked.

The likelihood of a hypothesis, $L(H)$, is proportional to the probability of the data under that hypothesis, $p(D|H)$, the proportionality constant being arbitrary. The principle of maximum likelihood states that the hypothesis with greatest likelihood is that for which the probability of the observations is maximized. In the present case, this maximum is obtained by finding that value of the recombination frequency between the two loci, which maximizes the probability of the experimental data, $p(D|r)$. To obtain this maximum, an iterative procedure is applied. The value $\hat{r}$, for which this maximum is obtained, is the maximum likelihood estimate of the recombination frequency.

As with all estimates derived from a limited sample of experimental data, a significant sampling error is associated with estimations of recombination frequency, and therefore whether or not the two loci are linked cannot be inferred by simple examination of the estimate of recombination frequency. Rather, one must perform a statistical test, contrasting the hypothesis of linkage with that of independent segregation. The likelihood of the latter hypothesis is proportional to the probability of the observations when the recombination frequency is taken as 0.5. The relative likelihoods of the two competing hypotheses can be formally expressed by the ratio of the two likelihoods, $p(D|\hat{r})/p(D|0.5)$, which measures odds in favor of linkage.

Although such a ratio is a valid measure of support for an hypothesis, it does not correspond to a significance level in the classical sense: an odds ratio of 100:1 does not mean a significance level of 0.01. To obtain a significance level, the distribution of the likelihood ratio must be known and a bound must be derived, yielding the probability that the test statistic exceeds that bound under the null hypothesis. In large samples, twice the natural logarithm of the likelihood ratio, $2\log_e[p(D|\hat{r})/p(D|0.5)]$ follows a χ^2 distribution, with 1 df for the single-parameter case.

LOD SCORE

To detect linkage, it is customary to assess significance by computing a very closely related statistic, $\log[p(D|\hat{r})/p(D|0.5)]$, and to infer linkage when this statistic exceeds 3.0. This statistic, or lod score (Morton, 1955), finds its origin in the theory of sequential tests, used to reach a decision as additional data are sequentially obtained. The significance bound of 3.0 was derived by taking into account the fact that any two loci have a certain probability of being on the same chromosome. The wide acceptance of lod scores, however, stems from other considerations: as multiple tests are performed between pairs of loci, the proposed bound has been found empirically to provide a reasonable hedge against the false assertion of linkage.

Together with the maximum-likelihood estimate of the recombination frequency and its associated lod score, it is customary to report a lod score table (Morton, 1955), where the lod score is computed for a set of defined recombination values. Through this convention, published results from independent studies can be combined without reference to the raw genetic data.

CONFIDENCE LIMITS

The estimate of the recombination frequency derived from a linkage test admits some margin of error. Confidence intervals in the Neyman–Pearson sense are based on estimates of standard errors. In linkage analysis, however, because of small sample sizes, such confidence limits are generally not trustworthy. A preferred alternative consists of deriving empirical bounds from the distribution of the observations. A one-lod-unit support limit is derived by finding the two values of the recombination frequency for which the maximum lod score is decreased by one unit (Conneally et al., 1985). Given that a lod score of 3 is usually required to declare significant linkage between autosomal loci, a three-lod-unit interval is sometimes also calculated to correspond more directly to the duality of significance testing and confidence intervals in standard statistical theory. The rationale for this approach is discussed in Chapter 4 of Ott (1991).

It is also possible to use simulation-based methods to generate empirical confidence intervals for r (Chiano and Yates, 1994; Nemesure et al., 1995), using techniques known as *Jacknifing* and *Bootstrapping* (Efron and Tibshirani, 1993). These offer improved accuracy at the cost of a greater computational workload.

PROBABILITY CALCULATIONS

In the simple case of codominant traits in a phase-known backcross, recombination events are directly identified in the offspring, and the probability distribution of the observations is given by the binomial distribution

$$\binom{n}{m} r^m (1 - r)^{n-m}$$

reaching its maximum for $\hat{r} = m/n$. When phase is unknown, assuming equal prior probabilities for each phase, the probability distribution of the offspring is a linear combination of two binomial distributions. Most simple situations that can be encountered in nuclear families have been treated in detail by Morton (1955).

In the general case, where dominance or extended familial structures may be considered, probability calculations will involve three types of probabilities: the prior probability of a genotype in an ancestor in the pedigree; the probability of a phenotype given a genotype; and the probability of a genotype in the offspring given parental genotypes. The last probability is given by elementary mendelian rules. Specification of prior probabilities requires estimates of allelic frequencies in the population from which the data have been sampled; rough estimates are sufficient for this purpose. Phenotype probabilities incorporate phenomena such as dominance, incomplete penetrance, and phenocopies.

INCOMPLETE PENETRANCE AND PHENOCOPIES

The concept of incomplete penetrance is primarily used to characterize the inheritance of mendelian conditions that do not occur ineluctably in individuals at risk. A penetrance can be associated with each genotype at the corresponding locus, specifying the probability that an individual of this genotype will express the disease. Delayed onset or gender-specific morbid risks can be incorporated in the model. The lower the penetrance of the genotypes that impart risk, the smaller the amount of information provided by unaffected family members. Phenocopies consist of the rare occurrence of a clinical syndrome undistinguishable from the inherited condition, but resulting from other causes. A phenocopy can be incorporated in the genetic model by assuming that individuals with a normal genotype have a small probability of expressing the disease. The power of linkage analysis is significantly affected by phenocopies when they account for more than a small percentage of cases.

Ideally, penetrances are estimated by formal segregation analysis of families ascertained from the population through a well-defined sampling scheme (reviewed in Elston and Rao, 1978). Usually their calculation also requires an estimate of the prevalence of the disease in the reference population. For many rare conditions, however, limited data may resolve the issue of dominance without providing reliable estimates of penetrances. In those situations linkage analysis can still be performed with approximate estimates of penetrance that have been derived from prevalence data, empirical recurrence risks in families, and limited data on age of onset or gender-specific morbid risks. The careful investigator will take the precaution of verifying that his or her inference of linkage does not critically depend on the assumed penetrances, by testing linkage over a reasonable range of numerical values.

Most computer programs for linkage analysis incorporate an assumption of incomplete penetrance and phenocopies. While the parameters that specify the mode of inheritance of the phenotype of interest are held fixed when tests of linkage are performed, such parameters could also be estimated together with the recombination frequency. That is, linkage and segregation analysis could be performed jointly. However, this strategy imposes a significant analytical penalty and stringent sampling conditions, as the mode of ascertainment and construction of pedigrees from initial probands profoundly affects the inference of modes of inheritance.

Although unaffected individuals do not contribute significant information about segregation at the test locus under reduced penetrance, their genotypes at the marker locus can sometimes contribute critical information on the genotypes of diseased parents. This fact should be borne in mind when one is investigating pedigrees.

THE EFFECT OF GENDER ON RECOMBINATION

Variation in recombination frequencies between sexes is a common feature in most species examined. In the human, recombination usually occurs at a higher frequency in females than in males. Furthermore, this differential effect appears variable from one chromosomal region to another, with a density of crossing-over being two- to fourfold higher in females than in males, the larger ratios being seen particularly near the centromere (Broman et al., 1998). It is also becoming increasingly clear that in some chromosomal regions (e.g., near the telomere) the converse is true. As a result, there is a great deal of variability in the female to male ratios of genetic lengths of the chromosomes, from 1.2:1 for chromosomes 15 and 19, to 2:1 for chromosome 8 (Broman et al., 1998). This phenomenon is poorly understood, and observations on chiasma occurrence in spermatogenesis and oogenesis fail to substantiate the genetic observations (reviewed in White and Lalouel, 1987). In light of the available observations, it is reasonable to assume that both the density and the distribution of crossing-over differ in the two sexes.

What is the implication of this effect on linkage analysis? The estimation and test procedures reviewed above can be extended to include gender-specific recombination frequencies. Indeed, the test of linkage can be formulated in terms of these two parameters. The consequence, however, is that a formal likelihood ratio test now includes 2 df; the power to detect linkage may be reduced by this effect and the conventional bound of 3.0 may not be appropriate. In the absence of a thorough statistical investigation of this issue, most investigators feel that the effect of gender may be neglected for the purpose of linkage detection. Indeed, to carry out the linkage analysis separately for males and females would effectively halve the number of meioses available for each study, counteracting any benefit gained from the increase in precision of the sex-specific genetic maps. Once linkage is detected, however, gender-specific recombination frequencies may be estimated separately and the significance of the effect of gender may be formally tested by a likelihood ratio test. The probability of the data is maximized with respect to both r_m and r_f, and it is contrasted to the maximum obtained under the hypothesis of equal recombination frequencies in the two sexes. The likelihood ratio statistic $2 \log_e [p(D|\hat{r}_m, \hat{r}_f)/p(D|r)]$ can be referred to a χ^2 table with 1 df.

AETIOLOGIC HETEROGENEITY

Defining inherited conditions solely on the basis of clinical manifestations may obscure distinct etiologies. Unless the phenotype reflects allelic differences at a single locus, etiologic heterogeneity may drastically affect linkage analysis. The analytical approach depends on whether heterogeneity occurs within or among pedigrees. When two independent causes account for affected individuals within a pedigree, heterogeneity can be handled through the concept of phenocopy, as discussed above. The more common the disorder, the greater the proportion of phenocopies may become; while power decreases drastically with an increasing proportion of phenocopies, quantification through formal analysis or extensive simulations is not at hand.

Heterogeneity within a pedigree is unlikely when the inherited condition under study is rare. However, independently ascertained pedigrees may reflect the segregation of different loci, possibly obscuring all evidence for genetic linkage. This problem can be circumvented by seeking evidence of linkage within one or within each of several large pedigrees. Statistical methods, however, offer two other alternatives. When heterogeneity is to be tested with respect to a predefined partition of the data, standard likelihood theory provides a test of this partition. The data may be subdivided according to clinical symptoms, origin, sampling units, or other a priori criteria. Maximum likelihood estimation is carried out for each subset, as well as for the entire sample. A likelihood ratio test is constructed, contrasting the product of the maximized probabilities in each subset to the maximum probability obtained for the total sample $2 \log_e [\Pi_i p(D_i|r_i)/p(D|r)]$. Under the hypothesis of homogeneity, this statistic follows a χ^2 distribution with $n-1$ df for this one parameter case, where n is the number of classes into which the data have been partitioned. Equivalently, this test can be expressed in terms of lod scores: $2 \log_{10} [\Sigma_i z_i (r_i) - z(r)]$. This test was first used by Morton (1956) to demonstrate genetic heterogeneity in elliptocytosis. When applied to a collection of nuclear families segregating elliptocytosis, it indicated significant heterogeneity of recombination with respect to the Rh factor locus on chromosome 1, leading Morton to conclude that an Rh-linked locus accounts for only a portion of cases of elliptocytosis. In a more recent application of the heterogeneity test, two pedigrees segregating spastic paraplegia, an X-linked condition in some families, appeared heterogeneous in their linkage relationship to two markers on the X chromosome that are unlinked to each other (Kenwrick et al., 1986; Keppen et al., 1987). In one pedigree, spastic paraplegia was accompanied by mental retardation and other manifestations, suggesting that "pure" and "complicated" forms of X-linked spastic paraplegia may have distinct genetic etiologies. It is possible that the same locus was involved in the expression of spastic paraplegia in both pedigrees, albeit associated with a structural alteration in the long arm of the X chromosome in the complicated form.

Another test of heterogeneity can be used when the alternative to homogeneity is that the families examined belong to two etiologic classes, one linked and the other unlinked to the marker locus (Smith, 1963; Ott, 1983). Assuming that a proportion m of the families exhibit linkage while $1-m$ are unlinked, the probability of the observations can be expressed in terms of two parameters, the recombination fraction r for the linked form and the admixture proportion, m. A likelihood ratio test can be formulated, contrasting the likelihood obtained when both parameters are estimated to that obtained under the hypothesis of homogeneity, where m is fixed to unity and only the recombination fraction is estimated. This yields a

χ^2 with 1 *df*. The two parameters *m* and *r* can be estimated simultaneously or they can be obtained by analysis of the lod-score tables (Ott, 1991). For tests of locus heterogeneity involving more than two independent sampling units, greater power is expected of the admixture test than of the predivided sample test, because of the smaller degree of freedom allowed in computing the statistics.

Although heterogeneity makes the detection of linkage more difficult, the investigator can also take advantage of these two tests to infer the etiologic significance of particular clinical, biological, or epidemiological features of an inherited condition.

MULTILOCUS LINKAGE ANALYSIS

As the number of known DNA markers increased, extensive genetic maps have been constructed for most human chromosomes. Mapping of marker loci is best achieved by following the joint segregation of several allelic series, all characterized in the same sample of families. Indeed, multilocus analysis is more efficient than pairwise analysis to determine gene order, to detect linkage, and to estimate recombination frequencies.

Multipoint analyses are based on more complex probability models, expressed in terms of multiple between-loci recombination fractions. Maximum likelihood methods, however, still apply and are used to estimate the recombination parameters in the presence of uninformative meioses and unknown phase. The resulting calculations are computationally intensive, but can be carried out by packages such as VITESSE (O'Connell and Weeks, 1995). For further details and examples, see Chapter 6 of Ott (1991).

The presence of multiple loci also raises the spectre of interference effects (the inhibition of recombination at a given point by the presence of recombinations in adjacent intervals). Such positive interference would obscure the relationship between recombination and genetic distance. When this phenomenon was examined in three-point tests (Lathrop et al., 1985), the following conclusions were reached: (1) while interference can indeed be estimated, the power to detect significant departure from independence is low; and (2) the bias in the estimate of a recombination frequency that results from neglecting interference is, at most, 7% of the recombination frequency; this maximum occurs for loose linkage. In light of the sample sizes generally achieved in humans, it was concluded that interference could be ignored in most practical applications.

The use of several linked markers imparts greater power to the detection of linkage. For example, three-point experiments with complete information can be five times as effi-

cient as two-point experiments (Lathrop et al., 1985). In general, though, linkage experiments do not yield the maximum information expected from the pedigrees sampled: the markers used do not have maximal heterozygosity, and therefore they will not identify uniquely all segregating chromosomes. The chance distribution of heterozygosity is such that each marker of a linkage group may add further information on linkage to a test locus. This is illustrated by experience in linkage studies on multiple polyposis coli, where combining the information contributed by several loci increased confidence in linkage by two orders of magnitude over the support obtained with each marker singly (Leppert et al., 1987). Genetic maps now available are leading to efficient detection of linkage. Multilocus information also yields more precise estimates of recombination frequencies than can be obtained by using only pairs of loci.

Genetic maps

One can efficiently construct a genetic map by collecting genotypic information on polymorphic loci (*markers*) in a common panel of reference families. Nuclear pedigrees are ideally suited for this purpose (White et al., 1985a). For this reason, a panel of 60 test families has been made available by the Centre d'Etude du Polymorphisme Humain in Paris (Dausset, 1986) to investigators carrying out linkage studies with DNA markers.

To construct a genetic map of a set of linked loci, the most likely order of the loci must be established by multilocus linkage analysis. Because sampling errors are inevitable, support for this best order must be evaluated by testing critical alternate orders. As the number of loci increases, the number of possible orders becomes so large that the likelihood of each one cannot be evaluated. Consequently, construction of a linkage map consists of establishing partial order for subsets of loci, adding loci and testing unresolved orders until a most likely order has been established with sufficient confidence (see Lathrop et al., 1988 for an example of this strategy).

As an example, a primary genetic map of chromosome 17 is presented in Figure 8.7. The map consists of 21 loci derived from 27 RFLPs, and it includes eight highly informative VNTR loci. (The average heterozygosity among all 21 loci in the panel of reference families was 58%; it was 77% for the VNTRs.) The map covers the whole chromosome, spanning 218 cM in males and 279 cM in females. While the average chiasma density does not differ in the

Fig. 8.7. Sex-specific genetic maps of chromosome 17, with physical localizations of selected markers indicated on the karyogram. Maps are scaled in centimorgans, under the assumption of a variable sex ratio in each interval. θ = recombination fraction. (From Nakamura et al., 1988, with permission.)

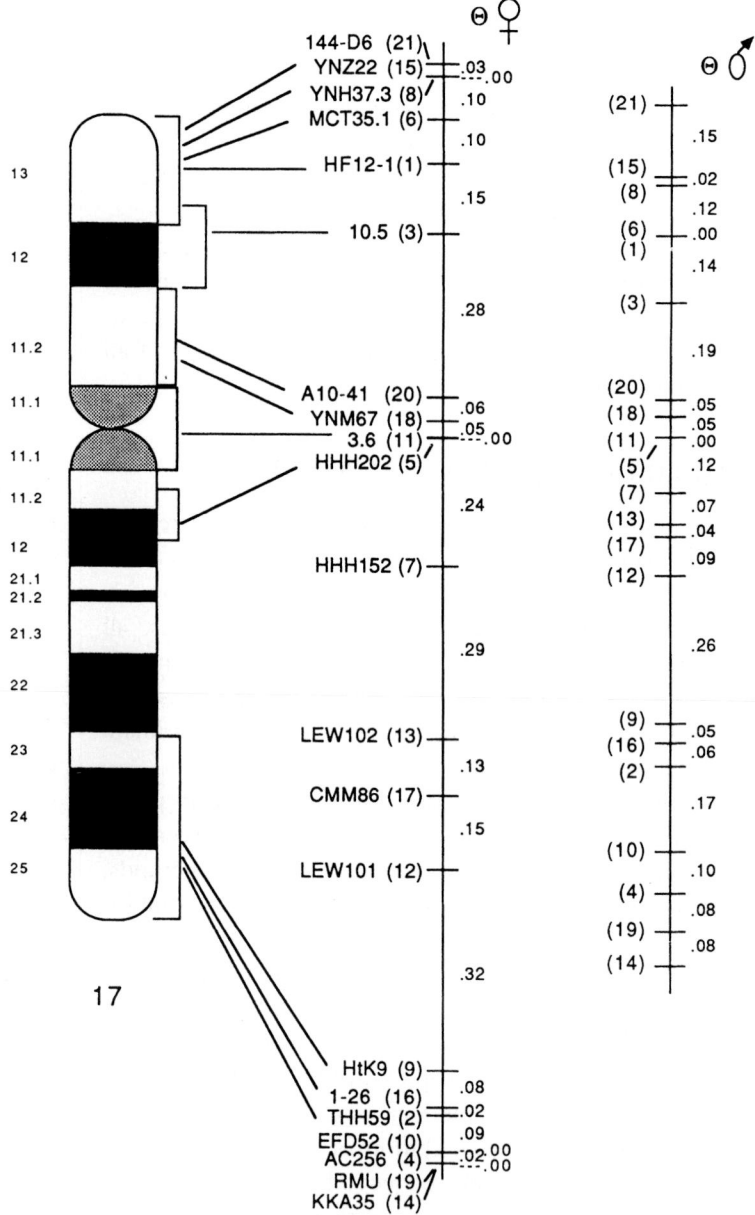

two sexes, there is significant variation in recombination frequencies between the sexes in the intervals defined by the loci on this map; in particular, more recombination events have occurred in males within both telomeric regions. Consequently, a separate map has been reported for each sex (Nakamura et al., 1988). Because six markers – YNZ22, MCT35.1, YNM67, CMM86, THH59, and RMU – span the entire chromosome in a continuous linkage group, a linkage analysis with only these six markers would require, at most, 35 phase-known meioses to detect significant linkage for any new locus on chromosome 17.

As the example illustrates, the complete specification of a genetic map includes (1) the linear order of the loci along the chromosome; (2) the estimates of the recombination frequencies for each interval of the map (whenever it is suggested by the data, gender-specific recombination rates are derived so that a separate map can be reported for each sex); and the support in favor of the reported order, arrived at by documenting the odds in favor of the reported order versus critical alternatives. Further support for the placement of each locus on the map can be documented by depicting ranges of uncertainty. As mentioned earlier, maps of increasing marker density are continually being refined.

Mapping genetic diseases

With the DNA markers now available, any genetic disease segregating in a simple mendelian fashion can be added to the human gene map by linkage analysis, provided sufficient familial data are available. The latter issue can be assessed by computing expected lod scores for the familial structures sampled (e.g., Skolnick et al., 1984), or for general pedigrees by relying on computer simulations (Ott, 1989; Weeks et al., 1990). One can also invoke simple arguments to assess the potential value of family resources for the detection of linkage. For a disease with incomplete penetrance, a pedigree with 10 affected individuals could yield a lod score of 3 for complete linkage only if phase were known in all sibships including these individuals, and if the marker used were fully informative. In practice this situation is unlikely, and therefore between 15 and 20 affected individuals within a pedigree may actually be required. Looser linkage would require an even larger number of informative individuals.

Mapping a disease by linkage is only a step toward the ultimate goal of identifying the gene that harbors mutation(s) leading to expression of the disease. For disorders of unclear inheritance or likely heterogeneity, the confirmation of genetic etiology provided by a mapped gene is a significant scientific inference. The weaker our knowledge of the molecular basis of the disease, the greater is the relevance of linkage analysis.

Linkage also offers a unique opportunity to infer or refute the role of a known gene in disease etiology. In this "candidate-gene" approach, the pathophysiology of a disease may focus our suspicion on one or several known genes. If polymorphisms have been identified in cloned sequences from these candidate loci, the cloned sequences can be used as probes in linkage tests.

Prior knowledge may or may not be available with regard to the likely localization of the mutant gene at the origin of a disease. The mutation leading to Duchenne muscular dystrophy was expected to be on the short arm of the X chromosome because of the rare occurrence of the condition in females who presented a particular chromosomal translocation; the report of a 5q deletion in a patient with nonfamilial Gardner syndrome oriented the search for the gene responsible for familial adenomatous polyposis toward that region of the chromosome (Bodmer et al., 1987; Leppert et al., 1987). On the other hand, Huntington disease (Gusella et al., 1983), cystic fibrosis (CF) (Tsui et al., 1985; Wainwright et al., 1985; White et al., 1985b), type I (von Recklinghausen) neurofibro-

matosis (Barker et al., 1987; Seizinger et al., 1987), and multiple endocrine neoplasia (Simpson et al., 1987) were localized to chromosomes 4, 7, 17, and 10, respectively, in the absence of any prior information. The general linkage strategy is regularly providing new information about the chromosomal localization of a rapidly increasing number of inherited diseases.

LINKAGE BETWEEN A MARKER AND A DISEASE: AN EXAMPLE

Tight linkage observed between CF and an RFLP at the *MET* oncogene locus (White et al., 1985b) illustrates an application of the linkage strategy to an autosomal recessive disease with complete penetrance. At least one parent was heterozygous for the diallelic marker in 12 of 13 independently ascertained nuclear families that had at least two affected children. Linkage analysis yielded a lod score of 8.65 at a recombination value of 0, indicating no evidence of recombination. This corresponds to odds of 4×10^8: 1 in favor of complete linkage over independent segregation. In each family the lod score was maximum for complete linkage, therefore no heterogeneity was evident in this set of families. The one unit support limit on the estimate of recombination was 0.05. Assuming complete linkage, the parental phases could be determined from the offspring genotypes, yielding marginally significant evidence of allelic association between the *CF* mutation and allele 1 at the *MET* locus ($\chi^2 = 3.86$, 1 *df, p* = .05). This linkage disequilibrium was confirmed in a larger series (Beaudet et al., 1986). The gene involved was identified ultimately by positional cloning (Kerem et al., 1989).

The data reported in Table 8.3 are useful in assessing the contribution of each family to the linkage evidence. If we assume that all parents are heterozygotes at the *CF* locus, all but two families are single backcrosses for the marker. In these families, each affected offspring contributes terms equal to r and $(1 - r)$ under each parental phase, respectively. In the absence of recombination, the parental phase can be established from a single affected individual, and each additional individual contributes two units to the odds ratio, or 0.301 to the lod score. Families 1415 and 1427 are double intercrosses. In such families, after phase has been inferred each additional affected offspring homozygous at the marker locus contributes $(1 - r)^2$ to the lod score, or 0.602 lod units. While less informative, unaffected offspring can still contribute some information in an intercross, affected sibling of genotype 12 contributes $2(1 - r + r^2)$, or 0.125, to the total lod score. This can be verified by comparing families 1415 and 1427.

Table 8.3. Genetic Linkage Between Cystic Fibrosis and the *MET* Locus

Family	Parental Genotype	Number of Affected Children (Genotypes)	Number of Normal Sibs (Genotypes)	Lod Score at r = 0
1409	12 × 11	3 (11)		0.60
1414	12 × 22	3 (12)		0.60
1415	12 × 12	3 (11)	1 (12)	1.33
1422	12 × 11	3 (12)		0.60
1425	12 × 11	5 (12)	2 (12, 11)	1.15
1426	22 × 12	3 (12)		0.60
1427	12 × 12	3 (11)	4 (12)	1.70
1438	11 × 12	2 (11)		0.30
1442	12 × 11	3 (11)		0.60
1446	11 × 12	3 (11)		0.60
774	11 × 12	2 (11)		0.30
1378	22 × 12	3 (22)	2 (22)	0.25
1436	11 × 22	3 (12)		0.00

Reprinted by permission from Nature *(White et al., 1985b,* Nature *318: 382–384), copyright 1985, Macmillan Magazines Ltd.*

USING THE MAP

The availability of detailed genetic maps of human chromosomes has significantly enhanced the efficiency of linkage analysis. Ideally spaced markers can be selected for testing, and linkage can be sought by utilizing simultaneously all markers of a linkage group (Lathrop et al., 1984).

Adenomatous polyposis coli can serve as an example. It is an autosomal dominant inherited predisposition to colon cancer where subjects at risk present hundreds of polyps in the colon. A case report of a person with these symptoms and an interstitial deletion of the long arm of chromosome 5 (Herrera et al., 1986) was followed by evidence of linkage in segregating families (Bodmer et al., 1987; Leppert et al., 1987). Genotypes for 16 DNA markers were determined in a reference panel of 59 normal nuclear pedigrees, and a genetic map was constructed. Five pedigrees with multiple cases of familial polyposis coli were ascertained and tested for genotypes at nine of the marker loci. Autosomal inheritance with incomplete penetrance was assumed, and the likely localization of the mutant gene was sought by the method of location scores (Lathrop et al., 1984). A likelihood ratio was computed for various locations of the putative mutant gene along the map, contrasting the probability of the data when the test locus was at each location against the corresponding probability when the test locus was assumed to be unlinked to all markers of the map, using all available markers jointly. The odds for linkage were increased by two orders of magnitude with this multilocus test over the pairwise test between the disease and the closest marker. Figure 8.8 summarizes the results of the

study. The gene was subsequently isolated (Groden et al., 1991; Joslyn et al., 1991).

Application to diagnosis

Molecular techniques are contributing powerful diagnostic tools to medical practice. By identifying genotypes at risk, DNA markers can be used to confirm a clinical diagnosis, to detect preclinical cases, or to carry out prenatal diagnosis. The inference can be direct or indirect. By direct inference, we mean that the mutation at the origin of a disorder can be detected directly in the patient.

Sickle-cell anemia offers a paradigm. The mutation responsible for the synthesis of the abnormal hemoglobin HbS can be identified directly in genomic DNA by Southern blot analysis or by hybridization with specific oligomers (Conner et al., 1983). When the mutation itself cannot be determined, diagnosis can be based on site polymorphisms in its vicinity. The diagnostic strategy may rely on demonstrated linkage disequilibrium between clinical phenotype and site polymorphisms, or it may use documented linkage between DNA markers and the condition. In the former case, the site polymorphisms may be in the defective gene itself, or they may be in DNA sequences in its proximity, like the markers for CF.

When linkage has been demonstrated between a putative gene and DNA markers, the probability that an individual in a family has a given genotype can be computed by a simple extension of the probabilities used in linkage analysis. For

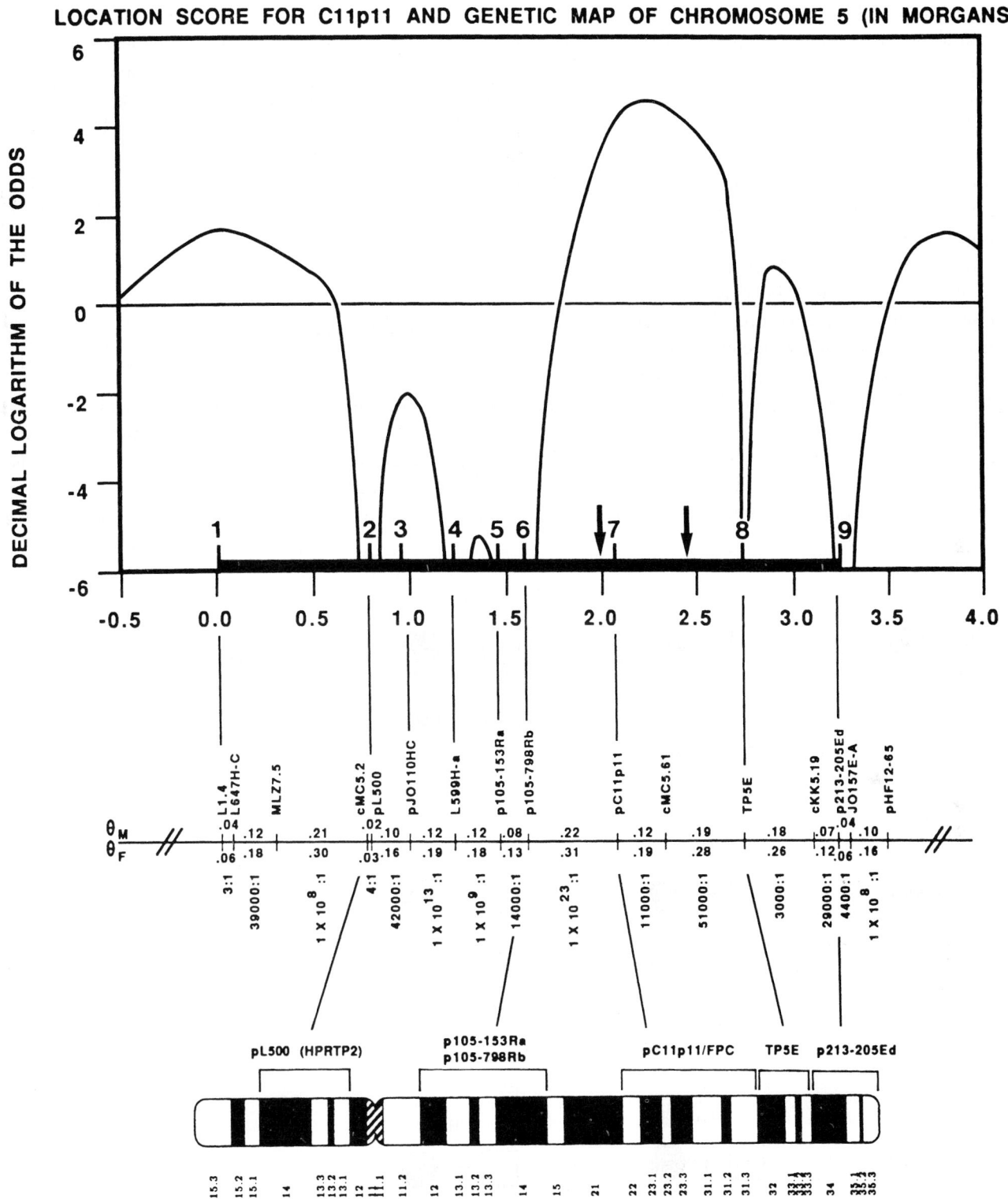

Fig. 8.8. Genetic linkage map of 16 DNA markers on chromosome interval 5, with location scores (*top*) for the *FPC-GS* gene on the female map. Two arrows on the abscissa indicate the 95% confidence boundaries for the location of the *FPC-GS* locus. The genetic map (*centered*), also scaled to female genetic distance, indicates estimates of recombination distance (θ) between markers for males (*above line*) and females (*below line*). Genotypes were obtained in a panel of 59 normal reference families and the most likely gene order was determined under the assumption of a constant ratio of male: female map distance along the entire chromosome. The physical localizations of selected probes are indicated on the ideogram of chromosome 5. (Reprinted with permission from Leppert et al., 1987, Science 238: 1411–1413. Copyright 1987, American Association for the Advancement of Science.)

example, the probability that an individual has genotype G at the test locus, given the information available on clinical phenotypes and DNA markers in the pedigree, I, is given by

$$p(G\backslash I) = \frac{p(G,I)}{\sum_i p(G_i, I)}$$

Therefore the algorithm used for linkage analysis can be applied to the calculation of genetic risks. Genetic models of inheritance must be specified for all loci used, including allelic frequencies in the reference population. In the absence of complete linkage, the ideal situation consists of two closely linked markers flanking the test locus; this is illustrated in Figure 8.9, which documents the efficiency of flanking markers and the critical role of phase information. A single affected individual (a) contributes no information; however, an unaffected sib (b), an affected sib (c), or an affected grandparent (d) can contribute information. While a diallelic system may be informative (e), it also may not, hence the high premium on multiallelic systems (f).

Flanking markers afford more information than a single marker (g), but a recombination event between markers can reduce (h) or even cancel (i) all available information. Allelic association and linkage must be jointly considered in some instances. The same method applies, but haplotype frequencies must be incorporated.

Genetic diagnosis raises multiple ethical issues; although outside the scope of this chapter, they will continue to challenge clinicians and researchers alike.

Toward gene isolation

Mapping of a putative gene at the origin of an inherited condition may be the first step toward its eventual identification. The initial discovery of linkage usually yields loose bounds on the possible localization of the gene. However, these bounds can be further reduced by linkage analysis of a larger series of

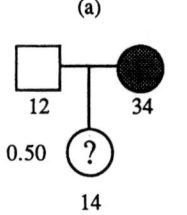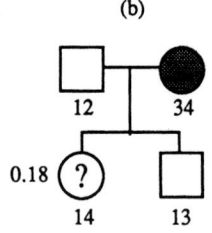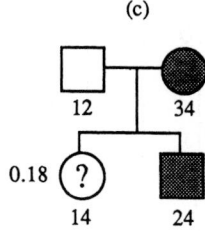
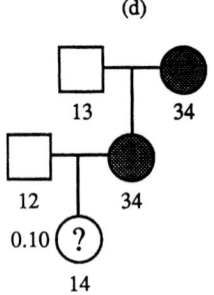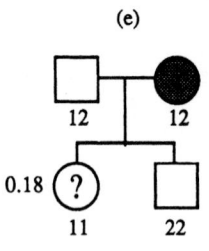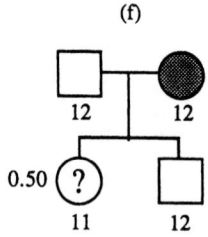
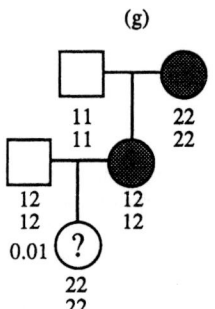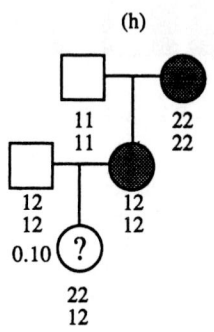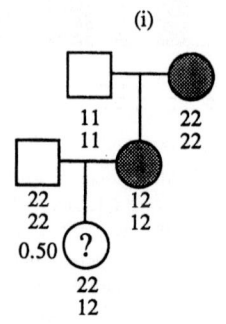

Fig. 8.9. Genetic risks for a rare autosomal dominant condition with complete penetrance. In each case, we report the probability that the individual at risk (question mark within the symbol) is of the normal genotype. A recombination frequency of 0.10 is assumed between the test locus and each marker. Filled-in symbols indicate affected individuals (see text for discussion).

segregating families or by testing new markers that map in the incriminated region. Thus, after the initial discovery of linkage between CF and the markers MET and pJ3.11, seven centers collaborated in a further characterization of the linkage relationship between CF and the two markers in 211 families (Beaudet et al., 1986). The location of the *CF* gene was narrowed to within an interval of about 3 cM, the markers appearing to flank the *CF* locus with odds of 10:1. Further mapping of the region, with a total of six DNA markers, established stronger support yet for this order, with odds of 800:1 against the next most likely alternative. Eventually, the gene was isolated from this region (Kerem et al., 1989).

Genetic mapping by analysis of linkage has entered a new era. Advances in cloning technologies raise the promise that the combination of statistical genetics and molecular biology will lead to the elucidation of the etiology of numerous inherited disorders whose biochemical causes are not yet understood.

Acknowledgements

This chapter is an updated version of the one that appeared in the 3rd Edition of this work. The original was written by Drs Jean-Marc Lalouel and Raymond L. White of the University of Utah, USA.

REFERENCES

Barker D, Wright E, Nguyen K et al. (1987) Gene for von Recklinghausen neurofibromatosis is in the pericentromeric region of chromosome 17. Science 236:1100–1102

Beaudet A, Bowcock A, Buchwald M et al. (1986) Linkage of cystic fibrosis to two tightly linked DNA markers: joint report from a collaborative study. Am J Hum Genet 39: 681–693

Bell GI, Karam JH, Rutter WJ (1981) Polymorphic DNA region adjacent to the 5′ end of the human insulin gene. Proc Nat Acad Sci USA 78:5759–5763

Bell G, Selby M, Rutter W (1982) The highly polymorphic region near the human insulin gene is composed of simple tandemly repeating sequences. Nature 295:31–35

Bodmer W, Bailey C, Bodmer J et al. (1987) Localization of the gene for familial adenomatous polyposis on chromosome 5. Nature 328:614–616

Botstein D, White R, Skolnick M, Davis R (1980) Construction of a genetic linkage map in man using restriction fragment length polymorphisms. Am J Hum Genet 32:314–331

Broman KW, Murray JC, Sheffield VC, White RL, Weber JL (1998) Comprehensive human genetic maps: Individual and sex-specific variation in recombination. Am J Hum Genet 63:861–869

Buetow KH, Edmonson MN, Cassidy AB (1999) Reliable identification of large numbers of candidate SNPs from public EST data. Nature Genet 21:323–325

Chiano MN, Yates JRW (1994) Bootstrapping in human genetic linkage. Ann Hum Genet 58:129–143

Conneally PM, Edwards JH, Kidd KK et al. (1985) Report of the committee on methods of linkage analysis and reporting. Cytogenet Cell Genet 40:356–359

Conner B, Reyes A, Morin C et al. (1983) Detection of sickle cell B5-globin allele by hybridization with synthetic oligonucleotides. Proc Nat Acad Sci USA 80:278–282

Cotterman CW (1969) Factor-union phenotype systems. In Morton NE (ed): Computer Applications in Genetics. University of Hawaii Press, Honolulu, pp. 1–19

Dausset J (1986) Le centre d'étude du polymorphisme humain. Presse Med 15:1801–1802

Dib C, Faure S, Fizames C et al. (1996) A comprehensive genetic map of the human genome based on 5,264 microsatellites. Nature 380:152–154

Edwards AWF (1984) Likelihood. Cambridge University Press, Cambridge, UK

Efron B, Tibshirani RJ (1993) An Introduction to the Bootstrap. Chapman and Hall, NY

Elston RC, Rao DC (1978) Statistical methods in human genetics. Annu Rev Bioeng 7:253–286

Goldfarb M, Shimizu K, Perucho M, Wigler M (1982) Isolation and preliminary characterization of a human transforming gene from T24 bladder carcinoma cells. Nature 296:404–409

Groden J, Thliveris A, Samowitz W et al. (1991) Identification and characterization of the familial adenomatous polyposis coli gene. Cell 66:589–600

Gusella J, Wexler N, Conneally P et al. (1983) A polymorphic DNA marker genetically linked to Huntington's disease. Nature 306:234–238

Haldane JBS (1919) The combination of linkage values, and the calculation of distance between the loci of linked factors. J Genet 8:299–309

Herrera L, Kakati S, Gibas L et al. (1986) Brief clinical report: Gardner syndrome in a man with an interstitial deletion of 5q. Am J Med Genet 25:473–476

HGBASE (2000) Human Genic Bi-Allelic Sequence database by Uppsala University and Interactiva Biotechnologie GmbH. Release 6. http://hgbase.interactiva.de/

Jeffreys A, Wilson V, Thein S (1985) Hypervariable "minisatellite" regions in human DNA. Nature 314:67–73

Joslyn G, Carlson M, Thliveris A et al. (1991) Identification of deletion mutations and three new genes at the familial polyposis locus. Cell 66:601–613

Kenwrick S, Ionasescu V, Ionasescu G et al. (1986) Linkage studies of X-linked recessive spastic paraplegia using DNA probes. Hum Genet 73:264–266

Keppen L, Leppert M, O'Connell P et al. (1987) Etiological heterogeneity in X-linked spastic paraplegia. Am J Hum Genet 41:933–943

Kerem B, Rommens JM, Buchanan JA et al. (1989) Identification of the cystic fibrosis gene: Genetic analysis. Science 245:1073–1080

Kornberg A (1980) DNA Replication. WH Freeman, San Francisco, p.19

Kruglyak L (1997) The use of a genetic map of biallelic markers in linkage studies. Nat Genet 17:21–24

Lander E, Botstein D (1987) Homozygosity mapping: A way to map human recessive traits with the DNA of inbred children. Science 236:1567–1570

Lathrop GM, Lalouel JM, Julier C, Ott J (1984) Strategies for multilocus linkage analysis in humans. Proc Nat Acad Sci USA 81:3443–3446

Lathrop GM, Lalouel JM, Julier C, Ott J (1985) Multilocus linkage analysis in humans: Detection of linkage and estimation of recombination. Am J Hum Genet 37:482–498

Lathrop GM, Farrall M, O'Connell P et al. (1988) Refined linkage map of chromosome 7 in the region of the cystic fibrosis gene. Am J Hum Genet 42:38–44

Leppert M, Dobbs M, Scambler P et al. (1987) The gene for familial polyposis coli maps to the long arm of chromosome 5. Science 238:1411–1413

Litt M, Luty JA (1989) A hypervariable microsatellite revealed by in vitro amplification of a dinucleotide repeat within the cardiac muscle actin gene. Am J Hum Genet 44:397–401

Morton NE (1955) Sequential tests for the detection of linkage. Am J Hum Genet 7:277–318

Morton NE (1956) The detection and estimation of linkage between the genes for elliptocytosis and the Rh blood types. Am J Hum Genet 8:80–96

Murray JC, Buetow KH, Weber JL et al. (1994) A comprehensive human linkage map with centimorgan density. Science 265:2049–2054

Nakamura Y, Leppert M, O'Connell P et al. (1987) Variable number of tandem repeat (VNTR) markers for human gene mapping. Science 235:1616–1622

Nakamura Y, Lathrop M, O'Connell P et al. (1988) A mapped set of DNA markers for human chromosome 17. Genomics 2:302–309

Nemesure BB, Greenberg DA, Mendell NR (1995) Simulation study comparing interval estimates for the recombination fraction. Genet Epidemiology 12:351–359

O'Connell JR, Weeks DE (1995) The VITESSE algorithm for rapid exact multilocus linkage analysis via genotype set-recoding and fuzzy inheritance. Nat Genet 11:402–408

Ott J (1974) Estimation of the recombination fraction in human pedigrees: Efficient computation of the likelihood for human linkage studies. Am J Hum Genet 26:588–597

Ott J (1983) Linkage analysis and family classification under heterogeneity. Ann Hum Genet 47:311–320

Ott J (1989) Computer-simulation methods in human linkage analysis. Proc Nat Acad Sci USA 86:4175–4178

Ott J (1991) Analysis of Human Genetic Linkage, Revised Edition. Johns Hopkins University Press, Baltimore

Proudfoot N, Gil A, Maniatis T (1982) The structure of the human zeta-globin gene and a closely linked, nearly identical pseudogene. Cell 31:553–563

Renwick JH (1968) Ratios of female to male recombination fractions in man. Bull Eur Soc Hum Genet 2:7–14

Seizinger B, Rouleau G, Ozelius L et al. (1987) Genetic linkage of von Recklinghausen neurofibromatosis to the nerve growth factor receptor gene. Cell 49:589–594

Simpson N, Kidd K, Goodfellow P et al. (1987) Assignment of multiple endocrine neoplasia type 2a to chromosome 10 by linkage. Nature 328:528–530

Skolnick M, Bishop DT, Cannings C, Hasstedt S (1984) The impact of RFLPs on human gene mapping. In Rao DC, Elston RC, Kuller LH (eds): Genetic Epidemiology of Coronary Heart Disease: Past, Present and Future. Alan R Liss, New York, pp. 271–292

Smith CAB (1953) The detection of linkage in human genetics. J R Stat Soc Ser B 15:153–184

Smith CAB (1963) Testing for heterogeneity of recombination values in human genetics. Ann Hum Genet 27:175–182

Southern E (1975) Detection of specific sequences among DNA fragments separated by gel electrophoresis. J Mol Biol 98:503–517

Tsui LC, Buchwald M, Barker D et al. (1985) Cystic fibrosis locus defined by a genetically linked polymorphic DNA marker. Science 230:1054–1057

The Utah Marker Development Group (1995) A collection of ordered tetranucleotide-repeat markers from the human genome. Am J Hum Genet 57:619–628

Wainwright B, Scambler P, Schmidtke J et al. (1985) Localization of cystic fibrosis locus to human chromosome 7cen-q22. Nature 318:384–386

Weber JL, May PE (1989) Abundant class of human DNA polymorphisms which can be typed using the polymerase chain reaction. Am J Hum Genet 44:388–396

Weeks DE, Ott J, Lathrop GM (1990) SLINK: a general simulation program for linkage analysis. Am J Hum Genet 47:A204

White R, Lalouel J-M (1987) Investigation of genetic linkage in human families. Adv Hum Genet 16:121–228

White R, Leppert M, Bishop T et al. (1985a) Construction of linkage maps with DNA markers for human chromosomes. Nature 313:101–105

White R, Woodward S, Leppert M et al. (1985b) A closely linked genetic marker for cystic fibrosis. Nature 318:382–384

Wyman A, White R (1980) A highly polymorphic locus in human DNA. Proc Nat Acad Sci USA 77:6754–6758

Chromosomal basis of inheritance

J. R. Korenberg
T. K. Mohandas

Introduction

DNA, the genetic material in humans, is packaged into a set of chromosomes as in other eukaryotes. Chromosomes are the vehicles of inheritance as they contain virtually all of the DNA of the cell with the exception of the small fraction present in the mitochondria. Consequently, the chromosomes of a cell are also the linear representation of a single copy of all the DNA defining an individual's genome. Finally, as the visible transmitters of genetic information, chromosomes can be seen and studied under the light microscope. The structure, function and behavior of chromosomes are, therefore, of much interest and importance. Chromosomes are derived in equal numbers from mother and father. Each ovum and sperm contains a set of 23 different chromosomes, which is the haploid number (n) of chromosomes in humans. The diploid fertilized egg and virtually every cell of the organism arising from it has two haploid sets of chromosomes resulting in the diploid human chromosome number (2n) of 46. The human karyotype consists of 22 pairs of autosomes and a pair of sex chromosomes. The correct chromosome number in humans was determined and confirmed only in 1956 (Ford and Hamerton, 1956; Tjio and Levan, 1956).

In recent years, it has become apparent that chromosomal landmarks including bands reflect important distinctions in the functional organization of chromosome regions and in the molecular structure that underlies them. Moreover, these structural features of chromosomes also predispose them to rearrangements that are associated with disease states. The behavior of chromosomes in meiotic cell divisions provides the basis for the Mendelian laws of inheritance whereas the abnormal behavior of chromosomes in cell division leads to abnormalities of chromosome number. Recent advances in sequencing the human genome now provide the opportunity to determine the DNA sequences underlying chromosomal landmarks and therefore to determine the molecular basis of chromosomal events in development, disease and evolution. In this chapter, we will examine the current understanding of the structure, molecular organization and behavior of human chromosomes and explore how these features contribute to chromosomal diseases.

Methods for studying human chromosomes

Technical innovations in the past fifty years have revolutionized the study of human chromosomes. Chromosomes are normally visible only during cell division as they become condensed in preparation for orderly division. Therefore, chromosomes can be studied only in cells that are dividing in vivo or in vitro. Dividing cells are sufficiently common in some tissues in vivo to permit the direct study of chromosomes. This is true of meiotic divisions in testis and embryonic ovary, and of mitotic divisions in the bone marrow, some epithelia, and tumors. However, cell culture methods have greatly extended the range of tissue and cell types from which dividing cells can be obtained in vitro. These include small lymphocytes, fibroblasts from skin and other tissues, and cells from amniotic fluid or chorionic villi. Viable cells can even be obtained for a number of hours after death of an individual or spontaneous abortion of an embryo. It is thus possible to carry out chromosome studies in a wide range of clinical situations.

The introduction of a short-term peripheral blood culture technique (Moorhead et al., 1960) provided a reliable way for obtaining human chromosome preparations of good quality for human cytogenetic investigations and for clinical diagnosis. In this widely used technique, T-lymphocytes from a small sample of peripheral blood are stimulated to divide in culture with the lectin, phytohemagglutinin (PHA). The blood culture is initiated in a suitable culture medium and within two to three days the stimulated leukocytes provide very large numbers of dividing cells. These are blocked in metaphase by adding a mitotic spindle poison, such as colchicine, to the culture for a few minutes. Treatment of the cells with a hypotonic solution swells the cells, which allows spreading of the chromosomes. This makes it possible to prepare well-spread, flattened metaphase chromosome preparations on glass slides suitable for microscopic analysis using chromosome banding methods and molecular cytogenetic techniques.

HUMAN CHROMOSOME IDENTIFICATION

In the early days of human cytogenetic investigations, chromosomes were stained with Giemsa or a similar dye yielding uniform staining along their lengths. Based on these studies, human chromosomes were classified according to their size and morphology. Two regions in metaphase chromosomes are less contracted and appear as much less stained primary and secondary constrictions. The primary constriction is the centromere (Figs. 9.1 and 9.2), where the sister chromatids of a replicated chromosome are held together until the anaphase stage of cell division. Based on the position of their centromeres, human chromosomes are classified as metacentric, for which the centromere is at or

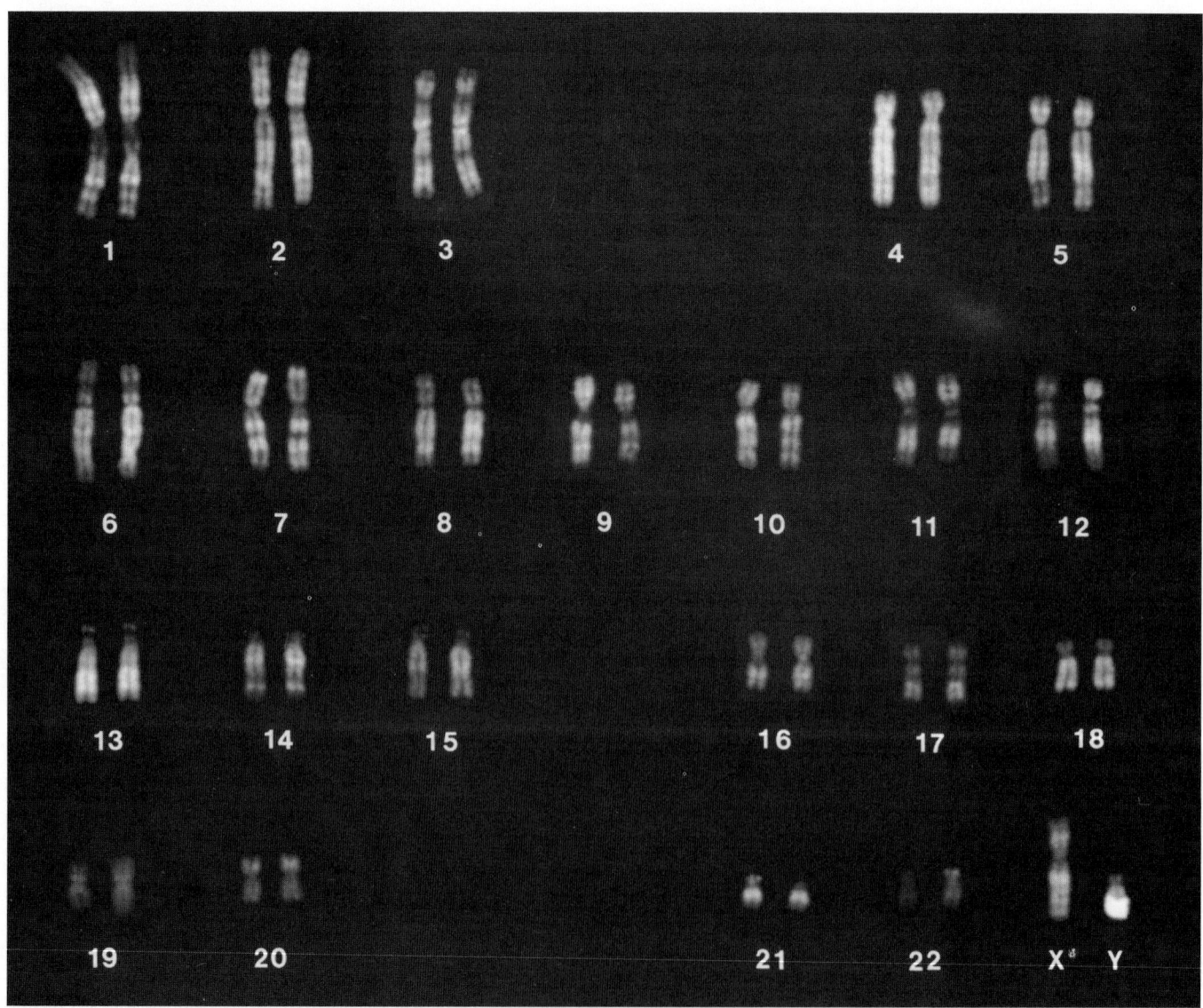

Fig. 9.1. Q-band karyotype of a male cell. Note the identical pattern of fluorescence banding of the two homologous chromosomes in each pair, the intense fluorescence of the distal part of the Y chromosome.

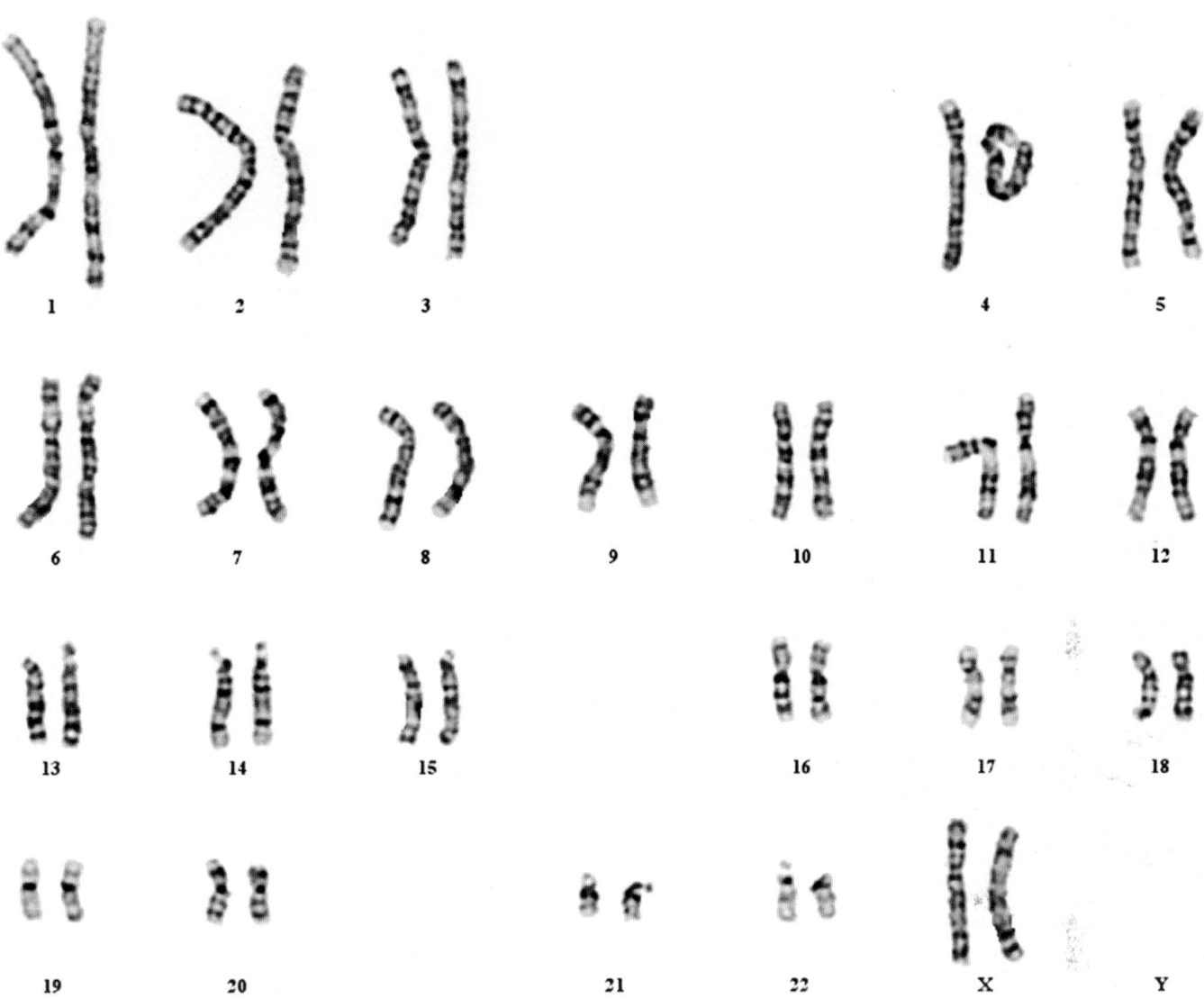

Fig. 9.2. G-band karyotype of a female cell. The banding pattern is identical to that seen by quinacrine fluorescence, except for an additional band adjacent to the centromeres of numbers 1 and 16.

near the middle of the chromosome, submetacentric, for which the centromere is located significantly off center, or acrocentric, for which the centromere is very close to one end. For all categories, the short arm of the chromosome is referred to as "p" for petite, and the long arm as "q". In addition to the centromere or primary constriction, up to five pairs of the acrocentric chromosomes (13–15, 21, 22) may exhibit secondary constrictions (see Fig. 9.6). These mark the site of each cluster of ribosomal RNA (rRNA) genes and are called nucleolus organizer regions (NORs) because, at telophase, nucleoli are formed at a subset of these sites that are transcriptionally active. The rRNA genes remain in a moderately extended state at metaphase, reflecting the late shutoff of these genes in prophase and the rapid re-initiation of their transcription after the anaphase separation of sister chromatids. A rare exception to these characteristic features of chromosomes is called "double minutes" (dm) (Stark et al., 1989), found in tumors and in certain in vitro artificial selective systems. As illustrated in Figure 9.9F, these are chromosomal fragments without centromeres that consist of genomic reduplications carrying multiple copies of genes advantageous to the proliferation of the particular cell. Consequently, they do not attach to the mitotic apparatus and are found in variable copy number. Such chromosomal fragments can be useful for cancer diagnosis and prognosis (Pauletti et al., 1996) and may provide clues to the growth of cells and the pathways of tumorigenesis.

CHROMOSOME BANDING

The conventional (Giemsa) staining without pretreatment does not allow complete identification of individual chromosomes. This was provided by the next major technical innovation in human cytogenetics which came in 1970, when Caspersson and colleagues discovered that human chromosomes stained with quinacrine mustard, a fluorescent DNA-binding compound, and examined under ultra violet light, show characteristic variation of fluorescence intensity along the length of each chromosome, producing a banded appearance (Caspersson et al., 1970). Each chromosome could then be identified by its characteristic quinacrine (Q)-banding pattern (Fig. 9.1). Subsequently, a large number of techniques have been developed that reveal banding patterns reflecting the underlying structural features of chromosomes. One group of procedures, the general banding techniques, produces the full range of bands along each chromosome allowing identification of individual chromosomes. General banding techniques of practical importance are G-banding and R-banding. A second group of banding techniques produces much more restricted staining of specific subsets of chromosome bands and include C-banding and NOR-staining. A technique that differentially stains the two sister chromatids of a chromosome is also of particular interest. Chromosome banding methods of interest are discussed in the following sections.

Although Q-banding was the method first employed for human chromosome identification, it is rarely used today for routine chromosome analysis in clinical cytogenetic laboratories, as simpler methods have become available that do not require the use of a fluorescence microscope. A banding pattern that is almost identical to the Q-banding pattern can be produced by treatment of chromosomes with a denaturing agent or a proteolytic enzyme, prior to staining them with Giemsa. In the most consistent and commonly used version of this technique, chromosomes are treated with a dilute solution of trypsin followed by staining with Giemsa (Seabright, 1971). The resulting Giemsa(G)-banding is the most widely used technique for human chromosome identification in clinical cytogenetics laboratories today (Figs. 9.2 and 9.3). The G-banding patterns are also readily captured and analyzed by the automated karyotyping systems used in most clinical cytogenetics laboratories. As an extension of the G-banding technique, methods are now in use for obtaining longer, less condensed prometaphase chromosomes which exhibit twice as many G-bands (about 800 bands per haploid set) as the usual metaphase chromosome preparations (about 400 bands per haploid set), providing greater precision to cytogenetic analysis (Yunis, 1976).

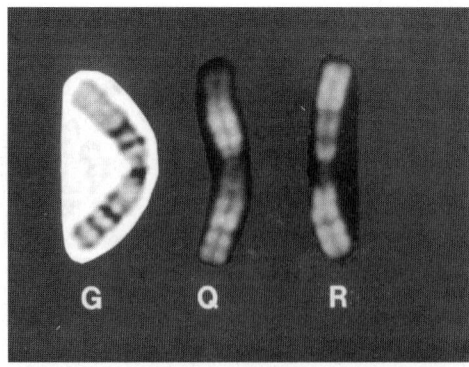

Fig. 9.3. Comparison of Q, G and R-banding patterns of human chromosome 1 from three different cells. Note that Q and G-banding patterns are similar, whereas the staining pattern following R-banding is the reverse of Q and G.

A less commonly used general banding technique is one that produces a Reverse (R)-banding pattern. Many techniques have been developed which produce this pattern, in which the staining intensity of each band is the reverse of that seen with Q- or G-banding (Fig. 9.3). R-banding of the highest resolution is obtained by a combination of chromomycin, that emits fluorescence most strongly in the R-bands, and distamycin A, that quenches fluorescence in G-bands. The commonly used method to generate R-bands is to subject chromosome preparations to moderate heat (~85°C in the presence of high salt) before staining them with Giemsa. An alternative R-banding technique, that also sheds some light on the mechanism of chromosome banding, is based on the differential replication timing of chromosome bands (Dutrillaux et al., 1973). In this technique, growing cells are exposed to the thymidine analog, bromodeoxyuridine (BrdU) during the S phase of the cell cycle and examined following staining with the fluorochrome, acridine orange (AO). Cells that incorporate BrdU into their DNA at the late stage of the S phase are selected for observation. With acridine orange staining, the BrdU-containing chromosomal regions appear dull (G or Q bands), whereas the early replicating regions that have incorporated thymidine fluoresce brightly giving a reverse or R-banding pattern (Figs. 9.3 and 9.4). Thus, the R-bands on chromosomes represent regions that replicate their DNA early in the synthetic period. The inactivated, late replicating X chromosome in females (see below) is also stained differentially (dull) from the active X chromosome following this replication banding protocol (Fig. 9.4).

The C-banding method selectively stains the areas located around the centromeres of all chromosomes and on the distal long arm of the Y chromosome (Arrighi and Hsu, 1971). The largest C-bands usually occur on chromosomes

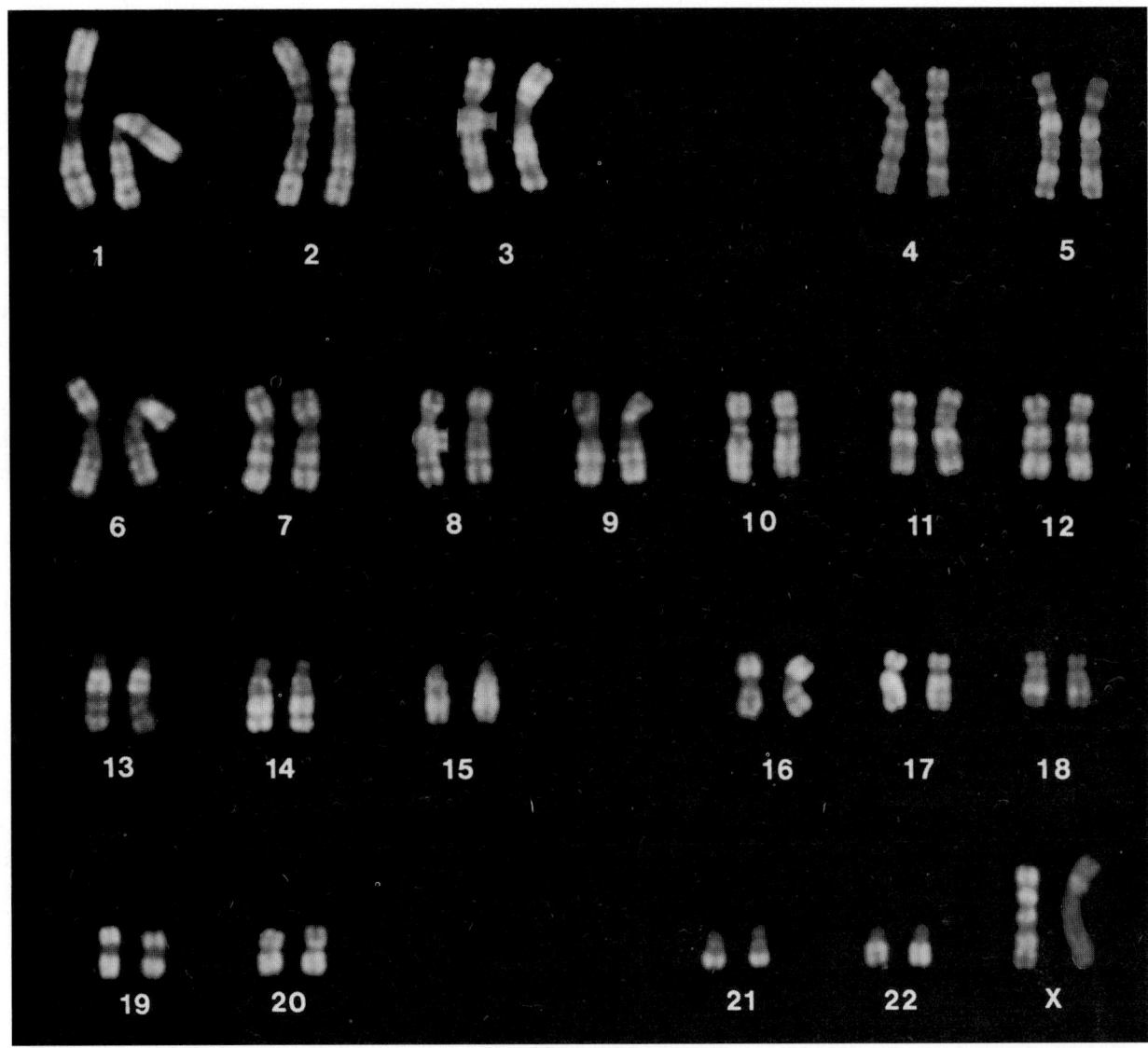

Fig. 9.4. R-banded karyotype following incorporation of BrdU into the late replicating regions of the chromosome. The early replicating R-band regions have incorporated thymidine and fluoresce brightly. The late replicating Q/G band regions have incorporated BrdU resulting in faint flourescence. Note that the inactive, late replicating X chromosome is also faintly fluorescent.

1, 9, and 16 and the Y in regions that contain highly repetitive, non-transcribed DNA. To elicit C-bands, metaphase chromosome preparations are treated with sodium hydroxide or barium hydroxide followed by Giemsa staining (Fig. 9.5). This alkali treatment extracts most of the DNA from chromosomes but leaves the protein-DNA complexes consisting of highly repetitive DNA sequences in the C-band regions. The size of the C-band on a given chromosome is usually constant in all the cells of an individual but is highly variable from person to person reflecting variations in the amount of heterochromatic DNA present at the centromeric regions. Such C-band heteromorphisms on chromosomes are transmitted from parent to offspring as simple

Mendelian dominant traits. These variations in chromosome morphology are not associated with any known phenotypic effects (see below) but are useful as markers in various clinical and epidemiological studies of chromosome abnormalities.

AgNOR or Silver staining uses a silver nitrate solution to selectively stain the sites of *transcriptionally active* ribosomal RNA genes which are located in the satellite stalk regions on the short arms of human acrocentric chromosomes (Goodpasture et al., 1976). These nucleolar organizing regions may also be manifested as secondary constrictions with conventional Giemsa stain. Silver staining regions are usually present on 6 to 8 of the 10 acrocentric

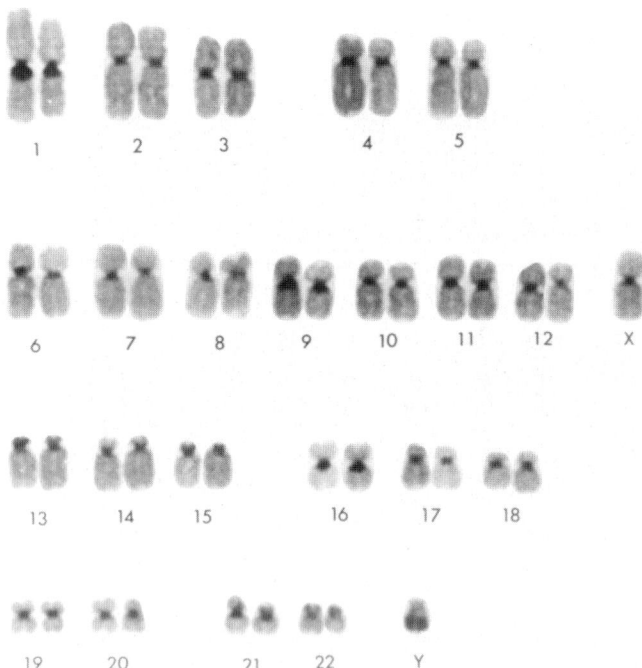

Fig. 9.5. C-band karyotype of a male cell. Identification of individual chromosomes is probably not accurate in every case as C-banding stains only a subset of bands. The largest C-bands are seen on chromosomes 1,9,16, and the Y. The sizes of C-bands vary, even within homologous pairs (e.g., chromosomes 1,6,9 and 16).

chromosomes, 13, 14, 15, 21, and 22 (Fig. 9.6), although they may be seen on as few as three and as many as all ten of these chromosomes. The sizes of the AgNORs are highly variable in the human population, although the size of each AgNOR in the cells of one individual is quite consistent and usually remains unchanged from one generation to the next. AgNOR staining is useful in characterizing rearranged chromosomes involving the human acrocentric chromosomes. The mechanism of AgNOR staining is based on the oxidation of nucleolar nonhistone proteins with $AgNO_3$ by which Ag^+ is reduced to black native silver. Interestingly,

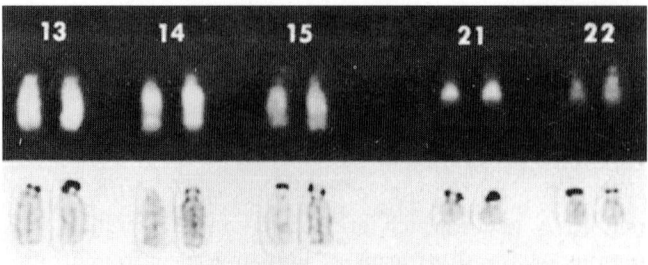

Fig. 9.6. Partial double karyotype of the acrocentric chromosomes from a single cell, stained first by Q banding to identify each chromosome, and then by the AgNOR technique to show the sites of the ribosomal RNA genes (nucleolus organizer regions) and their relative transcriptional activity.

the acrocentric chromosomes show association of their satellite stalk regions even in metaphase chromosome preparations, reflecting the functional association of these sites in the formation of the nucleolus in the interphase nucleus. This association of the nucleolar organizing regions is considered to be a factor responsible for the high incidence of exchanges or Robertsonian translocations involving the short arms of acrocentric chromosomes.

Sister Chromatid Exchange (SCE) is an extension of the replication banding technique using BrdU incorporation to produce differential staining of the two sister chromatids of the metaphase chromosome. This requires BrdU incorporation into DNA throughout two successive rounds of DNA replication. At the end of the first round of DNA replication, the two newly synthesized strands of DNA in the double-stranded helix will contain BrdU, but the two template strands will not. At the second round of DNA replication, two new double-stranded helices will be produced, of which one will have BrdU incorporated on both strands and the other will have BrdU substitution in only one strand of the DNA double helix. When the chromosomes containing singly (TB) and doubly (BB) substituted chromatids are stained with the DNA binding flurochrome, Hoechst 33258, and exposed to UV light, they show differential sister chromatid staining, with the bifilarly substituted chromatid staining paler (Latt, 1973). Staining of these BrdU incorporated chromosomes with Giemsa produces darkly stained and lightly stained sister chromatids (Korenberg and Friedlander, 1974) (Fig. 9.7). Therefore, exchanges of material between sister chromatids or sister chromatid exchanges (SCEs) are readily visible at high resolution following this staining protocol. The differential sister chromatid staining observed following the SCE protocol is a rather remarkable cytological demonstration of the semi-conservative replication of DNA. It also demonstrates that each chromosome is composed of a single very long duplex of DNA. Further, it shows that exchanges between the two sister chromatids take place in somatic cells that could potentially have mutagenic effects. SCE is used to diagnose diseases associated with chromosomal instability in clinical cytogenetic laboratories. For example, SCE analysis is a diagnostic test for Bloom's syndrome, a rare autosomal recessive disease caused by mutations in a DNA helicase of the RecQ family that catalyze the unwinding of duplex nucleic acid molecules (van Brabant et al., 2000). It is characterized by growth deficiency, predisposition to neoplasia and chromosome instability in somatic cells. The frequency of spontaneous SCEs in cells from patients with Bloom's syndrome is markedly increased. SCE analysis is also used

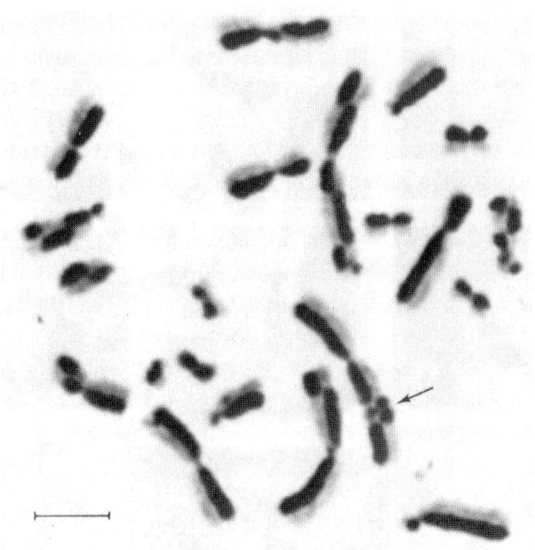

Fig. 9.7. Sister chromatid exchanges shown in Chinese hamster ovary cell. Cells grown for two generations in BrdU are heated at 88°C for 10 minutes in 1.0 M NaH2PO4, pH 8.0, rinsed in distilled water and stained with Giemsa. Dark segments TB; light ones; BB. Note multiple exchanges at arrow.

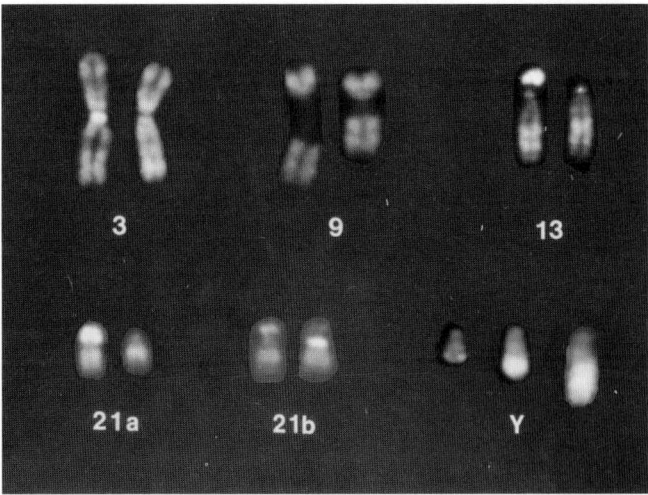

Fig. 9.8. Examples of human chromosome polymorphisms following Q-banding. A homologous pair from the same cell is shown for chromosomes 3, 9, 13, and 21. The Y chromosomes are from three different normal males. Note the extra q-bright band at the centromere of a chromosome 3, the large pericentromeric heterochromatic region on a chromosome 9, large bright satellites on a chromosome 13 and 21(a), and bright short arm on a chromosome 21 (b). The Y chromosomes show variation in the length of the brightly fluorescent heterochromatin in the long arm.

to monitor the effects of potentially mutagenic or carcinogenic agents that enhance the rate of sister chromatid exchanges.

CHROMOSOME POLYMORPHISMS

Heritable variations in human chromosome morphology have been recognized since the beginning of human cytogenetic investigations. As already noted, these normal variations in chromosome morphology are called *chromosome polymorphisms*. With the exception of these variable regions, human chromosomes are largely invariant at the cytogenetic level. However, with the introduction of banding techniques, a larger number of chromosome polymorphisms were revealed. In all cases, these variations were seen in chromosomal regions that are now known to consist largely of highly reiterated DNA. This includes the centromeres and pericentromeric blocks of heterochromatin found in 1q, 9q, 16q, and the long arm of the Y as well as the short arms and chromosomal satellite regions of 13, 14, 15, 21 and 22. The techniques most useful in this regard are Q-banding and C-banding (Figs. 9.8 and 9.5). For example, enlarged quinacrine-bright satellites and an elongated stalk are relatively common on the acrocentric chromosomes. Moreover, the Y chromosome also shows marked variations in the amount of heterochromatin, comprised largely of repetitive DNA sequences, in the distal part of its long arm and consequently, in the overall length of the Y. This can be

shown by any of the general banding techniques or by C-banding but is perhaps most dramatically seen with Q-banding because the polymorphic segment on the distal Y fluoresces brightly (Fig. 9.8).

Chromosome polymorphisms are transmitted unchanged from parent to child in a dominant fashion and are useful markers for genetic studies. For example, before the advent of DNA polymorphisms, chromosome heteromorphisms were used to determine the parental origin of the extra chromosome in trisomy 21 (Down syndrome) or the extra set of chromosomes in triploid conceptuses with 69 chromosomes. A well known example of the use of a chromosome polymorphism in human genetics is that of a variant centromeric region on human chromosome 1, which was used as a marker to establish linkage with the Duffy blood group locus (Donahue et al., 1968). This assignment of Duffy to chromosome I was the first assignment of a human gene to a specific autosome.

In summary, there are striking variations in the amount of the highly repetitive, clustered, simple DNA sequences found in the heteochromatic regions of chromosomes, that manifest as chromosome polymorphisms. With higher resolution molecular cytogenetic techniques, further, more subtle variation may be found along chromosome arms in the normal population. Chromosome polymorphisms are now rarely used as markers in genetic studies; however, an understanding that these are normal heteromorphisms is critical for the interpretation of results in the clinical cytogenetics laboratory.

IN SITU HYBRIDIZATION

Molecular hybridization in situ of labeled, single-stranded DNA probes to denatured (single-stranded) DNA in otherwise standard chromosome spreads is a powerful method for mapping genes and for identifying chromosomal rearrangements. In situ hybridization with radioactive probes labeled with tritiated nucleotides was introduced first but provides low resolution. In situ hybridization results of high resolution are attained with DNA probes that are generated by incorporating nucleotides conjugated to biotin or digoxigenin. Signals may then be detected using avidin or antibodies to digoxigenin that are covalently linked to any one of a number of fluorescent dyes. Alternatively, fluoresceinated nucleotides can be incorporated *directly* into the probe, obviating the need for a secondary detection step. The direct methods for signal production yield less intense signals but higher signal to noise ratios and are therefore of use clinically for tissues that tend to produce higher background. The sites of hybridization are visualized under a fluorescence microscope with suitable filter combinations. The introduction of this fluorescence in situ hybridization (FISH) technique (Pinkel et al., 1986; Lichter et al., 1988;) marked the beginning of the era of molecular cytogenetics.

The availability of highly sensitive CCD (charge coupled device) cameras for capturing FISH images and computer-assisted image analysis has made FISH a routine technique in cytogenetics laboratories for investigational and diagnostic studies. FISH is now one method of choice for determining the chromosomal location of a cloned segment of DNA (Fig. 9.9) and may be integrated with sequence based methods. Mapping by FISH requires precise identification of chromosome band with which can be accomplished by counterstaining the chromosomes a suitable fluorescent dye generating R or G banding pattern (Korenberg et al., 1995). One significant limitation for gene mapping by FISH is the size of the DNA probe. Results are routinely obtained with DNA probes that are at least 2 kb long but can vary up to hundreds of kb.

A DNA probe of known chromosomal location can be used in a FISH assay to detect subtle chromosomal rearrangements involving that locus, which may be undetectable by the analysis of banded chromosomes (Fig. 9.9). It is in this context that the FISH technique is most often employed in clinical cytogenetics laboratories today. As reviewed elsewhere (Chs. 4–6), a number of microdeletion syndromes have now been identified, which can be diagnosed reliably by the use of

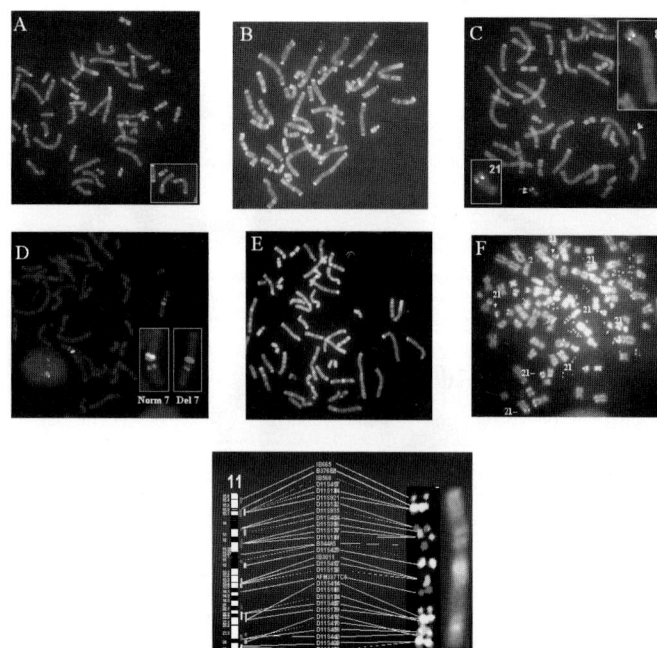

Fig. 9.9. Fluorescence in situ hybridization (see Plate 9.9).

A. Centromeric regions of human chromosomes shown by fluorescence in situ hybridization (FISH) using the DNA from a bacterial artificial chromosome (BAC) containing sequences homologous to all centromeres. Inset shows centromere specific hybridization to single chromosomal array of alpha satellite sequence.

B. Telomeric regions of all human chromosomes shown by fluorescence in situ hybridization using an oligonucleotide probe for the telomere sequence, TTAGGG.

C. A subtle chromosomal rearrangement that translocates the terminal band of chromosome 21 to the short arm of chromosome 8 is shown by two color FISH with two single copy BAC probes containing DNA sequences from chromosome 21. Signals are seen on the normal 21 and the derivative 8.

D. A deletion of chromosome band 7q11.2 in Williams syndrome is shown on one homolog using BAC DNAs containing the gene for elastin (green) and for a flanking duplicated region (pink).

E. Duplications that are below the level of cytogenetic detection are found in the chromosome arms in the normal population using a BAC whose DNA markers nonetheless map it uniquely.

F. Gene amplification of the myc oncogene on dm (double minute) chromosome fragments (green) is shown in a highly aneuploid lymphoma specimen by using FISH with a BAC carrying myc. Chromosome numbers are noted.

G. Molecular cytogenetic analysis of chromosome 11 using 28 BAC DNAs, each linked to a specific STS (sequence tagged site) (Korenberg et al., 1999). Such analyses can now provide visual definition of molecular breakpoints in single cells, in order to define characteristic changes or genes involved in cancer and germline rearrangements. Probes were each labelled directly with one of 5 fluorescent tags and then hybridized simultaneously. (See Plate 9.9C-F.)

FISH using DNA probes from the region that is commonly deleted in these patients (Fig. 9.9D).

The availability of chromosome specific probes for FISH studies has increased dramatically in recent years as a result of the efforts to construct a complete physical map and sequence the entire human genome. Simultaneous hybridization of a library or array of DNA probes from a specific human chromosome or segment results in a continuous signal along the length of that chromosome or region, giving it a "painted" appearance. Such chromosome painting technology is a valuable tool for identification of interchromosomal rearrangements. Recently, techniques have also been developed to label these chromosome specific painting probes with combinations of flurochromes such that each human chromosome will have a characteristic fluorescent tag. Use of a cocktail of such painting probes in a single hybridization reaction followed by computerized image processing generates a rather spectacular image in which each pair of chromosomes in a metaphase appears in a different color (Schrock et al., 1996). This has been facilitated by the definition of large arrays of bacterial artificial chromosomes (BACs) that span the entire human genome and carry known DNA sequences (Korenberg et al., 1999). This new generation of FISH methods for chromosome analysis has provided a direct link between DNA sequence and chromosome landmarks. Each BAC (and consequently its associated DNA sequence) can be labeled with a distinct color and hybridized simultaneously with 24 or more distinct BACs. The pattern of colors then reflects the order of the linked DNA sequences and can be used as a sensitive indicator of the position of chromosomal rearrangements and thereby of the candidate genes involved in the clinical phenotype associated with the chromosomal rearrangement. This multicolor FISH technique has enhanced the precision of diagnostic cytogenetics to new levels.

Molecular cytogenetic studies employing FISH have an additional advantage in that dividing cells are not always necessary for their use. For example, chromosome-specific α-satellite probes hybridize to the corresponding highly repetitive sequences at the centromeric region of particular chromosomes and permit rapid determination of the copy number of that chromosome in large numbers of dividing or interphase nuclei. This approach has been successfully used for the rapid prenatal diagnosis of chromosomal aneuploidies from uncultured amniotic fluids and also for the diagnosis of aneuploidy involving specific chromosomes in neoplastic cells (Fig. 9.9E). FISH has also made invaluable contributions to the analysis of organization of DNA in human chromosomes, thus increasing our understanding of the structure of chromosomes.

Chromosome structure

Although the structure of human and other eukaryotic chromosomes is not understood in complete detail, recent investigations have provided insights into several aspects of chromosome structure at the molecular level. The haploid human genome consists of about 3×10^9 base pairs (bp) of DNA. Since 3000 base pairs of naked DNA are 1 μm long, the total length of the haploid human genome is about 1 meter, whereas the nucleus itself is no more than 10 μm in diameter. It is immediately apparent that all of this DNA needs to be packaged into manageable-sized chromosomes. The DNA of the cell nucleus is packaged in a hierarchic fashion of ever-larger supercoils superimposed on a linear pattern of differential condensation. The first level of this packaging, and thus the fundamental unit of chromosome organization, is a regularly repeating protein-DNA complex called the nucleosome. The basic structural features of the

Table 9.1. Characteristics of chromosome bands

Characteristic	R-bands	Q- or G- bands	C-bands
Location	Chromosome arms	Chromosome arms	Centromeres, distal Y
Type of DNA sequences	Unique, some repetitive	Repetitive, some unique	Highly repetitive satellite
Base composition	GC-rich	AT-rich	AT-rich, some GC-rich
5-methylcytosine content	Moderate	Low	High
Type of chromatin	Euchromatin	Heterochromatin	Heterochromatin
Meiotic (pachytene) morphology	Inter-chromosome	Chromomere	–
Replication	Early S	Mid to late S	Late S
Transcription	High	Low	Absent
Gene density	High	Low	Absent
CpG-rich islands	Many	Few	Absent
Repeats	SINES-rich	LINES-rich	–
Acetylated histones	High	Low	Absent

nucleosome were established in the early 1970s and have been confirmed by recent high-resolution analysis of its crystal structure (Kornberg and Lorch, 1999). The nucleosome has the same design in all eukaryotes and consists of a cylindrical core of about 11 nm in diameter and 6 nm in height made up of two molecules each of the four core histones: H2A, H2B, H3, and H4 with 146 bp of DNA wrapped around it. A "linker" DNA of about 60 bp in length connects adjacent nucleosomes. Each nucleosome is also associated with one molecule of histone H1 that is located in the region of the linker DNA and is thought to play a key role in the coiling of chromatin.

The next higher level of packaging is the chromatin fiber, visible by standard electron microscopy. This is a superhelix, 25 to 30 nm in diameter, composed of nucleosomes and histone H1. The 30 nm fiber is the basic component of interphase chromatin and metaphase chromosomes. Short, AT-rich matrix attachment regions (MARs) occur about every 30 to 150 kb which anchor the DNA to proteins of the nuclear matrix of the interphase nucleus. Topoisomerase II, an enzyme that induces transient double-strand breaks in DNA, and permits uncoiling of the two strands of the DNA duplex is one of the two major matrix proteins. Thus MARs appear to provide not only a site for attachment of chromatin in the interphase nucleus, but also a site for topological changes in DNA. The MARs are also the site for attachment of the chromatin fiber to the non-histone protein scaffold of the metaphase chromosome (hence also referred to scaffold attachment regions or SARs) which also has Topoisomerase II as one of its components (Hart and Laemmli, 1998). The 30-nm chromatin fiber forms a complex with nonhistone proteins and is further organized to produce the condensed metaphase chromosome. The details of this higher order structure are not well understood at the molecular level. However, it is clear that each chromosome contains only a single very long duplex of DNA with an estimated packaging ratio of about 1:10,000 (length of metaphase chromosome: DNA Helix). In prometaphase chromosome complements with about 800 bands per haploid set, the average band contains about four million base pairs (4 mb) of DNA. At the highest level of compaction, the metaphase-anaphase chromosomes are transcriptionally inert, but most easily movable by the spindle apparatus during cell division.

GENOME ORGANIZATION OF CHROMOSOMAL LANDMARKS

Understanding the mechanism(s) of chromosome banding was of particular interest from the outset as it was appreci-ated that banding reflected an underlying organization of chromosomes. In fact, Caspersson and colleagues discovered chromosome banding using quinacrine mustard while experimenting with various DNA-binding fluorescent dyes in order to determine variations in the amount of DNA per nucleus in cancer versus normal cells. The banding pattern immediately established dyes as probes of chromosome structure and DNA composition. Almost contemporaneously, Britten and Kohne (1968) discovered that the human genome contained a large fraction of DNA sequences of variable size each of which was present in more than one copy. It was subsequently found that these were organized as families of repeated sequences ranging from simple sequences of 5–10 bp with millions of copies that were arranged largely in tandem, to sequences of 200–6,000 base pairs with one hundred to one million copies that were interspersed among the remaining largely single copy DNA. The DNA of some of these simple sequence families is of such extreme base composition (A+T versus G+C) that it yields distinct bands, called "satellites" that lie separate from the remaining distribution in density gradient centrifugation. In the ensuing 30 years, specific families of repeated sequences have been shown to correspond to the specific chromosomal landmarks defined previously by staining. Understanding the DNA sequences has led to gradual elucidation of the molecular basis of chromosomal functions. Localization of specific sequences called alpha and beta satellites, to the centromeric region, other simple sequences to the telomeric region, and different families of interspersed repeats to the G-bands, R-bands and T bands (a subset of R bands located at the telomeric regions) have been of particular interest and are discussed below.

CHROMOSOME BANDING REVEALS GENOME SEQUENCE ORGANIZATION

Quinacrine associates directly with DNA by intercalating between base pairs. Although quinacrine binds equally well to DNA of any base composition, its fluorescence is enhanced in regions containing uninterrupted runs of AT base pairs, and is quenched in regions with more frequent GC-base pairs. In the Q-banding pattern of human chromosomes (Fig. 9.1), the intensity of fluorescence is generally proportional to the AT-richness of the DNA (Korenberg and Engels, 1978). However, the highly AT-rich satellite DNA which is concentrated at the C-bands of chromosomes 1, 9, 15, and 16 has interspersed GC base pairs and usually fails to show bright Q-banding. That on the Y, in contrast, has no such GC pairs and is intensely fluorescent. Thus Q-banding is related both to base composition and base interspersion that result in the differential fluorescence or quenching of signals produced by the fluorescent dye. DNA-protein interactions may also be important in the generation of Q-bands.

G-banding is produced most commonly by treatment of chromosomal preparations with the proteolytic enzyme, trypsin. Giemsa stains DNA primarily by intercalating between adjacent base pairs in double-stranded regions. G-bands result from the degradation of chromosomal proteins by trypsin, which modifies the interaction of chromosomal DNA with the Giemsa dyes. Since the fixative used in standard chromosome preparation methods, methanol: acetic acid (3:1), removes some of the histone proteins, it is the degradation of the nonhistone proteins that appears to be critical for the production of G-bands. The DNA-protein interactions at the G-band positive regions apparently render these sites resistant to denaturation by the enzyme.

The commonly used method to generate R-bands is to subject chromosome preparations to moderate heat (~85 C in the presence of high salt) before staining them with Giemsa. The heat pretreatment is thought to selectively denature the more AT-rich DNA sequences which have a lower thermal stability than GC base pairs and to result in altered DNA structure upon renaturation. Therefore, after chromosomes are exposed to moderate heat, Giemsa stains the unaffected GC-rich double-stranded DNA regions producing R-banding. R-bands can also be produced by the replication banding technique, which demonstrates that R-band positive regions contain early replicating DNA. It also follows that G-band and Q-band positive regions contain AT-rich DNA that replicates relatively late in the cell cycle (Korenberg and Engels, 1978).

Fluorescence in situ hybridization (FISH) studies have shown that the G-band and R-band regions differ in the type of interspersed repeated DNA sequences located in them (Korenberg and Rykowski, 1988). Interspersed repeated sequences are classified as SINES (short interspersed repeated sequences) or LINES (long interspersed repeated sequences). The major human SINE is the Alu DNA sequence family, which has a consensus sequence of about 300 bp and present in about 1,000,000 copies accounting for an estimated 7–8% of the human genome. The major human LINE sequence family is L1 or Kpn1 which has a consensus sequence of about 6 kb and is present in about 100,000 copies accounting for an estimated 7–8% of the human genome. A majority of the LINE elements have variable truncations of the consensus 5′ end. FISH analysis using Alu and L1 DNA as probes demonstrated that G-band regions are rich in LINEs whereas R-band regions are dominated by SINEs (Korenberg and

Rykowski, 1988). A comparison of the characteristics of Q/G, R and C bands is presented in Table 9.1.

The DNA structure of C bands has also been found by in situ hybridization and DNA sequencing to consist of alpha satellite (discussed below) sequences at the centromeres of human chromosomes and of different families of simple sequence satellite DNAs at the large peri-centromeric blocks of chromosomes 1, 9, 16 and distal Yq. Recent in silico studies (Smit, 1996) have defined further families of repetitive DNA based on large scale sequence but these have not yet been associated with functional or structural landmarks of chromosomes. In contrast, recent studies employing in situ hybridization have revealed that the human genome also includes highly homologous duplications of DNA in the range of hundreds of kb that are located both in the peri-centromeric regions and in the chromosome arms. Although some of these are known to predispose to genomic deletions and duplications, their significance for chromosome function is otherwise unknown.

Also related to simple sequences are chromosomal regions called fragile sites that remain stretched at metaphase after various treatments that limit DNA replication (Sutherland et al., 1998). Fragile sites are classified as rare (inherited) or common (constitutional) and are further subdivided according to the conditions under which they are induced, for example, folate or amphidicolin sensitive. Several fragile sites have now been cloned and sequenced. These studies have shown that the expression of rare, inherited fragile sites is associated with repeat expansions (Sutherland et al., 1998). The first folate sensitive rare fragile site to be characterized was the one associated with the Fragile X syndrome (FMR1) which was shown to result from the expansion and methylation of a CGG trinucleotide repeat. Other folate sensitive fragile sites also result from expansion of trinucleotide repeats. A distamycin sensitive rare fragile site on chromosome 16 has been shown to involve the expansion of a 33 bp AT-rich minisatellite (Sutherland et al., 1998). In contrast, sequencing of constitutional fragile sites has not revealed any characteristic DNA sequences at these sites (Krummel et al., 2000).

FUNCTIONAL ORGANIZATION OF CHROMOSOMES

Chromatin is classified into euchromatin and heterochromatin. Euchromatin consists of active genes; however, not all genes in euchromatic regions are active at any given time. Therefore, location in euchromatin is currently thought to be necessary but not sufficient for gene activity. Euchromatin is dispersed in the interphase nucleus and replicates its DNA early in the S phase of the cell cycle. Heterochromatin consists predominantly of inactive genetic material, replicates its DNA late in the S phase, and is condensed in the interphase nucleus. Heterochromatin is further classified into constitutive heterochromatin and facultative heterochromatin. Constitutive heterochromatin consists of highly repetitious simple sequence DNA, remains transcriptionally inactive, and is located at specific regions of the chromosomes such as the centromere and the distal long arm of the human Y chromosome. Facultative heterochromatin also remains condensed in the interphase nucleus, replicates its DNA late in the S phase and is largely transcriptionally inactive. However, it is not inactive permanently, does not consist exclusively of repetitious DNA, and can become transcriptionally active. The inactive X chromosome in the human female is a good example of facultative heterochromatin. However, location in facultative heterochromatin does not exclude transcription altogether, as several genes on the inactive X chromosome are expressed (see below).

As already noted, the R-band positive regions of human chromosomes have characteristics of euchromatin in that they replicate their DNA in early S and have high transcriptional activity due in part to high gene density (Table 9.1). The G-band positive regions, on the other hand, are more heterochromatic as they replicate their DNA in late S and are low in transcriptional activity associated with low gene density. Confirmation of the relative paucity of genes in G bands has come from the recent complete genomic sequence of chromosome 21 which revealed less than 10% of genes located in the G band, q21 and more than 90% of genes located in the similarly sized R band, q22 (Hattori et al., 2000). The C-band positive regions consist of constitutive heterochromatin with no known functional genes. The facultative heterochromatin of the inactive X chromosome replicates its DNA in late S phase (Fig. 9.4), and forms the condensed Barr body in the interphase nucleus. Consequently, there is a general relationship of functional properties (time of replication during the S phase and transcriptional status or gene density) with chromosome band classes characterized by differential condensation and staining characteristics (Holmquist, 1992). However, the features that are correlated with chromosome band classes also include some of the basic characteristics of chromosomal cellular biology, in that G bands condense earlier during mitotic prophase and during meiotic prophase, also forming the more condensed regions called chromomeres that appear during pachnema, the time of crossing over. Combining these basic attributes of chromosome mechanics with new data on genomic DNA sequence may help to elucidate the mechanisms underlying the functional properties.

Recent investigations have provided insights into the molecular organization of two specialized structures on chromosomes, the centromere and the telomere, which are of particular interest and are summarized below.

THE CENTROMERE

As already noted, each chromosome has a primary constriction, the centromere where the sister chromatids of a replicated chromosome are held together until the anaphase stage of cell division. A sub-domain of the centromere is the kinetochore, a protein-DNA complex that serves as the attachment site for the spindle fibers essential for chromosome movement and segregation during mitosis and meiosis. The structure of the centromere has been a focus of molecular cytogenetic investigations in recent years. The best characterized eukaryotic centromere is that of the budding yeast, *Saccharomyces cerevisiae*. In this organism, a short sequence of about 125 bp specifies the centromere of each of the chromosomes. The nucleotide sequence and organization of this centromere DNA is conserved among the different chromosomes in the budding yeast. The search for a similar specific sequence in the larger and more complex centromeres of higher eukaryotes has not been successful. Rather, the centromeres in these organisms consist of large arrays of repeated DNA sequences. In human centromeres the arrays consist of tandem, head-to-tail repeats of a 171-bp monomer that is further organized into higher order repeats (Willard, 1998). The array size of this α-satellite repeat ranges in size from 300 kb to 9000 kb on human chromosomes with the average being 2000–4000 kb. The sequence of the basic 171-bp unit is sufficiently divergent among human chromosomes, so that with very few exceptions, centromere specific α-satellite DNA probes can generate fluorescent signals on specific chromosomes in a FISH assay (Fig. 9.9A). This is useful from a practical standpoint for identifying and determining the copy number for specific human chromosomes in cells.

Several lines of evidence implicate a critical role for α-satellite DNA in centromere function. Although there are other repeated sequences in the centromeric heterochromatin, α-satellite is the only one localized to the centromeres of all normal human chromosomes. Moreover, recent studies have shown that human artificial chromosome constructs containing α-satellite DNA are able to form functional centromeres (Grimes and Cooke, 1998). However, independent evidence from rearranged chromosomes suggests that the presence of α-satellite DNA alone is not sufficient for the formation of an active centromere.

Many cases of rearranged human chromosomes containing two centromeric regions have been identified. A true dicentric chromosome with two primary constrictions would be unstable during cell division as spindle fiber attachment occurs independently at the two centromeres, if these are sufficiently far apart. The two centromeres on a single chromatid (daughter chromosome) could then be pulled toward opposite poles of the spindle, breaking the chromosome. However, many dicentric chromosomes with two blocks of alpha satellite DNA and C-band regions are stable and show only one primary constriction indicating that only one of the two centromeres is active. Such stable dicentric chromosomes, referred to as pseudodicentrics, indicate that the presence of α-satellite DNA alone is not sufficient for the formation of an active centromere. They also suggest that specification of a centromere is at least in part *epigenetic*, a heritable change not dependent on the nucleotide sequence alone. In addition, several human marker chromosomes have been characterized that originate from normal human chromosomes but lack α-satellite DNA sequences (Choo, 1997). As these chromosomes are mitotically stable, presence of α-satellite DNA is not an absolute requirement for functional centromeres. Thus, although normal human centromeres are composed of α-satellite DNA, it appears to be neither necessary nor sufficient for centromere formation.

Recent investigations have identified several proteins associated with centromeres that have contributed to our understanding of centromere structure and function (Craig et al., 1999). A group of these proteins are constitutively associated with centromeres while others are associated with centromeres only during part of the cell cycle and are involved in chromosome movement during division. The centromere specific proteins were initially identified as autoantigens in patients with certain autoimmune diseases, such as the CREST form of scleroderma. The major constitutive centromere proteins identified by this strategy are CENP-A, CENP-B, and CENP-C. The location of these proteins at centromeres has been determined by immunofluorescence microscopy using antibodies specific for these proteins. CENP-A is a 17-kD histone H3-like protein, which may participate in producing centromere-specific nucleosomes and altered chromatin structure. CENP-A is detected at all *functional* centromeres, including the neocentromeres lacking α-satellite DNA present on marker chromosomes. CENP-B is an 80-kD protein that binds to a specific 17-bp sequence, the CENP-B box, in α-satellite DNA and is found, as expected, even at the inactive centromere of pseudodicentric chromosomes. CENP-C, a 140-kD protein, is also found at active centromeres, where it is located in the proteinaceous kinetochore. CENP-C shares homology with a domain of the Mif2 protein of yeast that is essential for normal chromosome segregation. CENP-E is a 275-kD kinesin-related protein that is associated with centromeres and mitotic spindle and is thought to be involved in chromosome movement. Localization of these proteins by immunofluorescence has been employed as a strategy to localize and characterize the active centromeres on structurally abnormal chromosomes.

Analysis of centromere-associated DNAs in other organisms with complex centromeres, such as *Schizosaccharomyces pombe*, *Drosophila* and mice, has shown that they are also composed of repeats of monomer subunits and are relatively A-T rich as the human α-satellite DNA. However, the nucleotide sequences of these centromere-specific DNAs are not homologous. These observations have lead to the suggestion that the centromere may be specified by an epigenetic mechanism (Murphy and Karpen, 1998). The molecular basis of this epigenetic mechanism is unknown. It has been suggested that some sequences may be favored as sites for the assembly of centromeres because of their repetitive nature, the chromatin structure, their replication timing and/or affinity for centromere-specific proteins (Willard, 1998). It may be that the location of the a-satellite DNA is simply the more favorable site for the assembly of the centromere. The suppression of activity of the second centromere on a dicentric chromosome suggests that a developmental mechanism analogous to X-inactivation may exist for centromeres, such that there is a single active centromere per chromosome. The molecular basis of this exclusion is unknown.

THE TELOMERE

Telomeres are special DNA-protein structures that are present at the ends of linear chromosomes and prevent fusion of chromosome ends and maintain chromosome integrity. The concept of the telomere was developed from early genetic and cytological observations that the broken ends of chromosomes are unstable and often fuse with other broken ends. Molecular techniques have now shown that telomeres in eukaryotes consist of tandem repeats of a simple sequence and an unknown number of proteins. In humans and other vertebrates, the sequence of the basic repeat is 5′-TTAGGG-3′ on one strand of the DNA and 5′-CCCTAA-3′ on the complementary strand. The G-rich strand runs 5′–3′ towards the end of the chromosome, with a short single-stranded G-rich overhang (Blackburn, 1991). The length of the telomeric sequence averages about 15,000 to 20,000 bp on human chromosomes and is replicated by its own polymerase, called telomerase. In the absence of telomerase, each round of DNA replication leaves 50–200 bp of DNA unreplicated at the 3′ end as the DNA replication machinery works only in the 5′ to 3′ direction and requires an RNA primer. Telomerase has a short RNA molecule as a component, which provides the template for synthesizing the G-rich repeating sequence. Telomere-associated proteins regulate telomerase activity and maintain the length of telomeres (Blasco et al., 1999). Telomerase is present in early embryonic cells and cancer cells, but not in most somatic cells. As a result, somatic cells, but not cancer cells, lose telomeric sequences with each division. This is considered to be one factor contributing to the finite life span of most somatic cells and indefinite growth potential of cancer cells.

Telomere sequence oligonucleotides can be used as probes in FISH assays to produce signals at the telomeric regions of human chromosomes (Fig. 9.9B). This technique is useful for determining the presence or absence and position of telomeres on structurally abnormal human chromosomes. Recent studies have also shown that telomere sequences can be added to certain deleted chromosomes, thus stabilizing these broken ends (Flint et al., 1994). The DNA sequences at these broken sites are thought to permit the addition of telomere sequences by telomerase to "heal" these broken ends.

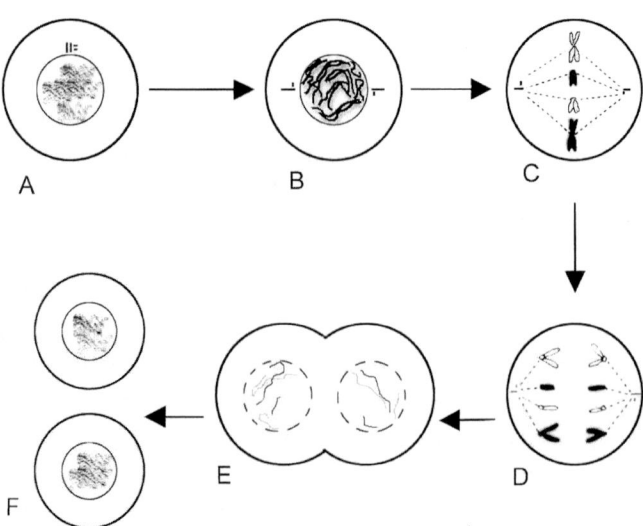

Fig. 9.10. Diagramatic representation of mitosis showing only two pairs of hemologous chromosomes. Note that at the end of mitosis, the two daughter cells have identical chromosome complements. The major events in mitosis. (A) G2 interphase. (B) Prophase. (C) Metaphase. (D) Anaphase. (E) Telophase. (F) G1 interphase.

Chromosomes in cell division

Cell division and proliferation are central to growth and development of multicellular organisms. The major events in the cell cycle are replication and segregation of chromosomes. Cell division also ensures proper segregation and partitioning of the genetic material into daughter cell, thus providing the basis for Mendelian laws of inheritance. Further, abnormalities in chromosome disjunctio during cell division leads to changes of chromosome number in the daughter cells. Finally, abnormalities of chromosome transactions during cell division are the cause of many structural chromosome changes. The cytological aspects of mitosis and meiosis, the two forms of cell division in eukaryotes have been described in great detail in numerous studies in the past. However, the explosive growth of molecular biology in the last twenty years has brought the study of mitosis and meiosis to the forefront again, as the new methodologies provide characterization of the mechanisms of cell division at the molecular level. These investigations have elucidated biochemical aspects of cell cycle biology and chromosome mechanics, which are discussed in recent reviews (Nurse, 2000). This section describes the essential features of mitosis and meiosis relevant to inheritance. Knowledge of these features is crucial for understanding the Mendelian laws of inheritance, construction of genetic maps, and the origin of chromosomal aberrations.

MITOSIS

In somatic cells, and in cells of the germline prior to the time they undergo their first specialized meiotic divisions, nuclear division takes place by a process called mitosis. In mitosis, the duplicated chromosomes of a single cell are separated by an equational division to produce two daughter cells with identical chromosome constitutions. The salient features of mitosis are summarized in Figure 9.10. In cells with a generation time of 18 to 24 hours, mitosis takes about one hour and is divided into four major stages: prophase, metaphase, anaphase, and telophase.

In the initial phase of mitosis, prophase the chromosomes become visible as a result of condensation that continues throughout prophase. Each chromosome has already undergone replication during the preceding interphase, generating two sister chromatids that will become daughter chromosomes. The sister chromatids are closely held together along their length until anaphase separations. The nucleoli, which are present throughout interphase, regress as a result of the shutoff of ribosomal RNA synthesis and processing. The centrioles, duplicate during the S-phase occupy positions at opposite ends of the cell move apart and defining the poles of the mitotic spindle.

Metaphase is initiated with the dissolution of the nuclear membrane. The chromosomes continue their condensation but still fairly long in early metaphase (promctaphase). The chromosomes become attached to microtubules of the spindle at their centromeres and undergo movements that lead to their alignment in the equatorial plane of the spindle. At this stage, the chromosomes have reached their maximum state of condensation.

Anaphase begins after the chromosomes are fully aligned on the metaphase plate. Each pair of sister chromatids separates as cohesion is last, first along the arms and finally at the centromere of each chromosome. The resultant daughter chromosomes move toward opposite poles of the spindle as a result of microtubule dynamics and the action of motor proteins. Recent investigations in lower eukaryotes have identified several proteins involved in the cohesion of the sister chromatids through metaphase to ensure correct segregation of daughter chromosomes at anaphase (Hirano et al., 2000).

At telophase, each set of daughter chromosomes arrives at the centriole at the ends of the mitotic spindle. Reconstitution of the nuclear membrane begins, and ribosomal RNA (rRNA) synthesis is initiated. Cytokinesis, the division of the cytoplasm, follows telophase and leads to the formation of two genetically identical daughter cells.

MEIOSIS

Meiosis is a specialized cell division in germ cells that generates gametes with the haploid set of 23 chromosomes. The final gametic set includes single representatives of each of the 23 chromosomes pairs that is selected at random. The details of meiosis and gamete formation are somewhat different in males and females, but the basic features are the same in both and are of fundamental importance. Meiosis accounts for the major principles of Mendelian genetics: segregation, independent assortment, and recombination of linked genes. Recombination or crossing over, is the exchange of genetic material between homologous non-sister chromatids, a process that adds to genetic diversity by generating new combinations of genes.

Meiosis consists of two cell divisions (Meiosis I and II) and is distinguished from mitosis by the following:

1. *Homologous pairing.* Maternal and paternal homologues of each chromosome are replicated and then undergo exact pairing along their lengths during prophase of

Meiosis I. Such a paired unit is called a bivalent because there are only two centromeres, although it is composed of four chromatids. When pairing of homologues fails, each of the resulting pairs of sister chromatids (a single homologue) is called a univalent. The pairing of homologous chromosomes is mediated by the formation of a special protein-rich tripartite pairing structure, the synaptonemal complex (SC), which has a central element flanked by two lateral elements. The lateral elements and the central element are held together by transverse filaments. Initially the synaptonemal complex was characterized by ultrastructural analysis. More recent studies have characterized three of the protein components of the mammalian synaptonemal complex, *SCP1*, *SCP2* and *SCP3*. *SCP1* is a component of the transverse filaments. *SCP2* and *SCP3* are components of the lateral elements and play important roles in chromosome synapsis (Yuan et al., 2000).

2. *Recombination (crossing over).* Crossing over occurs at the four-strand stage between any two of the four chromatids of a bivalent. However, it results in recombination of flanking markers only when the two chromatids involved are derived from different members of the homologous pair. Because this means that only one half of the cross over events can be detected genetically, this explains why the maximum recombination frequency between any two markers is only 50%. The probability of recombination increases with the physical distance between two chromosomal sites and therefore provides a basis of the genetic map.

3. *Segregation of maternal and paternal homologues.* Centromeres do not divide at the first meiotic division (MI). Instead, the members of a homologous pair go to opposite poles at anaphase of the first meiotic division. This accounts for Mendel's first law, the segregation of homologous genetic units. The segregation of maternal and paternal homologues in each bivalent chromosome pair occurs independently of the segregation in all the other bivalents. That is, the segregation of chromosome 1 homologues is independent of that of chromosome 2 homologues and so on. This accounts for Mendel's second law of independent assortment of genes. Meiosis I also leads to a reduction in the number of chromosomes from the diploid number, 2n = 46, to the haploid number, n = 23 in the gametes.

4. *Mitosis of the haploid set with centromere division.* The second meiotic division, MII, occurs without a preceding round of DNA synthesis and chromosome duplication. In Meiosis II, the two chromatids of a chromosome move to opposite daughter cells.

Meiotic prophase is rather prolonged and can be subdivided into five stages on the basis of condensation of chromosomes and the extent of homologous pairing: leptonema, zygonema, pachynema, diplonema, and diakinesis. In leptonema, the chromosomes are seen as long threads and the homologues are not paired. Chromosomal condensation continues and pairing of homologues (synapsis) begins at zygonema and is completed at pachynema, the stage at which recombination occurs (Fig. 9.11). The synaptonemal complex is fully formed at this stage, and there are recombination nodules at intervals along its length. These are thought to be enzyme complexes that mediate genetic recombination via DNA breakage and repair. Chiasmata or cruciform structures become visible at the more condensed diplonema stage as cohesion is lost along the chromosome arms except at each chiasma, the point of interchange of genetic material between homologous chromosomes.

Chiasmata are still visible at diakinesis, the stage of maximal condensation, can be used to determine the frequency as well as location of recombination. Chiasmata, like their underlying recombination events, play an important role in the normal segregation (disjunction) of homologues and each pair of homologues has at least one chiasma. Moreover, failure of chiasma formation predisposes to nondisjunction of homologues as the two univalents can move to the poles independently and may go to the same pole. The X and Y chromosomes pair at their distal short arms, but even in this small region, there appears to be obligate crossing over between X and Y in every meiosis (see below).

The MII division resembles an ordinary mitotic division, except for the presence of a single set of 23 duplicated chromosomes, each with two chromatids held together at their centromeres as well as along their lengths. Also, MII is not strictly a genetically equational division as the two chromatids of a chromosome may not be identical as a result of genetic exchange(s) with a non-sister chromatid. At the end of the two meiotic divisions, each primary oocyte or spermatocyte has given rise to four haploid products (Fig. 9.11E). Their fate is rather different in males and females as discussed below.

Much remains to be learned about the molecular details of mitosis and meiosis. The genes involved in mitosis and meiosis are just beginning to be identified and characterized. Recent studies have illustrated the role of DNA mismatch repair genes in meiosis. Mutations in one of these genes, *MLH1*, occur in families with hereditary non-polyposis colon cancer. Mice deficient in *Mlh1*, generated from targeted disruption of this gene, are infertile in addition to exhibiting microsatellite instability (Baker et al., 1996). Spermatocytes of these mice show high levels of prematurely separated chromosomes and arrest in the first division of meiosis. In addition, immunolocalization experiments appear to place *Mlh1* protein at sites of crossing over on meiotic chromosomes suggesting that *Mlh1* is involved in

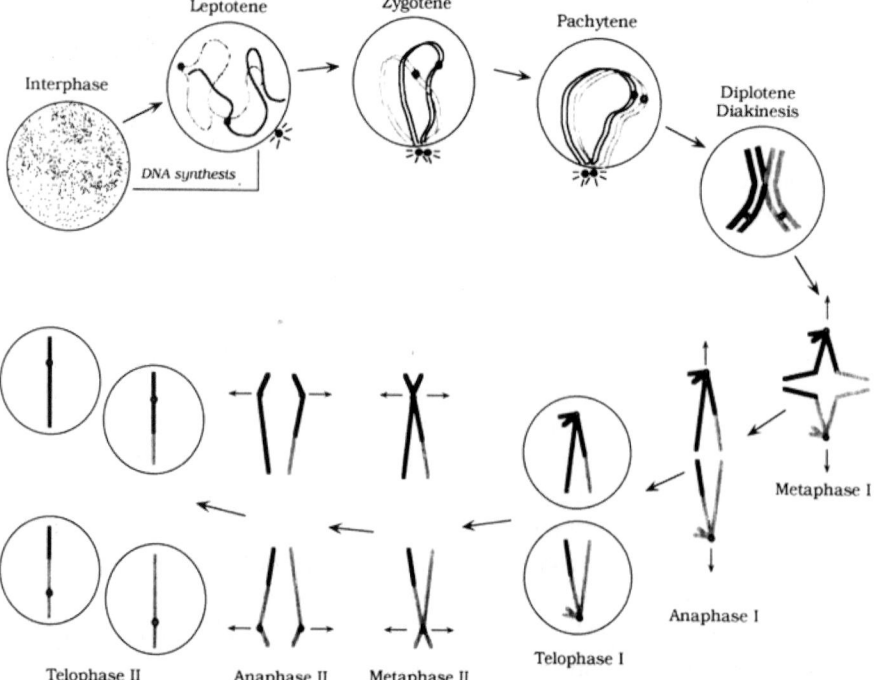

Fig. 9.11. Diagramatic representation of meiosis showing one pair of homologous chromosomes that form a single chiasma. In each homologous pair, the light chromosome was inherited from one parent and the dark chromosome from the other. Note that crossing over occurs at the four strand stage during parenchyma and this results in the exchange of genetic material betwen homologs. Note also that at the end of meiosis I, in telophase I, only one member of each homologous pair is segregated to a given daughter cell, thereby reducing the number of chromosomes per cell to the haploid level. The meiosis II, at telophase II, after the sister chromatids separate, the products are not likely to be genetically identical due to previous crossing over.

chiasma formation and stabilization of bivalents. Similarly, mice deficient in the Atm gene, the mouse homologue of human *ATM* gene responsible for ataxia telangiectasia, are also sterile (Xu et al., 1996). Analysis of meiotic chromosomes in the spenmatocytes of these mice show abnormal synapsis and chromosome fragmentation. The product of the Atm gene, which plays a role in DNA repair, also localizes to the paired axes of meiotic chromosomes. In summary, abnormalities of genes and processes associated with meiosis are also responsible for both germline and acquired genetic disease.

SPERMATOGENESIS AND OOGENESIS

In the human male, the production of sperm begins at puberty and continues throughout life. Undifferentiated stem cells of the germ line, the spermatogonia, are abundant in the seminiferous tubules of the testis and show a high rate of mitotic activity throughout the adult life of a normal male. Of the two types of spermatogonia, only type A can differentiate into primary spermatocytes that then enter meiosis, whereas type B are the long-lived progenitors and can divide to generate daughter cells of both types A and B. In meiosis, each diploid spermatocyte gives rise to four haploid cells, each of which differentiates into a functional sperm. The entire process, from spermatogonium to sperm, takes about 70 days. The rate of sperm production may be as high as 50 to 100 million per day over many years and thus the parental spermatogonia undergo many successive mitoses. It is estimated that the number of mitoses before sperm production in a 20-year old male is about 200, while in a 45-year old it is about 800 (Crow, 1997). This provides the opportunity for the occurrence of more adverse genetic change with age in males, which is reflected in an increased mutation rate for certain inherited diseases. The phenomenon emphasizes the origin of genetic disease risk in the developmental and structural features of human chromosomes.

The behavior of germline cells in the female is quite different from that in the male. By about the fourth month of prenatal development, about 7 million oogonia have begun to develop into primary oocytes and to enter meiosis. Of the approximately one million remaining at birth, only about 400 are ovulated as eggs. Primary oocytes proceed only as far as prophase of the first meiotic division by the time of birth, where they remain until ovulation. This suspended stage of prophase occurs after pachynema, is referred to as dictyonema, and lasts from birth until after puberty, when small cohorts of the germ cells progress further into meiosis. The first meiotic division is stimulated by ovulation and is an unequal division in that most of the cytoplasm remains in the ovum and very little is pinched off to enter the first polar body containing one set of homologues. The mitotic apparatus remains close to the plasma membrane and sperm penetration of the ovum stimulates the second meiotic division, leading to formation of the second polar body that contains a haploid set of chromosomes. It is estimated that the number of divisions from a zygote to an egg is about 30 in the female.

It is of interest to note that the frequency of point mutations and structural chromosomal changes are in general higher in male gametes and increases with age. In contrast, changes of chromosome number in female gametes and also increase with age. This increased mutation rate in males is attributed mainly to the much larger number of cell divisions in the male germ line. In contrast, errors of disjunction seen with maternal age appear to be related to the 13–50 years the occytes spend in prophase before chromosome segregation. Recent genetic mapping studies indicate that the number as well as the positioning of cross over events influence meiotic segregation of chromosomes (Hassold and Sherman, 2000). However, it is not known why these patterns of recombination are associated with normal chromosome segregation in younger women but less so after age 35–40 years when fertility decreases with the approaching menopause. Moreover, the molecular causes underlying non-disjunction are still not understood and solving this mystery may result in novel approaches to prevent aneuploidy both in the germline and soma.

Sex chromosomes and sex determination

Sex chromosomes of the human chromosome complement are of special interest, as they determine sex of the human embryo. Also, the sex chromosome pair, the X and Y, is heteromorphic (different in size and morphology) in humans. The Y chromosome is significantly smaller than the X chromosome and contains a large block of heterochromatin on its long arm comprised of non-coding repetitious DNA. This leaves only a short segment of chromosome capable of carrying functional genes. The finding of heteromorphic sex chromosomes in humans, an XX pair in females and an XY pair in males, suggested a chromosomal basis for sex determination in the early twentieth century. However, the dominant role of Y chromosome in male sex determination became evident only in 1959 when cytogenetic studies showed that individuals with a complete set of autosomes and a single X chromosomes developed as females whereas individuals with two X chromosomes and a Y chromosome developed as males (Ford et al., 1959; Jacobs and Strong, 1959). We now know that individuals with as many as 4 X chromosomes and a Y also develop as males. The number of X chromosomes or its ratio to the number of autosomes is not important for human male sex determination. The Y chromosome, thus, carries a dominant determinant for testis development.

Unlike autosomal pairs of chromosomes, the heteromorphic X and Y are not completely homologous. There are two regions of complete homology between the X and Y that reside at the distal ends of their short and long arms covering approximately 2600 and 320 kb of DNA respectively (Rappold et al., 1993). Other regions of X and Y show discontinuous or partial homology reflecting the joined evolutionary history of these chromosomes. The X and Y chromosomes pair during meiosis at the distal ends of their short arms. There is also obligatory crossing over, usually a single one, in this region of pairing which is probably essential for correct segregation of the sex chromosomes. As a result of this crossing over, female offspring of males can inherit DNA sequences from the Y chromosome distal to the point of exchange and vice versa. Thus genetic markers in this region of pairing and exchange between the X and Y segregate independently of sexual phenotype and hence this region is called the pseudoautosomal region.

THE Y CHROMOSOME AND SEX DETERMINATION

Identification of the testis-determining factor (TDF) on the human Y chromosome has been of much interest since the role of the Y in male sex determination was established. Early cytogenetic investigations in individuals with structurally abnormal Y chromosomes showed that the TDF resided on the short arm of Y. The isolation and molecular characterization of this gene was made possible by studies of a naturally occurring sex-reversed condition, the XX male. Cytogenetic and molecular investigations of XX males showed that the majority of them resulted from an unequal exchange between the X and Y, such that the TDF is transferred from the Y to the X chromosome. By identifying the minimal region of Y necessary for male determination from independent XX males, and searching this region for candidate genes, the *SRY* (sex determining region on Y) gene was identified. Later studies confirmed that *SRY* is the long sought TDF (Goodfellow and Lovell-Badge, 1993). *SRY* resides just proximal to the pseudoautosomal region on the Y. *SRY* encodes a protein with a DNA-binding motif consisting of a 79-amino acid high-mobility-group domain,

called the HMG box. This domain of *SRY* is fairly highly conserved among mammals, but the remainder of the *SRY* gene shows rapid evolutionary change, leading to amino acid substitutions and large changes in the size of the gene product. The molecular details of how *SRY* directs the embryonic gonad to the testicular pathway are still under investigation. Recent molecular dissection of other conditions that result in sex reversal has allowed the identification of some of the other genes involved in the sex-determining pathway (Roberts et al., 1999; Swain and Lovell-Badge, 1999). Not surprisingly, many of these are autosomal and not sex-linked genes.

THE X CHROMOSOME

The heteromorphic nature of the sex chromosome pair in humans immediately raises the question of dosage difference for X-linked genes in the human male and female. The answer to this question was provided by observations on the behavior of the two X chromosomes and the expression patterns of X-linked genes in human and other mammalian females. These findings indicated that there were differences in the functional organization of the two X chromosomes in mammalian females. Early cytological studies demonstrated that a sex chromatin body (now called the Barr body) was present in female interphase cells, but not in male cells. Moreover, the amount of certain X-linked gene products, such as the enzyme glucose-6-phosphate dehydrogenase (G6PD), was no different in individuals with one, two or even more X chromosomes. Also, studies on the timing of DNA replication in diploid cells indicated that the DNA in one X chromosome replicated in synchrony with the DNA of the autosomes, while that of any additional X chromosomes replicated late in the synthetic phase. Thus, the number of Barr bodies equals the number of late replicating X chromosomes.

Based on the observation that female mice heterozygous for X-linked genes show mosaicism for the expression of these genes, Lyon in 1961 proposed the single active X hypothesis (Lyon, 1993), which offers an explanation for the gender specific behavior of the X chromosome and X-linked genes. According to this hypothesis, commonly referred to as the Lyon hypothesis, the somatic cells of all mammals undergo a process of chromosome differentiation early in embryogenesis that leaves a single active X chromosome per cell. All additional X chromosomes are inactivated by a process that renders them heterochromatic and capable of forming a Barr body. Thus, diploid somatic cells of individuals with three X chromosomes have two Barr bodies, while those of individuals with four X chromosomes have three Barr bodies. The initial choice for inactivation of an X is random in a normal female. However, this differentiation is fixed, so that all the descendants of a cell in which the maternal X was inactivated initially will have the maternal X in the inactive state, while the descendants of a cell in which the paternal X was inactivated will have that X in the inactive state. Every XX individual is thus a genetic mosaic consisting of cells in which the maternal X is active and cells in which the paternal X is active

Proof of the single active X hypothesis has come from various studies. One of these is single cell cloning of cells from skin biopsies of females heterozygous for *G6PD* A and B electrophoretic variants, which serve as markers for the two X chromosomes in these individuals. Each colony of cells derived from a single somatic cell contains either the *G6PD A* variant or the *G6PD B* variant, but not both. The single active X hypothesis readily explains chromosome behavior and dosage compensation for X-linked gene products in males and females.

The phenomenon of X-chromosome inactivation has been a subject of much interest and investigation in mammalian biology. This interest in X-inactivation derives from the fact that it is a relatively unique epigenetic process of gene regulation at the level of the chromosome. It is epigenetic, because the inactivated X chromosome does not undergo any permanent changes in its DNA sequence and can be reactivated, as it does in female germ cells. Genes from the inactive X chromosome can also be reactivated experimentally in cultured cells (Mohandas et al., 1981). Further, attention has been focused on X-inactivation as means of understanding broader aspects of chromatin, specifically the structure and function of facultative heterochromatin. Finally, the burden of human X-linked diseases and X-chromosome abnormalities has generated an interest in X-inactivation for a better understanding of the pathogenesis and ultimately the treatment of these conditions.

Investigations in the last two decades have provided some insights into the molecular mechanism of X chromosome inactivation. It is now clear that X is maintained in the inactive state by DNA methylation. Studies of several genes have shown that cytosine residues in their 5′ promoter regions are methylated when they reside on an inactive X, and unmethylated on an active X (Riggs and Pfeifer, 1992). Methylated DNA interacts with chromosomal proteins differently compared to unmethylated DNA and such protein-DNA interactions could account for the transcriptional silencing of genes on the inactivated X. The nature of these interactions remains to be fully elucidated. Recent studies employing immunofluorescent labeling of human metaphase chromosomes with antibodies specific for acety-

lated isoforms of nucleosome core histones (H2A, H3, H3 and H4) have shown that the inactive X chromosome is hypoacetylated linking methylation and histone acetylation in control of gene expression from the inactive X (Jeppesen and Tumer, 1994; Keohane et al., 1998). Examination of histone H4 acetylation status at the individual gene level has also shown hypoacetylation in the promoter regions of X-inactivated genes (Gilbert and Sharp, 1999). Immunofluorescence microscopy indicates that underacetylation of histone H4, which has been studied most widely, appears to be a general feature of heterochromatin.

Initiation of X-inactivation, which must also include counting the number of X's in a cell and its spreading along the X, is still not completely understood. An exciting finding in this regard has been that of the *XIST* (X inactive specific transcript) gene which is expressed exclusively from the inactive X and not from the active X (Brown et al., 1991). *XIST* is expressed only as an RNA molecule and is a highly useful cellular marker for the presence of an inactive X. *XIST* is located in the proximal long arm of the human X chromosome in a region called the X-inactivation center, which is invariably present on all X chromosomes that undergo inactivation including those with structural rearrangements. Recent transgenic experiments indicate that *XIST* is necessary and sufficient for initiation of X-inactivation. However, molecular details of how *XIST* mediates X-inactivation are still under investigation (Lee and Jaenisch, 1997; Brockdorff, 1998). Recently, it has been suggested that spreading of inactivation along the X may be mediated by long interspersed sequences (LINE-1 elements or L1) based on the finding that the X chromosome is enriched about two-fold for L1 repetitive elements (Bailey et al., 2000; Lyon, 2000). Enrichment of the human X for L1 elements was also noted in the earlier FISH studies using L1 as the probe (Korenberg and Rykowski, 1988). It is also of interest that the paired X and Y chromosomes in the spermatocytes form a condensed body referred to as the sex vesicle, which resembles the Barr body. This observation has led to the suggestion that the X may be inactivated in spermatocytes. Consistent with this suggestion, recent molecular studies have shown XIST expression, a hallmark of an inactive X, in mouse spermatocytes (Richler et al., 1992; Salido et al., 1992).

It is now well established that not all genes on the X chromosome are subject to X-inactivation. Early studies established that the genes for the XG blood group and for the enzyme steroid sulfatase (deficiency of which causes X-linked ichthyosis) escape X-inactivation (Race and Sanger 1975; Shapiro et al., 1979). More recent studies evaluating a large number of known genes as well as anonymous expressed sequences from the X chromosome estimate that as many as 20% of X-linked genes may escape X-inactivation (Carrel et al., 1999). A majority of these genes that escape inactivation is located on the short arm of the X chromosome; but they are also present on the long arm and are interspersed with genes that undergo inactivation. As expected, the genes in the pseudoautosomal region escape X-inactivation; these have homologues on the Y chromosome and dosage compensation is not a requirement for these genes. However, there are genes on the X that escape X-inactivation for which there is no functional homologue on the Y, thus resulting in an increased dose in the female. In contrast, there is no known example of a gene that undergoes inactivation for which there is a functional homologue on the Y at present. These differences between the X and Y reflect the evolutionary history of the sex chromosomes. It is thought that the heteromorphic sex chromosomes of today evolved from a homomorphic autosome-like pair with progressive loss of genes from the Y and incorporation of the corresponding genes on the X into the X-inactivation system. The genes that escape inactivation on the X may be essential for normal female development in two doses or they may have simply failed to be incorporated into the X-inactivation system with no adverse consequences. The non-inactivated genes thus have implications for the pathogenesis of sex chromosome disorders and sex-linked inheritance. The abnormal development associated with X chromosome aneuploidy is most readily explained by dosage inequities in these genes that escape inactivation. Identification of the specific genes involved in these diseases is, therefore, of great interest and is a focus of ongoing investigations.

Uniparental disomy and imprinting

It has been appreciated for some time that one paternal and one maternal set of chromosomes are required for the normal development of the embryo. In rare cases, a pregnancy arises in which an ovum undergoes some degree of embryonic development by a process of parthenogenesis or androgenesis; i.e., the cells are solely of maternal origin (parthenogenesis) or of paternal origin (androgenesis). Ovarian teratomas appear to be the result of parthenogenetic development of ova that have not undergone the second meiotic division. The cells are thus diploid and XX. Referring to Figure 9.11 may help in understanding that these parthenogenetic cells will be homozygous for all genes except those distal to a recombination event. In contrast, some pregnancies which terminate in spontaneous abortion, are associated with the presence of a hydatidiform

mole, an abnormal development of extra-embryonic tissue. Many of these moles are diploid and XX (rarely XY), with both sets of chromosomes of paternal origin. The mechanism of production of such androgenetic conceptuses is unknown. They may arise by extrusion of the female pronucleus from the fertilized egg, with diploidizaton of the male-derived chromosome set. Understanding the origin and functional capacities of such abnormal products will help to elucidate the nature of gene and chromosome function in human development.

One of the most interesting novel concepts to emerge from these and other studies in the mouse is that of genomic imprinting, which provides an explanation for the abnormal development of parthenogenetic and androgenetic embryos. Genomic imprinting refers to a process by which maternal and paternal alleles of specific genes or chromosomal regions are differentially marked during gametogenesis such that they are expressed differently in the embryo (Bartolomei and Tilghman, 1997). One allele of the imprinted gene is usually active, while the other is inactive. Thus the paternal and maternal copies are not functionally equal for all genes and therefore both a maternal copy and a paternal copy are required for normal development. Like X-chromosome inactivation, genomic imprinting is also an epigenetic phenomenon in that the imprinted gene does not undergo any permanent change and the imprint is reversible. Thus a female who begins life with a maternally and paternally imprinted allele at a locus will produce gametes that exhibit only maternal imprint even on her own paternal chromosome. Similarly, males produce only gametes with the male specific imprint. In other words, during gametogenesis the parental imprint is erased and reset in a sex specific manner. Like X-chromosome inactivation, maintenance of the imprint in the somatic cells is mediated by DNA methylation.

Imprinting is known to affect only a small number of genes and chromosomal regions in the human genome. Imprinting thus differs from X-inactivation in that it does not affect a whole or most of a chromosome. Moreover, even within an imprinted chromosomal region, individual genes located within a few hundred kilobases of DNA may show differential imprinting. As a result, a gene may be inactive on the maternal chromosome and active on the paternal chromosome while a neighboring gene exhibits the opposite imprinting being active on the maternal chromosome and inactive on the paternal chromosome. Imprinting also shows tissue specific variation for certain genes. Thus, the Angelman syndrome (AS) gene, *UBE3A*, on chromosome 15 is expressed from both chromosomes (biallelic expression) in somatic cells but is expressed only from the maternal chromosome in the brain. X-chromosome inactivation in females is different from imprinting in this regard in that is presumed to be present in all somatic cells.

Although imprinting affects only a few chromosomal regions, imprinted genes contribute to genetic diseases. Analysis of these disease states has led to the discovery of uniparental disomy (UPD), a novel form of chromosomal inheritance in which both chromosomes of a pair are inherited from the same parent (Ledbetter and Engel, 1995). In the case of Prader-Willi syndrome (PWS), about 70% of the patients have a deletion in the proximal long arm of the paternally inherited chromosome 15. In normal individuals population the PWS critical gene(s) are transcribed only from the paternal homologue. Therefore, with the deletion of the PWS critical region on the paternal 15, PWS patients are completely deficient for the products of these imprinted genes. The remaining 30% of PWS patients have two chromosome 15's derived from their mother and none from their father. In the absence of a paternal 15 these patients also lack the expression of PWS critical gene(s). A likely mechanism for the origin of this UPD is the conception of a fetus with trisomy for chromosome 15 with two chromosomes from the mother and one from the father. Trisomy 15 is usually lethal and will lead to miscarriage. However, loss of a 15 in an occasional cell during early embryogenesis, will allow that cell line to proliferate and result in a viable fetus. If the sole paternal chromosome is the one that is lost in this "trisomy rescue", the resulting infant will have maternal UPD and PWS. Alternatively, UPD could arise from the rescue of a monosomic conceptus, by duplication of the single homologue. Maternal and paternal UPDs for many of the human chromosomes have now been identified. Several of these result in normal phenotype presumably because the chromosome does not harbor any imprinted gene(s) (Ledbetter and Engel, 1995). However, these individuals may be at risk for being homozygous for recessive genes. The possible role of UPD, a unique form of chromosomal inheritance, in disease states of unknown etiology is being investigated.

Chromosome abnormalities

Human cytogenetics has grown during the past four decades because of continuing technical advances and the high incidence of chromosomal abnormalities in the human population. It is estimated that the frequency of significant chromosome abnormalities among livebirths is about 1/150. It is well documented that about 50% of first trimester pregnancy losses are due to chromosome abnormalities, mostly numerical anomalies. Thus chromosome aberrations have a significant impact as causes of pregnancy wastage, congenital malformations, mental retardation, abnormalities of sex differentiation, and behavioral problems, as discussed in detail elsewhere in this volume. Acquired chromosomal changes play a significant role in carcinogenesis and in tumor progression.

Changes in chromosome number are far more common than changes in structure as causes of clinically significant abnormalities. However, structural changes such as translocations and inversions pose a much more serious familial recurrence risk for chromosome abnormalities. This is due to aberrant segregation of chromosomes during meiosis in clinically normal carriers of these balanced rearrangements.

NUMERICAL CHROMOSOME ABNORMALITIES

As already noted, errors in chromosome dysfunction during mitosis or meiosis can give rise to numerical changes in chromosomes in the resulting individual. Aneuploidy is the most common clinically significant chromosome abnormality in humans occurring in 3–4% of all clinically recognized pregnancies. Aneuploidy refers to a chromosome number that is more or less than an exact multiple of the haploid set. Aneuploidy for a human autosome is usually a trisomy that results from meiotic nondisjunction. Monosomy for an autosome is rarely seen in livebirths or even in spontaneous abortuses presumably due to lethality in very early gestation. The availability of highly polymorphic DNA markers has allowed the determination of the origin of the extra chromosome in many trisomic conditions seen in liveborns and spontaneous abortuses. In the case of trisomy 21, for example, about 95% of the cases result from maternal meiotic error in chromosome segregation. About 75% of this maternal nondisjunction occurs in meiosis I (Antonarakis, 1998). In Meiosis I non-disjunction, both homologues of a chromosome move to the same pole during anaphase I instead of moving to opposite poles, giving rise to a daughter cell with two copies of the chromosome and the other with none. The latter product is never recovered because of lethality associated with monosomy. In the case of Meiosis II non-disjunction, the two sister chromatids of a homologue move to the same pole, again giving rise to a daughter cell with two copies of the chromosome and the other with none. The common autosomal trisomies (21, 18 and 13) seen among livebirths and their associated phenotypes, are discussed in Chapter 44.

Aneuploidy can also result from segregation errors in mitosis. Nondisjunction or anaphase lag during early embryonic mitotic divisions often leads to chromosome mosaicism, the presence of two or more populations of cells derived from a single zygote but that differ in their chromosome constitution. If, at separation of sister chromatids during anaphase, one daughter chromosome lags behind, it may be excluded from the nucleus of a daughter cell. If the cell is able to proliferate, the result may be a 2n/2n-1 mosaic where "n" equals the haploid number of chromosomes. If both sister chromatids go to one pole of the mitotic spindle, one daughter cell will have 2n+1 chromosomes, and the other 2n-1. Such nondisjunctional mosaics can therefore be totally aneuploid. However, unless nondisjunction occurs at the first cleavage division after fertilization, euploid (2n) cells can also be present, and may even predominate. A mosaic is distinct from a chimera in that the latter is an individual whose cells have arisen from more than one fertilized egg. For example, anastomosis of placental blood vessels in twin pregnancies produces, on rare occasions, individuals chimeric for genetically different myeloid and lymphoid cells. Also, there are rare individuals with genotypic and phenotypic indications of their chimeric origin having two cell types such as XX and XY.

Monosomy is rarely seen for a whole autosome, but is a common abnormality of the sex chromosomes resulting from a paternal or maternal non-disjunction leading to a karyotype of 45 chromosomes with a single X chromosome. Although this is the most common aneuploidy found in about 20% of chromosomally abnormal first trimester abortions, the prevalence at birth decreases to high 1/2500 live female births. The cause of the fetal lethality in 45X pregnancies is unknown. Non-disjunction of the X chromosome also leads to individuals with extra X chromosomes. In fact, numerical abnormalities of sex chromosomes are the most common of all chromosome abnormalities and the phenotypes associated with them are less severe than those of the autosomes due primarily to X-chromosome inactivation and the low gene content of the Y chromosome. Thus in an individual with 3, 4 or 5 X chromosomes all but one X is inactivated, thus maintaining the dosage correct for most X-linked genes and reducing the severity of the phenotype. However, genes that escape X-chromosome inactivation have an increased or decreased dosage in individuals with X chromosome aneuploidy. Abnormal development associated with numerical abnormalities of the sex chromosomes is most readily explained by the dosage inequities in these genes that escape inactivation. Abnormalities associated with sex chromosomes are discussed in detail in Chapter 45.

STRUCTURAL CHROMOSOME ABNORMALITIES

Recurrent, non-random chromosomal rearrangements associated with disease states have led to the hypothesis that the sequence and/or organization of DNA at specific chromosomal sites may predispose them to rearrangements. Recent molecular characterization of many chromosomal regions, including some that are predisposed to rearrangements, has provided support for this hypothesis. For example, a combination of FISH and sequencing of large chromosomal regions has shown that there are many duplications of DNA segments consisting of coding and/or non-coding regions in the human genome reflecting the role of gene and genome duplication in evolution. These include locally duplicated families of genes, low copy repeats (LCRs) consisting of highly homologous sequences interspersed with other sequences and inverted repeats. A recent analysis of the DNA sequence of human chromosome 22 has identified 8 copies of an LCR specific to that chromosome, each of which contain a set of genes or pseudogenes (Dunham et al., 1999). Rearrangements mediated by these low copy repeats have been shown to be the basis of a number of related genetic conditions (Edelman et al., 1999a). One of these structural changes is an interstitial deletion in the proximal region of chromosome 22 which is usually undetectable by conventional light microscopic analysis. This microdeletion is associated with the DiGeorge and Velocardiofacial syndromes (discussed in Ch. 46). Although other factors beyond sequence homology are likely involved, a molecular mechanism for the origin of this microdeletion is misalignment of homologous non-sister chromatids during meiotic pairing at the interspersed LCR sequences that flank the commonly deleted region, followed by crossing over. In other words, an LCR pairs with a highly homologous LCR upstream or downstream of it rather than its true homologue on the non-sister chromatid. The DNA on both chromatids may loop out to accommodate such local mispairing. If there is a cross over in the mispaired region, this will result in one chromatid with duplication of the sequences between the two LCRs and one with a deletion of the corresponding sequences Alternatively, deletions and duplications mediated by these repetitive DNA sequences could also result from aberrant intra-chromosomal recombination or unequal exchanges between sister chromatids (SCEs) (Hu and Worton, 1992; Lupski, 1998; Edelman et al., 1999a). Detailed molecular analysis of the deletion breakpoints in patients with the 22q11.2 deletion syndrome has shown that they are located in the LCRs consistent with the above models (Edelman et al., 1999a; Shaikh et al., 2000).

Microdeletions or microduplications mediated by locally duplicated chromosomal regions (duplicons) have now been shown to be the molecular basis of a number of diseases. Some of the best studied examples include Williams syndrome at 7q11.2 (Ch. 46), Prader-Willi and Angelman syndromes at 15q11.2 (Ch. 46), Charcot-Marie-Tooth disease type 1A (CMT1A) and HNPP at 17p11.2. Although the number of duplicated sites and the extent to which they vary within the normal population is unknown, future studies will determine the evolutionary origin of these duplicons as well as their role in both germline and acquired human diseases.

Another clinically important structural chromosome abnormality is an exchange of segments between two (or rarely more than two) chromosomes, called a reciprocal translocation. The majority of the constitutional reciprocal translocations is balanced and do not functionally disrupt genes at or near the breakpoints. Therefore constitutional carriers of balanced translocations usually have a normal phenotype. However, homologous pairing of balanced translocation chromosomes in their germ cells produce a quadrivalent of four chromosomes leading to abnormal segregation and genetically unbalanced gametes (see Ch. 46 for more details). Therefore, translocation carriers are at increased risk for having offspring with chromosome imbalance. Chromosome inversions are intra-chromosomal rearrangements generated by breakage and inversion of a DNA segment and like reciprocal translocations are also usually balanced. However, carriers of inversions are predisposed to generating gametes that are unbalanced as a result of pairing of homologous segments, followed by crossing over within the inverted segment.

The recurrence of several structural chromosome abnormalities, particularly among the acquired chromosome changes in neoplastic diseases, suggests that certain chromosomal sites may be prone to such rearrangements. Translocations are a particularly important group of these acquired chromosome abnormalities associated with neoplasia. Organizational aspects of the chromosome predisposing to these structural rearrangements are currently under investigation. Recent analysis of the breakpoint regions of the recurrent constitutional 11; 22 reciprocal translocation [t(11;22)(q23;q11)] show that they occur in palindromic AT rich regions on both chromosomes (Edelman et al., 1999b; Kurahashi et al., 2000), implicating these sequences in the origin of this exchange. Interestingly, on chromosome 22 the breakpoint is located in one of the LCRs, which is also implicated in the origin of the 22q11.2 deletions. Whether similar sequences are involved in the origin of other translocations remains to be determined. The ability to rapidly sequence regions around breakpoints of independent translocations may ultimately elucidate the molecular mechanism(s) underlying these rearrangements. With the availability of the complete sequence of the human genome, it is expected that structural features predisposing to chromosomes rearrangements will be elucidated.

Concluding remarks and challenges

In this chapter, we have outlined the structural and behavioral aspects of human chromosomes and their relationship to disease states.

We have seen that the normal behaviors of chromosomes during meiosis and mitosis are related to particular structural features. These include but are not limited to the centromeres in anaphase separation, ribosomal gene clusters at secondary constrictions to the nucleolus, the inactive X chromosome to the interphase Barr Body, and chromosome band classes to the chromomeres of pachytene meiosis as well as to replication timing during DNA synthesis. Accordingly, the gross structural landmarks of visible chromosomes provide clues to the existence of underlying associated functions and the emergence of the human genome sequence will provide the tools with which to explore these crucial mechanisms in human development and disease.

We have begun to understand the DNA sequences that are associated with chromosomal landmarks, such as centromeres, telomeres, chromosome bands and fragile sites. However, we still do not understand the role of such sequences in producing the associated functional correlates. For example, which sequences are critical for centromere function and how do dicentric chromosomes decide which will function? Most enigmatic, what is the origin of chromosome bands and in what manner do the interspersed repeated sequences, Alu and L1 relate to the correlated functions (Table 9.1). What is the function of these band domains in meiosis? In what way might the chromatin organization of G versus R bands limit their transcriptional potential? Further, what is the molecular organization of a band border that must maintain a forked junction for a time during DNA synthesis, and does this structure have consequences for regional chromosomal instability?

We have also begun to understand that the organization of some duplicated DNA sequences predisposes the chromosomes that carry them to germline rearrangements such as local deletions, duplications and inversions. However, we do not understand the mechanisms that initially led to the local duplications, nor the sequences or structures responsible for the continued instability.

Acquired structural chromosome changes play a critical role in carcinogenesis and in tumor progression. Yet we do not appreciate the chromosomal mechanisms by which these changes occur, their commonality of sequences, or whether they are similar to germline events. Answers to these questions could provide novel approaches to disease prevention or treatments.

Many new insights have come from understanding the structure and function of the human X chromosome and genomic imprinting. However, we do not know to what extent the remainder of the genome may contain imprinted or partially imprinted genes whose parental origin determines in part tissue specific expression. Might such "epigenetic" phenomena provide another mechanism for both normal human variation and disease susceptibility?

Much remains to be learned about the molecular aspects of chromosome structure and behavior. It is anticipated that the human genome sequence and its functional characterization will provide the tools with which to approach these problems and define a new frontier for the role of chromosomes in human disease.

REFERENCES

Antonarakis SE (1998) Ten years of genomics, chromosome 21, and Down syndrome. Genomics 51:1–16

Arrighi FE, Hsu TC (1971) Localization of heterochromatin in human chromosomes. Cytogenetics 10:81–86

Bailey JA, Carrel L, Chakravarti A, Eichler EE (2000) Molecular evidence of a relationship between LINE1 elements and X chromosome inactivation: The Lyon repeat hypothesis. Proc Natl Acad Sci USA 97:6634–6639

Baker SM, Plug AW, Prolla TA et al. (1996) Involvement of mouse *Mlh1* in DNA mismatch repair and meiotic crossing over. Nature Genet 13:336–342

Bartolomei MS, Tilghman SM (1997) Genomic imprinting in mammals. Ann Rev Genet 31:493–525

Blackburn EH (1991) Structure and function of telomeres. Nature 350:569–573

Blasco MA, Gasses SM, Lingner J (1999) Telomeres and telomerase. Genes and Development 13:2353–2359

Britten RJ and Kohne DE (1968) Repeated sequences in DNA. Science, 161:529–540

Brockdorff N (1998) The role of *Xist* in X-inactivation. Curr Opin Genet Dev 8:328–333

Brown CJ, Balllabio A, Rupert JL et al. (1991) A gene from the region of the human X-chromosome inactivation centre is expressed exclusively from the inactive X chromosome. Nature 349:38–44

Carrel L, Cottle AA, Goglin KC et al. (1999) A first generation X-inactivation profile of the human X chromosome. Proc Natl Acad Sci 96:14440–14444

Caspersson T, Zech L, Johansson C, Modest EJ (1970) Identification of human chromosomes by DNA-binding fluorescent reagents. Chromosoma 30:215–227

Choo KHA (1997) Centromere DNA dynamics: Latent centromeres and neocentromere formation. Am J Hum Genet 61:1225–1233

Craig JM, Earnshaw WC, Vagnarelli P (1999) Mammalian centromeres: DNA sequence, protein composition, and role in cell cycle progression. Exp Cell Res 246:249–262

Crow JF (1997) The high spontaneous mutation rate: Is it a health risk? Proc Natl Acad Sci USA 94:8380–8386

Dobson MJ, Pearlman RE, Karaiskakis A et al. (1994) Synaptonemal complex proteins: Occurrence, epitope mapping and chromosome disjunction. J Cell Sci 107:2749–2760

Donahue RP, Bias WB, Renwick JH, McKusick VA (1968) Probable assignment of the Duffy blood group locus to chromosome 1 in Man. Proc Nat Acad Sci USA 61:949–955

Dunham I, Shimizu N, Roe BA et al. (1999) The DNA sequence of human chromosome 22. Nature 402:489–495

Dutrillaux B, Laurent C, Couturier J, Lejeune J (1973) Coloration par l'acridine orange de chromosomes prealablement traites par le 5-bromadeoxyuridine (BUDR). C. R. Acad. Sci.- D: Sciences Naturelles (Paris) 276(24):3179–3181

Edelman L, Pandita RK, Spiteri E et al. (1999a) A common molecular basis for rearrangement disorders on chromosome 22q11. Hum Mol Genet 8:1157–1167

Edelman L, Spiteri E, McCain N et al. (1999b) A common breakpoint on 11q23 in carriers of the t(11;22) translocation. Am J Hum Genet 65:1608–1616

Flint J, Craddock CF, Villegas A et al. (1994) Healing of broken human chromosomes by the addition of telomeric rpeats. Am J Hum Genet 55:505–512

Ford CE, Hamerton JL (1956) The chromosomes of man. Nature 178:1020–1023

Ford CE, Jones KW, Polani PE et al. (1959) A sex chromosome anomaly in a case of gonadal dysgenesis (Turner's syndrome) Lancet 1:711–713

Gilbert SL, Sharp PA (1999) Promoter-specific hypoacetylation of X-inactivated genes. Proc Natl Acad Sci USA 96:13825–13830

Goodfellow PH, Lovell-Badge R (1993) SRY and sex determination in mammals. Annu Rev Genet 27:71–92

Goodpasture C, Bloom SE, Hsu TC, Arrighi FE (1976) Human nucleolus organizers: The satellites or the stalks? Am J Hum Genet 28:559–566

Grimes B, Cooke H (1998) Engineering mammalian chromosomes. Hum Mol Genet 7:1635–1640

Hart CM, Laemmli UK (1998) Facilitation of chromatin dynamics by SARs. Curr opin Genet Dev 8:519–525

Hattori M, Fujiyama A, Taylor TD, Watanabe H, Yada T et al. (2000) The DNA sequence of Human Chromosome 21. Nature 405:311–319

Hassold T, Sherman S (2000) Down syndrome: Genetic recombination and the origin of the extra chromosome 21. Clin Genet 57:95–100

Hirano T (2000) Chromosome cohesion, condensation and speration. Annu Rev Biochem 69:115–144

Holmquist, GP, Chromosome bands, their chromatin flavors and their functional features (1992) Am J Hum Genet 51; 17–37

Hu X, Worton R (1992) Partial gene duplication as a cause of human disease. Hum Mut 1:3–12

Jackson DA (1995) Nuclear organization: Uniting replication foci, chromatin domains and chromosome structure. Bioessays 17:587–591

Jacobs PA, Strong JA (1959) A case of human intersexuality having a possible XXY sex-determining mechanism. Nature 183:302–303

Jeppesen P, Tumer BM (1994) The inactive X chromosome in female mammals is distinguished by lack of histone H4 acetylation, a cytogenetic marker for gene expression. Cell 74:281–289

Keohane AM, Lavender JS, O'Neill LP, Turner BM (1998) Histone acetylation and X inactivation. Dev Genet 22:65–73

Korenberg JR, Engels WR (1978) Base ratio, DNA content, and quinacrine-brightness of human chromosomes. Proceedings of the National Academy of Sciences, 75(7):3382–3386

Korenberg JR, Friedlander EF (1974) Giemsa technique for the detection of sister chromatid exchanges. Chromosoma, 48:355–360

Korenberg JR, Rykowski MC (1988) Human genome organization: Alu, Lines, and the molecular structure of the metaphase chromosome bands. Cell 53:391–400

Korenberg JR, Chen X-N, Adams MD, Venter J (1995) Toward a cDNA map of the human genome. Genomics, 29(2):364–370

Korenberg JR, Chen X-N, Sun-Y et al. (1999) Human Genome Anatomy: BACs integrating the Genetic and Cytogenetic Maps for bridging genome and biomedicine. Genome Res 9:10 994–1001

Kornberg RD, Lorch Y (1999) Twenty-five years of the nucleosome, fundamental particle of the eukaryote chromosome. Cell 98:285–294

Krummel KA, Roberts LR, Kwakami M et al. (2000) The characterization of common fragile site FRA16D and its involvement in multiple myeloma translocations. Genomics 69:37–46

Kurahashi H, Shaikh TH, Hu P et al. (2000) Regions of genomic instability on 22q11 and 11q23 as the etiology for the recurrent constitutional t(11;22). Hum Mol Genet 9:1665–1670

Latt SA (1973) Microfluorometric detection of deoxyribonucleic acid replication in human metaphase chromosomes. Proc Natl Acad Sci USA 70:3395–3399

Ledbetter DH, Engel E (1995) Uniparental disomy in humans: Development of an imprinting map and its implications for prenatal diagnosis. Hum Mol Genet 4:1757–1764

Lee JT, Jaenisch R (1997) The (epi)genetic control of mammalian X-chromosome inactivation. Curr Opin Genet Dev 7:274–280

Lichter P, Cremer T, Borden J et al. (1988) Delineation of individual human chromosomes in metaphase and interphase cells by in situ suppression hybridization using recombinant DNA libraries. Hum Genet 80:224–234

Lupski JR (1998) Genomic disorders: Structural features of the genome can lead to DNA rearrangements and human disease traits. Trends Genet 14:417–422

Lyon MF (1993) Epigenetic inheritance in mammals. Trends Genet 9:123–128

Lyon MF (2000) LINE-1 Elements and X chromosome inactivation: A function for "junk" DNA? Proc Natl Acad Sci USA 97:6248–6249

Mohandas T, Sparkes RS, Shapiro LJ (1981) Reactivation of an inactive human X chromosome: Evidence for X-inactivation by DNA methylation. Science 211:393–396

Moorhead PS, Nowell PC, Mellman WJ et al. (1960) Chromosome preparations of leukocytes cultured from peripheral blood. Exp Cell Res 20:613–616

Murphy TD, Karpen GH (1998) Centromeres take flight: Alpha satellite and the quest for the human centromere. Cell 93:317–320

Nurse P (2000) The incredible life and times of biological cells. Science 289:1711–1716

Pauletti G, Godolthin W, Press MF, Slamon DJ (1996) Detection and quantitation of HER-2/neu gene amplification in human breast cancer archival material using fluorescence in situ hybridization. Oncogene 13:63–72

Pinkel D, Straume T, Gray JW (1986) Cytogenetic analysis using quantitative, high-sensitivity, fluorescence hybridization. Proc Natl Acad Sci USA 83:2934–2938

Race R, Sanger R (1975) Blood Groups in Man, Blackwell, London

Rappold GA (1993) The pseudoautosomal regions of the human sex chromosomes. Hum Genet 92:315–324

Richler C, Soreq H, Wahrman J (1992) X inactivation in mammalian testis is correlated with inactive X-specific transcription. Nature Genet 2:192–195

Riggs AD, Pfeifer GP (1992) X-chromosome inactivation and cell memory. Trends Genet 8:169–174

Roberts LM, Shen J, Ingraham HA (1999) New solutions to an ancient riddle: Defining the differences between adam and eve. Am J Hum Genet 65:933–942

Salido EC, Yen PH, Mohandas TK, Shapiro LJ (1992) Expression of the X-inactivation-associated gene XIST during spermatogenesis. Nature Genet 2:196–199

Seabright M (1971) Rapid banding technique for human chromosomes. Lancet 2:971–972

Schrock E, duManoir S, Veldman T et al. (1996) Multicolor spectral karyotyping of human chromosomes. Science 273:494–497

Shaikh TH, Kurahashi H, Saitta SC et al. (2000) Chromosome 22-specific low copy repeats and the 22q11.2 deletion syndrome: Genome organization and deletion endpoint analysis. Hum Mol Genet 9:489–501

Shapiro LJ, Mohandas T, Weiss R, Romeo G (1979) Non-inactivation of an X-chromosome locus in Man. Science 204:1224–1226

Smit AFA (1996) The origin of interspersed repeats in the human genome. Curr Opin Genet Dev 6:43–748

Stark GR, Debatisse M, Giulotto E and Wahl GM (1989) Recent progress in understanding mechanisms of mammalian DNA amplification. Cell 57:901–908

Sutherland GR, Baker E, Richards RI (1998) Fragile sites still breaking. Trends in Genet 14:51–506

Swain A and Lovell-Badge R (1999) Mammalian sex determination: A molecular drama. Genes Dev 13:755–767

Tjio JH, Levan A (1956) The chromosome number of man. Hereditas 42:1–6

van Brabant AJ, Stan R, Ellis NA (2000) DNA helicases, genomic instability and human genetic disease. Ann Rev Genomics Hum Genet 1:409–459

Warburton D, Yu C, Stein Z (1979) Mosaic autosomal trisomy in cultures from spontaneous abortions. Am J Hum Genet 30:609–618

Willard HF (1998) Centromeres: The missing link in the development of human artificial chromosomes. Curr Opin Genet Dev 8:219–225

Xu Y, Ashley T, Brainerd EE et al. (1996) Targeted disruption of ATM leads to growth retardation, chromosomal fragmentation during meiosis, immune defects and thymic lymphoma. Genes Dev 10:2411–2422

Yuan L, Liu JG, Zhao et al. (2000) The murine SCP3 gene is required for synaptonemal complex assembly, chromosome synapsis, and male fertility. Cell 5:73–83

Yunis JJ (1976) High resolution of human chromosomes. Science 191:1268–1270

Morbid anatomy of the human genome

10

Victor A. McKusick
Joanna S. Amberger

Microscopic studies of the human chromosomes, dating particularly from 1956 when the correct diploid number in humans was determined, and the mapping of genes on chromosomes have provided medical genetics with an anatomic basis. Charles Scriver has referred to it as the neo-Vesalian basis of medical genetics and of medicine in general, because the impact has been comparable to that of Andreas Vesalius' *De Corporis humani fabrica* (1543) on the evolution of modern medicine.

When we speak of gene mapping, we use a cartographic metaphor; however, an anatomic metaphor is equally appropriate: the anatomy of the human genome. One then can speak of the morbid anatomy, the comparative anatomy and evolution, the functional anatomy, the developmental anatomy, and, of particular interest to health professionals, the applied anatomy of the human genome.

The complete DNA sequence of the human genome is the ultimate anatomic base for medicine. The precise chromosomal location of many disease related genes is now possible through searching of the complete human sequence provided by the Human Genome Project.

At this point, the specific chromosomal sites of more than 1879 disease-related genes are known. In some cases the information is solely that a particular disease phenotype is genetically linked to DNA markers at a specific chromosomal site, and no direct information is available on the gene that is mutant. But for 1123 of the 1879 disease-related loci, the gene has been cloned and at least one disease-related mutation identified. (In addition, about 100 other genes have been related to disease by their identification as partners in translocation fusion genes causing neoplastic disorders, most often leukemia or lymphoma but also some solid tumors such as Ewing sarcoma.)

Many loci (genes) are the site of more than one phenotypically distinct disorder (allelic disorders), witness the different hematologic diseases caused by different mutations in the beta-globin gene (HBB; MIM# 141900). For this reason, the total number of distinct disorders caused by mutations at these 1123 loci is 1521.

Table 10.1 lists, chromosome-by-chromosome, the 1879 loci with which pathologic phenotypes are associated. Table 10.2 is an alphabetized listing of 2460 clinical disorders that have been mapped to those loci; it serves, in effect, as an index for Table 10.1[1]. Many disorders are caused by mutations in any one of two or more genes. In such instances, the clinical phenotype is described in an entry with a MIM number preceded by a number sign (#) and the gene containing the disease-related mutations(s) is described in a separate entry with a MIM number preceded by an asterisk (*).

The morbid (disease-related) gene loci on each chromosome are listed in Table 10.1 in order of chromosomal position from the telomere of the short arm to the telomere of the long arm, and in numerical sequence from chromosome 1 to chromosome 22, followed by the X and Y chromosomes. (Gene maps of the mitochondrial chromosome are presented elsewhere.)

[1] Detailed information on the clinical phenotype of each disorder, its genetics including mapping, and its molecular basis is provided in Victor A McKusick's *Mendelian Inheritance in Man: A Catalog of Human Genes and Genetic Disorders* (Johns Hopkins University Press, 1998, 12th edn.) and its continuously updated online version OMIM. The six-digit MIM numbers in the tables refer to entries in MIM and OMIM. OMIM is authored and edited primarily in the McKusick-Nathans Institute of Genetic Medicine at Johns Hopkins Hospital, Baltimore, MD 21287–4922 with assistance from an international group of experts. OMIM is available on the World Wide Web from the National Center for Biotechnology Information of the National Library of Medicine, Bethesda, MD (http://www.ncbi.nlm.nih.gov/omim/).

The fields in Table 10.1 are as follows (from left to right):

A. **Chromosomal location:** The bands given are inclusive. They are stated with the short-arm telomeric limit first, e.g., 5p14-p13 (not 5p13-p14) and 5q31-q33.
B. **Gene symbol:** The symbol approved by the Nomenclature Committee of the Human Gene Mapping Workshops and its HUGO-sponsored successor organization is given first. Other literature symbols are included for the convenience of the user.
C. **Title:** Gene or locus name.
D. **MIM#:** Unique identification number of the entry in *Mendelian Inheritance in Man* that describes the locus or gene. In general, one entry per gene locus has been created; see comment under "Disorder" for a qualification to this statement. Presently, the MIM numbers have six digits. Those numbers beginning with "3" refer to entries in the X-linked catalog; autosomal loci have numbers beginning with a "1" or a "2", depending on whether the entry was originally created on the basis of an autosomal dominant or an autosomal recessive phenotype, respectively. All new entries referring to autosomal loci created since May 1994 have a MIM number beginning with "6," regardless of the inheritance of any associated phenotype. The entries in the Y chromosome and mitochondrial chromosome catalogs have numbers beginning with "4" and "5", respectively.
E. **Disorder(s):** This field lists the disorders caused by mutations in the particular gene. The number in parentheses after the name of the disorder indicates whether the phenotype was positioned by mapping the wildtype gene (**1**), by mapping the disease phenotype itself (**2**), or whether the gene has been mapped and its molecular basis elucidated (**3**). Brackets surround "nondiseases" (aberrations of laboratory measurements or innocent variations), e.g., [dysalbuminemic hyperthyroxinemia]; braces indicate susceptibilities, e.g., {vivax malaria, susceptibility to}. For some disorders, a MIM entry number is given after the disorder; this indicates that there is a separate, #-sign labeled entry describing the disease phenotype in addition to the asterisked locus entry denoted in the MIM# field (see above). This "disorder" field constitutes the "Morbid Anatomy of the Human Genome" and is the basis for the alphabetical listing in Table 10.2.
F. **Mouse:** This field gives the chromosomal location of the homologous locus in the mouse. The symbol for the mouse gene is given in parentheses. Sometimes two symbols are given: a phenotype-based symbol and a symbol derived from the fundamental biochemical defect.

Table 10.1. The morbid anatomy of the human genome (by chromosome)

Location	Symbol	Title	MIM#	Disorder	Mouse
1pter-p36.13	CCV	Cataract, congenital, Volkmann type	115665	Cataract, congenital, Volkmann type (2)	
1pter-p36.13	ENO1, PPH	Enolase-1, alpha	172430	Enolase deficiency (1)	4 (Eno1)
1pter-p36.1	CTPP, CPP, CTPA	Cataract, posterior polar	116600	Cataract, posterior polar (2)	
1pter-p33	HMGCL	3-hydroxy-3-methylglutaryl-Coenzyme A lyase	246450	HMG-CoA lyase deficiency (3)	4 (Hmgcl)
1p36.3	MTHFR	Methylenetetrahydrofolate reductase	236250	Homocystinuria due to MTHFR deficiency (3)	4 (Mthfr)
1p36.3-p36.2	NB, NBS	Neuroblastoma (neuroblastoma suppressor)	256700	Neuroblastoma (2)	
1p36.3-p36.2	PLOD	Procollagen-lysine, 2-oxoglutarate 5-dioxygenase (lysine hydroxylase)	153454	Ehlers-Danlos syndrome, type VI, 225400 (3)	4 (Plod)
1p36.3-p34.1	C1QA	Complement component-1, q subcomponent, alpha polypeptide	120550	Clq deficiency, type A (3)	
1p36.3-p34.1	C1QB	Complement component-1, q subcomponent, beta polypeptide	120570	Clq deficiency, type B (3)	(C1qb)
1p36.3-p34.1	C1QG	Complement component-1, q subcomponent, gamma polypeptide	120575	C1q deficiency, type C (3)	
1p36.2-p36.12	PAX7	Paired box homeotic gene-7	167410	Rhabdomyosarcoma, alveolar, 268220 (3)	4 (Pax7)
1p36.2-p36.1	GLC3B	Glaucoma 3, primary infantile, B	600975	Glaucoma 3, primary infantile, B (2)	
1p36.2-p34	EPB41, EL1	Erythrocyte surface protein band 4.1	130500	Elliptocytosis-1 (3)	4 (Elp1)
1p36.1	ECE1	Endothelin converting enzyme 1	600423	Hirschsprung disease, cardiac defects, and autonomic dysfunction (3)	
1p36.1	HSPG2, PLC, SJS, SJA, SJS1	Heparan sulfate proteoglycan of basement membrane (perlecan)	142461	Schwartz-Jampel syndrome, type 1, 255800 (3)	4 (Plc)
1p36.1-p35	SDHB, SDH1, SDHIP	Succinate dehydrogenase complex, subunit B, iron sulfur (Ip)	185470	?Myopathy due to succinate dehydrogenase deficiency (1)	
1p36.1-p34	ALPL, HOPS	Alkaline phosphatase, liver/bone/kidney	171760	Hypophosphatasia, infantile, 241500 (3); Hypophosphatasia, childhood, 241510 (3); ?Hypophosphatasia, adult, 146300 (1)	4 (Akp2)
1p36	ALDH4, P5CDH	Aldehyde dehydrogenase-4 (delta-1-pyrroline 5-carboxylate dehydrogenase)	239510	Hyperprolinemia, type II (3)	
1p36	BRCD2	Breast cancer, ductal	211420	Breast cancer, ductal (2)	
1p36	CLCNKB	Chloride channel, kidney, B	602023	Bartter syndrome, type 3 (3)	
1p36	CMM, MLM, DNS	Cutaneous malignant melanoma/dysplastic nevus	155600	Malignant melanoma, cutaneous (2)	
1p36	IBD7	Inflammatory bowel disease 7	605225	Inflammatory bowel disease 7 (2)	
1p36	PCBC, CAPB	Prostate cancer-brain cancer susceptibility	603688	{Prostate cancer-brain cancer susceptibility} (2)	
1p36	TP73	p53-related protein	601990	?Neuroblastoma (1)	
1p36-p35	CMT2A	Charcot-Marie-Tooth neuropathy-2A (hereditary motor sensory neuropathy II)	118210	Charcot-Marie-Tooth neuropathy-2A (2)	
1p36-p35	GALE	UDP galactose-4-epimerase	230350	Galactose epimerase deficiency (3)	

continued

Table 10.1. The morbid anatomy of the human genome (by chromosome) (*continued*)

Location	Symbol	Title	MIM#	Disorder	Mouse
1p36-p35	RSMD1, MDRS1	Muscular dystrophy, congenital, with early spine rigidity	602771	Muscular dystrophy, congenital, with early spine rigidity (2)	
1p36-p34.1	SCCD	Schnyder crystalline corneal dystrophy	121800	Corneal dystrophy, crystalline, Schnyder (2)	
1p35.1	GJB3, CX31, DFNA2	Gap junction protein, beta-3	603324	Erythrokeratodermia variabilis, 133200 (3); Deafness, autosomal dominant 2, 600101 (3); Deafness, autosomal recessive (3)	
1p35.1	GJB4, CX30.3	Gap junction protein, beta-4	605425	Erythrokeratodermia variabilis with erythema gyratum repens, 133200 (3)	
1p35	PLA2G2A, PLA2B, PLA2L, MOM1	Phospholipase A2, group IIA, platelets, synovial fluid	172411	{?Colorectal cancer, resistance to} (1)	4 (Pla2g2a)
1p35-p34.3	CSF3R, GCSFR	Colony-stimulating factor-3 receptor (granulocyte)	138971	Kostmann neutropenia, 202700 (3)	
1p35-p34.3	LCK	Lymphocyte-specific protein tyrosine kinase	153390	SCID due to LCK deficiency (1)	4 (Lck)
1p35-p31.3	SLC2A1, GLUT1	Solute carrier family 2 (facilitated glucose transporter), member 1	138140	Glucose transport defect,) blood-brain barrier (3)	
1p34.1-p32	FH3	Hypercholesterolemia, familial, 3	603776	Hypercholesterolemia, familial, 3 (2)	
1p34.1-p32	PTOS1	Ptosis, congenital 1, autosomal dominant	178300	Ptosis hereditary congenital, 1 (2)	
1p34	DFNA2	Deafness, autosomal dominant 2	600101	Deafness, autosomal dominant 2 (2)	
1p34	ELAVL4, HUD, PNEM	Embryonic lethal, abnormal vision, Drosophila, homolog of, like-4 (Hu antigen D)	168360	Neuropathy, paraneoplastic sensory (1)	4 (Hud)
1p34	FUCA1	Fucosidase, alpha-L- 1, tissue	230000	Fucosidosis (3)	4 (Fuca)
1p34	KCNQ4, DFNA2	Potassium voltage-gated channel, KQT-like subfamily, member 4	603537	Deafness, autosomal dominant 2, 600101 (3)	
1p34	MPL, TPOR, MPLV	Myeloproliferative leukemia virus, homolog of	159530	Thrombocytopenia, congenital amegakaryocytic, 604498 (3)	
1p34	UROD	Uroporphyrinogen decarboxylase	176100	Porphyria cutanea tarda (3); Porphyria, hepatoerythropoietic (3)	4 (Urod)
1p34-p32	MEB	Muscle-eye-brain disease	253280	Muscle-eye-brain disease (2)	
1p33-p32.2	COL9A2, EDM2	Collagen IX, alpha-2 polypeptide	120260	Epiphyseal dysplasia, multiple, type 2, 600204 (3); Intervertebral disc disease, 603932 (3)	4 (Col9a2)
1p32	C8A	Complement component-8, alpha polypeptide	120950	C8 deficiency, type I (2)	
1p32	C8B	Complement component-8, beta polypeptide	120960	C8 deficiency, type II (3)	4 (C8b)
1p32	CPT2	Carnitine palmitoyltransferase II	600650	Myopathy due to CPT II deficiency, 255110 (3); CPT deficiency, hepatic, type II, 600649 (3)	
1p32	HNMT	Histamine N-methyltransferase	605238	{Asthma, susceptibility to} (3)	
1p32	PPT1, CLN1	Palmitoyl-protein thioesterase 1	600722	Ceroid lipofuscinosis, neuronal-1, infantile, 256730 (3); Ceroid lipofuscinosis, neuronal, variant juvenile type, with granular osmiophilic deposits (3)	

continued

Table 10.1. The morbid anatomy of the human genome (by chromosome) (*continued*)

Location	Symbol	Title	MIM#	Disorder	Mouse
1p32	PTCH2	Patched, Drosophila, homolog of, 2	603673	Medulloblastoma, 155255 (3); Basal cell carcinoma, 109400 (3)	4 (Ptch2)
1p32	RAD54L, HR54, HRAD54	RAD54, S. cerevisiae, homolog-like	603615	Lymphoma, non-Hodgkin (3); Breast cancer, invasive intraductal (3); Colon adenocarcinoma (3)	
1p32	TAL1, TCL5, SCL	T-cell acute lymphocytic leukemia-1	187040	Leukemia-1, T-cell acute lymphocytic (3)	4 (Scl)
1p32-q12	M1S1	Membrane component, chromosome 1, surface marker 1 (40 kD glycoprotein, identified by monoclonal antibody GA733)	137290	Corneal dystrophy, gelatinous drop-like, 204870 (3)	
1p31	ACADM, MCAD	Acyl-Coenzyme A dehydrogenase, C-4 to C-12 straight chain	201450	Acyl-CoA dehydrogenase, medium chain, deficiency of (3)	3 (Acadm)
1p31	AIR	Acute insulin response	601676	Acute insulin response (2)	
1p31	ARHI	Ras homolog gene family, member I	605193	Ovarian cancer (1)	
1p31	BSND	Bartter syndrome, infantile, with sensorineural deafness	602522	Bartter syndrome, infantile, with sensorineural deafness (2)	
1p31	DBT, BCATE2	Dihydrolipoamide branched chain transacylase (E2 component of branched chain keto acid dehydrogenase complex)	248610	Maple syrup urine disease, type II (3)	
1p31	RPE65, RP20	Retinal pigment epithelium-specific protein, 65 kD	180069	Leber congenital amaurosis-2, 204100 (3); Retinal dystrophy, autosomal recessive, childhood-onset (3); Retinitis pigmentosa-20 (3)	3 (Rpe65)
1p31-p21	AVSD, AVCD	Atrioventricular canal defect 1	600309	Atrioventricular canal defect-1 (2)	
1p22	BCL10	B-cell leukemia/lymphoma 10	603517	Lymphoma, MALT (3); Lymphoma, follicular (3); Mesothelioma (3); Germ cell tumor (3); Sezary syndrome (3); Colon cancer (3)	
1p22	DPYD, DPD	Dihydropyrimidine dehydrogenase	274270	Thymine-uraciluria (3); {Fluorouracil toxicity, sensitivity to} (3)	
1p22	UOX	Urate oxidase	191540	[Urate oxidase deficiency] (1)	
1p22-p21	VMGLOM	Venous malformations with glomus cells (glomus tumors, multiple)	138000	Glomus tumors, multiple (2)	
1p21	AGL, GDE	Amylo-1, 6-glucosidase, 4-alpha-glucanotransferase (glycogen debranching enzyme)	232400	Glycogen storage disease IIIa (3); Glycogen storage disease IIIb (3)	
1p21	CHRNB2, EFNL3	Cholinergic receptor, nicotinic, beta polypeptide-2	118507	Epilepsy, nocturnal frontal lobe, 3, 605375 (3)	3 (Acrb2)
1p21	COL11A1, STL2	Collagen XI, alpha-1 polypeptide	120280	Stickler syndrome, type II, 604841 (3); Marshall syndrome, 154780 (3)	3 (Col11a1)
1p21	OPTA2	Osteopetrosis, autosomal dominant, type II	166600	Osteopetrosis, AD, type II (2)	
1p21-p13	ABCA4, ABCR, STGD1, FFM, RP19	ATP-binding transporter, retina-specific	601691	Stargardt disease-1, 248200 (3); Retinitis pigmentosa-19, 601718 (3); Cone-rod dystrophy 3 (3); Macular dystrophy, age-related, 2, 153800 (3); Fundus flavimaculatus, 248200 (2)	

continued

Table 10.1. The morbid anatomy of the human genome (by chromosome) (*continued*)

Location	Symbol	Title	MIM#	Disorder	Mouse
1p21-p13	AMPD1	Adenosine monophosphate deaminase-1, muscle	102770	Myoadenylate deaminase deficiency (3)	3 (Ampd1)
1p21-p13.3	WS2B	Waardenburg syndrome, type 2B	600193	Waardenburg syndrome, type 2B (2)	
1p13.2	NRAS	Neuroblastoma RAS viral (v-ras) oncogene homolog	164790	Colorectal cancer (3)	3 (Nras)
1p13.1	HSD3B2	Hydroxy-delta-5-steroid dehydrogenase, 3 beta- and steroid delta-isomerase, type 2 (adrenal, gonadal)	201810	3-beta-hydroxysteroid dehydrogenase, type II, deficiency (3)	3 (Hsd3b2)
1p13	TSHB	Thyroid-stimulating hormone, beta polypeptide	188540	Hypothyroidism, nongoitrous (3)	3 (Tshb)
1p13	VUR	Vesicoureteral reflux	193000	Vesicoureteral reflux (2)	
1p13-p12	HMGCS2	3-hydroxy-3-methylglutaryl-Coenzyme A synthase 2	600234	HMG-CoA synthase-2 deficiency (1)	
1p13-q23	RP18	Retinitis pigmentosa-18	601414	Retinitis pigmentosa-18 (2)	
1p	CSE, DYT9	Choreoathetosis/spasticity, episodic (paroxysmal choreoathetosis/spasticity)	601042	Choreoathetosis/spasticity, episodic (2)	
1p	PCHC	Pheochromocytoma	171300	Pheochromocytoma (2)	
1cen-q21	PSORS4	Psoriasis susceptibility 4	603935	{Psoriasis, susceptibility to} (2)	
1q	HFE2	Hemochromatosis, type 2	602390	Hemochromatosis, type 2 (2)	
1q11-q21	LGMD1B	Limb-girdle muscular dystrophy-1B, autosomal dominant	159001	Muscular dystrophy, limb-girdle, type 1B (2)	
1q12-q24	CORD8	Cone-rod dystrophy 8	605549	Cone-rod dystrophy 8 (2)	
1q21	AF1Q	ALL1-fused gene from chromosome 1q	604684	Leukemia, acute myelomonocytic (3)	
1q21	ARNT	Aryl hydrocarbon receptor nuclear translocator	126110	Leukemia, acute myeloblastic (3)	3 (Arnt)
1q21	CTSK	Cathepsin K	601105	Pycnodysostosis, 265800 (3)	
1q21	FLG	Filaggrin	135940	?Ichthyosis vulgaris, 146700 (1)	3 (flg)
1q21	GBA	Glucosidase, acid beta	230800	Gaucher disease (3); Gaucher disease with cardiovascular calcification (3)	3 (Gba)
1q21	LOR	Loricrin	152445	Vohwinkel syndrome with ichthyosis, 604117 (3); Erythrokeratoderma, progressive symmetric, 602036 (3)	3 (lor)
1q21	MCKD1	Medullary cystic kidney disease 1, autosomal dominant	174000	Medullary cystic kidney disease 1 (2)	
1q21	PKLR, PK1	Pyruvate kinase, liver and RBC type	266200	Anemia, hemolytic, due to PK deficiency (3)	3 (Pk1)
1q21	PRCC, RCCP1	Papillary renal cell carcinoma, translocation-associated	179755	Renal cell carcinoma, papillary, 1, 605074 (3)	
1q21	RFH1, AORF	Renal failure, progressive, with hypertension	161900	Nephropathy-hypertension (2)	
1q21	SDHC, PGL3	Succinate dehydrogenase complex, subunit C, integral membrane protein, 15 kD	602413	Paragangliomas, familial nonchromaffin, 3, 605373 (3)	
1q21	SPTA1	Spectrin, alpha, erythrocytic-1	182860	Elliptocytosis-2 (3); Pyropoikilocytosis (3); Spherocytosis, recessive (3)	1 (Spnal)
1q21-q22	FY, GPD	Duffy blood group	110700	{Vivax malaria, susceptibility to} (1)	1 (Fy, Darc)

continued

Table 10.1. The morbid anatomy of the human genome (by chromosome) (*continued*)

Location	Symbol	Title	MIM#	Disorder	Mouse
1q21-q22	NTRK1, TRKA, MTC	Neurotrophic tyrosine kinase, receptor, type 1	191315	Insensitivity to pain, congenital, with anhidrosis, 256800 (3); Medullary thyroid carcinoma, familial, 155240 (3)	
1q21-q22	SCZD9	Schizophrenia susceptibility locus, chromosome 1q-related	604906	{Schizophrenia}, 181500 (2)	
1q21-q23	APCS, SAP	Amyloid P component, serum	104770	{?Amyloidosis, secondary, susceptibility to} (1)	1 (Sap)
1q21-q23	APOA2	Apolipoprotein A-II	107670	Apolipoprotein A-II deficiency (3)	1 (Apoa2)
1q21-q23	DFNA7	Deafness, autosomal dominant 7	601412	Deafness, autosomal dominant 7 (2)	
1q21-q23	FCGR2A, IGFR2, CD32	Fc fragment of IgG, low affinity IIa, receptor for (CD32)	146790	{Lupus nephritis, susceptibility to} (3)	1 (Ly17, Cd32)
1q21-q23	HYPLIP1	Hyperlipidemia, familial combined, 1	602491	Hyperlipidemia, familial combined, 1 (2)	3 (Hyplipl)
1q21-q23	MHP2	Migraine, familial hemiplegic, 2	602481	Migraine, familial hemiplegic, 2 (2)	
1q21.1	GJAB, CX50, CAE1	Gap junction membrane channel protein alpha-8 (connexin 50)	600897	Cataract, zonular pulverulent-1, 116200 (3)	3 (Gja8)
1q21.1-q21.3	RFX5	Regulatory factor X, 5 (influences HLA class II expression)	601863	MHC class II deficiency, complementation group C, 209920 (3)	
1q21.2	LMNA, LMN1, EMD2, FPLD, CMD1A	Lamin A/C	150330	Emery-Dreifuss muscular dystrophy, AD, 181350 (3); Cardiomyopathy, dilated, 1A, 115200 (3); Lipodystrophy, familial partial, 151660 (3); Emery-Dreifuss muscular dystrophy, AR, 604929 (3)	
1q21.2-q21.3	FCGR1A, IGFR1, CD64	Fc fragment of IgG, high affinity Ia, receptor for (CD64)	146760	[IgG receptor I, phagocytic, familial deficiency of] (1)	3 (Fcgr1)
1q22	FCGR2B, CD32	Fc fragment of IgG, low affinity IIb, receptor for	604590	Lymphoma, progression of (3)	
1q22	MPZ, CMT1B	Myelin protein zero	159440	Charcot-Marie-Tooth neuropathy-1B, 118200 (3); Dejerine-Sottas disease, myelin P-zero-related, 145900 (3); Hypomyelination, congenital (3)	1 (Mpp)
1q22	PPOX	Protoporphyrinogen oxidase	600923	Porphyria variegata, 176200 (3)	
1q22-q23	CD3Z, TCRZ	CD3Z antigen, zeta polypeptide (TiT3 complex)	186780	CD3, zeta chain, deficiency (1)	1 (T3z, Cd3z)
1q22-q23	TPM3, NEM1	Tropomyosin 3	191030	Nemaline myopathy 1, autosomal dominant, 161800 (3)	1 (Tpm3)
1q23	F5	Coagulation factor V (proaccelerin, labile factor)	227400	Hemorrhagic diathesis due to factor V deficiency (1); {Thromboembolism susceptibility due to factor V Leiden} (3)	1 (Cf5)
1q23	FCGR3A, CD16, IGFR3	Fc fragment of IgG, low affinity III, receptor for (CD16)	146740	{Lupus erythematosus, systemic, susceptibility}, 152700 (1); Neutropenia, alloimmune neonatal (3); {Viral infections, recurrent} (3)	
1q23	PBX1	Pre-B cell leukemia transcription factor-1	176310	Leukemia, acute pre-B-cell (2)	1 (Pbx)
1q23	TNFSF6, APT1 LG1, FASL	Tumor necrosis factor ligand superfamily, member 6	134638	{Systemic lupus erythematosus, susceptibility}, 152700 (3)	1 (Fas1)

continued

Table 10.1. The morbid anatomy of the human genome (by chromosome) (*continued*)

Location	Symbol	Title	MIM#	Disorder	Mouse
1q23-q25	AT3	Antithrombin III	107300	Antithrombin III deficiency (3)	1 (At3)
1q23-q25	FMO3	Flavin-containing monooxygenase 3	136132	[Fish-odor syndrome], 602079 (3)	
1q23-q25	SELE, ELAM1	Selectin E (endothelial leukocyte adhesion molecule-1)	131210	{Atherosclerosis, susceptibility to} (2)	1 (Elam)
1q23-q25	SELP, GRMP	Selectin P (granulocyte membrane protein, 140 kD; antigen CD62)	173610	Platelet alpha/delta storage pool deficiency (1)	1 (Grmp)
1q23.3	SLC19A2, THTR1	Solute carrier family 19 (folate transporter), member 2	603941	Thiamine-responsive megaloblastic anemia syndrome, 249270 (3)	
1q23.3-q24	HCA2	Hypercalciuria, absorptive, 2	605329	Hypercalciuria, absorptive, 2 (2)	
1q24	DFNM1	Deafness, nonsyndromic, modifier 1	605429	[Deafness, nonsyndromic, modifier 1] (2)	
1q24-q25	ABL2, ABLL, ARG	Abelson murine leukemia viral (v-abl) oncogene homolog 2 (arg, Abelson-related gene)	164690	Leukemia, acute myeloid, with eosinophilia (1)	1 (Abll)
1q24-q25	PRCA1, HPC1	Prostate cancer, hereditary, 1	601518	Prostate cancer, hereditary, 1, 176807 (2)	
1q24.3-q25.2	MYOC, TIGR, GLCIA, JOAG, GPOA	Myocilin (trabecular meshwork-induced glucocorticoid response protein)	601652	Glaucoma 1A, primary open angle, juvenile-onset, 137750 (3); Glaucoma 1A, primary open angle, recessive (3)	1 (Tigr)
1q25	NCF2	Neutrophil cytosolic factor-2, 65 kD	233710	Chronic granulomatous disease due to deficiency of NCF-2 (3)	1 (Ncf2)
1q25-q31	ARMD1	Macular degeneration, age-related, 1	603075	Macular degeneration, age-related, 1 (2)	
1q25-q31	HRPT2	Hyperparathyroidism 2, with jaw tumor	145001	Hyperparathyroidism-jaw tumor syndrome (2); Hyperparathyroidism, familial primary, 145000 (2)	
1q25-q31	LAMC2, LAMNB2, LAMB2T	Laminin, gamma-2 (nicein, 100 kD; kalinin, 105 kD; BM600, 100 kD)	150292	Epidermolysis bullosa, Herlitz junctional type, 226700 (3)	
1q25-q31	PDCN, NPHS2, SRN1	Podocin	604766	Nephrotic syndrome, steroid-resistant, 600995 (3)	
1q25-q31	PRG4, CACP, MSF, SZP	Proteoglycan 4 (megakaryocyte stimulating factor)	604283	Camptodactyly-arthropathy-coxa vara-pericarditis syndrome, 208250 (3)	
1q25-q31	SRN1	Nephrotic syndrome, idiopathic, steroid-resistant	600995	Nephrotic syndrome, idiopathic, steroid-resistant (2)	
1q31	BOS2	Branchiootic syndrome 2	120502	Branchiootic syndrome 2 (2)	
1q31	EBR2A	Epidermolysis bullosa 2A, junctional Herlitz	226450	Epidermolysis bullosa inversa, junctional (2)	
1q31	MCPH5	Microcephaly, primary autosomal recessive, 5	605481	Microcephaly, primary autosomal recessive, 5 (2)	
1q31-q32	CHIT	Chitotriosidase	600031	[Chitotriosidase deficiency] (3)	
1q31-q32	PTPRC, CD45, LCA	Protein tyrosine phosphatase, receptor type, c polypeptide	151460	{Multiple sclerosis, susceptibility to}, 126200 (3); Severe combined immunodeficiency due to PTPRC deficiency (3)	1 (Ly5)
1q31-q32.1	CRB1, RP12	Crumbs, Drosophila, homolog of, 1	604210	Retinitis pigmentosa-12, autosomal recessive, 600105 (3)	
1q31-q32.1	F13B	Coagulation factor XIII, B polypeptide	134580	Factor XIIIB deficiency (3)	1 (F13b)
1q31-q42	PHA2A, PHA2	Pseudohypoaldosteronism type II	145260	Pseudohypoaldosteronism, type II (2)	
1q31-q42	PSEN2, AD4, STM2	Presenilin 2	600759	Alzheimer disease-4 (3)	

continued

Table 10.1. The morbid anatomy of the human genome (by chromosome) (*continued*)

Location	Symbol	Title	MIM#	Disorder	Mouse
1q32	CACNA1S, CACNL1A3, CCHL1A3	Calcium channel, voltage-dependent, L type, alpha 1S subunit	114208	Hypokalemic periodic paralysis, 170400 (3); {Malignant hyperthermia susceptibility 5}, 601887 (3)	1 (Cchlla3, mdg)
1q32	CMD1D, CMPD2	Cardiomyopathy, dilated-1D, autosomal dominant	601494	Cardiomyopathy, familial, dilated-2 (2)	
1q32	CR1, C3BR	Complement component (3b/4b) receptor-1	120620	CR1 deficiency (1); {?SLE susceptibility} (1)	
1q32	GFND	Glomerulopathy with fibronectin deposits	601894	Glomerulopathy, fibronectin (2)	
1q32	HF1, CFH, HUS	H factor-1 (complement factor H)	134370	Factor H deficiency (1); Membroproliferative glomerulonephritis (1); Hemolytic-uremic syndrome, 235400 (3); Nephropathy, chronic hypocomplementemic (3)	1 (Cfh)
1q32	LAMB3	Laminin, beta-3 (nicein, 125 kD; kalinin, 140 kD; BM600, 125 kD)	150310	Epidermolysis bullosa, Herlitz junctional type, 226700 (3); Epidermolysis bullosa, generalized atrophic benign, 226650 (3)	
1q32	MCP, CD46	Membrane cofactor protein (CD46, trophoblast-lymphocyte cross-reactive antigen)	120920	{Measles, susceptibility to} (1)	
1q32	PPS	Popliteal pterygium syndrome	119500	Popliteal pterygium syndrome (3)	
1q32	REN	Renin	179820	[Hyperproreninemia] (3)	1 (Ren1)
1q32	TNNT2, CMH2	Troponin-T2, cardiac	191045	Cardiomyopathy, familial hypertrophic, 2, 115195 (3)	
1q32	VWS, LPS, PIT	van der Woude syndrome (lip pit syndrome)	119300	van der Woude syndrome (2)	
1q32-q44	PKP1	Plakophilin-1	601975	Ectodermal dysplasia/skin fragility syndrome, 604536 (3)	
1q41	RMD1	Rippling muscle disease 1	600332	Rippling muscle disease-1 (2)	
1q41	USH2A	Usherin	276901	Usher syndrome, type 2A (3)	
1q41-q42	SLEB1, SLE1	Systemic lupus erythematosus, susceptibility to, 1	601744	{Systemic lupus erythematosus, susceptibility to, 1}, 152700 (2)	1 (Nba2)
1q42	ADPRT, PPOL	ADP-ribosyltransferase NAD (+)	173870	?Xeroderma pigmentosum (1)	
1q42	MDC1B	Muscular dystrophy, congenital, 1B	604801	Muscular dystrophy, congenital, 1B (2)	
1q42-q43	AGT	Angiotensinogen	106150	{Hypertension, essential, susceptibility to} (3); {Preeclampsia, susceptibility to} (3)	8 (Agt)
1q42-q43	ARVD2	Arrhythmogenic right ventricular dysplasia-2 (arrhythmogenic right ventricular cardiomyopathy)	600996	Arrhythmogenic right ventricular dysplasia-2 (2)	
1q42-q43	HRD	Hypoparathyroidism-retardation-dysmorphism syndrome (Sanjad-Sakati syndrome)	241410	Hypoparathyroidism-retardation-dysmorphism syndrome (2)	
1q42-q43	KCS, KCS1	Kenny-Caffey syndrome-1	244460	Kenny-Caffey syndrome-1 (2)	

continued

Table 10.1. The morbid anatomy of the human genome (by chromosome) (*continued*)

Location	Symbol	Title	MIM#	Disorder	Mouse
1q42.1	ACTA1, ASMA, NEM2, NEM1	Actin, alpha-1, skeletal muscle	102610	Myopathy, nemaline, 161800, 256030 (3); Myopathy, actin (3)	8 (Actsk1)
1q42.1	EBAF, TGFB4, LEFTY1	Transforming growth factor, beta-4 (endometrial bleeding-associated factor; LEFTY A)	601877	Left-right axis malformation (3)	1 (lefty1)
1q42.1	EPHX1	Epoxide hydroxylase 1, microsomal xenobiotic	132810	?Fetal hydantoin syndrome (1); Diphenylhydantoin toxicity (1)	1 (Eph1)
1q42.1	FH	Fumarate hydratase	136850	Fumarase deficiency (3)	
1q42.1-q43	RYR2, VTSIP	Ryanodine receptor-2 (cardiac)	180902	Ventricular tachycardia, stress-induced polymorphic, 604772 (3)	13 (Ryr2)
1q42.1-q42.2	CHS1, LYST	Lysosomal trafficking regulator	214500	Chediak-Higashi syndrome (3)	13 (Lyst, bg)
1q42.2-q43	PCAP, PRCA2	Predisposing for prostate cancer	602759	Prostate cancer, hereditary, 2, 176807 (2)	
1q43	MTR	5-methyltetrahydrofolate-homocysteine methyltransferase 1	156570	Methylcobalamin deficiency, cb1 G type (3)	13 (Mtr)
1q44	MWS	Muckle-Wells syndrome	191900	Muckle-Wells syndrome (2)	
1q44	FCU	Cold urticaria, familial	120100	Cold urticaria, familial (2)	
Chr.1	GNPAT, DHAPAT	Glyceronephosphate O-acyltransferase	602744	Chondrodysplasia punctata, rhizomelic, type 2, 222765 (3)	
Chr.1	PEX10, NALD	Peroxisome biogenesis factor 10	602859	Zellweger syndrome, 214100 (3); Adrenoleukodystrophy, neonatal, 202370 (3)	
2p25.3	D2S448, MG50, D2S448E	Melanoma associated gene	600134	?Melanoma (1)	
2p25	TPO, TPX	Thyroid peroxidase	274500	Thyroid iodine peroxidase deficiency (1); Goiter, congenital (3); Hypothyroidism, congenital (3)	12 (Tpo)
2p25-p22	ETM2	Tremor, familial essential, 2	602134	Tremor, familial essential, 2 (2)	
2p24	APOB	Apolipoprotein B (including Ag(x) antigen)	107730	Hypobetalipoproteinemia (3); Abetalipoproteinemia (3); Hyperbetalipoproteinemia, 144400 (3); Apolipoprotein B-100, ligand-defective, 144010 (3)	12 (Apob)
2p24-p23	ODED, MODED	Oculodigitoesophagoduodenal syndrome	164280	Oculodigitoesophagoduodenal syndrome (2)	
2p23.3	POMC	Proopiomelanocortin (adrenocorticotropin/beta-lipotropin)	176830	ACTH deficiency (1); Obesity, adrenal insufficiency, and red hair (3)	12 (Pomc1)
2p23.3-p23.2	KHK	Ketohexokinase (fructokinase)	229800	[Fructosuria] (1)	
2p23	HADHA, MTPA	Hydroxyacyl-Coenzyme A dehydrogenase/3-ketoacyl-Coenzyme A thiolase/enoyl-Coenzyme A hydratase (trifunctional protein), alpha subunit	600890	LCHAD deficiency (3); Trifunctional protein deficiency, type 1 (3); HELLP syndrome, maternal, of pregnancy (3); Fatty liver, acute, of pregnancy (3)	
2p23	HADHB	Hydroxyacyl-Coenzyme A dehydrogenase/3-ketoacyl-Coenzyme A thiolase/enoyl-Coenzyme A hydratase (trifunctional protein), beta subunit	143450	Trifunctional protein deficiency, type II (3)	
2p23	SRD5A2	Steroid-5-alpha-reductase, alpha polypeptide-2 (3-oxo-5 alpha-steroid delta 4-dehydrogenase alpha-2)	264600	Pseudovaginal perineoscrotal hypospadias (3)	

continued

Table 10.1. The morbid anatomy of the human genome (by chromosome) (*continued*)

Location	Symbol	Title	MIM#	Disorder	Mouse
2p23-p22	OTOF, DFNB9, NSRD9	Otoferlin	603681	Deafness, autosomal recessive 9, 601071 (3)	
2p23-p22	XDH	Xanthine dehydrogenase (xanthine oxidase)	278300	Xanthinuria, type I (3)	17 (Xd)
2p22-p21	CYP1B1, GLC3A	Cytochrome P450, subfamily I, dioxin-inducible, polypeptide 1	601771	Glaucoma 3A, primary infantile, 231300 (3)	
2p22-p21	MSH2, COCA1, FCC1	mutS, E. coli, homolog of, 2	120435	Colorectal cancer, hereditary, nonpolyposis, type 1 (3); Ovarian cancer (3); Muir-Torre syndrome, 158320 (3)	
2p22-p21	SPG4, SPAST	Spastin	604277	Spastic paraplegia-4, 182601 (3)	
2p21	ABCG5	ATP-binding cassette, subfamily G, member 5	605459	Sitosterolemia, 210250 (3)	
2p21	ABCG8	ATP-binding cassette, subfamily G, member 8	605460	Sitosterolemia, 210250 (3)	
2p21	GF1, HGF	Gingival fibromatosis, hereditary, 1	135300	Fibromatosis, gingival (2)	
2p21	LHCGR	Luteinizing hormone/choriogonadotropin receptor	152790	Precocious puberty, male, 176410 (3); Pseudohermaphroditism, male, with Leydig cell hypoplasia (3); Hypogonadotropic hypogonadism (3); Micropenis (3); Leydig cell adenoma, with precocious puberty (3)	
2p21	SIX3, HPE2	Sine oculis homeo box, Drosophila, homolog of, 3	603714	Holoprosencephaly-2, 157170 (3)	17 (Six3)
2p21-p16	FSHR, ODG1	Follicle stimulating hormone receptor	136435	Ovarian dysgenesis, hypergonadotropic, with normal karyotype, 233300 (3)	
2p16.3	SLC3A1, ATR1, D2H, NBAT	Solute carrier family 3 (cystine, dibasic and neutral amino acid transporters), member 1	104614	Cystinuria, 220100 (3)	
2p16	CNC2	Carney complex, type II	605244	Carney complex, type II (2)	
2p16	EFEMP1, FBNL, DHRD	EGF-containing fibulin-like extracellular matrix protein 1 (fibrillin-like)	601548	Doyne honeycomb degeneration of retina, 126600 (3)	
2p16	MSH6, GTBP, HNPCC5	MutS, E. coli, homolog of, 6	600678	{Cancer susceptibility} (3); Endometrial carcinoma (3)	
2p16-p15	DYX3	Dyslexia, specific, 3	604254	Dyslexia, specific, 3 (2)	
2p15	PEX13, ZWS, NALD	Peroxisome biogenesis factor 13 (peroxin 13)	601789	Zellweger syndrome, 214100 (3); Adrenoleukodystrophy, neonatal, 202370 (3)	
2p13.3-p13.1	DYSF, LGMD2B	Dysferlin	603009	Muscular dystrophy, limb-girdle, type 2B, 253601 (3); Miyoshi myopathy, 254130 (3); Myopathy, distal, with anterior tibial onset (3)	6 (Dysf)
2p13	ALMS1, ALSS	Alstrom syndrome	203800	Alstrom syndrome (2)	
2p13	OFC2	Orofacial cleft-2	602966	Orofacial cleft-2 (2)	
2p13	PEE1, PREG1	Preeclampsia/eclampsia	189800	Preeclampsia (2)	
2p13	PARK3	Parkinson disease, type 3	602404	Parkinson disease, type 3 (2)	
2p13	WDM	Welander distal myopathy	604454	Welander distal myopathy (2)	

continued

Table 10.1. The morbid anatomy of the human genome (by chromosome) (*continued*)

Location	Symbol	Title	MIM#	Disorder	Mouse
2p13-p12	GCS1	Glucosidase I	601336	Glucosidase I deficiency (3)	
2p12	EIF2AK3, PEK, PERK, WRS	Eukaryotic translation initiation factor 2-alpha kinase 3	604032	Wolcott-Rallison syndrome, 226980 (3)	
2p12	GGCX	Gamma-glutamyl carboxylase	137167	Vitamin K-dependent coagulation defect, 277450 (3)	
2p12	IGKC	Immunoglobulin kappa constant region	147200	[Kappa light chain deficiency] (3)	6 (Igkc)
2p12-p11.2	SFTPB, SFTB3	Pulmonary surfactant-associated protein B, 18 kD	178640	Pulmonary alveolar proteinosis, congenital, 265120 (3)	6 (Sftp3)
2cen-q13	ATP6B1, VPP3	ATPase, H+ transporting, lysosomal, beta polypeptide, 58 kD (vacuolar proton pump, subunit 3)	192132	Renal tubular acidosis with deafness, 267300 (3)	8 (Atp6b1)
2cen-q13	GLC1B	Glaucoma 1, open angle, B (adult-onset)	137760	Glaucoma 1B, primary open angle, adult onset (2)	
2q11	CNGA3, CNG3, ACHM2	Cyclic nucleotide-gated channel, alpha-3	600053	Achromatopsia-2, 216900 (3)	
2q11-q13	DL, ED3, EDA3	Downless, mouse, homolog of	604095	Ectodermal dysplasia, hypohidrotic, autosomal dominant, 129490 (3); Ectodermal dysplasia, hypohidrotic, autosomal recessive, 224900 (3)	
2q12	ZAP70, SRK, STD	Zeta-chain associated protein kinase, 70 kD (syk-related tyrosine kinase)	176947	Selective T-cell defect (3)	1 (Zap70)
2q12-q13	OADIP, DIPOA	Osteoarthritis of distal interphalangeal joints	140600	?Osteoarthritis of distal interphalangeal joints (2)	
2q12-q14	PAX8	Paired box homeotic gene-8	167415	Hypothyroidism, congenital, due to thyroid dysgenesis or hypoplasia (3)	2 (Pax8)
2q13	NPHP1, NPH1	Nephronophthisis-1 gene	256100	Nephronophthisis, juvenile (3)	
2q13-q14	PROC	Protein C (inactivator of coagulation factors Va and VIIIa)	176860	Thrombophilia due to protein C deficiency (3); Purpura fulminans, neonatal (1)	
2q14	BUB1	Budding uninhibited by benzimidazoles 1, S. cerevisiae, homolog of (mitotic checkpoint gene BUB1)	602452	Colorectal cancer with chromosomal instability (3)	2 (Bub1)
2q14-q21	LCO	Liver cancer oncogene	165320	?Hepatocellular carcinoma (1)	
2q14-q22	CMDIH	Cardiomyopathy, dilated, 1H	604288	Cardiomyopathy, dilated, 1H (2)	
2q14.1	MERTK	Mer tyrosine kinase protooncogene	604705	Retinitis pigmentosa, MERTK-related, 268000 (3)	
2q21	ERCC3, XPB	Excision-repair cross-complementing rodent repair deficiency, complementation group 3	133510	Xeroderma pigmentosum, group B (3); Trichothiodystrophy (3)	
2q21-q31	SCP	Spastic cerebral palsy, symmetric, autosomal recessive	603513	Spastic cerebral palsy, symmetric (2)	
2q22	NEB	Nebulin	161650	Nemaline myopathy 2, autosomal recessive, 256030 (3)	2 (Neb)
2q22-q23	CACNB4	Calcium channel, voltage-dependent, beta 4 subunit	601949	Epilepsy, juvenile myoclonic, 254770 (3); Epilepsy, generalize idiopathic, 600669 (3); Ataxia, episodic (3)	2 (Cacnb4)
2q23-q24	FEB3	Convulsions, familial febrile, 3	604403	Convulsions, familial febrile, 3 (2)	
2q23-q24.3	DFNA16	Deafness, autosomal dominant 16	603964	Deafness, autosomal dominant 16 (2)	

continued

Table 10.1. The morbid anatomy of the human genome (by chromosome) (*continued*)

Location	Symbol	Title	MIM#	Disorder	Mouse
2q24	ABCB11, BSEP, SPGP, PFIC2	ATP-binding cassette, subfamily B, member 11 (bile salt export pump)	603201	Progressive intrahepatic cholestasis-2, 601847 (3)	
2q24	SCNIA, GEFSP2	Sodium channel, voltage-gated, type I, alpha polypeptide	182389	Epilepsy, generalized, with febrile seizures plus, type 2, 604233 (3)	2 (Scnla)
2q24	SPG13	Spastic paraplegia 13, autosomal dominant	605280	Spastic paraplegia-13 (2)	
2q24-q31	MPRM	Myopathy, proximal, with early respiratory muscle involvement (Edstrom myopathy)	603689	Myopathy, proximal, with early respiratory muscle involvement (2)	
2q24-q32	CHRNA1	Cholinergic receptor, nicotinic, alpha polypeptide-1, muscle	100690	Myasthenic syndrome, slow-channel congenital, 601462 (3)	2 (Acra)
2q24-q32	MMDK, MDK	Mesomelic dysplasia, Kantaputra type	156232	Mesomelic dysplasia, Kantaputra type (2)	
2q24.1	GPD2	Glycerol-3-phosphate dehydrogenase 2 (mitochondrial)	138430	{Diabetes mellitus, type II} (3)	
2q24.3	TTN	Titin	188840	Cardiomyopathy, familial hypertrophic, 9 (3)	2 (Ttn)
2q31	AGPS, ADHAPS	Alkylglycerone-phosphate synthase	603051	Rhizomelic chondrodysplasia punctata, type 3, 600121 (3)	
2q31	BBS5	Bardet-Biedl syndrome 5	603650	Bardet-Biedl syndrome 5 (2)	
2q31	CMDIG	Cardiomyopathy, dilated, 1G	604145	Cardiomyopathy, dilated, 1G (2)	
2q31	COL3A1	Collagen III, alpha-1 polypeptide	120180	Ehlers-Danlos syndrome, type IV, 130050 (3); Ehlers-Danlos syndrome, type III, 130020 (3); Aneurysm, familial arterial (3)	1 (Col3a1)
2q31	COL5A2	Collagen V, alpha-2 polypeptide	120190	Ehlers-Danlos syndrome, type I, 130000 (3)	
2q31	DURS2	Duane retraction syndrome 2	604356	Duane retraction syndrome 2 (2)	
2q31	IDDM7	Insulin-dependent diabetes mellitus-7	600321	{Diabetes mellitus, insulin-dependent, 7} (2)	
2q31	TMD	Tibial muscular dystrophy	600334	Tibial muscular dystrophy (2)	
2q31-q32	HOXD13, HOX4I, SPD	Homeo box-D13	142989	Synpolydactyly, type II, 186000 (3)	2 (Hox4.9)
2q31-q33	PMS1, PMSL1	Postmeiotic segregation increased, S. cerevisiae, like 1	600258	Colorectal cancer, hereditary nonpolyposis, type 3 (3)	
2q32	CPI, CPI, CPO	Cleft palate, isolated	119540	Cleft palate, isolated (2)	
2q32	NEUROD1, NIDDM	Neurogenic differentiation 1	601724	Diabetes mellitus, type II, 125853 (3)	2 (Neurod)
2q32	WSS	Wrinkly skin syndrome	278250	Wrinkly skin syndrome (2)	
2q32.1-q32.3	ARVD4	Arrhythmogenic right ventricular dysplasia-4	602087	Arrhythmogenic right ventricular dysplasia-4 (2)	
2q33	ALS2	Amyotrophic lateral sclerosis-2, juvenile recessive	205100	Amyotrophic lateral sclerosis, juvenile recessive (2)	
2q33	BMPR2, PPH1	Bone morphogenetic receptor, type II	600799	Pulmonary hypertension, familial primary, 178600 (3)	
2q33	IDDM12	Insulin-dependent diabetes mellitus-12	601388	{Diabetes mellitus, insulin-dependent, 12} (2)	

continued

Table 10.1. The morbid anatomy of the human genome (by chromosome) (*continued*)

Location	Symbol	Title	MIM#	Disorder	Mouse
2q33-q34	CHRNG, ACHRG	Cholinergic receptor, nicotinic, gamma polypeptide	100730	Myasthenia gravis, neonatal transient (2)	1 (Acrg)
2q33-q34	NDUFS1	NADH dehydrogenase (ubiquinone), Fe-S protein-1, 75 kD	157655	Lactic acidosis due to defect in iron-sulfur cluster of complex I (1)	
2q33-q35	CRYGC, CRYG3, CZP1, CAE1	Crystallin, gamma C	123680	Cataract, Coppock-like, 604307 (3); Cataract, variable zonular pulverulent (3)	
2q33-q35	CRYGD, CRYG4	Crystallin, gamma D	123690	Cataracts, punctate, progressive juvenile-onset (3); Cataract, crystalline aculeiform, 115700 (3)	1 (Crygd, Lop2)
2q33-q35	ICR2B, LI2	Ichthyosis congenita IIB	601277	Ichthyosis, lamellar, type 2 (2)	
2q33-q35	PCC, CCP	Cataract, polymorphic congenital, autosomal dominant nonnuclear	601286	Cataract, polymorphic congenital (2)	
2q33-q35	PNKD, FPD1, PDC, DYT8	Paroxysmal nonkinesiogenic dyskinesia	118800	Choreoathetosis, familial paroxysmal (2)	
2q33-q37	FLNMS	Finnish lethal neonatal metabolic syndrome	603358	Finnish lethal neonatal metabolic syndrome (2)	
2q33-qter	CYP27A1, CYP27, CTX	Cytochrome P450, subfamily XXVIIA, polypeptide 1 (sterol 27-hydroxylase)	213700	Cerebrotendinous xanthomatosis (3)	1 (Cyp27)
2q34	FN1	Fibronectin-1	135600	?Ehlers-Danlos syndrome, type X, 225310 (1)	1 (Fn1)
2q34	IDDM13	Insulin-dependent diabetes mellitus-13	601318	{Diabetes mellitus, insulin-dependent, 13} (2)	
2q34	TCL4	T-cell leukemia/lymphoma-4	186860	Leukemia/lymphoma, T-cell (2)	
2q34-q35	ACADL, LCAD	Acyl-Coenzyme A dehydrogenase, long chain	201460	Acyl-CoA dehydrogenase, long chain, deficiency of (3)	1 (Acad1)
2q34-q36	BJS, PTD	Bjornstad syndrome (pili torti and deafness)	262000	Bjornstad syndrome (2)	
2q34-q36	SDTY1, SD1	Syndactyly, type I	185900	Syndactyly, type 1 (2)	
2q35	CPS1	Carbamoyl-phosphate synthetase 1, mitochondrial	237300	Carbamoylphosphate synthetase I deficiency (3)	1 (Cps)
2q35	DES, CMD1I	Desmin	125660	Myopathy, desmin-related, cardioskeletal, 601419 (3); Cardiomyopathy, dilated, II, 604765 (3)	1 (Des)
2q35	PAX3, WS1, HUP2, CDHS	Paired box homeotic gene-3	193500	Waardenburg syndrome, type I (3); Waardenburg syndrome, type III, 148820 (3); Rhabdomyosarcoma, alveolar, 268220 (3); Craniofacial-deafness-hand syndrome, 122880 (3)	1 (Sp)
2q35	NRAMP1, NRAMP	Natural resistance-associated macrophage protein	600266	?Resistance/susceptibility to TB, etc. (1)	1 (Nramp)
2q35-q36	BDA1	Brachydactyly, type A1	112500	Brachydactyly, type A1 (2)	
2q36	IRS1	Insulin receptor substrate-1	147545	{Diabetes mellitus, noninsulin-dependent} (3)	1 (Irs1)
2q36-q37	AGXT, SPAT	Alanine-glyoxylate aminotransferase, liver-specific peroxisomal	604285	Hyperoxaluria, primary, type 1, 259900 (3)	
2q36-q37	COL4A3	Collagen IV, alpha-3 polypeptide (Goodpasture antigen)	120070	Alport syndrome, autosomal recessive, 203780 (3)	

continued

Table 10.1. The morbid anatomy of the human genome (by chromosome) *(continued)*

Location	Symbol	Title	MIM#	Disorder	Mouse
2q36-q37	COL4A4	Collagen IV, alpha-4 polypeptide	120131	Alport syndrome, autosomal recessive, 203780 (3); Hematuria, familial benign (3)	
2q36-q37	GCG	Glucagon	138030	[?Hyperproglucagonemia] (1)	2 (Gcg)
2q37	BDE	Brachydactyly type E	113300	?Brachydactyly type E (2)	
2q37	BDMR	Brachydactyly-mental retardation syndrome	600430	Brachydactyly-mental retardation syndrome (2)	
2q37	COL6A3	Collagen VI, alpha-3 polypeptide	120250	Bethlem myopathy, 158810 (3)	1 (Col6a3)
2q37	SLEB2	Systemic lupus erythematosus, susceptibility to, 2	605218	{Systemic lupus erythematosus, susceptibility to, 2}, 152700 (2)	
2q37.1	SAG	S-antigen; retina and pineal gland (arrestin)	181031	Oguchi disease-1, 258100 (3)	1 (Sag)
2q37.3	CAPN10	Calpain-10	605286	{Diabetes mellitus, non-insulin dependent, 1}, 601283 (3)	
Chr.2	ITGA6	Integrin, alpha-6	147556	Epidermolysis bullosa, junctional, with pyloric stenosis, 226730 (3)	
Chr.2	LSFC	Leigh syndrome, French-Canadian type	220111	Leigh syndrome, French-Canadian type (2)	
Chr.2	UGT1A, UGT1, UGT1A1, GNT1	UDP glycosyltransferase 1A	191740	Crigler-Najjar syndrome, type I, 218800 (3); [Gilbert syndrome], 143500 (3)	1 (Ugt1)
3p26.2	OGG1	8-hydroxyguanine DNA glycosylase	601982	Renal cell carcinoma, clear cell, 144700 (3)	6 (Ogg1)
3p26-p25	VHL	von Hippel-Lindau syndrome	193300	von Hippel-Lindau syndrome (3); Renal cell carcinoma (3)	
3p26-p24.2	MYMY	Moyamoya disease	252350	Moyamoya disease (2)	
3p25.3	FANCD, FACD, FAD	Fanconi anemia, complementation group D	227646	Fanconi anemia, type D (2)	
3p25	CAV3, LGMD1C	Caveolin-3	601253	Muscular dystrophy, limb-girdle, type IC (3)	
3p25	BTD	Biotinidase	253260	Biotinidase deficiency (3)	
3p25	PPARG, PPARG1, PPARG2	Peroxisome proliferator activated receptor, gamma	601487	Obesity, severe, 601665 (3); [Obesity, protection against] (3); Diabetes mellitus, insulin-resistant, with acanthosis nigricans and hypertension, 604367 (3)	
3p25	XPC, XPCC	Xeroderma pigmentosum, complementation group C	278720	Xeroderma pigmentosum, group C (3)	6 (Xpc)
3p25-p24.2	MFS2	Marfan-like connective tissue disorder	154705	Marfan-like connective tissue disorder (2)	
3p25-p22	CMD1E, CDCD2, CMPD2	Cardiomyopathy, dilated, 1E, autosomal dominant	601154	Cardiomyopathy, dilated, 1E (2)	
3p24.3	THRB, ERBA2, THR1	Thyroid hormone receptor, beta (avian erythroblastic leukemia viral (v-erb-a) oncogene homolog-2)	190160	Thyroid hormone resistance, 274300, 188570 (3)	
3p24.2	COLQ, EAD	Collagenic tail of endplate acetylcholinesterase	603033	Endplate acetylcholinesterase deficiency, 603034 (3)	
3p24.2-p23	USH2B	Usher syndrome, type IIB	276905	Usher syndrome, type IIB (2)	

continued

Table 10.1. The morbid anatomy of the human genome (by chromosome) (*continued*)

Location	Symbol	Title	MIM#	Disorder	Mouse
3p23	ARVD5, ARVC5	Arrhythmogenic right ventricular dysplasia-5	604400	Arrhythmogenic right ventricular dysplasia-5 (2)	
3p23-p22	ACAA1	Acetyl-Coenzyme A acyltransferase 1 (peroxisomal 3-oxoacyl-Coenzyme A thiolase)	604054	Pseudo-Zellweger syndrome, 261510 (1)	
3p23-p21	SCLC1	Small-cell cancer of lung	182280	Small-cell cancer of lung (2)	
3p22	TGFBR2, HNPCC6	Transforming growth factor, beta receptor II, 70–80 kD	190182	Colon cancer (3); Colorectal cancer, familial nonpolyposis, type 6 (3); Esophageal cancer, 133239 (3)	
3p22-p21.3	CTNNB1	Catenin (cadherin-associated protein), beta 1, 88 kD	116806	Colorectal cancer (3); Hepatoblastoma (3); Pilomatricoma (3); Ovarian carcinoma, endometrioid type (3)	9 (Catnb)
3p22-p21.3	DLEC1, DLC1	Deleted in lung and esophageal cancer 1	604050	Lung cancer, 211980 (1); Esophageal cancer, 133239 (1)	
3p22-p21.1	FHBL2	Hypobetalipoproteinemia, familial, 2	605019	Hypobetalipoproteinemia, familial, 2 (2)	
3p22-p21.1	PTHR1, PTHR	Parathyroid hormone receptor-1	168468	Metaphyseal chondrodysplasia, Murk Jansen type, 156400 (3)	
3p21.33	GLB1	Galactosidase, beta-1	230500	GM1-gangliosidosis (3); Mucopolysaccharidosis IVB (3)	9 (Bgl)
3p21.31	CACT, CAC	Carnitine-acylcarnitine translocase	212138	Carnitine-acylcarnitine translocase deficiency (3)	
3p21.3	COL7A1	Collagen VII, alpha-1 polypeptide	120120	Epidermolysis bullosa dystrophica, dominant, 131750 (3); Epidermolysis bullosa dystrophica, recessive, 226600 (3); Epidermolysis bullosa, pretibial, dominant and recessive, 131850 (3); Epidermolysis bullosa dystrophica, Bart type, 132000 (3); Epidermolysis bullosa dystrophica, generalized atrophic benign, 226650 (3); Epidermolysis bullosa dystrophica, localisata variant (3); Transient bullous dermolysis of the newborn, 131705 (3); Epidermolysis bullosa pruriginosa, autosomal recessive, 604129 (3)	
3p21.3	GPX1	Glutathione peroxidase-1	138320	Hemolytic anemia due to glutathione peroxidase deficiency (1)	
3p21.3	MLH1, COCA2	mutL, E. coli, homolog of, 1	120436	Colorectal cancer, hereditary nonpolyposis, type 2 (3); Turcot syndrome with glioblastoma, 276300 (3); Muir-Torre family cancer syndrome, 158320 (3); Leukemia (3)	
3p21.3-p21.2	HYAL1	Hyaluronoglucosaminidase 1	601492	Mucopolysaccharidosis type IX (3)	9 (Hyal1)
3p21.2-p21.1	AMT	Aminomethyltransferase (glycine cleavage system protein T)	238310	Hyperglycinemia, nonketotic, 2 (1)	
3p21.2-p21.1	HESX1, RPX	Homeo box gene expressed in ES cells	601802	Septooptic dysplasia, 182230 (3)	14 (Hesx1)
3p21.1	ARP	Arginine-rich protein	601916	Pancreatic cancer (2)	
3p21.1-p14.1	LRS1, LAR1	Larsen syndrome 1, autosomal dominant	150250	Larsen syndrome, autosomal dominant (2)	

continued

Table 10.1. The morbid anatomy of the human genome (by chromosome) (*continued*)

Location	Symbol	Title	MIM#	Disorder	Mouse
3p21.1-p12	SCA7, OPCA3	Spinocerebellar ataxia 7 gene	164500	Spinocerebellar ataxia-7 (3)	
3p21	AGS1	Aicardi-Goutieres syndrome 1	225750	Aicardi-Goutieres syndrome 1 (2)	
3p21	CMKBR2, CCR2	Chemokine (C-C) receptor 2	601267	{HIV infection, susceptibility/resistence to} (3)	
3p21	CMKBR5, CCCKR5	Chemokine (C-C) receptor 5	601373	{HIV infection, susceptibility/resistance to} (3)	
3p21	GNA12, GNA12B, GIP	Guanine nucleotide-binding protein (G protein), alpha-inhibiting activity polypeptide-2	139360	Pituitary ACTH-secreting adenoma (3); Ventricular tachycardia, idiopathic, 192605 (3)	9 (Gnai2)
3p21	IECN2, NCIE2	Ichthyosiform erythroderma, congenital, nonbullous, 2	604780	Ichthyosiform erythroderma, congenital, nonbullous, 2 (2)	
3p21	GNAT1	Guanine nucleotide-binding protein (G protein), alpha-transducing (transducin) activity polypeptide-1	139330	Night blindness, congenital stationary (3)	9 (Gnat1)
3p21	SCN5A, LQT3, IVF, HB2	Sodium channel, voltage-gated, type V, alpha polypeptide	600163	Long QT syndrome-3, 603830 (3); Brugada syndrome, 601144 (3); Heart block, progressive, 2, 604559 (3); Heart block, nonprogressive, 604559 (3); Ventricular fibrillation, idiopathic, 603829 (3)	
3p21-p14	DFNB6	Deafness, autosomal recessive 6	600971	Deafness, autosomal recessive 6 (2)	?9 (sr)
3p14.3	TKT	Transketolase	277730	{Wernicke-Korsakoff syndrome, susceptibility to} (1)	
3p14.1-p12.3	MITF, WS2A	Microphthalmia-associated transcription factor	156845	Waardenburg syndrome, type IIA, 193510 (3); Waardenburg syndrome/ocular albinism, digenic, 103470 (3); Tietz syndrome, 103500 (3)	6 (mi)
3p13-p12	BBS3	Bardet-Biedl syndrome 3	600151	Bardet-Biedl syndrome 3 (2)	
3p12	GBE1	Glycogen branching enzyme	232500	Glycogen storage disease IV (3)	
3p11.1-q11.2	DMT1	Dementia, familial, nonspecific	600795	Dementia, familial, nonspecific (2)	
3p11.1-q11.2	PROS1	Protein S, alpha	176880	Protein S deficiency (3)	
3p11	POU1F1, PIT1	POU domain, class 1, transcription factor 1 (Pit1, growth hormone factor 1)	173110	Pituitary hormone deficiency, combined (3)	16 (Pit1, dw)
3p	MYL3	Myosin, light polypeptide-3, alkali; ventricular, skeletal, slow	160790	Cardiomopathy, hypertrophic,	9 (Mylc)
3q	DFNB15	Deafness, autosomal recessive 15	601869	Deafness, autosomal recessive 15 (2)	
3q	DM2	Myotonic dystrophy 2	602668	Myotonic dystrophy 2 (2)	
3q12	CPO	Coproporphyrinogen oxidase	121300	Coproporphyria (3); Harderoporphyrinuria (3)	
3q13	ETM1, FET1	Tremor, familial essential, 1	190300	Tremor, familial essential, 1 (2)	
3q13	FIH	Hypoparathyroidism	146200	Hypoparathyroidism, familial (2)	
3q13	UMPS, OPRT	Uridine monophosphate synthetase (orotate phosphoribosyl transferase and orotidine-5'-decarboxylase)	258900	Oroticaciduria (3)	
3q13-q22	CMT2B	Charcot-Marie-Tooth neuropathy 2B	600882	Charcot-Marie-Tooth neuropathy-2B (2)	

continued

Table 10.1. The morbid anatomy of the human genome (by chromosome) (*continued*)

Location	Symbol	Title	MIM#	Disorder	Mouse
3q13.1	HMSNO, HMSNP	Neuropathy, hereditary motor and sensory, Okinawa type	604484	Neuropathy, hereditary motor and sensory, Okinawa type (2)	
3q13.1	MHS4	Malignant hyperthermia susceptibility 4	600467	{Malignant hyperthermia susceptibility 4} (2)	
3q13.3	DRD3	Dopamine receptor D3	126451	{?Schizophrenia, susceptibility to} (2)	
3q13.3-q21	CASR, HHC1, PCAR1	Calcium-sensing receptor	601199	Hypocalciuric hypercalcemia, type I, 145980 (3); Neonatal hyperparathyroidism, 239200 (3); Hypocalcemia, autosomal dominant, 601198 (3)	
3q13.3-q21	TRH	Thyrotropin-releasing hormone	275120	Thyrotropin-releasing hormone deficiency (1)	6 (Trh)
3q21	ATOD	Dermatitis, atopic	603165	Dermatitis, atopic (2)	
3q21	PSORS5	Psoriasis susceptibility 5	604316	{Psoriasis susceptibility} (2)	
3q21	TF	Transferrin	190000	Atransferrinemia (1)	9 (Trf)
3q21-q22	MBS2	Moebius syndrome 2	601471	Moebius syndrome-2 (2)	
3q21-q22	PCCB	Propionyl Coenzyme A carboxylase, beta polypeptide	232050	Propionicacidemia, type II or pccB type (3)	
3q21-q23	HGD, AKU	Homogentisate 1,2-dioxygenase (homogentisate oxidase)	203500	Alkaptonuria (3)	16 (aku)
3q21-q23	LTF	Lactotransferrin	150210	?Lactoferrin-deficient neutrophils, 245480 (1)	9 (Ltf)
3q21-q24	ATP2C1, BCPM, HHD	ATPase, Ca(2+)-sequestering	604384	Hailey-Hailey disease, 169600 (3)	
3q21-q24	GLC1C	Glaucoma 1, open angle, C	601682	Glaucoma 1C, primary open angle (2)	
3q21-q24	RHO, RP4	Rhodopsin	180380	Retinitis pigmentosa-4, autosomal dominant (3); Retinitis pigmentosa, autosomal recessive (3); Night blindness, congenital stationery, rhodopsin-related (3)	6 (Rho)
3q21-q25	AGTR1, AGTR1A, AT2R1	Angiotensin receptor 1	106165	Hypertension, essential, 145500 (3)	
3q21-q25	BFSP2, CP49, CP47	Beaded filament structural protein 2 (cytoskeletal protein, 49 kD)	603212	Cataract, juvenile-onset, 604219 (3); Cataract, congenital, 604219 (3)	
3q21-q25	USH3	Usher syndrome-3	276902	Usher syndrome, type 3 (2)	
3q22	NPHP3, NPH3	Nephronophthisis, adolescent	604387	Nephronophthisis, adolescent (2)	
3q22-q23	BPES, BPES1	Blepharophimosis, epicanthus inversus, and ptosis 1	110100	Blepharophimosis, epicanthus inversus, and ptosis, type 1 (2)	
3q22.1-q24	SCKL	Seckel syndrome	210600	Seckel syndrome (2)	
3q23-q24	CP	Ceruloplasmin	117700	[Hypoceruloplasminemia, hereditary] (1); Hemosiderosis, systemic, due to aceruloplasminemia (3)	9 (Cp)
3q25-q26	SI	Sucrase-isomaltase	222900	Sucrose intolerance (3)	3 (Sis)
3q25.1	MLF1	Myeloid leukemia factor-1	601402	Leukemia, myeloid, acute (1)	
3q25.2-q27	CCM3	Cerebral cavernous malformations-3	603285	Cerebral cavernous malformations-3 (2)	

continued

Table 10.1. The morbid anatomy of the human genome (by chromosome) (*continued*)

Location	Symbol	Title	MIM#	Disorder	Mouse
3q26	EVI1	Ectropic viral integration site-1 (oncogene EVI1)	165215	3q21q26 syndrome (1)	3 (Evi1)
3q26	MDS1	Myelodysplasia syndrome-1	600049	Myelodysplasia syndrome-1 (3)	
3q26	SERPINI1, PI12	Protease inhibitor 12	602445	Encephalopathy, familial, with neuroserpin inclusion bodies, 604218 (3)	
3q26.1-q26.2	BCHE, CHE1	Butyrylcholinesterase	177400	Apnea, postanesthetic (3)	
3q26.1-q26.3	SLC2A2, GLUT2	Solute carrier family 2 (facilitated glucose transporter), member 2	138160	{Diabetes mellitus, noninsulin-dependent} (3); Fanconi-Bickel syndrome, 227810 (3)	
3q26.3	CDL1	Cornelia de Lange syndrome 1	122470	?Cornelia de Lange syndrome (2)	
3q26.3	PIK3CA	Phosphatidylinositol 3-kinase, catalytic, alpha polypeptide	171834	Ovarian cancer (1)	
3q26.3-q27	THPO, MGDF, MPLLG, TPO	Thrombopoietin (megakaryocyte growth and development factor)	600044	Thrombocythemia, essential, 187950 (3)	16 (Thpo)
3q27	BCL6	B-cell CLL/lymphoma-6	109565	Lymphoma, B-cell (2); Lymphoma, diffuse large cell (3)	16 (Bcl6)
3q27	CLDN16, PCLN1	Claudin 16 (paracellin 1)	603959	Hypomagnesemia, primary, 248250 (3)	
3q27	EHHADH, PBFE	Enoyl-Coenzyme A, hydratase/3-hydroxyacyl Coenzyme A dehydrogenase	261515	Peroxisomal bifunctional enzyme deficiency (1)	
3q27	HRG	Histidine-rich glycoprotein	142640	Thrombophilia due to HRG deficiency (3); ?Thrombophilia due to elevated HRG (1)	
3q27	KNG	Kininogen	228960	[Kininogen deficiency] (3)	
3q27	LMS	Limb-mammary syndrome	603543	Limb-mammary syndrome (2)	
3q27	LVWM, CACH	Leukoencephalopathy with vanishing white matter	603896	Leukoencephalopathy with vanishing white matter (2)	
3q27	TP63, KET, EEC3, SHFM4	Tumor protein p63	603273	Ectrodactyly, ectodermal dysplasia, and cleft lip/palate syndrome 3, 604292 (3); Split-hand/foot malformation, type 4, 605289 (3)	16 (Trp63)
3q27-q28	SPG14	Spastic paraplegia 14, autosomal recessive	605229	Spastic paraplegia 14, autosomal recessive (2)	
3q28	LPP	Lipoma-preferred-partner gene	600700	Lipoma (1)	
3q28-q29	OPA1	Optic atrophy 1 gene	605290	Optic atrophy 1, 165500 (3)	?16 (Bst)
Chr.3	GP9	Glycoprotein IX, platelet	173515	Bernard-Soulier syndrome, type C (3)	
4p16.3	CRBM	Cherubism	118400	Cherubism (2)	
4p16.3	DFNA6	Deafness, autosomal dominant 6	600965	Deafness, autosomal dominant 6 (2)	
4p16.3	FGFR3, ACH	Fibroblast growth factor receptor-3	134934	Achondroplasia, 100800 (3); Hypochondroplasia, 146000 (3); Thanatophoric dysplasia, types I and II, 187600 (3); Crouzon syndrome with acanthosis nigricans (3); Muencke syndrome, 602849 (3); Bladder cancer, 109800 (3); Cervical cancer, 603956 (3)	5 (Fgfr3)

continued

Table 10.1. The morbid anatomy of the human genome (by chromosome) (*continued*)

Location	Symbol	Title	MIM#	Disorder	Mouse
4p16.3	HD, IT15	Huntingtin	143100	Huntington disease (3)	5 (Hdh)
4p16.3	IDUA, IDA	Iduronidase, alpha-L-	252800	Mucopolysaccharidosis Ih (3); Mucopolysaccharidosis Is (3); Mucopolysaccharidosis Ih/s (3)	5 (Idua)
4p16.3	PDE6B, PDEB, CSNB3	Phosphodiesterase-6B, cGMP-specific, rod, beta	180072	Night blindness, congenital stationary, type 3, 163500 (3); Retinitis pigmentosa, autosomal recessive (3)	5 (Pdeb, rd)
4p16.3	WHCR	Wolf-Hirschhorn syndrome chromosome region	194190	Wolf-Hirschhorn syndrome (2)	
4p16.2-p12	PROML1, AC133	Prominin, mouse, homolog-like 1	604365	Retinal degeneration, autosomal recessive, prominin-related (3)	
4p16.1	MSX1, HOX7, HYD1	msh, Drosophila, homeo box homolog of, 1 (formerly homeo box 7)	142983	Hypodontia, autosomal dominant, 106600 (3); Hypodontia with orofacial cleft, 106600 (3)	5 (Hox7)
4p16.1	WFS1, WFRS, WFS	Wolframin	222300	Wolfram syndrome (3)	
4p16	CRSA, CRS3	Craniosynostosis, Adelaide type	600593	Craniosynostosis, Adelaide type (2)	
4p16	EVC	Ellis-van Creveld syndrome gene	604831	Ellis-van Creveld syndrome, 225500 (3); Weyers acrodental dysostosis, 193530 (3)	
4p16-p15.2	SLEB3	Systemic lupus erythematosus, susceptibility to, 3	605480	{Systemic lupus erythematosus, susceptibility to, 3}, 152700 (2)	
4p15.31	QDPR, DHPR	Quinoid dihydropteridine reductase	261630	Phenylketonuria due to dihydropteridine reductase deficiency (3)	5 (Qdpr)
4p15.3	HLN2	Huntington-like neurodegenerative disorder 2	604802	Huntington-like neurodegenerative disorder 2 (2)	
4p14	UCHL1	Ubiquitin C-terminal esterase L1	191342	Parkinson disease, familial, 168600 (3)	
4p15	PARK4	Parkinson disease #4, autosomal dominant Lewy body	605543	Parkinson disease #4, autosomal dominant Lewy body, (2)	
4p13-q12	TAPVR1	Total anomalous pulmonary venous return	106700	Total anomalous pulmonary venous return (2)	
4p12-cen	CNGA1, CNCG1	Cyclic nucleotide gated channel, alpha 1	123825	Retinitis pigmentosa, autosomal recessive (3)	5 (Cncg)
4p	MHW1	Mental health wellness 1	603663	{Mental health wellness-1} (2)	
4p	STGD4	Stargardt disease 4	603786	Stargardt disease 4 (2)	
4q	DTDP2	Dentin dysplasia, Shields type II	125420	Dentin dysplasia, type II (2)	
4q	MHW2	Mental health wellness 2	603664	{Mental health wellness-2} (2)	
4q	PSORS3	Psoriasis susceptibility 3	601454	{Psoriasis susceptibility 3} (3)	
4q11-q12	CHIC2, BTL	Cysteine-rich hydrophobic domain 2 (Brx-like gene translocated in leukemia)	604332	{Leukemia, acute myeloid} (3)	
4q11-q13	AFP, HPAFP	Alpha-fetoprotein	104150	[AFP deficiency, congenital] (1); [Hereditary persistence of alpha-fetoprotein] (3)	5 (Afp)
4q11-q13	ALB	Albumin	103600	Analbuminemia (3); [Dysalbuminemic hyperthyroxinemia] (3); [Dysalbuminemic hyperzincemia], 194470 (3)	5 (Alb1)

continued

Table 10.1. The morbid anatomy of the human genome (by chromosome) (*continued*)

Location	Symbol	Title	MIM#	Disorder	Mouse
4q11-q13	JPD	Periodontitis, juvenile	170650	Periodontitis, juvenile (2)	
4q11-q21	AIH2	Amelogenesis imperfecta-2, hypocalcification, autosomal dominant	104500	Amelogenesis imperfecta-2, hypoplastic local type (2)	
4q12	SGCB, LGMD2E	Sarcoglycan, beta (43 kD dystrophin-associated glycoprotein)	600900	Muscular dystrophy, limb-girdle, type 2E, 604286 (3)	
4q12	KIT, PBT	Hardy-Zuckerman 4 feline sarcoma (v-kit) oncogene	164920	Piebaldism (3); Mast cell leukemia (3); Mastocytosis with associated hematologic disorder (3); Germ cell tumors, 273300 (3)	5 (Kit; W)
4q13-q21	DGI1	Dentinogenesis imperfecta-1	125490	Dentinogenesis imperfecta-1 (2)	
4q21	HIES	Hyper-IgE syndrome	147060	Hyper-IgE syndrome (2)	
4q21	SLC4A4, NBC1, KNBC, SLC4A5	Solute carrier family 4, sodium bicarbonate cotransporter, member 4	603345	Renal tubular acidosis, proximal, with ocular abnormalities, 604278 (3)	
4q21	SNCA, NACP, PARK1	Synuclein, alpha (non A4 component of amyloid precursor)	163890	Parkinson disease, type 1, 601508 (3)	
4q21-q23	GNPTA	UDP-N-acetylglucosamine-lysosomal-enzyme N-acetylglucosamine phosphotransferase	252500	Mucolipidosis II (1); Mucolipidosis III (1)	
4q21-q23	PKD2, PKD4	Polycystin-2	173910	Polycystic kidney disease, adult, type II (3)	5 (Pkd2)
4q21-q25	RAP1GDS1	RAP1, GTP-GDP dissociation stimulator 1	179502	Lymphocytic leukemia, acute T-cell (3)	
4q21.2	GNRHR	Gonadotropin-releasing hormone receptor	138850	Hypogonadotropic hypogonadism (3)	5 (Gnrhr)
4q22	ADH2	Alcohol dehydrogenase (class I), beta polypeptide	103720	{Alcoholism, susceptibility to} (1)	
4q22-q24	MTP	Microsomal triglyceride transfer protein, 88 kD	157147	Abetalipoproteinemia, 200100 (3)	3 (Mtp)
4q22-q24	WFS2	Wolfram syndrome 2	604928	Wolfram syndrome 2 (2)	
4q22-q25	MANBA, MANB1	Mannosidase, beta A, lysosomal	248510	Mannosidosis, beta-(3)	3 (Bmn)
4q23	TYS, HRZ	Sclerotylosis	181600	Huriez syndrome (2)	
4q25	IF	I factor (complement component I)	217030	C3b inactivator deficiency (3)	
4q25-q26	PITX2, IDG2, RIEG1, RGS, IGDS2	Paired-like homeodomain transcription factor-2	601542	Rieger syndrome, 180500 (3); Iridogoniodysgenesis syndrome-2, 137600 (3)	
4q25-q27	LQT4	Long QT syndrome-4	600919	Long QT syndrome-4 with sinus bradycardia (2)	
4q26-q27	IL2	Interleukin-2	147680	Severe combined immunodeficiency due to IL2 deficiency (1)	3 (Il2)
4q27-q31	FOP	Fibrodysplasia ossificans progressiva	135100	Fibrodysplasia ossificans progressiva (2)	
4q28	FGA	Fibrinogen, alpha polypeptide	134820	Dysfibrinogenemia, alpha type, causing bleeding diathesis (3); Dysfibrinogenemia, alpha type, causing recurrent thrombosis (3); Amyloidosis, hereditary renal, 105200 (3); Afibrinogenemia, 202400 (3)	

continued

Table 10.1. The morbid anatomy of the human genome (by chromosome) (*continued*)

Location	Symbol	Title	MIM#	Disorder	Mouse
4q28	FGB	Fibrinogen, beta polypeptide	134830	Dysfibrinogenemia, beta type (3); Afibrinogenemia, congenital, 202400 (3); Thrombophilia, dysfibrinogenemic (3)	
4q28	FGG	Fibrinogen, gamma polypeptide	134850	Dysfibrinogenemia, gamma type (3); Hypofibrinogenemia, gamma type (3); Thrombophilia, dysfibrinogenemic (3)	3 (Fgg)
4q28-q31	ASMD	Anterior segment mesenchymal dysgenesis	107250	Anterior segment mesenchymal dysgenesis (2)	
4q28-q31	HCL2, RHC	Hair color 2, red	266300	[Hair color, red] (2)	
4q31	DFNB26	Deafness, autosomal recessive 26	605428	Deafness, autosomal recessive 26 (2)	
4q31.1	NR3C2, MLR, MCR	Nuclear receptor subfamily 3, group C, member 2 (mineralocorticoid receptor; aldosterone receptor)	600983	Pseudohypoaldosteronism type I, autosomal dominant, 177735 (3); Hypertension, early-onset, autosomal dominant, with exacerbation in pregnancy, 605115 (3)	
4q32-q33	AGA	Aspartylglucosaminidase	208400	Aspartylglucosaminuria (3)	8 (Aga)
4q32-qter	ETFDH	Electron transfer flavoprotein: ubiquinone oxidoreductase	231675	Glutaricaciduria, type IIC (3)	3 (Etfdh)
4q32.1	HVBS6	Hepatitis B virus integration site-6	142380	Hepatocellular carcinoma (3)	
4q33-qter	HCA	Hypercalciuria, absorptive	143870	Hypercalciuria, absorptive (2)	
4q35	BHD, BFHD	Beukes familial hip dysplasia	142669	Hip dysplasia, Beukes type (2)	
4q35	F11	Coagulation factor XI (plasma thromboplastin antecedent)	264900	Factor XI deficiency (3)	8 (cf11)
4q35	FSHMD1A, FSHD1A	Facioscapulohumeral muscular dystrophy-1A	158900	Facioscapulohumeral muscular dystrophy-1A (2)	?8 (myd)
4q35	KLKB1, KLK3	Kallikrein B plasma 1 (Fletcher factor)	229000	Fletcher factor deficiency (1)	8 (Kal3)
4q35-qter	BCD	Bietti crystalline corneoretinal dystrophy	210370	Bietti crystalline corneoretinal dystrophy (2)	
4q35	SLC25A4, ANT1, T1, PEO3	Solute carrier family 25 (mitochondrial carrier) member 4 (adenine nucleotide translocator-1, skeletal muscle)	103220	Progressive external ophthalmoplegia, type 3, 601227 (3)	8 (Ant1)
Chr.4	LAG5	Leukocyte antigen group 5	151450	Neutropenia, neonatal alloimmune (1)	
5p15.3	SLC6A3, DAT1	Solute carrier family 6 (neurotransmitter transporter, dopamine), member 3	126455	{Attention-deficit hyperactivity disorder, susceptibility to}, 143465 (2)	13 (Dat1)
5p15.3-p15.2	MTRR	Methionine synthase reductase	602568	Homocystinuria-megaloblastic anemia, cb1 E type, 236270 (3)	
5p15.2	CTNND2, NPRAP	Catenin, delta-2	604275	Mental retardation in cri-du-chat syndrome, 123450 (2)	
5p15.2-p14.1	CMDJ	Craniometaphyseal dysplasia, Jackson type	123000	Craniometaphyseal dysplasia (2)	
5p15	CCAL2, CPPDD	Chondrocalcinosis 2 (calcium pyrophosphate dihydrate deposition disease)	118600	Chondrocalcinosis, familial articular (2)	
5p15	PTC	Phenylthiocarbamide taste	171200	[Phenylthiocarbamide tasting] (2)	
5p15	SDHA, SDH2, SDHF	Succinate dehydrogenase complex, subunit A, flavoprotein	600857	Leigh syndrome (3)	

continued

Table 10.1. The morbid anatomy of the human genome (by chromosome) (*continued*)

Location	Symbol	Title	MIM#	Disorder	Mouse
5p14	FST, FS	Follistatin	136470	Polycystic ovary syndrome, 184700 (2)	
5p14-p12	NPR3, ANPRC	Natriuretic peptide receptor C	108962	?Hypertension, salt-resistant (1)	
5p13.2-q11.1	AMACR	Alpha-methylacyl-CoA racemase	604489	Alpha-methylacyl-CoA racemase deficiency (3)	
5p13.1-p12	GDNF	Glial cell line derived neurotrophic factor	600837	Hirschsprung disease, 142623 (3)	
5p13	C6	Complement component-6	217050	C6 deficiency (1); Combined C6/C7 deficiency (1)	15 (C6)
5p13	C7	Complement component-7	217070	C7 deficiency (1)	15 (C7)
5p13	C9	Complement component-9	120940	C9 deficiency (3)	
5p13	IL7R	Interleukin-7 receptor	146661	Severe combined immunodeficiency, T-cell negative, B-cell/natural killer cell-positive type, 600802 (3)	
5p13	SCOT, OXCT	Succinyl CoA:3-oxoacid CoA transferase	245050	Ketoacidosis due to SCOT deficiency (3)	
5p13-p12	GHR	Growth hormone receptor	600946	Laron dwarfism, 262500 (3); Short stature, idiopathic (3); Short stature, autosomal dominant, with normal serum growth hormone binding protein (3)	15 (Ghr)
5p	MHS6	Malignant hyperthermia susceptibility 6	601888	{Malignant hyperthermia susceptibility 6} (2)	
5q	MPD2, CMT2C, HMSN2C	Myopathy, distal, with vocal cord and pharyngeal weakness	158580	Myopathy, distal 2 (2)	
5q	PROP1	Prophet of Pit1, paired-like homeodomain transcription factor	601538	Pituitary hormone deficiency, combined (3)	11 (df, Prop1)
5q11	MOCS2, MPTS	Molybdenum cofactor synthesis-2	603708	Molybdenum cofactor deficiency, type B, 252150 (3)	
5q11-q12	MSH3	mutS, E. coli, homolog of, 3	600887	Endometrial carcinoma (3)	13 (Msh3)
5q11-q13	ARSB	Arylsulfatase B	253200	Maroteaux-Lamy syndrome, several forms (3)	13 (As1)
5q11.1	NDUFS4, AQDQ	NADH dehydrogenase (ubiquinone) Fe-S protein 4, 18 kD (NADH-coenzyme Q reductase)	602694	Complex I deficiency (3)	
5q11.2	KFS	Klippel-Feil syndrome	214300	?Klippel-Feil syndrome (2)	
5q11.2-q13.2	DHFR	Dihydrofolate reductase	126060	?Anemia, megaloblastic, due to DHFR deficiency (1)	13 (Dhfr)
5q11.2-q13.3	SCZD1	Schizophrenia susceptibility locus, chromosome 5-related	181510	{?Schizophrenia}, 181500 (2)	
5q12.2-q13.3	SMN1	Survival of motor neuron 1, telomeric	600354	Spinal muscular atrophy-1, 253300 (3); Spinal muscular atrophy-2, 253550 (3); Spinal muscular atrophy-3, 253400 (3)	13 (Smn)
5q13	HEXB	Hexosaminidase B, beta polypeptide	268800	Sandhoff disease, infantile, juvenile, and adult forms (3); Spinal muscular atrophy, juvenile (3)	13 (Hex2)
5q13-q14	WGN1, ERVR	Wagner syndrome (erosive vitreoretinopathy)	143200	Wagner syndrome (2); Erosive vitreoretinopathy (2)	

continued

Table 10.1. The morbid anatomy of the human genome (by chromosome) (*continued*)

Location	Symbol	Title	MIM#	Disorder	Mouse
5q13.3	RASA1, GAP	RAS p21 protein activator 1 (GTPase activating protein)	139150	Basal cell carcinoma (3)	13 (Gap)
5q14-q15	FEB4	Convulsions, familial febrile, 4	604352	Convulsions, familial febrile, 4 (2)	
5q14-q21	USH2C	Usher syndrome, type 2C	605472	Usher syndrome, type 2C (2)	
5q15-q21	PCSK1, NEC1, PC1, PC3	Proprotein convertase subtilisin/kexin type 1	162150	Obesity with impaired prohormone processing, 600955 (3)	13 (Nec1)
5q2	HSD17B4	Hydroxysteroid (17-beta) dehydrogenase 4	601860	D-bifunctional protein deficiency (3)	
5q21	MCC	Mutated in colorectal cancers	159350	Colorectal cancer (3)	18 (Mcc)
5q21-q22	APC, GS, FPC	Adenomatous polyposis coli	175100	Gardner syndrome (3); Adenomatous polyposis coli (3); Colorectal cancer (3); Desmoid disease, hereditary, 135290 (3); Turcot syndrome, 276300 (3); Adenomatous polyposis coli, attenuated (3); Gastric cancer, 137215 (3); Adenoma, periampullary (3)	18 (Min, Apc)
5q23	ADAMTS2, NPI	A disintegrin-like and metalloproteinase with thrombospondin type 1 motif, 2 (procollagen I N-proteinase)	604539	Ehlers-Danlos syndrome, type VIIC, 225410 (3)	11 (Adamts2)
5q23	DTR, DTS, HBEGF, HEGFL	Diphtheria toxin receptor (heparin-binding EGF-like growth factor)	126150	{Diphtheria, susceptibility to} (1)	18 (Hegfl)
5q23-q31	FBN2, CCA	Fibrillin-2	121050	Contractural arachnodactyly, congenital (3)	18 (Fbn2)
5q23-q31	ITGA2, CD49B, BR	Integrin, alpha-2 (CD49B; alpha-2 subunit of VLA-2 receptor; platelet antigen BR)	192974	Neonatal alloimmune thrombocytopenia (2); ?Glycoprotein Ia deficiency (2)	
5q23-q31	UBE2B, RAD6B	Ubiquitin-conjugating enzyme E2B (RAD6 homolog)	179095	?Male infertility (1)	
5q23.3-q31.2	LOX	Lysyl oxidase	153455 219100	Cutis laxa, recessive, type I, (1)	18 (Lox)
5q31	ACS2	Long-chain acyl-CoA synthetase 2	604443	Myelodysplastic syndrome (3); Myelogenous leukemia, acute (3)	
5q31	DIAPH1, DFNA1, LFHL1	Diaphanous, Drosophila, homolog of, 1	602121	Deafness, autosomal dominant nonsyndromic sensorineural, 1, 124900 (3)	
5q31	GRAF	GTPase regulator associated with the focal adhesion kinase pp125	605370	Leukemia, juvenile myelomonocytic (3)	
5q31	NR3C1, GCR, GRL	Nuclear receptor subfamily 3, group C, member 1 (glucocorticoid receptor)	138040	Cortisol resistance (3)	18 (Grl1)
5q31	POU4F3, BRN3C	POU domain, class 4, transcription factor-3	602460	Deafness, autosomal dominant 15, 602459 (3)	18 (pou4f3)
5q31	TGFBI, CSD2, CDGG1, CSD, BIGH3	Transforming growth factor, beta-induced, 68 kD	601692	Corneal dystrophy, Groenouw type I, 121900 (3); Corneal dystrophy, lattice type I, 122200 (3); Corneal dystrophy, Reis-Bucklers type, 121900 (3); Corneal dystrophy, Avellino type (3); Corneal dystrophy, lattice type IIIA (3)	

continued

Table 10.1. The morbid anatomy of the human genome (by chromosome) (*continued*)

Location	Symbol	Title	MIM#	Disorder	Mouse
5q31	TTID, MYOT	Myotilin (titin immunoglobulin domain protein)	604103	Muscular dystrophy, limb-girdle, type 1A, 159000 (3)	
5q31-q33	BHR1	Bronchial hyperresponsiveness-1 (bronchial asthma)	600807	Bronchial asthma (2)	
5q31-q33	EOS	Eosinophilia, familial	131400	Eosinophilia, familial (2)	
5q31-q33	HCI, HEMC	Hemangioma, capillary infantile	602089	Hemangioma, capillary infantile (2)	
5q31-q33	PFBI	Plasmodium falciparum blood infection levels	248310	{Plasmodium falciparum parasitemia, intensity of} (2)	
5q31-q33	PPP2R2B	Protein phosphatase 2, regulatory subunit B, beta	604325	Spinocerebellar ataxia 12, 604326 (3)	
5q31-q33	SM1	Schistosoma mansoni infection, susceptibility/resistance to	181460	{Schistosoma mansoni infection, susceptibility/resistance to} (2)	
5q31.1	IGES	Immunoglobulin E concentration, serum	147061	?{Allergy and asthma susceptibility} (2)	
5q31.1	IRF1, MAR	Interferon regulatory factor-1	147575	Macrocytic anemia, refractory, of 5q- syndrome, 153550 (3); Myelodysplastic syndrome, preleukemic (3); Myelogenous leukemia, acute (3); Gastric cancer, 137215 (3); Nonsmall cell lung cancer (3)	11 (Irf1)
5q31.1-q33.1	IL12B, NKSF2	Interleukin-12B (natural killer cell stimulatory factor-2, cytotoxic lymphocyte maturation factor-2, p40)	161561	BCG and salmonella infection, disseminated, 209950 (1)	11 (Il12b)
5q31.2-q31.3	EPD, PDE	Epilepsy, pyridoxine-dependent	266100	Epilepsy, pyridoxine-dependent (2)	
5q31.2-q34	PDE6A, PDEA	Phosphodiesterase-6A, cGMP-specific, rod, alpha	180071	Retinitis pigmentosa, autosomal recessive (3)	18 (Pde6a)
5q31.3-q33.1	GM2A	GM2 ganglioside activator protein	272750	GM2-gangliosidosis, AB variant (3)	11 (Gm2a)
5q32	CMTND	Charcot-Marie-Tooth neuropathy, demyelinating	601596	Charcot-Marie-Tooth neuropathy, demyelinating (2)	
5q32	GLRA1, STHE	Glycine receptor, alpha-1 polypeptide	138491	Startle disease/hyperekplexia, autosomal dominant, 149400 (3); Startle disease, autosomal recessive (3); Hyperekplexia and spastic paraparesis (3)	11 (spd)
5q32	SPINK5, LEKTI	Serine protease inhibitor, Kazal type, 5	605010	Netherton syndrome, 256500 (3)	
5q32-q33.1	SLC26A2, DTD, DTDST, D5S1708	Solute carrier family 26 (sulfate transporter), member 2 (diastrophic dysplasia sulfate transporter)	222600	Diastrophic dysplasia (3); Atelosteogenesis II, 256050 (3); Achondrogenesis Ib, 600972 (3); Epiphyseal dysplasia, multiple, 226900 (3)	
5q32-q33.1	TCOF1, MFD1	Treacher Collins-Franceschetti syndrome-1 (TREACLE)	154500	Treacher Collins mandibulofacial dysostosis (3)	18 (Tcof1)
5q32-q34	ADRB2	Adrenergic, beta-2-, receptor, surface	109690	{Asthma, nocturnal, susceptibility to} (3); {Obesity, susceptibility to} (3)	18 (Adrb2)
5q33	SGCD, SGD, LGMD2F	Sarcoglycan, delta (35 kD dystrophin-associated glycoprotein)	601411	Muscular dystrophy, limb-girdle, type 2F, 601287 (3)	
5q33-qter	F12, HAF	Coagulation factor XII (Hageman factor)	234000	Factor XII deficiency (3)	

continued

Table 10.1. The morbid anatomy of the human genome (by chromosome) (*continued*)

Location	Symbol	Title	MIM#	Disorder	Mouse
5q33.1	SLC22A5, OCTN2, CDSP, SCD	Solute carrier, family 22 (organic cation transporter), member 5	603377	Carnitine deficiency, systemic primary, 212140 (3)	11 (jvs)
5q33.2-q33.3	CSF1R, FMS	Colony-stimulating factor-1 receptor; oncogene FMS (McDonough feline sarcoma)	164770	Myeloid malignancy, predisposition to (3)	18 (Fim2)
5q34	CSX	Cardiac-specific homeo box	600584	Atrial septal defect with atrioventricular conduction defects, 108900 (3)	17 (Csx)
5q34-q35	MSX2, CRS2, HOX8	msh, Drosophila, homeo box homolog of, 2	123101	Craniosynostosis, type 2, 604757 (3); Parietal foramina 1, 168500 (3)	
5q35	AMCN, AMCN1	Arthrogryposis multiplex congenital, neurogenic	208100	Arthrogryposis multiplex congenita, neurogenic (2)	
5q35	LTC4S	Leukotriene C4 synthase	246530	Leukotriene C4 synthase deficiency (1)	
5q35	NPM1	Nucleophosmin 1 (nucleolar phosphoprotein B23, numatrin)	164040	Leukemia, acute promyelocytic, NPM/RARA type (3)	
5q35.1-q35.3	B4GALT7, XGALT1, XGPT1	Xylosylprotein 4-beta-galactosyl transferase, polypeptide 7	604327	Ehlers-Danlos syndrome, progeroid form, 130070 (3)	
5q35.3	FLT4, VEGFR3, PCL	fms-related tyrosine kinase-4 (vascular endothelial growth factor receptor 3)	136352	Lymphedema, hereditary I, 153100 (3)	11 (Flt4)
Chr.5	AP3B1, ADTB3A, HPS	Adaptor-related protein complex 3, beta 1 subunit (adaptin, beta-3a)	603401	Hermansky-Pudlak syndrome, 203300 (3)	
Chr.5	CKN1	Cockayne syndrome 1, classical	216400	Cockayne syndrome-1 (3)	
Chr.5	SPINK1, PSTI, PCTT, TATI	Serine protease inhibitor, Kazal type I (pancreatic secretory trypsin inhibitor)	167790	Pancreatitis, hereditary, 167800 (3)	
6p25	FOXC1, FKHL7, FREAC3	Forkhead, Drosophila, homolog-like 7	601090	Iridogoniodysgenesis, 601631 (3); Anterior segment mesenchymal dysgenesis (3); Rieger anomaly (3); Axenfeld anomaly (3); Iris hypoplasia and glaucoma (3)	13 (Fkh17, ch, Mf1)
6p25	IRF4, MUM1	Interferon regulatory factor-4 (multiple myeloma oncogene-1)	602028	Multiple myeloma (3)	
6p25-p24	F13A1, F13A	Coagulation factor XIII, A polypeptide	134570	Factor XIIIA deficiency (3)	
6p24.3	OFC1, CL	Orofacial cleft-1 (cleft lip with or without cleft palate; isolated cleft palate)	119530	Orofacial cleft-1 (2)	
6p24	DSP, KPPS2, PPKS2	Desmoplakin	125647	Keratosis palmoplantaris striata II (3)	
6p23	ATX1, SCA1	Ataxin-1	601556	Spinocerebellar ataxia-1, 164400 (3)	13 (Sca1, Atx1)
6p23	DEK, D6S231E	DEK oncogene	125264	Leukemia, acute nonlymphocytic (2)	
6p23	SCZD3	Schizophrenia susceptibility locus, chromosome 6-related	600511	{Schizophrenia}, 181500 (2)	
6p22.3	TPMT	Thiopurine S-methyltransferase	187680	6-mercaptopurine sensitivity (3)	
6p22	SSADH	Succinic semialdehyde dehydrogenase	271980	Succinic semialdehyde dehydrogenase deficiency (3)	
6p22-p21	BCKDHB, E1B	Branched chain keto acid dehydrogenase E1, beta polypeptide	248611	Maple syrup urine disease, type Ib (3)	
6p22-p21	FANCE, FACE	Fanconi anemia, complementation group E gene	600901	Fanconi anemia, complementation group E (3)	

continued

Table 10.1. The morbid anatomy of the human genome (by chromosome) (*continued*)

Location	Symbol	Title	MIM#	Disorder	Mouse
6p21.3	ABCB3, TAP2, RING11, PSF2	ATP-binding cassette, subfamily B, member 3	170261	Bare lymphocyte syndrome, type I, due to TAP2 deficiency (1)	17 (Ham2)
6p21.3	AS, ANS	Ankylosing spondylitis	106300	Ankylosing spondylitis (2)	
6p21.3	ASD1, ASD2	Atrial septal defect, secundum type	108800	Atrial septal defect, secundum type (2)	
6p21.3	C2	Complement component-2	217000	C2 deficiency (3)	17 (C2)
6p21.3	C4A, C4S	Complement component-4A	120810	C4 deficiency (3)	17 (C4)
6p21.3	C4B, C4F	Complement component-4B	120820	C4 deficiency (3)	17 (C4)
6p21.3	COL11A2, STL3	Collagen XI, alpha-2 polypeptide	120290	Stickler syndrome, type III, 184840 (3); OSMED syndrome, 215150 (3); Weissenbacher-Zweymuller syndrome, 277610 (3); Deafness, nonsyndromic sensorineural 13, 601868 (3)	17 (Col11a2)
6p21.3	CYP21A2, CYP21, CA21H	Cytochrome P450, subfamily XXIA, polypeptide 2 (steroid 21-hydroxylase)	201910	Adrenal hyperplasia, congenital, due to 21-hydroxylase deficiency (3)	17 (Cyp21)
6p21.3	DYX2, DYLX2, DLX2	Dyslexia 2	600202	Dyslexia, specific, 2 (2)	
6p21.3	GLYS1	Renal glucosuria-1	233100	[Renal glucosuria] (2)	
6p21.3	HFE	Hemochromatosis	235200	Hemochromatosis (3); Porphyria variegata, 176200 (3)	13 (Mr2, Hfe)
6p21.3	HLA-DPB1	Major histocompatibility complex, class II, DP beta-1	142858	{Beryllium disease, chronic, susceptibility to} (3)	
6p21.3	HLA-DR1B	Major histocompatibility complex, class II, DR beta-1	142857	{Pemphigoid, susceptibility to} (2)	
6p21.3	HTSS	Hypotrichosis simplex of scalp	146520	Hypotrichosis simplex of scalp (2)	
6p21.3	IDDM1	Insulin-dependent diabetes mellitus-1	222100	{?Diabetes mellitus, insulin-dependent-1} (2)	
6p21.3	IGAD1	Immunoglobulin A deficiency	137100	Immunoglobulin A deficiency (2)	
6p21.3	MOCS1, MOCOD	Molybdenum cofactor synthesis-1	603707	Molybdenum cofactor deficiency, type A, 252150 (3)	
6p21.3	NEU1, NEU, SIAL1	Neuraminidase 1 (lysosomal sialidase; sialidase 1)	256550	Sialidosis, type I (3); Sialidosis, type II (3)	17 (Neu1)
6p21.3	PBLT	Panbronchiolitis, diffuse	604809	Panbronchiolitis, diffuse (2)	
6p21.3	PDB	Paget disease of bone	167250	?Paget disease of bone (2)	
6p21.3	PSORS1	Psoriasis susceptibility 1	177900	{Psoriasis susceptibility-1} (2)	
6p21.3	RWS	Ragweed sensitivity	179450	?Ragweed sensitivity (2)	
6p21.3	TNF, TNFA	Tumor necrosis factor (cachectin)	191160	{Malaria, cerebral, susceptibility to} (3)	17 (Tnfa)
6p21.3	TNXA, HXBL, TNX	Tenascin XA	600261	Ehlers-Danlos-like syndrome (3)	
6p21.3	TULP1, RP14	Tubby-like protein-1	602280	Retinitis pigmentosa-14, 600132 (3)	
6p21.3-p21.2	LAP	Laryngeal adductor paralysis	150270	?Laryngeal adductor paralysis (2)	
6p21.2-p12	PLA2G7, PAFAH	Phospholipase A2, group VII (platelet-activating factor acetylhydrolase)	601690	Platelet-activating factor acetylhydrolase deficiency (3); {Asthma and atopy, susceptibility to}, 147070 (3)	
6p21.1	GUCA1A, GCAP	Guanylate cyclase activator 1A, retina	600364	Cone dystrophy-3, 602093 (3)	
6p21.1	PEX6, PXAAA1, PAF2	Peroxisomal biogenesis factor 6 (peroxisomal AAA-type ATPase 1)	601498	Peroxisomal biogenesis disorder, complementation group 4 (3)	17 (Pxaaa1)

continued

Table 10.1. The morbid anatomy of the human genome (by chromosome) (*continued*)

Location	Symbol	Title	MIM#	Disorder	Mouse
6p21.1-p12	PKHD1, ARPKD	Polycystic kidney and hepatic disease-1, autosomal recessive	263200	Polycystic kidney disease, autosomal recessive (2)	
6p21.1-p11	RHAG, RH50A	Rhesus blood group-associated glycoprotein	180297	Anemia, hemolytic, Rh-null, regulator type, 268150 (3); Rh-mod syndrome (3)	
6p21.1-cen	RDS, RP7	Retinal degeneration, slow (peripherin)	179605	Retinitis pigmentosa-7, peripherin-related (3); Retinitis punctata albescens (3); Macular dystrophy (3); Retinitis pigmentosa, digenic (3); Butterfly dystrophy, retinal (3); Macular dystrophy, vitelliform (3); Retinitis pigmentosa with bull's-eye maculopathy (3); Foveomacular dystrophy, adult-onset, with choroidal neovascularization (3); Pattern dystrophy of retina (3)	17 (rds)
6p21	HMGIY	High-mobility group (nonhistone chromosomal) protein isoforms I and Y	600701	?Lipoma (1)	
6p21	MUT, MCM	Methylmalonyl Coenzyme A mutase	251000	Methylmalonicaciduria, mutase deficiency type (3)	17 (Mut)
6p21	RUNX2, CBFA1, PEBP2A1, AML3	Runt-related transcription factor 2	600211	Cleidocranial dysplasia, 119600 (3); Dental anomalies, isolated (3)	17 (Cbfa1)
6p12	GCLC, GLCLC	Glutamate-cysteine ligase, catalytic subunit	230450	Hemolytic anemia due to gamma-glutamylcysteine synthetase deficiency (1)	9 (Glclc)
6p12	NYS2, NYSA	Nystagmus-2, autosomal dominant	164100	Nystagmus-2, autosomal dominant (2)	
6p12	TFAP2B, CHAR	Transcription factor AP-2 beta (activating enhancer-binding protein 2 beta)	601601	Char syndrome, 169100 (3)	1 (Tfap2b)
6p	GSE, CD	Gluten-sensitive enteropathy (celiac disease)	212750	Celiac disease (2)	
6p	PUJO	Pelviureteric junction obstruction	143400	Pelviureteric junction obstruction (2)	
6cen-q14	CORD7	Cone-rod dystrophy 7	603649	Cone-rod dystrophy-7 (2)	
6p	IBD3	Inflammatory bowel disease 3	604519	Inflammatory bowel disease 3 (2)	
6p	EJM1	Epilepsy, juvenile myoclonic 1	254770	Epilepsy, juvenile myoclonic (2)	
6q	MPSH	Mixed polyposis syndrome, hereditary	601228	Mixed polyposis syndrome, hereditary (2)	
6q11-q16	LCA5	Leber congenital amaurosis, type V	604537	Leber congenital amaurosis 5 (2)	
6q13-q15	OA3, OAR	Ocular albinism, autosomal recessive	203310	?Ocular albinism, autosomal recessive (2)	
6q13-q26	SCZD5	Schizophrenia susceptibility locus, chromosome 6q-related	603175	{Schizophrenia}, 181500 (2)	
6q14	ELOVL4, ADMD, STGD2, STGD3	Elongation of very long chain fatty acids 4	605512	Stargardt disease 3, 600110 (3); Macular dystrophy, autosomal dominant, chromosome 6-linked, 600110 (3)	
6q14-q15	SLC17A5, SIASD, SLD	Solute carrier family 17 (sodium phosphate), member 5	604322	Salla disease, 604369 (3); Sialic acid storage disorder, infantile, 269920 (3)	
6q14-q16.2	PBCRA, CRAPB	Progressive bifocal chorioretinal atrophy	600790	Chorioretinal atrophy, progressive bifocal (2)	

continued

Table 10.1. The morbid anatomy of the human genome (by chromosome) (*continued*)

Location	Symbol	Title	MIM#	Disorder	Mouse
6q14-q16.2	MCDR1	Macular dystrophy, retinal, 1, North Carolina type	136550	Macular dystrophy, North Carolina type (2)	
6q14-q21	RP25	Retinitis pigmentosa-25	602772	Retinitis pigmentosa-25 (2)	
6q16.3-q21	SIM1	Single-minded, Drosophila, homolog of, 1	603128	Obesity, severe (3)	10 (Sim1)
6q21	IDDM15	Insulin-dependent diabetes mellitus-15	601666	{Diabetes mellitus, insulin-dependent, 15} (2)	
6q21-q22	CMDR	Craniometaphyseal dysplasia, autosomal recessive	218400	Craniometaphyseal dysplasia, autosomal recessive (2)	
6q21-q22.3	COL10A1	Collagen X, alpha-1 polypeptide	120110	Metaphyseal chondrodysplasia, Schmid type (3); Spondylometaphyseal dysplasia, Japanese type (3)	10 (Col10a1)
6q22-q23	ENPP1, PDNP1, NPPS, M6S1, PCA1	Ectonucleotide pyrophosphatase/ phosphodiesterase 1 (Ly-41 antigen, mouse, homolog of)	173335	Ossification of posterior longitudinal ligament of spine, 602475 (3)	10 (Ly41, Pca1)
6q22-q23	IGAN	IgA nephropathy	161950	Nephropathy, IgA type (2)	
6q22-q23	LAMA2, LAMM	Laminin, alpha-2 (merosin)	156225	Muscular dystrophy, congenital merosin-deficient (3)	10 (dy, Lamm)
6q22-q23	SM2	Hepatic fibrosis susceptibility due to Schistosoma mansoni infection	604201	{Hepatic fibrosis susceptibility due to Schistosoma mansoni infection} (2)	
6q22-q23	WISP3, PPAC, PPD	Wnt-1 inducible signaling pathway protein 3	603400	Arthropathy, progressive pseudorheumatoid, of childhood, 208230 (3)	
6q22-q24	ODDD, SDTY3, ODOD	Oculodentodigital dysplasia (syndactyly type III)	164200	Oculodentodigital dysplasia (2); Syndactyly, type III, 186100 (2)	
6q22-q24	PEX7, RCDP1	Peroxisomal biogenesis factor-7	601757	Rhizomelic chondrodysplasia punctata, type 1, 215100 (3)	
6q22.3-q23.1	HPFH	Hereditary persistence of fetal hemoglobin, heterocellular	142470	[Hereditary persistence of fetal hemoglobin, heterocellular] (2)	
6q22.2-q23.3	DFNA10	Deafness, autosomal nonsyndromic sensorineural, 10	601316	Deafness, autosomal dominant 10 (2)	
6q23	ARG1	Arginase, liver	207800	Argininemia (3)	
6q23	CMD1F, CDCD3	Cardiomyopathy, dilated-1F, autosomal dominant	602067	Cardiomyopathy, dilated, 1F (2)	
6q23-q24	CMD1J	Cardiomyopathy, dilated, 1J	605362	Cardiomyopathy, dilated, 1J (2)	
6q23-q24	IFNGR1	Immune interferon, receptor for	107470	Mycobacterial infection, atypical, familial disseminated, 209950 (3); BCG infection, generalized familial (3); {Tuberculosis, susceptibility to} (3)	10 (Ifgr)
6q23-q24	PEX3	Peroxisomal biogenesis factor-3	603164	Zellweger syndrome, 214100 (3)	
6q24	EPM2A, MELF, EPM2	Laforin	254780	Epilepsy, myoclonic, Lafora type (3)	
6q24	TNDM, DMTN	Diabetes mellitus, transient neonatal	601410	{Diabetes mellitus, transient neonatal} (2)	
6q24-q27	IDDM5	Insulin-dependent diabetes mellitus-5	600320	{Diabetes mellitus, insulin-dependent, 5} (2)	
6q25-q26	RCD1	Retinal cone dystrophy-1	180020	?Retinal cone dystrophy-1 (2)	
6q25-q27	IDDM8	Insulin-dependent diabetes mellitus-8	600883	{Diabetes mellitus, insulin-dependent, 8} (2)	

continued

Table 10.1. The morbid anatomy of the human genome (by chromosome) (*continued*)

Location	Symbol	Title	MIM#	Disorder	Mouse
6q25.1	ESR1, ESR	Estrogen receptor 1	133430	Breast cancer (1); Estrogen resistance (3)	10 (Esr)
6q25.2-q27	PRKN, PARK2, PDJ	Parkin	602544	Parkinson disease, juvenile, type 2, 600116 (3)	
6q25.3-q26	ACAT2	Acetyl-Coenzyme A acetyltransferase 2 (acetoacetyl Coenzyme A thiolase)	100678	?ACAT2 deficiency (1)	
6q26	IGF2R, MPRI	Insulin-like growth factor-2 receptor (mannose-6-phosphate receptor, cation-independent)	147280	Hepatocellular carcinoma (3)	17 (Igf2r)
6q26	PLG	Plasminogen	173350	Plasminogen Tochigi disease (3); Thrombophilia, dysplasminogenemic (1); Plasminogen deficiency, types I and II (1); Conjunctivitis, ligneous, 217090 (3)	17 (Plg)
6q26-q27	ST8, OVCS	Suppression of tumorigenicity-8, ovarian	167000	Ovarian cancer, serous (2)	
6q27	LPA	Apolipoprotein Lp (a)	152200	{Coronary artery disease, susceptibility to} (1)	
6q27	TBP	TATA box binding protein	600075	Complex neurologic disorder, 117200 (3)	
Chr.6	GCNT2	Glucosaminyl (N-acetyl) transferase 2, I-branching enzyme	600429	[Ii blood group, 110800] (1)	
Chr.6	PBCA	Pancreatic beta cell, agenesis of	600089	?Diabetes mellitus, insulin-dependent, neonatal (2)	
Chr.6	POLH, XPV	Polymerase, DNA, eta	603968	Xeroderma pigmentosum, variant type, 278750 (3)	
7p22	PMS2, PMSL2	Postmeiotic segregation increased, S. cerevisiae, 2, homolog of	600259	Turcot syndrome with glioblastoma, 276300 (3); Colorectal cancer, hereditary nonpolyposis, type 4 (3)	
7p21.3-p21.2	CRS, CSO	Craniosynostosis, type I	123100	Craniosynostosis, type 1 (2)	
7p21	IL6, IFNB2, BSF2	Interleukin-6 (interferon, beta-2)	147620	Osteopenia/osteoporosis, 166710 (2)	5 (Il6)
7p21	TWIST, ACS3, SCS	TWIST, Drosophila, homolog of	601622	Saethre-Chotzen syndrome, 101400 (3)	12 (Twist)
7p21-p15	MDDC	Macular dystrophy, dominant cystoid	153880	Macular dystrophy, dominant cystoid (2)	
7p21-p13	BPES2	Blepharophimosis, epicanthus inversus, and ptosis 2	601649	Blepharophimosis, epicanthus inversus, and ptosis, type 2 (2)	
7p15.1-p13	RP9	Retinitis pigmentosa-9	180104	Retinitis pigmentosa-9 (2)	
7p15	DFNA5	Deafness, autosomal dominant 5	600994	Deafness, autosomal dominant 5 (3)	6 (Dfna5)
7p15-p14	GHRHR	Growth hormone releasing hormone receptor	139191	Growth hormone deficient dwarfism (3)	6 (Lit, Ghrhr)
7p15-p14.2	HOXA11, HOX1I	Homeo box-A11	142958	Radioulnar synostosis with amegakaryocytic thrombocytopenia, 605432 (3)	
7p15-p14.2	HOXA13, HOX1J	Homeo box-A13	142959	Hand-foot-uterus syndrome, 140000(3)	6 (Hoxa13, Hd)
7p15-p13	CCM2	Cerebral cavernous malformations-2	603284	Cerebral cavernous malformations-2 (2)	
7p15-p13	GCK	Glucokinase (hexokinase-4)	138079	MODY, type 2, 125851 (3); Hyperinsulinism, familial, 602485 (3)	

continued

Table 10.1. The morbid anatomy of the human genome (by chromosome) (*continued*)

Location	Symbol	Title	MIM#	Disorder	Mouse
7p15-p11.2	WTSL, WT5	Wilms tumor suppressor locus	601583	{Wilms tumor susceptibility-5} (2)	
7p14	AQP1, CHIP28, CO	Aquaporin-1 (channel-forming integral protein, 28 kD)	107776	Colton blood group, 110450 (3); [Aquaporin-1 deficiency] (3)	6 (Aqp1)
7p14	CMT2D	Charcot-Marie-Tooth neuropathy, neuronal type, D	601472	Charcot-Marie-Tooth neuropathy-2D (2)	
7p14-p13	OGDH	Oxoglutarate dehydrogenase (lipoamide)	203740	Alpha-ketoglutarate dehydrogenase deficiency (1)	
7p13	GLI3, PAPA, PAPB	GLI-Kruppel family member GLI3 (oncogene GL13)	165240	Greig cephalopolysyndactyly syndrome, 175700 (3); Pallister-Hall syndrome, 146510 (3); Polydactyly, preaxial, type IV, 174700 (3); Polydactyly, postaxial, types A1 and B, 174200 (3)	13 (Xt)
7p13-p12.3	PGAM2, PGAMM	Phosphoglycerate mutase, muscle form	261670	Myopathy due to phosphoglycerate mutase deficiency (3)	
7p12	ZNFN1A1, IK1, LYF1	Zinc finger protein, subfamily 1A, 1 (Ikaros)	603023	Leukemia, acute lymphoblastic (3)	11 (Ikaros)
7p12-p11.2	GRB10, RSS	Growth factor receptor-bound protein-10	601523	Russell-Silver syndrome, 180860 (3)	11 (Grb1)
7p	GHS	Goldenhar syndrome	141400	?Goldenhar syndrome (2)	
7p	SMAD1	Spinal muscular atrophy, distal, with upper limb predominance	600794	Spinal muscular atrophy, distal, with upper limb predominance (2)	
7cen-q11.2	ASL	Argininosuccinate lyase	207900	Argininosuccinicaciduria (3)	5 (Asl)
7q	AUT	Autism, susceptibility to	209850	{Autism, susceptibility to} (2)	
7q	LGMD1D	Limb-girdle muscular dystrophy-1D, autosomal dominant	603511	Muscular dystrophy, limb-girdle, type 1D (2)	
7q11.2	CD36	CD36 antigen (collagen type I)	173510	[Macrothrombocytopenia] (1); Platelet glycoprotein IV deficiency (3)	
7q11.2	ELN	Elastin	130160	Supravalvar aortic stenosis, 185500 (3); Williams-Beuren syndrome, 194050 (3); Cutis laxa, 123700 (3)	5 (Eln)
7q11.2-q21	CCM1, CAM, KRIT1	KREV interaction trapped 1	604214	Cerebral cavernous malformations-1, 116860 (3)	
7q11.2-q21.3	EEC1	Ectrodactyly, ectodermal dysplasia, cleft lip/palate, 1	129900	?EEC syndrome-1 (2)	
7q11.23	NCF1	Neutrophil cytosolic factor-1, 47 kD	233700	Chronic granulomatous disease due to deficiency of NCF-1 (3)	
7q11.23	PTPN12, PTPG1	Protein tyrosine phosphatase, 12 nonreceptor-type,)	600079	Colon cancer (3)	5 (Ptpn12
7q21	DYT11	Dystonia 11, myoclonic	605408	Dystonia 11, myoclonic (2)	
7q21	EPO	Erythropoietin	133170	?Erythremia (1)	5 (Epo)
7q21-q22	MHS3	Malignant hyperthermia susceptibility 3	154276	{Malignant hyperthermia susceptibility 3} (2)	
7q21-q22	PEX1, ZWS1	Peroxisome biogenesis factor-1	602136	Zellweger syndrome-1, 214100 (3); Adrenoleukodystrophy, neonatal, 202370 (3); Refsum disease, infantile, 266510 (3)	
7q21.1	ABCB4, PGY3, MDR3	ATP-binding cassette, subfamily B, member 4 (P-glycoprotein-3/multiple drug resistance-3)	171060	Cholestasis, progressive familial intrahepatic, type III, 602347 (3); Cholestasis, familial intrahepatic, of pregnancy, 147480 (3)	

continued

Table 10.1. The morbid anatomy of the human genome (by chromosome) (*continued*)

Location	Symbol	Title	MIM#	Disorder	Mouse
7q21.1	ABCB1, PGY1, MDR1	ATP-binding cassette, subfamily B, member 1 (P-glycoprotein-1/multiple drug resistance-1)	171050	Colchicine resistance (3)	5 (Pgy1)
7q21.11	GUSB	Glucuronidase, beta-	253220	Mucopolysaccharidosis VII (3)	5 (Gus)
7q21.2-q21.3	SHFM1, SHFD1, SHSF1	Split hand/foot malformation (ectrodactyly) type 1	183600	Split hand/foot malformation, type 1 (2)	
7q21.3	CALCR, CRT	Calcitonin receptor	114131	{Osteoporosis, postmenopausal, susceptibility}, 166710 (3)	
7q21.3	PON1, PON, ESA	Paraoxonase-1	168820	{Coronary artery disease, susceptibility to} (3)	6 (Pon1)
7q21.3	PON2	Paraoxonase-2	602447	{Coronary artery disease, susceptibility to} (3)	
7q21.3	SLC25A13, CTLN2	Solute carrier family 25 (mitochondrial carrier, citrin), member 13	603859	Citrullinemia, adult-onset type II, 603471 (3)	
7q21.3-q22	PAI1, PLANH1	Plasminogen activator inhibitor, type I	173360	Thrombophilia due to excessive plasminogen activator inhibitor (1); Hemorrhagic diathesis due to PAI1 deficiency (1)	
7q22	MUC3A	Mucin 3A, intestinal	158371	{Ulcerative colitis, susceptibility to}, 191390 (1)	
7q22	RELN, RL	Reelin	600514	Lissencephaly syndrome, Norman-Roberts type, 257320 (3)	5 (r1)
7q22	TFR2	Transferrin receptor 2	604720	Hemochromatosis, 604250 (3)	
7q22-q31.1	SLC26A3, DRA, CLD	Solute carrier family 26 (sulfate transporter), member 3	126650	?Colon cancer (1); Chloride diarrhea, congenital, Finnish type, 214700 (3)	
7q22.1	COL1A2	Collagen I, alpha-2 polypeptide	120160	Osteogenesis imperfecta, 3 clinical forms, 166200, 166210, 259420 (3); Ehlers-Danlos syndrome, type VIIA2, 130060 (3); Osteoporosis, idiopathic, 166710 (3); Marfan syndrome, atypical (3)	6 (Cola2)
7q3	CMH6	Cardiomyopathy, hypertrophic 6	600858	Cardiomyopathy, familial hypertrophic with Wolff–Parkinson–White syndrome (2)	
7q31	DFNB14	Deafness, autosomal recessive 14	603678	Deafness, autosomal recessive 14 (2)	
7q31	DFNB17	Deafness, autosomal recessive 17	603010	Deafness, autosomal recessive 17 (2)	
7q31	MET	Oncogene MET	164860	Renal cell carcinoma, papillary, familial and sporadic, 605074 (3); Hepatocellular carcinoma, childhood type, 114550 (3)	6 (Met)
7q31	SLC26A3, DRA, DFNB4	Solute carrier family 26 (sulfate transporter), member 3	274600	Pendred syndrome (3); Deafness, autosomal recessive 4, 600791 (3); Enlarged vestibular aqueduct, 603545 (3)	
7q31	SPCH1	Speech-language disorder-1	602081	Speech-language disorder-1 (2)	
7q31-q32	DLD, LAD, PHE3	Dihydrolipoamide dehydrogenase (E3 component of pyruvate dehydrogenase complex, 2-oxo-glutarate complex)	246900	Lipoamide dehydrogenase deficiency (3)	12 (Dld)
7q31-q32	SMOH, SMO	Smoothened, Drosophila, homolog of	601500	Basal cell carcinoma, sporadic (3)	
7q31-q34	BPGM	2,3-bisphosphoglycerate mutase	222800	Hemolytic anemia due to bisphosphoglycerate mutase deficiency (1)	
7q31-q35	RP10	Retinitis pigmentosa-10, autosomal dominant	180105	Retinitis pigmentosa-10 (2)	
7q31.1-q31.3	LAMB1	Laminin, beta-1	150240	?Cutis laxa, marfanoid neonatal type (1)	1 (Lamb1)

continued

Table 10.1. The morbid anatomy of the human genome (by chromosome) (*continued*)

Location	Symbol	Title	MIM#	Disorder	Mouse
7q31.2	CFTR, ABCC7, CF, MRP7	Cystic fibrosis transmembrane conductance regulator (ATP-binding cassette, subfamily C, member 7)	602421	Cystic fibrosis, 219700 (3); Congenital bilateral absence of vas deferens, 277180 (3); Sweat chloride elevation without CF (3); {Pancreatitis, idiopathic} (3); {Hypertrypsinemia, neonatal} (3)	6 (Cftr)
7q31.3	AASS	Alpha-aminoadipic semialdehyde synthase	605113	Hyperlysinemia, 238700 (3); Saccharopinuria, 268700 (1)	
7q31.3	LEP, OB	Leptin (murine obesity homolog)	164160	Obesity, severe, due to leptin deficiency (3); Obesity, morbid, with hypogonadism (3)	6 (ob)
7q31.3-q32	BCP, CBT	Blue cone pigment	190900	Colorblindness, tritan (3)	6 (Bcp)
7q33-q34	ATP6N1B, VPP2, RTA1C, RTADR	ATPase, H+ transporting, lysosomal, noncatalytic accessory protein 1B	605239	Renal tubular acidosis, distal, autosomal recessive, 602722 (3)	
7q34	TBXAS1	Thromboxane A synthase 1, platelet	274180	Thromboxane synthase deficiency (2)	6 (Tbxas1)
7q34-q36	DFNB13	Deafness, autosomal recessive 13	603098	Deafness, autosomal recessive 13 (2)	
7q35	CLCN1	Chloride channel-1, skeletal muscle	118425	Myotonia congenita, recessive, 255700 (3); Myotonia congenita, dominant, 160800 (3); Myotonia levior, recessive (3)	6 (adr, Clc1)
7q35	PRSS1, TRY1	Protease, serine, 1 (trypsin 1)	276000	Trypsinogen deficiency (1); Pancreatitis, hereditary, 167800 (3)	6 (Try1)
7q35-q36	GLC1F	Glaucoma 1, open angle, F	603383	Glaucoma 1F (2)	
7q35-q36	GPDS1, PDS1	Glaucoma-related pigment dispersion syndrome-1	600510	Pigment dispersion syndrome (2)	
7q35-q36	KCNH2, LQT2, HERG	Potassium channel, voltage-gated, subfamily H, member 2 (human ether-a-go-go-related gene)	152427	Long QT syndrome-2 (3)	
7q36	C7orf2, ACHP, LMBR1	Limb region 1, mouse, homolog of	605522	Acheiropody, 200500 (3)	5 (Lmbr1)
7q36	HLXB9, HOXHB9, SCRA1	Homeo box-HB9	142994	Currarino syndrome, 176450 (3)	
7q36	HPFH2	Hereditary persistence of fetal hemoglobin, heterocellular, Indian type	142335	?Hereditary persistence of fetal hemoglobin, heterocellular, Indian type (2)	
7q36	NOS3	Nitric oxide synthase 3, endothelial cell	163729	{Preeclampsia, susceptibility to, 189800} (2); {Coronary spasm, susceptibility to} (3)	5 (Nos3)
7q36	SCRA1	Sacra1 agenesis, autosomal dominant (Currarino triad)	176450	Sacral agenesis-1 (2)	
7q36	SHH, HPE3, HLP3	Sonic hedgehog, Drosophila, homolog of	600725	Holoprosencephaly-3, 142945 (3)	
7q36	TPTPS, TPT	Triphalangeal thumb-polysyndactyly syndrome	190605	Triphalangeal thumb-polysyndactyly syndrome (2)	
8pter-p22	CLN8, EPMR	CLN8 gene	600143	Epilepsy, progressive, with mental retardation (2)	8 (mnd)
8pter-p22	MCPH1	Microcephaly, primary autosomal recessive 1	251200	Microcephaly, autosomal recessive 1 (2)	
8p23.1	MASL1	Malignant fibrous histiocytoma-amplified sequences with leucinerich tandem repeats-1	605352	Malignant fibrous histiocytoma (2)	
8p23-p22	KWE	Keratolytic winter erythema	148370	Keratolytic winter erythema (2)	

continued

Table 10.1. The morbid anatomy of the human genome (by chromosome) (*continued*)

Location	Symbol	Title	MIM#	Disorder	Mouse
8p22	LPL, LIPD	Lipoprotein lipase	238600	Hyperlipoproteinemia I (1); Lipoprotein lipase deficiency (3); Chylomicronemia syndrome, familial (3); Combined hyperlipemia, familial (3)	8 (Lp1)
8p22	N33	Putative prostate cancer tumor suppressor	601385	?Prostate cancer (1)	
8p22-p21.3	ASAH, AC	N-acylsphingosine amidohydrolase (acid ceramidase)	228000	Farber lipogranulomatosis (3)	
8p22-p21.3	PDGFRL, PDGRL, PRLTS	Platelet-derived growth factor receptor-like	604584	Hepatocellular cancer, 114550 (3); Colorectal cancer, 114500 (3)	
8p22-p21	TNFRSF10B, DR5, TRAILR2	Tumor necrosis factor receptor superfamily, member 10B	603612	Squamous cell carcinoma, head and neck, 601400 (3)	
8p21.2	HR, AU	Hairless, mouse, homolog of	602302	Alopecia universalis, 203655 (3); Atrichia with papular lesions, 209500 (3)	14 (hr)
8p21.1	GSR	Glutathione reductase	138300	Hemolytic anemia due to glutathione reductase deficiency (1)	8 (Gr1)
8p21.1	GULOP, GULO	Gulonolactone (L-) oxidase pseudogene	240400	Scurvy (3)	
8p21	MUHH	Hypotrichosis, Marie Unna type	146550	Hypotrichosis, Marie Unna type (2)	
8p21	NEFL, CMT2E	Neurofilament, light polypeptide	162280	Charcot-Marie-Tooth disease, type 2E (3)	14 (Nf1)
8p21	SCZD6	Schizophrenia susceptibility locus, chromosome 8p-related	603013	{Schizophrenia}, 181500 (2)	
8p21-p11.2	GNRH1, LNRH	Gonadotropin-releasing hormone-1 (leutinizing-releasing hormone)	152760	?Hypogonadotropic hypogonadism due to GNRH deficiency, 227200 (1)	14 (Gnrh)
8p21-q22	DYT6	Dystonia-6 (torsion dystonia, adult onset, of mixed type)	602629	Dystonia-6, torsion (2)	
8p12	PLAT, TPA	Plasminogen activator, tissue type	173370	Plasminogen activator deficiency (1)	8 (Plat)
8p12-p11.2	RECQL3, WRN	RecQ protein-like 3	604611	Werner syndrome, 277700 (3)	8 (wrn)
8p12-q13	SPG5A	Spastic paraplegia-5A, autosomal recessive	270800	Spasticparaplegia-5A (2)	
8p11.2	ANK1, SPH2	Ankyrin-1, erythrocytic	182900	Spherocytosis-2 (3)	8 (nb)
8p11.2	STAR	Steroidogenic acute regulatory protein	600617	Lipoid adrenal hyperplasia, 201710 (3)	
8p11.2-p11.1	FGFR1, FLT2	Fibroblast growth factor receptor-1 (fms-related tyrosine kinase-2)	136350	Pfeiffer syndrome, 101600 (3); Jackson-Weiss syndrome, 123150 (3)	
8q	CCAL1	Chondrocalcinosis 1	600668	Chondrocalcinosis with early-onset osteoarthritis (2)	
8q11	PRKDC, HYRC1, DNPK1	Protein kinase, DNA-activated, catalytic polypeptide (hyperradiosensitivity of murine SCID mutation, complementing-1)	600899	?Severe combined immunodeficiency, type I, 202500 (1)	16 (scid)
8q11-q13	RP1, ORP1	Oxygen-regulated photoreceptor protein-1 (retinitis pigmentosa-1)	603937	Retinitis pigmentosa-1, 180100 (3)	
8q12	SGPA, PSA	Salivary gland pleomorphic adenoma	181030	Salivary gland pleomorphic adenoma (2)	
8q13	CRH	Corticotropin releasing hormone	122560	ACTH deficiency, 201400 (2)	3 (Crh)
8q13	DURS1, DUS	Duane retraction syndrome 1	126800	Duane syndrome (2)	

continued

Table 10.1. The morbid anatomy of the human genome (by chromosome) (*continued*)

Location	Symbol	Title	MIM#	Disorder	Mouse
8q13-q21	FEB1	Convulsions, familial febrile, 1	602476	Convulsions, familial febrile, 1 (2)	
8q13-q21.1	CMT4A	Charcot-Marie-Tooth neuropathy-4A, autosomal recessive	214400	Charcot-Marie-Tooth neuropathy-4A (2)	
8q13.1-q13.3	TTPA, TTP1, AVED	Tocopherol, alpha, transfer protein	600415	Ataxia with isolated vitamin E deficiency, 277460 (3)	
8q13.3	EYA1, BOR	Eyes absent, Drosophila, homolog of, 1	601653	Branchiootorenal syndrome, 113650 (3); Branchiootic syndrome (3); Anterior segment anomalies and cataract (3); Branchiootorenal syndrome with cataract, 113650 (3)	
8q21-q22	CNGB3, ACHM3	Cyclic nucleotide-gated channel, beta-3	605080	Achromatopsia-3, 262300 (3)	
8q21	CYP11B1, P450C11	Cytochrome P450, subfamily XIB, polypeptide I (11-beta-hydroxylase; corticosteroid methyl-oxidase II (CMO II)	202010	Adrenal hyperplasia, congenital, due to 11-beta-hydroxylase deficiency (3); Aldosteronism, glucocorticoid-remediable (3)	
8q21	CYP11B2	Cytochrome P450, subfamily XIB, polypeptide 2	124080	CMO II deficiency (3)	
8q21	NBS1, NBS	Nibrin	602667	Nijmegen breakage syndrome, 251260 (3)	
8q21.1	PXMP3, PAF1, PMP35, PEX2	Peroxisomal membrane protein-3, 35 kD	170993	Zellweger syndrome-3 (3); Refsum disease, infantile form, 266510 (3)	
8q21.3	CYP7B1	Oxysterol 7-alpha-hydroxylase	603711	Giant cell hepatitis, neonatal, 231100 (3)	
8q21.3	DECR1	2, 4-dienoyl CoA reductase	222745	?DECR deficiency (2)	
8q21.3-q22	RAD54B	RAD54, S. cerevisiae, homolog of, B	604289	Lymphoma, non-Hodgkin (3); Colon adenocarcinoma (3)	
8q22	CA2	Carbonic anhydrase II	259730	Renal tubular acidosis-osteopetrosis syndrome (3)	3 (Car2)
8q22	DPYS, DHP	Dihydropyrimidinase	222748	Dihydropyrimidinuria (3)	
8q22-q23	COH1	Cohen syndrome 1	216550	Cohen syndrome (2)	
8q22.2	SGM1, KFSL	Segmentation syndrome 1 (Klippel-Feil syndrome with laryngeal malformation)	148900	Klippel-Feil syndrome with laryngeal malformation (2)	
8q23	GLC1D	Glaucoma 1, open angle, D	602429	Glaucoma 1D, primary open angle (2)	
8q23-q24	SPG8	Spastic paraplegia-8	603563	Spastic paraplegia-8 (2)	
8q23.3-q24.11	MEBA, BAFME	Myoclonic epilepsy, benign adult familial	601068	Epilepsy, myoclonic, benign adult familial (2)	
8q24	EBS1	Epidermolysis bullosa simplex-1, Ogna	131950	Epidermolysis bullosa, Ogna type (2)	
8q24	ECA1	Epilepsy, childhood absence, 1	600131	Epilepsy, childhood absence, 1 (2)	
8q24	EGI	Epilespy, generalized, idiopathic	600669	Epilepsy, generalized, idiopathic (2)	
8q24	KCNQ3, EBN2, BFNC2	Potassium voltage-gated channel, KQT-like subfamily, member-3	602232	Epilepsy, benign neonatal, type 2, 121201 (3)	
8q24	PLEC1, PLTN	Plectin 1, intermediate filament binding protein, 500 kD	601282	Muscular dystrophy with epidermolysis bullosa simplex, 226670 (3)	
8q24	VMD1	Macular dystrophy, atypical vitelliform	153840	Macular dystrophy, atypical vitelliform (2)	
8q24.1	THM	Tibial hemimelia	275220	?Tibial hemimelia (2)	

continued

Table 10.1. The morbid anatomy of the human genome (by chromosome) (*continued*)

Location	Symbol	Title	MIM#	Disorder	Mouse
8q24.1	TRC8, RCA1, HRCA1	Translocation-related gene on chromosome 8	603046	Renal cell carcinoma, 144700 (3)	
8q24.11-q24.13	EXT1	Exostoses, multiple, 1	133700	Exostoses, multiple, type 1 (3); Chondrosarcoma, 215300 (3)	15 (Ext1)
8q24.11-q24.13	LGCR, LGS, TRPS2	Langer-Giedion syndrome chromosome region	150230	Langer-Giedion syndrome (2)	
8q24.12	TRPS1	Trichorhinophalangeal syndrome type I zinc finger protein	604386	Trichorhinophalangeal syndrome, type I, 190350 (3)	
8q24.12-q24.13	MYC	Avian myelocytomatosis viral (v-myc) oncogene homolog	190080	Burkitt lymphoma, 113970 (3)	15 (Myc)
8q24.2-q24.3	TG	Thyroglobulin	188450	Hypothyroidism, hereditary congenital (3); Goiter, adolescent multinodular (1); Goiter, nonendemic, simple (3)	15 (Tgn; cog)
8q24.3	NDRG1	N-myc downstream-regulated gene 1	605262	Neuropathy, hereditary motor and sensory, Lom type, 601455 (3)	
8q24.3	RECQL4, RTS, RECQ4	RecQ protein-like 4 (DNA helicase, RecQ-like, type 4)	603780	Rothmund-Thomson syndrome, 268400 (3)	
8qter	MDM	Meleda disease (mal de Meleda)	248300	Meleda disease (2)	
9p24.3	DMRT1, DMT1	Double sex and mab-3-related transcription factor-1	602424	XY sex reversal (1)	
9p24	SLC1A1, EAAC1	Solute carrier family 1, member 1 (high-affinity glutamate transporter; excitatory amino acid carrier 1)	133550	?Dicarboxylicaminoaciduria, 222730 (1)	
9p24	OVC	Oncogene OVC (ovarian adenocarcinoma oncogene)	164759	Ovarian carcinoma (2)	
9p24	SRA2, TDFA	Sex-reversal, autosomal, 2 (testis-determining factor, autosomal)	154230	XY sex reversal (2)	
9p23	TYRP1, CAS2, GP75	Tyrosinase-related protein 1	115501	Albinism, brown, 203290 (1); Albinism, rufous, 278400 (3)	4 (b; trp1)
9p22	GLDC, HYGN1, GCSP	Glycine dehydrogenase (decarboxylating; glycine decarboxylase, glycine cleavage system protein P)	238300	Hyperglycinemia, nonketotic, 1 (3)	19 (Gldc)
9p22	IFNA1, IFNA@	Interferon, alpha-1	147660	Interferon, alpha, deficiency (1)	4 (Ifa)
3p25	ST11, PETS1	Suppression of tumorigenicity 11, pancreas	602011	?Pancreatic endocrine tumors (1)	
9p22-p21	DMSMFH, BDMF	Diaphyseal medullary stenosis with malignant fibrous histiocytoma	112250	Diaphyseal medullary stenosis with malignant fibrous histiocytoma (2)	
9p22-p21	LALL	Lymphomatous acute lymphoblastic leukemia	247640	Leukemia, acute lymphoblastic (2)	
9p21	CDKN2A, MTS1, P16, MLM, CMM2	Cyclin-dependent kinase inhibitor 2A (p16, inhibits CDK4)	600160	Melanoma, 155601 (3)	4 (Cdkn2a)
9p21	MFT, TEM	Trichoepithelioma, multiple familial	601606	Trichoepithelioma, multiple familial (2)	
9p21	TEK, TIE2, VMCM	TEK tyrosine kinase, endothelial	600221	Venous malformations, multiple cutaneous and mucosal, 600195 (3)	4 (tek)
9p21-p13	DNAI1	Dynein, axonemal, intermediate chain 1	604366	Immotile cilia syndrome-1, 242650 (3)	

continued

Table 10.1. The morbid anatomy of the human genome (by chromosome) (*continued*)

Location	Symbol	Title	MIM#	Disorder	Mouse
9p21-q21	AMCD1, DA1	Arthrogryposis multiplex congenita, distal, type 1	108120	Arthrogryposis multiplex congenita, distal, type 1 (2)	
9p13	CHH	Cartilage-hair hypoplasia	250250	Cartilage-hair hypoplasia (2)	
9p13	GALT	Galactose-1-phosphate uridyltransferase	230400	Galactosemia (3)	4 (Galt)
9p13	XRCC9, FANCG	X-ray repair, complementing defective, in Chinese hamster, 9	602956	Fanconi anemia, complementation group G (3)	
9p13-p12	AMDM	Acromesomelic dysplasia, Maroteaux type	602875	Acromesomelic dysplasia, Maroteaux type (2)	
9p12-p11	GNE, GLCNE	UDP-N-acetylglucosamine 2-epimerase/N-acetylmannosamine kinase	603824	Sialuria, 269921 (3)	
9p12-q12	ACP	Cerebral palsy, ataxic, autosomal recessive	605388	Cerebral palsy, ataxic, autosomal recessive (2)	
9p11	MROS	Melkersson-Rosenthal syndrome	155900	?Melkersson-Rosenthal syndrome (2)	
9p1-q1	IBM2	Inclusion body myopathy, autosomal recessive	600737	Inclusion body myopathy, autosomal recessive (2)	
9cen	GRHPR, GLXR	Glyoxylate reductase/hydroxypyruvate reductase	604296	Hyperoxaluria, primary, type II, 260000 (3)	
9q12-q22.2	HOMG, HSH, HMGX	Hypomagnesemia with secondary hypocalcemia	602014	Hypomagnesemia with secondary hypocalcemia (2)	
9q13	CMD1B, CMPD1, FDC	Cardiomyopathy, dilated-1B, autosomal dominant	600884	Cardiomyopathy, familial dilated 1B (2)	
9q13	FRDA, FARR	Frataxin	229300	Friedreich ataxia (3); Friedreich ataxia with retained reflexes (3)	
9q13-q21	DFNB7	Deafness, autosomal recessive 7	600974	Deafness, autosomal recessive 7 (2)	?19 (dn)
9q13-q21	GSM1, GSP	Geniospasm 1	190100	Geniospasm (2)	
9q21	CHAC	Choreoacanthocytosis	200150	Choreoacanthocytosis (2)	
9q21	GNAQ	Guanine nucleotide-binding protein (G protein), q	600998	Bleeding diathesis due to GNAQ deficiency (1)	
9q21-q22	ALSFTD	Amyotrophic lateral sclerosis with frontotemporal dementia	105550	Amyotrophic lateral sclerosis with frontotemporal dementia (2)	
9q21.3-q22	HPLH1	Hemophagocytic lymphohistiocytosis, familial, 1	603552	Hemophagocytic lymphohistiocytosis, familial, 1 (2)	
9q22	CSMF	Chondrosarcoma, extraskeletal myxoid, fused to EWS in	600542	Chondrosarcoma, extraskeletal myxoid (1)	
9q22	FOXE1, FKHL15, TITF2, TTF2	Forkhead box E1 (thyroid transcription factor-2)	602617	Bamforth-Lazarus syndrome, 241850 (3)	4 (Tiff2)
9q22	HSD17B3, EDH17B3	Hydroxysteroid (17-beta) dehydrogenase 3	264300	Pseudohermaphroditism, male, with gynecomastia (3)	
9q22	ROR2, BDB1, BDB, NTRKR2	Receptor tyrosine kinase-like orphan receptor 2	602337	Brachydactyly, type B1, 113000 (3); Robinow syndrome, autosomal recessive, 268310 (3)	13 (Ror2)
9q22-q31	ABCA1, ABC1, HDLDT1, TGD	ATP-binding cassette 1	600046	Tangier disease, 205400 (3); HDL deficiency, familial, 604091 (3)	
9q22-q31	NPHP2, NPH2	Nephronophthisis-2 (infantile)	602088	Nephronophthisis, infantile (2)	
9q22.1-q22.3	HSN1, HSAN1	Hereditary sensory neuropathy, type 1	162400	Neuropathy, hereditary sensory and autonomic, type 1 (2)	
9q22.2-q22.3	FBP1	Fructose-bisphosphatase 1	229700	Fructose-bisphosphatase deficiency (1)	

continued

Table 10.1. The morbid anatomy of the human genome (by chromosome) (*continued*)

Location	Symbol	Title	MIM#	Disorder	Mouse
9q22.3	ALDOB	Aldolase B, fructose-bisphosphatase	229600	Fructose intolerance (3)	4 (Aldo2)
9q22.3	FANCC, FACC	Fanconi anemia, complementation group C	227645	Fanconi anemia, type C (3)	13 (Facc)
9q22.3	PTCH, NBCCS, BCNS	Patched, Drosophila, homolog of	601309	Basal cell nevus syndrome, 109400 (3); Basal cell carcinoma, sporadic (3)	13 (Ptc)
9q22.3	XPA	Xeroderma pigmentosum, complementation group A	278700	Xeroderma pigmentosum, group A (3)	4 (Xpa)
9q31	FCMD	Fukuyama congenital muscular dystrophy	253800	Muscular dystrophy, Fukuyama congenital (3); ?Walker-Warburg syndrome, 236670 (2)	
9q31	MSSE, ESS1	Epithelioma, self-healing, squamous 1, Ferguson-Smith type	132800	Epithelioma, self-healing, squamous 1, Ferguson-Smith type (2); ?Basal cell carcinoma (2)	
9q31	NBCCS, BCNS	Nevoid basal cell carcinoma syndrome	109400	Basal cell nevus syndrome (2)	
9q31	TAL2	T-cell acute lymphocytic leukemia-2	186855	Leukemia-2, T-cell acute lymphoblastic (3)	4 (Tal2)
9q31-q33	DYS	Dysautonomia (Riley-Day syndrome, hereditary sensory autonomic neuropathy type III)	223900	Dysautonomia, familial (2)	
9q31-q34.1	LGMD2H	Limb-girdle muscular dystrophy 2H	254110	Muscular dystrophy, limb-girdle, type 2H (2)	
9q32	AFD1, AFDN	Acrofacial dysostosis-1, Nager type	154400	?Acrofacial dysostosis, Nager type (2)	
9q32	DEC1	Deleted in esophageal cancer 1	604767	Esophageal squamous cell carcinoma, 133239 (1)	
9q32-q33	TLR4	Toll-like recpetor-4	603030	Endotoxin hyporesponsiveness (3)	
9q33	FTZF1, FTZ1, SF1	Fushi tarazu factor, Drosophila, homolog of, 1	184757	Sex reversal, XY, with adrenal failure (3)	2 (Ftzf1)
9q33-q34	SARDH, SARD, SAR	Sarcosine dehydrogenase	604455	[Sarcosinemia], 268900 (2)	2 (sar)
9q34	ALAD	Aminolevulinate, delta-, dehydratase	125270	Porphyria, acute hepatic (3); {Lead poisoning, susceptibility to} (3)	4 (Lv)
9q34	ALS4	Amyotrophic lateral sclerosis-4, juvenile dominant	602433	Amyotrophic lateral sclerosis-4, juvenile dominant (2)	
9q34	AOA	Ataxia-oculomotor apraxia syndrome	208920	Ataxia-oculomotor apraxia (2)	
9q34	ASS	Argininosuccinate synthetase	603470	Citrullinemia, 215700 (3)	2 (Ass1)
9q34	BSCL	Berardinelli-Seip congenital lipodystrophy	269700	Berardinelli-Seip congenital lipodystrophy (2)	
9q34	DBH	Dopamine-beta-hydroxylase	223360	Dopamine-beta-hydroxylase deficiency (1)	2 (Dbh)
9q34	DYT1	Dystonia-1, torsion, autosomal dominant	128100	Dystonia-1, torsion (3)	
9q34	GSN	Gelsolin	137350	Amyloidosis, Finnish type, 105120 (3)	2 (Gsn)
9q34	LCCS	Lethal congenital contracture syndrome	253310	Lethal congenital contracture syndrome (2)	
9q34	MCPH3	Microcephaly, primary autosomal recessive, 3	604804	Microcephaly, primary autosomal recessive, 3 (2)	
9q34	SURF1	Surfeit-1	185620	Leigh syndrome, due to COX deficiency, 256000 (3)	2 (Surf)

continued

Table 10.1. The morbid anatomy of the human genome (by chromosome) *(continued)*

Location	Symbol	Title	MIM#	Disorder	Mouse
9q34	TSC1	Hamartin (tuberous sclerosis 1 gene)	605284	Tuberous sclerosis-1, 191100 (3)	
9q34.1	ABL1	Abelson murine leukemia viral (v-abl) oncogene homolog 1	189980	Leukemia, chronic myeloid (3)	2 (Ab1)
9q34.1	AK1	Adenylate kinase-1	103000	Hemolytic anemia due to adenylate kinase deficiency (3)	2 (Ak1)
9q34.1	C5	Complement component-5	120900	C5 deficiency (1)	2 (Hc)
9q34.1	CRAT, CAT1	Carnitine acetyltransferase	600184	?Carnitine acetyltransferase deficiency (1)	
9q34.1	D9S46E, CAN, CAIN, NUP214	CAIN gene	114350	Leukemia, acute myeloid (2)	2 (D2H9S46E)
9q34.1	ENG, END, HHT1, ORW	Endoglin	131195	Hereditary hemorrhagic telangiectasia-1, 187300 (3)	2 (Eng)
9q34.1	EPB72	Erythrocyte membrane protein band 7.2 (stomatin)	133090	?Stomatocytosis I, 185000 (1)	2 (Epb7.2)
9q34.1	LMX1B, NPS1	LIM homeo box transcription factor 1, beta	602575	Nail-patella syndrome, 161200 (3); Nail-patella syndrome with open-angle glaucoma, 137750 (3)	2 (Lmx1b)
9q34.2-q34.3	COL5A1	Collagen V, alpha-1 polypeptide	120215	Ehlers-Danlos syndrome, type II, 130010 (3); Ehlers-Danlos syndrome, type I, 130000 (3)	2 (Col5al)
9q34.3	JBTS1	Joubert syndrome-1	213300	Joubert syndrome-1 (2)	
9q34.3	LHX3	LIM/homeodomain protein LHX3	600577	Pituitary hormone deficiency, combined, with rigid cervical spine, 262600 (3)	2 (Lhx3)
9q34.3	NOTCH1, TAN1	Notch, Drosophila, homolog of, 1, translocation-associated	190198	Leukemia, T-cell acute lymphoblastic (2)	2 (Notchl)
10pter-p11.2	PHYH, PAHX	Phytanoyl-CoA hydroxylase	602026	Refsum disease, 266500 (3)	
10pter-p11.2	RDPA	Refsum disease, adult, with increased pipecolicacidemia	600964	Refsum disease, adult, with increased pipecolicacidemia (2)	
10pter-q11	ST12, PAC1	Suppression of tumorigenicity 12, prostate	601188	Prostate adenocarcinoma (2)	
10p15.1-p14	HDR	Hypoparathyroidism, sensorineural deafness, renal dysplasia	146255	HDR syndrome (2)	
10p15	GATA3, HDR	GATA-binding protein-3	131320	Hypoparathyroidism, sensorineural deafness, and renal dysplasia, 146255 (3)	2 (Gata3)
10p15-p14	IL2RA, IL2R	Interleukin-2 receptor	147730	Interleukin-2 receptor, alpha chain, deficiency of (3)	2 (Il2ra)
10p14-p13	DGCR2, DGS2	DiGeorge syndrome chromosome region-2	601362	DiGeorge syndrome/velocardiofacial syndrome complex-2 (2)	
10p14-p12	ARVD6	Arrhythmogenic right ventricular dysplasia-6	604401	Arrhythmogenic right ventricular dysplasia-6 (2)	
10p12	AF10	ALL1 fused gene from chromosome 10	602409	Leukemia, acute myeloid (3); Leukemia, acute T-cell lymphoblastic (3)	
10p12-p11.2	THC2	Thrombocytopenia 2	188000	Thrombocytopenia-2 (2)	
10p12.1	CUBN, IFCR, MGA1	Cubilin (intrinsic factor-cobalamin receptor)	602997	Megaloblastic anemia-1, 261100 (3)	
10p11-q11	IDDM10	Insulin-dependent diabetes mellitus-10	601942	{Diabetes mellitus, insulin-dependent, 10} (2)	

continued

Table 10.1. The morbid anatomy of the human genome (by chromosome) (*continued*)

Locationa	Symbol	Title	MIM#	Disorder	Mouse
10p	OB10	Obesity, susceptibility to, on chromosome 10	603188	{Obesity, susceptibility to}, 601665 (2)	
10p	SCIDA	Severe combined immunodeficiency, Athabascan type	602450	Severe combined immunodeficiency, Athabascan type (2)	
10q11	ERCC6, CKN2, COFS	Excision repair cross complementing rodent repair deficiency, complementation group 6	133540	Cockayne syndrome-2, type B (3); Cerebrooculofacioskeletal syndrome, 214150 (3)	
10q11.1	SDF1	Stromal cell-derived factor 1	600835	{AIDS, resistance to} (3)	
10q11.2	RET, MEN2A	RET transforming sequence; oncogene RET	164761	Multiple endocrine neoplasia IIA, 171400 (3); Medullary thyroid carcinoma, 155240 (3); Multiple endocrine neoplasia IIB, 162300 (3); Hirschsprung disease, 142623 (3)	
10q11.2-q21	MBL2, MBL, MBP1	Mannose-binding lectin 2, soluble (opsonic defect)	154545	{Chronic infections, due to opsonin defect} (3)	14 (Mbl1)
10q21	D10S170, H4, TST1, PTC, TPC	RET-activating gene H4	601985	Thyroid papillary carcinoma, 188550 (1)	
10q21	RNANC, NCRNA	Retinal nonattachment, nonsyndromic congenital	221900	Retinal nonattachment, nonsyndromic congenital (2)	
10q21-q22	CDH23, USH1D	Cadherin-23	605516	Usher syndrome, type 1D, 601067 (3)	10 (Cdh23, v)
10q21-q22	DFNB12	Deafness, autosomal recessive 12	601386	Deafness, autosomal recessive 12 (2)	
10q21-q23	CMD1C, CMPD3	Cardiomyopathy, dilated-1C, autosomal dominant	601493	Cardiomyopathy, dilated 1C (2)	
10q21.1-q22.1	EGR2, KROX20	KROX-20, Drosophila, homolog of (early growth response-2)	129010	Neuropathy, congenital hypomyelinating, 1, 605253 (3)	10 (Krox20; Egr2)
10q21.3-q22.1	MBS3	Moebius syndrome 3	604185	Moebius syndrome-3 (2)	
10q22	HK1	Hexokinase-1	142600	Hemolytic anemia due to hexokinase deficiency (3)	10 (Hk1)
10q22	MAT1A, MATA1, SAMS1	Methionine adenosyltransferase I, alpha	250850	Hypermethioninemia, persistent, autosomal dominant, due to methionine adenosyltransferase I/III deficiency (3); Methionine adenosyltransferase deficiency, autosomal recessive (3)	
10q22	PCBD, DCOH	Pterin-4a-carbinolamine dehydratase (dimerization cofactor of hepatic nuclear factor 1-alpha)	126090	Hyperphenylalaninemia due to pterin-4a-carbinolamine dehydratase deficiency, 264070 (3)	10 (Dcoh)
10q22	PRF1, HPLH2	Perforin	170280	Hemophagocytic lymphohistiocytosis, familial, 2, 603553 (3)	10 (Prf1)
10q22.1	PSAP, SAP1	Prosaposin (sphingolipid activator protein-1)	176801	Metachromatic leukodystrophy due to deficiency of SAP-1 (3); Gaucher disease, variant form (3)	10 (Psap)
10q23	RGR	Retinal G protein coupled receptor	600342	Retinitis pigmentosa, autosomal recessive (3); Retinitis pigmentosa, autosomal dominant (3)	
10q23-q24	ATPSK2	ATP sulfurylase/APS kinase 2	603005	SEMD, Pakistani type (3)	19 (Atpsk2, bm)
10q23-q24	UFS	Urofacial syndrome (Ochoa syndrome)	236730	Urofacial syndrome (2)	
10q23.1-q23.3	HPS1	Hermansky-Pudlak syndrome gene	604982	Hermansky-Pudlak syndrome, 203300 (3)	19 (ep, ru)

continued

Table 10.1. The morbid anatomy of the human genome (by chromosome) (*continued*)

Location	Symbol	Title	MIM#	Disorder	Mouse
10q23.2	BLNK, SLP65	B-cell linker protein (SH2 domain-containing leukocyte protein, 65 kD)	604515	Hypoglobulinemia and absent B cells (3)	
10q23.2	NMSR, HMSNR	Neuropathy, hereditary motor and sensory, Russe type	605285	Neuropathy, motor and sensory, Russe type (2)	
10q23.3	GLUD1	Glutamate dehydrogenase-1	138130	Hyperinsulinism-hyperammonemia syndrome (3)	14 (Glud)
10q23.3	PTEN, MMAC1	Phosphatase and tensin homolog (mutated in multiple advanced cancers 1)	601728	Cowden disease, 158350 (3); Lhermitte-Duclos syndrome (3); Bannayan-Zonana syndrome, 153480 (3); Endometrial carcinoma (3); Polyposis, juvenile intestinal, 174900 (3); Prostate cancer (3); Bannayan-Riley-Ruvalcaba syndrome (3)	19 (Pten)
10q23.3-q24.1	EPT	Epilepsy, partial	600512	Epilepsy, partial (2)	
10q23.3-q24.1	SPG9	Spastic paraplegia-9 (spastic paraparesis with amyotrophy, cataracts and gastroesophageal reflux)	601162	Spastic paraplegia-9 (2)	
10q23.3-q24.3	PEO1, PEO	Progressive external ophthalmoplegia, type 1	157640	PEO with mitochondrial DNA deletions, type I (2)	
10q24	ABCC2, CMOAT	ATP-binding cassette, subfamily C, member 2 (canalicular multispecific organic anion transporter)	601107	Dubin-Johnson syndrome, 237500 (3)	19 (Cmoat)
10q24	AD6	Alzheimer disease 6	605526	Alzheimer disease 6, 104300 (2)	
10q24	CDB2, CDTB	Corneal dystrophy, Thiel-Behnke type	602082	Corneal dystrophy, Thiel-Behnke type (2)	
10q24	CYP2C9	Cytochrome P450, subfamily IIC (mephenytoin 4-hydroxylase), polypeptide 9	601130	Tolbutamide poor metabolizer (3); Warfarin sensitivity, 122700 (3)	
10q24	HOX11, TCL3	Homeo box-11 (T-cell leukemia-3 associated breakpoint, homologous to Drosophila Notch)	186770	Leukemia, T-cell acute lymphocytic (2)	
10q24	IOSCA, SCA8	Infantile-onset spinocerebellar ataxia	271245	Spinocerebellar ataxia, infantile-onset, with sensory neuropathy (2)	
10q24	RBP4	Retinol-binding protein-4, interstitial	180250	Retinol binding protein, deficiency of (3)	19 (Rbp4)
10q24	SHFM3, DAC	Split hand/foot malformation, type 3 (dactylin)	600095	Split hand/foot malformation, type 3 (2)	19 (Dac)
10q24-q25	LIPA	Lipase A, lysosomal acid, cholesterol esterase	278000	Wolman disease (3); Cholesteryl ester storage disease (3)	19 (Lip1)
10q24.1	TNFRSF6, APT1, FAS, CD95	Tumor necrosis factor receptor superfamily, member 6	134637	{Autoimmune lymphoproliferative syndrome} (3)	19 (Fas1)
10q24.1-q24.3	CYP2C, CYP2C19	Cytochrome P450, subfamily IIC (mephenytoin 4'-hydroxylase)	124020	Mephenytoin poor metabolizer (3)	19 (P4502c)
10q24.3	COL17A1, BPAG2	Collagen XVII, alpha-1 polypeptide	113811	Epidermolysis bullosa, generalized atrophic benign, 226650 (3)	19 (Bpag2)
10q24.3	CYP17, P450C17	Cytochrome P450, subfamily XVII (steroid 17-alpha-hydroxylase)	202110	Adrenal hyperplasia, congenital, due to 17-alpha-hydroxylase deficiency (3)	19 (Cyp17)

continued

Table 10.1. The morbid anatomy of the human genome (by chromosome) (*continued*)

Location	Symbol	Title	MIM#	Disorder	Mouse
10q24.3	PYCS, GSAS	Pyrroline-5-carboxlate synthetase	138250	?P5CS deficiency (1)	
10q24.3-q25.1	PAX2	Paired box homeotic gene-2	167409	Optic nerve coloboma with renal disease, 120330 (3)	19 (Pax2)
10q25	IDDM17	Insulin-dependent diabetes mellitus-17	603266	{Diabetes mellitus, insulin-dependent, 17} (2)	
10q25	MXI1	MAX-interacting protein 1	600020	Prostate cancer, 176807 (3); Neurofibrosarcoma (3)	19 (Mxi1)
10q25	PITX3	Paired-like homeodomain transcription factor-3	602669	Anterior segment mesenchymal dysgenesis and cataract, 107250 (3); Cataract, congenital (3)	19 (Pitx3)
10q25.2-q26.3	UROS	Uroporphyrinogen III synthase	263700	Porphyria, congenital erythropoietic (3)	7 (Uros)
10q25.3	TCF7L2, TCF4	Transcription factor 7-like 2	602228	Colorectal cancer, 114500 (3)	
10q25.3-q26.1	DMBT1	Deleted in malignant brain tumors 1	601969	Glioblastoma multiforme, 137800 (3); Medulloblastoma, 155255 (3)	
10q26	DEC	Deleted in endometrial carcinoma	602084	Endometrial carcinoma (2)	
10q26	FGFR2, BEK, CFD1, JWS	Fibroblast growth factor receptor-2 (bacteria-expressed kinase)	176943	Crouzon syndrome, 123500 (3); Jackson-Weiss syndrome, 123150 (3); Beare-Stevenson cutis gyrata syndrome, 123790 (3); Pfeiffer syndrome, 101600 (3); Apert syndrome, 101200 (3); Saethre-Chotzen syndrome (3); Antley-Bixler syndrome (3); Craniosynostosis, nonspecific (3)	7 (Fgfr2)
10q26	OAT	Ornithine aminotransferase	258870	Gyrate atrophy of choroid and retina with ornithinemia, B6 responsive or unresponsive (3)	7 (Oat)
10q26.1	EMX2	Empty spiracles, Drosophila, homolog of, 2	600035	Schizencephaly (3)	19 (Emx2)
10q26.1	PNLIP	Pancreatic lipase	246600	Pancreatic lipase deficiency (1)	
Chr.10	GLC1E	Glaucoma 1, open angle, E	602432	Glaucoma 1E, primary open angle, adult-onset (2)	
Chr.10	NODAL	Nodal, mouse, homolog of	601265	Situs ambiguus (3)	10 (nodal)
Chr.10	USH1F	Usher syndrome-1F, autosomal recessive, severe	602083	Usher syndrome, type IF (2)	
11pter-p13	AMPD3	Adenosine monophosphate deaminase-3, isoform E	102772	[AMP deaminase deficiency, erythrocytic] (3)	7 (Ampd3)
11p15.5	AMCD2B, DA2B, FSSV	Arthrogryposis multiplex congenita, distal, type 2B (Freeman-Sheldon syndrome variant)	601680	Arthrogryposis multiplex congenita, distal, type 2B (2)	
11p15.5	CDKN1C, KIP2, BWS	Cyclin-dependent kinase inhibitor 1C (p57, Kip2)	600856	Beckwith-Wiedemann syndrome, 130650 (3)	7 (Kip2)
11p15.5	CLN2	Ceroid-lipofuscinosis, neuronal 2, late infantile (Jansky-Bielschowsky disease)	204500	Ceroid-lipofuscinosis, neuronal 2, classic late infantile (2)	
11p15.5	DRD4	Dopamine receptor D4	126452	Autonomic nervous system dysfunction (3); [Novelty seeking personality], 601696 (1)	
11p15.5	IDDM2	Insulin-dependent diabetes mellitus-2	125852	{Diabetes mellitus, insulin-dependent, 2} (2)	

continued

Table 10.1. The morbid anatomy of the human genome (by chromosome) (*continued*)

Location	Symbol	Title	MIM#	Disorder	Mouse
11p15.5	KCNQ1, KCNA9, LQT1, KVLQT1	Potassium voltage-gated channel, KQT-like subfamily, member 1	192500	Long QT syndrome-1 (3); Jervell and Lange-Nielsen syndrome, 220400 (3)	
11p15.5	HBB	Hemoglobin beta	141900	Sickle cell anemia (3); Thalassemias, beta-(3); Methemoglobinemias, beta- (3); Erythremias, beta- (3); Heinz body anemias, beta- (3); HPFH, deletion type (3)	7 (Hbb)
11p15.5	HBD	Hemoglobin delta	142000	Thalassemia, delta- (3); Thalassemia due to Hb Lepore (3)	
11p15.5	HBG1	Hemoglobin, gamma A	142200	HPFH, nondeletion type A (3)	
11p15.5	HBG2	Hemoglobin, gamma G	142250	HPFH, nondeletion type G (3)	
11p15.5	HRAS	Harvey rat sarcoma viral (v-Ha-ras) oncogene homolog	190020	Bladder cancer, 109800 (3)	7 (Hras1)
11p15.5	INS	Insulin	176730	Diabetes mellitus, rare form (1); MODY, one form (3); Hyperproinsulinemia, familial (3)	6 (Ins1); 7 (Ins2)
11p15.5	MTACR1, WT2	Multiple tumor associated chromosome region-1	194071	Wilms tumor, type 2 (2); Adrenocortical carcinoma, hereditary, 202300 (2)	
11p15.5	SLC22A1L, BWSCR1A, IMPT1	Solute carrier family 22, member 1-like (Beckwith-Wiedemann region 1A; organic-cation transporter-like 2)	602631	Breast cancer, 114480 (3); Rhabdomyosarcoma, 268210 (3); Lung cancer, 211980 (3)	
11p15.5	TH, TYH	Tyrosine hydroxylase	191290	Segawa syndrome, recessive (3)	7 (Th)
11p15.4	LDHA, LDH1	Lactate dehydrogenase A	150000	Exertional myoglobinuria due to deficiency of LDH-A (3)	7 (Ldh1)
11p15.4-p15.1	SMPD1, NPD	Sphingomyelin phosphodiesterase-1, acid lysosomal	257200	Niemann-Pick disease, type A (3); Niemann-Pick disease, type B (3)	7 (Smpd1)
11p15.3-p15.1	PTH	Parathyroid hormone	168450	Hypoparathyroidism, autosomal dominant (3); Hypoparathyroidism, autosomal recessive (3)	7 (Pth)
11p15.2-p15.1	CALCA, CALC1	Calcitonin/calcitonin-related polypeptide, alpha	114130	Osteoporosis (3)	7 (Calc)
11p15.2-p15.1	TSG101	Tumor susceptibility gene 101	601387	Breast cancer (3)	
11p15.1	ABCC8, SUR, PHHI, SUR1	ATP-binding cassette, subfamily C, member 8 (sulfonylurea receptor)	600509	Persistent hyperinsulinemic hypoglycemia of infancy, 256450 (3)	
11p15.1	KCNJ11, BIR, PHHI	Potassium inwardly-rectifying channel, subfamily J, member 11	600937	Persistent hyperinsulinemic hypoglycemia of infancy, 256450 (3)	
11p15.1	USH1C	Harmonin (Usher syndrome 1C gene)	605242	Usher syndrome, type 1C, 276904 (3)	
11p15.1-p14	DFNB18	Deafness, autosomal recessive 18	602092	Deafness, autosomal recessive 18 (2)	
11p15	AA	Atrophia areata	108985	Atrophia areata (2)	
11p15	CMT4B2	Charcot-Marie-Tooth disease, type 4B, form 2	604563	Charcot-Marie-Tooth disease, type 4B, form 2 (2)	
11p15	FANCF	Fanconi anemia, complementation group F	603467	Fanconi anemia, complementation group F (3)	
11p15	LMO1, RBTN1, RHOM1	LIM domain only 1 (rhombotin 1)	186921	Leukemia, T-cell acute lymphoblastic (2)	7 (Ttg1)
11p15	NUP98	Nucleoporin, 98 kD	601021	Leukemia, lymphycytic, acute T-cell (1)	
11p14-p13	HVBS1	Hepatitis B virus integration site-1	114550	Hepatocellular carcinoma (1)	

continued

Table 10.1. The morbid anatomy of the human genome (by chromosome) (*continued*)

Location	Symbol	Title	MIM#	Disorder	Mouse
11p13	CAT	Catalase	115500	Acatalasemia (3)	2 (Cas1)
11p13	CD59, MIC11	CD59 antigen (p18–20)	107271	CD59 deficiency (3)	15 (Ly6)
11p13	FSHB	Follicle-stimulating hormone, beta polypeptide	136530	?Male infertility, familial (1)	2 (Fshb)
11p13	LMO2, RBTNL1, RHOM2, TTG2	LIM domain only 2 (rhombotin-like 1)	180385	Leukemia, acute T-cell (2)	
11p13	PAX6, AN2	Paired box homeotic gene-6	106210	Aniridia (3); Peters anomaly, 603807 (3); Cataract, congenital, with late-onset corneal dystrophy (3); Foveal hypoplasia, isolated, 136520 (3); Ectopia pupillae, 129750 (3); Keratitis, 148190 (3); Eye anomalies, multiplex (3)	2 (Sey)
11p13	PDX1	Pyruvate dehydrogenase complex, lipoyl-containing component X	245349	Lacticacidemia due to PDX1 deficiency (3)	
11p13	RAG1	Recombination activating gene-1	179615	Severe combined immunodeficiency, B cell-negative, 601457 (3); Reticulosis, familial histiocytic, 267700 (3); Omenn syndrome, 603554 (3)	2 (Rag1)
11p13	RAG2	Recombination activating gene-2	179616	Severe combined immunodeficiency, B cell-negative, 601457 (3); Omenn syndrome, 603554 (3)	2 (Rag2)
11p13	TCL2	T-cell leukemia/lymphoma-2	151390	Leukemia, acute T-cell (2)	
11p13	WT1	Wilms tumor-1	194070	Wilms tumor, type 1 (3); Denys-Drash syndrome (3); Frasier syndrome, 136680 (3)	2 (Wt1)
11p12-p11.2	MAPK8IP1, IB1	Mitogen-activated protein kinase 8-interacting protein 1	604641	Diabetes mellitus, noninsulin-dependent, 125853 (3)	
11p12-p11	ACP2	Acid phosphatase 2, lysosomal	171650	?Lysosomal acid phosphatase deficiency (1)	2 (Acp2)
11p12-p11	DDB2	Damage-specific DNA binding protein 2, 48 kD	600811	Xeroderma pigmentosum, group E, DDB-negative subtype, 278740 (3)	
11p12-p11	EXT2	Exostoses, multiple, 2	133701	Exostoses, multiple, type 2 (3)	2 (Ext2)
11p11.2	ALX4, PFM2	Aristaless-like 4, mouse, homolog of	605420	Parietal foramina 2, 168500 (3)	
11p11.2	MYBPC3, CMH4	Myosin-binding protein C, cardiac	600958	Cardiomyopathy, familial hypertrophic, 4, 115197 (3)	
11p11.2	KAI1, ST6, CD82, SAR2	Kangai 1 (suppression of tumorigenicity 6, prostate)	600623	Prostate cancer, 176807 (2)	
11p11-q11	SCA5	Spinocerebellar ataxia 5	600224	Spinocerebellar ataxia-5 (2)	
11p11-q12	F2	Coagulation factor II (thrombin)	176930	Hypoprothrombinemia (3); Dysprothrombinemia (3)	2 (Cf2)
11p	HYPLIP2	Hyperlipidemia, combined, 2	604499	Hyperlipidemia, combined, 2 (2)	
11p	NNO1	Nanophthalmos 1	600165	Nanophthalmos-1 (2)	
11q	OASF, OA	Osteoarthritis susceptibility, female-specific	165720	{Osteoarthritis susceptibility, female-specific} (2)	
11q11-q13.1	C1NH	Complement component-1 inhibitor	106100	Angioedema, hereditary (3)	2 (C1nh)

continued

Table 10.1. The morbid anatomy of the human genome (by chromosome) *(continued)*

Location	Symbol	Title	MIM#	Disorder	Mouse
11q12-q13	DDB1	Damage-specific DNA binding protein 1, 127 kD	600045	Xeroderma pigmentosum, group E, subtype 2 (1)	19 (Ddb1)
11q12-q13	DHCR7, SLOS	Delta-7-dehydrocholesterol reductase	602858	Smith-Lemli-Opitz syndrome, type I, 270400 (3); Smith-Lemli-Opitz syndrome, type II, 268670 (3)	
11q12-q13	HBM	High bone mass	601884	[High bone mass] (2)	
11q12-q13	IGER, APY	IgE responsiveness, atopic	147050	Atopy (2)	
11q12-q13	OPPG	Osteoporosis-pseudoglioma syndrome	259770	Osteoporosis-pseudoglioma syndrome (2)	
11q13	BBS1	Bardet-Biedl syndrome 1	209901	Bardet-Biedl syndrome 1 (2)	
11q13	CCND1, PRAD1	Cyclin D1	168461	Parathyroid adenomatosis 1 (2); Centrocytic lymphoma (2); Multiple myeloma, 254500 (2)	
11q13	CPT1A	Carnitine palmitoyltransferase I, liver	600528	CPT deficiency, hepatic, type I, 255120 (3)	
11q13	GIF	Gastric intrinsic factor	261000	Anemia, pernicious, congenital, due to deficiency of intrinsic factor (1)	19 (Gif)
11q13	IDDM4	Insulin-dependent diabetes mellitus-4	600319	{Diabetes mellitus, insulin-dependent, 4} (2)	
11q13	MEN1	Menin	131100	Multiple endocrine neoplasia I (3); Hyperparathyroidism, AD, 145000 (3); Prolactinoma, hyperparathyroidism, carcinoid syndrome (3); Carcinoid tumor of lung (3); Parathyroid adenoma, sporadic (3); Lipoma, sporadic (3); Angiofibroma, sporadic (3); Adrenal adenoma, sporadic (3)	19 (Men1)
11q13	MKS2	Meckel syndrome, type 2	603194	Meckel syndrome, type 2 (2)	
11q13	MS4A1, FCER1B	Membrane-spanning 4-domains, subfamily A, member 1 (Fc fragment of IgE, high affinity I, receptor for, beta polypeptide)	147138	{Asthma, atopic, susceptibility to} (3)	
11q13	NDUFS8	NADH dehydrogenase (ubiquinone) Fe-S protein 8, 23 kD (NADH-coenzyme Q reductase)	602141	Leigh syndrome, 256000 (3)	
11q13	NDUFV1, UQOR1	NADH dehydrogenase (ubiquinone) flavoprotein 1, 51 kD	161015	Leigh syndrome, 256000 (3); Alexander disease, 203450 (3)	
11q13	NUMA1	Nuclear mitotic apparatus protein-1	164009	Leukemia, acute promyelocytic, NUMA/RARA type (3)	
11q13	PYGM	Phosphorylase, glycogen, muscle	232600	McArdle disease (3)	19 (Pygm)
11q13	ROM1, ROSP1	Rod outer segment membrane protein-1	180721	Retinitis pigmentosa, digenic (3)	19 (Rosp1)
11q13	RT6	RT6 antigen, rat, homolog of	180840	? {Susceptibility to IDDM} (1)	7 (Rt6)
11q13	SMTPHN	Somatotrophinoma	102200	Somatotrophinoma (2)	
11q13	ST3	Suppression of tumorigenicity-3 (tumor-suppressor gene, HELA cell type)	191181	Cervical carcinoma (2)	
11q13	VMD2	Vitelliform macular dystrophy (Best disease)	153700	Macular dystrophy, vitelliform type (3)	
11q13	VRNI	Vitreoretinopathy, neovascular inflammatory	193235	Vitreoretinopathy, neovascular inflammatory (2)	

continued

Table 10.1. The morbid anatomy of the human genome (by chromosome) (*continued*)

Location	Symbol	Title	MIM#	Disorder	Mouse
11q13-q21	SMARD1	Spinal muscular atrophy with respiratory distress 1	604320	Spinal muscular atrophy with respiratory distress 1 (2)	
11q13-q23	EVR1, FEVR	Exudative vitreoretinopathy-1, autosomal dominant (Criswick-Schepens syndrome)	133780	Vitreoretinopathy, exudative, familial (2)	
11q13.1	PGL2	Paraganglioma or familial glomus tumors 2	601650	Paraganglioma, familial nonchromaffin, 2 (2)	
11q13.2	FEOM2, CFEOM2	Fibrosis of extraocular muscles, congenital, 2, autosomal recessive	602078	Fibrosis of extraocular muscles, congenital, 2 (2)	
11q13.3	BCL1	B-cell CLL/lymphoma-1	151400	Leukemia/lymphoma, B-cell, 1 (2)	
11q13.3-q13.5	FOLRI	Folate receptor-1, adult	136430	{?Congenital anomalies, susceptibility to} (2)	
11q13.4-q13.5	PC	Pyruvate carboxylase	266150	Pyruvate carboxylase deficiency (3)	19 (Pc)
11q13.4-q13.5	TCIRG1, TIRC7, OC116, OPTB1	T-cell immune regulator 1	604592	Osteopetrosis, recessive, 259700 (3)	19 (oc)
11q13.5	MYO7A, USH1B, DFNB2, DFNA11	Myosin VIIA	276903	Usher syndrome, type 1B (3); Deafness, autosomal recessive 2, neurosensory, 600060 (3); Deafness, autosomal dominant 11, neurosensory, 601317 (3)	7 (sh1, Myo7a)
11q14	CALM, CLTH	Clathrin assembly lymphoid-myeloid leukemia gene	603025	Leukemia, acute myeloid (3); Leukemia, acute T-cell lymphoblastic (3)	
11q14-q21	SCZD2	Schizophrenia susceptibility locus, chromosome 11-related	603342	{?Schizophrenia}, 181500 (2)	
11q14-q21	TYR	Tyrosinase	203100	Albinism, oculocutaneous, type IA (3); Waardenburg syndrome/ocular albinism, digenic, 103470 (3)	7 (Tyr)
11q14.1-q14.3	CTSC, CPPI, PALS, PLS, HMS	Cathepsin C	602365	Papillon-Lefevre syndrome, 245000 (3); Haim-Munk syndrome, 245010 (3)	7 (Ctsc)
11q21-q22	FSGS2	Focal segmental glomerulosclerosis 2	603965	Glomerulosclerosis, focal segmental, 2 (2)	
11q21	MRE11A, MRE11, ATLD	Meiotic recombination 11, S. cerevisiae, homolog A of	600814	Ataxia-telangiectasia-like disorder, 604391 (3)	
11q22	MTMR2, CMT4B	Myotubularin-related protein 2	603557	Charcot-Marie-Tooth disease, type 4B, 601382 (3)	
11q22-q24	PPP2R1B	Protein phosphatase 2, structural/regulatory subunit A, beta	603113	Lung cancer, 211980 (3)	
11q22-q24	TECTA, DFNA8, DFNA12, DFNB21	Tectorin, alpha	602574	Deafness, autosomal dominant 8, 601543 (3); Deafness, autosomal dominant 12, 601842 (3); Deafness, autosomal recessive 21, 603629 (3)	
11q22-qter	ANC	Anal canal carcinoma	105580	?Anal canal carcinoma (2)	
11q22.3	ATM, ATA, AT1	Ataxia-telangiectasia mutated (includes complementation groups A, C, D, and E)	208900	Ataxia-telangiectasia (3); T-cell prolymphocytic leukemia, sporadic (3); Lymphoma, B-cell non-Hodgkin, somatic (3); {Breast cancer, susceptibility to} (3); Lymphoma, mantel cell (3)	9 (Atm)
11q22.3-q23.1	ACAT1	Acetyl-Coenzyme A acetyltransferase-1 (acetoacetyl Coenzyme A thiolase)	203750	3-ketothiolase deficiency (3)	

continued

Table 10.1. The morbid anatomy of the human genome (by chromosome) (*continued*)

Location	Symbol	Title	MIM#	Disorder	Mouse
11q22.3-q23.1	CRYAB, CRYA2	Crystallin, alpha B	123590	Myopathy, desmin-related, cardioskeletal, 601419 (3)	
11q22.3-q23.3	PTS	6-pyruvoyltetrahydropterin synthase	261640	Phenylketonuria due to PTS deficiency (3)	
11q23	APOA1	Apolipoprotein A-I	107680	ApoA-I and apoC-III deficiency, combined (3); Hypertriglyceridemia, one form (3); Hypoalphalipoproteinemia (3); Corneal clouding, autosomal recessive (3); Amyloidosis, 3 or more types (3)	9 (Apoal)
11q23	APOC3	Apolipoprotein C-III	107720	Hypertriglyceridemia (3)	
11q23	BRCA3	Breast cancer, 11; 22 translocation associated	600048	Breast cancer-3 (2)	
11q23	CD3E	CD3E antigen, epsilon polypeptide (TiT3 complex)	186830	Immunodeficiency, T-cell receptor/CD3 complex (3)	9 (T3 e)
11q23	CD3G	CD3G antigen, gamma polypeptide (TiT3 complex)	186740	Immunodeficiency due to defect in CD3-gamma (3)	9 (T3 g)
11q23	DRD2	Dopamine receptor D2	126450	Dystonia, myoclonic, 159900 (3)	
11q23	ECB2	Erythrocytosis, autosomal recessive benign	263400	Erythrocytosis, autosomal recessive benign (2)	
11q23	FXYD2, ATP1G1, HOMG2	FXYD domain-containing ion transport regulator 2 (sodium-potassium-ATPase, gamma polypeptide)	601814	Hypomagnesemia-2, renal, 154020 (3)	
11q23	G6PT1	Glucose-6-phosphate transporter-1	602671	Glycogen storage disease Ib, 232220 (3); Glycogen storage disease Ic, 232240 (3)	
11q23	GTS	Gilles de la Tourette syndrome	137580	Tourette syndrome (2)	
11q23	JBS	Jacobsen syndrome	147791	Jacobsen syndrome (2)	
11q23	MLL, HRX, HTRX1	Myeloid/lymphoid or mixed-lineage leukemia (trithorax, Drosophila, homolog)	159555	Leukemia, myeloid/lymphoid or mixed-lineage (2)	9 (All1)
11q23	SDHD, PGL1	Succinate dehydrogenase complex, subunit D, integral membrane protein	602690	Paragangliomas, familial nonchromaffin, 1, 168000 (3)	
11q23	TCPT	Thrombocytopenia, Paris-Trousseau type (deletion 11q23 syndrome)	188025	?Thrombocytopenia, Paris-Trousseau type (2)	
11q23	TSG11	Tumor suppressor gene on chromosome 11	603040	{Nonsmall cell lung cancer} (2)	
11q23-q24	HVEC, PVRL1, PVRR1, PRR1	Herpesvirus entry mediator C (poliovirus receptor-related 1; nectin)	600644	Ectodermal dysplasia, Margarita Island type, 225060 (3); Zlotogora-Ogur syndrome, 225000 (3); Cleft lip/palate ectodermal dysplasia syndrome, 225000 (3)	
11q23-q25	HLS	Hydrolethalus syndrome	236680	Hydrolethalus syndrome (2)	
11q23.1	PLZF	Promyelocytic leukemia zinc finger	176797	Leukemia, acute promyelocytic, PL2F/RARA type (3)	
11q23.1	PORC	Porphyria, acute, Chester type	176010	Porphyria, Chester type (2)	
11q23.3	ARHGEF12, LARG, KIAA0382	Rho guanine nucleotide exchange factor 12, leukemia-associated	604763	Leukemia, acute myeloid (3)	

continued

Table 10.1. The morbid anatomy of the human genome (by chromosome) (*continued*)

Location	Symbol	Title	MIM#	Disorder	Mouse
11q23.3	HYALP, HDLD3	Hypoalphalipoproteinemia, primary	605201	Hypoalphalipoproteinemia, primary (2)	
11q23.3	HMBS, PBGD, UPS	Hydroxymethylbilane synthase	176000	Porphyria, acute intermittent (3); Porphyria, acute intermittent, nonerythroid variant (3)	9 (Ups)
11q24	KCNJ1, ROMK1	Potassium inwardly-rectifying channel, subfamily J, member 1	600359	Bartter syndrome, type 2 (3)	
11q25	HJCD	Histiocytosis with joint contractures and sensorineural deafness	602782	Faisalabad histiocytosis (2)	
11q25-qter	DFNB20	Deafness, autosomal recessive 20	604060	Deafness, autosomal recessive 20 (2)	
12pter-p12	CD4	CD4 antigen (p55)	186940	[CD4+ lymphocyte deficiency] (2); {Lupus erythematosus, susceptibility to} (2)	6 (Ly4)
12p13.31	DRPLA	Atrophin 1	125370	Dentatorubro-pallidoluysian atrophy (3)	6 (Drpla)
12p13.3	FGF23, ADHR, HPDR2	Fibroblast growth factor 23	605380	Hypophosphatemic rickets, autosomal dominant, 193100 (3)	
12p13.3	PXR1, PEX5, PTS1R	Peroxisome receptor 1	600414	Adrenoleukodystrophy, neonatal, 202370 (3)	
12p13.3	VWF, F8VWF	Coagulation factor VIII VWF (von Willebrand factor)	193400	von Willebrand disease (3)	6 (Vwf)
12p13.3-p12.3	A2M	Alpha-2-macroglobulin	103950	Emphysema due to alpha-2-macroglobulin deficiency (1); {Alazheimer disease, susceptibility to} (3)	6 (A2 m)
12p13.3-p11.2	ACLS	Acrocallosal syndrome	200990	?Acrocallosal syndrome (2)	
12p13.2	TNFRSF1A , TNFR1, TNFAR, FPF	Tumor necrosis factor receptor superfamily, member 1A	191190	Periodic fever, familial, 142680 (3)	6 (Tnfr2)
12p13.2-q24.1	IBD2	Inflammatory bowel disease-2	601458	Inflammatory bowel disease-2 (2)	
12p13.1-p12.3	MGP	Matrix Gla protein	154870	Keutel syndrome, 245150 (3)	6 (Mglap)
12p13	AICDA, AID, HIGM2	Activation-induced cytidine deaminase	605257	Immunodeficiency with hyper-IgM, type 2, 605258 (3)	
12p13	C1R	Complement component-1, r subcomponent	216950	C1r/C1s deficiency, combined (1)	
12p13	C1S	Complement component-1, s subcomponent	120580	C1r/C1s deficiency, combined (1); C1s deficiency, isolated (3)	
12p13	ETV6, TEL	ETS variant gene-6 (TEL oncogene)	600618	Leukemia, acute lymphoblastic (1)	
12p13	GNB3	Guanine nucleotide-binding protein, beta polypeptide-3	139130	{Hypertension, essential, susceptibility to}, 145500 (3)	6 (Gnb3)
12p13	KCNA1, AEMK, EA1	Potassium voltage-gated channel, shaker-related subfamily, member 1	176260	Episodic ataxia myokymia syndrome, 160120 (3)	6 (Kcnal)
12p13	MPE	Malignant proliferation, eosinophil	131440	?Eosinophilic myeloproliferative disorder (2)	
12p13	PHA2C	Pseudohypoaldosteronism, type IIC	605232	Pseudohypoaldosteronism, type IIC (2)	
12p13	SCNN1A	Sodium channel, nonvoltage-gated 1, alpha	600228	Pseudohypoaldosteronism, type I, 264350 (3)	6 (Scnn1)

continued

Table 10.1. The morbid anatomy of the human genome (by chromosome) (*continued*)

Location	Symbol	Title	MIM#	Disorder	Mouse
12p13	TPI1	Triosephosphate isomerase-1	190450	Hemolytic anemia due to triosephosphate isomerase deficiency (3)	6 (Tpi1)
12p12.2	GYS2	Glycogen synthase-2, liver	138571	Glycogen storage disease, type 0, 240600 (3)	
12p12.2-p12.1	LDHB	Lactate dehydrogenase B	150100	Lactate dehydrogenase-B deficiency (3)	6 (Ldh2)
12p12.2-p11.2	HTNB	Hypertension with brachydactyly	112410	Hypertension with brachydactyly (2)	
12p12.1	KRAS2, RASK2	Kirsten rat sarcoma-2 viral (v-Ki-ras2) oncogene homolog	190070	Colorectal adenoma (1); Colorectal cancer (1)	6 (Kras2)
12p12.1-p11.2	PTHLH	Parathyroid hormone-like hormone	168470	?Humoral hypercalcemia of malignancy (1)	6 (Pthlh)
12p12	BCAT1, BCT1	Branched chain aminotransferase-1, cytosolic	113520	?Hyperleucinemia-isoleucinemia or hypervalinemia (1)	6 (Bcat1)
12p11.23-q13.12	AD5	Alzheimer disease, familial, type 5	602096	Alzheimer disease-5 (2)	
12p11.2-q12	FEOM1, CFEOM1, FEOM1	Fibrosis of extraocular muscles, congenital, 1, autosomal dominant	135700	Fibrosis of extraocular muscles, congenital, 1 (2)	
12q11-q13	KRT2A, KRT2E	Keratin-2A	600194	Ichthyosis bullosa of Siemens, 146800 (3)	
12q11-q13	PPKB	Palmoplantar keratoderma, Bothnia type	600231	Palmoplantar keratoderma, Bothnia type (2)	
12q11-q14	ACVRL1, ACVRLK1, ALK1, HHT2	Activin A receptor, type II-like kinase 1	601284	Hereditary hemorrhagic telangiectasia-2, 600376 (3)	
12q12-q14	VDR	Vitamin D (1, 25-dihydroxyvitamin D3) receptor	601769	Rickets, vitamin D-resistant, 277440 (3); ?Osteoporosis, involutional (1)	
12q13	AAAS, AAA	Aladin	605378	Achalasia-addisonianism-alacrimia syndrome, 231550 (3)	
12q13	AMHR2, AMHR	Anti-Mullerian hormone receptor, type II	600956	Persistent Mullerian duct syndrome, type II, 261550 (3)	15 (Amhr)
12q13	AQP2	Aquaporin-2 (collecting duct)	107777	Diabetes insipidus, nephrogenic, autosomal recessive, 222000 (3); Diabetes insipidus, nephrogenic, autosomal dominant, 125800 (3)	
12q13	KRTHB1, HB1	Keratin, hair, basic, 1	602153	Monilethrix, 158000 (3)	
12q13	KRTHB6, HB6	Keratin, hair, basic, 6	601928	Monilethrix, 158000 (3)	
12q13	ITGA7	Integrin, alpha-7	600536	Myopathy, congenital (3)	
12q13	KRT1	Keratin-1	139350	Epidermolytic hyperkeratosis, 113800 (3); Keratoderma, palmoplantar, nonepidermolytic (3); Cyclic ichthyosis with epidermolytic hyperkeratosis (3)	15 (Krt2)
12q13	KRT3	Keratin-3	148043	Meesmann corneal dystrophy, 122100 (3)	
12q13	KRT4, CYK4	Keratin-4	123940	White sponge nevus, 193900 (3)	
12q13	KRT5	Keratin-5	148040	Epidermolysis bullosa simplex, Koebner, Dowling-Meara, and Weber-Cockayne types, 131900, 131760, 131800 (3)	

continued

Table 10.1. The morbid anatomy of the human genome (by chromosome) (*continued*)

Location	Symbol	Title	MIM#	Disorder	Mouse
12q13	KRT6A	Keratin-6A	148041	Pachyonychia congenita, Jadassohn-Lewandowsky type, 167200 (3)	
12q13	KRT6B, PC2	Keratin-6B	148042	Pachyonychia congenita, Jackson-Lawler type, 167210 (3)	
12q13	KRT18	Keratin-18	148070	{?Liver disease, susceptibility to, from hepatotoxins or viruses} (1)	
12q13	MIP, AQPO	Major intrinsic protein of lens fiber	154050	Cataract, polymorphic and lamellar, 604219 (3)	10 (Mip)
12q13	SPG10	Spastic paraplegia 10, autosomal dominant	604187	Spastic paraplegia-10 (2)	
12q13-q14	RDH5	Retinol dehydrogenase-5	601617	Fundus albipunctatus, 136880 (3)	
12q13-q15	GAS41	Glioma-amplified sequence-41	602116	Glioma (1)	
12q13-q21	ENUR2	Enuresis, nocturnal, 2	600808	Enuresis, nocturnal, 2 (2)	
12q13.1	DHH	Desert hedgehog, Drosophila, homolog of	605423	Gonadal dysgenesis, 46XY, partial, with minifascicular neuropathy (3)	
12q13.1-q13.2	DDIT3, GADD153, CHOP10	DNA-damage-inducible transcript-3	126337	Myxoid liposarcoma (3)	
12q13.11-q13.2	COL2A1	Collagen II, alpha-1 polypeptide	120140	Stickler syndrome, type I, 108300 (3); SED congenita (3); Kniest dysplasia (3); Achondrogenesis-hypochondrogenesis, type II, 200610 (3); Osteoarthrosis, precocious (3); Wagner syndrome, type II (3); SMED Strudwick type, 184250 (3); Spondyloepiphyseal dysplasia, congenita, 183900 (3); Osteoarthritis with mild chondrodysplasia (3); Hypochondrogenesis (3); Kniest dysplasia, 156550 (3); Spondylometaphyseal dysplasia, 184252 (3); Wagner syndrome, 143200 (3); Spondyloperipheral dysplasia, 271700 (3); Epiphyseal dysplasia, multiple, with myopia and conductive deafness, 132450 (3)	
12q13.3	PFKM	Phosphofructokinase, muscle type	232800	Glycogen storage disease VII (3)	
12q13.3-q15	SPPM, SPMD	Scapuloperoneal syndrome, myopathic type	181430	Scapuloperoneal syndrome, myopathic type (2)	
12q14	CDK4, CMM3	Cyclin-dependent kinase 4	123829	Melanoma (3)	
12q14	CYP27B1, PDDR, VDD1	Cytochrome P450, subfamily XXVIIB, polypeptide 1	264700	Pseudovitamin D deficiency rickets 1 (3)	
12q14	GNS, G6S	N-acetylglucosamine-6-sulfatase	252940	Sanfilippo syndrome, type D (1)	
12q14	IFNG	Interferon, gamma	147570	Interferon, immune, deficiency (1)	10 (Ifg)
12q15	HMGIC, BABL, LIPO	High-mobility group protein HMGI-C	600698	Lipoma (3); Salivary adenoma (3); Uterine leiomyoma (3); ?Lipomatosis, mutiple, 151900 (2)	10 (pg, Hmgic)
12q21	MYF6	Myogenic factor-6	159991	Myopathy, centronuclear, 160150 (3); Becker muscular dystrophy modifier, 310200 (3)	10 (Myf6)

continued

Table 10.1. The morbid anatomy of the human genome (by chromosome) (*continued*)

Location	Symbol	Title	MIM#	Disorder	Mouse
12q21-q23	MYP3	Myopia, high grade, autosomal dominant 2	603221	Myopia-3 (2)	
12q21.3-q22	KERA, CNA2	Keratocan	603288	Cornea plana congenita, recessive, 217300 (3)	10 (Kera)
12q22	MGCT	Male germ cell tumor	273300	Male germ cell tumor (2)	
12q22-q23	HAL, HSTD	Histidine ammonia-lyase (histidase)	235800	[Histidinemia] (1)	10 (Hstd)
12q22-q24.1	IGF1	Insulin-like growth factor-1, or somatomedin C	147440	Growth retardation with deafness and mental retardation (3)	10 (Igf1)
12q22-qter	ACADS, SCAD	Acyl-Coenzyme A dehydrogenase, C-2 to C-3 short chain	201470	Acyl-CoA dehydrogenase, short-chain, deficiency of (3)	5 (Bcd1)
12q23-q24	SMAL	Spinal muscular atrophy, congenital nonprogressive, of lower limbs	600175	Spinal muscular atrophy, congenital nonprogressive, of lower limbs (2)	
12q23-q24.1	ATP2A2, ATP2B, DAR	ATPase, Ca++ dependent, slow-twitch, cardiac muscle-2	108740	Darier disease, 124200 (3)	11 (Atpb2)
12q23-q24.3	MYL2	Myosin, light polypeptide-2, regulatory, cardiac, slow	160781	Cardiomyopathy, hypertrophic, mid-left ventricular chamber type (3)	
12q24	ATX2, SCA2	Ataxin-2	601517	Spinocerebellar ataxia-2, 183090 (3)	
12q24	BDC	Brachydactyly, type C	113100	Brachydactyly, type C (2)	
12q24	MVK, MVLK	Mevalonate kinase	251170	Mevalonicaciduria (3); Hyperimmunoglobulinemia D and periodic fever syndrome, 260920 (3)	
12q24	NS1, CFC	Noonan syndrome 1	163950	Noonan syndrome-1 (2); Cardiofaciocutaneous syndrome, 115150 (2)	
12q24	SMA4, HMN2	Spinal muscular atrophy-4	158590	Spinal muscular atrophy-4 (2)	
12q24-qter	HPD	4-hydroxyphenylpyruvate dioxygenase	276710	Tyrosinemia, type III (3)	
12q24.1	PAH, PKU1	Phenylalanine hydroxylase	261600	Phenylketonuria (3); [Hyperphenylalaninemia, mild] (3)	10 (Pah)
12q24.1	BCL7A, BCL7	B-cell CLL/lymphoma-7A	601406	B-cell non-Hodgkin lymphoma, high-grade (3)	
12q24.1	TBX3	T-box 3	601621	Ulnar-mammary syndrome, 181450 (3)	5 (Tbx3)
12q24.1	TBX5	T-box 5	601620	Holt-Oram syndrome, 142900 (3)	5 (Tbx5)
12q24.1-q24.31	SPSMA	Scapuloperoneal spinal muscular atrophy, New England type	181405	Scapuloperoneal spinal muscular atrophy, New England type (2)	
12q24.2	ALDH2	Aldehyde dehydrogenase-2, mitochondrial	100650	Alcohol intolerance, acute (3); {?Fetal alcohol syndrome} (1)	4 (Aldh2)
12q24.2	TCF1, HNF1A, MODY3	Interferon production regulator factor (HNF1), albumin proximal factor	142410	MODY, type 3, 600496 (3); {Diabetes mellitus, noninsulin-dependent, 2}, 601407 (2); {Diabetes mellitus, insulin-dependent} (3)	5 (Tcf1)
Chr.12	LYZ	Lysozyme	153450	Amyloidosis, renal, 105200 (3)	
13q11	GJA3, CX46, CZP3, CAE3	Gap junction protein, alpha-3, 46kD (connexin 46)	121015	Cataract, zonular pulverulent-3, 601885 (3)	14 (Gja3)
13q11-q12	GJB2, CX26, DFNB1, PPK	Gap junction protein, beta-2, 26kD (connexin 26)	121011	Deafness, autosomal recessive 1, 220290 (3); Deafness, autosomal dominant 3, 601544 (3); Vohwinkel syndrome, 124500 (3); Keratoderma, palmoplantar, with deafness, 148350 (3)	14 (Gjb2)

continued

Table 10.1. The morbid anatomy of the human genome (by chromosome) (*continued*)

Location	Symbol	Title	MIM#	Disorder	Mouse
13q11-q12	ZNF198, SCLL, RAMP, FIM	Zinc finger protein-198	602221	Stem-cell leukemia/lymphoma syndrome (3)	
13q12	GJB6, CX30, DFNA3, HED, ED2	Gap junction protein, beta-6 (connexin-30)	604418	Deafness, autosomal dominant nonsyndromic sensorineural 3, 601544 (3); Ectodermal dysplasia 2, hidrotic, 129500 (3)	
13q12	SACS, ARSACS	Sacsin	604490	Spastic ataxia, Charlevoix-Saguenay type, 270550 (3)	1 (Sacs)
13q12	SGCG, LGMD2C, DMDA1, SCG3	Sarcoglycan, gamma (35 kD dystrophin-associated glycoprotein)	253700	Muscular dystrophy, limb-girdle, type 2C (3)	
13q12.1	IPF1	Insulin promoter factor 1, homeodomain transcription factor	600733	Pancreatic agenesis, 260370 (3); MODY, type IV (3)	5 (Ipf1)
13q12.2-q13	MBS, MBS1	Moebius syndrome	157900	?Moebius syndrome (2)	
13q12.3	BRCA2	Breast cancer-2, early onset	600185	Breast cancer 2, early onset (3); Pancreatic cancer (3)	5 (Brca2)
13q13-q14.3	ENUR1	Enuresis, nocturnal, 1	600631	Enuresis, nocturnal, 1 (2)	
13q14	D13S25, DBM	Disrupted in B-cell neoplasia	109543	Leukemia, chronic lymphocytic, B-cell (2)	
13q14	GER	Gastroesophageal reflux	109350	Gastroesophageal reflux (2)	
13q14	ITM2B, BRI, ABRI, FBD	Integral membrane protein 2B (BRI gene)	603904	Dementia, familial British, 176500 (3); Dementia, familial Danish, 117300 (3)	
13q14	RFXAP	Regulatory factor X-associated protein	601861	Bare lymphocyte syndrome type II, 209920 (3)	
13q14	RIEG2, RGS2	Rieger syndrome, type 2	601499	Rieger syndrome, type 2 (2)	
13q14	SLC25A15, ORNT1, HHH	Solute carrier family 25 (mitochondrial carrier), member 15 (ornithine transporter 1)	603861	Hyperornithinemia-hyperammonemia-homocitrullinemia syndrome, 238970 (3)	
13q14.1	FKHR	Forkhead, Drosophila, homolog of, 1	136533	Rhabdomyosarcoma, alveolar, 268220 (3)	
13q14.1-q14.2	RB1	Retinoblastoma-1	180200	Retinoblastoma (3); Osteosarcoma, 259500 (2); Bladder cancer, 109800 (3); Pinealoma with bilateral retinoblastoma (2)	14 (Rb1)
13q14.12-q14.2	DICE1	Deleted in cancer 1	604331	{Nonsmall cell lung cancer} (2)	
13q14.3-q21.1	ATP7B, WND	ATPase, Cu++ transporting, beta polypeptide	277900	Wilson disease (3)	8 (Atp7b)
13q21	BRCA4, BRCAX	Breast cancer, type 4	605365	Breast cancer, type 4 (2)	
13q21	SCA8	Spinocerebellar ataxia 8	603680	Spinocerebellar ataxia 8 (3)	
13q21-q32	PAPA2	Postaxial polydactyly, type A2	602085	Postaxial polydactyly, type A2 (2)	
13q21.1-q32	CLN5	Ceroid-lipofuscinosis, neuronal-5	256731	Ceroid-lipofuscinosis, neuronal-5, variant late infantile (3)	
13q22	EDNRB, HSCR2	Endothelin receptor type B	131244	Hirschsprung disease-2, 600155 (3)	
13q31-q32	MCOR	Microcoria, congenital	156600	Microcoria, congenital (2)	
13q32	PCCA	Propionyl Coenzyme A carboxylase, alpha polypeptide	232000	Propionicacidemia, type I or pccA type (3)	14 (Pcca)
13q32	SCZD7	Schizophrenia susceptibility locus, chromosome 13q-related	603176	{Schizophrenia}, 181500 (2)	
13q32	ZIC2, HPE5	ZIC family member 2	603073	Holoprosencephaly-5 (3)	

continued

Table 10.1. The morbid anatomy of the human genome (by chromosome) (*continued*)

Location	Symbol	Title	MIM#	Disorder	Mouse
13q33	ERCC5, XPG	Excision-repair, complementing defective, in Chinese hamster, number 5	133530	Xeroderma pigmentosum, group G, 278780 (3)	1 (Ercc5)
13q33	SLC10A2, NTCP2	Solute carrier family 10 (sodium/bile acid cotransporter family), member 2	601295	Bile acid malabsorption, primary (3)	8 (Slc10a2)
13q34	F7	Coagulation factor VII	227500	Factor VII deficiency (3); {Myocardial infarction, decreased susceptibility to} (3)	
13q34	F10	Coagulation factor X	227600	Factor X deficiency (3)	8 (Cf10)
13q34	ING1	Inhibitor of growth 1	601566	Squamous cell carcinoma, head and neck, 601400 (3)	
13q34	RHOK, RK, GRK1	Rhodopsin kinase	180381	Oguchi disease-2, 258100 (3)	
Chr.13	BRCD1	Breast cancer, ductal, suppressor-1	211410	Breast cancer, ductal (2)	
14q	BCH	Chorea, hereditary benign	118700	Chorea, hereditary benign (2)	
14q	BGCI, IBGC	Basal ganglia calcification, idiopathic (Fahr disease)	213600	Basal ganglia calcification, idiopathic (2)	
14q	MNG1	Multinodular goiter-1	138800	Goiter, multinodular, 1 (2)	
14q	MPD1	Myopathy, distal 1	160500	Myopathy, distal (2)	
14q11-q12	DAD1	Defender against cell death 1	600243	Temperature-sensitive apoptosis (1)	14 (Dad1)
14q11.1-q11.2	NRL, D14S46E	Neural retina leucine zipper	162080	Retinitis pigmentosa, autosomal dominant (3)	14 (Nr1)
14q11.2	RSCIS	Radiation sensitivity/chromosome instability syndrome, autosomal dominant	605463	Radiation sensitivity/chromosome instability syndrome, autosomal dominant (1)	
14q11.2	SLC7A7, LPI	Solute carrier family 7 (cationic amino acid transporter, y+ system), member 7	603593	Lysinuric protein intolerance, 222700 (3)	
14q11.2	TCRA	T-cell antigen receptor, alpha polypeptide	186880	Leukemia/lymphoma, T-cell (3)	14 (Tcra)
14q11.2	TGM1, ICR2, LI1	Transglutaminase-1 (K polypeptide epidermal type I, protein-glutamine gamma-glutamyltransferase)	190195	Ichthyosis, lamellar, autosomal recessive, 242300 (3); Ichthyosiform erythroderma, congenital, 242100 (3)	
14q11.2-q13	PABPN1, PABP2, PAB2	Poly(A)-binding protein, nuclear 1	602279	Oculopharyngeal muscular dystrophy, 164300 (3); Oculopharyngeal muscular dystrophy, autosomal recessive, 257950 (3)	
14q11.2-q24.3	SPG3A	Spastic paraplegia-3A	182600	Spastic paraplegia-3A (2)	
14q12	DFNB5	Deafness, autosomal recessive 5	600792	Deafness, autosomal recessive 5 (2)	
14q12	MYH7, CMH1	Myosin, heavy polypeptide-7, cardiac muscle, beta	160760	Cardiomyopathy, familial hypertrophic, 1, 192600 (3); ?Central core disease, one form (3)	
14q12-q13	COCH, DFNA9	Cochlin	603196	Deafness, autosomal dominant 9, 601369 (3); Meniere disease, 156000 (3)	12 (Coch5B2)
14q12-q13	PAX9	Paired box homeotic gene-9	167416	Oligodontia, 604625 (3)	
14q12-q22	ARVD3	Arrhythmogenic right ventricular dysplasia-3	602086	Arrhythmogenic right ventricular dysplasia-3 (2)	
14q13	TITF1, NKX2A, TTF1	Thyroid transcription factor 1 (NK-2, Drosophila, homolog of, A)	600635	Goiter, familial, due to TTF-1 defect (1)	
14q13	TMIP	Tetramelic mirror-image polydactyly	135750	?Tetramelic mirror-image polydactyly (2)	

continued

Table 10.1. The morbid anatomy of the human genome (by chromosome) (*continued*)

Location	Symbol	Title	MIM#	Disorder	Mouse
14q13.1	NP	Nucleoside phosphorylase	164050	Nucleoside phosphorylase deficiency, immunodeficiency due to (3)	14 (Np1, 2)
14q21	MGAT2, CDGS2	Mannosyl (alpha-1, 6-)-glycoprotein beta-1, 2-N-acetylglucosaminyl-transferase	602616	Carbohydrate-deficient glycoprotein syndrome, type II, 212066 (3)	
14q21-q22	DFNA23	Deafness, autosomal dominant nonsyndromic sensorineural 23	605192	Deafness, autosomal dominant 23 (2)	
14q21-q22	PYGL	Phosphorylase, glycogen, liver	232700	Glycogen storage disease VI (3)	12 (Pygl)
14q22-q23.2	SPTB	Spectrin, beta, erythrocytic	182870	Elliptocytosis-3 (3); Spherocytosis-1 (3); Anemia, neonatal hemolytic, fatal and near-fatal (3)	12 (Sptb1)
14q22.1-q22.2	GCH1, DYT5	GTP cyclohydrolase 1	600225	Phenylketonuria, atypical, due to GCH1 deficiency, 233910 (1); Dystonia, DOPA-responsive, 128230 (3)	
14q23-q24	ARVD1	Arrhythmogenic right ventricular dysplasia-1	107970	Arrhythmogenic right ventricular dysplasia-1 (2)	
14q24	LCA3	Leber congenital amaurosis, type III	604232	Leber congenital amaurosis, type III (2)	
14q24-qter	CTAA1	Cataract, anterior polar 1	115650	?Cataract, anterior polar-1 (2)	
14q24.3	CHX10, HOX10	C. elegans ceh-10 homeo domain-containing homolog	142993	Microphthalmia, cataracts, and iris abnormalities (3)	12 (Hox10)
14q24.3	GSTZ1, MAAI	Glutathione S-transferase, zeta-1 (maleylacetoacetate isomerase)	603758	Tyrosinemia, type Ib (1)	
14q24.3	HE1, NPC2	Epididymal secretory protein HE1	601016	Niemann-pick disease, type C2 (3)	
14q24.3	MMSDH	Methylmalonate semialdehyde dehydrogenase	603178	Methylmalonate semialdehyde dehydrogenase deficiency (3)	
14q24.3	PSEN1, AD3	Presenilin 1	104311	Alzheimer disease-3 (3)	
14q24.3-q31	IDDM11	Insulin-dependent diabetes mellitus-11	601208	{Diabetes mellitus, insulin-dependent, 11} (2)	
14q24.3-q31	MJD, SCA3	Machado-Joseph disease (spinocerebellar ataxia 3, olivopontocerebellar ataxia 3, autosomal dominant); ataxin-3	109150	Machado-Joseph disease (3)	
14q31	GALC	Galactosylceraminidase	245200	Krabbe disease (3)	12 (tw)
14q31	TSHR	Thyroid-stimulating hormone receptor	603372	Hypothyroidism, congenital, due to TSH resistance, 275200 (3); Thyroid adenoma, hyperfunctioning (3); Graves disease, 275000 (1); Hyperthroidism, congenital (3)	12 (Tshr)
14q32	CKBE	Creatine kinase, ectopic expression	123270	[Creatine kinase, brain type, ectopic expression of] (2)	
14q32	MCOP	Microphthalmia, autosomal recessive	251600	Microphthalmia, autosomal recessive (2)	
14q32	USH1A, USH1	Usher syndrome-1A, autosomal recessive, severe	276900	Usher syndrome, type 1A (2)	
14q32.1	CBG	Corticosteroid-binding globulin	122500	[Transcortin deficiency] (1)	
14q32.1	PCI, PLANH3	Protein C inhibitor (plasminogen activator inhibitor-3)	601841	Protein C inhibitor deficiency (2)	

continued

Table 10.1. The morbid anatomy of the human genome (by chromosome) *(continued)*

Location	Symbol	Title	MIM#	Disorder	Mouse
14q32.1	PI, AAT	Protease inhibitor (alpha-1-antitrypsin)	107400	Emphysema-cirrhosis (3); Hemorrhagic diathesis due to "antithrombin" Pittsburgh (3); Emphysema (3)	12 (Aat)
14q32.1	SERPINA3, AACT, ACT	Alpha-1-antichymotrypsin	107280	Alpha-1-antichymotrypsin deficiency (3); Cerebrovascular disease, occlusive (3)	
14q32.1	TCL1A, TCL1	T-cell lymphoma/leukemia 1A	186960	Leukemia/lymphoma, T-cell (2)	
14q32.1	TCL1B, TML1	T-cell lymphoma/leukemia 1B	603769	Leukemia/lymphoma, T-cell (2)	
14q32.33	IGHG2	Constant region of heavy chain of IgG2	147110	IgG2 deficiency, selective (3)	
14q32.33	IGHM, MU	Constant region of heavy chain of IgM	147020	Agammaglobulinemia, 601495 (3)	
14q32.33	IGHR	Immunoglobulin heavy chain regulator	144120	?Hyperimmunoglobulin G1 syndrome (2)	
Chr.14	ACHM1, RMCH1	Achromatopsia-1	603096	Achromatopsia-1 (2)	
Chr.14	MPS3C	Mucopolysaccharidosis, type IIIC	252930	?Sanfilippo syndrome, type C (2)	
15q	CHLS	Cholestasis-lymphedema syndrome	214900	Cholestasis-lymphedema syndrome (2)	
15q	HYT2	Hypertension, essential, susceptibility to, 2	604329	Hypertension, essential, susceptibility to, 2 (2)	
15q11	PWCR, PWS	Prader-Willi syndrome chromosome region	176270	Prader-Willi syndrome (2)	
15q11-q13	AHO2	Albright hereditary osteodystrophy-2	103581	?Albright hereditary osteodystrophy-2 (2)	
15q11-q13	BCL8	B-cell CLL/lymphoma-8	601889	Lymphoma, diffuse large cell (3)	
15q11-q13	NDN	Necdin	602117	Prader-Willi syndrome, 176270 (3)	7 (Ndn)
15q11-q13	UBE3A, ANCR	Ubiquitin protein ligase E3A	601623	Angelman syndrome (3)	
15q11-q15	EYCL3	Eye color 3, brown	227220	[Eye color, brown] (2)	
15q11-q15	HCL3	Hair color 3, brown	601800	[Hair color, brown] (2)	
15q11.1	SPG6	Spastic paraplegia-6	600363	Spastic paraplegia-6 (2)	
15q11.2-q12	OCA2, P, PED, D15S12	Oculocutaneous albinism II (pink-eye dilution, murine, homolog of)	203200	Albinism, oculocutaneous, type II (3); Albinism, ocular, autosomal recessive (3)	7 (p)
15q11.2-q13.1	HTGS	Hypertriglyceridemia, familial	145750	{Hypertriglyceridemia, susceptibility to} (2)	
15q12	SNRPN	Small nuclear ribonucleoprotein polypeptide N	182279	Prader-Willi syndrome, 176270 (3)	7 (Snrpn)
15q13-q15	ACCPN	Agenesis of corpus callosum and peripheral neuropathy (Andermann syndrome)	218000	Andermann syndrome (2)	
15q13-q15	SPG11	Spastic paraplegia 11, autosomal recessive	604360	Spastic paraplegia-11 (2)	
15q14	ACTC	Actin, alpha, cardiac muscle	102540	Cardiomyopathy, dilated, 115200 (3); Cardiomyopathy, familial hypertrophic, 192600 (3)	2 (Actc1)
15q14	CHRNA7	Cholinergic receptor, nicotinic, alpha polypeptide-7	118511	Schizophrenia, neurophysiologic defect in (2)	7 (Acra7)
15q14	EJM2, JME	Epilepsy, juvenile myoclonic 2	604827	Epilepsy, juvenile myoclonic (2)	
15q14-q15	IVD	Isovaleryl Coenzyme A dehydrogenase	243500	Isovalericacidemia (3)	

continued

Table 10.1. The morbid anatomy of the human genome (by chromosome) (*continued*)

Location	Symbol	Title	MIM#	Disorder	Mouse
15q14-q21.3	SCA11	Spinocerebellar ataxia 11	604432	Spinocerebellar ataxia-11 (2)	
15q15	EPB42	Erythrocyte surface protein band 4.2	177070	Spherocytosis, hereditary, Japanese type (3)	2 (Epb4.2)
15q15	SCZD10	Schizophrenia susceptibility locus, chromosome 15q-related	605419	{Schizophrenia}, 181500 (2)	
15q15-q21	MCPH4	Microcephaly, primary autosomal recessive 4	604321	Microcephaly, primary autosomal recessive 4 (2)	
15q15-q21.1	SLC12A1, NKCC2	Solute carrier family 12 (sodium/potassium/chloride transporters), member 1	600839	Bartter syndrome, 241200 (3)	2 (Slc12a1)
15q15.1-q15.3	CDAN1, CDA1	Congenital dyserythropoietic anemia, type I	224120	Dyserythropoietic anemia, contenital, type I (2)	
15q15.1-q21.1	ALS5	Amytrophic lateral sclerosis-5, juvenile recessive	602099	Amytrophic lateral sclerosis-5, juvenile recessive (2)	
15q15.1-q21.1	CAPN3, CANP3	Calpain, large polypeptide L3	114240	Muscular dystrophy, limb-girdle, type 2A, 253600 (3)	2 (Canp3)
15q15.3	SORD, SORD1	Sorbitol dehydrogenase	182500	?Cataract, congenital (2)	2 (Sdh1)
15q21	CDAN3, CDA3	Congenital dyserythropoietic anemia, type III	105600	Dyserythropoietic anemia, congenital, type III (2)	
15q21	DYX1	Dyslexia-1	127700	Dyslexia-1 (2)	
15q21	MYO5A, MYH12	Myosin, heavy polypeptide kinase	160777	Griscelli syndrome-type pigmentary dilution with mental retardation, 214450 (3)	9 (d, Myh12)
15q21	RAB27A, RAM	Ras-associated protein RAB27A	603868	Griscelli syndrome, 214450 (3)	
15q21-q22	B2M	Beta-2-microglobulin	109700	Hemodialysis-related amyloidosis (1)	2 (B2m)
15q21-q22	DFNB16	Deafness, autosomal recessive 16	603720	Deafness, autosomal recessive 16 (2)	
15q21-q23	CLN6	Ceroid-lipofuscinosis, neuronal 6, late infantile, variant	601780	Ceroid-lipofuscinosis, neuronal-6, variant late infantile (2)	
15q21-q23	LIPC	Lipase, hepatic	151670	Hepatic lipase deficiency (3)	9 (Hl)
15q21.1	CYP19, ARO	Cytochrome P450, subfamily XIX (aromatization of androgens)	107910	Gynecomastia, familial, due to increased aromatase activity (1); Virilization, maternal and fetal, from placental aromatase deficiency (3)	9 (Cyp19)
15q21.1	FBN1, MFS1	Fibrillin-1	134797	Marfan syndrome, 154700 (3); Shprintzen-Goldberg syndrome, 182212 (3); Ectopia lentis, familial (3)	2 (Fbn1)
15q21.1	HNPCC7	Colorectal cancer, hereditary nonpolyposis, type 7	604940	{Colorectal cancer, susceptibility to, 2} (2)	
15q22	PML, MYL	Promyelocytic leukemia, inducer of	102578	Leukemia, acute promyelocytic, PML/RARA type (3)	9 (Pm1)
15q22-qter	MPI, PMI1	Mannosephosphate isomerase (phosphomannose isomerase 1)	154550	Carbohydrate-deficient glycoprotein syndrome, type Ib, 602579 (3)	9 (Mpi1)
15q22.1	TPM1, CMH3	Tropomyosin 1, alpha	191010	Cardiomyopathy, familial hypertrophic, 3, 115196 (3)	9 (Tpm1)
15q22.3-q23	BBS4	Bardet-Biedl syndrome 4	600374	Bardet-Biedl syndrome 4 (2)	
15q23	NR2E3, PNR, ESCS	Nuclear receptor subfamily 2, group E, member 3	604485	Enhanced S-cone syndrome, 268100 (3); Retinitis pigmentosa, late onset, 268000 (3)	9 (rd7)

continued

Table 10.1. The morbid anatomy of the human genome (by chromosome) (*continued*)

Location	Symbol	Title	MIM#	Disorder	Mouse
15q23-q24	CYP11A, P450SCC	Cytochrome P450, subfamily XIA (cholesterol side chain cleavage enzyme)	118485	?Polycystic ovary syndrome, 184700 (2)	9 (Cyp11a)
15q23-q24	HEXA, TSD	Hexosaminidase A, alpha polypeptide	272800	Tay-Sachs disease (3); GM2-gangliosidosis, several forms (3); [Hex A pseudodeficiency] (3)	9 (Hexa)
15q23-q25	ETFA, GA2	Electron transfer flavoprotein, alpha polypeptide	231680	Glutaricaciduria, type IIA (1)	13 (Etfa)
15q23-q25	FAH	Fumarylacetoacetase	276700	Tyrosinemia, type I (3)	
15q24	CHRNA3	Cholinergic receptor, neuronal nicotinic, alpha polypeptide-3	118503	?Megacystis-microcolon-intestinal hypoperistalsis syndrome, 249210 (1)	9 (Acra3)
15q24	ENFL2	Epilepsy, nocturnal frontal lobe, type 2	603204	Epilepsy, nocturnal frontal lobe, type 2 (2)	
15q24	MRST	Mental retardation, severe, with spasticity and tapetoretinal degeneration	602685	Mental retardation, severe, with spasticity and tapetoretinal degeneration (2)	
15q24-q26.1	PAPAS	Pyogenic sterile arthritis, pyoderma gangrenosum, and acne (PAPA syndrome)	604416	PAPA syndrome (2)	
15q25-q26	FHCB1, ARH1	Hypercholesterolemia, familial, autosomal recessive	603812	Hypercholesterolemia, familial, autosomal recessive (2)	
15q26	IDDM3	Insulin-dependent diabetes mellitus-3	600318	{Diabetes mellitus, insulin-dependent, 3} (2)	
15q26	RLBP1	Retinaldehyde-binding protein-1, cellular	180090	Retinitis pigmentosa, autosomal recessive (3)	7 (Rlbp1)
15q26.1	RECQL2, BLM, BS	RecQ protein-like 2	604610	Bloom syndrome, 210900 (3)	
15q26.1-qter	OTS	Otosclerosis	166800	Otosclerosis (2)	
16pter-p13.3	HBA1	Hemoglobin alpha-1	141800	Thalassemias, alpha- (3); Methemoglobinemias, alpha- (3); Erythremias, alpha- (3); Heinz body anemias, alpha- (3)	11 (Hba)
16pter-p13.3	HBA2	Hemoglobin alpha-2	141850	Thalassemia, alpha- (3); Erythrocytosis (3); Heinz body anemia (3); Hemoglobin H disease (3); Hypochromic microcytic anemia (3)	11 (Hba)
16pter-p13.3	HBHR, ATR1	Alpha-thalassemia/mental retardation syndrome, type 1	141750	Alpha-thalassemia/mental retardation syndrome, type 1 (1)	
16p13.3	ABAT, GABAT	4-aminobutyrate aminotransferase	137150	GABA-transaminase deficiency (3)	
16p13.3	AXIN1, AXIN	Axis inhibitor 1	603816	Hepatocellular carcinoma, 114550 (3)	
16p13.3	CATM	Cataract, congenital, with microphthalmia	156850	Cataract, congenital, with microphthalmia (2)	
16p13.3	CREBBP, CBP, RSTS	CREB binding protein	600140	Rubenstein-Taybi syndrome, 180849 (3)	
16p13.3	PKDTS	Polycystic kidney disease, infantile severe, with tuberous sclerosis	600273	Polycystic kidney disease, infantile severe, with tuberous sclerosis (3)	
16p13.3	TSC2	Tuberin (tuberous sclerosis 2 gene)	191092	Tuberous sclerosis-2, 191100 (3); Lymphangioleiomyomatosis, somatic (3)	17 (Tsc2)
16p13.3-p13.2	PMM2, CDG1	Phosphomannomutase 2	601785	Carbohydrate-deficient glycoprotein syndrome, type I, 212065 (3)	

continued

Table 10.1. The morbid anatomy of the human genome (by chromosome) (*continued*)

Location	Symbol	Title	MIM#	Disorder	Mouse
16p13.3-p13.13	ERCC4, XPF	Excision-repair, complementing defective, in Chinese hamster, number 4	133520	Xeroderma pigmentosum, group F, 278760 (3)	
16p13.3-p13.12	PKD1	Polycystin-1	601313	Polycystic kidney disease, adult type I, 173900 (3)	17 (Pkd1)
16p13.3-p12.1	MHAC	Microhydranencephaly	605013	Microhydranencephaly (2)	
16p13.11	SAH	SA (rat hypertension-associated) homolog	145505	{?Hypertension, essential} (1)	
16p13.1	ABCC6, ARA, ABC34, MLP1, PXE	ATP-binding cassette, subfamily C, member 6	603234	Pseudoxanthoma elasticum, autosomal recessive, 264800 (3); Pseudoxanthoma elasticum, autosomal dominant, 177850 (3)	
16p13	EIM	Infantile myoclonic epilepsy	605021	Epilepsy, myoclonic, infantile (2)	
16p13	HAGH, GLO2	Hydroxyacyl glutathione hydrolase; glycoxalase II	138760	[Glyoxalase II deficiency] (1)	
16p13	MEFV, MEF, FMF	Pyrin (marenostrin)	249100	Familial Mediterranean fever (3)	16 (Mefv)
16p13	MHC2TA, C2TA	MHC class II transactivator	600005	MHC class II deficiency, complementation group A, 209920 (3)	
16p13-p12	SCNN1B	Sodium channel, nonvoltage-gated 1, beta	600760	Liddle syndrome, 177200 (3); Pseudohypoaldosteronism, type I, 264350 (3)	7 (Scnn1b)
16p13-p12	SCNN1G, PHA1	Sodium channel, nonvoltage-gated 1, gamma	600761	Liddle syndrome, 177200 (3); Pseudohypoaldosteronism, type I, 264350 (3)	7 (Scnn1g)
16p12.3-p12.1	RP22	Retinitis pigmentosa-22	602594	Retinitis pigmentosa-22 (2)	
16p12.1	CLN3, BTS	Ceroid-lipofuscinosis, neuronal-3, juvenile (Batten disease)	204200	Ceroid-lipofuscinosis, neuronal-3, juvenile (3)	7 (Cln3)
16p12.1-p11.2	IL4R, IL4RA	Interleukin-4 receptor	147781	{Atopy, susceptibility to} (3)	7 (Il4r)
16p12.1-p11.2	MVP, PMV	Mitral valve prolapse, familial	157700	Mitral valve prolapse, familial (2)	
16p12.1-p11.2	PHKG2	Phosphorylase kinase, gamma 2 (testis/liver)	172471	Glycogenosis, hepatic, autosomal (3)	
16p12	ATP2A1, SERCA1	ATPase, Ca++ transporting, fast-twitch, 1	108730	Brody myopathy, 601003 (3)	7 (Atp2a1)
16p12	MCKD2, ADMCKD2	Medullary cystic kidney disease 2, autosomal dominant	603860	Medullary cystic kidney disease 2 (2)	
16p12-q12	ICCA	Infantile convulsions and paroxysmal choreoathetosis	602066	Convulsions, infantile and paroxysmal choreoathetosis (2)	
16p12-q13	IBD1	Inflammatory bowel disease-1 (Crohn disease)	266600	Inflammatory bowel disease-1 (2)	
16p12-q21	ACUG, BLAU	Arthrocutaneouveal granulomatosis (Blau syndrome)	186580	Arthrocutaneouveal granulomatosis (2)	
16p11.2	SLC5A2, SGLT2	Solute carrier family 5 (sodium/glucose cotransporter), member 2	182381	?Renal glucosuria, 233100 (1)	
16p11.2-q12.1	PKC, DYT10	Paroxysmal kinesigenic choreoathetosis	128200	Paroxysmal kinesigenic choreoathetosis (2)	
16q	WT3	Wilms tumor-3	194090	Wilms tumor, type 3 (2)	
16q12-q13	CYLD1, CDMT, EAC	Cylindromatosis gene	605018	Cylindromatosis, familial, 132700 (3)	
16q12-q13	PHKB	Phosphorylase kinase, beta polypeptide	172490	Phosphorylase kinase deficiency of liver and muscle, autosomal recessive, 261750 (3)	

continued

Table 10.1. The morbid anatomy of the human genome (by chromosome) (*continued*)

Location	Symbol	Title	MIM#	Disorder	Mouse
16q12-q13	SBS	Spiegler-Brooke syndrome	605041	Spiegler-Brooke syndrome (2)	
16q12.1	HYD2	Hypodontia, autosomal recessive	602639	Hypodontia, autosomal recessive (2)	
16q12.1	SALL1, HSAL1, TBS	Sal-like 1	602218	Townes-Brocks syndrome, 107480 (3)	
16q12.2	SLC6A2, NAT1, NET1	Solute carrier family 6 (neurotransmitter transporter, noradrenalin), member 2, cocaine- and antidepressant-sensitive	163970	Orthostatic intolerance, 604715 (3)	8 (Slc6a2)
16q13	SLC12A3, NCCT, TSC	Solute carrier family 12 (sodium/potassium/chloride transporters), member 3	600968	Gitelman syndrome, 263800 (3)	
16q13-q22.1	CES1, SES1	Carboxylesterase 1 (monocyte/macrophage serine esterase 1)	114835	?Monocyte carboxylesterase deficiency (1)	8 (Ces1)
16q21	BBS2	Bardet-Bied1 syndrome 2	209900	Bardet-Biedl syndrome 2 (2)	
16q21	CETP	Cholesteryl ester transfer protein, plasma	118470	[CETP deficiency] (3)	
16q22	AMLCR2	Acute myeloid leukemia chromosome region 2	602439	Leukemia, acute myelogenous (2)	
16q22	CBFB	Core-binding factor, beta subunit	121360	Myeloid leukemia, acute, M4Eo subtype (2)	
16q22	CHST6, MCDC1	Carbohydrate sulfotransferase-6 (GlcNAc-6-sulfotransferase, corneal)	605294	Macular corneal dystrophy, 217800 (3)	
16q22	CIRH1A, NAIC	North American Indian childhood cirrhosis	604901	Cirrhosis, North American Indian childhood type (2)	
16q22	HSD11B2, HSD11K	Hydroxysteroid (11-beta) dehydrogenase 2	218030	Apparent mineralocorticoid excess, hypertension due to (3); Hypertension, mild low-renin (3)	
16q22-q24	ALDOA	Aldolase A, fructose-bisphosphatase	103850	Aldolase A deficiency (3)	
16q22.1	CDH1, UVO	Cadherin-1 (E-cadherin; uvomorulin)	192090	Endometrial carcinoma (3); Ovarian carcinoma (3); Breast cancer, lobular (3); Gastric cancer, familial, 137215 (3)	8 (Um)
16q22.1	CTM	Cataract, Marner type	116800	Cataract, Marner type (2)	
16q22.1	DIA4, NMOR1	Diaphorase-4	125860	{Benzene toxicity, susceptibility to} (3); {Leukemia, post-chemotherapy, susceptibility to} (3)	8 (Nmor1)
16q22.1	HP	Haptoglobin	140100	[Anhaptoglobinemial] (3); [Hypohaptoglobinemia] (3)	8 (Hp)
16q22.1	LCAT	Lecithin-cholesterol acyltransferase	245900	Norum disease (3); Fish-eye disease (3)	8 (Lcat)
16q22.1	SCA4	Spinocerebellar ataxia 4	600223	Spinocerebellar ataxia-4 (2)	
16q22.1-q22.3	TAT	Tyrosine aminotransferase, cytosolic	276600	Tyrosinemia, type II (3)	8 (Tat)
16q23-q24	DHS	Dehydrated hereditary stomatocytosis	194380	Dehydrated hereditary stomatocytosis (2); Pseudohyperkalemia, familial, 177720 (2)	
16q24	CYBA	Cytochrome b-245, alpha polypeptide	233690	Chronic granulomatous disease, autosomal, due to deficiency of CYBA (3)	
16q24	MLYCD, MCD	Malonyl-CoA decarboxylase	248360	Malonyl-CoA decarboxylase deficiency (3)	

continued

Table 10.1. The morbid anatomy of the human genome (by chromosome) (*continued*)

Location	Symbol	Title	MIM#	Disorder	Mouse
16q24.1	GAN, GAN1	Gigaxonin	605379	Giant axonal neuropathy-1, 256850 (3)	
16q24.2-q24.3	FEOM3	Fibrosis of extraocular muscles, congenital, 3	604361	Fibrosis of extraocular muscles, congenital, 3 (2)	
16q24.3	APRT	Adenine phosphoribosyltransferase	102600	Urolithiasis, 2, 8-dihydroxyadenine (3)	8 (Aprt)
16q24.3	FANCA, FACA, FA1, FA, FAA	Fanconi anemia, complementation group A	227650	Fanconi anemia, type A (3)	
16q24.3	GALNS, MPS4A	Galactosamine (N-acetyl)-6-sulfate sulfatase	253000	Mucopolysaccharidosis IVA (3)	
16q24.3	LD	Lymphedema with distichiasis	153400	Lymphedema with distichiasis (2)	
16q24.3	MC1R	Melanocortin-1 receptor (alpha melanocyte-stimulating hormone receptor)	155555	{UV-induced skin damage, vulnerability to} (3); [Red hair/fair skin] (3)	8 (Mc1r)
16q24.3	PGN, SPG7	Paraplegin	602783	Spastic paraplegia-7 (3)	
Chr.16	CTH	Cystathionase	219500	[Cystathioninuria] (1)	
17pter-p13	ASPA	Aspartoacylase (aminoacylase-2)	271900	Canavan disease (3)	
17pter-p12	GP1BA	Glycoprotein Ib, platelet, alpha polypeptide	231200	Bernard-Soulier syndrome (3)	
17pter-p12	PLI	Alpha-2-plasmin inhibitor	262850	Plasmin inhibitor deficiency (3)	
17p13.3	BCPR	Breast cancer-related regulator of TP53	113721	Breast cancer (1)	
17p13.3	MDCR, MDS	Miller-Dieker syndrome chromosome region	247200	Miller-Dieker lissencephaly syndrome (2)	11 (Mds)
17p13.3	PAFAH1B1, LIS1	Platelet-activating factor acetylhydrolase, isoform 1B, alpha subunit	601545	Lissencephaly-1 (3); Subcortical laminar heterotopia (3)	
17p13.3	RP13	Retinitis pigmentosa-13	600059	Retinitis pigmentosa-13 (2)	
17p13.1	AIPL1, LCA4	Arylhydrocarbon-interacting receptor protein-like 1	604392	Leber congenital amaurosis, 604393 (3)	
17p13.1	GUCY2D, GUC2D, LCA1, CORD6	Guanylate cyclase 2D, membrane, retina-specific	600179	Leber congenital amaurosis, type I, 204000 (3); Cone-rod dystrophy 6, 601777 (3)	
17p13.1	TP53	Tumor protein p53	191170	Colorectal cancer, 114500 (3); Li-Fraumeni syndrome (3)	11 (Trp53)
17p13	CTAA2	Cataract, anterior polar 2	601202	Cataract, anterior polar-2 (2)	
17p13	CTNS	Cystinosis	219800	Cystinosis, nephropathic (3)	
17p13	MGI, FIMG	Myasthenia gravis, familial infantile	254210	Myasthenia gravis, familial infantile (2)	
17p13	SLC2A4, GLUT4	Solute carrier family 2 (facilitated glucose transporter), member 4	138190	{Diabetes mellitus, noninsulin-dependent} (3)	
17p13-p12	CORD5	Cone rod dystrophy 5	600977	Cone dystrophy, progressive (2)	
17p13-p12	SCOD1, SCO1	Cytochrome oxidase-deficient 1, S. cerevisiae, homolog of	603644	Hepatic failure, early onset, and neurologic disorder (3)	
17p12	BRKS, TLH1	Telopeptide lysyl hydroxylase, bone-specific	259450	Bruck syndrome (2)	
17p12-p11.2	COX10	Cytochrome c oxidase, subunit X	602125	Encephalopathy, progressive mitochondrial, with proximal renal tubulopathy due to cytochrome c oxidase deficiency (3)	

continued

Table 10.1. The morbid anatomy of the human genome (by chromosome) (*continued*)

Location	Symbol	Title	MIM#	Disorder	Mouse
17p12-p11	CHRNB1, ACHRB	Cholinergic receptor, nicotinic, beta polypeptide-1, muscle	100710	Myasthenic syndrome, slow-channel congenital, 601462 (3)	11 (Acrb)
17p11.2	ALDH10, SLS, FALDH	Aldehyde dehydrogenase-10 (fatty aldehyde dehydrogenase)	270200	Sjogren-Larsson syndrome (3)	
17p11.2	MYO15, DFNB3	Myosin XV	602666	Deafness, autosomal recessive 3, 600316 (3)	11(sh2, Myo15)
17p11.2	PMP22, CMT1A	Peripheral myelin protein-22	601097	Charcot-Marie-Tooth neuropathy-1A, 118220 (3); Dejerine-Sottas disease, 145900 (3); Neuropathy, recurrent, with pressure palsies, 162500 (3); Charcot-Marie-Tooth disease with deafness, 118300 (3)	11 (Tr)
17p11.2	SMCR	Smith-Magenis syndrome chromosome region	182290	Smith-Magenis syndrome (2)	
17p11.2-p11.1	ACADVL, VLCAD	Acyl-Coenzyme A dehydrogenase, very long chain	201475	VLCAD deficiency (3)	11 (Acadvl)
17p	CACD	Choroidal dystrophy, central areolar	215500	Choroidal dystrophy, central areolar (2)	
17p	HPC2, ELAC2	Prostate cancer, hereditary, 2	605367	{Prostate cancer, susceptibility to} (3)	
17p	RCD2	Retinal cone dystrophy-2	601251	Retinal cone dystrophy 2 (2)	
17cen-q21.3	TCF2, HNF2	Transcription factor-2, hepatic; LF-B3; variant hepatic nuclear factor	189907	MODY, type V, 604284 (3); MODY5 with non-diabetic renal disease and Mullerian aplasia (3); MODY5 with nephron agenesis (3)	11 (Hnf2)
17q	HYT1	Hypertension, essential, susceptibility to, 1	603918	{Hypertension, essential, susceptibility to, 1}, 145500 (2)	
17q	PSORS2, PSS1	Psoriasis susceptibility 2	602723	{Psoriasis susceptibility-2} (2)	
17q11-q12	WHN	Winged helix nude	600838	T-cell immunodeficiency, congenital alopecia, and nail dystrophy (3)	
17q11-qter	ITGB4	Integrin, beta-4	147557	Epidermolysis bullosa, junctional, with pyloric atresia, 226730 (3); Epidermolysis bullosa, generalized atrophic benign, 226650 (3)	
17q11.1-q11.2	TAF2N, RBP56	TATA box-binding protein-associated factor 2N (RNA-binding protein 56)	601574	Chondrosarcoma, extraskeletal myxoid (1)	
17q11.1-q12	CRYBA1, CRYB1	Crystallin, beta A1	123610	Cataract, congenital zonular, with sutural opacities, 600881 (3)	11 (Cryba1)
17q11.1-q12	SLC6A4, HTT	Solute carrier family 6 (neurotransmitter transporter, serotonin), member 4	182138	Anxiety-related personality traits (3)	11 (Htt)
17q11.2	BLMH, BMH	Bleomycin hydrolase	602403	{Alzheimer disease, susceptibility to} (3)	
17q11.2	NF1, VRNF, WSS	Neurofibromin (neurofibromatosis, type I)	162200	Neurofibromatosis, type 1 (3); Watson syndrome, 193520 (3); Leukemia, juvenile myelomonocytic (3); Melanoma, desmoplastic neurotropic (2)	
17q11.2	VBCH	Van Buchem disease	239100	Van Buchem disease (2)	
17q11.2-q12	SCYA5, D17S136E, TCP228	Small inducible cytokine A5 (RANTES)	187011	{HIV-1 disease, delayed progression of} (2)	
17q11.2-q24	MHS2	Malignant hyperthermia susceptibility 2	154275	{Malignant hyperthermia susceptibility 2} (2)	

continued

Table 10.1. The morbid anatomy of the human genome (by chromosome) (*continued*)

Location	Symbol	Title	MIM#	Disorder	Mouse
17q12	KRT12	Keratin-12	601687	Meesmann corneal dystrophy, 122100 (3)	
17q12	RARA	Retinoic acid receptor, alpha polypeptide	180240	Leukemia, acute promyelocytic (1)	11 (Rara)
17q12	TCAP, LGMD2G	Telethonin	604488	Muscular dystrophy, limb-girdle, type 2G, 601954 (3)	
17q12-q21	KRT9, EPPK	Keratin-9	144200	Epidermolytic palmoplantar keratoderma (3)	
17q12-q21	KRT14	Keratin-14	148066	Epidermolysis bullosa simplex, Koebner, Dowling-Meara, and Weber-Cockayne types, 131900, 131760, 131800 (3); Epidermolysis bullosa simplex, recessive, 601001 (3)	
17q12-q21	KRT16	Keratin-16	148067	Pachyonychia congenita, Jadassohn-Lewandowsky type, 167200 (3); Nonepidermolytic palmoplantar keratoderma, 600962 (3)	
17q12-q21	KRT17, PC2, PCHC1	Keratin-17	148069	Pachyonychia congenita, Jackson-Lawler type, 167210 (3); Steatocystoma multiplex, 184500 (3)	
17q12-q21	SOST	Sclerosteosis	269500	Sclerosteosis (2)	
17q12-q21	WT4	Wilms tumor-4	601363	Wilms tumor, type 4 (2)	
17q12-q21.33	SGCA, ADL, DAG2, LGMD2D	Sarcoglycan, alpha (50 kD dystrophin-associated glycoprotein; adhalin)	600119	Muscular dystrophy, Duchenne-like, type 2 (3); Adhalinopathy, primary (1)	
17q21	ACACA, ACAC, ACC1	Acetyl-Coenzyme A carboxylase, alpha	200350	Acetyl-CoA carboxylase deficiency (1)	
17q21	BRCA1, PSCP	Breast cancer-1 gene	113705	Breast cancer-1 (3); Ovarian cancer (3); Breast-ovarian cancer (3); Papillary serous carcinoma of the peritoneum (3)	11 (Brca1)
17q21	G6PC, G6PT	Glucose-6-phosphatase, catalytic	232200	Glycogen storage disease I (3)	
17q21	GFAP	Glial fibrillary acidic protein	137780	Alexander disease, 203450 (3)	11 (Gfap)
17q21	HCRT, OX	Hypocretin	602358	Narcolepsy, 161400 (3)	
17q21	JUP, DP3, PDGB	Junction plakoglobin	173325	Naxos disease, 601214 (3)	11 (Jup, Pkgb)
17q21	NAGLU	N-acetylglucosaminidase, alpha-	252920	Sanfilippo syndrome, type B (3)	
17q21	PHB	Prohibitin	176705	Breast cancer, sporadic (3)	
17q21	PPND	Parkinsonism-dementia with pallidopontonigral degeneration	168610	Parkinsonism-dementia with pallidopontonigral degeneration (2)	
17q21-q22	GPSC	Gliosis, familial progressive subcortical	221820	Gliosis, familial progressive subcortical (2)	
17q21-q22	KRT10	Keratin-10	148080	Epidermolytic hyperkeratosis, 113800 (3)	
17q21-q22	KRT13	Keratin-13	148065	White sponge nevus, 193900 (3)	
17q21-q22	PHA2B	Pseudohypoaldosteronism type II	601844	Pseudohypoaldosteronism type II (2)	
17q21-q22	PNMT, PENT	Phenylethanolamine N-methyltransferase	171190	?Hypertension, essential, 145500 (1)	
17q21-q22	PTLAH, FPAH	Patella aplasia or hypoplasia	168860	Patella aplasia or hypoplasia (2)	

continued

Table 10.1. The morbid anatomy of the human genome (by chromosome) (*continued*)

Location	Symbol	Title	MIM#	Disorder	Mouse
17q21-q22	SLC4A1, AE1, EPB3	Solute carrier family 4, anion exchanger, member 1 (erythrocyte membrane protein band 3, Diego blood group)	109270	[Acanthocytosis, one form] (1); [Elliptocytosis, Malaysian-Melanesian type] (3); Spherocytosis, hereditary (3); Hemolytic anemia due to band 3 defect (3); Renal tubular acidosis, distal, 179800 (3)	
17q21.31-q22	COL1A1	Collagen I, alpha-1 polypeptide	120150	Osteogenesis imperfecta, 4 clinical forms, 166200, 166210, 259420, 166220 (3); Ehlers-Danlos syndrome, types I and VIIA, 130000, 130060 (3); Osteoporosis, idiopathic, 166710 (3); {Dissection of cervical arteries, susceptibility to} (3)	11 (Col1a1)
17q21.1	MAPT, MTBT1, DDPAC, MSTD	Microtubule-associated protein tau	157140	Dementia, frontotemporal, with parkinsonism, 601630 (3)	
17q21.3	NME1, NM23	Non-metastatic cells 1, protein (NM23A) expressed in	156490	Neuroblastoma (3)	
17q21.3-q22	DLX3, TDO	Distal-less homeo box-3	600525	Trichodontoosseous syndrome, 190320 (3)	
17q21.32	ITGA2B, GP2B, CD41B	Integrin, alpha-2b (platelet glycoprotein IIb of IIb/IIIa complex, antigen CD41B)	273800	Glanzmann thrombasthenia, type A (3); Thrombocytopenia, neonatal alloimmune (1)	
17q21.32	ITGB3, GP3A	Integrin, beta-3 (platelet glycoprotein IIIa; antigen CD61)	173470	Glanzmann thrombasthenia, type B (3)	
17q21.32	RCCP3	Renal cell carcinoma, papillary, 3	605075	Renal cell carcinoma, papillary, 3 (2)	
17q22	NOG, SYM1, SYNS1	Noggin, mouse, homolog of	602991	Symphalangism, proximal, 185800 (3); Synostoses syndrome, multiple, 1, 186500 (3)	
17q22	RP17	Retinitis pigmentosa-17	600852	Retinitis pigmentosa-17 (2)	
17q22-q23	MKS1, MKS	Meckel syndrome, type 1	249000	Meckel syndrome, type 1 (2)	
17q22-q23	MUL	Mulibrey nanism gene	253250	Mulibrey nanism, 253250 (3)	
17q22-q23.2	PRKCA, PKCA	Protein kinase C, alpha polypeptide	176960	Pituitary tumor, invasive (3)	11(Pkca)
17q22-q24	CSH1, CSA, PL	Chorionic somatomammotropin hormone-1	150200	[Placental lactogen deficiency] (1)	13(Pl1)
17q22-q24	GH1, GHN	Growth hormone-1	139250	Isolated growth hormone deficiency, Illig type with absent GH and Kowarski type with bioinactive GH (3)	11(Gh)
17q23	ACE, DCP1, ACE1	Angiotensin I converting enzyme (dipeptidyl carboxypeptidase-1)	106180	{Myocardial infarction, susceptibility to} (3); {Alzheimer disease, susceptibility to}, 104300 (3)	
17q23-q24	AXIN2	Axis inhibitor 2 (conductin, mouse, homolog of)	604025	Colorectal cancer, 114500 (3)	
17q23-q24	PRKAR1A, TSE1, CNC1, CAR	Protein kinase, cAMP-dependent, regulatory, type I, alpha	188830	Carney complex, type 1, 160980 (3); Myxoma, intracardiac, 255960 (3)	11(Tse1)
17q23-qter	APOH	Apolipoprotein H (beta-2-glycoprotein I)	138700	[Apolipoprotein H deficiency] (3)	11(Apoh)
17q23.1	MPO	Myeloperoxidase	254600	Myeloperoxidase deficiency (3)	11 (Mpo)
17q23.1-q25.3	SCN4A, HYPP, NAC1A	Sodium channel, voltage-gated, type IV, alpha polypeptide	603967	Hyperkalemic periodic paralysis, 170500 (3); Paramyotonia congenita, 168300 (3); Myotonia congenita, atypical, acetazolamide-responsive (3); Cramps, familial, potassium-aggravated (3)	

continued

Table 10.1. The morbid anatomy of the human genome (by chromosome) (*continued*)

Location	Symbol	Title	MIM#	Disorder	Mouse
17q24	CCA1	Cataract, congenital, cerulean type	115660	Cataract, cerulean, type 1 (2)	
17q24	GALK1	Galactokinase-1	604313	Galactokinase deficiency with cataracts, 230200 (3)	11(Glk)
17q24	SSTR2	Somatostatin receptor-2	182452	Lung cancer, small cell (3)	11(Sstr2)
17q24	TOC, TEC	Tylosis with esophageal cancer	148500	Tylosis with esophageal cancer (2)	
17q24.3-q25.1	SOX9, CMD1, SRA1	SRY (sex-determining region Y)-box 9	114290	Campomelic dysplasia with autosomal sex reversal (3)	11 (Ts, Sox9)
17q25	ACOX1, ACOX	Acyl-Coenzyme A oxidase 1	264470	Adrenoleukodystrophy, pseudoneonatal (2)	
17q25	DFNA20	Deafness, autosomal dominant 20	604717	Deafness, autosomal dominant 20 (2)	
17q25	GCGR	Glucagon receptor	138033	Diabetes mellitus, type II (3)	
17q25	MSF, MSF1	MLL septin-like fusion gene	604061	Leukemia, acute myeloid, therapy-related (1); Ovarian carcinoma (1)	
17q25	NAPB	Neuralgic amyotrophy with predilection for brachial plexus	162100	Neuralgic amyotrophy with predilection for brachial plexus (2)	
17q25.2-q25.3	GAA	Glucosidase, acid alpha-	232300	Glycogen storage disease II (3)	
17q25.3	SGSH, MPS3A, SFMD	N-sulfoglucosamine sulfohydrolase (sulfamidase)	252900	Sanfilippo syndrome, type A (3)	11 (Sgsh)
Chr.17	CHRNE	Cholinergic receptor, nicotinic, epsilon polypeptide	100725	Myasthenic syndrome, slow-channel congenital, 601462 (3)	
18p11.32	MCL	Multiple hereditary cutaneous leiomyoma	150800	?Leiomyoma, multiple hereditary cutaneous (2)	
18p11.32-p11.23	HTS	Hypotrichosis simplex	605389	Hypotrichosis simplex (2)	
18p11.31	MYP2	Myopia, high grade, autosomal dominant 1	160700	Myopia-2 (2)	
18p11.31-p11.2	NDUFV2	NADH dehydrogenase (ubiquinone) flavoprotein 2, 24 kD	600532	{Parkinson disease, susceptibility to}, 168600 (3)	
18p11.3	TGIF, HPE4	TG-interacting factor	602630	Holoprosencephaly-4, 142946 (3)	
18p11.2	MC2R	Melanocortin-2 receptor (ACTH receptor)	202200	Glucocorticoid deficiency, due to ACTH unresponsiveness (1)	18 (Mc2r)
18p	DYT7	Dystonia-7 (torsion dystonia, adult-onset, focal)	602124	Dystonia-7, torsion (2)	
18p	MAFD1, BPAD, MD1	Major affective disorder 1	125480	Bipolar affective disorder (2)	
18p	SCZD8	Schizophrenia susceptibility locus, chromosome 18-related	603206	{Schizophrenia}, 181500 (2)	
18q	OHDS	Orthostatic hypotensive disorder of Streeten	143850	Orthostatic hypotensive disorder of Streeten (2)	
18q11-q12	LCFS2	Lynch cancer family syndrome II	114400	?Lynch cancer family syndrome II (2)	
18q11-q12	NPC1, NPC	Niemann-Pick disease, type C	257220	Niemann-Pick disease, type C1 (3); Niemann-Pick disease, type D, 257250 (3)	18 (spm)
18q11.2	LAMA3	Laminin, alpha-3 (nicein, 150 kD; kalinin, 165 kD; BM600, 150 kD; epilegrin)	600805	Epidermolysis bullosa, junctional, Herlitz type (3)	

continued

Table 10.1. The morbid anatomy of the human genome (by chromosome) (*continued*)

Location	Symbol	Title	MIM#	Disorder	Mouse
18q11.2	SSXT, SYT	Synovial sarcoma, translocated to X chromosome	600192	Sarcoma, synovial (1)	
18q11.2-q12.1	TTR, PALB	Transthyretin (prealbumin)	176300	Amyloid neuropathy, familial, several allelic types (3); [Dystransthyretinemic hyperthyroxinemia] (3); Amyloidosis, senile systemic (3); Carpal tunnel syndrome, familial (3)	18 (Palb)
18q12.1-q12.2	DSG1	Desmoglein-1	125670	Keratosis palmoplantaris striata I, 148700 (3)	18 (Dsg1)
18q12.2-q12.3	OPA4	Optic atrophy-4	605293	Optic atrophy-4 (2)	
18q21	ATP8B1, FIC1, BRIC, PFIC1	ATPase, class I, type 8B, member 1	602397	Cholestasis, progressive familial intrahepatic-1, 211600 (3); Cholestasis, benign recurrent intrahepatic, 243300 (3)	
18q21	IDDM6	Insulin-dependent diabetes mellitus-6	601941	{Diabetes mellitus, insulin-dependent, 6} (2)	
18q21-q22	LOH18CR1, OSTS	Loss of heterozygosity, 18, chromosomal region 1 (osteosarcoma tumor suppressor)	603045	Osteosarcoma, 259500 (2)	
18q21.1	MADH4, DPC4, SMAD4, JIP	Mothers against decapentaplegic, Drosophila, homolog of, 4	600993	Pancreatic cancer (3); Polyposis, juvenile intestinal, 174900 (3)	
18q21.1-q21.3	CORD1, CRD1	Cone rod dystrophy 1, autosomal dominant	600624	Cone rod retinal dystrophy-1 (2)	
18q21.3	BCL2	B-cell CLL/lymphoma-2	151430	Leukemia/lymphoma, B-cell, 2 (2)	1 (Bc12)
18q21.3	CNSN	Carnosinemia (carnosinase)	212200	Carnosinemia (2)	
18q21.3	DCC	Deleted in colorectal carcinoma	120470	Colorectal cancer (3)	18 (Dcc)
18q21.3	FECH, FCE	Ferrochelatase	177000	Protoporphyria, erythropoietic (3); Protoporphyria, erythropoietic, recessive, with liver failure (3)	
18q21.3	FVT1	Follicular lymphoma, variant translocation 1	136440	Lymphoma/leukemia, B-cell, variant (1)	
18q21.3-q22	LMAN1, ERGIC53, F5F8D, MCFD1	Lectin, mannose-binding, 1	601567	Combined factor V and VIII deficiency, 227300 (3)	
18q22	MC4R	Melanocortin-4 receptor	155541	Obesity, autosomal dominant (3)	
18q22.1	TNFRSF11A, RANK, ODFR, OFE	Tumor necrosis factor receptor superfamily, member 11A	603499	Osteolysis, familial expansile, 174810 (3); Paget disease of bone, 602080 (3)	
18q23	CYB5	Cytochrome b5	250790	Methemoglobinemia due to cytochrome b5 deficiency (3)	
18q23-qter	CCFDN	Congenital cataract, facial dysmorphism, and neuropathy syndrome	604168	Congenital cataract, facial dysmorphism, and neuropathy syndrome (2)	
19p13.3	ATCAY, CLAC	Ataxia, cerebellar, Cayman type	601238	Cerebellar ataxia, Cayman type (2)	
19p13.3	ELA2	Elastase-2, neutrophil	130130	Cyclic hematopoiesis, 162800 (3)	10 (Ela2)
19p13.3	FEB2	Convulsions, familial febrile, 2	602477	Convulsions, familial febrile, 2 (2)	
19p13.3	FUT6	Fucosyltransferase 6 (alpha (1,3) fucosyltransferase)	136836	Fucosyltransferase-6 deficiency (3)	
19p13.3	GAMT	Guanidinoacetate methyltransferase	601240	GAMT deficiency (3)	10 (Gamt)
19p13.3	HHC2, FHH2	Hypocalciuric hypercalcemia-2	145981	Hypocalciuric hypercalcemia, type II (2)	

continued

Table 10.1. The morbid anatomy of the human genome (by chromosome) (*continued*)

Location	Symbol	Title	MIM#	Disorder	Mouse
19p13.3	MDRV	Muscular dystrophy with rimmed vacuoles	601846	Muscular dystrophy with rimmed vacuoles (2)	
19p13.3	NRTN, NTN	Neurturin	602018	Hirschsprung disease, 142623 (3)	17 (Nrtn)
19p13.3	STK11, PJS, LKB1	Serine/threonine protein kinase-11	602216	Peutz-Jeghers syndrome, 175200 (3)	10 (Stk11)
19p13.3	TBXA2R	Thromboxane A2 receptor	188070	Bleeding disorder due to defective thromboxane A2 receptor (3)	10 (Tbxa2r)
19p13.3	TCF3, E2A	Transcription factor-3 (E2A immunoglobulin enhancer-binding factors E12/E47)	147141	Leukemia, acute lymphoblastic (1)	
19p13.3-p13.2	AMH, MIF	Anti-Mullerian hormone	600957	Persistent Mullerian duct syndrome, type I, 261550 (3)	10 (Amh)
19p13.3-p13.2	ATHS, ALP	Atherosclerosis susceptibility (lipoprotein associated)	108725	{Atherosclerosis, susceptibility to} (2)	
19p13.3-p13.2	C3	Complement component-3	120700	C3 deficiency (3)	17 (C3)
19p13.3-p13.2	EPOR	Erythropoietin receptor	133171	[Erythrocytosis, familial], 133100 (3)	9 (Epor)
19p13.3-p13.2	ICAM1	Intercellular adhesion molecule-1	147840	{Malaria, cerebral, susceptibility to} (3)	9 (Icam1)
19p13.3-p13.2	MCOLN1, ML4	Mucolipin 1	605248	Mucolipidosis IV, 252650 (3)	
19p13.2	GCDH	Glutaryl-Coenzyme A dehydrogenase	231670	Glutaricaciduria, type I (3)	8 (Gcdh)
19p13.2	INSR	Insulin receptor	147670	Leprechaunism, 246200 (3); Rabson-Mendenhall syndrome, 262190 (3); Diabetes mellitus, insulin-resistant, with acanthosis nigricans (3)	8 (Insr)
19p13.2	LDLR, FHC, FH	Low density lipoprotein receptor	143890	Hypercholesterolemia, familial (3)	9 (Ldlr)
19p13.2	TCO	Thyroid carcinoma, nonmedullary, with cell oxyphilia	603386	Thyroid carcinoma, nonmedullary, with cell oxyphilia (2)	
19p13.2-p13.1	INLNE	Ichthyosis, nonlamellar and nonerythrodermic, congenital, autosomal recessive	604781	Ichthyosis, nonlamellar and nonerythrodermic, congenital (2)	
19p13.2-p13.1	LYL1	Lymphoblastic leukemia derived sequence-1	151440	Leukemia, T-cell acute lymphoblastoid (2)	8 (Lyl1)
19p13.2-p13.1	NOTCH3, CADASIL, CASIL	Notch, Drosophila, homolog of, 3	600276	Cerebral arteriopathy with subcortical infarcts and leukoencephalopathy,125310 (3)	17 (Notch3)
19p13.2-p12	SLC5A5, NIS	Solute carrier family 5 (sodium iodide symporter), member-5	601843	Hypothyroidism, congenital, 274400 (3)	
19p13.2-q13.3	LPSA, D19S381E	Oncogene liposarcoma (DNA segment, single copy, expressed, probes MC15, MC6)	164953	Liposarcoma (1)	
19p13.1	COMP, EDM1, MED, PSACH	Cartilage oligomeric matrix protein	600310	Pseudoachondroplasia, 177170 (3); Epiphyseal dysplasia, multiple 1, 132400 (3)	
19p13.1	IL12RB1	Interleukin-12 receptor, beta-1	601604	{Mycobacterial and salmonella infections, susceptibility to} (3)	
19p13.1	JAK3, JAKL	Janus kinase 3 (Janus kinase, leukocyte)	600173	SCID, autosomal recessive, T-negative/B-positive type (3)	
19p13	CACNA1A, CACNL1A4, SCA6	Calcium channel, voltage-dependent, P/Q type, alpha 1A subunit	601011	Hemiplegic migraine, familial, 141500 (3); Episodic ataxia, type 2, 108500 (3); Spinocerebellar ataxia-6, 183086 (3); Cerebellar ataxia, pure (3)	8 (tg, Cacl1a4)

continued

Table 10.1. The morbid anatomy of the human genome (by chromosome) (*continued*)

Location	Symbol	Title	MIM#	Disorder	Mouse
19p13	NDUFS7, PSST	NADH dehydrogenase (ubiquinone) Fe-S protein 7, 20 kD (NADH-coenzyme Q reductase)	601825	Leigh syndrome, 256000 (3)	
19p13	PSORS6	Psoriasis susceptibility 6	605364	{Psoriasis, susceptibility to}, 177990 (3)	
19p13	SH3GL1, EEN	SH3 domain GRB2-like 1 (Extra 11–19 leukemia fusion gene)	601768	Leukemia, acute myeloid (1)	
19p12	RFXANK	Regulatory factor X, ankyrin repeat-containing	603200	MHC class II deficiency, complementation group B, 209920 (3)	
19p12-q12	LI3	Ichthyosis congenita III	604777	Ichthyosis, lamellar, type 3 (2)	
19p	EXT3	Exostoses, multiple, 3	600209	Exostoses, multiple, type 3 (2)	
19cen-q12	MAN2B1, MANB	Mannosidase, alpha, class 2B, member 1	248500	Mannosidosis, alpha-, types I and II (3)	8 (Man2b1)
19cen-q13.11	PEPD	Peptidase D (prolidase)	170100	Prolidase deficiency (3)	7 (Pep4)
19cen-q13.2	AD2	Alzheimer disease-2, late-onset	104310	Alzheimer disease-2, late onset (2)	
19q	BFIC	Benign familial infantile convulsions	601764	Benign familial infantile convulsions (2)	
19q13	ACTN4, FSGS1, FSGS	Actinin, alpha-4	604638	Glomerulosclerosis, focal segmental, 1, 603278 (3)	
19q13	BCAT2, BCT2	Branched chain aminotransferase-2, mitochondrial	113530	?Hypervalinemia or hyperleucine-isoleucinemia (1)	7(Bcat2)
19q13	BCL3	B-cell CLL/lymphoma-3	109560	Leukemia/lymphoma, B-cell, 3 (2)	7 (Bcl3)
19q13	DFNA4	Deafness, autosomal dominant 4	600652	Deafness, autosomal dominant 4 (2)	
19q13	DLL3, SCDO1	Delta, Drosophila, homolog of	602768	Spondylocostal dysostosis, autosomal recessive, 1, 277300 (3)	7 (Dll3)
19q13	DYT12, RDP	Dystonia-12	128235	Dystonia-12 (2)	
19q13	HHC3, FBH3	Hypercalcemia, familial benign, 3 (hypercalcemia, familial benign, Oklahoma type)	600740	Hypercalciuric hypercalcemia, type III (2)	
19q13	OFC3	Orofacial cleft-3	600757	Orofacial cleft-3 (2)	7 (Cebpa)
19q13	SPG12	Spastic paraplegia 12, autosomal dominant	604805	Spastic paraplegia-12 (2)	
19q13.1	SLC7A9, CSNU3	Solute carrier family 7 (cationic amino acid transporter, y+ system), member 9	604144	Cystinuria, type III (3); Cystinuria, type II (3)	
19q13.1	GPI	Glucose phosphate isomerase; neuroleukin	172400	Hemolytic anemia due to glucosephosphate isomerase deficiency (3); Hydrops fetalis, one form (1)	7 (Gpi1)
19q13.1	NPHN, NPHS1	Nephrin	602716	Nephrosis-1, congenital, Finnish type, 256300 (3)	
19q13.1	RYR1, MHS, CCO	Ryanodine receptor-1, skeletal	180901	{Malignant hyperthermia susceptibility 1}, 145600 (3); Central core disease, 117000 (3)	7 (Ryr)
19q13.1	SCN1B	Sodium channel, voltage-gated, type I, beta polypeptide	600235	Generalized epilepsy with febrile seizures plus (3)	
19q13.1	TGFB1, DPD1, CED	Transforming growth factor, beta-1	190180	Camurati-Engelmann disease, 131300 (3)	7 (Tgfb1)

continued

Table 10.1. The morbid anatomy of the human genome (by chromosome) (*continued*)

Location	Symbol	Title	MIM#	Disorder	Mouse
19q13.1	TYROBP, PLOSL	TYRO protein tyrosine kinase-binding protein	604142	Polycystic lipomembranous osteodysplasia with sclerosing leukenencephalophathy, 221770 (3)	
19q13.1-q13.2	AKT2	Murine thymoma viral (v-akt) homolog-2	164731	Ovarian carcinoma, 167000 (2)	7(Akt2)
19q13.1-q13.2	BCKDHA, MSUD1	Branched chain keto acid dehydrogenase E1, alpha polypeptide	248600	Maple syrup urine disease, type Ia (3)	
19q13.1-q13.2	MCPH2	Microcephaly, primary autosomal recessive 2	604317	Microcephaly, autosomal recessive 2 (2)	
19q13.1-q13.3	CMT4F	Charcot-Marie-Tooth disease, type 4F	605260	Charcot-Marie-Tooth disease, type 4F (2)	
19q13.2	APOE	Apolipoprotein E	107741	Hyperlipoproteinemia, type III (3); {Myocardial infarction susceptibility} (3)	7 (Apoe)
19q13.2	APOC2	Apolipoprotein C-II	207750	Hyperlipoproteinemia, type Ib (3)	
19q13.2	CYP2A6, CYP2A3	Cytochrome P450, subfamily IIA, phenobarbital-inducible, polypeptide 6	122720	Coumarin resistance, 122700 (3); {Nicotine addiction, protection from} (3)	
19q13.2	RPS19, DBA	Ribosomal protein S19	603474	Anemia, Diamond-Blackfan, 105650 (3)	
19q13.2-q13.3	DMPK, DM, DMK	Dystrophia myotonica-protein kinase	605377	Myotonic dystrophy, 160900 (3)	7 (Dm15)
19q13.2-q13.3	ERCC2, EM9	Excision repair cross complementing rodent repair deficiency, complementation group-2	126340	Xeroderma pigmentosum, group D, 278730 (3); Trichothiodystrophy, 601675 (3)	7 (Ercc2)
19q13.2-q13.3	HB1, PFHB1	Heart block, progressive familial, type I	113900	Heart block, progressive familial, type I (2)	
19q13.2-q13.3	LIG1	Ligase I, DNA, ATP-dependent	126391	DNA ligase I deficiency (3)	7 (Lig1)
19q13.2-q13.3	OPA3, MGA3	Optic atrophy 3 (Iraqi-Jewish "optic atrophy plus")	258501	3-methylglutaconicaciduria, type III (2)	
19q13.2-q13.3	PVR, PVS	Polio virus receptor	173850	{Polio, susceptibility to} (2)	9 (Pvs)
19q13.2-q13.4	CFM1	Cystic fibrosis modifier-1	603855	Meconium ileus in cystic fibrosis, susceptibility to (2)	7 (Cfm1)
19q13.3	CRX, CORD2, CRD	Cone-rod homeo box-containing gene	602225	Cone-rod retinal dystrophy-2, 120970 (3); Leber congenital amaurosis due to defect in CRX, 204000 (3); Retinitis pigmentosa, late-onset dominant (3)	
19q13.3	ETFB	Electron transfer flavoprotein, beta polypeptide	130410	Glutaricaciduria, type IIB (3)	7 (Etfb)
19q13.3	GYSI, GYS	Glycogen synthase	138570	{Diabetes mellitus, noninsulin-dependent} (2)	
19q13.3-q13.4	BAX	BCL2-associated X protein	600040	Colorectal cancer (3); T-cell acute lymphoblastic leukemia (3)	7 (Bax)
19q13.3-q13.4	FTL	Ferritin, light chain	134790	Hyperferritinemia-cataract syndrome, 600886 (3)	7 (Ftl1)
19q13.3-q13.4	HYDM	Hydatidiform mole	231090	Hydatidiform mole (2)	
19q13.3-q13.4	SCA13	Spinocereballar ataxia 13	605259	Spinocereballar ataxia-13 (2)	
19q13.3-qter	KTGNR	Kartagener syndrome	244400	Kartagener syndrome (2)	

continued

Table 10.1. The morbid anatomy of the human genome (by chromosome) (*continued*)

Location	Symbol	Title	MIM#	Disorder	Mouse
19q13.32	LHB	Luteinizing hormone, beta polypeptide	152780	Hypogonadism, hypergonadotropic (3); ?Male pseudohermaphroditism due to defective LH (1)	7(Lhb)
19q13.4	RP11	Retinitis pigmentosa-11, autosomal dominant	600138	Retinitis pigmentosa	11 (2)
19q13.4	TNN13	Troponin-I, cardiac	191044	Cardiomyopathy, familial hypertrophic (3)	7 (Tnni3)
19q13.4	TNNT1, ANM	Troponin-T1, skeletal, slow	191041	Nemaline myopathy, Amish type, 605355 (3)	
19q13.4-qter	SCA14	Spinocerebellar ataxia-14	605361	Spinocerebellar ataxia-14 (2)	
Chr.19	EEC2	Ectrodactyly, ectodermal dysplasia, cleft lip/palate-2	602077	Ectrodactyly, ectodermal dysplasia, cleft lip/palate-2 (2)	
20pter-p12	PRNP, PRIP	Prion protein (p27–30)	176640	Creutzfeldt-Jakob disease, 123400 (3); Gerstmann-Straussler disease,137440 (3); Insomnia, fatal familial (3)	2 (Prnp)
20p13	AVP, AVRP, VP	Arginine vasopressin (neurophysin II, antidiuretic hormone)	192340	Diabetes insipidus, neurohypophyseal, 125700 (3)	2 (Avp)
20p13	CHED2	Congenital hereditary endothelial dystrophy of cornea	121700	Congenital hereditary endothelial dystrophy of cornea (2)	
20p13-p12.3	NBIA1	Neurodegeneration with brain iron accumulation 1 (Hallervorden-Spatz syndrome)	234200	Neurodegeneration with brain iron accumulation (2)	
20p12	MKKS, HMCS, KMS, MKS, BBS6	McKusick-Kaufman syndrome gene	604896	McKusick-Kaufman syndrome, 236700 (3); Bardet-Biedl syndrome, type 6, 605231 (3)	
20p12	JAG1, AGS, AHD	Jagged 1	601920	Alagille syndrome, 118450 (3)	
20p12-q12	CTPP3, CPP3	Cataract, posterior polar 3	605387	Cataract, posterior polar-3 (2)	
20p11.2	CST3	Cystatin C	604312	Cerebral amyloid angiopathy, 105150 (3)	2 (Cst3)
20p11.2	THBD, THRM	Thrombomodulin	188040	Thrombophilia due to thrombomodulin defect (3); {Myocardial infarction, susceptibility to} (3)	2 (Thbd)
20p11.2-q11.2	PPCD, PPD	Posterior polymorphous corneal dystrophy	122000	Corneal dystrophy, posterior polymorphous (2)	
20p	HLN1	Huntington-like neurodegenerative disorder 1	603218	Huntington-like neurodegenerative disorder 1 (2)	
20p	ITPA	Inosine triphosphatase-A	147520	[Inosine triphosphatase deficiency] (1)	2 (Itp)
20q11.2	CDAN2, HEMPAS	Congenital dyserythropoietic anemia II	224100	Congenital dyserythropoietic anemia II (2)	
20q11.2	DNMT3B, ICF	DNA methyltransferase 3B	602900	Immunodeficiency-centromeric instability-facial anomalies syndrome, 242860 (3)	
20q11.2	GDF5, CDMP1	Growth/differentiation factor-5 (cartilage-derived morphogenetic protein-1)	601146	Acromesomelic dysplasia, Hunter-Thompson type, 201250 (3); Brachydactyly, type C, 113100 (3); Chondrodysplasia, Grebe type, 200700 (3)	2 (bp)

continued

Table 10.1. The morbid anatomy of the human genome (by chromosome) (*continued*)

Location	Symbol	Title	MIM#	Disorder	Mouse
20q11.2	GHRH, GHRF	Growth hormone releasing hormone (somatocrinin)	139190	?Isolated growth hormone deficiency due to defect in GHRF (1); Gigantism due to GHRF hypersecretion (1)	
20q11.2	GSS, GSHS	Glutathione synthetase	601002	Hemolytic anemia due to glutathione synthetase deficiency, 231900 (3); 5-oxoprolinuria, 266130 (3)	
20q12-q13	SRC, ASV, SRC1	Protooncogene SRC, Rous sarcoma	190090	Colon cancer, advanced (3)	2 (Src)
20q12-q13.1	HNF4A, TCF14, MODY1	Hepatocyte nuclear factor 4, alpha (transcription factor-14)	600281	MODY, type 1, 125850 (3); {Diabetes mellitus, noninsulin-dependent}, 125853 (3)	2 (Hnf4a)
20q12-q13.1	NIDDM3	Noninsulin-dependent diabetes mellitus 3	603694	Diabetes mellitus, noninsulin-dependent, 3 (2)	
20q13.1	PPGB, GSL, NGBE, GLB2, CTSA	Protective protein for beta-galactosidase (cathepsin A)	256540	Galactosialidosis (3)	2 (Ppgb)
20q13.11	ADA	Adenosine deaminase	102700	Severe combined immunodeficiency due to ADA deficiency (3); Hemolytic anemia due to ADA excess (1)	2 (Ada)
20q13.11	GRD2	Graves disease, susceptibility to, 2	603388	{Graves disease, susceptibility to, 2} (2)	
20q13.11-q13.2	OQTL	Obesity quantitative trait locus (Obesity susceptibility locus on chromosome 20)	602025	{Obesity/hyperinsulinism, susceptibility to} (2)	
20q13.2	GNAS1, GNAS, GPSA	Guanine nucleotide-binding protein (G protein), alpha-stimulating activity polypeptide-1	139320	Pseudohypoparathyroidism, type Ia, 103580 (3); McCune-Albright polyostotic fibrous dysplasia, 174800 (3); Somatotrophinoma (3); Pituitary ACTH secreting adenoma (3)	2 (Gnas)
20q13.2-q13.3	CHRNA4, ENFL1	Cholinergic receptor, nicotinic, alpha polypeptide-4	118504	Epilepsy, nocturnal frontal lobe, 1, 600513 (3)	2 (Acra4)
20q13.2-q13.3	EDN3	Endothelin-3	131242	Shah-Waardenburg syndrome, 277580 (3)	2 (Edn3)
20q13.3	COL9A3, EDM3	Collagen IX, alpha-3 polypeptide	120270	Epiphyseal dysplasia, multiple, 3, 600969 (3); Epiphyseal dysplasia, multiple, with myopathy (3)	
20q13.3	KCNQ2, EBN1	Potassium voltage-gated channel, KQT-like subfamily, member 2	602235	Epilepsy, benign, neonatal, type 1, 121200 (3)	
20q13.3	PHP1B	Pseudohypoparathyroidism, type IB	603233	Pseudohypoparathyroidism, type IB (2)	
20q13.31	PCK1	Phosphoenolpyruvate carboxykinase-1 (soluble)	261680	?Hypoglycemia due to PCK1 deficiency (1)	2 (Pck1)
21q11.2	TAM, MST	Myeloproliferative syndrome, transient (transient abnormal myelopoiesis)	159595	Leukemia, transient, of Down syndrome (2)	
21q21	APP, AAA, CVAP, AD1	Amyloid beta (A4) precursor protein	104760	Amyloidosis, cerebroarterial, Dutch type (3); Alzheimer disease-1, APP-related (3); Schizophrenia, chronic (3)	16 (App)
21q21	PRSS7, ENTK	Protease, serine, 7 (enterokinase)	226200	Enterokinase deficiency (1)	
21q21	USH1E	Usher syndrome-1E, autosomal recessive, severe	602097	Usher syndrome, type 1E (2)	
21q22.1	HLCS, HCS	Holocarboxylase synthetase	253270	Multiple carboxylase deficiency, biotin-responsive (3)	16 (Hlcs)

continued

Table 10.1. The morbid anatomy of the human genome (by chromosome) (*continued*)

Location	Symbol	Title	MIM#	Disorder	Mouse
21q22.1	KCNE2, MIRP1	Potassium voltage-gated channel, Isk-related family, member 2	603796	Long QT syndrome-6 (3)	
21q22.1	SOD1, ALS1	Superoxide dismutase-1, soluble	147450	Amytrophic lateral sclerosis, due to SOD1 deficiency, 105400 (3)	16 (Sod1)
21q22.1-q22.2	IFNGR2, IFNGT1, IFGR2	Interferon gamma receptor-2 (interferon gamma transducer 1)	147569	Mycobacterial infection, atypical, familial disseminated, 209950 (3)	16 (Ifgr2)
21q22.1-q22.2	KCNE1, JLNS, LQT5	Potassium voltage-gated channel, Isk-related subfamily, member 1	176261	Jervell and Lange-Nielsen syndrome, 220400 (3); Long QT syndrome-5 (3)	
21q22.3	AIRE, APECED	Autoimmune regulator	240300	Autoimmune polyglandular disease, type I (3)	
21q22.3	CBS	Cystathionine beta-synthase	236200	Homocystinuria, B6-responsive and nonresponsive types (3)	17 (Cbs)
21q22.3	COL6A1	Collagen VI, alpha-1 polypeptide	120220	Bethlem myopathy, 158810 (3)	10 (Col6a1)
21q22.3	COL6A2	Collagen VI, alpha-2 polypeptide	120240	Bethlem myopathy, 158810 (3)	10 (Col6a2)
21q22.3	CRYAA, CRYA1	Crystallin, alpha A	123580	Cataract, congenital, autosomal dominant (3)	17 (Cryal)
21q22.3	CSTB, STFB, EPM1	Cystatin B (stefin B)	601145	Epilepsy, progressive myoclonic 1, 254800 (3)	
21q22.3	DFNB10	Deafness, neurosensory, autosomal recessive 10	605316	Deafness, neurosensory, autosomal recessive 10 (2)	
21q22.3	DCR, DSCR	Down syndrome chromosome region	190685	Down syndrome (1)	
21q22.3	HPE1	Holoprosencephaly-1, alobar	236100	Holoprosencephaly-1 (2)	
21q22.3	ITGB2, CD18, LCAMB, LAD	Integrin, beta-2 (antigen CD18 (p95), lymphocyte function-associated antigen-1; macrophage antigen, beta polypeptide)	600065	Leukocyte adhesion deficiency, 116920 (3)	7 (Ly15)
21q22.3	KNO, KS	Knobloch syndrome	267750	Knobloch syndrome (2)	
21q22.3	PFKL	Phosphofructokinase, liver type	171860	Hemolytic anemia due to phosphofructokinase deficiency (1)	17 (Pfk1)
21q22.3	RUNX1, CBFA2, AML1	Runt-related transcription factor 1 (aml1 oncogene)	151385	Leukemia, acute myeloid (1); Platelet disorder, familial, with associated myeloid malignancy, 601399 (3)	
21q22.3	TMPRSS3, ECHOS1, DFNB8, DFNB10	Transmembrane protease, serine 3	605511	Deafness, autosomal recessive 8, childhood onset, 601072 (3); Deafness, autosomal recessive 10, congenital, 605316 (3)	
22q11	CECR, CES	Cat eye syndrome	115470	Cat eye syndrome (2)	
22q11	CTHM	Conotruncal cardiac anomalies	217095	?Conotruncal cardiac anomalies (2)	
22q11	DGCR, DGS, VCF	DiGeorge syndrome chromosome region (velocardiofacial syndrome)	188400	DiGeorge syndrome (2); Velocardiofacial syndrome, 192430 (2)	
22q11	HCF2, HC2	Heparin cofactor II	142360	Thrombophilia due to heparin cofactor II deficiency (3)	
22q11	NAGA	Acetylgalactosaminidase, alpha-N- (alpha-galactosidase B)	104170	Schindler disease (3); Kanzaki disease (3); NAGA deficiency, mild (3)	
22q11	SMARCB1, SNF5, INI1, RDT	SWI/SNF related, matrix associated, actin dependent regulator of chromatin, subfamily b, member 1	601607	Rhabdoid tumors (3); Rhabdoid predisposition syndrome, familial (3)	
22q11-q12	FPEVF	Epilepsy, partial, with variable foci	604364	Epilepsy, partial, with variable foci (2)	

continued

Table 10.1. The morbid anatomy of the human genome (by chromosome) (*continued*)

Location	Symbol	Title	MIM#	Disorder	Mouse
22q11-q13	SCZD4	Schizophrenia susceptibility locus, chromosome 22-related	600850	{Schizophrenia}, 181500 (2)	
22q11.1-q11.2	GGT1, GTG	Gamma-glutamyltransferase-1	231950	Glutathioninuria (1)	
22q11.1	GGT2	Gamma-glutamyltransferase-2	137181	[Gamma-glutamyltransferase, familial high serum] (2)	
22q11.2	GP1BB	Glycoprotein Ib, platelet, beta polypeptide	138720	Bernard-Soulier syndrome, type B, 231200 (2); Giant platelet disorder, isolated (3))	16 (Gp1bb
22q11.2	MYH9, MHA, FTNS, DFNA17	Myosin, heavy polypeptide-9, nonmuscle	160775	May-Hegglin anomaly, 155100 (3); Fechtner syndrome, 153640 (3); Sebastian syndrome, 605249 (3); Deafness, autosomal dominant 17, 603622 (3)	
22q11.2	OGS2, BBBG2, GBBB2	Opitz G syndrome, type II	145410	Opitz G syndrome, type II (2)	
22q11.2	PRODH	Proline dehydrogenase (proline oxidase)	239500	Hyperprolinemia, type I (1)	
22q11.2-q12.2	CRYBB2, CRYB2	Crystallin, beta-B2	123620	Cataract, cerulean, type 2, 601547 (3)	5 (Crybb2)
22q11.21	IGLL1, IGO, IGL5	Immunoglobulin lambda-like polypeptide 1 (immunoglobulin omega peptide)	146770	Agammaglobulinemia, autosomal recessive (3)	
22q11.2-qter	TCN2, TC2	Transcobalamin II	275350	Transcobalamin II deficiency (3)	11 (Tcn2)
22q11.21	BCR, CML, PHL	Breakpoint cluster region	151410	Leukemia, chronic myeloid (3)	10 (Bcr)
22q12	EWSR1, EWS	Ewing sarcoma breakpoint region-1	133450	Ewing sarcoma (3); Neuroepithelioma (2)	
22q12	HMOX1	Heme oxygenase, decycling, 1	141250	Heme oxygenase-1 deficiency (3)	
22q12.1	CHK2, RAD53	Checkpoint kinase 2	604373	Li-Fraumeni syndrome, 151623 (3)	
22q12.1-q13.2	TIMP3, SFD	Tissue inhibitor of metalloproteinase-3	188826	Sorsby fundus dystrophy, 136900 (3)	
22q12.2	NEFH	Neurofilament, heavy polypeptide	162230	{Amyotrophic lateral sclerosis, susceptibility to}, 105400 (3)	11 (Nfh)
22q12.2	NF2	Neurofibromatosis-2 (bilateral acoustic neuroma); merlin	101000	Neurofibromatosis, type 2 (3); Meningioma, NF2-related, sporadic (3) Schwannoma, sporadic (3); Neurolemmomatosis (3); Malignant mesothelioma, sporadic (3)	11 (Nf2)
22q12.2-q13.1	CSF2RB	Colony-stimulating factor-2 receptor, beta, low-affinity	138981	Pulmonary alveolar proteinosis, 265120 (3)	
22q12.3-q13.1	LARGE	Acetylglucosaminyltransferase-like protein	603590	?Meningioma (2)	
22q12.3-q13.1	PDGFB, SIS	Platelet-derived growth factor, beta polypeptide (oncogene SIS)	190040	Meningioma, SIS-related (3); Dermatofibrosarcoma protuberans (3); Giant-cell fibroblastoma (3)	15 (Pdgfb)
22q12.3-q13.2	RAC2	Ras-related C3 botulinum toxin substrate 3 (rho family, small GTP-binding protein Rac2)	602049	Neutrophil immunodeficiency syndrome (3)	
22q12.3-qter	MGCR, MN1	Meningioma chromosome region	156100	Meningioma (2)	
22q13	EP300	E1A-binding protein, 300 kD	602700	Colorectal cancer, 114500 (3)	
22q13	SCA10	Spinocerebellar ataxia 10 gene	603516	Spinocerebellar ataxia-10 (3)	

continued

Table 10.1. The morbid anatomy of the human genome (by chromosome) (*continued*)

Location	Symbol	Title	MIM#	Disorder	Mouse
22q13	SCO2	SCO2, S. cerevisiae, homolog of	604272	Cardioencephalomyopathy, fatal infantile, due to cytochrome c oxidase deficiency, 604377 (3)	
22q13	SOX10, WS4	SRY (sex-determining region Y)-box-10	602229	Waardenburg-Shah syndrome, 277580 (3); Yemenite deaf-blind hypopigmentation syndrome, 601706 (3); Waardenburg-Shah syndrome, neurologic variant (3)	15 (Sox10, Dom)
22q13-qter	ACR	Acrosin	102480	?Male infertility due to acrosin deficiency (2)	15 (Acr)
22q13.1	ADSL	Adenylosuccinate lyase	103050	Adenylosuccinase deficiency (1); Autism, succinylpurinemic (3)	15 (Ads1)
22q13.1	CYP2D@, CYP2D, P450C2D	Cytochrome P450, subfamily IID	124030	{?Parkinsonism, susceptibility to} (1); Debrisoquine sensitivity (3)	15(Cyp2d)
22q13.1	SLC5A1, SGLT1	Solute carrier family 5 (sodium/glucose transporter), member 1	182380	Glucose/galactose malabsorption (3)	
22q13.31-qter	ARSA	Arylsulfatase A	250100	Metachromatic leukodystrophy (3)	15(As2)
22q13.31-qter	DIA1	Diaphorase (NADH); cytochrome b-5 reductase	250800	Methemoglobinemia, type I (3); Methemoglobinemia, type II (3)	15 (Dia1)
22q13.32-qter	ECGF1	Endothelial cell growth factor-1, platelet-derived	131222	Myoneurogastrointestinal encephalomyopathy syndrome, 603041 (3)	
22qter	LVM, VL	Leukoencephalopathy, vacuoliting megalencephalic, with subcortical cysts	604004	Leukoencephalopathy, vacuoliting megalencephalic, with subcortical cysts (2)	
Xpter-p22.32	SHOX, GCFX, SS, PHOG	Growth control factor, X-linked (pseudoautosomal homeo box-containing osteogenic gene)	312865	Short stature, idiopathic familial (3); Leri-Weill dyschondrosteosis, 127300 (3); Langer mesomelic dysplasia, 249700 (3)	
Xpter-p22.32	HDPA	Hodgkin disease, susceptibility, pseudoautosomal	300221	{Hodgkin disease susceptibility, pseudoautosomal} (2)	
Xp22.33	VSPA	Visuospatial/perceptual abilities	313000	Turner syndrome-associated neurocognitive phenotype (2); [Visuospatial/perceptual abilities] (2)	
Xp22.32	CSF2RA	Colony-stimulating factor-2 receptor, alpha, low-affinity, granulocyte-macrophage	306250	Leukemia, acute myeloid, M2 type (1)	19 (Csf2ra)
Xp22.32	STS, ARSC1, ARSC, SSDD	Steroid sulfatase, microsomal (arylsulfatase C, isozyme S)	308100	Ichthyosis, X-linked (3); Placental steroid sulfatase deficiency (3)	X, Y (Sts)
Xp22.31	MLS, MIDAS	Microphthalmia with linear skin defects	309801	Microphthalmia with linear skin defects (2); Microphthalmia, dermal aplasia, and sclerocornea (2)	
Xp22.3	ARSE, CDPX1, CDPXR	Arylsulfatase E	300180	Chondrodysplasia punctata, X-linked recessive, 302950 (3); Chondrodysplasia punctata, brachytelephalangic, 302940 (3)	
Xp22.3	EMWX	Episodic muscle weakness, X-linked	300211	Episodic muscle weakness, X-linked (2)	
Xp22.3	KAL1, KMS, ADMLX	Kallmann syndrome-1 sequence (anosmin-1)	308700	Kallmann syndrome (3)	
Xp22.3	MRX49	Mental retardation, X-linked-49	300114	Mental retardation, X-linked-49 (2)	

continued

Table 10.1. The morbid anatomy of the human genome (by chromosome) (*continued*)

Location	Symbol	Title	MIM#	Disorder	Mouse
Xp22.3	OA1	Ocular albinism-1, Nettleship-Falls type	300500	Ocular albinism, Nettleship-Falls type (3)	X(Oa1)
Xp22.3	OASD	Ocular albinism and sensorineural deafness	300650	Ocular albinism with sensorineural deafness (2)	
Xp22.3-p22.2	OFD1	Oral-facial-digital syndrome 1	311200	Oral-facial-digital syndrome 1 (2)	
Xp22.3-p22.1	AMELX, AMG, AIH1, AMGX	Amelogenin	301200	Amelogenesis imperfecta (3)	X (Amel)
Xp22.3-p21.3	MRX29	Mental retardation, X-linked-29	300077	Mental retardation, X-linked 29 (2)	
Xp22.3-p21.1	NHS	Nance-Horan cataract-dental syndrome	302350	Nance-Horan syndrome (2)	?X (Xcat)
Xp22.3-p21.1	POLA	Polymerase (DNA directed), alpha	312040	?N syndrome, 310465 (1)	X(Pola)
Xp22.2	CMTX2	Charcot-Marie-Tooth disease, X-linked-2, recessive	302801	Charcot-Marie-Tooth neuropathy, X-linked-2, recessive (2)	
Xp22.2	FCP1, FCPX, FCP	F-cell production 1	305435	Heterocellular hereditary persistence of fetal hemoglobin, Swiss type (2)	
Xp22.2-p22.13	KFSD	Keratosis follicularis spinulosa decalvans	308800	Keratosis follicularis spinulosa decalvans (2)	
Xp22.2-p22.1	PDHA1, PHE1A	Pyruvate dehydrogenase, E1-alpha polypeptide-1	312170	Pyruvate dehydrogenase deficiency (3)	X(Pdha1)
Xp22.2-p22.1	PHEX, HYP, HPDR1	Phosphate regulating gene with homologies to endopeptidases on the X chromosome	307800	Hypophosphatemia, hereditary (3)	X (Phex, Gy)
Xp22.2-p22.1	PHKA2, PHK	Phosphorylase kinase deficiency, liver (glycogen storage disease type VIII)	306000	Glycogenosis, X-linked hepatic, type I (3); Glycogenosis, X-linked hepatic, type II (3)	
Xp22.2-p22.1	PRTS, MRXS1	Partington syndrome (mental retardation, X-linked, syndromic-1, with dystonic movements, ataxia, and seizures)	309510	Mental retardation, X-linked, syndromic-1, with dystonic movements, ataxia, and seizures (2)	
Xp22.2-p22.1	RPS6KA3, RSK2, MRX19	Ribosomal protein S6 kinase, 90 kD, polypeptide 3	300075	Coffin-Lowry syndrome, 303600 (3); Mental retardation, X-linked nonspecific, type 19 (3)	
Xp22.2-p22.1	RS1, XLRS1	Retinoschisis	312700	Retinoschisis (3)	
Xp22.2-p22.1	SEDL, SEDT	Sedlin	300202	Spondyloepiphyseal dysplasia tarda, 313400 (3)	
Xp22.13-p21.1	MEHMO	MEHMO syndrome (Mental retardation, epileptic seizures, hypogonadism and hypogenitalism, microcephaly, and obesity)	300148	MEHMO syndrome (2)	
Xp22.11-p21.2	GDXY, TDFX, SRVX	Gonadal dysgenesis, XY female type	306100	Gonadal dysgenesis, XY female type (2)	
Xp22.1	PIGA	Phosphatidylinositol glycan, class A	311770	Paroxysmal nocturnal hemoglobinuria (3)	X (Piga)
Xp22.1-p21.3	IL1RAPL, MRX1, MRX21	Il-1 receptor accessory protein-like	300206	Mental retardation, X-linked 1, non-dysmorphic, 309530 (3)	
Xp22.1-p21.3	ISSX	Infantile spasm syndrome, X-linked	308350	Infantile spasm syndrome, X-linked (2)	
Xp22	AGMX2, XLA2, IMD6	Agammaglobulinemia, X-linked 2 (with growth hormone deficiency)	300310	Agammaglobulinemia, type 2, X-linked (2)	X (Xid)
Xp22	AIC	Aicardi syndrome	304050	Aicardi syndrome (2)	
Xp22	CFNS, CFND	Craniofrontonasal syndrome	304110	Craniofrontonasal dysplasia (2)	

continued

Table 10.1. The morbid anatomy of the human genome (by chromosome) (*continued*)

Location	Symbol	Title	MIM#	Disorder	Mouse
Xp22	DFN6	Deafness, X-linked 6, sensorineural	300066	Deafness, X-linked 6, sensorineural (2)	
Xp22	MID1, OGS1, BBBG1, GBBB1, OSX	Midline-1	300000	Opitz G syndrome, type I (3)	X (Mid1)
Xp22	MNG2	Multinodular goiter-2	300273	Goiter, multinodular, 2 (2)	
Xp22	SGBS2	Simpson-Golabi-Behmel syndrome, type 2	300209	Simpson-Golabi-Behmel syndrome, type 2 (2)	
Xp22-p21	PDR	Pigment disorder, reticulate	301220	Partington syndrome II (2)	
Xp22-q12	MRX58	Mental retardation, X-linked nonspecific, 58	300210	Mental retardation, X-linked nonspecific, 58 (2)	
Xp21.3-p21.2	DAX1, AHC, AHX, NROB1	DSS-AHC critical region on the X chromosome, gene 1	300200	Adrenal hypoplasia, congenital, with hypogonadotropic hypogonadism (3); Dosage-sensitive sex reversal, 300018 (3)	X (Ahch)
Xp21.3-p21.2	GK	Glycerol kinase deficiency	307030	Glycerol kinase deficiency (3); Hyperglycerolemia (3)	X (Gyk)
Xp21.3-p21.2	RP6	Retinitis pigmentosa-6, X-linked recessive	312612	?Retinitis pigmentosa-6 (2)	
Xp21.2	DFN4	Deafness 4, congenital sensorineural	300030	Deafness, X-linked 4, congenital sensorineural (2)	
Xp21.2	DMD, BMD	Dystrophin (muscular dystrophy, Duchenne and Becker types)	310200	Duchenne muscular dystrophy (3); Becker muscular dystrophy (3); Cardiomyopathy, dilated, X-linked (3)	X (Dmd)
Xp21.2-p21.1	XK	Kell blood group precursor	314850	McLeod phenotype (3)	
Xp21.1	CYBB, CGD	Cytochrome b-245, beta polypeptide	306400	Chronic granulomatous disease, X-linked (3)	X (Cybb)
Xp21.1	OTC	Ornithine transcarbamylase	311250	Ornithine transcarbamylase deficiency (3)	X (spf; Otc)
Xp21.1	RPGR, RP3, CRD, RP15	Retinitis pigmentosa GTPase regulator	312610	Retinitis pigmentosa-3 (3); Cone-rod dystrophy, 300029 (3)	
Xp21.1-q22	WTS, MRXS6	Wilson-Turner syndrome (mental retardation, X-linked, syndromic-6, with gynecomastia and obesity)	309585	Mental retardation, X-linked, syndromic-6, with gynecomastia and obesity (2)	
Xp21	GTD	Gonadotropin deficiency	306190	?Gonadotropin deficiency (2); ?Cryptorchidism (2)	
Xp21	SRS, MRSR	Snyder-Robinson X-linked mental retardation syndrome	309583	Mental retardation, Snyder-Robinson type (2)	
Xp21-q13	MRX9	Mental retardation, X-linked-9	309549	Mental retardation, X-linked 9 (2)	
Xp11.4	COD1, PCDX	Cone dystrophy-1, X-linked	304020	Cone dystrophy, progressive X-linked, 1 (2)	
Xp11.4	NDP, ND	Norrin	310600	Norrie disease (3); Exudative vitreoretinopathy, X-linked, 305390 (3); Coats disease, 300216 (3)	X (Ndp)
Xp11.4-p11.23	AIED, OA2	Aland island eye disease (ocular albinism, Forsius-Eriksson type)	300600	Ocular albinism, Forsius-Eriksson type (2)	
Xp11.4-p11.23	PFC, PFD	Properdin P factor, complement	312060	Properdin deficiency, X-linked (3)	X (Pfc)
Xp11.4-p11.21	OPA2	Optic atrophy, X-linked	311050	Optic atrophy, X-linked (2)	
Xp11.4-p11.2	RENS1, MRXS8	Renpenning syndrome-1	309500	Renpenning syndrome-1 (2)	

continued

Table 10.1. The morbid anatomy of the human genome (by chromosome) (*continued*)

Location	Symbol	Title	MIM#	Disorder	Mouse
Xp11.4	CSNB1, NYX	Nyctalopin	300278	Night blindness, congenital stationary, type 1, 310500 (3)	
Xp11.3	RP2	Retinitis pigmentosa-2, X-linked recessive	312600	Retinitis pigmentosa-2 (2)	
Xp11.3-p11.21	MRX50	Mental retardation, X-linked nonspecific, type 50	300115	Mental retardation, X-linked nonspecific, type 50 (2)	
Xp11.3-q11.2	AMCX1	Arthrogryposis multiplex congenita, X-linked (spinal muscular atrophy, infantile, X-linked)	301830	Arthrogryposis, X-linked (spinal muscular atrophy, infantile, X-linked) (2)	
Xp11.3-q21.3	MRXSSD	Siderius X-linked mental retardation syndrome	300263	Mental retardation syndrome, X-linked, Siderius type (2)	
Xp11.3-q13.3	MRX14	Mental retardation, X-linked-14	300062	Mental retardation, X-linked 14 (2)	
Xp11.3-q22	MRXS7	Mental retardation, X-linked, syndromic 7	300218	Mental retardation, X-linked, syndromic 7 (2)	
Xp11.23	CACNA1F, CSNB2	Calcium channel, voltage-dependent, alpha-1F subunit	300110	Night blindness, congenital stationary, X-linked, type 2, 300071 (3)	
Xp11.23	GATA1, GF1, ERYF1, NFE1	GATA-binding protein-1 (globin transcription factor-1)	305371	Dyserythropoietic anemia with thrombocytopenia (3)	X (Gf1)
Xp11.23	MAOA	Monoamine oxidase A	309850	Brunner syndrome (3)	X (Maoa)
Xp11.23-p11.22	EBP, CDPX2, CPXD, CPX	Emopamil-binding protein	30025	Chondrodysplasia punctata, X-linked dominant, 302960 (3)	X (Bpa)
Xp11.23-p11.22	WAS, IMD2, THC	Wiskott-Aldrich syndrome	301000	Wiskott-Aldrich syndrome (3); Thrombocytopenia, X-linked, 313900 (3)	X (Wasp, ?sf)
Xp11.23-q13.3	FOXP3, IPEX, AIID, XPID, PIDX	Forkhead box P3 (scurfin)	300292	Autoimmunity-immunodeficiency syndrome, X-linked, 304930 (3)	X (sf, Foxp3)
Xp11.22	CLCN5, CLCK2, NPHL2, DENTS	Chloride channel-5	300008	Dent disease, 300009 (3); Nephrolithiasis, type I, 310468 (3); Hypophosphatemia, type III (3); Proteinuria, low molecular weight, with hypercalciuric nephrocalcinosis (3)	X (Clcn5)
Xp11.22	TFE3	Transcription factor for IgH enhancer	314310	Renal cell carcinoma, papillary, 1, 605074 (3)	X (Tfe3)
Xp11.21	ALAS2, ASB, ANH1	Aminolevulinate, delta-, synthase-2	301300	Anemia, sideroblastic/hypochromic (3)	X (Alas)
Xp11.21	FGD1, FGDY, AAS	Faciogenital dysplasia (Aarskog-Scott syndrome)	305400	Aarskog-Scott syndrome (3)	X (Fgdy)
Xp11.21-q21.3	CLA2, OPCA	Cerebellar ataxia-2	302500	Cerebellar ataxia-2 (2)	
Xp11.2	CAMR, MRXS10	Chorioathetosis with mental retardation and abnormal behavior	300220	Chorioathetosis with mental retardation and abnormal behavior (2)	
Xp11.2	SSX1, SSRC	Synovial sarcoma, X breakpoint 1	312820	Sarcoma, synovial (3)	
Xp11.2	SSX2	Sarcoma, synovial, X breakpoint 2	300192	Sarcoma, synovial (1)	
Xp11	IDDMX	Diabetes mellitus, insulin-dependent, X-linked, susceptibility to	300136	{Diabetes mellitus, insulin-dependent, X-linked} (2) (2)	
Xp11	MRXA	Mental retardation, X-linked nonspecific, with aphasia	309545	?Mental retardation, X-linked nonspecific, with aphasia (2)	

continued

Table 10.1. The morbid anatomy of the human genome (by chromosome) (*continued*)

Location	Symbol	Title	MIM#	Disorder	Mouse
Xp11-q21	MRX20	Mental retardation, X-linked-20	300047	Mental retardation, X-linked 20 (2)	
Xp11-q21	PRS, MRXS2	Prieto syndrome (mental retardation, X-linked, syndromic-2, with dysmorphism and cerebral atrophy)	309610	Mental retardation, X-linked, syndromic-2, with dysmorphism and cerebral atrophy (2)	
Xp11-q21.3	SHS, MRXS3	Sutherland-Haan syndrome (mental retardation, X-linked, syndromic-3, with spastic diplegia)	309470	Mental retardation, X-linked, syndromic-3, with spastic diplegia (2)	
Xp	CCT	Cataracts, congenital total	302200	?Cataract, congenital total (2)	
Xp	SMAX2	Spinal muscular atrophy, X-linked lethal infantile	300021	Spinal muscular atrophy, X-linked lethal infantile (2)	
Xq	CGF1	Cognitive function-1, social	300082	[Social cognition] (2)	
Xq	MTBS	Mycobacterium tuberculosis, susceptibility to infection by	300259	{Tuberculosis, susceptibility to} (2)	
Xq	MFTS	Migraine, familial typical, susceptibility to	300125	{Migraine, familial typical, susceptibility to, 1} (2)	
Xq11	TM4SF2, MXS1, A15	Transmembrane 4 superfamily, member 2	300096	Mental retardation, X-linked nonspecific (3)	
Xq11-q12	AR, DHTR, TFM, SBMA, KD	Androgen receptor (dihydrotestosterone receptor)	313700	Androgen insensitivity, several forms, 300068 (3); Spinal and bulbar muscular atrophy of Kennedy, 313200 (3); Prostate cancer (3); Perineal hypospadias (3); Breast cancer, male, with Reifenstein syndrome (3)	X (Tfm)
Xq11.2	SPG16	Spastic paraplegia-16, X-linked, complicated	300266	Spastic paraplegia-16, X-linked, complicated (2)	
Xq12	OPHN1	Oligophrenin-1	300127	Mental retardation, X-linked, 60 (3)	
Xq12-q13	ATP7A, MNK, MK, OHS	ATPase, Cu++ transporting, alpha polypeptide	300011	Menkes disease, 309400 (3); Occipital horn syndrome, 304150 (3); Cutis laxa, neonatal (3)	X (Mnk)
Xq12-q13.1	ED1, EDA, HED	Ectodermal dysplasia-1, anhidrotic	305100	Ectodermal dysplasia-1, anhidrotic (3)	X (Ta)
Xq12-q21.31	FGS1	FG syndrome 1	305450	FG syndrome (2)	
Xq13	ATRX, XH2, XNP, MRXS3	ATR-X gene (helicase 2; X-linked nuclear protein)	300032	Alpha-thalassemia/mental retardation syndrome, 301040 (3); Juberg-Marsidi syndrome, 309590 (3); Sutherland-Haan syndrome, 309470 (3); Smith-Fineman-Myers syndrome, 309580 (3)	X (Xh2)
Xq13	IL2RG, SCIDX1, SCIDX, IMD4	Interleukin-2 receptor, gamma	308380	Severe combined immunodeficiency, X-linked, 300400 (3); Combined immunodeficiency, X-linked, moderate, 312863 (3)	X (Il2rg)
Xq13	PGK1, PGKA	Phosphoglycerate kinase-1	311800	Hemolytic anemia due to PGK deficiency (3); Myoglobinuria/hemolysis due to PGK deficiency (3)	X (Pgk1)
Xq13	PHKA1	Phosphorylase kinase, muscle, alpha polypeptide	311870	Muscle glycogenosis (3)	X (Phka)
Xq13-q21	WWS	Wieacker-Wolff syndrome	314580	Wieacker-Wolff syndrome (2)	

continued

Table 10.1. The morbid anatomy of the human genome (by chromosome) (*continued*)

Location	Symbol	Title	MIM#	Disorder	Mouse
Xq13-q22	MCS, MRXS4	Miles-Carpenter syndrome (mental retardation, X-linked, syndromic-4, with congenital contractures and low fingertip arches)	309605	Mental retardation, X-linked, syndromic-4, with congenital contractures and low fingertip arches (2)	
Xq13.1	DYT3	Torsion dystonia-parkinsonism, Filipino type	314250	Dystonia-3, torsion, with parkinsonism, Filipino type (2)	
Xq13.1	GJB1, CX32, CMTX1	Gap junction protein, beta-1, 32 kD (connexin 32)	304040	Charcot-Marie-Tooth neuropathy, X-linked-1, dominant, 302800 (3)	X (Gjb1)
Xq13.1-q13.3	ABCB7, ABC7, ASAT	ATP-binding cassette-7	300135	Anemia, sideroblastic, with ataxia, 301310 (3)	X (Abc7)
Xq13.2	MRXSAB	Abidi X-linked mental retardation syndrome	300262	Mental retardation syndrome, X-linked, Abidi type (2)	
Xq13.2	XIC, XCE, XIST	X chromosome controlling element (X-inactivation center)	314670	X-inactivation, familial skewed (3)	X (Xce)
Xq21	AHDS	Allan-Herndon-Dudley mental retardation syndrome	309600	Allan-Herndon syndrome (2)	
Xq21	POF1, POF	Premature ovarian failure-1	311360	Ovarian failure, premature (2)	
Xq21.1	POU3F4, DFN3	POU domain, class 3, transcription factor 4	300039	Deafness, X-linked 3, conductive, with stapes fixation, 304400 (3)	X (Pou3f4)
Xq21.2-q24	ARTS	Arts syndrome	301835	Arts syndrome (2)	
Xq21.2	CHM, TCD	Choroideremia	303100	Choroideremia (3)	X (rep1)
Xq21.3	CPX	Cleft palate and/or ankyloglossia	303400	Cleft palate, X-linked (2)	
Xq21.3-q22	BTK, AGMX1, IMD1, XLA, AT	Bruton agammaglobulinemia tyrosine kinase	300300	Agammaglobulinemia, type 1, X-linked (3); ?XLA and isolated growth hormone deficiency, 307200 (3)	X (xid, Btp)
Xq21.3-q22	MGC1, MGCN	Megalocornea-1, X-linked	309300	Megalocornea, X-linked (2)	
Xq21.3-q24	PAK3	p21-activated kinase-3	300142	Mental retardation, X-linked 30 (3)	
Xq22	DFN2	Deafness, X-linked 2, perceptive, congenital	304500	Deafness, X-linked 2, perceptive congenital (2)	
Xq22	DIAPH2, DIA	Diaphanous, Drosophila, homolog of, 2	300108	Premature ovarian failure, 311360 (3)	
Xq22	EFMR	Epilepsy, female restricted, with mental retardation (Juberg-Hellman syndrome)	300088	Epilepsy, female restricted, with mental retardation (2)	
Xq22	GLA	Galactosidase, alpha	301500	Fabry disease (3)	X (Ags)
Xq22	PLP, PMD	Proteolipid protein	312080	Pelizaeus-Merzbacher disease (3); Spastic paraplegia-2, 312920 (3)	X (Plp(jp))
Xq22	TIMM8A, DFN1, DDP, MTS, DDP1	Translocase of inner mitochondrial membrane 8, yeast, homolog of, A	304700	Deafness, X-linked 1, progressive (3); Mohr-Tranebjaerg syndrome (3); Jensen syndrome, 311150 (3)	
Xq22-q24	PRPS1	Phosphoribosyl pyrophosphate synthetase-1	311850	Phosphoribosyl pyrophosphate synthetase-related gout (3)	
Xq22-q28	AIH3	Amelogenesis imperfecta-3, hypomaturation or hypoplastic type	301201	?Amelogenesis imperfecta-3, hypoplastic type (2)	
Xq22.2	TBG	Thyroxine-binding globulin	314200	[Euthyroidal hyper- and hypothyroxinemia] (1)	
Xq22.3	AMMECR1	Alport syndrome, mental retardation, midface hypoplasia, and elliptocytosis chromosomal region gene 1	300195	Alport syndrome, mental retardation, midface hypoplasia, and elliptocytosis, 300194 (2)	

continued

Table 10.1. The morbid anatomy of the human genome (by chromosome) (*continued*)

Location	Symbol	Title	MIM#	Disorder	Mouse
Xq22.3	COL4A5, ATS, ALSN	Collagen IV, alpha-5 polypeptide	303630	Alport syndrome, 301050 (3)	X(Col4a5)
Xq22.3	COL4A6	Collagen IV, alpha-6 polypeptide	303631	Leiomyomatosis, diffuse, with Alport syndrome, 308940 (3)	
Xq22.3-q23	DCX, DBCN, LISX	Doublecortin	300121	Lissencephaly, X-linked, 300067 (3); Subcortical laminal heteropia, X-linked, 300067 (3)	X (Dcx)
Xq23-q24	MRX23	Mental retardation, X-linked-23	300046	Mental retardation, X-linked 23, nonspecific (2)	
Xq24	LAMP2, LAMPB	Lysosome-associated membrane protein-2	309060	Glycogen storage disease IIb, 300257 (3)	X(Lamp2)
Xq24-q26.1	NAMSD, CMT2D, NADMR	Neuropathy, axonal motor-sensory, with deafness and mental retardation (Cowchock syndrome)	310490	Cowchock syndrome (2)	
Xq24-q27	BZX	Bazex syndrome	301845	Bazex syndrome (2)	
Xq24-q27.1	HTC2, HCG, CGH	Hypertrichosis, congenital generalized	307150	Hypertrichosis, congenital generalized (2)	
Xq24-q27.1	MRGH	Mental retardation with isolated growth hormone deficiency	300123	Mental retardation with isolated growth hormone deficiency (2)	
Xq24-q27.1	PTOS2, PTOSX	Ptosis, hereditary congenital 2	300245	Ptosis, hereditary congenital 2 (2)	
Xq24-q27.3	MRSA	Mental retardation, X-linked, South African type	300243	Mental retardation, X-linked, South African type (2)	
Xq25	SH2D1A, LYP, IMD5, XLP, XLPD	SH2 domain protein 1A	308240	Lymphoproliferative syndrome, X-linked (3)	X (Sh2d1a)
Xq25-q26	PHP, GHDX, PHPX	Panhypopituitarism, X-linked	312000	Panhypopituitarism, X-linked (2)	
Xq25-q26.1	THAS, TAS	Thoracoabdominal syndrome	313850	Thoracoabdominal syndrome (2)	
Xq25-q27	PGS, MRXS5	Pettigrew syndrome (mental retardation, X-linked, with Dandy-Walker malformation, basal ganglia disease, and seizures)	304340	Mental retardation, X-linked, syndromic-5, with Dandy-Walker malformation, basal ganglia disease, and seizures (2)	
Xq26	ARHGEF6, MRX46, COOL2	Rho guanine nucleotide exchange factor-6	300267	Mental retardation, X-linked nonspecific, type 46 (3)	
Xq26	GPC3, SDYS, SGBS1	Glypican 3	300037	Simpson-Golabi-Behmel syndrome, type 1, 312870 (3)	
Xq26	GUST	Gustavson mental retardation syndrome (with microcephaly, optic atrophy, deafness)	309555	Gustavson syndrome (2)	
Xq26	SHFM2, SHFD2	Split hand/foot malformation, type (ectrodactyly) 2	313350	Split hand/foot malformation, type 2 (2)	
Xq26	TNFSF5, CD40LG, HIGM1, IGM	Tumor necrosis factor ligand superfamily, member 5	308230	Immunodeficiency, X-linked, with hyper-IgM (3)	X(CD40l)
Xq26-q27	HPT, HPTX, HYPX	Hypoparathyroidism	307700	Hypoparathyroidism, X-linked (2)	
Xq26-q27	NYS1	Nystagmus 1, congenital	310700	Nystagmus 1, congenital (2)	
Xq26-q27	RP24	Retinitis pigmentosa-24	300155	Retinitis pigmentosa-24 (2)	
Xq26-q27	SMRXS	Shashi X-linked mental retardation syndrome	300238	Mental retardation, X-linked, Shashi type (2)	
Xq26-q27.2	HPRT1, HPRT	Hypoxanthine phosphoribosyltransferase 1	308000	Lesch-Nyhan syndrome (3); HPRT-related gout (3)	X(Hprt)

continued

Table 10.1. The morbid anatomy of the human genome (by chromosome) (*continued*)

Location	Symbol	Title	MIM#	Disorder	Mouse
Xq26-qter	INDX	Immunoneurologic syndrome X-linked, of Wood, Black, and Norbury	300076	Wood neuroimmunologic syndrome (2)	
Xq26.1	OCRL, LOCR, OCRL1	Oculocerebrorenal syndrome of Lowe	309000	Lowe syndrome (3)	
Xq26.2	ZIC3, HTX1, HTX	Zic family member-3	300265	Heterotaxy, X-linked visceral, 306955 (3)	
Xq26.3	BFLS	Borjeson-Forssman-Lehmann syndrome	301900	Borjeson-Forssman-Lehmann syndrome (2)	
Xq26.3-q27.1	ADFN, ALDS	Albinism-deafness syndrome	300700	Albinism-deafness syndrome (2)	
Xq27	COD2	Cone dystrophy-2, X-linked	300085	Cone dystrophy, progressive X-linked, 2 (2)	
Xq27	TGCT1	Testicular germ cell tumor 1	300228	Testicular germ cell tumor (2)	
Xq27-q28	ANOP1	Anophthalmos-1 (with mental retardation but without anomalies)	301590	?Anophthalmos-1 (2)	
Xq27-q28	HPCX	Prostate cancer, hereditary, X-linked	300147	{Prostate cancer susceptibility, X-linked} (2)	
Xq27.1-q27.2	F9, HEMB	Coagulation factor IX (plasma thromboplastic component)	306900	Hemophilia B (3); Warfarin sensitivity (3)	X (Cf9)
Xq27.3	FMR1, FRAXA	Fragile X mental retardation-1	309550	Fragile X syndrome (3)	X (Fmr1)
Xq27.3-q28	ODPF	Osseous dysplasia, digital, with facial pigmentary defects and multiple frenula	300244	Osseous dysplasia, digital, with facial pibmentary defects and multiple frenula (2)	
Xq28	ABCD1, ALD, AMN	ATP-binding cassette, subfamily D, member 1	300100	Adrenoleukodystrophy (3); Adrenomyeloneuropathy (3)	X (Ald)
Xq28	AVPR2, DIR, DI1, ADHR	Arginine vasopressin receptor-2	304800	Diabetes insipidus, nephrogenic (3)	
Xq28	CBBM, BCM	Blue-monochromatic colorblindness (blue cone monochromacy)	303700	Colorblindness, blue monochromatic (3)	
Xq28	CVD1, XMVD	Cardiac valvular dysplasia-1 (myxomatous valvular dystrophy, X-linked)	314400	Cardiac valvular dysplasia-1 (2)	
Xq28	DKC1, DKC	Dyskerin	300126	Dyskeratosis congenita-1, 305000 (3); Hoyeraal-Hreidarsson syndrome, 300240 (3)	
Xq28	EMD, EDMD	Emery-Dreifuss muscular dystrophy	310300	Emery-Dreifuss muscular dystrophy (3)	
Xq28	F8, F8C, HEMA	Coagulation factor VIII, procoagulant component	306700	Hemophilia A (3)	X (Cf8)
Xq28	FLNA, FLN1, ABPX, NHBP	Filamin A, alpha (actin-binding protein-280)	300017	Heterotopia, periventricular, 300049 (3)	X (Fln1)
Xq28	FMR2, FRAXE, MRX2	Fragile site, X-linked, E	309548	Mental retardation, X-linked, FRAXE type (3)	
Xq28	FRAXF	Fragile site, folic acid type, rare, fra (X) (q28)	300031	Mental retardation, X-linked, FRAXF type (3)	
Xq28	G6PD, G6PD1	Glucose-6-phosphate dehydrogenase	305900	G6PD deficiency (3); Favism (3); Hemolytic anemia due to G6PD deficiency (3)	X (G6pd)
Xq28	GDI1, RABGD1A, MRX41, MRX48	GDP dissociation inhibitor 1	300104	Mental retardation, X-linked nonspecific, 309541 (3)	
Xq28	HMS1, GAY1	Homosexuality, male	306995	[?Homosexuality, male] (2)	

continued

Table 10.1. The morbid anatomy of the human genome (by chromosome) (*continued*)

Location	Symbol	Title	MIM#	Disorder	Mouse
Xq28	GCP, CBD	Green cone pigment	303800	Colorblindness, deutan (3)	X (Rsvp)
Xq28	IDS, MPS2, SIDS	Iduronate 2-sulfatase (Hunter syndrome)	309900	Mucopolysaccharidosis II (3)	X (Ids)
Xq28	IKBKG, NEMO, FIP3, IP2	Inhibitor of kappa light polypeptide gene enhancer in B cells, kinase of, gamma (NF-kappa-B essential modulator)	300248	Incontinentia pigmenti, type II, 308310 (3); Ectodermal dysplasia, hypohidrotic, with immune deficiency, 300291 (3)	X (?Str)
Xq28	IPOX, CIIPX	Intestinal pseudoobstruction, neuronal, primary idiopathic	300048	Intestinal pseudoobstruction, neuronal, X-linked (2)	
Xq28	L1CAM, CAML1, HSAS1	L1 cell adhesion molecule	308840	Hydrocephalus due to aqueductal stenosis, 307000 (3); MASA syndrome, 303350 (3); Spastic paraplegia, 312900 (3)	X (L1cam)
Xq28	MAFD2, MDX	Major affective disorder-2	309200	?Manic-depressive illness, X-linked (2)	
Xq28	MEAX, XMEA	Myopathy, X-linked, with excessive autophagy	310440	Myopathy, X-linked, with excessive autophagy (2)	
Xq28	MECP2, RTT	Methyl-CpG-binding protein-2	300005	Rett syndrome, 312750 (3); Mental retardation, X-linked, with progressive spasticity, 300279 (3); Rett syndrome, preserved speech variant, 312750 (3)	X (Mecp2)
Xq28	MRSD, CHRS	Mental retardation-skeletal dysplasia	309620	Mental retardation-skeletal dysplasia (2)	
Xq28	MRX72	Mental retardation, X-linked-72	300271	Mental retardation, X-linked-72 (2)	
Xq28	MRXSA	Armfield X-linked mental retardation syndrome	300261	Mental retardation syndrome, X-linked, Armfield type (2)	
Xq28	MRXSL	Lubs X-linked mental retardation syndrome	300260	Mental retardation syndrome, X-linked, Lubs type (2)	
Xq28	MTM1, MTMX	Myotubularin	310400	Myotubular myopathy, X-linked (3)	
Xq28	MYP1, BED	Myopia, X-linked (Bornholm eye disease)	310460	Myopia-1 (2); Bornholm eye disease (2)	
Xq28	NSDHL	NAD (P) H steroid dehydrogenase-like protein	300275	CHILD syndrome, 308050 (3)	X (Nsdh1)
Xq28	OPD1	Otopalatodigital syndrome, type I	311300	Otopalatodigital syndrome, type I (2)	
Xq28	PPMX	Mental retardation with psychosis, pyramidal signs, and macroorchidism	300055	Mental retardation with psychosis, pyramidal signs, and macroorchidism (2)	
Xq28	RCP, CBP	Red cone pigment	303900	Colorblindness, protan (3)	X (Rsvp)
Xq28	TAZ, EFE2, BTHS, CMD3A	Tafazzin	302060	Endocardial fibroelastosis-2 (2); Barth syndrome (3); Cardiomyopathy, X-linked dilated, 300069 (3); Noncompaction of left ventricular myocardium, isolated, 300183 (3)	
Xq28	TKCR, TKC	Torticollis, keloids, cryptorchidism and renal dysplasia	314300	Goeminne TKCR syndrome (2)	
Xq28	TKTL1, TKT2, TKR	Transketolase-like 1	300044	{?Wernicke-Korsakoff syndrome, susceptibility to} (1)	
Xq28	WSN, BGMR	Waisman syndrome (basal ganglion disorder with mental retardation)	311510	Waisman parkinsonism-mental retardation syndrome (2)	

continued

Table 10.1. The morbid anatomy of the human genome (by chromosome) (*continued*)

Location	Symbol	Title	MIM#	Disorder	Mouse
Chr.X	HAEX	Angioneurotic edema, hereditary, with normal C1-inhibitor concentration and function	300268	Angioneurotic edema, hereditary, X-linked (2)	
Chr.X	IMAGE	Intrauterine growth retardation, metaphyseal dysplasia, adrenal hypoplasia congenita, and genital anomalies	300290	IMAGE syndrome (2)	
Chr.X	RFMN	Roifman syndrome	300258	Roifman syndrome (2)	
Yp11.3	SRY, TDF	Sex-determining region Y (testis determining factor)	480000	Gonadal dysgenesis, XY type (3)	Yp (Tdy, Sry)
Yq11	AZF1, SP3	Azoospermia factor 1	415000	?Sertoli-cell-only syndrome (1)	
Yq11	DAZ	Deleted in azoospermia	400003	?Sertoli-cell-only syndrome (1)	17 (dazla)
Yq11.2	USP9Y, DFFRY	Ubiquitin-specific protease-9, Y chromosome (Drosophila fat facets related, Y-linked)	400005	Azoospermia (3)	

Table 10.2. The morbid anatomy of the human genome (alphabetical by disorder)

Disorder	MIM#	Location
3q21q26 syndrome (1)	165215	3q26
Aarskog-Scott syndrome (3)	305400	Xp11.21
Abetalipoproteinemia, 200100 (3)	157147	4q22-q24
Abetalipoproteinemia (3)	107730	2q24
[Acanthocytosis, one form] (1)	109270	17q21-q22
?ACAT2 deficiency (1)	100678	6q25.3-q26
Acatalasemia (3)	115500	11p13
Acetyl-CoA carboxylase deficiency (1)	200350	17q21
Achalasia-addisonianism-alacrimia syndrome, 231550 (3)	605378	12q13
Acheiropody, 200500 (3)	605522	7q36
Achondrogenesis Ib, 600972 (3)	222600	5q32-q33.1
Achondrogenesis-hypochondrogenesis, type II, 200610 (3)	120140	12q13.11-q13.2
Achondroplasia, 100800 (3)	134934	4p16.3
Achromatopsia-1 (2)	603096	Chr. 14
Achromatopsia-2, 216900 (3)	600053	2q11
Achromatopsia-3, 262300 (3)	605080	8q21-q22z
Achromatopsia-3, 262300 (3)	605080	8q21-q22
?Acrocallosal syndrome (2)	200990	12p13.3-p11.2
?Acrofacial dysostosis, Nager type (2)	154400	9q32
Acromesomelic dysplasia, Hunter-Thompson type, 201250 (3)	601146	20q11.2
Acromesomelic dysplasia, Maroteaux type (2)	602875	9p13-p12
ACTH deficiency (1)	176830	2p23.3
ACTH deficiency, 201400 (2)	122560	8q13
Acute insulin response (2)	601676	1p31
Acyl-CoA dehydrogenase, long chain, deficiency of (3)	201460	2q34-q35
Acyl-CoA dehydrogenase, medium chain, deficiency of (3)	201450	1p31
Acyl-CoA dehydrogenase, short-chain, deficiency of (3)	201470	12q22-qter
Adenoma, periampullary (3)	175100	5q21-q22
Adenomatous polyposis coli (3)	175100	5q21-q22
Adenomatous polyposis coli, attenuated (3)	175100	5q21-q22
Adenylosuccinase deficiency (1)	103050	22q13.1
Adhalinopathy, primary (1)	600119	17q12-q21.33
Adrenal adenoma, sporadic (3)	131100	11q13
Adrenal hyperplasia, congenital, due to 11-beta-hydroxylase deficiency (3)	202010	8q21
Adrenal hyperplasia, congenital, due to 17-alpha-hydroxylase deficiency (3)	202110	10q24.3
Adrenal hyperplasia, congenital, due to 21-hydroxylase deficiency (3)	201910	6p21.3
Adrenal hypoplasia, congenital, with hypogonadotropic hypogonadism (3)	300200	Xp21.3-p21.2
Adrenocortical carcinoma, hereditary, 202300 (2)	194071	11p15.5
Adrenoleukodystrophy (3)	300100	Xq28
Adrenoleukodystrophy, neonatal, 202370 (3)	602859	Chr. 1
Adrenoleukodystrophy, neonatal, 202370 (3)	600414	12p13.3
Adrenoleukodystrophy, neonatal, 202370 (3)	601789	2p15
Adrenoleukodystrophy, neonatal, 202370 (3)	602136	7q21-q22
Adrenoleukodystrophy, pseudoneonatal (2)	264470	17q25
Adrenomyeloneuropathy (3)	300100	Xq28
Afibrinogenemia, 202400 (3)	134820	4q28
Afibrinogenemia, congenital, 202400 (3)	134830	4q28
[AFP deficiency, congenital] (1)	104150	4q11-q13
Agammaglobulinemia, 601495 (3)	147020	14q32.33
Agammaglobulinemia, autosomal recessive (3)	146770	22q11.21
Agammaglobulinemia, type 1, X-linked (3)	300300	Xq21.3-q22
Agammaglobulinemia, type 2, X-linked (2)	300310	Xp22
Aicardi syndrome (2)	304050	Xp22
Aicardi-Goutieres syndrome 1 (2)	225750	3p21
{AIDS, resistance to} (3)	600835	10q11.1
Alagille syndrome, 118450 (3)	601920	20p12
Albinism, brown, 203290 (1)	115501	9p23
Albinism, ocular, autosomal recessive (3)	203200	15q11.2-q12

continued

Table 10.2. The morbid anatomy of the human genome (alphabetical by disorder) (*continued*)

Disorder	MIM#	Location
Albinism, oculocutaneous, type IA (3)	203100	11q14-q21
Albinism, oculocutaneous, type II (3)	203200	15q11.2-q12
Albinism, rufous, 278400 (3)	115501	9p23
Albinism-deafness syndrome (2)	300700	Xq26.3-q27.1
?Albright hereditary osteodystrophy-2 (2)	103581	15q11-q13
Alcohol intolerance, acute (3)	100650	12q24.2
{Alcoholism, susceptibility to} (1)	103720	4q22
Aldolase A deficiency (3)	103850	16q22-q24
Aldosteronism, glucocorticoid-remediable (3)	202010	8q21
Alexander disease, 203450 (3)	161015	11q13
Alexander disease, 203450 (3)	137780	17q21
Alkaptonuria (3)	203500	3q21-q23
Allan-Herndon syndrome (2)	309600	Xq21
{?Allergy and asthma susceptibility} (2)	147061	5q31.1
Alopecia universalis, 203655 (3)	602302	8p21.2
Alpha-1-antichymotrypsin deficiency (3)	107280	14q32.1
Alpha-ketoglutarate dehydrogenase deficiency (1)	203740	7p14-p13
Alpha-methylacyl-CoA racemase deficiency (3)	604489	5p13.2-q11.1
Alpha-thalassemia/mental retardation syndrome, 301040 (3)	300032	Xq13
Alpha-thalassemia/mental retardation syndrome, type 1 (1)	141750	16pter-p13.3
Alport syndrome, 301050 (3)	303630	Xq22.3
Alport syndrome, autosomal recessive, 203780 (3)	120070	2q36-q37
Alport syndrome, autosomal recessive, 203780 (3)	120131	2q36-q37
Alport syndrome, mental retardation, midface hypoplasia, and elliptocytosis, 300194 (2)	300195	Xq22.3
Alstrom syndrome (2)	203800	2p13
Alzheimer disease 6, 104300 (2)	605526	10q24
{Alzheimer disease, susceptibility to}, 104300 (3)	106180	17q23
{Alzheimer disease, susceptibility to} (3)	103950	12p13.3-p12.3
{Alzheimer disease, susceptibility to} (3)	602403	17q11.2
Alzheimer disease-1, APP-related (3)	104760	21q21
Alzheimer disease-2, late onset (2)	104310	19cen-q13.2
Alzheimer disease-3 (3)	104311	14q24.3
Alzheimer disease-4 (3)	600759	1q31-q42
Alzheimer disease-5 (2)	602096	12p11.23-q13.12
Amelogenesis imperfecta (3)	301200	Xp22.3-p22.1
Amelogenesis imperfecta-2, hypoplastic local type (2)	104500	4q11-q21
?Amelogenesis imperfecta-3, hypoplastic type (2)	301201	Xq22-q28
[AMP deaminase deficiency, erythrocytic] (3)	102772	11pter-p13
Amyloid neuropathy, familial, several allelic types (3)	176300	18q11.2-q12.1
Amyloidosis, 3 or more types (3)	107680	11q23
Amyloidosis, cerebroarterial, Dutch type (3)	104760	21q21
Amyloidosis, Finnish type, 105120 (3)	137350	9q34
Amyloidosis, hereditary renal, 105200 (3)	134820	4q28
Amyloidosis, renal, 105200 (3)	153450	Chr.12
{?Amyloidosis, secondary, susceptibility to} (1)	104770	1q21-q23
Amyloidosis, senile systemic (3)	176300	18q11.2-q12.1
Amyotrophic lateral sclerosis, juvenile recessive (2)	205100	2q33
{Amyotrophic lateral sclerosis, susceptibility to}, 105400 (3)	162230	22q12.2
Amyotrophic lateral sclerosis with frontotemporal dementia (2)	105550	9q21-q22
Amyotrophic lateral sclerosis-4, juvenile dominant (2)	602433	9q34
Amytrophic lateral sclerosis, due to SOD1 deficiency, 105400 (3)	147450	21q22.1
Amytrophic lateral sclerosis-5, juvenile recessive (2)	602099	15q15.1-q21.1
?Anal canal carcinoma (2)	105580	11q22-qter
Analbuminemia (3)	103600	4q11-q13
Andermann syndrome (2)	218000	15q13-q15
Androgen insensitivity, several forms, 300068 (3)	313700	Xq11-q12
Anemia, Diamond-Blackfan, 105650 (3)	603474	19q13.2
Anemia, hemolytic, due to PK deficiency (3)	266200	1q21

continued

Table 10.2. The morbid anatomy of the human genome (alphabetical by disorder) (*continued*)

Disorder	MIM#	Location
Anemia, hemolytic, Rh-null, regulator type, 268150 (3)	180297	6p21.1-p11
?Anemia, megaloblastic, due to DHFR deficiency (1)	126060	5q11.2-q13.2
Anemia, neonatal hemolytic, fatal and near-fatal (3)	182870	14q22-q23.2
Anemia, pernicious, congenital, due to deficiency of intrinsic factor (1)	261000	11q13
Anemia, sideroblastic, with ataxia, 301310 (3)	300135	Xq13.1-q13.3
Anemia, sideroblastic/hypochromic (3)	301300	Xp11.21
Aneurysm, familial arterial (3)	120180	2q31
Angelman syndrome (3)	601623	15q11-q13
Angioedema, hereditary (3)	106100	11q11-q13.1
Angiofibroma, sporadic (3)	131100	11q13
Angioneurotic edema, hereditary, X-linked (2)	300268	Chr.X
[Anhaptoglobinemia] (3)	140100	16q22.1
Aniridia (3)	106210	11p13
Ankylosing spondylitis (2)	106300	6p21.3
?Anophthalmos-1 (2)	301590	Xq27-q28
Anterior segment anomalies and cataract (3)	601653	8q13.3
Anterior segment mesenchymal dysgenesis (2)	107250	4q28-q31
Anterior segment mesenchymal dysgenesis (3)	601090	6p25
Anterior segment mesenchymal dysgenesis and cataract, 107250 (3)	602669	10q25
Antithrombin III deficiency (3)	107300	1q23-q25
Antley-Bixler syndrome (3)	176943	10q26
Anxiety-related personality traits (3)	182138	17q11.1-q12
Apert syndrome, 101200 (3)	176943	10q26
Apnea, postanesthetic (3)	177400	3q26.1-q26.2
ApoA-I and apoC-III deficiency, combined (3)	107680	11q23
Apolipoprotein A-II deficiency (3)	107670	1q21-q23
Apolipoprotein B-100, ligand-defective, 144010 (3)	107730	2p24
[Apolipoprotein H deficiency] (3)	138700	17q23-qter
Apparent mineralocorticoid excess, hypertension due to (3)	218030	16q22
[Aquaporin-1 deficiency] (3)	107776	7p14
Argininemia (3)	207800	6q23
Argininosuccinicaciduria (3)	207900	7cen-q11.2
Arrhythmogenic right ventricular dysplasia-1 (2)	107970	14q23-q24
Arrhythmogenic right ventricular dysplasia-2 (2)	600996	1q42-q43
Arrhythmogenic right ventricular dysplasia-3 (2)	602086	14q12-q22
Arrhythmogenic right ventricular dysplasia-4 (2)	602087	2q32.1-q32.3
Arrhythmogenic right ventricular dysplasia-5 (2)	604400	3p23
Arrhythmogenic right ventricular dysplasia-6 (2)	604401	10p14-p12
Arthrocutaneouveal granulomatosis (2)	186580	16p12-q21
Arthrogryposis multiplex congenita, distal, type 1 (2)	108120	9p21-q21
Arthrogryposis multiplex congenita, distal, type 2B (2)	601680	11p15.5
Arthrogryposis multiplex congenita, neurogenic (2)	208100	5q35
Arthrogryposis, X-linked (spinal muscular atrophy, infantile, X-linked) (2)	301830	Xp11.3-q11.2
Arthropathy, progressive pseudorheumatoid, of childhood, 208230 (3)	603400	6q22-q23
Arts syndrome (2)	301835	Xq21.2-q24
Aspartylglucosaminuria (3)	208400	4q32-q33
{Asthma and atopy, susceptibility to}, 147070 (3)	601690	6p21.2-p12
{Asthma, atopic, susceptibility to} (3)	147138	11q13
{Asthma, nocturnal, susceptibility to} (3)	109690	5q32-q34
{Asthma, susceptibility to} (3)	605238	1p32
Ataxia, episodic (3)	601949	2q22-q23
Ataxia with isolated vitamin E deficiency, 277460 (3)	600415	8q13.1-q13.3
Ataxia-oculomotor apraxia (2)	208920	9q34
Ataxia-telangiectasia (3)	208900	11q22.3
Ataxia-telangiectasia-like disorder, 604391 (3)	600814	11q21
Atelosteogenesis II, 256050 (3)	222600	5q32-q33.1
{Atherosclerosis, susceptibility to} (2)	131210	1q23-q25
{Atherosclerosis, susceptibility to} (2)	108725	19p13.3-p13.2

continued

Table 10.2. The morbid anatomy of the human genome (alphabetical by disorder) (*continued*)

Disorder	MIM#	Location
Atopy (2)	147050	11q12-q13
{Atopy, susceptibility to} (3)	147781	16p12.1-p11.2
Atransferrinemia (1)	190000	3q21
Atrial septal defect, secundum type (2)	108800	6p21.3
Atrial septal defect with atrioventricular conduction defects, 108900 (3)	600584	5q34
Atrichia with papular lesions, 209500 (3)	602302	8p21.2
Atrioventricular canal defect-1 (2)	600309	1p31-p21
Atrophia areata (2)	108985	11p15
{Attention-deficit hyperactivity disorder, susceptibility to}, 143465 (2)	126455	5p15.3
Autism, succinylpurinemic (3)	103050	22q13.1
{Autism, susceptibility to} (2)	209850	7q
{Autoimmune lymphoproliferative syndrome} (3)	134637	10q24.1
Autoimmune polyglandular disease, type I (3)	240300	21q22.3
Autoimmunity-immunodeficiency syndrome, X-linked, 304930 (3)	300292	Xp11.23-q13.3
Autonomic nervous system dysfunction (3)	126452	11p15.5
Axenfeld anomaly (3)	601090	6p25
Azoospermia (3)	400005	Yq11.2
Bamforth-Lazarus syndrome, 241850 (3)	602617	9q22
Bannayan-Riley-Ruvalcaba syndrome (3)	601728	10q23.3
Bannayan-Zonana syndrome, 153480 (3)	601728	10q23.3
Bardet-Biedl syndrome 1 (2)	209901	11q13
Bardet-Biedl syndrome 2 (2)	209900	16q21
Bardet-Biedl syndrome 3 (2)	600151	3p13-p12
Bardet-Biedl syndrome 4 (2)	600374	15q22.3-q23
Bardet-Biedl syndrome 5 (2)	603650	2q31
Bardet-Biedl syndrome, type 6, 605231 (3)	604896	20p12
Bare lymphocyte syndrome, type I, due to TAP2 deficiency (1)	170261	6p21.3
Bare lymphocyte syndrome, type II, 209920 (3)	601861	13q14
Barth syndrome (3)	302060	Xq28
Bartter syndrome, 241200 (3)	600839	15q15-q21.1
Bartter syndrome, infantile, with sensorineural deafness (2)	602522	1p31
Bartter syndrome, type 2 (3)	600359	11q24
Bartter syndrome, type 3 (3)	602023	1p36
Basal cell carcinoma, 109400 (3)	603673	1p32
?Basal cell carcinoma (2)	132800	9q31
Basal cell carcinoma (3)	139150	5q13.3
Basal cell carcinoma, sporadic (3)	601500	7q31-q32
Basal cell carcinoma, sporadic (3)	601309	9q22.3
Basal cell nevus syndrome, 109400 (3)	601309	9q22.3
Basal cell nevus syndrome (2)	109400	9q31
Basal ganglia calcification, idiopathic (2)	213600	14q
Bazex syndrome (2)	301845	Xq24-q27
B-cell non-Hodgkin lymphoma, high-grade (3)	601406	12q24.1
BCG and salmonella infection, disseminated, 209950 (1)	161561	5q31.1-q33.1
BCG infection, generalized familial (3)	107470	6q23-q24
Beare-Stevenson cutis gyrata syndrome, 123790 (3)	176943	10q26
Becker muscular dystrophy (3)	310200	Xp21.2
Becker muscular dystrophy modifier, 310200 (3)	159991	12q21
Beckwith-Wiedemann syndrome, 130650 (3)	600856	11p15.5
Benign familial infantile convulsions (2)	601764	19q
{Benzene toxicity, susceptibility to} (3)	125860	16q22.1
Berardinelli-Seip congenital lipodystrophy (2)	269700	9q34
Bernard-Soulier syndrome (3)	231200	17pter-p12
Bernard-Soulier syndrome, 231200 (2)	138720	22q11.2
Bernard-Soulier syndrome, 231200 (3)	173515	Chr. 3
{Beryllium disease, chronic, susceptibility to} (3)	142858	6p21.3
3-Beta-hydroxysteroid dehydrogenase, type II, deficiency (3)	201810	1p13.1
Bethlem myopathy, 158810 (3)	120250	2q37

continued

Table 10.2. The morbid anatomy of the human genome (alphabetical by disorder) (*continued*)

Disorder	MIM#	Location
Bethlem myopathy, 158810 (3)	120220	21q22.3
Bethlem myopathy, 158810 (3)	120240	21q22.3
Bietti crystalline corneoretinal dystrophy (2)	210370	4q35-qter
Bile acid malabsorption, primary (3)	601295	13q33
Biotinidase deficiency (3)	253260	3p25
Bipolar affective disorder (2)	125480	18p
Bjornstad syndrome (2)	262000	2q34-q36
Bladder cancer, 109800 (3)	190020	11p15.5
Bladder cancer, 109800 (3)	180200	13q14.1-q14.2
Bladder cancer, 109800 (3)	134934	4p16.3
Bleeding diathesis due to GNAQ deficiency (1)	600998	9q21
Bleeding disorder due to defective thromboxane A2 receptor (3)	188070	19p13.3
Blepharophimosis, epicanthus inversus, and ptosis, type 1 (2)	110100	3q22-q23
Blepharophimosis, epicanthus inversus, and ptosis, type 2 (2)	601649	7p21-p13
Bloom syndrome, 210900 (3)	604610	15q26.1
Borjeson-Forssman-Lehmann syndrome (2)	301900	Xq26.3
Bornholm eye disease (2)	310460	Xq28
Brachydactyly, type A1 (2)	112500	2q35-q36
Brachydactyly, type B1, 113000 (3)	602337	9q22
Brachydactyly, type C, 113100 (3)	601146	20q11.2
Brachydactyly, type C (2)	113100	12q24
?Brachydactyly, type E (2)	113300	2q37
Brachydactyly-mental retardation syndrome (2)	600430	2q37
Branchiootic syndrome 2 (2)	120502	1q31
Branchiootic syndrome (3)	601653	8q13.3
Branchiootorenal syndrome, 113650 (3)	601653	8q13.3
Branchiootorenal syndrome with cataract, 113650 (3)	601653	8q13.3
Breast cancer (1)	113721	17p13.3
Breast cancer (1)	133430	6q25.1
Breast cancer, 114480 (3)	602631	11p15.5
Breast cancer 2, early onset (3)	600185	13q12.3
Breast cancer (3)	601387	11p15.2-p15.1
Breast cancer, ductal (2)	211420	1p36
Breast cancer, ductal (2)	211410	Chr. 13
Breast cancer, invasive intraductal (3)	603615	1p32
Breast cancer, lobular (3)	192090	16q22.1
Breast cancer, male, with Reifenstein syndrome (3)	313700	Xq11-q12
Breast cancer, sporadic (3)	176705	17q21
{Breast cancer, susceptibility to} (3)	208900	11q22.3
Breast cancer, type 4 (2)	605365	13q21
Breast cancer-1 (3)	113705	17q21
Breast cancer-3 (2)	600048	11q23
Breast-ovarian cancer (3)	113705	17q21
Brody myopathy, 601003 (3)	108730	16p12
Bronchial asthma (2)	600807	5q31-q33
Bruck syndrome (2)	259450	17p12
Brugada syndrome, 601144 (3)	600163	3p21
Brunner syndrome (3)	309850	Xp11.23
Burkitt lymphoma, 113970 (3)	190080	8q24.12-q24.13
Butterfly dystrophy, retinal (3)	179605	6p21.1-cen
C1q deficiency, type A (3)	120550	1p36.3-p34.1
C1q deficiency, type B (3)	120570	1p36.3-p34.1
C1q deficiency, type C (3)	120575	1p36.3-p34.1
C1r/C1s deficiency, combined (1)	216950	12p13
C1r/C1s deficiency, combined (1)	120580	12p13
C1s deficiency, isolated (3)	120580	12p13
C2 deficiency (3)	217000	6p21.3
C3 deficiency (3)	120700	19p13.3-p13.2

continued

Table 10.2. The morbid anatomy of the human genome (alphabetical by disorder) (*continued*)

Disorder	*MIM#*	*Location*
C3b inactivator deficiency (3)	217030	4q25
C4 deficiency (3)	120810	6p21.3
C4 deficiency (3)	120820	6p21.3
C5 deficiency (1)	120900	9q34.1
C6 deficiency (1)	217050	5p13
C7 deficiency (1)	217070	5p13
C8 deficiency, type I (2)	120950	1p32
C8 deficiency, type II (3)	120960	1p32
C9 deficiency (3)	120940	5p13
Campomelic dysplasia with autosomal sex reversal (3)	114290	17q24.3-q25.1
Camptodactyly-arthropathy-coxa vara-pericarditis syndrome, 208250 (3)	604283	1q25-q31
Camurati-Engelmann disease, 131300 (3)	190180	19q13.1
Canavan disease (3)	271900	17pter-p13
{Cancer susceptibility} (3)	600678	2p16
Carbamoylphosphate synthetase I deficiency (3)	237300	2q35
Carbohydrate-deficient glycoprotein syndrome, type I, 212065 (3)	601785	16p13.3-p13.2
Carbohydrate-deficient glycoprotein syndrome, type Ib, 602579 (3)	154550	15q22-qter
Carbohydrate-deficient glycoprotein syndrome, type II, 212066 (3)	602616	14q21
Carcinoid tumor of lung (3)	131100	11q13
Cardiac valvular dysplasia-1 (2)	314400	Xq28
Cardioencephalomyopathy, fatal infantile, due to cytochrome c oxidase deficiency, 604377 (3)	604272	22q13
Cardiofaciocutaneous syndrome, 115150 (2)	163950	12q24
Cardiomopathy, hypertrophic, mid-ventricular chamber type (3)	160790	3p
Cardiomyopathy, dilated, 115200 (3)	102540	15q14
Cardiomyopathy, dilated, 1A, 115200 (3)	150330	1q21.2
Cardiomyopathy, dilated 1C (2)	601493	10q21-q23
Cardiomyopathy, dilated, 1E (2)	601154	3p25-p22
Cardiomyopathy, dilated, 1F (2)	602067	6q23
Cardiomyopathy, dilated, 1G (2)	604145	2q31
Cardiomyopathy, dilated, 1H (2)	604288	2q14-q22
Cardiomyopathy, dilated, 1I, 604765 (3)	125660	2q35
Cardiomyopathy, dilated, 1J (2)	605362	6q23-q24
Cardiomyopathy, dilated, X-linked (3)	310200	Xp21.2
Cardiomyopathy, familial dilated 1B (2)	600884	9q13
Cardiomyopathy, familial dilated-2 (2)	601494	1q32
Cardiomyopathy, familial hypertrophic, 1, 192600 (3)	160760	14q12
Cardiomyopathy, familial hypertrophic, 192600 (3)	102540	15q14
Cardiomyopathy, familial hypertrophic, 2, 115195 (3)	191045	1q32
Cardiomyopathy, familial hypertrophic, (3)	191044	19q13.4
Cardiomyopathy, familial hypertrophic, 3, 115196 (3)	191010	15q22.1
Cardiomyopathy, familial hypertrophic, 4, 115197 (3)	600958	11p11.2
Cardiomyopathy, familial hypertrophic, 9 (3)	188840	2q24.3
Cardiomyopathy, familial hypertrophic with Wolff-Parkinson-White syndrome (2)	600858	7q3
Cardiomyopathy, hypertrophic, mid-left ventricular chamber type (3)	160781	12q23-q24.3
Cardiomyopathy, X-linked dilated, 300069 (3)	302060	Xq28
Carney complex, type 1, 160980 (3)	188830	17q23-q24
Carney complex, type II (2)	605244	2p16
?Carnitine acetyltransferase deficiency (1)	600184	9q34.1
Carnitine deficiency, systemic primary, 212140 (3)	603377	5q33.1
Carnitine-acylcarnitine translocase deficiency (3)	212138	3p21.31
Carnosinemia (2)	212200	18q21.3
Carpal tunnel syndrome, familial (3)	176300	18q11.2-q12.1
Cartilage-hair hypoplasia (2)	250250	9p13
Cat eye syndrome (2)	115470	22q11
?Cataract, anterior polar-1 (2)	115650	14q24-qter
Cataract, anterior polar-2 (2)	601202	17p13
Cataract, cerulean, type 1 (2)	115660	17q24
Cataract, cerulean, type 2, 601547 (3)	123620	22q11.2-q12.2

continued

Table 10.2. The morbid anatomy of the human genome (alphabetical by disorder) (*continued*)

Disorder	MIM#	Location
?Cataract, congenital (2)	182500	15q15.3
Cataract, congenital (3)	602669	10q25
Cataract, congenital, 604219 (3)	603212	3q21-q25
Cataract, congenital, autosomal dominant (3)	123580	21q22.3
?Cataract, congenital total (2)	302200	Xp
Cataract, congenital, Volkmann type (2)	115665	1pter-p36.13
Cataract, congenital, with late-onset corneal dystrophy (3)	106210	11p13
Cataract, congenital, with microphthalmia (2)	156850	16p13.3
Cataract, congenital zonular, with sutural opacities, 600881 (3)	123610	17q11.1-q12
Cataract, Coppock-like, 604307 (3)	123680	2q33-q35
Cataract, crystalline aculeiform, 115700 (3)	123690	2q33-q35
Cataract, juvenile-onset, 604219 (3)	603212	3q21-q25
Cataract, Marner type (2)	116800	16q22.1
Cataract, polymorphic and lamellar, 604219 (3)	154050	12q13
Cataract, polymorphic congenital (2)	601286	2q33-q35
Cataract, posterior polar (2)	116600	1pter-p36.1
Cataract, posterior polar-3 (2)	605387	20p12-q12
Cataract, variable zonular pulverulent (3)	123680	2q33-q35
Cataract, zonular pulverulent-1, 116200 (3)	600897	1q21.1
Cataract, zonular pulverulent-3, 601885 (3)	121015	13q11
Cataracts, punctate, progressive juvenile-onset (3)	123690	2q33-q35
CD3, zeta chain, deficiency (1)	186780	1q22-q23
[CD4+ lymphocyte deficiency] (2)	186940	12pter-p12
CD59 deficiency (3)	107271	11p13
Celiac disease (2)	212750	6p
Central core disease, 117000 (3)	180901	19q13.1
?Central core disease, one form (3)	160760	14q12
Centrocytic lymphoma (2)	168461	11q13
Cerebellar ataxia, Cayman type (2)	601238	19p13.3
Cerebellar ataxia, pure (3)	601011	19p13
Cerebellar ataxia-2 (2)	302500	Xp11.21-q21.3
Cerebral amyloid angiopathy, 105150 (3)	604312	20p11.2
Cerebral arteriopathy with subcortical infarcts and leukoencephalopathy, 125310 (3)	600276	19p13.2-p13.1
Cerebral cavernous malformations-1, 116860 (3)	604214	7q11.2-q21
Cerebral cavernous malformations-2 (2)	603284	7p15-p13
Cerebral cavernous malformations-3 (2)	603285	3q25.2-q27
Cerebral palsy, ataxic, autosomal recessive (2)	605388	9p12-q12
Cerebrooculofacioskeletal syndrome, 214150 (3)	133540	10q11
Cerebrotendinous xanthomatosis (3)	213700	2q33-qter
Cerebrovascular disease, occlusive (3)	107280	14q32.1
Ceroid lipofuscinosis, neuronal, variant juvenile type, with granular osmiophilic deposits (3)	600722	1p32
Ceroid lipofuscinosis, neuronal-1, infantile, 256730 (3)	600722	1p32
Ceroid-lipofuscinosis, neuronal-2, classic late infantile (2)	204500	11p15.5
Ceroid-lipofuscinosis, neuronal-3, juvenile (3)	204200	16p12.1
Ceroid-lipofuscinosis, neuronal-5, variant late infantile (3)	256731	13q21.1-q32
Ceroid-lipofuscinosis, neuronal-6, variant late infantile (2)	601780	15q21-q23
Cervical cancer, 603956 (3)	134934	4p16.3
Cervical carcinoma (2)	191181	11q13
[CETP deficiency] (3)	118470	16q21
Char syndrome, 169100 (3)	601601	6p12
Charcot-Marie-Tooth disease, type 2E (3)	162280	8p21
Charcot-Marie-Tooth disease, type 4B, 601382 (3)	603557	11q22
Charcot-Marie-Tooth disease, type 4B, form 2 (2)	604563	11p15
Charcot-Marie-Tooth disease, type 4F (2)	605260	19q13.1-q13.3
Charcot-Marie-Tooth disease with deafness, 118300 (3)	601097	17p11.2
Charcot-Marie-Tooth neuropathy, demyelinating (2)	601596	5q32
Charcot-Marie-Tooth neuropathy, X-linked-1, dominant, 302800 (3)	304040	Xq13.1
Charcot-Marie-Tooth neuropathy, X-linked-2, recessive (2)	302801	Xp22.2

continued

Table 10.2. The morbid anatomy of the human genome (alphabetical by disorder) (*continued*)

Disorder	MIM#	Location
Charcot-Marie-Tooth neuropathy-1A, 118220 (3)	601097	17p11.2
Charcot-Marie-Tooth neuropathy-1B, 118200 (3)	159440	1q22
Charcot-Marie-Tooth neuropathy-2A (2)	118210	1p36-p35
Charcot-Marie-Tooth neuropathy-2B (2)	600882	3q13-q22
Charcot-Marie-Tooth neuropathy-2D (2)	601472	7p14
Charcot-Marie-Tooth neuropathy-4A (2)	214400	8q13-q21.1
Chediak-Higashi syndrome (3)	214500	1q42.1-q42.2
Cherubism (2)	118400	4p16.3
CHILD syndrome, 308050 (3)	300275	Xq28
[Chitotriosidase deficiency] (3)	600031	1q31-q32
Chloride diarrhea, congenital, Finnish type, 214700 (3)	126650	7q22-q31.1
Cholestasis, benign recurrent intrahepatic, 243300 (3)	602397	18q21
Cholestasis, familial intrahepatic, of pregnancy, 147480 (3)	171060	7q21.1
Cholestasis, progressive familial intrahepatic, type III, 602347 (3)	171060	7q21.1
Cholestasis, progressive familial intrahepatic-1, 211600 (3)	602397	18q21
Cholestasis-lymphedema syndrome (2)	214900	15q
Cholesteryl ester storage disease (3)	278000	10q24-q25
Chondrocalcinosis, familial articular (2)	118600	5p15
Chondrocalcinosis with early-onset osteoarthritis (2)	600668	8q
Chondrodysplasia, Grebe type, 200700 (3)	601146	20q11.2
Chondrodysplasia punctata, brachytelephalangic, 302940 (3)	300180	Xp22.3
Chondrodysplasia punctata, rhizomelic, type 2, 222765 (3)	602744	Chr.1
Chondrodysplasia punctata, X-linked dominant, 302960 (3)	300205	Xp11.23-p11.22
Chondrodysplasia punctata, X-linked recessive, 302950 (3)	300180	Xp22.3
Chondrosarcoma, 215300 (3)	133700	8q24.11-q24.13
Chondrosarcoma, extraskeletal myxoid (1)	601574	17q11.1-q11.2
Chondrosarcoma, extraskeletal myxoid (1)	600542	9q22
Chorea, hereditary benign (2)	118700	14q
Choreoacanthocytosis (2)	200150	9q21
Choreoathetosis, familial paroxysmal (2)	118800	2q33-q35
Choreoathetosis/spasticity, episodic (2)	601042	1p
Chorioathetosis with mental retardation and abnormal behavior (2)	300220	Xp11.2
Chorioretinal atrophy, progressive bifocal (2)	600790	6q14-q16.2
Choroidal dystrophy, central areolar (2)	215500	17p
Choroideremia (3)	303100	Xq21.2
Chronic granulomatous disease, autosomal, due to deficiency of CYBA (3)	233690	16q24
Chronic granulomatous disease due to deficiency of NCF-1 (3)	233700	7q11.23
Chronic granulomatous disease due to deficiency of NCF-2 (3)	233710	1q25
Chronic granulomatous disease, X-linked (3)	306400	Xp21.1
{Chronic infections, due to opsonin defect} (3)	154545	10q11.2-q21
Chylomicronemia syndrome, familial (3)	238600	8p22
Cirrhosis, North American Indian childhood type (2)	604901	16q22
Citrullinemia, 215700 (3)	603470	9q34
Citrullinemia, adult-onset type II, 603471 (3)	603859	7q21.3
Cleft lip/palate ectodermal dysplasia syndrome, 225000 (3)	600644	11q23-q24
Cleft palate, isolated (2)	119540	2q32
Cleft palate, X-linked (2)	303400	Xq21.3
Cleidocranial dysplasia, 119600 (3)	600211	6p21
CMO II deficiency (3)	124080	8q21
Coats disease, 300216 (3)	310600	Xp11.4
Cockayne syndrome-1 (3)	216400	Chr.5
Cockayne syndrome-2, type B (3)	133540	10q11
Coffin-Lowry syndrome, 303600 (3)	300075	Xp22.2-p22.1
Cohen syndrome (2)	216550	8q22-q23
Colchicine resistance (3)	171050	7q21.1
Cold urticaria, familial (2)	120100	1q44
Colon adenocarcinoma (3)	603615	1p32
Colon adenocarcinoma (3)	604289	8q21.3-q22

continued

Table 10.2. The morbid anatomy of the human genome (alphabetical by disorder) (*continued*)

Disorder	MIM#	Location
?Colon cancer (1)	126650	7q22-q31.1
Colon cancer (3)	603517	1p22
Colon cancer (3)	190182	3p22
Colon cancer (3)	600079	7q11.23
Colon cancer, advanced (3)	190090	20q12-q13
Colorblindness, blue monochromatic (3)	303700	Xq28
Colorblindness, deutan (3)	303800	Xq28
Colorblindness, protan (3)	303900	Xq28
Colorblindness, tritan (3)	190900	7q31.3-q32
Colorectal adenoma (1)	190070	12p12.1
Colorectal cancer (1)	190070	12p12.1
Colorectal cancer, 114500 (3)	602228	10q25.3
Colorectal cancer, 114500 (3)	604025	17q23-q24
Colorectal cancer, 114500 (3)	191170	17p13.1
Colorectal cancer, 114500 (3)	602700	22q13
Colorectal cancer, 114500 (3)	604584	8p22-p21.3
Colorectal cancer (3)	164790	1p13.2
Colorectal cancer (3)	120470	18q21.3
Colorectal cancer (3)	600040	19q13.3-q13.4
Colorectal cancer (3)	116806	3p22-p21.3
Colorectal cancer (3)	159350	5q21
Colorectal cancer (3)	175100	5q21-q22
Colorectal cancer, familial nonpolyposis, type 6 (3)	190182	3p22
Colorectal cancer, hereditary, nonpolyposis, type 1 (3)	120435	2p22-p21
Colorectal cancer, hereditary nonpolyposis, type 2 (3)	120436	3p21.3
Colorectal cancer, hereditary nonpolyposis, type 3 (3)	600258	2q31-q33
Colorectal cancer, hereditary nonpolyposis, type 4 (3)	600259	7p22
{?Colorectal cancer, resistance to} (1)	172411	1p35
{Colorectal cancer, susceptibility to, 2} (2)	604940	15q21.1
Colorectal cancer with chromosomal instability (3)	602452	2q14
Colton blood group, 110450 (3)	107776	7p14
Combined C6/C7 deficiency (1)	217050	5p13
Combined factor V and VIII deficiency, 227300 (3)	601567	18q21.3-q22
Combined hyperlipemia, familial (3)	238600	8p22
Combined immunodeficiency, X-linked, moderate, 312863 (3)	308380	Xq13
Complex I deficiency (3)	602694	5q11.1
Complex neurologic disorder, 117200 (3)	600075	6q27
Cone dystrophy, progressive (2)	600977	17p13-p12
Cone dystrophy, progressive X-linked, 1 (2)	304020	Xp11.4
Cone dystrophy, progressive X-linked, 2 (2)	300085	Xq27
Cone dystrophy-3, 602093 (3)	600364	6p21.1
Cone-rod dystrophy 3 (3)	601691	1p21-p13
Cone-rod dystrophy, 300029 (3)	312610	Xp21.1
Cone-rod dystrophy 6, 601777 (3)	600179	17p13.1
Cone-rod dystrophy 8 (2)	605549	1q12-q24
Cone-rod dystrophy-7 (2)	603649	6cen-q14
Cone-rod retinal dystrophy-1 (2)	600624	18q21.1-q21.3
Cone-rod retinal dystrophy-2, 120970 (3)	602225	19q13.3
{?Congenital anomalies, susceptibility to} (2)	136430	11q13.3-q13.5
Congenital bilateral absence of vas deferens, 277180 (3)	602421	7q31.2
Congenital cataract, facial dysmorphism, and neuropathy syndrome (2)	604168	18q23-qter
Congenital dyserythropoietic anemia II (2)	224100	20q11.2
Congenital hereditary endothelial dystrophy of cornea (2)	121700	20p13
Conjunctivitis, ligneous, 217090 (3)	173350	6q26
?Conotruncal cardiac anomalies (2)	217095	22q11
Contractural arachnodactyly, congenital (3)	121050	5q23-q31
Convulsions, familial febrile, 1 (2)	602476	8q13-q21
Convulsions, familial febrile, 2 (2)	602477	19p13.3

continued

Table 10.2. The morbid anatomy of the human genome (alphabetical by disorder) (*continued*)

Disorder	MIM#	Location
Convulsions, familial febrile, 3 (2)	604403	2q23-q24
Convulsions, familial febrile, 4 (2)	604352	5q14-q15
Convulsions, infantile and paroxysmal choreoathetosis (2)	602066	16p12-q12
Coproporphyria (3)	121300	3q12
Cornea plana congenita, recessive, 217300 (3)	603288	12q21.3-q22
Corneal clouding, autosomal recessive (3)	107680	11q23
Corneal dystrophy, Avellino type (3)	601692	5q31
Corneal dystrophy, crystalline, Schnyder (2)	121800	1p36-p34.1
Corneal dystrophy, gelatinous drop-like, 204870 (3)	137290	1p32-q12
Corneal dystrophy, Groenouw type I, 121900 (3)	601692	5q31
Corneal dystrophy, lattice type I, 122200 (3)	601692	5q31
Corneal dystrophy, lattice type IIIA (3)	601692	5q31
Corneal dystrophy, posterior polymorphous (2)	122000	20p11.2-q11.2
Corneal dystrophy, Reis-Bucklers type, 121900 (3)	601692	5q31
Corneal dystrophy, Thiel-Behnke type (2)	602082	10q24
?Cornelia de Lange syndrome (2)	122470	3q26.3
{Coronary artery disease, susceptibility to} (1)	152200	6q27
{Coronary artery disease, susceptibility to} (3)	168820	7q21.3
{Coronary artery disease, susceptibility to} (3)	602447	7q21.3
{Coronary spasm, susceptibility to} (3)	163729	7q36
Cortisol resistance (3)	138040	5q31
Coumarin resistance, 122700 (3)	122720	19q13.2
Cowchock syndrome (2)	310490	Xq24-q26.1
Cowden disease, 158350 (3)	601728	10q23.3
CPT deficiency, hepatic, type I, 255120 (3)	600528	11q13
CPT deficiency, hepatic, type II, 600649 (3)	600650	1p32
CR1 deficiency (1)	120620	1q32
Cramps, familial, potassium-aggravated (3)	603967	17q23.1-q25.3
Craniofacial-deafness-hand syndrome, 122880 (3)	193500	2q35
Craniofrontonasal dysplasia (2)	304110	Xp22
Craniometaphyseal dysplasia (2)	123000	5p15.2-p14.1
Craniometaphyseal dysplasia, autosomal recessive (2)	218400	6q21-q22
Craniosynostosis, Adelaide type (2)	600593	4p16
Craniosynostosis, nonspecific (3)	176943	10q26
Craniosynostosis, type 1 (2)	123100	7p21.3-p21.2
Craniosynostosis, type 2, 604757 (3)	123101	5q34-q35
[Creatine kinase, brain type, ectopic expression of] (2)	123270	14q32
Creutzfeldt-Jakob disease, 123400 (3)	176640	20pter-p12
Crigler-Najjar syndrome, type I, 218800 (3)	191740	Chr.2
Crouzon syndrome, 123500 (3)	176943	10q26
Crouzon syndrome with acanthosis nigricans (3)	134934	4p16.3
?Cryptorchidism (2)	306190	Xp21
Currarino syndrome, 176450 (3)	142994	7q36
Cutis laxa, 123700 (3)	130160	7q11.2
?Cutis laxa, marfanoid neonatal type (1)	150240	7q31.1-q31.3
Cutis laxa, neonatal (3)	300011	Xq12-q13
Cutis laxa, recessive, type I, 219100 (1)	153455	5q23.3-q31.2
Cyclic hematopoiesis, 162800 (3)	130130	19p13.3
Cyclic ichthyosis with epidermolytic hyperkeratosis (3)	139350	12q13
Cylindromatosis, familial, 132700 (3)	605018	16q12-q13
[Cystathioninuria] (1)	219500	Chr. 16
Cystic fibrosis, 219700 (3)	602421	7q31.2
Cystinosis, nephropathic (3)	219800	17p13
Cystinuria, 220100 (3)	104614	2p16.3
Cystinuria, type II (3)	604144	19q13.1
Cystinuria, type III (3)	604144	19q13.1
Darier disease, 124200 (3)	108740	12q23-q24.1
D-bifunctional protein deficiency (3)	601860	5q2

continued

Table 10.2. The morbid anatomy of the human genome (alphabetical by disorder) (*continued*)

Disorder	MIM#	Location
Deafness, autosomal dominant 10 (2)	601316	6q22.2-q23.3
Deafness, autosomal dominant 11, neurosensory, 601317 (3)	276903	11q13.5
Deafness, autosomal dominant 12, 601842 (3)	602574	11q22-q24
Deafness, autosomal dominant 13, 601868 (3)	120290	6p21.3
Deafness, autosomal dominant 15, 602459 (3)	602460	5q31
Deafness, autosomal dominant 16 (2)	603964	2q23-q24.3
Deafness, autosomal dominant 17, 603622 (3)	160775	22q11.2
Deafness, autosomal dominant 2 (2)	600101	1p34
Deafness, autosomal dominant 2, 600101 (3)	603324	1p35.1
Deafness, autosomal dominant 2, 600101 (3)	603537	1p34
Deafness, autosomal dominant 20 (2)	604717	17q25
Deafness, autosomal dominant 23 (2)	605192	14q21-q22
Deafness, autosomal dominant 3, 601544 (3)	121011	13q11-q12
Deafness, autosomal dominant 4 (2)	600652	19q13
Deafness, autosomal dominant 5 (3)	600994	7p15
Deafness, autosomal dominant 6 (2)	600965	4p16.3
Deafness, autosomal dominant 7 (2)	601412	1q21-q23
Deafness, autosomal dominant 8, 601543 (3)	602574	11q22-q24
Deafness, autosomal dominant 9, 601369 (3)	603196	14q12-q13
Deafness, autosomal dominant 1, 124900 (3)	602121	5q31
Deafness, autosomal dominant 3, 601544 (3)	604418	13q12
Deafness, autosomal recessive 1, 220290 (3)	121011	13q11-q12
Deafness, autosomal recessive 10 (2)	605316	21q22.3
Deafness, autosomal recessive 10, congenital, 605316 (3)	605511	21q22.3
Deafness, autosomal recessive 12 (2)	601386	10q21-q22
Deafness, autosomal recessive 13 (2)	603098	7q34-q36
Deafness, autosomal recessive 14 (2)	603678	7q31
Deafness, autosomal recessive 15 (2)	601869	3q
Deafness, autosomal recessive 16 (2)	603720	15q21-q22
Deafness, autosomal recessive 17 (2)	603010	7q31
Deafness, autosomal recessive 18 (2)	602092	11p15.1-p14
Deafness, autosomal recessive 2, 600060 (3)	276903	11q13.5
Deafness, autosomal recessive 20 (2)	604060	11q25-qter
Deafness, autosomal recessive 21, 603629 (3)	602574	11q22-q24
Deafness, autosomal recessive 26 (2)	605428	4q31
Deafness, autosomal recessive (3)	603324	1p35.1
Deafness, autosomal recessive 3, 600316 (3)	602666	17p11.2
Deafness, autosomal recessive 4, 600791 (3)	274600	7q31
Deafness, autosomal recessive 5 (2)	600792	14q12
Deafness, autosomal recessive 6 (2)	600971	3p21-p14
Deafness, autosomal recessive 7 (2)	600974	9q13-q21
Deafness, autosomal recessive 8, childhood onset, 601072 (3)	605511	21q22.3
Deafness, autosomal recessive 9, 601071 (3)	603681	2p23-p22
[Deafness, nonsyndromic, modifier 1] (2)	605429	1q24
Deafness, X-linked 1, progressive (3)	304700	Xq22
Deafness, X-linked 2, perceptive congenital (2)	304500	Xq22
Deafness, X-linked 3, conductive, with stapes fixation, 304400 (3)	300039	Xq21.1
Deafness, X-linked 4, congenital sensorineural (2)	300030	Xp21.2
Deafness, X-linked 6, sensorineural (2)	300066	Xp22
Debrisoquine sensitivity (3)	124030	22q13.1
?DECR deficiency (2)	222745	8q21.3
Dehydrated hereditary stomatocytosis (2)	194380	16q23-q24
Dejerine-Sottas disease, 145900 (3)	601097	17p11.2
Dejerine-Sottas disease, myelin P-zero-related, 145900 (3)	159440	1q22
Dementia, familial British, 176500 (3)	603904	13q14
Dementia, familial Danish, 117300 (3)	603904	13q14
Dementia, familial, nonspecific (2)	600795	3p11.1-q11.2
Dementia, frontotemporal, with parkinsonism, 601630 (3)	157140	17q21.1

continued

Table 10.2. The morbid anatomy of the human genome (alphabetical by disorder) (*continued*)

Disorder	MIM#	Location
Dent disease, 300009 (3)	300008	Xp11.22
Dental anomalies, isolated (3)	600211	6p21
Dementia, frontotemporal, with parkinsonism, 601630 (3)	157140	17q21.1
Dent disease, 300009 (3)	300008	Xp11.22
Dental anomalies, isolated (3)	600211	6p21
Dentatorubro-pallidoluysian atrophy (3)	125370	12p13.31
Dentin dysplasia, type II (2)	125420	4q
Dentinogenesis imperfecta-1 (2)	125490	4q13-q21
Denys-Drash syndrome (3)	194070	11p13
Dermatitis, atopic (2)	603165	3q21
Dermatofibrosarcoma protuberans (3)	190040	22q12.3-q13.1
Desmoid disease, hereditary, 135290 (3)	175100	5q21-q22
Diabetes insipidus, nephrogenic (3)	304800	Xq28
Diabetes insipidus, nephrogenic, autosomal dominant, 125800 (3)	107777	12q13
Diabetes insipidus, nephrogenic, autosomal recessive, 222000 (3)	107777	12q13
Diabetes insipidus, neurohypophyseal, 125700 (3)	192340	20p13
{Diabetes mellitus, insulin-dependent, 10} (2)	601942	10p11-q11
{Diabetes mellitus, insulin-dependent, 11} (2)	601208	14q24.3-q31
{Diabetes mellitus, insulin-dependent, 12} (2)	601388	2q33
{Diabetes mellitus, insulin-dependent, 13} (2)	601318	2q34
{Diabetes mellitus, insulin-dependent, 15} (2)	601666	6q21
{Diabetes mellitus, insulin-dependent, 17} (2)	603266	10q25
{Diabetes mellitus, insulin-dependent, 2} (2)	125852	11p15.5
{Diabetes mellitus, insulin-dependent} (3)	142410	12q24.2
{Diabetes mellitus, insulin-dependent, 3} (2)	600318	15q26
{Diabetes mellitus, insulin-dependent, 4} (2)	600319	11q13
{Diabetes mellitus, insulin-dependent, 5} (2)	600320	6q24-q27
{Diabetes mellitus, insulin-dependent, 6} (2)	601941	18q21
{Diabetes mellitus, insulin-dependent, 7} (2)	600321	2q31
{Diabetes mellitus, insulin-dependent, 8} (2)	600883	6q25-q27
?Diabetes mellitus, insulin-dependent, neonatal (2)	600089	Chr. 6
{Diabetes mellitus, insulin-dependent, X-linked} (2) (2)	300136	Xp11
{Diabetes mellitus, insulin-dependent-1} (2)	222100	6p21.3
Diabetes mellitus, insulin-resistant, with acanthosis nigricans (3)	147670	19p13.2
Diabetes mellitus, insulin-resistant, with acanthosis nigricans and hypertension, 604367 (3)	601487	3p25
{Diabetes mellitus, non-insulin dependent, 1}, 601283 (3)	605286	2q37.3
{Diabetes mellitus, noninsulin-dependent}, 125853 (3)	604641	11p12-p11.2
{Diabetes mellitus, noninsulin-dependent}, 125853 (3)	600281	20q12-q13.1
{Diabetes mellitus, noninsulin-dependent} (2)	138570	19q13.3
{Diabetes mellitus, noninsulin-dependent, 2}, 601407 (2)	142410	12q24.2
{Diabetes mellitus, noninsulin-dependent} (3)	138190	17p13
{Diabetes mellitus, noninsulin-dependent} (3)	147545	2q36
{Diabetes mellitus, noninsulin-dependent} (3)	138160	3q26.1-q26.3
{Diabetes mellitus, noninsulin-dependent}, 3 (2)	603694	20q12-q13.1
Diabetes mellitus, rare form (1)	176730	11p15.5
{Diabetes mellitus, transient neonatal} (2)	601410	6q24
{Diabetes mellitus, type II}, 125853 (3)	601724	2q32
{Diabetes mellitus, type II} (3)	138033	17q25
{Diabetes mellitus, type II} (3)	138430	2q24.1
Diaphyseal medullary stenosis with malignant fibrous histiocytoma (2)	112250	9p22-p21
Diastrophic dysplasia (3)	222600	5q32-q33.1
?Dicarboxylicaminoaciduria, 222730 (1)	133550	9p24
DiGeorge syndrome (2)	188400	22q11
DiGeorge syndrome/velocardiofacial syndrome complex-2 (2)	601362	10p14-p13
Dihydropyrimidinuria (3)	222748	8q22
Diphenylhydantoin toxicity (1)	132810	1q42.1
{Diphtheria, susceptibility to} (1)	126150	5q23
{Dissection of cervical arteries, susceptibility to} (3)	120150	17q21.31-q22

continued

Table 10.2. The morbid anatomy of the human genome (alphabetical by disorder) (*continued*)

Disorder	MIM#	Location
DNA ligase I deficiency (3)	126391	19q13.2-q13.3
Dopamine-beta-hydroxylase deficiency (1)	223360	9q34
Dosage-sensitive sex reversal, 300018 (3)	300200	Xp21.3-p21.2
Down syndrome (1)	190685	21q22.3
Doyne honeycomb degeneration of retina, 126600 (3)	601548	2p16
Duane retraction syndrome 2 (2)	604356	2q31
Duane syndrome (2)	126800	8q13
Dubin-Johnson syndrome, 237500 (3)	601107	10q24
Duchenne muscular dystrophy (3)	310200	Xp21.2
[Dysalbuminemic hyperthyroxinemia] (3)	103600	4q11-q13
[Dysalbuminemic hyperzincemia], 194470 (3)	103600	4q11-q13
Dysautonomia, familial (2)	223900	9q31-q33
Dyserythropoietic anemia, congenital, type III (2)	105600	15q21
Dyserythropoietic anemia, congenital, type I (2)	224120	15q15.1-q15.3
Dyserythropoietic anemia with thrombocytopenia (3)	305371	Xp11.23
Dysfibrinogenemia, alpha type, causing bleeding diathesis (3)	134820	4q28
Dysfibrinogenemia, alpha type, causing recurrent thrombosis (3)	134820	4q28
Dysfibrinogenemia, beta type (3)	134830	4q28
Dysfibrinogenemia, gamma type (3)	134850	4q28
Dyskeratosis congenita-1, 305000 (3)	300126	Xq28
Dyslexia, specific, 2 (2)	600202	6p21.3
Dyslexia, specific, 3 (2)	604254	2p16-p15
Dyslexia-1 (2)	127700	15q21
Dysprothrombinemia (3)	176930	11p11-q12
Dystonia 11, myoclonic (2)	605408	7q21
Dystonia, DOPA-responsive, 128230 (3)	600225	14q22.1-q22.2
Dystonia, myoclonic, 159900 (3)	126450	11q23
Dystonia-1, torsion (3)	128100	9q34
Dystonia-12 (2)	128235	19q13
Dystonia-3, torsion, with parkinsonism, Filipino type (2)	314250	Xq13.1
Dystonia-6, torsion (2)	602629	8p21-q22
Dystonia-7, torsion (2)	602124	18p
[Dystransthyretinemic hyperthyroxinemia] (3)	176300	18q11.2-q12.1
Ectodermal dysplasia 2, hidrotic, 129500 (3)	604418	13q12
Ectodermal dysplasia, hypohidrotic, autosomal dominant, 129490 (3)	604095	2q11-q13
Ectodermal dysplasia, hypohidrotic, autosomal recessive, 224900 (3)	604095	2q11-q13
Ectodermal dysplasia, hypohidrotic, with immune deficiency, 300291 (3)	300248	Xq28
Ectodermal dysplasia, Margarita Island type, 225060 (3)	600644	11q23-q24
Ectodermal dysplasia-1, anhidrotic (3)	305100	Xq12-q13.1
Ectodermal dysplasia/skin fragility syndrome, 604536 (3)	601975	1q32-q44
Ectopia lentis, familial (3)	134797	15q21.1
Ectopia pupillae, 129750 (3)	106210	11p13
Ectrodactyly, ectodermal dysplasia, and cleft lip/palate syndrome 3, 604292 (3)	603273	3q27
Ectrodactyly, ectodermal dysplasia, cleft lip/palate-2 (2)	602077	Chr.19
?EEC syndrome-1 (2)	129900	7q11.2-q21.3
Ehlers-Danlos syndrome, progeroid form, 130070 (3)	604327	5q35.1-q35.3
Ehlers-Danlos syndrome, type I, 130000 (3)	120190	2q31
Ehlers-Danlos syndrome, type I, 130000 (3)	120215	9q34.2-q34.3
Ehlers-Danlos syndrome, type II, 130010 (3)	120215	9q34.2-q34.3
Ehlers-Danlos syndrome, type III, 130020 (3)	120180	2q31
Ehlers-Danlos syndrome, type IV, 130050 (3)	120180	2q31
Ehlers-Danlos syndrome, type VI, 225400 (3)	153454	1p36.3-p36.2
Ehlers-Danlos syndrome, type VIIA2, 130060 (3)	120160	7q22.1
Ehlers-Danlos syndrome, type VIIC, 225410 (3)	604539	5q23
?Ehlers-Danlos syndrome, type X, 225310 (1)	135600	2q34
Ehlers-Danlos syndrome, types I and VIIA, 130000, 130060 (3)	120150	17q21.31-q22
Ehlers-Danlos-like syndrome (3)	600261	6p21.3
[Elliptocytosis, Malaysian-Melanesian type] (3)	109270	17q21-q22

continued

Table 10.2. The morbid anatomy of the human genome (alphabetical by disorder) (*continued*)

Disorder	MIM#	Location
Elliptocytosis-1 (3)	130500	1p36.2-p34
Elliptocytosis-2 (3)	182860	1q21
Elliptocytosis-3 (3)	182870	14q22-q23.2
Ellis-van Creveld syndrome, 225500 (3)	604831	4p16
Emery-Dreifuss muscular dystrophy (3)	310300	Xq28
Emery-Dreifuss muscular dystrophy, AD, 181350 (3)	150330	1q21.2
Emery-Dreifuss muscular dystrophy, AR, 604929 (3)	150330	1q21.2
Emphysema (3)	107400	14q32.1
Emphysema due to alpha-2-macroglobulin deficiency (1)	103950	12p13.3-p12.3
Emphysema-cirrhosis (3)	107400	14q32.1
Encephalopathy, familial, with neuroserpin inclusion bodies, 604218 (3)	602445	3q26
Encephalopathy, progressive mitochondrial, with proximal renal tubulopathy due to cytochrome c oxidase deficiency (3)	602125	17p12-p11.2
Endocardial fibroelastosis-2 (2)	302060	Xq28
Endometrial carcinoma (2)	602084	10q26
Endometrial carcinoma (3)	601728	10q23.3
Endometrial carcinoma (3)	192090	16q22.1
Endometrial carcinoma (3)	600678	2p16
Endometrial carcinoma (3)	600887	5q11-q12
Endotoxin hyporesponsiveness (3)	603030	9q32-q33
Endplate acetylcholinesterase deficiency, 603034 (3)	603033	3p24.2
Enhanced S-cone syndrome, 268100 (3)	604485	15q23
Enlarged vestibular aqueduct, 603545 (3)	274600	7q31
Enolase deficiency (1)	172430	1pter-p36.13
Enterokinase deficiency (1)	226200	21q21
Enuresis, nocturnal, 1 (2)	600631	13q13-q14.3
Enuresis, nocturnal, 2 (2)	600808	12q13-q21
Eosinophilia, familial (2)	131400	5q31-q33
?Eosinophilic myeloproliferative disorder (2)	131440	12p13
Epidermolysis bullosa dystrophica, Bart type, 132000 (3)	120120	3p21.3
Epidermolysis bullosa dystrophica, dominant, 131750 (3)	120120	3p21.3
Epidermolysis bullosa dystrophica, generalized atrophic benign, 226650 (3)	120120	3p21.3
Epidermolysis bullosa dystrophica, localisata variant (3)	120120	3p21.3
Epidermolysis bullosa dystrophica, recessive, 226600 (3)	120120	3p21.3
Epidermolysis bullosa, generalized atrophic benign, 226650 (3)	150310	1q32
Epidermolysis bullosa, generalized atropic benign, 226650 (3)	113811	10q24.3
Epidermolysis bullosa, generalized atrophic benign, 226650 (3)	147557	17q11-qter
Epidermolysis bullosa, Herlitz junctional type, 226700 (3)	150292	1q25-q31
Epidermolysis bullosa, Herlitz junctional type, 226700 (3)	150310	1q32
Epidermolysis bullosa inversa, junctional (2)	226450	1q31
Epidermolysis bullosa, junctional, Herlitz type (3)	600805	18q11.2
Epidermolysis bullosa, junctional, with pyloric atresia, 226730 (3)	147557	17q11-qter
Epidermolysis bullosa, junctional, with pyloric stenosis, 226730 (3)	147556	Chr.2
Epidermolysis bullosa, Ogna type (2)	131950	8q24
Epidermolysis bullosa, pretibial, dominant and recessive, 131850 (3)	120120	3p21.3
Epidermolysis bullosa pruriginosa, autosomal recessive, 604129 (3)	120120	3p21.3
Epidermolysis bullosa simplex, Koebner, Dowling-Meara, and Weber-Cockayne types, 131900, 131760, 131800 (3)	148040	12q13
Epidermolysis bullosa simplex, Koebner, Dowling-Meara, and Weber-Cockayne types, 131900, 131760, 131800 (3)	148066	17q12-q21
Epidermolysis bullosa simplex, recessive, 601001 (3)	148066	17q12-q21
Epidermolytic hyperkeratosis, 113800 (3)	139350	12q13
Epidermolytic hyperkeratosis, 113800 (3)	148080	17q21-q22
Epidermolytic palmoplantar keratoderma (3)	144200	17q12-q21
Epilepsy, benign, neonatal, type 1, 121200 (3)	602235	20q13.3
Epilepsy, benign neonatal, type 2, 121201 (3)	602232	8q24
Epilepsy, childhood absence, 1 (2)	600131	8q24
Epilepsy, female restricted, with mental retardation (2)	300088	Xq22

continued

Table 10.2. The morbid anatomy of the human genome (alphabetical by disorder) (*continued*)

Disorder	MIM#	Location
Epilepsy, generalized idiopathic, 600669 (3)	601949	2q22-q23
Epilepsy, generalized, idiopathic (2)	600669	8q24
Epilepsy, generalized, with febrile seizures plus, type 2, 604233 (3)	182389	2q24
Epilepsy, juvenile myoclonic (2)	604827	15q14
Epilepsy, juvenile myoclonic (2)	254770	6p
Epilepsy, juvenile myoclonic, 254770 (3)	601949	2q22-q23
Epilepsy, myoclonic, benign adult familial (2)	601068	8q23.3-q24.11
Epilepsy, myoclonic, infantile (2)	605021	16p13
Epilepsy, myoclonic, Lafora type (3)	254780	6q24
Epilepsy, nocturnal frontal lobe, 1, 600513 (3)	118504	20q13.2-q13.3
Epilepsy, nocturnal frontal lobe, 3, 605375 (3)	118507	1p21
Epilepsy, nocturnal frontal lobe, type 2 (2)	603204	15q24
Epilepsy, partial (2)	600512	10q23.3-q24.1
Epilepsy, partial, with variable foci (2)	604364	22q11-q12
Epilepsy, progressive myoclonic 1, 254800 (3)	601145	21q22.3
Epilepsy, progressive, with mental retardation (2)	600143	8pter-p22
Epilepsy, pyridoxine-dependent (2)	266100	5q31.2-q31.3
Epiphyseal dysplasia, multiple 1, 132400 (3)	600310	19p13.1
Epiphyseal dysplasia, multiple, 226900 (3)	222600	5q32-q33.1
Epiphyseal dysplasia, multiple, 3, 600969 (3)	120270	20q13.3
Epiphyseal dysplasia, multiple, type 2, 600204 (3)	120260	1p33-p32.2
Epiphyseal dysplasia, multiple, with myopathy (3)	120270	20q13.3
Epiphyseal dysplasia, multiple, with myopia and conductive deafness, 132450 (3)	120140	12q13.11-q13.2
Episodic ataxia, type 2, 108500 (3)	601011	19p13
Episodic ataxia/myokymia syndrome, 160120 (3)	176260	12p13
Episodic muscle weakness, X-linked (2)	300211	Xp22.3
Epithelioma, self-healing, squamous 1, Ferguson-Smith type (2)	132800	9q31
Erosive vitreoretinopathy (2)	143200	5q13-q14
?Erythremia (1)	133170	7q21
Erythremias, alpha- (3)	141800	16pter-p13.3
Erythremias, beta- (3)	141900	11p15.5
Erythrocytosis (3)	141850	16pter-p13.3
Erythrocytosis, autosomal recessive benign (2)	263400	11q23
[Erythrocytosis, familial], 133100 (3)	133171	19p13.3-p13.2
Erythrokeratoderma, progressive symmetric, 602036 (3)	152445	1q21
Erythrokeratodermia variabilis, 133200 (3)	603324	1p35.1
Erythrokeratodermia variabilis with erythema gyratum repens, 133200 (3)	605425	1p35.1
Esophageal cancer, 133239 (1)	604050	3p22-p21.3
Esophageal cancer, 133239 (3)	190182	3p22
Esophageal squamous cell carcinoma, 133239 (1)	604767	9q32
Estrogen resistance (3)	133430	6q25.1
[Euthyroidal hyper- and hypothyroxinemia] (1)	314200	Xq22.2
Ewing sarcoma (3)	133450	22q12
Exertional myoglobinuria due to deficiency of LDH-A (3)	150000	11p15.4
Exostoses, multiple, type 1 (3)	133700	8q24.11-q24.13
Exostoses, multiple, type 2 (3)	133701	11p12-p11
Exostoses, multiple, type 3 (2)	600209	19p
Exudative vitreoretinopathy, X-linked, 305390 (3)	310600	Xp11.4
Eye anomalies, multiplex (3)	106210	11p13
[Eye color, brown] (2)	227220	15q11-q15
Fabry disease (3)	301500	Xq22
Facioscapulohumeral muscular dystrophy-1A (2)	158900	4q35
Factor H deficiency (1)	134370	1q32
Factor VII deficiency (3)	227500	13q34
Factor X deficiency (3)	227600	13q34
Factor XI deficiency (3)	264900	4q35
Factor XII deficiency (3)	234000	5q33-qter
Factor XIIIA deficiency (3)	134570	6p25-p24

continued

Table 10.2. The morbid anatomy of the human genome (alphabetical by disorder) (*continued*)

Disorder	MIM#	Location
Factor XIIIB deficiency (3)	134580	1q31-q32.1
Faisalabad histiocytosis (2)	602782	11q25
Familial Mediterranean fever (3)	249100	16p13
Fanconi anemia, complementation group E (3)	600901	6p22-p21
Fanconi anemia, complementation group F (3)	603467	11p15
Fanconi anemia, complementation group G (3)	602956	9p13
Fanconi anemia, type A (3)	227650	16q24.3
Fanconi anemia, type C (3)	227645	9q22.3
Fanconi anemia, type D (2)	227646	3p25.3
Fanconi-Bickel syndrome, 227810 (3)	138160	3q26.1-q26.3
Farber lipogranulomatosis (3)	228000	8p22-p21.3
Fatty liver, acute, of pregnancy (3)	600890	2p23
Favism (3)	305900	Xq28
Fechtner syndrome, 153640 (3)	160775	22q11.2
{?Fetal alcohol syndrome} (1)	100650	12q24.2
?Fetal hydantoin syndrome (1)	132810	1q42.1
FG syndrome (2)	305450	Xq12-q21.31
Fibrodysplasia ossificans progressiva (2)	135100	4q27-q31
Fibromatosis, gingival (2)	135300	2p21
Fibrosis of extraocular muscles, congenital, 1 (2)	135700	12p11.2-q12
Fibrosis of extraocular muscles, congenital, 2 (2)	602078	11q13.2
Fibrosis of extraocular muscles, congenital, 3 (2)	604361	16q24.2-q24.3
Finnish lethal neonatal metabolic syndrome (2)	603358	2q33-q37
Fish-eye disease (3)	245900	16q22.1
[Fish-odor syndrome], 602079 (3)	136132	1q23-q25
Fletcher factor deficiency (1)	229000	4q35
{Fluorouracil toxicity, sensitivity to} (3)	274270	1p22
Foveal hypoplasia, isolated, 136520 (3)	106210	11p13
Foveomacular dystrophy, adult-onset, with choroidal neovascularization (3)	179605	6p21.1-cen
Fragile X syndrome (3)	309550	Xq27.3
Frasier syndrome, 136680 (3)	194070	11p13
Friedreich ataxia (3)	229300	9q13
Friedreich ataxia with retained reflexes (3)	229300	9q13
Fructose intolerance (3)	229600	9q22.3
Fructose-bisphosphatase deficiency (1)	229700	9q22.2-q22.3
[Fructosuria] (1)	229800	2p23.3-p23.2
Fucosidosis (3)	230000	1p34
Fucosyltransferase-6 deficiency (3)	136836	19p13.3
Fumarase deficiency (3)	136850	1q42.1
Fundus albipunctatus, 136880 (3)	601617	12q13-q14
Fundus flavimaculatus, 248200 (2)	601691	1p21-p13
G6PD deficiency (3)	305900	Xq28
GABA-transaminase deficiency (3)	137150	16p13.3
Galactokinase deficiency with cataracts, 230200 (3)	604313	17q24
Galactose epimerase deficiency (3)	230350	1p36-p35
Galactosemia (3)	230400	9p13
Galactosialidosis (3)	256540	20q13.1
[Gamma-glutamyltransferase, familial high serum] (2)	137181	22q11.1
GAMT deficiency (3)	601240	19p13.3
Gardner syndrome (3)	175100	5q21-q22
Gastric cancer, 137215 (3)	175100	5q21-q22
Gastric cancer, 137215 (3)	147575	5q31.1
Gastric cancer, familial, 137215 (3)	192090	16q22.1
Gastroesophageal reflux (2)	109350	13q14
Gaucher disease (3)	230800	1q21
Gaucher disease, variant form (3)	176801	10q22.1
Gaucher disease with cardiovascular calcification (3)	230800	1q21
Generalized epilepsy with febrile seizures plus (3)	600235	19q13.1

continued

Table 10.2. The morbid anatomy of the human genome (alphabetical by disorder) (*continued*)

Disorder	MIM#	Location
Geniospasm (2)	190100	9q13-q21
Germ cell tumor (3)	603517	1p22
Germ cell tumors, 273300 (3)	164920	4q12
Gerstmann-Straussler disease, 137440 (3)	176640	20pter-p12
Giant axonal neuropathy-1, 256850 (3)	605379	16q24.1
Giant cell hepatitis, neonatal, 231100 (3)	603711	8q21.3
Giant platelet disorder, isolated (3)	138720	22q11.2
Giant-cell fibroblastoma (3)	190040	22q12.3-q13.1
Gigantism due to GHRF hypersecretion (1)	139190	20q11.2
[Gilbert syndrome], 143500 (3)	191740	Chr.2
Gitelman syndrome, 263800 (3)	600968	16q13
Glanzmann thrombasthenia, type A (3)	273800	17q21.32
Glanzmann thrombasthenia, type B (3)	173470	17q21.32
Glaucoma 1A, primary open angle, juvenile-onset, 137750 (3)	601652	1q24.3-q25.2
Glaucoma 1A, primary open angle, recessive (3)	601652	1q24.3-q25.2
Glaucoma 1B, primary open angle, adult onset (2)	137760	2cen-q13
Glaucoma 1C, primary open angle (2)	601682	3q21-q24
Glaucoma 1D, primary open angle (2)	602429	8q23
Glaucoma 1E, primary open angle, adult-onset (2)	602432	Chr.10
Glaucoma 1F (2)	603383	7q35-q36
Glaucoma 3, primary infantile, B (2)	600975	1p36.2-p36.1
Glaucoma 3A, primary infantile, 231300 (3)	601771	2p22-p21
Glioblastoma multiforme, 137800 (3)	601969	10q25.3-q26.1
Glioma (1)	602116	12q13-q15
Gliosis, familial progressive subcortical (2)	221820	17q21-q22
Glomerulopathy, fibronectin (2)	601894	1q32
Glomerulosclerosis, focal segmental, 1, 603278 (3)	604638	19q13
Glomerulosclerosis, focal segmental, 2 (2)	603965	11q21-q22
Glomus tumors, multiple (2)	138000	1p22-p21
Glucocorticoid deficiency, due to ACTH unresponsiveness (1)	202200	18p11.2
Glucose transport defect, blood-brain barrier (3)	138140	1p35-p31.3
Glucose/galactose malabsorption (3)	182380	22q13.1
Glucosidase I deficiency (3)	601336	2p13-p12
Glutaricaciduria, type I (3)	231670	19p13.2
Glutaricaciduria, type IIA (1)	231680	15q23-q25
Glutaricaciduria, type IIB (3)	130410	19q13.3
Glutaricaciduria, type IIC (3)	231675	4q32-qter
Glutathioninuria (1)	231950	22q11.1-q11.2
Glycerol kinase deficiency (3)	307030	Xp21.3-p21.2
Glycogen storage disease I (3)	232200	17q21
Glycogen storage disease Ib, 232220 (3)	602671	11q23
Glycogen storage disease Ic, 232240 (3)	602671	11q23
Glycogen storage disease II (3)	232300	17q25.2-q25.3
Glycogen storage disease IIb, 300257 (3)	309060	Xq24
Glycogen storage disease IIIa (3)	232400	1p21
Glycogen storage disease IIIb (3)	232400	1p21
Glycogen storage disease IV (3)	232500	3p12
Glycogen storage disease, type 0, 240600 (3)	138571	12p12.2
Glycogen storage disease VI (3)	232700	14q21-q22
Glycogen storage disease VII (3)	232800	12q13.3
Glycogenosis, hepatic, autosomal (3)	172471	16p12.1-p11.2
Glycogenosis, X-linked hepatic, type I (3)	306000	Xp22.2-p22.1
Glycogenosis, X-linked hepatic, type II (3)	306000	Xp22.2-p22.1
?Glycoprotein Ia deficiency (2)	192974	5q23-q31
[Glyoxalase II deficiency] (1)	138760	16p13
GM1-gangliosidosis (3)	230500	3p21.33
GM2-gangliosidosis, AB variant (3)	272750	5q31.3-q33.1
GM2-gangliosidosis, several forms (3)	272800	15q23-q24

continued

Table 10.2. The morbid anatomy of the human genome (alphabetical by disorder) (*continued*)

Disorder	MIM#	Location
Goeminne TKCR syndrome (2)	314300	Xq28
Goiter, adolescent multinodular (1)	188450	8q24.2-q24.3
Goiter, congenital (3)	274500	2p25
Goiter, familial, due to TTF-1 defect (1)	600635	14q13
Goiter, multinodular, 1 (2)	138800	14q
Goiter, multinodular, 2 (2)	300273	Xp22
Goiter, nonendemic, simple (3)	188450	8q24.2-q24.3
?Goldenhar syndrome (2)	141400	7p
Gonadal dysgenesis, 46XY, partial, with minifascicular neuropathy (3)	605423	12q13.1
Gonadal dysgenesis, XY female type (2)	306100	Xp22.11-p21.2
Gonadal dysgenesis, XY type (3)	480000	Yp11.3
?Gonadotropin deficiency (2)	306190	Xp21
Graves disease, 275000 (1)	603372	14q31
{Graves disease, susceptibility to, 2} (2)	603388	20q13.11
Greig cephalopolysyndactyly syndrome, 175700 (3)	165240	7p13
Griscelli syndrome, 214450 (3)	603868	15q21
Griscelli syndrome-type pigmentary dilution with mental retardation, 214450 (3)	160777	15q21
Growth hormone deficient dwarfism (3)	139191	7p15-p14
Growth retardation with deafness and mental retardation (3)	147440	12q22-q24.1
Gustavson syndrome (2)	309555	Xq26
Gynecomastia, familial, due to increased aromatase activity (1)	107910	15q21.1
Gyrate atrophy of choroid and retina with ornithinemia, B6 responsive or unresponsive (3)	258870	10q26
Hailey-Hailey disease, 169600 (3)	604384	3q21-q24
Haim-Munk syndrome, 245010 (3)	602365	11q14.1-q14.3
[Hair color, brown] (2)	601800	15q11-q15
[Hair color, red] (2)	266300	4q28-q31
Hand-foot-uterus syndrome, 140000 (3)	142959	7p15-p14.2
Harderoporphyrinuria (3)	121300	3q12
HDL deficiency, familial, 604091 (3)	600046	9q22-q31
HDR syndrome (2)	146255	10p15.1-p14
Heart block, nonprogressive, 604559 (3)	600163	3p21
Heart block, progressive, 2, 604559 (3)	600163	3p21
Heart block, progressive familial, type I (2)	113900	19q13.2-q13.3
Heinz body anemia (3)	141850	16pter-p13.3
Heinz body anemias, alpha- (3)	141800	16pter-p13.3
Heinz body anemias, beta- (3)	141900	11p15.5
HELLP syndrome, maternal, of pregnancy (3)	600890	2p23
Hemangioma, capillary infantile (2)	602089	5q31-q33
Hematuria, familial benign (3)	120131	2q36-q37
Heme oxygenase-1 deficiency (3)	141250	22q12
Hemiplegic migraine, familial, 141500 (3)	601011	19p13
Hemochromatosis (3)	235200	6p21.3
Hemochromatosis, 604250 (3)	604720	7q22
Hemochromatosis, type 2 (2)	602390	1q
Hemodialysis-related amyloidosis (1)	109700	15q21-q22
Hemoglobin H disease (3)	141850	16pter-p13.3
Hemolytic anemia due to ADA excess (1)	102700	20q13.11
Hemolytic anemia due to adenylate kinase deficiency (3)	103000	9q34.1
Hemolytic anemia due to band 3 defect (3)	109270	17q21-q22
Hemolytic anemia due to bisphosphoglycerate mutase deficiency (1)	222800	7q31-q34
Hemolytic anemia due to G6PD deficiency (3)	305900	Xq28
Hemolytic anemia due to gamma-glutamylcysteine synthetase deficiency (1)	230450	6p12
Hemolytic anemia due to glucosephosphate isomerase deficiency (3)	172400	19q13.1
Hemolytic anemia due to glutathione peroxidase deficiency (1)	138320	3p21.3
Hemolytic anemia due to glutathione reductase deficiency (1)	138300	8p21.1
Hemolytic anemia due to glutathione synthetase deficiency, 231900 (3)	601002	20q11.2
Hemolytic anemia due to hexokinase deficiency (3)	142600	10q22
Hemolytic anemia due to PGK deficiency (3)	311800	Xq13

continued

Table 10.2. The morbid anatomy of the human genome (alphabetical by disorder) (*continued*)

Disorder	MIM#	Location
Hemolytic anemia due to phosphofructokinase deficiency (1)	171860	21q22.3
Hemolytic anemia due to triosephosphate isomerase deficiency (3)	190450	12p13
Hemolytic-uremic syndrome, 235400 (3)	134370	1q32
Hemophagocytic lymphohistiocytosis, familial, 1 (2)	603552	9q21.3-q22
Hemophagocytic lymphohistiocytosis, familial, 2, 603553 (3)	170280	10q22
Hemophilia A (3)	306700	Xq28
Hemophilia B (3)	306900	Xq27.1-q27.2
Hemorrhagic diathesis due to "antithrombin" Pittsburgh (3)	107400	14q32.1
Hemorrhagic diathesis due to factor V deficiency (1)	227400	1q23
Hemorrhagic diathesis due to PAI1 deficiency (1)	173360	7q21.3-q22
Hemosiderosis, systemic, due to aceruloplasminemia (3)	117700	3q23-q24
Hepatic failure, early onset, and neurologic disorder (3)	603644	17p13-p12
{Hepatic fibrosis susceptibility due to Schistosoma mansoni infection} (2)	604201	6q22-q23
Hepatic lipase deficiency (3)	151670	15q21-q23
Hepatoblastoma (3)	116806	3p22-p21.3
Hepatocellular cancer, 114550 (3)	604584	8p22-p21.3
Hepatocellular carcinoma (1)	114550	11p14-p13
?Hepatocellular carcinoma (1)	165320	2q14-q21
Hepatocellular carcinoma, 114550 (3)	603816	16p13.3
Hepatocellular carcinoma (3)	142380	4q32.1
Hepatocellular carcinoma (3)	147280	6q26
Hepatocellular carcinoma, childhood type, 114550 (3)	164860	7q31
Hereditary hemorrhagic telangiectasia-1, 187300 (3)	131195	9q34.1
Hereditary hemorrhagic telangiectasia-2, 600376 (3)	601284	12q11-q14
[Hereditary persistence of alpha-fetoprotein] (3)	104150	4q11-q13
[Hereditary persistence of fetal hemoglobin, heterocellular] (2)	142470	6q22.3-q23.1
?Hereditary persistence of fetal hemoglobin, heterocellular, Indian type (2)	142335	7q36
Hermansky-Pudlak syndrome, 203300 (3)	604982	10q23.1-q23.3
Hermansky-Pudlak syndrome, 203300 (3)	603401	Chr. 5
Heterocellular hereditary persistence of fetal hemoglobin, Swiss type (2)	305435	Xp22.2
Heterotaxy, X-linked visceral, 306955 (3)	300265	Xq26.2
Heterotopia, periventricular, 300049 (3)	300017	Xq28
[Hex A pseudodeficiency] (3)	272800	15q23-q24
[High bone mass] (2)	601884	11q12-q13
Hip dysplasia, Beukes type (2)	142669	4q35
Hirschsprung disease, 142623 (3)	164761	10q11.2
Hirschsprung disease, 142623 (3)	602018	19p13.3
Hirschsprung disease, 142623 (3)	600837	5p13.1-p12
Hirschsprung disease, cardiac defects, and autonomic dysfunction (3)	600423	1p36.1
Hirschsprung disease-2, 600155 (3)	131244	13q22
[Histidinemia] (1)	235800	12q22-q23
{HIV infection, susceptibility/resistance to} (3)	601373	3p21
{HIV infection, susceptibility/resistence to} (3)	601267	3p21
{HIV-1 disease, delayed progression of} (2)	187011	17q11.2-q12
HMG-CoA lyase deficiency (3)	246450	1pter-p33
HMG-CoA synthase-2 deficiency (1)	600234	1p13-p12
{Hodgkin disease susceptibility, pseudoautosomal} (2)	300221	Xpter-p22.32
Holoprosencephaly-1 (2)	236100	21q22.3
Holoprosencephaly-2, 157170 (3)	603714	2p21
Holoprosencephaly-3, 142945 (3)	600725	7q36
Holoprosencephaly-4, 142946 (3)	602630	18p11.3
Holoprosencephaly-5 (3)	603073	13q32
Holt-Oram syndrome, 142900 (3)	601620	12q24.1
Homocystinuria, B6-responsive and nonresponsive types (3)	236200	21q22.3
Homocystinuria due to MTHFR deficiency (3)	236250	1p36.3
Homocystinuria-megaloblastic anemia, cbl E type, 236270 (3)	602568	5p15.3-p15.2
[?Homosexuality, male] (2)	306995	Xq28
Hoyeraal-Hreidarsson syndrome, 300240 (3)	300126	Xq28

continued

Table 10.2. The morbid anatomy of the human genome (alphabetical by disorder) (*continued*)

Disorder	MIM#	Location
HPFH, deletion type (3)	141900	11p15.5
HPFH, nondeletion type A (3)	142200	11p15.5
HPFH, nondeletion type G (3)	142250	11p15.5
HPRT-related gout (3)	308000	Xq26-q27.2
?Humoral hypercalcemia of malignancy (1)	168470	12p12.1-p11.2
Huntington disease (3)	143100	4p16.3
Huntington-like neurodegenerative disorder 1 (2)	603218	20p
Huntington-like neurodegenerative disorder 2 (2)	604802	4p15.3
Huriez syndrome (2)	181600	4q23
Hydatidiform mole (2)	231090	19q13.3-q13.4
Hydrocephalus due to aqueductal stenosis, 307000 (3)	308840	Xq28
Hydrolethalus syndrome (2)	236680	11q23-q25
Hydrops fetalis, one form (1)	172400	19q13.1
Hyperbetalipoproteinemia, 144400 (3)	107730	2p24
Hypercalciuria, absorptive (2)	143870	4q33-qter
Hypercalciuria, absorptive, 2 (2)	605329	1q23.3-q24
Hypercalciuric hypercalcemia, type III (2)	600740	19q13
Hypercholesterolemia, familial (3)	143890	19p13.2
Hypercholesterolemia, familial, 3 (2)	603776	1p34.1-p32
Hypercholesterolemia, familial, autosomal recessive (2)	603813	15q25-q26
Hyperekplexia and spastic paraparesis (3)	138491	5q32
Hyperferritinemia-cataract syndrome, 600886 (3)	134790	19q13.3-q13.4
Hyperglycerolemia (3)	307030	Xp21.3-p21.2
Hyperglycinemia, nonketotic, 1 (3)	238300	9p22
Hyperglycinemia, nonketotic, 2 (1)	238310	3p21.2-p21.1
Hyper-IgE syndrome (2)	147060	4q21
?Hyperimmunoglobulin G1 syndrome (2)	144120	14q32.33
Hyperimmunoglobulinemia D and periodic fever syndrome, 260920 (3)	251170	12q24
Hyperinsulinism, familial, 602485 (3)	138079	7p15-p13
Hyperinsulinism-hyperammonemia syndrome (3)	138130	10q23.3
Hyperkalemic periodic paralysis, 170500 (3)	603967	17q23.1-q25.3
?Hyperleucinemia-isoleucinemia or hypervalinemia (1)	113520	12p12
Hyperlipidemia, combined, 2 (2)	604499	11p
Hyperlipidemia, familial combined, 1 (2)	602491	1q21-q23
Hyperlipoproteinemia I (1)	238600	8p22
Hyperlipoproteinemia, type Ib (3)	207750	19q13.2
Hyperlipoproteinemia, type III (3)	107741	19q13.2
Hyperlysinemia, 238700 (3)	605113	7q31.3
Hypermethioninemia, persistent, autosomal dominant, due to methionine adenosyltransferase I/III deficiency (3)	250850	10q22
Hyperornithinemia-hyperammonemia-homocitrullinemia syndrome, 238970 (3)	603861	13q14
Hyperoxaluria, primary, type I, 259900 (3)	604285	2q36-q37
Hyperoxaluria, primary, type II, 260000 (3)	604296	9cen
Hyperparathyroidism, AD, 145000 (3)	131100	11q13
Hyperparathyroidism, familial primary, 145000 (2)	145001	1q25-q31
Hyperparathyroidism-jaw tumor syndrome (2)	145001	1q25-q31
Hyperphenylalaninemia due to pterin-4a-carbinolamine dehydratase deficiency, 264070 (3)	126090	10q22
[Hyperphenylalaninemia, mild] (3)	261600	12q24.1
[?Hyperproglucagonemia] (1)	138030	2q36-q37
Hyperproinsulinemia, familial (3)	176730	11p15.5
Hyperprolinemia, type I (1)	239500	22q11.2
Hyperprolinemia, type II (3)	239510	1p36
[Hyperproreninemia] (3)	179820	1q32
Hypertension, early-onset, autosomal dominant, with exacerbation in pregnancy, 605115 (3)	600983	4q31.1
{?Hypertension, essential} (1)	145505	16p13.11
?Hypertension, essential, 145500 (1)	171190	17q21-q22
Hypertension, essential, 145500 (3)	106165	3q21-q25
{Hypertension, essential, susceptibility to, 1}, 145500 (2)	603918	17q

continued

Table 10.2. The morbid anatomy of the human genome (alphabetical by disorder) (*continued*)

Disorder	MIM#	Location
{Hypertension, essential, susceptibility to}, 145500 (3)	139130	12p13
{Hypertension, essential, susceptibility to, 2} (2)	604329	15q
{Hypertension, essential, susceptibility to} (3)	106150	1q42-q43
Hypertension, mild low-renin (3)	218030	16q22
?Hypertension, salt-resistant (1)	108962	5p14-p12
Hypertension with brachydactyly (2)	112410	12p12.2-p11.2
Hyperthroidism, congenital (3)	603372	14q31
Hypertrichosis, congenital generalized (2)	307150	Xq24-q27.1
Hypertriglyceridemia (3)	107720	11q23
Hypertriglyceridemia, one form (3)	107680	11q23
{Hypertriglyceridemia, susceptibility to} (2)	145750	15q11.2-q13.1
{Hypertrypsinemia, neonatal} (3)	602421	7q31.2
?Hypervalinemia or hyperleucine-isoleucinemia (1)	113530	19q13
Hypoalphalipoproteinemia (3)	107680	11q23
Hypoalphalipoproteinemia, primary (2)	605201	11q23.3
Hypobetalipoproteinemia (3)	107730	2p24
Hypobetalipoproteinemia, familial, 2 (2)	605019	3p22-p21.1
Hypocalcemia, autosomal dominant, 601198 (3)	601199	3q13.3-q21
Hypocalciuric hypercalcemia, type I, 145980 (3)	601199	3q13.3-q21
Hypocalciuric hypercalcemia, type II (2)	145981	19p13.3
[Hypoceruloplasminemia, hereditary] (1)	117700	3q23-q24
Hypochondrogenesis (3)	120140	12q13.11-q13.2
Hypochondroplasia, 146000 (3)	134934	4p16.3
Hypochromic microcytic anemia (3)	141850	16pter-p13.3
Hypodontia, autosomal dominant, 106600 (3)	142983	4p16.1
Hypodontia, autosomal recessive (2)	602639	16q12.1
Hypodontia with orofacial cleft, 106600 (3)	142983	4p16.1
Hypofibrinogenemia, gamma type (3)	134850	4q28
Hypoglobulinemia and absent B cells (3)	604515	10q23.2
?Hypoglycemia due to PCK1 deficiency (1)	261680	20q13.31
Hypogonadism, hypergonadotropic (3)	152780	19q13.32
Hypogonadotropic hypogonadism (3)	152790	2p21
Hypogonadotropic hypogonadism (3)	138850	4q21.2
?Hypogonadotropic hypogonadism due to GNRH deficiency, 227200 (1)	152760	8p21-p11.2
[Hypohaptoglobinemia] (3)	140100	16q22.1
Hypokalemic periodic paralysis, 170400 (3)	114208	1q32
Hypomagnesemia, primary, 248250 (3)	603959	3q27
Hypomagnesemia with secondary hypocalcemia (2)	602014	9q12-q22.2
Hypomagnesemia-2, renal, 154020 (3)	601814	11q23
Hypomyelination, congenital (3)	159440	1q22
Hypoparathyroidism, autosomal dominant (3)	168450	11p15.3-p15.1
Hypoparathyroidism, autosomal recessive (3)	168450	11p15.3-p15.1
Hypoparathyroidism, familial (2)	146200	3q13
Hypoparathyroidism, sensorineural deafness, and renal dysplasia, 146255 (3)	131320	10p15
Hypoparathyroidism, X-linked (2)	307700	Xq26-q27
Hypoparathyroidism-retardation-dysmorphism syndrome (2)	241410	1q42-q43
?Hypophosphatasia, adult, 146300 (1)	171760	1p36.1-p34
Hypophosphatasia, childhood, 241510 (3)	171760	1p36.1-p34
Hypophosphatasia, infantile, 241500 (3)	171760	1p36.1-p34
Hypophosphatemia, hereditary (3)	307800	Xp22.2-p22.1
Hypophosphatemia, type III (3)	300008	Xp11.22
Hypophosphatemic rickets, autosomal dominant, 193100 (3)	605380	12p13.3
Hypoprothrombinemia (3)	176930	11p11-q12
Hypotrichosis simplex (2)	605389	18p11.32-p11.23
Hypothyroidism, congenital, 274400 (3)	601843	19p13.2-p12
Hypothyroidism, congenital (3)	274500	2p25
Hypothyroidism, congenital, due to thyroid dysgenesis or hypoplasia (3)	167415	2q12-q14
Hypothyroidism, congenital, due to TSH resistance, 275200 (3)	603372	14q31

continued

Table 10.2. The morbid anatomy of the human genome (alphabetical by disorder) (*continued*)

Disorder	MIM#	Location
Hypothyroidism, hereditary congenital (3)	188450	8q24.2-q24.3
Hypothyroidism, nongoitrous (3)	188540	1p13
Hypotrichosis, Marie Unna type (2)	146550	8p21
Hypotrichosis simplex of scalp (2)	146520	6p21.3
Ichthyosiform erythroderma, congenital, 242100 (3)	190195	14q11.2
Ichthyosiform erythroderma, congenital, nonbullous, 2 (2)	604780	3p21
Ichthyosis bullosa of Siemens, 146800 (3)	600194	12q11-q13
Ichthyosis, lamellar, autosomal recessive, 242300 (3)	190195	14q11.2
Ichthyosis, lamellar, type 2 (2)	601277	2q33-q35
Ichthyosis, lamellar, type 3 (2)	604777	19p12-q12
Ichthyosis, nonlamellar and nonerythrodermic, congenital (2)	604781	19p13.2-p13.1
?Ichthyosis vulgaris, 146700 (1)	135940	1q21
Ichthyosis, X-linked (3)	308100	Xp22.32
[IgG receptor I, phagocytic, familial deficiency of] (1)	146760	1q21.2-q21.3
IgG2 deficiency, selective (3)	147110	14q32.33
[Ii blood group, 110800] (1)	600429	Chr. 6
IMAGE syndrome (2)	300290	Chr. X
Immotile cilia syndrome-1, 242650 (3)	604366	9p21-p13
Immunodeficiency due to defect in CD3-gamma (3)	186740	11q23
Immunodeficiency, T-cell receptor/CD3 complex (3)	186830	11q23
Immunodeficiency with hyper-IgM, type 2, 605258 (3)	605257	12p13
Immunodeficiency, X-linked, with hyper-IgM (3)	308230	Xq26
Immunodeficiency-centromeric instability-facial anomalies syndrome, 242860 (3)	602900	20q11.2
Immunoglobulin A deficiency (2)	137100	6p21.3
Inclusion body myopathy, autosomal recessive (2)	600737	9p1-q1
Incontinentia pigmenti, type II, 308310 (3)	300248	Xq28
Infantile spasm syndrome, X-linked (2)	308350	Xp22.1-p21.3
Inflammatory bowel disease 3 (2)	604519	6p
Inflammatory bowel disease 7 (2)	605225	1p36
Inflammatory bowel disease-1 (2)	266600	16p12-q13
Inflammatory bowel disease-2 (2)	601458	12p13.2-q24.1
[Inosine triphosphatase deficiency] (1)	147520	20p
Insensitivity to pain, congenital, with anhidrosis, 256800 (3)	191315	1q21-q22
Insomnia, fatal familial (3)	176640	20pter-p12
Interferon, alpha, deficiency (1)	147660	9p22
Interferon, immune, deficiency (1)	147570	12q14
Interleukin-2 receptor, alpha chain, deficiency of (3)	147730	10p15-p14
Intervertebral disc disease, 603932 (3)	120260	1p33-p32.2
Intestinal pseudoobstruction, neuronal, X-linked (2)	300048	Xq28
Iridogoniodysgenesis, 601631 (3)	601090	6p25
Iridogoniodysgenesis syndrome-2, 137600 (3)	601542	4q25-q26
Iris hypoplasia and glaucoma (3)	601090	6p25
?Isolated growth hormone deficiency due to defect in GHRF (1)	139190	20q11.2
Isolated growth hormone deficiency, Illig type with absent GH and Kowarski type with bioinactive GH (3)	139250	17q22-q24
Isovalericacidemia (3)	243500	15q14-q15
Jackson-Weiss sydnrome, 123150 (3)	136350	8p11.2-p11.1
Jackson-Weiss syndrome, 123150 (3)	176943	10q26
Jacobsen syndrome (2)	147791	11q23
Jensen syndrome, 311150 (3)	304700	Xq22
Jervell and Lange-Nielsen syndrome, 220400 (3)	192500	11p15.5
Jervell and Lange-Nielsen syndrome, 220400 (3)	176261	21q22.1-q22.2
Joubert syndrome-1 (2)	213300	9q34.3
Juberg-Marsidi syndrome, 309590 (3)	300032	Xq13
Kallmann syndrome (3)	308700	Xp22.3
Kanzaki disease (3)	104170	22q11
[Kappa light chain deficiency] (3)	147200	2p12
Kartagener syndrome (2)	244400	19q13.3-qter

continued

Table 10.2. The morbid anatomy of the human genome (alphabetical by disorder) (*continued*)

Disorder	MIM#	Location
Kenny-Caffey syndrome-1 (2)	244460	1q42-q43
Keratitis, 148190 (3)	106210	11p13
Keratoderma, palmoplantar, nonepidermolytic (3)	139350	12q13
Keratoderma, palmoplantar, with deafness, 148350 (3)	121011	13q11-q12
Keratolytic winter erythema (2)	148370	8p23-p22
Keratosis follicularis spinulosa decalvans (2)	308800	Xp22.2-p22.13
Keratosis palmoplantaris striata I, 148700 (3)	125670	18q12.1-q12.2
Keratosis palmoplantaris striata II (3)	125647	6p24
Ketoacidosis due to SCOT deficiency (3)	245050	5p13
3-Ketothiolase deficiency (3)	203750	11q22.3-q23.1
Keutel syndrome, 245150 (3)	154870	12p13.1-p12.3
[Kininogen deficiency] (3)	228960	3q27
?Klippel-Feil syndrome (2)	214300	5q11.2
Klippel-Feil syndrome with laryngeal malformation (2)	148900	8q22.2
Kniest dysplasia, 156550 (3)	120140	12q13.11-q13.2
Kniest dysplasia (3)	120140	12q13.11-q13.2
Knobloch syndrome (2)	267750	21q22.3
Kostmann neutropenia, 202700 (3)	138971	1p35-p34.3
Krabbe disease (3)	245200	14q31
Lactate dehydrogenase-B deficiency (3)	150100	12p12.2-p12.1
Lactic acidosis due to defect in iron-sulfur cluster of complex I (1)	157655	2q33-q34
Lacticacidemia due to PDX1 deficiency (3)	245349	11p13
?Lactoferrin-deficient neutrophils, 245480 (1)	150210	3q21-q23
Langer mesomelic dysplasia, 249700 (3)	312865	Xpter-p22.32
Langer-Giedion syndrome (2)	150230	8q24.11-q24.13
Laron dwarfism, 262500 (3)	600946	5p13-p12
Larsen syndrome, autosomal dominant (2)	150250	3p21.1-p14.1
?Laryngeal adductor paralysis (2)	150270	6p21.3-p21.2
LCHAD deficiency (3)	600890	2p23
{Lead poisoning, susceptibility to} (3)	125270	9q34
Leber congenital amaurosis 5 (2)	604537	6q11-q16
Leber congenital amaurosis, 604393 (3)	604392	17p13.1
Leber congenital amaurosis due to defect in CRX, 204000 (3)	602225	19q13.3
Leber congenital amaurosis, type I, 204000 (3)	600179	17p13.1
Leber congenital amaurosis, type III (2)	604232	14q24
Leber congenital amaurosis-2, 204100 (3)	180069	1p31
Left-right axis malformation (3)	601877	1q42.1
Leigh syndrome, 256000 (3)	602141	11q13
Leigh syndrome, 256000 (3)	161015	11q13
Leigh syndrome, 256000 (3)	601825	19p13
Leigh syndrome (3)	600857	5p15
Leigh syndrome, due to COX deficiency, 256000 (3)	185620	9q34
Leigh syndrome, French-Canadian type (2)	220111	Chr. 2
?Leiomyoma, multiple hereditary cutaneous (2)	150800	18p11.32
Leiomyomatosis, diffuse, with Alport syndrome, 308940 (3)	303631	Xq22.3
Leprechaunism, 246200 (3)	147670	19p13.2
Leri-Weill dyschondrosteosis, 127300 (3)	312865	Xpter-p22.32
Lesch-Nyhan syndrome (3)	308000	Xq26-q27.2
Lethal congenital contracture syndrome (2)	253310	9q34
Leukemia (3)	120436	3p21.3
Leukemia, acute lymphoblastic (1)	600618	12p13
Leukemia, acute lymphoblastic (1)	147141	19p13.3
Leukemia, acute lymphoblastic (2)	247640	9p22-p21
Leukemia, acute lymphoblastic (3)	603023	7p12
Leukemia, acute myeloblastic (3)	126110	1q21
Leukemia, acute myelogenous (2)	602439	16q22
Leukemia, acute myeloid (1)	601768	19p13
Leukemia, acute myeloid (1)	151385	21q22.3

continued

Table 10.2. The morbid anatomy of the human genome (alphabetical by disorder) (*continued*)

Disorder	MIM#	Location
Leukemia, acute myeloid (2)	114350	9q34.1
Leukemia, acute myeloid (3)	602409	10p12
Leukemia, acute myeloid (3)	603025	11q14
Leukemia, acute myeloid (3)	604763	11q23.3
{Leukemia, acute myeloid} (3)	604332	4q11-q12
Leukemia, acute myeloid, M2 type (1)	306250	Xp22.32
Leukemia, acute myeloid, therapy-related (1)	604061	17q25
Leukemia, acute myeloid, with eosinophilia (1)	164690	1q24-q25
Leukemia, acute myelomonocytic (3)	604684	1q21
Leukemia, acute nonlymphocytic (2)	125264	6p23
Leukemia, acute pre-B-cell (2)	176310	1q23
Leukemia, acute promyelocytic (1)	180240	17q12
Leukemia, acute promyelocytic, NPM/RARA type (3)	164040	5q35
Leukemia, acute promyelocytic, NUMA/RARA type (3)	164009	11q13
Leukemia, acute promyelocytic, PL2F/RARA type (3)	176797	11q23.1
Leukemia, acute promyelocytic, PML/RARA type (3)	102578	15q22
Leukemia, acute T-cell (2)	180385	11p13
Leukemia, acute T-cell (2)	151390	11p13
Leukemia, acute T-cell lymphoblastic (3)	602409	10p12
Leukemia, acute T-cell lymphoblastic (3)	603025	11q14
Leukemia, chronic lymphocytic, B-cell (2)	109543	13q14
Leukemia, chronic myeloid (3)	151410	22q11.21
Leukemia, chronic myeloid (3)	189980	9q34.1
Leukemia, juvenile myelomonocytic (3)	162200	17q11.2
Leukemia, juvenile myelomonocytic (3)	605370	5q31
Leukemia, lymphycytic, acute T-cell (1)	601021	11p15
Leukemia, myeloid, acute (1)	601402	3q25.1
Leukemia, myeloid/lymphoid or mixed-lineage (2)	159555	11q23
{Leukemia, post-chemotherapy, susceptibility to} (3)	125860	16q22.1
Leukemia, T-cell acute lymphoblastic (2)	186921	11p15
Leukemia, T-cell acute lymphoblastic (2)	190198	9q34.3
Leukemia, T-cell acute lymphoblastoid (2)	151440	19p13.2-p13.1
Leukemia, T-cell acute lymphocytic (2)	186770	10q24
Leukemia, transient, of Down syndrome (2)	159595	21q11.2
Leukemia-1, T-cell acute lymphocytic (3)	187040	1p32
Leukemia-2, T-cell acute lymphoblastic (3)	186855	9q31
Leukemia/lymphoma, B-cell, 1 (2)	151400	11q13.3
Leukemia/lymphoma, B-cell, 2 (2)	151430	18q21.3
Leukemia/lymphoma, B-cell, 3 (2)	109560	19q13
Leukemia/lymphoma, T-cell (2)	186960	14q32.1
Leukemia/lymphoma, T-cell (2)	603769	14q32.1
Leukemia/lymphoma, T-cell (2)	186860	2q34
Leukemia/lymphoma, T-cell (3)	186880	14q11.2
Leukocyte adhesion deficiency, 116920 (3)	600065	21q22.3
Leukoencephalopathy, vacuoliting megalencephalic, with subcortical cysts (2)	604004	22qter
Leukoencephalopathy with vanishing white matter (2)	603896	3q27
Leukotriene C4 synthase deficiency (1)	246530	5q35
Leydig cell adenoma, with precocious puberty (3)	152790	2p21
Lhermitte-Duclos syndrome (3)	601728	10q23.3
Liddle syndrome, 177200 (3)	600760	16p13-p12
Liddle syndrome, 177200 (3)	600761	16p13-p12
Li-Fraumeni syndrome, 151623 (3)	604373	22q12.1
Li-Fraumeni syndrome (3)	191170	17p13.1
Limb-mammary syndrome (2)	603543	3q27
Lipoamide dehydrogenase deficiency (3)	246900	7q31-q32
Lipodystrophy, familial partial, 151660 (3)	150330	1q21.2
Lipoid adrenal hyperplasia, 201710 (3)	600617	8p11.2
Lipoma (1)	600700	3q28

continued

Table 10.2. The morbid anatomy of the human genome (alphabetical by disorder) (*continued*)

Disorder	MIM#	Location
?Lipoma (1)	600701	6p21
Lipoma (3)	600698	12q15
Lipoma, sporadic (3)	131100	11q13
?Lipomatosis, mutiple, 151900 (2)	600698	12q15
Lipoprotein lipase deficiency (3)	238600	8p22
Liposarcoma (1)	164953	19p13.2-q13.3
Lissencephaly syndrome, Norman-Roberts type, 257320 (3)	600514	7q22
Lissencephaly, X-linked, 300067 (3)	300121	Xq22.3-q23
Lissencephaly-1 (3)	601545	17p13.3
{?Liver disease, susceptibility to, from hepatotoxins or viruses} (1)	148070	12q13
Long QT syndrome-1 (3)	192500	11p15.5
Long QT syndrome-2 (3)	152427	7q35-q36
Long QT syndrome-3, 603830 (3)	600163	3p21
Long QT syndrome-4 with sinus bradycardia (2)	600919	4q25-q27
Long QT syndrome-5 (3)	176261	21q22.1-q22.2
Long QT syndrome-6 (3)	603796	21q22.1
Lowe syndrome (3)	309000	Xq26.1
Lung cancer, 211980 (1)	604050	3p22-p21.3
Lung cancer, 211980 (3)	603113	11q22-q24
Lung cancer, 211980 (3)	602631	11p15.5
Lung cancer, small cell (3)	182452	17q24
{Lupus erythematosus, susceptibility to} (2)	186940	12pter-p12
{Lupus erythematosus, systemic, susceptibility}, 152700 (1)	146740	1q23
{Lupus nephritis, susceptibility to} (3)	146790	1q21-q23
Lymphangioleiomyomatosis, somatic (3)	191092	16p13.3
Lymphedema, hereditary I, 153100 (3)	136352	5q35.3
Lymphedema with distichiasis (2)	153400	16q24.3
Lymphocytic leukemia, acute T-cell (3)	179502	4q21-q25
Lymphoma, B-cell (2)	109565	3q27
Lymphoma, B-cell non-Hodgkin, somatic (3)	208900	11q22.3
Lymphoma, diffuse large cell (3)	601889	15q11-q13
Lymphoma, diffuse large cell (3)	109565	3q27
Lymphoma, follicular (3)	603517	1p22
Lymphoma, MALT (3)	603517	1p22
Lymphoma, mantel cell (3)	208900	11q22.3
Lymphoma, non-Hodgkin (3)	603615	1p32
Lymphoma, non-Hodgkin (3)	604289	8q21.3-q22
Lymphoma, progression of (3)	604590	1q22
Lymphoma/leukemia, B-cell, variant (1)	136440	18q21.3
Lymphoproliferative syndrome, X-linked (3)	308240	Xq25
?Lynch cancer family syndrome II (2)	114400	18q11-q12
Lysinuric protein intolerance, 222700 (3)	603593	14q11.2
?Lysosomal acid phosphatase deficiency (1)	171650	11p12-p11
Machado-Joseph disease (3)	109150	14q24.3-q31
Macrocytic anemia, refractory, of 5q- syndrome, 153550 (3)	147575	5q31.1
[Macrothrombocytopenia] (1)	173510	7q11.2
Macular corneal dystrophy, 217800 (3)	605294	16q22
Macular degeneration, age-related, 1 (2)	603075	1q25-q31
Macular dystrophy (3)	179605	6p21.1-cen
Macular dystrophy, age-related, 2, 153800 (3)	601691	1p21-p13
Macular dystrophy, atypical vitelliform (2)	153840	8q24
Macular dystrophy, autosomal dominant, chromosome 6-linked, 600110 (3)	605512	6q14
Macular dystrophy, dominant cystoid (2)	153880	7p21-p15
Macular dystrophy, North Carolina type (2)	136550	6q14-q16.2
Macular dystrophy, vitelliform (3)	179605	6p21.1-cen
Macular dystrophy, vitelliform type (3)	153700	11q13
{Malaria, cerebral, susceptibility to} (3)	147840	19p13.3-p13.2
{Malaria, cerebral, susceptibility to} (3)	191160	6p21.3

continued

Table 10.2. The morbid anatomy of the human genome (alphabetical by disorder) (*continued*)

Disorder	MIM#	Location
Male germ cell tumor (2)	273300	12q22
?Male infertility (1)	179095	5q23-q31
?Male infertility due to acrosin deficiency (2)	102480	22q13-qter
?Male infertility, familial (1)	136530	11p13
?Male pseudohermaphroditism due to defective LH (1)	152780	19q13.32
Malignant fibrous histiocytoma (2)	605352	8p23.1
{Malignant hyperthermia susceptibility 1}, 145600 (3)	180901	19q13.1
{Malignant hyperthermia susceptibility 2} (2)	154275	17q11.2-q24
{Malignant hyperthermia susceptibility 3} (2)	154276	7q21-q22
{Malignant hyperthermia susceptibility 4} (2)	600467	3q13.1
{Malignant hyperthermia susceptibility 5}, 601887 (3)	114208	1q32
{Malignant hyperthermia susceptibility 6} (2)	601888	5p
Malignant melanoma, cutaneous (2)	155600	1p36
Malignant mesothelioma, sporadic (3)	101000	22q12.2
Malonyl-CoA decarboxylase deficiency (3)	248360	16q24
?Manic-depressive illness, X-linked (2)	309200	Xq28
Mannosidosis, alpha-, types I and II (3)	248500	19cen-q12
Mannosidosis, beta- (3)	248510	4q22-q25
Maple syrup urine disease, type Ia (3)	248600	19q13.1-q13.2
Maple syrup urine disease, type Ib (3)	248611	6p22-p21
Maple syrup urine disease, type II (3)	248610	1p31
Marfan syndrome, 154700 (3)	134797	15q21.1
Marfan syndrome, atypical (3)	120160	7q22.1
Marfan-like connective tissue disorder (2)	154705	3p25-p24.2
Maroteaux-Lamy syndrome, several forms (3)	253200	5q11-q13
Marshall syndrome, 154780 (3)	120280	1p21
MASA syndrome, 303350 (3)	308840	Xq28
Mast cell leukemia (3)	164920	4q12
Mastocytosis with associated hematologic disorder (3)	164920	4q12
May-Hegglin anomaly, 155100 (3)	160775	22q11.2
McArdle disease (3)	232600	11q13
McCune-Albright polyostotic fibrous dysplasia, 174800 (3)	139320	20q13.2
McKusick-Kaufman syndrome, 236700 (3)	604896	20p12
McLeod phenotype (3)	314850	Xp21.2-p21.1
{Measles, susceptibility to} (1)	120920	1q32
Meckel syndrome, type 1 (2)	249000	17q22-q23
Meckel syndrome, type 2 (2)	603194	11q13
Meconium ileus in cystic fibrosis, susceptibility to (2)	603855	19q13.2-q13.4
Medullary cystic kidney disease 1 (2)	174000	1q21
Medullary cystic kidney disease 2 (2)	603860	16p12
Medullary thyroid carcinoma, 155240 (3)	164761	10q11.2
Medullary thyroid carcinoma, familial, 155240 (3)	191315	1q21-q22
Medulloblastoma, 155255 (3)	603673	1p32
Medulloblastoma, 155255 (3)	601969	10q25.3-q26.1
Meesmann corneal dystrophy, 122100 (3)	148043	12q13
Meesmann corneal dystrophy, 122100 (3)	601687	17q12
?Megacystis-microcolon-intestinal hypoperistalsis syndrome, 249210 (1)	118503	15q24
Megaloblastic anemia-1, 261100 (3)	602997	10p12.1
Megalocornea, X-linked (2)	309300	Xq21.3-q22
MEHMO syndrome (2)	300148	Xp22.13-p21.1
?Melanoma (1)	600134	2p25.3
Melanoma, 155601 (3)	600160	9p21
Melanoma (3)	123829	12q14
Melanoma, desmoplastic neurotropic (2)	162200	17q11.2
Meleda disease (2)	248300	8qter
?Melkersson-Rosenthal syndrome (2)	155900	9p11
Membroproliferative glomerulonephritis (1)	134370	1q32
Meniere disease, 156000 (3)	603196	14q12-q13

continued

Table 10.2. The morbid anatomy of the human genome (alphabetical by disorder) (*continued*)

Disorder	MIM#	Location
?Meningioma (2)	603590	22q12.3-q13.1
Meningioma (2)	156100	22q12.3-qter
Meningioma, NF2-related, sporadic (3) Schwannoma, sporadic (3)	101000	22q12.2
Meningioma, SIS-related (3)	190040	22q12.3-q13.1
Menkes disease, 309400 (3)	300011	Xq12-q13
{Mental health wellness-1} (2)	603663	4p
{Mental health wellness-2} (2)	603664	4q
Mental retardation in cri-du-chat syndrome, 123450 (2)	604275	5p15.2
Mental retardation, severe, with spasticity and tapetoretinal degeneration (2)	602685	15q24
Mental retardation, Snyder-Robinson type (2)	309583	Xp21
Mental retardation syndrome, X-linked, Abidi type (2)	300262	Xq13.2
Mental retardation syndrome, X-linked, Armfield type (2)	300261	Xq28
Mental retardation syndrome, X-linked, Lubs type (2)	300260	Xq28
Mental retardation syndrome, X-linked, Siderius type (2)	300263	Xp11.3-q21.3
Mental retardation with isolated growth hormone deficiency (2)	300123	Xq24-q27.1
Mental retardation with psychosis, pyramidal signs, and macroorchidism (2)	300055	Xq28
Mental retardation, X-linked 1, non-dysmorphic, 309530 (3)	300206	Xp22.1-p21.3
Mental retardation, X-linked 14 (2)	300062	Xp11.3-q13.3
Mental retardation, X-linked 20 (2)	300047	Xp11-q21
Mental retardation, X-linked 23, nonspecific (2)	300046	Xq23-q24
Mental retardation, X-linked 29 (2)	300077	Xp22.3-p21.3
Mental retardation, X-linked 30 (3)	300142	Xq21.3-q24
Mental retardation, X-linked, 60 (3)	300127	Xq12
Mental retardation, X-linked 9 (2)	309549	Xp21-q13
Mental retardation, X-linked, FRAXE type (3)	309548	Xq28
Mental retardation, X-linked, FRAXF type (3)	300031	Xq28
Mental retardation, X-linked nonspecific (3)	300096	Xq11
Mental retardation, X-linked nonspecific, 309541 (3)	300104	Xq28
Mental retardation, X-linked nonspecific, 58 (2)	300210	Xp22-q12
Mental retardation, X-linked nonspecific, type 19 (3)	300075	Xp22.2-p22.1
Mental retardation, X-linked nonspecific, type 46 (3)	300267	Xq26
Mental retardation, X-linked nonspecific, type 50 (2)	300115	Xp11.3-p11.21
?Mental retardation, X-linked nonspecific, with aphasia (2)	309545	Xp11
Mental retardation, X-linked, Shashi type (2)	300238	Xq26-q27
Mental retardation, X-linked, South African type (2)	300243	Xq24-q27.3
Mental retardation, X-linked, syndromic 7 (2)	300218	Xp11.3-q22
Mental retardation, X-linked, syndromic-1, with dystonic movements, ataxia, and seizures (2)	309510	Xp22.2-p22.1
Mental retardation, X-linked, syndromic-2, with dysmorphism and cerebral atrophy (2)	309610	Xp11-q21
Mental retardation, X-linked, syndromic-3, with spastic diplegia (2)	309470	Xp11-q21.3
Mental retardation, X-linked, syndromic-4, with congenital contractures and low fingertip arches (2)	309605	Xq13-q22
Mental retardation, X-linked, syndromic-5, with Dandy-Walker malformation, basal ganglia disease, and seizures (2)	304340	Xq25-q27
Mental retardation, X-linked, syndromic-6, with gynecomastia and obesity (2)	309585	Xp21.1-q22
Mental retardation, X-linked, with progressive spasticity, 300279 (3)	300005	Xq28
Mental retardation, X-linked-49 (2)	300114	Xp22.3
Mental retardation, X-linked-72 (2)	300271	Xq28
Mental retardation-skeletal dysplasia (2)	309620	Xq28
Mephenytoin poor metabolizer (3)	124020	10q24.1-q24.3
6-Mercaptopurine sensitivity (3)	187680	6p22.3
Mesomelic dysplasia, Kantaputra type (2)	156232	2q24-q32
Mesothelioma (3)	603517	1p22
Metachromatic leukodystrophy (3)	250100	22q13.31-qter
Metachromatic leukodystrophy due to deficiency of SAP-1 (3)	176801	10q22.1
Metaphyseal chondrodysplasia, Murk Jansen type, 156400 (3)	168468	3p22-p21.1
Metaphyseal chondrodysplasia, Schmid type (3)	120110	6q21-q22.3
Methemoglobinemia due to cytochrome b5 deficiency (3)	250790	18q23
Methemoglobinemia, type I (3)	250800	22q13.31-qter

continued

Table 10.2. The morbid anatomy of the human genome (alphabetical by disorder) (*continued*)

Disorder	MIM#	Location
Methemoglobinemia, type II (3)	250800	22q13.31-qter
Methemoglobinemias, alpha- (3)	141800	16pter-p13.3
Methemoglobinemias, beta- (3)	141900	11p15.5
Methionine adenosyltransferase deficiency, autosomal recessive (3)	250850	10q22
Methylcobalamin deficiency, cb1 G type (3)	156570	1q43
Methylmalonate semialdehyde dehydrogenase deficiency (3)	603178	14q24.3
Methylmalonicaciduria, mutase deficiency type (3)	251000	6p21
3-Methylglutaconicaciduria, type III (2)	258501	19q13.2-q13.3
Mevalonicaciduria (3)	251170	12q24
MHC class II deficiency, complementation group A, 209920 (3)	600005	16p13
MHC class II deficiency, complementation group B, 209920 (3)	603200	19p12
MHC class II deficiency, complementation group C, 209920 (3)	601863	1q21.1-q21.3
Microcephaly, autosomal recessive 1 (2)	251200	8pter-p22
Microcephaly, autosomal recessive 2 (2)	604317	19q13.1-q13.2
Microcephaly, primary autosomal recessive, 3 (2)	604804	9q34
Microcephaly, primary autosomal recessive, 4 (2)	604321	15q15-q21
Microcephaly, primary autosomal recessive, 5 (2)	605481	1q31
Microcoria, congenital (2)	156600	13q31-q32
Microhydranencephaly (2)	605013	16p13.3-p12.1
Micropenis (3)	152790	2p21
Microphthalmia, autosomal recessive (2)	251600	14q32
Microphthalmia, cataracts, and iris abnormalities (3)	142993	14q24.3
Microphthalmia, dermal aplasia, and sclerocornea (2)	309801	Xp22.31
Microphthalmia with linear skin defects (2)	309801	Xp22.31
Migraine, familial hemiplegic, 2 (2)	602481	1q21-q23
{Migraine, familial typical, susceptibility to, 1} (2)	300125	Xq
Miller-Dieker lissencephaly syndrome (2)	247200	17p13.3
Mitral valve prolapse, familial (2)	157700	16p12.1-p11.2
Mixed polyposis syndrome, hereditary (2)	601228	6q
Miyoshi myopathy, 254130 (3)	603009	2p13.3-p13.1
MODY, one form (3)	176730	11p15.5
MODY, type I, 125850 (3)	600281	20q12-q13.1
MODY, type II, 125851 (3)	138079	7p15-p13
MODY, type III, 600496 (3)	142410	12q24.2
MODY, type IV (3)	600733	13q12.1
MODY, type V, 604284 (3)	189907	17cen-q21.3
MODY5 with nephron agenesis (3)	189907	17cen-q21.3
MODY5 with non-diabetic renal disease and Mullerian aplasia (3)	189907	17cen-q21.3
?Moebius syndrome (2)	157900	13q12.2-q13
Moebius syndrome-2 (2)	601471	3q21-q22
Moebius syndrome-3 (2)	604185	10q21.3-q22.1
Mohr-Tranebjaerg syndrome (3)	304700	Xq22
Molybdenum cofactor deficiency, type A, 252150 (3)	603707	6p21.3
Molybdenum cofactor deficiency, type B, 252150 (3)	603708	5q11
Monilethrix, 158000 (3)	602153	12q13
Monilethrix, 158000 (3)	601928	12q13
?Monocyte carboxylesterase deficiency (1)	114835	16q13-q22.1
Moyamoya disease (2)	252350	3p26-p24.2
Muckle-Wells syndrome (2)	191900	1q44
Mucolipidosis II (1)	252500	4q21-q23
Mucolipidosis III (1)	252500	4q21-q23
Mucolipidosis IV, 252650 (3)	605248	19p13.3-p13.2
Mucopolysaccharidosis Ih (3)	252800	4p16.3
Mucopolysaccharidosis Ih/s (3)	252800	4p16.3
Mucopolysaccharidosis II (3)	309900	Xq28
Mucopolysaccharidosis Is (3)	252800	4p16.3
Mucopolysaccharidosis IVA (3)	253000	16q24.3
Mucopolysaccharidosis IVB (3)	230500	3p21.33

continued

Table 10.2. The morbid anatomy of the human genome (alphabetical by disorder) (*continued*)

Disorder	MIM#	Location
Mucopolysaccharidosis type IX (3)	601492	3p21.3-p21.2
Mucopolysaccharidosis VII (3)	253220	7q21.11
Muencke syndrome, 602849 (3)	134934	4p16.3
Muir-Torre family cancer syndrome, 158320 (3)	120436	3p21.3
Muir-Torre syndrome, 158320 (3)	120435	2p22-p21
Mulibrey nanism, 253250 (3)	253250	17q22-q23
Multiple carboxylase deficiency, biotin-responsive (3)	253270	21q22.1
Multiple endocrine neoplasia I (3)	131100	11q13
Multiple endocrine neoplasia IIA, 171400 (3)	164761	10q11.2
Multiple endocrine neoplasia IIB, 162300 (3)	164761	10q11.2
Multiple myeloma, 254500 (2)	168461	11q13
Multiple myeloma (3)	602028	6p25
{Multiple sclerosis, susceptibility to}, 126200 (3)	151460	1q31-q32
Muscle glycogenosis (3)	311870	Xq13
Muscle-eye-brain disease (2)	253280	1p34-p32
Muscular dystrophy, congenital, 1B (2)	604801	1q42
Muscular dystrophy, congenital merosin-deficient (3)	156225	6q22-q23
Muscular dystrophy, congenital, with early spine rigidity (2)	602771	1p36-p35
Muscular dystrophy, Duchenne-like, type 2 (3)	600119	17q12-q21.33
Muscular dystrophy, Fukuyama congenital (3)	253800	9q31
Muscular dystrophy, limb-girdle, type 1A, 159000 (3)	604103	5q31
Muscular dystrophy, limb-girdle, type 1B (2)	159001	1q11-q21
Muscular dystrophy, limb-girdle, type 1D (2)	603511	7q
Muscular dystrophy, limb-girdle, type 2A, 253600 (3)	114240	15q15.1-q21.1
Muscular dystrophy, limb-girdle, type 2B, 253601 (3)	603009	2p13.3-p13.1
Muscular dystrophy, limb-girdle, type 2C (3)	253700	13q12
Muscular dystrophy, limb-girdle, type 2E, 604286 (3)	600900	4q12
Muscular dystrophy, limb-girdle, type 2F, 601287 (3)	601411	5q33
Muscular dystrophy, limb-girdle, type 2G, 601954 (3)	604488	17q12
Muscular dystrophy, limb-girdle, type 2H (2)	254110	9q31-q34.1
Muscular dystrophy, limb-girdle, type IC (3)	601253	3p25
Muscular dystrophy with epidermolysis bullosa simplex, 226670 (3)	601282	8q24
Muscular dystrophy with rimmed vacuoles (2)	601846	19p13.3
Myasthenia gravis, familial infantile (2)	254210	17p13
Myasthenia gravis, neonatal transient (2)	100730	2q33-q34
Myasthenic syndrome, slow-channel congenital, 601462 (3)	100725	Chr. 17
Myasthenic syndrome, slow-channel congenital, 601462 (3)	100710	17p12-p11
Myasthenic syndrome, slow-channel congenital, 601462 (3)	100690	2q24-q32
{Mycobacterial and salmonella infections, susceptibility to} (3)	601604	19p13.1
Mycobacterial infection, atypical, familial disseminated, 209950 (3)	147569	21q22.1-q22.2
Mycobacterial infection, atypical, familial disseminated, 209950(3)	107470	6q23-q24
Myelodysplasia syndrome-1 (3)	600049	3q26
Myelodysplastic syndrome (3)	604443	5q31
Myelodysplastic syndrome, preleukemic (3)	147575	5q31.1
Myelogenous leukemia, acute (3)	604443	5q31
Myelogenous leukemia, acute (3)	147575	5q31.1
Myeloid leukemia, acute, M4Eo subtype (2)	121360	16q22
Myeloid malignancy, predisposition to (3)	164770	5q33.2-q33.3
Myeloperoxidase deficiency (3)	254600	17q23.1
Myoadenylate deaminase deficiency (3)	102770	1p21-p13
{Myocardial infarction, decreased susceptibility to} (3)	227500	13q34
{Myocardial infarction susceptibility} (3)	107741	19q13.2
{Myocardial infarction, susceptibility to} (3)	106180	17q23
{Myocardial infarction, susceptibility to} (3)	188040	20p11.2
Myoglobinuria/hemolysis due to PGK deficiency (3)	311800	Xq13
Myoneurogastrointestinal encephalomyopathy syndrome, 603041 (3)	131222	22q13.32-qter
Myopathy, actin (3)	102610	1q42.1
Myopathy, centronuclear, 160150 (3)	159991	12q21

continued

Table 10.2. The morbid anatomy of the human genome (alphabetical by disorder) (*continued*)

Disorder	MIM#	Location
Myopathy, congenital (3)	600536	12q13
Myopathy, desmin-related, cardioskeletal, 601419 (3)	123590	11q22.3-q23.1
Myopathy, desmin-related, cardioskeletal, 601419 (3)	125660	2q35
Myopathy, distal (2)	160500	14q
Myopathy, distal 2 (2)	158580	5q
Myopathy, distal, with anterior tibial onset (3)	603009	2p13.3-p13.1
Myopathy due to CPT II deficiency, 255110 (3)	600650	1p32
Myopathy due to phosphoglycerate mutase deficiency (3)	261670	7p13-p12.3
?Myopathy due to succinate dehydrogenase deficiency (1)	185470	1p36.1-p35
Myopathy, nemaline, 161800, 256030 (3)	102610	1q42.1
Myopathy, proximal, with early respiratory muscle involvement (2)	603689	2q24-q31
Myopathy, X-linked, with excessive autophagy (2)	310440	Xq28
Myopia-1 (2)	310460	Xq28
Myopia-2 (2)	160700	18p11.31
Myopia-3 (2)	603221	12q21-q23
Myotonia congenita, atypical, acetazolamide-responsive (3)	603967	17q23.1-q25.3
Myotonia congenita, dominant, 160800 (3)	118425	7q35
Myotonia congenita, recessive, 255700 (3)	118425	7q35
Myotonia levior, recessive (3)	118425	7q35
Myotonic dystrophy, 160900 (3)	605377	19q13.2-q13.3
Myotonic dystrophy 2 (2)	602668	3q
Myotubular myopathy, X-linked (3)	310400	Xq28
Myxoid liposarcoma (3)	126337	12q13.1-q13.2
Myxoma, intracardiac, 255960 (3)	188830	17q23-q24
?N syndrome, 310465 (1)	312040	Xp22.3-p21.1
NAGA deficiency, mild (3)	104170	22q11
Nail-patella syndrome, 161200 (3)	602575	9q34.1
Nail-patella syndrome with open-angle glaucoma, 137750 (3)	602575	9q34.1
Nance-Horan syndrome (2)	302350	Xp22.3-p21.1
Nanophthalmos-1 (2)	600165	11p
Narcolepsy, 161400 (3)	602358	17q21
Naxos disease, 601214 (3)	173325	17q21
Nemaline myopathy 1, autosomal dominant, 161800 (3)	191030	1q22-q23
Nemaline myopathy 2, autosomal recessive, 256030 (3)	161650	2q22
Nemaline myopathy, Amish type, 605355 (3)	191041	19q13.4
Neonatal alloimmune thrombocytopenia (2)	192974	5q23-q31
Neonatal hyperparathyroidism, 239200 (3)	601199	3q13.3-q21
Nephrolithiasis, type I, 310468 (3)	300008	Xp11.22
Nephronophthisis, adolescent (2)	604387	3q22
Nephronophthisis, infantile (2)	602088	9q22-q31
Nephronophthisis, juvenile (3)	256100	2q13
Nephropathy, chronic hypocomplementemic (3)	134370	1q32
Nephropathy, IgA type (2)	161950	6q22-q23
Nephropathy-hypertension (2)	161900	1q21
Nephrosis-1, congenital, Finnish type, 256300 (3)	602716	19q13.1
Nephrotic syndrome, idiopathic, steroid-resistant (2)	600995	1q25-q31
Nephrotic syndrome, steroid-resistant, 600995 (3)	604766	1q25-q31
Netherton syndrome, 256500 (3)	605010	5q32
Neuralgic amyotrophy with predilection for brachial plexus (2)	162100	17q25
?Neuroblastoma (1)	601990	1p36
Neuroblastoma (2)	256700	1p36.3-p36.2
Neuroblastoma (3)	156490	17q21.3
Neurodegeneration with brain iron accumulation (2)	234200	20p13-p12.3
Neuroepithelioma (2)	133450	22q12
Neurofibromatosis, type 1 (3)	162200	17q11.2
Neurofibromatosis, type 2 (3)	101000	22q12.2
Neurofibrosarcoma (3)	600020	10q25
Neurolemmomatosis (3)	101000	22q12.2

continued

Table 10.2. The morbid anatomy of the human genome (alphabetical by disorder) (*continued*)

Disorder	MIM#	Location
Neuropathy, congenital hypomyelinating, 1, 605253 (3)	129010	10q21.1-q22.1
Neuropathy, hereditary motor and sensory, Lom type, 601455 (3)	605262	8q24.3
Neuropathy, hereditary motor and sensory, Okinawa type (2)	604484	3q13.1
Neuropathy, hereditary sensory and autonomic, type 1 (2)	162400	9q22.1-q22.3
Neuropathy, motor and sensory, Russe type (2)	605285	10q23.2
Neuropathy, paraneoplastic sensory (1)	168360	1p34
Neuropathy, recurrent, with pressure palsies, 162500 (3)	601097	17p11.2
Neutropenia, alloimmune neonatal (3)	146740	1q23
Neutropenia, neonatal alloimmune (1)	151450	Chr.4
Neutrophil immunodeficiency syndrome (3)	602049	22q12.3-q13.2
{Nicotine addiction, protection from} (3)	122720	19q13.2
Niemann-Pick disease, type A (3)	257200	11p15.4-p15.1
Niemann-Pick disease, type B (3)	257200	11p15.4-p15.1
Niemann-Pick disease, type C1 (3)	257220	18q11-q12
Niemann-Pick disease, type C2 (3)	601016	14q24.3
Niemann-Pick disease, type D, 257250 (3)	257220	18q11-q12
Night blindness, congenital stationary (3)	139330	3p21
Night blindness, congenital stationary, type 1, 310500 (3)	300278	Xp11.4
Night blindness, congenital stationary, type 3, 163500 (3)	180072	4p16.3
Night blindness, congenital stationary, X-linked, type 2, 300071 (3)	300110	Xp11.23
Night blindness, congenital stationery, rhodopsin-related (3)	180380	3q21-q24
Nijmegen breakage syndrome, 251260 (3)	602667	8q21
Noncompaction of left ventricular myocardium, isolated, 300183 (3)	302060	Xq28
Nonepidermolytic palmoplantar keratoderma, 600962 (3)	148067	17q12-q21
{Nonsmall cell lung cancer} (2)	603040	11q23
{Nonsmall cell lung cancer} (2)	604331	13q14.12-q14.2
Nonsmall cell lung cancer (3)	147575	5q31.1
Noonan syndrome-1 (2)	163950	12q24
Norrie disease (3)	310600	Xp11.4
Norum disease (3)	245900	16q22.1
[Novelty seeking personality], 601696 (1)	126452	11p15.5
Nucleoside phosphorylase deficiency, immunodeficiency due to (3)	164050	14q13.1
Nystagmus 1, congenital (2)	310700	Xq26-q27
Nystagmus-2, autosomal dominant (2)	164100	6p12
Obesity, adrenal insufficiency, and red hair (3)	176830	2p23.3
Obesity, autosomal dominant (3)	155541	18q22
Obesity, morbid, with hypogonadism (3)	164160	7q31.3
[Obesity, protection against] (3)	601487	3p25
Obesity, severe (3)	603128	6q16.3-q21
Obesity, severe, 601665 (3)	601487	3p25
Obesity, severe, due to leptin deficiency (3)	164160	7q31.3
{Obesity, susceptibility to} (3)	109690	5q32-q34
{Obesity, susceptibility to}, 601665 (2)	603188	10p
{Obesity/hyperinsulinism, susceptibility to} (2)	602025	20q13.11-q13.2
Obesity with impaired prohormone processing, 600955 (3)	162150	5q15-q21
Occipital horn syndrome, 304150 (3)	300011	Xq12-q13
?Ocular albinism, autosomal recessive (2)	203310	6q13-q15
Ocular albinism, Forsius-Eriksson type (2)	300600	Xp11.4-p11.23
Ocular albinism, Nettleship-Falls type (3)	300500	Xp22.3
Ocular albinism with sensorineural deafness (2)	300650	Xp22.3
Oculodentodigital dysplasia (2)	164200	6q22-q24
Oculodigitoesophagoduodenal syndrome (2)	164280	2p24-p23
Oculopharyngeal muscular dystrophy, 164300 (3)	602279	14q11.2-q13
Oculopharyngeal muscular dystorphy, autosomal recessive, 257950 (3)	602279	14q11.2-q13
Oguchi disease-1, 258100 (3)	181031	2q37.1
Oguchi disease-2, 258100 (3)	180381	13q34
Oligodontia, 604625 (3)	167416	14q12-q13
Omenn syndrome, 603554 (3)	179615	11p13

continued

Table 10.2. The morbid anatomy of the human genome (alphabetical by disorder) (*continued*)

Disorder	MIM#	Location
Omenn syndrome, 603554 (3)	179616	11p13
Opitz G syndrome, type I (3)	300000	Xp22
Opitz G syndrome, type II (2)	145410	22q11.2
Optic atrophy 1, 165500 (3)	605290	3q28-q29
Optic atrophy, X-linked (2)	311050	Xp11.4-p11.21
Optic atrophy-4 (2)	605293	18q12.2-q12.3
Optic nerve coloboma with renal disease, 120330 (3)	167409	10q24.3-q25.1
Oral-facial-digital syndrome 1 (2)	311200	Xp22.3-p22.2
Ornithine transcarbamylase deficiency (3)	311250	Xp21.1
Orofacial cleft-1 (2)	119530	6p24.3
Orofacial cleft-2 (2)	602966	2p13
Orofacial cleft-3 (2)	600757	19q13
Oroticaciduria (3)	258900	3q13
Orthostatic hypotensive disorder of Streeten (2)	143850	18q
Orthostatic intolerance, 604715 (3)	163970	16q12.2
OSMED syndrome, 215150 (3)	120290	6p21.3
Osseous dysplasia, digital, with facial pibmentary defects and multiple frenula (2)	300244	Xq27.3-q28
Ossification of posterior longitudinal ligament of spine, 602475 (3)	173335	6q22-q23
?Osteoarthritis of distal interphalangeal joints (2)	140600	2q12-q13
{Osteoarthritis susceptibility, female-specific} (2)	165720	11q
Osteoarthritis with mild chondrodysplasia (3)	120140	12q13.11-q13.2
Osteoarthrosis, precocious (3)	120140	12q13.11-q13.2
Osteogenesis imperfecta, 3 clinical forms, 166200, 166210, 259420 (3)	120160	7q22.1
Osteogenesis imperfecta, 4 clinical forms, 166200, 166210, 259420, 166220 (3)	120150	17q21.31-q22
Osteolysis, familial expansile, 174810 (3)	603499	18q22.1
Osteopenia/osteoporosis, 166710 (2)	147620	7p21
Osteopetrosis, AD, type II (2)	166600	1p21
Osteopetrosis, recessive, 259700 (3)	604592	11q13.4-q13.5
Osteoporosis (3)	114130	11p15.2-p15.1
Osteoporosis, idiopathic, 166710 (3)	120150	17q21.31-q22
Osteoporosis, idiopathic, 166710 (3)	120160	7q22.1
?Osteoporosis, involutional (1)	601769	12q12-q14
{Osteoporosis, postmenopausal, susceptibility}, 166710 (3)	114131	7q21.3
Osteoporosis-pseudoglioma syndrome (2)	259770	11q12-q13
Osteosarcoma, 259500 (2)	180200	13q14.1-q14.2
Osteosarcoma, 259500 (2)	603045	18q21-q22
Otopalatodigital syndrome, type I (2)	311300	Xq28
Otosclerosis (2)	166800	15q26.1-qter
Ovarian cancer (1)	605193	1p31
Ovarian cancer (1)	171834	3q26.3
Ovarian cancer (3)	113705	17q21
Ovarian cancer (3)	120435	2p22-p21
Ovarian cancer, serous (2)	167000	6q26-q27
Ovarian carcinoma (1)	604061	17q25
Ovarian carcinoma, 167000 (2)	164731	19q13.1-q13.2
Ovarian carcinoma (2)	164759	9p24
Ovarian carcinoma (3)	192090	16q22.1
Ovarian carcinoma, endometrioid type (3)	116806	3p22-p21.3
Ovarian dysgenesis, hypergonadotropic, with normal karyotype, 233300 (3)	136435	2p21-p16
Ovarian failure, premature (2)	311360	Xq21
5-Oxoprolinuria, 266130 (3)	601002	20q11.2
?P5CS deficiency (1)	138250	10q24.3
Pachyonychia congenita, Jackson-Lawler type, 167210 (3)	148042	12q13
Pachyonychia congenita, Jackson-Lawler type, 167210 (3)	148069	17q12-q21
Pachyonychia congenita, Jadassohn-Lewandowsky type, 167200 (3)	148041	12q13
Pachyonychia congenita, Jadassohn-Lewandowsky type, 167200 (3)	148067	17q12-q21
?Paget disease of bone (2)	167250	6p21.3
Paget disease of bone, 602080 (3)	603499	18q22.1

continued

Table 10.2. The morbid anatomy of the human genome (alphabetical by disorder) (*continued*)

Disorder	MIM#	Location
Pallister-Hall syndrome, 146510 (3)	165240	7p13
Palmoplantar keratoderma, Bothnia type (2)	600231	12q11-q13
Panbronchiolitis, diffuse (2)	604809	6p21.3
Pancreatic agenesis, 260370 (3)	600733	13q12.1
Pancreatic cancer (2)	601916	3p21.1
Pancreatic cancer (3)	600185	13q12.3
Pancreatic cancer (3)	600993	18q21.1
?Pancreatic endocrine tumors (1)	602011	3p25
Pancreatic lipase deficiency (1)	246600	10q26.1
Pancreatitis, hereditary, 167800 (3)	167790	Chr.5
Pancreatitis, hereditary, 167800 (3)	276000	7q35
{Pancreatitis, idiopathic} (3)	602421	7q31.2
Panhypopituitarism, X-linked (2)	312000	Xq25-q26
PAPA syndrome (2)	604416	15q24-q26.1
Papillary serous carcinoma of the peritoneum (3)	113705	17q21
Papillon-Lefevre syndrome, 245000 (3)	602365	11q14.1-q14.3
Paragangliomas, familial nonchromaffin, 2 (2)	601650	11q13.1
Paragangliomas, familial nonchromaffin, 1, 168000 (3)	602690	11q23
Paragangliomas, familial nonchromaffin, 3, 605373 (3)	602413	1q21
Paramyotonia congenita, 168300 (3)	603967	17q23.1-q25.3
Parathyroid adenoma, sporadic (3)	131100	11q13
Parathyroid adenomatosis 1 (2)	168461	11q13
Parietal foramina 1, 168500 (3)	123101	5q34-q35
Parietal foramina 2, 168500 (3)	605420	11p11.2
Parkinson disease 4, autosomal dominant, Lewy body (2)	605543	4p15
Parkinson disease, familial, 168600 (3)	191342	4p14
Parkinson disease, juvenile, type 2, 600116 (3)	602544	6q25.2-q27
{Parkinson disease, susceptibility to}, 168600 (3)	600532	18p11.31-p11.2
Parkinson disease, type 1, 601508 (3)	163890	4q21
Parkinson disease, type 3 (2)	602404	2p13
{?Parkinsonism, susceptibility to} (1)	124030	22q13.1
Parkinsonism-dementia with pallidopontonigral degeneration (2)	168610	17q21
Paroxysmal kinesigenic choreoathetosis (2)	128200	16p11.2-q12.1
Paroxysmal nocturnal hemoglobinuria (3)	311770	Xp22.1
Partington syndrome II (2)	301220	Xp22-p21
Patella aplasia or hypoplasia (2)	168860	17q21-q22
Pattern dystrophy of retina (3)	179605	6p21.1-cen
Pelizaeus-Merzbacher disease (3)	312080	Xq22
Pelviureteric junction obstruction (2)	143400	6p
{Pemphigoid, susceptibility to} (2)	142857	6p21.3
Pendred syndrome (3)	274600	7q31
PEO with mitochondrial DNA deletions, type 1 (2)	157640	10q23.3-q24.3
Perineal hypospadias (3)	313700	Xq11-q12
Periodic fever, familial, 142680 (3)	191190	12p13.2
Periodontitis, juvenile (2)	170650	4q11-q13
Peroxisomal bifunctional enzyme deficiency (1)	261515	3q27
Peroxisomal biogenesis disorder, complementation group 4 (3)	601498	6p21.1
Persistent hyperinsulinemic hypoglycemia of infancy, 256450 (3)	600509	11p15.1
Persistent hyperinsulinemic hypoglycemia of infancy, 256450 (3)	600937	11p15.1
Persistent Mullerian duct syndrome, type I, 261550 (3)	600957	19p13.3-p13.2
Persistent Mullerian duct syndrome, type II, 261550 (3)	600956	12q13
Peters anomaly, 603807 (3)	106210	11p13
Peutz-Jeghers syndrome, 175200 (3)	602216	19p13.3
Pfeiffer syndrome, 101600 (3)	176943	10q26
Pfeiffer syndrome, 101600 (3)	136350	8p11.2-p11.1
Phenylketonuria (3)	261600	12q24.1
Phenylketonuria, atypical, due to GCH1 deficiency, 233910 (1)	600225	14q22.1-q22.2
Phenylketonuria due to dihydropteridine reductase deficiency (3)	261630	4p15.31

continued

Table 10.2. The morbid anatomy of the human genome (alphabetical by disorder) (*continued*)

Disorder	MIM#	Location
Phenylketonuria due to PTS deficiency (3)	261640	11q22.3-q23.3
[Phenylthiocarbamide tasting] (2)	171200	5p15
Pheochromocytoma (2)	171300	1p
Phosphoribosyl pyrophosphate synthetase-related gout (3)	311850	Xq22-q24
Phosphorylase kinase deficiency of liver and muscle, autosomal recessive, 261750 (3)	172490	16q12-q13
Piebaldism (3)	164920	4q12
Pigment dispersion syndrome (2)	600510	7q35-q36
Pilomatricoma (3)	116806	3p22-p21.3
Pinealoma with bilateral retinoblastoma (2)	180200	13q14.1-q14.2
Pituitary ACTH secreting adenoma (3)	139320	20q13.2
Pituitary ACTH-secreting adenoma (3)	139360	3p21
Pituitary hormone deficiency, combined (3)	173110	3p11
Pituitary hormone deficiency, combined (3)	601538	5q
Pituitary hormone deficiency, combined, with rigid cervical spine, 262600 (3)	600577	9q34.3
Pituitary tumor, invasive (3)	176960	17q22-q23.2
[Placental lactogen deficiency] (1)	150200	17q22-q24
Placental steroid sulfatase deficiency (3)	308100	Xp22.32
Plasmin inhibitor deficiency (3)	262850	17pter-p12
Plasminogen activator deficiency (1)	173370	8p12
Plasminogen deficiency, types I and II (1)	173350	6q26
Plasminogen Tochigi disease (3)	173350	6q26
{Plasmodium falciparum parasitemia, intensity of} (2)	248310	5q31-q33
Platelet alpha/delta storage pool deficiency (1)	173610	1q23-q25
Platelet disorder, familial, with associated myeloid malignancy, 601399 (3)	151385	21q22.3
Platelet glycoprotein IV deficiency (3)	173510	7q11.2
Platelet-activating factor acetylhydrolase deficiency (3)	601690	6p21.2-p12
{Polio, susceptibility to} (2)	173850	19q13.2-q13.3
Polycystic kidney disease, adult type I, 173900 (3)	601313	16p13.3-p13.12
Polycystic kidney disease, adult, type II (3)	173910	4q21-q23
Polycystic kidney disease, autosomal recessive (2)	263200	6p21.1-p12
Polycystic kidney disease, infantile severe, with tuberous sclerosis (3)	600273	16p13.3
Polycystic lipomembranous osteodysplasia with sclerosing leukenencephalophathy, 221770 (3)	604142	19q13.1
?Polycystic ovary syndrome, 184700 (2)	118485	15q23-q24
Polycystic ovary syndrome, 184700 (2)	136470	5p14
Polydactyly, postaxial, types A1 and B, 174200 (3)	165240	7p13
Polydactyly, preaxial, type IV, 174700 (3)	165240	7p13
Polyposis, juvenile intestinal, 174900 (3)	601728	10q23.3
Polyposis, juvenile intestinal, 174900 (3)	600993	18q21.1
Popliteal pterygium syndrome (3)	119500	1q32
Porphyria, acute hepatic (3)	125270	9q34
Porphyria, acute intermittent (3)	176000	11q23.3
Porphyria, acute intermittent, nonerythroid variant (3)	176000	11q23.3
Porphyria, Chester type (2)	176010	11q23.1
Porphyria, congenital erythropoietic (3)	263700	10q25.2-q26.3
Porphyria, cutanea tarda (3)	176100	1p34
Porphyria, hepatoerythropoietic (3)	176100	1p34
Porphyria variegata, 176200 (3)	600923	1q22
Porphyria variegata, 176200 (3)	235200	6p21.3
Postaxial polydactyly, type A2 (2)	602085	13q21-q32
Prader-Willi syndrome, 176270 (3)	602117	15q11-q13
Prader-Willi syndrome, 176270 (3)	182279	15q12
Prader-Willi syndrome, (2)	176270	15q11
Precocious puberty, male, 176410 (3)	152790	2p21
Preeclampsia (2)	189800	2p13
{Preeclampsia, susceptibility to, 189800} (2)	163729	7q36
{Preeclampsia, susceptibility to} (3)	106150	1q42-q43
Premature ovarian failure, 311360 (3)	300108	Xq22
Progressive external ophthalmoplegia, type 3, 601227 (3)	103220	4q35

continued

Table 10.2. The morbid anatomy of the human genome (alphabetical by disorder) (*continued*)

Disorder	MIM#	Location
Progressive intrahepatic cholestasis-2, 601847 (3)	603201	2q24
Prolactinoma, hyperparathyroidism, carcinoid syndrome (3)	131100	11q13
Prolidase deficiency (3)	170100	19cen-q13.11
Properdin deficiency, X-linked (3)	312060	Xp11.4-p11.23
Propionicacidemia, type I or pccA type (3)	232000	13q32
Propionicacidemia, type II or pccB type (3)	232050	3q21-q22
Prostate adenocarcinoma (2)	601188	10pter-q11
?Prostate cancer (1)	601385	8p22
Prostate cancer, 176807 (2)	600623	11p11.2
Prostate cancer, 176807 (3)	600020	10q25
Prostate cancer (3)	601728	10q23.3
Prostate cancer (3)	313700	Xq11-q12
Prostate cancer, hereditary, 1, 176807 (2)	601518	1q24-q25
Prostate cancer, hereditary, 2, 176807 (2)	602759	1q42.2-q43
{Prostate cancer, susceptibility to} (3)	605367	17p
{Prostate cancer, susceptibility, X-linked} (2)	300147	Xq27-q28
{Prostate cancer-brain cancer susceptibility} (2)	603688	1p36
Protein C inhibitor deficiency (2)	601841	14q32.1
Protein S deficiency (3)	176880	3p11.1-q11.2
Proteinuria, low molecular weight, with hypercalciuric nephrocalcinosis (3)	300008	Xp11.22
Protoporphyria, erythropoietic (3)	177000	18q21.3
Protoporphyria, erythropoietic, recessive, with liver failure (3)	177000	18q21.3
Pseudoachondroplasia, 177170 (3)	600310	19p13.1
Pseudohermaphroditism, male, with gynecomastia (3)	264300	9q22
Pseudohermaphroditism, male, with Leydig cell hypoplasia (3)	152790	2p21
Pseudohyperkalemia, familial, 177720 (2)	194380	16q23-q24
Pseudohypoaldosteronism, type I, 264350 (3)	600228	12p13
Pseudohypoaldosteronism, type I, 264350 (3)	600760	16p13-p12
Pseudohypoaldosteronism, type I, 264350 (3)	600761	16p13-p12
Pseudohypoaldosteronism type I, autosomal dominant, 177735 (3)	600983	4q31.1
Pseudohypoaldosteronism, type II (2)	145260	1q31-q42
Pseudohypoaldosteronism type II (2)	601844	17q21-q22
Pseudohypoaldosteronism, type IIC (2)	605232	12p13
Pseudohypoparathyroidism, type Ia, 103580 (3)	139320	20q13.2
Pseudohypoparathyroidism, type IB (2)	603233	20q13.3
Pseudovaginal perineoscrotal hypospadias (3)	264600	2p23
Pseudovitamin D deficiency rickets 1 (3)	264700	12q14
Pseudoxanthoma elasticum, autosomal dominant, 177850 (3)	603234	16p13.1
Pseudoxanthoma elasticum, autosomal recessive, 264800 (3)	603234	16p13.1
Pseudo-Zellweger syndrome, 261510 (1)	604054	3p23-p22
{Psoriasis susceptibility} (2)	604316	3q21
{Psoriasis susceptibility 3} (3)	601454	4q
{Psoriasis, susceptibility to}, 177900 (3)	605364	19p13
{Psoriasis, susceptibility to} (2)	603935	1cen-q21
{Psoriasis susceptibility-1} (2)	177900	6p21.3
{Psoriasis susceptibility-2} (2)	602723	17q
Ptosis, hereditary congenital, 1 (2)	178300	1p34.1-p32
Ptosis, hereditary congenital 2 (2)	300245	Xq24-q27.1
Pulmonary alveolar proteinosis, 265120 (3)	138981	22q12.2-q13.1
Pulmonary alveolar proteinosis, congenital, 265120 (3)	178640	2p12-p11.2
Pulmonary hypertension, familial primary, 178600 (3)	600799	2q33
Purpura fulminans, neonatal (1)	176860	2q13-q14
Pycnodysostosis, 265800 (3)	601105	1q21
Pyropoikilocytosis (3)	182860	1q21
Pyruvate carboxylase deficiency (3)	266150	11q13.4-q13.5
Pyruvate dehydrogenase deficiency (3)	312170	Xp22.2-p22.1
Rabson-Mendenhall syndrome, 262190 (3)	147670	19p13.2
Radiation sensitivity/chromosome instability syndrome, autosomal dominant (1)	605463	14q11.2

continued

Table 10.2. The morbid anatomy of the human genome (alphabetical by disorder) (*continued*)

Disorder	MIM#	Location
Radioulnar synostosis with amegakaryocytic thrombocytopenia, 605432 (3)	142958	7p15-p14.2
?Ragweed sensitivity (2)	179450	6p21.3
[Red hair/fair skin] (3)	155555	16q24.3
Refsum disease, 266500 (3)	602026	10pter-p11.2
Refsum disease, adult, with increased pipecolicacidemia (2)	600964	10pter-p11.2
Refsum disease, infantile, 266510 (3)	602136	7q21-q22
Refsum disease, infantile form, 266510 (3)	170993	8q21.1
Renal cell carcinoma, 144700 (3)	603046	8q24.1
Renal cell carcinoma (3)	193300	3p26-p25
Renal cell carcinoma, clear cell, 144700 (3)	601982	3p26.2
Renal cell carcinoma, papillary, 1, 605074 (3)	179755	1q21
Renal cell carcinoma, papillary, 1, 605074 (3)	314310	Xp11.22
Renal cell carcinoma, papillary, 3 (2)	605075	17q21.32
Renal cell carcinoma, papillary, familial and sporadic, 605074 (3)	164860	7q31
[Renal glucosuria] (2)	233100	6p21.3
?Renal glucosuria, 233100 (1)	182381	16p11.2
Renal tubular acidosis, distal, 179800 (3)	109270	17q21-q22
Renal tubular acidosis, distal, autosomal recessive, 602722 (3)	605239	7q33-q34
Renal tubular acidosis, proximal, with ocular abnormalities, 604278 (3)	603345	4q21
Renal tubular acidosis with deafness, 267300 (3)	192132	2cen-q13
Renal tubular acidosis-osteopetrosis syndrome (3)	259730	8q22
Renpenning syndrome-1 (2)	309500	Xp11.4-p11.2
?Resistance/susceptibility to TB, etc. (1)	600266	2q35
Reticulosis, familial histiocytic, 267700 (3)	179615	11p13
Retinal cone dsytrophy 2 (2)	601251	17p
?Retinal cone dystrophy-1 (2)	180020	6q25-q26
Retinal degeneration, autosomal recessive, prominin-related (3)	604365	4p16.2-p12
Retinal dystrophy, autosomal recessive, childhood-onset (3)	180069	1p31
Retinal nonattachment, nonsyndromic congenital (2)	221900	10q21
Retinitis pigmentosa, autosomal dominant (3)	600342	10q23
Retinitis pigmentosa, autosomal dominant (3)	162080	14q11.1-q11.2
Retinitis pigmentosa, autosomal recessive (3)	600342	10q23
Retinitis pigmentosa, autosomal recessive (3)	180090	15q26
Retinitis pigmentosa, autosomal recessive (3)	180380	3q21-q24
Retinitis pigmentosa, autosomal recessive (3)	180072	4p16.3
Retinitis pigmentosa, autosomal recessive (3)	123825	4p12-cen
Retinitis pigmentosa, autosomal recessive (3)	180071	5q31.2-q34
Retinitis pigmentosa, digenic (3)	180721	11q13
Retinitis pigmentosa, digenic (3)	179605	6p21.1-cen
Retinitis pigmentosa, late onset, 268000 (3)	604485	15q23
Retinitis pigmentosa, late-onset dominant (3)	602225	19q13.3
Retinitis pigmentosa, MERTK-related, 268000 (3)	604705	2q14.1
Retinitis pigmentosa, with bull's-eye maculopathy (3)	179605	6p21.1-cen
Retinitis pigmentosa-1, 180100 (3)	603937	8q11-q13
Retinitis pigmentosa-10 (2)	180105	7q31-q35
Retinitis pigmentosa-11 (2)	600138	19q13.4
Retinitis pigmentosa-12, autosomal recessive, 600105 (3)	604210	1q31-q32.1
Retinitis pigmentosa-13 (2)	600059	17p13.3
Retinitis pigmentosa-14, 600132 (3)	602280	6p21.3
Retinitis pigmentosa-17 (2)	600852	17q22
Retinitis pigmentosa-18 (2)	601414	1p13-q23
Retinitis pigmentosa-19, 601718 (3)	601691	1p21-p13
Retinitis pigmentosa-2 (2)	312600	Xp11.3
Retinitis pigmentosa-20 (3)	180069	1p31
Retinitis pigmentosa-22 (2)	602594	16p12.3-p12.1
Retinitis pigmentosa-24 (2)	300155	Xq26-q27
Retinitis pigmentosa-25 (2)	602772	6q14-q21
Retinitis pigmentosa-3 (3)	312610	Xp21.1

continued

Table 10.2. The morbid anatomy of the human genome (alphabetical by disorder) (*continued*)

Disorder	MIM#	Location
Retinitis pigmentosa-4, autosomal dominant (3)	180380	3q21-q24
?Retinitis pigmentosa-6 (2)	312612	Xp21.3-p21.2
Retinitis pigmentosa-7, peripherin-related (3)	179605	6p21.1-cen
Retinitis pigmentosa-9 (2)	180104	7p15.1-p13
Retinitis punctata albescens (3)	179605	6p21.1-cen
Retinoblastoma (3)	180200	13q14.1-q14.2
Retinol binding protein, deficiency of (3)	180250	10q24
Retinoschisis (3)	312700	Xp22.2-p22.1
Rett syndrome, 312750 (3)	300005	Xq28
Rett syndrome, preserved speech variant, 312750 (3)	300005	Xq28
Rhabdoid predisposition syndrome, familial (3)	601607	22q11
Rhabdoid tumors (3)	601607	22q11
Rhabdomyosarcoma, 268210 (3)	602631	11p15.5
Rhabdomyosarcoma, alveolar, 268220 (3)	167410	1p36.2-p36.12
Rhabdomyosarcoma, alveolar, 268220 (3)	136533	13q14.1
Rhabdomyosarcoma, alveolar, 268220 (3)	193500	2q35
Rhizomelic chondrodysplasia punctata, type 1, 215100 (3)	601757	6q22-q24
Rhizomelic chondrodysplasia punctata, type 3, 600121 (3)	603051	2q31
Rh-mod syndrome (3)	180297	6p21.1-p11
Rickets, vitamin D-resistant, 277440 (3)	601769	12q12-q14
Rieger anomaly (3)	601090	6p25
Rieger syndrome, 180500 (3)	601542	4q25-q26
Rieger syndrome, type 2 (2)	601499	13q14
Rippling muscle disease-1 (2)	600332	1q41
Robinow syndrome, autosomal recessive, 268310 (3)	602337	9q22
Roifman syndrome (2)	300258	Chr.X
Rothmund-Thomson syndrome, 268400 (3)	603780	8q24.3
Rubenstein-Taybi syndrome, 180849 (3)	600140	16p13.3
Russell-Silver syndrome, 180860 (3)	601523	7p12-p11.2
Saccharopinuria, 268700 (1)	605113	7q31.3
Sacral agenesis-1 (2)	176450	7q36
Saethre-Chotzen syndrome, 101400 (3)	601622	7p21
Saethre-Chotzen syndrome (3)	176943	10q26
Salivary adenoma (3)	600698	12q15
Salivary gland pleomorphic adenoma (2)	181030	8q12
Salla disease, 604369 (3)	604322	6q14-q15
Sandhoff disease, infantile, juvenile, and adult forms (3)	268800	5q13
Sanfilippo syndrome, type A (3)	252900	17q25.3
Sanfilippo syndrome, type B (3)	252920	17q21
?Sanfilippo syndrome, type C (2)	252930	Chr.14
Sanfilippo syndrome, type D (1)	252940	12q14
Sarcoma, synovial (1)	600192	18q11.2
Sarcoma, synovial (1)	300192	Xp11.2
Sarcoma, synovial (3)	312820	Xp11.2
[Sarcosinemial], 268900 (2)	604455	9q33-q34
Scapuloperoneal spinal muscular atrophy, New England type (2)	181405	12q24.1-q24.31
Scapuloperoneal syndrome, myopathic type (2)	181430	12q13.3-q15
Schindler disease (3)	104170	22q11
{Schistosoma mansoni infection, susceptibility/resistance to} (2)	181460	5q31-q33
Schizencephaly (3)	600035	10q26.1
{Schizophrenia}, 181500 (2)	604906	1q21-q22
{?Schizophrenia], 181500 (2)	603342	11q14-q21
{Schizophrenia}, 181500 (2)	603176	13q32
{Schizophrenia}, 181500 (2)	605419	15q15
{Schizophrenia}, 181500 (2)	603206	18p
{Schizophrenia}, 181500 (2)	600850	22q11-q13
{Schizophrenia}, 181500 (2)	181510	5q11.2-q13.3
{Schizophrenia}, 181500 (2)	603175	6q13-q26

continued

Table 10.2. The morbid anatomy of the human genome (alphabetical by disorder) (*continued*)

Disorder	MIM#	Location
{Schizophrenia}, 181500 (2)	600511	6p23
{Schizophrenia}, 181500 (2)	603013	8p21
Schizophrenia, chronic (3)	104760	21q21
Schizophrenia, neurophysiologic defect in (2)	118511	15q14
{?Schizophrenia, susceptibility to} (2)	126451	3q13.3
Schwartz-Jampel syndrome, type 1, 255800 (3)	142461	1p36.1
SCID, autosomal recessive, T-negative/B-positive type (3)	600173	19p13.1
SCID due to LCK deficiency (1)	153390	1p35-p34.3
Sclerosteosis (2)	269500	17q12-q21
Scurvy (3)	240400	8p21.1
Schwannoma, sporadic (3)	101000	22q12.2
Sebastian syndrome, 605249 (3)	160775	22q11.2
Seckel syndrome (2)	210600	3q22.1-q24
SED congenita (3)	120140	12q13.11-q13.2
Segawa syndrome, recessive (3)	191290	11p15.5
Selective T-cell defect (3)	176947	2q12
SEMD, Pakistani type (3)	603005	10q23-q24
Septooptic dysplasia, 182230 (3)	601802	3p21.2-p21.1
?Sertoli-cell-only syndrome (1)	415000	Yq11
?Sertoli-cell-only syndrome (1)	400003	Yq11
Severe combined immunodeficiency, Athabascan type (2)	602450	10p
Severe combined immunodeficiency, B cell-negative, 601457 (3)	179615	11p13
Severe combined immunodeficiency, B cell-negative, 601457 (3)	179616	11p13
Severe combined immunodeficiency due to ADA deficiency (3)	102700	20q13.11
Severe combined immunodeficiency due to IL2 deficiency (1)	147680	4q26-q27
Severe combined immunodeficiency due to PTPRC deficiency (3)	151460	1q31-q32
Severe combined immunodeficiency, T-cell negative, B-cell/natural killer cell-positive type, 600802 (3)	146661	5p13
?Severe combined immunodeficiency, type I, 202500 (1)	600899	8q11
Severe combined immunodeficiency, X-linked, 300400 (3)	308380	Xq13
Sex reversal, XY, with adrenal failure (3)	184757	9q33
Sezary syndrome (3)	603517	1p22
Shah-Waardenburg syndrome, 277580 (3)	131242	20q13.2-q13.3
Short stature, autosomal dominant, with normal serum growth hormone binding protein (3)	600946	5p13-p12
Short stature, idiopathic (3)	600946	5p13-p12
Short stature, idiopathic familial (3)	312865	Xpter-p22.32
Shprintzen-Goldberg syndrome, 182212 (3)	134797	15q21.1
Sialic acid storage disorder, infantile, 269920 (3)	604322	6q14-q15
Sialidosis, type I (3)	256550	6p21.3
Sialidosis, type II (3)	256550	6p21.3
Sialuria, 269921 (3)	603824	9p12-p11
Sickle cell anemia (3)	141900	11p15.5
Simpson-Golabi-Behmel syndrome, type 1, 312870 (3)	300037	Xq26
Simpson-Golabi-Behmel syndrome, type 2 (2)	300209	Xp22
Sitosterolemia, 210250 (3)	605459	2p21
Sitosterolemia, 210250 (3)	605460	2p21
Situs ambiguus (3)	601265	Chr.10
Sjogren-Larsson syndrome (3)	270200	17p11.2
{?SLE susceptibility} (1)	120620	1q32
Small-cell cancer of lung (2)	182280	3p23-p21
SMED Strudwick type, 184250 (3)	120140	12q13.11-q13.2
Smith-Fineman-Myers syndrome, 309580 (3)	300032	Xq13
Smith-Lemli-Opitz syndrome, type I, 270400 (3)	602858	11q12-q13
Smith-Lemli-Opitz syndrome, type II, 268670 (3)	602858	11q12-q13
Smith-Magenis syndrome (2)	182290	17p11.2
[Social cognition] (2)	300082	Xq
Somatotrophinoma (2)	102200	11q13
Somatotrophinoma (3)	139320	20q13.2

continued

Table 10.2. The morbid anatomy of the human genome (alphabetical by disorder) (*continued*)

Disorder	MIM#	Location
Sorsby fundus dystrophy, 136900 (3)	188826	22q12.1-q13.2
Spastic ataxia, Charlevoix-Saguenay type, 270550 (3)	604490	13q12
Spastic cerebral palsy, symmetric (2)	603513	2q21-q31
Spastic paraplegia 14, autosomal recessive (2)	605229	3q27-q28
Spastic paraplegia, 312900 (3)	308840	Xq28
Spastic paraplegia-10 (2)	604187	12q13
Spastic paraplegia-11 (2)	604360	15q13-q15
Spastic paraplegia-12 (2)	604805	19q13
Spastic paraplegia-13 (2)	605280	2q24
Spastic paraplegia-16, X-linked, complicated (2)	300266	Xq11.2
Spastic paraplegia-2, 312920 (3)	312080	Xq22
Spastic paraplegia-3A (2)	182600	14q11.2-q24.3
Spastic paraplegia-4, 182601 (3)	604277	2p22-p21
Spastic paraplegia-5A (2)	270800	8p12-q13
Spastic paraplegia-6 (2)	600363	15q11.1
Spastic paraplegia-7 (3)	602783	16q24.3
Spastic paraplegia-8 (2)	603563	8q23-q24
Spastic paraplegia-9 (2)	601162	10q23.3-q24.1
Speech-language disorder-1 (2)	602081	7q31
Spherocytosis, hereditary (3)	109270	17q21-q22
Spherocytosis, hereditary, Japanese type (3)	177070	15q15
Spherocytosis, recessive (3)	182860	1q21
Spherocytosis-1 (3)	182870	14q22-q23.2
Spherocytosis-2 (3)	182900	8p11.2
Spiegler-Brooke syndrome (2)	605041	16q12-q13
Spinal and bulbar muscular atrophy of Kennedy, 313200 (3)	313700	Xq11-q12
Spinal muscular atrophy, congenital nonprogressive, of lower limbs (2)	600175	12q23-q24
Spinal muscular atrophy, distal, with upper limb predominance (2)	600794	7p
Spinal muscular atrophy, juvenile (3)	268800	5q13
Spinal muscular atrophy with respiratory distress 1 (2)	604320	11q13-q21
Spinal muscular atrophy, X-linked lethal infantile (2)	300021	Xp
Spinal muscular atrophy-1, 253300 (3)	600354	5q12.2-q13.3
Spinal muscular atrophy-2, 253550 (3)	600354	5q12.2-q13.3
Spinal muscular atrophy-3, 253400 (3)	600354	5q12.2-q13.3
Spinal muscular atrophy-4, (2)	158590	12q24
Spinocereballar ataxia-13 (2)	605259	19q13.3-q13.4
Spinocerebellar ataxia 12, 604326 (3)	604325	5q31-q33
Spinocerebellar ataxia 8 (3)	603680	13q21
Spinocerebellar ataxia, infantile-onset, with sensory neuropathy (2)	271245	10q24
Spinocerebellar ataxia-1, 164400 (3)	601556	6p23
Spinocerebellar ataxia-10 (3)	603516	22q13
Spinocerebellar ataxia-11 (2)	604432	15q14-q21.3
Spinocerebellar ataxia-14 (2)	605361	19q13.4-qter
Spinocerebellar ataxia-2, 183090 (3)	601517	12q24
Spinocerebellar ataxia-4 (2)	600223	16q22.1
Spinocerebellar ataxia-5 (2)	600224	11p11-q11
Spinocerebellar ataxia-6, 183086 (3)	601011	19p13
Spinocerebellar ataxia-7 (3)	164500	3p21.1-p12
Split hand/foot malformation, type 1 (2)	183600	7q21.2-q21.3
Split hand/foot malformation, type 2 (2)	313350	Xq26
Split hand/foot malformation, type 3 (2)	600095	10q24
Split-hand/foot malformation, type 4, 605289 (3)	603273	3q27
Spondylocostal dysostosis, autosomal recessive, 1, 277300 (3)	602768	19q13
Spondyloepiphyseal dysplasia, congenita, 183900 (3)	120140	12q13.11-q13.2
Spondyloepiphyseal dysplasia tarda, 313400 (3)	300202	Xp22.2-p22.1
Spondylometaphyseal dysplasia, 184252 (3)	120140	12q13.11-q13.2
Spondylometaphyseal dysplasia, Japanese type (3)	120110	6q21-q22.3
Spondyloperipheral dysplasia, 271700 (3)	120140	12q13.11-q13.2

continued

Table 10.2. The morbid anatomy of the human genome (alphabetical by disorder) (*continued*)

Disorder	MIM#	Location
Squamous cell carcinoma, head and neck, 601400 (3)	601566	13q34
Squamous cell carcinoma, head and neck, 601400 (3)	603612	8p22-p21
Stargardt disease 3, 600110 (3)	605512	6q14
Stargardt disease 4 (2)	603786	4p
Stargardt disease-1, 248200 (3)	601691	1p21-p13
Startle disease, autosomal recessive (3)	138491	5q32
Startle disease/hyperekplexia, autosomal dominant, 149400 (3)	138491	5q32
Steatocystoma multiplex, 184500 (3)	148069	17q12-q21
Stem-cell leukemia/lymphoma syndrome (3)	602221	13q11-q12
Stickler syndrome, type I, 108300 (3)	120140	12q13.11-q13.2
Stickler syndrome, type II, 604841 (3)	120280	1p21
Stickler syndrome, type III, 184840 (3)	120290	6p21.3
?Stomatocytosis I, 185000 (1)	133090	9q34.1
Subcortical laminal heteropia, X-linked, 300067 (3)	300121	Xq22.3-q23
Subcortical laminar heterotopia (3)	601545	17p13.3
Succinic semialdehyde dehydrogenase deficiency (3)	271980	6p22
Sucrose intolerance (3)	222900	3q25-q26
Supravalvar aortic stenosis, 185500 (3)	130160	7q11.2
?{Susceptibility to IDDM} (1)	180840	11q13
Sutherland-Haan syndrome, 309470 (3)	300032	Xq13
Sweat chloride elevation without CF (3)	602421	7q31.2
Symphalangism, proximal, 185800 (3)	602991	17q22
Syndactyly, type I (2)	185900	2q34-q36
Syndactyly, type III, 186100 (2)	164200	6q22-q24
Synostoses syndrome, multiple, 1, 186500 (3)	602991	17q22
Synpolydactyly, type II, 186000 (3)	142989	2q31-q32
{Systemic lupus erythematosus, susceptibility}, 152700 (3)	134638	1q23
{Systemic lupus erythematosus, susceptibility to, 1}, 152700 (2)	601744	1q41-q42
{Systemic lupus erythematosus, susceptibility to, 2}, 152700 (2)	605218	2q37
{Systemic lupus erythematosus, susceptibility to, 3}, 152700 (2)	605480	4p16-p15.2
Tangier disease, 205400 (3)	600046	9q22-q31
Tay-Sachs disease (3)	272800	15q23-q24
T-cell acute lymphoblastic leukemia (3)	600040	19q13.3-q13.4
T-cell immunodeficiency, congenital alopecia, and nail dystrophy (3)	600838	17q11-q12
T-cell prolymphocytic leukemia, sporadic (3)	208900	11q22.3
Temperature-sensitive apoptosis (1)	600243	14q11-q12
Testicular germ cell tumor (2)	300228	Xq27
?Tetramelic mirror-image polydactyly (2)	135750	14q13
Thalassemia, alpha- (3)	141850	16pter-p13.3
Thalassemia, delta- (3)	142000	11p15.5
Thalassemia due to Hb Lepore (3)	142000	11p15.5
Thalassemias, alpha- (3)	141800	16pter-p13.3
Thalassemias, beta- (3)	141900	11p15.5
Thanatophoric dysplasia, types I and II, 187600 (3)	134934	4p16.3
Thiamine-responsive megaloblastic anemia syndrome, 249270 (3)	603941	1q23.3
Thoracoabdominal syndrome (2)	313850	Xq25-q26.1
Thrombocythemia, essential, 187950 (3)	600044	3q26.3-q27
Thrombocytopenia, congenital amegakaryocytic, 604498 (3)	159530	1p34
Thrombocytopenia, neonatal alloimmune (1)	273800	17q21.32
?Thrombocytopenia, Paris-Trousseau type (2)	188025	11q23
Thrombocytopenia, X-linked, 313900 (3)	301000	Xp11.23-p11.22
Thrombocytopenia-2 (2)	188000	10p12-p11.2
{Thromboembolism susceptibility due to factor V Leiden} (3)	227400	1q23
?Thrombophilia due to elevated HRG (1)	142640	3q27
Thrombophilia due to excessive plasminogen activator inhibitor (1)	173360	7q21.3-q22
Thrombophilia due to heparin cofactor II deficiency (3)	142360	22q11
Thrombophilia due to HRG deficiency (3)	142640	3q27
Thrombophilia due to protein C deficiency (3)	176860	2q13-q14

continued

Table 10.2. The morbid anatomy of the human genome (alphabetical by disorder) (*continued*)

Disorder	MIM#	Location
Thrombophilia due to thrombomodulin defect (3)	188040	20p11.2
Thrombophilia, dysfibrinogenemic (3)	134830	4q28
Thrombophilia, dysfibrinogenemic (3)	134850	4q28
Thrombophilia, dysplasminogenemic (1)	173350	6q26
Thromboxane synthase deficiency (2)	274180	7q34
Thymine-uraciluria (3)	274270	1p22
Thyroid adenoma, hyperfunctioning (3)	603372	14q31
Thyroid carcinoma, nonmedullary, with cell oxyphilia (2)	603386	19p13.2
Thyroid hormone resistance, 274300, 188570 (3)	190160	3p24.3
Thyroid iodine peroxidase deficiency (1)	274500	2p25
Thyroid papillary carcinoma, 188550 (1)	601985	10q21
Thyrotropin-releasing hormone deficiency (1)	275120	3q13.3-q21
?Tibial hemimelia (2)	275220	8q24.1
Tibial muscular dystrophy (2)	600334	2q31
Tietz syndrome, 103500 (3)	156845	3p14.1-p12.3
Tolbutamide poor metabolizer (3)	601130	10q24
Total anomalous pulmonary venous return (2)	106700	4p13-q12
Tourette syndrome (2)	137580	11q23
Townes-Brocks syndrome, 107480 (3)	602218	16q12.1
Transcobalamin II deficiency (3)	275350	22q11.2-qter
[Transcortin deficiency] (1)	122500	14q32.1
Transient bullous dermolysis of the newborn, 131705 (3)	120120	3p21.3
Treacher Collins mandibulofacial dysostosis (3)	154500	5q32-q33.1
Tremor, familial essential, 1 (2)	190300	3q13
Tremor, familial essential, 2 (2)	602134	2p25-p22
Trichodontoosseous syndrome, 190320 (3)	600525	17q21.3-q22
Trichoepithelioma, multiple familial (2)	601606	9p21
Trichorhinophalangeal syndrome, type I, 190350 (3)	604386	8q24.12
Trichothiodystrophy (3)	133510	2q21
Trichothiodystrophy, 601675 (3)	126340	19q13.2-q13.3
Trifunctional protein deficiency, type I (3)	600890	2p23
Trifunctional protein deficiency, type II (3)	143450	2p23
Triphalangeal thumb-polysyndactyly syndrome (2)	190605	7q36
Trypsinogen deficiency (1)	276000	7q35
{Tuberculosis, susceptibility to} (2)	300259	Xq
{Tuberculosis, susceptibility to} (3)	107470	6q23-q24
Tuberous sclerosis-1, 191100 (3)	605284	9q34
Tuberous sclerosis-2, 191100 (3)	191092	16p13.3
Turcot syndrome, 276300 (3)	175100	5q21-q22
Turcot syndrome with glioblastoma, 276300 (3)	120436	3p21.3
Turcot syndrome with glioblastoma, 276300 (3)	600259	7p22
Turner syndrome-associated neurocognitive phenotype (2)	313000	Xp22.33
Tylosis with esophageal cancer (2)	148500	17q24
Tyrosinemia, type I (3)	276700	15q23-q25
Tyrosinemia, type Ib (1)	603758	14q24.3
Tyrosinemia, type II (3)	276600	16q22.1-q22.3
Tyrosinemia, type III (3)	276710	12q24-qter
{Ulcerative colitis, susceptibility to}, 191390 (1)	158371	7q22
Ulnar-mammary syndrome, 181450 (3)	601621	12q24.1
[Urate oxidase deficiency] (1)	191540	1p22
Urofacial syndrome (2)	236730	10q23-q24
Urolithiasis, 2, 8-dihydroxyadenine (3)	102600	16q24.3
Usher syndrome, type 1A (2)	276900	14q32
Usher syndrome, type 1B (3)	276903	11q13.5
Usher syndrome, type 1C, 276904 (3)	605242	11p15.1
Usher syndrome, type 1D, 601067 (3)	605516	10q21-q22
Usher syndrome, type 1E (2)	602097	21q21
Usher syndrome, type 2A (3)	276901	1q41

continued

Table 10.2. The morbid anatomy of the human genome (alphabetical by disorder) (*continued*)

Disorder	*MIM#*	*Location*
Usher syndrome, type 2C (2)	605472	5q14-q21
Usher syndrome, type 3 (2)	276902	3q21-q25
Usher syndrome, type IF (2)	602083	Chr.10
Usher syndrome, type IIB (2)	276905	3p24.2-p23
Uterine leiomyoma (3)	600698	12q15
{UV-induced skin damage, vulnerability to} (3)	155555	16q24.3
Van Buchem disease (2)	239100	17q11.2
van der Woude syndrome (2)	119300	1q32
Velocardiofacial syndrome, 192430 (2)	188400	22q11
Venous malformations, multiple cutaneous and mucosal, 600195 (3)	600221	9p21
Ventricular fibrillation, idiopathic, 603829 (3)	600163	3p21
Ventricular tachycardia, idiopathic, 192605 (3)	139360	3p21
Ventricular tachycardia, stress-induced polymorphic, 604772 (3)	180902	1q42.1-q43
Vesicoureteral reflux (2)	193000	1p13
{Viral infections, recurrent} (3)	146740	1q23
Virilization, maternal and fetal, from placental aromatase deficiency (3)	107910	15q21.1
[Visuospatial/perceptual abilities] (2)	313000	Xp22.33
Vitamin K-dependent coagulation defect, 277450 (3)	137167	2p12
Vitreoretinopathy, exudative, familial (2)	133780	11q13-q23
Vitreoretinopathy, neovascular inflammatory (2)	193235	11q13
{Vivax malaria, susceptibility to} (1)	110700	1q21-q22
VLCAD deficiency (3)	201475	17p11.2-p11.1
Vohwinkel syndrome, 124500 (3)	121011	13q11-q12
Vohwinkel syndrome with ichthyosis, 604117 (3)	152445	1q21
von Hippel-Lindau syndrome (3)	193300	3p26-p25
von Willebrand disease (3)	193400	12p13.3
Waardenburg syndrome, type 2B (2)	600193	1p21-p13.3
Waardenburg syndrome, type I (3)	193500	2q35
Waardenburg syndrome, type IIA, 193510 (3)	156845	3p14.1-p12.3
Waardenburg syndrome, type III, 148820 (3)	193500	2q35
Waardenburg syndrome/occular albinism, digenic, 103470 (3)	203100	11q14-q21
Waardenburg syndrome/ocular albinism, digenic, 103470 (3)	156845	3p14.1-p12.3
Waardenburg-Shah syndrome, 277580 (3)	602229	22q13
Waardenburg-Shah syndrome, neurologic variant (3)	602229	22q13
Wagner syndrome, 143200 (3)	120140	12q13.11-q13.2
Wagner syndrome (2)	143200	5q13-q14
Wagner syndrome, type II (3)	120140	12q13.11-q13.2
Waisman parkinsonism-mental retardation syndrome (2)	311510	Xq28
?Walker-Warburg syndrome, 236670 (2)	253800	9q31
Warfarin sensitivity, 122700 (3)	601130	10q24
Warfarin sensitivity (3)	306900	Xq27.1-q27.2
Watson syndrome, 193520 (3)	162200	17q11.2
Weissenbacher-Zweymuller syndrome, 277610 (3)	120290	6p21.3
Welander distal myopathy (2)	604454	2p13
Werner syndrome, 277700 (3)	604611	8p12-p11.2
{?Wernicke-Korsakoff syndrome, susceptibility to} (1)	300044	Xq28
{Wernicke-Korsakoff syndrome, susceptibility to} (1)	277730	3p14.3
Weyers acrodental dysostosis, 193530 (3)	604831	4p16
White sponge nevus, 193900 (3)	123940	12q13
White sponge nevus, 193900 (3)	148065	17q21-q22
Wieacker-Wolff syndrome (2)	314580	Xq13-q21
Williams-Beuren syndrome, 194050 (3)	130160	7q11.2
{Wilms tumor susceptibility-5} (2)	601583	7p15-p11.2
Wilms tumor, type 1 (3)	194070	11p13
Wilms tumor, type 2 (2)	194071	11p15.5
Wilms tumor, type 3 (2)	194090	16q
Wilms tumor, type 4 (2)	601363	17q12-q21
Wilson disease (3)	277900	13q14.3-q21.1

continued

Table 10.2. The morbid anatomy of the human genome (alphabetical by disorder) (*continued*)

Disorder	MIM#	Location
Wiskott-Aldrich syndrome (3)	301000	Xp11.23-p11.22
Wolcott-Rallison syndrome, 226980 (3)	604032	2p12
Wolf-Hirschhorn syndrome (2)	194190	4p16.3
Wolfram syndrome 2 (2)	604928	4q22-q24
Wolfram syndrome (3)	222300	4p16.1
Wolman disease (3)	278000	10q24-q25
Wood neuroimmunologic syndrome (2)	300076	Xq26-qter
Wrinkly skin syndrome (2)	278250	2q32
Xanthinuria, type I (3)	278300	2p23-p22
?Xeroderma pigmentosum (1)	173870	1q42
Xeroderma pigmentosum, group A (3)	278700	9q22.3
Xeroderma pigmentosum, group B (3)	133510	2q21
Xeroderma pigmentosum, group C (3)	278720	3p25
Xeroderma pigmentosum, group D, 278730 (3)	126340	19q13.2-q13.3
Xeroderma pigmentosum, group E, DDB-negative subtype, 278740 (3)	600811	11p12-p11
Xeroderma pigmentosum, group E, subtype 2 (1)	600045	11q12-q13
Xeroderma pigmentosum, group F, 278760 (3)	133520	16p13.3-p13.13
Xeroderma pigmentosum, group G, 278780 (3)	133530	13q33
Xeroderma pigmentosum, variant type, 278750 (3)	603968	Chr.6
X-inactivation, familial skewed (3)	314670	Xq13.2
?XLA and isolated growth hormone deficiency, 307200 (3)	300300	Xq21.3-q22
XY sex reversal (1)	602424	9p24.3
XY sex reversal (2)	154230	9p24
Yemenite deaf-blind hypopigmentation syndrome, 601706 (3)	602229	22q13
Zellweger syndrome, 214100 (3)	602859	Chr.1
Zellweger syndrome, 214100 (3)	601789	2p15
Zellweger syndrome, 214100 (3)	603164	6q23-q24
Zellweger syndrome, 214100 (3)	602136	7q21-q22
Zellweger syndrome, 214100 (3)	170993	8q21.1
Zlotogora-Ogur syndrome, 225000 (3)	600644	11q23-q24

Mitochondrial genes in degenerative diseases, cancer and aging

Douglas C. Wallace
Marie T. Lott

A wide variety of degenerative diseases have now been associated with mitochondrial defects. These can result from mutations in either the mitochondrial DNA (mtDNA) or the nuclear DNA (nDNA). Some mtDNA mutations result in idiosyncratic symptoms, such as the missense mutations that cause Leber's hereditary optic neuropathy (LHON) (Wallace et al., 1988a); while others give variable multi-system presentations, such as the deletion mutations causing chronic progressive external ophthalmoplegia (CPEO) (Holt et al., 1988).

Mitochondrial diseases can be transmitted by both maternal and mendelian modes of inheritance, as well as by novel combinations of the two. This genetic complexity results from the fact that the mitochondrion is assembled from perhaps a 1000 genes dispersed across the mitochondrial and nuclear genomes. In addition, mitochondrial diseases frequently have a delayed onset and a progressive course, probably resulting from the accumulation of somatic mtDNA mutations in post-mitotic tissues. Somatic mtDNA mutations also contribute to cancer and aging.

Mitochondrial diseases frequently affect the central nervous system (CNS), skeletal muscle, heart, renal and/or endocrine systems, though any organ system may be involved. This phenotypic complexity results from the central role played by the mitochondria in a variety of cellular processes which include generation of cellular energy by oxidative phosphorylation (OXPHOS), production of toxic reactive oxygen species (ROS) as a by-product of OXPHOS, and regulation of the initiation of apoptosis through the activation of the mitochondrial permeability transition pore (mtPTP).

Mitochondrial biology

The typical human cell contains several hundred mitochondria with their characteristic double membrane structure (Figure 11.1). The outer membrane is smooth, but the inner membrane is highly folded forming structures called cristae. The large surface area of the inner mitochondrial membrane accommodates the enzymes of the mitochondrial energy generating apparatus, OXPHOS.

MITOCHONDRIAL PROCESSES: ENERGY PRODUCTION, ROS GENERATION, AND APOPTOSIS

OXPHOS is composed of five multi-polypeptide enzyme complexes. Complexes I, II, III, and IV make up the electron transport chain (ETC), while complex V is the ATP synthase (Figure 11.1). Dietary carbohydrates and fats are transported to the mitochondria where they are oxidized by the tricarboxylic acid (TCA) cycle and the β-oxidation pathways, respectively. This liberates CO_2 and hydrogen atoms, the latter being transferred to soluble NAD^+ to generate $NADH + H^+$ or to FAD bound within enzymes to yield $FADH_2$. $NADH + H^+$ is oxidized by complex I (NADH: ubiquinone oxidoreductase, EC 1.6.5.3) and the electrons transported through flavin mononucleotide (FMN) and multiple iron-sulfur centers until they are transferred to ubiquinone (CoQ_{10}). CoQ_{10} is subsequently reduced to ubisemiquinone ($CoQ_{10}H^.$), then to ubiquinol ($CoQ_{10}H_2$). CoQ_{10} is also reduced to $CoQ_{10}H_2$ by succinate through complex II (succinate: ubiquinone oxidoreductase, EC 1.3.5.1) and by electrons from fatty acid oxidation *via* the electron transfer flavoprotein (ETF) together with

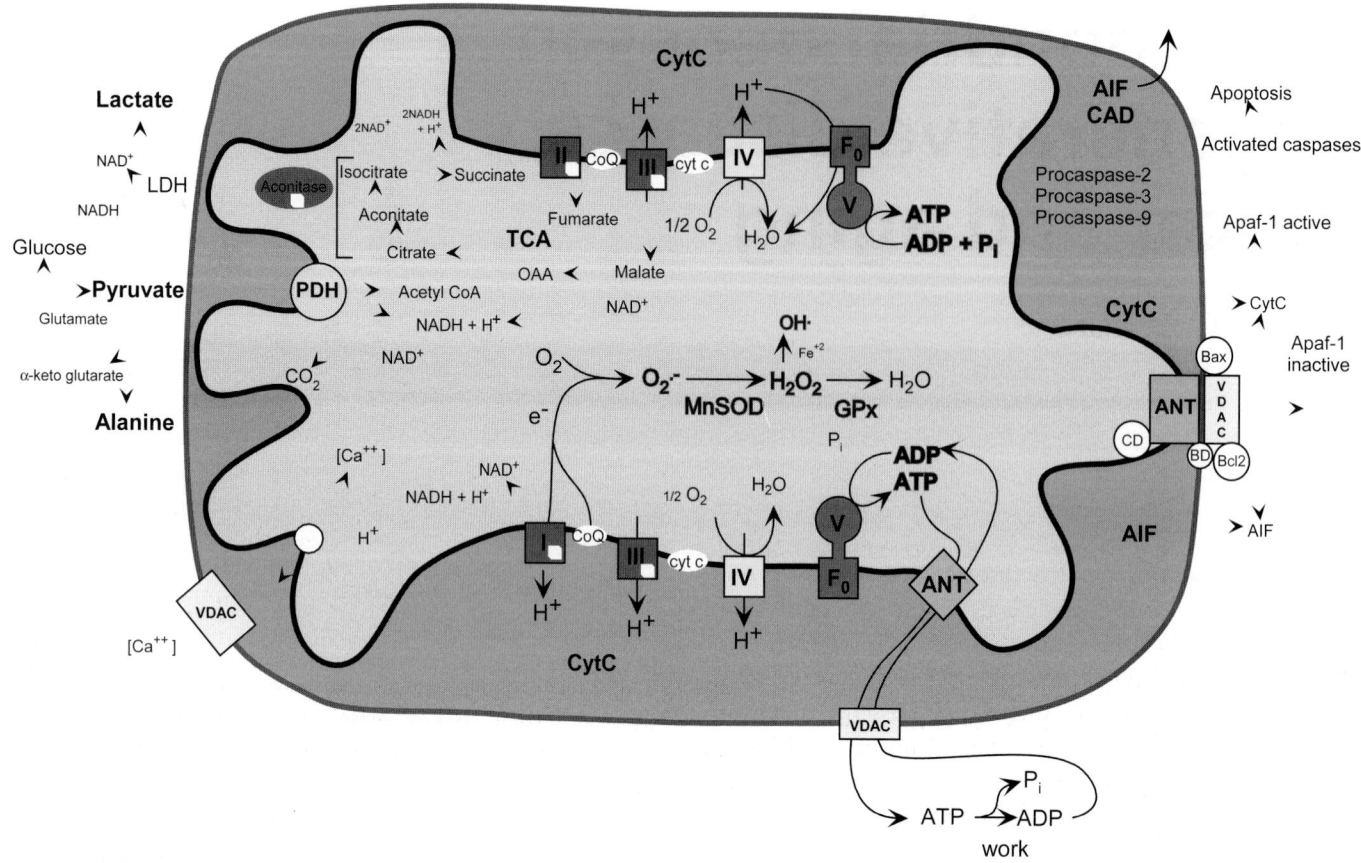

Fig. 11.1. Diagram of a mitochondrion, illustrating the relationships between mitochondrial oxidative phosphorylation and (a) the production of energy (ATP), (b) the generation of reactive oxygen species (ROS), and (c) the initiation of apotosis through activation of the mitochondrial permeability transition pore (mtPTP). The respiratory enzyme complexes involved in OXPHOS are complex I (NADH: ubiquinone oxidoreductase), complex II (succinate:ubiquinone oxidoreductase), complex III (ubiquinol:cytochrome c oxidoreductase), complex IV (cytochrome c oxidase), and complex V (H-translocating ATP synthase). Pyruvate from glucose enters the mitochondria *via* pyruvate dehydrogenase (PDH), generating acetyl CoA, which enters the tricarboxylic acid (TCA) cycle by combining with oxaloacetate (OOA). *cis*-Aconitase converts citrate to isocitrate. All enzymes containing an iron-sulfur cluster are designated with a cube. Lactate dehydrogenase (LDH) converts excess pyruvate plus NADH to lactate. Small molecules diffuse through the outer membrane via the voltage-dependent anion channels (VDAC) or porin. VDACs together with the adenine nucleotide translocator (ANT), Bax, and cyclophilin D (CD) are thought to come together at the mitochondrial inner and outer membrane contact points to create the mtPTP. Bax is pro-apoptotic and is thought to interact with the anti-apoptotic protein BCL-2 and the benzodiazepine receptor (BD). The opening of the mtPTP is associated with the release of cytochrome c, AIF (apoptosis initiating factor), CAD (caspase-activated DNAase), and the procaspases 2, 3, and 9. In the cytosol, cytochrome c activates Apaf-1 which actives procaspace-2 and 9. The activated caspases activate caspases 3, 6, 7, and CAD. The caspases degrade the cytoplasm while AIF and CAD migrate to the nucleus and degrade the chromatin. (Modified from Wallace, 1999).

the ETF dehydrogenase (EC 1.5.5.1). Both succinate dehydrogenase and ETF dehydrogenase contain a FAD and one or more iron sulfur centers. $CoQ_{10}H_2$ ferries the electrons through the inner membrane to complex III (ubiquinol: ferrocytochrome c oxidoreductase, EC 1.10.2.2 or the bc_1 complex). Within this complex, the electrons move through the Q cycle, cytochrome b, cytochrome $c1$, and the Rieske iron-sulfur components. The electrons are then transferred from complex III to cytochrome c, which is loosely associated with the exterior of the inner membrane. Cytochrome c transfers the electrons to complex IV (ferrocytochrome c: oxygen oxidoreductase, EC1.9.3.3.1 or cytochrome c oxidase, COX). Within this complex the electrons are trans-

ferred through the CuA and CuB centers and cytochromes a and a_3 and ultimately combine with $\frac{1}{2} O_2$ to give H_2O. The energy that is released in this controled oxidation of the electrons is used to pump protons from inside the mitochondrial matrix across the inner membrane into the inter-membrane space through complexes I, III, and IV. The resulting electrochemical gradient, $\Delta\rho$, which involves both ΔpH ($\Delta\mu^{H+}$) and electrostatic potential ($\Delta\Psi$) differences, serves as a source of potential energy for synthesizing adenosine triphosphate (ATP). ATP is synthesized by complex V (ATP phosphohydrolase (H⁺-transporting), EC 3.6.1.34, or ATP synthase, ATPsyn) which contains three distinctive components: the base, F_0; the stalk; and the hexagonal head, F_1. As protons move back through the proton channel in F_0, they cause the central axle of the ATPsyn to spin within the hexagonal array of 3α and 3β subunits, causing them to change their conformation. This causes ADP and P_i to bind, be condensed into ATP, and to be released into the matrix. Matrix ATP is exchanged for cytosolic ADP by the adenine nucleotide translocator (ANT) (Wallace, 1992a; 1992b; 1995a) (Figure 11.1).

Each of the ETC complexes incorporates multiple electron carriers. Complexes I, II, and III encompass several Fe-S centers, as does aconitase of the TCA cycle. Complexes III and IV encompass the cytochromes (Wallace, 1992a; 1992b; 1999).

Since the ETC is coupled to ATP synthesis through $\Delta\Psi$, mitochondrial oxygen consumption is regulated by the matrix concentration of ADP. In the absence of ADP, oxygen consumption is slow (state IV respiration). However, when ADP is added, it is transported into the matrix by the ANT, and oxygen consumption goes up as the ATP synthase utilizes the proton gradient to phosphorylate ADP back to ATP (state III respiration). The ratio of state III and state IV respiration is called the respiratory control ratio (RCR) and the amount of molecular oxygen consumed relative to the ADP phosphorylated is the P/O ratio. The addition of uncouplers such as 2,4-dinitrophenol (DNP) and FCCP collapse $\Delta\Psi$ and permit the ETC and oxygen consumption to run at their maximum rates.

The mitochondria are also the primary source of endogenous reactive oxygen species (ROS). The first of the ROSs, superoxide anion (O_2^-) is generated by the transfer of one electron from the ETC to O_2 (Figure 11.1). Ubisemiquinone, localized at the CoQ binding sites of complexes I, II, and III, appears to be the primary electron donor (Boveris and Turrens, 1980; Ksenzenko et al., 1983; Turrens et al., 1985).

Mitochondrial O_2^- is converted to H_2O_2 by manganese superoxide dismutase (MnSOD) and the resulting H_2O_2 is reduced to water by glutathione peroxidase-1 (GPx1) in brain, liver and kidney, and possibly by catalase in heart and muscle. However, H_2O_2, in the presence of reduced transition metals can also be converted to the highly reactive hydroxyl radical ($\cdot OH$). The Fe-S centers of the TCA cycle and the ETC are the major targets of ROS reactivity. Hence the mitochondria are particularly sensitive to oxidative stress (Bandy and Davison, 1990; Goldhaber and Weiss, 1992; Rotig et al., 1997; Wallace, 1999; Yan et al., 1997).

Superoxide production and H_2O_2 generation are highest when the ETC is more reduced (state IV respiration) and lowest when it is more oxidized (state III respiration) (Boveris, 1984; Boveris et al., 1972; Cadenas and Boveris,

1980; Chance et al., 1979; Loschen et al., 1974). Since ubisemiquinone is probably the primary electron donor for O_2^- generation, ROS production will be maximized under physiological condition that maximize the concentration of ubisemiquinone. Hence, mitochondria with primarily oxidized ubiquinone would produce minimal ROS species. Similarly, mitochondria with completely reduced ubiquinol would produce less ROS. However, a predominantly though not completely reduced ETC would have the maximum ubisemiquinone and hence maximal ROS production. This then explains why blocking electron flow through the ETC with drugs such as antimycin A, which inhibits complex III, stimulates ROS production, and why adding uncouplers further stimulates ROS production (Boveris et al., 1972; Cadenas and Boveris, 1980; Ksenzenko et al., 1983; Loschen et al., 1974).

The mitochondria are also the major regulators of apoptosis, which is initiated though the opening of mtPTP (Figure 11.1). The mtPTP is thought to be composed of the inner membrane ANT, the outer membrane voltage dependent anion channel (VDAC) or porin, Bax, Bcl2, cyclophilin D, and the benzodiazepine receptor (Green and Reed, 1998; Petit et al., 1996; Zoratti and Szabo, 1995). When the mtPTP opens, $\Delta\Psi$ collapses and ions equilibrate between the matrix and cytosol, causing the mitochondria to swell. Ultimately, this disrupts the outer membrane, releasing the contents of the inter-membrane space into the cytosol. The inter-membrane space contains a number of cell death-promoting factors, including cytochrome c; procaspases-2, 3, and 9; apoptosis initiating factor (AIF) and caspase-activated DNase (CAD) (Earnshaw, 1999; Liu et al., 1996; Mancini et al., 1998; Susin et al., 1999a; 1999b). On release, cytochrome c activates the cytosolic Apaf-1 which activates the procaspases destroying the cytoplasm. AIF and CAD are transported to the nucleus where they degrade the chromatin (Wallace, 1999). The mtPTP can be stimulated to open by uptake of excessive Ca^{2+} which binds to cyclophilin D; increased oxidative stress; decreased mitochondrial $\Delta\Psi$; and ANT ligands such as atractyloside. It is inhibited from opening by ADP (Green and Reed, 1998; Liu et al., 1996). Thus, disease states which inhibit OXPHOS and increase ROS production also increase the propensity of the cell to undergo apoptosis (Brustovetsky and Klingenberg, 1996; Green and Reed, 1998; Marzo et al., 1998).

STRESS RESPONSE AND THE MITOCHONDRIA

The mitochondria interact with the cellular stress response pathways to globally regulate cellular functions, survival and proliferation. One major rapid acting cellular regulator is the short half-life nitric oxide (NO). NO is generated from arginine by nitric oxide synthase (NOS). There are three cytosolic NOS isoforms: neuronal NOS (nNOS), inducible NOS (iNOS) and endothelial NOS (eNOS) which is expressed in activated macrophages. NOS has recognition sites for calmodulin, NADPH, FAD, FMN, and uses heme and tetrahydiobiopterin as oxidation-reduction cofactors. nNOS is tethered to NMDA receptors in neurons by the PSD-95 protein. Hence, when NMDA receptors are activated by glutamate permitting Ca^{2+} to flow into the cytosol. This immediately activates nNOS *via* calmodulin (Knowles, 1997; Snyder et al., 1998). The NO generated by NOS can react with superoxide anion O_2^- to give the highly reactive peroxynitrite anion ($ONOO^-$). This can be protonated to give peroxynitrous acid (ONOOH) (Radi et al., 1997).

The mitochondria has its own mitochondria-specific NOS (mtNOS), which may be attached to the mitochondrial inner membrane (Ghafourifar and Richter, 1997; Richter et al., 1999). Mitochondrial NO has been shown to reversibly inhibit complex IV (COX) causing a reduction in $\Delta\Psi$ and Ca^{2+} release from the mitochondrion (Richter et al., 1997). Mitochondrial NO can also react with O_2^- to generate peroxynitrite ($ONOO^-$) which can inactivate mitochondrial creatine phosphokinase (mtCPK) (Stachowiak et al, 1998), active the mitochondrial release cytochrome c (Ghafourifar et al., 1999), inhibit other respiratory complexes (Brown et al., 1997a) and possibly activate poly (ADP-ribose) polymerase (PARP) (Szabo, 1997).

The heme oxygenases (HO) degrade heme by cleaving the porphyrin ring and generating biliverdin and carbon monoxide (CO). Biliverdin is rapidly reduced to bilirubin by biliverdin reductase. The bilirubin-biliverdin oxido-reductase system provides a potent anti-oxidant mechanism for protecting the cell (Synder et al., 1998). There are two HOs enzymes. HO1 is the most abundant form, is highly concentrated in the spleen, and degrades heme from senescent red blood cells. HO1 is induced by heme, oxidative stress, and agents that induce heat shock proteins. HO2 is a non inducible form localized in the brain and testis (Snyder et al., 1998). Both CO and NO function in neuronal transmission of signals to target cells such as the intestine (Zakhary et al., 1997) and are involved in endothelial cell-dependent relaxation (Zakhary et al., 1996). Interestingly, CO, like NO, is a potent inhibitor of COX. However, NO has a very short half-life and must be produced close to the target where as CO is extremely stable and can diffuse large distances. Hence, the products of the HO2 may regulate mitochondrial energetics through the CO and with mitochondrial ROS through bilirubin-biliverdin antioxidant system.

Another stress-response enzyme is poly (ADP-ribose) polymerase (PARP). PARP is a nuclear DNA enzyme which is activated by fragments of DNA resulting from DNA damage. Utilizing NAD^+ as a substrate, it transfers 50 or more ADP-ribose moieties to nuclear proteins such as histones and PARP itself. Massive DNA damage results in excessive activation of PARP, which leads to the depletion of NAD^+. The resynthesis of NAD^+ from ATP then markedly depletes cellular ATP leading to death (Synder et al., 1998). Mice in which the PARP gene has been genetically inactivated show remarkable resistance to cellular stress such as cerebral ischemia (stroke) (Eliasson et al., 1997; Takahashi et al., 1999) and streptozotocin-induced diabetes (Pieper et al., 1999).

The nuclear protein, p53, is also activated by DNA damage and can initiate programed cell death. This pathway has been shown to be mediated through mitochondrial release of cytochrome c, which in turn activates Apaf-1 and caspase 9. The p53 initiation of mitochondrial cytochrome c release requires the intervention of pro-apoptotic protein Bax. Hence, DNA damage activates p53, which activates Bax, which causes mitochondrial cytochrome c release, which initiates apoptosis (Schuler et al., 2000).

Another nuclear protein, SIR2, uses NAD^+ as a cofactor to diacetylate histones. Diacetylated histones keep silent genes, such as proto-oncogenes, turned off (Lin et al., 2000). Depletion of NAD^+ would inactivate SIR2, permitting histones to be acetylated, and silent genes to be illegitimately expressed (Lin et al., 2000).

Finally, mitochondrially generated H_2O_2 may be augmented by ROS production from the cytosolic NADPH oxidases. NADPH oxidases reduce O_2 to generate superoxide anion in the cytosol. The best characterized of the NADPH oxidases is the macrophage "oxidative burst" complex involved in generating the O_2^- to kill engulfed microorganisms. However, an additional NADPH oxidase, Mox1, is a homologue of the gp91phox catalytic subunit of the phagocyte NADP oxidase. Mox1 generates O_2^-, and over-expression of Mox1 in NIH3T3 cells increases the cellular mitotic rate, transformation frequency, and tumorgenicity (Suh et al., 1999a). The mitogenic activity of Mox1 can be neutralized by overexpression of catalase. Hence, the, cell growth signal must be H_2O_2 (Arnold et al., 2001). The fact that H_2O_2 is a mitogenic signal for the cell nucleus is of great importance for the mitochondria, since H_2O_2 is the only mitochondrial ROS that it stable enough to defuse to the nucleus.

Acting together, these various enzymes form an integrated metabolic network with the mitochondrion.

Production of NO by NOS and CO by HO provide short-term and long-term inhibitors of complex IV, and hence mitochondrial ATP production. Inhibition of the mitochondrial ETC also increases O_2^- production, which is converted to H_2O_2 by mitochondrial MnSOD. Mitochondrial H_2O_2 can diffuse to the nucleus where at low concentrations it can act as a mitogen. However, excessive mitochondrial generation of H_2O_2 can overwhelm the antioxidant defenses of the cytosol (catalase, glutathione peroxidase, and bilirubin) and cause nDNA damage. Nuclear DNA damage can mutagenize proto-oncogenes, causing their activation. Excessive DNA damage also activates PARP, which degrades NAD^+. Depletion of NAD^+ inactivates SIR2 which causes the depression of inactive nDNA genes including proto-oncogenes. Hence, the introduction of mitochondrial metabolites with these stress response systems can mediate both programed cell death and neoplastic transformation.

MITOCHONDRIAL OXPHOS COMPLEXES

Complex I (NADH dehydrogenase, NDH)

OXPHOS complex I is composed of approximately 42 polypeptides, seven (MTND1, 2, 3, 4, 4L, 5 and 6) of which are encoded by the mtDNA. These encompass three flavoproteins (FPs), seven iron-sulfur proteins (ISPs), and over 24 hydrophobic proteins (Galante and Hatefi 1979; Anderson et al., 1981, Oliver and Wallace 1982; Arizmendi et al, 1992; Attardi et al, 1986; Chomyn et al, 1983, 1985, 1986; Skehel et al., 1998; Smeitink and van den Heuvel 1999; Walker 1995; Walker et al., 1992; Wallace et al., 1999b).

Complex I oxidizes NADH and reduces CoQ_{10} and uses the energy released to pump protons across the mitochondrial inner membrane. Electrons from NADH are transferred through FMN and up to nine iron sulfur centers, including N-1a, N-1b, N-2, N-3, N-4 and N-5 (Ohnishi, 1979; Ragan, 1987). The overall structure of complex I is slipper shaped, with the foot lying in the membrane and the ankle extending into the mitochondrial matrix (Grigorieff, 1998; Guenebaut et al., 1998).

The bovine complex I consists of a globular hydrophilic region containing the NADH binding site, FMN, and all ISPs; a 30 Å diameter stalk, and a hydrophobic membrane component. The overall molecular mass is 890 kDa. The hydrophilic globular component and stalk are 175Å and have a mass of about 520 kDa. The hydrophobic component is 200Å long and has a mass of about 370 kDa (Grigorieff, 1998). The complex can be split into two major components, Iα and Iβ, by the detergent lauryl-dimethylamine oxide (LDAO). The Iα component can oxidize NADH and reduce ubiquinone, and contains the NADH binding site, FMN, and all of the known Fe-S centers. The Iβ component has no enzymatic activity, is hydrophobic, and probably represents the membrane bound component. The Iα consists of 23 polypeptides including polypeptides the 75 kDa protein which contains two iron sulfur centers, the 51 kDa which forms the NADH and FMN binding sites and also binds a tetranuclear iron-sulfur center, the 24 kDa contains a binuclear iron-sulfur center, and the TYKY, PSST, and PGIV polypeptides which bind the redox centers (Hatefi, 1985; Pilkington and Walker, 1989; Toda et al., 1989; Chow et al., 1991; Duncan et al., 1992; Spencer et al., 1992; de Coo et al., 1995; Hattori et al., 1995; Walker, 1995). The Iβ fragment contains 17 polypeptides, 13 of which contain at least one membrane-spanning segment, two of which are ND4 and ND5 (Fearnley et al., 1994; Walker, 1992; 1995). Thus, most of the mtDNA-encoded polypeptides probably reside in the foot-shaped membrane component IB.

Respiratory complex I can also be subfractionated by treatment with the chaotrophic anion perchlorate into three fragments: the flavoprotein fragment, iron-protein fragment, and hydrophobic fragment (Ragan, 1987). The flavoprotein fragment encompasses FMN, six iron atoms, and the 51 kDa, 24 kDa, and 10 kDa polypeptides (Belogrudov and Hatefi, 1994; Walker, 1995). The iron-protein fragment contains nine or ten iron atoms (Ragan et al., 1982a,b), a 15 kDa protein which may be a ubiquinone-binding protein (Suzuki and Ozawa, 1986), and the ND6 polypeptide may also be located in this fragment (Chomyn et al., 1986) and involved in CoQ_{10} binding (Jun et al., 1996). The hydrophobic fragment probably contains the majority of the mtDNA-encoded polypeptides, including MTND1, MTND3 and MTND4L (Chomyn et al., 1986; Ragan, 1987) and may also contain MTND2, MTND4, and MTND5. The hydrophobic fragment may also encompass the iron-sulfur centers which donate electrons to CoQ_{10} (Ragan, 1987; Ahmed and Krishnamoorthy, 1992). MTND6 may also occupy the CoQ_{10} binding site, since mutations in the MTND6 gene are associated with optic atrophy and dystonia (Jun et al., 1994) and also alter the efficiency of electron transfer to CoQ_{10} (Jun et al., 1996).

The actual mechanism of electron transfer and protein pumping for complex I is unknown. The redox differential across complex I is from −320 mV for NADH to +60 mV for CoQ_{10}. The approximate redox potentials for selected iron-sulfur centers are N–1 ($\approx$ −305 mV), N–4 ($\approx$ −245 mV), N–2 ($\approx$ −20 mV). Hence, N–1 and N–4 are closest to NADH/FMN and N–2 is closest to CoQ_{10}.

Complex I is affected by a wide variety of inhibitors, the best known of which are the rotenone and its derivatives. One notable example of considerable clinical and experimental significance is the activated form of 1-methyl-4-phenyl-1,2,3,4,-tetrahydropyridine (MPTP), 1-methyl-4-phenylpyridinium (MPP$^+$). Exposure to MPTP in both humans and other mammals results in the selective destruction of basal ganglia neurons and induction of parkinsonism (Degli Esposti, 1998; Wallace, 1997).

Complex II (succinate dehydrogenase, SDH)

Complex II oxidizes succinate to fumarate and transfers the electrons to CoQ$_{10}$. The enzyme is composed of four subunits: a 70 kDa flavoprotein (FP), a 27 kDa iron-sulfur protein (ISP), a 15 kDa membrane polypeptide and a 5–7 kDa membrane polypeptide.

All four complex II subunits are nuclear encoded. The 70 kDa flavoprotein contains the succinate binding site and a covalently bound FAD moiety (Hirawake et al., 1994; Morris et al., 1994); the 27 kDa iron sulfur protein contains three iron sulfur clusters (center 1 [2Fe-2S]$^{2+,1+}$, center 2 [4Fe-4S]$^{2+,1+}$, and center 3 [3Fe-4S]$^{1+,0}$) which transport electrons to CoQ$_{10}$ (Kita et al., 1990). CoQ$_{10}$ is bound to the two membrane-intrinsic subunits, CII-3 (Cochran et al., 1994) and CII-4. A b_{560} type heme is also associated with to CII-3 (SDHD) and CII-4 (SDHC) (Hirawake et al., 1997), but its function is unclear (Clarkson et al., 1991; Cochran et al., 1994; Davis and Hatefi, 1971a; 1971b; Hatefi and Galante, 1980). However, in *Caenorhabditis elegans* the *mev*-1 mutant alters the amino acid sequence of the CII-3 (SDHD) subunit which greatly increases ROS production and decreases lifespan, suggesting that the cytochrome b_{560} may function to stabilize or dismutate ubisemiquinone (CoQ$_{10}$H$^-$) (Ishii et al., 1998).

Complex III (bc_1 complex)

Complex III is composed of 11 polypeptides, one (cytochrome *b*, MTCYB) encoded by the mtDNA (Schagger et al., 1986; Gonzalez-Halphen et al., 1988). The crystal structure of complex III has been determined and revealed that complex III functions as a dimer, with a monomer mass of 240 kDa (Iwata et al., 1998; Nishikimi et al, 1988a; 1998b; Saraste, 1999). This enzyme oxidizes ubiquinol (CoQ$_{10}$H$_2$), reduces ferricytochrome *c* to ferrocytochrome *c*, and uses the energy released to pump protons across the mitochondrial inner membrane *via* the Q cycle. The polypeptides of complex III include two core proteins (subunit I and subunit II), MTCYB (subunit III),

cytochrome c_1 (subunit IV), the "Rieske" iron-sulfur protein (ISP) (subunit V), and seven smaller polypeptides, subunits 6 to 11. Cytochrome *b*, cytochrome c_1 and the Rieske ISP provide the major redox centers of the enzyme (Iwata et al., 1998).

The "Rieske" ISP and cytochrome c_1 are on the intermembrane side of the enzyme, and both contain one membrane-spanning domain. The heme cytochrome c_1 is covalently bound to Cys37 and Cys40 and its ligands are His41 and Met160 (Weiss et al., 1987; Gonzalez-Halphen et al., 1988; Trumpower and Gennis, 1994). Subunit 8, or the "acidic/hinge protein," lies above cytochrome c_1 and the two form the docking site for cytochrome *c*. The Rieske ISP encompasses a single 2Fe-2S iron-sulfur center and changes conformation, switching from intermediate ("int"), to "*b*", to "c_1" forms. In this process, its relationship to the adjacent cytochrome c_1 changes, facilitating directional electron flow. In the c_1 state, the iron-sulfur center is adjacent to the heme of cytochrome c_1, in the "int" state the iron-sulfur center is displaced from both cytochromes c_1 and *b*, and in the *b* state it interacts with cytochrome *b*.

The central core of the transmembrane domain is composed of cytochrome *b*. Cytochrome *b* has a low potential heme, b_L (b_{566}), and the high potential heme, b_H (b_{562}). Heme b_L is close to the intermembrane side, while heme b_H is on the matrix side.

The matrix side of the enzyme is composed of the core 1 and core 2 proteins, together with subunits 6 and 9. Subunit 9 is generated by metalloprotease cleavage of the NH$_2$-terminal 78 amino acids of the nascent "Rieske" ISP. Core 1 shows sequence homology to the mitochondrial processing protease β-MPP and core 2 to α-MPP and probably catalyze the cleavage.

Proton translocation of complex III is linked to electron transport through the intermediates of CoQ$_{10}$ oxidation-reduction in the proton-motive Q cycle (Mitchell, 1976; Hatefi, 1985; Wikstrom and Krab, 1986; Trumpower and Gennis, 1994). Complex III has two CoQ$_{10}$ binding sites, one on the cytoplasmic side (Q$_o$ or Q$_p$ site) and one on the matrix side (Q$_i$ or Q$_N$ site) of the inner membrane. Q$_p$ is on the intermembrane side close to heme b_L and binds the inhibitor myxothiazole, while Q$_n$ is close to heme b_H on the matrix side and binds the inhibitor Antimycin A (Wikstrom et al., 1981; Saraste 1984; Degli Esposti et al., 1993; Trumpower and Gennis 1994; Iwata et al., 1998).

CoQ$_{10}$H$_2$ binds to the Q$_o$ site and transfers one electron to the Rieske ISP, which passes it on to cytochrome c_1. The resulting ubisemiquinone donates the other electron to the adjacent b_L heme located on the cytoplasmic side of the membrane. The transfer of the two electrons from $CoQ_{10}H_2$ releases the two ubiquinol protons to the outside of the mitochondrial membrane. The electron at the b_L heme is then transported to the more matrix b_H heme where it is transferred to CoQ_{10} at Q_i site to generate ubisemiquinone. A second molecule of $CoQ_{10}H_2$ is oxidized as above, and the resulting b_H electron is donated to the ubisemiquinone at the Q_i site. This reduced quinone then combines with two protons from the matrix to generate ubiquinone, $CoQ_{10}H_2$. Hence two protons are transported through the membrane for each pair of electrons that exits Complex III (Hosler et al., 1993).

The Q cycle is driven by the conformational changes of the Rieske ISP. When complex III is oxidized, the Rieske ISP is in the "int" state. When $CoQ_{10}H_2$ binds to the Q_0 site in cytochrome b, the $CoQ_{10}H_2$ is deprotonated to $CoQ_{10}H^-$, which overcomes the activation barrier. This pulls the ISP to the "b" position. An electron is transferred to the Rieske ISP while it is adjacent to the $CoQ_{10}H^-$ (ubisemiquinone) in the "b" conformation. The second electron from $CoQ_{10}H^-$ is then transferred to heme b_L, weakening the interaction between the quinone and the Rieske ISP, permitting the ISP to move to the "c_1" state. Here it transfers the electron to cytochrome c_1, and the ISP moves to the "int" state. The cytochrome c_1 electron moves on to cytochrome c and the heme b_L electron moves on to the heme b_H site (Iwata et al., 1998).

The proteins, cDNAs and gene structures and chromosome locations for complex III are described in Table 11.1.

Cytochrome c

Cytochrome c ferries electrons along the outer mitochondrial membrane from complex III to complex IV. It contains a single covalently bound heme and is encoded by two isoform genes, a systemic cytochrome c and a testes cytochrome c (Evans and Scarpulla, 1988; Limbach and Wu, 1985; Virbasius and Scarpulla, 1988; Cuticchia, 1995).

Complex IV (cytochrome c oxidase, COX)

Complex IV is composed of 13 polypeptides, three (COI, COII, and COIII) encoded by the mtDNA. The remaining nuclear polypeptides have been designated IV, Va, Vb, VIa, VIb, VIc, VIIa, VIIb, VIIc and VIII (Kadenbach et al., 1983).

The crystal structure of complex IV (Tsukihara et al., 1996; Saraste, 1999) has revealed that it is a functional dimer with a minimal monomer molecular mass of 204 kDa. Complex IV collects electrons from reduced cytochrome c (ferrocytochrome c), transfers them to CuA, then to cytochrome a, then to the bimetallic cytochrome a_3/CuB active site and then to oxygen to give water, concurrently pumping four protons across the mitochondrial inner membrane (Anderson et al., 1981, 1982; Capaldi, 1990; Hosler et al., 1993; Fetter et al., 1995; Gennis and Ferguson-Miller, 1995; Tsukihara et al., 1996).

Complex IV encompasses two hemes a ($a + a_3$); three copper ions, two for CuA and one for CuB; one magnesium and one zinc ion. The two copper ions forming the binuclear center, CuA, are associated with mtDNA subunit II (COII), while the two hemes and CuB (heme a and heme a_3-CuB) form a trinuclear center associated with mtDNA subunit I (COI). Electron flow is from cytochrome c to CuA, then to heme a, and then to the heme a_3-CuB binuclear center where oxygen is reduced to water (Gennis and Ferguson-Miller, 1995; Tsukihara et al., 1995; 1996). Molecular oxygen (O_2) binds to the a_3-CuB binuclear center and electron transfer to O_2 is probably linked to proton transport. Complex IV uses four electrons to reduce O_2 and four protons from the matrix to generate 2 H_2O. Four additional protons are transferred from the matrix, across the mitochondrial membrane, possibly in the proximity of heme a_3 (Rousseau et al., 1993).

The three mtDNA encoded subunits form the core of the monomer, with the nuclear encoded subunits surrounding it. COI has 12 membrane-spanning domains (I to XII) which associate in three sets of four transmembrane helixes forming three "comma-shaped" spokes radiating out from the center. COII has two transmembrane domains which lie on one side of COI, while COIII has seven transmembrane domains which lie on the opposite site of COI from COII. Finally, seven of the ten nDNA subunits (IV, VIa, VIc, VIIa, VIIb, VIIc, and VIII) have one membrane-spanning domain, which surround the core COI, COII, and COIII subunits in the membrane. The remaining three nDNA subunits Va, Vb, and VIb do not have transmembrane domains. Subunits Va and Vb lie on the matrix side and subunit VIb on the cytosolic side of complex IV.

Subunits II, VIa and VIb appear to form the 25 Å diameter cytochrome c binding site composed of acidic residues which interact with the basic residues of cytochrome c (Tsukihara et al., 1996). The CuA coppers form a Cu-Cu bond and lie near the outside of the membrane, at the interface of COII and COI. The heme a and heme a_3-CuB centers are located 13Å into the membrane. Heme a and heme a_3 are close together, perpendicular to the membrane, and at a 104° angle relative to each other. Heme a_3 is 4.5Å from the magnesium atom and is located close to the trinuclear center, at the interface between COII and COI and

Table 11.1. Reported mitochondrial DNA missense diseases

Locus	Disease	Allele	np	Nucleotide change	AA change	Ho	He	Status	References
MTND1	MELAS	3308C	3308	T-C	M-T	–	+	Prov	Campos et al. (1997)
MTND1	NIDDM	3316A	3316	G-A	A-T	+	–	Prov	Nakagawa et al. (1995) Brown et al. (1992c, 1995)
MTND1	LHON	3394C	3394	T-C	Y-H	+	–	Prov	Howell et al. (1995), Johns et al. (1992a), Obayashi et al. (1992)
MTND1	NIDDM	3394C	3394	T-C	Y-H	+	–	P.M.	Thomas et al. (1996)
MTND1	ADPD	3397G	3397	A-G	M-V	+	–	Prov	Shoffner et al. (1993a), Wallace et al. (1992a)
MTND1	LHON	3460A	3460	G-A	A-T	+	+	Cfrm	Brown et al. (1992c), Howell et al. (1991a), Howell et al. (1992), Huoponen et al. (1993), Huoponen et al. (1991), Johns (1992), Johns & Neufeld (1993a), Johns et al. (1992b), Majander et al. (1991), Norby (1993)
MTND1	LHON	4136G	4136	A-G	Y-C	+	–	Prov	Howell et al. (1995), Howell et al. (1991b), Obermaier- Kusser et al. (1994), Riordan-Eva & Harding (1995)
MTND1	LHON	4160C	4160	T-C	L-P	+	–	Prov	Hanefeld et al.)1994) Howell et al. (1995), Howell et al. (1991b), Mackey (1994), Riordan-Eva & Harding (1995)
MTND1	LHON	4216C	4216	T-C	Y-H	+	–	Cfrm	Brown et al. (1995), Brown et al. (1992b), Hanefeld et al. (1994), Howell et al. (1995), Johns & Berman (1991), Mackey & Howell (1992), Obermaier-Kusser et al. (1994), Oostra et al. (1994), Salmaggi et al. (1994)
MTND2	LHON	4917G	4917	A-G	D-N	+	–	Cfm	Brown et al. (1995), Hanefeld et al. (1994), Howell et al. (1995), Johns (1992), Johns & Berman (1991), Obermaier-Kusser et al. (1994), Oostra et al. (1994)
MTND2	LHON	5244A	5244	G-A	G-S	–	+	Prov	Brown et al. (1995), Brown et al. (1992b), Hanefeld et al. (1994), Riordan-Eva & Harding (1995)
MTND2	AD	5460A	5460	G-A	A-T	+	+	P.M.	Kosel et al. (1994), Lin et al. (1992) Petruzzella et al. (1992)
MTND2	AD	5460T	5460	G-T	A-S	+	+	Prov	Kosel et al. (1994), Lin et al. (1992), Petruzzella et al. (1992)

continued

Table 11.1. Reported mitochondrial DNA missense diseases (*continued*)

Locus	Disease	Allele	np	Nucleotide change	AA change	Ho	He	Status	References
MTCO1	LHON	7444A	7444	G-A	Term-K	+	–	Prov	Brown et al. (1995), Brown et al. (1992c), Brown et al. (1992d), Hanefeld et al. (1994), Huoponen et al. (1993), Johns & Neufeld (1993b), Newman et al. (1995), Reynier et al. (1994a)
MTATP6	NARP	8993G	8993	T-G	L-R	–	+	Cfrm	Ciafaloni et al. (1993), Harding et al. (1992a). Holt et al. (1990), Obayashi et al. (1992), Ortiz et al. (1993), Puddu et al. (1993), Santorelli et al. (1993), Shoffner, et al. (1992), Tatuch et al. (1992), Tatuch & Robinson (1993)
MTATP6	NARP/ Leigh Disease	8993C	8993	T-C	L-P	–	+	Cfrm	Chakrapani, et al. (1998), De Vries et al. (1993), Mak et al. (1998), Santorelli et al. (1994)
MTATP6	LHON	9101C	9101	T-C	I-T	+	–	Prov	Lamminen et al. (1995)
MTATP6	FBSN	9176C	9176	T-C	L-P	+	+	Prov	Thyagarajan et al. (1995)
MTCO3	LHON	9438A	9438	G-A	G-S	+	–	Prov	Brown et al. (1994), Howell (1994), Johns (1994), Johns & Neufeld (1993b), Johns et al. (1994), Newman et al. (1994), Newman et al. (1995), Oostra, et al. (1995a)
MTCO3	LHON	9738T	9738	G-T	A-T	+	–	Prov	Johns et al. (1994) Johns & Neufeld (1993b),
MTCO3	LHON	9804A	9804	G-A	A-T	+	–	Prov	Newman et al. (1995) Manfredi et al. (1994),
MTCO3	PEM; MELAS	9957C	9957	T-C	F-L	–	+	Prov	Manfredi et al. (1995a) Lertrit et al. (1992),
MTND4	MELAS	11084G	11084	A-G	T-A	+	+	P.M.	Sakuta et al. (1993b)
MTND4	LHON	11696G	11696	A-G	V-I	–	–		De Vries et al. (1996)
MTND4	LHON	11778A	11778	G-A	R-H	+	+	Cfrm	Bolhuis et al. (1990), Holt et al. (1989b), Hotta et al. (1989), Huoponen et al. (1990), Johns (1990), Lott et al. (1990), Singh et al. (1989), Vilkki et al. (1989), Wallace et al. (1988a), Yoneda et al. (1989)
MTND4	DM	12026G	12026	A-G	I-V	+	–	Prov	Tawata et al. (1998)

continued

Table 11.1. Reported mitochondrial DNA missense diseases (*continued*)

Locus	Disease	Allele	np	Nucleotide change	AA change	Ho	He	Status	References
MTND5	LHON	13708A	13708	G-A	A-T	+	−	Prov	Brown et al. (1992b), Brown et al. (1992c), Haferkamp et al. (1994), Hanefeld et al. (1994), Johns (1992), Johns & Berman (1991), Johns & Neufeld (1993a), Johns & Neufeld (1991), Johns et al. (1992a), Mackey & Howell (1992)
MTND5	LHON	13730A	13730	G-A	G-E	−	+	Prov	Howell et al. (1993a), Riordan-Eva & Harding (1995)
MTND6	LDYT	14459A	14459	G-A	A-V	+	+	Cfrm	Brown et al. (1995), Jun et al. (1994), Jun et al. (1996), Riordan-Eva & Harding (1995), Shoffner et al. (1995b)
MTND6	LHON	14482G	14482	A-G	M-I	−	−	Prov	Howell et al. (1998)
MTND6	LHON	14498T	14498	C-T	Y-C	+	−	Prov	Wissinger et al. (1997)
MTND6	LHON	14484C	14484	T-C	M-V	+	+	Cfrm	Brown et al. (1992c), Govan et al. (1994), Hanefeld et al. (1994), Johns et al. (1993a), Johns & Neufeld (1993a), Johns et al. (1992a), Mackey & Howell (1992), Mackey (1994), Obermaier-Kusser et al. (1994), Oostra et al. (1994)
MTND6	LHON	14596A	14596	G-A	I-M	−	+	Prov	De Vries et al. (1996)
MTCYB	PD/ MELAS	14787del4	14787	CTCC-del	I-frameshift	−	+	Prov	de Coo et al. (1999)
MTCYB	MM	15059A	15059	G-A	G-Term	−	+	Prov	Andreu et al. (1999)
MTCYB	LHON	15257A	15257	G-A	D-N	+	−	Prov	Brown et al. (1992b), Haferkamp et al. (1994), Hanefeld et al. (1994), Heher & Johns (1993), Howell et al. (1993b), Huoponen et al. (1993), Johns & Neufeld (1993a), Johns & Neufeld (1991), Johns et al. (1993b), Mackey & Howell (1992)
MTCYB	MM	15762A	15762	G-A	G-E	−	+	Prov	Andreu et al. (1998)
MTCYB	LHON	15812A	15812	G-A	V-M	+	−	Prov	Brown et al. (1995), Brown et al. (1992b), Haferkamp et al. (1998), Hanefeld et al. (1994), Howell et al. (1995), Johns & Neufeld (1991), Mackey & Howell (1992), Obermaier-Kusser et al. (1994)

ligated to both, directly between CuA and heme a_3. The Zn is associated with the nuclear encoded subunits Vb on the matrix side of the enzyme bound to with cysteine residues (Capaldi, 1990; Hosler et al., 1993; Gennis and Ferguson-Miller, 1995; Tsukihara et al., 1995).

Complex IV has two hydrophobic proton-conducting channels, D (Asp91) and K (Lys319), named after conserved amino acids which form the matrix sides of the channels. Channel D ends at the conserved Glu242 in the middle of the membrane which resides in a hydrophobic cavity extending towards the binuclear heme-copper center and is required for proton translocation. The K channel also ends at the binuclear center. Protons for both water formation and proton pumping move through these channels.

Proton pumping involves reduction of both metals (a3 and CμB) at the active site with two electrons and two protons taken up. Oxygen then reacts, initially forming oxygen intermediate. An additional electron is acquired creating the peroxy state. Then three protons are acquired generating the ferryl intermediate and creating a H_2O and translocating two protons. A fourth electron is then accepted, resulting in a second water indecules and transport of two additional protons. The overall reaction involves oxidation of four electrons, generation of two H_2O molecules, and translocation of four protons (Saraste, 1999; Wikstrom, 1998).

While COIII is a universal component of all cytochrome c oxidase enzymes, its function is unclear. It does bind dicyclohexyicarbodiimide (DCCD) (Prochaska et al., 1981).

The functions of the ten nuclear-encoded subunits are still unclear. Two of the human subunits (VIa and VIIa) have two isoenzymes, one systemic and the other heart and muscle specific (Lomax and Grossman, 1989; Capaldi, 1990) which can be regulated at both the transcriptional and posttranscriptional levels (Preiss and Lightowlers, 1993). Complementary cDNAs have been cloned for all of the human COX genes (Zeviani et al., 1987; 1988; Otsuka et al., 1988; Rizzuto et al., 1988; 1989; Fabrizi et al., 1989; Taanman et al., 1989; Koga et al., 1990; Arnaudo et al., 1992; Sadlock et al., 1993;). Many of the genes have also been assigned to chromosomes (Darras et al., 1987; Rizzuto et al., 1989, Lomax et al., 1990, 1991; Taanman et al., 1991a; 1991b; Arnaudo et al., 1992; Bachman et al., 1997; Hofmann et al., 1998;).

A number of adenine nucleotide binding sites have been identified in complex IV, at least some of which can alter the kinetics of the enzyme. Five nucleotide binding sites have been found on complex IV: one between subunits I and III on the cytosolic side of the enzyme, two in subunit IV, one each on the cytosolic and matrix ends of the mole-

cule; and two in subunit IVa, again cytosolic and matrix. In addition, three lower affinity binding sites have been detected for ADP (Napiwotzki et al., 1997; Taanman et al., 1994; Tsukihara et al., 1996). Nucleotide binding to the matrix side of subunit VIa changes the H^+/e^- stoichiometry, while nucleotide binding to the cytosolic domain of subunit IV affects the affinity of cytochrome c (Anthony et al., 1993; Arnold and Kadenbach, 1997; 1999; Napiwotzki and Kadenbach, 1998; Napiwotzki et al., 1997).

Complex IV is sensitive to a variety of common toxic chemicals. These include cyanide and azide which form a bridge between cytochrome a_3 and CuB and thiocyanate and formate which bind other locations in the binuclear center (Palmer, 1993).

The complex structure of the respiratory complexes suggest that the assembly of active complexes requires the action of additional gene products. This has been shown to be the case for complex IV, where an additional protein, SURF-1, is required for generating normal human complex IV (COX) activity. Mutations in the SURF-1 gene have been found to be the primary cause of COX-deficient Leigh's syndrome (Tiranti et al., 1998b; Zhu et al., 1998). SURF-1 is 25.6% homologous with the yeast gene SHY-1. While the human SURF-1 mutation gives a specific COX defect, the yeast SHY-1 mutation is more pleiotropic. Hence, it has been suggested that SURF-1 may function in the assembly or maintenance of an active holoenzyme COX complex (Tiranti et al., 1998b; Zhu et al., 1998).

Two additional proteins, SCO1 and SCO2 are involved in insertion of the copper atoms into the copper centers of complex IV. Mutations in both of these genes have been associated with complex IV deficiency and mitochondrial disease (Dickinson et al., 2000; Papadopoulou et al., 1999; Valnot et al., 2000).

Complex V (H⁺-translocating ATP synthase, ATPsyn)

Complex V encompasses 16 polypeptides, two (ATPase6 and ATPase8) encoded by the mtDNA(Walker, 1995). This H^+-translocating ATP synthase utilizes the electrochemical gradient ($\Delta\rho = \Delta\Psi + \Delta\mu^{pH}$) generated by complexes I, III, and IV to catalyze the condensation of ATP and Pi to make ATP. This enzyme uses a rotary catalytic mechanism which is close to 100% efficient.

The F_o component of the enzyme is based in the mitochondrial inner membrane, with the enzyme extending into the matrix in a lollipop involving a 45 Å long stalk, and a 90–100 Å diameter barrel (F_1). The F_1, as isolated, is composed of five subunits α, β, γ, δ, and ε, with amino acid lengths in cow of 510, 482, 272, 146, and 50 amino acid residues, respectively. The ratio of these subunits in the F1 particle is 3:3:1:1:1, with a total mass of about 370 kDa (Hatefi, 1985). The α and β subunits are highly homologous, 20% identical, and form a hexagonal array of alternating α and β subunits. While both α and β subunits bind nucleotides, only the β subunits are catalytic. The crystal structure for the F_1 shows that the α and γ subunits form a hollow barrel into which the γ subunit projects up from the stalk to form an axle (Abrahams et al., 1994).

Based on the concept of rotary catalysis, complex V has been divided into two functional components: a "rotor" and a "stator" (Elston et al., 1998; Ogilvie et al., 1998; Wang and Oster, 1998). The rotor consists of a hydrophobic wheel of 12 "c" (ATP9) subunits lying in the plane of the inner membrane which rotates with its axle extending into the matrix. The axle is composed of the ε subunit at the base and the γ projecting up into the F1 barrel. The "stator" is composed of a base made by the "a" subunit (ATP6) embedded in the membrane, adjacent to the "c" subunit wheel. The "a" (ATP6) subunit anchors a pair of "b" subunits that project out of the membrane and bind to the δ subunit of F_1 which is attached to an α subunit of the α-β barrel. Thus, the Fo subunit "a" (ATP6) is linked to the 3α:3β barrel in a static structure through the "b" subunits and δ.

The stator subunit "a" (ATP6) and rotor subunit "c" (ATP9) interface mediates the proton flux from the intermembrane space to the matrix, thus driving the rotor's rotation and causing the γ axel to spin within the α and β subunit barrel. As the "c" subunit rotor spins past the "a" subunit stator, the rotor's axle, ending in the γ subunit, rotates inside the hollow α and β barrel. As it spins, the γ subunit makes two contacts with the β subunit, thus mediating the two components of the catalytic cycle. This generates sequential conformational changes in the β subunit nucleotide binding sites which bind ADP + P_i, condense it to ATP, and release the ATP into the matrix (Elston et al., 1998; Wang and Oster, 1998).

The mechanism by which the proton motive force drives rotation of the 12 subunit "c" (ATP9) rotor past the subunit "a" (ATP6) of the stator is highly conserved. All ATP synthases have a key negative charge in the "c" subunit in the middle of the membrane. This is Asp61 of the "c" subunit of the bacterial enzyme and Glu58 of the "ATP6" subunit of the mammalian enzyme. This carboxylate group faces outward from the wheel adjacent to the opposing face of the stator subunit "a" (ATP6) and also the hydrophobic core of the membrane's lipid bilayer. The stator subunit "a" (ATP6) has a opposing positive charge, Arg210 for the bac-

terial subunit "c" and Arg159 for the mammalian subunit ATP6. This positive charge is offset 0.52 nm from the plane of carboxyl groups, such that it exerts electrostatic attraction against the Asp61 of "c" or the Glu58 of ATP9 without being capable of forming a salt bridge to stop rotation. The stator subunit "c" has two half proton channels which penetrate half way into the membrane from opposite sides, but are offset from each other. One half channel is open to the proton-rich intermembrane space. The other to the proton poor (alkaline) matrix. In the presence of an electrochemical gradient, the half channel open to the inner membrane space conducts a proton to protonate the carboxyl group of subunit "c" (Asp61) or subunit ATP9 (Glu58), neutralizing its charge and permitting the subunit to rotate into the hydrophobic lipid bilayer without energetic inhibition. The protonated subunit "c" rotates all of the way around the wheel until it returns to the subunit "a" or "ATP6" stator, where it encounters the other half well opening to the negatively charged and alkaline matrix. In this environment, the proton leaves subunit "c" (Asp61) or "ATP9" (Glu58) and enters the matrix. The exposed negative charge of the Asp61 of "c" or the Glu58 of "ATP9" is then attracted to the displaced positive charge of the Arg210 of "a" or the Arg159 of "ATP6" causing the Asp61 or Glu58 carboxyl group of "c" or "ATP9" to rotate until it reenters the environment of the half channel of the proton-rich intermembrane space, where it is again reprotonated (Hartzog and Cain, 1994; Elston et al., 1998; Fillingame et al., 1998; Wang and Oster, 1998). The stoicheometry of proton translocation to ATP synthesis is 4H+/ATP. Given that there are three β subunit active sites, three ATPs indecules are synthesized per rotation of the rotor. Hence, 12 H+ must be bound for each complete turn of the wheel. Given that each subunit "c" or "ATP9" has only one carboxylate group, then the wheel must have 12 spokes provided by 12 "c" (ATP9) subunits.

In the F_1 barrel, the three α and three β subunits are capped by β-pleated sheets. Just below this cap is a hydrophobic ring forming a bearing in which the C-terminal end of the γ subunit rotates (Abrahams et al., 1994). Below the β-sheet, and in the middle of the α and β subunits, are the nucleotide binding sites. The conformational change and nucleotide binding sites of the β subunits are dynamic. The three β subunits sequentially go through three states: "O" or open with very low affinity for ligands and catalytically inactive; "L" or loose with the capacity to binding the ligands ADP and P_i, but catalytically inactive; and "T" or tight with the ligands tightly bound associated with catalysis. These three states are generated as the asymmetric γ subunit interacts with the interior side of the β subunits (Boyer, 1993).

The binding affinity of the β subunit for adenine nucleotides is modified by sequential changes in the β subunit conformation mediated by two "catches" that interact with the rotating γ subunit. The "major catch" is a loop that protrudes into the interior of the 3α:3β barrel. This is encountered as the γ subunit rotates from βTP (triphosphate or (T) tight) to βE (empty or (O) open). The βE conformation differs from the βTP (triphosphate or (T) tight) and βDP (diphosphate or (L) loose) conformation in that part of the nucleotide binding site is rotated 30°. The "minor catch" separates βDP (diphosphate, loose) from βTP (triphosphate, tight) (Bullough et al., 1989; Zhuo et al., 1993; Abrahams et al., 1994). These molecular interactions create a catalytic engine driven by elastic forces rather than thermal effects, which permits the near 100% efficiency (Wang and Oster, 1998; Saraste, 1999).

A number of the nuclear encoded complex V subunit cDNA and genomic clones have been reported. The cDNAs include the ATP synthase α subunit (Breen, 1988; Walker et al., 1989; Kataoka and Biswas, 1991); ATPsynβ (Ohta and Kagawa, 1986; Wallace et al., 1987), ATPsynδ (Jordan and Breen, 1992), F_0 subunit b (Higuti et al., 1991), F_0 subunit F6 (Javed et al., 1991), and F_0 subunit 9 or c which has three isoforms (Gay and Walker, 1985; Farrell and Nagley, 1987; Dyer and Walker, 1993; Higuti et al, 1993; Yan et al., 1994). The genomic clones include the ATPsynα (Akiyama et al., 1994; Jabs et al., 1994), ATPsynβ (Ohta et al., 1988; Neckelmann et al., 1989; Haraguchi et al., 1994), ATPsynγ (Matsuda et al., 1993; Jabs et al., 1994; Cuticchia, 1995), and ATPsynγ which generates two alternative mRNAs, heart-muscle and systemic (Matsuda et al., 1993). This is accomplished through the loss of exon 9 associated with the synthesis of a *trans*-acting factor which is inducible by high extracellular pH through a protein kinase C signaling mechanism (Endo et al., 1994)

Adenine nucleotide translocator (ANT) and uncoupling protein (Ucp)

The mitochondrial anion carrier protein family functions to transport solutes through the mitochondrial inner membrane. This group of related proteins has a tripartite repeating domain, each domain of about 100 amino acid residues, all of which function as homodimers. This family includes two classes of carriers of particular relevance to bioenergetics, the ADP/ATP carriers (AAC) or adenine nucleotide translocators (ANT) and the uncoupling proteins (UCP).

The adenine nucleotide translocators exchange matrix ATP for cytosolic ADP. ANT proteins are derived by multiple isoform genes. In humans there are three tissue-specific isoforms (Stepien et al., 1992): a heart-muscle specific isoform (*ANT1*) located at the chromosome 4q35 locus (Neckelmann et al., 1987; Houldsworth and Attardi, 1988; Cozens et al., 1989; Li et al., 1989; Wijmenga et al., 1992, 1993; Haraguchi et al., 1993; Giraud et al., 1998), an inducible isoform (*ANT2*) located at Xq24 (Battini et al., 1987; Houldsworth and Attardi, 1988; Chen et al., 1990; Ku et al., 1990; Schiebel et al., 1994), and a systemic isoform (*ANT3*) located in the pseudoautosomal region at Xp22.3 (Houldsworth and Attardi, 1988; Schiebel et al., 1993; Slim et al., 1993; Giraud et al., 1998). In mouse there are only two *ANT* genes (*Ant1* and *Ant2*), homologues of the human ANT1 and ANT2 proteins (Levy et al., 2000). Mouse *Ant1* maps to chromosome 8, syntenic with human 4q35 (Graham et al., 1997; Mills et al., 1996), while mouse *Ant2* maps to regions A-D of X chromosome, syntenic to human Xq24 (Ellison et al., 1996).

The uncoupling proteins form a proton channel through the inner membrane, thus depolarizing the electrochemical gradient and uncoupling electron transport from ATP synthesis. The uncoupler protein 1 (UCP1) is primarily associated with brown adipose tissue (BAT), where it functions in thermal regulation. It is strongly induced by cold stress through a β-adrenergic response pathway (Jacobsson et al., 1985; Kozak, et al., 1988; Cassard et al., 1990; Fleury et al., 1997). Uncoupler protein-2 (UCP2) has 59% amino acid identity with UCP1, and is widely expressed in adult human tissues with mRNA levels being highest in skeletal muscle. It is also up-regulated in white fat in response to an increased fat diet. In mouse it has been linked to quantitative trait locus for hyperinsulinemia and obesity (Fleury et al, 1997). Uncoupler protein-3 (UCP3) is 57% identical with UCP1 and 73% identical with UCP2. UPC3 is also widely expressed in adult tissues, and at particularly high levels in skeletal muscle. Moreover, it is hormonally regulated, being induced in skeletal muscle by thyroid hormone, in white fat by β3-adrenergic agonists, and also regulated by dexamethasone, leptin, and starvation. *UCP3* is located adjacent to *UCP2* in human chromosome 11q13 and mouse chromosome 7 (Boss et al., 1997; Gong et al., 1997; Solanes et al., 1997; Vidal-Puig et al., 1997).

MITOCHONDRIAL PROTEIN IMPORT

The mitochondrion is assembled from 13 mtDNA-encoded polypeptides and approximately 1000 nuclear-encoded polypeptides. These polypeptides are synthesized on cytosolic 80 S ribosomes and vectorally transported into the mitochondrion *via* receptor binding to the outer membrane and transfer through a mitochondrial inner membrane import pore. Once inside the mitochondrial matrix, the proteins are folded and assembled by the chaperone proteins mtHSP70 and mtHSP60 (Roise, 1988; Pfanner and Neupert, 1990; Glick and Schatz, 1991; Glick et al, 1992; Pfanner et al., 1991) (Figure 11.2).

The mitochondrial protein import apparatus encompasses a set of outer and inner membrane complexes. The Tom complexes function to transport proteins across the outer membrane while the Tim complexes function to transport proteins across the inner membrane (Schatz, 1996; Schatz and Dobberstein, 1996; Neupert, 1997) (Figure 11.2).

Proteins to be imported into the mitochondrion have embedded into their structure specific mitochondrial targeting sequences. Most proteins to be imported into the mitochondrial matrix have an amino terminal targeting peptide which is amphiphilic and basic (usually due to an excess of arginine residues). These amino terminal targeting peptides are cleaved from the protein on import. Other proteins can have internal targeting sequences.

While in the cytosol, proteins destined for mitochondrial import interact with cytosolic chaparones. These include members of the cytosolic 70 kDa heat-shock protein (hsp70) family, which bind to non-native proteins. In addition, there is at least one cytosolic chaperone specific for mitochondrial proteins. This is the heterochimeric mitochondrial import stimulating factor (MSF) which specifically binds matrix targeting signals. Both Hsp70 and MSF are ATPases (Neupert, 1997; Schatz, 1996; Schatz and Dobberstein, 1996).

The mitochondrial proteins, presumably maintained in a random conformation by the chaperone proteins, then interact with the receptor complexes on the mitochondrial

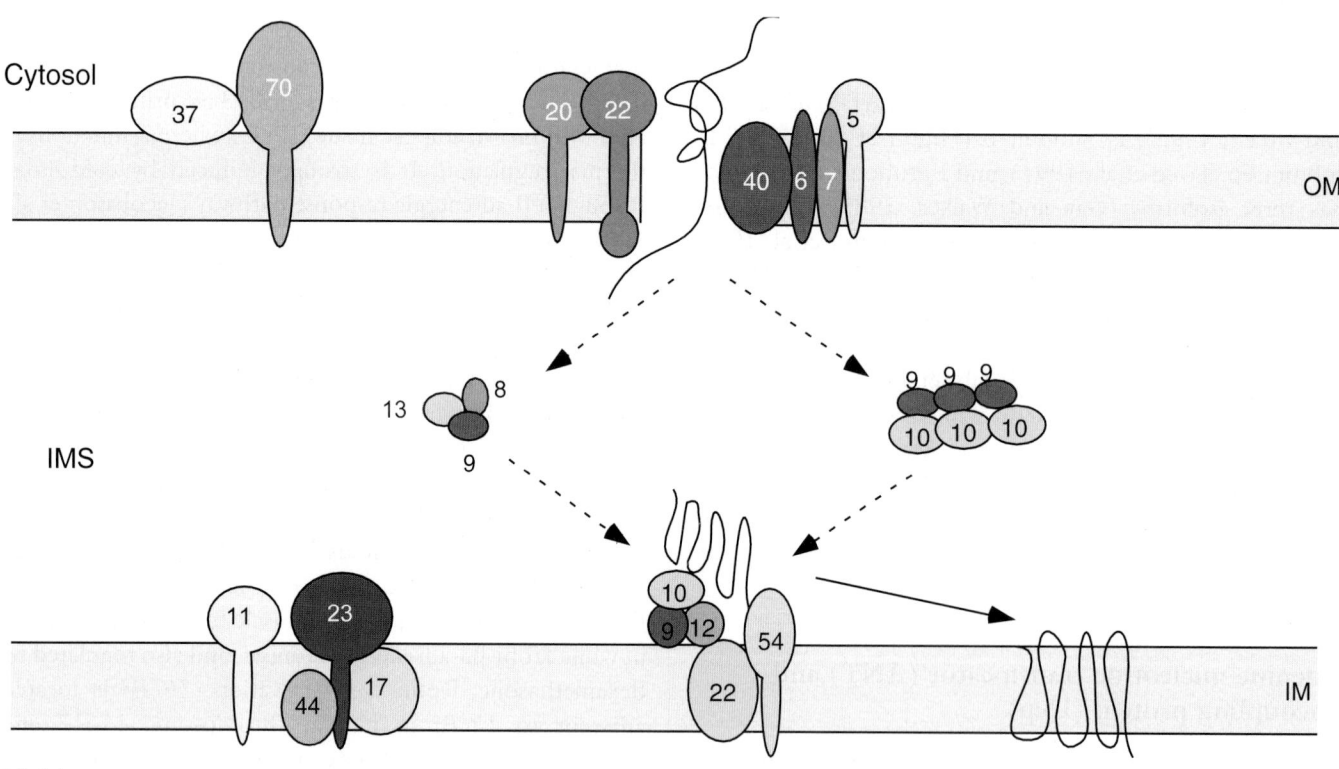

Fig. 11.2. Proteins thought to be involved in the import of cytosolically synthesized polypeptides through the outer and inner mitochondrial membranes. The outer membrane Tom (transport across the outer membrane) complexes consist of two main receptor complexes and the general insertion pore (GIP) complex. Receptor complex Tom20 + Tom22 binds proteins with amino-terminal targeting peptides and feeds them through the GIP, of which Tom22 is thought to be a component. Tom37 + Tom70 are thought to bind proteins with internal targeting sequences and to transfer them to Tom20 + Tom22. The central channel protein of the GIP is thought to be Tom40; with Tom5, Tom6, and Tom7 also being important components. Proteins with amino-terminal targeting peptides destined for the matrix are transferred from the intermembrane space domain of Tom22 to the Tim complex. Tim23 is the central channel protein, and Tim44 binds to the preprotein as it emerges from the Tim23 channel on the matrix side. Anion carrier proteins destined for integration into the mitochondrial inner membrane, such as the ANT, follow a different pathway. As they emerge into the intermembrane space they interact with either of two soluble complexes (Tim8 + Tim9 + Tim13) or (3 Tim9 + 3 Tim10). These soluble complexes transport the protein through the intermembrane space to the other Tim complex, which is composed of Tim9 + Tim10 + Tim12 + Tim22 + Tim54. (Reprinted from Wallace and Murdock, 1999, which was adapted from Koehler et al., 1998a,b.)

outer membrane. Two receptor complexes have been identified: Tom20 + Tom22 and Tom37 + Tom70. Current thinking is that Tom20 + Tom22 binds to proteins with amino-terminal targeting peptides. The Tom37 + Tom70 complex is thought to interact with proteins with internal targeting sequences, such as the inner membrane carrier proteins like ANT and UCP. The Tom37 + Tom70 complex then interacts with the Tom20 + Tom22 complex through a 34 amino acid "tetratrico-peptide" motifs, and the Tom20 + Tom22 complex transfers the protein to the general insertion pore (GIP) (Schatz, 1996; Schatz and Dobberstein, 1996; Neupert, 1997).

The outer membrane GIP is probably composed of Tom40, Tom22, Tom5, Tom6, and Tom7 (Dekker et al., 1998). Tom40 is deeply embedded in the outer membrane and forms a 22Å hydrophilic transmembrane channel (Hill et al., 1998). Tom22 functions both as a key component of the receptor complex and as well as an integral part of the GIP channel (Schatz, 1996; Schatz and Dobberstein, 1996; Neupert, 1997; Dekker et al., 1998).

Once a protein traverses the outer membrane, it can either proceed through the inner membrane to the matrix or be inserted directly into the inner membrane. Proteins destined for the matrix with an amino-terminal targeting sequence are electrostatically attracted to the inner membrane import complex consisting of Tim23, Tim11, Tim14, and Tim 17, and possibly Tim33. The Tim23 protein is central to this channel and in the presence of $\Delta\Psi$, it dimerizes, possibly providing a gating mechanism for the channel. On the matrix side, the Tim23, Tim11, Tim14, and Tim17 complex interacts with an inner membrane complex consisting of Tim44, mtHsp70, and MGE. Tim44 interacts with the preprotein as it emerges from the Tim23 pore and also binds mtHsp70. mtHsp70 then interacts with the preprotein and promotes its import, in conjunction with the hydrolysis of ATP. The interaction of Tim44 and mtHsp70 is regulated by adenine nucleotides and also by the nucleotide exchange factor (MGE) which regulates Tim44-mtHsp70 dissociation (Roise, 1988; Pfanner and Neupert, 1990; Glick and Schatz, 1991; Pfanner et al., 1991; Glick et al., 1992; Schatz, 1996; Schatz and Dobberstein, 1996; Neupert, 1997).

Once in the matrix, the targeting peptides are cleaved off by the mitochondrial processing peptidase (MPP) consisting of two subunits, α-MPP and the catalytic β-MPP. A subset of preproteins have a second cleavage by the mitochondrial intermediate peptidase (MIP). Once in the matrix, proteins in are folded by chaperones complexes mtHsp70, MD5 and MGE and Hsp60 and Hsp10. Mitochondrial cyclophilins, which are sensitive to ciclosporin A, can also act as folding

catalysts (Schatz, 1996; Schatz and Dobberstein, 1996; Neupert, 1997).

Mitochondrial inner membrane transport proteins such as the ANTs and UCPs follow a different pathway. Once they enter the intermembrane space *via* the Tom complex, they interact with one of two soluble complexes. One complex involves three Tim9 and three Tim10 subunits, while the other involves one each of Tim8, Tim9, and Tim13 polypeptides. These complexes deliver the carrier protein to a 300 kDa complex composed of Tim54, Tim22, Tim12, Tim10, and Tim9, bound to the outer face of the inner membrane. The polypeptides Tim8, Tim9, Tim10, Tim12, and Tim13 all belong to the same gene family which contains a distinctive duplicated C(N3)C motif reminiscent of a Zn finger (Koehler et al., 1998a; 1999; Sirrenberg et al., 1998; Wallace and Murdock, 1999).

MITOCHONDRIAL GENETICS

Each human cell contains hundreds of cytoplasmic mitochondria and thousands of mtDNAs. The cytoplasmic location and high copy number of the mitochondria result in the mtDNA having a unique genetics.

Mitochondrial genes and genomes

The mtDNA is a 16,569 nucleotide pair (np), closed circular molecule, located within the mitochondrial matrix. It codes for 13 key polypeptides of OXPHOS as well as the structural RNAs of mitochondrial protein synthesis including the small (12 S) and large (16 S) rRNAs as well as 22 tRNAs (Figure 11.3). These 22 tRNAs interpret the mitochondrial genetic code through the use of modified wobble codon rules. Certain mitochondrial tRNAs also have modified anticodons which alter the mitochondrial genetic code. In particular, the anticodon of the tryptophan tRNA is modified so that it reads both the normal tryptophan codon (UGG) as well as the opal stop codon (UGA). Similarly, the methionine tRNA recognizes both AUG and AUA as methionine. Finally, the "universal" arginine codons AGA and AGG are utilized as stop codons in the mtDNA (Wallace 1982; Shoffner and Wallace 1995).

The 13 polypeptides of the mtDNA include seven (ND1, 2, 3, 4, 4L, 5, 6) of the 42 subunits of complex I, one (cytb) of the 11 subunits of complex III, three (COI, II, III) of the 13 subunits of complex IV and two (ATP6 and 8) of the 16 subunits of complex V. The mtDNA also contains an approximately 1121 nucleotide pair (np) control region that encompasses the heavy (H) and light (L)-strand promoters (P_H and P_L) and the H-strand origin

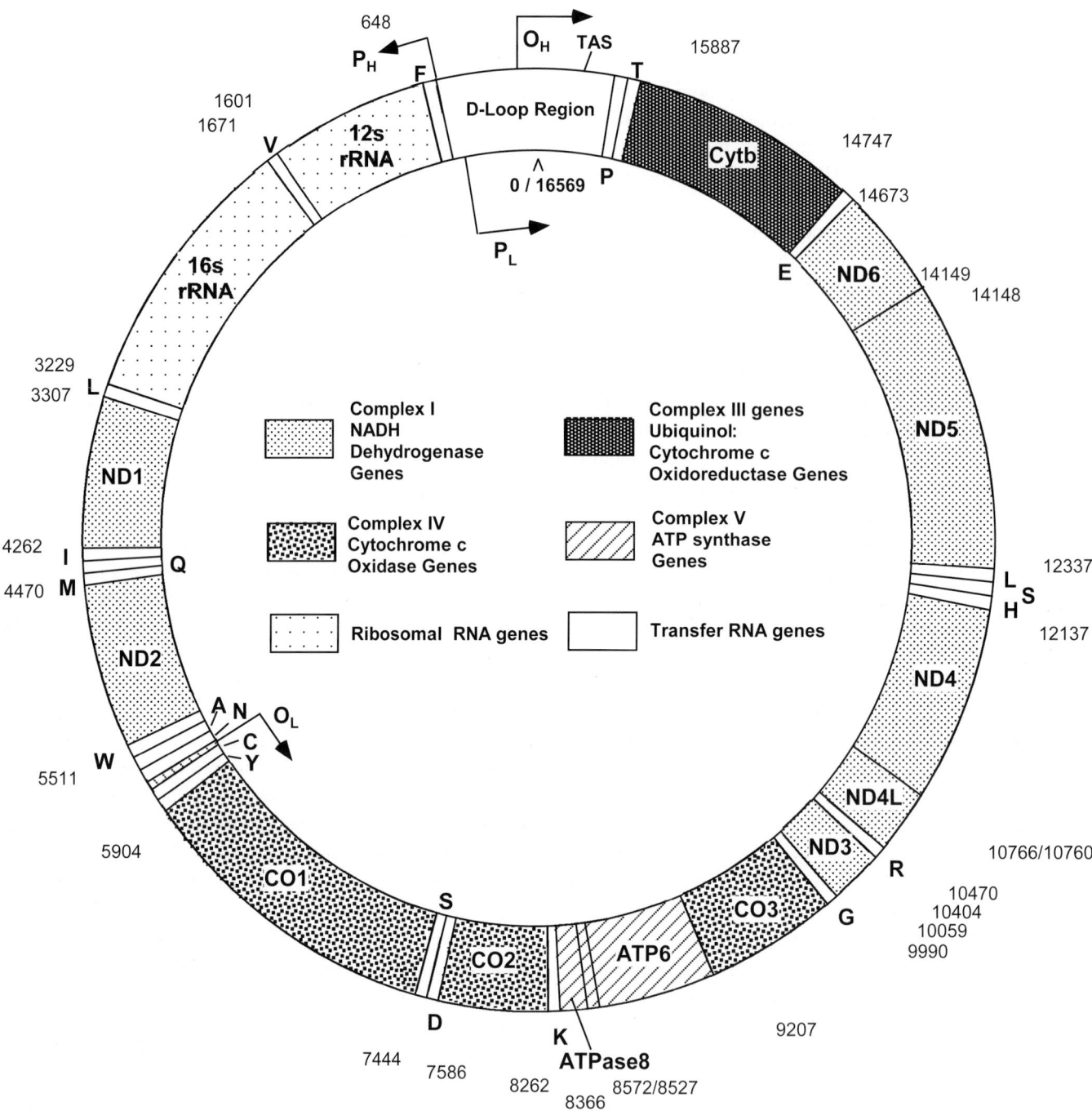

Fig. 11.3. The human mtDNA map. The mtDNA encompasses 16,569 nps with numbering starting at O_H and proceeding counterclockwise around the circular map. The function of each gene is identified by shading according to the designations within the circle. The first and last nucleotides of the rRNAs and mRNA genes are given on the external ares. The tRNA genes are indicated by the letter of their cognate amino acid. The names for the genes are O_H, MTOHR; CSBI-III, MTCSB 1–3; P_L, MTLSP; P_H, MTHSP1; F, tRNA^{Phe} or MTTF; 12 S rRNA, MTRNR1; V, tRNA^{Val} or MTTV; 16 S rRNA, MTRNR2; L, tRNA$^{Leu(UUR)}$ or MTTL1 (which also contains the transcription terminator); ND1, MTND1; 1, tRNA^{Ile} or MTT1; Q, tRNA^{Gly} or MTTQ; M, tRNA^{Mer} or MTTM; ND2, MTND2; N, tRNA^{Trp} or MTTW; A, tRNA^{Ala} or MTTA; N, tRNA^{Asp} or MTTN; OL, MTOLR; C, tRNA^{Cys} or MTTC; Y, tRNA^{Tyr} or MTTY; COI, MTCO1; S, tRNA$^{Ser(UCN)}$ or MTTS1; D, tRNA^{Asp} or MTTD; COII or MTCO2; K, tRNA^{Lys} or MTTK; ATP8, MTATP8; ATP6, MTATP6; COIII, MTCO3; G, tRNA^{Gly} or MTTG; ND3, MTND3; R, tRNA^{Arg} or MTTR; ND4, MTND4L; ND4, MTND4; H, tRNA^{His} or MTTH; S or tRNA$^{Ser(AGY)}$ or MTTS2; L, tRNA$^{Leu(CUN)}$ or MTTL2; ND5, MTND5; ND6, MTND6; E, tRNA^{Glu} or MTTE; Cytb, MTCYB; T, tRNA^{Thr} or MTTT; P or tRNA^{Pro} or MTTP; TAS, termination-associated sequence or MTTAS. (www.gen.emory.edu/mitomap.html)

of replication (O_H). The L-strand origin (O_H) is located on the other side of the circle in a cluster of five tRNA genes (WANCY).

DNA replication initiates at O_H using an RNA primer generated from the L-strand transcript. The L-strand transcript initiates at the adjacent L-strand promoter (P_L) and is cleaved by the nuclear-encoded RNase MRP at runs of G nucleotides in the conserved sequence blocks CSBIII, CSBII, and CSBI, primarily after CSBI (Chang and Clayton, 1987a; 1987b; 1989; Clayton, 1994). The resulting 3′-OH is utilized by DNA polymerase γ as a primer to synthesize a 7 S DNA. The 7 S DNA ends at the termination associated sequence (TAS) at the end of the control region. The TAS binds to a specific factor which may regulate this replication pause site (Madsen et al., 1993). This newly synthesized region of the H-strand displaces the parental H-strand to create the displacement-loop (D-loop) (Doda et al., 1981; Madsen et al., 1993). The 7 S DNA is subsequently utilized as a primer to synthesize a new H-strand. From the 7 S DNA, H-strand synthesis proceeds two-thirds of the way around the mtDNA, displacing the parental H-strand until it reaches the light strand origin (O_L). Once exposed on the displaced H-strand, O_L folds into a stem-loop structure and L-strand synthesis initiates and proceeds back along the H-strand template. Consequently, mtDNA replication is bi-directional but asynchronous (Clayton, 1982).

MtDNA transcription initiates from the two promoters in the control region, one for each strand: P_L and P_H, P_H is responsible for transcribing the two rRNA genes, 13 tRNAs genes and 12 of the protein coding genes. P_L transcribes the ND6 protein gene, nine tRNAs and also generates the primers for H-strand replication at O_H (Wallace, 1999). Both promoters are associated with a binding site for a nuclear-encoded mitochondrial transcription factor (Tfam). Tfam is a high mobility group DNA-binding protein with two DNA-binding domains and a carboxyl terminal tail essential for transcription (Fisher et al., 1987; Milatovich et al., 1991; Parisi and Clayton, 1991; Dairaghi et al., 1995). It binds with higher affinity to P_L than P_H, consistent with their relative transcription frequencies (Ghivizzani et al., 1993; Ikeda et al., 1994). Tfam also binds with a 40 to 50 base periodicity throughout the D-loop, with CSBII and CSBIII being unbound and CSBI being strongly bound. The Tfam phasing downstream from CSBI on the H-strand DNA corresponds to DNA synthesis initiation sites suggesting that Tfam may help define the transitions between RNA and DNA (Ghivizzani et al., 1994).

Transcription from both promoters proceeds around the mtDNA circle creating a poly-cistronic RNA. The tRNA genes, which punctuate the larger rRNA and mRNA sequences, then fold within the transcript and are cleaved out by an RNaseP-like activity. The freed mRNAs and rRNAs are post-transcriptionally polyadenylated; and the tRNAs are modified and the 3′ terminal CCA added (Attardi et al., 1982; Attardi and Montoya, 1983; Clayton, 1984; Wallace et al., 1995a).

The rRNAs are present in about a 50–1 with the mRNAs. This differential transcription is accomplished in part by a transcriptional terminator (5′-TGGCAGAGCCCGG-3′) located within the tRNA[Leu(UUR)] gene, immediately downstream from the 16 S rRNAs in the direction of H-strand transcription from P_H. This terminator is bi-directional, thus accounting for the reduction in read-through of the H-strand promoter as well as the termination of the L-strand transcripts prior to its reaching the rRNA genes (Christianson and Clayton, 1986; 1988; Ghivizzani et al., 1993).

The mtDNA mRNAs are translated on mitochondrial 55 S ribosomes (mitoribosomes) composed of a large 39 S and small 28 S subunit. These ribosomes have a smaller amount of rRNA than bacterial or eukaryotic ribosomes but a larger number of ribosomal proteins (Hamilton and O'Brien, 1974; Matthews et al., 1982; O'Brien et al., 1990). MtDNA mRNAs lack the traditional Shine-Dalgarno sequence for ribosome binding and generally start with the initiation codon at the 5′ end. Translation is thought to initiate with the binding of the small subunit to a 40-base region of the mRNA. The ribosome then moves back to the 5′ end to initiate translation. The mRNA has been proposed to wrap around the ribosome thus limiting polysome formation (Liao and Spremulli 1990; Shoffner and Wallace 1995).

The mitoribosomes are sensitive to the bacterial ribosome inhibitor chloramphenicol (CAP), but resistant to the cytosolic 80 S ribosome inhibitors cycloheximide and emetine. They are also relatively insensitive to the aminoglycoside antibodies such as streptomycin and gentamycin (Wallace, 1982).

Mitochondria are semiautonomous

Because the mitochondria retain their own self-replicating genome and associated replication, transcription, and translation systems they behave as semiautonomous organisms within the human cell cytoplasm. This was first demonstrated through studies of cultured mammalian cells selected for resistance to the mitochondrial ribosome inhibitor CAP. CAP-resistant (CAP[R]) cells were enucleated by treatment with cytochalasin B to disaggregate the cytoskeleton and suspension in a centrifugal field to pull the dense nucleus from the cells, thus creating plasma membrane bound nuclear (karyoplast) and cytoplasmic fragments (cytoplast), the latter encapsulating the mitochondria and mtDNAs. The CAP^R cytoplasts were then fused to CAP-sensitive (CAP^S) cells and the resulting cytoplasmic hybrids or cybrids were shown to acquire the CAR^R genotype and phenotype (Bunn et al., 1974; Wallace et al., 1975; 1976). By this cybrid transfer procedure, CAP resistance could be transferred from cell to cell and was linked to restriction fragment length polymorphisms (RFLPs) in the mtDNA (Wallace, 1981), as well as to mtDNA encoded protein polymorphisms (Oliver and Wallace, 1982). Subsequent sequencing of CAP-R mtDNAs revealed that CAP resistance was due to single nucleotide changes in the peptidyltransferase region of the 16 S rRNA (MTRNR1) near the 3′ end: a T to C transition at np 2991 or a C to a transversion at np 2939 (Blanc et al., 1981a).

Cybrid transfer of mtDNAs can be facilitated by removing the mtDNAs of the recipient cell prior to fusion. This can be accomplished by fusing the cytoplast to a karyoplast to yield a reconstituted cell (Ege et al., 1974), by destroying the resident mitochondria by treating the recipient cell with the mitochondrial poison rhodamine-6G (R6G) (Ziegler and Davidson, 1981; Trounce and Wallace, 1996), or by curing the recipient cell of its resident mtDNAs by growth in the mtDNA replication inhibitor ethidium bromide (EtBr) (King and Attardi, 1989). Cells that have been cured of their resident mtDNAs using EtBr are designated ρ^0 cells. They become auxotrophic for uridine (Desjardins et al, 1985) and require high glucose for energy and pyruvate to maintain redox balance through oxidation of NADH + H$^+$ *via* lactate dehydrogenase to give lactate (King and Attardi, 1988). The ρ^0 recipient cells have provided a powerful tool for studying the biochemical basis of mtDNA disease mutations by permitting demonstration that a specific biochemical defect in a patient cell line can be transferred along with the patient mtDNAs to a ρ^0 cell having a different set of nuclear genes (King and Attardi, 1988; Chomyn et al., 1994; Trounce et al., 1994; 1996; Jun et al., 1996).

Mitochondrial are maternally inherited

The human mtDNA is strictly maternally inherited (Case and Wallace, 1981; Giles et al., 1980). This is due in large measure to the fact that the mammalian egg contains about 100 000 mitochondria and mtDNAs, while the sperm contains in the order of 100 mtDNAs (Chen et al., 1995a; Michaels et al., 1982). The sperm mtDNAs are contributed to the zygote at fertilization and will persist in interspecific crosses (Gyllensten et al., 1991). However, in intraspecific crosses the sperm mitochondria are selectively eliminated (Kaneda et al., 1995). This has been correlated with the dis-

covery that the sperm mitochondria are decorated with ubiquitin, which presumably marks them for degradation upon entrance into the oocytes (Sutovsky et al., 1999). This destruction of sperm mitochondria and mtDNAs can also be demonstrated by injecting sperm into ρ^0 somatic cells (Manfredi et al., 1997).

Heteroplasmy and replicative segregation

When a mutation arises in a cellular mtDNA, it creates a mixed intracellular population of mutant and normal molecules known as heteroplasmy. When a cell divides, it is a matter of chance whether the mutant mtDNAs will be partitioned into one daughter cell or another. Thus over time the percentage of mutant mtDNAs in different cell lineages can drift toward either pure mutant or normal (homoplasmy), a process known as replicative segregation. In somatic cell hybrids between transformed human cell lines, the direction of segregation appears to be random (Wallace, 1986). However, in crosses between HeLa cells and either diploid fibroblasts (White and Bunn, 1984; Hayashi et al., 1986; Miranda et al., 1989) or lymphoblastoid cell lines (Wallace et al., 1976), the HeLa mtDNAs are preferentially lost, even when selected for using CAP resistance. The reason for this directional replicative segregation is unknown. However, it may have clinical significance since it has been reported that in five out of seven ρ^0 cybrids heteroplasmic for the pathogenic tRNA mutation MTTL1*MELAS3243G (Goto et al., 1990), the wild-type mtDNAs were selectively lost and the mutant mtDNAs preferentially retained (Yoneda et al., 1992). This directional segregation may also involve nuclear genes. In a another study, using the same osteosarcoma 143B TK⁻ρ^0 recipient cell, one out of 14 heteroplasmic cybrids segregated toward mutant mtDNAs, while the others remained stable. By contrast, using a different ρ^0 recipient cell (A549, B2), five out of 25 heteroplasmic cybrids segregated to wild-type mtDNAs (Dunbar et al., 1995). Preferential growth of cells with wild-type mtDNAs has also been observed during cybrid clone isolation (Shoubridge, 1995) and in propagation of heteroplasmic fibroblasts (Matthews et al., 1995). Hence, the rules governing the directionality of mtDNA segregation and the factors which influence it still remain to be elucidated.

Threshold expression

Different tissues and organs rely on mitochondrial energy generation to different extents. This has been well established through studies of respiratory inhibitor toxicity in mammals, including primates. Acute respiratory toxicity can result in unconsciousness, while chronic toxicity can result in optic atrophy, basal ganglia degeneration, cardiac and renal failure (Wallace, 1987). Studies on maternal pedigrees harboring heteroplasmic mtDNA mutations indicate that as the percentage of mutant mtDNAs increases, and energy production declines. Ultimately, the percentage of mutant mtDNAs crosses a threshold resulting in clinical manifestations. Observations from many cases now indicate that the bioenergetic expression thresholds for human organs are, in decreasing order, the central nervous system, heart and skeletal muscle, renal system, endocrine system and liver (Wallace, 1988; 1994b; 1995b; Shoffner et al., 1990x). The pathophysiological bases of these organ thresholds is still unclear. However, current data suggests that three major processes of the mitochondria are relevant: decline in energy production, increase in ROS production, and initiation of apoptosis which eventually removes sufficient cells from the organ that the organ malfunctions resulting in disease.

While the mechanism for threshold expression may vary in different contexts, genetic studies have repeatedly shown that the difference in mitochondrial function between normal and defective cells can be quite small. In somatic cell hybrids between CAP^R and CAP^S cells, as little as 10% CAP^R mtDNAs are required for the cell to survive and grow in CAP (Wallace, 1986). Similarly, in diseases resulting from mtDNA tRNA mutations, the percentage of mutant mtDNAs must be high before the biochemical and clinical expression threshold is exceeded. In families harboring the MTTK*MERRF8344G mutation (Shoffner et al., 1990), it has been observed that individuals in the 20 to 40 year range require at least 85% mutant mtDNAs for symptoms to appear (Wallace et al., 1988b; Shoffner et al., 1990; Wallace, 1993). This is consistent with data from cultured somatic cells in which the percentage of MTTK*MERRF8344G or MTTLI*MELAS 3243G mutant mtDNAs must exceed 90% before both protein synthesis and O$_2$ consumption decline (Attardi et al., 1995).

Part of the threshold effect is explained by "respiratory control theory." It is well established that certain of the respiratory complexes can be strongly inhibited without reducing the respiration rate. This results from the fact that the various respiratory complexes have different degrees of excess respiratory capacity, relative to the overall electron flux rate through the respiratory chain. For example, complex I activity must be reduced by more than 70% before oxygen consumption or ATP production are perturbed (Letellier et al., 1994; Malgat et al., 1995; Jun et al., 1996). Hence, a mutation in a mtDNA complex I subunit

would have to increase to a relatively high percentage of the cellular mtDNAs before it would significantly impede mitochondrial respiration and energy production.

mtDNA complementation

The mitochondria and mtDNAs within a cell also appear to fuse and fusion permitting the mtDNA genomes to complement each other in *trans*. This was first demonstrated by fusing two human cells together to form hybrids, one cell carrying the CAP^R mutation linked to a ND3 protein polymorphism (MV-1) and the other carrying a CAP^S mtDNA linked to the other ND3 allele (MV-2). When the mitochondrial translation products of the hybrids were selectively labeled by growth in [^{35}S]methionine together with emetine to block cytosolic protein synthesis, both MV-1 and MV-2 were synthesized in proportion to the percentage of the two mtDNAs. Moreover, when the mitochondrial proteins were labeled in the presence of both emetine and CAP, both proteins were still labeled in proportion to the parental genomes. This implies that in these hybrids the CAP^R mtDNA ribosomes were able to translate the ND3 mRNAs from the CAP^S mtDNAs suggesting the genomes occupied the same mitochondrial structures (Oliver and Wallace, 1982).

Intracellular mtDNA complementation has also been demonstrated in cells heteroplasmic for the pathogenic tRNA mutations MTTL1*MERRF 8344G. In cybrids derived from heteroplasmic cells, as little as 10% of normal mtDNAs was able to restore oxygen consumption and mitochondrial protein synthesis. However, when essentially homoplasmic MTTL1*MELAS3243G genomes were mixed with homoplasmic MTTK*MERRF8344G genomes by two-step cybrid selection; complementation was not observed for either oxygen consumption or mitochondrial translation (Attardi et al., 1995). Hence, the majority of evidence supports intracellular mitochondrial fusion and mtDNA complementation, but further research is required to adequately describe this phenomenon.

mtDNA recombination

Over the past several years, the evidence has been accumulating that mtDNAs may recombine when mixed within somatic cells. While recombination in cultured mammalian cells is infrequent (Zuckerman et al., 1984), evidence for the inter-conversion of duplicated and deleted mtDNA molecules with the same breakpoint junction within patient tissues has suggested that intra-molecular recombination may be relatively frequent (Poulton and Holt, 1994). Introduction of a deleted mtDNA into the mouse female germline resulted in a strain of mice in which maternal descendants harbored the deleted and normal mtDNAs, but also developed duplicated molecules which seem to be the combination of the deleted and normal molecules (Inoue et al., 2000).

However, evidence for recombination has not been found between different human mtDNA lineages. Initial studies of mtDNA haplotypes from different populations revealed a high degree of linkage disequilibrium throughout the mtDNA (Merriwether et al., 1991), and in Native American populations where only five primary mtDNA lineages compose all of the tribal mtDNAs, no authentic recombinants have been identified in hundreds of mtDNAs that have been analyzed (Schurr et al., 1990). Recently, studies of mtDNA haplotypes have purported to demonstrate the loss of linkage disequilibrium within mtDNA lineages (Awadalla et al., 1999), but the analysis of the data has been question (Jorde and Bamshad, 2000; Kivisild and Villems, 2000; Kumar et al., 2000). Furthermore, analysis of complete mtDNA sequences has not substantiated this loss of linkage disequilibrium (Ingman et al., 2000). Hence, recombination between human mtDNA lineages probably does not occur. This is likely to be the product of the elimination of the sperm mitochondria and mtDNAs by the oocyte through ubiquitin-mediated degradation. As a result, different mtDNA lineages are physically kept separate and never come into physical contact to recombine.

mtDNA's high mutation rate

The mtDNA mutation rate is much higher than that of nuclear genes (Brown et al., 1979). Comparison of the sequence diversity of mtDNA and nDNA genes that function in the same enzymes indicates that mtDNA genes evolve about 10 to 17 times faster than nDNA genes (Neckelmann et al., 1987; Wallace et al., 1987). This high sequence evolution rate has resulted in the accumulation of a broad spectrum of mtDNA sequence polymorphisms in different female lineages in the human population. While mtDNA polymorphisms are prevalent, they must be neutral to become established by genetic drift in the population. However, mutations are random and the majority of the nucleotides in the mtDNA have a coding function. Hence, a high percentage of the *de novo* mtDNA mutations must be deleterious. These mutations may be either base substitutions or rearrangements, and they may occur in either the female germline or in early development resulting in systemic distribution and disease (Brown and Wallace, 1994a). Alternatively, they may occur in the body's tissues throughout life and accumulate as a heterogeneous array of mutations in post-mitotic tissues

(Wallace, 1994b; Walker et al., 1995). Whatever their source, these deleterious mtDNA mutations must be eliminated by selection and they are the molecular basis for the high frequency of mtDNA diseases that we observe in the clinic. A regularly updated compendium of known mtDNA sequence variants is available at our website MITOMAP (www.gen.emory.edu/mitomap.html) (Kogelnik et al., 1996).

POLYMORPHIC MTDNA VARIATION IN HUMAN POPULATIONS

Since the mtDNA is strictly maternally inherited, the mtDNA sequence can only evolve by the sequential accumulation of base substitutions along radiating maternal lineages. This means that mtDNA variation should correlate with the geographic origin of the individual. This was proven to be the case by demonstrating that Africans, Asians, and Europeans each had distinctive continent-specific *Hpa*I mtDNA restriction site polymorphisms (RSPs) (Denaro et al., 1981). Further characterization of restriction site polymorphisms revealed that all mtDNA types were fit into a single tree (Johnson et al., 1983), with the greatest mtDNA variation and root of the tree being in Africa (Cann et al., 1987; Johnson et al., 1983; Merriwether et al., 1991) and with specific branches radiating into the different continents (Wallace et al., 1999a). The sequence variation found in a particular mtDNA is designated the mtDNA haplotype, and a group of related haplotypes is call the haplogroup. Haplogroups are defined by ancient sequence polymorphisms that arose early in the radiation of a particular branch of the mtDNA tree (Wallace et al., 1999a). The structure and radiation of the mtDNA tree has been confirmed in two studies of complete mtDNA sequences that have confirmed the African origin of mtDNA and the continental branching order of African to Asian to European, with a coalescence time of 149,000 (95% CL of 81,000–231,000) years before present (YBP) (Wallace et al., 1999a; Ingman et al., 2000) (Figure 11.4).

Continent-specific studies of mtDNA variation have revealed that African mtDNAs were the most diverse and thus ancient, with an overall age of about 150,000 YBP. African mtDNAs share a *Dde*I site at np 10394 and have been shown to fall into three major haplogroups: L1 (oldest), L2 and L3 (youngest). L1 and L2 represent about 76% of all African mtDNAs and are defined by a *Hpa*I restriction site at np 3592. The !Kung of South Africa and the Biaka Pygmies of west-central Africa are concentrated in L1 and are the closest to the root of the human tree, while and the Asian macro-haplogroup M and Eurasian macro-

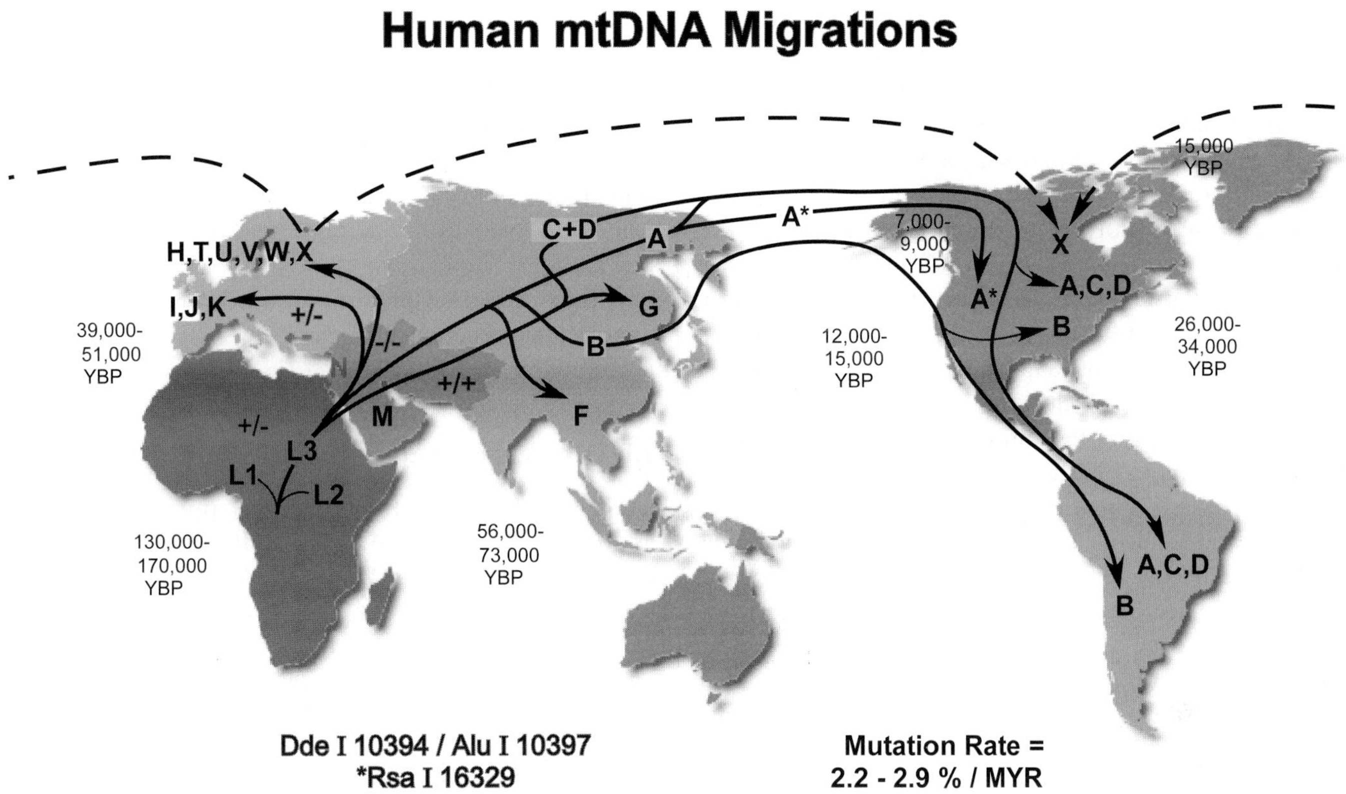

Human mtDNA Migrations

Fig. 11.4. Global migration of human mtDNAs and the origins of the continent specific lineages.

haplogroup N lineages radiate from L3 and give rise to all Eurasian mtDNAs (Chen et al., 1995c; 2000). The Asian mtDNAs separated from African L mtDNAs 50,000 to 70,000 YBP and are divided into two major macro-haplogroups N, which has lost the *Dde*I site at np 10,394, and M which has gained an adjacent *Alu*I site at np 10,397. Thus N is 10,394 negative and 10,397 negative (−/−), while M is 10,394 positive and 10,397 positive (+/+). From macro-haplogroup N radiate a variety of Asian haplogroups including A, B, F, and Y and from M radiate other haplogroups including C, D, E, G, and Z (Ballinger et al., 1992a; Torroni et al., 1994c). European mtDNAs, are derived from L3 and N. Those that have the *Dde*I site at np 10394 include haplogroups H (about 45%), T, U, V, W and X (about 2%). Those that lack the *Dde*I 10394 site include haplogroups I, J (about 9%), and K. Europeans separated from Africans about 40,000–50,000 YBP (Torroni et al., 1994b; 1996b) (Figure 11.4).

As Asians migrated northeast into Siberia, the amount of mtDNA diversity declined due to genetic drift. Ultimately, Siberia mtDNAs were reduced to haplogroups A, C, D, G, Y, and Z (Torroni et al., 1993b; Starikovskaya et al., 1998; Schurr et al., 1999). From Siberia A, C, and D crossed the Bering land bridge about 20,000–30,000 YBP giving rise to the Paleo-Indians. A subsequent migration brought

haplogroup B, defined by a 9 np deletion between nps 8271–8281, to the Americas where it mixed with A, D, and C. Later migrations from Chukotka, carrying a modified A, founded the Na-Déné populations about 7000–9500 YBP. A subsequent migration from Chukotka brought modified haplotypes A and D to give rise to the Eskimos and Aleuts (Schurr et al., 1990; Torroni et al., 1992; 1993a; 1993b; 1994a; 1994d; Torroni and Wallace, 1995). Analysis of Siberian and Native American Y chromosome variation has revealed similar migration patterns (Lell et al., 1997).

In addition to Asian haplogroups A, B, C, and D, 25% of the mtDNAs of the Great Lakes Ojibwa belong to European haplogroup X. However, the Native American haplogroup X mtDNAs separated from their European counterparts about 15,000 YBP. Hence, they may represent an ancient European migration to the New World as well (Brown et al., 1998) (Figure 11.4).

Mitochondrial diseases resulting from systemic mutations

Mitochondrial diseases can be manifest with either stereotypical symptoms such as Leber's hereditary optic neuropathy (LHON) or Leigh's syndrome or as complex multisystem degenerative diseases such as the mitochondrial encephalomyopathies. Moreover, mitochondrial diseases can result from mtDNA mutations, nDNA mutations, and the faulty interaction of the two genetic systems. As a result, the classification, diagnosis, prognosis, and therapeutics of mitochondrial diseases is particularly problematic.

The variable phenotypes of mitochondrial diseases is the result of the mitochondria's central role in multiple cellular processes and its complex genetics. Among the cellular functions of the mitochondria are the production of cellular energy, generation of ROS, and initiation of apoptosis.

MtDNA mutations include both base substitutions and rearrangements. Base substitution mutations can be either missense mutations affecting protein coding genes, or protein synthesis mutations altering tRNA and rRNA genes. Rearrangement mutations remove a portion of the mtDNA, generally eliminating one or more tRNAs or rRNAs. Pathogenic nDNA mutations can alter respiratory complex structural genes, assembly genes, anti-oxidant genes, or mtDNA replication and repair genes.

Because of these pathophysiological and genetic complexities, the same mitochondrial disease phenotype can often be caused by a variety of different mtDNA or nDNA mutations. Alternatively, a variety of different phenotypes can be generated by the same mutation.

Here, we will discuss mitochondrial disease from the phenotypic perspective, since that is what confronts the clinician. We will then discuss the various genetic changes that can cause that phenotype (Wallace, 1992a; 1992b; 1994b; 1995a).

LEBER'S HEREDITARY OPTIC NEUROPATHY (LHON)

LHON is a form of acute or subacute, bilateral, central vision loss associated with the degeneration of the retinal ganglion cell layer and optic nerve and resulting in central scotoma. The age of onset is generally in the 20s and 30s, though onset of symptoms can occur from childhood to late adulthood. Typically, the onset and progression of blindness is relatively rapid, with both eyes developing vision loss during the same period. The disease is frequently familial, and in all familial cases the affected individuals are related through the maternal lineage. There is a predilection for males to be affected with the ratio of affected males to females reaching 4:1 in some instances (Erickson, 1972; Newman, 1993; Newman and Wallace, 1990; Riordan-Eva et al, 1995). While most mtDNA LHON pedigrees manifest primarily LHON, the more severe mutations can exhibit other neurodegenerative disease symptoms. A typical pedigree showing the maternal inheritance of LHON is presented in Figure 11.5.

Since the discovery of the first LHON mtDNA mutation, MTND4*LHON11778A, in 1988 (Wallace et al., 1988a), LHON has been shown to be due primarily to mtDNA mutations. Over 20 missense mutations have been associated with LHON patients (Table 11.2), however, only four "primary" mutations are common causes of LHON (Table 11.2). The remaining mutations are either rare pathogenic mutations or are polymorphisms associated with the European haplogroup J, which has been shown to increase the penetrance of the milder LHON mutations (Brown et al., 1995; Torroni et al., 1997).

LHON as the primary clinical manifestation

Three of the "primary" mutations primarily manifest as LHON. These are MTND4*LHON11778A (Wallace et al., 1988a), MTND1*LHON3460A (Howell et al., 1991a; Huoponen et al., 1991; 1993), and MTND6*LHON14484C (Johns et al., 1992a; Mackey and Howell, 1992) (Table 11.24). These mutations represent strong risk factors for developing LHON; have been observed in multiple unrelated LHON families; rarely co-occur with each other; and have not been detected in a large number of control mtDNAs (Brown and Wallace, 1994b; Brown et al., 1995; Howell et al., 1995; Howell, 1997). Together, these three mutations account for roughly 90% of European patients, with MTND4*LHON11778A encompassing about 50% of cases and the MTND1*LHON3460A and MTND6*LHON14484C mutations each encompassing roughly 15% (Table 11.2). In Asia, the MTND4*LHON11778A mutation accounts for 95% of patients (Mashima et al., 1993).

*MTND4*LHON11778A*

The MTND4*LHON11778A mutation converts the highly conserved ND4 codon 340 from an arginine to a histidine residue (Wallace et al., 1988a). This mutation typically displays variable expression in families, with males being predominantly affected, and is heteroplasmic in about 14% of cases (Newman et al., 1991). The MTND4*LHON11778A mutation also has a highly variable penetrance. Among MTND4*LHON11778A families, about 33–60% of maternal relatives are affected, with 82% of the affected individuals being male and 18% female (Newman et al., 1991; Brown and Wallace, 1994a). Furthermore, only about 4% of affected individuals experience visual recovery.

Of the affected individuals, the mean age of onset is 27.6 years, with a range of onset from eight to 60 years. About 58% of patients show additional ophthalmological features

Maternal Lineage of Family with
Leber's Hereditary Optic Neuropathy

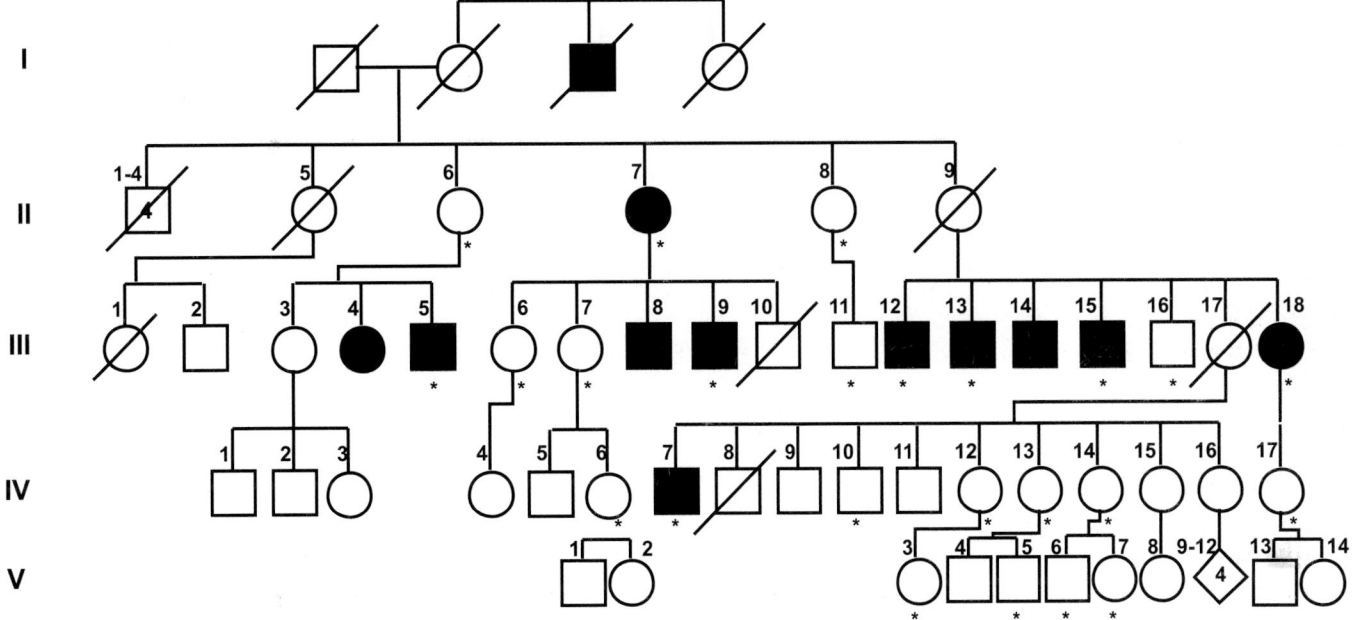

Shaded symbols indicate affected individuals. Asterisks indicate individuals examined.

Fig. 11.5. Maternally inherited pedigree of LHON due to the MTND4*LHON11778A mutation. Affected individuals (filled symbols) experience acute onset optic atrophy and central vision loss, generally as young adults. Even though the mutation is essentially homoplasmic, penetrance among maternal relatives is highly variable. Moreover, males are about three to four times more likely to lose their vision than females (Newman et al., 1991; Wallace et al., 1988a).

including peripapillary telangiectasias, microangiopathy, disk pseudo-edema, and vascular tortuosity. A total of 55% of patients have a simultaneous onset of vision loss in both eyes, while the overall mean inter-ocular interval is 1.8 months, and the maximum interval is about nine months. Once vision loss begins, it can progress rapidly or slowly. The mean length of progression for the MTND4*LHON11778A mutation is 3.7 months, with a range of 0 to 24 months. In about 98% of cases, the final visual acuity is 20/200 or worse, while only 2% are better than 20/200 (Newman et al., 1991). Most cases are limited to optic atrophy, although a variety of other mild abnormalities have been associated with this mutation. These include cardiac conduction defects such as abnormal QT interval (Ortiz et al., 1992), skeletal abnormalities, and other neurological signs (Newman, 1993).

In one patient the MTND4*LHON11778A mutation has been associated with Wolfram syndrome, which included diabetes mellitus, optic atrophy, sensorineural deafness (Pilz et al., 1994).

Some biochemical studies on the MTND4*LHON11778A mutation have reported complex I enzymatic defects ranging from 0–50%. However, most studies have found no statistically significant reduction in complex I activity (Larsson et al, 1991; Majander et al, 1991; Degli Esposti et al., 1994; Smith et al, 1994; Carelli et al., 1997; Brown et al., 2000). In contrast, most studies have observed a reduction in mitochondrial respiration using complex I-linked substrates of 30–50%, while respiration rates using succinate are normal (Larsson et al., 1991; Majander et al., 1991; 1996; Brown et al., 2000). When the MTND4*LHON11778A mtDNAs are transferred to a different nuclear background by cybrid transfer, the respiration defect is transferred indicating that the respiration defect is linked to the mtDNA mutation (Vergani et al., 1995; Hofhaus et al., 1996; Brown et al., 2000). The MTND4*LHON11778A mutation has also been reported to have an increased resistance to rotenone, a complex I inhibitor which acts as a ubiquinone antagonist. The mutant enzyme also has an altered affinity for ubiquinone analogs, though other groups have not detected

Table 11.2. Leber's hereditary optic neuropathy (LHON) disease mutations

No.[a]	Mutation	Class[b]	Other neurol. disease	Amino acids[c] Change	Cons	Approx. % European patients	% Controls	Het.[e]	Penetrance[f] % Relatives	% Males	% Recovery[g]	References
1	MTND6*LDYT14459A	Primary	+/-	A72V	M	Rare	0	+	61	58	Low	Jun et al. (1994), Shoffner et al. (1995b)
2	MTND4*LHON11778A	Primary	+/-	R340H	H	50	0	+/-	33-60	82	4	Mashima et al. (1993), Newman et al. (1991), Wallace et al. (1988a)
3	MTND1*LHON3460A	Primary	+/-	A52T	M	15	0	+/-	14-75	40-80	22	Howell et al. (1991a), Huoponen et al. (1991)
4	MTND6*LHON14484C	Primary	-	M64V	L	15	0	+/-	27-80	68	37-50	Brown et al. (1992b), Howell et al. (1991b), Johns et al. (1992a)
5	MTND2*LHON5244A	Primary	-	G259S	H	Rare	0	+	NA	NA	UN	Brown et al. (1995)
6	MTND5*LHON13730A	Primary	-	G465E	M	Rare	0	+	NA	NA	Yes	Howell et al. (1993a)
7	MTCO3*LHON9804A	Primary ?	-	A200T	H	1.5	0	-	UN	UN	UN	Johns and Neufeld (1993b)
8	MTND3*LHON10663C	Primary ?	-	V65A	L	Rare	0	-	56	60	UN	Brown et al. (1995)
9	MTATP6*LHON9101C	Primary ?	-	I192T	L	Rare	0	-	NA	NA	UN	Brown et al. (1995)
10	MTND4*LDYT11696G	Primary ?	+/-	V312I	L	Rare	0	-	UN	UN	UN	De Vries et al. (1996)
11	MTND6*LHON14482G	Primary ?	-	M64I	L	Rare	0	-	UN	89	UN	Howell et al. (1998)
12	MTND6*LHON14498T	Primary ?	-	Y59C	M	Rare	0	+	31	50	UN	Wissinger et al. (1997)
13	MTND6*LHON14568T	Primary ?	-	G36S	L	Rare	0	-	NA	NA	UN	Wissinger et al. (1997)
14	MTND6*LDYT14596A	Primary ?	+/-	I26M	M	Rare	0	+	UN	UN	UN	De Vries et al. (1996)
15	MTCYB*LHON15257A	Intermediate	-	D171N	H	9	0.4	-	NA	NA	NA	Brown et al. (1995), Brown et al. (1992c), Johns and Neufeld (1991)
16	MTND5*LHON13708A	Secondary	-	A458T	M	30	6	-	NA	NA	NA	Brown et al. (1992c), Johns and Berman (1991)
17	MTND1*LHON3394C	Secondary	-	Y30H	H	Rare	0.9	-	NA	NA	NA	Brown et al. (1992b)

Table 11.2. continued

No.[a]	Mutation	Class[b]	Other neurol. disease	Amino acids[c] Change	Cons	Approx. % European patients	% Controls	Het.[e]	Penetrance[f] % Relatives	% Males	% Recovery[g]	References
18	MTND1*LHON4160C	Secondary	++	L285P	H	Rare	0	–	76	54	0	Howell et al. (1991b)
19	MTND1*LHON4216C	Secondary	–	Y304H	L	~40	13	–	NA	NA	NA	Brown et al. (1992c), Johns and Berman (1991)
20	MTND2*LHON4917G	Secondary	–	D150N	H	3	3	–	NA	NA	NA	Johns and Berman (1991)
21	MTCO1*LHON7444A	Secondary		Ter->K	NA	5	1		NA	NA	UN	Brown et al. (1992d)
22	MTCO3*LHON9438A	Secondary	–	G78S	H	2.5	4.6	–	NA	UN	NA	Johns and Neufeld (1993b)
23	MTCYB*LHON15812A	Secondary	–	V357M	M	4	0.1	–	NA	NA	NA	Brown et al. (1992c)

[a] The first ten LHON-associated mtDNA mutations are listed in order of estimated severity (see the text).
[b] C, confirmed; NC, not confirmed; A, ambiguous. A question mark in classification indicates transient assignment pending more data.
[c] H, high amino acid conservation; M, moderate; L, low; NA, not applicable; Ter, termination codon.
[d] M, multiple background haplotypes; F, few; UN, unknown; 1*, one reported case or family. Mutant association numbers refer to numbers in column one of this table.
[e] Het., Heteroplasmy
[f] NA, not applicable; UN, unknown; penetrance estimate for the 10,663 mutation is from a single LHON family which does not harbor a common primary LHON mutation by complete mtDNA sequence analysis.
[g] Low, anecdotal low degree of vision recovery; UN, unknown; NA, not applicable

this alteration in rotenone sensitivity (Degli Esposti et al., 1994; Majander et al., 1996; Carelli et al., 1997). These observations have led to the postulation that the MTND4*LHON11778A mutation alters the complex I interaction with ubiquinone. Alternatively, the amino acid change has been hypothesized to compromise the enzyme's energy conserving (proton translocation) function, or to destabilize ubisemiquinone intermediates promoting the production of ROS. The absence of an enzymological defect in the presence of a clear respiration defect might be due to a defect in proton translocation or to an alternation of co-enzyme Q affinity which is masked in the enzyme assays by the use of coenzyme Q analogue at non-physiological concentrations as electron acceptors.

MTND1*LHON3460A

The MTND1*LHON3460A mutation changes a moderately conserved alanine residue at codon 52 in the ND1 gene to a threonine residue and has been observed to be heteroplasmic in a number of families (Howell et al., 1991a; Huoponen et al., 1991; 1993). Generally, the clinical manifestations of this mutation are confined to LHON, and only occasionally is the MTND1*LHON3460A mutation associated with other neurological signs, though patients harboring this mutation can manifest multiple sclerosis (Kellar-Wood et al., 1994; Nikoskelainen et al., 1995). Virtually every MTND1*LHON3460A family is due to an independent mutation (Brown et al., 1995), and a small percentage of the families are heteroplasmic (Brown and Wallace, 1994a). The number of affected maternal relatives has varied widely in different studies, but can approach 75% (Johns et al., 1992b; Harding et al., 1995), with between 40% and 80% of all affected individuals being male. Approximately 22% of affected individuals with the MDND1*LHON3460A have been reported to experience visual recovery (Johns et al., 1993a).

The MTND1*LHON3460A mutation is associated with markedly reduced complex I activity, and a reduction in respiration. In multiple studies of patient cells, the MTND1*LHON3460A mutation has been found to be associated with a 60 to 80% reduction in the complex I specific activity (Howell et al., 1991a; Majander et al., 1991; Smith et al., 1994; Carelli et al., 1997; Brown et al., 2000). Despite the pronounced reduction in complex I activity, ATP synthesis in MTND1*LHON3460A mitochondria is not compromised (Cock et al., 1999). Respiration studies have shown a roughly 30% reduction in maximal respiration rates using complex I-linked substrates (Majander et al., 1996; Brown et al., 2000). In cybrid transfer experiments, the complex I defect transfers faithfully (Brown et al., 2000), although nuclear genetic backgrounds may alter the magnitude of the functional defect found in cybrids (Cock et al., 1998). When complex I activity has been titrated with ubiquinone analogs/derivatives, a substrate-inhibition pattern was observed (Cock et al., 1998). This suggests that the primary biochemical defect is in altered ubiquinone binding affinity, which would be in line with the proposal that both the ND1 and ND6 polypeptides are components of the ubiquinone binding site.

MTND6*LHON14484C

Finally, the MTND6*LHON14484C mutation changes the weakly conserved methionine residue at codon 64 in the ND6 protein to a valine residue. This mutation is generally homoplasmic in LHON families (Johns et al., 1992a; Mackey and Howell, 1992), having been reported to be heteroplasmic in only a few pedigrees (Biousse et al., 1997).

Clinically, the penetrance of the MTND6*LHON14484C mutation is comparable with that of the other primary LHON mutations, resulting in symptoms in 27–80% of maternal relatives. Also, the male to female ratio of affected individuals is similarly high compared to that for the MTND4*LHON-11778A and MTND1*LHON3460A mutations (Johns et al., 1993a; Harding et al., 1995; Riordan-Eva et al., 1995). While most MTND6*LHON14484C families are likely to be independent mutations, the strong association with haplogroup J perhaps indicates that the MTND6*LHON14484C is less capable of causing LHON alone than are the MTND4*LHON11778A and MTND1*LHON3460A mutations (Torroni et al., 1990; Brown et al., 1997b). Moreover, the MTND6*LHON14484C mutation is only rarely heteroplasmic (Biousse et al., 1997), suggesting that the mutation is sufficiently mild that most of the mtDNAs must be mutant before a phenotype is likely.

The MTND6*LHON14484C mutation is additionally noteworthy for the tendency of patients to experience visual recovery. Fully 37–50% of patients with this mutation report visual improvement 11.3 (Johns et al., 1993a; Riordan-Eval et al., 1995). Thus, the MTND6*LHON14484C mutation has the lowest pathogenicity of the primary LHON mutations and may be pathogenic only when present in certain mtDNA contexts.

The biochemical defect of the MTND6*LHON14484C mutation has proven very difficult to detect. Thus the functional defects associated with this mutation may match the milder genetic and clinical signature of this mutation. In our enzyme and respiration analysis on patient lymphoblasts and cybrids and we found that the specific activity of complex I was essentially normal, through maximal respiration rates were reduced 15–20% with complex I-linked substrates (Brown et al., 2000). Similarly, in separate, independent studies, no reduction in complex I activity in was found in MTND6*LHON14484C positive patient fibroblasts (Cock et al., 1995; Carelli et al., 1999), although another study has reported a severe (65%) reduction in complex I activity and an associated 20% reduction in complex I-linked ATP synthesis in their patients (Oostra et al., 1995b). One study of platelet mitochondria implicated this mutation in complex I-ubiquinone interactions, since the mitochondria hard increased sensitivity to the complex I product inhibitors mixothiazol and $NBQH_2$ (Carelli et al., 1999). While additional studies will be needed to reach a consensus concerning the functional defects of this mutation, it is apparent that the biochemical defect of the MTND6*LHON14484C mutation is milder than that of the MTND1*LHON3460A, MTND4*LHON11778A, and MTND6*LDYT14459A mutations.

Additional potentially causal mutations for LHON

Eight other "mutants" have features that suggest that they maybe rare causal mutations of LHON. However, the causal nature of these variants is difficult to establish since they have generally only been reported in one paper or family (Table 11.2).

One of these rare mutations nicely legitimates the pathogenicity of the MTND6*LHON14484C mutation. This MTND6*LHON14482G mutation alters the same codon as the MTND6*LHON14484C mutation, but converts the methionine at codon 64 to an isoleucine instead of a valine (Howell, 1998).

Two of the rare mutations, MTND2*LHON5244A (Brown et al., 1992c) and MTND5*LHON13730A (Howell et al., 1993a), altered conserved amino acids and were heteroplasmic. Hence, they are likely to be pathogenic mutations. Three other mutations, MTCO3*LHON9804A (Johns and Neufeld, 1993b), MTND4L*LHON10663C (Brown et al., 1995) and MTATP6*LHON 9101C (Lamminen et al., 1995) were homoplasmic. Hence the pathogenicity of these mutants is unclear. The MTCO3*LHON9804 mutation changed the conserved alanine residue at codon 200 in the COIII polypeptide to a threonine. It was reported in 1.5% of LHON patients without other known primary mutations, but not in any of the controls surveyed (Johns and Neufeld, 1993b). The MTND4L*LHON10663C mutation was found to change a poorly conserved valine to an alanine residue at amino acid 65

in the ND4L polypeptide. However, this mutation was found in two independent LHON patients, and was not detected in a large number of ethnic group or haplotype-matched controls. The two MTND4L*LHON10663C-positive patients both had haplogroup J mtDNA haplotypes, incorporating the MTND1*LHON4216C, MTND5*LHON13708A and MTCYB*LHON15257A variants. One of the patients also harbored the heteroplasmic MTND2*LHON5244A mutation. Determination of the complete mtDNA sequence for the other patient, the proband of a three-generation LHON pedigree, revealed no other candidate mutations (Brown et al., 1995). This would imply that either the MTND4L*LHON10663C mutation, haplogroup J or both are required to precipitate the clinical phenotype. Finally, the MTATP6*LHON9101C mutation converts the poorly conserved isoleucine at amino acid 192 in the MTATP6 polypeptide to a threonine. This mutation was not found in 100 geographically matched controls and was associated with a Complex V biochemical defect (Lamminen et al., 1995).

Of the two remaining potentially causal mutations, the MTND6*LHON14498T (Wissinger et al., 1997) and MTND6*LHON14568T (Wissinger et al., 1997) mutations were both found in individual LHON pedigrees.

The MTND1*LHON4160 mutation was found together with the MTND6*LHON14484C mutation in the mtDNA of a large pedigree with acute-onset optic atrophy as well as other neurological symptoms (Howell et al., 1991b). Hence, this mutation may augment the pathogenicity of the MTND6*LHON14484C mutation. The pathogenicity of the MTND6*LHON14484C mutation has also been underscored by its co-occurrence with the MTND4*LHON11778A mutation (Riordan-Eva et al., 1995).

LHON and the haplogroup J background

Analysis of the background mtDNA haplotypes in LHON families harboring the various primary mutations has shown that most families are new mutations. However, many European LHON patients with *LHON* mutations are also associated with mtDNA haplogroup J. It is now clear that haplogroup J is also an important risk factor for LHON, thus explaining the frequent association of its polymorphic markers with LHON.

In two studies, haplotype analysis was performed on LHON patients of European decent harboring the three common "primary" mutations: MTND4*LHON11778A, MTND1*LHON3460A, and MTND6*LHON14484C (Brown et al., 1995; Torroni et al., 1997) (Figure 11.6). These studies revealed that patients harboring the

MtDNA Phylogenetic Tree
of Caucasian LHON Patients

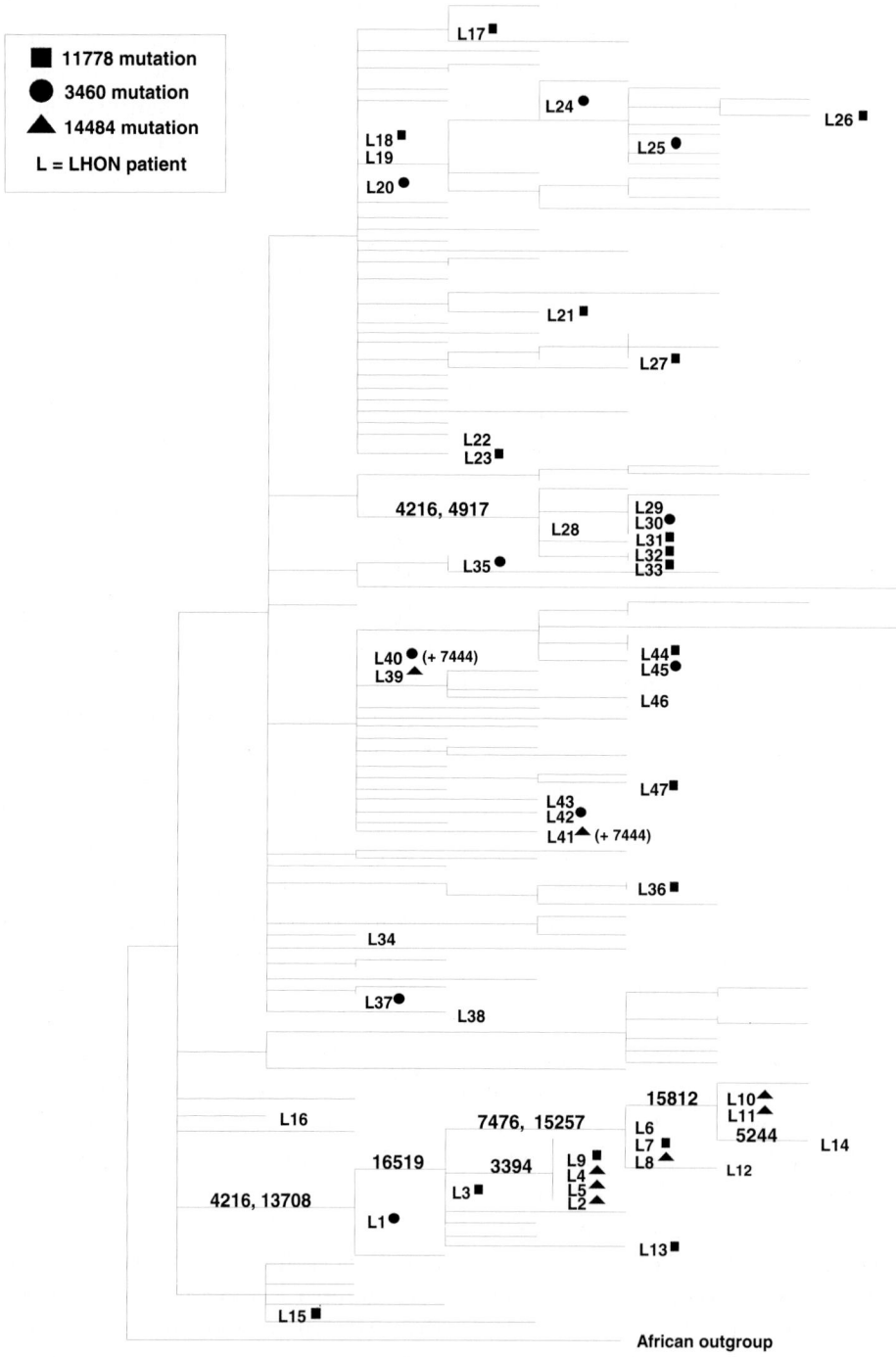

Fig. 11.6. Phylogenetic tree of Caucasian mtDNAs from 47 LHON patients (L1-L47, bold) and 175 Caucasian controls obtained from the United States and Canada. Haplotypes were determined by RFLP analysis using the entire mtDNA. For the patients, all mtDNA haplotypes are shown and the presence of a common primary mutation is indicated (see the key). Additional mutations of interest are noted in parentheses. Multiple occurrences of the three common primary LHON mutations are indicated by their presence in independent mtDNA lineages, and, when occurring within the same large mtDNA lineage, by the presence of intermediate haplotypes lacking LHON mutations. The numbers in large, bold characters on branches indicate mutations that define specific groups of mtDNAs but are not necessarily the mutational steps used to create the phylogeny. The horizontal branch lengths are proportional to the number of mutational events that separate haplotypes. From Brown et al. (1995), Hum Mutat 6: 311–325. © 1995. Reprinted by permission of Wiley-Liss Inc., a subsidiary of John Wiley and Sons, Inc.

MTND1*LHON3460A and MTND4*LHON11778A mutations had a variety of different mtDNA background haplotypes that are dispersed throughout the European mtDNA haplogroups. Thus, most European LHON families must be the result of new independent mutational events (Brown et al., 1995; Torroni et al., 1997). On the other hand, most patients harboring the MTND6*LHON14484C mutation clustered together on a single mtDNA lineage, haplogroup J. Still, the patient mtDNAs with the MTND6*LHON14484C mutation were interspersed with haplogroup J mtDNAs which lacked this mutation, and some of the MTND6*LHON14484C mutation patients were on totally different mtDNA lineages (Brown et al., 1995; Biousse et al., 1997) (Figure 11.6). In fact, in one case the MTND6*LHON14484C mutation was found to be associated with the African haplogroup L mtDNA (Torroni et al., 1996a). Hence, most MTND6*LHON14484C mutation families must also be independent mutational events.

Since the MTND6*LHON14484C mutation is not shared among the haplogroup J mtDNAs by descent, then the onset of blindness for the MTND6*LHON14484C mutation must also require the co-occurrence of haplogroup J. This conclusion is supported by the fact that 80% MTND6*LHON14484C of LHON patients are haplogroup J, and the 37% of MTND4*LHON11778A LHON patients are also haplogroup J, while only 9% of the general European population is haplogroup J (Brown et al., 1997b). Hence, haplogroup J must augment the pathogenicity of the milder primary LHON mutations.

Haplogroup J is defined by two mtDNA variants: MTND5*LHON13708A and MTND1*LHON4216C (Johns et al., 1992a; 1993a; Obermaier-Kusser et al., 1994; Oostra et al., 1994; Brown et al., 1995; Howell et al., 1995; Riordan-Eva et al., 1995) (Table 11.2). The MTND5*LHON13708A mutation converts a moderately conserved alanine residue at codon 458 in the ND5 protein to a threonine residue (Johns and Neufeld, 1991; Brown et al., 1992c), while the MTND1*LHON4216C mutation converts a weakly conserved tyrosine residue at codon 304 in the ND1 protein to a histidine residue (Johns and Neufeld, 1991; Brown et al., 1992c). These are the only mtDNA variants that are consistently found in the multiple haplogroup J mtDNAs that have been sequenced in association with LHON, suggesting that they must be important in the physiological effect (Brown et al., 1992b). In addition to these common variants, haplogroup J is divided into several sub-lineages with distinctive variants that have also been correlated with LHON. Two of the branches are defined by the MTCYB*LHON15257A variant and by the MTND1*LHON3394C variant.

The MTCYB*LHON15257A mutation is always associated with the haplogroup J MTND1*LHON4216C and MTND5*LHON13708A variants, and defines one branch of the haplogroup J tree (Table 11.2). It converts a highly conserved aspartate residue at codon 171 in the cytochrome b gene to an asparagine residue (Brown et al., 1992c). The haplogroup J MTCYB*LHON15257A lineage is further subdivided by the presence or absence of the MTCYB*LHON15812A variant (Brown et al., 1992c). Therefore, these variants are either secondary markers of haplogroup J or further augment the effect of the basic MTND1*LHON4216C and MTND5*LHON13708A variants.

The MTND1*LHON3394C variant defines a second sublineage of haplogroup J that is prevalent in French Canadians. The MTND1*LHON3394C variant changes the highly conserved tyrosine residue at codon 30 in the ND1 protein to a histidine residue. In most LHON patients, MTCYB*LHON15257A and MTND1*LHON3394C LHON variants are usually associated with the primary MTND6*LHON14484C mutation. Hence, the relative contribution of all of these haplogroup J polymorphisms to the onset of blindness remains to be clarified (Brown et al., 1992b; 1992c).

While all haplogroup J mtDNAs harbor the MTND1*LHON4216C and the MTND5*LHON13708A variants, the MTND1*LHON4216C variant can also be associated with the MTND2*LHON4917G missense variant. The MTND2*LHON4917G variant changes a highly conserved aspartate residue at codon 150 in the ND2 protein to an asparagine (Brown et al., 1995). The sharing of the MTND1*LHON4216C between these two lineages raises the possibility that the two lineages may be sub-branches of a common macro-haplogroup which predisposes individuals to LHON (Howell et al., 1995). If so, then the pathogenic significance of the MTND1*LHON4216C variant might be greater than the mild amino acid substitution might suggest. Alternatively, the predisposition to LHON might be caused by MTND5*LHON13708A on the one lineage and MTND2*LHON4917 on the other.

The MTCO1*LHON7444A mutation changes the termination codon of the COI polypeptide, extending the polypeptide by three charged amino acids (Brown et al., 1992d). However, this mutation is unlikely to be pathogenicity, since both reported cases with this mutation also harbored a primary mutation, either the MTND6*LHON14484C or the MTND1*LHON3460A mutations (Brown et al., 1995). The MTCO3*LHON9438A variant was reported in about 2.5% of European patients and to change a highly conserved glycine residue to a serine residue (Johns and Neufeld,

1993b). However, the MTCO3*LHON9438A variant is always homoplasmic, has also been found in a low frequency in African and African-American controls (Brown et al., 1994), and has been found to co-occur with the MTND4*LHON11778A mutation (Oostra et al., 1995a). Hence, it is unlikely to contribute substantially to the pathophysiology of LHON.

Possible pathophysiological mechanisms of LHON

The pathophysiology mechanism by which the LHON mutations cause acute onset vision loss in young adults remains a mystery. One respiratory defect that ties many of LHON mutations together is an inhibition in the transfer of electrons from complex I to CoQ_{10}. A faulty interaction between CoQ_{10} and complex I has been suggested for the MTND6*LHON14484C mutation (Carelli et al., 1999), implying that the region of ND6 around codons 64–72 may be involved in CoQ_{10} interaction with complex I. Furthermore, five other pathogenic missense mutations have been found in this same region of ND6, which encompasses the most evolutionarily conserved transmembrane helix (helix c) as well as a region similar to the ubiquinone-reacting domain of cytochrome *b* in complex III (Carelli et al., 1999). These are the MTND6*LDYT14459A mutation which changes codon 72 (Jun et al., 1994), MTND6*LHON-14482C mutation which alters codon 64, the MTND6*LHON14498T mutation which alters codon 59, the MTND6*LHON-14568T mutation which affects codon 36, and the MTND6*LDYT14596A mutation which changes codon 26 (Table 11.2). Moreover, the biochemical defects of the MTND6*LDYT14459A and MTND1*LHON3460A mutations are similar, suggesting a common mechanism and ND1 is also thought to be important in electron transfer to CoQ_{10}. Finally, the MTND4*LHON11778A mutation has been associated with altered rotenone binding and thus of CoQ_{10} (Degli Esposti et al., 1994; Majander et al., 1996; Carelli et al., 1997). Thus, all of the primary LHON mutations have been implicated in problems with CoQ_{10} interaction with complex I. Such a defect might be difficult to accurately evaluate given the difficulties with assaying complex I with the physiological substrate, CoQ_{10}, necessitating the use of the CoQ_{10} analogues such as DB. The possibility that all of these mutations impair electron transfer to CoQ_{10} is supported by the observation that all of the primary LHON and LDYT mutations that have been studied (MTND6*LDYT14459A, MTND4*LHON11778A, MTND1*LHON3460A, and MTND6*LHON14484C) show at least a partial defect in complex 1-linked respiration, with reductions in maximal respiration rates for the various mutations ranging from 15% to 40%. It is possible that even the small reduction in respiration observed for the MTND6*LHON14484C mutation might reflect a significant defect in electron transfer within the mitochondria under physiological conditions.

Assuming that the primary defect of most LHON mutations is the inhibition of the electron transport chain between complex I and CoQ_{10}, then the pathophysiological basis of the disease might either be chronic energy deficiency or increased ROS generation. If increased ROS production and oxidative stress have a role in LHON, then this might contribute to the pathology of LHON in two ways. It is possible that chronic oxidative stress to the retinal ganglion cells and optic nerve might damage the mtDNA and degrade mitochondrial function to such an extent that ultimately the neuronal mtPTP is activated and the cells undergo a wave of programmed cell death. Such a model is attractive because it explains how a chronic disease could result in a sudden onset of symptoms with a precipitous course.

Alternatively, the increased mitochondrial production of ROS might inactivate the vasodilator NO, resulting in chronic vasoconstriction, ischemia and death of the retinal ganglion cells. A common set of preclinical findings in LHON families includes microangiopathy, retinal vessel telangiectasias, and tortuous vessels, consistent with LHON being due to a retinal vasculopathy. NO is a natural vasodilator, and it is acutely sensitive to inactivation by ROS (Bandy and Davison, 1990). If the LHON mutations inhibit the electron transport chain and increase mitochondrial ROS production, then it is possible that these ROS chronically deplete the retinal vascular NO, causing vasoconstriction and ultimately resulting in the spasmodic constriction of the retinal blood vessels, depriving the retinal ganglia cells of oxygen and nutrients. This would lead to ischemia and neuronal death. Thus sudden onset of vision loss would be envisioned as a form of a retinal stroke.

While it will be difficult to define the pathophysiology of mitochondrial ophthalmological disease in human studies, it is likely that more progress will be made using mouse models for mitochondrial disease. If LHON is the result of increased oxidative stress, then mice lacking mitochondrial anti-oxidant defenses should be more prone to ophthalmological decline.

LHON, multiple sclerosis, and dystonia

While most LHON cases present with isolated optic atrophy, certain pedigrees manifest additional neurological symptoms, which have suggested additional diseases that may be of mitochondrial origin. Prominent among the LHON-associated symptoms are a multiple sclerosis-like presentation and movement disorders (Novotny et al., 1986; Nikoskelainen et al., 1995; Riordan-Eva et al., 1995).

Multiple sclerosis as a manifestation of LHON

An association between some primary LHON mutations and a multiple sclerosis-like demyelinating disease has been repeatedly reported. About 1–2% of female patients from LHON pedigrees with the MTND4*LHON11778A mutation have been diagnosed with multiple sclerosis-like demyelination disease (Newman et al., 1991; Harding et al., 1992b; Flanigan and Johns, 1993; Hanefeld et al., 1994; Kellar-Wood et al., 1994; Olsen et al., 1995). Eight females with the MTND4*LHON11778A mutation have been described which presented with LHON but subsequently developed clinical and/or neuroradiological signs consistent with multiple sclerosis (Harding et al., 1992b). A number of other similar cases exhibited an association between either the MTND4*LHON11778A or the MTND1*LHON3460A mutations and multiple sclerosis, mostly in females (Kellar-Wood et al., 1994; Nikoskelainen et al., 1995), but also in males (Nikoskelainen et al., 1995; Olsen et al., 1995). Surprisingly, though the MTND4*LHON11778A mutation accounts for greater than 90% of Japanese LHON cases, no association has been found between this mutation and multiple sclerosis in the Japanese population (Nishimura et al., 1995). However, LHON mutation associations with multiple sclerosis have been evident only when patients are ascertained through LHON presentation (with or without family history) or through multiple sclerosis patients with early and prominent optic nerve involvement (Kellar-Wood et al., 1994). Given the rare population frequency of both LHON and multiple sclerosis diseases, it is likely that their frequent coincidence reflects a related cause. It is possible that neuronal cell lysis resulting from the mitochondrial defect releases cellular proteins which initiate the auto-immune response (Chalmers et al., 1995, Olsen et al., 1995).

LHON and Dystonia

There is increasing evidence that mitochondrial defects are a common feature of dystonia (Figure 11.7). Biochemical analysis of an isolated case of idiopathic dystonia, putaminal lesions, and myopathy revealed a partial complex III defect (Nigro et al., 1990). Moreover, complex I defects were observed in the platelet mitochondria of a wide variety of

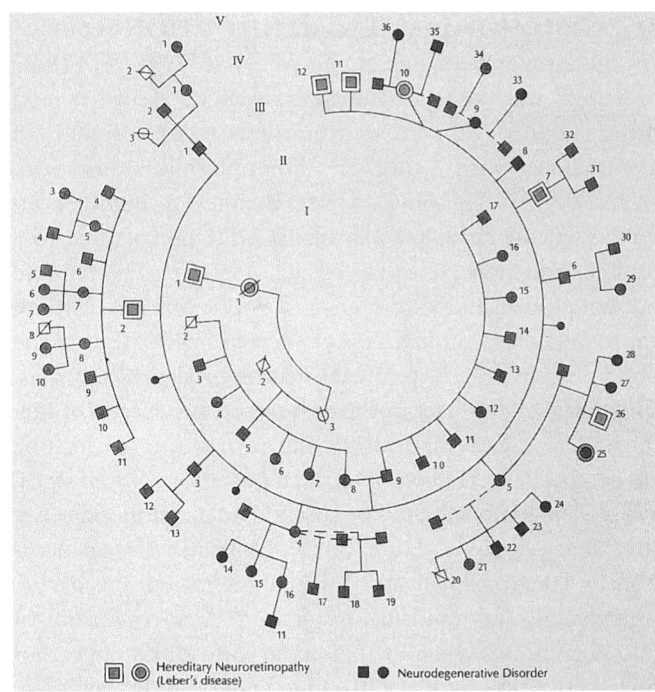

Fig. 11.7. Hispanic family with maternally inherited LHON and/or dystonia due to the heteroplasmic mtDNA mutation at MTND6*LDYT14459A. Individuals with LHON experience acute onset optic atrophy and central vision loss, generally as young adults. Individuals with neurodegenerative disease have a much earlier age on onset and experience gait disturbance, rigidity, pseudobulbar syndrome, impaired intelligence, short stature, and frequently infantile bilateral striatal necrosis (IBSN). (Reproduced Novotny et al., 1986.) (See Plate 11.7.)

dystonia patients, with the average complex I activity of generalized or segmental dystonia patients being reduced 62% while that from focal dystonia patients was reduced 37% (Benecke et al., 1992).

MTND4*LHON11778A and movement disorders

A number of LHON pedigrees harboring the MTND4*LHON11778A mutation include patients which also develop movement disorders. One individual, which lost his vision at 37, developed cerebellar-extrapyramidal tremor and left-side rigidity associated with bilateral basal ganglia lesions at age 38 (Larsson et al., 1991). A second MTND4*LHON11778A patient which suffered visual loss at 23, showed pyramidal signs including spastic paraparesis, inexhaustible patellar and ankle clonus, diffuse muscle weakness and multiple periventricular and subcortical hyper-intensities on MRI compatible with demyelinating disease (Vergani et al., 1995). A third mother and son exhibited ataxia associated with cerebellar and pontine atrophy (Funakawa et al., 1995).

MTND6*LHON14484C + MTND1*LHON4160C

In another large pedigree, the MTND6*LHON14484C mutation was associated with movement disorders and other neurodegenerative symptoms when present in association with another homoplasmic mutation, MTND1*LHON4160C, which changes a highly conserved leucine at codon 285 of the ND1 polypeptide to a proline and was (Howell et al., 1991b). The clinical presentation included sudden onset optic atrophy with an approximately twofold excess of affected males. Beyond the optic atrophy, there were two neurological presentations. The first had an onset in the first or second decade of life, starting as a gait abnormality and progressing to include ataxia, spasticity, tremor, dysarthria, posterior column signs, and skeletal deformities. The second had a childhood onset (five to ten years), with severe encephalitic disease occasionally resulting in death. Initial signs include headache, convulsions, and abnormal respiration. A novel feature of this later presentation is that some individuals appear to fully recover (Wallace, 1970). One branch of the pedigree, with less severe symptoms was found to have a second homoplasmic mutation, MTND1*LHON4136G, which was hypothesized to be protective (Howell et al., 1991b). Biochemical analysis of platelet derived mitochondria from four subjects revealed an 80% average reduction in rotenone-sensitive NADH-CoQ oxidoreductase specific activity (Parker et al., 1989b).

MTND6*LDYT14459A

The MTND6*LDYT14459A mutation has been shown to cause LHON and/or early onset generalized dystonia (Novotny et al., 1986; Jun et al, 1994; Shoffner et al., 1995b). The MTND6*LDYT14459A mutation is relatively rare, having been reported in several independent pedigrees (Jun et al., 1994; Shoffner et al., 1995b). This mutation changes the highly conserved alanine at codon 72 in the ND6 polypeptide to a valine and can manifest as two very different phenotypes: LHON and/or generalized dystonia (Figure 11.7). This mutation has been found to be heteroplasmic in at least some family members in every pedigree studied (Table 11.2) (Jun et al., 1994; Shoffner et al., 1995b). The dystonia generally has an early onset and includes gait disturbance and rigidity of the lower extremities, which advances with age to include the upper extremities (Novotny et al., 1986). Bilateral basal ganglia degeneration (bilateral striatal necroses) is also a common finding in the dystonia patients (Figure 11.8).

Evidence for the independent origin of the different family mutations is clear for the MTND6*LDYT14459A mutation. The mutation was first identified in a large Hispanic family, which proved to harbor a Native American haplogroup D mtDNA (Jun et al., 1994). Subsequently, the same mutation was found in an African-American LHON family with a haplogroup L1 mtDNA and in a European dystonia patient with a haplogroup I mtDNA (Jun et al., 1994; Shoffner et al., 1995b). Since mtDNA

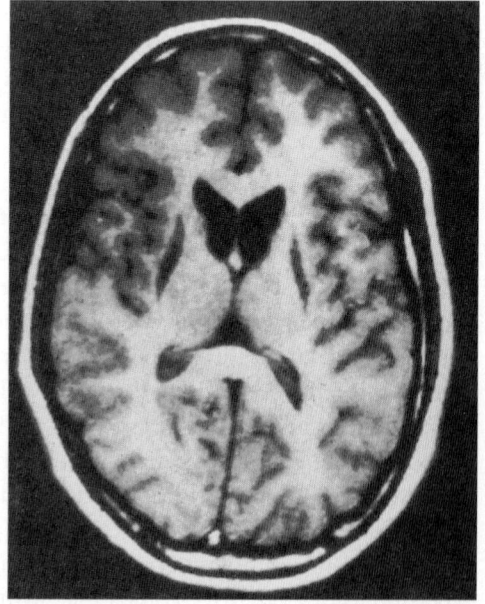
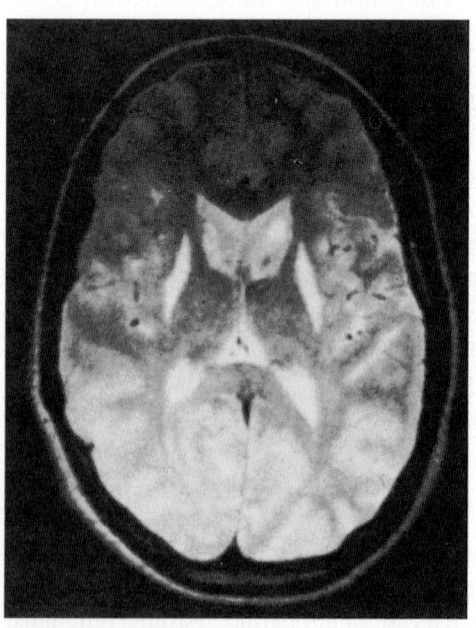

A   B

Fig. 11.8. Magnetic resonance image of the head of patient IV24 in Fig. 11.4 showing bilateral striatel necrosis. The left-hand panel is a T_1 image (cellular material light). The right panel is a T_2 image (aqueous areas light). The lesions are the symmetrical fusiform lesions below and to the left and right of the ventricles. Reprinted from Wallace (1999) Mitochondrial diseases in man and mouse. Science 238: 1482–1488. © 1999 American Association for the Advancement of Science).

haplotypes of these three families encompasses most of the world's mtDNA sequence diversity, it was not possible that the MTND6*LDYT14459A mutations are related through a common ancestor. Rather, all three MTND6*LDYT14459A mutations must have arisen recently and independently, a conclusion consistent with the fact that all three families were heteroplasmic. Hence, this mutation must be the cause of this disease (Jun et al., 1994; Shoffner et al., 1995b). Moreover, two additional complex I mutations, MTND4*LDYT11696G and MTND6*LDYT14596A, had similar presentations of large maternal pedigrees with LHON and dystonia, the MTND6*LDYT14596A mutation also being heteroplasmic (De Vries et al., 1996).

While the MTND6*LDYT14459A mutation has consistently been associated with neurological disease, the symptoms have differed among patients with different mtDNA backgrounds. This suggests that genetic background might also influence these mutations. In the five generation Hispanic pedigree with the background mtDNA haplogroup D, among 42 maternal relatives, 19% had LHON, 31% had dystonia and bilateral striatal necrosis, and 2% had both (Novotny et al., 1986). Its penetrance among maternal relatives is about 61%, with 58% of the affected individuals being male, and there is no record of an affected individual recovering. The mean age of onset of dystonia was four years, with a range of one and a half to nine years. The motor system was primarily involved and resulted in gait disturbance and rigidity of the lower extremities, which advanced with age to include the upper extremities. Patients also developed pseudo-bulbar syndrome (swallowing and speech problems), impaired intelligence, short stature and myopathic features. These symptoms were often associated with bilateral striatal necrosis (Novotny et al., 1986), the loss of cells in the striatum, putamen and caudate. In the African-American pedigree with backgroup haplogroup L1, the mother and daughter both developed LHON, but on MRI scan the daughter was found to have unilateral basal ganglia degeneration. Finally, the singleton European male with haplogroup I mtDNA had dystonia and bilateral striatal necrosis (Jun et al., 1994, Shoffner et al., 1995b).

Analysis of MTND6*LDYT14459A patient skeletal muscle mitochondria has revealed that complex I activity is essentially eliminated (Shoffner et al., 1995b). In contrast, biochemical analysis of OXPHOS enzymes and respiration in mitochondria isolated from Epstein-Barr virus (EBV)-transformed lymphoblastoid cell lines of MTND6*LDYT14459A patients revealed a 55% reduction in complex I-specific activity when normalized to citrate synthase or mitochondrial protein (Jun et al., 1996). This defect could be transferred along with the mutant mtDNAs

to p^0 lymphoblastoid cells in cybrid experiments (Jun et al., 1996). In contrast to the greater than 50% reduction in complex I specific activity, the overall mitochondrial respiration rate using complex I substrates was not significantly reduced. This implies that the complex I defect alone is not sufficient to be rate-limiting, consistent with respiratory control theory (Letellier et al., 1994; Malgat et al., 1995).

Kinetic analysis of the MTND6*LDYT14459A complex I defect revealed that the V_{max} for NADH is reduced, but the K_m is not (Jun et al., 1996). Furthermore, the enzyme activity with increased decyl-ubiquinone (DB), a CoQ_{10} analogue, showed a maximum activity at 5 mM and then declined as DB was increased to 10 mM, a result in marked contrast to the steady increase in activity seen in the control enzyme over this same concentration range. Finally, there was a marked product inhibition of the enzyme by 5 mM DBH_2 with the specific activity being inhibited 71%. These data suggest that the MTND6*LDYT14459A mutation may alter the CoQ_{10} binding site of complex I (Jun et al., 1996). Hence, the MTND6*LDYT1459A mutation places MTND6 near the CoQ_{10} binding site.

Dystonia and nDNA mitochondrial genes

Mutations in mitochondrial genes of the nDNA have also been shown to cause neurodegenerative diseases including dystonia and hereditary spastic paraplegia (HSP).

The Mohr-Tranebjaerg Syndrome, which presents in early childhood with sensorineural hearing loss that can progress to dystonia, spasticity, mental deterioration, paranoia and cortical blindness. Those patients which develop the movement disorder characteristically exhibit progressive degeneration of the basal ganglia, corticospinal tract, and brain stem. The gene responsible for Mohr-Tranebjaerg syndrome was identified on the X chromosome through a patient with a 10 bp deletion in exon 2 of the gene. The identity of the gene was confirmed in a second family found to harbor a 1 bp deletion in exon 1. The gene, designated DFN-1, generates a 1167 np cDNA encoding a 97 amino acid, 11 kDa polypeptide, designated DDP1p. The predicted polypeptide has a high homology to a Schizosaccharomyces pombe gene of unknown function (Jin et al., 1996) (Table 11.3).

The mouse homologue of the DDP1 cDNA was first isolated by applying differential display to the skeletal muscle mRNAs of Antl −/− knockout mice. Since a variety of energy genes had been found to be induced in this system, the discovery that a homology of DDP1 is unregulated in Ant1 −/− muscle provided preliminary evidence that this gene was involved in mitochondrial biogenesis and assembly (Wallace and Murdock, 1999). A role for proteins of the

Table 11.3. Nuclear OXPHOS gene disease mutations

Phenotype	Gene funtion	Mutation	Chromosome	Reference
Metaphyseal chondrodysplasia or cartilage-hair hypoplasia [MIM #250250]	RNA of RNAse MRP	Promoter deletions, RNA:A70G, G262T, G193A, 98insTG	9q13	Ridanpaa et al. (2001)
Leigh syndrome	PDH–E1α	Multiple	X	Matthews et al. (1993)
Leigh syndrome	Complex I–NDUFS8 N-2 FeS	P79L, R102H	9q33.2–34.11	Loeffen et al. (1998), Smeitink and van den Heuvel (1999)
Leigh syndrome	*Complex I–NDUFS7*	V122M	11q13.1–13.3	Smeitink and van den Heuvel (1999)
Leigh syndrome	*Complex I– NDUFS7*	V122M	11q13.1–13.3	Smeitink and van den Heuvel (1999)
Pediatric hypotonia, retardation, convulsions, brain and basal ganglia atrophy	Complex I–NDUFS4 18 kDa protein	5 bp duplication	5	van den Heuvel et al. (1998)
Pediatric hypotonia, vomiting, strabismus, myoclonus, CNS atrophy	Complex I–NDUFVI	R59X, T423M	11q13	Smeitink and van den Heuvel (1999)
Pediatric hypotonia, vomiting, strabismus, myoclonus, CNS atrophy	Complex I–NDUFVI	R59X, T423M	11q13	Smeitink and van den Heuvel (1999)
Pediatric myoclonic epilepsy, CNS atrophy	Complex I–NDUFVI	A341V	11q13	Smeitink and van den Heuvel (1999)
Leight syndrome	*Complex II–Fp subuni*	R554W	5p16	Bourgeron et al (1995)
Leigh syndrome	Complex IV–SURF1	Q251X, C762T, 37ins17, 516+2T→G, 550delAG, 868insT, 312insATdel10, insAT, 845delCT, 722delCC, 326insATdel10, 855delCT, 882insT	9q34	Tiranti et al. (1998b), Zhu et al. (1998)
Neonatal cardioencephalo-myopathy	ComplexIV–SCO2	E140K, S225F, R171W, null	22q13	Papadopoulou et al. (1999)
Neonatal hepatic failure and encephalopathy	Complex IV–SCO1	C520T, P174L Frameshift	17q12–13	Valnot et al. (2000)
Neonatal tubulopathy and encephalopathy	Complex IV–COX10	N204K	17q13.1–q11.1	Valnot et al. (2000)
AD-PEO	ANT1-unstable mtDNA	A114P V289M	4q34–35	Kaukonen et al. (1995)
AD-PEO	mtDNA stability	Unknown	3p14.2–21.2 10q23.3–24.3	Suomalainen et al. (1995), Zeviani et al. (1990)
Spastic paraplegia	ATPase protease	Δ gene, 784del2 2228insA	16q24.3	Casari et al. (1998)
Mohr-Tranebjaerg syndrome, deafness and dystonia	DFN-1, mitochondrial import	Δ gene, 183del10, 151delT	Xq21–22	Jin et al. (1996), Koehler et al. (1999), Wallace and Murdock (1999)
Friedreich ataxia, neuropathy, cardiomyopathy, diabetes	frataxin, mito. Fe transport, ROS toxicity	Trinuc.* Repeat, Structural	9q13	Campuzano et al. (1996), Rotig et al. (1997)

continued

Table 11.3. Nuclear OXPHOS gene disease mutations (*continued*)

Phenotype	Gene funtion	Mutation	Chromosome	Reference
MNGIE	Thymidine phosphorylase	E289A, G145R, K222S, G153S, 4196insC, g4090a, del16bp, g3867c skip E9, t1504c skip E4	22q13.32–qter	Nishino et al. (1999)
MtDNA depletion	MtDNA copy control (?)	Unknown	Unknown	Bodnar et al. (1993, 1995), Boustany et al. (1983), Figarella-Branger et al. (1992), Mazziotta et al. (1992) Moraes et al. (1991), Poulton et al. (1995c), Telerman-Toppet et al. (1992), Tritschler et al. (1992)

* trinucleotide repeat
MNGIE, mitochondrial neurogastrointestinal encephalomyopathy

DDP1 structure in mitochondrial protein import was demonstrated by studies of the yeast mitochondrial import proteins. While studying the *Saccharomyces cerevisiae* import pathway for mitochondrial inner membrane carrier proteins such as the ANT (yeast ACC), the Tim8p family of proteins was discovered to be located in the mitochondrial intermembrane space (Koehler et al., 1999). This family includes Tim8p, Tim9p, Tim10p, Tim12p and Tim13p, all of which are similar in size and contain a distinctive duplicated $C(N)_3C$ motif, reminiscent of a Zn finger protein. Surprisingly, the DDP1 protein of the Mohr-Tranebjaerg syndrome was found to have the same duplicated $C(N)_3C$ motif as the Tim8p family protein. Moreover, synthetic DDP1 is incorporated into the mitochondrial intermembrane space in yeast and haptin-tagged DDP1 is specifically localized to yeast and mammalian mitochondrial (Koehler et al., 1999). Recent data indicated that duplicated $C(N)_3C$ motif is found in a large family of mitochondrial proteins, and that the DDP1 polypeptide may be involved in mitochondrial fission (Blackstone, 2001, personal communication).

The demonstration that the DDP1 protein is involved in mitochondrial bioenergetics or biogenesis indicates that the underlying defect of the Mohr-Tranebjaerg syndrome is probably energy deficiency in the neurons. This is particularly satisfying, since deafness and dystonia associated with basal ganglia degeneration have also been linked to mtDNA mutations. Thus, both nDNA and mtDNA mutations can cause the same phenotype.

Another neurological phenotype associated with a mitochondrial defect is HSP. HSP, in the "pure" form, presents primarily with progressive weakness and spasticity of the lower limbs. However, in the "complicated" form, symptoms can include mental retardation, peripheral neuropathy, amyotrophy, ataxia, retinitis pigmentosa, optic atrophy, deafness and ichthyosis. Muscle histology of patients in one mutant family revealed RRFs, which were SDH hyperreactive and contained packed abnormal mitochondria. HSP was initially found to be linked to the paraplegin gene on chromosome 16q24.3 in a large Italian family. The paraplegin gene consists of five exons extending over 10.8 kb of genomic sequence. The index family was found to harbor a complex rearrangement in the gene, possibly associated with the interactions of multiple Alu repeat elements. Paraplegin mutations have also been observed in two additional families: a homozygous 2 bp deletion causing a frameshift that abolished 60% of the protein and a single A insertion which created a frameshift and stop codon, two amino acids downstream, thus removing the C-terminal 57 amino acid residues. The paraplegin protein is an 88 kDa polypeptide with a 40–45 amino acid residue targeting peptide. It shows homology to a subfamily of adenosine triphosphatases (AAA proteins) which are yeast mitochondrial metalloproteases. In yeast such proteins have both protease and chaperon-like activities (Casari et al., 1998). Thus, the paraplegin protein may function in the assembly and degradation of mitochondrial enzyme complexes.

PARKINSON'S DISEASE (PD) AND HUNTINGTON'S DISEASE (HD)

Many factors undoubtedly contribute to the etiology of PD (Schapira, 1995a), but both biochemical and genetic data indicate that one of these factors may be defects in mitochondrial function. PD is clinically characterized by bradykinesia, rigidity, and tremor associated with the death of the dopaminergic neurons in the substantia nigra. Clinical symptoms are generally noted when approximately 80% of the dopaminergic neurons are lost. Neuropathologically, PD patient neurons contain characteristic Lewy bodies (Schapira 1992; 1994b; 1995b).

Chromosomal genetics of Parkinson disease

PD is clinically and genetically heterogeneous. A hereditary component for PD has long been suspected, though classical twin studies have been unsuccessful at defining the extent of the heritable component (Johnson et al., 1990). Occasional pedigrees show a clear autosomal dominant inheritance, including two large kindreds reported from a single Italian village which exhibit an early onset (mean age of 46.5 years) and rapid course (average length of 9.7 years) disease (Golbe et al., 1990).

Two chromosomal PD genes have been identified. The best studied of these encodes α-synuclein, a major constituent of Lewy bodies. A codon 209 mutation has been identified in PD patients (Polymeropoulos et al., 1997; Spillantini et al., 1997; Kruger et al., 1998). α-synuclein, like Aβ in Alzheimer's disease, can undergo self-oligomerization in the presence of Cu^{2+} or Aβ25–35 peptide. Oxidation of α-synuclein by exposure to Cu^{++} and H_2O_2 also stimulates its aggregation (Paik et al, 2000). The other gene is parkin, causing autosomal recessive juvenile-onset PD. Parkin is a ubiquitous protein, abundant in the brain, that functions as a ubiquitin-protein ligase (Kitada et al., 1998; Shimura et al., 2000). Parkin mutations may therefore adversely effect protein degradation and clearance leading to aggregation and neuronal death (Kaytor and Warren, 1999).

Association studies have demonstrated that defects in the cytochrome p450 mono-oxygenase, debrisoquine 4-hydroxylase (CYP2D6), are also at increased frequency in PD patients. The presence of a mutant allele increases the risk of PD about 2.54-fold (Armstrong et al., 1992; Smith et al., 1992; Rempfer et al., 1994). An association has also been reported between a monoamine oxidase B (MAO-B) allele and PD (Kurth et al., 1993), though this has not been confirmed (Schapira, 1995a). Thus, it would appear that an inability to effectively detoxify environmental toxins may contribute to some extent to a predisposition for PD.

MtDNA mutations in PD

MtDNA mutations have also been linked to PD in three families. One maternal pedigree harboring the MTND4*LHON11778A mutation encompassed four individuals with the akinesis and rigidity typical of parkinsonism. At least one of the affected individuals responded to levodopa. Ophthalmoplegia and ptosis were seen in one family member, though none of the maternal relatives presented with the optic atrophy. Sequencing the entire mtDNA revealed only the 11778 mutation. In addition, the α-synuclein codon 209 mutation, parkin mutations, and SCA3 (Machado-Joseph) repeat expansion were all ruled out. Hence, it would appear that the MTND4*LHON11778A mutation is the primary cause of parkinsonism in this family (Simon et al., 1999).

A second large maternal pedigree exhibited tremor, rigidity, PD and sensory neural deafness with or without aminoglycoside induction. Sequencing the entire mtDNA of this pedigree revealed the deafness mutation MTRNR1*DEAF1555G (Shoffner et al., 1994). Additional biochemical studies have suggested that a partial nDNA complex I defect may also be segregating in this family (unpublished data). Hence, the 1555 mutation may be only one component of the etiology of PD in this family. A third patient presented with pediatric onset parkinsonism and encephalomyopathy. This individual had a 5 bp deletion in her mtDNA COI gene (Comi et al., 1998).

To identify other mtDNA mutations that might be associated with PD, the mtDNAs of three PD patients have been sequenced. This revealed multiple sequence variants, one of which was a missense mutation at np 7237 (A to T) in the *MTCO1* gene which altered a conserved amino acid. However, none of the variants was found to be a consistent feature among all of the patients (Ozawa et al., 1991a), and a survey of 19 Lewy-body positive PD patients failed to reveal the COI np 7237 mutation (Lucking et al., 1995). The complete sequence of a third PD patient mtDNA revealed two novel mutations: a G to A transition at np 1709 in the *MTRNR2* gene and an A to G missense mutation at np 15851 in the *MTCYB* gene which changed a weakly conserved isoleucine to a valine. Neither of these mutations were found in numerous controls (Brown et al., 1996), and the np 15851 variant had previously been found in a hypertrophic cardiomyopathy patient (Obayashi et al., 1992). These and other PD mtDNA sequencing projects have revealed a variety of novel mtDNA variants, but each patient harbors a different array of variants (Mizuno, 1995) (#1218) (Johns, 1991) (#1277). Hence, either mtDNA mutations are not an important component of the etiology of PD or any one of a variety of mtDNA mutations might contribute to PD through interaction with other genetic and environmental factors.

Mitochondrial defects in PD

Substantial biochemical evidence has implicated mitochondrial defects in PD. PD can be induced in both humans and animals by a contaminant of illicitly synthesized meperidine, 1-methyl-4-phenyl-1, 2, 3, 6-tetrahydropyridine (MPTP) (Langston et al., 1983). MPTP is oxidized by monoamine oxidase (MAO) B to its active form 1-methyl-4-phenylpyridiniumoin (MPP$^+$). MPP$^+$ is actively taken up the dopaminergic neurons of the substantia nigra through the dopamine transporter and electrostatically attracted to the mitochondria like other lipophilic cationic compounds (Singer et al., 1987; Schapira, 1994b; Mizuno et al., 1995). The selective concentration of MPP$^+$ within dopaminergic neurons and their mitochondria raises the intra-mitochondrial concentration of MPP$^+$ several hundred-fold into the mM range. At these concentrations MPP$^+$ reversibly inhibits mitochondrial complex I and respiration by NADH-linked substrates. The inhibition of complex I occurs at a site between the highest-potential Fe-S cluster and CoQ, the same site which binds barbiturates, rotenone, and piericidin A (Singer et al., 1987; Schapira, 1994b; Mizuno et al, 1995). While incubation of complex I with 10 mM MPP$^+$ for 15 minutes can reversibly inhibit 40% of complex I, prolonged incubation can irreversibly inhibit the enzyme up to 78% and this effect can be inhibited by oxygen radical scavengers. This suggests that part of the MPP$^+$ effect is the induction of oxygen radical damage through inhibition of complex I (Cleeter et al., 1992; Schapira, 1994b). The importance of ROSs in the toxicity of MPP$^+$ is supported by the increased sensitivity of MnSOD deficient mice to MPTP. Mice with mutations at the T-associated maternal effect (Tme) locus have a deletion in the mitochondrial MnSOD. Mice with 50% of the normal MnSOD, when exposed to MPTP, show massive basal ganglia toxicity relative to mice with elevated MnSOD levels (Cortopassi and Wang, 1995).

MPP$^+$ at 2 mM can also inhibited the NADH-linked α-ketoglutarate dehydrogenase by 55%. This effect interacts with the complex I inhibition to result in an overall inhibition of state III mitochondrial respiration of 88% (Mizuno et al., 1987; 1995).

Evidence that MPP$^+$ induces PD through inhibition of complex I led to the investigation of OXPHOS enzyme levels in PD patients. The first report that PD patients harbored complex I defects involved an analysis of substantia nigra homogenates from autopsy patients which revealed a 39% reduction in complex I + III activity and a 30% reduction in complex I activity (Schapira et al., 1989; 1990a). Two subsequent studies reported a 30–37% reduction in complex I activity (Mann et al., 1992a) and a 24–35% reduction in complex I + III activity (Janetzky et al., 1994). The cortex, cerebellum, tegmentum, caudate nucleus and globus pallidus were reported to not show a significant decrease in complex I (Schapira, 1992; 1994a). Isolated mitochondria from PD brains showed a significant reduction in complex III activity in the striatum (33%), but not in complex I (Mizuno et al., 1990), but striatal complex I activity was found to be reduced 25% in a second study (Mizuno et al., 1989).

Immunohistochemical staining in the medial, central, and lateral parts of the substantia nigra revealed 40%, 32%, and 37% reductions, respectively, in the melanin-containing neurons, with a significant proportion of neurons weakly or barely staining with complex I antibodies. Complex III and IV staining was not reduced in PD patients, though several of the patients had reduced complex II staining (Hattori et al., 1991). Western blot analysis of complex I polypeptides in PD brains revealed a preferential loss of 30, 25 and 24 kDa proteins (Mizuno et al., 1989), though this was not confirmed in a similar study (Schapira et al., 1990a). While inconsistencies remain, the collective data suggest that PD appear to have a partial complex I defect in their substantia nigra neurons.

To determine if this substantia nigra defect was systemic, OXPHOS enzymes have been analyzed in platelets and skeletal muscle. Platelets have some of the same biochemical features as the dopaminergic neurons of the substantia nigra. They express MAO-B and have specific amine-uptake mechanisms which could concentrate cytotoxic compounds such as MPP$^+$ (Schapira, 1994b). In the first platelet study, mitochondria were prepared by Percoll gradients and complex I was found to be reduced an average 54% (Parker et al., 1989a). In subsequent studies of platelet mitochondria, complex I was reported to be reduced 14–16% (Krige et al., 1992), complex I about 50% and complex IV about 30%, with the decline of the two complexes being coordinated and declining with age (Benecke et al., 1993). However, respiration rates and complex I + III activities were not significantly reduced in another study, though the complex I + III activity was reduced 33% (Bravi et al., 1992). In studies of total platelet homogenates, complex I activity was found to be reduced 25% in one study (Yoshino et al., 1992), but not reduced in another study (Mann et al., 1992a). Hence, the collective platelet data support the possibility of a systemic defect in a portion of PD patients.

Studies of PD patient skeletal muscle OXPHOS enzymes have also suggested a systemic complex I defect. The first report on OXPHOS activities on isolated skeletal muscle mitochondria from PD patients reported a 40% reduction in complex I, a 49% reduction in complex II, and a 40% reduction in complex IV. These reductions were supported by reduced concentrations of cytochromes $a+a_3$, b and c (Bindoff et al., 1989). In a subsequent study of six PD patients, three had complex I reductions of between 86 and

92% with an overall mean reduction of 65%, one also had a complex IV defect, and four had increased mitochondrial fragility (Shoffner et al., 1991b; Wallace et al., 1992b). Muscle mitochondria isolated from PD autopsy tissue showed a 49% reduction in complex I + III activity (Nakagawa-Hattori et al., 1992), and a study of a mitochondria fraction isolated from frozen muscle showed a 70% reduction in complex I activities, with treated PD patients reduced 71%, untreated PD patients reduced 68%, and multisystem atrophy patients reduced 75% (Blin et al., 1994). However, these complex I values may be aberrantly low because of the lability of complex I activity in mitochondria isolated from frozen tissue (Zheng et al., 1990). On the other hand, two other studies have failed to find OXPHOS enzyme defects in PD skeletal muscle: one using mitochondria isolated from fresh biopsies (Mann et al., 1992a) and the other using homogenates of needle biopsies or mitochondria isolated from fresh biopsies (DiDonato et al., 1993). Thus, the association between complex I defects in skeletal muscle mitochondria and PD remains ambiguous.

That mitochondrially generated ROS are involved in PD pathology is suggested by a 33% induction of MnSOD activity in the substantia nigra of PD patients, with no induction of Cu/ZnSOD. Malondialdehyde, an indicator of chronic lipid peroxidation, was significantly increased in the substantia nigra of PD patients and acutely generated hydroperoxides were increased tenfold in PD patients. Reduced glutathione was decreased 40% in the substantia nigra of PD patients and also in subjects with presymptomatic Lewy body disease (Jenner et al., 1992). Hence, these data support a role for mitochondrially generated oxidative damage in PD.

The increased mitochondrial ROS production seen in PD might be expected to damage mitochondrial proteins, lipids and mtDNA. Consequently, we might expect to see an increase in mtDNA rearrangement mutations in PD patient tissue. This prediction has been examined in several instances (Ikebe et al., 1990; Ozawa et al., 1990, Schapira et al., 1990b, Mann et al., 1992b, DiDonato et al., 1993, Sandy et al., 1993, Shan et al., 1995). This data will be discussed under Section III. Somatic mtDNA Mutations in Degenerative Disease, Cancer and Aging.

Mitochondrial defects in Huntington disease

Huntington disease (HD), like PD, is a pathology of the basal ganglia associated with movement disorders as well as cognitive loss and psychiatric manifestations. The disease has an autosomal dominant mode of inheritance and is caused by a CAG repeat expansion in the huntingtin gene located on chromosomal 4p16.3. This repeat expansion causes the expansion of a poly-glutamine stretch within the huntingtin protein (The Huntington's Disease Collaborative Research Group, 1993). HD is one of five neurodegenerative diseases which are caused by a pathologic intra-protein poly-glutamine expansion, including Kennedy spinal bulbar muscular atrophy (SBMA), spinocerebellar ataxia type 1 (SCAI), dentatorubral-pallidoluysian atrophy (DRPLA), and Machado-Joseph disease (MJD) (Barinaga 1996).

A number of physiological studies have implicated defects in energy metabolism in the pathophysiology of HD. Position emission tomography (PET) studies of striatal glucose consumption in 20 symptomatic HD patients, 20 controls, and 27 chorea-free patients revealed a marked reduction in all patients (Kuwert et al., 1993). Cortical glucose metabolism of HD patients is also reduced. Patients with symptoms for less than five years had a 15% decrease in frontal and partial cortex metabolism, while 16 patients with symptoms for longer than five years had a 25% to 30% decrease in metabolic rate for all cortical regions except the temporal lobe (Martin et al., 1992). HD patients also had a significant increase in lactate levels of the occipital cortex relative to controls. Lactate to N-acetylaspartate (NAA) ratios of the occipital cortex of HD patients was 12.5 ($\pm$4.8) versus 3.9 ($\pm$1.5) for controls, and in the basal ganglia it was 15.9 ($\pm$12.9) in HD patients versus 4.3 ($\pm$1). Two asymptomatic individuals with a 96% chance of carrying the HD gene had normal lactate/NAA ratios (Jenkins et al., 1993). These results are consistent with a generalized energy deficit in the brains of HD patients which becomes apparent when symptoms appear and gets progressively worse as the symptoms become more severe.

Biochemical analysis of mitochondria isolated from frozen HD brain revealed a significant reduction in oxygen utilization using succinate as a substrate in the presence of rotenone. Moreover, the COX-specific activity in the caudate but not the cortex was reduced in HD patients, and the cytochrome $a + a_3$ content was also reduced (Brennan et al., 1985). Tissue homogenates from the caudate nucleus of HD patients revealed a 53–56% decrease in complex II, a 55–59% reduction in complex III, and a 32–38% reduction in complex IV, but the complex I activity was normal (Gu et al., 1996). Interestingly, treatment of rodents or primates with the complex II inhibitor, 3-nitropropionic acid (3NP), creates a HD like phenotype (Beal, 1994).

Analysis of platelet mitochondria from HD patients revealed a reduction in complex I of 72% (Parker et al., 1990a). However, an independent study of platelet homogenates did not reveal a significant defect in any of the respiratory complexes (Gu et al., 1996). The platelet complex I defect did not transfer with the mtDNA in cybrid experiments, consistent with the known nuclear location of the HD mutation (Swerdlow et al., 1999). Hence, current biochemical data support a generalized brain metabolic defect which progresses with the disease, but the systemic nature of the defect remains to be proven.

Recently, it has been discovered that the mutant Huntingtin protein with the polyglutamine expansion binds other proteins. The first target protein to be identified and characterized is the Huntingtin-associated protein I (HAP1) of unknown function (Li et al., 1995a). The distribution and subcellular localization of HAP1 correlates well with nuclear nitric oxide synthase (nNOS), which has been associated with excitotoxic neuronal damage by glutamate involving N-methyl-D-aspartate (NMDA) receptors (Li et al., 1996). Moreover, impairment of OXPHOS reduces the threshold for NMDA induced neuronal death (Beal, 1994).

The poly-glutamine expansion of huntingtin can also bind to glyceraldehyde-3-phosphate dehydrogenase (GAPDH), a key enzyme in glycolysis (Burke et al., 1996) inhibiting enzyme activity (Roses; 1996). GAPDH has also been shown to interact with the SCA1 product (Barinaga, 1996; Roses, 1996). Since the brain relies primarily on glycolysis to generate pyruvate for mitochondrial oxidation, inhibition of GAPDH would strongly inhibit mitochondrial energy metabolism.

The apparent mitochondrial defect in HD brains raises the possibility of increased mitochondrial ROS production and mtDNA damage. Consistent with this hypothesis, the common 5 kb deletion was found to be elevated nine-fold in the cortex of HD patients, relative to age-matched controls (Horton et al., 1995). Increased mitochondrial ROS production would also be expected to sensitize the mtPTP. This was also confirmed through study of the mtPTP of HD patient lymphoblasts. HD lymphoblast mitochondria were much more sensitive to cyanide-induced mitochondrial membrane depolarization. The cyanide-induced depolarization was inhibited by cyclosporin A and the sensitivity of the HD mitochondrial was directly proportion to the number huntingtin CAG repeats, above 60. The HD cells were also more sensitive to induction of apoptosis by staurosporin. Staurosporin-induced cells showed increased DNA degradation, nuclear fragmentation, and activation of caspase-3 and 9, but not 8 (Sawa et al., 1999). Thus, there is increasing evidence that the pathophysiology of HD might also include defects in mitochondria energy production and/or ROS production, thus predisposing neurons to premature apoptosis.

RETINITIS PIGMENTOSA (RP) AND LEIGH'S SYNDROME

Pigmentary retinopathy, neurodegeneration, and Leigh's syndrome have been associated with mutations in the mtDNA MTATP6 gene, as well as with mutations in several nDNA genes involved in the assembly of the respiratory complexes.

Leigh's syndrome (subacute necrotizing encephalomyopathy) has an average age of onset of about one and a half years with a mean duration of illness until death of about five years. Clinical manifestations include ataxia, hypotonia, spasticity, developmental delay and regression, optic atrophy, nystagmus, respiratory abnormalities and ophthalmoplegia. The myopathy is generally non-specific and includes fat accumulations. Occasional patients can show liver involvement, cardiomyopathy and mitochondrial myopathy including ragged-red muscle fibers (RRFs) and mitochondria with paracrystalline inclusions, although most patients have normal muscle fiber and mitochondria morphology. A common observation is the abrupt worsening of the patient's clinical and metabolic status with infections or fibril episodes. A common neuroradiological finding of end stage patients is the bilateral degeneration of the basal ganglion, readily observed by CT and MRI analysis. Brain pathology classically reveals basal ganglia necrosis associated with marked vascular proliferation in the brain stem (Shoffner and Wallace, 1995).

Current estimates of the proportion of cases resulting from the known biochemical and molecular defects (Dahl 1998) include: (1) about 18% mtDNA mutations: (2) about 10% pyruvate dehydrogenase defects (Kretzchmar et al., 1987; Robinson et al., 1987; Matthews et al., 1993); (3) about 19% complex I defects (Robinson et al., 1987; Loeffen et al., 1998); (4) about 18% complex IV defects including SURF-1 mutations (DiMauro et al., 1987; Miranda et al., 1989; Tiranti et al., 1998b; Zhu et al., 1998); and (5) about 35% other causes, including complex II (Bourgeron et al., 1995) and pyruvate carboxylase defects (Hommes et al., 1968). The fact that so many different mitochondrial bioenergetic defects can cause the same lethal phenotype, Leigh's syndrome, indicates that the clinical manifestations of Leigh's syndrome represent the common clinical end point for the most severe mitochondrial OXPHOS defects.

While the clinical presentation for Leigh's syndrome is relatively constant, regardless of the molecular defect, the clinical manifestations of other family members can vary greatly depending on the nature of the genetic defect. Generally, in families resulting from a nuclear gene mutation, the clinical presentation of affected family members is similar to that of the proband. Thus for X-linked Leigh's due to PDH E1α mutations, males are primary affected and should have a similarly severe phenotype. Likewise, Leigh's patients resulting from recessive mutations in nuclear genes will have similar phenotypes in affected family members, with consanguineous marriages being more common. By contrast, Leigh's syndrome resulting from heteroplasmic mtDNA mutations will be associated with highly variable clinical presentations among maternal relatives, depending on the percentage of mutant mtDNAs inherited by each family member.

mtDNA mutations in RP and Leigh's syndrome

The three main mtDNA mutations associated with retinitis pigmentosa and Leigh's syndrome are MTATP6*NARP8993G (Holt et al., 1990; Ortiz et al., 1993; Santorelli et al., 1993; Shoffner et al., 1992; Tatuch et al., 1992), MTATP6*NARP8993C (De Vries et al., 1993; Santorelli et al., 1994), and MTATP6*FBSN9176C (Thyagarajan et al., 1995). Leigh's syndrome has also been observed in individuals harboring the protein synthesis mutations MTTK*MERRF8344G (Berkovic et al., 1989, 1991) and MTTL1*MELAS3243G (Shoffner and Wallace, 1995) (Table 11.1).

The first description of maternally inherited retinitis pigmentosa came with the report of the MTATP6*NARP8993G mutation. MTATP6*NARP8993G pedigrees are invariably maternally inherited and heteroplasmic (Holt et al., 1990). The initial three generation pedigree included individuals who presented with neurogenic muscle weakness, ataxia, and retinitis pigmentosa, hence the acronym "NARP". The severity of the symptoms varied markedly between individuals and generally correlated with the percentage of mutant mtDNAs harbored by the individual. Neurodegenerative symptoms included generalized seizures, axonal sensory neuropathy, dementia, corticospinal tract degeneration, and cerebellar and brainstem atrophy (Holt et al., 1990). This later clinical feature can manifest as olivopontocerebellar atrophy on MRI. One individual presented with mental retardation, macular degeneration, and spicular retinitis pigmentosa (Ortiz et al., 1993). Subsequently, families harboring the MTATP6*NARP8993G mutation were also found to encompass individuals presenting with Leigh's syndrome (Houstek et al., 1995; Makela-Bengs et al., 1995; Shoffner et al, 1992; Tatuch et al., 1992; Tulinius et al., 1995).

The variability in clinical presentation of the MTATP6*NARP8993G and C mutations is primarily due to the replicative segregation of the heteroplasmic mtDNA mutation. In a typical MTATP6*NARP8993G pedigree symptoms can ranged from mild salt and pepper retinitis pigmentosa; through olivopontocerebellar atrophy; to a pediatric cerebellar ataxia, and lethal Leigh's syndrome. Generally, adults with retinitis pigmentosa harbor about 75% mutant mtDNAs, while children with lethal Leigh's syndrome have in excess of 90% mutant (Ortiz et al., 1993).

The pathophysiology of the MTATP6*NARP8993G and C mutations has been elucidated through the biochemical analysis of patient mitochondria isolated from cultured cells, and through studies of the mechanism of ATP synthesis by the ATP synthase. The MTTP6*NARP8993G and C mutations change the highly conserved leucine 156 in the ATP6 polypeptide to an arginine or proline, respectively. Biochemical analysis of the MTATP6*NARP8993G mutation in patient lymphoblasts or fibroblasts has revealed a 30–50% reduction in the rate of ATP synthesis (Houstek et al., 1995; Makela-Bengs et al., 1995; Tatuch and Robinson, 1993). Moreover, in patient lymphoblasts and in their *trans*-mitochondrial cybrids, there was a 30–40% reduction in the rate of maximal (state III) respiration and a comparable reduction in ADP/O ratios (Trounce et al., 1994). Thus, the MTATP6*NARP8993G mutation results in a significant defect in ATP synthesis.

Correlating the position and nature of the amino acid changes caused by the MTATP6*NARP8993G and C mutations with recent data on the rotor-stator mechanism of the ATP synthase indicates that the MTATP6*NARP8993 G and C mutations must compromise the ATP synthase proton channel. The highly conserved leucine at ATP6 amino acid 156 is analogous to the *Escherichia coli* amino acid 207. This forms the base of α-helix 4 in the bacterial protein "a", the homologue of ATP6. Leucine 156 (bacterial 207) is on the same face of the helix as arginine 159 (bacterial 210). Arginine 159 (bacterial 210) is thought to provide the positive charge which pulls the negatively charged, deprotonated glutamate 58 (bacterial aspartate 61) from the matrix-space half proton channel around to the intermembrane-space half proton channel. Arginine 159 (bacterial 210) is displaced from the glutamate 58 (aspartate 61) so as to provide attraction, without forming a salt bridge and blocking rotation of the ATP9 (subunit c) protein wheel. However, conversion of leucine 156 to an arginine residue adds a second positive charge on the ATP6 ("a")/ATP9 ("c") interface, and conversion of leucine 156 to a proline residuce disrupts the α-helix and presumably the interface between ATP6 ("a") and ATP9 ("c"). Hence, both mutations would stall the rotor, block the proton channel, and inhibit ATP synthesis.

Two other pathogenic missense mutations have also been localized in the MTATP6 gene. These are MTATP6*FBSN9176C and MTATP6*LHON9101C

(Table 11.1) mutations. The MTATP6*FBSN9176C variant changes the highly conserved leucine residue at codon 217 to a proline residue, while the MTATP6*LHON9101C changes the weakly conserved leucine residue at amino acid 192 to a threonine residue. These mutations are 61 and 36 codons away from the MTATP6*NARP8993G and C mutations respectively. In *E. coli*, mutations in the "c" subunit (ATP9) which change aspartate 61 to aglycine residue can be suppressed by mutations in the "a" subunit (ATP6) at Ala217, IIe221 and Leu224. Moreover, mutations at Gly218 and His214 of protein "a" (ATP6) result in uncoupling proton translocation from ATP synthesis, while the double mutant Gly218 to Lys plus His245 to Gly restores activity (Hartzog and Cain, 1994). This implies that the region of human ATP6 around amino acid 197 (bacteria 245) may also be important in coupling the proton gradient to ATP synthesis. Thus, the MTATP6*LHON9101C mutation affecting ATP6 amino acid 192 (approximately bacterial 240) and the MTATP6*FBSN9176C mutation affecting ATP6 amino acid 217 (bacterial 256) flank the bacterial His 245 and hence might also alter the integrity of the ATP synthase proton channel. Hence, all of the pathogenic ATP6 missense mutation appear to affect the ATP synthase proton channel and thus inhibit the coupling of the proton gradient to the synthesis of ATP.

The observation that the MTATP6*LHON9101C mutation causes LHON and not retinitis pigmentosa and Leigh's syndrome, like the other ATP6 mutations, may provide further insight into the pathophysiology of LHON. Mice in which the heart-muscle isoform of ANT (ANT1) has been genetically inactivated can not import adequate ADP into the heart and skeletal muscle mitochondria to provide substrate for the ATP synthase. This inhibits the use of the ATP synthase proton channel which blocks the depolarization $\Delta\Psi$. Hyperpolarization of $\Delta\Psi$ then inhibits the electron transport chain and diverts the excess electrons into ROS production (Esposito et al., 1999; Graham et al., 1997). Assuming that the ATP6 mutations also block the ATP synthase proton channel, then the MTATP6*LHON9101C mutation might also increase ROS production and oxidative stress. This would support the hypothesis that LHON is the product of chronic oxidative stress acting on the retinal ganglia cells or the vascular endothelial cell-generated NO.

nDNA mutations in RP and Leigh's syndrome

Mutations in a number of nuclear genes can also cause Leigh's syndrome in association with retinitis pigmentosa (Table 11.2). These include mutations in the X-linked Elα subunit of pyruvate dehydrogenase (Matthews et al., 1993),

in the autosomal NDUFS8 N-2 iron-sulfur center protein and the DNUFS7 protein of complex I (Loeffen et al., 1998; Smeitink and van den Heuvel, 1999), in the autosomal flavoprotein subunit of complex II (Bourgeron et al., 1995), and in the autosomal SURF-1 gene associated with complex IV defects (Tiranti et al., 1998b; Zhu et al., 1998).

The best-described Leigh's patient with a complex I gene mutation was the product of a compound heterozygote for mutations in the complex I subunit NDUFS8 (TYKY). NDUFS8 (TYKY) contains two 4Fe-4S ferrodoxin consensus motifs, potentially forming the binding site for the N-2 iron sulfur cluster. The missense mutations in the two alleles were Pro79Leu and Arg102His (Loeffen et al., 1998). The other two Leigh's syndrome complex I cases had the same genotype. This was a homozygous missense mutation in the NDUFS7 gene causing a Val122Met substitution (Smeitink and van den Heuvel, 1999) (Table 11.3).

The Leigh's syndrome complex II mutation altered the flavoprotein gene on chromosome 5p15 and was observed in two siblings. The proband had isolated complex II deficiency in skeletal muscle, cultured skin fibroblasts and circulating lymphocytes, with the enzyme showing a heightened sensitivity to oxaloacetate, the physiological inhibitor. The causal mutation was a C to T transition at nucleotide 1684 in the cDNA resulting in an Arg544Trp substitution in a highly conserved domain of the protein. Both siblings were homozygous mutant, while the two parents were heterozygotes (Bourgeron et al., 1995) (Table 11.3).

Multiple Leigh's syndrome families with complex IV deficiency have been found to harbor mutations in the *SURF-1* gene on chromosome 9q34. The SURF-1 protein appears to be involved in the assembly or maintenance of an active complex IV. The reported *SURF-1* mutations have included nonsense mutations, missense mutations, and frame-shift mutations resulting from small insertions and deletions (Tiranti et al., 1998b; Zhu et al., 1998).

Four additional pathogenic mutations have been reported in nDNA complex I subunits in children with progressive degenerative disease. These children had a variety of symptoms, many reminiscent of Leigh's syndrome, including hypotonia, feeding problems, vomiting, strabismus, myoclonic epilepsy, and MRI findings including basal ganglia abnormalities and atrophy. The complex I genes affected are for the NDUFS4–18 kDa protein (5 bp duplication) (van den Heuvel et al., 1998); the NDUFV1 protein (two compound heterozygotes for Arg59Stop + Thr423Met), and the NDUFV1 protein (Ala341 Val) (Smeitink and van den Heuvel, 1999).

The most detailed report of a nDNA complex I mutation patient involved the 18 kDa NDUFS4 mutation resulting from 5 bp duplication. This child presented with hypotonia, mental retardation, convulsions, and brain and basal ganglia degeneration. The patient was found to be homozygous for a 5 bp duplication which resulted in a frameshift at codon Lys158, causing a change in the amino acid sequence of the protein from amino acid 178 to the end. This frameshift destroyed a consensus phosphorylation site and extended the protein 14 amino acid residues. The 18 kDa complex I gene was mapped to chromosome 5 (van den Heuvel et al., 1998) (Table 11.3).

MITOCHONDRIAL MYOPATHY AND THE ENCEPHALOMYOPATHIES

A wide spectrum of mitochondrial base substitution mutations have been identified which cause mitochondrial myopathy and encephalomyopathy. Mitochondrial myopathy involves progressive muscle weakness in association with a distinctive muscle pathology detected by Gomori modified trichrome staining. Trichrome staining reveals turquoire-muscle fibers that tear on sectioning and have aggregates of red staining material, generally in the subsarcolemmal regions. This red material is aggregates of highly abnormal mitochondria, often containing precipitates, membrane whorls, or paracrystalline arrays (Figure 11.9). The paracrystalline structures contain mitochondrial creatine phosphokinase (mtCPK) (Wallace, 1992a; Stadhouders et al., 1994). Such muscle fibers are called ragged red muscle fibers (RRFs). The best characterized mitochondrial encephalomyopathies are the myoclonic epilepsies and ragged red fiber disease (MERRF) and mitochondrial encephalomyopathy, lacticacidosis and stroke-like episodes (MELAS) (DiMauro and Bonilla, 1997).

Progressive muscle weakness and associated with mtDNA cytochrome b mutations

Progressive muscle weakness with or without the RRF of mitochondrial myopathy has been repeatedly observed in patients with complex III defects and mtDNA cytb mutations (Table 11.1). Two patients have been reported with missense mutations. The first was a 29 year old male with progressive muscle weakness and exercise intolerance associated with complex III deficiency. This individual had a T14766C mutation which changed the highly conserved glycine 290 to an aspartate residue (G290D). The proband had 90% mutant mtDNAs in his muscle, but no mutant in blood. The blood of his mother or sister also lacked mutant (Dumoulin et al., 1996).

The second missense mutation involved a 38 year old female with progressive muscle weakness, exercise intoler-

ance and lactic acidosis. Using ^{32}P-NMR she was also found to have a marked inhibition of recovery in her muscle PCr/Pi ratio following exercise. Her cytochrome b gene harbored a cytb G15762A mutation which changed the highly conserved glycine 339 to a glutamate residue (G339E). The patient's muscle contained 85% mutant mtDNAs, but the mutation could not be detected in her blood or that of her maternal relatives.

Two patients were found to have cytochrome b nonsense mutations. The first of these as a young woman with marked exercise intolerance and mitochondrial myopathy associated with complex III deficiency. She had a heteroplasmic nonsense mutation the cytochrome b gene (Kennaway et al., 1998). In an effort to circumvent the block in her ETC transport chain, this patient was treated with ascorbate and menadione. This metabolic therapy substantially improved the patient's capacity for PCr/Pi recovery following exercise (Eleff et al., 1984).

The second case was a 27-year-old male with progressive muscle weakness, exercise intolerance, and episodic myoglobinuria. He had a marked decrease in complex III and RRFs, as detected by SDH staining, which were COX positive. Molecular analysis of his cytochrome b gene revealed a G15059A mutation which converted glycine 190 to a stop codon, truncating the terminal 244 amino acid residues of the protein. The patient was heteroplasmic, with 63% mutant in muscle, but no mutant in blood. Furthermore, his RRFs were about 81% mutant while his non-RRFs were about 35% mutant. This mutation could not be detected in his mother or sister (Andreu et al., 1999).

While progressive muscle weakness was the primary symptom of patients with cytochrome b missense and nonsense mutations, it was a secondary manifestation of a patient harboring a 4 bp mtDNA deletion in cytochrome b. This boy first manifested fine motor coordination problems at six and showed fatigue and regressive behavior by 14, along with tremor, stimulus-responsive myoclonus, lactic acidosis, cardiac conduction defects, and diffuse cerebral and cerebellar atrophy. At 20 he was experiencing short episodes of disturbed consciousness, episodes of status epilepticus, tonic-clonic seizures, a stroke-like episode associated with cortical blindness and parieto-occipital cerebral infarcts. Muscle biopsy revealed a complex III defect associated with a single RRF and aggregates of subsarcolemmal mitochondria. Analysis of his mtDNA cytochrome b gene revealed a 14787del4 mutation resulting in a frame shift from codon 13, which terminated the protein at codon 50. In muscle, approximately 95% of the mtDNAs were mutant, while blood, hair follicles, oral mucosa and fibroblasts were about 60% of the mtDNAs were mutant (de

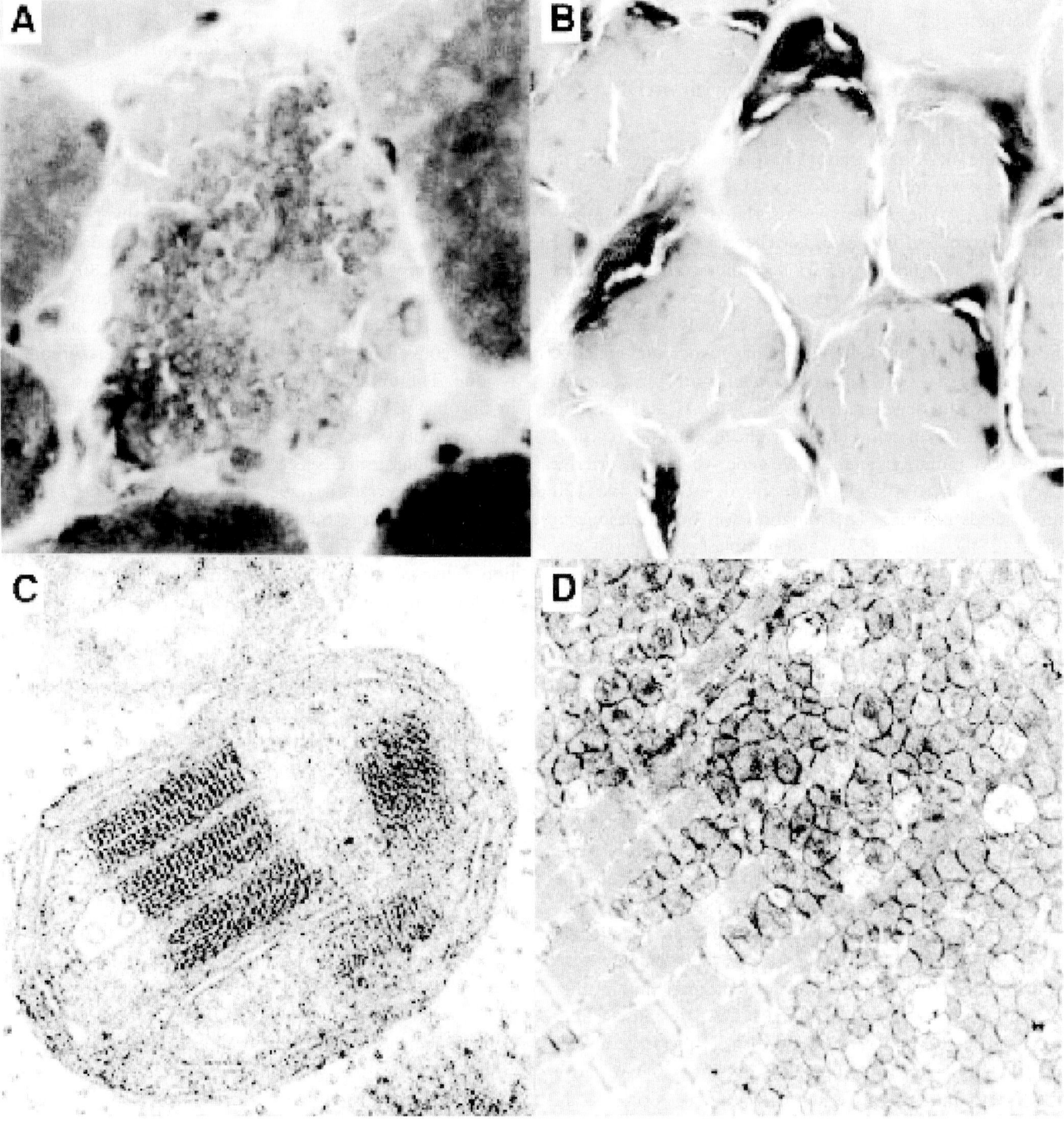

Fig. 11.9. Mitochondrial myopathy in man and mouse. (a) and (c) Skeletal muscle samples from a patient with myoclonic epilepsy and ragged-red-fiber disease (MERRF), which is caused by a mutation in the mitochondrially encoded tRNA^{Lys} gene (Shoffner et al., 1990; Wallace et al., 1998b) (b) and (d) Skeletal muscle samples from a mouse with mitochondrial myopathy and hypertrophic cardiomyopathy resulting from the targeted inactivation of the gene encoding the heart-muscle isoform of the adenine nucleotide translocator (ANT1) (Graham et al., 1997). Frozen sections showing a (a) single fiber or (b) several fibers were stained with Gomori modified trichrome to show the ragged-red muscle fibers (RRFs). Electron micrographs show (c) an abnormal mitochondrion with paracrystalline arrays in a human RRF, and (d) the abnormal proliferation of mitochondria and degeneration of the contractile elements in a mouse RRF. From Wallace (1999) Mitochondrial diseases in man and mouse. Science 283: 1482–1488. © 1999 American Association for the Advancement of Science.

Coo et al., 1999). Hence, this patient had a more general-ized distribution of the mutant mtDNAs and a more severe phenotype.

Encephalomyopathies associated with mtDNA *COX* gene mutations

Pathogenic mtDNA mutations have also been identified in all three of the mtDNA subunits, COI, COII, and COIII (Table 11.1). The phenotypes associated with these muta-tions are complex. Two cases have been reported with COI mutations. The first was a 21 year old woman who had developed bilateral cataracts at three years; sensorineural hearing loss at seven; and muscle weakness with 90% of muscle fibers being COX deficient, myoclonic epilepsy, cerebellar ataxia, optic atrophy, cerebellar atrophy, bilateral basal ganglion degeneration, lactic acidosis and elevated serum creatine kinase by age 21. Molecular analysis revealed a G6930A mutation in the *COI* gene which converted a glycine codon to a stop codon and deleted the last 170 amino acids residues. The mutation was heteroplasmic in blood (27%), muscle (75%) and myoblasts (33%), but was not detected in the blood of the mother or sister. Cybrids harboring the mutation had reduced growth rate on galac-tose and diminished COX activity (Bruno et al., 1999).

The second COI mutation patient had a very different phenotype. She exhibited upper motor neuron disease at one year which progressed to spastic paraparesis at 29 years. MRI revealed bilateral corticobulbar track lesions, muscle histochemistry revealed RRFs and mitochondrial COX-deficiency, and physiological studies mild lactic acidosis. Molecular analysis revealed the deletion of one of two adja-cent 5 bp repeats encompassing np 6015 to 6024. This generated a stop codon, six codons downstream from the deletion, resulting in a 42 amino acid residue instead of the 513 amino acid residue product. The patients' muscle was heteroplasmic for the mutation, 47% and 69% on successive muscle biopsies, while the muscle of the patients' mother and three sisters lacked the mutation. Single muscle fiber mutation analysis revealed that normal fibers were 29% mutant, COX-deficient fibers 38% mutant, COX-negative fibers 69% mutant, and RRFs 91% mutant (Comi et al., 1998).

Two patients have been reported with mutations in *COII*. The first case was a 14-year-old boy with a history of muscle weakness and fatigue. He was thin and had elevated serum lactate. Histochemical analysis revealed severe COX deficiency in 97% of fibers, though no RRFs on trichrome stain. Other clinical and physiological findings were normal. Polarographic analysis of muscle mitochondria revealed a

COX deficiency, and histochemical studies revealed a severe reduction in COIII. Molecular analysis revealed a T7671A mutation which change the highly conserved methionine residue at codon 30 to a lysine residue (M30K). The muta-tion was heteroplasmic in muscle, but was not detected in myoblasts. It was present at 4.5% to 6% in peripheral blood (Rahman et al., 1999).

The second patient developed progressive ataxia at five years of age, and was wheel chair bound with mild distal wasting, cognitively impairment optic atrophy, pigmentary retinopathy, and decreased color vision by age 25 years. A muscle biopsy revealed he had 15% RRF and 80% COX-negative fibers. Molecular analysis revealed a heteroplasmic T7587C mutation in the second base of the initiation codon converting it from a methionine to a threonine residue. The mutation was present in 91% of muscle, 89% in fibroblasts, and 36% in blood. In single fiber analysis, COX activity was severely reduced in fibers with over 55–65% mutant mtDNAs (Clark et al., 1999).

Finally, two cases have been reported with *COIII* muta-tions, one a chain termination mutation and the other a 15 bp microdeletion. The patient with the stops codon muta-tion collapsed after vigorous exercise at 17 years of age, experiencing confusion and headache. She developed episodic myalgia by age 21, which progressed to increased fatigue and regular headaches, following three pregnancies. This progressed to periodic stuporous states with elevated lactate and creatine kinase and frequent migraine-type headaches. Muscle histology revealed COX-negative fibers but no RRFs, and muscle mitochondrial COX activity was 20% of control while cytochrome aa_2 content was 17%. Molecular analysis revealed a G9952A mutation in the *COIII* gene, which changed a tryptophane codon to a stop codon 13 amino acid residues form the C-terminal end. The mutation was heteroplasmia, being present in 57% of the mtDNAs in two independent tests. In COX-negative fibers the proportion of mutant was 56%, but in COX-positive fibers it was 10% (Hanna et al., 1998b).

The second patient with a COIII mutation was a 15-year-old female with periodic muscle cramps, elevated cre-atine kinase and myoglobinuria associated with decreased caloric intakes. Histochemical analysis revealed many RRFs with 64% COX-negative fibers. Muscle mitochondrial COX activity was reduced 86% and cytochromes a and a_2 were also reduced. Molecular analysis revealed a 15 bp deletion in *COIII* removing the intervening sequence between two direct repeats. This mutation was heteroplas-mic with the mutation being present at 92% in muscle, 1% in leukocytes and absent in fibroblasts. In muscle, COX-positive fibers had 25% mutant mtDNAs, COX-deficient fibers 97% and COX-deficient RRFs 99%. The mutant mtDNA was not detected in the mother's leukocytes (Kennaway et al., 1994; 1995). These observations demonstrate that heteroplasmic missense mutations can result in a wide spectrum of the symptoms associated with mitochondrial encephalomyopathes.

Mitochondrial myopathy associated with mtDNA tRNA mutations

MM can also be the primary clinical presentation in mtDNA tRNA mutations (Table 11.4). One tRNA$^{Leu\ (UUR)}$ mutation, MTTL1*MM3250C, converted a weakly conserved T to a C base. This mutation was associated with fatigability and RRFs, with one individual having respiratory muscle weakness, and elevated lactate with exercise. The mutation was heteroplasmic and varying percentages of mutant mtDNAs in skeletal muscle were associated with complex I and IV defects (Goto et al., 1992b).

A second tRNA$^{Leu\ (UUR)}$ mutation, MTTL1*MM3302G, was reported in two independent families. This heteroplasmic mutation changes the highly conserved penultimate 3′ A to a G base. The first individual exhibited a progressive muscle weakness as a young adult (Bindoff et al., 1993), while the second exhibited an early onset and rapidly progressive weakness and degeneration of the scapular flexor and extensor muscles resulting in a striking inability to hold the head erect against any lateral pressure (Shoffner et al., 1993b). Both mutations were heteroplasmic and associated with skeletal muscle RRFs and OXPHOS enzyme defects. However, analysis of mitochondrial protein synthesis in lymphoblast and fibroblast cell lines failed to reveal a mitochondrial protein synthesis defect. Analysis of tRNA$^{Leu(UUR)}$ processing by monitoring the RNA 19 (16 S rRNA + tRNA$^{Leu\ (UUR)}$ + ND1), 16 S rRNA, tRNA$^{Leu\ (UUR)}$ and ND1 transcripts led to the proposal that this mutation causes a defect in the processing of the tRNA$^{Leu(UUR)}$ in the skeletal muscle, but not in lymphocytes and fibroblasts, presumably due to tissue-specific tRNA processing enzyme (Bindoff et al., 1993). Additional studies are required to substantiate this hypothesis, but if true it provides a novel mechanism for tissue-specific defects in mutations changing highly conserved nucleotides.

A mutation in tRNA^{Pro}, MTTP*MM15990A, converts the proline anticodon UGG (codon CCA) to a serine anticodon UGA (codon UCA), rendering the mutant tRNA nonfunctional. This mutation caused classical MM without extraocular muscle involvement in a seven-year-old patient harboring 85% muscle mutant mtDNA in skeletal muscle. The mutation only affected mitochondrial protein synthesis

of cultured cells when present in greater than 90% of the mtDNAs (Moraes et al., 1993a; Ionasescu et al., 1994).

Hypertrophic cardiomyopathy and myopathy associated with mtDNA mutations

Hypertrophic cardiomyopathy with MM in children and adults has been associated with a number of tRNA mutations (Table 11.4). Hypertrophic cardiomyopathy an infant has been associated with a tRNA^{Ile} mutation, MTTI*FICP4317G (Tanaka et al., 1990). This infant died at one year old of severe hypertrophic cardiomyopathy together with a skeletal muscle necrosis and a complex I and IV deficiency in the heart (Tanaka et al., 1990). While the mutation was proposed to alter the TΨC loop by creating a new G-C base-pair, the mutation was not reported to be heteroplasmic and only 28 controls were screened. Hence, the etiology of this mutation requires confirmation.

A pedigree of infantile hypertrophic cardiomyopathy was associated with a tRNA$^{Leu\ (UUR)}$ mutation, MTTL1*MMC3303T. This mutation was found in two infants who died at 10 weeks and nine months of age, and was observed to be heteroplasmic (Silvestri et al., 1994).

A tRNA^{Ile} mutation, MTTI*FICP4269G, has been observed in an 18 year old who died with hypertrophic cardiomyopathy, mitochondrial myopathy, renal disease, hearing loss, generalized seizures and mental retardation. The mutation was heteroplasmic in the mother and proband, was associated with morphological changes of the mitochondria in cultured cells, and resulted in a protein synthesis defect in cybrids derived from patient fibroblasts (Taniike et al., 1992; Hayashi et al., 1994).

A heteroplasmic tRNA^{Ile} mutation has been associated with adult-onset hypertrophic cardiomyopathy with slow progression. This mutation, MTTI*MICM4300G, was found in a maternally inherited pedigree in which three maternal relatives were diagnosed with hypertrophic cardiomyopathy and several other maternal relatives exhibited mild clinical and electrocardiographic indications of hypertrophic cardiomyopathy (Casali et al., 1995). Although RRFs were found in the patient's skeletal muscle, no OXPHOS biochemical defects were detected in cardiac or skeletal muscle.

The tRNA$^{Leu\ (UUR)}$ mutation, MTTL1*MMC3260G, associated with hypertrophic cardiomyopathy, has been reported in two independent pedigrees, (Zeviani et al., 1991; Sweeney et al., 1993a). Individuals harboring the MTTL1*MMC3260G mutation manifest symptoms of congestive heart failure as young adults, ultimately leading to hypertrophy with disorganized cardiomyocytes, fibrosis,

Table 11.4 Reported mitochondrial DNA protein synthesis diseases

Locus	Disease	Allele	np	RNA	Ho	He	Status	References
MTTF	MELAS	583A	583	TRNA Phe	–	+	Prov	Hanna et al. (1998a)
MTTG	Myoglobinuria	606G	606	TRNA Phe	–	+	Prov	Chinnery et al. (1997b)
MTTF	MM	618C	618	tRNA Phe	–	+	Prov	Kleinle et al. (1998)
MTRNR1	DM	1310T	1310	12S	+	–	Prov	Tawata et al. (1998)
MTRNR1	DM	1438G	1438	12S	+	–	Prov	Tawata et al. (1998)
MTRNR1	DEAF	1555G	1555	rRNA 12S	+	–	Cfrm	Fischel-Ghodsian et al. (1993), Hutchin et al. (1993), Matthijs et al. (1994), Prezant et al. (1993), Shoffner et al. (1994), Tono et al. (1998), Tulinius et al. (1995), Usami et al. (1998)
MTTV	AMDF	1606A	1606	tRNA Val	–	+	Prov	Tiranti et al. (1998a)
MTTV	MELAS	1642A	1642	tRNA Val	–	+	Prov	de Coo et al. (1998)
MTRNR2	Rett Syndrome	2835T	2835	rRNA 16S	–	+	Prov	Cardaioli et al. (1999), Tang et al. (1997)
MTRNR2	ADPD	3196A	3196	rRNA 16S	+	+	Prov	Shoffner et al. (1993a), Wallace et al. (1992a)
MTTL1	MELAS	3243G	3243	tRNA Leu (UUR)	–	+	Cfrm	Ciafaloni et al. (1991), Enter et al. (1991), Goto et al. (1990), Hammans et al. (1991), Hess et al. (1991), Ino et al. (1990), Johns and Hurko (1991), Kobayashi et al. (1990), Kobayashi et al. (1991), Poulton et al. (1988)
MTTL1	DM/DMDF	3243G	3243	tRNA Leu (UUR)	–	+	Cfrm	Alcolado et al. (1994b), Alcolado and Thomas (1995), Campos et al. (1995), Gerbitz et al. (1995), Hammans et al. (1995), Kadowaki et al. (1995), Manouvrier et al. (1995), Massin et al. (1995), van den Ouweland et al. (1994), van den Ouweland et al. (1992b)
MTTL1	MM	3243T	3243	tRNA Leu(UUR)	–	+	Prov	Shaag et al. (1997)
MTTL1	CPEO	3243G	3243	TRNA Leu(UUR)	–	+	Cfrm	Jean-Francois et al. (1994), Moraes et al. (1993c)
MTTL1	MM	3250C	3250	tRNA Leu (UUR)	–	+	Prov	Goto et al. (1992b)
MTTL1	MM	3251G	3251	tRNA Leu (UUR)	–	+	Prov	Sweeney et al. (1993b)
MTTL1	MELAS	3252G	3252	tRNA Leu (UUR)	–	+	Prov	Goto (1995), Morten et al. (1993)
MTTL1	MM	3254G	3254	tRNA Leu (UUR)	–	+	Prov	Kawarai et al. (1997)
MTTL1	MELAS	3256T	3256	tRNA Leu (UUR)	–	+	Cfrm	Moraes et al. (1993b), Sato et al. (1994),

continued

Table 11.4 Reported mitochondrial DNA protein synthesis diseases (*continued*)

Locus	Disease	Allele	np	RNA	Ho	He	Status	References
MTTL1	MMC	3260G	3260	tRNA Leu (UUR)	–	+	Cfrm	Mariotti et al. (1994), Sweeney et al. (1993a), ZeviaNni et al. (1991)
MTTL1	DM	3264C	3264	tRNA Leu (UUR)	–	+	Prov	Suzuki et al. (1997)
MTTL1	MELAS	3271C	3271	tRNA Leu (UUR)	–	+	Conf	Goto (1995), Goto et al. (1991), Hayashi et al. (1993), Koga et al. (1995), Sakuta et al. (1993a), Takeda et al. (1998), Tokunaga et al. (1993)
MTTL1	PEM	3271delT	3271	tRNA Leu (UUR)	–	+	Prov	Shoffner et al. (1995a)
MTTL1	DM	3271C	3271	tRNA Leu (UUR)	–	+	Prov	Tsukuda et al. (1997)
MTTL1	Myopathy	3288G	3288	TRNA Leu(UUR)	–	+	Prov	Hadjigeorgiou et al. (1999)
MTTL1	MELAS	3291C	3291	tRNA Leu (UUR)	–	+	Prov	Goto (1995), Goto et al. (1994)
MTTL1	MM	3302G	3302	tRNA Leu (UUR)	–	+	Cfrm	Bindoff et al. (1993), Howell et al. (1995), Shoffner et al. (1993b)
MTTL1	MMC	3303T	3303	tRNA Leu (UUR)	+	+	Prov	Silvestri et al. (1994)
MTTI	FICP	4269G	4269	tRNA Ile	–	+	Prov	Hayashi et al. (1994), Taniike et al. (1992)
MTTI	CPEO	4274C	4274	tRNA Ile	–	+	Prov	Chinnery et al. (1997a)
MTTI	CPEO	4285C	4285	tRNA Ile	–	+	Prov	Silvestri et al. (1996)
MTTI	MHCM	4295G	4295	TRNA Ile	–	+	Prov	Merante et al. (1996)
MTTI	CPEO/MS	4298A	4298	tRNA Ile	–	+	Prov	Taylor et al. (1998)
MTTI	MICM	4300G	4300	tRNA Ile	–	+	Prov	Casali et al. (1995)
MTTI	CPEO	4309A	4309	tRNA Ile	–	+	Prov	Franceschina et al. (1998)
MTTI	FICP	4317G	4317	tRNA Ile	nd	nd	Prov	Ito et al. (1992), Tanaka et al. (1990)
MTTI	Mitochondrial Encephalocardio myopathy	4320T	4320	tRNA Ile	–	+	Prov	Santorelli et al. (1995)
MTTQ	ADPD	4336C	4336	tRNA Gln	+	–	Cfrm	Cortopassi and Hutchin (1994), Hutchin and Cortopassi (1995), Leroy and Norby (1994), Shoffner et al. (1993a), Wallace et al. (1992a)
MTTM	MM	4409C	4409	tRNA Met	–	+	Prov	Vissing et al. (1998)
MTTM	MM	4450A	4450	tRNA Met	–	+	Prov	Sternberg et al. (1998)
MTTW	MM	5521A	5521	tRNA Trp	–	+	Prov	Silvestri et al. (1998)
MTTW	MILS	5537insT	5537	tRNA Trp	–	+	Prov	Santorelli et al. (1997)
MTTW	DEMCHO	5549A	5549	tRNA Trp	–	+	Prov	Nelson et al. (1995)
MTTN	CPEO	5692G	5692	tRNA Asn	–	+	Prov	Munscher et al. (1993a), Seibel et al. (1994)
MTTN	CPEO, MM	5703G	5703	tRNA Asn	–	+	Prov	Hao and Moraes (1997), Moraes et al. (1993b)
MTTC	Mitochondrial Encephalopathy	5814C	5814	tRNA Cys	–	+	Prov	Manfredi et al. (1996), Stemberg et al. (1998)

continued

Table 11.4 Reported mitochondrial DNA protein synthesis diseases (*continued*)

Locus	Disease	Allele	np	RNA	Ho	He	Status	References
MTTSI	DEAF	7445G	7445	tRNA Ser (UCN)	+	+	Prov	Guan et al. (1998), Reid et al. (1994a,b), Vernham et al. (1994)
MTTS1	PEM/AMDF	7472insC	7472	tRNA Ser (UCN)	+	+	Cfrm	Jaksch et al. (1998a,b), Schuelke et al. (1998), Tiranti et al. (1995)
MTTSI	MM	7497A	7497	tRNA Ser (UCN)	+	+	Prov	Jaksch et al. (1998b)
MTTSI	SNHL	7511C	7511	tRNA Ser(UCN)	+	+	Prov	Sue et al. (1999)
MTTSI	PEM/ MERME	7512C	7512	tRNA Ser (UCN)	+	+	Prov	Jaksch et al. (1998a,b), Nakamura et al. (1995)
MTTD	MEPR	7543G	7543	tRNA Asp	–	+	Prov	Shtilbans et al. (1999)
MTTK	DMDF	8296G	8296	tRNA Lys	–	+	Prov	Kameoka et al. (1998a,b)
MTTK	MNGIE	8313A	8313	tRNA Lys	–	+	Prov	Verma et al. (1997)
MTTK	Mitochondrial Encephalopathy	8328A	8328	tRNA Lys	–	+	Prov	Houshmand et al. (1999)
MTTK	CPEO+Myoclonus	8328A	8328	tRNA Lys	–	+	Prov	Tiranti et al. (1999)
MTTK	MERRF	8344G	8344	tRNA Lys	–	+	Cfrm	Berkovic et al. (1991), Hammans et al. (1991), Lauber et al. (1991), Noer et al. (1991), Seibel et al (1991), Shoffner et al. (1990), Shoffner et al. (1991a), Tanno et al. (1991), Wallace et al. (1988b), Yoneda et al. (1990)
MTTK	MERRF	8356C	8356	tRNA Lys	–	+	Cfrm	Masucci et al. (1995) Silvestri et al. (1992), Zeviani et al. (1993)
MTTK	MERRF	8363A	8363	tRNA Lys	–	+	Prov	Ozawa et al. (1997)
MTTG	MHCM	9997C	9997	tRNA Gly	nd	+	Prov	Merante et al. (1994)
MTTG	CIPO	10006G	10006	tRNA Gly	nd	nd	Prov	Lauber et al. (1991), Munscher et al. (1993a)
MTTG	PEM	10010C	10010	tRNA Gly	–	+	Prov	Bidooki et al. (1997)
MTTG	GER/SIDS	100446	10044	tRNA Gly	–	+	Prov	Santorelli et al. (1996)
MTTS1	CIPO	12246G	12246	tRNA Ser (AGY)	nd	nd	Prov	Lauber et al. (1991), Munscher et al. (1993a)
MTTS2	DMDF	12258A	12258	tRNA Ser (AGY)		+	Prov	Lynn et al. (1998)
MTTL2	CPEO	12308G	12308	tRNA Leu (CUN)	nd	nd	P.M.	Houshmand et al. (1994), Lauber et al. (1991), Marzuki et al. (1991), Merante et al. (1994), Moraes et al. (1993b), Noer et al. (1991), van den Ouweland et al, (1992a)
MTTL2	CPEO	12311C	12311	tRNA Leu (CUN)	+	+	Prov	Hattori et al. (1994), Sato et al. (1994)

continued

Table 11.4 Reported mitochondrial DNA protein synthesis diseases (*continued*)

Locus	Disease	Allele	np	RNA	H o	H e	Status	References
MTTL2	CPEO	12315A	12315	tRNA Leu (CUN)	–	+	Prov	Fu et al. (1996)
MTTL2	MM	12320G	12320	tRNA Leu (CUN)	–	+	Prov	Weber et al. (1997) Hanna et al. (1995)
MTTE	MM+DM	14709C	14709	tRNA Glu	–	+	Conf	Hao et al. (1995), Vialettes et al. (1997)
MTATT	MM	15915A	15915	tRNA Thr	–	+	Prov	Nishino et al. (1996), Seki et al. (1997) Brown et al. (1992a),
MTTT	LIMM	15923G	15923	tRNA Thr	nd	–	Prov	Yoon et al. (1991), Yoon et al. (1993) Brown et al. (1992a)
MTTT	LIMM	15924G	15924	tRNA Thr	nd	–	P.M.	Ozawa et al. (1991b), Yoon et al. (1991)
MTTT	MM	15940delT	15940	tRNA Thr	+	–	Prov	Seneca et al. (1998)
MTTP	MM	15990T	15990	tRNA Pro	–	+	Prov	Ionasescu et al. (1994), Moraes et al. (1993a)

and cardiac conduction defects (Wolff-Parkinson-White syndrome). Other clinical manifestations in the maternal lineage included insulin-dependent diabetes mellitus and cataracts. This heteroplasmic mutation has been shown to segregate along the maternal lineage and the percent mutant mtDNAs has been shown to correlate with the level of skeletal muscle complex I deficiency, oxygen consumption and clinical severity (Zeviani et al., 1991). Transmitochondrial cybrids harboring the MTTL1*MMC3260G mutation prepared from patient myoblasts have been found to have defective protein synthesis and mitochondrial respiration (Mariotti et al., 1994) confirming the pathogenicity of this mutation.

A heteroplasmic tRNA^{Gly} mutation, MTTG*MHCM-9997C, has been reported in associated with maternally transmitted hypertrophic cardiomyopathy in a single, multi-generation family. This mutation changes a highly conserved base, has not been observed in controls, and results in multiple OXPHOS enzyme defects (Merante et al., 1994). Finally, cardiomyopathy is often seen in association with the classical MTTK*MERRF8344G and MTTL1*MELAS3243G mutations (Goto, 1995).

Encephalomyopathies associated with mtDNA mutations

The mitochondrial encephalomyopathies combine MM with a complex array of neurodegenerative disease symptoms. Most of the mitochondrial encephalomyopathies are the product of mtDNA tRNA or rRNA gene mutations (Table 11.4). These mitochondrial protein synthesis mutations often affect multiple tissues, although the central nervous system, heart, skeletal muscle, kidney and endocrine system are most often compromised. The nature and extent of the clinical symptoms can vary markedly based on the nature of the mutation and the degree of heteroplasmy in the affected tissues. The more severe protein synthesis mutations are frequently associated with elevated serum, urine or cerebral spinal fluid lactate, alanine and/or other organic and amino acids.

The most severe mitochondrial encephalomyopathies are frequently isolated cases which appear spontaneously. This may be because that mutation is sufficiently deleterious that affected individuals do not survive long enough to reproduce. An example of such cases was a patient with progressive mitochondrial encephalomyopathy with cerebral calcifications (Fahr's disease) associated with the deletion of one of the Ts in the anticodon stem of the tRNA$^{Leu (UUR)}$ gene (MTTL1*PEM3271ΔT) (Shoffner et al., 1995a). This heteroplasmic mutation was initially manifest at five years of age with progressive hearing loss leading to deafness by age 18 years. Seizures occurred in childhood, and the disease progressed into young adulthood to include mitochondrial myopathy (RRFs), retinitis pigmentosa, glaucoma, hypogonadism, dementia, and severe cerebral calcifications. The patient died at 28 years of age as a result of tonic/clonic seizures, renal failure, and sepsis. The percentage of mutant mtDNAs was about 75% in the patient's skeletal muscle, but the mutant was absent in the mother's peripheral blood. Hence, this appears to be a new mutation that arose in the female germline which segregated sufficiently rapidly to give a lethal phenotype.

Somewhat milder tRNA mutations can result in maternally inherited mitochondrial encephalomyopathies such as MERRF and MELAS. MERRF typically presents with myoclonic epilepsy and mitochondrial myopathy. Myoclonic epilepsy is an uncontrolled periodic jerking, frequently beginning focally but progressing over the course of the disease to generalized cyclic muscle contractions. These are associated with high amplitude voltage spikes on electromyographic (EMG) analysis and with marked slowing of electroencephalographic (EEG) wave activity (Rosing et al., 1985; Wallace et al., 1988a).

While a pedigree might first be identified by a patient with MERRF, careful clinical examination frequently reveals individuals along the maternal lineage with a variety of other less severe clinical presentations. These can include subclinical electrophysiological changes such as hyperexcitable visual evoked response (VER) and clinically related slowing and variability in somatosensory evoked response (SSER), sensorneural hearing loss, ataxia, renal dysfunction, mitochondrial myopathy, diabetes, cardiomyopathy and dementia (Rosing et al., 1985; Wallace et al., 1988a; Suzuki et al., 1994b; Shoffner and Wallace, 1995). Anterior and posterior cervical lipomas are also frequently seen in severely affected MERRF patients (Berkovic et al., 1991; Larsson et al., 1995; Shoffner and Wallace, 1995).

MERRF is most frequently associated with mutations in the tRNA^{Lys} gene. Approximately 80 to 90% of cases result from the MTTK*MERRF8344G mutation (Wallace et al., 1988a; Shoffner and Wallace, 1990), while many of the remaining cases are due to the MTTK*MERRF8356C mutation (Silvestri et al., 1992; Zeviani et al., 1993). Occasionally, other tRNA mutations can also result in MERRF, most notably the MTTL1*MELAS3243G mutation (Morgan-Hughes et al., 1995). The MTTK*MERRF8344G mutation changes a highly conserved A to a G in the TΨC loop of tRNA^{Lys} gene, while the MTTK*MERRF8356C converts a T to a C base disrupting an A-U base-pair at the base of the TΨC loop. MERRF mutations are heteroplasmic in families.

A detailed analysis of the associations between clinical presentation, biochemical defect, and mtDNA genotype in one large MTTK*MERRF8344G family revealed a strong correlation between genotype and phenotype, when age was taken into account (Shoffner and Wallace, 1990; Wallace et al., 1994). Among the 19–24 year olds of this family, an individual with 15% normal mtDNAs in skeletal muscle had normal muscle mitochondrial energy capacity as determined by the anaerobic threshold in exercise stress tests (θ_{an}), normal OXPHOS enzyme activities, and normal phenotype, exhibiting only mild electrophysiological changes. By contrast, 20 year olds with only about 5% normal muscle mtDNA had reduced mitochondrial energy capacity and more severe symptoms, with the proband having less than 25% normal muscle energy capacity and the complete MERRF syndrome. Similarly, maternal relatives in the 40 to 50 year age range who retained about 10% normal mtDNAs showed higher muscle energy capacity and milder phenotypes than comparably aged individuals with half that level of normal mtDNAs, the latter exhibiting reduced energy metabolism and more severe symptoms. Finally, among two maternal relatives in the 60 to 70 year range, an individual with 27% normal mtDNAs had significant residual mitochondrial energy capacity and mild to moderate symptoms, while the other individual with 16% normal mtDNAs had complete MERRF syndrome. Most striking, however, was the difference between the 19 year old with 15% normal mtDNAs and no clinical symptoms and the 60 year old with 16% normal mtDNAs and severe disease. The much more severe clinical problems of the older subject with the sample mtDNA genotype reflects a general feature of mtDNA diseases; they showed a delayed onset and they progress with age (Wallace et al., 1994).

A severe mitochondrial protein synthesis defect has been found to be associated with the MTTK*MERRF8344G mutation in patient skeletal muscle (Noer et al., 1991), myoblasts/myotubes (Chomyn et al., 1991; Boulet et al., 1992) and fibroblasts (Seibel et al., 1991). The translation defect results in a general reduction in the rate of protein synthesis most affecting the larger mitochondrial polypeptides, together with the generation of abnormal translation products. This results from a 50–60% decrease in tRNA^{Lys} aminoacylation (Enriquez et al., 1995). Accompanying the translation defect is a reduction in mitochondrial O_2 consumption and electron transport chain enzyme activity (Wallace et al., 1988b). Protein synthesis abnormalities and OXPHOS defects have been unambiguously assigned to both the MTTK*MERRF8344G and MTTK*MERRF8356C mutations by cybrid transfer using both patient myoblasts (MTTK*MERRF8344G only) (Chomyn et al., 1991) and fibroblasts (Masucci et al., 1995). It is postulated that the reduction of mitochondria protein synthesis results in a lowering of the steady-state levels of OXPHOS enzyme complexes, perhaps due to premature termination of translation at lysine codons.

The MELAS pedigrees often present through a patient who has experienced a stroke-like episode. Generally this first occurs between the ages of five to 15 years, though it can occur any time from infancy to adulthood. Muscle biopsy of such patients usually reveals mitochondrial myopathy (Pavlakis et al., 1984). In addition, maternal relatives can exhibit a wide variety of complex clinical problems involving the CNS, muscle, heart, renal, and endocrine systems. MELAS can be caused by a variety of mtDNA tRNA mutations, most of which are in the tRNA$^{Leu\,(UUR)}$ gene. By far the most common MELAS mutation is MTTL1*MELAS3243G (Kobayashi et al., 1990; Goto et al., 1992a). Additional MELAS mutations include MTTL1*MELAS3252G (Morten et al., 1993), MTTL1*MELAS3256T (Sato et al., 1994), and MTTL1*MELAS3271C (Goto et al., 1991). In addition to these mutations, other tRNA mutations, including the MTTK*MERRF8344G mutation, can give a MELAS like phenotype. Some mtDNA tRNA mutations, such as the MTTL1*MELAS3256T and the MTTS1 *MERME7512C mutations, can give rise to a MERRF/ MELAS overlap syndrome (Moraes et al., 1993b; Sato et al., 1994; Nakamura et al., 1995). One missense mutation, MTND4*MELAS11084G, has also been associated with a MELAS pedigree (Lertrit et al., 1992), but more recent studies suggest that this may be an Asian polymorphism (Sakuta et al., 1993b). A second missense mutation, G13513A, in the ND5 gene has also been associated with MELAS. This mutation changes a highly conserved asparagine to an aspartate and is heteroplasmic (Manfredi et al, 1995a). Hence, this mutation strongly implicates severe complex I defects as the cause of mitochondrial myopathy and stroke-like episodes.

Like the MTTK*MERRF8344G mutation, both the MTTL1*MELAS3243G and the MTTL1*MELAS3271C mutations result in a marked defect in mitochondrial protein synthesis. This is most dramatically demonstrated in cybrid studies performed with patient myoblasts (Chomyn et al., 1992; King et al., 1992) and fibroblasts (King et al., 1992; Koga et al., 1995). Invariably, the MELAS mutations cause a generalized reduction in the rate of mitochondrial protein synthesis of up to 70% (Chomyn et al., 1992) and a concomitant reduction in the steady-state levels of mitochondrial proteins when the proportion of mutant mtDNAs is greater than about 94%. Cybrid cell lines with greater than 94% MTTL1*MELAS3243G and MTTL1*MELAS3271C mutant mtDNAs can also have oxygen consumption rates reduced up to 70% (Chomyn et al, 1992; King et al., 1992; Koga et al., 1995), although to a lesser degree in the MTTL1*MELAS3271C cybrid lines (Koga et al., 1995). Histological and immunohistochemical analyses (Moraes et al., 1992) have revealed a reduction in the levels of gene products in patient skeletal muscle harboring the MTTL1*MELAS3243G mutation.

The translation of the larger mitochondrial encoded gene products appear to be most severely compromised and preferential defects in complex I and/or complex IV are frequently observed in skeletal muscle ((Obermaier-Kusser et al., 1991; Goto et al., 1992a; De Vries et al., 1994; Mariotti et al., 1995) for MTTL1*MELAS3243G patients.

The actual pathophysiological mechanism by which the MTTL1*MELAS3243G mutation results in MELAS remains unclear. Because the 3243 nucleotide lies within the transcriptional terminator sequence for the rRNA genes, it is possible that this mutation perturbs the transcriptional processes. In *in vitro* experiments, diminished affinity for the mitochondrial transcription terminator protein (mTERM) for the mutant terminator sequence has been reported (Hess et al., 1991). This was related to an impairment of transcript termination for the 16 S rRNA gene, and possibly altering the rRNA/mRNA ratio. Some studies have confirmed a reduced affinity of mTERM for the mutant termination sequence (Chomyn et al., 1992) and, in some cases, reduced transcriptional termination (Suomalainen et al., 1993), but others have found no evidence of abnormal termination, altered rRNA production, or a MELAS-specific perturbation in rRNA to mRNA ratios (Moraes et al., 1992; Koga et al., 1993; Suomalainen et al., 1993; Tokunaga et al., 1993). Moreover, the MTTL1*MELAS3271C mutation is not found within the transcription termination sequence, yet still results in MELAS. This suggests that the primary cause of MELAS is altered mitochondrial translation. One proposal is that the MTTL1*MELAS3243G and MTTL1*MELAS3271C mutations alter transcript processing. Cybrids harboring these mutants have been reported to accumulate RNA processing intermediate RNA 19, which corresponds to a transcript containing the contiguous 16 S rRNA + tRNA$^{Leu(UUR)}$ + ND1 genes (King et al., 1992; Koga et al., 1995).

The spectrum of clinical manifestations associated with maternal relatives of MELAS patients is best characterized for the MTTL1*MELAS3243G mutation (Moraes et al., 1992; Goto, 1995; Hammans et al., 1995; Mariotti et al., 1995; Shoffner and Wallace, 1995). In addition to strokes, patients harboring this mutation can be prone to migraine headaches and focal or generalize seizures, ataxia, myoclonus, sensory neural deafness, retinopathy, and dementia. They can experience fatigability, myopathy, renal failure, myalgia, and ophthalmoplegia, and develop hypertrophic or dilated cardiomyopathy and cardiac conduction defects. In rare cases, this mutation has also been associated with peripheral neuropathy plus rhabdomyolysis (Hara et al., 1994), demyelinating polyneuropathy (Rusanen et al., 1995), and ischemic colitis (Hess et al., 1995). By far the most dramatic alternative phenotype of the MTTL1*MELAS3243G mutation is type II diabetes mellitus with or without sensory neural hearing loss (van den Ouweland et al., 1992a). It is now well established that diabetes mellitus is by far the most common clinical presentation of the MTTL1*MELAS3243G mutation (see below).

The pathophysiology of mitochondrial stroke is quite different from that of stroke associated with vascular occlusion. CT and MRI analysis frequently reveals infarcts in the posterior temporal, parietal, and occipital lobes. These frequently overlap several large vessel vascular beds, and can be transitory, often resolving along with the clinical signs. It has been hypothesized that these infarcts are due to transient OXPHOS dysfunction within the brain parenchyma, rather than vascular events (Pavlakis et al., 1984; Shoffner and Wallace, 1994; 1995). Alternatively, they might be the product of vascular spasm, the contraction extending along a extended region of the cortical vasculature inhibiting blood flow and causing ischemia. This hypothesis is supported by extensive post mortem analysis of the cortical vasculature of MTTL1*MELAS3243G and MTTL1*MELAS3271C mutation patients (Hayashi et al., 1993; Sakuta et al, 1993a; Tokunaga et al., 1993; Goto 1995). Histochemical and electron microscopic analysis of MELAS patient vessels have revealed accumulations of abnormal mitochondria in the vascular endothelial cells and vascular smooth muscle cells. The mitochondria are frequently pycnotic, contain mitochondrial occlusions, and stain extensively for succinate dehydrogenase (complex II) which is associated with a large increase in both mutant and normal mtDNAs (Ohama et al, 1987; Sakuta and Nonaka, 1989; Goto et al., 1992a; Tokunaga et al., 1993). The increased complex II activity implies a compensatory induction in mitochondrial biogenesis in response to a vascular cell OXPHOS deficiency.

Patients with mitochondrial protein synthesis defects resulting from the MTTL1*MELAS3243G mutation or mtDNA deletions show striking increases in immunohistochemical staining of their RRFs for the mitochondrial MnSOD and weakly increased staining for the cytosolic Cu/ZnSOD. Moreover, the MnSOD staining is strongly positive in the subsarcolemmal region and shows a coarsely granular, reticular, or diffuse pattern between the myofibrils. Interestingly, the MELAS RRFs which are MnSOD positive are frequently still COX positive, while the CPEO MnSOD-positive fibers are generally COX negative (Ohkoshi et al., 1995). Hence, mitochondrial protein synthesis defects are associated with MnSOD and Cu/ZnSOD induction and hence increased ROS production. Partial defects in respiratory complex I are associated with induction of the mitochondrial MnSOD, suggesting increased oxygen radical production (Pitkanen and Robinson, 1996).

Vascular blood flow is regulated by the contraction and dilation of the vascular smooth muscle cells, which in turn is regulated by diffusable effectors synthesized and released by the vascular endothelial cells, specifically, the vasodilator nitric oxide or NO. NO is rapidly inactivated by superoxide anion (O_2^-) and other reactive oxygen species (Nakazono et al, 1991; Seccombe et al., 1994).

The increased production of ROS should deplete the NO, causing loss of vasodilatory activity. The resulting vasoconstriction could in some instances be sufficient to block blood flow and cause a stroke. Later fluctuations in superoxide production would permit increased NO production and vasodilation, partially restoring blood flow.

After stroke-like episodes, the most common clinical presentation of the MTTL1*MELAS3243G mutation is ophthalmoplegia, ptosis, and mitochondrial myopathy. Chronic progressive external ophthalmoplegia (CPEO) is also the most common presentation of mtDNA rearrangement syndromes. Since every pathogenic rearrangement that has been studied to date alters or removes one or more tRNA genes (Wallace et al., 1999b), mtDNA rearrangement mutations also cause protein synthesis defects. Hence, ophthalmoplegia, ptosis, and mitochondrial myopathy are common presentations of severe defects in mitochondrial energy production.

MITOCHONDRIAL MYOPATHY ASSOCIATED WITH NDNA MUTATIONS (MNGIE) AND MTDNA DEPLETION

Mutations in two nDNA mitochondrial genes cause mitochondrial myopathy through the destabilization or loss of the mtDNA. These are the mitochondrial neurogastrointestinal encephalomyopathy (MNGIE) syndrome and the mtDNA depletion syndrome (Table 11.3). MNGIE is associated with mitochondrial myopathy including RRFs and abnormal mitochondria; decreased respiratory chain activity; and multiple mtDNA deletions, mtDNA depletion or both. This autosomal recessive disease has been linked to multiple mutations in the nuclear thymidine phosphorylase (TP) gene. While the disease is caused by TP mutations, the clinical symptoms are probably the result of the destruction of the mtDNA. Hence, it has been hypothesized that inactivation of TP alters cellular thymidine pools which are important in mtDNA maintenance (Nishino et al., 1999).

Mitochondrial depletion is associated with early childhood, frequently lethal, respiratory failure, lactic acidosis, and selective organ failure involving muscle (mitochondrial myopathy), heart, liver, or kidney. A total of 18 cases have been reported, 11 of which are male, giving a male: female ratio of 1.55:1 (Bodnar et al., 1993; Figarella-Branger et al., 1992; Mazziotta et al., 1992; Moraes et al., 1991; Poulton et al., 1995c; Telerman-Toppet et al., 1992; Tritschler et al., 1992; Vu et al., 1998). About half of the depletion families encompass other clinically affected individuals. In one case, two affected siblings who died at 12 weeks and $2\frac{1}{2}$ months of age as a result of respiratory failure associated with generalized hypotonia, PEO, and severe lactic acidosis had a second cousin through the maternal grandfather who died at age nine months of age as a result of hepatic failure (Boustany et al., 1983). This implies that the inheritance is chromosomal, either autosomal recessive or autosomal dominant with incomplete penetrance.

In mtDNA depletion syndrome, organ failure is associated with a severe diminution of the level of the mtDNA relative to nDNA in the affected tissue. This has been documented by molecular hybridization of mtDNA and 18 S rRNA sequences to Southern blots of *Pvu*II digests followed by determining the ratio of hybridization by densitometry (Moraes et al., 1991; Tritschler et al., 1992) or by dot-blot hybridization using a [^{35}S]dCTP-labeled mtDNA probe and [^{32}P]dCTP-labeled arginosuccinate synthetase gene probe (Poulton et al., 1995c). Depletion has been confirmed by demonstrating the loss of mtDNA gene products and loss of cytoplasmic mtDNA by immuno-histochemistry (Moraes et al., 1991; Tritschler et al., 1992).

The age of onset and severity of symptoms varies among patients, and this has been loosely correlated with the severity of the depletion. In one series of ten patients, individuals exhibiting symptoms shortly after birth and dying in the first year of life had between 2% and 17% residual mtDNA in the affected organ, while individuals who exhibited symptoms after the first year and lived for three or more years had between 14% and 34% of the normal mtDNA (Mazziotta et al., 1992; Moraes et al., 1991; Tritschler et al., 1992). This association is less clear in another series of patients, although one complexity is the rapid rise in the mtDNA:nDNA ratio during the first two to three years of life (Poulton et al., 1995c).

The reason for organ-specific DNA depletion is unknown. However, the fact that the disease is hereditary and that in the same family different individuals have different affected organs implies that the disease is due to a nuclear mutation which controls mtDNA copy number. A lack of regulation of copy number would then permit replicative segregation to generate cell lineages which had severely reduced or lost their mtDNAs, resulting in depleted organs. This concept is supported by somatic cell genetic experiments. Skin fibroblasts from one depletion patient were found to retain less than 2% of control mtDNAs, be deficient in OXPHOS enzymes, and require pyruvate and uridine to grow, in effect to be functionally ρ^0. When these cells were enucleated and the cytoplasms fused to a ρ^0 recipient cell line, the cybrids acquired the patient's mtDNA, but at a normal mtDNA:nDNA ratio. Hence, the nucleus, not the mtDNA, must regulate the mtDNA:nDNA ratio (Bodnar et al., 1993). Propagation of the patient's fibroblast in culture resulted in the gradual diminution in mtDNA and increased reliance on uridine and pyruvate for growth (Bodnar et al., 1995). Hence, mtDNA depletion appears to be a nuclear deficit in either mtDNA copy control or replication.

NEONATAL CARDIOMYOPATHY, ENCEPHALOMYOPATHY AND TUBULOPATHY ASSOCIATED WITH NDNA MUTATIONS

Neonatal multisystem degenerative diseases have also been associated with mutations in three COX assembly genes: *SCO1*, *SCO2*, and *COX10* (Table 11.3). Infants with lethal hypertrophic cardiomyopathy, lactic acidosis, neurodegeneration and atrophy, and hepatomegaly associated with a complex IV defect have been found to harbor mutations in the complex IV assembly gene *SCO2* (Table 11.3). To date, patients with pathogenic *SCO2* mutations always have one allele with the E140K missense mutation. The other allele has been either a null allele or another missense mutation, e.g. S225F or R171W (Papadopoulou et al., 1999). Interestingly, in the yeast model system the equivalent of the E140K mutation does not significantly reduce complex IV activity, while the S225F results in respiratory deficiency. Yeast with the S225F mutation assembles complex IV without the mtDNA subunit COII. This suggested that SCO2 is involved in the insertion of Cu^{2+} into the Cu_A site of the mtDNA COII subunit (Dickinson et al., 2000). Hence, *SCO2* mutations like *SURF1* mutations result in defects in the assembly of complex IV, COX.

Infants with hepatic failure and encephalomyopathy have been identified with mutations is a second complex IV Cu^{2+} incorporation enzyme SCO1 (Table 11.3). Patients have been found to have compound heterozygous mutations including frameshift and missense mutations. Two identified missense mutations are C250T and P174L, the latter mutation being thought to affect the copper binding domain (CXXXC) of the enzyme (Valnot et al., 2000).

Another infant has been described with ataxia, severe hypotonia, ptosis, pyramidal syndrome, status epilepticus, and proximal tubulopathy due to a mutation in the *COX10* gene (Table 11.3). The patient progressed and died at two years of age. He had an older sister who died at five years of age as a result of mitochondrial encephalopathy associated with complex IV deficiency, and a younger sister who had progressive neurological deterioration and died at three years of age. Genetic analysis revealed that these patients were homozygous for a deleterious missense mutation (N204K) in the COX10 enzyme. The parents were both heterozygous for this mutation. *COX10* encodes the heme A:farnesyltransferase enzyme and the patients have a 50% reduction in complex IV subunits III and IVc and a >97% reduction in subunit II (Valnot et al., 2000).

OPHTHALMOPLEGIA, PTOSIS AND MITOCHONDRIAL MYOPATHY

Ophthalmoplegia and ptosis is a common manifestation of mitochondrial disorders. When associated with mitochondrial myopathy, these clinical manifestations are a reliable indicator of severe mitochondrial myopathy. Mitochondrial patients with ophthalmoplegia, ptosis, and mitochondrial myopathy can have a wide range of additional symptoms. Patients with milder disorders may present with only ophthalmoplegia, ptosis, and mitochondrial myopathy, with an age of onset ranging from the late 20s up to late adulthood and a relatively mild course. Such patients are said to have "chronic progressive external ophthalmoplegia" (CPEO). By contrast, other patients can present with ophthalmoplegia, ptosis, and mitochondrial myopathy prior to age 20 and experience multiple additional symptoms including retinitis pigmentosa and at least one of the following: cardiac conduction defects, cerebellar ataxia, or elevated cerebral spinal fluid protein above 100 mg/dl (Rowland, 1983; Poulton et al., 1995a). These patients are said to have the Kearns-Sayre Syndrome (KSS). Other symptoms which may be observed in KSS or CPEO patients can include optic atrophy, hearing loss, seizures, dementia, cardiomyopathy, cardiac dysrhythmias, renal failure, endocrine disorders including diabetes mellitus, respiratory failure, lactic acidosis (Ota et al., 1994; Shoffner and Wallace, 1995), chronic diarrhea and villous atrophy in early childhood (Cormier-Daire et al., 1994).

Approximately 83% of KSS and 47% of CPEO patients are the product of mtDNA rearrangements (Moraes et al., 1989). The great majority of these cases are new spontaneous mutations derived from a single clonal event such that all of the affected tissues of the patient are heteroplasmic for normal mtDNAs plus rearranged mtDNAs with a single unique breakpoint junction. Presumably, most of these mutations arose in the oocyte or early in development. A few cases, however, involve rearrangements which

can also be detected at low levels in the mother and/or other maternal relatives (Poulton et al., 1991).

Most of the remaining cases are the of various mtDNA tRNA point mutations, including the tRNA mutations MTTL1*MELAS3243G (Goto et al., 1990, Johns and Hurko, 1991; Schon et al., 1994; Goto, 1995) and MTTN*CPEO5692G (Seibel et al., 1994) (Table 11.4). A small percentage of patients with progress external ophthalmoplegia (PEO) harbor multiple mtDNA rearrangements caused by the inheritance of autosomal dominant or recessive nuclear mutations which predispose the mtDNAs to rearrangements (Zeviani et al., 1989) (Table 11.3).

Ophthalmoplegia associated with mtDNA mutations

The mtDNA rearrangements associated with CPEO and KSS can include deletions, insertions, or a combination of the two (Poulton and Holt, 1994). The first mtDNA rearrangements were recognized in skeletal muscle of patients with mitochondrial myopathy (Holt et al., 1988). Subsequent analysis of a large number of patients revealed that mtDNA rearrangements could be associated with four interrelated phenotypes: the KSS, CPEO, Pearson's marrow/pancreas syndrome, and maternally inherited diabetes mellitus and deafness.

Chronic progressive ophthalmoplegia (CPEO) and the Kearns-Sayre syndrome (KSS) associated with mtDNA rearrangement mutations

In addition to ophthalmoplegia and ptosis, patients with CPEO and KSS due to mtDNA rearrangements have a progressive severe mitochondrial myopathy (Figure 11.10). Additional histological analysis of CPEO and KSS muscle has revealed bands of COX-deficient (COX⁻) and SDH-hyper-reactive (SDH⁺) activity along the muscle fibers. These COX⁻ and SDH⁺ fibers generally correspond to regions of mitochondrial proliferation and RRFs, high levels of mutant mtDNA, and induction of nDNA and mtDNA OXPHOS gene expression (Heddi et al., 1993, 1994; 1999; Mita et al., 1989; Shoubridge et al., 1990).

The great majority of KSS and CPEO cases are due to spontaneous mtDNA rearrangements (Schon et al., 1994; Wallace et al., 1995a). Of the 89 different break points which have been reported, 80% were flanked by direct repeats of four to 16 nucleotides, 7% involved direct repeats of four to six nucleotides, and 12% did not involve a direct repeat (Wallace et al., 1995a). Hence, the majority of rearrangements involve a region of homology suggesting

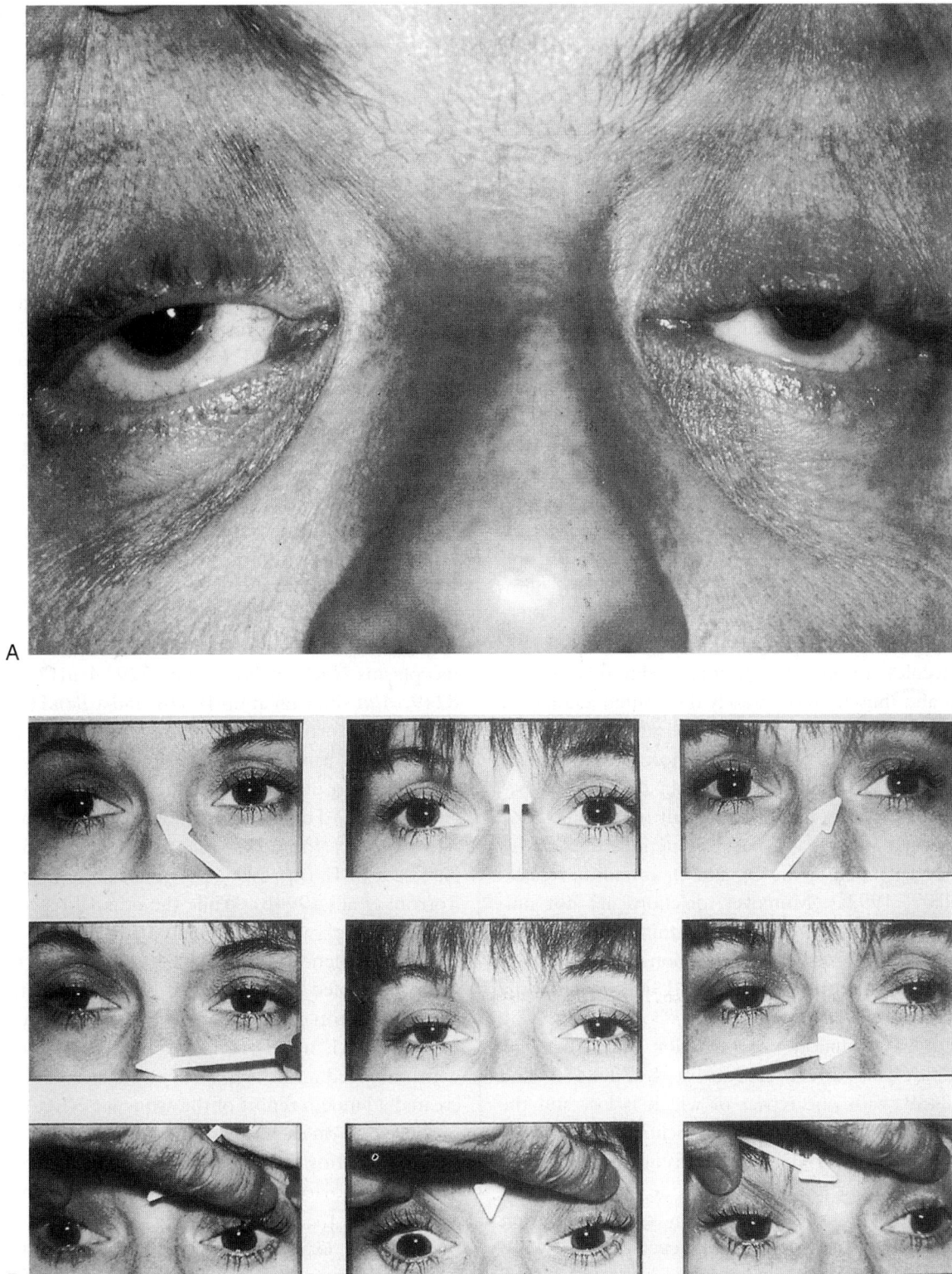

Fig. 11.10. (a) Severe ptosis in a patient with CPEO. In this photograph, patient was asked to look directly upward while eyelids were manually lifted by examiner. (b) Ophthalmoplegia in a 37-year-old woman with CPEO and mitochondrial myopathy. Ocular motility is shown in nine cardinal positions, *arrows* indicating the requested direction of gaze. Note mild bilateral ptosis and omnidirectional ophthalmoparesis. (Photograph courtesy of Nancy J. Newman, MD, Emory University School of Medicine.)

some type of sequence associated rearrangement mechanism. Many KSS patients harbor an inter-related family of rearranged molecules, all of which share a common breakpoint junction. These frequently include, in addition to normal mtDNAs, a duplicated mtDNA, a deletion monomer which retains only the duplicated region, and a deletion dimer containing two copies of the inserted sequence (Poulton et al, 1993; 1995a).

Duplications may predispose individuals to the more severe disease, since in one survey all ten KSS patients were found to have duplications as well as deletions, while all eight CPEO patients harbored only deletion monomers (Poulton et al., 1994). Furthermore, the amount of the duplicated molecule in the KSS patients appears to correlate with the duplication size. The larger the duplication, the lower the level of duplicated molecules. Moreover, the patients with the smallest duplications (largest deletions) also had deletion dimers. As the disease progresses in skeletal muscle, the normal and duplicated mtDNAs decline while the deletion dimers increase; and the patients harboring duplications are more likely to develop diabetes mellitus than those with only deletions (Poulton et al., 1995a). These observations have lead to the speculation that duplicated molecules are propagated more readily than deleted molecules and thus are more widely distributed among the tissues. Hence, patients harboring duplications have more organ systems affected and hence more severe disease (Brockington et al., 1995; Poulton et al., 1995a).

While a wide variety of rearrangement breakpoints have been mapped, the great majority of deletions tend to fall into two areas defined by the O_H and O_L origins of replication (Wallace, 1992a). Moreover, deletions are not uniformly distributed. Approximately one-third to one-half of all deletion events occur at the common deletion breakpoint between nucleotide pairs 8469:13447 joining the mtDNA genes MTND5 and MTATP8, and removing 4977 nps. This "common" 5 kb deletion occurs between two 13 base-pair direct repeats at 8470–8482 and 13447–13459, with one repeat of which is lost and the other retained (Holt et al., 1989a; Schon et al., 1989; Shoffner et al., 1989). Two other frequently observed rearrangements bring together nucleotide pairs 7841 and 13905 in the MTCO2 and MTND5 genes, removing 6063 np at a six to eight base direct repeat; and between nucleotide pairs 8648:16085 in gene MTATP6 and MTTP removing 7436 np at 12 np direct repeat (Wallace et al., 1995a). The increased frequency of deletions at these breakpoints suggests a predominant rearrangement mechanism. In one case of the common 4977 np deletion, the break occurred one nucleotide outside the direct repeat.

This permitted a demonstration that the upstream 13447–13459 repeat was retained while the downstream 8470–8482 repeat was lost. Since this corresponds to the direction of H-strand replication, it was proposed that one mechanism for mtDNA rearrangement was slip mispairing. As replication proceeds, a new H-strand is synthesized along the L-strand template starting from O_H and moving down in nucleotide numbers from 16,569 np, with the parental H-stand being displaced as a single stranded loop. Direct repeats in the parental H-strand are thus exposed and can base-pair with downstream homologous repeats exposed on the L-strand by the replicating fork. Breakage of the single-stranded H-strand on the downstream side of the base-paired repeat would create an 3′-OH gap, which would permit reinitiation of replication continuing along the template, beginning downstream of the L-strand repeat and skipping the intervening mtDNA (Shoffner et al., 1989; Lestienne et al., 1995).

Slip-mispairing has been confirmed as an important mutational mechanism in the mtDNA through studies of a spontaneous mtDNA mutation that occurs in the D-loop of a specific European haplogroup I mtDNA lineage. Haplogroup I is defined by the novel restriction site polymorphisms *Hae*II site loss at np 4529, *Ava*II site gain at np 8249, *Alu*I site gain at np 10028, and a *Bam*HI site gain at np 16389 (Torroni et al., 1994b). Individuals that harbor this mtDNA haplotype are prone to develop a heteroplasmic a 270 np duplication in the D-loop between np 302 and np 567. This tandem duplication duplicates P_H (np 545–567), P_L (np 392–445), CSBIII (np 346–363), and part of CSBII (np 299–315) (Brockington et al., 1993; Torroni et al., 1994b). While the original report proposed that this duplication predisposed mtDNA to subsequent large scale deletions (Brockington et al., 1993), this has not been confirmed (Torroni et al., 1994b; Manfredi et al., 1995b; Poulton et al., 1995a). Subsequent analysis revealed haplogroup I mtDNAs harbored a germline mutation which inserted a run of C nucleotides at np 568–573. This created a tandem repeat of the sequence 5′-ACCCCCCCC … CCCC-3′ on each side of duplicated region. Every individual harboring this germline mutation was found to be heteroplasmic for the duplication in all somatic tissues tested. Since the duplicated regions are tandemly arrayed, the simplest explanation for this self-generating D-loop duplication is slip-mispairing (Torroni et al., 1994b). While predisposition to this duplication does not appear to be pathogenic *per se*, it has been found to be present at relatively high levels (32%) in one patient with mitochondrial myopathy including RRFs and partial COX deficiency. This patient also had a small percentage of mtDNAs with this region triplicated (Manfredi et al., 1995b). This observation could suggest that either the duplication can be toxic at high levels or alternatively that the duplicated mtDNA is preferentially amplified in mitochondrial myopathy due to the presence of the additional promoters and O_H.

Alternative deletion mechanisms that have been proposed include topoisomerase II cleavage (Lestienne et al., 1995) and homologous recombination. Putative topoisomerase II recognition sequences have been observed in the vicinity of certain mtDNA deletions and proposed to play a role in removal of sequences (Mita et al., 1990; Blok et al., 1995). Recombination is likely to play an important role since it is now established that many rearrangement patients harbor a complex array of related molecules including duplication molecules, deletion monomers and deletion dimers suggesting that they may be interconverted by a recombinational process (Poulton et al., 1993; 1994; Poulton and Holt, 1994). MtDNA recombination has now been confirmed in somatic cell hybrids between two cell lines harboring non-overlapping CPEO deletions, both of which retained O_H and O_L. In the hybrids, the mtDNAs complemented each other to give respiratory competence and a few cell lines have been found to contain recombinant molecules involving the coalescence of the two deleted molecules (Davidson et al., 1995). Hence, mtDNA recombination does occur in cultured human cells, though in this experiment its frequency was very low.

The pathophysiology of KSS and CPEO resulting from spontaneous mtDNA rearrangements appears to be the result of a protein synthesis defect combined with the stochastic distribution of the mutant molecules during development. All KSS and CPEO associated deletions studied to date remove at least one structural RNA (tRNA or rRNA) essential for mitochondrial protein synthesis. Cytoplasmic transfer of deleted molecules from patient cells to ρ^0 HeLa cells confirmed that the deleted molecules caused a defect in mitochondrial protein synthesis. In cybrids with up to 60% deleted mtDNAs, the normal mtDNAs complimented in *trans* permitting high respiration and synthesis rates of the mtDNA-encoded polypeptides. However, above the 60% mutant mtDNA threshold, mitochondrial respiration, protein synthesis, and the level of the individual mitochondrial polypeptides declined precipitously, ultimately falling to zero (Hayashi et al., 1991). This threshold effect on protein synthesis for deletion mutations explains why KSS and CPEO, like the pathogenic tRNA mutations, are frequently associated with mitochondrial myopathy and RRFs. Analysis of the tissue distribution of mtDNA deletions in KSS and CPEO patients at autopsy has revealed that the rearranged molecules are broadly distributed throughout the tissues of the body (Shanske et al., 1990; Poulton et al, 1995b; Brockington et al., 1995). The interesting exception is blood, which is commonly devoid of the mtDNA deletions (Holt et al., 1988; Shoffner et al., 1989; Brockington et al., 1995; Poulton et al., 1995b), though duplications have been found (Poulton et al., 1995a). Hence, molecular diagnosis of KSS and CPEO generally requires a muscle biopsy.

The time in development when pathogenic mtDNA deletions arise is not yet known. However, their broad tissue distribution would imply a mutation in the oocyte or very early in development. This is supported by surveys of the mtDNAs of human oocytes left over from *in vitro* fertilization clinics which have revealed that many oocytes do harbor deletions. Eight at of 15 oocytes harbored the common 4977 np deletion, confirming that deletions must occur early in development (Chen et al., 1995b; Keefe et al., 1995). The maximum number of molecules containing the 5 kb deletion was 171 molecules, or about 0.1% (Chen et al., 1995b). Moreover, a survey of oocytes from women of different ages revealed that of women less than 38 years, 28% of the oocytes had the common deletion while for women older than 38, 93% of the oocytes had this deletion. Consequently, the mean age of women without oocyte deletions was 31.4 years, while that of women with deletions was 37.7 years (Keefe et al., 1995). This correlates with a marked increase in ovarian mtDNA deletions at menopause, about age 45 (Kitagawa et al., 1993). Thus, it appears that mtDNA rearrangements may arise in the oocyte or early in development, and the frequency of mtDNA rearrangement syndromes may increase with maternal age at conception.

Molecular histological analysis of the distribution of deleted mtDNAs in skeletal muscle of KSS and CPEO patients has revealed that the levels of mtDNA deletions increase with age (Larsson et al., 1990; Fassati et al., 1994; Poulton et al., 1995a), and that the deleted molecules are not uniformly distributed along the length of the muscle fiber. Staining muscle fibers for COX and SDH has revealed that the COX levels vary from normal to absent and that the SDH staining is normal where COX is normal, but greatly increased in COX-negative regions (Muller-Hocker 1990). *In situ* hybridization and regional PCR amplification have shown that regions which are COX-negative have increased levels of the deleted mtDNAs and a coordinate induction of mtDNA transcripts from the undeleted genes. By contrast, the COX-positive regions have predominantly normal mtDNAs (Mita et al., 1989; Shoubridge et al., 1990; Moraes et al., 1995). These observations imply that the deleted mtDNAs are initially scattered along the muscle fiber, but that as the individual ages, there is a selectively amplification of the deleted molecules, ultimately reaching a high enough concentration to inhibit mitochondrial protein synthesis and cause COX-deficiency.

The mechanism by which the deleted mtDNAs are selectively amplified remains unknown, though two hypothesis have been put forward. The first hypothesis is that the deleted molecules are shorter and thus have a replicative advantage (Wallace 1992a). Mitochondrial proteins and mtDNAs are known to be continuously, albeit slowly, turned over in post-mitotic tissues (Neubert et al., 1968; Gross et al., 1969; Kadenbach, 1969; Menzies and Gold, 1971). Hence repeated replication cycles might favor shorter deleted mtDNAs or duplicated molecules with extra origins. The alternative hypothesis is that the nuclei adjacent to mutant mtDNAs and mitochondria sense the OXPHOS defect of the mutant mitochondria and attempt to compensate by inducing mtDNA replication and mitochondrial biogenesis in the surrounding mitochondria. Coordinate induction of nuclear and mtDNA OXPHOS gene expression has been documented in skeletal muscle of patients with both mtDNA rearrangement and tRNA mutations (Heddi et al., 1993; 1994; 1999), and since skeletal muscles are synctia, each nucleus controls a particular cytosolic domain (Pavlath et al., 1989). If nDNA OXPHOS gene expression is modulated by a mitochondrial substrate, such as NADH, then inhibition of the ETC by a mtDNA mutation would cause a local rise in NADH and concomitant increase in mitochondrial gene expression in the adjacent nucleus. Such a process could be a mediated *via* a nuclear transcription factor which activates OXPHOS gene expression. Such a factor has been identified which binds to the REBOX sequence element located 5′ to a variety of nuclear bioenergetic genes and possibly also in the D-loop of the mtDNA. The binding of the REBOX-binding factor (RBF) is stimulated by a reducing environment (Chung et al., 1992a; Haraguchi et al., 1994). Thus in cells with partial respiratory deficiency, increased NADH could activate RBF to bind to the REBOX element and thus stimulate the nucleus to induce the biogenesis of the surrounding mitochondria, including the associated mutant mtDNA. The resulting increase in number of mutant mtDNAs would further increase the NADH and stimulate the nuclear gene expression, creating a self perpetuating feedback loop which would preferentially amplified the mutant mtDNAs (Wallace, 1994a; 1994b). Whatever the mechanism, it would appear that it is the regional bioenergetic defect caused by the selective amplification of the mutant mtDNAs that causes the progressive decline muscle function in KSS and CPEO.

CPEO associated with mtDNA base substitution mutations

A variety of mtDNA tRNA base substitution mutations have also been found to cause ophthalmoplegia, ptosis, and mitochondrial myopathy (Table 11.4). The tRNA mutation which is the most common cause of ophthalmoplegia is the MELAS mutation, MTL1*MELAS3243G (Johns and Hurko, 1991; Schon et al., 1994; Goto, 1995; Hammans et al., 1995; Mariotti et al., 1995). In a survey of 28 KSS and 109 PEO patients, 28 KSS patients had deletions and one harbored the MTTL1*MELAS3243G mutation, while of the PEO patients 46 (42%) harbored mtDNA deletions while 15 (14%) harbored the MTTL1*MELAS3243G mutation. One additional PEO patient had the MTTK*MERRF8344G mutation. KSS and CPEO patients which harbor mtDNA tRNA mutations are generally members of larger maternal pedigrees with several variously affected family members (Moraes et al., 1993c).

In addition to the MTTLI*MELAS3243G mutation, other tRNA base substitution mutations which present with CPEO are the tRNA(Asn) mutations MTTN*CPEO5692G (Seibel et al., 1994) and MTTN*CPEO5703G (Moraes et al, 1993b); the tRNA(Ile) mutation MTTI*CPEO4298A (Taylor et al., 1998); and the tRNA(Leu(CUN)) mutations MTTL2*CPEO12308G (Lauber et al., 1991), MTTL2*-CPEO12311G (Hattori et al., 1994), and MTTL2*CPEO-12315A (Fu et al., 1996). Ophthalmoplegia is also a major clinical feature of the tRNA(Glu) mutation at MTTG*CIPO-1000GG (Lauber et al., 1991), and the tRNA(Ser(AGY)) mutation at MTTS1*CIPO12246G (Lauber et al., 1991). Ophthalmoplegia is also a major clinical feature of the tRNA(Glu) mutation at MTTG*CIPO10006G (Lauber et al., 1991) and the tRNA(Ser(AGY)) mutation at MTTS1*CIPO-12246G (Lauber et al., 1991). Ophthalmoplegia is also an occasional symptom for a variety of other deleterious mtDNA tRNA mutations, including the MTTK*MERRF8344G mutation (Moraes et al., 1993c) and potentially others of the tRNA(Leu(UUR)) MELAS mutations (Goto, 1995). As is the case for mtDNA rearrangement mutations, milder renditions of the CPEO mutations can also cause diabetes mellitus and deafness. This phenotype is a common presentation of patients harboring 5% to 30% of the MTTL1*MELAS3243G mutation (Gerbitz et al., 1995; Goto, 1995).

The clear demonstration that both the MELAS and MERRF tRNA mutations inhibit mitochondrial protein synthesis indicates that this is the underlying mechanism that causes ophthalmoplegia, ptosis, and mitochondrial myopathy. This would also explain the origin of the symptoms in the CPEO and KSS patients with mtDNA rearrangements, since every pathogenic rearrangement that has been studied to date alters or removes one or more tRNA genes (Wallace et al., 1999b). Hence, the rearrangement mutations would also cause protein synthesis defects, a result confirmed by cybrid studies of CPEO patient deletion cell lines. Hence, ophthalmoplegia, ptosis, and mitochondrial myopathy must result from primary defects in mitochondrial protein synthesis. Since the mtDNA encodes seven subunits of complex I and three complex IV subunits, these would be the OXPHOS enzymes likely to be most affected. This is observed. Hence, ophthalmoplegia, ptosis, and mitochondrial myopathy probably, reflect severe defects in mitochondrial energy production.

PEO associated with nDNA mutations

While most ophthalmoplegia, ptosis, and mitochondrial myopathy patients are the result of spontaneous mtDNA rearrangement mutations and thus have no family history (Shoffner et al., 1989; Larsson et al., 1992), approximately 6% of PEO cases have been found to harbor multiple deletions and show a clear autosomal dominant inheritance pattern. Such families are known as autosomal dominant-PEO (AD-PEO) (Zeviani et al., 1989; 1990; Cormier et al., 1991b; Moraes et al., 1993c) (Table 11.3).

In AD-PEO, each affected individual has a different array of mtDNA deletions. This demonstrates that it is a nuclear mutation which increases the tendency toward deletion that is inherited, not the deletion itself (Cormier et al., 1991b; Zeviani et al., 1989, 1990). Clinically, the mean age of onset of AD-PEO is 26 years, which is older than the average spontaneous CPEO case. In addition to PEO, these patients experience proximal muscle atrophy and weakness in about 62% of patients, hearing loss in 25%, and ataxia in 17% of cases. Cardiac and retinal involvement are rare, and the most common cause of death is respiratory failure (Kawai et al., 1995). Multiple deletions have also been found in four patients with RRFs but atypical neurological symptoms. Two individuals presented with Parkinsonism, one with ptosis, a third with exercise intolerance and limb weakness, and a fourth with elevated blood creatine phosphokinase (Checcarelli et al., 1994). The nature of the deletions in multiple deletion syndrome is similar to that found in spontaneous deletion patients. Among the 81 deletions reported from multiple deletion syndrome patients, 96% are encompassed by direct repeats of four to 13 nucleotides, while 4% involve indirect repeats of 4 bp (Wallace et al., 1995a). Moreover, patients show multiple deletions in tissues throughout the body (Suomalainen et al., 1992).

Efforts to localize the nuclear gene mutations responsible for multiple deletion syndrome have employed extended families and linkage analysis. At least three loci are currently known. One Finnish locus has been linked to chromosome 10q23.3–24.3 (Suomalainen et al., 1995; Zeviani et al., 1995), and a second Italian locus to chromosome 4q34–35, with a few families remaining unlinked (Table 11.1) (Kaukonen et al., 1995; 1996). The mutant gene at the 4q34–35 locus has been identified as the *ANT1*. Two missense mutations have been identified, one that was found in five Italian families with a common background haplotype, suggesting that they are related by descent. This mutation changes a highly conserved alanine at codon 114 to a proline residue. The second mutation was identified in a single individual and changed the valine at codon 289 to a methionine residue (Kaukonen et al., 2000). The nature of the mutant genes at the 10q23.3–24.3 locus is currently unknown, though the structural genes for the *Tfam* and the mt*SSB* loci have been excluded (Zeviani et al., 1995). Additional autosomal recessive PEO pedigrees with multiple deletions have also been identified. Presumably, these represent additional loci involved in mtDNA maintenance (Carrozzo et al., 1998).

PEARSON'S MARROW/PANCREAS SYNDROME

A more severe form of the CPEO/KSS mtDNA rearrangement syndrome presents in the first five years of life with pancytopenia (loss of all blood cells). This condition is known as the Pearson's marrow/pancreas syndrome. Pearson's patients develop a severe transfusion-dependent, macrocytic anemia with varying degrees of neutropenia and thrombocytopenia. The bone marrow of Pearson's patients shows extensive vacuolization of erythroid and myeloid precursors, hemosiderosis and ringed sideroblasts. Pearson's patients generally die due to complications of the bone marrow dysfunction or transfusions. In addition to pancytopenia, many Pearson's patients develop exocrine pancreatic insufficiency, hepatic failure, renal failure, and other neuromuscular problems (Pearson et al., 1979; Cormier et al., 1991a; Kapsa et al., 1994; Rotig et al., 1995; Shoffner and Wallace, 1995; Smith et al., 1995). Analysis of circulating white blood cells has revealed a generalized respiratory defect in association with mtDNA rearrangements, both deletions and duplications. As with most CPEO and KSS patients, Pearson's patients are generally isolated cases, suggesting mutational events early in development (Rotig et al., 1988; 1989; 1993; 1991). Moreover, autopsy analysis of Pearson's patients has revealed that the mtDNA rearrangements are not simply localized to the bone marrow, but are systemic (Cormier et al., 1990; De Vries et al, 1992), and the rare Pearson's patients which spontaneously recover the ability to make blood cells and survive, ultimately progress to a KSS-like phenotype (McShane et al., 1991; Poulton et al., 1995a; Rotig et al., 1995). These observations suggest that the Pearson's Marrow/Pancreas Syndrome and CPEO-KSS are the same disease, with the phenotypic differences resulting from the distribution of the rearranged molecules in the different tissues. This interpretation is supported by the observation that some Pearson's patients including patients which have progressed to KSS harbor duplications as well as deletions (Poulton et al, 1994; 1995a). One explanation for the difference between Pearson's Syndrome and KSS/CPEO is that in Pearson's syndrome the rearranged mtDNAs are widely distributed and include all of the bone marrow precursor cells. As the bone marrow stem cells replicate, the rearranged mtDNAs accumulate until there is insufficient energy for further proliferation and/or maturation. At this point the rearranged molecules are prevalent in the peripheral blood and blood cell production declines leading to pancytopenia. By contrast, in KSS/CPEO patients or in Pearson's syndromes that survive and progress to KSS, the rearranged molecules may be distributed such that a portion of the bone marrow precursor cells are free of mutant mtDNAs. As the stem cells containing rearranged molecules decline in their replicative potential, the cells having only normal mtDNAs continue to proliferate and ultimately supplant the mutant cells and repopulate the bone marrow. At this point, the patient loses the rearranged mtDNAs in the circulating white blood cells, but still retains rearranged mtDNAs in other organs. These later mutant mtDNAs exert their effects later in life leading to the multisystem diseases of KSS and CPEO.

DIABETES MELLITUS

Diabetes mellitus with and without deafness is a common presentation for patients harboring mitochondrial protein synthesis mutations. While this phenotype has been found in patients harboring both rearrangement (Ballinger et al., 1992b; 1994) and tRNA base substitution (Suzuki et al., 1994a; van den Ouweland et al., 1992b; 1994) mutations. The MTTLI*MELAS3243G mutation is by far the most common known cause of mtDNA-associated diabetes mellitus (Gerbitz et al., 1995).

Diabetes mellitus patients are commonly divided into two idiopathic forms: type I or insulin-dependent diabetes mellitus (IDDM) and type II or non-insulin dependent diabetes mellitus (NIDDM). Type I IDDM patients have a childhood to adult-onset, are insulin dependent making little, if any, insulin and showing no insulin response to glucose, have normal glucagon secretion, are prone to ketoacidosis and generally thin, and show a 40% concordance in identical twins. In Caucasians, 95% of the IDDM patients carry the HLA-DR3 and/or DR4 alleles as compared to 50% of the general population, and they make anti-islet cell, insulin, and glutamic acid decarboxylase (GAD) antibodies suggesting an autoimmune process. By contrast, type II NIDDM patients generally have mid-life onset after age 40, make insulin and have variable insulin response to glucose such that they can be managed by diet or drugs, have normal glucagon secretion, are not prone to ketoacidosis and may be obese, and show a 90% concordance in identical twins. NIDDM patients show no HLA association and do not have anti-islet cell, insulin, or GAD antibodies. These features have been interpreted as indicating that the causes of NIDDM have a strong genetic component (Gerbitz et al., 1995).

Two factors suggested that the inheritance of type II diabetes might have a mtDNA component (Wallace, 1992a). Early epidemiological studies of diabetes mellitus patients revealed that as the age-of-onset of the proband increases, the probability that the mother will be the affected parent also increases, reaching a ratio of 3:1 for mean age-of-onset of 46 years. Moreover, the maternal transmission can be sustained for several generations (Dorner et al., 1975; 1987; Dorner and Mohnike, 1976; Pimentel, 1979; Freinkel et al., 1986). This trend has been recently confirmed in Britain for 1326 type II diabetic subjects in which 183 had affected parents of which 125 (68%) were the mother, as well as for French and Turkish studies (Alcolado and Thomas, 1995). The second indication that mtDNA mutations might cause diabetes mellitus comes from the observation that many patients with known mtDNA mutations either present with diabetes mellitus or have maternal relatives with the disease. This association was first clearly demonstrated for KSS patients with mtDNA duplications. The smaller the duplication, and larger the reciprocal deletion, the more likely the patient is to have diabetes mellitus (Dunbar et al., 1993; Poulton et al., 1989a; 1989b; 1994; 1995b). Diabetes mellitus has also been repeatedly observed in family members of patients harboring the MTTL1*MELAS3243G mutation (Suzuki et al., 1994a).

Type II diabetes caused by a MtDNA rearrangements

The first proof that type II diabetes mellitus could be caused by a mtDNA mutation came from the study of a large African-American pedigree which showed maternal inheritance of diabetes and deafness and harbored a mtDNA duplication and reciprocal deletion (Ballinger et al., 1992b, 1994). Since that observation, diabetes mellitus has been found to be a common clinical manifestation in patients with mtDNA duplications, generally in association with KSS (Poulton et al., 1995a; 1995b).

In the initial African-American family with Type II diabetes mellitus and sensorineural hearing loss, the maternal relatives developed hearing loss in their twenties and thirties and Type II diabetes mellitus in their thirties and forties. Occasional individuals in the rearrangement pedigree experienced stroke-like episodes associated with cortical and brain stem lucencies on MRI examination. None of the patients had ophthalmoplegia or ptosis, nor did they have mitochondrial myopathy as detected by muscle histology. However, detailed biochemical analysis of several family members revealed a generalized OXPHOS defect in the skeletal muscle. Physiological analysis indicated that all maternal relatives developed an insulin-dependent diabetes mellitus, with some individuals developing diabetic ketoacidosis. Glucose tolerance tests revealed that severely affected individuals were unable to respond to hyperglycemia with increase insulin production from β cells or decreased glycogen production from α cells (Ballinger et al., 1994).

The mtDNA rearrangement in this maternally inherited pedigree consisted of three main types of mtDNA molecules: (a) normal mtDNAs; (b) duplicated mtDNAs containing an insertion of 6.1 kb of the mtDNA encompassing from np 4389 in the tRNA^{Gln} gene to np 14,822 in the *MTCYB* gene and including the ND1, 16 S rRNA, 12 S rRNA, and part of the *MTCYB* genes, as well as the tRNA^{Ile}, tRNA$^{Leu(UUR)}$, tRNA^{Val}, tRNA^{Phe}, tRNA^{Pro}, and tRNA^{Thr} genes, and the D-loop including O$_H$; and (c) finally deleted mtDNAs which lack 10.4 kb of mtDNA including 11 of the 13 OXPHOS genes; 15 of 22 tRNAs, $-$O$_L$, and 75 bp of the 5′ end of the *MTCYB* gene. The deleted molecules appear to be present as a dimer of about 12 kb, and the rearrangement is encompassed by a 10 bp direct repeat (5′-CACCCCATCC-3′). Lymphoblastoid cell lines carrying this rearrangement exhibit a partial protein synthesis defect. Extended propagation results in the selective enrichment for the duplicated molecules and loss of the deleted and normal mtDNAs. Moreover, white blood cells from patients have an excess of duplicated molecules while the post-mitotic muscle had a higher proportion of deleted than duplicated mtDNAs. These results suggest that the duplicated molecules with the extra O$_H$ are preferentially replicated and hence transmitted through the germline, and

that the deleted molecules are generated from the duplicated molecules through a recombinational process in post-mitotic tissues. While the deleted molecules have only one origin O$_H$, it is possible that they could also replicate. If the two components of the dimers were arrayed in a head to tail position, then there would be an O$_H$ for each strand (Ballinger et al., 1992b; 1994).

This pedigree is remarkable in that it harbored the same type of duplication and deletion dimer molecular defect that has been documented for diabetes mellitus in association with KSS patients and Pearson's Syndrome patients which progress to KSS (Poulton et al., 1989a; 1993; 1994; 1995a; 1995b), yet none of the patients exhibited evidence of ptosis, ophthalmoplegia, or mitochondrial myopathy. In another family a patient has been described with dystonia, external ophthalmoplegia, slowly progressive proximal muscle weakness, no RRFs on muscle biopsy though showing mitochondrial hyperplasia, and diabetes mellitus which developed at age 36 years and was treated with insulin. This individual also showed normal and duplicated mtDNAs, with the duplication encompassing nucleotides 13445 to 3318 and flanked by imperfect direct repeats at nps 3318–3337 and 13445–13462. This duplication duplicated the 12 S and 16 S rRNAs, ND6 and MTCYB genes, O$_H$ and the encompassed tRNAs; and was found in 15% of the proband's muscle mtDNA, 80% of his blood mtDNA, and 40% of his mother's blood mtDNA (Dunbar et al., 1993). In a second family, the child presented at eight years of age with diabetes mellitus and occasional episodes of ketoacidosis, which progressed on to CPEO and mitochondrial myopathy, with the individual dying at age 20 years of cardiac dysrhythmia. The patient harbored a family of mtDNA molecules including normal, duplicated, deleted, and deletion dimers which were widely distributed among her tissues including her pancreas (Poulton et al., 1995b). Thus, these two families have similar duplications to the maternally inherited diabetes mellitus and deafness family and also had diabetes without or without RRFs, but the patients did have ophthalmoplegia. This implies that mtDNA rearrangement syndromes represent a phenotypic continuum with isolated diabetes mellitus and deafness being the mildest presentation, CPEO and KSS intermediate, and Pearson's marrow/pancreas syndrome the most severe.

The diabetes mellitus and deafness can also be associated with mtDNA base substitutions in protein synthesis genes, particularly the MTLL1*MELAS3243G mutation. However, the phenotypes of the mtDNA rearrangements and, induced diabetes and deafness are somewhat different in that the rearrangement patients are more frequently insulin requiring diabetics (Ballinger et al., 1992b; Poulton et al., 1995b). In one case this has been associated with the loss of pancreatic β cells (Poulton et al., 1995b).

Because of the clinical variability of the mtDNA rearrangement syndromes, diabetes mellitus together with mtDNA rearrangements can be associated with a spectrum of other clinical symptoms. A 5 kb deletion has been identified in an infant with diabetic ketoacidosis, rickets, and de Toni-Debre-Fanconi syndrome (Luder and Barash, 1994) and a 5778 np deletion was detected by PCR in patients with diabetic amyotrophy, diabetic myoatrophy and nephropathy, and diabetic fatty liver, though this deletion was not confirmed by Southern blot and the same deletion was found at lower levels in controls (Hinokio et al., 1995). Finally, one patient has been reported with Wolfram's syndrome including early-onset diabetes mellitus, optic atrophy, and deafness in association with a 7.6 kb mtDNA deletion (Rotig et al., 1993), though analysis of another Wolfram's patient failed to reveal a mtDNA defect (Jackson et al., 1994).

Type II diabetes caused by mtDNA base substitutions

The most common mtDNA mutation associated with diabetes mellitus is the MTLL1*MELAS3243G mutation (van denOuweland et al., 1992b; 1994; Suzuki et al., 1994a; Gerbitz et al., 1995). The MTTL1*MELAS3243G mutation has been found at about 1.4% in IDDM and NIDDM patients (Gerbitz et al., 1995). The frequency is higher for NIDDM if the mother is also affected (5.7%), and much higher if the patients have both NIDDM and sensorineural hearing loss, being 60% (3/5) in a Japanese study (Kadowaki et al., 1995) and 10% (2/20) in a British study (Alcolado and Thomas, 1995). While the great majority of diabetes mellitus MTTL1*MELAS3243G patients have a primarily NIDDM presentation, many either present with or progress to IDDM (Gerbitz et al., 1995; Kadowaki et al., 1995). Furthermore, slowly progressive IDDM has been associated with the MTTL1*MELAS3243G mutation, and in one study of islet-cell antibody positive patients with progressive NIDDM, the MTTL1*MELAS3243G mutation was found in three of 27 (11%) of the patients suggesting that islet cell loss and subsequent auto-antibody production can also be associated with mitochondrial defects (Oka et al., 1993; 1995). These and other observations have led to a delineation of the characteristics MTTL1*MELAS3243G diabetes mellitus which include maternal transmission; variable clinical phenotype including NIDDM, slowly progressive IDDM and IDDM; young to middle age onset; tendency toward progression;

and association with sensorineural hearing loss. Moreover, many of these patients are lean, require insulin, but are less prone to ketoacidosis. They show a delayed insulin response to glucose and impaired glucagon secretion, and they may or may not have auto-antibodies to pancreatic islet cells (Oka, 1994; Gerbitz et al., 1995; Kadowaki et al., 1995). The MTTL1*MELAS3243G mutation is invariably heteroplasmic in diabetes mellitus patients, and generally present a lower percentage mutant than commonly found in MELAS patients, frequently in the range of 5–30% in blood, with levels potentially higher in muscle and fibroblasts (van den Ouweland et al., 1992b; Suzuki et al, 1994a). Indeed, it is not uncommon that blood cells will lack the mutation even though it is present in post-mitotic tissues. Hence, this cause of diabetes mellitus is probably under-diagnosed.

Due to the systemic nature of the MTTL1*MELAS3243G mutation, it is not uncommon for patients presenting with diabetes mellitus to also exhibit additional clinical manifestations. Examples include diabetes mellitus with diabetic amyotrophy (Suzuki et al., 1994a), diabetes mellitus with diarrhea and abdominal pain involving 37% mutant mtDNAs in blood and 70% mutant mtDNAs in gastric and rectal mucosa and skeletal muscle (Kishimoto et al., 1995), and diabetes mellitus with post-insulin treatment neuropathy (Suzuki et al., 1994c).

Other mtDNA tRNA mutations have also been associated with type II diabetes mellitus. One three generation pedigree presented with diabetes mellitus and deafness and harbored the MTTK*MERRF8344G mutation, with mutant mtDNA levels ranging from 12% to 28% in peripheral blood cells (Suzuki et al., 1994b). However, this MERRF mutation is not a common cause of diabetes mellitus, since the mutation was not found in a survey of several hundred Japanese diabetes mellitus patients (Kadowaki et al., 1995). A new mtDNA missense mutation has recently been reported in Japanese NIDDM patients. This G-to-A transition at np 3316 in the MTND1 gene converts a moderately conserved non-polar alanine readuce to a polar threonine readuce. A survey of patients and controls revealed that this mutation was present in 3.4% of patients but 1% of controls (Nakagawa et al., 1995). Additional studies will be needed to confirm the clinical relevance of this mutation.

Diabetes mellitus is also seen in Wolfram's syndrome, which is characterized by diabetes insipidus, diabetes mellitus, optic atrophy, and deafness (DIDMOAD). Other less common endocrine and neurological symptoms include hypogonadism, atonic bladder, ataxia, insomnia, seizures, and psychiatric disorders (Gerbitz et al., 1995). One patient diagnosed with Wolfram's syndrome including diabetes mellitus, optic atrophy, and sensorineural deafness was found to harbor the MTND4*LHON11778A mutation (Pilz et al., 1994) and another case of Wolfram syndrome was found to contain a 7.6 kb and mtDNA deletion (Rotig et al., 1993). However, sequence analysis of the blood cell tRNAs from two other Wolfram patients failed to reveal any disease specific mutations (van den Ouweland et al., 1992a). Hence, the role of mtDNA protein synthesis mutations in Wolfram's syndrome remains unclear (Gerbitz et al., 1995).

Myopathy and diabetes

Myopathy with diabetes mellitus has been associated with a heteroplasmic MTTE*MDM14709G mutation in two families (Hanna et al., 1995; Hao et al., 1995) one of which also presented with mental retardation and cerebellar ataxia (Hanna et al., 1995). Histological and/or immunohistochemical analysis of patient skeletal muscle revealed the classic signs of myopathy: ragged red fibers, COX-negative fibers, abnormal mitochondrial morphology and paracrystalline inclusions. Biochemically, this tRNA^{Glu} mutation caused a reduction in complex I and IV specific activities and, in myoblasts, resulted in a mitochondrial protein synthesis defect (Hanna et al., 1995).

Pathophysiology of diabetes and deafness

The biochemical basis of mitochondrial diabetes mellitus is still unclear. Defects in the glucose sensor and/or insulin secretory pathway (Alcolado et al., 1994a; Suzuki et al., 1994a; Gerbitz et al., 1995, Kadowaki et al., 1995) and/or decreased insulin sensitivity (Ballinger et al., 1994; Kanamori et al., 1994; 1995; Odawara et al., 1995; Walker et al., 1995) have been proposed.

This defect in the "glucose sensor" is similar to that seen in maturity onset diabetes of the young (MODY) (Figure 11.11). MODY results from mutations in the pancreatic islet cell glucokinase gene. The K_m of the islet cell glucokinase is higher than that of other cellular hexokinases, and hence glucokinase is only active during hyperglycemia (German, 1993; Gidh-Jain et al., 1993; Stoffel et al., 1992a; 1993). Since most of the cellular glucokinase is attached to the mitochondrial outer membrane by porin, and porin interacts with the ANT of the inner membrane (Malaisse-Lagae and Malaisse, 1988; Adams et al., 1991; Gelb et al., 1992), it is possible that glucose sensing involves the linkage between glucokinase and OXPHOS through this trans-mitochondrial membrane macromolecular complex. Hence, mutations in either the glucokinase gene, which binds glucose during hyperglycemia, or mitochondrial OXPHOS which provides the ATP for glucose phosphoryl-

ation could affect the ability of the pancreas to respond to hyperglycemia (McCabe, 1994; Wallace, 1994a).

In addition to phosphorylation of glucose by β-cell glucokinase, mitochondrial ATP generation may also play a role in insulin secretion through regulation of the β-cell, plasma membrane, ATP-sensitive K$^+$ channel (Figure 11.11). At low ATP/ADP ratios, the K$^+$ channel is leaky and the plasma membrane transmembrane potential remains high. However, during active glucose oxidation, mitochondrial ATP production goes up, the cytosolic ATP to ADP ratio increases, the ATP-sensitive K$^+$ channel closes, and this causes the plasma membrane to depolarize. The depolarization of the β-cell plasma membrane activates the voltage-sensitive Ca^{2+} channel. This causes Ca^{2+} to flow into the cytosol, which activates fusion of the insulin-containing vesicles causing release of insulin (Wollheim, 2000).

The importance of the mitochondrial oxidation of NADH to generate ATP in insulin secretion has been demonstrated by the fact that elimination of mtDNAs from rat insulinoma cell line (INS-s) resulted in the complete abolition of the insulin secreting capacity of the β-cells (Wollheim, 2000) and inhibition of the mitochondrial NADH shuttle results in inhibition of β-cells insulin secretion (Eto et al., 1999). The importance of the ATP-sensitive K$^+$ channel in insulin secretion has been confirmed by creating knockout and knockin mice with altered ATP-sensitive K$^+$ channel (Koster et al., 2000).

Based on this data, mitochondrial function appears to play an integral role in insulin phosphorylate secretion: first, by keeping the ATP-binding site of glucokinase charged and primed to phosphorylate glucose when its concentration exceeds the glucokinase K_m and second, to generate ATP through the OXPHOS to regulate the ATP-sensitive K$^+$ channel. Since mtDNA mutations would inhibit the ETC, this would reduce mitochondrial ATP generation and block plasma membrane depolarization and insulin secretion (Figure 11.11).

In addition to mtDNA mutations, nDNA mutations in mitochondrial functions might also play an important role in diabetes. MODY has been associated with a number of nDNA mutations. MODY2 is due to glucokinase mutations and accounts for 10–65% of cases. MODY1 is a rare form due to mutations in hepatic nuclear factor (HNF)-4α. MODY3 accounts for 20–75% of cases; results in post-pubertal diabetes, obesity, dyslipidaemia, and arterial hypertension and is due to mutations in HNF-1α. The rare MOD4 results from mutations in the insulin promoter factor (IPF)-1. HNF-4α is a member of the steroid/thyroid hormone receptor superfamily and acts as an upstream regulator of HNF-1α. HNF-1α is a transcription factor

Metabolic Basis of Diabetes Mellitus

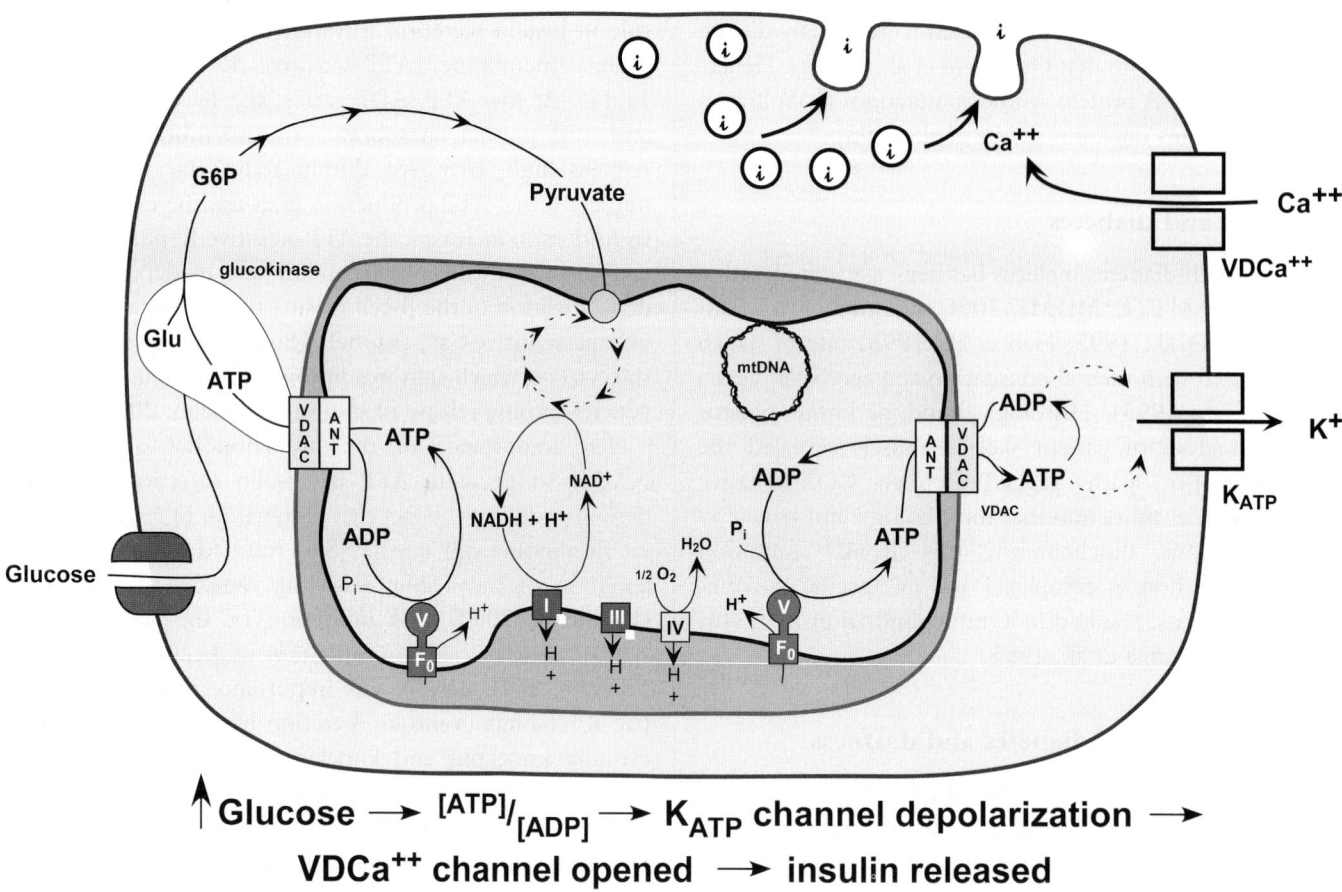

$$\uparrow \text{Glucose} \longrightarrow [ATP]/_{[ADP]} \longrightarrow K_{ATP} \text{ channel depolarization} \longrightarrow$$

$$\text{VDCa}^{++} \text{ channel opened} \longrightarrow \text{insulin released}$$

Fig. 11.11. Proposed metabolic involvement of the mitochondria in regulation of insulin secretion by the β cells of the pancrease. Abbrevation are the same as those detailed in the legend to Fig. 11.1.

involved in the tissue-specific regulation of liver and pancreatic islet genes (Velho and Froguel, 1998). However, HNF-1α is also important in regulating nDNA encoded mitochondrial gene expression and the GLUT 2 glucose transporter (Wollheim, 2000). Type II diabetes has been associated with a Pro12A1 polymorphism in the peroxisome proliferator-activated receptor γ gene (PPARγ) (Altshuler et al., 2000). PPARγ might play a role in the regulation of peroxisome and mitochondrial number and structure.

In addition to defects in insulin release, patients with mitochondrial defects also show insulin-resistance, which may precede the defect in insulin secretion (Gebhart et al., 1996). This could reflect the systemic nature of the OXPHOS defect, which would inhibit the cellular effects of glucose uptake. Finally, diabetic hyperglycemia is associated with a variety of secondary pathological changes affecting small vessels, arteries, and peripheral nerves. These changes are associated with: (a) glucose induced activation of protein kinase C isoforms; (b) formation of glucose-derived advanced glycation end-products (AGFs); (c) increased glucose flux through the aldose reductase pathway; and (d) activation of NFκB. In cultured vascular endothelial cells, all of these processes can blocked by inhibition of complex II (SDH) by thenoyltrifluoroacetone, (TTFA), uncoupling OXPHOS with carbonyl cyanide m-chlorophenylhydrazone (CCCP), induction of uncoupling protein-1 (Ucp1), or induction of mitochondrial MnSOD. Hence, all of the pathological effects of hyperglycemia are mediated through mitochondrial ROS production. Since NFκB is involved in induction of the expression of stress-response genes such as MnSOD, mitochondrial regulation of NFκB activation may have broad effects on cellular metabolism (Nishikawa et al., 2000).

MATERNALLY INHERITED DEAFNESS AND/OR AMINOGLYCOSIDE-INDUCED DEAFNESS

Maternally inherited deafness and/or aminoglycoside-induced deafness has been associated with three protein synthesis mutations: a 12 S rRNA mutation, MTRNR1*-DEAF1555G; and two tRNA^{Ser} mutations, MTTS1*-DEAF7445G and MTTS1*AMDF7472Cins. The MTRNR1*DEAF1555G mutation, though consistently homoplasmic, has now been confirmed in several independent studies (Fischel-Ghodsian et al., 1993; Hutchin et al., 1993; Prezant et al., 1993; Matthijs et al., 1994; Shoffner and Wallace, 1994). Individuals harboring this mutation were first observed in a large Middle Eastern pedigree featuring sensorineural hearing loss along the maternal lineage. The maternal transmission with variable penetrance was hypothesized to be the combination of the maternally transmitted MTRNR1*DEAF1555G mutation acting together with an autosomal recessive nuclear gene (Fischel-Ghodsian et al., 1993). Subsequent studies in China and elsewhere have shown that individuals harboring this mutation are acutely sensitive to aminoglycoside inhibition. The mutation occurs at the end of a stem and loop structure in the small rRNA subunit, adding a terminal base-pair and thus making the mitochondrial ribosome more like a bacterial ribosome at the aminoglycoside binding site (Hutchin et al., 1993). Pedigrees harboring this mutation have occasionally been observed to manifest other neurological signs including the extrapyramidal signs of tremors and rigidity seen in Parkinson's disease (Shoffner and Wallace, 1994). Despite the alteration of rRNA structure, a protein synthesis defect has not been reported for this mutation.

Maternally transmitted bilateral sensorineural hearing loss has also been observed in the absence of the MTRNR1*DEAF1555G in one family. A complete sequence of this family's mtDNA revealed a novel homoplasmic tRNA^{Ser} mutation, MTTS1*DEAF7445G (Reid et al, 1994a; 1994b; Vernham et al., 1994). This mutation was subsequently reported to heteroplasmic within the family (Verham et al., 1994).

A third mtDNA tRNA mutation, MTTS1*AMDF-7472Cins, has been found in a maternally inherited pedigree featuring progressive, bilateral hearing loss as the most common clinical manifestation. Ataxia due to cerebellar dysfunction and myoclonus were also prominent in the family (Tiranti et al., 1995). This mutation involves the insertion of a C base within a homopolymeric stretch of six C nucleotides, was found to be heteroplasmic in the family, was not found in nearly 400 controls, resulted a complex I biochemical deficiency, and likely alters the conformation of the TψC stem-loop. Cybrid studies confirmed the pathogenicity of this mutation and there was a correlation between proportion of mutant mtDNA and clinical manifestations in blood (Tiranti et al., 1995).

DEMENTIAS AS MITOCHONDRIAL DISEASES

Patients harboring mtDNA mutations may also develop progressive dementia. One patient with progressive cognitive decline, dementia, deafness, ataxia and chorea was found to be heteroplasmic for a tRNA^{Trp} mutation, MTTW*DEMCHO5549A. Postmortem analysis of the brain revealed diffuse and moderate neuronal loss in the cortex and basal ganglia with gliosis present throughout the brain. RRFs and COX-negative staining fibers were evident upon skeletal muscle analysis, as were morphologically abnormal mitochondria upon electron microscopy of skeletal muscle. A complex I defect was detected in mitochondrial respiration assays. Hence, this tRNA^{Trp} mutation demonstrates that respiratory defects can cause dementia (Nelson et al., 1995). This has been substantiated by the identification of the tRNA^{Gln} gene mutation at np 4336, MTTQ*ADPD4336G, which has been associated with about 5% of late-onset Alzheimer's disease (AD) (Shoffner et al., 1993a; Hutchin and Cortopassi, 1995; Egensperger et al., 1997) (Table 11.4)

The biology and genetics of Alzheimer's disease

Alzheimer's disease (AD) is the most common recognized form of late-onset dementia (St George-Hyslop 2000). Clinically, AD has been split into early onset and late-onset forms, divided roughly at age 65. Early onset AD has been associated with mutations in at least three autosomal dominant loci: amyloid precursor protein (APP) on chromosome 21, presenilin (PS) 1 on chromosome 14, and PS2 on chromosome 1. APP is processed by "secretase" proteolytic cleavage. A number of APP mutations have been identified which cause the inappropriate processing of APP into the toxic Aβ40 and 42 peptides. The presenilins have been implicated in secretase processing of APP, with defects in these proteins favoring the accumulation of the Aβ peptides. Current evidence indicates that PS1 may be the APP γ-secretase or alternatively a cofactor or important in the trafficking of γ-secretase (Wolfe et al., 1999). Multiple pathogenic PS1 missense mutations have been identified which account for the majority of early onset cases and 2% of the total AD cases (Schellenberg et al., 1992; Selkoe, 1995; Sherrington et al., 1995). In addition, two homologous genes encoding the β-secretase activity have been cloned, BACE 1 and 2 (Saunders et al., 1999). Tissue-specific transcription levels (Vassar et al., 1999; Bennett et al., 2000) and genetic mapping studies (Saunders et al., 1999) further implicate Aβ production in AD.

The excessive deposition of Aβ in AD brains has generated the "amyloid cascade hypothesis" of AD. Aβ is envisioned as perturbing cellular homeostasis, possibly through altering Ca^{2+} metabolism or generating toxic ROS. The increased ROS stimulate neurofibrillary tangle formation which fills and ultimately kills the cell (Hardy and Higgins, 1992). Strong support for this hypothesis comes from observations that all three autosomal dominant AD genes increase production of toxic Aβ peptides. Considerable evidence has implicated the Aβ peptide in increasing cellular calcium permeability, either directly or indirectly through Ca^{2+} or K^+ channels (Barger et al., 1993; Etcheberrigaray et al., 1994; Fukuyama et al., 1994). Aβ might also increase the sensitivity of AD cell mitochondria to oxygen radical generation and Ca^{2+} toxicity (Kumar et al., 1994). Moreover, Aβ has been shown to bind Zn^{2+} and Cu^{2+} and in that form to aggregate and actually generate ROS, particularly H_2O_2 (Bush et al., 1994; Atwood et al., 1998, 2000; Huang et al., 1999). Since increased oxidative damage in AD brains is well documented (DiCiero Miranda et al., 2000; Rottkamp et al., 2000), it is very possible that the pathophysiology of amyloid accumulation could be the result of increased neuronal oxidative stress.

Late-onset AD is also genetically heterogeneous with several loci now implicated in this disease. The best studied of these encodes the ApoE gene (Pericak-Vance et al., 1991; Roses et al., 1994). Multiple other loci have recently been associated with late-onset AD; including *BACE2*, *TNFα* (Tanzi, pers and communication), a locus on chromosome 12 (Scott et al., 2000) and α2-macroglobulin (*A2M*) (Blacker et al., 1998; Tanzi, 1999), although this is controversial. In addition, several groups have associated the interleukin-1 gene with AD (Tanzi, 1999; Du et al., 2000; Grimaldi et al., 2000; Licastro et al., 2000; Nicoll et al., 2000; Rogers, 2000). Another late-onset AD locus on chromosome 10 appears to be related to the insulin degrading enzyme (IDE), which may be involved in the degradation of Aβ (Perez et al., 2000; Vekrellis et al., 2000). A related enzyme, neprolysin, has recently been directly implicated in Aβ degradation. Suppression of neprolysin in normal rat brain elevates Aβ deposition (Iwata et al., 2000), and the human neprolysin gene is polymorphic (Comings et al., 1999).

Mitochondrial defects in AD

AD is associated with protein aggregation and oxidative stress, with Aβ peptide in the presence of Cu^{2+} actually gen-erating H_2O_2. Both diseases are associated brain and systemic mitochondrial OXPHOS defects and specific mtDNA mutations have been linked to some cases. Since the mitochondria play a pivotal role in energy production, calcium homeostasis, ROS metabolism, and apoptosis; the mitochondria may provide a common element that could provide a unified pathophysiological mechanism for AD.

Multiple studies have implicated mitochondrial OXPHOS defects in both AD and PD. Histological analysis of AD brains has revealed alterations in mitochondrial morphology in apparently normal dendrites from the superficial cortical layers which include increased matrix density and paracrystalline inclusions in the intercristal space (Saraiva et al., 1985). PET studies of AD patients have observed decreased glucose transport suggesting a bioenergetic defect (Jagust et al., 1991), and analysis of brain sections from AD patients has revealed a 30% reduction in pyruvate dehydrogenase activity (Sorbi et al, 1983; Sheu et al., 1985) and a 42% reduction in the ADP to O_2 ratio suggesting the partial uncoupling of OXPHOS (Sims et al., 1987). Chronic inhibition of complex IV in rats by infusion of sodium azide impairs both spatial and non-spatial learning in rats (Bennett et al., 1992), and significant reductions in glucose and glutamine oxidation and calcium accumulation have been reported for AD skin fibroblasts (Peterson and Goldman, 1986). Normal skin fibroblasts treated with the OXPHOS uncoupler carbonyl cyanide m-chlorophenyl-hydrazone, show a tenfold increase in epitopes recognized by antibodies to paired bilateral filaments and a 157-fold increase in the protein detected by the AD-specific monoclonal antibody 50 (Blass et al., 1990). Finally, ROS have been implicated in AD, both in damaging neurons and catalyzing the aggregation of the Aβ peptide (Benzi and Moretti, 1995; Mattson, 1995).

AD patient materials have repeatedly been reported to have partial defects in respiratory complex IV (COX) in both platelet and brain mitochondria (Parker et al., 1990b, 1994; Kish et al., 1992; Mutisya et al., 1994; Maurer et al., 2000). These complex IV defects have been proposed to be associated with mtDNA defects, based on their apparent ability to be transferred from AD patients to cultured cells by fusion of patient platelets to $ρ^0$ Ntera/Dl neurons or the neuroblastoma SH-SY5Y. AD platelet cybrids have been reported to have reduced complex IV activity, increased ROS production and reduced Ca^{2+} capacity (Sheehan et al., 1997; Swerdlow et al., 1997; Cassarino et al., 1998), though the validity of these experiments has been questioned (Schon et al., 1998).

Histochemical staining of COX in AD brains revealed marked reduction in activities in the dentate gyrus and the hippocampal subfields CA1>CA2>CA4 (Simonian and Hyman, 1993). Defects in mitochondrial respiration (Sims et al, 1987) and in pyruvate dehydrogenase (Sorbi et al., 1983; Sheu et al., 1985) have also been reported. Consistent with these biochemical defects, levels for several, but not all, nDNA and mtDNA OXPHOS gene transcripts are reduced in AD brain (Simonian and Hyman, 1994; Chandrasekaran et al., 1996, 1997; Hatanpaa et al., 1996). This down-regulation of specific mitochondrial mRNA levels is paralleled by the down-regulation of a variety of genes encoding proteins relevant to AD pathology, as detected by DNA microarray (chip) analysis. Down-regulated genes included phosphatases/kinases, cytoskeletal proteins, synaptic proteins, and glutamate and dopamine receptors. By contrast, the cathepsin D mRNA is up-regulated in tangle containing cells (Ginsberg et al., 2000).

The potential importance of the mitochondria and oxidative stress in AD has been demonstrated by treating brain synaptosomes and cultured astrocytes with Aβ peptides. Treatment of a nucleate and mitochondria-rich cortical synaptosomes with Aβ, Fe^{2+}, or the complex II inhibitor 3-nitropropionic acid (3NP) reduced glucose and glutamate uptake, reduced mitochondrial ΔΨ, increased mitochondrial ROS generation, and stimulated expression of the stress proteins HAP70, HSP60, and GRP78. Moreover, the deleterious effects of these agents were substantially reduced in dietary restricted animals (Guo et al., 2000). Amyloid precursor protein (APP) binds to heme oxygenase-2 (HO-2). The heme oxygenases degrade bilirubin to generate an anti-oxidant and carbon monoxide (CO). The binding of APP to HO-2 inhibits its anti-oxidant effects, and this inhibition is greatly accentuated if the APP harbors familial AD mutations (Takahashi et al., 2000; Takahashi and Snyder, 2000). Treatment of cortical astrocytes with Aβ peptides induces HO-1 which degrades heme and results in the sequestration of non heme iron by the mitochondria and the activation of the mtPTP. These astrocyte effects are inhibited by concurrent treatment with dexamethasone, which suppresses HO-1 induction, and ciclosporin A, which stabilizes the mtPTP (Ham and Schipper, 2000). The induction of HO-1 subsequently results in the induction of the MnSOD, and this induction can be blocked by anti-oxidants including ascorbic acid, melatonin, and reservation (Frankel et al., 2000). These results directly link Aβ peptide toxicity to mitochondrial oxidative stress and the activation of the mtPTP, at least in part through the mediation of HO-1. HO-1 is a stress response protein that degrades heme into CO plus biliverdin. Biliverdin, in turn, is converted to bilirubin which has free radical scavenging properties. CO is thought to bind and inhibit mitochondrial

COX, blocking the ETC and increasing mitochondrial ROS production. The degradation of the heme releases iron, which appears to be taken up by the mitochondria through the mtPTP. The excess intra-mitochondrial iron then stimulates ·OH production *via* the Fenton reaction, and the increased mitochondrial oxidative stress is compensated by the induction of the MnSOD. While the reason for the specific toxicity of the Aβ peptides for the CA1 layer of the hippocampus is not yet clear, one possibility could lie with the cell and tissue-specific modulation of the mtPTP in both iron uptake and the induction of apoptosis. Such regulation would require the tissue specific expression of a protein that interacts with the mtPTP. Such a protein is PRAX-1, which is expressed at high levels in the CA1 neurons and specifically binds to the mitochondrial benzodiazepine receptor (MBR) of the mtPTP. PRAX-1 is a 1857 amino acid texture protein that links two MBRs and thus mtPTPs together through their C-terminal peptides. Moreover, PRAX-1 has a long N-terminal end that contains three proline-rich domains, two glutamate-rich domains, a *src* homology 3 domain, and mitochondrial-targeting sequence and three nuclear-targeting signals. Thus PRAX-1 has all of the characteristics that might be expected for a protein coordinated the actions of the mtPTP with other structures in the CA1 cells (Galiegue et al., 1999).

AD associated with mtDNA mutations

If the mitochondrial plays an important role in AD, then one might expect that the some mtDNA sequence variants might influence the onset and progression of PD. This hypothesis is supported by studies indicating that the probability of inheriting AD from the mother is 1.7 to 3.6 time more likely than inheriting the disease from the father (Duara et al., 1993; Edland et al., 1996). This strong maternal bias in transmission of AD suggests that some mtDNA variants may be risk factors for AD. This concept has been supported by showing that the mitochondrial OXPHOS defects AD patients can be transferred with the cytoplasm in transmitochondrial cybrids (Ghosh et al., 1999).

One MtDNA variant associated with AD is an A to G mutation in the tRNA^{Gln} gene at np 4336. This variant was found in 5.2% of AD and PD patients (3.2% AD, 6.8% AD + PD, and 3% PD), but between 0.4 and 0.7% of controls (Shoffner et al., 1993a). In one confirmatory study, the np 4336 mutant was found in 6% of AD patients and 0.3% of controls (Cortopassi and Hutchin, 1994), and in the other this mutation was found in 3.6% AD and 8.7% PD cases but in 0 of 100 controls (Egensperger et al., 1997). By contrast, one report did not find the np 4336 mutation in either their patient or control population (Mayr-Wohlfart et al., 1997) and in a second study found that the np 4336 mutation was at a lower frequency in their AD patients (0.6%) than their controls (4%) (Wragg et al., 1995). Not surprisingly, these Caucasian variants have not been found in a survey of Japanese AD patients (Tanno et al., 1998). In the initial survey of AD and PD patient mtDNAs, several additional variants were found including a missense mutation in ND1 at np 3397, a 16 S rRNA mutation, and an insertion in the 12 S rRNA gene at np 956–965 (Shoffner et al., 1993a) (Tables 11.1 and 4). A mitochondrial role in AD was further corroborated by the demonstration of a 15-fold elevated cortical somatic mtDNA mutation level in AD brains versus age matched controls (Corral-Debrinski et al., 1994). However, this elevation of somatic mtDNA rearrangements has not be confirmed in some other studies (Bonilla et al., 1999; Chang et al., 2000). One of these later studies may have failed to detect the increase in mtDNA deletions because they examined patients over age 70 years of age (Chang et al., 2000), and the mtDNA deletions are lost in older patients presumably due to the apoptotic destruction of the cells with the highest proportion of deletions.

A mtDNA A-to-G transition in the ND2 gene at np 5460 variants has also been reported to be associated with AD (Lin et al., 1992), but was subsequently found to be a polymorphism (Petruzzella et al., 1992; Kosel et al., 1994; Schnopp et al., 1996). Regional sequencing of the mtDNAs of French Canadian AD patients and controls found one mtDNA lineage that was at increased risk for AD. This lineage harbored the cytb 15812 amino acid polymorphism (Chagnon et al., 1999), which has been shown is a maker for the Caucasian mtDNA haplogroup J (Torroni et al., 1994b; 1996b). The complete sequence of two other mtDNAs of AD patients have been reported, one harboring this mtDNAs haplotype and another harboring the np 4336 mutation (Brown et al., 1996).

METAPHYSEAL CHONDRODYSPLASIA OR CARTILAGE-HAIR HYPOPLASIA DUE TO RNASE MRP MUTATIONS

Metaphyseal chondrodysplasia or cartilage-hair hypoplasia (CHH) (MIM #250250) is an autosomal recessive disorder associated with disproportionate short stature, hypoplastic hair, ligamentous laxity, defective immunity, hypoplastic anemia, and neuronal dysplasia of the intestine. These problems can be manifest as congenital megacolon (Hirschsprung's disease) and predisposition to lymphomas and other cancers. The disease is remarkable in its clinical variability within and between pedigrees. This disease is the result of mutations in the RNA component of the mitochondrial RNase *MRP*, a gene transcribed by RNA polymerase III and located on chromosome 9p13 (Table 11.3). Two classes of mutations have been identified: deletions between the promoter and the transcription start site which result in null mutants and base substitutions in the structure RNA. Four structural mutations have been identified, two which alter bases in single strand loops and a base substitution and a two base insertion that affect double stranded components of the RNA (Ridanpaa et al., 2001). The pathophysiology of this disease is currently unknown, since the RNAse MRP functions in both the nucleolus and in processing the mtDNA L-strand transcript to generate primers for mtDNA L-strand synthesis. However, it is interesting that many of the symptoms associated with this disease are also see in other mitochondrial diseases. Hence, it is possible that mitochondrial deficiency may play an important role in this disease process.

MULTIFACTORIAL DISEASES AND THE MTDNA

Certain multifactorial diseases may also have a mtDNA component. Several common multifactorial diseases including diabetes mellitus, epilepsy, and stroke have already been correlated with a mtDNA defects. Other diseases have been suggested to have a mitochondrial component based on family studies and or genetic epidemiological analysis.

Genetic epidemiological studies have also revealed a maternal bias in the transmission of epilepsy and seizures (Ottman et al., 1985). In one study population, individuals with seizures up to age 25 years had affected mothers in 8.7% of cases, but affected fathers in 2.4%. Furthermore, the earlier the seizures occurred in the parent, the more likely that seizures would occur in the child (Ottman et al., 1988). Since seizures are common clinical presentations of mtDNA tRNA mutations such as MTTL1*MELAS 3243G and MTTK*MERRF8344G, it would seem logical that additional mtDNA protein synthesis mutations might contribute to seizures.

Hypertension, stroke, and migraine might also be affected by mtDNA mutations. Migraine and stroke are common presentations form tDNA protein synthesis mutations such as MTTL1*MELAS3243G (Shoffner and Wallace, 1995). Moreover, histological analysis of MTTL1*MELAS3243G patient blood vessels has revealed marked morphological changes in vascular endothelial and smooth muscle cells, and increase numbers of enlarged mitochondria with abnormal crystalline arrays (Ohama et al., 1987; Sakuta and Nonaka, 1989; Goto et al., 1992a; Tokunaga et al., 1993). Comparable strongly SDH-positive and COX-negative blood vessels have also been observed for the MTTK*MERRF 8344G mutation (Hasegawa et al., 1993). Since inhibition of the respiratory chain is known to increase oxygen radical production (Bandy and Davison, 1990; Wallace, 1992a; 1992b), and oxygen radicals are known to inactivate the vasodilator NO (Nakazono et al., 1991; Seccombe et al., 1994), it is logical that mtDNA mutations could contribute to increased blood pressure.

MtDNA mutations may also play a role in psychiatric disorders. Two independent patients with progressive external ophthalmoplegia associated with multiple deletion syndrome have been reported to have affective disorder including depression, apathy, fatigue, and insomnia (Ciafaloni et al., 1991) and severe psychiatric disturbance principally involving depression and irritability was observed in several members of the large LHON plus neurological disease pedigree (Wallace, 1970) subsequently found to harbor the MTND6*LHON14484C and MTND1*LHON4160C mutations (Howell et al., 1991b). An extensive genetic epidemiological analysis of bipolar affective disorder (BPAD) pedigrees revealed that there was a higher than expected frequency of affected mothers of probands, a 2.3 to 2.8-fold increased risk of illness for maternal relatives, and a 1.3 to 2.5-fold increased risk of illness for offspring of affected mothers. Moreover, ten pedigrees were observed in which disease transmission was almost exclusively matrilineal. However, sequencing of the mtDNA from these pedigrees did not reveal a common mtDNA mutation to which BPAD could be ascribed (McMahon et al., 1995; 2000).

Somatic mtDNA mutations in degenerative diseases, cancer and aging

A common feature of many mtDNA diseases is that they have a delayed onset and they progress. Since patients born with base substitution mutations more or less retain the heteroplasmic genotype they are born with, it is unclear why expression should be delayed. We have hypothesized that the reason for the delay is that most inherited mitochondria mutations are insufficient to suppress mitochondrial OXPHOS enough to cross the expression thresholds. However, subsequent accumulation of somatic mutations in post-mitotic tissues exacerbates the inherited OXPHOS defect and ultimately leads to phenotypic expression. Rearrangements with the accumulation of both mtDNA base substitution and rearrangement mutations in post-mitotic tissues with age, consistent with this hypothesis

mitochondrial OXPHOS enzyme levels have been observed to decline with age. Hence, somatic mtDNA mutations may be important in both the onset and progression of mtDNA diseases as well as the aging and senescence process (Wallace, 1992a; 1992b; 1995a).

AGE-RELATED ACCUMULATION OF SOMATIC MTDNA MUTATIONS

The age-related accumulation of somatic mtDNA mutations in post-mitotic human tissues correlates with the age-related decline in mitochondrial OXPHOS enzymes. OXPHOS enzyme activities have been shown to decline with age in human and primate skeletal muscle (Cooper et al., 1992; Torroni et al., 1993b; Boffoli et al, 1994) liver (Yen et al., 1989) and brain (Bowling et al., 1993). The common 5 kb (4977 np) deletion has been quantified in these same tissues (Cortopassi and Arnheim, 1990) and shown to accumulate with age in skeletal muscle (Simonetti et al., 1992; Lezza et al, 1994), heart (Corral-Debrinski et al., 1991; 1992b; Hayakawa et al., 1993), extraocular muscle (Muller-Hocker et al., 1993), the basal ganglia and cerebral cortex of the brain (Corral-Debrinski et al., 1992a; Soong et al., 1992), and other tissues (Cortopassi et al., 1992; Zhang et al., 1992). The highest levels of the common deletion are found in the brain, where deletion levels increase over 10,000-fold from young to old individuals with maximum levels of the 5 kb deletion exceeding 10% in the basal ganglia of 80 year olds and 2–3% in the cortex. By contrast, less than 0.0001% of the 5 kb deletion accumulates with age in the human cerebellum (Corral-Debrinski et al., 1992a; Soong et al., 1992; Hamblet and Castora, 1995) (Figure 11.12).

The accumulation of the 5 kb deletion appears to be but the "tip-of-the-iceberg." Using long-extension PCR (Cheng et al., 1994) to amplify the entire mtDNA in a single fragment, skeletal muscle mtDNAs from subjects under 40 years of age were found to generate virtually all full-length mtDNA molecules. By contrast, skeletal muscle mtDNAs of subjects older than age 75 years of age gave very little full-length molecules, but instead gave a wide variety of smaller length PCR products suggesting extensive mtDNA rearrangement (Melov et al., 1995) (Figure 11.13). Similar results were obtained in a second less extensive study (Reynier and Malthiery, 1995). In an attempt to estimate the amount of rearrangement mtDNA in skeletal muscle, undigested mtDNA was run on agarose gels and analyzed by Southern blotting and hybridization with a total mtDNA probe. Parallel lanes included CPEO-KSS patient DNAs with known levels of the 5 kb deletion. The

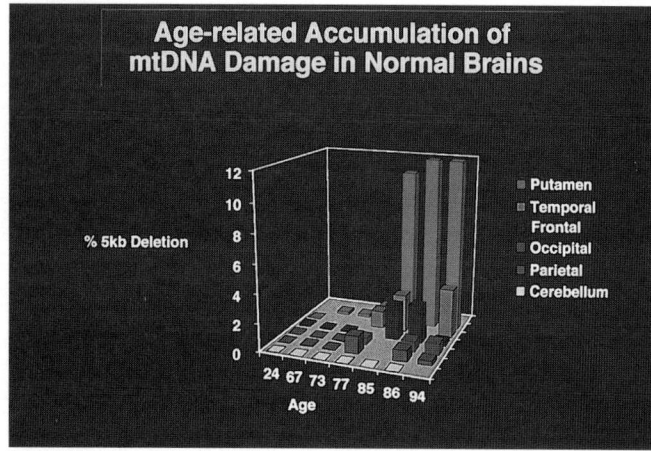

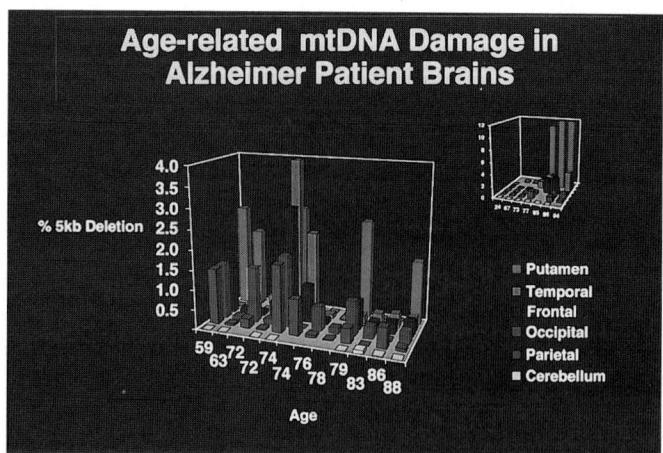

Fig. 11.12. Levels of the common 5-kb deletion in different regions of the brains of normal controls and Alzheimer's disease patients Normal individuals (left-hand panel) experience an exponential increase in mtDNA deletions in the cortex and putamen after age 75 years. AD patients (right-hand panel). have high levels of deletion in the cortex prior to age 75 which are subsequently lost after age 75 years, possibly due to apoptosis (Reproduced from Corral-Debrinski et al., 1992a, 1994). (See Plate 11.2.)

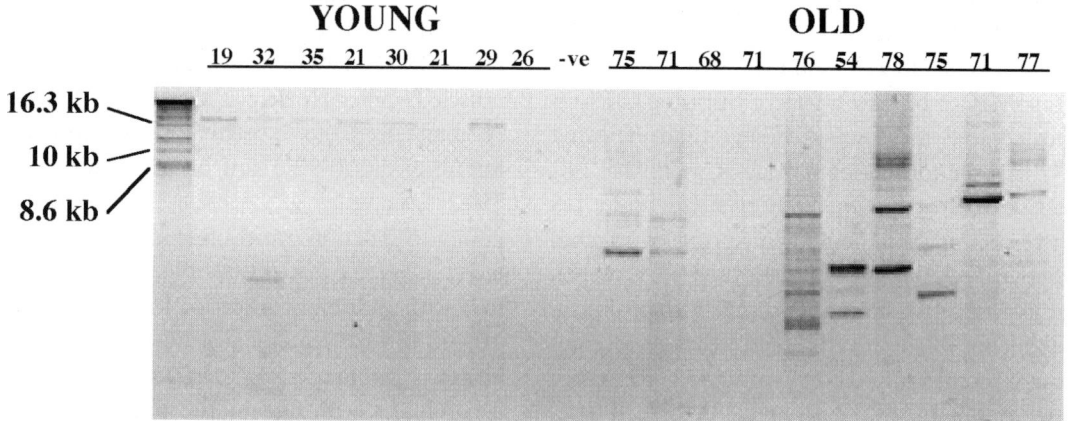

Fig. 11.13. Increased mtDNA rearrangements in human skeletal muscle with aging. The individual designations and the ages of the subjects are given above each lane. Each lane contains the long extension-polymerase chain reaction (LX-PCR) products of the individual using PCR primers located within the MTCYB gene separated by 333 nucleotide pairs, and with the 3′ ends pointing away from each other. Normal mtDNAs give a 16.3 kb product, but rearranged molecules are shorter. The LX-PCR products were separated by field-inversion gel electrophoresis, transferred to Hybaid N filters, and hybridized to digoxigenin0-labeled, full-length, mtDNA probe. Melov et al. (1995), Reproduced from Nucl Acid Res 23: 4122–4126. © Oxford University Press.

Southern blots from younger subjects gave complex patterns indicating that muscle mtDNA must harbor a wide range of mtDNA conformations including different levels of super-coiled, nicked, and concatenated molecules. In addition, the two KSS-CPEO samples had two extra bands, one migrating slightly faster than the linearized 16.5 kb mtDNA at 11.5 kb, consistent with lineralized deleted mtDNA; and the other migrating faster than any of the slower migrating super-coiled, nicked, and concatenated molecule bands and probably representing super-coiled, or nicked deleted mtDNA. The muscle mtDNAs of the old subjects had all of the same bands as the younger subjects, but in addition all of these samples had an additional diffuse band in the same region as the patient's super-coiled or nicked rearranged mtDNA. This suggests that elderly individuals may accumulate a significant level of heterogeneously rearranged mtDNA molecules (Melov et al., 1995). This same phenomenon has been observed in mouse, where long extension PCR revealed increased mtDNA in those rearrangements in old mouse hearts, but not in those of young mouse. Southern blots of undigested mtDNA revealed the accumulation of a novel mtDNA band which is recent in old but not young animals. Moreover, this band is eliminated by caloric restriction (Melov et al., 1998). Similar age-related accumulation of mtDNA rearrangements has been documented in chimp heart (Melov et al., 1997).

In addition to mtDNA rearrangements, base substitutions also accumulate with age in post-mitotic tissues. However, the specific mtDNA mutations differ between tissues. Significant accumulations of the pathologic MTTK*MERRF 8344G, MTTL1*MELAS 3243G, and MTTG*CIP010006G mutations have been reported in old but not young individuals detected by allele-specific PCR (Munscher et al., 1993a; 1993b; Rieger et al., 1993). However, more specific and sensitive analytical techniques have failed to substantiate the accumulation of the mutations (Murdock et al., 2000). A more general survey of mtDNA base substitutions in brain using denaturing gradient gels electrophoresis (DGGE), cloning, and sequencing revealed a spectrum of point mutations, and single base insertions and deletions in the D-loop, with 35–41% of the molecules differing in at least one position. Heteroplasmic mutants were much less common in coding regions. Point mutations were observed to increase 2.5-fold and insertion-deletions tenfold between ages 28 and 96–99 years. Two distinctive control region base substitution mutations were T146C and T195C (Jazin et al., 1995). Using a similar technique to analyze the mtDNAs from diploid fibroblasts cultured from individuals of various ages also revealed distinctive control region variants including T146C, T152C, T195C, A249G, T285C, A368G, 383i, and T414G. The most prevalent variant was T414G located at the *Tfam* binding site adjacent to LSP. This variant was found in 50% of the fibroblast cultures derived from patients over 65, but not seen in the cultures of younger individuals. In some individuals, the percentage of mutant mtDNAs excluded 50% (Michikawa et al., 1999). Using a sensitive and specific protein nucleic acid (PNA) detection system, this mutation was detected in skeletal muscle of individuals 35 years old, but surprisingly was not detected in any of the DNA samples from the brains of subjects up to 95 year old (Murdock et al., 2000). Hence, these mutations appear to be tissue specific.

Analysis of the distribution of somatic mtDNA mutations in aging skeletal muscle indicates that individual mutations are regionally localized and thus may be clonally amplified, just as CPEO-KSS rearrangement mutations are differentially distributed along muscle fibers. Histological analysis of muscle tissues from old subjects has revealed periodic COX-positive and negative regions (Muller-Hocker, 1990; Muller Hocker et al., 1992). Each COX-negative region was found through in situ hybridization to contain either a specific mtDNA deletion clone or to be deficient in mtDNA (Muller-Hocker et al., 1993). Similar analysis of individual cardiomyocytes from human hearts has indicated that individual cells have high levels of specific mtDNA rearrangements, while other cells have only normal mtDNA (Khrapko et al., 1999). This implies that individual somatic mtDNA mutations arise spontaneously and randomly in cells, but once they occur, they are selectively replicated in that all result in respiratory deficiency. This replication phase would be exponential and might explain why the frequency of specific mtDNA deletions appears to increase exponentially with time (Corral-Debrinski et al., 1991; 1992a; 1992b; Simonetti et al., 1992).

The origin of the high rate of mtDNA mutations is unknown. However, one likely source of new mutations is the generation and subsequent resolution of DNA oxidation products including thymine glycols and 8-hydroxy-2′-deoxyquanosine (8-OHdG) (Corral-Debrinski et al., 1992a; Soong et al., 1992; Hamblet and Castora, 1995; Ozawa, 1995). The 8-OHdG product is the most common form of oxidative DNA damage, though it may not be the main mtDNA mutagen, since mtDNA base substitutions show a 20-fold bias toward transitions over transversions (Brown et al, 1982) while 8-OHdG is thought to increase the transversion rate (Wood et al., 1990; Cheng et al., 1992; Tudek et al., 1993). MtDNA oxidation products might also cause replication errors increasing the rate of mtDNA rearrangement mutations.

The mtDNA seems to be particularly prone to oxygen radical damage. The mitochondrial respiratory chain is the major source of reactive oxygen species generation, and the mtDNA is attached to the mitochondrial inner membrane in close proximity to the OXPHOS complexes, it (Richter, 1988). This preferential mtDNA oxidative damage has been confirmed in several studies. In young rats, the mtDNA has been reported to contain approximately 16-fold more 8-OHdG than does nDNA, and this increases another threefold in older rats (Chung et al, 1992b; Ames et al., 1993). Current estimates place the differential 8-OHdG levels of the mtDNA at tenfold above the nDNA (Richter, 1988). Similarly, mtDNA 8-OHdG levels in human brain were tenfold higher than nDNA and increased with age (Mecocci et al., 1994). Levels of 8-OHdG have been reported to increase with age in the mtDNAs of human diaphragm, heart muscle (Hayakawa et al., 1992, 1993) and brain (Mecocci et al., 1993) and 8-OHdG and the 7.4 kb deletion to increase with age by the same exponential kinetics in human hearts (Hayakawa et al., 1993; Ames et al., 1995).

The preferential accumulation of oxidation damage in the mtDNA might imply that the mtDNA is deficient in DNA repair. While the mtDNA cannot repair thymine dimers (Clayton et al., 1974), the mitochondria do contain uracil DNA glycosylase (Anderson and Friedberg, 1980),

AP endonuclease (Tomkinson et al., 1988) and enzymes to repair pyrimidine glycols (Tomkinson et al., 1990). A variety of other repair activities have been detected by treating cultured cells with DNA damaging agents, purifying genomic DNA, digesting with endonucleases specific for each type of damage, and using Southern blots of alkaline agarose gels to monitor the removal of the endonuclease sensitive sites from post-treatment cell. By this procedure, it has been found that the mitochondria cannot repair pyrimidine dimers, but they can repair 8-OHdG and adducts for 4NQO and monofunctional alkylating agents. The mitochondria cannot repair cis-platinum intra-strand cross-links, consistent with an absence of thymidine dimer repair, but can repair cis-platinum inter-strand cross-links suggesting recombinational repair (Bohr, 1991; LeDoux et al., 1992, 1993; Pettepher et al., 1991; Pirsel and Bohr, 1993; Snyderwine and Bohr, 1992; Wallace et al., 1995b). It is surprising that the mitochondria would retain active repair systems, yet experience such a high degree of preferential damage. Presumably, the level of repair is set to be sufficient to keep the mtDNAs intact until after reproductive age, at which point sustaining the parents tissues is no longer necessary.

IDIOPATHIC SIDEROBLASTIC ANEMIA

Somatic mtDNA mutations may arise in specific cell types and result in distinctive clinical presentations. One possible example of such a phenomenon is idiopathic sideroblastic anemia. Sideroblastic anemia is characterized by the inadequate formation of heme and the excessive accumulation of iron in erythroblastoid mitochondria. A common finding is anemia associated with ring sideroblasts, which are also seen in Pearsons marrow/pancreas syndrome. Sideroblastic anemia is associated with the accumulation of protoporphyrin IX and the deposition of Fe^{3+} in the mitochondria. To make heme, iron must be in the reduced Fe^{2+} form to be inserted in protoporphyrin IX by ferrochelatase, and the reduction of iron occurs via the ETC. Hence, it has been proposed that sideroblastic anemia may be the result of mitochondrial defects (Gattermann et al., 1997). This concept has been supported the discovery of two novel mtDNA COI missense mutations in patients with sideroblastic anemia. The first patient was found to have a T6721C mutation which changed a highly conserved methionine 273 to a threonine residue. This mutation was heteroplasmic in the myeloid lineage, but was not present in other tissues of the patient or in the mother or daughter. The second patient was found to have a T6742C mutation which converted the conserved isoleucine 280 to a threo-

nine residue. This mutation was also heteroplasmic. Hence, it would appear that these somatic mutations arose in the bone marrow can resulted in the physiological malfunction of the descendent cells (Gattermann et al., 1997).

ISCHEMIC HEART DISEASE AND DILATED CARDIOMYOPATHY

Ischemic heart disease results from the development of atherosclerotic plagues on the coronary arteries of the heart. When the arteries constrict, the plaques occlude the artery blocking blood flow to the heart and starving the heart mitochondria for oxygen (ischemia). In the absence of oxygen, the electron transport chain stops and since fatty acids and hence reducing equivalents are abundant, the electron carriers become fully reduced. On dilation of the coronary artery, blood flows back into the heart supplying oxygen (reperfusion). At this point, electrons contained in reduced ubisemiquinone can be donated directly to oxygen to give a burst of superoxide anion which is rapidly converted to H_2O_2 and ·OH. Within one minute of reperfusion in experimental systems, 95% of the ·OH is located in the mitochondria (Das et al., 1989). These cyclic bursts of oxygen radicals damage heart mitochondrial membranes, proteins, and DNA.

A high degree of mtDNA damage in chronically ischemic hearts has been confirmed by quantifying the common 5 kb deletion. Individuals with dilated cardiomyopathy due to chronic ischemia-reperfusion were found to have between 8 and 2200-fold more mtDNA deletion than age-matched controls. Moreover, the levels of the 7436 bp and 10423 bp deletions went up concurrently with the 5 kb deletion and the ischemic hearts showed a coordinate induction of the nuclear OXPHOS genes for ANT1, ANT3, and ATPsynβ and the mtDNA genes for MTCYB, MTRNR (12 S rRNA) and MTRNR2 and (16 S rRNA) (Corral-Debrinski et al., 1991; 1992b). These data suggest that chronic cardiac ischemia and reperfusion results in a severe destruction of the cardiac mtDNAs and probably a decline in bioenergetic capacity. This in turn is compensated for by the induction of mitochondrial biogenesis. Elevated mtDNA 5 kb deletion has also been observed in patients with idiopathic dilated cardiomyopathy (Corral-Debrinski et al., 1991) and multiple different rearrangements were detected by whole genome-PCR amplification in 18 out of 40 dilated cardiomyopathy endomyocardial biopsies (Li et al., 1995c) and in myocardium (Reynier and Malthiery, 1995). Similarly, increased rearrangement and base substitution mutations have been reported in the hearts of sudden infant death syndrome children (Gerbitz and Jaksch, 1994) and 212 different deletions have been found in the heart of a child with familial dilated cardiomyopathy versus only five in a control heart. Furthermore, both this patient and a patient with hypertrophic cardiomyopathy were found to have a 12 S rRNA A-to-G transition at np 827 which alters a conserved nucleotide (Ozawa, 1995). Consequently, it is possible that mitochondrial energy depletion may be an important factor in cardiac failure.

NEURODEGENERATIVE DISEASES: PD, HD AND AD

Since PD, HD and AD have all been associated with mitochondrial OXPHOS defects and increased ROS production, it is possible that they might also be associated with an increased mtDNA somatic mutation rate. If this is true, then it is possible that the premature accumulation of mtDNA mutations might contribute to these diseases and may even be a major factor in the pathophysiology of these diseases. The examine this possibility somatic mtDNA mutations have been sought in these diseases in a variety of studies.

Parkinson's disease and Huntington disease

The role of somatic mtDNA mutations in PD is currently unclear. Testing for the presence of the 5 kb deletion in five PD patients, ages 51–77, and six controls, ages 38–73, revealed detectable deletion in the striatum while all five PD patients, while only the two oldest controls had detectable striatum deletions (Ikebe et al., 1990). Quantification of the striatal 5 kb deletion levels in a 73 year old patient and a 38 year old control revealed a tenfold higher deletion levels (Ozawa et al., 1990), but this difference was probably due to age differences. Analysis of the 5 kb deletion in substantia nigra (Mann et al., 1992b) and in skeletal muscle (DiDonato et al., 1993) failed to reveal a difference. Unfortunately, none of these studies took into account the effects of neuronal loss by apoptosis.

The 5 kb deletion has also been detected in the platelets of older PD patients, but in age-matched controls (Sandy et al, 1993), though this deletion was not detected in the platelets of early-onset PD patients (Shan et al., 1995). Hence, it remains unclear whether the mtDNA somatic mutation rate is increased in PD.

MtDNA deletion levels have been observed to be elevated in the cortical regions of HD patients. The 5 kb deletion levels of the frontal and temporal cortical lobes of 22 Huntington's patients were found to be increased 5 and 11-fold, respectively, relative to age-matched controls. The occipital lobe of the cortex and the putamen were not significantly different, though the lack of deletions in the HD putamens could reflect the severe neuronal loss of the basal ganglia neurons associated with terminal HD (Horton et al., 1995). In another study, analysis of the 5 kb deletion levels in the putamen, cortex, and caudate of three HD patients, ages 36–39, and three controls, ages 27–42, revealed no difference in the caudate, while the HD patients had 1000-fold less 5 kb deletion in the putamen and cortex than to controls (Chen et al., 1995a). Such a striking reduction in brain somatic mtDNA mutations might best be explained by the selective apoptosis and loss of cells with the highest levels of mtDNA deletion. Hence, the overall percentage of mutant mtDNA would decline, but at the expense of extensive cell loss in the tissue (Kokoszka et al., 2001).

ALZHEIMER DISEASE

As mentioned above, Alzheimer disease and movement disorders have also been associated with OXPHOS defects and specific mtDNA mutations. Since defects in OXPHOS would inhibit the electron transport chain, this could reduce electron flow, and increase oxygen radical generation, possibly causing increased somatic mtDNA mutation rates in selected regions of the brain. Consistent with this hypothesis, the mtDNAs of AD brains have been found to have 20-fold higher 8-OHdG levels than nDNA, and there is a significant threefold increase in 8-OHdG levels in the mtDNAs of AD parietal cortex relative to controls (Mecocci et al., 1994). This increase in oxidative damage has been correlated with an approximately 15-fold increase in the 5 kb deletion in the cortical regions of AD patients who died prior to age 75 years, relative to age matched controls; but a fivefold decrease of cortical deletions of patients who died after age 75 years of age, relative to age-matched controls (Corral-Debrinski et al., 1994). This suggests that many Alzheimer patients have an elevated mtDNA somatic mutation rate, and when the neurons accumulate sufficient mutant mtDNAs, they die resulting in loss of the mutant mtDNAs and associated dementia.

SOMATIC MTDNA MUTATIONS IN OTHER COMPLEX DISEASE

Somatic mtDNA mutations are being sought in the context of an increasing number of degenerative conditions. MtDNA deletions have been reported to be increased in aging and seen exposed skin (Pang et al., 1994; Yang et al., 1994), in the livers of alcoholics (Fromenty et al., 1995), in the ovaries of postmenopausal women (Kitagawa et al., 1993) and in reduced sperm mobility (Kao et al., 1995). These observations support the hypothesis that the accumulation of somatic mtDNA mutations may be associated with a wide range of degenerative processes.

LATE-ONSET MITOCHONDRIAL MYOPATHY, INCLUSION BODY MYOSITIS AND POLYMYALGIA RHEUMATICA

Late-onset mitochondrial myopathy (LOMM), inclusion body myositis (IBM), and polymyalgia rheumatic (PMR) appear to be degenerative muscle diseases associated with an increase frequency of somatic mtDNA mutations. LOMM is associated with late-onset (> 69 years of age) insidious proximal muscle (limb-girdle) weakness with fatigability, mainly in the lower extremities, and only subtle craniobulbar involvement such as ptosis. Histological analysis of muscle revealed increased numbers of RRFs (0.7%), SDH-hyperreactive fibers (2%) and COX-negative fibers (1.7%), with some patients having 5% of their fibers SDH-hyperreactive or COX-negative and with 80% of the SDH-hyperactive fibers being COX-negative. MtDNA analysis by Southern blot ruled out a common mtDNA deletion, but PCR amplification revealed a variety of different deletions at low frequencies. *In situ* hybridization of mtDNA transcripts revealed that many of the fibers had large accumulations of rRNA and mRNA transcripts, and most of these fibers were COX-negative and SDH-hyperreactive. Moreover, most fibers with accumulations of rRNA, ND2 and COI mRNAs, had much lower levels of COII and COIII mRNA consistent with mtDNA deletions. ^{31}P-Magnetic Resonance Spectroscopy showed that the patients had an average muscle PCr/Pi ratio of 6.4 ($\pm$ 1.2) mM, significantly less than controls at 9.1 ($\pm$ 1.5) mM. These data are consistent with an increase frequency of random mtDNA mutations in the skeletal muscle of these patients. Approximately 27% of the myopathies diagnosed in patients over 69 have this defect (Johnston et al., 1995).

IBM seems to have a very similar etiology to LOMM. IBM is a chronic inflammatory muscle disease with an insidious onset between 50 and 70 years of age. It is associated with distal muscle weakness in the upper extremities and proximal muscle weakness in the lower extremities, with poor response to anti-inflammatory drugs. Histological analysis of muscle reveals inflammatory infiltrates of T-lymphocytes in muscle fibers, the presence of "rimmed vacuoles," RRFs and COX-negative fibers. Southern blot analysis of mtDNAs only rarely shows detectable rearrangements (Oldfors et al., 1993), but PCR reveals multiple heterogeneous mtDNA rearrangements with the 5 kb deletion being commonly found (Oldfors et al., 1995). COX-negative and SDH-hyperreactive fibers are present in all patients and range in frequency from 0.5 to 5%. *In situ* hybridization shows that these fibers have high levels of ND2 mRNA but generally low levels of ND6 and/or MTCYB mRNAs consistent with the presence of mtDNA deletions (Oldfors et al., 1993; 1995).

PMR may also have a similar etiology. PMR is associated with stiffness and pain chiefly in the scapular and pelvic girdles, associated with inflammatory syndrome which responds to corticosteroid treatment. Analysis of muscle biopsies from PMR patients have revealed mitochondrial OXPHOS defects and RRFs. Long extension PCR analysis of the deltoid muscle mtDNAs from ten patients, ages 51 to 90 years, revealed that all contained multiple deletions, with the number of bands ranging from two to 15. No deletions were found in three control muscles, ages 39, 40, and 47 years of age, though several deletions were found in 81 and 84 year old controls (Reynier and Malthiery, 1995; Reynier et al., 1994b). These data suggest that LOMM, IBM, and PMR may all be the product of increased muscle mtDNA mutation rates.

SOMATIC MUTATIONS IN CANCER

Somatic mtDNA mutations have also been identified in various solid tumors. The first definitively pathologic mtDNA mutation to be identified in a cancer cell was a 264 bp deletion in the ND1 subunit of a renal cell carcinoma. This deletion removed np 3323 to 3588 and was flanked on both sides by a CCT repeat. The in-frame deletion resulted in a ND1 mtDNA of diminished size and removed amino acids 7 through to 94 of the ND1 polypeptide. Approximately 50% of the mtDNAs of the tumor were deleted, while the deletion was absent in non-tumor DNA (Horton et al., 1996).

Subsequently, a variety of mtDNA base substitutions have been found in cancer mtDNAs. Analysis of colorectal cancer cell lines revealed mtDNA mutations in seven out of 10 samples. Twelve of the mutants were present in the cell lines and tumors but not in the patients normal tissue. Eight of these were in protein coding genes and four were in rDNA genes. Eleven were base substitutions and one was a one base-pair insertion. One of the base substitutions G6264A crated a stop codon in the COI gene G121 Ter. The insertion mutation added an additional A at np 12418 in the ND5 gene resulting in a frame shift after amino acid 28 (K28 frameshift). The remaining base substitutions involved missense mutations, one each in COII and COIII, two in cytb, and one each in ND1 and ND46. There was also one mutation in the 12 S rRNA and three mutations in the 16 S rRNA. Surprisingly, 10 out of the 12 mutations were homoplasmic, suggesting that they were strongly selected in the tumor tissues. The selective advantage of these mutant mtDNAs was demonstrated by fusing tumor cell lines with mutant mtDNAs to cell lines with more normal mtDNA. Consistently, the mtDNA shifted to the mutant form, frequently within 15 to 60 days of fusion. Hence, the deleterious mtDNA mutations must have a strong intracellular advantage over the normal genomes (Polyak et al., 1998).

Somatic mtDNA mutations were sought in 14 bladder, 13 head and neck, and 14 lung tumors. This revealed 39 acquired somatic mutations in 64% of the bladder, 46% of head and neck, and 43% in lung tumors. Most of these mutations were either small changes in the control region or synonymous base substitutions in the coding region. Only four of the mutations were likely to be of functional significance. One bladder cancer had a deletion in the cytochrome b gene at np 15642 which removed seven amino acids resides Another bladder cancer had a missense mutation in ND3, T10321C, which changed a valine to an alanine residue. Two of the head and neck tumors also had novel missense mutations: C10822T changing a threonine to a methionine residue in ND1, and G11150A converting an alanine to threonine residue in the ND4 gene. Surprisingly, most of the novel mtDNA mutations were essentially homoplasmic, suggesting that the deleterious mutations were strongly selected for the cell (Fliss et al., 2000).

A study of prostate cancers also revealed mtDNA mutations. Cancerous and normal epithelia cells were collected from eight radial prostatectomy specimens using laser capture microscopy. The DNA was isolated and regions sequenced. Five of the tumors were found to harbor novel mutations which altered the amino acid sequence of mtDNA genes. One tumor was homoplasmic for a COI chain termination mutation G5949A which changed a glycine codon to a stop codon. This mutation was homoplasmic in the tumor but was not found in the patient's normal tissue. This same tumor contained two other germline missense mutations, one in cytochrome b, A14769G, which changed a conserved asparagine to a serine residue and the other in ATPase 6, T8932C, changing a proline to a serine residue. These two mutations were present in both the tumor and normal epithelia of the patient. The novel missense mutations in the COI gene of the other prostate tumors were also present in both the tumor and surrounding epithelia (Petros et al., 2001).

Nuclear mutations in mitochondrial genes have also been found in certain tumors. Autosomal dominant non-chromoffin paragangliomas (PGLs) are commonly derived from the carotid body, a highly vascular small organ located at the bifurcation of the common carotid artery in the neck. This organ plays a central role in acute adaptation to hypoxia. These tumors are inherited as autosomal dominants with variable penetrance. Three loci are known: PGL1, 2, and 3. The gene involved in PGL1 has been identified as subunit D of complex II (SDHD), which encodes the cytochrome by membrane component of complex I. A variety of mutations have been identified including non-sense mutations in the signal peptide (codons 36 and 38) and missense mutations (H102L, P81L, and D92Y). PGL1 has an unusual transmission, being inherited from affected fathers but not affected mothers, but this could not be explained by imprinting of a parental SDHD gene (Baysal et al., 2000).

The gene for PGL3 has also been identified, and this turns out to be $SDHC$, the other membrane subunit of complex II. One autosomal dominant family was found to have a germline G958A mutation, which changed the initiation codon to a stop codon. This mutation was associated with loss of heterozygosity at the other allele in all tumors (Niemann and Muller, 2000).

The pathophysiological role of these mitochondrial gene mutations is suggested by the study of the mev-1 mutant in the nematode worm $C.$ $elegans$. The mev-1 mutant affects the cytochrome b (SDHD) locus of complex II, and is thus equivalent to PGL-1. These mev-1 worms have greatly elevated levels of oxidative damage, are sensitive to oxygen, and have a 37% reduction in lifespan (Ishii et al., 1998). The reduction in lifespan can be corrected by growing the worms in the catalytic anti-oxidant EUK-134 (Melov et al., 2000). Hence, one possible consequence of the PGL1 and PGL3 mutations could be to increase mitochondrial ROS production. This would increase the mitochondria secretion of H_2O_2 which could then act as a mitogen resulting in the hyperproliferation of the cells.

The mitogen hypothesis for mitochondrial ROS has been supported in studies of prostate cancer cells in which the resident mtDNAs have been substituted with mtDNAs harboring known pathogenic mtDNA mutations. The PC-3 prostate cancer cell line was cured of its resident mtDNAs by R6G treatment and was then fused to cytoplasts carrying the ATP6 NARP T8993G mutation or its wildtype counterpart T89993T. The prostate cancer cells with the 8993G mutant mtDNAs were found to grow 50% faster than their companion cells with the wild-type 8993T mtDNA. The mutant cell lines also had a four-fold reduction in apoptosis, decreased apoptotic chromosomal degradation, and elevated cellular ROS production. Subcutaneous injection of the PC-3 cybrids into nude mice revealed that the 8993G mutant tumors grew much faster than the 8993T wild-type tumors, with the mutant giving mean tumor volumes that were ten times that of the 8993T wild-type. These data prove that partial respiratory deficiency in solid tumors greatly accelerates the tumor growth rate (Petros et al., 2001). Hence, this selective replicative advantage could readily explain the rapid segregation somatic mtDNA mutations to homoplasmy.

Since the PGL tumors and the PC-3 cybrids strongly implicate increased mitochondrial ROS production as the source of the growth stimulation, the growth advantage must be due to the mitochondrial production of H_2O_2. Hence, mutation in mtDNA or nDNA OXPHOS enzymes would stimulate cellular transformations in exactly the same way that Mox1 gene over-expression transforms NIH3T3 cells (Arnold et al., 2001; Suh et al., 1999b).

Animal models of mitochondrial disease

To investigate the pathophysiology of mitochondrial disease, mitochondrial gene mutations have been introduced into the mouse.

MOUSE MODELS OF MTDNA DISEASE

Several approaches have been used to introduce genetically distinctive mtDNAs into the mouse female germline. To date two basic procedures have been successful: (a) fusion of enucleated cell cytoplasts baring mutant mtDNA to undifferentiated mouse female stem cells, injection of the stem cell cybrids into mouse blastocysts, and implantation of the chimeric embryos into a foster mother; and (b) fusion of cytoplasts from mutant cells directly to mouse single cell embryos and implantation of the embryos into the oviduct of pseudopregnant females. The former method has permitted the creation of mouse strains baring deleterious base substitution mutations (Sligh et al., 2000), while the later has been used to create mouse strains harboring mtDNA deletions (Inoue et al., 2000).

ES cells and base substitution mutations

The first attempt to utilize the cybrid technique to introduce mutant mtDNAs into mouse stem cells involved the fusion of the cytoplasts from CAP^R B16 melanoma cells to

the teratocarcinoma cell line OTT6050. The resulting teratocarcinoma cybrids were injected into blastocysts and five chimeric animals were generated with 10–15% chimerism in various organs. However, no direct evidence was obtained that the CAP^R mtDNA was present in the transgenic mice (Watanabe et al., 1978).

More recent efforts have focused on mouse female embryonic stem (ES) cell lines. In two independent experiments, CAP^R mouse cell lines were enucleated and the cytoplasts fused to female ES cells. CAR^R ES cell cybrids were isolated, injected into blastocysts, and chimeric mice generated with tissues have low percentages of chimerism detectable levels of CAP^R mtDNAs (Levy et al., 1999; Marchington et al., 1999). In one of these studies, the CAP^S mtDNAs in the ES cells were removed prior to cytoplast fusion by treatment with R6G (Levy et al., 1999). This greatly enriched for the CAP^R mtDNAs in the ES cell cybrids, as detected using the *Mae* III and *Tai*I restriction site polymorphism generated by the CAP^R T-to-C transition at np 2433 in the 16 S rRNA gene (Blanc et al., 1981b).

These studies were extended by identifying a female ES cell that would produce fertile oocytes. The successful ES cell line CC9.3.1. was then used to recover the mtDNAs from the brain of NZB mice and introduce them into the female germline of mice which formerly harbored only the "common haplotype" mtDNA. Most inbred strains of mice from North American had the same founding female, and thus have the same mtDNA haplotype. By contrast, NZB mice were inbred in New Zealand and their mtDNAs differ from this "common haplotype" by 108 nucleotide substitutions (Ferris et al., 1982), one of which creates a *Bam*HI restriction site polymorphism. To transfer the mtDNAs of the NZB mice into cultured cells, the brain of an NZB mouse was homogenized, and the synaptic boutons with their resident mitochondria were isolated by Percoll gradient as synaptosomes. These synaptosomes were fused to the mouse mtDNA-deficient (ρ°) cell line LMEB4 (Trounce et al, 2000). Synaptosome cybrids were recovered having the LMEB4 nucleus and the NZB mtDNA, designated the LMEB4(mtNZB) cybrids (Trounce et al., 2000). Next, the LMEB4(mtNZB) cybrids were enucleated and the cytoplasts fused to R6G-treated CC9.3.1 cells. This generated the CC9.3.1 (mtNZB) cybrids which were injected into C57B1/6 (B6) embryos and mice with a high degree of chimerism generated. One female chimeric mouse, heteroplasmic for the NZB and the "common haplotype" mtDNAs, was matted with two different B6 males and the heteroplasmic mtDNAs were transferred to all of the seven and ten offspring, respectively. A female of the next generation was matted to a B6 male and transmitted the heteroplasmic mtDNAs to her seven progeny, while a heteroplasmic male mated to two B6 females did not transmit the NZB mtDNAs to any of his sixteen offspring. Hence, this experiment established that exogenous mtDNA mutations could be introduced into the female mouse germline, and subsequently be maternally transmitted through repeated generations (Sligh et al., 2000).

Using this same procedure CAP^R mtDNAs from the mouse 501–1 cell line were introduced into chimeric mice. The resulting CAP^R chimeric animals developed bilateral nuclear cataracts, reduced rod and cone excitation detected by electroretinograms (ERG), and retinal hamartomatous growths emanating from the optic nerve heads. Several of the chimeric females when matted were able to transmit the CAP^R mtDNAs to their progeny in either the homoplasmic or heteroplasmic state. The resulting CAP^R progeny either died in utero or in the neonatal period. Mice born alive exhibited striking growth retardation, progressive myopathy with myofibril disruption and loss, dilated cardiomyopathy, and abnormal heart and muscle mitochondria morphology (Sligh et al., 2000). These phenotypes are remarkably similar to those seen in the patient with the single base deletion in the anti-codon stem of the tRNA$^{Leu(UUR)}$. Hence, deleterious mtDNA protein synthesis mutations can cause mitochondrial disease in the mouse with a severity and nature analogous to those seen in humans.

Single cell embryos and rearrangement mutations

The alternative successful approach for introducing mutant mtDNAs into the mouse female germline has involved introduction of variant mtDNAs directly into mouse single cell embryos, either by microinjection of mitochondria or fusion of cytoplasts. Microinjection *Mus spretus* mitochondria of into *Mus musculus domesticus* embryos has resulted in chimeric embryos, but the mutant mtDNAs appear to be lost by replicative segregation early in pre-implantation development (Irwin et al., 1999; Pinkert et al., 1997). Fusion of cytoplasts from mouse oocytes harboring one mtDNA type (NZB/BINJ) with single cell embryos harboring a different mtDNA type (C57BL/6 or BALB/c) has resulted in heteroplasmic mice. These mice permitted the analysis of mitochondrial replicative segregation through the germline, and have revealed that heteroplasmic mixtures of the NZB and "common haplotype" mtDNAs undergo directional replicative segregation in different adult tissues. However, these animals have not been found to have an abnormal phenotype (Jenuth et al., 1996; 1997; Meirelles and Smith, 1998). Heteroplasmic animals have also been generated by fusing membrane bound karyoplasts containing a zygote nucleus and a portion of the oocyte cytoplasm with enucleated eggs (Meirelles and Smith, 1997; 1998).

These studies have been extended to include the fusion of cultured cell cytoplasts to single cell embryos. Synaptosome cybrids, heteroplasmic for a 4696 bp deletion, were enucleated and the cytoplasts fused to pronucleus-stage embryos, which were then and implanted into the oviducts of pseudopregnant females. The 4696 bp deletion used removed six tRNAs and seven structural genes. This procedure resulted in 24 animals having 6–42% deleted mtDNAs in their muscle. Females with 6–13% deleted mtDNA were mated and the rearranged mtDNAs were transmitted through three successive generations, with the percentage of deleted mtDNAs increasing with successive generations to a maximum of 90% deletion in the muscle of some animals. While mtDNA duplications were not observed in the original synaptosome cybrid cells, they were found in the in the post-mitotic tissues of the animals. This raises the possibility that the maternal transmission of the rearranged mtDNA was through a duplicated mtDNA intermediate, as proposed for the human maternally-inherited mtDNA rearrangement pedigree presenting with diabetes mellitus and deafness (Ballinger et al., 1992b; 1994). While RRFs were not observed in these animals, fibers with greater than 85% mutant mtDNAs were COX-negative, and many fibers had aggregates of subsarcolemmal mitochondria. The heart tissue of heteroplasmic animals were also a mosaic of COX-positive and COX-negative fibers, and the amount of lactic acid in peripheral blood was proportional to the amount of mutant mtDNA in the muscle tissues. Mice with predominantly mutant mtDNAs in their muscle tissue died within 200 days with systemic ischemia and enlarged kidneys with granulated surfaces and dilation of the proximal and distal renal tubules. These animals also developed high concentrations of blood urea and creatinine (Inoue et al., 2000). Hence, mtDNA deletion mutations can also cause disease in mice, but the phenotypes and inheritance patterns are somewhat different from those seen in most human mtDNA rearrangement patients.

The generation of mouse strains harboring a mtDNA base substitution or large deletion mutations now provide mouse models for a range of mtDNA diseases. However, the severity of the phenotypes that were observed in the two mouse mtDNA mutant strains prepared to date were the converse of those traditionally seen in humans. In humans, many base substitution mutations in protein synthesis genes are maternally inherited and usually are compatible with maturation to at least late childhood, while most deletion mutations are spontaneous and patients with a high percentage mutant are severely affected in childhood. The converse was seen for the mice. The CAP^R base substitution resulted in mice which were neonatal lethal, while the "deletion" mutation was maternally inherited and gave viable animals with up to 90% deleted mtDNAs. These aberrant findings could be explained in two ways. On possibility is that the mtDNA mutations introduced into the mouse are qualitatively different from those generally encountered in human families resulting in differences that are more apparent than real. For example, no clinically relevant 16 S rRNA mutation has been reported in humans, so they may be as lethal in man as they are in mouse. Also, mtDNA duplications can be maternally-inherited in humans and the mouse rearrangement may be a duplication. Hence, more analogous to the human maternally-inherited diabetes and deafness than to Pearson's marrow/pancreas syndrome. Still, this later possibility doesn't explain the high levels of rearranged mtDNAs that accumulated in the mouse nor the low level of duplicated molecules that were reported. The alternative possibility is that the mouse may be more tolerant of mitochondrial defects than humans. This alternative is supported by the mouse's greater tolerance of ANT1-deficiency (Graham et al., 1997) then is seen in human (Kaukonen et al., 2000). Many different mtDNA mutations will need to be introduced into the mouse before these alternatives can be distinguished.

MOUSE MODELS OF NDNA MITOCHONDRIAL MUTATIONS

Three different classes of nDNA-encoded mitochondrial gene mutations have now been reported for the mouse: mutations in the biosynthetic apparatus gene *Tfam*; mutations in the mitochondrial bioenergetic genes *Ant1 and Unc2*, and mutations in the mitochondrial anti-oxidant genes *GPx1* and *Sod2* (MnSOD).

Tfam-deficient mice

Genetic inactivation of the nuclear-encoded mitochondrial transcription factor, Tfam, may provide a model for the mtDNA deletion syndrome. This follows from the importance of Tfam directed transcription from the P_L promoter for the initiation of mtDNA H-strand replication.

The *Tfam* gene was inactivated in tissues by bracketing the terminal two exons of the gene with loxP sites, designated *Tfam^{loxP}*. The *Tfam* gene was then inactivated by crossing +/*Tfam^{loxP}* animals with animals bearing the *Cre*

recombinase driven by the β-actin promoter. The resulting heterozygous +/*Tfam$^-$* animals were viable and reproductively competent, while the homozygous *Tfam–/–* animals were embryonic lethals (Larsson et al., 1998). The *Tfam* heterozygous animals had a 50% reduction in *Tfam* transcripts and protein, a 34% reduction in mtDNA copy number, a 22% reduction in mitochondrial transcripts, and a partial reduction in the COI protein in heart, but not liver. The homozygous *Tfam–/–* mutant animals died between embryonic days E8.5 and E10.5, with a complete absence of Tfam protein, and either a severely reduced or a complete absence of mtDNA. The mitochondria in the *Tfam–/–* animals were enlarged with abnormal cristae and were deficient in COX but not SDH (Larsson et al., 1998).

To determine the effect of mtDNA depletion in heart and skeletal muscle, the homozygous *Tfam^{loxP}* allele was combined with the *Cre* recombinase gene driven by the mmtCPK promoter, resulting in the selective destruction of the *Tfam* genes in those tissues. While the hearts of 18.5 day embryos had reduced levels of Tfam, they appeared to be otherwise morphologically and biochemically normal. However, after birth, the mutant animals proved to be postnatal lethals, dying at a mean age of 20 days of dilated cardiomyopathy. Under anesthesia, the animals developed cardiac conduction defects with a prolongation of the PQ interval and intermittent atrioventricular block. This was associated with a reduction in Tfam protein and mtDNA transcript levels in heart and muscle, a reduction in heart mtDNA to 26% a reduction in skeletal muscle mtDNA to 60% and a reduction of respiratory complexes I and IV but not complex II. Histochemical analysis of the hearts revealed a mosaic staining pattern with some cardiomyocytes being COX-negative and SDH-hyper-reactive (Wang et al., 1999).

To examine the importance of mtDNA depletion in diabetes, the homozygous *Tfam^{loxP}* allele was combined with a rat insulin promoter driven *Cre* recombinase (*RIP-Cre*). This resulted in the deletion of the *Tfam* gene in most of the β-cells of the pancreas by seven days of age. The Tfam-depleted β-cells were found to have greatly reduced COX staining, with normal SDH staining, and to contain highly abnormal giant mitochondria. The mutant mice developed diabetes with increased blood glucose, both fasting and non-fasting, starting at about five weeks. They subsequently showed a progressive decline in β-cell mass, reaching a minimum at 14 weeks, and a decreased ratio of endocrine to exocrine pancreatic tissue. Thus, mitochondrial diabetes progresses through two stages. The younger animals were diabetic because their β-cells could not secrete insulin, but the older animals were diabetic because they lost many of their β-cells. The secondary loss of the β-cells did not seem to be the product of apoptosis, however, since the number of TUNEL positive cells were not increased in the mutant animals. The mitochondria of the mutant islets showed decreased hyperpolarization and the intracellular Ca^{2+} oscillations were severely dampened in response to glucose, but not to K^+-induced Ca^{2+} modulation (Silva et al., 2000). These data support a central role for the mitochondria in the β-cell signal transduction pathway leading to insulin release. Glucose up-take provides substrate for increased mitochondrial ATP production raising the cellular ATP/ADP ratio. The elevated ATP/ADP ratio causes the closure of the ATP-dependent K^+-channels, depolarizing the plasma membrane. Depolarization of the plasma membrane opens the voltage-dependent L-type Ca^{2+} channels which increases intracellular Ca^{2+} and stimulates the exocytosis of the insulin containing secretory granules. Mitochondrial defects which inhibit oxidation of pyruvate thus inhibit ATP production and block insulin release. Hence mitochondrial function must be a central factor in the regulation of blood insulin levels.

Ant1-deficient mice

The genetic inactivation of the mouse nDNA *Ant1* gene may provide a model for the mtDNA multiple deletion syndrome, since both result from the inactivation of the human ANT1 gene (Graham et al., 1997; Kaukonen et al., 2000). Analysis of the *Ant1*−/− mouse has also provided important insights into the significance of depleting cellular ATP; inhibiting the ETC, and increasing mitochondrial ROS production in the pathophysiology of mitochondrial disease.

ANT1-deficient [$Ant1^{tm2Mgr}$ (−/−)] mice are viable, though they developed classical mitochondrial myopathy and hypertrophic cardiomyopathy. They also develop elevated serum lactate, alanine, succinate, and citrate, consistent with the inhibition of the ETC and the TCA cycle (Graham et al., 1997).

The mouse *Ant1* isoform gene is expressed at high levels in skeletal muscle and heart and at lower levels in brain, while the mouse *Ant2* gene is expressed in all tissues but skeletal muscle (Levy et al., 2000). Consequently, mice mutant in *Ant1* have a complete deficiency of ANT in skeletal muscle, a partial deficiency in heart, but normal ANT levels in liver; an expectation supported by the relative ADP-stimulation of respiration in mitochondrial isolated from these three tissues (Graham et al., 1997).

The skeletal muscle of *Ant1*−/− animals exhibit classic RRFs and increased SDH and COX staining in the type I oxidative muscle fibers (Fig. 11.9). These elevated OXPHOS enzyme activities correlate with a massive proliferation of giant mitochondria in the skeletal muscle fibers, degeneration of the contractile fibers, and a marked exercise fatigability. The hearts of the ANT1-deficient mice also exhibited a striking hypertrophic cardiomyopathy, associated with a significant proliferation of cardiomyocyte mitochondria. The proliferation of mitochondria in the *Ant1*−/− mouse skeletal muscle is associated with the coordinate up-regulation of genes involved in energy metabolism including most mtDNA transcripts and the nDNA complex I 18 kDa and complex IV COXVa and COXVb transcripts; genes involved in apoptosis including the muscle Bcl-2 homologue Mcl-1; and genes potentially involved in mitochondrial biogenesis such as SKD3 (Murdock et al., 1999).

The inhibition of ADP/ATP exchange would deprive the ATP synthase of substrate, block proton transport through ATP synthase membrane channel and result in the hyperpolarization of Δψ inhibiting the ETC. The inhibition of the ETC would re-direct the electrons to O_2 to generate O_2^-, and the increased oxidative stress should damage the mtDNA. Consistent with this expectation, the mitochondrial H_2O_2 production rate was found to be increased six to eight fold in the ANT1-deficient skeletal muscle and heart mitochondria, levels comparable to those obtained for control mitochondria inhibited by Antimycin A. In skeletal muscle, where the respiratory defect was complete, the increased oxidative stress was paralleled by a six fold increase in mitochondrial MnSOD and a three fold increase in mitochondrial GPx1. In heart, where the respiratory defect was incomplete, GPx1 was also increased three fold, but MnSOD was not increased (Esposito et al., 1999). Hence, inhibition of OXPHOS was associated with increased ROS, and the increased ROS was countered by an induction of anti-oxidant defenses, if the oxidative stress was sufficiently severe.

The increased ROS production would also be expected to increase mitochondrial macromolecular damage. This was confirmed by the analyses of the mtDNA rearrangements in the hearts. The hearts of 16–20 month ANT1-deficient mice had much higher levels of mtDNA rearrangements than did age-matched controls. In fact, the level of heart mtDNA rearrangements in middle-aged *Ant1*−/− animals was comparable to that seen in the hearts of very old (32 months) normal mice. Surprisingly, the mtDNAs of the skeletal muscle showed substantially less mtDNA rearrangements than the heart. However, this could be the consequence of the strong induction of MnSOD in skeletal muscle, which was not the case in heart (Esposito et al., 1999).

The phenotypic, biochemical and molecular analysis of the *Ant1−/−* mice have confirmed that they have many of the features of patients with adPEO. These include mitochondrial myopathy with fatigability and multiple mtDNA deletions. Hence, this *Ant1−/−* mouse model may provide valuable insights into the pathophysiological basis of adPEO. There is one striking difference between these two systems, however. In humans, the ANT1 mutation is dominant, while in mouse it is recessive. There are two possible explanations for this difference. The human and mouse ANT1 mutations might be functionally different. The human mutations are missense mutations while the mouse mutations are nulls mutations. Since the ANTs peptides function as dimers, an aberrant ANT1 polypeptide could bind to normal subunits and result in a non-functional complex. Hence, only one-quarter of all of the ANT1 complexes might be active. This would render the human biochemical defect similarly severe to that of the mouse. Alternatively, the mouse might be less sensitive to OXPHOS defects than humans. One way to distinguish these two hypotheses would be to prepare a transgenic mouse harboring the same *Ant1* gene mutations as found in the adPEO patients. These mice could then be crossed onto an *Ant1+/−* heterozygous background and the phenotype analyzed. If the *Ant1+/−* transgenic mice develop myopathy and multiple deletions, then the mutation must be acting as a dominant negative. If not, then the mouse must be less sensitive to mitochondrial defects.

Comparison of the human and mouse *Ant1* mutants may also provide some insight into the cause of the mtDNA rearrangements. Two alternative hypotheses have been suggested. In the first, the ANT1-deficiency has been proposed to alter the mitochondrial nucleotide precursor pools thus perturbing replication (Kaukonen et al., 2000). This is analogous to the proposal for why the cytosolic TP-deficiency causes multiple deletions in the MINGIE syndrome (Nishino et al., 1999). The difficulty with this hypothesis is that in the mouse the ANT1-deficiency in the muscle is much more sever than that in the heart, yet the heart accumulated many more mtDNA deletions than did the skeletal muscle. The alternative hypothesis is that the inhibition of the ETC caused by the ANT1-defect increases ROS production and this acts as a mutagen leading to rearrangements of the mtDNAs. This possibility is more consistent with the data since the anti-oxidant defenses in the skeletal muscle are much more strongly induced than those of the heart. Hence, the heart mtDNAs would be more vulnerable to oxidative damage and prone to rearrangements.

These studies on the *Ant1−/−* mice have demonstrated the importance of ATP deficiency in skeletal muscle and

heart pathology, and have suggested that increased mitochondrial ROS production is also an important factor in the pathophysiology of mitochondrial disease. Since evaluation of *Ant1* resulted in increased ROS production due to the hyperpolarization of $\Delta\psi$ and the associated inhibition of the ETC, it would follow that reduction of the mitochondrial inner membrane proton leak would also stimulate mitochondrial ROS generation.

Ucp-deficient mouse

The mitochondrial inner membrane permeability to protons is normally regulated by the uncoupler proteins (Ucp). Mammals have three uncoupler genes Ucp 1, 2, 4. Ucp1 is primarily associated with brown fat where it functions in thermogenics. Mice exposed to cold dramatically induce Ucp1 mRNA and protein expression. This introduces a proton channel in the mitochondrial inner membrane, short circuits $\Delta\psi$, and rapidly burns brown fat to make heat (Nicholls and Locke, 1984; Jacobsson et al., 1985; Ridley et al, 1986; Reichling et al., 1987; Kozak et al., 1988). Mice with knockout mutations of Ucp1 are cold sensitive, though not obese (Enerback et al., 1997).

Ucp2 and Ucp3 are more systemically expressed. Mice lacking either of these two proteins exhibit increased mitochondrial ROS production, consistent with an increased $\Delta\psi$ and associated inhibition of the ETC (Arsenijevic et al., 2000; Vidal-Puig et al., 2000). The Ucp2 knockout mice are particularly informative in this regard. These animals are not obese and have a normal response to cold. However, they have a marked increased resistance to *Toxoplasma gondii* infection, which forms cysts in the brain. *Ucp1+/+* mice succumb to infection between 28 and 51 days, while *Ucp1−/−* mice survive over 80-days. *Toxoplasma* is eliminated by macrophages by oxidative burst, and *Ucp2−/−* macrophages produced more ROS than *Ucp2+/+* macrophages. This is associated with an elevated expression of interluckin-1B (Il16) and MnSOD. Therefore, it is possible that *Ucp2−/−* mutation increases mitochondrial ROS production (Arsenijevic et al., 2000). It follows that mice deficient in the mitochondrial anti-oxidant genes *GPx1* and *Sod2* (MnSOD) should also show disease symptoms. Accordingly, mice deficient in GPx1 and MnSOD have been prepared and analyzed.

Gpx1-deficient mouse

To increase the level of mitochondrial H_2O_2 production, the mouse GPx1 gene has been inactivated by homologous recombination. However, to understand the resulting phenotype of this mutation can be understood by taking into account inter-tissue and intro-cellular distribution of GPx1. The tissue and cellular distribution of *Gpx1* was studied in two ways: insertion of a reporter cassette (β-galactosidase) into the *Gpx1* gene driven by the endogenous *GPx1* promoter and preparation of GPx1-specific antibodies and their use in Western blot analysis. These studies revealed that GPx1 is strongly expressed in the liver, brain and renal cortex, but very weakly expressed in the heart and skeletal muscle. Furthermore, the GPx1 protein was found in both the cytosol and the mitochondrial of liver and kidney but only found in the cytosol of the heart. Hence, the major physiological and phenotypic consequences of the *GPx1* knockout should be found in the brain, liver and kidney, but not in the heart and skeletal muscle.

GPx1–/– mice are viable, but experience a 20% reduction in body mass which suggests chronic growth retardation. Consistent with the *GPx1* expression profile, liver mitochondria of GPx1-deficient animals secreted fourfold more H_2O_2 then wild-type mitochondrial, while mutant heart mitochondria secreted the same levels of H_2O_2 as controls. Physiological analysis revealed that the RCR and the power output (state III rate times P/O ratio) levels were reduced by one-third in the *GPx1*–/– liver mitochondria but were normal in heart mitochondria (Esposito et al., 2000). Thus, excessive mitochondrial H_2O_2 production in the brain, liver and kidney appears to be only mildly deleterious to the animal.

Sod2-deficient mouse

The importance of O_2^- production to mitochondrial and mtDNA integrity, mice with different levels of MnSOD were generated by using different number of copies of the T-associated maternal effect (Tme) locus. This locus deletes the mitochondrial MnSOD gene, *Sod2*. Since this locus can only be transmitted through males, but not females, it is possible to breed mice with 50%, 100%, 150%, and 200% of the normal MnSOD level. When these animals are treated with the complex I inhibitor MPTP, a drug known to induce Parkinsonism by selectively killing neurons of the substantial nigra, the mice with 50% MnSOD activity show massive basal ganglia toxicity when compared to mice with normal or elevated MnSOD levels (Cortopassi and Wang, 1995).

To further investigate the importance of mitochondrial O_2^- in the pathophysiology of disease, the MnSOD gene has been insertionally inactivated ES cells. Two mouse strains lacking *Sod2* have been reported: *Sod2*[tmlCje] (Li et al., 1995b) and *Sod2*[tmlLeb] (Lebovitz et al., 1996). The *Sod2*[tmlCje]

mutation was originally studied on the CD1 background and resulted in death due to dilated cardiomyopathy at about eight days of age (Li et al., 1995b; Melov et al., 1998). The *Sod2*[tmlLeb] mutation was studied on the B6 background and resulted in death after about 18 days associated with injury to the neuronal mitochondria and degeneration of the large neurons, particularly in the basal ganglia and brain stem (Lebovitz et al., 1996). While inactivation of the mitochondrial MnSOD has proven to be lethal early in life, the inactivation of either the cytosolic Cu/ZnSOD (Reaume et al., 1996) or extra-cellular Cu/ZnSOD (Carlsson et al., 1995) genes were found to have little effect on the viability or fecundity of the animals. Hence, mitochondrial toxicity of O_2^- is far more deleterious to mammals than is the toxicity of cytosolic or extra-cellular O_2^-. Hence, the mitochondria must be both the major source and target for O_2^- toxicity.

Mice harboring the *Sod2*[tmlCje] mutation have been extensively characterized. To determine the effects of acute O_2^- toxicity, *Sod2*[tm1Cje] homozygous (–/–) mutant mice have been analyzed. In addition to causing neonatal death due to dilated cardiomyopathy (Li et al., 1995b; Melov et al., 1998), these animals developed a massive lipid deposition in the liver and a marked deficiency in SDH (complex II) in the hearts, as determined by histochemical analysis (Li et al., 1995b) and direct biochemical assays (Melov et al., 1999). In addition to complex II deficiency in heart and muscle, *Sod2*–/– mice also had partial complex I and citrate synthetase defects in the heart. However, the most striking enzyme deficiency was in mitochondrial aconitase which was almost entirely inactivated in heart and brain. Thus the increased mitochondrial O_2^- appears to have inactivated all of the mitochondrial Fe-S center containing enzymes, thus blocking the TCA cycle and ETC chain (Melov et al., 1999). This would inhibit mitochondrial fatty acid oxidation causing fat to accumulate in the liver and energy starvation in the heart leading to dilation and failure.

Respiration studies on *Sod2*[tm1Cje] homozygous (–/–) liver mitochondria have revealed a 40% reduction in state III respiration, consistent with impaired ETC activity. Moreover, while ADP increased the respiration rate about 1.6-fold (state III), subsequent addition of uncoupler did not increase the respiration above the state IV rate. Mitochondrial from these neonatal animals also showed a marked increased tendency toward activation of the mtPTP (Kokoszka et al., 2001). These observations are interpreted as indicating that acute exposure of the mitochondria to high levels of O_2^- has sensitized the mtPTP. Consequently, the transient reduction in Δψ caused by ADP-stimulated respiration activates the mtPTP causing the release of mitochondrial matrix cofactors and the inter-membrane cytochrome c thus disrupting respiration (Cai et al., 2000). Similar respiratory defects have been reported for the "senescence accelerated mouse" (Nakahara et al., 1998), suggesting that this animal may also suffer from increased mitochondrial oxidative stress.

The increased mitochondrial oxidative stress of the $Sod2-/-$ animals also resulted in the development of a methylglutaconic aciduria, associated with reduced liver HMG-CoA lyase activity. These animals also had increased oxidative damage to their DNA, with the greatest extent and level of base adducts being found in the heart followed by the brain and then the liver (Melov et al., 1999). This later observation adds credence to the hypothesis that the primary cause of mtDNA rearrangement mutations in aging and the adPEO patients is oxidative damage to the mtDNA.

To determine the effects of chronic O_2^- toxicity, $Sod2^{tm1Cje}$ heterozygotes (+/−) animals were studied. These animals had approximately 50% of the normal MnSOD protein, and thus a partial reduction in anti-oxidant capacity. Studies of three month old $Sod2-/-$ animals on a B6 background revealed increased oxidative damage to mitochondrial proteins and mtDNA; reduced activity of mitochondrial glutathione, aconitase and complex I; and an increased mitochondrial predilection to undergo mtPTP transition on exposure to t-butylhydroperoxide (Williams et al., 1998). Studies of young (five months), middle aged (10–15 months) and old (20–25 months) $Sod2 +/−$ mice on the CD1 background revealed that $\Delta\psi$ was reduced throughout life by the chronic oxidative stress, and that $\Delta\psi$ declined in parallel in both the heterozygous mutant and normal animals with old age. State IV respiration rates were elevated in the $Sod2 +/−$ animals, while the state III respiration was inhibited. Moreover, the state IV levels in normal animals increased and the state III rates declined with age. These data are consistent with chronic O_2^- exposure partially inactivating the Fe-S center enzymes in the TCA cycle and ETC and an increasing proton leak of the inner membrane short-circuiting $\Delta\psi$. They also indicate that normal animals develop the same mitochondrial defects as the $Sod2 +/−$ animals, but at a later age. Hence, the aging phenomena are the same for the two genotypes, but the increased O_2^- exposure increased the rate of aging in the $Sod2 +/−$ animals.

Analysis of oxidative damage in $Sod2 +/−$ versus −/− animals revealed that total cellular and mitochondrial lipid peroxidation of the $Sod2 +/−$ animals peaked at high levels in the middle aged animals, but then fell precipitously in old age. By contrast, lipid peroxidation remained low in the normal animals during middle age, but then increased toward the heterozygote levels in older animals. Analysis of the Ca^{2+} sensitivity of the mtPTPs in the $Sod2 +/−$ animals revealed that the heterozygous mitochondria were much more prone to transition than the normal mitochondria. Furthermore, the Ca^{2+} sensitivity of the mtPTP transition increased in older animals for both genotypes. TUNEL staining of hepatocytes of the older animals revealed that the apoptosis rates of the older heterozygous animals were three to fourfold higher that those of older controls, and that the average OXPHOS enzyme specific activity in isolated mitochondria was higher in the mutants than the normals. All of these observations suggest that increased mitochondrial oxidative stress of the $Sod2 +/−$ animals caused the premature accumulation of mitochondrial damage, inhibition the Fe-S center enzymes, increase in the inner membrane proton leakage, damage to the mitochondrial macromolecules, and sensitization of the mtPTP. Ultimately the most affected cells undergo mtPTP transition, killing the cells with the most mitochondrial damage. The removal of these damaged cells increases the overall average of the mitochondrial enzyme specific activities, but also results in the loss of functional cell causing a decline in overall tissue function (Kokoszka et al., 2001). Thus, chronic mitochondrial oxidative damage does have a significant deleterious effect on mitochondria and hence must play a central role in the progression of mitochondrial diseases and aging.

ANTI-OXIDANT TREATMENTS IN ANIMAL MODELS OF MITOCHONDRIAL DISEASE

The advent of mouse models of mitochondrial disease now provides the opportunity for investigating the efficacy and mechanism of new therapeutics. The most productive studies to date have been conducted on the $Sod2^{tm1Cje}$ −/− mouse on the CD1 background, which has proven to be a powerful system for screening for anti-oxidant drugs. The most effective of these have been the catalytic anti-oxidants or SOD mimetics, such as MnTBAP (Manganese 5,10,15,20-tetrakis (4-benzoic acid) porphyrin). Peritoneal injection of MnTBAP into $Sod2 -/-$ animals rescued them from the lethal dilated cardiomyopathy, reduce the liver lipid deposition, and extend the mean lifespan of the animals to about 16 days of age. However, MnTBAP does not cross the blood-brain barrier, and by 12 days of age the MnTBAP-treated animals began to exhibit gait disturbances which progressed by 21 days of age to ataxia, dystonia, repetitive movements, tremor and immobility. Histological analysis of the brains of these mice revealed a symmetrical spongiform encephalopathy, together with glial fibrillary acid protein deposition, in regions of the cortex and brainstem (Melov et al., 1998). This suggests that the increased mitochondrial ROS production is extremely toxic to the brain, possibly causing neuronal apoptosis. Therefore, the *Sod2 −/−* mouse has permitted the demonstration of the efficacy of MnTBAP as a mitochondrial anti-oxidant drug. Moreover, the effectiveness of MnTBAP treatment prove that the toxic entry in the *Sod2 −/−* mice is the over-production of O^-_2.

To determine if mitochondrial ROS toxicity was also an important factor in aging, the short-lived nematode worm (*C. elegans*) was treated with the SOD mimetic EUK134, which is similar in action to MnTBAP. The *mev-1* mutant of *C. elegans* has a 30% reduction in life span due to a defect in the mitochondrial complex II (SDH) which greatly increases its mitochondrial ROS production. Treatment of *mev-1* animals with EUK134 restored to their life span to normal. Furthermore, EUK134-treatment of normal *C. elegans* increased their life span 50% to a level comparable to the *age-1* mutant (Melov et al., 2000). Hence, mitochondrial ROS toxicity also appears to be an important factor in limiting life span, at least of *C. elegans*, and drugs that are effective in ameliorating the symptoms of pathogenic mitochondrial mutations might also be helpful in delaying the onset and progression of symptoms in degenerative diseases and aging.

Mitochondrial paragigm for degenerative diseases, cancer and aging

These observations provide strong evidence that the mitochondrial play a central role in degenerative diseases, cancer and aging. These diverse effects can be interrelated to each other through the cellular redox state as maintained by the mitochondria through oxidation and reduction of NAD^+ and $NADH + H^+$ (Figure 11.14). Dietary calories enter the mitochondria where they provide reducing equivalents which reduce NAD^+ to $NADH + H^+$. $NADH + H^+$ is then reoxidized by the mitochondrial to generate $\Delta\psi$, and $\Delta\psi$ is used by the mitochondria to synthesize ATP from cytosolic $ADP + P_1$ or to take up cations such as Ca^{2+}. When cellular work levels are high, ATP is actively hydrolyzed, resulting in increased cellular ADP which is transported into the matrix by the ANT. The increased matrix ADP is rephosphorylated at the expense of $\Delta\psi$, driving the oxidation of $NADH + H^+$ to NAD^+ by the ETC. When dietary calories exceed the cellular work load, all ADP becomes phosphorylated to ATP, $\Delta\psi$ becomes hyperpolarized, and NAD^+

becomes progressively reduced to $NADH + H^+$. The excess of reducing equivalents of NADH reduce the ETC, which stimulates the transfer of electrons to O_2 to give O^-_2. The mitochondrial O^-_2, along with mitochondrial NO production, reacts with and damages mitochondrial membranes, proteins, and DNA. The increased O^-_2 is also converted to H_2O_2 by mitochondrial MnSOD, and the excess H_2O_2 diffuses to the nucleus where in mutagenizes the nDNA and activates the PARP protein to begin degrading NAD^+. As somatic mtDNA mutations accumulate, they further inhibit the mitochondrial ETC and stimulate ROS production. Moreover, injury to the plasma membrane or stimulation of NMDA-receptors in neurons by glutamate increases cytosolic Ca^{2+}, which is subsequently concentrated in the mitochondria. The increased Ca^{2+} binding to the cyclophilin D, elevated oxidative stress, and decreased $\Delta\psi$ all impinge on the mtPTP ultimately leading to permeability transition and cell loss due to apoptosis. This cell loss results in tissue and organ decline and system failure.

The reduction of cellular NAD^+, both by reduction to $NADH + H^+$ and degradation by PARP, leads to the inhibition of the nuclear chromatin silencing protein SIR2. SIR2 uses NAD^+ as a substrate to cleave acetyl groups from histones, thus keeping "off" genes inactive (Lin et al., 2000). In the absence of active SIR2 nucleosome histones become increasingly acetylated. This results in the progressive illegitimate transcription of normally "off" genes, a characteristic feature of aging tissues. This process not only activates structural proteins, it could also actives otherwise inactive proto-oncogenes. This transcriptional activation, the associated H_2O_2 mutagenesis of the proto-oncogenes, and the mitogenic stimulation of the H_2O_2 would progressively increase in probability for developing cancer as the individual ages.

This model now explains why caloric restriction not only increases longevity but also decreases cancer risks. By reducing caloric intake and balancing reducing equivalents with the work-related hydrolysis of ATP, the NAD^+ would remain oxidized. This would remove excess electrons from producing ROS, thus minimizing oxidative stress, mutagenesis of the mtDNA, cell loss by apoptosis, and nDNA damage and activation by H_2O_2. The protection of the NAD^+ pool would also assure that SIR2 remains maximally active, thus suppressing oncogene activation.

Thus mitochondrial disease, cancer, and aging can now be envisioned as the interaction of two mitochondrial genetic factors: (a) the inheritance of a deleterious mtDNA or nDNA mutations in a mitochondrial gene; and (b) the age-related accumulation of somatic mtDNA mutations causing mitochondrial decline, increased ROS production

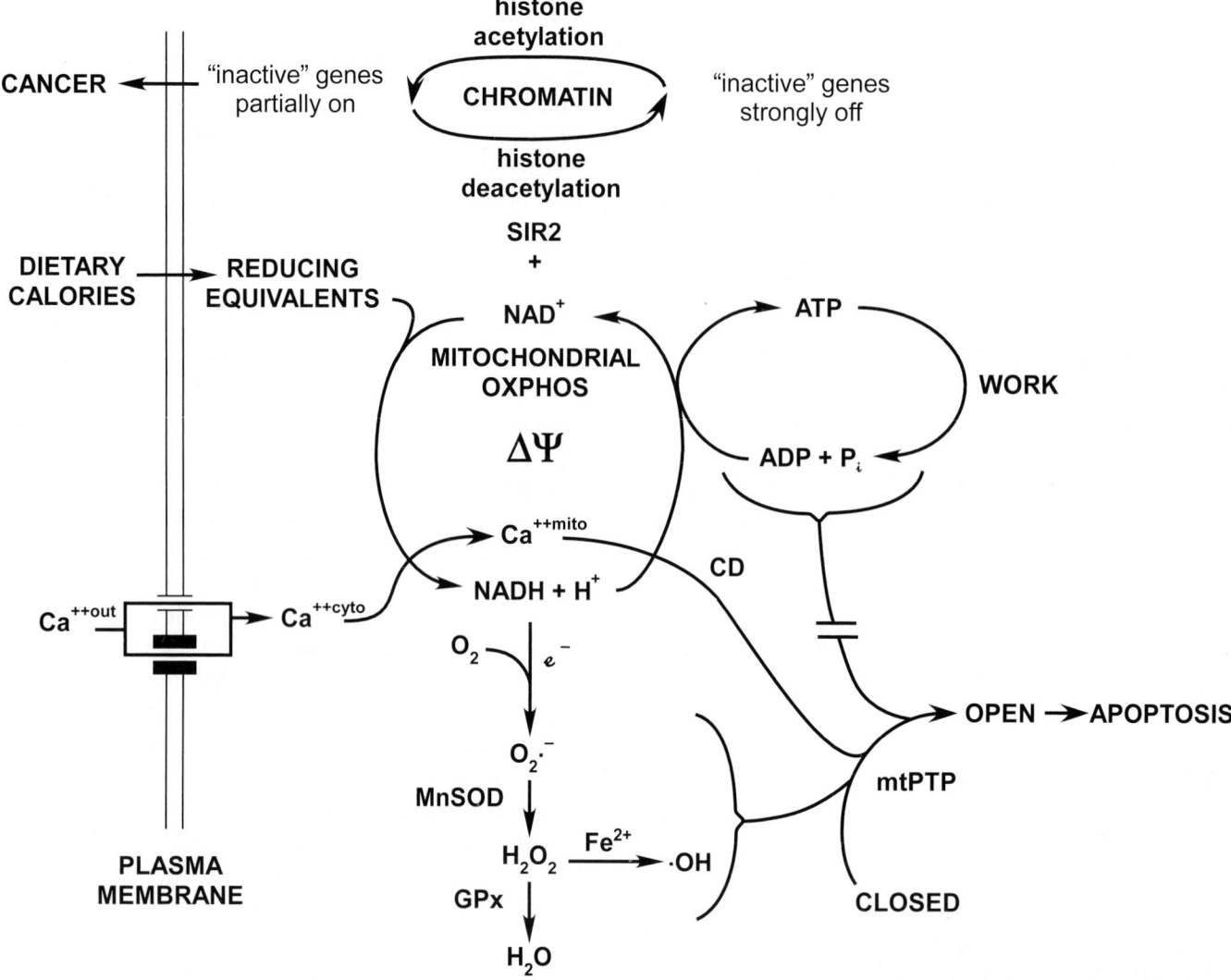

Fig. 11.14. Metabolic pathway showing the central role of mitochondrial NADH oxidation-reduction in regulation ATP production, ROS generation, apoptosis, and neoplastic transformation leading to cancer.

and apoptosis. It is envisioned that each individual is born with an array of nDNA and mtDNA alleles that determine their initial bioenergetic capacity. If the individual inherits an energetic genotype then he will have a high initial energy capacity, well above the minimum energetic thresholds required by his tissues. However, if he inherits a deleterious mutation, then his initial energetic capacity will be lower and ROS production higher. As the individual ages, somatic mtDNA mutations will accumulate in post-mitotic cells that further erode his tissue's energy production and increase ROS output. Ultimately, the combined effects of the inherited and somatic mitochondrial defects will push the tissue's energetic capacity below the bioenergetic threshold resulting in apoptosis and organ failure, and will activate nDNA proto-oncogenes resulting in cancer (Figure 11.15).

This pathophysiological mechanism suggests that mitochondrial disease, cancer, and aging, might all be treated by common strategies. These could include augmentation of energy production, removal of toxic ROS with drugs like MnTBAP, and/or inhibition of the mtPTP and postponement of cell loss due to apoptosis. Hopefully, such approaches might improve the clinical status of mitochondrial disease and cancer patients, in the not-to-distant future.

ACKNOWLEDGEMENTS

This work was supported by National Institutes of Health grants GM46915, NS21328, NS37167, HL45572, HL64017, AG13154, and AG10130 awarded to D.C.W.

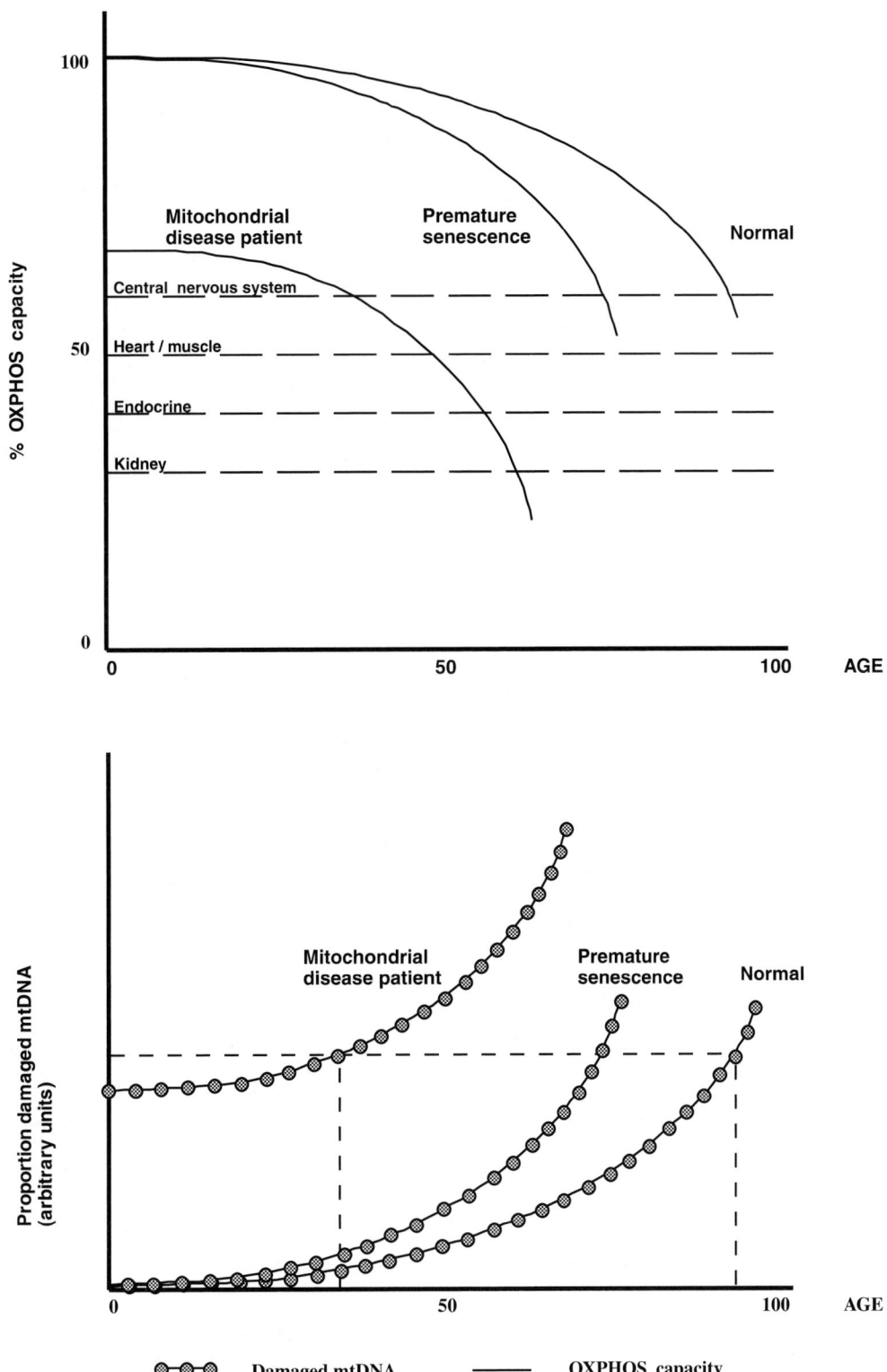

Fig. 11.15. Hypothesis relating the acquisition of mitochondrial DNA (mtDNA) mutations (inherited and somatic) to the age-related decline of oxidative phosphorylation (OXPHOS) and the progression of OXPHOS diseases and senescence. The dashed horizontal lines in both panels represent tissue-specific expression thresholds. The top panel shows the age-related decline of OXPHOS in individuals born with a normal OXPHOS genotype, a mutant OXPHOS gene, and an increased mtDNA somatic mutation rate. The bottom panel shows the relative levels of defective mtDNA with age for each of these individuals. Reproduced from Wallace (1995a) Mitochondical DNA variation in human evolution, degenerative disease, and aging. Am J Hum Genet 57: 201–223. © University of Chicago Press.

BIBLIOGRAPHY

Abrahams JP, Leslie AG, Lutter R, Walker JE (1994) Structure at 2.8 A resolution of F_1-ATPase from bovine heart mitochondria. Nature 370:621–628

Adams V, Griffin L, Towbin J, Gelb B, Worley K, McCabe ER (1991) Porin interaction with hexokinase and glycerol kinase: metabolic microcompartmentation at the outer mitochondrial membrane. Biochem Med Metabol Biol 45:271–291

Ahmed I, Krishnamoorthy G (1992) The non-equivalence of binding sites of coenzyme quinone and rotenone in mitochondrial NADH-CoQ reductase. FEBS Letters 300:275–278

Akiyama S, Endo H, Inohara N, Ohta S, Kagawa Y (1994) Gene structure and cell type-specific expression of the human ATP synthase alpha subunit. Biochim Biophys Acta 1219:129–140

Alcolado JC, Thomas AW (1995) Maternally inherited diabetes mellitus: the role of mitochondrial DNA defects. Diabet Med 12:102–108

Alcolado JC, Clark PM, Rees A, Hales CN (1994a) Insulin resistance and impaired glucose tolerance [letter; comment]. Lancet 344:1293–1294

Alcolado JC, Majid A, Brockington M et al. (1994b) Mitochondrial gene defects in patients with NIDDM. Diabetologia 37:372–376

Altshuler D, Hirschhorn JN, Klannemark M et al. (2000) The common PPARgamma Pro12Ala polymorphism is associated with decreased risk of type 2 diabetes. Nat Genet 26:76–80

Ames BN, Shigenaga MK, Hagen TM (1993) Oxidants, antioxidants, and the degenerative diseases of aging. Proc Natl Acad Sci USA 90:7915–7922

Ames BN, Shigenaga MK, Hagen TM (1995) Mitochondrial decay in aging. Biochim Biophys Acta 1271:165–170

Anderson CT, Friedberg EC (1980) The presence of nuclear and mitochondrial uracil-DNA glycosylase in extracts of human KB cells. Nucl Acids Res 8:875–888

Anderson S, Bankier AT, Barrell BG et al. (1981) Sequence and organization of the human mitochondrial genome. Nature 290:457–465

Anderson S, deBruijn MHL, Coulson AR, Eperon IC, Sanger F, Young IG (1982) Complete sequence of bovine mitochondrial DNA. Conserved features of the mammalian mitochondrial genome. J Mol Biol 156:683–717

Andreu AL, Bruno C, Shanske S et al. (1998) Missense mutation in the mtDNA cytochrome b gene in a patient with myopathy. Neurology 51:1444–1447

Andreu AL, Bruno C, Dunne TC et al. (1999) A nonsense mutation (G15059A) in the cytochrome b gene in a patient with exercise intolerance and myoglobinuria. Ann Neurol 45:127–130

Anthony G, Reimann A, Kadenbach B (1993) Tissue-specific regulation of bovine heart cytochrome-c oxidase activity by ADP via interaction with subunit VIa. Proc Natl Acad Sci USA 90:1652–1656

Arizmendi JM, Skehel JM, Runswick MJ, Fearnley IM, Walker JE (1992) Complementary DNA sequences of two 14.5 kDa subunits of NADH:ubiquinone oxidoreductase from bovine heart mitochondria. Complementation of the primary structure of the complex? FEBS Letters 313:80–84

Armstrong M, Daly AK, Cholerton S, Bateman DN, Idle JR (1992) Mutant debrisoquine hydroxylation genes in Parkinson's disease. Lancet 339:1017–1018

Arnaudo E, Hirano M, Seelan RS et al. (1992) Tissue-specific expression and chromosome assignment of genes specifying two isoforms of subunit VIIa of human cytochrome c oxidase. Gene 119:299–305

Arnold S, Kadenbach B (1997) Cell respiration is controlled by ATP, an allosteric inhibitor of cytochrome-c oxidase. Eur J Biochem 249:350–354

Arnold S, Kadenbach B (1999) The intramitochondrial ATP/ADP-ratio controls cytochrome c oxidase activity allosterically. FEBS Letters 443:105–108

Arnold RS, Shi J, Murad E et al. (2001) Hydrogen Peroxide Mediates the Cell Growth and Transformation Caused by the Mitogenic Oxidase Nox1. Submitted

Arsenijevic D, Onuma H, Pecqueur C et al. (2000) Disruption of the uncoupling protein-2 gene in mice reveals a role in immunity and reactive oxygen species production. Nat Genet 26:435–439

Attardi G, Montoya J (1983) Analysis of human mitochondrial RNA. Methods Enzymol 97:435–469

Attardi G, Chomyn A, Montoya J, Ojala D (1982) Identification and mapping of human mitochondrial genes. Cytogenet Cell Genet 32:85–98

Attardi G, Chomyn A, Doolittle RF, Mariottini P, Ragan CI (1986) Seven unidentified reading frames of human mitochondrial DNA encode subunits of the respiratory chain NADH dehydrogenase. Cold Spring Harbor Symp Quant Biol 1:103–114

Attardi G, Yoneda M, Chomyn A (1995) Complementation and segregation behavior of disease-causing mitochondrial DNA mutations in cellular model systems. Biochim Biophys Acta 1271:241–248

Atwood CS, Moir RD, Huang X et al. (1998) Dramatic aggregation of Alzheimer abeta by Cu(II) is induced by conditions representing physiological acidosis. J Biol Chem 273:12817–12826

Atwood CS, Huang X, Khatri A et al. (2000) Copper catalyzed oxidation of Alzheimer A βeta. Cell Mol Biol 46:777–783

Awadalla P, Eyre-Walker A, Smith JM (1999) Linkage disequilibrium and recombination in hominid mitochondrial DNA. Science 286:2524–2525

Bachman NJ, Riggs PK, Siddiqui N, Makris GJ, Womack JE, Lomax MI (1997) Structure of the human gene (COX6A2) for the heart/muscle isoform of cytochrome c oxidase subunit VIa and its chromosomal location in humans, mice, and cattle. Genomics 42:146–151

Ballinger SW, Schurr TG, Torroni A et al. (1992a) Southeast Asian mitochondrial DNA analysis reveals genetic continuity of ancient mongoloid migrations [published erratum appears in Genetics (1992) Apr;130(4):957]. Genetics 130:139–152

Ballinger SW, Shoffner JM, Hedaya EV et al. (1992b) Maternally transmitted diabetes and deafness associated with a 10.4 kb mitochondrial DNA deletion. Nat Genet 1:11–15

Ballinger SW, Shoffner JM, Gebhart S, Koontz DA, Wallace DC (1994) Mitochondrial diabetes revisited [letter]. Nat Genet 7:458–459

Bandy B, Davison AJ (1990) Mitochondrial mutations may increase oxidative stress: implications for carcinogenesis and aging? Free Rad Biol Med 8:523–539

Barger SW, Smith-Swintosky VL, Rydel RE, Mattson MP (1993) Beta-Amyloid precursor protein mismetabolism and loss of calcium homeostasis in Alzheimer's disease. Ann NY Acad Sci 695:158–164

Barinaga M (1996) An intriguing new lead on Huntington's disease. Science 271:1233–1234

Battini R, Ferrari S, Kaczmarek L, Calabretta B, Chen ST, Baserga R (1987) Molecular cloning of a cDNA for a human ADP/ATP carrier which is growth-regulated. J Biol Chem 262:4355–4359

Baysal BE, Ferrell RE, Willett-Brozick JE et al. (2000) Mutations in SDHD, a mitochondrial complex II gene, in hereditary paraganglioma. Science 287:848–851

Beal MF (1994) Neurochemistry and toxin models in Huntington's disease. Curr Opin Neurol 7:542–547

Belogrudov G, Hatefi Y (1994) Catalytic sector of complex I (NADH:ubiquinone oxidoreductase): subunit stoichiometry and substrate-induced conformation changes. Biochemistry 33:4571–4576

Benecke R, Strumper P, Weiss H (1992) Electron transfer complex I defect in idiopathic dystonia. Ann Neurol 32:683–686

Benecke R, Strumper P, Weiss H (1993) Electron transfer complexes I and IV of platelets are abnormal in Parkinson's disease but normal in Parkinson-plus syndromes. Brain 116:1451–1463

Bennett BD, Babu-Khan S, Loeloff R et al. (2000) Expression analysis of BACE2 in brain and peripheral tissues. J Biol Chem 275:20647–20651

Bennett MC, Diamond DM, Stryker SL, Parks JK, Parker WD, Jr., (1992) Cytochrome oxidase inhibition: A novel animal model of Alzheimer's disease. J Geriatr Psych Neurol 5:93–101

Benzi G, Moretti A (1995) Are reactive oxygen species involved in Alzheimer's disease? Neurobiology of Aging 16:661–674

Berkovic SF, Carpenter S, Evans A et al. (1989) Myoclonus epilepsy and ragged-red fibres (MERRF). I. A clinical, pathological, biochemical, magnetic resonance spectrographic and positron emission tomographic study. Brain 112:1231–1260

Berkovic SF, Shoubridge EA, Andermann F, Andermann E, Carpenter S, Karpati G (1991) Clinical spectrum of mitochondrial DNA mutation at base pair 8344 [letter; comment]. Lancet 338:457

Bidooki SK, Johnson MA, Chrzanowska-Lightowlers Z, Bindoff LA, Lightowlers RN (1997) Intracellular mitochondrial triplasmy in a patient with two heteroplasmic base changes. Am J Hum Genet 60:1430–1438

Bindoff LA, Birch-Machin M, Cartlidge NEF, Parker WD, Jr., Turnbull DM (1989) Mitochondrial function in Parkinson's disease. Lancet 2:49

Bindoff LA, Howell N, Poulton J et al. (1993) Abnormal RNA processing associated with a novel tRNA mutation in mitochondrial DNA. A potential disease mechanism. J Biol Chem 268:19559–19564

Biousse V, Brown MD, Newman NJ et al. (1997) De novo 14484 mitochondrial DNA mutation in monozygotic twins discordant for Leber's hereditary optic neuropathy. Neurology 49:1136–1138

Blacker D, Wilcox MA, Laird NM et al. (1998) Alpha-2 macroglobulin is genetically associated with Alzheimer disease. Nat Genet 19:357–360

Blanc H, Adams CW, Wallace DC (1981a) Different nucleotide changes in the large rRNA gene of the mitochondrial DNA confer chloramphenicol resistance on two human cell lines. Nucl Acids Res 9:5785–5795

Blanc H, Wright CT, Bibb MJ, Wallace DC, Clayton DA (1981b) Mitochondrial DNA of chloramphenicol-resistant mouse cells contains a single nucleotide change in the region encoding the 3' end of the large ribosomal RNA. Proc Natl Acad Sci USA 78:3789–3793

Blass JP, Baker AC, Ko L, Black RS (1990) Induction of Alzheimer antigens by an uncoupler of oxidative phosphorylation. Arch Neurol 47:864–869

Blin O, Desnuelle C, Rascol O et al. (1994) Mitochondrial respiratory failure in skeletal muscle from patients with Parkinson's disease and multiple system atrophy. J Neurol Sci 125:95–101

Blok RB, Thorburn DR, Thompson GN, Dahl HH (1995) A topoisomerase II cleavage site is associated with a novel mitochondrial DNA deletion. Hum Genet 95:75–81

Bodnar AG, Cooper JM, Holt IJ, Leonard JV, Schapira AH (1993) Nuclear complementation restores mtDNA levels in cultured cells from a patient with mtDNA depletion. Am J Hum Genet 53:663–669

Bodnar AG, Cooper JM, Leonard JV, Schapira AH (1995) Respiratory-deficient human fibroblasts exhibiting defective mitochondrial DNA replication. Biochem J 305:817–822

Boffoli D, Scacco SC, Vergari R, Solarino G, Santacroce G, Papa S (1994) Decline with age of the respiratory chain activity in human skeletal muscle. Biochim Biophys Acta 1226:73–82

Bohr VA (1991) Gene specific DNA repair. Carcinogenesis 12:1983–1992

Bolhuis PA, Bleeker-Wagemakers EM, Ponne NJ et al. (1990) Rapid shift in genotype of human mitochondrial DNA in a family with Leber's hereditary optic neuropathy. Biochem Biophys Res Commun 170:994–997

Bonilla E, Tanji K, Hirano M, Vu TH, DiMauro S, Schon EA (1999) Mitochondrial involvement in Alzheimer's disease. Biochim Biophys Acta 1410:171–182

Boss O, Samec S, Paoloni-Giacobino A et al. (1997) Uncoupling protein-3: a new member of the mitochondrial carrier family with tissue-specific expression. FEBS Letters 408:39–42

Boulet L, Karpati G, Shoubridge EA (1992) Distribution and threshold expression of the tRNA^Lys mutation in skeletal muscle of patients with myoclonic epilepsy and ragged-red fibers (MERRF). Am J Hum Genet 51:1187–1200

Bourgeron T, Rustin P, Chretien D et al. (1995) Mutation of a nuclear succinate dehydrogenase gene results in mitochondrial respiratory chain deficiency. Nat Genet 11:144–149

Boustany RN, Aprille JR, Halperin J, Levy H, DeLong GR (1983) Mitochondrial cytochrome deficiency presenting as a myopathy with hypotonia, external ophthalmoplegia, and lactic acidosis in an infant and as fatal hepatopathy in a second cousin. Ann Neurol 14:462–470

Boveris A (1984) Determination of the production of superoxide radicals and hydrogen peroxide in mitochondria. Methods Enzymol 105:429–435

Boveris A, Turrens JF (1980) Production of superoxide anion by the NADH-dehydrogenase of mamalian mitochondria. In Bannister JV, Hill HAO (eds): Chemical and Biochemical Aspects of Superoxide and Superoxide Dismutase. Developments in Biochemistry. Elsevier-North Holland, N Y, 11A, p84–91

Boveris A, Oshino N, Chance B (1972) The cellular production of hydrogen peroxide. Biochem J 128:617–630

Bowling AC, Mutisya EM, Walker LC, Price DL, Cork LC, Beal MF (1993) Age-dependent impairment of mitochondrial function in primate brain. J Neurochem 60:1964–1967

Boyer PD (1993) The binding change mechanism for ATP synthase–some probabilities and possibilities. Biochim Biophys Acta 1140:215–250

Bravi D, Anderson JJ, Dagani F et al. (1992) Effect of aging and dopaminomimetic therapy on mitochondrial respiratory function in Parkinson's disease. Move Disord 7:228–231

Breen GA (1988) Bovine liver cDNA clones encoding a precursor of the alpha-subunit of the mitochondrial ATP synthase complex. Biochem Biophys Res Commun 152:264–269

Brennan WA, Jr., Bird ED, Aprille JR (1985) Regional mitochondrial respiratory activity in Huntington's Disease brain. J Neurochem 44:1948–1950

Brockington M, Sweeney MG, Hammans SR, Morgan-Hughes JA, Harding AE (1993) A tandem duplication in the D-loop of human mitochondrial DNA is associated with deletions in mitochondrial myopathies. Nat Genet 4:67–71

Brockington M, Alsanjari N, Sweeney MG, Morgan-Hughes JA, Scaravilli F, Harding AE (1995) Kearns-Sayre syndrome associated with mitochondrial DNA deletion or duplication: a molecular genetic and pathological study. J Neurol Sci 131:78–87

Brown GC, McBride AG, Fox EJ, McNaught KS, Borutaite V (1997a) Nitric oxide and oxygen metabolism. Biochem Soc Trans 25:901–904

Brown MD, Torroni A, Shoffner JM, Wallace DC (1992a) Mitochondrial tRNA^Thr mutations and lethal infantile mitochondrial myopathy [letter]. Am J Hum Genet 51:446–447

Brown MD, Voljavec AS, Lott MT, MacDonald I, Wallace DC (1992b) Leber's hereditary optic neuropathy: A model for mitochondrial neurodegenerative diseases. FASEB J 6:2791–2799

Brown MD, Voljavec AS, Lott MT, Torroni A, Yang C-C, Wallace DC (1992c) Mitochondrial DNA complex I and III mutations associated with Leber's hereditary optic neuropathy. Genetics 130:163–173

Brown MD, Yang C-C, Trounce I, Torroni A, Lott MT, Wallace DC (1992d) A mitochondrial DNA variant, identified in Leber hereditary optic neuropathy patients, which extends the amino acid sequence of cytochrome c oxidase subunit I. Am J Hum Genet 51:378–385

Brown MD, Torroni A, Huoponen K, Chen YS, Lott MT, Wallace DC (1994) Pathological significance of the mtDNA COX III mutation at nucleotide pair 9438 in Leber hereditary optic neuropathy [letter]. Am J Hum Genet 55:410–412

Brown MD, Wallace DC (1994a) Molecular basis of mitochondrial DNA disease. J Bioenerg Biomembr 26:273–289

Brown MD, Wallace DC (1994b) Spectrum of mitochondrial DNA mutations in Leber's hereditary optic neuropathy. Journal 2:138–145

Brown MD, Torroni A, Reckord CL, Wallace DC (1995) Phylogenetic analysis of Leber's hereditary optic neuropathy mitochondrial DNA's indicates multiple independent occurrences of the common mutations. Hum Mutat 6:311–325

Brown MD, Shoffner JM, Kim YL et al. (1996) Mitochondrial DNA sequence analysis of four Alzheimer's and Parkinson's disease patients. Am J Hum Genet 61:283–289

Brown MD, Sun F, Wallace DC (1997b) Clustering of Caucasian Leber hereditary optic neuropathy patients containing the 11778 or 14484 mutations on an mtDNA lineage. Am J Hum Genet 60:381–387

Brown MD, Hosseini SH, Torroni A et al. (1998) mtDNA Haplogroup X: an ancient link between Europe/Western Asia and North America? Am J Hum Genet 63:1852–1861

Brown MD, Trounce I, Jun AS, Allen JC, Wallace DC (2000) Functional analysis of lymphoblast and cybrid mitochondria containing the 3460, 11778, or 14484 Leber's Hereditary Optic Neuropathy mtDNA mutation. J Biol Chem 275:39831–39836

Brown WM, George M, Wilson AC (1979) Rapid evolution of animal mitochondrial DNA. Proc Natl Acad Sci USA 76:1967–1971

Brown WM, Prager EM, Wan A, Wilson AC (1982) Mitochondrial DNA sequences in primates: Tempo and mode of evolution. J Mol Evol 18:225–239

Bruno C, Martinuzzi A, Tang Y et al. (1999) A stop-codon mutation in the human mtDNA cytochrome c oxidase I gene disrupts the functional structure of complex IV. Am J Hum Genet 65:611–620

Brustovetsky N, Klingenberg M (1996) Mitochondrial ADP/ATP carrier can be reversibly converted into a large channel by Ca2+. Biochemistry 35:8483–8488

Bullough DA, Ceccarelli EA, Roise D, Allison WS (1989) Inhibition of the bovine-heart mitochondrial FI-ATPase by cationic dyes and amphipathic peptides. Biochim Biophys Acta 975:377–383

Bunn CL, Wallace DC, Eisenstadt JM (1974) Cytoplasmic inheritance of chlormaphenicol resistance in mouse tissue culture cells. Proc Natl Acad Sci USA 71:1681–1685

Burke JR, Enghild JJ, Martin ME et al. (1996) Huntingtin and DRPLA proteins selectively interact with the enzyme GAPDH. Nat Med 2:347–350

Bush AI, Pettingell WH, Jr., Paradis MD, Tanzi RE (1994) Modulation of A beta adhesiveness and secretase site cleavage by zinc. J Biol Chem 269:12152–12158

Cadenas E, Boveris A (1980) Enhancement of hydrogen peroxide formation by protophores and ionophores in antimycin-supplemented mitochondria. Biochem J 188:31–37

Cai J, Wallace DC, Zhivotovsky B, Jones DP (2000) Separation of cytochrome c-dependent caspase activation from thiol-disulfide redox change in cells lacking mitochondrial DNA [In Process Citation]. Free Radic Biol Med 29:334–342

Campos Y, Bautista J, Gutierrez-Rivas E et al. (1995) Clinical heterogeneity in two pedigrees with the 3243 bp tRNA$^{Leu(UUR)}$ mutation of mitochondrial DNA. Acta Neurol Scand 91:62–65

Campos Y, Martin MA, Rubio JC, Gutierrez del Olmo MC, Cabello A, Arenas J (1997) Bilateral striatal necrosis and MELAS associated with

a new T3308C mutation in the mitochondrial ND1 gene. Biochem Biophys Res Commun 238:323–325

Campuzano V, Montermini L, Molto MD et al. (1996) Friedreich's ataxia: autosomal recessive disease caused by an intronic GAA triplet repeat expansion (see comments). Science 271:1423–1427

Cann RL, Stoneking M, Wilson AC (1987) Mitochondrial DNA and human evolution. Nature 325:31–36

Capaldi RA (1990) Structure and function of cytochrome c oxidase. Annu Rev Biochem 59:569–596

Cardaioli E, Dotti MT, Hayek G, Zappella M, Federico A (1999) Studies on mitochondrial pathogenesis of Rett syndrome: ultrastructural data from skin and muscle biopsies and mutational analysis at mtDNA nucleotides 10463 and 2835 [letter]. J Submicrosc Cytol Pathol 31:301–304

Carelli V, Ghelli A, Ratta M et al. (1997) Leber's hereditary optic neuropathy: biochemical effect of 11778/ND4 and 3460/ND1 mutations and correlation with the mitochondrial genotype. Neurology 48:1623–1632

Carelli V, Ghelli A, Bucchi L et al. (1999) Biochemical features of mtDNA 14484 (ND6/M64V) point mutation associated with Leber's hereditary optic neuropathy. Ann Neurol 45:320–328

Carlsson LM, Jonsson J, Edlund T, Marklund SL (1995) Mice lacking extracellular superoxide dismutase are more sensitive to hyperoxia. Proc Natl Acad Sci USA 92:6264–6268

Carrozzo R, Hirano M, Fromenty B et al. (1998) Multiple mtDNA deletions features in autosomal dominant and recessive diseases suggest distinct pathogeneses. Neurology 50:99–106

Casali C, Santorelli FM, D'Amati G, Bernucci P, DeBiase L, DiMauro S (1995) A novel mtDNA point mutation in maternally inherited cardiomyopathy. Biochem Biophys Res Commun 213:588–593

Casari G, De Fusco M, Ciarmatori S et al. (1998) Spastic paraplegia and OXPHOS impairment caused by mutations in paraplegin, a nuclear-encoded mitochondrial metalloprotease. Cell 93:973–983

Case JT, Wallace DC (1981) Maternal inheritance of mitochondrial DNA polymorphisms in cultured human fibroblasts. Somatic Cell Genet 7:103–108

Cassard AM, Bouillaud F, Mattei MG et al. (1990) Human uncoupling protein gene: structure, comparison with rat gene, and assignment to the long arm of chromosome 4. J Cell Biochem 43:255–264

Cassarino DS, Swerdlow RH, Parks JK, Parker WD, Jr., Bennett JP, Jr. (1998) Cyclosporin A increases resting mitochondrial membrane potential in SY5Y cells and reverses the depressed mitochondrial membrane potential of Alzheimer's disease cybrids. Biochem Biophys Res Commun 248:168–173

Chagnon P, Gee M, Filion M, Robitaille Y, Belouchi M, Gauvreau D (1999) Phylogenetic analysis of the mitochondrial genome indicates significant differences between patients with Alzheimer disease and controls in a French-Canadian founder population. Am J Med Genet 85:20–30

Chakrapani A, Heptinstall L, Walter J (1998) A family with Leigh syndrome caused by the rarer T8993C mutation. J Inherit Metabol Dis 21:685–686

Chalmers RM, Robertson N, Kellar-Wood H, Compston DA, Harding AE (1995) Sequence of the human homologue of a mitochondrially encoded murine transplantation antigen in patients with multiple sclerosis. J Neurol 242:332–334

Chance B, Sies H, Boveris A (1979) Hydroperoxide metabolism in mammalian organs. Phys Rev 59:527–605

Chandrasekaran K, Hatanpaa K, Brady DR, Rapoport SI (1996) Evidence for physiological down-regulation of brain oxidative phosphorylation in Alzheimer's disease. Exp Neurol 142:80–88

Chandrasekaran K, Hatanpaa K, Rapoport SI, Brady DR (1997) Decreased expression of nuclear and mitochondrial DNA-encoded genes of oxidative phosphorylation in association neocortex in Alzheimer disease. Mol Brain Res 44:99–104

Chang DD, Clayton DA (1987a) A mammalian mitochondrial RNA processing activity contains nucleus-encoded RNA. Science 235:1178–1184

Chang DD, Clayton DA (1987b) A novel endoribonuclease cleaves at a priming site of mouse mitochondrial DNA replication. EMBO J 6:409–417

Chang DD, Clayton DA (1989) Mouse RNAase MRP RNA is encoded by a nuclear gene and contains a decamer sequence complementary to a conserved region of mitochondrial RNA substrate. Cell 56:131–139

Chang SW, Zhang D, Chung HD, Zassenhaus HP (2000) The frequency of point mutations in mitochondrial DNA is elevated in the Alzheimer's brain. Biochem Biophys Res Commun 273:203–208

Checcarelli N, Prelle A, Moggio M et al. (1994) Multiple deletions of mitochondrial DNA in sporadic and atypical cases of encephalomyopathy. J Neurol Sci 123:74–79

Chen ST, Chang CD, Huebner K et al. (1990) A human ADP/ATP translocase gene has seven pseudogenes and localizes to chromosome X. Som Cell Mol Genet 16:143–149

Chen X, Bonilla E, Sciacco M, Schon EA (1995a) Paucity of deleted mitochondrial DNAs in brain regions of Huntington's disease patients. Biochim Biophys Acta 1271:229–233

Chen X, Prosser R, Simonetti S, Sadlock J, Jagiello G, Schon EA (1995b) Rearranged mitochondrial genomes are present in human oocytes. Am J Hum Genet 57:239–247

Chen YS, Torroni A, Excoffier L, Santachiara-Benerecetti AS, Wallace DC (1995c) Analysis of mtDNA variation in African populations reveals the most ancient of all human continent-specific haplogroups. Am J Hum Genet 57:133–149

Chen YS, Olckers A, Schurr TG, Kogelnik AM, Huoponen K, Wallace DC (2000) mtDNA variation in the South African Kung and Khwe and their genetic relationships to other African populations. Am J Hum Genet 66:1362–1383

Cheng KC, Cahill DS, Kasai H, Nishimura S, Loeb LA (1992) 8-Hydroxyguanine, an abundant form of oxidative DNA damage, causes G—T and A—C substitutions. J Biol Chem 267:166–172

Cheng S, Higuchi R, Stoneking M (1994) Complete mitochondrial genome amplification. Nat Genet 7:350–351

Chinnery PF, Johnson MA, Taylor RW, Durward WF, Turnbull DM (1997a) A novel mitochondrial tRNA isoleucine gene mutation causing chronic progressive external ophthalmoplegia. Neurology 49:1166–1168

Chinnery PF, Johnson MA, Taylor RW, Lightowlers RN, Turnbull DM (1997b) A novel mitochondrial tRNA phenylalanine mutation presenting with acute rhabdomyolysis. Ann Neurol 41:408–410

Chomyn A, Mariottini P, Gonzalez-Cadavid N et al. (1983) Identification of the polypeptides encoded in the ATPase 6 gene and in the unassigned reading frames 1 and 3 of human mtDNA. Proc Natl Acad Sci USA 80:5535–5539

Chomyn A, Mariottini P, Cleeter WJ et al. (1985) Six unidentified reading frames of human mitochondrial DNA encode components of the respiratory-chain NADH dehydrogenase. Nature 314:592–597

Chomyn A, Cleeter WJ, Ragan CI, Riley M, Doolittle RF, Attardi G (1986) URF6, last unidentified reading frame of human mtDNA, codes for an NADH dehydrogenase subunit. Science 234:614–618

Chomyn A, Meola G, Bresolin N, Lai ST, Scarlato G, Attardi G (1991) In vitro genetic transfer of protein synthesis and respiration defects to mitochondrial DNA-less cells with myopathy-patient mitochondria. Mol Cell Biol 11:2236–2244

Chomyn A, Martinuzzi A, Yoneda M et al. (1992) MELAS mutation in mtDNA binding site for transcription termination factor causes defects in protein synthesis and in respiration but no change in levels of upstream and downstream mature transcripts. Proc Natl Acad Sci USA 89:4221–4225

Chomyn A, Lai ST, Shakeley R, Bresolin N, Scarlato G, Attardi G (1994) Platelet-mediated transformation of mtDNA-less human cells:

analysis of phenotypic variability among clones from normal individuals and complementation behavior of the tRNA^{Lys} mutation causing myoclonic epilepsy and ragged red fibers. Am J Hum Genet 54:966–974

Chow W, Ragan I, Robinson BH (1991) Determination of the cDNA sequence for the human mitochondrial 75-kDa Fe-S protein of NADH-coenzyme Q reductase. Eur J Biochem 201:547–550

Christianson TW, Clayton DA (1986) In vitro transcription of human mitochondrial DNA: accurate termination requires a region of DNA sequence that can function bidirectionally. Proc Natl Acad Sci USA 83:6277–6281

Christianson TW, Clayton DA (1988) A tridecamer DNA sequence supports human mitochondrial RNA 3'-end formation in vitro. Mol Cell Biol 8:4502–4509

Chung AB, Stepien G, Haraguchi Y, Li K, Wallace DC (1992a) Transcriptional control of nuclear genes for the mitochondrial muscle ADP/ATP translocator and the ATP synthase beta subunit. Multiple factors interact with the OXBOX/REBOX promoter sequences. J Biol Chem 267:21154–21161

Chung MH, Kasai H, Nishimura S, Yu BP (1992b) Protection of DNA damage by dietary restriction. Free Radic Biol Med 12:523–525

Ciafaloni E, Ricci E, Servidei S et al. (1991) Widespread tissue distribution of a tRNA$^{Leu(UUR)}$ mutation in the mitochondrial DNA of a patient with MELAS syndrome. Neurology 41:1663–1665

Ciafaloni E, Santorelli FM, Shanske S et al. (1993) Maternally inherited Leigh syndrome. J Pediatr 122:419–422

Clark KM, Taylor RW, Johnson MA et al. (1999) An mtDNA mutation in the initiation codon of the cytochrome C oxidase subunit II gene results in lower levels of the protein and a mitochondrial encephalomyopathy. Am J Hum Genet 64:1330–1339

Clarkson GH, Neagle J, Lindsay JG (1991) Topography of succinate dehydrogenase in the mitochondrial inner membrane. A study using limited proteolysis and immunoblotting. Biochem J 273:719–724

Clayton DA (1982) Replication of animal mitochondrial DNA. Cell 28:693–705

Clayton DA (1984) Transcription of the mammalian mitochondrial genome. Annu Rev Biochem 53:573–594

Clayton DA (1994) A nuclear function for RNase MRP. Proc Natl Acad Sci USA 91:4615–4617

Clayton DA, Doda JN, Friedberg EC (1974) The absence of a pyrimidine dimer repair mechanism in mammalian mitochondria. Proc Natl Acad Sci USA 71:2777–2781

Cleeter MW, Cooper JM, Schapira AH (1992) Irreversible inhibition of mitochondrial complex I by 1-methyl-4-phenylpyridinium: evidence for free radical involvement. J Neurochem 58:786–789

Cochran B, Capaldi RA, Ackrell BA (1994) The cDNA sequence of beef heart C$_{II-3}$, a membrane-intrinsic subunit of succinate-ubiquinone oxidoreductase. Biochim Biophys Acta 1188:162–166

Cock HR, Cooper JM, Schapira AH (1995) The 14484 ND6 mtDNA mutation in Leber hereditary optic neuropathy does not affect fibroblast complex I activity [letter]. Am J Hum Genet 57:1501–1502

Cock HR, Tabrizi SJ, Cooper JM, Schapira AH (1998) The influence of nuclear background on the biochemical expression of 3460 Leber's hereditary optic neuropathy. Ann Neurol 44:187–193

Cock HR, Cooper JM, Schapira AH (1999) Functional consequences of the 3460-bp mitochondrial DNA mutation associated with Leber's hereditary optic neuropathy. J Neurol Sci 165:10–17

Comi GP, Bordoni A, Salani S et al. (1998) Cytochrome c oxidase subunit I microdeletion in a patient with motor neuron disease. Ann Neurol 43:110–116

Comings DE, Dietz G, Johnson JP, MacMurray JP (1999) Association of the enkephalinase gene with low amplitude P300 waves. Neuroreport 10:2283–2285

Cooper JM, Mann Vm, Schapira AHV (1992) Analyses of mitochondrial respiratory chain function and mitochondrial DNA deletion in human skeletal muscle: Effect of ageing. J Neurol Sci 113:91–98

Cormier V, Rotig A, Quartino AR et al. (1990) Widespread multissue deletions of the mitochondrial genome in the Pearson marrow-pancreas syndrome. J Pediatr 117:599–602

Cormier V, Rotig A, Bonnefont JP et al. (1991a) Pearson's syndrome. Pancytopenia with exocrine pancreatic insufficiency: New mitochondrial disease in the first year of childhood. Archives Francaises de Pediatric 48:171–178

Cormier V, Rotig A, Tardieu M, Colonna M, Saudubray JM, Munnich A (1991b) Autosomal dominant deletions of the mitochondrial genome in a case of progressive encephalopathy. Am J Hum Genet 48:643–648

Cormier-Daire V, Bonnefont JP, Rustin P et al. (1994) Mitochondrial DNA rearrangements with onset as chronic diarrhea with villous atrophy. J Pediatr 124:63–70

Corral-Debrinski M, Stepien G, Shoffer JM, Lott MT, Kanter K, Wallace DC (1991) Hypoxemia is associated with mitochondrial DNA damage and gene induction. JAMA 266:1812–1816

Corral-Debrinski M, Horton T, Lott MT, Shoffner JM, Beal MF, Wallace DC (19992a) Mitochondrial DNA deletions in human brain: Regional variability and increase with advanced age. Nat Genet 2:324–329

Corral-Debrinski M, Shoffner JM, Lott MT, Wallace DC (1992b) Association of mitochondrial DNA damage with aging and coronary atherosclerotic heart disease. Mutation Res 275:168–180

Corral-Debrinski M, Horton T, Lott MT et al. (1994) Marked changes in mitochondrial DNA deletion levels in Alzheimer brains. Genomics 23:471–476

Cortopassi GA, Arnheim N (1990) Detection of a specific mitochondrial DNA deletion in tissues of older humans. Nucl Acids Res 18:6927–6933

Cortopassi GA, Hutchin TP (1994) Germline inheritance of a rare mtDNA variant leads to greatly increased risk for Alzheimer's disease. (Abstract 857). Journal 55:A149

Cortopassi G, Wang E (1995) Modelling the effects of age-related mtDNA mutation accumulation; complex I deficiency, superoxide and cell death. Biochim Biophys Acta 1271:171–176

Cortopassi GA, Shibata D, Soong NW, Arnheim N (1992) A pattern of accumulation of a somatic deletion of mitochondrial DNA in aging human tissues. Proc Natl Acad Sci USA 89:7370–7374

Cozens AL, Runswick MJ, Walker JE (1989) DNA sequences of two expressed nuclear genes for human mitochondrial ADP/ATP translocase. J Mol Biol 206:261–280

Cuticchia AJ (1995) Human Gene Mapping (1994), a Compendium. Journal

Dahl HH (1998) Getting to the nucleus of mitochondrial disorders: Identification of respiratory chain-enzyme genes causing Leigh syndrome [editorial; comment]. Am J Hum Genet 63:1594–1597

Dairaghi DJ, Shadel GS, Clayton DA (1995) Addition of a 29 residue carboxyl-terminal tail converts a simple HMG box-containing protein into a transcriptional activator. J Mol Biol 249:11–28

Darras BT, Zeviani M, Schone EA, Francke U (1987) Sequences homologous to cytochrome c oxidase subunit IV are located on human chromosome 14q21-qter and 16q22-q24. Journal 46:603

Das DK, George A, Liu XK, Rao PS (1989) Detection of hydroxyl radical in the mitochondria of ischemic-reperfused myocardium by trapping with salicylate. Biochem Biophys Res Commun 165:1004–1009

Davidson M, King MP, Koga Y, Zhang L, Schon EA (1995) Physical communication between mammalian mitochondria: a genetic approach. (Abstract PS111). Journal 23

Davis KA, Hatefi Y (1971a) Spectral and reconstitution properties of cytochromes b in complexes II and 3. Biochem Biophys Res Commun 44:1338–1344

Davis KA, Hatefi Y (1971b) Succinate dehydrogenase. I. Purification, molecular properties, and substructure. Biochemistry 10:2509–2516

de Coo R, Buddiger P, Smeets H et al. (1995) Molecular cloning and characterization of the active human mitochondrial NADH:ubiquinone oxidoreductase 24-kDa gene (NDUFV2) and its pseudogene. Genomics 26:461–466

de Coo IF, Sistermans EA, de Wijs IJ et al. (1998) A mitochondrial tRNA(Val) gene mutation (G1642A) in a patient with mitochondrial myopathy, lactic acidosis, and stroke-like episodes. Neurology 50:293–295

de Coo IF, Renier WO, Ruitenbeek W et al. (1999) A 4-base pair deletion in the mitochondrial cytochrome b gene associated with parkinsonism/MELAS overlap syndrome. Ann Neurol 45:130–133

De Vries DD, Buzing CJM, Ruitenbeek W et al. (1992) Myopathology and a mitochondrial DNA deletion in the Pearson marrow and pancreas syndrome. Neuromuscular Disorders 2:185–195

De Vries DD, Van Engelen BG, Gabreels FJ, Ruitenbeek W, Van Oost BA (1993) A second missense mutation in the mitochondrial ATPase 6 gene in Leigh's syndrome. Ann Neurol 34:410–412

De Vries D, De Wijs I, Ruitenbeek W et al. (1994) Extreme variability of clinical symptoms among sibs in a MELAS family correlated with heteroplasmy for the mitochondrial A3243G mutation. J Neurol Sci 124:77–82

De Vries DD, Went LN, Bruyn GW et al. (1996) Genetic and biochemical impairment of mitochondrial complex I activity in a family with Leber hereditary optic neuropathy and hereditary spastic dystonia. Am J Hum Genet 58:703–711

Degli Esposti M (1998) Inhibitors of NADH-ubiquinone reductase: An overview. Biochim Biophys Acta 1364:222–235

Degli Esposti M, DeVries S, Crimi M, Ghelli A, Patarnello T, Meyer A (1993) Mitochondrial cytohrome b: Evolution and structure of the protein. Biochim Biophys Acta 1143:243–271

Degli Esposti M, Carelli V, Ghelli A et al. (1994) Functional alterations of the mitochondrially encoded ND4 subunit associated with Leber's hereditary optic neuropathy. FEBS Letters 352:375–379

Dekker PJ, Ryan MT, Brix J, Muller H, Honlinger A, Pfanner N (1998) Preprotein translocase of the outer mitochondrial membrane: molecular dissection and assembly of the general import pore complex. Mol Cell Biol 18:6515–6524

Denaro M, Blanc H, Johnson MJ et al. (1981) Ethnic variation in Hpa 1 endonuclease cleavage patterns of human mitochondrial DNA. Proc Natl Acad Sci USA 78:5768–5772

Desjardins P, Frost E, Morais R (1985) Ethidium bromide-induced loss of mitochondrial DNA from primary chicken embryo fibroblasts. Mol Cell Biol 5:1163–1169

DiCiero Miranda M, de Bruin VM, Vale MR, Viana GS (2000) Lipid peroxidation and nitrite plus nitrate levels in brain tissue from patients with Alzheimer's disease. Gerontology 46:179–184

Dickinson EK, Adams DL, Schon EA, Glerum DM (2000) A human SCO2 mutation helps define the role of Sco1p in the cytochrome oxidase assembly pathway. J Biol Chem 275:26780–26785

DiDonato S, Zeviani M, Giovannini P et al. (1993) Respiratory chain and mitochondrial DNA in muscle and brain in Parkinson's disease patients. Neurology 43:2262–2268

DiMauro S, Bonilla E (1997) Mitochondrial Encephalomyopathies. In Rosenberg RN, Prusiner SB, DiMauro S and Barchi RL (eds): The Molecular and Genetic Basis of Neurological Disease. Butterworth-Heinemann, Boston, p201–235

DiMauro S, Servidei S, Zeviani M et al. (1987) Cytochrome c oxidase deficiency in Leigh syndrome. Ann Neurol 22:498–506

Doda JN, Wright CT, Clayton DA (1981) Elongation of displacement-loop strands in human mouse mitochondrial DNA is arrested near specific template sequences. Proc Natl Acad Sci USA 78:6116–6120

Dorner G, Mohnike A (1976) Further evidence for a predominantly maternal transmission of maturity-onset type diabetes. Endokrinologie 68:121–124

Dorner G, Mohnike A, Steindel E (1975) On possible genetic and epigenetic modes of diabetes transmission. Endokrinologie 66:225–227

Dorner G, Plagemann A, Reinagel H (1987) Familial diabetes aggregation in type I diabetics: Gestational diabetes an apparent risk factor for increased diabetes susceptibility in the offspring. Experimental and Clinical Endocrinology 89:84–90

Du Y, Dodel RC, Eastwood BJ et al. (2000) Association of an interleukin 1 alpha polymorphism with Alzheimer's disease. Neurology 55:480–483

Duara R, Lopez-Alberola RF, Barker WW et al. (1993) A comparison of familial and sporadic Alzheimer's disease. Neurology 43:1377–1384

Dumoulin R, Sagnol I, Ferlin T, Bozon D, Stepien G, Mousson B (1996) A novel gly290asp mitochondrial cytochrome b mutation linked to a complex III deficiency in progressive exercise intolerance. Molecular and Cellular Probes 10:389–391

Dunbar DR, Moonie PA, Swingler RJ, Davidson D, Roberts R, Holt IJ (1993) Maternally transmitted partial direct tandem duplication of mitochondrial DNA associated with diabetes mellitus. Human Molecular Genetics 2:1619–1624

Dunbar DR, Moonie PA, Jacobs HT, Holt IJ (1995) Different cellular backgrounds confer a marked advantage to either mutant or wild-type mitochondrial genomes. Proc Natl Acad Sci USA 92:6562–6566

Duncan AM, Chow W, Robinson BH (1992) Localization of the human 75-kDal Fe-S protein of NADH-coenzyme Q reductase gene (NDUFS1) to 2q33—-q34. Cytogenet Cell Genet 60:212–213

Dyer MR, Walker JE (1993) Sequences of members of the human gene family for the c subunit of mitochondrial ATP synthase. Biochem J 293:51–64

Earnshaw WC (1999) Apoptosis. A cellular poison cupboard [news]. Nature 397:387, 389

Edland SD, Silverman JM, Peskind ER, Tsuang D, Wijsman E, Morris JC (1996) Increased risk of dementia in mothers of Alzheimer's disease cases: evidence for maternal inheritance. Neurology 47:254–256

Ege T, Krondahl U, Ringertz NR (1974) Introduction of nuclei and micronuclei into cells and enucleated cytoplasms by Sendai virus induced fusion. Experimental Cell Research 88:428–432

Egensperger R, Kosel S, Schnopp NM, Mehrein P, Graeber MB (1997) Association of the mitochondrial tRNA(A4336G) mutation with Alzheimer's and Parkinson's diseases. Neuropathology and Applied Neurobiology 23:315–321

Eleff S, Kennaway NG, Buist NR et al. (1984) ^{31}P NMR study of improvement in oxidative phosphorylation by vitamins K$_3$ and C in a patient with a defect in electron transport at complex III in skeletal muscle. Proc Natl Acad Sci USA 81:3529–3533

Eliasson MJ, Sampei K, Mandir AS et al. (1997) Poly(ADP-ribose) polymerase gene disruption renders mice resistant to cerebral ischemia. Nat Med 3:1089–1095

Ellison JW, Li X, Francke U, Shapiro LJ (1996) Rapid evolution of human pseudoautosomal genes and their mouse homologs. Mammalian Genome 7:25–30

Elston T, Wang H, Oster G (1998) Energy transduction in ATP synthase. Nature 391:510–513

Endo H, Matsuda C, Kagawa Y (1994) Exclusion of an alternatively spliced exon in human ATP synthase gamma-subunit pre-mRNA requires de novo protein synthesis. J Biol Chem 269:12488–12493

Enerback S, Jacobsson A, Simpson EM et al. (1997) Mice lacking mitochondrial uncoupling protein are cold-sensitive but not obese. Nature 387:90–94

Enriquez JA, Chomyn A, Attardi G (1995) MtDNA mutation in MERRF syndrome causes defective aminoacylation of tRNA^{Lys} and premature translation termination. Nat Genet 10:47–55

Enter C, Muller-Hocker J, Zierz S et al. (1991) A specific point mutation in the mitochondrial genome of Caucasians with MELAS. Hum Genet 88:233–266

Erickson RP (1972) Leber's optic atrophy, a possible example of maternal inheritance. Am J Hum Genet 24:348–349

Esposito LA, Melov S, Panov A, Cottrell BA, Wallace DC (1999) Mitochondrial disease in mouse results in increased oxidative stress. Proc Natl Acad Sci USA 96:4820–4825

Esposito LA, Kokoszka JE, Waymire KG, Cottrell B, MacGregor GR, Wallace DC (2000) Mitochondrial oxidative stress in mice lacking the glutathione peroxidase-1 gene. Free Rad Biol Med 28:754–766

Etcheberrigaray R, Ito E, Kim CS, Alkon DL (1994) Soluble beta-amyloid induction of Alzheimer's phenotype for human fibroblast K+ channels. Science 264:276–279

Eto K, Tsubamoto Y, Terauchi Y et al. (1999) Role of NADH shuttle system in glucose-induced activation of mitochondrial metabolism and insulin secretion. Science 283:981–985

Evans MJ, Scarpulla RC (1988) The human somatic cytochrome c gene: Two classes of processed pseudogenes demarcate a period of rapid molecular evolution. Proc Natl Acad Sci USA 85:9625–9629

Fabrizi GM, Rizzuto R, Nakase H, Mita S, Kadenbach B, Schon EA (1989) Sequence of a cDNA specifying subunit VIa of human cytochrome c oxidase. Nucl Acids Res 17:6409

Farrell LB, Nagley P (1987) Human liver cDNA clones encoding proteolipid subunit 9 of the mitochondrial ATPase complex. Biochem Biophys Res Commun 144:1257–1264

Fassati A, Bordoni A, Amboni P et al. (1994) Chronic progressive external ophthalmoplegia: A correlative study of quantitative molecular data and histochemical and biochemical profile. J Neurol Sci 123:140–146

Fearnley IM, Skehel JM, Walker JE (1994) Electrospray ionization mass spectrometric analysis of subunits of NADH:ubiquinone oxidoreductase (complex I) from bovine heart mitochondria. Biochem Soc Trans 22:551–555

Ferris SD, Sage RD, Wilson AC (1982) Evidence from mtDNA sequences that common laboratory strains of inbred mice are descended from a single female. Nature 295:163–165

Fetter JR, Qian J, Shapleigh J et al. (1995) Possible proton relay pathways in cytochrome c oxidase. Proc Natl Acad Sci USA 92:1604–1608

Figarella-Branger D, Pellissier JF, Scheiner C, Wernert F, Desnuelle C (1992) Defects of the mitochondrial respiratory chain complexes in three pediatric cases with hypotonia and cardiac involvement. J Neurol Sci 108:105–113

Fillingame RH, Girvin ME, Jiang W, Valiyaveetil F, Hermolin J (1998) Subunit interactions coupling H+ transport and ATP synthesis in F$_1$F$_0$ ATP synthase. Acta Physiologica Scandinavica. Supplementum 643:163–168

Fischel-Ghodsian N, Prezant TR, Bu X, Oztas S (1993) Mitochondrial ribosomal RNA gene mutation in a patient with sporadic aminoglycoside ototoxicity. American J Otolaryngol 14:399–403

Fisher RP, Topper JN, Clayton DA (1987) Promoter selection in human mitochondria involves binding of a transcription factor to orientation-independent upstream regulatory elements. Cell 50:247–258

Flanigan KM, Johns DR (1993) Association of the 11778 mitochondrial DNA mutation and demyelinating disease. Neurology 43:2720–2722

Fleury C, Neverova M, Collins S et al. (1997) Uncoupling protein-2: a novel gene linked to obesity and hyperinsulinemia. Nat Genet 15:269–272

Fliss MS, Usadel H, Caballero OL et al. (2000) Facile detection of mitochondrial DNA mutations in tumors and bodily fluids. Science 287:2017–2019

Franceschina L, Salani S, Bordoni A et al. (1998) A novel mitochondrial tRNA(Ile) point mutation in chronic progressive external ophthalmoplegia [letter]. J Neurol 245:755–758

Frankel D, Mehindate K, Schipper HM (2000) Role of heme oxygenase-1 in the regulation of manganese superoxide dismutase gene expression in oxidatively-challenged astroglia. J Cell Physiol 185:80–86

Freinkel N, Metzger BE, Phelps RL et al. (1986) Gestational diabetes mellitus: a syndrome with phenotypic and genotypic heterogeneity. Horm Metabol Res 18:427–430

Fromenty B, Grimbert S, Mansouri A et al. (1995) Hepatic mitochondrial DNA deletion in alcoholics: Association with microvesicular steatosis. Gastroenterology 108:193–200

Fu K, Hartlen R, Johns T, Genge A, Karpati G, Shoubridge EA (1996) A novel heteroplasmic tRNAleu(CUN) mtDNA point mutation in a sporadic patient with mitochondrial encephalomyopathy segregates rapidly in skeletal muscle and suggests an approach to therapy. Human Molecular Genetics 5:1835–1840

Fukuyama R, Wadhwani KC, Galdzicki Z, Rapoport SI, Ehrenstein G (1994) Beta-amyloid polypeptide increases calcium-uptake in PC12 cells: a possible mechanism for its cellular toxicity in Alzheimer's disease. Brain Research 667:269–272

Funakawa I, Kato H, Terao A et al. (1995) Cerebellar ataxia in patients with Leber's hereditary optic neuropathy. J Neurol 242:75–77

Galante YM, Hatefi Y (1979) Purification and molecular and enzymic properties of mitochondrial NADH dehydrogenase. Archives of Biochemistry and Biophysics 192:559–568

Galiegue S, Jbilo O, Combes T et al. (1999) Cloning and characterization of PRAX-1. A new protein that specifically interacts with the peripheral benzodiazepine receptor. J Biol Chem 274:2938–2952

Gattermann N, Retzlaff S, Wang YL et al. (1997) Heteroplasmic point mutations of mitochondrial DNA affecting subunit of cytochrome c oxidase in two patients with acquired idiopathic sideroblastic anemia. Blood 90:4961–4972

Gay NJ, Walker JE (1985) Two genes encoding the bovine mitochondrial ATP synthase proteolipid specify precursors with different import sequences and are expressed in a tissue-specific manner. EMBO J 4:3519–3524

Gebhart SS, Shoffner JM, Koontz D, Kaufman A, Wallace D (1996) Insulin resistance associated with maternally inherited diabetes and deafness. Metabolism 45:526–531

Gelb BD, Adams V, Jones SN, Griffin LD, MacGregor GR, McCabe ER (1992) Targeting of hexokinase 1 to liver and hepatoma mitochondria. Proc Natl Acad Sci USA 89:202–206

Gennis R, Ferguson-Miller S (1995) Structure of cytochrome c oxidase, energy generator of aerobic life. Science 269:1063–1064

Gerbitz KD, Jaksch M (1994) Mitochondrial DNA, aging and sudden infant death syndrome. European J Clin Chem Clin Biochem 32:487–488

Gerbitz KD, van den Ouweland JM, Maassen JA, Jaksch M (1995) Mitochondrial diabetes mellitus: A review. Biochim Biophys Acta 1271:253–260

German MS (1993) Glucose sensing in pancreatic islet beta cells: The key role of glucokinase and the glycolytic intermediates. Proc Natl Acad Sci USA 90:1781–1785

Ghafourifar P, Richter C (1997) Nitric oxide synthase activity in mitochondria. FEBS Letters 418:291–296

Ghafourifar P, Schenk U, Klein SD, Richter C (1999) Mitochondrial nitric-oxide synthase stimulation causes cytochrome c release from isolated mitochondria. Evidence for intramitochondrial peroxynitrite formation. J Biol Chem 274:31185–31188.

Ghivizzani SC, Madsen CS, hauswirth WW (1993) In organello footprinting. Analysis of protein binding at regulatory regions in bovine mitochondrial DNA. J Biol Chem 268:8675–8682

Ghivizzani SC, Madsen CS, Nelen MR, Ammini CV, Hauswirth WW (1994) In organello footprint analysis of human mitochondrial DNA: Human mitochondrial transcription factor A interactions at the origin of replication. Mol Cell Biol 14:7717–7730

Ghosh SS, Swerdlow RH, Miller SW, Sheeman B, Parker WD, Jr., Davis RE (1999) Use of cytoplasmic hybrid cell lines for elucidating the role of mitochondrial dysfunction in Alzheimer's disease and Parkinson's disease. Annals of the New York Academy of Science 893:176–191

Gidh-Jain M, Takeda J, Xu LZ et al. (1993) Glucokinase mutations associated with non-insulin-dependent (type 2) diabetes mellitus have decreased enzymatic activity: Implications for structure/function relationships. Proc Natl Acad Sci USA 90:1932–1936

Giles RE, Blanc H, Cann HM, Wallace DC (1980) Maternal inheritance of human mitochondrial DNA. Proc Natl Acad Sci USA 77:6715–6719

Ginsberg SD, Hemby SE, Lee VM, Eberwine JH, Trojanowski JQ (2000) Expression profile of transcripts in Alzheimer's disease tangle-bearing CA1 neurons. Ann Neurol 48:77–87

Giraud S, Bonod-Bidaud C, Wesolowski-Louvel M, Stepien G (1998) Expression of human ANT2 gene in highly proliferative cells: GRBOX, a new transcriptional element, is involved in the regulation of glycolytic ATP import into mitochondria. J Mol Biol 281:409–418

Glick B, Schatz G (1991) Import of proteins into mitochondria. Annual Review of Genetics 25:21–44

Glick BS, Beasley EM, Schatz G (1992) Protein sorting in mitochondria. Trends in Biochemical Sciences 17:453–459

Golbe LI, Di Iorio G, Bonavita V, Miller DC, Duvoisin RC (1990) A large kindred with autosomal dominant Parkinson's disease. Ann Neurol 27:276–282

Goldhaber JI, Weiss JN (1992) Oxygen free radicals and cardiac reperfusion abnormalities. Hypertension 20:118–127

Gong DW, He Y, Karas M, Reitman M (1997) Uncoupling protein-3 is a mediator of thermogenesis regulated by thyroid hormone, beta3-adrenergic agonists, and leptin. J Biol Chem 272:24129–24132

Gonzalez-Halphen D, Lindorfer MA, Capaldi RA (1988) Subunit arrangement in beef heart complex III. Biochemistry 27:7021–7031

Goto Y (1995) Clinical features of MELAS and mitochondrial DNA mutations. Muscle and Nerve 3:S107–S112

Goto Y, Nonaka I, Horai S (1990) A mutation in the tRNA$^{Leu(UUR)}$ gene associated with the MELAS subgroup of mitochondrial encephalomyopathies. Nature 348:651–653

Goto Y, Nonaka I, Horai S (1991) A new mtDNA mutation associated with mitochondrial myopathy, encephalopathy, lactic acidosis and stroke-like episodes (MELAS). Biochim Biophys Acta 1097:238–240

Goto Y, Horai S, Matsuoka T et al. (1992a) Mitochondrial myopathy, encephalopathy, lactic acidosis, and stroke-like episodes (MELAS): A correlative study of the clinical features and mitochondrial DNA mutation. Neurology 42:545–550

Goto Y, Tojo M, Tohyama J, Horai S, Nonaka I (1992b) A novel point mutation in the mitochondrial tRNA$^{Leu(UUR)}$ gene in a family with mitochondrial myopathy. Ann Neurol 31:672–675

Goto Y, Tsugane K, Tanabe Y, Nonaka I, Horai S (1994) A new point mutation at nucelotide pair 3291 of the tRNA$^{Leu(UUR)}$ gene in a patient with mitochondrial myopathy, encephalopathy, lactic acidosis, and stroke-like episodes (MELAS). Biochem Biophys Res Commun 202:1624–1630

Govan GG, Smith PR, Kellar-Wood H, Schapira AH, Harding AE (1994) HLA class II genotypes in Leber's hereditary optic neuropathy. J Neurol Sci 126:193–196

Graham B, Waymire K, Cottrell B, Trounce IA, MacGregor GR, Wallace DC (1997) A mouse model for mitochondrial myopathy and cardiomyopathy resulting from a deficiency in the heart/skeletal muscle isoform of the adenine nucleotide translocator. Nat Genet 16:226–234

Green DR, Reed JC (1998) Mitochondria and apoptosis. Science 281:1309–1312

Grigorieff N (1998) Three-dimensional structure of bovine NADH:ubiquinone oxidoreductase (complex 1) at 22 A in ice. J Mol Biol 277:1033–1046

Grimaldi LM, Casadei VM, Ferri C et al. (2000) Association of early-onset Alzheimer's disease with an interleukin- lalpha gene polymorphism. Ann Neurol 47:361–365

Gross NJ, Getz GS, Rabinowitz M (1969) Apparent turnover of mitochondrial deoxyribonucleic acid and mitochondrial phospholipids in the tissues of the rat. J Biol Chem 244:1552–1562

Gu M, Gash MT, Mann VM, Javoy-Agid F, Cooper JM, Schapira AH (1996) Mitochondrial defect in Huntington's disease caudate nucleus. Ann Neurol 39:385–389

Guan MX, Enriquez JA, Fischel-Ghodsian N et al. (1998) The deafness-associated mitochondrial DNA mutation at position 7445, which affects tRNASer(UCN) precursor processing, has long-range effects on NADH dehydrogenase subunit ND6 gene expression. Mol Cell Biol 18:5868–5879

Guenebaut V, Schlitt A, Weiss H, Leonard K, Friedrich T (1998) Consistent structure between bacterial and mitochondrial NADH:ubiquinone oxidoreductase (complex I). J Mol Biol 276:105–112

Guo Z, Ersoz A, Butterfield DA, Mattson MP (2000) Beneficial effects of dietary restriction on cerebral cortical synaptic terminals: Preservation of glucose and glutamate transport and mitochondrial function after exposure to amyloid beta-peptide, iron, and 3-nitropropionic acid. J Neurochem 75:314–320

Gyllensten U, Wharton D, Josefsson A, Wilson AC (1991) Paternal inheritance of mitochondrial DNA in mice. Nature 352:255–257

Hadjigeorgiou GM, Kim SH, Fischbeck KH et al. (1999) A new mitochondrial DNA mutation (A3288G) in the tRNA(Leu(UUR)) gene associated with familial myopathy. J Neurol Sci 164:153–157

Haferkamp O, Scheuerle A, Schlenk R, Melzner I, Pavenstadt-Grupp I, Rodel G (1994) Mitochondrial complex I and III mutations and neutral-lipid storage in activated mononuclear macrophages and neutrophils: a case presenting with necrotizing myopathy, poikiloderma atrophicans vasculare, and xanthogranulomatous bursitis. Human Pathology 25:419–423

Haferkamp O, Rosenau W, Scheuerle A, Pietrczyk C, Skowronek P, Rodel G (1998) Disseminated neocortical and subcortical encephalopathy (DNSE) with widespread activation of brain macrophages: A new dementia disorder? Autopsy reports of two postmenopausal women from families with mitochondrial DNA mutations. Clinical Neuropathology 17:85–94

Ham D, Schipper HM (2000) Heme oxygenase-1 induction and mitochondrial iron sequestration in astroglia exposed to amyloid peptides. Cell Mol Biol 46:587–596

Hamblet NS, Castora FJ (1995) Mitochondrial DNA deletion analysis: A comparison of PCR quantitative methods. Biochem Biophys Res Commun 207:839–847

Hamilton MG, O'Brien TW (1974) Ultracentrifugal characterization of the mitochondrial ribosome and subribosomal particles of bovine liver: Molecular size and composition. Biochemistry 13:5400–5403

Hammans SR, Sweeney MG, Brockington M, Morgan-Hughes JA, Harding AE (1991) Mitochondrial encephalopathies: Molecular genetic diagnosis from blood samples. Lancet 337:1311–1313

Hammans SR, Sweeney MG, Hanna MG, Brockington M, Morgan-Hughes JA, Harding AE (1995) The mitochondrial DNA transfer RNA[Leu(UUR)] A→G[(3243)] mutation. A clinical and genetic study. Brain 118:721–734

Hanefeld FA, Ernst BP, Wilichowski E, Christen HJ (1994) Leber's hereditary optic neuropathy mitochondrial DNA mutations in childhood multiple sclerosis. Neuropediatrics 25:331

Hanna MG, Nelson I, Sweeney MG et al. (1995) Congenital encephalomyopathy and adult-onset myopathey and diabetes mellitus: Different phenotypic associations of a new heteroplasmic mtDNA tRNA glutamic acid mutation. Am J Hum Genet 56:1026–1033

Hanna MG, Nelson IP, Morgan-Hughes JA, Wood NW (1998a) MELAS: A new disease associated mitochondrial DNA mutation and evidence for further genetic heterogeneity. J Neurol, Neurosurgery & Psychiatry 65:512–517

Hanna MG, Nelson IP, Rahman S et al. (1998b) Cytochrome c oxidase deficiency associated with the first stop-codon point mutation in human mtDNA. Am J Hum Genet 63:29–36

Hao H, Moraes CT (1997) A disease-associated G5703A mutation in human mitochondrial DNA causes a conformational change and a marked decrease in steady-state levels of mitochondrial tRNA(Asn). Mol Cell Biol 17:6831–6837

Hao H, Bonilla E, Manfredi G, DiMauro S, Moraes CT (1995) Segregation patterns of a novel mutation in the mitochondrial tRNA glutamic acid gene associated with myopathy and diabetes mellitus. Am J Hum Genet 56:1017–1025

Hara H, Wakayama Y, Kouno Y, Yamada H, Tanaka M, Ozawa T (1994) Acute peripheral neuropathy, rhabdomyolysis, and severe lactic acidosis associated with 3243 A to G mitochondrial DNA mutation. J Neurol, Neurosurgery and Psychiatry 57:1545–1546

Haraguchi Y, Chung AB, Torroni A et al. (1993) Genetic mapping of human heart-skeletal muscle adenine nucleotide translocator and its relationship to the facioscapulohumeral muscular dystrophy locus. Genomics 16:479–485

Haraguchi Y, Chung AB, Neill S, Wallace DC (1994) OXBOX and REBOX, overlapping promoter elements of the mitochondrial F_0F_1-ATP synthase beta subunit gene. OXBOX/REBOX in the ATPsyn beta promoter. J Biol Chem 269:9330–9334

Harding AE, Holt IJ, Sweeney MG, Brockington M, Davis MB (1992a) Prenatal diagnosis of mitochondrial DNA8993 T-G disease. Am J Hum Genet 50:629–633

Harding AE, Sweeney MG, Miller DH et al. (1992b) Occurrence of a multiple sclerosis-like illness in women who have a Leber's heditary optic neuropathy mitochondrial DNA mutation. Brain 115:979–989

Harding AE, Sweeney MG, Govan GG, Riordan-Eva P (1995) Pedigree analysis in Leber hereditary optic neuropathy families with a pathogenic mtDNA mutation. Am J Hum Genet 57:77–86

Hardy JA, Higgins GA (1992) Alzheimer's disease: The amyloid cascade hypothesis. Science 256:184–185

Hartzog PE, Cain BD (1994) Second-site suppressor mutations at glycine 218 and histidine 245 in the alpha subunit of F_1F_0 ATP synthase in Escherichia coli. J Biol Chem 269:32313–32317

Hasegawa H, Matsuoka T, Goto Y, Nonaka I (1993) Cytochrome c oxidase activity is deficient in blood vessels of patients with myoclonus epilepsy with ragged-red fibers. Acta Neuropathologica (Berlin) 85:280–284

Hatanpaa K, Brady DR, Stoll J, Rapoport SI, Chandrasekaran K (1996) Neuronal activity and early neurofibrillary tangles in Alzheimer's disease. Ann Neurol 40:411–420

Hatefi Y (1985) The mitochondrial electron transport and oxidative phosphorylation system. Annu Rev Biochem 54:1015–1069

Hatefi Y, Galante YM (1980) Isolation of cytochrome b560 from complex II (succinateubiquinone oxidoreductase) and its reconstitution with succinate dehydrogenase. J Biol Chem 255:5530–5537

Hattori N, Tanaka M, Ozawa T, Mizuno Y (1991) Immunohistochemical studies on complexes I, II, III, and IV of mitochondria in Parkinson's disease. Ann Neurol 30:563–571

Hattori N, Suzuki H, Wang Y et al. (1995) Structural organization and chromosomal localization of the human nuclear gene (NDUFV2) for the 24-kDa iron-sulfur subunit of complex 1 in mitochondrial respiratory chain. Biochem Biophys Res Commun 216:771–777

Hattori Y, Goto Y, Sakuta R, Nonaka I, Mizuno Y, Horai S (1994) Point mutations in mitochondrial tRNA genes: sequence analysis of chronic progressive external ophthalmoplegia (CPEO). J Neurol Sci 125:50–55

Hayakawa M, Hattori H, Sugiyama S, Ozawa T (1992) Age-associated oxygen damage and mutations in mitochondrial DNA in human hearts. Biochem Biophys Res Commun 189:979–985

Hayakawa M, Sugiyama S, Hattori K, Takasawa M, Ozawa T (1993) Age-associated damage in mitochondrial DNA in human hearts. Molecular and Cellular Biochemistry 119:95–103

Hayashi J, Werbin H, Shay JW (1986) Effects of normal human fibroblast mitochondrial DNA on segregation of HeLaTG Mitochondrial DNA and on tumorigenicity of HeLaTG cells. Cancer Research 46:4001–4006

Hayashi J, Ohta S, Kikuchi A, Takemitsu M, Goto Y, Nonaka I (1991) Introduction of disease-related mitochondrial DNA deletions into HeLa cells lacking mitochondrial DNA results in mitochondrial dysfunction. Proc Natl Acad Sci USA 88:10614–10618

Hayashi J, Ohta S, Takai D et al. (1993) Accumulation of mtDNA with a mutation at position 3271 in tRNA$^{Leu(UUR)}$ gene introduced from a MELAS patient to HeLa cells lacking mtDNA results in progressive inhibition of mitochondrial respiratory function. Biochem Biophys Res Commun 197:1049–1055

Hayashi J, Ohta S, Kagawa Y et al. (1994) Functional and morphological abnormalities of mitochondria in human cells containing mitochondrial DNA with pathogenic point mutations in tRNA genes. J Biol Chem 269:19060–19066

Heddi A, Lestienne P, Wallace DC, Stepien G (1993) Mitochondrial DNA expression in mitochondrial myopathies and coordinated expression of nuclear genes involved in ATP production. J Biol Chem 268:12156–12163

Heddi A, Lestienne P, Wallace DC, Stepien G (1994) Steady state levels of mitochondrial and nuclear oxidative phosphorylation transcripts in Kearns-Sayre syndrome. Biochim Biophys Acta 1226:206–212

Heddi A, Stepien G, Benke PJ, Wallace DC (1999) Coordinate induction of energy gene expression in tissues of mitochondrial disease patients. J Biol Chem 274:22968–22976

Heher KL, Johns DR (1993) A maculopathy associated with the 15257 mitochondrial DNA mutation. Archives of Ophthalmology 111:1495–1499

Hess J, Burkhard P, Morris M, Lalioti M, Myers P, Hadengue A (1995) Ischaemic colitis due to mitochondrial cytopathy [letter]. Lancet 346:189–190

Hess JF, Parisi MA, Bennett JL, Clayton DA (1991) Impairment of mitochondrial transcription termination by a point mutation associated with the MELAS subgroup of mitochondrial encephalomyopathies. Nature 351:236–239

Higuti T, Tsurumi C, Osaka F et al. (1991) Molecular cloning of cDNA for the import precursor of human subunit B of H(+)-ATP synthase in mitochondria. Biochem Biophys Res Commun 178:1014–1020

Higuti T, Kawamura Y, Kuroiwa K, Miyazaki S, Tsujita H (1993) Molecular cloning and sequence of two cDNAs for human subunit c of H$^+$-ATP synthase in mitochondria. Biochim Biophys Acta 1173:87–90

Hill K, Model K, Ryan MT et al. (1998) Tom40 forms the hydrophilic channel of the mitochondrial import pore for preproteins [see comment]. Nature 395:516–521

Hinokio Y, Suzuki S, Komatu K et al. (1995) A new mitochondrial DNA deletion associated with diabetic amyotrophy, diabetic myoatrophy and diabetic fatty liver. Muscle and Nerve 3:S142–149

Hirawake H, Wang H, Kuramochi T, Kojima S, Kita K (1994) Human complex II (succinate-ubiquinone oxidoreductase): cDNA cloning of the flavoprotein (Fp) subunit of liver mitochondria. J Biochem 116:221–227

Hirawake H, Taniwaki M, Tamura A, Kojima S, Kita K (1997) Cytochrome b in human complex II (succinate-ubiquinone oxidoreductase): cDNA cloning of the components in liver mitochondria and chromosome assignment of the genes for the large (SDHC) and small (SDHD) subunits to Iq21 and 11q23. Cytogenet Cell Genet 79:132–138

Hofhaus G, Johns DR, Hurko O, Attardi G, Chomyn A (1996) Respiration and growth defects in transmitochondrial cell lines carrying the 11778 mutation associated with Leber's hereditary optic neuropathy. J Biol Chem 271:13155–13161

Hofmann S, Lichtner P, Schuffenhauer S, Gerbitz KD, Meitinger T (1998) Assignment of the human genes coding for cytochrome c oxidase subunits Va (COX5A), VIc (COX6C) and VIIc (COX7C) to chromosome bands 15q25, 8q22→q23 and 5q14 and of three pseudogenes (COX5API, COX6CPI, COX7CPI) to 14q22, 16p12

and 13q14→q21 by FISH and radiation hybrid mapping. Cytogenet Cell Genet 83:226–227

Holt IJ, Harding AE, Morgan-Hughes JA (1988) Deletions of muscle mitochondrial DNA in patients with mitochondrial myopathies. Nature 331:717–719

Holt IJ, Harding AE, Morgan-Hughes JA (1989a) Deletions of muscle mitochondrial DNA in mitochondrial myopathies: Sequence analysis and possible mechanisms. Nucl Acids Res 17:4465–4469

Holt IJ, Miller DH, Harding AE (1989b) Genetic heterogeneity and mitochondrial DNA heteroplasmy in Leber's hereditary optic neuropathy. J Med Genet 26:739–743

Holt IJ, Harding AE, Petty RK, Morgan-Hughes JA (1990) A new mitochondrial disease associated with mitochondrial DNA heteroplasmy. Am J Hum Genet 46:428–433

Hommes FA, Polman HA, Reerink JD (1968) Leigh's encephalomyelopathy: An inborn error of gluconeogenesis. Archives of Disease in Childhood 43:423–426

Horton TM, Graham BH, Corral-Debrinski M et al. (1995) Marked increase in mitochondrial DNA deletion levels in the cerebral cortex of Huntington's Disease patients. Neurology 45:1879–1883

Horton TM, Petros JA, Heddi A et al. (1996) Novel mitochondrial DNA deletion found in a renal cell carcinoma. Genes, Chromosomes & Cancer 15:95–101

Hosler JP, Ferguson-Miller S, Calhoun MW et al. (1993) Insight into the active-site structure and function of cytochrome oxidase by analysis of site-directed mutants of bacterial cytochrome aa_3 and cytochrome bo. J Bioenerg Biomembr 25:121–136

Hotta Y, Hayakawa M, Saito K, Kanai A, Nakajima A, Fujiki K (1989) Diagnosis of Leber's optic neuropathy by means of polymerase chain reaction amplification. Am J Ophthalmol 108:601–602

Houldsworth J, Attardi G (1988) Two distinct genes for ADP/ATP translocase are expressed at the mRNA level in adult human liver. Proc Natl Acad Sci USA 85:377–381

Houshmand M, Larsson NG, Holme E, Oldfors A, Tulinius MH, Andersen O (1994) Automatic sequencing of mitochondrial tRNA genes in patients with mitochondrial encephalomyopathy. Biochim Biophys Acta 1226:49–55

Houshmand M, Lindberg C, Moslemi AR, Oldfors A, Holme E (1999) A novel heteroplasmic point mutation in the mitochondrial tRNA(Lys) gene in a sporadic case of mitochondrial encephalomyopathy: de novo mutation and no transmission to the offspring. Hum Mutat 13:203–209

Houstek J, Klement P, Hermanska J et al. (1995) Altered properties of mitochondrial ATP-synthase in patients with a T→G mutation in the ATPase 6 (subunit a) gene at position 8993 of mtDNA. Biochim Biophys Acta 1271:349–357

Howell N (1994) Mitochondrial gene mutations and human diseases: A prolegomenon [editorial]. Am J Hum Genet 55:219–224

Howell N (1997) Leber hereditary optic neuropathy: How do mitochondrial DNA mutations cause degeneration of the optic nerve? J Bioenerg Biomembr 29:165–173

Howell N (1998) Leber hereditary optic neuropathy: Respiratory chain dysfunction and degeneration of the optic nerve. Vision Research 38:1495–1504

Howell N, Bindoff LA, McCullough DA et al. (1991a) Leber hereditary optic neuropathy: identification of the same mitochondrial ND1 mutation in six pedigrees. Am J Hum Genet 49:939–950

Howell N, Kubacka I, Xu M, McCullough DA (1991b) Leber hereditary optic neuropathy: Involvement of the mitochondrial ND1 gene and evidence for an intragenic suppressor mutation. Am J Hum Genet 48:935–942

Howell N, McCullough D, Bodis-Wollner I (1992) Molecular genetic analysis of a sporadic case of Leber hereditary optic neuropathy [letter]. Am J Hum Genet 50:443–446

Howell N, Halvorson S, Burns J, McCullough DA, Poulton J (1993a) When does bilateral optic atrophy become Leber hereditary optic atrophy? [letter]. Am J Hum Genet 53:959–963

Howell N, Kubacka I, Halvorson S, Mackey D (1993b) Leber's hereditary optic neuropathy: The etiological role of a mutation in the mitochondrial cytochrome b gene [letter]. Genetics 133:133–136

Howell N, Kubacka I, Halvorson S, Howell B, McCullough DA, Mackey D (1995) Phylogenetic analysis of the mitochondrial genomes from Leber hereditary optic neuropathy pedigrees. Genetics 140:285–302

Howell N, Bogolin C, Jamieson R, Marenda DR, Mackey DA (1998) mtDNA mutations that cause optic neuropathy: How do we know? [letter]. Am J Hum Genet 62:196–202

Huang X, Atwood CS, Hartshorn MA et al. (1999) The A beta peptide of Alzheimer's disease directly produces hydrogen peroxide through metal ion reduction. Biochemistry 38:7609–7616

Huoponen K, Vilkki J, Savontaus ML, Aula P, Nikoskelainen EK (1990) Analysis of mitochondrial ND4 gene DNA sequence in Finnish families with Leber hereditary optic neuroretinopathy. Genomics 8:583–585

Huoponen K, Vilkki J, Aula P, Nikoskelainen EK, Savontaus ML (1991) A new mtDNA mutation associated with Leber hereditary optic neuroretinopathy. Am J Hum Genet 48:1147–1153

Huoponen K, Lamminen T, Juvonen V, Aula P, Nikoskelainen E, Savontaus JL (1993) The spectrum of mitochondrial DNA mutations in families with Leber hereditary optic neuroretinopathy. Hum Genet 92:379–384

Hutchin T, Cortopassi G (1995) A mitochondrial DNA clone is associated with increased risk for Alzheimer disease. Proc Natl Acad Sci USA 92:6892–6895

Hutchin T, Haworth I, Higashi K et al. (1993) A molecular basis for human hypersensitivity to aminoglycoside antibiotics. Nucl Acids Res 21:4174–4179

Ikebe S, Tanaka M, Ohno K et al. (1990) Increase of deleted mitochondrial DNA in the striatum in Parkinson's disease and senescence. Biochem Biophys Res Commun 170:1044–1048

Ikeda S, Sumiyoshi H, Oda T (1994) DNA binding properties of recombinant human mitochondrial transcription factor 1. Cell Mol Biol 40:489–493

Ingman M, Kaessmann H, Paabo S, Gyllensten U (2000) Mitochondrial genome variation and the origin of modern humans. Journal 408:708–713

Ino H, Tanaka M, Ohno K et al. (1990) Mitochondrial leucine tRNA mutation in a mitochondrial encephalomyopathy [letter; comment]. Lancet 337:234–235

Inoue K, Nakada K, Ogura A et al. (2000) Generation of mice with mitochondrial dysfunction by introducing mouse mtDNA carrying a deletion into zygotes. Journal 26:176–181

Ionasescu VV, Hart M, DiMauro S, Moraes CT (1994) Clinical and morphologic features of a myopathy associated with a point mutation in the mitochondrial tRNA^{Pro} gene. Neurology 44:975–977

Irwin MH, Johnson LW, Pinkert CA (1999) Isolation and microinjection of somatic cell-derived mitochondria and germline heteroplasmy in transmitochondrial mice. Transgenic Research 8:119–123

Ishii N, Fujii M, Hartman PS et al. (1998) A mutation in succinate dehydrogenase cytochrome b causes oxidative stress and ageing in nematodes. Nature 394:694–697

Ito T, Hattori K, Obayashi T, Tanaka M, Sugiyama S, Ozawa T (1992) Mitochondrial DNA mutations in cardiomyopathy. Japanese Circulation Journal 56:1045–1053

Iwata N, Tsubuki S, Takaki Y et al. (2000) Identification of the major Abetal-42-degrading catabolic pathway in brain parenchyma: Suppression leads to biochemical and pathological deposition. Nat Med 6:143–150

Iwata S, Lee JW, Okada K et al. (1998) Complete structure of the 11-subunit bovine mitochondrial cytochrome bc1 complex. Science 281:64–71

Jabs EW, Thomas PJ, Bernstein M, Coss C, Ferreira GC, Pedersen PL (1994) Chromosomal localization of genes required for the terminal steps of oxidative metabolism: Alpha and gamma subunits of ATP synthase and the phosphate carrier. Hum Genet 93:600–602

Jackson MJ, Bindoff LA, Weber K et al. (1994) Biochemical and molecular studies of mitochondrial function in diabetes insipidus, diabetes mellitus, optic atrophy, and deafness. Diabetes Care 17:728–733

Jacobsson A, Stadler U, Glotzer MA, Kozak LP (1985) Mitochondrial uncoupling protein from mouse brown fat. Molecular cloning, genetic mapping, and mRNA expression. J Biol Chem 260:16250–16254

Jagust WJ, Seab JP, Huesman RH et al. (1991) Diminished glucose transport in Alzheimer's disease: Dynamic PET studies. J Cerebr Blood Flow Metab 11:323–330

Jaksch M, Hofmann S, Kleinle S et al. (1998a) A systematic mutation screen of 10 nuclear and 25 mitochondrial candidate genes in 21 patients with cytochrome c oxidase (COX) deficiency shows tRNA (Ser)(UCN) mutations in a subgroup with syndromal encephalopathy. J Med Genet 35:895–900

Jaksch M, Klopstock T, Kurlemann G et al. (1998b) Progressive myoclonus epilepsy and mitochondrial myopathy associated with mutations in the tRNA(Ser(UCN)) gene. Ann Neurol 44:635–640

Janetzky B, Hauck S, Youdim MB et al. (1994) Unaltered aconitase activity, but decreased complex I activity in substantia nigra pars compacta of patients with Parkinson's disease. Neuroscience Letters 169:126–128

Javed AA, Ogata K, Sanadi DR (1991) Human mitochondrial ATP synthase: cloning cDNA for the nuclear-encoded precursor of coupling factor 6. Gene 97:307–310

Jazin EE, Cavelier L, Eriksson I, Oreland L, Gyllensten U (1995) Estimation of the total amount of mitochondrial DNA sequence heteroplasmy in human brain. Abstract P 031. Journal 142

Jean-Francois MJ, Lertrit P, Berkovic SF et al. (1994) Heterogeneity in the phenotypic expression of the mutation in the mitochondrial tRNA$^{Leu(UUR)}$ gene generally associated with the MELAS subset of mitochondrial encephalomyopathies. Austr NZ J Med 24:188–193

Jenkins BG, Koroshetz WJ, Beal MF, Rosen BR (1993) Evidence for impairment of energy metabolism in vivo in Huntington's disease using localized ^{1}H NMR spectroscopy. Neurology 43:2689–2695

Jenner P, Dexter DT, Sian J, Schapira AH, Marsden CD (1992) Oxidative stress as a cause of nigral cell death in Parkinson's disease and incidental Lewy body disease. Ann Neurol 32 Suppl:S82–87

Jenuth JP, Peterson AC, Fu K, Shoubridge EA (1996) Random genetic drift in the female germline explains the rapid segregation of mammalian mitochondrial DNA. Nat Genet 14:146–151

Jenuth JP, Peterson AC, Shoubridge EA (1997) Tissue-specific selection for different mtDNA genotypes in heteroplasmic mice. Nat Genet 16:93–95

Jin H, May M, Tranebjaerg L et al. (1996) A novel X-linked gene, DDP, shows mutations in families with deafness (DFN-1), dystonia, mental deficiency and blindness. Nat Genet 14:177–180

Johns DR (1990) The molecular genetics of Leber's hereditary optic neuropathy. Archives of Ophthalmology 108:1405–1407

Johns DR (1992) Mitochondrial ND-1 mutation in Leber hereditary optic neuropathy [letter]. Am J Hum Genet 50:872–874

Johns DR (1994) Reply to Brown et al. ("Pathological significance of the mtDNA COX III mutation at nucleotide pair 9438 in Leber hereditary optic neuropathy", Am. J. Hum. Genet. 55:410, (1994)). Journal 55:410–412

Johns DR, Berman J (1991) Alternative, simultaneous complex I mitochondrial DNA mutations in Leber's hereditary optic neuropathy. Biochem Biophys Res Commun 174:1324–1330

Johns DR, Hurko O (1991) Mitochondrial leucine tRNA mutation in neurological diseases [letter]. Lancet 337:927–928

Johns DR, Neufeld MJ (1991) Cytochrome b mutations in Leber hereditary optic neuropathy. Biochem Biophys Res Commun 181:1358–1364

Johns DR, Neufeld M (1993a) Pitfalls in the molecular genetic diagnosis of Leber hereditary optic neuropathy (LHON). Am J Hum Genet 53:916–920

Johns DR, Neufeld MJ (1993b) Cytochrome c oxidase mutations in Leber hereditary optic neuropathy. Biochem Biophys Res Commun 196:810–815

Johns DR, Neufeld MJ, Park RD (1992a) An ND-6 mitochondrial DNA mutation associated with Leber hereditary optic neuropathy. Biochem Biophys Res Commun 187:1551–1557

Johns DR, Smith KH, Miller NR (1992b) Leber's hereditary optic neuropathy. Clinical manifestations of the 3460 mutation. Archives of Ophthalmology 110:1577–1581

Johns DR, Heher KL, Miller NR, Smith KH (1993a) Leber's hereditary optic neuropathy. Clinical manifestations of the 14484 mutation. Archives of Ophthalmology 111:495–498

Johns DR, Smith KH, Savino PJ, Miller NR (1993b) Leber's hereditary optic neuropathy. Clinical manifestations of the 15257 mutation. Archives of Ophthalmology 100:981–986

Johns DR, Neufeld MJ, Hedges TR (1994) Mitochondrial DNA mutations in Cuban optic and peripheral neuropathy. J Neuro-ophthalmol 14:135–140

Johnson MJ, Wallace DC, Ferris SD, Rattazzi MC, Cavalli-Sforza LL (1983) Radiation of human mitochondria DNA types analyzed by restriction endonuclease cleavage patterns. J Mol Evol 19:255–271

Johnson WG, Hodge SE, Duvoisin R (1990) Twin studies and the genetics of Parkinson's disease-a reappraisal. Move Disord 5:187–194

Johnston W, Karpati G, Carpenter S, Arnold D, Shoubridge EA (1995) Late-onset mitochondrial myopathy. Ann Neurol 37:16–23

Jordan EM, Breen GAM (1992) Molecular cloning of an import precursor of the delta-subunit of the human mitochondrial ATP synthase complex. Biochim Biophys Acta 1130:123–126

Jorde LB, Bamshad M (2000) Questioning evidence for recombination in human mitochondrial DNA. Science 288:1931

Jun AS, Brown MD, Wallace DC (1994) A mitochondrial DNA mutation at np 14459 of the ND6 gene associated with maternally inherited Leber's hereditary optic neuropathy and dystonia. Proc Natl Acad Sci USA 91:6206–6210

Jun AS, Trounce IA, Brown MD, Shoffner JM, Wallace DC (1996) Use of transmitochondrial cybrids to assign a complex I defect to the mitochondrial DNA-encoded NADH dehydrogenase subunit 6 gene mutation at nucleotide pair 14459 that causes Leber hereditary optic neuropathy and dystonia. Mol Cell Biol 16:771–777

Kadenbach B (1969) Half-lives of cytochrome c from various organs of the rat. Journal 186:399–401

Kadenbach B, Jarausch J, Hartmann R, Merle P (1983) Separation of mammalian cytochrome c oxidase into 13 polypeptides by a sodium dodecyl sulfate-gel electrophoretic procedure. Analytical Biochemistry 129:517–521

Kadowaki T, Sakura H, Otabe S et al. (1995) A subtype of diabetes mellitus associated with a mutation in the mitochondrial gene. Muscle and Nerve 3:S137–141

Kameoka K, Isotani H, Tanaka K et al. (1998a) Novel mitochondrial DNA mutation in tRNA(Lys) (8296A→G) associated with diabetes. Biochem Biophys Res Commun 245:523–527

Kameoka K, Isotani H, Tanaka K, Kitaoka H, Ohsawa N (1998b) Impaired insulin secretion in Japanese diabetic subjects with an A-to-G mutation at nucleotide 8296 of the mitochondrial DNA in tRNA(Lys) [letter]. Diabetes Care 21:2034–2035

Kanamori A, Tanaka K, Umezawa S et al. (1994) Insulin resistance in mitochondrial gene mutation. Diabetes Care 17:778–779

Kanamori A, Tanaka K, Umezawa S, Matoba K, Fujita Y, Yajima Y (1995) Response to Walker et al. (Insulin sensitivity and mitochondrial gene mutation). Diabetes Care 18:274–275

Kaneda H, Hayashi J, Takahama S, Taya C, Lindahl KF, Yonekawa H (1995) Elimination of paternal mitochondrial DNA in intraspecific crosses during early mouse embryogenesis. Proc Natl Acad Sci USA 92:4542–4546

Kao S, Chao HT, Wei YH (1995) Mitochondrial deoxyribonucleic acid 4977-bp deletion is associated with diminished fertility and motility of human sperm. Biology of Reproduction 52:729–736

Kapsa R, Thompson GN, Thorburn DR et al. (1994) A novel mtDNA deletion in an infant with Pearson syndrome. J Inherit Metabol Dis 17:521–526

Kataoka H, Biswas C (1991) Nucleotide sequence of a cDNA for the alpha subunit of human mitochondrial ATP synthase. Biochim Biophys Acta 1089:393–395

Kaukonen J, Amati P, Suomalainen A et al. (1995) Identification of a second autosomal locus predisposing to multiple deletions of mitochondrial DNA. (Abstract 1246). Journal 57:A216

Kaukonen J, Juselius JK, Tiranti V et al. (2000) Role of adenine nucleotide translocator 1 in mtDNA maintenance. Science 289:782–785

Kaukonen JA, Amati P, Suomalainen A et al. (1996) An autosomal locus predisposing to multiple deletions of mtDNA on chromosome 3p. Am J Hum Genet 58:763–769

Kawai H, Akaike M, Yokoi K et al. (1995) Mitochondrial encephalomyopathy with autosomal dominant inheritance: A clinical and genetic entity of mitochondrial diseases. Muscle and Nerve 18:753–760

Kawarai T, Kawakami H, Kozuka K et al. (1997) A new mitochondrial DNA mutation associated with mitochondrial myopathy: tRNA(Leu)(UUR) 3254C-to-G. Neurology 49:598–600

Kaytor MD, Warren ST (1999) Aberrant protein deposition and neurological disease. J Biol Chem 274:37507–37510

Keefe DL, Niven-Fairchild T, Powell S, Buradagunta S (1995) Mitochondrial deoxyribonucleic acid deletions in oocytes and reproductive aging in women. Fertility and Sterility 64:577–583

Kellar-Wood H, Robertson N, Govan GG, Compston DA, Harding AE (1994) Leber's hereditary optic neuropathy mitochondrial DNA mutations in multiple sclerosis. Ann Neurol 36:109–112

Kennaway NG, Burton MD, Hall RE et al. (1994) Mitochondrial myopathy and cytochrome c oxidase (COX) deficiency associated with a 15 bp deletion in the gene for COX subunit III. (Abstract 827). Journal 44 Suppl 2:A335

Kennaway NG, Keightley JA, Burton M, Hoffbuhr K, Buist NRM (1995) Single fiber analysis of muscle from a patient with a microdeletion in the gene for cytochrome c oxidase (COX) subunit III. (Abstract FC084). Journal 64

Kennaway NG, Keightley JA, Burton MD, Quan F, Libby BD, Buist NMR (1998) Mitochondrial encephalomyopathy associated with a nonsense mutation in the cytochrome b (Abstract). In UCSD Mitochondrial Medicine Conference. San Diego, California, USA. February 19–21, 1998. Molecular Genetics and Metabolism 63:49

Khrapko K, Bodyak N, Thilly WG et al. (1999) Cell-by-cell scanning of whole mitochondrial genomes in aged human heart reveals a significant fraction of myocytes with clonally expanded deletions. Nucl Acids Res 27:2434–2441

King MP, Attardi G (1988) Injection of mitochondria into human cells leads to a rapid replacement of the endogenous mitochondrial DNA. Cell 52:811–819

King MP, Attardi G (1989) Human cells lacking mtDNA: Repopulation with exogenous mitochondria by complementation. Science 246:500–503

King MP, Koga Y, Davidson M, Schon EA (1992) Defects in mitochondrial protein synthesis and respiratory chain activity segregate with the tRNA$^{Leu(UUR)}$ mutation associated with mitochondrial myopathy, encephalopathy, lactic acidosis, and stroke-like episodes. Mol Cell Biol 12:480–490

Kish SJ, Bergeron C, Rajput A et al. (1992) Brain cytochrome oxidase in Alzheimer's disease. J Neurochem 59:776–779

Kishimoto M, Hashiramoto M, Kanda F, Tanaka M, Kasuga M (1995) Mitochondrial mutation in diabetic patient with gastrointestinal symptoms. Lancet 345:452

Kita K, Oya H, Gennis RB, Ackrell BA, Kasahara M (1990) Human complex II (succinate-ubiquinone oxidoreductase): cDNA cloning of iron sulfur (Ip) subunit of liver mitochondria. Biochem Biophys Res Commun 166:101–108

Kitada T, Asakawa S, Hattori N et al. (1998) Mutations in the parkin gene cause autosomal recessive juvenile parkinsonism. Nature 392:605–608

Kitagawa T, Suganuma N, Nawa A et al. (1993) Rapid accumulation of deleted mitochondrial deoxyribonucleic acid in postmenopausal ovaries. Biology of Reproduction 49:730–736

Kivisild T, Villems R (2000) Questioning evidence for recombination in human mitochondrial DNA. Science 288:1931

Kleinle S, Schneider V, Moosmann P, Brandner S, Krahenbuhl S, Liechti-Gallati S (1998) A novel mitochondrial tRNA(Phe) mutation inhibiting anticodon stem formation associated with a muscle disease. Biochem Biophys Res Commun 247:112–115

Knowles RG (1997) Nitric oxide biochemistry. Biochem Soc Trans 25:895–901.

Kobayashi Y, Momoi MY, Tominaga K et al. (1990) A point mutation in the mitochondrial tRNA$^{Leu(UUR)}$ gene in MELAS (mitochondrial myopathy, encephalopathy, lactic acidosis and stroke-like episodes). Biochem Biophys Res Commun 173:816–822

Kobayashi Y, Momoi MY, Tominaga K et al. (1991) Respiration-deficient cells are caused by a single point mutation in the mitochondrial tRNA$^{Leu(UUR)}$ gene in mitochondrial myopathy, encephalopathy, lactic acidosis, and stroke-like episodes (MELAS). Am J Hum Genet 49:590–599

Koehler CM, Jarosch E, Tokatlidis K, Schmid K, Schweyen RJ, Schatz G (1998a) Import of mitochondrial carriers mediated by essential proteins of the intermembrane space. Science 279:369–373

Koehler CM, Merchant S, Oppliger W et al. (1998b) Tim9p, an essential partner subunit of Tim10p for the import of mitochondrial carrier proteins. EMBO J 17:6477–6486

Koehler CM, Leuenberger D, Merchant S, Renold A, Junne T, Schatz G (1999) Human deafness dystonia sydrome is a mitochondrial disease. Proc Natl Acad Sci USA 96:2141–2146

Koga Y, Fabrizi GM, Mita S et al. (1990) Sequence of a cDNA specifying subunit VIIc of human cytochrome c oxidase. Nucl Acids Res 18:684

Koga Y, Davidson M, Schon EA, King MP (1993) Fine mapping of mitochondrial RNAs derived from the mtDNA region containing a point mutation associated with MELAS. Nucl Acids Res 21:657–662

Koga Y, Davidson M, Schon EA, King MP (1995) Analysis of cybrids harboring MELAS mutations in the mitochondrial tRNA$^{Leu(UUR)}$ gene. Muscle and Nerve 3:S119–123

Kogelnik AM, Lott MT, Brown MD, Navathe SB, Wallace DC (1996) MITOMAP: A human mitochondrial genome database. Nucl Acids Res 24:177–179

Kokoszka JE, Coskun P, Esposito L, Wallace DC (2001) Increased mitochondrial oxidative stress in the Sod2+/– mouse results in the age-related decline of mitochondrial function culminating in increased apoptosis. Proc Natl Acad Sci USA February 27, 98(5):2278–2283.

Kosel S, Egensperger R, Mehraein P, Graeber MB (1994) No association of mutations at nucleotide 5460 of mitochondrial NADH dehydrogenase with Alzheimer's disease. Biochem Biophys Res Commun 203:745–749

Koster JC, Marshall BA, Ensor N, Corbett JA, Nichols CG (2000) Targeted overactivity of beta cell K(ATP) channels induces profound neonatal diabetes. Cell 100:645–654.

Kozak LP, Britton JH, Kozak UC, Wells JM (1988) The mitochondrial uncoupling protein gene. Correlation of exon structure to transmembrane domains. J Biol Chem 263:12274–12277

Kretzchmar HA, DeArmond SJ, Koch TK et al. (1987) Pyruvate dehydrogenase complex deficiency as a cause of subacute necrotizing encephalopathy (Leigh's disease). Pediatrics 79:370–373

Krige D, Carroll MT, Cooper JM, Marsden CD, Schapira AH (1992) Platelet mitochondrial function in Parkinson's Disease. Ann Neurol 32:782–788

Kruger R, Kuhn W, Muller T et al. (1998) Ala30Pro mutation in the gene encoding alpha-synuclein in Parkinson's disease [letter]. Nat Genet 18:106–108

Ksenzenko M, Konstantinov AA, Khomutov GB, Tikhonov AN, Ruuge EK (1983) Effect of electron transfer inhibitors on superoxide generation in the cytochrome bc1 site of the mitochondrial respiratory chain. FEBS Letters 155:19–24

Ku DH, Kagan J, Chen ST, Chang CD, Baserga R, Wurzel J (1990) The human fibroblast adenine nucleotide translocator gene. Molecular cloning and sequence. J Biol Chem 265:16060–16063

Kumar S, Hedrick P, Dowling T, Stoneking M (2000) Questioning evidence for recombination in human mitochondrial DNA. Science 288:1931.

Kumar U, Dunlop DM, Richardson JS (1994) Mitochondria from Alzheimer's fibroblasts show decreased uptake of calcium and increased sensitivity to free radicals. Life Sciences 54:1855–1860

Kurth JH, Kurth MC, Poduslo SE, Schwankhaus JD (1993) Association of a monoamine oxidase B allele with Parkinson's disease. Ann Neurol 33:368–372

Kuwert T, Lange HW, Boecker H et al. (1993) Striatal glucose consumption in chorea-free subjects at risk of Huntington's disease. J Neurol 241:31–36

Lamminen T, Majander A, Juvonen V et al. (1995) A mitochondrial mutation at nt 9101 in the ATP synthase 6 gene associated with deficient oxidative phosphorylation in a family with Leber hereditary optic neuroretinopathy [letter]. Am J Hum Genet 56:1238–1240

Langston JW, Ballard P, Tetrud JW, Irwin I (1983) Chronic parkinsonism in humans due to a product of meperidine-analog synthesis. Science 219:979–980

Larsson NG, Holme E, Kristiansson B, Oldfors A, Tulinius M (1990) Progressive increase of the mutated mitochondrial DNA fraction in Kearns-Sayre syndrome. Pediatr Res 28:131–136

Larsson NG, Andersen O, Holme E, Oldfors A, Wahlstrom J (1991) Leber's hereditary optic neuropathy and complex I deficiency in muscle. Ann Neurol 30:701–708

Larsson NG, Eiken HG, Boman H, Holme E, Oldfors A, Tulinius MH (1992) Lack of transmission of deleted mtDNA from a woman with Kearns-Sayre Syndrome to her child. Am J Hum Genet 50:360–363

Larsson NG, Tulinius MH, Holme E, Oldfors A (1995) Pathogenetic aspects of the A8344G mutation of mitochondrial DNA associated with MERRF syndrome and multiple symmetric lipomas. Muscle and Nerve 3:S102–106

Larsson NG, Wang J, Wilhelmsson H et al. (1998) Mitochondrial transcription factor A is necessary for mtDNA maintenance and embryogenesis in mice. Nat Genet 18:231–236

Lauber J, Marsac C, Kadenbach B, Seibel P (1991) Mutations in mitochondrial tRNA genes: a frequent cause of neuromuscular diseases. Nucl Acids Res 19:1393–1397

Lebovitz RM, Zhang H, Vogel H et al. (1996) Neurodegeneration, myocardial injury, and perinatal death in mitochondrial superoxide dismutase-deficient mice. Proc Natl Acad Sci USA 93:9782–9787

LeDoux SP, Wilson GL, Beecham EJ, Stevnsner T, Wassermann K, Bohr VA (1992) Repair of mitochondrial DNA after various types of DNA damage in Chinese hamster ovary cells. Carcinogenesis 13:1967–1973

LeDoux SP, Wilson GL, Bohr VA (1993) Mitochondrial DNA repair and cell injury. In Jones DP, Lash L (eds): Mitochondrial Dysfunction, Methods in Toxicology. Academic Press, NY, 2, pp. 461–476

Lell JT, Brown MD, Schurr TG et al. (1997) Y chromosome polymorphisms in native American and Siberian populations:

identification of native American Y chromosome haplotypes. Hum Genet 100:536–543

Leroy D, Norby S (1994) A new human mtDNA polymorphism: tRNA^Gln/4336 T(C). Clinical Genetics 45:109–110

Lertrit P, Noer AS, Jean-Francois MJ et al. (1992) A new disease-related mutation for mitochondrial encephalopathy lactic acidosis and strokelike episodes (MELAS) syndrome affects the ND4 subunit of the respiratory complex I. Am J Hum Genet 51:457–468

Lestienne P, Bataille N, Lucas-Heron B (1995) Role of the mitochondrial DNA and calmitine in myopathies. Biochim Biophys Acta 1271:159–163

Letellier T, Heinrich R, Malgat M, Mazat JP (1994) The kinetic basis of threshold effects observed in mitochondrial diseases:a systemic approach. Biochem J 302:171–174

Levy SE, Waymire KG, Kim YL, MacGregor GR, Wallace DC (1999) Transfer of chloramphenicol-resistant mitochondrial DNA into the chimeric mouse. Transgenic Research 8:137–145

Levy SE, Chen Y-S, Graham BH, Wallace DC (2000) Expression and sequence analysis of the mouse adenine nucleotide translocase 1 and 2 genes. Journal 254:57–66

Lezza AM, Boffoli D, Scacco S, Cantatore P, Gadaleta MN (1994) Correlation between mitochondrial DNA 4977-bp deletion and respiratory chain enzyme activities in aging human skeletal muscles. Biochem Biophys Res Commun 205:772–779

Li K, Warner CK, Hodge JA et al. (1989) A human muscle adenine nucleotide translocator gene has four exons, is located on chromosome 4, and is differentially expressed. J Biol Chem 264:13998–14004

Li XJ, Li SH, Sharp AH et al. (1995a) A huntingtin-associated protein enriched in brain with implications for pathology. Nature 378:398–402

Li XJ, Sharp AH, Li SH, Dawson TM, Snyder SH, Ross CA (1996) Huntingtin-associated protein (HAP1): Discrete neuronal localizations in the brain resemble those of neuronal nitric oxide synthase. Journal 93:4839–4844

Li Y, Huang TT, Carlson EJ et al. (1995b) Dilated cardiomyopathy and neonatal lethality in mutant mice lacking manganese superoxide dismutase. Nat Genet 11:376–381

Li YY, Hengstenberg C, Maisch B (1995c) Whole mitochondrial genome amplification reveals basal level multiple deletions in mtDNA of patients with dilated cardiomyopathy. Biochem Biophys Res Commun 210:211–218

Liao HX, Spremulli LL (1990) Effects of length and mRNA secondary structure on the interaction of bovine mitochondrial ribosomes with messenger RNA. J Biol Chem 265:11761–11765

Licastro F, Pedrini S, Ferri C et al. (2000) Gene polymorphism affecting alpha1-antichymotrypsin and interleukin-1 plasma levels increases Alzheimer's disease risk. Ann Neurol 48:388–391

Limbach KJ, Wu R (1985) Characterization of a mouse somatic cytochrome c gene and three cytochrome c pseudogenes. Nucl Acids Res 13:617–631

Lin F, Lin R, Wisniewski HM et al. (1992) Detection of point mutations in codon 331 of mitochondrial NADH dehydrogenase subunit 2 in Alzheimer's brains. Biochem Biophys Res Commun 182:238–246

Lin SJ, Defossez PA, Guarente L (2000) Requirement of NAD and SIR2 for life-span extension by calorie restriction in Saccharomyces cerevisiae. Science 289:2126–2128

Liu X, Kim CN, Yang J, Jemmerson R, Wang X (1996) Induction of apoptotic program in cell-free extracts: Requirement for dATP and cytochrome c. Cell 86:147–157

Loeffen J, Smeitink J, Triepels R et al. (1998) The first nuclear-encoded complex 1 mutation in a patient with Leigh Syndrome. Am J Hum Genet 63:1598–1608

Lomax MI, Grossman LI (1989) Tissue-specific genes for respiratory proteins. Trends in Biochemical Sciences 14:501–503

Lomax MI, Welch MD, Darras BT, Francke U, Grossman LI (1990) Novel use of a chimpanzee pseudogene for chromosomal mapping of human cytochrome c oxidase subunit IV. Gene 86:209–216

Lomax MI, Hsieh CL, Darras BT, Francke U (1991) Structure of the human cytochrome c oxidase subunit Vb gene and chromosomal mapping of the coding gene and of seven pseudogenes. Genomics 10:1–9

Loschen G, Azzi A, Richter C, Flohe L (1974) Superoxide radicals as precursors of mitochondrial hydrogen peroxide. FEBS Letters 42:68–72

Lott MT, Voljavec AS, Wallace DC (1990) Variable genotype of Leber's hereditary optic neuropathy patients. Am J Ophthalmol 109:625–631

Lucking CB, Kosel S, Mehraein P, Graeber MB (1995) Absence of the mitochondrial A7237T mutation in Parkinson's disease. Biochem Biophys Res Commun 211:700–704

Luder A, Barash V (1994) Complex I deficiency with diabetes, Fanconi syndrome and mtDNA deletion. J Inherit Metabol Dis 17:298–300

Lynn S, Wardell T, Johnson MA et al. (1998) Mitochondrial diabetes: Investigation and identification of a novel mutation. Diabetes 47:1800–1802

Mackey D, Howell N (1992) A variant of Leber hereditary optic neuropathy characterized by recovery of vision and by an unusual mitochondrial genetic etiology. Am J Hum Genet 51:1218–1228

Mackey DA (1994) Three subgroups of patients from the United Kingdom with Leber hereditary optic neuropathy. Eye 8:431–436

Madsen CS, Ghivizzani SC, Hauswirth WW (1993) Protein binding to a single termination-associated sequence in the mitochondrial DNA D-loop region. Mol Cell Biol 13:2162–2171

Majander A, Huoponen K, Savontaus ML, Nikoskelainen E, Wikstrom M (1991) Electron transfer properties of NADH:ubiquinone reductase in the ND1/3460 and the ND4/11778 mutations of the Leber hereditary optic neuroretinopathy (LHON). FEBS Letters 292:289–292

Majander A, Finel M, Savontaus ML, Nikoskelainen E, Wikstrom M (1996) Catalytic activity of complex I in cell lines that possess replacement mutations in the ND genes in Leber's hereditary optic neuropathy. Eur J Biochem 239:201–207

Mak SC, Chi CS, Tsai CR (1998) Mitochondrial DNA 8993 T > C mutation presenting as juvenile Leigh syndrome with respiratory failure. J Child Neurol 13:349–351

Makela-Bengs P, Suomalainen A, Majander A et al. (1995) Correlation between the clinical symptoms and the proportion of mitochondrial DNA carrying the 8993 point mutation in the NARP syndrome. Pediatr Res 37:634–639

Malaisse-Lagae F, Malaisse WJ (1988) Hexose metabolism in pancreatic islets: regulation of mitochondrial hexokinase binding. Biochem Med Metabol Biol 39:80–89

Malgat M, Letellier T, Jouaville SL, Mazat JP (1995) Value of control theory in the study of cellular metabolism – biomedical implications. Journal 3:165–175

Mancini M, Nicholson DW, Roy S et al. (1998) The caspase-3 precursor has a cytosolic and mitochondrial distribution: Implications for apoptotic signaling. J Cell Biol 140:1485–1495

Manfredi G, Bonilla E, Schon EA, DiMauro S, Moraes C (1994) A mitochondrial DNA missense mutation in the cytochrome oxidase subunit III gene associated with a progressive encephalopathy. Journal 4:17

Manfredi G, Schon EA, Moraes CT et al. (1995a) A new mutation associated with MELAS is located in a mitochondrial DNA polypeptide-coding gene. Neuromuscular Disorders 5:391–398

Manfredi G, Servidei S, Bonilla E et al. (1995b) High levels of mitochondrial DNA with an unstable 260-bp duplication in a patient with a mitochondrial myopathy. Neurology 45:762–768

Manfredi G, Schon EA, Bonilla E, Moraes CT, Shanske S, DiMauro S (1996) Identification of a mutation in the mitochondrial tRNA (Cys) gene associated with mitochondrial encephalopathy. Hum Mutat 7:158–163

Manfredi G, Thyagarajan D, Papadopoulou LC, Pallotti F, Schon EA (1997) The fate of human sperm-derived mtDNA in somatic cells. Am J Hum Genet 61:953–960.

Mann VM, Cooper JM, Krige D, Daniel SE, Schapira AH, Marsden CD (1992a) Brain, skeletal muscle and platelet homogenate mitochondrial function in Parkinson's disease. Brain 115:333–342

Mann VM, Cooper JM, Schapira AHV (1992b) Quantitation of a mitochondrial DNA deletion in Parkinson's disease. FEBS Letters 299:218–222

Manouvrier S, Rotig A, Hannebique G et al. (1995) Point mutation of the mitochondrial tRNA^Leu gene (A 3243 G) in maternally inherited hypertrophic cardiomyopathy, diabetes mellitus, renal failure, and sensorineural deafness. J Med Genet 32:654–656

Marchington DR, Barlow D, Poulton J (1999) Transmitochondrial mice carrying resistance to chloramphenicol on mitochondrial DNA: developing the first mouse model of mitochondrial DNA disease. Nat Med 5:957–960

Mariotti C, Tiranti V, Carrara F, Dallapiccola B, DiDonato S, Zeviani M (1994) Defective respiratory capacity and mitochondrial protein synthesis in transformant cybrids harboring the tRNA^Leu(UUR) mutation associated with maternally inherited myopathy and cardiomyopathy. J Clin Invest 93:1102–1107

Mariotti C, Savarese N, Suomalainen A et al. (1995) Genotype to phenotype correlations in mitochondrial encephalomyopathies associated with the A3243G mutation of mitochondrial DNA. J Neurol 242:304–312

Martin WR, Clark C, Ammann W, Stoessl AJ, Shtybel W, Hayden MR (1992) Cortical glucose metabolism in Huntington's disease. Neurology 42:223–229

Marzo I, Brenner C, Zamzami N et al. (1998) Bax and adenine nucleotide translocator cooperate in the mitochondrial control of apoptosis. Science 281:2027–2031

Marzuki S, Noer AS, Letrit P et al. (1991) Normal variants of human mitochondrial DNA and translation products: the building of a reference data base. Hum Genet 88:139–145

Mashima Y, Hiida Y, Oguchi Y, Kudoh J, Shimizu N (1993) High frequency of mutations at position 11778 in mitochondrial ND4 gene in Japanese families with Leber's hereditary optic neuropathy. Hum Genet 92:101–102

Massin P, Guillausseau PJ, Vialettes B et al. (1995) Macular pattern dystrophy associated with a mutation of mitochondrial DNA. Am J Ophthalmol 120:247–248

Masucci JP, Davidson M, Koga Y, Schon EA, King MP (1995) In vitro analysis of mutations causing myoclonus epilepsy with ragged-red fibers in the mitochondrial tRNA^Lys gene: two genotypes produce similar phenotypes. Mol Cell Biol 15:2872–2881

Matsuda C, Endo H, Ohta S, Kagawa Y (1993) Gene structure of human mitochondrial ATP synthase gamma-subunit. Tissue specificity produced by alternative RNA splicing. J Biol Chem 268:24950–24958

Matthews DE, Hessler RA, Denslow ND, Edwards JS, O'Brien TW (1982) Protein composition of the bovine mitochondrial ribosome. J Biol Chem 257:8788–8794

Matthews PM, Brown RM, Morten K, Marchington D, Poulton J, Brown G (1995) Intracellular heteroplasmy for disease-associated point mutations in mtDNA: Implications for disease expression and evidence for mitotic segregation of heteroplasmic units of mtDNA. Hum Genet 96:261–268

Matthews PM, Marchington DR, Squier M, Land J, Brown RM, Brown GK (1993) Molecular genetic characterization of an X-linked form of Leigh's syndrome. Ann Neurol 33:652–655

Matthijs G, Claes S, Longo-Mbenza B, Cassiman JJ (1994) Teenage onset non-syndromic deafness associated with a mutation and a polymorphism in the mitochondrial 12S ribosomal RNA gene in a large Zairese pedigree. Journal 55:A23 (abstract)

Mattson MP (1995) Free radicals and disruption of neuronal ion homeostasis in AD: a role for amyloid beta-peptide? Neurobiology of Aging 16:679–682

Maurer I, Zierz S, Moller H (2000) A selective defect of cytochrome c oxidase is present in brain of Alzheimer disease patients. Journal 21:455–462

Mayr-Wohlfart U, Rodel G, Henneberg A (1997) Mitochondrial tRNA(Gln) and tRNA(Thr) gene variants in Parkinson's disease. European J Med Res 2:111–113

Mazziotta MR, Ricci E, Bertini E et al. (1992) Fatal infantile liver failure associated with mitochondrial DNA depletion. J Pediatr 121:896–901

McCabe ER (1994) Microcompartmentation of energy metabolism at the outer mitochondrial membrane: Role in diabetes mellitus and other diseases. J Bioenerg Biomembr 26:317–325

McMahon FJ, Chen YS, Patel S et al. (2000) Mitochondrial DNA sequence diversity in bipolar affective disorder. American J Psych 157:1058–1064

McMahon FJ, Stine OC, Meyers DA, Simpson SG, DePaulo JR (1995) Patterns of maternal transmission in bipolar affective disorder. Am J Hum Genet 56:1277–1286

McShane MA, Hammans M, Sweeney I et al. (1991) Pearson Syndrome and mitochondrial encephalomyopathy in patient with a deletion of mtDNA. Am J Hum Genet 48:39–42

Mecocci P, MacGarvey U, Kaufman AE et al. (1993) Oxidative damage to mitochondrial DNA shows marked age-dependent increases in human brain. Ann Neurol 34:609–616

Mecocci P, MacGarvey U, Beal MF (1994) Oxidative damage to mitochondrial DNA is increased in Alzheimer's disease. Ann Neurol 36:747–751

Meirelles FV, Smith LC (1997) Mitochondrial genotype segregation in a mouse heteroplasmic lineage produced by embryonic karyoplast transplantation. Genetics 145:445–451

Meirelles FV, Smith LC (1998) Mitochondrial genotype segregation during preimplantation development in mouse heteroplasmic embryos. Genetics 148:877–883

Melov S, Shoffner JM, Kaufman A, Wallace DC (1995) Marked increase in the number and variety of mitochondrial DNA rearrangements in aging human skeletal muscle [published erratum appears in Nucleic Acids Res (1995) Dec 11;23(23):4938]. Nucl Acids Res 23:4122–4126

Melov S, Hinerfeld D, Esposito L, Wallace DC (1997) Multi-organ characterization of mitochondrial genomic rearrangements in ad libitum and caloric restricted mice show striking somatic mitochondrial DNA rearrangements with age. Nucl Acids Res 25:974–982

Melov S, Schneider JA, Day BJ et al. (1998) A novel neurological phenotype in mice lacking mitochondrial manganese superoxide dismutase. Nat Genet 18:159–163

Melov S, Coskun P, Patel M et al. (1999) Mitochondrial disease in superoxide dismutase 2 mutant mice. Proc Natl Acad Sci USA 96:846–851

Melov S, Ravenscroft J, Malik S et al. (2000) Extension of life-span with superoxide dismutase/catalase mimetics. Journal 289:1567–1569

Menzies RA, Gold PH (1971) The turnover of mitochondria in a variety of tissues of young adult and aged rats. J Biol Chem 246:2425–2429

Merante F, Tein I, Benson L, Robinson BH (1994) Maternally inherited hypertrophic cardiomyopathy due to a novel T-to-C transition at nucleotide 9997 in the mitochondrial tRNA(glycine) gene. Am J Hum Genet 55:437–446

Merante F, Myint T, Tein I, Benson L, Robinson BH (1996) An additional mitochondrial tRNA(Ile) point mutation (A-to-G at nucleotide 4295) causing hypertrophic cardiomyopathy. Hum Mutat 8:216–222

Merriwether DA, Clark AG, Ballinger SW et al. (1991) The structure of human mitochondrial DNA variation. J Mol Evol 33:543–555

Michaels GS, Hauswirth WW, Laipis PJ (1982) Mitochondrial DNA copy number in bovine oocytes and somatic cells. Developmental Biology 94:246–251

Michikawa Y, Mazzucchelli F, Bresolin N, Scarlato G, Attardi G (1999) Aging-dependent large accumulation of point mutations in the human mtDNA control region for replication. Science 286:774–779

Milatovich A, Parisi MA, Poulton J, Clayton DA, Francke U (1991) Sequences homologous to MTTF1, mitochondrial transcription factor 1, are located on human chromosomes 7 (7pter-cen), 10, and 11 (11cen-qter). Journal 58:1929

Mills KA, Ellison JW, Mathews KD (1996) The Antl gene maps near Klk3 on proximal mouse chromosome 8. Mammalian Genome 7:707

Miranda AF, Ishii S, DiMauro S, Shay JW (1989) Cytochrome c oxidase deficiency in Leigh's syndrome: genetic evidence for a nuclear DNA-encoded defect. Neurology 39:697–702

Mita S, Schmidt B, Schon EA, DiMauro S, Bonilla E (1989) Detection of "deleted" mitochondrial genomes in cytochrome-c oxidase-deficient muscle fibers of a patient with Kearns-Sayre syndrome. Proc Natl Acad Sci USA 86:9509–9513

Mita S, Rizzuto R, Moraes CT et al. (1990) Recombination via flanking direct repeats is a major cause of large-scale deletions of human mitochondrial DNA. Nucl Acids Res 18:561–567

Mitchell P (1976) Possible molecular mechanisms of the protomotive function of cytochrome systems. J Theoret Biol 62:327–347

Mizuno Y, Saitoh T, Sone N (1987) Inhibition of mitochondrial alpha-ketoglutarate dehydrogenase by 1-methyl-4-phenylpyridinium ion. Biochem Biophys Res Commun 143:971–976

Mizuno Y, Ohta S, Tanaka M et al. (1989) Deficiencies in complex 1 subunits of the respiratory chain in Parkinson's disease. Biochem Biophys Res Commun 163:1450–1455

Mizuno Y, Suzuki K, Ohta S (1990) Postmortem changes in mitochondrial respiratory enzymes in brain and a preliminary observation in Parkinson's disease. J Neurol Sci 96:49–57

Mizuno Y, Ikebe S, Hattori N et al. (1995) Role of mitochondria in the etiology and pathogenesis of Parkinson's disease. Biochim Biophys Acta 1271:265–274

Moraes CT, DiMauro S, Zeviani M et al. (1989) Mitochondrial DNA deletions in progressive external ophthalmoplegia and Kearns-Sayre syndrome. N Engl J Med 320:1293–1299

Moraes CT, Shanske S, Tritschler HJ et al. (1991) MtDNA depletion with variable tissue expression: a novel genetic abnormality in mitochondrial disease. Am J Hum Genet 48:492–501

Moraes CT, Ricci E, Bonilla E, DiMauro S, Schon EA (1992) The mitochondrial tRNA$^{Leu(UUR)}$ mutation in mitochondrial encephalomyopathy, lactic acidosis, and strokelike episodes (MELAS): genetic, biochemical, and morphological correlations in skeletal muscle. Am J Hum Genet 50:934–949

Moraes CT, Ciacci F, Bonilla E, Ionasescu V, Schon EA, DiMauro S (1993a) A mitochondrial tRNA anticodon swap associated with a muscle disease. Nat Genet 4:284–288

Moraes CT, Ciacci F, Bonilla E et al. (1993b) Two novel pathogenic mitochondrial DNA mutations affecting organelle number and protein synthesis. Is the tRNA$^{Leu(UUR)}$ gene an etiologic hot spot? J Clin Invest 92:2906–2915

Moraes CT, Ciacci F, Silverstri G et al. (1993c) Atypical clinical presentations associated with the MELAS mutation at position 3243 of human mitochondrial DNA. Neuromuscular Disorders 3:43–50

Moraes CT, Sciacco M, Ricci E et al. (1995) Phenotype-genotype correlations in skeletal muscle of patients with mtDNA deletions. Muscle and Nerve 3:S150–S153

Morgan-Hughes JA, Sweeney MG, Cooper JM et al. (1995) MtDNAdiseases: Correlation of genotype to phenotype. Biochim Biophys Acta 1271:135–140

Morris AA, Farnsworth L, Ackrell BA, Turnbull DM, Birch-Machin MA (1994) The cDNA sequence of the flavoprotein subunit of human heart succinate dehydrogenase. Biochim Biophys Acta 1185:125–128

Morten KJ, Cooper JM, Brown GK, Lake BD, Pike D, Poulton J (1993) A new point mutation associated with mitochondrial encephalomyopathy. Human Molecular Genetics 2:2081–2087

Muller-Hocker J (1990) Cytochrome c oxidase deficient fibres in the limb muscle and diaphragm of man without muscular disease: An age-related alteration. J Neurol Sci 100:14–21

Muller-Hocker J, Schneiderbanger K, Stefani FH, Kadenbach B (1992) Progressive loss of cytochrome c oxidase in the human extraocular muscles in ageing—a cytochemical-immunohistochmeical study. Mutation Research 275:115–124

Muller-Hocker J, Seibel P, Schneiderbanger K, Kadenbach B (1993) Different in situ hybridization patterns of mitochondrial DNA in cytochrome c oxidase-deficient extraocular muscle fibres in the elderly. Virchows Arch A, Pathological Anatomy and Histopathology 422:7–15

Munscher C, Muller-Hocker J, Kadenbach B (1993a) Human aging is associated with various point mutations in tRNA genes of mitochondrial DNA. Biological Chemistry Hoppe Seyler 374:1099–1104

Munscher C, Rieger T, Muller-Hocker J, Kadenbach B (1993b) The point mutation of mitochondrial DNA characteristic for MERRF disease is found also in healthy people of different ages. FEBS Letters 317:27–30

Murdock D, Boone BE, Esposito L, Wallace DC (1999) Up-regulation of nuclear and mitochondrial genes in the skeletal muscle of mice lacking the heart/muscle isoform of the adenine nucleotide translocator. J Biol Chem 274:14429–14433

Murdock DG, Christacos NC, Wallace DC (2000) The age-related accumulation of a mitochondrial DNA control region mutation in muscle, but not brain, detected by a sensitive PNA-directed PCR clamping based method. Nucl Acids Res 28:4350–4355

Mutisya EM, Bowling AC, Beal MF (1994) Cortical cytochrome oxidase activity is reduced in Alzheimer's disease. J Neurochem 63:2179–2184

Nakagawa Y, Ikegami H, Yamato E et al. (1995) A new mitochondrial DNA mutation associated with non-insulin-dependent diabetes mellitus [published erratum appears in Biochim Biophys Res Commun 209:664–668, 1995]. Biochem Biophys Res Commun 209:664–668

Nakagawa-Hattori Y, Yoshino H, Kondo T, Mizuno Y, Horai S (1992) Is Parkinson's disease a mitochondrial disorder? J Neurol Sci 107:29–33

Nakahara H, Kanno T, Inai Y et al. (1998) Mitochondrial dysfunction in the senescence accelerated mouse (SAM). Free Rad Biol Med 24:85–92

Nakamura M, Nakano S, Goto Y et al. (1995) A novel point mutation in the mitochondrial tRNA$^{Ser(UCN)}$ gene detected in a family with MERRF/MELAS overlap syndrome. Biochem Biophys Res Commun 214:86–93

Nakazono K, Watanabe N, Matsuno K, Sasaki J, Sato T, Inoue M (1991) Does superoxide underlie the pathogenesis of hypertension? Proc Natl Acad Sci USA 88:10045–10048

Napiwotzki J, Kadenbach B (1998) Extramitochondrial ATP/ADP-ratios regulate cytochrome c oxidase activity via binding to the cytosolic domain of subunit IV. Biological Chemistry 379:335–339

Napiwotzki J, Shinzawa-Itoh K, Yoshikawa S, Kadenbach B (1997) ATP and ADP bind to cytochrome c oxidase and regulate its activity. Biological Chemistry 378:1013–1021

Neckelmann N, Li K, Wade RP, Shuster R, Wallace DC (1987) cDNA sequence of a human skeletal muscle ADP/ATP translocator: lack of a leader peptide, divergence from a fibroblast translocator cDNA, and coevolution with mitochondrial DNA genes. Proc Natl Acad Sci USA 84:7580–7584

Neckelmann N, Warner CK, Chung A et al. (1989) The human ATP synthase beta subunit gene: Sequence analysis, chromosome assignment, and differential expression. Genomics 5:829–843

Nelson I, Hanna MG, Alsanjari N, Scaravilli F, Morgan-Hughes JA, Harding AE (1995) A new mitochondrial DNA mutation associated with progressive dementia and chorea: A clinical, pathological, and molecular genetic study. Ann Neurol 37:400–403

Neubert D, Oberdisse E, Bass R (1968) Biosynthesis and degradation of mammalian mitochondrial DNA. In Slater EC, Tager JM, Papa S, Quagliarello E (eds): Biochemical Aspects of the Biogenesis of Mitochondria. Adriatica Editrice, Bari, pp. 103–128

Neupert W (1997) Protein import into mitochondria. Annu Rev Biochem 66:863–917

Newman NJ (1993) Leber's hereditary optic neuropathy. New genetic considerations. Arch Neurol 50:540–548

Newman NJ, Wallace DC (1990) Mitochondria and Leber's hereditary optic neuropathy. Am J Ophthalmol 109:726–730

Newman NJ, Lott MT, Wallace DC (1991) The clinical characteristics of pedigress of Leber's hereditary optic neuropathy with the 11778 mutation. Am J Ophthalmol 111:750–762

Newman NJ, Torroni A, Brown MD et al. (1994) Epidemic neuropathy in Cuba not associated with mitochondrial DNA mutations found in Leber's hereditary optic neuropathy patients. Am J Ophthalmol 118:158–168

Newman NJ, Torroni A, Brown MD et al. (1995) Cuban optic neuropathy [letter; comment]. Neurology 45:397

Nicholls DG, Locke RM (1984) Thermogenic mechanisms in brown fat. Phys Rev 64:1–64.

Nicoll JA, Mrak RE, Graham DI et al. (2000) Association of interleukin-1 gene polymorphisms with Alzheimer's disease. Ann Neurol 47:365–368

Niemann S, Muller U (2000) Mutations in SDHC cause autosomal dominant paraganglioma, type 3. Nat Genet 26:268–270

Nigro MA, Martens ME, Awerbuch GI, Peterson PL, Lee CP (1990) Partial cytochrome b deficiency and generalized dystonia. Pediatric Neurology 6:407–410

Nikoskelainen EK, Marttila RJ, Huoponen K et al. (1995) Leber's "plus": neurological abnormalities in patients with Leber's hereditary optic neuropathy. J Neurol, Neurosurgery and Psychiatry 59:160–164

Nishikawa T, Edelstein D, Du XL et al. (2000) Normalizing mitochondrial superoxide production blocks three pathways of hyperglycaemic damage. Nature 404:787–790

Nishikimi M, Ohta S, Suzuki H et al. (1988a) Nucleotide sequence of a cDNA encoding the precursor to human cytochrome cl. Nucl Acids Res 16:3577

Nishikimi M, Suzuki H, Yamaguchi M, Matsukage A, Yoshida MC, Ozawa T (1988b) Assignment of the human cytochrome cl gene to chromosome 8. Biochem Int 16:655–660

Nishimura M, Obayashi H, Ohta M, Uchiyama T, Hao Q, Saida T (1995) No association of the 11778 mitochondrial DNA mutation and multiple sclerosis in Japan. Neurology 45:1333–1334

Nishino I, Seki A, Maegaki Y et al. (1996) A novel mutation in the mitochondrial tRNAThr gene associated with a mitochondrial encephalomyopathy. Biochem Biophys Res Commun 225:180–185

Nishino I, Spinazzola A, Hirano M (1999) Thymidine phosphorylase gene mutations in MNGIE, a human mitochondrial disorder. Science 283:689–692

Noer AS, Sudoya H, Lertrit P et al. (1991) A tRNA(Lys) mutation in the mtDNA is the causal genetic lesion underlying myoclonic epilepsy and ragged-red fiber (MERRF) syndrome. Am J Hum Genet 49:715–722

Norby S (1993) Screening for the two most frequent mutations in Leber's hereditary optic neuropathy by duplex PCR based on allele-specific amplification. Hum Mutat 2:309–313

Novotny EJ, Singh G, Wallace DC et al. (1986) Leber's disease and dystonia: a mitochondrial disease. Neurology 36:1053–1060

Obayashi T, Hattori K, Sugiyama S et al. (1992) Point mutations in mitochondrial DNA in patients with hypertrophic cardiomyopathy. American Heart Journal 124:1263–1269

Obermaier-Kusser B, Paetzke-Brunner J, Enter C et al. (1991) Respiratory chain activity in tissues from patients (MELAS) with a point mutation of the mitochondrial genome (tRNALeu(UUR)). FEBS Letters 286:67–70

Obermaier-Kusser B, Lorenz B, Schubring S et al. (1994) Features of mtDNA mutation patterns in European pedigrees and sporadic cases with Leber hereditary optic neuropathy. Am J Hum Genet 55:1063–1066

O'Brien TW, Denslow ND, Anders JC, Courtney BC (1990) The translation system of mammalian mitochondria. Biochim Biophys Acta 1050:174–178

Odawara M, Asakura Y, Tada K, Tsurushima Y, Yamashita K (1995) Mitochondrial gene mutation as a cause of insulin resistance. Diabetes Care 18:275

Ogilvie I, Wilkens S, Rodgers AJ, Aggeler R, Capaldi RA (1998) The second stalk: The delta-b subunit connection in ECF1F0. Acta Physiologica Scandinavica. Supplementum 643:169–175

Ohama E, Ohara S, Ikuta F, Tanaka K, Nishizawa M, Miyatake T (1987) Mitochondrial angiopathy in cerebral blood vessels of mitochondrial encephalomyopathy. Acta Neuropathologica (Berlin) 74:226–233

Ohkoshi N, Mizusawa H, Shiraiwa N, Shoji S, Harada K, Yoshizawa K (1995) Superoxide dismutases of muscle in mitochondrial encephalomyopathies. Muscle and Nerve 18:1265–1271

Ohnishi T (1979) Mitochondrial iron-sulfur flavohydrogenases. Jouranl 1

Ohta S, Kagawa Y (1986) Human F1-ATPase: Molecular cloning of cDNA for the beta subunit. J Biochem 99:135–141

Ohta S, Tomura H, Matsuda K, Kagawa Y (1988) Gene structure of the human mitochondrial adenosine triphosphate synthase beta subunit. J Biol Chem 263:11257–11262

Oka Y (1994) NIDDM–genetic marker; glucose transporter, glucokinase, and mitochondria gene. Diabetes Research and Clinical Practice 24:S117–121

Oka Y, Katagiri H, Yazaki Y, Murase T, Kobayashi T (1993) Mitochondrial gene mutation in islet-cell-antibody -positive patients who were initially non-insulin-dependent diabetics. Lancet 342:527–528

Oka Y, Katagiri H, Ishihara H, Asano T, Kikuchi M, Kobayashi T (1995) Mitochondrial diabetes mellitus–glucose-induced signaling defects and beta-cell loss. Muscle and Nerve 3:S131–136

Oldfors A, Larsson NG, Lindberg C, Holme E (1993) Mitochondrial DNA deletions in inclusion body myositis. Brain 116:325–336

Oldfors A, Moslemi AR, Fyhr IM, Holme E, Larsson NG, Lindberg C (1995) Mitochondrial DNA deletions in muscle fibers in inclusion body myositis. J Neuropathol and Exp Neurol 54:581–587

Oliver NA, Wallace DC (1982) Assignment of two mitochondrially synthesized polypeptides to human mitochondrial DNA and their use in the study of intracellular mitochondrial interaction. Mol Cell Biol 2:30–41

Olsen NK, Hansen AW, Norby S, Edal AL, Jorgensen JR, Rosenberg T (1995) Leber's hereditary optic neuropathy associated with a disorder indistinguishable from multiple sclerosis in a male harbouring the mitochondrial DNA 11778 mutation. Acta Neurol Scand 91:326–329

Oostra RJ, Bolhuis PA, Wijburg FA, Zorn-Ende G, Bleeker-Wagemakers EM (1994) Leber's hereditary optic neuropathy: Correlations between mitochondrial genotype and visual outcome. J Med Genet 31:280–286

Oostra RJ, Van den Bogert C, Nijtmans LG et al. (1995a) Simultaneous occurrence of the 11778 (ND4) and the 9438 (COX III) mtDNA mutations in Leber hereditary optic neuropathy: Molecular, biochemical, and clinical findings [letter]. Am J Hum Genet 57:954–957

Oostra RJ, Van Galen MJ, Bolhuis PA, Bleeker-Wagemakers EM, Van den Bogert C (1995b) The mitochondrial DNA mutation ND6/14484C associated with Leber hereditary optic neuropathy, leads to deficiency of complex 1 of the respiratory chain. Biochem Biophys Res Commun 215:1001–1005

Ortiz RG, Newman NJ, Manoukian SV, Diesenhouse MC, Lott MT, Wallace DC (1992) Optic disk cupping and electrocardiographic abnormalities in an American pedigree with Leber's hereditary optic neuropathy. Am J Ophthalmol 113:561–566

Ortiz RG, Newman NJ, Shoffner JM, Kaufman AE, Koontz DA, Wallace DC (1993) Variable retinal and neurologic manifestations in patients harboring the mitochondrial DNA 8993 mutation. Archives of Ophthalmology 111:1525–1530

Ota Y, Miyake Y, Awaya S, Kumagai T, Tanaka M, Ozawa T (1994) Early retinal involvement in mitochondrial myopathy with mitochondrial DNA deletion. Retina 14:270–276

Otsuka M, Mizuno Y, Yoshida M, Kagawa Y, Ohta S (1988) Nucleotide sequence of cDNA encoding human cytochrome c oxidase subunit Vlc. Nucl Acids Res 16:10916

Ottman R, Hauser WA, Susser M (1985) Genetic and maternal influences on susceptibility to seizures. An analytic review. Am J Epidemiol 122:923–939

Ottman R, Annegers JF, Hauser WA, Kurland LT (1988) Higher risk of seizures in offspring of mothers than of fathers with epilepsy. Am J Hum Genet 43:257–264

Ozawa M, Nishino I, Horai S, Nonaka I, Goto YI (1997) Myoclonus epilepsy associated with raggedred fibers: a G-to-A mutation at nucleotide pair 8363 in mitochondrial tRNA(Lys) in two families. Muscle & Nerve 20:271–278

Ozawa T (1995) Mechanism of somatic mitochondrial DNA mutations associated with age and diseases. Biochim Biophys Acta 1271:177–189

Ozawa T, Tanaka M, Ikebe S, Ohno K, Kondo T, Mizuno Y (1990) Quantitative determination of deleted mitochondrial DNA relative to normal DNA in parkinsonian striatum by a kinetic PCR analysis. Biochem Biophys Res Commun 172:483–489

Ozawa T, Tanaka M, Ino H et al. (1991a) Distinct clustering of point mutations in mitochondrial DNA among patients with mitochondrial encephalomyopathies and with Parkinson's disease. Biochem Biophys Res Commun 176:938–946

Ozawa T, Tanaka M, Sugiyama S et al. (1991b) Patients with idiopathic cardiomyopathy belong to the same mitochondrial DNA gene family of Parkinson's disease and mitochondrial encephalomyopathy. Biochem Biophys Res Commun 177:518–525

Paik SR, Shin HJ, Lee JH (2000) Metal-catalyzed oxidation of alpha-synuclein in the presence of Copper(II) and hydrogen peroxide. Archives of Biochemistry and Biophysics 378:269–277

Palmer G (1993) Current issues in the chemistry of cytochrome c oxidase. J Bioenerg Biomembr 25:145–151

Pang CY, Lee HC, Yang JH, Wei YH (1994) Human skin mitochondrial DNA deletions associated with light exposure. Archives of Biochemistry and Biophysics 312:534–538

Papadopoulou LC, Sue CM, Davidson MM et al. (1999) Fatal infantile cardioencephalomyopathy with COX deficiency and mutations in SCO2, a COX assembly gene. Nat Genet 23:333–337

Parisi MA, Clayton DA (1991) Similarity of human mitochondrial transcription factor 1 to high mobility group proteins. Science 252:965–969

Parker WD, Jr., Boyson SJ, Parks JK (1989a) Abnormalities of the electron transport chain in idiopathic Parkinson's disease. Ann Neurol 26:719–723

Parker WDJ, Oley CA, Parks JK (1989b) A defect in mitochondrial electron-transport activity (NADH-coenzyme Q oxidoreductase) in Leber's hereditary optic neuropathy. N Engl J Med 320:1331–1333

Parker WD, Jr., Boyson SJ, Luder AS, Parks JK (1990a) Evidence for a defect in NADH: ubiquinone oxidoreductase (complex I) in Huntington's disease. Neurology 40:1231–1234

Parker WD, Jr., Filley CM, Parks JK (1990b) Cytochrome oxidase deficiency in Alzheimer's disease. Neurology 40:1302–1303

Parker WD, Jr., Parks J, Filley CM, Kleinschmidt-DeMasters BK (1994) Electron transport chain defects in Alzheimer's disease brain. Neurology 44:1090–1096

Pavlakis SG, Phillips PC, DiMauro S, De Vivo DC, Rowland LP (1984) Mitochondrial myopathy, encephalopathy, lactic acidosis, and strokelike episodes: a distinctive clinical syndrome. Ann Neurol 16:481–488

Pavlath GK, Rich K, Webster SG, Blau HM (1989) Localization of muscle gene products in nuclear domains. Nature 337:570–573

Pearson HA, Lobel JS, Kocoshis SA et al. (1979) A new syndrome of refractory sideroblastic anemia with vacuolization of marrow precursors and exocrine pancreatic function. J Pediatr 95:976

Perez A, Morelli L, Cresto JC, Castano EM (2000) Degradation of soluble amyloid beta-peptides 1–40, 1–42, and the Dutch variant 1–40Q by insulin degrading enzyme from Alzheimer disease and control brains. Neurochemical Research 25:247–255

Pericak-Vance MA, Bebout JL, Gaskell PCJ et al. (1991) Linkage studies in familial Alzheimer disease: evidence for chromosome 19 linkage. Am J Hum Genet 48:1034–1050

Peterson C, Goldman JE (1986) Alterations in calcium content and biochemical processes in cultured skin fibroblasts from aged and Alzheimer donors. Proc Natl Acad Sci USA 83:2758–2762

Petit PX, Susin SA, Zamzami N, Mignotte B, Kroemer G (1996) Mitochondria and programmed cell death: back to the future. FEBS Letters 396:7–13

Petros JA, Hosseini SH, Amin MB et al. (2001) Mitochondrial DNA Mutations Increase the Tumorigenicity of Prostate Cancer Cells. Submitted

Petruzzella V, Chen X, Schon EA (1992) Is a point mutation in the mitochondrial ND2 gene associated with Alzheimer's disease? Biochem Biophys Res Commun 186:491–497

Pettepher CC, LeDoux SP, Bohr VA, Wilson GL (1991) Repair of alkali-labile sites within the mitochondrial DNA of RINr 38 cells after exposure to the nitrosourea streptozotocin. J Biol Chem 266:3113–3117

Pfanner N, Neupert W (1990) The mitochondrial protein import apparatus. Annu Rev Biochem 59:331–353

Pfanner N, Sollner T, Neupert W (1991) Mitochondrial import receptors for precursor proteins. Trends in Biochemical Sciences 16:63–67

Pieper AA, Brat DJ, Krug DK et al. (1999) Poly(ADP-ribose) polymerase-deficient mice are protected from streptozotocin-induced diabetes. Proc Natl Acad Sci USA 96:3059–3064

Pilkington SJ, Walker JE (1989) Mitochondrial NADH-ubiquinone reducatase: complementary DNA sequences of import precursors of the bovine and human 24-kDa subunit. Biochemistry 28:3257–3264

Pilz D, Quarrell OW, Jones EW (1994) Mitochondrial mutation commonly associated with Leber's hereditary optic neuropathy observed in a patient with Wolfram syndrome (DIDMOAD). J Med Genet 31:328–330

Pimentel E (1979) Some aspects of the genetics and etiology of spontaneous diabetes mellitus. Acta Diabetolgica Latina 16:193–201

Pinkert CA, Irwin MH, Johnson LW, Moffatt RJ (1997) Mitochondria transfer into mouse ova by microinjection. Transgenic Research 6:379–383

Pirsel M, Bohr VA (1993) Methyl methanesulfonate adduct formation and repair in the DHFR gene andin mitochondrial DNA in hamster cells. Carcinogenesis 14:2105–2108

Pitkanen S, Robinson BH (1996) Mitochondrial complex I deficiency leads to increased production of superoxide radicals and induction of superoxide dismutase. J Clin Invest 98:345–351

Polyak K, Li Y, Zhu H et al. (1998) Somatic mutations of the mitochondrial genome in human colorectal tumours. Nat Genet 20:291–293

Polymeropoulos MH, Lavedan C, Leroy E et al. (1997) Mutation in the alpha-synuclein gene identified in families with Parkinson's disease. Science 276:2045–2047

Poulton J, Holt (1994) Mitochondrial DNA: Does more lead to less? Nat Genet 8:313–315

Poulton J, Turnbull DM, Mehta AB, Wilson J, Gardiner RM (1988) Restriction enzyme analysis of the mitochondrial genome in mitochondrial myopathy. J Med Genet 25:600–605

Poulton J, Deadman ME, Gardiner RM (1989a) Duplications of mitochondrial DNA in mitochondrial myopathy. Lancet 1:236–240

Poulton J, Deadman ME, Gardiner RM (1989b) Tandem direct duplications of mitochondrial DNA in mitochondrial myopathy: analysis of nucleotide sequence and tissue distribution. Nucl Acids Res 17:10223–10229

Poulton J, Deadman ME, Ramacharan S, Gardiner RM (1991) Germ-line deletions of mtDNA in mitochondrial myopathy. Am J Hum Genet 48:649–653

Poulton J, Deadman ME, Bindoff L, Morten K, Land J, Brown G (1993) Families of mtDNA rearrangements can be detected in patients with mtDNA deletions: duplications may be a transient intermediate form. Human Molecular Genetics 2:23–30

Poulton J, Morten KJ, Weber K, Brown GK, Bindoff L (1994) Are duplications of mitochondrial DNA characteristic of Kearns-Sayre syndrome? Human Molecular Genetics 3:947–951

Poulton J, Morten KJ, Marchington D et al. (1995a) Duplications of mitochondrial DNA in Kearns-Sayre syndrome. Muscle and Nerve 3:S154–158

Poulton J, O'Rahilly S, Morten KJ, Clark A (1995b) Mitochondrial DNA, diabetes and pancreatic pathology in Kearns-Sayre syndrome. Diabetologia 38:868–871

Poulton J, Sewry C, Potter CG et al. (1995c) Variation in mitochondrial DNA levels in muscle from normal controls. Is depletion of mtDNA in patients with mitochondrial myopathy a distinct clinical syndrome? J Inherit Metabol Dis 18:4–20

Preiss T, Lightowlers RN (1993) Post-transcriptional regulation of tissue-specific isoforms. A bovine cytosolic RNA-binding protein, COLBP, associates with messenger RNA encoding the liver-form isopeptides of cytochrome c oxidase. J Biol Chem 268:10659–10667

Prezant TR, Agapian JV, Bohlman MC et al. (1993) Mitochondrial ribosomal RNA mutation associated with both antibiotic-induced and non-syndromic deafness. Nat Genet 4:289–294

Prochaska LJ, Bisson R, Capaldi RA, Steffens GC, Buse G (1981) Inhibition of cytochrome c oxidase function by dicyclohexylcarbodiimide. Biochim Biophys Acta 637:360–373

Puddu P, Barboni P, Mantovani V et al. (1993) Retinitis pigmentosa, ataxia, and mental retardation associated with mitochondrial DNA mutation in an Italian family. Br J Ophthalmol 77:84–88

Radi R, Castro L, Rodriguez M, Cassina A, Thomson L (1997) Free Radical Damage to Mitochondria. In Beal MF, Howell N and Bodis-Wollner I (eds): Mitochondria and Free Radicals in Neurodegenerative Diseases. Wiley-Liss, NY, pp. 57–89

Ragan CI (1987) Structure of NADH-ubiquinone reductase (Complex 1). Journal 15:1

Ragan CI, Galante YM, Hatefi Y (1982a) Purification of three iron-sulfur proteins from the iron-protein fragment of mitochondrial NADH-ubiquinone oxidoreductase. Biochemistry 21:2518–2524

Ragan CI, Galante YM, Hatefi Y, Ohnishi T (1982b) Resolution of mitochondrial NADH dehydrogenase and isolation of two iron-sulfur proteins. Biochemistry 21:590–594

Rahman S, Taanman JW, Cooper JM et al. (1999) A missense mutation of cytochrome oxidase subunit II causes defective assembly and myopathy. Am J Hum Genet 65:1030–1039

Reaume AG, Elliott JL, Hoffman EK et al. (1996) Motor neurons in Cu/Zn superoxide dismutase-deficient mice develop normally but exhibit enhanced cell death after axonal injury. Nat Genet 13:43–47

Reichling S, Ridley RG, Patel HV, Harley CB, Freeman KB (1987) Loss of brown adipose tissue uncoupling protein mRNA on

deacclimation of cold-exposed rats. Biochem Biophys Res Commun 142:696–701

Reid FM, Vernham GA, Jacobs HT (1994a) Complete mtDNA sequence of a patient in a maternal pedigree with sensorineural deafness. Human Molecular Genetics 3:1435–1436

Reid FM, Vernham GA, Jacobs HT (1994b) A novel mitochondrial point mutation in a maternal pedigree with sensorineural deafness. Hum Mutat 3:243–247

Rempfer R, Crook R, Houlden H et al. (1994) Parkinson's disease, but not Alzheimer's disease, Lewy body variant associated with mutant alleles at cytochrome P450 gene. Lancet 344:815

Reynier P, Malthiery Y (1995) Accumulation of deletions in mtDNA during tissue aging: analysis by long PCR. Biochem Biophys Res Commun 217:59–67

Reynier P, Figarella-Branger D, Serratrice G, Charvet B, Malthiery Y (1994a) Association of deletion and homoplasmic point mutation of the mitochondrial DNA in an ocular myopathy. Biochem Biophys Res Commun 202:1606–1611

Reynier P, Pellissier JF, Harle JR, Malthiery Y (1994b) Multiple deletions of the mitochondrial DNA in polymyalgia rheumatica. Biochem Biophys Res Commun 205:375–380

Richter C (1988) Do mitochondrial DNA fragments promote cancer and aging?. FEBS Letters 241:1–5

Richter C, Ghafourifar P, Schweizer M, Laffranchi R (1997) Nitric oxide and mitochondrial Ca2+. Biochem Soc Trans 25:914–918.

Richter C, Schweizer M, Ghafourifar P (1999) Mitochondria, nitric oxide, and peroxynitrite. Methods Enzymol 301:381–393

Ridanpaa M, van Eenennaam H, Pelin K et al. (2001) Mutations in the RNA Component of RNase MRP Cause a Pleiotropic Human Disease, Cartilage-Hair Hypoplasia. Cell 104:195–203

Ridley RG, Patel HV, Gerber GE, Morton RC, Freeman KB (1986) Complete nucleotide and derived amino acid sequence of cDNA encoding the mitochondrial uncoupling protein of rat brown adipose tissue: lack of a mitochondrial targeting presequence. Nucl Acids Res 14:4025–4035.

Rieger T, Munscher C, Seibel P, Muller-Hocker J, Kadenbach B (1993) Detection of small amounts of mutated mitochondrial DNA by allele-specific PCR (AS-PCR). Journal 4:121–127

Riordan-Eva P, Harding AE (1995) Leber's hereditary optic neuropathy: the clinical relevance of different mitochondrial DNA mutations. J Med Genet 32:81–87

Riordan-Eva P, Sanders MD, Govan GG, Sweeney MG, Da Costa J, Harding AE (1995) The clinical features of Leber's hereditary optic neuropathy defined by the presence of a pathogenic mitochondrial DNA mutation. Brain 118:319–337

Rizzuto R, Nakase H, Zeviani M, DiMauro S, Schon EA (1988) Subunit Va of human and bovine cytochrome c oxidase is highly conserved. Gene 69:245–256

Rizzuto R, Nakase H, Darras B et al. (1989) A gene specifying subunit VIII of human cytochrome c oxidase is localized to chromosome 11 and is expressed in both muscle and non-muscle tissues. J Biol Chem 264:10595–10600

Robinson BH, De Meirleir L, Glerum M, Sherwood G, Becker L (1987) Clinical presentation of mitochondrial respiratory chain defects in NADH-coenzyme Q reductase and cytochrome oxidase: clues to pathogenesis of Leigh disease. J Pediatr 110:216–222

Rogers J (2000) An IL-I alpha susceptibility polymorphism in Alzheimer's disease:new fuel for the inflammation hypothesis. Neurology 55:464–465

Roise D (1988) Import of proteins into mitochondria. Progress in Clinical and Biological Research 282:43–53

Roses AD (1996) From genes to mechanisms to therapies: Lessons to be learned from neurological disorders. Nat Med 2:267–269

Roses AD, Pericak-Vance MA, Saunders AM, Schmechel D, Goldgaber D, Strittmatter W (1994) Complex genetic disease: Can genetic strategies in Alzheimer's disease and new genetic mechanisms be applied to epilepsy? Epilepsia 35:S20–28

Rosing HS, Hopkins LC, Wallace DC, Epstein CM, Weidenheim K (1985) Maternally inherited mitochondrial myopathy and myoclonic epilepsy. Ann Neurol 17:228–237

Rotig A, Colonna M, Blanche S et al. (1988) Deletion of blood mitochondrial DNA in pancytopenia. Lancet 2:567–568

Rotig A, Colonna M, Bonnefont JP et al. (1989) Mitochondrial DNA deletion in Pearson's marrow-pancreas syndrome. Lancet 1:902–903

Rotig A, Cormier V, Koll F et al. (1991) Site-specific deletions of the mitochondrial genome in the Pearson marrow-pancreas syndrome. Genomics 10:502–504

Rotig A, Cormier V, Chatelain P et al. (1993) Delection of mitochondrial DNA in a case of early-onset diabetes mellitus, optic atrophy, and deafness (Wolfram syndrome, MIM 222300). J Clin Invest 91:1095–1098

Rotig A, Bourgeron T, Chretien D, Rustin P, Munnich A (1995) Spectrum of mitochondrial DNA rearrangements in the Pearson marrow-pancreas syndrome. Human Molecular Genetics 4:1327–1330

Rotig A, de Lonlay P, Chretien D et al. (1997) Aconitase and mitochondrial iron-sulphur protein deficiency in Friedreich ataxia. Nat Genet 17:215–217

Rottkamp CA, Nunomura A, Raina AK, Sayre LM, Perry G, Smith MA (2000) Oxidative stress, antioxidants, and Alzheimer disease. Alzheimer Disease and Associated Disorders 14:S62–S66

Rousseau DL, Ching Y, Wang J (1993) Proton translocation in cytochrome c oxidase: redox linkage through proximal ligand exchange on cytochrome a3. J Bioenerg Biomembr 25:165–176

Rowland LP (1983) Molecular genetics, pseudogenetics, and clinical neurology. Neurology 33:1179–1195

Rusanen H, Majamaa K, Tolonen U, Remes AM, Myllyla R, Hassinen IE (1995) Demyelinating polyneuropathy in a patient with the tRNA$^{Len(UUR)}$ mutation at base pair 3243 of the mitochondrial DNA. Neurology 45:1188–1192

Sadlock JE, Lightowlers RN, Capaldi RA, Schon EA (1993) Isolation of a cDNA specifying subunit VIIb of human cytochrome c oxidase. Biochim Biophys Acta 1172:223–225

Sakuta R, Nonaka I (1989) Vascular involvement in mitochondrial myopathy. Ann Neurol 25:594–601

Sakuta R, Goto Y, Horai S, Nonaka I (1993a) Mitochondrial DNA mutations at nucleotide positions 3243 and 3271 in mitochondrial myopathy, encephalopathy, lactic acidosis, and stroke-like episodes: a comparative study. J Neurol Sci 115:158–160

Sakuta R, Goto Y, Nonaka I, Horai S (1993b) An A-to-G transition at nucleotide pair 11084 in the ND4 gene may be an mtDNA polymorphism [letter; comment]. Am J Hum Genet 53:964–965

Salmaggi A, Carrara F, Zeviani M (1994) Remarkable recovery of visual function in a patient with Leber's optic neuropathy and multiple mutations of mitochondrial DNA. Int J Neurosci 77:261–266

Sandy MS, Langston JW, Smith MT, DiMonte DA (1993) PCR analysis of platelet mtDNA: lack of specific changes in Parkinson's disease. Move Disord 8:74–82

Santorelli FM, Shanske S, Macaya A, DeVivo DC, DiMauro S (1993) The mutation at nt 8993 of mitochondrial DNA is a common cause of Leigh's syndrome. Ann Neurol 34:827–834

Santorelli FM, Shanske S, Jain KD, Tick D, Schon EA, DiMauro S (1994) A T-C mutation at nt 8993 of mitochondrial DNA in a child with Leigh syndrome. Neurology 44:972–974

Santorelli FM, Mak SC, Vazquez-Acevedo M et al. (1995) A novel mitochondrial DNA point mutation associated with mitochondrial encephalocardiomyopathy. Biochem Biophys Res Commun 216:835–840

Santorelli FM, Schlessel JS, Slonim AE, DiMauro S (1996) Novel mutation in the mitochondrial DNA tRNA glycine gene associated with sudden unexpected death. Pediatric Neurology 15:145–149

Santorelli FM, Tanji K, Sano M et al. (1997) Maternally inherited encephalopathy associated with a single-base insertion in the mitochondrial tRNA Trp gene. Ann Neurol 42:256–260

Saraiva AA, Borges MM, Madeira MD, Tavares MA, Paula-Barbosa MM (1985) Mitochondrial abnormalities in cortical dendrites from patients with Alzheimer's disease. J Submicroscop Cytol 17:459–464

Saraste M (1984) Location of haem-binding sites in the mitochondrial cytochrome b. FEBS Letters 166:367–372

Saraste M (1999) Oxidative phosphorylation at the fin de siecle. Science 283:1488–1493

Sato W, Hayasaka K, Shoji Y et al. (1994) A mitochondrial tRNA(Leu)(UUR) mutation at 3,256 associated with mitochondrial myopathy, encephalopathy, lactic acidosis, and stroke-like episodes (MELAS). Biochemistry and Molecular Biology International (Sydney) 33:1055–1061

Saunders AJ, Kim T-W, Tanzi RE (1999) BACE Maps to Chromosome 11 and a BACE Homolog, BACE2, Reside in the Obligate Down Syndrome Region of Chromosome 21. Journal 286:1255

Sawa A, Wiegand GW, Cooper J et al. (1999) Increased apoptosis of Huntington disease lymphoblasts associated with repeat length-dependent mitochondrial depolarization. Nat Med 5:1194–1198

Schagger H, Link TA, Engel WD, von Jagow G (1986) Isolation of the eleven protein subunits of the bcl complex from beef heart. Methods Enzymol 126:224–237

Schapira AH (1995a) Nuclear and mitochondrial genetics in Parkinson's disease. J Med Genet 32:411–414

Schapira AH, Cooper JM, Dexter D, Jenner P, Clark JB, Marsden CD (1989) Mitochondrial complex I deficiency in Parkinson's disease. Lancet 1:1269

Schapira AH, Cooper JM, Dexter D, Clark JB, Jenner P, Marsden CD (1990a) Mitochondrial complex I deficiency in Parkinson's disease. J Neurochem 54:823–827

Schapira AH, Holt IJ, Sweeney M, Harding AE, Jenner P, Marsden CD (1990b) Mitochondrial DNA analysis in Parkinson's disease. Move Disord 5:294–297

Schapira AHV (1992) Mitochondrial abnormalities in neurodegeneration and normal aging. In DiMauro S, Wallace DC (eds): Mitochondrial DNA in Human Pathology. Raven Press, NY, pp. 159–172

Schapira AHV (1994a) Evidence for mitochondria dysfunction in Parkinson's disease – a critical appraisal. Move Disord 9:125–138

Schapira AHV (1994b) Mitochondrial dysfunction in neurodegenerative disorders and aging. In Schapira AHV, DiMauro S (eds): Mitochondrial disorders in neurology. Butterworth-Heinemann Oxford, pp. 227–244

Schapira AHV (1995b) The role of mitochondrial dysfunction in neurodegenerative disease. In Esser K, Martin GM (eds): Molecular Aspects of Aging. John Wiley, Chichester, pp. 241–251

Schatz G (1996) The protein import system of mitochondria. J Biol Chem 271:31763–31766

Schatz G, Dobberstein B (1996) Common principles of protein translocation across membranes. Science 271:1519–1526

Schellenberg GD, Bird TD, Wijsman EM et al. (1992) Genetic linkage evidence for a familial Alzheimer's disease locus on chromosome 14. Science 258:668–671

Schiebel K, Weiss B, Wohrle D, Rappold G (1993) A human pseudoautosomal gene, ADP/ATP translocase, escapes X-inactivation whereas a homologue on Xq is subject to X-inactivation. Nat Genet 3:82–87

Schiebel K, Mertz A, Winkelmann M, Nagaraja R, Rappold G (1994) Localization of the adenine nucleotide translocase gene ANT2 to chromosome Xq24-q25 with tight linkage to DXS425. Genomics 24:605–606

Schnopp NM, Kosel S, Egensperger R, Graeber MB (1996) Regional heterogeneity of mtDNA heteroplasmy in parkinsonian brain. Clinical Neuropathology 15:348–352

Schon EA, Rizzuto R, Moraes CT, Nakase H, Zeviani M, DiMauro S (1989) A direct repeat is a hotspot for large-scale deletion of human mitochondrial DNA. Science 244:346–349

Schon EA, Hirano M, DiMauro S (1994) Mitochondrial encephalomyopathies: Clinical and molecular analysis. Journal 26:291–299

Schon EA, Shoubridge EA, Moraes CT (1998) Cybrids in Alzheimer's disease: a cellular model of the disease? [letter; comment]. Neurology 51:326–327

Schuelke M, Bakker M, Stoltenburg G, Sperner J, von Moers A (1998) Epilepsia partialis continua associated with a homoplasmic mitochondrial tRNA(Ser(UCN)) mutation. Ann Neurol 44:700–704

Schuler M, Bossy-Wetzel E, Goldstein JC, Fitzgerald P, Green DR (2000) p53 induces apoptosis by caspase activation through mitochondrial cytochrome c release. J Biol Chem 275:7337–7342

Schurr TG, Ballinger SW, Gan YY et al. (1990) Amerindian mitochondrial DNAs have rare Asian mutations at high frequencies, suggesting they derived from four primary maternal lineages. Am J Hum Genet 46:613–623

Schurr TG, Sukernik RI, Starikovskaya YB, Wallace DC (1999) Mitochondrial DNA variation in Koryaks and Itel'men: Population replacement in the Okhotsk Sea-Bering Sea region during the Neolithic. Am J Phys Anthropol 108:1–39

Scott WK, Grubber JM, Conneally PM et al. (2000) Fine mapping of the chromosome 12 late-onset Alzheimer disease locus: Potential genetic and phenotypic heterogeneity. Am J Hum Genet 66:922–932

Seccombe JF, Pearson PJ, Schaff HV (1994) Oxygen radical-mediated vascular injury selectively inhibits receptor-dependent release of nitric oxide from canine coronary arteries. J Thor Cardiovasc Surg 107:505–509

Seibel P, Degoul F, Bonne G et al. (1991) Genetic biochemical and pathophysiological characterization of a familial mitochondrial encephalomyopathy (MERRF). J Neurol Sci 105:217–224

Seibel P, Lauber J, Klopstock T, Marsac C, Kadenbach B, Reichmann H (1994) Chronic progressive external ophthalmoplegia is associated with a novel mutation in the mitochondrial tRNA^Asn gene Biochem Biophys Res Commun 204:482–489

Seki A, Nishino I, Goto Y, Maegaki Y, Koeda T (1997) Mitochondrial encephalomyopathy with 15915 mutation: Clinical report. Pediatric Neurology 17:161–164

Selkoe DJ (1995) Alzheimer's disease. Missense on the membrane. Nature 375:734–735

Seneca S, Lissens W, Liebaers J et al. (1998) Pitfalls in the diagnosis of mtDNA mutations [letter]. J Med Genet 35:963–964

Shaag A, Saada A, Steinberg A, Navon P, Elpeleg ON (1997) Mitochondrial encephalomyopathy associated with a novel mutation in the mitochondrial tRNA(leu)(UUR) gene (A3243T). Biochem Biophys Res Commun 233:637–639

Shan DE, Yeh SI, Wan YC, Wei YH (1995) Absence of 4,977-bp deletion of blood cell mitochondrial DNA in patients with young-onset Parkinson's disease. Acta Neurol Scand 91:149–152

Shanske S, Moraes CT, Lombes A et al. (1990) Widespread tissue distribution of mitochondrial DNA deletions in Kearns-Sayre syndrome. Neurology 40:24–28

Sheehan JP, Swerdlow RH, Miller SW et al. (1997) Calcium homeostasis and reactive oxygen species production in cells transformed by mitochondria from individuals with sporadic Alzheimer's disease. J Neurosci 17:4612–4622

Sherrington R, Rogaev EI, Liang Y et al. (1995) Cloning of a gene bearing missense mutations in early-onset familial Alzheimer's disease. Nature 375:754–760

Sheu KF, Kim YT, Blass JP, Weksler ME (1985) An immunochemical study of the pyruvate dehydrogenase deficit in Alzheimer's disease brain. Ann Neurol 17:444–449

Shimura H, Hattori N, Kubo S et al. (2000) Familial Parkinson disease gene product, parkin, is a ubiquitin-protein ligase. Nat Genet 25:302–305

Shoffner JM, Wallace DC (1990) Oxidative phosphorylation diseases. Disorders of two genomes. In Harris H, Hirschhorn K (eds): Advances in Hum Genet. Plenum , 19, pp. 267–330

Shoffner JM, Wallace DC (1994) Oxidative phosphorylation diseases and mitochondrial DNA mutations: Diagnosis and treatment. Annual Review of Nutrition 14:535–568

Shoffner JM, Wallace DC (1995) Oxidative phosphorylation diseases. In Scriver CR, Beaudet AL, Sly WS, Valle D (eds): The Metabolic and Molecular Basis of Inherited Disease. McGraw-Hill, NY, pp.1535–1609

Shoffner JM, Lott MT, Voljavec AS, Soueidan SA, Costigan DA, Wallace DC (1989) Spontaneous Kearns-Sayre/chronic external ophthalmoplegia plus syndrome associated with a mitochondrial DNA deletion: a slip-replication model and metabolic therapy. Proc Natl Acad Sci USA 86:7952–7956

Shoffner JM, Lott MT, Lezza AM, Seibel P, Ballinger SW, Wallace DC (1990) Myoclonic epilepsy and ragged-red fiber disease (MERRF) is associated with a mitochondrial DNA tRNA^Lys mutation. Cell 61:931–937

Shoffner JM, Lott MT, Wallace DC (1991a) MERRF: A model disease for understanding the principles of mitochondrial genetics. Revue Neurologique (Paris) 147:431–435

Shoffner JM, Watts RL, Juncos JL, Torroni A, Wallace DC (1991b) Mitochondrial oxidative phosphorylation defects in Parkinson Disease. Ann Neurol 30:332–339

Shoffner JM, Fernhoff MD, Krawiecki NS et al. (1992) Subacute necrotizing encephalopathy: oxidative phosphorylation defects and the ATPase 6 point mutation. Neurology 42:2168–2174

Shoffner JM, Brown MD, Torroni A et al. (1993a) Mitochondrial DNA variants observed in Alzheimer disease and Parkinson disease patients. Genomics 17:171–184

Shoffner JM, Krawiecki N, Cabell MF, Torroni A, Wallace DC (1993b) A novel tRNA^Leu(UUR) mutation in childhood mitochondrial myopathy. Journal 53:949

Shoffner JM, Brown M, Huoponen K et al. (1994) A mtDNA mutation associated with maternally inherited Parkinson's disease (PD) and deafness. Journal 55:A242 (abstract 1417)

Shoffner JM, Bialer MG, Pavlakis SG et al. (1995a) Mitochondrial encephalomyopathy associated with a single nucleotide pair deletion in the mitochondrial tRNA^Leu(UUR) gene. Neurology 45:286–292

Shoffner JM, Brown MD, Stugard C et al. (1995b) Leber's hereditary optic neuropathy plus dystonia is caused by a mitochondrial DNA point mutation in a complex I subunit. Ann Neurol 38:163–169

Shoubridge EA (1995) Segregation of mitochondrial DNAs carrying a pathogenic point mutation (tRNA^Leu3243) in cybrid cells. Biochem Biophys Res Commun 213:189–195

Shoubridge EA, Karpati G, Hastings KEM (1990) Deletion mutants are functionally dominant over wild-type mitochondrial genomes in skeletal muscle fiber segments in mitochondrial disease. Cell 62:43–49

Shtilbans A, El-Schahawi M, Malkin E, Shanske S, Musumeci O, DiMauro S (1999) A novel mutation in the mitochondrial DNA transfer ribonucleic acid Asp gene in a child with myoclonic epilepsy and psychomotor regression. J Child Neurol 14:610–613

Silva JP, Kohler M, Graff C et al. (2000) Impaired insulin secretion and beta-cell loss in tissue-specific knockout mice with mitochondrial diabetes. Nat Genet 26:336–340

Silvestri G, Moraes CT, Shanske S, Oh SJ, DiMauro S (1992) A new mtDNA mutation in the tRNA^Lys gene associated with myoclonic epilepsy and ragged red fibers (MERRF). Am J Hum Genet 51:1213–1217

Silvestri G, Santorelli FM, Shanske S et al. (1994) A new mtDNA mutation in the tRNA$^{Leu(UUR)}$ gene associated with maternally inherited cardiomyopathy. Hum Mutat 3:37–43

Silvestri G, Servidei S, Rana M et al. (1996) A novel mitochondrial DNA point mutation in the tRNA(Ile) gene is associated with progressive external ophtalmoplegia. Biochem Biophys Res Commun 220:623–627

Silvestri G, Rana M, DiMuzio A, Uncini A, Tonali P, Servidei S (1998) A late-onset mitochondrial myopathy is associated with a novel mtDNA point mutation in the tRNA(Trp) gene. Neuromuscular Disorder 8:291–295

Simon DK, Pulst SM, Sutton JP, Browne SE, Beal MF, Johns DR (1999) Familial multisystem degeneration with parkinsonism associated with the 11778 mitochondrial DNA mutation. Neurology 53:1787–1793

Simonetti S, Chen X, DiMauro S, Schon EA (1992) Accumulation of deletions in human mitochondrial DNA during normal aging: Analysis by quantitative PCR. Biochim Biophys Acta 1180:113–122

Simonian NA, Hyman BT (1993) Functional alterations in Alzheimer's disease: Diminution of cytochrome oxidase in the hippocampal formation. J Neuropathol and Exp Neurol 52:580–585

Simonian NA, Hyman BT (1994) Functional alterations in Alzheimer's disease: selective loss of mitochondrial-encoded cytochrome oxidase mRNA in the hippocampal formation. J Neuropathol and Exp Neurol 53:508–512

Sims NR, Finegan JM, Blass JP, Bowen DM, Neary D (1987) Mitochondrial function in brain tissue in primary degenerative dementia. Brain Research 436:30–38

Singer TP, Castagnoli N, Jr., Ramsay RR, Trevor AJ (1987) Biochemical events in the development of parkinsonism induced by 1-methyl-4-phenyl-1,2,3,6-tetrahydropyridine. J Neurochem 49:1–8

Singh G, Lott MT, Wallace DC (1989) A mitochondrial DNA mutation as a cause of Leber's hereditary optic neuropathy. N Engl J Med 320:1300–1305

Sirrenberg C, Endres M, Folsch H, Stuart RA, Neupert W, Brunner M (1998) Carrier protein import into mitochondria mediated by the intermembrane proteins Tim10/Mrs11 and Tim 12/Mrs5. Nature 391:912–915

Skehel JM, Fearnley IM, Walker JE (1998) NADH:ubiquinone oxidoreductase from bovine heart mitochondria: sequence of a novel 17.2-kDa subunit. FEBS Letters 438:301–305

Sligh JE, Levy SE, Waymire KG et al. (2000) Maternal germ-line transmission of mutant mtDNAs from embryonic stem cell-derived chimeric mice. Proc Natl Acad Sci USA 97:14461–14466

Slim R, Levilliers J, Ludecke HJ et al. (1993) A human pseudoautosomal gene encodes the ANT3 ADP/ATP translocase and escapes X-inactivation. Genomics 16:26–33

Smeitink J, van den Heuvel L (1999) Protein Biosynthesis '99. Human mitochondrial complex I in health and disease. Am J Hum Genet 4:1505–1510

Smith CA, Gough AC, Leigh PN et al. (1992) Debrisoquine hydroxylase gene polymorphism and susceptibility to Parkinson's disease (published erratum appears in Lancet 1992;340(8810):64). Lancet 339:1375–1377

Smith OP, Hann IM, Woodward CE, Brockington M (1995) Pearson's marrow/pancreas syndrome: Haematological features associated with deletion and duplication of mitochondrial DNA. British J Haematol 90:469–472

Smith PR, Cooper JM, Govan GG, Harding AE, Schapira AH (1994) Platelet mitochondrial function in Leber's hereditary optic neuropathy. J Neurol Sci 122:80–83

Snyder SH, Jaffrey SR, Zakhary R (1998) Nitric oxide and carbon monoxide: Parallel roles as neural messengers. Brain Research. Brain Research Reviews 26:167–175

Snyderwine EG, Bohr VA (1992) Gene-and strand-specific damage and repair in Chinese hamster ovary cells treated with 4-nitroquinoline 1-oxide. Cancer Research 52:4183–4189

Solanes G, Vidal-Puig A, Grujic D, Flier JS, Lowell BB (1997) The human uncoupling protein-3 gene. Genomic structure, chromosomal localization, and genetic basis for short and long form transcripts. J Biol Chem 272:25433–25436

Soong NW, Hinton DR, Cortopassi G, Arnheim N (1992) Mosaicism for a specific somatic mitochondrial DNA mutation in adult human brain. Nat Genet 2:318–323

Sorbi S, Bird ED, Blass JP (1983) Decreased pyruvate dehydrogenase complex activity in Huntington and Alzheimer brain. Ann Neurol 13:72–78

Spencer SR, Taylor JB, Cowell IG, Xia CL, Pemble SE, Ketterer B (1992) The human mitochondrial NADH:ubiquinone oxidoreductase 51-kDa subunit maps adjacent to the glutathione S-transferase Pl–1 gene on chromosome 11q13. Genomics 14:1116–1118

Spillantini MG, Schmidt ML, Lee VM, Trojanowski JQ, Jakes R, Goedert M (1997) Alpha-synuclein in Lewy bodies [letter]. Nature 388:839–840

St George-Hyslop PH (2000) Molecular genetics of Alzheimer's disease. Biological Psychiatry 47:183–199

Stachowiak O, Dolder M, Wallimann T, Richter C (1998) Mitochondrial creatine kinase is a prime target of peroxynitrite-induced modification and inactivation. J Biol Chem 273:16694–16699

Stadhouders AM, Jap PHK, Winkler H-P, Eppenberger HM, Wallimann T (1994) Mitochondrial creatine kinase: A major constituent of pathological inclusions seen in mitochondrial myopathies. Proc Natl Acad Sci USA 91:5089–5093

Starikovskaya EB, Sukernik RI, Schurr TG, Kogelnik AM, Wallace DC (1998) Mitochondrial DNA diversity in Chukchi and Siberian Eskimos: implications for genetic history of ancient Beringia and peopling of the New World. Am J Hum Genet 63:1473–1491

Stepien G, Torroni A, Chung AB, Hodge JA, Wallace DC (1992) Differential expression of adenine nucleotide translocator isoforms in mammalian tissues and during muscle cell differentiation. J Biol Chem 267:14592–14597

Sternberg D, Danan C, Lombes A et al. (1998) Exhaustive scanning approach to screen all the mitochondrial tRNA genes for mutations and its application to the investigation of 35 independent patients with mitochondrial disorders. Human Molecular Genetics 7:33–42

Stoffel M, Froguel P, Takeda J et al. (1992a) Human glucokinase gene: Isolation, characterization, and identification of two missense mutations linked to early-onset non-insulin-dependent (type 2) diabetes mellitus [published erratum appears in Proc Natl Acad Sci USA, 1992,89(21):10562]. Proc Natl Acad Sci USA 89:7698–7702

Stoffel M, Patel P, Lo YM et al. (1992b) Missense glucokinase mutation in maturity-onset diabetes of the young and mutation screening in late-onset diabetes. Nat Genet 2:153–156

Stoffel M, Bell KL, Blackburn CL et al. (1993) Identification of glucokinase mutations in subjects with gestational diabetes mellitus. Diabetes 42:937–940

Sue CM, Tanji K, Hadjigeorgiou G et al. (1999) Maternally inherited hearing loss in a large kindred with a novel T7511C mutation in the mitochondrial DNA tRNA(Ser(UCN)) gene. Neurology 52:1905–1908

Suh YA, Arnold RS, Lassegue B et al. (1999a) Cell transformation by the superoxide-generating oxidase Mox1. Nature 401:79–82

Suh YA, Arnold RS, Lassegue B et al. (1999b) Cell transformation by the superoxide-generating oxidase Mox1. Nature 401:79–82.

Suomalainen A, Majander A, Haltia M et al. (1992) Multiple deletions of mitochondrial DNA in several tissues of a patient with severe retarded depression and familial progressive external ophthalmoplegia. J Clin Invest 90:61–66

Suomalainen A, Majander A, Pihko H, Peltonen L, Syvanen AC (1993) Quantification of tRNA³²⁴³⁽ᴸᵉᵘ⁾ point mutation of mitochondrial DNA in MELAS patients and its effects on mitochondrial transcription. Human Molecular Genetics 2:525–534

Suomalainen A, Kaukonen J, Amati P et al. (1995) An autosomal locus predisposing to deletions of mitochondrial DNA. Nat Genet 9:146–151

Susin SA, Lorenzo HK, Zamzami N et al. (1999a) Mitochondrial release of caspase-2 and -9 during the apoptotic process. J Exp Med 189:381–394

Susin SA, Lorenzo HK, Zamzami N et al. (1999b) Molecular characterization of mitochondrial apoptosis-inducing factor. Nature 397:441–446

Sutovsky P, Moreno RD, Ramalho-Santos J, Dominko T, Simerly C, Schatten G (1999) Ubiquitin tag for sperm mitochondria. Nature 402:371–372

Suzuki H, Ozawa T (1986) An ubiquinone-binding protein in mitochondrial NADH-ubiquinone reductase (Complex I). Biochem Biophys Res Commun 138:1237–12422

Suzuki S, Hinokio Y, Hirai S et al. (1994a) Pancreatic beta-cell secretory defect associated with mitochondrial point mutation of the tRNA^Leu(UUR) gene: A study in seven families with mitochondrial encephalomyopathy, lactic acidosis and stroke-like episodes (MELAS). Diabetologia 37:818–825

Suzuki S, Hinokio Y, Hirai S et al. (1994b) Diabetes with mitochondrial gene tRNA^Lys mutation. Diabetes Care 17:1428–1432

Suzuki Y, Kadowaki H, Katagiri H et al. (1994) c Posttreatment neuropathy in diabetic subjects with mitochondrial tRNA^Leu mutation. Diabetes Care 17:777–778

Suzuki Y, Suzuki S, Hinokio Y et al. (1997) Diabetes associated with a novel 3264 mitochondrial tRNA(Leu)(UUR) mutation. Diabetes Care 20:1138–1140

Sweeney MG, Brokington M, Weston MJ, Morgan-Hughes JA, Harding AE (1993a) Mitochondrial DNA transfer RNA mutation Leu⁽ᵁᵁᴿ⁾ A-G 3260: a second family with myopathy and cardiomyopathy. Quarterly J Med 86:435–438

Sweeney MG, Bundey S, Brockington M, Poulton KR, Winer JB, Harding AE (1993b) Mitochondrial myopathy associated with sudden death in young adults and a novel mutation in the mitochondrial DNA leucine transfer RNA⁽ᵁᵁᴿ⁾ gene. Quarterly J Med 86:709–713

Swerdlow RH, Parks JK, Cassarino DS et al. (1997) Cybrids in Alzheimer's disease: a cellular model of the disease?. Neurology 49:918–925

Swerdlow RH, Parks JK, Cassarino DS et al. (1999) Characterization of cybrid cell lines containing mtDNA from Huntington's disease patients. Biochem Biophys Res Commun 261:701–704

Szabo C (1997) Role of poly(ADP-ribose) synthetase activation in the suppression of cellular energetics in response to nitric oxide and peroxynitrite. Biochem Soc Trans 25:919–924

Taanman JW, Schrage C, Ponne N, Bolhuis P, de Vries H, Agsteribbe E (1989) Nucleotide sequence of cDNA encoding subunit VIb of human cytochrome c oxidase. Nucl Acids Res 17:1766

Taanman JW, Schrage C, Bokma E, Reuvekamp P, Agsteribbe E, De Vries H (1991a) Nucleotide sequence of the last exon of the gene for human cytochrome c oxidase subunit VIb and its flanking regions. Biochim Biophys Acta 1089:283–285

Taanman JW, van der Veen AY, Schrage C, de Vries H, Buys CH (1991b) Assignment of the gene coding for human cytochrome c oxidase subunit VIb to chromosome 19, band q13.1, by fluorescence in situ hybridisation. Hum Genet 87:325–327

Taanman JW, Turina P, Capaldi RA (1994) Regulation of cytochrome c oxidase by interaction of ATP at two binding sites, one on subunit VIa. Biochemistry 33:11833–11841

Takahashi M, Snyder SH (2000) Interaction of amyloid precursor proteins and heme oxygenase. Alzheimer Disease and Associated Disorders 14:S67–S71

Takahashi K, Pieper AA, Croul SE, Zhang J, Snyder SH, Greenberg JH (1999) Post-treatment with an inhibitor of poly(ADP-ribose) polymerase attenuates cerebral damage in focal ischemia. Brain Research 829:46–54

Takahashi M, Dore S, Ferris CD et al. (2000) Amyloid precursor proteins inhibit heme oxygenase activity and augment neurotoxicity in Alzheimer's disease. Neuron 28:461–473

Takeda A, Chiba S, Takaaki I, Tanamura A, Yamaguchi Y, Takeda N (1998) Cell cycle of myocytes of cardiac and skeletal muscle in mitochondrial myopathy. Japanese Circulation Journal 62:695–699

Tanaka M, Ino H, Ohno K et al. (1990) Mitochondrial mutation in fatal infantile cardiomyopathy. Lancet 336:1452

Tang J, Qi Y, Bao XH, Wu XR (1997) Mutational analysis of mitochondrial DNA of children with Rett syndrome. Pediatric Neurology 17:327–330

Taniike M, Fukushima H, Yanagihara I et al. (1992) Mitochondrial tRNA^Ile mutation in fatal cardiomyopathy. Biochem Biophys Res Commun 186:47–53

Tanno Y, Yondea M, Nonaka I, Tanaka K, Miyatake T, Tsuji S (1991) Quantitation of mitochondrial DNA carrying tRNA^Lys mutation in MERRF patients. Biochem Biophys Res Commun 179:880–885

Tanno Y, Okuizumi K, Tsuji S (1998) mtDNA polymorphisms in Japanese sporadic Alzheimer's disease. Neurobiology of Aging 19:S47–51

Tanzi RE (1999) A genetic dichotomy model for the inheritance of Alzheimer's disease and common age-related disorders. J Clin Invest 104:1175–1179

Tatuch Y, Robinson BH (1993) The mitochondrial DNA mutation at 8993 associated with NARP slows the rate of ATP synthesis in isolated lymphoblast mitochondria. Biochem Biophys Res Commun 192:124–128

Tatuch Y, Christodoulou J, Feigenbaum A et al. (1992) Heteroplasmic mtDNA mutation (T-G) at 8993 can cause Leigh disease when the percentage of abnormal mtDNA is high. Am J Hum Genet 50:852–858

Tawata M, Ohtaka M, Iwase E, Ikegishi Y, Aida K, Onaya T (1998) New mitochondrial DNA homoplasmic mutations associated with Japanese patients with type 2 diabetes. Diabetes 47:276–277

Taylor RW, Chinnery PF, Bates MJ et al. (1998) A novel mitochondrial DNA point mutation in the tRNA(Ile) gene: Studies in a patient presenting with chronic progressive external ophthalmoplegia and multiple sclerosis. Biochem Biophys Res Commun 243:47–51

Telerman-Toppet N, Biarent D, Bouton JM et al. (1992) Fatal cytochrome c oxidase-deficient myopathy of infancy associated with mtDNA depletion. Differential involvement of skeletal muscle and cultured fibroblasts. J Inherit Metabol Dis 15:323–326

The Huntington's Disease Collaborative Research Group (1993) A novel gene containing a trinucleotide repeat that is expanded and unstable on Huntington's disease chromosomes. Cell 72:971–983

Thomas AW, Edwards A, Sherratt EJ, Majid A, Gagg J, Alcolado JC (1996) Molecular scanning of candidate mitochondrial tRNA genes in type 2 (non-insulin dependent) diabetes mellitus. J Med Genet 33:253–256

Thyagarajan D, Shanske S, Vazquez-Memije M, De Vivo D, DiMauro S (1995) A novel mitochondrial ATPase 6 point mutation in familial bilateral striatal necrosis. Ann Neurol 38:468–472

Tiranti V, Chariot P, Carella F et al. (1995) Maternally inherited hearing loss, ataxia and myoclonus associated with a novel point mutation in mitochondrial tRNA^Ser(UCN) gene. Human Molecular Genetics 4:1421–1427

Tiranti V, D'Agruma L, Pareyson D et al. (1998a) A novel mutation in the mitochondrial tRNA(Val) gene associated with a complex neurological presentation. Ann Neurol 43:98–101

Tiranti V, Hoertnagel K, Carrozzo R et al. (1998b) Mutations of SURF-1 in Leigh Disease associated with cytochrome c oxidase deficiency. Am J Hum Genet 63:1609–1621

Tiranti V, Carrara F, Confalonieri P et al. (1999) A novel mutation (8342G – >A) in the mitochondrial tRNA(Lys) gene associated with progressive external ophthalmoplegia and myoclonus. Neuromuscular Disorders 9:66–71

Toda H, Hosokawa Y, Nishikimi M, Suzuki H, Kato K, Ozawa T (1989) Cloning and sequencing of a cDNA encoding the precursor to the 24 kDa iron-sulfur protein of human mitochondrial NADH dehydrogenase. International J Biochem 21:1161–1168

Tokunaga M, Mita S, Sakuta R, Nonaka I, Araki S (1993) Increased mitochondrial DNA in blood vessels and ragged-red fibers in mitochondrial myopathy, encephalopathy, lactic acidosis, and stroke-like like episodes (MELAS). Ann Neurol 33:275–280

Tomkinson AE, Bonk RT, Kim J, Bartfeld N, Linn S (1990) Mammalian mitochondrial endonucleasse activities specific for ultraviolet-irradiated DNA. Nucl Acids Res 18:929–935

Tomkinson AE, Bonk R, T., Linn S (1988) Mitochondrial endonuclease activities specific for apurinic/apyrimidinic sites in DNA from mouse cells. J Biol Chem 263:12532–12537

Tono T, Ushisako Y, Kiyomizu K et al. (1998) Cochlear implantation in a patient with profound hearing loss with the A1555G mitochondrial mutation. Am J Otol 19:754–757

Torroni A, Petrozzi M, D'Urbano L et al. (1997) Haplotype and phylogenetic analyses suggest that one European-specific mtDNA background plays a role in the expression of Leber hereditary optic neuropathy by increasing the penetrance of the primary mutations 11778 and 14484. Am J Hum Genet 60:1107–11021

Torroni A, Wallace DC (1995) MtDNA haplogroups in Native Americans [see also comment: Am. J. Hum. Genet. 56:1236–1238, 1995]. Am J Hum Genet 56:1234–1236

Torroni A, Semino O, Scozzari R et al. (1990) Y chromosome DNA polymorphisms in human populations: Differences between Caucasoids and Africans detected by 49a and 49f probes. Annals of Hum Genet 54:287–296

Torroni A, Schurr TG, Yang C-C et al. (1992) Native American mitochondrial DNA analysis indicates that the Amerind and the Nadene populations were founded by two independent migrations. Genetics 130:153–162

Torroni A, Schurr TG, Cabell MF et al. (1993a) Asian affinities and continental radiation of the four founding Native American mtDNAs. Am J Hum Genet 53:563–590

Torroni A, Sukernik RI, Schurr TG et al. (1993b) MtDNA variation of aboriginal Siberians reveals distinct genetic affinities with Native Americans. Am J Hum Genet 53:591–608

Torroni A, Chen Y, Semino O et al. (1994a) MtDNA and Y-chromosome polymorphisms in four native American populations from southern Mexico. Am J Hum Genet 54:303–318

Torroni A, Lott MT, Cabell MF, Chen Y, Laverge L, Wallace DC (1994b) MtDNA and the origin of Caucasians. Identification of ancient Caucasian-specific haplogroups, one of which is prone to a recurrent somatic duplication in the D-loop region. Am J Hum Genet 55:760–776

Torroni A, Miller JA, Moore LG et al. (1994c) Mitochondrial DNA analysis in Tibet. Implications for the origin of the Tibetan population and its adaptation to high altitude. Am J Phys Anthropol 93:189–199

Torroni A, Neel JV, Barrantes R, Schurr TG, Wallace DC (1994d) A mitochondrial DNA "clock" for the Amerinds and its implication for timing their entry into North America. Proc Natl Acad Sci USA 91:1158–1162

Torroni A, Carelli V, Petrozzi M et al. (1996a) Detection of the mtDNA 14484 mutation on an African-specific haplotype: Implications about its role in causing Leber hereditary optic neuropathy. Am J Hum Genet 59:248–252

Torroni A, Huoponen K, Francalacci P et al. (1996b) Classification of European mtDNAs from an analysis of three European populations. Genetics 144:1835–1850

Tritschler H-J, Andreetta F, Moraes CT et al. (1992) Mitochondrial myopathy of childhood associated with depletion of mitochondrial DNA. Neurology 42:209–217

Trounce I, Wallace DC (1996) Production of transmitochondrial mouse cell lines by cybrid rescue of rhodamine-6G pre-treated L-cells. Som Cell Mol Genet 22:81–85

Trounce I, Neill S, Wallace DC (1994) Cytoplasmic transfer of the mtDNA nt 8993 TG (ATP6) point mutation associated with Leigh syndrome into mtDNA-less cells demonstrates cosegregation with a decrease in state III respiration and ADP/O ratio. Proc Natl Acad Sci USA 91:8334–8338

Trounce IA, Kim YL, Jun AS, Wallace DC (1996) Assessment of mitochondrial oxidative phosphorylation in patient muscle biopsies, lymphoblasts, and transmitochondrial cell lines. Methods Enzymol 264:484–509

Trounce I, Schmiedel J, Yen HC et al. (2000) Cloning of neuronal mtDNA variants in cultured cells by synaptosome fusion with mtDNA-less cells. Nucl Acids Res 28:2164–2170

Trumpower BL, Gennis RB (1994) Energy transduction by cytochrome complexes in mitochondrial and bacterial respiration: The enzymology of coupling electron transfer reactions to transmembrane proton translocation. Annu Rev Biochem 63:675–716

Tsukihara T, Aoyama H, Yamashita E et al. (1995) Structures of metal sites of oxidized bovine heart cytochrome c oxidase at 2.8 A. Science 269:1069–1074

Tsukihara T, Aoyama H, Yamashita E et al. (1996) The whole structure of the 13-subunit oxidized cytochrome c oxidase at 2.8 A. Science 272:1136–1144

Tsukuda K, Suzuki Y, Kameoka K et al. (1997) Screening of patients with maternally transmitted diabetes for mitochondrial gene mutations in the tRNA[Leu(UUR)] region. Diabet Med 14:1032–1037

Tudek B, Laval J, Boiteux S (1993) SOS-independent mutagenesis in lacZ induced by methylene blue plus visible light. Mol Gen Genet 236:433–439

Tulinius MH, Houshmand M, Larsson NG et al. (1995) De novo mutation in the mitochondrial ATP synthase subunit 6 gene (T8993G) with rapid segregation resulting in Leigh syndrome in the offspring. Hum Genet 96:290–294

Turrens JF, Boveris A (1980) Generation of superoxide anion by the NADH dehydrogenase of bovine heart mitochondria. Biochem J 191:421–427

Turrens JF, Alexandre A, Lehninger AL (1985) Ubisemiquinone is the electron donor for superoxide formation by complex III of heart mitochondria. Archives of Biochemistry and Biophysics 237:408–414

Usami S, Abe S, Shinkawa H, Kimberling WJ (1998) Sensorineural hearing loss caused by mitochondrial DNA mutations: special reference to the A1555G mutation. J Commun Disord 31:423–434; quiz 434–435

Valnot I, Osmond S, Gigarel N et al. (2000) Mutations in SC01 gene causes mitochondrial cytochrome c oxidase deficiency presenting as neonatal-onset hepatic failure and encephalopathy. Journal 67:Abstract #60

van den Heuvel L, Ruitenbeek W, Smeets R et al. (1998) Demonstration of a new pathogenic mutation in human complex I deficiency: a 5-bp duplication in the nuclear gene encoding the 18-kD (AQDQ) subunit. Am J Hum Genet 62:262–268

van den Ouweland JM, Bruining GJ, Lindhout D, Wit JM, Veldhuyzen BF, Maassen JA (1992a) Mutations in mitochondrial tRNA genes: non-linkage with syndromes of Wolfram and chronic progressive external ophthalmoplegia. Nucl Acids Res 20:679–682

van den Ouweland JM, Lemkes HHP, Ruitenbeek W et al. (1992b) Mutation in mitochondrial tRNA^Leu(UUR) gene in a large pedigree with maternally transmitted type II diabetes mellitus and deafness. Nat Genet 1:368–371 van den Ouweland JM, Lemkes HH, Trembath RC et al. (1994) Maternally inherited diabetes and deafness is a distinct subtype of diabetes and associates with a single point mutation in the mitochondrial tRNA$^{Leu(UUR)}$ gene. Diabetes 43:746–751

Vassar R, Bennett BD, Babu-Khan S et al. (1999) Beta-secretase cleavage of Alzheimer's amyloid precursor protein by the transmembrane aspartic protease BACE. Science 286:735–741

Vekrellis K, Ye Z, Qiu WQ et al. (2000) Neurons regulate extracellular levels of amyloid beta-protein via proteolysis by insulin-degrading enzyme. J Neurosci 20:1657–1665

Velho G, Froguel P (1998) Genetic, metabolic and clinical characteristics of maturity onset diabetes of the young. European J Endocrinol 138:233–239

Vergani L, Martinuzzi A, Carelli V et al. (1995) MtDNA mutations associated with Leber's hereditary optic neuropathy: Studies on cytoplasmic hybrid (cybrid) cells. Biochem Biophys Res Commun 210:880–888

Verma A, Piccoli DA, Bonilla E, Berry GT, DiMauro S, Moraes CT (1997) A novel mitochondrial G8313A mutation associated with prominent initial gastrointestinal symptoms and progressive encephaloneuropathy. Pediatr Res 42:448–454

Vernham GA, Reid FM, Rundle PA, Jacobs HT (1994) Bilateral sensorineural hearing loss in members of a maternal lineage with mitochondrial point mutation. Clinical Otolaryngology 19:314–319

Vialettes BH, Paquis-Flucklinger V, Pelissier JF et al. (1997) Phenotypic expression of diabetes secondary to a T14709C mutation of mitochondrial DNA. Comparison with MIDD syndrome (A3243G mutation): A case report. Diabetes Care 20:1731–1737

Vidal-Puig A, Solanes G, Grujic D, Flier JS, Lowell BB (1997) UCP3: an uncoupling protein homologue expressed preferentially and abundantly in skeletal muscle and brown adipose tissue. Biochem Biophys Res Commun 235:79–82

Vidal-Puig AJ, Grujic D, Zhang CY et al. (2000) Energy metabolism in uncoupling protein 3 gene knockout mice. J Biol Chem 275:16258–16266

Vilkki J, Savontaus ML, Nikoskelainen EK (1989) Genetic heterogeneity in Leber hereditary optic neuroretinopathy revealed by mitochondrial DNA polymorphism. Am J Hum Genet 45:206–211

Virbasius JV, Scarpulla RC (1988) Structure and expression of rodent genes encoding the testis-specific cytochrome *c*. Differences in gene structure and evolution between somatic and testicular variants. J Biol Chem 263:6791–6796

Vissing J, Salamon MB, Arlien-Soborg P et al. (1998) A new mitochondrial tRNA(Met) gene mutation in a patient with dystrophic muscle and exercise intolerance. Neurology 50:1875–1878

Vu TH, Sciacco M, Tanji K et al. (1998) Clinical manifestations of mitochondrial DNA depletion. Neurology 50:1783–1790

Walker JE (1992) The NADH:ubiquinone oxidoreductase (complex I) of respiratory chains. Quarterly Reviews of Biophysics 25:253–324

Walker JE (1995) Determination of the structures of respiratory enzyme complexes from mammalian mitochondria. Biochim Biophys Acta 1271:221–227

Walker JE, Powell SJ, Vinas O, Runswick MJ (1989) ATP synthase from bovine mitochondria: Complementary DNA sequence of the import precursor of a heart isoform of the alpha subunit. Biochemistry 28:4702–4708

Walker JE, Arizmendi JM, Dupuis A et al. (1992) Sequences of 20 subunits of NADH:ubiquinone oxidoreductase from bovine heart mitochondria. Application of a novel strategy for sequencing proteins using the polymerase chain reaction. J Mol Biol 226:1051–1072

Walker M, Taylor RW, Stewart MW et al. (1995) Insulin sensitivity and mitochondrial gene mutation [letter; comment]. Diabetes Care 18:273–275

Wallace DC (1970) A new manifestation of Leber's disease and a new explanation for the agency responsible for its unusual pattern of inheritance. Brain 93:121–132

Wallace DC (1981) Assignment of the chloramphenicol resistance gene to mitochondrial deoxyribonucleic acid and analysis of its expression in cultured human cells. Mol Cell Biol 1:697–710

Wallace DC (1982) Cytoplasmic inheritance of chloramphenicol resistance in mammalian cells. In: Shay JW (ed): Techniques in Somatic Cell Genet. Plenum, NY, 12, pp. 159–187

Wallace DC (1986) Mitochodrial genes and disease. Hospital Practice (Office Edition) 21:77–87, 90–92

Wallace DC (1987) Maternal genes: mitochondrial diseases. In: McKusick VA, Roderick TH, Mori J, Paul MW (ed): Medical and Experimental Mammalian Genetics: A Perspective. A.R. Liss, March of Dimes Foundation, NY, 23, pp. 137–190

Wallace DC (1992a) Diseases of the mitochondrial DNA. Annu Rev Biochem 61:1175–1212

Wallace DC (1992b) Mitochondrial genetics: A paradigm for aging and degenerative diseases? Science 256:628–632

Wallace DC (1993) Mitochondrial diseases: Genotype versus phenotype. Trends in Genetics 9:128–133

Wallace DC (1994a) Mitochondrial DNA mutations in diseases of energy metabolism. J Bioenerg Biomembr 26:241–250

Wallace DC (1994b) Mitochondrial DNA sequence variation in human evolution and disease. Proc Natl Acad Sci USA 91:8739–8746

Wallace DC (1995a) (1994) William Allan Award Address. Mitochondrial DNA variation in human evolution, degenerative disease, and aging. Am J Hum Genet 57:201–223

Wallace DC (1995b) Mitochondrial DNA mutations in human disease and aging. In Esser K, Martin GM (ed): Molecular Aspects of Aging. John Wiley, NY, pp. 163–177

Wallace DC (1997) Mitochondrial DNA mutations and bioenergetic defects in aging and degenerative diseases. In Rosenberg RN, Prusiner SB, DiMauro S, Barchi RL (ed): The Molecular and Genetic Basis of Neurological Disease. Butterworth-Heinemann, Boston, pp. 237–269

Wallace DC (1999) Mitochondrial diseases in man and mouse. Science 283:1482–1488

Wallace DC, Murdock DG (1999) Mitochondria and dystonia: the movement disorder connection? Proc Natl Acad Sci USA 96:1817–1819

Wallace DC, Bunn CL, Eisenstadt JM (1975) Cytoplasmic transfer of chloramphenicol resistance in human tissue culture cells. J Cell Biol 67:174–188

Wallace DC, Pollack Y, Bunn CL, Eisenstadt JM (1976) Cytoplasmic inheritance in mammalian tissue culture cells. In Vitro 12:758–776

Wallace DC, Ye JH, Neckelmann SN, Singh G, Webster KA, Greenberg BD (1987) Sequence analysis of cDNAs for the human and bovine ATP synthase β-subunit: mitochondrial DNA genes sustain seventeen times more mutations. Curr Genet 12:81–90

Wallace DC, Singh G, Lott MT et al. (1988a) Mitochondrial DNA mutation associated with Leber's hereditary optic neuropathy. Science 242:1427–1430

Wallace DC, Zheng X, Lott MT et al. (1988b) Familial mitochondrial encephalomyopathy (MERRF): Genetic, pathophysiological, and biochemical characterization of a mitochondrial DNA disease. Cell 55:601–610

Wallace DC, Shoffner JM, Brown MD, Torroni A, Lott MT, Cabell M (1992a) Mitochondrial DNA mutations associated with Alzheimer's and Parkinson's disease. Journal 51:A30

Wallace DC, Shoffner JM, Watts RL, Juncos JL, Torroni A (1992b) Mitochondrial oxidative phosphorylation defects in Parkinson's disease. Ann Neurol 32:113–114

Wallace DC, Lott MT, Shoffner JM, Ballinger S (1994) Mitochondrial DNA mutations in epilepsy and neurological disease. Epilepsia 35:S43–S50

Wallace DC, Lott MT, Brown MD, Huoponen K, Torroni A (1995a) Report of the committee on human mitochondrial DNA. In: Cuticchia AJ (ed) Human Gene Mapping (1994), a Compendium. The Johns Hopkins University Press, Baltimore, p910–954

Wallace DC, Richter C, Bohr VA et al. (1995b) Group Report: The Role of Bioenergetics and Mitochondrial DNA Mutations in Aging and Age-Related Diseases. In: Esser K and Martin GM (ed) Molecular Aspects of Aging. John Wiley & Sons Ltd., New York, p199–225

Wallace DC, Brown MD, Lott MT (1999a) Mitochondrial DNA variation in human evolution and disease. Gene 238:211–230

Wallace DC, Lott MT, Kogelnik AM, Brown MD, Navathe SB (1999b) MITOMAP: A Human Mitochondrial Genome Database. Journal

Wang H, Oster G (1998) Energy transduction in the F1 motor of ATP synthase. Nature 396:279–282

Wang J, Wilhelmsson H, Graff C et al. (1999) Dilated cardiomyopathy and atrioventricular conduction blocks induced by heart-specific inactivation of mitochondrial DNA gene expression. Nat Genet 21:133–137

Watanabe T, Dewey MJ, Mintz B (1978) Teratocarcinoma cells as vehicles for introducing specific mutant mitochondrial genes into mice. Proc Natl Acad Sci USA 75:5113–5117

Weber K, Wilson JN, Taylor L et al. (1997) A new mtDNA mutation showing accumulation with time and restriction to skeletal muscle. Am J Hum Genet 60:373–380

Weiss H, Linke P, Haiker H, Leonard K (1987) Structure and function of the mitochondrial ubiquinol:cytochrome c reductase and NADH:ubiquinone reductase. Biochem Soc Trans 15:100–102

White FA, Bunn CL (1984) Segregation of mitochondrial DNA in human somatic cell hybrids. Mol Gen Genet 197:453–460

Wijmenga C, Hewitt JE, Sandkuijl LA et al. (1992) Chromosome 4q DNA rearrangements associated with facioscapulohumeral muscular dystrophy. Nat Genet 2:26–30

Wijmenga C, Winokur ST, Padberg GW et al. (1993) The human skeletal muscle adenine nucleotide translocator gene maps to chromosome 4q35 in the region of the facioscapulohumeral muscular dystrophy locus. Hum Genet 92:198–203

Wikstrom M (1998) Proton translocation by bacteriorhodopsin and heme-copper oxidases. Curr Opin Struct Biol 8:480–488

Wikstrom M, Krab K (1986) The semiquinone cycle. A hypothesis of electron transfer and proton translocation in cytochrome bc-type complexes. J Bioenerg Biomembr 18:181–193

Wikstrom M, Krab K, Saraste M (1981) Proton-translocating cytochrome complexes. Annu Rev Biochem 50:623–655

Williams MD, Van Remmen H, Conrad CC, Huang TT, Epstein CJ, Richardson A (1998) Increased oxidative damage is correlated to altered mitochondrial function in heterozygous manganese superoxide dismutase knockout mice. J Biol Chem 273:28510–28515

Wissinger B, Besch D, Baumann B et al. (1997) Mutation analysis of the ND6 gene in patients with Lebers hereditary optic neuropathy. Biochem Biophys Res Commun 234:511–515

Wolfe MS, Xia W, Ostaszewski BL, Diehl TS, Kimberly WT, Selkoe DJ (1999) Two transmembrane aspartates in presenilin-1 required for presenilin endoproteolysis and gamma-secretase activity. Nature 398:513–517

Wollheim CB (2000) Beta-cell mitochondria in the regulation of insulin secretion: A new culprit in type II diabetes. Diabetologia 43:265–277

Wood ML, Dizdaroglu M, Gajewski E, Essigmann JM (1990) Mechanistic studies of ionizing radiation and oxidative mutagenesis: Genetic effects of a single 8-hydroxyguanine (7-hydro-8-oxoguanine) residue inserted at a unique site in a viral genome. Biochemistry 29:7024–7032

Wragg MA, Talbot CJ, Morris JC, Lendon CL, Goate AM (1995) No association found between Alzheimer's disease and a mitochondrial tRNA glutamine gene variant. Neuroscience Letters 201:107–110

Yan LJ, Levine RL, Sohal RS (1997) Oxidative damage during aging targets mitochondrial aconitase [published erratum appears in Proc Natl Acad Sci USA (1998) Feb 17;95(4):1968]. Proc Natl Acad Sci USA 94:11168–11172

Yan WL, Lerner TJ, Haines JL, Gusella JF (1994) Sequence analysis and mapping of a novel human mitochondrial ATP synthase subunit 9 cDNA (ATP5G3). Genomics 24:375–377

Yang G, Chan PH, Chen J et al. (1994) Human copper-zinc superoxide dismutase transgenic mice are highly resistant to reperfusion injury after focal cerebral ischemia. Stroke 25:165–170

Yen TC, Chen YS, King KL, Yeh SH, Wei YH (1989) Liver mitochondrial respiratory functions decline with age. Biochem Biophys Res Commun 165:944–1003

Yoneda M, Tsuji S, Yamauchi T et al. (1989) Mitochondrial DNA mutation in family with Leber's hereditary optic neuropathy. Lancet 1:1076–1077

Yoneda M, Tanno Y, Horai S, Ozawa T, Miyatake T, Tsuji S (1990) A common mitochondrial DNA mutation in the tRNA^{Lys} of patients with myoclonus epilepsy associated with ragged-red fibers. Biochem Int 21:789–796

Yoneda M, Chomyn A, Martinuzzi A, Hurko O, Attardi G (1992) Marked replicative advantage of human mtDNA carrying a point mutation that causes the MELAS encephalomyopathy. Proc Natl Acad Sci USA 89:11164–11168

Yoon KL, Aprille JR, Ernst SG (1991) Mitochondrial tRNA^{Thr} mutation in fatal infantile respiratory enzyme deficiency. Biochem Biophys Res Commun 176:1112–1115

Yoon KL, Ernst SG, Rasmussen C, Dooling EC, Aprille JR (1993) Mitochondrial disorder associated with newborn cardiopulmonary arrest. Pediatr Res 33:433–440

Yoshino H, Nakagawa-Hattori Y, Kondo T, Mizuno Y (1992) Mitochondrial complex I and II activities of lymphocytes and platelets in Parkinson's disease. J Neur Trans Parkinsons Dis Dement sect 2:27–34

Zakhary R, Gaine SP, Dinerman JL, Ruat M, Flavahan NA, Snyder SH (1996) Heme oxygenase 2: Endothelial and neuronal localization and role in endothelium-dependent relaxation. Proc Natl Acad Sci USA 93:795–798

Zakhary R, Poss KD, Jaffrey SR, Ferris CD, Tonegawa S, Snyder SH (1997) Targeted gene deletion of heme oxygenase 2 reveals neural role for carbon monoxide. Proc Natl Acad Sci USA 94:14848–14853

Zeviani M, Nakagawa M, Herbert J et al. (1987) Isolation of a cDNA clone encoding subunit IV of human cytochrome c oxidase. Gene 55:205–217

Zeviani M, Sakoda S, Sherbany AA et al. (1988) Sequence of cDNAs encoding subunit Vb of human and bovine cytochrome c oxidase. Gene 65:1–11

Zeviani M, Servidei S, Gellera C, Bertini E, DiMauro S, DiDonato S (1989) An autosomal dominant disorder with multiple deletions of mitochondrial DNA starting at the D-loop region. Nature 339:309–311

Zeviani M, Bresolin N, Gellera C et al. (1990) Nucleus-driven multiple large-scale deletions of the human mitochondrial genome: A new autosomal dominant disease. Am J Hum Genet 47:904–914

Zeviani M, Gellera C, Antozzi C et al. (1991) Maternally inherited myopathy and cardiomyopathy: Association with mutation in mitochondrial DNA tRNA$^{Leu(UUR)}$. Lancet 338:143–147

Zeviani M, Muntoni F, Savarese N et al. (1993) A MERRF/MELAS overlap syndrome associated with a new point mutation in the mitochondrial DNA tRNA^{Lys} gene. Eur J Hum Genet 1:80–87

Zeviani M, Amati P, Comi G, Fratta G, Mariotti C, Tiranti V (1995) Searching for genes affecting the structural integrity of the mitochondrial genome. Biochim Biophys Acta 1271:153–158

Zhang C, Baumer A, Maxwell RJ, Linnane AW, Nagley P (1992) Multiple mitochondrial DNA deletions in an elderly human individual. FEBS Letters 297:4–8

Zheng XX, Shoffner JM, Voljavec AS, Wallace DC (1990) Evaluation of procedures for assaying oxidative phosphorylation enzyme activities in mitochondrial myopathy muscle biopsies. Biochim Biophys Acta 1019:1–10

Zhu Z, Yao J, Johns T et al. (1998) SURF1, encoding a factor involved in the biogenesis of cytochrome c oxidase, is mutated in Leigh syndrome. Nat Genet 20:337–343

Zhuo S, Paik SR, Register JA, Allison WS (1993) Photoinactivation of the bovine heart mitochondrial F1-ATPase by [14C]dequalinium cross-links phenylalanine-403 or phenylalanine-406 of an alpha subunit to a site or sites contained within residues 440–459 of a beta subunit. Biochemistry 32:2219–2227

Ziegler ML, Davidson RL (1981) Elimination of mitochondrial elements and improved viability in hybrid cells. Somatic Cell Genet 7:73–88

Zoratti M, Szabo I (1995) The mitochondrial permeability transition. Biochim Biophys Acta 1241:139–176

Zuckerman SH, Solus JF, Gillespie FP, Eisenstadt JM (1984) Retention of both parental mitochondrial DNA species in mouse-Chinese hamster somatic cell hybrids. Som Cell Mol Genet 1984:85–91

Genetic analysis of complex traits

12

Niall H. Anderson
Anna F. Dominiczak

Introduction

Success in identifying the genes responsible for many classic monogenetic disorders has implied that it may be possible to apply similar methods of molecular and statistical genetics to unravel the genetic basis of common disorders, such as diabetes, hypertension, and asthma. Such disorders are often described as *complex traits* or *multifactorial disorders* because they are diseases whose susceptibility is determined by multiple genetic and environmental factors acting in combination. The benefits of successful genetic studies of complex traits are clear and numerous. These would include new understanding of etiology based on knowledge of the molecular mechanisms of disease, improved diagnosis and therapy for genetically defined subsets of patients, the discovery of genetic markers related to disease complications, and the ability to target drug treatments to populations with specific genetic susceptibilities (sometimes described as pharmacogenomics).

Much of the success of an investigation of a multifactorial disorder depends on the design of the study and on the suitability of the underlying model or method of statistical analysis. The degree and pattern of epistasis (gene-gene interaction) and gene-environment interaction strongly influences the probability of detecting susceptibility loci. In addition, late age of onset and genetic heterogeneity are complicating factors for many such complex traits. Standard positional cloning strategies that require mapping of the susceptibility loci to regions of the order of 1 Mb of DNA are unlikely to be effective in such circumstances, and a combination of alternative approaches must be adopted to identify the genes that are responsible for the susceptibility to multifactorial disease. This chapter reviews some of these approaches and illustrates how they are being used in practice to investigate the genetic determinants of essential hypertension.

Interested readers may wish to refer to some of the many other available reviews of the genetic analysis of complex traits. General overviews are provided by, amongst others, Thomson and Esposito (1999), Lander and Schork (1994), Weeks and Lathrop (1995) and Zhang et al. (1997), while Lifton (1995), Dominiczak et al. (1998; 2000) and Gavras et al. (1999) consider particular areas related to hypertension.

Basic concepts

Many different study designs and methods of analysis can be used in the search for complex trait susceptibility loci, but all fundamentally involve evaluating the frequency of co-inheritance of disease with specific genes, markers, or regions of DNA. Linkage analysis of a Mendelian disorder depends upon the use of specific inheritance models parameterized by disease allele frequencies and penetrances. However, for a multifactorial disorder, this type of model does not encompass the full complexity of the etiology. Therefore, the analysis procedure will either have to assume robustness of the model to departures from the relevant assumptions, or an alternative approach that assesses the association between disease and allele sharing within pairs or groups of relatives will have to be used. The latter type of strategy is usually referred to as "nonparametric" or "model-free" and will form the basis of discussion in this chapter. It should be noted, however, that although nonparametric methods do not assume a specific genetic model,

410

the pattern of observed allele sharing will be affected by the pedigree structure and the underlying genetic mechanism through parameters such as penetrance, allele frequencies, locus heterogeneity, and the distance from the susceptibility locus. The result is that some assumptions about the inheritance pattern are made, often implicitly, even by a nonparametric method (Whittemore, 1996; Elston, 1998a).

IDENTITY BY DESCENT

Two alleles (one from each of a pair of related individuals) are said to be identical by state (IBS) if they are of the same type, i.e., have the same sequence of DNA. If both relatives inherited the IBS allele from the same ancestral allele, they are further described as being identical by descent (IBD). Figure 12.1 shows two hypothetical families that exemplify these concepts. If family members are affected with a genetic disease, they will exhibit IBD for alleles near a susceptibility locus more frequently than would be expected under Mendelian segregation. Similarly, unaffected family members will also show average increased IBD, since they will have inherited DNA variants not associated with disease more often than would be expected. Conversely, two family members with contrasting disease status (one affected and one unaffected) have an expectation of decreased IBD.

In practice, IBD is not measured directly; rather, it is estimated from similarities of alleles at marker loci. Obviously, the probability that similar alleles are IBD depends on a number of factors, such as the number of links between relatives and the genotypes of the individuals making up the links. The latter may be partially unknown. If a marker locus is highly polymorphic, that is, many different allelic variants are found in the population of reference, there is a strong probability that IBS is due to IBD. As the number of alleles becomes very large, it becomes increasingly likely that similarities must be due to IBD. Therefore, the most commonly used dense genetic linkage maps are those consisting of highly polymorphic microsatellite markers, such as the maps constructed by the Généthon group (Dib et al., 1996) or from the collaborative efforts of many laboratories (Murray et al., 1994). Microsatellite markers are highly variable and have many alleles, and are widely distributed through the genome, so that information from many markers can be pooled to estimate IBD from a single region. In addition, microsatellites are easy to characterize by polymerase chain reaction (PCR) methods.

The development of techniques and equipment for greater automation and higher throughput of PCR-based methods has prompted investigation of the feasibility of using large numbers of single nucleotide polymorphisms (SNPs) as genetic markers (Kruglyak, 1997a). The lower polymorphism rate of the SNPs would be compensated by their greater availability (estimated at 1 per 1000 base pairs), and the speed and efficiency of automated genotyping procedures would be increased by only having to perform a plus/minus assay. The success of SNP-based designs will depend on achieving sufficiently dense maps: Kruglyak (1997a) suggested that a dense map of SNPs at 1 cM intervals would provide an efficient tool for initial genome screens in linkage studies. Although this strategy is not yet feasible at time of writing, developments in marker identification are proceeding rapidly: see, for example, Buetow et al. (1999) and HGBASE (2000).

QUALITATIVE OR QUANTITATIVE PHENOTYPES?

Linkage analysis of a monogenic disorder is normally conducted on a qualitative phenotype, usually defined as a dichotomy between "affected" or "not affected". A multifactorial disorder may be defined in the same way, e.g., "hypertensive" or "normotensive", but it is also common to use a quantitative variable for the phenotype in this case. Often there will be a natural continuous measurement that will represent the phenotype with high fidelity, such as blood pressure for essential hypertension. This may then enable phenotypic observations to be made with greater precision than in the qualitative case, so that the statistical analysis should have greater power, either because of clearer

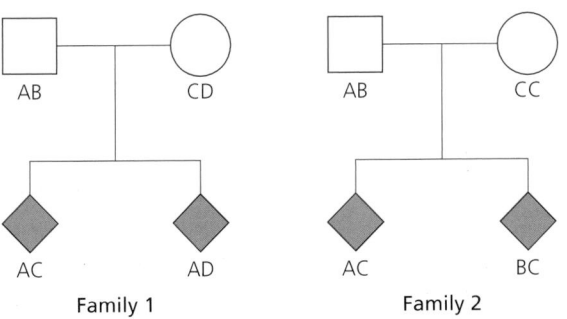

Fig. 12.1. Examples of IBS and IBD. In family 1, the A allele in both offspring has been inherited from the same paternal allele, and these two copies of A are therefore IBD. As the offspring receive different alleles from their mother, in total the siblings share 1 allele IBD. In family 2, the offspring have a common C allele inherited from their mother, but different paternal alleles. As the mother is homozygous, it is not clear whether these C alleles are copies of one particular maternal C, and therefore it is only possible to categorize them as IBS.

discrimination between cases and unaffecteds or because individuals with the most extreme phenotypes can be selected. Alternatively, the continuous measurement may be an *intermediate phenotype* for the condition of interest – a measurement that may represent an earlier stage in the etiology of the condition that is under the control of fewer genetic and environmental factors. Thus, it may be easier to detect the factors influencing the intermediate phenotype than the multifactorial disorder itself.

An example of an intermediate phenotype for essential hypertension is the level of circulating angiotensinogen. Plasma angiotensinogen has been shown to be significantly correlated with blood pressure in human subjects, and greater in hypertensive subjects or offspring of hypertensive parents than in normotensives (discussed in Jeunemaitre et al., 1992). A number of studies, including Jeunemaitre et al. (1992) and Caulfield et al. (1994), have shown an association between the *M235T* variant of the angiotensinogen gene (*AGT*) and hypertension, and that *M235T* is associated with increased levels of plasma angiotensinogen. In addition, studies in mouse strains with different numbers of gene copies have proven to be very powerful in this area (Smithies, 1997). Mice with one, two or three copies of the *AGT* gene have shown parallel increases of plasma angiotensinogen and blood pressure as a function of the number of copies of the gene (Smithies and Kim, 1994; Smithies and Maeda, 1995).

Kuntz et al. (1997) surveyed 11 different association studies of the *AGT M235T* variant, and although the meta analysis supported the relationship with hypertension, 6 of the individual studies did not. A more recent multi-center study, based on an analysis of linkage rather than association, reached similar negative conclusions (Brand et al., 1998). This apparent heterogeneity may indicate that *AGT* itself is not responsible for the functional changes that affect blood pressure, but that it lies close to (is in *linkage disequilibrium* with) a mutation that is responsible. Indeed, Inoue et al. (1997) demonstrated that the *AGT M235T* variant is in tight linkage disequilibrium with a guanine to adenosine transition at −6 base pairs upstream of the initiation site of transcription, and that this transition may result in an increased transcription rate.

Lessons from single-gene traits

A promising aid to the genetic dissection of multifactorial disorders has been the study of corresponding single gene syndromes, since these can be addressed by standard linkage and positional cloning techniques. Although most monogenetic syndromes are relatively rare, the genes involved may provide biological insight that will focus attention on the most promising candidate mechanisms for the more common multifactorial variants.

This process can be exemplified by considering recent research in three monogenic forms of salt-sensitive hypertension that have an early presentation and cause moderate to severe hypertension (Lifton, 1996; Luft, 1998). Glucocorticoid-remediable aldosteronism (GRA) is an autosomal dominant trait that results from the formation of a chimeric gene from the regulatory region and the first exons of the 11β-hydroxylase gene (*CYP11B1*) and exons of the aldosterone-synthase gene (*CYP11B2*) on chromosome 8. The result is to bring secretion of aldosterone under the control of adrenocorticotropic hormone (ACTH), rather than angiotensin II. Salt and water reabsorption is then increased, there is an expansion of plasma volume and blood pressure rises. Apparent mineralocorticoid excess (AME) is a rare autosomal recessive disorder that is characterized by low levels of aldosterone, in contrast to the high levels seen in GRA. AME results from mutations in the gene for the type 2 isoform of 11β-hydroxysteroid dehydrogenase (*11βHSD2*) on chromosome 16q22 that prevent 11βHSD2 from converting cortisol to cortisone. A second autosomal dominant disorder, Liddle's syndrome, shows a similar pathogenesis to GRA and AME, but antagonism of the mineralocorticoid receptor has no effect on blood pressure in this case. The syndrome results from mutations in the beta and gamma subunits of the amiloride-sensitive epithelial sodium channel gene (*ENaC*) on chromosome 16p12.2-13.11.

The common element in these monogenic conditions is that the mutations are in genes regulating salt reabsorption in the kidney, thus suggesting that attention should be focused on the genetics of the renin-angiotensin system. This has been a theme of recent research into essential hypertension, and has shown some benefits to date. The investigation of Liddle's syndrome inspired recent work that discovered an association between the T594M variant of the beta subunit of the *ENaC* and salt-sensitivity and hypertension in a UK black population of Afro-Caribbean descent (Baker et al., 1998).

Experimental models of complex traits

The use of a rat or mouse model of a complex trait such as hypertension allows a degree of experimental control impossible with a human population. Control over the breeding process allows (some) influence over the segregation of particular genetic factors, and the importance of environmental factors can be reduced or enhanced at will. Thus, an animal model of the trait of interest should have reduced genetic heterogeneity in comparison to the trait in humans and should allow easier dissection of the genetic influences. Equally, it should be possible to investigate more complex phenotypes and interactions in experimental forms of the trait (Lander and Schork, 1994).

Again taking hypertension as the exemplar, a typical approach is to study an F_2 intercross of inbred normotensive and hypertensive rat strains (see Fig. 12.2) using a "genome-wide scan". The F_2 progeny are phenotyped via tail-cuff plethysmography (Rapp, 2000) or radio-telemetry monitoring (Davidson et al., 1995), and genotyped with a panel of polymorphic microsatellite markers covering the rat genome. A genetic map is then produced and statistical modelling accomplished by software packages such as Mapmaker (Lander et al., 1987; Paterson et al., 1988) or Map Manager (Manly and Olson, 1999). A large number of regions of the rat genome, known as quantitative trait loci (QTLs), that seem to be associated with blood pressure have been detected in a variety of crosses with this technique (Dominiczak et al., 1998), with the QTLs discovered

to date being distributed across 15 different chromosomes. These regions are summarized in Table 12.1.

The QTLs inferred in this way are typically between 20 and 30 cM wide. They are therefore each likely to contain many genes that may be implicated in the development of hypertension. There are two main choices for the next stage of the process of identifying the causal mutations. The first of these is to breed congenic strains that contain different small, component regions of the QTL by a backcross breeding strategy that introduces small regions from the QTL area from the hypertensive strain into the normotensive background, and vice versa (Rapp and Deng, 1995). Although generally a slow procedure, requiring 8–12 generations of breeding, it is possible to shorten the time required by screening animals with densely spaced microsatellite markers to select those with the most favourable genetic background (Jeffs et al., 2000). The effects of the different components can then be compared to infer the role of the captured genes. The eventual goal is to produce a series of congenic animals containing progressively smaller chromosomal regions until positional cloning of a causal gene may be possible.

Rapp et al. (1998) provided the first evidence of an interaction between 2 QTLs in mammalian genetics by constructing a double congenic strain that placed low blood pressure loci from chromosomes 2 and 10 simultaneously onto the Dahl salt-sensitive rat genetic background. The resulting congenic animals showed significant blood pressure differences to the corresponding single congenic strains, and to the Dahl parental strain. This study shows the utility of experimental approaches to complex traits, and in particular the task of disentangling multiple interacting factors.

The second approach to identifying causal mutations, the feasibility of which has only recently been demonstrated, is to examine with large panels of microsatellite markers regions of the human genome that are homologous to the area covered by the QTL in the rat for linkage or association with hypertension. (This is sometimes referred to as *comparative mapping*). Using this methodology, Julier et al. (1997) examined areas homologous to a major QTL on rat chromosome 10 within subjects from a European population, and discovered significant linkage between familial essential hypertension and a region 18 cM proximal to the *ACE* gene on human chromosome 17. Baima et al. (1999) were able to replicate this result in a US population, and narrowed the region of interest to under 2 cM. Clearly, further systematic investigation of this region is required, but comparative mapping offers a powerful approach to the analysis of complex traits.

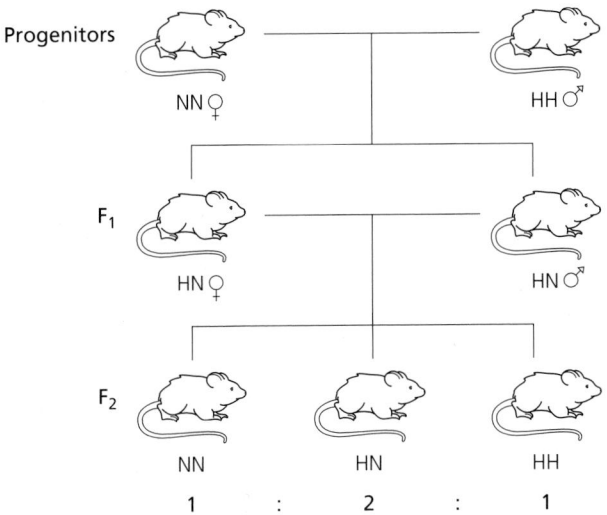

Fig. 12.2. One half of a reciprocal genetic cross with two inbred (homozygous) rat strains. NN represents the genotype at each locus for a normotensive strain, HH the genotype for hypertensive animals and HN represents a heterozygote. F_1 is the first filial generation, and F_2 the second. The ratio of each genotype expected in the F_2 generation is indicated at the bottom of the breeding plan. A second cross would also usually be undertaken starting with NN males and HH females, arriving at an F_2 generation with a similar distribution of genotypes, but each male F_2 having a Y chromosome that originated from the normotensive strain (rather than the hypertensive strain, as here).

Table 12.1. Quantitative Trait Loci for Blood Pressure in Rat Models of Essential Hypertension

Chr	Rat Strain	Central Gene/Marker	Lod Score	Reference
1	WKY × SHRSP$_{Izm}$	Lsn, My12	4.5	Nara et al. (1993)
	WKY × SHR	Sa	–	Samani et al. (1993)
	WKY × SHR	Mt1pa	–	Samani et al. (1993)
	WKY$_{Hd}$ × SHRSP$_{Hd}$	Sa	–	Lindpaintner et al. (1993)
	Lewis × Dahl SS	D1Mco1, Cytp450	3.4	Gu et al. (1996)
	Lewis × Dahl SS	Sa	2.5	Gu et al. (1996)
	ACI × FHH	Mt1pa	4.2	Brown et al. (1996)
	Sabra HR × Sabra HP	D1Mit2, Sa	4.9	Yagil et al. (1998)
	Sabra HR × Sabra HP	D1Mit1, Cytp450	4.7	Yagil et al. (1998)
	Donryu × SHR	D1mit3	4.3	Innes et al. (1998)
2	Lyon N × Lyon H	Cpb	7.0	Dubay et al. (1993)
	WKY × Dahl SS	Nakα1	3.4	Deng et al. (1994b)
	MNS × Dahl SS	Camk	2.6	Deng et al. (1994b)
	RI (BN × SHR)	D2N35	–	Pravenec et al. (1995)
	BN × SHR	Mt1pb	3.0	Schork et al. (1995)
	BN × SHR	Gca	6.3	Schork et al. (1995)
	BN × SHR	R598	3.0	Schork et al. (1995)
	BN × GH	Gca	–	Harris et al. (1995)
	WKY × SHRSP$_{Gla}$	D2Mit6	3.4	Clark et al. (1996)
	WKY × SHRSP$_{Gla}$	D2Wox7	3.1	Clark et al. (1996)
	WKY × SHR	D2Mit14	5.6	Samani et al. (1996)
	Lewis × Dahl SS	D2mco19	2.9	Garrett et al. (1998)
3	WKY × SHRSP$_{Izm}$	D3Mgh16	–	Matsumoto et al. (1996)
	WKY × SHRSP$_{Gla}$	D3Mgh16	5.6	Clark et al. (1996)
	WKY × SHRSP$_{Izm}$	D3Mgh12	6.2	Nara et al. (1996)
	Lewis × Dahl SS	D3Mgh16	3.0	Garrett et al. (1998)
4	WKY × SHR	Npy, Spr	–	Katsuya et al. (1993)
	RI (BN × SHR)	I1–6	–	Pravenec et al. (1995)
	BN × SHR	Npy2	4.6	Schork et al. (1995)
5	Lewis × Dahl SS	Glutb, Et2	–	Deng et al. (1994a)
	WKY × SHR	Mitr1678, Anf, Bnf	4.2	Zhang et al. (1996)
	Lewis × Dahl SS	Edn2	4.5	Garrett et al. (1998)
8	BN × SHR	R850	5.1	Schork et al. (1995)
10	WKY × SHRSP$_{Hd}$	Ace	–	Hilbert et al. (1991)
	WKY × SHRSP$_{Hd}$	Ace	5.1	Jacob et al. (1991)
	WKY × Dahl SS	Nos2	2.3	Deng & Rapp (1995)
	MNS × Dahl SS	Nos2	6.3	Deng & Rapp (1995)
	MNS × Dahl SS	Ace	4.8	Deng & Rapp (1995)
	BN × GH	Ace	–	Harris et al. (1995)
	Lewis × Dahl SS	D10Wox6	5.5	Garrett et al. (1998)
13	Lyon N × Lyon H	Renin	5.6	Dubay et al. (1993)
	WKY × SHR	D13Mit2	5.7	Samani et al. (1996)
16	BN × SHR	R220	4.3	Schork et al. (1995)
17	Sabra HR × Sabra HP	D17Mgh5	3.4	Yagil et al. (1998)
18	WKY × SHRSP$_{Hd}$	Rr1094	3.2	Jacob et al. (1991)
19	RI (BN × SHR)	D19Mit7	–	Pravenec et al. (1995)
20	RI (BN × SHR)	HSP70	–	Hamet et al. (1992)
X	WKY × SHRSP$_{Hd}$	Per-Ha2/Per-Ha7	–	Hilbert et al. (1991)
Y	WKY × SHR	–	–	Ely et al. (1993)

The normotensive/control strain is cited first on all occasions. WKY: Wistar-Kyoto; SHRSP$_{Izm}$: stroke-prone spontaneously hypertensive$_{Izumo}$; SHR: spontaneously hypertensive rat; Dahl SS: Dahl salt-sensitive; ACI: AxC9935 Irish; FHH: fawn-hooded hypertensive; Sabra HR: Sabra hypertension-resistant; Sabra HP: Sabra hypertension-prone; Lyon N: Lyon normotensive; Lyon H: Lyon hypertensive; MNS: Milan normotensive; RI (BN × SHR): recombinant inbred strains derived from normotensive Brown-Norway and SHR; GH: New Zealand genetically hypertensive; SHRSP$_{Gla}$: SHRSP$_{Glasgow}$; SHRSP$_{Hd}$: SHRSP$_{Heidelberg}$.

The following represent markers with known genes. Lsn: Leukosianin; My12: myosin short chain; Mt1pa: metallothionein 1, psuedogene A; Cytp450: cytochrome P450 cluster; Cpb: carboxypeptidase; Nakα: Na$^+$-K$^+$-ATPase α1; Camk: calmodulin dependent protein kinase II-delta; Mt1pb: metallothionein 1, psuedogene B; Gca: guanylylcyclase A/atrial natriuretic factor receptor; Npy: Neuropeptide Y; Spr: substance P receptor; IL6: interleukin 6; Npy2: Neuropeptide Y2; Glutb: glucose transporter type 2; Et2: endothelin-2; Anf: atrial natriuretic factor; Bnf: brain natriuretic factor; Ace: Angiotensin-converting enzyme; Nos2: inducible nitric oxide synthase: HSP70: Heat shock protein 70. Per-Ha2/Per-Ha7 are minisatellite bands. The remaining symbols represent anonymous microsatellite markers.

Statistical methods

AFFECTED SIB-PAIRS AND RELATED DESIGNS

One of the most commonly used experimental designs for genetic studies of complex traits is a collection of pairs of siblings who are both affected by the condition of interest, possibly along with any available parent to confirm IBD. Known as the Affected Sib Pairs (ASP) design, the analysis proceeds by comparing the proportions of 0, 1 or 2 alleles inherited IBD at each locus to the proportions that would be expected under the null hypothesis of no linkage (0.25, 0.5 and 0.25 respectively). If a given locus were to be related to the disorder, we would expect to see ASPs sharing more alleles IBD than would otherwise be expected. This is usually referred to as a "nonparametric" or "model-free" analysis, although as noted above, this is simply in the sense that an explicit set of genetic parameters is not defined before carrying out the analysis and cannot be estimated from the results (Farrall, 1997): full genetic models are implicit in all allele-sharing methods (Whittemore, 1996).

There are a number of approaches to the analysis of ASP data, some of which have been reviewed by Weeks and Lathrop (1995) and Sham (1998). These can be categorized into methods based around χ^2 statistics or those using likelihood methods. In the former group, the analyses are founded on counting the numbers of alleles in different categories. For example, the ordinary Pearson χ^2 statistic can be used to compare observed and expected numbers of sib-pairs sharing 0, 1 or 2 alleles IBD, or the mean test of Knapp et al. (1995) can be used to test whether the overall proportion of IBD alleles is equal to 0.5. The analyses in the second category, likelihood methods, were introduced to deal with missing data problems (e.g., an absence of parental data) that affect the identification of IBD status (Risch, 1990b; Holmans, 1993). The likelihood is usually parameterized in terms of the probabilities of a sib-pair having 0 or 1 alleles IBD, with the probability of 2 alleles IBD being a function of the first two. This type of method has been implemented in several computer packages; for example, MAPMAKER/SIBS (Kruglyak and Lander, 1995) will carry out both single marker and multipoint ASP likelihood analyses.

If there are other affected or unaffected siblings in the sample of pedigrees, then ASP tests are not entirely appropriate in their standard form. Modifications have been proposed to correct for the inclusion of multiple sib-pairs within a single pedigree, for example, but these tend to be heuristics without a rigorous theoretical justification (Sham, 1998). It is perhaps better in these circumstances to consider generalized analyses based on allele sharing within members of pedigrees, rather than siblings only. The affected pedigree member (APM) method of Weeks and Lange (1988, 1992) analyses all pairs of individuals in a pedigree based on IBS information, rather than IBD. It was used successfully by Caulfield et al. (1994) to support the finding of linkage of *AGT* to hypertension (originally found by ASP methods) as discussed above. However, APM depends on an arbitrary weighting function expressed in terms of the allele frequencies at the locus under examination, and is therefore sensitive to misspecification of these frequencies (Weeks and Lathrop, 1995).

It is thought that IBD-based methods will generally have better power than those using IBS only, and a number of authors have developed techniques for analyzing relative pairs using IBD information, either directly (such as Curtis and Sham, 1994) or by modifying APM (Davies et al., 1996). It may also be desirable to examine patterns of IBD sharing within pedigrees of more varied numbers of generations, types of relatives and numbers of affected individuals. This situation was considered by Kruglyak et al. (1996), who developed methods for carrying out multipoint analyses within general pedigrees of moderate size, and implemented them in the GENEHUNTER software package. Kong and Cox (1997) demonstrated that the main test for linkage within GENEHUNTER was conservative, and proposed a more acceptable alternative, now included in an updated version of the package called GENEHUNTER-PLUS.

The discussion of ASP methods thus far has considered qualitative traits only (e.g., hypertensive/normotensive). However, it is also possible to develop statistical techniques for allele sharing designs for quantitative traits. The most commonly used method is that due to Haseman and Elston (1972), which models the square of the difference in blood pressures, say, between siblings as a linear function of the number of alleles shared IBD. As with the discussion above, if it is necessary or desirable to look at relative pairs or groups other than ASPs, corresponding generalizations have been proposed for the quantitative trait case (e.g., Amos and Elston, 1989; Olson and Wijsman, 1993). The MAPMAKER/SIBS and GENEHUNTER software packages referred to above also have facilities for analyzing quantitative traits (Kruglyak and Lander, 1995; Kruglyak et al., 1996).

Use of a quantitative trait also offers the possibility of increasing power by employing different sampling schemes.

Cardon and Fulker (1994) suggested that a more powerful test could be achieved by ascertaining sib pairs through a single proband with an extreme trait value, while Risch and Zhang (1995, 1996) proposed the use of extremely discordant sib pairs; for example, one sib from the top 5% of the population distribution of systolic blood pressure, the other from the lowest 10%. In both cases, the designs offer the possibility of having to genotype many fewer individuals as part of a genome wide scan than with ASPs, with considerable savings in financial and logistical resources. However, large numbers of individuals would still have to be screened in order to find pairs with the necessary characteristics.

Jeunemaitre et al. (1992) carried out an ASP study on 2 sibships collected in France and the USA to investigate the *AGT* gene's role in essential hypertension. The ascertainment criteria for probands were onset before age 60, a DBP of at least 95 mm Hg and an absence of secondary hypertension. A total of 379 sib pairs were obtained from 132 sibships of 2 or more affected siblings collected in the USA and 83 sibships from France. Using a mean test approach, there was no evidence of linkage between *AGT* and hypertension in the US sample ($p = 0.11$), but there was significant linkage in the French sibship ($p < 0.05$), and also when the two samples were pooled ($p = 0.02$). When the analysis was restricted to siblings with more severe hypertension (those receiving 2 or more antihypertensive agents or with a DBP of at least 100 mm Hg), stronger evidence for linkage with *AGT* was found in both samples individually (USA $p < 0.01$, France $p < 0.02$) and overall ($p < 0.001$).

The discordant sib pair approach proposed by Risch and Zhang (1995) was recently adopted by Krushkal et al. (1999), who undertook a genome-wide scan for loci influencing extreme systolic blood pressure. By careful examination of a US population, 69 discordant sib pairs with one member in the age and sex-specific 80th percentile of SBP and the other in the corresponding 20th percentile were identified within 55 pedigrees. All available pedigree members were genotyped for 359 microsatellite markers on the autosomes. Four regions of possible linkage were identified on chromosomes 2, 5, 6 and 15: 2p22.1-21, 5q33.3-34, 6q23.1-24.1 and 15q25.1-26.1. These areas contain a number of candidate genes that are involved in systems controlling vascular smooth muscle tone, natriuresis and the renin-angiotensin system.

Whether qualitative or quantitative traits are of interest, at the design stage of a study it will be necessary to consider in detail the likely availability and extent of pedigrees. In late onset disorders, for example, pedigrees are often very flat, because the parents of probands are unlikely to be available.

Thus, a collection of either two affected or extremely discordant sibs may be more suitable in this situation. The latter option might be preferred if the prevalence of the condition is very low, and it is therefore less likely that two affected individuals could be found in the same family. If, however, pedigrees are likely to have greater depth, a collection of individuals of more general types (parents, unaffected siblings) may repay the extra sampling effort required, as the genetic information gathered can be used to infer phase and IBD status, even if the planned analysis is to be made solely on ASPs (Farrall, 1997).

Another important design criterion is the power to detect linkage between a marker and the hypothesized susceptibility locus. This will depend on factors including the distance from marker to susceptibility locus, marker heterozygosity, sample size, and the size of effect due to the locus. This latter term is conventionally represented in the power calculation by λ_s, the relative risk of the disease for the sibling of a proband compared to an individual in the population (Risch, 1990a). This sibling relative risk can be estimated from epidemiological data, and represents the total familial influence on the complex trait. It is usual to assume that this is entirely a genetic effect, and that this total risk can be divided into a set of risks corresponding to all of the susceptibility loci affecting the disease using, for example, a multiplicative model

$$\lambda_s = \lambda_1 \lambda_2 \ldots \lambda_N$$

where λ_i is a relative risk for the i th susceptibility locus. The power or sample size can then be estimated from results in Risch (1990a). The calculation is usually simplified by assuming that each λ_i is equal, that the marker is completely polymorphic and that the recombination fraction between marker and susceptibility locus is zero. As these assumptions will rarely be true in practice, it is hoped that the power lost by departures from these conditions will be offset by use of a multipoint analysis. For discussion of this issue, see Risch (1990a), Kruglyak and Lander (1995) and Weeks and Lathrop (1995).

STUDIES OF ALLELIC ASSOCIATION/ LINKAGE DISEQUILIBRIUM

An alternative strategy for detecting loci implicated in the development of complex traits is to attempt to map them by an *association* or *linkage disequilibrium* study. The rationale for this type of design is based on the assumption that a mutation in a founder of the population of interest is still causative for the disease (Kruglyak, 1997b). We assume that in a small region close to the mutation, alleles present in the founder haplotype will have been maintained in the same haplotype at meiosis and passed down through succeeding generations, relatively unaffected by recombination, so that in the present day there will be an association at the population level of those alleles and disease state. Thus, there will be what is usually described as allelic association (also called linkage disequilibrium) between alleles for markers near a causative locus and the alleles at that locus. An association study attempts to detect this allelic association using a set of markers distributed around the susceptibility locus, and thus localize the gene contributing to the disease.

Clearly, this is a rather different assumption to that made by linkage analysis, whether carried out by assuming Mendelian inheritance models or by using the ASP approach. In that case, associations between specific alleles only hold within families, because of a lack of recombination between marker and causative locus, and there is no assumption that the same allele is related to disease over the entire population. However, the underlying principle used for mapping is similar for the two strategies, in that affected individuals should possess similar alleles near a susceptibility gene: the difference lies in the degree of relatedness of the individuals involved (Kruglyak, 1997b).

It is thought that the size of the regions over which allelic association may hold in practice will be small: probably less than 2 cM (Chapman and Wijsman, 1998). Therefore, association studies tend to be regarded as *fine mapping* studies, in which susceptibility loci will be localized to small genomic regions. This has normally been regarded as a second-stage or refinement procedure that is carried out after using linkage analysis to identify a broader putative susceptibility region in an initial study. However, there is increasing interest in the possibility of carrying out genome-wide association studies without first localizing such a region, using very dense maps of biallelic SNPs (Kruglyak, 1997a; Risch and Merikangas, 1996). As discussed above, the main limiting factor on the feasibility of such a study would be the ability to characterize sufficient SNP markers across the genome. Halushka et al. (1999) and Cargill et al. (1999) examined sequence variation in many different candidate genes for cardiovascular disorders and detected large numbers of possible SNPs in both coding and non-coding regions. A similar study by Cambien et al. (1999) examined the patterns of allelic association between proposed SNPs, and detected a number of instances of strong linkage disequilibrium, including some haplotypes in almost complete disequilibrium. These studies offer support to the concept of genome-wide association studies, but validation in practice is still required. Uncertainty over the likely scale of linkage disequilibrium in

possibly heterogeneous general populations means that it may be that this method will be most successful in studies within genetically isolated populations (Jorde, 1995; Chapman and Wijsman, 1998; Wright et al., 1999).

Within the general framework of association studies there are a number of specific experimental designs that can be used. If it is of interest to estimate linkage disequilibrium between two loci with relatively common alleles, then it is possible to use the EH computer program (Terwilliger and Ott, 1994) to do so, providing that random mating can be assumed (so that the markers are in Hardy-Weinberg equilibrium). In a more commonly used design, a set of unrelated cases will be compared to a set of controls drawn from the same population. Standard statistical methods of analysis for case-control studies, such as calculation of odds ratios or χ^2 tests, can be used, but when the markers used become highly polymorphic, the associated contingency tables become very sparse and the χ^2 approximations are likely to break down. An analysis contrasting each allele individually against all of the others at the relevant marker would be one possible solution, but this would introduce a multiple comparisons problem requiring a correction to each significance level or a simulation-based test (Sham and Curtis, 1995). Likelihood methods, such as that of Terwilliger (1995), may then offer more reliable analyses. It is also common for there to be a degree of heterogeneity in the results from several case-control studies of the same disorder. The meta analysis of association between the *AGT 235T* variant and hypertension (Kuntz et al., 1997) discussed earlier exemplifies this problem.

Linkage disequilibrium need not only result from the preservation of founder haplotypes near a susceptibility locus, however. Other possible mechanisms include random genetic drift (random changes in allele frequencies between generations due to sampling variability), founder effects (rapid growth of genetically isolated populations leading to large regions of allelic association), new mutations, selection (particular alleles enhancing or decreasing reproductive fitness) and population admixture (population subgroups with different patterns of allele frequencies combined into a single study population). The last of these factors is of most concern for case-control studies, as the differences in allele frequencies in the subgroups may induce an apparent allelic association in the admixed population. Thus, the comparability of the control group to the cases is critical to the interpretation of the study.

One way of avoiding the problem of population admixture is to use family-based controls, and in particular parents or siblings. The haplotype relative risk (HRR) method of Falk and Rubinstein (1987) uses a set of simplex families (two parents plus one affected offspring). Each family provides two alleles transmitted from the parents to the child (regarded as the case genotype), and two alleles that were not transmitted (the control genotype). The analysis then employs standard techniques for case-control studies (the HRR is strictly an odds ratio, and estimates a relative risk). In this way, the controls have exactly the same ethnic and genetic background as the cases, so that worries over admixture problems should be removed. Based on the same principles as HRR, the Transmission/Disequilibrium Test (TDT) of Spielman et al. (1993) uses the fact that the transmitted and non-transmitted alleles from a given parent are paired observations, so that in the case of a biallelic locus it examines preferential transmission of one (identifiable) allele over the other in all heterozygous parents by McNemar's Test. The procedure is demonstrated for the trivial case of one simplex family in Figure 12.3 and Table 12.2. The TDT is thought to be a test of both linkage and allelic association simultaneously, although there has been considerable discussion in the literature regarding the conditions under which this holds (reviewed in Elston, 1998b and Schaid, 1998). However, in essence, allelic association will only affect the distribution of parents' marker genotypes in relation to population frequencies, and therefore the frequency of transmission of alleles to offspring can only be affected if the marker is close to (in linkage with) a susceptibility locus.

The TDT has been applied successfully in areas related to diabetes. For example, the original proposal of the design in Spielman et al. (1993) demonstrated linkage between the "class 1" allele adjacent to the insulin gene on chromosome 11q and insulin-dependent diabetes mellitus, although conventional ASP methods had been unable to detect this. Since then, a number of studies have identified genomic regions of interest for diabetes with the same methodology. In the field of hypertension, there have been few applications of the TDT as yet. Niu et al. (1999) did use this approach, however, to study the *AGT* M235T and T174M polymorphisms in 335 hypertensive/parent trios from a Chinese rural population. They found no linkage with hypertension in the sample as a whole or in age, sex or disease severity strata.

Many generalizations of the TDT have been proposed to cover situations involving multiallelic markers (e.g., Schaid, 1996; Lazzeroni and Lange, 1998), in preference to repeated TDT analyses of individual alleles compared to the remainder. Adaptations to deal with quantitative traits, rather than the dichotomy of disease status, have also been proposed (e.g., Allison, 1997). A third area considered is that of using unaffected siblings rather than parents to provide control information. The TDT analysis can be seriously biased if one parent is missing (Curtis and Sham, 1995), and is clearly impossible if both parents are unavailable, as would typically be the case with a late-onset disease. Spielman and Ewens (1998) considered an adapted procedure, called S-TDT, that compares marker allele frequencies between affected individuals and one or more unaffected siblings (providing they have different genotypes). Furthermore, when a sample contains a mixture of simplex families and sibships without parents, a combined TDT/S-TDT analysis can be attempted (Spielman and Ewens, 1998). Similar tests were proposed by Boehnke and Langefeld (1998) and Horvath and Laird (1998). Indeed, the idea of combining information from a variety of sources within families is appealing and undoubtedly one that will see further development in the future, perhaps along the lines of the general score statistic for detecting associations with mixtures of simplex families or sibships proposed by Schaid and Rowland (1998).

A type of quantitative TDT based around discordant sib pairs (thus combining several of the ideas described above) was used by Krushkal et al. (1998) to examine the long arm of chromosome 5 (5q31.1-qter) for regions of linkage to SBP. The sample used was that of a complementary

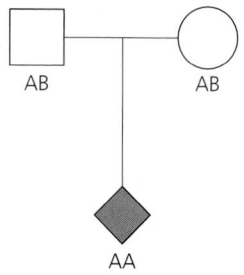

Fig. 12.3. Example of the transmission/disequilibrium test (TDT) for a single simplex family of two heterozygous parents and one affected child typed at a single biallelic marker. The A allele is transmitted twice, once by each parent, and AA (the child's genotype) forms the "case". The B allele is never transmitted, and so the "control" is BB. The data from the family are analyzed in Table 12.2.

Table 12.2. TDT Analysis of Single Family in Fig. 12.3

		Allele Not Transmitted	
		A	B
Allele Transmitted	A	0	2
	B	0	0

The counts in the two discordant cells (A transmitted & B not transmitted or B transmitted & A not transmitted) are analyzed by McNemar's Test. The test statistic = $(2-0)^2/(2+0) = 2$, and is compared to a χ^2 distribution with 1 df.

discordant sib pair analysis described in the previous section of this chapter and Krushkal et al. (1999), drawn from a US population with siblings in the top and bottom 20% of SBP distribution. The proposed test statistic contrasted differences in SBP between subjects receiving different parental alleles in the upper tail with the corresponding differences of their siblings from the lower tail. Three markers of 8 tested near the α_{1B} adrenergic receptor and dopamine receptor type 1A genes exhibited moderately significant linkage to SBP ($0.01 < p < 0.05$) by this TDT approach, the same region having been implicated by the previous linkage analysis.

The power of the TDT and related methods has been examined by theoretical and simulation techniques (e.g., Kaplan et al., 1997; Knapp, 1999). Power can be reduced if there are few parents heterozygous at markers in linkage with the susceptibility locus within an otherwise acceptably sized sample. Similarly, if the amount of allelic association between disease and marker alleles is small even if the loci are tightly linked, any variant of family-control association analysis will have low power. It is also clear that using sibs rather than parents as controls will give, in general, a less powerful test (Spielman and Ewens, 1998), in a situation where a choice of control relatives is available. On a more global scale, Risch and Merikangas (1996) estimated that a genome-wide association study based on a dense SNP map should have considerably greater power to localize disease susceptibility loci than a similar study directed towards linkage detection with a sample of affected sib pairs. As Schaid, (1998) comments, map density and strength of linkage disequilibrium will be key parameters in determining the success of such a study, but this and other related approaches should provide useful insights into the etiology of complex traits.

OTHER METHODS

In the discussion within this chapter so far, two of the main methodological families for dissecting the genetic factors influencing complex traits have been considered. However, there are other approaches that can be adopted. For example, a number of researchers advocate the use of standard "model-based" linkage analysis for multifactorial disorders, by fitting a range of different possible inheritance models at any given locus (see, for example, Greenberg et al., 1997). The asymptotic probability of a false positive will not be increased by using an "incorrect" model in this way, providing that the parameters of either the disease or the marker models are known. This allows explicit control over and testing of models and parameters in the analysis,

but there are still strong assumptions being made, and the behaviour of false positive probabilities in the finite sample case requires further investigation.

To try to overcome this type of limitation, complex segregation analysis has been proposed as a method of estimating the parameters of the genetic model before carrying out linkage analysis (Morton and MacLean, 1974; Lalouel et al., 1983; Bonney, 1984). The segregation models can incorporate both major gene and polygenic and/or residual familial factors and can include gene-gene interactions. Ascertainment corrections are normally necessary to adjust the model for the influence of the sampling strategy, which usually involves selection based on the phenotype or disease status of some family members. Alternatively, the segregation and linkage analyses can be combined into a joint procedure (Bonney et al., 1988). Application of this simultaneous modelling approach to families from Jamaica suggested that a number of genetic factors other than the *ACE* gene might also contribute to the regulation of serum ACE concentrations, a possible intermediate phenotype for essential hypertension (McKenzie et al., 1995).

When a quantitative trait is the phenotype of interest, an alternative approach to analysis is available via the "variance components" approach (Amos, 1994; Blangero and Almasy, 1997). The variance of the phenotype is modelled as a sum of terms representing the effects of quantitative trait loci, the effects of many genes of small effect (*polygenes*) and random environmental variability. It is also possible to include a variety of gene-gene and gene-environment interactions, along with covariates or age of onset effects. The method is available in multipoint versions and can be applied to general pedigrees. It has been implemented in a software package called SOLAR (Almasy and Blangero, 1998), although simpler analyses can be undertaken within some standard statistical packages. Although, multivariate normality is assumed within each pedigree, simulation results suggest that the method is robust to many types of departure from this distributional form (Allison et al., 1999). Further simulation studies suggest that the variance components approach has greater power than affected sib pair designs for quantitative traits (Williams and Blangero, 1999).

Technical issues

SIGNIFICANCE

Classification of linkage results as significant is not, in itself, an entirely straightforward matter. In the case of parametric linkage analysis for a monogenic disorder, a lod score of 3 is often judged to be significant. This corresponds to a p-value of approximately $p = 0.0001$ in a one-sided test with one degree of freedom. The theoretical argument for such a stringent criteria of linkage is the low prior probability of linkage between two genes (discussed in Ott, 1991, pp. 65–76). Based on a sequential significance testing argument outlined in Morton (1955), the rate of false-positive linkage (i.e., the frequency with which the lod score exceeds 3 by chance over the genome) associated with this critical value has been shown to be close to 5%.

There has been considerable recent debate over the methodology appropriate to the situation of a genome-wide scan for a multifactorial disorder, much of it prompted by the contribution of Lander and Kruglyak (1995). These authors proposed the use of more stringent criteria to achieve a whole experiment significance level of 5% assuming that a genome-wide screen with a dense map of completely informative markers was underway, that there was no interference between recombination events, and that a single phenotype was being evaluated. Using extreme value theory, an expression for the required individual locus p-value was obtained in terms of the number of chromosomes in the organism, the total length of the genome and the total rate of recombination. For an affected sib pair study, this gave a pointwise significance level of 0.00002, equivalent to a Lod score of 3.6.

The assumptions underlying the calculations of Lander and Kruglyak (1995) have a noticeable effect on the final critical value obtained, which has been shown both on theoretical grounds (Morton, 1998) and by simulation studies (Rogus et al., 1999, Zhao et al., 1999). For example, markers with a heterozygosity of less than 100% lead to a greater false-positive rate than that predicted with the assumed, fully informative markers. By contrast, a nondense map will decrease the false-positive rate. Thus, the formulation of Lander and Kruglyak (1995) is conservative; this was also demonstrated in the simulations of Rogus et al. (1999) and Zhao et al. (1999), although the effect can be small in many cases. An additional complication is that it will often be necessary to examine different models and methods of analysis, which will complicate the issue of assigning critical values even further (Curtis, 1996). As Witte et al. (1996) comment, there is a tendency for thresholds to be interpreted too literally, and it seems that a more sophisticated interpretation of Lod scores is needed. The "traditional" value of 3 for declaring significance may well be suitable for a number of situations and underlying mechanisms (Morton, 1998), but as the assumed mechanisms become more complex it is likely that the critical value will have to increase. Thus, it would seem to be necessary to move away from reliance on a single threshold significance level, and to develop further methods of assessing significance that allow more explicitly for the influences of study design, assumed (or implicit) inheritance models and extent of multiple testing. The Lod score or p-value would then be interpreted more explicitly as a measure of the evidence accumulated in favour of trait/locus linkage, conditional on the previously mentioned factors.

An alternative approach to the issue of critical values and power is to set significance levels to control the relative number of true and false positive linkages that may be observed in a given study. The key measure for this purpose would be the *reliability* – the proportion of true positives amongst the total number of linkages detected (Morton, 1998). For example, if five regions of potential linkage are detected, four true positive and one false positive results might be considered acceptable, since most follow-up work would then be devoted to regions that contained susceptibility loci. On the other hand, four regions of false positive linkage compared to only one of true linkage would probably be unacceptable. Weller et al. (1998) demonstrate the utility of this approach in searching for quantitative trait loci.

REPLICATION

Ultimately, the principal criterion by which linkage results are judged (prior to gene identification) is replication. However, a number of factors may cause difficulties in achieving this. It may be possible (indeed, quite likely) that there will be subtle ascertainment differences between populations studied for multifactorial disorders. Furthermore, there may be genetic heterogeneity between these populations. Even if there is no such heterogeneity, it is unlikely that any single study would have sufficient power to detect all of the susceptibility loci involved in a complex trait, thus we might expect to detect different subsets of the loci in different replicates. We would also expect sampling variability to affect the location estimates of the contributing loci, raising the possibility of a replicate study indicating the presence of an independent second factor on the same chromosome as the first, when in fact there is only one such locus. Roberts et al. (1999) present simulation results that indicate that such large effects seem to be feasible, and also derive a variety of procedures for estimating standard errors for locus positions to quantify these effects. It is clear that more consideration will have to be given to such issues in the future.

Conclusions

We have reviewed a number of the main types of experimental design and statistical method, and indicated some of the key concepts, involved in the genetic analysis of complex traits. We can make no claim to having covered all of the possible techniques, nor to have given a full account of the principles underpinning each of the ideas that has been discussed. However, we hope that the material will provide a useful introduction to this rapidly expanding area and that it may also point out some of the inherent problems.

In practice, it is very unlikely that there will be an obvious, optimal method for a given disease of interest. Real life applications will require the synthesis of information from any and all available sources to discern clues to the extent of genetic involvement in the condition's etiology, the likely number of loci, possible models for the mechanism of inheritance, evidence of locus heterogeneity and possible interactions. The likely extent of linkage disequilibrium will give some indication of the feasibility of an association-based approach, while epidemiological data on the condition will be required to assess the availability of pedigree members for collection, so that the merit of ASP or general pedigree-based approaches can be considered.

Once design issues are resolved, the choice of analysis method can then be considered, and hopefully tailored to give acceptable power for the chosen design.

In the near future, technological developments may change the character of complex trait studies quite dramatically. The Human Genome Mapping Project is nearing completion, which will offer an unparalleled resource for mapping qualitative and quantitative trait loci for multifactorial disorders. Equally, methods such as cDNA microarray analysis of gene expression (Duggan et al., 1999), used successfully in recent experimental studies (Aitman et al., 1999), may offer an alternative strategy to those considered in this chapter. We await developments with interest.

Acknowledgements

The British Heart Foundation (BHF) Blood Pressure Group is supported by Programme and Project Grants from the BHF (RG/97009 and PG/96175), as well as by an MRC Cooperative Group Grant (G9800025) and a Project Grant from the Wellcome Trust (057306/99). Thanks to Nicholas Brain for assistance with production of the figures for this chapter, and to Dr Cervantes D. Negrin for his assistance with Table 12.1.

REFERENCES

Aitman TJ, Glazier AM, Wallace CA et al. (1999) Identification of *Cd36* (*Fat*) as an insulin-resistance gene causing defective fatty acid and glucose metabolism in hypertensive rats. Nat Genet 21:76–83

Allison DB (1997) Transmission-disequilibrium tests for quantitative traits. Am J Hum Genet 60:676–690

Allison DB, Neale MC, Zannolli R et al. (1999) Testing the robustness of the likelihood-ratio test in a variance-component quantitative-trait loci-mapping procedure. Am J Hum Genet 65:531–544

Almasy L, Blangero J (1998) Multipoint quantitative-trait linkage analysis in general pedigrees. Am J Hum Genet 62:1198–1211

Amos CI (1994) Robust variance-component approach for assessing genetic linkage in pedigrees. Am J Hum Genet 54:535–543

Amos CI, Elston RC (1989) Robust methods for the detection of genetic linkage for quantitative data from pedigrees. Genet Epidem 6:349–360

Baima J, Nicolaou M, Schwartz F et al. (1999) Evidence for linkage between essential hypertension and a putative locus on human chromosome 17. Hypertension 34:4–7

Baker EH, Dong YB, Sagnella GA et al. (1998) Association of hypertension with T594M mutation in β-subunit of epithelial sodium channels in black people resident in London. Lancet 351:1388–1392

Blangero J, Almasy L (1997) Multipoint oligogenic linkage analysis of quantitative traits. Genet Epidem 14:959–964

Boehnke M, Langefeld CD (1998) Genetic association mapping based on discordant sib pairs: the discordant-alleles test. Am J Hum Genet 62:950–961

Bonney GE (1984) On the statistical determination of major gene mechanisms in continuous human traits: regressive models. Am J Med Genet 18:731–749

Bonney GE, Lathrop GM, Lalouel JM (1988) Combined linkage and segregation analysis using regressive models. Am J Hum Genet 43:29–37

Brand E, Chatelain N, Keavney B et al. (1998) Evaluation of the angiotensinogen locus in human essential hypertension: A European study. Hypertension 31:725–729

Brown DM, Provoost AP, Daly MJ et al. (1996) Renal disease susceptibility and hypertension are under independent genetic control in the fawn-hooded rat. Nat Genet 12:44–51

Buetow KH, Edmonson MN, Cassidy AB (1999) Reliable identification of large numbers of candidate SNPs from public EST data. Nat Genet 21:323–325

Cambien F, Poirier O, Nicaud V et al. (1999) Sequence diversity in 36 candidate genes for cardiovascular disorders. Am J Hum Genet 65:183–191

Cardon LR, Fulker DW (1994) The power of interval mapping of quantitative trait loci, using selected sib pairs. Am J Hum Genet 55:825–833

Cargill M, Altshuler D, Ireland J et al. (1999) Characterization of single-nucleotide polymorphisms in coding regions of human genes. Nat Genet 22:231–238

Caulfield M, Lavender P, Farrall M et al. (1994) Linkage of the angiotensinogen gene to essential hypertension. N Eng J Med 330:1629–1633

Chapman NH, Wijsman EM (1998) Genome screens using linkage disequilibrium tests: Optimal marker characteristics and feasibility. Am J Hum Genet 63:1872–1885

Clark JS, Jeffs B, Davidson AO et al. (1996) Quantitative trait loci in genetically hypertensive rats: Possible sex specificity. Hypertension 28:898–906

Curtis D (1996) Genetic dissection of complex traits. Nature Genet 12:356–357

Curtis D, Sham PC (1994) Using risk calculation to implement an extended relative pairs analysis. Ann Hum Genet 58:151–162

Curtis D, Sham PC (1995) A note on the application of the transmission disequilibrium test when a parent is missing. Am J Hum Genet 56:811–812

Davidson AO, Schork N, Jaques BC et al. (1995) Blood-pressure in genetically hypertensive rats – influence of the Y-chromosome. Hypertension 26:452–459

Davies S, Schroeder M, Goldin LR, Weeks DE (1996) Nonparametric simulation-based statistics for detecting linkage in general pedigrees. Am J Hum Genet 58:867–880

Deng AY, Rapp JP (1995) Locus for the inducible, but not constitutive, nitric oxide synthase cosegregates with blood pressure in the Dahl salt-sensitive rat. J Clin Invest 95:2170–2177

Deng AY, Dene H, Pravenec M, Rapp JP (1994a) Genetic-mapping of 2 new blood-pressure quantitative trait loci in the rat by genotyping endothelin system genes. J Clin Invest 93:2701–2709

Deng AY, Dene H, Rapp JP (1994b) Mapping of a quantitative trait locus for blood pressure on rat chromosome 2. J Clin Invest 94:431–436

Dib C, Faure S, Fizames C et al. (1996) A comprehensive genetic map of the human genome based on 5,264 microsatellites. Nature 380:152–154

Dominiczak AF, Jeffs B, Connell JMC (1998) New genetic concepts in hypertensive cardiovascular disease. Current Opinion in Cardiology 13:304–311

Dominiczak AF, Negrin CD, Clark JS et al. (2000) Genes and hypertension: from gene mapping in experimental models to vascular gene transfer strategies. Hypertension 35:164–172

Dubay C, Vincent M, Samani NJ et al. (1993) Genetic determinants of diastolic and pulse pressure map to different loci in Lyon hypertensive rats. Nat Genet 3:354–358

Duggan DJ, Bittner M, Chen Y et al. (1999) Expression profiling using cDNA microarrays. Nat Genet 21 (supplement):10–14

Elston RC (1998a) Methods of linkage analysis – and the assumptions underlying them. Am J Hum Genet 63:931–934

Elston RC (1998b) Linkage and association. Genet Epidem 15:565–576

Ely DL, Daneshvar H, Turner ME et al. (1993) The hypertensive Y-chromosome elevates blood-pressure in F2 normotensive rats. Hypertension 21:1071–1075

Falk CT, Rubinstein P (1987) Haplotype relative risks: an easy reliable way to construct a proper control sample for risk calculations. Ann Hum Genet 51:227–233

Farrall M (1997) LOD wars: the affected-sib-pair paradigm strikes back! Am J Hum Genet 60:735–737

Garrett MR, Dene H, Walder R et al. (1998) Genome scan and congenic strains for blood pressure QTL using Dahl salt-sensitive rats. Genome Research 8:711–723

Gavras I, Manolis A, Gavras H (1999) Genetic epidemiology of essential hypertension. J Hum Hypertension 13:225–229

Greenberg DA, Hodge SE, Vieland VJ, Spence MA (1997) Affecteds-only linkage methods are not a panacea. Am J Hum Genet 58:892–895

Gu L, Dene H, Deng AY et al. (1996) Genetic mapping of two blood pressure quantitative trait loci on rat chromosome 1. J Clin Invest 97:777–788

Halushka MK, Fan JB, Bentley K et al. (1999) Patterns of single-nucleotide polymorphisms in candidate genes for blood-pressure homeostasis. Nat Genet 22:239–247

Hamet P, Kong D, Pravenec M et al. (1992) Restriction-Fragment-Length-Polymorphism of *Hsp70*-gene, localized in the RT1-complex, is associated with hypertension in spontaneously hypertensive rats. Hypertension 19:611–614

Harris EL, Phelan EL, Thompson CM et al. (1995) Heart mass and blood pressure have separate genetic determinants in the New Zealand genetically hypertensive (GH) rats. J Hypertension 134:397–404

Haseman JK, Elston RC (1972) The investigation of linkage between a quantitative trait and a marker locus. Behavior Genet 2:3–19

HGBASE (2000) Human Genic Bi-Allelic Sequences database by Uppsala University and Interactiva Biotechnologie GmbH. Release 6. http://hgbase.interactiva.de/

Hilbert P, Lindpaintner K, Beckmann JS et al. (1991) Chromosomal mapping of the genetic loci associated with blood pressure regulation in hereditary hypertensive rats. Nature 353:521–529

Holmans P (1993) Asymptotic properties of affected-sib-pair linkage analysis. Am J Hum Genet 52:362–374

Horvath S, Laird NM (1998) A discordant-sibship test for disequilibrium and linkage: No need for parental data. Am J Hum Genet 63:1886–1897

Innes BA, McLaughlin MC, Kapuscinski MK et al. (1998) Independent genetic susceptibility to cardiac hypertrophy in inherited hypertension. Hypertension 31:741–746

Inoue I, Nakajima T, Williams CS et al. (1997) A nucleotide substitution in the promoter of human angiotensinogen is associated with essential hypertension and affects basal transcription. J Clin Invest 99:1786–1797

Jacob HJ, Lindpaintner K, Lincoln SE et al. (1991) Genetic mapping of a gene causing hypertension in stroke-prone spontaneously hypertensive rat. Cell 67:213–224

Jeffs B, Negrin CD, Graham D et al. (2000) Applicability of a "speed" congenic strategy to dissect blood pressure quantitative trait loci on rat chromosome 2. Hypertension 35:179–187

Jeunemaitre X, Soubrier F, Kotelevtsev YV et al. (1992) Molecular basis of human hypertension: Role of angiotensinogen. Cell 71:169–180

Jorde LB (1995) Linkage disequilibrium as a gene-mapping tool. Am J Hum Genet 56:11–14

Julier C, Delepine M, Keavney B et al. (1997) Genetic susceptibility for human familial essential hypertension in a region of homology with blood pressure linkage on rat chromosome 10. Hum Molec Genet 6:2077–2085

Kaplan NL, Martin ER, Weir BS (1997) Power studies for the transmission/disequilibrium tests with multiple alleles. Am J Hum Genet 60:691–702

Katsuya T, Higaki J, Zhao Y et al. (1993) A neuropeptide-Y locus on chromosome-4 cosegregates with blood-pressure in the spontaneously hypertensive rat. Biochemical and Biophysical Research Communications 192:261–267

Knapp M (1999) A note on power approximations for the transmission/disequilibrium test. Am J Hum Genet 64:1177–1185

Knapp M, Seuchter SA, Baur MP (1995) Linkage analysis in nuclear families, I: Optimality criteria for affected sib-pair tests. Hum Heredity 44:37–43

Kong A, Cox NJ (1997) Allele-sharing models: LOD scores and accurate linkage tests. Am J Hum Genet 61:1179–1188

Kruglyak L (1997a) The use of a genetic map of biallelic markers in linkage studies. Nature Genet 17:21–24

Kruglyak L (1997b) What is significant in whole-genome linkage disequilibrium studies? Am J Hum Genet 61:810–812

Kruglyak L, Lander E (1995) Complete multipoint sib pair analysis of qualitative and quantitative traits. Am J Hum Genet 57:439–454

Kruglyak L, Daly MJ, Reeve-Daly MP, Lander ES (1996) Parametric and nonparametric linkage analysis: A unified multipoint approach. Am J Hum Genet 58:1347–1363

Krushkal J, Xiong M, Ferrell R et al. (1998) Linkage and association of adrenergic and dopamine receptor genes in the distal portion of the long arm of chromosome 5 with systolic blood pressure variation. Hum Molec Genet 7:1379–1383

Krushkal J, Ferrell R, Mockrin SC et al. (1999) Genome-wide linkage analyses of systolic blood pressure using highly discordant siblings. Circulation 99:1407–1410

Kuntz R, Kreutz R, Beige J et al. (1997) A meta-analysis of 11 case-control association studies of the AGT 235T-variant with essential hypertension. Hypertension 30:1331–1337

Lalouel JM, Rao DC, Morton NE, Elston RC (1983) A unified model for complex segregation analysis. Am J Hum Genet 35:816–826

Lander E, Green P, Abrahamson J et al. (1987) MAPMAKER: An interactive computer package for constructing primary genetic linkage maps of experimental and natural populations. Genom 1:174–181

Lander ES, Kruglyak L (1995) Genetic dissection of complex traits: Guidelines for interpreting and reporting linkage results. Nature Genet 11:241–247

Lander ES, Schork NJ (1994) Genetic dissection of complex traits. Sci 265:2037–2048

Lazzeroni LC, Lange K (1998) A conditional inference framework for extending the transmission/disequilibrium test. Hum Hered 48:67–81

Lifton RP (1995) Genetic determinants of human hypertension. Proc Nat Ac Sci USA 92:8545–8551

Lifton RP (1996) Molecular genetics of human blood pressure variation. Sci 272:676–680

Lindpaintner K, Hilbert P, Ganten D et al. (1993) Molecular-genetics of the SA-gene – cosegregation with hypertension and mapping to rat chromosome-1. J Hypertension 11:19–23

Luft FC (1998) Molecular genetics of human hypertension. J Hypertension 16:1871–1878

McKenzie CA, Julier C, Forrester T et al. (1995) Segregation and linkage analysis of serum angiotensin I converting enzyme levels: Evidence for two quantitative trait loci. Am J Hum Genet 57:1426–1435

Manly KF, Olson JM (1999) Overview of QTL mapping software and introduction to Map Manager QT. Mammalian Genome 10:327–334

Matsumoto C, Nara Y, Ikeda K et al. (1996) Cosegregation of the new region on chromosome 3 with salt-induced hypertension in female F2 progeny from stroke-prone spontaneously hypertensive and Wistar-Kyoto rats. Clin Exper Pharm Physiol 23:1028–1034

Morton NE (1955) Sequential tests for the detection of linkage. Am J Hum Genet 7:277–318

Morton NE (1998) Significance levels in complex inheritance. Am J Hum Genet 62:690–697

Morton NE, MacLean CJ (1974) Analysis of family resemblance. III. Complex segregation analysis of quantitative traits. Am J Hum Genet 26:489–503

Murray JC, Buetow KH, Weber JL et al. (1994) A comprehensive human linkage map with centimorgan density. Sci 265:2049–2054

Nara Y, Nabika T, Ikeda K et al. (1993) Basal high blood pressure cosegregates with the loci on chromosome 1 in the F2 generation from crosses between normotensive Wistar Kyoto rats and strokeprone spontaneously hypertensive rats. Biochemical and Biophysical Research Communications 194:1344–1351

Nara Y, Ikeda K, Mashimo T et al. (1996) A new candidate locus for basal high blood pressure in male and female stroke-prone SHR (SHRSP/Izm). J Hypertension 14:511

Niu T, Yang J, Wang B et al. (1999) Angiotensinogen gene polymorphisms M235T/T174M – no excess transmission to hypertensive Chinese. Hypertension 33:698–702

Olson JM, Wijsman EM (1993) Linkage between quantitative trait and marker loci: Methods using all relative pairs. Genet Epidem 10:87–102

Ott J (1991) Analysis of Human Genetic Linkage, Revised Edition. Johns Hopkins University Press, Baltimore

Paterson A, Lander E, Lincoln S et al. (1988) Resolution of quantitative traits into Mendelian factors using a complete RFLP linkage map. Nature 335:721–726

Pravenec M, Gauguier D, Schott J-J et al. (1995) Mapping of quantitative trait loci for blood pressure and cardiac mass in the rat by genome scanning of recombinant inbred strains. J Clin Invest 96:1973–1978

Rapp JP (2000) Genetic analysis of inherited hypertension in the rat. Physiological Reviews 80:135–172

Rapp JP, Deng A (1995) Detection and positional cloning of blood pressure quantitative trait loci: Is it possible? Hypertension 25:1121–1128

Rapp JP, Garrett MR, Deng AY (1998) Construction of a double congenic strain to prove an epistatic interaction on blood pressure between rat chromosomes 2 and 10. J Clin Invest 101:1591–1595

Risch N (1990a) Linkage strategies for genetically complex traits II: The power of affected relative pairs. Am J Hum Genet 46:229–241

Risch N (1990b) Linkage strategies for genetically complex traits III: The effect of marker polymorphism on analysis of affected relative pairs. Am J Hum Genet 46:242–253

Risch N, Merikangas K (1996) The future of genetic studies of complex human diseases. Sci 273:1516–1517

Risch N, Zhang H (1995) Extreme discordant sib pairs for mapping quantitative trait loci in humans. Sci 268:1584–1589

Risch N, Zhang H (1996) Mapping quantitative trait loci with extreme discordant sib pairs: Sampling considerations. Am J Hum Genet 58:836–843

Roberts SB, MacLean CJ, Neale MC et al. (1999) Replication of linkage studies of complex traits: An examination of variation in location estimates. Am J Hum Genet 65:876–884

Rogus JJ, Cai TX, Wei LJ (1999) Issues in genomic screening: Critical values, sample sizes and the ability to detect linkage. Genet Epidem 17 (SI):S697–S701

Samani NJ, Lodwick D, Vincent M et al. (1993) A gene differentially expressed in the kidney of the spontaneously hypertensive rat cosegregates with increased blood-pressure. J Clin Invest 92:1099–1103

Samani NJ, Gauguier D, Vincent M et al. (1996) Analysis of quantitative trait loci for blood pressure on rat chromosome 2 and 13. Hypertension 28:1118–1122

Schaid DJ (1996) General score tests for associations of genetic markers with disease using cases and their parents. Genet Epidem 13:423–449

Schaid DJ (1998) Transmission disequilibrium, family controls, and great expectations. Am J Hum Genet 63:935–941

Schaid DJ, Rowland C (1998) Use of parents, sibs, and unrelated controls for detection of associations between genetic markers and disease. Am J Hum Genet 63:1492–1506

Schork RJ, Krieger JE, Trolliet MR et al. (1995) A biometrical genome search in rats reveals the multigenic basis of blood pressure variation. Genome Research 5:164–172

Sham P (1998) Statistics in Human Genetics. Arnold, London

Sham PC, Curtis D (1995) An extended transmission/disequilibrium test (TDT) for multiallele marker loci. Ann Hum Genet 59:323–336

Smithies O (1997) A mouse view of hypertension. Hypertension 30:1318–1324

Smithies O, Kim HS (1994) Targeted gene duplication and disruption for analyzing quantitative genetic traits in mice. Proc Nat Ac Sci USA 91:3612–3615

Smithies O, Maeda N (1995) Gene targeting approaches to complex genetic diseases: Atherosclerosis and essential hypertension. Proc Nat Ac Sci USA 92:5266–5272

Spielman RS, McGinnis RE, Ewens WJ (1993) Transmission test for linkage disequilibrium: The insulin gene region and insulin-dependent diabetes mellitus (IDDM). Am J Hum Genet 52:506–516

Spielman RS, Ewens WJ (1998) A sibship test for linkage in the presence of association: The sib transmission/disequilibrium test. Am J Hum Genet 62:450–458

Terwilliger JD (1995) A powerful likelihood method for the analysis of linkage disequilibrium between trait loci and one or more polymorphic marker loci. Am J Hum Genet 56:777–787

Terwilliger JD, Ott J (1994) Handbook of Human Genetic Linkage. Johns Hopkins, Baltimore

Thomson G, Esposito MS (1999) The genetics of complex diseases. Trends in Genet 15:M17–M20

Weeks DE, Lange K (1988) The affected-pedigree-member method of linkage analysis. Am J Hum Genet 42:315–326

Weeks DE, Lange K (1992) A multilocus extension of the affected-pedigree-member method of linkage analysis. Am J Hum Genet 50:859–868

Weeks D, Lathrop GM (1995) Polygenic disease: methods for mapping complex disease traits. Trends in Genet 11:513–519

Weller JI, Song JZ, Heyen DW et al. (1998) A new approach to the problem of multiple comparisons in the genetic dissection of complex traits. Genet 150:1699–1706

Whittemore AS (1996) Genome scanning for linkage: An overview. Am J Hum Genet 59:704–716

Williams JT, Blangero J (1999) Comparison of variance components and sibpair-based approaches to quantitative trait linkage analysis in unselected samples. Genet Epidem 16:113–134

Witte JS, Elston RC, Schork N (1996) Genetic dissection of complex traits. Nat Genet 12:355–356

Wright AF, Carothers AD, Piratsu M (1999) Population choice in mapping genes for complex diseases. Nat Genet 23:397–404

Yagil C, Sapojnikov M, Kreutz R et al. (1998) Salt susceptibility maps to chromosome 1 and 17 with sex specificity in the Sabra rat model of hypertension. Hypertension 31:119–124

Zhang L, Summers KM, West MJ (1996) Cosegregation of genes on chromosome 5 with heart weight and blood pressure in genetic hypertension. Clin Exper Hypertension 18:1073–1087

Zhang HP, Zhao HY, Merikangas K (1997) Strategies to identify genes for complex diseases. Ann Med 29:493–498

Zhao LP, Prentice R, Shen FM, Hsu L (1999) On the assessment of statistical significance in disease-gene discovery. Am J Hum Genet 64:1739–1753

Population genetics

Bronya J.B. Keats
Stephanie L. Sherman

Introduction

With advances in the application of molecular techniques to studies of the human genome, the genetic composition of populations can be examined in detail. Different mutations in the same gene are known to cause diseases such as cystic fibrosis, Tay-Sachs, phenylketonuria, hemophilia A, and familial hypercholesterolemia. The frequencies of these disease alleles often differ among populations. Normal variation within and among populations is also a result of differences in allele frequencies. The principles of population genetics attempt to explain the genetic diversity in present populations and the changes in allele and genotype frequencies over time. Population genetic studies may provide insight into the value of carrier screening programs and the effect of medical intervention on the population frequency of a disease. Allele and genotype frequencies depend on factors such as mating patterns, population size and distribution, mutation, migration, and selection. By making specific assumptions about these factors, Hardy (1908) and Weinberg (1908) independently formulated the Hardy–Weinberg law. This fundamental principle of population genetics provides a model for calculating genotype frequencies from allele frequencies for a random mating population in equilibrium.

Hardy–Weinberg law

The allele frequencies at a locus can always be calculated from the genotype frequencies, but the converse is not necessarily true. The Hardy–Weinberg law states that for a single autosomal locus in a large population in which

(1) mating takes place at random with respect to genotype, (2) allele frequencies are the same in males and females, and (3) mutation, selection, and migration are negligible, genotype frequencies can be calculated from allele frequencies after one generation regardless of the allele and genotype frequencies in the initial population. On the other hand, for a single X-linked locus or for any set of loci considered jointly, the establishment of this relationship between allele and genotype frequencies takes more than one generation.

AUTOSOMAL LOCUS

Consider a locus with two alleles, A_1 and A_2, and suppose the population frequencies of the three genotypes, A_1A_1, A_1A_2, A_2A_2 are p_{11}, p_{12}, p_{22}, respectively, where $p_{11} + p_{12} + p_{22} = 1$. Then, in this initial population, the frequency of A_1 is $p_{11} + \frac{1}{2}p_{12}$ and the frequency of A_2 is $p_{22} + \frac{1}{2}p_{12}$. Random mating is approximately equivalent to random union of gametes. Thus, random mating within this initial population results in the following genotype frequencies in the next generation:

$$\text{Frequency of } A_1A_1 = (p_{11} + \tfrac{1}{2}p_{12})^2$$
$$\text{Frequency of } A_1A_2 = 2(p_{11} + \tfrac{1}{2}p_{12})(p_{22} + \tfrac{1}{2}p_{12})$$
$$\text{Frequency of } A_2A_2 = (p_{22} + \tfrac{1}{2}p_{12})^2$$

The genotype frequencies in this second generation may be different from those in the first generation. However, calculation of the allele frequencies from the genotype frequencies in the second generation gives

$$
\begin{aligned}
&\text{Frequency of } A_1 \\
&= (p_{11} + \tfrac{1}{2}p_{12})^2 + (p_{11} + \tfrac{1}{2}p_{12})(p_{22} + \tfrac{1}{2}p_{12}) \\
&= p_{11}(p_{11} + p_{12} + p_{22}) + \tfrac{1}{2}p_{12}(p_{11} + p_{12} + p_{22}) \\
&= p_{11} + \tfrac{1}{2}p_{12}
\end{aligned}
$$

Similarly, the frequency of A_2 is $p_{22} + \frac{1}{2}$ which is equal to $1 - (p_{11} + \frac{1}{2}p_{12})$. These allele frequencies are identical to those in the first generation. In other words, if the allele frequencies are $p = p_{11} + \frac{1}{2}p_{12}$ and $q = 1 - p = p_{22} + \frac{1}{2}p_{12}$, then after one generation of random mating, the genotype frequencies are p^2, $2pq$, and q^2. These frequencies are the Hardy–Weinberg proportions and the population is said to be in Hardy–Weinberg equilibrium.

Table 13.1 presents a numerical example, in which the initial population comprises 20, 40, and 140 individuals with genotypes A_1A_1, A_1A_2, and A_2A_2, respectively. The genotype frequencies are:

$$\text{Frequency } A_1A_1 = p_{11} = 20/200 = .10$$
$$\text{Frequency } A_1A_2 = p_{12} = 40/200 = .20$$
$$\text{Frequency } A_2A_2 = p_{22} = 140/200 = .70$$

and, therefore, the allele frequencies are:

$$\text{Frequency } A_1 = .10 + \frac{1}{2}(.20) = .2$$
$$\text{Frequency } A_2 = .70 + \frac{1}{2}(.20) = .8$$

Random union of gametes results in the following genotype frequencies in the next generation:

$$\text{Frequency } A_1A_1 = .2^2 = .04$$
$$\text{Frequency } A_1A_2 = 2(.2)(.8) = .32$$
$$\text{Frequency } A_2A_2 = .8^2 = .64$$

Note that these genotype frequencies are different from those in the initial population. To confirm that these results are correct, Table 13.1 shows the genotype frequencies in the offspring that result from each of the six possible mating types. For example, all the offspring of the mating, $A_1A_1 \times A_1A_1$, must be A_1A_1, while for the mating type, $A_1A_1 \times A_1A_2$, each of the two offspring genotypes, A_1A_1 and A_1A_2, has a probability of one-half. Summing the columns in Table 13.1 gives the frequencies of each of the genotypes in the second generation. These frequencies are the same as those obtained by random union of gametes, and the allele frequencies calculated from these genotype frequencies are:

$$\text{Frequency } A_1 = .04 + \frac{1}{2}(.32) = .2$$
$$\text{Frequency } A_2 = .64 + \frac{1}{2}(.32) = .8$$

Repeating these steps will give identical genotype and allele frequencies in the third generation to those in the second generation. Note that only the genotype frequencies change in the establishment of equilibrium; the allele frequencies in the initial population remain the same in subsequent generations.

The chi-square goodness-of-fit test may be used to determine whether the observed numbers of each genotype are significantly different from those expected under Hardy–Weinberg equilibrium. The total number of individuals is 200, so the expected numbers for the three genotypes are $(.2)^2 200 = 8$, $2(.2)(.8)200 = 64$, and $(.8)^2 200 = 128$, compared with the observed numbers of 20, 40, and 140. The test value is $[(20-8)^2/8 + (40-64)^2/64 + (140-128)^2]/128 = 28$. This value is compared to the chi-square distribution with one degree of freedom. (There are three classes, but the total number of individuals is known and the allele frequencies are known. Thus, there is only one independent class and one degree of freedom.) In general, the number of degrees of freedom is equal to the number of observed classes minus the number of alleles. The 99.9th percentile of the chi-square distribution with one degree of freedom is 10.83. Thus, the observed numbers of each genotype in the initial population are significantly different at the 1% level from those expected under Hardy–Weinberg equilibrium. However, after one generation of random mating the observed and expected numbers are the same.

Calculation of allele frequencies from genotype frequencies is straightforward when all three genotypes are observable, but, in the case of recessive diseases, such as cystic fibrosis, only two phenotype classes are observed. However, if equilibrium is assumed, the frequency of affected individuals is q^2; thus, the square root of this frequency is the frequency of the disease allele. The frequency of heterozygotes (carriers) is $2(1 - q)q$, and the proportion of carriers among unaffected individuals in the population is

$$[2(1 - q)q]/(1 - q^2) = 2q/(1 + q)$$

For example, in populations of European ancestry, the frequency of cystic fibrosis is estimated to be $1/2,000$ (Boat et al., 1989); thus, the frequency of the abnormal allele is .022 and the frequency of the normal allele is .978. The frequency of heterozygotes is therefore $2 \times .022 \times .978$, which is about $1/23$. That is, approximately 4% of the population

Table 13.1. Establishment of Equilibrium in One Generation for an Autosomal Locus

Mating	Frequency	Offspring Genotype Frequencies		
		A_1A_1	A_1A_2	A_2A_2
$A_1A_1 \times A_1A_1$	$(.1)^2$	$(.1)^2$	0	0
$A_1A_1 \times A_1A_2$	$2(.1)(.2)$	$(.1)(.2)$	$(.1)(.2)$	0
$A_1A_1 \times A_2A_2$	$2(.1)(.7)$	0	$2(.1)(.7)$	0
$A_1A_2 \times A_1A_2$	$(.2)^2$	$\frac{1}{4}(.2)^2$	$\frac{1}{2}(.2)^2$	$\frac{1}{4}(.2)^2$
$A_1A_2 \times A_2A_2$	$2(.2)(.7)$	0	$(.2)(.7)$	$(.2)(.7)$
$A_2A_2 \times A_2A_2$	$(.7)^2$	0	0	$(.7)^2$
Total	1	.04	.32	.64

are carriers, but less than .1% are affected. Several different mutations have been described in the cystic fibrosis gene. Each one of these is an abnormal allele; thus, the frequency of .022 is actually the sum of the frequencies of all the abnormal alleles at the cystic fibrosis locus.

The Hardy–Weinberg principle may be extended to more than two alleles. In general, for n alleles, A_1, A_2, ..., A_n with frequencies p_1, p_2, ..., p_n the genotype frequencies are p_i^2 for homozygotes, A_iA_i and $2p_ip_j$ for heterozygotes, A_iA_j. The heterozygosity value (H) for a locus is the total frequency of heterozygotes, and it may be written as

$$H = \Sigma 2p_ip_j = 1 - \Sigma p_i^2.$$

For two alleles, the maximum heterozygosity is .5, for 5 alleles it is .8, and for 10 alleles it is .9. In other words, for a locus to have a heterozygosity of 80%, it must have at least 5 alleles. (The maximum heterozygosity is reached when the alleles have equal frequencies.)

Example:

Suppose a locus has 5 alleles (designated 1, 2, 3, 4, 5) with frequencies .5, .3, .1, .08, .02. What are the genotype frequencies when Hardy–Weinberg equilibrium is established? What is the heterozygosity value (H) at this locus?

With n alleles, there are n(n+1)/2 genotypes. Thus, for 5 alleles there are 15 genotypes. The frequencies of the five homozygotes, 1-1, 2-2, 3-3, 4-4, 5-5, are .25, .09, .01, .0064, .0004, respectively. The frequencies of the 10 heterozygotes, 1-2, 1-3, 1-4, 1-5, 2-3, 2-4, 2-5, 3-4, 3-5, 4-5, are .3, .1, .08, .02, .06, .048, .012, .016, .004, .0032, respectively.

$$\text{Heterozygosity (H)} = 1 - (.25 + .09 + .01 + .0064 + .0004)$$
$$= .6432$$

X-LINKED LOCUS

The genotype frequencies at a locus on the X chromosome differ in the two sexes because males have only one X chromosome, while females have two X chromosomes. Thus, in males the genotype frequency is equal to the allele frequency. For Hardy–Weinberg equilibrium, the allele frequencies in males must be equal to those in females. Suppose the frequency of the A_1 allele is p_m in males and p_f in females in the first generation. By the principles of X-linked inheritance, the frequency of this allele in males in the second generation must be p_f because males get their X chromosomes from their mothers. By contrast, in females in the second generation the frequency of the A_1 allele is $\frac{1}{2}(p_m + p_f)$ because females get one X chromosome from each parent. The difference between the male and female fre-

quencies in this generation is $p_f - \frac{1}{2}(p_m + p_f) = \frac{1}{2}(p_f - p_m)$, which is one half of the difference in the first generation. Similarly, in the third generation, the male allele frequency is $\frac{1}{2}(p_m + p_f)$, while the female frequency is $\frac{1}{4}p_m + \frac{3}{4}p_f$, and the difference is $\frac{1}{4}(p_f - p_m)$. With each generation the difference between the male and female frequencies becomes smaller and equilibrium is reached when they are the same. The equilibrium allele frequency of A_1 is equal to $\frac{2}{3}p_f + \frac{1}{3}p_m$ in both sexes. Table 13.2 shows the approach to equilibrium for an X-linked locus when the initial allele frequencies are 0.33 in males and 0.57 in females. With each generation, the difference between the frequencies in males and females is reduced, and they approach the equilibrium frequency of $\frac{1}{3}(.33) + \frac{2}{3}(.57) = .49$. If the frequencies of the two alleles at the locus (A_1 and A_2) are $p = 1/3p_m + 2/3p_f$ and $q = 1 - p$, the equilibrium genotype frequencies are p and q in males and p^2, 2pq, and q^2 in females. Table 13.3 gives the frequency of each possible mating type and the expected offspring genotype frequencies for males and females. Summing these genotype frequencies shows that the equilibrium frequencies are maintained in the next generation.

Example:

Suppose the frequency of an allele at an X-linked locus is .03 in males and .06 in females. What is the equilibrium allele frequency? Furthermore, suppose that this allele is responsible for a recessive trait. What are the equilibrium frequencies of this trait in males and females, and what is the frequency of heterozygous (carrier) females?

Table 13.2. Approach to Equilibrium for a Locus on the X Chromosome

Generation	p_m	p_f
0	.33	.57
1	.57	.45
2	.45	.51
3	.51	.48
4	.48	.495
5	.495	.4875
6	.4875	.49125
7	.49125	.489375
8	.489375	.4903125
9	.4903125	.48984375
10	.48984375	.490078125
11	.490078125	.4899609375
12	.4899609375	.49001953125
.		
.		
.		
Equilibrium	.49	.49

Table 13.3. Genotype Equilibrium Frequencies for an X-Linked Locus

Mating frequency (Male × Female)		Offspring Genotype Frequencies				
		Male		Female		
		A_1	A_2	A_1A_1	A_1A_2	A_2A_2
$A_1 \times A_1A_1$	p^3	p^3	0	p^3	0	0
$A_1 \times A_1A_2$	$2p^2q$	p^2q	p^2q	p^2q	p^2q	0
$A_1 \times A_2A_2$	pq^2	0	pq^2	0	pq^2	0
$A_2 \times A_1A_1$	p^2q	p^2q	0	0	p^2q	0
$A_2 \times A_1A_2$	$2pq^2$	pq^2	0	0	pq^2	pq^2
$A_2 \times A_2A_2$	q^3	0	q^3	0	0	q^3
Total		p	q	p^2	$2pq$	q^2

Table 13.4. Joint Genotype Frequencies for Two Loci

Genotype	Frequency	Equilibrium Frequency
$A_1A_1B_1B_1$	g_{11}^2	$p_1^2q_1^2$
$A_1A_1B_1B_2$	$2g_{11}g_{12}$	$2p_1^2q_1q_2$
$A_1A_1B_2B_2$	g_{12}^2	$p_1^2q_2^2$
$A_1A_2B_1B_1$	$2g_{11}g_{21}$	$2p_1p_2q_1^2$
$A_1A_2B_1B_2$	$2g_{11}g_{22} + 2g_{12}g_{21}$	$4p_1p_2q_1q_2$
$A_1A_2B_2B_2$	$2g_{12}g_{22}$	$2p_1p_2q_2^2$
$A_2A_2B_1B_1$	g_{21}^2	$p_2^2q_1^2$
$A_2A_2B_1B_2$	$2g_{21}g_{22}$	$2p_2^2q_1q_2$
$A_2A_2B_2B_2$	g_{22}^2	$p_2^2q_2^2$

The equilibrium frequency of the allele is $\frac{1}{3}$ (.03) + $\frac{2}{3}$ (.06) = .05. Thus, the frequency of males with the trait is .05 and the frequency of females with the trait is $(.05)^2$ = .0025. The frequency of carrier females is $2(.05)(.95)$ = .095.

TWO LOCI

Equilibrium is reached after one generation of random mating for a single autosomal locus, and over several generations for an X-linked locus. However, the approach to equilibrium may be much longer for two loci, and the number of generations depends on the recombination fraction. Suppose the first locus has alleles A_1 and A_2, with frequencies p_1 and p_2, and the second locus has alleles B_1 and B_2, with frequencies q_1 and q_2, respectively. The four possible gametes are A_1B_1, A_1B_2, A_2B_1, A_2B_2; let their frequencies in the population be g_{11}, g_{12}, g_{21}, g_{22}, where $p_1 = g_{11} + g_{12}$, $p_2 = g_{21} + g_{22}$, $q_1 = g_{11} + g_{21}$, and $q_2 = g_{12} + g_{22}$. Allowing these gametes to unite at random gives the genotype frequencies in the next generation (Table 13.4). Now consider the gametic output of this population. In doing so we must take into account the fact that the frequency of gametes produced by the double heterozygote ($A_1A_2B_1B_2$) depends on the recombination fraction, θ. If the phase is A_1B_1/A_2B_2, A_1B_1 and A_2B_2 are nonrecombinants, and A_1B_2 and A_2B_1 are recombinants. Conversely, if phase is A_1B_2/A_2B_1, A_1B_2 and A_2B_1 are nonrecombinants, and A_1B_1 and A_2B_2 are recombinants. Therefore, the frequency of A_1B_1 gametes from double heterozygotes is $g_{11}g_{22}(1-\theta) + g_{12}g_{21}\theta$. In addition, all the gametes produced by individuals with the genotype $A_1A_1B_1B_1$, and one-half of those produced by individuals with the genotypes $A_1A_1B_1B_2$ and $A_1A_2B_1B_1$ will be A_1B_1. Thus, the total frequency of A_1B_1 gametes in this generation is $g_{11}^2 + g_{11}g_{12} + g_{11}g_{21} + g_{11}g_{22}(1-\theta) + g_{12}g_{21}\theta$, which may be written as $g_{11} - \theta D$, where $D = g_{11}g_{22} - g_{12}g_{21}$. D is called the coefficient of linkage disequilibrium and is a measure of allelic

association. Similar calculations may be done for each of the gametic types and the frequencies obtained are $g_{12} + \theta D$, $g_{21} + \theta D$, and $g_{22} - \theta D$ for A_1B_2, A_2B_1, and A_2B_2, respectively.

If the loci are unlinked, $\theta = 1/2$, and the change in gametic frequency from one generation to the next is $\frac{1}{2}$ D. For linked loci the change is θD. Thus, the more closely two loci are linked, the slower is the approach to equilibrium. The coefficient of linkage disequilibrium after t generations may be written as

$$D_t = (1 - \theta) D_{t-1} = (1 - \theta)^t D_0$$

which approaches zero as t tends to infinity.

At equilibrium, D is equal to zero and the genotype and gametic frequencies are products of the allele frequencies (Table 13.4). The gametic frequencies may be written as $g_{11} = p_1q_1 + D$, $g_{12} = p_1q_2 - D$, $g_{21} = p_2q_1 - D$, and $g_{22} = p_2q_2 + D$. Each of these gametic frequencies must be greater than or equal to zero. Thus, D must be greater than or equal to both $-p_1q_1$ and $-p_2q_2$, and D must be less than or equal to both p_1q_2 and p_2q_1. These results may be written as

$$D_{min} = \max (-p_1q_1, -p_2q_2)$$

$$D_{max} = \min (p_1q_2, p_2q_1)$$

For two loci each with two alleles D must lie between −.25 and .25, and it can reach these extreme values only if the frequencies of the four alleles are .5. Thus, the value of D is dependent on allele frequencies, meaning that D values for different pairs of loci are not comparable. The value of the standardized measure, $D' = D/D_{extreme}$, where $D_{extreme}$ = $-D_{min}$ if D < 0 and D_{max} if D > 0, is less dependent on the allele frequencies and lies between −1 and 1.

Linkage disequilibrium studies were helpful in defining the precise location of the cystic fibrosis locus (Kerem et al., 1989); they are particularly useful in refining the flanking markers for a disease locus in populations that grew from a small number of founders with very little migration into the population. For example, the Usher syndrome type I locus in the Acadian population of southwestern Louisiana was localized to a small region on chromosome 11 by linkage disequilibrium analysis (Keats et al., 1994). Individuals in this population are the descendants of a small group of Acadians who moved to southwestern Louisiana, when they were expelled from the Nova Scotia region of Canada by the British in 1755. The new population remained a relatively isolated, cohesive group.

The statistic, δ, is another measure of linkage disequilibrium that is useful for estimating the location of a disease locus if a single mutation is likely. The formula is

$$\delta = (P_D - P_N)/(1 - P_N)$$

where P_D is the frequency of the associated allele on disease chromosomes and P_N is the frequency of this allele on normal chromosomes (Bengtsson and Thomson, 1981). This value represents an estimate of the proportion of disease chromosomes bearing the original associated allele. If there is a single mutation, the proportion of chromosomes carrying this mutation is the same for all marker loci, so differences in δ across loci should largely represent effects of recombination. Thus, δ can be used to determine the most likely location of the disease locus among a set of tightly linked marker loci and also to estimate the age of the mutation in the population. Using this approach, Risch et al. (1995) refined the location of the idiopathic torsion dystonia locus on chromosome 9 and estimated its age to be approximately 350 years in the Ashkenazi Jewish population.

Linkage disequilibrium is one possible explanation for association between a phenotype and a marker allele in a population. In this case the disease locus is tightly linked to the marker locus. However, population association does not imply tight linkage, and vice versa. Other possible reasons for association are pleiotropy (multiple effects of the same gene), such as the association between stomach cancer and the A allele of the ABO blood group and departures from random mating due to events such as racial admixture, inbreeding, and assortative mating.

Examples:

1. Suppose the frequencies of the gametes A_1B_1, A_1B_2, A_2B_1, A_2B_2 are .5, .1, .3, .1, respectively. What is the value of D after one generation of random mating if (1) the two loci are unlinked, and (2) the recombination fraction between the two loci is .01?

The value of D in the original population is $(.5)(.1) - (.1)(.3) = .02$. After one generation, $D = (1 - .5)(.02) = .01$ if the two loci are unlinked, and $D = (1 - .01)(.02) = .0198$ if the recombination fraction is .01.

2. How many generations are required for the value of D to be one-half its initial value?

$D_t/D_0 = (1 - \theta)^t = \frac{1}{2}$; therefore, $t = \log(\frac{1}{2})/\log(1-\theta)$.

Thus, for θ equal to .3, .1, .01, and .001, the numbers of generations required are approximately 2, 7, 69, and 693, respectively. Note that for unlinked loci D is halved in one generation as seen in example 1.

Factors that affect Hardy–Weinberg equilibrium

The assumption of a large, random mating population is fundamental to Hardy–Weinberg equilibrium. If mating is not at random, the allele frequencies at a locus (say, p and q) in the population do not change from one generation to the next but the genotype frequencies are not p^2, $2pq$, and q^2. Evolutionary forces such as random genetic drift, mutation, selection, and migration, however, will change allele frequencies (and consequently genotype frequencies) from one generation to the next.

FACTORS THAT AFFECT GENOTYPE FREQUENCIES BUT NOT ALLELE FREQUENCIES

Random mating has been assumed so far in all the derivations. If gametes do not unite at random, the genotype frequencies are not in Hardy–Weinberg proportions and cannot be derived simply from allele frequencies. Consanguinity and inbreeding are the most important examples. The frequency of homozygotes is increased at the expense of heterozygotes. Assortative mating may also lead to genotype frequencies that are significantly different from Hardy–Weinberg expectations. However, allele frequencies do not change.

Consanguinity and inbreeding

Individuals who are related are consanguineous and the offspring of matings between such individuals are said to be inbred. Inbreeding increases the frequency of homozygous genotypes and decreases the frequency of heterozygous genotypes in the population. The offspring of consanguineous marriages have an increased risk over that of the general population of having recessive disorders. The increase in risk depends on the population frequency of the disease allele and the degree of relationship between the parents. In cultures in which uncle-niece and first- and second-cousin marriages are encouraged, recessive disorders that are rare in most populations may be relatively common. However, the occurrence of a recessive disease that is relatively frequent in Caucasian populations, such as cystic fibrosis, is rarely the result of inbreeding. The coefficient of inbreeding for a child of a consanguineous marriage is the probability that the child receives two alleles at a given locus that were both from the same ancestor and are, thus, identical by descent (autozygous). For example, half first cousins share a grandparent in common. The probability that a child of half first cousins is homozygous by descent at a locus is $(\frac{1}{2})^5 = 1/32$. In general, the inbreeding coefficient for an individual is $(\frac{1}{2})(n_1+n_2+1)$, where n_1 and n_2 are the numbers of generations separating the individuals in the consanguineous mating from their common ancestor. (This formula assumes that the common ancestor is not inbred.) The parents of half first cousins are both separated from their common grandparent by two generations. Thus, the exponent is $2 + 2 + 1 = 5$. Table 13.5 gives the estimated proportion of alleles shared by consanguineous individuals that are identical by descent as well as the coefficient of inbreeding (F) for the offspring of these consanguineous matings. If a child is inbred through more than one line of descent, the total coefficient of inbreeding is the sum of each of the separate coefficients. For example, first cousins are related through two grandparents. Thus, the inbreeding coefficient for the offspring of first cousins is $(\frac{1}{2})^5 + (\frac{1}{2})^5 = (\frac{1}{2})^4 = 1/16$. The coefficient of inbreeding is also an estimate of the proportion of loci at which an individual is autozygous.

The coefficient of inbreeding for X-linked loci depends on the number of males in the lines of descent and is always zero for male offspring, because they have only one X chromosome. In order to calculate the inbreeding coefficient for daughters of first cousins, four possibilities need to be considered for the first cousins: their fathers are brothers, their mothers are sisters, or the father of the male cousin and the mother of the female cousin are siblings, and vice versa. If the fathers are brothers, the first cousins cannot share any X-linked alleles in common because the male first cousin did not inherit an X chromosome from his father. Thus, female offspring of this type of first cousin mating are not inbred for X-linked loci and have an inbreeding coefficient of zero. Similarly, if the first cousins are offspring of a brother and a sister with the father being the son of the brother and the mother being the daughter of the sister, the inbreeding coefficient for their daughters is zero because the first cousins cannot share any X-linked alleles in common. On the other hand, if the mothers of the first cousins are sisters then the inbreeding coefficient for X-linked loci in their daughters is greater than that for autosomal loci because a male transmits the X chromosome he received from his mother to all his daughters. Thus, the inbreeding coefficient in this situation is $(\frac{1}{2})^3 + (\frac{1}{2})^4 = 3/16$. The fourth possibility is that the first cousins are offspring of a brother and sister, with the sister being the mother of the male and the brother being the father of the female. In this case, the inbreeding coefficient for X-linked loci in female offspring is $(\frac{1}{2})^3 = 1/8$.

Genotype frequencies in inbred populations cannot be calculated from the allele frequencies alone, but they can be obtained if the average inbreeding coefficient in the population is known. The amount of inbreeding in the population may be measured in terms of the decrease in heterozygosity relative to a random mating population. If the allele frequencies at a locus are p and q, then under random mating the frequency of heterozygotes is 2pq. Suppose the frequency of heterozygotes in the inbred population is H. Then the inbreeding coefficient for the population is $F = (2pq - H)/2pq$. Therefore, $H = 2pq - 2pqF$. The frequencies of the two types of homozygotes in the inbred population can then be calculated to be $p^2 + pqF$ and $q^2 + pqF$. If the inbreeding coefficient is zero (i.e., random mating) the genotype frequencies are those expected for Hardy–Weinberg equilibrium. On the other hand, if there is complete inbreeding ($F = 1$), the frequency of heterozygotes is zero and the population consists only of homozygotes with frequencies of p and q. However, note that the allele frequencies will not change from one generation to the next, regardless of the value of the inbreeding coefficient in the population.

Table 13.5. Proportion of Alleles Shared by Related Individuals that are Identical by Descent and the Inbreeding Coefficient (F) in the Offspring of Various Types of Consanguineous Matings

Type of Mating	Proportion of Shared Alleles	F
Parent-offspring	1/2	1/4
Brother-sister	1/2	1/4
Half sibs	1/4	1/8
Uncle-niece, Aunt-nephew	1/4	1/8
First cousins	1/8	1/16
Double first cousins	1/4	1/8
Half first cousins	1/16	1/32
First cousins once removed	1/16	1/32
Second cousins	1/32	1/64
Second cousins once removed	1/64	1/128
Third cousins	1/128	1/256

Example:

Suppose the frequency of an autosomal recessive disease is 1/40,000 in the general population. What is the expected frequency of the disease among the offspring of first cousins?

The frequency of the deleterious allele is 1/200, the square root of the frequency of the disease. The inbreeding coefficient for offspring of first-cousin marriages is 1/16. Thus, the frequency of the disease among the offspring of first cousins is 1/40,000 + (199/200)(1/200)(1/16) = 1/2977.

Assortative mating

Assortative mating is the tendency for people to choose mates who are more similar (positive) or dissimilar (negative) to themselves in phenotype characteristics than would be expected by chance. If these characteristics are genetically determined, positive assortative mating may increase homozygosity in the population. An important difference between inbreeding and positive assortative mating is that inbreeding affects all loci, while assortative mating affects only those that play a role in the phenotype characteristics that are similar. Clinical examples of positive assortative matings are those between individuals who are profoundly hearing impaired or blind, which in some cases may be attributable to the same genotypes.

FACTORS THAT AFFECT ALLELE FREQUENCIES

Evolutionary forces such as random genetic drift, mutation, selection, and migration change the allele frequencies in a population. Important examples of each of these forces have been documented in human populations, and they are likely to become more relevant as knowledge of the genetic structure of populations at the DNA level increases.

Random genetic drift

The Hardy–Weinberg principle assumes that population size is large, and this assumption is probably valid for many present-day populations. However, if the population size is small, allele frequencies may change from one generation to the next by chance alone. This change is a consequence of sampling in small populations and is called random genetic drift. The sample is the set of gametes that contributes to the next generation. Suppose this sample consists of $2N$ gametes (N individuals) and consider a locus with two alleles, A_1 and A_2. The $2N+1$ possible values of the frequency of A_1 are

$$0, \tfrac{1}{2}N, \tfrac{2}{2}N, \tfrac{3}{2}N, ..., (2N-1)/2N, 2N/2N$$

The probability that the number of A_1 alleles in the population is k ($0 \le k \le 2N$) depends on the population size and the frequencies, p and q, of A_1 and A_2, respectively, in the previous generation. It may be written as

$$\Pr(k) = \binom{2N}{k} p^k q^{2N-k}$$

Thus, if N and p are known, the probability of a particular frequency of A_1 in the next generation may be calculated. For example, if $N = 50$ and $p = .5$, the probability that the frequency of A_1 in the next generation is less than .4 or greater than .6 is .023, while the probability that it is between .45 and .55 is .682. The probability that A_1 will either be lost or become fixed in the population in the next generation is extremely small but is greater than zero. If $N = 50$ and $p = .01$, the probability that A_1 will be lost in the next generation is .37, and the probability that it will have a frequency of greater than .05 is .002. The precise change in allele frequency from one generation to the next cannot be predicted because drift is a random process. However, over a number of generations, drift can lead to the loss of some alleles from the population, with others becoming fixed. If a large number of populations are considered, the average behavior of allele frequencies can be predicted. The probability that a new allele in a population will eventually become fixed is $1/2N$, the frequency of the allele in the population at the time it arose. If the allele is to become fixed in the population, the average time to fixation is approximately $4N$ generations. After a large enough number of generations of random genetic drift, every allele in a population can be traced back to a single allele in the initial ancestral population. All other alleles in the initial population will have been lost. This concept is known as *coalescence* and has been used to predict that all human mitochondrial DNA mtDNA traces back to an African population about 200,000 years ago (Cann et al., 1987).

The effect of random genetic drift in a population may be similar to inbreeding in that both processes can result in a deficiency of heterozygotes and excess of homozygotes. This effect arises in a population that consists of several subpopulations. Each subpopulation may be in Hardy–Weinberg equilibrium but the total population is not. An extreme example is the case where there are two subpopulations with all individuals having the genotype A_1A_1 in one subpopulation and all having A_2A_2 in the other. Both of these subpopulations are in Hardy–Weinberg equilibrium but the total population has no heterozygotes. When the population size is drastically reduced (a bottleneck) the genetic drift is known as a founder effect. Examples of this effect due to new colonization by a small subset of a population or environmental disasters such as plague and famine abound in history. Founder effect explains the relatively high frequency of diseases such as Usher syndrome type I in the Acadian population of southwestern Louisiana (Keats et al., 1994) and idiopathic torsion dystonia in the Ashkenazi Jewish population (Risch et al., 1995).

Example:

Suppose a new mutation arises in a population of size 500. What is the probability that this allele will be lost in the next generation? What is the probability that it will eventually become fixed in the population?

The total number of gametes in the population is 1000. Thus, the frequency of the new allele is .001, and the probability that it will be lost in the next generation is $[1000!/(0!)(1000)!]\,(.999)^{1000}\,(.001)^0 = .37$. The probability that this new allele will eventually become fixed in the population is $1/1000$.

Mutation

When mutations occur in the germ cells, they may be passed on to the next generation. The change in the DNA may be a single nucleotide substitution, or it may involve many nucleotides, such as in the case of an insertion or deletion. Many hemoglobinopathies are due to point mutations that cause the replacement of an amino acid (missense), and consequently an abnormal protein product. The most common mutation causing Tay-Sachs disease is a 4-base pair (bp) insertion (frameshift) while the ΔF508 mutation in the cystic fibrosis gene is a 3-bp deletion.

The source of genetic variation in a population is mutation. Mutation rates in humans have been estimated to be on the order of 10^{-4} to 10^{-6} per gene per generation (Neel et al., 1986). The rate of nucleotide substitutions is estimated to be one in 10^8 per generation, implying that 30 nucleotide mutations would be expected in each human gamete.

Most new mutations are lost due to chance. However, new mutations arise in each generation, and some become established in the population. Suppose μ is the mutation rate from A_1 to A_2 per generation. If the frequencies of A_1 and A_2 are p_t and q_t, respectively, in generation t, then in the (t+1) generation the frequency of A_2 is

$$q_{t+1} = q_t + \mu p_t = q_t + \mu(1 - q_t) = \mu + (1 - \mu)\,q_t$$

assuming no back mutation.

Similarly, $q_t = \mu + (1 - \mu)\,q_{t-1}$, $q_{t-1} = \mu + (1 - \mu)\,q_{t-2}$, etc. By substitution, q_t may be written in terms of q_0, the frequency of A_2 in the initial generation:

$$q_t = 1 - (1 - \mu)^t\,(1 - q_0)$$

$$\text{or } (1 - \mu)^t = (1 - q_t)/(1 - q_0) = p_t/p_0$$

Because μ is very small, $(1 - \mu)^t$ is approximately equal to $e^{-t\mu}$. Thus, the number of generations required to change the frequency of A_2 from q_0 to q_t is inversely proportional to the mutation rate. Also note that as t gets larger and larger, q_t gets closer and closer to 1. In other words, if mutation from A_1 to A_2 is the only force acting to change the allele frequencies, then A_2 will eventually become fixed in the population. The change in allele frequency from one generation to the next is $q_{t+1} - q_t = \mu(1 - q_t)$, meaning that the change in allele frequency is greater for smaller frequencies of A_2.

So far we have considered mutation in only one direction. Now suppose the mutation rate from A_1 to A_2 is μ and the reverse rate from A_2 to A_1 is v. Then the change in the frequency of A_2 per generation is $\mu p - vq$ and equilibrium is reached when this change is equal to zero. Thus, the equilibrium frequencies are $p = v/(\mu + v)$ and $q = \mu/(\mu + v)$. This equilibrium is stable meaning that if the frequencies are disturbed, they will eventually return to their equilibrium values as long as no other forces are affecting them.

Mutation rates have been estimated for a number of autosomal dominant disorders, such as neurofibromatosis type I, which has the high rate of 10^{-4}, and tuberous sclerosis, with a rate of about 10^{-5}. Some of these disorders (e.g., achondroplasia, for which the mutation rate is estimated to be 10^{-5}), have reduced fitness, which is discussed in the next section.

Examples:

1. How many generations will be required to change the frequency of A_2 (a) from .1 to .2, (b) from .8 to .9, if the mutation rate from A_1 to A_2 is 10^{-4}?

The number of generations is

$$\begin{aligned} t &= 1/\mu[\ln(1 - q_0) - \ln(1 - q_t)] \\ &= 1/\mu[\ln(.9) - \ln(.8)] \\ &= 1/\mu(.1178) \end{aligned}$$

Therefore, for a mutation rate of 10^{-4}, 1,178 generations are required, while for a mutation rate of 10^{-5}, 11,780 generations are required to change the frequency of A_2 from .1 to .2. On the other hand, to change the frequency from .8 to .9 requires 6,932 generations if the mutation rate is 10^{-4}, and 69,315 generations if the mutation rate is 10^{-5}.

2. Suppose the mutation rate from A_1 to A_2 is 10^{-4} and the reverse rate is 10^{-5}. What is the equilibrium frequency of A_1?

The equilibrium frequency of A_1 is $10^{-5}/(10^{-4} + 10^{-5}) = .091$. However, to reach this equilibrium frequency may take tens of thousands of generations, depending on the initial allele frequencies.

Selection

The fitness of an individual is defined as ability to survive and reproduce. The process by which the frequencies of genotypes in individuals with greater fitness increase in the population is natural selection. It acts to decrease the frequencies of disadvantageous alleles, and consequently, the frequencies of the less fit genotypes are also decreased. The relative fitness is defined as $1 - s$, where s is the selection coefficient against the deleterious genotype. Thus, the most fit genotype has a relative fitness of 1 (and a selection coefficient of 0).

Consider the situation where there are three genotypes, A_1A_1, A_1A_2, A_2A_2, at a locus with relative fitnesses of 1, 1, $1 - s$, respectively. That is, there is selection against the A_2A_2 homozygote. (If $s = 1$ the selection is complete, meaning that individuals with the A_2A_2 genotype do not reproduce.) Table 13.6 shows the change in allele frequencies from one generation to the next. In the case in which $s = 1$, the frequencies after t generations can be written in terms of the initial allele frequencies. Substituting in the formula given in Table 13.6 shows that when the A_2A_2 homozygote does not reproduce, the number of generations required to reduce the frequency of A_2 to one-half its initial value is equal to the reciprocal of its initial value. Thus, if the frequency of A_2 is .01, it will take 100 generations of complete selection against the A_2A_2 homozygote to reduce the frequency of A_2 to .005. In other words, lack of reproduction of individuals with a rare recessive disease does not lead to a rapid reduction in the frequency of the deleterious allele from one generation to the next.

Now consider the situation in which there is partial selection against the A_2A_2 genotype. The allele frequencies after t generations cannot be written in terms of the initial frequencies but the decrease in the frequency of the A_2 allele from one generation to the next can be calculated. This decrease is equal to $sq^2(1 - q)/(1 - sq^2)$, and the number of generations required to change the frequency of A_2 from its initial value to a new value can be approximated. For example, if $s = .001$ and the initial frequency of A_2 is .01, more than 100,000 generations will be required to reduce the frequency to .005. This example makes the point that even if the selective disadvantage of a genotype is very small the allele frequencies in the population will gradually change. For the same selection coefficient ($s = .001$), 11,665 generations are required to reduce the frequency of A_2 from .7 to .1. If there is selection against the heterozygous genotype (A_1A_2) as well as the A_2A_2 genotype, with $s = .001$ for A_2A_2 and $s = .0005$ for A_1A_2, then 6156 generations are required to reduce the frequency of A_2 from .7 to .1.

In the case in which there is selection favoring the heterozygote over both homozygotes, an equilibrium state is reached for the allele frequencies. Table 13.7 shows the change in allele frequencies from one generation to the next. At equilibrium, $s_1p = s_2q$, so that

$$p = s_2/(s_1 + s_2) \text{ and } q = s_1/(s_1 + s_2)$$

This equilibrium is stable and is called a balanced polymorphism. This type of selection is known as overdominance. If, on the other hand, selection is against the heterozygote, the equilibrium is unstable, and the selection is known as underdominance. The equilibrium frequencies are the same, but if a disturbance occurs such that $q > s_1/(s_1 + s_2)$, q will increase further rather than returning to its equilibrium value. The reverse is also true, so eventually one allele or the other will be eliminated.

Table 13.6. Selection Against the A_2A_2 Genotype at an Autosomal Locus

Genotype	A_1A_1	A_1A_2	A_2A_2
Frequency before selection	p^2	$2pq$	q^2
Relative fitness	1	1	$1-s$
Frequency after selection	p^2	$2pq$	$q^2(1-s)$

After one generation of selection,
  Freq. $A_1 = (p^2+pq)/[p^2+2pq+q^2(1-s)] = p/(1- sq^2)$
  Freq. $A_2 = (pq+(1-s)q^2)/(1-sq^2)$

If $s=1$ (that is, complete selection against the A_2A_2 genotype), then:
After one generation of selection,
  Freq. $A_1 = (p^2+pq)/(p^2+2pq) = 1/(1+q)$
  Freq. $A_2 = pq/(p^2+2pq) = q/(1+q)$

After t generations of selection,
  Freq. $A_1 = (1+(t-1)q)/(1+tq)$
  Freq. $A_2 = q/(1+tq)$

Table 13.7. Selection Favoring the Heterozygous Genotype at an Autosomal Locus

Genotype	A_1A_1	A_1A_2	A_2A_2
Frequency before selection	p^2	$2pq$	q^2
Relative fitness	$1-s_1$	1	$1-s_2$
Frequency after selection	$p^2(1-s_1)$	$2pq$	$q^2(1-s_2)$

After one generation of selection,
  Freq. $A_1 = (p-s_1p^2)/(1-s_1p^2-s_2q^2)$
  Freq. $A_2 = (q-s_2q^2)/(1-s_1p^2-s_2q^2)$

The change in the frequency of A_2 from one generation to the next is $pq(s_1p-s_2q)/(1-s_1p^2-s_2q^2)$. Equating this quantity to zero gives the equilibrium allele frequencies, which are
  Freq. $A_1 = s_2/(s_1+s_2)$
  Freq. $A_2 = s_1/(s_1+s_2)$

Let us now consider a balance between mutation and selection. Suppose the mutation rate from A_1 to A_2 is μ, and the relative fitnesses of the genotypes A_1A_1, A_1A_2, A_2A_2, are 1, 1, $1-s$, respectively. As shown in Table 13.6, the frequency of A_1 after selection is $p/(1-sq^2)$. Thus, the increase in frequency of A_2 due to mutation from A_1 to A_2 is $\mu p/(1-sq^2)$, while the decrease due to selection is $sq^2(1-q)/(1-sq^2)$. At equilibrium, $\mu p/(1-sq^2) = sq^2(1-q)/(1-sq^2)$, which simplifies to $q = \sqrt{(\mu/s)}$. This equilibrium is stable and $q = \sqrt{(\mu)}$ when $s = 1$. Thus, for a lethal recessive disease and a mutation rate of 10^{-6}, the equilibrium frequency of the deleterious allele is 1/1000.

In the case of a deleterious dominant phenotype, the fitness of both the homozygote and the heterozygote is reduced. With selection coefficients of $1-s$, $1-s$, 1, the increase in the frequency of A_1 due to mutation is equal to the decrease due to selection when $q = \mu/s$, which reduces to $q = \mu$ for $s = 1$. If individuals with a dominant disease do not reproduce, the frequency of the deleterious allele in the next generation is equal to the mutation rate. Examples of such disorders are atelosteogenesis and thanatophoric dysplasia, which are both lethal forms of short-limbed dwarfism. In the case of achondroplasia, fitness is not zero, but it is considerably lower than one, and is estimated to be about .2. Thus, the equilibrium frequency of the deleterious allele is $10^{-5}/.8 = 1.25 \times 10^{-5}$ or slightly higher than the mutation rate.

Selection against genotypes at loci on the X chromosome needs to be tabulated separately for males and females because males have only one allele at an X-linked locus. Table 13.8 shows the case in which the A_2A_2 genotype and the A_2 genotype are selected against in females and males, respectively. The decrease in frequency of A_2 due to reduced fitness in females is extremely small compared with the decrease due to reduced fitness in males. Thus, we will only consider males. The loss of A_2 alleles is equal to $sq(1-q)/(1-sq)$, which is q if $s = 1$. In other words, if selection is complete, all male A_2 alleles are lost in each generation. Because males have only one allele and females have two, this loss represents one-third of the A_2 alleles in the population. If the mutation rate from A_1 to A_2 is μ, the increase in frequency of A_2 due to mutation in males is $\mu p/(1-sq)$. But mutation in males represents only one-third of the mutations that are occurring in the population. Thus, increase in frequency due to mutation balances decrease due to selection when $3\mu p/(1-sq) = sq(1-q)/(1-sq)$, which reduces to $q = 3\mu/s$. For an X-linked recessive lethal, $s = 1$, and $\mu = q/3$. In other words, one-third of the deleterious alleles in the population, and, thus, one-third of cases of diseases such as Duchenne muscular dystrophy, are new mutations. In less severe X-linked disorders, the proportion of cases that are new mutations is not as high; for example, the relative fitness of individuals with hemophilia A is about 70%. Therefore, the proportion that are new mutations is $.3q/3$, meaning that about 10% of cases are new mutations. Of course, during the initial years of the AIDS epidemic when blood was not being screened for HIV, the relative fitness of hemophiliacs was considerably lower than 70%. The effect of this transient reduction on the frequency of hemophilia A will be seen in future generations.

Example:

Suppose the relative fitnesses of the genotypes A_1A_1, A_1A_2, A_2A_2 are .8, 1, .1, respectively. What are the equilibrium frequencies of the two alleles?

The heterozygote has a selective advantage in this population. At equilibrium, the frequencies of A_1 and A_2 are $.9/1.1 = .82$ and $.2/1.1 = .18$, respectively. Even though selection against the A_2A_2 homozygote is quite extreme, the equilibrium frequency of A_2 is relatively high because of overdominance. If the relative fitnesses were .9, 1, .7, the frequencies of A_1 and A_2 would be .75 and .25, respectively.

Migration (gene flow)

Migration introduces new alleles into the population and, like mutation, increases heterozygosity. In general, migration rates tend to be much higher than mutation rates, so migration is much more effective than mutation in counterbalancing the effects of genetic drift.

Comparison of alleles in different ethnic groups demonstrates the contribution of gene flow to the present population gene pools. For example, the common mutations in phenylalanine hydroxylase that cause phenylketonuria (PKU) are most likely to be of Celtic origin (Woolf et al.,

---

Table 13.8. X-linked locus: Selection Against the A_2A_2 Genotype in Females and the A_2 Genotype in Males

Females			
Genotype	A_1A_1	A_1A_2	A_2A_2
Frequency before selection	p^2	$2pq$	q^2
Relative fitness	1	1	$1-s$
Frequency after selection	p^2	$2pq$	$q^2(1-s)$

Males		
Genotype	A_1	A_2
Frequency before selection	p	q
Relative fitness	1	$1-s$
Frequency after selection	p	$q(1-s)$

After one generation of selection in males,
  Freq. $A_1 = p/(1-sq)$
  Freq. $A_2 = (q-sq)/(1-sq)$

1975). These same mutations have been found in many different populations throughout the world probably reflecting the migrations of the Celts.

As an example of the effect of gene flow on allele frequencies, suppose the frequency of an allele at an autosomal locus is 40% in one population and is not present in another population of equal size. Then the frequency of homozygotes for this allele is 16% in the first population and zero in the second. If these two populations fuse and undergo random mating, the frequency of the allele in the combined population is $(.4 + 0)/2 = .2$, and the frequency of homozygotes is 4%. The frequency of homozygotes in this combined population is considerably smaller than the average of the two populations (8%). This example illustrates the reduction in homozygosity, and consequently the increase in heterozygosity that results from gene flow between populations.

In general, suppose two populations have allele frequencies of p_1 and q_1 and p_2 and q_2. Then the frequency of heterozygotes in the mixed population is $p_1q_1 + p_2q_2$. After one generation of random mating, the frequency of heterozygotes is $p_1q_2 + p_2q_1$, which is always greater than $p_1q_1 + p_2q_2$.

Applications in population genetics

The evolutionary forces that govern the frequencies of genotypes and alleles provide us with the tools to understand the genetic structure of populations. The reasons why some disease mutations are relatively common in some ethnic groups but not in others can be deduced. This ethnic diversity, in disease alleles is also found for alleles at many loci throughout the genome. By examining this genetic diversity evolutionary patterns can be inferred. In addition, ethnic differences in allele frequencies have been the subject of a number of scientific disagreements concerning the use of DNA testing in forensics.

ETHNIC DIVERSITY OF DISEASE ALLELES

The existence of different disease alleles among ethnic groups is significant both for understanding the origins of the disease in a population and for estimating recurrence risks that will depend on ethnicity. More than one mutation has been found to be responsible in almost all diseases for which the deleterious gene has been identified.

The thalassemias have relatively high frequencies in many different populations, presumably due to the heterozygotes having a selective advantage (increased relative fitness) over the homozygotes against malaria. Mutations in the genes encoding both the α-chain (chromosome 16) and the β-chain (chromosome 11) of hemoglobin cause thalassemia. Most of the β-thalassemia mutations are single base pair substitutions as opposed to the α-thalassemias, in which complete genes are deleted. Kazazian (1990) reviewed the thalassemias and described more than 80 β-chain point mutations that cause β-thalassemia. These mutations have a wide ethnic distribution, with several different common alleles found in Mediterranean, African, and southeast Asian populations.

The most common mutation in the hexosaminidase-A α-subunit gene (chromosome 15) causing Tay-Sachs disease in the Ashkenazi Jewish population is a 4-bp insertion in exon 11. It is found in 80% of mutant alleles in this population but in less than 20% in other populations. Triggs-Raine et al. (1990) reported that three alleles account for 99% of mutations in the Ashkenazi Jewish population. The frequency of Tay-Sachs alleles is also relatively high in French Canadians. Two different mutant alleles have been described in this population. Members of several Acadian families in southwestern Louisiana were found with Tay-Sachs disease (McDowell et al., 1992). In 11 of 12 disease alleles, the mutation was the 4-bp insertion that is the most frequent mutant allele in the Ashkenazi Jewish population.

Other diseases, such as gyrate atrophy and familial hypercholesterolemia, show similar ethnic diversity in the distribution of mutant alleles. Founder effect (random genetic drift), mutation rate, selection, and gene flow determine the frequencies of mutations in different populations.

FORENSICS

DNA markers such as variable number of tandem repeat (VNTR) loci provide valuable information for forensics, but the validity of the results has been questioned. One concern has arisen from the variation in allele frequencies among ethnic groups. Databases such as that of the FBI may contain genotype data for mixtures of diverse subgroups; thus, the allele frequencies may not be representative of the ethnic group to which the suspect belongs (Lewontin and Hartl, 1991). Lander (1989, 1991) argued that this mixing of subgroups means that the data are not in equilibrium, and, thus, inferences from these data are not valid. To counter this argument, Devlin and Risch (1992) analyzed the data for two VNTR loci in the databases used for forensic inference. They estimated the allele frequencies and found that they were quite similar in the black, white, and Hispanic databases. In addition, they demonstrated that errors in the estimated genotype frequencies are minimal and that there is no evidence for deviation from Hardy–Weinberg equilibrium.

EVOLUTIONARY PATTERNS

Various types of DNA marker alleles have been analyzed in studies of population structure and evolution. In fact, before the introduction of DNA markers similar studies were done using blood group and protein polymorphisms. Analyses such as those by Cavalli-Sforza et al. (1988) and by Nei and Roychoudhury (1993) suggested an African origin for human populations based on differences in allele frequencies for blood group and protein markers. A similar study extended this work using DNA microsatellite markers (Bowcock et al., 1994), while Cann et al. (1987) analyzed variation in mtDNA. Batzer et al. (1994) examined the frequencies of presence or absence of *Alu* elements in 16 populations. The evolutionary tree suggested four major groupings, consisting of Africa, Europe, Asia/Americas, and Australia/New Guinea, with the most likely origin being the African branch.

Advances in technology (PCR amplification of small amounts of DNA) and identification of new polymorphisms in the mtDNA have extended these findings by further delineating the four major groups. In addition, these new studies have helped to determine the origins of Native Americans: four Asian-derived Native American haplogroups and now a fifth mtDNA type have been identified (Brown et al., 1998).

Recently, evolutionary studies using the Y chromosome have added insight concerning the origin of humans. The paternally-inherited Y chromosome provides a counterpart to the maternally-inherited mtDNA. Similar to the mtDNA, most of the Y chromosome does not undergo meiotic recombination and therefore accumulates mutations sequentially along paternal lineages. Initially, the Y chromosome was thought to have few genes and to be relatively devoid of polymorphisms. However, a systematic search of the non-recombining region of the Y chromosome resulted in the identification of 12 new genes (Lahn and Page, 1997). This discovery led to extended analyses of DNA sequence variation (for review, see Jobling and Tyler-Smith, 1995) and to the identification of single nucleotide polymorphisms (SNPs, see discussion below) (Underhill et al., 1997). The recent availability of such markers has made the Y chromosome an important molecular anthropological tool.

GENOME VARIATION

The advances of the Human Genome Project have renewed appreciation and interest in the study of naturally occurring variation in the human genome. About 90% of human DNA variation is due to single nucleotide base changes (Collins et al., 1998). Single nucleotide polymorphisms are defined as loci with alleles that differ at a single base, with the rarer allele having a frequency of at least 1% in a random set of individuals in a population. There are major initiatives to identify over 500,000 SNPs and to develop automated methods to genotype large populations. Clearly, these new tools will impact the field of population genetics. Moreover, the knowledge gained from these studies will be applicable to many genetic disciplines including forensics, pharmacogenetics and complex disease research (for a review, see Brookes, 1999).

Although the identification of SNPs and their population characteristics is in its infancy, some basic properties are known. On average, a single base pair difference between two human genomes is observed every 1000 base pairs. But the odds of finding a difference may be as much as a 100 fold greater in some regions of the genome than in others (Li and Sadler, 1991; Cargill et al., 1999; Halushka et al., 1999). For example, the likelihood of finding a difference is much higher in non-coding regions than in coding regions. (A SNP in a coding region is sometimes called a cSNP.) Also, the frequencies of the two alleles vary considerably among loci; based on these frequencies some of the loci will be SNPs and others will not.

Most SNPs found in the human genome are thought to have originated long after speciation, but before the separation into different human populations (Mountain et al., 1992). This explains the observation that human SNPs are usually not shared with primates but are common to all populations; only about 15% are thought to be "private" (Barbujani et al., 1997). Also, only a few of the SNP alleles that were present when humans moved out of Africa have become fixed (either 0% or 100%) at this point in time.

Earlier in this chapter the concept of linkage disequilibrium was described and it was mentioned that studies exploiting this phenomenon have been helpful in defining the precise location of disease genes. SNPs are likely to be valuable for such studies, as well as for analyses that seek to reconcile genome variation with population histories of bottlenecks, admixture, and migration. SNPs provide the population geneticist with a much larger set of densely mapped polymorphisms with low mutation rates to better study these phenomena.

The usefulness of SNPs as a tool for identification of genes involved in the etiology of human disorders, specifically complex disorders, is currently being explored both methodologically (Terwilliger, 1998; Kruglyak, 1999) and empirically (Nickerson et al., 1999). The properties of the SNPs potentially make them more applicable than other types of polymorphisms primarily because of the large number of them in the genome, their relatively low mutation rates and the ability to automate their genotyping. Various strategies have been proposed including both direct and indirect association studies. The direct strategy would involve examining all SNPs found in the coding and regulatory regions of the genome in patients and appropriate controls. The indirect approach would eliminate the need to characterize functional variants and instead rely on association between disease and any SNPs located near a susceptibility allele. This strategy depends on linkage disequilibrium between the SNP and the susceptibility gene.

Ongoing studies are examining essential issues concerning required number and density of markers and structure of the study population. For example, Kruglyak (1999) used population simulation studies to estimate the extent of linkage disequilibrium surrounding common variants in the general human population as well as isolated populations. Two main findings were identified: 1) a useful level of linkage disequi-

librium is unlikely to extend beyond about 3 kb in the general population, indicating the need for approximately 500,000 SNPs in an indirect association study, and 2) the extent of linkage disequilibrium is similar in isolated populations unless the founding bottleneck is very narrow or the frequency of the variant allele is less than 5%. Empirical studies of linkage disequilibrium are just beginning, but current evidence suggests that degree of linkage disequilibrium is extremely variable and is highly dependent on the particular evolutionary histories of the individual SNPs in each population (Clark et al., 1998; Nickerson et al., 1999).

The availability of characterized SNPs and automated technology for their detection will significantly enhance collaborative efforts between population geneticists and molecular geneticists. As with any advance in knowledge, old important questions may be answered, but at the same time, thousands of interesting new questions will arise.

Summary

1. Hardy–Weinberg equilibrium at a single autosomal locus is established in one generation of random mating.

2. The carrier frequency for a rare, autosomal recessive disease is approximately twice the square root of the disease frequency in the population.

3. Equilibrium at an X-linked locus is not reached in one generation. The equilibrium allele frequency is two-thirds of the frequency in females plus one-third of the frequency in males.

4. A population that is in equilibrium with respect to two loci considered jointly must be in equilibrium with respect to each locus separately, but the converse is not true.

5. Linkage does not imply linkage disequilibrium and vice versa. In other words, D may be zero for linked loci, and D may be different from zero for unlinked loci.

6. The effect of inbreeding in a population is to increase the frequency of homozygotes and decrease the frequency of heterozygotes. The genotype frequencies are not in Hardy–Weinberg proportions, but the allele frequencies are not affected.

7. Random genetic drift is the change in allele frequencies that occurs from one generation to the next in small populations by chance. The eventual result of random drift is fixation or loss of each allele in the initial population. Like inbreeding, random

genetic drift can lead to an excess of homozygotes at the expense of heterozygotes.

8. Founder effect is a special case of random genetic drift in which population size is severely reduced by such events as famine, and disease epidemics, or migration of a small subset of individuals to a new homeland.

9. Mutations are the source of variation in a population and lead to changes in allele frequencies and increased heterozygosity. However, mutation pressure alone is a very weak evolutionary force.

10. The effect of selection on allele frequencies depends on the relative fitnesses of the genotypes. In general, selection will lead to the eventual loss of an allele, but a large number of generations of selection may be required. However, if selection favors the heterozygote over both homozygotes, equilibrium allele frequencies will be reached.

11. Migration (gene flow), like mutation, increases heterozygosity in a population. It can lead to substantial changes in allele frequencies over short periods of time.

12. Ethnic diversity in allele frequencies is a result of mutation, random genetic drift, selection, and gene flow. Analysis of this diversity provides inferences about evolutionary patterns. In addition, population genetic studies provide insight into the mechanisms by which certain disease alleles have become more frequent in some populations than in others.

REFERENCES

Barbujani G, Magagni A, Minch E et al. (1997) An apportionment of human DNA diversity. Proc Natl Acad Sci 94:4516–4519

Batzer MA, Stoneking M, Alegria-Hartman M et al. (1994) African origin of human-specific polymorphic Alu insertions. Proc Natl Acad Sci USA 91:12288–12292

Bengtsson BO, Thomson G (1981) Measuring the strength of associations between HLA antigens and diseases. Tissue Antigens 18:356–363

Boat TF, Welsh MJ, Beaudet AL (1989) Cystic Fibrosis. 6th edn. In Scriver CR, Beaudet AL, Sly WS, Valle D (eds): The metabolic basis of inherited desease. McGraw-Hill, NY pp 2649–2680

Bowcock AM, Ruiz-Linares A, Tomfohrde J et al. (1994) High resolution of human evolutionary trees with polymorphic microsatellites. Nature 368:455–457

Brookes AJ (1999) The essence of SNPs. Gene 234:177–186

Brown MD, Hosseini SH, Torroni A et al. (1998) mtDNA haplogroup X: An ancient link between Europe/Western Asia and North America. Am J Hum Genet 63:1852–1861

Cann RL, Stoneking M, Wilson AC (1987) Mitochondrial DNA and human evolution. Nature 325:31–36

Cargill M, Altshuler D, Ireland J et al. (1999) Characterization of single-nucleotide polymorphisms in coding regions of human genes. Nature Genet 22:231–238

Cavalli-Sforza LL, Piazza A, Menozzi P, Mountain J (1988) Reconstruction of human evolution: Bringing together genetic, archaeological, and linguistic data. Proc Natl Acad Sci USA 85:6002–6006

Clark AG, Weiss KM, Nickerson DA et al. (1998) Haplotype structure and population genetic inferences from nucleotide-sequence variation in human lipoprotein lipase. Am J Hum Genet 63:595–612

Collins FS, Brooks LD, Chakravarti A (1998) A DNA polymorphism discovery resource for research on human genetic variation. Genome Res 8:1229–1231

Devlin B, Risch N (1992) A note on Hardy–Weinberg equilibrium of VNTR data by using the Federal Bureau of Investigation's fixed-bin method. Am J Hum Genet 51:549–553

Halushka MK, Fan JB, Bentley K et al. (1999) Patterns of single-nucleotide polymorphisms in candidate genes for blood-pressure homeostasis. Nature Genet 22:239–247

Hardy GH (1908) Mendelian proportions in a mixed population. Science 28:41–50

Jobling MA, Tyler-Smith C (1995) Fathers and sons: The Y chromosome and human evolution. Trends Genet 1:449–456

Kazazian HH (1990) The thalassemia syndromes: Molecular basis and prenatal diagnosis in 1990. In Miescher LA, Jaffe ER (eds): Seminars in Hematology. W B Saunders, Philadelphia pp 209–228

Keats BJB, Nouri N, Pelias MZ et al. (1994) Tightly linked flanking microsatellite markers for the Usher syndrome type I locus on the short arm of chromosome 11. Am J Hum Genet 54:681–686

Kerem B, Rommens JM, Buchanan JA et al. (1989) Identification of the cystic fibrosis gene: Genetic analysis. Science 245:1073–1080

Kruglyak L (1999) Prospects for whole-genome linkage disequilibrium mapping of common disease genes. Nature Genet 22:139–144

Lahn BT, Page DC (1997) Functional coherence of the human Y chromosome. Science 278:675–680

Lander ES (1989) DNA fingerprinting on trial. Nature 339:501–505

Lander ES (1991) Research on DNA typing catching up with courtroom application. Am J Hum Genet 48:819–823

Lewontin RC, Hartl D (1991) Population genetics in forensic DNA typing. Science 254:1745–1750

Li W, Sadler LA (1991) Low nucleotide diversity in man. Genetics 129:513–523

McDowell GA, Mules EH, Fabacher P et al. (1992) The presence of two different infantile Tay-Sachs disease mutations in a Cajun population. Am J Hum Genet 51:1071–1077

Mountain JL, Lin AA, Bowcock AM et al. (1992) Evolution of modern humans: Evidence from nuclear DNA polymorphisms. Philos Trans R Soc Lond 337:159–165

Neel JV, Satoh C, Goriki K et al. (1986) The rate with which spontaneous mutation alters the electrophoretic mobility of polypeptides. Proc Natl Acad Sci USA 83:389–393

Nei M, Roychoudhury AK (1993) Evolutionary relationships of human populations on a global scale. Mol Biol Evol 10:927–943

Nickerson DA, Taylor SL, Weiss KM et al. (1999) DNA sequence diversity in a 9.7-kb region of the human lipoprotein lipase gene. Nature Genet 19:233–240

Risch N, de Leon D, Ozelius L et al. (1995) Genetic analysis of idiopathic torsion dystonia in Ashkenazi Jews and their recent descent from a small founder population. Nature Genet 9:152–159

Terwilliger JD (1998) Linkage disequilibrium mapping of complex disease: fantasy or reality? Curr Opin Biotechnol 9:587–594

Triggs-Raine BL, Feigenbaum ASJ, Natowicz M et al. (1990) Screening for carriers of Tay-Sachs disease among Ashkenazi Jews. N Engl J Med 323:6–12

Underhill PA, Jin L, Lin AA et al. (1997) Detection of numerous Y chromosome biallelic polymorphisms by denaturing high-performance liquid chromatography. Genome Res 7:996–1005

Weinberg W (1908) On the demonstration of heredity in man. In Boyer SH (ed): 1963 Papers on Human Genetics. Prentice-Hall, Englewood Cliffs, NJ

Woolf LM, McBean MS, Woolf FM et al. (1975) Phenylketonuria as a balanced polymorphism: The nature of the heterozygote advantage. Ann Hum Genet 38:461–469

Pathogenetics of disease

Edmond A. Murphy
Reed. E. Pyeritz

Introduction

To wrest from nature the secrets which have perplexed philosophers in all ages, to track to their sources the causes of disease, to correlate the vast stores of knowledge, that they may be quickly available for the prevention and cure of disease—these are our ambitions.

Sir William Osler, 1902

The great ease with which molecular information can be collected on the genomes of higher organisms will tempt many. We can inevitably expect vast compendia of sequences but, without functional reference, these compendia will be uninterpretable, like an undeciphered ancient language. Many people and many computers will play games with these sequences, but we will have to find out by experiment what the sequences do and how the products they make participate in the physiology and development of the organism. Thus, although the analysis of the genotype has been taken care of, we still need better ways of analyzing phenotypes. Many of us are ultimately interested in the causal analysis of development and the reduction of the complex phenotypes of higher organisms to the level of gene products. This is still the major problem of biology. We must understand what cells can do because all of what we are is generated by cells growing, moving and differentiating.

Sydney Brenner, 1973

The effort spent on the identification of genes is likely to prove only a small fraction of that required to work out their normal function in the tissues in which they are expressed. Yet that is where clues to the treatment and prophylaxis of disease are most likely to arise.

John Maddox, 1994

Ontogeny is the process whereby the fetus ordinarily develops. Research on the topic long antedates the explicit definition of genetic mechanisms, which we now take so much for granted. When the organism has matured, it has a scope of ordinary operation as it meets the common day-to-day demands of the environment; this operation constitutes the subject matter of physiology. Disorders constitute *pathophysiology*. All studies of the operation of the organism, ordinary or extraordinary, must be set in these perspectives. At the outset, then, it will be best to define four terms that are fundamental to everything that follows. All deal with the causation of phenotypes, and they are distinguished as to method and scope of enquiry.

Etiology is the study of the causes of a phenomenon and, in the medical context, of disease. Its method is to discover the association between factors that are thought to be causes and certain features that we wish to explain. The goal and method of the discipline are strictly empirical ("blackbox"), with at best minor interest in discerning the actual mechanisms involved. For instance, there is a heavily documented etiologic relationship between plasma cholesterol level and the incidence of atherosclerosis. But whether the former causes the latter or the relationship is more oblique is as yet unresolved.

Pathogenesis is the study of the mechanisms by which the etiologic factors are converted into diseased states. For instance, the etiologic role of dietary fat in atherosclerosis has been ascribed to the infiltration of cholesterol into the arterial wall (the insudation theory); to the stimulation of organization and repair of small arterial thrombi (the encrustation theory); to the promotion of cellular and humoral immune processes within the arterial wall, and to secondary accumulation of cholesterol in areas of minor initial damage. Study of these rival or, perhaps complementary, explanations falls within the domain of pathogenesis.

Genetic etiology is a more specialized topic that deals with the properties of the genetic causal factors of disease and how they behave. Mendel's laws, which were formulated before anything was known of the genes and their mechanisms, are arguably the high point of genetic etiology. A positive family history for atherosclerosis is widely recognized as an important risk factor in the cause of atherosclerosis, with no appeal to explicit mechanisms, even genetic (see Ch. 23). Yet there are undoubted genetic versions, such as the Werner syndrome (OMIM *277700), an autosomal recessive with premature aging and accelerated atherosclerosis.

Pathogenetics, a condensation of "genetic pathogenesis", is the study of how anomalies in the genome are converted into phenotypic disorders. Atherosclerosis has many genetic and nongenetic causes (see Ch. 53). Its pathogenesis has occupied decades of intensive study costing billions of dollars, and it can be fairly stated that its pathogenesis is still uncertain (Ross, 1993; Libby, 2000). One explicit instance of progress in an etiological component is familial hypercholesterolemia, an autosomal dominant disorder (OMIM *143890) associated with precocious atherosclerosis. A pathologic mutation in the *LDLR* gene causes one of five types of defects in the cellular receptor for low density lipoprotein (Table 14.1); the result of any such mutation is disruption of cholesterol homeostasis and overt disease of early onset in nearly all instances. This understanding was the first major insight into the pathogenetics of this complex phenotype and was recognized with the Nobel Prize in Physiology or Medicine to Brown and Goldstein in 1985 (Motulsky, 1986).

Table 14.1. Effects of mutations in *LDLR* on the gene product

Mutation class	Consequence
Null	No receptor protein
Transport defective	No or reduced receptor at cell surface
Binding defective	Normal receptor number, but absent or reduced binding of LDL particles
Internalization defective	Normal receptor number and LDL binding; absent or decreased endocytosis of LDL
Recycling defective	Normal receptor number, LDL binding, and endocytosis; no or reduced release of LDL and recycling of receptor to cell surface

In this chapter, our emphasis has been and will be on disease. However, we stress the relationship of genetic processes to ordinary developmental mechanisms and maintenance of the healthy body, known as *orthogenetics*. One such concern is preserving an intact vascular system. Minor leaks in the vascular tree are mended by the hemostatic plug, comprising platelets and fibrin. At times, this mechanism may become exuberant, resulting in thrombosis, which may occlude a strategic blood vessel. In turn, the thrombus may be covered by endothelium, with its remains, sealed in the arterial wall, perhaps converted into an atheromatous lesion. This gradation points out the perils of drawing sharp boundaries between so-called normal and abnormal states, boundaries that are neither necessary nor illuminating. Precise definition of a disorder, although an important question in its own right, is a luxury that we cannot afford here (Childs, 1999; Ch. 2). For this reason, orthogenetics and pathogenetics are best seen as parts of a single continuous field of enquiry (Wolf, 1995). Understanding the phenotype comes from the interactions among the insights from many disciplines.

Physiologic homeostasis

Homeostasis, a mainstay of physiology, is a concept attributed to Bernard (1872), studied and named by Cannon (1932), and cast in formal terms by Wiener (1948). It involves cybernetic devices that maintain the inner environment of the organism in a state that favors normal functioning. Despite its cardinal role in both normal and disturbed physiology, homeostasis has been astonishingly neglected in medical genetics. To avoid confusion, we call it "Bernard-Cannon homeostasis". (Enlightenment has not been helped by the metaphorical appropriation of the term homeostasis by population geneticists and ontogenists.) Its characteristic pattern is to offset departures of a measurable characteristic, such as body temperature, glucose concentration, or blood pressure, from a steady state that is in some sense optimal (the *homing value*). The size and direction of the response varies with the perturbation, features that put it beyond the scope of the methods most quantitative geneticists use, which are founded on Galton-Fisher theory (Fisher, 1918).

Here we can attempt only a brief sketch of the topic (Murphy and Pyeritz, 1986). Two main structures characterize the response of a homeostatic system to a perturbation. One structure is the precise disturbance to which it is responding. Some models suppose that the response is to the current information only. Others suppose the system to be responding as well to data recorded indefinitely far into the past. The second structure is the form of the response. It will always be of opposite sign to the displacement. If its size is some multiple, b, times the displacement raised to some power, k, it is of order k. If k = 1, the process is linear; if k = 0, it is of zero order. Intermediate values of k are processes of fractional order; and higher values are quadratic, cubic, quartic, or of non-integer or mixed orders, and so forth. The zero-order process is the simplest and resembles a simple domestic thermostat.

What lends special interest to biologic processes lies in that innocuous phrase "current information". Messages travel at finite velocities. In cosmic terms, transmission through nerves is slow, through hormones considerably slower. So the information is at best always somewhat out of date: a *lag time* (L) may or may not be fixed and homogeneous. For instance, the sensors monitoring blood gases lie some way downstream from the apparatus that modifies them, the lungs. The latest information will be out of date by at least 10 seconds (the transit time). Sometimes delay is gross. The response of red cell production to high altitude takes weeks. Lag introduces new and important features not present where the response is instantaneous. For example, in a linear system if the product bL exceeds $\pi/2$, a wild (ever-amplifying) oscillation results that, left unchecked, would destroy the whole organism. If bL is negative, feedback is positive, which would also be fatal in most physiologic systems. Thus, both extremes are harmful. Darwinian selection will constrain the actual value well between these limits, but that state is not proof against pathologic length-ening of L during life, such as happens in some forms of type II diabetes mellitus.

Systems of fractional order are metastable: minute departures from the homing value set up perpetual oscillation, the amplitude of which depends on b, L, and K, but in no way on the initial displacement. While oscillation vitiates the primary stabilizing goal of homeostasis, it is a simple, reliable generator for rhythmical processes. It may explain how success in various physiologic maneuvers (e.g., breathing of the newborn, menarche and menopause, electric shock in ventricular fibrillation) stands or falls by whether the first step can be provoked. Much the same argument would explain bipolar mood disorder and particularly those puzzling, so-called endogenous depressions in which the initiating factor may be so trivial as to be totally overlooked (Murphy, 1987).

Processes with k > 1 have a property that is very rare, perhaps unique, in biologic models. If not large enough to cause wild oscillation, a perturbation causes a finite number of oscillations only, such as occurs in unsustained clonus (Murphy, 1990).

Much of the detailed workings of homeostatic systems depend on enzymes, receptors and ligands, all of which exhibit genetic variation. Perturbations are a fact of life, and physiologic homeostasis to correct them is ubiquitous. No reasonable system can correct them fully and instantaneously. Furthermore, as we have seen in the control of periodic functions, other competing benefits of homeostasis are to be considered. We attempt in Table 14.2 to give a brief summary of the advantages and disadvantages of the various types of functions. Wherever there is an inescapable

Table 14.2. Some broad patterns of response in physiologic homeostasis

Pattern of system	Generating specifications		
	L	*b*	*k*
Monotonic amplification (positive feedback)	Any	<0	Any
Pure drift	Any	0	Any
Monotonic decay	0	0	Any
Fast decay for big perturbations	Small	Large	Large
Fast decay for small perturbations	Small	Large	Fractional
Perpetual steady oscillation	>0	Any	<1
	$\dfrac{\pi}{2b}$	>0	1
Damped oscillation[a]	$\dfrac{1}{eb}$ to $\dfrac{\pi}{eb}$	>0	1
Temporary oscillation, then decay	Moderate	Moderate	>1
Wild oscillation		Otherwise	

[a] *L may assume values only in the open interval shown.*

lag, there will be added difficulties in achieving a prompt response without undesirable overshoot and perhaps even total loss of control. Optimal states may be very complicated, which we consider difficult to develop by wholly random evolution. This fruitful field in the genetic exploration of disease has been largely and deplorably neglected.

Ontogenesis of anatomic structures: angular homeostasis

A colleague from the humanities identifies a fundamental problem. "A novel is half a million words long and one line thick. How can a novel be coherently written?" This evocative image is the very nub of the pathogenetic challenge for large and complex structures. How is a linear (single-dimensional) code "one nucleotide thick" in the genome to be translated into the fetus? The objective involves three dimensions in space and one in time. That the whole must be carefully orchestrated is self-evident. (The linear genetic code certainly has spatial orientation; however this levorotatory optical asymmetry cannot convey any genetic information, since the essence of a code is the possibility of an alternative and no dextrorotatory alternative is known).

Perfect assembly of a spatial structure is rarely enough: it must commonly be adequately matured by a specified ontogenic time-line. Development of the lips and palate calls for exquisite timing. Even in genetic etiology, the ontogenic phenomenon of "time windows" indicates some state of minimal precision. This complex feat of organizing form and timing may perhaps be achieved by "dead-reckoning," by rigorous specifications and a relentless timetable. However, there is evidence that the system is more robust than that, because of what Waddington (1957) called homeorrhesis. This process in ontogeny, which we call angular homeostasis, is akin to Bernard-Cannon homeostasis (Murphy et al., 1988, 1990). In it, discrepancies between the current, and the ideal, states of ontogeny are discerned and corrected. There is plenty of biological evidence from age-old observations of tropisms and taxisms and from modern studies of target-tracking and predation to make the whole strategy highly plausible. What exactly the cybernetic details are and how they operate are little understood. We await with enthusiasm the casting of homeotic gene function in expressly and explicitly quantitative chemical terms (Krumlauf, 1994; Akam, 1998). But the greater efficiency that continuous sensing and correction enjoys over unbending protocol is evident to anyone who has experience of both the minutely directed process of parking a car and of firing a gun at a moving target, where the path of the bullet, once fired, is beyond correction.

If usual development is difficult to reconcile with a linear code of instruction, so too is maldevelopment. In this "post-genome" era, a variety of approaches will be required to address both the normal and the abnormal (Pandey and Mann, 2000; Risch, 2000).

Example

Phenotypes associated with aneuploidy, and more recently with "contiguous gene deletions" have stimulated considerable debate about pathogenesis (see Ch. 44 and 46). On the one hand are those who hold to the reductionist position that the phenotype reflects, in essence, mass action of too much or too little of the products of the affected genes. One result is the attempt to identify, for example, the gene or genes on chromosome 21 responsible for the cardiovascular malformations in the Down syndrome. On the other hand are those who see the phenotypes as the result of complex interplays among multiple genes, which are being expressed in a local environment that is asynchronous with normal development (Kurnit et al., 1987; Optiz and Gilbert-Barness, 1990).

Example

However it may be coded, the ontogeny of the fetal heart seems to be a matter of the direction of cellular growth rather than purely of molecular behavior. It is not at all obvious how connected these two levels of organization are. The details are puzzling: Take lateralization and the visceral asymmetry. There have been attempts to account for the dextrocardia of Kartagener syndrome and analogous mutant strains of mice by supposing cardiac lateralization a mendelian recessive trait (with levocardia dominant). However, as with all arguments from anomalies, it is not valid to infer from the effects of abnormality in one gene what is or is not a sufficient controlling factor for the normal state. (Nobody would argue from the fact that phenylketonuria causes mental retardation that this one locus, if intact, is sufficient to ensure normal intelligence.) Homozygous mice for the *iv* mutation show a defect of lateralization similar to that in Kartegener syndrome; one-half have situs inversus (Layton, 1976). A similar conclusion emerges from segregation analysis in humans (Moreno and Murphy, 1981). It suggests that the dextrocardia is due to random behavior following failure of the normal lateralization, not a *reversal* of it. However, at a different mouse locus, *ivf*, a homozygous mutant causes invariant dextrocardia (Yokoyama et al., 1993). We must then regard these two superficially similar states as quite different phenomena. Considerable effort has been spent on trying to explain the dextrocardia in Kartagener syndrome by an aberrant dynein molecule.

Considerable progress has been achieved in defining molecular defects associated with human syndromes involving heterotaxy (Ch. 47). For example, an X-linked, multiple malformation syndrome (OMIM#306955) is due to mutations in a gene, *ZIC3*, that has a structure consistent with it encoding a zinc-finger transcription factor (Gebbia et al., 1997). The homologous gene, *zic3*, in the mouse is involved in the bent tail phenotype. Heterozygosity for loss-of-function mutations in the *CFC1* gene, which encodes a protein involved in a signalling pathway (termed Nodal) that is highly conserved in vertebrate evolution, leads to relaxation of visceral asymmetry (Bamford et al., 2000).

Control of the asymmetry of the heart gives a foretaste of the larger problem but scarcely gets to grips with the major issues. Whatever the mechanisms, the development of the fetal heart, although patently complex, is both high reliable and avidly conserved.

Example

Several dozen disorders with at least some claim to be mendelian have developmental anomalies of both the heart and the hand. Now there is a communality of the region of the spinal cord representing these two ontogenic regions; and it is tempting to locate the germ of the syndromal association in it. But there are at least nagging difficulties in that view. The most disturbing is the detail of the phenotype in Ellis-van Creveld syndrome (McKusick et al., 1964) (OMIM*225500). It is autosomal recessive, with transmission in the Old Order Amish of Lancaster Co., Pennsylvania, undisturbed over 13 generations. The pleiotropy extends beyond heart and hand, and we have to explain other features, such as the hexadactyly in the feet in a substantial minority of cases, the characteristically short tibias, the disturbed architecture of the ankle joints in most, natal teeth and dysplastic dentition and nails. Ruiz-Perez and colleagues (2000) discovered the gene, termed *EVC*, that had previously been mapped to 4p16. The function of the protein encoded by *EVC* has not yet been determined, but the gene is expressed in embryologic tissues affected in the condition: skeleton and myocardium. Interestingly, *EVC* is also transcribed in tissues not clinically affected, including lung and kidney. Whether the role of *EVC* in these organs is minimal, or the pathologic changes have thus far been unrecognized is unclear. Polydactyly and cardiac septal defects in a father and his daughter, but not

the short stature typical of Ellis-van Creveld was found to be due to a different mutation in *EVC*.

But even if one fascinating condition is soon to be explained pathogenetically at the molecular level, many others may demand a disconcertingly new outlook in an unfamiliar and little explored field. For example, several serious proposals by various writers attempt highly economical genetical explanations for polydactyly (Shubin and Alberch, 1986). In general, they demand the belief forced on us by several family studies on congenital heart disease, that what is inherited is a morphogenesis rather than a morphology (Boughman et al., 1987; Pyeritz and Murphy, 1989). So little is known about these fields that an extensive theory and methodology may be the first demand, and empirical studies may have to pay attention to critical but unfamiliar details.

Example

Coding the laterality of the brain is a more perplexing problem than ever. For the choice now does not seem to be an anatomic one et al, but a question of which information and which kinds of mental process shall be assigned to the left side and to the right. Wholly indifferent, random assignment is theoretically possible (Laland et al., 1995). However, although the facts have been distorted in the past by social prejudice, there still seems to be a higher rate of "left brain dominance," and although the patterns are not altogether clear, there is evidence that genetic factors are at work. The genetics of handedness, as a surrogate for cerebral dominance, has been studied for decades. According to one hypothesis, mothers tend to support infants using their left arm, perhaps so to sooth them with the sound of the maternal heart. Thus, mothers who were by nature right-handed (dextral) would find some evolutionary favor (Huheey, 1977). While 93% of diverse populations are dextral over centuries (Coren and Porac, 1977), the prevalence of left-handedness decreases with age (Halpern and Coren, 1991). Whether sinistrality itself reduces life span, or serves as a marker for underlying neuropathology (perhaps related to cerebral dominance) remains unclear.

As to the vastly more complex problem of how the brain is constructed out of linearly arranged genetic instructions, the only mechanical model that comes to mind—and it is a feeble one—is the process of simultaneously loading and configuring a language on to a computer. Present general theory of the construction and operation of the brain taxes the imagination to the limit. But one, especially if a geneticist, cannot help but be impressed by the reliability of the system.

ELABORATENESS OF REPAIR

One is struck by the reciprocal relationship between onto-genic robustness and recuperative power. The brain is the most highly organized structure but, while having some functional capacity to recuperate from damage by the fluidity in allocating space to functions, only recently has it been shown to have any regenerative power of parenchymal cells at all. The structure of the kidney may be less critical than that of the heart but, like the heart, it has little capacity to repair damage to its architecture. Anatomically at least, the liver is both less critically structured and more robust but has much greater forces of recuperation. Tissues such as skin, bone marrow, spermatagonia, and intestinal endothelium are still less elaborate and are therefore so ready for regeneration as to be notorious sites of sensitivity to mutagens.

LIFE HISTORY

A natural feature of the impact of a disorder is how it affects well-being, fertility, and length of life. These three, although distinct, are obviously connected; yet the traditional methods of analysis pay little attention to the fact. Discussions on fitness make much of the fact that clinical, genetic, evolutionary, athletic, and moral fitness are so different that they must be discussed separately. Indeed, excellence in the one may go with mediocrity, even total incompetence in another. The superathlete may be sterile and morally bankrupt. The puny may live a long life free of disability. The fertile may be negligent in the care of their progeny. But it is absurd to suppose the several types of fitness totally unconnected. The issues are too large to deal with here, and we consider only the relationship between clinical fitness and length of life.

It is useful to distinguish between the unfolding of a disease and the impact of its complications. The wholly static disorders are mostly trivial: red-green colorblindness, tone-deafness, pentosuria, synophrys, and the like. The usual pattern of deterioration may vary greatly. In severe cardiac malformations, the disability is evident at birth or soon after. Even so, major complications such as pulmonary hypertension and reversals of flow through a patent ductus arteriosus or an atrial septal defect may occur late. In hereditary polyposis coli, it is the course of the disease itself—the long latent phase, progressive polyposis, malignancy—that is the chief concern, while other complications (except those due to therapy) are minor. By contrast, Alzheimer disease (OMIM*104300) often appears so late that it is often obscured by intercurrent and competing diseases. Indeed, until recently "senile dementia" was viewed by some as a concomitant of aging, and not as a disease. But while the duration of Alzheimer disease averages perhaps 5 years depending on diagnostic finesse and management, it is surprisingly difficult to find evidence that the patients ever have neurological deaths. They seem to die of the complications (e.g., trauma, intercurrent infections, and malnutrition) that occur at much increased risk.

The notion that well-being is eroded by overt catastrophes (e.g., strokes) or those imperceptible insults (e.g., chronic pyelonephritis) that we identify as "wear and tear" is so appealing that we are led, almost unconsciously, to accept multistage models (belonging to the broad Erlangian class). Where the genetic disorder becomes manifest early (as in Duchenne muscular dystrophy), the competing risks are small, and the pattern of deterioration is dominated by a single class of insults, with the typical survivorship curve positively skewed (i.e., has a long tail to the right). When the disease is late, the patient shows the characteristic multiplex pathology so familiar to the geriatrician: damage in several bodily systems, so that it is often difficult to say which is the final cause of death. The survivorship is then often negatively skewed. That class of survivorship in which death is due to whichever of several partially damaged systems fails first is a "bingo" model, usually given some qualifying term denoting the structure of the decay in the individual systems (e.g., bingo-gamma, bingo-logistic). It is a common state that flagrantly violates the assumptions underlying Galton-Fisher theory. We shall have more to say about these models in discussing pathways.

Disease and malformation

Conventionally we distinguish malformations from diseases. Both terms are indefinite but that need not concern us unduly. However, other challenges cannot be escaped so easily. It is a truism among pathologists that disease occurs only in the living. On the one hand, a cadaver cannot undergo poisoning, suppuration, or neoplasia. On the other hand, instantaneous death by catastrophe of a healthy person may occur without any disease even being started. Disease comprises both a *disruption* and *reaction* to it: homeostasis; inflammation and its sequelae (resolution, repair, and regrowth); curtailment of activities, whether voluntary or by invalidism; and diverse concealing devices ranging from epistasis to psychoneurosis.

There are various ways of exploring these devices, but they call for some circumspection about topics that we shall now address.

NOSOLOGIC DISPARITY

Deep problems arise from the (usually implicit) assumption that diseases, although diverse, are sufficiently similar and well defined to be subject to a homogeneous set of systematic methods of inquiry. Yet this claim is suspect. Sometimes disease connotes the primordial injury itself (burns, hypothermia, trauma), sometimes the symptoms of reaction to it (the cold sweat of hypoglycemia; the rigor of sepsis); sometimes rejection of the injurious cause (diarrhea and vomiting; allergy); sometimes a spontaneous loss of function (facial palsy; pneumothorax); sometimes loss of regulation (chorea, tremor, epilepsy); sometimes perversion of function (malignant hyperthermia; intractable hypertension); sometimes disorganization of the mind (schizophrenia); sometimes homeostasis that is too lax (postural hypotension) or too strict (dystonia); sometimes immune deficiency and sometimes immune excess, and much more. These types are so disparate and involve such diverse dynamic processes, or lack of them, as to challenge the taxonomist. They discredit facile generalities, let alone any all-purpose mathematical models, such as an analytic geneticist might hope to apply.

The starting point of any pathogenetic inquiry must be the idiosyncrasies of the disease itself, what is known about its ingredients, its pathogenesis, its evolution in both the Darwinian and the clinical sense, its prognosis, and its treatment. Formal (i.e., conceptual and mathematical) modeling is important; indeed, it is arguable that the genetics of no disorder is understood until a testable working model has been established. The etiologist may make some progress with black-box methods (i.e., descriptors that propose no explanation). But for almost nothing, one gets almost nothing: data without a model are a muddle. Mathematics without data is a myth.

Proper genetic allegiance conforms the model to the biology, and not the converse. Fascination with robust, all-purpose models is understandable. But models that describe equally accurately a wide variety of processes are by that very fact ill-equipped to distinguish among crucially competing models. If the model will fit almost any data, why, almost any data will fit the model. This risk is all too real. Theory of numerical analysis shows that a model may fit a process well, although its mathematical form has no similarity whatsoever to that of the process. In a reductionistic age, such promiscuously robust models merely obstruct useful inquiry.

This general misgiving demands that ultimately every model in pathogenesis be tailor-made. That does not mean that no two diseases are alike, or that the understanding of one throws no light on another, or that even a good model may not be improved by further experience.

THREE CHIMERAS

In coming to grips with pathogenetics, we must purge it of some misleading notions, half-implicit in the sense that they are often invoked without ever being expressly defined or examined.

Chimera 1: the genetic unit is the gene

It is widely believed that genetics is an "atomic" science in the sense that genetic processes involve indecomposable units to be used in formulating any coherent theory. There is much merit in that view. The snag is that there is neither agreement nor explicit disagreement as to what exactly that unit shall be. At various times it has been identified as the ovum and sperm, the chromosome, the haplotype, certain types of genes (operators, regressors and repressors), the common gene and various functional subtypes of it (the muton, the recon, the cistron, the peptidon), the intron and the exon, the codon, the nucleotide. All have appeal in their several ways and have particular triumphs. Main candidates at least have not been advanced on trivial grounds. But as cosmic candidates, as counterparts of the photon and quarks, all are superficial and hasty. Moderated use of narrow ideas, if recognized as such, does little harm and may prove useful. But if ever precarious claims for the primacy of any one lead to discarding any of the others, there may be serious danger. Ten years ago, it was still fashionable to deride "anticipation" as pure artifact and to dismiss as irrelevant the sex of the parent from whom a mutant autosomal gene is inherited. Interference in recombination of genes is still being treated as a phenomenon that can be falsified and authenticated, whereas it is far better seen as a discrepancy between the empirical facts and an inadequate model of crossing over. In each such case, there was a premature decision as to what the point of the point shall be.

The etiologic compactness of the radical genetic flaw is important, but so is that of the device that promulgates it. Many flaws are biochemical genetic traits expressed at the molecular level; some flaws are chromosomal (e.g., trisomies and deletions), others are expressed at a cellular level, and yet others are expressed in entire tissues. It is beside the point whether all these flaws ultimately prove to involve nucleotide changes, as the coarseness of the phenotype will also reflect the coarseness of the executive device. Ultimately, aneuploidy may be traced to a nucleotide defect, but its phenotype behaves like a chromosomal defect that is quite unlike pleiotropy. Total anomalous pulmonary venous return (TAPVR; OMIM* 106700) seems to be a matter of where cells grow, migrate, and die rather than of how polypeptides fold, but perhaps the two concepts can be reconciled. Now that one locus has been mapped (to 4p13–q12), partial resolution is in sight (Bleyl et al., 1995). Molecular dissection of the cat eye syndrome (OMIM#115470), which includes TAPVR in many cases, will provide a separate but potentially related solution. This "contiguous gene syndrome" is due to tetrasomy for multiple loci at 22q11 (McTaggert et al., 1998).

At an artificial level, the intent of much genetic engineering is to introduce changes at the level of an enzyme or a structural protein that nevertheless has to be promulgated at the level of a cell or even a whole organ (as in transplantation of a kidney in Fabry disease or of a liver in familial hypercholesterolemia). If nothing else, the form of these many procedures should underline the inadequacy of shallow conceptions of the "ultimate genetic unit."

Chimera 2: disease as a foreign invasion

A common notion, fostered by centuries of puzzlement over the nature of cancer, epilepsy, psychoses, and the like, is that a disease is like an invasion of the body from the exterior. In the face of the harsh realities of microbiology, parasitology, and environmental poisoning, this view may not be dismissed. But where all components of a disease are genetically transmissible, we recognize that the stuff of disease is very much the familiar stuff of health in some way distorted or impoverished (Scriver, 1984; Childs, 1999; Ch. 2). Sound pathogenetics not only allows, but demands, at least as much attention be paid to orthogenetics, the study of normal processes, as that given to disease. Indeed it would be better intellectually (though impractical politically) to draw no distinction whatsoever between health and disease throughout the whole enquiry until the final stages, where practical decisions are made about policy.

Chimera 3: unrecognized demons of orthogenetics and pathogenetics

An elusive but false image is that geneticists may ignore the organization behind the phenotype, that we have fully solved the problem of genetics when we have accounted in detail for the production of the raw material. This is a particular reductionist fallacy, that etiology is all-important and pathogenesis a minor detail. Those who review the superb precision with which the etiology of sickle cell disease was resolved in 1959 and since refined to the nucleotide level must be struck by how lamentably little progress we have made since in understanding the resulting sickle cell crisis,

the susceptibility to infections by the *Pneumococcus* and *Salmonella*, the risk of thrombosis, retarded growth, and much more. These are the characteristic phenotype and, it may be added, the concrete features on which genetic and Darwinian selection operate. The gap comes in ignoring the task of assembling the components; or (equivalently) by supposing that it may be allotted to a kind of Clerk-Maxwell demon with transcendent properties neither susceptible to, nor worthy of, rational exploration. Whatever merits such a view may possess—and we know of none—it certainly has no heuristic value. For historical reasons, if no other, sickle-cell disease will be remembered for two main reasons. The one is that for close to 40 years after its first and remarkable etiological analysis, pathogenesis of this disorder with an elaborate range of clues was almost wholly neglected. The other even more surprising result is how complex the clues have proved to be. It is yet further evidence that the pathogenesis should be handled properly.

Limited scope of Galton-Fisher theory

For many bodily characteristics, health is the avoidance of extremes. Diseases may then result from excess or deficiency, and the dynamic reactive component will aim to restore the optimal. Now, in Galton-Fisher theory, any variable genetic component becomes fixed in magnitude at conception. By contrast, the responses of health and disease are perpetually exercised in a fashion variable in both degree and direction, in accordance with the size and sign of each perturbation. It is scarcely surprising that Galton-Fisher theory, so useful in static traits, is irrelevant to most diseases. From time to time, Galton-Fisher theory has furnished more refined descriptors such as Pearson's threshold model in congenital heart disease. But it is difficult to cite any instance in which these maneuverings have led to yet deeper questions and understanding of disease, its cause, its pathogenesis, or its genotypic fate at large (genetic population dynamics). History demands that clinical geneticists not discard Galton-Fisher theory altogether. However, we believe this theory too restricted to be of much interest in pathogenetics or orthogenetics, and it often obfuscates enquiry.

RELICS OF THE PEARSONIAN-BATESONIAN DEBATE

The original conflict between the Pearsonians (in the Galtonian tradition) and the Batesonians (in the Mendelian tradition) was at first thought irreconcilable. Fisher's reformulation recast them in more unified terms. There were two serious gaps left that we have been slowly and painfully discarding since the time of the epochal papers on the specific chemistry of the gene. Fisher's argument was centered on the mean and variance of binomial and multinomial variables, which are strictly not genes but statistical properties of genes. It solved the problem but the questions resulting were much more intransigent. Linkage analysis and its analytical difficulties notwithstanding, it is an analogous mathematical descriptor. The elaborate formal theories for it have never had a rationale with a literal meaning. Linkage is now so refined and reconciled with detailed gene assignment that the false character of linkage anatomy scarcely matters any more. But we can make allowance for the fact that even in combining small linkage intervals, Fisher's binomial assumption may yet prove misleading (because of non-additivity, etc., in particular cases) and require special handling.

MULTI-VARIATE NORMAL DISTRIBUTIONS AND THE THRESHOLD MODEL

Galton's reconciliation with Mendel was based on multivariate normal theory and we know of many instances—arguably the great number of instances—in which the assumptions are in fact sound. Fisher recognized this fact very well and specified it in assumptions. But many papers in clinical medicine on "the inheritance" of quantitative aspects of disease have fallen into methodological disrepute without having ever been repudiated formally. We suggest that (like linkage analysis) Pearsonian quantitation of disease be treated as a descriptor of statistical properties of genetic disease and no longer as either an explanation or an account of it. It is only fair to Pearson's explicit warning (which has been widely ignored) that "quantitative genetics" should not be applied to putative "threshold traits" when no threshold has been identified, has been the object of sound surmise, or both. Even so the assumption of approximate Gaussian normality calls for some serious justification. As understanding of disorders gradually improves, the need for approximations becomes harder and harder to justify. We suggest that the now outmoded practice should be abandoned.

Example

Outside of a few disorders of connective tissue, attempts to find a genetic component in mild scoliosis have been unsuccessful (Axenovich et al., 1999). But reinvestigation in terms of laxity of postural control rather than mean angles might tell a very different story.

Example

Many details suggest that most type II diabetes mellitus at its outset is due to neither defective nor deficient insulin, but to impaired insulin regulation. Arguably, hyperglycemia and hypoglycemia are the same condition in different phases, as illustrated by potentially rapid oscillations between the two states in "brittle" diabetes. That interpretation of two apparently opposite disorders as a manifestation of instability of a single trait is not so startling as it may first appear. Besides the obvious precedent of bipolar mood disorder, there are many analogues, such as postural hypotension, dysautonomia, and anorexia-bulimia (Hebebrand and Remschmidt, 1995), but all such conditions would be inaccessible to Galton-Fisher theory, centered as it is on the first two moments of the Gaussian distribution as a gauge of the variation of means. Galton-Fisher theory is not sensitive to variation in tolerances as a segregating trait. Purely technical use of Galton-Fisher theory in almost purely genetic bipolar disease may yield a heritability at or close to zero and lead to the mistaken conclusion that it is nongenetic. Diabetes occurring early in life is usually type I and insulin-dependent, and its etiology has long been recognized to have both environmental and multiple genetic components (Ch. 83). One of these genes is the insulin locus, at which variation in tandemly repeated sequences $5'$ to the coding sequence affects the capacity for regulating insulin transcription (Bennet et al., 1995; Kennedy et al., 1995).

Nature and nurture reconsidered

Part of the notorious "Nature-Nurture" vision of medicine (that is, the image that disease is in origin either genetic or environmental or between them) was that it was suggested (we presume as a pun) for making sure that in the consequences nothing is overlooked. We have serious doubts that even at its best it was ever an illuminating axis. One merely has to think of whether scurvy is a vitamin deficiency or (so far as we know) an inborn error of metabolism. In a fair-skinned population at the equator sunburn is almost purely environmental. In a mixed population of pure fair-skinned and pure black-skinned it will be almost purely genetic. That radical and basically meaningless anomaly is well known. There is also the hidden and unsatisfactory notion of not only anomalous division into classes that are exclusive and exhaustive. This dichotomy is not only logically incoherent but also practically unsound. The difficulties lie in the uneven logic. An environmental disease requires at the very least a black-box empirical proof. Empirically, a mendelian trait must either powerfully follow from birth the pattern of mendelian inheritance or it must be shown to be due to an inherited polypeptide anomaly or various combinations of them. Again, a chromosomal trait must at some scale be cytologically evident from birth. Where a "multifactorial" trait is concerned, however, scarcely any proof at all is called and only the feeblest criteria. Inevitably, then, anything that is discarded from lists of empirical causes, mendelian traits and chromosomal anomalies will too often, sometimes alarmingly often, be treated as some non-specific assembly of disorders likely (especially if occurring in early life) due to "genes," a claim that is almost disprovable. Consider a few telling consequences.

Homosexuality has been declared a mendelian trait although its frequency is continually being identified as high, even preposterously high because it must severely impede reproduction and play havoc with the most fundamental principles of linkage.

It has for long been called into question whether hysteria exists at all. We cite two quite independent classical studies by Slater and Glithero (1965) and Slavney (1990). Its very existence is in question. Yet, though still equivocal, "it" remains very common.

Organization in ontogenesis

Although the notions of *organization* and *entropy* are rather elusive in the context of genetic diseases, they are of some value in classifying them and in offsetting the problem of nosological disparity. Entropy is low when random rearrangement of the parts in a sample space would make a big difference to the whole. The entropy of Raphael's *School of Athens*, constructed brush stroke by brush stroke, is low, that of a garbage landfill high. In pathology, the standards of resolution are mostly and advisedly low; and a natural caution leads us to avoid the term *entropy*, even in its least formal senses. We prefer to use the term *organization*. Nevertheless, in what follows entropy may be a helpful image to bear in mind. It is an unexplored question whether rigorous use of the idea of entropy in disease is possible and useful.

In *ontogenesis* (normal development), we have to address three major descriptive gauges: the scale of manufacture, the geographic concentration of the product (whether homogeneous or focal), and the scope of the promulgating mechanism. These topics are not to be confused. Synthesis of a chemical is a fine level of manufacture, a chromosome or an organelle is intermediate, and a cell or larger structure is coarse. Fine-structure components diffuse easily and, to conserve local concentrations, usually require active metabolism. Intermediate structures spread less easily and tend to be more stable; the nucleus of a cell is an excellent example. Cells that in ontogeny aggregate into organs or that migrate as part of their function require their own motive or anchoring devices and readily remain highly localized. However, the most refined product may yet have coarse expression, because of the system of propagation.

Example

Wilson disease (OMIM*277900) is a refined, well-identified chemical perturbation. But because copper concentrates in the liver, eyes, and nervous system, clinical changes are concentrated at these sites and spare other organs. These very crude characterizations may help impart order to our classification of the mechanisms of pathogenetics in what follows.

Pathogenetics of refined traits

The most important process known in genetics is generating the primary sequence of the polypeptide. It is attained by the elaborate apparatus of genetic coding, transcription, and translation, which is highly conserved in evolutionary time, but the high organization largely ends at that stage. Once formed, the polypeptide assumes its secondary and higher structure by processes that are little understood; aside from post-translational modifications catalyzed by enzymes, there seems little need to direct them. The polypeptide quickly assumes a stable low-energy state. Whether it ever becomes completely fixed is not readily established. But in or near that state, it functions most efficiently. The subsequent fate of the polypeptide may be largely random.

Example

The theory of red cell survival suggests that the cell is eventually destroyed by random wear and tear and the hemoglobin with it. But it has been well shown that survival of the whole is still shortened by some mutant forms of the primary structure of hemoglobin or of components of the erythrocyte wall.

The speed at which the polypeptide is made is certainly important. For instance, sickle hemoglobin is manufactured more slowly than the wild type, such as to lead to a representation in the heterozyote in the ratio 2–3 to 1. Furthermore, in heterozygotes, A and S hemoglobins tend to be concentrated in particular cells. However, one does not ordinarily regard translation (as opposed to transcription) primarily as a timed or quantitative process.

Where the components are interchangeable (e.g., β_A and β_S globins), systems are appropriately described by their corporate properties. Where the numbers are large (e.g., numbers of erythrocytes), the usual device is the probabilistic model; and where the numbers are even larger (e.g., molecules) deterministic methods greatly simplify the analysis with negligible loss of accuracy. However, whatever the value of deterministic models in microbial populations, they have little place in studies of human beings; even in molecular studies, they must be handled with circumspection. This is a major difference between classic population genetics and the highly individualized character of medical genetics.

Pathways and multiple-stage processes

Two highly refined approaches have much in common and may, in certain circumstances, be united by a single theory. There is much to be gained by dealing with them interchangeably in stochastic and chemical terms, by seeing the usual dynamics as probabilistic. However, we shall first treat them separately.

SIMPLE PATHWAYS

The simplest possible process involves synthesis of B from A by enzyme ab (Fig. 14.1). There are three potential deleterious consequences:

Precursor toxicity: Because ab fails, A accumulates and proves harmful. Alkaptonuria (OMIM*203500) is such a disorder, as are most enzymopathies in catabolic pathways, such as lysosomal storage disorders.

Product deficit: Because ab fails, B is reduced or absent. Examples include the various forms of albinism due to failure to produce pigment (e.g., OMIM*203100) and

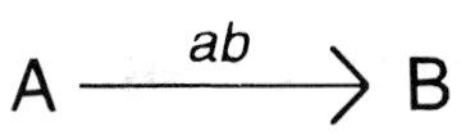

Fig. 14.1. An enzyme, ab, catalyzes coversion of substrate A to product B.

most enzymopathies involving post-translational processing of proteins. In a few mammalian species, the inability due to deficiency of one enzyme to synthesize ascorbic acid is another example. This example raises the fundamental issue of whether deficiency of this enzyme in all humans excludes it from the category of "disease".

Combined product deficit and precursor excess: The glycogen storage disorders are examples (e.g., OMIM*232200). The glycogen that accumulates disrupts cellular and tissue processes, while failure to release glucose from glycogen leads to hypoglycemia. Phenylketonuria (OMIM*261600) is another such example; phenylalanine is toxic in excess, and synthesis of tyrosine is impaired, resulting in the pleiotropic manifestations of phenylalanine hydroxylase deficiency.

Let us extend this elemental pattern to the three-step process: $A \rightarrow B \rightarrow C$ (Fig. 14.2) If A is absent, then B is lacking, and C cannot be synthesized. This suppression is *epistasis*; the gene governing the first step is epistatic to that governing the second. The classic example in humans is the rather trivial Bombay blood-group phenomenon (OMIM *211100) in which the failure to generate H substance destroys all means of expressing the ABO blood group phenotype.

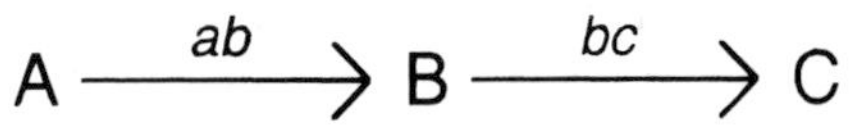

Fig. 14.2. An enzyme, ab, catalyzes coversion of substrate A to intermediate B, which is converted to final product C by enzyme bc. A defect in ab impairs production of C. The gene specifying ab is epistatic to that encoding bc.

Example

Consider a typical multistage metabolic pathway, such as the synthesis of cholesterol or thyroid hormone. Each step is under the control of an enzyme. It will be at once evident that total failure at one or more steps means total blockade of later stages and substrate accumulates before the first failed step. The gene for the enzyme at any step is therefore epistatic to all subsequent steps. The combined effect of defects in all genes will be the same as that of any (nonempty) subset of defective genes. In this it is quite different from the usual additivity of traits in Galton-Fisher theory.

BRANCHING PATHWAYS

We distinguish two kinds of branching pathways: the open and the closed. In the open type (Fig. 14.3A), the branches do not rejoin and pool their products; thus, they compete for substrate and the flow through each is correspondingly

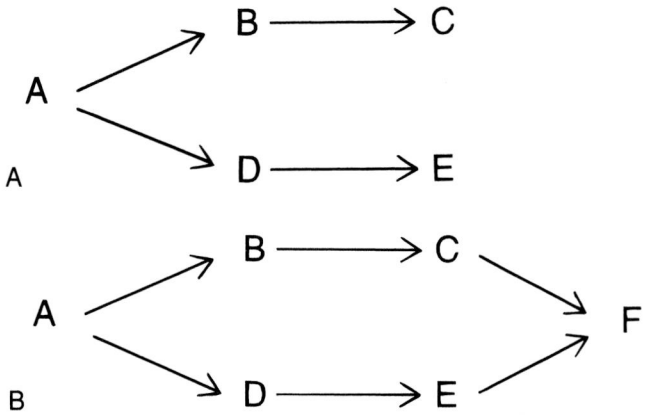

Fig. 14.3. Metabolic pathways with branches. (A) Open, branched pathway. (B) Closed, branched pathway.

decremented. In the closed type (Fig. 14.3B), the paths rejoin, the result is a *parastasis*; two or more pathways run in parallel which accelerates the entire process and acts as a failsafe device should some of them fail. This scheme can be used to advantage in treatment, such as by promoting remethylation of homocystineine to methionine through an alternative pathway dependent on the cofactor betaine (see Ch. 88). Those classic *inborn errors of metabolism* that lack adequate alternate pathways are the most severe clinically. Their rarity argues that metabolic processes without auxiliary paths are the exception and the selective disadvantages may explain why.

On the other hand, a defect in one branch of a pathway may generate all or most of its pathology by leading to overflow through the alternative branch. For example, a defect in the enzyme hypoxanthine-guanine phophoribosyl transferase (HPRT; OMIM*308000)) leads to overproduction of phosphoribosylpyrophosphate. This in turn drives overproduction of purines, which leads to hyperuricemia, hyperuricosuria, and gout (see Ch. 90).

PATHWAYS WITH FEEDBACK

Metabolic pathways may be actively regulated in some cases by demands downstream. Negative feedback, positive feedback, or both, can achieve a desired rate of processing or level of synthesis. This represents a form of physiologic homeostasis. Production of most hormones involves feedback at multiple levels. For example, estrogen is secreted by ovarian follicular cells in response to the anterior pituitary hormone follicle-stimulating hormone (FSH); estrogen in turn feeds back on both the hypothalamus, to inhibit production of gonadotropin releasing hormone, and on the anterior pituitary, to inhibit release of FSH, thereby modulating estrogen production and preparing the endometrium

for implantation. Once an embryo implants in the endometrium, synthesis of chorionic gonadotropin signals the ovary to continue production of progesterone, which maintains the endometrium as a nurturing environment for continuing the pregnancy.

MULTIPLE-HIT PROCESSES

A metabolic process involving several steps may, where necessary, be viewed in more quantitative terms. In the synthesis of insulin in response to a carbohydrate load, (n + p) steps are involved, but physiologic impact occurs only in the final p (potent) steps where physiologically active forms reside. The lag time for the response, then, is that for the transit through the system, and the first n (neutral) components, the inert precursors are neither here nor there. In this sense, what matters is only the process as a whole, and permutations of the components do not matter.

Example

At a more clinical level, one may cite the proposals that the onset of Alzheimer disease (Breitner et al., 1986) and aortic dissection in Marfan syndrome (Murphy et al., 1987) are multiple-hit processes.

MULTIPLE-COMPARTMENT MODELS

To deal with chemical processes in the foregoing fashion has certain uses, notably in understanding steady-state processes. Where changes need to be more rapid, however, we must take a more quantitative approach. Many of the processes of converting one class of compound into another are of so-called zero-order kinetics, that is, other things being equal, the rate of transfer equals the concentration of the substrate multiplied by the Michaelis constant, m. In a system without replenishment of substrate, these conditions define the negative exponential process and the mean time for conversion, *the waiting time*, is precisely $1/m$. This pattern may be viewed under two aspects: first as a chemist sees it, deterministically conforming to the law of mass action; or second as a probabilist sees it, a random exponential (one-hit) process in which every eligible molecule is at a fixed instantaneous hazard of change. As long as the number of molecules remains large, the distinction hardly matters. But the probabilistic model is more appealing because of its wider relevance in biology (e.g., when the number of decaying items—molecules, body cells, recurrent bodily insults—is small, and random uncertainty may no longer be safely ignored). Assuming that each step operates independently, the transit time through the metabolic chain is then the sum (or strictly convolution) of the waiting times of each step. The whole is termed a *multiple-hit process*. Its mean value is the sum of the waiting times, that is, the sum of the reciprocals of the Michaelis constants. (Throughout this discussion, the reader may be struck by the precise analogy to the corporate properties of the resistances in an electric circuit.)

It will be clear that the smaller any particular Michaelis constant compared to constants for steps elsewhere in the chain, the larger its reciprocal and the greater its impact on the whole transit time. Moreover, other things being equal, for any given variation in m, the smaller the mean, the larger the variation in its reciprocal, and the more sensitively the impact of variations in it will be detected. At some, quite arbitrarily small, value of m and large value for its reciprocal, this dominating step is termed the rate-limiting step; viewed genetically, if this step is itself mendelian, the whole will be termed mendelian. It will be evident that the conventional distinction between mendelian and galtonian ("multifactorial") traits is both vague and arbitrary.

Practical pathogenetics

When the defect in a genetic disorder is described at the level of the mutation, the object is at, or very close to, the genotype, and the field of inquiry is etiology. Anything more remote from the mutation represents phenotype and at least the first layer of complexity in the pathogenetics. Thus, the resolution or sensitivity of the methods being brought to bear on the investigation of how the disorder arises determines how closely the mutation can be approached. The clinician has long had to deal with crude tools—stethoscope, tape measure, electrocardiogram (ECG), radiograph, urinalysis—to define the phenotype; what generally results is a perception of pathogenesis that is shallow, often complex, even confused. At the bedside, and even in the clinical laboratory, one usually sees only the leaves on the pathogenetic tree. Advances in clinical chemistry, biochemical genetics, cytogenetics, immunology, non-invasive and invasive imaging of many types, and pathology have all led to a more radical, hence sensitive, discernment of what is wrong with the patient and elucidation of pathogenesis. All these advances have facilitated in brushing aside the leaves and clambering part way down branches toward the trunk of the pathogenetic tree (Fig. 14.4).

This figure also illustrates a fundamental characteristic of many human phenotypes termed *pleiotropy*. This word

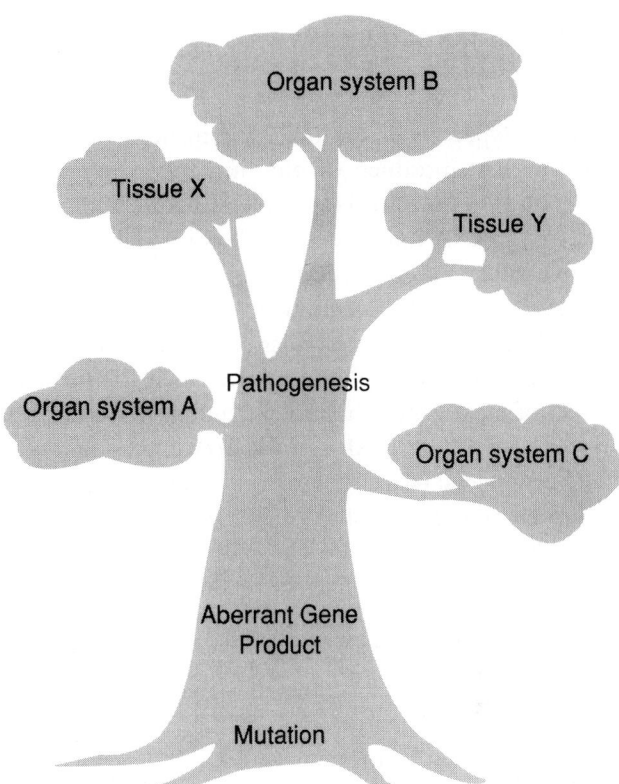

Fig. 14.4. Pathogenetic tree for a mendelian condition. Leaves correspond to the phenotypic features, detectable to bedside investigation. Branches represent the pathogenetic pathways leading to organ- and tissue-specific pathology. Trunk corresponds to the gene product. Roots indicate the cause, in this case, the mutation.

encompasses several concepts in biology; here it refers to multiple, even seemingly unrelated, aspects of the same syndrome. Indeed, *syndrome* embodies this notion of several clinical properties "running together". Each of the leaves on the pathogenetic tree represents an aspect of the phenotype, connected through the limbs of pathogenesis. The analogy breaks down in that while all leaves appear similar, the clinical details of the phenotype may be quite diverse. For example, the dislocated lens, elongated digits, dural ectasia and aortic root aneurysm are cardinal manifestations of Marfan syndrome, but outwardly bear no connection to each other (Ch. 149). These features are all rooted in mutations in the gene encoding a large structureal protein (*FBN 1*), and at the first level of pathogenesis, share defects in an extracellular structure, the microfibril (corresponding to the trunk in the figure). However, microfibrils vary structurally and functionally in different organs and tissues, so each of the limbs of the tree heads in its own direction. The molecular bases of pleiotropy are as diverse as the features of some syndromes (Pyeritz, 1989), and suffuse much of the next section.

Molecular pathogenetics

The phenotype can be explored systematically, beginning with the first product of the mutant gene, mRNA (Table 14.3). Various defects in the structure and amount of a given mRNA can be described, albeit only with considerable effort and sophistication in techniques. The thalassemias (see Ch. 68) constitute one group of diseases that beautifully illustrate the molecular pathology of mRNA.

It is more feasible and instructive to focus on the stable product of most genes, the protein, and describe the types of molecular pathology that arises from mutation. In the most fundamental terms, a mutation can affect the quantity of a protein, the quality of a protein, and occasionally both aspects (Scriver et al., 2001). The quantity of a protein synthesized by a gene is regulated at the level of transcription, by promoters, enhancers, and other locus control elements, and at the level of translation (see Ch. 4). Mutations in any of a number of sites *cis* and *trans* to the gene of interest can affect the amount of protein produced. Usually, but not always, production from mutant alleles is decreased. One class of mutation that has garnered considerable attention is expansion of a trinucleotide repeat within or, more commonly, outside the actual coding sequence (see Ch. 5). The number of repeats is inversely proportional to transcription of the gene. Furthermore, the more the repeats the more severe the phenotypic change.

A change in the primary structure, the amino acid sequence, of a protein may alter its function (i.e., the quality of the protein). The study of diverse variants of the same protein has greatly advanced the understanding of molecular pathogenetics and, given a certain sophistication to the "new" field of endeavor, investigating authentic relationships between genotype and phenotype. This inquiry calls for a new commitment to meaning and the authenticity of the descriptors, matters that are much more sophisticated than the correlations and coefficients that have dominated classic Galton-Fisher theory. The latter may lead to such paradoxic results as that a nearly perfect correspondence between genotype and phenotype may nevertheless yield a zero correlation and hence zero heritability. How the quality of a protein can be affected depends, in the first instance, on its normal function.

A mutation can change both quality and quantity of a protein. For example, a change in primary sequence might affect the stability of the protein and lead to enhanced (or retarded) degradation. In some situations, the amount of the mutant protein is crucial to the severity of the phenotype, especially in the dominant-negative scenario detailed below.

Proteins can be classified into three nonoverlapping classes based on function: (1) those whose essential functions involve interactions with small molecules, such as enzymes, receptors, and transporters; (2) those that perform regulatory roles, such as transcription factors and hormones; and (3) those that function in complex systems, often in a structural role, and often in association with other proteins. Table 14.4 lists some examples.

Most proteins have one or more domains associated with specific functions. Not surprisingly, proteins in the same class often have domains in common, and there is remarkable conservation of sequences among domains. For example, transcription factors all have one or more amino acid sequence motifs—leucine zipper, zinc finger—that facilitate binding of the protein to DNA sequences. Cellular receptor molecules have domains that enable interaction with the lipid bilayer of the cell membrane, an extracellular domain that binds a ligand, and often a domain that resides in the cytoplasm, perhaps exhibiting kinase activity. Some molecules have many domains, some of which are composed of dozens of repeated motifs, witness fibrillin (see Ch. 149), Lp(a) (see Ch. 91) and plasminogen (see Ch. 48). The conservation of domains has facilitated discovery of the cause of numerous diseases through positional cloning. Thus, when a newly identified open reading frame is sequenced and found to be a strong candidate for the cause of the disorder, generally through identification of a mutation, the logical question is what the function of the protein encoded by the

Table 14.3. Exploration of the phenotype by increasing level of complexity

mRNA

Translated protein

Post-translationally modified protein

Localization of gene product

Macromolecular aggregate

Cellular metabolism

Tissue/organ function or structure

Clinical manifestations

Table 14.4. Classification of proteins based on function

Function	Examples
Interaction with small molecules	Enzymes
Regulation	Peptide hormones, transcriptional regulators
Structure	Collagens, fibrillins

gene might be. If the coding sequence specifies an amino acid motif typical of a zinc finger, the protein is likely to be a transcription factor. This process is aided considerably by large databases that incorporate knowledge of genetic sequences and protein structure and function from both humans and all other organisms.

Proteins that interact with themselves (to form multimers) or with other proteins are subject to enhancement of a pathologic effect when one copy of their gene is mutant. Even though the patient is heterozygous for the mutation, the defective protein, by interacting with the product of its normal allele, or the products of other, nonmutant genes, consumes these normal proteins; the result is a much more severe phenotype than would be expected from having half-normal levels of the normal protein. This is termed the dominant-negative effect, and is rather common. The irony is that a "more severe" mutation, such as one that eliminates transcription from the mutant allele altogether (i.e., a null allele), has less effect on phenotype than does a missense mutation that leads to normal transcription and translation of a mutant protein.

Example

In Marfan syndrome, most mutations in the *FBN1* gene are missense mutations that result in substitution of a single amino acid. The mutant protein, which constitutes 50% of the total fibrillin-1 protein being produced, combines freely with the normal monomers, resulting in virtually no normal microfibrils being produced (see Ch. 149) (Dietz and Pyeritz, 1994; 2001).

Within each of the three classes of proteins, a mutation can have one of four consequences: quantitative increase or decrease in function and qualitative gain or loss of function. Each of these consequences can have a number of molecular explanations.

A quantitative increase in function is most likely due to a regulatory mutation. An example is loss of sensitivity to inhibition, such as by a repressor molecule. A mutation could also affect the active site of an enzyme such that its V_{max} was increased or the binding site of a hormone, such that the K_M was lowered.

A quantitative decrease in function could operate by the converse of any of the mechanisms in the previous paragraph. The extreme of the spectrum of decreased function is loss of function, perhaps the easiest to conceptualize, and certainly the most prevalent consequence. For example, most inborn errors of metabolic pathways result from an enzymatic failure. The enzymopathy can be due to a mutation in or around the locus encoding that enzyme, resulting

in a qualitative or quantitative defect as described above, to abnormal post-translational processing of the nascent enzyme, to abnormal subcellular localization or extracellular trafficking, to altered affinities for substrates or cofactors, or to altered responsiveness to allosteric regulators of activity. Other examples of loss-of-function phenotypes include familial hypercholesterolemia due to many of the defects in the LDL receptor and cancers due to defects in tumor suppresser genes such as the retinoblastoma or neurofibromatosis type I genes. Strains of mice bearing gene "knockouts" represent specified loss of function mutations; these are especially popular tools for studying development and neoplasia.

Quantitative and qualitative loss of function clearly overlap. A mutation that reduces the ability of an enzyme to bind substrate also might lead to enhanced degradation and a reduced steady-state amount of the protein molecule.

Mutations that cause a gain in function, that is, a function not intrinsic to the wild-type protein, are less common. The diverse familial amyloidoses are examples, in which a change in amino acid sequence of one or another protein (e.g., transthyretin) results in enhanced stability of the protein and abnormal tissue deposition (Ch. 76).

The least commonly recognized molecular phenotype, also qualitative, is a change in function. One example is the product of the fusion of the *BCR* and the *ABL* genes in chronic myelogenous leukemia (Ch. 72). Another example is the p53 protein, which when mutated in some ways, assumes regulatory capabilities foreign to the normal product.

As useful as these protein phenotypes are for classification (and education), there are limitations in making the intellectual leap to the next level of pathogenetic complexity. For example, gene knockout mutations are relatively easy to generate in mice, and increasingly in other species. Many investigators see this technique as a facile way to isolate the physiologic role of a particular gene product, to generate an animal model of a given disease, or to serve as the background strain into which a defined mutation is introduced (Harvey et al., 1995). There is no question that the approach has been brilliantly successful in a number of instances. However, the pitfalls have been underemphasized. For example, some mice homozygous for the absence of transforming growth factor-β_1 were born normal in appearance and survived, both unexpected results given the prominent role of this cytokine in many aspects of development (Letterio et al., 1994). The reason is "rescue" of the embryo by maternal TGF-β_1 that presumably crosses the placenta in sufficient quantity to replace the deficient fetal sources. But at a more fundamental level, the "null" mutant animal cannot be viewed as an artificial isolated system focused on that deficient gene product. Rather, the mutant strain is a complex homeostatic system capable of responding to loss of a specific protein, even compensating for it. Thus, if the null strain shows no phenotype, it would be inappropriate to conclude that the missing protein is not important to the physiology of a given system (physiologic or developmental) (Ward, 1995).

The actual effect of the mutation may be loss of function at the protein level but gain of function at the cellular level. For example, the Rett syndrome (OMIM#312750) is a pleiotropic, severe necrologic disorder that primarily affects girls. The cause is mutation of the *MECP2* locus, which encodes a protein that represses transcription of other genes (Dragich et al., 2000). Mutations that inactivate the MECP2 protein result in enhanced or inappropriate production of proteins in various tissues, most obviously the brain.

Conclusions

The prognosis of a disease is largely a matter of pathogenesis. For instance, its age of onset, the rapidity of its course, and the vulnerable points at which disease and complications may occur all depend on details that in principle, as much as in fact, may be difficult to infer even from the most detailed knowledge of the basic defect. Some knowledge of the prognosis may be come from "black-box" empirical enquiries: the natural history of myotonic dystrophy, for instance; but this course calls for extensive data, and there may be disturbing discrepancies between one study and another not readily reconciled. If the pathogenesis is understood, even partially, more incisive methods may be available, including direct measurements of the progress of components of the disease. For instance, the pathogenesis of familial polyposis coli is not clearly established, but currently the course of this disease and its response to treatment are easier to study than Alzheimer dementia. Refined studies at the molecular level make for very precise statements about etiology. It is tempting, but rather treacherous to view pathogenesis in the same way. But where the concern lies in either the assessment of morbidity or the study of the populational and eugenic behavior of the mutant, to attach too much weight to refined biochemistry may push the precision of the statement at the expense of its significance. For the overt clinical pattern and the target of selection are very coarse matters; the many modifying factors, which to the basic scientist are largely a nuisance, may have important attenuating effects on the course of the disorder.

Many advances in therapeutics have resulted from largely empiric reasoning as to choosing an approach, but from an understanding of natural history in judging whether the therapy was successful. A more rational approach to targeting therapy is based on an understanding of pathogenesis. Some fondly held the hope of circumventing "indirect" therapies for genetic disorders by simply replacing the defective gene. But considerable experience has amply shown the general fallacy in this approach. Until the molecular pathogenesis of a disorder is elucidated, the effects of simply adding back, or even replacing a gene that should have been functioning perhaps from conception will be as empiric as anything physicians had available in the eighteenth century.

REFERENCES

Akam M (1998) Hox genes, homeosis and the evolution of segment identity: No need for hopeless monsters. Int JDevel Biol 42(3 Spec No):445–51

Axenovich TI, Zaidman AM, Zorkoltseva IV et al. (1999) Segregation analysis of idiopathic scoliosis: demonstration of a major gene effect. Am J Med Genet 86:389–394

Bamford RN, Roessler E, Burdine RD et al. (2000) Loss-of-function mutations in the EGF-CFC gene *CFC1* are associated with human left-right laterality defects. Nature Genet 26:365–369

Bennet ST, Lucassen AM, Gough SCL et al. (1995) Susceptibility to human type 1 diabetes at IDDM2 is determined by tandem repeat variation at the insulin gene minisatellite locus. Nature Genet 9:284–292

Bernard C (1872) De la physiologie générale. Hachette, Paris

Bleyl S, Nelson L, Odelberg SJ et al. (1995) A gene for familial total anomalous pulmonary venous return maps to chromosome 4p 13-q12. Am J Hum Genet 56:408–415

Boughman JA, Berg KA, Astemborski JA et al. (1987) Familial risks of congenital heart defect assessed in a population-based epidemiologic study. Am J Med Genet 26:839–849

Breitner JCS, Folstein MF, Murphy EA (1986) Familial aggregation in Alzheimer dementia. I. A model for the age-dependent expression of an autosomal dominant gene. J Psychiatr Res 20:31–43

Brenner S (1973) Human genetics: Possibilities and relatives, Ciba Foundation Symposium. Excerpta Medica 66:1–3

Cannon WB (1932) The Wisdom of the Body. Norton, N Y

Childs B (1999) Genetic Medicine: A Logic of Disease. Johns Hopkins Univ Press, Baltimore

Childs B. Valle D, Jimenez-Sanchez G (2001) The inborn error and biohemical individuality. In Scriver CR, Beaudet AL, Sly WS, Valle D (eds) The Metabolic and Molecular Bases of Inherited Disease, 8th edn. N Y: McGraw-Hill, pp 155–174

Coren S, Porac C (1977) Fifty centuries of right-handedness: The historic record. Science 198:631–632

Dietz HC, Pyeritz RE (1994) Molecular genetic approaches to investigating cardiovascular disease. Annu Rev Physiol 56:763–796

Dietz HC, Pyeritz RE (2001) Marfan syndrome and related disorders. In Scriver CR, Beaudet AL, Sly WS, Valle D (eds): The Metabolic and Molecular Bases of Inherited Disease, 8th edn. N Y: McGraw-Hill, 5287–5312

Dragich J, Houwink-Manville I, Schanen C (2000) Rett syndrome: A surprising result of mutation in *MECP2*. Hum Molec Genet 9:2365–2375

Fisher RA (1918) The correlation between relatives on the supposition of mendelian inheritance. Trans R Soc (Edinb) 52:399–433

Gebbia M, Ferrero GB, Pilia G et al. (1997) X-linked situs abnormalities result from mutations in *ZIC3*. Nature Genet 17:305–308

Halpern DF, Coren S (1991) Handedness and life span. N Engl J Med 324:998

Harvey M, Vogel H, Morris D et al. (1995) A mutant p53 transgene accelerates tumor development in heterozygous but not nullizygous p53-deficient mice. Nature Genet 9:305

Hebebrand J, Remschmidt H (1995) Anorexia nervosa viewed as an extreme weight condition: genetic implications. Hum Genet 95:1

Huheey JE (1977) Concerning the origin of handedness in humans. Behav Genet 7:29–32

Kennedy GC, German MS, Rutter WJ (1995) The minisatellite in the diabetes susceptibility locus *IDDM2* regulates insulin transcription. Nature Genet 9:293–298

Krumlauf R (1994) *Hox* genes in vertebrate development. Cell 78:191–201

Kurnit DM, Layton WM, Matthysse S (1987) Genetics, chance and morphogenesis. Am J Hum Genet 41:979–995

Laland KN, Kumm J, Van Horn JD, Feldman MW (1995) A gene-culture model of human handedness. Behav Genet 25:433–445

Layton WM Jr (1976) Random determination of a developmental process: reversal of normal visceral asymmetry in the mouse. J Hered 67:336–338

Letterio JJ, Geiser AG, Kulkarni AB et al. (1994) Maternal rescue of transforming growth factor-β_1 null mice. Science 264:1936

Libby P (2000) Changing concepts of atherogenesis. J Intern Med 247:349–58

Maddox J (1994) Genes and patent law. Nature 371:270

McKusick VA (1999) Mendelian Inheritance in Man 12th edn. Johns Hopkins University Press, Baltimore

McKusick VA, Egeland JA, Eldridge R, Krusen DE (1964) Dwarfism in the Amish. I. The Ellis-van Creveld syndrome. Bull Johns Hopkins Hosp 115:306–336

McTaggert KE, Budarf ML, Driscoll DA et al. (1998) Cat eye syndrome chromosome breakpoint clustering: Identification of two intervals also associated with 22q11 deletion syndrome breakpoints. Cytogenet Cell Genet 81:222–228

Moreno A, Murphy EA (1981) Inheritance of Kartegener syndrome. Am J Med Genet 8:305–313

Motulsky AG (1986) The 1985 Nobel Prize in Physiology or Medicine. Science 231:126–129

Murphy EA (1987) A geneticist's approach to psychiatric disease. Psychol Med 17:805–815

Murphy EA (1990) Dynamics of quantifiable homeostasis. VIII. Processes that oscillate finitely many times. Am J Med Genet 35:552–560

Murphy EA, Pyeritz RE (1986) Homeostasis. VII. A conspectus. Am J Med Genet 24:735–751

Murphy EA, Berger KR, Trojak JE, Pyeritz RE (1987) The bingo model of survivorship. V. The problems of conformation to the empirical evidence. Am J Med Genet 28:703–717

Murphy EA, Berger KR, Trojak JE, Sagawa Y (1988) Angular homeostasis. V. Some issues in genetics, ontogeny and evolution. Am J Med Genet 31:963–979

Murphy EA, Berger KR, Pyeritz RE, Sagawa Y (1990) Angular homeostasis. VI. Threshold processes with bivariate liabilities. Am J Med Genet 36:115–121

Opitz JM, Gilbert-Barness EF (1990) Reflections on the pathogenesis of Down syndrome. Am J Med Genet 7(Suppl):38–51

Osler W (1902) Chauvinism in Medicine. Montreal Med J 31:684–699

Pandey A, Mann M (2000) Proteomics to study genes and genomes. Nature 405:837–846

Pyeritz RE, Murphy EA (1989) Genetics and congenital heart disease: Perspectives and prospects. J Am Coll Cardiol 13:1458–1468

Risch NJ (2000) Searching for genetic determinants in the new millennium. Nature 405:847–856

Ross R (1993) The pathogenesis of atherosclerosis: A perspective for the 1990s. Nature 362:801–809

Ruiz-Perez VL, Ide SE, Strom TM et al. (2000) Mutations in a new gene in Ellis-van Creveld syndrome and Weyers acrodental dysostosis. Nature Genet 24:283–286

Scriver CR (1984) An evolutionary view of disease in man. Proc R Soc Lond 220B:273–298

Shubin NH, Alberch P (1986) A morphogenetic approach to the origin and basic organization of the tetrapod limb. Evol Biol 20:319–387

Slater ET, Glithero E (1965) A follow-up of patients diagnosed as suffering from "hysteria". J Psychosom Res 9:9–13

Waddington CH (1957) The Strategy of the Genes. Allen & Unwin, London

Ward PA (1995) Adhesion molecule knockouts: One step forward and one step backward. J Clin Invest 95:15–25

Wiener N (1948) Cybernetics or Control and Communication in the Animal and the Machine John Wiley & Sons, N Y

Wolf U (1995) The genetic contribution to the phenotype. Human Genetics 95:127

Yokoyama T, Copeland NG, Jenkins NA et al. (1993) Reversal of left-right asymmetry: A situs inversus mutation. Science 260:679–682

Genetic epidemiology

Neil J. Risch

Introduction

The term genetic epidemiology was originally coined by Neel and Schull (1954) to describe the confluence of two fields required for the study of common diseases, their population distribution and etiology. Human genetics has always held the frequency and ethnic distribution of mendelian syndromes as a major interest, as well as the general understanding of the genetic basis for more common, complex conditions. On the other hand, epidemiology also concerns itself with the etiology and population distribution of disease, including the discovery and evaluation of risk factors, inherited and otherwise. Historically, the two fields had little overlap or interaction, and limited exchange of ideas, concepts and methodology. Over the past two decades, however, as epidemiologic methods have become more formalized and revolutions in molecular genetics have enormously enhanced the possibility of identifying specific genes and their effects, the hybrid field of genetic epidemiology has acquired a new status and importance in placing together the myriad puzzle pieces of a complex disease phenotype. Numerous books have been written on this topic, for the past decade this field has had its own journal, Genetic Epidemiology, and there is now an International Genetic Epidemiology Society.

Because of its hybrid nature, genetic epidemiology draws from several distinct related fields: population genetics, quantitative genetics, epidemiology and biostatistics. Indeed, the study of the population distribution and ethnic variation of human genetic (mendelian) diseases is the essence of human population genetics, details of which can be found in Chapter 14. On the other side, understanding the genetic and non-genetic contributions to complex,

common diseases also draws from study designs classic to human genetics, but more recently given an epidemiologic framework. Such designs include family, twin, adoption, linkage and marker-association studies. Several other chapters in this text overlap with the current one in this regard (in particular, Chs 7, 8, 13 and 19).

The heart of genetic epidemiology is understanding the genetic and environmental contributors to a disease, and how they relate to one another. An essential part of this endeavor is identification and description of the genetic component. We begin with a discussion of genes and their effects.

Measurement of gene effects

There are different ways of conceptualizing the magnitude of the effect of a genetic variant on an observed trait. First, it is important to make a distinction between quantitative traits (i.e., those measured on a continuous scale, such as height or weight) and qualitative or discrete traits (such as affected and normal). For the former, gene effects can be measured in terms of the difference in average trait value between genotypes. As an example, we consider the effect of ApoE genotype on total serum cholesterol. There are three common ApoE alleles, labeled E2, E3 and E4. In Caucasians, the frequencies of these alleles are .08, .77 and .15, respectively. In Table 15.1 are given the average total serum cholesterols for the six common ApoE genotypes, along with the standard deviation for each genotype. As can be seen from the table, the largest difference occurs between the genotypes E4/E4 and E2/E2. The difference in mean values between these genotypes is 0.76 standard

Table 15.1. Mean (± S D) Total Serum Cholesterol for Six ApoE Genotypes

ApoE Genotype	N	Cholesterol
E4/E4	23	203 ± 33
E3/E4	202	199 ± 36
E3/E3	627	195 ± 32
E2/E4	30	189 ± 36
E2/E3	110	182 ± 33
E2/E2	8	178 ± 47

(Data from Menzel et al., 1983.)

deviations, assuming an average standard deviation of 33. Similarly, the difference in mean values for the most common E3/E3 genotype and the E4/E4 homozygote is 0.24 standard deviations. The difference between genotypes in standard deviations is sometimes referred to as displacement.

An alternative measure of the magnitude of gene effect relates to variance. For a quantitative trait, the variance, or the average squared deviation from the mean is a measure of the amount of variability of the trait in the population. Geneticists often like to decompose the trait variance into components due to various effects. It is then possible to calculate the proportion of the total variance due to a particular effect.

There are standard biometrical methods for calculating the variance attributable to a segregating gene. Here we provide the simplest example. Consider a two-allele locus with alleles A and B. Suppose individuals with genotype AA have a mean trait value of M_{AA}, individuals of genotype AB have mean M_{AB} and similarly those with genotype BB have mean M_{BB}. Let p be the population frequency of allele A and q = 1 − p the frequency of B. Then it is straightforward to show that the population variance due to this locus is given by

$$V_G = 2pq \left[p(M_{AA} - M_{AB}) + q(M_{AB} - M_{BB}) \right]^2 + \left[pq(M_{AA} + M_{BB} - 2M_{AB}) \right]^2$$

(e.g., see Falconer, 1989). The first term in the above sum is called the additive genetic variance V_A and the second term is the dominance variance V_D. If the total population variance of the trait is V_T, then the proportion of the total variance due to this locus is simply V_G/V_T. For example, for the ApoE locus and total serum cholesterol, Davignon et al. (1988) estimated that 7% of the total population variance of serum cholesterol is attributable to the ApoE locus.

Displacement and proportion of the total variance are both useful measures of gene effect, but they are not the same. Notice that in the formula for the genetic variance given above that allele frequencies enter into the equation; this is not the case for displacement. Thus, an allele can have a large displacement, even several standard deviations, but contribute little to the variance because it is infrequent in the population. For example, mutations in the gene for the low density lipoprotein receptor (LDL-R) have a very large displacement. In one family, Leppert et al. (1986) estimated the mean total cholesterol of carriers to be 360 compared with 209 for the noncarriers, a difference (or displacement) of about 3.5 standard deviations. However, because of their low population frequency, such mutations contribute only 1% of the total phenotypic variance (Davignon et al., 1988).

Sometimes gene effects are referred to as major loci or minor loci. To some extent these distinctions are subjective and unclear, because genes of any magnitude can and do exist. Some have used a cut-off of a displacement of at least one standard deviation between homozygotes to define a major locus (Morton, 1982). In terms of variance, one might consider any gene contributing at least 10% of the total population variance as a major locus. These characterizations have more to do with what is detectable in segregation, linkage or association studies. The two different measures of gene effect become important when designing linkage studies, as will be described below.

Of course, it is typical that several or many genetic loci contribute to the total variation in a continuous trait. In this case, one can conceive of the proportion of the total trait variance attributable to the action of all contributing loci. This proportion is usually called the broad heritability and denoted by the letter H. The total genetic variance can be broken into several components; for example, the additive and dominance variances as described above, and also variance attributable to interactive (nonadditive) effects of contributing loci. Interactive effects among loci is referred to as epistasis, and there are numerous types of epistatic variance components depending on the number of loci involved (e.g., Kempthorne, 1969). The proportion of total variance attributable to just the additive genetic variance components is referred to as the narrow heritability. Absent from the above characterization of heritability is a discussion of possible interaction effects between genes and environmental components. Such interactions make separation of genetic and environmental variance components difficult.

The term polygenic, or multifactorial, has been used to describe traits which have no major gene components, but rather are due to the combined contribution of numerous small and equal genetic and environmental effects. To some extent, the notion polygenic is misleading, because we know that gene effects underlying a trait are of variable magnitude. A more modern conceptualization of a polygenic trait is one without a single gene contributing the majority of the genetic variance. Indeed, this is not truly a modern notion, but rather goes back decades to when "polygenic" traits were first dissected using chromosomal markers (Thoday, 1967).

Discrete (e.g., affected, unaffected) outcomes also lend themselves to the notion of magnitude of gene effect. For a classic mendelian phenotype, one whose variation is attributable entirely to the segregation of a single gene, the trait is fully explained by that locus. On the other hand, many discrete traits cannot be explained on such a simple basis, and are in fact due to the contributions of multiple genes and environmental factors. One approach to the conceptualization of such traits is the liability model. According to this model, there is a latent (unobserved) continuous variable called liability, which is normally distributed in the population, along with a threshold. Anyone whose liability value exceeds the threshold is affected, while those below the threshold are normal. By transforming discrete traits to the continuous liability-threshold model, all the genetic variance and heritability concepts derived for continuous traits can be applied to liability. For example, it is possible to define the heritability of liability to a discrete trait by estimating the various variance components of the quantitative trait, liability. These estimates are usually obtained from recurrence risks in family members of an affected individual.

With the advent of modern molecular genetic technology, the polygenic threshold model has diminished in popularity. This is because there is now the potential to identify the individual genetic contributors to a disease phenotype and understand the interactive effects of these genes. Indeed, this endeavor is likely to remain one of the major thrusts of human genetics for the twenty-first century.

For discrete traits, a typical measure of the effect of a single contributing locus is the genotype-specific relative risk, that is the ratio of risk for disease for an individual carrying a predisposing genotype compared to a reference genotype. In this sense, genotype relative risks are defined in a completely analogous way to any inherited or non-inherited exposures in epidemiology; here, the genotype is the exposure (Khoury et al., 1993).

Aside from mendelian syndromes, where genotype relative risks approach infinity (for example, if the predisposing locus is absolutely necessary), the HLA complex of loci on chromosome 6p has so far been associated with the largest genetic risk ratios. For example, the allele DR2 is associated with a relative risk of 36 with narcolepsy for heterozygous

individuals and 292 for homozygotes (Mignot et al., 1994), while the B27 allele has a very strong association with ankylosing spondylitis (RR = 116 for heterozygotes, RR = 197 for homozygotes) (Kidd et al., 1977). Numerous other diseases, mostly of an autoimmune nature, are associated with specific HLA alleles; such diseases include type 1 diabetes, multiple sclerosis, coeliac disease, and Graves disease.

A more recent example of the characterization of genotype relative risks for a disease has been given for the effect of ApoE on late-onset Alzheimer disease (AD) (Corder et al., 1993; Saunders et al., 1993). Here, the E4 allele appears to increase the risk, while the E2 allele decreases the risk for disease, in an age-dependent fashion. Corder et al. (1994) estimated a genotypic relative risk of 19.3 for E4 homozygotes and 4.4 for E4/E3 heterozygotes compared to E3 homozygotes, combining across all age of onset groups. However, they also found that these relative risks were greatest at early ages (before 70) and lowest at late ages (after 80). These relative risks are quite large, and thus from an epidemiological perspective ApoE represents a major risk factor for late onset AD.

Familial aggregation

The first line of evidence that genetic factors may be involved in the etiology of a disease or trait is the observation that it "runs in families". Geneticists refer to such clustering as familial aggregation. While the notion of a trait running in families appears simple, several different approaches to demonstrating familial aggregation can and have been employed, each with its own attendant advantages and disadvantages. Here we describe the primary study designs that geneticists and epidemiologists use.

Generally, there are two approaches to demonstrating familial aggregation: (1) Show that the risk for the trait among the relatives of affected individuals (cases) is greater than among some comparison group; this comparison group can be a predetermined population prevalence, an unrelated control group (for example, spouses or acquaintances of the cases) or the relatives of a group of unaffected individuals comparable to the cases (controls). (2) Show that the proportion of cases with an affected relative (positive family history) exceeds the same proportion among a suitable control group. Which of these approaches is employed is an analysis issue, but also depends somewhat on the design of the family study.

Because there are inherent biases in obtaining information about family members, modern studies generally employ control groups to equalize potential errors and biases. There are three common ways information about relatives is obtained: (1) by eliciting this information from the index subjects. This is referred to as family history because information about relatives is indirect and by history only; sometimes, information will be obtained from a second reporter on the family as well; (2) by interviewing the relatives themselves; this is called family study; and (3) by sending questionnaires to the relatives; this is similar to (2), but generally does not involve direct contact of the relatives with study personnel.

The primary advantage of family history is that it is efficient and inexpensive. Information about a sizeable number of relatives can be obtained simply by interviewing the index subjects. The main disadvantages of family history are that it is unreliable and potentially biased. It has been well documented that sensitivity of family history (i.e., identification of true cases) decreases with the distance of the genetic relationship (e.g., going from first to second or third degree relatives). Also, when subtleties of diagnosis are involved, family history can lead to incorrect diagnosis as well as general underreporting. To reduce this problem, some studies will use a second informant aside from the index case. While this often improves the information content, it does not entirely eliminate the unreliability. To some extent biases are reduced by using comparable methods to obtain family history information from the cases and controls, but they cannot be eliminated entirely. It is conceivable that affected individuals or those with the trait have greater awareness of the same disease state or trait in their relatives than would someone without the disease or trait. Thus, what would appear as evidence of familial aggregation would actually be greater awareness on the part of affected individuals.

A critical issue in obtaining information about relatives, and one that is often overlooked, is blindness on the part of study investigators in making diagnostic assessments on relatives. Specifically, if the investigator is aware of whether the subject being interviewed is a relative of a case or control, an inherent bias can enter into the assessment process, with a tendency to overdiagnose relatives of cases and underdiagnose relatives of controls. Thus, interviewers should be unaware of the subject's status. Of course, blindness is generally not possible with the family history method, because interviewers know whether they are interviewing a case or control, and the case awareness bias cannot be eliminated.

Often controls will be matched to the cases on relevant criteria, such as demographic variables (age, sex, ethnicity) to eliminate confounding. From an epidemiologic standpoint, this makes sense in a family history design, because

information about cases and controls, including family history, is compared. It makes less sense in a family interview study, because it is the relatives who are being compared, and these relatives have not been matched. Matching cases and controls will lead to matching of relatives for some variables (e.g., ethnicity), but not others (e.g., age, sex). Furthermore, cases are generally not matched to controls for *number* of relatives. These characteristics lead to special problems in data analysis, as described below.

There are two approaches to analyzing data from family studies. The first is based on comparing the proportion of index cases who have a positive family history to the same proportion among control subjects. From an epidemiologic perspective, this would be a "case-control" type analysis, and allows for the simultaneous consideration of potential confounding variables such as age, sex, ethnicity and so on. The major difficulty in this approach is in defining "positive family history". If only a single relative is considered (e.g., mother), then there is no problem because the outcome is simply dichotomous (e.g., mother affected or not). However, when there are multiple relatives evaluated, it is unclear how to define positive family history. For example, suppose information is obtained for both parents and all siblings (all first-degree relatives) of index cases and controls. Usually, positive family history is then defined as at least one first-degree relative affected. However, this outcome will be strongly confounded with the *number* of first-degree relatives. For example, a proband with four sibs will be more likely to have a positive family history than one with a single sib. A related problem is that for diseases with variable and/or late age of onset, positive family history will depend on the ages of the relatives, which again is not taken into account. Thus, a proband with older relatives is more likely to have a positive family history than one with younger relatives.

The second limitation is that when more than one relative is affected, such information cannot be used directly. For example, the variable "family history" would be recorded the same if a proband had three affected relatives as if he had one. While this does not generally lead to a directional bias, it does not allow for maximal use of the information.

The second method of analysis is a cohort analysis. In this case, it is the proportion of relatives who are affected among the cases that is contrasted with the same proportion among the controls. Because rates are being calculated for the relatives directly, the denominator is the total number of relatives, and so variable number of relatives across subjects is not a confounder. Also, age of the relatives can be included in the analysis by calculating age specific risks for the case and control relatives, for example, by life-table analysis or survival methods. Also, since the numerator is the total number affected, for cases with multiple affected relatives, all can be included directly. Finally, while matching of cases to controls only leads to direct matching of relatives for certain variables (e.g., ethnicity), it is still possible to adjust for potential confounders, such as sex or age, by stratified analysis when calculating rates in relatives. A potential disadvantage of this approach is that trait status may not be independent among the relatives of individual cases (or controls); however, under the null hypothesis of no familial aggregation, these relatives would be independent, and so the test is not biased.

As recent examples, we consider familial aggregation studies of breast cancer. Mettlin et al. (1990) examined the distribution of family history reported by 779 breast cancer cases and 1558 controls obtained from Roswell Park Memorial Institute, Buffalo, New York. These data are reproduced in Table 15.2. The cases and controls were also stratified by age at onset or current age, dichotomized at age 55. Defining positive family history as at least one first-degree relative (mother, sister or daughter) affected with breast cancer, 144 of 779 breast cancer cases, or 18.5%, reported a positive family history, compared to 191 of 1558 controls, or 12.3%. These values give a relative risk (odds ratio) of breast cancer associated with a positive family history of 1.62. When probands were dichotomized at age 55, the relative risk actually appeared greater for the over age 55 group, 1.88, compared with the earlier onset group, 1.34.

Onset of breast cancer is highly age-dependent with most cases occurring after age 50. Thus, younger probands are likely to have younger relatives who have not experienced as much risk as the relatives of older probands. This fact can confound studies evaluating family history characteristics of probands.

As a second example, we consider the results of Claus et al. (1990). These authors analyzed the family history data from the Cancer and Steroid Hormone (CASH) study, a multicenter epidemiologic case-control study of the risk of breast, ovarian and endometrial cancer associated with usage of steroid hormones (Wingo et al., 1988). All cases and controls were asked about family history in first-degree relatives, including mothers and sisters. In this study, the relatives were treated as a cohort, and age-specific cumulative risks were calculated for mothers and sisters of cases and controls. The probands were stratified into four groups based on their age of onset. The results are reproduced in Figures 15.1 and 15.2. The case's age of onset had a significant effect on risk of disease in relatives: the earlier the age of onset, the greater the risk. The lack of such an age effect (using age at interview) among the controls suggests this effect is real and not the result of proband age-associated reporting bias. Furthermore, these data demonstrate an increased disease incidence in relatives of cases (of all ages) versus the relatives of controls. This is true even for cases with onset between 50 and 54, although the effect is least in this group.

Sometimes it is also useful to examine family recurrence patterns in light of who in the family is already affected. For

Table 15.2. Case-Control Analysis of Breast Cancer Risk by Family History, for 779 Breast Cancer Cases and 1,558 Controls form Roswell Park Memorial Institute

	Age <55		Age ≥55		Total	
	Cases	Controls	Cases	Controls	Cases	Controls
Total	358	716	421	842	779	1558
FH+	58	90	86	101	144	191
FH−	300	626	335	741	635	1367
RR	1.34	1.00	1.88	1.00	1.62	1.00

FH+ = at least one first degree relative with breast cancer; FH− = no first degree relative with breast cancer; RR = relative risk. (From Mettlin et al., 1990, with permission.)

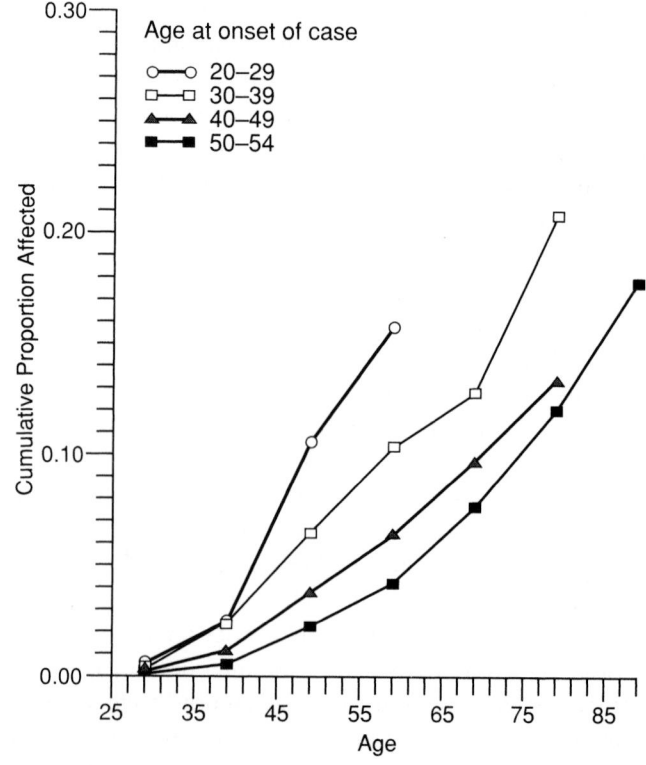

Fig. 15.1. Observed cumulative risk of breast cancer for mothers and sisters of white cases by age at onset of the case, Cancer and Steroid Hormone Study, 1980–1982. (From Claus et al., 1990, with permission.)

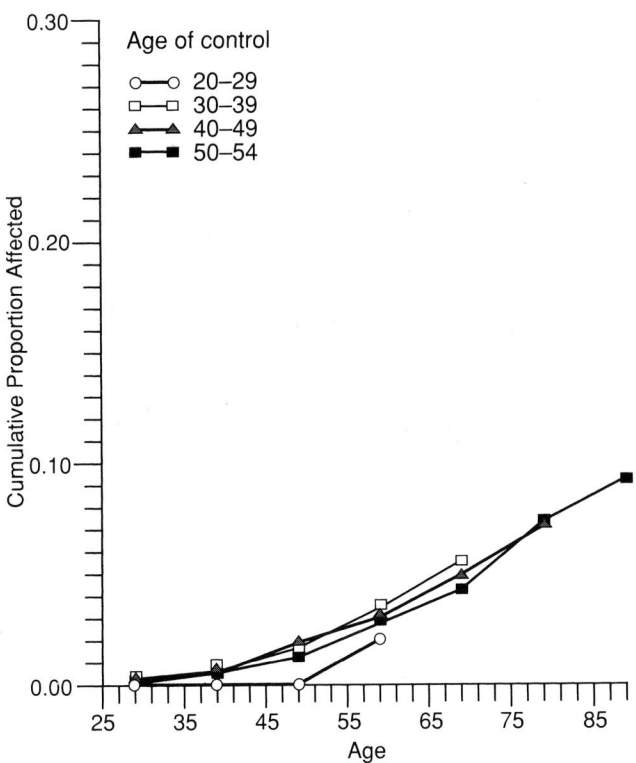

Fig. 15.2. Observed cumulative risk of breast cancer for mothers and sisters of white controls by current age of control, Cancer and Steroid Hormone Study, 1980–1982. (From Claus et al., 1990, with permission.)

Table 15.3. Cumulative Risk (in Percent) of Breast Cancer in Sisters of breast Cancer Cases by Mother's Breast Cancer Status, CASH study

	Sister with	
Age of Sister	Mother Affected	Mother Unaffected
29	0.71	0.04
34	2.27	0.34
39	4.95	0.84
44	7.94	1.94
49	12.20	3.01
54	15.92	4.03
59	15.92	5.67
64	25.26	7.94
69	25.26	11.17

(From Claus et al., 1990, with permission.)

example, Claus et al. (1990) also examined the risk to sisters of CASH breast cancer cases stratified by whether the mother of the case was also affected. The results from this analysis are given in Table 15.3. It is clear from this table that the age-specific cumulative risk to sisters is substantially greater if the mother of the proband is also affected (up to sevenfold at early ages, threefold at later ages). These results, along with those in Figure 15.1, were used to suggest that the inheritance of susceptibility to breast cancer is largely due to the effect of a rare autosomal dominant gene conferring early onset of disease with high penetrance, but that the large majority of breast cancer cases have no such inherited susceptibility (Schwartz et al., 1985; Newman et al., 1988; Claus et al., 1990, 1991). This conjecture was ultimately confirmed by the finding of linkage of early onset breast cancer to chromosome 17q (Hall et al., 1990) and 13q (Wooster et al., 1994) and the subsequent cloning of the 17q-linked and 13q-linked genes, *BRCA1* (Miki et al., 1994) and *BRCA2* (Wooster et al., 1995).

Family studies can also be used to determine whether common genetic factors underlie distinct clinical phenotypes. This is done by searching for coaggregation of different diseases or traits within the same family. A classic example of this analysis was given by Smith (1976) for the

related birth defects anencephaly and spina bifida. This author showed that parents who had a child with anencephaly were at increased risk of having a subsequent child with spina bifida. The reverse was also true, that a previous child with spina bifida increased the risk for a later anencephalic child. These results strongly suggested a common genetic etiology for the two defects.

More recently, Schildkraut et al. (1989) used the CASH study data to determine the degree to which common genetic factors underlie breast, ovarian and endometrial cancers. These authors found that the first-degree relatives (mothers and sisters) of the breast cancer probands were at increased risk of breast and ovarian cancer but not endometrial cancer. Similarly, the relatives of the ovarian cancer probands were at increased risk of ovarian and of breast cancer, but not endometrial cancer. The relatives of the endometrial cancer cases were only at increased risk of endometrial cancer. This risk ratios are reproduced in Table 15.4. The greatest risk ratios are for site-specific recurrence, but there is also clearly an inherited correlation between breast and ovarian cancer. This conclusion has subsequently been verified through the identification of *BRCA1* on chromosome 17q and *BRCA2* on chromosome 13q, which increase the risk of both breast and ovarian cancer (Narod et al., 1995; Gayther et al., 1997).

Similarly, subclassification of a disease into discrete subgroups, and the analysis of these subgroups in family studies, can provide clues to the genetic relatedness of these subgroups. Also, if one subgroup appears to be clinically "more severe", it is possible to determine whether the genetic contribution to the "severe" form is greater than the "milder" form by examining recurrence risks in the relatives of probands with the different forms. As an

Table 15.4. Age-Adjusted Relative Risks of Breast, Ovarian, and Endometrial Cancer in First-Degree Relatives (Mothers and Sisters) of Breast, Ovarian and Endometrial Cancer Cases; CASH study

Proband Dx	Relative Dx	RR
Breast	Breast	2.1
	Ovary	1.7
	Endometrium	0.9
Ovary	Breast	1.2
	Ovary	2.8
	Endometrium	1.1
Endometrium	Breast	1.2
	Ovary	0.6
	Endometrium	2.7

From Schildkraut et al., 1989, with permission.)

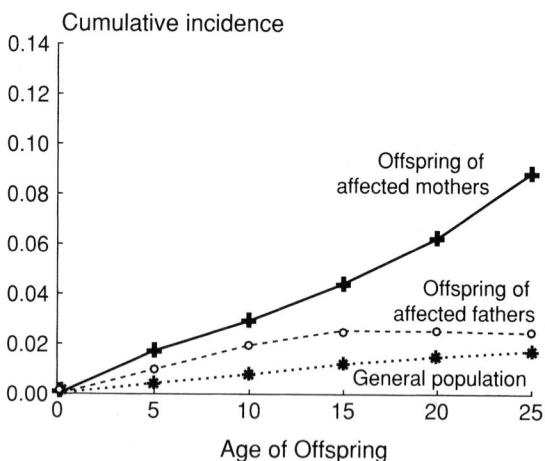

Fig. 15.3. Comparison of risk of epilepsy among the offspring of female epileptic probands and male epileptic probands. (From Ottman, 1988, with permission.)

example, we consider the birth defect cleft lip, which can occur as an isolated malformation or in conjunction with a cleft palate (CL + P). Such clefts can occur as a unilateral manifestation (i.e., only one side affected), or bilaterally (both sides affected). Either phenomenon, palate involvement or bilaterality could be considered as clinically more severe. To further complicate the situation, the palate is more likely to be involved if the defect is bilateral, that is, the conditions are correlated. In a meta analysis of various data sets, Mitchell and Risch (1993) showed that when bilaterality of the proband's defect was considered simultaneously with palate involvement, there was an increased recurrence risk in sibs associated with bilaterality but not palate involvement. Thus, bilaterality does appear to be associated with a greater genetic predisposition than a unilateral defect.

Sex-specific patterns of recurrence in family studies can provide insights regarding unusual genetic phenomena, such as X-linked inheritance, genomic imprinting or mitochondrial inheritance. For example, Ottman et al. (1988) have shown an increased risk of epilepsy among the offspring of female epileptic probands compared with the offspring of male probands (see Fig. 15.3). This phenomenon has been repeatedly seen, but apparently is not consistent with any, as yet defined, genetic inheritance pattern such as X-linkage or mitochondrial inheritance.

Finally, it needs to be mentioned that family studies are only the first line of evidence that genetic factors may be involved in the trait under study. Familial aggregation is a necessary, but not sufficient condition to infer a genetic basis. For example, numerous traits aggregate in families, such as wealth, religion or language, but it is unlikely that genes play much of a role in such clustering.

Twin studies

The biological and genetic basis for twinning is described in detail in Chapter 19. To review, identical, or monozygotic (MZ) twins share 100% of their genetic material in common, while fraternal, or dizygotic (DZ) twins share, on average, 50% of their genetic material in common. The 50% is only an average, because segregation of genes in meioses can lead to greater or less than 50% identity, but in general it will be quite close to one-half. The study of the relative similarity of monozygotic twins versus dizygotic twins has been the basis of an entire research discipline for the past century; a plethora of diseases and traits have been subjected to this paradigm.

In the twin study design, the similarity between MZ twins is compared with the similarity between DZ twins. But how is similarity defined? For discrete traits (such as diseases), it is defined by concordance, which means the proportion of twin pairs that both have the trait. There are two type of concordance rates – pairwise and probandwise. The difference has to do with the method by which the twins were identified. Generally, only pairs where at least one twin has the trait of interest are considered. Concordant pairs are those where both twins have the trait of interest; discordant pairs are those where one twin has the trait, the other does not. Pairwise concordance is defined as the simple proportion of all pairs (concordant plus discordant) that are concordant. This is always the simplest statistic to calculate. Comparing pairwise concordances for MZ versus DZ twins is usually the easiest statistical approach for demonstrating a genetic contribution to the trait (i.e., by showing that the MZ concordance is greater than the

DZ concordance). However, pairwise concordance is not a useful statistic for estimating the *magnitude* of the genetic contribution; for this, the probandwise concordance is preferable. In essence, the probandwise concordance is simply the recurrence risk of the trait in the co-twin of a proband. The notion of proband relates to how the twins were initially ascertained, and is identical to its use in segregation analysis as described in Chapter 7. The logic is as follows. Any individual who is the co-twin of a proband is counted, both in the numerator and denominator. So, for a discordant twin pair, only the twin without the trait is counted, because (s)he is a co-twin of a proband (the affected twin); the affected twin cannot be counted, because s(he) is not the co-twin of a proband. Concordant pairs are more complicated. If both twins of such a pair are probands, then both can be counted in the numerator and denominator, because both are co-twins of probands. However, if only one twin is a proband, only the non-proband twin can be counted, because only that individual is the co-twin of a proband.

In practice, the difficulty lies in defining which of the twins are probands. If only one twin was initially identified, and the second twin's trait status determined as part of the study, proband status is straightforward – only the first twin is a proband. If both twins were initially identified, then both are potential probands, but this depends on the assumption that each twin would have appeared even if the co-twin had not; often, this is impossible to know. In population-based twin studies, where all twins are identified independent of the trait, the issue of defining probands is simplified, as all twins with the trait can be considered to be probands.

A manufactured example is given in Table 15.5. A total of 100 MZ and 100DZ twin pairs has been identified. According to the table, 16 of the 100 MZ twin pairs are concordant, giving a pairwise concordance of 16%. By contrast, 5 of 100 DZ pairs are concordant, or a pairwise concordance of 5%. To calculate probandwise concordance of MZ pairs, we note that four concordant pairs get counted twice, so we get a probandwise concordance of $(8 + 12)/(8 + 12 + 84) = 20/104 = 19\%$. Similarly, for DZ pairs, we get $(2 + 4)/(2 + 4 + 95) = 6/101 = 6\%$.

Twin studies are also employed in the investigation of quantitative traits, such as height, weight, intelligence quotient, and so on. Instead of concordance rate, the intraclass correlation for the twin pairs is calculated. As for discrete traits, a higher MZ correlation than DZ correlation is taken as evidence for a genetic component.

There are numerous caveats in interpreting a higher MZ than DZ concordance as evidence of a genetic etiology. Some have to do with the manner in which the twins are ascertained, others with the assumptions underlying the design itself. Many twin studies are based on volunteers, often in response to advertment. It is known that volunteer studies lead to an excess of MZ and female twin pairs; also, because the trait under study is described in the solicitation, it is also possible that concordant twin pairs are more likely to volunteer than discordant ones, leading to an inflation of the concordance rate. If the bias toward concordant pairs is greater among MZ twins than DZ twins, the study design will be compromised, because the evidence for heritability comes from a higher MZ than DZ concordance. The studies with the least potential for bias are those that are population based, where all twins are surveyed independent of the trait of interest.

The genetic evidence from twin studies comes from the excess concordance, or correlation, for MZ twins compared to DZ twins; this is because MZ twins share more of their genetic constitution than do DZ twins. However, the critical assumption being made is that MZ twins do *not* share any non-genetic or environmental factors underlying the trait to a greater extent than do DZ pairs. While MZ and DZ twins may share similar life experiences due to common gestation, age and parentage, it is still conceivable that MZ twins share their environments to a greater extent than do DZ twins. For example, it is known that MZ twins tend to stay in closer contact and live closer to each other throughout life than do DZ twins.

Despite the caveats, twin studies have been used quite extensively and effectively to implicate (or not) a genetic component for a range of physical characteristics, disease states, and behavioral traits. There is vast literature on the use of twins in behavioral genetics research. As an example, Gottesman (1991) reviewed the literature on twin studies of schizophrenia and found consistency across studies for higher MZ than DZ concordance rates (Table 15.6), although there were substantial differences in concordance rates across studies, probably due to different diagnostic procedures. These data have been interpreted to provide strong evidence for a genetic contribution to schizophrenia.

Because twin studies are a special type of family study, they can also be used to address issues of etiologic heterogeneity, genetic relatedness of distinct phenotypes, and age of onset issues. For example, Marenberg et al. (1994) analyzed the Swedish Twin Cohort (a population-based twin study of

Table 15.5. Example of Data Derived from a Twin Study

Zygosity	Concordant		Discordant
	2 Probands	1 Proband	
MZ	4	12	84
DZ	1	4	95

Table 15.6. Modern Twin Studies of Schizophrenia

Country (year)	MZ		DZ	
	N	Probandwise Concordance	N	Probandwise Concordance
Finland (1963/1971)	17	.35	20	.13
Norway (1967)	55	.45	90	.15
Denmark (1973)	21	.56	41	.27
United Kingdom (1966/1987)	22	.58	33	.15
United States (1969/1983)	164	.31	277	.06

(From Gottesman, 1991, with permission.)

Table 15.7. Risk Ratios for Death from CVD by Age at CVD Death in Cotwins

Age at Death	Males		Females	
	MZ	DZ	MZ	DZ
36–55	13.4	4.3		
56–65	8.1	2.6	14.9	2.2
66–75	4.3	1.7	3.9	1.9
76–85	1.9	1.4	2.2	1.4
≥86	0.9	0.7	1.1	1.0

(From Marenberg et al., 1994, with permission.)

7310 MZ twin pairs and 13,694 DZ twins pairs) for cardiovascular disease (CVD) mortality. In this analysis, age at CVD death was divided into age intervals, and hazard rates for CVD mortality in the co-twin were calculated. The results (Table 15.7) showed hazards elevated at early ages of CVD mortality in the co-twin and then decreasing at later ages for both MZ and DZ twins. However, the ratio of hazards for MZ versus DZ twins also showed an age effect, with a high ratio at early ages that decreased at later ages. These results were interpreted as demonstrating the importance of genetic factors in causing early CVD mortality, and the lessening effect of these factors with increasing age.

In summary, twin studies are a valuable part of the genetic epidemiologist's arsenal of study designs. If done and interpreted carefully, they can provide important evidence regarding the genetic contribution to a trait or disease.

Adoption studies

Adoption studies provide a powerful approach for separating the contributions of genetic versus shared environmental effects to a disease or trait. The rationale of adoption studies is that when a child is adopted away at birth, separation is created between his/her genetic and environmental (rearing) contributions from a biological parent. Thus, by looking at various family constellations and relationships involving adoptees, it is possible to separately estimate the effects of genes and shared environment.

In general, in adoption studies, two comparisons can be made: the recurrence rates in non-biological (adopted) relatives who shared a common rearing environment (design 1); and the recurrence rates in biological relatives who shared no common environment (design 2). Design 1 is usually easier to execute because it does not require identification of biological relatives of adoptees. A typical example of design 1 was recently given by Ebers et al. (1995) for multiple sclerosis (MS), the first adoption study for any presumed autoimmune disease. These authors screened a population of 15,000 Canadian MS patients and identified adoptees as well as non-adopted cases who had adopted (i.e., non-biological) siblings or had adopted children themselves. This provided a total of 1201 non-biological relatives (470 parents, 345 sibs, 386 children) who had shared a common rearing environment with the proband. Out of the total of 1201 relatives of MS cases, only a single additional case of MS was identified, a rate identical to the population prevalence. Using age-adjusted rates observed for biological first-degree relatives from a previous Canadian study, the authors estimated that approximately 25 additional MS cases would have been identified had these relatives been biological. The low rate of MS in the reared-together non-biological relatives, comparable to population prevalence, provides evidence that the familial aggregation observed for this disease is genetic in origin.

Adoption studies of type 2 are often difficult, if not impossible to perform because adoptees usually do not know their biological relatives, and the sealing of adoption records makes the identification of these relatives untenable. One country in which such studies have been possible is Denmark because of a national registry system of all births, which allows the subsequent identification of biological relatives of all adopted individuals. This registry, along with another national registry of psychiatric inpatients, was used quite effectively by Seymour Kety and his colleagues (1975) to construct an adoption study of schizophrenia using design 2. These authors identified 34 schizophrenic adoptees from the Copenhagen area and created a control group of 34 non-schizophrenic adoptees from the same area. The biological relatives of the 34 schizophrenic adoptees were identified from the population registry, as were the biological relatives of the non-schizophrenic adoptees. Psychiatric interviews were then conducted with these relatives, where the interviewer was blinded to the status of the relative (i.e., relative of schizophrenic or non-schizophrenic adoptee). Out of a total of 173 biological relatives of the schizophrenic adoptees, 5 were found to be schizophrenic. By contrast, none of the biological relatives of the non-schizophrenic adoptees were so affected. Because these biological relatives shared no rearing environment in common, the authors concluded that familial aggregation of schizophrenia is genetic in origin. This study was subsequently expanded to include the rest of Denmark, with similar results to the first study; the rate of schizophrenia in the biological relatives of the schizophrenia adoptees was 10-fold greater than in the relatives of the control adoptees (Kety et al., 1994).

Another variant of this adoption design was previously performed by Leonard Heston (1966). In this study, 47 schizophrenic women who had given birth to a child in a state mental hospital were identified; for comparison, the author identified 50 non-schizophrenic mothers from the same hospital who had also given up their children for adoption. He then followed up these children to determine their mental status. Of the 47 biological children of the schizophrenic mothers, 5, or 11%, were found to be schizophrenic. By contrast, only 1 of the 50 children, or 2%, of the non-schizophrenic mothers were schizophrenic. Because neither group of children had shared a rearing environment with the biological mother, the author was able to conclude that the familial recurrence of schizophrenia has a genetic origin.

Again, because adoption studies are a special type of family study, where the separation of genetic and environmental contributions is possible, such studies are especially useful for defining the genetic relatedness of various phenotypes. For example, the Danish Adoption Study of Schizophrenia has provided excellent material for defining psychiatric conditions genetically related to schizophrenia. Reanalyzing all the psychiatric interview data from the original study with DSM III-R criteria, Kendler et al. (1994) found that certain non-schizophrenic psychotic disorders and non-psychotic personality disorders aggregated in the biological relatives of the schizophrenic adoptees. In particular, schizoaffective disorder (mainly schizophrenic) and schizotypal personality disorder were found to be genetically related to schizophrenia.

Although up to this point we have only discussed discrete outcomes (e.g., diseases), the adoption design can and has also been used to study continuous traits. For example, the same Danish Population Registry was used to show a genetic contribution to weight, and in particular human obesity (Stunkard et al., 1986).

Another useful variant of the adoption study design is the focus on half-sibs. Because over the past several decades divorce has become more common, the prevalence of half-sibs, i.e., those who share only one biological parent, has also increased. This phenomenon allows for the comparison of several distinct types of relationships. For example, some half-sibs will be raised together in the same household by the shared biological parent, while others will be raised in different households. Thus, in similar fashion to the adoption study design, half-sibs raised together can be contrasted to half-sibs raised apart. As an additional comparison, full sibs from the same families can also be considered. On average, half sibs share 25% of their genetic material in common, compared to 50% for full sibs. If a trait under study is genetically determined, then the half-sib recurrence (or correlation) should be less than that for full sibs, and the rates for half-sibs raised together or apart should be the same. By contrast, if the trait were environmentally determined, then the rates for half sibs raised together should be greater than for those raised apart, while the rate for full sibs raised together should be similar to the rate for half-sibs raised together.

Half-sib studies generally have less power than adoption studies based on full sibs because the genetic correlation for full sibs is twice as large. Nonetheless, because of the difficulty in performing adoption studies of biological relatives raised apart, half-sib studies will likely continue to play an important role in genetic epidemiology (Tierney et al., 1994).

Perhaps the most powerful of all genetic-epidemiologic study designs combines the adoption and twin paradigms. In this case, the usual twin design of contrasting MZ and DZ twins is extended to include the study of twins who were adopted into separate homes at birth, and thus shared no rearing environment in common. Thus, with this approach there are four groups of twins: MZ twins reared together, MZ twins reared apart, DZ twins reared together and DZ twins reared apart. Under a purely genetic hypothesis, the concordance (or correlation) between MZ twins should be the same whether they were reared together or apart, and similarly for DZ twins; however, the concordance between MZ twins should be greater than for DZ twins. According to an environmental hypothesis, the twins reared together (MZ or DZ) should have the largest concordances, while those raised apart should have lower values. Of course, the rarity of twins separated at birth makes this design feasible only for traits that are very common, or continuous traits. An example of the application of this design is the study of Hanson et al. (1991) on the genetic basis of allergy and asthma. This study was based on 34 pairs of MZ twins raised together, 53 pairs of MZ twins raised apart, 29 pairs of DZ twins raised together and 21 pairs of DZ twins raised apart. For asthma, none of the DZ pairs were found to be concordant, while 4 discordant pairs were found, 2 each in the raised together and raised apart groups. For the MZ twins raised apart, 4 concordant pairs were found and 1 discordant pair, for a probandwise concordance of 89%. For the MZ twins raised together, 2 concordant pairs were found and 1 discordant pair, for a probandwise concordance of 80%. The similarly high concordance rates for MZ twins raised together or apart (80–89%) and low rates for DZ twins (0%) suggests the importance of genetic susceptibility factors for this condition, although the numbers are small.

Such studies can also be employed for common, quantitative traits. For example, Stunkard et al. (1990) recently used the twin-adoption design to provide further support for a strong genetic component to body mass index and human obesity. They found similarly high correlations in body mass index for MZ twins raised apart or together, and much lower, but similar correlations for the DZ twins raised apart or together.

Characterizing the genetic component

The study designs described so far provide useful insights regarding the relative importance of genetic factors to the trait or disease of interest, but they cannot identify the specific factors involved. The advent of sophisticated molecular genetic methods over the last two decades, however, has now raised the prospect that many genes underlying susceptibility to a range of conditions and traits, common and rare, will be identified. Indeed, numerous such genes have already been found.

To date, the primary mode of gene identification has been positional cloning, where the initial indication of a gene's location is determined by linkage analysis. Linkage analysis is discussed in detail in Chapter 8; here we describe its relevance in genetic epidemiology. The great majority of genes identified through linkage analysis and positional cloning are those that underlie mendelian traits or syndromes, i.e., those that have a simple dominant, recessive or X-linked pattern of inheritance. Diseases with mendelian inheritance patterns tend to be quite rare.

Genetic epidemiology also tends to focus on common familial diseases without clear mendelian inheritance patterns. The reason for the lack of simple inheritance patterns for these diseases is that the genetic basis is not attributable to the effect of a single gene, but rather likely due to the combined effect of multiple contributing loci. It is important to have some idea of the genetic basis for a phenotype of interest before undertaking a linkage study because the optimal design of the study will depend on such information.

For some common diseases with complex inheritance patterns there exist subsets that appear to have a mendelian (usually autosomal dominant) pattern. Often, these subsets are syndromic in the sense that they are associated with distinct clinical features. Most prominent among these are mendelian cancer syndromes, such as those for colon cancer and breast cancer. In each case, most tumors are not due to an inherited susceptibility; however, in a small proportion of cases, the cancer susceptibility seems to be inherited in an autosomal dominant fashion, with multiple generations affected. For breast cancer, these pedigrees are generally associated with early onset of disease; for colon cancer, a similar story prevails. To date, two dominant breast cancer susceptibility genes have been cloned (Miki et al., 1994; Wooster et al., 1995).

The dominant colon cancer syndromes show some interesting clinical differences. Familial adenomatous polyposis is due to a gene on chromosome 5 (Groden et al., 1991; Kinzler et al., 1991) and leads to a colon lined with polyps, causing increased risk of colon cancer. The other colon cancer genes identified, those on chromosomes 2p, 2q, 3p and 7p, are homologous DNA mismatch repair enzymes, and are associated with a clinically more typical picture, but are still associated with relatively early age of onset (Fishel et al., 1993; Leach et al., 1993; Bronner et al., 1994; Nicolaides et al., 1994; Papadopoulos et al., 1994).

Another striking example of this phenomenon exists with Alzheimer disease (AD). This disease occurs with high frequency among the elderly, but rarely strikes before the sixth decade of life. Yet numerous pedigrees with apparent autosomal dominant inheritance of AD occurring with early onset have been found, giving rise to the eponym Familial Alzheimer Disease (FAD). These pedigrees have been used to clone three different FAD genes, one on chromosome 21 (Goate et al., 1991), one on chromosome 14 (Sherrington et al., 1995) and one on chromosome 1 (Levy-Lahad et al., 1995a, b).

When mendelian subsets of a common disease exist, especially when they are autosomal dominant, by far the best strategy for linkage analysis is a parametric, lod score approach using extended pedigrees likely to harbor these mutations. How can one know before hand that such dominant genes exist? First, as in the cases of breast and colon cancer, or FAD, if "dominant appearing" pedigrees exist and such pedigrees have "clinically" distinct character, for example early age of onset, such evidence is highly suggestive. However, it is possible that dominant families exist but are clinically typical; confidence that these families are segregating a dominant susceptibility gene a priori is usually less compelling.

Another approach that has been used to implicate the role of autosomal dominant susceptibility genes is complex segregation analysis (see Ch. 7). While the results of such analyses are often ambiguous, it has been successfully employed in breast cancer, where the analyses suggested a rare autosomal dominant susceptibility gene with high penetrance and early age of onset (Williams and Anderson, 1984; Bishop et al., 1988; Newman et al., 1988; Claus et al., 1991).

Accounting for the mendelian disease subsets still leaves us with a vast array of common diseases with a likely complex genetic pattern of inheritance involving multiple genes with interactive effects. What is the best way to identify the genes underlying these disorders? Often, for such diseases, it is far easier to find families with a small number of affected members, such as relative pairs; for example, sib pairs, avuncular pairs or cousin pairs. Such families lend themselves quite easily to linkage analysis using "non-parametric" methods based on identity by descent (Risch, 1990 a,b,c) or identity by state (Weeks and Lange, 1988; Bishop and Williamson, 1990). Such methods are considered "robust" because they do not depend on the precise mode of inheritance; rather, they depend on a gene having a sufficient effect to lead to excess allele sharing by affected relatives. In fact, Risch (1990 a,b,c) has shown how to characterize the effect of a susceptibility gene in terms of risk ratios for relatives compared to population prevalence attributable to that gene (a measure of familial aggregation). These ratios were termed λ_R (for example, λ_S for sibs, λ_C for cousins); he also showed that identity by descent, and thus power to detect linkage at a disease locus is directly related to λ_R.

Studies of numerous complex diseases, using full genome screens with affected relative pair designs are now beginning to appear. The first such studies were of type 1 diabetes (Davies et al., 1994; Hashimoto et al., 1994), although the number of families included in these studies was relatively small. Both of these studies suggested evidence for additional susceptibility loci for this disease aside from the HLA and INS loci (previously known), but these results were not strongly statistically significant and have not been confirmed in subsequent studies (Concannon et al., 1998). In any event, these studies have demonstrated that there is only a single gene with large effect underlying type 1 diabetes, the HLA region of chromosome 6p, and that other contributing loci have much smaller effects.

The second mode of gene identification is the candidate gene approach. While sometimes candidate genes are identified after a linkage search has narrowed the location to a small chromosomal region, here we mean genes whose function are known are candidates for a trait or disease independent of their chromosomal location. The primary method for studying the role of a candidate gene is the association study, whereby allele frequencies are compared between affected and unaffected individuals. Because population stratification can induce an artifactual association (see Ch. 14), more recent studies focus on alleles possessed by parents not transmitted to affected offspring as controls (Falk and Rubinstein, 1987; Terwilliger and Ott, 1992; Spielman et al., 1993; Thomson, 1995) or unaffected sibs (Penrose et al., 1939; Clarke et al., 1956; Curtis, 1997; Boehnke and Langefeld, 1998; Risch and Teng, 1998; Schaid and Rowland, 1998; Spielman and Ewens, 1998) to eliminate this problem. When a polymorphism in a candidate gene influences the risk of disease, association studies can be far more powerful than linkage studies, provided the causative polymorphism or one in strong linkage disequilibrium with it is used (Risch, 1987; Greenberg, 1993). For example, numerous association studies have shown that polymorphism at a *VNTR* locus flanking the insulin gene (*INS*) on chromosome 11p influences the risk of type 1 diabetes; however, the effect is not sufficiently strong to detect with linkage studies using non-associated markers (Risch, 1987; Spielman et al., 1993). Because many of the genes underlying common, familial non-mendelian diseases are likely to have only minor effects, we can predict that in the future most of those genes will be determined through association studies, as more and more candidate genes are identified through the human genome initiative (Risch and Merikangas, 1996). Also, the prospect of typing a large number of simple nucleotide polymorphisms (SNPs) leads to alternative marker based approaches for controlling for population stratification (Devlin and Roeder, 1999; Pritchard and Rosenberg, 1999), obviating the need for related controls.

Gene-environment interaction

Ultimately, genetic epidemiology attempts to understand both the genetic and environmental factors that determine a trait or disease, and how these factors relate to one another. Ruth Ottman (1990) has detailed the variety of ways that genetic and environmental factors can interact to create a disease phenotype. She describes five models with specific examples. For the first model, the genetic variant causes an increase in the expression of the risk factor, which leads to disease; the example given is PKU, where homozygosity for PKU mutations causes a high blood phenylalanine level, leading to mental retardation. In the second example, the gene effect is to exacerbate the effect of the risk factor; here the example is the genetic disease xeroderma pigmentosum; affected individuals are at increased sensitivity to UV irradiation for skin cancer risk. In the third model, the risk factor exacerbates the direct effect of the genotype; for example, the intake of barbiturates increases the risk of skin problems in individuals with the genetic disease porphyria variegata. For the fourth example, both the genotype and risk factor are required to elevate risk of a disease outcome; the example for this case is G6PD deficiency, and fava bean consumption, where both are necessary to lead to hemolytic anemia. In the final model, the genotype and risk factor each independently influence risk; the example is cigarette smoking and alpha-1-antitrypsin deficiency, each of which alone, or conjointly elevates the risk of emphysema. The above examples involve mendelian disease genes. Ultimately, common, complex disease phenotypes are influenced by a range of genetic variants, many of which are common. Dissecting out specific gene effects, how they interact with each other as well as with defined environmental variables remains as the major challenge facing genetic epidemiologists in the coming decades. Cardiovascular disease is a prime example of such complexity (Sing and Reilly, 1993).

Gene-environment interactions can be evaluated in the context of typical epidemiologic study designs, such as case-control studies or cohort studies. These approaches are most powerful when specific genes influencing risk have been identified. Genotypes can then be included as any other risk factor, and interactive effects between risk factors considered. In such cases, it should also be feasible to distinguish among various models, for example those described by Ottman (1990). Even when specific gene effects have not been identified, it is still possible to examine gene-environment interactions. A surrogate for genetic predisposition is family history, which, for example, could be considered in a case-control study as a contributing risk factor characteristic of cases and controls. However, in many cases, family history is likely to be only poorly correlated with actual genetic susceptibility, greatly reducing the power to detect or distinguish models of interaction.

To date, few genes for common diseases or traits have been identified. As more of these loci are found and environmental concomitants as well, the goals of genetic epidemiology will reach fruition.

REFERENCES

Bishop DT, Williamson JA (1990) The power of identity-by-state methods for linkage analysis. Am J Hum Genet 46:254–265

Bishop DT, Cannon-Albright L, McLellan T et al. (1988) Segregation and linkage analysis of nine Utah breast cancer pedigrees. Genet Epidemiol 5:151–170

Boehnke M, Langefeld C (1998) Genetic association mapping based on discordant sib pairs: The discordant alleles test. Am J Hum Genet 62:950–961

Bronner CE, Baker SM, Morrison PT et al. (1994) Mutation in the DNA mismatch repair gene homologue hMLH1 is associated with hereditary non-polyposis colon cancer. Nature 368:258–261

Clarke CA, Edwards JW, Haddock DRW et al. (1956) ABO blood groups and secretor character in duodenal ulcer. Br Med J 2:725–731

Claus EB, Risch N, Thompson WD (1990) Age of onset as an indicator of familial risk of breast cancer. Am J Epidemiol 131:961–972

Claus EB, Risch N, Thompson WD (1991) Genetic analysis of breast cancer in the Cancer and Steroid Hormone Study. Am J Hum Genet 48:232–242

Concannon P, Gogolin-Ewens KJ, Hinds DA et al. (1998) A second-generation screen of the human genome for susceptibility to insulin-dependent diabetes mellitus. Nat Genet 19:292–296

Corder EH, Saunders AM, Strittmatter WJ et al. (1993) Gene dose of apolipoprotein type 4 allele and the risk of Alzheimer disease in late onset families. Science 261:921–923

Corder EH, Saunders AM, Risch NJ et al. (1994) Apolipoprotein E-type 2 allele decrease the risk of late onset Alzheimer disease. Nature Genet 7:180–184

Curtis D (1997) Use of siblings as controls in case-control association studies. Ann Hum Genet 61:319–333

Davies JL, Kawaguchi Y, Bennett ST et al. (1994) A genome wide search for human type 1 diabetes susceptibility genes. Nature 371:130–136

Davignon J, Gregg RE, Sing CF (1988) Apolipoprotein E polymorphism and atherosclerosis. Arteriolsclerosis 8:1–21

Devlin B, Roeder K (1999) Genomic control for association studies. Biometrics 55:997–1004

Ebers GC, Sadovnick AD, Risch N (1995) A genetic basis for familial aggregation in multiple sclerosis. Nature 377:150–151

Falconer DS (1989) Introduction to Quantitative Genetics, 3rd edn. Longman, NY

Falk CT, Rubinstein P (1987) Haplotype relative risks: an easy reliable way to construct a proper control sample for risk calculations. Ann Hum Genet 51:227–233

Fishel R, Lescoe MK, Rao MRS et al. (1993) The human mutator gene homolog MSH2 and its association with hereditary nonpolyposis colorectal cancer. Cell 75:1027–1038

Gayther SA, Mangion J, Russell P et al. (1997) Variations of risks of breast and ovarian cancer associated with different germline mutations of the BRCA2 gene. Nat Genet 15:103–105

Goate A, Chartier-Harlin M-C, Mullan M et al. (1991) Segregation of a missense mutation in the amyloid precursor protein gene with familial Alzheimer's disease. Nature 349:704–706

Gottesman II (1991) Schizophrenia Genesis: The Origins of Madness. WH Freeman, NY

Greenberg DA (1993) Linkage analysis of "necessary" disease loci versus "susceptibility" loci. Am J Hum Genet 52:135–143

Groden J, Thliveris A, Samowitz W et al. (1991) Identification and characterization of the familial adenomatous polyposis coli gene. Cell 66:589–600

Hall JM, Lee MK, Newman B et al. (1990) Linkage of early-onset familial breast cancer to chromosome 17q21. Science 250:1684–1689

Hanson B, McGue M, Roitman-Johnson B et al. (1991) Atopic disease and immunoglobulin E in twins reared apart and together. Am J Hum Genet 48:873–879

Hashimoto L, Habita C, Beressi JP et al. (1994) Genetic mapping of a susceptibility locus for insulin-dependent diabetes mellitus on chromosome 11q. Nature 371:161–164

Heston LL (1966) Psychiatric disorders in foster home reared children of schizophrenic mothers. Br J Psychiatry 112:819–825

Kempthorne O (1969) An Introduction to Genetic Statistics. Iowa State University Press, Ames, IA

Kendler KS, Gruenberg AM, Kinney DK (1994) Independent diagnosis of adoptees and relatives as defined by DSM-III in the provincial and national samples of the Danish Adoption Study of Schizophrenia. Arch Gen Psychiatry 51:456–468

Kety SS, Rosenthal D, Wender PH et al. (1975) Mental illness in the biological and adoptive families of adopted individuals who have become schizophrenic: A preliminary report based on psychiatric interviews. In Fieve RR, Rosenthal D, Brill H. (eds): Genetic Research in Psychiatry. Johns Hopkins University Press, Baltimore pp. 147–165

Kety SS, Wender PH, Jacobsen B et al. (1994) Mental illness in the biological and adoptive relatives of schizophrenic adoptees: Replication of the Copenhagen Study in the rest of Denmark. Arch Gen Psychiatry 51:442–455

Khoury MJ, Beaty TH, Cohen BH (1993) Fundamentals of Genetic Epidemiology. OUP, NY

Kidd KK, Bernoco K, Carbonara AO et al. (1977) Genetic analysis of HLA associated diseases: The "illness-susceptible" gene frequency and sex ratio in ankylosing spondylitis. In Dausset J, Svejgaard A (eds): HLA and Disease. pp. 72–80

Kinzler KW, Nilbert MC, Su L-K et al. (1991) Identification of FAP locus genes from chromosome 5q21. Science 53:661–665

Leach FS, Nicolaides NC, Papadopoulos N et al. (1993) Mutations of a MutS homolog in hereditary nonpolyposis colorectal cancer. Cell 75:1215–1225

Leppert MF, Hasstedt SJ, Holm T et al. (1986) A DNA probe for the LDL receptor gene is rightly linked to hypercholesterolemia in a pedigree with early coronary disease. Am J Hum Genet 39:300–306

Levy-Lahad E, Wijsman EM, Nemens E et al. (1995a) A familial Alzheimer's disease locus on chromosome 1. Science 269:970–973

Levy-Lahad E, Wasco W, Poorkaj W et al. (1995b) "Candidate gene for the chromosome 1 familial Alzheimer's disease locus. Science 269:973–977

Marenberg M, Risch N, Berkman L et al. (1994) Genetic susceptibility to death from coronary heart disease: The Swedish twin registry. N Engl J Med 330:1041–1046

Menzel HJ, Kladetzky RG, Assmann G (1983) Apolipoprotein E polymorphism and coronary artery disease. Arteriosclerosis 3:310–315

Mettlin C, Corghan I, Natarajan N, Lane W (1990) The association of age and familial risk in a case-control study of breast cancer. Am J Epidemiol 131:973–986

Mignot E, Lin X, Arrigoni J et al. (1994) DQB1*0602 and DQA1*0102 (DQ1) are better markers than DR2 for narcolepsy in Caucasian and black Americans. Sleep 17:S60–S67

Miki Y, Swensen J, Shattuck-Eidens D et al. (1994) A strong candidate for the breast and ovarian cancer susceptibility gene BRCA1. Science 266:66–71

Mitchell LE, Risch N (1993) Correlates of genetic risk for non-syndromic cleft lip with or without cleft palate. Clin Genet 43:255–260

Morton NE, (1982) Outline of Genetic Epidemiology. S. Karger, Basel

Narod SA, Ford D, Devilee P et al. (1995) An evaluation of genetic heterogeneity in 145 breast-ovarian cancer families. Am J Hum Genet 56:254–264

Neel JV, Schull WJ (1954) Human Heredity. University of Chicago Press, Chicago

Newman B, Austin MA, Lee M, King MC (1988) Inheritance of human breast cancer: Evidence for autosomal dominant transmission in high risk families. Proc Natl Acad Sci 85:3044–3048

Nicolaides NC, Papadopoulos N, Liu B et al. (1994) Mutations of two PMS homologues in hereditary nonpolyposis colon cancer. Nature 371:75–80

Ottman R (1990) An epidemiologic approach to gene-environment interaction. Genet Epidemiol 7:177–186

Ottman R, Annegers JF, Hauser WA, Kurland LT (1988) Higher risk of seizures in offspring of mothers than of fathers with epilepsy. Am J Hum Genet 43:257–264

Papadopoulos N, Nicolaides NC, Wei YF et al. (1994) Mutation of a MurL homolog in hereditary colon cancer. Science 263:1625–1629

Penrose LS (1939) Some practical considerations in testing for genetic linkage in sib data. Ohio J Science 39:291–296

Pritchard JK, Rosenberg NA (1999) Use of unlinked genetic markers to detect population stratification in association studies. Am J Hum Genet 65:220–228

Risch N (1987) Assessing the role of HLA-linked and unlinked determinants of disease. Am J Hum Genet 40:1–14

Risch N (1990a) Linkage strategies for genetically complex traits. I. Multilocus models. Am J Hum Genet 46:222–228

Risch N (1990b) Linkage strategies for genetically complex traits. II. The power of affected relative pairs. Am J Hum Genet 46:229–241

Risch N (1990c) Linkage strategies for genetically complex traits. III. The effect of marker polymorphism on the analysis of affected relative pairs. Am J Hum Genet 46:242–253

Risch N, Merikangas K (1996) The future of genetic studies of complex human diseases. Science 273:1516–1517

Risch N, Teng J (1998) The relative power of family-based and case-control designs for association studies of complex human diseases. I. DNA pooling. Genome Res 8:1273–1288

Saunders AM, Strittmatter WJ, Schmechel D et al. (1993) Association of apolipoprotein E allele e4 with late-onset familial and sporadic Alzheimer's disease. Neurology 43:1467–1472

Schaid DJ, Rowland C (1998) Use of parents, sibs and unrelated controls for detection of associations between genetic markers and disease. Am J Hum Genet 63:1492–1506

Schildkraut J, Risch N, Thompson WD (1989) Evaluating genetic association among ovarian, breast and endometrial cancer: Evidence for a breast-ovarian relationship. Am J Hum Genet 45:521–529

Schwartz AG, King MC, Belle SH et al. (1985) Risk of breast cancer to relatives of young breast cancer patients. JNCI 75:665–668

Sherrington R, Rogaev EI, Liang Y et al. (1995) Cloning of a gene bearing missense mutations in early-onset familial Alzheimer's disease. Nature 375:754–760

Sing CF, Reilly SL (1993) Genetics of common diseases that aggregate, but do not segregate, in families. In Sing CF, Hanis CL (eds): Genetics of Cellular, Individual, Family and Population Variability. OUP, NY pp. 140–164

Smith C (1976) Statistical resolution of genetic heterogeneity in familial disease. Ann Hum Genet 39:281–290

Spielman RS, McGinnis RE, Ewens WJ (1993) Transmission test for linkage disequilibrium: The insulin gene region and insulin dependent diabetes mellitus. Am J Hum Genet 52:506–516

Spielman RS, Ewens WJ (1998) A sibship based test for linkage in the presence of association: The sib transmission/disequilibrium test. Am J Hum Genet 62:450–458

Stunkard AJ, Sorensen TIA, Hanis C et al. (1986) An adoption study of human obesity. N Engl J Med 314:193–198

Stunkard AJ, Harris JR, Pedersen NL, McCleam GE (1990) The bodymass index of twins who have been reared apart. N Engl J Med 322:1483–1487

Terwilliger JD, Ott J (1992) A haplotype-based "haplotype relative risk" approach to detecting allelic associations. Hum Hered 42:337–346

Thoday JM (1967) New insights into continuous variation. In Crow JF, Neel JV (eds): Proceedings of the Third International Congress on Human Genetics. Johns Hopkins University Press, Baltimore

Thomson G (1995) Mapping disease genes: Family-based association studies. Am J Hum Genet 57:487–498

Tierney C, Merikangas K, Risch N (1994) Feasibility of half-sibling designs for detecting a genetic component to a disease. Genet Epidemiol 11:523–538

Weeks DE, Lange K (1988) The affected pedigree-member method of linkage analysis. Am J Hum Genet 42:315–322

Williams WR, Anderson DE (1984) Genetic epidemiology of breast cancer: Segregation analysis of 200 Danish pedigrees. Genet Epidemiol 1:7–20

Wingo PA, Ory H, Layde PM, Lee NC, Cancer and Steroid Hormone Group (1988) The evaluation of the data collection process for a multi-center population based case-control design. Am J Epidemiol 128:206–217

Wooster R, Neuhausen SL, Mangion J et al. (1994) Localization of a breast cancer susceptibility gene, BRCA2 to chromosome 13q12-13. Science 265:2088–2090

Wooster R, Bignell G, Lancaster J et al. (1995) Identification of the breast cancer susceptibility gene BRCA2. Nat 378:789–792

Human developmental genetics

Jeffrey E. Ming
Maximilian Muenke

Introduction

Human congenital malformations often have a genetic contribution. Abnormal expression of a gene or genes during embryonic development can have significant consequences. Thus, understanding the genetic basis of normal development of the human embryo is essential for understanding the mechanism by which birth defects arise. In this chapter, we will first present some basic principles of development. Next, an overview of human embryonic development will be presented. We will then discuss in greater detail development of two regions, the limb and brain, and consider how abnormal development can give rise to human clinical conditions.

It has long been apparent to embryologists that the development of higher vertebrate embryos (including avian, rodent, and primate species) is very similar. The brain of a chick is grossly identifiable as a brain and has a similar overall structure and function as a human brain. This basic commonality suggests that many of the pathways involved in development in different species are similar. Many of the fundamental elements of developmental pathways are conserved not only among higher vertebrates, but also in lower vertebrates and invertebrates. Thus, many of the seminal discoveries in embryology have been derived from studies of the fly, worm, and frog, and studies using zebrafish, chick, mouse, and other animal models have provided key insights into human development. Although whether human development is governed by the precise mechanisms identified in animal models has not always been conclusively established, much of what has been learned in animal models has validity for human conditions. In this chapter, we will frequently draw on data derived from animal studies to gain insight into the genetic basis of human malformation syndromes.

Principles of patterning and development

The human body begins development as a single cell and undergoes a remarkable series of growth and differentiation steps to achieve the adult form. Clearly, a defined program must guide how the different organs form. Not only must the brain develop into a different organ than the limb or the heart, but each distinguishable functional region of the brain must be established in a specific fashion. The specification of the distinct anatomic and functional identities of different areas of each organ is critical for normal development. In addition, there must also be very specific programing in that not only does each person's brain contain the same general functional capabilities, but they are organized in the same fashion in different people. That is, not only is there the capacity for integrating visual signals coming from the eyes in the brain, but the location of the region of the brain involved in this process is the same in all people.

Several basic principles are important for understanding the potential role of different genes in development.

1. Developmental effects are mediated along cascades of signals, or pathways. A secreted factor will interact with its receptor, which will then initiate an intracellular sequence of events, culminating in a change in the cell's state. The pathway often results in activation or suppression of the activity of transcription factors, which can affect the expression of a number of genes.

2. The same factor may have many different functions. A given protein may be involved in the development of a number of different organ systems, and it may have different

roles and/or be expressed at multiple time points within a single organ. For example, the secreted factor Sonic Hedgehog is involved in the development of the nervous system, eyes, face, lungs, gut, and other organ systems. In the nervous system, it appears to have both differentiation and proliferation-inducing activities.

3.   The expression pattern of many genes is restricted both spatially and temporally. The activation of a gene in a specific region at a specific time can determine the fate of a cell, whether and where it will move, how it will interact with other cells, and other important aspects of becoming a specific cell.

4.   The concentration of a given protein to which a cell is exposed can determine the type of cell it becomes. A morphogen can induce different cell fates depending on its concentration. Many morphogens are secreted factors, and cells close to the source of the factor and that are exposed to the highest concentration of the factor adopt one fate, while cells further away from the source and exposed to a lower concentration develop another fate. For example, the type of neuron a cell becomes in the ventral spinal neural tube depends largely on the concentration of Sonic Hedgehog to which it is exposed.

5.   The degree of activation of a pathway in a given cell is dependent on the net effect of the inducers and inhibitors to which the cell is exposed. The fate of a cell depends not only on whether a pathway is activated, but also on the degree to which this or other pathways are suppressed. Both a secreted factor and its inhibitors may be present in the same tissue, and the factor may repress cells from adopting the fate induced by another factor. Methods of inhibition include direct binding and thus inactivation of a factor, competition for the same receptor, affecting the intracellular pathway, or activation of a competing pathway which has a different effect on the cell's development.

6.   There may be functional redundancy among factors for a given pathway, such that a given process may be induced by multiple factors. In this situation, "knocking out" the gene in animal models may not demonstrate all of the roles a gene/protein has, because other factors can take over the role of the missing gene. Thus, caution must be used in interpreting negative results when a gene is inactivated.

7.   The cumulative effects of mutations in several genes and environmental factors may determine the severity of a specific anomaly. While it is well known that many birth defects (e.g., cleft palate, spina bifida) and other medical conditions generally have complex inheritance patterns and depend on the level of activity of specific genes and environmental influences, this principle is also true for "single-gene" disorders. Each developmental pathway involves a number of different proteins and other molecules, and the formation of many tissues involves more than one pathway. It is the cumulative functional activity of the components of these pathways that determines the phenotype. Results of targeted gene disruption in "knockout" mice and the finding that a number of congenital anomaly syndromes are due to single gene defects indicate that decreased activity of a single gene can lead to dramatic developmental anomalies. However, even in these cases there are other contributing factors. For example, the phenotype of a knockout mouse often depends on the strain background employed. In humans, expressivity of a condition is often variable, especially in autosomal dominant conditions, even within families with the same genetic defect. The large number of identified teratogens also indicates the importance of environmental factors. Thus, while for many conditions the activity of a single gene may well have the greatest impact on the phenotype, the contribution of other genes or non-genetic factors are also important.

Overview of normal development

Development generally proceeds in a very orderly fashion in that the different organs form at specific times during the pregnancy. A critical window of development can be established for many organ systems, and environmental insults at specific times will affect most substantially those regions that are undergoing their critical period of development at that time.

THE FIRST TWO WEEKS OF DEVELOPMENT

Following fertilization, the resulting zygote undergoes a series of mitotic cleavage divisions. These cells are called blastomeres. This process gives rise to a solid ball of cells termed the morula (approximately three days after conception). Fluid accumulates to form a cavity within the morula, transforming it into a blastocyst (or blastula). As the amniotic cavity develops, the inner cell mass (embryoblast) of the blastocyst will form the embryo, while the outer cell mass will form the extraembryonic tissues, including part of the placenta.

At about six days, the blastocyst implants into the uterine lining. The inner cell mass forms two flat oval cell layers, or the bilaminar germ disc. The long axis of this structure becomes the cranial-caudal axis of the body. The two germ layers are termed the hypoblast and the epiblast. The epiblast will give rise to the three germ layers of the embryo and the cells of the hypoblast will line the blastocyst/yolk sac cavity.

GASTRULATION

Gastrulation which begins during the third week of gestation is the process by which the epiblast forms the mesoderm and endoderm of the three-layered embryo. Gastrulation occurs during the third week of gestation. All of the different tissues of the mature organism are derived from a specific layer (Table 16.1). The ectoderm, that layer of the epiblast that remains following gastrulation, gives rise to the epidermis, the nervous system, the majority of the eye and the connective tissue in the head. The endoderm gives rise to the epithelial lining of the gastrointestinal and respiratory tracts. The mesoderm gives rise to connective tissue outside of the head, most of the cardiovascular system, bone, and genitourinary tracts.

Gastrulation is initiated by the formation of the primitive streak on the surface of the epiblast. The streak originates at the caudal aspect of the dorsal side of the embryonic disk and elongates by the addition of cells to the caudal end. The primitive streak is a narrow groove and the cranial end forms the node. The primitive streak defines the rostral-caudal and dorsal-ventral axes. Gastrulation is the result of movement of cells originating in the epiblast and migrating to the primitive streak (Fig. 16.1). Invagination of these cells beneath the surface of the epiblast gives rise to mesenchymal cells, the mesoderm, that migrate to a position between the epiblast and hypoblast. The endoderm is formed by cells that migrate through the primitive streak, detaching from the epiblast, and displacing the hypoblast

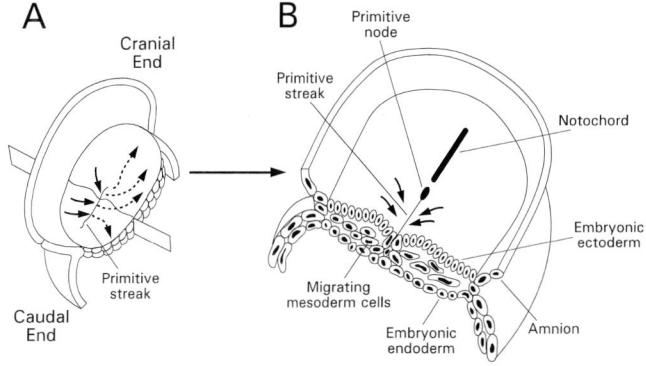

Fig. 16.1. Gastrulation gives rise to the three germ layers. Dorsal (A) and transverse (B) views of the embryonic disc during the third week. Arrows indicate movement of cells to the primitive streak and then below the ectoderm as the embryonic mesoderm.

layer. As previously mentioned, the ectoderm is formed from the remaining epiblast cells.

One important mesodermal structure that is formed is the notochord, a median cell population along the cranial-caudal axis. The notochord is formed from mesenchymal cells derived from the node of the primitive streak. The rostral limit of migration of the cells forming the notochord is the prechordal plate. The notochord induces the overlying embryonic ectoderm to form neural tissue. Thus, by the end of the third week of human development, the three basic germ layers have been established, and organogenesis commences.

DEVELOPMENT OF SPECIFIC ORGAN SYSTEMS

In this section we will briefly describe the formation of some of the organ systems of the body to illustrate the dynamic and fluid processes which underlie development. Developmental processes occur in three-dimensional space, along the three major body axes: cranial-caudal, dorsal-ventral, and left-right (Fig. 16.2). Malformations arising from abnormal development will be noted. In the next section, we will discuss the organogenesis of several organ systems and then focus on two regions, the brain and the limb, as examples of the complex interactions and regulation which occur during organogenesis.

SKELETON

Cartilage and bones of the body and limbs are formed from mesoderm. Bones of the face are derived from the neural crest, which arises from ectoderm. The axial skeleton of the

Table 16.1. Derivatives of the three germ layers

Ectoderm derivatives	Epidermis of skin
	Central nervous system (brain and spinal cord)
	All peripheral nerve tissue (neural crest)
	Some bones of the face
	Retina
	Pituitary gland, adrenal medulla
	Sensory epithelia of the eye, ear, nose
Endoderm derivatives	Epithelial parts of:
	Thyroid and parathyroid glands
	Respiratory tract
	Gastrointestinal tract, liver, pancreas
	Terminal part of urogenital systems
Mesoderm derivatives	Connective tissues
	Cartilage and bone
	Blood cells (red and white)
	All muscle types (cardiac, skeletal, smooth)
	Lining of body cavities (pericardial, pleural, peritoneal)
	Cardiovascular system
	Testes, ovaries
	Kidneys, adrenal cortex, spleen

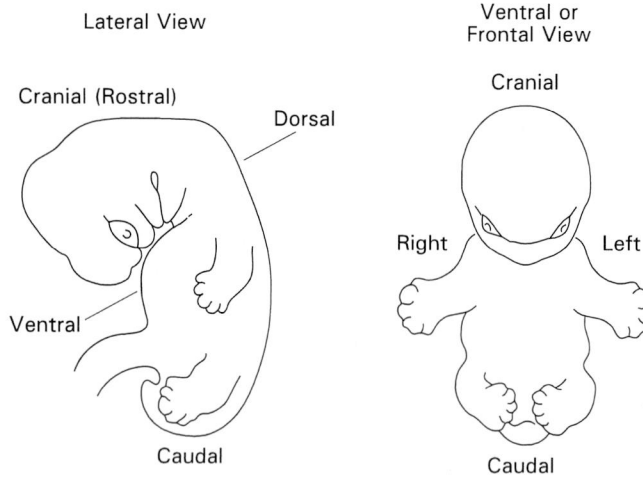

Lateral View

Cranial (Rostral)

Dorsal

Ventral

Caudal

Ventral or
Frontal View

Cranial

Right   Left

Caudal

Fig. 16.2. Embryonic body axes

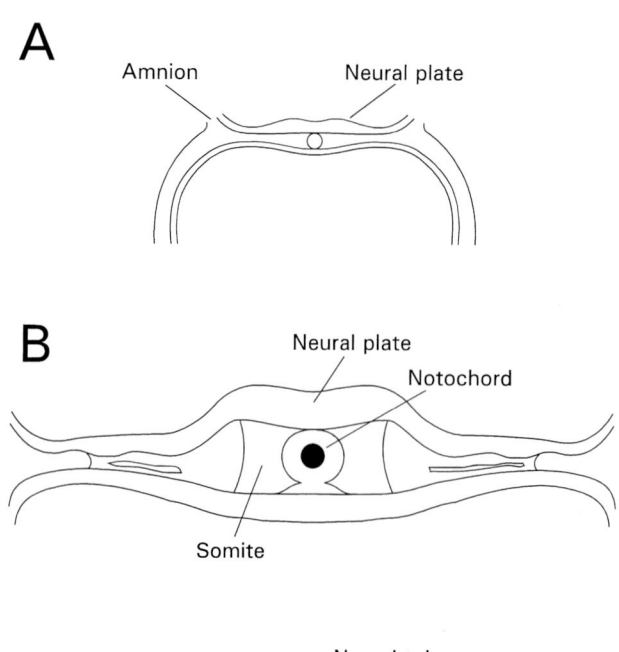

A

Amnion   Neural plate

B

Neural plate

Notochord

Somite

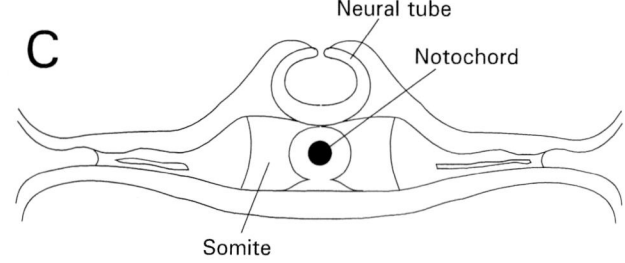

C

Neural tube

Notochord

Somite

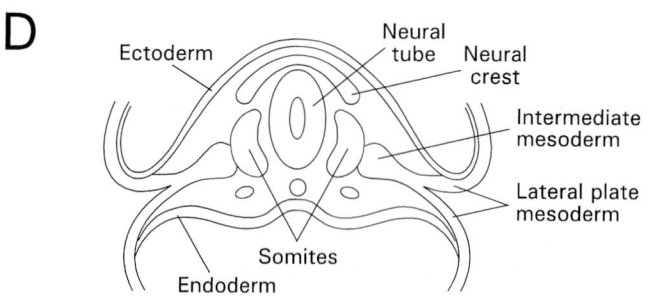

D

Ectoderm   Neural tube   Neural crest

Intermediate mesoderm

Lateral plate mesoderm

Somites

Endoderm

Fig. 16.3. Transverse sections showing neural tube formation. The neural plate gives rise to neural folds which fuse to form the neural tube.

body is formed from paraxial mesoderm, which is organized as columns on either side of the notochord. This mesoderm segments into somites. The somites then differentiate into dermatome, myotome, and sclerotome. The sclerotome is in a ventromedial position near the developing neural tube and forms the vertebrae and contributes to the ribs. The vertebrae are formed during weeks 5–6 of gestation. Each vertebral body is formed by sclerotome cells derived from two somite levels—the caudal half of one sclerotome fuses with the cranial half of the subsequent sclerotome. The ribs then grow out from ventrally migrating cells derived from the sclerotome. The dorsolateral region of the somite forms the dermamyotome. The myotome forms myoblasts, which will form muscle. The dermatome forms the dermis of the skin.

The skull can be divided into the neurocranium, which surrounds the brain, and the viscerocranium, which forms the bones of the face. Craniofacial bones are derived from a combination of neural crest derived cells (which form the bones of the face) and mesoderm (which form at least some of the bones of the neurocranium). The bones of the limbs, the appendicular skeleton, are derived from lateral plate mesoderm. The development of the limbs will be discussed in detail in a subsequent section.

BRAIN AND SPINAL CORD

All neural tissue is derived from the neurectoderm. Ectoderm is induced by the notochord to form neurectoderm, which thickens into the neural plate (Fig. 16.3). The plate rises up into neural folds, which subsequently fuse to form the neural tube. Fusion of the neural tube begins in the occipital region, the progresses both cranially and cau-

dally. Congenital anomalies of the spinal cord can result from defective closure of the neural tube during the fourth week of development. These neural tube defects may also affect overlying tissue including the menings, muscles, and skin.

The cells at the crest of the neural folds, which become the most dorsal region of the neural tube following fusion, give rise to the neural crest cells (Fig. 16.3). The neural tube goes on to form the central nervous system (the brain and spinal cord), while the neural crest forms many elements of the peripheral nervous system, including the cranial, spinal, and autonomic ganglia. Additionally, in the trunk neural crest cells differentiate into melanocytes.

In the spinal portion of the neural tube, the cells lining the central canal make up the ventricular zone, which gives rise to primitive nerve cells, or neuroblasts, which will form neurons. The marginal zone is initially composed of the nerve fibers of the neuroblasts and will become the white matter as axons grow into it. The intermediate zone (mantle) is derived from the ventricular zone and lies between the ventricular zone and the marginal zone. It will form the gray matter. A groove, the sulcus limitans, separates the spinal cord into the dorsal alar plate and the ventral basal plate. A similar overall organization can be recognized in the brain as well, especially in the hindbrain and midbrain.

The developing brain consists of three primary brain vesicles that give rise to the forebrain, midbrain, and hindbrain (Table 16.2). Five secondary brain vesicles are formed as the forebrain and hindbrain are subdivided. The rostral portion of the forebrain, the telencephalon, consists of a median region and two lateral diverticula which will give rise to the cerebral hemispheres. The cerebral hemispheres expand and cover the midbrain and hindbrain. The central lumen of the neural tube dilates as the ventricles enlarge. The cerebral hemispheres are connected by fiber bundles across the midline, or commisures. The largest commisure is the corpus callosum.

The dorsal and ventral regions of the neural tube give rise to distinct cell types. The dorsal alar plate gives rise to the afferent (sensory) portion of the spinal cord. The ventral basal plate gives rise to the motor horn of the spinal cord. As will be discussed in detail in a later section, the induction of dorsal-ventral specification involves signals derived from neighboring tissues, the ventral notochord and the dorsal non-neural ectoderm.

HEART

A functioning cardiovascular system is required once the oxygenation needs of the embryo cannot be met because of the embryo's growing size. Although the neural crest provides some cells to the heart, the majority of the tissues of the heart are derived from mesoderm. The bilateral endocardial tubes arise from mesoderm and fuse to form the heart tube. As these endothelial tubes fuse, the primordial myocardium form from the adjacent mesoderm adjacent to the endocardial tubes. As the tube enlarges, constrictions mark the division into the truncus arteriosus, bulbus cordis, ventricle, atrium, and sinus venosus, from rostral to caudal (Fig. 16.4). The bulbis cordis is incorporated into the mature right ventricle. The conus cordis, derived from the bulbis cordis, along with the truncus arteriosus form the outflow tracts of the ventricles. The sinus venosus receives venous blood. As the heart tube grows, it bends and forms the cardiac loop. The looping results in the different parts of the heart assuming their correct relative spatial orientations. The heart tube loops such that the cranial portion moves ventrally and to the right, while the atria move dorsally and to the left. The result is that the atrium and sinus venosus lie dorsal to the truncus arteriosus, bulbis cordis, and ventricle.

The AV canal connects the common atrium and the early embryonic ventricle. The AV canal is divided by endocardial cushions which arise at the superior and inferior borders of the canal in the fourth week. The cushions also form the AV valves. The endocardial cushions grow across the AV canal and fuse, creating left and right AV canals. Regions of the endocardial cushions then fuse with both atrial and ventricular septa. If both atrial and ventricular septa and the medial AV valve leaflets are incomplete due to failure of fusion of the cushions, a persistent AV canal can result, as may sometimes be seen in association with trisomy 21 (Down syndrome). In the atria, the

Table 16.2. Adult derivatives of the embryonic brain vesicles

Primary brain vesicles	Secondary brain vesicles	Derivatives
Prosencephalon (forebrain)	Telencephalon	Cerebral hemispheres Basal ganglia
	Diencephalon	Thalamus Hypothalamus Pituitary gland (neurohypophysis)
Mesencephalon (midbrain)	Mesencephalon	Midbrain
Rhombencephalon (hindbrain)	Metencephalon	Cerebellum Pons
	Myelencephalon	Medulla oblongata

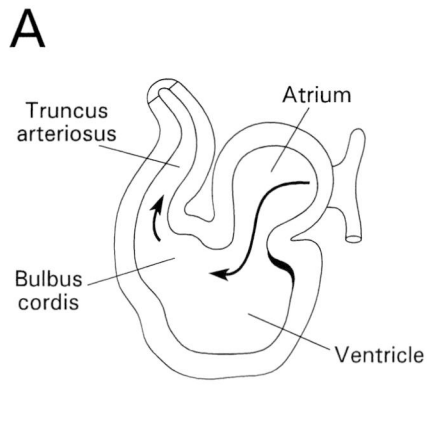

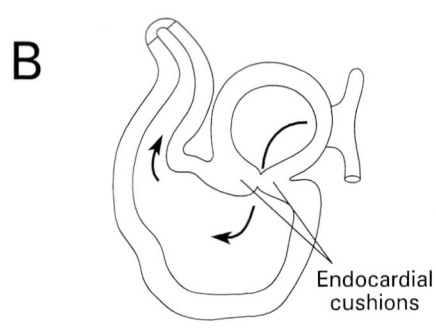

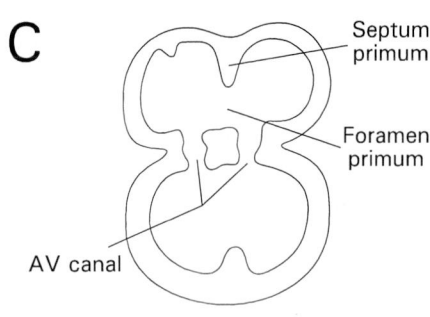

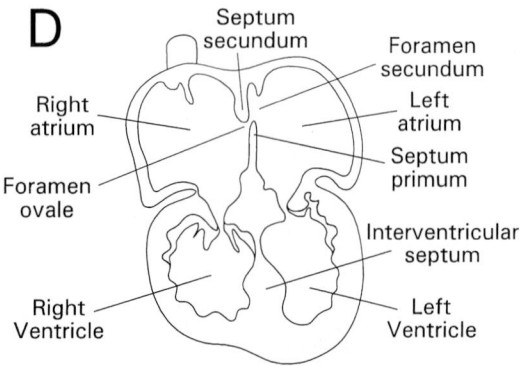

Fig. 16.4. Development and septation of the heart. A, B. Sagittal sections of the heart. C, D. Coronal sections of the heart. Arrows indicate flow of blood through the heart.

septum primum, a thin membrane, grows from the dorsal roof of the common atrium toward the atrioventricular (AV) canal (Fig. 16.4). Its forward edge creates an opening between the septum and the endocardial cushions, the ostium primum. As the ostium primum is being closed by fusion of the septum primum and the fused endocardial cushion tissue, perforations form in the septum primum by programed cell death. The coalescence of these holes forms the ostium secundum. A septum secundum then forms to the right of the septum primum, growing from the roof of the atrium, covering the ostium secundum. However, the septum secundum forms an incomplete division of the atria. The opening between the two septa is the foramen ovale (Fig. 16.4). Defects in closure of the ostium primum or ostium secundum result in atrial septal defects. Ostium secundum defects are relatively common and can be due to defects in formation of the septum primum or the septum secundum.

The muscular interventricular septum is formed, for the most part, as a result of cavitation of the right and left ventricular chambers. Final closure of the ventricular septum is brought about by fusion of the muscular septum with endocardial cushion tissue. This tissue also fuses with the aorticopulmonary septum. This final region of ventricular septation is the membranous part of the interventricular septum. Ventricular septal defects are the most common congenital heart defect, and membranous defects are the most common form.

The truncus arteriosus divides to form the proximal portion of the aorta and pulmonary artery. The septum between these great vessels form by fusion of the bilateral ridges. Neural crest cells migrate from the pharyngeal arches to participate in the formation of this septum. Failure of the ridges to fuse results in persistent truncus arteriosus. This is usually associated with a ventricular septal defect. Unequal division of the outflow vessels can lead to tetralogy of Fallot, which is characterized by 1) right ventricle outflow obstruction, resulting from a narrow pulmonary orifice, 2) ventricular septal defect, 3) overriding aorta, and 4) hypertrophy of the right ventricle.

GASTROINTESTINAL SYSTEM

The epithelial lining of the GI tract is derived from endoderm. Mesoderm forms the connective tissue and smooth muscle components. The primitive gut is bounded by the oropharyngeal membrane rostrally and the cloacal membrane caudally. The mesodermally-derived and endodermally-derived components induce each other's development. The different functional portions of the GI tract (e.g., stomach, small intestine, large intestine) are partly due to regional differences in these interactions.

The foregut, midgut, and hindgut are each supplied by different blood vessels. The foregut gives rise to the pharynx, respiratory system, the liver, esophagus, stomach, and proximal duodenum. The respiratory diverticulum forms from the ventral surface of the endodermal tube. A division must form between the developing esophagus and trachea. An error in normal development of the tracheo-esophageal septum can lead to esophageal atresia. Diverticula that will form the liver, biliary apparatus, and the pancreas arise from the distal portion of the foregut.

The midgut forms the distal part of the duodenum, the jejunum, the ileum, the cecum and appendix, the ascending colon, and the proximal two-thirds of the transverse colon. The connection between the midgut and the yolk sac (the vitelline duct) is located within the umbilical cord. Rapid growth of the midgut forms a loop of gut. At the sixth week, the midgut then grows outside of the abdominal cavity into the umbilical cord and the yolk stalk. This physiologic herniation of the midgut is required for normal growth of the intestines as there is insufficient space in the abdominal cavity at this time to contain the growing intestines. During the tenth week, the midgut returns to the embryonic abdomen. Abnormalities in the retraction process resulting in persistence of the herniation of the midgut into the umbilical cord can result in omphalocele.

The hindgut gives rise to the distal one-third of the transverse colon, the descending colon, the rectum, and the proximal portion of the anal canal. It also gives rise to the epithelium of the bladder and most of the urethra. The caudal part of the hindgut is continuous with the cloaca which is divided by the urogenital septum into the urogenital sinus (which gives rise to the bladder and urethra), and the rectum. Incomplete septation of the hindgut can cause a persistent cloaca.

The endodermal tube is initially hollow. Many parts of it then become solid as the endodermal epithelium rapidly proliferates. Recanalization reopens the lumen by weeks 8–10. Stenosis or atresia of the GI tract can result from failure to recanalize, especially in the proximal duodenum. More caudal atresias or stenosis may be due to compromise of the vascular supply, resulting in narrowing of the lumen.

The distal foregut and midgut undergo a series of rotations to reach their adult orientation. The stomach rotates such that the dorsal side forms the greater curvature while the ventral side forms the lesser curvature. Thus, the original left side becomes ventral while the original right side becomes dorsal. Rotation of the stomach causes the duodenum to adopt a C-shaped loop. While the midgut loop is in the umbilical cord and outside of the abdominal cavity, it begins to rotate around the axis of the superior mesenteric artery. A total rotation of 270 degrees counterclockwise occurs, and this rotation fixes the placement of the stomach, duodenum, and intestines. Abnormal rotation can result in twisting of the intestines (volvulus) and may compromise the blood supply to that region.

URINARY SYSTEM

The urinary and internal genital systems have a common origin, being derived primarily from the intermediate mesoderm. Growth of the mesoderm creates the urogenital ridge, which forms on either side of the dorsal aorta. It gives rise to the nephrogenic cord and the genital ridge. Three successive pairs of kidneys form from this mesoderm. They are termed the pronephros, mesonephros, and metanephros. The metanephros gives rise to the adult kidney. The pronephros is rudimentary. In addition to the mesonephric duct, the mesonephric kidney gives rise to the mesonephric tubules, which open into the mesonephric duct. The permanent kidney begins to form at five weeks gestation and becomes functional towards the end of the first trimester. It arises from inductive interactions between the ureteric bud (a mesonephric diverticulum) and the metanephric cap (metanephric mesoderm). The cells of the cap form small vesicles, which give rise eventually to the nephron, the excretory unit of the kidney. The ureteric bud forms the collecting system of the kidney, as well as the ureters. The kidneys initially develop in the pelvic region ventral to the sacrum but assume a position in the abdomen by the ninth week. This "migration" is primarily due to growth of the abdomen and pelvis, and the kidneys come to lie in the abdomen and move further apart.

Between 4–7 weeks, the urorectal septum divides the cloaca into the anorectal canal and the urogenital sinus. The urogenital sinus gives rise to the urinary bladder and prostatic and membranous portions of the urethra and becomes connected to the rest of the urinary system.

The kidneys may be united at their lower poles, forming a single horseshoe kidney. Horseshoe kidneys do not ascend properly (pelvic kidney). Renal agenesis is due to degeneration of the ureteric bud. Without the bud, the metanephric cap does not develop and no nephrons are formed.

Limb development

Higher vertebrates have two sets of distinguishable paired limbs: forelimbs and hindlimbs. Although the precise form of the limbs varies between species, they share a common morphologic pattern. There is a single proximal long bone (in humans, the humerus in the arm and the femur in the leg), a middle pair of long bones (ulna and radius in the arm, tibia and fibula in the leg), then the carpal (hand) or tarsal (foot) bones, with the phalanges of the digits being most distal (Fig 16.5). The ordered development of the limb must produce correct orientation in three planes: proximal-distal (shoulder-fingers), anterior-posterior (thumb-little finger), and dorsal-ventral (back of hand-palm). How these axes are established and maintained depend on the precise coordination of multiple molecules.

The bones and connective tissues of the limbs are derived from lateral plate mesoderm. Initiation of limb bud outgrowth involves members of the fibroblast growth factor (FGF) family. Fgf can induce development of limbs when applied to the lateral region of the chick embryo (Cohn et al., 1995, 1997; Ohuchi et al., 1995). That is, Fgf is sufficient to specify cells to give rise to limbs that normally would not. Fgf is capable of inducing either forelimb or hindlimb, depending on the position of its ectopic expression. *Fgf10* is expressed in the lateral plate mesoderm prior to the onset of limb budding (Crossley et al., 1996; Vogel et al., 1996; Ohuchi et al., 1997). As the bud arises, an apical ridge which espresses *Fgf8* forms in the ectoderm overlying the bud (the apical ectodermal ridge, or AER) (Fig. 16.5).

The forelimb and hindlimb are morphologically quite distinct. The signals specifying whether a forelimb or a hindlimb forms and the position of the limb relative to the rest of the body appears to correlated with the expression of a number of genes of the Hox 9 family (Cohn et al.,

1997), a group of transcriptional regulators. In addition, the T-box genes (*Tbx* genes), which encode another family of transcription factors, are differentially regulated in fore-limb vs. hindlimb (Gibson-Brown et al., 1998; Isaac et al., 1998; Logan et al., 1998; Ohuchi et al., 1998). *Tbx4* is expressed in the hindlimb, while *Tbx5* is expressed in the forelimb. Ectopic Fgf can induce *Tbx4* or *Tbx5* expression consistent with the identity of the limb. *Pitx1*, which can induce *Tbx4* expression encodes a bicoid-like transcription factor, and is also expressed in the early hindlimb. Expression of *Pitx1* ectopically in the forelimb can induce hindlimb identity (Logan and Tabin, 1999; Szeto et al., 1999). The *Pitx1* knockout mouse has abnormalities of the hindlimb (Lanctot et al., 1999; Szeto et al., 1999).

LONGITUDINAL GROWTH OF THE LIMB

For outgrowth of the limb from the bud a specialized region of ectoderm, the apical ectodermal ridge (AER) is essential. It forms at the tip of the limb bud along the dorsal-ventral boundary of the bud (Fig. 16.5). The position and maintenance of the AER appears to depend on signals from the underlying mesenchyme. The AER itself is also the source of secreted factors that allow for longitudinal outgrowth of the limb. Excision of the AER causes the limb to stop growing distally, resulting in a truncation defect, i.e., loss of distal structures (Saunders, 1948; Summerbell, 1974). The structures that are lost depend on the timing of the removal of the AER. If the AER is removed early, the limb is severely truncated, while later removal results in loss only of more distal structures. Three Fgfs are known to be expressed in the AER: *Fgf4* poster-

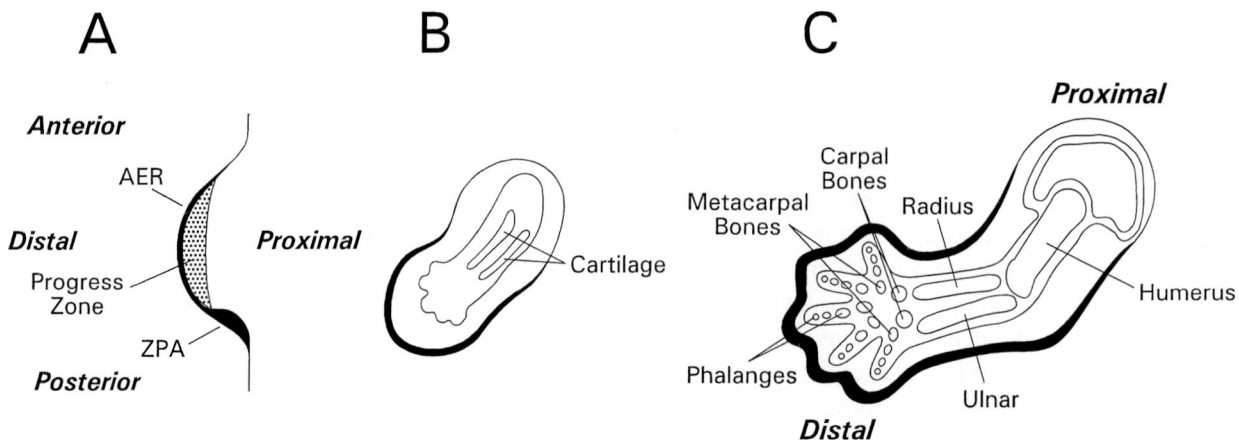

Fig. 16.5. Longitudinal sections of a developing upper limb. The apical ectodermal ridge (AER) and the zone of polarizing activity (ZPA) are involved in proximal-distal and antero-posterior specification.

iorly, and *Fgf2* and *Fgf8* throughout the ridge (Niswander and Martin, 1992; Crossley and Martin, 1995; Mahmood et al., 1995; Savage and Fallon, 1995). Adding back any of these Fgfs after AER excision results in rescue of the limb with preservation of the normal limb patterning (Niswander et al., 1993; Fallon et al., 1994; Vogel et al., 1996).

The progress zone is a region of rapidly proliferating undifferentiated mesenchyme that lies beneath the AER. This region specifies proximal-distal identity in the developing limb. The proximal-distal identity of the bone that is formed in the limb is governed according to the amount of time that a given cell has spent in the progress zone (Summerbell et al., 1973). That is, if a cell has spent only a short time in the zone, a proximal bone (e.g., humerus) will form. Conversely, those cells which exit from the zone last and have spent the most time in the zone will form distal elements (e.g., distal phalanges). A number of genes that are expressed in the progress zone and are induced by Fgfs. Cells must somehow measure the time spent in the progress zone and thus obtain their positional identity.

DORSAL-VENTRAL SPECIFICATION

Signaling by the dorsal and ventral ectoderm of the early limb bud regulates dorsal-ventral axis specification (MacCabe et al., 1974). Dorsal identity is controlled at least in part by *Wnt7a*, and null mutations in the mouse results in ventralization of distal dorsal aspects of the limb (Parr and McMahon, 1995). Wnt7a induces expression of *Lmx1* in the underlying mesenchyme. Mutations in the *Lmx1b* gene result in partial loss of dorsal structures (Chen et al., 1998). Ectopic expression of either *Wnt7a* or the LIM homeobox gene *Lmx1* in the chick can induce ventral tissues to become dorsal, resulting in a mirror-image dorsal limb (Riddle et al., 1995; Vogel et al., 1995). The homeobox gene *Engrailed-1* (*En1*) appears to be important for ventral specification. Loss of *En1* expression causes dorsal specification of the ventral limb with ventral expansion of the dorsal markers *Wnt7a* and *Lmx1*, resulting in a double dorsal limb (Loomis et al., 1996; Cygan et al., 1997). However, in the *Wnt7a* knockout, *En1* expression is not altered (Parr and McMahon, 1995). This implies that limb cells have a ventral identity unless signaled by Wnt7a or Lmx1 to acquire a dorsal fate. En1 preserves ventral identity by suppression of *Wnt7a* expression in the ectoderm (Logan et al., 1997), and subsequently *Lmx1* expression is confined to the dorsal limb mesenchyme (Logan et al., 1997). In addition, En1 seems to play a role in restricting

the AER to the apex of the bud (Loomis et al., 1996; Logan et al., 1997)

ANTERIOR-POSTERIOR PATTERNING

In humans, the anterior digit is the first digit, or thumb, and the posterior digit is the fifth digit. Anterior-posterior patterning is controlled by a region of mesenchyme at the posterior margin of the limb bud termed the zone of polarizing activity (ZPA) (Fig. 16.5). The ZPA confers posterior identity on limb mesenchyme cells, with the cells closest to the ZPA acquiring the most posterior fate. Transplantation of an ectopic ZPA to the anterior margin of the chick limb bud results in mirror-image duplication of the digits. That is, normal 2–3–4 pattern of digits is replaced by a 4–3–2–2–3–4 pattern. This pattern is presumably the result of cells at a greater distance from the ZPA being exposed to a lower concentration of a morphogen than those closer to the ZPA. The concentration of the morphogen reflects the distance from the ZPA. The implication is that the specification of which particular digit will form at a given site is dependent on a certain threshold for activation. This model explains why mirror-image duplications would result from application of a second ectopic ZPA, as there would be two sources of the morphogen. This model would also predict that application of an increased amount of the morphogen at a given position would induce more posterior development. When two ZPAs are grafted onto a wing bud, one at the apex and one at the anterior portion, only the more posterior digits are formed (Wolpert and Hornbruch, 1981).

The properties of the ZPA suggest the presence of a morphogen gradient, and the soluble factor Shh has been shown to play a role. The effect of the ZPA in determining digit identity in the chick can be mimicked by the application of Sonic Hedgehog (Shh) (Riddle et al., 1993). Shh signaling is dose-dependent, as would be predicted for a morphogen. Limbs exposed to beads soaked in high concentrations of Shh specify a more posterior digit, while progressively lower concentrations induce correspondingly more anterior digits (Yang et al., 1997). Application of retinoic acid to the anterior margin can also induce mirror-image duplication and mimic ZPA signaling (Tickle et al., 1982). It has subsequently been shown that retinoic acid has been shown to activate Shh (Riddle et al., 1993). Application of retinoic acid inhibitors results in loss of Shh expression in the posterior limb bud (Helms et al., 1996; Stratford et al., 1996). Thus, retinoic acids anterior-posterior axis patterning effects could be mediated by Shh, and Shh may be the actual morphogen which specifies position across that axis of the limb.

Retinoic acid can also induce expression of *Hoxb8* in the limb (Lu et al., 1997), and ectopic *Hoxb8* expression in the mouse can result in ectopic Shh expression (Charite et al., 1994). *Hoxb8* is normally expressed in the lateral plate mesoderm with an anterior expression boundary at the posterior region of the forelimb bud in chick and mouse (Charite et al., 1994; Lu et al., 1997; Stratford et al., 1997). Thus, it appears that Hoxb8 may specify the position of the ZPA in the limb in the lateral plate mesoderm. Activation of expression of regulatory genes at the 5′ region of the Hoxa and Hoxd clusters is controlled by patterning cues, and the patterns of expression map out different regions of the limb bud (Izpisua-Belmonte and Duboule, 1992). At least 23 different Hox genes are expressed during chick limb development (Nelson et al., 1996). *Hoxa* and *Hoxd* are expressed in both the forelimb and hindlimb. Expression of the Hox genes is very dynamic.

Maintenance of Shh expression and the ZPA can be regulated by Fgf4 from the AER (Laufer et al., 1994; Niswander et al., 1994). Shh also maintains *Fgf4* expression in the AER. In this way, proximal-distal and anterior-posterior patterning are linked. Mutant mice null for *Shh* have proximal structures in the limbs but not distal ones, indicating that Shh does play a role in maintaining proximal-distal outgrowth but not in initiating limb growth. Although Fgf4 can maintain *Shh* expression in the AER, Fgf4 may not be required as evidenced by a conditional knockout of Fgf4 that still had *Shh* expression in the AER (Moon et al., 2000). It is possible that there is functional redundancy between different Fgf family members.

Bmp2 is expressed in pattern overlapping *Shh* expression (Riddle et al., 1993; Francis et al., 1994). Bmp2 can induce *Fgf4* expression anteriorly in the AER (Francis-West et al., 1995; Duprez et al., 1996). Shh can induce *Bmp2* expression, and *Bmp7* expression is induced in a dose-dependent fashion (Yang et al., 1997). BMP signaling may be quite complex as at least *Bmp2*, *Bmp7*, and *Bmp4* are expressed in the limb, and the molecules may also form heterodimers.

HUMAN LIMB ANOMALIES

The studies demonstrating that a variety of factors are involved in specific patterns in limb development have been supported by the findings of specific genetic defects in a number of human malformation syndromes. For example, Holt-Oram syndrome, which is associated with upper extremity malformations and congenital heart disease, can be caused by mutation in *TBX5* (Basson et al., 1997; Li et al., 1997). Interestingly, *Tbx5* is expressed in the forelimb but the not hindlimb of chicks and mice. The ulnar-

mammary syndrome features upper limb anomalies and is due to mutations in *TBX3*, which is expressed mainly in the forelimb (Bamshad et al., 1997). Mutations in *GLI3*, a zinc-finger protein which is part of the Shh pathway, have been identified in several human conditions: Greig syndrome (associated with polysyndactyly), Pallister-Hall syndrome (characterized by polysyndactyly and hypothalamic and anal malformations), and isolated post-axial polydactyly (Vortkamp et al., 1991; Kang et al., 1997; Wild et al., 1997).

Type II polysyndactyly can be caused by mutations in the *HOXD13* gene in which there is an expansion of the polyalanine stretch (Muragaki et al., 1996; Goodman et al., 1997). Mutations in *HOXA13* can cause hand-foot genital syndrome (Mortlock and Innis, 1997). Mutations in *Hoxa13* cause reduced digit size (Scott, 1997). The nail and the patella are dorsal structures in the limb, and the human nail-patella syndrome can be caused by mutations in *LMX1B* (Dreyer et al., 1998; Vollrath et al., 1998). As noted previously, expression of Lmx1 is involved in specification of dorsal structures in chicks and mice.

Development of the brain

The brain is an extraordinarily complex organ, and regulation of its development is correspondingly intricate. The embryonic central nervous system originates from ectoderm and forms a hollow tube, the neural tube. The rostral region of the tube will form the brain, while more caudal regions form the spinal cord. The brain may be divided from rostral to caudal into three regions: the forebrain (prosencephalon, which is further subdivided into telencephalon and diencephalon), the midbrain (mesencephalon), and hindbrain (rhombencephalon, which is subdivided into the metencephalon and myelencephalon). Each region of the presumptive brain gives rise to specific derivatives (Table 16.2). We will focus primarily on patterning of the forebrain, or prosencephalon.

ANTERIOR-POSTERIOR PATTERNING

Anterior-posterior (or rostral-caudal) segmentation of the neural tube creates boundaries or compartments referred to as neuromeres. Neuromeres of the hindbrain are designated rhombomeres. The midbrain is formed from a mesencephalic neuromere, and there are likely to be six forebrain neuromeres (Figdor and Stern, 1993; Rubenstein et al., 1994). Each neuromere gives rise to specific structures. Cell movement between the neuromeres is restricted by either physical or chemical barriers. The anterior-posterior segmentation is best understood in the hindbrain. For example, *Hox* genes are expressed in a precise pattern in the specific rhombomeres. The rhombomeric compartments confer specific developmental properties to the cells within each rhombomere. Expression of the *Hox* clusters precedes rhombomere formation. They become progressively restricted such that the expression pattern coincides with rhombomere borders (Wilkinson et al., 1989; Studer et al., 1994). The expression patterns form an ordered set of domains along the anterior-posterior axis (Lumsden and Krumlauf, 1996).

In the forebrain, anterior-posterior patterning may be mediated in part by prechordal mesendoderm. *Goosecoid*, a homeobox gene, is expressed in the prechordal plate (mesoderm) but not the notochord (Izpisua-Belmonte et al., 1993). Conversely, the homeobox gene *Not* is required for function of the zebrafish notochord but not the prechordal mesendoderm (Talbot et al., 1995). Placement of prechordal tissues under uncommitted ectoderm induces formation of a forebrain-like vesicle (Pera and Kessel, 1997). Thus, the prechordal mesendoderm and the notochord may have different inducing capabilities, and various anterior-posterior regions of the neural tube have different competencies. When anterior neural plate is exposed to Shh or prechordal mesendoderm, the ventral forebrain marker Nkx2.1 is induced, but posterior neural plate does not respond in this way (Shimamura and Rubenstein, 1997).

The *Otx* genes may also play a role in anterior-posterior patterning of the neuraxis. These genes are homologues of the Drosophila homeobox gene *Otd* (orthodenticle). The *Otx* genes are expressed in the forebrain and midbrain. Mice null mutant for *Otx1* or *Otx2* have abnormalities affecting the forebrain, midbrain, and rostral hindbrain (Acampora et al., 1995; Acampora et al., 1996; Matsuo et al., 1995).

VENTRAL PATTERNING OF THE FOREBRAIN

Except for the most rostral portion of the neural tube, the median portion of its ventral side is adjacent to the notochord, which is derived from mesoderm (Fig. 16.6). The prosencephalon is flanked on the ventral side to the prechordal mesendoderm (the prechordal plate) (Seifert et al., 1993; Sulik et al., 1994). The prechordal mesendoderm is critical for normal patterning of the ventral forebrain and the eyes. Prechordal mesendoderm can induce expression of ventrally-restricted genes such as *Nkx2.1* (Shimamura et al., 1995). If notochord tissue is implanted ectopically to the dorsal or lateral portion of the neural tube, a second

floor plate forms, and motor neuron differentiation occurs (van Straaten et al., 1988). Transplantation of prechordal mesendoderm to an ectopic location induces ectopic *Nkx2.1* expression in the neural plate (Pera and Kessel, 1997; Shimamura and Rubenstein, 1997). In *Nkx2.1* null mutant mice, cells which normally give rise to the ventral globus pallidus instead acquire the characteristics of the dorsal striatum (Sussel et al., 1999). Zebrafish mutants, including one-eyed pinhead (*oep*), cyclops (*cyc*), knypek, and trilobite, which have abnormal prechordal mesendoderm, have defective forebrain and eye development (Schier et al., 1996; 1997; Marlow et al., 1998). The *oep* mutants have ventral forebrain deficits and cyclopia. *Cyc* mutants lack ventral forebrain structures and have cyclopia. The *oep* protein is required for signaling by the cyclops product, which appears to be related to Nodal, a member of the TGF-β family of secreted factors (Feldman et al., 1998; Rebagliati et al., 1998; Sampath et al., 1998). Double heterozygotes for *Nodal* and *Smad2* have ventral forebrain defects, cyclopia, and a proboscis (Nomura and Li, 1998).

These results suggested that the prechordal mesendoderm is the source of a factor which is required for normal ventral forebrain patterning. Sonic Hedgehog (Shh) was noted to be expressed in the prechordal mesendoderm (as well as in the notochord) (Echelard et al., 1993; Shimamura and Rubenstein 1997). Shh has been implicated in specifying ventral cell fate at multiple levels of the neuraxis (Marti et al., 1995a,b; Chiang et al., 1996), including the spinal cord (Roelink et al., 1994), hindbrain, midbrain (Hynes et al., 1995), and forebrain (Ericson et al., 1995; Pera and Kessel, 1997; Shimamura and Rubenstein, 1997; Kohtz et al., 1998).

Based on studies in the spinal cord, different concentrations of Shh can induce different neuronal cell types, with the highest concentration of Shh inducing the anatomically most ventral cells (Tanabe and Jessell, 1996). Shh signaling can induce expression of a number of transcription factors, including *Nkx2.1* (Ericson et al., 1995; Dale et al., 1997; Shimamura and Rubenstein, 1997), while repressing factors normally expressed in the dorsal neural tube. The critical role of Shh in patterning the developing forebrain was confirmed by studies of the null *Shh* mouse. Ventral neural cell fates are missing throughout the neuraxis (Chiang et al., 1996). The eye field failed to divide, resulting in a single midline cyclopic eye. The forebrain did not express ventral markers but instead expressed markers characteristic of dorsal telencephalon. In addition, the cerebral hemispheres failed to develop as separate left and right halves, but instead had a single holosphere. The similar human condition is known as holoprosencephaly. A similar finding occurs in chickens in which the prechordal mesendoderm had been removed (Pera and Kessel, 1997).

The zinc finger protein Gli2 is a component of the Shh signaling pathway. Null mutant mice for *Gli2* have ventral defects, lack of floorplate differentiation, and have a single central incisor (Hardcastle et al., 1998; Matise et al., 1998). These defects are consistent with midline defects. In contrast, the severe defects such as holoprosencephaly or cyclopia were not seen *Gli2−/−* in mice.

DORSAL PATTERNING OF THE FOREBRAIN

Dorsal identity in the neural tube is induced by the bone morphogenetic proteins (BMPs), a group of secreted factors in the transforming growth factor-β superfamily (Fig. 16.6). The BMPs are expressed in the non-neural ectoderm (Dickinson et al., 1995; Liem et al., 1995; Furuta et al., 1997), including tissue around the dorsal region of the forebrain (Golden et al., 1999; Streit and Stern, 1999) in the dorsal roof of the forebrain (Shimamura and Rubenstein, 1995; Furuta et al., 1997). BMPs may act to specify dorsal cell fates at several levels of the neuraxis (Liem et al., 1995; Furuta et al., 1997; Muhr et al., 1997; Golden et al., 1999; Lee et al., 2000). The BMPs can induce expression of dorsally-expressed genes such as *Msx1* (Shimamura and Rubenstein, 1995; Furuta et al., 1997). The expression of other factors, such as *BF1*, which is involved in growth of the telencephalon, is repressed (Furuta et al., 1997). Mutants of

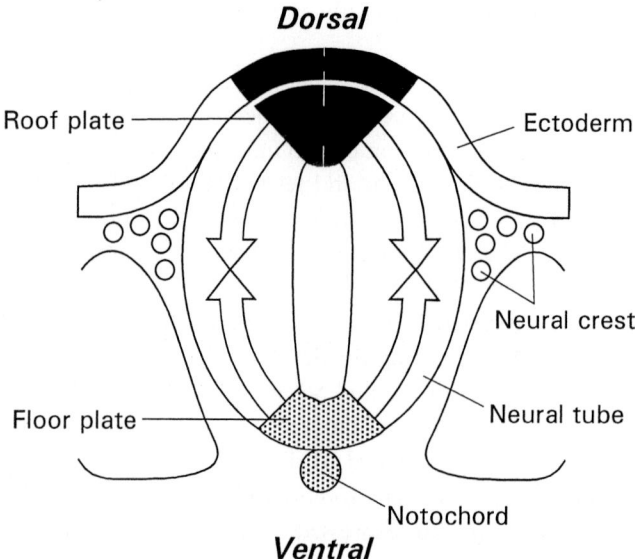

Fig. 16.6. Cross-section of the developing neural tube showing dorsal-ventral patterning. Distinct signals emanate from the overlying ectoderm and roof plate dorsally and the notochord and floor plate ventrally to specify dorsal-ventral fate.

BF1 have a very hypoplastic telencephlon with absent ventral cell types and absent basal ganglia (Xuan et al., 1995).

Mice mutant for individual BMPs have not shown decreased dorsal cell types in the telencephalon, possibly because of overlap of expression and function in this region. The extra-toes (xt) mouse has a mutation in *Gli3*, which encodes a zinc-finger DNA-binding protein which is part of the Shh signaling pathway. These mice have abnormalities in dorsally derived telencephalic structures such as the cerebral cortex, choroid plexus, and olfactory bulbs (Frantz, 1994). Dorsal telencephalic development is also abnormal in mice mutant for other genes known to be expressed in the dorsal region: *Pax6* (Schmahl et al., 1993; Stoykova et al., 1996; Warren and Price, 1997), and *Emx* genes (Pellegrini et al., 1996; Qiu et al., 1996; Yoshida et al., 1997).

DORSAL-VENTRAL PATTERNING DEFECTS AND HUMAN HOLOPROSENCEPHALY

Human holoprosencephaly (HPE) is a condition with a single cerebral vesicle instead of two distinct hemispheres. HPE is associated with marked craniofacial and eye abnormalities including midline cleft lip/palate, a single midline eye (cyclopia, synophthalmia) and nasal anomalies (Ming and Muenke, 1998; Muenke and Beachy, 2001). Familial HPE with autosomal dominant inheritance has been linked to DNA markers in chromosome region 7q36 (Muenke et al., 1994). A number of recurrent chromosomal abnormalities are seen in association with HPE (Roessler and Muenke, 1998). Several patients have rearrangements of 7q36, and it was determined that the human *Sonic Hedgehog* (*SHH*) gene maps close to the breakpoints in these patients with HPE (Belloni et al., 1996). In addition, the brain and craniofacial anomalies present in human HPE resemble those seen in the *Shh* null mutant mouse. In fact, mutations in *SHH* have been found in a significant number of patients with HPE (Roessler et al., 1996; 1997; Nanni et al., 1999; Odent et al., 1999). Because a number of the mutations are predicted to lead to premature truncation of the protein and some patients with deletions of 7q36 encompassing *Shh* have HPE, it is likely that the underlying mechanism is haploinsufficiency.

The SHH protein undergoes an intramolecular cleavage to form the mature protein (Porter et al., 1995), and the amino-terminal product is responsible for the biological activity (Beachy et al., 1997). The cleavage is mediated by addition of a cholesterol moiety to the carboxy-terminal residue of the amino-terminal half of Shh (Fig. 16.7) (Porter et al., 1996a; 1996b). Interestingly, treatment of

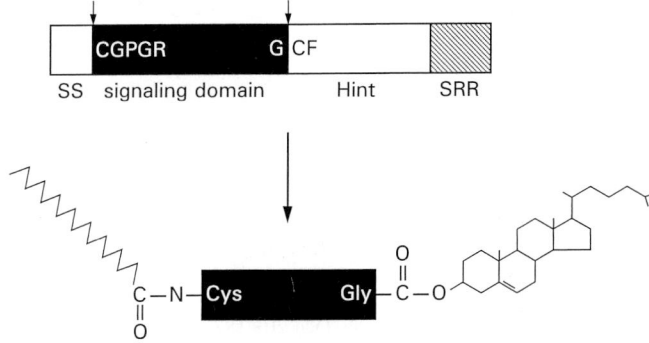

Fig. 16.7. Autoprocessing and lipid modification of the Sonic hedgehog (Shh) signaling protein. Following cleavage of the signal sequence (SS), Shh undergoes an autoprocessing reaction that results in cleavage between Gly and Cys of a conserved Gly-Cys-Phe (GCF) tripeptide, and attachment of cholesterol to the carboxy-terminus of the amino-terminal cleavage product. *Abbreviations*: SS, signal sequence; Hint, Hint processing domain module found in *Hedgehog* proteins and *inteins*, and involved in formation of a thioester intermediate; SRR, sterol recognition module of the processing domain (for details see text and Muenke and Beachy, 2000).

animals with inhibitors of cholesterol biosynthesis can result in HPE (Binns et al., 1963; Roux 1964; 1966; Dehart et al., 1997; Lanoue et al., 1997). In addition, mice with a null mutation for *Megalin*, which is involved in cholesterol transport in the body, also have HPE (Willnow et al., 1996). Moreover, a subset of children with Smith-Lemli-Opitz syndrome, a condition featuring multiple congenital anomalies, have HPE (Kelley et al., 1996). The condition is due to a defect in 7-dehydrocholesterol reductase, which results in accumulation of the precursor to cholesterol and decreased cholesterol production. Thus, the lack of production of cholesterol is also associated with HPE.

Studies in the chick have also demonstrated that exposure of the telencephalon to recombinant BMPs can also result in a phenotype like holoprosencephaly (Golden et al., 1999). The chicks had cyclopia, a proboscis, and single cerebral hemispheres and ventricle. There was increased cell death in the ventral telencephalon and loss of ventral cell types. These defects are likely to reflect the ectopic actions of the dorsalizing activity of the BMPs.

Thus, one mechanism underlying HPE is perturbed dorsal-ventral patterning and lack of development of the ventral telencephalon. This can occur by loss of function of the prechordal plate, as shown in animal models including the chick and zebrafish, loss of the ventralizing activity of Shh in mouse or human, or overexpression of the dorsalizing BMP factors in the chick.

Other genes have also been identified that cause HPE in humans. These include *SIX3* (Wallis et al., 1999), *ZIC2* (Brown et al., 1998), and *TGIF* (Gripp et al., 2000). However, the role of these genes in dorsal-ventral patterning of the telencephalon is not yet clear. It is likely that there may be several mechanisms for causing holoprosencephaly, as there is not a known effect of some of these genes on ventral specification. The studies with cholesterol biosynthesis inhibitors and the finding that prenatal exposure to certain agents (e.g., ethanol, infants of diabetic mothers, vitamin A analogues) increase the risk for holoprosencephaly and/or the associated craniofacial malformations indicate there are likely to be environmental influences as well (Sulik et al., 1982, 1995). The severity of the phenotype may well depend on the interaction of several genetic and environmental factors.

Conclusion

Development of the body is an extremely complex and tightly regulated process. Precise regulation of gene expression is critical for normal development. Recent exciting findings in a number of animal models have shed substantial insight into the pathways, cells, and molecules that are important for development. The demonstration of mutations in several genes important in development in human genetic conditions further substantiates the importance of these pathways. In addition, the identification of genes involved in human diseases has fueled studies on the function of these genes in animal studies. Further understanding of these developmental processes in both humans and animal models will undoubtedly lead to a greater understanding of both normal embryonic development and insight into the conditions that arise when abnormal development ensues.

REFERENCES

Acampora D, Mazan S, Lallemand Y et al. (1995) Forebrain and midbrain regions are deleted in Otx2-/- mutants due to a defective anterior neuroectoderm specification during gastrulation. Development 121:3279–3290

Acampora D, Mazan S, Avantaggiato V et al. (1996) Epilepsy and brain abnormalities in mice lacking the Otx1 gene. Nature Genet 14:218–222

Bamshad M, Lin RC, Law DJ et al. (1997) Mutations in human TBX3 alter limb, apocrine and genital development in ulnar-mammary syndrome. Nature Genet 16:311–315

Basson CT, Bachinsky DR, Lin RC et al. (1997) Mutations in human TBX5 cause limb and cardiac malformation in Holt-Oram syndrome. Nat Genet 15:30–35

Beachy PA, Cooper MK, Young (1997) Multiple roles of cholesterol in Hedgehog protein biogenesis and signalling. Cold Spring Harb Symp Quant Biol 62:191–204

Belloni E, Muenke M, Roessler E et al. (1996) Identification of Sonic hedgehog as a candidate gene responsible for holoprosencephaly. Nat Genet 14(3):353–356

Binns W, James LF, Shupe JL et al. (1963) A congenital cyclopian-type malformation in lambs induced by maternal ingestion of a range plant, Veratrum californicum. Am J Vet Res 24:1164–1175

Brown SA, Warburton D, Brown LY et al. (1998) Holoprosencephaly due to mutations in ZIC2, a homologue of Drosophila odd-paired. Nat Genet 20(2):180–3

Charite J, de Graaff W, Shen S et al. (1994) Ectopic expression of Hoxb-8 causes duplication of the ZPA in the forelimb and homeotic transformation of axial structures. Cell 78:589–601

Chen H, Lun Y, Ovchinnikov D et al. (1998) Limb and kidney defects in Lmxlb mutant mice suggest an involvement of LMX1B in human nail patella syndrome. Nat Genet 19:51–55

Chiang C, Litingtung Y, Lee E et al. (1996) Cyclopia and defective axial patterning in mice lacking Sonic hedgehog gene function. Nature 383:407–413

Cohn MJ, Izpisúa-Belmonte JC, Abud H et al. (1995) Fibroblast growth factors induce additional limb development from the flank of chick embryos. Cell 80:739–746

Cohn MJ, Patel K, Krumlauf R et al. (1997) Hox9 genes and vertebrate limb specification. Nature 387:97–101

Crossley PH, Martin GR (1995) The mouse Fgf8 gene encodes a family of polypeptides and is expressed in regions that direct out-growth and patterning in the developing embryo. Development 121:439–451

Crossley PH, Minowada G, MacArthur CA et al. (1996) Roles for FGF8 in the induction, initiation, and maintenance of chick limb development. Cell 84:127–136

Cygan JA, Johnson RL, McMahon AP (1997) Novel regulatory interactions revealed by studies of murine limb pattern in Wnt-7a and En-1 mutants. Development 124:5021–5032

Dale, JK, Vesque C, Lints TJ et al. (1997) Cooperation of BMP7 and SHH in the induction of forebrain ventral midline cells by prechordal mesoderm. Cell 90:257–269

Dehart DB, Lanoue L, Tint GS, Sulik KK (1997) Pathogenesis of malformations in a rodent model for Smith–Lemli–Opitz syndrome. Am J Med Genet 68:328–337

Dickinson ME, Selleck MAJ, McMahon AP et al. (1995) Dorsalization of the neural tube by the non-neural ectoderm. Development 121:2099–2106

Dreyer SD, Zhou G, Baldini A et al. (1998) Mutations in LMX1B cause abnormal skeletal patterning and renal dysplasia in nail patella syndrome. Nat Genet 19:47–50

Duprez DM, Kostakopoulou K, Francis-West P et al. (1996) Activation of Fgf-4 and HoxD gene expression by BMP-2 expressing cells in the developing chick limb. Development 122:1821–1828

Durand B, Gao F-B, Raff M (1997) Accumulation of the cyclin-dependent kinase inhibitor p27/kip1 and the timing of oligodendrocyte differentiation. Embo J 16:306–317

Echelard Y, Epstein DJ, St-Jacques B et al. (1993) Sonic hedgehog, a member of a family of putative signaling molecules, is implicated in the regulation of CNS polarity. Cell 75:1417–1430

Ericson J, Muhr J, Placzek M et al. (1995) Sonic hedgehog induces the differentiation of ventral forebrain neurons: A common signal for ventral patterning within the neural tube. Cell 81:747–756

Fallon JF, Lopez A, Ros MA et al. (1994) FGF-2:apical ectodermal ridge growth signal for chick lumb development. Science 264:104–107

Feldman B, Gates MA, Egan ES et al. (1998) Zebrafish organizer development and germ-layer formation require Nodal-related signals. Nature 395:181–185

Figdor MC, Stern CD (1993) Segmental organization of embryonic diencephalon. Nature 363:630–634

Francis PH, Richardson MK, Brickell PM et al. (1994) Bone morphogenetic proteins and a signaling pathway that controls patterning in the developing chick limb. Development 120:209–218

Francis-West P, Robertson KE, Ede DA et al. (1995) Expression of genes encoding bone morphogenetic proteins and sonic hedgehog in talpid (ta3) limb buds: Their relationships in the signaling cascade involved in limb patterning. Dev Dyn 203:187–197

Frantz T (1994) Extra-toes (Xt) homozygous mutant mice demonstrate a role for the Gli-3 gene in the development of the forebrain. Acta Anat 150:38–44

Furuta Y, Piston DW Hogan BL (1997) Bone morphogenetic proteins (BMPs) as regulators of dorsal forebrain development. Development 124:2203–2212

Gibson-Brown JJ, Agulnik SI, Silver LM et al. (1998) Involvement of T-box genes Tbx2-Tbx5 in vertebrate limb specification and development. Development 125:2499–2509

Golden JA, Bracilovic A, McFadden KA et al. (1999) Ectopic bone morphogenetic proteins 5 and 4 in the chicken forebrain lead to cyclopia and holoprosencephaly. Proc Natl Acad Sci USA 96:2439–2444

Goodman FR, Mundlos S, Muragaki Y et al. (1997) Synpolydactyly phenotypes correlate with size of expansions in HOXD13 polyalanine tract. Proc Natl Acad Sci USA 94:7458–7463

Gripp KW, Wotton D, Edwards MC et al. (2000) Mutations in TGIF cause holoprosencephaly and link NODAL signalling to human neural axis determination. Nat Genet 25(2):205–8

Hardcastle Z, Mo R, Hui CC et al. (1998) The Shh pathway in tooth development: Defects in Gli2 and Gli3 mutants. Development 125:2803–2811

Helms JA, Kim CH, Eichele G et al. (1996) Retinoic acid signaling is required during early chick limb development. Development 122:1385–1394

Hynes M, Porter JA, Chiang C et al. (1995) Induction of midbrain dopaminergic neurons by Sonic hedgehog. Neuron 15:35–44

Isaac A, Rodriguez-Esteban C, Ryan A et al. (1998) Tbx genes and limb identity in chick embryo development. Development 125:1867–1875

Izpisua-Belmonte J-C, Duboule D (1992) Homeobox genes and pattern formation in the vertebrate limb. Dev Biol 152:26–36

Izpisua-Belmonte JC, De Robertis EM, Storey KG, Stern CD (1993) The homeobox gene goosecoid and the origin of organizer cells in the early chick blastoderm. Cell 74:645–659

Kang S, Graham JM Jr, Olney AH et al. (1997) GLI3 frameshift mutations cause autosomal dominant Pallister-Hall syndrome. Nat Genet 15:266–268

Kelley RL, Roessler E, Hennekam RC et al. (1996) Holoprosencephaly in RSH/Smith-Lemli-Opitz syndrome: Does abnormal cholesterol metabolism affect the function of Sonic Hedgehog? Am J Med Genet 66(4):478–84

Kohtz JD, Baker DP, Corte G et al. (1998) Regionalization within the mammalian telencephalon is mediated by changes in responsiveness to sonic hedgehog. Development 125:5079–5089

Laufer E, Nelson CE, Johnson RL et al. (1994) Sonic hedgehog and Fgf-4 act through a signaling cascade and feed-back loop to integrate growth and patterning of the developing limb bud. Cell 79:993–1003

Lanctot C, Moreau A, Chamberland M et al. (1999) Hindlimb patterning and mandible development require the Ptxl gene. Development 126:1805–1810

Lanoue L, Dehart DB, Hinsdale ME et al. (1997) Limb, genital, CNS and facial malformations result from gene/environment-induced cholesterol deficiency: Further evidence for a link to sonic hedgehog. Am J Med Genet 73:24–31

Lee KJ, Dietrich P, Jessell, TM (2000) Genetic ablation reveals that the roof plate is essential for dorsal interneuron specification. Nature 403:734–740

Li QY, Newbury-Ecob RA, Terret JA et al. (1997) Holt-Oram syndrome is caused by mutations in TBX5, a member of the Brachyury (T) family. Nature Genet 15:21–29

Liem KF, Tremml G, Roelink H et al. (1995) Dorsal differentiation of neural plate cells induced by BMP-mediated signals from epidermal ectoderm. Cell 82:969–979

Logan C, Hornbruch A, Campbell I et al. (1997) The role of *Engrailed* in establishing the dorsoventral axis of the chick limb. Development 124:2317–2324

Logan M, Tabin CJ (1999) Role of Pitx1 upstream of Tbx4 in specification of hindlimb identity. Science 283:1736–1739

Logan M, Simon HG, Tabin C (1998) Differential regulation of T-box and homeobox transcription factors suggests roles in controlling chick limb-type identity. Development 125:2825–2835

Loomis CA, Harris E, Michaud J et al. (1996) The mouse *Engrailed-1* gene and ventral limb patterning. Nature 382:360–363

Lu HC, Revelli JP, Goerïng L et al. (1997) Retinoid signaling is required for the establishment of a ZPA and for the expression of Hoxb-8, a mediator of ZPA formation. Development 124:1643–1651

Lumsden A, Krumlauf R (1996) Patterning the vertebrate neuraxis. Science 274:1109–1115

MacCabe JA, Errick J, Saunders JW (1974) Ectodermal control of the dorsoventral axis in the leg bud of in the chick embryo. Dev Biol 39:69–82

Mahmood R, Bresnick J, Hornbruch A et al. (1995) A role for FGF-8 in the initiation and maintenance of vertebrate limb bud outgrowth. Curr Biol 5:797–806

Marlow F, Zwartkruis F, Malicki J (1998) Functional interactions of genes mediating convergent extension, knypek and trilobite, during the partitioning of the eye primordium in zebrafish. Dev Biol 203(2):382–99

Marti E, Bumcrot DA, Takada R (1995a) Requirement of 19K form of Sonic hedgehog for induction of distinct ventral cell types in CNS explants. Nature 25;375(6529):322–5

Marti E, Takada R, Bumcrot DA et al. (1995b) Distribution of Sonic hedgehog peptides in the developing chick and mouse embryo. Development 121:2537–2547

Matise MP, Epstein DJ, Park HL et al. (1998) Gli2 is required for induction of floor plate and adjacent cells, but not most ventral neurons in the mouse central nervous system. Development 125:2759–2770

Matsuo I, Kuratani S, Kimura C et al. (1995) Mouse Otx2 functions in the formation and patterning of rostral head. Genes Dev 9:2646–2658

Ming JE, Muenke M (1998) Holoprosencephaly: from Homer to Hedgehog. Clin Genet 53:155–163

Moon AM, Boulet AM Capecchi MR (2000) Normal limb development in conditional mutants of Fgf4. Development 127:989–996

Mortlock DP, Innis JW (1997) Mutation of HOXA13 in hand-foot-genital syndrome. Nat Genet 156:179–180

Muenke M, Beachy PA (2001) Holoprosencephaly. In Scriver CR, Beaudet AL, Sly WS et al. (eds): The Metabolic and Molecular Bases of Inherited Disease. 8th edn., Ch. 250, pp. 6203–6230

Muenke M, Gurrieri F, Bay, C et al. (1994) Linkage of a human brain malformation, familial holoprosencephaly, to chromosome 7q36 and evidence for genetic heterogeneity. Proc Natl Acad Sci USA 91:8102–8106

Muhr J, Jessell T, Edlund T (1997) Assignment of early caudal identity to neural plate cells by a signal from caudal paraxial mesoderm. Neuron 19:487–502

Muragaki Y, Mundlos S, Upton J et al. (1996) Altered growth and branching patterns in synpolydactyly caused by mutations in HOXD13. Science 272:548–551

Nanni L, Ming JE, Bocian M et al. (1999) The mutational spectrum of the sonic hedgehog gene in holoprosencephaly: SHH mutations cause a significant proportion of autosomal dominant holoprosencephaly. Hum Mol Genet 8(13):2479–88

Nelson CE, Morgan BA, Burke AC et al. (1996) Analysis of Hox gene expression in the chick limb bud. Development 122:1449–66

Niswander L, Martin GR (1992) Fgf-4 expression during gastrulation, myogenesis, limb and tooth development in the mouse. Development 114:755–768

Niswander L, Tickle C, Vogel A et al. (1993) FGF-4 replaces the apical ectodermal ridge and directs outgrowth and patterning of the limb. Cell 75:579–587

Niswander L, Jeffrey S, Martin GR (1994) A positive feedback loop coordinates growth and patterning in the vertebrate limb. Nature 371 (6498):609–12

Noji S, Nohno T, Koyama E et al. (1991) Retinoic acid induces polarizing activity but is unlikely to be a morphogen in the chick limb bud. Nature 350:83–86

Nomura M, Li E (1998) Smad2 role in mesoderm formation, left-right patterning and craniofacial development. Nature 393:786–790

Odent S, Attié-Bitach T, Blayau M et al. (1999) Expression of the Sonic hedgehog (SHH) gene during early human development and phenotypic expression of new mutations causing holoprosencephaly. Hum Mol Genet 8:1683–1689

Ohuchi H, Nakagawa T, Yamauchi M et al. (1995) An additional limb can be induced from the flank of the chick embryo by FGF4. Biochem Biophys Res Commun 209:809–816

Ohuchi H, Nakagawa T, Yamamoto A et al. (1997) The mesenchymal factor, FGF10, initiates and maintains the outgrowth of the chick limb bud through interaction with FGF8, an apical ectodermal factor. Development 124:2235–2244

Ohuchi H, Takeuchi J, Yoshioka H et al. (1998) Correlation of wing-leg identity in ectopic FGF-induced chimeric limbs with the differential expression of chick Tbx5 and Tbx4. Development 125:51–60

Parr BA, McMahon AP (1995) Dorsalizing signal Wnt-7a required for normal polarity of D-V and A-P axes of mouse limb. Nature 374:350–353

Pellegrini M, Mansouri A, Simeone A et al. (1996) Dentate gyrus formation requires Emx2. Development 122:3893–3898

Pera EM, Kessel M (1997) Patterning of the chick forebrain anlage by the prechordal plate. Development 124:4153–4162

Porter JA, von Kessler DP, Ekker SC et al. (1995) The product of hedgehog autoproteolytic cleavage active in local and long-range signalling. Nature 374:363–366

Porter JA, Ekker SC, Park W-J et al. (1996a) Hedgehog patterning activity: role of a lipophilic modification mediated by the carboxy-terminal autoprocessing domain. Cell 86:21–34

Porter JA, Young KE, Beachy PA (1996b) Cholesterol modification of Hedgehog signaling proteins in animal development. Science 274:255–259

Qiu M, Anderson S, Chen S et al. (1996) Mutation of the Emx-1 homeobox gene disrupts the corpus callosum. Dev Biol 178:174–178

Rebaglianti MR, Toyama R, Haffter P et al. (1998) Cyclops encodes a Nodal-related factor involved in midline signaling. Proc Natl Acad Sci USA 95:9932–9937

Riddle RD, Johnson RL, Laufer E et al. (1993) Sonic hedgehog mediates the polarizing activity of the ZPA. Cell 75:1401–1416

Riddle RD, Ensini M, Nelson C et al. (1995) Induction of LIM homeobox gene *Lmx-1* by WNT7a establishes dorsoventral pattern in the vertebrate limb. Cell 83:631–640

Roelink H, Augsberger A, Heemskerk J et al. (1994) Floor plate and motor neuron induction by vhh-1, a vertebrate homolog of hedgehog expressed by the notochord. Cell 76:761–775

Roessler E, Muenke M (1998) Holoprosencephaly: A paradigm for the complex genetics of brain development. J Inher Metab Dis 21:481–497

Roessler E, Belloni E, Gaudenz K et al. (1996) Mutations in the human Sonic Hedgehog gene cause holoprosencephaly. Nat Genet 14:357–60

Roessler E, Belloni E, Gaudenz K et al. (1997) Mutations in the C-terminal domain of Sonic Hedgehog cause holoprosencephaly. Hum Mol Genet 6(11):1847–53

Roux C (1964) Teratogenic effect of triparanol in animals. CR Soc Biol 21:451–464

Roux C (1966) Teratogenic effect in the rat of an inhibitor of cholesterol synthesis, AY9944. CR Soc Biol 160:1353–1357

Rubenstein JLR, Beachy PA (1998) Patterning of the embryonic forebrain. Curr Opin Neurobiol 8:18–25

Rubenstein JLR, Martinez S, Shimamura K et al. (1994) The prosomereic model: A proposal for the organization of the embryonic forebrain. Science 266:578–580

Sampath K, Rubinstein AL, Cheng AM et al. (1998) Induction of the zebrafish ventral brain and floorplate requires cyclops/nodal signalling. Nature 395:185–189

Saunders JW (1948) The proximo-distal sequence of origin of the parts of the chick wing and the role of the ectoderm. J Exp Zool 108:363–402

Savage MP, Fallon JF (1995) FGF-2 mRNA and its antisense message are expressed in a developmentally specific manner in the chick limb bud and mesonephros. Dev Dyn 202:343–353

Schier AF, Neuhauss SCF, Harvey M et al. (1996) Mutations affecting the development of the embryonic zebrafish brain. Development 123:165–178

Schier AF, Neuhauss SC, Helde KA (1997) The one-eyed pinhead gene functions in mesoderm and endoderm formation in zebrafish and interacts with no tail. Development 124:327–342

Schmahl W, Knoedlseder M, Favor J et al. (1993) Defects of neuronal migration and pathogenesis of cortical malformations are associated with Small eye (Sey) in the mouse, a point mutation at the Pax-6-locus. Acta Neuropathol 86:126–135

Scott MP (1997) Hox genes, arms and the man. Nature Genet 15:117–118

Seifert R, Jacob M, Jacob HJ (1993) The avian prechordal head region: a morphological study. J Anat 183:75–89

Shimamura K, Rubenstein JLR (1997) Inductive interactions direct early regionalization of the mouse forebrain. Development 124:2709–2718

Shimamura K, Hartigan DJ, Martinez S et al. (1995) Longitudinal organization of the anterior neural plate and neural tube. Development 121:3923–3933

Shimamura K, Martinez S, Puelles L et al. (1997) Patterns of gene expression in the neural plate and neural tube subdivide the embryonic forebrain into transverse and longitudinal domains. Dev Neurosci 19:88–96

Stoykova A, Walther C, Fritsch R et al. (1996) Forebrain patterning defects in Pax6/Small eye mutant mice. Development 122:3453–3465

Stratford T, Horton C, Maden M (1996) Retinoic acid is required for the initiation of outgrowth in the chick limb bud. Curr Biol 6:1124–1233

Stratford TH, Kostakopoulou K, Maden M (1997) Hoxb-8 has a role in establishing early anteroposterior polarity in chick forelimb but not hindlimb. Development 124:4225–4234

Streit A, Stern CD (1999) Establishment and maintenance of the border of the neural plate in the chick: Involvement of FGF and BMP activity. Mech Dev 82:51–66

Studer M, Popperl H, Marshall H et al. (1994) Role of a conserved retinoic acid response element in rhombomere restriction of Hoxb-1. Science 265:1728–1732

Sulik KK, Johnston MC (1982) Embryonic origin of holoprosencephaly: Interrelationship of the developing brain and face. Scan Electr Microsc I:309–322

Sulik K, Dehart DB, Inagaki T et al. (1994) Morphogenesis of the murine node and notochordal plate. Dev Dyn 201:260–278

Sulik KK, Dehart DB, Rogers JM, Chernoff N (1995) Teratogenicity of law doses of all-*trans* retinoic acid in pre-somite mouse embryos. Teratology 51:398–403

Summerbell D (1974) A quantitative analysis of the effect of excision of the AER from the chick limb-bud. J Embryol Exp Morphol 32:651–660

Summerbell D, Lewis J, Wolpert L (1973) Positional information in chick limb morphogenesis. Nature 224:492–496

Sussell L, Marin O, Kimura S et al. (1999) Loss of Nkx2.1 homeobox gene function results in a ventral to dorsal molecular respecification within the basal telencephalon: evidence for a transformation of the pallidum into the striatum. Development 126:3359–3370

Szeto DP, Rodriguez-Esteban C, Ryan AK et al. (1999) Role of the Bicoid-related homeodomain factor Pitx1 in specifying hindlimb morphogenesis and pituitary development. Genes Dev 13:484–494

Talbot WS, Trevarrow B, Halpern ME et al. (1995) A homeobox gene essential for zebrafish notochord development. Nature 378:150–157

Tanabe Y, Jessell TM (1996) Diversity and pattern in the developing spinal cord. Science 274:1115–1123

Thaller C, Eichele G (1987) Identification and spatial distribution of retinoids in the developing chick limb bud. Nature 327:625–628

Tickle C, Alberts B, Wolpert L et al. (1982) Local application of retinoic acid to the limb bond mimics the action of the polarizing region. Nature 296:564–566

van Straaten HW, Hekkung JW, Wiertz-Hoessels EJ et al. (1988) Effect of differentiation of a floor plate area in the neural tube of the chick embryo. Anat Embryol (Berl) 177:317–324

Vogel A, Rodriguez C, Warnken W et al. (1995) Dorsal cell fate specified by chick Lmx1 during vertebrate limb development. Nature 378:716–720

Vogel A, Rodriguez C, Izpisúa-Belmonte JC (1996) Involvement of FGF-8 in initiation, outgrowth and patterning of the vertebrate limb. Development 122:1737–1750

Vollrath D, Jaramillo-Babb VL, Clough MV et al. (1998) Loss of function mutations in the LIM-homeodomain gene, LMX1B, in nail-patella syndrome. Nat Genet 7:1091–1098

Vortkamp A, Gessler M, Grzeschik KH (1991) GLI3 zinc-finger gene interrupted by translocations in Greig syndrome families. Nature 352:539–540

Wallis DE, Roessler E, Hehr U et al. (1999) Mutations in the homeodomain of the human SIX3 gene cause holoprosencephaly. Nat Genet 22(2):196–8

Wanek N, Gardiner DM, Muneoka K (1991) Conversion by retinoic acid of anterior cells into ZPA cells in the chick wing bud. Nature 350:81–83

Warren N, Price DJ (1997) Roles of Pax-6 in murine diencephalic development. Development 12:1573–1582

Wilkinson DG, Bhatt S, Cook M et al. (1989) Segmental expression of Hox-2 homoeobox-containing genes in the developing mouse hindbrain. Nature 341:405–409

Wild A, Kalff-Suske M, Vortkamp A et al. (1997) Point mutations in human GLI3 cause Greig syndrome. Hum Mol Genet 6:1979–1984

Willnow TE, Hilpert J, Armstrong SA et al. (1996) Defective forebrain development in mice lacking gp330/megalin. Proc. Natl Acad Sci USA 93:8460–8464

Wolpert L, Hornbruch A (1981) Positional signalling along the antero-posterior axis of the chick wing: The effect of multiple polarizing region grafts. J Embryol Exp Morphol 63:145–159

Xuan S, Baptista CA, Balas G et al. (1995) Winged helix transcription factor BF-1 is essential for the development of the cerebral hemispheres. Neuron 14:1141–1152

Yang Y, Drossopoulou G, Chuang PT et al. (1997) Relationship between dose, distance and time in Sonic Hedgehog-mediated regulation of anteroposterior polarity in the chick limb. Development 124:4393–4404

Yoshida M, Suda Y, Matsuo I et al. (1997) Emx1 and Emx2 functions in development of dorsal telencephalon. Development 124:101–111

Human malformations

17

Jill Clayton-Smith
Dian Donnai

Introduction

The complex transition from a single fertilized ovum to a normally formed human being depends upon a series of precisely timed genetic and environmental interactions. Reproductive failure is more common than success with less than half of all conceptions reaching a stage of development compatible with extrauterine life. About 15–20% of stillborn babies have a major malformation, and 2–3% of all livebirths have a detectable birth defect (Knox and Lancashire, 1991). Over the centuries, many explanations for human malformations have been suggested, including supernatural forces, mechanical effects and maternal behavior and experiences during pregnancy. Recent studies have proven that genetic factors, and their interplay with the environment during the period of embryogenesis, are more likely to be the cause of birth defects. Cascades of developmental genes which act sequentially and involve complicated feedback loops to regulate gene expression have now begun to be elucidated (Epstein, 1995). In some circumstances it has been possible to demonstrate that environmental factors such as maternal diet and medications taken during pregnancy influence some of these pathways. These discoveries have come about both through the study of specific birth defects and malformation syndromes in humans and animals, and by the detailed observation of the early stages of normal human development. In this way it has been possible to compare normal and abnormal developmental processes, observe the precise timing of occurrence of birth defects and suggest possible mechanisms for further investigation.

Embryologic milestones

Embryogenesis is a complex process determined by both genetic and environmental factors. The stage of embryogenesis at which these act influences the type of malformation which results. Important embryologic milestones are summarized in Figure 17.1. The development of the human embryo can be divided into three periods.

PREIMPLANTATION PERIOD

The preimplantation period includes ovulation and fertilization until the end of the second week of development. During this stage, the zygote undergoes cleavage by a series of mitotic divisions. The resulting bundle of cells divides into an outer cell mass, the trophoblast, and an inner cell mass or blastocyst, which gives rise to the embryo. At the end of this period, the uteroplacental circulation begins. Errors that occur during this early stage of embryogenesis are more likely to cause the death of the embryo than give rise to malformations.

EMBRYONIC PERIOD

This lasts from the third to the eighth week postconception, and during this period the cells differentiate to form the different tissues and organs of the embryo. As a result, the shape of the embryo changes greatly. At the end of this period, the main external features of the body are recognizable. Most major malformations arise during this critical period of organogenesis.

The onset of the embryonic period is heralded by gastrulation. During this important process, the three germ layers

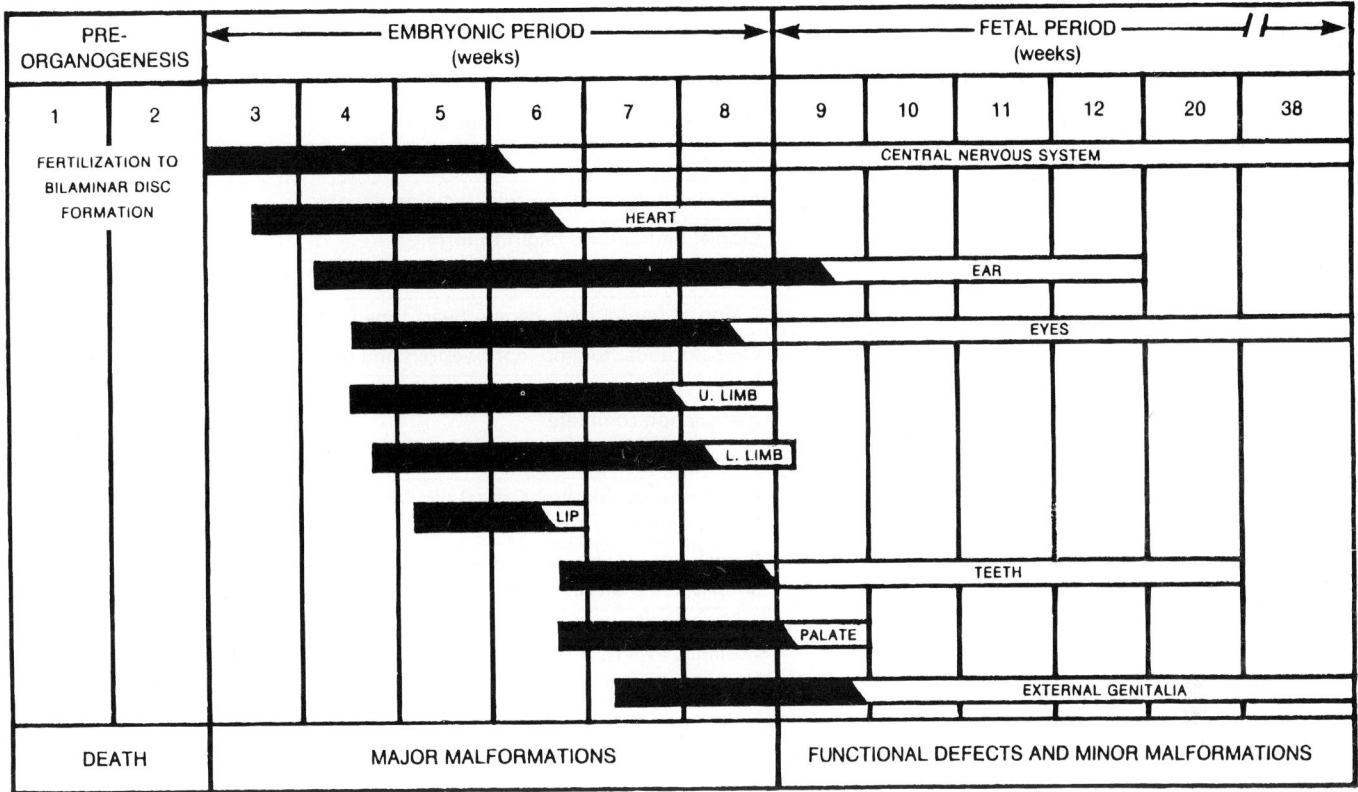

Fig. 17.1. Susceptibility to teratogenesis for different organ systems. Solid bar indicates highly sensitive periods. (From Sadler, 1989, with permission.)

of the embryo—the ectoderm, mesoderm, and endoderm—are defined. Completion of gastrulation establishes important relationships between cells of the three germ cell layers so that differentiation of the organ systems can then proceed.

Ectoderm forms the central and peripheral nervous system, skin, hair, nails, pituitary, sweat glands, tooth enamel, and sensory epithelium of the ear, nose, and eye.

Mesoderm gives rise to the vascular and urogenital systems, adrenal glands, and spleen. Some mesodermal cells become organized into collections known as somites, which have a segmental arrangement and differentiate into muscle, cartilage, bone, and subcutaneous tissue.

Endoderm forms the lining of the gastrointestinal and respiratory tracts, the lining of the eustachian tube, and the thyroid, parathyroids, liver, and pancreas.

Neural crest cells initially form the most lateral part of the ectoderm, which ultimately gives rise to the nervous system and is therefore known as the neural plate. Neural crest cells migrate from the neuroectoderm to enter the underlying mesoderm and they eventually give rise to many different tissues including spinal and some cranial nerve ganglia, melanocytes, Schwann cells, adrenal medulla, and the cells forming the truncoconal cushions of the heart. They also form the bones and connective tissues of the craniofacial structures (Johnston, 1975). Failure of migration of neural

crest cells has been implicated in many malformation syndromes, including those associated with craniofacial malformations, congenital heart defects, and pigmentary disturbances. During the third week of development, neurulation occurs. During this process, the edges of the neural plate become elevated to form neural folds, and the depressed region between them forms the neural groove. The neural folds approach each other in the midline and fuse. Fusion of the folds to form the neural tube begins in the neck region of the embryo initially and proceeds in both directions, but recent studies have suggested that there are multiple closure sites (Van Allen et al., 1993). The cephalic end of the tube (the anterior neuropore) closes on day 25 and the caudal end (the posterior neuropore) closes on day 27. Neurulation is then complete. The narrow caudal end of the neural tube forms the spinal cord and the broader cephalic end the brain vesicles. Neurulation abnormalities give rise to the group of malformations known as neural tube defects. These include anencephaly and spina bifida, which are among the commonest major malformations.

FETAL PERIOD

The last stage of development lasts from the third month until birth. Few, if any malformations arise during this period,

Table 17.1. Main milestones of the embryonic period of development

Days Post Conception	Length of Embryo (mm)	Tissues/Organs Forming
13		Uteroplacental circulation begins
14–15	0.2	Gastrulation begins
16–18	0.4	Notochord, basis of the axial skeleton appears
19–20	1.5	Cranial neural folds begin to form
20–21	2.5	Neural folds elevate, neural tube, basis of CNS forms, embryo folds
22–23	3.5	Fusion of neural folds begins, heart tube forms and begins to fold
24–25	4	Cephalocaudal folding, optic vesicles and otic placodes appear
26–27	4.5	Neurulation complete, upper limb buds appear, branchial arches form, gastrulation complete
28–30	5	Hindlimb buds appear, otic vesicle forms; lens placode appears
31–35	7–10	Paddle-shaped forelimbs; nasal pits form Kidney appears
36–42	10–14	Digital rays present in hand and foot plates; external auricle forms; umbilical herniation begins
43–49	13–22	Digital rays separate; nipples and eyelids form; maxillary and medial nasal swellings fuse to form; upper lip Four-chambered heart complete
50–56	20–30	Fingers and toes free; face looks human; tail disappears

which is devoted mainly to maturation of the tissues and organs and rapid growth of the body. The central nervous system (CNS) may, however, be vulnerable to problems as its development is ongoing during this time. The most rapid growth in length of the fetus occurs during the fourth and fifth months of intrauterine life and increase in fetal weight occurs mainly during the eighth and ninth months. The growth of the head slows down in comparison with the rest of the body, and the face assumes more normal human features.

When attempting to ascertain the cause or timing of a specific malformation, referral back to the embryonic origin of the organ or tissue involved is often helpful. This is particularly true in the case of multiple congenital abnormalities, in which the structures involved may have a common embryologic origin.

In summary, most major congenital malformations arise during the embryonic period of development. Many good embryologic texts are available documenting the events of this period in detail. The main milestones are summarized in Table 17.1.

Frequencies of common malformations

The frequency of different types of malformation can be ascertained from various sources, including government records, birth defect registries, and registration of deaths and stillbirths. The accuracy of these data is influenced by inadequate reporting, failure to make diagnoses in malformed babies, or incorrect diagnoses. There may also be biased ascertainment of cases from some sections of the population. In some cultures, for example, postmortem examination is unacceptable on moral or religious grounds and, thus, internal malformations may remain undiscovered. Pooled data from many different studies probably give the best indication of the prevalence of particular malformations. The frequency of several common malformations is shown in Table 17.2. Prevalence of certain malformations

Table 17.2. Estimated birth prevalence of common handicapping malformations

Type of malformation	Prevalence per 1000 births (United Kingdom)
Anencephaly	1.6
Spina bifida aperta	2.0
Congenital cardiac defects	6.9
Cleft lip with or without cleft palate	1.2
Pyloric stenosis	3–4
Talipes	6.2
Congenital dislocation of hip	3.2

(Data from Leck, 1993.)

may vary between populations; for example, the incidence of neural tube defects is significantly lower in Japan than in the United Kingdom. There is also variation between ethnic groups and neural tube defects are two to three times commoner in white than in black Americans. This has led people to question whether dietary factors, environmental pollution, and lifestyles are associated with the causation of malformations. Malformations are also more frequent in twins, especially monozygotic twins (Schinzel et al., 1979).

Two types of study can be used to study the incidence of major malformations. The direct approach is to examine the frequency of malformations in embryos and early fetuses removed during termination of pregnancy for a reason other than fetal abnormality. This approach will miss fetuses that are aborted spontaneously. The indirect approach is to collect data on malformations in fetuses that have been spontaneously and therapeutically aborted as well as on livebirths. Again, not all the products of spontaneous abortion will be available for examination. A Japanese study that was carried out using the direct approach documented the presence of an external malformation in 4.2% of 6- to 8-week embryos, 1.9% of which had a chromosomal defect. A London study of spontaneous abortions at eight to 28 weeks gestation showed isolated malformations in 4.7% and multiple problems in a further 4.9% (Leck, 1993). In 32% of cases there was an empty gestational sac; 40% of those karyotyped had a chromosomal abnormality, confirming that only a small proportion of embryos with a chromosomal abnormality will survive until birth.

Definitions

MALFORMATION

Malformations are morphologic abnormalities of organs or parts of the body that arise because of abnormal developmental processes. Structures may fail to form altogether, may form incompletely, or may develop with the wrong configuration from the outset. Most malformations will have occurred by eight weeks gestation, when organogenesis is complete. In general, those initiated earlier during organogenesis are more complex.

MALFORMATION SEQUENCE

Malformation sequence refers to a pattern of multiple defects that result from a single primary malformation (e.g.,

spina bifida). A primary malformation sets off a chain of events that may result in hydrocephalus, talipes deformity of the foot, and congenital dislocation of the hip.

DEFORMATION

Deformations are alterations in the shape or position of body parts due to mechanical forces acting over a prolonged period. They result in loss of alignment or body symmetry. Deformations evolve after the period of organogenesis is complete during the later part of pregnancy. The mechanical forces responsible for these deformations are usually external (e.g., constraint within an unusually shaped uterus), but they are occasionally internal (e.g., in the case of fetal edema). Whatever the cause, there is generally lack of fetal movement. Deformations are relatively common anomalies that occur in approximately 2% of newborns. The incidence of deformations is higher in first pregnancies, which are associated with unstretched uterine and abdominal muscles and in pregnancies associated with oligohydramnios, since amniotic fluid protects the fetus from constraining forces. Following birth, infants with deformities may lie or can easily be folded into their prenatal postures. Provided the deforming forces have not been too longstanding, deformations may be reversed postnatally, often by physiotherapy alone. Common deformations include talipes deformities, plagiocephaly, and congenital dislocation of the hip.

DISRUPTION

Disruptions are the result of destructive processes that alter a structure after it has formed normally. Disruptions can lead to loss or division of body parts, abnormal fusion of body parts, or alterations in shape. Aberrant tissue bands following amnion rupture, for example, may lead to limb amputations and extensive facial clefting (Higginbottom, 1979). It is important to make the distinction between a disruption and a malformation, as the former are generally sporadic occurrences with a low recurrence risk, whereas the latter may not be.

APLASIA/HYPOPLASIA AND DYSPLASIA

Aplasia refers to the absence of a tissue or an organ due to absent cellular proliferation. Insufficient cellular proliferation leading to undergrowth is termed *hypoplasia*, and *hyperplasia* refers to the formation of an excessive mass of tissue due to an increase in the cell number above normal.

Dysplasia describes the disorganization of a cell structure itself or disordered organization of cells within tissues or of tissues within a particular structure.

MAJOR AND MINOR ANOMALIES

A *major anomaly* has significant medical and social or cosmetic consequences for the individual concerned (e.g., cleft lip or abdominal wall defect). It cannot be considered to be due to normal variation within the population. Major anomalies are recognizable at birth in 2% to 3% liveborn infants, and a further 2% of infants will be discovered to have a major anomaly (e.g., heart or renal defect) by five years of age.

A *minor anomaly* poses no significant problems to health and tends not to have cosmetic or social implications. These include such features as epicanthic folds, thick lips, or slanting palpebral fissures. They are found relatively frequently within the general population. However, it has been suggested that an abnormality must occur at a frequency of 4% or more in the general population before it can be considered a normal variant, whereas a minor congenital anomaly occurs less frequently than this. Minor congenital anomalies are easily recognizable at birth but, unlike major anomalies, they may resolve spontaneously and decrease in frequency with time.

Although minor anomalies have fewer adverse implications for the individuals concerned, recognition of these minor features is important because the presence of two or more minor anomalies suggests the presence of a major anomaly and should prompt a search for one. Minor anomalies may also provide clues to the timing of the insult during embryogenesis and are an aid to diagnosis in infants with multiple congenital anomaly syndromes.

SYNDROME

A *syndrome* is the term used to describe a pattern of features that arise from several different errors in morphogenesis but that nevertheless tend to be seen together. (The word *syndrome* is derived from the Greek, literally translated as "running together.") The various features of a syndrome usually have a common, specific etiology. Many different multiple congenital anomaly syndromes have now been delineated (Winter and Baraitser, 2000) (OMIM) and, although some have a recognizable mendelian, chromosomal, or environmental cause, many remain for which the etiology is unknown. In many cases, the syndromes exhibit marked variability in phenotype and may be difficult to diagnose with certainty in the absence of specific tests.

ASSOCIATION

Association is the term used to describe the occurrence of two or more features seen together more frequently than would be expected by chance alone but that are not known to have a common cause. One of the best known associations is the CHARGE association in which coloboma, heart defects, atresia choanae, retarded growth and development and ear abnormalities may be seen together (Pagon et al., 1981). Not all features need to be present for the diagnosis of an association to be made, and there may also be additional features. Identification of one component of a syndrome or an association should always prompt the search for other features.

Genetic causes of malformations

The precise cause of many malformations and malformation syndromes are still not known. However, careful clinical delineation coupled with molecular and cytogenetic investigations has resulted in the elucidation of the mechanisms underlying an increasing number of disorders. Chromosomal aneuploidy is shown to be a frequent causative factor especially since the advent of techniques to detect subtle translocations and deletions. Mutated single genes can be responsible for both single malformations and for multiple malformation syndromes. Environmental factors may interact with particular genetic variations. It is artificial therefore to completely separate genetic and environmental causes although it can be helpful to recognize the separate components to facilitate detection and/or prevention.

SINGLE MALFORMATIONS

Most birth defects are single, and the affected person is the only affected member of the family. However, the genetic contribution to such malformations has long been recognized, and specific genes involved are increasingly being identified. Factors that suggested a partly genetic basis for common malformations such as neural tube defects and cleft lip and palate were the observed increase in risk for first-degree relatives and a lesser, although still greater than background, risk for second- and third-degree relatives. Also, in malformations in which the frequency between the sexes is unequal, the recurrence risk was found to be greater if the proband was of the lesser affected sex.

Interaction of genetic and environmental factors

Environmental factors contributing to the occurrence of certain malformations have been identified. Not all embryos

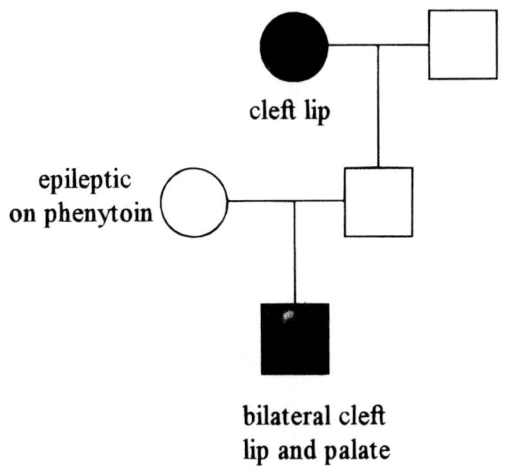

Fig. 17.2. Familial occurrence of cleft lip, demonstrating the balance between genetic and environmental factors.

subjected to a particular environmental influence have a malformation, and it is assumed that only those who have a genetic predisposition are affected. Perhaps there is a balance between the "level" of genetic susceptibility and the "strength" of the environmental influence. The family illustrated in Figure 17.2 may reflect this balance, with a paternal grandmother who had a cleft lip, a mother who was prescribed phenytoin during pregnancy, and a child who had a bilateral cleft lip and palate. A further example is the role of folic acid in reducing recurrence risk of neural tube defects in susceptible mothers after the birth of an affected child (MRC Vitamin Study Research Group, 1991).

Monogenic causes of single malformations

Rarely, single malformations have a unifactorial genetic cause with no apparent environmental contribution and with a high penetrance. Such conditions include the autosomal dominant forms of cleft lip and palate, polydactyly and cataracts. Even in these families, there may be variations in the severity of effects, and the occasional unaffected obligatory carrier.

MULTIPLE MALFORMATIONS

When a child is born with several malformations there is an urgent need to find a precise diagnosis in order to manage and treat the baby appropriately. A diagnosis will also allow prognosis and causative factors to be discussed with the parents. A systematic approach to diagnosis includes:

1. History—family, past obstetric and pregnancy history.
2. Examination—behavior, size and proportions, specific anomalies.

3. Measurements.
4. Investigations—may include chromosomal or DNA analysis, metabolic studies, X-rays or scans.
5. Photographs—for record purposes. Written records cannot capture "gestalt".

Once examination and investigations are complete a diagnostic synthesis is then appropriate. With experience certain patterns may be recognized. Various computerized systems exist to help in syndrome identification and to provide rapid access to relevant literature.

CHROMOSOMAL CAUSES OF MALFORMATIONS

Autosomal aneuploidy

Aneuploidies cause malformations by disturbing the action of multiple genes. By definition, aneuploidies cause gene dosage abnormalities, either reduced in the case of monosomy or deletion, or increased in trisomies or duplications. Specific patterns and malformations associated with aneuploidy are discussed in Chapter 44 to 46. A number of different hypotheses have been proposed to explain the underlying mechanisms of the clinical effects observed in aneuploidy. The so-called "reductionist" or "additive" model proposes that the phenotypes are the result of the direct action of the genes from the involved chromosome or segment; if only all the genes and their actions were recognized and understood, the phenotype could be predicted (Epstein, 1988). The "developmental instability" hypothesis argues that there are more similarities than differences between the various aneuploid phenotypes and that an imbalance of a large number of gene products amplifies the instability inherent in many epigenetic pathways involved in development (Shapiro, 1983).

Microdeletions

As cytogenetic techniques have improved, smaller chromosomal duplications and deletions can be detected but many recurrent pattern malformation syndromes suspected to have a chromosomal basis have no visible abnormality with conventional microscopy. Further studies using the technique of fluorescent in situ hybridization (FISH) have revealed submicroscopic deletions in many clinically delineated syndromes. Such syndromes include Prader-Willi syndrome and Angelman syndromes with deletions at 15q11–13 (Buiting et al., 1995), Di George syndrome with deletions at 22q11.23 and Williams syndrome with deletions at 7q11.23 (Ewart et al., 1993). Recent studies have shown that small chromosomal rearrangements involving the terminal bands of chromosomes (subtelomeric regions) are an important cause of mental retardation. A recent systematic study revealed that just over 7% of children with moderate to severe mental retardation had such an abnormality (Knight et al., 1999).

Sex chromosome aneuploidy

Clinical effects of sex chromosome aneuploidy can range from minimal to lethal and depend on the specific defect and on other influences such as X inactivation and mosaicism. There may be no structural malformations in males with 47,XXY or 47, XYY or in girls with 47, XXX. In conceptuses with a 45, X karyotype it is not fully understood what determines whether the pregnancy will abort, as most do in the first or second trimester with generalized hydrops, or whether the child will survive with relatively few effects other than short stature and streak gonads. Females with Turner syndrome may have structural abnormalities such as horseshoe kidney, coarctation of the aorta and minor skeletal abnormalities such as short fourth metacarpals. Aberrant X inactivation has been demonstrated in individuals with structural X chromosomal abnormalities and physical and developmental disabilities. For example, the minute ring in females with a karyotype 46,Xr(X) and developmental problems has been shown to be lacking the XIST locus (Wolff et al., 1994). Females with X-autosome translocations may be abnormal because of disruption of a single gene locus, or as a result of faulty X inactivation resulting in functional disomy for a portion of the X chromosome (Gustashaw et al., 1994).

SINGLE GENE CAUSES OF MALFORMATIONS

Hundreds of multiple malformation syndromes are inherited as single gene traits. Many are well delineated and the range of phenotypic features well documented, whereas others, particularly where only a few reports have been published, require further delineation. Diagnosis is often by pattern recognition and pedigree analysis, although for some disorders diagnosis is possible by molecular or biochemical investigations or on radiologic or histologic features.

Classification of multiple congenital anomaly syndromes has often been on the basis of the tissues or organs involved, e.g., ectodermal dysplasias and skeletal dysplasias. Disorders may also be classified according to the specific malformations seen, e.g., the first arch syndromes, the short rib/polydactyly syndromes. This type of classification has proved particularly helpful in elucidation of the molecular defects in skeletal dysplasias. Spranger (1985) proposed families of syndromes on the basis of the pattern of the skeletal elements involved. Subsequently, for example, the family which included hypochondroplasia, achondroplasia and thanatophoric dysplasias was shown to be caused by several mutations in the same gene (fibroblast growth factor receptor 3).

Autosomal dominant disorders

These may show variable clinical expressivity, e.g., in Waardenburg's syndrome type 1 due to PAX3 haploinsufficiency, the presence and extent of deafness and pigmentary defects may vary markedly within affected members in a kindred. For disorders where the mutation confers a gain of function on the gene product there is less variation within a kindred, e.g., in synpolydactyly due to HOXD13 mutations.

Autosomal recessive disorders

For many of the rare autosomal recessive multiple malformation syndromes there is an increased rate of parental consanguinity. Many inborn errors of metabolism are inherited in this way and an increasing number are now known to be associated with structural malformations. Smith-Lemli-Opitz syndrome which is characterized by polydactyly, syndactyly, cleft palate, cardiac, renal and genital defects is now known to be due to a defect in cholesterol biosynthesis.

X-linked recessive disorders

There are a number of well described X-linked recessive disorders with multiple malformations where exclusively males are affected or where females are more mildly affected. The X-linked disorder ATRX consists of severe mental retardation, facial and genital abnormalities; carrier females in general have no signs or symptoms. However, in Coffin-Lowry syndrome where there is severe mental retardation and skeletal abnormalities with characteristic face and digital abnormalities, males are more severely affected, but carrier females can also have significant features.

X-linked dominant disorders

Many of these disorders are lethal in utero in affected males and hence only affected females are born. Clinical effects are often asymmetrical, this asymmetry reflects mosaicism due to X-inactivation. For example, in Goltz syndrome skeletal and ectodermal features are usually asymmetrical.

MOSAICISM

The phenomenon of mosaicism, by its very nature, results in enormous variability in phenotype between one individual and another. There are, however, common themes in terms of clinical features that can apply to virtually any type of mosaicism and are useful in suggesting further investigations. These clinical features include asymmetry, joint contractures, pigmentary or other skin changes, hair and teeth anomalies, pin point pupils and seizures. Chromosomal mosaicism can be divided into disorders usually seen in the full form such as Down syndrome or Turner syndrome, and into disorders which are lethal in the full form and survival is due to the mosaic state. Such conditions include trisomy 8,12p tetrasomy and diploid/triploid mosaicism. Pigmentary mosaicism (a better term than hypomelanosis of Ito) is a description of a clinical phenotype of skin pigmentary changes (hypo- and hyperpigmentation) that follow Blaschko's lines. Lymphocyte chomosome analysis is usually normal, but in approximately 30% of patients there is detectable chromosomal mosaicism when cells from skin fibroblast cultures are analyzed.

The clinical effects of single gene mosaicism depend on the nature of the mutation and the timing of the mutation and which tissues are involved. These factors can result in a mild phenotype, a segmental phenotype or a patchy phenotype. Examples of a mild phenotype include instances of individuals with mild Osteogenesis Imperfecta who may themselves have a child with a severe form. Segmental phenotypes are well described for neurofibromatosis type 1 and a patchy phenotype is observed in McCune-Albright syndrome where a mutation in the alpha subunit of a G protein that stimulates adenyl cyclase has been described in mosaic form.

Human malformations arising as a result of environmental factors

Environmental factors may be wholly or partly responsible for some recognizable human malformations. These factors may be inherent in the maternal environment (e.g., acetylcholine receptor antibodies in a mother with myasthenia gravis giving rise to congenital contractures in the fetus) or may be extraneous agents such as drugs or infections. The main categories of environmental agents that cause problems are documented in Table 17.3. Many human malformations are not solely genetically determined, but arise because of the interplay of both genetic and environmental factors. Neural tube defects are a good example of multifactorial inheritance. Although there is an inherited predisposition to neural tube defect, it has been shown that the rate of recurrence in susceptible individuals can be halved by maternal treatment with folic acid (MRC Vitamin Study research Group, 1991).

TERATOGENS

A teratogen is an environmental agent that can cause abnormalities of form or function in an exposed fetus. For teratogenic effects to occur, the environmental agent must gain access to the fetus. Certain agents present in the maternal circulation cannot gain access to the fetus because of their size, means of transport or binding properties. The effects of a teratogen are dependent on several different factors.

Timing of exposure

There are two possible outcomes if exposure to the teratogen occurs before the stage of cell differentiation; this is likely to result in embryonic death or, if only a few cells are injured the loss would be compensated for, and no abnormalities will be apparent. During the stage of organ differentiation, teratogens produce numerous malformations. The type of malformation is dependent on which organ is susceptible at exposure. In general, an organ goes through its most susceptible stage early in its differentiation. Later in gestation, during the fetal period, susceptibility to teratogenic agents decreases. Only a small number of organs,

Table 17.3. Genes responsible for specific human malformations or malformation syndromes

Gene	Type of gene product	Chromosome	Disorder
PAX 3	Transcription factor	2q	Waardenburg Syndrome (Tassabehji et al., 1992)
GLI 3	Transcription factor	7p13	polydactyly, Grieg syndrome (Vortkamp et al., 1991)
GNAS1	Signal transducer	20q13	McCune Albright Syndrome (Schwindinger et al., 1992)
FGFR3	Receptor	4p16	Achondroplasia (Schiang et al., 1994)
L1CAM	Cell adhesion molecule	Xq28	X-linked hydrocephalus (Rosenthal et al., 1992)
CX 43	Gap junction protein	6q21–23	cardiac anomalies (Britz-Cunningham et al., 1995)
ARSE	Enzyme	X p22.3	X-linked recessive chondrodysplasia punctata (Franco et al., 1995)
FBN 1	Structural protein	15q 21	Marfan syndrome (Dietz and Pyeritz, 1995)

including the cerebellum, cerebral cortex, and urogenital structures, continue with their differentiation and therefore remain susceptible to the action of teratogenic factors. Insults that are mechanical in nature, however, can produce structural abnormalities later in gestation but these are, strictly speaking, deformations rather than malformations.

Dose and interaction with other environmental factors

For some, but not all, teratogens there is clearly a dose-related effect, with higher doses giving rise to more malformations. The potency of some teratogens can be increased in the presence of other environmental factors. The teratogenicity of some anticonvulsants is increased, for example, if used in combination with another drug.

Maternal Genetic Factors

Some teratogens increase the frequency of malformations that would otherwise occur sporadically. The incidence of cleft lip and palate is increased, for example, in pregnancies exposed to phenytoin (Hanson and Smith, 1975). In this instance genetic and environmental factors are additive in the causation of a multifactorial malformation. There is also differing "host susceptibility" to some teratogenic agents; for example, a specified dose of sodium valproate will cause malformations in the fetus of one mother, but not in that of another. This finding suggests that different mothers have different thresholds for fetal malformation and this work has been borne out by the observations that women with epilepsy off medication and diabetic mothers have an increased risk of having a child with malformations over and above that of the general population (Dieterich et al., 1980).

Teratogens produce their effects by causing cell death, by altering tissue growth (giving rise to hypoplasia, dysplasia) and by interfering with cellular differentiation. Because these are all general effects, a teratogen may affect more than one tissue, different teratogens may produce common effects, reflecting a disturbance in basic processes. Exposure to both alcohol and to sodium valproate can, for example, lead to dysmorphic facial features with underdevelopment of the mid-face and philtrum (Sulik, 1986; Sulik et al., 1988; Winter et al., 1987). This is thought to be due to death of differentiating cells in this area. Some teratogens do, however, produce a characteristic pattern of growth and morphogenesis; for example, methotrexate exposure gives rise to dysplasia of the skull bones and short limbs (Gellis and Feingold, 1979). The reader is referred to Chapter 39 for further details of specific teratogenic effects.

The identification of an environmental factor as the cause of a malformation is important from the point of view of genetic counseling. Most of these exposures are sporadic, with a low risk of recurrence in future pregnancies. Those due to mechanical constraint may recur but often improve in subsequent pregnancies as the uterus becomes more distensible. Those caused by maternal disease can be recurrent, but attempts may be made to minimize the effects (e.g., of maternal autoantibodies) but should be sought if the pattern of malformations suggests a teratogenic etiology. Information regarding ingestion of some drugs and alcohol is often difficult to elicit but a history of exposure to noxious agents should be sought if the clinical features in the child are suggestive. In the case of congenital infections, a history of maternal infection is not always present, as some infections may be asymptomatic in the mother, yet still give rise to significant effects in the fetus.

Women who are seen for preconceptual counseling are advised to eat a balanced diet and to ensure an adequate daily folic acid intake (400 µg/day) from the time of planning the pregnancy until 12 weeks gestation (Department of Health Expert Advisory Group, 1992). They should also check that they are rubella immune. Once pregnant, they are advised to avoid all drugs that are not strictly essential, as well as cigarette smoking and radiation. Recent guidelines have also suggested that pregnant women should not eat unpasteurized dairy products because of the risk of contracting infection with *Listeria monocytogenes* and should not include liver in their diet because vitamin A, known to be teratogenic, is found in high concentrations in some animal livers.

Developmental biology and birth defects

In recent years an increased understanding of the basic mechanisms of cell biology and the study of developmental processes in lower organisms have facilitated the identification of the molecular basis of many inherited disorders in humans (Epstein, 1995). This has been aided by the development of improved techniques for cytogenetic and molecular genetic analysis.

ANIMAL MODELS

Genetic models for many human malformations exist in the mouse and in other species. These mutants may be spontaneous or engineered, e.g., by targeted gene disruption. The body plan for many species is essentially the same. There is conserved synteny of genetic information with correlation between expression patterns of specific genes in humans and other species such as the fruit fly, mice and zebra fish. This has enabled researchers to focus on chromosomal regions in the human based on knowledge of homologous genes in other species. Homologous areas of the gene maps for man and mouse have been well documented in the Oxford Grid (Searle et al., 1994). It has thus been possible to identify cytogenetic and molecular genetic abnormalities in a variety of different genes which are involved in human developmental processes (Winter, 1988). One such example is the mouse which is heterozygous for the *Twist* gene. This mouse has skull and limb anomalies which resemble those seen in Saethre-Chotzen syndrome, an autosomal dominant craniosynostosis. Recognition of the phenotype in the mouse led to a search for mutations in the homologous *TWIST* gene in humans at chromosome 7p21–22 and these were subsequently identified (El Ghouzzi et al., 1997). Animal models are also useful in studying the teratogenic effects of various experimental agents.

CLASSIFICATION OF GENES GIVING RISE TO BIRTH DEFECTS

Birth defects may be caused by mutations in many different types of gene. One of the main groups of genes involved are genes encoding transcription factors, which contain specific nucleotide sequences (motifs) which are important as recognition sequences for DNA binding. Once bound, transcription factors regulate gene expression, and are thus essential for developmental control. Mutations in genes which encode signal transducers, receptors involved in the transfer of information within and between cells may also give rise to human malformations, along with abnormalities in enzymes, transporter molecules and structural proteins. Two further types of protein which may be disrupted to cause birth defects are gap junction proteins which are essential for correct functioning of intercellular communication and cell adhesion molecules which are involved in cell migration. Table 17.3 gives examples of genes now known to be responsible for specific human malformations or malformation syndromes.

PATHOGENIC EFFECTS OF MUTATIONS

Mutations may act in different ways to cause their effects. A loss of function mutation results in absence or several reduction of the total amount of protein and may result from a variety of mechanisms, including deletion of the entire gene, premature truncation of the protein product or replacement of an essential amino acid. In some circumstances where mutations lead to overexpression of a gene or switching on of a receptor there may be a **gain of function**. This is the case with activating mutations of the *GNAS1* gene which cause upregulation of cyclic AMP production in McCune Albright syndrome (Shwindinger et al., 1992). Gene expression may also be altered by other mechanisms such as increased gene dosage and disturbances of methylation or imprinting. One such example is that of *MeCP2* mutations in Rett syndrome, a neurodevelopmental disorder (Amir et al., 1999). *MeCP2* is able to bind to methylated DNA and thereby silence transcription of other genes. Failure of binding of *MeCP2* due to mutation is thought to result in excessive transcription from genes which are normally silenced and thereby gives rise to the symptomatology of Rett syndrome.

Chromosomal aneuploidy and birth defects

Chromosomal aneuploidy is a major cause of human malformation and recent studies have demonstrated the frequent occurrence of submicroscopic chromosomal deletions and duplications as a cause of mental retardation, dysmorphic features and structural birth defects (Flint et al., 1995). Chromosome maps correlating different chromosome deletions and duplications with types of birth defect have been compiled. (Brewer et al., 1998; 1999) The mechanisms whereby chromosomal aneuploidies cause birth defects include haploinsufficiency, an increase in gene dosage or disruption of a gene lying at a chromosomal breakpoint. There are, however, some instances where cytogenetic abnormalities may affect expression of genes distal to the breakpoints involved via a "position effect" which may involve alteration of chromatin structure in that region.

Gene/environment interactions and birth defects

Some genetic abnormalities give rise to birth defects which are very similar to those resulting from exposure to known teratogens. The fetal warfarin syndrome, which is associated with characteristic epiphyseal stippling of the bones (chondrodysplasia punctata), has a phenotype resembling that seen in patients with mutations of the arylsulphatase E gene (Franco et al., 1995). It has been shown that warfarin may specifically interfere with the *ARSE* pathway, hence the similarity in phenotype. It has recently been suggested that infants of mothers exposed to anti-epileptic drugs in utero have a higher level of homozygosity for a common mutation causing lower activity of MTHFR, an enzyme involved in the metabolism of folate (Dean et al., 1999). Genetic/environmental interactions therefore merit consideration as a cause of birth defects, especially as in these cases prevention may be possible with manipulation of the diet or environment.

Developmental pathways

Developmental pathways of sequentially acting genes are now beginning to be elucidated to explain the aetiology of human malformations. Figure 17.3 demonstrates one such pathway involving the Sonic Hedgehog (*Shh*) gene. Abnormalities of this signalling pathway may give rise to holoprosencephaly (Ming and Muenke, 1998). It is expected that our understanding of such pathways will increase over the next few years. Further work will also

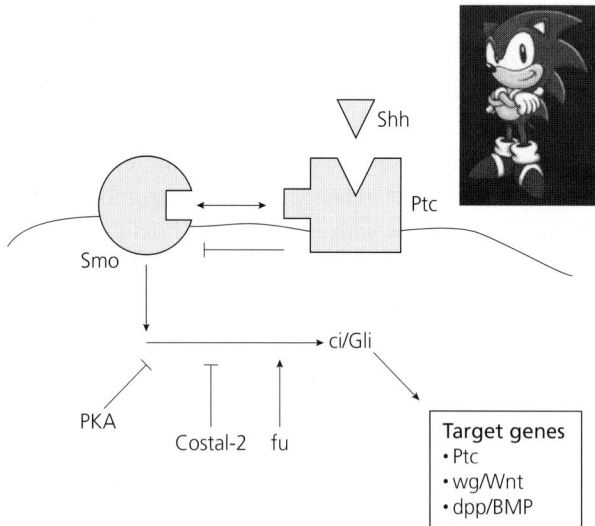

Fig. 17.3. The Sonic Hedgehog (Shh) signaling pathway. Patched (Ptc) is the receptor for Shh. Smoothened (Smo), another transmembrane protein, initiates the intracellular events that result in expression of the target genes. Ptc (red) opposes the actions of Shh (blue) by inhibiting Smo (green) in the absence of Shh. When Shh binds to Ptc. Smo is released from repression, and signal transduction occurs. There are several other proteins identified in *Drosophila* which exert positive (fused) or negative (costal2, Protein kinase A (PKA)) influences. Ultimately, the effects of the different factors converge on the zinc-finger transcription factor cubitus interruptus (ci) in *Drosophila*, or the GLI factors in humans. Target genes of Shh include *Ptc*, *wingless* (*wg*), and *decapentaplegic* (*dpp*). The human homologues of the latter two genes are the *WNT* family and the transforming growth factor-B family members, the bone morphogenetic proteins (*BMPs*). Not all of the components of the pathway have identified human homologues. Note that "Sonic the Hedgehog" (insert: "Sonic the Hedgehog" is a trademark of SEGA), who inspired the naming of the *SHH* gene, has synophthalmia with a nose-like structure below the eyes. (From Ming and Muenke, Holoprosencephaly: From Homer to hedgehog. Clin Genet 1998; **53**: 155–163, © 1998 Munksgaard International Publishers Ltd., Copenhagen, Denmark.)

focus on other genes which are known to cause birth defects in lower species but where no human counterpart has yet been identified.

Management of special needs of individuals with malformations, and their families

DIAGNOSIS AND PROVISION OF INFORMATION

Arriving at a diagnosis is important for appropriate clinical management of a child with malformations. The natural history of the condition and the long-term implications for the child can be considered and associated complications may be detected or screened for. Only with a diagnosis can the parents' questions about what the problem is, why it happened, what it means for the child and whether it could happen again be answered. In the absence of a diagnosis parents will continue to seek this, often with multiple referrals, and it may make it harder for them to come to terms with the child's problem. If a diagnosis cannot be reached then this should be clearly explained to the parents and appropriate follow up and re-evaluations arranged. Where a diagnosis is made, particularly if it is of a rare condition, then follow up by clinical geneticists can also be very useful because of their expertise and access to knowledge about natural history of the condition. For many conditions, or groups of conditions, there are specific or broad family support groups. Information about these should be given to appropriate families. Increasingly for many conditions there are web-based resources. Not all of these are comprehensive or even accurate so the genetic team have a role to play in evaluation and interpretation of such information for the family.

SUPPORT AND COUNSELING

The birth of a child with a malformation places severe stress on parents and other family members. There is usually an initial sense of shock, followed by a period of adjustment. Parental adjustments vary considerably: anger, disappointment, denial and guilt are all common emotions at this time. The stresses imposed on parents may be helped by understanding the cause and implications of the malformation. Genetic counseling gives the family the opportunity to ask questions and to consider recurrence risks and available options. The genetic team have a major role to play in future pregnancies together with obstetric and pediatric services. The needs of the extended family also should be considered. Parents of a malformed child who has died need special help which may involve input by specialist bereavement counselors. Genetic counseling should then be given at an appropriate time.

EDUCATIONAL

Children with malformations with or without intellectual disability have special educational needs and the clinical genetic team have an important role in provision of information about the condition to assist in assessing appropriate educational resources. Geneticists also have a role in educating other health care professionals and non-medical professionals. Many geneticists with particular expertise are associated with lay support groups.

MULTIDISCIPLINARY MEDICAL MANAGEMENT

For those individuals with many disabilities, involvement of multiple medical specialists can pose major problems. Not only are the family faced with numerous hospital appointments but they may be given conflicting information. There is an overwhelming need for co-ordination of medical services and very often it is the pediatrician who fulfils this co-ordinating role. It is helpful for the various specialists involved if there is readily accessible information, and clinical geneticists may be able to provide this. Management guidelines and care pathways are useful and have been developed for some of the commoner conditions. Full information should be given to the primary care team and where the first language of a family is not that of the clinicians, interpreters should be readily available.

SOCIAL CARE

Individuals with disabilities have needs which extend beyond medical care and the clinical genetics team can provide information in a clearly understood format to help the patient obtain appropriate benefits, employment and housing.

REFERENCES

Amir RE, Van den Veyver IB, Wan M et al. (1999) Rett syndrome is caused by mutations in X-linked MECP2, encoding methyl-CpG-binding protein 2. Nat Genet 23; 185–189

Brewer C, Holloway S, Zawalnyski P et al. (1998) A Chromosomal deletion map of human malformations. Am J Hum Genet 63:1153–1159

Brewer C, Holloway S, Zawalnyski P et al. (1999) A chromosomal duplication map of malformations: Regions of suspected haplo and trilethality—and tolerance of segmental aneuploidy—in humans. Am J Hum Genet 64:1702–1708

Britz-Cunningham SH, Shah MM, Zuppan CW et al. (1995) Mutations of the Connexin43 gap-junction gene in patients with heart malformations and defects of laterality. New Eng J Med 332 (20) 1323–1329

Buiting K, Saitoh S, Gros S et al. (1995) Inherited microdeletions in the Angelman and Prader-Willi syndromes define an imprinting centre on human chromosome 15. Nature Genet 9:395–400

Dean JCS, Moore SJ, Osborne A et al. (1999) Fetal anticonvulsant syndrome and mutation in the maternal MTHFR gene. Clin Genet 56:216–220

Department of Health Expert Advisory Group (1992) Folic Acid and the Prevention of Neural Tube Defects. Health Publications Unit, Heywood Lancashire

Dieterich E, Steveling A, Lukas A et al. (1980) Congenital anomalies in children of epileptic mothers and fathers. Neuropediatrics 11:274–283

Dietz HC, Pyeritz RE (1995) Mutations in the human gene for fibrillin—1 (FBN1) in the Marfan syndrome and related disorders. Hum Mol Genet 4:1799–1809

El Ghouzzi V, LeMerrer M, Perrin-Schmidt F et al. (1997) Mutations of the TWIST gene in Saethre-Chotzen syndrome. Nat Genet 15:42–46

Epstein CJ (1988) Mechanisms of the effects of aneuploidy in mammals. Ann Rev Genet 22:51–75

Epstein CJ (1995) The new dysmorphology: Application of insights from basic developmental biology to the understanding of human birth defects. Proc Natl Accad Sci USA 92:8566–8573

Ewart AK, Morris CA, Atkinson D et al. (1993) Hemizygosity at the elastin locus in a developmental disorder, Williams syndrome. Nat Genet 5:11–16

Flint J, Wilkie AOM, Buckle V et al. (1995) The detection of subtelomeric chromosome rearrangements in idiopathic mental retardation. Nat Genet 9:132–140

Franco B, Rappold GA, Andria G et al. (1995) A cluster of sulfatase genes on Xp22.3: Mutations in chondrodysplasia punctata (CDPX) and implications for warfarin embryopathy. Cell 81:15–25

Gellis SS, Feingold M (1979) Aminopterin embryopathy syndrome. Am J Dis Child 133:1189–1190

Gustashaw KM, Zurcher V, Dickerman LH et al. (1994) Partial X chromosome trisomy with functional disomy of Xp due to failure of X inactivation. Am J Med Genet 53:39–45

Hanson JW, Smith DW (1975) The fetal hydantoin syndrome. J Pediatr 87:285–290

Higginbottom MC (1979) The amniotic band disruption complex: Timing of amnion rupture and variable spectra of consequent defects. J Pediatr 95:544–549

Johnston MC (1975) The neural crest in abnormalities of the face and brain. Birth Defects 7:1

Knight SL, Regan R, Nicod A et al. (1999) Subtle chromosomal rearrangements in children with unexplained mental retardation. Lancet 354:1676–1681

Knox EG, Lancashire RJ (1991) Epidemiology of Congenital Malformations. Her Majesty's Stationary Office, London

Leck I (1993) The Contribution of epidemiologic studies to understanding human malformations. In Stevenson RE, Hall JG, Goodman RM (eds): Human Malformations and Related Anomalies. No. 27:1. 65–93 Oxford Monographs on Medical Genetics, Oxford

Ming JE, Muenke M (1998) Holoprosencephaly: From Homer to Hedgehog. Clin Genet 53:155–163

MRC Vitamin Study Research Group (1991) Prevention of neural tube defects: Results of the Medical Research Council Vitamin Study. Lancet 338:131

OMIM: McKusick VA. "Online Mendelian Inheritance in Man" http://www.ncbi.nlm.nih.gov/omim/

Pagon RA, Graham JM Jr, Zonana J, Yong SL (1981) Coloboma, congenital heart disease and choanal atresia with multiple anomalies: CHARGE association. J Pediatr 99:223–227

Rosenthal A, Jouet M, Kenwrick S (1992) Aberrant splicing of neural cell adhesion molecule L1 mRNA in a family with X-linked hydrocephalus. Nat Genet 2:107–112

Sadler TW (1989) Langman's Medical Embryology, 6th edn. Williams & Wilkins, Baltimore

Schiang R, Thompson LM, Zhu Y et al. (1994) Mutations in the transmembrane domain of FGFR3 cause the most common form of dwarfism—achondroplasia. Cell 78:335–342

Schinzel AAGL, Smith DW, Miller JR (1979) Monozygotic twinning and structural defects. J Pediatr 95:921–930

Schwindinger WF, Francomano CA, Levine MA (1992) Identification of a mutation in the gene encoding the alpha subunit of the stimulatory G protein of adenylyl cyclase in McCune Albright syndrome. Proc Nat Acad Sci USA 89: 5152–5156

Searle AG, Edwards JH, Hall JG (1994) Mouse homologues of human hereditary disease. J Med Genet 31:1–19

Shapiro BL (1983) Down syndrome—a disruption of homeostasis. Am J Med Genet 14:241–269

Spranger J (1985) Pattern recognition in bone dysplasias. Prog Clin Biol Res 200:315–42

Sulik KK (1986) Fetal alcohol syndrome and di George anomaly: critical ethanol exposure periods for craniofacial malformations as illustrated in an animal model. Am J Med Genet, suppl. 2:97–112

Sulik KK, Cook CS, Webster WS (1988) Teratogens and craniofacial malformations: Relationships to cell death. Development 103:213

Tassabehji M, Read AP, Newton VE et al. (1992) Waardenburg's syndrome patients have mutations in the human homologue of the Pax 3 paired box gene. Nature 355:635–636

Van Allen MI, Kalousek DK, Chernoff GF et al. (1993) Evidence for multi-site closure of the neural tube in humans. Am J Med Genet 47:723–743

Vortkamp A, Gessler M, Grzeschik K-H (1991) GLI3 zinc-finger gene interrupted by translocations in Grieg syndrome families. Nature 352:539–540

Winter RM (1988) Malformation syndromes: A review of mouse human homology: J Med Genet 25:480–487

Winter RM, Baraitser M (2000) London Dysmorphology Database. Oxford Medical Databases, Oxford University Press, Oxford

Winter RM, Donnai D, Burn J, Tucker SM (1987) Fetal valproate syndrome: Is there a recognizable phenotype? J Med Genet 24:692–695

Wolff DJ, Brown CJ, Schwartz S et al. (1994) Small marker X chromosomes lack the X inactivation centre: Implications for karyotype/phenotype correlations. Am J Hum Genet 55:87–95

Twins and twinning

Judith G. Hall

18

Introduction

Humans have always been fascinated by twins. They are the makings of legends and the essence of old wives' tales. Mythology is full of tales of twins. Romulus and Remus, said to be the founders of Rome, were twins who were supposedly nursed by a she-wolf. The two brightest stars in the Gemini constellation Castor and Pollux are named after a pair of mythologic twins. Conjoined or "siamese" twins have also fascinated humans. They used to be part of circuses and sideshows, where they were displayed as oddities or "freaks of nature." The most famous pair of conjoined twins were Chang and Eng, a pair of conjoined twins that came from Siam (hence the term "siamese twins") and were exhibited in an American circus for many years.

Throughout history, different cultures have had different attitudes regarding twins. In some, the birth of twins was thought to be good luck and to predict times of abundance, giving the family a special place in the community. In other cultures they were thought to be a bad omen, and both the twins and the mother were often rejected by the community or even killed. With time, twins have become less of an oddity and more of a tool for scientific research (Hall, 1996; Martin et al., 1997).

The importance of twins in genetic studies was first recognized by Sir Francis Galton, who in 1875 suggested the study of twins as a model for investigating the differences between the environmental and genetic effects on disease. He proposed that the comparison of the concordance rates for a specific trait or disorder between monozygotic (MZ) twins and dizygotic (DZ) twins would allow the distinction between inherited and environmental effects. The proposal is based on the assumption that MZ twins are identical

genetically. During the past few years, advances in molecular and developmental genetics have uncovered a number of mechanisms, including imprinting, mosaicism, cytoplasmic inheritance, and uniparental disomy associated with discordance of monozygotic twins. These observations raise doubts about Galton's basic premises and have challenged the classic twin method. The purpose of this chapter is to review these new developments and their implications for twins, twin studies, and the twinning process itself.

Determining zygosity

Twins can be either dizygotic (fraternal) or monozygotic (identical). Dizygotic twins (DZ) are the result of two different ova fertilized by two different sperm. Monozygotic twins (MZ) are the result of one ovum fertilized by one sperm that divides to form two embryos (Burn and Corney, 1988). In the past, the only way of differentiating between MZ and DZ twins at birth was their sex and appearance. If twins were of unlike sex, they were said to be DZ, and if they were like-sexed and looked identical, they were said to be MZ. Although not always reliable, placentation was another means of establishing zygosity (Burn and Corney, 1988). Other methods that have been used to differentiate between MZ and DZ twins include blood types, blood protein polymorphisms, HLA typing, and dermatoglyphic studies that document finger and palm prints and creases. More recently DNA studies have been used to establish zygosity. Zygosity testing is important for medical reasons such as disease predisposition and transplantation donation (St Clair et al., 1998).

The first to propose a reliable statistical approach to establish zygosity was Weinberg (1901), who used the

"Weinberg differential method" to estimate the number of MZ and DZ twin pairs. The method assumes that all MZ twins are like-sexed. It also assumes that in DZ pairs the sex of twin pairs occurs at random, so that one-half are like-sexed and one-half are unlike-sexed (i.e., in one-fourth of DZ twin pairs, both are female, in one-half there will be male/female pairs, and in one-fourth both twins are male). Thus, if A is the number of like-sexed twins and B is the number of unliked-sexed twin pairs observed, the estimated proportion of MZ twin pairs would be (A − B) (A + B), and the estimated proportion of DZ twins pairs would be 2B/(A + B).

The Weinberg method has been questioned by new evidence that shows that unlike-sexed twins are not always DZ as when one is 46XY and the other 45X (Edwards et al., 1966; Dellapicola et al., 1985; Kurosawa et al., 1992). Placentation, which was thought to be a reliable indicator of zygosity, is not always accurate, since a single placenta is only expected in 60–70% of liveborn MZ twins (Machin et al., 1996; van Dijk et al., 1996); and very rarely a single placenta is seen with dizygotic twins and may lead to vascular compromise or chimerism (Phelan et al., 1998; Langlois 1999). Machin et al. (1996), using DNA studies to determine zygosity, has found an excess of same sex twins among DZ twin pairs. Today, sex, placentation, cord blood type, HLA antigens, and DNA fingerprinting are all used to differentiate between MZ and DZ twin pairs. However, DNA fingerprinting has become the most accurate method to differentiate between MZ and DZ twins (Derom et al., 1985; Hill and Jeffreys, 1985; Akane et al., 1991). Microsatellite analysis may be a rapid method as well (Becker et al., 1997). Fibroblast DNA analysis may be more accurate than blood studies since in DZ twinning chimerism of blood supply is known to occur.

Twins in genetic studies

The classic twin study methods (Bouchard et al., 1990) rely on the assumption that MZ twins are genetically identical; therefore, any discordance between them is due to environmental influences, whereas differences within DZ twin pairs are though to be a combination of both genetic and environmental factors. For the most part, the assumption that MZ twins are identical genetically is probably correct; however, there are major exceptions.

There are many types of studies in which twins can provide valuable information. The purpose of twin studies is to obtain results that are applicable not only to twins but to the whole human population. However, when using twin methodologies, it is necessary to determine whether twin and nontwin populations differ in the trait under study, since any differences may alter the validity of the conclusion (Doyle et al., 1990). In studies that compare the differences between MZ and DZ twins with regard to a specific trait and then subsequently draw conclusions for the general population, it is necessary to know whether nongenetic factors act differently on MZ and DZ twins, since it is assumed that MZ and DZ twins are exposed to the same pre- and postnatal environmental factors. Machin et al. 1999 suggest the intra uterine blood supplies to each individual of the MZ twin pair may be markedly different. Nevertheless, studies of MZ twins reared apart have been helpful in establishing the significance of genetic and environmental factors regarding susceptibility to complex psychiatric disorders like schizophrenia (Casanova et al., 1990), nightmares (Hublin et al., 1999), and manic depressive disorders (Hublin et al., 1999), as well as to measure the extent of genetic as compared to environmental contribution in disorders with multifactorial inheritance. Thus twin studies may help to sort out the genetic aspects of a variety of complex traits (Neale and Kendler, 1995; Martin et al., 1997; Box et al., 1997).

Structural defects in twins

Both MZ and DZ twins are known to have an increased risk of structural defects compared to singletons (Bryan and Little, 1987; Mastroiacovo et al., 1999). Deformations are particularly increased because two growing fetuses share the space usually meant for one. However, all anatomic sites are involved. Nevertheless structural defects in MZ twins are three times more frequent than among DZ twins and two to three times more frequent than in singletons (Kallen, 1986; Schinzel et al., 1979; Doyle et al., 1990). The structural defects seen in MZ twins can be divided into three groups (Table 18.1) based on the type of process producing them. Because of the high rate of structural anomalies in twins, and the high rate of conversion of a twin pregnancy to a singleton (see below), many singletons born with congenital anomalies may have started as a twin.

Incidence of twins

The incidence of MZ twins has been thought to be constant throughout the world. By contrast, the incidence of

Table 18.1 Structural defects in monozygotic twins

Associated with the twinning process or due to incomplete splitting of the embryo	Due to shared vascular connections or to In utero death of second twin	Due to fetal constraint or crowding in utero
Conjoined twins Fetus in fetu Fetus papyraceous	Acardia (TRAP sequence) Asplenia Microcephaly, hydrocephaly Intestinal atresia Aplasia cutis Terminal limb defects Gastroschisis Disseminated intravascular coagulation	Craniosynostosis Positional defects of the foot Bowing of the limbs Contractures

DZ twins varies from population to population (Nylander, 1981), with a higher prevalence in some areas, such as Nigeria (Nylander, 1979; Little and Thompson, 1988) and a lower prevalence in other areas, such as Japan (Imaizumi and Inouye, 1982; Imaizumi, 1990). The prevalence of MZ twins has been reported to be remarkably constant and has not been observed to be affected by environmental or maternal factors. The incidence of twins (the combination of MZ and DZ) in North America is estimated at 10 to 15 in every 1000 births, that is, roughly 1 in every 80 births (Nylander, 1975). This means that 1 in every 40 people in North America is born a twin. There does seem to be seasonal variation with peaks in March to June and September in the Northern Hemisphere (Fellman and Eriksson, 1999).

Data from several countries suggest that the MZ birth rate may be increasing (Bressers et al., 1987; Bryan, 1994; Murphy and Hey, 1997). Czeizel et al. (1994) have shown that periconceptual vitamin supplementation increased the incidence of twin births by almost twofold. The mechanism for increased live birth of twins is unclear, but may reflect improvement in the living environment and better nutrition in the general population. The number of twin conceptions is harder to assess, since studies have shown that at least 70% of twin pregnancies diagnosed by ultrasound examination before the tenth week miscarry or convert to singleton (Taylor et al., 1984; Landy et al., 1986). The disappearance of a co-twin has been termed the "vanishing twin."

Vanishing twin

Ultrasound studies done early in pregnancy have shown that at least 10% of twin pregnancies are either lost early in pregnancy by miscarriage or are reduced to singletons (Szymonowicz et al., 1986; Sampra et al., 1990; Landy et al., 1986; Machin et al., 1999). Several studies have also

shown that the number of twins in spontaneous abortuses is three times more frequent than that seen in live births (Livingston and Poland, 1980; Uchida et al., 1983). Nevertheless, the rate of vanishing twins is hard to assess. Higher rates are seen in ultrasound studies done before the tenth week of gestation. Estimates of vanishing twin rates vary, depending on the time (i.e., how early) and the number of ultrasound scans. Several investigators have confirmed that the number of twins at delivery is considerably less than the number of twin conceptions seen on ultrasound examination in early pregnancy (Jeanty et al., 1981; Landy et al., 1986; Sebire et al., 1997). Jauniaux et al. (1986) reported that only 29% of women with twin pregnancies diagnosed before 10 weeks gestation give birth to twins. This suggests a 70% loss or reduction rate. Twin pregnancies resulting from in vitro fertilization have also shown that the number of twins seen at birth is lower than that seen on ultrasound in early pregnancy (Levi, 1976).

The greatest "disappearance" rate of the co-twin recognized by ultrasound examination seems to occur during the first trimester. The earliest loss may not be detectable. Some of the mechanisms that have been suggested for the vanishing twin include vascular compromise, life-threatening malformations, spontaneous mutations incompatible with life (Landy et al., 1986) and cord entanglement (Sebire et al., 1997).

Dizygotic twins

DZ twins are derived from the fertilization of two ova by two sperm and may be of the same or different sex (Benirschke and Kim, 1973). Their genetic contribution is different since it comes from two different ova and two different sperm (Bulmer, 1970) (e.g., two siblings who happen to be in the same uterus at the same time). DZ twinning is a common occurrence in animals. Mammals are known to have sizable litters, generally due to polyovulation, making every member of a litter a DZ twin.

TYPES

Multiple ovulation, that is, the release of more than one ovum from the ovaries is necessary for DZ twinning. Women who have given birth spontaneously (i.e., without the use of fertility drugs) to DZ twins are known to have higher levels of follicle-stimulating hormone (FSH) and luteinizing hormone (LH) than are found in those who delivered singletons (Nylander, 1973). This evidence has led to the now established association of increased levels of FSH and LH and DZ twinning.

DZ twins produced by the fertilization of multiple ova may be the result of *superfecundation*. Superfecundation occurs when two different ova are fertilized by two different sperm in more than one act of coitus, either during one ovarian cycle or in subsequent cycles. Very few documented reports have been published. In a case reported by Archer (1810), one twin was white and the other black; in another case (Gedda, 1961), the twins were significantly discordant in size and development at birth. A recent study by Wenk et al. (1992) reviews the frequency of documented cases of superfecundation (Girela et al., 1997). DZ twins may also arise from superfetation. *Superfetation* occurs when a second fertilized ovum implants in a uterus already containing a pregnancy of at least one month (Bulmer, 1970). Superfetation has been suggested in some cases in whom the twins are markedly discordant for birthweight, supposedly due to different gestational ages (Bulmer, 1970; Scrimgeour and Baker, 1974). *Polar body twins* are another type of DZ twins, thought to arise from the simultaneous fertilization of the meiotic products of the same primary oocyte—the oocyte and a polar body—by two different sperm (Scrimgeour and Baker, 1974). Polar body twinning has not yet been reported in liveborn DZ twins but has been suggested in one case as a cause for acardia (Beiber et al, 1981).

PLACENTATION

By definition, DZ twins would be expected to have two placentas, and two chorions, and two amnions, that is, be diamniotic dichorionic (Machin et al., 1999). However, placentas in DZ conceptions may fuse and look like one placenta. In cases of fused placentas, DZ twins often have vascular connections (Phelan et al., 1998). Van Dijk et al. (1966) have demonstrated chimerism in 8% of DZ twins using sensitive immunology techniques, suggesting those

DZ twins will have immunologic tolerance and be good transplantation donors for each other. Careful pathologic and histologic examination of the placenta and other membranes will help establish the zygosity of a twin pregnancy (Machin et al., 1996; Machin et al., 1999).

INCIDENCE

The incidence of DZ twins varies from country to country (Little and Thompson, 1988). However, because of the lack of accurate distinction between MZ and DZ twins, most countries report combined twinning rates. If the MZ twinning rate is constant, the variation is thought to reflect DZ twinning rates. Asia has the lowest reported twinning rate (2 to 7 per 1000 births) (Imaizumi, 1990). A slightly higher twinning rate has been reported in Europe (9 to 20 per 1000 births). The highest twinning rate is seen in the black African population, where it is estimated to be 45 to 50 per 1000 births (Nylander, 1979). The DZ twinning rate in North America is generally estimated at 7 to 11 per 1000 births (Nylander, 1981). However, seasonal variation certainly does occur (Fellman and Eriksson, 1999) with the high birth rate of twins in spring and summer. The DZ twinning rate is closely related to maternal age, parity, height, weight, and gonadotropin levels. An increased DZ twinning rate is seen with increasing maternal age and peaks around the age of 35 to 39 years; higher parity is also independently associated with a higher DZ twinning rate (MacGillivray et al., 1988). Tall, heavy women are more likely to give birth to DZ twins than are short, thin women (Nylander, 1971; Campbell et al., 1974). DZ twinning has been associated with relatively high levels of gonadotrophin leading to excess ovulation. Recently smoking has been suggested to play a role (James, 1997). No substantial variation in DZ twinning rates has been reported with regard to social class. In North America, approximately 1 in 100 births has been of DZ twins and 1 in 50 individuals was born as a DZ twin.

Lewis et al. (1996), using the Australian twin registry, have shown a major genetic contribution to the occurrence of DZ twinning. They point out that multiple ovulation does not always result in a live born DZ twin because of the high loss rate of one of the twins; however, increased multiple ovulation is likely to lead to increased fertility. A gene for increased fertility therefore could be expected to have a selective advantage. They suggest that a single gene responsible for DZ twinning would be expected to be quite frequent in the general population. Meulemans et al. (1996) have analyzed their European twin data and also suggest a single autosomal dominant gene model for DZ twinning.

In the future and even presently in some areas (Murphy et al., 1997) the incidence of DZ twins is likely to increase because of better techniques for successful in vitro fertilization and the use of fertility drugs. However, it appears the spontaneous/natural rate of DZ twinning is decreasing, perhaps secondary to decreasing parity and maternal age.

FAMILIAL DIZYGOTIC TWINNING

There are many reports of familial DZ twinning (Parisi et al., 1983). The female members of these families are thought to have an inherited predisposition to multiple ovulation and in turn have a higher number of DZ twin pairs when compared to the general population (Meulemans et al., 1996). An established association between higher gonadotropin levels and higher incidence of DZ twins in certain families is thought to be the basis for familial DZ twinning. However, there is controversy as to whether this is an autosomal, maternal or paternal effect (Lewis et al., 1996; Lichtenstein et al., 1998). It is possible that some genetic disorders predispose to dizygotic twinning (Healey et al., 1997).

Monozygotic twins

MZ or "identical" twins are the result of the fertilization of one ovum by one sperm. The single fertilized ovum (zygote) then divides into two embryos; both embryos are thought to have the same genetic contribution and in the past have been expected to be genetically "identical." However, with new molecular genetic techniques, it has become clear that some MZ twins are not completely identical, either genetically or phenotypically. Monozygotic twinning is rare among non-humans where most multiple births represent polyovulation rather than splitting of a zygote.

TYPES OF PLACENTATION

The type of placentation in MZ twins is thought to correspond to the stage in embryonic life during which the twinning occurred (Table 18.2); the later the timing of the event, the more likely the twins are to be monochorionic, monoamniotic, or even conjoined (Benirschke and Kim, 1973; Machin et al., 1999). There are a number of different types of placentation according to the number of chorionic membranes and amniotic sacs. MZ twins may have separate or contiguous placentas and may be monochorionic monoamniotic (extremely rare with a poor outcome because of tangled umbilical cords—<1%), monochorionic diamniotic (almost uniformly with vascular connections—about 70%), or dichorionic diamniotic (with separate or contiguous placentas—about 30%). There is likely to be increased loss (of the pregnancy or of one twin) among the types of placentas with vascular connections (Lage et al., 1989; Sebire et al., 1997). In the case of contiguous placentas, MZ twins often share vascular connections and circulation. Seventy-five percent of MZ twins surviving to birth are thought to have had vascular connections in utero (van Dijk et al., 1996).

INCIDENCE

The incidence of MZ twins in humans has been thought to be constant throughout the world, at 3 to 4 in every 1000 births (Nylander, 1979; Imaizumi, 1990). This means that approximately 1 in 300 births has been a MZ twin birth and 1 in 150 individuals has been born as a MZ twin. The rate of MZ twinning appears to be unaffected by maternal age, parity, height, or weight (Bressers et al., 1987). Although temperature, delay from the time of ovulation until fertilization or implantation, oxygen supply, and various teratogenic agents have been shown to affect MZ twinning rates in other animals (Kaufman and O'Shea, 1978), no such factors have been associated with MZ twinning rates in humans. A recent association between an increase of twin births (both MZ and DZ) and periconceptual vitamin supplementation, specifically folic acid, has been reported by Czeizel et al. (1994) suggesting adequate maternal nutrition is important for survival to birth for twins—e.g., loss or conversion to singleton may occur with inadequate nutrition. An increase in MZ twin births has been seen with in vitro fertilization, perhaps related to puncture of the zona pellucida (Edwards et al., 1986).

Table 18.2 Types of monozygotic twins according to placentation

Types of placentation in MZ twins	Time of division after fertilization (days)	MZ twin pregnancies surviving at birth (%)
Dichorionic diamniotic	<3	25
Monochorionic diamniotic	4–6	70–75
Monoamniotic monochorionic	7–13	1–2

FAMILIAL MONOZYGOTIC TWINNING

A few families have been reported in which MZ twinning occurs more frequently than expected (Harvey et al., 1977). This has been termed "familial MZ twinning." Interestingly, there does not seem to be an increase in congenital anomalies among the MZ twins in these families. Because familial MZ twinning has been reported to be inherited from both the maternal and paternal side of the family it has also been suggested that it may be caused by a single gene effect that is unaffected by the sex of the parent transmitting the gene (Michels and Ricardi, 1978; Shapiro et al., 1978). However, the data from Lichtenstein et al. (1998) have suggested there is no paternal effect on familial monozygotic twinning. Familial monozygotic twinning could be related to an inherited defect in the zona pellucida leading to early hatching—a similar mechanism to that proposed for the increased rate of MZ twinning seen in in vitro fertilization.

ANOMALIES ASSOCIATED WITH MONOZYGOTIC TWIN CONCEPTIONS AND OBSERVED DIFFERENCES BETWEEN THE MEMBERS OF AN MZ PAIR OF TWINS

Twin pregnancies and twins are at risk for a variety of obstetrical, perinatal and neonatal medical problems not covered in this text. However, MZ twins are known to have a higher incidence of all types of congenital anomalies which are covered (Table 18.1), but some anomalies are unique to the MZ twinning process itself. Most of these unique anomalies are thought to be due to defects in the completion of the development of the embryo, such as conjoined twins (Machin and Sperber, 1987; Machin, 1993; Machin, 1996; Stockard, 1921; Guttmacher, 1967) and fetus in fetu (Kimmel, 1950; Lord, 1956); to vascular aberrations such as acardia (Van Allen et al., 1983; Nance, 1981; Métneki et al., 1996); and vascular accidents such as terminal limb defects and death of the co-twin (Saier et al., 1975); and fetal constraint (which occurs in both types of twins) (Table 18.3). The intra uterine environment may be different for the two MZ twins because of the number of cells allocated to each twin, the timing of the twinning event and the placental vascular supply to each twin (Machin, 1996; Machin et al., 1999). Interestingly, in utero studies of monozygotic twin behavior have recently shown clear differences in activity and responsiveness before 20 weeks of the pregnancy (Piontelli et al., 1999).

It is becoming clear by studying MZ twin pairs that a number of neurologic, immunologic, and structural aspects of embryogenesis appear to be independent of genetic factors. Steinmetz et al. (1994) have described the discordance in brain surface anatomy in MZ twins. Wolf et al. (1995) and Trejo et al. (1995) have shown differences in the immune response between MZ twins in spite of exposure to very similar in utero and post birth environments. Somatic changes have been observed to occur in the course of development of the MZ twins leading to differences between the MZ twins in telomere size (Slagboom et al., 1994), the fragile X triplet repeat expansion (Tuckerman et al., 1985), and Alu band variants (Huang et al., 1995).

MIRROR-IMAGE TWINS

A disturbance of laterality is regarded as a diagnostic feature of mirror-imaging in MZ twins. Approximately 10% of liveborn MZ twins have some form of mirror-image features. Although very rare, MZ twins with situs inversus or with different handedness are also regarded as mirror-image twins (Sommer et al., 1999). Much more common differ-

Table 18.3 Anomalies exclusive to monozygotic twins

Anomaly	Description	Reference
Fetus in fetu	Small parasitic dead twin attached to a normal twin. Often confused with a tumor. Generally located at the origin of the superior mesenteric vessels. Other sites have been reported.	Kimmel et al. (1950) Lord (1956) MacGillivray et al. (1975)
Fetus papyraceous	Mummified dead fetus usually attached to the placenta and present with a normal or more viable twin.	Saier et al. (1975) Lage et al. (1989)
Acardia	Twin with an absent or rudimentary or nonfunctioning heart and whose circulation has been sustained by a normal twin. Associated with a higher rate of chromosomal anomalies.	Schinzel et al. (1979) Van Allen et al. (1983)
Conjoined twins	Incomplete twins resulting from an abnormality of the twinning process. They are derived from a single zygote and are always of the same sex. Incidence varies from 1–20,000 to 1–100,000. Females make up 80% of conjoined twins.	Guttmacher (1967) Bulmer (1970) Machin and Sperber (1987 Machin (1993)

ences are minor asymmetries of facial features, such as the side of upsweep of the head hair or eyebrow, one-sided ptosis, or side of eruption of the first tooth (Boklage, 1987a; Cidis et al., 1997; Sperber et al., 1994). A very interesting hypothesis regarding mirror-image twins was made by Boklage (1981a; 1981b; 1987b), suggesting that MZ twinning requires readjustment of the body axis plan. Sperler et al. (1994) suggest mirror image twinning may occur relatively late in embryonic development after the orientation of axis of the zygote has been established.

SEX RATIO IN MONOZYGOTIC TWINS

The sex ratio—the proportion of males to the combination of males and females—among MZ twins is lower than among DZ twins or singletons (James, 1975; 1980) (Table 18.4). Conjoined twins have an even lower sex ratio than that of MZ twins (Benirschke and Kim, 1973; Zake, 1984) meaning there is an excess of female conjoined twins. Tsunoda et al. (1985) showed in mice that female embryos are behind male embryos in the number of cells present at a specific stage in early development, suggesting that female conceptions may be at higher risk, because of their delayed development, for late splitting of the embryo leading to the excess of conjoined and MZ twins.

ETIOLOGY OF MONOZYGOTIC TWINNING

The etiology of MZ twinning in humans is unknown, but several mechanisms have been proposed. Stockard (1921) suggested that MZ twinning may be due to lack of oxygen prior to implantation that caused developmental arrest and splitting in the zygote. His work was supported by the finding that the implantation of the ovum is delayed in the armadillo which results in monozygotic quadruplets or octuplets (Storrs and Williams, 1968) and by studies in rabbit and roe deer showing that twinning in these animals is also associated with delayed implantation (Bulmer, 1970). These findings suggested that MZ twinning is associated with disturbance of development clocks or thresholds and that delayed fertilization or delayed implantation may play a role in MZ twinning.

Table 18.4 Sex ratio in twins

	DZ twins and singletons	All MZ twins	Conjoined twins	Sacral teratomas
Sex ratio (M/(M + F)	0.514	0.496	0.23	0.25

(From James, 1980, with permission.)

On the basis of observations of a higher than expected incidence of MZ twins following in vitro fertilization (Yovich et al., 1984; Derom et al., 1987), Edwards et al. (1986) suggested that abnormalities or rupture of the zona pellucida may lead to herniation of the blastocyst and predispose to MZ twinning. Boklage (1981b; 1987a; 1987b) pointed out that differentiation of the chorion occurs at approximately the fourth day after fertilization and that, in monochorionic MZ twins, the physical separation of two embryos is unlikely if the zona is still intact when the chorion begins to develop. Boklage suggested that if the zona is intact, rather than a physical separation of the MZ twins, there may be "developmental" separation rendering two groups of cells within a morula that organize themselves separately and continue with embryogenesis separately.

Other investigators have suggested that twinning itself may be a type of congenital anomaly or an abnormality of development with the "twinning" fertilized egg (i.e., a fertilized egg resulting in twins) developing at a different rate and in a different way, as compared to a "normal" fertilized egg (i.e., an egg resulting in a singleton). There must be a relatively narrow window during which MZ twinning can occur (normally only up until 11 to 13 days postfertilization, when the primitive streak forms), and there are a number of different events taking place during postfertilization, including hatching, implantation, genomic imprinting, and X-inactivation (Fig. 18.1). If the twinning zygote is maturing at a different rate than the normal zygote, the timing for all these events may be different and even in a different order from the predicted normal timing for singletons.

The finding that mammalian female embryos are somewhat behind male embryos in the number of cells present at a certain stage during early stages of embryonic development (Tsunoda et al., 1985) and the fact that there is a slightly higher incidence of female MZ twins, particularly among conjoined twins, in which the twinning process is assumed to occur relatively late in the very early embryonic developmental process, support the suggestion that MZ twinning is somehow related to delayed implantation and that the timing of different developmental clocks plays a critical role in MZ twinning.

Several authors have suggested that skewed X-chromosomal inactivation may play a role in female MZ twinning if, during embryogenesis, two different foci were to arise—one expressing the maternal X, the other expressing the paternal X. A number of female MZ twins have been discordant for a variety of X-linked recessive diseases, suggesting, and often demonstrating, non-random X-inactivation (Table 18.5). Goodship et al. (1996) have tested the hypothesis that skewed X-inactivation can trigger MZ twinning in females by study-

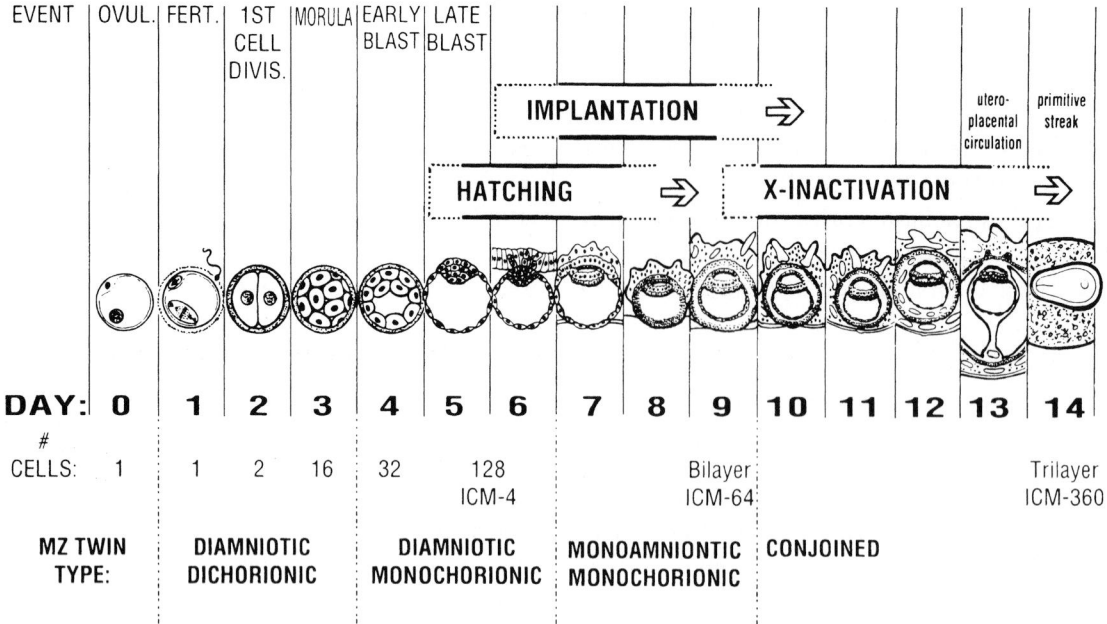

Fig. 18.1. Process of monozygotic twinning during postfertilization.

ing umbilical cord tissue in female MZ twins. They observed random X-inactivation in most pairs of female MZ twins, but some showed marked skewing. Thus, it would appear that skewed X-inactivation does not explain all female monozygote twinning, but could be responsible for the excess of MZ female twins. Interestingly, Tan et al. (1993) have shown that X-inactivation occurs at different times in different tissues post-implantation in the mouse embryo. These findings suggest that X-inactivation occurs at the time of tissue differentiation; thus, X-inactivation in blood and skin may not be representative of the rest of the tissue in an organism. To properly determine the exact role of X-inactivation in female MZ twinning, it would be necessary to study many different tissues. Bamforth et al. (1996) have studied the parent-of-origin of X-inactivation in placental membranes and umbilical cords in twins and triplets. The chorion did show asymmetric X-inactivation in MZ dichorionic twins. Of course, the chorion is not representative of the whole embryo but may represent processes which occurred early in development. The study also suggested that "connected" monozygous twins may react differently from "unconnected" ones, reflecting the importance of timing in the MZ twinning process.

There are many reports of discordance in the expression of genetic material in MZ twins (Table 18.5). Discordant MZ twins for X-linked traits such as Duchenne muscular dystrophy (Burn et al., 1986; Goodship et al., 1996), autosomal traits, and chromosomal anomalies have all been reported (Haskins-Olney et al., 1988). These observations have suggested that, in addition to familial MZ twinning and rupture

of the zona pellucida-induced MZ twinning, some cases of MZ twinning may occur because of a discordance in the expression of genetic information, not only by discordance of X inactivation, but by many other genetic mechanisms as well, including genomic imprinting, loss of imprinting, the development of uniparental disomy, changes in chromosome number, mitochondrial mutations (Hall, 1996; Cote and Gyftodimov, et al., 1991) and telomere crossover (Shaffer et al., 1999). This discordance would be expected to arise early in development among cells from a single zygote. A discordance of expression of genetic information could then lead to division of the zygote into two separate embryos during a specific period, early in development, perhaps from the stage of eight cells to approximately 360 cells in the inner cell mass, when differentiation and primitive streak formation begins. After birth, this discordance of genetic information could be mosaic in each twin, but it could be present to different degrees in the two different twins sufficient to cause observable phenotypical discordance. In other words, genetic discordance or differences in the expression of genetic information should be suspected in cases of discordant MZ twins.

Conclusion

In the field of twins and twinning, there is still a great deal to be learned. The development of new DNA molecular

Table 18.5 Reported discordance in monozygotic twins

Adrenal hyperplasia	Kanjilal et al. (1989)
Aglossia-adactylia	Robinow et al. (1978)
Aicardi syndrome	Costa et al. (1990)
Alzheimer disease	Creasey et al. (1989); Kumar et al. (1991)
Amniotic bands	Donnenfeld et al. (1985)
Amyoplasia	Hall et al. (1983)
Amyotrophic lateral sclerosis	Jokelainen et al. (1978)
Anorchia	Aynsley-Green et al. (1976)
Asplenia	Wilkinson et al. (1979)
Beckwith-Wiedemann syndrome	Bose et al. (1985); Litz et al. (1988); Haskins-Olney et al. (1988); Clayton-Smith et al. (1992)
Biliary atresia	Strickland et al. (1985)
Coeliac disease	Henker et al. (1989)
Cleft lip ± cleft palate	Hunter and Dijkman (1977); Cronin and Hunter (1980); Nystrom and Ranta (1988)
Cloverleaf skull	Corsello et al. (1992)
Congenital heart disease	Stoll et al. (1984)
Cutaneous mastocytosis	Cainelli et al. (1983)
Diabetes	Johnston et al. (1988)
Duane retraction syndrome	Kaufman et al. (1989)
Duchenne muscular dystrophy	Burn et al. (1986); Chotkow et al. (1987); Richards et al. (1990); Lupski et al. (1991)
Endocardial fibroelastosis	Lazda (1998)
Factor IX deficiency	Kitchens (1987)
Fibular aplasia	Halal (1991)
Fragile X syndrome	Kruyer et al. (1993)
G syndrome	Young et al. (1988)
Genital anomalies	Berry et al. (1984)
Gerstmann-Strüssler-Scheinker disease	Hamasaki et al. (1998)
Goldenhar syndrome	Boles et al. (1987)
Gonadal dysgenesis	Karp et al. (1991)
Handedness	Boklage (1981a)
Hirschsprung disease	Moore et al. (1979); Hanon and Boston (1988)
Hunter disease	Clarke et al. (1991)
Hypothyroidism	Retting et al. (1980)
Kallmann	Hipkin et al. (1990)
Kleeblattschadel anomaly	Horton et al. (1983)
Lipodystrophy	Lampert et al. (1984)
McCune-Albright	Endo et al. (1991)
Multiple sclerosis	Kinnunen et al. (1988)
Myasthenia gravis	Lefvert et al. (1989)
Neural tube defects	Schinzel et al. (1979); Putz and Rehder (1985)
Neuroblastoma	Kushner and Helson (1985)
Oculo-oto-radial syndrome	ElHiolu and Berry (1997)
Oral-facial-digital syndrome, type 1	Shotelersuk et al. (1999)
Proteus syndrome	Saul et al. (1990)
Renal agenesis	Klinger et al. (1997)
Rheumatoid arthritis	Singal et al. (1989)
Rubinstein-Taybi syndrome	Kajii et al. (1981)
Russell-Silver syndrome	Samn et al. (1990)
Sex	Perlman et al. 1990, Arizawa et al. (1988)
Schimmelpenning-Feuerstein-Mims syndrome	Schworm et al. (1996)
Schizophrenia	Casanova et al. (1990); Lewis et al. (1991)
Scleroderma	Dustoor et al. (1987)
Skeletal dysplasia	Stoll et al. (1984)

continued

Table 18.5 Reported discordance in monozygotic twins (*continued*)

Sotos syndrome	Brown et al (1998)
Symbrachydactyly	Shiono and Ogino (1980)
Sudden infant death syndrome	Beal (1989)
Trisomy 1	Watson et al. 1990
Trisomy 13 (phenotype)	Naor et al. (1987); Loevy et al. (1985)
Trisomy 18 (phenotype)	Mulder et al. (1989); Schlessel et al. (1990)
Trisomy 21	Rogers et al. (1989); Gilgenkrantz and Janot (1983)
Tuberous sclerosis	Briliant et al. (1982); Kondo et al. (1991)
Urinary tract anomalies	Johnstone and Benirschke (1976)
Ullrich-Turner syndrome	Perlman et al. (1990); Kaplowitz et al. (1991)
VATER	King et al. (1977)

and cytogenetic techniques; the use of prenatal diagnosis such as chorionic villi sampling, amniocentesis, and ultrasound examination in humans; as well as embryopathology and histology advances all give clues to the understanding of MZ and DZ twins and the twinning process.

Twins will continue to be useful in the study of complex disorders. Determining zygosity is of medical importance since MZ twins are an excellent source for transplantation between the MZ twins. Perhaps some DZ twins will tolerate transplantation better because of shared in utero connections. MZ twins are much more prone to developing the same diseases and MZ pregnancies are at risk for a number of specific medical problems.

In the future, determination of zygosity at birth will be expected. It will also be standard practice to document placental connections and vascular supplies in order to establish in utero environmental differences in individual twins.

REFERENCES

Akane A, Matsubara K, Shiono H et al. (1991) Diagnosis of twins zygosity by hypervariable RFLP markers. Am J Med Genet 41:96–98

Archer J (1810) Facts illustrating a disease peculiar to the female children of negro slaves. Med Reposit 1:319–323

Arizawa M, Suehara N, Takemura T et al. (1988) Monozygotic twins discordant for sex. Acta Obstet Gynecol Jpn 40:1479–1482

Aynsley-Green A, Zachmann M, Illig R et al. (1976) Congenital bilateral anorchia in childhood: A clinical, endocrine and therapeutic evaluation of twenty-one cases. Clin Endocrinol 5:381–391

Bamforth F, Machin G, Innes M (1996) X-chromosome inactivation is mostly random in placental tissues or tissues of female monozygotic twins and triplets. Am J Med Genet 61:209–215

Beal S (1989) Sudden infant death syndrome in twins. Pediatrics 84:1038–1044

Becker A, Busjahn A, Faulhaber HD et al. (1997) Twin zygosity. Automated determination with microsatellites. J Reprod Med 42:260–266

Beiber FR, Nance WE, Morton CC et al. (1981) Genetic studies of an acardiac monster: Evidence of polar body twinning in man. Science 213:775–777

Benirschke K, Kim CK (1973) Multiple pregnancy. N Engl J Med 288:1276–1284, 1329–1336

Berry SA, Johnson DE, Thopsom TR (1984) Agenesis of the penis, scrotal raphe and anus in one of monoamniotic twins. Teratology 29:173–176

Boklage CE (1981a) On the distribution of nonrighthandedness among twins and their families. Acta Genet Med Gemellol 30:167–187

Boklage CE (1981b) On the timing of monozygotic twinning events. In Gedda L, Parisi P, Nance WE (eds): Twin Research. Vol. 3. Twin Biology and Multiple Pregnancy. Alan R. Liss, N Y, pp.155–165

Boklage CE (1987a) Invited editorial essay: Twinning, nonrighthandedness and fusion malformations: Evidence for heritable elements in common. Am J Med Genet 28:67–84

Boklage CE (1987b) The organization of the oocyte and embryogenesis in twinning and fusion malformations. Acta Genet Med Gemellol 36:421–431

Boles DJ, Bodurtha J, Nance WE (1987) Goldenhar complex in discordant monozygotic twins: A case report and review of the literature. Am J Med Genet 28:103–109

Bose B, Wilhie RA, Madlom M (1985) Wiedemann-Beckwith syndrome in one of monozygotic twins. Arch Dis Child 60:1191–1192

Bouchard TJ, Lykken DT, McGue M (1990) Sources of human psychological differences; The Minnesota study of twins reared apart. Science 250:223–228

Box NF, Wyeth JR, O'Gorman LE et al. (1997) Characterization of melanocyte stimulating hormone receptor variant alleles in twins with red hair. Hum Mol Genet 6:1891–1897

Bressers WMA, Eriksson AW, Kostense PJ (1987) Increasing trend in monozygotic twinning rate. Acta Genet Med Gemellol 36:397–399

Brilliant MH, Cleve H, Edwards JH et al. (1990) Cell lines from monozygotic twins discordant for tuberous sclerosis display protein and DNA differences. Am J Hum Genet 47:A210

Brown WT, Wisniewski KE, Sudhalter V et al. (1998) Identical twins discordant for Sotos syndrome. Am J Med Genet 79:329–333

Bryan E (1994) Trends in twinning rates. Lancet 343:1151–1152

Bryan E, Little J (1987) Congenital anomalies in twins. Clin Obstet Gynecol 1:697–721

Bulmer M (1970) The biology of twinning in man. Clarendon Press, Oxford

Burn J, Corney G (1988) Zygosity determination and the types of twinning. In MacGillivray I, Campbell DM, Thompson B (eds): Twinning and Twins. John Wiley & Sons, Chichester, UK pp. 7–25

Burn J, Povey S, Boyd Y et al. (1986) Duchenne muscular dystrophy in one of monozygotic twin girls. J Med Genet 23:494–500

Cainelli T, Marchesi L, Pasquali F et al. (1983) Monozygotic twins discordant for cutaneous mastocytosis. Arch Dermatol 119:1021–1022

Campbell DM, Campbell AL, MacGillivray I (1974) Maternal characteristic of women having twin pregnancies. J Biosoc Sci 6:463–469

Casanova MF, Zito M, Goldberg T et al. (1990) Shape distortion of the corpus callosum of monozygotic twins discordant for schizophrenia. Schizophr Res 3:155–156

Chotkow JG, Hyser CL, Edwards JA et al. (1987) Monozygotic female twin carriers discordant for the clinical manifestations of Duchenne muscular dystrophy. Neurology 37:1147–1151

Cidis MB, Warshowsky JH, Goldrich SG et al. (1997) Mirror-image optic nerve dysplasia with associated anisometropia in identical twins. J Am Optom Assoc 68:325–329

Clarke JTR, Greer WL, Srasber PM et al. (1991) Hunter disease (Mucopolysaccharidosis Type II) associated with unbalanced activation of the X chromosomes in a karyotypically normal girl. Am J Hum Genet 49:289–297

Clayton-Smith J, Read AP, Donnai D (1992) Monozygotic twinning and Wiedemann-Beckwith syndrome. Am J Med Genet 42:633–637

Corsello G, Maresi E, Rossi C et al. (1992) Thanatophoric dysplasia in monozygotic twins discordant for cloverleaf skull: Prenatal diagnosis, clinical and pathological findings. Am J Med Genet 42:122–126

Costa T, Greer W, Duckworth-Rysiecki G et al. (1990) Monozygotic twins discordant for Aicardi syndrome. Am J Hum Genet, suppl. 47:A53

Cote GN, Gyftodimou J (1991) Twinning and mitotic crossing-over, some possibilities and their implications. Am J Med Genet 49:120–130

Creasey H, Jorm A, Longley W et al. (1989) Monozygotic twins discordant for Alzheimer's disease. Neurology 39:1474–1476

Cronin DG, Hunter WS (1980) Craniofacial morphology in twins discordant for cleft lip and/or palate. Cleft Palate J 17:116–126

Czeizel A, Metneki J, Dudas I (1994) Higher rate of multiple births after periconceptual vitamin supplementation. Lancet 330:23–24

Dellapicola B, Stomeo C, Ferranti G et al. (1985) Discordant sex in one of three monozygotic triplets. J Med Genet 22:6–11

Derom C, Bakker J, Vlietnick R (1985) Zygosity determination in newborn twin using DNA variants. J Med Genet 22:279–284

Derom C, Vlientnick R, Derom R et al. (1987) Increased monozygotic twinning rate after ovulation induction. Lancet 1:1236–1238

Donnenfeld AE, Dunn LK, Rose NC (1985) Discordant amniotic band sequence in monozygotic twins. Am J Med Genet 20:685–694

Doyle PE, Beral V, Botting B, Wale CJ (1990) Congenital malformations in twins in England and Wales. J Epidemiol Community Health 45:43–48

Dustoor MM, McInerney MM, Mazanec DJ et al. (1987) Abnormal lymphocyte function in scleroderma: a study on identical twins. Clin Immunol Immunopathol 44:20–30

Edwards JH, Dent T, Kahn J (1966) Monozygotic twins of different sex. J Med Genet 3:117–118

Edwards RG, Mettler L, Walters DE (1986) Identical twins and in vitro fertilization. J In Vitro Fertil Embryo Trans 3:114–117

ElHiolu N, Berry AC (1997) Monozygotic twins discordant for the oculo-oto-radial syndrome (IVIC syndrome). Genet Counseling 4:201–206

Endo M, Yamada Y, Nijikawa N (1991) Monozygotic twins discordant for the major signs of McCune-Albright syndrome. Am J Med Genet 41:216–220

Fellman J, Eriksson AW (1999) Statistical analysis of the seasonal variation in the twinning rate. Twin Research 2:22–29

Galton F (1875) The history of the twins as a criterion of the relative powers of nature and nurture. J Anthropol Inst

Gedda L (1961) Twins in history and science. Charles C Thomas, Springfield, Illinois

Gilgenkrantz S, Janot C (1983) Monozygotic twins discordant for trisomy 21 or chimeric dizygotic twins? Am J Med Genet 15:159–160

Girela E, Rodrigo MD, Lorente JA et al. (1997) Indisputable double paternity in dizygous twins. Fertil Steril 67:1159–1161

Goodship J, Carter J, Burn J (1996) X-inactivation patterns in monozygotic and dizygotic female twins. Am J Med Genet 64:205–208

Guttmacher AF (1967) Teratology of conjoined twins. Birth Defects 3:3–7

Halal F (1991) Monozygotic twins discordant for fibular aplasia. Am J Med Genet 41:434–437

Hall JG (1996) Twinning: Mechanisms and genetic implications. Current Opinion in Genetics & Development 6:343–347

Hall JG, Reed SD, McGillivray BC et al. (1983) Part II. Amyoplasia: Twinning in amyoplasia—a specific type of arthrogryposis with an apparent excess of discordantly affected identical twins. Am J Med Genet 15:591–599

Hamasaki S, Shirabe S, Tsuda R et al. (1998) Discordant Gerstmann-Strussler-Scheinker disease in monozygotic twins. Lancet 352:1358–1360

Hanon RJ, Boston VE (1988) Discordant Hirschprung's disease in monozygotic twins: A clue to pathogenesis. J Pediatr Surg 23:1034–1035

Harvey MAS, Huntley RMC, Smith DW (1977) Familial monozygotic twinning. J Pediatr 90:246–250

Haskins-Olney A, Buehler BA, Waziri (1988) Wiedemann-Beckwith syndrome in apparently discordant monozygotic twins. Am J Med Genet 29:491–499

Healey SC, Duffy DL, Martin NG et al. (1997) Letter to the Editor. Is fragile X syndrome a risk factor for dizygotic twinning? Am J Med Genet 72:245–246

Henker J, Fischer R, Gebhardt B (1989) Discordant manifestation of coeliac disease in monozygotic twins. Klin Pediatr 201:136–138

Hill AVS, Jeffreys AJ (1985) Use of minisatellite DNA probes for determination of twin zygosity at birth. Lancet 2:1394

Hipkin LJ, Casson IF, Davis JC (1990) Identical twins discordant for Kallman syndrome. J Med Genet 27:198–199

Horton WA, Harris DJ, Collins DL (1983) Discordance for the Kleeblattschadel anomaly in monozygotic twins with thanatophoric dysplasia. Am J Med Genet 15:97–101

Huang B, Meyer JM, Jackson-Cook CK (1995) Heritability and heteromorphic distributions of alu 1 chromosome banding variants in twins. Am J Med Genet 57:429–436

Hublin C, Kaprio J, Partinen M et al. (1999) Nightmares: Familial aggregation and association with psychiatric disorders in a nationwide twin cohort. Am J Med Genet 88:329–336

Hunter WS, Dijkman DJ (1977) The timing of height and weight in twins discordant for cleft of the lip and/or palate. Cleft Palate J 14:158–166

Imaizumi Y (1990) Triplets and higher order multiple births in Japan. Acta Genet Med Gemellol 39:295–306

Imaizumi Y, Inouye E (1982) Analysis of multiple birth in Japan. Jpn J Hum Genet 27:227–234

James WH (1975) Sex ratio in twin births. Ann Hum Biol 2:365–378

James WH (1980) Sex ratio and placentation in twins. Ann Hum Biol 7:273–276

James WH (1997) An hypothesis on the association between maternal smoking and dizygotic twinning. Hum Reprod 12:1391–1392

Jauniaux E, Elkazen N, Leroy F (1986) Clinical and morphologic aspects of the vanishing twin phenomenon. Obstet Gynecol 68:577–581

Jeanty P, Rodesch F, Verhoogen C (1981) The vanishing twin. Ultrasonics 2:25–30

Johnston C, Alviggi L, Millward BA et al. (1988) Alterations in T-lymphocyte subpopulations in type 1 diabetes. Exploration of the genetic influence in identical twins. Diabetes 37:1484–1488

Johnstone H, Benirschke K (1976) Monozygotic twins discordant for urinary tract anomalies and presenting as hydramnios. Obstet Gynecol 47:610–614

Jokelainen M, Palo J, Lokki J (1978) Monozygotic twins discordant for amyotrophic lateral sclerosis. Eur Neurol 17:296–299

Kajii T, Hagiwara K, Tsukahara M et al. (1981) Monozygotic twins discordant for Rubinstein-Taybi syndrome. J Med Genet 18:312–314

Kallen B (1986) Congenital malformations in twins: a population study. Acta Genet Gemellol 33:61–69

Kanjilal D, Verma RS, Glass L et al. (1989) Congenital adrenal hyperplasia in monozygotic twins with variable clinical manifestations. Jpn J Hum Genet 34:231–234

Kaplowitz PB, Bodurtha J, Brown J et al. (1991) Monozygotic twins discordant for Ullrich-Turner syndrome. Am J Med Genet 11:596–575

Karp L, Bryant JI, Tagatz G et al. (1975) The occurrence of gonadal dysgenesis with monozygotic twinning. J Med Genet 12:78–82

Kaufman MH, O'Shea KS (1978) Induction of monozygotic twinning in the mouse. Nature 276:707–709

Kaufman LW, Folk ER, Miller MT (1989) Monozygotic twins discordant for Duane's retraction syndrome. Arch Ophthalmol 107:324–325

Kimmel DL, Moyer EK, Pearle et al. (1950) Cerebral tumour containing five human fetuses: Case of fetus in fetu. Anatomical Record 106:141–165

Kinnunen E, Juntunen J, Ketonen L et al. (1988) Genetic susceptibility to multiple sclerosis. A co-twin study of a nationwide series. Arch Neurol 45:1108–1011

King SL, Ladda RL, Shochat SJ (1977) Monozygotic twins concordant for tracheo-esophageal fistula and discordant for the VATER association. Acta Pediatr Scand 66:783–785

Kitchens CS (1987) Discordance in a pair of identical twin carriers of factor IX deficiency. Am J Hematol 24:225–228

Klinger G, Merlob P, Aloni D et al. (1997) Normal pulmonary function in a monoamniotic twin discordant for bilateral renal agenesis: report and review. Am J Med Genet 73:76–79

Kondo S, Yanashina U, Sato N, Asu K (1991) Discordant expression of tuberous sclerosis in monozygotic twins. J Dermatol 18:178–180

Kruyer H, Mila M, Glover G et al. (1993) Monozygotic twins discordant for the fragile X syndrome. Am J Hum Genet, Suppl. 53:4465

Kumar A, Schapiro MB, Grady CL et al. (1991) Anatomic, metabolic, neuropsychological and molecular genetic studies of three pairs of identical twins discordant for dementia of the Alzheimer's type. Arch Neurol 48:160–168

Kurosawa K, Kuromaru R, Imazumi K et al. (1992) Monozygotic twins with discordant sex. Acta Med Gemellol 41:301–310

Kushner BH, Helson L (1985) Monozygotic siblings discordant for neuroblastoma: Etiologic implications. J Pediatr 107:405–409

Lage JM, Vanmarter LJ, Mikhail E (1989) Vascular anastomoses in fused, dichorionic twin placentas resulting in twin transfusion. Placenta 10:55–59

Lampert RP, Edwards JG, Young RS (1984) Partial lipodystrophy in one of twins. Proc Greenwood Genet 3:53–55

Landy HJ, Weiner S, Corson SL (1986) The "vanishing twin" ultrasonographic assessment of fetal disappearance in the first trimester. Am J Obstet Gynecol 155:14–20

Langlois S (1999) Personal communication

Lazda EJ (1998) Endocardial fibroelastosis in growth-discordant monozygotic twins. Pediatric and Developmental Pathology 1:522–527

Lefvert AK, Pirskanen R, Eng H et al. (1989) B cell and autoantibody repertoire in a pair of monozygotic twins discordant for myasthenia gravis. Clin Immunol Immunopathol 53:161–170

Levi S (1976) Ultrasonic assessment of the high rate of human multiple pregnancy in the first trimester. J Clin Ultrasound 4:3–7

Lewis CM, Healey SC, Martin NG (1996) Genetic contribution to DZ twinning. Am J Med Genet 61:237–246

Lewis SW, Chitkara B, Reveley AM (1991) Obsessive-compulsive disorder and schizophrenia in three identical twins. Psychol Med 21:135–141

Lichtenstein P, Kallen B, Koster M (1998) No paternal effect on monozygotic twinning in the Swedish twin registry. Twin Research 1:212–215

Little J, Thompson B (1988). Descriptive epidemiology. In MacGillivray I, Campbell DM, Thompson B (eds): Twinning and Twins. John Wiley & Sons, Chichester, UK, pp. 37–66.

Litz CE, Taylor KA, Taylor JSQ et al. (1988) Absence of detectable chromosomal molecular abnormalities in monozygotic twins discordant for the Wiedemann-Beckwith syndrome. Am J Med Genet 30:821–833

Livingston JE, Poland BJ (1980) A study of spontaneously aborted twins. Teratology 21:139–148

Loevy HT, Miller M, Rosenthal IM (1985) Discordant monozygotic twins with trisomy 13. Acta Genet Med Gemellol 34:185–188

Lord JM (1956) Intra abdominal fetus-in-fetu. J Pathol Bacteriol 72:627–641

MacGillivray I, Samphier M, Little J (1988). Factors affecting twinning. pp. 67–97. In MacGillivray I, Campbell DM, Thompson B (eds): Twinning and Twins. John Wiley & Sons, Chichester, UK

MacGillivray I, Campbell DM (1978) The physical characteristics and adaptations of women with twin pregnancies. In Gedda L, Parisi P, Nance WE (eds): Twin Research. Clinical Studies. Alan R. Liss, N Y p. 81–91.

Machin GA, Sperber GH (1987) Invited Editorial comment: Lessons from conjoined twins. Am J Med Genet 28:89–97

Machin GA (1993) Conjoined twins: Implications for blastogenesis. Blastogenesis normal and abnormal. March of Dimes Original Article Series. 29:141–179

Machin GA (1996) Some causes of genotypic and phenotypic discordance in monozygotic twin pairs. Am J Med Genet 61:216–228

Machin G, Still K, Lalani T (1996) Correlations of placental vascular anatomy and clinical outcomes in 69 monochorionic twin pregnancies. Am J Med Genet 61:229–236

Machin GA, Keith LG, Bamforth et al. (1999) An atlas of multiple pregnancy. Biology and pathology. Parthenon Publishing, NY

Martin N, Boomsma D, Machin G (1997) A twin-pronged attack on complex traits. Nat Genet 17:387–392

Mastroiacovo P, Castilla EE, Arpino C, et al. (1999) Congenital malformations in twins: An international study. Am J Med Genet 83:117–124

Métneki J, Czeizel AE, Evans JA (1996) Congenital limb reduction defects in twins. Eur J Pediatr 155:483–490

Meulemans WJ, Lewis CM, Boomsma DI et al. (1996) Genetic modelling of dizygotic twinning in pedigrees of spontaneous dizygotic twins. Am J Med Genet 61:258–263

Michels VV, Ricardi VM (1978) Twin recurrence and amniocentesis; male and MZ heritability factors. Birth Defects, 14:201–212

Moore TC, Landers DB, Lachman RS et al. (1979) Hirschprung's disease discordant in monozygotic twins: A study of possible environmental factors in the production of colonic aganglionosis. J Pediatr Surg 14:158–161

Mulder AF, van Eyck J, Groenendaal F, Wladimiroff JW (1989) Trisomy 18 in monozygotic twins. Hum Genet 83:300–301

Murphy M, Hey K (1997) Twinning rates. Lancet 349:1398–1399

Nance WE (1981) Malformations unique to the twinning process. In Gedda L, Parisi P, Nance WE (eds): Twin Research. Vol 3. Twins Biology and Multiple Pregnancy. Alan R. Liss, N Y, pp. 123–130.

Naor N, Amir Y, Cohen T, Davidson S (1987) Trisomy 13 in monozygotic twins discordant for major congenital anomalies. J Med Genet 24:500–502

Neale MC, Kendler KS (1995) Models of comorbidity for multifactorial disorders. Am J Hum Genet 57:935–953

Nylander PPS (1971) Biosocial aspects of multiple births. J Biosoc Sci, suppl 3:29–34

Nylander PPS (1973) Serum levels of gonadotrophins in relation to multiple pregnancy in Nigeria. J Obstet Gynaecol Br Common 80:651–654

Nylander PPS (1975) Frequency of multiple births. In MacGillivray I, Nylander PPS, Corney G (eds): Human Multiple Reproduction. WB Saunders, London, pp. 87–98.

Nylander PPS (1979) The twinning incidence in Nigeria. Acta Genet Med Gemellol 36:397–402

Nylander P (1981) The factors that influence twinning rates. Acta Genet Med Gemellol 30:189–202

Nystrom M, Ranta R (1988) Dental age and assymmetry in the formation of mandibular teeth in twins concordant and discordant for oral clefts. Scand J Dent Res 96:393–398

Parisi P, Gatti M, Prinzi G et al. (1983) Familial incidence of twinning. Nature 304:626–628

Perlman EJ, Stetten G, Tuck-Muller C et al. (1990) Sexual discordance in MZ twins. Am J Med Genet 37:551–557

Phelan MC, Geer JS, Blackburn WR (1998) Vascular anastomoses leading to amelia and cutis aplasia in a dizygotic twin pregnancy. Clin Genet 52:126–130

Piontelli A, Bocconi L, Boschetto C et al. 1999 Differences and similarities in the intra-uterine behaviour of monozygotic and dizygotic twins. Twin Research 2:264–273

Putz B, Rehder H (1985) Anencephaly in one monoamniotic monochorionic twin and encephalocele in the other. Am J Med Genet 21:631–635

Retting KR, Vargas A, Reitter E, Root WA (1980) Discordance for congenital athyrotic hypothyroidism in one monozygotic twin. Clin Pediatr 68:63–65

Richards CS, Watkins SC, Hoffman EP et al. (1990) Skewed X-inactivation in a female MZ twins results in Duchenne muscular dystrophy. Am J Hum Genet 46:672–668

Robinow M, Marsh JL, Edgerton MT et al. (1978) Discordance in monozygotic twins for aglossia-adactylia, and possible clues to the pathogenesis of the syndrome. Birth Defects 14:223–230

Rogers JG, Voullaire L, Gold H (1982) Monozygotic twins discordant for trisomy 21. Am J Med Genet 11:143–146

Saier F, Burden D, Cavanagh D (1975) Fetus papyraceous: An unusual case with congenital anomaly of the surviving fetus. Obstet Gynecol 45:217–220

St. Clair DM, St. Clair JB, Swainson CP et al. (1998) Twin zygosity testing for medical purposes. Am J Med Genet 77:412–414

Samn M, Lewis K, Blumberg B (1990) Monozygotic twins discordant for the Russell-Silver syndrome. Am J Med Genet 37:543–545

Sampra JS, Hampton N, Fitzgibbon MN et al. (1990) The second twin. Lancet 336:342–343

Saul RA, Schwartz CE, Stevenson RE (1990) DNA evidence for somatic mosaicism in monozygotic twins discordant for *Proteus* syndrome. Proc Greenwood Genet Ctr 9:12–15

Schinzel AGL, Smith DW, Miller JR (1979) Monozygotic twinning and structural defects. J Pediatr 95:921–930

Schlessel JS, Brown WT, Lysikiewicz A et al. (1990) Monozygotic twins with trisomy 18: a report of discordant phenotype. J Med Genet 27:640–642

Schworm HD, Jedele KB, Holinski E et al. (1996) Discordant monozygotic twins with the Schimmelpenning-Feuerstein-Mims syndrome. Clin Genet 50:393–397

Scrimgeour JB, Baker TG (1974) A possible cause of superfetation in man. J Reprod Fertil 36:69–73

Sebire NJ, Snijders RJM, Hughes K et al. (1997) The hidden mortality of monochorionic twin pregnancies. Br J Obstet Gynaecol 104:1203–1207

Shaffer LG, Kashortk C, Bacino CA et al. (1999) Letter to the Editor. Caution: Telomere crossing. Am J Med Genet 87:278–280

Shapiro LR, Zemek L, Shulman MJ (1978) Genetic etiology for monozygotic twinning. Birth Defects 14:219–225

Shotelersuk V, Tifft CJ, Vacha S et al. (1999) Discordance of oral-facial-digital syndrome type 1 in monozygotic twin girls. Am J Med Genet 86:269–273

Shiono H, Ogino T (1980) A discordant case of monozygotic twins with symbrachydactyly. Acta Genet Med Gemellol 29:241–245

Singal DP, D'Souza M, Reid B et al. (1989) Molecular analysis of the HLA-D region and the T-cell antigen receptor beta-chain genes in monozygotic twins discordant for rheumatoid arthritis. Transplant Proc 21:623–624

Slagboom PE, Droog S, Boomsma DI (1994) Genetic determination of telomere size in humans: A study of three age groups. Am J Hum Genet 55:876–882

Sommer IEC, Ramsey NF, Bouma A et al. (1999) Cerebral mirror-imaging in a monozygotic twin. Lancet 354:1445–1446

Sperber GH, Machin GA, Bamforth FJ (1994). Mirror-image dental fusion and discordance in monozygotic twins. Am J Med Genet 51:41–45

Steinmetz H, Herzog A, Huang Y et al. (1994). Discordant brain-surface anatomy in monozygotic twins. N Engl J Med 331:952–959

Stockard CR (1921) Developmental rate and structural expression. I. An experimental study of twins, double monsters and single deformities and the interaction among embryonic organs during their origin and development. Am J Anat 28:115–277

Stoll C, Roth MP, Dott B et al. (1984) Discordance for skeletal and cardiac defect in monozygotic twins. Acta Genet Med Gemellol 33:51–56

Storrs EE, Williams RJ (1968) A study of monozygous quadruplet armadillos in relation to mammalian inheritance. Biochemistry 60:910–914

Strickland AD, Shannon K, Cola DC (1985) Biliary atresia in two sets of twins. J Pediatr 107:418–422

Szymonowicz W, Preston H, Yu VYH (1986) The surviving monozygotic twin. Arch Dis Child 61:454–458

Tan SS, Williams EA, Tam PPL (1993) X-chromosome inactivation occurs at different times in different tissues of the post-implantation mouse embryo. Nat Genet 3:170–174

Taylor MB, Anderson RL, Golbus MS (1984) One hundred twin pregnancies in a prenatal diagnosis program. Am J Med Genet 18:419–422

Trejo V, Derom C, Vlietinck et al. (1995) X-chromosome inactivation patterns correspond with fetal-placental anatomy in monozygotic twin pairs: Implications for immune relatedness and concordance for autoimmunity. Mol Med 1:62–70

Tsunoda Y, Tokunaga T, Susie T (1985) Altered sex ratio of live young after transfer of fast and slow developing mouse embryos. 12:301–304

Tuckerman E, Webb T, Bunday SE (1985). Frequency and replication status of the fragile X, fra(X)(q27–28), in a pair of monozygotic twins of markedly differing intelligence. J Med Genet 22:85–91

Uchida IA, Freeman VCP, Gedeon M (1983) Twining rate in spontaneous abortions. Am J Hum Genet 35:987–990

Van Allen MI, Smith DW, Hepard TH (1983) Twin reversed arterial perfusion (TRAP) sequence: A study of 14 pregnancies with acardius. Semin Pathol 7:285–293

van Dijk, BA, Boomsma DI, de Man AJM (1996) Blood group chimerism in human multiples is not rare. Am J Med Genet 61:264–268

Watson WJ, Katz VL, Albright SG et al. (1990) Monozygotic twins discordant for trisomy 1. Obstet Gynecol 76:949–951

Weinberg W (1901) Contribution on the physiology and pathology of multiple birth in man. Pflugers Arch Physiol 88:346

Wenk RE, Tonz T, Brooks M, Chiatari FA (1992) How frequent is heteropaternal superfecundation? Acta Genet Med Gemellol 41:43–47

Wilkinson JL, Holt PA, Dickson DF et al. (1979) Asplenia syndrome in one of monozygotic twins. Eur J Cardiol 10:301–304

Wolf HM, Haurber I, Gulle H et al. (1995) Twin boys with major histocompatibility complex class II deficiency but inducible immune responses. N Engl J Med 332:86–90

Young ID, Dalgleish R, MacKay EH et al. (1988) Discordant expression of the G syndrome in monozygotic twins. Am J Med Genet 29:863–869

Yovich JL, Stanger JD, Granang A et al. (1984) Monozygotic twins from in vitro fertilization. Fertil Steril 41:833–837

Zake EZ (1984) Case reports of 16 sets of conjoined twins from an Uganda hospital. Acta Genet Med. Gemeloll 33:25–26

The molecular biology of cancer

Edward S. Tobias
Donald M. Black

19

Introduction

Cancer is a genetic disease, arising from the progressive accumulation of mutations that promote the clonal selection of cells with increasingly deregulated growth. Studies from many different fields, including tumor virology, chemical carcinogenesis, molecular biology, somatic cell genetics, and genetic epidemiology, have all provided fundamental insights into the genetic basis of cancer. Most of these alterations are somatically acquired, but some are inherited. During the last three decades many of the genetic targets of the mutations have been identified. However, except for one or two notable examples, little is known about the precise combination of genetic alterations required to produce a particular type of tumor and of what determines the tissue specificity of these changes. Moreover, the cancer phenotype is a result of complex gene interactions, not only involving the known cancer gene products but also a multitude of other proteins. A great many "modifier" and low penetrance cancer susceptibility genes are still to be discovered. The individual impact of any one of these genes is likely to be small compared to that of the known cancer genes, but collectively their variant alleles may hugely influence an individual's cancer risk. Additionally, all these interactions are subject to modification by poorly understood environmental factors. The disentangling of all such interrelations clearly poses a tough challenge to cancer biologists.

Cancer genes fall into three broad classes: proto-oncogenes, which are positive regulators of cell proliferation and survival; tumor suppressor genes, which are negative regulators; and DNA repair genes, which are responsible for the detection and repair of genetic damage. The coordinated regulation of these gene classes is responsible for maintaining tissue homeostasis; cancer reflects a fundamental breakdown in this control. The types of alteration that occur in proto-oncogenes and tumor suppressor genes display intrinsic differences. Point mutations in proto-oncogenes are usually missense and tend to activate—or give new functions to—the gene product. Alternatively, proto-oncogenes can be subject either to amplification or to translocations that place them under the control of active promoter sequences or that generate a fusion product with new or constitutive function. Oncogenes are thus proto-oncogenes which have undergone gain-of-function alterations that act in a positive fashion to promote tumorigenesis. Tumor suppressor genes, on the other hand, are subject to loss of function alterations, most commonly through deletions or through point mutations which truncate the protein product or alter a crucial functional domain. These differences partially account for the dominant transforming ability of oncogenes and the recessiveness (at the cellular level) of tumor suppressors. Many of the cellular genes affected by inherited and somatic mutations in human cancer are discussed in greater detail below.

Finally, recent studies have highlighted the critical role of mutations involving the third class of genes in the cancer process, i.e., the DNA repair genes. As with the tumor suppressor genes, loss of function mutations in these genes is the basis for their role in tumorigenesis. However, they differ from tumor suppressor genes in critical ways. The protein products of some tumor suppressor genes may transduce growth-inhibitory signals or activate differentiation pathways. Other tumor suppressor proteins may mediate programmed cell death (apoptosis) following DNA damage or cell cycle perturbations. In contrast, inactivation of DNA repair genes probably does not directly affect the normal processes controlling growth. Rather, their inactivation appears to result in an increased rate of mutations in a variety of cellular genes, including proto-oncogenes and tumor suppressor genes, in affected cells. Because the accumulation of mutations in these two classes of growth-regulating genes appears to be the rate-limiting step in tumorigenesis, inactivation of DNA damage recognition and repair genes greatly accelerates the process of tumor progression.

Given the enormous progress that has been made in furthering our understanding of the genetic alterations present in cancer cells, this chapter does not attempt to review all of the various mutations in oncogenes and tumor suppressor genes that have been identified to date in human cancers. Rather, the primary aims of this chapter are fivefold: (1) to review the historical basis underlying the search for genetic alterations in human cancers; (2) to address the relationship between cancer-causing retroviruses and cellular proto-oncogenes involved in cancer, as well as the relationships between DNA tumor viruses and tumor suppressor gene products; (3) to review the strategies for identifying oncogenic alleles in human cancer and some of the most common and instructive oncogenic alterations elucidated in human cancers; (4) to review the roles of a number of tumor suppressor genes which are associated with inherited cancer syndromes; and (5) to address the molecular biology of some of the more common inherited cancer syndromes resulting from defects in DNA repair genes.

A genetic basis for cancer

An inherited basis for some cancers in humans and other animals has been hypothesized for over a century. Broca was perhaps the first to describe an inherited cancer syndrome (Broca, 1866). In 1866, he described a family with many members affected by breast and liver cancer and suggested that some inherited aberration within the affected tissue allowed tumors to form. Subsequent studies of mammary tumor formation in inbred strains of mice led Haaland to propose in the early 1900s that tumorigenesis behaved in a formal sense as a mendelian genetic trait (Haaland, 1911). Similarly, Warthin's studies of four families with markedly increased cancer rates led him to propose in 1913 that susceptibility to several cancer types appeared to be transmitted as an autosomal dominant mendelian trait (Warthin, 1913). Although these and other studies were consistent with the proposal that a genetic basis for cancer might account for familial clustering of cancer, other explanations for these observations were possible (e.g., clustered exposure to environmental or dietary agents). Moreover, it

was argued that the majority of cancers arose as sporadic or isolated cases.

The proposal that cancer might result from somatic alterations in the genetic material of cells was first advanced by Boveri (Boveri, 1929). He had previously noted that abnormal mitotic divisions and atypical cell masses could be seen in sea urchin eggs fertilized by two sperm. He reasoned that the abnormal masses bore significant similarity to tumors, and thus he hypothesized that cancer might result from cellular aberrations that produced abnormal mitotic figures. Nevertheless, Boveri's studies provided few insights into the genetic or cellular mechanisms that might give rise to abnormalities in the regulation of cell division.

Therefore, the studies of Peyton Rous can be seen as a particularly critical turning point in the search for a genetic basis for cancer development because they provided the first mechanistic insights into the pathogenesis of cancer. In 1911 Rous demonstrated that sarcomas in the chicken (*Galus galus*) could be induced following inoculation with a cell-free filtrate obtained from an independent chicken sarcoma (Rous, 1911). Nearly 70 years later, it was conclusively demonstrated that the Rous sarcoma virus (RSV) is a retrovirus that induces cancers in chickens because it harbors an altered version of a cellular proto-oncogene known as the *src* gene (Stehelin et al., 1976). Though retroviruses have thus far been implicated in the causation of a limited number of forms of human cancer (e.g., acute T-cell leukemia), as reviewed below, their study has acquired a much larger significance by providing experimental access to the genetic underpinnings of tumorigenesis.

Viral oncogenes

RNA TUMOR VIRUSES AND THE IDENTIFICATION OF PROTO-ONCOGENES

RNA tumor viruses (also known as retroviral tumor viruses) can be divided into two classes: acute and chronic transforming viruses. The identification of oncogenes began with studies of acutely transforming retroviruses. Although not oncogenic in humans, these can rapidly induce tumors in animals and transform cells *in vitro*. In contrast to the chronic transforming viruses, the genomes of the acute transforming viruses contain nucleic acid sequences that have been acquired or transduced from the host cell as a result of genetic recombination. The host-derived sequences are termed *viral oncogenes* (*v-onc* genes), and these sequences, although not necessary for the replication of the virus, are directly responsible for its rapid transforming activity (Varmus, 1984; Bishop 1985; 1987; 1991; Cantley et al., 1991; Hunter, 1991). Characterization of the *v-onc* genes present in various acute transforming viruses has led to the identification of more than 20 different cellular genes that have been transduced by various tumor viruses (Table 19.1).

There is no reason to believe that proto-oncogenes are unique in their capacity to be transduced by retroviruses; rather, the proto-oncogenes represent a unique class of genes because of their biologic properties. Transduction of other classes of genes does not give rise to acute transforming viruses. Hence, because of their vital role in the generation of acute transforming viruses, the proto-oncogenes might be presumed to represent at least part of the genetic repertoire that might underlie cancer. Moreover, because the *v-onc* genes harbored by the acute transforming viruses represent mutated versions of their corresponding cellular proto-oncogene, comparison of the two sequences might be expected to provide insights into the means by which

oncogenic variant alleles are generated by somatic mutations, such as by point mutation, chromosomal translocation, or gene amplification. Subsequent to the discovery that *v-src* has a counterpart in the cellular gene *c-src* (Stehelin et al., 1976), it has transpired that nearly all retroviral oncogenes are transduced cellular proto-oncogenes whose expression and activity is increased as a consequence of the transduction process. The acute transforming viruses cause tumors at the site of inoculation after short latency periods (e.g., a few weeks in newborn animals), and they are also able to transform cells in culture. The chronic transforming viruses are capable of producing tumors only in hosts in which the virus can replicate. The tumors arise after relatively long latency periods and at specific tissue sites, irrespective of the inoculation site. The differences in the properties of the two classes of viruses can be traced to differences in their genetic content.

The chronic transforming viruses transform cells by random integration of a DNA copy of the virus, termed the *provirus*, into the host cell genome. The provirus can affect

Table 19.1. Retroviral oncogenes and tumors

V-ONC gene	*RNA tumor virus*	*Species of origin*	*Major disease*
Growth factor family			
V-SIS	SSV	Wooly monkey	Glioma/sarcoma
	PI-FeSV	Cat	Sarcoma
Integral membrane tyrosine kinases			
V-FMS	SM-FeSV	Cat	Sarcoma
V-ERBB	AEV-H, AEV-ES4	Chicken	Erythroleukemia, sarcoma
V-KIT	HZ4-FeSV	Cat	Sarcoma
V-ROS	UR2	Chicken	Sarcoma
Membrane associated tyrosine kinases			
V-SRC	RSV	Chicken	Sarcoma
V-FGR	Gr-FeSV	Cat	Sarcoma
V-YES	Y73/ESV	Chicken	Sarcoma
F-FPS	FuSV/PRCII	Chicken	Sarcoma
V-ABL	Ab-MLV	Mouse	Leukemia
V-ABL	HZ2-FeSV	Cat	Sarcoma
Serine-threonine kinases			
V-MOS	Mo-MSV	Mouse	Sarcoma
V-RAF	MSV-3611	Mouse	Sarcoma
RAS Family			
V-H-RAS	Ha-MSV	Rat	Sarcoma
V-K-RAS	Ki-MSV	Rat	Sarcoma
Nuclear proteins			
V-MYC	MC29	Chicken	Carcinoma, myeloid leukemia
V-MYB	E26	Chicken	Erythroleukemia
V-FOS	FBJ-MSV	Mouse	Osteosarcoma
V-SKI	SKV770	Chicken	Carcinoma
V-REL	REV-T	Turkey	Lymphatic leukemia
V-ETS	E26	Chicken	Erythroleukemia
V-ERBA	AEV-ES4	Chicken	Erythroblastosis

(Modified from Weinberg, 1994, with permission.)

Table 19.2. Cellular genes activated by chronic transforming retroviruses

Gene	Disease	Virus	Animal
myc	Bursal lymphoma	ALV, CSF, REV	Chicken
	T-cell lymphoma	MLV	Mouse
	T-cell lymphoma	FeLV	Cat
erbb (egfr)	Erythroleukemia	ALV	Chicken
myb	Lymphosarcoma	MLV	Mouse
h-ras	Nephroblastoma	MAV	Chicken
mos	Plasmacytoma	IAP	Mouse
il2	T-cell lymphoma	GaLV	Ape
il3	Myelomonocytic leukemia	IAP	Mouse
intl	Mammary cancer	MMTV	Mouse
int2	Mammary cancer	MMTV	Mouse
evi1	Myeloid lymphoma	MCF-MLV	Mouse
evi2	Myeloid lymphoma	MCF-MLV	Mouse
pim1	T-cell lymphoma	M-MLV	Mouse

(Modified from Perkins and Van de Woude, 1993, with permission.)

the genes in the region of the host chromosome where it integrates. If a proto-oncogene is contained in the region, provirus integration can alter the structure and/or expression of the proto-oncogene and thus contribute to tumorigenesis. The relatively long latency of the tumorigenic process for the chronic transforming viruses reflects the low probability that any one integration event will specifically affect a proto-oncogene. Nevertheless, given infection of enough cells, transformation will likely occur, with leukemias and lymphomas being the most prominent tumor types generated by these chronic transforming viruses. Several of the proto-oncogenes that are altered by chronic transforming viruses in animal tumors are also affected in a subset of human tumors by somatic mutations (Varmus, 1984; Bishop, 1985; 1987; 1991; Cantley et al., 1991; Hunter, 1991) (Table 19.2).

DNA TUMOR VIRUSES

Many DNA viruses, of the adenovirus, herpesvirus, poxvirus and papovavirus families, also encode oncoproteins. However, the transforming genes rarely have proto-oncogene homologues within the normal genome. Chronic transforming retroviruses (such as mouse mammary tumor virus and avian leukosis virus) also possess no cellular sequences. As mentioned above, these viruses induce neoplastic transformation after a latency period of months or years, via the integration of proviral DNA in such a way as to activate specific host target genes: cellular genes are

either brought under the control of the viral LTR or are fused to viral sequences with the consequent production of novel proteins (Hayward et al., 1981). This knowledge led to the prospective use of insertional mutagenesis as a means of identifying novel proto-oncogenes that are consistent targets for proviral insertion (Nusse and Varmus, 1982). It was suggested that *spontaneous* alteration of any of these genes might account for tumors – including most human tumors – whose initiation is virus independent. The finding that around one in five tumors possesses genomic sequences with intrinsic transforming ability supported this hypothesis (Shih et al., 1981). Indeed, tumor gene transfer experiments identified oncogenes already known to be the cellular counterparts of various retroviral oncogenes, in addition to several novel genes (many of which belonged to the *src* and *ras* superfamilies). The presence of activating alterations in many of these cellular genes was subsequently demonstrated (Santos et al., 1982; Tabin et al., 1982; Taparowsky et al., 1982). Other oncogenes were identified directly through their association with translocations, which caused activation either by the generation of new fusion products or by bringing the proto-oncogene under the transcriptional control of nearby enhancer elements (Adams et al., 1983; Gale and Canaani, 1984). Probes and primers derived from the oncogenes identified in these various ways were then used to isolate further, homologous, genes by cross-hybridization or the use of the polymerase chain reaction. In general, while the RNA tumor viruses promote tumor development by harboring or generating oncogenic alleles, several of the DNA tumor viruses, such as simian type 40 virus (SV40), human papillomaviruses, and adenoviruses, primarily contribute to tumorigenesis by inactivating or inhibiting the activities of tumor suppressor proteins (Marshall, 1991; Weinberg, 1991). Several of the specific interactions of DNA tumor virus proteins with tumor suppressor proteins are addressed below in detail in the discussion of tumor suppressor gene products.

Oncogenic alleles in human cancers

The precise location of oncogenic mutations often gave the first indication of the important functional domains of the protein (McKay et al., 1986). Genetic, biochemical and cellular studies in both humans and model organisms have further illuminated the functions of these genes. The majority of proto-oncogenes are now known to be components of signal transduction pathways, which are responsible for translating extracellular signals into nuclear changes in gene expression. Activation of proto-oncogenes (and inactivation of tumor suppressor genes) results in the deregulation of these pathways, such that aspects of cellular behavior – for example proliferation and survival – become autonomous. Proto-oncogenes have been discovered at most stages of the signal transduction pathways, acting as (among others) ligands, receptors, membrane-associated tyrosine kinases, lipid kinases, cytoplasmic regulators, G proteins, kinases, transcription factors and transcriptional co-activators. A small subset of proto-oncogenes are more directly involved in cellular proliferation and survival, and function as components of the cell cycle or anti-apoptotic machinery. *CCND1* and *CDK4*, encoding cyclin D1 and cyclin dependent kinase 4 (CDK4), respectively, have both been found to be activated in tumors (Hall and Peters, 1996). The anti-apoptotic gene *Bcl-2* is another target for activation, and was first identified at the breakpoint of translocations in follicular lymphomas (Bakhshi et al., 1985; Tsujimoto et al., 1985). An important consequence of oncogenic activation, therefore, is to uncouple cell proliferation and survival from regulation by extrinsic factors. This can be achieved either by constitutive activation of mitogenic signalling pathways or through direct stimulation of cell cycle progression or cellular survival.

Certain oncogenes are important in the advanced stages of tumorigenesis. A variety of proto-oncogenes are involved in the regulation of the actin cytoskeleton, of cell adhesion, and of the extracellular matrix. Deregulation of these facets via oncogene activation promotes the cell migration and substrate-independence required for tumor cell invasion and metastasis. Other oncogenes are thought to have a role in the process of angiogenesis, the induction of new blood vessel growth from existing vessels. This process is probably essential if solid tumors are to enlarge beyond around one cubic millimetre.

Proto-oncogene activation probably contributes to the development of all sporadic cancers. Activating *germline* mutations in proto-oncogenes are likely, in general, to be lethal, but mutations in a limited number of proto-oncogenes are heritable and give rise to familial cancer syndromes. Germ-line mutations in *MET*, *RET* and *CDK4*, for example, are respectively responsible for hereditary papillary renal cancer, multiple endocrine neoplasia type 2 (MEN2), and some cases of familial melanoma (Mulligan et al., 1993; Zuo et al., 1996; Schmidt et al., 1997). However, the majority of cancer syndromes are caused by germline mutations in tumor suppressor genes, where, in contrast to proto-oncogene mutations, loss of the remaining wild-type allele is the initiating transforming event. Even here, progression to full tumorigenicity requires further mutations in additional, prob-ably multiple, proto-oncogenes and tumor suppressors. It should be stressed that although the study of the oncogenes carried by acute transforming retroviruses has led to the identification of many genes with critical roles in cell growth, only a subset of these genes are frequently affected by somatic mutations in human cancer. In addition, as reviewed below, several oncogenes that are frequently activated in human cancer involve gene sequences that are not known to be harbored by acute transforming viruses. Many of the oncogenic alleles often observed in human cancers are summarized in Table 19.3.

ONCOGENES IDENTIFIED BY DNA TRANSFECTION

DNA transfection techniques were first used to study and identify the transforming genes of RNA and DNA tumor viruses. In these assays, DNA from primary human tumors or tumor-derived cell lines is transferred into non-tumorigenic recipient cells, and cells that acquire morphologic changes and lose contact inhibition of their growth (so-called "focus formation") are studied further (Fig. 19.1). The human tumor-derived DNA sequences that are sufficient for mediating transformation can ultimately be recovered and characterized by serial passaging of DNA from a focus.

In seminal studies using the DNA transfection approach, the research groups of Robert Weinberg, Jeffrey Cooper, and Michael Wigler identified the first oncogenic allele in human cancer. This oncogenic allele was a mutated *H-RAS* gene in the human bladder cancer cell line known as EJ or T24 (Krontiris and Cooper, 1981; Perucho et al., 1981; Der et al., 1982; Parada et al., 1982; Shih and Weinberg, 1982). Their observation was particularly notable because *RAS* genes had previously been identified by characterization of the cellular homologues of the *v-onc* genes in the Harvey and Kirsten rat sarcoma viruses (*h-ras* and *k-ras*, respectively). Subsequent studies established that the "activated" *H-RAS* allele in the bladder cancer cell line differed from a normal copy of the gene by a single nucleotide substitution (Capon et al., 1983a). This nucleotide substitution, from G to T, resulted in a single amino acid change from glycine to valine at codon 12. Additional DNA transfection studies established that about 10% to 15% of human tumors and tumor cell lines possessed *H-RAS*, *K-RAS*, or *N-RAS* alleles with mutations (Capon et al., 1983b; Shimizu et al., 1983a; 1983b; Barbacid, 1987). *N-RAS* is a third closely related *RAS* gene family member that was first identified as a transforming allele in a human neuroblastoma (Shimizu et al., 1983b). *RAS* gene mutations are particularly prominent in several common cancer types (Bos,

Table 19.3. Representative oncogenic alleles in human cancers

Gene	Activation mechanism	Protein properties	Tumor type
K-RAS	Point mutation	p21 GTPase	Pancreatic, colrectal, lung (adeno) and other cancers, leukemia
N-RAS	Point mutation	p21 GTPase	Myeloid leukemia
H-RAS	Point mutation	p21 GTPase	Bladder and other cancers
EGFR (ERBB)	Amplification, rearrangement	Growth factor receptor	Gliomas, carcinomas
NEU (ERBB2)	Amplification	Growth factor receptor	Breast, ovarian, and other carcinomas
MYC	Chromosome translocation amplification	Transcription factor	Burkitt's lymphoma; SSCL; other cancers
N-MYC	Amplification	Transcription factor	Neuroblastoma, SCCL
L-MYC	Amplification	Transcription factor	SCCL
BCL2	Chromosome translocation	Anti-apotosis protein	B-cell lymphoma (follicular type)
CYCD1	Amplification, chromosome translocation	Cyclin D (G1 phase?)	Breast cancer, B-cell lymphoma, various carcinomas
BCR-ABL	Chromosome translocation	Chimeric nonreceptor tyrosine kinase	CML, ALL (T cell)
RET	Rearrangement	Chimeric receptor tyrosine kinase	Thyroid cancer (papillary)
TRK	Rearrangement	Chimeric receptor tyrosine kinase	Colorectal cancer
HST	Amplification	Growth factor (FGF-like)	Gastric cancer
APL-RARA	Chromosome translocation	Chimeric transcription factor	Acute promyelocytic leukemia
E2A-PBX1	Chromosome translocation	Chimeric transcription factor	Pre-B-ALL
MDM2	Amplification	p53 binding protein (nuclear)	Sarcomas
GL1	Amplification	Transcription factor	Sarcomas, gliomas
TTG	Chromosome translocation	Transcription factor	T-ALL
CDK4	Amplification	Cyclin-dependent kinase	Sarcomas, gliomas

Abbreviations: ALL, acute lymphoid leukemia; CML, chronic myeloid leukemia; SCLL, small cell lung cancer.

1989), and the mutational spectrum and functional significance of *RAS* gene mutations in several types of cancer are addressed below.

Several other oncogenic alleles that are not members of the *RAS* gene family have also been identified by the DNA transfection approach. Moreover, several of these genes identified are not related to the *v-onc* genes of the acute transforming viruses. Among the genes identified are *NEU, TRK, RET, MET, MAS, HST,* and *KS3* (Bishop, 1991; Hunter, 1991; Weinberg, 1994). With the exception of the *MAS* oncogene, which appears to be an integral membrane protein, the others are members of the tyrosine kinase growth factor receptor family (*NEU, MET, RET,* or *TRK*) or the fibroblast growth factor family (*HST, KS3*). Despite the successes of the DNA transfection approach in the identification of novel oncogenic alleles in human cancer, the approach is very labor intensive and has failed to detect a number of oncogenic alleles present in human cancers, in large part because the mutant alleles failed to cause morphologic transformation of rodent fibroblasts, the recipient cells typically used in the assays. Moreover, the approach has often identified mutant alleles that were generated during the in vitro manipulations of the tumor-derived DNA. Such alleles represent an experimental artifact, because they did not actually exist in the cancers from which the DNA was prepared.

ONCOGENES IDENTIFIED BY STUDY OF CHROMOSOMAL TRANSLOCATIONS

The nonrandom chromosomal alterations observed in cancer cells have proven particularly valuable for the identification of oncogenic alleles. In many cases, a strong correlation has been established between a particular chromosomal abnormality and the type of tumor, and even its specific histopathologic subtype. Over the past two decades, standard karytotypic analyses have identified an enormous number of specific chromosomal abnormalities in leukemias and lymphomas, perhaps in large part, because these malignancies can be induced to divide in culture more readily than many solid tumors (Solomon et al., 1991). Nevertheless, nonrandom chromosomal aberrations are increasingly being detected in solid tumors using either standard karyotypic analysis or recently developed fluorescence

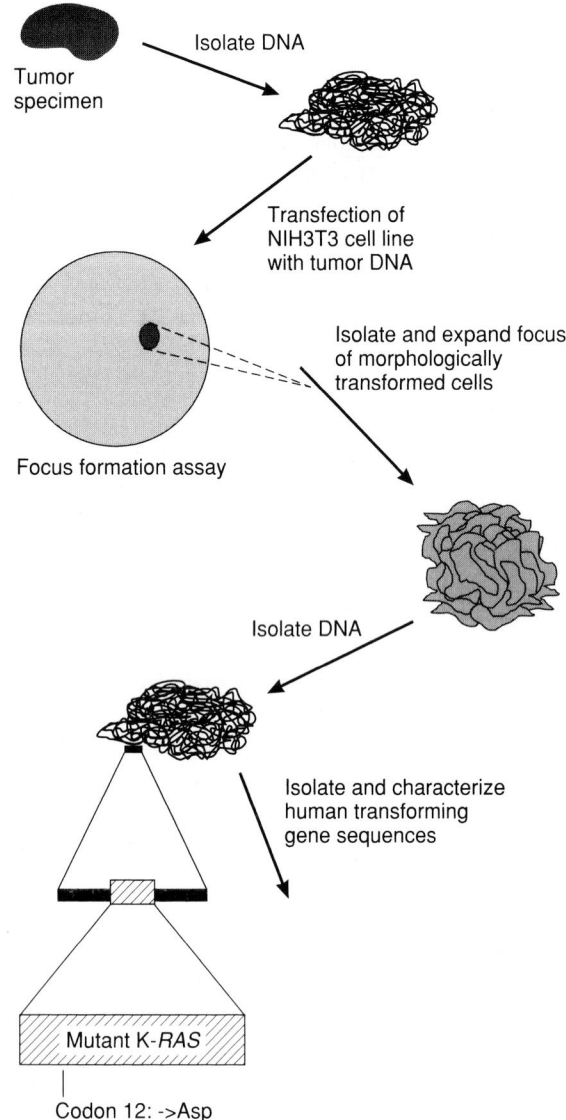

Tumor
specimen

Isolate DNA

Transfection of
NIH3T3 cell line
with tumor DNA

Focus formation assay

Isolate and expand focus
of morphologically
transformed cells

Isolate DNA

Isolate and characterize
human transforming
gene sequences

Mutant K-*RAS*

Codon 12: ->Asp

Fig. 19.1. Schematic representation of a DNA transfection assay for oncogenic alleles. DNA is isolated from primary human tumor specimen (or in some cases a tumor cell line). The purified DNA preparation is then transferred into the mouse NIH3T3 fibroblast cell line or another immortal rodent cell line. The NIH3T3 cells have an unlimited life span in culture, but grow as a monolayer in tissue culture and their growth is inhibited by cell contact. If the tumour DNA contains a "transforming" gene or oncogenic allele, then the cell taking up the oncogenic DNA sequences may fail to be inhibited by cell-cell contact. This cell may then continue its growth to form a "focus" of highly refractile cells that have lost their contact-inhibition. The transformed focus of cells can be isolated from the non transformed NIH3T3 cells, and subsequently expanded into a large population of cells. The DNA can then be isolated from the transformed NIH3T3 cells. The specific human tumour-derived DNA sequences responsible for transformation of the NIH3T3 cells can eventually be identified by serial DNA transfection and focus formation assays. In each round of selection, fewer nonspecific human DNA sequences are taken up by the NIH3T3 cells, and the specific human sequences mediating transformation are therefore enriched. In many cases, the transforming genes in human cancers are mutant *K-RAS* genes, and substitutions at codon 12 are the most common oncogenic alteration (see text). (From Fearon, 1995, with permission.)

in situ hybridization-based approaches, and several oncogenic alleles generated by specific chromosomal abnormalities in solid tumors have been characterized (Solomon et al., 1991).

Many of the chromosomal abnormalities in lymphomas and lymphoid leukemias involve translocation between an immunoglobulin (Ig) or T-cell receptor (TCR) locus and a novel gene (Bishop, 1991; Solomon et al., 1991). Sequence analysis of the translocation joint sequences has revealed that the canonical heptamer-nonamer sequences used by the recombinase system during normal somatic rearrangement of the *Ig* and *TCR* genes have probably been used to generate the translocation, as a result of a recombination error. The translocation juxtaposes the novel sequences present at the chromosomal break point with a TCR or an Ig locus. This juxtaposition can alter the normal structure and/or expression pattern of a gene(s) present near the break point. For example, a gene that is normally expressed only in neural tissues or in developing embryonic tissues may be activated. The altered gene expression presumably leads to abnormalities in the proliferation and/or differentiation of the affected cells. In addition, because many of the translocations in lymphomas or leukemias involve Ig or TCR locus sequences, the proximity of the novel gene to the well-characterized Ig or TCR locus sequences has often allowed the novel gene to be identified rapidly by standard molecular cloning approaches. Among the genes that have been found to be commonly activated in lymphoid tumors by juxtaposition with Ig or TCR locus sequences are *MYC* and *BCL2* (Bishop, 1991; Solomon et al., 1991). Both the *MYC* and the *BCL2* genes are discussed in greater detail below. Other genes that have been found to be activated in lymphoid tumors by juxtaposition with the Ig and TCR loci are transcription factors, such as the *TTG1*, *LYL1*, and *SCL1* genes, and a cell cycle regulatory protein known as PRAD1, BCL1, or cyclin D1 (Tsujimoto et al., 1984; Cleary, 1991; Motokura et al., 1991; Solomon et al., 1991; Lammie et al., 1992).

A number of other translocation break points that do not involve the Ig or TCR loci have also been characterized in hematopoietic malignancies. Many of these other translocations, while deregulating gene expression, also generate novel chimeric proteins by fusing gene sequences from one side of the break point to gene sequences on the other side of the break point. The first example of such an oncogenic allele encoding a chimeric protein was provided by the elucidation of the molecular basis of the Philadelphia chromosome. The Philadelphia chromosome was first described by Nowell and Hungerford in 1960, as a result of their karyotypic analysis of bone marrow cells from a patient with

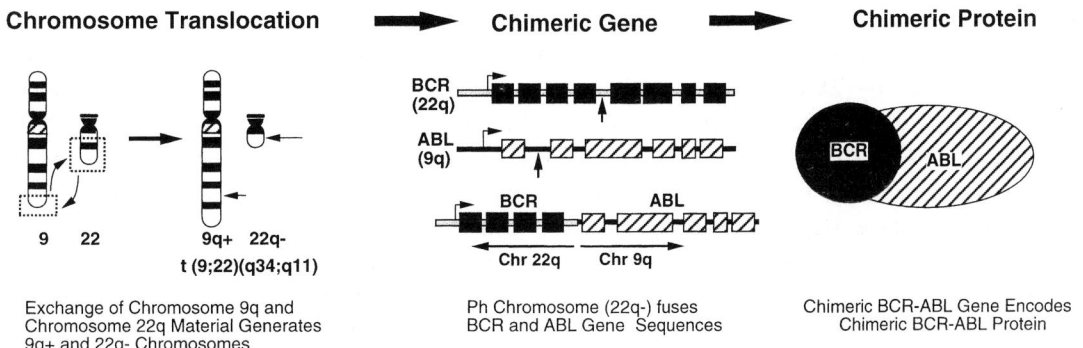

Chromosome Translocation → **Chimeric Gene** → **Chimeric Protein**

Exchange of Chromosome 9q and Chromosome 22q Material Generates 9q+ and 22q- Chromosomes

Ph Chromosome (22q-) fuses BCR and ABL Gene Sequences

Chimeric BCR-ABL Gene Encodes Chimeric BCR-ABL Protein

Fig. 19.2. Philadelphia chromosome translocation [t(9;22) (q34;q11)] fuses *BCR* and *ABL* gene sequences and results in the synthesis of a chimeric BCR-ABL protein. (From Fearon, 1995, with permission.)

chronic myelogenous leukemia (CML) (Nowell and Hungerford, 1960). Subsequent studies in the 1970s established that the Philadelphia chromosome was generated by a translocation involving chromosomes 9 and 22 (Rowley, 1973). The Philadelphia chromosome can be identified by cytogenetic studies in the vast majority of patients with CML, as well as in some adult and pediatric patients with lymphoid leukemia. The translocation fuses chromosome 9q sequences from the *ABL* gene, a cellular homologue of a *v-onc* gene, to sequences from chromosome 22q (de Klein et al., 1982; Heisterkamp et al., 1983; Groffen et al., 1984) (Fig. 19.2). The novel sequences on chromosome 22q are termed the *BCR* (for break point cluster region) gene. The resultant chimeric BCR-ABL protein retains the active protein kinase sequences from the *ABL* gene but replaces the ABL regulatory sequences with BCR sequences. The net result is the generation of a protein kinase with altered structure and function (Lugo et al., 1990).

Other oncogenic alleles encode chimeric transcription factors with altered structure and function. For example, in pre-B acute leukemia, translocations involving chromosome 1q and chromosome 19p, i.e., t(1;19) (q23;p13), can be detected. This translocation has been characterized in detail and has been found to fuse *E2A* gene sequences from chromosome 19 to *PBX1* gene sequences from chromosome 1 (Kamps et al., 1990; Nourse et al., 1990). Both genes encode transcription factors, but the *PBX1* gene is not normally expressed in lymphoid or hematopoietic cells. The intriguing aspect of the chimeric transcription factor generated is that it has an altered structure and altered transcriptional regulatory activity. In addition, because the PBX1 protein is not normally expressed in lymphoid cells and the PBX1 sequences necessary for specific DNA binding are retained in the chimeric protein, the expression of genes regulated by PBX1 is altered. A second chimeric transcription factor that combines *E2A* elements with those of another transcription factor

has also been characterized in leukemia. In this case, the transcriptional regulatory domain of *E2A* has been fused to the DNA binding sequences of a transcription factor (HLF) that is normally expressed in hepatocytes and renal cells (Inaba et al., 1992). Presumably, the unscheduled expression of a chimeric transcription factor, such as the E2A-HLF chimeric protein, alters the normal regulatory circuits controlling early B-lymphocyte growth and differentiation. Furthermore, the frequent generation of chimeric transcription factors in leukemia lends support to the notion that aberrant transcriptional control of gene expression is a primary event in human leukemia.

ONCOGENES IDENTIFIED BY DNA AMPLIFICATION

Several oncogenic alleles have been identified because they are contained within DNA sequences amplified in tumor cells. In some cases, the amplified DNA sequences were first revealed in karyotypic analyses as extrachromosomal elements termed *double minute chromosomes* (DMs) or as novel banding regions on chromosomes termed *homogeneously staining regions* (HSRs). DMs and HSRs contain from 20 to several hundred copies of a chromosomal region of several hundred thousand base-pairs. Biologic selection for the generation and maintenance of the amplified DNA sequences in the tumor cells is thought to be driven by the increased copy number and increased expression of a target gene or genes within the larger region of amplified DNA. Further detailed molecular genetic characterization of the amplified sequences is necessary to identify the specific target(s) genes in the larger region of amplified DNA. In some cases, a cellular homologue of a known *v-onc* gene is thought to be the target gene present in the amplified DNA. In other cases, characterization of the amplified DNA sequences has led to the identification of novel oncogenic alleles.

Among the cellular homologues of *v-onc* genes affected by DNA amplification in human tumors are the *MYC, MYB*, epidermal growth factor receptor (*EGFR*), and *c-erbB2* (also known as *HER2* or *NEU*) genes (Bishop, 1991; Solomon et al., 1991; Weinberg, 1994). The *MYC* and *MYB* genes encode transcription factors, and the *EGFR* and *NEU* genes encode transmembrane receptor tyrosine kinase proteins. *MYC* is discussed in more detail below, as is the *c-erbB2* (*HER2/NEU*) gene. Other novel cellular proto-oncogenes that have been identified because they are present within the amplified DNA sequences include two genes, *N-MYC* and *L-MYC*, that are closely related to *MYC*, the *GLI* gene, the *MDM2* gene (see the *p53* tumor suppressor gene section), the *cyclin D1/PRAD1* gene (also activated by chromosomal translocation as noted above), and several genes encoding growth factors (e.g., *HST, INT2*) (Bishop, 1991; Fakharzadeh et al., 1991; Kinzler et al., 1987; Lammie et al., 1991; Momand et al., 1993; Nau et al., 1985; Oliner et al., 1992; Schwab et al., 1983; Solomon et al., 1991; Weinberg, 1994). Because the DNA amplifications involve several hundred thousand base-pairs, in some tumors more than one cellular proto-oncogene may be contained in the amplified sequences. One example of DNA amplifications affecting several proto-oncogenes is the amplification of chromosome 12q sequences in a subset of sarcomas. These amplifications often involve and activate the expression of the *MDM2, GLI*, and *CDK4* (see the p105-RB function section below) genes (Khatib et al., 1993).

Many candidate oncogenes have been identified by comparative genome hybridization (Kallioniemi et al., 1992) and, recently, by studying changes in global gene expression in human solid tumors (Gray and Collins, 2000). Additionally, candidate oncogenes have been found to be amplified in certain tumor types. For example, telomerase activity has been linked to cellular immortality and tumor progression and is a potential target for chemotherapy (Lavelle et al., 2000). The human telomerase RNA gene (*hTERC*) was mapped to chromosome 3q26.2–q27, a region frequently subject to copy number gains in human tumors (Soder et al., 1997). Increased copy numbers of the *hTERC* locus were also observed with up to ten copies per nucleus and hybridizations with a chromosome 3 centromeric probe indicated that polysomy and isochromosome 3q formation may contribute to this, supporting the role of telomerase in human cancer and the notion that telomerase may be reactivated in some human tumor types (Soder et al., 1997).

RAS gene alterations

The initial DNA transfer studies using DNA from a variety of human tumor types provided evidence that mutations in one of the three highly related *RAS* genes were present in about 10% to 15% of all human cancers (Barbacid, 1987). The *K-RAS* gene was found to be a more common target for mutations than either the *H-RAS* or *N-RAS* genes. In addition, *K-RAS* codon 12 was a particularly frequent target for point mutations, though mutations affecting codons 13 and 61 were seen in a small subset of cases. Subsequent studies have used PCR-based techniques to identify RAS gene mutations in a wide spectrum of human cancers (Bos, 1989; Bishop, 1991). Despite the fact that the *H-RAS* gene was identified first, it is mutated in only a small subset of tumors, perhaps most frequently in bladder cancer, where about 10% of cases have *H-RAS* mutations. *K-RAS* mutations are seen in about 50% of colorectal cancers, about 70% to 90% of pancreatic cancers, and about 30% of adenocarcinomas of the lung. *N-RAS* mutations have been detected in about 20% to 30% of acute nonlymphocytic leukemias but are infrequent in epithelial cancers.

Each of the *RAS* genes encodes a guanine nucleotide-binding protein with a molecular mass of 21,000 Da (often termed p21). A large body of evidence gathered from biochemical and genetic studies has implicated the RAS proteins in the transduction of growth and differentiation signals from activated transmembrane receptors to downstream protein kinases (Bourne et al., 1990; Boguski and McCormick, 1993; Lowy and Willumsen, 1993; McCormick, 1993). The oncogenic mutations at codons 12, 13, and 61 of the *RAS* genes reduce the ability of the RAS protein to hydrolyze guanosine triphosphate (GTP) to guanosine diphosphate. Biochemical studies have established that, while mutant RAS proteins exhibit minor reductions in their intrinsic guanosine triphosphatase (GTPase) activity, the major defect is a marked decrease in their ability to interact with the GTPase-activating protein (termed RAS-GAP). Hence, the RAS protein remains in the GTP-bound or active state, and the normal regulation of cell growth is altered.

Ras mediates a wide variety of signal transduction, especially from the cell surface receptor tyrosine kinases. Upon receptor activation by ligand, receptor tyrosine kinases, such as EGFR, PDGFR, IGFR and heterotrimeric G proteins-coupled receptors, SoS (ubiquitous GEF) is recruited to the plasma membrane where it catalyzes the exchange of GTP for GDP on Ras. The association of SoS with the receptor tyrosine kinases is mediated by a membrane attachment domain of SoS and the SH2 and SH3-domain-containing adaptor protein Grb2 (Byrne et al., 1996). In some receptors, such as NGFR, SoS and Grb2 are associated with these receptors *via* tyrosine-phosphorylated Shc proteins. Serpentine (i.e., G protein-coupled) receptors activate Ras by releasing a subunit of the heterotrimeric G protein complexes (van Biesen et al., 1995). This subunit activates PI-3 kinase, which by a pathway involving Src or a Src-like tyrosine kinase, induces the tyrosine phosphorylation of Shc and subsequently SoS-mediated activation of Ras (Lopez-Ilasaca et al., 1997).

Ras activation leads to the activation of multiple signalling pathways. However, the mechanisms of activation as well as the direct effects of activation of the downstream pathways are not fully understood in most cases. Nevertheless, Ras activation in immortalised cells results in proliferation (entry into S phase of the cell cycle) via the activation of cyclin D1 through the Ras/Raf/MAPK pathway (Aktas et al., 1997; Mittnacht et al., 1997; Peeper et al., 1997), differentiation and cellular transformation.

In addition to the many studies carried out to address the role of the *RAS* mutations in the pathogenesis of cancer, several studies suggest that *RAS* mutations may have clinical significance. As noted above, *K-RAS* mutations are present in about 30% of adenocarcinomas of the lung (Bos, 1989), and patients whose tumors harbor a mutant *K-RAS* gene may have a poorer prognosis than those whose tumors do not (Slebos et al., 1990). Though *K-RAS* mutation appears to be a useful prognostic marker in adenocarcinoma of the lung, no evidence suggests that it has prognostic utility in colorectal or other cancer types. *K-RAS* mutations may, however, prove useful for diagnostic purposes in some tumor types. Preliminary findings suggest that *K-RAS* mutations may be an adjunctive marker in the diagnosis of pancreatic cancer by fine needle aspiration (Urban et al., 1993). In addition, *K-RAS* gene mutations have been detected in stool specimens from patients with colorectal cancers and large adenomas (Sidransky et al., 1992). Initial studies suggested that *K-RAS* mutation might be a sensitive and specific marker for the diagnosis of pancreatic cancer or the early detection of colorectal tumors. However, the identification of *K-RAS* mutations in colonic hyperplastic polyps and aberrant crypt foci, as well as in pancreatic ductal hyperplasias and pancreatitis (Caldas et al., 1994; DiGiuseppe et al., 1994; Brentnall et al., 1995;), suggests that detection of *K-RAS* mutation may provide a useful screening tool but will not, alone, establish a diagnosis of cancer or even a precancerous lesion.

Given the prevalence of *RAS* gene mutations in specific cancer types and cancer in general, there is great interest in identifying agents that specifically affect RAS-dependent growth regulatory pathways in cells. The studies demonstrating that genetic inactivation of the mutant *K-RAS* gene inhibits tumor cell growth provide the proof-in-principle that inhibition of the altered signaling of the mutant RAS protein may have a marked effect on tumor growth in the patient. Studies of the effectiveness of RAS-targeted agents, such as farnesyltransferase inhibitors, are currently underway.

There is now mounting evidence that some mutations in *RAS* are associated with more aggressive tumor phenotypes than others. *In vivo*, the RASCAL study, which has collected data from colorectal cancer patients in many countries came to the conclusion that the codon 12 G to T mutation in Ki-*ras* but not the G to A mutation is associated with an increased risk of relapse and mortality (Andreyev et al. 1998). *In vitro*, Seeburg et al. (1984) have shown that valine-12 is more transforming than aspartate-12. In addition, a similar association between the valine substitution and poor prognosis has been reported for patients with lung cancer (Keohavong et al. 1996).

The RAS protein

Much is known about the tertiary structures of Ras protein molecules (Sprang 1997). The nucleotide sits in a crevice at the surface and three regions closely surrounding the di- or triphosphate part can be distinguished: the P-loop, which binds the triphosphates, and switch I and switch II, which are the regions which change conformation between the GTP and GDP-bound forms. The P-loop (residues to 10–17), containing the GxxxxGKS/T sequence motif, has the same 3D structure in a wide variety of proteins including GTPases, ATPases and kinases. Functionally it can be regarded as a triphosphate-binding site because several amide groups lie together in an anion hole (Dreusicke and Schulz 1986) or "nest" (Sayle and Milner-White 1995) that neatly accommodates the triphosphate by multiple hydrogen bonding to the oxygen atoms. In Ras the sequence is GxGxxGKS and it is the second glycine which represents residue 12.

The effector region, also called switch I, comprising residues 30 to 40, which are mostly exposed at the surface, is found by genetic analysis to be the most important in determining the transducing effect of Ras. It shows differences in conformation between the GDP and GTP-bound forms of the protein. The nature of the downstream signalling proteins for Ras has been controversial, but it is clear that Raf is a major effector protein (Moodie et al. 1993; Wittinghofer and Nassar 1996). However, other proteins, including GAP, neurofibromin, RalGDS and PI-3 kinase bind to this region of Ras and may also act as effectors. Although the area to which they bind overlaps the Raf effector region, their binding sites on Ras are distinct (Winkler et al. 1997).

The switch II region (residues 60 to 70) contains the Gln61 residue that is of interest because its amide side-chain has been found to be necessary for the catalysis of GTP hydrolysis (Pai et al., 1990) and the region exhibits relatively large conformational changes. Switch II has also been shown to be important in binding of Raf-1 cysteine-rich domain (residues 139–184). Mutation in switch I (T35A and E37G) or switch II of Ras (G60A and Y64W) resulted in diminished binding of Ras to the Ras-binding domain of Raf-1 (residues 55–131) or the Raf-1 cysteine-rich domain (139–184), respectively (Drugan et al., 1996). Both of these interactions of Ras with the Raf-1 domains are necessary for transformation by Ras and for activation of Raf-1 (Hu et al., 1995; Drugan et al., 1996).

MYC gene alterations and cancer

The *MYC* gene is the cellular homologue of a *v-onc* gene present in the MC29 and several other highly oncogenic avian retroviruses. When expressed at high levels, it is capable of transforming some rodent fibroblast cell lines (reviewed by Weinberg, 1989), but it was not identified as an oncogene through DNA transfection studies. Rather, the *MYC* gene was first found to be activated in human cancers as a result of chromosomal translocation in Burkitt's lymphoma (Bishop, 1991; Solomon et al., 1991). It is most commonly activated by a chromosome 8:14 translocation, in which Ig heavy chain sequences on chromosome 14 are fused to sequences at or near the *MYC* gene locus on chromosome 8. The *MYC* gene is also activated by fusion with light chain sequences in the subset of cases with chromosome 2:8 or 8:22 translocations. While the break points in and around the *MYC* gene may vary widely in different tumors, the consistent feature of all cases is that the normal regulation of *MYC* gene expression is altered by the translocation, causing either higher expression or unregulated expression with regard to particular phases of the cell cycle.

As noted above, in addition to translocations that deregulate *MYC* expression, the *MYC* gene is affected by DNA amplification in several tumor types. It is frequently amplified in small cell carcinoma of the lung (SCCL) and is much less frequently amplified in a wide spectrum of epithelial cancers, including breast and colorectal carcinomas (Little et al., 1983; DePinho et al., 1991). The *N-MYC* and *L-MYC* genes each encode proteins that are closely related to the protein encoded by *MYC*, and these genes were initially identified, in large part, because they are amplified in tumors. The *N-MYC* and *L-MYC* genes are activated by DNA amplification in SCCL, and about 30% to 40% of

SCCL cases have amplification of *MYC*, *N-MYC*, or *L-MYC* (DePinho et al., 1991). The *N-MYC* gene is also affected by DNA amplification in other tumor types, including neuroblastomas and glioblastomas (Brodeur et al., 1984; Fuller and Bigner, 1992). In neuroblastoma, *N-MYC* gene amplification is often seen in higher stage (i.e., stage 3 and 4) tumors. Moreover, patients whose lower stage neuroblastomas (i.e., stage 2) have *N-MYC* amplification appear to have a much worse prognosis than those whose tumors do not (Schwab and Amler, 1990).

Many studies have focused on the function of the *MYC* gene products in the regulation of cell growth and apoptosis. Studies have revealed that each of the MYC proteins functions as a transcription factor by binding to specific DNA sequences, following dimerization with a protein termed MAX (Blackwood and Eisenman, 1991; Kato and Dang, 1992; Marcu et al., 1992). Each of the MYC proteins has a unique pattern of expression in development and subtle functional differences in *in vitro* assays. Therefore each of the MYC proteins may have a unique function in regulating the expression of specific genes. Approximately 30 putative MYC target genes have recently been identified (Dang, 1999). Some of these encode proteins likely to play a role in mediating MYC functions. In addition to MAX, a large number of proteins which interact with the C-terminal domain of MYC have been identified, including YY-1, AP-2, BRCA-1, TFII-I and MIZ-1 (Sakamuro and Prendergast, 1999). Proteins that interact with the N-terminal domain of MYC include the Rb-related protein p107, and also BIN1, TRRAP, MM-1, AMY-1, Pam and alpha-tubulin (Sakamuro and Prendergast, 1999). Studies in transgenic and knockout mice have recently given insights into the balance between proliferation and apoptosis in MYC-induced carcinogenesis. An outsanding feature of these experiments is the demonstration that the balance between oncogene-induced proliferation and apoptosis in a given tissue can be a critical determinant in the initiation and maintenance of the tumor (Pelengaris et al., 2000).

The *NEU* gene

The *NEU* gene (also known as the *HER2* or *c-erbB-2* gene) was initially identified through transfection studies using purified DNA from chemically induced neuro/glioblastomas of neonatal rats (Shih et al., 1981). Further studies revealed that a single amino acid substitution within the transmembrane region accounted for the transforming activity of the *NEU* alleles identified from the tumors compared to normal *NEU* alleles (Bargmann et al., 1986). In addition, based on the characterization of the *NEU* gene sequences and the biochemical studies of the NEU protein, it was established that the *NEU* gene encoded a protein with a great deal of similarity to the epidermal growth factor receptor (EGFR) (reviewed by Dougall et al., 1994). Specifically, the *NEU* gene encodes a phosphoprotein with a molecular mass of about 185,000 Da (hence it is sometimes termed p185). The extracellular domain of the NEU protein is roughly 40% identical with the EGFR protein. The protein has a single membrane-spanning domain, and the tyrosine kinase cytoplasmic domain sequences exhibit a high degree of similarity to the corresponding region of the EGFR protein. The human *NEU* gene has been localized to chromosome 17q.

Although the *NEU* gene was initially identified as an oncogenic allele through DNA transfection studies, the gene is most commonly affected by gene amplification and overexpression of its RNA and protein in primary human cancers, including carcinomas of the breast, ovary, and stomach (Bishop, 1991; Dougall et al., 1994). Studies of primary tumors from patients with node-negative breast cancer have provided evidence that patients with amplification and overexpression of the *NEU* gene fare more poorly than those whose tumors do not have *NEU* gene amplification and overexpression (Press et al., 1993; Slamon et al., 1987; 1989).

Like the *EGFR* gene, *NEU* is believed to encode a peptide hormone receptor, and much attention has focused on the identification of ligands (reviewed by Dougall et al., 1994). While EGFR ligands like EGF and transforming growth factor-alpha (TGF-alpha) will stimulate tyrosine phosphorylation of NEU, they do not do so by binding to NEU. Rather, they appear to modulate NEU activity by virtue of the formation of heterodimers by EGFR and NEU. The EGF agonists activate the kinase activity of EGFR, which can then activate NEU by phosphorylation. Recent studies have identified another class of potential ligands for NEU termed the heregulins or NEU differentiation factors (NDFs). However, other studies have suggested that these proteins do not bind specifically to NEU. Rather, the NDFs appear to interact with other transmembrane receptors that share similarity with both EGFR and NEU.

As mentioned above, although *NEU* mutations are rarely, if at all, found in human cancers, wild-type *NEU* has been often found to be either amplified at the genomic level and/or found to be overexpressed at the protein level. In the majority of cases overexpression correlates with tumor chemo-resistance and poor patient prognosis (Klapper et al., 2000a,b). *NEU* amplification has been most extensively addressed in the domain of breast cancer biology, in which *NEU* is amplified with a 20–30% incidence. This has

motivated the development of therapies designed to subvert *NEU* expression. Specifically, the cancer-inhibitory potential of antibodies to NEU was realized as far back as 1984, when mice bearing tumors with an active form of the rodent NEU were treated with specific anti-NEU antibodies (Dougall et al., 1994; Drebin et al., 1988). However, only within the last few years has this realization yielded a method to treat cancer patients (Baselga et al., 1996). Although antibodies conjugated to toxins, radionucleotides and prodrugs show promising results in animal models, it is important to note that even naked forms of antibodies to NEU are active in arresting tumorigenic growth of NEU-overexpressing cells. Experiments performed on various systems suggest that these antibodies can induce differentiation of rapidly dividing breast cancer cells to growth-arrested cells (Bacus et al., 1992). Likewise, it has been reported that anti-NEU antibodies down-regulate expression of angiogenic growth factors in tumor cells, both in vitro and in animal models (Petit et al., 1997). Furthermore, NEU-mediated resistance to the cytotoxic effects of the tumor necrosis factor can be significantly reduced by monoclonal antibodies to NEU (Hudziak et al., 1988). Mechanistically, the antibodies appear to act by removing NEU from the cell surface. It has previously been shown that the oncogenic activity of NEU necessitates its localization at the plasma membrane. In line with blocking NEU action by preventing its oncogenic interaction with other surface-localized NEU proteins, the tumor-inhibitory potential of specific antibodies (Hurwitz et al., 1995) or certain combinations of anti-NEU antibodies correlates with the efficiency of antibody-induced down-regulation of NEU. Consistent with this notion is the observation that antibody bivalence is essential for inhibitory activity. However, effects mediated by the Fc portion of these antibodies also contribute to their tumor-arresting activity (Clynes et al., 2000). Because bivalent antibodies to NEU share partial agonistic activity, their ability to down-regulate surface NEU may relate to kinase activation. Indeed, some recent evidence suggests that auto-phosphorylation of NEU and subsequent recruitment of c-Cbl are necessary for antibody-induced down-regulation of NEU (Klapper et al., 2000b). As a consequence of down-regulation, antibodies to NEU elevate p27 and the Rb-related protein p130, resulting in a reduction in the number of cells in the S phase of the cell cycle (Sliwkowski et al., 1999). In independent studies, NEU-inhibitory antibodies curtailed the levels of p21 in cells overexpressing NEU, although levels of cyclin D1 remained relatively unchanged (Pietras et al., 1999). When examining all known cyclin D members, it was found that cyclins D2 and D3 decreased dramatically

(Lane et al., 2000; Neve et al., 2000). Thus the downstream effects of NEU blocking antibodies translate to signals that inhibit progression through the cell cycle and can explain their potential clinical benefit.

BCL2 gene alterations, cancer, and cell death

The *BCL2* (B-cell lymphoma/leukemia-2) gene was identified because it was activated in a B-cell malignancy by a translocation [t(14;18) (q32;q21)] between the Ig heavy chain gene locus on chromosome 14q and chromosome 18q. This translocation juxtaposed *BCL2* gene sequences on 18q with the powerful Ig regulatory elements (Tsujimoto et al., 1985; Cleary et al., 1986; Solomon et al., 1991). The result, in B cells containing such translocations, was overproduction of *BCL2* mRNAs and their encoded proteins. Translocations activating *BCL2* gene expression can be noted in the majority of follicular non-Hodgkin's B-cell lymphomas (Yunis et al., 1989; Bishop, 1991; Solomon et al., 1991). Although some studies suggest that *BCL2* gene expression may be increased in other cancer types, specific gene defects (such as chromosomal translocation) that might be responsible for such gene activation have not yet been described in these tumors.

BCL2 encodes a protein with a molecular mass of about 25,000 Da. When first characterized, the predicted protein product of the *BCL2* gene did not show significant similarity to other known proteins. Hence, little was known of its function (reviewed by Reed, 1994). The first clues to BCL2 function were provided by studies demonstrating that constitutive expression of BCL2 in interleukin-3 (IL-3)-dependent lymphoid cells prolonged their in vitro survival when they were cultured in the absence of IL-3 (Vaux et al., 1988). The constitutive expression of BCL2 in the cells, however, did not result in concomitant cell proliferation. Because it was known that lymphokines, such as IL-3, and other colony-stimulating factors help to maintain hematopoietic cell survival in vitro, the results were consistent with the notion that BCL2 might prevent programmed cell death or apoptosis. The ability of *BCL2* to prevent cell death without affecting the rate of cell proliferation suggested that *BCL2* defined a new category of oncogene (Hockenbery et al., 1990). Cancers presumably arise, at least in part, because of excess cell accumulation. Such excess cell accumulation may result from an increased rate of cell proliferation, a decreased rate of cell death, or a combination of the two processes. Thus, while many of the oncogenic alleles in human cancer may increase the rate of cell proliferation, others such as *BCL2* are likely to affect the pathways regulating cell death.

The mechanism by which BCL2 regulates cell death has received increasing attention and a number of proteins with structural similarity to BCL2 have been discovered during the past five years (Bernardi et al., 2001). Some of these promote cell survival and possess three or four regions with extensive amino acid sequence similarity to BCL2 (BCL2-homology regions BH1-BH4) (Strasser et al., 2000). More distantly related family members contain two or three BH regions and enhance apoptosis under conditions of stress. The most potent inducers of cell death are a group of proteins that possess only a BH3 region and otherwise bear no resemblance to the BCL2 family or any other presently known protein (Huang and Strasser, 2000). Targeting of BCL2 family members to the outer mitochondrial membrane plays a critical role in apoptosis signaling. In general terms, antiapoptotic members of the BCL2 family tend to inhibit the release of mitochondrial proteins, whereas proapoptotic members favor release. The precise mechanisms for cytochrome *c* release, as well as the mechanistic link with BCL2 proteins have not been elucidated as yet (Di Lisa and Bernardi, 1998). Pro-apoptotic and anti-apoptotic members of the BCL2 protein family can physically interact (Oltvia and Korsmeyer, 1994), but it is presently unknown whether this interaction occurs in the form of dimers or as part of a conglomerate of molecules. Remarkably little overall sequence similarity is needed for similar function among the pro-apoptotic BCL2 family members. However, the possession of a BH3 region may be a defining characteristic for the subfamily (Bernardi et al., 2001).

Tumor suppressor genes

As reviewed above, the identification of oncogenic alleles in human tumors has been facilitated by several of their properties, including the prior identification of the *v-onc* genes, the characterization of sequences present at translocation break points, and the ability of oncogenes to generate tumorigenic growth properties when transferred to non-tumorigenic recipient cells. In contrast, the direct identification of tumor suppressor genes has proven far more difficult, because functional strategies for their identification have a number of practical problems. For example, although the successful transfer of a tumor suppressor gene to a tumor cell would be expected to suppress at least some of the altered growth properties of the tumor cell, such as anchorage-independent growth, lack of contact inhibition, unlimited life span, or tumorigenicity, the identification of suppressed cells in a background of fully transformed cells has proven to be a particularly difficult experimental task. Thus, the strategies to identify tumor suppressor genes and the specific alterations in these genes in human cancers have been, by necessity, more circuitous.

HISTORICAL BASIS FOR THE EXISTENCE OF TUMOR SUPPRESSOR GENES

The studies of Henry Harris and his colleagues formed the basis for the concept that the ability of cells to generate a tumor is a recessive trait, resulting, at least in part, from the inactivation of a class of cellular genes termed tumor suppressor genes (Harris, 1988). These investigators first established that hybrids generated from the fusion of fully malignant murine tumor cells with nontumorigenic murine cells were often nontumorigenic when injected into mice. The hybrid cells, however, often reverted to tumorigenicity when passaged in culture, and the tumorigenic revertants had chromosome losses detected when compared to the nontumorigenic hybrids. The interpretation of Harris and his colleagues i.e., that malignancy could be suppressed in somatic cell hybrids between tumorigenic and nontumorigenic cells, subsequently received support from many additional studies of somatic cell hybrids generated from the fusion of normal and tumorigenic rodent cells, as well as normal and malignant human cells. Hybrids retaining both sets of parental chromosomes were suppressed, with tumorigenic segregants arising most commonly after the loss of specific chromosomes from the normal parent. Moreover, tumorigenicity could be suppressed even if activated oncogenes, such as mutated *RAS* genes, were expressed in the hybrids (Stanbridge and Cavanee, 1989).

The observation that the reversion to malignancy of the hybrids was associated with the loss of specific chromosomes contributed by the nontumorigenic cells suggested that specific chromosomes might be sufficient for suppression of tumorigenicity. Furthermore, the findings suggested that tumors must arise, in part, through the inactivation of a class of cellular genes termed tumor suppressor genes. Evidence supporting the proposal that specific tumor suppressor genes might be sufficient for suppression of the tumorigenic phenotype was initially provided by studies in which single chromosomes were transferred using a technique known as microcell-mediated chromosome transfer (Weissman et al., 1987; Oshimura et al., 1990; Trent et al., 1990). For example, the tumorigenicity of some cervical cancer cells or rhabdomyosarcoma cells has been shown to be suppressed following transfer of human chromosome 11. However, there is some cell-type specificity to the ability of a particular chromosome to suppress tumori-

genicity, because chromosome 11 fails to suppress the tumorigenicity of some neuroblastoma and renal cell cancer cells (Table 19.4). Furthermore, although the ability of the cells to form tumors in immunocompromised (nude) mice and to grow in an anchorage-independent fashion may be suppressed following single-chromosome transfer, other traits characteristic of the parental tumor cells (e.g. unlimited life span in culture) are still retained in the suppressed hybrids. The observation that not all properties of the parental tumor cells can be suppressed by a single chromosome (and perhaps a single tumor suppressor gene) is clearly consistent with the proposal that tumors arise as the result of multiple genetic alterations.

While the somatic cell genetic studies of tumorigenesis reviewed above did not lead directly to the identification of tumor suppressor genes, they did provide persuasive evidence that a subset of the mutations in human cancers must be in genes of this type. In addition, concurrent with the initial cell fusion experiments of Harris and his colleagues, other epidemiological and genetic studies also suggested an important role for the inactivation of cellular genes in cancer development. Many of these studies were first carried out on retinoblastoma, and some of the critical observations from these studies are reviewed below.

THE RETINOBLASTOMA GENE

Retinoblastoma: a paradigm for tumor suppressor gene identification

The relative rarity of retinoblastoma belies the importance of observations gleaned through study of this tumor. Indeed, many of the concepts and techniques used to identify and characterise tumor suppressor genes and inherited and somatic genetic alterations in cancer were first established through studies of the genetic basis of retinoblastoma.

Retinoblastoma is a paediatric tumor that occurs sporadically in many patients but also occurs in some families in a pattern consistent with autosomal dominant inheritance. Knudson's analysis of the age-specific incidence of retinoblastoma led him to propose that two distinct mutagenic events were necessary for the development of retinoblastoma in all patients (Knudson, 1971; 1985). Knudson's hypothesis is thus often termed "the two-hit hypothesis". He proposed that in those patients with the inherited form of the disease, one mutation was present in the germline and in all cells of the body. A second mutational event occurring in any one of the developing retinoblasts would then lead to the generation of a retinoblastoma. Thus, in a patient with the inherited

Table 19.4. Summary of selected familial cancer syndromes

Syndrome	Tumor	Associated cancers/traits	Chromosome location	Cloned gene	Proposed gene/protein function
Familial retinoblastoma	Retinoblastoma	Osteosarcoma	13q14	RB1	Cell cycle regulation, and transcriptional regulation (E2F-mediated)
Familial polyposis	Colorectal cancer	Intestinal polyposis, duodenal tumors Gardner syndrome Jaw osteomas Desmoid tumors Turcot's syndrome Medulloblastoma	5q21	APC	Regulation of level of transcriptional activator, beta - catenin
Li-Fraumeni syndrome	Sarcomas, breast cancer	Brain tumors, leukemia, lymphoma, others	17q13	p53	Transcriptional regulation, response to DNA damage and other cellular stresses, cell cycle control, and apoptosis
Hereditary non-polyposis colorectal cancer	Colorectal cancer	Endometrial, ovarian, hepato-biliary, and urinary tract cancer	2p16 3p21 Others	hMSH2 hMLH1 Others	DNA mismatch repair
Neurofibromatosis type 1	Neurofibromas	Neurofibrosarcoma, brain tumors	17q11	NF1	GAP for RAS proteins and microtubule binding
Familial Wilms tumor	Wilms tumor	WAGR Wilms Aniridia Genitourinary Abns. Mental retardation Denys-Drash syndrome	11p13	WT1	Transcriptional regulation
Beckwith-Wiedemann	Wilms tumor	Exomphalos, macroglossia, gigantism, hepatoblastoma, adreno-cortical cancer	11p15	CDKNIC	Cell cycle regulator
Gorlin syndrome	Basal cell carcinomas	Jaw cysts, palmar and plantar pits, medulloblastomas, ovarian fibromas	9q22	PTCH	Receptor for sonic hedgehog
Neurofibromatosis type 2	Acoustic neuromas	Meningioma, gliomas, ependymomas	22q12	NF2	Links cell membrane to cytoskeleton?
Familial breast cancer	Breast cancer	Ovarian cancer	17q21 13q12	BRCA1 BRCA2	Double-strand break repair of DNA
von Hippel-Lindau	Renal cancer, pheochromocytomas	Retinal angiomas, hemangioblastomas	3p25	VHL	Indirect regulator of transcription of hypoxia-inducible genes
Familial melanoma	Melanoma	Pancreatic cancer, dysplasic nevi, atypical moles	9p21	p16INK4A	Inhibitor of CDK4 and CDK6 cyclin dependent kinases; cell cycle regulation
Multiple endocrine neoplasia type 1	Pancreatic islet cell	Parathyroid hyperplasia pituitary adenomas	11q13	MEN1	Transcriptional repressor

continued

Table 19.4. Summary of selected familial cancer syndromes (*continued*)

Syndrome	Tumor	Associated cancers/traits	Chromosome location	Cloned gene	proposed gene/protein function
Multiple endocrine neoplasia type 2	Medullary thyroid cancer	Type 2A Pheochromocytoma Parathyroid hyperplasia Type 2B Pheochromocytoma Mucosal hamartoma	10q11	*RET*	Receptor tyrosine kinase
Ataxia telangiectasia	Lymphoma	Cerebellar ataxia, immunodeficiency, breast cancer in heterozygotes?	11q22	*ATM*	DNA repair, cell cycle arrest
Blooms syndrome	Solid tumors, leukemia	Immunodeficiency, small stature	15q26	*BLM*	DNA helicase
Xeroderma pigmentosum	Skin cancer	Pigmentation abnormalities, hypogonadism	Seven complementation groups	*XPA* to *XPG*	Nucleotide excision repair
Fanconi anemia	AML	Pancytopenia, skeletal abnormalities	Multiple complementation groups	*FANCA* to *FANCG*	DNA repair

form of the disease, one or more retinoblastomas might be likely to develop. However, the number of retinoblastomas arising in an inherited case might well be expected to vary from none to three or four, depending on the frequency of second mutations. With this model, Knudson could account for the absence of disease in some patients known to harbor the predisposing mutation (i.e., skipped generations), as well as the presence of bilateral or multifocal disease in some affected family members. In those with the sporadic form of retinoblastoma, Knudson proposed that both mutational events were somatic and arose in the same developing retinoblast. The very reduced probability that two somatic mutations would occur in the same retinoblast was consistent with the low prevalence of retinoblastoma in the general population. Although each of the two mutational events could have been predicted to affect different genes, Knudson subsequently proposed that the two mutational events affect the two parental copies of a retinoblastoma tumor suppressor gene (subsequently referred to here as the *RB1* gene). Thus, while retinoblastoma could be inherited as a dominant trait at the phenotypic level, at the cellular level, mutations in the *RB1* gene were predicted to be recessive such that both parental copies of the gene would need to be inactivated in a cell for a retinoblastoma to develop.

The significance of Knudson's hypothesis should not be underestimated. The two-hit hypothesis not only served as a framework for considering the mechanisms through which inherited and somatic genetic mutations might interact in tumor development, but it also linked the notion of recessive genetic determinants for human cancer development to the somatic cell genetic observations demonstrating that the ability to form tumors is often a recessive trait.

Cytogenetic studies of peripheral blood lymphocytes from retinoblastoma patients provided the first clues to the location of the retinoblastoma predisposition gene (Francke, 1976). In about 5% of patients with retinoblastoma, interstitial deletions involving band q14 of chromosome 13 were identified in peripheral blood lymphocytes or normal skin fibroblasts. It was thus hypothesised that a gene predisposing to retinoblastoma development must reside at 13q14. Subsequent studies noted that the levels of esterase D, an enzyme of unknown physiological function, were reduced in normal cells from some patients with germline chromosomal deletions involving 13q14, as compared to karyotypically normal family members (Sparkes et al., 1980). Therefore, in at least a subset of patients with deletions of chromosome band 13q14, the deletions were likely to affect not only one copy of the *RB1* gene but also the esterase D gene and perhaps several other genes.

Further examination of the esterase D locus in those with retinoblastoma yielded several other critical insights into the genetics of retinoblastoma. Analysis of the segregation patterns of polymorphic esterase D isozymes in several retinoblastoma kindreds in which the affected members lacked cytogenetic alterations of 13q14 provided strong evidence for genetic linkage between the esterase D locus and the retinoblastoma predisposition gene (Sparkes et al., 1983). In addition, studies of esterase D proved particularly illustrative in a child with inherited retinoblastoma who had no detectable cytogenetic alteration in her normal cells (Benedict et al., 1983). Though a cytogenetic alteration was not apparent, this child was noted to have an approximately 50% reduction of esterase D levels in peripheral blood cells. Of even greater interest, tumor cells from this patient had no detectable esterase D activity, despite having one copy of chromosome 13. Based on these observations, Benedict, Sparkes, and their colleagues proposed that in all cells of the patient, one copy of chromosome 13 was affected by a submicroscopic deletion. This submicroscopic deletion inactivated one copy of the *RB1* gene and one copy of the esterase D gene. During tumor development, the normal copy of chromosome 13 was lost, leaving only the defective chromosome 13 in the tumor cells. Based on their findings in this patient, these investigators concluded that the predisposing mutation in the patient, the submicroscopic 13q deletion involving the *RB1* gene and the esterase D gene, was recessive at the cellular level. The effect of the predisposing mutation could be observed, however, by inactivation of the remaining normal copy of the *RB1* gene, such as by its loss in the tumor cells. These studies thus provided the first direct experimental evidence supporting Knudson's two-hit hypothesis for retinoblastoma development.

To establish the generality of this two-hit model for retinoblastoma, Cavenee, White, and their colleagues undertook studies of additional cases of inherited retinoblastoma as well as sporadic cases, using DNA probes from chromosome 13 (Cavenee et al., 1983). The probes detected DNA sequence polymorphisms and thus allowed the two parental copies of chromosome 13 to be distinguished from one another in normal and tumor tissues from each patient. Following comparison of the parental alleles present in the paired normal and tumor samples from each patient, Cavenee and co-workers demonstrated that loss of heterozygosity (i.e., the loss of one parental chromosome) for chromosome 13 had occurred during the development of more than 60% of retinoblastomas studied. They also demonstrated that loss of heterozygosity (LOH, also termed allelic loss) could occur by a number of different mechanisms (Fig. 19.3). The unmasking of the recessive predisposing mutations at the retinoblastoma locus, whether the mutation had been inherited or had arisen somatically, occurred through the same chromosomal

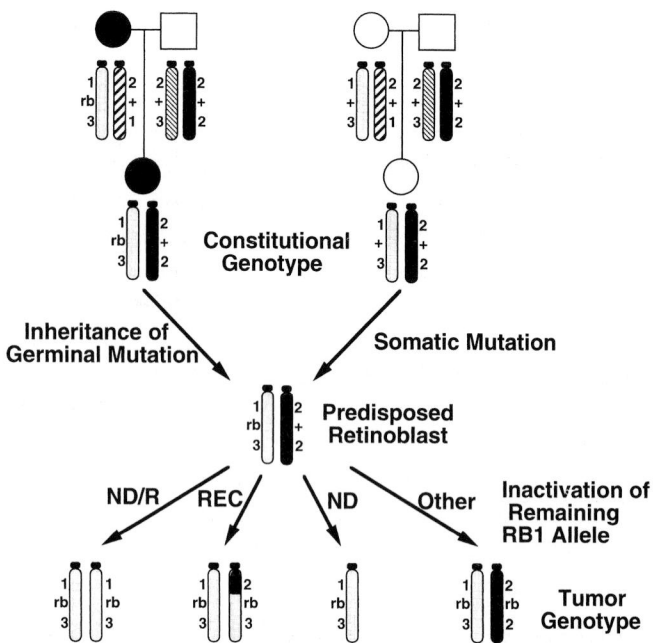

Fig. 19.3. Chromosomal mechanisms that result in loss of heterozygosity for alleles at the retinoblastoma predisposition (*RB1*) locus at chromosome band 13q14. In the inherited form of the disease (top left), the affected daughter inherits a mutant *RB1* allele (*rb*) from her affected mother and a normal *RB1* allele (+) from her father. Thus, she has one wild-type *RB1* allele and one mutant *RB1* allele in all her cells (constitutional genotype *rb/*+). The two copies of chromosome 13 in her normal cells (one from each parent) can be distinguished using polymorphic DNA markers flanking the *RB1* locus (the various polymorphic alleles are designated by a number). A retinoblastoma can arise after inactivation of the remaining wild-type *RB1* allele. Among the genetic mechanisms found to inactivate the remaining wild-type *RB1* allele during tumor development are: chromosome nondisjunction and reduplication of the remaining copy of chromosome 13 (ND/R); mitotic recombination (REC); nondisjunction (ND); and other more localized mutations that inactivate the remaining *RB1* allele (OTHER). In the non-inherited (sporadic) form of the disease, a somatic mutation arises in a developing retinal cell and inactivates one of the *RB1* alleles. A retinoblastoma will develop if the remaining *RB1* allele is inactivated by one of the mechanisms shown (From Cavenee et al., 1986.) Recessive mutant genes predisposing to human cancer. Mutation Research 168:3.

mechanisms. Furthermore, the study of inherited cases confirmed that the chromosome 13 homologue retained in tumor cells that had suffered chromosome 13 LOH was always derived from the affected parent (Cavenee et al., 1985; Hansen and Cavanee, 1987).

Previous epidemiological studies had established that patients with the inherited form of retinoblastoma were also predisposed to the development of osteosarcomas, with these lesions most often arising in areas that had been exposed to radiotherapy. Study of chromosome 13q LOH in osteosarcomas arising in patients with retinoblastoma, as well as in apparently sporadic cases of osteosarcoma, revealed that the majority of osteosarcomas studied had undergone LOH for the 13q region containing the *RB1* gene (Hansen et al., 1985; Hansen and Cavanee, 1987). Such findings established a genetic link between retinoblastoma and osteosarcoma.

The studies of chromosome 13q LOH in retinoblastomas and osteosarcomas were therefore particularly instructive. They provided definitive evidence in support of Knudson's hypothesis and illustrated the multiple chromosomal mechanisms that could unmask pre-existing recessive mutations at a tumor suppressor locus. The studies also established that similar genetic mechanisms could account for both inherited and sporadic cases of a particular type of cancer. Finally, the DNA-based studies provided genetic evidence that inactivation of the same tumor suppressor gene was responsible, at least in part, for the development of two distinct tumor types.

Molecular cloning and mutational analysis of the retinoblastoma gene

The molecular cloning of the *RB1* gene was greatly facilitated by the identification of a chromosome 13q14 DNA marker that detected rearrangements in Southern blot analysis of two retinoblastomas and the complete loss of both retinoblastoma alleles in a third case (Dryja et al., 1986). Following its identification, it was established that *RB1* is a large gene with 27 exons, spanning more than 200 kb of genomic DNA (Friend et al., 1986; Fung et al., 1987; Lee et al., 1987a). It has been estimated that 90% of individuals with a germline *RB1* mutation will develop retinoblastoma (Musarella and Gallie, 1987).

The cloning of the *RB1* gene allowed definitive studies of the inherited and somatic mutations present in the gene. Although gross deletions, of either inherited or somatic origin, affect the *RB1* gene in a subset of retinoblastomas and osteosarcomas, most of these tumors do not have gross alterations of the gene. In fact, most mutations inactivating the *RB1* gene are point mutations or small insertions and deletions that result in premature truncation of the protein product (Goddard et al., 1988; Dunn et al., 1989; Yandell et al., 1989). However, several missense and splicing mutations have also been identified in primary retinoblastomas and osteosarcomas. Almost all *RB1* tumorigenic mutations result in the disruption or loss of the "pocket" domain of the pRB protein (Brehm and Kouzarides, 1999) that is required for interaction with E2F protein and viral oncoproteins (see below). In general, no clear genotype-phenotype association has yet emerged. As predicted by the Knudson hypothesis and the studies of 13q LOH, both *RB1* alleles are inactivated in retinoblastomas and osteosarcomas.

In addition to the identification of germline and somatic mutations that inactivate the *RB1* gene in retinoblastomas and osteosarcomas, functional evidence indicates that the *RB1* gene can suppress aspects of the tumorigenic phenotype when a cloned copy is introduced into retinoblastoma or osteosarcoma cells growing in culture (Huang et al., 1988a,b,c). At least in some cases, successful transfer of a normal copy of the *RB1* gene to retinoblastoma or osteosarcoma cells results in changes in cell morphology and the suppression of growth in culture or in nude (immunocompromised) mice.

Since its initial cloning in 1986, *RB1* mutations have been extensively analysed in many tumor types other than retinoblastoma and osteosarcoma. Some of these studies were motivated by observations that 13q LOH was prevalent in other tumor types. The mutations inactivating the *RB1* gene in other tumor types are similar to those in retinoblastomas and osteosarcomas and include frameshift and nonsense mutations that result in a truncated and often unstable protein (Harbour et al., 1988; Lee et al., 1988; Horowitz et al., 1989; Bookstein et al., 1990; Scheffner et al., 1991). However, the prevalence of mutations in the *RB1* gene varies markedly from one tumor type to another. For example, *RB1* mutations have been observed in nearly 100% of small cell carcinomas of the lung and in about 10% to 20% of breast, bladder, pancreatic, and prostate carcinomas, while less than 5% of primary colorectal carcinomas have *RB1* mutations.

At least at first glance, the identification of somatic *RB1* mutations in tumor types other than retinoblastoma and osteosarcoma is somewhat puzzling. Patients with germline mutations in the *RB1* gene are at elevated risk (relative to the general population) of developing a rather limited spectrum of tumors, including retinoblastoma, osteosarcoma, and occasionally soft tissue sarcoma and melanoma. Patients with germline mutations in the *RB1* gene do not, however, appear to be at elevated risk for the development of other tumor types in which somatic *RB1* mutations are relatively common. Given that the *RB1* gene is ubiquitously expressed in adult tissues and that its inactivation apparently contributes in some fashion to the development of a number of common human cancer types, it is not yet clear why those with germline *RB1* mutations are not predisposed to a greater variety of cancer types. Nevertheless, the data suggest that in some cell types, such as retinoblasts, the *RB1* gene is one of the primary controlling elements in growth regulation, while in other cell types, such as mammary and prostatic epithelial cells, the growth regulatory pathways in which the *RB1* gene plays a role may be more redundant.

The cloning of the *RB1* gene ushered in a new era in the management of patients and families with inherited cancer syndromes. Those individuals who carried germline mutations could now be identified and closely followed, while those who had not inherited a specific *RB1* mutation possessed by a parent could be spared anxiety and frequent clinical examinations.

Function of the retinoblastoma protein (pRB)

The protein product of the *RB1* gene, pRB (also termed RB or p105-RB), is a nuclear phosphoprotein of 928 amino acids residues with a molecular mass of about 105 kDa (Lee et al., 1987b). The first critical insights into the function of pRB were provided by the studies of Ed Harlow and his colleagues (Whyte et al., 1988). They demonstrated that the E1A oncoprotein of the murine DNA tumor virus adenovirus type 5 complexed with pRB. Prior studies had established that E1A had many functions, including cell immortalization, induction of DNA synthesis, cooperation with other oncoproteins in transformation, and regulation of viral and host gene transcription. The studies of the Harlow group suggested that the complexing of pRB with E1A might account for some of E1A's effects on cells. Furthermore, they provided compelling evidence that the binding of E1A to pRB not only was physiologically significant but was absolutely critical to E1A's ability to mediate neoplastic transformation. In particular, they demonstrated that mutant E1A proteins that were unable to bind pRB were also unable to transform cells (Whyte et al., 1989).

The significance of this physical interaction between a tumor suppressor gene product and a DNA tumor virus oncogene product was reinforced by the subsequent demonstration that several other DNA tumor virus proteins could bind to pRB (DeCaprio et al., 1988; Dyson et al., 1989), including simian virus type 40 (SV40) large T antigen and the E7 protein of human papillomavirus (HPV) type 16 (Fig. 19.4). Mutations that inactivated the transforming activities of these proteins were found to inactivate their ability to complex with pRB. In addition, while HPV E7 proteins from the "high-risk" viruses (i.e., those strongly associated with cancer development), such as HPV types 16 and 18, were shown to complex tightly with pRB, HPV E7 proteins from "low-risk" viruses (e.g., HPV types 6 and 11) showed reduced binding to pRB. It is now recognised that these viral proteins interact, via their LXCXE motif, with the so-called "pocket" domain of pRB, the 3-D structure of which has now been solved (Lee et al., 1998).

Although the DNA tumor virus proteins inactivate the function of pRB by complexing with it, the function of pRB

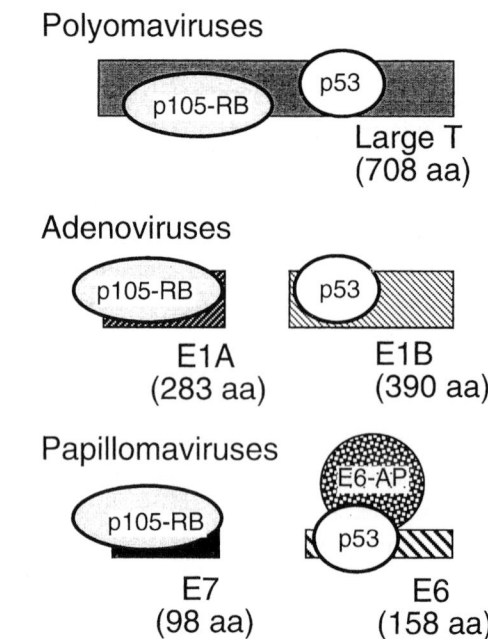

Fig. 19.4. Schematic representation of the interactions between the proteins encoded by DNA tumor viruses and tumour suppressor gene products. Large T antigen from polyomaviruses (such as simian virus 40 [SV40]) binds both the retinoblastoma protein (pRB) and the p53 protein. For the adenoviruses and the high risk human papillomaviruses (HPV types 16 and 18), different viral protein products complex with pRB and p53. A cellular protein known as E6-associated protein (E6-AP) is involved in the complexing and degradation of p53 by the HPV E6 protein (Modified from Werness et al., 1990, with permission.)

is apparently physiologically inactivated by protein phosphorylation during the normal progression through the cell cycle (Buchkovich et al., 1989; Chen et al., 1989). Indeed, pRB appears to be in a predominantly unphosphorylated or hypophosphorylated state in the G1 phase of the cell cycle and maximally phosphorylated in G2 (Fig. 19.5). The critical phosphorylation events regulating the function of pRB are likely to be mediated at the boundary between the G1 and S (DNA synthesis) phases of the cell cycle by protein complexes that consist of a protein known as a cyclin (especially cyclins D1 and E) and another protein known as a cyclin-dependent kinase (CDK). There are 16 potential CDK phosphorylation sites on pRB, and it appears that different cyclin/CDK complexes phosphorylate distinct subsets of sites, possibly in response to different growth factor signalling pathways (Mittnacht, 1998). These phosphorylation events at the G1-S boundary reduce the ability of pRB to bind to certain cellular proteins, including the members of a family of at least six transcriptional regulatory proteins known as the E2F proteins (Helin et al., 1992; 1993; Kaelin, et al., 1992; Nevins, 1992; Weintraub et al., 1992; Helin, 1998). When it is not phosphorylated, pRB complexes with and prevents the E2F protein from

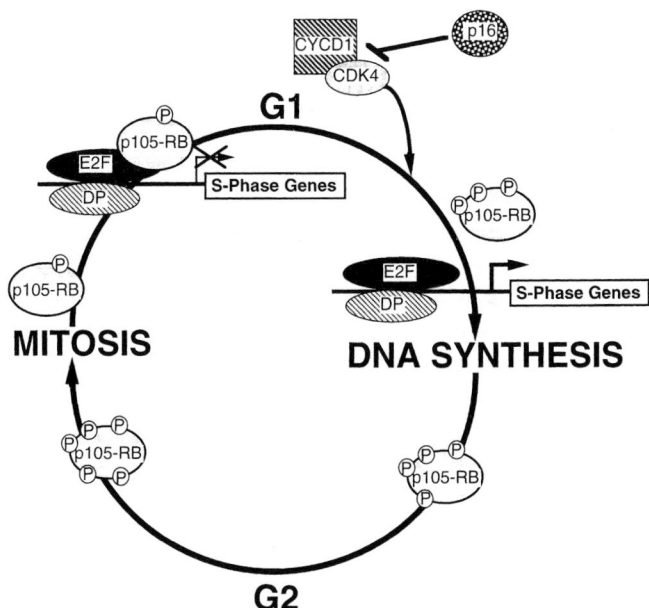

Fig. 19.5. Retinoblastoma protein function is regulated during the cell cycle by phosphorylation. The retinoblastoma protein (pRB) is hypophosphorylated in the G1 phase of the cell cycle, and phosphorylation (P) of specific sites appears to increase during progression through the cell cycle. One of the protein complexes that is likely to phosphorylate pRB prior to DNA synthesis (S-phase) includes a cyclin (CYC) and a cyclin dependent kinase (CDK) (probably, cyclin D1 and CDK4). The p16INK4a protein appears to inhibit CDK4 activity by interfering with the binding of CDK4 to cyclin D1. When pRB is hyposphosphorylated it can complex with E2F transcriptional regulatory proteins, and actively repress transcription. E2F dimerises with a DP protein and regulates the transcription of several genes involved in DNA synthesis, including DNA polymerase α, thymidine kinase, p19-ARF, cyclin E and dihydrofolate reductase. Other cellular targets for regulation by pRB are not well defined. The pRB protein is dephosphorylated at or near anaphase. (From Fearon, 1995.) Oncogeats and humour suppressor genes in Clinical Oncology (Abel off et al. eds).

activating gene expression, although it is now recognised that the latter remains bound to the promoter of its target gene (Zwicker et al., 1996). This inhibition of E2F-mediated transcriptional activation is not simply due to masking by pRB of the activation domain of E2F. Rather, pRB, bound to E2F, shuts off transcription in an active way. A currently favored hypothesis is that pRB recruits a histone de-acetylase (HDAC) protein, leading to local changes in chromatin structure which result in transcriptional repression of the gene to which the E2F protein is bound (Luo et al., 1998; Magnaghi-Jaulin et al., 1998; Brehm et al., 1999). The transcriptional repressor complex of E2F-pRB-HDAC is believed to be disrupted by binding of viral oncoprotein to pRB, mutation of pRB, or, physiologically, by phosphorylation of pRB (Brehm and Kouzarides, 1999). In the resulting nonrepressed state, the E2F protein, heterodimerised with one of at least two members of the DP protein family, can activate the expression of its target gene

(Fig. 19.5). Further support for the role of pRB in regulating transcription through chromatin remodeling has been provided by the detection of complexes containing pRB together with HDAC and the nucleosome disrupting proteins, hSWI/SNF (Zhang et al., 2000).

The E2F target genes include a number of genes that are likely to play a critical role in the cell's transition into S phase, including DNA polymerase alpha, thymidine kinase, dihydrofolate reductase and ARF. In fact, it may be the increased expression of the latter, and the consequent stabilization of *TP53* protein (see below) which causes the apoptosis that normally follows deregulation of the pRB pathway (Adams and Kaelin, 1998). Increasing evidence suggests that pRB may also bind to other cellular proteins. For instance the C-domain of pRB, located C-terminal to the pocket domain, binds to C-ABL (the function of which it inhibits) and to MDM2. In fact, given that MDM2 is a critical regulator of *TP53* (see below) and that a trimeric complex of pRB-MDM2-*TP53* has been detected, it has been proposed that pRB and *TP53* may act together in regulating apoptosis (Yap et al., 1999). In addition, pRB binds to and inhibits TAF250 kinase (Siegert and Robbins, 1999), a component of the important TFIID transcription factor complex, and this interaction may therefore contribute to the transcriptional repression by pRB discussed above. However, the interactions between these other proteins and pRB, and especially the physiological significance of these interactions, are not yet well characterised.

Several other nuclear phosphoproteins with important roles in growth regulation share significant similarity with the retinoblastoma protein, including proteins known as p107 and p130 (Ewen et al., 1991; Cobrinik et al., 1993; Hannon et al., 1993; Li et al., 1993; Eckner et al., 1994), which, together with pRB, are known as the "pocket proteins". These pRB-related proteins may have physiological functions that are closely related to those of pRB and have, in fact, also been found to complex with the E1A, SV40 large T antigen, and HPV E7 DNA tumor virus proteins. However, no evidence indicates that either inherited or somatic mutations in the genes encoding these proteins are prevalent in any forms of human cancer. Future studies will undoubtedly provide insights into the means by which loss of function of pRB, but apparently not of the other pocket proteins, contributes to tumorigenesis.

THE *TP53* TUMOR SUPPRESSOR GENE

The p53 protein was first identified in the late 1970s because it formed a tight complex with the SV40 large T antigen. It was named p53 because it is a phosphoprotein with a relative molecular mass of about 53,000 (Lane and Crawford, 1979; Linzer and Levine, 1979; Lane and Benchimol, 1990). Subsequent studies established that the p53 protein formed complexes with other polyomavirus large T antigens and the adenovirus E1B oncoprotein (Sarnow et al., 1982; Lane and Benchimol, 1990) (Fig. 19.4). While the p53 protein was present in small amounts in normal cells and was metabolically labile, high levels of p53 protein were present in many tumors and tumor cell lines. In addition, transfection of *TP53* expression constructs was shown to immortalize some cells. Furthermore, *TP53* appeared to cooperate with some oncogenes, such as mutated *H-RAS*, to transform primary rat embryonic fibroblasts cells to immortal, tumorigenic cells (Jenkins et al., 1984; Parada et al., 1984; Eliyahu et al., 1988; Weinberg, 1989). The initial interpretations of these observations were that *TP53* functioned in a positive fashion to participate in tumorigenesis. That is, *TP53* appeared to be an oncogene.

Other observations, however, suggested that *TP53* was not likely to be an oncogene. For example, in Friend virus-induced mouse erythroleukaemias, the *TP53* gene was found to be a frequent target site for viral integration, and many of the integration events led to *TP53* inactivation (Mowat et al., 1985; Lane and Benchimol, 1990). Rearrangements and deletions that appeared to completely inactivate *TP53* were also observed in the HL60 human promyelocytic leukaemia line and in several human osteosarcomas (Wolf et al., 1984; Masuda et al., 1987). Furthermore, re-examination of the cellular transformation studies revealed that the cloned murine *TP53* genes used in the aforementioned transformation assays were not wild-type but contained point mutations in their coding sequences (Eliyahu et al., 1988; Hinds et al., 1989). Both the wild-type murine and human *TP53* genes were shown to be incapable of mediating transformation in collaboration with *RAS* oncogenes, and the wild-type *TP53* gene was found to inhibit the transforming ability of mutated *TP53* and other oncogenes.

Inactivation of the *TP53* gene in human cancer

Evidence that the *TP53* gene might be frequently inactivated in human cancers was initially provided by studies demonstrating that loss of heterozygosity for chromosome 17p alleles was common in a number of tumor types, particularly colorectal cancer (Fearon et al., 1987; Vogelstein et al., 1988; Baker et al., 1989). Because the *TP53* gene was contained in the 17p region frequently affected by LOH, sequence analysis of the *TP53* alleles retained in colorectal tumors with 17p LOH was carried out. This analysis identified point muta-

tions in the great majority of cases. Subsequent analysis of other tumor types with 17p LOH, including breast, lung, bladder, and brain tumors also revealed frequent mutations in the *TP53* coding region (Nigro et al., 1989).

Mutations in *TP53* are very prevalent in a wide spectrum of human cancers. Indeed, *TP53* is believed to be one of the most commonly mutated genes in human cancer (reviewed by Greenblatt et al., 1994). Complete loss of functional *TP53* occurs in over 50% of human tumors, through point mutation of one allele and loss of the other allele (Lane, 1999). The overwhelming majority of the mutations identified are located in the central region of the *TP53* coding sequences and result in the synthesis of a p53 protein with a missense substitution (Fig. 19.6). Detailed characterization of the mutations present in *TP53* has revealed that the pattern of DNA base substitutions is distinctly different in different types of cancer (Greenblatt et al., 1994). For example, the majority of *TP53* mutations in human colorectal cancers appear to arise as a result of deamination of methylated cytosine bases. In contrast, many of the *TP53* mutations seen in lung cancers may have arisen as a result of direct interactions of *TP53* gene sequences with carcinogens present in tobacco smoke. In addition, in squamous cell skin cancers arising in ultraviolet light-exposed areas, a sizable fraction of the *TP53* mutations observed may have resulted from the generation of pyrimidine dimer premutagenic lesions.

Although *TP53* is frequently inactivated in human cancers by somatic mutations, in some cancer types the function of p53 is inactivated by other mechanisms (Vogelstein and Kinzler, 1992). For example, in cervical cancers, the main known risk factor is infection with the so-called "high-risk" or cancer-associated human papillomaviruses (HPVs) (i.e., HPV types 16 and 18) (Werness et al., 1990). The E6 proteins encoded by the high-risk HPVs bind a cellular protein called E6-AP (for E6-associated protein). This complex binds p53 and mediates its degradation via the ubiquitin pathway (Huibregtse et al., 1991) (Fig. 19.4). Cancer-associated HPVs are present in the vast majority of cervical cancers, and only a small subset of cervical cancers have somatic *TP53* mutations (Scheffner et al., 1991; Kessis et al., 1993; Greenblatt et al., 1994; Park et al., 1994). In the rare instances when a cancer-associated HPV E6 protein and a cellular *TP53* mutation are present, the cancers may behave more aggressively (Crook and Vousden, 1992). In a subset of soft tissue sarcomas, a cellular protein known as MDM2 is overexpressed as a result of gene amplification involving sequences on chromosome 12q (Oliner et al., 1992; Vogelstein and Kinzler, 1992; Momand et al., 1993). When expressed at high levels, the *MDM2* gene functions as an oncogene (Fakharzadeh et al., 1991). It is of particular note

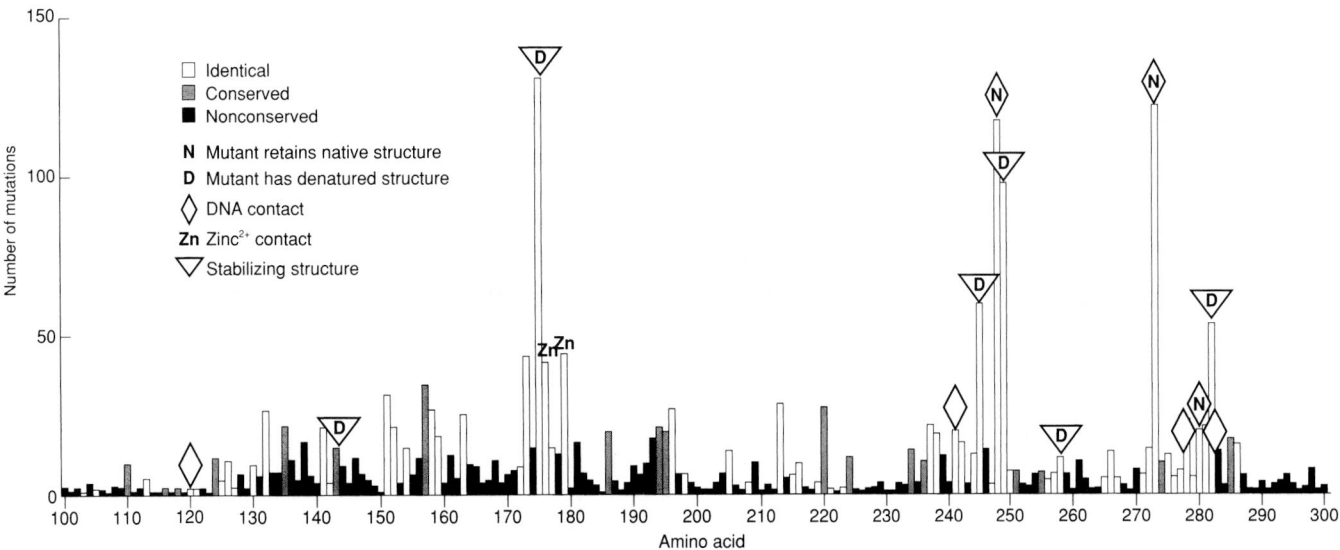

Fig. 19.6. Structure-function comparison for the central regions of p53. Codons 100–300 encode the site-specific DNA-binding core domain of the protein. The number of missense mutations identified at each codon in studies of human tumors is indicated. Some mutations inactivate p53 function while either retaining overall structural stability of the protein (N) or disrupting global stability (D). Other mutations affect specific p53 protein sequences involved in DNA binding, Zn^{2+} atom contacts, or stabilizing protein structure. Amino acids that are identical, conserved, or not conserved among p53 proteins of diverse species are indicated. Many mutations occur at amino acids that are identical or conserved in p53 proteins of many species. (From Friend, 1994).

that the MDM2 protein can bind to and inactivate the p53 protein. Thus, it appears that one of the mechanisms by which overexpression of the MDM2 protein promotes cancer cell growth is by complexing and inactivating p53. In fact, MDM2 is the key physiological regulator of the level of p53, masking its trans-activation domain, and also ensuring that p53 is a short-lived protein. MDM2 achieves this by interacting with p53's N-terminus and acting as a ubiquitin ligase, thus promoting p53's destruction (Lane and Hall, 1997). Responses of p53 *in vivo* are believed to require the stabilization of the protein, principally through reduced MDM2 binding. This occurs, for example, following (a) phosphorylation of serine 15 or serine 20 in its N terminus following either the activation of the checkpoint kinase CHK2 (Chehab et al., 2000; Hirao et al., 2000; Shieh et al., 2000), DNA-dependent protein kinase (DNA-PK) (Woo et al., 1998) and ataxia-telangiectasia mutated (ATM) (Banin et al., 1998) in response to DNA damage (e.g., by gamma-irradiation); or (b) transcriptional activation of p14/19ARF caused by oncogene activation (Zindy et al., 1998). It is by binding via its amino terminus to MDM2, that p14/19ARF, which is encoded by an alternative reading frame (ARF) at the same locus as the p16INK4a cyclin-dependent kinase (CDK) inhibitor, prevents MDM2 from inducing degradation of p53 (Pomerantz, 1998). In addition to the stabilization of p53, activation of the protein appears to also require the acetylation of residues at its C terminus: lysine 320 by PCAF and lysine 382 by p300 (Sakaguchi et al., 1998).

In addition to the somatic mutations of the *TP53* gene in different tumor types, inherited *TP53* gene mutations have been identified in the majority of individuals with the Li-Fraumeni syndrome (LFS), as well as in a small subset of pediatric patients with soft tissue sarcomas or osteosarcomas who do not meet more strict criteria for LFS (Malkin et al., 1990; Birch et al., 1994). Individuals affected by LFS are at a very elevated risk for the development of a number of tumor types, including soft tissue sarcomas, osteosarcomas, brain tumors, leukemias, and breast carcinomas. As was previously noted for inherited mutations in the *RB1* gene, the association of inherited *TP53* mutations with markedly increased cancer risk provides compelling evidence that *TP53* inactivation plays a critical role in cancer development. Given the ubiquitous expression of *TP53* in adult tissues, the basis of the tissue-specificity of *TP53*-related tumorigenesis remains to be elucidated. Recently, in LFS families possessing wild-type *TP53* genes, heterozygous germ-line mutations have been found in the *CHK2* gene, supporting the importance of inactivation of the *TP53* pathway in this human cancer predisposition syndrome (Bell et al., 1999).

TP53 function

The p53 nuclear phosphoprotein functions in transcriptional regulation, though it may also have other functions (reviewed by Friend, 1994; Vogelstein and Kinzler, 1992). The central core domain of the 393 amino acid protein binds

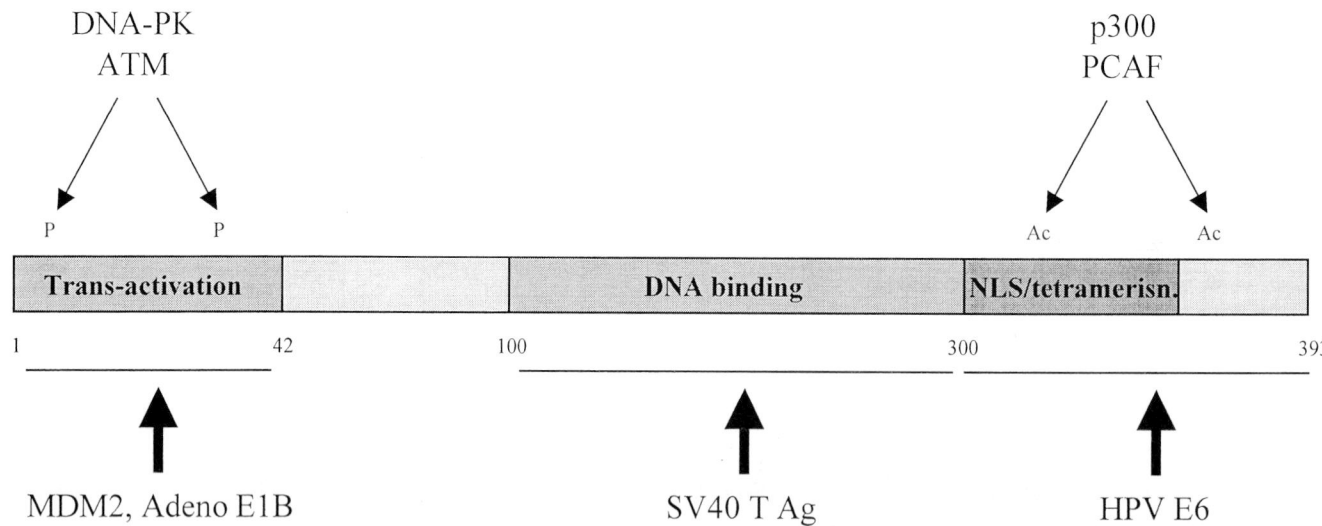

Fig. 19.7. The p53 regions involved in transcriptional activation, sequence-specific DNA binding, nuclear localization/tetramerization, and binding by DNA tumor virus proteins have been localised and are indicated. In addition, the locations of a few key sites in the amino or carboxyl termini of the protein that are phosphorylated (P) or acetylated (Ac) are indicated.

to specific DNA sequences, and its aminoterminal sequences have a transcriptional activation function (Fig. 19.7) (Cho et al., 1994; Friend, 1994). The carboxy-terminal sequences appear to be critical to the ability of the p53 protein to form homo-dimers and tetramers with itself. p53 has been implicated in the positive regulation of several genes with critical roles in the control of the cell cycle, including the *p21/WAF1/CIP1* gene, which regulates CDK activity, and the *GADD45* (for growth arrest DNA damage inducible) gene (Kastan et al., 1992; El-Deiry et al., 1993; Harper et al., 1993) (Fig. 19.8). Other p53-induced genes have been identified, including *14–3–3 sigma*, which, like p53-induced *GADD45* (Zhan et al., 1999), is reported to lead to cell cycle arrest in G2 (Hermeking et al., 1997), and the pro-apoptotic protein, Bcl-2-associated protein X (BAX) (Miyashita et al., 1995; Polyak et al., 1997). The transcription of *MDM2* is also positively regulated by p53, while that of ARF is reported to be repressed by p53 (Stott et al., 1998), providing negative feedback control. This explains the detectable increase in p53 protein levels in tissues possessing mutated *TP53* that is transcriptionally inactive. The vast majority of the mutations identified in *TP53* alleles of human tumors inactivate the DNA-binding activity of the p53 protein. Based on its three-dimensional structure, many of the mutations affect amino acids involved in p53's contact with DNA (Cho et al., 1994; Friend, 1994). In other cases, the mutations generate misfolded p53 proteins that can no longer bind to the specific DNA recognition sequence (Fig. 19.6).

Other studies suggest that p53 may also function as a repressor of transcription and that this may contribute to the biological effects of p53. For example p53 has been reported to repress expression of (a) the growth-promoting genes *C-FOS, C-MYC, IL2, IL4, IL6* and the insulin receptor: (b) the transcription factors, TBP, SP1, the oestrogen receptor and hypoxia-inducible factor, and (c) the anti-apoptotic factor, BCL-2 (El-Deiry, 1998). This repressive effect is believed to be mediated by the C-terminal region of p53 (Shaulian et al., 1995) but, unlike p53's ability to activate transcription, is probably not sequence-specific (El-Deiry, 1998).

Several cellular functions for p53 have been identified (Vogelstein and Kinzler, 1992; Fisher, 1994; Friend, 1994; Prives, 1994). In some circumstances, p53 acts at the G1/S checkpoint of the cell cycle, controlling the cell's decision to synthesise DNA. At other times, it appears to exert important control over the cell's decision to undergo programmed cell death (i.e. apoptosis). Of great additional interest, particularly with regard to cancer pathogenesis and therapy, is that several studies have demonstrated that p53 has a critical role in the cellular response to DNA damage (Kastan et al., 1991; Lane, 1992; Fisher, 1994). Specifically, cells with wild-type p53 function appear to arrest in the G1 phase of the cell cycle in response to DNA damage. Presumably, cells arrested in G1 can repair the damaged DNA template before synthesizing new DNA. Cells lacking functional p53 fail to arrest and replicate a damaged DNA template.

One of the goals of a number of ongoing drug-discovery programs is to identify small-molecule chemotherapeutic agents that might restore or enhance wild-type p53 function in cancer cells. These agents might then be used either by themselves or in combination with conventional cytotoxic agents or radiotherapy. For instance, microinjection of a plasmid encoding a peptide mimicking the MDM2

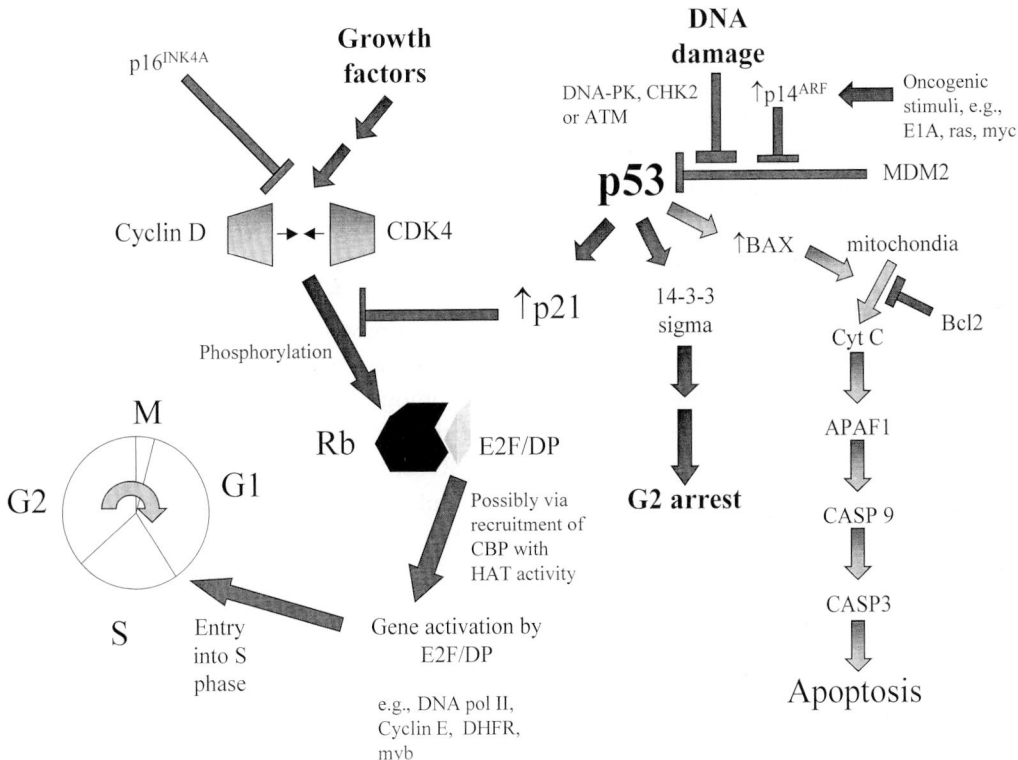

Fig. 19.8. Simplified representation of some of the upstream regulatory factors to which p53 responds and some of its principal effects, including cell cycle control and programmed cell death.

binding site of p53 leads to stabilisation of p53 and induction of the p53 response, by preventing the normal MDM2-p53 interaction (Lane, 1999). Furthermore, gene therapy clinical trials are currently evaluating the Onyx-015 E1B-attenuated adenovirus, which is reported to replicate preferentially in *TP53* mutant cells (Bischoff et al., 1996; Ganly et al., 2000; Rogulski et al., 2000).

Homologues of p53

Two homologues of p53 have been identified, p73 (Kaghad et al., 1997) and p63 (also known as Ket, p40, p51 and p73L) (Osada et al., 1998). At least when overexpressed, both proteins mimic the ability of p53 to bind DNA and to induce gene transcription and apoptosis. However, p73 and p63 are more closely related to each other than either is to p53 (Kaelin, 1999). In addition, neither *p73* nor *p63* are commonly mutated in human cancer. Moreover, unlike p53-deficient mice, mice lacking p73 or p63 are not prone to tumors (Yang et al., 2000). Interestingly, however, mutations in *p63* have recently been identified in the ectrodactytly, ectodermal dysplasia and facial clefting (EEC) developmental syndrome (Celli et al., 1999). In eight out of

nine cases, these mutations appeared to abolish the DNA-binding capacity of the protein (Celli et al., 1999). Even more recently, evidence has emerged that *p73* may, too, play a role in normal development. Specifically, it appears that it participates in a *TP53*-independent E2F1-triggered apoptotic pathway, and, in fact, is a direct transcriptional target of E2F1 (Stiewe and Putzer, 2000).

THE ADENOMATOUS POLYPOSIS COLI TUMOR SUPPRESSOR GENE

Hereditary colorectal cancer syndromes have long been recognised. The syndromes are usually divided into polyposis and nonpolyposis types. The polyposis types are those in which hundreds and sometimes even a thousand or more benign tumors (polyps) arise before the development of cancer. In the nonpolyposis types, very few polyps are noted, despite the very elevated risk of cancer. The nonpolyposis colorectal cancer syndromes are addressed later in this chapter. The most common of the polyposis syndromes is known as familial adenomatous polyposis (FAP), or adenomatous polyposis coli (APC). This syndrome is an autosomal dominant disorder characterised by the development of hundreds of adenomatous polyps in the colon and rectum of affected individuals by early adulthood and congenital hypertrophy of the retinal pigment epithelium (CHRPE). A variant of this syndrome, Gardner syndrome, is a closely related disease characterised by polyposis and extracolonic manifestations such as desmoid tumors, osteomas and sebaceous cysts.

The initial observation that led to the localization of the *APC* gene was the demonstration by Herrera and Sandberg and co-workers in 1986 of an interstitial deletion on chromosome 5q in a patient with hundreds of adenomatous polyps (Herrera et al., 1986). Subsequent linkage analysis studies confirmed that in multiple kindreds with FAP or the related Gardner syndrome, the polyposis phenotype segregated with markers near 5q21 (Bodmer et al., 1987; Leppert et al., 1987). An intense research effort over the next four years identified the specific gene responsible for predisposition to polyposis: the *APC* gene (Groden et al., 1991; Joslyn et al., 1991; Kinzler et al., 1991; Nishisho et al., 1991). *APC* is a relatively large gene with at least 15 exons and encodes a very large protein of 2843 amino acid residues and approximately 300 kDa that is expressed in many adult tissues. The predicted protein product shows little similarity to other proteins and is localized in the cytoplasm. It binds to beta-catenin, an abundant protein, much of which is normally bound to the cell-cell adhesion protein, E-cadherin. The beta-catenin-APC interaction occurs via two motifs on APC: one consists of three 15 amino acid residue repeats located between residues 1020 and 1169 (Rubinfeld et al., 1993; Su et al., 1993), while the other consists of seven 20 amino acid residue repeats located between residues 1324 and 2075, which can be phosphorylated by the serine kinase, glycogen synthase kinase 3 (GSK3) (Munemitsu et al., 1995; Rubinfeld et al., 1996).

APC function and WNT signaling

In normal cells, as a member of a cytoplasmic complex that also contains constitutively active GSK3 and the recently discovered scaffolding protein, AXIN, APC promotes the phosphorylation and subsequent proteosomal degradation of beta-catenin (Behrens et al., 1998; Hart et al., 1998). However, if this phosphorylation of beta-catenin by GSK3 is inhibited, free beta-catenin accumulates. Such inhibition can occur either as a result of Wingless (WNT) signaling via the Frizzled receptor and the Dishevelled (DSH) protein (Moon and Miller, 1997), or through loss of functional APC, as occurs in more than 80% of sporadic colorectal cancers (Kinzler and Vogelstein, 1996). Some of this excess

beta-catenin moves into the nucleus where it forms a complex with T cell factor 4 (TCF4), which then induces the transcription (Korinek et al., 1997; Morin et al., 1997) of growth promoting genes (Korinek et al., 1997; Morin et al., 1997; Peifer, 1997) including c-*MYC* (He et al., 1998). Recently, mutations in *AXIN* and in beta-catenin have been detected in some hepatocellular carcinomas and in APC-wild type colon tumors, respectively (Roose and Clevers, 1999; Satoh et al., 2000). The *APC* gene has thus been proposed to act as a "gatekeeper", a gene which normally functions to maintain correct cell numbers by directly inhibiting abnormal cell proliferation or by promoting cell death (Kinzler and Vogelstein, 1997).

Recent evidence indicates that beta-catenin/TCF4 complex also induces the expression of the nuclear hormone receptor named peroxisome-proliferator-activated receptor delta (PPAR-delta) (He et al., 1999). This protein, following its activation by a ligand, can then induce the expression of other, unidentified, genes. Interestingly, nonsteroidal inflammatory drugs (NSAIDs), which may reduce the risk of colorectal cancer (Smalley et al., 1997), appear to reduce the binding of PPAR-delta to DNA (He et al., 1999). This may occur by a cyclooxygenase-2 (COX-2)-independent mechanism, or by the inhibition of the COX-2-mediated production of PPAR-delta ligands such as eicosanoids, or by a combination of COX-2-dependent and -independent mechanisms. Importantly, this inhibition of PPAR-delta function appears to promote apoptosis of colon cancer cells (He et al., 1999).

APC gene mutations

In the vast majority of individuals affected by FAP or Gardner syndrome, germline mutations can be identified in one of the two *APC* alleles (Miyoshi et al., 1992a,b; Nagase et al., 1992; Powell et al., 1993). The germline mutations in *APC* studied thus far generally appear to inactivate the protein. The mutations include gross deletions of the gene in a minority of cases, but, in the majority of cases, cause truncation by creating frameshifts or premature stop codons. The second hit, present in most colorectal adenomas in FAP patients, is generally another truncating mutation, though, more rarely, is allele loss (Ichii et al., 1993). Interestingly, the nature of the second hit appears to be dependent upon that of the first hit. Thus allele loss occurs as the second hit when the germline mutation lies within the mutation cluster region (MCR) i.e., codons 1286–1513. This is particularly true when the germline mutation is close to codon 1300, while truncating second hit mutations are preferentially selected when the first mutation lies outside the MCR (Lamlum et al., 1999; Rowan et al., 2000). The *APC* gene may therefore be regarded as a "nonclassical" tumor suppressor gene.

A genotype-phenotype correlation has emerged regarding the location of germline mutations within the *APC* gene. Classical polyposis is associated with mutations between codons 169 and 1403 (Nagase et al., 1993; Dobbie et al., 1996) with the occurrence of CHRPE being associated with mutations situated between codons 463 and 1387 (Olschwang et al., 1993; Wallis et al., 1994; Caspari et al., 1995). Particularly profuse polyposis in APC may occur with germ-line mutations lying between codons 1285 and 1465, including the most common germ-line *APC* mutation, at codon 1309 (Gayther et al., 1994). In contrast, mutations located proximal to codon 157 of APC appear to correlate with an attenuated phenotype in which there are fewer polyps and a later age of onset of colorectal cancer (Leppert et al., 1990; Spirio et al. 1993). A predisposition to extracolonic tumors, which is especially evident in those with Gardner syndrome, appears to be associated with mutations located distal to codon 1403 of APC (Caspari et al., 1995; Davies et al., 1995; Dobbie et al., 1996). The studies reviewed above have provided definite support for the proposal that loss of function mutations in the *APC* gene lead to predisposition to adenomatous polyps of the colon and rectum. In addition, a mouse model of intestinal tumorigenesis resulting from the inactivation of one allele of the murine homologue of the *APC* gene has also been described. This model is known as the Min (for multiple intestinal neoplasia) mouse (Moser et al., 1990; Su et al., 1992). Whereas FAP and Gardner syndrome patients develop adenomatous polyps of the colon and rectum, the Min mouse develops adenomatous polyps predominantly in the small intestine. Although the site in the gastrointestinal tract at which most polyps arise differs from that seen in human polyposis patients, the Min mouse, nevertheless, should prove to be a very useful system for furthering our understanding of the pathogenesis of polyposis and colorectal tumors.

Familial polyposis is a relatively uncommon cause of colorectal cancer in the general population, and thus, germline inactivation of the *APC* gene is an infrequent predisposing factor to colorectal cancer. However, somatic inactivation of the *APC* gene appears to be critical in the development of the majority of sporadic colorectal adenomas and carcinomas (Miyoshi et al., 1992b; Powell et al., 1992). The chromosome 5q region containing the *APC* gene is affected by LOH in the majority of colorectal adenomas and carcinomas from patients without polyposis (Solomon et al., 1987; Fearon and Vogelstein, 1990). Since the identification of the *APC* gene in 1991, detailed analyses of somatic *APC* mutations have been carried out (Fig. 19.9). The somatic mutations identified in sporadic tumors have a similar spectrum and distribution to the germline mutations observed in those with FAP or Gardner syndromes. Present findings suggest that more than 70% of colorectal tumors and adenomatous polyps, regardless of their size or histopathological features, harbor a specific somatic mutation in one or both of their *APC* alleles (Kinzler and Vogelstein, 1996). Gastric cancers are among the other tumor types that have been found to harbor mutations in the *APC* gene (Horii et al., 1992; Tamura et al., 1994). In addition, *APC* gene inactivation may also be involved in the genesis of other tumor types. For example patients with Turcot syndrome (in most cases, an allelic variant of FAP) are predisposed to the development of intestinal polyps and, also, primary brain tumors (Hamilton et al., 1995). Finally, a low penetrance mutation in the *APC* gene, I1307K, has been identified, that is found almost exclusively in Ashkenazi Jews (Laken, 1997) (see section entitled "Predisposition to Colorectal Cancer by Low Penetrance Genes"). It was detected in 10.4% of Ashkenazi Jewish colorectal cancer patients, in 28% of the 25 patients with a positive family history of colorectal neoplasia, and in 6% of unaffected Ashkenazi Jews (Laken, 1997).

THE NEUROFIBROMATOSIS TYPE 1 TUMOR SUPPRESSOR GENE

Type 1 neurofibromatosis (NF1) or von Recklinghausen disease has a prevalence of between 1 in 2500 and 1 in 5000 (Huson et al., 1989). It is a dominantly inherited syndrome whose principal manifestations involve tissues derived from the neural crest. In addition to neurofibromas and café-au-lait spots, NF1 patients are at increased risk of developing phaeochromocytomas, optic gliomas, neurofibrosarcomas, and primary brain tumors (Ponder, 1990). The *NF1* gene was localized to the pericentromeric region of chromosome 17q by linkage analyses carried out on several large kindreds with NF1 (Barker et al., 1987; Seizinger et al., 1987c). Subsequently, karyotype analysis led to the identification of two patients with NF1 and constitutional chromosomal translocations involving band 17q11.2 (Fountain et al., 1989; O'Connell et al., 1989). Intensive molecular genetic analyses then focused on this region, and in 1991, the *NF1* gene was identified (Cawthon et al., 1990; Viskochil et al., 1990; Wallace et al., 1990). *NF1* is a large gene comprising 60 exons, spanning over 400 kb, and encoding a very large protein product with a molecular mass of greater than 300 kDa (Viskochil et al., 1993). The estimated new mutation rate of 1 in

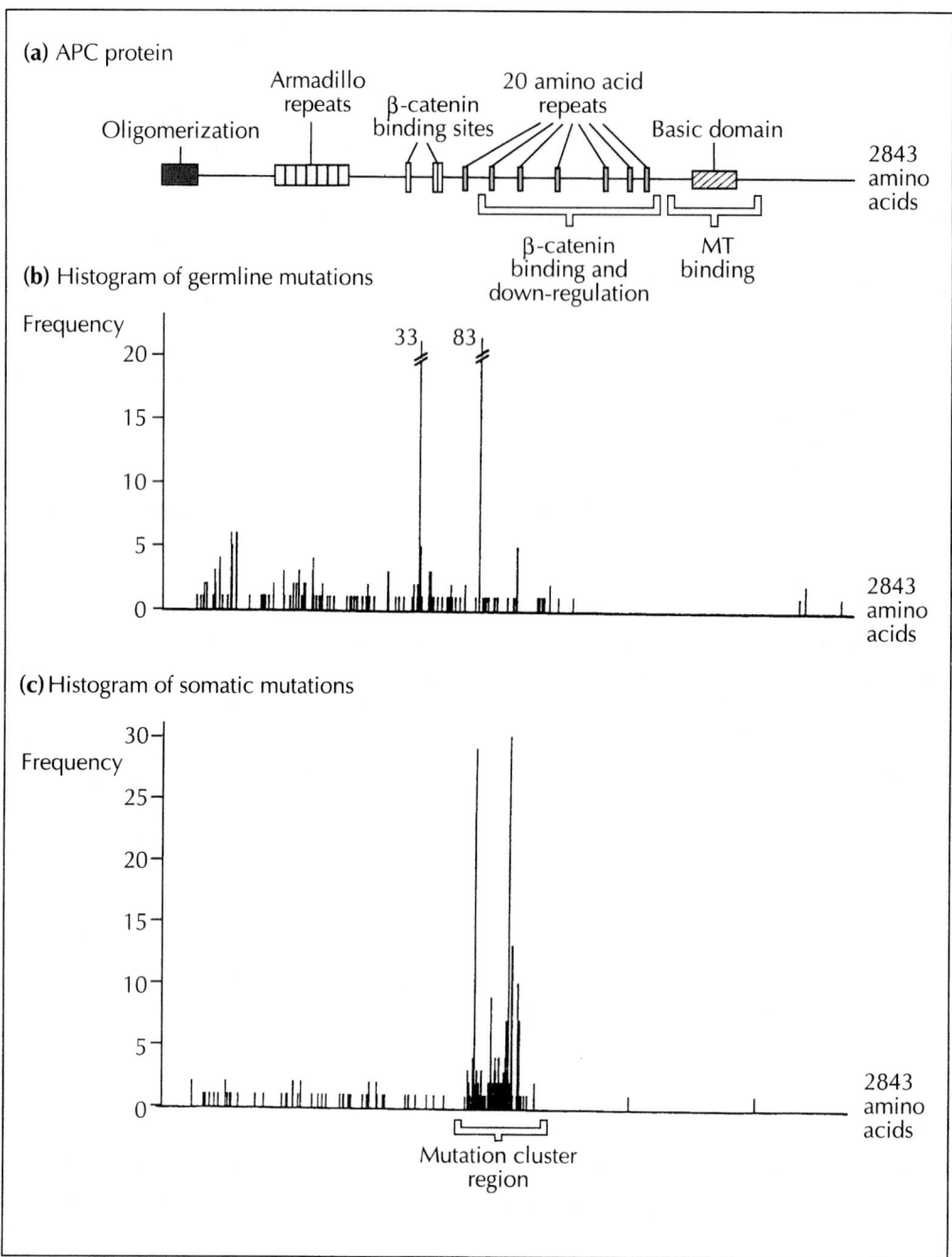

(a) APC protein

Oligomerization

Armadillo repeats

β-catenin binding sites

20 amino acid repeats

Basic domain

2843 amino acids

β-catenin binding and down-regulation

MT binding

(b) Histogram of germline mutations

Frequency

33 83

2843 amino acids

(c) Histogram of somatic mutations

Frequency

2843 amino acids

Mutation cluster region

Fig. 19.9. Schematic representation of the APC protein with histograms of the germline and somatic mutations. (A) The relative positions of known and presumed structural features of the 2843 amino acid APC protein. (B) and (C) Histograms of the germline and somatic mutations identified in the *APC* gene. The relative positions of the *APC* mutations are indicated on the horizontal axis and the frequency of their occurrence is indicated on the vertical axis. The germline mutations are distributed throughout the 5′ half of the gene. The somatic mutations appear to cluster in a region termed the mutation cluster region. (Modified from Polakis, 1995, with permission.)

10,000 is one of the highest for a human disorder and most mutations are paternal in origin, although there is no significant paternal age effect (Jadayel et al., 1990). Comprehensive mutation analysis of the gene is currently laborious on account of the gene's size and large number of exons, the presence of several *NF1* pseudogenes and the wide spectrum of genetic lesions, including gross rearrangements and distinct point mutations. More than 200 mutations have been described. A recent exhaustive mutation analysis identified mutations in 64 (95%) of 67 unrelated

NF1 patients, of whom 37 had nonsense or frameshift mutations and 19 possessed splice mutations (Messiaen et al., 2000). There is no clear genotype-phenotype correlation at present, other than the association of dysmorphic features, increased numbers of neurofibromas and significant developmental delay (in addition to the typical NF1 manifestations) with gross *NF1* gene deletions (Upadhyaya et al., 1998).

In addition to germline *NF1* gene mutations in those with neurofibromatosis, somatic mutations inactivating the *NF1* gene have been found in a subset of other solid tumor types, including colorectal cancer, melanoma, neuroblastoma, and in some bone marrow specimens from those with the myelodysplastic syndrome (Johnson et al., 1993; Seizinger, 1993; The et al., 1993; Viskochil et al., 1993). Recent studies suggest that, in benign neurofibromas, in accordance with the Knudson model of tumor suppressor gene function, the normal copy of the *NF1* gene often undergoes LOH (John et al., 2000) or point mutation (Eisenbarth et al., 2000). Moreover in benign neurofibromas the Schwann cells, but not the fibroblasts, generally exhibit loss of *NF1* transcript and of neurofibromin, indicating that the abnormal cell in neurofibromas is the Schwann cell (Rutkowski et al. 2000). As was noted above for the *RB1*, *TP53*, and *APC* genes, the *NF1* gene is expressed ubiquitously. Therefore, the basis for the tissue specificity of the malignant tumors seen in neurofibromatosis patients (predominantly neurofibrosarcomas and primary brain tumors) is unclear. In segmental NF1, where the cutaneous manifestations are restricted to a particular body region, it is generally believed that a post-zygotic mutation is responsible, giving rise to somatic mosaicism. In fact, one such mutation has now been identified, a microdeletion detected by FISH (Tinschert et al., 2000).

The protein encoded by the *NF1* gene is termed neurofibromin. It is localized in the cytoplasm of the cell and bears considerable similarity to the catalytic domains of GTPase-activating proteins (GAPs) (Wigler, 1990; Xu et al., 1990; DeClue et al., 1992). One of the best studied GAPs is RAS-GAP, which has been shown to stimulate the (regulatory) GTPase activity of wild-type K-RAS, H-RAS, and N-RAS proteins (see section entitled "Oncogenic Alleles in Human Cancers" above). In addition to the predicted similarity of the neurofibromin protein to GAPs, recent studies have shown that neurofibromin can, indeed, stimulate the GTPase activity of both yeast and mammalian RAS proteins. This activity of neurofibromin might be envisaged, *in vivo*, to help to prevent over-activity of the RAS signalling proteins in the pathway which promotes cell proliferation. Thus, loss of neurofibromin would be expected to result in the abnormal persistence of the GTP-bound (i.e., active) form of RAS. The mechanisms by which *NF1* mutations alter cell growth are still not completely understood, however, and might also involve interactions of neurofibromin with components of the cytoskeleton such as microtubules (Gregory et al., 1993) and intermediate filaments (Koivunen et al., 2000).

THE *INK4A* GENE

Loss of heterozygosity affecting chromosome 9p has been seen frequently in a wide spectrum of tumors, including melanomas, gliomas, leukaemias and non-small cell lung, bladder and head and neck cancers. A subset of such tumors were found to have homozygous deletions affecting the 9p21 region. In addition to the frequent somatic alterations on 9p in cancers, linkage studies of some families with inherited melanoma established that a melanoma predisposition gene mapped to 9p (reviewed by Goldstein and Tucker, 1995).

These findings motivated efforts to define a more limited region of chromosome 9p that was presumed to contain a tumor suppressor gene affected by both germline and somatic mutations. One of the genes identified in this region of 9p as a result of positional cloning efforts was termed *MTS1* (multiple tumor suppressor 1) (Kamb et al., 1994a). Sequence analysis of the *MTS1* gene revealed that it was identical to a previously identified gene, *p16*. The *p16* (*CDKN2*) gene was originally identified because it encoded a protein that functions as a specific inhibitor of cyclin-dependent kinases CDK4 and CDK6. Subsequent studies have revealed that mutations of one *p16* allele are present in some patients with inherited melanoma, as well as in some families with inherited melanoma and pancreatic cancer (Hussussian et al., 1994; Kamb et al., 1994b; Wainwright, 1994; Whelan et al., 1995). Somatic mutations in *p16* have been found in a significant fraction of many different cancer types, including but not limited to melanomas, gliomas, pancreatic and bladder cancers, and leukaemias. In some of these tumors, deletions of the *p16* gene were also found to involve a nearby gene, *p15*, that encodes a protein closely related to *p16*. In some tumors, mutations have been found that appear to inactivate *p15* but not *p16* (Shimizu and Sekiya, 1995).

The *p16* gene has been shown to encode a second unique protein (in addition to the p16 protein) as the result of an alternative reading frame; this protein is termed p14[ARF] in humans and p19[ARF] in mouse. The *p16* gene, therefore, encodes two separate products, and its name has now been changed to *INK4A*. Both the p16[INK4a] and p19^{ARF} proteins have been found to have growth suppressive functions (Quelle et al., 1995). Hence, there may be strong selection for simultaneous inactivation of both proteins during tumor development. Homozygous deletion of the gene may be a particularly efficient means to achieve this goal in a number of tumor types.

The prevalence and nature of *p16INK4a* mutations appear to vary markedly from one tumor type to another, and the gene appears to be more frequently mutated in tumor cell lines adapted for culture than in primary tumors. This finding may reflect the fact that *p16INK4a* inactivation may provide an additional growth advantage to cultured tumor cells. Homozygous deletion is a particularly common mechanism by which *p16INK4a* has been found to be inactivated in some primary human tumors and tumor cell lines (Cairns et al., 1995). Other studies suggest that *p16INK4a* (and similarly *p19INK4a*) expression may be lost in some tumor types as a result of methylation of the gene's regulatory sequences (i.e. promoter/enhancer elements) (Herman et al., 1995; Merlo et al., 1995), a situation that in several other genes often results in the loss of gene expression. In fact, the finding of *p16INK4a* inactivation by DNA methylation led to the study of DNA methylation as a general mechanism for inactivation of tumor suppressor gene function during tumorigenesis. As discussed above for the *RB1* and *TP53* genes, the frequent inactivation of the *p16INK4a* gene in a wide spectrum of human cancers underscores the importance of proper control of the cell cycle in normal cell growth and in the suppression of the neoplastic phenotype.

p16^{INK4A} AND p14^{ARF}/p19^{ARF} FUNCTION

p16^{INK4a} is a CDK inhibitor that maintains pRB in its growth-suppressive, hypophosphorylated state (Alcorta et al., 1996; Hara et al., 1996). In contrast to p21^{WAF1}, whose expression in replicating fibroblasts increases sharply just before the onset of replicative senescence but then declines, p16^{INK4a} expression increases gradually to a sustained, greatly elevated level in the later stages of senescence. Thus, while p21^{WAF1} may be responsible for the induction of senescence, p16^{INK4a} may be essential for its maintenance (Stein et al., 1999). The upstream effector of p16^{INK4a} is still unknown but its expression is clearly *TP53*-independent. However, it has been shown that treating fibroblasts with agents that induce double strand breaks results in both p16^{INK4a} enrichment and premature senescence (Robles and Adami, 1998). It is plausible, therefore, that p16^{INK4a} is also induced in response to a DNA damage signal from eroded telomeres.

Another recent study indicates that p16^{INK4a} (and p14/p19^{ARF}) is under the transcriptional control of the Polycomb-group protein Bmil, which represses transcription by packaging DNA into higher-order chromatin (Jacobs et al., 1999). Fibroblasts from mice that lack *bmil* express very high levels of p16^{INK4a} and undergo premature senescence, suggesting that downregulation of this gene could play a crucial role in the induction of p16^{INK4a} in normal senescence. It has been difficult to demonstrate conclusively that p16^{INK4a} is essential for senescence. This is partly because deletion of the *INK4a* locus affects the overlapping gene encoding p14^{ARF}, which has also been implicated in cell cycle arrest (Quelle et al., 1995). However, *p16^{INK4a}* expression is clearly very frequently lost by mutation, deletion or promoter silencing in both immortal tumor cell lines and in vitro immortalized, nontumorigenic cell lines (Vogt et al., 1998). Furthermore, loss of the protein by methylation of its promoter is associated with the increased lifespan of a subset of normal human breast epithelial cells (Brenner et al., 1998). Treatment of these cells with the methylation inhibitor 5-aza-2-deoxycytidine restores *INK4a* expression and induces premature senescence. Re-expression of p16^{INK4a} in this manner can also induce senescence in an oral squamous cell carcinoma cell line and in immortalized human fibroblasts (Vogt et al., 1998). In fact, further evidence is now emerging for the specific involvement in human replicative senescence of p16^{INK4a} rather than p14^{ARF}. In a recent study of keratinocytes, no p14^{ARF} protein was detected in senescent cells and no p16^{INK4a}-independent deletions or mutations of *p14^{ARF}* were observed in neoplastic cells (Munro et al., 1999). p14^{ARF} exerts its growth inhibitory effects through the inhibition of mdm2-induced degradation of *TP53* (Stott et al., 1998) (Fig. 19.8). The fact, then, that *TP53* levels do not increase during senescence also argues against a role of p14^{ARF} in replicative senescence in humans, and suggests that p16^{INK4a} is indeed the target of losses at the INK4a locus in immortal cell lines. The role of p16^{INK4a} in pRB-mediated replicative senescence is further emphasised by the fact that loss of function of p16^{INK4a} or pRB, but not of both together, occurs in most immortal cell lines (Kamb et al., 1994a).

Surprisingly, species-dependent variations in the regulation of replicative senescence by p16^{INK4a} and p14^{ARF}/p19^{ARF} also exist. Mouse and human cells, the cell types in which most senescence research has been carried out, appear to differ in both the way that senescence is triggered and in the actual effector pathways. While the primary "mitotic clock" in human cells is believed to be progressive erosion of telomeres, the telomere dynamics of rodent cells are such that this clock can be of little functional significance. As discussed above, there is little direct evidence in human cells for the involvement in replicative senescence of p14^{ARF}, despite its role in the inhibition of mdm2-induced degradation of *TP53* and the fact that its ectopic expression induces growth arrest. However, this is not the case for the murine homologue p19^{ARF}, which accumulates greatly as rodent fibroblasts approach senescence (Zindy et al., 1998). A mouse knockout of *p19*^{ARF} in which the coding sequence of p16^{INK4a} is unaffected has now been generated (Kamijo et al., 1997). Significantly, embryonic fibroblasts derived from these mice do not undergo senescence. This is reflected by the fact that establishment of mouse embryonic fibroblast cultures is usually accompanied by loss of function of just p19^{ARF} or *TP53*. These differences in the trigger of senescence and in the effector mechanisms may be functionally related: while in humans senescence may be largely triggered by telomeric attrition and subsequent, p14^{ARF}-independent activation of *TP53*, a different trigger in mice could result in the p19^{ARF}-mediated *TP53* response. Consistent with this, there is no evidence for the involvement of p19^{ARF} in DNA damage signaling to the cell cycle machinery (Stott et al., 1998). Species-dependent differences in the effector pathways of senescence also account for variations in the stringency of senescence. While inactivation of the p19/*TP53* pathway is enough for murine cells to escape senescence, human cells invariably need to disrupt, at least, both the *TP53*/p21 and p16^{INK4a}/pRB pathways. Perhaps in consequence, human cells very rarely spontaneously immortalize in culture whereas rodent cells do so much more easily. The existence of "back-up" senescence pathways in human cells is probably a reflection of the importance of cancer avoidance mechanisms in long-lived animals.

Oncogene activation of p14^{ARF}/p19^{ARF}

It has been known for several years that adenovirus 5 *E1A* and *myc* expression can lead to stabilization of *TP53* and apoptosis (Lowe and Ruley, 1993; Hermeking and Eick, 1994). More recently, it has been demonstrated that ectopic expression of oncogenic *ras* or *raf*, or constitutive activation of *MEK*, can induce senescence in primary cells (Serrano et al., 1997; Lin et al., 1998). These cellular responses to oncogene expression are partly mediated by upregulation of p19^{ARF} and (probably) the human homologue p14^{ARF} (de Stanchina et al., 1998; Zindy et al., 1998), whose inhibition of mdm2-induced degradation of *TP53* causes upregulation of the CDK inhibitor p21^{WAF1} (Kamijo et al., 1998; Stott et al., 1998). Inactivation of

either *TP53* or p19^{ARF} is sufficient for murine, but not human, fibroblasts to escape ras-induced arrest (Serrano et al., 1997; Palmero et al., 1998). It has recently been shown that p14^{ARF} is transcriptionally activated by un-sequestered E2F, thus providing the missing molecular link between hyper-proliferative signalling and ARF induction and revealing further inter-relations between the *TP53* and pRB pathways (Bates et al., 1998). However, p16^{INK4a} is also induced during ras and raf-induced senescence, and in human cells may be the main senescence effector (Serrano et al., 1997; Zhu et al., 1998). Again, inactivation of p16^{INK4a} is sufficient for evasion of senescence in murine cells but not in human cells (Serrano et al., 1997).

The induction of senescence or apoptosis by oncogenes may represent an *in vivo* safeguard against inappropriate proliferative signals, and thus represent a mechanism of tumor suppression. However, the precise relevance of oncogene-induced senescence to tumorigenesis remains uncertain. Oncogene expression (rather than telomeric shortening) may, in some tumors, provide the selective pressure for events such as *TP53* or *p16*^{INKa} mutation that disable the senescence and apoptotic pathways. Consistent with this view, *ras* mutation does sometimes precede *TP53* or *INK4A* mutation during tumorigenesis (Fearon and Vogelstein, 1990). In the model system of skin carcinogenesis, however, ras activation is an early event while immortalization occurs much later (Balmain et al., 1984). It is also possible that the cellular response to the artifically high levels of ras and raf induced by ectopic expression using heterologous promoters has little in vivo relevance.

WT1, THE WILMS TUMOR SUPPRESSOR GENE AT CHROMOSOME 11p13

Similar to retinoblastoma, and despite its relative rarity compared to common adult tumors, Wilms tumor has provided a number of critical insights into tumor suppressor gene identification and function. The first findings to suggest the contribution of a gene at 11p13 to the development of Wilms tumor were those of Miller and co-workers (Miller et al., 1964). They noted an association between aniridia, a congenital absence of the iris, and Wilms tumor. Further studies confirmed that a rare complex of developmental abnormalities, including aniridia, genitourinary malformations, and mental retardation, was associated with a high (more than 30%) probability of developing Wilms tumor, hence the WAGR (Wilms tumor with aniridia, genitourinary malformations, and retardation) syndrome. Similar to the situation seen in some patients with inherited retinoblastoma and deletion of chromosome 13q14 sequences, some patients with WAGR syndrome were found to have constitutional deletions involving one copy of chromosome 11, at band p13 (Riccardi et al., 1980). Based on these data, it was inferred that one of the genes involved in Wilms tumorigenesis, the *WT1* gene, must reside at 11p13.

The *WT1* gene was identified in 1990 by virtue of mutations in the gene in patients with the WAGR syndrome, as well as somatic mutations in the gene in tumors from a minority of patients with unilateral Wilms tumor and no associated congenital malformations (Bonetta et al., 1990; Call et al., 1990; Gessler et al., 1990; Haber and Housman, 1992). The *WT1* gene is encoded by ten exons. The mRNA produced is subject to a complex pattern of alternative splicing, and the mRNAs encode four proteins with molecular masses of 45,000 to 49,000 (Coppes et al., 1994). Based on the predicted amino acid sequence, the WT1 proteins appear to function in transcriptional regulation, and evidence has been obtained that the WT1 protein may suppress the expression of several growth-inducing genes, including the early growth response (*EGR1*), insulin-like growth factor II (*IGF2*), and platelet-derived growth factor A chain (*PDGFA*) genes (Haber et al., 1991). The ability of the WT1 protein to regulate the expression of growth-inducing genes may account, at least in part, for the function of *WT1* as a tumor suppressor gene. Unlike other tumor suppressor genes, such as *RB1* and *TP53*, the expression of the *WT1* gene appears to be restricted to embryonic kidney cells and a subset of other cell types. Very recently, a clue to the normal role of WT1 has been provided by the report that WT1 trans-activates the E-cadherin promoter (Hosono et al., 2000). Recent data suggest that WT1 may also regulate gene expression through interactions with RNA, probably via a role in gene splicing (Davies et al., 1998). In addition, WT1 binds to a variety of proteins, including *TP53*. Again, the physiological relevance of many of these interactions remains unclear (Little et al., 1999).

Although *WT1* gene inactivation contributes to the development of some Wilms tumors, a large body of evidence supports the proposal that Wilms tumors may arise through mutations in genes other than the *WT1* gene (reviewed by Haber and Housman, 1992). First, chromosome 11p allelic losses in Wilms tumors have been localized, and, in many cases, they involve band 11p15, but not band 11p13 and the *WT1* gene. Second, the 11p15 region harbors a gene responsible for Beckwith-Wiedemann syndrome, a congenital syndrome characterized by hyperplasia of the kidneys and endocrine pancreas, macroglossia, hemihypertrophy and a predisposition to embryonic tumors such as hepatoblastoma and Wilms tumor. Finally, linkage studies of three families with dominant inheritance of Wilms tumor have excluded

linkage of the susceptibility locus in these families to any part of chromosome 11p. *In toto*, the data suggest that there are at least three different genes that, when mutated in the germline, can predispose an individual to Wilms tumor (the *WT1* gene, the Wiedemann-Beckwith gene, and a non-11p gene) (Grundy et al., 1995). Whether a combination of inherited and somatic mutations in more than one of these genes (or even all three) is required for the development of Wilms tumor, or whether alternative genetic pathways for the development of Wilms tumor exist, remains to be resolved. Interestingly, while some studies support the hypothesis that WT1 plays a tumor suppressing, anti-proliferative role, other analyses suggest that the wild-type protein can promote proliferation and suppress apoptosis (Yamagami et al., 1998). Moreover, the over expression of wild-type WT1 in acute myeloid leukemia has been proposed by some, though not others, to be an indicator of poor prognosis and drug resistance.

THE *NF2* GENE AND SCHWANNOMIN

Neurofibromatosis type 2 (NF2), also known as central neurofibromatosis, is an autosomal dominant disorder that is genetically and clinically distinct from NF1 (Ponder, 1990; Seizinger, 1993) and is approximately ten times less common. The hallmark of NF2 is the occurrence of bilateral schwannomas affecting the vestibular branch of the eighth cranial nerve (acoustic neuromas). In addition, NF2 patients are also at risk for the development of other tumors, including cranial and spinal meningiomas, spinal schwannomas, and ependymomas. The *NF2* gene was localised to chromosome 22q in the late 1980s by a combination of linkage analyses and LOH studies (Seizinger et al., 1986; 1987b; Evans et al., 1992). The gene was identified in 1993 using a positional cloning approach (Seizinger et al., 1987a; Rouleau et al., 1993; Trofatter et al., 1993). It spans 110 kb and comprises 16 constitutive and one alternatively spliced exon (Rouleau et al., 1993; Trofatter et al., 1993). The gene is widely expressed both in terms of tissues and individual cell types. Germline mutations inactivating the *NF2* gene have been observed in those with NF2, and patients with truncating mutations generally have an earlier onset and increased number of tumors (Evans et al., 1998). Mutation detection in classically affected unrelated patients with NF2 has been relatively difficult with detection rates of 43% (Evans et al., 1998), 56% (Ruttledge et al., 1996), and 66% (Parry et al., 1996). The difficulty might, in part, be due to the relatively high frequency of large deletions, which have been reported to account for as many as 33% of NF2 gene alterations (Zucman-Rossi et al., 1998). Somatic mutations in the gene have been detected in up to 60% of sporadic schwannomas (Bruder et al., 1999) and also in 70% and 83% of sporadic fibroblastic and transitional meningiomas, respectively (Wellenreuther et al., 1995). Mutations of the *NF2* gene have also been detected in up to 30% of melanomas and 41% of malignant mesotheliomas (Bianchi et al., 1995; Kley et al., 1995; De Vitis et al., 1996). Interestingly, a recent analysis of tumors for both LOH and mutations found that the majority of patients presenting with unilateral vestibular schwannomas and histories suggestive of NF2, but who do not fulfil the classical NF2 criteria, do not have germline mutations in the *NF2* gene (Wu et al., 1998).

The *NF2* gene encodes a protein, named schwannomin (or merlin), that bears strong similarity to a family of cytoskeletal proteins that are thought to act as linker proteins that connect integral membrane proteins to scaffolding proteins of the filamentous submembrane lattice (Trofatter et al., 1993; Mangeat et al., 1999). These "ERM" linker proteins, ezrin, radixin and moesin, each possess an N-terminal FERM domain, a long alpha-helical central region, and a charged C-terminal domain that binds to F-actin and can interact, intra-molecularly, with the N-terminal region. The intramolecular interaction but not the F-actin binding is a property of schwannomin (L Huang et al., 1998; Koga et al., 1998) and appears to be necessary for the protein's tumor suppressor function (Gutmann et al., 1999). The presence of the alpha-helical central region may permit schwannomin to form a stable interaction, as a coiled-coil, with another ERM protein or with other proteins such as the novel coiled-coil protein, SCHIP-1 (Goutebroze et al., 2000). The homology of schwannomin and ERM proteins suggests a number of possible mechanisms by which *NF2* gene alterations might affect cell shape, cell-cell interactions, and tumor growth. Very recently, schwannomin has been found to interact with the hepatocyte growth factor (HGF)-regulated tyrosine kinase substrate (HRS) by yeast two-hybrid analysis (Scoles et al., 2000), but the precise mechanism by which *NF2* gene inactivation leads to tumorigenesis remains unclear at present.

THE *VHL* GENE

VHL syndrome is a rare, dominantly inherited disorder that predisposes individuals to the development of hemangioblastomas of the central nervous system and retina, as well as renal cell carcinomas and phaeochromocytomas. The *VHL* gene was assigned to chromosome 3p by linkage analysis, and LOH studies were used to establish that the gene behaves as a typical tumor suppressor, as defined by Knudson's model, wherein both alleles are inactivated

during tumorigenesis (Seizinger et al., 1988). A positional cloning approach was successfully employed to identify the *VHL* gene in 1993 (Latif et al., 1993), germline inactivating mutations in which are responsible for VHL (reviewed by Kaelin and Maher, 1998). Somatic mutations in the *VHL* gene have also been detected in most sporadic renal cell carcinomas of the clear cell type but not in other histological subtypes of renal cell carcinoma. Interestingly, at least 20% of sporadic clear cell renal cancers do not harbor a detectable mutation in the *VHL* gene. In many of these cases, the *VHL* gene may be inactivated by methylation of its transcriptional regulatory sequences (Herman et al., 1994), as noted above for the *p16INK4a* gene. Therefore the *VHL* gene plays a critical role in the pathogenesis of the most common form of adult renal cancer. In other tumor types, however, inactivation of the *VHL* gene by somatic mutations or methylation appears to be uncommon.

Initial studies demonstrated that the *VHL* gene encodes a 213 amino acid residue protein, pVHL, that complexes with the B and C subunits of the elongin transcriptional elongation factor, forming a heterotrimeric protein complex that appeared to regulate transcriptional elongation by RNA polymerase II (Aso et al., 1995; Duan et al., 1995; Kibel et al., 1995). However, no regulation of transcriptional elongation by pVHL has been shown in vivo. Rather, pVHL appears to participate in a regulatory mechanism that normally prevents inappropriate accumulation of a transcription factor that stimulates the transcription of hypoxia-responsive genes such as vascular endothelial growth factor (*VEGF*) (Maxwell et al., 1999). The VHL protein comprises two domains. Its alpha domain functions as a platform upon which a complex is assembled, including elongin C, elongin B, Cul2 and Rbx1 (known, collectively, as the VCB-Cul2 complex). Moreover, the pVHL beta domain has very recently been shown to bind to the oxygen-dependent degradation domain of the alpha subunit of the transcription factor known as hypoxia inducible factor (HIF) 1 (Ohh et al., 2000). By structural comparisons of the VCB-Cul2 complex with the yeast SCF complex, and by extensive studies of pVHL activity, it is now recognised that (1) HIF1-alpha, under normoxic conditions, undergoes ubiquitin-mediated degradation; (2) the ubiquitination of HIF1-alpha is dependent on its interaction with the ubiquitination machinery of the VCB-Cul2 complex (which functions as an E3 ubiquitin ligase) via the beta domain of pVHL; (3) this ubiquitination is disabled either in hypoxic conditions or as a consequence of most *VHL* mutations; and (4) this disabling leads to HIF1-alpha accumulation and the activation of hypoxia-responsive genes such as *VEGF*, which is an important factor in tumor angiogenesis (Maxwell et al., 1999; Stebbins et al., 1999; Ohh et al., 2000).

Nevertheless, at the time of writing, many questions remain unanswered. It is unclear precisely how hypoxia inhibits HIF1-alpha ubiquitination, especially as the HIF1-alpha interaction with pVHL appears not to be blocked (Maxwell et al., 1999). In addition, the basis of the differing VHL phenotypes, and the identity of other possible pVHL-interacting proteins, remain to be determined.

HEREDITARY BREAST CANCER AND THE *BRCA1* AND *BRCA2* GENES

It has long been known that family history is a major contributor to breast cancer risk and that the risk is greatest in those who have a history of breast cancer in one or more first-degree relatives. However, it was not until the late 1980s that definitive evidence was obtained that the predisposition to premenopausal breast cancer in some families could be attributed to a highly penetrant autosomal dominant allele. Subsequently, Hall, King, and their co-workers reported in 1990 that one such gene, now termed *BRCA1* (for breast cancer predisposition gene 1), mapped to chromosome 17q21 (Hall et al., 1990). Other investigators subsequently provided evidence that the *BRCA1* locus was associated with susceptibility to both breast and ovarian cancer (Narod et al., 1991; Easton et al., 1993). On account of the intensive research efforts that were focused on the chromosome 17q region thought to contain the gene, *BRCA1* was ultimately identified in 1994 (Futreal et al., 1994; Miki et al., 1994).

While germline mutations in the *BRCA1* gene account for around 50% of the families in which four or more members are affected by breast cancer at an early age, approximately 30% of such kindreds have been attributed to mutations of another highly penetrant autosomal dominant susceptibility gene termed *BRCA2*. The *BRCA2* gene was mapped to chromosome 13q12–13 in 1994 (Wooster et al., 1994) and was subsequently identified (Wooster et al., 1995). Mutations in *BRCA1* and *BRCA2* appear to confer, in the high-risk families studied, similar "lifetime" risks of female breast cancer, of 85% and 84% by age 70, respectively (Rahman and Stratton, 1998). However, the risk of ovarian cancer appears considerably higher in those with *BRCA1* mutations than in those with *BRCA2* mutations, at 44% and 27%, respectively (Ford et al., 1994; 1998). Conversely, the risk of breast cancer in males with a *BRCA2* mutation (around 6%) is substantially higher than in males with a *BRCA1* mutation. The risks of other cancers are not yet clear, but may include prostate and colon cancer for

BRCA1 (Ford et al., 1994). For *BRCA2* mutation carriers, statistically significant increases in risk were observed for malignant melanoma and for prostate, pancreatic, gallbladder, bile duct and stomach cancer (Breast Cancer Linkage Consortium, 1999). Perhaps not suprisingly, in population-based studies, the penetrances of *BRCA1* and *BRCA2* mutations appear to be significantly lower than in high-risk families, presumably on account of the presence or absence of risk modifying genes (see section entitled "*BRCA1* and *BRCA2* mutations and cancer predisposition").

Structure and function of the BRCA1 protein

The *BRCA1* gene contains 24 exons, of which the first is non coding, with exon 11 encompassing about half of the coding sequence (Miki et al., 1994). It encodes a 220 kDa nuclear protein of 1863 amino acid residues, which appears to interact with a variety of proteins that have diverse cellular functions (Fig. 19.10).

At its amino terminus is a zinc-binding RING finger domain. Ring fingers are evolutionarily conserved structures consisting of two loops held together at their base by eight histidine or cystine residues and two zinc ions. They can function, rather like the pVHL protein complex, as ubiquitin-protein ligases or E3s (Joazeiro et al., 1999 Lorick et al., 1999;). In addition, the RING finger of BRCA1 can bind to the RING finger of another protein designated BRCA1-associated RING domain 1 (BARD1) (Wu et al., 1996). The significance of the BRCA1 RING domain is not yet clear although it has been reported recently that the BRCA1-BARD1 complex inhibits polyadenylation by binding to the polyadenylation factor, CStF-50 and may thus prevent inappropriate RNA processing at sites of DNA repair (Kleiman and Manley, 1999).

Located in the central portion of *BRCA1* are three putative nuclear localization signals (NLS). Two of these regions of highly charged, basic residues were found to interact with a component of the NLS receptor complex, importin-alpha, in a yeast two-hybrid screen using *BRCA1* as the bait (Chen et al., 1996). Located at the extreme C terminus are two BRCT (BRCA1 C-terminal) repeats. BRCT domains are evolutionarily conserved regions, of approximately 95 amino acids residues, whose 3D structure suggests a role in protein-protein interactions and which are found in many proteins involved in DNA repair and cell cycle control (Zhang et al., 1998). While almost all identified mutations in *BRCA1* result in a truncated product, yielding little functional information, a few missense mutations have been found (Breast Cancer Information Core database). These are located predominantly within either

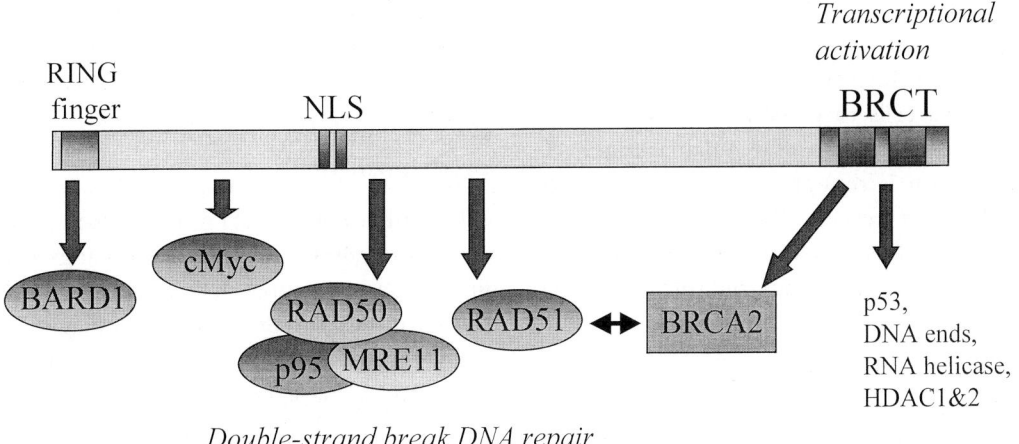

Double-strand break DNA repair

Fig. 19.10. Possible functional regions of the BRCA1 protein. The protein is large, comprising 1863 amino acids, and is believed to participate in the repair of double-strand breaks in DNA. Several additional regions have been described for the protein, a number of which are indicated.

the RING finger domain or the BRCT repeats, providing support for the functional importance of these regions.

The normal role of BRCA1 in tumor suppression may involve DNA repair, transcriptional regulation, cell-cycle control or apoptosis. Most likely, its role involves a combination of two or more of these individual functions. Evidence that it is involved in DNA repair includes the observation that BRCA1-deficient embryonic stem (ES) cells are hypersensitive to both ionising radiation and hydrogen peroxide (Gowen et al., 1998) and that such cells have impaired transcription-coupled DNA repair (Gowen et al., 1998) and homology-directed chromosomal double-strand break (DSB) repair (Moynahan et al., 1999). Moreover, the BRCT domains of BRCA1 have recently been reported to bind to the ends of linear DNA fragments, independent of the DNA sequence (Yamane and Tsuruo, 1999), although, as mentioned above, they may also participate in protein-protein interactions. Previous studies have found that BRCA1 interacts, through the C-terminal end of the region encoded by exon 11, with both RAD51 and RAD50 (Zhong et al., 1999). RAD51 is the human homologue of the yeast RecA protein, which functions in homologous recombination and DNA damage repair (Scully et al., 1997). Significantly, RAD51 is known to form a complex with both BRCA1 and BRCA2 during DNA repair (Chen et al., 1999). Similarly, upon induction of DNA damage, RAD50 forms a complex with BRCA1, MRE11 and p95/NIBRIN (the protein encoded by the gene mutated in Nijmegen breakage syndrome) (Trujillo et al., 1998). This complex is believed to function, in yeast, in DSB repair, homologous recombination, nonhomologous end joining and telomere maintenance (Haber, 1998).

In summary, BRCA1 appears to help to maintain genomic integrity, principally by promoting homologous-directed DNA double-strand break repair.

With regard to transcriptional regulation by BRCA1, a region between amino acids 1142 and 1646 (Chen et al., 1996) and a domain encompassing the carboxy-terminal residues 1760–1863 (Chapman and Verma, 1996; Chen et al., 1996; Monteiro et al., 1996) have been shown to possess transactivation activity. Specific DNA binding by BRCA1 has not yet been demonstrated. However, evidence is accumulating that BRCA1 functions as a transcriptional regulator by interacting with other proteins, including sequence-specific binding proteins. For instance, BRCA1 interacts with both the transcriptional transactivator, c-MYC (Wang et al., 1998), whose activity it inhibits, and RNA helicase A (Anderson et al., 1998). Furthermore, a recent report indicates that the BRCT domain, located between amino acids 1536 and 1863 of BRCA1, can also bind to components of the histone deacteylase complex (HDAC) (Yarden and Brody, 1999). The implied function of BRCA1 in the regulation of chromatin remodelling could, theoretically, contribute to transcription, replication, recombination or DNA repair. This BRCA1 C-terminal region also interacts with *TP53*, appearing to stimulate its transcriptional activation of the p21 gene (Chai et al., 1999), and with the RNA pol II holoenzyme, itself (Anderson et al., 1998). In fact, in human cells the cell cycle arrest that occurs following ectopic expression of BRCA1 appears to be mediated by transactivation of the *p21* promoter (Somasundaram, 1997). Another gene that is involved in cell-cycle regulation, *GADD45*, is also transcriptionally up-regulated in response to BRCA1 (Harkin et al., 1999). Finally, BRCA1 also appearss to function as a negative transcriptional regulator as it represses oestrogen-induced transcriptional activation mediated by the oestrogen receptor, ERa1pha.

Exposure of normal cells to gamma irradiation causes phosphorylation of BRCA1 and this DNA damage-induced BRCA1 phosphorylation is thought to be at least partly mediated by ATM (Cortez et al., 1999). Finally, the proposed roles of BRCA1 in DNA repair and in transactivation may not be mutually exclusive. In fact, the role of BRCA1 in DNA repair may be closely linked to its role as a transcriptional regulator.

Structure and function of the BRCA2 protein

The *BRCA2* gene, which comprises 27 exons, encodes a nuclear protein of 3418 amino acid residues and 384 kDa, which is almost twice the size of *BRCA1* (Wooster et al., 1995). Like in *BRCA1*, exon 1 is non-coding and exon 11 is particularly large. As with *BRCA1*, it is not yet entirely clear how loss of function of the protein leads to tumorigenesis, although there are several clues. A role in DNA repair appears particularly likely. Like the BRCA1 protein, BRCA2 can bind to RAD51. Again, the region involved is encoded by exon 11, though in BRCA2 the RAD51-interacting region contains four of the eight copies of a motif of 30–80 amino acids known as the BRC repeat (Bignell et al., 1997; Wong et al., 1997). Furthermore, cells of BRCA2 knockout mice exhibit an increased sensitivity to genotoxic agents (Friedman et al., 1998) but normal apoptotic and cell cycle checkpoint activation (Patel et al., 1998) thus further implicating BRCA2 in DNA repair.

Located at the carboxyl terminus of BRCA2 are three nuclear localization signals, suggesting that disease-causing mutations, which tend to cause truncation upstream of this position, would all result in an abnormal cytoplasmic localisation of the mutant protein. At the amino terminus of BRCA2 is a region that interacts with the transcriptional co-activator protein PCAF (p300/CBP-associated factor), which possesses histone acetylase activity (Fuks et al., 1998). In addition, studies in yeast indicate that the BRCA2 exon3 product can activate transcription when fused to a DNA-binding domain (Milner et al., 1997). Thus, although less well supported than for BRCA1, the crucial normal function of BRCA2 may involve transcriptional regulation in addition to DNA repair and maintenance of genomic integrity. An interesting paradox is that homozygous BRCA2 truncation, alone, in mice leads to proliferative arrest rather than tumorigenicity. In fact, recent studies in mice suggest that BRCA2-induced tumorigenesis may require the co-inactivation of one or more cell cycle regulators that normally respond to mitotic

spindle disruption, such as the mitotic checkpoint kinases, Bub1 and Mad3L (Lee et al., 1999).

BRCA1 and *BRCA2* mutations and cancer predisposition

While studies of *BRCA1* mutations in breast cancer patients are still ongoing, a number of findings have emerged. By linkage and mutation analyses of nearly 237 families with four or more cases of breast cancer diagnosed before age 60 (or at any age in male cases), germline mutations of *BRCA1* and *BRCA2* have been implicated in 52% and 32%, respectively, overall (Ford et al., 1998). Moreover, germline *BRCA1* mutations were thought to account for the cancer predisposition in as many as 81% of those families affected by both breast and ovarian cancer (Fig. 19.11). In contrast, *BRCA2* mutations were thought to be responsible for approximately 76% of families in which there is at least one case of male breast cancer (Ford et al., 1998). A sizeable variety of germline mutations in the *BRCA1* gene have been identified, and around 95% are predicted to result in the synthesis of a truncated BRCA1 protein. Most mutations have been identified in only one or two families, but a limited number have been seen recurrently. Of particular note, a population survey of Ashkenazi Jews, selected without regard to family history of cancer, has demonstrated that about 1% carry the *BRCA1* 185de1AG frameshift mutation (Struewing et al., 1995). This mutation, or one of two other Ashkenazi founder mutations, the *BRCA1* 5382insC and the *BRCA2* 6174delT, is found in 2.5% of individuals in this population group. Together, they account for at least half of the "high risk" breast or breast/ovarian cancer families. Similarly, 0.6% of Icelanders carry the 999de15 *BRCA2* mutation, which accounts for almost all hereditary breast cancer in Iceland (Foulkes, 1998).

Notably, population-based studies of the penetrance of the Ashkenazi founder *BRCA1* mutation 185de1AG (Struewing et al., 1997) and the Icelandic founder *BRCA2* mutation 999de15 (Thorlacius et al., 1998) have suggested lower breast cancer penetrances (of 56% and 37% by age 70, respectively) than the previous pedigree-based studies. The differences are likely to be due to the presence or absence of as-yet unidentified important risk-modifying genes which may well serve to increase the risk when a gene carrier is a member of a family with several affected members. Interestingly, truncating mutations located towards the 5′ end (proximal to codon 1435) of *BRCA1* (Gayther et al., 1995) or within the ovarian cancer cluster region (OCCR) bounded by codons 1000 and 2000, approximately, within exon 11 of *BRCA2* (Gayther et al.,

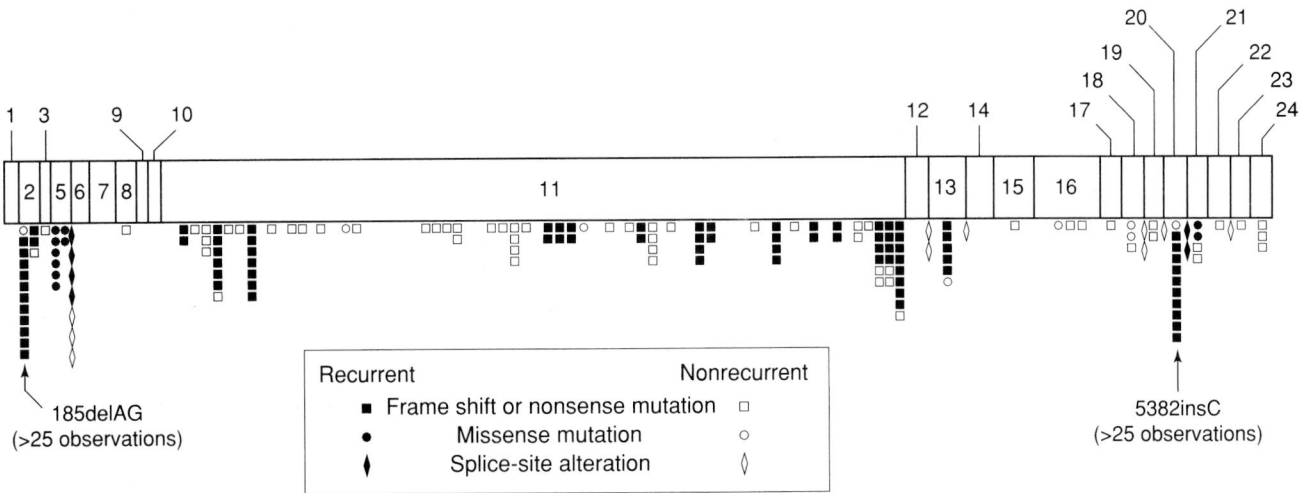

Fig. 19.11. Germline mutations reported in the *BRCA1* gene, predominantly from families with a high incidence of breast and/or ovarian cancer. The numbers correspond to *BRCA1* exons; there is no exon 4. The nature of the mutations and whether they have been seen in more than one apparently unrelated individual (i.e. recurrent) are indicated. (From Collins, 1996.)

1997; Ford et al., 1998) appear to confer greater risks of ovarian cancer than mutations situated elsewhere in these genes.

Surprisingly, very few sporadic tumors have been found to harbor detectable somatic pathogenic mutations in *BRCA1* or *BRCA2* (Szabo and King, 1995; Miki et al., 1996). This has raised questions regarding the role of these genes in sporadic breast and ovarian cancers. However, it now appears that promoter hypermethylation, rather than somatic mutation, may represent an important mechanism by which at least *BRCA1* is inactivated in certain types of sporadic tumors. *BRCA1* promoter hypermethylation was observed in 67%, 55% and 12% of sporadic medullary, mucinous and ductal breast carcinomas, respectively (Esteller et al., 2000). In addition, *BRCA1* hypermethylation was detected in 20% of sporadic ductal breast tumors showing *BRCA1* LOH, suggesting that in these tumors, one allele might be lost by deletion, while the other is silenced by aberrant methylation (Esteller et al., 2000).

Study of the pathology of sporadic and hereditary breast cancers has revealed some intriguing differences. For instance, the histology of breast cancers in *BRCA1* germline mutation carriers is more often of higher grade malignancy and more frequently of medullary type than in sporadic cases (Armes 1998; Breast Cancer Linkage Consortium, 1999). Despite the higher grade and a higher rate of ipsilateral and contralateral second primary breast tumors, however, the prognosis of *BRCA1* hereditary breast cancer appears to be no worse than for non-hereditary cases (Watson et al., 1998).

CANDIDATE TUMOR SUPPRESSOR GENES

The identification of specific germline mutations inactivating gene function in those with inherited predisposition to cancer provides compelling evidence that the particular gene functions as a tumor suppressor gene. Frequent somatic mutations in the tumor suppressor gene in sporadic cancers of various types serve to highlight the significance of the gene in the development of more common sporadic cancers. Nonetheless, it seems reasonable to suspect that some tumor suppressor genes with critical roles in human cancer may not give rise to an obvious cancer predisposition phenotype even when present in mutant form in the germline. Indeed, many of the tumor suppressor genes that are commonly inactivated in many forms of human cancer (e.g. *TP53*, *p16INK4a*, *RB1*) predispose those with germline mutations to only a very limited subset of tumors. One approach to identify those tumor suppressor genes that may contribute to cancer predominantly through somatic mutation has been to identify and analyse chromosomal regions for which allelic losses can be frequently observed in sporadic cancers of a particular type.

E-cadherin

E-cadherin is a calcium-dependent, epithelial cell adhesion molecule whose function is critical for normal epithelial development and is lost during the growth of most if not all human epithelial cancers (Christofori and Semb, 1999). The protein is also known to form a complex with beta-catenin, a protein which interacts with APC and also, by signalling to the TCF4 transcription factor, activates growth-promoting genes such as c-*MYC* (see section entitled "APC Function and WNT Signalling"). Inactivation of the alleles of the *E-CADHERIN* tumor suppressor gene may occur by deletion, point mutation or promoter hypermethylation. Germline *E-CADHERIN* mutations have been identified in a minority of familial gastric cancers, such as in the three gastric cancer kindreds of Maori origin (Guilford et al., 1998). However, more recently, such mutations have been found not only in non-Maori familial gastric cancer, but also in a member of such a family who had early-onset colorectal cancer (Richards et al., 1999). Interestingly, *E-CADHERIN* promoter hypermethylation has been detected on both alleles of the gene in two patients with sporadic leukaemia (Melki et al., 2000) as has been previously observed for *hMLH1* in sporadic colorectal cancers (Veigl et al., 1998). In many sporadic human cancers, loss of E-cadherin expression occurs late in the process of tumorigenesis and is associated with metastasis. This fact, together with its role as a cell-cell specific recognition receptor, suggests that the protein functions as an "invasion suppressor" (Richards et al., 1999).

As already mentioned, a recent report indicates that *E-CADHERIN* is transcriptionally activated by the *WT1* tumor suppressor gene product by direct binding of WT1 to the *E-CADHERIN* promoter, raising the possibility that altered *E-CADHERIN* expression might play a role in Wilms tumor pathogenesis (Hosono et al., 2000).

The role of DNA damage repair genes in inherited cancer syndromes

Tumor suppressor genes have been defined in this chapter as the class of genes that are inactivated by germline and somatic mutations in cancers and that normally have active roles in the regulation of cell growth in response to growth-inhibitory or differentiation signals. Though they are also inactivated in cancer cells, the DNA damage repair genes can be viewed as having more indirect roles in the processes controlling growth. Loss of function mutations in these genes are presumed to have little direct effect on cell growth. Rather, their inactivation appears, in affected cells, to increase the rate of mutations in cellular genes, including proto-oncogenes and tumor suppressor genes.

Several cancer predisposition syndromes have been described that result from germline mutations inactivating genes involved in DNA damage repair. These include xeroderma pigmentosum, Werner syndrome, Bloom syndrome, Nijmegen breakage syndrome, ataxia telangectasia, and the hereditary nonpolyposis colorectal cancer syndromes. The principal mechanisms of DNA repair include mismatch repair of mis-paired bases (mainly from errors arising in DNA replication), repair by homologous reombination (or by end-joining) of double-strand breaks (induced, for example, by X-rays), nucleotide excision repair of UV-induced intra-strand pyrimidine dimers, and base excision repair of small base modifications caused, for example, by oxygen radicals and alkylating agents.

HEREDITARY NON-POLYPOSIS COLORECTAL CANCER AND MISMATCH REPAIR

Familial clustering of colorectal cancer has long been noted. In fact, a genetic component is likely to be a primary factor in at least 10% of colorectal cancer cases (Lynch and de la Chapelle, 1999). Hereditary nonpolyposis colorectal cancer (HNPCC), probably accounts for about 5–8% of all colorectal cancer (CRC) patients (Lynch and de la Chapelle, 1999). At least ten fold less frequent than HNPCC (Lynch et al., 1993) is familial adenomatous polyposis, which, as reviewed above, is a rare syndrome (with an approximate incidence of 1 in 10,000) that results from germline mutations in the *APC* gene.

The diagnosis of the HNPCC syndromes on a clinical basis alone is problematic for two reasons. Firstly, for a common malignancy like CRC, there is a likelihood of clustering within families by chance. Secondly, there is a lack of overt premalignant clinical characteristics, such as polyposis. Nevertheless, strict diagnostic criteria for HNPCC have been published, the Amsterdam criteria II (Vasen et al., 1999): (1) exclusion of familial polyposis in the CRC cases, if any, and verification of tumor types by pathological examination; (2) HNPCC-associated cancer in at least three relatives, one of them being a first-degree relative of the other two; (3) two or more successive generations affected; and, in addition, (4) at least one of the affected individuals should be less than 50 years of age at the time of diagnosis. For these strict criteria, the "HNPCC-associated cancer" was defined as cancer of the colon or rectum, the endometrium, small bowel, ureter or renal pelvis. These tumors were considered to be the most specific for HNPCC, having the highest relative risks. It was acknowledged, however, that gastric, ovarian, brain, hepatobiliary and sebaceous skin tumors are also associated with the syndrome, despite not being included in the Amsterdam criteria II (Vasen et al., 1999). These criteria represent a modification (by the International Collaborative Group on HNPCC) of the original "Amsterdam" criteria, in which only CRCs were included (Vasen et al., 1991a,b). Nevertheless, the modified criteria remain relatively strict and are designed primariliy as selection criteria for collaborative studies. They "are not intended to serve as a guide to exclude suspected families from genetic counselling and mutation analysis" (Vasen et al., 1999). The HNPCC kindreds were often previously categorized as either Lynch syndrome I (CRC only) or Lynch syndrome II (colorectal and other tumors). The more inclusive term HNPCC is often used now to encompass both syndromes and distinguishes them from the polyposis syndromes. In HNPCC, compared to sporadic cases, the CRCs show a predilection for the proximal colon, have a better prognosis, a tendency to be of mucinous type with a lymphoid aggregation at the tumor margin, and, on immunohistochemistry, to exhibit loss of hMLH1, hMSH2 or hMSH6 protein expression. Furthermore, the adenomas that occur in HNPCC tend to be larger, have a villous growth pattern and to be more dysplastic than those arising in the general population (Vasen et al., 1999).

Genes responsible for HNPCC

Studies from the mid-1980s attempted to localize the genes responsible for HNPCC. No evidence was obtained to link the HNPCC syndrome to any known tumor suppressor genes (such as *APC*, *TP53*, or *RB1*). Thus, a search of the entire genome for the HNPCC gene(s) was carried out. Several different genes responsible for the HNPCC syndromes have since been identified, predominantly by linkage analysis of large kindreds, including a gene at chromosome 2p16 (*hMSH2*) and one at chromosome 3p21 (*hMLH1*) that together account for the majority of HNPCC cases (Fishel et al., 1993; Leach et al., 1993; Lindblom et al., 1993; Peltomaki et al., 1993; Bronner et al., 1994; Papadopoulos et al., 1994). Based on studies of highly related genes from bacteria and yeast, the protein products of the *hMSH2* and *hMLH1* genes (homologues of the bacterial mismatch repair enzymes MutS and MutL, respectively) were predicted to be involved in the recognition and repair of DNA mismatches in humans. Additional mismatch repair (MMR) genes have been identified, the MutL homologues, *hPMS1* and *hPMS2* (Nicolaides et al., 1994), and, more recently, two MutS homologues, *hMSH6* (Palombo et al., 1995) and *hMSH3* (Risinger et al., 1994), which both encode proteins that heterodimerise with hMSH2.

Approximately 50% of those families who satisfy the original Amsterdam criteria have mutations in either the *hMLH1* or *hMSH2* genes (Dunlop et al., 1997; Wijnen et al., 1997) with mutations in *hPMS1*, *hPMS2* or *hMSH6* (also known as *GTBP*) being detected much less frequently. In contrast to germline mutations in *hMLH1*, 49% of which are nonsense or frameshift, 83% of germline mutations in

hMSH2 are truncating (Peltomaki and Vasser, 1997). Moreover, genomic deletions of *hMSH2* (but not of *hMLH1*) account for a significant proportion (6.5%) of Dutch HNPCC families defined by the Amsterdam criteria, suggesting that a thorough mutation analysis of this gene should include Southern analyses (Wijnen et al., 1998).

Interestingly, as many as 28% of patients with very early onset CRC (<30 years), unselected for family history, possess a germline mutation in a MMR gene (Farrington et al., 1998). In these early onset cases, the determination of replication error (RER) status by screening for microsatellite instability (MSI) (the accumulation of different-sized alleles of microsatellite sequences in tumor DNA) appears to be useful in predicting the presence of a germline mutation in a MMR gene (Farrington et al., 1998). The positive predictive value of the analysis was 63%, with a sensitivity of 12/14 cases (86%) (Farrington et al., 1998).

Although MSI is present in cancers in nearly all patients with HNPCC, in sporadic CRC cases, in general, MSI is observed in only 10–15% (Ionov et al., 1993). In these sporadic tumors with MSI, however, somatic mutations in MMR genes are found in only around 25% (Borresen et al., 1995). The most common mechanism of MMR gene inactivation in at least sporadic endometrial and gastric cancers with MSI, in contrast, is hypermethylation of the CpG island at the *hMLH1* promoter, followed by loss or hypermethylation of the second allele (Leung et al., 1999; Simpkins et al., 1999).

The mismatch repair system

The roles of the protein products of the genes involved in HNPCC are becoming clearer (Sancar, 1999). Mispaired bases, usually arising from replication errors, are initially recognized by a complex of two MutS-related proteins. Generally, single base mispairs are recognized by a MutS alpha heterodimer consisting of hMSH2/hMSH6, while insertion/deletion loops are recognized by hMSH2/hMSH3 (MutS beta). The DNA-bound MutS heterodimer subsequently interacts with a heterodimeric complex of MutL-related proteins (hMLH1/hPMS1 or hMLH1/hPMS2). Following the assembly of this large protein complex, a portion of the DNA strand containing the mismatched base is excised by an exonuclease that proceeds from a "nick" made up to 2 kb from the mismatch. Finally, the excised tract is repaired with correctly pairing bases by DNA polymerase delta.

Interestingly, patients with HNPCC whose tumors show no or mild MSI (i.e., "MSI-low") often possess germline *hMSH6* mutations (Wu et al., 2000). This finding presumably reflects the predominant involvement of *hMSH6* in repair of mismatches, rather than of the insertion/deletion events that give rise to MSI. An important implication of this finding is that when HNPCC is suspected, absence of MSI does not completely exclude the possibility that a MMR gene mutation is present.

In cells with one normal and one mutant allele of a DNA mismatch repair gene, DNA repair is not, for the most part, impaired. However, inactivation of the remaining allele can occur as a result of a somatic event, usually allelic loss, in an initiated cell population during tumor development. Once the cell loses this vital component of its self-protection mechanism, it acquires a so-called "mutator phenotype". Hundreds of errors may then arise and fail to be repaired during each cell division. Complete inactivation of an MMR gene may, therefore, promote tumorigenesis through a failure to recognize and repair the multiple point mutations that arise subsequently. Although many of these mutations may be detrimental to cell growth and survival, a subset of the mutations are likely to activate oncogenes or inactivate other tumor suppressor genes. For instance, genes which have been identified as being frequently mutated in tumors with a MMR defect include those encoding the transforming growth factor beta type II receptor, the E2F4 transcription factor, the IGF-II receptor and the Bax proapoptotic protein (Markowitz et al., 1995; Souza et al., 1996; Rampino et al., 1997; Fujiwara et al., 1998).

Cancer predisposition in MMR gene mutation carriers

As mentioned above, in addition to CRC, HNPCC mutation carriers are at a significantly increased risk of other cancers. A recent study of 360 Finnish mutation carriers found them to have a significantly increased risk of colorectal (standardized incidence ratio (SIR) of 68, with a cumulative incidence of 82% by age 70), endometrial (SIR 62, 60% in women), ovarian (SIR 13, 12% in women), biliary tract (SIR 9.1, 2.0%), bladder/ureter/urethra (SIR 7.6, 4.0%), gastric (SIR 6.9, 13%), kidney (SIR 4.7, 3.3%) and CNS (SIR 4.5, 3.7%) cancers (Aarnio et al., 1999). The ovarian cancers were predominantly cystadenocarcinomas, while the CNS tumors were most commonly glioblastoma multiforme. Only four breast cancers occurred, with an SIR of 1.4 that was not statistically significant. The 360 carriers were from 50 families, most of whom possessed the same *hMLH1* mutation and only three had an *hMSH2* mutation. Interestingly in females, by age 70, the incidence of endometrial cancer (60%) exceeded that of CRC (54%), while in men, the incidence of CRC was said to be 100%. These figures were thus higher than those of Dunlop et al. (1997) who, studying 67 mutation carriers (predominantly of *hMSH2*), found that the incidences of endometrial and CRC in females (by age 70) were 42% and 30%, respectively, while the incidence of the latter in males was 74%.

Predisposition to colorectal cancer by low penetrance genes

Many apparently familial CRCs that are not due to FAP or HNPCC, may be predisposed to by low-penetrance gene mutations or polymorphisms. An example of the latter is the polymorphism in the *APC* gene, the T to A transversion at nucleotide 3920, which results in substitution of a lysine in place of an isoleucine at codon 1307 (I1307K). More importantly, it creates a small hypermutable region of the gene, by converting an AAATAAAA sequence to an AAAAAAAA sequence, that is then susceptible to single adenine insertion or deletion (Laken et al., 1997). Large-scale clinical studies are currently underway, which will hopefully determine the magnitude of any I1307K-associated increase in CRC risk. The polymorphism, which is found almost exclusively in Ashkenazi Jews, appears to be associated with an increased number, *per patient*, of colorectal adenomatous polyps and possibly also CRCs (Frayling et al., 1998; Woodage et al., 1998; Gryfe et al., 1999). It may partially explain the reportedly increased incidence of CRC in Ashkenazi Jews (9–15% lifetime risk) (Laken et al., 1997; Rozen et al., 1999).

ATAXIA TELANGIECTASIA

The DNA mismatch repair genes are not the only genes involved in DNA damage recognition and repair that have been found to be responsible for cancer predisposition syndromes. Ataxia telangiectasia (AT) is an autosomal recessive disorder primarily affecting the central nervous and immune systems. The condition is characterised by cerebellar degeneration, immunodeficiency, radiation sensitivity, cell cycle abnormalities, chromosomal instability, and a striking predisposition to leukaemias and lymphomas. There are conflicting data regarding whether heterozygosity for an AT mutation confers an increased risk of breast cancer. Thus while a fourfold increased risk was reported in one study of 99 AT families (Athma et al., 1996) in which the precise mutations were not described, several studies have not found such an association. For example, no increase in truncating *AT* mutations was found in the germline DNA of 401 women with early onset breast cancer compared to 202 control subjects. Mutations were detected in 0.5% and 1% of these individuals, respectively (FitzGerald et al., 1997). While there may indeed be a predisposition to breast cancer, it is currently difficult to quantify, and is probably less than predicted previously (Inskip et al., 1999; Khanna et al., 2000).

Originally, AT was thought to be genetically heterogeneous, with four complementation groups attributed to different genes. Using positional cloning strategies, *ATM* (for AT, mutated), the gene on chromosome 11q responsible for AT, was identified (Savitsky et al., 1995). Surprisingly, *ATM* was found to be mutated in the germline of patients from all four complementation groups, indicating that it was the sole gene responsible for this disorder (Savitsky et al., 1995). The *ATM* gene, which possesses 66 exons and is located at 11q22-23, is widely expressed and has a transcript size of 12 kb (Savitsky et al., 1995). It encodes a protein exhibiting similarity, through a kinase domain located in its C-terminal region, to several yeast and mammalian phosphatidylinositol-3 kinases involved in DNA damage recognition and cell cycle control. Its kinase domain, however, possesses protein, rather than phospholipid, kinase activity. Although the precise mechanism by which ATM is activated is currently unclear, its protein kinase activity has been observed to increase dramatically following double-strand breaks such as those induced by ionising radiation (Banin et al., 1998; Canman et al., 1998). Phosphorylation of *TP53* directly by ATM occurs on Ser15 (Banin et al., 1998; Canman et al., 1998). However, although this direct phosphorylation is critical for the apoptotic activity of *TP53*, the mechanism by which stabilisation of *TP53* is induced by ATM is indirect (Chehab et al., 1999). It occurs by ATM's activation of Chk2/hCds1 which, in turn, phosphorylates *TP53* on Ser20 preventing *TP53*'s degradation by MDM2 (Chehab et al., 1999; Caspari, 2000) (Fig. 19.8). In addition to this role in inducing cell-cycle arrest following DNA damage, ATM is implicated in signalling to the repair machinery. For instance, in response to double-strand breaks it appears to be required for the activation of both the BRCA1/Rad51 complex (Cortez et al., 1999) and the nibrin/Mre11/Rad50 complex (see the section entitled "Nijmegen breakage syndrome" below).

BLOOM SYNDROME AND WERNER SYNDROME

Bloom syndrome (BS) is a progressive autosomal recessive disorder characterized by small stature, sun sensitivity, immunodeficiency, chromosome instability, and striking predisposition to cancer. Cells from patients with BS show an abnormally high incidence of sister chromatid exchanges (SCEs). *BLM*, the gene responsible for BS, was identified (Ellis et al., 1995) by taking advantage of the fact that some patients with BS have a minor population of phenotypically normal cells. These cells fail to exhibit the BS phenotype because of somatic intragenic recombinations within the target gene that effectively restore a wild-type allele. Based on this "somatic crossover point mapping" a 250 kb segment of the genome containing the BS gene was identified. A gene within the region (*BLM*) was found that contains truncating mutations in patients with BS. *BLM* encodes a 1417 amino acid residue protein with homology to the RecQ helicases, proteins that are believed to have a role in DNA repair and/or replication. The BLM protein contains seven conserved helicase motifs (Ellis et al., 1995) and appears to exist as a hexameric ring structure surrounding a central hollow (Karow et al., 1999). The normal function of BLM in human cells remains to be determined, although recent findings suggest that the SCEs arise principally by excessive homologous recombination that is normally suppressed by BLM (Wang et al., 2000). Thus BLM, and perhaps other disease-associated RecQ helicases, may act as anti-recombinases, disrupting recombination intermediates. Interestingly, mutations of other genes in this helicase family (*XPB*, *XPD* and *ERCC6*) have been identified in patients with xeroderma pigmentosum and Cockayne syndrome, two other human diseases characterized by a strong predisposition to cancer.

Werner syndrome (WS) is a rare autosomal recessive disorder characterized by premature aging, with an early onset of age related diseases such as atherosclerosis and, in addition, tumors such as soft-tissue sarcomas. The causative gene, *WRN*, has now been identified and its function studied (Yu et al., 1996; Gray et al., 1997; Suzuki et al., 1997). Like the Bloom syndrome gene, it encodes an ATP-dependent DNA helicase, with 3′–5′ directionality, that is homologous to the *E. coli* protein RecQ and which unwinds double-stranded DNA (Gray et al., 1997; Suzuki et al., 1997). The WRN protein has been found to interact with the multifunctional replication protein A (RPA) (Brosh et al., 1999) and also with *TP53* (Blander et al., 1999). In addition to helicase and ATPase activity, the WRN protein possesses a 3′–5′ exonuclease function (Fry and Loeb, 1998; S Huang et al., 1998; Shen et al., 1998). Cells from WS patients, unlike those from BS patients, do not show increased SCEs, though both groups of cells do exhibit genomic instability. The physiological function of WRN may be to facilitate reconstruction of genomic structure following DNA damage or the resolution of aberrant DNA structures during DNA synthesis

(Shen and Loeb, 2000). It also appears to participate in *TP53*-mediated apoptosis, in view of the observed attenuation of *TP53*-mediated apoptosis in WS fibroblasts and its restoration by WRN expression (Spillare et al., 1999). Such a role in apoptosis might, therefore, contribute to the cancer predisposition of WS patients.

Recently, patients with Rothmund-Thomson syndrome, another rare autosomal recessive disorder associated with genomic instability, premature ageing and a predisposition to neoplasia, have been found to have mutations in another RecQ helicase gene, *RECQL4* (Kitao et al., 1999).

NIJMEGEN BREAKAGE SYNDROME

Nijmegen breakage syndrome (NBS) is another rare autosomal recessive DNA repair disorder. Like in both AT and BS, there is chromosomal instability, immunodeficiency, and a predisposition to cancer. Unlike in AT, however, neurological features are rare, and the serum alphafetoprotein is not raised. In addition to those feautures mentioned above, microcephaly with relatively preserved mental development, typical facial appearance, growth retardation and X-ray hypersensitivity are characteristic, with café au lait spots, vitiligo, clinodactyly and syndactyly being additional important features (Weemaes et al., 2000). The sister chromatid exchanges, characteristic of BS, are not, however, a feature of either AT or NBS. Although the first patient with NBS was not described until 1981 (Weemaes et al., 1981), the defective gene, *NBS-1*, has already been cloned (Matsuura et al., 1998; Varon et al., 1998). *NBS-1* is located on chromosome 8q21 and encodes a protein, named nibrin. Sequence analysis revealed two amino terminal domains, a forkhead associated domain (FHA) and a breast cancer carboxy terminal domain (BRCT) domain, both of which had previously been found in DNA damage responsive cell cycle checkpoint proteins (Matsuura et al., 1998; Varon et al., 1998). Further evidence for the role of nibrin in the repair of DNA damage was provided by the finding that it forms a heterotrimeric complex with hMRE11 and hRAD50, which participate in double strand break (DSB) DNA repair (Carney et al., 1998). This complex is recruited to DSB sites to process the DNA in preparation for repair (Paull and Gellert, 1999).

The similarity between the chromosomal instability observed in at least AT and NBS can now be partly explained at the protein level. The protein kinase, ATM, which is activated by DSBs, is now known to phosphorylate not only *TP53* (Banin et al., 1998; Canman et al., 1998), CHK2 (Matsuoka et al., 1998), and BRCA1 (Cortez et al., 1999), but also nibrin (Gatei et al., 2000; Lim et al., 2000;

Wu et al., 2000; Zhao et al., 2000). Phosphorylation of nibrin by ATM occurs at four sites, serine residues 278, 343, 397 and 615, and phosphorylation of all four appears necessary for the cellular response to DNA damage (Wu et al., 2000; Zhao et al., 2000). Thus in the presence of damaged DNA, ATM normally functions not only by activating cell-cycle checkpoints (by phosphorylating CHK2 and *TP53*) and thus preventing duplication of damaged DNA but also by activating the repair of the damage. The possibility that nibrin may also be activated by other kinases, perhaps in response to other signals, remains to be fully investigated.

With regard to mutations, 45 out of 55 patients in the NBS registry, were recently reported to possess a founder truncating 5 bp *NBS-1* deletion, 657–661 delACAAA, but no specific genotype-phenotype relationship is yet apparent (International NBS Study Group, 2000).

XERODERMA PIGMENTOSUM AND NUCLEOTIDE EXCISION REPAIR

Xeroderma pigmentosum (XP) is one of three rare recessive syndromes with cutaneous photosensivity (XP, Cockayne syndrome and the photosensitive form of trichothiodystrophy) that result from a defect in the nucleotide excision repair (NER) DNA repair mechanism. The role of NER is to remove helix-distorting bulky adducts, such as the UV-induced cyclobutane pyrimidine dimer (CPD) formed between adjacent pyrimidines in the same DNA strand. Cockayne syndrome (CS), in addition to cutaneous photosensitivity, comprises a growth defect, cataracts, progressive neurological degeneration, sensorineural hearing loss, pigmentary retinopathy and dental caries (Nance and Berry, 1992). Trichothiodystrophy (TTD), sulfur-deficient brittle hair, is a feature of a group of syndromes that comprise, in addition, cutaneous photosensitivity, intellectual impairment and other features such as ichthyosis and neutropenia (Tolmie et al., 1994). The cutaneous hallmarks of XP are parchment skin and freckles on the sun-exposed areas of skin. Moreover, XP patients have a 1000-fold increased risk of skin cancer, predominantly basal cell and squamous cell carcinomas, with melanomas occurring less frequently. The mean age of onset of skin tumor is eight years. Patients with CS or TTD, in contrast, have not been reported to have an increased risk of skin cancer.

Cell fusion experiments have defined seven complementation groups for XP (XP-A to XP-G), two for CS (CS-A and CS-B), and three for TTD (TTD-A, XP-B and XP-D). The corresponding genes (with the current exception of TTD-A) have now been cloned and the function of their products has been partly determined. There are two tightly regulated NER pathways, together involving a total of more than 30 proteins and both of which are defective in XP: global genome repair (GGR) and the less widespread (but often more rapid) transcription-coupled repair (TCR) (Berneburg et al., 2000; de Boer and Hoeijmakers, 2000). In general, NER proceeds by the following steps: (a) DNA damage recognition (involving *XP-C* in GGR, and *CS-A* and *B* in TCR); (b) local chromatin unwinding (involving the zinc-finger protein, XP-A, and the two helicase subunits of the transcription initiation factor TFIIH, *XP-B* and *XP-D*); (c) excision of 24–32 nucleotides of the damaged strand by incisions made at sites flanking the lesion (by the 5′ and 3′ endonucleases XP-F and XP-G); and finally (d) gap-filling by DNA polymerase and DNA ligase (Sugasawa et al., 1998; de Boer and Hoeijmakers, 2000).

Many patients in the XP-A, XP-B, XP-D and XP-G groups (in which, typically, both TCR and GGR NER activities are deficient) tend to have more severe NER deficiencies, while patients in the XP-C group (who have deficient GGR but not TCR) tend to have either absent or late-onset neurological symptoms. Genotype-phenotype correlations are becoming increasingly defined. For instance, in XP-A patients CNS effects are particularly associated with mutations affecting the DNA binding region. Marked variation exists between cases in the XP-D complementation group, different point mutations in the *XP-D* gene causing XP, combined XP/CS or TTD. It has been postulated that *XP-D* gene mutations that only block the NER function of the protein lead to XP, while the mutations which abrogate XP-D's function in basal transcription may cause nonphotosensitive TTD and mutations affecting both functions may cause typical TTD (Bootsma and Hoeijmakers, 1993). Consistent with this hypothesis is the disease-specificity of the mutations. Furthermore, it has since been reported that the clinical severity of the TTD phenotype does not correlate with the level of the repair deficiency, per se (Botta et al., 1998).

THE *RET* GENE AND MULTIPLE ENDOCRINE NEOPLASIA TYPE 2

Unlike most inherited cancer predisposition syndromes, multiple endocrine neoplasia type 2 (MEN 2) results from the activation of a proto-oncogene, *RET*, rather than tumor suppressor gene inactivation (Takahashi et al., 1988). *RET*, which maps to 10q11.2 and comprises 21 exons spanning >60 kb, encodes a transmembrane tyrosine kinase (Takahashi et al., 1988). Its extracellular portion comprises a cadherin-like domain in addition to a cysteine-rich motif, while its intracellular region contains two tyrosine kinase sub-

domains. The protein forms part of a receptor complex whose ligands include glial cell line-derived neurotrophic factor (GDNF), neurturin and persephin (Airaksinen et al., 1999). The ligand specificity is dictated by the presence in the complex of GDNF family receptor (GFR) alpha proteins (Jing et al., 1996; Treanor et al., 1996; Klein et al., 1997). Ligand binding by the receptor induces its dimerization and the activation of its tyrosine kinase (Ponder, 1999). This, in turn, leads to its autophosphorylation on tyrosine residues and the subsequent activation of signalling cascades including the Ras/mitogen-activated protein kinase pathway (Ohiwa et al., 1997). The receptor plays an important role during the development of the kidney and enteric nervous system with GDNF acting to promote the growth of the ureteric bud and to protect the enteric neurons from apoptotic cell death (Durbec et al., 1996; Airaksinen et al., 1999).

Germline gain of function mutations in *RET* are linked to three dominantly inherited related cancer predisposition syndromes: multiple endocrine neoplasia type 2A and 2B (MEN 2A and MEN 2B) and familial medullary thyroid cancer (FMTC) (Mulligan et al., 1993; Hofstra et al., 1994; van Heyningen, 1994; Ponder, 1999). Individuals affected by FMTC simply show familial clustering of MTCs. In those with MEN 2A, however, MTCs are often accompanied by phaeochromocytomas and parathyroid hyperplasia. The most severe syndrome (MEN 2B) is characterized by the features of MEN 2A in addition to ganglioneuromas of the lips, tongue, and colon. In contrast to the gain-of-function point mutations in *RET* associated with these conditions, loss-of-function *RET* mutations cause Hirschprung's disease (Romeo et al., 1994).

The different MEN 2 and FMTC phenotypes are associated with different spectra of predisposing *RET* mutations. Missense mutations affecting a conserved cysteine residues (Cys 609, 611, 618, 620 or 634) in the cysteine-rich region of the extracellular domain of RET have been found, by the International *RET* Mutation Consortium, in 98% of 203 MEN 2A families and in 79% of 30 FMTC families tested (Eng et al., 1996). It is presumed that these cysteine residues normally form intramolecular disulfide bonds and that the mutation of such a residue leaves an unpaired cysteine which then forms an intermolecular disulphide bond with an adjacent mutated RET molecule (Ponder, 1999). It is envisaged that the resulting homodimerization of the receptor leads to constitutive receptor activation. Cysteine 634 is far more commonly mutated in MEN 2A than in FMTC (Eng et al., 1996). However, the basis for the phenotypic difference between FMTC and MEN 2A patients is not yet clear, although it may result from differing levels of receptor activation (Ponder, 1999).

In contrast, the mutations found in those with MEN 2B (and in some FMTC families) occur in one of the intracellular tyrosine kinase domains. In particular, a germline mutation involving the replacement of methionine 918 by a threonine residue, is found in almost all MEN 2B cases (Gimm et al., 1997; Smith et al., 1997). This Met residue is situated in the substrate recognition pocket within the catalytic core of the tyrosine kinase (Carlson et al., 1994). Its substitution leads to altered substrate specificity, with, for example, reduced binding to Grb2, and, presumably, aberrant cellular signalling (Liu et al., 1996). The intracellular FMTC-associated mutations, at codons 768, 790, 791, 804, 844 and 891, cause receptor activation in the absence of ligand binding and dimerisation (Ponder, 1999).

Finally, somatic *RET* mutations are uncommon in sporadic phaeochromocytoma (Eng et al., 1995) but somatic codon 918 *RET* mutations have been detected in 25% of sporadic MTC (Wohllk et al., 1996) and germline *RET* mutations have been reported in 6%–23% of apparently sporadic cases of MTC (Wohllk et al., 1996; Shirahama et al., 1998; Uchino et al., 1998).

THE *PTEN* GENE

An extensive linkage analysis involving a genome scan of 12 classical Cowden syndrome (CS) families, localised the CS gene to 10q23 (Nelen et al., 1996). In addition, frequent LOH at this locus was found in follicular thyroid tumors, suggesting that the putative CS gene was a tumor suppressor (Marsh et al., 1997a,b). Subsequently, two independent groups isolated a novel gene at this locus (Li et al., 1997; Steck et al., 1997). Sequence analysis predicted that the gene would encode a protein with homology to the cytoskeletal proteins, tensin and auxilin, and that the protein would contain a protein tyrosine and serine/threonine phosphatase domain (Li et al., 1997; Steck et al., 1997). The new gene was named *PTEN* for phosphatase and tensin homologue deleted on chromosome ten. Germline mutations in the *PTEN* gene have since been found in both CS and another related dominantly inherited disorder, Bannayan-Zonana (or Bannayan-Riley-Ruvalcaba) syndrome (Liaw et al., 1997; Marsh et al., 1997; 1999; Nelen et al., 1997). In addition, somatic mutations have been found in various human sporadic tumor types, including glioblastoma, and cancer of the endometrium, prostate, kidney and breast (Kong et al., 1997; Steck et al., 1997; Tashiro et al., 1997). In fact, mutations of *PTEN* are believed to occur early in endometrial carcinogenesis, as they are found in more than 20% of complex atypical hyperplasia (Levine et al., 1998). In common with many other TSGs (although not *TP53*), the majority of mutations result in

protein truncation (Han et al., 2000). Although the mutations are scattered over the entire gene, clustering is observed in the phosphatase core motif in exon 5 and in the phosphorylation sites in exons 7 and 8 (Liaw et al., 1997; Lynch et al., 1997; Marsh et al., 1998). Interestingly, specific germline *PTEN* mutations may give rise to either CS or Bannayan-Riley-Ruvalcaba syndrome, even within the same family, (Celebi et al., 2000; Perriard et al., 2000).

The tumor suppressor function of the PTEN protein, the first TSG to be identified in the phosphatase family, appears to depend on its lipid phosphatase, rather than its protein phosphatase, activity (Furnari et al., 1998; Myers et al., 1998;). In particular, its critical activity is the dephosphorylation of the lipid second messengers phosphatidylinositol 3,4-bisphosphate and phosphatidylinositol 3,4,5-trisphosphate (PIP3), at position 3 on the inositol ring, thus antagonizing the phosphoinositide 3-kinase (PI3K) signaling pathway. Mice that are homozygous and heterozygous for PTEN mutations show embryonic lethality and hyperplasia/dysplasia, respectively (Suzuki et al., 1998). Notably, in the heterozygous mice, the tissue distribution of the hyperplasia resembled that of CS and Bannayan-Zonana (Suzuki et al., 1998). Cells derived from the embryos of the homozygous PTEN knock-out mice show elevated levels of PIP3 and constitutively increased activity of the PKB/Akt enzyme (Stambolic et al., 1998), consistent with the role of PTEN in the inhibition of the PI3K pathway. Moreover, they exhibit a reduced sensitivity to apoptosis, implicating PTEN in the negative regulation of cell survival (Stambolic et al., 1998).

Summary and future directions

Although a genetic basis for the development of cancer has long been hypothesized, it is only in the past 25 years or so that significant experimental support for this hypothesis has been obtained. As reviewed in this chapter, we now know that germline and somatic mutations in three classes of genes, i.e., oncogenes, tumor suppressor genes, and DNA damage recognition and repair genes, play a primary role in the pathogenesis of cancer. However, as noted at the outset of this chapter, given the enormous progress that has been made in furthering our understanding of the genetic basis of cancer, it is not possible to review in detail all of the various mutations in oncogenes and tumor suppressor genes that have been identified in human cancers. Nor is it possible to describe all of the studies that have been carried out to address the cellular functions of various oncogene and tumor suppressor gene protein products. Rather, the primary goals of the chapter have been: (1) to provide an overview of the experimental strategies used to characterize specific genetic alterations in cancer; (2) to review some of the most prevalent and/or most informative genetic alterations in human cancer that have been elucidated; (3) to highlight some of the relationships between specific genetic alterations and clinical aspects of cancer; and (4) to review the current thinking regarding the normal cellular functions of the genes involved.

Undoubtedly, many novel discoveries on the genetic basis of cancer await. Additional oncogenes and tumor suppressor genes remain to be identified, and further studies will no doubt be facilitated by the recent elucidation of the sequence of the human genome. Importantly, genes that modify the risk of cancer development in individuals predisposed to cancer also await discovery. In addition, the relationships between dietary and environmental factors and genetic alterations in cancer will need to be addressed if we hope to prevent or at least delay the development of cancer. An optimistic view is that future studies of the genetic basis

of cancer not only will provide further insights into the pathogenesis of cancer but will lead to the development of important new diagnostic tools and therapeutic agents for the clinical management of patients with cancer. An exciting recent development is the use of cDNA microarrays for transcriptional profiling, whereby the levels of expression of thousands of gene sequences can be compared between different tissues. The application of this technology has already permitted the molecular sub-classification of diffuse large B-cell lymphoma (Alizadeh et al., 2000) and malignant melanoma (Bittner et al., 2000). It has also led to the recent finding that the gene-expression patterns in breast tumors with germline *BRCA1* mutations, *BRCA2* mutations, and sporadic tumors differ significantly from each other (Hedenfalk et al., 2001). Despite the current complexity of the analyses, such methodology might in the future prove to be invaluable in the classification of tumors for diagnostic and prognostic purposes and perhaps also for the prediction of the response to chemotherapy.

REFERENCES

Aarnio M, Sankila R, Pukkala E et al. (1999) Cancer risk in mutation carriers of DNA-mismatch-repair genes. Int J Cancer 81:214–218

Adams JM, Gerondakis S, Webb E, Corcoran LM, Cory S (1983) Cellular myc oncogene is altered by chromosome translocation to an immunoglobulin locus in murine plasmacytomas and is rearranged similarly in human Burkitt lymphomas. Proc Natl Acad Sci USA 80:1982–1986

Adams PD, Kaelin WG (1998) Negative control elements of the cell cycle in human tumors. Curr Opin Cell Biol 10:791–7

Airaksinen MS, Titievsky A, Saarma M (1999) GDNF family neurotrophic factor signaling: four masters, one servant? Mol Cell Neurosci 13:313–25

Aktas H, Cai H, Cooper GM (1997) Ras links growth factor signaling to the cell cycle machinery via regulation of cyclin D1 and the Cdk inhibitor p27KIP1. Mol Cell Biol 17:3850–3857

Alcorta DA, Xiong Y, Phelps D, Hannon G, Beach D, Barrett JC (1996) Involvement of the cyclin-dependent kinase inhibitor p16 (INK4a) in replicative senescence of normal human fibroblasts. Proc Natl Acad Sci USA 93:13742–13747

Anderson SF, Schlegel BP, Nakajima T et al. (1998) BRCA1 protein is linked to the RNA polymerase II holoenzyme complex via RNA helicase A. Nat Genet 19:254–6

Andreyev HJ, Norman AR, Cunningham D, Oates JR, Clarke PA (1998) Kirsten ras mutations in patients with colorectal cancer: The multicenter "RASCAL" study. J Natl Cancer Inst 90:675–684

Armes JE, Egan AJ, Southey MC et al. (1998) The histologic phenotypes of breast carcinoma occurring before age 40 years in women with and without BRCA1 or BRCA2 germline mutations: A population-based study. Cancer 83:2335–45

Aso T, Lane WS, Conaway JW, Conaway RC (1995) Elongin (SIII): A multisubunit regulator of elongation by RNA polymerase II. Science 269:1439–1443

Athma P, Rappaport R, Swift M (1996) Molecular genotyping shows that ataxia-telangiectasia heterozygotes are predisposed to breast cancer. Cancer Genet Cytogenet 92:130–4

Bacus SS, Stancovski I, Huberman E et al. (1992) Tumor-inhibitory monoclonal antibodies to the HER-2/Neu receptor induce differentiation of human breast cancer cells. Can Res 52:2580–2589

Baker S, Fearon E, Nigro J et al. (1989) Chromosome 17 deletions and TP53 gene mutations in colorectal carcinomas. Science 244:217–221

Balmain A, Ramsden M, Bowden GT, Smith J (1984) Activation of the mouse cellular Harvey-ras gene in chemically induced benign skin papillomas. Nature 307:658–660

Banin S, Moyal L, Shieh S et al. (1998) Enhanced phosphorylation of TP53 by ATM in response to DNA damage. Science 281:1674–7

Barbacid M (1987) Ras genes. Annu Rev Biochem 56:779–827

Bargmann CI, Hung MC, Weinberg RA (1986) Multiple independent activations of the neu oncogene by a point mutation altering the transmembrane domain of p185. Cell 45:649–657

Barker D, Wright E, Nguyen K et al. (1987) Gene for von Recklinghausen neurofibromatosis is in the pericentromeric region of chromosome 17. Science 236:1100–1102

Baselga J, Tripathy D, Mendelsohn J et al. (1996) Phase II study of weekly intravenous recombinant humanized anti-p185HER2 monoclonal antibody in patients with HER2/neu-overexpressing metastatic breast cancer. J Clin Oncol 14:737–744

Bates S, Phillips AC, Clark PA, Stot, F. Peters G, Ludwig RI, Vousden KH (1998) p14ARF links the tumor suppressors RB and TP53. Nature 395:124–125

Becker KF, Atkinson MJ, Reich U et al. (1994) E-cadherin gene mutations provide clues to diffuse type gastric carcinomas. Cancer Res 54:3845–3852

Behrens J, Jerchow BA, Wurtele M et al. (1998) Functional interaction of an axin homolog, conductin, with beta-catenin, APC, and GSK3beta. Science 280:596–9

Bell DW, Varley JM, Szydlo TE et al. (1999) Heterozygous germ line hCHK2 mutations in Li-Fraumeni syndrome. Science 286:2528–31

Benedict WF, Murphree AL, Banerjee A et al. (1983) Patient with chromosome 13 deletion: Evidence that the retinoblastoma gene is a recessive cancer gene. Science 219:973–975

Bergmann L, Miething C, Maurer U et al. (1997). High levels of Wilms tumor gene (wt1) mRNA in acute myeloid leukemias are associated with a worse long-term outcome. Blood 90:1217–1225

Bernardi P, Petronilli V, Di Lisa F, Forte M (2001) A mitochondrial perspective on cell death. Trends Biochem Sci 26:112–117

Berneburg M, Lowe JE, Nardo T et al. (2000) UV damage causes uncontrolled DNA breakage in cells from patients with combined features of XP-D and Cockayne syndrome. Embo J 19:1157–66

Bianchi AB, Mitsunaga SI, Cheng JQ et al. (1995) High frequency of inactivating mutations in the neurofibromatosis type 2 gene (NF2) in primary malignant mesotheliomas. Proc Natl Acad Sci USA 92:10854–10858

Bignell G, Micklem G, Stratton MR et al. (1997) The BRC repeats are conserved in mammalian BRCA2 proteins. Hum Mol Genet 6:53–8

Birch JM, Hartley AL, Tricker KJ et al. (1994) Prevalence and diversity of constitutional mutations in the TP53 gene among 21 Li-Fraumeni families. Cancer Res 54:1298–1304

Birchmeier W, Hulsken J, Behrens J (1995) Adherens junction proteins in tumor progression. Cancer Surv 24:129–140

Bischoff JR, Kirn DH, Williams A et al. (1996) An adenovirus mutant that replicates selectively in TP53-deficient human tumor cells. Science 274:373–6.

Bishop JM (1985) Viral oncogenes. Cell 52:301–354

Bishop JM (1987) The molecular genetics of cancer. Science 235:305–311

Bishop JM (1991) Molecular themes in oncogenesis. Cell 64:235–248

Blackwood EM, Eisenman RN (1991) Max: A helix-loop-helix zipper protein that forms a sequence-specific DNA-binding complex with Myc. Science 251:1211–1217

Blander G, Kipnis J, Leal JF et al. (1999) Physical and functional interaction between TP53 and the Werner's syndrome protein. J Biol Chem 274:29463–9

Bodmer W, Bailey C, Bodmer J et al. (1987) Localization of the gene for familial adenomatous polyposis on chromosome 5. Nature 328:614–619

Boguski MS, McCormick F (1993) Proteins regulating Ras and its relatives. Nature 366:643–654

Bonetta L, Kuehn SE, Huang A et al. (1990) Wilms tumortumor locus on 11p13 defined by multiple CpG island-associated transcripts. Science 250:994–997

Bookstein R, Shew J, Chen P et al. (1990) Suppression of tumortumorigenicity of human prostate carcinoma cells by replacing a mutated Rb gene. Science 247:712–715

Bootsma D, Hoeijmakers JH (1993) DNA repair. Engagement with transcription. Nature 6425:114–5

Borresen AL, Lothe RA, Meling GI et al. (1995) Somatic mutations in the hMSH2 gene in microsatellite unstable colorectal carcinomas. Hum Mol Genet 4:2065–72

Bos JL (1989) Ras oncogenes in human cancer: A review. Cancer Res 49:4682–4689

Botta E, Nardo T, Broughton BC et al. (1998) Analysis of mutations in the XPD gene in Italian patients with trichothiodystrophy: Site of mutations correlates with repair deficiency, but gene dosage appears to determine clinical severity. Am J Hum Genet 63:1036–48

Bourne HR, Sanders DA, McCormick F (1990) The GTPase superfamily: a conserved switch for diverse cell functions. Nature 348:125–132

Boveri T (1929) The Origin of Malignant TumorTumours. Williams & Wilkins, Baltimore

Breast Cancer Linkage Consortium (1999) Cancer risks in BRCA2 mutation carriers. J Natl Cancer Inst 91:1310–6

Brenner AJ, Stampfer MR, Aldaz CM (1998) Increased p16 expression with first senescence arrest in human mammary epithelial cells and extended growth capacity with p16 inactivation. Oncogene 17:199–205

Brehm A, Kouzarides T (1999) Retinoblastoma protein meets chromatin. Trends Biochem Sci 24:142–5

Brehm A, Miska E, Reid J et al. (1999) The cell cycle-regulating transcription factors E2F-RB. Br J Cancer 80 Suppl 1:38–41

Brenner AJ, Stampfer MR, Aldaz CM (1998) Increased p16 expression with first senescence arrest in human mammary epithelial cells and extended growth capacity with p16 inactivation. Oncogene 17:199–205

Brentnall TA, Chen R, Lee JG et al. (1995) Microsatellite instability and K-ras mutations associated with pancreatic adenocarcinoma and pancreatitis. Cancer Res 55:4264–4267

Broca PP (1866) Traite des Tumeurs. Asselin, Paris

Brodeur GM, Seeger RC, Schwab M et al. (1984) Amplification of N-myc in untreated human neuroblastomas correlates with advanced disease stage. Science 224:1121–1124

Bronner CE, Baker SM, Morrison PT et al. (1994) Mutation in the DNA mismatch repair gene homologue hMLH1 is associated with hereditary non-polyposis colon cancer. Nature 368:258–260

Brosh RM, Orren DK, Nehlin JO et al. (1999) Functional and physical interaction between WRN helicase and human replication protein A. J Biol Chem 274:18341–50

Bruder CE, Ichimura K, Tingby O et al. (1999) A group of schwannomas with interstitial deletions on 22q located outside the NF2 locus shows no detectable mutations in the NF2 gene. Hum Genet 104:418–24

Buchkovich K, Duffy LA, Harlow E (1989) The retinoblastoma protein is phosphorylated during specific phases of the cell cycle. Cell 58:1097–1105

Byrne JL Paterson HE, Marshall CJ (1996) P21Ras activation by the guanine nucleotide exchange factor Sos, requires the Sos/Grb2 interaction and a second ligand-dependent signal involving the Sos N-terminus. Oncogene 13:2055–2065

Cairns P, Polascik TJ, Eby Y et al. (1995) Frequency of homozygous deletion at p16INK4a/cdkn2 in primary human tumours. Nature Genet 11:210–212

Caldas C, Hahn SA, Hruban RH et al. (1994) Detection of K-ras mutations in the stool of patients with pancreatic adenocarcinoma and pancreatic ductal hyperplasia. Cancer Res 54:3568–3573

Call K, Glaser T, Ito C et al. (1990) Isolation and characterization of a zinc finger polypeptide gene at the human chromosome 11 Wilms' tumortumour locus. Cell 60:509–520

Canman CE, Lim DS, Cimprich KA et al. (1998) Activation of the ATM kinase by ionizing radiation and phosphorylation of TP53. Science 281:1677–9

Cannon-Albright L, Skolnick M, Bishop T et al. (1988) Common inheritance of susceptibility to colonic adenomatous polyps and associated colorectal cancers. N Engl J Med 319:533–537

Cantley LC, Auger KR, Carpenter et al. (1991) Oncogenes and signal transduction. Cell 64:281–302

Capon DJ, Chen EY, Levinson AD et al. (1983a) Complete nucleotide sequences of the T24 human bladder carcinoma oncogene and its normal homologue. Nature 302:33–37

Capon DJ, Seeburg PH, McGrath JP et al. (1983b) Activation of Ki-ras2 gene in human colon and lung carcinomas by two different point mutations. Nature 304:507–513

Carlson KM, Dou S, Chi D et al. (1994) Single missense mutation in the tyrosine kinase catalytic domain of the RET protooncogene is associated with multiple endocrine neoplasia type 2B. Proc Natl Acad Sci USA 91:1579–83

Carney JP, Maser RS, Olivares H et al. (1998) The hMrel1/hRad50 protein complex and Nijmegen breakage syndrome: linkage of double-strand break repair to the cellular DNA damage response. Cell 93:477–86

Caspari R, Olschwang S, Friedl W et al. (1995) Familial adenomatous polyposis: Desmoid tumours and lack of ophthalmic lesions (CHRPE) associated with APC mutations beyond codon 1444. Hum Mol Genet 4:337–40

Caspari T (2000) How to activate *TP53*. Curr Biol 10:R315–7

Cavenee WK, Dryja TP, Phillips RA et al. (1983) Expression of recessive alleles by chromosomal mechanisms in retinoblastoma. Nature 305:779–784

Cavenee WK, Hansen MF, Nordenskjold M et al. (1985) Genetic origin of mutations predisposing to retinoblastoma. Science 228:501–503

Cavenee W, Koufos A, Hansen M (1986) Recessive mutant genes predisposing to human cancer. Mutat Res 168:3

Cawthon R, Weiss R, Xu G et al. (1990) A major segment of the neurofibromatosis type 1 gene: cDNA sequence, genomic structure, and point mutations. Cell 62:193–201

Celebi JT, Ping XL, Zhang H et al. (2000) Germline PTEN mutations in three families with Cowden syndrome. Exp Dermatol 9:152–6

Celli J, Duijf P, Hamel BC et al. (1999) Heterozygous germline mutations in the *TP53* homolog p63 are the cause of EEC syndrome. Cell 99:143–53

Chai YL, Cui J, Shao N et al. (1999) The second BRCT domain of BRCA1 proteins interacts with *TP53* and stimulates transcription from the p21WAF1/CIP1 promoter. Oncogene 18:263–8

Chapman MS, Verma IM (1996) Transcriptional activation by BRCA1. Nature 382:678–9

Chehab NH, Malikzay A, Stavridi ES, Halazonetis TD (1999) Phosphorylation of Ser-20 mediates stabilization of human *TP53* in response to DNA damage. Proc Natl Acad Sci USA 96:13777–82

Chehab NH, Malikzay A, Appel M, Halazonetis TD (2000) Chk2/hCds1 functions as a DNA damage checkpoint in G(1) by stabilizing *TP53*. Genes Dev 14:278–88

Chen CF, Li S, Chen Y et al. (1996) The nuclear localization sequences of the BRCA1 protein interact with the importin-alpha subunit of the nuclear transport signal receptor. J Biol Chem 271:32863–8

Chen JJ, Silver D, Cantor S et al. (1999) BRCA1, BRCA2, and Rad51 operate in a common DNA damage response pathway. Cancer Res 59:1752s–1756s

Chen PL, Scully P, Shew JY et al. (1989) Phosphorylation of the retinoblastoma gene product is modulated during the cell cycle and cellular differentiation. Cell 58:1193–1198

Chen YM, Chen CF, Riley DJ et al. (1995) Aberrant subcellular localization of BRCA1 in breast cancer. Science 270:789–791

Cho YJ, Gorina S, Jeffrey PD et al. (1994) Crystal structure of a *TP53* tumourtumour suppressor DNA complex—understanding tumourtumourigenic mutations. Science 265:346–355

Christofori G, Semb H (1999) The role of the cell-adhesion molecule E-cadherin as a tumour-suppressor gene. Trends Biochem Sci 24:73–6

Clarke AR, Robanus Maaridag E, van Roon M et al. (1992) Requirement for a functional Rb-1 gene in murine development. Nature 359:328–330

Cleary ML (1991) Oncogenic conversion of transcription factors by chromosomal translocations. Cell 66:619–622

Cleary ML, Smith SD, Sklar J (1986) Cloning and structural analysis of cDNAs for bcl-2 and a hybrid bcl-2/immunoglobulin transcript resulting from the t(14;18) translocation. Cell 47:19–28

Clynes RA, Towers TL, Presta LG, Ravetch JV (2000) Inhibitory Fc receptors modulate in vivo cytoxicity against tumor targets. Nat Med 6:443–446

Cobrinik D, Whyte P, Peeper DS et al. (1993) Cell cycle-specific association of E2F with the p130 E1A-binding protein. Genes Dev 7:2392–2404

Collins FS (1996) BRCA1—lots of mutations, lots of dilemmas. N Engl J Med 334:186–188

Coppes MJ, Haber DA, Grundy PE (1994) Genetic events in the development of Wilms' tumourtumour. N Engl J Med 331:586–590

Cortez D, Wang Y, Qin J, Elledge SJ (1999) Requirement of ATM-dependent phosphorylation of BRCA1 in the DNA damage response to double-strand breaks. Science 286:1162–6

Crook T, Vousden KH (1992) Properties of *TP53* mutations detected in primary and secondary cervical cancers suggest mechanisms of metastasis and involvement of environmental carcinogens. EMBO J 11:3935–3940

Dang CV (1999) c-Myc target genes involved in cell growth, apoptosis, and metabolism. Mol Cell Biol 19:1–11

Davies DR, Armstrong JG, Thakker N et al. (1995) Severe Gardner syndrome in families with mutations restricted to a specific region of the APC gene. Am J Hum Genet 57:1151–8

Davies RC, Calvio C, Bratt E et al. (1998) WT1 interacts with the splicing factor U2AF65 in an isoform-dependent manner and can be incorporated into spliceosomes. Genes Dev 12:3217–3225

de Boer J, Hoeijmakers JH (2000) Nucleotide excision repair and human syndromes. Carcinogenesis 21:453–60

de Klein A, van Kessel AG, Grosveld G et al. (1982) A cellular oncogene is translocated to the Philadelphia chromosome in chronic myelocytic leukaemia. Nature 300:765–767

de Stanchina E, McCurrach ME, Zindy F et al. (1998) E1A signaling to *TP53* involves the p19 (ARF) tumor suppressor. Genes Dev 12:2434–2442

De Vitis LR, Tedde A, Vitelli F et al. (1996) Analysis of the neurofibromatosis type 2 gene in different human tumors of neuroectodermal origin. Hum Genet 97:638–41

DeCaprio JA, Ludlow JW, Figge J et al. (1988) SV40 large tumortumour antigen forms a specific complex with the product of the retinoblastoma susceptibility gene. Cell 54:275–283

DeClue JE, Papageorge AG, Fletcher JA et al. (1992) Abnormal regulation of mammalian p21ras contributes to malignant tumortumour growth in von Recklinghausen (type 1) neurofibromatosis. Cell 69:265–273

DePinho RA, Schreiber-Agus N, Alt FW (1991) Myc family oncogenes in the development of normal and neoplastic cells. Adv Cancer Res 57:1–46

Der CJ, Krontiris TG, Cooper GM (1982) Transforming genes of human bladder and lung carcinoma cell lines are homologous to the ras genes of Harvey and Kirsten sarcoma viruses. Proc Natl Acad Sci USA 79:3637–3640

Dietrich WF, Lander ES, Smith JS et al. (1993) Genetic identification of Mom-1, a major modifier locus affecting Min-induced intestinal neoplasia in the mouse. Cell 75:631–639

DiGiuseppe JA, Hruban RH, Offerhaus GJ (1994) Detection of K-ras mutations in mucinous pancreatic duct hyperplasia from a patient with a family history of pancreatic carcinoma. Am J Pathol 144:889–895

Di Lisa E, Bernardi P (1998) Mitochondrial function as a determinant of recovery or death in cell response to injury. Mol Cell Biochem. 184:379–391

Dobbie Z, Spycher M, Mary JL et al. (1996) Correlation between the development of extracolonic manifestations in FAP patients and mutations beyond codon 1403 in the APC gene. J Med Genet 33:274–80

Dougall WC, Qian X, Peterson NC et al. (1994) The neu-oncogene: signal transduction pathways, transformation mechanisms and evolving therapies. Oncogene 9:2109–2123

Drebin JA, Link VC, Greene MI (1988) Monoclonal antibodies reactive with distinct domains of the neu oncogene-encoded p185 molecule exert synergistic anti-tumortumour effects in vivo. Oncogene 2:273–277

Dreusicke D, Schulz GE (1986) The glycine-rich loop of adenylate kinase forms a giant anion hole. FEBS Lett 208:301–304

Drugan JK, Khosravi-Far R, White MA, Der CJ, Sung YJ, Hwang YW, Campbell SL (1996) Ras interaction with two distinct binding domains in Raf-1 may be required for Ras transformation. J Biol Chem 271:233–237

Dryja TP, Rapaport JM, Joyce JM, Petersen RA (1986) Molecular detection of deletions involving band q14 of chromosome 13 in retinoblastomas. Proc Natl Acad Sci USA 83:7391–7394

Duan DR, Pause A, Burgess WH et al. (1995) Inhibition of transcription elongation by the VHL tumortumour suppressor protein. Science 269:1402–1406

Dunlop MG, Farrington SM, Carothers AD et al. (1997) Cancer risk associated with germline DNA mismatch repair gene mutations. Hum Mol Genet 6:105–10

Dunn JM, Phillips RA, Zhu X et al. (1989) Mutations in the RB1 gene and their effects on transcription. Mol Cell Biol 9:4596–4604

Durbec PL, Larsson-Blomberg LB, Schuchardt A et al. (1996) Common origin and developmental dependence on c-ret of subsets of enteric and sympathetic neuroblasts. Development 122:349–58

Dyson N, Howley P, Munger K, Harlow E (1989) The human papillomavirus—16 E7 oncoprotein is able to bind to the retinoblastoma gene product. Science 243:934–937

Easton DF, Bishop DT, Ford D, Crockford GP (1993) Genetic linkage analysis in familial breast and ovarian cancer: Results from 214 families. The Breast Cancer Linkage Consortium. Am J Hum Genet 52:678–701

Eckner R, Ewen ME, Newsome D et al. (1994) Molecular cloning and functional analysis of the adenovirus E1A-associated 300-kD protein (p300) reveals a protein with properties of a transcriptional adaptor. Genes Dev 8:869–884

Eisenbarth I, Beyer K, Krone W, Assum G (2000) Toward a survey of somatic mutation of the NF1 gene in benign neurofibromas of patients with neurofibromatosis type 1. Am J Hum Genet 66:393–401

El-Deiry WS (1998) Regulation of TP53 downstream genes. Semin Cancer Biol 8:345–57

El-Deiry WS, Tokino T, Velculescu VE et al. (1993) Wafl, a potential mediator of TP53 tumortumour suppression. Cell 75:817–825

Eliyahu D, Goldfinger N, Pinhasi-Kimhi O et al. (1988) Meth A fibrosarcoma cells express two transforming mutant TP53 species. Oncogene 3:313–321

Ellis NA, Groden J, Ye TZ et al. (1995) The Bloom's syndrome gene product is homologous to RecQ helicases. Cell 83:655–66

Eng C, Crossey PA, Mulligan LM et al. (1995) Mutations in the RET proto-oncogene and the von Hippel-Lindau disease tumour suppressor gene in sporadic and syndromic phaeochromocytomas. J Med Genet 32:934–7

Eng C, Clayton D, Schuffenecker I et al. (1996) The relationship between specific RET proto-oncogene mutations and disease phenotype in multiple endocrine neoplasia type 2. International RET mutation consortium analysis. JAMA 276:1575–9

Esteller M, Silva JM, Dominguez G et al. (2000) Promoter hypermethylation and BRCA1 inactivation in sporadic breast and ovarian tumors. J Natl Cancer Inst 92:564–9

Evans DG, Huson SM, Donnai D et al. (1992) A genetic study of type 2 neurofibromatosis in the United Kingdom. I. Prevalence, mutation rate, fitness, and confirmation of maternal transmission effect on severity. J Med Genet 29:841–846

Evans DG, Trueman L, Wallace A et al. (1998) Genotype/phenotype correlations in type 2 neurofibromatosis (NF2): Evidence for more severe disease associated with truncating mutations. J Med Genet 35:450–5

Ewen ME, Xing YG, Lawrence JB, Livingston DM (1991) Molecular cloning, chromosomal mapping, and expression of the cDNA for p107, a retinoblastoma gene product-related protein. Cell 66:1155–1164

Fakharzadeh SS, Trusko SP, George DL (1991) TumorTumourigenic potential associated with enhanced expression of a gene that is amplified in a mouse tumortumour cell line. EMBO J 10:1565–1569

Farrington SM, Lin-Goerke J, Ling J et al. (1998) Systematic analysis of hMSH2 and hMLH1 in young colon cancer patients and controls. Am J Hum Genet 63:749–59

Fearon ER (1993) K-ras gene mutation as a pathogenetic and diagnostic marker in human cancer. J Natl Cancer Inst 85:1978–1980

Fearon ER (1995) Oncogenes and tumour suppressor genes. p. 11. In Abeloff MD, Armitage JO, Lichter AS, Niederhuber JE (eds): Clinical Oncology. Churchill Livingstone, New York

Fearon ER, Hamilton S, Vogelstein B (1987) Clonal analysis of human colorectal tumours. Science 238:193–197

Fearon ER, Vogelstein B (1990) A genetic model for colorectal tumourigenesis. Cell 61:759–767

Fearon ER, Vogelstein B (1993) Tumour suppressor genes. In Holland JF, Frei E III, Bast RC Jr et al. (eds): Cancer Medicine, 3rd edn. Lea & Febiger, Philadelphia

Fishel R, Lescoe MK, Rao MRS et al. (1993) The human mutator gene homolog MSH2 and its association with hereditary nonpolyposis colon cancer. Cell 75:1027–1038

Fisher DE (1994) Apoptosis in cancer therapy: Crossing the threshold. Cell 78:539–542

Fitzgerald MG, MacDonald DJ, Krainer M et al. (1996) Germ-line BRCA1 mutations in Jewish and non-Jewish women with early-onset breast cancer. N Engl J Med 334:143–149

FitzGerald MG, Bean JM, Hegde SR et al. (1997) Heterozygous ATM mutations do not contribute to early onset of breast cancer. Nat Genet 15:307–10

Ford D, Easton DF, Bishop DT et al. (1994) Risks of cancer in BRCA1-mutation carriers. Breast Cancer Linkage Consortium. Lancet 343:692–5

Ford D, Easton DF, Stratton M et al. (1998) Genetic heterogeneity and penetrance analysis of the BRCA1 and BRCA2 genes in breast cancer families. The Breast Cancer Linkage Consortium. Am J Hum Genet 62:676–89

Foulkes WD (1998) BRCA1 and BRCA2: Penetrating the clinical arena. Lancet 352:1325–6

Fountain JW, Wallace MR, Bruce MA et al. (1989) Physical mapping of a translocation breakpoint in neurofibromatosis. Science 244:1085–1087

Francke U (1976) Retinoblastoma and chromosome 13. Cytogenet Cell Genet 16:131–134

Franken SM, Scheidig AJ, Krengel U et al. (1993) Three-dimensional structures and properties of a transforming and a nontransforming glycine-12 mutant of p21H-ras. Biochemistry 32:8411–8420

Frayling IM, Beck NE, Ilyas M et al. (1998) The APC variants I1307K and E1317Q are associated with colorectal tumors, but not always with a family history. Proc Natl Acad Sci USA 95:10722–7

Friedman LS, Thistlethwaite FC, Patel KJ et al. (1998) Thymic lymphomas in mice with a truncating mutation in Brca2. Cancer Res 58:1338–43

Friend S (1994) TP53: A glimpse at the puppet behind the shadow play. Science 265:334–335

Friend SH, Bernards R, Rogelj S et al. (1986) A human DNA segment with properties of the gene that predisposes to retinoblastoma and osteosarcoma. Nature 323:643–646

Fry M, Loeb LA (1998) The three faces of the WS helicase. Nat Genet 19:308–9

Fujiwara T, Grimm EA, Mukhopadhyay T et al. (1994) Induction of chemosensitivity in human lung cancer cells in vivo by adenovirus-mediated transfer of the wild-type TP53 gene. Cancer Res 54:2287–2291

Fujiwara T, Stolker JM, Watanabe T et al. (1998) Accumulated clonal genetic alterations in familial and sporadic colorectal carcinomas with widespread instability in microsatellite sequences. Am J Pathol 153:1063–78

Fuks F, Milner J, Kouzarides T (1998) BRCA2 associates with acetyltransferase activity when bound to P/CAF. Oncogene 17:2531–4

Fuller GN, Bignel SH (1992) Amplified cellular oncogenes in neoplasms of the human central nervous system. Mutat Res 276:299–306

Fung YK, Murphree AL, T'Ang A et al. (1987) Structural evidence for the authenticity of the human retinoblastoma gene. Science 236:1657–1661

Furnari FB, Huang HJ, Cavenee WK (1998) The phosphoinositol phosphatase activity of PTEN mediates a serum-sensitive G1 growth arrest in glioma cells. Cancer Res 58:5002–8

Futreal PA, Liu QY, Shattuckeidens D et al. (1994) BRCA1 mutations in primary breast and ovarian carcinomas. Science 266:120–122

Ganly I, Kirn D, Eckhardt SG et al. (2000) A phase I study of Onyx-015, an E1B attenuated adenovirus, administered intratumorally to patients with recurrent head and neck cancer. Clin Cancer Res 6:798–806

Gatei M, Young D, Cerosaletti KM et al. (2000) ATM-dependent phosphorylation of nibrin in response to radiation exposure. Nat Genet 25:115–9

Gayther SA, Wells D, SenGupta SB et al. (1994) Regionally clustered APC mutations are associated with a severe phenotype and occur at a high frequency in new mutation cases of adenomatous polyposis coli. Hum Mol Genet 3:53–6

Gayther SA, Warren W, Mazoyer S et al. (1995) Germline mutations of the BRCA1 gene in breast and ovarian cancer families provide evidence for a genotype-phenotype correlation. Nat Genet 11:428–33

Gayther SA, Mangion J, Russell P et al. (1997) Variation of risks of breast and ovarian cancer associated with different germline mutations of the BRCA2 gene. Nat Genet 15:103–5

Geitvik GA, Hoyheim B, Gedde-Dahl T et al. (1987) The Kidd (JK) blood group locus assigned to chromosome 18 by close linkage to a DNA-RFLP. Hum Genet 77:205–209

Gessler M, Poustka A, Cavenee W et al. (1990) Homozygous deletion in Wilms tumours of a zinc-finger gene identified by chromosome jumping. Nature 343:774–778

Giaretti W, Monaco R, Pujic N, Rapallo A, Nigro S, and Geido E (1996) Intratumor heterogeneity of K-ras2 mutations in colorectal adenocarcinomas: association with degree of DNA aneuploidy. Am J Pathol 149:237–245

Goddard AD, Balakier H, Canton M et al. (1988) Infrequent genomic rearrangement and normal expression of the putative RB1 gene in retinoblastoma tumours. Mol Cell Biol 8:2082–2088

Goldstein AM, Tucker MA (1995) Genetic epidemiology of familial melanoma. Dermatol Clin 13:605–612

Goutebroze L, Brault E, Muchardt C et al. (2000) Cloning and characterization of SCHIP-1, a novel protein interacting specifically with spliced isoforms and naturally occurring mutant NF2 proteins. Mol Cell Biol 20:1699–712

Gowen LC, Avrutskaya AV, Latour AM et al. (1998) BRCA1 required for transcription-coupled repair of oxidative DNA damage. Science 281:1009–12

Gray JW, Collins C (2000) Genome changes in gene expression in human solid tumors. Carcinogen 21:443–452

Gray MD, Shen JC, Kamath-Loeb AS et al. (1997) The Werner syndrome protein is a DNA helicase. Nat Genet 17:100–3

Greenblatt MS, Bennett WP, Hollstein M, Harris CC (1994) Mutations in the TP53 tumour suppressor gene: clues to cancer etiology and molecular pathogenesis. Cancer Res 54:4855–4878

Gregory PE, Gutmann DH, Mitchell A et al. (1993) Neurofibromatosis type 1 gene product (neurofibromin) associates with microtubules. Somat Cell Mol Genet 19:265–74

Grieco M, Santoro M, Berlingieri MT et al. (1990) PTC is a novel rearranged form of the ret proto-oncogene and is frequently detected in vivo in human thyroid papillary carcinomas. Cell 60:557–563

Groden J, Thliveris A, Samowitz W et al. (1991) Identification and characterization of the familial adenomatous polyposis coli gene. Cell 66:589–600

Groffen J, Stephenson JR, Heisterkamp N et al. (1984) Philadelphia chromosomal breakpoints are clustered within a limited region, bcr, on chromosome 22. Cell 36:93–99

Grundy P, Coppes MJ, Haber D (1995) Molecular genetics of Wilms tumourtumour. Hematol Oncol Clin North Am 9:1201–1215

Gryfe R, Di Nicola N, Lal G et al. (1999) Inherited colorectal polyposis and cancer risk of the APC I1307K polymorphism. Am J Hum Genet 64:378–84

Guilford P, Hopkins J, Harraway J et al. (1998) E-cadherin germline mutations in familial gastric cancer. Nature 392:402–5

Gutmann DH, Sherman L, Seftor L et al. (1999) Increased expression of the NF2 tumor suppressor gene product, merlin, impairs cell motility, adhesionand spreading. Hum Mol Genet 8:267–75

Haaland M (1911) Spontaneous tumours in mice. Sci Rep Invest Imp Cancer Res Fund 4:1

Haber DA, Housman DE (1992) The genetics of Wilms' tumourtumour. Adv Cancer Res 59:41–68

Haber DA, Sohn RL, Buckler AJ et al. (1991) Alternative splicing and genomic structure of the Wilms tumour gene WT1. Proc Natl Acad Sci USA 88:9618–9622

Haber JE (1998) The many interfaces of Mrell. Cell 95:583–6

Hall JM, Lee MK, Newman B et al. (1990) Linkage of early onset breast cancer to chromosome 17q21. Science 250:1684–1689

Hamilton SR, Liu B, Parsons RE (1995) The molecular basis of Turcots syndrome. N Engl J Med 332:839–847

Han SY, Kato H, Kato S et al. (2000) Functional evaluation of PTEN missense mutations using in vitro phosphoinositide phosphatase assay. Cancer Res 60:3147–51

Hannon GJ, Demetrick D, Beach D (1993) Isolation of the Rb-related p130 through its interaction with CDK2 and cyclins. Genes Dev 7:2378–2391

Hansen MF, Cavanee WK (1987) Genetics of cancer predisposition. Cancer Res 47:5518–5527

Hansen MF, Koufos A, Gallie BL (1985) Osteosarcoma and retinoblastoma: a shared chromosomal mechanism revealing recessive predisposition. Proc Natl Acad Sci USA 82:6216–6220

Hara E, Smith R, Parry D, Tahara H, Stone S, Peters G (1996) Regulation of p16CDKN2 expression and its implications for cell immortalization and senescence. Mol Cell Biol 16:859–67

Harbour JW, Lai SL, Whang-Peng J et al. (1988) Abnormalities in structure and expression of the human retinoblastoma gene in SCLC. Science 241:353–357

Harkin DP, Bean JM, Miklos D et al. (1999) Induction of GADD45 and JNK/SAPK-dependent apoptosis following inducible expression of BRCA1. Cell 97:575–86

Harper JW, Adami GR, Wei N et al. (1993) The p21 cdk-interacting protein cipl is a potent inhibitor of G1 cyclin-dependent kinases. Cell 75:805–816

Harris H (1988) The analysis of malignancy in cell fusion: the position in 1988. Cancer Res 48:3302–3306

Hart MJ, de los Santos R, Albert IN et al. (1998) Downregulation of beta-catenin by human Axin and its association with the APC tumor suppressor, beta-catenin and GSK3 beta. Curr Biol 8:573–81

Hayward WS, Neel BG, Astrin SM (1981) Activation of a cellular onc gene by promoter insertion in ALV-induced lymphoid leukosis. Nature 290:475–80

He TC, Sparks AB, Rago C et al. (1998) Identification of c-MYC as a target of the APC pathway. Science 281:1509–12

He TC, Chan TA, Vogelstein B, Kinzler KW (1999) PPARdelta is an APC-regulated target of nonsteroidal anti-inflammatory drugs. Cell 99:335–45

Heisterkamp N, Stephenson JR, Groffen J et al. (1983) Localization of the c-abl oncogene adjacent to a translocation break point in chronic myelocytic leukaemia. Nature 306:239–242

Helin, K (1998) Regulation of cell proliferation by the E2F transcription factors. Curr Opin Genet Dev 8:28–35

Helin K, Lees JA, Vidal M et al. (1992) A cDNA encoding a pRB-binding protein with properties of the transcription factor E2F. Cell 70:337–350

Helin K, Wu CL, Fattaey AR (1993) Heterodimerization of the transcription factors E2F-1 and DP-1 leads to cooperative transactivation. Genes Dev 7:1850–1861

Hemminki A, Markie D, Tomlinson I et al. (1998) A serine/threonine kinase gene defective in Peutz-Jeghers syndrome. Nature 391:184–7

Herman JG, Latif F, Weng Y et al. (1994) Silencing of the VHL tumortumour-suppressor gene by DNA methylation in renal carcinoma. Proc Natl Acad Sci USA 91:9700–9704

Herman JG, Merlo A, Mao L et al. (1995) Inactivation of the cdkn2/p16INK4a/mts1 gene is frequently associated with aberrant DNA methylation in all common human cancers. Cancer Res 55:4525–4530

Hermeking H, Eick D (1994) Mediation of c-Myc-induced apoptosis by TP53. Science 265:2091–2093

Hermeking H, Lengauer C, Polyak K et al. (1997) 14-3-3 sigma is a TP53-regulated inhibitor of G2/M progression. Mol Cell 1:3–11

Herrera L, Kakati S, Gibas L et al. (1986) Gardner syndrome in a man with an interstitial deletion of 5q. Am J Med Genet 25:473–476

Hinds PW, Finlay C, Levin AJ (1989) Mutation is required to activate the TP53 gene for cooperation with the ras oncogene and transformation. J Virol 63:739–746

Hirao A, Kong YY, Matsuoka S et al. (2000) DNA damage-induced activation of TP53 by the checkpoint kinase Chk2. Science 287:1824–7

Hockenbery D, Nunez G, Milliman C et al. (1990) Bcl-2 is an inner mitochondrial membrane protein that blocks programmed cell death. Nature 348:334–336

Hofstra RM, Landsvater RM, Ceccherini I et al. (1994) A mutation in the RET proto-oncogene associated with multiple endocrine neoplasia type 2B and sporadic medullary thyroid carcinoma. Nature 367:375–376

Horii A, Nakatsuru S, Miyoshi Y et al. (1992) The APC gene, responsible for familial adenomatous polyposis, is mutated in human gastric cancer. Cancer Res 52:3231–3233

Horowitz JM, Yandell DW, Park SH et al. (1989) Point mutational inactivation of the retinoblastoma antioncogene. Science 243:937–940

Hosono S, Gross I, English MA et al. (2000) E-cadherin is a WT1 target gene. J Biol Chem 275:10943–53

Hu CD, Kariya K, Tamada M, Akasaka K, Shirouzu M, Yokoyama S, Kataoka T (1995) Cysteine-rich region of Raf-1 interacts with activator domain of post-translationally modified Ha-Ras. J Biol Chem 270, 30274–30277

Huang DC, Strasser A (2000) BH3-Only proteins-essential initiators of apoptotic cell death. Cell 103:839–942

Huang HS, Yee J, Shew J et al. (1988) Suppression of the neoplastic phenotype by replacement of the Rb gene in human cancer cells. Science 242:1563–1566

Huang L, Ichimaru E, Pestonjamasp K et al. (1998) Merlin differs from moesin in binding to F-actin and in its intra- and intermolecular interactions. Biochem Biophys Res Commun 248:548–53

Huang S, Li B, Gray MD et al. (1998) The premature ageing syndrome protein, WRN, is a 3′→5′ exonuclease. Nat Genet 20:114–6

Hudziak RM, Lewis GD, Shalaby MR, Eessalu TE, Aggarwal BB, Ullrich A, Shepard HM (1988) Amplified expression of the HER2/ERBB2 oncogene induces resistance to tumor necrosis factor alpha in NIH 3T3 cells. Proc Natl Acad Sci USA 85:5102–5106

Huibregtse JM, Scheffner M, Howley PM (1991) A cellular protein mediates association of TP53 with the E6 oncoprotein of human papillomavirus types 16 or 18. EMBO J 10:4129–4135

Hunter T (1991) Cooperation between oncogenes. Cell 64:249–270

Hurwitz E, Stancovski I, Sela M, Yarden Y (1995) Suppression and promotion of tumor growth by monoclonal antibodies to ErbB-2 differentially correlate with cellular uptake. Proc Natl Acad Sci USA 92:3353–3357

Huson SM, Compston DA, Clark P, Harper PS (1989) A genetic study of von Recklinghausen neurofibromatosis in south east Wales. I. Prevalence, fitness, mutation rate, and effect of parental transmission on severity. J Med Genet 26:704–11

Hussussian CJ, Struewing JP, Goldstein AM (1994) Germline p16INK4a mutations in familial melanoma. Nat Genet 8:15–21

Ichii S, Takeda S, Horii A et al. (1993) Detailed analysis of genetic alterations in colorectal tumors from patients with and without familial adenomatous polyposis (FAP). Oncogene 8:2399–405

Inaba T, Roberts WM, Shapiro LH (1992) Fusion of the leucine zipper gene HLF to the E2A gene in human acute B-lineage leukemia. Science 257:531–534

Inskip HM, Kinlen LJ, Taylor AM et al. (1999) Risk of breast cancer and other cancers in heterozygotes for ataxia-telangiectasia. Br J Cancer 79:1304–7

Ionov Y, Peinado MA, Malkhosyan S et al. (1993) Ubiquitous somatic mutations in simple repeated sequences reveal a new mechanism for colonic carcinogenesis. Nature 363:558–61

Jacks T, Fazeli A, Schmitt EM et al. (1992) Effects of an Rb mutation in the mouse. Nature 359:295–300

Jacobs JJ, Kieboom K, Marino S, DePinho RA, van Lohuizen M (1999) The oncogene and Polycomb-group gene bmi-1 regulates cell proliferation and senescence through the ink4a locus. Nature 397:164–168

Jadayel D, Fain P, Upadhyaya M et al. (1990) Paternal origin of new mutations in von Recklinghausen neurofibromatosis. Nature 343:558–9

Jenkins JR, Rudge K, Currie GA (1984) Cellular immortalization by a cDNA clone encoding the transformation-associated phosphoprotein TP53. Nature 312:651–654

Jenne DE, Reimann H, Nezu J et al. (1998) Peutz-Jeghers syndrome is caused by mutations in a novel serine threonine kinase. Nat Genet 18:38–43

Jing S, Wen D, Yu Y et al. (1996) GDNF-induced activation of the ret protein tyrosine kinase is mediated by GDNFR-alpha, a novel receptor for GDNF. Cell 85:1113–24

Joazeiro CA, Wing SS, Huang H et al. (1999) The tyrosine kinase negative regulator c-Cbl as a RING-type, E2-dependent ubiquitin-protein ligase. Science 286:309–312

John AM, Ruggieri M, Ferner R, Upadhyaya M (2000) A search for evidence of somatic mutations in the NF1 gene. J Med Genet 37:44–9

Johnson MR, Look AT, DeClue JE et al. (1993) Inactivation of the NF1 gene in human melanoma and neuroblastoma cell lines without impaired regulation of GTP Ras. Proc Natl Acad Sci USA 90:5539–5543

Joslyn G, Carlson M, Thliveris A et al. (1991) Identification of deletion mutations and three new genes at the familial polyposis locus. Cell 66:601–613

Kaelin WG, Jr (1999) The emerging TP53 gene family. J Natl Cancer Inst 91:594–8

Kaelin WG, Maher ER (1998) The VHL tumour-suppressor gene paradigm. Trends Genet 14:423–6

Kaelin WG, Jr, Krek W, Sellers WR et al. (1992) Expression cloning of a cDNA encoding a retinoblastoma-binding protein with E2F-like properties. Cell 70:351–364

Kaghad M, Bonnet H, Yang A et al. (1997) Monoallelically expressed gene related to TP53 at 1p36, a region frequently deleted in neuroblastoma and other human cancers. Cell 90:809–19

Kallioniemi A, Kallioniemi OP, Sudar D, Rutovitz D, Gray JW, Waldman F and Pinkel D (1992) Comparative genomic hybridization for molecular cytogenetic analysis of solid tumors. Science 258:818–821

Kamb A, Gruis NA, Weaver-Feldhaus J et al. (1994a) A cell cycle regulator potentially involved in genesis of many tumortumour types. Science 264:436–440

Kamb A, Shattuck-Eidens D, Eeles R et al. (1994b) Analysis of the p16INK4a gene (CDKN2) as a candidate for the chromosome 9p melanoma susceptibility locus. Nat Genet 8:23–26

Kamijo T, Zindy F, Roussel MF et al. (1997) Tumor suppression at the mouse INK4a locus mediated by the alternative reading frame product p19ARF. Cell 91:649–659

Kamps MP, Murre C, Sun XH, Baltimore D (1990) A new homeobox gene contributes the DNA binding domain of the t(1;19) translocation protein in pre-B ALL. Cell 60:547–555

Karow JK, Newman RH, Freemont PS, Hickson ID (1999) Oligomeric ring structure of the Bloom's syndrome helicase. Curr Biol 9:597–600

Kastan MB, Onyekwere O, Sidransky D et al. (1991) Participation of TP53 protein in the cellular response to DNA damage. Cancer Res 51:6304–6311

Kastan M, Zhan Q, El-Diery W et al. (1992) A mammalian cell cycle checkpoint pathway utilizing TP53 and GADD45 is defective in ataxia-telangiectasia. Cell 71:587–598

Kato GJ, Dang CV (1992) Function of the c-myc oncoprotein. FASEB J 6:3065–3072

Kessis T, Slebos R, Han S et al. (1993) TP53 gene mutations and mdm2 amplification are uncommon in primary carcinomas of the uterine cervix. Am J Pathol 143:1398–1405

Keohavong P, DeMichele MAA, Melacrinos AC, Landreneau RJ, Weyant RJ, Siegfried JM (1996) Detection of K-ras Mutations in Lung Carcinomas: Relationship to Prognosis. Clin Cancer Res 2:411–418

Khanna KK (2000) Cancer risk and the ATM gene: a continuing debate. J Natl Cancer Inst 92:795–802

Khatib ZA, Matsushime H, Valentine M et al. (1993) Coamplification of the CDK4 gene with MDM2 and GLI in human sarcomas. Cancer Res 53:5535–5541

Kibel A, Iliopoulos O, DeCaprio JA et al. (1995) Binding of the von Hippel-Lindau tumortumour suppressor protein to Elongin B and C. Science 269:1444–1446

King-Underwood L, Pritchard-Jones K (1998) Wilms' tumor (WT1) gene mutations occur mainly in acute myeloid leukemia and may confer drug resistance. Blood 91:2961–2968

Kinzler K, Nilbert M, Su L et al. (1991) Identification of FAP locus genes from chromosome 5q21. Science 253:661–665

Kinzler KW, Vogelstein, B (1996) Lessons from hereditary colorectal cancer. Cell 87:159–70

Kinzler KW, Vogelstein B (1997) Cancer-susceptibility genes. Gatekeepers and caretakers. Nature 386:761–3

Kinzler KW, Bigner SH, Bigner DD et al. (1987) Identification of an amplified, highly expressed gene in a human glioma. Science 236:70–73

Kitao S, Shimamoto A, Goto M et al. (1999) Mutations in RECQL4 cause a subset of cases of Rothmund-Thomson syndrome. Nat Genet 22:82–4

Klapper LN, Vaisman N, Hurwitz E, Pinkas KR, Yarden Y (2000a) Biochemical and clinical implications of the ErbB/HER signaling network of growth factor receptors. Adv Cancer Res 77:25–79

Klapper LN, Waterman H, Sela M, Yarden Y (2000b) Tumor-inhibitory antibodies to HER-2/ErbB-2 may act by recruiting c-Cbl and enhancing ubiquitination of HER-2. Cancer Res 60(13):3384–8

Kleiman FE, Manley JL (1999) Functional interaction of BRCA1-associated BARD1 with polyadenylation factor CstF-50. Science 285:1576–9

Klein RD, Sherman D, Ho WH et al. (1997) A GPI-linked protein that interacts with Ret to form a candidate neurturin receptor. Nature 387:717–21

Kley N, Whaley J, Seizinger BR (1995) Hereditary tumortumour syndromes, tumortumour suppressor genes, nervous system, and disorders. Neurofibromatosis type 2 and von Hippel-Lindau disease—from gene cloning to function. Glia 15:297–307

Knudson A (1971) Mutation and cancer: Statistical study of retinoblastoma. Proc Natl Acad Sci USA 68:820–823

Knudson A (1985) Hereditary cancer, oncogenes, and antioncogenes. Cancer Res 45:1437–1443

Koga H, Araki N, Takeshima H et al. (1998) Impairment of cell adhesion by expression of the mutant neurofibromatosis type 2 (NF2) genes which lack exons in the ERM-homology domain. Oncogene 17:801–10

Koivunen J, Yla-Outinen H, Korkiamaki T et al. (2000) New function for NF1 tumor suppressor. J Invest Dermatol 114:473–9

Kong D, Suzuki A, Zou TT et al. (1997) PTEN1 is frequently mutated in primary endometrial carcinomas. Nat Genet 17:143–4

Korinek V, Barker N, Morin PJ et al. (1997) Constitutive transcriptional activation by a beta-catenin-Tcf complex in APC-/- colon carcinoma. Science 275:1784–7

Krontiris TG, Cooper GM (1981) Transforming activity of human tumortumour DNAs. Proc Natl Acad Sci USA 78:1181–1184

Laken SJ, Petersen GM, Gruber SB et al. (1997) Familial colorectal cancer in Ashkenazim due to a hypermutable tract in APC. Nat Genet 17:79–83

Lamlum H, Ilyas M, Rowan A et al. (1999) The type of somatic mutation at APC in familial adenomatous polyposis is determined by the site of the germline mutation: A new facet to Knudson's "two-hit" hypothesis. Nat Med 5:1071–5

Lammie GA, Fantl V, Smith R et al. (1991) D11S287, a putative oncogene on chromosome 11q13, is amplified and expressed in squamous cell and mammary carcinomas and linked to BCL-1. Oncogene 6:439–444

Lammie GA, Smith R, Silver J et al. (1992) Proviral insertions near cyclin D1 in mouse lymphomas: A parallel for BCL1 translocations in human B-cell neoplasms. Oncogene 7:2381–2387

Lane D, Benchimol S (1990) TP53: Oncogene or anti-oncogene? Genes Dev 4:1–8

Lane D, Crawford L (1979) T antigen is bound to a host protein in SV40-transformed cells. Nature 278:261–263

Lane DP (1992) TP53, guardian of the genome. Nature 358:15–16

Lane DP (1999) Exploiting the TP53 pathway for cancer diagnosis and therapy. Br J Cancer 80 Suppl 1:1–5

Lane DP, Hall PA (1997) MDM2—arbiter of TP53's destruction. Trends Biochem Sci 22:372–4

Lane HA, Beuvink I, Motoyama AB, Daly JM, Neve RM, Hynes NE (2000) ErbB2 potentiates breast tumor proliferation through modulation of p27 (Kip1)-Cdk2 complex formation: Receptor overexpression does not determine growth dependency. Mol Cell Biol 20:3210–3223

Latif F, Tory K, Gnarra J et al. (1993) Identification of the von Bippel-Lindau disease tumortumour suppressor gene. Science 260:1317–1320

Lavelle F, Riou JF, Laoui A et al. (2000) Telomerase: A therapeutic target for the third millennium? Crit Rev Oncol Hemat 34:111–126

Leach FS, Nicolaides NC, Papadopoulos N et al. (1993) Mutations of a muts homolog in hereditary nonpolyposis colorectal cancer. Cell 75:1215–1226

Lee EY, To H, Shew JY et al. (1988) Inactivation of the retinoblastoma susceptibility gene in human breast cancers. Science 241:218–221

Lee EY, Chang CY, Hu N et al. (1992) Mice deficient for Rb are nonviable and show defects in neurogenesis and haematopoiesis. Nature 359:288–294

Lee JO, Russo AA, Pavletich NP (1998) Structure of the retinoblastoma tumour-suppressor pocket domain bound to a peptide from HPV E7. Nature 391:859–65

Lee W, Shew J, Hong F et al. (1987b) The retinoblastoma susceptibility gene encodes a nuclear phosphoprotein associated with DNA binding activity. Nature 329:642–645

Lee WH, Bookstein R, Hong F et al. (1987a) Human retinoblastoma susceptibility gene: cloning, identification and sequence. Science 235:1394–1399

Lee WH, Trainer AH, Friedman LS et al. (1999) Mitotic checkpoint inactivation fosters transformation in cells lacking the breast cancer susceptibility gene, Brca2. Mol Cell 4:1–10

Leppert M, Dobbs M, Scambler P et al. (1987) The gene for familial polyposis coli maps to the long arm of chromosome 5. Science 238:1411–1414

Leppert M, Burt R, Hughes JP et al. (1990) Genetic analysis of an inherited predisposition to colon cancer in a family with a variable number of adenomatous polyps. N Engl J Med 322:904–908

Leung SY, Yuen ST, Chung LP et al. (1999) hMLH1 promoter methylation and lack of hMLH1 expression in sporadic gastric carcinomas with high-frequency microsatellite instability. Cancer Res 59:159–64

Levine RL, Cargile CB, Blazes MS et al. (1998) PTEN mutations and microsatellite instability in complex atypical hyperplasia, a precursor lesion to uterine endometrioid carcinoma. Cancer Res 58:3254–8

Li J, Yen C, Liaw D et al. (1997) PTEN, a putative protein tyrosine phosphatase gene mutated in human brain, breast, and prostate cancer. Science 275:1943–7

Li Y, Graham C, Lacy S (1993) The adenovirus ElA-associated 130-kD protein is encoded by a member of the retinoblastoma gene family and physically interacts with cyclins A and E. Genes Dev 7:2366–2377

Liaw D, Marsh DJ, Li J et al. (1997) Germline mutations of the PTEN gene in Cowden disease, an inherited breast and thyroid cancer syndrome. Nat Genet 16:64–7

Lim DS, Kim ST, Xu B et al. (2000) ATM phosphorylates p95/nbs1 in an S-phase checkpoint pathway. Nature 404:613–7

Lin AW, Barradas M, Stone JC, van Aelst L, Serrano M and Lowe SW (1998) Premature senescence involving TP53 and p16 is activated in response to constitutive MEK/MAPK mitogenic signaling. Genes Dev 12:3008–3019

Lindblom A, Tannergard P, Werelius B, Nordenskjold M (1993) Genetic mapping of a second locus predisposing to hereditary non-polyposis colon cancer. Nature Genet 5:279–282

Linzer D, Levine A (1979) Characterization of a 54K dalton cellular SV40 tumortumour antigen present in SV40-transformed cells and uninfected embryonal carcinoma cells. Cell 17:43–52

Little CD, Nau MM, Carney DN (1983) Amplification and expression of the c-myc oncogene in human lung cancer cell lines. Nature 306:194–196

Little M, Holmes G and Walsh P (1999) WT1: What has the last decade told us? Bioessays 21:191–202

Liu X, Vega QC, Decker RA et al. (1996) Oncogenic RET receptors display different autophosphorylation sites and substrate binding specificities. J Biol Chem 271:5309–12

Lopez-Ilasaca M, Crespo P, Pellici PG, Gutkind JS, Wetzker R (1997) Linkage of G protein-coupled receptors to the MAPK signaling pathway through PI 3-kinase gamma. Science 275:394–397

Lorick KL, Jensen JP, Fang S et al. (1999) RING fingers mediate ubiquitin-conjugating enzyme (E2)-dependent ubiquitination. Proc Natl Acad Sci USA 96:11364–9

Lowe SW, Ruley HE (1993) Stabilization of the TP53 tumor suppressor is induced by adenovirus 5 E1A and accompanies apoptosis. Genes Dev 7:535–545

Lowy DR, Willumsen BM (1993) Function and regulation of ras. Annu Rev Biochem 62:851–891

Lugo TG, Pendergast AM, Muller AJ, Witte ON (1990) Tyrosine kinase activity and transformation potency of bcr-abl oncogene products. Science 247:1079–1082

Luo RX, Postigo AA, Dean DC (1998) Rb interacts with histone deacetylase to repress transcription. Cell 92:463–73

Lynch ED, Ostermeyer EA, Lee MK et al. (1997) Inherited mutations in PTEN that are associated with breast cancer, cowden disease, and juvenile polyposis. Am J Hum Genet 61:1254–60

Lynch HT, de la Chapelle A (1999) Genetic susceptibility to non-polyposis colorectal cancer. J Med Genet 36:801–18

Lynch H, Schuelke G, Kimberling W et al. (1985) Hereditary nonpolyposis colorectal cancer (Lynch syndromes I and II). II. Biomarker studies. Cancer 56:939–951

Lynch HT, Smyrk TC, Watson P et al. (1993) Genetics, natural history, tumortumour spectrum, and pathology of hereditary nonpolyposis colorectal cancer: An updated review. Gastroenterology 104:1535–1549

McKay IA, Paterson H, Brown R, Toksoz D, Marshall CJ, Hall A (1986) N-ras and human cancer. Anticancer Res 6, 483–90

Magnaghi-Jaulin L, Groisman R, Naguibneva I et al. (1998) Retinoblastoma protein represses transcription by recruiting a histone deacetylase. Nature 391:601–5

Maher ER, Webster AR, Moore AT (1995) Clinical features and molecular genetics of Von Hippel-Lindau disease. Ophthalmic Paediatr Genet 16:79–84

Malkin D, Li FP, Strong LC et al. (1990) Germ line TP53 mutations in a familial syndrome of breast cancer, sarcomas, and other neoplasms. Science 250:1233–1238

Mangeat P, Roy C, Martin M (1999) ERM proteins in cell adhesion and membrane dynamics. Trends Cell Biol 9:187–92

Marcu KB, Bossone SA, Patel AJ (1992) Myc function and regulation. Annu Rev Biochem 61:809–860

Markowitz S, Wang J, Myeroff L et al. (1995) Inactivation of the type II TGF-beta receptor in colon cancer cells with microsatellite instability. Science 268:1336–8

Marsh DJ, Dahia PL, Zheng Z et al. (1997a) Germline mutations in PTEN are present in Bannayan-Zonana syndrome. Nat Genet 16:333–4

Marsh DJ, Zheng Z, Zedenius J et al. (1997b) Differential loss of heterozygosity in the region of the Cowden locus within 10q22–23 in follicular thyroid adenomas and carcinomas. Cancer Research 57:500–3

Marsh DJ, Coulon V, Lunetta KL et al. (1998) Mutation spectrum and genotype-phenotype analyses in Cowden disease and Bannayan-Zonana syndrome, two hamartoma syndromes with germline PTEN mutation. Hum Mol Genet 7:507–15

Marsh DJ, Kum JB, Lunetta KL et al. (1999) PTEN mutation spectrum and genotype-phenotype correlations in Bannayan-Riley-Ruvalcaba syndrome suggest a single entity with Cowden syndrome. Hum Mol Genet 8:1461–72

Marshall C (1991) TumorTumour suppressor genes. Cell 64:313–326

Masuda H, Miller C, Koeffler HP (1987) Rearrangement of the TP53 gene in human osteogenic sarcomas. Proc Natl Acad Sci USA 84:7716–7719

Matsuoka S, Huang M, Elledge SJ (1998) Linkage of ATM to cell cycle regulation by the Chk2 protein kinase. Science 282:1893–7

Matsuura S, Tauchi H, Nakamura A et al. (1998) Positional cloning of the gene for Nijmegen breakage syndrome. Nat Genet 19:179–81

Maxwell PH, Wiesener MS, Chang GW et al. (1999) The tumour suppressor protein VHL targets hypoxia-inducible factors for oxygen-dependent proteolysis. Nature 399:271–5

McCormick F (1993) Signal transduction. How receptors turn Ras on. Nature 363:15–16

Melki JR, Vincent PC, Brown RD, Clark SJ (2000) Hypermethylation of E-cadherin in leukemia. Blood 95:3208–13

Merajver SD, Pham TM, Caduff RF et al. (1995) Somatic mutations in the BRCA1 gene in sporadic ovarian tumours. Nature Genet 9:439–443

Merlo A, Herman JG, Mao L et al. (1995) 5′ CPG island methylation is associated with transcriptional silencing of the tumour suppressor p16INK4a/cdkn2/mts1 in human cancers. Nature Med 1:686–692

Messiaen LM, Callens T, Mortier G et al. (2000) Exhaustive mutation analysis of the NF1 gene allows identification of 95% of mutations and reveals a high frequency of unusual splicing defects. Hum Mutat 15:541–55

Miki Y, Swensen J, Shattuckeidens D et al. (1994) A strong candidate for the breast and ovarian cancer susceptibility gene BRCA1. Science 266:66–71

Miki Y, Katagiri T, Kasumi F et al. (1996) Mutation analysis in the BRCA2 gene in primary breast cancers. Nat Genet 13:245–7

Miller RW, Fraumeni JF Jr, Manning MD (1964) Association of Wilms' tumortumour with aniridia, hemihypertrophy, and other congenital abnormalities. N Engl J Med 270:922

Milner J, Ponder B, Hughes-Davies L et al. (1997) Transcriptional activation functions in BRCA2. Nature 386:772–3

Mittnacht S (1998) Control of pRB phosphorylation. Curr Opin Genet Dev 8:21–7

Mittnacht S, Paterson H, Olson MF, Marshall CJ (1997) Ras signalling is required for inactivation of the tumour suppressor pRb cell-cycle control protein. Curr Biol 7:219–221

Miyashita T, Reed JC (1995) Tumor suppressor TP53 is a direct transcriptional activator of the human BAX gene. Cell 80:293–9

Miyoshi Y, Ando H, Nagase H et al. (1992a) Germ-line mutations of the APC gene in 53 familial adenomatous polyposis patients. Proc Natl Acad Sci USA 89:4452–4456

Miyoshi Y, Nagase H, Ando H et al. (1992b) Somatic mutations of the APC gene in colorectal tumortumours: mutation cluster region in the APC gene. Hum Mol Genet I:229–233

Momand J, Zambetti GP, Olson DC et al. (1993) The MDM2 oncogene product forms a complex with the TP53 protein and inhibits TP53 mediated transactivation. Cell 691:1237–1245

Monteiro AN, August A, Hanafusa H (1996) Evidence for a transcriptional activation function of BRCA1 C-terminal region. Proc Natl Acad Sci USA 93:13595–9

Moodie SA, Willumsen BM, Weber MJ, Wolfman A (1993) Complexes of Ras.GTP with Raf-1 and mitogen-activated protein kinase kinase. Science 260:1658–1661

Moon RT, Miller JR (1997) The APC tumor suppressor protein in development and cancer. Trends Genet 13:256–8

Morin PJ, Sparks AB, Korinek V et al. (1997) Activation of beta-catenin-Tcf signaling in colon cancer by mutations in beta-catenin or APC [see comments]. Science 275:1787–90

Moser A, Pitot H, Dove W (1990) A dominant mutation that predisposes to multiple intestinal neoplasia in the mouse. Science 247:322–324

Moser AR, Mattes EM, Dove WF et al. (1993) APC^{Min}, a mutation in the murine APC gene, predisposes to mammary carcinomas and focal alveolar hyperplasias. Proc Natl Acad Sci USA 90:8977–8981

Motokura T, Bloom T, Kim HG et al. (1991) A novel cyclin encoded by a bcll-linked candidate oncogene. Nature 350:512–515

Mowat M, Cheng A, Kimura N et al. (1985) Rearrangements of the cellular TP53 gene in erythroleukaemic cells transformed by Friend virus. Nature 314:633–636

Moynahan ME, Chiu JW, Koller BH, Jasin M (1999) BRCA1 controls homology-directed DNA repair. Mol Cell 4:511–8

Mulligan LM, Kwok JB, Healey CS et al. (1993) Germ-line mutations of the RET proto-oncogene in multiple endocrine neoplasia type 2A. Nature 363:458–460

Munemitsu S, Albert I, Souza B et al. (1995) Regulation of intracellular beta-catenin levels by the adenomatous polyposis coli (APC) tumor-suppressor protein. Proc Natl Acad Sci USA 92:3046–50

Munro J, Stott FJ, Vousden KH, Peters G, Parkinson EK (1999) Role of the alternative INK4A proteins in human keratinocyte senescence: evidence for the specific inactivation of p16INK4A upon immortalization. Cancer Res 59:2516–2521

Musarella MA, Gallie BL (1987) A simplified scheme for genetic counseling in retinoblastoma. J Pediatr Ophthalmol Strabismus 24:124–5

Myers MP, Pass I, Batty IH et al. (1998) The lipid phosphatase activity of PTEN is critical for its tumor supressor function. Proc Natl Acad Sci USA 95:13513–8

Nagase H, Nakamura Y (1993) Mutations of the APC (adenomatous polyposis coli) gene. Hum Mutat 2:425–434

Nagase H, Miyoshi Y, Horii A et al. (1992) Correlation between the location of germ-line mutations in the APC gene and the number of colorectal polyps in familial adenomatous polyposis patients. Cancer Res 52:4055–4057

Nance MA, Berry SA (1992) Cockayne syndrome: review of 140 cases. Am J Med Genet 42:68–84

Narod SA, Feunteun J, Lynch HT et al. (1991) Familial breast-ovarian cancer locus on chromosome 17q12–q23. Lancet 338:82–83

Nau MM, Brooks BJ, Battey J et al. (1985) L-myc, a new myc-related gene amplified and expressed in huamn small cell lung cancer. Nature 318:69–73

Nelen MR, Padberg GW, Peeters EA et al. (1996) Localization of the gene for Cowden disease to chromosome 10q22–23. Nat Genet 13:114–6

Nelen MR, van Staveren WC, Peeters EA et al. (1997) Germline mutations in the PTEN/MMAC1 gene in patients with Cowden disease. Hum Mol Genet 6:1383–7

Neve RM, Sutterluty H, Pullen N, Lane HA, Daly JM, Krek W, Hynes NE (2000) Effects of oncogenic ErbB2 on G1 cell cycle regulators in breast tumour cells. Oncogene 19:1647–1656

Nevins JR (1992) E2F: A link between the Rb tumortumour suppressor protein and viral oncoproteins. Science 258:424–429

Nicolaides NC, Papadopoulos N, Liu B et al. (1994) Mutations of two PMS homologues in hereditary nonpolyposis colon cancer. Nature 371:75–80

Nigro JM, Baker SJ, Preisinger AC et al. (1989) Mutations in the TP53 gene occur in diverse human tumour types. Nature 342:705–708

Nishisho I, Nakamura Y, Miyoshi Y et al. (1991) Mutations of chromosome 5q21 genes in FAP and colorectal cancer patients. Science 253:665–669

Nourse J, Mellentin JD, Galili N et al. (1990) Chromosomal translocation t(1;19) results in synthesis of a homeobox fusion mRNA that codes for a potential chimeric transcription factor. Cell 60:535–545

Nowell PC, Hungerford DA (1960) A minute chromosome in human granulocytic leukemia. Science 132:1497

Nusse R, Varmus HE (1982) Many tumors induced by the mouse mammary tumor virus contain a provirus integrated in the same region of the host genome. Cell 31:99–109

O'Connell P, Leach R, Cawthon RM et al. (1989) Two NF1 translocations map within a 600-kilobase segment of 17q11.2. Science 244:1087–1088

Ohh M, Park CW, Ivan M et al. (2000) Ubiquitination of hypoxia-inducible factor requires direct binding to the beta-domain of the von Hippel-Lindau protein. Nat Cell Biol 2:423–7

Ohiwa M, Murakami H, Iwashita T et al. (1997) Characterization of Ret-Shc-Grb2 complex induced by GDNF, MEN 2A, and MEN 2B mutations. Biochem Biophys Res Commun 237:747–51

Oliner JD, Kinzler KW, Meltzer PS et al. (1992) Amplification of a gene encoding a TP53-associated protein in human sarcomas. Nature 358:80–83

Olschwang S, Tiret A, Laurent-Puig P et al. (1993) Restriction of ocular fundus lesions to a specific subgroup of APC mutations in adenomatous polyposis coli patients. Cell 75:959–68

Oltvai ZN, Korsmeyer SJ (1994) Checkpoints of dueling dimers foil death wishes. Cell 79:189–192

Osada M, Ohba M, Kawahara C et al. (1998) Cloning and functional analysis of human p51, which structurally and functionally resembles TP53. Nat Med 4:839–43

Oshimura M, Kugoh H, Koi M et al. (1990) Transfer of a normal human chromosome 11 suppresses tumortumourigenicity of some but not all tumortumour cell lines. J Cell Biochem 42:135–142

Pai EF, Krengel U, Petsko GA, Goody RS, Kabsch W, Wittinghofer A (1990) Refined crystal structure of the triphosphate conformation of H-ras p21 at 1.35 A resolution: implications for the mechanism of GTP hydrolysis. Embo J 9:2351–2359

Papadopoulos N, Nicolaides NC, Wei Y-F et al. (1994) Mutation of a mutL homolog in hereditary colon cancer. Science 263:1625–1629

Parada LF, Tabin CJ, Shih C, Weinberg RA (1982) Human EJ bladder carcinoma oncogene is homologue of Harvey sarcoma virus ras gene. Nature 297:474–478

Parada LF, Land H, Weinberg RA et al. (1984) Cooperation between gene encoding TP53 tumour antigen and ras in cellular transformation. Nature 312:649–651

Park DJ, Wilczynski SP, Paquette RL et al. (1994) P53 mutations in HPV-negative cervical carcinoma. Oncogene 9:205–210

Patel KJ, Yu VP, Lee H et al. (1998) Involvement of BRCA2 in DNA repair. Mol Cell 1:347–57

Paull TT, Gellert M (1999) Nbs1 potentiates ATP-driven DNA unwinding and endonuclease cleavage by the Mre11/Rad50 complex. Genes Dev 13:1276–88

Peeper DS, Upton TM, Ladha MH, Neuma E, Zalvide J, Bernards R, DeCaprio JA and Ewen ME (1997) Ras signalling linked to the cell-cycle machinery by the retinoblastoma protein. Nature 386:177–181

Peifer M (1997) Beta-catenin as oncogene: the smoking gun [comment]. Science 275:1752–3

Pelengaris S, Rudolph B and Littlewood T (2000) Action of Myc in vivo—proliferation and apoptosis. Current Opin Genet Develop 10:100–105

Peltomaki P, Sistonen P, Mecklin JP et al. (1991) Evidence supporting exclusion of the DCC gene and a portion of chromosome 18q as the locus for susceptibility to hereditary nonpolyposis colorectal carcinoma in five kindreds. Cancer Res 51:4135–4140

Peltomaki P, Aaltonen L, Sistonen P et al. (1993) Genetic mapping of a locus predisposing to human colorectal cancer. Science 260:810–812

Peltomaki P, Vasen HF (1997) Mutations predisposing to hereditary nonpolyposis colorectal cancer: Database and results of a collaborative study. The International Collaborative Group on Hereditary Nonpolyposis Colorectal Cancer. Gastroenterology 113:1146–58

Perkins AS, Van de Woude GF (1993) Principles of molecular cell biology of cancer: Oncogenes. In DeVita VT Jr, Hellman S, Rosenberg SA (eds): Cancer: Principles and Practice of Oncology,. 3rd edn. JB Lippincott, Philadelphia

Perriard J, Saurat JH, Harms M (2000) An overlap of Cowden's disease and Bannayan-Riley-Ruvalcaba syndrome in the same family. J Am Acad Dermatol 42:348–50

Perucho M, Goldfarb M, Shimizu K et al. (1981) Human-tumortumour-derived cell lines contain common and different transforming genes. Cell 27:467–476

Petit AM, Rak J, Hung MC, Rockwell P, Goldstein N, Fendly B, Kerbel RS (1997) Neutralizing antibodies against epidermal growth factor and ErbB-2/neu receptor tyrosine kinases down-regulate vascular endothelial growth factor production by tumor cells in vitro and in vivo: angiogenic implications for signal transduction therapy of solid tumors. Am J Pathol 151:1523–1530

Pierceall WE, Woodard AS, Morrow JS et al. (1995) Frequent alterations in e-cadherin and alpha- and beta-catenin expression in human breast cancer cell lines. Oncogene 11:1319–1326

Pietras RJ, Poen JC, Gallardo D, Wongvipat PN, Lee HJ, Slamon DJ (1999) Monoclonal antibody to HER-2/neureceptor modulates repair of radiation-induced DNA damage and enhances radiosensitivity of human breast cancer cells overexpressing this oncogene. Cancer Res 59:1347–1354

Polakis P (1995) Mutations in the APC gene and their implications for protein structure and function. Curr. Opin. Genet Devel. 5:66

Polyak K, Xia Y, Zweier JL et al. (1997) A model for TP53-induced apoptosis. Nature 389:300–5

Pomerantz J, Schreiber-Agus N, Liegeois NJ et al. (1998) The INK4A tumor suppressor gene product, p19ARF, interacts with MDM2 and neutralizes MDM2's inhibition of TP53. Cell 92:713–23

Ponder B (1990) Neurofibromatosis gene cloned. Nature 346:703–704

Ponder, BA (1999) The phenotypes associated with ret mutations in the multiple endocrine neoplasia type 2 syndrome. Cancer Res 59:1736s–1741s; discussion 1742s

Powell SM, Zilz N, Beazerbarclay Y et al. (1992) APC mutations occur early during colorectal tumortumourigenesis. Nature 359:235–237

Powell SM, Petersen GM, Krush AJ et al. (1993) Molecular diagnosis of familial adenomatous polyposis. N Engl J Med 329:1982–1987

Press MF, Pike MC, Chazin VR et al. (1993) Her-2/neu expression in node-negative breast cancer: direct tissue quantitation by computerizeised image analysis and association of overexpression with increased risk of recurrent disease. Cancer Res 53:4960–4970

Pretlow TP, Brasitus TA, Fulton NC et al. (1993) K-ras mutations in putative preneoplastic lesions in human colon. J Natl Cancer Inst 85:2004–2007

Prives C (1994) How loops, B sheets, and α helices help us to understand TP53. Cell 78:543–546

Quelle DE, Zindy F, Ashmun RA, Sherr CJ (1995) Alternative reading frames of the ink4a tumortumour suppressor gene encode two unrelated proteins capable of inducing cell cycle arrest. Cell 83:993–1000

Rahman N, Stratton MR (1998) The genetics of breast cancer susceptibility. Annu Rev Genet 32:95–121

Rampino N, Yamamoto H, Ionov Y et al. (1997) Somatic frameshift mutations in the BAX gene in colon cancers of the microsatellite mutator phenotype. Science 275:967–9

Rauscher FJ (1993) The WT1 Wilms tumortumour gene product—a developmentally regulated transcription factor in the kidney that functions as a tumortumour suppressor. FASEB J 7:896–903

Reed JC (1994) Bcl-2 and the regulation of programmed cell death. J Cell Biol 124:1–6

Riccardi VM, Hittner HM, Francke U et al. (1980) The aniridia-Wilms' tumortumour association: The clinical role of chromosome bank 11p13. Cancer Genet Cytogenet 2:131

Richards FM, McKee SA, Rajpar MH et al. (1999) Germline E-cadherin gene (CDH1) mutations predispose to familial gastric cancer and colorectal cancer. Hum Mol Genet 8:607–10

Risinger JI, Berchuck A, Kohler MF, Boyd J (1994) Mutations of the E-cadherin gene in human gynecologic cancers. Nat Genet 7:98–102

Robles SJ, Adami GR (1998) Agents that cause DNA double strand breaks lead to p16INK4a enrichment and the premature senescence of normal fibroblasts. Oncogene 16:1113–1123

Rogulski KR, Freytag SO, Zhang K et al. (2000) In vivo antitumor activity of ONYX-015 is influenced by TP53 status and is augmented by radiotherapy. Cancer Res 60:1193–6

Romeo G, Ronchetto P, Luo Y et al. (1994) Point mutations affecting the tyrosine kinase domain of the RET proto-oncogene in Hirschsprung's disease. Nature 367:377–8

Roose J, Clevers H (1999) TCF transcription factors: Molecular switches in carcinogenesis. Biochim Biophys Acta 1424:M23–37

Rouleau GA, Merel P, Lutchman M et al. (1993) Alteration in a new gene encoding a putative membrane-organizing protein causes neuro-fibromatosis type 2. Nature 363:515–521

Rous P (1911) A sarcoma of the fowl transmissable by an agent separable from the tumor cells. J Exp Med 13:397

Rowan AJ, Lamlum H, Ilyas M et al. (2000) APC mutations in sporadic colorectal tumors: A mutational "hotspot" and interdependence of the "two hits". Proc Natl Acad Sci USA 97:3352–7

Rowley JD (1973) A new consistent chromosomal abnormality in chronic myelogenous leukaemia identified by quinacrine fluorescence and Giemsa staining. Nature 243:290–293

Rozen P, Shomrat R, Strul H et al. (1999) Prevalence of the I1307K APC gene variant in Israeli Jews of differing ethnic origin and risk for colorectal cancer. Gastroenterology 116:54–7

Rubinfeld B, Souza B, Albert I et al. (1993) Association of the APC gene product with beta-catenin. Science 262:1731–1734

Rubinfeld B, Albert I, Porfiri E et al. (1996) Binding of GSK3beta to the APC-beta-catenin complex and regulation of complex assembly [see comments]. Science 272:1023–6

Rutkowski JL, Wu K, Gutmann DH et al. (2000) Genetic and cellular defects contributing to benign tumor formation in neurofibromatosis type 1. Hum Mol Genet 9:1059–66

Ruttledge MH, Andermann AA, Phelan CM et al. (1996) Type of mutation in the neurofibromatosis type 2 gene (NF2) frequently determines severity of disease. Am J Hum Genet 59:331–42

Sakaguchi K, Herrera JE, Saito S et al. (1998) DNA damage activates TP53 through a phosphorylation-acetylation cascade. Genes Dev 12:2831–41

Sakamuro D, Prendergast GC (1999) New Myc-interacting proteins: a second Myc network emerges. Oncogene 18:2942–2954

Santos E, Tronick SR, Aaronson SA, Pulciani S, Barbacid M (1982) T24 human bladder carcinoma oncogene is an activated form of the normal human homologue of BALB- and Harvey-MSV transforming genes. Nature 298:343–347

Sarnow P, Ho Y, Williams J, Levine A (1982) Adenovirus E1b-58kd tumortumour antigen and SV40 large tumortumour antigen are physically associated with the same 54 kd cellular protein in transformed cells. Cell 28:387–394

Satoh S, Daigo Y, Furukawa Y et al. (2000) AXIN1 mutations in hepatocellular carcinomas, and growth suppression in cancer cells by virus-mediated transfer of AXIN1. Nat Genet 24:245–50

Savitsky K, Barshira A, Gilad S et al. (1995) A single ataxia telangiectasia gene with a product similar to PI-3 kinase. Science 268:1749–1753

Sayle RA, Milner-White EJ (1995) RASMOL: biomolecular graphics for all. Trends Biochem Sci 20:374

Scheffner M, Münger K, Byrne JC, Howley PM (1991) The state of the TP53 and retinoblastoma genes in human cervical carcinoma cell lines. Proc Natl Acad Sci USA 88:5523–5527

Schmidt L, Duh FM, Chen F et al. (1997) Germline and somatic mutations in the tyrosine kinase domain of the MET proto-oncogene in papillary renal carcinomas. Nat Genet 16:68–73

Schwab M, Amler LC (1990) Amplification of cellular oncogenes: A predictor of clinical outcome in human cancer. Genes Chromosom Cancer 1:181–193

Schwab M, Alitalo K, Klempnauer KH et al. (1983) Amplified DNA with limited homology to myc cellular oncogene is shared by human neuroblastoma cell lines and a neuroblastoma tumour. Nature 305:245–248

Scoles DR, Huynh DP, Chen MS et al. (2000) The neurofibromatosis 2 tumor suppressor protein interacts with hepatocyte growth factor-regulated tyrosine kinase substrate. Hum Mol Genet 9:1567–74

Scully R, Chen J, Plug A et al. (1997) Association of BRCA1 with Rad51 in mitotic and meiotic cells. Cell 88:265–75

Seeburg PH, Colby WW, Capon DJ, Goeddel DV, Levinson AD (1984) Biological properties of human c-Ha-ras1 genes mutated at codon 12. Nature 312:71–75

Seizinger BR (1993) NF1: A prevalent cause of tumortumourigenesis in human cancers? Nat Genet 3:97–99

Seizinger BR, Martuza RL, Gusella JF (1986) Loss of genes on chromosome 22 in tumortumourigenesis of human acoustic neuroma. Nature 322:644–647

Seizinger BR, de la Monte S, Atkins L et al. (1987a) Molecular genetic approach to human meningioma: loss of genes on chromosome 22. Proc Natl Acad Sci USA 84:5419–5423

Seizinger BR, Rouleau G, Ozelius LJ et al. (1987b) Common pathogenetic mechanism for three tumortumour types in bilateral acoustic neurofibromatosis. Science 236:317–319

Seizinger BR, Rouleau GA, Ozelius LJ et al. (1987c) Genetic linkage of von Recklinghausen neurofibromatosis to the nerve growth factor receptor gene. Cell 49:589–594

Seizinger BR, Rouleau GA, Ozelius LJ et al. (1988) Von Hippel-Lindau disease maps to the region of chromosome 3 associated with renal cell carcinoma. Nature 332:268–269

Serrano M, Lin AW, McCurrach ME, Beach D, Lowe SW (1997) Oncogenic ras provokes premature cell senescence associated with accumulation of TP53 and p16INK4a. Cell 88:593–602

Shannon KM, O'Connell P, Martin GA et al. (1994) Loss of the normal NF1 allele from the bone marrow of children with type 1 neurofibromatosis and malignant myeloid disorders. N Engl J Med 330:597–601

Shaulian E, Haviv I, Shaul Y, Oren M (1995) Transcriptional repression by the C-terminal domain of TP53. Oncogene 10:671–80

Shen JC, Loeb LA (2000) The Werner syndrome gene: the molecular basis of RecQ helicase-deficiency diseases. Trends Genet 16:213–20

Shen JC, Gray MD, Oshima J et al. (1998) Werner syndrome protein. I. DNA helicase and dna exonuclease reside on the same polypeptide. J Biol Chem 273:34139–44

Shieh SY, Ahn J, Tamai K et al. (2000) The human homologs of checkpoint kinases Chk1 and Cds1 (Chk2) phosphorylate TP53 at multiple DNA damage-inducible sites. Genes Dev 14:289–300

Shih C, Weinberg RA (1982) Isolation of a transforming sequence from a human bladder carcinoma cell line. Cell 29:161–169

Shih C, Padhy LC, Murray M, Weinberg RA (1981) Transforming genes of carcinomas and neuroblastomas introduced into mouse fibroblasts. Nature 290:261–264

Shimizu T, Sekiya T (1995) Loss of heterozygosity at 9p21 loci and mutations of the MTS1 and MTS2 genes in human lung cancers. Int J Cancer 63:616–620

Shimizu K, Birnbaum D, Ruley MA et al. (1983a) Structure of the Ki-ras gene of the human lung carcinoma cell line Calu-1. Nature 304:497–500

Shimizu K, Goldfarb M, Perucho M, Wigler M (1983b) Isolation and preliminary characterization of the transforming gene of a human neuroblastoma cell line. Proc Natl Acad Sci USA 80:383–387

Shirahama S, Ogura K, Takami H et al. (1998) Mutational analysis of the RET proto-oncogene in 71 Japanese patients with medullary thyroid carcinoma. J Hum Genet 43:101–6

Shirasawa S, Furuse M, Yokoyama N, Sasazuki T (1993) Altered growth of human colon cancer cell lines disrupted at activated Ki-ras. Science 260:85–88

Sidransky D, Tokino T, Hamilton SR et al. (1992) Identification of RAS oncogene mutations in the stool of patients with curable colorectal tumortumours. Science 256:102–105

Siegert JL, Robbins PD (1999) Rb inhibits the intrinsic kinase activity of TATA-binding protein-associated factor TAFII250. Mol Cell Biol 19:846–54

Simpkins SB, Bocker T, Swisher EM et al. (1999) MLH1 promoter methylation and gene silencing is the primary cause of microsatellite instability in sporadic endometrial cancers. Hum Mol Genet 8:661–666

Slamon DJ, Clark GM, Wong SG et al. (1987) Human breast cancer: correlation of relapse and survival with amplification of the HER-2/neu oncogene. Science 235:177–182

Slamon DJ, Godolphin W, Jones LA et al. (1989) Studies of the HER-2/neu proto-oncogene in human breast and ovarian cancer. Science 244:707–712

Slebos RJ, Kibdelaar RE, Dalesio O (1990) K-ras oncogene activation as a prognostic marker in adenocarcinoma of the lung. N Engl J Med 323:561–565

Sliwkowski MX, Lofgren JA, Lewis GD, Hotaling TE, Fendly BM, Fox JA (1999) Nonclinical studies addressing the mechanism of action of trastuzumab (Herceptin). Semin Oncol 26:60–70

Smalley WE, DuBois RN (1997) Colorectal cancer and nonsteroidal anti-inflammatory drugs. Adv Pharmacol 39:1–20

Soder AI, Hoare SF, Muir S, Going JJ, Parkinson EK, Keith WN (1997) Amplification, increased dosage and in situ expression of the telomerase RNA gene in human cancer. Oncogene 14:1013–1021

Solomon E, Voss R, Hall V et al. (1987) Chromosome 5 allele loss in human colorectal carcinomas. Nature 328:616–619

Solomon E, Borrow J, Goddard AD (1991) Chromosome aberrations and cancer. Science 254:1153–1160

Somasundaram K, Zhang H, Zeng YX et al. (1997) Arrest of the cell cycle by the tumor-suppressor BRCA1 requires the CDK-inhibitor p21WAF1/CiP1. Nature 389:187–90

Souza RF, Appel R, Yin J et al. (1996) Microsatellite instability in the insulin-like growth factor II receptor gene in gastrointestinal tumours. Nat Genet 14:255–257

Sparkes RS, Sparkes MC, Wilson MG et al. (1980) Regional assignment of genes for human esterase D and retinoblastoma to chromosome band 13q14. Science 208:1042–1044

Sparkes RS, Murphree AL, Lingua RW et al. (1983) Gene for hereditary retinoblastoma assigned to human chromosome 13 by linkage to esterase D. Science 219:971–973

Spillare EA, Robles AI, Wang XW et al. (1999) TP53-mediated apoptosis is attenuated in Werner syndrome cells. Genes Dev 13:1355–1360

Spirio L, Olschwang S, Groden J et al. (1993) Alleles of the APC gene: an attenuated form of familial polyposis. Cell 75:951–957

Sprang SR (1997) G protein mechanisms: Insights from structural analysis. Annu Rev Biochem 66:639–678

Stambolic V, Suzuki A, de la Pompa JL et al. (1998) Negative regulation of PKB/Akt-dependent cell survival by the tumor suppressor PTEN. Cell 95:29–39

Stanbridge EJ, Cavanee WK (1989) Heritable cancer and tumortumour suppressor genes: a tentative connection. In Weinberg RA (ed): Oncogenes and the Molecular Origins of Cancer. Cold Spring Harbor Laboratory, Old Spring Harbor, N Y, p. 281.

Stebbins CE, Kaelin WG, Pavletich NP (1999) Structure of the VHL-ElonginC-ElonginB complex: Implications for VHL tumor suppressor function. Science 284:455–461

Steck PA, Pershouse MA, Jasser SA et al. (1997) Identification of a candidate tumour suppressor gene, MMAC1, at chromosome 10q23.3 that is mutated in multiple advanced cancers. Nat Genet 15:356–362

Stehelin D, Varmus HE, Bishop JM, Vogt PK (1976) DNA related to the transforming gene(s) of avian sarcoma viruses is present in normal avian DNA. Nature 260:170–173

Stein GH, Drullinger LF, Soulard A, Dulic V (1999) Differential roles for cyclin-dependent kinase inhibitors p21 and p16 in the mechanisms of senescence and differentiation in human fibroblasts. Mol Cell Biol 19:2109–2117

Stott FJ, Bates S, James MC et al. (1998) The alternative product from the human CDKN2A locus, p14(ARF), participates in a regulatory feedback loop with TP53 and MDM2. Embo J 17:5001–5014

Strasser A, O'Connor L, Dixit VM (2000) Apoptosis signaling. Annu Rev Biochem 69:217–245

Struewing JP, Abeliovich D, Peretz T et al. (1995) The carrier frequency of the BRCA1 185delAG mutation is approximately 1 percent in Ashkenazi Jewish individuals. Nature Genet 11:198–200

Struewing JP, Hartge P, Wacholder S et al. (1997) The risk of cancer associated with specific mutations of BRCA1 and BRCA2 among Ashkenazi Jews. N Engl J Med 336:1401–1408

Su LK, Kinzler KW, Vogelstein B et al. (1992) Multiple intestinal neoplasia caused by a mutation in the murine homolog of the APC gene. Science 256:668–670

Su LK, Vogelstein B, Kinzler KW (1993) Association of the APC tumortumor suppressor protein with catenins. Science 262:1734–1737

Sugasawa K, Ng JM, Masutani C et al. (1998) Xeroderma pigmentosum group C protein complex is the initiator of global genome nucleotide excision repair. Mol Cell 2:223–232

Suzuki A, de la Pompa JL, Stambolic V et al. (1998) High cancer susceptibility and embryonic lethality associated with mutation of the PTEN tumor suppressor gene in mice. Curr Biol 8:1169–1178

Suzuki N, Shimamoto A, Imamura O et al. (1997) DNA helicase activity in Werner's syndrome gene product synthesized in a baculovirus system. Nucleic Acids Res 25:2973–2978

Szabo CI, King MC (1995) Inherited breast and ovarian cancer. Hum Mol Genet 4:1811–1817

Tabin CJ, Bradley SM, Bargmann CI et al. (1982) Mechanism of activation of a human oncogene. Nature 300:143–149

Takahashi M, Buma Y, Iwamoto T et al. (1988) Cloning and expression of the ret proto-oncogene encoding a tyrosine kinase with two potential transmembrane domains. Oncogene 3:571–578

Tamura G, Maesawa C, Suzuki Y et al. (1994) Mutations of the APC gene occur during early stages of gastric adenoma development. Cancer Res 54:1149–1151

Taparowsky E, Suard Y, Fasano O et al. (1982) Activation of the T24 bladder carcinoma transforming gene is linked to a single amino acid change. Nature 300:762–765

Tashiro H, Blazes MS, Wu R et al. (1997) Mutations in PTEN are frequent in endometrial carcinoma but rare in other common gynecological malignancies. Cancer Res 57:3935–3940

The I, Murthy AE, Hannigan GE et al. (1993) Neurofibromatosis type 1 gene mutations in neuroblastoma. Nat Genet 3:62–66

Thorlacius S, Struewing JP, Hartge P et al. (1998) Population-based study of risk of breast cancer in carriers of BRCA2 mutation. Lancet 352:1337–1339

Tinschert S, Naumann I, Stegmann E et al. (2000) Segmental neurofibromatosis is caused by somatic mutation of the neurofibromatosis type 1 (NF1) gene. Eur J Hum Genet 8:455–459

Tolmie JL, de Berker D, Dawber R et al. (1994) Syndromes associated with trichothiodystrophy. Clin Dysmorphol 3:1–14

Treanor JJ, Goodman L, de Sauvage F et al. (1996) Characterization of a multicomponent receptor for GDNF. Nature 382:80–383

Trent JM, Stanbridge EJ, McBride HL et al. (1990) TumorTumourigenicity in human melanoma cell lines controlled by introduction of human chromosome 6. Science 247:568–571

Trofatter JA, MacCollin MM, Rutter JL et al. (1993) A novel moesin-, ezrin-, radixin-like gene is a candidate for the neurofibromatosis 2 tumortumour suppressor. Cell 72:791–800

Trofatter JA, MacCollin MM, Rutter JL et al. (1993) A novel moesin-, ezrin-, radixin-like gene is a candidate for the neurofibromatosis 2 tumor suppressor. Cell 75:826

Trujillo KM, Yuan SS, Lee EY, Sung P (1998) Nuclease activities in a complex of human recombination and DNA repair factors Rad50, Mre11, and p95. J Biol Chem 273:21447–21450

Tsujimoto Y, Yunis J, Onorato-Showe L et al. (1984) Molecular cloning of the chromosomal breakpoint of B-cell lymphomas and leukemias with the t(11;14) chromosome translocation. Science 224:1403–1406

Tsujimoto Y, Cossman J, Jaffe E, Croce CM (1985) Involvement of the bcl-2 gene in human follicular lymphoma. Science 228:1440–1443

Uchino S, Noguchi S, Adachi M et al. (1998) Novel point mutations and allele loss at the RET locus in sporadic medullary thyroid carcinomas. Jpn J Cancer Res 89:411–418

Upadhyaya M, Shen M, Cherryson A et al. (1992) Analysis of mutations at the neurofibromatosis 1 (NF1) locus. Hum Mol Genet 1:735–740

Upadhyaya M, Ruggieri M, Maynard J et al. (1998) Gross deletions of the neurofibromatosis type 1 (NF1) gene are predominantly of maternal origin and commonly associated with a learning disability, dysmorphic features and developmental delay. Hum Genet 102:591–597

Urban T, Ricci S, Grange JD et al. (1993) Detection of c-Ki-ras mutation by PCR/RFLP analysis and diagnosis of pancreatic adenocarcinomas. J Natl Cancer Inst 85:2008–2012

van Biesen T, Hawes BE, Luttrell DK, Krueger MK, Touhara K, Porfiri E, Sakaue M, Luttrell LM, and Lefkowitz RJ (1995) Receptor-tyrosine-kinase- and G beta gamma-mediated MAP kinase activation by a common signalling pathway. Nature 376:781–784

van Heyningen V (1994) One gene—four syndromes Nature 367:319–320

Varmus HE (1984) The molecular genetics of cellular oncogenes. Annu Rev Genet 18:553–612

Varon R, Vissinga C, Platzer M et al. (1998) Nibrin, a novel DNA double-strand break repair protein, is mutated in Nijmegen breakage syndrome. Cell 93:467–76

Vasen HFA, Mecklin JP, Meera Kahn P, Lynch HT (1991a) Hereditary non-polyposis colorectal cancer. Lancet 338:877

Vasen HF, Mecklin JP, Khan P, Lynch HT (1991b) The International Collaborative Group on Hereditary Non-Polyposis Colorectal Cancer (ICG-HNPCC). Dis Colon Rectum 34:424–425

Vasen HF, Watson P, Mecklin JP, Lynch HT (1999) New clinical criteria for hereditary nonpolyposis colorectal cancer (HNPCC, Lynch syndrome) proposed by the International Collaborative group on HNPCC. Gastroenterology 116:1453–1456

Vaux DL, Cory S, Adams JM (1988) Bcl-2 gene promotes haemopoietic cell survival and cooperates with c-myc to immortalize pre-B cells. Nature 335:440–442

Veigl ML, Kasturi L, Olechnowicz J et al. (1998) Biallelic inactivation of hMLH1 by epigenetic gene silencing, a novel mechanism causing human MSI cancers. Proc Natl Acad Sci USA 95:8698–702

Viskochil D, Buchberg A, Xu G (1990) Deletions and a translocation interrupt a cloned gene at the neurofibromatosis type 1 locus. Cell 62:187–192

Viskochil D, White R, Cawthon R (1993) The neurofibromatosis type 1 gene. Annu Rev Neurosci 16:183–205

Vogelstein B, Kinzler KW (1992) TP53 Function and dysfunction. Cell 70:523–526

Vogelstein B, Fearon E, Hamilton S (1988) Genetic alterations during colorectal-tumour development. N Engl J Med 319:525–532

Vogt M, Haggblom C, Yeargin J, Christiansen-Weber T, Haas M (1998) Independent induction of senescence by p16INK4a and p21CIP1 in spontaneously immortalized human fibroblasts. Cell Growth Differ 9:139–146

Wainwright B (1994) Familial melanoma and p16INK4a—a hung jury. Nat Genet 8:3–5

Wallace MR, Marchuk DA, Andersen LB et al. (1990) Type 1 neurofibromatosis gene: Identification of a large transcript disrupted in three NF1 patients. Science 249:181–186

Wallis YL, Macdonald F, Hulten M et al. (1994) Genotype-phenotype correlation between position of constitutional APC gene mutation and CHRPE expression in familial adenomatous polyposis. Hum Genet 94:543–8

Wang Q, Zhang H, Kajino K, Greene MI (1998) BRCA1 binds c-Myc and inhibits its transcriptional and transforming activity in cells. Oncogene 17:1939–48

Wang W, Seki M, Narita Y et al. (2000) Possible association of BLM in decreasing DNA double strand breaks during DNA replication. Embo J 19:3428–3435

Warthin AS (1913) Heredity with reference to carcinoma. Arch Intern Med 12:546

Watson P, Marcus JN, Lynch HT (1998) Prognosis of BRCA1 hereditary breast cancer. Lancet 351:304–305

Weemaes CM, Hustinx TW, Scheres JM et al. (1981) A new chromosomal instability disorder: The Nijmegen breakage syndrome. Acta Paediatr Scand 70:557–564

Weemaes CM, Hustinx TW, Scheres JM et al. (2000) Nijmegen breakage syndrome. The International Nijmegen Breakage Syndrome Study Group. Arch Dis Child 82:400–446

Weinberg R (1989) Oncogenes, antioncogenes, and the molecular basis of multistep carcinogenesis. Cancer Res 49:3713–3721

Weinberg RA (1991) TumorTumour suppressor genes. Science 254:1138–1146

Weinberg RA (1994) Oncogenes and tumortumour suppressor genes. CA 44:160–170

Weintraub SJ, Prater CA, Dean DC (1992) Retinoblastoma protein switches the E2F site from positive to negative element. Nature 358:259–261

Weissman BE, Saxon PJ, Pasquale SR et al. (1987) Introduction of a normal human chromosome 11 into a Wilms' tumortumour cell line controls its tumortumourigenic expression. Science 236:175–180

Wellenreuther R, Kraus JA, Lenartz D et al. (1995) Analysis of the neurofibromatosis 2 gene reveals molecular variants of meningioma. Am J Pathol 146:827–832

Werness BA, Levine AJ, Howley PM (1990) Association of human papillomavirus types 16 and 18 E6 proteins with TP53. Science 248:76–79

Whelan AJ, Bartsch D, Goodfellow PJ (1995) A familial syndrome of pancreatic cancer and melanoma with a mutation in the cdkn2 tumortumour-suppressor gene. N Engl J Med 333:975–977

Whyte P, Buchkovich KJ, Horowitz JM (1988) Association between an oncogene and an anti-oncogene: The adenovirus E1A proteins bind to the retinoblastoma gene product. Nature 334:124–129

Whyte P, Williamson NM, Harlow E (1989) Cellular targets for transformation by the adenovirus E1A proteins. Cell 56:67–75

Wigler MH (1990) Oncoproteins. GAPs in understanding Ras. Nature 346:696–697

Wijnen J, Khan PM, Vasen H et al. (1997) Hereditary nonpolyposis colorectal cancer families not complying with the Amsterdam criteria show extremely low frequency of mismatch-repair-gene mutations. Am J Hum Genet 61:329–335

Wijnen J, van der Klift H, Vasen H et al. (1998) MSH2 genomic deletions are a frequent cause of HNPCC. Nat Genet 20:326–328

Winkler DG, Johnson JC, Cooper JA, and Vojtek AB (1997) Identification and characterization of mutations in Ha-Ras that selectively decrease binding to cRaf-1. J Biol Chem 272:24402–24409

Wittinghofer A, and Nassar N (1996) How Ras-related proteins talk to their effectors. Trends Biochem Sci 21:488–491

Wohllk N, Cote GJ, Bugalho MM et al. (1996) Relevance of RET proto-oncogene mutations in sporadic medullary thyroid carcinoma. J Clin Endocrinol Metab 81:3740–3745

Wolf D, Admon S, Oren M, Rotter V (1984) Major deletions in the gene encoding the TP53 tumortumour antigen cause lack of TP53 expression in HL-60 cells. Proc Natl Acad Sci USA 82:790–794

Wong AK, Pero R, Ormonde PA et al. (1997) RAD51 interacts with the evolutionarily conserved BRC motifs in the human breast cancer susceptibility gene brca2. J Biol Chem 272:31941–31944

Woo RA, McLure KG, Lees-Miller SP et al. (1998) DNA-dependent protein kinase acts upstream of TP53 in response to DNA damage. Nature 394:700–704

Woodage T, King SM, Wacholder S et al. (1998) The APCI1307K allele and cancer risk in a community-based study of Ashkenazi Jews. Nat Genet 20:62–5

Wooster R, Neuhausen SL, Mangion J et al. (1994) Localization of a breast cancer susceptibility gene, BRCA2, to chromosome 13q12–13. Science 265:2088–2090

Wooster R, Bignell G, Lancaster J et al. (1995) Identification of the breast cancer susceptibility gene BRCA2. Nature 378:789–792

Wu CL, Thakker N, Neary W et al. (1998) Differential diagnosis of type 2 neurofibromatosis: Molecular discrimination of NF2 and sporadic vestibular schwannomas. J Med Genet 35:973–977

Wu LC, Wang ZW, Tsan JT et al. (1996) Identification of a RING protein that can interact in vivo with the BRCA1 gene product. Nat Genet 14:430–440

Wu X, Ranganathan V, Weisman DS et al. (2000) ATM phosphorylation of Nijmegen breakage syndrome protein is required in a DNA damage response. Nature 405:477–482

Xu GF, O'Connell P, Viskochil D et al. (1990) The neurofibromatosis type 1 gene encodes a protein related to GAP. Cell 62:599–608

Yamagami T, Ogawa H, Tamaki H, et al. (1998) Suppression of Wilms' tumor gene (WT1) expression induces G2/M arrest in leukemic cells. Leuk Res 22:383–384

Yamane K, Tsuruo T (1999) Conserved BRCT regions of TopBP1 and of the tumor suppressor BRCA1 bind strand breaks and termini of DNA. Oncogene 18:5194–5203

Yandell DW, Campbell TA, Dayton SH et al. (1989) Oncogenic point mutations in the human retinoblastoma gene: their application to genetic counseling. N Engl J Med 321:1689–1695

Yap DB, Hsieh JK, Chan FS, Lu X (1999) mdm2: A bridge over the two tumour suppressors, TP53 and Rb. Oncogene 18:7681–7689

Yarden RI, Brody LC (1999) BRCA1 interacts with components of the histone deacetylase complex. Proc Natl Acad Sci USA 96:4983–4988

Yu CE, Oshima J, Fu YH et al. (1996) Positional cloning of the Werner's syndrome gene. Science 272:258–262

Yunis JJ, Mayer MG, Arnesen MA et al. (1989) bcl-2 and other genomic alterations in the prognosis of large-cell lymphoma. N Engl J Med 320:1047–1054

Zhan Q, Antinore MJ, Wang XW et al. (1999) Association with Cdc2 and inhibition of Cdc2/Cyclin B1 kinase activity by the TP53-regulated protein Gadd45. Oncogene 18:2892–900

Zhang HS, Gavin M, Dahiya A et al. (2000) Exit from G1 and S phase of the cell cycle is regulated by repressor complexes containing HDAC-Rb-hSWI/SNF and Rb-hSWI/SNF. Cell 101:79–89

Zhang X, Morera S, Bates PA et al. (1998) Structure of an XRCC1 BRCT domain: A new protein-protein interaction module. EMBO J 17:6404–6411

Zhao S, Weng YC, Yuan SS et al. (2000) Functional link between ataxiatelangiectasia and Nijmegen breakage syndrome gene products. Nature 405:473–7

Zhong Q, Chen CF, Li S et al. (1999) Association of BRCA1 with the hRad50-hMrell-p95 complex and the DNA damage response. Science 285:747–50

Zhu J, Woods D, McMahon M, Bishop, JM (1998) Senescence of human fibroblasts induced by oncogenic Raf. Genes Dev 12:2997–3007

Zindy F, Eischen CM, Randle DH et al. (1998) Myc signaling via the ARF tumor suppressor regulates TP53-dependent apoptosis and immortalization. Genes Dev 12:2424–2433

Zucman-Rossi J, Legoix P, Der Sarkissian H et al. (1998) NF2 gene in neurofibromatosis type 2 patients. Hum Mol Genet 7:2095–101

Zuo L, Weger J, Yang Q, et al. (1996) Germline mutations in the p16INK4a binding domain of CDK4 in familial melanoma. Nat Genet 12:97–99

Zwicker J, Liu N, Engeland K et al. (1996) Cell cycle regulation of E2F site occupation in vivo. Science 271:1595–1597

The biologic basis of aging: implications for medical genetics

George M. Martin

Introduction

Evolutionary biology has provided a robust theory to explain *why* we age, but we have much less confidence that we understand *how* we age, by which we mean the proximal molecular mechanisms of aging. Medical geneticists are in a good position to advance our knowledge of such mechanisms. The first strategy is the time-honored approach of mapping, cloning and characterizing the relevant gene actions underlying important late-onset disorders of aging, such as dementias of the Alzheimer type, atherosclerosis, ocular cataracts, type 2 diabetes mellitus, osteoporosis, osteoarthritis, and cancer. Here is where we can show the most progress. Genetic analysis has the potential of identifying the earliest stages of a pathogenetic pathway; these can be viewed as basic aging mechanisms that "set the stage" for the emergence of such important geriatric disorders in subsets of vulnerable subjects. The second strategy is to investigate the genetic basis for *unusually well preserved* structure and function during the latter half of the usual life span. Unfortunately, medical geneticists have been too preoccupied with disease and, with some notable exceptions, other human geneticists have not shown a strong inclination to investigate late-life phenotypes. The result is a paucity of information. Given the new statistical and molecular tools at our disposal, one hopes that this situation will change in the near future.

What is aging?

Some gerontologists, particularly those interested in the aging of plants (Leopold, 1978), sharply differentiate between the terms *aging* and *senescing*. Senescent changes, they would argue, are those structural and functional changes that occur near the end of the life cycle of a cell, tissue, organ, or organism and are associated with the impending death of the tissue or organism. By contrast, the term *aging* would be used for any change in structure or function throughout the life cycle.

In other words, some would argue that "aging begins at birth". Most gerontologists who work with mammals and human subjects, however, use the two terms more or less interchangeably. While none would deny the importance of development in the determination of the subsequent life history of an organism, they are concerned, as we are, with declines in structure and function that gradually and insidiously unfold after the organism has achieved the young, mature adult phenotype. At the level of populations, these functional declines translate into an exponential increase in the force of mortality over unit time—the hazard function or instantaneous mortality rate (Gavrilov and Gavrilova, 1991). This is the famous Gompertz relationship (Gompertz, 1825). This was modified by Makeham (Makeham, 1860), who included a constant, A, to account for kinetic departures presumed to have resulted from causes of death during the early life history that were age independent. The Gompertz-Makeham equation can thus be given as the sum of two types of mortalities, age-independent, and age-dependent, the latter exhibiting exponential kinetics over the adult life span:

$$\mu_x = A + Re^{\alpha}x$$

where μ_x is the force of mortality at a given age x; A is the Makeham constant; and R is the hypothetical value for the force of mortality at birth, the lowest force of mortality (or the Y intercept in a graphic plot of age (X axis) versus force

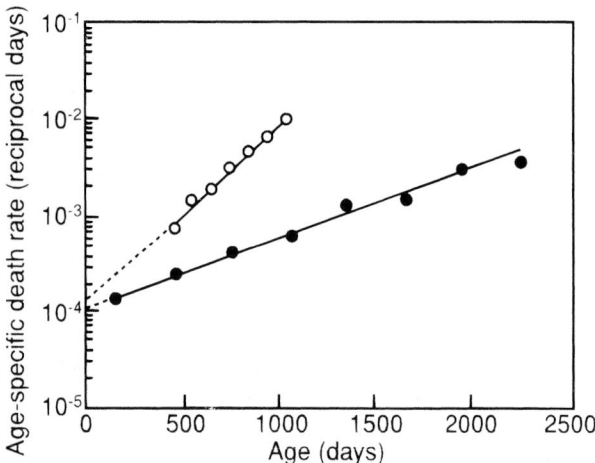

Fig. 20.1. Gompertz function plot of the age-specific mortality rates for combined sexes of two different murine species of contrasting maximum life span potentials but of comparable size. Both species were wild-type and randomly bred from small cohorts captured near the Argonne National Laboratories (Argonne, IL) by the late George A Sacher. They were housed under essentially identical conditions (caging, bedding, humidity, temperature, diet) in adjacent animal rooms with no special efforts to establish specific pathogen-free conditions (G A Sacher, personal communication to GMM). The longer lived species (●). *Peromyscus leucopus*, was found to have a maximum life span of about eight years, approximately twice that of *Mus musculus* (○). (From Sacher, 1978, with permission.)

have also been seen for very aged individuals in human populations (Vaupel et al., 1998). Perhaps this observation might also be explained by behavioral changes, (e.g., a more protective environment) in extreme old age. It will nevertheless be prudent to explore various non-Gompertzian models of mortality in human populations, as it has been claimed that such standard models may not adequately describe mortality at extreme ages (Manton et al., 1994; Wilson, 1994).

Observations of exponential increases in the force of mortality within populations should not lead one to conclude that underlying processes of aging or incidences of geriatric diseases necessarily exhibit exponential kinetics. Most physiologic declines, at least in cross-sectional studies, exhibit linear declines, the slopes of which are variable (Fig. 20.2). Many major diseases of late life, however, show exponential increases in age-specific incidence and prevalence, although there may be slight declines in age-specific incidence at very advanced ages, raising the question of selection for genotypic resistance against specific late-life disorders. Alzheimer disease serves as a good example (Ritchie and Kildea, 1995). Figure 20.3 summarizes the results of twelve studies of the age-specific prevalence of late-life dementias, most of which are due to dementias of the Alzheimer type (Katzman and Kawas, 1998).

of mortality (Y axis) (Fig. 20.1); e is an exponent; and α is a constant representing the slope of the graphical plot (Fig. 20.1).

Figure 20.1 illustrates differing rates of exponential increases in the force of mortality for two non-inbred wild-type murine species despite comparable values for R. These two species, *Peromyscus leucopus* and *Mus musculus*, are of approximately the same size and were housed and fed throughout their lifetimes under identical conditions (Sacher, 1978). The maximum life span of *Peromyscus* sp. was found to be about eight years, about twice that of *Mus* sp. These data illustrate the importance of genetic factors in the determination of approximate life potential. Given the considerable evolutionary distance between these two species (at least 15 million years) (Sarich, 1985), this is not a surprising result.

Experiments employing very large populations of aging cohorts of fruit flies, and medflies have recently been reported as showing dramatic departures from Gompertz kinetics within the oldest cohorts, with apparent decreases in the force of mortality at very advanced ages (Carey et al. 1992; Curtsinger et al., 1992). Very aged flies, however, may become virtually immobilized and may therefore be protected from environmental hazards related, for example, to attempts at flight. Declines in age-specific mortality rates

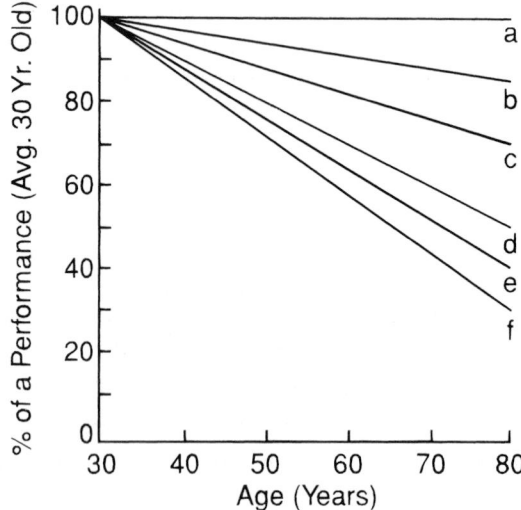

Fig. 20.2. Linear declines of functional assays for several different human physiological parameters as studied cross-sectionally by the late Nathan W Shock and colleagues. The values are expressed as percentages of the average performances of healthy 20- to 35-year-old male subjects. (a) Fasting blood glucose. (b) Nerve conduction velocity. (c) Cardiac index (resting). (d) Vital capacity and renal blood flow. (e) Maximum breathing capacity. (f) Maximum work rate and maximum oxygen uptake. (Adapted from Shock, 1977, with permission.)

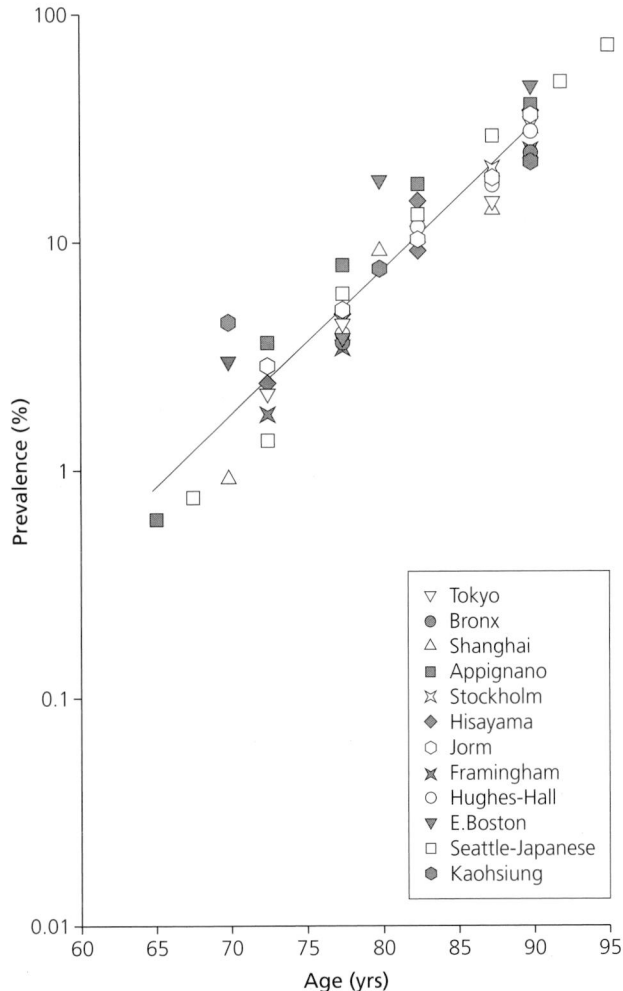

Fig. 20.3. Evidence for exponential increases in the age-specific prevalence of dementia in twelve independent studies. The majority of such cases are attributable to dementia of the Alzheimer type (From Katzman and Kawas, 1998, with permission).

Longitudinal studies of physiologic parameters may exhibit striking variations among individuals (Nelson and Dannefer, 1992). Figure 20.4 illustrates the case of a measure of renal function. By this measure, some individuals show no evidence of a decline in renal function (Lindeman et al., 1985; Lindeman, 1990). Are any of these varied patterns of functional decline (or lack of decline) in apparently normal aging human subjects determined, in part, by constitutional differences in the genotype? Essentially no research has been carried out to address this important question. Medical geneticists have an obvious bias in favor of the discovery of mutations and deleterious allelic variants. There is a great need to define allelic variants that, in ordinary environments, are associated with the maintenance of enhanced structure and function during aging. One such example may be the *ApoE ε2* allele, the prevalence of which is significantly increased in centenarians (Schachter et al., 1994). The *APOE ε2* results are understandable, in that there is evidence that carriers are provided with some protection against Alzheimer disease (Benjamin et al., 1994; Talbot et al., 1994). Surprisingly, however, in the same study, centenarians also exhibited a higher prevalence of homozygosity for the *ACE DD* genotype, one that is known to be associated with a higher risk of myocardial infarction. This raises the interesting possibility of a differential gene action of the angiotensin I-converting enzyme (ACE), dipeptidyl carboxypeptidase-1, in young and old subjects, either regarding an effect on blood pressure or on some other function. In neither example, however, can one exclude a role for a tightly linked gene in linkage disequilibrium.

When considering the senescent phenotype at the cellular level of analysis, it is convenient to consider two broad categories of cell types. The first class consists of families of cells, subsets of which retain the capability to undergo semi-conservative DNA synthesis and cytokinesis. Such populations of cells can potentially maintain homeostasis, via compensatory proliferation, subsequent to age-associated cell loss. The second class consists of obligately postreplicative (i.e., terminally differentiated) cells. These include almost all adult central nervous system (CNS) neurons. (Primary sensory olfactory neurons constitute an exception to this rule, as do putatively rare neural stem cells [Reynolds and Weiss, 1992; Gage, 2000].) A great deal of attention has been devoted to a cell culture model whereby normal diploid human somatic cells can be observed to undergo an attenuation of replicative capacity, with eventual cessation of proliferation, the *Hayflick limit* (Hayflick and Moorhead, 1961). Such cultures are characterized by a great deal of clonal heterogeneity of growth potential, but all individual clones undergo replicative attenuation. The resulting postreplicative cells have exceedingly large cytoplasmic volumes and somewhat enlarged nuclei. A very large number of biochemical alterations have been catalogued in such *senescent cells* (Hayflick, 1980), including aggregates of pigments with properties of lipofuscins—the so-called *age pigments*—thought to result, in part, via peroxidation of lipids (see below). Unfortunately, however, most of these alterations have been described in fibroblast-like cells from the fetal lung or from fetal or adult skin, so that it has been difficult to determine the degree of concordance of such markers with what can be observed with homologous cell types in vivo. The degree to which the replicative potentials of skin fibroblast cells decline after the achievement of the adult stature is clouded by the mass culture methodologies utilized for such studies (Martin et al, 1970; Cristofalo et al., 1998). The bulk of the evidence,

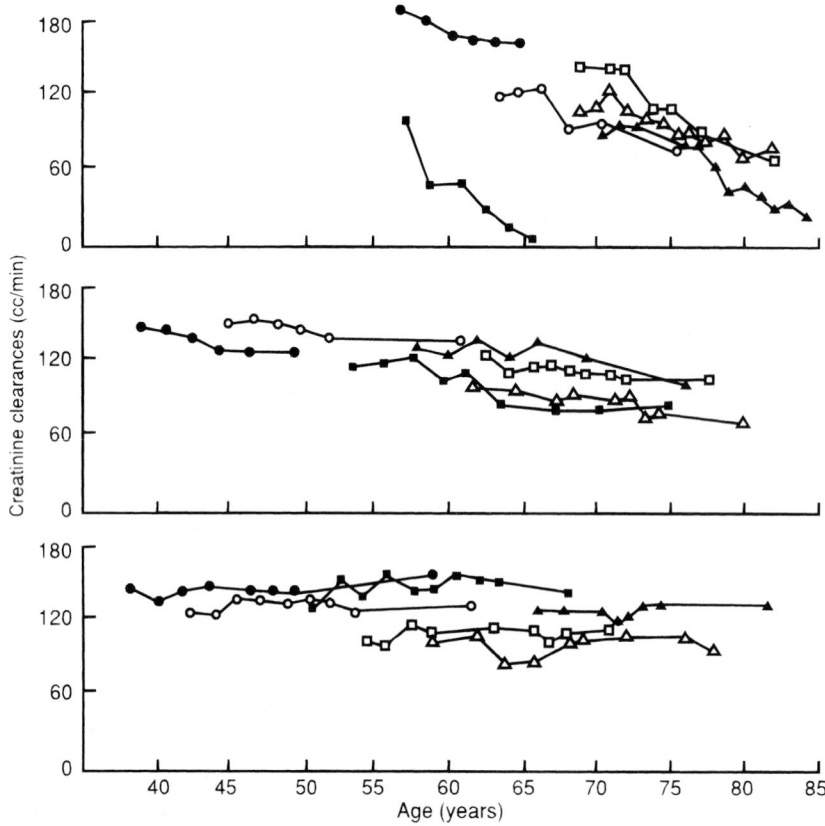

Fig. 20.4. Longitudinal studies of creatinine clearance (an approximate measure of the glomerular filtration rate) for a representative sample of a subset of 446 clinically normal male volunteers in the Baltimore Longitudinal Study of Aging of the National Institute on Aging followed between 1958 and 1981. The results could be classified in one of three major patterns. The top panel illustrates substantial rates of decline in this measure of renal function for six representative subjects who were followed for eight to 14 years. The middle panel illustrates a pattern of slight, but significant decline for six representative subjects followed for 11 to 22 years. For the six representative subjects in the bottom panel, who were followed for periods of 15 to 21 years, there were no apparent declines in this measure of renal function. (From Lindeman et al., 1985, with permission.)

however, does indicate that a variety of mammalian somatic cell types exhibit declines in replicative potentials throughout the adult life span as measured both in-vitro and in-vivo (e.g., Li et al., 1996; Wolf and Pendergrass, 1999). Moreover, the findings of a striking limitation of replicative life span for the case of the Werner syndrome (progeria of the adult) (see below) have been particularly well documented (reviewed by Tollefsbol and Cohen, 1984). While some cell types have vast reserves of replicative potential, for example, cells capable of repopulating the erythropoietic lineage (Harrison et al., 1984), there could well be multifocal regions in which such limited replication could play a critical role in the pathogenesis of major age-related pathologies. A potential example is the role of the limited regenerative potential of arterial endothelial cells in the pathogenesis of atherosclerotic lesions, especially at arterial branch points (Chang and Harley, 1995). Paradoxically, the pathologist will typically observe, side by side with evidence of atrophy, hyperplastic foci in various tissues of aging human subjects and other aging mammals (Martin, 1979).

This raises the question of some type of proliferative deregulation that accompanies aging. Such proliferative deregulation could set the stage for neoplastic processes. It could also play a role in the pathogenesis of atherosclerosis, which includes a conspicuous proliferative component of myointimal cells (Martin et al., 1975). The loss of replicative potential per se may be less significant than the gradual changes in gene expression that accompany such declines and the potential impact of even a few replicatively deficient cells on the surrounding tissues (Campisi, 1997). Changes in gene expression may be associated with an increased probability of mitotic errors (Ly et al., 2000).

The interest in Alzheimer's disease has fueled a great deal of new research on the aging of neurons and other cell types within the CNS. Although the subject is controversial, there is no convincing evidence that any of the neuropathologic parameters that are classically associated with dementia of the Alzheimer type are qualitatively unique. They can also be found, to a lesser degree, in the brains of "normal"-aged subjects. Thus, it is commonplace to find the occasional neuritic plaque, neurofibrillary tangle, and deposit of β-amyloid (in blood vessels and in association with neuritic plaques) in the brains of subjects who were considered to have no significant cognitive impairments during life. Similarly, postmortem anatomic and neuro-chemical data are consistent with a gradual depletion in the nigrostriatal dopaminergic system during "normative" aging. In at least some populations, however, this age-related loss could not be confirmed using positron emission tomography (Sawle et al., 1990). An increased rate of loss is presumed responsible for the emergence of Parkinson's disease. Do variations in the constitutional genotype modulate the rate of loss? Earlier, largely negative twin studies are now being reevaluated because of certain methodologic flaws; certainly, there are well-documented pedigrees in which Parkinson's disease (with the characteristic neuro-pathological hallmark of Lewy bodies) segregate as auto-somal dominants (Duvoisin, 1993). Mutations in the alpha-synuclein, parkin, and ubiquitin carboxy-terminal hydrolase L1 genes have been linked to a few instances of familial Parkinson's disease (reviewed by Solano et al., 2000).

There is very strong evidence indicating a major role for the constitutional genotype in the susceptibility to various familial and "sporadic" forms of Alzheimer's disease. In addition to the apparent protection by the ε2 allele of *ApoE* noted above, individuals carrying the ε4 allele, particularly homozygotes, are clearly at elevated risk of the disease (Corder et al., 1993). *ApoE* ε4 may act as an age-of-onset modifier for the common relatively late onset forms of the disorder. Current evidence supports the hypothesis that the ApoE protein acts pathogenetically via the modulation of the metabolism of the beta amyloid precursor protein, including the rate of formation of amyloid aggregates. The *ApoE* ε3 dimer is a particularly potent inhibitor of a stage of amyloidogenesis prior to a nucleation event (Evans et al., 1995). Thus, the elevated risk of subjects with *ApoE* ε4 alleles may merely reflect a deficiency of a more effective inhibitor of amyloidogenesis. There are alternative or addi-tional explanations, however. The ε4 allele is probably asso-ciated with diminished neuronal plasticity and repair, perhaps as a result of alterations in lipid homeostasis (Krzywkowski et al., 1999). This important subject is con-sidered in much more detail in Chapter 108. The layman's perception that aging is accompanied by a global loss of neurons is certainly incorrect. Only selected regions of the nervous system appear to be particularly susceptible.

The other type of terminally differentiated cell type that has received special attention by gerontologists is the mult-inucleated skeletal muscle cell. Structural and functional declines in skeletal muscle vary from muscle to muscle, with weight-bearing muscles more susceptible; the rates of these declines accelerate after about age 70 (Carmeli and Reznick, 1994). At least some proportion of the pathology is likely to be related to denervation atrophy.

Disuse atrophy is also an important component, as evi-denced by the significant gains in muscle strength in even very aged subjects following a modest conditioning regimen (McMurdo and Rennie, 1994). Old skeletal muscle is also more susceptible to contraction-induced injury and is less subject to repair via satellite cell-mediated regeneration (Brooks and Faulkner, 1994).

Many postreplicative aging cell types gradually accumu-late a mixture of complex fluorescent pigments called lipo-fuscins. These are likely to vary in composition from tissue to tissue. Lipofuscins of the retina, for example, are thought to consist, in part, of the reaction products of retinaldehyde with a membrane lipid, phosphatidylethanolamine (Wolf, 1993). Cardiac lipofuscins appear to involve the action of tyrosinase (Qiao et al., 1993). Most investigators believe that all lipofuscins are the products of lipid peroxidation reactions. They could therefore be regarded as evidence in support of theories of aging that invoke oxidative alter-ations of macromolecules. That lipofuscins are markers of some underlying aging process is supported by three lines of evidence. First, they appear to be almost invariable fea-tures of aging in an amazing variety of organisms, including certain strains of fungi under certain growth conditions (e.g., *Podospora anserina* and *Neurospora crassa*), parame-cia, nematodes, snails, fruit flies, house flies, frogs, parrots, house mice, rats, guinea pigs, cats, dogs, pigs, monkeys, and humans) (for references, see Martin, 1987; Lopez-Torres et al., 1993). Second, quantitative studies of their rates of accumulation in the hearts of dogs and humans indicate appropriate correlations with the life span poten-tials of those species (Martin, 1977). (No such correlations have been observed, however, among cardiac tissues from a group of primates of contrasting life spans [Nakano et al., 1993). Third, age-related increases in concentrations of at least some classes of lipofuscins are blunted by caloric restriction, an intervention known to increase life span in mammals (Rao et al., 1990; Katz et al., 1993).

The importance of extracellular aging has been empha-sized by the late Robert R Kohn (Kohn, 1978). Long-lived proteins, such as lens crystallins and collagens, are particularly susceptible to a variety of posttranslational alterations. Diabetics, who have many progeroid features, are particularly susceptible to glycation of proteins (Monnier et al., 1992). Alterations of the proteoglycans of cartilage are thought to be central events in the genesis of osteoarthritis, one of the most prevalent of the senescent phenotypes (Hardingham and Bayliss, 1990). Modified matrix components could perturb cell-matrix interactions and hence change cell function. Such a scenario has been suggested to play a role in the genesis of atherosclerosis (Robert et al., 1992). It remains to be seen which of the numerous human mutations involving matrix proteins can inform us as to pathogenetic mechanisms in the normative aging of the extracellular environment.

Why do we age?

Evolutionary biologists believe that they have an answer to the ultimate cause of aging in age-structured populations (i.e., populations that consist, at any given time, of cohorts of varying chronological ages) (Charlesworth, 1980). Simply put, we age because senescent phenotypes escape the force of natural selection (Rose, 1991). For human populations, the late William Hamilton showed that the force of natural selection for or against alleles that do not reach phenotypic expression until about the age around 45 years is essentially nil (Martin et al., 1996a). There is no good evidence that aging evolved because it was adaptive for the species or for the individual. Essentially all population geneticists who have considered this issue have concluded that aging is nonadaptive.

In terms of gene action, two ideas currently dominate the field. The first suggestion, championed by the late Peter Medawar, implicated an accumulation of constitutional mutations that did not reach phenotypic expression until late in the life course, when the force of natural selection would be attenuated (Medawar, 1952). In thinking about the evolutionary history of such mutations, one can imagine that a subset, during some earlier epoch, may indeed have had some negative effects upon reproductive fitness, but that these effects were subject to selection for suppressor mutations that progressively delayed the age of phenotypic expression (Medawar, 1952); eventually, however, the delayed age of expression would be such that there could be little or no influence of natural selection. The second dominant idea was first clearly enunciated by George C Williams (1957) and has been referred to as *antagonistic pleiotropy* by Michael R Rose (1991). This idea invokes sets of alleles selected because of positive effects during the early life history, but that are paradoxically responsible for deleterious phenotypes late in the life course. As one potential example, Williams speculated that alleles selected because of enhanced incorporation of calcium into bones might be responsible for forms of cal-

cific arteriosclerosis, when acting over long periods. Medical geneticists are in a good position to suggest a number of other examples, and perhaps to provide compelling supportive evidence. Such research has the potential to illuminate the most basic aspects of the aging problem.

Another conceptual formulation, one that overlaps with what has been discussed above, is that there is, inevitably, a tradeoff of energetic resources expended by an organism for purposes of reproduction and resources devoted to the maintenance of the macromolecular integrity of the organism. Examples include repair of DNA, scavenging of abnormal proteins, and replacement of effete somatic cells—the *disposable soma theory* of Tom Kirkwood (Kirkwood and Rose, 1991). These ideas can be generalized as life history "optimization" theories of aging (Partridge and Barton, 1993).

Experimental evidence in *Drosophila* sp. supports both optimization theories and the mutation accumulation theory of aging (reviewed by Partridge and Barton, 1993). The relative quantitative contributions of each theory, however, particularly in *Homo sapiens*, are completely unknown. As pointed out by Partridge and Barton (1993), the resolution of this issue has potentially profound implications for the future life history of our species. If optimization mechanisms predominate, any life span extensions may be offset by the tradeoff of lower early fertility, delayed maturation, and potential increases in early life history morbidity and mortality. If mutation accumulation mechanisms prevail, enhanced life span attributable to the elimination of such constitutional mutations would presumably have few effects on early life span structure and function. Given a major role for optimization theories, a continuation of the present secular trends of elective delays in the ages of reproduction in the developed societies would predict the emergence, by indirect selection, of increased life spans and related declines in early fertility after several centuries of continued evolution of our species. However, it has been well documented that advanced parental age is associated with increases in germ line mutations. Of particular relevance to our interest in late-life disorders is the evidence that there is a large paternal age effect for point mutations (reviewed by Crow, 1999). Such secular trends could therefore be associated with increases in germ line mutations, with potential deleterious effects in subsequent generations. An interesting potential specific example, from the US Framingham study, is the evidence showing a paternal age effect on the risk that a son will develop cancer of the prostate (Zhang et al., 1999).

At a more fundamental level, one can ask why one observes such striking variations in the life spans of various mammalian species. While such variation is obviously related to the constitutional genotype, it does not necessarily follow that aging is "programmed"—at least in the sense of concerted, determinative, sequential gene action comparable to what one observes in development. The most satisfying idea invokes differential impacts of environmental hazards (e.g., accidents, predation, drought, starvation, infectious diseases) during the emergence and maintenance of various species. This is nicely articulated in a popular book by Austad (1999). Species with comparatively high hazard functions would be expected to evolve life history strategies that emphasize rapid maturation, high fecundity, early fecundity, and short life spans. An attenuation of those hazards could set the stage for the emergence of sibling species with a more leisurely rate of maturation, lower early fecundity and longer life spans. One of the few field biology studies to examine this idea has in fact provided strong support for that hypothesis (Austad, 1993b).

The evolutionary formulations of the nature of aging have a number of interesting and important implications, in addition to those noted above. Let us summarize some of these propositions:

1. *Stochastic processes.* These are likely to play a major role in senescence. This follows from the conclusion that one is not dealing with a determinative sequence of concerted gene action but rather with an epiphenomenon of selection for gene action designed for reproductive fitness. Consider the analogy with a space craft engineered to function for a given period of time in order to complete a specific mission. Engineering specifications for indefinite maintenance of the craft would be prohibitively expensive or impossible. One would therefore anticipate an element of chance as to which components will initially exhibit structural and functional failures and when such failures will be detectible with the available diagnostic facilities. Many major geriatric diseases of humans (e.g., cancer, strokes, coronary thrombosis) are surely based on stochastic events. For the case of malignant neoplasms, selection for a series of random somatic mutations are keys to the understanding of the pathogenesis. Overall longevity also is subject, in part, to stochastic laws. There are numerous examples in which investigators have rigorously controlled both environment and genotype, yet have observed marked variations in longevity. The most convincing example comes from studies of *Caenorhabditis elegans*, which can be grown in chemically defined medium in suspension cultures, thus ensuring rigorous control of the environment (Vanfleteren et al., 1998).

2. *Polygenic basis.* There is a polygenic basis for aging. There is no reason to believe that the optimization theories or mutation accumulation theories involve only a few genes. Indeed, for the case of the successful experiments involving indirect selection for increased life spans in genetically heterogeneous wild-type stocks of *Drosophila melanogaster*, genetic analysis indicated genes on all of the major chromosomes (Luckinbill et al., 1988). Martin (1978) has estimated (as an upper limit) that allelic variation or mutation at close to 7% of loci of the human genome has the potential to modulate varying aspects of the senescent phenotype. A different and more conservative estimate—the number of genes likely to have evolved in the hominoid lineage leading to humans (and thus could be associated with the increased life span of *Homo sapiens*)—gave a figure of 0.6% of functional genes (Cutler, 1975). Neither estimate can be characterized as *oligogenic*.

3. *Multiple mechanisms.* There are likely to be multiple mechanisms of aging, although there would be selective pressure toward some degree of synchronization of the ages of expression of phenotypic effects resulting from independent mechanisms. This proposition follows from the randomness of the accumulated constitutional mutations and from the great variety of types of gene action that could be involved in "tradeoff" types of gene action. Against this proposition, however, is the fact that a single environmental manipulation—caloric restriction—regularly leads to life span extension in rodents, at least those that have been selected for the easy life of the laboratory setting (reviewed by Masoro, 1998). We have little information on the effects of caloric restriction in the wild, however. The life course histories of organisms whose evolutionary history reflected exceptionally high environmental hazard functions, such as the mice and rats used for most of the calorie-restriction experiments, are quite distinct from those of the higher primates (Austad, 1993). It is therefore not at all clear that caloric restriction would make a significant impact on the life span potentials of human subjects. We shall have to await the outcome of current research in Rhesus and squirrel monkeys (reviewed by Roth et al., 1999) to know how likely such an effect will obtain for our species. Meanwhile, common sense tells us that we should avoid gluttony!

4. *Species specificity.* There is likely to be a degree of species specificity in relevant gene action. We have already developed certain of these arguments, but let us consider an extended argument. If aging is in fact an

epiphenomenon—a by-product of selection for alleles ensuring an optimal degree of reproductive fitness in a given environment—there is no a priori reason to expect identical scenarios of gene action among very different species. Consider the striking differences in the behavioral patterns among different species that lead to successful matings. There are surely a wide variety of different loci involved, and those that are operative in fruit flies must surely differ from those that are relevant for man! Nevertheless, it is quite possible that there are a number of common mechanisms among groups of related species (including all mammals), and it is even conceivable that such global mechanisms as oxidative damage to macromolecules underlay the aging of all or most organisms (see, for example, the above discussion on lipofuscins). This is the rationale for carrying out comparative gerontologic research.

5. *Intraspecific variations.* There are likely to be significant intraspecific variations in phenotypic patterns of aging, particularly in humans. This also follows from many of the arguments discussed above. Given its polygenic nature, the likelihood of a variety of mechanisms, a strong stochastic component, the realization that one is dealing with alterations in all body systems, and the enormous genetic and environmental heterogeneity in our species, one would certainly predict substantial differences in the way aging plays out in individual subjects. Every clinician has witnessed this phenomenon first hand. While differential impacts of the environment are likely to be partially responsible for such variations, the challenge for medical geneticists is to dissect out specific major and minor genetic factors responsible for particularly favorable or unfavorable nature-nurture interactions.

6. *Plasticity.* The life span of a species should exhibit a degree of plasticity. This follows directly from the arguments on the nature of gene action in aging discussed above and from the experimental results in *Drosophila* sp. Nonetheless, there are likely to be some severe constraints on such plasticity—constraints related to the basic architecture of the organism. We do not expect a fruit fly to live as long as a mouse without essentially creating a new species.

How do we age?

We now turn to a more systematic consideration of the present state of our knowledge concerning the underlying molecular mechanisms of aging. In contrast to the reasonably satisfying evolutionary explanations for *why* we age, there is no consensus as to *how* we age, although the research programs of a growing number of investigators appear to be motivated by the theory that oxidative damage to macromolecules, including those mediated by chemical free radicals (the "free radical theory of aging") (Harman, 1994) are of paramount importance. At a more fundamental level, while evolutionary theory would predict multiple mechanisms of aging, investigators who emphasize caloric restriction as a route to enhanced longevity would argue for a small number of proximal mechanisms of aging (Weindruch and Walford, 1988; Masoro, 1998).

ALTERATIONS IN PROTEINS

In 1963, Orgel introduced the protein synthesis error catastrophe theory of aging (Orgel, 1963; 1970). It was proposed that transcriptional and/or translational errors in the synthesis of proteins that were themselves used for the synthesis of proteins (e.g., DNA-dependent RNA polymerases, ribosomal proteins) could result in an exponential cascade of errors involving essentially all proteins, leading to cell and organismal death. Biosynthetic errors in protein synthesis appear to be rare, however, even in old organisms (Rothstein, 1989). Although most gerontologists have abandoned this theory, very few tests of the theory have been carried out with postreplicative cells in vivo (Rabinovitch and Martin, 1982). By contrast, there is a growing body of evidence indicating the prevalence of post-translational modifications in proteins in aging tissues, although, of the more than 140 major and minor known modifications of proteins, only a few have been studied in aging cells, tissues and organisms (Rattan et al., 1992). Beginning with a classic paper on senescent nematodes by Gershon and Gershon (1970), many studies have demonstrated an accumulation of immunologically detectable, but enzymatically inactive, enzyme molecules in various mammalian tissues (Rothstein, 1982; 1989). These may result from a variety of post-translational modifications, including subtle conformational changes (Rothstein, 1989). There is currently a great deal of interest in oxidative alterations. Metal-catalyzed oxidation systems have the potential to inactivate enzymes oxidatively via attacks on the side chains of certain amino acids, with the formation of carbonyl derivatives (Stadtman and Berlett, 1998). The side chains of histidine, arginine, lysine, and proline are particularly susceptible (Amici et al., 1989). The sulfhydryl groups of methionine are also susceptible to oxidation (Stadtman, 1988).

Other post-translational changes that can be observed in aging cells include racemization, deamidation, isomerization, phosphorylation, and glycation (reviewed by Stadtman, 1988; Gracy, et al., 1990; Rattan et al., 1992).

Many gerontologists believe that glycation, the spontaneous nonenzymatic reaction of glucose with proteins and nucleic acids, may be a major factor in the development of certain age decrements, as well as complications of diabetes mellitus (reviewed by Baynes and Monnier, 1989; Lee and Cerami, 1992). Glycation is the slow, spontaneous reaction of the aldehydic form of glucose with free amino groups to form a Schiff base, which subsequently rearranges to form a stable Amadori product. Subsequent reactions, possibly involving oxygen radicals, generate more complex products referred to as advanced glycosylation end (AGE) products. Certain of these compounds, including pentosidine, have been characterized. Antibodies to the AGE products have been generated and used to map their distribution to neuritic plaques and tangles and to other sites (Yan et al., 1994). Because the levels of AGE products increase with age and with elevated blood glucose, cross-link proteins and change their physical and biologic properties, they are thought to underlie the development of atherosclerosis, cataracts, and peripheral neuropathies. In addition, macrophage receptors bind to the AGE products and initiate the secretion of inflammatory cytokines such as the tumor necrosis factor (Kirstein et al., 1992). Thus, glycation represents a progressive age change linked to age-associated disabilities. Support for these ideas have come from experiments in aging dogs, in which it was possible to reverse myocardial stiffness and improve cardiac function by the administration of an experimental compound known to break the cross-links associated with the formation of advanced glycation endproducts (Asif et al., 2000).

Calorically restricted rodents, which have substantially increased life span, exhibit evidence of both enhanced defenses against reactive oxygen species (Laganiere and Yu, 1989; Lee and Yu, 1990) and reduced levels of protein glycation (associated with decreased levels of plasma glucose) (Masoro et al., 1989). Such results suggest that both the free radical theory of aging (Harman, 1994) and the glycation theory of aging may be operative and potentially synergistic (Kristal and Yu, 1992). A number of different types of amyloids accumulate in mammalian tissues during aging. In their advanced states, they are detected extracellularly as protein aggregates associated with proteoglycans and other proteins. Each type is derived from a different precursor protein. These include the beta amyloid protein of Alzheimer's disease and the aging brain (Naslund et al., 1994); a transthyretin-derived amyloid in peripheral nerve

tissues, autonomic nervous system, choroid plexus, cardiovascular system, and kidneys (Takahashi et al., 1991); atrial amyloid derived from the atrial natriuretic peptide (Johansson et al., 1987); the amylin-derived amyloid in the pancreatic islets of Langerhans (Edwards and Morley, 1993); systemic amyloid AA, derived from apolipoprotein A-II (Higuchi et al., 1991); and possibly unique types of amyloid in the anterior pituitary gland (Tashima et al., 1988), intervertebral discs (Wullbrand et al., 1990), the aortic intima and media (Mucchiano et al., 1992), aortic heart valves (Yokota et al., 1994), and the adrenal cortex (Eriksson and Westermark, 1990). In certain of these conditions, mutations or polymorphic variants in the precursor protein greatly accelerate the rates of deposition of the derivative amyloids.

It is a challenge for the future to discover common denominators underlying this remarkable propensity of mammalian tissues to accumulate these different types of abnormal proteins. Obvious approaches would include more detailed studies of alterations in protein turnover with age (including the turnover of amyloid deposits) and how such turnover might be modulated by endocrine and neuroendocrine factors. Another promising and relatively new area of research seeks to define gene products that function in the repair of altered proteins. An example is the catalysis of the transfer of a methyl group from S-adenosylmethionine to L-aspartyl and D-aspartyl residues by protein carboxyl methyltransferases (ED 2.1.1.77). These enzymes have the potential to repair abnormal proteins via the conversion of L-isoaspartyl residues to L-aspartyl residues (Mudgett and Clarke, 1993). This enzyme is polymorphic in humans, raising the question of the differential repair of such classes of altered proteins during aging in human populations (Tsai and Clarke, 1994).

ALTERATIONS IN DNA

Nuclear DNA

Epigenetic events

Given the fact that, for most genetic loci, only two alleles are present, nuclear DNA would appear to be a particularly vulnerable target for damage during aging. Historically, the first specific type of somatic "mutational" theory of aging was proposed by a physicist, Leo Szilard (1959). He envisioned random "hits" that would inactivate entire chromosomes or chromosome arms. In modern terms, such inactivations could conceivably be associated with epigenetic events such as methylation of cytosines, as for the case of the random inactivation of one of the two X chromosomes of the human female during embryonic development (reviewed by Gartler et al., 1992) and the processes of parental genomic imprinting (reviewed by Surani, 1994). There is no good evidence of widespread heterochromatizations or inactivation of large chromatin domains during aging. In fact, at least for the case of mice, there is evidence of a *reactivation* of certain gene loci on a previously inactive X chromosome during aging (Cattanach, 1974; Wareham et al., 1987). No such reactivation could be demonstrated for the case of the *HPRT* locus of heterozygous human females (Migeon et al., 1988). At the molecular level, global losses of 5-methyl cytosine have been demonstrated in aging fibroblast cultures (Wilson and Jones, 1983) and in tissues of two species of aging rodents (Wilson et al., 1987), but there have been few studies of altered methylation in specific domains of specific genes during aging. In one such study, hypermethylation was mapped to the proximal 5′ spacer domain of ribosomal DNA genes of aging mice; silver stains of cytogenetic preparations revealed that the ribosomal gene cluster on chromosome 16 was preferentially inactivated (Swisshelm et al., 1990). It remains to be seen, however, whether this remarkable result reflects some developmental, adaptive process in laboratory mice or in the particular strain of mice investigated, as the biochemical changes were observed as early as six months. A form of gene-specific methylation of CpG islands has clearly been established to progress steadily into old age in human subjects. It is associated with the silencing of the estrogen receptor gene of a subset of cells of the colonic mucosa (Issa et al., 1994). A striking finding in that study was that, of a set of 45 colorectal human tumors examined, including those in very early stages of oncogenesis, estrogen receptor expression was either diminished or absent. Moreover, the introduction and expression of an estrogen receptor gene in a line of colon carcinoma cells resulted in marked growth suppression. This important paper therefore demonstrates a link between a presumably epigenetically based, progressive repression of a specific gene during aging and the susceptibility to the development of a common type of cancer of aging.

Using the yeast model of replicative aging, Lenny Guarente and his colleagues have highlighted a key role of NAD-dependent histone deacetylation in the regulation of energy metabolism, genomic silencing and aging (Imai et al., 2000). There are mouse homologues of the yeast *Sir2* gene, which was shown to be a histone deacetylase.

There is a great deal of evidence for a variety of other changes in gene expression throughout the life span, but it remains to be seen which of these alterations are of primary significance to one or more aging processes and which are merely epiphenomena. One such approach is to explore the effects of caloric restriction (Heydari and Richardson, 1992). Assessments of global changes in mRNA expression have now been made for the case of the skeletal muscle of aging cohorts of control and calorically restricted mice (Lee et al., 1999). The picture suggests that aging muscle exhibits a marked stress response, with lowered expression of metabolic and biosynthetic genes. These alterations are ameliorated in the calorically restricted mice. It will of course be important to evaluate such changes at the protein level. We can conclude, however, that the study of epigenetic events will continue to be of major importance to the science of gerontology (Holliday, 1990).

Mutational events

In 1961, a now classic paper appeared casting doubt on the validity of somatic mutational theories of aging (Clark and Rubin, 1962). Taking advantage of the occurrence, in nature, of a species of wasps, males of which exist as either haploid or diploid organisms, it was found that there was no difference in the life spans of these organisms. As expected, however, the haploid wasps were much more susceptible to the effects of ionizing radiation. These results were strong evidence against a role for recessive mutations in insects. They did not rule out, however, some role for a combination of dominant and recessive mutations in the aging of such organisms. Moreover, those experiments tell us nothing about the role of somatic mutations of replicating populations of cells in the limitation of life span, since wasps and other insects, with the exception of gonadal tissues, consist of postreplicative cells. For the case of such replicating populations of cells, there is now compelling evidence that somatic mutations constitute a link between the biology of aging and the biology of cancer. Thus, while much more data are required, there are reasonable correlations of species-specific life spans and rates of development of various neoplasms (see references in Martin, 1991). Clearly, among those genes that evolved in association with the relatively long life spans of *Homo sapiens* (the longest-lived of all mammalian species), there must be loci conferring enhanced genomic stability in comparison, for example, with those of *Mus musculus domesticus* (Smith, 1994). Moreover, there may be considerable species differences in the patterns of somatic mutation.

For mice, for example, there is evidence of a marked susceptibility to cytologically detectible chromosomal mutations during aging (Martin et al., 1985), while in comparable cell types (renal tubular epithelial cells) there is little evidence for the accumulation of mutations (presumably intragenic) at the *HPRT* locus, a target chosen because of the lack of evidence for selection against such mutations in renal tissue (Horn et al., 1984). Mutations have been shown to accumulate at the *HPRT* locus of T lymphocytes and in the renal tubular epithelial cells of aging human subjects, however, with higher frequencies of mutation being observed in the epithelial cell type (Trainor et al., 1984; Martin et al., 1996b). The lymphocyte study showed that deletions were relatively common (Turner et al., 1985). Such accumulations could be attributable to chronologic time, rather than to intrinsic biologic aging. We will require additional research in mammals of contrasting life span potentials to address this question; an approach using comparable transgenic reporter constructs (Lee et al., 1994) may be promising if these could be comparably buffered from position effects.

Microarray hybridization experiments on a few strains of human fibroblasts from donors of varying ages and from subjects with Progeria (the Hutchinson-Gilford syndrome) suggest that mitotic misregulation may be of importance in human aging (Ly et al., 2000). It will be important to extend such studies to replicating cells in vivo.

We will also need to re-evaluate the question of genomic instability in populations of postreplicative cells such as neurons. Evidence that this may prove to be a productive line of research comes from a remarkable series of experiments with the Brattleboro rat, a model of diabetes insipidus caused by homozygosity for a single base pair deletion in the vasopressin gene (van Leeuwen, 1992; Evans et al., 1994; van Leeuwen et al., 1994). During aging of these animals, frameshift reversions were detected, thus establishing the phenomenon of somatic mutations in nondividing neuronal cells. Another line of research deserving additional attention is the potential mutagenic effects of glycation of DNA (reviewed by Lee and Cerami, 1992).

Telomeric DNA

The most robust age changes noted in the nuclear genome of normal somatic cells are alterations in telomere length (Harley et al., 1990; Lindsey et al., 1991; Allsopp et al., 1992; Vaziri et al., 1993; Counter et al., 1994). Telomeres have a highly repetitive structure (TTAGGG in humans and mice) that extends for many thousand of nucleotides at the ends of chromosomes. The telomeres stabilize chromosomal structure and their loss leads to various cytologic aberrations and the arrest of cell division. Current concepts suppose that telomeres in cells of the germ line and in many neoplastic cells (Kim et al., 1994) are added to the ends of

chromosomes de novo by a unique enzyme referred to as telomerase, which uses an associated RNA to code for the hexanucleotide repeats. It appears that telomerase is lost from the progeny of the stem cells and the telomeres are then duplicated during cell division by DNA polymerase. It is characteristic of DNA polymerase that it fails to copy some 50 to 200 terminal bases of the trailing strand and the telomeres are shortened by this amount with every cell division (Levy et al., 1992). The shortening of telomeres is strikingly apparent when one examines the telomeric/subtelomeric DNA isolated by appropriate restriction enzyme cleavage from normal human fibroblasts which have undergone high numbers of cell divisions in culture.

A mechanism of clonal senescence has been proposed, based upon loss of telomeric repeats (Wright and Shay, 1992). The hypothesis attempts to reconcile observations of the loss of telomeric repeats in serially passaged cell cultures with (1) the observations of reproducible alterations in gene action associated with the exit from the mitotic cell cycle in senescent cells (Seshadri and Campisi, 1990; Stein et al., 1990); (2) experiments indicating the dominance of the senescent phenotype in hybrid synkaryons between normal somatic cells and cells of indefinite proliferative potential (Bunn and Tarrant, 1980; Pereira-Smith and Smith, 1983); and (3) evidence that exit from the cell cycle is an active process associated with the appearance of inhibitors (Spiering and Smith, 1991). Wright and Shay (1992) proposed that, as a result of the shortening of telomeric repeats, a region of heterochromatization eventually reaches a contiguous chromatin domain encompassing a gene coding for a repressor of a program of gene action that removes the cell from the mitotic cell cycle. Could this type of gene action be comparable to the "checkpoints" hypothesized to underlay the transient cell cycle arrest following DNA damage (Hartwell and Kastan, 1994)? More research will be required to address this issue. There are likely to be differences as well as similarities (Fig. 20.5).

In both conditions, critical effectors are cyclin-dependent kinases activated by their cyclin partners that phosphorylate negative regulators of the cell cycle, such as the retinoblastoma protein, to permit DNA synthesis. It is well known that damage to DNA will cause cells to cease DNA synthesis and cell division and that the p53 tumor suppressor gene has an important role in arresting DNA synthesis under these circumstances. Still another protein known by various names, including p21, WAF-1, and SDI-1 (reviewed by Hunter, 1993), has been found to be induced by p53 and to bind to the cdc kinase/cyclin/PCNA complex and block its kinase activity. The p21 protein is elevated in senescent cells (Noda et al., 1994), while p53 levels

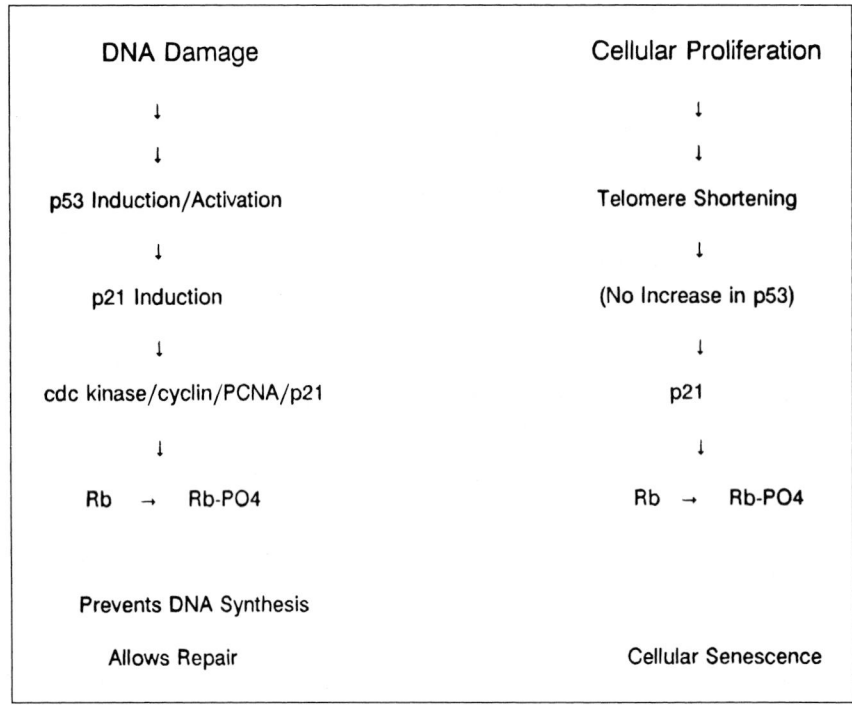

Fig. 20.5. Simplified summarization of the regulation of mitotic cell cycle arrest after DNA damage and in association with the clonal senescence of cultures of proliferating normal diploid somatic cells.

may be normal or depressed. Given the fact that telomere length plays an important role in stabilizing chromosomal structure and possibly their association with the nuclear matrix, it seems possible that telomere shortening induces cellular senescence via the activation of the p21 gene. In support of this concept is the demonstration that p21 arrests cellular proliferation when introduced into cultured cells and that the SV40 large antigen, known to retard cellular senescence, reverses p21 arrest. Taken together, the data suggest that the p21 protein could be the key mediator of cell cycle arrest in cellular senescence and that it is activated as a result of the shortening of the telomeres.

A similar decline in telomere length is observed in DNA isolated from the cells of persons of increasing age (Lindsey et al., 1991; Vaziri et al., 1993). Given the importance of telomeres to chromosomal stability, it is possible that this accounts in part for the increase in chromosomal aberrations seen in cells from old donors and in cultured cells maintained for many generations in culture. It is not established, however, whether the shortening of telomeres is in fact an important cause of aging or merely one of many biomarkers of aging. At a more fundamental level, it is possible that the cell culture model of replicative failure, with which most of the molecular studies on "cellular aging" have been carried out, may have evolved as a mechanism for the normal regulation of cell growth and development (Martin,

1993). Even so, such replicative decline could have important consequences for aging, in keeping with the antagonistic pleiotropic gene action idea discussed above. In any case, medical geneticists should be aware that twin studies have demonstrated that individual differences in telomere restriction fragment lengths are to a large extent genetically determined, with heritability estimated at 78% (Slagboom et al., 1994). It remains to be seen to what extent polymorphisms at loci regulating basal lengths of telomeres and their rates of decline can influence various aspects of human aging and late-life disease (Martin, 1994).

The vital role of telomerase in maintaining telomere length and permitting sustained replication has received very strong support from transfection experiments using the catalytic subunit of telomerase (Bodnar et al., 1998). It has since been possible to use this methodology to "immortalize" primary cultures from a variety of human donors, including those with genetic disorders (Ouellette et al., 2000). This should greatly expedite research on human biochemical and somatic cell genetics.

MITOCHONDRIAL DNA

Considerable attention is now being directed to changes in mitochondrial DNA (mtDNA) that might underlie age deficits in metabolism and muscle and nerve function (reviewed by Wallace, 1997). This is based in part on a growing number of observations that various types of mtDNA mutations accumulate, to varying degrees, in multiple tissues of aging human subjects and in the tissues of other aging mammals. Most of the assays were for large deletions, but tandem duplications and point mutations have also been reported.

mtDNA (reviewed by Gilham, 1994) is a closed circular DNA of some 16,569 nucleotides that codes for some of the mitochondrial proteins plus the tRNAs and rRNAs used for mitochondrial protein synthesis. Other components of the mitochondria are coded for by nuclear genes and are transported to the mitochondria. Essentially all mtDNA molecules are maternal in origin; thus, mtDNA genetic diseases are maternally transmitted.

Based on the frequency and consistent location of common specific age-related deletions, one can postulate that the sequences between the direct repeats are looped out following damage to the DNA by a slip replication mechanism. The damage to mtDNA molecules may be initiated by oxygen radicals generated as a by-product of the oxidative phosphorylation reactions carried out by the mitochondria. The proximity of mtDNA to the sources of oxygen radicals, plus the lack of associated histones, would make mtDNA more vulnerable than nuclear DNA. While certain forms of DNA repair are lacking in mitochondria, other lesions appear to be repaired (LeDoux al, 1992). Thus, the age changes observed could be due to increased damage and/or reduced repair.

For human subjects, accumulations of mtDNA mutations have been documented in tissues which contain large numbers of postreplicative or slowly replicating cells, such as skeletal muscles (Katayama et al., 1991; Simonetti et al., 1992; Cooper et al., 1992; Munscher et al., 1993; Lee et al., 1994; Hsieh et al., 1994), brain (Corral-Debrinski et al, 1992 Soong et al., 1992), heart (Corral-Debrinski et al., 1992b; Hayakawa et al., 1992; Takeda et al., 1993), liver (Yen et al., 1992), and ovary (Suganuma et al., 1993).

In spite of the fact that there are substantial increases in mtDNA damage with age, only a small proportion of the total mtDNA molecules are affected. Indeed, no clear consensus exists as to whether oxidative phosphorylation declines with age. Thus, some investigators doubt that the alterations occurring in mtDNA are a significant factor underlying aging and/or age-associated diseases. Alternatively, it has been proposed that damaged mtDNA molecules preferentially replicate as a local adaptive response to energetic deficits created by impaired mitochondria. An alternative hypothesis is that damaged mtDNA molecules accumulate because they generate fewer altered proteins and are thus less likely to be targeted for turnover; this theory has been referred to as the "survival of the slowest" (de Grey, 1999). Thus, as in the genetic mtDNA diseases, it is proposed that the altered DNA molecules are concentrated by a focal expansion in individual cells, nerves, and muscle fibers and lead to the death of such cells, perhaps through apoptosis. An increase in mtDNA damage may therefore cause the progressive depletion of single cells without causing major alterations in the remaining cells in the tissue, which would be affected individually and later. Clearly, such a mechanism could play an important role in the decline of CNS function, in the development of frailty, in impaired wound healing, and in other age-associated declines by depleting cells from these tissues.

GERMLINE MUTATIONS

Medical geneticists are well aware of the increased risk to the conceptus of chromosomal types of mutations (mainly aneuploidies) as functions of maternal age. This is, of course, the basis for the clinical practice of recommending amniocentesis and prenatal diagnosis for pregnant women over the age of 35. The relationship of paternal age to the increased risk of certain types of mutations has also been well-documented (Vogel and Rathenberg, 1975) and has been mentioned above in a different context. Suffice it to say that, from the point of view of the pathobiology of aging, we remain ignorant of the underlying mechanisms. These important subjects have in fact received substantially less attention by the gerontologic community than the question of somatic mutation and aging.

ALTERATIONS IN LIPIDS

Given the seminal importance of membranes in cell biology, alterations in the structure of membrane lipids could constitute a primary mechanism of age-related cellular dysfunction and cell death. Most research in this field has addressed the issue of lipid peroxidation, an integral component of the free radical theory of aging (Harman, 1994). Aspects of this idea have been discussed above, including the ubiquitous nature of lipofuscin pigments as a biologic marker of aging. A second line of research in this field has emphasized age-related increases, in various cell types, of the cholesterol-to-phospholipid ratios of plasma cell membranes, with a consequent decrease in membrane fluidity. At least in some cell types, however, such as neurons of the dorsal root ganglia, the decline in membrane fluidity, as measured by lateral diffusion coefficients, is related to development rather than to postmaturational aging (Horie et al., 1986).

Progeroid syndromes of humans

Having reviewed the present state of our knowledge of the biology and pathobiology of aging, we can now consider spontaneous mutations in man that may modulate the aging phenotype. As we have seen, however, evolutionary theory would argue that no single mutation or polymorphism is likely to modulate all aspects of the senescent phenotype. In a systematic survey of several editions of McKusick's catalog of the mendelian inheritance of humans, it was indeed concluded that no single mutation has yet been identified that could be characterized as a *global progeria* (Martin, 1978). A number of mutations, however, could be characterized as "segmental progeroid mutations" in that multiple segments of the complex senescent phenotype of man appear to have been affected. The prototype for this group is the Werner syndrome (progeria of the adult) (McKusick, 1994) (*WRN*). A translation of Otto Werner's original manuscript and reprints of subsequent classical reviews together with other contributions are available in monograph form (Salk et al., 1985). More recent reviews are available (Goto, 1997; Martin et al., 1999). Homozygous affected individuals appear to be normal at birth and typically do not come to the attention of physicians until about the time of puberty, when they fail to enjoy the usual adolescent growth spurt. The full-blown syndrome includes premature graying and thinning of the hair of the scalp, thinning of body hair, atrophic tight skin, with pigmentation abnormalities, bilateral ocular cataracts, hypogonadism, osteoporosis, diabetes mellitus, varying forms of arteriosclerosis (e.g., atherosclerosis, medial calcinosis, arteriosclerosis, calcific changes of heart valves), soft tissue calcification, chronic ulcerations of the skin overlying the malleoli and Achilles tendon, and a variety of benign and malignant neoplasms. There is a characteristic weak, high-pitched, squeaky or hoarse voice and a body habitus, usually characterized by very thin extremities, but with adequate or increased adiposity of the abdominal fat pad. Death occurs at a median age of 47–48 years, usually from a myocardial infarction or a neoplasm. As for the case of other rare, autosomal recessives, there is an increased prevalence of parental consanguinity. Fertility is substantially decreased in homozygotes. There is no clearly established clinical phenotype in heterozygous carriers, although there are anectodal reports of premature graying of hair in some potential carriers and a provocative report suggesting that family members may be collectively more susceptible to malignant neoplasms (Goto et al., 1981). Consistent with that possibility is a report that lymphoblastoid cell lines

from proven heterozygous carriers indicate a degree of susceptibility to a genotoxic agent (4-nitroquinoline-1-oxide) that is intermediate to that found in wild type and homozygous affected siblings (Ogburn et al., 1997). These observations are of considerable potential public health significance, as the prevalence of the heterozygous carriers, at least in Japan, is greater than 0.6%; screening for a full set of mutations is likely to give a larger number of carriers (Satoh et al., 1999). Diagnostic criteria for the identification of what are now known to be null mutations at the *WRN* locus were developed by the University of Washington International Registry of Werner Syndrome and are given in Nakura et al. 1994) and in Table 20.1.

The *WRN* mutation was mapped to the short arm of chromosome 8 by Goto et al. (1992) and confirmed by Schellenberg and colleagues, who used the method of homozygosity mapping (Schellenberg et al., 1992). Linkage

Table 20.1 Criteria for the diagnosis of Werner syndrome as employed by the University of Washington International Registry of Werner Syndrome

Cardinal signs

1. Bilateral cataracts
2. Characteristic dermatological pathology (tight skin, atrophic skin, pigmentary alterations, ulceration, hyperkeratosis, regional subcutaneous atrophy) and characteristic facies ("bird" facies)
3. Short stature
4. Paternal consanguinity (3rd cousin or greater) or affected sibling
5. Premature graying and/or thinning of scalp hair
6. Elevation of 24-h urinary hyaluronic acid, when test is available

Further signs and symptoms

1. Diabetes mellitus
2. Hypogonadism (secondary sexual underdevelopment, diminished fertility, testicular or ovarian atrophy)
3. Osteoporosis
4. Osteosclerosis of distal phalanges of fingers and/or toes (X-ray diagnosis)
5. Soft tissue calcification
6. Evidence of premature atherosclerosis (e.g., history of myocardial infarction)
7. Mesenchymal neoplasms, rare neoplasms, or multiple neoplasms
8. Voice changes (high pitched, squeaky, or hoarse voice)
9. Flat feet

Inclusive diagnostic classifications are as follows. Definite: all cardinal signs (including no. 6 when test is available) and any two others. Probable: the first three cardinal signs and any two others. Possible: either cataracts or dermatological alteration and any four others. Exclusion of diagnosis: a) onset of signs and symptoms before adolescence (except short stature, since current data on preadolescent growth patterns are inadequate); b) absence of hyaluronic aciduria. (Modified from Nakura et al., 1994, with permission.)

disequilibrium studies have provided evidence for several distinct haplotypes in the Japanese and Caucasian populations (Yu et al., 1994). The *WRN* mutation was shown to involve a member of the RecQ family of DNA helicases, now known as the Werner helicase (Yu et al., 1996). In addition to a central helicase domain, the gene encodes an exonuclease domain, but the precise role or roles of the protein in DNA transactions is not known. There are lines of evidence that support roles in replication, repair, recombination and transcription.

Somatic cells from homozygotes exhibit a sharply limited replicative potential (Martin et al., 1970) and have been characterized as mutator strains on the basis of cytogenetic analysis (Salk et al., 1981), fluctuation analysis (Fukuchi et al., 1989), and a host cell plasmid mutagenesis assay (Runger et al., 1994). Werner syndrome thus provides support for an important role of somatic mutation/instability in aging and late-life disorders. It is possible that the mechanisms underlying these disabilities are distinct from those that obtain in most aging human subjects. For example, Werner syndrome fibroblasts that have undergone in vitro replicative senescence retain the inducibility of c-*fos* expression after a mitogenic stimulus, in contrast to the case for control fibroblast strains (Oshima et al., 1995). There are also discordances at the clinical level. For example, the long bones of the limbs, especially of the lower limbs, are particularly vulnerable to osteoporosis, whereas in ordinary aging the vertebral column is particularly vulnerable, especially in females. There also appear to be disproportionate numbers of neoplasms derived from mesenchymal cells in Werner syndrome patients, whereas epithelium-derived neoplasms are by far the commonest class associated with aging in most individuals. There is also a peculiar osteosclerosis of the distal phalanges that is not seen during ordinary aging (Goto et al., 1989).

Some evolutionary biologists would argue that the Werner syndrome is a poor model of aging, in that it is clear that it would not fit the definition of a set of phenotypes that have escaped the force of natural selection (Rose, 1991). That criticism is even more pertinent for the case of classic Progeria (Hutchinson-Gilford syndrome) (Brown, 1990), expressed within the first decade of life, and which has a number of features that are different from usual aging (Martin, 1978; Hamer et al., 1988). One should keep in mind, however, that for each of these loci identified by such strong phenotypes, there are likely to be allelic variants that result in more subtle phenotypes that do indeed escape the force of natural selection. Indeed, for some populations, there may well be alleles at such loci that result in enhanced structure and function during the posterproductive periods of the life histories of human subjects. A challenge for the medical geneticist is to discover such alleles. This will involve a departure from the traditional disease-oriented focus, which introduces ascertainment bias to the investigation of genetic aspects of the biology of aging. Some suggestions for an experimental design to identify genetic factors associated with unusually successful aging have been published (Martin, 1998).

REFERENCES

Allsopp RC Vaziri H, Patterson C et al. (1992) Telomere length predicts replicative capacity of human fibroblasts. Proc Natl Acad Sci USA 89:10114–10118

Amici A, Levine RL, Tsai L, Stadtman ER (1989) Conversion of amino acid residues in proteins and amino acid homopolymers to carbonyl derivatives by metal-catalyzed oxidation reactions. J Biol Chem 264:3341–3346

Asif M, Egan J, Vasan S et al. (2000) An advanced glycation endproduct cross-link breaker can reverse age-related increases in myocardial stiffness. Proc Natl Acad Sci USA 97:2809–2813

Austad SN (1993a) FRAR course on laboratory approaches to aging. The comparative perspective and choice of animal models in aging research. Aging (Milano.) 5:259–267

Austad SN (1993b) Retarded senescene in an unsular population of Virginia opossums (*Didelphis virginiana*). J Zool Lond 229:695–708

Austad SN (1999) Why We Age: What Science if Discovering about the Body's Journey Through Life. John Wiley & Sons, N Y

Baynes JW, Monnier VM et al., eds. (1989) The Maillard reaction in aging, diabetes, and nutrition. Proceedings of an NIH conference. Bethesda, Maryland, September 22–23, 1988. Dedicated to John E. Hodge on the occasion of his 75th birthday. Prog Clin Biol Res 304:1–410

Benjamin R, Leake A, McArthur FK et al. (1994) Protective effect of apoE epsilon 2 in Alzheimer's disease [letter; comment]. Lancet 344:473

Bodnar AG, Ouellette M, Frolkis M et al. (1998) Extension of life-span by introduction of telomerase into normal human cells. Science 279:349–352

Brooks SV, Faulkner JA (1994) Skeletal muscle weakness in old age: Underlying mechanisms. Med Sci Sports Exerc 26:432–439

Brown WT (1990) Genetic diseases of premature aging as models of senescence. Annu Rev Gerontol Geriatr 10:23–42

Bunn CL, Tarrant GM (1980) Limited lifespan in somatic cell hybrids and cybrids. Exp Cell Res 127:385–396

Campisi J (1997) Aging and cancer: The double-edged sword of replicative senescence. J Am Geriatr Soc 45:482–488

Carey JR, Liedo P, Orozco D, Vaupel JW (1992) Slowing of mortality rates at older ages in large medfly cohorts. Science 258:457–461

Carmeli E, Reznick AZ (1994) The physiology and biochemistry of skeletal muscle atrophy as a function of age. Proc Soc Exp Biol Med 206:103–113

Cattanach BM (1974) Position effect variegation in the mouse. Genet Res 23:291–306

Chang E, Harley CB (1995) Telomere length and replicative aging in human vascular tissues. Proc Natl Acad Sci USA 92:11190–11194

Charlesworth B (1980) Evolution in Age-Structured Populations. Cambridge University Press, Cambridge

Clark AM, Rubin MA (1962) The modification by X-irradiation of the life span of haploids and diploids of the wasp, *Habrobracon* sp. Radiat Res 15:244–253

Cooper JM, Mann VM, Schapira AH (1992) Analyses of mitochondrial respiratory chain function and mitochondrial DNA deletion in human skeletal muscle: effect of ageing. J Neurol Sci 113:91–98

Corder EH, Saunders AM, Strittmatter WJ et al. (1993) Gene dose of apolipoprotein E type 4 allele and the risk of Alzheimer's disease in late onset families. Science 261:921–923

Corral-Debrinski M, Horton T, Lott MT et al. (1992a) Mitochondrial DNA deletions in human brain: Regional variability and increase with advanced age. Nat Genet 2:324–329

Corral-Debrinski M, Shoffner JM, Lott MT, Wallace DC (1992b) Association of mitochondrial DNA damage with aging and coronary atherosclerotic heart disease. Mutat Res 275:169–180

Counter CM, Botelho FM, Wang P et al. (1994) Stabilization of short telomeres and telomerase activity accompany immortalization of Epstein-Barr virus-transformed human B lymphocytes. J Virol 68:3410–3414

Cristofalo VJ, Allen RG, Pignolo RJ (1998) Relationship between donor age and the replicative lifespan of human cells in culture: a reevaluation. Proc Natl Acad Sci USA 95:10614–10619

Crow JF (1999) Spontaneous mutation in man. Mutat Res 437:5–9

Curtsinger JW, Fukui HH, Townsend DR, Vaupel JW (1992) Demography of genotypes: Failure of the limited life-span paradigm in Drosophila melanogaster. Science 258:461–463

Cutler RG (1975) Evolution of human longevity and the genetic complexity governing aging rate. Proc Natl Acad Sci USA 72:4664–4668

de Grey ADNJ (1999) The Mitochondrial Free Radical Theory of Aging. R.G. Landes Co., Austin

Duvoisin RC (1993) The genetics of Parkinson's disease. A review. Adv Neurol 60:306–315

Edwards BJ, Morley JE (1993) Amylin. Life Sci 51:1899–1912

Eriksson L, Westermark P (1990) Age-related accumulation of amyloid inclusions in adrenal cortical cells. Am J Pathol 136:461–466

Evans DA, van der Kleij AA, Sonnemans MA et al. (1994) Frameshift mutations at two hotspots in vasopressin transcripts in post-mitotic neurons. Proc Natl Acad Sci USA 91:6059–6063

Evans KC, Berger EP, Cho CG et al. (1995) Apolipoprotein E is a kinetic but not a thermodynamic inhibitor of amyloid formation: implications for the pathogenesis and treatment of Alzheimer disease. Proc Natl Acad Sci USA 92:763–767

Fukuchi K, Martin GM, Monnat RJ, Jr. (1989) Mutator phenotype of Werner syndrome is characterized by extensive deletions Proc Natl Acad Sci USA 86:5893–5897

Gage FH (2000) Mammalian neural stem cells. Science 287:1433–1438

Gartler SM, Dyer KA, Goldman MA (1992) Mammalian X chromosome inactivation. Mol Genet Med 2:121–160

Gavrilov LAD, Gavrilova NS (1991) The Biology of Life Span: A Quantitative Approach. Harwood Academic, N Y

Gershon H, Gershon D (1970) Detection of inactive enzyme molecules in ageing organisms. Nature 227:1214–1217

Gilham NW (1994) Organelle Genes and Genomes. Oxford University Press, New York

Gompertz B (1825) On the nature of the function of the law of human mortality and on a new mode of determining life contingencies. Philos Trans R Soc Lond Biol 115:513–585

Goto M (1997) Hierarchical deterioration of body systems in Werner's syndrome: Implications for normal ageing. Mech Ageing Dev 98:239–254

Goto M, Tanimoto K, Horiuchi Y, Sasazuki T (1981) Family analysis of Werner's syndrome: A survey of 42 Japanese families with a review of the literature. Clin Genet 19:8–15

Goto M, Kindynis P, Resnick D, Sartoris DJ (1989) Osteosclerosis of the phalanges in Werner syndrome. Radiology 172:841–843

Goto M, Rubenstein M, Weber J et al. (1992) Genetic linkage of Werner's syndrome to five markers on chromosome 8. Nature 355:735–738

Gracy RW, Yuksel KU, Chapman ML, Dimitrijevich SD (1990) Isoprotein changes in aging: biochemical basis and physiological consequences. Isozymes: Structure, Function, and USe in Biology and Medicine. Wiley-Liss, N Y

Hamer L, Kaplan F, Fallon M (1988) The musculoskeletal manifestations of progeria. A literature review. Orthopedics 11:763–769

Hardingham T, Bayliss M (1990) Proteoglycans of articular cartilage: Changes in aging and in joint disease. Semin. Arthritis Rheum. 20:12–33

Harley CB, Futcher AB, Greider CW (1990) Telomeres shorten during ageing of human fibroblasts. Nature 345:458–460

Harman D (1994) Free-radical theory of aging. Increasing the functional life span. Ann. N.Y.Acad. Sci. 717:1–15

Harrison DE, Astle CM, Lerner C (1984) Ultimate erythropoietic repopulating abilities of fetal, young adult, and old adult cells compared using repeated irradiation. J Exp Med 160:759–771

Hartwell LH, Kastan MB (1994) Cell cycle control and cancer. Science 266:1821–1828

Hayakawa M, Hattori K, Sugiyama S, Ozawa T (1992) Age-associated oxygen damage and mutations in mitochondrial DNA in human hearts. Biochem Biophys Res Commun 189:979–985

Hayflick L (1980) Call ageing. Annu Rev Gerontol Geriatr 1:26–67

Hayflick L, Moorhead PS (1961) The serial cultivation of human diploid cell strains. Exp Cell Res 25:585–621

Heydari AR, Richardson A (1992) Does gene expression play any role in the mechanism of the antiaging effect of dietary restriction? Ann NY Acad Sci 663:384–395

Higuchi K, Naiki H, Kitagawa K et al. (1991) Mouse senile amyloidosis. ASSAM amyloidosis in mice presents universally as a systemic age-associated amyloidosis. Virchows Arch. B Cell Pathol Incl Mol Pathol 60:231–238

Holliday R (1990) DNA methylation and epigenetic inheritance. Philos Trans R Soc Lond B Biol Sci 326:329–338

Horie H, Kawasaki Y, Takenaka T (1986) Lateral diffusion of membrane lipids changes with aging in C57BL mouse dorsal root ganglion neurons from a fetal stage to an aged stage. Brain Res 377:246–250

Horn PL, Turker MS, Ogburn CE et al. (1984) A cloning assay for 6-thioguanine resistance provides evidence against certain somatic mutational theories of aging. J Cell Physiol 121:309–315

Hsieh RH, Hou JH, Hsu HS, Wei YH (1994) Age-dependent respiratory function decline and DNA deletions in human muscle mitochondria. Biochem Mol Biol Int 32:1009–1022

Hunter T (1993) Braking the cycle. Cell 75:839–841

Imai S, Armstrong CM, Kaeberlein M, Guarente L (2000) Transcriptional silencing and longevity protein Sir2 is an NAD-dependent histone deacetylase. Nature 403:795–800

Issa JP, Ottaviano YL, Celano P et al. (1994) Methylation of the oestrogen receptor CpG island links ageing and neoplasia in human colon. Nat Genet 7:536–540

Johansson B, Wernstedt C, Westermark P (1987) Atrial natriuretic peptide deposited as atrial amyloid fibrils. Biochem Biophys Res Commun 148:1087–1092

Katayama M, Tanaka M, Yamamoto H et al. (1991) Deleted mitochondrial DNA in the skeletal muscle of aged individuals. Biochem Int 25:47–56

Katz ML, White HA, Gao CL et al. (1993) Dietary restriction slows age pigments accumulation in the retinal pigment epithelium. Invest Ophthalmol Vis Sci 34:3297–3302

Katzman R, Kawas C (1998) Risk factors for Alzheimer's disease. Neuroscience News 1:27–34

Kim NW, Piatyszek MA, Prowse KR et al. (1994) Specific association of human telomerase activity with immortal cells and cancer. Science 266:2011–2015

Kirkwood TB, Rose MR (1991) Evolution of senescence: late survival sacrificed for production. Phil Trans Ray Soc Lond ser B Biol Sci 332:15–24

Kirstein M, Aston C, Hintz R, Vlassara H (1992) Receptor-specific induction of insulin-like growth factor I in human monocytes by advanced glycosylation end product-modified proteins. J Clin Invest 90:439–446

Kohn RR (1978) Extracellular aging. Principles of Mammalian Aging, 2nd edn. Prentice-Hall, Englewood Cliffs, NJ

Kristal BS, Yu BP (1992) An emerging hypothesis: Synergistic induction of aging by free radicals and Maillard reactions. J Gerontol 47:B107–B114

Krzywkowski P, Ghribi O, Gagne J et al. (1999) Cholinergic systems and long-term potentiation in memory-impaired apolipoprotein E-deficient mice. Neuroscience 92:1273–1286

Laganiere S, Yu BP (1989) Effect of chronic food restriction in aging rats. II. Liver cytosolic antioxidants and related enzymes. Mech Ageing Dev 48:221–230

LeDoux SP, Wilson GL, Beecham EJ et al. (1992) Repair of mitochondrial DNA after various types of DNA damage in Chinese hamster ovary cells. Carcinogenesis 13:1967–1973

Lee AT, Cerami A (1992) Role of glycation in aging. Ann N Y Acad Sci 663:63–70

Lee AT, DeSimone C, Cerami A, Bucala R (1994) Comparative analysis of DNA mutations in lacI transgenic mice with age. FASEB J. 8:545–550

Lee CK, Klopp RG, Weindruch R, Prolla TA (1999) Gene expression profile of aging and its retardation by caloric restriction. Science 285:1390–1393

Lee DW, Yu BP (1990) Modulation of free radicals and superoxide dismutases by age and dietary restriction. Aging (Milano.) 2:357–362

Lee HC, Pang CY, Hsu HS, Wei YH (1994) Ageing-associated tandem duplications in the D-loop of mitochondrial DNA of human muscle. FEBS Lett. 354:79–83

Leopold AC (1978) The biological significance of death in plants. In Behnke JA, Finch CE, Moment GB (eds): The Biology of Aging. Plenum Press, N Y

Levy MZ, Allsopp RC, Futcher AB et al. (1992) Telomere end-replication problem and cell aging. J Mol Biol 225:951–960

Li Y, Deeb B, Pendergrass W, Wolf N (1996) Cellular proliferative capacity and life span in small and large dogs. J Gerontol A Biol Sci Med Sci 51:B403–B408

Lindeman RD (1990) Overview: Renal physiology and pathophysiology of aging. Am J Kidney Dis 16:275–282

Lindeman RD, Tobin J, Shock NW (1985) Longitudinal studies on the rate of decline in renal function with age. J Am Geriatr Soc 33:278–285

Lindsey J, McGill NI, Lindsey LA et al. (1991) In vivo loss of telomeric repeats with age in humans. Mutat Res 256:45–48

Lopez-Torres M, Perez-Campo R, Fernandez A et al. (1993) Brain glutathione reductase induction increases early survival and decreases lipofuscin accumulation in aging frogs. J Neurosci Res 34:233–242

Luckinbill LS, Graves JL, Reed AH, Koetsawang S (1988) Localizing genes that defer senescence in Drosophila melanogaster. Heredity 60 (Pt 3):367–374

Ly DH, Lockhart DJ, Lerner RA, Schultz PG (2000) Mitotic misregulation and human aging. Science 287:2486–2492

McKusick VA (1994) Mendelian Inheritance in Man: A Catalog of Human Genes and Genetic Disorders, 11th edn. Johns Hopkins University Press, Baltimore

McMurdo ME, Rennie LM (1994) Improvements in quadriceps strength with regular seated exercise in the institutionalized elderly. Arch Phys Med Rehabil 75:600–603

Makeham WM (1860) On the law of mortality and the construction of annuity tables. J Inst Actuaries 8:301–310

Manton KG, Stallard E, Woodbury MA, Dowd JE (1994) Time-varying covariates in models of human mortality and aging: multidimensional generalizations of the Gompertz. J Gerontol 49:B169–B190

Martin GM (1977) Cellular aging—postreplicative cells. A review (Part II). Am J Pathol 89:513–530

Martin GM (1978) Genetic syndromes in man with potential relevance to the pathobiology of aging. Birth Defects Orig Artic Ser 14:5–39

Martin GM (1979) Proliferative homeostasis and its age-related aberrations. Mech Ageing Dev 9:385–391

Martin GM (1987) Interactions of aging and environmental agents: The gerontological perspective. Prog Clin Biol Res 228:25–80

Martin GM (1991) Genetic and environmental modulatins of chromosomal stability: Their roles in aging and oncogenesis. Ann N Y Acad Sci 621:401–417

Martin GM (1993) Clonal attenuation: Causes and consequences. J Gerontol 48:B171–B172

Martin GM (1994) Genetic modulation of telomeric terminal restriction-fragment length: relevance for clonal aging and late-life disease. Am J Hum Genet 55:866–869

Martin GM (1998) Toward a genetic analysis of unusually successful neural aging. In Wang E, Snyder DS (eds): Handbook of the Aging Brain. Academic Press, N Y, p. 125

Martin GM, Sprague CA, Epstein CJ (1970) Replicative life-span of cultivated human cells. Effects of donor's age, tissue, and genotype. Lab Invest 23:86–92

Martin GM, Ogburn CE, Sprague CA (1975) Senescence and vascular disease. Adv Exp Med Biol 61:163–193

Martin GM, Smith AC, Ketterer DJ et al. (1985) Increased chromosomal aberrations in first metaphases of cells isolated from the kidneys of aged mice. Isr J Med Sci 21:296–301

Martin GM, Austad SN, Johnson TE (1996a) Genetic analysis of ageing: Role of oxidative damage and environmental stresses. Nat Genet 13:25–34

Martin GM, Ogburn CE, Colgin LM et al. (1996b) Somatic mutations are frequent and increase with age in human kidney epithelial cells. Hum Mol Genet 5:215–221

Martin GM, Oshima J, Gray MD, Poot M (1999) What geriatricians should know about the Werner syndrome. J Am Geriatr Soc 47:1136–1144

Masoro EJ (1998) Influence of caloric intake on aging and on the response to stressors. J Toxicol Environ Health B Crit Rev 1:243–257

Masoro EJ, Katz MS, McMahan CA (1989) Evidence for the glycation hypothesis of aging from the food-restricted rodent model. J Gerontol 44:B20–B22

Medawar PB (1952) An Unsolved Problem of Biology. HK Lewis, London

Migeon BR, Axelman J, Beggs AH (1988) Effect of ageing on reactivation of the human X-linked HPRT locus [see comments]. Nature 335:93–96

Monnier VM, Sell DR, Nagaraj RH et al. (1992) Maillard reaction-mediated molecular damage to extracellular matrix and other tissue proteins in diabetes, aging, and uremia. Diabetes 41 Suppl 2:36–41

Mucchiano G, Cornwell GG, III, Westermark P (1992) Senile aortic amyloid. Evidence for two distinct forms of localized deposits. Am J Pathol 140:871–877

Mudgett MB, Clarke S (1993) Characterization of plant L-isoaspartyl methyltransferases that may be involved in seed survival: Purification, cloning, and sequence analysis of the wheat germ enzyme. Biochemistry 32:11100–11111

Munscher C, Muller-Hocker J, Kadenbach B (1993) Human aging is associated with various point mutations in tRNA genes of mitochondrial DNA. Biol Chem Hoppe Seyler 374:1099–1104

Nakano M, Mizuno T, Gotoh S (1993) Accumulation of cardiac lipofuscin in crab-eating monkeys (*Macaca fasicularis*): The same rate of lipofuscin accumulation in several species of primates. Mech Ageing Dev 66:243–248

Nakura J, Wijsman EM, Miki T et al. (1994) Homozygosity mapping of the Werner syndrome locus (WRN). Genomics 23:600–608

Naslund J, Schierhorn A, Hellman U et al. (1994) Relative abundance of Alzheimer A beta amyloid peptide variants in Alzheimer disease and normal aging. Proc Natl Acad Sci USA 91:8378–8382

Nelson EA, Dannefer D (1992) Aged heterogeneity: Fact or fiction? The fate of diversity in gerontological research. Gerontologist 32:17–23

Noda A, Ning Y, Venable SF et al. (1994) Cloning of senescent cell-derived inhibitors of DNA synthesis using an expression screen. Exp Cell Res 211:90–98

Ogburn CE, Oshima J, Poot M et al. (1997) An apoptosis-inducing genotoxin differentiates heterozygotic carriers for Werner helicase mutations from wild-type and homozygous mutants. Hum Genet 101:121–125

Orgel LE (1963) The maintenance of the accuracy of protein synthesis and its relevance to ageing. Proc Natl Acad Sci USA 49:517–521

Orgel LE (1970) The maintenance of the accuracy of protein synthesis and its relevance to ageing: a correction. Proc Natl Acad Sci USA 67:1476

Oshima J, Campisi J, Tannock TC, Martin GM (1995) Regulation of c-fos expression in senescing Werner syndrome fibroblasts differs from that observed in senescing fibroblasts from normal donors. J Cell Physiol 162:277–283

Ouellette MM, McDaniel LD, Wright WE et al. (2000) The establishment of telomerase-immortalized cell lines representing human chromosome instability syndromes [In Process Citation]. Hum Mol Genet 9:403–411

Partridge L, Barton NH (1993) Optimality, mutation and the evolution of ageing. Nature 362:305–311

Pereira-Smith OM, Smith JR (1983) Evidence for the recessive nature of cellular immortality. Science 221:964–966

Qiao JH, Welch CL, Xie PZ et al. (1993) Involvement of the tyrosinase gene in the deposition of cardiac lipofuscin in mice. Association with aortic fatty streak development. J Clin Invest 92:2386–2393

Rabinovitch PS, Martin GM (1982) Encephalomyocarditis virus as a probe of errors in macromolecular synthesis in aging mice. Mech Ageing Dev 20:155–163

Rao G, Xia E, Nadakavukaren MJ, Richardson A (1990) Effect of dietary restriction on the age-dependent changes in the expression of antioxidant enzymes in rat liver. J Nutr 120:602–609

Rattan SI, Derventzi A, Clark BF (1992) Protein synthesis, posttranslational modifications, and aging. Ann N Y Acad Sci 662:48–62

Reynolds BA, Weiss S (1992) Generation of neurons and astrocytes from isolated cells of the adult mammalian central nervous system. Science 255:1707–1710

Ritchie K, Kildea D (1995) In senile dementia "age-related" or "ageing-related"?—evidence from meta-analysis of dementia prevalence in the oldest old. Lancet 346:931–934

Robert L, Jacob MP, Labat-Robert J (1992) Cell-matrix interactions in the genesis of arteriosclerosis and atheroma. Effect of aging. Ann N Y Acad Sci 673:331–341

Rose MR (1991) Evolutionary Biology of Aging. Oxford University Press, New York

Roth GS, Ingram DK, Lane MA (1999) Calorie restriction in primates: will it work and how will we know? J Am Geriatr Soc 47:896–903

Rothstein M (1982) Biochemical Approaches to Aging. Academic Press

Rothstein M (1989) An overview of age-related changes in proteins. Prog Clin Biol Res 287:259–267

Runger TM, Bauer C, Dekant B et al. (1994) Hypermutable ligation of plasmid DNA ends in cells from patients with Werner syndrome. J Invest Dermatol 102:45–48

Sacher GA (1978) Evolution of longevity and survival characteristics in mammals. In Schneider EL (ed): The Genetics of Aging. Plenum Press, New York

Salk D, Au K, Hoehn H, Martin GM (1981) Cytogenetics of Werner's syndrome cultured skin fibroblasts: Variegated translocation mosaicism. Cytogenet Cell Genet 30:92–107

Salk D et al., eds. (1985) Werner's syndrome and human aging. Proceedings of a United States-Japan cooperative seminar, December 10–12, 1982, Kobe, Japan. Adv Exp Med Biol 190:1–656

Sarich VM (1985) Of molecules, comparative anatomy, and the fossil record: The evolutionary messages cannot conflict, abstracted. Am J Phys Anthropol 66:224

Satoh M, Imai M, Sugimoto M et al. (1999) Prevalence of Werner's syndrome heterozygotes in Japan [letter]. Lancet 353:1766

Sawle GV, Colebatch JG, Shah A et al. (1990) Striatal function in normal aging: Implications for Parkinson's disease. Ann Neurol 28:799–804

Schachter F, Faure-Delanef L, Guenot F et al. (1994) Genetic associations with human longevity at the APOE and ACE loci. Nat Genet 6:29–32

Schellenberg GD, Martin GM, Wijsman EM et al. (1992) Homozygosity mapping and Werner's syndrome. Lancet 339:1002

Seshadri T, Campisi J (1990) Repression of c-fos transcription and an altered genetic program in senescent human fibroblasts. Science 247:205–209

Shock NW (1977) Systems integration. In Finch CE, Hayflick L (eds): Handbook of the Biology of Aging. Van Nostrand-Reinhold, N Y

Simonetti S, Chen X, DiMauro S, Schon EA (1992) Accumulation of deletions in human mitochondrial DNA during normal aging: Analysis by quantitative PCR. Biochim Biophys Acta 1180:113–122

Slagboom PE, Droog S, Boomsma DI (1994) Genetic determination of telomere size in humans: A twin study of three age groups. Am J Hum Genet 55:876–882

Smith SS (1994) Species-specific differences in tumorigenesis and senescence. Trends Genet 10:305–306

Solano SM, Miller DW, Augood SJ et al. (2000) Expression of alpha-synuclein, parkin, and ubiquitin carboxy-terminal hydrolase L1 mRNA in human brain: Genes associated with familial Parkinson's disease. Ann Neurol 47:201–210

Soong NW, Hinton DR, Cortopassi G, Arnheim N (1992) Mosaicism for a specific somatic mitochondrial DNA mutation in adult human brain. Nat Genet 2:318–323

Spiering AL, Smith JR (1991) Negative growth effectors and cellular senescence. Mutat Res 256:263–269

Stadtman ER (1988) Protein modification in aging. J Gerontol 43:B112–B120

Stadtman ER, Berlett BS (1998) Reactive oxygen-mediated protein oxidation in aging and disease. Drug Metab Rev 30:225–243

Stein GH, Beeson M, Gordon L (1990) Failure to phosphorylate the retinoblastoma gene product in senescent human fibroblasts. Science 249:666–669

Suganuma N, Kitagawa T, Nawa A, Tomoda Y (1993) Human ovarian aging and mitochondrial DNA deletion. Horm Res 39 Suppl 1:16–21

Surani MA (1994) Genomic imprinting: control of gene expression by epigenetic inheritance. Curr Opin Cell Biol 6:390–395

Swisshelm K, Disteche CM, Thorvaldsen J et al. (1990) Age-related increase in methylation of ribosomal genes and inactivation of chromosome-specific rRNA gene clusters in mouse. Mutat Res 237:131–146

Szilard L (1959) On the nature of the aging process. Proc Natl Acad Sci USA 45:30–45

Takahashi K, Yi S, Kimura Y, Araki S (1991) Familial amyloidotic polyneuropathy type 1 in Kumamoto, Japan: A clinicopathologic, histochemical, immunohistochemical, and ultrastructural study. Hum Pathol 22:519–527

Takeda N, Tanamura A, Iwai T et al. (1993) Mitochondrial DNA deletion in human myocardium. Mol Cell Biochem 119:105–108

Talbot C, Lendon C, Craddock N et al. (1994) Protection against Alzheimer's disease with apoE epsilon 2. Lancet 343:1432–1433

Tashima T, Kitamoto T, Tateishi J et al. (1988) Incidence and characterization of age related amyloid deposits in the human anterior pituitary gland. Virchows Arch A Pathol Anat Histopathol 412:323–327

Tollefsbol TO, Cohen HJ (1984) Werner's syndrome: an underdiagnosed disorder resembling premature aging. Age 7:75–88

Trainor KJ, Wigmore DJ, Chrysostomou A et al. (1984) Mutation frequency in human lymphocytes increases with age. Mech Ageing Dev 27:83–86

Tsai W, Clarke S (1994) Amino acid polymorphisms of the human L-isoaspartyl/D-aspartyl methyltransferase involved in protein repair. Biochem Biophys Res Commun 203:491–497

Turner DR, Morley AA, Haliandros M et al. (1985) In vivo somatic mutations in human lymphocytes frequently result from major gene alterations. Nature 315:343–345

van Leeuwen FW (1992) Mutant vasopressin precursor producing cells of the homozygous Brattleboro rat as a model for co-expression of neuropeptides. Prog Brain Res 92:149–155

van Leeuwen FW, Evans DA, Meloen R, Sonnemans MA (1994) Differential neurophysin immunoreactivities in solitary magnocellular neurons of the homozygous Brattleboro rat indicate an altered neurophysin moiety. Brain Res 635:328–330

Vanfleteren JR, De Vreese A, Braeckman BP (1998) Two-parameter logistic and Weibull equations provide better fits to survival data from isogenic populations of Caenorhabditis elegans in axenic culture than does the Gompertz model. J Gerontol A Biol Sci Med Sci 53:B393–B403

Vaupel JW, Carey JR, Christensen K et al. (1998) Biodemographic trajectories of longevity. Science 280:855–860

Vaziri H, Schachter F, Uchida I et al. (1993) Loss of telomeric DNA during aging of normal and trisomy 21 human lymphocytes. Am J Hum Genet 52:661–667

Vogel F, Rathenberg R (1975) Spontaneous mutation in man. Adv Hum Genet 5:223–318

Wallace DC (1997) Mitochondrial DNA in aging and disease. Sci Am 277:40–47

Wareham KA, Lyon MF, Glenister PH, Williams ED (1987) Age related reactivation of an X-linked gene. Nature 327:725–727

Weindruch R, Walford RL (1988) The Retardation of Aging and Disease by Dietary Restriction. Charles C. Thomas, Springfield, IL

Williams GC (1957) Pleiotropy, natural selection, and the evolution of senescence. Evolution 11:398–411

Wilson DL (1994) The analysis of survival (mortality) data: fitting Gompertz, Weibull, and logistic functions. Mech Ageing Dev 74:15–33

Wilson VL, Jones PA (1983) DNA methylation decreases in aging but not in immortal cells. Science 220:1055–1057

Wilson VL, Smith RA, Ma S, Cutler RG (1987) Genomic 5-methyldeoxycytidine decreases with age. J Biol Chem 262:9948–9951

Wolf G (1993) Lipofuscin, the age pigment. Nutr Rev 51:205–206

Wolf NS, Pendergrass WR (1999) The relationships of animal age and caloric intake to cellular replication in vivo and in vitro: a review. J Gerontol A Biol Sci Med Sci 54:B502–B517

Wright WE, Shay JW (1992) Telomere positional effects and the regulation of cellular senescence. Trends Genet 8:193–197

Wullbrand A, Saeger W, Missmahl HP et al. (1990) Amyloid in intervertebral discs of surgery and autopsy material. A new class of amyloid? Virchows Arch A Pathol Anat Histopathol 416:335–341

Yan SD, Chen X, Schmidt AM et al. (1994) Glycated tau protein in Alzheimer disease: a mechanism for induction of oxidant stress. Proc Natl Acad Sci USA 91:7787–7791

Yen TC, Pang CY, Hsieh RH et al. (1992) Age-dependent 6 kb deletion in human liver mitochondrial DNA. Biochem Int 26:457–468

Yokota T, Okabayashi H, Ishihara T et al. (1994) Immunohistochemical and pathological characteristics of dystrophic amyloid in surgically excised cardiac valves. Pathol Int 44:182–185

Yu CE, Oshima J, Fu YH et al. (1996) Positional cloning of the Werner's syndrome gene. Science 272:258–262

Yu CE, Oshima J, Goddard KA et al. (1994) Linkage disequilibrium and haplotype studies of chromosome 8p 11.1–21.1 markers and Werner syndrome. Am J Hum Genet 55:356–364

Zhang Y, Kreger BE, Dorgan JF (1999) Parental age at child's birth and son's risk of prostate cancer. The Framingham Study. Am J Epidemiol 150:1208–1212

Pharmacogenetics and pharmacogenomics

21

Daniel W. Nebert
Lucia F. Jorge-Nebert

Introduction

When a patient receives a particular dose of prescribed drug, or any over-the-counter medication, the response is very often quite different from one individual to the next. We now realize that this is because each individual has his own unique "pharmacogenetic profile"—just as each of us has his own distinct pattern of DNA fragments by PCR analysis or unique thumb print (the latter two being useful in criminology). The response to many pharmaceuticals is, likewise, determined by one's genetic constitution.

This subject has been central to the field of *pharmacogenetics* for more than five decades (Motulsky, 1957; Vesell, 1972; Evans, 1994; Meyer, 1994; Kalow and Bertilsson, 1994; Nebert, 1997a; 1997b; 1999; 2000b, Weber, 1997; Caraco, 1998; Kleyn and Vesell, 1998; Weinshilboum et al., 1999). Pharmacogenetics is defined as "the study of heritable variability in drug response" (Vogel, 1959). The recently coined term *pharmacogenomics* refers to the field of new drug development based on our rapidly increasing knowledge of all genes in the human genome. The two terms pharmacogenetics and pharmacogenomics, however, are often used interchangeably.

It should be emphasized that this field has exploded in recent years, and therefore this chapter must be regarded very clearly as "simply a snapshot in time." During the several months in preparing this chapter, we have encountered more than a dozen new findings that helped in updating and understanding more clearly one or another of the pharmacogenetic disorders being described.

Adverse drug reactions have been reported to rank between the fourth and sixth leading causes of death in the US (Lazarou et al., 1998). Adverse drug reactions include: dose-dependent, *dose-independent* (this includes *idiosyncratic drug reactions* and allergic reactions), dose- and time-dependent (cumulative), time-related, withdrawal, and *unexpected failure of therapy* (Edwards, 2000). Advances in the fields of pharmacogenetics and pharmacogenomics should help significantly in reducing the morbidity and mortality caused by idiosyncratic drug reactions and unexpected failure of therapy.

The term "polymorphism" has been very confusing in the field of pharmacogenetics (Arias et al., 1991). A *polymorphism* is defined as the presence of two or more subgroups in any species population. During the past six decades, E.B. Ford and, more recently, Harry Harris (1980) stated that a polymorphism exists when the "commonest identifiable allele has a frequency no greater than 0.99 …". When a minor allele has a frequency of 0.01 or greater, this is a "*polymorphic variant*," and if a minor allele has a frequency of less than 0.01, this is a "*rare variant*." Considering the Hardy-Weinberg distribution ($p^2 + 2pq + q^2 = 1$), therefore, q represents the sum of the variant alleles and, if $q = 0.01$, this means that the percentage of individuals homozygous for an autosomal recessive trait will be 0.01%, or one in 10,000. A polymorphism implies, of course, the manifestation of two or more allelic variants of a gene responsible for the trait (phenotype).

In this chapter, a few fundamental aspects of pharmacology are briefly reviewed. Next, numerous examples of pharmacogenetic differences, many of them possibly the causes of drug-induced morbidity or mortality, are presented; these will be discussed in light of the innumerable recently discovered allelic variants in pharmacogenetically relevant genes. In many cases, ethnic differences in these pharmacogenetic traits will also be briefly described. Interethnic variability is a feature that has a genetic basis and is increasingly recognized to have clinical significance in many instances. Finally, we discuss the realization that all diseases—including pharmacogenetic diseases—are *multifactorial, polygenic* traits. In other words, all pharmacogenetic differences, as well as all gene-environment interactions, represent to varying degrees *multiplex phenotypes* (i.e., traits that are caused by at least two and usually many more than two major genes, and dozens if not hundreds of modifier genes, plus effects of the environment).

Fundamental aspects of pharmacology

The objective of the administration to a patient of most drug products is to maintain the plasma levels of the active principle (drug) in the *therapeutic range* (Fig. 21.1). If the dose of drug is too small, the interval of administration inadequate, the bioavailability of the drug product low, or the active principle (drug) extensively metabolized and quickly excreted, then the plasma drug level might not reach the minimum effective concentration. This would lead to an absence of the expected therapeutic response (*therapeutic failure*). On the contrary, if the dose of the drug is too large, its interval of administration too short, or the active principle poorly metabolized or excreted, this can lead to adverse drug reactions. These reactions are due to the accumulation of the drug at levels that reach the minimum toxic concentration in blood, as well as in critical target organs.

PHARMACOKINETICS AND PHARMACODYNAMICS

Pharmacokinetics reflects what the body does to the drug, whereas pharmacodynamics reflects what the drug does to the target tissue(s) (Fig. 21.2). The end result of all of the pharmacokinetic and pharmacodynamic processes is a therapeutic effect (or therapeutic failure) of the drug, or, an unwanted toxicity (adverse drug reaction).

Variations in the drug pharmacokinetic phase encompass the processes of uptake or *absorption*, binding and *distribution*, biotransformation or *metabolism*, and *excretion*. Pharmacokinetic differences have generally been monitored by blood determinations of the active drug (or metabolite) and less often by urinary (or saliva, sweat, fecal) determinations of the active drug and/or metabolites. For most systemic drugs, the concentration of the (unbound, or free) active principle in blood is proportional to the concentration of active principle in the target tissue. There are numerous pharmacogenetic differences in genes participating in metabolism and distribution (binding, transport), whereas there are fewer known pharmacogenetic defects in genes governing the processes of absorption and excretion.

Variations in the pharmacodynamic phase can occur in the processes of drug binding to receptors and signaling pathways. Gene differences thus might be seen in: receptors at the cell surface, cytoplasm and nucleus; tissue- and cell type-specific transcription factors and signal transduction pathways; nucleic acid and protein repair processes; and cell infrastructure (e.g., nuclear matrix, membranes, and subcellular organelles such as Golgi bodies or peroxisomes).

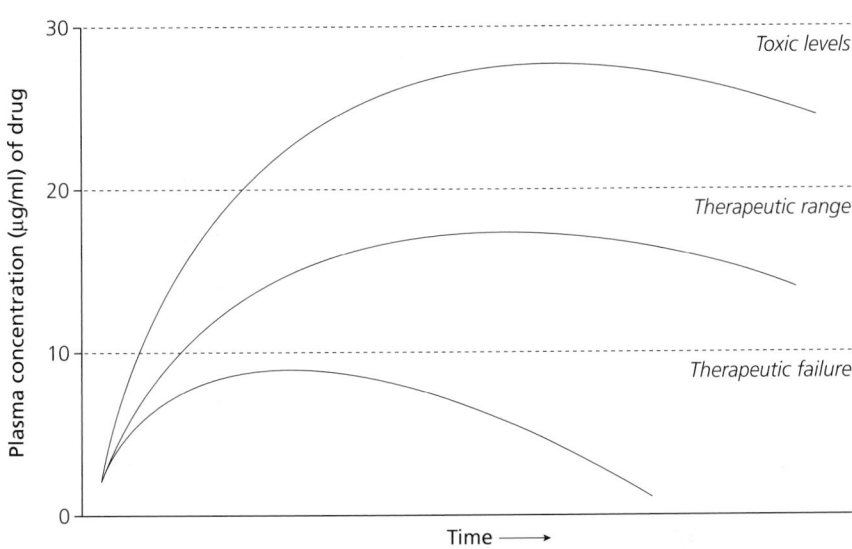

Fig. 21.1. Theoretical plasma concentration curves for any drug, as a function of time after oral administration of the dose. In this hypothetical case, the horizontal line at 10 μg/ml is the minimum effective concentration; the horizontal line at 20 μg/ml is the minimum toxic concentration.

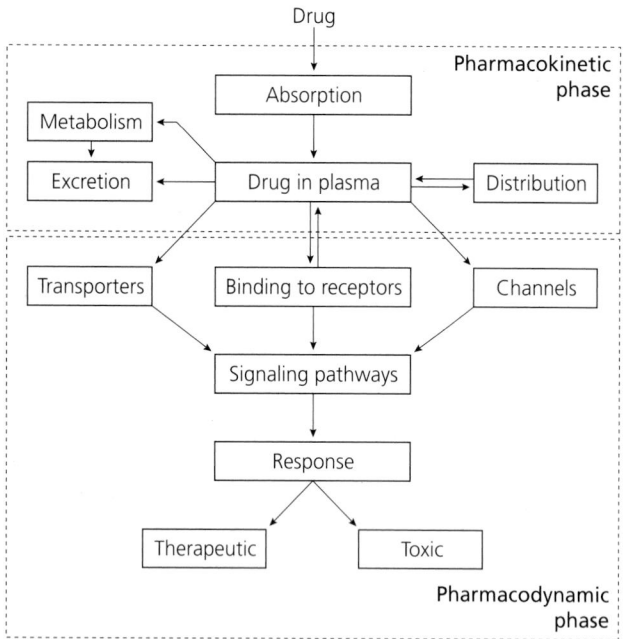

Fig. 21.2. The processes involved in the pharmacokinetic phase, and the processes involved in the pharmacodynamic phase, of any pharmaceutical agent.

Until the last decade or two, what happened in the pharmacodynamic phase—especially after drug binding to its receptor—was largely considered a "black box." As drug-signaling pathways have now become much better understood, the field of pharmacodynamics has advanced quickly.

Historically, variations in pharmacokinetics—reflected in abnormal plasma drug levels—led to the elucidation of genetic differences in drug-metabolizing enzymes (DMEs) and, in a few cases, differences in receptor or transporter proteins. This was because blood samples are easier to obtain than tissue biopsies. Thus, genetic variations due to differences in the processes of pharmacokinetics have been quite well characterized, while differences and variability at the pharmacodynamic level remain largely an unknown area of study.

As described throughout this chapter, variations in pharmacokinetics or pharmacodynamics (Fig. 21.2) among individuals, all of which can be ascribed to genetic differences, can range from 10- to more than 40-fold. It is now clear that all pharmacogenetic differences are polygenic and multifactorial, i.e., traits are caused by at least two and usually many more than two major genes, and dozens if not hundreds of modifier genes, plus effects of the environment. This means that, at one time or another, perhaps every gene in the human genome is capable of being a "susceptibility" gene; thus, a drug or metabolite can interact (directly or indirectly) with its gene product as an agonist

or antagonist, or as an activator or inhibitor. The complete sequence of the human genome, with all its genes, was reported during 2001. Hence, the field of pharmacogenomics will be examining the effect of allelic variants of all candidate genes in a drug's pharmacokinetic and pharmacodynamic pathways, thereby leading to new drug discovery and drug design to prevent adverse drug reactions. The ultimate goal of pharmacogeneticists is to offer the clinician the choice to select the dosage and frequency of administering a drug, based on that patient's genotype (DNA sequence variation), rather than on monitoring plasma drug levels or on waiting for a favorable therapeutic response, as is currently done today.

There are many ways in which one might classify pharmacogenetic defects. Table 21.1 shows one such classification and lists more than ten dozen pharmacogenetic differences. Slightly more than half of those understood at a molecular level represent polymorphisms in DMEs, and most of the others reflect differences in receptor, transporter and channel genes. To reiterate what was stated above, historically, it has been easier to examine for differences in metabolism than, for example, kinase/phosphatase signal cascades or transcription-factor interactions in effecting gene expression. As we come to understand more pharmacodynamic processes, it is anticipated that as many pharmacogenetic differences will be found in those as in any of the above-mentioned pharmacokinetic processes.

THERAPEUTIC "WINDOW"

For drugs with a relatively narrow *therapeutic window* (Fig. 21.1), the minimum effective concentration (in the blood or target tissue) is close to the minimum toxic concentration [in whatever tissue(s) toxicity occurs]. Due to minor fluctuations, dependent on the dose and the frequency of administration, such a drug will tend to cause more adverse reactions. It therefore follows that this narrow therapeutic window causes a narrow *therapeutic index*, i.e., the dose causing toxicity is not much greater than that needed for effectiveness.

Most pharmacogenetic studies are successful because they exploit drugs having narrow therapeutic windows. If a drug shows a wide therapeutic window, it is unlikely to cause toxicity in a significant portion of any human population; therefore, this would be of little concern to public health, and the need to prevent adverse drug events would be small. For example, if the dose causing toxicity is 20 times greater than the dose needed to be effective, and genetic differences in handling this drug are no greater than 4-fold across the entire human population, this drug would

Table 21.1. One possible classification of human pharmacogenetic disorders

A. Less enzyme/defective protein
1. N-acetylation (*NAT2, NAT1*)
2. Glucose-6-phosphate dehydrogenase (*G6PD*)
3. Hereditary methemoglobinemias; hemoglobinopathies
4. NADH-cytochrome b_5 reductase
5. P450 monooxygenases (oxidation deficiencies), debrisoquine (*CYP2D6*), S-mephenytoin (*CYP2C19 & CYP2C9*), nifedipine (*CYP3A4*), coumarin and nicotine (*CYP2A6*), theophylline (*CYP1A2*), acetaminophen (*CYP2E1*), *CYP1A1, CYP2B6*
6. Null mutants of glutathione transferase, mu class (*GSTM1*); theta class (*GSTT1*)
7. Sulfotransferases (*SULT*)
8. Thiopurine methyltransferase (*TPMT*)
9. Thiol methyltransferase (*THMT*)
10. Catechol O-methyltransferase (*COMT*)
11. Histamine N-methyltransferase (*HNMT*)
12. Paraoxonase, sarinase deficiency (*PON1*)
13. UDP glucuronosyltransferases (Gilbert's disease, *UGT1A1*; (S)-oxazepam, *UGT2B7*)
14. NAD(P)H:quinone oxidoreductase (*NQO1*)
15. Microsomal, soluble epoxide hydrolases (*EPHX1, EPHX2*)
16. Atypical alcohol dehydrogenase (*ADH*)
17. Aldehyde dehydrogenase (*ALDH2*)
18. Defect in converting aldophosphamide to carboxyphosphamide (*ALDH1A1?*)
19. Alpha-one (α_1)-antitrypsin (*PI*)
20. Alpha-one (α_1)-antichymotrypsin (*ACT*)
21. Angiotensin-converting enzyme (*DCP1*, ACE) and sensitivity to ACE inhibitors
22. Hypocatalasemia (*CAT*)
23. Dihydropyrimidine dehydrogenase (*DPYD*) and fluorouracil toxicity
24. Succinylcholine-induced apnea, butyrylcholinesterase (*BCHE*)
25. Fish odour syndrome (*FMO3*)
26. Glucocorticoid-remediable aldosteronism (*CYP11B1, CYP11B2*)
27. Dubin-Johnson syndrome; multispecific organic anion transporter (*MOAT, MRP*)
28. γ-Aminolevulinate synthase (*ALAS2*) and pyridoxine (vitamin B6)-responsive sideroblastic anemia
29. Adriamycin- and 5-fluorouracil-induced apoptosis in colon cancer cells, dependent on *TP21, TP53* gene expression
30. *TP53* mutations, response to doxorubicin but not 5-fluorouracil
31. Surfactant protein (*SFTPA1, SFTPB, SFTPC, SFTPD*) deficiencies and lung toxicity
32. Lactose intolerance

B. Alteration in receptor, transporter or channel protein
1. Inability to taste phenylthiourea
2. Coumarin anticoagulant resistance (receptor-based?)
3. Long-QT syndrome (KVLQT1, HERG, *KCBMB1, KCNMB2, SCN5A*)
4. Androgen resistance
5. Estrogen resistance
6. Cushing syndrome from low doses of dexamethasone
7. Insulin resistance
8. Rhodopsin variants; dominant form of retinitis pigmentosa
9. Vasopressin resistance (*AVPR2*)
10. Malignant hyperthermia/general anesthesia (defect in Ca^{++}-release channel ryanodine receptor) (*RYR1*)
11. Cyanocobalamine (vitamin B_{12} malabsorption), absence of intrinsic factor
12. β-Adrenergic receptors (*ADRB1, ADRB2, ADRB3*) and sensitivity to β-agonists in asthmatics
13. Angiotensin II T1 receptor and vascular reactivity to phenylephrine or response to ACE inhibitors
14. Aquaporin-5 (*AQP5*), bronchial hyperresponsiveness to methacholine in asthma patients
15. Sulfonylurea receptor (*ABCC8*) and responsiveness to sulfonylurea hypoglycemic agents
16. Altered serotonin receptors (*HTR*) and transporter (*SLC6A4*) and response to neuroleptics such as clozapine
17. Altered dopamine transporter (*SLCG3*)
18. Dopamine receptors (*D2DR, D4DR*)
19. Dopamine D3 receptor (*D3DR*) and risk of drug-induced tardive dyskinesia
20. Nicotine α 7 receptor (*CHRNA7*) and vulnerability to psychology.
21. Methylenetetrahydrofolate reductase transporter and risk of acute lymphocytic leukemia, neural tube defects
22. Resistance to tuberculosis, other infections, and *NRAMP1*
23. *CCR5* (β-chemokine receptor) and resistance to HIV
24. Cholesteryl ester transfer protein (*CETP*) and pravastatin efficacy in coronary atherosclerosis patients
25. Defective drug transporters (*e.g. MDR1*), resistance to chemotherapeutic agents
26. Cystinuria (defect in amino-acid transporter, *SLC3A1*)

continued

Table 21.1. One possible classification of human pharmacogenetic disorders (*continued*)

C. Change in response due to enzyme induction, overexpression
   1. Porphyrias (*esp.* cutanea tarda)
   2. Aryl hydrocarbon receptor (*AHR*) (*CYP1A1, CYP1A2, CYP1B1* inducibility)
      Cancer, immunosuppression, birth defects, chloracne, porphyria, (?)eye toxicity, (?)ovarian toxicity
   3. Licorice-induced pseudoaldosteronism (*HSD11B1*)
   4. Mineralocorticoid excess with hypertension (*HSD11B2*)
   5. *c-ERBB2* overexpression and adjuvant therapy for early-stage breast cancer
   6. Thymidylate kinase overexpression; resistance to methotrexate, 5-fluorouracil
   7. Dihydrofolate reductase overexpression; resistance to methotrexate, 5-fluorouracil

D. Disorders of unknown etiology
   1. Corticosteroid (eye drops)-induced glaucoma
   2. Halothane-induced hepatitis
   3. Chloramphenicol-induced aplastic anemia
   4. Phenytoin-induced gingival overgrowth
   5. Fetal hydantoin syndrome
   6. Methotrexate-induced toxicity in juvenile rheumatoid arthritis
   7. *L*-DOPA-induced dyskinesis in Parkinson disease
   8. Glucosidation of amobarbital
   9. Chlorpropamide-alcohol flushing syndrome
   10. Aminoglycoside antibiotic-induced deafness
   11. Myocardial toxicity by anthracyclines (adriamycin, doxorubicin)
   12. Bleomycin-induced pulmonary toxicity
   13. Beryllium-induced lung disease
   14. Hepatitis B vaccine resistance
   15. Retinoic acid resistance and acute promyelocytic leukemia
   16. Thrombophilia (activated protein C resistance)
   17. Fructose intolerance
   18. Beeturia; red urine after eating beets
   19. Malodorous urine after eating asparagus
   20. Reproductive disadvantage in ΔF508 cystic fibrosis heterozygotes who smoke cigarettes (*CFTR*)
   21. Apolipoprotein E and decreased response of Alzheimer patients to tacrine
   22. Binding to TP53 and pifithrin-α protection from γ-irradiation antitumor therapy
   23. High risk of cerebral vein thrombosis in defective prothrombin (*F2*) heterozygotes
   24. High risk of cerebral vein thrombosis in users of oral contraceptives

The genes (when known to be associated, or strongly suspected of being associated, with the pharmacogenetic difference) are italicized and are usually denoted in parentheses.

be of little concern to the pharmacogeneticist. On the other hand, if the dose causing toxicity is only three times greater than the dose for efficacy, and pharmacogenetic differences in handling this drug are 30-fold, this drug would be an important candidate to study, in order to prevent adverse drug reactions leading to morbidity and mortality.

PHASE I AND PHASE II METABOLISM

Virtually all therapeutic agents are metabolized by "Phase I" (functionalization), followed by "Phase II" (conjugation) DMEs (Fig. 21.3). The function of Phase I DMEs is to insert or activate a functional (generally polar) group on the drug substrate. The human genome is expected to contain several thousand metabolism genes. One major class of Phase I DMEs comprises the cytochromes P450 (CYPs), which have been probably the most thoroughly studied of all pharmacologically relevant enzymes. At the

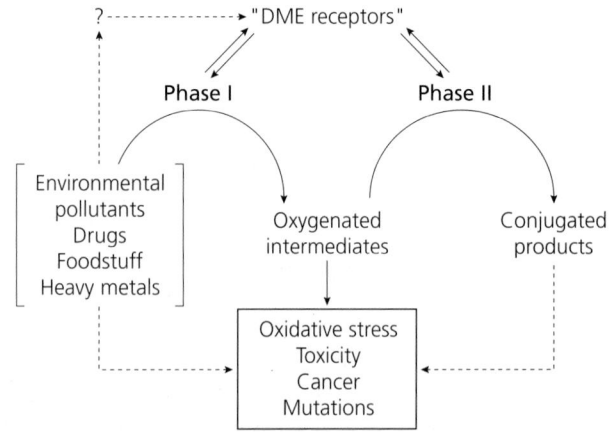

Fig. 21.3. Theoretical scheme of the Phase I and Phase II drug-metabolizing enzymes (DMEs) and the receptors that sometimes up-regulate or down-regulate DME levels. Certain environmental pollutants, drugs, foodstuff and heavy metals interact with DME receptors, or other "reception" pathways, to up- or down-regulate DME gene expression. (Modified from Nebert et al., 1996.)

present time, there are 55 known human *CYP* genes, with the possibility of one or two additional ones that might still be discovered (Nebert and Nelson, 2001; Nelson, 2001). Interestingly, four P450 enzymes handle probably greater than 80% of all commonly prescribed and over-the-counter medications: CYP2C9, CYP2C19, CYP2D6 and CYP3A4. CYP1A2, CYP2A6, CYP2B6, CYP2E1, CYP3A5 and CYP4A11 also metabolize a few drugs. CYP1A1, CYP1A2, CYP1B1, CYP2E1 and CYP3A4 appear to be primarily responsible for detoxifying (in some cases) or metabolically activating (in most cases) environmental carcinogens (Gonzalez, 1997). Other examples of Phase I DMEs include flavin-containing monooxygenases (FMOs), hydroxylases, peroxidases, lipooxygenases, cyclooxygenases, monoamine oxidases, dioxygenases, reductases, and dehydrogenases.

The function of Phase II DMEs is to conjugate the Phase I products, usually inserting a highly polar conjugation moiety on the polar moiety produced by Phase I enzymes (Fig. 21.3). Examples of Phase II DMEs include glucuronyl, sulfate, glutathione, acyl, amine, acetyl, and methyl transferase reactions. Research for the past five decades has concentrated largely on Phase I and Phase II DMEs. As described above, we now know that pharmacogenetic differences can include virtually every gene involved in any of the drug pharmacokinetic and pharmacodynamic processes.

PLASMA DRUG HALF-LIVES

In the late 1960s comparisons of the half-life of drug clearance were carried out in monozygotic versus dizygotic twins. The "heritability index" was calculated as the variance within pairs of dizygotic twins (V_d) minus the variance within pairs of monozygotic twins (V_m) divided by the variance within pairs of dizygotic twins (V_d). An heritability index of 1.0 would mean "purely genetic," while an heritability index of less than 0.50 or less than zero would mean predominantly environmental factors. From twin studies—with dicoumarol, phenylbutazone, desipramine, halothane, nortriptyline, oxyphenylbutazone, and antipyrine—the main conclusion was that drug clearance rates always reflect a strong genetic component (Vesell, 1972). Three decades later, we can appreciate that these observations reflect, for the main part, allelic differences in two or more DMEs in the same metabolic pathway for each of these drugs, and this will be amply covered in this chapter. Thus, Phase I and Phase II "rapid" versus "slow" DMEs are the principal effectors of plasma drug clearance. These findings underscore one of the themes of this chapter, that some pharmacogenetic differences can be explained largely on the basis of one gene, while many other variations are polygenic and multifactorial.

PHARMACOGENETIC DIFFERENCES CAN OCCUR IN ANY TISSUE

A common misconception, possibly stemming from the way pharmacology and toxicology has been taught during the past several decades, is that DMEs exist largely—if not completely—in the liver; this could not be further from the truth (Nebert, 1999; Nebert and Nelson, 2001). CYP3A4, the most abundant hepatic cytochrome P450, is also present in large concentrations in the gastrointestinal tract. Many DMEs are located in the lung and kidney. Many Phase I and Phase II DMEs exist in the vascular endothelial cells and contribute to the arachidonic acid cascade, cell division, inflammatory response, cell migration, bronchoconstriction, vasodilation, and numerous other homeostatic mechanisms. DMEs exist in the choroid plexus, substantia nigra, vasculature, and basically any other cell of the brain and play roles in neuroendocrine functions. Phenytoin oxidation (due principally to CYP2C9 and CYP2C19) is as much as 50-fold greater in the human oral mucosa than in liver (Zhou et al., 1996). Some DMEs exist at high concentrations in the nasal mucosa (Gu et al., 1998). Clinical geneticists must therefore keep in mind that variability in drug response (efficacy, toxicity) can occur in any tissue and need not be determined by DMEs or drug receptors or transporters located solely in the liver.

What follows is a series of examples of pharmacogenetic differences, which are often causes of drug-induced toxicity. The latest knowledge about allelic variants is included. The examples are taken approximately in the order that they appear in Table 21.1. Due to space limitations, only selected examples will be expanded upon, but the remainder are discussed in detail in one or another of the reviews cited at the beginning of this chapter.

Examples due to less enzyme or defective protein

N-ACETYLATION POLYMORPHISM

Originally called the "isoniazid acetylation polymorphism," this defect was first identified in the late 1940s when patients who converted to a positive tuberculin test were routinely treated with isoniazid. A high incidence of peripheral neuropathy was found among those taking isoniazid. Hence, this is an example of the therapeutic drug reaching toxic levels (Fig. 21.1) in many individuals. By giving isoniazid and measuring plasma levels six hours later (Fig. 21.4), individuals could be phenotyped as "slow acetylators" (clearing the drug slowly) or "rapid acetylators" (clearing the drug

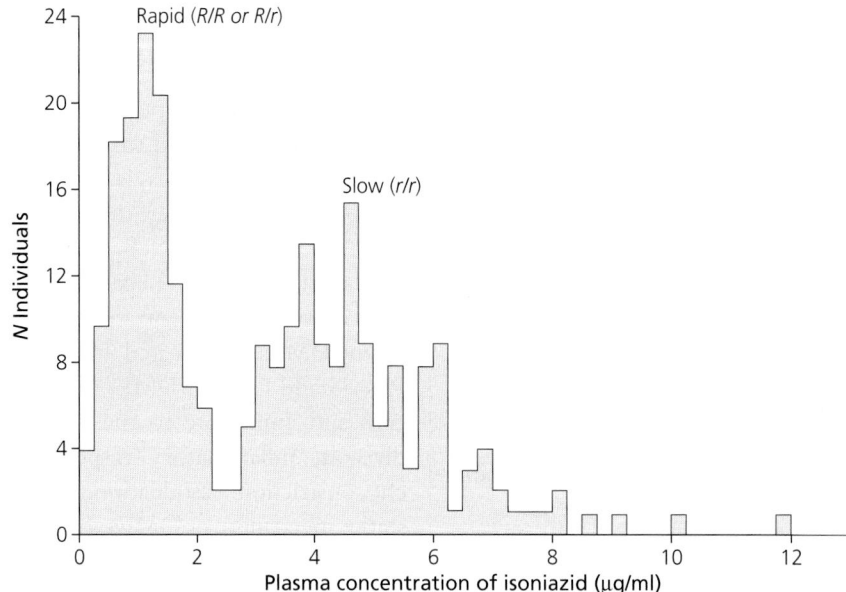

Fig. 21.4. Plasma isoniazid concentrations six hours after the drug was given. Results were obtained in 267 members of 53 complete family units. All subjects received approximately 9.8 mg isoniazid per kg body weight. (Redrawn from Evans et al., 1960.)

quickly). The parents of slow acetylator children were found to be also slow acetylators. In other words, slow acetylators are homozygous for the putative "slow-acetylator (r) allele," whereas rapid acetylators are either heterozygous or homozygous for the "rapid (R) allele." Hence, the *slow phenotype* is inherited as an autosomal recessive trait. Frequency of the r allele was found to be about 0.72 in the United States, meaning that about one in every two individuals (using the Hardy–Weinberg equation, $q^2 = 0.72 \times 0.72 = 0.518$) is homozygous for r/r and thus shows the slow-acetylator trait. This is an example of a Phase II DME polymorphism.

Two human *N*-acetyltransferase functional genes (*NAT1, NAT2*) and one pseudogene (*NATP*) have been localized to the same region on chromosome 8pter-q11. The rapid- and slow-acetylator phenotypes reflect the *NAT2* gene, encoding the NAT2 enzyme which has a 10-times-lower Km than NAT1 for isoniazid and other amines. Several *NAT2* slow-acetylator variant alleles were found to encode a stable protein having little or no enzymic activity, or an unstable protein (Blum et al., 1990).

The *NAT2* gene was originally thought to be "intronless" (Blum et al., 1990), but a small noncoding first exon—about 8 kb upstream from the coding exon 2—was then found (Ebisawa and Deguchi, 1991). Three major *NAT2* slow-acetylator alleles exist: *NAT2*5B* and *NAT2* 6A* are common in Caucasians; *NAT2*6A* and *NAT2*7A* are common in Asians. There are at least two dozen other, relatively rare, *NAT2* alleles (Hein et al., 2001). Large ethnic

differences exist in the frequency of the rapid-acetylator (consensus, reference, wild-type) allele and slow-acetylator variant alleles (Table 21.2). The slow-acetylation frequency ranges worldwide from less than 10% in Japanese populations to more than 90% in some Mediterranean peoples (Kalow and Bertilsson, 1994). This polymorphism is the first of many pharmacogenetic polymorphisms that were somewhat of a dilemma for the "pure" geneticist: the predominant allele in one ethnic group is often not the predominant allele in another ethnic group; thus, which allele should be regarded as the "wild-type?" The rapid acetylator trait is regarded as that encoded by the consensus (reference, wild-type) allele (*NAT2*4*), and the slow acetylator trait is encoded by the many polymorphic and rare variant alleles.

Table 21.2. Frequency of the slow N-acetylator *NAT2* alleles (q) in different ethnic populations

Population	Number of studies	Mean
Eskimo	4	0.23
South Pacific Islands	5	0.35
Korean/Chinese/Japanese	14	0.37
North and South American Indian	10	0.50
African (excluding Kung, 0.18)	19	0.71
Central and West Asian	22	0.74
European	50	0.75
Egyptian	2	0.96

(Data modified and condensed from Evans, 1992)

An increasing number of alleles has also been uncovered in the nearby *NAT1* gene (which encodes NAT1, an *N*-acetyltransferase having substrate specificities different from that for NAT2). There are many *NAT1* allelic variants that exhibit diminished NAT1 activity (Hein et al., 2001).

The NAT2 slow-acetylator phenotype has been shown to be associated with a more than four-fold increased risk of breast cancer among postmenopausal women who are cigarette smokers (Ambrosone et al., 1996). This genotype-phenotype relationship seems feasible, because cigarette smoke contains nitrosamines that are probably metabolized by NAT2. Thus, the *NAT2* gene appears to be a modifier gene for environmentally-caused breast cancer.

The associations of acetylation phenotypes with toxicity or cancer have received considerable attention. Besides isoniazid-induced *peripheral neuropathy*, hydralazine and procainamide cause *drug-related lupus syndrome* in slow acetylators. Sulfonamides that can be *N*-acetylated (e.g., sulfasalazine) produce *hemolytic anemia* in slow acetylators. The following drugs have major *differences in clearance* between slow and rapid acetylators, but, because of large therapeutic indices, usually do not manifest blatant toxicities: aminoglutethimide, dapsone, phenelzine, nitrazepam, and clonazepam. The slow-acetylator phenotype shows a three-fold lower incidence of colorectal carcinoma but a higher incidence (odds ratio of 16.7) of urinary bladder cancer (Gonzalez and Idle, 1994; Weber, 1997). Both occupational exposure to arylamines and cigarette smoking are required, however, in conjunction with the slow-acetylator phenotype, for development of bladder cancer, and no relationship is found between acetylator phenotype and smoking-related bladder cancer in the absence of exposure to arylamines or cigarette smoking.

GLUCOSE-6-PHOSPHATE DEHYDROGENASE (*G6PD*) POLYMORPHISM

In Croton, southern Italy, about 510 B.C., Pythagoras is believed to be the first to describe the "dangers of eating the fava bean," because many individuals in that area who ate fava beans often experienced painful hemolytic crises (i.e., developed hemolytic anemia). Now we know that this disease (favism) is associated with G6PD deficiency, and the incidence of that disease in Sardinia and parts of southern Italy is as high as one in three.

There are several stories about how the G6PD polymorphism was discovered. One story concerns a World War II observation that certain soldiers, especially African-Americans—who were taking the antimalarial drug primaquine and flying in troop transport aircraft at more than 8000 feet altitude (lowered pO_2)—were reported to develop painful acute hemolytic crises. This led to the discovery of low red blood cell G6PD activity and decreased GSH concentrations in affected individuals (Carson et al., 1956). Subsequently, it was found that this enzyme is extremely polymorphic, that almost one in ten African-Americans have the *A*-type of G6PD deficiency, that more than two dozen commonly prescribed drugs in addition to primaquine cause hemolytic anemia in G6PD-deficient patients (Table 21.3), and that G6PD deficiency is inherited as an X-linked recessive trait and currently affects probably more than 500 million people worldwide.

This is an example of an enzyme polymorphism having an indirect effect on drug toxicity. G6PD is an enzyme in the hexose monophosphate shunt, one of the principal sources of NADPH generation (which restores oxidized glutathione, GS-SG, to its reduced form, GSH) in the normal red cell and many other tissues. Many drugs and their metabolites can put a burden on GSH levels, and this can lead to a GSH deficiency in G6PD-deficient patients who have little GSH reserves to spare. GSH deficiency in the red cell results in membrane fragility and hemolysis—hence, hemolytic anemia. Thiozalsulfone was the first arylamine sulfa drug shown to cause a bimodal distribution of hemolytic anemia in the treated population, due to G6PD differences. The *G6PD* gene has several hundred allelic variants, a large number of which cause one or more amino acid changes. The *G6PD* gene is located on the X chromosome, which is consistent with G6PD deficiency being transmitted as an X-linked recessive trait; this means that a "carrier" mother and a healthy father will have children displaying one of four possibilities: a healthy female, a carrier female, a healthy male, and an afflicted male. As with the *NAT2* polymorphism, many amino-acid mutations in G6PD cause lowered enzyme activity; however, in contrast to NAT2 activity, it appears that the complete absence of G6PD activity is incompatible with life. Interestingly, there is a

Table 21.3. Partial list of drugs and chemicals that have clearly been Shown to cause clinically significant hemolytic anemia in G6PD-deficient patients

Acetanilide	Primaquine
Methylene blue	Sulfacetamide
Nalidixic acid	Sulfamethoxazole
Naphthalene	Sulfaniliamide
Niridazole	Sulfapyridine
Nitrofurantoin	Thiazolesulfone
Pamaquine	Toluidine blue
Pentaquine	Trinitrotoluene
Phenacetin	
Phenylbutazone	

(Modified and condensed, from Nebert and Weber, 1990)

more than 100-fold difference in the incidence of G6PD deficiency between Ashkenazic (0.4%) and Sephardic (53%) Jewish males (Nebert and Weber, 1990).

SYNERGY BETWEEN TWO PHARMACOGENETIC DIFFERENCES

Toxicity by a drug or other environmental agent can be greatly exaggerated by the combination of two pharmaco-genetic phenotypes in the same individual. For example, aniline dye workers exhibited varying degrees of "apparent exposure in the work place," depending on their G6PD and acetylator phenotypes. Table 21.4 shows that the quantity of hemoglobin adducts among workers exposed to aniline was much greater in individuals having the combined G6PD-deficiency + slow-acetylator phenotype, as compared with the other possible combinations of these traits.

Figure 21.5 illustrates the multiple pathways of aniline metabolism, involving NAT2 and G6PD, which would explain the clinical findings in Table 21.4. Aniline-hemoglobin adducts are the result of a P450-mediated arene oxide, which is highly reactive and binds covalently to various cellular proteins (and probably nucleic acids as well). The arene oxide can decompose nonenzymatically to *para*- or *ortho*-hydroxyaniline, both of which are excreted and are not particularly toxic. Glutathione conjugation of the arene oxide by a glutathione S-transferase (followed by γ-glutamyltranspeptidase, cysteinylglycinase and N-acetyltransferase actions) is one major route of detoxification. N-acetylation of aniline's amino group is another route of detoxification. Both of these products are no longer toxic and readily excreted. Hence, a poor acetylator combined with G6PD deficiency (i.e., decreases in two major routes of detoxification) stacks the cards in favor of a build-up of aniline-hemoglobin adducts.

The data in Table 21.4 suggest that, although individuals might be exposed to the same level of an occupationally hazardous chemical or other environmental pollutant or

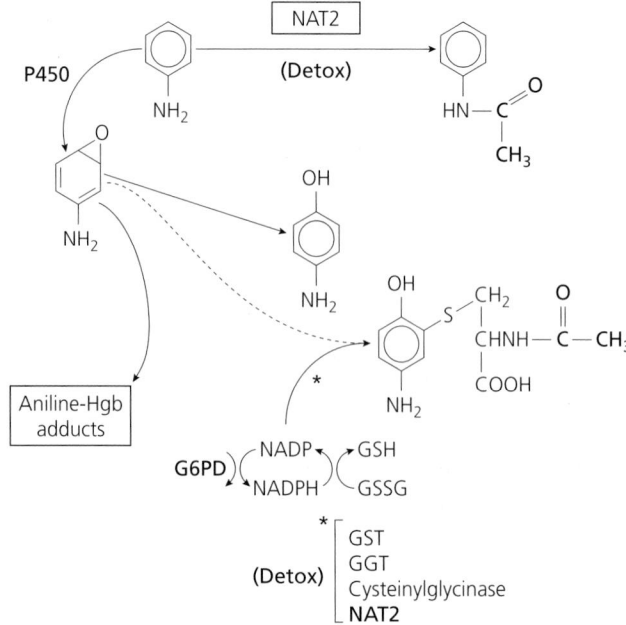

Fig. 21.5. Metabolic pathways of aniline, leading to N-acetylated aniline, *p*-hydroxyaniline, the *m*-mercapturic acid derivative of *p*-hydroxyaniline, and the reactive aniline arene oxide that can bind covalently to many cellular macromolecules such as hemoglobin. Hgb, hemoglobin. The *o*-hydroxyaniline formation, which occurs to a much lesser extent than *p*-hydroxy-, is not shown.

mixture, the risk of an adverse health effect may vary by one or more orders of magnitude—due to interindividual genetic differences. This example is important in occupational medicine, and also a warning to those who rely on biomarkers as "indicators of exposure." In this case, striking differences are seen, not because of the amount of exposure to an occupationally hazardous chemical in the work place, but rather due to the underlying genetic predisposition of each individual worker.

METHEMOGLOBINEMIAS, HEMOGLOBINOPATHIES

Abnormalities in the globin protein can lead to heme iron being more easily oxidized from Fe^{++} to Fe^{+++}, thereby causing methemoglobinemia, or to the protein being more unstable and subject to oxidative stress attack by nucleophilic metabolites, thereby causing hemolytic anemia. This is an example of an indirect pharmacogenetic effect.

The occurrence of hemolytic anemia after ingestion of medications by a Swiss father and daughter led to the discovery of the unstable hemoglobin Zürich. The father had a serious hemolytic episode following ingestion of sulfamethoxypyridazine. Following the initial discovery, several other structural hemoglobin variants—typically based on

Table 21.4. Aniline-hemoglobin (Hgb) adducts in chemical dye workers

Aniline-Hgb adducts	Acetylator status		G6PD deficiency	
	Fast	Slow	No	Yes
2	+		+	
3	+			+
20		+	+	
100		+		+

(Modified and condensed from Lewalter and Korallus, 1985.)

one or more amino-acid changes in the globin molecule—were found to be associated with drug-induced anemia, jaundice, and hemolytic crises. Severity of clinical manifestations in these disorders is related to the amount of unstable globin chain produced and the stability of residual chains that are present in excess. In some cases of hemoglobinopathy, the drug (or especially its metabolites) oxidizes the Fe^{++} to Fe^{+++}, i.e., causing methemoglobinemia. Many of the same drugs and chemicals shown in Table 21.3 can cause methemoglobinemia in patients with a particular hemoglobinopathy. In some instances, cigarette smoking has a protective effect against hemolysis; the high affinity of carbon monoxide (in the smoke) for the heme, can stabilize hemoglobin against the effects of sulfonamides and other drugs (Evans, 1994).

NADH-CYTOCHROME B_5 REDUCTASE

This is another example of an indirect pharmacogenetic effect. Heterozygotes for a functionally inadequate variant form of NADH-cytochrome b_5 reductase (which has also been called methemoglobin reductase and NADH diaphorase) have been reported to develop methemoglobinemia following a standard dose of certain drugs or exposure to particular environmental chemicals. Chlorzoxazone, 7-ethoxycoumarin, aniline and N-nitrosodimethylamine are especially potent in this regard, participating in large part via CYP2E1 (Yamazaki et al., 1996).

About 3% of hemoglobin is converted to methemoglobin daily, and about 1% is in the methemoglobin form normally at any given time; hence, there must be a dynamic equilibrium between the oxidizing and reducing factors affecting the heme iron. The reducing mechanism is an electron-transport chain from NADH to methemoglobin that requires cytochrome b_5 and cytochrome b_5 reductase. Allelic variants leading to the absence of the cytochrome, or deficiency of the reductase, can cause drug-induced methemoglobinemia (Nagai et al., 1993).

CYP1A2 STRUCTURAL GENE POLYMORPHISM

This is an example of a Phase I DME polymorphism. A number of drugs (e.g., zoxazolamine, acetaminophen, phenacetin, theophylline and caffeine) are substrates for this P450 enzyme (Eaton et al., 1995). CYP1A2 also metabolizes many environmental aromatic amine procarcinogens, including tobacco smoke-specific dibenzo[c,g]carbazole and nitrosamines such as 4-(methylnitrosamino)-1-(3-pyridyl)-1-butanone (NNK), and numerous food-derived heterocyclic amines generated from the frying of meat and fish. There is suggestive evidence of an association between diets of fried meats and certain forms of cancer; metabolic activation of these environmental chemicals largely by CYP1A2 appears to be responsible for their mutagenic and tumorigenic properties (Felton et al., 1997). Difuranocoumarins, such as the mycotoxin aflatoxin B_1, and nitrated polycyclic aromatic hydrocarbons, such as 6-nitrochrysene and 1,3-dinitropyrene in diesel exhaust particles, are CYP1A2 substrates. Interestingly, 6-nitrochrysene is activated to the proximate carcinogen by CYP1A2, whereas 1,3-dinitropyrene is detoxified by CYP1A2 (Shimada and Guengerich, 1990). Occupationally hazardous arylamines, including 4-aminobiphenyl, 2-naphthylamine, benzidine and methylene-*bis*-2-chloroaniline, are known to cause bladder tumors and are (at least partially) CYP1A2 substrates. CYP1A1 metabolism (Butler et al., 1989) and CYP1B1 metabolism in certain tissues (Shimada et al., 1996) might contribute, however, to the activation of some of these above-mentioned chemicals.

Endogenous substrates of CYP1A2 include estradiol (Aoyama et al., 1990) and uroporphyrinogen (Sinclair et al., 1998). There is no known physiological function of estrogen 2-hydroxylation. Nevertheless, clearance of estradiol or an alteration in the estradiol metabolite profile appears to contribute to one's risk of breast cancer (Nebert, 1993). Uroporphyrinogen oxidation by high levels of basal CYP1A2 may contribute to porphyria cutanea tarda (Smith et al., 2001), and this subject will be covered in detail later in the chapter.

There are two distinctly different human *CYP1A2* gene polymorphisms (Eaton et al., 1995; Nebert et al., 1996). The *CYP1A2* structural gene polymorphism is described here. The *CYP1A2* inducibility polymorphism (governed by the aromatic hydrocarbon (AH) receptor) is described in the "Enzyme Induction" section later.

The human *CYP1A2* gene is located close to the *CYP1A1* gene on chromosome 15 (Corchero et al., 2001). Numerous studies have shown interindividual differences between 30- and more than 60-fold in CYP1A2 transcription, mRNA levels, protein levels, and enzyme activity. The fact that transcription, translation and enzyme activity levels always go hand-in-hand suggests that there might be no amino-acid change in the human CYP1A2 protein responsible for the low versus high basal activity, and this is what has been found so far. In other words, 12 mutant alleles have been described, yet none is associated with these striking interindividual differences in CYP1A2 activity. Five of the variant alleles result in amino-acid changes (Oscarson et al., 2001).

Although some studies have shown a log normal distribution of the interindividual differences in CYP1A2 protein or activity, AH receptor-mediated induction of CYP1A2 by cigarette smoke is a confounding variable. Hence, if data from smokers and nonsmokers are analyzed separately, a polymodal distribution has been found in three separate laboratories (Eaton et al., 1995; Nebert et al., 1996).

Two *Cyp1a2(-/-)* knockout mouse lines have been created (Pineau et al., 1995; Liang et al., 1996). These mice show no abnormal phenotype—other than absence of the *Cyp1a2* gene and its mRNA and protein and, as expected, the absence of metabolism of CYP1A2 substrates. High- and low-activity human *CYP1A2* alleles are being placed into *Cyp1a2(-/-)* mice; these lines should be helpful in elucidating the role of human CYP1A2 in environmental toxicity and cancer. An intriguing increase in the incidence of hydronephrotic kidney disease, as the *Cyp1a2(-/-)* mouse ages, is also under investigation in the Nebert laboratory.

In summary, no DNA test is yet available for detecting the *CYP1A2* structural gene polymorphism, although greater than 60-fold differences exist in various populations studied. Many of these investigations have been confusing, however, because they did not exclude the variable of cigarette smoking, which (described later) represents a distinctly different polymorphism involving differences in the AH receptor. As this chapter goes to press, it can be stated that the genetic basis of the *CYP1A2* structural gene polymorphism has been extensively investigated (Yokoi et al., 1995), but not delineated yet.

MULTIPLE PHARMACOGENETIC DIFFERENCES IN SAME METABOLIC PATHWAY

For the CYP1A2 phenotype, three CYP1A2 substrates are commonly used—phenacetin (Distlerath et al., 1985; Sesardic et al., 1988), theophylline (Robson et al., 1988), and caffeine (Butler et al., 1989; Kalow and Tang, 1991; Horn et al., 1995). The caffeine metabolic pathways (Fig. 21.6) are another example of more than one pharmacogenetic difference contributing to the clearance of the same drug. If an individual has a high-CYP1A2 phenotype and is a rapid acetylator, his half-life of caffeine clearance might be two hours. If another person has a low-CYP1A2 phenotype and is a slow acetylator, his caffeine half-life might be 12 hours. We all know someone who drinks a lot of coffee with little "caffeine effect," while others remain jittery for 12 hours from the caffeine in a single cup of coffee. Because cigarette smoking induces CYP1A2 levels—irrespective of the *CYP1A2* structural gene polymorphism—the caffeine half-life in an individual having a combined high-CYP1A2/rapid acetylator phenotype might be shortened further to 30 minutes, thus

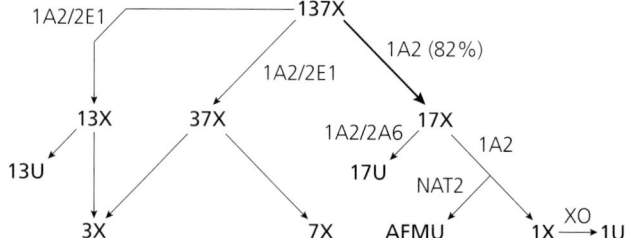

Fig. 21.6. Caffeine metabolic pathways, 137X, 17X, 1X=1,3,7-trimethyl, 1,7-dimethyl and 1-methylxanthine, respectively. 17U, 1U=1,7-dimethyl and 1-methyluric acid, respectively. AFMU=5-acetylamino-6-formyl-amino-3-methyluracil. In addition to other P450 reactions (CYP2A6, CYP2E1), and xanthine oxidase (XO) that metabolizes 1X to 1U, the specific reactions of CYP1A2 and N-acetyltransferase (NAT2) are shown.

providing an answer as to why the usual cigarette smoker requires a lot of coffee to feel the caffeine effect!

Additional enzymes (CYP2A6, CYP2E1 and xanthine oxidase) also contribute to the clearance of caffeine (Fig. 21.6). The *CYP2A6* and *CYP2E1* polymorphisms are described later. A low-activity versus high-activity phenotype in any (or all) of these three enzymes might further complicate the picture. This subject—the fact that all pharmacogenetic disorders actually represent polygenic traits—will be taken up in greater detail toward the end of this chapter.

CYP2D6 DEBRISOQUINE/SPARTEINE (DRUG OXIDATION) POLYMORPHISM

The debrisoquine/sparteine polymorphism (Fig. 21.7A) was discovered independently about the same time by two groups. Robert L Smith in England studied debrisoquine, while Michel Eichelbaum in Germany studied sparteine metabolism. This is another example of a Phase I DME polymorphism.

Smith noticed that the antihypertensive agent debrisoquine caused an unexpectedly high incidence of adverse drug reactions. Smith reasoned that the combination of a narrow therapeutic index (described earlier) and an underlying genetic variation in the way individual patients metabolize the drug might be responsible for this high incidence of undesirable responses. Smith and three laboratory colleagues took the prescribed dose and measured their urinary levels of metabolites. Besides becoming hypotensive himself, from ingesting the "usual" dosage of debrisoquine, Smith found that his urinary 4-hydroxy metabolite was about 20-fold less than that of his three colleagues. A larger population was subsequently screened (Fig. 21.7B). Poor metabolizers (PMs) of debrisoquine, such as Smith, were found to represent 6% to 10% of Caucasians, as compared

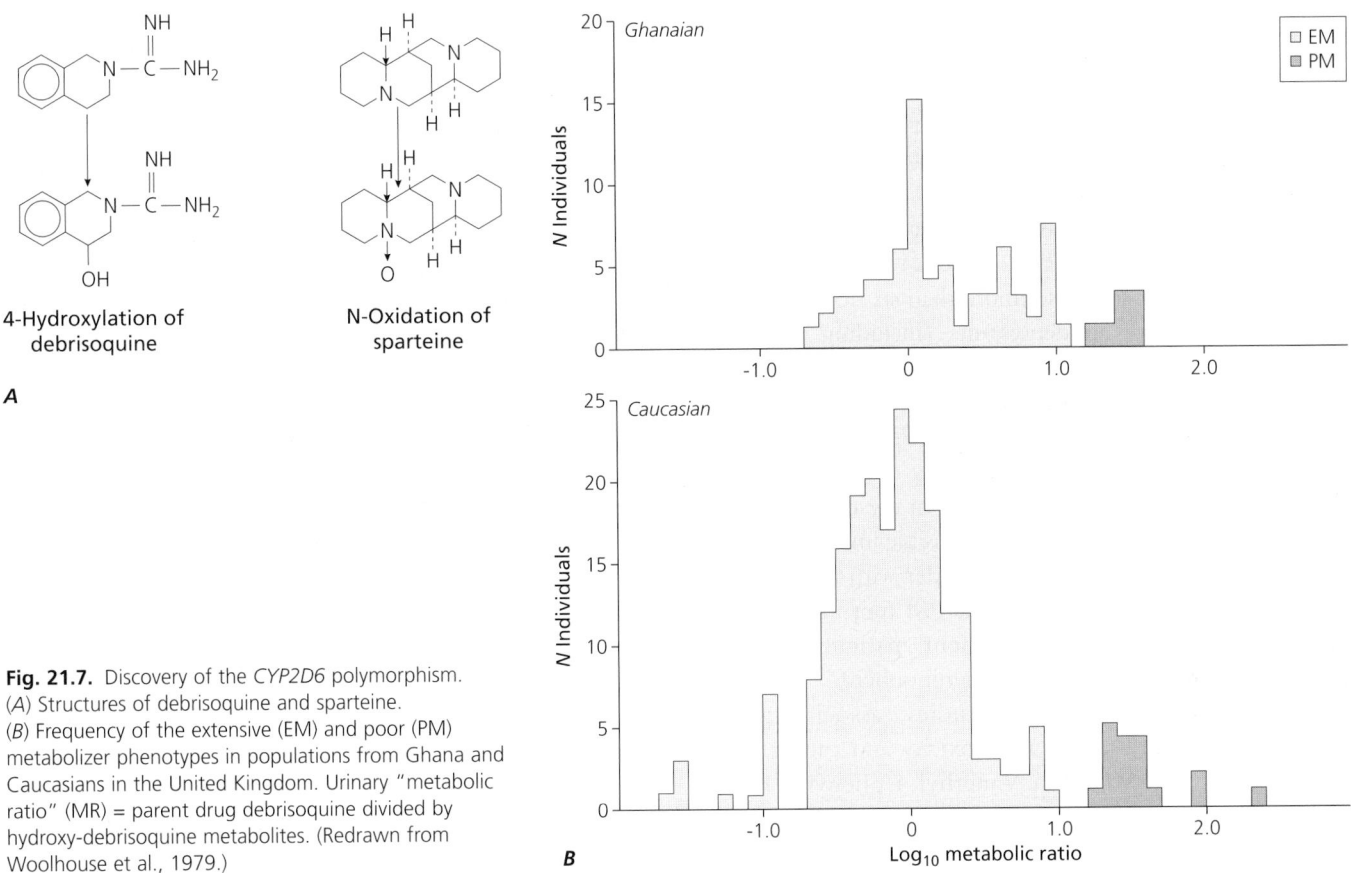

Fig. 21.7. Discovery of the *CYP2D6* polymorphism. (*A*) Structures of debrisoquine and sparteine. (*B*) Frequency of the extensive (EM) and poor (PM) metabolizer phenotypes in populations from Ghana and Caucasians in the United Kingdom. Urinary "metabolic ratio" (MR) = parent drug debrisoquine divided by hydroxy-debrisoquine metabolites. (Redrawn from Woolhouse et al., 1979.)

with extensive metabolizers (EMs) who handle the drug 10 to more than 40 times more efficiently (Idle and Smith, 1979). PM frequencies are about 5% in African populations and less than 1% in Asians. This is another example of a striking difference in the incidence of PM individuals between two ethnic groups.

The Eichelbaum laboratory investigated the oxytocic drug sparteine, which was known to occasionally cause excessive uterine contraction in women. The conversion of the drug to two different dehydrosparteines was quantitated by the urinary concentration ratio of sparteine to dehydrosparteines, and these data showed a bimodal distribution (Eichelbaum et al., 1979).

The DME responsible for the debrisoquine/sparteine polymorphism was shown to be a cytochrome P450, and the gene was named *CYP2D6*. The cloning of *CYP2D6*, and characterization of several mutant alleles (Gonzalez et al., 1988), is believed to represent a landmark study in that it brought descriptive pharmacogenetics for the first time to the cutting edge of molecular biology and genetics (Nebert, 1997b). PM alleles code for a defective protein and/or incorrect splicing of the gene transcript, or even complete deletion of the gene—resulting in lowered, or

completely absent, enzyme activity. The *CYP2D6* gene is located on chromosome 22q13.1 near the *SIS* proto-oncogene. Interestingly, an "ultra-rapid metabolizer" (UM) phenotype has also been found—and shown to be due to amplification of the *CYP2D6* gene as many as 13 times (Meyer, 1994). The incidence of the UM phenotype is about 0.8% in Caucasians, 21% in Saudi Arabians, and 29% in Ethiopians (Ingleman-Sundberg et al., 1999); the reason for these ethnic differences is not known.

A unified nomenclature system for the human *CYP2D6* alleles was initiated (Daly et al., 1996), which has been recommended to become standard for the allelic nomenclature of all human genes (Nebert, 2000b). The *CYP2D6*1* allele is the consensus sequence (wild-type, EM), and currently there are more than 70 allelic variants reported—both low activity and no activity, as well as extremely high activity. The most common alleles in Caucasians are: the *CYP2D6*4* series (splicing defects), the *CYP2D6*5* allele (deletion of the entire gene), and the *CYP2D6*6* series (nucleotide deletions leading to codon frameshifts). All of these result in either no enzyme protein or a very unstable truncated protein, i.e., no enzymic activity. The *CYP2D6*4* allelic frequency is 0.23 and is Caucasian-specific. The

CYP2D6*17 (R296C mutation) and *CYP2D6*29* (four amino acid changes) alleles are African-specific. The *CYP2D6*10* series (P34S mutation, causing an unstable protein and altered substrate specificity) is Asian-specific and the most common variant allele among Chinese (Oscarson et al., 2001).

Many prescribed drugs, as well as over-the-counter drugs, are metabolized by CYP2D6 (Table 21.5). The debrisoquine "panel" now comprises more than six dozen drugs—tricyclics and other antidepressants (including serotonin reuptake inhibitors and monoamine oxidase inhibitors), neuroleptics, antiarrhythmics and antihypertensives (including β-blockers), and opiates. The *CYP2D6* polymorphism appears to be important in the handling of more than 20% of all commonly prescribed drugs. From the drugs listed in Table 21.5, one can appreciate the possible important interactions of one pharmacogenetic disorder with another. For example, is the CYP2D6 EM versus PM trait important in determining which G6PD-deficient patients develop hemolytic anemia when taking acetaminophen?

Numerous epidemiological studies, associating the *CYP2D6* allelic differences with toxicity and cancer, have been reported. MPTP (*N*-methyl-4-phenyl-1,1,3,6-tetrahydropyridine, formed as a by-product during the illicit manufacture of a meperidine analog), and similar compounds, can cause Parkinsonian tremors in humans; MPTP inhibits CYP2D6-mediated metabolism in vitro.

Individuals having the PM phenotype also appear to have a 2- to 2.5-fold increased risk of developing Parkinson disease (Nebert and McKinnon, 1994). Fourteen mothers were treated with flecainide for fetal atrial tachycardias associated with intrauterine cardiac failure; 12 of the 14 fetuses responded by conversion to sinus rhythm, whereas one of the 12 fetuses subsequently died in utero (Allan et al., 1991). Because the incidence of the CYP2D6 PM trait is about one in 12 Caucasians, could such in utero toxicity reflect the CYP2D6 phenotype of the fetus, the mother, or both? The EM phenotype appears to be correlated with an increased incidence of tumors in the bladder, liver, pharynx, and stomach—and especially cigarette smoking-induced lung cancer (Nebert and Weber, 1990). These data suggest that enhanced CYP2D6-mediated metabolism of one or more unknown dietary or other environmental agents, i.e., formation of a reactive intermediate (Phase I effect), might play a role in cancer initiation and/or promotion in the above-named tissues.

Possible relationships between the PM phenotype and decreased tolerance to chronic pain, differences in the morphine metabolism in the brain, and variations in tendency for opiate addiction have also been described in the literature. At least two studies have implicated a relationship between CYP2D6 and dopamine neurotransmission in the brain. Differences between EM and PM individuals' personality, creativity, and organizational skills have even been

Table 21.5. Major drug substrates of CYP2D6

Alprenolol	Dexfenfluramine	Methoxyamphetamine	Phenacetin
Amiflamine	Dextromethorphan	Methoxyphenamine	Phenformine
Amitriptyline	Dihydrocodeine	Metiamide	Promethazine
Aprindine	Dolasetron	Methylendioxymethamphetamine ("ecstasy")	Propafenone
Atenolol	Encainide	Metoprolol	Propranolol
Brofaromine	Ethylmorphine	Mexiletine	Remoxipride
(Bufuralol)	Flecainide	Mianserin	Risperidone
Bunitrolol	Flunarizine	Minaprine	(Sparteine)
Bupranolol	Fluoxetine	Nicergoline	Tamoxifen
Carvedilol	Fluperlapine	Norcodeine	Thioridazine
Chloroquine	Fluvoxamine	Nortriptyline	Timolol
Chlorpropamide	Guanoxan	*N*-Propylajmaline	Tolferodine
Cinnarizine	Halofantrine	Ondansetron	Tomoxetine
Clomipramine	Haloperidol	Otycodone	Tramadol
Clozapine	Hydrocodone	Oxycodone	Tropisetron
Codeine	Imipramine	Paroxetine	Venlafaxine
(Debrisoquine)	Indoramin	Perhexiline	Zuclopenthixol
Desipramine	Maprotiline	Perphenazine	
Desmethylcitalopram*			

* this metabolite of the drug citalopram is the CYP2D6 substrate.
Bufuralol, debrisoquine and sparteine are listed here only for historical importance, because none of the three is still used clinically. For some of these drugs, the metabolism by CYP2D6 is not the only, or not the major, pathway. For some, the clinical relevance of the CYP2D6 polymorphism is questionable, or dependent on additional variables such as drug-drug interactions and disease. Drug inhibitors of CYP2D6 include chinidin, fluoxetin, levomepromazine, lobelin, methadone, paroxetine, quinidine and trifluperidol. Alkaloid inhibitors of CYP2D6 include ajmalicine, berberine, coniine, ergotamine, gramine, harmaline, laudanosine, sempervirine, vincamine and vinblastine (Meyer, 2000; Ingelman-Sundberg, 2001a).

reported, suggesting further that CYP2D6 might metabolize substances critical to central nervous system function (Kalow and Bertilsson, 1994).

CYP2C9 POLYMORPHISM

CYP2C9 metabolizes fluoxetine, phenytoin, losartan, tolbutamide, torsemide, S-warfarin, cyclophosphamide, ifosfamide, and numerous nonsteroid anti-inflammatory drugs (NSAIDs). Compared with patients having one or two consensus (wild-type) alleles (*CYP2C9*1*), individuals who are homozygous for the variant alleles *CYP2C9*2* (R144C), and especially *CYP2C9*3* (I359L), have very low enzyme activity. Patients having the CYP2C9 poor metabolizer (PM) trait are reported to be more sensitive to commonly prescribed doses of all the above-mentioned drug substrates (Goldstein and de Morais, 1994; Streetman et al., 2000). This is another example of a Phase I DME polymorphism.

Ethnic differences in the *CYP2C9*3* allelic frequency were reported as 0.06 in Caucasians, 0.005 in Africans, and 0.026 in Chinese (Sullivan-Klose et al., 1996). An additional variant, *CYP2C9*4*, an I359T mutation causing low activity, has recently been found, but its effect on enzyme activity has not yet been characterized (Imai et al., 2000).

Is there an endogenous substrate(s) for CYP2C9, or is this purely an enzyme that metabolizes drugs and various plant metabolites? In the coronary artery endothelium of the pig, β-naphthoflavone-inducible CYP2C was shown to mediate 11,12-epoxyeicosatrienoic acid formation (Fisslthaler et al., 1999). The effects of particular eicosanoids include: vasoconstriction and vasodilation, bronchoconstriction and bronchodilation, cell migration and division, and phagocytosis. It seems likely that one or more of the human vascular CYP2C enzymes might carry out critical-life functions similar to those in the pig (Nebert and Dieter, 2000).

S-MEPHYTOIN (*CYP2C19*) POLYMORPHISM

CYP2C19 preferentially metabolizes S-mephenytoin, omeprazole, diazepam, propranolol, citalopram, proguanil/chloroguanil, imipramine, amitriptyline, mephobarbital, and hexobarbital, and (among many other drugs) phenytoin to a lesser extent. As described for the other polymorphisms above, the CYP2C19 PM individual requires a lower dose of these drugs for efficacy than the CYP2C19 EM individual, and the PM individual is more prone than the EM person to toxicity, if both are given the "recommended" prescribed dose of such drugs and especially if the drug has a narrow therapeutic index. Two reference (wild-type) EM alleles (*CYP2C19*1A, *1B*) and nine PM mutant alleles have now

been described; all nine of these variants exhibit little or no enzyme activity (Oscarson et al., 2001). This is another example of a Phase I DME polymorphism.

The frequency of *CYP2C19* PM individuals ranges between 2% and 5% in Caucasians and between 13% and 23% in Asians. More specifically, the frequency of the *CYP2C19*2A* and *2B* alleles (which cause splicing defects) is 2–5% in Caucasians, yet 20–30% in Asians; the frequency of the *CYP2C19*3* allele (premature stop codon) is exclusively Asian and ranges between 13% and 23% (Goldstein and de Morais, 1994). As with the *CYP2D6* polymorphism, the *CYP2C19* polymorphism is also an example of a striking difference in the incidence of PM individuals between two ethnic groups.

NIFEDIPINE (*CYP3A4*) POLYMORPHISM

There are three members in the *CYP3A* subfamily (CYP3A4, 3A5 and 3A7). About half of all commonly prescribed and over-the-counter medications are metabolized principally by the CYP3A enzymes. More than twelve dozen CYP3A4 substrates are listed in Table 21.6. Note that some drugs listed in Table 21.6 as CYP3A4 substrates are also listed in Table 21.5 as CYP2D6 substrates (or inhibitors). Variations in CYP3A4 catalytic activity are obviously extremely important in issues of bioavailability and drug–drug interactions. This is another example of a Phase I DME polymorphism.

CYP3A4 is the most abundantly expressed of all CYP enzymes (approximately 30–40% of the total CYP content in human adult liver and small intestine). CYP3A5 is expressed at a much lower level than CYP3A4 in the liver, but is the main CYP3A enzyme in the kidney. CYP3A7 is the major CYP isoform detected in the endometrium and embryonic, fetal and newborn liver, but is also detectable at low levels in adult liver (Nebert and Nelson, 2001).

Substrate specificity for the individual enzymes, and CYP3A inducibility by numerous drugs and dietary moieties, has made it very difficult to characterize the impact of distinct *CYP3A* polymorphisms on drug-induced toxicity. The *CYP3A4* gene is known to be inducible by barbiturates, glucocorticoids, and rifampicin (in patients as well as in isolated hepatocytes), and the 5′-untranslated region includes the putative basal transcription element, hepatocyte nuclear factor HNF4, TP53, AP-3, glucocorticoid regulatory element, pregnane X receptor, and estrogen receptor response elements (Guengerich, 1999). That the gene is up- and down-regulated by so many factors will make dissection of pharmacogenetically relevant diseases extremely difficult. Also, profound changes occur in the activity of

Table 21.6. Major drug substrates of CYP3A4

Acetaminophen	Diazepam	Itraconazole	*R*-Warfarin
Alfentanil	Diltiazem	Ketoconazole	Rapamycin
Alprazolam	Disopyramide	Lansoprazole	Rifabutin
Amiodarone	Docetaxel	Lidocaine	Rifampin
Amitriptyline	Dolasetron	Loratadine	Ritonavir
Amlodipine	Donepezil	Losartan	Salmeterol
Anastrozole	Doxorubicin	Lovastatin	Saquinavir
Astemizole	Ebastine	Methadone	Sertindole
Atorvastatin	Enalapril	Mibefradil	Sertraline
Bepridil	Ergot alkaloids	Miconazole	Sildenafilcitrate
Budesonide	Erythromycin	Midazolam	Simvastatin
Busulfan	Estradiol	Mirtazapine	Sufentanil
Cannabinoids	Estrogens, oral	Navelbine	Sulfamethoxazole
Carbamazepine	Ethinylestradiol	Nefazodone	Tacrolimus
Cerivastatin	Ethosuximide	Nelfinavir	Tamoxifen
Chlorpromazine	Ethylmorphine	Nevirapine	Taxol
Cimetidine	Etoposide	Nicardipine	Toremifene
Cisapride	Felodipine	Nifedipine	Temazepam
Citalopram	Fenbendazole	Nimodipine	Teniposide
Clarithromycin	Fentanyl	Nisoldipine	Terfenadine
Clindamycin	Fexofenadine	Nitrendipine	Testosterone
Clomipramine	Finasteride	Nordazepam	Tetrahydrocannabinol
Clonazepam	FK506	Omeprazole	Theophylline
Cocaine	Fluconazole	Ondansetron	Tiagabine
Codeine	Flutamide	Oral contraceptives	Tretinoin
Cortisol	Gestodene	Paclitaxel	Triazolam
Cyclobenzaprine	Glyburide	Pimozide	Troleandomycin
Cyclophosphamide	Granisetron	Potassium carenoate	Verapamil
Cyclosporine (A & G)	Hydrocodone	Pravastatin	Vinblastine
Dapsone	Hydrocortisone	Prednisone	Vinca alkaloids
Delavirdine	Ifosfamide	Progesterone	Vincristine
Dexamethasone	Imipramine	Proguanil	Vindesine
Digitoxin	Indinavir	Propafenone	Zatosetron
Dihydroergotamine	Isotretinoin (and other retinoids)	Quinidine	Zileuton
Dextromethorphan	Isradipine	Quinine	Zonisamide

For some of these drugs, the metabolism by CYP3A4 is not the only, or not the major, pathway. In many instances, the contribution of CYP3A5 is also not clear. For some, the clinical relevance of the CYP3A4 polymorphism is questionable, or dependent on additional variables such as drug-drug interactions and disease (Ingelman-Sundberg, 2001b). Help with this list was kindly provided also by Patrick Maurel.

CYP3A isoforms during all stages of development (de Wildt et al., 1999).

More than 30-fold interindividual differences in CYP3A4 and 3A5 mRNA and protein expression and enzyme activity exist, suggesting that genetic polymorphisms will be clinically very important (Guengerich, 1999). Although some mutant alleles have been identified, the impact of these mutations on the pharmacokinetics of CYP3A substrates remains to be established. The *CYP3A4*2* (S222P mutation), *CYP3A4*3* (M445T mutation), *CYP3A4*4* (I118V mutation), *CYP3A4*5* (P218R mutation), *CYP3A4*6* (frameshift), and *CYP3A5*2* (T398N mutation) alleles have all been reported, but which alleles lead to little or no CYP3A enzymic activity is not yet clear (Oscarson et al., 2001). Variant alleles of *CYP3A5* and *CYP3A7* were recently described (Kuehl et al., 2001).

The abundance of CYP3A4, and the vast array of drugs as CYP3A substrates, make the *CYP3A4* polymorphism of extreme clinical importance. The complex interplay between basal genetic (constitutive) expression and inducibility by endogenous, as well as exogenous agents, however, makes this polymorphism difficult to understand and resolve at the present time.

COUMARIN AND NICOTINE (*CYP2A6*) POLYMORPHISM

Both the anticoagulant coumarin, and nicotine in tobacco, are metabolized principally by CYP2A6. The CYP1A2 substrates—caffeine (Fig. 21.6) and tobacco smoke-specific nitrosamines such as NNK—are also CYP2A6 substrates. Besides the normal-activity consensus allele, *CYP2A6*1*, eight mutant alleles have been characterized. The *CYP2A6*1X2* represents a gene duplication (meaning higher activity), and the *CYP2A6*2* allele (L160H mutation), the *CYP2A6*4* series (gene deletions), and the *CYP2A6*5* allele (G479V mutation) all result in no CYP2A6 activity (Oscarson et al., 2001). This is an example of a Phase I DME polymorphism. The effects of the *CYP2A6* polymorphism on smoking behavior and addiction are under intense investigation (Sellers and Tyndale, 2000). Marked differences in the *CYP2A6*2* and *3* allelic frequencies in Caucasians, Asians and Amerindians have also been noted (Nowak et al., 1998).

CYP2E1 POLYMORPHISM

CYP2E1 monooxygenates a number of drugs (e.g., chlorzoxazone, acetaminophen, halothane) and numerous procarcinogens (e.g., vinyl chloride, vinyl bromide, dimethylnitrosamine and diethylnitrosamine, acrylonitrile, urethane, styrene, benzene, carbon tetrachloride, chloroform, and trichloroethylene). Therefore, it was exciting to find, but perhaps came as no surprise, that the *Cyp2e1(-/-)* knockout mouse is extremely resistant to benzene toxicity (Valentine et al., 1996). Acetone is an endogenous substrate for CYP2E1. Interestingly, CYP2E1 metabolism is induced by alcohol, acetone and fasting.

Interindividual differences in hepatic CYP2E1 protein content in patient samples are as much as 12-fold (Snawder and Lipscomb, 2000). Nine mutant *CYP2E1* alleles have been identified so far (Oscarson et al., 2001), with *CYP2E1*2* (R76H mutation) being the only one demonstrated experimentally to encode lowered enzymic activity. This is an example of a Phase I DME polymorphism. The *CYP2E1*5* series (mutations in the 5′ flanking region and proposed to increase the transcription rate) has been reported to be associated with increased CYP2E1 activity, and a possible risk factor in nasopharyngeal cancer (Hildesheim et al., 1997). Further work on this allele is needed, however, to prove that CYP2E1*5 mRNA levels and enzyme activity are indeed augmented.

CYP2B6 POLYMORPHISM

This Phase I enzyme is present in liver, lung and breast epithelium. CYP2B6-expressing cells were found to be more sensitive than control cells to the cytotoxicity and mutagenicity of cyclophosphamide, aflatoxin B_1, and NNK (Code et al., 1997). *CYP2B6* substrates also include *S*-mephenytom and buprorion. CYP2B6 is thus a widely expressed CYP that can contribute to a broad range of drug metabolism and procarcinogen activation reactions (Elkins and Wrighton, 1999). Besides the consensus (reference, wild-type) *CYP2B6*1* allele, six mutant alleles—all with one or more amino-acid changes—have recently been reported (Oscarson et al., 2001); studies are in progress to determine whether each of these allelic variants affect the CYP2B6 enzymic activity and, if so, how much.

CYP1A1 STRUCTURAL GENE POLYMORPHISM

As described above for the *CYP1A2* polymorphism, the polymorphism in the *CYP1A1* structural gene is distinctly different from that in the AH receptor-mediated inducibility of CYP1A1 by dioxin and polycyclic hydrocarbons. To date, the allelic variants of *CYP1A1* include *CYP1A1*2A* (*Msp* I site 450 bp 3′-ward of the last exon), *CYP1A1*2B* (I462V), *CYP1A1*2C* (*Msp* I site plus I462V), *CYP1A1*3* (nucleotide change in the 3′ noncoding region), *CYP1A1*4* (T461N), *CYP1A1*5* (R464S), and *CYP1A1*6* (M3311) (Oscarson et al., 2001). In Japan, the *CYP1A1*2A* allele appears to be associated with a higher incidence of cigarette smoking-induced lung cancer, especially when combined with the *GSTM1* (glutathione transferase mu) null mutation (Table 21.7). A similar result was found in China (Song

Table 21.7. Relative risk estimate of lung cancer types in Japanese Patients having the combined genotypes for the *CYP1A1* and *GSTM1* genes

CYP1A1: GSTM1:	Ile/Ile		Ile/Val		Val/Val*	
	+	–	+	–	+	–**
Lung cancer	1.0	1.7	1.7	1.4	2.3	5.8
Kreyberg I	1.0	1.8	1.3	1.8	1.6	7.9
Squamous cell CA	1.0	2.3	1.2	1.5	2.0	9.1
Kreyberg II (adenocarcinoma)	1.0	1.6	2.2	1.0	3.1	3.5

* Ile-462 versus Val-462 in the CYP1A1 protein.
** "+" and "–" denotes presence and deletion, respectively, of the GSTM1 gene. (Modified and condensed from Hayashi et al., 1992.)

et al., 2001), but no such association exists in other ethnic groups—Norwegians, Caucasian Americans and African Americans, Finns, and Eastern Mediterraneans (Nebert et al., 1996). There is usually (but not always) linkage disequilibrium between the *Msp* I site and the I462V mutation (Wedlund et al., 1994).

Studies have shown that cDNA-expressed CYP1A1 enzyme activity for polycyclic hydrocarbon metabolism in vitro is not different, however, between the *CYP1A1*1* wild-type and *CYP1A1*2* allelic products (Zhang et al., 1996; Persson et al., 1997). In contrast, differences in steroid metabolism by *CYP1A1* mutant alleles have been noted (Schwarz et al., 2000). It is possible that, in Asian populations but not in Caucasian or African populations, the *CYP1A1*2* allelic series is in linkage disequilibrium with another mutation important for *CYP1A1* inducibility, or another gene involved in tumorigenesis. The recent localization of the human *CYP1A1* and *CYP1A2* genes, head-to-head and less than 25 kb apart on chromosome 15 (Corchero et al., 2001), suggests *CYP1A2* as a candidate gene for this ethnic difference.

GLUTATHIONE *S*-TRANSFERASE (*GST*) POLYMORPHISMS

GSTs add glutathione to a large number of drug and chemical metabolites (e.g., acetaminophen, paracetamol, adriamycin, chlorambucil, aflatoxin B$_1$, aniline, dichloromethane, or 1-chloro-2,4-dinitrobenzene, and numerous polycyclic hydrocarbon epoxides and arene oxides). While usually considered a Phase II detoxification enzyme (Fig. 21.2), GSTs can also be involved in metabolic potentiation (Monks et al., 1990). Five *GST* families (*GSTA, GSTM, GSTP, GSTS,* and *GSTT*) had been characterized for many years (Hayes and Pulford, 1995), and then a sixth family (*GSTZ*) was recently discovered (Cornett et al., 1999). There are one or more genes in each of these six human *GST* families.

Human populations show relatively high frequencies for the deletion of the *GSTM1* or *GSTT1* gene (so-called "null alleles" *GSTM1*0, GSTT1*0*), and frequencies range between 20% and 50% and differ among ethnic populations. Numerous studies have shown associations between one or the other deleted *GST* gene and enhanced or diminished risk of cancer or toxicity, depending upon the etiologic agent (Nebert et al., 1999) (Table 21.7). Duplications leading to two gene copies of *GSTM1* on one chromosome have been reported (McLellan et al., 1997). The *GSTP1*2* allele (I105V mutation, low-activity for certain substrates), and the *GSTP1*3* allele (A114V mutation, with normal activity) have been described. In mice having the entire

Gstp gene cluster disrupted, a more than three-fold increase in papillomas was observed following topical treatment with 7,12-dimethylbenzo[a]anthracene and promotion with phorbol ester. This study was among the first to prove the importance of the GST Phase II enzymes in preventing toxicity caused by drugs or preventing cancer caused by certain chemicals (Henderson et al., 1998).

SULFOTRANSFERASE (*SULT1*) POLYMORPHISMS

Sulfotransferases can be membrane-bound or cytosolic. The membrane-bound forms include as substrates: the keratans, chondroitins and glucosamines (*CHST* genes); heparans (*HS2ST* and *HS3ST* genes); cerebroside and carbohydrates. These are not to be confused with the cytosolic sulfotransferases.

Soluble sulfotransferases (SULTs) are Phase II DMEs that catalyze the sulfate conjugation of many hormones, catecholamine neurotransmitters, drugs, and foreign chemicals (Weinshilboum et al., 1997). The sulfate donor is 3′-phosphoadenosine-5′-phosphosulphate (PAPS). These reactions result in enhanced renal excretion of the sulfate-conjugated reaction products, but (as described above for the GSTs) they can also lead to the formation of reactive metabolites. Two separate PAPS synthase genes (*PAPSS1, PAPSS2*) have recently been identified (Xu et al., 2000), with pharmacogenetic studies now underway.

SULT enzymes are members of an emerging gene superfamily, which presently includes the phenol (P-SULT), estrogen (E-SULT), hydroxysteroid (HS-SULT), and, in plants, flavonol (F-SULT) families, i.e., members that share at least 45% amino acid sequence identity. Currently there are five known human cytosolic *SULT* genes: three P-SULTs (now named *SULT1A1, SULT1A2* and *SULT1A3*), one E-SULT, and one HS-SULT. The genes have all been cloned, and chromosomal localizations reported for all five genes. There is a high degree of structural homology, with conservation of the locations of most intron/exon splice junctions. The *SULT1A* cluster is located on chromosome 16p (Dooley, 1999). Besides the phenol-preferring SULT1A1, either SULT1A2 or SULT1A3 is the monoamine neurotransmitter-preferring enzyme (Dooley, 1998).

Human SULT activity varies among individuals, and functionally significant genetic polymorphisms have begun to be reported (Raftogianis et al., 1997). Ethnic differences for the *SULT1A1*1, *2* and *3* alleles and the *SULT1A2*1, *2* and *3* alleles have recently been reported (Carlini et al., 2001). Knowledge of the molecular biology of the cytosolic SULTs, when placed within a context provided by decades of biochemical research, promises soon to enhance significantly our understanding of the regulation of the sulfate conjugation of hormones, neurotransmitters, and drugs (Weinshilboum et al., 1997).

THIOPURINE METHYLTRANSFERASE (*TPMT*) POLYMORPHISM

TPMT is a Phase II enzyme that plays a major role in the detoxification of 6-mercaptopurine (6MP), commonly used in chemotherapy for acute lymphocytic leukemia. The frequencies of the *high/high*, *high/low*, and *low/low* genotypes appear to be about 88%, 11% and 0.4%, respectively, in Caucasians. This means that, when given the "usual dosage" of 6MP, one out of approximately 300 patients might die as the result of too much of the chemotherapeutic drug, 11% would have a high probability of being cured of their disease, and 88% patients would have relapses in their leukemia due to undertreatment, i.e., metabolic inactivation of 6MP is too extensive (Fig. 21.8).

This pharmacogenetic disorder is very dramatic, because it can lead to life-or-death clinical situations. Because the TPMT defect can lead to dire consequences, acute lymphocytic leukemia patients are now routinely phenotyped for TPMT activity (or genotyped for the *TPMT* variant alleles) prior to the initiation of 6MP chemotherapy.

High/high patients are then usually given a four-times-larger dose, and *low/low* patients are given a 10- to 15-times-smaller dose—leading to a much better cure rate and survival rate for childhood leukemia (Weinshilboum et al., 1999).

At least eight PM allelic variants have been characterized for the *TPMT* gene. The consensus (wild-type, reference) *TPMT*1* allele encodes the enzyme having normal activity. The mutant alleles include *TPMT*2, *3A, *3B, *3C, *3D, *4, *5, *6*), resulting in very low or negligible catalytic activity. *TPMT*3A* is the most common variant in Caucasians and is not found in Chinese. The *TPMT*3C* allele, second most frequent amongst Caucasians, is the most common in Asians (Nebert et al., 1999).

Azathioprine is another TPMT substrate (Fig. 21.8). Azathioprine is widely used as an immunosuppressant in conditions as diverse as systemic lupus erythematosus and organ transplantation. Again, as with 6MP, the one in 300 homozygous low-TPMT individual is highly susceptible to azathioprine toxicity.

THIOL METHYLTRANSFERASE

"*THMT*" is suggested as the name for the thiol methyltransferase gene, because *TMT* already has been chosen for the transmembrane tryptase gene. THMT is a membrane-bound Phase II enzyme that methylates aliphatic sulfhydryl

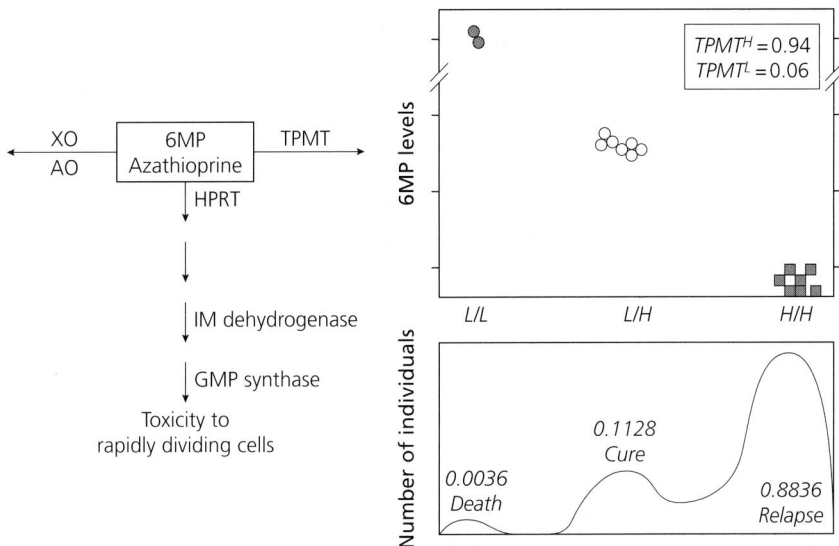

Fig. 21.8. Diagram of 6-mercaptopurine (6MP) or azathioprine toxicity (which can occur in all cells but more so in rapidly-dividing malignant cells, due to disruption of purine biosynthesis), and the response of acute lymphocytic leukemia patients given the "common dose" of 6MP. Xanthine oxidase (XO), adenine oxidase (AO), and TPMT (thiopurine methyltransferase) are all enzymes that detoxify 6MP and azathioprine. Toxicity of these agents occurs much more readily in individuals homozygous for the low-activity allele, TMPT^L, than the high-activity allele, TMPT^H. Allelic frequencies for TMPT^H and TMPT^L in a Caucasian population in southern Minnesota are 0.94 and 0.06, respectively. About three in 1000 Caucasians are homozygous for the *L/L* genotype, 13% are heterozygotes, and 88% are homozygous for the *H/H* genotype.

compounds. Family data, examined by means of co-mingling and segregation analyses, have revealed the existence of a major gene polymorphism with allelic frequencies of 0.42 for high activity and 0.58 for low activity—with the likelihood of more than one gene responsible for this enzymic activity. Probable substrates for THMT include captopril, N-acetylcysteine, 7α-thiospirolactone, and D-penicillamine. Red blood cell THMT activity has been associated with Parkinson disease and juvenile rheumatoid arthritis. Much more work is needed to resolve the *THMT* polymorphism, which is without any doubt different from the *TPMT* polymorphism (Evans, 1994).

CATECHOL O-METHYLTRANSFERASE (COMT)

COMT, a Phase II enzyme well known for its activity in methylating epinephrine and norepinephrine after they are released from nerve fibers, is widely distributed in the body. COMT can methylate a variety of catechols, and its activity in erythrocytes is based on the methylation of 3,4-dihydroxybenzoic acid.

Twin and family studies indicate that there is a major gene effect in the control of red blood cell COMT activity with two alleles, *COMT^L* and *COMT^H*. The gene has been located at chromosome 22q11.2. There is a correlation between activity in internal organs and red cells, indicating similar genetic control. For reasons not clear, liver activities are one-third higher in males than in females.

The antiparkinsonism drug *L*-DOPA is biotransformed by O-methylation to 3-O-methyl-*L*-DOPA, which has a long half-life and accumulates in the CNS. The plasma ratio 3-O-methyl-*L*-DOPA to L-DOPA is correlated with red cell COMT activity. Approximately 75% of Parkinson disease patients treated with *L*-DOPA develop severe dyskinesia within five years (Table 21.1), whereas the other 25% of the population benefit greatly from this drug. Parkinson disease patients who do not respond to *L*-DOPA have high plasma 3-O-methyl-*L*-DOPA levels. It had been proposed that the *COMT^H/COMT^H* genotype might be more likely than the *COMT^L/COMT^L* genotype to develop dyskinesia and to have less clinical response on *L*-DOPA, due to greater 3-O-methyl-*L*-DOPA production (Evans, 1994); however, no association has been found between *COMT* allelic differences and *L*-DOPA-induced dyskinesia in Parkinson disease patients (Tan et al., 2000). Nor has any association been found between *COMT* allelic differences and early-onset alcoholism (Hallikainen et al., 2000) or attention-deficit hyperactivity disorder (Tahir et al., 2000). The *COMT* polymorphism needs to be understood, and the importance of this polymorphism in pharmacogenetic, or other, diseases remains to be determined.

HISTAMINE N-METHYLTRANSFERASE (HNMT)

HNMT, a Phase II enzyme ubiquitous in virtually all tissues, catalyzes the N-methylation of histamine and structurally related compounds [(R)α-methylhistamine is a substrate, SKF91488 is a specific inhibitor]. Complex segregation analysis of red-cell HNMT activity in 241 individuals in 51 nuclear families showed the presence of mendelian major gene segregation (Price et al., 1993). The *HNMT* gene has been cloned and localized to chromosome 2. Common DNA sequence variants include the T105I mutation and a polymorphic $(CA)_n$ repeat in intron 5. Whereas an association between the T105I allele and asthma has been reported (Yan et al., 2000b), no correlation between either the T105I mutation or the polymorphic $(CA)_n$ repeat in intron 5 with schizophrenia was found (Yan et al., 2000a).

PARAOXONASE (PON1) POLYMORPHISM

Paraoxon is the P450-mediated metabolite of parathion, an organophosphate insecticide. Paraoxon and the nerve gas sarin are substrates for PON1 (Fig. 21.9). Three paraoxonases (PON1, 2, 3)—also called "calcium-dependent

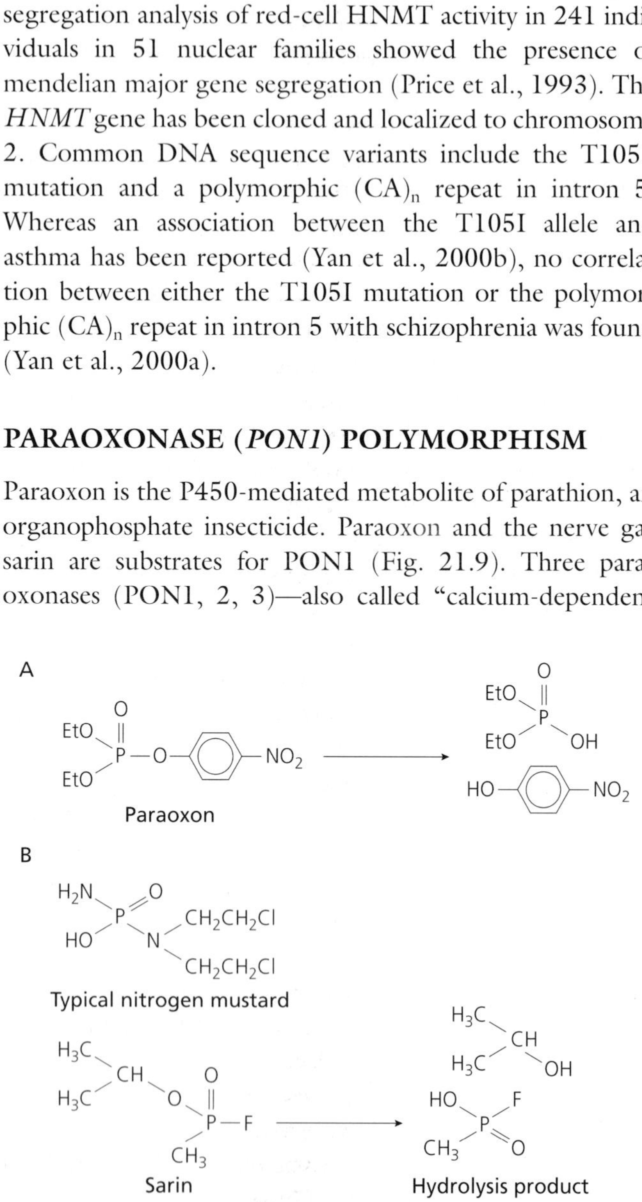

Fig. 21.9. Esterase-mediated pathways of organophosphate substrates. (A) Metabolism of paraoxon by human plasma paraoxonase. The polymorphism leading to low activity is caused mostly by the *PON1* R192Q mutation. (B) A typical nitrogen mustard gas, and sarin, both having structures and phosphate-containing products similar to those of the paraxon pathway.

A-esterases"—are found in human plasma. For a long time, it had been believed that these Phase I DMEs must exist for some reason other than detoxifying organophosphates (which were first synthesized in the twentieth century). PON1 is now known to be an apoJ high-density-lipoprotein (HDL)-associated enzyme that plays a role in cardiovascular homeostasis, yet PON1 also hydrolyzes many toxic organophosphates.

Two common variant PON1 alleles have been identified. The *PON1*2* allele (R192Q mutation) and the *PON1*3* allele (L55M) are both assiociated clinically with low activity of the enzyme. Frequencies of the *high/high, high/low,* and *low/low* PON1 phenotypes are approximately 50%, 40% and 10%, respectively, in Caucasians. As with every pharmacogenetic disorder described above, there exist striking ethnic differences worldwide. The R192Q mutation affects the catalytic efficiency (V_m/K_m) of PON1: for the hydrolysis of paraoxon, the Arg-192 is 10 times better than the Gln-192 enzyme; for chlorpyrifos oxon, soman and sarin, Arg-192 is 1.5 times better than the Gln-192 enzyme; and the Arg- and Gln-192 enzymes are equally efficient in hydrolyzing diazoxon and phenylacetate. Three DNA sequence variants in the *PON1* promoter region and four in the 3' noncoding region have recently been identified; at least some of these affect PON1 activity (Brophy et al., 2001).

The organophosphates allegedly used as biological warfare, and pyridostigmine used as a prophylactic agent against possible nerve gas attack, have caused speculation that the *PON1* polymorphism might have some association with the "Gulf War Syndrome" (Nebert, 1994). Striking variations in illness were found in some, but not other, soldiers who fought in this 1991 war, and it is presumed that entire platoons of soldiers were equally exposed (Mackness et al., 1998; Furlong, 2000). The low-activity PON1 individual (having a slower rate of sarin hydrolysis than intermediate- or high-activity PON1 individuals), appears to have been more protected against neurologic symptom complexes in Gulf War veterans.

There are several clinical epidemiological studies about associations of high or low PON1 activity with heart disease. *Pon1(-/-)* knockout mice were found to be more susceptible to diazoxon and chlorpyrifos oxon toxicity, as well as atherosclerosis (Shih et al., 1998), and *Pon1(-/-)/Apoe(-/-)* double-knockout mice show increased lipoprotein oxidation and atherosclerosis (Shih et al., 2000). Interestingly, the *Pon1(-/-)* mice showed no increase in sensitivity to paraoxon. The catalytic efficiencies of the Arg- and Gln-192 enzymes clearly explain these observations.

The enzyme functions of PON2 are not yet understood. Rabbit PON3, on the other hand, was recently found to be an HDL-associated enzyme with very limited arylesterase and no paraoxonase activities. PON3 rapidly hydrolyzes lactones such as the statin prodrugs (e.g., lovestatin) and protects LDL better than PON1 from oxidation (Draganov et al., 2000). A C311S mutation associated with low PON3 activity was recently described. No human *PON2* polymorphism has yet been reported.

UDP GLUCURONOSYLTRANSFERASE (*UGT*) POLYMORPHISMS

The UGTs are Phase II enzymes that catalyze the addition of a glycosyl group from a nucleotide sugar to a drug or chemical substrate (e.g., glucuronic acid to *p*-nitrophenol, benzo[a]pyrene dihydrodiol or arene oxide, or 2-hydroxyestradiol). A nomenclature system (McKinnon and Mackenzie, 2001) has been devised, assigning gene names to animals, plants, yeast and bacteria. To date, humans have four *UGT* subfamilies.

The human *UGT1* gene is particularly fascinating in that it spans more than 500 kb on chromosome 2, with at least 13 promoters/first exons (including several pseudogenes) that appear to be differentially spliced and ligated to exons 2 through 5; these genes are named *UGT1A1, 1A2, … 1A13* where the *UGT1A1* promoter/first exon is closest to exon 2, and *UGT1A13* is the 5'-most promoter/first exon. Each first exon encodes about half the protein, and also determines substrate specificity. One or another promoter/first exon is inducible by phenobarbital, pregnenolone 16α-carbonitrile, dexamethasone, and dioxin or polycyclic hydrocarbons. Several of the 13 promoters/first exons are pseudogenes. Defects in bilirubin conjugation represent mutations in *UGT1A1*, which are responsible for Gilbert's disease and the Crigler-Najjar syndrome. More than 30 human *UGT1A1* variant alleles, all associated with clinical hyperbilirubinemia of one form or another, have been named (Mackenzie et al., 1997). The importance of all the *UGT1* allelic variants in drug toxicity has not yet been thoroughly explored.

Enzymes of the UGT2B family conjugate steroid hormones, bile acids, and some foreign chemicals. The *UGT2B* cluster on human chromosome 4q13 contains at least three active genes and a number of pseudogenes (Riedy et al., 2000). Mutant alleles include a D458E mutation in the *UGT2B4* gene, an H268Y mutation in the *UGT2B7* gene, and a D85Y mutation in the *UGT2B15* gene. Striking differences in allelic frequencies were reported between Caucasians and Asians (Lampe et al., 2000). Proof that changes in these mutant enzymic activities are associated with any of these amino-acid alterations—remains to be done.

NAD(P)H:QUINONE OXIDOREDUCTASE (*NQO1*) POLYMORPHISM

NQO1 (previous names include DT diaphorase and aminoazo reductase) is a Phase I DME that catalyzes the 2- or 4-electron reduction of various endogenous and environmental quinones (e.g., α-tocopherol quinone, coenzyme Q, menadione). For years, inhibitors of NQO1 metabolism had been known to predispose to toxicity or cancer in laboratory animals; also, the *Nqo1(-/-)* knockout mouse is more sensitive to toxicity caused by several drug and environmental quinones.

The *NQO1*2* allele encodes a P187S mutation, exhibiting negligible NQO1 activity. The frequency of homozygotes for the *NQO1*2* allele is about 4% in a British population. Individuals homozygous for the *NQO1*2* allele show an increased risk of renal cell and urothelial carcinoma, as well as a more than 7-fold greater risk of bone marrow toxicity following benzene exposure (Ross, 1998). The relevance of this *NQO1* polymorphism to various pharmaceutical agents has not yet been reported.

MICROSOMAL, SOLUBLE EPOXIDE HYDROLASES (*EPHX1, EPHX2*)

Epoxides and arene oxides are converted to dihydrodiols by way of epoxide hydrolase (EH), regarded as Phase I DMEs. In mammals, epoxide hydrolases include microsomal (mEH, EPHX1), soluble (sEH, EPHX2), leukotriene A_4 hydrolase, cholesterol epoxide hydrolase, and hepoxilin hydrolase (Beetham et al., 1995). The microsomal EH (EPHX1) is responsible for dihydrodiol formation of numerous drug epoxide and arene oxide substrates. The *Ephx1(-/-)* knockout mouse is resistant to 7,12-dimethylbenzo[a]anthracene (DMBA)-induced toxicity and cancer. These data establish in an intact animal model that mEH is a key genetic determinant in DMBA toxicity and carcinogenesis through its role in production of the ultimate carcinogenic metabolite of DMBA, the 3,4-diol-1,2-epoxide (Miyata et al., 1999).

There are two human mutant alleles that cause lowered EH activity—*EPHX1*2* (Y113H mutation) and *EPHX1*3* (H139R mutation) (Nebert et al., 1999). The *EPHX1* gene maps to the long arm of chromosome 1. The consensus (reference, wild-type) *EPHX1*1* allele encodes the mEH having the highest activity and occurs in about 40% of Caucasians. The low-activity *EPHX1*2* allele appears to be correlated with an increased risk of hepatocellular carcinoma, presumably due to the decreased capacity to detoxify aflatoxin B_1 (McGlynn et al., 1995). Drug toxicity associated with *EPHX1* or *EPHX2* polymorphisms have not yet been reported.

ALCOHOL DEHYDROGENASE (ADH), ALDEHYDE DEHYDROGENASE (*ALDH*) POLYMORPHISMS

Ethanol is oxidized to acetaldehyde in large part by alcohol dehydrogenase (ADH), which, in turn, is metabolized by aldehyde dehydrogenase (ALDH) to acetic acid. These are Phase I DMEs. Initial reports of genetic variation in ADH activity (von Wartburg et al., 1965) and in ALDH activity (Harada et al., 1978) paved the way to molecular biologic and genetic studies that have elucidated the following genotypes. Three *ADH* genes encode subunits α, $β_1$, $β_2$, $β_3$, $γ_1$, and $γ_2$. Since the ADH molecule is a dimer, this results in 21 possible different dimers in the human population; the $β_2$ "atypical" subunit, prominent in Asians, produces the most significant change (with several times faster metabolism).

To date, 17 human *ALDH* genes have been described, and numerous mutant alleles have been reported for *ALDH1B1, ALDH2, ALDH3A1, ALDH3A2, ALDH4A1* and *ALDH9A1* (Vasiliou et al., 1999; Vasiliou, 2001). The *ALDH2*2* variant allele (E487K mutation) is of particular pharmacogenetic importance. The clinical signs of ALDH2 deficiency—which is associated with the "ethanol-induced facial flushing" syndrome—is caused by a build-up of the toxic acetaldehyde. Disulfiram, the drug used to curb alcoholism, inhibits ALDH2 activity and causes the same build-up of toxic acetaldehyde as does the *ALDH2*2* mutation; thus, individuals with the genetic defect, or those taking disulfiram, handle ethanol similarly. Metronidazole and other nitroimidazoles are also ALDH2 inhibitors.

ALDH comprises four subunits (Fig. 21.10); even if one subunit is defective, the whole tetramer is catalytically inactive. This means that ALDH2 deficiency is inherited as an

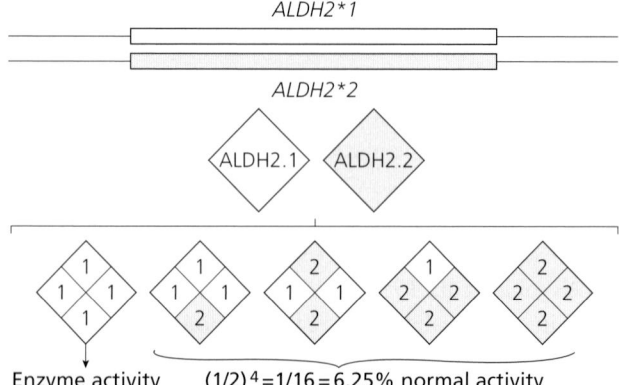

Fig. 21.10. Diagram to explain how the *ALDH2*1/*2* heterozygote exhibits ALDH activity that is only 6.25% of normal. There are five possible combinations of the two allelic products, to produce the active tetramer enzyme. Thus, ALDH2 deficiency is inherited as an autosomal dominant trait.

Table 21.8. Distribution of ALDH2 isozyme deficiency in different populations

Population	Percent deficient in ALDH2
Japanese	44
Central, East and Southeast Asian	30–50
South American Indian	40–45*
North American Indian	2–5
European, Near-East, and African	0

*Mutation is different from that in Asians and North American Indians.
(Data modified and condensed from Goedde and Agarwal, 1986.)*

autosomal dominant trait. In an *ALDH2*1/*2* heterozygote, since there is actually a one-in-16 chance of four ALDH2.1 normal subunits combining in the cytoplasm, the ALDH2 enzyme activity would theoretically be about 6.25% of that found in the *ALDH2*1/*1* homozygote.

There are striking ethnic differences in ALDH2 deficiency (Table 21.8). The incidence of the defect is as high as about one-in-two in some Asian subpopulations, yet is not seen among Africans or Caucasians. Intriguingly, a different *ALDH2* allele, causing the same lack of ALDH activity, occurs in South American Amerindians (Kalow and Bertilsson, 1994), probably due to a founder effect or genetic bottleneck. These findings have led some to speculate that ALDH2 deficiency arose only in populations that traditionally have not used ethanol (i.e., Asians have boiled water for at least the last 30 centuries), as compared with populations that have used alcohol for many centuries for enjoyment and food preservation.

HYPOCATALASEMIA

This is among the earliest pharmacogenetic disorders described. The discovery of "acatalasemia" occurred because of the clinical use of hydrogen peroxide, which, although not a drug in the usual sense, has been used as a therapeutic chemical to sterilize wounds. In 1946 an oral surgeon, treating a peculiar form of gangrene spreading from the upper jaw to the maxillary sinuses, poured hydrogen peroxide on the wound. The tissues and blood, instead of being bright red and bubbling, turned brownish black without any bubbles. The surgeon then determined that the patient's blood had no detectable catalase activity, a Phase I DME. The proband had seven siblings; four of them had suffered the oral gangrene syndrome and were acatalasemic, whereas the other three were normal (Takahara, 1952).

Acatalasemia has since been shown to be due to a number of abnormal alleles of the catalase (*CAT*) gene,

located on chromosome 11p12–13. Although acatalasemia (more accurately called hypocatalasemia) has been found in at least nine ethnic groups, attention has generally been paid to the Japanese and Swiss varieties. The percentage of normal CAT activity is higher in Swiss than in Japanese (Ogata, 1991). Individuals having hypocatalasemia appear to be otherwise healthy.

DIHYDROPYRIMIDINE DEHYDROGENASE (*DPYD*) POLYMORPHISM

The pyrimidine analog 5-fluorouracil (5FU) is used as an antimetabolite in the treatment of various solid tumors. More than 80% of an administered 5FU dose is degraded by DPYD, making this enzyme an important determinant in 5FU therapy. 5FU toxicity has been unpredictable—characterized by myelosuppression, gastrointestinal and neurologic toxicity, and often, death. Patients particularly sensitive to 5FU were found to have a deficiency in blood monocyte DPYD activity, a Phase I DME. This has led to cloning of the *DPYD* gene and discovery of mutant alleles. Heterozygotes (having the normal allele and a mutant allele) exhibit intermediate levels of DPYD activity and significantly increased sensitivity to 5FU therapy. At last count, 17 DNA sequence variants have been reported, although most have not yet been demonstrated to have clinical relevance (Collie-Duguid et al., 2000). Because this is a life-and-death situation, similar to that seen for the *TPMT* polymorphism described above, many medical centers now require that the DPYD phenotype be determined before 5FU therapy is begun in the cancer patient.

BUTYRYLCHOLINESTERASE (*BCHE*) POLYMORPHISM

This polymorphism has a history of almost five decades, and is associated with experimental findings on the clinical condition "atypical succinylcholine-induced apnea." Soon after the introduction of succinylcholine into clinical practice as a short-term muscle relaxant in 1951, the occasional patient suffered prolonged muscle paralysis, and, consequently, apnea. A number of plasma cholinesterase variants, associated with this rare Phase I DME disorder, were described during the 1950s and 1960s (Evans, 1994).

The enzyme is now called butyrylcholinesterase (BCHE), which, similar to PON1, may play a role in the Gulf War syndrome. BCHE is known to scavenge low doses of organophosphorus (e.g., paraoxon) and carbamate pesticides (e.g., carbaryl) and, in this way, to protect the individual from the toxic effects of these poisons.

Homozygotes for the consensus (reference, wild-type) *BCHE*1 allele comprise 76% of Caucasians, whereas 24% carry at least one variant allele. Most of the variant *BCHE* alleles cause decreased enzyme activity. The most important clinical variant is the D70G mutation. In vitro studies have demonstrated that the atypical enzyme reacts more slowly with any positively-charged toxicant (e.g., physostigmine, echothiophate); this would leave more of the toxicant available for reaction with acetylcholinesterase in nerve synapses, thereby predicting that individuals with atypical BCHE would be less protected. It has been postulated that persons having *BCHE* variant alleles might be at higher risk for pesticide toxicity (Lockridge and Masson, 2000).

There is considerable interethnic variability in the *BCHE* allelic frequencies. In Caucasians, the average frequency of "E^a_1" is about 0.017, meaning the homozygote occurs at a rate of one in 3460 persons ($1/0.017^2$). In African and Asian populations, the allelic frequency is about 0.0002. The "E^f_1" allele is very rare in most populations, but 0.0021 in Europeans (Evans, 1994).

FISH ODOR SYNDROME (*FMO3* POLYMORPHISM)

Some individuals carry a smell that resembles that of rotting fish, due to the presence of trimethylamine (TMA) in their body fluids. In the affected patient, the smell is accentuated by the consumption of fish, egg yolk, liver, and soybeans, from which TMA can be produced in the body. The disease can lead to mental depression, failing grades in school, inability to socialize, and even suicide.

The metabolic defect is the failure to biotransform TMA to its odorless N-oxide. Persons affected in this way are autosomal recessive. The use of a TMA-loading test disclosed two heterozygotes among 169 healthy Caucasian volunteers. A population of 156 subjects with suspected body malodor was tested with the TMA loading test, and 11 were found to have the fish odor syndrome. The parents

of six of these probands were found to be heterozygotes (Ayesh et al., 1993).

Trimethylaminuria is now known to be caused by mutations in the flavin-containing monooxygenase-3 (*FMO3*) gene (Dolphin et al., 1997). Four other *FMO* genes (*FMO1, FMO2, FMO4, FMO5*) are part of a five-gene cluster on chromosome 1q23–q25. The other genes encode FMOs having substrate specificities distinct from that of FMO3. A major variant allele (P135L mutation) appears to be responsible for fish odour syndrome, because this has been shown to result in total loss of FMO3 activity. Basarab et al. (1999) reported two additional mutations, V143E and E158K, the former not being characterized yet and the latter causing some 10% decrease in enzyme activity. A total of 18 single-nucleotide polymorphisms (SNPs) in the *FMO3* gene have now been identified, all resulting in amino-acid changes (Ian R Phillips, in preparation).

Examples of alteration in receptor, transporter, or channel protein

PHENYLTHIOUREA NONTASTER POLYMORPHISM

Back in the 1930s, chemists typically tasted each chemical that they used or synthesized. Snyder (1932) was curious that some, but not other, of his laboratory colleagues could not taste phenylthiourea (PTU) as "bitter." He went on to publish an incredibly large study of 800 families, including 2043 children! By means of a dilution series test, he showed that the children having both "PTU-nontaster" parents exhibited almost exclusively the nontaster phenotype (Table 21.9). Snyder thus concluded that the nontaster trait is autosomal recessively inherited, and the US incidence of the nontaster homozygote was about 30%. This report has been regarded (Nebert, 1997b) as the "first example of a pharmacogenetic study."

Table 21.9. Inheritance of the inability to taste phenylthiourea

| Parents | Number of families | Offspring | | Fraction of nontasters | |
		Taster	Nontaster	Observed*	Expected*
T × T	425	929	130	0.123	0.127
T × NT	289	483	278	0.366	0.357
NT × NT	86	5	218	0.978	1.0

* Expected frequency of the nontaster phenotype (for chi-square analysis), based on the assumption that this is an autosomal recessive trait. (Modified and condensed from Snyder, 1932.)
T, "taster." NT, "nontaster."

Recently, while mining genomic data, several laboratories independently found a new superfamily of between 50 and 90 taste receptors (G-protein-coupled receptors, GPCRs)—as clusters spread out on three different chromosomes—in both the human and the mouse (Adler et al., 2000; Chandrashekar et al., 2000; Matsunami et al., 2000). Not only the variant alleles responsible for the PTU-nontaster phenotype are part of this *GPCR* superfamily, but taste receptors that detect all grades of bitter, sweet, salty, sour, and umami (ability to taste glutamate) are also members of this taste receptor superfamily. The clinical relevance of the PTU-nontaster and other nontasters remains to be seen, although knowledge about the inability (of a certain percentage of the population) to taste saccharin, aspartame, and other dietary additives might be of commercial value.

COUMARIN (ANTICOAGULANT) RESISTANCE

Rare families have been described in which otherwise healthy members display resistance to coumarin anticoagulant drugs, and this is inherited as an autosomal dominant trait. Numerous possibilities—such as interaction with other drugs, absorption, or unusual pharmacokinetics—were shown not to apply. All experimental evidence points to the existence of an abnormal receptor molecule, concerned with vitamin K metabolism, or action with a greatly lowered affinity for warfarin (O'Reilly, 1970; Holt and Freytes, 1983). Vitamin K deprivation lowers the plasma prothrombin activity much more quickly in the warfarin-resistant patient than in the normal individual, and larger amounts of vitamin K_1 are required to restore it to a physiological level. This observation matches precisely the findings in warfarin-resistant rats. On the strength of this evidence, it has been suggested that human hereditary coumarin anticoagulant resistance might reflect a mutant form of vitamin K 2,3-epoxide reductase (Evans, 1994).

LONG-QT SYNDROME

The incidence in the US of sudden cardiac death, commonly considered to be due to arrhythmias, is more than 300,000 persons per year. In young persons in whom no structural heart disease can be identified, drug-induced long-QT syndrome is a prevalent disorder of uncertain etiology that predisposes to sudden death. Multiple genes causing long-QT syndromes have been identified thus far, all of which encode ion channels in cardiac muscle (Li et al., 2000). These include: two potassium channel alpha subunits, named KvLQT1 and HERG; two potassium channel beta subunits, minK and MiRP1; and one sodium channel gene (*SCN5A*). These channel proteins also exist in many other tissues besides cardiac muscle. KvLQT1 is a shaker-like voltage-gated potassium channel, which can form a complex with KCNE1; the emerging family of KCNE1-related peptides includes KCNE1, KCNE2 and KCNE3. Blockade of the HERG channel by certain fluoroquinolone antibacterials has been associated with prolongation of the QT interval and, on rare occasions, ventricular arrhythmia. In contrast to HERG, the KvLQT1/minK K(+) channel is not a target for block by the fluoroquinolones (Kang et al., 2001).

KCNE2 encodes MinK-related peptide 1 (MiRP1), a subunit of the cardiac potassium channel I(Kr) that has been previously associated previously with long-QT syndrome. In 98 patients with drug-induced long-QT syndrome, three individuals with sporadic mutations and one patient with sulfamethoxazole-associated long-QT syndrome revealed a single-nucleotide polymorphism (SNP) in the *KCNE2* gene. This SNP was found in approximately 1.6% of the general population. Whereas mutant channels showed diminished potassium flux at baseline and wild-type drug sensitivity, the mutant channel protein was normal at baseline but inhibited by sulfamethoxazole at therapeutic levels that did not affect wild-type channels (Sesti et al., 2000). It is anticipated that many additional genetic variants in the genes responsible for these long-QT syndrome-related channel proteins will be uncovered during the next several years (Chiang and Roden, 2000).

MALIGNANT HYPERTHERMIA (*RYR* POLYMORPHISM)

Malignant hyperthermia is an uncommon complication of general anesthesia or emergency intubation that formerly carried a high mortality. Many inhalational and muscle-relaxing agents have been incriminated as precipitating the event. The clinical features of malignant hyperthermia include muscular rigidity, rapidly developing pyrexia, tachycardia, increased oxygen consumption, cyanosis, rise in carbon dioxide production, respiratory acidosis, hyperkalemia, ventricular arrhythmia, metabolic (lactic) acidosis, myoglobin-induced renal tubular obstruction, and consumptive coagulopathy. Mortality has now fallen to less than 1% at most medical centers due to greater awareness, avoidance of precipitating factors, and prompt treatment with dantrolene, cooling, and steroids. Every patient undergoing surgery today is always queried by the anesthesiologist as to "whether any abnormal reaction to anesthesia has ever happened to a family member."

Malignant hyperthermia is caused by a rare variant allele. The incidence of malignant hyperthermia in North America has been estimated as 1 in 15,000 to 1 in 150,000. It appears to be less common in Africans and Asians than in Caucasians. At present, the mainstay of diagnosis is Kalow's *in vitro* muscle contracture test, in which a piece of quadriceps muscle is subjected to electrical stimulation and its contraction measured. Fresh specimens from the biopsy are exposed to halothane (as measured in the bath liquid) and caffeine. The modified protocol of the European Malignant Hyperpyrexia Group (1985) appears to be the most satisfactory. The results match well with clinical experiences of actual anesthesia.

Malignant hyperthermia appears to be usually inherited as a mendelian autosomal dominant character, but of variable penetrance. The breakthrough in the molecular genetics of malignant hyperthermia came about by realizing that the same condition, called "porcine stress syndrome," exists in pigs being brought to slaughter. If farmers wish to sell pigs for their meat, muscular rigidity is an unwanted side-effect. A mutant allele in the ryanodine receptor (*RYR1*) gene was first discovered in the pig. RYR1 is a calcium-release channel protein of large molecular weight (M_r=200,000). The *RYR1*2* allele (the R614C mutation), first found in the pig, has the same amino acid alteration found in several human families with members afflicted with malignant hyperthermia. The *RYR1*3* allele (R248G) was discovered next. Further studies have confounded the field, because three *RYR* genes have been found—two loci on human chromosome 17q, and another on 19q. Moreover, another *RYR1* mutation (R2434H, inherited myopathy) has a possible association with central core disease.

Mutations in the *RYR1* gene account for susceptibility to malignant hyperthermia in more than 50% of cases and, also, in the majority of central core disease cases. Currently, 22 mutations in the 15,117-bp coding region of the *RYR1* gene have been found to segregate with the malignant hyperthermia trait, whereas a much smaller number of these mutations is associated with central core disease. Functional analyses show that these mutations produce abnormalities that alter the RYR1 channel kinetics for calcium inactivation and make the channel hyper- and hypo-sensitive to activating and inactivating ligands, respectively. The likely deciding factors in determining whether a particular *RYR1* mutation results in malignant hyperthermia alone, or malignant hyperthermia plus central core disease, are: sensitivity of the mutant RYR proteins to agonists; the level of abnormal channel-gating caused by the mutation; the consequential decrease in the size of the calcium stored and able to be released; the increase in resting concentration of calcium; and the level of compensation achieved by the muscle with respect to maintaining calcium homeostasis (McCarthy et al., 2000).

From a diagnostic point of view, the ultimate goal of developing a simple DNA test, rather than a muscle biopsy assay, for routine diagnosis of malignant hyperthermia remains elusive. Attainment of this goal will require further detailed molecular genetic investigations aimed at solving the heterogeneity, incomplete penetrance, and discordance issues of this fascinating disease.

Examples of change in response due to enzyme induction

PORPHYRIAS

Essentially all types of porphyria are exacerbated by CYP inducers, because the heme synthesis pathway is stimulated in order to make more heme which, when combined with the apoproteins, results in more cytochromes P450. The porphyrias can be either inherited or acquired. The hereditary forms have defects (low or absent activity) in one or another of the eight enzymes of the heme biosynthetic pathway (Sassa, 2000). With the exception of the first enzyme (Fig. 21.11), an enzymatic defect at every step leads to tissue accumulation and excessive excretion of porphyrins and/or their precursors, such as δ-aminolevulinte and porphyrobilinogen. Heme, the final product of the biosynthetic pathway, is biologically important. On the other hand, porphyrins and their precursors appear not to be important, and sometimes can be toxic.

The three major erythropoietic porphyrias are congenital erythropoietic porphyria, hepatoerythropoietic porphyria, and erythropoietic protoporphyria. The tissue-specific expression of porphyrias is largely due to the tissue-specific control of heme pathway gene expression—particularly at the level of 5-aminolevulinate synthase, the first and the rate-limiting enzyme of heme biosynthesis.

Porphyria cutanea tarda (PCT) is the most common clinical form of porphyria. PCT can be inherited either as an autosomal dominant trait (familial, or type II), or more commonly, "acquired" by exposure to environmental chemicals or drugs (sporadic, or type I). The activity of uroporphyrinogen decarboxylase (UROD), in the heme biosynthetic pathway (Fig. 21.11), is decreased more than 50% in both types of PCT, leading to the urinary excretion of uroporphyrin isomers and decarboxylated analogues—as well as strikingly elevated uroporphyrin and coproporphyrin levels in the liver, skin, and feces.

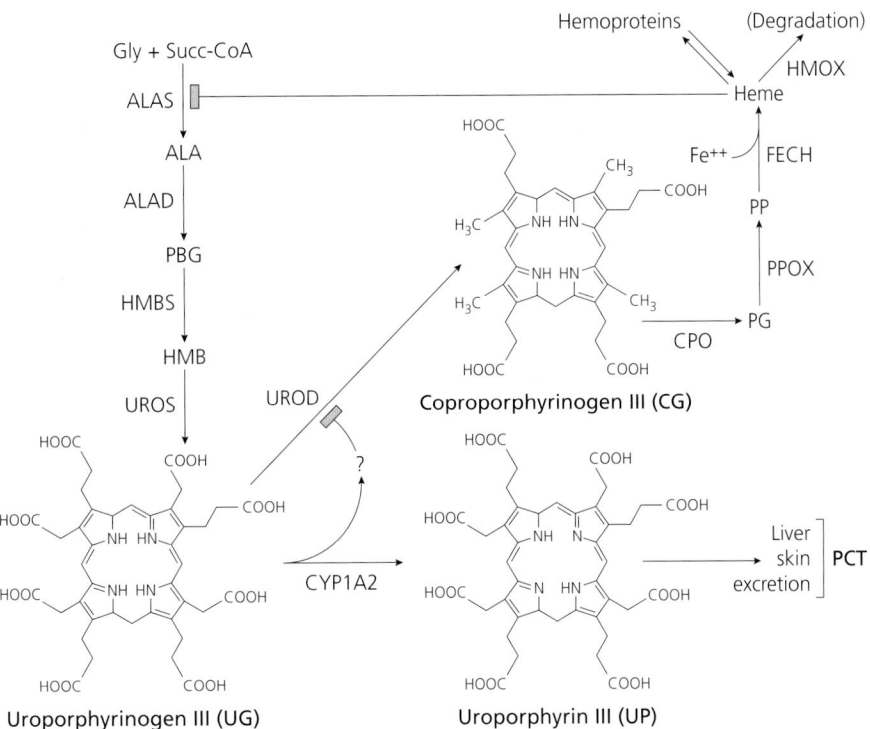

Fig. 21.11. Current understanding of the heme protein biosynthetic pathway. Gly, glycine. Succ-CoA, succinyl-coenzyme A. ALAS, 5-aminolevulinic acid synthase. ALA, 5-aminolevulinic acid. ALAD, 5-aminolevulinic acid dehydratase. PBG, porphobilinogen. HMBS, hydroxymethylbilane synthase. HMB, hydroxymethylbilane. UROS, uroporphyrinogen synthase. UG, uroporphyrinogen. CYP1A2, cytochrome P450 1A2. UP, uroporphyrin. UROD, uroporphyrinogen decarboxylase. CG, coproporphyrinogen. CPO, coproporphyrinogen oxidase. PG, protoporphyrinogen. PPOX, protoporphyrinogen oxidase. PP, protoporphyrin IX. FECH, ferrochelatase. HMOX, heme oxygenase. Decreasing levels of heme stimulate ALAS activity, whereas elevated heme levels repress ALAS activity. The UROD enzyme mediates the sequential removal of four carboxylic groups of the acetic acid side chains—from UG to hepta-, hexa-, penta-, and tetra-carboxylate porphyrinogen (this latter being CG); the naturally most abundant type III isomer of UG and precursor of heme is metabolized most rapidly. (Modified from Smith et al., 2001.)

In the heritable type II PCT, there are mutations in the *UROD* gene and lower levels of immunologically detectable UROD protein. Type I sporadic PCT, on the other hand, has no associated mutations in the *UROD* gene nor decreases in amount of UROD protein (Elder, 1998). In type II PCT, UROD activity is deficient in all tissues, whereas in type I PCT the enzyme deficiency is confined only to the liver. The onset of acquired PCT typically is either "spontaneous" (meaning the etiology is unknown), or, more commonly, occurs in conjunction with known precipitating factors—especially alcohol abuse, but also estrogen, drug use, viral hepatitis, or occupational exposure to halogenated environmental chemicals.

There is evidence for the involvement of aberrant iron metabolism in the development of both types of PCT (Elder, 1998). Mutations in the hemochromatosis (*HFE*) gene, which usually lead to an iron overload in the patient, have been correlated with increased risk of type I PCT (Bonkovsky et al., 1998). In addition, PCT has been associated with a wide variety of conditions that affect liver iron metabolism. A disease similar to sporadic type I PCT,

showing massive uroporphyria and liver damage, may develop following exposure to the CYP inducers hexachlorobenzene (Cain and Nigogosyan, 1963) or 2,3,7,8-tetrachlorodibenzo-*p*-dioxin (dioxin) (Jirasek et al., 1976).

Polyhalogenated aromatic hydrocarbons hexachlorobenzene and dioxin (Fig. 21.12), and nonhalogenated polycyclic aromatic hydrocarbons such as 3-methylcholanthrene, administered to mice, cause inhibition of UROD activity and uroporphyria, suggesting that mice treated with these chemicals might be useful as models of acquired type I PCT (de Matteis, 1998). Studies with the *Cyp1a2(-/-)* knockout mouse line (Sinclair et al., 1998) indicate that so-called sporadic type I environmentally-caused uroporphyria actually has an underlying genetic predisposition; CYP1A2 appears to be necessary but not sufficient. Hence, the level of CYP1A2 pushes the porphyrin pathway in favor of excess uroporphyrins, and CYP1A2 inhibits UROD and coproporphyrinogen formation by an as-yet-unknown mechanism (Fig. 21.11).

Because humans show greater than 60-fold differences in their levels of hepatic basal CYP1A2 (described earlier in

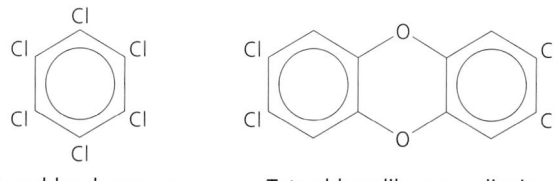

Fig. 21.12. Chemical structures of hexachlorobenzene and 2,3,7,8-tetrachlorodibenzo-p-dioxin (TCDD, dioxin). Both chemicals are dangerous environmental pollutants. Both (but dioxin is much more potent) induce CYP1A1, CYP1A2 and CYP1B1, which stimulates the heme biosynthesis and exacerbates porphyria in genetically susceptible individuals. Other enzymes (NQO1, UGT1A6, UGT1A7, GSTA1) are also induced by dioxin via the AH receptor.

this chapter), acquired type I PCT is expected to be influenced by an underlying genetic predisposition (Christiansen et al., 2000). Furthermore, in workers exposed to occupationally hazardous chemicals, or environmental chemicals that induce the level of CYP1A2 (such as cigarette smoke, described in the next section), the AH receptor-mediated control of CYP1A2 represents another genetic entity. Thus, basal and inducible levels of CYP1A2 are expected to be critical, in addition to exposure and smoking history, as to whether or not PCT develops (Sinclair et al., 1998).

ARYL HYDROCARBON RECEPTOR (*AHR*) POLYMORPHISM

The AHR is a ligand-activated transcription factor that controls a number of genes encoding DMEs, including among others the *CYP1A1* and *CYP1A2* genes (Whitlock, 1999; Nebert et al., 2000). AHR ligands include dioxin, halogenated aromatic hydrocarbons, and polycyclic hydrocarbons commonly found in cigarette smoke and combustion processes. Intriguingly, there appear to be *AHR* genes not only in all vertebrates (Hahn et al., 1998), but even in the nematode. Expression analysis of the *AHR* gene in *Caenorhabditis elegans* showed, however, that the nematode AHR has no ligand-binding properties (Powell-Coffman et al., 1998).

Inbred mice having a high-affinity receptor allele (*Ahr*[b1], *Ahr*[b2]. *Ahr*[b3]) are more sensitive to CYP1A1/1A2 inducibility at lower doses of AHR ligands and exhibit more toxicity and cancer, compared with that in resistant mice having only the low-affinity receptor (*Ahr*[d]) (Nebert, 1989). Differences similar to those found in mice are therefore expected to occur in human populations (Eaton et al., 1995; Nebert et al., 1996). More than a 12-fold variation in affinity of the human AHR has been found (Fig. 21.13). From numerous animal studies, the high-

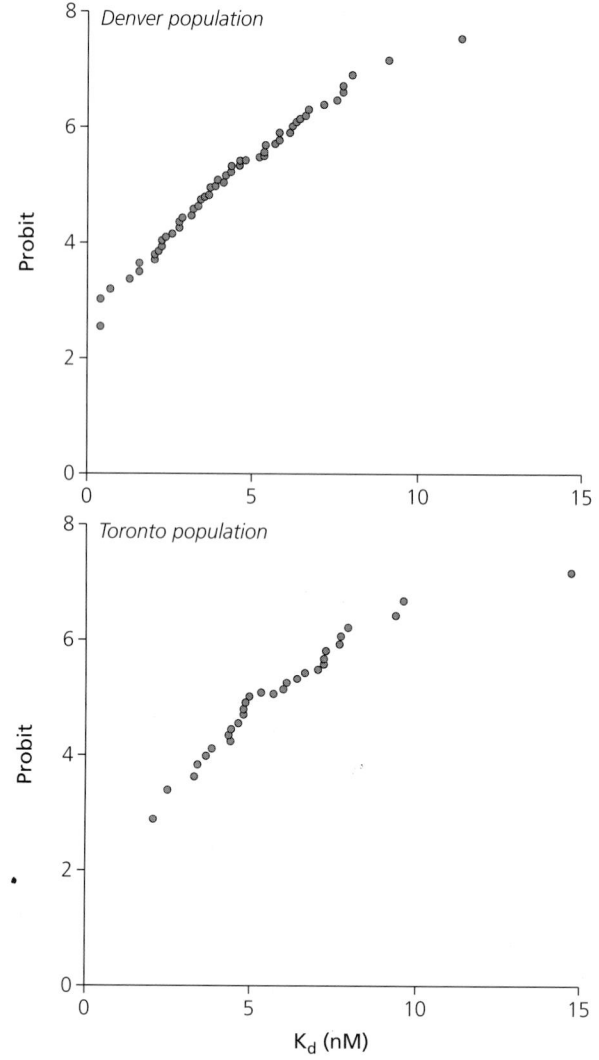

Fig. 21.13. Probit analysis of placenta cytosolic samples from 115 patients. The dissociation constant, Kd, for each patient was determined by Scatchard plot containing five concentrations of radiolabeled dioxin. Data generously provided by Allan B Okey. ("Variation in dioxin binding to the aryl hydrocarbon (AH) receptor: population studies in human placenta." Renehan E, Manchester DK, Parker NB et al., in preparation.)

affinity AHR has been shown to mediate more polycyclic hydrocarbon-induced toxicity and cancer than the low-affinity AHR (Nebert, 1989). It thus seems likely that a "high-affinity-AHR" individual might develop cigarette smoke-induced lung cancer after 20 or 40 pack-years of smoking, whereas a "low-affinity-AHR" individual might never develop cancer even after more than 100 pack-years of smoking.

To date, allelic variants of the human *AHR* gene include the L146P, W176R, T407I, P517S, R554K, D574N, V570I, and M786V mutations, plus the 2416delT leading to an additional 44 amino acids in the C-terminus (Daly et al., 1998; Smart and Daly, 2000; Wong et al., 2001). A small effect on AHR affinity was shown with the R554K mutation (Kawajiri et al., 1995). On the other hand, the D574N mutation, and gender, appear to be determinants of CYP1A1 activity inducibility (Smart and Daly, 2000). As described earlier, the interindividual variation in levels of induced CYP1A1 activity, associated with regulation by the AHR, appear to be more important than the *CYP1A1* structural gene polymorphism. A convenient assay, such as one that compares the AHR phenotype (CYP1A1 inducibility in a yeast two-hybrid system) with the *AHR* genotype (nucleotide sequencing) might prove useful for the large-scale screening of human populations (Maier et al., 1998).

The *Ahr(-/-)* knockout mouse is resistant to dioxin toxicity (Fernandez-Salguero et al., 1996) and benzo[a]pyrene-induced cancer (Shimizu et al., 2000). The *Ahr(-/-)* knockout mouse line, as it ages, displays impaired development of the liver and immune system, splenic atrophy, hyperkeratosis of the skin, and cataracts (Fernandez-Salguero et al., 1997). This mouse line might be helpful in delineating further the role of the AHR in toxicity and cancer, as well as its participation in critical-life functions.

Examples of unknown etiology

GLUCOCORTICOID EYE DROPS-INDUCED GLAUCOMA

Soon after steroid eye drops were introduced into ophthalmologic practice, it was noticed that about 5% of patients developed serious increased intraocular pressure (IOP). Frequency distribution histograms were bimodal or trimodal, and family studies gave results supporting the hypothesis that the IOP phenotype was inherited as an autosomal recessive trait (Armaly, 1968).

Activation of stress pathways and apoptosis pathways in human trabecular meshwork (HTM) cells is now being examined as a potential mechanism for glaucoma pathogenesis. The recent cloning of an "HTM gene" (Polansky et al., 2000), now called myocilin (*MYOC*) located on chromosome 1, may prove to be the etiology of certain types of glaucoma, including glucocorticoid-induced IOP. Glucocorticoids increase *MYOC* expression in HTM cells, whereas basic fibroblast growth factor (bFGF) and the thyroid hormone triiodothyronine (T3) inhibit these increases. Coding-region mutations in the *MYOC* gene are predicted to alter biosynthetic pathways and cellular homeostatic functions. Two mutations in particular, E323K and P370L, are currently under study.

HALOTHANE-INDUCED HEPATITIS

Halothane maintenance anesthesia causes a *dose-dependent* depression of liver function in every patient, while *dose-independent* halothane-induced liver toxicity can occur, although rarely. Familial aggregation of halothane-induced chemical hepatitis is well known and, thus, an underlying genetic predisposition must exist. Halothane (1,1,1,trichloro-2-propene oxide) is an epoxide hydrolase inhibitor. Halothane is oxidized by CYP2E1 and CYP2A6 to form trifluoroacetic acid, bromide and a reactive intermediate that can acetylate liver proteins (Spracklin et al., 1997). These protein neo-antigens stimulate an immune reaction that appears to cause halothane hepatitis (Furst et al., 1997).

As described earlier in this chapter, *CYP2E1* and *CYP2A6* polymorphisms exist. It is anticipated that epidemiological studies, attempting to relate the phenotype (dose-independent halothane toxicity) with DNA sequence variants in either or both of these P450 genes, will soon be carried out. As this book goes to press, however, the mechanism underlying this pharmacogenetic disorder remains unknown.

PHENYTOIN-INDUCED GINGIVAL OVERGROWTH

Phenytoin (PHT) has a high frequency of dose-related and idiosyncratic adverse effects, which reflect the complex pharmacokinetics, endocrine-mediated, and immune-mediated effects of the drug. The primary site-of-action of PHT is in the motor cortex, where the spread of seizure activity can be inhibited by a membrane potential-dependent blockade of Na^+ channels and perhaps presynaptic Ca^{2+} channels (Hassell et al., 2000).

As with halothane, PHT displays dose-dependent toxicity in most, and dose-independent toxicity in some, patients. Chronic PHT toxicity includes: peripheral neuropathy; impairment of motor, concentration and memory functions; gingival overgrowth; disturbances in bone formation (osteomalacia, rickets), thyroid function, and the pituitary-adrenal-gonadal axis; hematologic effects; immunosuppression; and birth defects. The fibrous overgrowth of the gingivae generally happens after at least 30–40 days of PHT therapy, with incidences ranging between 24% (Perlik et al., 1995) and 40% (Casetta et al., 1997). Whereas cyclosporin A and various calcium channel blockers can also cause gingival overgrowth, PHT is the most common drug that causes this condition. This form of PHT-induced toxicity has sometimes been erroneously termed "gingival hyperplasia," but there are no increases in cell number or DNA content, but rather enhanced extra-cellular tissue volume due to elevated amounts of collagen fibres and noncollagenous proteins. Concomitant administration of phenobarbital, primadone and carbamazepine—drugs that induce certain forms of CYP—have no effect on the severity of PHT-induced gingival overgrowth.

As mentioned earlier in this chapter, PHT Phase I metabolism in the human gingiva is as much as 50 times greater than that in liver. Gaedigk and coworkers (1994) postulated that defects in microsomal epoxide hydrolase (EPHX1) activity, and Zhou and coworkers (1996) postulated that PHT metabolic reactive intermediates (Fig. 21.14), might be responsible for PHT-induced gingival overgrowth. In other words, increases in CYP2C9/2C19-mediated oxidative metabolite formation, combined with decreases in EPHX1-mediated detoxification of PHT reactive intermediates, has been proposed as the cause of this toxicity.

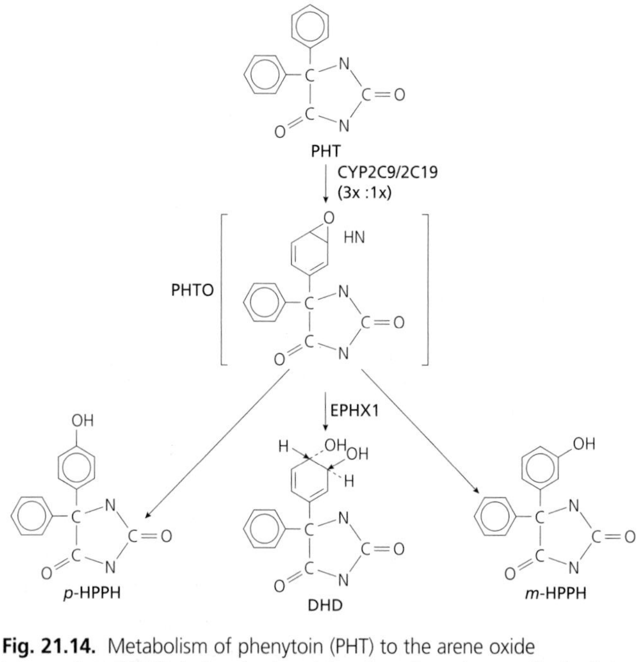

Fig. 21.14. Metabolism of phenytoin (PHT) to the arene oxide intermediate (PHTO, *in brackets*) and the phenolic and *trans*-dihydrodiol products. Arene oxide formation by CYP2C9 occurs three times faster than by CYP2C19 (Talas et al., 1999). The arene oxide is a substrate for EPHX1, resulting in 3,4-*trans*-dihydrodiol formation. The bottom three chemical structures shown for the *R* ring also occur for the *S* ring (not shown). The *p*-HPPH and *m*-HPPH (both *R* and *S* rings) also undergo further metabolism to catechols, methylcatechols, quinones, and conjugated products. The *R* ring (top) is beta to the N, whereas the *S* ring (left) is beta to the ketone. Formation of *p*-(R)-HPPH is 4.4 times higher in CYP2C9 EM than in PM patients, whereas no clear differences between EM and PM individuals were detected in formation of the *p*-(S)-HPPH, *m*-(R)-HPPH or *m*-(S)-HPPH. The *S* to *R* ratios are preserved in chronic-PHT treatment patients; the nonenzymic rearrangement to the *para*-hydroxy or *meta*-hydroxy can be influenced by the CYP enzyme active-site (Yasumori et al., 1999). Whether the parent nonmetabolized PHT or the arene oxide intermediate is responsible for gingival overgrowth or any other type of PHT toxicity has not yet been established.

The published literature is mixed with regard to whether DME allelic variants might correlate with gingival overgrowth. Some studies find no correlation, some find correlations favoring a PHT metabolite, and others find correlations favoring the nonmetabolized parent PHT as the causative agent in gingival overgrowth (McLaughlin et al., 1995; Ball et al., 1996). Hence, this metabolism hypothesis for gingival overgrowth has not yet been proven. Allelic variants in other candidate genes—sodium and calcium channel genes (Varadi et al., 1999; Kuo et al., 2000), PHT transporter genes (if they exist), c-*MYC* and *BCL2* (Saito et al., 2000)—might also be the primary cause of, or contribute to, PHT-induced gingival overgrowth.

FETAL HYDANTOIN SYNDROME

Another example of PHT toxicity is the fetal hydantoin syndrome (FHS), first described by Loughman and coworkers in 1973 (Buehler et al., 1994). Distinguishing features of FHS include craniofacial abnormalities, low-set ears, prominent lips, short up-turned nose, hypertelorism, wide mouth, ptosis or strabismus, distal digital hypoplasia, intrauterine growth retardation, and mental retardation. Hanson and coworkers (1976) found an 11% incidence of the full expression of FHS in the offspring of women receiving PHT alone, and an additional 30% of infants exhibiting various features of FHS. In a more recent prospective study of 500 single-therapy cases, the incidence of FHS in PHT-exposed offspring was 9.1% (Kaneko et al., 1999). Again, as with PHT-induced gingival overgrowth, FHS appears to be PHT *dose-independent* and caused by an underlying genetic predisposition.

As with PHT-induced gingival overgrowth, a number of mechanisms have been proposed for PHT-mediated birth defects, but none proven. These possibilities include: formation of PHT reactive intermediates by embryonic (or maternal?) CYP2C9 and CYP2C19 and/or prostaglandin H synthase, perhaps combined with deficient arene oxide detoxification (Wells et al., 1997); a glutathione *S*-transferase (Phase II enzyme) defect, leading to the build-up of the reactive PHT arene oxide; and increased requirements of folic acid in individuals who have an inherited deficiency of the methylenetetrahydrofolate reductase (MTHFR) enzyme (Parman et al., 1998). The *MTHFR* gene has two mutations (C677T and A1298C) that lower enzymic activity, as reviewed by De Marco and coworkers (2000).

GLUCOSIDATION OF AMOBARBITAL

Amobarbital was considered an attractive drug for pharmacokinetic studies because of its almost complete intestinal absorption, absence of a first-pass effect, elimination by first-order kinetics, small interindividual variation in binding to plasma proteins, four-fold interindividual variability in half-life, three-fold variability in clearance, and almost complete conversion to two urinary metabolites. Three out of 200 individuals exhibited a complete lack of amobarbital-*N*-glucoside formation. These included a pair of identical twins, plus a member of another family, in which *N*-glucosidation of amobarbital was deficient. The evidence indicated that this Phase II DME defect was inherited as an autosomal recessive trait. Asians produce more *N*-glucoamobarbital, whereas Caucasians produce more 3-hydroxyamobarbital. Other drugs (e.g., phenobarbital and sulfonamides) are glucosylated, but it is not known whether these biotransformations are controlled by the same gene(s) as that for amobarbital glucosylation (Tang, 1990). One or more of the *UGT* polymorphisms must be considered as the etiology of the *N*-glucosidation of amobarbital phenotype.

CHLORPROPAMIDE-ALCOHOL FLUSHING

After the sulfonylurea drug, chlorpropamide, was introduced for the treatment of diabetes, it was noticed that some persons showed a red face when they ingested ethanol while taking chlorpropamide. As described earlier, the *ALDH2*2* mutant allele (or inhibition of ALDH2 by disulfiram, metronidazole or other nitroimidazoles) is the cause of the ethanol-induced facial flushing syndrome. The chlorpropamide-alcohol flushing (CPAF) differs from the flush produced by alcohol alone, because many CPAF-positive individuals do not flush with alcohol alone; also, the ethanol-alone flush is more pronounced with increasing alcohol doses, whereas CPAF seems to be more dose-*in*dependent, often occurring after a relatively small dose of ethanol (Evans, 1994).

The genetics of the phenomenon have been investigated in twins and families. It has been suggested that CPAF is an autosomal dominant character, but this has not been unequivocally confirmed using any rigorously standardized tests. Because chlorpropamide is a CYP2D6 substrate (Table 21.5), the *CYP2D6* polymorphism might have an effect on the CPAF trait. The sulphonylurea drugs have been the mainstay of oral treatment for patients with diabetes mellitus since they were introduced. In general, they are well tolerated, with a low incidence of adverse effects (Harrower, 2000).

AMINOGLYCOSIDE ANTIBIOTIC-INDUCED DEAFNESS

A large study in China investigated the possibility that the well-known deafness produced by aminoglycoside anti-biotics could have a genetic basis. Deaf-mute probands, whose pathology could be ascribed to aminoglycoside toxicity, led to 36 informative pedigrees containing a total of 108 cases. In 22 of the pedigrees, the manner of transmission was believed to be the result of mitochondrial inheritance. Even though there was an approximately equal sex frequency of the aminoglycoside-induced deafness, apparently transmission was always through females. Affected males did not transmit the character to their offspring (Evans, 1994).

In 1993 a mutant allele that predisposes to aminoglycoside ototoxicity was described. Seventeen (33%) of patients with aminoglycoside ototoxicity carried the 1555A>G mutation in their mitochondrial 12S ribosomal RNA gene. Studies of an Italian family with five maternally related family members who went deaf after aminoglycosides led to the identification of another mutation, 961delT, in the mitochondrial 12S ribosomal RNA gene. However, analysis of this gene in 41 additional patients with aminoglycoside ototoxicity did not reveal any mutations in the coding region (Fischel-Ghodsian, 1999). To date, unfortunately, these studies have not yet led to a clear understanding of the pathophysiology of aminoglycoside toxicity, or to prevention of the disease.

URINARY SMELL AFTER ASPARAGUS INGESTION

For centuries it has been known that some who have eaten asparagus claim that their urine has a peculiar smell. Numerous sulfur-containing compounds have been found in urine after asparagus ingestion, including *S*-methylthio-acrylate and *S*-methyl-3-(methylthio)thiopropionate; volatile compounds collected above the odorous urine include methanethiol, *bis*-(methylthio)methane, dimethyl-sulfide, dimethylsulfoxide, and dimethylsulfome. There is some dispute as to whether the addition of these compounds to urine reproduces the characteristic odor (Waring et al., 1987). It has been suggested that the reduced sulfur compounds (sulfides and disulfides) give the pungency to the aroma, whilst the partially oxidized sulfones and sulfoxides add a sweetness. These phenomena may have relevance to pharmacogenetics, because the biotransformation of sulfur-containing drugs may be mediated by the same mechanisms as those involved in asparagus metabolism (Evans, 1994).

There are two possibilities that might explain the urinary smell after ingesting asparagus. First, some persons, but not others, might excrete a chemical(s) derived from asparagus that causes the smell. Mitchell and coworkers (1987) showed experimentally that this was the case in 43% of 800 volunteers and that the trait was inherited as autosomal dominant. The second possibility is that everyone might excrete the chemical(s) in their urine, but only some people can smell this as a particular odor. Lison et al. (1980) proved experimentally that this was the case and concluded that the detection of this odor constitutes a specific "smell hypersensitivity." All of those who could smell the odor in their own urine could also smell it in the urine of anyone who had eaten asparagus—whether or not that person was able to smell it himself. Thresholds for detecting the odor appeared to be bimodal in distribution, with 10% of 307 subjects tested able to smell it at high dilutions, suggesting a genetically determined specific hypersensitivity (Lison et al., 1980).

We thus conclude that neither the genetic basis nor the genetic heritability of this trait has been established. Given the recent discovery of the olfactory cluster of G-protein-coupled receptors spread out on three different chromosomes—as described earlier in this chapter (Matsunami et al., 2000; Adler et al., 2000; Chandrashekar et al., 2000)—these receptors might play a role in the mechanism underlying pharmacogenetic differences in the urinary smell after asparagus ingestion.

CEREBRAL VEIN THROMBOSIS AND ORAL CONTRACEPTIVE STEROIDS

Cerebral vein thrombosis (CVT) is a severe clinical problem that is perplexing to diagnose, difficult to manage, and has a poor prognosis. Among 23 cases of CVT consecutively admitted to the University of Parma between 1990 and 1997, 22 were female. Of these women, 15 (68%) were on low-estrogen (meaning less than 50 µg estrogen) oral contraceptive treatment. This percentage of oral contraceptive use by patients having CVT is much higher than that of the rest of the female population in Italy. Although some associations of oral contraceptive use were found with a factor V Leiden mutation in two cases, a deficiency of protein C in one case, and a deficiency of protein S in another, the underlying mechanism of this serious pharmacogenetic disorder remains completely obscure (Buccino et al., 1999).

Ethinyl estradiol is a common oral contraceptive steroid, and is metabolized largely by CYP3A4 (Table 21.6). Multiple environmental factors affect the pharmacokinetics of ethinyl estradiol, which is a common phenomenon seen with CYP3A4-specific drugs. There are large differences in ethinyl estradiol pharmacokinetics between groups of women in different countries. It is anticipated that the *CYP3A4* polymorphism might play a role in oral contraceptive-induced cerebral vein thrombosis.

Pharmacogenomics

WHY DO THESE POLYMORPHISMS PERSIST IN THE HUMAN POPULATION?

If an allele has a frequency of 0.001 (i.e., 0.1%) and represents an autosomal recessive trait, this means that (the Hardy-Weinberg $q^2 = 0.001 \times 0.001$) one in 1 million individuals will be an afflicted homozygote. Spontaneous mutations generally occur at rates between 1 in 10^6 and 1 in 10^8 bases of DNA. To a geneticist, therefore, any time an allele is found to exist in the population at frequencies of greater than 0.001, one should consider possible reasons for this. For example, as described earlier, the frequency of the slow-acetylator NAT2 phenotype is greater than 90% in Mediterraneans, glucose-6-phosphate dehydrogenase (G6PD) deficiency is 53% in Sephardic Jews, and the frequency of the *low/low* homozygote for thiopurine methyltransferase is 1 in 300. These represent Hardy-Weinberg distribution allelic frequencies of > 0.95, > 0.72, and 0.055, respectively. Why do these variant alleles remain at such high frequencies in human populations?

The *founder effect*, which is the overpropagation of a particular allele due to a genetic "bottleneck" (sparsity of breeding pairs due to geography, disease, or many other kinds of environmental factors), can explain increases in the frequency of a gene in local populations of recent origin. Neither spontaneous mutation nor the founder effect, however, can explain the striking interindividual differences or the geographic differences in DME alleles that have been described in this chapter. Possible selective pressures are therefore likely to include diet, climate and geography, and "balanced" polymorphisms (Nebert, 1997a). The other possible explanation (which has emerged only in the last couple of years because of the capacity of some laboratories to resequence quickly and inexpensively alleles of the same gene in dozens or hundreds of individuals) is that many, or all, genes are highly polymorphic.

ETHNIC DIFFERENCES

Differences in diet, which have evolved over thousands of years, might explain at least some of the striking variability in ethnic differences in allelic frequencies. Just as is true for all drugs and environmental pollutants, foodstuff (from which the development of most drugs has been derived) represents DME substrates (Nebert, 1997a).

How long might it take for the human genome to adapt to dietary selective pressures? By means of genetic drift and natural selection (random mutations, gene duplication, crossing-over events, etc.), new genes become fixed and passed on to the next generation because of an ecological advantage to the species; the response of the genome to environmental pressures, over many generations, has been described as "molecular drive" (Dover, 1986). It is becoming increasingly appreciated in evolutionary studies that such changes might occur slowly, or might occur rapidly in just a few generations—depending upon the selective pressures. If the population of a species decreases dramatically so that rare variants are more likely to reproduce, the distribution in that population would shift much more rapidly (Nebert, 1997a). The development, within a population, of individuals that are resistant to changes in their environment has been demonstrated experimentally in various organisms from prokaryotes to insects and vertebrates (Nebert and Dieter, 2000), but the mechanisms involved remain basically obscure. Depending on the organism studied, between 10 and 50 generations appear to be required. For humans, 10 to 50 generations would extrapolate to a range between 200 and 1000 years.

Most *Homo sapiens* ethnic groups have diverged from one another during the past 50,000 years (Nebert and Menon, 2001). Based on animal studies alone, 50,000 years is thus more than sufficient time for striking differences in pharmacogenetically relevant polymorphisms to have arisen from selective pressures due to tribal differences in diet or exposure to other environmental signals. It seems very likely that, for example, 5000 years of a diet principally of goat meat and milk products—compared with that principally of tropical fruit and fish—might result in tribal differences in variant alleles.

BALANCED POLYMORPHISMS

The high allelic frequencies seen in pharmacogenetically relevant genes, between individuals within any one ethnic group, also might represent the evolution of balanced polymorphisms. The classical example of a compensating, or "shared benefit," polymorphism is the sickle-cell trait. Whereas the homozygous carriers of this trait almost always fail to reproduce because of severe anemia, the much larger number of heterozygotes resist malaria better than wild-type homozygotes. There are several classes of diseases in which the homozygote bears the risks while the heterozygote is believed to retain a distinct survival advantage: (a) resistance to bacterial and viral pathogens, (b) improved prenatal survival, and (c) improved postnatal survival in response to particular environmental stresses (Rotter and Diamond, 1987).

Table 21.10 provides a list of several examples of what many accept as balanced polymorphisms. It is possible that at least some of the pharmacogenetic allelic differences described throughout this chapter might represent balanced polymorphisms, ones that we perhaps cannot appreciate at the present time—such as improved rates of implantation, prenatal growth, postnatal development in response to dietary selective pressures, or even resistance to bacterial, viral or fungal infections (Nebert, 1997a).

If pharmacogenetically relevant gene products are important for critical life functions, one would also reason that the presence of some of these defective alleles would be indistinguishable from an "inborn error of metabolism." That this is indeed the case is illustrated in Table 21.11. It is concluded, therefore, that many so-called "inborn errors of metabolism" are actually caused by DNA sequence variants, or deletions, of pharmacogenetically relevant genes.

GENETIC VARIABILITY THROUGHOUT THE HUMAN GENOME

Some have argued that the variability found in DME genes will not be seen in the rest of the human genome. This has proven to be false. Recent resequencing efforts have

---

Table 21.10. Proposed examples of a balanced polymorphism, or "shared benefit," seen in the heterozygote

- Sickle cell anemia—resistance to malaria
- Congenital adrenal hyperplasia—protection against *Hemophilus influenzae B* infections
- Glucose-6-phosphate dehydrogenase deficiency—resistance to malaria
- Tay-Sachs disease—resistance to tuberculosis
- High pepsinogen I (in gastric secretions)—resistance to tuberculosis
- Idiopathic hemochromatosis—protection against iron loss (menses)
- Noninsulin-dependent diabetes mellitus—protection against intermittent/limited food intake
- Cystic fibrosis—resistance to cholera toxin

(Extracted from the text of Rotter and Diamond, 1987.)

Table 21.11. List of several "inborn errors of metabolism," caused by fefects in DME genes

- Primary congenital glaucoma (buphthalmos), autosomal recessive eye disorder (mutations/deletions/insertions in the *CYP1B1* gene)
- Miller-Dieker lissencephaly, defects in the 45-kDa subunit of brain platelet-activating factor (PAF) acetylhydrolase, appears identical to the *LIS1* gene
- Congenital adrenal hyperplasia (CAH), autosomal recessive disorders involving CYP11A1, CYP11B1, CYP11B2, CYP17, and (most common) CYP21
- Vitamin D-dependent rickets, autosomal recessive (defect in 25-HO-D$_3$ 1α-hydroxylase, CYP27B1)
- Sjögren-Larsson syndrome (SLS), autosomal recessive disorder: mental retardation, ichthyosis, spastic diplegia or tetraplegia [point mutations/deletions/insertions in the microsomal fatty aldehyde dehydrogenase (*ALDH10*) gene]
- Smith-Lemli-Opitz syndrome (autosomal recessive disorder having facial dysmorphisms, mental retardation and multiple congenital anomalies), mutations in the 7-dehydrocholesterol reductase (*7DCR*) gene
- Progressive familial intrahepatic cholestasis (PFIC), heterogeneous group of autosomal recessive liver disorders leading to cirrhosis/liver failure before adulthood (mutations in the *MDR3* gene)

The last example is a drug transporter, rather than a DME, gene. (Summarized from Nebert and Dieter, 2000.)

demonstrated that the human genome is incredibly variable from one individual to the next, and that high allelic frequencies are definitely not restricted only to pharmacogenetically relevant genes. For example, a 9.7-kb region inside the human lipoprotein lipase (*LPL*) gene in 71 unrelated individuals revealed 88 variable sites. A 4-Mb region around the *APOE* gene has one single-nucleotide polymorphism (SNP) per 1100 bp of genomic sequence. Resequencing 24.1 kb of the *DCP1* gene in 11 unrelated individuals showed 78 variable sites. In 114 independent alleles from 106 genes, 560 SNPs were found. Sequencing 190 kb from 148 alleles in 74 unrelated individuals, 874 candidate SNPs were uncovered. Resequencing about 2 kb of the tryptase-1 (*TPS1*) gene and 1.8 kb of the *TPS2* gene in 32 individuals identified 38 SNPs. Large deletions (100 bp, 200 kb, 3 Mb) in the same chromosomal region from two individuals are being found. More than 1.2 million SNPs are available in public databases on the web (reviewed in Nebert, 1999; Nebert, 2000b). We thus conclude that one can expect high degrees of variability and large differences in DNA sequence variant frequencies, on a gene-by-gene basis, throughout the entire human genome.

ETHNIC DIFFERENCES IN PHARMACOGENETICS AND THE HUMAN GENOME PROJECT

Ethnic differences in allelic frequencies of pharmacogenetically relevant genes have been described throughout this chapter. We predict that ethnic differences are also going to create problems in the Human Genome Project. For example, the common reference (wild-type, consensus) sequence has been regarded for a long time as the *CYP2D6*1* (extensive metabolizer, EM) allele (Oscarson et al., 2001) and the *NAT2*4* (rapid acetylator) allele

(Hein et al., 2001). The Human Genome Database, on the other hand, contains the rare *CYP2D6*5* allele (in which the entire *CYP2D6* gene is deleted, PM) and the very rare *NAT2*12A* allele (rapid acetylator). Obviously, all information in the Human Genome Database will depend on whose DNA (and which allele) is sequenced.

ALL DISEASES (INCLUDING PHARMACOGENETIC DISORDERS) ARE POLYGENIC

Throughout this chapter, we have described four fundamental types of pharmacogenetic disorders, although, in reality, perhaps none is distinct from another (i.e., a gradient of responses is present), and this can apply to all human disease. Genes causing disease (including drug toxicity) can be: (a) *high-frequency high-penetrance* (e.g., *NAT2* alleles affecting plasma isoniazid clearance; or *HFE* mutations causing hereditary hemochromatosis), (b) *high-frequency low-penetrance* (*NAT2* alleles as a modifier of breast cancer risk; *NQO1* alleles and toxicity following benzene exposure); (c) *low-frequency low-penetrance* (*EPHX1* alleles and risk of nasopharyngeal cancer; *RYR1* mutations and central core disease), or (d) *low-frequency high-penetrance* (*RYR1* mutations and malignant hyperthermia; *DPYD* mutations and 5-fluorouracil sensitivity). If threshold models apply, they are not established for any of these disorders.

Can any of the pharmacogenetic differences (traits) described in this chapter truly be caused by solely one gene? Although generally thought of as "single-gene" traits, the *NAT2* polymorphism (Fig. 21.4) and the *CYP2D6* polymorphism (Fig. 21.7B), and others described throughout this chapter, must actually be regarded as *polygenic multifactorial* traits. If one examines closely the actual variability in plasma isoniazid clearance (Fig. 21.4) and in the metabolic ratio of debrisoquine metabolism (Fig. 21.7B), a continuous transition of individuals can be seen—from the slowest of the slow metabolizers to the fastest of the extensive metabolizers. The distributions are clearly bimodal, however. Thus, we must conclude that plasma isoniazid clearance and the metabolic ratio of debrisoquine metabolism are principally controlled by the *NAT2* and *CYP2D6* gene products but that genes modifying these traits also exist.

On the other hand, there are many phenotypes described throughout this chapter in which the variability is more or less Gaussian (i.e., not polymodal) and the mean variation between ethnic groups is no more than two- to three-fold, whereas differences between individuals—within an ethnic group—are 10- to more than 40-fold. This type of trait is the hallmark of *polygenic complex diseases*, i.e., traits reflecting two and usually many more than two genes, combined with dozens if not hundreds of modifier genes, plus environmental factors. Examples include plasma drug half-lives, phenytoin-induced gingival overgrowth, fetal hydantoin syndrome, and glucosidation of amobarbital. Fig. 21.15 illustrates two additional examples, out of hundreds of other studies reported in the literature (Kalow and Bertilsson, 1994). We thus conclude that pharmacogenetic differences might reflect: (a) predominantly a single gene, with some effect by modifier genes; or (b) a multiplex phenotype, representing two or more genes, plus effects of modifier genes and environmental factors.

An additional consideration involves *polyallelic inheritance*. The variability in affinity, as measured by a Scatchard plot for the AH receptor (Fig. 21.13), is an example. Either there exist cytosolic proteins that affect dioxin binding (in the *in vitro* assay) which differ between individuals, or the data must reflect polyallelic inheritance of the receptor protein itself. In other words, two or more amino-acid changes in the same protein (and each of the two alleles might produce different proteins) can lead to a *gradient* of responses, e.g., a receptor may exhibit two-fold or four-fold differences in affinity. The same can be true for enzymes; an enzyme might display 80% or 40% of normal activity. The enzymes encoded by the *NAT1, G6PD, CYP2D6, EPHX1* and *ALDH2* variant alleles are examples of polyallelic inheritance, i.e., the mutant enzymic activity is not zero but rather 6% or 50% of the normal wild-type activity.

Two further complexities (related to metabolism) are illustrated in Fig. 21.16 and Fig. 21.17. Just as a metabolic pathway goes from compound **A** to **B**, there often are enzymes that will take the compound **B** back to **A** (Fig. 21.16). Furthermore, there may be one gene or several genes encoding the DME activities that go in either direction (note that amitryptyline, codeine, dolasetron and tamoxifen are substrates for both CYP2D6 and CYP3A4 in Tables 21.5 and 21.6). Thus, there are genes that encode proteins responsible for the dihydrodiol dehydrogenase, alcohol dehydrogenase and aldoketoreductase activities (Fig. 21.16, *top*) and—as has been described above—undoubtedly multiple alleles for each gene, some of which will affect enzyme activity levels. Hence, if the patient is genetically an extensive metabolizer for the methyltransferase activity and a poor metabolizer for the N-demethylase activity (Fig. 21.16, *bottom*), his methyltransferase phenotype will appear to be even "higher."

The other complexity involves so-called "drug-drug interactions," which are likely to be greatly magnified by allelic differences in pharmacogenetically relevant genes (Fig. 21.17). Consider that the patient is taking drug **A** and drug **B** and that these two drugs compete for the same site of action. If the patient is, for example, a poor metabolizer (or poor affinity receptor, or poor transporter) for drug **B**, then the commonly prescribed dose of drug **B** will lead to abnormally elevated levels—thereby leading to an exaggerated drug-drug interaction, i.e., greater inhibition of the efficacy of drug **A**.

In the field of medical genetics, in general, it has become increasingly appreciated that even phenotypes of patients believed to have "simple" mendelian disorders virtually always represent multiplex traits—affected by thresholds, modifier genes, and environmental factors. Examples of Gaucher disease, phenylketonuria, congenital adrenal hyperplasia, and others were discussed by Dipple and McCabe (2000). Clearly, essentially all disease, as well as pharmacogenetic differences (traits of drug-efficacy or drug-toxicity), depict *multiplex phenotypes*.

NEED FOR A QUANTITATIVE PHENOTYPE

In the field of pharmacogenomics research, as with any other complex disease, therefore, it can be difficult to identify patients with an *unequivocal phenotype*. Because drug efficacy or toxicity always represents a *gradient*, one approach to quantitate the clinical phenotype would be to examine the extreme ends of a distribution, in much the same way as genetic studies have been done in the dissection and identification of genes responsible for blood pressure homeostasis (Jacob et al., 1991; Brown et al., 1996; Halushka et al., 1999). Patients who are arguably "intermediate" should not (at least, initially) be included, for the sake of reducing the complexity of the two subsets being studied. Hence, it is possible to examine relatively small numbers of highly informative patients having an unequivocal quantitative trait—following which one can attempt to

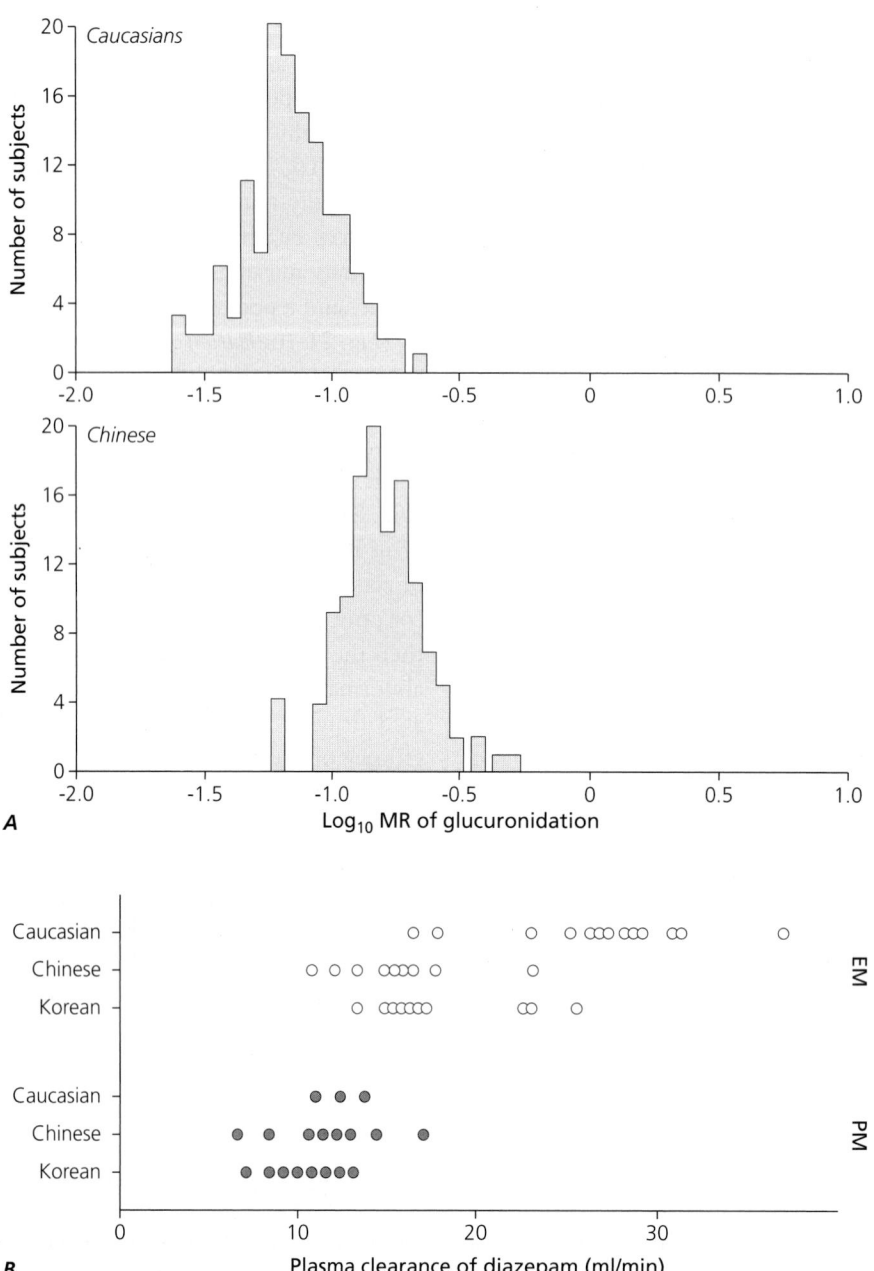

Fig. 21.15. Examples of interethnic differences in drug metabolism or clearance. (*A*) Frequency distributions of the $\log_{10}$ MR (metabolic ratio = parent drug divided by metabolite) of codeine glucuronidation. Total number of subjects, N = 149 and 133 for Caucasians and Chinese, respectively. (Redrawn from Yue et al., 1989). (*B*) Plasma clearance of diazepam in CYP2C19 EM and PM individuals from three ethnic groups. Total number of EM subjects, N = 13 Caucasian, 8 Chinese, and 9 Korean; total number of PM subjects, N = 3 Caucasian, 8 Chinese, and 8 Korean. (Redrawn from Bertilsson and Kalow, 1993.)

correlate the phenotype with a genotype. For example, selecting only patients from the top and bottom 2.5th percentile of a normalized blood-pressure distribution, Halushka and coworkers (1999) examined 75 candidate genes in 74 patients (148 alleles); the remaining 95% in the middle were not included in their study. It has been proposed (Nebert, 2000a) that the same approach can be highly successful in pharmacogenetic studies.

EXTREME DISCORDANT PHENOTYPE (EDP) METHODOLOGY

The principle of EDP methodology is presented in Fig. 21.18. As the dose of any drug under study is increased, more patients would be expected to show toxicity. Hence, as the dose of the drug is increased and the incidence of toxicity rises, there would be fewer in the population who are still

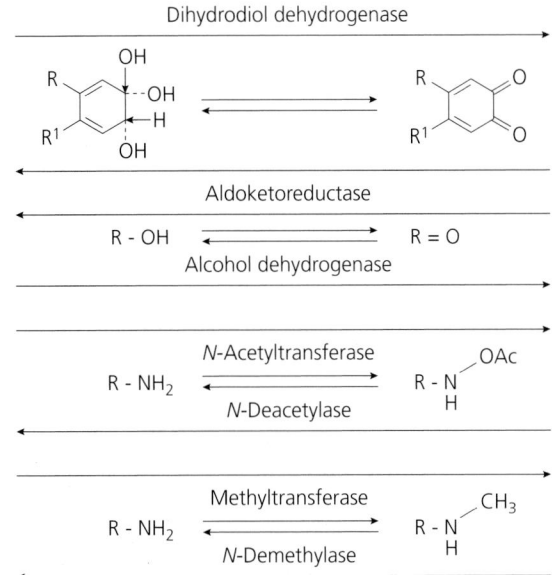

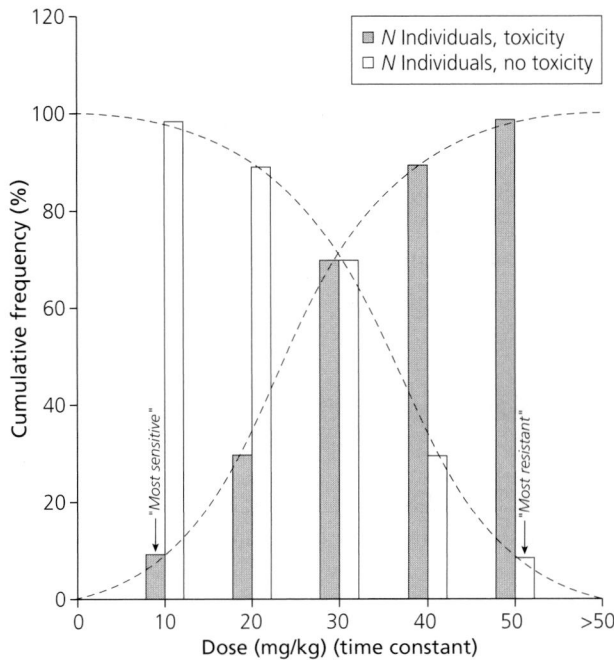

Fig. 21.16. Four examples of metabolic pathways catalyzed by drug-metabolizing enzymes (DMEs), illustrating that different DMEs can work in one or the other direction in the same pathway. (Reproduced with permission from Nebert, 2000b.)

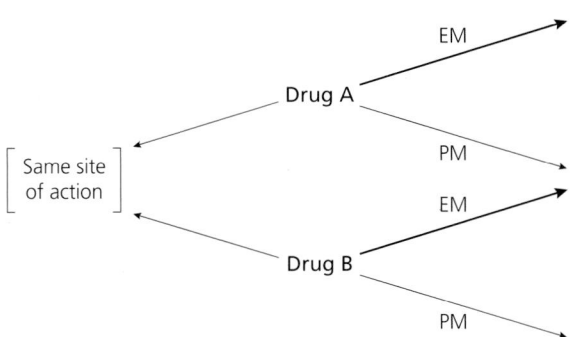

Fig. 21.18. Generic dose-response relationship from an idealized clinical population. The bars depict theoretical numbers of patients (exhibiting toxicity or no toxicity). The percent cumulative frequency is also plotted, as a function of drug dosage, in patients exhibiting a particular type of toxicity (increasing from *left* to *right*) versus patients showing no toxicity (increasing from *right* to *left*). The curves shown here are symmetrical but would not necessarily be expected to be symmetrical in the typical clinical population. Also, the dose (10 to > 50 mg/kg) is completely arbitrary, simply to make the point; this 5-fold dose range might easily be only two-fold for certain drugs. As discussed in the text, rigorous parameters for the unequivocal phenotype of "toxicity," versus "no toxicity," *must* be set beforehand. The same approach could also be used for drug efficacy—if rigorous quantitative endpoints were defined and established ahead of time. (Reproduced with permission from Nebert, 2000a.)

Fig. 21.17. Diagram of possible genetic effects on drug-drug interactions. EM, extensive-metabolizer phenotype. PM, poor-metabolizer phenotype. (Reproduced with permission from Nebert, 2000b.)

taking this drug and exhibit no toxicity. Those patients receiving the lowest doses who show an exaggerated toxic response (i.e., a dose-*in*dependent response) would be classified as the "*most sensitive*" trait, and those patients receiving the highest doses who exhibit no toxicity are classified as the "*most resistant*" trait. In order to identify the genes responsible for this difference, it is therefore very important to focus on these most-sensitive and most-resistant phenotype groups. Initially, one should disregard the vast majority of patients who are being given intermediate doses (of the drug under study) or who exhibit intermediate responses (showing no toxicity at low doses, or small degrees of toxicity at high doses). One might therefore select the "top 1%" and "bottom 1%"

extremes, and attempt to correlate a DNA sequence variant in candidate genes with the most-sensitive versus the most-resistant trait. This EDP approach has previously been carried out, in principle, in numerous pharmacogenetic studies—but not in the rigorous mathematically systematic way that was recently described (Nebert, 2000a).

From the list of pharmacogenetic differences (Table 21.1), there are many with the molecular mechanisms still unexplained. This proposed approach of EDP methodology is a realistic means for dissecting most, if not all, of these complex gene-drug interactions (Nebert, 2000a).

In principle, the EDP approach has been discussed in affected sib pairs (Risch and Zhang, 1995; 1996; McCarthy et al., 1998; Epstein et al., 2000). Selection of the most appropriate ethnic groups, and numbers of patients needed for an informative study, has also been described in detail (Kruglyak, 1999; Wright et al., 1999;

Pratt et al., 2000). For the EDP approach without using sib pairs, a random-mating diploid population is assumed, with non-overlapping generations. Further details concerning the statistical power of EDP methodology, choosing candidate genes, finding a DNA sequence variant between the "most sensitive" and "most resistant" phenotypes, and proving that a DNA sequence variant is responsible for the phenotype—have all been recently described (Nebert, 2000a).

Conclusions

Some general conclusions can be drawn from the foregoing account on both a theoretical level and a clinical level.

THEORETICAL

When a doctor gives a patient a dose of a drug medication, there is an element of uncertainty. In most cases, the desired effect occurs and nothing else transpires. However, in some instances, there may be an adverse reaction or lack of efficacy. There are many reasons for these reactions, but genetic factors are being shown again and again to play an important role.

These pharmacogenetic differences represent polymorphisms. One way in which a polymorphism may be demonstrated is by means of a frequency distribution histogram of a measurement of biotransformation or effect. If artifacts can be excluded, then the finding of a bimodal or trimodal frequency distribution curve may indicate the existence of different phenotypes (reflecting underlying differences in genotypes). Family studies are required to examine the type of inheritance and penetrance of the trait. Pharmacogenetic disorders that are not due primarily to a single gene (i.e., frequency distribution not polymodal), but are polygenic and multifactorial, are more difficult to study. In this case, extreme discordant phenotype (EDP) methodology is proposed as a means to define an unequivocal phenotype. One can then attempt to associate the "most sensitive" versus the "most resistant" traits with one or more genotypes; this can be done by the candidate-gene approach or by a genomic scan (quantitative trait loci, or QTL, analysis).

The knowledge in 2001 of all genes in the human genome, combined with the extensive single-nucleotide polymorphism (SNP) database now in place, will greatly facilitate genetic epidemiologic studies and clinical investigations. Direct genotyping will avoid the complicating

influences involved in determining an unequivocal trait, particularly when environmental and inducibility factors make phenotyping difficult.

When a drug is biotransformed by means of more than one pathway, it may be subject to the influence of more than one genetic polymorphism. In such a situation, it may be the individual who has a low metabolic capacity due to two or more genes, who will be the one most likely to develop an adverse reaction or toxicity.

A full understanding of the nature of a pharmacogenetic polymorphism would ideally require a detailed knowledge of the three-dimensional structure of the gene product (enzyme, receptor, transporter, transcription factor, component of a subcellular organelle). This is available only in very few examples.

Within a pharmacogenetic polymorphism, a particular phenotype may be at a disadvantage in one set of circumstances but at an advantage in a different set of circumstances. This bears some resemblance to the mechanism of Darwinian selection seen in many biologic systems.

CLINICAL

The initial step in the successful practice of medicine is to take a sound history. This may be particularly revealing when there is a mendelian dominant condition in the family.

Phenotyping tests have been applied with great benefit in some pharmacogenetic conditions, such as malignant hyperthermia, porphyrias, and glucose-6-phosphate dehydrogenase (G6PD) deficiency. It is now clear that direct genotyping tests will prove far less laborious.

It is worth emphasizing that, when an adverse drug reaction has been found to be common only in a phenotype that constitutes a segment of the population, it may not be logical to discard that drug completely. This is what happened, for example, with the useful antianginal drug perhexilene, which produced peripheral neuropathy and liver disease principally in CYP2D6 PM patients. As a result, about 95% of the population that was not particularly susceptible to these complications were denied the possible benefits of the drug. Many other examples exist. Theoretically, the employment of a phenotyping test would have been a more logical alternative approach. Giving a lower dose to the PM individual might also be a viable alternative.

From what we now know about the large interethnic variability in the distribution of pharmacogenetic alleles, it is possible for new adverse reactions or unsuspected lack of efficacy to occur when a drug is introduced for use in a new ethnic population. This means that careful postmarketing surveillance should accompany such an introduction.

It is accepted that there should be full metabolic accounting for any new drug. The fate of all drug molecules should be known, and biotransformations characterized. What is also clear is that this exercise should be undertaken in all major ethnic groups.

Clinical trials should be structured in such a way that all test groups contain adequate numbers of the different phenotypes within polymorphisms. This means that the use of sufficiently large numbers, and phenotyping tests, might also sometimes be appropriate.

ACKNOWLEDGEMENTS

We thank our colleagues for valuable discussions and a careful reading of this manuscript. The artistic help of Marian Miller with all the figures is gratefully appreciated. This work was funded in part by NIH Grants R01 ES06321, R01 ES08147, R01 ES10416, and P30 ES06096.

REFERENCES

Adler E, Hoon MA, Mueller KL et al. (2000) A novel family of mammalian taste receptors. Cell 100:693–702

Allan LD, Chita SK, Sharland GK et al. (1991) Flecainide in the treatment of fetal tachycardia. Br Heart J 65:46–48

Ambrosone CB, Freudenheim JL, Graham S et al. (1996) Cigarette smoking, N-acetyltransferase 2 genetic polymorphisms, and breast cancer risk. J Am Med Assoc 276:1494–1501

Aoyama T, Korzekwa K, Nagata K et al. (1990) Estradiol metabolism by complementary deoxyribonucleic acid-expressed human cytochrome P450s. Endocrinology 126:3101–3106

Arias TD, Jorge LF, Barrantes R (1991) Uses and misuses of definitions of genetic polymorphism. A perspective from population pharmacogenetics. Brit J Clin Pharmacol 31:117–119

Armaly MF (1968) Genetic factors related to glaucoma. Ann NY Acad Sci 151:861–875

Ayesh R, Mitchell SC, Zhang A, Smith RL (1993) The fish odour syndrome: Biochemical, familial, and clinical aspects. B Med J 307:655–657

Ball DE, McLaughlin WS, Seymour RA, Kamali F (1996) Plasma and saliva concentrations of phenytoin and 5-(4-hydroxyphenyl)-5-phenylhydantoin in relation to the incidence and severity of phenytoin-induced gingival overgrowth in epileptic patients. J Periodontol 67:597–602

Basarab T, Ashton GH, Menage HP, McGrath JA (1999) Sequence variations in the flavin-containing monooxygenase 3 gene (FMO3) in fish odour syndrome. Br J Dermatol 140:164–167

Beetham JK, Grant D, Arand M et al. (1995) Gene evolution of epoxide hydrolases and recommended nomenclature. DNA Cell Biol 14:61–71

Bertilsson L, Kalow W (1993) Why are diazepam metabolism and polymorphic S-mephenytoin hydroxylation associated with each other in white and Korean populations but not in Chinese populations? Clin Pharmacol Ther 53:608–610

Blum M, Grant DM, McBride W et al. (1990) Human arylamine N-acetyltransferase genes: isolation, chromosomal localization, and functional expression. DNA Cell Biol9:193–203

Bonkovsky HL, Poh-Fitzpatrick M, Pimstone N et al. (1998) Porphyria cutanea tarda, hepatitis C, and HFE gene mutations in North America. Hepatology 27:1661–1669

Brophy VH, Jampsa RL, Clendenning JB et al. (2001) Promoter polymorphism effects on paraoxonase (PON1) expression. Am J Hum Genet, 68:1428:1436.

Brown DM, Provoost AP, Daly MJ et al. (1996) Renal disease susceptibility and hypertension are under independent genetic control in the fawn-hooded rat. Nat Genet 12:44–51

Buccino G, Scoditti U, Pini M et al. (1999) Low-oestrogen oral contraceptives as a major risk factor for cerebral venous and sinus thrombosis: evidence from a clinical series. Ital J Neurol Sci 20:231–235

Buehler BA, Rao V, Finnell RH (1994) Biochemical and molecular teratology of fetal hydantoin syndrome. Neurol Clinics 1994 12:741–748

Butler MA, Iwasaki M, Guengerich FP, Kadlubar FF (1989) Human cytochrome P-450PA (P-450IA2), the phenacetin O-deethylase, is primarily responsible for the hepatic 3-demethylation of caffene and N-oxidation of carcinogenic arylamines. Proc Natl Acad Sci USA 86:7696–7700

Cain C, Nigogosyan G (1963) Acquired toxic porphyria cutanea tarda due to hexachlorobenzene. J Am Med Assoc 183:88–91

Caraco Y (1998) Genetic determinants of drug responsiveness and drug interactions. Therap Drug Monit 20:517–524

Carlini EJ, Raftogianis RB, Wood TC et al. (2001) Sulfation pharmacogenetics: SULT1A1 and SULT1A2 allele frequencies in Caucasian, Chinese and African-American subjects. Pharmacogenetics 11:57–68

Carson PE, Flanagan CL, Ickes CE, Alving AS (1956) Enzymatic deficiency in primaquine sensitive erythrocytes. Science 124:484–486

Casetta I, Granieri E, Desidera M et al. (1997) Phenytoin-induced gingival overgrowth: A community-based cross-sectional study in Ferrara, Italy. Neuroepidemiology 16:296–303

Chandrashekar J, Mueller KL, Hoon MA et al. (2000) T2Rs function as bitter taste receptors. Cell 100:703–711

Chiang CE, Roden DM (2000) The long QT syndromes: Genetic basis and clinical implications. J Am Col Cardiol 36:1–12

Christiansen L, Bygum A, Jensen A et al. (2000) Association between CYP1A2 polymorphism and susceptibility to porphyria cutanea tarda. Hum Genet 107:612–614

Code EL, Crespi BW Gonzalez F j, Chang TK, Waxman DJ Human cytochrome P450 2B6 : interivindual hepatic expression, substrate specify, and role in procarcinogen activation. Drug Meta Disp 25:985-993

Collie-Duguid ES, Etienne MC, Milano G, McLeod HL (2000) Known variant DPYD alleles do not explain DPD deficiency in cancer patients. Pharmacogenetics 10:217–223

Corchero J, Pimprale S, Kimura S, Gonzalez FJ (2001) Organization of the CYP1A cluster on human chromosome 15: Implications for gene regulation. Pharmacogenetics 11:1–6

Cornett R, James MO, Henderson GN et al. (1999) Inhibition of glutathione S-transferase zeta and tyrosine metabolism by dichloroacetate: A potential unifying mechanism for its altered biotransformation and toxicity. Biochem Biophys Res Comm 262:752–756

Daly AK, Brockmoller J, Broly F et al. (1996) Nomenclature for human CYP2D6 alleles. Pharmacogenetics 6:193–201

Daly AK, Fairbrother KS, Smart J (1998) Recent advances in understanding the molecular basis of polymorphisms in genes encoding cytochrome P450 enzymes. Toxicol Letters 102–103:143–147

De Marco P, Moroni A, Merello E et al. (2000) Folate pathway gene alterations in patients with neural tube defects. Am J Med Genet 95:216–223

de Matteis F (1998) Porphyria cutanea tarda of the toxic and sporadic varieties. Clin Dermatol 16:265–275

de Wildt SN, Kearns GL, Leeder JS, van den Anker JN (1999) Cytochrome P450 3A: Ontogeny and drug disposition. Clin Pharmacokin 37:485–505

Dipple KM, McCabe ERB (2000) Phenotypes of patients with "simple" Mendelian disorders are complex traits: thresholds, modifiers, and systems dynamics. Am J Hum Genet 66:1729–1735

Distlerath LM, Reilly PE, Martin MV et al. (1985) Purification and characterization of the human liver cytochromes P-450 involved in debrisoquine 4-hydroxylation and phenacetin O-deethylation, two prototypes for genetic polymorphism in oxidative drug metabolism. J Biol Chem 260:9057–9067

Dolphin CT, Janmohamed A, Smith RL et al. (1997) Missense mutation in flavin-containing monooxygenase-3 gene, FMO3, underlies fish-odour syndrome. Nat Genet 17:491–494

Dooley TP (1998) Cloning of the human phenol sulfotransferase gene family: Three genes implicated in the metabolism of catecholamines, thyroid hormones and drugs. Chem-Biol Interactions 109:29–41

Dooley TP (1999) Molecular biology of the human cytosolic sulfotransferase gene superfamily implicated in the bioactivation of minoxidil and cholesterol in skin. Exp Dermatol 8:328–329

Dover GA (1986) Molecular drive in multigene families: How biological novelties arise, spread and are assimilated. Trends Genet 2:159–165

Draganov DI, Stetson PL, Watson CE et al. (2000) Rabbit serum paraoxonase 3 (PON3) is a high density lipoprotein-associated lactonase and protects low density lipoprotein against oxidation. J Biol Chem 275:33435–33442

Eaton DL, Gallagher EP, Bammler TK, Kunze KL (1995) Role of cytochrome P450 1A2 in chemical carcinogenesis: Implications for human variability in expression and enzyme activity. Pharmacogenetics 5:259–274

Ebisawa T, Deguchi T (1991) Structure and restriction fragment length polymorphism of genes for human liver arylamine N-acetyl transferases. Biochem Biophys Res Comm 177:1252–1257

Edwards IR (2000) Adverse drug reaactions: definitions, diagnosis, and management. Lancet 356:1255–1259

Eichelbaum M, Spannbrücker N, Steincke B, Dengler HJ (1979) Defective N-oxidation of sparteine in man: A new pharmacogenetic defect. Europ J Clin Pharmacol 16:183–187

Elder GH (1998) Genetic defects in the porphyrias: Types and significance. Clin Dermatol 16:225–233

Elkins S, Wrighton SA (1999) The role of CYP2B6 in human xenobiotic metabolism. Drug Metab Res 31:719–754

Epstein MP, Duren WL, Boehnke M (2000) Improved inference of relationship for pairs of individuals. Am J Hum Genet 67:1219–1231

European Malignant Hyperthermia Group (1985) Laboratory diagnosis of malignant hyperthermia susceptibility (MHS). Br J Anaesth 57:1038

Evans DAP (1994) Pharmacogenetics. In Emery and Rimoin's Principles and Practice of Medical Genetics, 3rd edn. Harcourt, Churchill-Livingstone, New York, pp. 455–477,

Evans DAP, Manley K, McKusick VA (1960) Genetic control of isoniazid metabolism in man. Br Med J 2:485–498

Felton JS, Malfatti MA, Knize MG et al. (1997) Health risks of heterocyclic amines. Mutat Res 376:37–41

Fernandez-Salguero PM, Hilbert DM, Rudikoff S et al. (1996) Aryl-hydrocarbon receptor-deficient mice are resistant to 2,3,7,8-tetrachlorodibenzo-p-dioxin-induced toxicity. Toxicol Appl Pharmacol 140:173–179

Fernandez-Salguero PM, Ward JM, Sundberg JP, Gonzalez FJ (1997) Lesions of aryl-hydrocarbon receptor-deficient mice. Vet Pathol 34:605–614

Fischel-Ghodsian N (1999) Genetic factors in aminoglycoside toxicity. Ann N Y Acad Sci 884:99–109

Fisslthaler B, Popp R, Kiss L et al. (1999) Cytochrome P450 2C is an EDHF synthase in coronary arteries. Nature 401:493–497

Furlong CE (2000) PON1 status and neurologic symptom complexes in Gulf War veterans. Genome Res 10:153–155

Furst SM, Luedke D, Gaw HH et al. (1997) Demonstration of a cellular immune response in halothane-exposed guinea pigs. Toxicol Appl Pharmacol 143:245–255

Gaedigk A, Spielberg SP, Grant DM (1994) Characterization of the microsomal epoxide hydrolase gene in patients with anticonvulsant adverse drug reactions. Pharmacogenetics 4:142–153

Goedde HW, Agarwal DP (1986) Aldehyde oxidation: Ethnic variations in metabolism and response. Progr Clin Biol Res 214:113–138

Goldstein JA, de Morais SM (1994) Biochemistry and molecular biology of the human CYP2C subfamily. Pharmacogenetics 4:285–299

Gonzalez FJ (1997) The role of carcinogen-metabolizing enzyme polymorphisms in cancer susceptibility. Reprod Toxicol 11:397–412

Gonzalez FJ, Idle JR (1994) Pharmacogenetic phenotyping and genotyping. Present status and future potential. Clin Pharmacokin 26:59–70

Gonzalez FJ, Skoda RC, Kimura S et al. (1988) Characterization of the common genetic defect in humans deficient in debrisoquine metabolism. Nature 331:442–446

Gu J, Zhang QY, Genter MB et al. (1998) Purification and characterization of heterologously expressed mouse CYP2A5 and CYP2G1: Role in metabolic activation of acetaminophen and 2,6-dichlorobenzonitrile in mouse olfactory mucosal microsomes. J Pharmacol Exp Ther 285:1287–1295

Guengerich FP (1999) Cytochrome P-450 3A4: Regulation and role in drug metabolism. Annu Rev Pharmacol Toxicol 39:1–17

Hahn ME, Karchner SI, Shapiro MA, Perera SA (1997) Molecular evolution of two vertebrate aryl hydrocarbon (dioxin) receptors (AHR1 and AHR2) and the PAS family. Proc Natl Acad Sci USA 94:13743–13748

Hallikainen T, Lachman H, Saito T et al. (2000) Lack of association between the functional variant of the catechol-O-methyltransferase (COMT) gene and early-onset alcoholism associated with severe antisocial behavior. Am J Med Genet 96:348–352

Halushka MK, Fan JB, Bentley K et al. (1999) Patterns of single-nucleotide polymorphisms in candidate genes for blood-pressure homeostasis. Nat Genet 22:239–247

Hanson JW, Myrianthopoulos NC, Harvey MA, Smith DW (1976) Risks to the offspring of women treated with hydantoin anticonvulsants, with emphasis on the fetal hydantoin syndrome. J Pediatr 89:662–668

Harada S, Agarwal DP, Goedde HW (1978) Human liver alcohol dehydrogenase isoenzyme variations. Improved separation methods using prolonged high voltage starch-gel electrophoresis and isoelectric focusing. Hum Genet 40:215–220

Harris H (1980) Principles of Human Biochemical Genetics, 3rd edn. Elsevier/North Holland Biomedical, NY, p. 331.

Harrower AD (2000) Comparative tolerability of sulphonylureas in diabetes mellitus. Drug Safety 22:313–320

Hassell TM, Burtner AP, McNeal D, Smith RG (2000) Oral problems and genetic aspects of individuals with epilepsy. Periodontology 6:68–78

Hayashi S, Watanabe J, Kawajiri K (1992) High susceptibility to lung cancer analyzed in terms of combined genotypes of P450 IA1 and mu-class glutathione S-transferase genes. Jpn J Cancer Res 83:866–870

Hayes JD, Pulford DJ (1995) The glutathione S-transferase supergene family: Regulation of GST and the contribution of the isoenzymes to cancer chemoprotection and drug resistance. Crit Rev Biochem Mol Biol 30:445–600

Hein DW, Grant DM, Sim E (2001) Arylamine N-acetyltransferase (EC 2.3.1.5) Web site: http://www.louisville.edu/medschool/pharmacology/NAT.html/

Henderson CJ, McLaren AW, Moffat GJ et al. (1998) Pi-class glutathione S-transferase: regulation and function. Chemico-Biological Interactions 111–112:69–82

Hildesheim A, Anderson LM, Chen CJ et al. (1997) CYP2E1 genetic polymorphisms and risk of nasopharyngeal carcinoma in Taiwan. J Natl Cancer Institute 89:1207–1212

Holt RJ, Freytes CO (1983) Familial warfarin resistance. Drug Intelligent Clin Pharm 17:281–283

Horn EP, Tucker MA, Lambert G et al. (1995) A study of gender-based cytochrome P450 1A2 variability: a possible mechanism for the male excess of bladder cancer. Cancer Epidemiol, Biomark Prevention 4:529–533

Idle JR, Smith RL (1979) Polymorphisms of oxidation at carbon centers of drugs and their clinical significance. Drug Metab Rev 9:301–317

Imai J, Ieiri I, Mamiya K et al. (2000) Polymorphism of the cytochrome P450 (CYP) 2C9 gene in Japanese epileptic patients: genetic analysis of the CYP2C9 locus. Pharmacogenetics 10:85–89

Ingelman-Sundberg M (2001a) Cytochrome P450 2D6 (debrisoquine hydroxylase, CYP2D6). In, Encyclopaedia of Molecular Medicine, John Wiley, in press

Ingelman-Sundberg M (2001b) Pharmacogenetics, an opportunity for a safer and more efficient pharmacotherapy. J Internal Medicine, in press

Ingelman-Sundberg M, Oscarson M, McLellan RA (1999) Polymorphic human cytochrome P450 enzymes: an opportunity for individualized drug treatment. Trends Pharmacol Sci 20:342–349

Jacob HJ, Lindpaintner K, Lincoln SE et al. (1991) Genetic mapping of a gene causing hypertension in the stroke-prone spontaneously hypertensive rat. Cell 67:213–224

Jirasek L, Kalensky J, Kubec K et al. (1976) Chloracne, porphyria cutanea tarda, and other poisonings due to the herbicides. Hautarzt 27:328–333

Kalow W, Bertilsson L (1994) Interethnic factors affecting drug response. Advan Drug Res 23:1–53

Kalow W, Tang BK (1991) Use of caffeine metabolite ratios to explore CYP1A2 and xanthine oxidase activities. Clin Pharmacol Therap 50:508–519

Kaneko S, Battino D, Andermann E et al. (1999) Congenital malformations due to antiepileptic drugs. Epilepsy Res 33:145–158

Kang J, Wang L, Chen XL et al. (2001) Interactions of a series of fluoroquinolone antibacterial drugs with the human cardiac K+ channel HERG. Mol Pharmacol 59:122–126

Kawajiri K, Watanabe J, Eguchi H, Hayashi S (1995) Genetic polymorphisms of drug-metabolizing enzymes and lung cancer susceptibility. Pharmacogenetics 5:S70–S73

Kleyn PW, Vesell ES (1998) Genetic variation as a guide to drug development. Science 281:1820–1821

Kruglyak L (1999) Prospects for whole-genome linkage disequilibrium mapping of common disease genes. Nat Genet 22:139–144

Kuehl P, Zhang J, Lin Y, Lamba J, Assem M, Schuetz J, Watkins PB, Daly A, Wrighton SA, Hall SD, Maurel P, Relling M, Brimer C, Yasuda K, Venkataramanan R, Strom S, Thummel K, Boguski MS, Schuetz E 2001 Sequence diversity in CYP3A promoters and characterization of the genetic basis of polymorphic CYP3A5 expression. Nat Genet 27: 383-391

Kuo CC, Huang RC, Lou BS (2000) Inhibition of Na+ current by diphenhydramine and other diphenyl compounds: Molecular determinants of selective binding to the inactivated channels. Mol Pharmacol 57:135–143

Lampe JW, Bigler J, Bush AC, Potter JD (2000) Prevalence of polymorphisms in the human UDP-glucuronosyltransferase 2B family: UGT2B4(D458E), UGT2B7(H268Y), and UGT2B15(D85Y). Cancer Epidemiol, Biomark Prevent 9:329–333

Lazarou J, Pomeranz BH, Corey PN (1998) Incidence of adverse drug reactions in hospitalized patients: A meta-analysis of prospective studies. J Am Med Assoc 279:1200–1205

Lewalter J, Korallus U (1985) Blood protein conjugates and acetylation of aromatic amines. Interna Arch of Occup and Environ Health 56:179–196

Li H, Fuentes-Garcia J, Towbin JA (2000) Current concepts in long QT syndrome. Pediatr Cardiol 21:542–550

Liang HC, Li H, McKinnon RA et al. (1996) CypIa2(-/-) null mutant mice develop normally but show deficient drug metabolism. Proc Natl Acad Sci USA 93:1671–1676

Lison M, Blondheim SH, Melmed RN (1980) A polymorphism of the ability to smell urinary metabolites of asparagus. Br Med J 281:1676–1678

Lockridge O, Masson P (2000) Pesticides and susceptible populations: People with butyrylcholinesterase genetic variants may be at risk. Neurotoxicology 21:113–126

Mackenzie PI, Owens IS, Burchell B et al. (1997) The UDP glycosyltransferase gene superfamily: Recommended nomenclature update based on evolutionary divergence. Pharmacogenetics 7:255–269

Mackness B, Mackness MI, Arrol S et al. (1998) Effect of the human serum paraoxonase 55 and 192 genetic polymorphisms on the protection by high density lipoprotein against low density lipoprotein oxidative modification. FEBS Letters 423:57–60

Maier A, Micka J, Miller K et al. (1998) Aromatic hydrocarbon receptor polymorphism: Development of new methods to correlate genotype with phenotype. Environ Health Pers 106:421–426

Matsunami H, Montmayeur JP, Buck LB (2000) A family of candidate taste receptors in human and mouse. Nature 404:601–604

McCarthy MI, Kruglyak L, Lander ES (1998) Sib-pair collection strategies for complex diseases. Genet Epidemiol 15:317–340

McCarthy TV, Quane KA, Lynch PJ (2000) Ryanodine receptor mutations in malignant hyperthermia and central core disease. Hum Mutation 15:410–417

McGlynn KA, Rosvold EA, Lustbader ED et al. (1995) Susceptibility to hepatocellular carcinoma is associated with genetic variation in the enzymatic detoxification of aflatoxin B$_1$. Proc Nat Acad Sci USA 92:2384–2387

McKinnon RA, Mackenzie PI (2001) UDP glycosyltransferase gene superfamily. Web site: http://www.unisa.edu.au/pharm_medsci/gluc_trans/

McLaughlin WS, Ball DE, Seymour RA et al. (1995) The pharmacokinetics of phenytoin in gingival crevicular fluid and plasma in relation to gingival overgrowth. J Clin Periodontol 22:942–945

McLellan RA, Oscarson M, Alexandrie AK et al. (1997) Characterization of a human glutathione S-transferase mu cluster containing a duplicated GSTM1 gene that causes ultra-rapid enzyme activity. Mol Pharmacol 52:958–965

Meyer UA (1994) The molecular basis of genetic polymorphisms of drug metabolism. J Pharm Pharmacol 46:409–415

Meyer UA (2000) Pharmacogenetics. pp. In Carruthers et al. (eds)Melmon and Morelli's Clinical Pharmacology, 4th edn. McGraw-Hill, NY, 1179–1221

Mitchell SC, Waring RH, Land D, Thorpe WV (1987) Odorous urine following asparagus ingestion in man. Experientia 43:382–383

Miyata M, Kudo G, Lee YH et al. (1999) Targeted disruption of the microsomal epoxide hydrolase gene. Microsomal epoxide hydrolase is required for the carcinogenic activity of 7,12-dimethylbenz[a]anthracene. J Biol Chem 274:23963–23968

Monks TJ, Anders MW, Dekant W et al. (1990) Glutathione conjugate-mediated toxicities. Toxicol Appl Pharmacol 106:1–19

Motulsky AG (1957) Drug reactions, enzymes and biochemical genetics. J Am Med Assoc 165:835–837

Nagai T, Shirabe K, Yubisui T, Takeshita M (1993) Analysis of mutant NADH-cytochrome b$_5$ reductase: apparent "type III" methemoglobinemia can be explained as type I with an unstable reductase. Blood 81:808–814

Nebert DW (1989) The *Ah* locus: Genetic differences in toxicity, cancer, mutation, and birth defects. Crit Rev in Toxicol 20:153–174

Nebert DW (1993) Elevated estrogen 16α-hydroxylase activity: Is this a genotoxic or nongenotoxic biomarker in human breast cancer risk? J Natl Cancer Inst 85:1888–1891

Nebert DW (1997a) Polymorphisms in drug-metabolizing enzymes: What is their clinical relevance and why do they exist? Am J Hum Genet 60:265–271

Nebert DW (1997b) Pharmacogenetics: 65 candles on the cake. Pharmacogenetics 7:435–440

Nebert DW (1999) Pharmacogenetics and pharmacogenomics: Why is this relevant to the clinical geneticist? Clin Genet 56:247–258

Nebert DW (2000a) Extreme discordant phenotype methodology: An intuitive approach to clinical pharmacogenetics. Eur J Pharmacol 410:107–120

Nebert DW (2000b) Suggestions for the nomenclature of human alleles: Relevance to ecogenetics, pharmacogenetics and molecular epidemiology. Pharmacogenetics 10:279–290

Nebert DW, Dieter MZ (2000) The Evolution of drug metabolism. Pharmacol 61:124–135

Nebert DW, McKinnon RA (1994) Cytochrome P450: evolution and functional diversity. Prog Liver Dis 12:63–97

Nebert, Menon (2001) Pharmacogenomics, ethnicity, and susceptibility genes. Pharmacogenom in press

Nebert, Nelson (2001) Cytochrome P450 (*CYP*) superfamily. In Encyclopaedia of the Human Genome (on the web), article #667, Nature Publishing Group, London

Nebert DW, Weber WW (1990) Pharmacogenetics. In Pratt WB, Taylor PW(eds): Principles of Drug Action. The Basis of Pharmacology 3rd edn. Churchill Livingstone NY, pp. 469–531

Nebert DW, McKinnon RA, Puga A (1996) Human drug-metabolizing enzyme polymorphisms: Effects on risk of toxicity and cancer. DNA Cell Biol 15:273–280

Nebert DW, Ingelman-Sundberg M, Daly AK (1999) Genetic epidemiology of environmental toxicity and cancer susceptibility: human allelic polymorphisms in drug-metabolizing enzyme genes, their functional importance, and nomenclature issues. Drug Metab Rev 31:467–487

Nebert DW, Roe AL, Dieter MZ et al. (2000) Role of the aromatic hydrocarbon receptor and [*Ah*] gene battery in the oxidative stress response, cell cycle control, and apoptosis. Biochem Pharmacol 59:65–85

Nelson DR (2001) Cytochrome P450 gene superfamily Web site: http://drnelson.utmem.edu/cytochromeP450.html/

Nowak MP, Sellers EM, Tyndale RF (1998) Canadian Native Indians exhibit unique *CYP2A6* and *CYP2C19* mutant allele frequencies. Clin Pharmacol Ther 64:378–383

Ogata M (1991) Acatalasemia. Hum Genet 86:331–340

O'Reilly RA (1970) The second reported kindred with hereditary resistance to oral anticoagulant drugs. N Eng J Med 282:1448–1451

Oscarson M, Ingelman-Sundberg M, Daly AK, Nebert DW (2001) Human cytochrome P450 (*CYP*) alleles. Web site: http://www.imm.ki.se/CYPalleles/

Parman T, Chen G, Wells PG (1998) Free radical intermediates of phenytoin and related teratogens. Prostaglandin H synthase-catalyzed bioactivation, electron paramagnetic resonance spectrometry, and photochemical product analysis. J Biol Chem 273:25079–25088

Perlik F, Kolinova M, Zvarova J, Patzelova V (1995) Phenytoin as a risk factor in gingival hyperplasia. Therapeutic Drug Monit 17:445–448

Persson I, Johansson I, Ingelman-Sundberg M (1997) In vitro kinetics of two human CYP1A1 variant enzymes suggested to be associated with interindividual differences in cancer susceptibility. Biochem Biophys Res Comm 231:227–230

Pineau T, Fernandez-Salguero P, Lee SS et al. (1995) Neonatal lethality associated with respiratory distress in mice lacking cytochrome P450 1A2. Proc Natl Acad Sci 92:5134–5138

Polansky JR, Fauss DJ, Zimmerman CC (2000) Regulation of TIGR/*MYOC* gene expression in human trabecular meshwork cells. Eye 14:503–514

Powell-Coffman JA, Bradfield CA, Wood WB (1998) *Caenorhabditis elegans* orthologs of the aryl hydrocarbon receptor and its heterodimerization partner the aryl hydrocarbon receptor nuclear translocator. Proc Natl Acad Sci USA 95:2844–2849

Pratt SC, Daly MJ, Kruglyak L (2000) Exact multipoint quantitative-trait linkage analysis in pedigrees by variance components. Am J Hum Genet 66:1153–1157

Price RA, Scott MC, Weinshilboum RM (1993) Genetic segregation analysis of red blood cell (RBC) histamine N-methyltransferase (HNMT) activity. Genet Epidemiol 10:123–131

Raftogianis RB, Wood TC, Otterness DM et al. (1997) Phenol sulfotransferase pharmacogenetics in humans: Association of common *SULT1A1* alleles with TS-PST phenotype. Biochem Biophys Res Comm 239:298–304

Riedy M, Wang JY, Miller AP et al. (2000) Genomic organization of the *UGT2B* gene cluster on human chromosome 4q13. Pharmacogenetics 10:251–260

Risch N, Zhang H (1995) Extreme discordant sib pairs for mapping quantitative trait loci in humans. Science 268:1584–1589

Risch NJ, Zhang H (1996) Mapping quantitative trait loci with extreme discordant sib pairs: Sampling considerations. Am J Hum Genet 58:836–843

Robson RA, Miners JO, Matthews AP et al. (1988) Characterisation of theophylline metabolism by human liver microsomes. Inhibition and immunochemical studies. Biochem Pharmacol 37:1651–1659

Ross D (1998) Quinone reductases. In Guengerich FP(ed) : Vol. 3, Comprehensive Toxicology, Elsevier Science, Oxford, pp. 179–197

Rotter JI, Diamond JM (1987) What maintains the frequencies of human genetic diseases? Nature 329:289–290

Saito K, Mori S, Tanda N, Sakamoto S (2000) Immunolocalization of c-*MYC* and *BCL2* proto-oncogene products in gingival hyperplasia induced by nifedipine and phenytoin. J Periodontol 71:44–49

Sassa S (2000) Hematologic aspects of the porphyrias. Int J Hematol 71:1–17

Schwarz D, Kisselev P, Schunck WH et al. (2000) Allelic variants of human cytochrome P450 IA1 (*CYP1A1*): effect of T461N and I462V substitutions on steroid hydroxylase specificity. Pharmacogenetics 10:519–530

Sellers EM, Tyndale RF (2000) Mimicking gene defects to treat drug dependence. Ann N Y Acad Sci 909:233–246

Sesardic D, Boobis AR, Edwards RJ, Davies DS (1988) A form of cytochrome P450 in man, orthologous to form d in the rat, catalyses the O-deethylation of phenacetin and is inducible by cigarette smoking. Br J Clin Pharmacol 26:363–372

Sesti F, Abbott GW, Wei J et al. (2000) A common polymorphism associated with antibiotic-induced cardiac arrhythmia. Proc Nat Acad Sci USA 97:10613–10618

Shih DM, Gu L, Xia YR et al. (1998) Mice lacking serum paraoxonase are susceptible to organophosphate toxicity and atherosclerosis. Nature 394:284–287

Shih DM, Xia YR, Wang XP et al. (2000) Combined serum paraoxonase knockout/apolipoprotein E knockout mice exhibit increased lipoprotein oxidation and atherosclerosis. J Biol Chem 275:17527–17535

Shimada T, Guengerich FP (1990) Inactivation of 1,3-, 1,6-, and 1,8-dinitropyrene by cytochrome P-450 enzymes in human and rat liver microsomes. Cancer Res 50:2036–2043

Shimada T, Hayes CL, Yamazaki H et al. (1996) Activation of chemically diverse procarcinogens by human cytochrome P-450 1B1. Cancer Res 56:2979–2984

Shimizu Y, Nakatsuru Y, Ichinose M et al. (2000) Benzo[a]pyrene carcinogenicity is lost in mice lacking the aryl hydrocarbon receptor. Proc Natl Acad Sci USA 97:779–782

Sinclair PR, Gorman N, Dalton T et al. (1998) Uroporphyria produced in mice by iron and 5-aminolaevulinic acid does not occur in Cyp1a2(-/-) null mutant mice. BiochemJ 330:149–153

Smart J, Daly AK (2000) Variation in induced CYP1A1 levels: Relationship to CYP1A1, Ah receptor and GSTM1 polymorphisms. Pharmacogenetics 10:11–24

Smith AG, Clothier B, Carthew P et al. (2001) Protection of the Cyp1a2(-/-) null mouse against uroporphyria and hepatic injury following dioxin exposure. Toxicol Appl Pharmacol, in press

Snawder JE, Lipscomb JC (2000) Interindividual variance of cytochrome P450 forms in human hepatic microsomes: Correlation of individual forms with xenobiotic metabolism and implications in risk assessment. Regul Toxicol Pharmacol 32:200–209

Snyder LH (1932) Studies in human inheritance. IX. The inheritance of taste deficiency in man. Ohio J Sci 32:436–468

Song N, Tan W, Xing D, Lin D (2001) CYP1A1 polymorphism and risk of lung cancer in relation to tobacco smoking: a case-control study in China. Carcinogenesis 22:11–16

Spracklin DK, Hankins DC, Fisher JM et al. (1997) Cytochrome P450 2E1 is the principal catalyst of human oxidative halothane metabolism in vitro. J Pharmacol Exp Ther 281:400–411

Streetman DS, Bertino JS Jr, Nafziger AN (2000) Phenotyping of drug-metabolizing enzymes in adults: a review of in-vivo cytochrome P450 phenotyping probes. Pharmacogenetics 10:187–216

Stubbins MJ, Harries LW, Smith G et al. (1996) Genetic analysis of the human cytochrome P450 CYP2C9 locus. Pharmacogenetics 6:429–439

Sullivan-Klose TH, Ghanayem BI, Bell DA et al. (1996) The role of the CYP2C9 Leu359 allelic variant in the tolbutamide polymorphism. Pharmacogenetics 6:341–349

Tahir E, Curran S, Yazgan Y et al. (2000) No association between low- and high-activity catecholamine-methyl-transferase (COMT) and attention deficit hyperactivity disorder (ADHD) in a sample of Turkish children. Am J Med Genet 96:285–288

Takahara S (1952) Progressive oral gangrene probably due to lack of catalase in the blood (acatalasemia)—report of nine cases. Lancet 2:1101–1104

Talas G, Brown RA, McGrouter DA (1999) Role of phenytoin in wound healing—a wound pharmacology perspective. Biochem Pharmacol 57:1085–1094

Tan EK, Khajavi M, Thornby JI et al. (2000) Variability and validity of polymorphism association studies in Parkinson disease. Neurology 55:533–538

Tang BK (1990) Drug glucosidation. Pharmacol Therap 46:53–56

Valentine JL, Lee SS, Seaton MJ et al. (1996) Reduction of benzene metabolism and toxicity in mice that lack CYP2E1 expression. Toxicol Appl Pharmacol 141:205–213

Varadi G, Strobeck M, Koch S et al. (1999) Molecular elements of ion permeation and selectivity within calcium channels. Crit Rev Biochem Mol Bio 34:181–214

Vasiliou V (2001) Aldehyde dehydrogenase gene superfamily. Web site: http://www.uchsc.edu/sp/sp/alcdbase/aldhcov.html/

Vasiliou V, Bairoch A, Tipton KF, Nebert DW (1999) Eukaryotic aldehyde dehydrogenase (ALDH) genes: human polymorphisms, and recommended nomenclature based on divergent evolution and chromosomal mapping. Pharmacogenetics 9:421–434

Vesell ES (1972) Pharmacogenetics. N Eng J Med 287:904–909

Vogel F (1959) Moderne probleme der Humangenetik. Ergeb Inn Med Kinderheilk 12:52–125

von Wartburg JP, Papenberg J, Aebi H (1965) An atypical human alcohol dehydrogenase. Can J Biochem 43:889–898

Waring RH, Mitchell SC, Fenwick GR (1987) The chemical nature of the urinary odour produced by man after asparagus ingestion. Xenobiotica 17:1363–1371

Weber WW (1997) Pharmacogenetics. OUP,

Wedlund PJ, Kimura S, Gonzalez FJ, Nebert DW (1994) 1462V mutation in the human CYP1A1 gene: lack of correlation with either the Msp 11.9 kb (M2) allele or CYP1A1 inducibility in a three-generation family of east Mediterranean descent. Pharmacogenetics 4:21–26

Weinshilboum RM, Otterness DM, Aksoy IA et al. (1997) Sulfation and sulfotransferases 1: Sulfotransferase molecular biology: cDNAs and genes. FASEB J 11:3–14

Weinshilboum RM, Otterness DM, Szumlanski CL (1999) Methylation pharmacogenetics: Catechol O-methyltransferase, thiopurine methyltransferase, and histamine N-methyltransferase. Annul Rev Pharmacol Toxicol 39:19–52

Wells PG, Kim PM, Laposa RR et al. (1997) Oxidative damage in chemical teratogenesis. Mutation Res 396:65–78

Whitlock JP Jr (1999) Induction of cytochrome P450 1A1. Annul Rev Pharmacol Toxicol 39:103–125

Wong JMY, Harper PA, Meyer UA et al. (2001) Ethnic variability in the allelic distribution of human aryl hyddrocarbon receptor codon-554 assessment of variant receptor function in vitro. Pharmacogenetics 11:85–94

Woolhouse NM, Andoh B, Mahgoub A et al. (1979) Debrisoquine hydroxylation polymorphism among Ghanaians and Caucasians. Clin Pharmacol Ther 26:584–591

Wright AF, Carothers AD, Pirastu M (1999) Population choice in mapping genes for complex diseases. Nat Genet 23:397–404

Xu ZH, Otterness DM, Freimuth RR et al. (2000) Human 3′-phosphoadenosine 5′-phosphosulfate synthetase-1 (PAPSS1) and PAPSS2: gene cloning, characterization and chromosomal localization. Biochem Biophys Res Comm 268:437–44

Yamazaki H, Nakano M, Gillam EM et al. (1996) Requirements for cytochrome b5 in the oxidation of 7-ethoxycoumarin, chlorzoxazone, aniline, and N-nitrosodimethylamine by recombinant cytochrome P450 2E1 and by human liver microsomes. Biochem Pharmacol 52:301–309

Yan L, Szumlanski CL, Rice SR et al. (2000a) Histamine N-methyltransferase functional polymorphism: Lack of association with schizophrenia. Am J Med Genet 96:404–406

Yan L, Galinsky RE, Bernstein JA et al. (2000b) Histamine N-methyltransferase pharmacogenetics: Association of a common functional polymorphism with asthma. Pharmacogenetics 10:261–266

Yasumori T, Chen LS, Li QH et al. (1999) Human CYP2C-mediated stereoselective phenytoin hydroxylation in Japanese: Difference in chiral preference of CYP2C9 and CYP2C19. Biochem Pharmacol 57:1297–1303

Yokoi T, Sawada M, Kamataki T (1995) Polymorphic drug metabolism: Studies with recombinant Chinese hamster cells and analyses in human populations. Pharmacogenetics 5:S65–S69

Yue QY, Svensson JO, Alm C et al. (1989) Interindividual and interethnic differences in the demethylation and glucuronidation of codeine. Br J Clin Pharmacol 28:629–637

Zhang ZY, Fasco MJ, Huang L et al. (1996) Characterization of purified human recombinant cytochrome P450 1A1-Ile462 and -Val462: assessment of a role for the rare allele in carcinogenesis. Cancer Res 56:3926–3933

Zhou LX, Pihlstrom B, Hardwick JP et al. (1996) Metabolism of phenytoin by the gingiva of normal humans: The possible role of reactive metabolites of phenytoin in the initiation of gingival hyperplasia. Clin Pharmacol Therap 60:191–198

GENERAL PRINCIPLES

Genetic assessment and pedigree analysis

22

Helen M. Kingston

Introduction

There are many facets to genetic counseling, including diagnosis, investigation, risk assessment, information-giving, supportive counseling, and follow-up. The process often involves many members of a family and relates to a variety of health and reproductive issues from preconception to adulthood. The following definitions encompass the essential elements of genetic counseling. "An educational process that seeks to assist affected, and/or at risk individuals to understand the nature of the genetic disorder, its transmission, and the options open to them in management and family planning," (Kelly, 1986). "Genetic counselling is the process by which patients at risk of a disorder that may be hereditary, are advised of the consequences of the disorder, the probability of developing and transmitting it, and of the ways in which this may be prevented or ameliorated" (Harper, 1993);

To achieve these aims, an accurate diagnosis and detailed information regarding the family history are essential. The basis for establishing a diagnosis depends on medical history, examination, and investigation. The diagnostic information is combined with information obtained from the family pedigree to determine the mode of inheritance of the disorder and to calculate the risk of recurrence, so that family members can be appropriately counseled.

Genetic assessment

The basic techniques of history-taking, examination, and appropriately directed investigations apply to genetic dis-

orders as they do in any other branch of medicine. A situation almost unique to medical genetics, however, is that the person presenting for genetic counseling may not necessarily be clinically affected. When the affected relative cannot be examined in person, his or her medical records are essential to provide the information needed to reach or confirm a diagnosis.

HISTORY

A history, together with the family pedigree, is the foundation of the diagnostic process. The medical history taken from the affected individual follows conventional lines, but the emphasis placed on particular aspects will vary with the presenting disorder. In assessing children with congenital malformations, for example, specific information is needed concerning parental health and age at conception, early pregnancy history, exposure to potential teratogens, fetal growth and movement, and detailed birth history. Direct questioning will elicit information relevant to the presenting disorder that is not spontaneously volunteered. Associated anomalies in other family members should be documented, such as the presence or absence of pigmentary abnormalities affecting the skin and hair, heterochromatic irides, telecanthus, and deafness, in the relatives of a child presenting with features suggesting Waardenburg syndrome. The age of onset of symptoms in affected relatives should be documented, together with the age reached by apparently unaffected relatives.

Sufficient time and a suitable environment need to be provided for taking a genetic history, bearing in mind that the presence of congenital abnormalities and genetic disorders place considerable emotional burdens on parents and relatives who may find the process of history-taking upsetting or threatening. Gathering information must be presented as an impartial process that is not judgmental, since subsequent counseling will be affected by the rapport established between the consultand and the counselor.

EXAMINATION

The affected individual or individuals should be seen and examined before genetic counseling is given, if possible. Asymptomatic relatives should also be examined for mild or early disease. Full physical examination is required, although the medical and family history will indicate organ systems or anatomic regions requiring particular attention. Genetic disorders can affect any body system, and the clinical geneticist may need to rely on information provided by specialists in other disciplines, such as ophthalmology and neurology, to complete the clinical evaluation of the patient. In this respect, joint clinics held with other specialists may be very beneficial.

In the assessment of dysmorphic syndromes, detailed examination is the cornerstone of diagnosis and entails careful search for both major and minor congenital abnormalities. A systematic approach to detecting and documenting malformations, deformations, and disruptions in anatomic zones is described by Aase (1990). Selected measurements are an essential part of the examination, and standard tables and graphs are available for growth parameters in conditions such as Down syndrome, achondroplasia, and Marfan syndrome (Hall et al., 1989), as well as for normal ranges of body proportion and facial measurements, including inner canthal and interpupillary distance, ear length, and palm length (Jones, 1997; Hall et al., 1989). Good quality clinical photographs constitute an important component of the medical records.

INVESTIGATION

Appropriate investigation of affected individuals and family members is essential if correct genetic advice is to be given. Investigation may determine the primary diagnosis in affected individuals, identify affected relatives or carriers, and provide prenatal diagnosis. Investigation of the affected person is directed along conventional lines, according to the presenting signs and symptoms, and includes tests required to make a diagnosis, direct therapy, and screen for the presence of associated abnormalities. Radiology and ultrasound, biochemical analysis, karyotyping, and molecular analysis are frequently used. Investigation of family members to detect other affected individuals or to identify carriers of a particular gene mutation is an integral part of

the diagnostic and counseling process, and is often crucial to the distinction between familial disorders and new mutations, as well as identifying whether the mode of inheritance is autosomal dominant or autosomal recessive. Investigation of the extended family may identify distant relatives who are at high risk of producing affected children in familial chromosomal rearrangements or X-linked-recessive disorders, while close relatives may be at low, or negligible, risk.

All clinical geneticists have faced situations in which they are asked to counsel family members about recurrence risk after the affected member has died, and neither essential investigation nor autopsy had been performed, which often precludes a definitive diagnosis. Complete investigation is particularly important in relation to therapeutic termination of pregnancy, stillbirth, and neonatal deaths where there may be a reluctance to pursue further investigation which might increase emotional stress for the parents. To provide accurate information for future pregnancies it is essential to document all abnormalities; photographic records are often very helpful in addition to radiology, karyotyping, and detailed autopsy. In cases where a diagnosis cannot be reached despite all appropriate investigations, long-term storage of samples such as DNA and cell lines should be considered, as they may enable future diagnosis.

DIAGNOSIS

The process of history-taking, examination, investigation, and pedigree analysis often enables a genetic diagnosis to be reached, and the mode of inheritance to be clearly defined. This forms the basis for further counseling and investigation of family members at risk. However, a firm diagnosis may not be reached despite careful and complete assessment of the affected individual and the family, and it is difficult to precisely identify risk of recurrence within families where there is only a single affected individual or knowledge of the particular disorder is incomplete.

Diagnosis of genetic disease may be complicated by pleiotropic gene action, which results in multiple phenotypic expressions of a single gene and diverse presentation of a particular disorder within a family. Figure 22.1 illustrates this situation in a family presenting with varying manifestations of von Hippel-Lindau disease, in whom careful evaluation of the pedigree identified the unifying diagnosis.

Many children with dysmorphic features have an unrecognized disorder, and reassessment of the child after a period of time may enable diagnosis as the features of the disorder evolve. To assign the wrong diagnosis is much more harmful than to admit uncertainty. An inaccurate

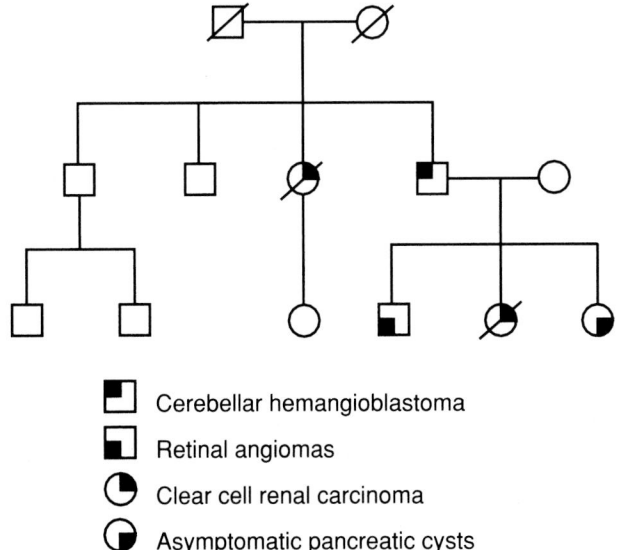

■ Cerebellar hemangioblastoma

◨ Retinal angiomas

◔ Clear cell renal carcinoma

◕ Asymptomatic pancreatic cysts

Fig. 22.1. Pedigree of a family presenting with different manifestations of von Hippel-Lindau disease.

symbols in pedigree construction, and the emergence of the pedigree as a central tool in eugenics. The use of the Mars (♂) and Venus (♀) symbols for males and females was already well established at the time of the Mendel's publications (Stern and Sherwood, 1966), and these symbols were incorporated into the pedigree style of Galton and Pearson (Pearson, 1912). The American Eugenics Record Office (ERO) adopted a pedigree style using square and circular symbols to represent males and females (Davenport, 1911), and the research committee of the Eugenics Education Society established in London, recognized the need for pedigree standardization and published guidelines recommending the use of these same symbols (Carr-Saunders et al., 1912–1913). This pedigree style was also used in Snyder's (1935) *The Principles of Heredity*, which was one of the earliest textbooks on human genetics.

Drawing a pedigree

The pedigree style currently used by most geneticists is very similar to that of the ERO, using, for example, the same symbols for consanguineous mating and twins with generations indicated by Roman numerals and individuals within each generation by Arabic numbers. Despite universal use of the pedigree as a method of recording information and as an analytical tool, there is still considerable variation in the use of symbols relating to both routine medical information (pregnancy, spontaneous abortion, and termination of pregnancy) and new reproductive technologies (artificial insemination by donor semen, donor ovum, and surrogate motherhood) (Bennett et al., 1993).

An example of a family pedigree is shown in Figure 22.2, using the symbols illustrated in Figure 22.3 and the working pedigree, containing further details, shown in Figure 22.4. When drawing a pedigree it is usually simplest to start with the person seeking advice (the *consultand*). Pedigree details are then completed for both sides of the family, including previous and subsequent generations. Conventionally, the paternal lineage is placed on the left and the maternal lineage on the right. Within sibships, individuals are listed from left to right in birth order. The affected person (*proband*), through whom the family has been ascertained, should be indicated by an arrow. The proband will not always be the consultand, who is often an apparently healthy relative seeking information about how the condition may affect him or her or their offspring.

Name, date of birth, and a summary of their medical details should be recorded for all family members. Further information, including medical records, will be required for affected individuals. Not all relevant information may be

diagnosis leads to false confidence, may prevent the detection of associated problems, and could result in erroneous advice being given about recurrence risk on which couples may base important reproductive decisions. The ability to discuss such cases with colleagues and consult databases (Bankier, 2000; Baraitser and Winter, 2000; Winter and Baraitser, 2000; Winter et al., 1984) is important. Literature searches can be performed via the Internet using Medline and a catalogue of known human mendelian characters, OMIM (Online Mendelian Inheritance in Man), created by Victor McKusick, is also accessible on the world wide web and as a book (McKusick, 1998).

PEDIGREE CONSTRUCTION

Accurate documentation of the family history is an essential part of genetic assessment, and the best method of recording this information is by constructing a family pedigree. Pedigrees are universally used in patients' genetic records, journal articles, and textbooks as the means of relaying information in an easily interpreted visual format. Pedigrees also provide the basis for calculations required for both recurrence risk estimation in individual families and linkage analysis in gene-mapping studies.

Historical aspects

The origin of the modern pedigree in human genetics has been reviewed by Resta (1993), tracing the function of the pedigree in genealogy, biology and sociology, the use of

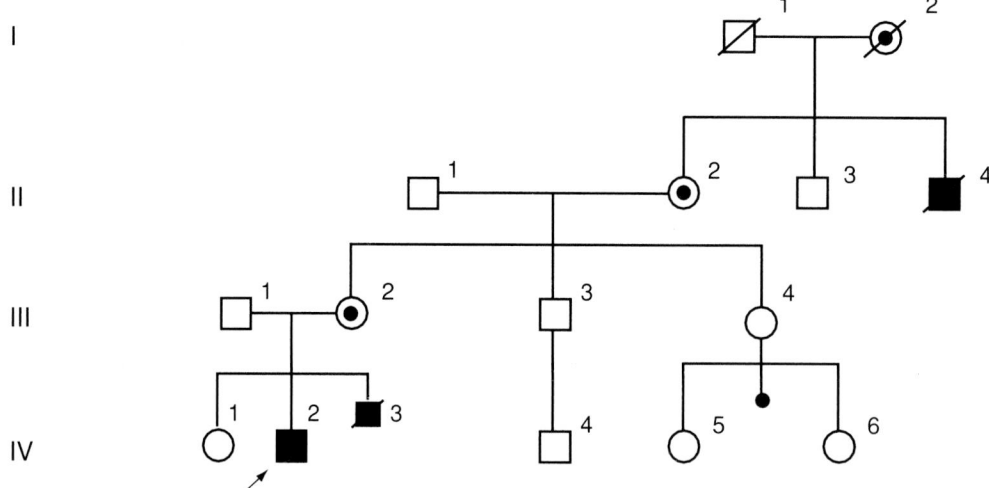

Fig. 22.2. Example of a formal pedigree illustrating X-linked-recessive inheritance of Duchenne muscular dystrophy.

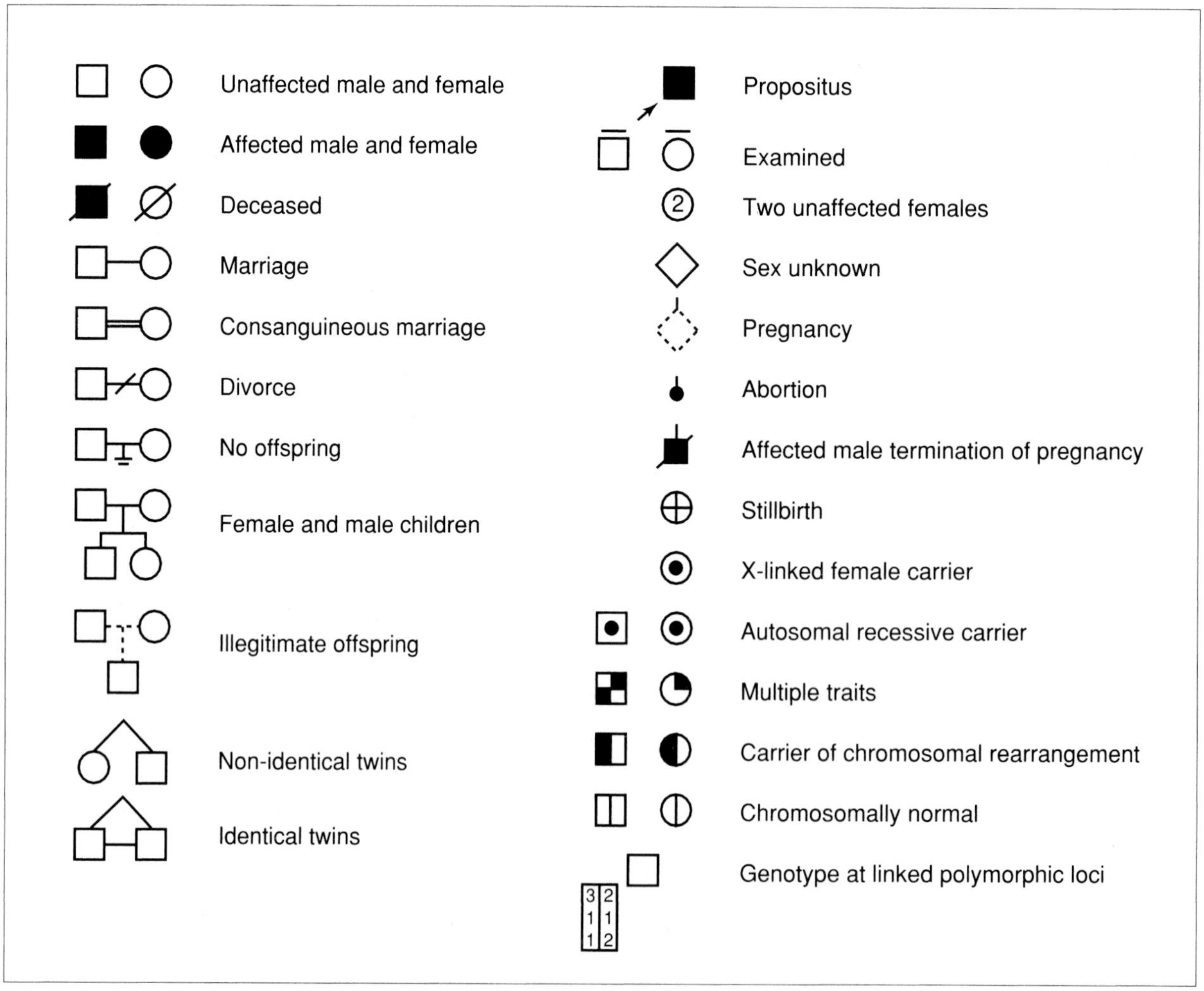

□ ○	Unaffected male and female	■ Propositus
■ ●	Affected male and female	□̶ ō̶ Examined
◪ ⊘	Deceased	② Two unaffected females
□⊢○	Marriage	◇ Sex unknown
□⊨○	Consanguineous marriage	◇ Pregnancy
□⊬○	Divorce	• Abortion
□⊤○	No offspring	◪ Affected male termination of pregnancy
	Female and male children	⊕ Stillbirth
		⊙ X-linked female carrier
	Illegitimate offspring	▣ ⊙ Autosomal recessive carrier
	Non-identical twins	◩ ◓ Multiple traits
	Identical twins	◧ ◑ Carrier of chromosomal rearrangement
		▯ ◒ Chromosomally normal
		□ Genotype at linked polymorphic loci

Fig. 22.3. Symbols commonly used in drawing a pedigree.

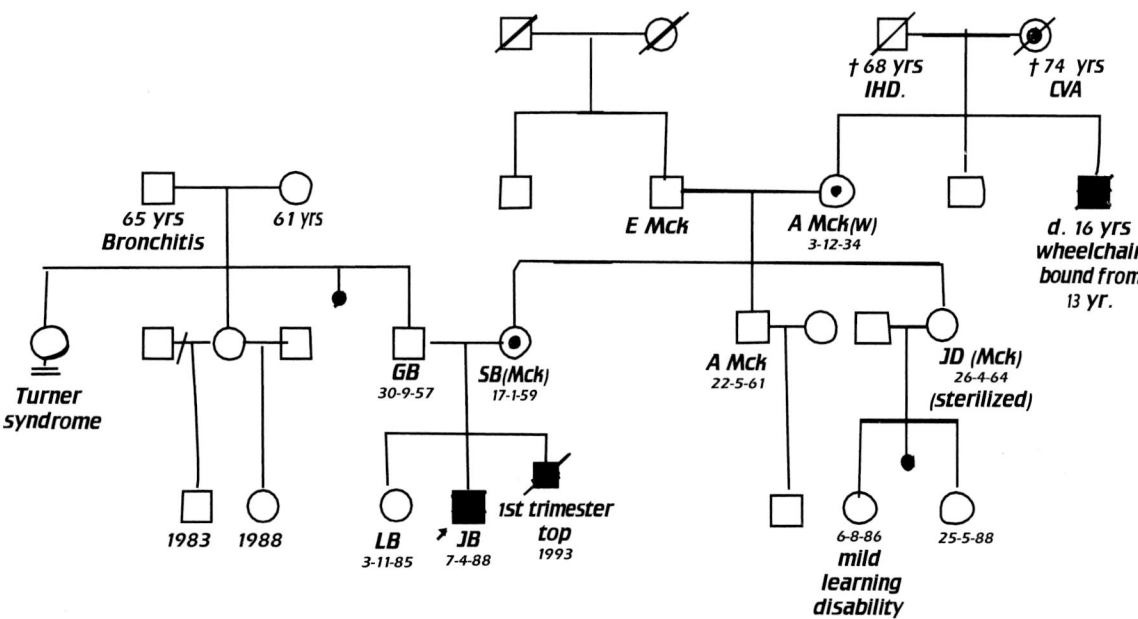

Fig. 22.4. Example of the working pedigree recording family data, from which the pedigree in Figure 22.2 was constructed.

volunteered by the consultand, indeed certain sensitive information – such as a previous termination of pregnancy or illegitimacy – may be deliberately withheld if the accompanying partner is not aware of it. Important details that should be asked about include assisted conception, previous miscarriages, stillbirths, terminations, children adopted into or out of the family, and consanguinity. Ethnic origin should be recorded, since some genetic conditions are more prevalent in particular ethnic groups, and this information may provide a clue to the likely diagnosis. The family history should be completed on both sides of the family for a consultand couple, even if the presenting condition is clearly traced to one side, since unrelated pregnancy losses or handicapping disorders may have occurred on the other side of the family that could have greater reproductive impact for the couple than the disorder for which they are seeking information.

VERIFICATION OF PEDIGREE INFORMATION

After a pedigree has been drawn up, it is necessary to check the accuracy of the information to avoid errors when calculating recurrence risks. A stated diagnosis needs to be confirmed either by examination of the affected person or by consulting medical records, the importance of which is illustrated by the pedigree example shown in Figure 22.5. The family history given by the consultand (II_4) was based on information provided by her sister (II_1) and indicated

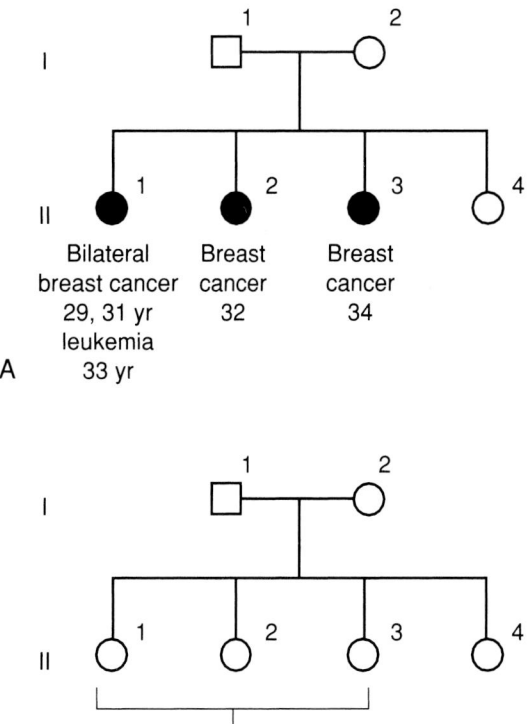

Fig. 22.5. (A) Family pedigree based on information supplied by II_1, **(B)** Family pedigree revised after consulting hospital records (see text).

that she was at high risk for developing breast cancer. The consultand's relatives were contacted and their hospital records obtained. The diagnosis of cancer was not confirmed in any of them, but a diagnosis of both Munchausen

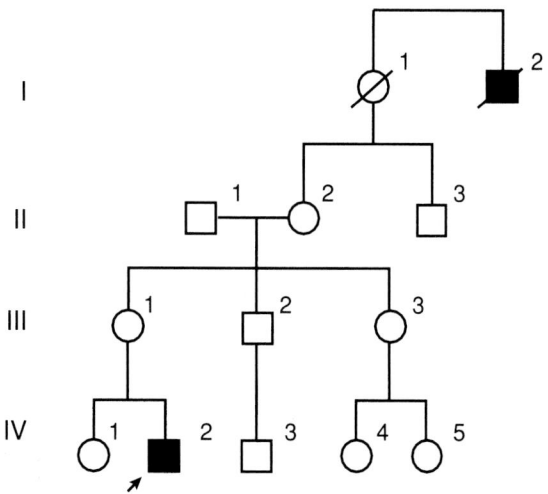

Fig. 22.6. Family pedigree of proband (IV₂) with Becker muscular dystrophy. The risk of carrier status in individual II₂ is affected by the presumptive diagnosis of Becker muscular dystrophy in individual I₂ (see text).

syndrome and Munchausen syndrome by proxy in II₁ became apparent. The consultand's risk of developing breast cancer was therefore no greater than the general population risk (Evans et al., 1996; Kerr et al., 1998).

Problems are encountered when an affected individual is no longer living and medical records cannot be traced. Policies regarding the storage of medical records vary from hospital to hospital in the United Kingdom. Some records are stored long term, others are stored on microfilm or microfiche, but in some cases files are destroyed after a period of time without a permanent record. An example of how this may affect counseling is shown in Figure 22.6. The proband (IV₂) was referred with a diagnosis of Becker muscular dystrophy based on clinical presentation, muscle biopsy, histology, and dystrophin analysis. The mutation within the dystrophin gene was not identified by DNA analysis. Individual I₂ had died at the age of 52, having been confined to a wheelchair for several years. No diagnosis had been reached in this individual who had died before Becker muscular dystrophy was delineated as a distinct disorder by Becker and Kiener in 1955. No medical records could be traced for this individual, and uncertainty about his diagnosis affected the assessment of carrier status in several female family members. Assuming that individual IV₂ was an isolated case, investigation of the family incorporating serum creatine kinase activity and DNA linkage analysis indicated that his maternal grandmother (II₂) had a 2% risk of carrier status. However, if individual I₂ is assumed to have had Becker muscular dystrophy also, then individual II₂ is an obligate carrier, and risks to individuals III₃, IV₄, and IV₅ are substantially increased.

Pedigree analysis

With the advent of mutation analysis in an increasing number of genetic disorders, risks to individuals may be identified in absolute terms. In many cases, however, risks are expressed in terms of probabilities or odds calculated from pedigree data, and these estimates of risk are transmitted to families as part of the counseling process. Careful evaluation of the pedigree and consideration of all possible modes of inheritance is crucial to accurate risk assessment.

COMMON MISCONCEPTIONS

It is important to recognize that there are many potential misconceptions concerning genetic disorders and risks that need to be identified and rectified to ensure that families understand the information they are given and can use it appropriately. Some common misconceptions and misinterpretations are as follows:

1. All genetic disorders are inherited and have a high recurrence risk.
2. All genetic disorders and their carrier state can be detected by chromosome analysis.
3. Absence of other affected members indicates that a disorder is not genetic/inherited.
4. A pattern observed in a family will be maintained, i.e., only females affected, even though the disorder is autosomal dominant.
5. Sex-linked inheritance must apply if only males or females are affected in the family.
6. A 1 in 4 recurrence risk means that only 1 of 4 children will be affected, and if the first child is affected, the next three will be unaffected.
7. A 1 in 20 risk for recurrence is interpreted as a 1 in 20 chance of a healthy child.
8. Confusion of odds, fractions, and percentage risks.
9. Confusion of carrier risk with risk of an affected child.
10. Physical or emotional upsets during pregnancy cause malformations.
11. Scientific explanations may be acknowledged but overruled by cultural beliefs.

It is important to remember that perception of risk may vary greatly. A 5% risk may be perceived as low by one individual, but unacceptably high by another. In general, perception of risk is affected by severity of the disorder. A high risk of a mild or treatable disorder may be accepted, whereas a low risk of a severe disorder has greater impact on reproductive decisions. It is often helpful to put risks into context by comparing them with the general population risk for the particular disorder, or the overall risk of 2% that any pregnancy might result in the birth of a child with a congenital or genetic abnormality.

HETEROGENEITY

One of the major problems encountered when assessing risk for genetic counseling is the occurrence of genetic heterogeneity (Childs and Der Kaloustian, 1968). This is the phenomenon by which a clinical phenotype results from different genetic defects, representing either mutations at separate loci (locus heterogeneity) or different mutations at a single locus (allelic heterogeneity). Heterogeneity may be detected by subtle differences in phenotype or documentation of different patterns of inheritance, but confirmation often relies on biochemical, physiologic, or molecular genetic analysis.

Different modes of inheritance have been documented for a number of clinically defined disorders with similar phenotypes. Autosomal-dominant, autosomal-recessive, and X-linked-recessive inheritance have been documented in hereditary spastic paraplegia (HSP) (Zatz et al., 1976; Harding, 1981), Charcot-Marie-Tooth disease (CMT) (also known as hereditary motor and sensory neuropathy) (Vance, 1991; Patel and Lupski, 1994), and retinitis pigmentosa (Inglehearn, 1998), for example. In addition, linkage studies and mutation analysis have demonstrated locus heterogeneity within the autosomal-dominant forms of HSP (Hazan et al., 1993; Fink et al., 1996) and CMT (Patell and Lupski, 1994; Nelis et al., 1999), as well as a number of other disorders, including tuberous sclerosis (The European Chromosome 16 Tuberous Sclerosis Consortium, 1993; Nellist et al., 1993; Janssen et al., 1994; Van-Slegtenhorst et al., 1997), adult polycystic kidney disease (Reeders et al., 1985; Peters et al., 1993; Coto et al., 1995), and malignant hyperthermia (Levitt et al., 1991; Deufel et al., 1992; Robinson et al., 1998). Locus heterogeneity is also well documented in recessive disorders such as HSP (Coutinho et al., 1999), and severe congenital deafness, in which the absence of affected offspring to parents who both have phenotypically identical autosomal-recessive deafness indicates the existence of separate loci (McKusick, 1992). Similar heterogeneity is observed in X-linked-recessive disorders, for example, X-linked retinitis pigmentosa (Chen et al., 1989; Teague et al., 1994; Bergen et al., 1995). The presence of genetic heterogeneity makes it difficult to determine risks of recurrence for disorders that follow both dominant and recessive inheritance if the mode of inheritance is not clearly defined by the family pedigree.

Linkage analysis within families is also complicated by locus heterogeneity, since demonstration of linkage between a polymorphic marker and the disease in a particular family does not necessarily prove that a mutation at the same locus is responsible.

Heterogeneity of disease causing mutations is the rule rather than the exception, and is clearly illustrated by the numerous mutations detected in the β-globin, cystic fibrosis, and collagen genes. This allelic heterogeneity complicates the identification of the underlying mutation in a particular affected individual. Phenotypic variation may also be attributed to allelic heterogeneity of mutations at a single locus. Hurler and Scheie syndromes are allelic variations of α-L-iduronidase deficiency (McKusick et al., 1972) and Duchenne and Becker muscular dystrophy, initially thought to be separate disorders, are both attributable to a variety of mutations with varying effect occurring within the dystrophin gene at Xp21 (Hoffmann et al., 1987; Monaco et al., 1988). Different mutations affecting the peripheral myelin protein (PMP 22) gene at 17p11.2 also result in different phenotypes, with CMT type 1A and hereditary neuropathy with liability to pressure palsies (HNPP) likely to be due to overexpression and underexpression of the gene, respectively (Patel and Lupski, 1994). In some cases different mutations within a single gene cause quite distinct phenotypes, for example, testicular feminization and Kennedy syndrome (X-linked spinobulbar muscular atrophy) are due to different mutations in the androgen receptor gene (La Spada et al., 1991; Griffin, 1992).

AUTOSOMAL-DOMINANT INHERITANCE

In families presenting with an autosomal-dominant disorder and a classical pedigree, as illustrated in Figure 22.7, mode of inheritance and risks of recurrence are easy to identify. The risk to each child of an affected individual is 50% regardless of sex, and the risk to children of unaffected relatives is not increased above the general population risk. In clinical practice, many factors influence the expression of dominantly transmitted genes and have an effect on estimation of risk. These include late or variable onset, reduced penetrance, variable expressivity, and gonadal mosaicism.

Late or variable onset

Problems are encountered in genetic counseling for disorders that have late or variable onset because it is difficult to know at what age unaffected persons can be reassured that they will not subsequently develop the disorder. This is

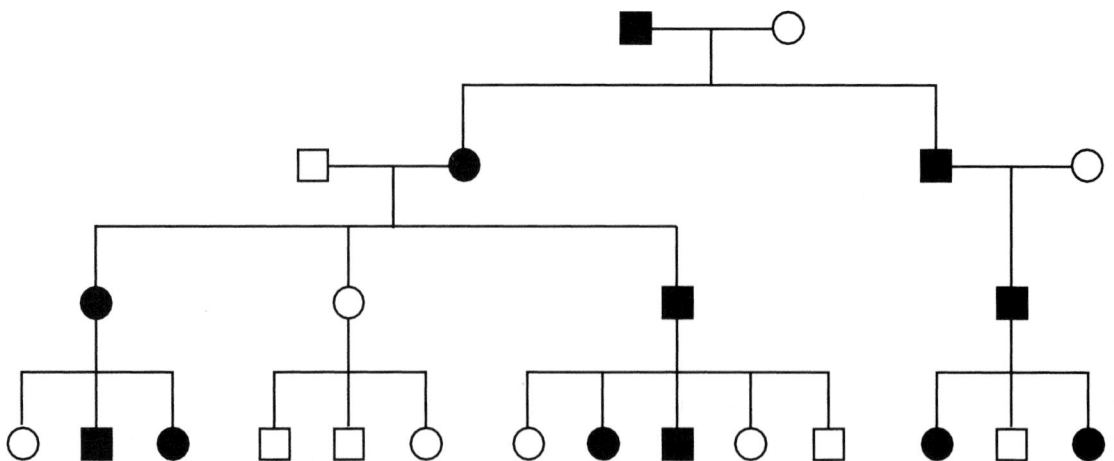

Fig. 22.7. Pedigree demonstrating typical autosomal-dominant inheritance of a disorder with transmission by affected males and females to offspring of both sexes.

particularly relevant to apparently healthy young adults at risk who wish to know their own genetic status before making reproductive decisions. Life tables to aid genetic counseling have been produced for Huntington's disease (Harper et al., 1979; Harper and Newcombe, 1992), which indicate the probability that a person possessing the gene will develop the disorder at a given age, and the risk of a healthy relative carrying the Huntington gene at different ages. Following the identification of an unstable CAG trinucleotide expansion in the Huntington disease gene, Brinkman et al., (1997) determined the likelihood of being affected by the disease by a particular age, for a specific CAG size. For many disorders, however, there is too much variation or too few data to enable the use of a disease specific life table. The uncertainty of a person's genetic status for late onset disorders may be overcome by the increasing availability of presymptomatic genetic testing, which can be achieved either by direct mutation analysis, as in Huntington disease (Harper, 1993), myotonic dystrophy (Suthers et al., 1992), and Charcot-Marie-Tooth disease (Patel and Lupski, 1994) or by linkage analysis, as in adult polycystic kidney disease (Elles et al., 1994).

Reduced penetrance

The penetrance of a gene relates to the proportion of individuals carrying the mutant gene who manifest the disorder. A small number of autosomal-dominant disorders demonstrate reduced penetrance, in which individuals known to carry the gene by virtue of having an affected parent and child remain unaffected themselves. Careful examination of apparently nonpenetrant individuals may reveal minor manifestations of the disorder, as in tuberous

sclerosis (Northrup et al., 1993) or biochemical abnormality in clinically unaffected individuals with acute porphyria (Waldenstrom, 1956). Age is also a relevant factor in penetrance, some disorders showing increasing penetrance with age, as in Huntington disease (Harper and Newcombe, 1992) and familial adenomatous polyposis (Evans et al., 1993), and others showing reducing penetrance, as in petit mal epilepsy (Metrakos and Metrakos, 1961). The various mechanisms underlying lack of penetrance are likely to be elucidated by molecular analysis. In familial retinoblastoma, for example, a somatic mutation affecting the normal retinoblastoma allele is required for tumor to develop in an individual inheriting the mutation in the heterozygous state (Knudson, 1971; Cavenee, 1986).

The penetrance (P) of a disorder is usually expressed as a proportion or percentage of the individuals carrying the gene who develop the disorder. If the P value is known for a particular condition, the risk to the offspring of an apparently unaffected individual can be calculated (Aylesworth and Kirkman, 1979; Pauli and Motulsky, 1981). In practice, the risk is usually less than 10%, since an unaffected relative is not likely to carry the gene if the penetrance is high, and a gene carrier is not likely to develop the disorder if the penetrance is low.

Variable expressivity

Expressivity relates to the degree to which an affected person manifests a particular disorder. Some autosomal-dominant disorders, such as achondroplasia, demonstrate virtually no variability, but this is an exception rather than the rule. Indeed, some disorders previously thought to represent separate conditions, such as familial adenomatous polyposis and Gardner syndrome, result from the variable effect of the same mutation within a single gene (Nishisho et al., 1991). The variability seen in autosomal-dominant disorders may present as both inter- and intrafamilial differences. Intrafamilial variability may reflect the action of modifying genes, as suggested for neurofibromatosis type 1 (Ponder et al., 1991), but interfamilial variability is more likely to be due to allelic heterogeneity at a single locus. A problem encountered in genetic counseling is that a mildly affected individual, such as a parent with only skin manifestations of tuberous sclerosis, may have a severely affected child. This situation is seen in other autosomal-dominant disorders, in that the mildly affected individuals are more likely to reproduce. Occasionally the mild phenotype will represent somatic mosaicism for the mutation in the affected individual, having arisen as a de novo post zygotic event. In the rare situations where homozygosity for dominant genes may occur, the phenotype is generally more severe with earlier onset (Pauli, 1983), as is demonstrated in homozygous familial hypercholesterolemia and achondroplasia. Huntington disease, however, is a notable exception in that an affected homozygote appears to be clinically indistinguishable from a heterozygote (Wexler et al., 1987).

Other factors that may contribute to phenotypic variability in autosomal-dominant disorders include sex-modifying genes, other modifying alleles, and environmental agents such as drugs and diet.

Anticipation

The variation seen in some autosomal-dominant disorders reflects an increase in severity in successive generations of a family. This phenomenon of anticipation is well recognized in myotonic dystrophy and has its basis in the unstable nature of the underlying mutation, which consists of a CTG trinucleotide repeat expansion (Aslanidis et al., 1992; Buxton et al., 1992; Harley et al., 1992). The size of the expansion can change between generations and generally correlates with severity of phenotype, the largest expansion being observed in maternally transmitted congenital cases. An unstable trinucleotide repeat expansion (CAG) is also the mutation underlying Huntington disease (the Huntington disease Collaborative Research Group, 1993). The size of the expansion again correlates with age of onset, but is not absolutely predictive in individual cases (Harper, 1993b; Trottier et al., 1994). Other autosomal-dominant disorders found to be due to a trinucleotide repeat expansion, in which the size of repeat correlates with the age of disease onset are dentatorubropallidoluysian atrophy (Koide et al., 1994; Nagafuchi et al., 1994), spinocerebellar ataxia (SCA) type 1 (Orr et al., 1993), SCA type 2 (Imbert et al., 1996; Pulst et al., 1996; Sanpei et al., 1996), SCA type 3 (Machado-Joseph disease) (Kawaguchi et al., 1994), SCA type 6 (Zhuchenko et al., 1997), SCA 7 (Abbas et al., 1997) and SCA 8 (Koob et al., 1999).

Genomic imprinting

Genomic imprinting is a phenomenon in which gene expression depends on parental origin (Surani, 1986; Hall, 1990). This modifies the transmission and expression of certain genetic diseases and should be borne in mind as a possible mechanism underlying disorders that do not follow typical mendelian inheritance. Imprinting is the likely explanation for the exclusive paternal transmission of familial dominant glomus tumors (van der Mey et al., 1989), the maternal transmission of familial cases of Angelman syndrome (Meijers-Heijboer et al., 1992; Chan et al., 1993) and the preponderance of maternal transmission in Beckwith–Wiedemann syndrome (Moutou et al., 1992; Schneid et al., 1993) and Albright's hereditary osteodystrophy (Davies and Hughes, 1993).

New mutations and gonadal mosaicism

De novo mutations are common in some autosomal-dominant disorders, and account for up to 80% of cases of achondroplasia, 50% of cases of neurofibromatosis type 1, and 60% of cases of tuberous sclerosis. Recurrence risks for the parents of isolated cases due to new mutation are not increased. However, if the disorder shows reduced penetrance and one parent is an unaffected heterozygote, or if one parent carries the mutation in mosaic form confined to germline cells, the recurrence risk will be increased – although less than 50%.

AUTOSOMAL-RECESSIVE INHERITANCE

In autosomal-recessive disorders the difficulty lies not with risk estimation, but in determining the underlying mode of inheritance, since these disorders usually present as isolated cases with little contributory information gleaned from the pedigree. Recurrence risk for the parents of a child with an autosomal-recessive disorder is 25%. Carrier risks to other relatives can be calculated from the pedigree, and carrier testing may be appropriate for disorders with a high gene frequency or when consanguineous marriages are planned. The risk to members of the extended family for having an affected child will depend on their own risk calculated from pedigree data and the population-based carrier risk appropriate to their

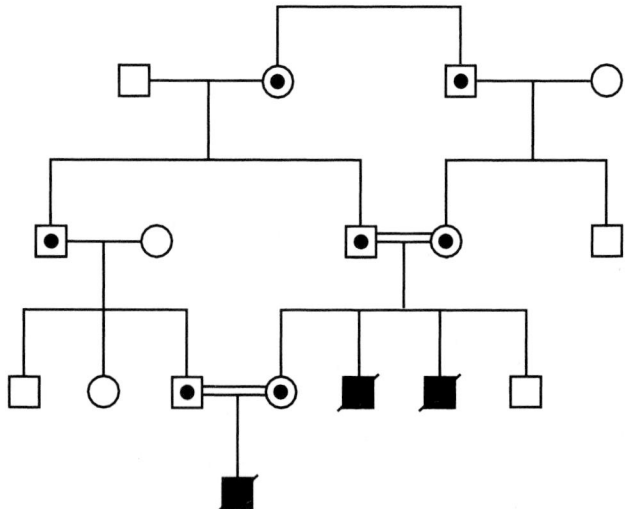

Fig. 22.8. Pedigree demonstrating occurrence of an autosomal-recessive inborn error of metabolism in separate sibships due to multiple consanguinity, giving the appearance of X-linked-recessive inheritance.

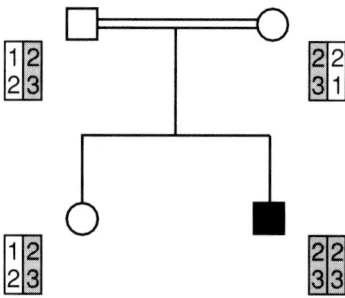

Fig. 22.9. Pedigree depicting inheritance of spinal muscular atrophy from consanguineous parents and haplotype with DNA markers at 5q13.

spouse. Higher risks in consanguineous marriages are dependent on the degree of relationship between the partners. In disorders of unknown genetic etiology, consanguinity suggests, but does not prove, an autosomal-recessive mode of inheritance. Extensive consanguinity within a family in which an autosomal-recessive mutation is segregating may give the appearance of autosomal-dominant or X-linked-recessive inheritance if an affected or carrier individual marries another carrier (Fig. 22.8). In rare autosomal-recessive disorders, a greater proportion of cases are observed in the offspring of consanguineous marriages, and inbred populations, such as the Amish of North America, may be notable for rare recessive disorders (McKusick, 1978).

On the assumption that everyone carries one gene for a serious nonlethal autosomal-recessive disorder, there is a 1 in 32 chance that the child of a first-cousin union will be homozygous by descent for a recessive gene derived from a common grandparent. In the affected offspring of consanguineous parents, the detection of homozygosity for several closely linked polymorphic markers can be useful in localizing autosomal-recessive genes by "homozygosity mapping" (Lander and Botstein, 1987; Pollak et al., 1993). In a given family, homozygosity for a tightly-linked marker at a particular locus, for example, the spinal muscular atrophy locus, in the affected offspring of consanguineous parents provides evidence that the causative mutation is at that locus (Fig. 22.9) and validated the use of linked markers in prenatal diagnosis prior to the identification of SMN gene deletions as the underlying cause of childhood onset SMA.

In exceptional cases, a recessive disorder may be due to uniparental isodisomy, resulting in a child inheriting two copies of a single parental chromosome carrying the mutant gene. This has been described, for example, in cystic fibrosis with maternal isodisomy for chromosome 7 (Spence et al., 1988; Voss et al., 1989) and chronic spinal muscular atrophy with paternal isodisomy for chromosome 5 (Suslak et al., 1993). The recurrence risk in these situations would be negligible. An autosomal-recessive disorder may potentially be due to the inheritance of a mutation from one parent, with a de novo mutation occurring at the same locus on the chromosome inherited from the other parent. This is likely to be a very rare phenomenon, but accounts for some cases of spinal muscular atrophy due to a predisposition to generate deletions in the 5q13 region involving the SMN gene (Melki et al., 1994; Rodrigues et al., 1995). The recurrence risk in this situation would relate to the risk of repeated de novo mutation. In other instances, the occurrence of two affected children with normal parents, suggesting autosomal-recessive inheritance, may actually be due to parental gonadal mosaicism for a dominant mutation, as described in lethal osteogenesis imperfecta (Cohen et al., 1990), or due to maternal disease as in recurrent congenital heart block in the offspring of mothers with systemic lupus erythematosis (Chameides et al., 1977; McCue et al., 1977) or congenital arthrogryposis associated with maternal myasthenia gravis (Dinger and Prager, 1993).

Recessive disorders demonstrate less variation in expression than autosomal-dominant disorders, and lack of penetrance is rare. Most variability appears to be due to genetic heterogeneity involving multiple alleles at a single locus, as in cystic fibrosis, or multiple loci, as in congenital deafness.

X-LINKED INHERITANCE

X-linked-recessive inheritance can be readily recognized from a characteristic pedigree, such as the one shown in Figure 22.10 with multiple affected males in different sibships. Male-to-male transmission never occurs, and the disorder does not recur in the descendants of unaffected

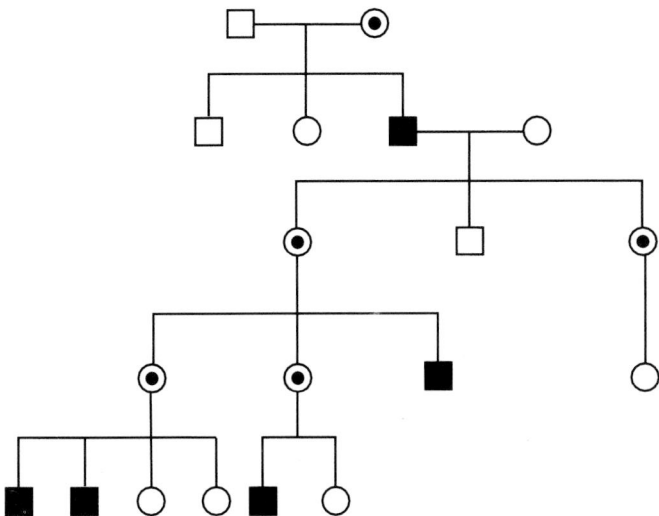

Fig. 22.10. Typical X-linked-recessive pedigree demonstrating inheritance of retinitis pigmentosa.

males, although a notable exception to this is the fragile X syndrome in which unaffected transmitting males carry a pre-mutation that can be transmitted through obligate carrier daughters to affected grandsons (Fu et al., 1991). For women carrying X-linked-recessive mutations, there is a 50% risk for sons being affected and for daughters being carriers. When affected males reproduce, all their daughters are obligate carriers, but sons are unaffected. X-linked-dominant or -intermediate inheritance is more difficult to identify, since the pedigree may contain both affected males and females and can appear to resemble autosomal-dominant inheritance (Fig. 22.11). In general, females are less severely affected than males, as seen, for example, in Coffin–Lowry syndrome, X-linked hypophosphatemia, and X-linked hereditary motor and sensory neuropathy. X-linked-dominant inheritance with lethality in males gives rise to pedigrees in which only females

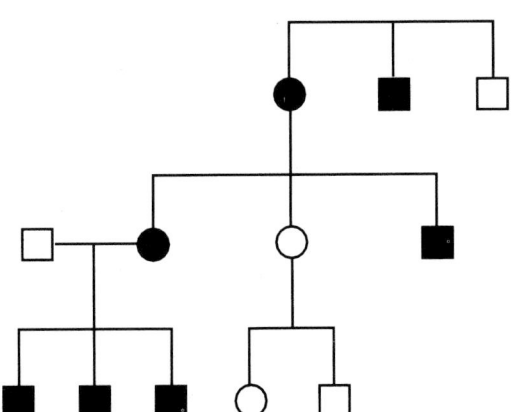

Fig. 22.11. Pedigree of X-linked Charcot-Marie-Tooth neuropathy with mild disease in heterozygous females simulating autosomal-dominant inheritance.

are affected, with an overall excess of females (female: male ratio, 2:1) due to early loss of affected male pregnancies (Wettke-Schäfer and Kantner, 1983). Examples of these disorders include orofaciodigital syndrome type I, focal dermal hypoplasia, and incontinentia pigmenti. In Rett syndrome, affected females do not reproduce and usually present as sporadic cases. Mutations in the X-linked MECP2 gene, which acts as a transcription regulator, have been found in girls with Rett syndrome (Amir et al., 1999).

In X-linked-recessive disorders, heterozygous females are generally unaffected, but careful clinical examination and investigation may reveal subtle abnormalities, such as the presence of pigmentary retinal changes in female carriers of X-linked retinitis pigmentosa. Some heterozygous females will manifest symptoms of the disorder due to unequal lyonization. Approximately 8% of female carriers of Duchenne muscular dystrophy are manifesting carriers (Moser and Emery, 1974) and lyonization explains the patchy expression of dystrophin demonstrated in muscle biopsies taken from manifesting carriers (Arahata et al., 1989). In some cases, fully affected females occur due to the concomitant presence of Turner syndrome (Ferrier et al., 1965) or an X/autosome translocation (Emery, 1994) disrupting the gene at Xp21 on the X chromosome that remains preferentially activated by virtue of its translocation to an autosome.

Pedigree analysis in families with more than one affected male enables the identification of obligate carriers. These are females who have an affected son and another affected maternal male relative, or who are daughters of an affected male. The prior genetic risk can be calculated for other female relatives, as shown in Figure 22.12. These risks can be incorporated into a bayesian calculation with other conditional pedigree information and the results of specific carrier tests as described in Chapter 25. Isolated cases of X-linked-recessive disorders require careful assessment, since they may be due to transmission of a mutant gene from an asymptomatic carrier mother associated with high recurrence risks, arise by new mutation with negligible recurrence risk, or represent gonadal mosaicism in the mother.

Mutations arising during meiosis may occur in male or female germ cells. If a particular mutation occurs largely in male germ cells, as in Lesch–Nyhan syndrome (Francke et al., 1976) and hemophilia A (Bröcker-Vriends et al., 1991) the majority of mothers of affected boys will be carriers and risks to sisters will be 50% regardless of how many unaffected brothers they have. In Duchenne muscular dystrophy the overall mutation rate appears to be equal in males and females, but most point mutations appear to occur in spermatogenesis, while most deletions arise in

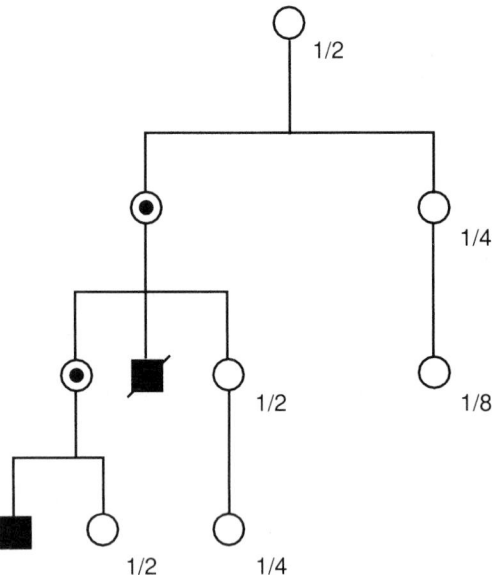

Fig. 22.12. Pedigree of Duchenne muscular dystrophy indicating obligate carrier females and the prior risk to other female relatives.

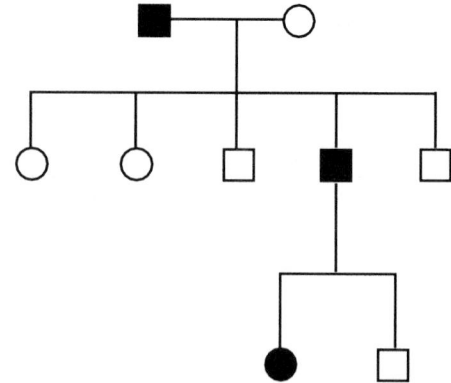

Fig. 22.13. Clustering of cases of cleft lip and palate in a family, suggesting autosomal-dominant inheritance.

oogenesis (Grimm et al., 1994). In isolated cases the recurrence risk is therefore higher in nondeletion cases, since these mothers are more likely to be carriers. A similar difference between male and female mutation rates is also seen in hemophilia B with a high male mutation rate for point mutations (Ketterling et al., 1993).

Mutations occurring during mitosis result in germline, somatic, or gonosomatic mosaicism. Maternal germline mosaicism is associated with an increased risk of recurrence for the mother of an isolated case, a phenomenon that appears to be relatively common in Duchenne muscular dystrophy (Bakker et al., 1989; Passos-Bueno et al., 1992; Van Essen et al., 1992) and has been reported in other disorders (Bröcker-Vriends et al., 1990). Gonadal mosaicism in healthy males is the most likely mechanism for transmission of a pathogenic mutation by a healthy male to more than one daughter (Darras and Francke, 1987).

MULTIFACTORIAL INHERITANCE

A large group of relatively common disorders have a considerable genetic predisposition, but do not follow clear-cut patterns of inheritance within families. These include many birth defects and chronic diseases of later life. Liability to these disorders appears to be due to the interaction of several genetic and environmental influences. Clusters of cases within a family may simulate a mendelian pattern of inheritance (Fig. 23.13). It is often difficult to be precise about recurrence risks in multifactorial disorders. The risk is greatest among first-degree relatives, is usually small for second-degree relatives, and often does not exceed the general population risk for third-degree relatives. The risk increases when multiple family members are affected. Risks are also affected by the incidence of the disorder in the general population and the sex of the patient and relatives in disorders that have unequal sex incidence, such as pyloric stenosis and Hirschsprung disease. The severity of the disorder also influences risk, for example, the recurrence risk is greater for bilateral cleft lip and palate than for unilateral cleft lip alone (Carter et al., 1982).

In many disorders, empirical risks have been derived from family studies that provide data on observed recurrences, as exemplified by Carter's (1961) original studies on pyloric stenosis. Risks derived in this way will be less accurate in disorders that are genetically heterogeneous and may not be applicable to populations different from those in which the family studies were performed. Nevertheless, empirical risks provide a useful basis for discussing levels of risk during genetic counseling. Risk tables for some of the common congenital malformations, such as cleft lip, with or without cleft palate, pyloric stenosis, and neural tube defects have been published (Bonaiti-Pellié and Smith, 1974), and empirical risk figures for a variety of disorders following multifactorial inheritance are given by Harper (1998).

When empirical data are not available, assessment of risk can be based on theoretical models in which the frequency of the disorder, its heritability (genetic as opposed to environmental predisposition), and the type and number of relatives affected are incorporated into the risk calculation (Smith, 1971; Curnow, 1972; Lange et al., 1976). A computer program RISKMF has been derived, using these parameters by Smith (1972), to estimate recurrence risks for disorders for which there are no empirical data source and multiple family members are affected. Table 22.1 summarizes some risk data derived from the RISKMF computer program.

Table 22.1. Recurrence Risks in Multifactorial Inheritance

Population Frequency (%)	Heritability (%)	Affected Parents								
		0			1			2		
		Affected Sibs			Affected Sibs			Affected Sibs		
		0	1	2	0	1	2	0	1	2
1	80	1.0	6.5	14.2	8.3	18.5	27.8	40.9	46.6	51.6
	50	1.0	3.9	8.4	4.3	9.3	15.1	14.6	20.6	26.3
	20	1.0	2.0	3.3	2.0	3.3	4.8	3.7	5.3	7.1
0.5	80	0.5	5.1	12.3	6.2	15.5	24.3	37.6	43.2	47.9
	50	0.5	2.7	6.4	2.8	6.9	11.8	11.2	16.6	22.0
	20	0.5	1.1	2.0	1.1	2.0	3.2	2.3	3.5	5.0
0.1	80	0.1	2.5	8.2	2.9	9.8	17.9	31.7	37.4	42.4
	50	0.1	1.0	3.2	1.0	3.4	6.9	6.6	10.9	15.3
	20	0.1	0.3	0.7	0.3	0.7	1.3	0.8	1.4	2.3

Considerable heterogeneity occurs within groups of disorders traditionally considered to be multifactorial or polygenic, such as diabetes, epilepsy, and congenital heart disease, with a proportion of cases attributable to single gene defects. Identification of a specific genetic etiology, such as the presence of a submicroscopic deletion at chromosome 22q11 in some cases of nonsyndromic congenital heart disease (Wilson et al., 1992; Goldmuntz et al., 1993) is important in providing genetic advice appropriate to a particular case. Hirschsprung disease provides a good example of a polygenic disorder in which involvement of several single loci have now been identified in a proportion of families. Data from initial family studies suggested sex-modified polygenic inheritance, and empirical recurrence risks have been produced for genetic counseling based on the sex of the index case and relative and the length of the aganglionic segment involved (Passarge, 1972; Harper, 1998). A mode of inheritance compatible with an incompletely penetrant autosomal-dominant gene was suggested in some families (Badner et al., 1990). Linkage to a gene on chromosome 10 was subsequently demonstrated (Angrist et al., 1993; Lyonnet et al., 1993) and mutations in the RET oncogene demonstrated (Luo et al., 1993, Edery 1994). Mutations in other genes, notably the endothelin receptor type B gene, have also been implicated (Puffenberger et al., 1994; Chakravarti, 1996). Thus in a subset of families with Hirschsprung disease there is a major unifactorial predisposition, a situation likely to be reflected in other multifactorial disorders.

CHROMOSOMAL DISORDERS

Factors that indicate the possibility of a familial chromosomal disorder in a pedigree include a family history of infertility, multiple spontaneous abortions, and malformed stillbirths or liveborn infants with multiple congenital malformations occurring in a pattern that does not conform to that of mendelian inheritance. Figure 22.14 illustrates a kindred in which there is segregration of a reciprocal translocation in both balanced and unbalanced form.

The majority of chromosomal disorders present as sporadic cases. Although very low, the recurrence risk is increased above the normal age-related risk. After the birth of a child with Down syndrome to a mother under the age of 35 years, the recurrence risk is 0.5% for trisomic Down syndrome and 1% for all chromosomal abnormalities. For other potentially viable autosomal trisomies, most age-related recurrence risk is also for the more common trisomy 21. Although often requested, parental chromosome analysis is not necessary. Many unbalanced structural abnormalities also arise de novo, but in these cases it is essential to perform parental karyotypes to identify carriers of balanced rearrangements and to extend investigations to other family members as appropriate. The possibility of a subtle rearrangement not detected by routine cytogenetic analysis but leading to recurrent chromosome inbalance in offspring, such as 4p-syndrome (Estabrooks et al., 1994), should be borne in mind and fluorescence in situ hybridisation (FISH) performed using appropriate probes.

It is difficult to give precise reproductive risks to a person known to carry a balanced reciprocal translocation. The risk of viable chromosome inbalance will depend on the size and origin of the unbalanced segment generated, and there is an association between the mode of ascertainment and the risk of recurrence (Jacobs et al., 1970; Petrosky and Borgaonkar, 1984; Daniel et al., 1988), although this is not absolute. Ascertainment through the live birth of an

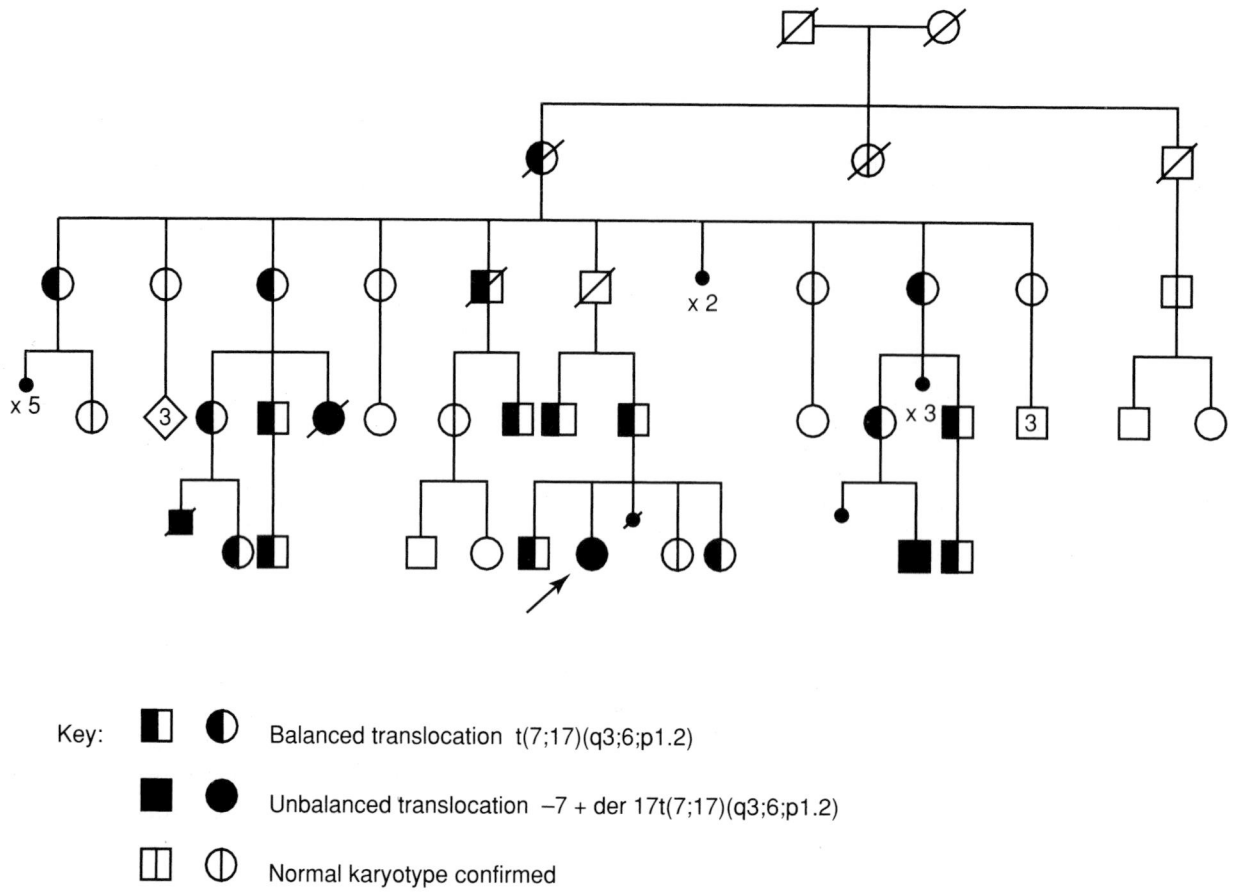

Key: ◧ ◑   Balanced translocation t(7;17)(q3;6;p1.2)

      ■ ●   Unbalanced translocation −7 + der 17t(7;17)(q3;6;p1.2)

      ◻ ◔   Normal karyotype confirmed

Fig. 22.14. Pedigree illustrating the segregation of balanced and unbalanced reciprocal translocation.

abnormal baby is associated with a higher risk than ascertainment through miscarriage or infertility. Information from an individual pedigree is seldom sufficient to derive a family-specific risk based on reproductive outcomes in known carriers, and estimation of risk is mainly based on the likely segregation pattern at meiosis and the chance of imbalance being viable (Gardner and Sutherland, 1989; Young, 1999). If one of the breakpoints has occurred in a terminal or acrocentric short-arm region, the potential imbalance will affect only a single segment, and risk estimates derived from an analysis of over 1000 pedigrees by Stengel-Rutkowski and colleagues (1988) can be used. For unbalanced products affecting two chromosomal segments that will consist of monosomy and trisomy, empirical data from collaborative studies based on the length of chromosome imbalance may be used (Daniel et al., 1988). Analysis of data from reciprocal translocations predisposing to the 3–1 segregation ascertained through a history of viable imbalance (Lindenbaum and Bobrow, 1975), which result in offspring with 45 or 47 chromosomes, suggested a high miscarriage rate with a risk of viable imbalance of 7% to 10% for female carriers and a lower risk for male carriers. The risk of a viable fetus with an unbalanced karyotype resulting from a parental robertsonian translocation varies from 3% to 15% depending on the chromosomes involved (Gosden, 1990), with the exception of t(21;21), which has a 100% risk.

Risks associated with parental pericentric inversions, as with reciprocal translocations, depend on the position of the breakpoint and the chromosome involved. Inversions affecting chromosomes 3, 4, 8, 13, and 18 are associated with high risk, and those involving chromosomes 1, 2, 5, 10, and Y are associated with low risk (Lilford and Gosden, 1990). For families ascertained through a viable recombinant, an overall recurrence risk of around 7% has been suggested (Sherman et al., 1986), and it seems reasonable to use a similar figure for other inversions considered likely to be viable. A very low risk of viable unbalanced offspring from parental paracentric inversions has been reported by a French collaborative study (Groupe Cytogénéticians, 1986).

MITOCHONDRIAL INHERITANCE

Mitochondrial diseases due to mitochondrial DNA mutations demonstrate matrilineal inheritance, since sperm do not contribute mitochondria to the zygote. Genetic assessment of mitochondrial diseases is complicated by the great variability of these disorders and a pedigree that is seldom conclusive of maternal transmission, since many cases are due to sporadic mitochondrial DNA mutations or are determined by nuclear genes. Clinical suspicion of a mitochondrial disease is backed up by appropriate investigations, which include fasting and postexercise serum lactate and pyruvate, cerebrospinal fluid lactate, computed tomography brain scan, and muscle biopsy for histochemistry, electron microscopy, biochemistry, and mitochondrial DNA mutation screen. Examples of disorders associated with mitochondrial DNA mutations are shown in Table 22.2 (see also Ch. 25).

In Leber's hereditary optic neuropathy (previously designated Leber's optic atrophy) the pattern of maternal inheritance has been well documented (Van Senus, 1963). The mitochondrial DNA mutation consisting of a point mutation in base pair 1178 of the *ND4* gene of complex I discovered by Wallace and coworkers (1988) was documented in several family members of the typical kindred shown in Figure 22.15. Women with the mutation will transmit it to all offspring, but only around one in two males and one in five females with the mutation develop loss of vision. An additional X-linked susceptibility gene has been postulated to explain these observations, but is not yet confirmed (Riordan-Eva and Harding, 1995). Affected and carrier males do not transmit the mutation to their offspring. A single cell contains many copies of the mitochondrial genome and heteroplasmy for the mutation is usual.

Table 22.2. Examples of Disorders due to Mitochondrial DNA Mutations

Disorder	Inheritance
Leber's hereditary optic neuropathy	Maternal
MELAS syndrome (mitochondrial myopathy with encephalopathy, lactic acidosis, and strokelike episodes)	Sporadic or maternal
MERRF syndrome (myoclonic epilepsy with ragged red fibers)	Sporadic or maternal
Progressive external ophthalmoplegia with mitochondrial myopathy (including Kearns-Sayre syndrome)	Usually sporadic
Diabetes and deafness (occasional cases)	Maternal

The proportion of mutant mitochondrial DNA in leukocytes is not a reliable indicator of which individuals will develop symptoms. As with other mitochondrial disorders, this presents problems in counseling asymptomatic individuals known to carry the mutation. The recurrence risks for mitochondrial disorders is difficult to determine. Large scale mitochondrial DNA deletions, as in Kearns–Sayre syndrome are usually sporadic, while point mutations, as in Leber's hereditary optic neuropathy, MELAS and MERRF, are more likely to be maternally transmitted.

ISOLATED CASES

Many patients presenting to the genetics clinic represent isolated cases within the family, and pedigree information

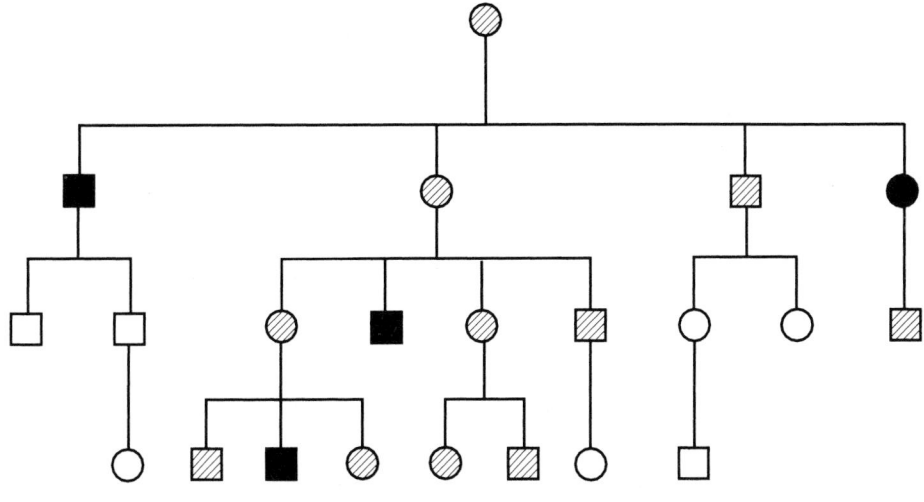

Key: ◼ ● Clinically affected
⬓ ◐ Asymptomatic mutation carrier

Fig. 22.15. Pedigree of Leber's hereditary optic neuropathy due to a mitochondrial DNA mutation demonstrating exclusively maternal transmission.

does not contribute to defining the mode of inheritance. Genetic advice in such cases depends on reaching a diagnosis in the affected individual and identifying the underlying etiology. Any of the following situations may apply:

1. The disorder may be due to an autosomal-dominant gene defect, arising by new mutation, transmitted through a nonpenetrant or very mildly affected parent, or by a clinically unaffected parent who carries a mosaic germline mutation. The situation may also represent nonpaternity. Risk to siblings varies between 0 and 50%, depending on the origin of the mutation, while risk to the offspring of the affected individual would be 50%.

2. The disorder may be caused by an autosomal-recessive gene defect with a 25% recurrence risk for siblings unless due to uniparental disomy or new mutation. If carrier state can be confirmed by molecular or biochemical analysis, cascade screening of other family members may be appropriate when the population carrier frequency is high or consanguineous marriages are planned.

3. The disorder may be due to an X-linked gene, usually presenting in a hemizygous male, but affecting females if the X inactivation pattern is skewed or the gene acts dominantly. Isolated cases may represent new mutations, which are frequent in lethal X-linked-recessive disorders, or may be transmitted by asymptomatic mothers who are carriers or who have germline mutations.

4. The disorder may be due to a mitochondrial DNA mutation representing a sporadic case or maternal transmission.

5. The disorder may be due to a chromosomal abnormality. Many of these, including the common trisomies due to nondisjunction, have a low risk of recurrence, but unbalanced karyotypes due to familial chromosomal rearrangements may carry high risks of recurrence, and investigation of relatives is required.

6. The disorder may be polygenic and recurrence risks depend on the disorder. These are based on empirical data derived from family studies.

7. The disorder may have a nongenetic etiology with no increase in the risk of recurrence, unless due to a teratogenic agent which further pregnancies will also be exposed to.

REFERENCES

Aase JM (1990) Diagnostic Dysmorphology. Plenum, NY

Abbas DG, Stevanin N, Dürr G et al. (1997) Cloning of the SCA 7 gene reveals a highly unstable CAG repeat expansion. Nat Genet 17:65–70

Amir RE, Van den Veyver IB, Wan M et al. (1999) Rett syndrome is caused by mutations in X-linked MECP2, encoding methyl-CpG-binding protein 2. Nat Genet 23:185–188

Angrist M, Kauffman E, Slaugenhaupt SA et al. (1993) A gene for Hirschsprung disease (megacolon) in the pericentromeric region of human chromosome 10. Nat Genet 4:351–356

Arahata K, Ishihara T, Kamakura K et al. (1989) Mosaic expression of dystrophin in symptomatic carriers of Duchenne's muscular dystrophy. N Engl J Med 320:138–142

Aslanidis C, Jansen G, Amemiya C et al. (1992) Cloning of the essential myotonic dystrophy region and mapping of the putative defect. Nature 355:548–551

Aylsworth AS, Kirkman HN (1979) Genetic counselling for autosomal dominant disorders with incomplete penetrance. Birth Defects Orig Art Ser 15:25–38

Badner JA, Sieber WK, Garver KL, Chakravarti A (1990) A genetic study of Hirschsprung disease. Am J Hum Genet 46:568–580

Bakker E, Veenema H, Den Dunnen JT et al. (1989) Germinal mosaicism increases the recurrence risk of 'new' Duchenne muscular dystrophy mutations. J Med Genet 26:553–559

Bankier A (2000) POSSUM (dysmorphology database and photo library). Murdoch Institute, Melbourne, Australia

Baraitser M, Winter RM (2000) London neurogenetics database. OUP, Oxford

Becker PE, Kiener F (1955) Ein neue X-chromosomale Muskeldystrophie. Arch Psychiatr Nervenk 193:427–448

Bennett RL, Steinhaus KA, Uhrich SB, O'Sullivan C (1993) The need for developing standardised family pedigree nomenclature. J Genet Counsel 2:261–273

Bergen AA, Van-den-Born LI, Schuurman EJ et al. (1995) Multipoint linkage analysis and homogeneity tests in 15 Dutch X-linked retinitis pigmentosa families. Ophthalmic Genet 16:63–70

Bonaiti-Pellié C, Smith C (1974) Risk tables for genetic counselling in some common congenital malformations. J Med Genet 11:374–377

Brinkman RR, Mezei MM, Theilmann J et al. (1997) The likelihood of being affected with Huntington disease by a particular age, for a specific CAG size. Am J Hum Genet 60:1202–1210

Bröcker-Vriends AHJT, Briët E, Dreesen JCFM et al. (1990) Somatic origin of inherited haemophilia A. Hum Genet 85:288–292

Bröcker-Vriends AHJT, Rosendaal FR, van Houwelingen JC et al. (1991) Sex ratio of the mutation frequencies in haemophilia A: Coagulation assays and RFLP analysis. J Med Genet 28:672–680

Buxton J, Shelbourne P, Davies J et al. (1992) Detection of an unstable fragment of DNA specific to individuals with myotonic dystrophy. Nature 355:547–548

Carr-Saunders AM, Greenwood M, Lidbetter EJ et al. (1912–13) The standardization of pedigrees: A recommendation. Eugen Rev 4:383–390

Carter CO (1961) The inheritance of congenital pyloric stenosis. Br Med Bull 17:251–254

Carter CO, Evans K, Coffey R et al. (1982) A three generation family study of cleft lip with or without cleft palate. J Med Genet 19:246–261

Cavenee WK (1986) The genetic basis of neoplasia: The retinoblastoma paradigm. Trends Genet 2:299–300

Chakravarti A (1996) Endothelin receptor-mediated signalling in Hirschsprung's disease. Hum Molec Genet 5:303–307

Chameides L, Truex RC, Velter V et al. (1977) Maternal systemic lupus erythematosus and congenital complete heart block. N Engl J Med 297:1204–1207

Chan C-TJ, Clayton-Smith J, Cheng X-J et al. (1993) Molecular mechanisms in Angelman syndrome: Survey of 93 patients. J Med Genet 30:895–902

Chen JD, Dickinson P, Gray R et al. (1989) Non-allelic mutations in X-linked retinitis pigmentosa. Clin Genet 35:338–342

Childs B, Der Kaloustian VM (1968) Genetic heterogeneity. N Engl J Med 279:1205–1212, 1267–1274

Cohen DH, Starman BJ, Blumberg B, Byers PH (1990) Recurrence of lethal osteogenesis imperfecta due to parental mosaicism for a dominant mutation in a human type I collagen gene (COL1A1). Am J Hum Genet 46:591–601

Coutinho P, Barros J, Zemmouri R et al. (1999) Clinical heterogeneity of autosomal recessive spastic paraplegias: analysis of 106 patients in 46 families. Arch Neurol 56:943–9

Coto E, Sanz-de-Castro S, Aguado S et al. (1995) DNA microsatellite analysis of families with autosomal dominant polycystic kidney disease types 1 and 2: evaluation of clinical heterogenicity between both forms of the disease. J Med Genet 32:442–445

Curnow RN (1972) The multifactorial model for the inheritance of liability to disease and its implications for relatives at risk. Biometrics 28:931–946

Daniel A, Hook EB, Wulf G (1988) Collaborative USA data on prenatal diagnosis for parental carriers of chromosome rearrangements: risks of unbalanced progeny. In Daniel A (ed): The Cytogenetics of Mammalian Autosomal Rearrangements. Wiley, NY

Darras BT, Francke U (1987) A partial deletion of the muscular dystrophy gene transmitted twice by an unaffected male. Nature 329:556–558

Davenport CB (1911) Heredity in Relation to Eugenics. Holt, NY

Davies SJ, Hughes HE (1993) Imprinting in Albright's hereditary osteodystrophy. J Med Genet 30:101–103

Deufel T, Golla A, Iles D et al. (1992) Evidence for genetic heterogeneity of malignant hyperthermia susceptibility. Am J Hum Genet 50:1151–1161

Dinger J, Prager B (1993) Arthrogryposis multiplex in a newborn of a myasthenic mother: Case report and literature. Neuromusc Disorders 3:335–339

Edery P, Pelet A, Mulligan LM et al. (1994) Long segment and short segment familial Hirschsprung's disease: Variable clinical expression at the RET locus. J Med Genet 31:602–606

Elles RG, Hodgkinson KA, Mallick NP et al. (1994) Diagnosis of adult polycystic kidney disease by genetic markers and ultrasonographic imaging in a voluntary family register. J Med Genet 31:115–120

Emery AEH (1994) Duchenne Muscular Dystrophy, 2nd edn. OUP, Oxford

Estabrooks LL, Lamb AN, Aylsworth AS et al. (1994) Molecular characterisation of chromosome 4p deletions resulting in Wolf-Hirschhorn syndrome. J Med Genet 31:103–107

The European Chromosome 16 Tuberous Sclerosis Consortium (1993) Identification and characterisation of the tuberous sclerosis gene on chromosome 16. Cell 75:1305–1315

Evans DGR, Guy SP, Thakker N et al. (1993) Nonpenetrance and late appearance of polyps in families with familial adenomatous polyposis. Gut 34:1389–1393

Evans DG, Kerr B, Cade D et al. (1996) Fictitious breast cancer family history (letter). Lancet 348 (9033):1034

Ferrier P, Bamatter F, Klein D (1965) Muscular dystrophy (Duchenne) in a girl with Turner's syndrome. J Med Genet 2:38–46

Fink JK, Heiman-Patterson T, Bird T et al. (1996) Hereditary spastic paraplegia: Advances in genetic research. Hereditary spastic paraplegia working group. Neurology 46:1507–1514

Francke U, Felsenstein J, Gartler SM et al. (1976) The occurrence of new mutants in the X-linked recessive Lesch-Nyhan disease. Am J Hum Genet 28:123–137

Fu Y-H, Kuhl DPA, Pizzuti A et al. (1991) Variation of the CGG repeat at the fragile X site results in genetic instability: Resolution of the Sherman paradox. Cell 67:1047–1058

Gardner RJM, Sutherland GR (1989) Chromosome Abnormalities and Genetic Counselling. OUP, Oxford

Goldmuntz E, Driscoll D, Budarf ML et al. (1993) Microdeletions of chromosomal region 22q11 in patients with congenital conotruncal defects. J Med Genet 30:807–812

Gosden C (1990) Prenatal diagnosis of chromosome anomalies. In Lilford R (ed): Prenatal Diagnosis and Prognosis. Butterworth, London

Griffin JE (1992) Androgen resistance: The clinical and molecular spectrum. N Engl J Med 326:611–618

Grimm T, Meng G, Liechti-Gallati S et al. (1994) On the origin of deletions and point mutations in Duchenne muscular dystrophy: Most deletions arise in oogenesis and most point mutations result from events in spermatogenesis. J Med Genet 31:183–186

Groupe de Cytogénéticiens Français (1986) Paracentric inversions in man. A French collaborative study. Ann Genet 29:169–176

Hall JG (1990) Genomic imprinting: Review and relevance to human diseases. Am J Hum Genet 46:857–873

Hall JG, Froster-Iskenius UG, Allanson JE (1989) Handbook of Normal Physical Measurements. OUP, Oxford

Harding AE (1981) Hereditary "pure" spastic paraplegia: A clinical and genetic study of 22 families. J Neurol Neurosurg Psychiatry 44:871–883

Harley HG, Brook JD, Rundle SA et al. (1992) Expansion of an unstable DNA region and phenotypic variation in myotonic dystrophy. Nature 355:545–546

Harper PS (1993) A specific mutation for Huntington's disease. J Med Genet 30:975–977

Harper PS (1998) Practical Genetic Counselling, 5th edn. Butterworth-Heinemann, Oxford, UK

Harper PS, Newcombe RG (1992) Age at onset and life table risks in genetic counselling for Huntington's disease. J Med Genet 29:239–242

Harper PS, Walker DA, Tyler A, Newcombe RG (1979) Huntington's chorea: The basis for long-term prevention. Lancet ii:346–349

Hazan J, Lamy C, Melki J (1993) Autosomal dominant familial spastic paraplegia is genetically heterogeneous and one locus maps to chromosome 14q. Nat Genet 5:163–167

Hoffmann EP, Brown RH Jr, Kunkel LM (1987) Dystrophin: The protein product of the Duchenne muscular dystrophy locus. Cell 51:919–928

The Huntington Disease Collaborative Research Group (1993) A novel gene containing a trinucleotide repeat that is expanded and unstable on Huntington's disease chromosomes. Cell 72:971–983

Imbert G, Saudou F, Yvert G et al. (1996) Cloning of a gene for spinocerebellar ataxia 2 reveals a locus with high sensitivity to expanded CAG/glutamine repeats. Nat Genet 14:285–291

Inglehearn CF (1998) Molecular genetics of human retinal dystrophies. Eye 12:571–579

Jacobs PA, Aitken J, Frackiewicz A et al. (1970) The inheritance of translocations in man: Data from families ascertained through a balanced heterozygote. Ann Hum Genet 34:119–131

Janssen B, Sampson J, van-der-Est M et al. (1994) Refined localization of TSC1 by combined analysis of 9q34 and 16p13 data in 14 tuberous sclerosis families. Hum Genet 94:437–440

Jones KL (1997) Smith's Recognizable Patterns of Human Malformation, 5th edn. WB Saunders, Philadelphia

Kawaguchi Y, Okamoto T, Taniwaki M et al. (1994) CAG expansions in a novel gene for Machado-Joseph disease at chromosome 14q32.1. Nat Genet 8:221–227

Kelly TE (1986) Clinical genetics and genetic counselling. Year Book, Chicago

Kerr B, Foulkes WD, Cade D et al. (1998) False family history of breast cancer in the family cancer clinic. Eur J Surg Oncol 24:275–279

Ketterling RP, Vielhaber E, Bottema CDK et al. (1993) Germline origins of mutation in families with haemophilia B: The sex ratio varies with the type of mutation. Am J Hum Genet 52:152–166

Knudson AG Jr (1971) Mutation and cancer: Statistical study of retinoblastoma. Proc Nat Acad Sci 68:820–823

Koide R, Ikeuchi T, Onodera O et al. (1994) Unstable expansion of CAG repeat in hereditary dentatorubral-pallidoluysian atrophy (DRPLA). Nat Genet 6:9–13

Koob MD, Moseley ML, Schut LJ et al. (1999) An untranslated CTG expansion causes a novel form of spinocerebellar ataxia (SCA 8). Nat Genet 21:379–384

Lander ES, Botstein D (1987) Homozygosity mapping: A way to map human recessive traits with the DNA of inbred children. Science 236:1567–1570

Lange K, Westlake J, Spence MA (1976) Extensions to pedigree analysis. II. Recurrence risk calculation under the polygenic threshold model. Hum Hered 26:337–348

La Spada AR, Wilson EM, Lubahn DB et al. (1991) Androgen receptor gene mutations in X-linked spinal and bulbar muscular atrophy. Nature 352:77–79

Levitt RC, Nourin N, Jedlicka AE et al. (1991) Evidence for genetic heterogeneity in malignant hyperthermia susceptibility. Genomics 11:543–547

Lilford RJ, Gosden C (1990) Chromosomes in prenatal diagnosis. In Lilford R (ed): Prenatal Diagnosis and Prognosis. Butterworth, London

Lindenbaum RH, Bobrow M (1975) Reciprocal translocations in man. 3:1 meiotic disjunction resulting in 47- or 45-chromosome offspring. J Med Genet 12:29–43

Luo Y, Ceccherini I, Pasini B et al. (1993) Close linkage of the RET protooncogene and boundaries of deletion mutations in autosomal dominant Hirchsprung's disease. Hum Molec Genet 2:1803–1808

Lyonnet S, Bolino A, Pelet A et al. (1993) A gene for Hirschsprung disease maps to the proximal long arm of chromosome 10. Nat Genet 4:346–350

McCue CM, Mantakas ME, Tengelstad JB, Ruddy S (1977) Congenital heart block in newborns of mothers with connective tissue disease. Circulation 56:82–90

McKusick VA (1978) Medical Genetic Studies of the Amish. Johns Hopkins University Press, Baltimore

McKusick VA (1992) Mendelian Inheritance in Man. Catalogs of Autosomal Dominant, Autosomal Recessive, and X-Linked Phenotypes. Johns Hopkins University Press, Baltimore

McKusick VA (1998) Mendelian Inheritance in Man, 12th edn. John Hopkins University Press, Baltimore

McKusick VA, Howell RR, Hussels IE et al. (1972) Allelism, nonallelism and genetic compounds among the mucopolysaccharidoses. Lancet i:993–996

Meijers-Heijboer EJ, Sandkuijl LA, Brunner HG et al. (1992) Linkage analysis with chromosome 15q 11–13 markers shows genomic imprinting in familial Angelman syndrome. J Med Genet 29:853–857

Melki J, Lefebvre S, Burglen L et al. (1994) De novo and inherited deletions of the 5q13 region in spinal muscular atrophies. Science 264:1474–1477

Metrakos K, Metrakos JD (1961) Genetics of convulsive disorders II. Genetic and electroencephalographic studies in centrencephalic epilepsy. Neurology 11:474–483

Monaco AP, Bertelson CJ, Liechti-Gallati S et al. (1988) An explanation for the phenotypic differences between patients bearing partial deletions of the DMD locus. Genomics 2:90–95

Moser H, Emery AEH (1974) The manifesting carrier in Duchenne muscular dystrophy. Clin Genet 5:271–284

Moutou C, Junien C, Henry I, Bonaiti-Pellie C (1992) Beckwith–Wiedemann syndrome: A demonstration of the mechanisms responsible for the excess of transmitting females. J Med Genet 29:217–220

Nagafuchi S, Yanagisaw H, Sato K et al. (1994) Dentatorubral and pallidoluysian atrophy expansion of an unstable CAG trinucleotide on chromosome 12p. Nat Genet 6:14–18

Nelis E, Haites N, Van Broeckhoven C (1999) Mutations in the peripheral myelin genes and associated genes in inherited peripheral neuropathies. Human Mutation 13:11–28

Nellist M, Brook-Carter PT, Connor JM et al. (1993) Identification of markers flanking the tuberous sclerosis locus on chromosome 9 (TSC1). J Med Genet 30:224–227

Nishisho I, Nakamura Y, Miyoshi Y et al. (1991) Mutations of chromosome 5q21 genes in FAP and colorectal cancer patients. Science 253:665–669

Northrup H, Wheless JW, Bertin TK, Lewis RA (1993) Variability of expression in tuberous sclerosis. J Med Genet 30:41–43

OMIM, Online Mendalian Inheritance in Man, word wide web URL: http://www.ncbi.nlm.nih.gov/omim/

Orr HT, Chung M, Banfi S et al. (1993) Expansion of an unstable trinucleotide CAG repeat in spinocerebellar ataxia type 1. Nat Genet 4:221–226

Passarge E (1972) Genetic heterogeneity and recurrence risk of congenital intestinal aganglionosis. Birth Defects Orig Art Ser 8:63–67

Passos-Bueno MR, Bakker E, Kneppers ALJ et al. (1992) Different mosaicism frequencies for proximal and distal Duchenne muscular dystrophy (DMD) mutations indicate difference in aetiology and recurrence risk. Am J Hum Genet 51:1150–1155

Patel PI, Lupski JR (1994) Charcot-Marie-Tooth disease: A new paradigm for the mechanism of inherited disease. Trends Genet 10:128–133

Pauli RM (1983) Dominance and homozygosity in man. Am J Med Genet 16:455–458

Pauli RM, Motulsky AG (1981) Risk counselling in autosomal disorders with undetermined penetrance. J Med Genet 15:339–345

Pearson K (1912) The Treasury of Human Inheritance. Dulau, London

Peters DJM, Spruit L, Saris JJ et al. (1993) Chromosome 4 localisation of a second gene for autosomal dominant polycystic kidney disease. Nat Genet 5:359–362

Petrosky DL, Borgaonkar D (1984) Segregation analysis in reciprocal translocation carriers. Am J Med Genet 19:137–159

Pollak MR, Chou Y-HW, Cerda JJ et al. (1993) Homozygosity mapping of the gene for alkaptonuria to chromosome 3q2. Nat Genet 5:201–204

Ponder M, Easton D, Huson S, Ponder BAJ (1991) Variation in expression of NF1: A twin study. Am J Hum Genet 49:3

Puffenberger EG, Hosada K, Washington SS et al. (1994) A misserise mutation of the endothelin-B receptor gene in multigenic Hirschsprung's disease. Cell 79:1257–1266

Pulst SM, Nechiporuk A, Nichiporuk T et al. (1996) Moderate expansion of a normally biallelic trinucleotide repeat in spinocerebellar ataxia type 2. Nat Genet 14:269–276

Reeders ST, Breuning MH, Davies KE et al. (1985) A highly polymorphic DNA marker linked to adult polycystic kidney disease on chromosome 16. Nature 317:542–544

Resta RG (1993) The crane's foot: the rise of the pedigree in human genetics. J Genet Counsel 2:235–260

Riordan-Eva P, Harding AE (1995) Leber's hereditary optic atrophy: The clinical relevance of different mitochondrial DNA mutations. J Med Genet 32:81–87

Robinson R, Curran JL, Hall WJ et al. (1998) Genetic heterogeneity and HOMOG analysis in British malignant hyperthermia families. J Med Genet 35:196–201

Rodrigues NR, Owen N, Talbot K (1995) Deletions in the survival motor neuron gene on 5q13 in autosomal recessive spinal muscular atrophy. Hum Molec Genet 4:631–634

Sanpei K, Takano H, Igarashi S et al. (1996) Identification of the spinocerebellar ataxia type 2 gene using a direct identification of repeat expansion and cloning technique, DIRECT. Nat Genet 14:277–284

Schneid H, Seurin D, Vazquez M-P et al. (1993) Parental allele specific methylation of the human insulin-like growth factor II gene and Beckwith–Wiedemann syndrome. J Med Gene 30:353–362

Sherman SL, Iselius L, Gallano P et al. (1986) Segregation analysis of balanced pericentric inversions in pedigree data. Clin Genet 30:87–94

Smith C (1971) Recurrence risks for multifactorial inheritance. Am J Hum Genet 23:578–588

Smith C (1972) Computer programme to estimate recurrence risks for multifactorial familial disease. BMJ 1:495–497

Snyder LE (1935) The Principles of Heredity. DC Heath, Indianapolis

Spence JE, Perciaccante RG, Greig GM et al. (1988) Uniparental disomy as a mechanism for human genetic disease. Am J Hum Genet 42:217–226

Stengel-Rutkowski S, Stene J, Gallano P (1988) Risk estimates in balanced parental reciprocal translocations: analysis of 1120 pedigrees. Monogr Ann Gn

Stern C, Sherwood ER (1966) The Origins of Genetics: A Mendel Source Book. Freeman, NY

Surani MAH (1986) Evidences and consequences of differences between maternal and paternal genomes during embryogenesis in the mouse. In Rossan J, Pederson RA (eds): Experimental Approaches to Mammalian Embryonic Development. Cambridge University Press, Cambridge

Suslak L, Dhamcharee V, Desposito F (1993) Uniparental isodisomy in an autosomal recessive disorder. J Genet Counsel 2:327

Suthers GK, Husan SM, Davies KE (1992) Instability versus predictability: The molecular diagnosis of myotonic dystrophy. J Med Genet 29:761–765

Teague PW, Aldred MA, Jay M et al. (1994) Heterogeneity analysis in 40 X-linked retinitis pigmentosa families. Am J Hum Genet 55:105–111

Trottier Y, Biancalana V, Mandel J-L (1994) Instability of CAG repeats in Huntington's disease: relation to parental transmission and age of onset. J Med Genet 31:377–382

Vance JM (1991) Hereditary motor and sensory neuropathies. J Med Genet 28:1–5

van der Mey AGL, Maaswinkle-Mooy PD, Cornelisse CJ et al. (1989) Genomic imprinting in hereditary glomus tumours: evidence for new genetic theory. Lancet ii:1291–1294

Van Essen AJ, Abbs S, Baiget M et al. (1992) Parental origin and germline mosaicism of deletions and duplications of the dystrophin gene: A European study. Hum Genet 88:249–257

Van Senus AHC (1963) Leber's disease in the Netherlands. Doc Ophthalmol 17:1–162

Van-Slegtenhorst M, de Hoogt R, Hermans C et al. (1997) Identification of the tuberous sclerosis gene TSC1 on chromosome 9q34. Science 277:805–808

Voss R, Ben-Simon E, Avital A et al. (1989) Isodisomy of chromosome 7 in a patient with cystic fibrosis: could uniparental disomy be common in humans? Am J Hum Genet 45:373–380

Waldenstrom J (1956) Studies on the incidence and heredity of acute porphyria in Sweden. Acta Genet Stat Med 6:122–131

Wallace DC, Singh G, Lott MT et al. (1988) Mitochondrial DNA mutation associated with Leber's hereditary optic neuropathy. Science 242:1427–1430

Wettke-Schäfer R, Kantner G (1983) X-linked dominant inherited diseases with lethality in hemizygous males. Hum Genet 64:1–23

Wexler NS, Young AB, Tanzi RE et al. (1987) Homozygotes for Huntington's disease. Nature 326:194–197

Wilson DI, Goodship JA, Burn J et al. (1992) Deletions within chromosome 22q11 in familial congenital heart disease. Lancet 340:573–575

Winter RM, Baraitser M, Douglas JM (1984) A computerised database for the diagnosis of rare dysmorphic syndromes. J Med Genet 21:121–123

Winter RM, Baraitser M (2000) London dysmorphology database and dysmorphology photo library. OUP, Oxford

Young ID (1999) Introduction to Risk Calculation in Genetic Counselling, 2nd edn. OUP, Oxford

Zatz M, Penha-Serrano C, Otta PA (1976) X-linked recessive type of pure spastic paraplegia in a large pedigree: absence of detectable linkage with Xg. J Med Genet 13:217–222

Zhuchenko O, Bailey J, Bonnen P et al. (1997) Autosomal dominant cerebellar ataxia (SCA 6) associated with small polyglutamine expansions in the αIA-voltage-dependent calcium channel. Nature Genet 15:62–69

Genetic risk assessment for common disease

23

Maren T. Scheuner
Ora Karp Gordon

Definition of common disease genetics

Common disease genetics refers to the study of genetic aspects of the leading causes of death and disability in the United States such as coronary heart disease, cancer and diabetes (Table 23.1) (Greenlee et al., 2000). By definition they are prevalent diseases, typically affecting more than 1 in 1000 individuals (King et al., 1992). They are chronic conditions that develop over decades, which have long been considered diseases of affluence occurring as a consequence of industrialization due to inactivity, excess calories, processed foods, tobacco, alcohol, radiation and pollution. However, there is increasing evidence that genes predispose to these diseases, including their etiology, natural history and response to therapy. However, a single genetic factor rarely acts alone in determining the disease process for these common disorders. This is in contrast to the classic paradigm of genetic disease, where a gene mutation is usually considered sufficient for disease expression, although single

Table 23.1. Ten leading causes of death, US, 1997

1. Heart Disease
2. Cancer
3. Cerebrovascular Diseases
4. Chronic Obstructive Lung Disease
5. Accidents
6. Pneumonia and Influenza
7. Diabetes Mellitus
8. Suicide
9. Diseases of Arteries
10. Nephritis

Greenlee et al., 2000

gene disorders are now recognized to have significant polygenic influences (Dipple et al., 2000).

Common diseases are complex, due to the interaction of multiple genetic and environmental risk factors, each of which may cause imbalance or disruption of crucial steps in pathways involved in metabolism and the cell cycle (i.e., cell growth, differentiation or apoptosis). For most common, chronic diseases, the genetic factors involved are thought to be prevalent and of low penetrance (Risch and Merikangas, 1996). Generally, the manifestation of a common disease may be considered as the interaction of unfavorable genetic and environmental factors with the lowest risk for those with favorable genotypes and few environmental risks (Fig. 23.1). In some individuals an offending environmental agent may play the most significant role in disease development whereas in others genetic susceptibilities may be most important. For example, endometrial cancer may occur primarily because of unopposed estrogen use which increases the relative risk 8-fold (Gruber and Thompson, 1996) or because of an *MSH2* gene mutation which is associated with a cumulative risk of 43% by age 80 (Aarnio et al., 1995). The environment and lifestyle of our Western society are generally unfavorable and contribute to the development of common chronic diseases. Given these pervasive unfavorable conditions, most individuals who develop a common, chronic disease, especially at an early age, are those who have the greatest degree of genetic susceptibility.

Because of the complex nature of common diseases, they are often heterogeneous, occurring as the result of several different abnormalities within a common pathway. Furthermore, the genetic variations within a common pathway contributing to a disease phenotype may be relatively frequent. Therefore, certain individuals will have

654

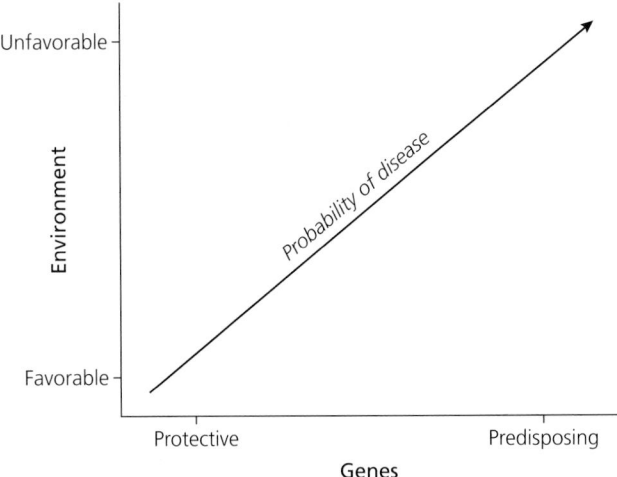

Fig. 23.1. Both genetic and environmental factors contribute to the development of common diseases such as coronary heart disease, diabetes and cancers. Disease is least likely for individuals who have genes that are protective rather than predisposing and who have favorable versus unfavorable environmental exposures. In Western cultures, unfavorable environmental factors such as inactivity, excess calories, processed foods, tobacco, alcohol, radiation and pollution are common place and nearly everyone encounters these exposures. Therefore, individuals who develop common diseases are generally those who have the greatest genetic predisposition.

more than one genetic risk factor for a common disease, which will increase the likelihood of being affected, typically with an earlier age of onset and possibly a more aggressive course. For example, inherited susceptibilities for deep vein thrombosis (DVT) include deficiencies of the natural anticoagulants (e.g., protein C, S, and antithrombin III), resistance to activated protein C (e.g., factor V Leiden) and prothrombin abnormalities (e.g., prothrombin G20210A mutation). The estimated frequencies of these hereditary hypercoagulable disorders ranges from 1 in 2500 for antithrombin deficiency to 1 in 25 for resistance to activated protein C due to the factor V Leiden mutation (Barrow and Jensen 1999; Kearon et al., 2000). Therefore, it is not unreasonable to suspect that in some cases of hereditary hypercoagualibilty more than one abnormality will contribute to the clinical phenotype. In fact it has been estimated that two or more inherited clotting disorders occur in 25% of cases with DVT and family history of DVT (Barrow et al., 2000).

An abnormality involving a specific pathway contributing to a common disease may have pleiomorphic effects. For example, hyperhomocysteinemia due to methylenetetrahydrofolate reductase (MTHFR) polymorphisms predisposes to cardiovascular disease, neural tube defects and unexplained recurrent embryo losses in early pregnancy (Eikelboom et al., 1999; Isotalo et al., 2000). The

apolipoprotein E genotypes contribute to serum cholesterol differences in the population and have been associated with cardiovascular disease risk as well as risk for Alzheimer disease (Wilson et al., 1996; Farrer et al., 1997). Recognizing these associations has important implications regarding informed consent when offering specific tests for the purpose of refining a diagnosis or for presymptomatic detection of disease.

Thus, the complexity underlying the genetic aspects of common diseases, including penetrance, heterogeneity, and pleiomorphic effects, poses significant challenges when applying genetic risk information clinically. With information about genetic aspects of common disease, genetic risk assessment becomes feasible. For patients, confirming a suspected genetic risk can be empowering and may relieve anxiety related to not knowing. Identifying a genetic risk might also improve the clinical management and prevention of a disease. Genetic risk assessment can also reassure individuals for whom a familial susceptibility has been excluded.

Application of genetic susceptibility information

The loss of life and productivity caused by common diseases, as well as the financial burden incurred by their treatment, seriously impacts the economy and often devastates families. To improve the public's health and quality of life and contain costs of health care services, there has been a significant trend toward an evidence-based approach to evaluation and management of disease (Guyatt et al., 2000). Evidence-based medicine (EBM) acknowledges that intuition, unsystematic clinical experience, and pathophysiologic rationale, are insufficient grounds for clinical decision-making, and stresses the examination of evidence from clinical research. Two fundamental principles of EBM are: (1) assessment of validity of research findings using a hierarchy of evidence to guide decision making and (2) when applying evidence, the benefits and risks, inconvenience, and costs associated with alternative management strategies should be considered, as well as the patient's values. Generally, an evidence-based approach is lacking in clinical genetics. This is due in part to the rarity of most genetic disorders and the inability to study large populations of affected individuals. In the field of common disease genetics the novelty of the available information and technology currently poses the greatest challenge to providing an evidence-based approach in clinical practice.

Most existing clinical guidelines for disease diagnosis, treatment and prevention do not recognize individual differences among patients, which may confound the ability to recognize benefit of a management or prevention strategy. This appears to be most evident in the field of prevention, where data supporting the efficacy and cost-effectiveness of current population-based guidelines for early detection and prevention of common diseases are for the most part controversial and incomplete. This contributes to a lack of consensus and limits the adoption of guidelines for disease prevention. Areas of debate include the appropriateness of mammography screening for women less than age 50 (Fletcher et al., 1993; Sickles and Kopans, 1995; Miller et al., 2000), the utility of prostate specific antigen screening (Woolf, 1995), the most effective screening method for colon cancer (Imperiale et al., 2000; Lieberman et al., 2000), the appropriateness of diabetes screening for both early detection and prevention of its associated complications (Singer et al., 1991; Knowler et al., 1995); and the long term benefits and risks of cholesterol screening and reduction (Assmann and Schulte, 1990; Goldman et al., 1992; Smith and Pekkanen, 1992; Hulley et al., 1993; Vince, 1994; Jacobson, 2000).

Because of the extensive biologic diversity and heterogeneity of common diseases it is not reasonable to expect that a single path could exist for every patient (Mirvis and Chang, 1997). Strict adherence to clinical guidelines may deny appropriate access to care for those patients who may benefit from alternative treatment or enhanced preventive strategies. Knowledge of genetic susceptibility to common diseases may identify important biologic differences that could lead to better disease management and prevention through use of targeted therapies and enhanced screening and prevention strategies based on a genetic susceptibility. For example, with respect to disease management, the molecular characterization of childhood leukemias directly affects treatment strategies. Acute lymphoblastic leukemia patients who have the MLL-AF4 or the BCR-ABL fusion in their lymphoblasts are often candidates for allogeneic hematopoietic stem cell transplantation during first remission, and patients with acute promyelocytic leukemia who carry the PML-RAR-alpha fusion respond to all-trans retinoic acid and have an excellent outcome when this is coupled with anthracyclines (Rubnitz and Pui, 1999). In the area of disease prevention, a few examples exist demonstrating the efficacy of enhanced screening and prevention for individuals with an inherited cancer susceptibility. Use of frequent colonoscopy followed by polypectomy beginning at a young age has been shown to be effective in reducing the incidence of colorectal cancer by more than half for family members in hereditary nonpolyposis colon cancer pedigrees (Jarvinen et al., 1995). Women who carry

BRCA mutations have a substantial reduction in the occurrence of a second primary breast cancer with use of tamoxifen and/or prophylactic bilateral oophorectomy (Rebbeck et al., 1999; Narod, 2000).

To date, the greatest impact of knowledge about a genetic susceptibility to a common, chronic disease has been in the field of preventive medicine. Because common diseases usually have a long indolent course that precedes overt symptoms and signs of disease, early detection and prevention are feasible (Fig. 23.2). Genetically susceptible individuals usually have the greatest risk for disease; therefore the positive predictive value of traditional screening tests increases (Morrison, 1992). Consequently, early detection strategies may be most cost-effective and certain screening tests may only be appropriate for such high-risk persons. For example, use of electron beam computed tomography for early detection of coronary artery disease might be most cost-effective if performed in those individuals having a genetic risk for premature coronary heart disease, as they have the greatest risk of developing clinical events (Nora et al., 1980). The cost-benefit of extraordinary preventive measures such as prophylactic surgery or use of a chemopreventive agent that has significant side effects and risks might also be greatest in genetically susceptible individuals. For example, women with an increased risk for breast cancer due to family history or the presence of a *BRCA* mutation can reduce their chances of breast cancer through use of tamoxifen (Fisher et al., 1998; Narod et al., 2000), bilateral mastectomy (Hartmann et al., 1999) or bilateral salpingo-oophorectomy (Rebbeck et al., 1999; Narod et al., 2000). None of these preventive strategies are recommended for the average risk woman.

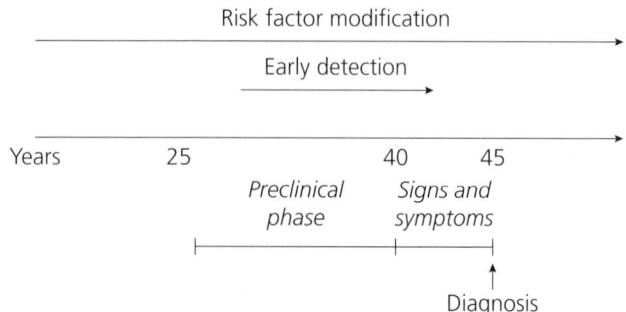

Fig. 23.2. Hypothetical time line of an individual predisposed to a common disease. Common diseases are usually chronic disorders that develop over decades with a lengthy preclinical phase. Early detection is often possible prior to signs and symptoms of disease. Early detection can lead to earlier treatment resulting in improved outcomes. Risk factor modification can also occur throughout the natural history of disease and is most likely to provide benefit early on for those with the greatest probability of developing disease.

Approaches to genetic risk assessment for common diseases

Genetic susceptibility to common disease can be assessed by several approaches, including DNA-based testing, phenotypic assessment of biochemical and physiological traits, as well as personal and family history collection. Each approach may be used in the clinical setting when performing risk assessment. Which approach is most cost-effective for identification of individuals with a genetic risk (case finding) is influenced by the prevalence of genetically determined disease, the attributable risk of a genetic factor for a common disease, as well as the accuracy, reliability and acceptability of the method for identification of genetically susceptible individuals. Generally, physiological and biochemical genetic traits (e.g., colonic polyps or serum cholesterol) are not unique to genetically determined disease, and they are, therefore, less powerful as initial markers for genetic risk assessment. Utilization of DNA markers as a sceening tool to identify individuals with genetic predisposition to common disease does not yet appear to be feasible due to the lack of data regarding the clinical validity of these tests (Scheuner, 2000). Generally, at this time molecular testing for a common disorder is limited to use in the context of a positive family history (National Advisory Council for Human Genome Research, 1994; American society of human Genetic, 1994; Hoskins et al., 1995).

The systematic collection of family history information currently appears to be the most appropriate approach for identification of individuals with a genetic susceptibility to most common diseases. A positive family history is common among many chronic conditions and it is quantitatively significant (King et al., 1992). Family history is also an accurate predictor of risk for several chronic conditions (Love et al., 1985; Acton et al., 1989; Kee et al., 1993; Bensen et al., 1999). The family history can reveal qualitative characteristics of disease risks, which are important when planning disease management and prevention strategies (Scheuner et al., 1997a). Furthermore, several studies have shown that knowledge regarding the risk related to a positive family history may improve prevention efforts (see below).

RECOGNIZING FAMILY HISTORY CHARACTERISTICS SUGGESTIVE OF AN INHERITED SUSCEPTIBILITY

Family history is one of the greatest risk factors for many common diseases with relative risks ranging from 2 to 10 times those of the general population as seen in Table 23.2. Furthermore, for most common diseases, an even greater increase in relative risk is associated with an increasing number of affected relatives, as well as earlier ages of disease onset. Qualitative characterization of risk can also be accomplished by reviewing the family history. Characteristics of a high-risk family history include multifocal or bilateral disease, higher rates of disease recurrence, and the occurrence of related diagnoses. For instance, different phenotypic subsets of cardiovascular disease or cancer may be revealed by the family history. Aggregation of atherosclerotic cardiovascular disease, hypertension, dyslipidemia (increased triglycerides and decreased HDL cholesterol), and impaired glucose tolerance or type 2 diabetes is suggestive of an underlying familial trait of insulin resistance, often referred to as syndrome X (Reaven, 1988). Altered hemostasis may be suspected in a pedigree that features multiple affected relatives with early onset of coronary artery disease and stroke or other thromboembolic events. The occurrence of different cancers within a family may be diagnostic of an inherited cancer syndrome such as hereditary non-polyposis colorectal cancer (HNPCC), which is characterized by susceptibility to early onset colon, gastric, endometrial, uroepithelial, ovarian and biliary tract cancers (Watson and Lynch, 1993). Recognition of these quantitative and qualitative familial disease risks has important implications for identifying family members at risk, arriving at the appropriate diagnosis, and for recommending appropriate genetic tests as well as individualized management and prevention for those individuals. For example, screening for evidence of glucose intolerance and dyslipidemia may be helpful in preventing disease in relatives from Syndrome X pedigrees. In families with HNPCC, relatives with an identified familial mutation might benefit from enhanced screening for early cancer detection and/or surgical prophylaxis or chemoprevention, or for those in whom the familial mutation is excluded reassurance that enhanced preventive strategies are not required.

ACCURACY OF FAMILY HISTORY INFORMATION

Accuracy of family history information has been investigated for coronary heart disease, diabetes, hypertension and several cancers. In assessing the reliability of reported family histories of myocardial infarction, Kee et al. (1993) performed a case-control study in which reported histories of first-degree relatives were validated using death certificates, physician records, and hospital records. In the 174 cases, the sensitivity, positive predictive value, and specificity of a reported history of myocardial infarction in first-degree relatives were 67.3%, 70.5%, and 96.5%, respectively. These values did not differ significantly from the corresponding figures for the

Table 23.2. Characteristics of familial forms of common disease

Disease	Prevalence of familial disease	Characteristics of "high-risk" families	Risk associated with family history	References
Coronary artery disease (CAD)	In families of male cases with myocardial infarction (MI) before age 45, 38% had first-degree relatives with premature CAD (before age 60). In families of male patients who had undergone coronary artery bypass graft surgery (CABG), 68% had at least one first-degree relative with CAD and 18% had three or more affected first-degree relatives. In female patients with CABG, 82% had at least one first-degree relative with CAD and 34% had three or more.	Early onset CAD (under 55 in males and 65 in females); multiple affected family members, especially females; multi-vessel disease; refractory to conventional risk factor modification; multiple family members with coronary artery disease, diabetes, hypertension, and lipid abnormalities.	Males with a parental history of MI or death from CAD have a 2-fold increase in risk of CAD even after adjustment for traditional risk factors. Females with a parental history of MI at or before age 60 have a 2.4-fold increased risk of non-fatal MI and 4.9-fold increased risk for fatal MI even after adjustment for traditional risk factors. Risk to first-degree relatives increased 5-fold if proband is male and less than age 60; 7-fold if proband is female and less than age 70. Heritability estimates for CAD before age 50 are estimated to be 90–100% and for later onset disease, 15–30%.	Scholtz et al., 1975; Colditz et al., 1991; Colditz et al., 1986; Thomas and Cohen, 1955; Rose, 1964; Slack and Evans, 1966; Rissanen, 1979; Scheuner and Alarcon, 1999.
Stroke	Thirty-eight percent to 47% of patients with stroke have first-degree relatives with history of stroke; 48–73% have first-degree relatives with history of ischemic heart disease	Early age of onset (under age 60 years), multiple family members with stroke and/or ischemic heart disease. Single gene disorders associated with ateriovenous malformation and cavernous angiomas; intracranial aneurysms (e.g., polycystic kidney disease, Ehleres-Danlos type IV, Marfan syndrome); hereditary forms of amyloid angiopathy or hypertension; and hereditary coagulopathies.	2-fold increase associated with first-degree relative affected with stroke. 2 to 3-fold increase associated with first-degree relative affected with ischemic heart disease.	Graffagnino et al., 1994; Kiely et al., 1993; Spriggs et al., 1990; Alberts, 1990.
Type 2 diabetes	In Hispanic families with type 2 diabetes, 29% have affected first-degree relatives; 13% have affected second-degree relatives; 11% have affected third-degree relatives.	Early onset of diabetes (between ages 25 and 40); multiple family members with diabetes; aggregation of other characteristics of insulin resistance including hypertension, dyslipidemia, premature atherosclerosis.	In Hispanic families, 2-fold increase associated with affected first-degree relatives, 1.3-fold increase with affected second-degree relatives. In Caucasian families, 3-fold increase associated withaffected first-degree relatives.	Mitchell et al., 1994; Keen and Track, 1968; Köbberling and Tattersall, 1982; Walker, 1999.
Osteoporosis	Forty-seven percent of females and 33% of males with osteoporosis have a family history.	No significant phenotypic differences between familial and non-familial cases including age at diagnosis, gender, osteoporosis-related fracture, and bone mineral density scores.	Maternal history of hip fracture associated with 2-fold increase in risk of hip fracture. 33% of mothers and 6% of fathers of cases are affected with osteoporosis. Heritability of peak bone mass at lumbar spine, 90% and at femoral neck, 70%.	Henderson et al., 2000; Evans et al., 1998; Pocock et al., 1987; Krall and Dawson-Hughes, 1993.
Breast cancer	Five to 20% of women with breast cancer report a family history of breast cancer, of these about half are consistent with a high familial risk.	Early onset breast cancer (typically before age 50), the occurrence of multiple family members with breast cancer, bilateral and/or multifocal disease and male breast cancer are features of an inherited	The risk of breast cancer in a woman with a first-degree relative with breast cancer is increased about 2.5-fold. Women with only a second-degree relative affected with breast cancer have a 1.8-fold increase	Slattery and Kerber, 1993; Hoskins et al., 1995; Anderson and Badzioch, 1993; Schildkraut et al., 1989;

	susceptibility due to a highly penetrant single gene mutation. The occurrence of other cancers in a breast cancer patient or her family members might suggest a known hereditary breast cancer syndrome such as thyroid cancer in Cowden syndrome, ovarian cancer in hereditary breast/ovary cancer, syndrome and CNS malignancies in Li-Fraumeni syndrome.	in breast cancer risk, and women whose nearest relative is a third-degree relative have a 1.35-fold increase compared to women without a family history. Women with a first-degree relative affected with bilateral breast cancer have about a 3-fold increase in breast cancer risk, and women with an affected first-degree male relative have a 2-fold increase in breast cancer risk. A family history of prostate, endometrial and ovarian cancer also increase the risk of breast cancer in first-degree relatives. The relative risk of breast cancer for Ashkenazi Jewish women with a first degree relative with breast cancer is 3.8 compared to non-Jewish women with a risk of about 1.7.	Claus et al., 1993; Scheuner et al., 1997a; Egan et al., 1996.
Ovarian cancer	Approximately 5% of ovarian cancer cases report a family history and about 20% of these familial cases are consistent with a high familial risk.	Ovarian cancer in at least two close family members may be consistent with an inherited susceptibility due to a highly penetrant single gene mutation. High risk/hereditary ovarian cancer may be classified as site-specific ovarian cancer, breast-ovary syndrome or hereditary nonpolyposis colon cancer, each accounting for approximately one-third of high-risk familial cases. Additional rare single gene disorders which feature ovarian cancers include Gorlin syndrome (ovarian fibrosarcomas), Peutz-Jeghers syndrome and Ollier's disease (sex chord tumors). — The relative risk of ovarian and breast cancer for first-degree relatives of cases with ovarian cancer is increased 2.8 and 1.6 fold, respectively. Among first-degree relatives of breast cancer cases the risk for ovarian cancer is increased 1.7-fold. The risk for ovarian cancer for Jewish women with an affected first-degree relative is increased 8.8-fold compared to a 3-fold risk for a non-Jewish woman.	Greggi et al., 1990; Houlston et al., 1992; Grover et al., 1973; Scheuner et al., 1997a; Schildkraut et al., 1989; Amos and Struewing, 1993; Steinberg et al., 1998.
Endometrial cancer	An estimated 13% of endometrial cancer cases have a family history of endometrial cancer and/or other cancers. About 50% of these familial cases have histories consistent with hereditary non-polyposis colorectal cancer syndrome (HNPCC), and about 12.5% of these familial cases have histories consistent with a high-risk, site-specific hereditary syndrome.	Two or more close relatives with endometrial cancer, especially at an early age (prior to menopause). Many high-risk families may have HNPCC featuring early onset colorectal cancer, and cancer of the stomach, bile duct, uroepithelium, and ovaries. — A family history of endometrial cancer in a first-degree relative is associated with about a 3-fold increase in endometrial cancer risk. There is a 1.9-fold increase in risk for colorectal cancer among endometrial cancer cases.	Sandles, et al., 1992; Boltenberg, et al., 1990; Gruber and Thompson, 1996;

continued

Table 23.2. Characteristics of familial forms of common disease (continued)

Disease	Prevalence of familial disease	Characteristics of "high-risk" Families	Risk associated with family history	References
Prostate cancer	Approximately 15% of prostate cancer is familial and about 33% of these familial cases are consistent with a high familial risk. Among 691 families ascertained through a single prostate cancer case, 14% had two affected first-degree relatives and 2% had 3 or more affected first-degree relatives.	Prostate cancer in two or more close relatives especially with early age of onset. Prostate cancer is within the spectrum of cancers associated with BRCA mutations, which feature increased risk for cancers of the breast, ovaries, colon, pancreas, stomach, bile duct, and melanoma.	Men with an affected father or brother have a 2-fold increase in prostate cancer risk. Men with two or three affected first-degree relatives have a 5 and 11-fold increase in risk, respectively.	Spitz et al., 1991; Steinberg et al., 1990; Carter et al., 1992
Colon cancer	Approximately 20 to 25% of colorectal cancer cases report a family history of colorectal cancer. About 0.5% of familial cases are high-risk, polyposis syndromes. About 25 to 50% of familial cases are consistent with a high-risk, hereditary nonpolyposis colorectal cancer (HNPCC) syndrome.	Early onset colon cancer and increased risk for synchronous and metachronous disease, family history of colon cancer and other syndrome associated malignancies. Polyposis syndromes may be classified according to the polyp type: adenomatous, hamartomatous, and juvenile. The cancer spectrum in HNPCC includes colorectal, endometrial, gastric, biliary tract, ovarian, and uroepithelial carcinoma. Some families may feature breast cancer; others may have sebaceous adenomas and keratoacanthoma (Muir-Torre syndrome). Turcot syndrome features central nervous system tumors and colorectal cancers associated with adenomatous polyposis or familial HNPCC.	There is a 3.2 to 3.5-fold increase in incidence and mortality from colorectal cancer in first-degree relatives of colon cancer cases.	Ponz de Leon et al., 1992; Eddy et al., 1987; Mecklin 1987; Stephenson et al., 1991; Woolf, 1958; Macklin 1960, Lovett, 1976

175 controls (68.5%, 73.8%, and 97.7%, respectively). In this study, only small differences were observed between odds ratios based on reported and verified data, indicating that neither misclassification nor recall bias had a substantial impact on the measurement of the effect of the family history. In a study assessing the accuracy of family history reports of diabetes, Hispanic and non-Hispanic white patients and controls were interviewed at clinic visits (Kahn et al., 1990). Verification of these reports was obtained by subsequently interviewing family members. There was complete agreement between the information given by the proband regarding diabetic status and answers given by the respective family members. The Family Heart Study also characterized the validity of reports of coronary artery disease, diabetes and hypertension by probands (Bensen et al., 1999). Using a relative's self report as a standard, the sensitivity of the proband's report for coronary artery disease was 85% and 81% for parents and siblings, respectively. The report for hypertension was 76% and 56% for these relatives, and for diabetes it was 87% and 72%, respectively. Most specificity values were above 90%.

Love and co-workers (1985) have studied the accuracy of patient reports of a family history of cancer. Verification of cancer histories was done by reviewing pathology and operative reports, hospital admission and discharge summaries, death certificates, and autopsy reports. Verification of negative histories was not performed. The accuracy of cancer site identification by the participant was 83.7% in first degree, 71.3% in second degree, and 71% in third degree relatives. Participants were correct in 91% and 89% of the cases for all relatives in which they reported breast and colon as the primary sites, respectively. For first-degree relatives, 94% of reported breast cancer cases and 93% of colon cancer cases were confirmed. For pancreas, lung, and liver as the primary cancer site, the accuracy rates of cancer reports were less at 75%, 60%, and 5%, respectively.

Overall, these studies suggest that a positive family history report can generally be used with a high degree of confidence for the identification of individuals who may be at increased risk for developing disease. The lower sensitivity values do indicate some under-reporting of disease in relatives; thus, a negative report should not be used as an indicator of a minimum or decreased disease risk (below the general population risk).

PREVALENCE OF FAMILY HISTORY OF COMMON DISEASE

Estimates for the frequency of family history reports among cases with several common diseases are available in the lit-erature (Table 23.2). However, knowledge of the prevalence of family history reports of common diseases among individuals within the population at large is necessary for shaping policy regarding genetic risk assessment for these conditions. The population frequency of average, moderate, or high risk family history reports for heart disease, stroke, hypertension, diabetes, and colon, breast, ovarian, endometrial and prostate cancers have been determined by reviewing pedigrees obtained by genetic counselors in a prenatal diagnosis clinic (Scheuner et al., 1997a). The population consisted of 400 "healthy", employed, middle-class people age 18 to 66 years. None of the consultands were seeking counseling because of a family history of one of the chronic disorders under study. Forty-three percent (170) reported a family history of at least one of the selected common disorders (130 individuals were at risk for one disorder, 33 were at risk for two, and seven were at risk for three). Depending on the specific disorder, most consultands had an average risk (general population risk) for any given disorder, approximately 5% to 15% were at moderate risk (2 to 3 times the population risk), and 1% to 10% were at high risk (risks approaching those associated with mendelian disorders). Family history of cardiovascular diseases, including coronary artery disease, stroke and syndrome X, were most common and reported by 34% of consultands. Family history of cancer was reported by 8% of the consultands and several individuals had histories suggestive of dominant cancer syndromes.

Genetic evaluation for common disease

A comprehensive genetic evaluation for common disease is comprised of several components: (1) Genetic risk assessment and diagnosis which often may include genetic testing, (2) genetic counseling reviewing perceptions, motivations and preferences pertaining to genetic risk assessment, (3) genetic education reviewing medical and genetic facts about a diagnosis, and (4) discussion of management and prevention options appropriate for a genetic risk. A genetic evaluation for common disease is generally performed by a team of professionals with expertise in genetics who work in collaboration with the patient and referring physician. In addition to important clinical implications of the genetic evaluation, this information may have significant psychological, social, reproductive, ethical and legal ramifications. Furthermore, the clinical information resulting from an evaluation usually has important health and possibly reproductive implications for multiple family members. Dealing with these genetic issues may be unfamiliar to non-geneticist physicians (Hoffman et al., 1993; Rowley et al., 1995; Suchard et al., 1999; Acheson et al., 2000). Most physicians lack the time it takes to provide genetic services (Suhr et al., 1995). Clinical genetic professionals routinely deal with these issues and can support the primary care provider or specialist in a consultative manner.

GENETIC RISK ASSESSMENT AND DIAGNOSIS

The genetic evaluation or risk assessment for common diseases typically begins with pedigree analysis. The pedigree structure is created and information for each family member is collected. Demographic information is documented including each relative's name, current age or age at death, locale, and ethnicity. Medical history is documented for each family member including age at diagnosis and known interventions or procedures. Information is also collected regarding important risk factors for a disease, such as smoking for heart disease or emphysema. Validation of the medical history of each family member is performed by reviewing records when possible.

After collecting the family history a qualitative assessment of disease risk can be performed which might include a differential diagnosis for identified familial traits. For example, when considering an inherited form of breast cancer there are at least six different genetic syndromes that can feature breast cancer, including site-specific breast cancer, breast-ovary syndrome, Li-Fraumeni syndrome, Cowden syndrome, Peutz-Jeghers syndrome and HNPCC (Hoskins et al., 1995). The types of cancers and other conditions reported in the family distinguish each of these syndromes. Mutations in different genes may underlie the genetic susceptibility in these syndromes and genetic testing can help to confirm a suspected diagnosis. Thus, estimation of the probability that genetic testing will provide information that will change the risk assessment and management and prevention of disease should also be discussed as part of the risk assessment and diagnosis process.

Quantitative risk assessment can also be performed for specific conditions relating to the family history using mathematical models or published estimates (Gail et al., 1989; Amos et al., 1992; Kerlikowske et al., 1992; Schildkraut et al., 1989). For example, in the case of breast cancer a woman's empiric risk based on the family history of breast and/or ovarian cancer can be provided and she can contrast this to the population risk and the risk that would be associated with an inherited cancer susceptibility mutation. However, most estimates using these models and

algorithms have limitations and they should not be the only means for risk assessment.

Thus, accurate genetic diagnosis and risk assessment requires the expertise of professionals who are familiar with the characteristics of genetic susceptibilities to common disease, the differential diagnosis of a suspected disease susceptibility, the resources available for determining disease risk based on a family history, as well as the likelihood that genetic testing may be useful in risk assessment, diagnosis and planning management and prevention.

GENETIC TESTING

Identification of appropriate tests that may be helpful in confirming a genetic diagnosis and refining genetic risk is the initial step in the genetic testing process. Genetic tests for assessing common diseases usually include DNA-based tests and biochemical tests. DNA-based testing is typically performed when assessing an inherited cancer susceptibility (Table 23.3), whereas biochemical testing is more often performed to assess a susceptibility to cardiovascular disease or diabetes (Table 23.4). DNA-based tests are usually performed in DNA isolated from white blood cells obtained via phlebotomy. Occasionally, DNA mutation analysis can be performed in archived tissue. This is most often considered when affected family members are deceased and founder mutations are known, such as in the case of Ashkenazi Jewish breast or ovarian cancer patients. Most commercial laboratories utilize PCR-based (polymerase chain reaction) methods to amplify the patient's DNA to be followed by sequencing or other methodologies. Sequencing is considered the gold standard for mutation analysis in most cases. However, even sequencing may miss rearrangements or large deletions of DNA or mutations in regulatory regions (Yan et al., 2000). Rarely, errors may occur with sample handling, contamination by airborne particles in the laboratory, or failure of the PCR technique.

When considering genetic testing, clinicians should choose the testing strategy that would be most informative for a patient and their family members (Fig. 23.3). Ideally genetic testing should begin in an affected family member. If an inherited susceptibility is present in the family, it is likely to be found in an affected individual. If a genetic risk factor is identified, then management and prevention strategies specific to that genetic risk can be recommended. Additionally, at-risk relatives can be tested and their genetic status can be known. Those who have not inherited the familial risk factor can be reassured. Those with the familial risk can enter into appropriate surveillance and prevention practices.

Table 23.3. Examples where clinical genetic testing is available for cancer susceptibility

Disorder	Gene	Locus	Available testing strategies
Ataxia telangectasia	ATM	11q22–q23	Linkage analysis and modified colony survival assay for radiosensitivity detects affected cases but not carriers.[1]
Hereditary breast/ovarian cancer	BRCA1 BRCA2	17q21 13q12	Testing available for the three Ashkenazi Jewish founder mutations. Testing for unknown mutations available by various techniques including protein truncation, conformation sensitive gel electrophoresis, single stranded conformational polymorphism, complete sequencing or a combination. Sequencing is available[1] and is considered gold standard but may miss large deletions (up to 30% of Dutch patients), insertions/duplications or rearrangements of DNA.
Familial adenomatous polyposis and Gardner syndrome	APC	5q21–q22	Protein truncation followed by other techniques with direct sequencing of abnormal gene products, detects 70% of mutations. Linkage analysis (99.5% sensitivity).
Hereditary nonpolyposis colorectal Cancer (HNPCC)	MLH MSH2 MSH6 PMS1 PMS2	3p21 2p21–22 2p16 2q31–q33 7p22	Testing only available for MLH1, MSH2 genes, which includes full exon screening with 40–70% detection rate. Microsatellite instability testing of tumor tissue and linkage analysis more widely available.
Cowden syndrome	PTEN	10q23.3	Sequencing of all nine exons (81% detection rate) with buccal swab testing available[1]. One lab provides research testing with clinical confirmation.
Li-Fraumeni syndrome	TP53	17p13	Sequencing of exons 5–8 (80% of mutations), with a 70% detection rate. One lab provides sequencing of all exons.
Peutz-Jegers syndrome	STK1I	19p13	Full sequencing of all nine exons, with 50+% mutation detection rate.[1]
Multiple endocrine neoplasia, Type 1	MEN1	11q13	Linkage widely available. Direct sequencing with 85% mutation detection rate.
Multiple endocrine neoplasia, Type 2A (MEN2A)	RET	10q11	90–95% of mutations found in one of five cysteine codons in the cysteine-rich extracellular domains (sequence analysis of exons 10 and 11).
Familial medullary thyroid cancer (FMTC)	RET	10q11	85–90% of mutations found within the extracellular cysteine-rich domain (sequence analysis of exons 10 and 11), or either of the two intracellular tyrosine kinase domains (sequence analysis of exons 13, 14, 15, 16).
Multiple endocrine neoplasia, Type 2B (MEN2B)	RET	10q11	95–98% of cases involves a mutation at codon 918 in exon 16 (sequence analysis). Almost half are new germline mutations.
Von Hipple Lindau	VHL	3p25–26	Southern blot and other methods followed by direct sequencing with 93% detection rate.
Familial atypical mole multiple Melanoma Syndrome (FAMMM)	CDK4 CDKN2A (p16) CMM	12q14 9p21 1p36	Sequencing of all exons and introns for p16 and CDK4 coding exons. No testing available for CMM.
Basal cell nevus (Gorlin) syndrome	PTCH	9q22	Linkage widely available. Exon screen by dideoxyfingerprinting (100% sensitivity for mutations found by full sequencing).[1]
Neurofibromatosis, Type 1	NF1	17q11	Linkage (99.9% sensitivity). Protein truncation testing followed by sequencing[1] (70% detection rate). Not currently available for prenatal testing. FISH available for deletion testing.[1]
Papillary renal cell	MET	7q31	Protein truncation followed by sequencing.[1]

From NIH GeneTests (www.genetests.org) and information provided directly by laboratory
[1] Single laboratory offering testing

Table 23.4. Metabolic risk factors for coronary artery disease

Disorder	Frequency in coronary artery disease patients (%)	Relative risk of coronary artery disease	Treatment
Small LDL cholesterol	50	3	Typically associated with insulin resistance. Weight loss and avoidance of high carbohydrate diets as excess carbohydrates will promote glycemic response and contribute to insulin resistance and the associated metabolic abnormalities. Niacin or fibrates can be effective in conversion to larger LDL cholesterol particle size.
Lipoprotein(a)	33	3	Niacin or estrogen (for women) and testosterone (for men) may decrease lipoprotein(a); however, generally resistant to treatment. Therefore, aggressive modification of other risk factors (e.g., high LDL cholesterol) is recommended. Antioxidants might be beneficial. Aspirin therapy may be beneficial.
Hyperhomocysteinemia	20–30	2–3	Folate, pyridoxine (B6) and vitamin B12 at doses titrated to homocysteine levels. Avoidance of high protein diet.
High LDL cholesterol	20	2–3	HMGCoA reductase inhibitor, resins, or niacin and low saturated fat diet to reach a target LDL cholesterol level of 100 mg/dL for patients with established atherosclerosis or in high-risk patients.
High triglycerides	15	2–3	Niacin and fibrates. Avoid alcohol and high fat diet.
Hypoalphalipoproteinemia	5	3	Niacin and fibrates might be beneficial.
Apo E4	20	1.4	Associated with elevated LDL cholesterol. For lowering of LDL cholesterol, these patients respond well to low fat diets.
Apo E2/E2 (Type III hyperlipoproteinemia)	2	2–3	Associated with elevated chylomicron remnants. Usually not penetrant unless other metabolic abnormalities present such as hypothyroidism, diabetes, or obesity. Fibrates may be beneficial in improving lipids.

Adapted from Superko (2000) www.BerkeleyHeartLab.com, with permission.

It is not always possible to test an affected family member, as they are often deceased and therefore unable to provide a blood sample, or not interested in testing, or unable to participate due to financial reasons. In this case, unaffected family members may participate in testing. Identification of a genetic risk factor may help in planning appropriate preventive strategies. Though unaffected individuals can initiate the testing process, a normal test result cannot be entirely reassuring for them in the absence of a known familial mutation because many genetic traits for an inherited susceptibility remain unknown. A normal test result can exclude the genetic risk factors that have been tested but not the possibility of an inherited susceptibility. In such a case, medical management would typically depend upon the empiric risks associated with the family history. To further clarify the situation, testing additional family members may be helpful.

Once a genetic testing strategy has been formulated, laboratories that can provide the testing are identified. Obtaining, processing and shipping the sample may also be necessary, as well as facilitation of the billing process (providing the most appropriate diagnostic codes and documenting medical necessity for testing when requested). Issues to consider when choosing a laboratory include methodology, analytic sensitivity and specificity, technical support, cost and turn-around time. Understanding which methodology is used is important since standards for many genetic tests currently do not exist. There is great variability in testing procedures for many conditions. Although clinical laboratories are required to participate in reviews and standardized mock patient analyses, there is no mechanism to revoke a laboratory's ability to offer a molecular test, even if they fail to make a correct diagnosis on multiple exam

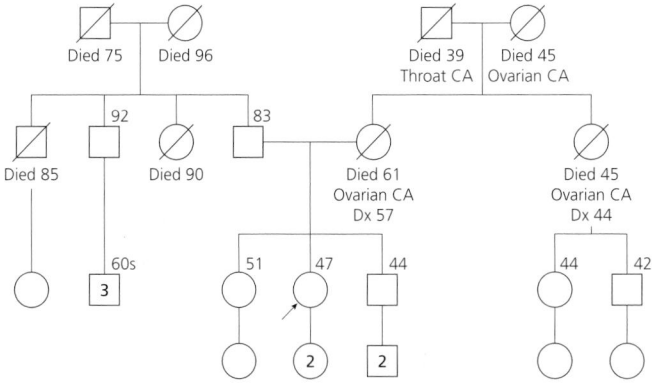

Fig. 23.3. Genetic testing strategies for evaluating an inherited susceptibility. The proband is a 47-year-old Ashkenazi Jewish woman with a family history consistent with hereditary site-specific ovarian cancer syndrome which is often but not always due to *BRCA* gene mutations. At age 36 she had prophylactic bilateral salpingo-oophroectomy. She has been using hormone replacement therapy (HRT) but became concerned that this might be contraindicated if she had a genetic susceptibility to breast cancer due to a *BRCA* mutation. She also had concerns regarding her daughters', sister's, and niece's risks for breast and ovarian cancer. No affected family members were living; therefore, she underwent *BRCA* testing to clarify her cancer risks. None of the three common Ashkenazi Jewish *BRCA* founder mutations were identified in her sample. This was reassuring with respect to her breast cancer risk since she has no family history of breast cancer and the most likely *BRCA* mutations had been excluded in her sample. However, without identification of a cancer gene mutation her maternal family history of ovarian cancer was unexplained. To interpret her negative result as a true negative, testing was performed in DNA extracted from her deceased mother's archived tumor block. A *BRCA1* 185delAG mutation was identified consistent with a germline mutation. Therefore the proband's and her daughters' risks for breast and ovarian cancer are not increased above the general population, and enhanced cancer surveillance, chemoprevention or prophylactic surgery are not indicated on the basis of a genetic predisposition. In addition, she can continue use of HRT for its benefits in alleviating menopausal symptoms, urogenital atrophy, osteoporosis and improvement in several cardiovascular risk factors. The proband's brother and sister can also undergo counseling and testing of the familial *BRCA* mutation to clarify their mutation status.

attempts (Grody, 2000, personal communication). As a result, clinicians need to be personally familiar with a given laboratory's protocol and accuracy.

An individual's genetic test results should be interpreted within the context of their family history, as penetrance estimates may vary depending upon the family history. The interpretation should incorporate a discussion of the impact of the results on their risk assessment, diagnosis and plans for management and prevention. Family members who might benefit from risk assessment and genetic testing should also be identified, and the clinician should facilitate communication between the index case and at-risk relatives as well as provide referrals to genetics professionals for relatives.

GENETIC COUNSELING AND EDUCATION

An important goal of genetic risk assessment for common disease is the development of individualized preventive strategies based on the genetic risk assessment, as well as the patient's personal medical history, lifestyle and preferences. The patients' participation in the process is vital to the success of the prevention plan. Generally, individuals are motivated to participate in genetic risk assessment with the hope that it will clarify the most appropriate plan for disease management and prevention, and for the benefit genetic information may have for their family members (Scheuner 2000). Common barriers to obtaining genetic risk information for common disease include fear of discrimination both in the work place and by insurers, cost, and uncertainty about the value of interventions (Hudson et al., 1995; Lerman et al., 1996; Croyle et al., 1997; Rothenberg et al., 1997).

Perception of susceptibility to disease, severity of disease, education level, knowledge about implications of identifying a risk, and internal and external cues to action influence compliance and adherence with prevention strategies (Bamberg et al., 1993). Genetic counseling is critical to delineating a patient's motivations and understanding of the genetic risk assessment process, and perceived barriers and benefits to learning of a genetic risk. Genetic counseling is a communication process that deals with the human problems associated with a genetic disorder or the risk of a genetic disorder occurring within a family (Fraser, 1974). The education component of genetic counseling helps an individual and family members to understand (1) the medical information available about the genetic risk or diagnosis including the probable course of the disorder including penetrance and variable expressivity, (2) the contribution of heredity to the disorder and the risk of occurrence in other family members and to future offspring, and (3) the options for dealing with the risk of occurrence and recurrence.

The genetic counseling process also helps the individual or family by (1) helping each family member choose the course of action that is most appropriate in view of their risk and the family's goals and values, (2) supporting decisions made by family members, (3) aiding the family members in adjustment to the disorder by discussing potential emotional concerns, helping them recognize and understand their emotions including anxiety, fear, and guilt, thereby facilitating their coping and adaptation process, and (4) identifying potential societal concerns that may arise as a consequence of participating in genetic risk assessment and/or testing, including possible stigmatization by friends and employers, potential discrimination by insurers and employers, and the financial costs resulting from testing and consequent prevention and management strategies.

Thus, genetic counseling ensures the opportunity to provide an informed consent, a necessary process including discussion of the potential benefits, risks and limitations regarding genetic risk assessment and testing (National advisory Council for human Genome Research, 1994; American Society of clinical Oncology, 1996; American Society of Human Genetic, 1996; geller et al., 1997; McKinnon et al., 1997)

MANAGEMENT AND PREVENTION STRATEGIES

Because the natural history of an inherited predisposition to common disease is generally different from sporadic cases with earlier ages of onset and susceptibility for additional conditions, recommendations for different management and prevention options are appropriate (NIH Consensus development panel on Ovarian cancer, 1995; Burke et al., 1997a; 1997b). These recommendations generally include enhanced surveillance at earlier ages and/or at more frequent intervals, prophylactic surgery, chemoprevention, lifestyle changes that can promote health and avoidance of aggravating factors specific to a genetic risk.

There is some evidence in the literature to support the efficacy of special strategies for early disease detection and prevention among individuals with a genetically susceptibility to cancer. Several studies suggest that prophylactic oophorectomy is useful in reducing the risk for ovarian and breast cancer among *BRCA* mutation carriers (Kerlikowske et al., 1992; Rebbeck et al., 1999; Narod et al., 2000). Prophylactic mastectomy is effective in reducing the risk of developing breast cancer (Hartmann et al., 1999). Tamoxifen has also been shown to reduce the incidence of breast cancer among high-risk women by about 50% (Fisher et al., 1998; Narod et al., 2000). Raloxifene might also be effective in reducing breast cancer incidence in women at risk (Cummings et al., 1999). Similar to the general population, women with a genetic susceptibility for ovarian cancer may reduce their ovarian cancer risks with oral contraceptive use. Narod and coworkers (1998) describe a 70% reduction in ovarian cancer risk among BRCA mutation carriers who used oral contraceptives for six or more years. Colonoscopy with polypectomy has been shown to reduce the incidence of colon cancer among members of HNPCC kindreds (Jarvinen et al., 1995). Improvement in most inherited cardiovascular risk factors is possible with several proven methods (Table 23.4). However, except for the risk factor of LDL cholesterol (Jacobson, 2000), data are lacking regarding the efficacy of preventing clinical cardiovascular events in individuals who have modified these risk factors.

The plan for management and prevention should be tailored to an individual's genetic risk while taking into consideration their personal medical history, family history, habits and preferences. Other disease risks that may influence decision making regarding options for risk reduction should be identified as part of the management and prevention plan (Fig. 23.4). For example, use of tamoxifen for breast cancer prevention might be contraindicated given a personal or family history of thrombophilia. In addition, as with any treatment plan, potential risks or complications that may result from the recommended management and prevention strategies must be recognized. For example, avoidance of long-term hormone replacement therapy (HRT) might be warranted for women with a genetic predisposition to breast cancer; however, estrogen deficiency may pose a significant risk for osteoporosis and have unfavorable effects on multiple cardiovascular risk factors. A meta-analysis of five studies has shown that women with family history of breast cancer who used HRT had a 3.4-fold increase in breast cancer risk. This was more than twice the 1.5-fold increase in risk of women who used HRT and did not have a family history of breast cancer (Steinberg et al., 1991). It is suspected that use of hormone replacement therapy might also contribute to an increased breast cancer risk in women with *BRCA* mutations, similar to that reported for women with a family history of breast cancer, although this remains to be proven. Thus, if long-term hormone replacement is not an option for a woman with an inherited risk for breast cancer, it is important that the competing concerns of osteoporosis and cardiovascular disease be addressed, and that alternatives to hormone replacement are explored (Fig. 23.5).

Finally, the recommendation for management and prevention options specific to an individual's genetic risk should be communicated in writing so the patient and referring physician can incorporate these recommendations into a plan for future health management. Plans for continued contact or follow-up with a genetics professional may be appropriate to review the individualized plan and updated personal and family history information can be obtained, with revision of the management and prevention plan as indicated. New information/technology available for genetic risk assessment or management and prevention of disease can also be discussed.

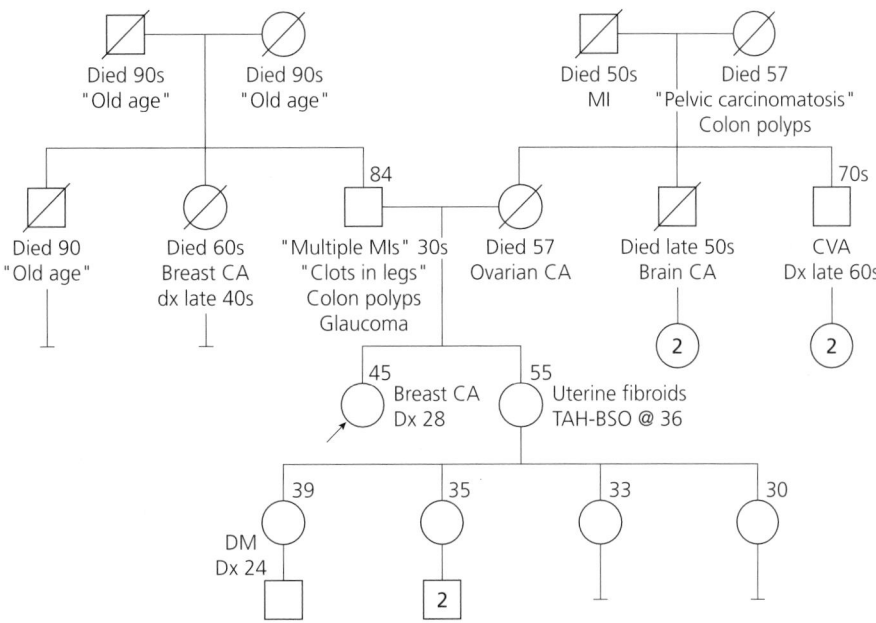

Fig. 23.4. Assessing competing risks when designing an individualized management and prevention plan. The proband is a 45-year-old Ashkenazi Jewish woman with personal and maternal family histories consistent with hereditary breast/ovary cancer syndrome. The *BRCA1* 185delAG mutation was identified in her sample. She was interested in use of tamoxifen for chemoprevention of breast cancer. The most significant medical risks associated with tamoxifen include deep vein thrombosis, pulmonary embolism and endometrial cancer (Fisher et al., 1998). The proband's father had history of recurrent "sudden death". Review of his records revealed recurrent pulmonary embolism now treated with chronic anticoagulation. He underwent an extensive thrombophilia evaluation and was found to be heterozygous for factor V Leiden. The proband did not inherit this mutation and tamoxifen was offered as an option for breast cancer prevention. The proband's sister had hysterectomy and bilateral salpingo-oophorectomy (TAH-BSO) at age 36 for menorrhagia due to uterine fibroids and had been on estrogen replacement for 20 years. She has both the *BRCA* and Factor V mutations. Continued use of estrogen was discouraged due to her breast cancer risk and tamoxifen was not recommended due to its prothrombotic effects. Subsequently, her two youngest daughters have proceeded with genetic counseling and testing. One has neither of these familial mutations. She has continued on her oral contraceptives for contraception and is reassured about her cancer and clotting risks. The other has only the factor V Leiden mutation. The manifestations of thrombosis were reviewed and she was advised to avoid use of hormonal preparations and prolonged episodes of immobilization.

Genetic risk assessment and utility of preventive services

Targeting high-risk, genetically susceptible individuals can improve the efficacy of preventive screening efforts by improving the predictive values of screening tests (Morrison, 1992), as well as improving participant compliance with recommended screening guidelines and therapies (Bamberg et al., 1993; Lynch et al., 1993; Stephenson et al., 1993). Several factors influence attitudes and behaviors regarding disease which can facilitate compliance, including perceived susceptibility, severity, benefits of screening, barriers to screening, and internal or external cues that trigger an initiation to act on a selected intervention (Bamberg et al., 1993). The impact of genetic risk information on preventive practices has been investigated for several common genetic conditions. Some evidence of this for colon cancer, breast cancer and coronary heart disease is reviewed below.

Using fecal occult blood testing and flexible sigmoidoscopy, colonic polyp and carcinoma detection rates increased two to three fold in the context of a positive family history (Rozen et al., 1987; Stephenson et al., 1993). This increase in detection has been projected to cause a 30% reduction in colon cancer mortality using fecal occult blood testing, and an 85% reduction in colon cancer mortality using either colonoscopy or barium enema in first degree relatives of colon cancer patients (Eddy et al., 1987). Jarvinen and co-workers (1995) have demonstrated that colorectal cancer incidence can be significantly reduced with periodic colonoscopy in at-risk family members from HNPCC pedigrees. In a ten-year, longitudinal study of 251 at-risk individuals from 22 hereditary nonpolyposis colorectal cancer pedigrees, only six of the 133 screened subjects (4.5%) versus 14 of the 118 (11.9%) control subjects developed colorectal cancer, corresponding to a significant reduction of 62% in the screening group (p=0.03), presumably due to polypectomies. Additionally, the tumor stage was more favorable in the screened group, with no deaths from colorectal cancer, compared with five colorectal cancer deaths among the 14 diseased control subjects. Regarding compliance issues, in a study comparing 159 siblings of newly diagnosed colorectal cancer patients and 194 control subjects, those with a family

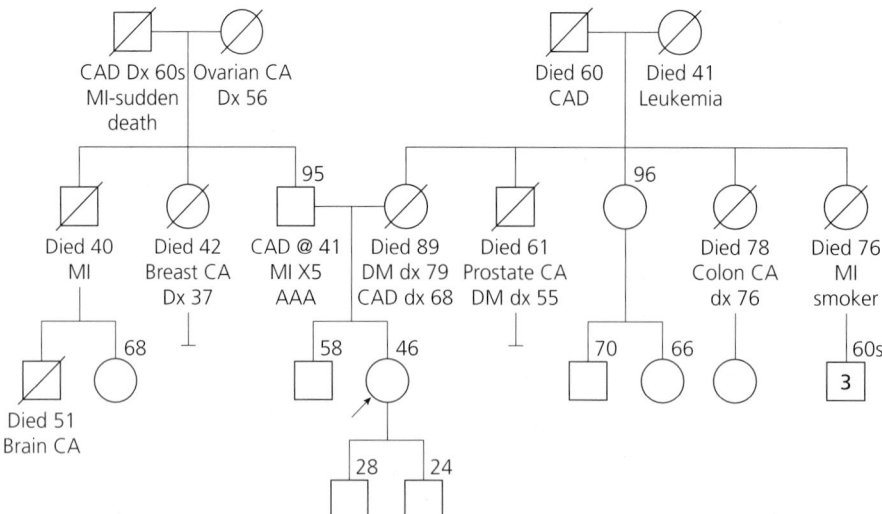

Fig. 23.5. Management of cardiovascular disease risks in women with an inherited susceptibility to breast cancer. The proband was experiencing menopausal symptoms and wished to use hormone replacement therapy (HRT) to alleviate these symptoms and for its benefits in improvement of cardiovascular risks. Her paternal family history is significant for early onset coronary heart disease and her maternal family history is consistent with Syndrome X. The proband underwent an evaluation for genetically determined cardiovascular disease risk factors. She had evidence of insulin resistance with an elevated fasting insulin of 16 uU/ml; an LDL gel electrophoresis demonstrating small, dense particles; and triglycerides of 143 mg/dl with an HDL cholesterol of 43 mg/dl. She also had two additional risk factors, an increased Lp(a) of 20 mg/dl (range 1–20) and elevated LDL cholesterol of 156 mg/dl. Use of HRT therapy might be beneficial in reducing Lp(a) and LDL cholesterol while improving insulin sensitivity (Barrett-Conner and Laakso, 1990). However, targeted therapies might be more effective in managing these risks, such as Niacin to lower LDL cholesterol, triglycerides and Lp(a), or use of thiazolidinedione-type drug for improving insulin sensitivity. However the proband had concerns about using HRT as she perceived having an increased breast cancer risk because her paternal family history is suggestive of hereditary breast/ovarian cancer syndrome due to early onset breast cancer in her aunt and ovarian cancer in her grandmother. The proband underwent *BRCA* sequence analysis and normal results were obtained. This provided reassurance regarding her empiric breast and ovarian cancer risks and use of HRT. Nonetheless, if she would prefer alternative therapies to HRT several options are available for management of her identified cardiovascular disease risk factors.

history in a first-degree relative (52%) were more likely to participate in fecal occult blood screening than those without such a history (38%) (Sandler et al., 1989). These findings were consistent with a similar study of siblings of colon cancer cases and control subjects; subjects with a family history were more likely to participate in fecal occult blood testing than those without a family history (60% 47%) (Blalock et al., 1990).

Kerlikowske and co-workers (1993) have demonstrated that family history reporting enhances the efficacy of breast cancer screening. In women age 40 years and older with a positive family history of breast cancer, positive predictive values for mammography were comparable to the group with the highest positive predictive value, women age 50 years and older. Considering the current debate surrounding the appropriateness of mammography screening for women age 40 to 50, this information has important implications for this group of high-risk women who have much to gain from mammography screening. With regard to enhancing compliance, a study of 501 Texas women found that a significantly greater percentage of women with a family history for breast cancer considered their perceived risk as moderate or great compared to those without a family history (79% 54%) and,

thus, would be more likely to participate in mammography screening (Vogel et al., 1990).

Several studies have shown that the family history can be a powerful influence in determining compliance with lipid screening and other preventive interventions for cardiovascular disease In a study that compared 69 freshmen college students with a family history for cardiovascular disease to 154 students without a family history, students without a family history were more likely to be smokers, to have parents who smoked, and they were less likely to exercise and to have had a blood cholesterol test (Tamragouri et al., 1986). In another study that utilized DNA markers in addition to the family history for definition of genetic risk for heart disease, increased compliance with recommended preventive guidelines was seen in those with genetic risk (Bamberg et al., 1990). Based on self-reports of having a blood cholesterol level rechecked, seeking advice from a physician or a dietician for weight loss and limiting fat and cholesterol intake, there was at least an 18% higher compliance rate and at least a four times greater likelihood of performing the behaviors in the group with genetic risk than the "non-genetic" risk group. When those subjects with a blood cholesterol level above 200 mg/dL were analyzed as a subgroup, the genetic risk group had a statistically significant higher compliance rate for having a blood cholesterol level rechecked than the non-genetic risk group (Bamberg et al., 1990).

Screening for identification of individuals at risk for coronary heart disease can also improve with integration of genetic risk information. Family history has been shown to be a greater predictor of risk for premature ischemic heart disease than the conventional risk factors including elevated serum cholesterol, inactivity, and smoking (Nora et al., 1980). The risk ratio for premature heart disease associated with having a first-degree relative with premature heart disease was 10.4 and this risk was more than twice the risk associated with having a serum cholesterol value greater than 270 mg/dL. This has significant implications for individuals with an inherited susceptibility since many would be missed with the current screening guidelines for coronary heart disease, which recommend measurement of total serum cholesterol and HDL cholesterol (Expert Panel on Detection, Evaluation, and Treatment of High Blood Cholesterol in Adults, 1993). In one study, only 38% of individuals with premature heart disease had abnormal lipid values (Genest et al., 1992); 19% had elevated Lp(a) values which would not be detected with routine cholesterol screening and only 3% had elevated LDL cholesterol values. Other genetic risk factors involving several different metabolic pathways may contribute to a predisposition to coronary heart disease (Cheng et al., 1999). Measuring these risks should aid in the identification of such individuals and in addition, modification of these risk factors might lead to a reduction in risk.

Genetic information and technology transfer

Participation in effective early detection and prevention strategies should have significant benefit for individuals with a genetic susceptibility to common diseases. Under-utilization of these services by genetically susceptible individuals has been documented (Scheuner et al., 1997b). A genetic risk assessment survey of 176 managed care members found that the only significant predictor of cholesterol screening was advanced age (p=0.05). Gender, ethnicity, time since last visit to the doctor, and family history of cardiovascular disease (heart disease, stroke, and carotid, aortic or peripheral vascular disease), diabetes, or a cholesterol abnormality were not predictive of who was likely to have had cholesterol checked. Similarly, participation in mammography, sigmoidoscopy, fecal occult blood testing and serum prostate-specific antigen testing was associated with older age rather than a cancer

family history. This included individuals from hereditary colon cancer and high-risk breast and ovarian cancer pedigrees. Among the respondents to the mailed genetic risk assessment survey, 53 charts from 15 primary care physicians selected randomly were reviewed for family history (Henderson and Scheuner, 1998).This included data collected from 223 patient visits (4.2 visits per patient) that occurred over the five-year period prior to the mailing of the survey. Among the charts reviewed, 39 belonged to subjects who gave self-reports of a family history of at least one common disease; the physician documented this family history in only 36%. The number of first-degree relatives that were reported by patients as having one of the conditions under study was 115, compared to only 23 documented by the physician. The corresponding number of self-reported affected second-degree relatives was 213, and the physicians documented only four. The type of disease did not influence the family history documentation by the physician; they were dismal across all disease categories.

Thus, the failure of the primary care physician to collect the appropriate family history data appears to be an important factor that precluded adequate genetic risk assessment and access to appropriate preventive services for subjects with a genetic susceptibility to many common, chronic conditions. Acheson et al. (2000) have found that family practice physicians discuss family history about half of the time during new patient visits, and only 22% of the time during established patient visits. This included discussion of "family issues" that might represent a broad range of topics in addition to medical issues. The quality of information collected was likely limited (although this was not determined) since the average duration of family history discussions was less than 2.5 minutes. Only 11% of patients' records included a family tree. This was probably due to the limited time available for a patient visit, 10 minutes. It is estimated that construction of a pedigree in the family practice setting obtained via semi-structured interview takes 15 to 20 minutes.

In a survey of 339 primary care providers in the United Kingdom the majority felt a need to provide genetic services (Suchard et al., 1999). However, only 29% felt sufficiently prepared to take family histories and draw pedigrees and only 15% felt prepared to counsel patients about genetic test results. Almost two-thirds would participate in training and education regarding genetics and would participate in providing genetic services, yet not all were willing to provide these services. For practitioners who do feel comfortable with transmitting genetic information, the increased time demands required to research the family history and provide genetic counseling (Surh et al., 1995) may act as disincentives to routinely offering adequate genetic risk assessment.

Thus, rather than providing comprehensive genetic services for patients with complex genetics service needs, the role of the primary care provider should include 1) identification of patients who may benefit from genetic services, 2) provision of basic genetic information to facilitate the referral process, 3) recognition of the special psychosocial issues for a family with a genetic condition, and 4) coordination of care and monitoring of health (Hayflick et al., 1998). Primary care providers' lack of general knowledge in genetics (Hoffman et al., 1993) may preclude appropriate referrals to genetic professionals for genetic risk assessment, counseling, and when appropriate, DNA testing (Hayflick et al., 1998). This is compounded by incentive arrangements that reward "gate-keeper" physicians to limit patient access to specialty referrals and treatments (Swartz and Brennan, 1996). Unfortunately, there are a limited number of professionals who are trained in genetics (Rowley et al., 1995), and this may be the most significant factor related to provision of clinical genetic services for common diseases. Clinicians may also be reluctant to pursue genetic risk assessment for their patients since evidence regarding the efficacy and utility of using genetic information in disease management and prevention is limited. This lack of evidence should not, however, deter clinicians from utilizing genetic information regarding common disease, as it clearly has value in providing risk information and in many instances can guide decision making for disease management and prevention.

The social, ethical and legal issues surrounding the clinical application of genetic risk assessment include confidentiality, privacy, stigmatization, discrimination, and cost, and these may act as barriers to gaining access to genetic information. Fear of discrimination by employers or insurers may be the greatest barrier to obtaining genetic information (Lerman et al., 1996), although the evidence regarding genetic discrimination of otherwise healthy individuals is minimal (Billings et al., 1992; Geller et al., 1996). Yet, because of the fear of discrimination, individuals may choose to bear the financial liability not only for an initial genetic risk assessment (which may include costly DNA testing), but also for the surveillance or therapeutic measures they undertake to reduce their disease risk. A study of semi-structured interviews with genetic counselors and geneticists has shown that the greatest deterrence to participation in genetic testing is for those individuals who do not wish to use their health insurance for reimbursement of testing and who cannot afford to pay for testing (Hall and Rich, 2000). There was little deterrence for participating in affordable testing or when the perceived need for immediate information was greater, as in the case of prenatal and pediatric genetic testing. Fear of discrimination was not reported in testing decisions for pediatric or prenatal situations, but was significant for adult-onset conditions.

Since 1990, there has been a steady rise in interest regarding regulating the use of genetic information by health insurers (Reilly, 1998). However, the impact of these bills is limited since most Americans have access to their health insurance through their employer and large employers do not customarily use genetic information as a means to evaluate employees entering the risk pool. Moreover, self-insuring employers can circumvent the state laws due to the Employee Retirement Income Security Act (Reilly, 1998). In 1996, the Health Insurance Portability and Accountability Act (HIPAA) became the first federal law to limit the use of genetic data by health insurers. It forbids group plans from using genetic predisposition to disease as a "pre-existing" condition that could delay or limit coverage (Reilly, 1997). However, existing laws have not greatly reduced the fear of discrimination.

Summary

Genetic factors play an important role in the etiology, natural history and response to therapy for many common diseases. Knowledge of a genetic susceptibility to a common disease may provide the basis for directing the most appropriate disease management and prevention. However, translational research that addresses the efficacy and cost-effectiveness of genetic services in the management and prevention of disease is needed. Currently, the family history is the best predictor of a genetic risk for common diseases. Additional markers of risk including biochemical studies and DNA testing help to qualify and quantify a genetic risk. Access to a sufficient number of professionals who are expert in the field of medical genetics and genetic counseling is likely the most important clinical issue related to the clinical applications of genetic information and technology.

Electronic-database information

The URLs for data in this chapter are as follows:

GeneDx, Inc. Rockville, MD, www.genedx.com for testing methodology information on Peutz-Jegers syndrome, Gorlin syndrome and Cowden syndrome

Genetests, http://www.genetests.org

Online Mendelian inheritance in Man (OMIM), http://www.ncbi.nlm.nih.gov/Omim

REFERENCES

Aarnio M, Mecklin J-P, Aaltonen L et al. (1995) Life-time risk of different cancers in hereditary nonpolyposis colorectal cancer (HNPCC) syndrome. Inter J Cancer 64:430–433

Acheson LS, Wiesner GL, Zyzanski SJ et al. (2000) Family history-taking in community family practice: Implications for genetic screening. Genet in Med 2:180–185

Acton RT, Go R, Roseman J (1989) Strategies for the utilization of genetic information to target preventive interventions.Proceedings of the 25th Annual Meeting of the Society of Prospective Medicine, Indianapolis, Indiana, pp. 88–100

Alberts MJ (1990) Genetic aspects of cerebrovascular disease. Current Concepts of Cerebrovascular Disease and Stroke 25:25–30

American Society of Clinical Oncology (ASCO) Subcommittee on Genetic Testing for Cancer Susceptibility (1996) Statement of ASCO: Genetic testing for cancer susceptibility. J Clin Oncol 14:1730–1736

American Society of Human Genetics (ASHG) Ad Hoc Committee on Genetic Testing for Breast and Ovarian Cancer (1994) Statement on genetic testing for breast and ovarian cancer predispostion. Am J Hum Genet 55:ii–iv

American Society of Human Genetics (1996) Statement on informed consent for genetic research. Am J Hum Genet 59:471–474

Amos CI, Shaw GL, Tucker MA, Hartge P (1992) Age at onset for familial epithelial ovarian cancer. J Am Med Assoc 268:1896–1899

Amos CI, Struewing JP (1993) Genetic epidemiology of epithelial ovarian cancer. Cancer 71:566–572

Anderson DE, Badzioch MD (1993) Familial breast cancer risks. Effects of prostate and other cancers. Cancer 72:114–119

Assmann G, Schulte H (1990) Primary prevention of coronary heart disease in the Federal Republic of Germany. Analysis of cost-effectiveness. Drugs 40 Supplement 1:33–37

Bamberg R, Acton RT, Roseman JM (1990) The effect of genetic risk information and health risk assessment on compliance with preventive behaviors. Health Education 21:26–32

Bamberg R, Acton RT, Roseman JM (1993) Health and genetics risk impact on preventive behaviors. pp. In Matzen RN, Lang RS (eds): Clinical Preventive Medicine. Mosby, St. Louis, 799–812

Barrett-Connor E, Laakso M (1990) Ischemic heart disease risk in postmenopausal women: Effects of estrogen use on glucose and insulin levels. Arteriosclerosis 10:531–534

Barrow DA, Jensen RL (1999) Thrombotic risk assessment: Annual risk, age at first event, and epidemiological impact of hereditary causes. Clin Hemostasis Rev 13:13–14

Bensen JT, Liese AD, Rushing JT et al. (1999) Accuracy of proband reported family history: The NHLBI Family Heart Study (FHS). Genet Epidemiol 17:141–150

Billings PR, Kohn MA, de Cuevas M et al. (1992) Discrimination as a consequence of genetic testing [see comments]. Am J Hum Genet 50:476–82

Blalock SJ, De Vellis BM, Afifi RA, Sandler RS (1990) Risk perceptions and participation in colorectal cancer screening. Health Psychology 9:792–806

Boltenberg A, Furgyik S, Kullander S (1990) Familial cancer aggregation in cases of adenocarcinoma corporis uteri. Acta Obstet Gynecol Scand 69:249–258

Burke W, Petersen G, Lynch P et al. for the Cancer Genetics Studies (1997a) Recommendations for follow-up care of individuals with an inherited predisposition to cancer. I. Hereditary nonpolyposis colon cancer. J Am Med Assoc 277:915–919

Burke W, Daly M, Garber J et al. for the Cancer Genetics Studies Consortium (1997b) Recommendations for follow-up care of individuals with an inherited predisposition to cancer. II. BRCA1 and BRCA2. J Am Med Assoc 277:997–1003

Carter BS, Beaty TH, Steinberg GD et al. (1992) Mendelian inheritance of familial prostate cancer. Proc Natl Acad Sci 89:3367–3371

Cheng S, Grow MA, Pallaud C et al. (1999) A multilocus genotyping assay for candidate markers of cardiovascular disease risk. Genome Research 9:936–949

Claus EB, Risch N, Thompson WD (1993) The calculation of breast cancer risk for women with a first degree family history of ovarian cancer. Breast Cancer Res and Treat 28:115–120

Colditz GA, Stampfer MJ, Willett WC et al. (1986) A prospective study of parental history of myocardial infarction and coronary heart disease in women. Am J Epidemiol 123:48–58

Colditz GA, Rimm EB, Giovannucci E et al. (1991) A prospective study of parental history of myocardial infarction and coronary artery disease in men. Am J Cardiol 67:933–938

Croyle RT, Smith K, Botkin JR et al. (1997) Psychological responses to BRCA1 mutation testing. Health Psychology 16:63–72

Cummings SR, Eckert S, Krueger KA et al. (1999) The effect of raloxifene on risk of breast cancer in postmenopausal women. Results of the MORE randomized trial. J Am Med Assoc 281:2189–2197

Dipple KM, Zhang YH, Havens J et al. (2000) "Simple" mendelian disorders are complex traits: Human glycreol kinase deficiency as a model. J Inherited Metabolic Dis 23 (Supplement 1):172

Eddy DM, Nugent FW, Eddy JF et al. (1987) Screening for colorectal cancer in a high-risk population, results of a mathematical model. Gastroenterol 92:682–92

Egan KM, Newcomb PA, Longnecker MP (1996) Jewish religion and risk of breast cancer. Lancet 347:1645–1646

Eikelboom JW, Lonn E, Genest J et al. (1999) Homocyste(e)ine and cardiovascular disease: A critical review of the epidemiologic evidence. Ann Int Med 131:363–375

Evans RA, Marel GM, Lancaster ED et al. (1998) Bone mass is low in relatives of osteoporotic patients. Ann Intern Med 109:870–873

Expert Panel on Detection, Evaluation, and Treatment of High Blood Cholesterol in Adults (1993) Summary of the second report of the National Cholesterol Education Program (NCEP) Expert Panel on Detection, Evaluation, and Treatment of High Blood Cholesterol in Adults (Adult Treatment Panel II). J Am Med Assoc 269:3015–3023

Farrer LA, Cupples LA, Haines JL et al. (1997) Effects of age, sex, and ethnicity on the association between apolipoprotein E genotype and Alzheimer disease: A meta-analysis. J Am Med Assoc 278:1349–1356

Fisher B, Costantino JP, Wickerham DL and other National Surgical Adjuvant Breast and Bowel Project Investigators (1998) Tamoxifen for prevention of breast cancer: Report of the National Surgical Adjuvant Breast and Bowel Project P-1 Study. J National Cancer Institute 90:1371–1388

Fletcher SW, Black W, Harris R et al. (1993) Report of the International Workshop on Screening for Breast Cancer. J National Cancer Institute 85:1644–56

Fraser FC (1974) Genetic counseling. Am J Hum Genet 26:636–659

Gail MH, Brinton LA, Byar DP et al. (1989) Projecting individualized probabilities of developing breast cancer for white females who are being examined annually. J Natl Cancer Inst 81:1879–1886

Geller LN, Alper JS, Billings PR et al. (1996) Individual, family, and societal dimensions of genetic discrimination: A case study analysis. Science & Engin Ethics 2:71–88

Geller G, Botkin JR, Green MJ et al. (1997) Genetic testing for susceptibility to adult-onset cancer. The process and content of informed consent. J Am Med Assoc 277:1467–1474

Genest JJ, Martin-Munley SS, McNamara JR et al. (1992) Familial lipoprotein disorders in patients with premature coronary artery disease. Circulation 85:2025–2033

Goldman L, Gordon DJ, Rifkind BM et al. (1992) Cost and health implications of cholesterol lowering. Circulation 85:1960–68

Graffagnino C, Gasecki AP, Doig GS, Hachinski VC (1994) The importance of family history in cerebrovascular disease. Stroke 25:1599–1604

Greenlee RT, Murray T, Bolden S, Wingo PA (2000) Cancer statistics 2000. CA Cancer Journal Clin 50:7–33

Greggi S, Genuardi M, Benedetti-Panici P et al. (1990) Analysis of 138 consecutive ovarian cancer patients: Incidence and characteristics of familial cases. Gynecologic Oncol 39:300–304

Grody W, Cutting G (2000) American College of Medical Genetics Policy Statement: Recommended Core Mutation Panel for Cystic Fibrosis Testing

Grover S, Quinn MA, Weideman P (1973) Patterns of inheritance of ovarian cancer. An analysis from an ovarian cancer screening program. Cancer 72:526–530

Gruber SB, Thompson WD (1996) A population-based study of endometrial cancer and familial risk in younger women. Cancer and Steroid Hormone Study Group. Cancer Epidemiol Biomark Prev 5:411–417

Guyatt GH, Haynes BR, Jaeschke RZ et al. for the Evidence-Based Medicine Working Group (2000) Users' guides to the medical literature: XXV. Evidence-based medcine: Principles for applying the users' guides to patient care. J Am Med Assoc 284:1290–1296

Hall MA, Rich S (2000) Patients' fear of genetic discrimination by health insurers: The impact of legal protections. Genet in Med 2:214–221

Hartmann LC, Schaid DJ, Woods JE et al. (1999) Efficacy of bilateral prophylactic mastectomy in women with a family history of breast cancer. N Eng J Med 340:77–84

Hayflick SJ, Eiff MP, Carpenter L, Steinberger J (1998) Primary care physicians' utilization and perceptions of genetics services. Genet in Med 1:13–21

Henderson LB, Scheuner MT (1998) Suboptimal family history collection: An obstacle to genetic risk assessment and prevention. Am J Hum Genet 63:A240

Henderson LB, Adams JS, Goldstein DR et al. (2000) A familial risk profile for osteoporosis. Genet in Med 2:222–225

Hoffman KJ, Tambor ES, Chase GA et al. (1993) Physician's knowledge of genetics and genetic tests. Acad Med 68:625–632

Hoskins KF, Stopfer JE, Calzone KA et al. (1995) Assessment and counseling for women with a family history of breast cancer. J Am Med Assoc 273:577–585

Houlston RS, Bourne TH, Davies A et al. (1992) Use of family history in a screening clinic for familial ovarian cancer. Gynecol Oncol 47:247–252

Hudson KL, Rothenberg KH, Andrews LB et al. (1995) Genetic discrimination and health insurance: An urgent need for reform. Science 270:391–393

Hulley SB, Newman TB, Grady D et al. (1993) Should we be measuring blood cholesterol levels in young adults? J Am Med Assoc 269:1416–1419

Imperiale TF, Wagner Dr, Lin CY et al. (2000) Risk of advanced proximal neoplasms in asymptomatic adults according to the distal colorectal findings. N Eng J Med 343:169–174

Isotalo PA, Wells GA, Donnelly JG (2000) Neonatal and fetal methylenetetrahydrofolate reductatase genetic polymorphisms: An examination of C677T and A1298C mutations. Am J Hum Genet 67:986–990

Jacobson TA (2000) "The lower the better" in hypercholesterolemia therapy: A reliable clinical Guideline? Ann Int Med 133:549–554

Jarvinen HJ, Mecklin J-P, Sistonen P (1995) Screening reduces colorectal cancer rate in families with hereditary nonpolyposis colorectal cancer. Gastroenterol 108:1405–1411

Kahn LB, Marshall JA, Baxter J et al. (1990) Accuracy of reported family history of diabetes mellitus. Results from San Luis Valley Diabetes Study. Diabetes Care 13:796

Kearon C, Crowther M, Hirsch J (2000) Management of patients with hereditary hypercoagulable disorders. Annual Rev Med 51:169–185

Kee F, Tiret L, Robo JY et al. (1993) Reliability of reported family history of myocardial infarction. BMJ 307:1528–1530

Keen H, Track NS (1968) Age of onset and inheritance of diabetes: The importance of examining relatives. Diabetologia 4:317–321

Kerlikowsk K, Brown JS, Grady DG (1992) Should women with familial ovarian cancer undergo prophylactic oophorectomy? Obstet Gynecol 80:700–707

Kerlikowske K, Grady D, Barclay J et al. (1993) Positive predicitive value of screening mammography by age and family history of breast cancer. J Am Med Assoc 270:2444–2450

Kiely DK, Wolf PA, Cupples A et al. (1993) Familial aggregation of stroke. The Framingham Study. Stroke 24:1366–1371

King RA, Rotter JI, Motulsky AG (1992) The approach to genetic bases of common diseases.In King RA, Rotter JI, Motulsky AG (eds): The Genetic Basis of Common Diseases. Oxford University Press, pp. 3–18,

Knowler WC, Narayan KMV, Hanson RL et al. (1995) Preventing non-insulin-dependent diabetes. Diabetes 44:483–488

Köbberling J, Tattersall R (1982) The genetics of diabetes mellitus. Academic Press, London.

Krall EA, Dawson-Hughes B (1993) Heritable and life determinants of bone mineral density. J Bone Miner Res 8:1–9

Lerman C, Narod S, Schulman K et al. (1996) BRCA1 testing in families with hereditary breast-ovarian cancer. A prospective study of patient decision making and outcomes. J Am Med Assoc 275:1885–1892

Lieberman DA, Weiss DG, Bond JH et al. (2000) Use of colonoscopy to screen asymptomatic adults for colorectal cancer. N Eng J Med 343:162–168

Love RR, Evans AM, Josten DM (1985) The accuracy of patient reports of a family history of cancer. J Chronic Disorders 38:289–93

Lovett E (1976) Family studies in cancer of the colon and rectum. Br J Surg 63:13–18

Lynch HT, Watson P, Conway TA et al. (1993) DNA screening for breast/ovarian cancer susceptibility based on linked markers. A family study. Arch Intern Med 153:1979–1985

McKinnon WC, Baty BJ, Bennett RL (1997) Predisposition genetic testing for late-onset disorders in adults. A position paper of the National Society of Genetic Counselors. JAMA. 278:1217–1220

Macklin MT (1960) Inheritance of cancer of the stomach and large intestine in man. J Natl Cancer Inst 24:551–571

Mecklin J-P (1987) Frequency of hereditary colorectal carcinoma. Gastroenterology 93:1021–25

Miller AB, To T, Baines CJ, Wall C (2000) Canadian National Breast Cancer Screening Study—2: 13-year results of randomized trial in women aged 50–59. J Nat Cancer Instit 92:1490–1499

Mirvis DM, Chang CF (1997) Managed care, managing uncertainty. Arch Intern Med 157:385–88

Mitchell BD, Kammerer CM, Reinhart LJ, Stern MP (1994) NIDDM in Mexican-Americcan families. Heterogeneity by age of onset. Diabetes Care 17:567–573

Morrison AS (1992) The feasibility of screening programs. In Morrison AS (ed.): Screening in Chronic Disease. Oxford University Press, pp. 148–167

Narod SA, Risch H, Moslehi R et al. for the Hereditary Ovarian Cancer Clinical Study Group (1998) Oral contraceptives and the risk of hereditary ovarian cancer. N Eng J Med 339:424–428

Narod SA, Brunet J, Ghadirian P et al. for the Hereditary Breast Cancer Study Group (2000) Tamoxifen and the risk of contralateral breast cancer in BRCA1 and BRCA2 mutation carriers: A case-control study. Lancet 356:1876–1881

National Advisory Council for Human Genome Research (1994) Statement on use of DNA testing for presymptomatic identification of cancer risk. J Am Med Assoc 271:785

NIH Consensus Development Panel on Ovarian Cancer (1995) Ovarian cancer. Screening, treatment, and follow-up. J Am Med Assoc 273:491–497

Nora JJ, Lortscher RH, Spangler RD et al. (1980) Genetic-epidemiologic study of early-onset ischemic heart disease. Circulation 61:503–508

Pocock NA, Eisman JA, Hopper JL et al. (1987) Genetic determinants of bone mass in adults: A twin study. J Clin Invest 80:706–710

Ponz de Leon M, Scapoli C, Zanghieri G et al. (1992) Genetic transmission of colorectal cancer: exploratory data analysis from a population based registry. J Med Genet 29:531–538

Reaven GM (1988) Role of insulin resistance in human disease. Diabetes 37:595–607

Reaven GM (1988) Banting lecture 1988. Role of insulin resistance in human disease. Diabetes 37:1595–1607

Rebbeck TR, Levin AM, Eisen A et al. (1999) Breast cancer risk after bilateral prophylactic oophorectomy in BRCA1 mutation carriers. J Natl Cancer Inst 91:1475–1479

Reilly PR (1997) Laws that regulate the use of genetic information. In Rothstein MA (ed): Genetic Secrets: Protecting Privacy and Confidentiality in the Genetic Era. Yale University Press, New Haven, CT, pp.369–391.

Reilly PR (1998) Genetic risk assessment and insurance. Genetic testing 2:1–2

Risch N, Merikangas K (1996) The future of genetic studies of complex human diseases. Science 273:1516–1517

Rissanen AM (1979) Familial occurrence of coronary heart disease: Effect of age at diagnosis. Am J Cardiol 44:60–66

Rose G (1964) Familial patterns in ischaemic heart disease. Br J Prev Soc Med 18:75–80

Rothenberg K, Fuller B, Rothstein M et al. (1997) Genetic information and the workplace: Legislative approaches and policy changes. Science 275:1755–1757

Rowley PT, Loader S, Sutera CJ, Kozyra A (1995) Prenatal genetic counseling for hemoglobinopathy carriers: A comparison of primary providers of prenatal care and professional genetic counselors. Am J Hum Genet 56:769–776

Rozen P, Fireman Z, Figer A, Legum C, Ron E, Lynch HT (1987) Family history of colorectal cancer as a marker of potential malignancy within a screening program. Cancer 60:248–254

Rubnitz JE, Pui C-H (1999) Molecular diagnostics in the treatment of leukemia. Current Opinion in Hematol 6:229

Sandler RS, DeVellis BM, Blalock SJ, Holland KL (1989) Participation of high-risk subjects in colon cancer screening. Cancer 63:2211–2215

Sandles LG, Shulman LP, Elias S et al. (1992) Endometrial carcinoma: Genetic analysis suggesting heritable site-specific uterine cancer. Gynecologic Oncol 47:167–171

Scheuner MT (2000) Validator of clinical genetic teste. genet med 2:155–156

Scheuner MT, Alarcon M (1999) Diabetes increases coronary artery disease (CAD) risk to relatives of female CAD cases. Am J Hum Genet 65:A49

Scheuner MT, Wang S-J, Raffel LJ et al. (1997a) Family history: A comprehensive genetic risk assessment method for the chronic conditions of adulthood. Am J Med Genet 71:315–324

Scheuner MT, Tran LT, Henderson LB, Goldstein DR (1997b) Utilization of preventive strategies by genetically susceptible individuals. Am J Hum Genet 61:A57.

Scheuner MT, Cheng LS-C, Hixon HEC, Rotter JI (2000) BRCA testing uptake and participation in ovarian cancer prevention in women at risk for an inherited ovarian cancer suceptibility. Genet Med 2:86

Schildkraut JM, Risch N, Thompson WD (1989) Evaluating genetic association among ovarian, breast, and endometrial cancer: Evidence for a breast/ovarian cancer relationship. Am J Hum Genet 45:521–529

Scholtz RI, Rosenman RH, Brand RJ (1975) The relationship of reported parental history to the incidence of coronary artery disease in the Western Collaborative Group Study. Am J Epidemiol 102:350–356

Sickles EA, Kopans DB (1995) Mammographic screening for women aged 40 to 49 years: the primary care practioner's dilemma. Ann Int Med 122:534–538

Singer DE, Samet JH, Coley CM, Nathan DM (1991) Screening for diabetes mellitus. In Eddy DM (ed.): Common Screening Tests. American College of Physicians, Philadelphia, PA, pp.154–178

Slack J, Evans KA (1966) The increased risk of death from ischaemic heart disease in first-degree relatives of 121 men and 96 women with ischaemic heart disease. J Med Genet 3:239–257

Slattery ML, Kerber RA (1993) A comprehensive evaluation of family history and breast cancer risk. JAMA 270:1563–1568

Smith GD, Pekkanen J (1992) Should there be a moratorium on the use of cholesterol lowering drugs? BMJ 304:431–434

Spitz MR, Currier RD, Fueger JJ et al. (1991) Familial patterns of prostate cancer: A case-control analysis. J Urol 146:1305–1307

Spriggs DA, French JM, Murdy JM et al. (1990) Historical risk factors for stroke: A case control study. Age and Ageing 19:280–287

Steinberg GD, Carter BS, Beaty TH et al. (1990) Family history and the risk of prostate cancer. Prostate 17:337–347

Steinberg KK, Thacker SB, Smith SJ et al. (1991) A meta-analysis of the effect of estrogen replacement therapy on the risk of breast cancer. J Am Med Assoc 265:1985–1990

Steinberg KK, Pernarelli JM, Marcus M et al. (1998) Increased risk for familial ovarian cancer among Jewish women: A population-based case-control study. Genet Epidemiol 15:51–59

Stephenson BM, Finan PJ, Gascoyne J et al. (1991) Frequency of familial colorectal cancer. Br J Surg 78:1162–66

Stephenson BM, Murday VA, Finan PJ et al. (1993) Feasibility of family based screening for colorectal neoplasia: Experience in one general surgical practice. Gut 34:96–100

Suchard MA, Yudkin P, Sinsheimer JS, Fowler GH (1999) General practitioners' views on genetic screening for common diseases. B J Gen Prac 49:45–6

Surh LC, Wright PG, Cappelli M et al. and the Molecular Study Group (1995) Delivery of molecular genetic services within a health care system: Time analysis of the clinical workload. Am J Hum Genet 56:760–768

Swartz K, Brennan TA (1996) Integrated health care, capitated payment, and quality: The role of regulation. Ann Int Med 124:442–48

Tamragouri RN, Martin RW, Cleavenger RL, Sieber WK Jr (1986) Cardiovascular risk factors and health knowledge among freshemen college students with a family history of cardiovascular disease. College Health 34:267–270

Thomas CB, Cohen BH (1955) The familial occurrence of hypertension and coronary artery disease with observations concerning obesity and diabetes. Ann Intern Med 42:90–127

Turk A (2000) Scientific, clinical, and economic rationale for combination therapy in managing asthma: A paradigm for managed care. Am J Managed Care 6:S916–S917

Vine DL (1994) Doubts about clinical impact of cholesterol reduction. American Family Physician 49:558, 560, 567

Vogel VG, Graves DS, Vernon SW et al. (1990) Mammographic screening of women with increased risk of breast cancer. Cancer 66:1613–20

Walker M (1999) Non-diabetic relatives: Characteristics and opportunities for intervention. In Hitman GA (ed). Type 2 Diabetes Prediction and Prevention. John Wiley, NY, pp.303–322

Watson P, Lynch HT (1993) Extracolonic cancer in hereditary nonpolyposis colorectal cancer. Cancer 71:677–685

Wilson PWF, Schaefer EJ, Larson MG, Ordovas JM (1996) Apolipoprotein E alleles and risk of coronary disease: A meta-analysis. Arteriosclerosis Thrombolic Vascular Biology 16:1250–1255

Woolf CM (1958) A genetic study of carcinoma of the large intestine. Am J Hum Genet 10:42–47

Woolf, SH (1995) Current concepts: Screening for prostate cancer with prostate-specific antigen—an examination of the evidence. N Eng J Med 333:1401–1405

Yan H, Papadopoulos N, Marra G et al. (2000) Conversion of diploidy to haploidy. Nature 403:723–724

Risk estimation in genetic counseling

24

Ian D. Young

Introduction

One of the most important components of the genetic counseling process is the provision of a risk figure. Whilst it is clearly essential that an individual's needs for support and counseling should not be neglected, it is also vital that information given should be correct and precise. Although true for some, it is not acceptable to assume that a consultand is simply concerned with whether a risk is high or low. The genetic counselor is obliged to ensure that an accurate risk estimate has been derived and that it is conveyed in a meaningful fashion.

The advent of sophisticated computer programs has greatly facilitated risk calculation, particularly in complex situations utilizing information provided by analysis with linked DNA markers. Without access to a program such as Linkage (Lathrop and Lalouel, 1984), risk calculation in large families or using multiple markers can be extremely laborious and exceedingly difficult. However, computer programs are not always as user-friendly as their compilers might wish us to believe, nor are they always readily available. Moreover it is clearly desirable that those who use this new technology should have a reasonable grasp of the basic principles involved so that they can assess intuitively, or with the help of paper and pencil, whether the answer appearing on the monitor is plausible.

Quantitative risks can be conveyed in several ways, for example, as fractions, decimals, percentages or odds. It is conventional to denote a probability as a proportion of 1, so that a value of 0.25 will be equivalent to 1/4, 25% or a risk of one in four. Alternatively, this can be expressed as odds of three to one against or one to three in favor of a particular event being observed.

Methods used in risk calculation

A knowledge of three basic principles will be sufficient to cater for most genetic counseling risk calculations. Two of these, the laws of addition and multiplication, will be familiar to many from their school days. The third and most complex is known as Bayes theorem. Although originally expounded well over 200 years ago, it has proved to be particularly useful for calculating genetic risks.

LAW OF ADDITION

Stated formally, the law of addition is as follows. If two (or more) events are *mutually exclusive*, and if the probability of event one occurring is $P1$ and of event two occurring is $P2$, then the probability of *either* the first event *or* the second event occurring equals $P1 + P2$. The key words in this definition are *mutually exclusive, either* and *or*. For example, twins can be *either* monozygotic (MZ) *or* dizygotic (DZ) and the probability that they will be *either* MZ *or* DZ equals 1.

LAW OF MULTIPLICATION

The law of multiplication deals with events that are *independent*. If the probability of one such event occurring is $P1$, and of another occurring is $P2$, then the probability of *both* the first *and* the second occurring equals $P1 \times P2$. Here the key words are *independent, both* and *and*. For example, for DZ twins born to parents who are both carriers of the same autosomal recessive disorder, the probability that *both* the first twin *and* the second twin will be affected equals $1/4 \times 1/4 = (1/16)$. Whether or not the

675

first twin is affected is irrelevant to the health of the second twin: these are *independent* events, so that the probability of both events occurring is the product rather than the sum of each probability.

EXAMPLE 1

Healthy parents have had a child with a severe autosomal recessive disorder. Aware of the recurrence risk of 1 in 4, they embark upon another pregnancy. During the early stages of this pregnancy, ultrasonography reveals the presence of twins. The parents now wish to know the probability that at least one twin will be affected by the autosomal recessive disorder.

To answer this question the risks are first calculated for the two mutually exclusive possibilities that the twins are either (1) monozygotic ($P = 1/3$) or (2) dizygotic ($P = 2/3$).

1. Monozygotic. In this situation the probability that both twins will be affected equals 1/4, that only one will be affected equals 0, and that both will be unaffected equals 3/4.
2. Dizygotic. If the twins are dizygotic then the genotype of one twin does not influence the genotype of the other twin, i.e., these events are independent. Therefore the probability that both twins will be affected equals 1/16 (i.e., $1/4 \times 1/4$), the probability that only one will be affected equals 3/8 [i.e., $(1/4 \times 3/4) + (3/4 \times 1/4)$] and the probability that both will be unaffected equals 9/16 (i.e., $3/4 \times 3/4$).

Using this combination of mutually exclusive and independent events the parents' question can now be answered. The overall probability that:

(a) both twins will be affected equals MZ ($1/3 \times 1/4$) plus DZ ($2/3 \times 1/16$) giving a total probability of 1/8;
(b) only one twin will be affected equals MZ ($1/3 \times 0$) plus DZ ($2/3 \times 3/8$) giving a total probability of 1/4;
(c) both twins will be unaffected equals MZ ($1/3 \times 3/4$) plus DZ ($2/3 \times 9/16$) giving a total probability of 5/8.

With this information, the parents can be reliably informed that there is a probability of $1/8 + 1/4 = 3/8$ that at least one of their unborn babies will be affected.

BAYES THEOREM

We are indebted to the Reverend Thomas Bayes for providing us with an extremely valuable means of quantifying

Table 24.1. Bayes Theorem for Quantifying Genetic Risks

Probability	Event A	Event B
Prior	a	b
Conditional	c	d
Joint	ac	bd
Posterior	$\dfrac{ac}{ac + bd}$	$\dfrac{bd}{ac + bd}$

genetic risks (Bayes, 1763 and 1958). In essence Bayes theorem offers a method for considering all possibilities or events and then weighting or "conditioning" these by incorporating information which sheds light on which is the most likely. The initial probability of each event is known as its *prior* probability and is based on "anterior" information such as the ancestral family history. The observations that modify these prior probabilities allow *conditional* probabilities to be derived from "posterior" information such as the results of linkage analysis or carrier tests. The resulting probability for each possibility or event is known as its *joint* probability. The overall final probability of each event, which is known as its *posterior* or *relative* probability, is obtained by dividing its joint probability by the sum of all the joint probabilities.

This potentially confusing statement of Bayes theorem may be more easily understood by referring to Table 24.1.

The easiest way to understand how these laws can be combined in practice is to consider the following relatively simple counseling situation.

EXAMPLE 2

II_2 in Figure 24.1 wishes to know the probability that she is a carrier of Duchenne muscular dystrophy. She has an affected brother and also had an affected maternal uncle. Consequently her mother is an obligatory carrier. This anterior information allows us to assign her prior probability of being a carrier as 1 in 2. Similarly her prior probability of not being a carrier also equals 1 in 2. These are mutually exclusive events and the sum of their probabilities equals 1.

This consultand (II_2) already has two unaffected sons. This is posterior information which points towards the woman not being a carrier. The conditional probability that a carrier would have two unaffected sons equals $1/2 \times 1/2$ ($= 1/4$), that is, the product of the individual probabilities of these two independent events. The conditional probability that II_2 would have two unaffected sons if she is not a carrier equals 1, that is, $1 \times 1 = 1$.

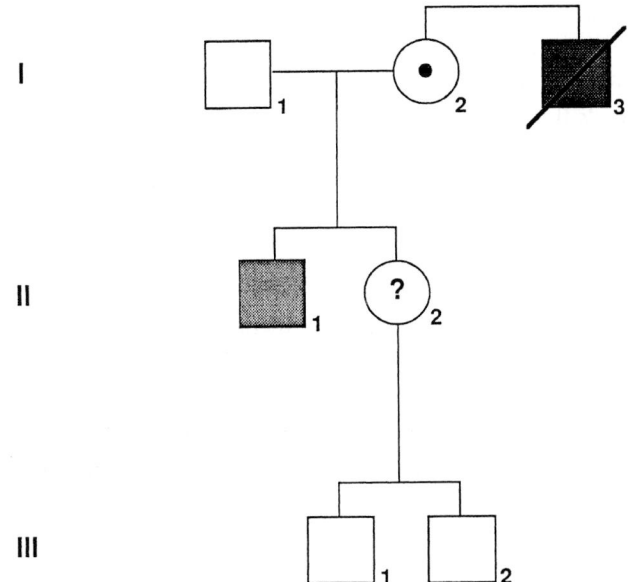

Fig. 24.1. See Examples 2 and 13. II_2 wishes to know the probability that she is a carrier of Duchenne muscular dystrophy.

All this information is now incorporated in a Bayesian table (Table 24.2). The posterior probability that II_2 is a carrier equals

$$\frac{1/8}{1/8 + 1/2} = 1/5$$

and the posterior probability that she is not a carrier equals

$$\frac{1/2}{1/8 + 1/2} = 4/5$$

Alternatively the posterior probability can be stated in the form of odds by comparing the joint probabilities, that is, the odds for being a carrier are 1 to 4 (which is the same as 1 *in* 5) and for not being a carrier are 4 to 1 (the same as 4 *in* 5).

Table 24.2. Calculating Carrier Risk for Duchenne Type Muscular Dystrophy for II_2 in Figure 24.1[a]

Probability	II_2 Is a Carrier	II_2 Is Not a Carrier
Prior	$\frac{1}{2}$	$\frac{1}{2}$
Conditional		
2 unaffected sons	$\frac{1}{4}$	1
Joint	$\frac{1}{8}$	$\frac{1}{2}$

[a] *See Example 2.*

Thus this exercise has provided a means of quantifying the extent to which the two unaffected sons have reduced their mother's risk of being a carrier, that is, from 1 in 2 to 1 in 5. Later in this chapter (see Examples 13 and 14) we shall see how additional information can be incorporated to further modify this risk.

Autosomal-dominant inheritance

Several factors can influence and complicate risk calculation in autosomal-dominant inheritance. These include reduced penetrance, delayed age of onset and the use of genetic polymorphisms (most commonly DNA "markers") linked to the disease locus. Each of these factors will be considered in turn.

REDUCED PENETRANCE

This refers to the phenomenon whereby only a proportion of individuals who harbour a mutant allele manifest signs or symptoms of the relevant disorder. The concept is rather unsatisfactory in that there is as yet no clear underlying explanation as to why one member of a family with a condition such as Treacher-Collins syndrome should be severely affected, when a heterozygous close relative may show absolutely no features. Presumably other genes, allelic or non-allelic, can somehow influence expression of the relevant mutant gene. Alternatively, expression of the mutant gene may require a second and somatic mutational event, which must occur within a specific organ and time-frame. Such an explanation might account for the reduction in penetrance seen in retinoblastoma (see Ch. 140), in which approximately only 80% of gene carriers develop a tumor. For this condition the penetrance (P) would therefore be said to equal 0.8.

Whatever the correct explanation, reduction in penetrance is a major problem when counseling for disorders in which this phenomenon is recognized. Two such situations are now considered.

EXAMPLE 3

In the example shown in Figure 24.2, II_1 wishes to know the probability that his newborn daughter, III_1, will develop a retinoblastoma. His father (I_1) underwent treatment for bilateral tumors in early childhood. Therefore II_1 began life with a risk of $1/2 \times P = 0.4$ that he would develop a tumor. The fact that he did not develop a tumor

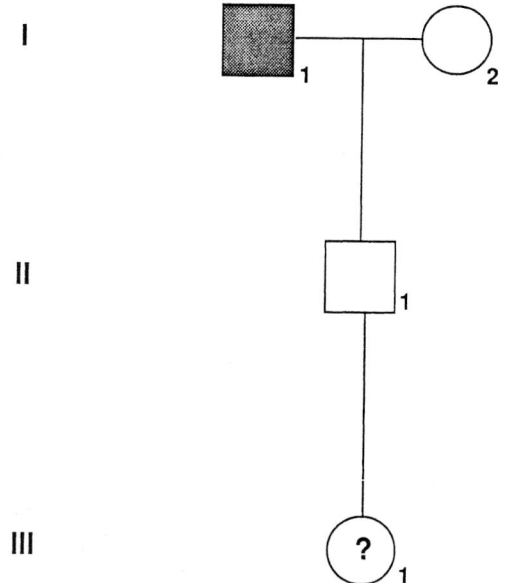

Fig. 24.2. See Example 3. II$_1$ wishes to know the probability that his daughter III$_1$ will develop her grandfather's disorder which shows autosomal-dominant inheritance with reduced penetrance.

does not mean that his daughter (III$_1$) is at negligible risk, as II$_1$ could be a nonpenetrant heterozygote. The precise risk to III$_1$ is determined by constructing a simple Bayesian table (Table 24.3). The posterior probability that II$_1$ is an example of nonpenetrance equals

$$\frac{1/2\ (1-P)}{1/2\ (1-P)+1/2} \quad \text{which simplifies to} \quad \frac{1-P}{2-P}$$

Therefore the risk that III$_1$ will develop the disorder can be calculated as her father's probability of heterozygosity multiplied by $P/2$, that is

$$\frac{P-P^2}{4-2P}$$

Table 24.3. Predicting Risk of Inheriting Retinoblastoma for II$_1$ in Figure 24.3.[a]

Probability	II$_1$ Is Heterozygous	II$_1$ Is Not Heterozygous
Prior	$\frac{1}{2}$	$\frac{1}{2}$
Conditional Not affected	$1-P$	1
Joint	$\frac{1}{2}(1-P)$	$\frac{1}{2}$

[a] See Example 3.

For a value of P equal to 0.8, the risk for tumor development in III$_1$ will be 0.067 (1 in 15). It has been shown in this situation that the maximum risk for III$_1$ arises when P equals 0.6 giving a probability for developing the disease of 0.086 (Pauli and Motulsky, 1981).

EXAMPLE 4

The simple pedigree shown in Figure 24.3 presents a much more difficult calculation. Healthy parents with no relevant positive family history have a single affected child (II$_1$). This could have occurred as the result of a new mutation or as a consequence of one of the parents being a nonpenetrant heterozygote. Germinal mosaicism in one of the parents represents a third possibility which is discussed towards the end of this chapter.

The risk that a future child (II$_2$ in Figure 24.3) will be affected can be calculated as follows. The prior probability that either I$_1$ or I$_2$ is heterozygous approximates to 4 pq where p and q are the frequencies of the normal and mutant genes respectively. (The derivation of this value of 4 pq may be better understood by referring to the paragraphs on Hardy-Weinberg law in the section on autosomal-recessive inheritance). The Bayesian calculation in Table 24.4 shows that the posterior probability that one of the parents is heterozygous equals

$$\frac{4pq(1-P)P/2}{4pq(1-P)P/2+2\mu P}$$

In practice the mutation rate (μ) is usually not known. This problem is resolved by substituting $I/2(1-f)$ for μ (Haldane, 1949), where I equals the incidence of the disorder (which in turn equals $2pq$) and f equals the fitness of heterozygotes. By making this substitution, the posterior

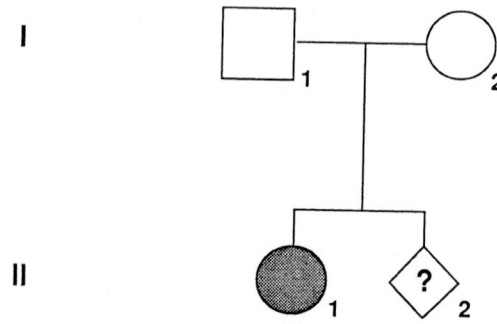

Fig. 24.3. See Example 4. II$_1$ has an autosomal-dominant disorder which shows reduced penetrance. What is the probability that II$_2$ will also be affected?

Table 24.4. Risk of Inheriting an Autosomal-Dominant Disorder With Reduced Penetrance[a]

Probability	One Parent Heterozygous	Neither Parent Heterozygous
Prior	$4pq$	$1 - 4pq \approx 1$
Conditional		
Parents are unaffected	$1 - P$	1
1 affected child	$\dfrac{P}{2}$	$2\mu P$
Joint	$4pq(1 - P)\dfrac{P}{2}$	$2\mu P$

[a] See Figure 24.3 and Example 4.

probability of heterozygosity in one of the parents neatly reduces to

$$\frac{1 - P}{2 - P - f}$$

(Friedman, 1985).

Emery (1986) has pointed out that in disorders with reduced penetrance, fitness is only assessed for affected heterozygotes and he has introduced a modification to the above approach giving a final risk that II_2 in Figure 24.3 will be affected of

$$\frac{P(1 - P)}{2(1 - Pf^a)}$$

where f^a is the fitness of affected individuals. Arguably, the presence of other healthy siblings should also be taken into account, as the greater the number of these individuals the more likely it becomes that the disease in the isolated case has resulted from a new mutation. Recurrence risks for a future sibling are provided in Table 24.5 for different values of fitness and penetrance given from 0 to 3 healthy siblings.

In practice these are extremely difficult counseling situations in which full family evaluation is essential. Germinal mosaicism, which is discussed elsewhere, simply adds to the problem. Increasingly the identification of underlying mutations in conditions such as retinoblastoma allows much more accurate counseling and renders the use of this theoretical approach unnecessary.

VARIABLE AGE OF ONSET

Many autosomal-dominant disorders do not manifest until late childhood or adult life. Examples are listed in Table 24.6. Details of families in which these conditions are segregating are often held on confidential and carefully maintained genetic registers which allow clinical and genetic information to be integrated and coordinated. One of the most useful roles fulfilled by these registers is to enable young family members to be informed of the risks that they themselves could develop the condition known to be running in the family.

EXAMPLE 5

In Figure 24.4, II_1 is aged 25 years and wishes to know the probability that he has inherited familial adenomatous polyposis (FAP) from his deceased father (I_1). Clearly II_1 has commenced life with a prior probability of one in two for inheriting the disorder. This risk can be modified by bowel examination and by a search for congenital hypertrophy of the retinal pigment epithelium (CHRPE) (Burn et al., 1991). Both of these investigations are undertaken and fortunately both yield negative results.

This information allows the prior probability of one in two to be modified as follows. The probability that a

Table 24.5. Recurrence Risks for a Sibling of an Isolated Case of a Disorder Showing Autosomal-Dominant Inheritance With Reduced Penetrance and Fitness

	Fitness															
	0.3				0.5				0.7				0.9			
	n				n				n				n			
Penetrance	0	1	2	3	0	1	2	3	0	1	2	3	0	1	2	3
0.6	0.146	0.12	0.095	0.074	0.171	0.145	0.119	0.094	0.207	0.183	0.156	0.130	0.261	0.247	0.23	0.209
0.7	0.133	0.1	0.072	0.05	0.162	0.125	0.093	0.067	0.206	0.169	0.132	0.099	0.284	0.258	0.255	0.189
0.8	0.105	0.072	0.046	0.029	0.133	0.086	0.061	0.039	0.182	0.133	0.092	0.061	0.286	0.24	0.189	0.14
0.9	0.070	0.036	0.021	0.012	0.082	0.049	0.028	0.016	0.122	0.076	0.045	0.026	0.237	0.171	0.113	0.07

n, number of healthy siblings (from Young, 1999, with permission)

Table 24.6. Autosomal-Dominant Disorders That Show Variable Age of Onset

von Hippel-Lindau disease
Huntington disease
Facioscapulohumeral muscular dystrophy
Familial adenomatous polyposis
Basal cell nevus syndrome
Tuberous sclerosis
Multiple endocrine adenomatosis
Retinoblastoma
Hypertrophic cardiomyopathy
Marfan syndrome
Polycystic renal disease, adult type
Hereditary motor and sensory neuropathy
Neurofibromatosis types I and II
Familial hypercholesterolemia
Myotonic dystrophy

Table 24.7. Variable Age of Onset and the Risk of Inheriting an Autosomal-Dominant Disorder[a]

Probability	II1 Is Heterozygous	II1 Is Not Heterozygous
Prior	$\frac{1}{2}$	$\frac{1}{2}$
Conditional		
No polyps at age 25	$\frac{1}{10}$	1
Less than 4 CHRPEs	$\frac{1}{10}$	1
Joint	$\frac{1}{200}$	$\frac{1}{2}$

CHRPE, congenital hypertrophy of the retinal pigment epithelium
[a] See Figure 24.4 and Example 5.

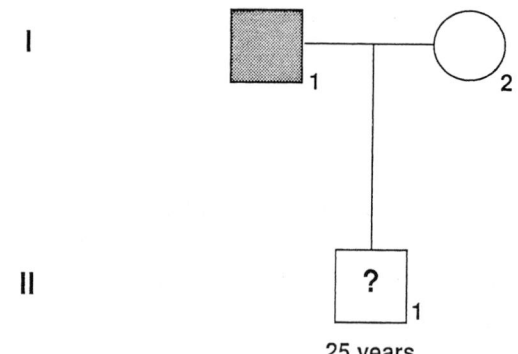

Fig. 24.4. See Example 5. II$_1$ wishes to know the probability that he has inherited an autosomal-dominant disorder showing variable age of onset.

I

II

? 1

25 years

25-year-old heterozygote would have no polyps at bowel examination is one in ten. The probability that he would have four or less CHRPEs is also one in ten. The Bayesian calculation shown in Table 24.7 yields a posterior probability of

$$\frac{1/200}{1/200 + 1/2} = 1/101$$

which is a probability of 1 in 101 that II$_1$ has inherited the gene for FAP and will go on to be affected. This is obviously a much more reassuring risk than the prevailing prior probability of one in two.

THE USE OF LINKED DNA MARKERS

The identification of the specific underlying mutation in disorders such as Huntington disease and myotonic dys-

trophy has enabled very precise prediction of disease status for individuals who are at risk because of a positive family history. However, for several of the disorders in Table 24.6, direct mutation analysis is not readily available either because the gene has not been identified or because the search for individual mutations in the gene is extremely laborious. Therefore for some families resort has to be made to the use of linked DNA markers using the technique of gene tracking described elsewhere (Ch. 8 and 29).

EXAMPLE 6

In some families the use of linked DNA markers is very straightforward. This applies particularly if the linkage phase can be established in the key individual who also happens to be heterozygous for the DNA marker allele. Consider III$_1$ in Figure 24.5. A and B represent allelic marker genes at a locus closely linked to the disease locus with a recombination fraction equal to θ. In the key individual, II$_2$, both the disease gene and the B marker have been inherited from I$_2$. Therefore in II$_2$ these genes must be on the same chromosome, that is, "in coupling". (It is important to note that this does not mean that the disease gene in I$_2$ is on the same chromosome as the B marker, as a crossover could have occurred during the meiosis which lead to formation of the gamete that resulted in II$_2$.)

Knowledge of the linkage phase in II$_2$ permits the disease status in III$_1$ to be predicted. If she inherits marker A from her mother, then the probability that she will be affected equals θ, that is, she will be affected only if a crossover occurs at maternal meiosis. If she inherits marker B from

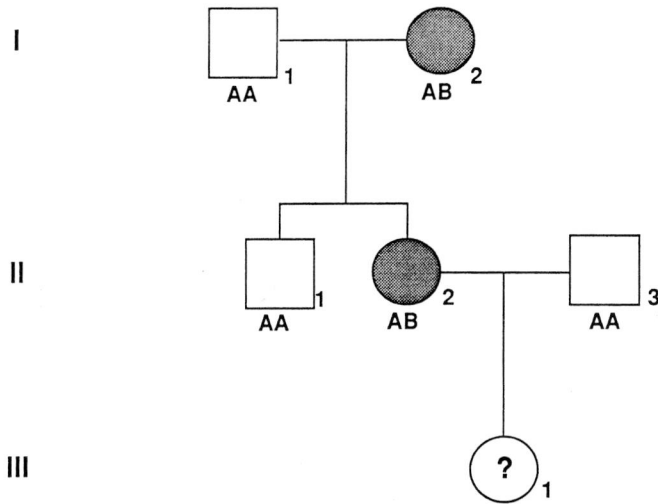

Fig. 24.5. See Example 6. What is the probability that III₁ will be affected if she inherits either marker A or marker B from her mother?

her mother, she will be affected unless a crossover occurs at maternal meiosis, that is, the probability that she will be affected equals $1 - \theta$.

EXAMPLE 7

If the linkage phase in the key individual is not known with certainty, then it may be possible to use information from another family member to establish which phase is more likely. In Figure 24.6 II₂ is at risk of developing a late onset autosomal-dominant disorder that affects his mother and sister. Once again A and B are alleles at a DNA locus closely linked to the disease locus. The linkage phase is known in II₁ (disease is in coupling with B), but for the reason discussed in the previous example, this is not known with certainty in I₂. Intuitively, the disease gene is *probably* in coupling with the B marker in I₂. We now have to construct a Bayesian table (Table 24.8) to quantify this intuition.

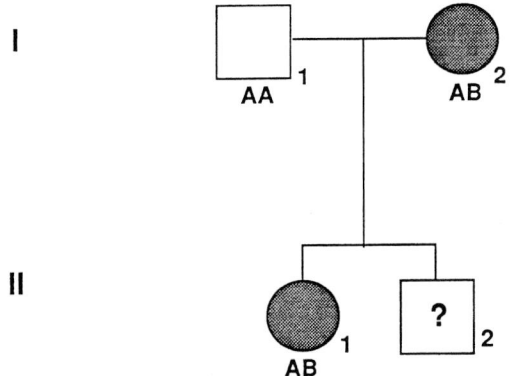

Fig. 24.6. See Example 7. What is the probability that II₂ will be affected if he inherits either marker A or marker B from his mother?

Table 24.8. Using Linked Markers in Autosomal-Dominant Inheritance[a]

Probability	Disease in I₂ in Coupling With A	Disease in I₂ in Coupling With B
Prior	$\dfrac{1}{2}$	$\dfrac{1}{2}$
Conditional II₁ has inherited B and is affected	θ	$1 - \theta$
Joint	$\dfrac{\theta}{2}$	$\dfrac{1-\theta}{2}$

[a] See Example 7.

From Table 24.8 it can be seen that the posterior probability that the disease gene is in coupling with the A marker in I₂ equals

$$\frac{\theta/2}{\theta/2 + 1 - \theta/2} = \theta.$$

Similarly, the probability that the disease gene is in coupling with the B marker equals $1 - \theta$. Now we can determine the risk for II₂. If he inherits marker A from his mother then the probability that he will also have inherited the disease gene equals the sum of

the probability that the disease gene in I₂ is in coupling with A (= θ) multiplied by $1 - \theta$, that is, $\theta (1 - \theta)$ plus

the probability that the disease gene in I₂ is in coupling with B (= $1 - \theta$) multiplied by θ, that is, $\theta (1 - \theta)$.

This gives a total probability of $2\theta - 2\theta^2$. By the same process it can be shown that the probability that II₂ will have inherited the disease gene if he inherits marker B from his mother equals $1 - 2\theta + 2\theta^2$. This example demonstrates that when the linkage phase in the transmitting parent is not known with certainty, the predictive error becomes greater. For a value of $\theta = 0.05$, the error rate for II₂ in Example 7 is close to 10%, in contrast with 5% for III₁ in Example 6.

The use of linked DNA markers has revolutionized genetic counseling over the last 10 years enabling carrier detection, prenatal diagnosis and preclinical diagnosis to be offered for most of the more common severe single gene disorders which present at a genetic clinic. If markers on either side of the disease locus ("flanking" or "bridging") are available, this greatly reduces the margin of error, but at the expense of a much more difficult calculation (Winter, 1985). Locus heterogeneity is an important obstacle to the application of linked markers, although some large families may yield sufficient information to indicate which disease locus is more likely to be implicated (Lau et al., 1988). Simple examples of how these aspects can be approached manually are considered elsewhere (Bridge, 1997; Young, 1999). More complex linkage calculations are much better handled by computer programs.

Autosomal-recessive inheritance

Traditionally, risk estimation for autosomal-recessive disorders has been regarded as being relatively straightforward. When parents have had an affected child it is reasonable to conclude that they are both carriers so that the risk to each future child is one in four. The probability that the healthy sibling of an affected patient is a carrier equals $2/3$. Risks to family members other than the siblings of an affected individual are usually very low.

Before considering specific examples, it is necessary to review one of the fundamental principles of population genetics which enables the incidence of carriers of any particular autosomal-recessive disorder to be established in the general population.

THE HARDY-WEINBERG LAW

If the frequency of the normal (wild-type) gene equals p, and the frequency of the abnormal (mutant) gene equals q so that $p + q = 1$, then the incidence of non-carriers, carriers and affected will be p^2, $2pq$ and q^2 respectively. This conclusion involves several assumptions:

1. A large randomly mating stable population.
2. Either a constant mutation rate, which balances out those genes lost due to death of affected homozygotes, or no new mutations and no selection against affected homozygotes.
3. No selection for or against carriers.

These assumptions are not always valid, but for practical counseling purposes these limitations can usually be ignored.

If the Hardy-Weinberg law applies, then the incidence (I) of carriers in the general population, which will equal the probability that a healthy member of that population is a carrier, will approximate to twice the square root of the disease incidence (q^2), that is

$I = 2 \times p \times q \approx 2q$ as p is very close to 1.

Therefore for conditions such as cystic fibrosis and phenylketonuria which have incidences of approximately one in 1600 and one in 10,000 respectively, the respective carrier incidences will be

$1/20$ that is, $(2 \times \sqrt{1/1,600})$ and $1/50$ that is, $(2 \times \sqrt{1/10,000})$.

RISKS TO OTHER FAMILY MEMBERS

As already indicated these are usually low. Relatives can often be reassured by presenting them with an estimate of their actual risk.

EXAMPLE 8

The brother (II_2) of a boy with cystic fibrosis wishes to know the probability that his first child will be affected (Fi. 24.7). His partner (II_3) is healthy and unrelated and has no family history of the disorder. The probability that II_2 is a carrier equals $2/3$. The probability that his partner is a carrier equals the incidence of carriers in the general population, that is, one in 20. Therefore the risk that their first child will be affected equals the probability that both prospective parents are carriers, that is, $(2/3 \times 1/20)$ multiplied by $1/4$, this being the probability that any two carriers will have an affected child. This gives an overall risk of

$2/3 \times 1/20 \times 1/4 = 1/120$

This example illustrates the general approach employed to calculate a risk figure when counseling for an autosomal-recessive disorder in the extended family. The probability that each partner is a carrier is calculated. The product of these independent probabilities is then multiplied by $1/4$ to arrive at the risk that their first child will be affected.

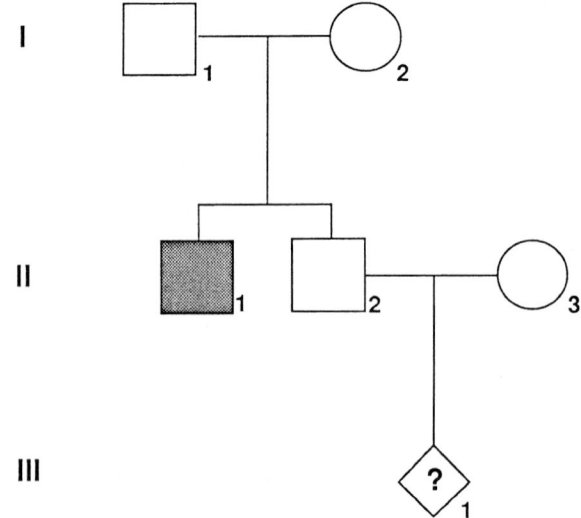

Fig. 24.7. See Example 8. What is the probability that III_1 will have the same autosomal-recessive disorder as his/her paternal uncle II_1?

EXAMPLE 9

In the family shown in Figure 24.8, individuals II_1 and II_2 have phenylketonuria, which shows a disease incidence of one in 10,000 and a carrier frequency of approximately one in 50. I_3 and I_4 already have two unaffected children and wish to know the probability that a future third child will be affected. These two healthy children have to be taken into account as their unaffected status influences the probability that both of their parents are carriers. A Bayesian table is constructed in Table 24.9.

The posterior probability that both I_3 and I_4 are carriers equals

$$9/(9 + 1584) = 1/177$$

Therefore the probability that their third child will be affected equals

$$1/177 \times 1/4 = 1/708$$

Consequently, the two healthy children have reduced their parents' risk of having an affected child from 1/400 to 1/708.

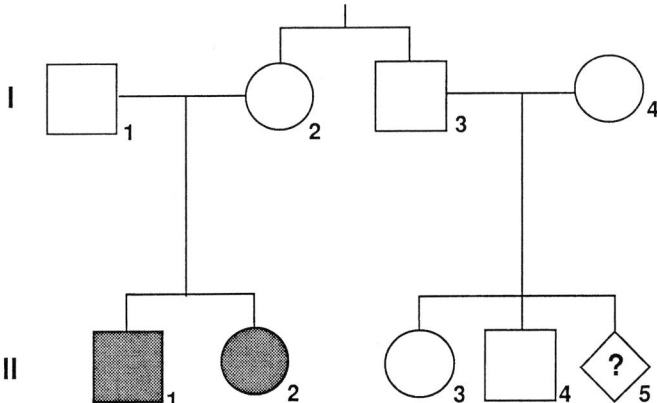

Fig. 24.8. See Example 9. What is the probability that II_5 will have the autosomal recessive-disorder which affects II_1 and II_2?

Table 24.9. Calculating the Probability of a Third Child Inheriting an Autosomal-Recessive Disorder.[a]

Probability	Both I_3 and I_4 Are Carriers	I_3 and I_4 Are Not Both Carriers
Prior	$\frac{1}{2} \times \frac{1}{50} = \frac{1}{100}$	$1 - \frac{1}{100} = \frac{99}{100}$
Conditional		
2 unaffected children	$\frac{9}{16}$	1
Joint	$\frac{9}{1600}$	$\frac{99}{100} = \frac{1584}{1600}$

[a] See Example 9 and Figure 24.8.

DIRECT MUTATION ANALYSIS AND MULTIPLE ALLELES

In the United Kingdom, approximately 75% of all cystic fibrosis carriers have an identical mutation/deletion known as ΔF508. At least 800 other mutations have been identified in this gene. This can lead to some quite difficult counseling situations.

EXAMPLE 10

In this example II_2 wishes to know the probability that she is a carrier of cystic fibrosis (Fig. 24.9). Both her father (I_1) and her affected brother (II_1) are deceased, and no material is available from either for DNA analysis. The mother (I_2) has been shown to carry ΔF508. The daughter (II_2) does not carry ΔF508.

Two methods are outlined to show how the risk of heterozygosity in II_2 can be determined. In the first a simple Bayesian table is constructed (see Table 24.10). This yields a posterior probability that II_2 is a carrier of

$$\frac{1/12}{1/12 + 1/3} = 1/5$$

The key point in this approach is the derivation of the conditional probability that II_2 is a carrier. One half of her potential carrier risk is removed as she does not carry ΔF508 which is carried by her mother. The prior probability that her father carried ΔF508 is 3/4, as this mutation accounts for 75% of all cystic fibrosis mutations in the relevant population. Therefore the remaining half of her potential carrier risk is diminished by this factor of 3/4. This leaves a conditional probability of 1/8 that II_2 is a carrier, that is, $1/2 \times 1/4$.

An alternative and perhaps simpler approach is to consider all of the possible parental genotypes, as shown in Table 24.11.

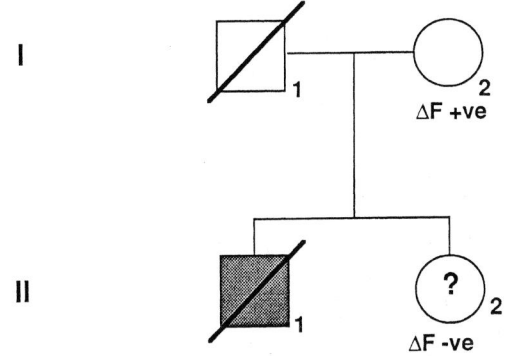

Fig. 24.9. See Example 10. What is the probability that II_2 is a carrier of cystic fibrosis?

Table 24.10. Calculating Carrier Risk for Cystic Fibrosis[a]

Probability	II$_2$ Is a Carrier	II$_2$ Is Not a Carrier
Prior	$\dfrac{2}{3}$	$\dfrac{1}{3}$
Conditional ΔF negative		
(mat) $\dfrac{1}{2} \times 0$		1
+ (pat) $\dfrac{1}{2} \times \dfrac{1}{4}$		
$= \dfrac{1}{8}$		
Joint	$\dfrac{1}{12}$	$\dfrac{1}{3}$

mat, maternal; pat, paternal
[a] See Example 10 and Figure 24.9.

Table 24.11. Possible Parental Genotypes in Example 10[a]

Probability	ΔF Father +	Mother +	ΔF Father −	Mother +
Prior	3		1	
Conditional II$_2$	C	NC	C	NC
Prior	$\dfrac{2}{3}$	$\dfrac{1}{3}$	$\dfrac{2}{3}$	$\dfrac{1}{3}$
Conditional ΔF negative	0	1	$\dfrac{1}{2}$	1
Joint	0	1	$\dfrac{1}{3}$	$\dfrac{1}{3}$

C, carrier; NC, noncarrier; +, positive; −, negative
[a] See also Figure 24.9.

From Table 24.11 the posterior probability that II$_2$ is a carrier is one in five: that is,

$$\frac{1/3}{5/3} = 1/5$$

This alternative approach of setting out all the possible genotypes tends to occupy more space, but is often less prone to error as derivation of a complex conditional probability becomes unnecessary.

The fact that II$_2$ tested negative for ΔF508 allows a new probability to be calculated for the likelihood that her father carried ΔF508. This is achieved by summing the joint probabilities for columns one and two in Table 24.11 (that is 1) and dividing this by the total of all the joint probabilities (5/3), giving a posterior probability of 3/5.

THE USE OF LINKED DNA MARKERS

The method used to determine risks for an autosomal-recessive disorder using linked DNA markers is essentially the same as that outlined in the previous section on autosomal-dominant inheritance. However, calculations are complicated by the fact that there are now two parents rather than one in whom a crossover can occur.

EXAMPLE 11

The first child (II$_1$) of healthy parents has an autosomal-recessive disorder for which a closely linked DNA marker is available. This marker identifies four alleles A, B, C and D. Both parents are heterozygous and the affected child has markers A and C. The parents wish to know the probability that a second child (II$_2$) will be affected given each of the four possible marker genotypes (AC AD BC BD) (Fig. 24.10).

The calculation is approached by establishing the posterior probabilities for the linkage phase in the parents based on the information provided by II$_1$. The Bayesian table constructed in Table 24.12 shows that the posterior probabilities for each of the parental genotypes are as indicated below:

Disease Alleles Coupled With		
I$_1$	I$_2$	Posterior probability
A	C	$(1 - \theta)^2$
A	D	$(1 - \theta)\theta$
B	C	$\theta(1 - \theta)$
B	D	θ^2

Based on this information the probability that II$_2$ will be affected given different genotypes can be calculated. If, for

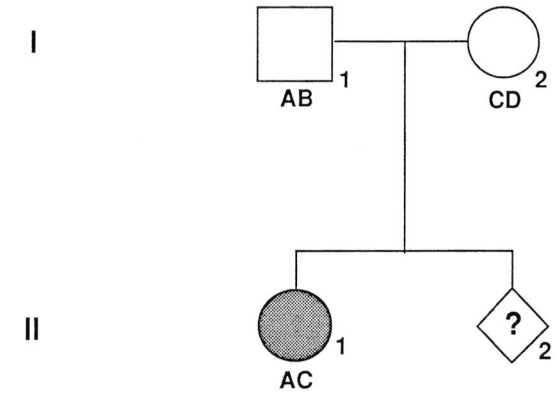

Fig. 24.10. See Example 11. What is the probability that II$_2$ will be affected given marker genotypes AC, AD, BC or BD?

Table 24.12. Linkage Phase of Disease Alleles in I_1 and I_2 in Figure 24.10[a]

Probability	$I_1(A)I_2(C)$	$I_1(A)I_2(D)$	$I_1(B)I_2(C)$	$I_1(B)I_2(D)$
Prior	$\dfrac{1}{4}$	$\dfrac{1}{4}$	$\dfrac{1}{4}$	$\dfrac{1}{4}$
Conditional II1 (AC) is affected	$(1-\theta)^2$	$(1-\theta)\,\theta$	$\theta\,(1-\theta)$	θ^2
Joint	$\dfrac{1}{4}(1-\theta)^2$	$\dfrac{1}{4}(1-\theta)\,\theta$	$\dfrac{1}{4}\theta(1-\theta)$	$\dfrac{1}{4}4\,\theta^2$

[a] See Example 11.

example, II_2 has an AC genotype then the overall probability that he/she will be affected equals the sum of

1. the probability if the disease alleles are in coupling with A in I_1 and C in I_2, that is, $(1-\theta)^2 \times (1-\theta)^2$ plus
2. the probability if the disease alleles are in coupling with A in I_1 and D in I_2, that is, $(1-\theta)\theta \times (1-\theta)\theta$ plus
3. the probability if the disease alleles are in coupling with B in I_1 and C in I_2, that is, $\theta(1-\theta) \times \theta(1-\theta)$ plus
4. the probability if the disease alleles are in coupling with B in I_1 and D in I_2, that is, $\theta^2 \times \theta^2$.

These four probabilities summate to $1 - 4\theta + 8\theta^2 - 8\theta^3 + 4\theta^4$, which approximates to $1 - 4\theta$.

Looked at very simply there are four meioses in which a single crossover could have occurred which would result in II_2 not being affected. By an equally lengthy process it can be shown that the probability that II_2 will be affected with an AD or BC genotype approximates to 2θ and with a BD genotype to $4\theta^2$. As with autosomal-dominant disorders, the use of flanking markers will greatly reduce the margin of error, although the associated calculations become formidably complex!

Sex-linked recessive inheritance

This pattern of inheritance has a well-deserved reputation for generating difficult risk calculations. In 1978, Bundey circulated 32 clinical geneticists in the United Kingdom seeking their assessment of risks in five relatively simple family trees. Only 7 of the 18 who were brave enough to respond gave correct answers for all the pedigrees. This occurred despite the earlier publication in 1975 of an authoritative textbook outlining the basic principles of risk calculation and describing in detail the practical application of Bayes theorem (Murphy and Chase, 1975).

Before considering specific examples it is necessary to establish the prior probability that any female is a carrier of a particular sex-linked recessive disorder. Towards this end, consider a multigeneration family and assume equal mutation rates (μ) in males and females. The mother in the first generation is not a carrier and affected males are unable to reproduce. In the second generation the probability that a female will be a carrier equals 2μ. In the third generation this value rises to 3μ, that is, half of the mother's probability of 2μ plus 2μ. By generation n this probability of heterozygosity will have reached 4μ. This then is the value of the prior probability that any female who does not have a positive family history will be a carrier of a sex-linked recessive disorder with zero fitness in affected males and equal mutation rates in the sexes.

RISK BASED ON SIMPLE PEDIGREE ANALYSIS

A simple example has already been considered in the introductory section on Bayes theorem (Example 2). A more complex pedigree is now considered.

Example 12

In the family shown in Figure 24.11, III_1 is an isolated case of a sex-linked recessive disorder such as Duchenne muscular dystrophy (DMD). Three females, II_2, II_6 and III_3, wish to know their probable carrier status. This is resolved by drawing up a large Bayesian table as shown in Table 24.13.

From Table 24.13 the posterior probability that I_2 is a carrier can be calculated as

$$\frac{\mu/16 + \mu^2/4}{\mu/16 + \mu^2/4 + \mu/2 + \mu} = 1/25$$

(Note that in this calculation $\mu^2/4$ is ignored, as this will represent a negligible quantity compared with the other

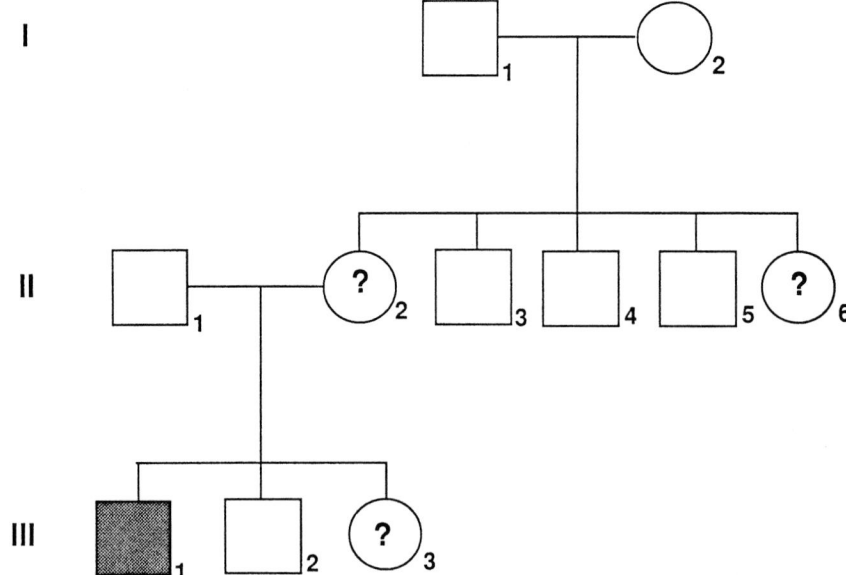

Fig. 24.11. See Example 12. II₂, II₆ and III₃ wish to know the probability that they are carriers of Duchenne muscular dystrophy.

Table 24.13. Probable Carrier Status for Females in Figure 24.11[a]

Probability	I_2 Is a Carrier		I_2 Is Not a Carrier	
Prior	4μ		$1 - 4\mu \approx 1$	
Conditional				
3 unaffected sons	$\frac{1}{8}$		1	
II_2	C	NC	C	NC
Prior	$\frac{1}{2}$	$\frac{1}{2}$	2μ	1
Conditional				
III_1 affected	$\frac{1}{2}$	μ	$\frac{1}{2}$	μ
III_2 unaffected	$\frac{1}{2}$	1	$\frac{1}{2}$	1
Joint	$\dfrac{\mu}{16}$	$\dfrac{\mu^2}{4}$	$\dfrac{\mu}{2}$	μ

C, carrier; NC, noncarrier
[a] See Example 12.

joint probabilities. In practical terms we are ignoring any option which involves two independent mutations).

This value of 1/25 can be used to determine the prior probability that II₆ is a carrier. This will be half her mother's posterior probability, that is, one in 50.

The Bayesian table also allows us to establish the posterior probability that II₂ is a carrier. This equals

$$\frac{\mu/16 + \mu/2}{\mu/16 + \mu^2/4 + \mu/2 + \mu} = 9/25$$

and the prior probability that III₃ is a carrier equals

$$9/25 \times 1/2 = 9/50$$

This example illustrates several important and useful practical points when using Bayes theorem.

1. All relevant information must be taken into account, but no information must ever be used more than once.
2. The individual who is seeking information is considered last. In the case of II₂ this was achieved by introducing her towards the lower half of the table and calculating probabilities assuming her to be either a carrier or not a carrier. This is necessary in the case of II₂ because the pedigree contains both anterior and posterior information which influences the probability that she is a carrier.
3. If an individual seeking information does not feature in the Bayesian table because that individual does not provide relevant information, then a technique involving a "dummy consultand" is employed. In the cases of II₆ and III₃, prior probabilities were obtained by determining posterior probabilities for their mothers and then halving these values. For this purpose these mothers are referred to as "dummy consultands". The dummy consultand is usually the nearest female ancestor common to both the affected male(s) and the female seeking information.

INCORPORATING LABORATORY RESULTS

For many sex-linked recessive conditions such as DMD and haemophilia, carrier tests show overlap between carriers and non-carriers. For example, in DMD serum creatine kinase is elevated in approximately two-thirds of all carriers, and statistical analysis of curves which overlap for normals and carriers allows a conditional probability to be obtained based on creatine kinase analysis alone. This can then be incorporated into a Bayesian table.

EXAMPLE 13

Consider once again individual II_2 in Figure 24.1. Creatine kinase assay has yielded a conditional probability of one to four that she is a carrier. This is included in the overall calculation (see Table 24.14).

The posterior probability that II_2 is a carrier is now $1/32 \div (1/32 + 1/2)$ which equals $1/17$.

THE USE OF LINKED DNA MARKERS

Linked DNA markers are now available for almost all sex-linked recessive disorders. Prior to the isolation of the DMD gene, these were particularly valuable in carrier detection, and in those families in which the disease mutation remains unknown they still provide a very useful means of determining probable carrier status.

The calculations involved are very similar to those described in the section on autosomal-dominant inheritance.

EXAMPLE 14

Once again we shall consider individual II_2 in Figure 24.1, which has been redrawn as Figure 24.12 to include the results obtained using a closely linked DNA marker which identifies two alleles, A and B. A large Bayesian table is constructed (Table 24.15) to take into account all relevant information.

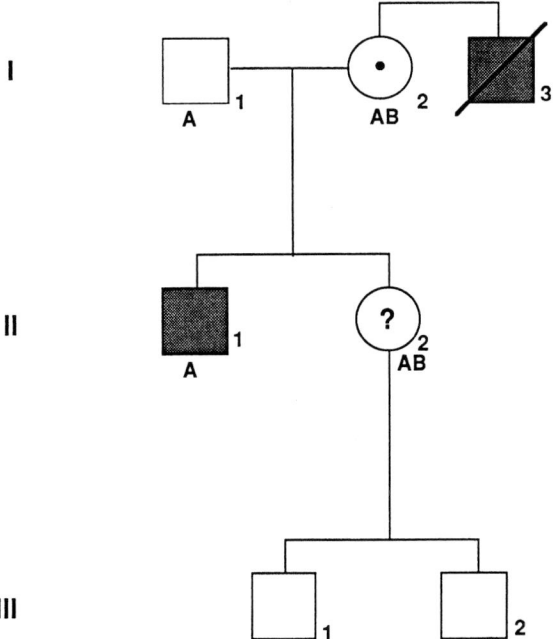

Fig. 24.12. See Example 14. This is the same pedigree as shown in Figure 24.1. Linkage analysis using DNA markers has now been undertaken.

This shows that the posterior probability that II_2 is a carrier can be calculated as

$$\frac{[\theta^2 (1 - \theta)^2]/4}{([\theta^2 (1 - \theta)^2]/4 + ([1 - 2\theta + 2\theta^2]/2)}$$

For a value of $\theta = 0.05$, this gives a posterior probability of $1/805$ that II_2 is a carrier. Inspection of Figure 24.12 reveals that at least two crossovers must have occurred if II_2 is a carrier. This accounts for the very low posterior probability which has been obtained.

This particular example illustrates how careful evaluation of the family pedigree can be incorporated with the results of biochemical tests and linkage analysis to modify a potential carrier's risk. For II_2 this was initially one in two. Pedigree analysis based on the two unaffected sons gave a risk of 1 in 5. Creatine kinase assay reduced this further to one in 17. Finally DNA studies resulted in a very dramatic reduction to a value of less than one in 800.

Germinal mosaicism

Traditionally it has been assumed that if a child inherits a mutant allele, this has occurred either because the transmitting parent is a full-blown carrier, or as the result of a new mutation having occurred during one of the meiotic

Table 24.14. Determination of Carrier Risk for II_2 in Figure 24.1 Incorporating Result of Creatine Kinase (CK) Assay[a]

Probability	II_2 Is a Carrier	II_2 Is Not a Carrier
Prior	$\frac{1}{2}$	$\frac{1}{2}$
Conditional		
CK assay	$\frac{1}{4}$	1
2 unaffected sons	$\frac{1}{4}$	1
Joint	$\frac{1}{32}$	$\frac{1}{2}$

[a] See Example 13.

Table 24.15. DNA Linkage Analysis and the Probability of Carrier Status for Duchenne Muscular Dystrophy[a]

Probability	Disease in I_2 Is in Coupling With A		Disease in I_2 Is in Coupling With B	
Prior	$\dfrac{1}{2}$		$\dfrac{1}{2}$	
Conditional				
II$_1$(A) affected	$1-\theta$		θ	
II$_2$ (inherits B from I_2)	C (Dis B)	NC	C (Dis B)	NC
Prior Conditional	θ	$1-\theta$	$1-\theta$	θ
Normal CK	$\dfrac{1}{4}$	1	$\dfrac{1}{4}$	1
III$_1$(A) unaffected	$1-\theta$	1	$1-\theta$	1
III$_2$(B) unaffected	θ	1	θ	1
Joint	$\dfrac{\theta^2(1-\theta)^2}{8}$	$\dfrac{(1-\theta)^2}{2}$	$\dfrac{\theta^2(1-\theta)^2}{8}$	$\dfrac{\theta^2}{2}$

C, Carrier; NC, noncarriers; Dis, disease.
[a] See Figure 24.12 and Example 14.

divisions which led to formation of the gamete that resulted in the child's conception. Recent studies have confirmed that there is a third possibility, in that the mutation could have occurred post-zygotically in the transmitting parent resulting in that individual being mosaic for the mutation. If this mitotic embryonic – as opposed to meiotic gametogenic – mutation occured in cells ancestral to, or in, the developing gonads, then this will have resulted in germinal (germline) mosaicism.

Analysis of families in which one child has Duchenne muscular dystrophy has revealed that in this disorder, germline mosaicism is a relatively frequent occurrence. For example, if a mother who does not have a deletion in either of her dystrophin genes has a deletion positive affected son, she cannot be reassured that the recurrence risk is negligible. In fact empiric studies indicate that there is a risk of between 14% and 20% that a future child who inherits the same dystrophin haplotype as the affected child will also inherit the deletion (Bakker et al., 1989; van Essen et al., 1992).

At present it is extremely difficult to quantify or calculate risks associated with germinal mosaicism as the proportion of mutations resulting in this phenomenon is not known.

Zlotogora (1998) has reviewed the relatively sparse literature on germinal mosaicism and has noted that this is relatively common in some disorders (e.g., Duchenne muscular dystrophy, facioscapulohumeral muscular dystrophy and hemophilia) and very rare in others (e.g., achondroplasia, Apert syndrome and multiple endocrine adenomatosis type 2). The reasons for these differences in mutation origin are not known. When counseling for disorders in which germinal mosaicism has been reported it is reasonable to use the recurrence risk tables derived by Van der Meulen et al., (1995) which incorporate information from DNA marker studies in affected and unaffected siblings. For Duchenne muscular dystrophy Grimm and colleagues (1990) have suggested that the recurrence risk to the sibling of an isolated case is approximately 36% instead of the traditionally quoted value of 33.3%. The important message to emerge from these studies is that for a condition such as Duchenne muscular dystrophy in which a definitive carrier test such as deletion analysis is available, an apparent noncarrier mother of an affected child should not be counseled on the basis of a negligible recurrence risk, and, if appropriate, she should be offered the option of prenatal diagnostic studies.

REFERENCES

Bakker E, Veenema H, Den Dunnen JT et al. (1989) Germinal mosaicism increases the recurrence risk for "new" Duchenne muscular dystrophy mutations. J Med Genet 26:553–559

Bayes T (1763 and 1958) An essay towards solving a problem in the doctrine of chances. Phil Trans 53:376–418 and Biometrika 45:296–315

Bridge PJ (1997) The Calculation of Genetic Risks, 2nd edn. Johns Hopkins University Press, Baltimore

Bundey S (1978) Calculation of genetic risks in Duchenne muscular dystrophy by geneticists in the United Kingdom. J Med Genet 15:249–253

Burn J, Chapman P, Delhanty J et al. (1991) The UK Northern Region genetic register for familial adenomatous polyposis coli: use of age of onset, congenital hypertrophy of the retinal pigment epithelium, and DNA markers in risk calculations. J Med Genet 28:289–296

Emery AEH (1986) Risk estimation in autosomal dominant disorders with reduced penetrance. J Med Genet 23:316–318

Friedman JM (1985) Genetic counseling for autosomal dominant diseases with a negative family history. Clin Genet 27:68–71

Grimm T, Müller B, Müller CR, Janka M (1990) Theoretical considerations on germline mosaicism in Duchenne muscular dystrophy. J Med Genet 27:683–687

Haldane JBS (1949) The rate of mutation of human genes. Hereditas 35:267–273

Lathrop GM, Lalouel JM (1984) Easy calculations of lod scores and genetic risks on small computers. Am J Hum Genet 36:460–465

Lau YL, Levinsky RJ, Malcolm S, Goodship J, Winter R, Pembrey M (1988) Genetic prediction in X-linked agammaglobinulaemia. Am J Med Genet 31:437–448

Murphy EA, Chase GA (1975) Principles of Genetic Counseling. Year Book Medical Publishers, Chicago

Pauli RM, Motulsky AG (1981) Risk counseling in autosomal dominant disorders with undetermined penetrance. J Med Genet 18:340–343

Van der Meulen MA, van der Meulen MJP, te Meerman GJ (1995) Recurrence risk for germinal mosaics revisited. J Med Genet 32:102–105

van Essen AJ, Abbs S, Baiget M et al. (1992) Parental origin and germline mosaicism of deletions and duplications of the dystrophin gene: A European study. Hum Genet 88:249–257

Winter RM (1985) The estimation of recurrence risks in monogenic disorders using flanking marker loci. J Med Genet 22:12–15

Young ID (1999) Introduction to Risk Calculation in Genetic Counseling, 2nd edn. OUP, Oxford

Zlotogora J (1998) Germ line mosaicism. Hum Genet 102:381–386

Cytogenetic analysis

25

Malcolm A. Ferguson-Smith
Kim Smith

Introduction

Cytogenetics is the study of chromosomes by microscopy. Because chromosomes carry the genetic material, an understanding of their behavior, structure, and function is essential to an understanding of genetics. Visible changes in the number and structure of chromosomes are associated with a broad spectrum of disease, and so the analysis of chromosomes under the microscope has become an important tool in medical genetics. This chapter describes the most useful techniques of those now available for chromosome analysis. Much can be seen by simple staining methods and light microscopy; for higher resolution, however, fluorescence microscopy and image analysis techniques are often required.

Milestones in human cytogenetics

Human chromosomes were probably first observed by Arnold in 1879 in dividing tumor cells. Hansemann in 1891 and Flemming in 1898 attempted to count the number of chromosomes in serial sections of dividing cells and obtained crude estimates of about 24. Quite different results were reported by de Winiwarter in 1912. He seems to have been the first to study sections of gonadal tissue, and he found counts of 47 in testes and 48 in ovary. He interpreted these results as indicating that, like some invertebrates, males had a single X chromosome and females had two. In 1921, Painter demonstrated in testis sections the presence of an additional small Y chromosome that was overlooked by de Winiwarter. Although he assumed that 48

was the correct chromosome number in both sexes, it is interesting to note that in his 1921 paper he states that he could count only 46 chromosomes in the clearest mitotic figures. In a paper published in 1923, Painter predicted the existence of individuals with unusual combinations of sex chromosomes, in particular intersexes with an XXY sex chromosome complement. No one seems to have tested this idea until 1942, when Severinghaus described an XY sex chromosome constitution in an XY female.

Largely as a result of the unfavorable material available for studying human chromosomes, there were few reports on this subject until the early 1950s. An important exception was a paper by Koller (1937) in which the X-Y pairing segment in human meiosis is described for the first time and the possibility of partial sex linkage raised.

The possibility that pathologic disorders might be due to abnormalities of chromosome number and structure seems to have been suggested first by Theodor Boveri. He described his theory on the origin of cancer from chromosomal aberrations in a classic monograph published in 1914. Then, 46 years later, the first specific chromosome abnormality associated with malignancy was described, namely, the Philadelphia chromosome in chronic myeloid leukemia (Nowell and Hungerford, 1960). Subsequent developments in cancer cytogenetics have fully confirmed the role of chromosome aberrations in the pathogenesis of cancer and established cytogenetic analysis as an essential component in classification and prognosis. With regard to constitutional chromosome abnormalities, Waardenburg in 1932 was one of the first to suggest that Down syndrome might be due to a numeric chromosome aberration resulting from nondisjunction. This may have prompted Mittwoch (1952) to study testis material from a case of Down syndrome. She counted an average of 24 bivalents in diakinesis and about 48 in spermatogonial mitoses and concluded that the chromosome number was normal. Had hypotonic pretreatment and control material from a normal individual been available, she might have appreciated that the number at diakinesis in Down syndrome was abnormal, with 23 bivalents plus one univalent.

Human cytogenetics became a practical proposition with the discovery in 1956 by Tjio and Levan that the correct chromosome number was 46 and not 48. Both were experienced cytologists who exploited the availability in their laboratory of fetal tissue culture from abortus material. Levan had earlier introduced into plant cytogenetics the use of colchicine to arrest and accumulate mitoses at metaphase, and he knew of the effect of hypotonic solutions to separate individual chromosomes from one another by pretreatment before fixation. The hypotonic technique had been discovered independently by three scientists, Hsu (1952) in the United States, Makino and Nishimura (1952) in Japan, and Hughes in England. Apparently, both Hsu and Makino made the discovery fortuitously, after mistakenly adding hypotonic instead of isotonic salt solution during the washing stage before fixation. Following fixation, the technique current at that time was to squash the dividing cells between the slide and coverslip so that the chromosomes could be spread in one optical plane. A variety of nuclear stains including aceto-orcein, Giemsa, and Feulgen were used to stain the chromosome preparations. All these methods, especially tissue culture, contributed to the rapid developments in human cytogenetics in the following years.

The chromosome number of 46 was soon confirmed in testis material by Ford and Hamerton (1956). Two years later, Ford et al. (1958) introduced a method for chromosome analysis using bone marrow samples that was suitable for clinical studies in that it exploited the presence of actively dividing cells in that material. At about the same time, Lejeune and his colleagues (1959) were reinvestigating the chromosomes in Down syndrome from fibroblast cultures. Their discovery of trisomy for one of the smallest autosomes was announced in 1958, although the description in nine patients was not published until early in 1959. Simultaneously, interest in the chromosomes of the Turner and Klinefelter syndromes was prompted by the paradoxical nuclear sex chromatin (Barr body) findings suggesting that amenorrheic women with Turner syndrome might be genetic males (Polani et al., 1954), and that infertile men with Klinefelter syndrome might be genetic females. The latter seemed to be confirmed by Ford et al. (1958), who found one Klinefelter patient to have an apparently normal female chromosome constitution on bone marrow preparations. This may have been the first XX male. However, it was soon found that Turner syndrome was usually associated with a 45, X chromosome complement (Ford et al., 1959) and that Klinefelter syndrome had a 47, XXY complement (Jacobs and Strong, 1959). The important conclusion from these studies was that human sex differentiation was determined by the Y chromosome and not by the number of X chromosomes.

It came as a surprise to clinicians that such gross numeric chromosome abnormalities could be associated with viability. There followed intense activity worldwide to determine whether other dysmorphic conditions were due to chromosomal abnormalities visible under the microscope. Trisomies 13 and 18 were quickly identified, followed by several instances of sex chromosomal mosaicism, translocation Down syndrome, and the deletion of the short arm of chromosome 5, which causes the cri du chat syndrome. The Philadelphia chromosome in chronic myeloid leukemia (Nowell and Hungerford, 1960) was a notable discovery at this time, because it supported the Boveri theory on the cause of malignancy.

The search for new examples of conditions that are due to chromosome aberrations was accompanied by strenuous attempts to simplify techniques and improve the identification of individual chromosomes so that smaller structural changes could be detected. The most important of these early technical developments was the introduction of phytohemagglutinin, which allowed chromosome preparations to be made within two to three days from peripheral blood samples (Moorehead et al., 1960). This reagent was originally used to clear red cells from preparations of lymphocytes, but it was found that T lymphocytes underwent transformation and division under its influence. When colchicine was used to accumulate lymphocytes in metaphase during short-term culture, air-dried drop preparations of metaphase chromosomes could be made far superior to any previous method. The simplicity of the technique, which is still in use almost unchanged, has undoubtedly been responsible for the widespread application of chromosome analysis throughout the world and for the growth of human cytogenetics as a diagnostic procedure in clinical medicine. In the 1960s, individual chromosomes were identified by characteristics such as total length, centromere index (length of short arm divided by total length), the presence of heterochromatic regions, and the pattern of DNA replication as revealed by pulse labeling with tritiated thymidine. These studies revealed considerable normal variation in chromosome size and centromere position, much of which was heritable and of no clinical significance. Only chromosomes 1, 2, 3, 9, 16, and the Y chromosome could be identified with certainty in any one metaphase by standard techniques. Chromosomal hetero-morphisms mainly involved the centromeres of chromosomes 1, 9, 16 (and occasionally chromosomes 3 and 4); the short arms and satellites of chromosomes 13, 14, 15, 21, and 22; and the distal heterochromatic region of the long arm of the Y chromosome.

Because of the limited availability of testicular biopsies and the virtual lack of access to ovarian tissue, meiotic chromosome analysis has contributed comparatively little to human cytogenetics and to the diagnosis of chromosome aberrations. However, much has been learned about the behavior of human chromosomes in meiosis, about the identification of bivalents at pachytene (especially the nucleolar chromosomes), about the pairing of chromosomal rearrangements, about the number and location of chiasmata, and about the extent of homologous and nonhomologous pairing of the X and Y chromosomes. Although the morphologic aspects of meiosis have been well studied, the biochemistry of synapsis and recombination is still largely unresolved.

In 1970 two new techniques were introduced that have had a major impact on modern cytogenetic analysis. The first was the demonstration by Pardue and Gall (1970) that isotopically labeled DNA probes could be annealed to complementary DNA sequences in cytologic preparations of chromosomes made by standard techniques, a procedure referred to as in situ hybridization (ISH). They demonstrated that mouse satellite DNA hybridized to the paracentric regions of mouse chromosomes. The chromosome preparations and DNA probes were denatured by alkali and heat, and the specific hybridization, which took place at lower temperature, was demonstrated by autoradiography. Pardue and Gall also noted that when the denatured chromosomes were stained by Giemsa, the paracentric regions were preferentially stained (C bands, see below). Various modifications of the denaturing and staining process by other workers following Pardue and Gall yielded chromosomes that showed patterns of differential staining along their length, which appeared specific for each chromosome. These experiments were extended and led to the second major development, the establishment of standard chromosome banding patterns, which have become the criteria for chromosome identification and classification in many species.

Even before chromosome denaturation was being used to produce various banding patterns, Caspersson et al. (1970) independently discovered that quinacrine compounds that intercalate in DNA could produce bright fluorescent bands visible along the chromosome using fluorescence microscopy. The quinacrine bands (Q bands) were at first more reproducible than those produced by denaturing and Giemsa staining but yielded virtually the same banding pattern and were equally useful for chromosome identification. A striking feature of Q-banding was that it preferentially stained the distal long arm of the Y chromosome, a feature that could be seen in interphase nuclei as a bright spot.

Modern cytogenetic analysis has evolved from these beginnings, the main ingredients being cell culture, colchicine treatment to accumulate metaphases, manipulations of the cell cycle to enhance chromosome morphology, hypotonic treatment to separate the chromosomes from one another, fixation in suspension followed by air drying, banding methods for chromosome identification, and in situ hybridization for the localization of specific DNA sequences.

The indications for cytogenetic analysis

The history of human cytogenetics over the past 40 years has been punctuated by the introduction of new technology followed by the identification of increasing numbers of aberrations, smaller in extent and often associated with less striking phenotypic changes. The indications for cytogenetic analysis have thus widened over the years. For example, the occurrence of a monogenic disorder associated with mild mental handicap may indicate the presence of a microdeletion detectable by modern techniques, or of DNA disruption at one of the breakage sites of a reciprocal translocation. A list of general indications for cytogenetic analysis includes the following:

1. Confirmation or exclusion of the diagnosis for known chromosomal syndromes
2. Unexplained psychomotor retardation with or without dysmorphic features
3. Abnormalities of sexual differentiation and development
4. Infertility
5. Monogenic disorders associated with mental retardation and or dysmorphic features
6. Recurrent miscarriage or stillbirth
7. Pregnancies shown to be at risk of aneuploidy from the results of maternal serum screening or fetal ultrasound scanning
8. Neoplastic conditions, particularly hematologic malignancies, for which the identification of specific chromosomal aberrations may be valuable in diagnosis and management

A classification of chromosomal abnormalities is provided later in this chapter, and full descriptions of the main chromosomal syndromes are given in Chapters 44, 45 and 46.

Tissue samples and cell culture

Chromosome preparations for analysis are made from dividing cells, either directly from tissue samples (e.g., bone marrow, testis, chorionic villi, neoplastic tissue) or following cell culture (biopsy of skin or almost any other living tissue including amniotic fluid cells). It is obvious that tissue preserved in a fixative is not suitable for making conventional chromosome preparations. It is imperative to use the correct sterile containers when sending biopsy and other tissues to the cytogenetics laboratory to ensure the cells remain viable and suitable for cell culture. The most widely used samples for routine analysis are samples of peripheral blood from which T-lymphocyte chromosomes are prepared. A 2- to 5-ml sample of venous blood, sent in either a sterile heparinized tube or in a tube containing sterile acid-citrate-dextrose (ACD), usually is sufficient for a wide variety of special staining techniques. Short-term, three-day cultures are routinely made from 0.25 ml of whole blood in 5 ml of defined tissue culture medium supplemented with fetal calf serum, mitotic stimulant (phytohemagglutinin), and antibiotics. Colcemid is added during the last two hours of culture to arrest and accumulate mitoses. Preferential collection of longer chromosomes can be achieved by synchronising the cell cycle via a DNA synthesis block, with chemicals such as thymidine. Cells in early metaphase can be collected during the peak of mitotic activity by adding colcemid for a shortened period of approximately 20 minutes. The cells are harvested by centrifugation, incubated for 10 minutes in hypotonic solution (potassium chloride or sodium citrate) to separate the chromosomes from one another, and then fixed in two changes of chilled glacial acetic acid/methanol (1:3) for about 30 minutes. Various modifications can be made during cell culture to induce fragile sites (fragile X syndrome), or to identify chromosomal breakage syndromes (Fanconi's anemia, Bloom syndrome, ataxia telangiectasia).

It is possible to collect mitotically active cells from some tissues such as bone marrow and chorionic villi by exposing the cells to colcemid for a short period of 1–2 hours followed by the usual harvesting procedures. For many tissues, such as skin biopsies, amniocytes and chorionic villi cells, chromosome preparations are prepared from cells cultured over a longer period as monolayer cultures. Cells can be grown on coverslips and processed "in situ" or grown in culture vessels and harvested using trypsin/EDTA to dislodge and disaggregate the cells. Exposure to colcemid, a hypotonic treatment and methanol/acetic acid fixation are essential steps in processing all cultures for chromosome preparations.

Air-dried preparations are made by placing a drop of the fixed cell suspension onto clean microscope slides and allowing the fixative to evaporate. The aim is to achieve the separation of chromosomes from one another and the spread of each metaphase in one optical plane and in one field under the microscope. The remaining fixed cell suspension may be kept at 4°C in a sealed tube in case additional slides are required.

It is possible to transfer cells directly from solid tissue, such as skin, onto microscope slides by touching a cut surface of the tissue repeatedly onto the slide and hence the name "touch preparations". These preparations are fixed in methanol/glacial acetic acid and, after treatment with RNase, are suitable for interphase in situ hybridization studies.

Conventional banding

For identification of normal chromosomes and detection of aberrations, the air-dried chromosome preparations must be stained appropriately. The rapid development of in situ hybridization for the identification of specific chromosomes and chromosome regions should not be allowed to overshadow the usefulness of conventional staining techniques, which continue to form the basis of modern cytogenetic analysis. Conventional banding is comparatively simple to achieve and is inexpensive in relation to the in situ hybridization methods. It is capable of unequivocally identifying every normal human chromosome and the origin of most of the larger chromosome rearrangements. Its performance in specificity for the identification of small chromosome segments is, however, poor; therefore, it should be used in conjunction with in situ methods. The following brief review of conventional banding techniques concentrates on the most valuable methods and their application for the identification of aberrations in particular circumstances. For each procedure, one tried and tested method is provided in the Annex at the end of the chapter; other protocols are readily available in a number of excellent reviews and manuals. Local safety rules must be applied for all techniques.

SOLID STAINING

The chromosomes are exposed to a Giemsa or similar stain that has an affinity for DNA, yielding a uniformly dark appearance to the chromatids. Though now of limited use, the solid staining technique still has applications in the investigation of fragile sites, in the study of chromosome breakage syndromes, and for scoring radiation damage. It is also a useful, simple, and often overlooked technique to use with marker chromosomes, in the determination of the extent of satellite polymorphism, and in the measurement of individual chromosomes.

G-BANDING

G-banding is the benchmark for the routine analysis of human chromosomes, producing a characteristic light and dark banding pattern along the chromosomes (Fig. 25.1). Each chromosome has a unique sequence of bar code-like stripes, allowing identification of individual homologues and the analysis of abnormalities of their structure by disruption of the normal banding pattern. Many methods have been published for the production of G bands, but most rely on proteolytic digestion of the chromosomes by trypsin followed by staining with either Giemsa or Leishman stain. Little is known of the precise nature of the mechanism of G-banding despite much conjecture. The dark bands contain mainly A-T rich DNA, and the light bands are G-C rich. Manipulation of the cell cycle to produce prometaphase chromosomes with between 400 and 700 G bands per haploid set provides a mechanism for high-resolution analysis of the structure of the chromosomes. This method can detect quite subtle changes, crucial for the identification of deletions, duplications, inversions, and translocations and for the determination of break points involved in such anomalies. Increasing the limits of resolution can itself be problematic, because it is possible to identify differences between homologues that are more likely to be examples of normal variation rather than clinically relevant abnormality. G-banding is often inconclusive in the identification of small supernumerary ring or marker chromosomes where bands are insufficient for pattern recognition. This is also true for some de novo rearrangements involving unbalanced translocations or duplications, and in such cases supplementary banding and in situ techniques are indicated.

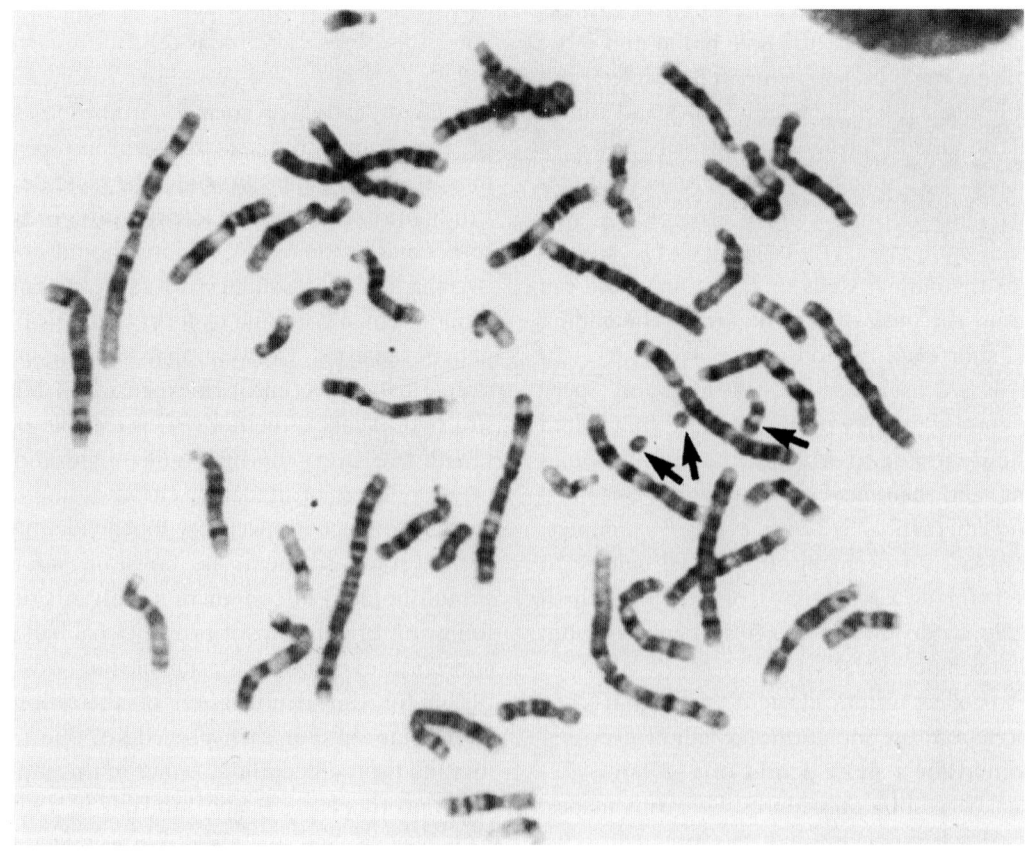

Fig. 25.1. G-banded metaphase with three marker chromosomes (whose origin from chromosomes 22, 11, and 14 cannot be identified by this technique).

REVERSE BANDING

A disadvantage of G-banding is in the definition of the light-staining telomeric regions. Therefore R-banding, resulting in the reverse of the banding pattern to that seen with G- and Q-banding, is sometimes employed. Various approaches have been employed to obtain this effect including heat treatment followed by Giemsa staining, incorporation of the thymidine analogue bromodeoxyuridine (BrdU) into the S phase of the cell cycle, and the use of various fluorochromes to produce an analogous pattern. This technique can be modified to give differential replication staining by exposing growing cells to BrdU at different stages of the cell cycle and is used for the identification of the late-replicating X chromosome often of use in the study of structurally abnormal X chromosomes.

Q-BANDING AND DAPI BANDING

The first of the stains to show a chromosome-specific differential banding pattern, quinacrine mustard, gives a rather unclear indistinct bright and dull fluorescence along the chromosome when exposed to ultraviolet light. The pattern fades quickly, though this is less of a problem with modern image capture facilities. The pattern reflects G-banding with brightly fluorescing AT-rich regions and dull GC-rich regions. Quinacrine mustard has now been replaced by the more effective quinacrine dyhydrochloride. Q-banding is particularly useful for the identification of the Y heterochromatic segment, which stains very brightly, and for the study of the satellite regions of the acrocentric chromosomes. A similar pattern is obtained using the fluorochrome 4'-6-diamidino-2-phenylindole (DAPI), which also highlights the centromeres of chromosomes 1, 9, and 16. The specificity of fluorochromes can be enhanced further by the application of fluorescent or nonfluorescent counterstains.

COUNTERSTAINING BANDING PATTERNS

The combination of a fluorescent primary stain and fluorescent or nonfluorescent counterstaining DNA ligand to quench the primary stain produces highly specific banding patterns of great clinical use. A particularly useful combination for the identification of chromosome 15-derived supernumerary markers is DAPI with distamycin A (DA) as the counterstain. The DAPI-DA staining results in brightly fluorescing centromeric regions of chromosome 1, 9, 16; a bright Yqh region; and a highlighted region on the proximal short arm of chromosome 15. This technique permits identification of a clinically important subgroup of marker chromosomes, with a high risk of abnormality.

C-BANDING

Constitutive heterochromatin is found at the centromeric region of all human chromosomes. The chromatin in this region has an increased proportion of highly repetitive satellite DNA compared with euchromatic regions and is more resistant to denaturation processes. Staining with Giemsa following heat and/or alkali denaturation results in darkly staining heterochromatic regions at the centromeres with lightly staining chromosome arms (Fig. 25.2). An exception is the Y chromosome, which, in addition to the darkly stained centromere, has a distinctive block of heterochromatin toward the end of the long arm. Several chromosomes, specifically, chromosomes 1, 9, and 16, show pronounced pericentromeric heteromorphisms of both the amount and position (inversion), of the C-band regions and can usefully be employed as heritable chromosomes markers.

AG-NOR STAINING

The satellite stalk regions of the acrocentric chromosomes contain multiple copies of 18s and 28s sequences coding for ribosomal RNA associated with the nucleolus organizer regions (NOR) of interphase nuclei. These areas of the karyotype can be preferentially stained by the application of silver nitrate solution, which in the presence of NOR precipitates specific proteins associated with the transcription of ribosomal cistrons in the preceding cell cycle. The staining pattern is consistent and heritable and allows identification of acrocentric-derived chromosomes (Fig. 25.3).

This technique is of particular use in the identification of bisatellited marker chromosomes and in the delineation of break points in translocations involving acrocentric chromosomes.

A variety of other stains and counterstains can be used to emphasize specific areas of the karyotype. All enable more precise definition of structurally abnormal chromosomes and are valuable ammunition in the cytogeneticist's arsenal. Excellent reviews of these techniques, together with their underlying mechanisms, have been produced by various authors; of special note is the publication by Verma and Babu on human chromosomes (1989).

Further ammunition to help elucidate the chromosomal abnormality is provided by DNA probes and fluorescence in situ hybridization studies and these will be discussed in a later section.

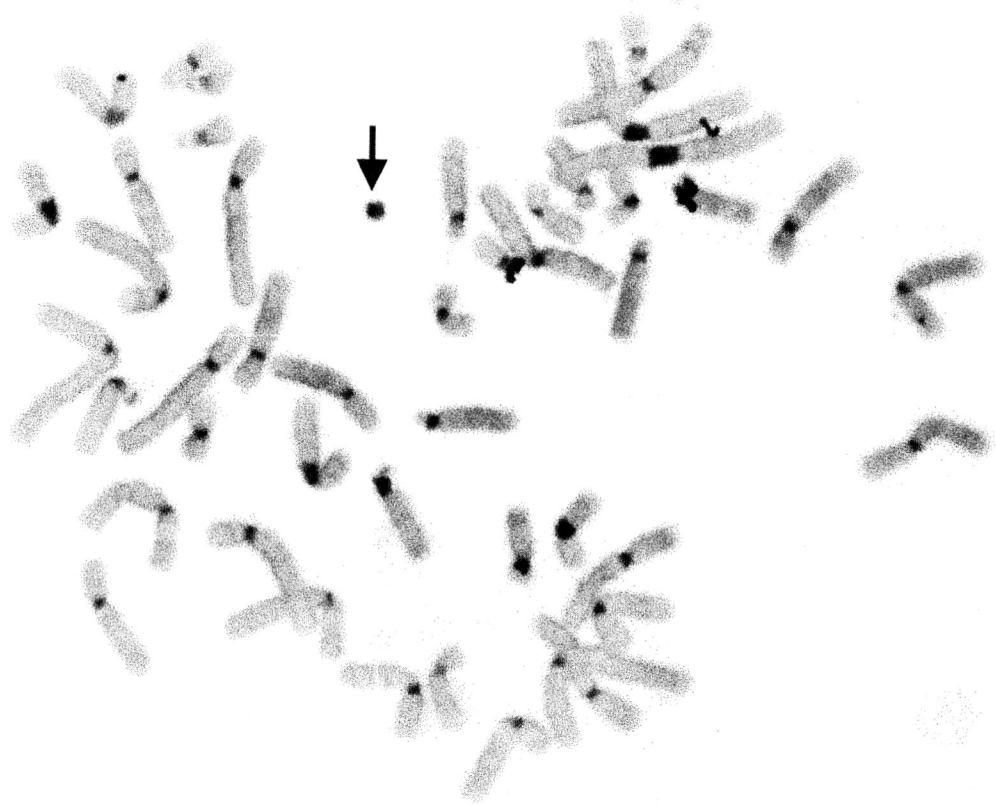

Fig. 25.2. C-banded metaphase preparation of a female with an additional heterochromatic ring chromosome. Note prominent centric heterochromatin of chromosomes 1, 9, and 16.

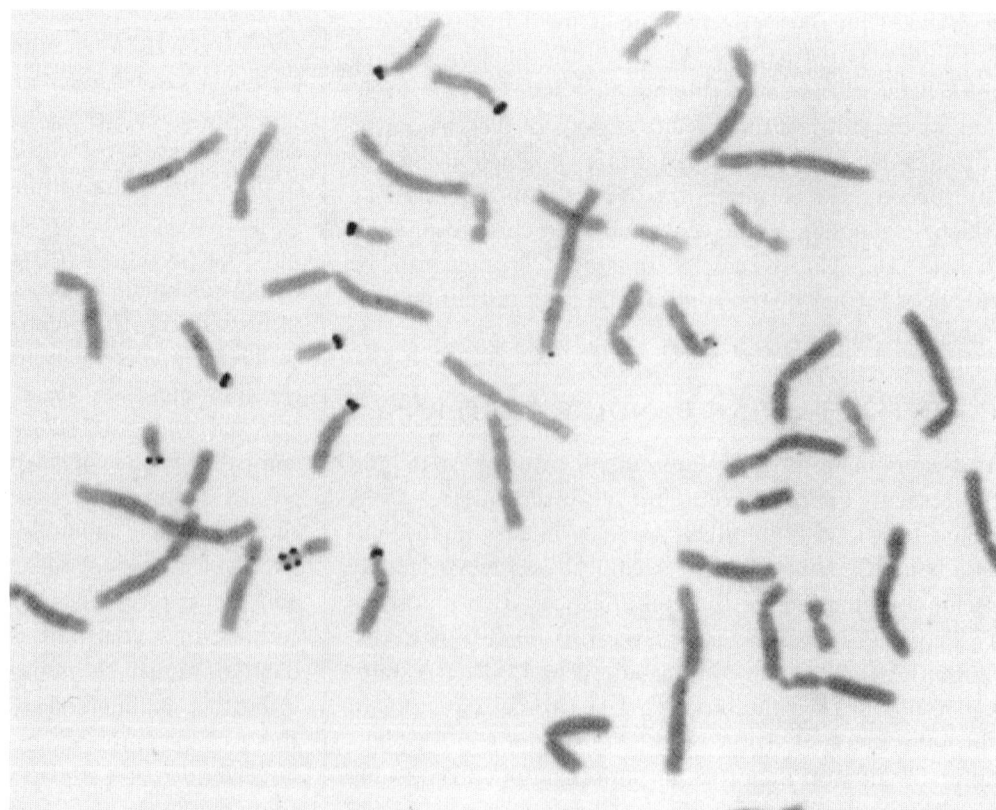

Fig. 25.3. Silver-stained partial metaphase preparation showing nucleolus organizer regions (NOR) of six large acrocentric and four small acrocentric chromosomes. Note duplication of NOR on one chromosome and variable staining intensity on others, reflecting variable NOR activity.

The normal human karyotype

Each species has a chromosome complement, characteristic in number and form. This is known as the *karyotype*, and the name is also used for a photographic preparation in which the stained chromosomes are arranged approximately in order of decreasing length. Conventional banding allows each normal human chromosome to be given its specific identity number. To make analysis easier, the banding pattern can be diagrammatically represented in the form of an idiogram (Fig. 25.4). About 400 distinct bands per haploid complement usually may be visible in any one metaphase preparation. In prometaphase cells, more than 550 bands may be resolved because the chromosomes are more extended; however, the centromere is less readily distinguished, and this can make the identification of some chromosomes difficult.

The International System for Human Cytogenetic Nomenclature (ISCN) was established in 1978 by a standing committee to provide a simple shorthand, based on the human banded idiogram, to describe any given chromosome aberration and the karyotype of any individual. In this nomenclature, which has been updated regularly, the number of chromosomes in the karyotype is given first, then the sex chromosome constitution, followed by a shorthand description for any abnormal chromosome. Thus, 46, XY is a normal male karyotype, and 47, XX, +21 is the karyotype of a female with Down syndrome. Parts of chromosomes or sites of chromosome rearrangement are identified using a simple numbering system specific for each chromosome band or sub-band. In this description, the chromosome identifier is given, followed by the designation for the chromosome arm, p (petit) for the short arm and q for the long arm, and then the number of the chromosome band involved in the rearrangement. The main landmarks of each chromosome are the centromere, cen, and the end of the arm, pter for the short arm and qter for the long arm. The most striking of the bands are the remaining landmarks, and these divide the arm into distinct regions. Each region is further subdivided into bands and sub-bands. Thus, band Xp21.2 is to be found in the short arm of the X chromosome in region 2, band 1, and sub-band 2. The shorthand for the exchange of chromosome fragments between 7p21.2 and, for example, 9q34.1 in a female individual would be given as 46, XX, t (7;9) (p21.2;q34.1), where t = translocation and the semicolon is used to separate the chromosomes and break points. These and other symbols used are listed in Table 25.1. The ISCN (1995) provides nomenclature to describe constitutional and acquired chromosome abnormalities and fluorescence in situ hybridization studies (further details of ISH nomenclature are given in the FISH section). Examples of the use of the shorthand are given in the following section where the classification of chromosome abnormalities is considered.

Chromosome analysis in normal individuals has revealed substantial variation in the karyotype that is without phenotypic effect. It is important to recognize and distinguish this normal variation from the abnormal chromosomal rearrangements that are clinically significant. The most striking of these variations, or heteromorphisms, occur at the centromeric regions of chromosomes 1, 9, and 16, at the short arms of chromosomes 13, 14, 15, 21, and 22, and at the distal end of the long arm of the Y chromosome. All these regions contain variable amounts of highly repetitive DNA (satellite DNA) composed largely of tandemly arranged repeats that are not transcribed. Unequal crossing-over within these repeats during meiosis may account for the variation, but this must occur rarely, because extreme examples of these heteromorphisms are invariably transmitted unchanged in pedigrees.

Table 25.1. The ISCN nomenclature: symbols and abbreviations used for describing Chromosome aberrations

Symbol	Definition
p	Short arm
q	Long arm
pter	Terminal of short arm
qter	Terminal of long arm
cen	Centromere
h	Heterochromation
add	Additional material of unknown origin
del	Deletion
der	Derivative of a translocation
dic	Dicentric
dup	Duplication
fra	Fragile site
i	Isochromosome
isodic	Isodicentric
inv	Inversion or inverted
r	Ring chromosome
rec	Recombinant from inversion or insertion
t	Translocation
upd	Uniparental disomy
mat	Maternal origin
pat	Paternal origin
mar	Marker chromosome of unknown origin
dir	Direct as opposed to inverted
::	Breakage with reunion
/	Mosaicism (separates clones)
+/–	Before a chromosome number, indicates gain or loss of that chromosome
;	Separates altered chromosomes and breakpoints involved in structural rearrangements
–	Indicates *from* and *to*

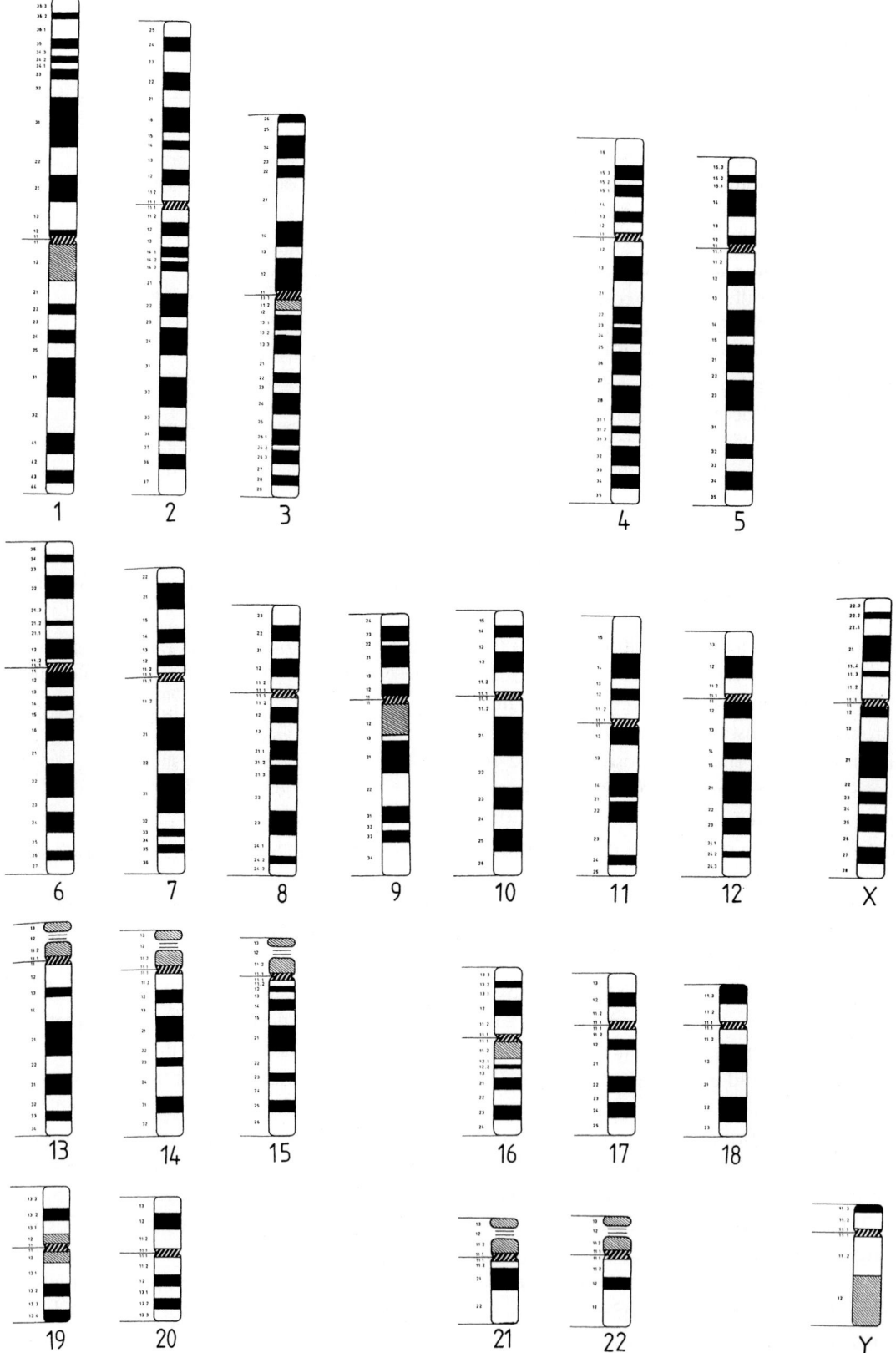

Fig. 25.4. Human idiogram based on G-banding pattern and showing the banding nomenclature according to the International System for Human Cytogenetic Nomenclature (ISCN, 1995). (A) Approximately 400 of the main G bands per haploid complement are shown, as seen in most banded metaphase preparations suitable for cytogenetic analysis.

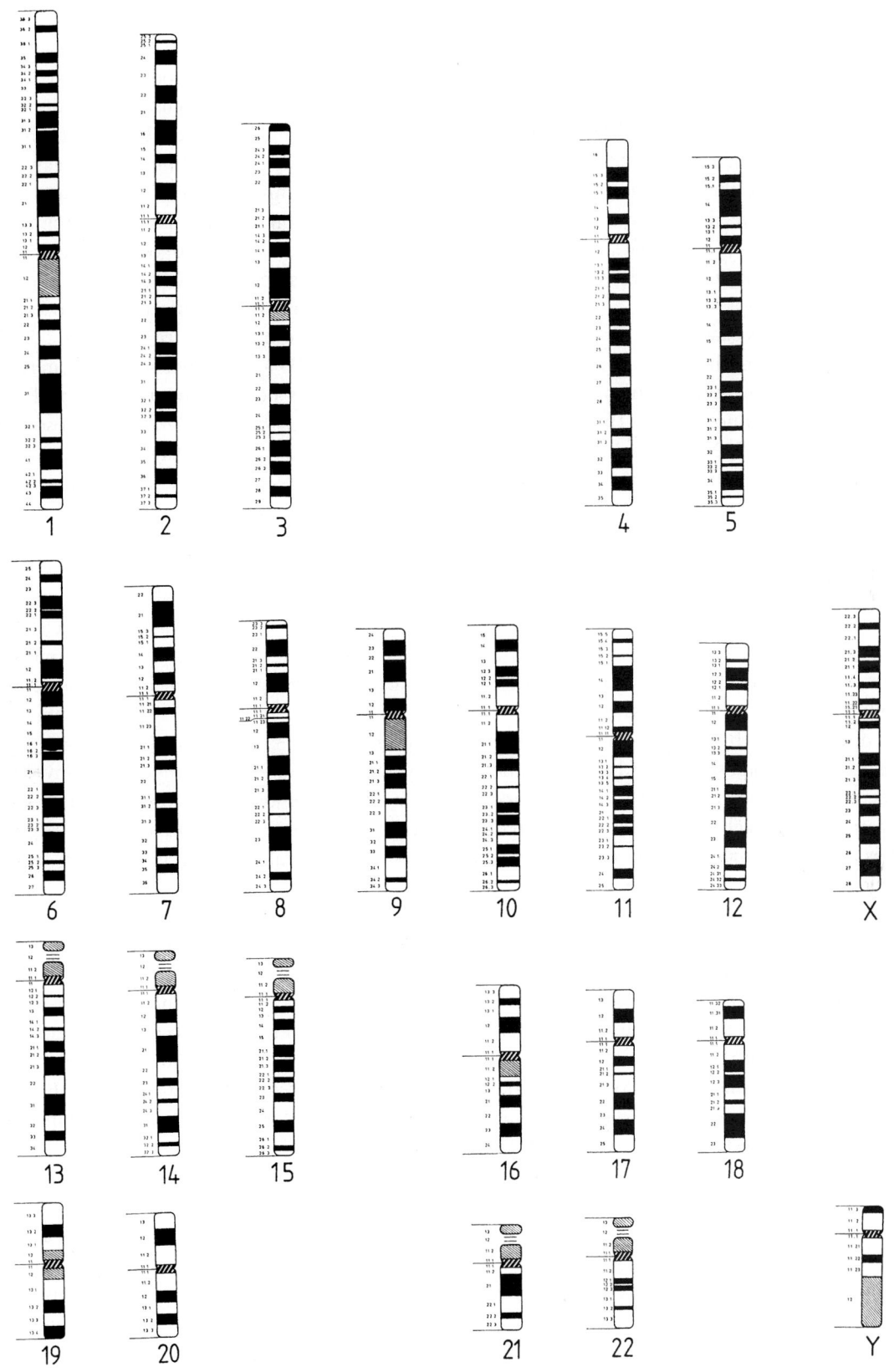

B

Fig. 25.4. *Continued* (B) Approximately 550 G-bands per haploid complement are shown, as seen in early metaphase preparations.

Chromosome abnormalities

Genetic mutations involve duplication, deletion, or rearrangement of DNA. The extent of the change varies from the gain or loss of a single nucleotide (a point mutation) to gain or loss of whole chromosomes. Those changes that are large enough to be detectable under the light microscope are classified as chromosome aberrations, but they differ from molecular mutations involving individual genes only in terms of scale.

As indicated earlier in this chapter, the first chromosome abnormalities discovered were the more obvious abnormalities of chromosome number, such as trisomy 21 (Down syndrome, 47, XY, +21), monosomy X (Turner syndrome 45, X), and triploidy (e.g., 69, XXX). The term *aneuploidy* refers to conditions with an increase or decrease in the diploid number of chromosomes, and *polyploidy* is used when the abnormal number is a multiple of the haploid number (23 in humans) exceeding the diploid complement. Nondisjunction and chromosome loss are the usual causes of aneuploidy, and errors of cell cleavage or multiple fertilization of the egg lead to polyploidy.

Nondisjunction leading to trisomy may occur at either of the parental meiotic divisions, and these alternatives can sometimes be distinguished by genetic marker studies. If the two copies of the chromosome derived from nondisjunction in one parent are heterozygous for DNA markers near the centromere, it is likely that the error occurred at the first meiotic division. If the two nondisjoined chromosomes are homozygous for centromeric markers and show only heterozygosity (that is due to crossing over) more distally, the nondisjunction probably occurred at the second meiosis. The failure of two homologous chromosomes to undergo synapsis in the first meiosis (nonconjunction) can be distinguished as a cause of trisomy from nondisjunction by marker studies that reveal the absence of crossing-over. If two of the three chromosomes share all genetic markers, the nondisjunction must have occurred in a mitotic division after fertilization. Mitotic nondisjunction is frequently associated with chromosomal mosaicism, that is, the presence of two or more cell lines with different chromosome complements in the individual.

Mosaicism is a relatively common finding associated with sex chromosome aneuploidy, for example, 45, X/46, XX. In trisomic embryos, the abnormality seems to tend to be corrected by loss of one of the trisomic chromosomes, often referred to as *trisomic rescue*, which results in a return to the disomic state. When the disomy is achieved by retaining both homologues from the parent in whom the nondis-junction arose with loss of the homologue from the other parent, the phenotype of the embryo may still be abnormal, depending on the chromosome involved. This outcome of trisomic rescue is known as uniparental disomy (UPD), and the associated phenotypic abnormality is the result of parental genomic imprinting during gametogenesis (see Chapter 46). Chromosomes 7, 11, 14, and 15 are examples of human chromosomes in which parental imprinting of certain genes is known to occur; uniparental disomy of these chromosomes is associated with phenotypic abnormality, whereas no such effect seems to occur when non-imprinted chromosomes are involved. The best known example is UPD for chromosome 15; maternal UPD occurs in one quarter of the patients with the Prader-Willi syndrome, while paternal UPD for chromosome 15 occurs in 2–5% of patients with Angelman syndrome. Genomic imprinting is associated with differential methylation of a number of gene loci in chromosome 15q12 during parental gametogenesis.

Structural abnormalities of the chromosome are due to chromosome breakage and abnormal reunion. This can be reproduced experimentally by treating cells with mutagenic agents including radiation. However, most spontaneous structural rearrangements in both somatic and germ cells probably arise from errors of recombination. Meiotic recombination is preceded by synapsis of homologous chromosomes, and this is thought to involve the recognition by one homologue of complementary sequences in the other homologue. Mismatching can occur during this process, particularly in regions with multiple tandem repeats of DNA sequences. Similarly, synapsis between homologous regions on nonhomologous chromosomes may lead to accidental recombination between nonhomologous chromosomes, thereby causing translocations.

Recombination can occur also between homologous chromosomes in somatic cells, and examples of somatic pairing and chromatid exchange are occasionally seen during routine chromosome analysis. Substantial molecular evidence indicates that unequal recombination resulting in deletion or duplication is a comparatively common event in tumors. Complex structural chromosomal rearrangements in tumors presumably arise in the same way.

Chromosome analysis of cell cultures exposed to irradiation reveals that when a chromosome breaks, two unstable ends are produced. Repair mechanisms within the cell usually ensure that the two ends are rejoined. However, when there is more than one break, rejoining of the correct ends is not assured, and abnormal chromosomes may result. Various combinations can occur, including acentric fragments, ring chromosomes, and multicentric chromosomes.

Chromatid aberrations, in which chromatids rather than whole chromosomes are seen to be involved in exchanges, are produced when breaks are induced during or after DNA synthesis. These studies show that somatic cells are capable of DNA repair and also that the ends of chromosomes are unstable unless they possess an organized telomere. Constitutional terminal deletions that are associated with a number of chromosomal syndromes (e.g., the cri du chat syndrome) must occur in such a way as to retain a functional telomere; some are generated by reciprocal translocation or interstitial deletion; in others, deletion continues down the chromosome until a DNA region homologous to telomeric sequences is reached, when the enzyme telomerase is able to synthesize a new telomere.

When a chromosome rearrangement occurs, there may be no loss or gain of chromosome material. The rearrangement is then regarded as balanced, and there should be no phenotypic effect. Sometimes, however, DNA may be disrupted or deleted at one of the break points of an apparently balanced rearrangement, leading to phenotypic abnormality. Most instances of this type occur as new mutations and are not transmitted.

Balanced chromosomal translocations may be inherited without obvious effect through many generations. However, unequal meiotic segregation may result in unbalanced gametes containing one or other of the translocation derivatives together with a normal homologue and capable of fertilization. Often, the resulting embryo is inviable, and miscarriage or stillbirth is the result. Alternatively, a liveborn infant is delivered who will have varying degrees of developmental abnormality depending on the nature of the chromosomal imbalance. Careful correlation between the phenotype and karyotype in many such cases over the years has led to the characterization of a large number of clinically distinguishable chromosomal syndromes, each associated with imbalance of a particular chromosome region. In general, deletions tend to have more serious phenotypic effects than duplications, and distal regions of the chromosome are more commonly involved than central regions. Understandably, smaller aberrations tend to be more viable and thus more often encountered than larger aberrations. The smaller the aberration, the less likely that it will be detectable by conventional banding techniques. Therefore, in recent years, molecular cytogenetic techniques based on ISH of DNA probes, such as sub-telomeric probes have played an increasing role in the identification of these conditions.

The various types of chromosomal aberration that are encountered in routine chromosome analysis are summarized and defined in the following discussion. Detailed descriptions of the phenotypes associated with particular aberrations are described in later chapters.

RECIPROCAL TRANSLOCATION

In reciprocal translocation, the exchange occurs at the ends of two nonhomologous chromosomes (Fig. 25.5 and Fig. 25.6B). When these chromosomes pair during meiosis, a cross-shaped quadrivalent is formed involving the two translocation chromosomes and their two normal partners. The homologous segments undergo recombination in the usual way, and chiasmata can be observed when the quadrivalent opens out into a ring or chain of four during the first meiotic metaphase (Fig. 25.7A). At the anaphase of first meiosis, the four chromosomes segregate into two pregametic cells. Twelve possible combinations of these four chromosomes can enter each gamete: all four chromosomes, none of the four chromosomes, four combinations of three chromosomes (3:1 segregation), and six combinations of two chromosomes (2:2 segregation). If one considers 2:2 segregation, only one possibility leads to a normal gamete, and only one to a gamete with the balanced translocation (alternate segregation). The other four options for segregation (adjacent segregation) result in unbalanced gametes, which might lead to chromosomally abnormal conceptions.

ROBERTSONIAN (CENTRIC FUSION) TRANSLOCATION

Exchanges occurring close to the centromere between two acrocentric chromosomes (chromosomes 13, 14, 15, 21, and 22) have some special features. In many cases, the exchange occurs between repeated elements within the

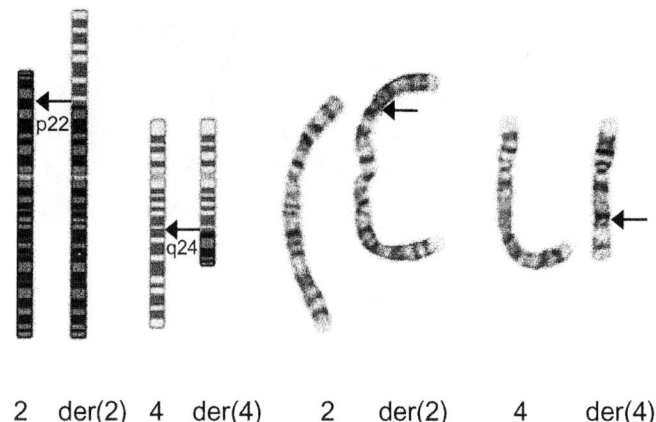

2   der(2)   4   der(4)   2   der(2)   4   der(4)

Fig. 25.5. A balanced reciprocal translocation involving the short arm of chromosome 2 and the long arm of chromosome 4; t (2;4) (p22:q24). G-banding.

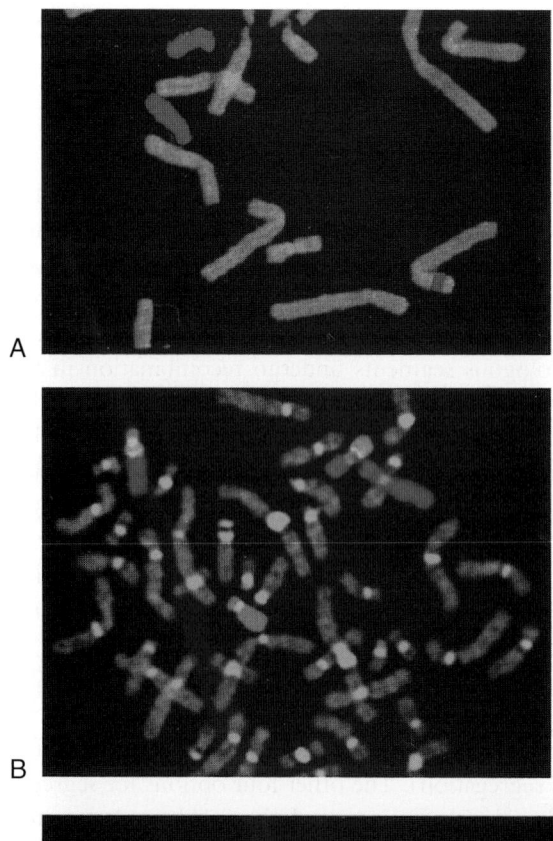

A

B

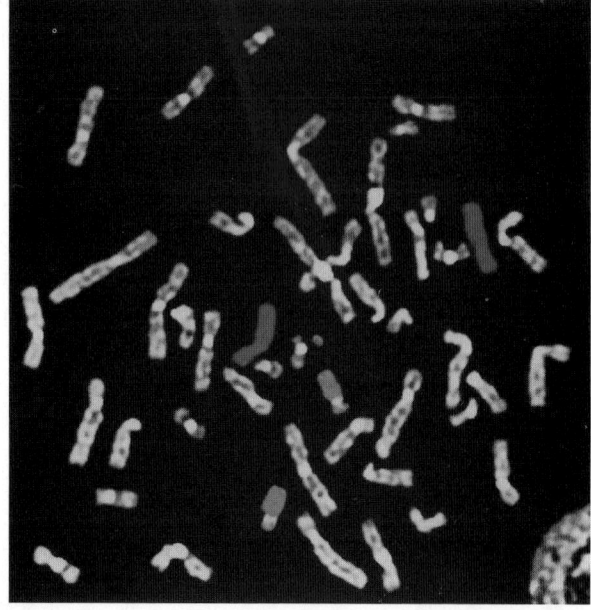

C

Fig. 25.6. Forward chromosome painting revealing (A) an insertional translocation of 18q12.3–18q21.2 (red) into 4p15.2, (B) a 46,XX, t(8;18)(q11.2;q12.2) reciprocal translocation, and (C) a small marker chromosome identified as a ring 8 chromosome in a preparation hybridized with chromosome-specific paint probes (CAMBIO) for chromosome 8 (red) and chromosome 18 (green). (See Plate 25.6.)

short arms, and the result is a dicentric chromosome and a tiny acentric fragment (containing the ribosomal genes but no other transcribed sequence). The acentric fragment is

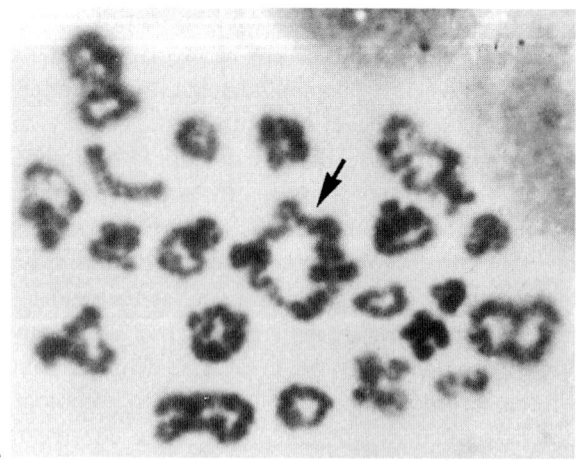

A

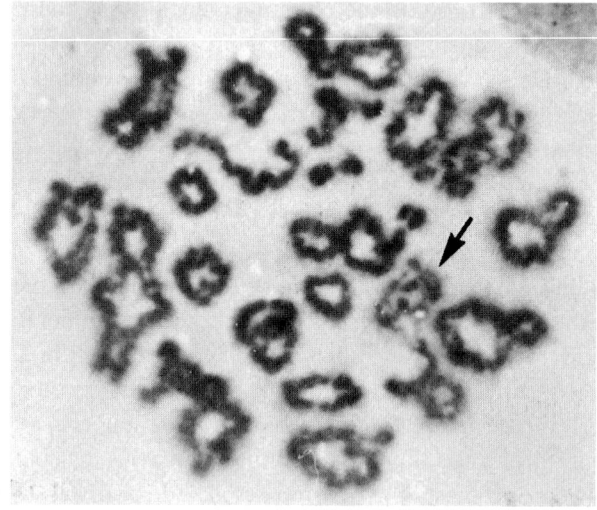

B

Fig. 25.7. (A) A ring quadrivalent (arrow) at the first meiotic division from an individual with a balanced reciprocal translocation between chromosomes 5p13 and 10q26. (B) A chain trivalent at the first meiotic division from an individual with a centric fusion translocation involving chromosomes 13 and 14 (arrow). (From Connor and Ferguson-Smith, 1993, with permission.)

readily eliminated from the cell, and so balanced carriers of Robertsonian translocations typically have only 45 chromosomes and show no phenotypic effects of chromosomal loss (sufficient ribosomal genes are present in the remaining acrocentrics). Robertsonian translocations are the most common type of translocations in humans; carriers occur in about 1 in 500 births. The most important categories are 45, t(13q14q) and 45, t(14q21q) because they can lead to unbalanced offspring with translocation trisomy 13 (Patau syndrome) and translocation trisomy 21 (Down syndrome), respectively. These abnormalities arise as a result of adjacent segregation from the trivalent formed during meiosis (Fig. 25.7B).

INSERTIONAL TRANSLOCATIONS

Insertional translocations are less common than reciprocal or centric fusion translocations. They may occur within a chromosome or between two chromosomes. The latter type of exchange requires three break points; two lead to an interstitial deletion of a chromosome fragment, which can then be inserted into the gap formed by the third break point (see Fig. 25.6A). The balanced carrier is healthy, but segregation of the two translocation derivatives during meiosis may lead to unbalanced offspring with either a deletion or a duplication of the inserted segment.

DELETIONS AND DUPLICATIONS

Deletions may be either interstitial such as the deletion of chromosome 15 associated with Prader-Willi and Angelman syndromes (e.g., 46, XY, del(15) (q11–q13) or terminal such as the deletion of part of the short arm of chromosome 5, i.e. 46, XX, del (5) (p15), which is found in the cri du chat syndrome. Because terminal deletions (Fig. 25.8) have stable ends, it is assumed that most result from an unbalanced terminal translocation, from the creation of a new telomere, or from an interstitial deletion. The latter requires two breaks with loss of the intervening segment. Interstitial deletions ranging in size from visible to sub-microscopic are now known to be important causes of microdeletion syndromes, listed in Table 25.2 and described in Chapter 46.

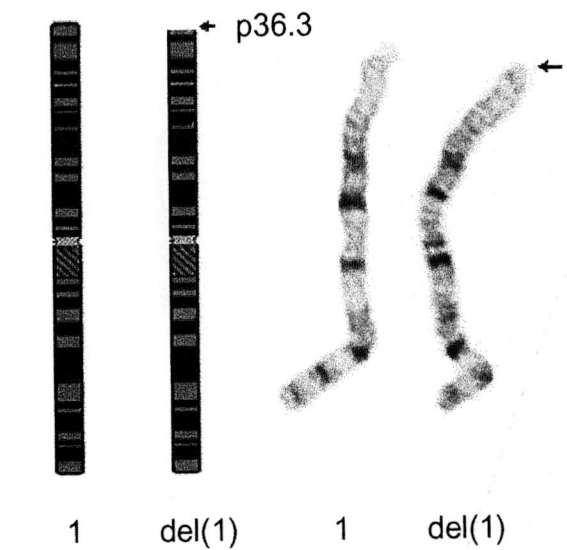

p36.3

1   del(1)   1   del(1)

Fig. 25.8. A subtle terminal deletion of chromosome 1, breakpoint p36.3.

Duplication is an intrachromosomal gain of chromatin (Fig. 25.9), lying in either the same linear orientation (direct duplication) or reverse orientation (inverted duplication) with respect to the centromere

RING CHROMOSOMES

Ring chromosomes (Fig. 25.2) may be associated with significant terminal deletions of DNA. They arise when breaks occur at both ends of a chromosome with reunion of the

Table 25.2. Microdeletion/microduplication syndromes

Chromosome band	Syndrome	Duplication/deletion	FISH probe available
4p16	Wolf-Hirschhorn	del	+
5p16	cri-du-chat	del	+
7p13	Greig cephalopolysyndactyly	del	+
7q11.23	Williams	del	+
7q34	Holoprosencephaly	del	−
8q24	Langer-Giedion	del	−
11p15	Beckwith-Wiedemann	dup	+
11q13	WAGR	del	+
13q14.11	Retinoblastoma	del	+
15q12	Prader-Willi/Angelman	del	+
16p13.3	α-Thalassemia/mentally retarded	del	+
16p13.3	Rubinstein-Taybi	del	+
17p13	Miller-Dieker	del	+
17p11.2	Smith-Magenis	del	+
17p11.2	Charcot-Marie-Tooth disease, 1A	dup	+
20p11.23	Alagille	del	−
22q11.2	Di George	del	+
22q11.2	Sprintzen	del	+
Xp22.3	Kalmann/ichthyosis	del	+
Xp21.2	DMD/MR/AH/GK	del	+
Xq21.1	Choroideremia/MR	del	+

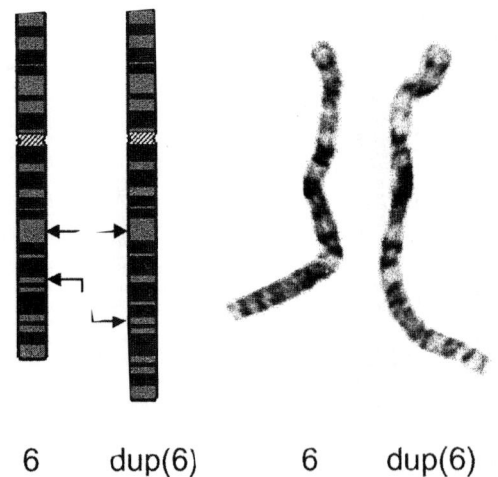

6   dup(6)   6   dup(6)

PLate 25.9. An inverted duplication involving the long arm of chromosome 6, breakpoints q21 and q23.1.

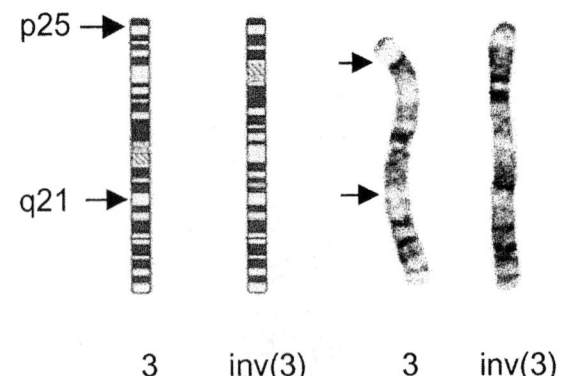

3   inv(3)   3   inv(3)

Plate 25.10. A pericentric inversion of chromosome 3, breakpoints p25 and q21.

proximal ends and loss of the distal telomeric fragments. They are seldom inherited (unless very small) and are a common feature in irradiated cells. Some are unstable, and sister chromatid exchange within a ring chromosome may generate dicentric double-sized rings. The instability of the dicentric ring may lead to further gain or loss, thereby adding to the phenotypic abnormality.

ISOCHROMOSOMES

Isochromosomes are abnormal chromosomes with duplication of one arm and loss of the other; they are usually metacentric, and each arm usually contains identical gene loci. The sex chromosomes are most commonly involved in isochromosome formation. Most arise from an isochromatid break and fusion above the centromere so that both centromeres are retained. They are thus isodicentric, or pseudoisodicentric because the activity of one of the two centromeres is usually suppressed. Isochromosomes for the long arm of the X, i.e. 46, X, idic (X) (p11.21) and for the long arm of the Y are found in some cases of Turner syndrome, and isochromosomes for the short arm of the Y are sometimes a cause of male infertility. Both are frequently associated with mosaicism for a 45, X cell line.

Inversions

Inversions arise from two breaks within the same chromosome with inversion through 180 degrees of the segment between the breaks, followed by reunion (Fig. 25.9). If the breaks occur on either side of the centromere, the inversion is pericentric (Fig. 25.10). If the breaks occur on the same side, the inversion is paracentric and the implications for

offspring are different. An inversion simply changes the order of gene loci within a chromosome and thus in itself may have no phenotypic effect. However, inversions interfere with synapsis during meiosis; one homologue may form a loop in the inverted region to pair with its homologue (Fig. 25.11B). If crossing-over occurs within a *paracentric* inversion, the recombinant chromosomes will be a dicentric chromosome and an acentric fragment. Both are unstable and tend not to be found in offspring. Crossing-over within a *pericentric* inversion results in recombinant chromosomes with duplication-deletions of the chromosome distal to the break points of the inversion. The closer the break points are to the ends of the chromosome, the smaller the imbalance. Because large imbalances tend to be lethal, inversions that result in abnormal offspring tend to have more distal break points.

Meiotic analysis

The nature of the various chromosome aberrations described above can be studied in meiotic preparations, but this is a research exercise and has little application in routine chromosome analysis. The study of male meiosis requires testicular biopsy from adult males, but female meiosis can be studied adequately only from fetal ovarian tissue. It follows that most experience of human meiotic chromosomes has been obtained from adult males.

The testis biopsy is best obtained by open operation during which a small incision is made in the tunica albuginea and a 3-mm³ biopsy taken from the material that exudes from the incision. Part of the material is used for air-dried chromosome preparations and part for surface-spread analysis of synaptonemal complexes (Moses et al., 1975).

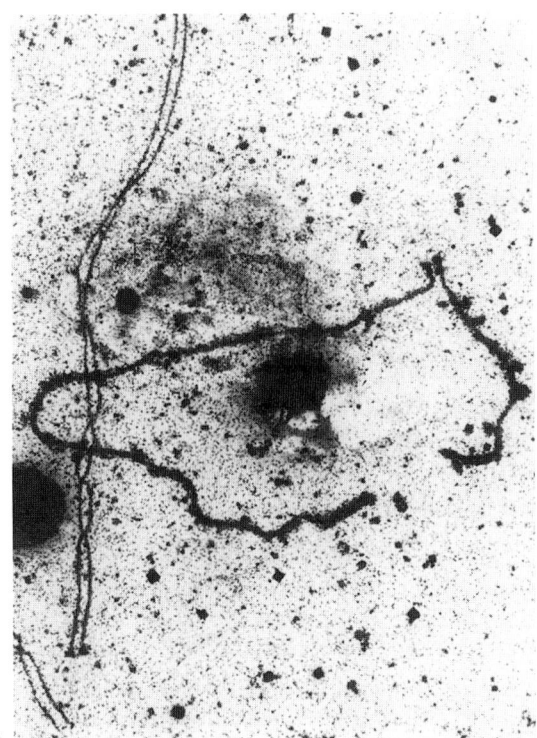
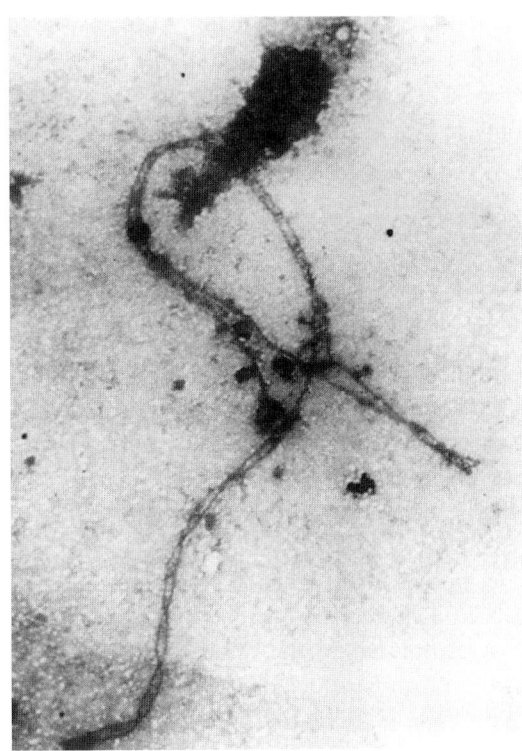

Fig. 25.11. (A) Electron microscopy preparation of human sex bivalent at pachytene, prepared by surface spreading technique. The X chromosome (left) and the Y chromosome (right) are attached to one another by their pairing segments (top). (Courtesy Dr Anne Chandley and from Connor and Ferguson-Smith, 1993, with permission.) (B) Chromosome 2 inversion heterozyote with break points at 2p11 and 2q13, prepared as in A, showing the inversion loop following synapsis. (Courtesy of Professor Maj Hultén.)

Because testis material deteriorates quickly on exposure to air, the preparations must be made immediately. Air-dried preparations are made from minced material treated in 1% hypotonic sodium citrate (10 to 15 minutes) followed by fixation in methanol glacial acetic acid (3:1 and containing 1% chloroform). Drop preparations are air dried on microscope slides and stained by 2% aceto-orcein or one of the fluorescent stains or by C-banding. Analysis of pachytene and diakinesis stages allows the detection of translocations (Fig. 25.7) and defects of synapsis (oligochiasmate maturation arrest).

In the surface-spreading technique, a drop of testis cells suspended in culture medium (and without hypotonic pretreatment) is added to a drop of sucrose solution (0.2 M) on a microscope slide. The cells are allowed to spread for 5 minutes before being fixed by adding drops of a 4% solution of paraformaldehyde until the slide is covered. The fixative is left for one hour and then rinsed in water and allowed to dry in air. The preparation is then stained under a sealed coverslip with a 50% solution of silver nitrate in 0.03% formalin at 60°C for one hour. After it is rinsed in water, the stained preparation is dried in air and mounted for light microscopy. The lateral elements of the synaptonemal complexes take up the silver stain and so allow the analysis of chromosome pairing during meiosis (Fig. 25.11A). The preparations are therefore suitable for the examination of structural abnormalities including translocations and inversions (Saadallah and Hulten, 1986) (Fig. 25.11B) at the prophase of first meiosis. Individual meiotic chromosomes are identified with difficulty unless hybridized with chromosome-specific painting probes.

Flow karyotyping

Conventional microscopy using chromosome preparations fixed to microscope slides must be regarded as the standard approach to chromosome analysis. However, it is not the only method, and the analysis of chromosomes in fluid suspension using the techniques of flow cytometry has had increasing application during the past 25 years since it was introduced by Gray et al. (1975).

The analysis of chromosomes by flow cytometry requires a dual laser fluorescent-activated cell sorter (FACS) in which the first laser is tuned to emit light at 364 nm to excite Hoechst 33258 fluorescence, and the second laser is tuned to emit light at 458 nm to excite Chromomycin A3 fluorescence. The fixed chromosome suspension in polyamine buffer is stained in a dilute mixture of the two stains. Hoechst 33258 has an affinity for A-T rich DNA, and Chromomycin A3 has an affinity for G-C rich DNA. The stained chromosomes are passed in a fluid stream sequentially through the two lasers at a speed of about 2000 chromosomes per second. The fluorescence excited by the two lasers in each chromosome is collected, measured by photomultipliers and stored by the FACS. After a few minutes several hundred thousand individual measurements of each of the 23 types of chromosome have been collected to generate a histogram, or flow karyotype, which separates the chromosomes into groups depending on their DNA content and base-pair ratio. The base-pair ratio is determined by the relative amounts of fluorescence generated by the two fluorescent stains. The result is a bivariate flow karyotype, in which the individual chromosomes are grouped by size into clusters (Fig. 25.12) each of which has a characteristic relationship to the others. A-T rich chromosomes tend to be above a diagonal line drawn through the middle of the clusters, while G-C rich chromosomes are below this line. Chromosomes 9–12 tend to sort in one cluster, as they have similar DNA contents and base pair-ratios, but all the other chromosomes resolve into separate groups. Sometimes individual homologues of the same chromosome pair may be separated from one another because of variation in amounts of hetrochromatin. The technique is useful for assessing variations in chromosomal size due to aberrations and heteromorphisms. The lower limit of resolution of DNA content is between 1 and 2 megabases.

The design of the FACS allows the sorting of chromosomes for collection into separate containers. This is achieved by breaking the fluid stream containing the dilute chromosome suspension into a series of droplets containing single chromosomes, each of which can be positively or negatively charged depending on the fluorescence profile of the chromosome within the droplet. As the charged droplet passes between two voltage plates, it is deflected into the appropriate container. The procedure is remarkably accurate, and it is a comparatively straightforward matter, if the preparation is good, to collect any number of chromosomes of one type without contamination. Chromosomes sorted in this way are commonly used for preparing chromosome-specific DNA libraries, reagents for chromosome mapping, and chromosome-specific paint probes.

The key to producing good flow karyotypes and pure chromosome-specific samples of uncontaminated chromosomes lies in the preparation of suitable chromosome suspensions. The first essential is a culture with a high mitotic index from which large numbers of undamaged chromosomes can be collected. Fibroblast cultures, short-term lymphocyte cultures, and lymphoblastoid cells lines have all been used with good success. Cultures may be treated for up to 16 hours with colcemid (0.1 µg/ml) to give a high yield of mitosis. Although the chromosomes can be abnormally contracted by such long-term exposure to colcemid, this does not seem to affect the quality of the preparation. Cells cultured in suspension (e.g., lymphoblastoid cell lines) can be used directly, but mitoses from monolayer cultures are best harvested by gentle agitation to shake off the cells in division. The cells are treated in hypotonic KCl (0.075 M) for 10 to 20 minutes and then resuspended in a polyamine buffer containing triton X-100. Chromosomes are released into suspension by 10 seconds of rapid vortexing, stained immediately in Chromomycin A3 (final concentration, 40 µg/ml) and Hoechst 33258 (final concentration, 2 µg/ml) followed by 2 hours of incubation at 4°C. Then, 15 minutes before flow analysis, sodium citrate (final concentration, 10 mM) and sodium sulphate (final concentration, 25 mM) are added to the sample. It is important to avoid excessive disruption of the mitotic cells because this leads to chromosome fragmentation, indicated by an unacceptable level of debris at the lower end of the flow karyotype. Cultures that contain a high proportion of

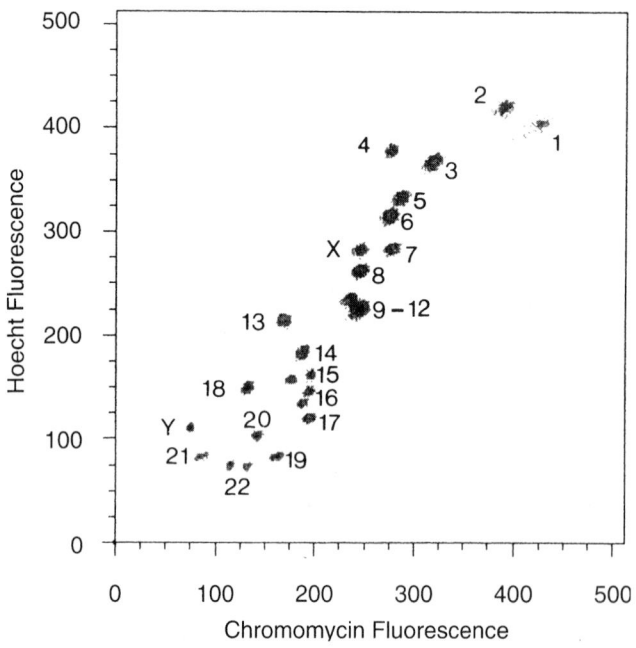

Fig. 25.12. Flow karyotype generated by fluorescence-activated chromosome sorting. Bivariate analysis of normal male by DNA content and base pair composition. Greater resolution is possible, including separation of homologues of chromosomes 15, 16 and 22 by virtue of centric heteromorphisms.

cells in anaphase or telophase may also lead to contamination of the chromosome peaks by the inclusion of chromatids in the preparation.

In situ hybridization

The ISH technique is based on the principle that when double-stranded DNA is heated it denatures into single-stranded DNA. On cooling, the single-stranded DNA reanneals with its complementary sequence into double-stranded DNA. If an appropriately labeled DNA sequence (probe) is denatured and added to denatured nuclei or chromosomes during the process of reannealing, some of that labeled DNA will hybridize to its complementary sequence in the chromosomal DNA. Detection of the labeled DNA will identify the site of hybridization and thus the region of chromosomal DNA complementary to the DNA sequence in the labeled probe. Thus, ISH may be used to map and order genes and other DNA sequences along the length of a chromosome.

In the early days of ISH, DNA probes were labeled with radioisotopes such as tritium (H^3) or radioactive iodine (^{125}I) and detected by autoradiography using photographic emulsion applied directly to the microscope slide. The scatter of radioactive disintegrations, revealed by silver grains in the developed emulsion, meant that the resolution was poor. The autoradiographs often had to be exposed for several weeks to achieve an adequate signal; therefore, it was not possible to tell whether the probe had hybridized satisfactorily until long after the experiment had been set up. These disadvantages, coupled with the hazards of radioisotopes and the need to count silver grains in a large number of cells to establish significant counts above background levels, led to the search for nonisotopic methods of labeling.

In situ hybridization was first used to map the chromosomal location of highly repetitive (satellite) DNA to the centromeric regions of mouse chromosomes (Pardue and Gall, 1970) and the moderately repetitive ribosomal DNA to the nucleolus organizing regions in the polytene chromosomes of Diptera (Pardue et al., 1970). Similar studies soon located these repetitive DNAs to the equivalent sites in human chromosomes (Henderson et al., 1972; Jones and Corneo, 1971). However, it was not possible to incorporate sufficient radioactivity in probes derived from single-copy DNA sequences to permit the more extensive application of ISH in gene mapping. This had to await the introduction of recombinant DNA techniques and the development of DNA sequences cloned in plasmids that could be heavily labeled. The early 1980s saw the first chromosomal localizations of single-copy DNA sequences by ISH (Gerhard et al., 1981; Harper and Saunders, 1981, Malcolm et al., 1981), and ISH soon became the method of choice for assigning a cloned DNA sequence to its position in the chromosomal map. It was quickly appreciated that ISH also had application in diagnostic cytogenetics, particularly for the detection of structural abnormalities beyond the resolution of conventional banding techniques.

The search for nonisotopic alternatives for labeling probes for ISH led first to the introduction of biotin (Langer et al., 1981) and then other haptens including acetylaminofluorene (Landegent et al., 1984), mercury (Bauman et al., 1983), digoxigenin (Heiles et al., 1988; Seibl et al., 1990), and sulphonate (Morimoto et al., 1987).

Biotin and digoxigenin have proved the most useful, and a variety of methods have been developed to detect both these labels in cytologic preparations using fluorescence or enzyme-linked reactions. Biotinylated probes are detected by fluorochromes or enzymes coupled to avidin, streptavidin, or antibiotin antibody. The enzymes most commonly used are alkaline phosphatase and horseradish peroxidase. The former depends on the production of the insoluble formezan from nitroblue tetrazolium chloride, and the signal is best seen using phase contrast optics (Garson et al., 1987). The peroxidase reaction uses the oxidation of diaminobenzidine to produce a dark brown insoluble complex that presents most clearly as a bright spot on reflection contrast microscopy (Landegent et al., 1985). The fluorochromes most commonly used are fluorscein isothiocyanate (FITC), tetramethyl rhodamine isothiocyanate (TRITC), amino methyl coumarin acetic acid (AMCA), and Texas red. With these reagents coupled to avidin, streptavidin, and various antibodies, including antibiotin, antidigoxigenin, antiavidin, and antibodies to these reagents, it is possible to build a strong fluorescence signal using several layers of fluorochrome-coupled antibodies.

In recent years, the indirect detection systems using antibodies have been replaced by direct labeling methods in which the fluorochromes such as FITC, Cy3, and Cy5 are coupled directly to the nucleotides (e.g., FITC-11-dUTP) that are used in the labeling of the DNA probes.

Enzyme-based detection systems have the advantage that the signal is permanent, whereas in fluorescence detection systems, the signal tends to fade on exposure to UV light in the fluorescence microscope. This fading can be reduced to a certain extent by the use of antifade agents in the mounting medium. However, the need for the detection of fluorescent signals of low luminosity and their rapid analysis has led to the development of sensitive cameras and sophisticated image analysis systems. These systems allow the fluorescence image to be digitized and acquired by a personal computer and archived onto optical disc or computer tape. The stored image is then available for image processing and analysis (see below). For many applications in diagnostic cytogenetics, however, the DNA probes are large enough to produce bright signals, and image processing is not essential. Digital fluorescence microscopy has particular application in multicolor FISH and in the detection of weak fluorescent signals.

Almost all types of DNA probe used in FISH applications in diagnostic cytogenetics contain interspersed repetitive elements that will hybridize to complementary sequences throughout the entire genome leading to a high level of background signals. This background can be suppressed effectively by preannealing unlabeled genomic or Cot-1 (enriched for highly repetitive sequences) DNA to the labeled probe before hybridizing the probe to the target DNA (Lichter et al., 1988). The unlabeled DNA acts as a competitor and will form duplexes rapidly with the repetitive DNA sequences within the probe. The low-copy DNA remaining in the probe will then be available to hybridize with complementary sequences in the target DNA. With many DNA probes the use of Cot-1 DNA may be avoided by allowing the probe to preanneal with itself before application to the target.

The current procedures for FISH use standard air-dried chromosome preparations, which are denatured by heating in 70% formamide at 65°C for 2 minutes before being placed in ice-cold 70% ethanol. This is followed by dehydrating through an ethanol series and air drying. The rapid cooling ensures that the denatured single-stranded DNA in the preparations does not reanneal. Meanwhile, the DNA probe is labeled by nick-translation, random primer extension, or amplification in the presence of labeled nucleotides using the polymerase chain reaction (PCR).

In the nick-translation method, DNase randomly nicks the double-stranded target DNA, and then DNA polymerase is used to fill in the nicked strand with newly synthesized DNA containing the hapten-dUTP. Similarly, in the PCR method, the labeled nucleotide is added to the reaction mixture. Probe-specific primers can be used for probe sequences of about 1 kilobase (kb), but larger sequences, for example, cosmid clones, are best labeled using degenerate oligonucleotide primed-PCR (DOP-PCR,) (Telenius et al., 1992). For hybridization, 50 to 100 ng of labeled DNA probe are prepared in 16 µl of hybridization buffer (containing formamide and dextran sulphate) together with 1 mg/ml of Cot-1 DNA. This mix is added to the dena-

tured slide preparation; covered with a coverslip, which is sealed with cow gum; and incubated at 37 to 43°C overnight. Following hybridization, the coverslip is removed, and the slide is washed for 10 minutes in 50% formamide and 1X SSC at 42°C.

The choice of detection method depends on the hapten used in the labeling of the DNA probe. If a biotinylated probe is used, detection involves treating the slide with fluresceinated avidin and fluresceinated antiavidin and incubating in detection buffer at 37°C for 30 minutes. Washing in three changes of detection buffer is followed by 4X SSC with 0.05% Tween20 for five minutes, dehydration through an ethanol series, and mounting in 1 mg/ml of DAPI in antifade solution. The slides are viewed using a fluorescence microscope equipped with a 50-watt mercury lamp; appropriate excitation and emission filters are chosen according to the fluorochromes used (Table 25.3). Each fluorochrome is excited by a different wavelength, and each emits a distinctive fluorescence. Multiple excitation/dichroic/bandpass filter blocks are available, which can be used in the microscope to observe simultaneously several fluorochromes excited by different wavelengths. This means that the blue DAPI counterstain can be used, for example, in conjunction with FITC (green) and TRITC (red) probe signals.

It is comparatively straightforward to use a three-color FISH system with conventional fluorescence microscopy along the lines outlined above. Additional fluorochromes are becoming available that add colors to the FISH armamentarium. However, the most satisfactory approach to obtaining multicolor FISH is by the technique of combinatorial-labeling, whereby mixtures of two to five fluorochromes are used to label each DNA probe. For example, different combinations of the three fluorochromes in each probe can give up to seven distinguishable color differences

Table 25.3. Fluorochromes used for FISH

	Wavelength (nm)	
	Excitation maximum	Emission maximum
Fluorescein isothiocyante (FITC)	495	525
Tetramethyl rhodamine isothiocyanate (TRITC)	543	570
Texas red	596	620
Amino methyl coumarin acetic acid (AMCA)	345	440
Cy5	650	674
4′,6-diamidino-2-phenylindole (DAP1)	372	456
Hoechst 33258	395	450
Propidium iodide	342,495	639

by digital fluorescence microscopy (Dauwerse et al., 1992; Ried et al., 1992). This exploits a sensitive monochromatic, cooled, charged coupled device (CCD) camera and computerized image processing. A gray-level image of the fluorescence of each fluorochrome is acquired sequentially and merged to provide a false color on the computer screen, which is chosen on the basis of the relative intensity of each of the three components. Because the three images must be aligned accurately in the merged image, a system to prevent registration errors has been found to be useful. Triple dichroic band-pass filters are used in the epifluorescence optical path, with individual excitation filters mounted in a computer-controlled motorized filter wheel in front of the lamp house. Filter changes can then be made without the risk of moving the stage or objectives. More complex filter sets are used when more than three fluorochromes are employed.

In addition to their use in multicolor FISH, the systems available for digital fluorescence microscopy and image processing allow image enhancement, color adjustment, image reversal, and a number of procedures that assist in chromosome measurement and analysis. The use of spatial filters and contrast adjustment is particularly useful in enhancing the weak banding patterns obtained using DAPI counterstaining. The combination of chromosome banding and multicolor FISH has added greatly to the resolution of problems in modern diagnostic cytogenetics.

DNA PROBES AND THEIR APPLICATIONS

The various classes of DNA probe have particular applications to problems in diagnostic cytogenetics.

Total genome probes

Total genome probes are prepared from DNA extracted from blood samples, cell cultures, or solid tissues and labeled appropriately. Chromosomes hybridized with these probes show an evenly distributed signal along their length, referred to as *chromosome painting*. A total genome probe can be used to identify human chromosome material in human:rodent interspecific somatic cell hybrids, including radiation-reduced cell hybrids.

Chromosome-specific painting probes

Chromosome-specific painting probes (Fig. 25.13) are genomic probes made either from chromosome-specific genomic libraries, from single chromosome-interspecific somatic cell hybrids, or from flow-sorted chromosomes. The latter produce probes with the highest resolution. The

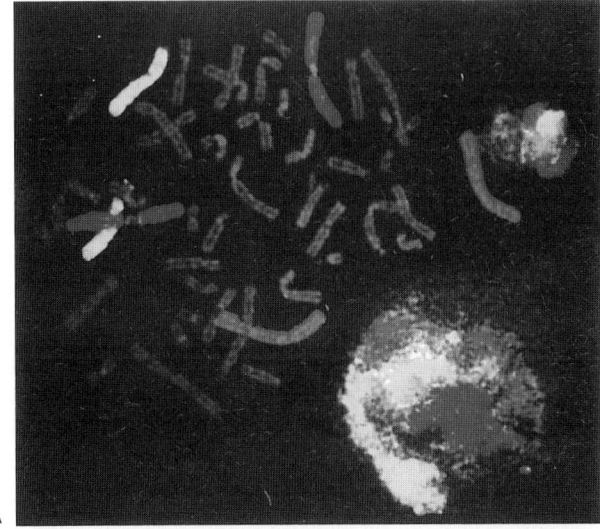

A

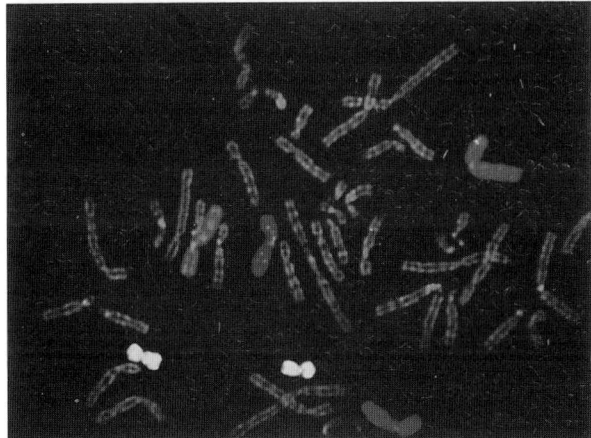

B

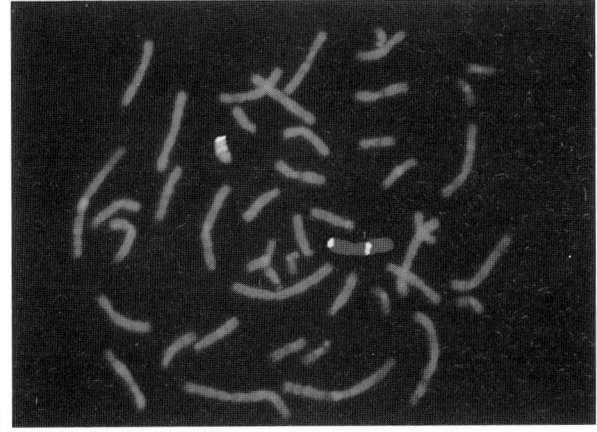

C

Fig. 25.13. Chromosome painting using chromosome specific probes (CAMBIO Ltd., Cambridge, England) from flow sorted chromosomes (DAPI counterstain). (A) Chromosome 1 (red), chromosome 2 (green), and chromosome 6 (yellow). Interphase nucleus reveals chromosome domains within nucleus. (B) Chromosome 7 (green), chromosome 11(red), and chromosome 20 (yellow). (C) X chromosome (red), Y chromosome (green). Note Y signal (yellow) on XY homologous regions of Xp (tip) and Xq (proximal third) and X signal (yellow) on XY homologous region of Yp (tip). (See Plate 25.13.)

human chromosomes in somatic cell hybrids can be specifically labeled in the presence of rodent chromosome by exploiting the presence of interspersed repeated sequences present only in human DNA. PCR primers made from Alu sequences can be used for this purpose (Lengauer et al., 1990; Lichter et al., 1990). All other sources used for chromosome-specific painting probes can be labeled by nick-translation or DOP-PCR. These paint probes are commercially available from several distributors and are used extensively in the analysis of chromosome rearrangements.

The origin of de novo balanced or unbalanced rearrangements can often be suggested by an altered banding pattern and definitive confirmation made by "forward" painting using the most likely chromosome-specific probes (Fig. 25.6). The alternative, where there is no suggestion that one chromosome is more likely to be involved than another, is to try the hybridization of panels of several chromosome paints until the correct one is identified. It is helpful to remember that most de novo unbalanced chromosomal duplications are intrachromosomal, and so the paint corresponding to the derivative chromosome should be tried first.

If there is access to chromosome sorting by FACS, the abnormal chromosome should be flow sorted and 300 to 500 chromosomes used to produce a DOP-PCR-amplified paint for "reverse" painting onto normal male metaphases (Carter et al., 1992). The various chromosomes involved in the rearrangement will be evident from the areas of hybridization revealed on the normal chromosomes by the paint probe.

Region-specific paint probes may be prepared from dissected chromosomes (Meltzer et al., 1992) or by coincidence painting (Bailey et al., 1993). Multicolor paint probes constructed from multiple yeast artificial chromosome (YAC) clones and regional microdissection libraries or from several radiation-reduced hybrids, each labeled with a different fluorochrome, have been used to produce a universal color bar code for every chromosome, which may help in chromosome identification using automated methods (Lengauer et al., 1993). Such bar code paints may have application in the identification of cancer chromosomes.

Several multicolour FISH systems are commercially available which, in one hybridization and using digital processing, can identify each chromosome in a different colour (Schröck et al., 1996; Speicher et al., 1996). Each system has similar resolution and most interchromosomal rearrangements can be readily identified. The technique could have wider application in diagnostic and cancer cytogenetics were it not for the prohibitively expensive fluorescence labels which put the method beyond the reach of most cytogenetic laboratories. Fig. 25.14 shows a metaphase prepared by M-FISH

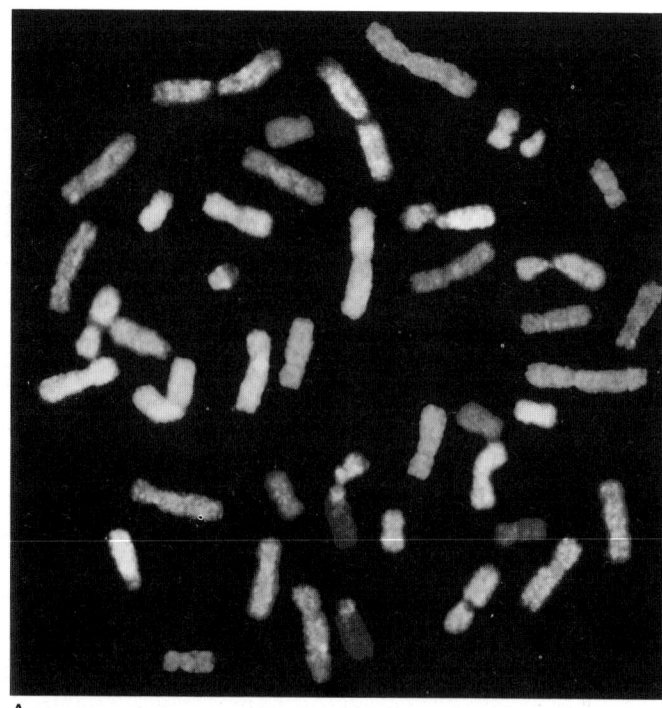

A

Fig. 25.14. Multicolor FISH analysis of a normal human male metaphase using combinatorial chromosome-specific painting probes produced with 5 fluorescent dyes. (A) Raw image of metaphase in pseudocolor, (B) Karyotype of raw image. (C) M-FISH karyotype after chromosome identification by computer. (See Plate 25.14.)

and Fig. 25.15 shows a modification of M-FISH, termed colour banding, which exploits a probe set prepared from gibbon chromosomes. In this modification the rearrangements which have occurred during the divergence of humans and lesser apes provide a reproducible pattern of colour bands along each chromosome. This permits the identification of regions within chromosomal arms and is helpful in detecting intrachromosomal aberrations such as inversions (Fig. 25.16) and duplications which cannot be distinguished by conventional M-FISH probes. Even higher resolution within each chromosome can be achieved by using up to 10 differently labelled microdissection probes.

In the application of paint probes, one of the disadvantages is that areas composed of repetitive elements, especially paracentric and telomeric regions, are not painted. This is due to the preannealing procedures which are designed to eliminate background due to DNA repeats. Analysis of these regions require the use of centromere-specific and telomere-specific probes (see below).

Chromosome-specific centromeric probes

Chromosome-specific centromeric probes are cloned from the alphoid-repetitive DNA that is located close to chro-

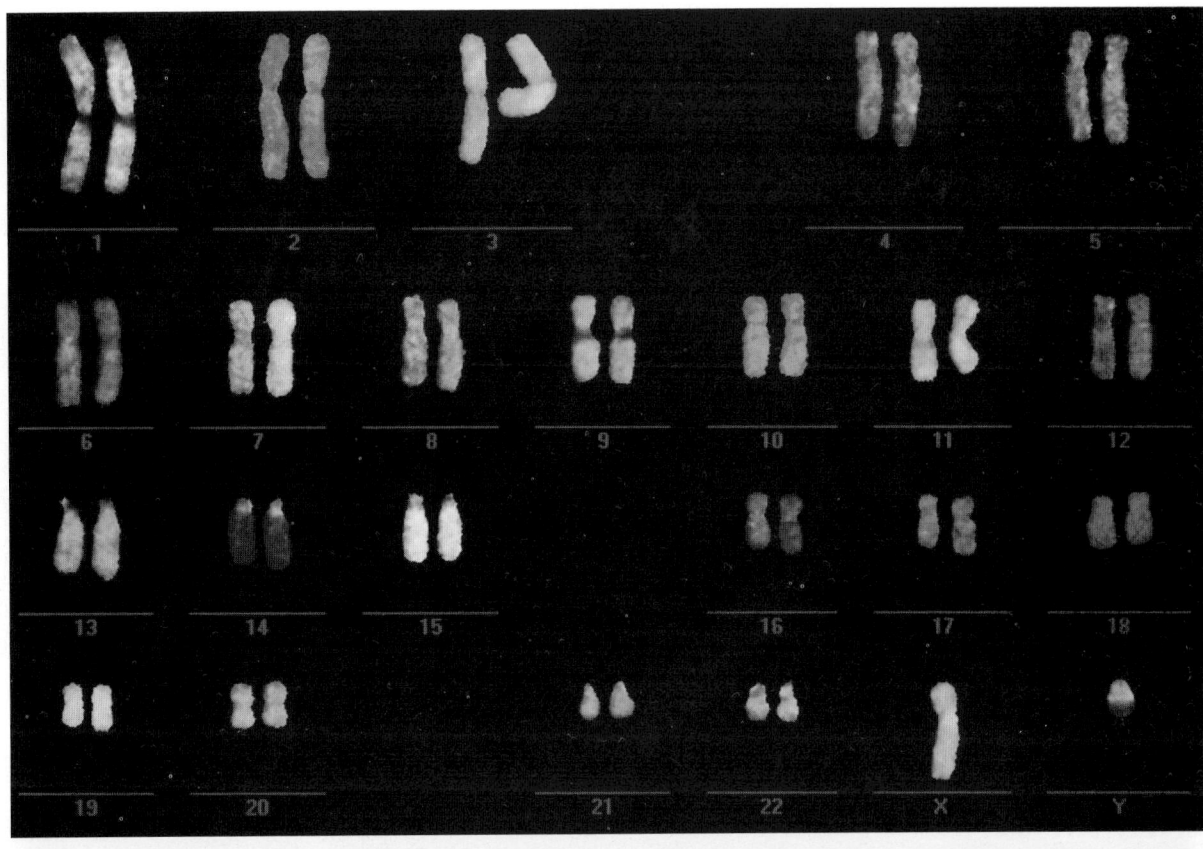

B

C

Fig. 25.14. (B) & (C) .

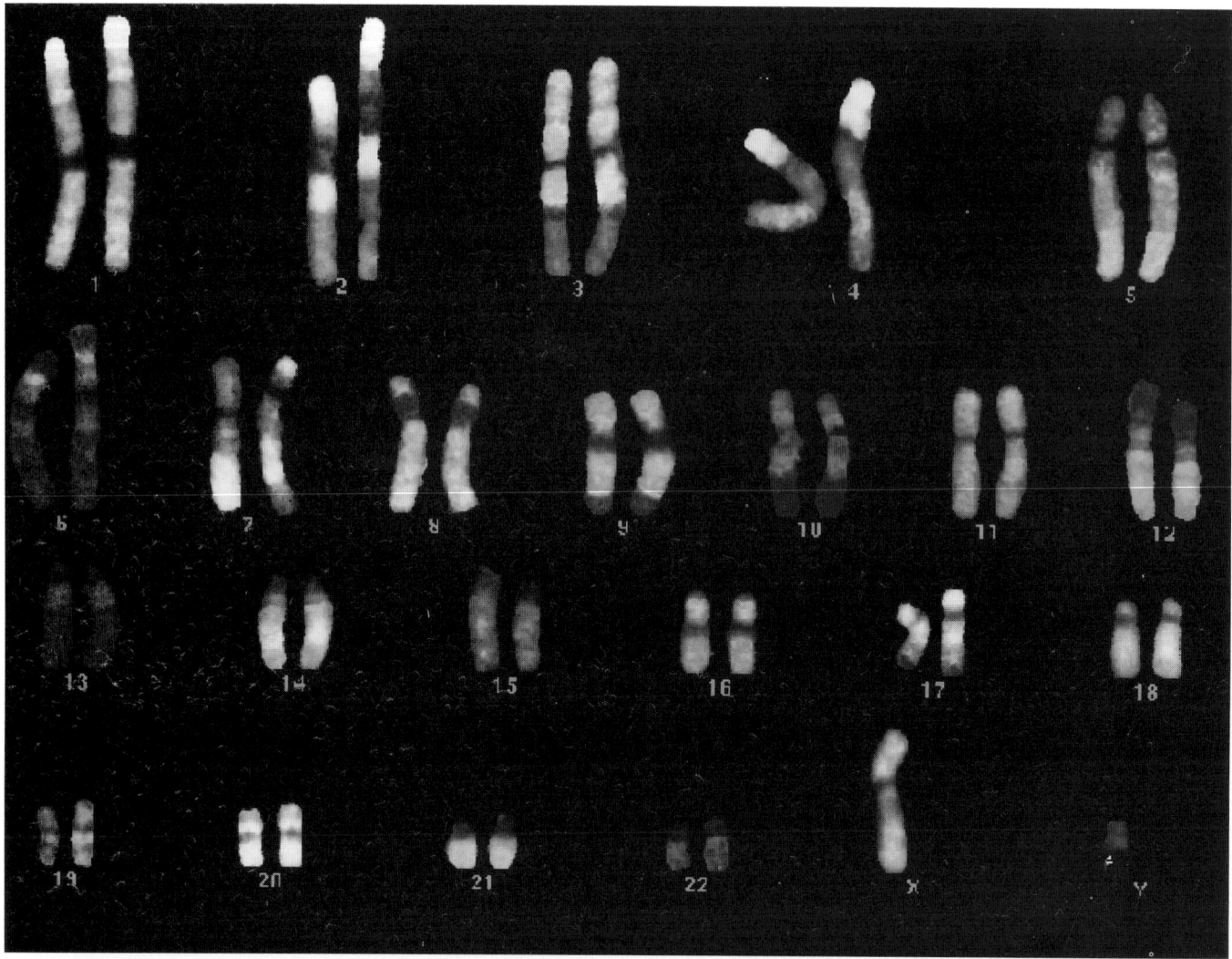

Fig. 25.15. Color banding of human male metaphase using chromosome-specific gibbon painting probes. Color bands reflect interchromosomal rearrangements arising during divergence of human and gibbon. Note large pericentric inversion of right homologue of chromosome 7. (See Plate 25.15.)

mosome centromeres. Almost all human centromeres have chromosome-specific sequences of this type. The exceptions are chromosomes 13 and 21, and 14 and 22; each pair shares indistinguishable sequences. The main application of centromeric probes is in the determination of chromosome copy number in interphase nuclei (Fig. 25.16). More than 80% of normal diploid nuclei will consistently show two specific signals representing the centromeres of each pair of chromosomes. They are used in aneuploidy detection in uncultured amniotic fluid cells, for preimplantation diagnosis of aneuploidy in cells from the blastocyst, for the diagnosis and detection of residual disease in the management of certain hematologic malignancies, and for the analysis of nondisjunctional abnormalities in sperm. In these copy number applications, YAC probes and cosmid contig probes are used for chromosomes 13, 14, 21, and 22

instead of centromeric probes (which are nonspecific for these chromosomes).

Single-copy DNA sequence probes

Thanks to the International Human Gene Project, a physical map of the human genome composed of a series of overlapping cloned DNA sequences along each chromosome is available in BAC or PAC vectors These clones act as reference markers along the chromosome and are also suitable for FISH (Fig. 25.16). Many other DNA sequences of interest, including sequences from known genes, have been cloned in yeast artificial chromosome (YAC) and cosmid vectors; both are suitable for FISH. YAC clones can accept inserts of up to 2 million base pairs and have the disadvantage that they may contain sequences from more than one

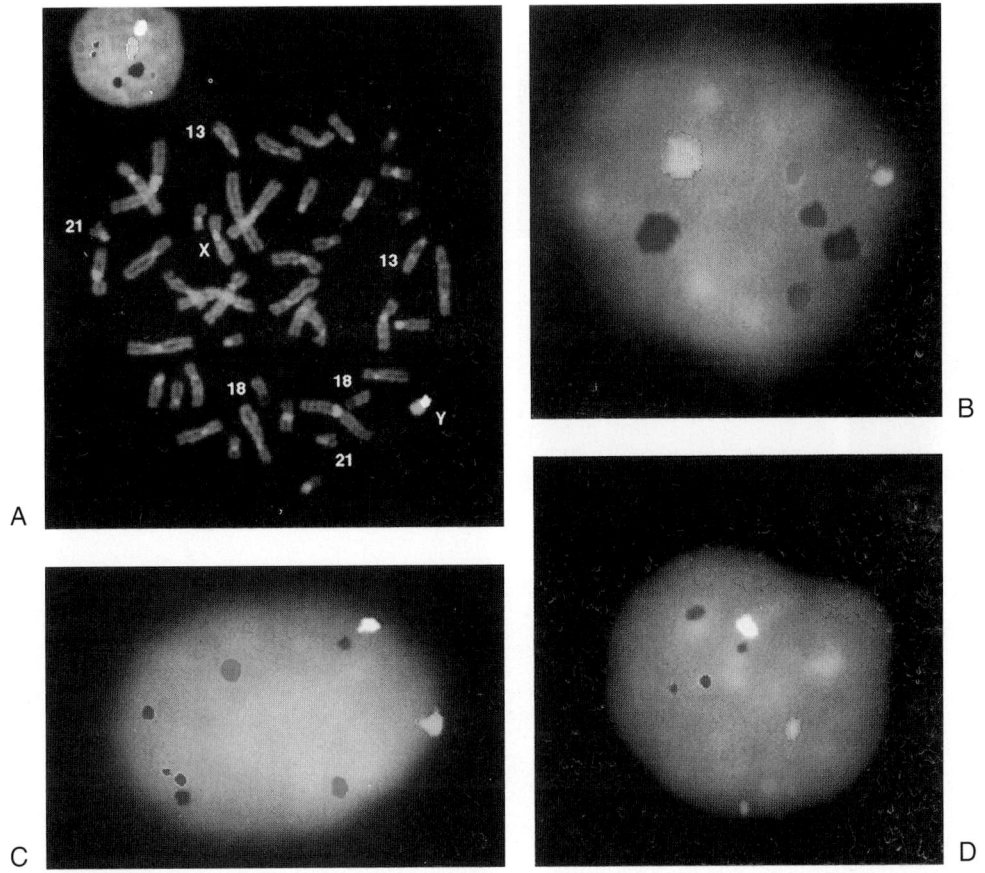

Fig. 25.16. FISH probes useful for determining chromosome copy number in interphase nuclei. (A) Lymphocyte metaphase showing centromeric probes for X chromosome (lilac), Y chromosome (yellow), and chromosome 18 (blue); a YAC clone marks chromosome 13 (green) and a contig of two overlapping cosmids marks chromosome 21 (red). (B) Uncultured amniotic fluid cell nucleus from a female fetus hybridized with the above probes revealing normal copy number of each chromosome. (C) As above, from male fetus with trisomy 21 (Down syndrome). (D) As above, from normal male fetus. (From Divane A, Carter NP, Spathas DH, Ferguson-Smith MA (1994) Rapid prenatal diagnosis of aneuploidy from uncultured amniotic fluid cells using five-colour fluorescence in situ hybridization. Prenatal Diagnosis 14:1061–1069, with permission.) (See Plate 25.16.)

chromosomal region (due to coligation) and seem more liable to lose parts of the insert through deletion. Cosmid clones can accept smaller inserts up to 40 kb and do not have these disadvantages. Both types of clone can be used as markers for gene loci, for the delineation of breakpoints and for the identification of deletions and duplications associated with chromosomal syndromes. For example, cosmid clones are widely used for the diagnosis of microdeletion syndromes (Table 25.2 and Fig. 25.17).

TELOMERE-SPECIFIC DNA PROBES

By far the majority of structural inter-chromosomal rearrangements involve the ends of chromosomes. G-banding and chromosome-specific paint probes are capable of identifying comparatively large (i.e. more than 2 Mb) duplications and deletions involving chromosome ends. As smaller unbalanced aberrations are much more likely to lead

to viable offspring than larger aberrations, it follows that many such conditions may be missed by conventional methods. Telomeric DNA probes specific for the ends of all human chromosomes have been developed to improve the identification of these cryptic aberrations (Ning et al., 1996). Subsequent results have confirmed the favourable expectations made for these probes. The production of chromosome-specific telomeric probes depends on the cloning (usually in cosmids) of unique subtelomeric sequences as near as possible (less than 300 Kb) to the ends of the chromosome. Multicolour FISH allows two or more chromosome-specific telomeric probes to be used in a specific hybridization (Fig. 25.18).

DNA FIBER-FISH

Because of the condensation of the chromosome fiber at metaphase, the fluorescent signals from two cosmid clones

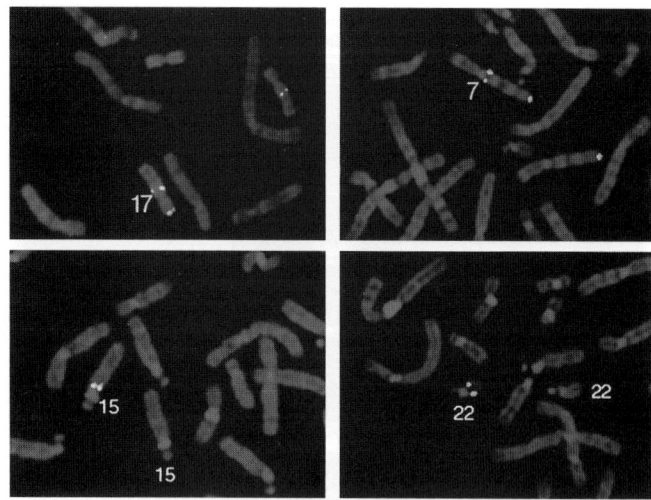

Fig. 25.17. The diagnosis of microdeletion syndromes using labeled cosmid clones (ONCOR, Gaithersburg, USA) that map into the region involved in the deletion. (A) Miller-Dieker syndrome. Chromosome 17 identified by cosmid clone in 17q. Note loss of signal at 17q13 in one homologue (*right*). (B) Williams syndrome. Chromosome 7 identified by cosmid clone at distal end of 7q. Note loss of signal at the elastin locus on 7q11.23 in one homologue (*lower*). (C) Prader-Willi syndrome. One homologue of chromosome 15 shows loss of signal at 15q12. (D) DiGeorge syndrome. One homologue of chromosome 22 shows loss of signal at 22q11. (See Plate 25.17.)

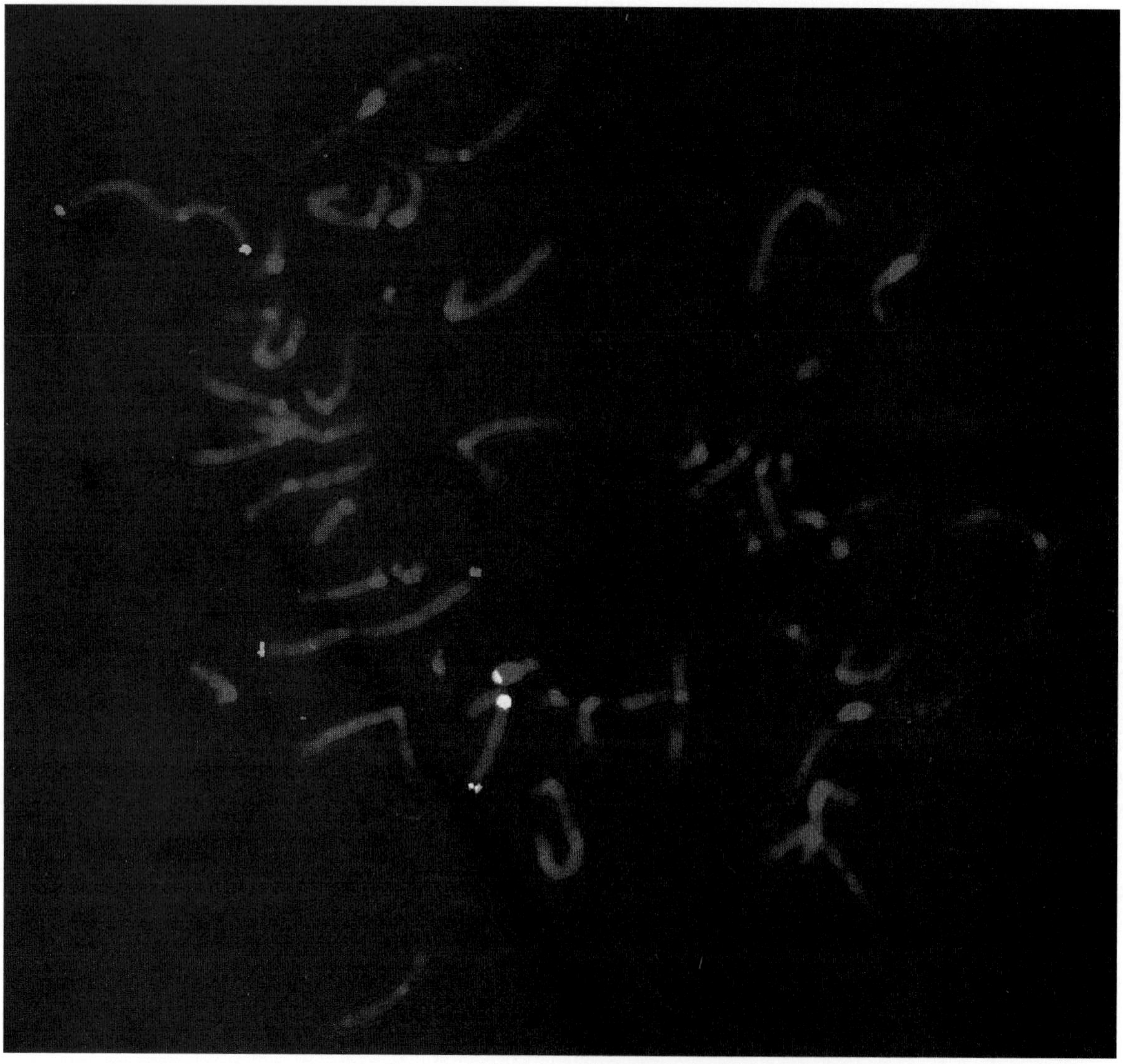

Fig. 25.18. Human metaphase showing telomeric probes for chromosome 2p (Spectrum Green), 2q (Spectrum Orange) and pairing regions of Xq and Yq (Spectrum Green + Spectrum Orange). X alpha centromeric probe (Spectrum Aqua) identifies the X centromere. (See Plate 25.18.)

hybridized to the same chromosome can be resolved only if they are more than 2 to 3 megabases apart. Because the chromosomes are 10 times more extended in interphase nuclei, the resolution at interphase is much better, and two cosmids more than 50 kb apart can usually be distinguished from one another (Trask, 1991). The order of several closely linked cosmids may be determined at interphase, provided they are more than 50 kb and less than 1 megabase apart (Van Den Engh et al., 1992). The latter restriction is due to the tendency of a chromosome to coil back on itself and also because the chromosome fiber forms loops radiating in all directions from the central chromosome scaffold. Various techniques have now been developed that release the chromosome fiber from its associated protein within the chromosome scaffold (Fidlerova et al., 1994; Parra and Windle, 1993; Wiegant et al., 1992). This permits DNA sequences to be hybridized directly onto extended chromosome fibers fixed on a microscope slide and analyzed by FISH (Fig. 25.19). The resolution of this technique is astonishing; sequences less than 5 kb apart can be separated readily, and distances down to 1 kb have been claimed (van Ommen et al., 1995).

Decondensation of chromatin by detergent and salt or alkaline solutions results in the release of loops of chromatin fibers of more than 200 μm in length from nuclei in air-dried fixed preparations. Typically, the chromatin loops out from the nucleus and forms a halo of DNA fibers

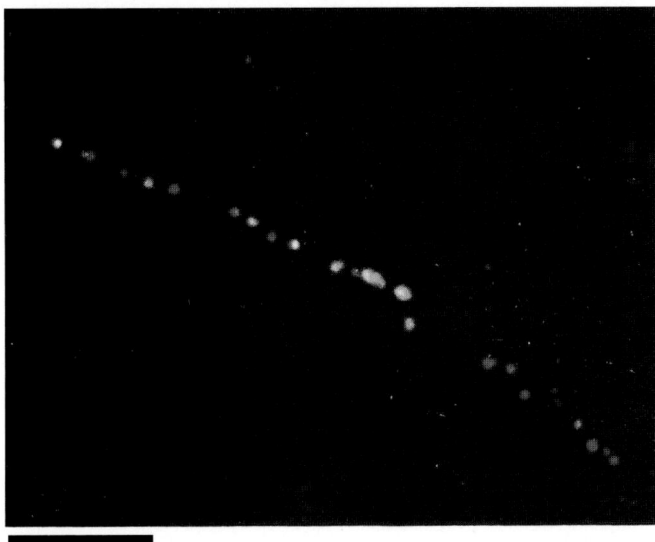

10μm

Fig. 25.19. Fiber-FISH. Decondensation of chromatin by alkali treatment of fixed nuclei and hybridization of closely linked labeled cosmid clones. Three cosmids from the HLA region labeled with FITC, Texas Red, and a 50:50 mixture of FITC and Texas Red, respectively. Each cosmid measures 35 kb and there is a 5 to 10 Kb gap between the red and green cosmids. (See Plate 25.19.)

around the nucleus. Where the loops are broken, the fibers are more extended and are seen as long thin filaments that radiate away from the nucleus. Fibers up to 10 megabases long have been achieved by using agarose-embedded cells treated with proteinase K and ribonuclease. The agarose is then melted and spread onto poly-l-lysine-coated microscope slides (Heiskanen et al., 1994). This method seems more robust than others used for fiber-FISH.

The analysis of extended DNA fibers by FISH has application both in the mapping and ordering of contiguous DNA sequences and, more recently, in the diagnosis of single gene aberrations using cosmid probes. One important example has been in the detection of carriers of intragenic gene deletions in X-linked Duchenne muscular dystrophy (Florijn et al., 1995). In this and similar situations, carrier detection by PCR techniques can be difficult, and the fiber-FISH method shows considerable promise.

FISH NOMENCLATURE

The Standing Committee for the ISCN has developed nomenclature to describe investigations and abnormalities detected by DNA probes. The observed chromosome banding is described by the standard nomenclature. This is followed by a period (.) and the abbreviation "ish" which precedes the description of the in situ hybridization findings. The abnormality identified by ish is described starting with the abbreviation for the type of abnormality followed, in separate parenthesis, by the chromosome(s), break point(s), and the loci for which probes were used, designated according to the Genome Data Base (GDB) and ordered from pter to qter. If no GDB locus is available, the name of the probe can be given instead. Capital letters are used for the locus, and + or − given immediately afterward indicates whether the locus has been identified as being present or absent, respectively. Thus, ish del (22) (q11.2q11.2) (D22S75−) indicates a deletion in the DiGeorge chromosome region, and ish dup (17) (p11.2p11.2) (CMT1A++) indicates a duplication at the Charcot-Marie-Tooth locus. If no abnormality is detected, the chromosomal location follows "ish" and the usual two copies of the probe are confirmed e.g. ish 22q11.2 (D22S75×2). The origin of a cryptic balanced translocation identified by forward painting is given as ish t(4: 11) (p16.3;p15) (wcp11+;wcp4+), where wcp is whole chromosome paint. Similarly, the origin of an extra marker chromosome revealed by reverse painting is given as 47, XY, +mar.rev ish der (18)t(12;18) (p13.3;p11.2). The ish nomenclature (Table 25.4) includes symbols appropriate for interphase FISH (nuc ish) and fiber-FISH (fib ish).

Table 25.4. Symbols and Abbreviations to Describe Chromosome Abnormalities Identified by In Situ Hybridization (ish)

Symbol	Definition
•	Full stop (period) separates conventional from ish observations
–	Absent from a given chromosome
+	Present in a given chromosome
+ +	Duplicated in a given chromosome
×	Multiplication sign—precedes the number of signals seen
;	Semicolon—separates probes on different derivative chromosomes
amp	Amplified signal
con	Adjacent signals
dim	Diminished signal intensity
enh	Enhanced signal intensity
fib ish	ISH using fiber DNA
fish	Fluorescence in situ hybridization
ish	Given without a prefix, applies to chromosomes
mv	Moved signal (from original location)
nuc ish	Interphase ISH
pcp	Parial chromosome paint
rev ish	Reverse painting, including comparative genomic hybridization
sep	Signals are separate
sp	Split signal
st	Stationary signal
wcp	Whole-chromosome paint

COMPARATIVE GENOMIC HYBRIDIZATION

An ingenious FISH technique has been developed for the cytogenetic analysis of tumor samples that is capable of identifying DNA amplifications of over 5 to 10 megabases, deletions in the order of 10 to 20 megabases, and the threefold to fivefold amplification of oncogenes in a single sample of tumor material (Kallionemi et al., 1992). The method, comparative genomic hybridization (CGH), is a development of reverse painting in which fluorescein-labeled total tumor DNA (green) and Texas red-labeled normal genomic reference DNA (red) are mixed and hybridized to normal metaphases. The relative amounts of tumor and normal DNA that anneal to a particular chromosome region depend on the number of copies of DNA complementary to that region in the test sample. If the test sample contains relatively more of a particular DNA than the reference sample, this will be revealed by an increased green/red fluorescence ratio in the complementary region; similarly, chromosomal deletion in the test sample is revealed by a decreased green/red fluo-

rescence ratio (Fig. 25.20). The method requires digital fluorescence microscopy in which the relative amounts of green and red fluorescence is measured along the length of the chromosome.

In addition to confirming the results of conventional chromosome analysis in neoplastic conditions, the CGH technique has already revealed many previously undetected aberrations consistently associated with specific tumours. Because the loss of tumor suppressor gene loci are frequently associated with deletion of large chromosome regions, it is not possible to map them precisely by CGH; it is possible only to define the smallest region within which to use gene cloning methods. CGH may have application in the detection of constitutional aneuploidy or in the origin of extra marker chromosomes, especially if it is possible to apply the method to single cell analysis as, for example, in preimplantation diagnosis.

CROSS-SPECIES CHROMOSOME PAINTING

The conservation of the genetic information during evolution is evident from comparative genetic mapping studies. The mammalian X chromosome is a particularly striking example because it contains virtually all the same transcribed genes in every mammalian species. Other genetic linkage groups show similar conservation between species indicating that during evolution whole groups of genes have been transmitted together over millions of years. In

Fig. 25.20. Comparative genomic hybridization (CGH) analysis of a small cell lung carcinoma (SCLC). (A) Hybridization of control DNA labeled with digoxigenin and visualized with TRITC (red) to a normal male metaphase. (B) The same metaphase hybridized with tumor DNA labeled with biotin and visualized with FITC (green). The images in (A) and (B) are merged in (C) and given false colors by image analysis to reveal areas of gain (green) and loss (red) of tumor DNA when the ratios of tumor DNA:control DNA are more than 1.5 and less than 0.5, respectively. Ratios between 0.5 and 1.5 are indicated in blue. (D) is the karyotype of this metaphase showing that the homologues of each chromosome have a consistent pattern. Fluorescence ratio along each chromosome are generated as illustrated in (E). In (F) ratios profiles for each chromosome have been determined derived from five metaphases of the same SCLC. The three vertical lines to the right of each chromosome idogram represent fluorescence ratios of 0.5, 1, and 1.5 (*from left to right*) between tumor and control DNA. The ratio profile (curve) represents the mean value of the five metaphases. The gray-shaded boxes represent chromosomal regions rich in heterochromatin that could not be interpreted due to abundance of repetitive DNA. All changes visible in (C) are confirmed by mean ration profile measurements. Note especially the loss of 3p, 5q, 10q, 13q, and 17p and the amplification of 3q, 5p, and 19q that are commonly observed in SCLC. (From Ried T, Peteersen I, Holtgrave-Grez H (1994) Mapping of multiple DNA gains and loses in primary small cell lung carcinomas by comparative genomic hybridization. Cancer Res 54:1801–1806, with permission. Courtesy of Dr. Thomas Reid). (See Plate 25.20.)

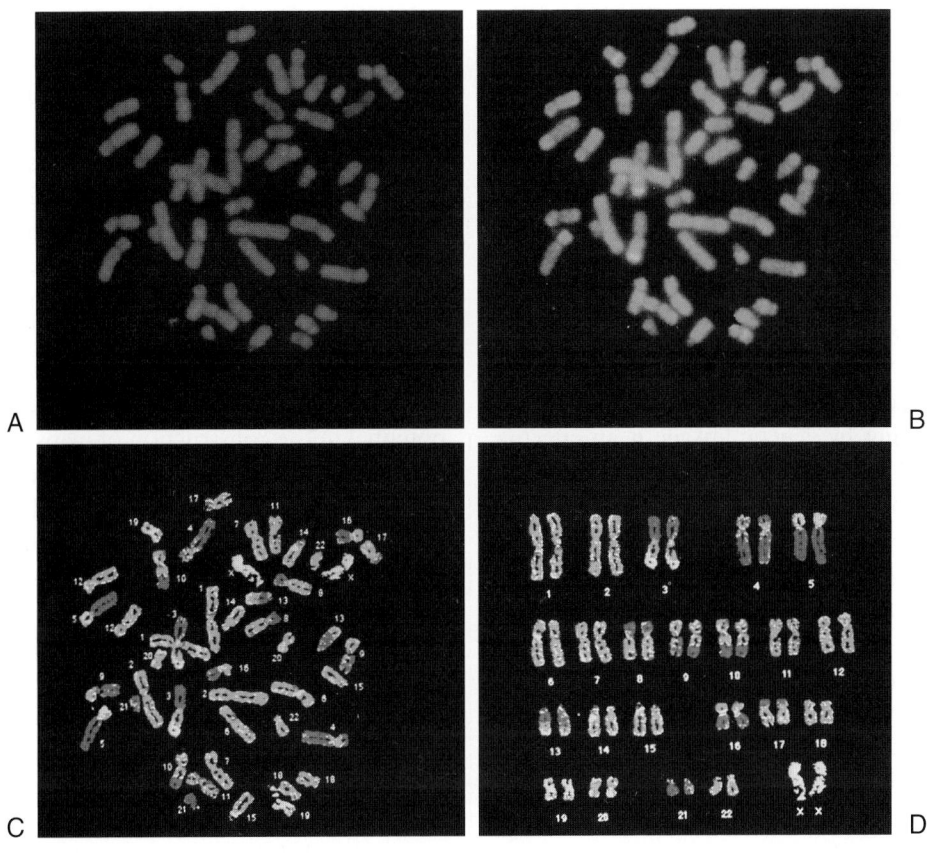

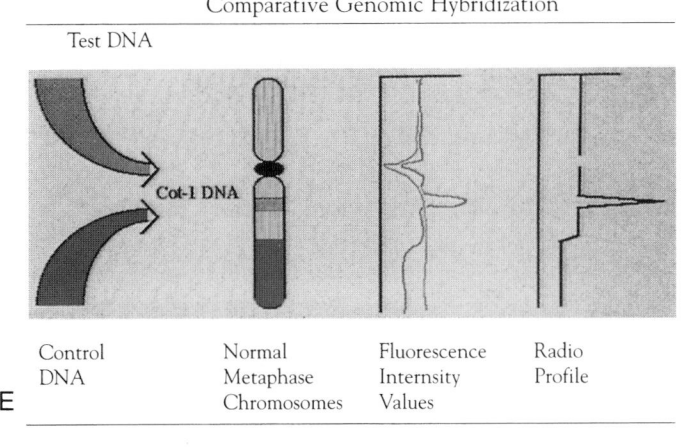

Comparative Genomic Hybridization

Test DNA

Control
DNA

Normal
Metaphase
Chromosomes

Fluorescence
Internsity
Values

Radio
Profile

E

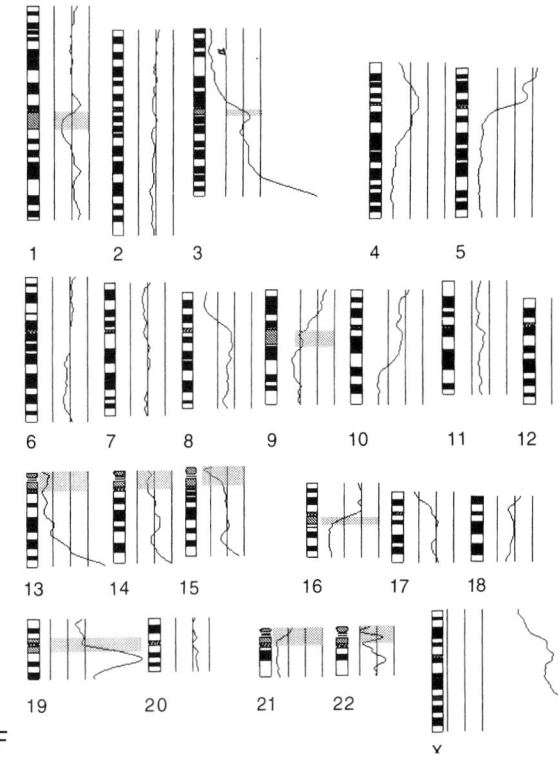

F

closely related species, these genetic linkage groups tend to be more extensive than in more distantly related species and represent large regions of individual chromosomes even whole chromosomes in some instances. Differences between species clearly are due to the occurrence of chromosomal rearrangements that have become fixed within populations as the result of a variety of factors, beyond the scope of this chapter, including migration and founder effect. Repetitive sequences diverge more rapidly than transcribed sequences, and, in fact, this divergence is invariably the most striking genetic difference between two closely related species. It is not known if this plays a role in speciation.

Comparative mapping by genetic linkage is an effective but laborious method for studying the evolution of karyotypes. The introduction of molecular cytogenetic methods in recent years now offers a new procedure for the rapid analysis of chromosome homology between species, which is leading to the construction of genetic maps of previously unmapped species and the identification of homologies with the human chromosome map (Wienberg et al., 1992). The current technique involves taking a chromosome-specific paint from one species and mapping the regions of homology by FISH in the other species. This is another application of reverse painting, which depends on the ability to sort chromosomes by FACS and to make chromosome-specific paints by the DOP-PCR method. Suppression by unlabeled competitor DNA is not always necessary in these experi-

ments, because the repetitive DNA may be sufficiently diverged between the two species to prevent cross-hybridization. Chromosome-specific paint probes are now available for a number of species, including the mouse (Rabbitts et al., 1995). Fig. 25.21A shows the flow karyotype of a C3H mouse, and Fig. 25.21B shows a chromosome-specific paint from mouse chromosome 11 that has been hybridized to a human metaphase Fig. 25.21C. Homology is demonstrated to human chromosome 17 and to parts of human chromosome 2, 5, 7, and 22, consistent with information obtained by comparative mapping studies.

Interspecies chromosome painting has considerable potential in the construction of maps of unmapped species, based on homologies between species with detailed maps (such as mouse and human). It also has relevance for medical genetics, in that information useful for the positional cloning of disease and other genes can be obtained from species in which disease traits are clearly familial. The many breeds of dogs and the genetic traits and disorders associated with particular breeds provide a case in point. The 39 pairs of dog chromosomes have now been sorted, and chromosome-specific paints are available which have led to a detailed description of the dog map including the assignment of genetic linkage and radiation hybrid groups to all the dog chromosomes (Sargan et al., 2000). A similar approach is in progress for many other species (Fig. 25.22).

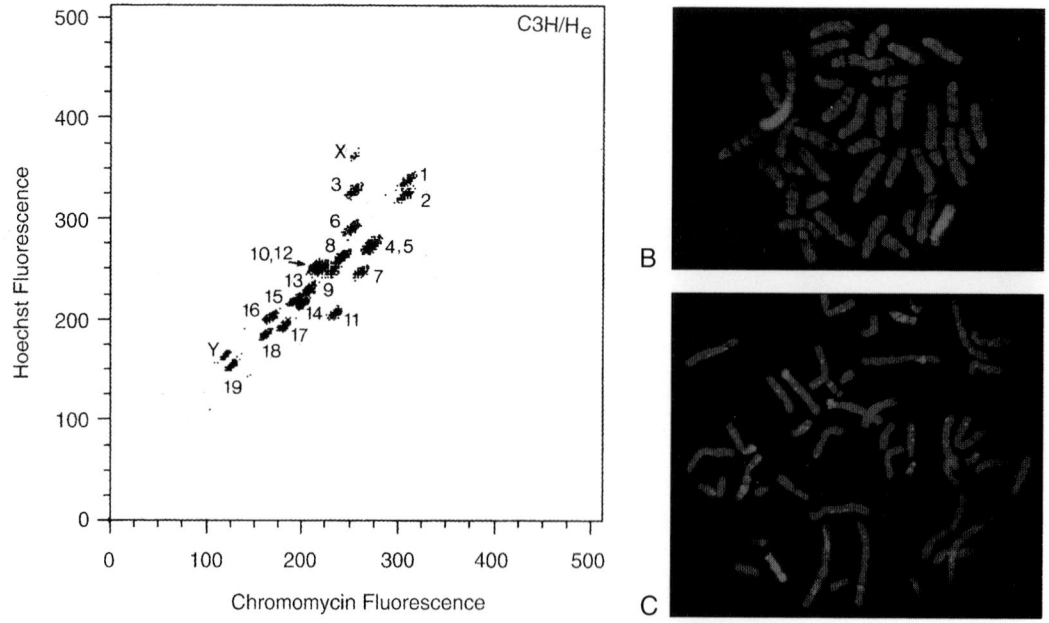

Fig. 25.21. Cross species chromosome painting. (A) Flow karyotype of male C3H/He mouse showing separation of most of the autosomes and the sex chromosomes. (B) Mouse chromosome specific paint probe (CAMBIO Ltd., Cambridge, England) from chromosome 11 and hybridized to male mouse metaphase. (C) Mouse chromosome 11 paint hybridized to male human metaphase showing cross-species homology of conserved DNA sequences on chromosomes 17, 2p, distal 5q, 7q, and 22q. (See Plate 25.21.)

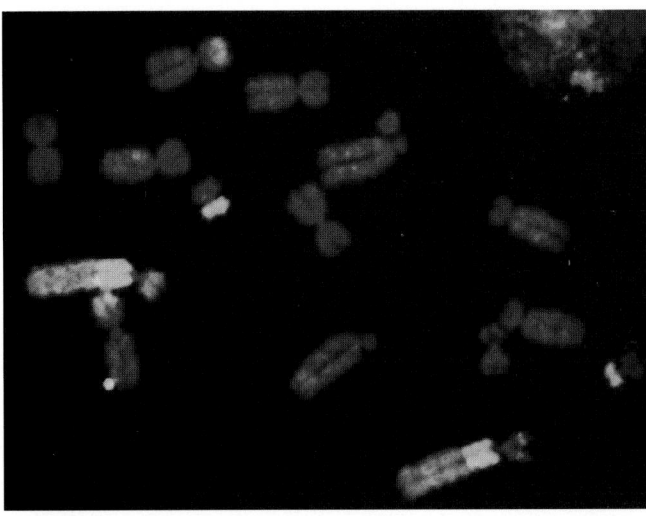

Fig. 25.22. Cross-species chromosome painting. Chromosomes 4 (red), 7 (green), and 9 (yellow) from the brush-tailed possum hybridized to chromosomes 1, 3, and 7 of the tammar wallaby. (From Rens et al, 1999, with permission.) (See Plate 25.22.)

Annex: some staining methods used in cytogenetic analysis

Protocol for Giemsa Solid Staining

Reagents
  Giemsa stain
  pH 6.8 buffer

Method
- Add 5 ml of Giemsa stain to 45 ml of buffer in a staining jar.

1. Place slides in stain for five minutes.
2. Rinse slides in distilled water.
3. Dry, mount, and examine.

Protocol for Trypsin Banding

Reagents
  Trypsin solution (Difco Bacto-trypsin reconstituted with 10 ml distilled water)
  Leishman stain
  Phosphate-buffered saline (PBS)
  Hank's balanced salt solution (2X)
  Buffer, pH 6.8
  Saline solution (0.85% NaCl)

Method
Age slides at either 60°C overnight or at 95°C for 90 minutes.
- Place Hank's balanced salt solution (2X) in a staining jar.
- Place 1 ml trypsin in 50 ml saline in a staining jar.

- Place Leishman stain (10 ml + 40 ml pH 6.8 buffer) in a staining jar.

1. Place slides in Hank's solution for five minutes.
2. Rinse slides in distilled water.
3. Place slides in trypsin solution for optimum time (5–20 seconds).
4. Rinse slides in saline solution.
5. Stain slides in Leishman stain for three to five minutes.
6. Rinse slides in distilled water.
7. Dry, mount, and examine.

Protocol for Reverse Banding

Reagents
  Acridine orange
  Phosphate buffer, pH 6.5

Method
- Place 50 ml of pH 6.5 phosphate buffer in a staining jar.
- Place 0.01% acridine orange solution in pH 6.5 phosphate buffer in a staining jar.

1. Incubate slides in phosphate buffer at 85°C for five to 10 minutes.
2. Place slides in acridine orange solution at room temperature for five minutes.
3. Rinse slides in pH 6.5 phosphate buffer at room temperature.
4. Mount in buffer and examine using fluorescence microscopy and appropriate excitation and barrier filters.

Protocol for Replication Banding

Reagents
  Bromodeoxyuridine
  Hoechst 33258 stain
  Giemsa stain
  Phosphate buffer, pH 6.8

Method

1. Establish standard lymphocyte cultures.
2. Six hours before harvest, add BrdU to a final concentration of 1×10^{-4}M.
3. Harvest according to standard protocol.
4. Place slides in Hoechst 33258 stain (1 μg/ml in pH 6.8 buffer) under a mercury vapor lamp for 30 minutes.
5. Rinse slides well in distilled water.
6. Place slides in 5% Giemsa stain in pH 6.8 buffer for three to five minutes.
7. Rinse slides well in distilled water.
8. Dry, mount, and examine.

Protocol for Q-Banding

Reagents

Quinacrine dihydrochloride
Methanol

Method

● Prepare fresh stain (0.25 g quinacrine dihydrochloride dissolved in 5 ml methanol + 50 ml distilled water) in a staining jar.

1. Place slides in stain for three to five minutes.
2. Rinse slides well in distilled water.
3. Mount in distilled water, and examine using fluorescence microscopy and appropriate excitation and barrier filters.

Protocol for DAPI-DA Staining

Reagents

Distamycin A (DA)
DAPI
MacIlvaine's buffer (pH 7)

Method

● Prepare a fresh solution of DA by dissolving 2 mg in 10 ml of MacIlvaine's buffer.
● Prepare stock solution of DAPI by dissolving 1 mg in 5 ml of distilled water, store at −20°C.
● Prepare working solution of DAPI by diluting 0.1 ml in 20 ml of MacIlvaine's buffer.

1. Place the slide in a petri dish, cover with DA solution, add a coverslip, and leave at room temperature for 30 minutes.
2. Take the slide out of the petri dish, remove the coverslip, and rinse with buffer.
3. Place the slide in a clean petri dish, flood it with DAPI working solution, add a coverslip, and leave it for 30 minutes in the dark.
4. Take the slide out of the petri dish, remove the coverslip, and rinse it with buffer.
5. Mount the slide in buffer, and examine it using fluorescence microscopy and appropriate excitation and barrier filters.

An almost identical banding pattern can be achieved with Hoechst 33258 and methyl green banding.

Protocol for C-Banding

Reagents

Giemsa stain
Hydrochloric acid
Barium hydroxide
Saline sodium citrate (SSC)
Buffer, pH 6.8

Method

● Place distilled water in four staining jars.
● Place Leishman stain (10 ml + 40 ml pH 6.8 buffer) in a staining jar.

1. Pretreat slides in 0.2 M hydrochloric acid for two to five minutes at room temperature.
2. Rinse slides well in distilled water.
3. Incubate slides in 5% barium hydroxide at 60°C for two to five minutes.
4. Rinse slides well in distilled water.
5. Incubate slides in 2X SSC at 60°C for two to five minutes.
6. Rinse slides well in distilled water.
7. Stain slides in Leishman stain for three to five minutes.
8. Rinse slides in distilled water.
9. Dry, mount, and examine.

Protocol for Ag-NOR Banding

Reagents

Leishman stain
Silver nitrate solution (50%)
Gelatin solution
Formic acid

Method

● Place gelatin solution (2 g gelatin in 99 ml of water, heat until dissolved, then add 1 ml of formic acid).
● Prepare 50% $AgNO_3$ in distilled water.
● Place Leishman stain (10 ml + 40 ml pH 6.8 buffer) in a staining jar.

1. Place four drops of $AgNO_3$ solution onto the slide, add one drop of gelatin solution, and cover with a coverslip.
2. Incubate the slide at 60°C for three minutes.
3. Remove the coverslip, and rinse it well in distilled water.
4. Place the slide in Leishman stain for two minutes.
5. Rinse the slide well in distilled water.
6. Dry, mount, and examine.

Acknowledgments

We are grateful to Patricia O'Brien, Fentang Yang, Willem Rens and colleagues from the Human Molecular Cytogenetics Group at the Centre for Veterinary Science and Zoe Broadfield, Debbie Morgan, Lionel Willatt and colleagues from the East Anglian Regional Cytogenetics Department for help with preparing the illustrations and for many helpful discussions.

REFERENCES

Arnold T (1879) Beobachtungen über Kerntheilungen in den Zellen der Geschwülste. Virchows Arch 78:279–301

Bailey DMD, Carter NP, de Vos D et al. (1993) Coincidence painting: A rapid method for cloning region specific DNA sequences. Nucleic Acids Res 21:5117–5123

Bauman JGJ, Weigant J, van Duijn P (1983) The development using poly (Hg-U) in a model system, of a new method to visualise hybridisation in fluorescence microscopy. J Histochem Cytochem 31:571–578

Boveri T (1914) Zür Frage der Entstehung maligner Tumoren. Jena, Verlag von Gustav Fischer (Translation by Boveri M (1929) The Origin of Malignant Tumours.) Williams & Wilkins, Baltimore

Carter NP, Ferguson-Smith MA, Perryman MT et al. (1992) Reverse chromosome painting: A method for the rapid analysis of aberrant chromosomes in clinical cytogenetics. J Med Genet 29:299–307

Caspersson T, Zech L, Johansson C (1970) Differential banding of alkylating fluorochromes in human chromosomes. Exp Cell Res 60:315–319

Connor JM, Ferguson-Smith MA (1993) Essential Medical Genetics., 4th edn. Blackwell Scientific, Oxford, England, pp. 56, 68.

Dauwerse JG, Wiegant J, Raap AK et al. (1992) Multiple colours by fluorescence in situ hybridisation using ratio labelled DNA probes create a molecular karyotype. Hum Molec Genet 1:593–598

de Winiwarter H (1912) Études sur la spermatogenèse humaine. Arch Biol (Liège) 27:91–189

Divane A, Carter NP, Spathas DH, Ferguson-Smith MA (1994) Rapid prenatal diagnosis of aneuploidy from uncultured amniotic fluid cells using five-colour fluorescence in situ hybridization. Prenat Diag 14;1061–1069

Fidlerova H, Senger G, Kost M et al. (1994) Two simple processes for releasing chromatin from routinely fixed cells for fluorescence in situ hybridisation. Cytogenet Cell Genet 65:203–205

Flemming W (1898) Ueber die Chromosomenzahl beim Menshen. Anatomischer Anzeiger 14:171–174

Florijn RJ, Blonden LAJ, Vrolijk J et al. (1995) High resolution DNA fibre-FISH genomic DNA mapping and colour bar coding of large genes. Hum Molec Genet 4:831–836

Ford CE, Hamerton JL (1956) The chromosomes of man. Nature 178:1020

Ford CE, Jacobs PA, Lajtha LG (1958) Human somatic chromosomes. Nature 181:1565–1568

Ford CE, Jones KW, Polani PE et al. (1959) A sex-chromosome anomaly in a case of gonadal dysgenesis (Turner's syndrome). Lancet 1:711–713

Garson JA, van den Berghe J, Kemshead JT (1987) Novel non-isotopic in situ hybridisation techniques detects small (1 kb) unique sequences in routinely banded human chromosomes: fine mapping of N-myc and B-NGF genes. Nucleic Acids Res 15:4761–4770

Gerhard DS, Kawasaki ES, Bancroft FC, Szabo P (1981) Localisation of a unique gene by direct hybridisation in situ. Proc Natl Acad Sci USA 78:3755–3759

Gray JW, Carrano AV, Steinmetz LL et al. (1975) Chromosome measurement and sorting by flow systems. Proc Natl Acad Sci USA 72:1231–1234

Hansemann D (1891) Über pathologische Mitosen. Virchows Arch 123:356

Harper ME, Saunders GF (1981) Localisation of single copy DNA sequences on G banded human chromosomes by in situ hybridisation. Chromosoma 83:431–439

Heiles HBJ, Genersch E, Kessler C et al. (1988) In situ hybridisation with digoxigenin-labelled DNA of papilloma viruses (HPV16/18) in HeLa and SiHa cells. Biotechniques 6:978–981

Heiskanen M, Karhu R, Hellster E (1994) High resolution mapping using fluorescence in situ hybridisation to extended DNA fibres prepared from agarose-embedded cells. Biotechniques 17:928–933

Henderson AS, Warburton D, Atwood KC (1972) Location of rDNA in the human chromosome complement. Proc Natl Acad Sci USA 69:3394–3398

Hsu TC (1952) Mammalian chromosomes in vitro. I. The karyotype of man. J Hered 43:167–172

ISCN (1985) An international system for human cytogenetics nomenclature. In Harnden DG, Klinger HP (eds). Published in Collaboration with Cytogenetics and Cell Genetics. Karger, Basel.

ISCN (1995) An international system for human cytogenetics nomenclature, 1995. In Mitelman F (ed) Published in Collaboration with Cytogenetics and Cell Genetics, S. Karger Inc., Farmington, USA.

Jacobs PA, Strong JA (1959) A case of human intersexuality having a possible XXY sex determining mechanism. Nature 183:302

Jones KW, Corneo G (1971) Location of satellite and homogeneous DNA sequences in human chromosomes. Nature 233:268

Kallioniemi A, Kallioniemi OP, Sudar D et al. (1992) Comparative genomic hybridisation for molecular cytogenetic analysis of solid tumours. Science 258:818–821

Koller PC (1937) The genetical and mechanical properties of sex chromosomes. III. Man. Proc Soc Edinburgh B 57:194–214

Landegent JE, Jansen in de Wal N, Baan RA (1984) 2-acetylaminofluorene-modified probes for the indirect hybridocytochemical detection of specific nucleic acid sequences. Exp Cell Res 153:61–72

Landegent JE, Jansen in de Wal N, Ploem JS et al. (1985) Sensitive detection of hybridocytochemical results by means of reflection contrast microscopy. J Histochem Cytochem 33:1241–1246

Langer PR, Waldrop AA, Ward DC (1981) Enzymatic synthesis of biotin labelled polynucleotides: novel nucleic acid affinity probes. Proc Natl Acad Sci USA 78:6633–6637

Lejeune J, Gautier M, Turpin R (1959) Les chromosomes somatique des enfants mongoliens. Comptes Rendus des Academy des Science, Paris 248:1721

Lengauer C, Riethman H, Cremer T (1990) Painting of human chromosomes with probes generated from hybrid cell lines by PCR with Alu and L1 primers. Hum Genet 86:1–6

Lengauer C, Speicher MR, Popp S et al. (1993) Chromosomal bar codes produced by multicolour fluorescence in situ hybridisation with multiple YAC clones and whole chromosome painting probes. Hum Molec Genet 2:505–512

Lichter P, Cremer T, Borden J et al. (1988) Delineation of individual human chromosomes in metaphase and interphase cells by in situ suppression hybridisation using recombinant DNA libraries. Hum Genet 80:224–234

Lichter P, Ledbetter S, Ledbetter D, Ward DC (1990) Fluorescence in situ hybridization with Alu and L1 polymerase chain reaction probes for rapid characterization of human chromosomes in hybrid cell lines. Proc Natl Acad Sci USA 87:6634–6638

Makino S, Nishimura I (1952) Water pre-treatment squash technique. Stain Technol 27:1–7

Malcolm S, Barton P, Murphy CS, Ferguson-Smith MA (1981) Chromosomal localisation of a single copy gene by in situ hybridisation: Human β-globin genes on the short arm of chromosome 11. Ann Human Genet 45:135–141

Meltzer PS, Guan XY, Burgess A, Trent JM (1992) Rapid generation of region specific probes by chromosome microdissection and their application. Nature Genet 1:24–28

Mittwoch U (1952) The chromosome complement in a mongolian imbecile. Ann Eugenics, Cambridge 17:37

Morimoto H, Monden T, Shimano T et al. (1987) Methods in laboratory investigation: Use of sulphonated probes for in situ detection of amylase in RNA in formalin-fixed paraffin sections of human pancreas and submaxillary gland. Lab Invest 57:734–741

Moorehead PS, Nowell PC, Mellman WJ et al. (1960) Chromosome preparations of leukocytes cultured from human peripheral blood. Exp Cell Res 20:613–616

Moses MJ, Counce SJ, Paulson DF (1975) Synaptonemal complex complement of man in spreads of spermatocytes, with details of the sex chromosome pair. Science 187:363–365

Nederlof PM, Van der Flier S, Wiegant J et al. (1990) Multiple fluorescence in situ hybridisation. Cytometry 11:126–131

Ning et al. (1996) A complete set of telomeric probes and their clinical applications. Nature Genetics 14:86–89

Nowell PC, Hungerford DA (1960) A minute chromosome in human chronic granulocytic leukemia. Science 132:1497

Painter TS (1921) The Y chromosome in mammals. Science 53:503

Painter TS (1923) Studies in mammalian spermatogenesis. II. The spermatogenesis in man. J Exp Zool 37:291

Pardue ML, Gall JG (1970) Chromosomal localisation of mouse satelitte DNA. Science 168:1356–1358

Pardue ML, Gerbie SA, Eckhardt RA, Gall JG (1970) Cytological localisation of DNA complementary to ribosomal RNA in polytene chromosomes in Diptera. Chromosoma 29:268–269

Parra I, Windle B (1993) High resolution visual mapping of stretched DNA by fluorescent hybridisation. Nature Genet 5:17–21

Polani PE, Hunter WF, Lennox B (1954) Chromosomal sex in Turner's syndrome with coarctation of the aorta. Lancet 2:120

Rabbitts P, Impey H, Heppel-Parton A et al. (1995) Chromosome specific paints from a high resolution flow karyotype of the mouse. Nature Genet 9:369–375

Rens W, O'Brien PCM, Yang F, Graves JAM, Ferguson-Smith MA (1999) Karyotype relationships between four distantly related marsupials. Chromosome Res 7:461–474

Ried T, Baldini A, Rand TC, Ward DC (1992) Simultaneous visualization of seven different DNA probes by in situ hybridization using combinatorial fluorescence and digital imaging microscopy. Proc Natl Acad Sci USA 89:1388–1392

Ried T, Peteersen I, Holtgrave-Grez H (1994) Mapping of multiple DNA gains and losses in primary small cell lung carcinomas by comparative genomic hybridization. Cancer Res 54:1801–1806

Saadalla N, Hulten M (1986) EM investigations of surface spread synaptonemal complexes in a human male carrier of a pericentric inversion inv(13) (p12q14): The role of heterosynapsis for spermatocyte survival. Ann Hum Genet 50:369–383

Sargan DR, Yang F, Squire M, Milne BS, O'Brien PMC, Ferguson-Smith MA (2000) Use of flow-sorted canine chromosomes in the assignment of canine linkage, radiation hybrid, and syntenic groups to chromosomes: Refinement and verification of the comparative map for dog and human. Genomics 69:182–195

Reid T, Peteersen I, Holtgrave-Grez H (1994) mapping of multiple DNA gains and loses in primary small cell lung carcinomas by comparative genomic hybridization. Cancer Res 54:1801–1806

Schröck E, du Mahoir S, Veldman T et al. (1996) Multicolour spectral karyotyping of human chromosomes. Science 273:494–497

Seibl R, Hoeltke H-J, Rüger R et al. (1990) Non-radioactive labeling and detection of nucleic acids. III. Aplication of the digoxigenin-system. Biol Chem Hoppe-Seyler 371:939–951

Severinghaus AE (1942) Sex chromosomes in a human intersex. Am J Anat 70:73–92

Speicher MR, Ballard SG, Ward DC (1996) Karyotyping human chromosomes by combinatorial multi-color FISH. Nature Genet 12:368–375

Telenius H, Pelmear AH, Tunnacliffe A et al. (1992) Cytogenetic analysis by chromosome painting using DOP-PCR amplified flow-sorted chromosomes. Genes Chromosomes Cancer 4:257–263

Tjio JH, Levan A (1956) The chromosome number of man. Hereditas 42:1–6

Trask BJ (1991) Fluorescence in situ hybridisation: applications in cytogenetics and gene mapping. Trends Genet 7:149–154

Van Den Engh G, Sachs R, Trask BJ (1992) Estimating genomic distance from DNA sequence location in cell nuclei by a random walk model. Science 257:1410–1412

Van Ommen GJB, Breuning MH, Rapp AK (1995) FISH in genome research and molecular diagnostics, Curr Opin Genet Dev 5:304–308

Verma RS, Babu A (1989) Human Chromosomes: Manual of Basic Techniques. Pergamon Press, NY

Waardenburg PJ (1932) Das menschliche Auge und seine Erbanlagen. Martinus Nijhoff, The Hague,p. 47.

Wiegant J, Kalle W, Mullenders L et al. (1992) High resolution in situ hybridisation using DNA halo preparations. Hum Molec Genet 1:587–591

Wienberg J, Stanyon R, Jauch A, Cremer T (1992) Homologies in human and Macaca fuscata chromosomes revealed by in situ suppression hybridisation with chromosome specific DNA libraries. Chromosoma 101:265–270

Diagnostic molecular genetics

26

Wayne W. Grody
David B. Seligson
Milhan Telatar

Introduction

There can be no question that we are in the midst of a revolution in clinical medicine, as profound in its own way as the early revelations of human anatomy and physiology and the germ theory of disease. The twenty-first century has already been christened the age of molecular medicine—the molecule in question being, of course, DNA. Molecular biology, which came to dominate basic life sciences research over the second half of the twentieth century, has now found inroads into clinical medicine as well. The development of new technologies, such as the polymerase chain reaction (PCR) and automated DNA sequencing, and the extraordinary productivity of the Human Genome Project in elucidating medically relevant targets for these techniques, have firmly ensconced patient DNA as a powerful new "analyte" in the clinical laboratory and as a valid substrate for therapeutic manipulation in the clinic.

While all areas of medicine have been impacted by these developments, it is medical genetics, as the specialty most directly attuned to the human genome, that is the first discipline to be entirely transformed by them. And if the promise of gene therapy remains somewhat elusive, such is not the case for gene diagnostics. In no other sector of medical practice does at least the question, if not always the actual execution, of molecular testing arise with virtually every patient seen. Not only is medical genetics by definition concerned with inherited alterations in the patient's genome which are detectable in this way, but much of its attention is directed at ascertaining recessive carrier states, fetal conditions which will not be expressed until after birth, and predisposition to adult-onset disorders before

they are symptomatic; such diagnoses often exhibit no other evidence of their presence than at the DNA level. For these reasons, medical geneticists and genetic counselors, as a group, tend to be significantly more facile and familiar with the applications and interpretation of molecular genetic tests than other clinicians. Nevertheless, keeping up with a field as rapidly evolving as this one, in which new techniques and disease genes (not to mention their associated ethical and societal dilemmas) are reported every week, can be a challenge for even the most dedicated specialist. That is why close two-way communication between the clinic and the laboratory is so essential, more so in medical genetics practice than in any other.

Indications for molecular genetic testing

Molecular genetics has a unique range of indications, most of which are quite different from the uses of traditional clinical laboratory testing and even molecular biologic testing in other disease classes (e.g., infectious disease, cancer). Most notably, as mentioned above, these procedures are often performed on healthy people who have no other signs or symptoms of the disease being tested. And even if they are symptomatic, the assay is not directed at a discrete lesion, as would be the case with a DNA test for an infection or a tumor. Since genetic disorders reflect heritable mutations in the germline, the test in most cases can be performed on any accessible body fluid or tissue. The most common specimen is whole blood, though saliva, buccal swab, dried blood spots, urine, etc. can be used, while amniocytes or chorionic villus samples are collected for prenatal diagnosis.

723

The technical approaches as well as the psychosocial and ethical implications of molecular genetic tests may vary substantially depending upon the reason for testing. The major indications are considered individually below.

DIAGNOSTIC TESTING

Most straightforward and least foreign to other areas of laboratory medicine are diagnostic molecular genetic tests performed on symptomatic patients. These are most often performed for diagnostic confirmation of a clinical impression, though they may also assist in differential diagnosis. In the latter regard, however, it should be kept in mind that gene-based tests are specific for the disease gene being tested, and even closely related disorders will not be detected when testing for a single one (e.g., the DNA test for spinocerebellar ataxia type 1 will not detect the mutations of spinocerebellar ataxia type 2). And while diagnostic tests do not typically carry the heavy ethical concerns of predictive tests, the uniqueness of genetic disease comes into play here as well, such that a positive test in the proband places other blood relatives at risk.

NEWBORN SCREENING

Newborn screening is in one sense a very early form of diagnostic testing, except that it is performed on large populations of infants who are not (yet) symptomatic, though the affected ones may well exhibit signs of the disease, biochemical or otherwise. The goal, of course, is to identify affected babies early in life so that treatment (dietary or pharmaceutical) can be initiated before irreversible damage occurs. Unfortunately, most of the classic autosomal recessive disorders screened in this setting, such as phenylketonuria and galactosemia, have so many causative mutations that molecular genetic testing would be less sensitive and far less cost-effective than testing by biochemical or enzymatic means. For most such disorders, the molecular tests, if available, are reserved for backup confirmation of indeterminate results, for further genotype-phenotype correlation, or for identification of DNA markers that could be used by the family for prenatal diagnosis in a subsequent pregnancy. However, as DNA-based methods become more comprehensive with the development of microarray technologies and less expensive through high-throughput automation, they may become the first-tier approach for certain newborn screens.

PRENATAL DIAGNOSIS

While classical cytogenetic analysis remains the most commonly performed mode of prenatal diagnosis, the advent of reliable molecular techniques has opened a new world of prenatal testing for single-gene defects. Even though some inborn errors of metabolism can be diagnosed by biochemical analysis of amniotic fluid, other disorders, such as the muscular dystrophies, do not produce such easily accessible analytes and would require far more invasive biopsy of the target tissue (e.g., fetal muscle) for examination of the gene product. Molecular genetic techniques obviate this need, since DNA containing the mutation of interest is readily obtainable from amniocytes or CVS specimens. However, given the time constraints of the prenatal setting, such an approach is usually not attempted unless there is prior knowledge of the identity of the parental mutation(s), at least in the case of disorders with extensive mutational heterogeneity.

A more recent variant of prenatal diagnosis now available in certain situations in preimplantation diagnosis, involving single-cell genetic analysis (using powerful PCR techniques) performed on blastomere biopsy of embryos produced by in vitro fertilization (IVF). Because of the difficulty and expense of the procedure, it is usually reserved for those couples who would be averse to abortion of an in utero pregnancy or who are already undergoing IVF for other obstetrical or infertility indications. Even more so than for traditional prenatal diagnosis, the exact identity of the mutation(s) in the parent (for a dominant disease) or both parents (for a recessive disease) must be known before embarking on this involved procedure. Still, despite its formidable prerequisites, preimplantation diagnosis has been used many times for pregnancies at risk for cystic fibrosis, thalassemia, and other disorders (Handyside et al., 1992; Sermon et al., 1999; Kuliev et al., 1999).

CARRIER SCREENING

Carrier screening is another type of laboratory testing unique to the genetics setting. The term is most properly used to denote testing for recessive mutations in the heterozygous state in otherwise healthy individuals. It may be indicated in two quite different situations: one in which an individual is at risk because of a positive family history for the disorder in question, the other in which the individual is at risk by virtue of belonging to an ethnic group in which the population frequency of one or more mutant alleles is particularly high. The first application is more accurately termed carrier *testing* rather than carrier screening, especially when the causative mutation in the family is already known. The second application is true screening, since it is performed on an entire population without respect to family history, and the likely mutation in any one individual being tested will not be known (unless the disorder has only a single mutation, as in sickle cell disease).

Because screening tests must be kept inexpensive in order to be cost-effective, screening strategies for disorders with mutational heterogeneity will often entail complex decisions regarding the number and type of mutations to be included in the test panel. Such debates have been waging for years in the case of cystic fibrosis (Grody, 1999). A decision must also be made whether molecular genetic testing, with its narrow focus on specific mutations, casts a wide enough net within the target population to justify using it in preference to biochemical or enzymatic screening methods which are often less expensive. In the case of cystic fibrosis, the carriers have no biochemical abnormalities that can be ascertained, so direct mutation testing is the only alternative. In the case of Tay-Sachs disease, even though there are a limited number of hexosaminidase-A mutations that account for most carriers in the Ashkenazi Jewish target population, enzymatic testing is still preferred for population screening because of its ease of use, low cost, and ability to capture carriers with uncommon mutations. Since recessive mutations are clinically significant only in the setting of reproduction, it follows that, whatever the approach, the ultimate goal of carrier testing and screening is to identify couples at risk (i.e., both the man and the woman are carriers) so they can be offered the opportunity for prenatal testing.

PRESYMPTOMATIC/PREDISPOSITION TESTING

Predictive DNA testing is the newest and, in some sense, the most problematic, of molecular genetic applications. It is applied primarily to adult- or late childhood-onset autosomal dominant disorders. It is never appropriate as a screening test, but is strictly reserved for individuals with a strong, usually parental, family history of the disorder, conferring upon them a 50% a priori risk of having inherited the mutant gene. Depending on the penetrance of the mutations being tested, predictive testing is further subdivided into presymptomatic testing and predisposition testing. The former is applied to those disorders with virtually complete penetrance, such as Huntington disease, in which a positive DNA test result is fully predictive of eventual symptomatology (though not necessarily indicative of severity or age of onset). The latter is applied to diseases with reduced penetrance, such as familial breast/ovarian cancer due to the *BRCA1* and *BRCA2* genes, in which a positive test result confers increased risk of eventual disease compared to the baseline population risk, but does not allow prediction that any particular patient will actually experience the disease. This situation makes genetic and clinical counseling much more difficult, especially for diseases like familial breast/ovarian cancer, in which risky or irreversible medical or surgical interventions may be initiated based on a positive DNA test result. And with both types of predictive testing there are significant psychosocial risks, since otherwise healthy adults are being given potentially devastating news about future disease. There are also risks of insurance or employment discrimination which beg the question of whether a nucleotide change predictive of future disease in a presently healthy person is to be considered a "preexisting condition". For all these reasons, predictive genetic testing has been the area most stringently subject to standardized protocols for informed consent, pre- and post-test genetic counseling, and psychosocial supportive services (Huntington's Disease Society of America 1989; American College of Medical Genetics 1999a).

Technical approaches to molecular genetic testing

SPECIMEN COLLECTION

Just as many of the applications are unique, so too the types of patient samples collected for molecular genetic testing may be different from those obtained for other types of clinical laboratory testing. Since germline mutations are present in every cell of the body, site-specific biopsy is not required and simple phlebotomy will suffice for most purposes (this is in contrast to the approach for laboratory diagnosis of infectious and neoplastic diseases, where a specific lesion must be sampled). Alternatively, the great sensitivity of the polymerase chain reaction (PCR) allows for genetic testing to be performed on minute samples of any readily accessible tissue or body fluid, including saliva, urine, etc. Newborn DNA screening can easily be performed on the same blood spots collected for biochemically-based screening. For prenatal diagnosis, either amniocytes or chorionic villus samples can be used, since both contain the full complement of fetal DNA. In addition, PCR-based single-cell genetic analysis now allows for preimplantation diagnosis on individual embryonic blastomeres, as discussed above, and some preliminary work has targeted fetal cells circulating in the maternal blood (Di Naro et al., 2000; Zhong et al., 2000), thus potentially obviating the need for any sort of invasive fetal sampling.

SELECTION OF TECHNIQUE

Once in hand, the specimen can be subjected to any of the molecular genetic techniques in the current armamentarium.

The choice of technique will depend upon the nature of the disease gene being studied (especially its size and complexity), the purpose of the test, and to some extent the condition of the specimen. Specimens that are extremely small, fixed, or degraded will require some sort of PCR-based analysis, since that technique is the most tolerant of suboptimal samples. Once amplified to abundant amount, the DNA is then amenable to further analysis by other techniques such as allele-specific oligonucleotide hybridization or DNA sequencing. Southern blotting, on the other hand, which is required for certain tests involving large genomic regions, requires intact DNA of high molecular weight in pristine enough condition to be digested efficiently with restriction endonucleases and to produce reproducible patterns on gel electrophoresis. This usually means at least a few milliliters of whole blood, or 1–2 dishes of cultured amniocytes, transported to the lab in a timely fashion. In either case the first step is typically the isolation of DNA from the specimen, for which a variety of commonly used methods and kits are available. For PCR-based tests, a crude preparation of DNA may be all that is needed; for Southern blotting, carefully prepared, highly purified DNA is required.

Detection of point mutations

For detection of a known point mutation or microdeletion/insertion, the patient DNA sample can be hybridized with allele-specific oligonucleotide (ASO) probes which contain either the wild type or mutant sequence within them. Since hybridization under high stringency can distinguish a single nucleotide change by mismatch of a probe with its target, using these ASO probes in pairs provides an internal control for accurately genotyping both heterozygotes and homozygotes. An alternative strategy capitalizes on the availability of a wide variety of bacterial restriction endonucleases with many different target recognition sequences. With a little investigation (made easy these days through the use of computer DNA sequence analysis programs), it will often be found that the mutation of interest either disrupts a preexisting restriction enzyme cleavage site or creates a new one in the target DNA. In that case the mutation can be detected by exposing the patient's PCR-amplified DNA to the specific restriction enzyme and analyzing the cleavage products (sometimes called amplified restriction fragment polymorphisms, or AmpFLPs) by polyacrylamide gel electrophoresis. The same thing can sometimes be done by Southern blot, since it too involves a restriction enzyme digestion step, though that approach is usually more unwieldy.

Detection of large deletions

Large deletions, while sometimes detectable by these methods, are usually more easily seen by Southern blot hybridization (signalled by absence of one or more expected hybridization bands). Alternatively, one can use differential PCR amplification, in which the failure of one or both of a pair of PCR primers to hybridize to the target DNA because of the deletion will result in absence of an expected PCR product. The only drawback to this technique is that there are many other technical reasons for PCR failure (of artifactual origin), and so appropriate internal PCR amplification controls must be included in the assay. Extremely large deletions may require the specialized technique of pulsed-field gel electrophoresis, which is amenable to very high molecular weight fragments, or fluorescence in situ hybridization (which is typically performed in the cytogenetics laboratory rather than the molecular genetics laboratory).

Detection of trinucleotide repeat expansions

To detect the trinucleotide repeat expansion mutations characteristic of fragile X syndrome, Huntington disease and other neuromuscular disorders, accurate sizing becomes important. Indeed, this is the most visible area of molecular genetic testing that approaches quantitative assay criteria, as opposed to the more qualitative observational assays for point mutations and deletions. If the expansion size is of moderate length, as in Huntington disease and the spinocerebellar ataxias, amplification and sizing of PCR products suffices. For larger expansions that are difficult or impossible to amplify, such as in fragile X syndrome, sizing by Southern blot analysis is required.

Detection of heterogeneous mutations

What about those disorders in which a wide range of point mutations has been reported, often spanning a very large gene? Such complex disorders present special problems to the laboratory in attempting to assure detection of a majority of the mutations; detection of all potential mutations is virtually impossible, even by complete DNA sequencing of the gene (since mutations may lie in noncoding regions, far upstream enhancers, etc.). Sequencing does cast the widest net and is therefore considered the "gold standard", but it is also the most cumbersome, and not easily adaptable to high-throughput screening tests. As a compromise, one can select a more limited test panel comprised of a few of the more commonly recurring mutations in the gene, recognizing at the outset that some fraction of carriers will go undetected.

These then become amenable to the ASO hybridization or restriction endonuclease strategies described above. In fact, a variation of the ASO approach in which the panel probes are arrayed on a paper strip or solid platform and hybridized with the patient's amplified DNA (the so-called a reverse dot blot) has become the preferred approach in this setting. This is the strategy currently used for cystic fibrosis testing and carrier screening in many laboratories. In some sense, it is but a rather crude version of the much more extensive DNA probe arrays now being incorporated into "DNA chips", a technology that has the potential to wed the convenience advantages of ASO dot blot hybridization with the comprehensive coverage of DNA sequencing.

DNA sequencing, because of its laboriousness and expense, is usually reserved for situations in which it is not clinically acceptable to overlook a pathologic mutation if one is present; an example would be predictive testing for *BRCA1/2* mutations of familial breast/ovarian cancer. In other cases, sequencing may be used for detection of even a limited number of mutations in a gene, provided they are localized to hot spots within one or a few exons. This strategy is used in our laboratory for diagnosis of familial Mediterranean fever, in which the majority of the mutations are located in exon 10 of the *MEFV* gene (Telatar and Grody, 2000). Either manual or automated DNA sequencing may be used, though the latter is preferable for sequencing of long stretches. For highly critical studies the sequencing is often performed in both directions (i.e., sequencing both strands of the double helix) for optimal quality control.

Because sequencing will detect any nucleotide change present—not just the previously known mutations in the gene—it becomes important to distinguish benign changes (polymorphisms) from pathologic ones. This is not as easy or straightforward as it may seem. While nonsense and frameshift mutations are usually quite obviously pathologic, especially if they occur in the 5′ half of the gene, missense mutations can bend the rules: even a mutation leading to an apparently conservative amino acid substitution may somehow disrupt transcription or somatic stability down the line (Gryfe et al., 1998), and a major amino acid substitution may not be deleterious if it lies within a static or nonessential domain of the protein.

Finally, there are the so-called mutation-scanning techniques. These can be used as a first-pass screen of a gene or gene fragment for the presence of point mutations, without the effort and expense of meticulous gene sequencing. These techniques capitalize on the altered three-dimensional topology of a mutant DNA fragment compared to the corresponding wild type fragment, an alteration which can be detected by differential migration through an electrophoresis gel. Single-strand conformation polymorphism (SSCP) and denaturing gradient gel electrophoresis (DGGE) do this for single-stranded or double-stranded DNA targets, respectively. However, because they are qualitative assays relying on poorly understood physicochemical behaviors of DNA fragments, they are never 100% sensitive (Orban et al., 2000). Furthermore, any abnormality detected must then be confirmed by DNA sequencing of the fragment for precise mutation location, identification and interpretation.

A rather different and more predictable mutation-scanning technique is the protein truncation test (PTT), in which a gene or exon is used as substrate for an in vitro transcription/translation assay and the polypeptide products are analyzed by acrylamide gel electrophoresis. Presence of a nonsense mutation (or a frameshift mutation leading to a stop codon downstream) will produce a shortened (truncated) polypeptide as compared to a wild type control. Of course, this technique will not pick up missense mutations, and so a substantial proportion of pathologic alterations in the gene under study will go undetected. Moreover, all of the mutation-scanning techniques are rather involved and finicky, making them more suitable as research tools than for routine clinical laboratory use at the present time.

Detection of unknown disease genes

All of the approaches listed above are direct mutation detection methods, which can only be used for disorders whose genes have been identified and cloned. Testing for diseases whose genes have not yet been identified but have at least been mapped to a particular chromosome requires linkage analysis, the use of polymorphic DNA markers to follow segregation of the mutant allele in a family group. This sort of testing requires collection of DNA specimens not only from the proband but also from multiple other affected and unaffected family members over two or three generations. Also required are polymorphic markers located sufficiently close to (or even inside) the disease gene so that false results due to crossing over are minimized. This is now readily possible thanks to the saturation of the human genome with polymorphic sites as a major thrust of the Human Genome Project, in which short tandem repeat markers, accessible by PCR, now outnumber the formerly used restriction fragment-length polymorphisms (RFLP) detected by Southern blot. Despite these recent advances, however, linkage analysis is not especially favored by diagnostic laboratories and instead is kept in reserve as a last resort for diseases with unknown or very large genes. Linkage analysis is always more cumbersome than direct mutation analysis, it has a higher risk of misleading results, and it requires family cooperation which may not always be feasible. It is also typically more expensive, and reimbursement becomes awkward when third-party payers see multiple individuals being tested under the same billable procedure. Most laboratories are only too happy to leave it behind the instant the identification of the disease gene is reported.

Molecular genetic diagnosis of particular diseases

CYSTIC FIBROSIS

It seems appropriate to begin the discussion of specific disease examples of molecular genetic testing with cystic fibrosis (CF), since over the last 10 years it has come to be viewed as the prototypic challenge in DNA testing for mutationally heterogeneous disorders. Because it has one of the highest carrier frequencies of any serious autosomal recessive disease, it has been discussed as a likely target for population screening ever since the causative gene was identified in 1989 (Riordan et al., 1989; Kerem et al., 1989). And because CF carriers have no detectable signs or symptoms to distinguish them from other members of the population, such screening could only be accomplished at the DNA level, making CF a "pure" molecular genetic disease from this standpoint. In addition, DNA testing for CF mutations allows for reliable prenatal diagnosis (provided the identity of both carrier mutations has been established in the parents) and for clinical diagnosis in cases where the manifestations or the sweat chloride levels are ambiguous.

However, as is now widely known, the CF gene and in some sense the disease itself have proven resistant to simplistic approaches. While approximately 70% of Caucasian carriers have the common △F508 mutation, the other 30% (and an even greater proportion in other racial and ethnic groups) may have any of over 800 other, much less common, mutations. This may not be such a problem in testing relatives of affected patients, especially when the mutations in the index case are already known, but it makes random population screening extremely difficult. The second most common mutation, G542X, has a frequency of only about 2%, and beyond the first six mutations the individual carrier frequencies fall below 1% (Cystic Fibrosis Genetic Analysis Consortium, 1994). Additional problems are raised by the extreme ethnic heterogeneity of the US target population, ethical issues surrounding prenatal testing for a disease of significant clinical variability, the notoriously poor correlation between individual CF mutations and phenotypic expression

(Cystic Fibrosis Genotype-Phenotype Consortium, 1993), and a perception of inadequate genetic counseling resources to handle the anticipated caseload of nationwide screening (Wilfond and Fost 1990; Grody 1999).

As discussed earlier, the most assured way to pick up any and all possible mutations in a large gene like *CFTR* (which spans 230 kb and 27 exons [Zielenski et al., 1991]) is DNA sequencing. But that is such a labor-intensive and expensive procedure that it would be entirely inappropriate for population screening. Screening requires a simpler procedure such as dot blot hybridization with ASO probes. But which ASO probes to use? Choosing a consensus panel of prevalent CF mutations is not an obvious undertaking, since all but one are rare, and the prevalences of individual mutations vary greatly according to ethnic group. Over the years laboratories have employed panels of 6, 16, 30 or over 70 mutations, with remarkable diversity in practice from lab to lab (Grody et al., 1998). Recently a core, pan-ethnic panel of 25 mutations (along with some associated polymorphisms) has been recommended by a subcommittee of the American College of Medical Genetics, in order to bring some uniformity to the field and to offer the most efficient strategy for screening in an ethnically diverse population like that of the United States (Grody et al., 2001). The criterion used for inclusion in the panel was ≥0.1% allele frequency in the general population as gauged by a large survey of CF patients (Cystic Fibrosis Foundation, 1998); in addition, some mutations especially prevalent in ethnic groups likely to be screened, such as the W1282X mutation in the Ashkenazi Jewish population and the 3120+1G→A mutation in African Americans, were included. The core panel should produce carrier detectability rates of about 97% in Ashkenazi Jews, 80% in non-Jewish Caucasians, 69% in African Americans, 57% in Hispanic Americans, and an uncertain though very low percentage in Asian Americans (Grody et al., 2001). At time of this writing, it is still unclear how well universal CF carrier screening will succeed in the United States as it has in the United Kingdom (Harris et al., 1993).

With sequencing not really an option, laboratories have developed other platforms to encompass whatever mutation panel is chosen. Some CF mutations can be differentiated by electrophoretic sizing and/or restriction endonuclease digestion of PCR products encompassing the codon in question (Chong and Thibodeau, 1990), though this approach becomes quite laborious when targeting more than a handful of mutations. Most laboratories have favored some sort of array technology, such as the reverse dot blot procedure introduced previously (Wall et al., 1995), with numerous variations and automations of this theme having evolved (DeMarchi et al., 1994; Shuber et al., 1997). Certainly a comprehensive microarray (DNA chip) would be ideally suited for CF mutation screening.

Another lesson from the CF gene story, since repeated in other diseases as well, is the broadening of clinical phenotype as novel mutations are detected in increasing numbers and varieties of patients. It was already known that some CF patients may have minimal lung disease (Cutting et al., 1990) or normal sweat chloride levels (Highsmith et al., 1994), but it later became apparent that there were individuals with mutations in the *CFTR* gene presenting with phenotypes not resembling classical CF at all. The gene has been implicated in such conditions as pancreatitis (Cohn et al, 2000) and sinusitis (Coltrera et al., 2000), but most important has been the association of certain *CFTR* mutation and polymorphism combinations with an isolated congenital malformation, bilateral absence of the vas deferens (Anguiano et al., 1992). Especially linked with this condition are the R117H mutation and an intronic polymorphism designated 5T (Gervais et al., 1993; Kiesewetter et al., 1993). One can imagine the genetic counseling complications entailed when these alleles, and others like them, are included in a carrier screening or prenatal testing program. But CF is certainly not unique in this regard, and that is why the lessons we learn from widespread molecular testing in this disease will be so relevant to many other applications in diagnostic molecular genetics.

FACTOR V LEIDEN AND THE HEREDITARY THROMBOPHILIAS

Like the CF carrier state, the Leiden mutation in the clotting factor V gene is a common enough allele (up to 7% in Caucasians [Ridker et al., 1997a]) that its DNA assay has been proposed as a screening test, if not in the general population then perhaps at least in those individuals already at risk for thrombosis due to environmental factors (surgery, paralysis, trauma, malignancy, oral contraceptive use). Indeed, the DNA test itself is very easy, since the Leiden mutation (R506Q) disrupts an *Mnl*I restriction endonuclease site present in the wild type gene (Gregg et al., 1997). There are even some newer automated methods that do not require either restriction digestion or PCR (Ryan et al., 1999). Yet, also analogous to CF, the biology of this gene in vivo and in large populations is somewhat more complex.

The R506Q substitution renders factor V resistant to cleavage by activated protein C (APC), a key mechanism for keeping the coagulation cascade in check. It is the major (but not the only) cause of thrombophilia due to APC resistance. It is best to think of factor V Leiden as a genotype and

APC resistance as the phenotype. As such, the latter can be diagnosed by functional coagulation assays on patient plasma, and some authorities feel that the functional assay is preferable over the DNA test as an initial diagnostic screen since it casts a wider net. On the other hand, recent technical modifications of the functional assay have made it almost entirely specific for the factor V Leiden etiology (Sun et al., 1994). In any event, the DNA test is certainly useful because of its lack of interference by anticoagulant therapy and its ability to reliably distinguish homozygotes from heterozygotes. The latter is important because heterozygotes have a 7-fold increased risk of venous thrombosis, while homozygotes have about an 80-fold increased risk (Ridker et al., 1995). But while these fold-risk estimates may seem high, it is important to remember that idiopathic thrombosis in otherwise healthy adults, especially young adults, is quite rare, so the absolute risk especially in heterozygotes is not particularly great. In fact, the lifetime risk of an adverse event in a carrier is less than the risk of complications from longterm anticoagulant therapy, which is the intervention presumably being considered in those testing positive. A similar risk differential can be stated for female carriers on oral contraceptives who, as a result of DNA testing, would be obligated to seek other, less effective methods of birth control, leading to the risk of adverse events in unintended pregnancies (Kuperminc et al., 1999). In view of these low-magnitude relative probabilities, it is understandable that notions of population screening of asymptomatic individuals for the factor V Leiden mutation remain controversial. The test remains useful, however, in differential diagnosis of otherwise unexplained thromboembolic events, with a positive result conferring some prognostic information as to risk of recurrence. It has become, in short order, the highest volume molecular genetic test in most diagnostic laboratories.

Factor V Leiden is but one of a group of disorders classified as hereditary thrombophilias. While some of the others, such as protein S deficiency, protein C deficiency and antithrombin III deficiency, are too rare and mutationally heterogeneous to become candidates for testing at the molecular level, there is one that approaches factor V Leiden in its indications and ease of testing. The prothrombin 20210A mutation (located in the 3′-untranslated region of the gene) leads to increased levels of prothrombin in the circulation and a phenotype similar to that of factor V Leiden (Poort et al., 1996). It too can be detected by restriction enzyme digestion of PCR products or by automated methods, including multiplex analysis with the factor V Leiden test. And since it, too, is relatively common (1–2% carrier frequency), it makes some sense to test for it at the same time as factor V Leiden, providing the same indications are present. Some laboratories also include in their thrombophilia DNA panel the 677C→T variant of the methylenetetrahydrofolate reductase gene, which leads to elevated plasma homocysteine levels through inhibition of the folate-mediated remethylation of that compound. This allele is very common, found in 30–40% of the general population (Kang et al., 1991). However, the phenotype is different than factor V Leiden and prothrombin 20210A, since elevated homocysteine is also associated with arterial (including coronary) thrombosis. For purposes of clinical decision-making, therefore, there does not seem to be a compelling reason to lump this test in with the other two. On the other hand, since all three of these carrier states are quite common, it is not unusual to see double (or even triple) mutants, with documented synergistic effects on thrombotic risk (Ridker et al., 1997b; Halbmayer et al., 1999). It should also be kept in mind that the prothrombin 20210A mutation has itself been implicated in myocardial infarction in women (Rosendaal et al., 1997).

The anticoagulant system is extremely complex, and no doubt there are other hereditary factors yet to be discovered. Even though factor V Leiden is a single, simple mutant allele, the thrombophilic state behaves more like a complex, multifactorial disease, with numerous gene products interacting with one another and with environmental stresses. Some time in the future we can probably anticipate the advent of a "thrombophilia DNA chip" for screening, much as the CF chip would be useful today. But for such a technology to be truly useful, we will need to achieve a much more thorough understanding of the biology of this complex system.

HEREDITARY HEMOCHROMATOSIS

Despite the greater attention paid of late to CF, hemochromatosis is actually the most common inherited single-gene disorder in people of northwest European ancestry. It is an autosomal recessive disease estimated to affect about 1 in 300 individuals in this population (Merryweather-Clarke et al, 1997). The disease locus was first mapped to the short arm of chromosome 6 by genetic linkage analysis (Jazwinska et al., 1993) and then isolated using an identity-by-descent positional cloning method in 1996 (Feder et al., 1996). The gene, originally called *HLA-H* but renamed as *HFE*, is located 4.5 megabases telomeric to the *HLA-A* locus and encodes a major histocompatibility complex class I-like protein.

Two missense mutations, C282Y and H63D, have been identified within the gene (Feder et al., 1996). Seventy to

100% of hereditary hemochromatosis cases in various studies are homozygous for the C282Y mutation which is carried by about 10% of Caucasian individuals (Press, 1999). The other mutation, H63D, is found in compound heterozygous form with C282Y in 3–5% of patients. These two mutations are in linkage disequilibrium and have not been found together on the same haplotype. However, considering the high carrier frequency of the H63D mutation in the general population (about 25%), its involvement in the pathogenesis of the disease remains controversial; it might represent a minor mutation of low penetrance or even a polymorphism (Risch, 1997). Definite evidence that homozygosity for the H63D mutation is associated with disease is so far lacking.

Most laboratories offering HFE mutation testing assay for both mutations. It is usually performed by PCR amplification of the two regions of the gene encompassing codons 282 and 63, followed by restriction digestion of the PCR products (Fig. 26.1). The C282Y mutation creates a restriction site for the enzyme *Rsa*I, and the H63D mutation abolishes the restriction site for the enzymes *Mbo*I, *Dpn*II or *Bcl*I. Molecular diagnostic testing for these mutations can be used to confirm the diagnosis of hemochromatosis in those with symptomatic disease and also, more importantly, to detect those with presymptomatic iron overload in whom future disease manifestations may then be prevented by simple measures (regular phlebotomy). Because of the high carrier frequency, easy therapeutic intervention, and irreversibility of organ damage if not diagnosed in time, hereditary hemochromatosis has been proposed as a target for population screening. It remains controversial, however,

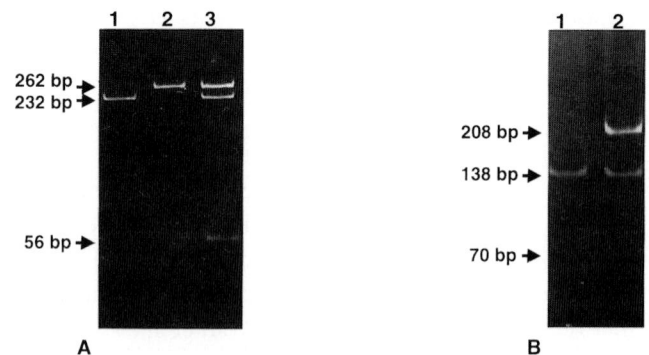

Fig. 26.1. PCR analysis of the C282Y and H63D mutations in the *HFE* gene associated with hereditary hemochromatosis. Panel A, *Rsa*I digestion of PCR products in which presence of the C282Y mutation creates a new restriction endonuclease cleavage site: 1, homozygote for C282Y; 2, normal; 3, heterozygote for C282Y. Panel B, *Dpn*II digestion of PCR products in which the presence of the H63D mutation abolishes a restriction endonuclease cleavage site: 1, normal; 2, heterozygote for H63D.

because of the reduced penetrance (about 70%) even in C282Y homozygotes (Crawford et al., 1998; Robson et al., 2000). There are also concerns about insurance and other discrimination in the huge number of individuals who would test positive. And it is not clear whether, analogous to the situation with factor V Leiden, the functional assay (in this case, serum ferritun and/or transferrin saturation) might be the more appropriate initial screening test.

HEREDITARY HEMOGLOBINOPATHIES

Hereditary hemoglobinopathies encompass a vastly heterogenous group of genetic disorders affecting globin protein structure and/or synthesis. Thus, while the globin genes are relatively small compared to those of other important medical genetic disorders, the approach to their molecular testing is quite varied.

Structural globin disorders

While the greatest incidence of sickle cell disease occurs in sub-Saharan Africa, the carrier frequency in the African-American population is 8%, making it potentially a significant target for DNA testing and screening, though socioeconomic factors have impeded such efforts thus far. This is ironic considering that sickle cell disease was the first human genetic disorder for which the molecular basis was described. Later, the β-globin gene was the first human gene to be cloned and its various mutations demonstrated. Over 300 point mutations in the β-globin gene have

now been identified ("Human Gene Mutation Database," http://www.uwcm.ac.uk/uwcm/mg/hgmd0/html), with the sickle cell mutation being the most common and most severe. While many of these can be identified by nonmolecular methods as well, it is important to remember that the number of structural variants that can be identified by standard hemoglobin electrophoresis represents a minority of the total number in existence, because only approximately one-third of them produce an altered charge in the hemoglobin molecule. In addition, in hyper-unstable hemoglobin syndromes, the protein may be so labile or short-lived that electrophoretic identification is hampered. In these cases, DNA analysis will be preferable.

The original DNA-based method for prenatal diagnosis of sickle cell disease used linkage analysis. An *Hpa*I restriction fragment length polymorphism (RFLP) downstream of the β-globin gene was linked to the sickle cell mutation in 87% of African-American HbS genes (Kan and Dozy, 1978). Now, of course, direct mutation detection strategies are preferred. This can be accomplished by hybridizing labeled ASO probes complementary to either the β^A or β^S allele to genomic DNA blotted or spotted onto a membrane (Conner et al., 1983). Alternatively, one can use either a Southern blot or PCR approach that capitalizes on disruption of a restriction endonuclease cleavage site by the HbS mutation. The mutation ablates an *Mst*II or *Dde*I restriction site in the gene, producing a larger fragment after enzyme digestion, as compared to normal DNA (Chang and Kan, 1982) (Fig. 26.2). This technique was recently used also for preimplantation diagnosis of sickle cell disease in biopsied blastomeres (Xu et al., 1999).

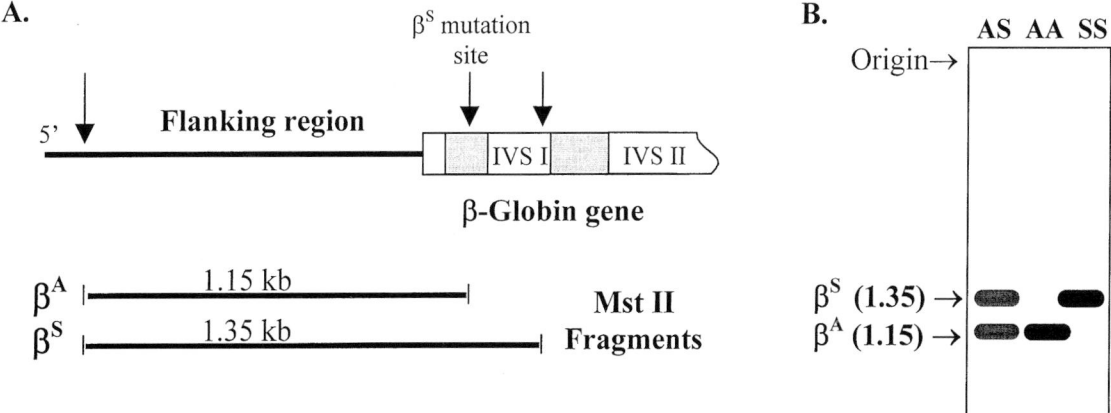

Fig. 26.2. Detection of the sickle cell disease missense mutation by restriction endonuclease digestion. Panel A, schematic diagram of the 5' portion of the β-globin gene containing the sickle cell disease mutation site in codon 6. *Mst*II restriction endonuclease cleavage sites are indicated by the arrows. The abolishment of one *Mst*II site by the β^s mutation results in an increase in size of the digest fragment from 1.15 to 1.35 kb. Panel B, schematic diagram of an electrophoretic gel or Southern blot in which the two fragments have been separated: AS, heterozygote HbS carrier; AA, normal control; SS, HbS homozygote. (Adapted from Chang and Kan, 1982, with permission.)

Other structurally abnormal hemoglobin disorders that may be detected in this fashion include HbE, HbD-Los Angeles, and several rarer variants (Akar et al., 1995; Johnson et al., 1992). The alternate mutation in codon 6 of β-globin causing HbC disease does not affect a restriction endonuclease recognition site, and therefore must be detected with ASO probes (Maggio et al., 1993) or ASO primers (amplification refractory mutation system [ARMS]). Multiplexing of ARMS primers to detect several globin mutations at once has been successfully attempted (Tan, 1994), as has competitive priming of fluorescently-labeled primers (Chehab and Kan, 1990). Other methods, such as ligase chain reaction (Barany, 1991), have also been used for this purpose.

Disorders of globin synthesis—the thalassemias

Widespread population-specific screening of carriers for autosomal recessive disorders was initiated first with the thalassemias. Experiences with thalassemia screening programs have resulted in a marked reduction in the birth rate of affected children in Greece, Cyprus, continental Italy, Sardinia, Taiwan, China (Guangzhou), and Southeast Asia (Cao et al., 1998; Alter, 1985). The thalassemias are a large and heterogeneous group of disorders of imbalanced hemoglobin synthesis with widely varied phenotypic expression. From the laboratory perspective, the most important ones are α- and β-thalassemia (and their respective intermediate subtypes).

α-thalassemia

α-Thalassemia is most commonly due to a deletion of one or more of the 4 α-globin genes ($\alpha_1 \alpha_2/\alpha_1 \alpha_2$). Deficits relate closely to gene dosage effects, and therefore dosage, and sometimes phase, analysis is an important component of the molecular diagnostic effort. Deletion of one α-globin gene, usually the α_2, is most common. These occur predominantly in two types, a 3.7-kb deletion ($-\alpha^{3.7}$), and a 4.2-kb deletion ($-\alpha^{4.2}$). The $-\alpha^{3.7}$ deletion is seen in individuals from Africa, the Mediterranean, the Middle East, and Oceania. It is also present in heterozygous form in up to 90% of the population of parts of India and Papua New Guinea. The $-\alpha^{4.2}$ deletion is seen in individuals from Southeast Asia and the Pacific Islands (Flint et al., 1998). A subset of patients in certain ethnic groups may have point mutations in the α-globin genes.

Since most α-thalassemias are thus due to sizable deletions, Southern blotting of endonuclease-digested genomic DNA can be used for diagnosis. The two α-globin genes

have divergence in their sequences in the 110-nucleotide-long 3′-untranslated region, allowing the presence of one or the other or both to be distinguished by their restriction digest pattern. However, one must be alert to the fact that patients with the $\alpha\alpha/-$ (thal-1) or $\alpha\alpha/\alpha-$ (silent carrier) genotype will show a normal blot pattern, having α_1 and α_2 genes both intact. For this reason, dosage analysis must also be performed. Rubin and Kan (1985) described a sensitive slot-blot method for determining how many α-globin genes are present for screening of deletional α-thalassemias and for prenatal diagnosis. Parallel serial dilutions of sample DNA was hybridized with α-globin-specific probes. The comparative intensity of the α-probed band with a band in a complementary β-probed slot (reflecting the total DNA present) distinguished the $\alpha\alpha/-$, $-\alpha/-$ and $-/-$ genotypes from one another. Alternatively, multiplex PCR strategies to differentiate the common $-\alpha^{3.7}$ and $-\alpha^{4.2}$ deletions and to detect junction fragments created by the various deletion combinations have been developed (Oron-Karni et al., 1998).

β-thalassemia

More than 180 different defects in the β-globin gene that result in β-thalassemia have been described (Huisman and Carver, 1998). Molecular diagnosis of the β-thalassemias is made complicated by this heterogeneity. For this reason, molecular testing is done in only a few specialized laboratories. Yet, despite marked heterogeneity at the molecular level, a unique spectrum of mutations is usually prevalent in a given population at risk for β-thalassemia. Less than 10 mutations usually encompass the majority of molecular lesions in the target population, making screening and prenatal diagnosis manageable. In fact, approximately 20 total mutations account for 80% of all the β-thalassemia alleles in the world (Weatherall and Clegg, 1999).

Most (about 95%) β-globin gene defects that result in β-thalassemia syndromes are due to point mutations, including small deletions (up to 17 bp) and insertions. About half of these mutations completely inactivate the β-globin gene (β⁰-thalassemia). This portion is caused by mutations in the initiation codon or splice junctions, or by nonsense or frameshift mutations. The β⁺-thalassemia mutations mainly affect transcription or mRNA processing, usually resulting from mutations located in the promoter region. Gross deletion (>24 bp) of the β-globin gene alone is quite rare, with fewer than 20 types seen (Kazazian 1990). The deletion may more often involve large portions of the β-globin gene cluster, resulting in δβ⁰- and δβ⁰-thalassemias. Depending on the number and variety of mutations expected, laboratories can choose any of a number of ASO or mutation scanning strategies (Cai and Kan, 1990; Cai et al., 1994).

TRINUCLEOTIDE REPEAT EXPANSION DISORDERS

Trinucleotide repeats are part of the tandem repeat families found throughout the genome. But unlike the more ubiquitous di- and tetranucleotide repeat polymorphisms, expansion of these triplet repeats to larger size can have a pathologic effect. Such expansion has been identified as a novel mutation mechanism in several human neuromuscular disorders that result from instability of the expanded repeat once it has reached a certain length (Timchenko and Caskey, 1999). The expansions are unstable mutations that tend to increase in size through successive generations, in contrast to repeat lengths in the normal range that are usually transmitted stably despite their polymorphic nature. The subsequent expansion of the repeat in descending generations does not adhere strictly to the rules of mendelian inheritance due to incomplete penetrance and/or variable expressivity. The severity of the diseases varies and correlates directly with increasing repeat length. Anticipation is the hallmark of the trinucleotide repeat disorders, where increasing severity and earlier onset occur in successive generations. Parent-of-origin effect (imprinting) is also a feature.

Despite their shared features, trinucleotide repeat disorders can be separated into two distinct groups, Type I and Type II (Paulson and Fischbeck, 1996). Type I is comprised of neurodegenerative disorders that are associated with neuronal loss in the brain, brainstem and spinal cord. The members of this group are Huntington disease (HD), spinobulbar muscular atrophy (SBMA), dentatorubral-pallidoluysian atrophy (DRPLA) and the spinocerebellar ataxias, SCA1, SCA2, SCA3 (MJD), SCA6, SCA7 and SCA12. Type I disorders are all autosomal dominant, except for SBMA which is X-linked. These diseases are caused by CAG repeat expansions in the coding regions of the genes, resulting in the insertion of abnormally long polyglutamine tracts in the mutant protein. This change in the protein leads to a gain-of-function defect that is ultimately damaging to neurons in which it is expressed. The magnitude of the intergenerational expansion is usually greater in male than female transmissions; the most severely affected individuals inherit the disease gene from their father. The Type II disorders, in contrast, show a variety of clinical features other than neurodegeneration, and involve repeat sequences other than CAG that are not in the coding regions of the genes. The sequence and expansion ranges of the repeats in the major trinucleotide disorders are summarized in Table 26.1.

Table 26.1. Mutation ranges for the trinucleotide repeat disorders

Disease	Repeat Unit	Normal Range	Premutation or Partial Penetrance Range*	Affected Range
SBMA	CAG	9–34	–	>34
HD	CAG	10–35	36–39	40–121
DRPLA	CAG	6–35	–	49–88
SCA1	CAG	6–34	–	39–81
SCA2	CAG	14–31	32–35	36–64
SCA3	CAG	12–37	–	64–84
SCA6	CAG	4–18	–	21–33
SCA7	CAG	<30	30–36	>36
SCA12	CAG	7–28	–	65–78
FraX	CGG	5–54	55–230	230–>1000
DM	CTG	5–37	38–49	50–>3000
FRDA	GAA	6–34	–	67–1700

Absence of a listing in this column does not necessarily mean that the disorder has no premutation range, only that it has not yet been documented or well defined.

Type I disorders

Spinobulbar muscular atrophy

SBMA, known also as Kennedy disease, is a motor neuron disorder characterized by progressive muscle weakness and atrophy in males (La Spada et al., 1991). The disease results from an expanded CAG repeat in the androgen gene located at Xq12. The number of CAG repeats ranges from nine to 34 in normal alleles. Affected males and carrier females have an allele with greater than 35 CAG repeats.

Huntington disease

An unstable CAG repeat in HD patients was reported in 1993 (Huntington's Disease Collaborative Research Group, 1993). The expansion lies in the 5′ coding region of the huntingtin gene on chromosome 4p16.3. The CAG repeat length at this locus in the normal population ranges from 10 to 35, whereas in HD patients it ranges from 36 to 121, with a reduced penetrance at repeat sizes of 36–39. Strong inverse correlations between repeat length and age of onset have been observed. Adult-onset patients usually have an expansion in the range of 40–55, whereas juvenile-onset patients have expansions above 60 that are often inherited from the father. Sizing of repeat lengths is readily accomplished by PCR amplification and gel electrophoresis, sometimes followed by blotting and probe hybridization to eliminate nonspecific fragments (Fig. 26.3).

Earlier PCR primer sets encompassed a neighboring nonpathologic CAG repeat, itself polymorphic, which led to inaccurate sizing. Newer PCR strategies do not include

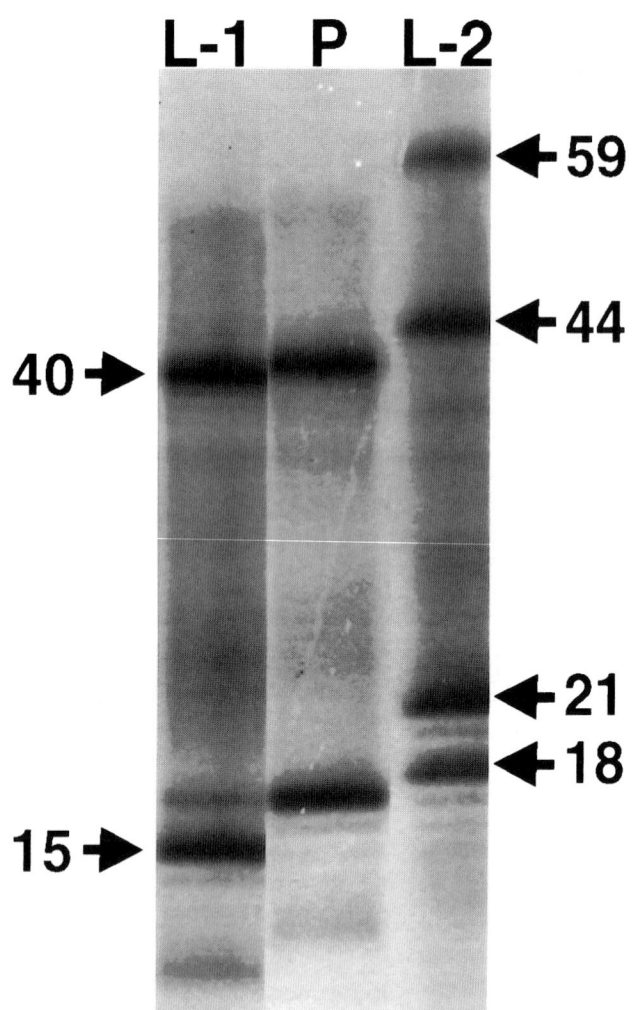

Fig. 26.3. PCR analysis of Huntington disease CAG trinucleotide repeat expansion. L-1, L-2, allelic sizing ladders; P, patient showing one normal allele of 17 CAG repeats and an expanded mutation allele of 41 repeats.

HD was the first genetic disorder to be a target of presymptomatic molecular testing. Because of the virtually 100% penetrance of the full CAG expansion and the lack of any preventive therapy, a positive result in this test represents particularly devastating news, carrying risks of depression, suicide, and discrimination (Almqvist et al., 1999). For these reasons, standard protocols for testing have been developed, emphasizing pre- and post-test psychosocial support and genetic counseling (Huntington's Disease Society of America, 1989).

Dentatorubral-pallidoluysian atrophy

DRPLA results in both ataxia and choreoathetosis, along with myoclonus, epilepsy and dementia, so it is sometimes considered in the differential diagnosis of HD. The gene is on chromosome 12p and encodes a cytoplasmic protein with a polyglutamine tract in the middle (Yazawa et al., 1995). The number of CAG repeats in unaffected individuals ranges from six to 35, whereas in patients with DRPLA it ranges from 49 to 88. Molecular sizing is done as for HD.

Spinocerebellar ataxias

The SCAs are a group of genetically diverse neurological conditions that share progressive deterioration in balance and coordination due to degeneration of the cerebellum and its afferent and efferent pathways (Rosenberg, 1995). Linkage studies identified multiple subtypes, six of which have thus far been found to have unstable CAG expansions (types 1, 2, 3, 6, 7 and 12). The relatively small size of the SCA expansions allows for PCR-based testing as for HD.

The *SCA1* gene is located on chromosome 6p22–23 and encodes ataxin-1 that is widely expressed in neurons and Purkinje cells (Servadio et al., 1995). The number of CAG repeats ranges from six to 34 in normal alleles and from 39 to 81 in disease-causing alleles. Normal alleles with 21 or more repeats may contain one to three interspersed CAT repeats, while disease-causing alleles show an uninterrupted CAG expansion, likely reflecting a pathogenetic mechanism for expansion due to replication error.

The gene responsible for SCA2 is mapped to chromosome 12q24 and encodes ataxin 2. In the ataxia clinic at our institution, SCA2 accounts for 13% of the autosomal dominant cerebellar ataxias, with an additional 6% for SCA1 and 23% for SCA3 (Geschwind et al., 1997). The number of CAG repeats in the *SCA2* gene ranges from 14 to 31 in normal alleles and 36 to 64 in the disease-causing alleles. CAG repeats between 32 and 35 are considered intermediate alleles, which may or may not be associated with phenotypic changes.

this repeat in the amplicon. However, the older primer set is still sometimes helpful for confirming two normal alleles when only a single band is seen on the primary screen, which could indicate either homozygosity for a normal allele or failure to amplify a very large expansion. Backup Southern blot is another way to distinguish these two possibilities (American College of Medical Genetics/American Society of Human Genetics Huntington Disease Genetic Testing Working Group, 1998). Another reported reason for observing only a single band is PCR failure due to a "null allele" at the primer hybridization site on the opposite chromosome (Williams et al., 2000). Needless to say, accurate sizing of the repeat number in this disease is extremely important, in part because of the emotionally charged nature of the test, but also since the difference in size between affected and intermediate or normal alleles is as little as three nucleotides.

SCA3, also known as Machado-Joseph disease (MJD), is a result of CAG expansion in the *MJD* gene at 14q32 (Kawaguchi et al., 1994). The unstable CAG repeat ranges from 12 to 37 in normal individuals, with expansion to 64–84 repeats in MJD patients.

SCA6 is caused by CAG repeat expansion in the human α1A voltage-dependent calcium channel subunit gene (*CACNA1A*) on chromosome 19p13 (Zhuchenko et al., 1997). The number of repeats ranges from four to 18 in the normal population and from 21 to 33 repeats in affected patients.

The CAG repeat expansion is located in the first exon of the *SCA7* gene on chromosome 3p21–p12 (David et al., 1997). Affected individuals usually have more than 37 CAG repeats in the mutated allele. The number of repeats ranges from four to 19 in normal alleles, with repeats of 30–36 being intermediate alleles.

In 1999 Holmes et al. identified a CAG repeat expansion on chromosome 5q31–q33 that is responsible for *SCA12* (Holmes et al., 1999). The repeat lies 133 nucleotides upstream of the transcription start site of the *PPP2R2B* gene. Unexpanded alleles range from seven to 28 repeats and expanded alleles are between 65 and 78 repeats.

Type II disorders

The Type II triplet repeat disorders include myotonic dystrophy (DM), fragile X syndrome (FraX) and Friedreich ataxia (FRDA). In contrast to the Type I group, these are multisystem disorders that are characterized by a constellation of symptoms involving many tissues. The repeat sequences are different in each, they are located in noncoding regions of the genes, and they are characterized by much larger expansions which may require Southern blot analysis for sizing. The expanding triplet repeats are located in the 5′-untranslated region of the *FMR1* gene in FraX, in the 3′-untranslated region of the *DMPK* gene in DM, and, remarkably, in the first intron of the frataxin gene in FRDA. The underlying molecular mechanism does not alter protein function but rather the expression of the gene.

Fragile X syndrome

The most common form of inherited mental retardation, fragile X syndrome is caused by a large expansion of CGG repeats in the 5′-UTR of the fragile X mental retardation (*FMR1*) gene. The larger expansions are associated with increased methylation of both the repeat and the adjacent CpG island, leading to transcriptional silencing of the gene. The expansion and the subsequent methylation account for

the presence of a fragile site (FRAXA) at chromosome Xq27.3 that results from a failure of normal chromatin condensation during mitosis.

Alleles of the CGG repeat can be classified as normal, premutation or full mutation based on the number of the repeats. In the normal population this repeat is highly polymorphic, ranging from five to 54 repeats, while in affected individuals the expansions range from about 230 to over 1000 repeats and are referred to as full mutations. The full mutation alleles are methylated and fail to express the *FMR1* mRNA and protein (FMRP). Southern blot sizing of the *FMR1* expansion also includes use of a methylation-sensitive restriction enzyme to determine methylation status (Fig. 26.4), especially important since some males with full but unmethylated expansion and no clinical symptoms have been reported (Smeets et al., 1995). In addition, use of the methylation-sensitive enzyme allows separation of the two *FMR1* alleles in females, since the one located on the inactive X chromosome will be resistant to digestion due to intrinsic (nonpathologic) methylation. This approach helps to avoid overlooking a very large expansion in a female when only a single normal band is observed on the first-pass Southern blot (using a methylation-insensitive enzyme) or PCR.

On the other hand, PCR is preferred for accurate sizing of premutations in carrier females, since the risk of expansion in offspring increases incrementally with increasing premutation lengths (Nolin et al., 1996). Difficulty in amplifying the GC-rich premutation alleles of fragile X patients can be overcome by the addition of dimethylsulfoxide, 7-deaza-dGTP and betaine to the PCR reaction.

Large expansions display mitotic instability, resulting in a mixture of allele sizes within a single individual. Premutation alleles ranging from about 55 to 230 are not typically associated with an abnormal phenotype or methylation, but they display instability in subsequent generations. These alleles may change in size when transmitted from either sex, invariably remaining within the premutation size range in male transmission, but expanding to full mutation size in female transmission. The presence and the location of the AGG triplets interspersed within the CGG repeats in the *FMR1* gene also play an important role in the stability of the repeat. An uninterrupted pure CGG repeat of greater than about 33–39 triplets appears to increase the instability of maternal alleles (Eichler et al., 1994).

Identification of some families that were cytogenetically positive for the fragile site on chromosome Xq27–28 but negative for *FMR1* expansion led to the discovery of two more fragile sites, FRAXE and FRAXF, both located distal to FRAXA (Nelson, 1995). Both involve GCC repeat expan-

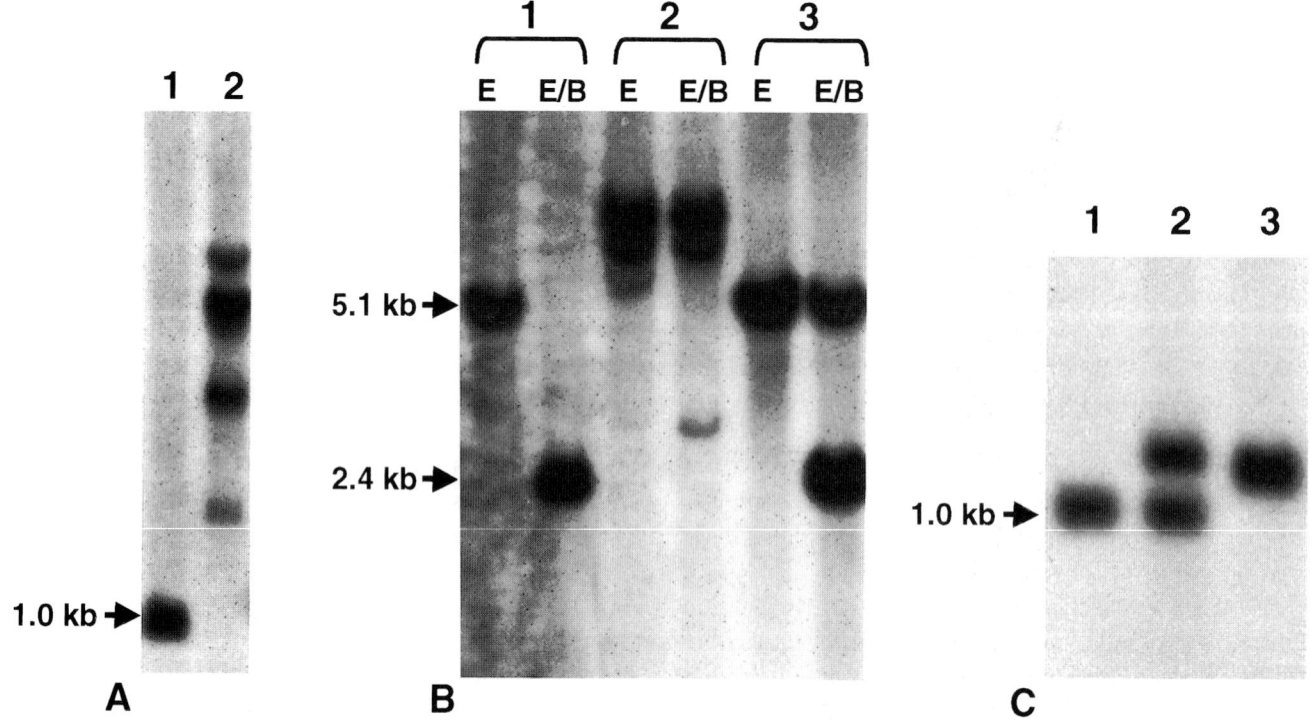

Fig. 26.4. Southern blot analysis of the *FMR1* gene of fragile X syndrome. Panel A, *Pst*I digestion and probing of genomic DNA: 1, normal control showing unexpanded allelic band at 1.0 kb; 2, patient with full CGG expansion mutation showing a spread of high molecular weight bands. Panel B, Southern blot methylation analysis by *Eco*RI and *Eco*RI/*Bss*HII double digestion (*Bss*HII is a methylation-sensitive restriction enzyme): 1, normal male showing single unexpanded, unmethylated allele; 2, affected male showing a single expanded and almost completely methylated allele; 3, normal female showing two unexpanded alleles, one of which is methylated due to X-inactivation. Panel C, *Pst*I digestion and probing of genomic DNA: 1, normal male; 2, female with one normal allele and one premutation allele; 3, premutation male.

sion, with FRAXE exhibiting mild mental retardation in the absence of the characteristic physical stigmata of FRAXA, and FRAXF showing no apparent clinical phenotype.

Myotonic dystrophy

Myotonic dystrophy is the most common inherited muscle disorder in adults, with effects in many other organ systems as well. The genetic basis for DM is an expanded CTG repeat in the 3-untranslated region of a protein kinase gene (*DMPK*) on chromosome 19q13 (Brook et al., 1992). The size of the expanded repeat and the severity of the disease tend to increase in successive generations. The normal repeat size is 5–37 copies, while expansions range from 50 to >3000 in affected individuals. CTG repeat lengths in the range of 38–49 are considered "premutations". In the range of 50–150 repeats, patients develop mild DM with cataract, mild myotonia, or diabetes mellitus, and they may have fully active lives and a normal or minimally shortened life span. In the range of 100 to 1500 repeats, patients usually develop classic DM with muscle weakness and wasting, myotonia, cataracts, and often cardiac conduction abnormalities with the age of onset typically in the twenties

and thirties. Most infants with congenital DM have greater than 1000 CTG repeats, with mental retardation (in 50–60% of cases) and early death. Infants with congenital DM nearly always inherit the expanded *DMPK* allele from the mother, but inheritance from the father is possible. Because of the large size of some DM expansions, Southern blot may be required for diagnosis.

Friedreich ataxia

Friedreich ataxia (FRDA), the only autosomal recessive among the triplet repeat disorders, is caused in 97% of patients by expansion of a GAA repeat in the first intron of the *FRDA* gene on chromosome 9q13, which encodes a 210 amino acid protein called frataxin (Campuzano et al., 1996). The level of frataxin protein expression is decreased in affected individuals with expanded repeats, presumably by an inhibitory effect of the intronic repeat on transcription (Sakamoto et al., 1999). The larger the repeat, the greater the effect on mRNA and protein levels. Normal individuals have 6–34 uninterrupted GAA repeats, and affected patients have 67–1700 repeats. Sizing can be accomplished by either PCR or Southern blot (Fig. 26.5).

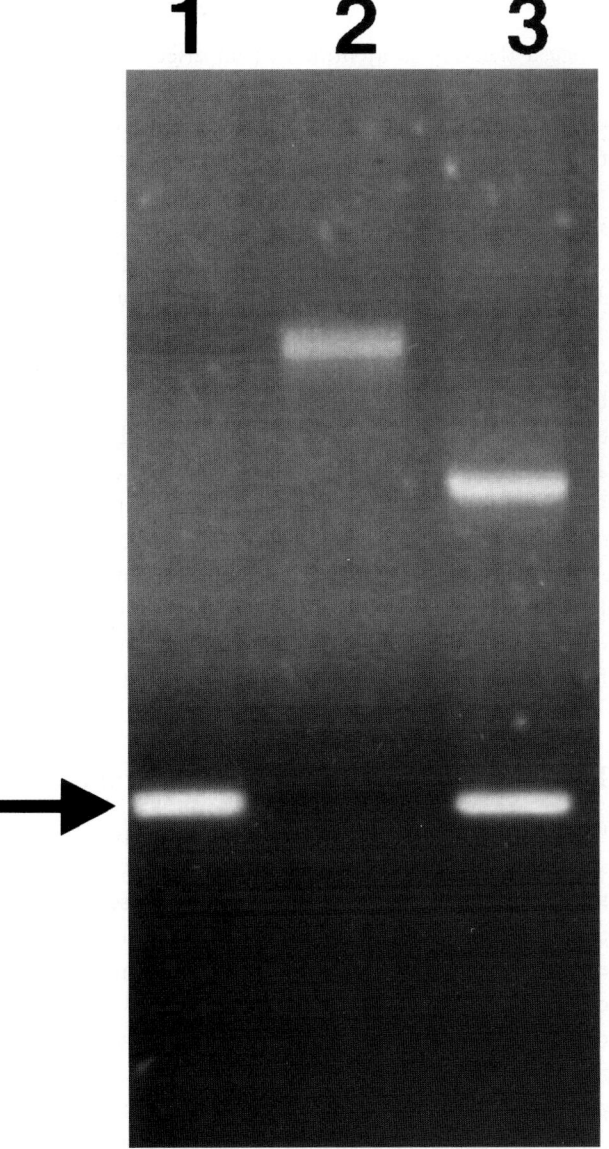

Fig. 26.5. PCR analysis of Friedreich ataxia GAA trinucleotide repeat expansion. Arrow indicates the size of PCR products generated from normal alleles. 1, normal; 2, homozygous expanded; 3, heterozygous.

Compound heterozygotes have been identified with a triplet expansion in one allele and either a nonsense mutation, missense point mutation, or initiation codon mutation in the other allele. This makes the results reporting rather complicated, since the methods used for repeat sizing will not pick up point mutations.

DUCHENNE AND BECKER MUSCULAR DYSTROPHIES

Duchenne (DMD) and Becker (BMD) muscular dystrophies are allelic forms of an X-linked neuromuscular dis-

order that affects about 1 in 3500 live male births. Both are caused by mutations arising in the gene encoding dystrophin, a cytoskeletal protein that underlies the plasma membrane of normal skeletal muscle (Suzuki et al., 1994). The dystrophin gene is located on the short arm of the X-chromosome (Xp21) and is the largest gene ever characterized, spanning about 2.4Mb and encoding at least 79 exons (Roberts at al., 1993). The gene has an unusually high rate of intragenic recombination of about 10–12% in normal pedigrees (Abbs et al., 1990). Recombination events appear to occur mostly in two hot spots located between exons 1–8 and exons 44–51 (Oudet et al., 1992). The majority of the mutations are intragenic deletions (~65%) or duplications (5%) (Forrest et al., 1988; Hu et al., 1988). The remaining one third of cases includes point mutations such as microdeletions, insertions, and substitutions. According to the frameshift hypothesis proposed by Monaco et al. (1988), a patient most likely develops a DMD phenotype if the mutation disrupts the reading frame, whereas a BMD phenotype results if the reading frame is maintained. This would explain the apparent paradox of even fairly large BMD deletions producing a mild phenotype. At the protein level (e.g., on Western blot), DMD is seen to be caused by the absence of detectable dystrophin, while muscle from BMD patients shows a protein of reduced size at less than 40% of normal levels (Hoffman et al., 1988).

Since DMD is a serious disorder for which at present there is no effective treatment, much emphasis has been given to prevention. This involves the ascertainment of women at risk of giving birth to affected sons, and the provision of genetic counseling and prenatal diagnosis. Accurate carrier detection and genetic counseling depend upon first identifying the mutation itself in the proband. The current strategy for DNA testing in this disorder was developed to attempt to circumvent problems arising from the unusual features of the gene, such as its very large size and the great variety of mutations. The approach will vary somewhat depending on the intent and indications for testing, as described in the following paragraphs.

Detection of large deletions in patients

Either Southern analysis or PCR can be used. The first method uses full-length or partial cDNA probes to detect deletions in about 60–70% of patients (Darras and Francke, 1988). This is a laborious approach, which may take several weeks to complete if multiple probes have to be tested sequentially. The second method uses two sets of multiplex PCR primers, each covering deletion hot spots in nine exons of the dystrophin gene (Chamberlain et al., 1988; Beggs et al., 1990). Deleted exons fail to be amplified and are recognized as absent bands on the electrophoretic gel of the PCR products (Fig. 26.6). Because the PCR method screens many regions of the gene simultaneously, it is dramatically faster than the Southern blot approach, with results possible in one day.

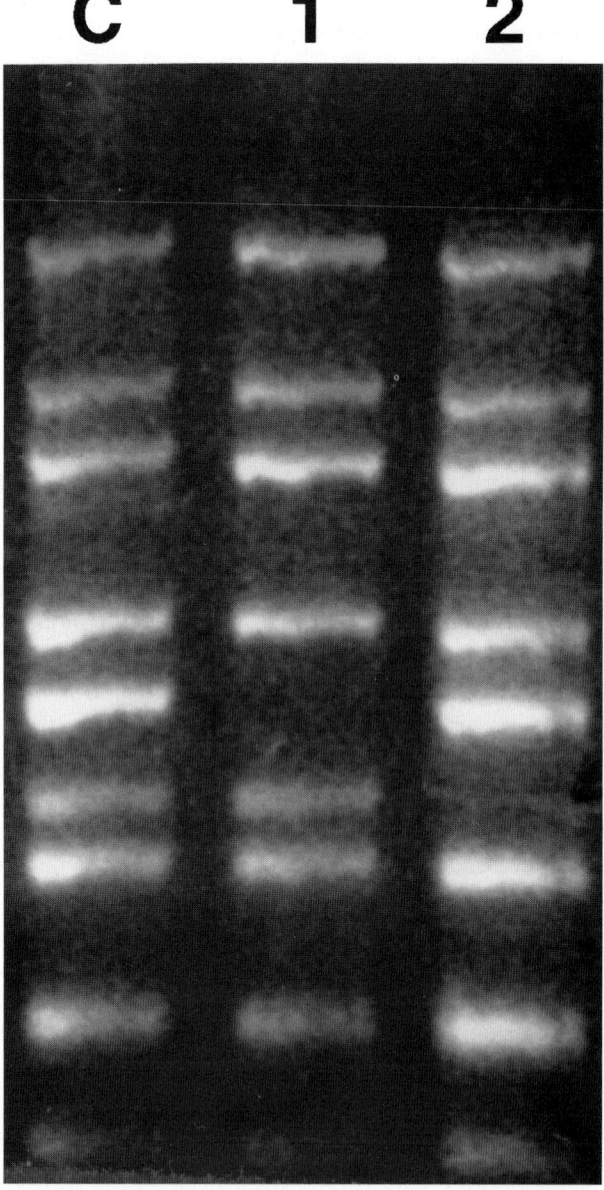

Fig. 26.6. Multiplex PCR for detection of dystrophin deletions in Duchenne/Becker muscular dystrophy, by the method of Beggs et al (1990). C, normal control showing PCR products corresponding to (from top to bottom of electrophoretic gel) promoter and exons 3, 43, 50, 13, 6, 47, 60 and 52; 1, patient positive for a deletion involving exon 13; 2, patient positive for a deletion involving exon 6.

Detection of large deletions in carriers

Once a deletion is identified in an affected patient, DNA samples from women at risk in the family can be tested for carrier status. The assay is complicated, however, by the existence of two X chromosomes, so the particular deletion must be detected by dosage analysis. The female's DNA is subjected to Southern analysis using the same probe that detects the deletion in the related patients. If done carefully, a deletion in one of her two dystrophin alleles results in autoradiographic bands with half the normal intensity (Mao and Cremer, 1989). Dosage analysis can also be performed by combining the multiplex PCR assay with capillary electrophoresis to measure the height and/or integrated area of each product peak. Alternatively, the deletion can be identified directly if a so-called "junction fragment" is observed in the Southern analysis (Yamagishi et al., 1996). A junction fragment arises as the result of fusion of the two DNA fragments flanking the deletion, producing a hybridizing band of abnormal size. Unfortunately, though, junction fragments are found in less than 5% of patients tested.

Detection of microlesions in patients and carriers

One-third of mutations in the dystrophin gene are base substitutions or microdeletions/insertions. Several methods have been used to screen the gene for these microlesions, including the mutation scanning techniques introduced earlier: SSCP, heteroduplex analysis, chemical mismatch cleavage, DGGE, and PTT (van Essen et al., 1997). Once the mutation is found in a patient, reliable carrier detection is then possible by sequencing only the region containing that particular mutation. And as in many other disease examples, carrier detection becomes much easier if the mutation creates or abolishes a restriction site in the DNA.

In families where the mutation cannot be detected, carrier risk needs to be assessed by serum creatine kinase (CK) levels in female relatives and linkage analysis using flanking and intragenic markers. Increased serum CK levels have been observed in two-thirds of DMD carriers, though also are seen in about 1 in 20 females in general population (Emery and King, 1971). Earlier linkage analysis protocols relied on RFLP markers flanking the dystrophin gene and were subject to false results because of the very high intragenic recombination rate. The introduction of four intragenic CA repeat markers improved the reliability of carrier detection and prenatal diagnosis in these families (Clemens et al., 1991). These markers can support the identification of deletion mutations, exclusion of maternal cell contamination in chorionic villus samples, confirmation of paternity, and mapping of dystrophin gene recombinations. Dystrophin immunochemistry in muscle biopsy tissue from the patient is important to confirm DMD when no dystrophin gene mutation is detected (Hoffman et al., 1988).

Female relatives of DMD and BMD patients (mothers, sisters, nieces, aunts and cousins) often request genetic counseling, genetic testing and prenatal diagnosis. As a first step, a pedigree analysis is helpful in evaluating the carrier status in a female. A woman with an affected son and with affected relatives from her maternal side is an obligate carrier (van Essen et al., 1997). A woman with one or more affected brothers but no affected offspring is a possible carrier. A woman with more than one affected son and no family history of muscular dystrophy is either a full carrier or a germline mosaic or a somatic mosaic including her germline (Bakker et al., 1987). Subsequent brothers and sisters of a patient with a new mutation have an estimated risk of 5–10% of inheriting the same germline mutation. Prenatal diagnosis is readily achieved by molecular detection of DNA deletions using chorionic villi or amniocytes, or by linkage analysis. In some cases, however, molecular methods fail to provide a definitive diagnosis and in such cases in utero fetal muscle biopsy for immunohistochemistry or Western blot may serve as a diagnostic option.

PRADER-WILLI AND ANGELMAN SYNDROMES

Despite their disparate clinical phenotypes and completely independent genes, these two disorders are forever linked in cytogenetics and molecular genetics laboratories because of their coincident deletion sites on chromosome 15q11–q13 and mirror-image imprinting mechanisms. About 70% of cases of both disorders are due to deletions at this locus, some of which are too small to be visible by chromosome banding though they may be detected by FISH (Nicholls, 1993). Most of the remainder are due to uniparental disomy (UPD) in Prader-Willi syndrome (PWS) and point mutations in Angelman syndrome (AS). About 10% of AS cases are due to an imprinting defect, while a smaller proportion (3–5%) are due to UPD. The small fraction of PWS cases not due to deletion or UPD apparently involve an imprinting defect. Owing to the imprinting phenomenon active at this locus, the AS gene (*UBE3A*) is expressed only on the maternally inherited chromosome 15 (Knoll et al., 1989), while the *PWS* gene (which is still not identified) is expressed only on the paternally inherited chromosome. Thus, loss of maternal *UBE3A* gene expression by either deletion or UPD for the paternal allele will produce AS, while loss of the paternal PWS gene by either deletion or

UPD for the maternal allele will produce AS. As mentioned, loss of *UBE3A* function through point mutation is also seen in AS, but whether or not it occurs in PWS will not be known until the gene is identified. And either disorder can also be produced by aberrant parental gene expression due to a primary imprinting defect.

Molecular genetic testing for these disorders is aimed at tracking the maternal and paternal alleles and determining whether one or the other is either missing (deletion) or duplicated (UPD); obviously, the UPD mechanism results in both duplication of one allele and loss of the other. The two parental alleles can be distinguished from one another because of the differential methylation that occurs at this locus, using either Southern blot following digestion of patient DNA with a methylation-sensitive restriction enzyme (van den Ouweland et al., 1995), or by methylation-sensitive PCR (Kosaki et al., 1997). A missing maternal allele (the upper band on the Southern blot, since it is not cleaved by the methylation-sensitive restriction enzyme) is diagnostic of AS, while a missing paternal allele (the lower band on Southern blot) indicates PWS (Fig. 26.7). Neither of these approaches can distinguish between the deletion and UPD mechanisms, however, though in actual practice the difference is not critical since both have very low recurrence risks. Documentation of UPD requires microsatellite analysis of chromosome 15 in the patient and parents, demonstrating homozygosity for the polymorphic alleles. PWS or AS caused by imprinting defects (presumably involving aberrant methylation) will also not be distinguished by these methods (though the tests will still be positive), which is unfortunate because those cases do have a much higher recurrence risk (Burger et al., 1997); but to prove that mechanism is really a research investigation. Yet another approach, at least for PWS, is by studying transcriptional expression of *SNRPN*, a gene located in the PWS-deleted region, using reverse transcription-PCR (RT-PCR) (Wevrick and Francke, 1996).

Familial cancer syndromes

The counseling and diagnosis of hereditary cancers represents a new paradigm for the specialty of medical genetics, and one with which it has yet to come completely to terms. Indeed, it is safe to say that it would not even be part of the specialty, remaining instead within the exclusive domain of oncologists, were it not for the advent of molecular diagnostic testing with all its risks and complexities. After all, familial cancers have always been with us, but they have come to the forefront of public consciousness only recently

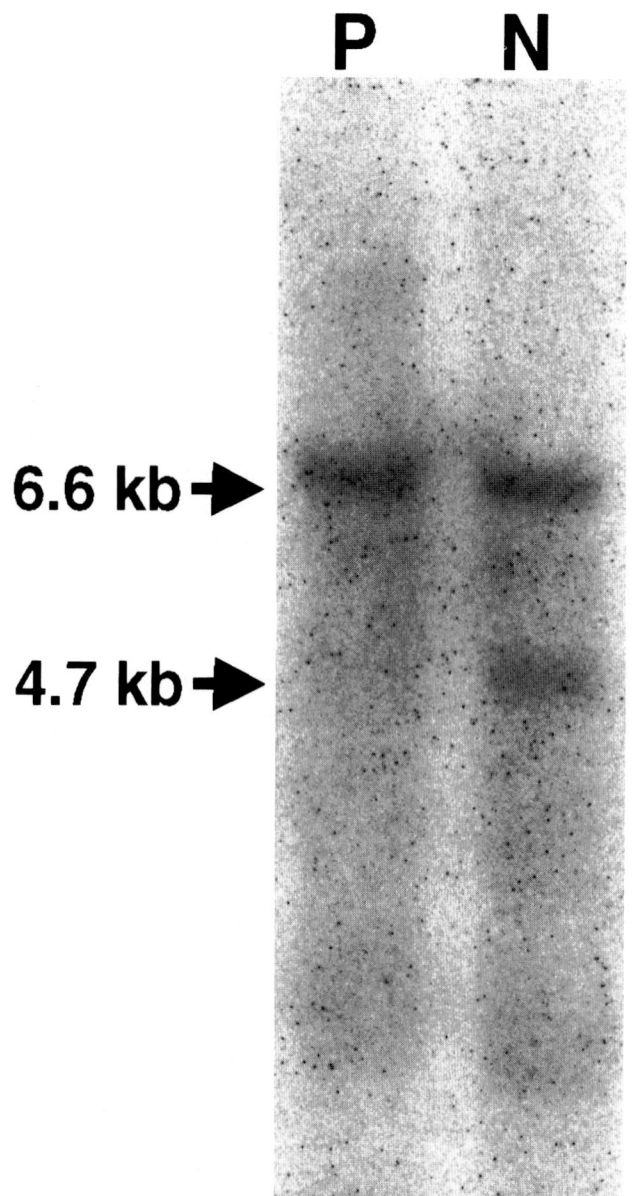

P   N

6.6 kb →

4.7 kb →

Fig. 26.7. Southern blot methylation analysis of the Prader-Willi/Angelman region on chromosome 15, using the PW71 (D15S63) probe (van den Ouweland et al, 1995). P, patient with Prader-Willi syndrome showing absence of the paternal allele (4.7 kb band); N, normal control showing presence of both paternal and maternal allelic bands.

because there are now predictive tests for at least some of them. In most cases these are not simple tests with clearcut results; extreme mutational heterogeneity and variable penetrance make their performance and interpretation quite difficult. These factors, and the ever-present risks of insurance discrimination and adverse psychosocial impact, have impelled internists, surgeons and oncologists to refer these cases to geneticists at the time DNA testing is considered, and have led to practice guidelines mandating pre- and post-test genetic counseling for some of them. Indeed, there are

documented cases of serious misinformation ensuing when these procedures are not followed (Giardello et al., 1997).

There are at least 35 strongly heritable syndromes in which various cancers are a primary manifestation (Lindor et al., 1998). This section will consider only those autosomal dominant forms for which DNA testing has become prevalent. All of them have in common a pathogenetic mechanism fitting the classical tumor suppressor gene model.

FAMILIAL BREAST/OVARIAN CANCER

While it was the retinoblastoma gene many years before that first defined the "two-hit" model of dominantly inherited cancer, it was the discovery of the *BRCA1* and *BRCA2* genes that really put familial cancer on the map for the medical genetics community and led to only the second routinely offered predictive genetic test after Huntington disease. In fact, the two tests are often discussed as instructive analogies for one another, yet they could hardly be more different. Mutations in the HD gene show virtually 100% penetrance, giving the DNA test an extraordinarily high predictive value, while *BRCA1/2* mutations may only be 50–85% penetrant in various families (Frank, 1999). HD has no prevention or treatment (yet), while breast cancer (and to a much lesser extent ovarian cancer) can be prevented in some cases by prophylactic surgery and/or medication, and screened for early detection. Breast cancer is one of the most common serious diseases in medicine, affecting roughly 1 in 9 women, though it is important to keep in mind that the *BRCA1/2* genes account for only 10% of this incidence at best. Finally, and most important from the perspective of this chapter, HD shows only a single species of easily detectable mutation (the CAG triplet repeat expansion), while *BRCA1/2* mutations are extremely heterogeneous and not yet completely characterized.

Because of its difficulty and expense, the potential risk of insurance discrimination, and the not uncommon finding of nucleotide changes of unknown significance within the gene (Shattuck-Eidens et al., 1997) imparting even more uncertainty to the patient than she had before the test, *BRCA* testing should never be undertaken lightly. There is a general consensus that testing not be encouraged unless the a priori risk of the proband testing positive exceeds 10%, and there are several formulas for making this estimation based on family history, ethnicity, and other factors (Shattuck-Eidens et al., 1997; Couch et al., 1997; Frank et al., 1998). And of course, testing of minors should not be considered outside of exceptional circumstances, since there is great risk of unnecessary stigmatization for a condition that has no symptomatic onset or clinical intervention until adulthood.

The *BRCA1/2* genes are very large and there are well over 200 mutations reported, spread diffusely across the length of both genes. In this sense they are similar, from a molecular testing point of view, to the *CFTR* gene. However, while the clinical impact of missing a carrier of a rare *CFTR* mutation in a population screening program does not justify the cost of sequencing the gene, the adverse consequences of missing a *BRCA* mutation in a presymptomatic test are great enough that full sequencing of both genes is justified despite the cost (assuming there was a strong enough family history to consider testing in the first place). Such methodology is available in only a few laboratories and is indeed quite expensive, especially considering that some women prefer to pay the cost out of pocket because of fears of insurance discrimination. Patients testing negative must be cautioned that even complete sequencing could potentially miss a mutation in an unusual location (outside the coding region), and also that it is possible the cancer in their family was due to a non-*BRCA* etiology.

There are two major exceptions to the need for complete gene sequencing in *BRCA* testing. One is the situation in which the mutation in the family is already known from prior testing of an index case (something which should always be sought, even if it means testing archival tissue from a deceased affected relative). The other is in the Ashkenazi Jewish population, in which three recurring mutations account for the vast majority (at least 90%) of *BRCA* carriers: 185delAG and 5382insC in BRCA1 and 174delT in BRCA2 (Struewing et al., 1997). Individuals in this ethnic group can be offered a limited screening panel using ASO probes or other simple methods at much reduced cost, though if they test negative in the absence of a known mutation in the index case, the difficult question of pursuing more comprehensive testing of low yield will come up.

In some respects *BRCA* testing is still in its infancy, and we are learning as we go along. Much longer clinical follow-up of women testing positive will be needed to determine the ultimate utility and predictive value of the test. In the meantime, very careful counseling regarding the risks and benefits of testing and the difficult clinical decisions that will ensue is absolutely essential.

HEREDITARY NON-POLYPOSIS COLON CANCER

Colon cancer is, like breast cancer, a common disease, and similarly about 10% of cases have a strong familial component. The dominant form of adult colon cancer, as distinguished from familial adenomatous polyposis, is hereditary non-polyposis colon cancer ([HNPCC], Lynch syndrome), characterized by predisposition to early-onset (average age 44 years) tumors mostly proximal to the splenic flexure. Some forms (Lynch II) are associated with other adenocarcinomas of the endometrium, ovary, small bowel, stomach, pancreas and other organs. Ascertainment of HNPCC families based on history is done using the Amsterdam criteria or its modifications (Lynch et al., 1997; Park et al., 1999).

At least five genes are known to be responsible for HNPCC: *hMSH2*, *hMLH1*, *hPMS1*, *hPMS2*, and *hMSH6*; the first two account for about 90% of the cases (Peltomaki and Vasen, 1997). The protein products of these genes are involved in DNA mismatch repair, producing the so-called "replication error" phenotype in tumor cells. The latter can be assayed in the molecular diagnostic laboratory by observing novel, nongermline bands in electrophoretic gels of short tandem repeat loci. Indeed, this is an easier test than searching for the many possible mutations in the five causative genes, though it is not entirely sensitive or specific for familial colon cancer. However, it may be helpful in determining if a colon tumor is due to HNPCC when the family history is incomplete or ambiguous (Lamberti et al., 1999). Direct mutation testing of the five dominant genes (or the two major ones) by PCR-amplification and sequencing is possible, but the number of genes and the extreme mutational heterogeneity of each makes the test technically difficult and expensive.

FAMILIAL ADENOMATOUS POLYPOSIS

This autosomal dominant syndrome is characterized by early onset (childhood or young adulthood) of large numbers of colonic polyps with high malignant potential, along with benign and malignant lesions in a number of other tissues. It is due to mutations in the *APC* gene, which are quite heterogeneous, though the majority are of the nonsense or frameshift class. For this reason the few laboratories offering this molecular test tend to begin with a protein truncation assay which picks up 70–80% of the mutations (Powell et al., 1993). This is one of the few predictive genetic tests acceptable for performance in children, because of the early onset of polyps and the onerous clinical surveillance procedures.

An unusual single nucleotide substitution, 11307K, creating a hypermutable tract in the *APC* gene, is found at high carrier frequency (6%) in the Ashkenazi Jewish population and seems to be associated with a two-fold increased risk of HNPCC-type colon cancer (not adenomatous polyposis) (Laken et al., 1997). The DNA test for this single mutation is easy, but the low penetrance of the alteration has kept the test in limbo since its discovery.

MULTIPLE ENDOCRINE NEOPLASIA

Multiple endocrine neoplasia (MEN) type 1 is characterized predominantly by neoplasms in the parathyroid, pancreas, adrenals, and pituitary. MEN type 2 features medullary thyroid cancer, pheochromocytoma, and hyperparathyroidism. A subtype, MEN2B, is further characterized by marfanoid habitus, ganglioneuromas and mucosal neuromas.

The gene for MEN2, the *RET* proto-oncogene, was discovered first, and DNA testing has proven quite valuable for at-risk family members. Indeed, the *RET* gene seems to be everything the *BRCA* genes are not: it contains a limited number of mutations localized to a few exons, and the penetrance is virtually 100%. In fact, most of the mutations in MEN2A are found in exons 10 and 11, with a single cysteine codon, #634, most commonly affected with every possible missense substitution of its three nucleotides. Less common mutations have also been found in exons 13 and 14 (Decker and Peacock, 1997). Furthermore, almost all cases of MEN2B, which have a unique presentation, show a single missense mutation at codon 918 in exon 16. Thus, molecular genetic testing for MEN2 is very straightforward, typically involving ASO probes or limited sequencing of the mutable exons to identify almost all carriers. Because the penetrance is so high and the highly aggressive medullary thyroid cancers can occur in childhood, *RET* gene analysis is another predictive genetic test indicated for use in presymptomatic children.

The MEN1 gene (designated simply *MEN1*) was identified more recently (Guru et al., 1998), and the range of mutations is still being explored. Testing is available in only a few laboratories.

Mitochondrial DNA disorders

Lastly, we must not forget about "the *other* human genome", the one that exists outside the nucleus, in those energy-generating organelles called mitochondria. Notwithstanding the emphasis of the Human Genome Project on identifying disease-associated associated genes in the nuclear genome, the mitochondrial genome is subject to pathogenic mutations as well, and thus is fair game for molecular diagnostic attention. In fact, the mutation or replication error rate of mitochondrial DNA is substantially higher than that of nuclear DNA, making the mitochondrial genome highly polymorphic between individuals and heteroplasmic within different cells and tissues of the same individual. This latter property in particular makes DNA-based diagnosis of mitochondrial disorders tricky and subtle. Because polymorphisms are usually homoplasmic and mutations are usually heteroplasmic, mitochondrial DNA diagnostic techniques must be of sufficient sensitivity to detect alterations in a fraction, or even a minority, of cells, yet of sufficient specificity and clinical predictive value to distinguish them from benign polymorphisms.

The 16.5-kb mitochondrial genome carries genes for 13 polypeptides (components of the respiratory chain), 22 tRNAs and two rRNAs, and mutations may be found in any one of them. Over 50 mutations are already catalogued, and it appears that many more are likely to be discovered (Kogelnik et al., 1996). In working up a patient with a suspected mitochondrial myopathy or neuropathy of unknown type, it would thus be optimal if the entire mitochondrial genome could be screened for mutations, either by DNA sequencing or by various mutation scanning techniques such as temperature gradient electrophoresis (Chen et al., 1999). But since this approach may be overly costly or otherwise impractical, a compromise is to test first for some of the recurring mutations associated with particular disorders, such as the 11778 mutation which is found in 50–70% of patients with Leber's hereditary optic atrophy or the 3243 mutation found in a large proportion of patients with MELAS (myopathy, encephalopathy, lactic acidosis and stroke-like episodes) (Schapira, 1993). Laboratories may therefore offer one or more core mutation panels to be employed as a first-tier test depending upon the clinical presentation of the patient, to be followed by another panel or a wider mutation scanning method if the first test is negative (Simon and Johns, 1999). The protocol requires close communication with the referring physician in order to decide which panel to utilize and just how far to pursue a mitochondrial etiology that may in fact never be found. In embarking on such testing, the phenomenon of heteroplasmy must always be at the top of one's mind, even from the point of specimen collection: mitochondrial DNA testing may require sampling of the affected tissue, rather than simple phlebotomy, in order to increase the chances of finding the causative mutation. And of course, with its great molecular heterogeneity yet limited genome size, mitochondrial genetics cries out for the advent of a practical "mitochondrial DNA chip".

Quality assurance, reimbursement and regulatory issues

All clinical laboratories in the United States must adhere to the Clinical Laboratory Improvement Amendment (CLIA) guidelines as a minimal level of quality assurance. Since all molecular genetic tests are considered "high complexity", the regulations for that category must be followed. A problematic loophole has arisen from the fact that molecular genetic tests had not been listed specifically in the existing CLIA regulations, but this situation is being rectified at time of this writing. For this reason, and because the CLIA regulations are seen as minimal standards, professional organizations have developed more detailed and rigorous practice guidelines. The most important are those of the American College of Medical Genetics (American College of Medical Genetics, 1999b), the College of American Pathologists (College of American Pathologists, 2000), and the National Committee for Clinical Laboratory Standards (NCCLS, 2000). The CAP checklist is particularly crucial since it is used for inspection and accreditation of those laboratories that choose to submit to this agency which has been granted "deemed" status under CLIA. It and the ACMG guidelines are continually updated to reflect changes in techniques and maturation of the discipline. They contain many guidelines unique to molecular diagnostic laboratories, addressing such issues as PCR contamination, communication with genetic counselors, informed consent, interpretation of mutational heterogeneity, molecular genetics personnel qualifications, appropriateness of test requests, and so on. While some have argued that it is not within the purview of laboratories to serve as gatekeepers for such matters as informed consent and appropriate test ordering, in practice it often falls to them since primary care providers may not be aware of such criteria.

Quality assurance (QA) encompasses all aspects of testing, from requisitions to specimen receipt through performance, interpretation and reporting. In addition, recent initiatives by governmental and professional organizations have focused increasing attention on the need to include pre- and post-analytic factors within overall QA for genetic tests, especially those of a predictive nature. Tests must be validated both analytically and clinically prior to introduction, though that is often easier said than done, particularly for predisposition tests that may take decades to establish clinical predictive value. Even analytic validation and basic quality control can become problematic with the most modern molecular genetic technologies. For instance, the CLIA regulations stipulate that positive and negative controls must be run for each analyte tested. But if the "analyte" of molecular genetics is considered to be a nucleotide or a mutation, and hundreds or thousands of different ones are tested simultaneously on a DNA chip, how can so many controls be included or even obtained (if the mutations are rare)?

Especially in a field with few, if any, manufactured test kits available, and most tests developed in-house by the individual laboratories (so-called "home brews"), concern

has arisen regarding proper oversight of the QC elements of these tests. While it technically has the authority, the U.S. Food and Drug Administration (FDA) has thus far chosen not to attempt to license the myriad of home brew tests, for practical reasons as much as anything. A partial compromise was recently reached by making allowances for the use of "analyte-specific reagents" (including DNA probes and PCR primers) which could be accepted as components of in-house tests without specific licensure as long as they have been internally validated by the laboratory (Garrett and Ferreira-Gonzalez, 1996).

Another important component of QA is proficiency testing. This involves the regular shipment to laboratories of specimen unknowns which are analyzed, reported, and sometimes graded. Just as for controls, CLIA mandates that laboratories participate in proficiency testing programs for each analyte they test, and if an organized formal program is not available, they must revert to other means such as informal sample exchanges with another laboratory. At present a fairly successful and ever-expanding national program exists, co-developed by the College of American Pathologists and the American College of Medical Genetics.

Reimbursement for molecular genetic testing has been a particularly frustrating issue for the laboratories. These tests tend to be relatively expensive to perform, and are often considered esoteric or experimental by third-party payers (and the fact that virtually none of them is FDA-approved provides another potential excuse to deny coverage). Furthermore, since they are frequently performed on healthy individuals, the usual diagnostic/symptomatic indications for clinical laboratory testing are often absent. The acceptance and updating of essential procedural billing codes that more realistically represent the range and workload effort of modern molecular techniques is a step in the right direction (Grody and Watson, 1997). But the insurance industry and federal health care underwriters need to be brought up to speed so they can appreciate the public health benefits of supporting these diagnostic modalities. Lastly, there is great concern that the whole field might be priced out of existence if mandatory royalties for use of patented genes and mutations in clinical laboratory tests inordinately add to the cost.

Internet resources for molecular genetic testing

With the Human Genome Project producing an overwhelming information load and new genetic tests appearing almost every week, print sources in this field can never be up to date, and even if they were, it is difficult and time-consuming to extract the information needed, especially to answer an urgent clinical question. Fortunately, the genetics revolution has occurred at the same time as the informatics revolution, so computer technology can be used for rapid searching of relevant information that is constantly updated. The internet offers many sites with useful medical genetics content; listed here are some of the key resources available to assist those ordering or performing molecular genetic tests.

Most readers of this book will already be familiar with the "Online Mendelian Inheritance in Man" (OMIM) (http://www.ncbi.nlm.nih.gov/omim), the most comprehensive and up-to-date catalog of human genetic disorders available, currently boasting over 10,000 entries. Each disease entry includes information on the mapping and structure of the involved gene where known) and its mutations. "GeneTests" (http://genetests.org), formerly called Helix, is the primary listing of genetic testing labs, searchable by disease. It is extremely useful for those facing a patient in need of an "orphan" genetic test for a rare disease, when one does not know where in the country (or the world) it might be offered. But it is also an excellent referral source for more routine molecular genetic tests as well. Contact information for each laboratory is provided in order to address indications and requirements for testing prior to sending a specimen. GeneTeats (http://geneclinics.org) is the newer sister site of GeneClinics, providing detailed background educational material on the major disorders subject to molecular genetic testing, including information on clinical manifestations, the molecular pathology of the gene, and interpretation of DNA test results. "GeneCards" (http://www.bioinformatics.weizman.ac.il/cards) is structured like an encyclopedia, with entries on human genes, their protein products, and their associated genetic disorders. Providing even finer detail, the "Human GeneMutationDatabase"(http://www.uwcm.ac.uk/uwcm/mg/ hgmd.html) is the most comprehensive, continually updated listing of molecular alterations, currently cataloging over 21,000 reported mutations in over 1000 human genes. For those who prefer a more newsy, conversational approach, "GeneSage" (http://www.genesage.com) is one of several new genetics-related internet sites featuring reports on the latest genetics news, information on genetic diseases, and a directory of genetic testing and clinical genetics resources.

The web sites of professional organizations can also be useful, both as starting points for additional links and as sources of educational programs. Most of the important ones are listed at "A World of Genetic Societies" (http://www.faseb.org/genetics), which contains links to the official sites for such organizations as the American Society of Human Genetics, the American College of Medical Genetics,

the National Society of Genetic Counselors, etc. The "National Coalition for Health Professional Education in Genetics" (http://www.nchpeg.org) serves as a clearing-house for a number of professionally-oriented genetics information websites. "The Genetic Alliance" (http://www.geneticalliance.org) is the best source for listings of patient support groups for genetic diseases, including many rare diseases, searchable by disease. The "College of American Pathologists" website (http://www.cap.org) contains the most up-to-date version of the Molecular Pathology laboratory inspection Checklist, and the website of the "American College of Medical Genetics" (http://www.faseb.org/genetics/acmg) features its own Standards and Guidelines document. Lastly, for those desiring a more basic introduction to the field, "The DNA Learning Center" (http://vector.cshl.org), based at Cold Spring Harbor Laboratories, contains multimedia tutorials on introductory molecular biology concepts and history of the discipline.

The future of molecular genetic testing: microarrays

Despite their birth in fits and starts, a bewildering variety of competing platforms, and a general sense that at time of this writing their hype exceeds their actual accomplishments, there can be little doubt that oligonucleotide microarrays, or "DNA chips", truly represent the wave of the future in molecular diagnostics. This is especially true for the screening of genetic diseases with many possible mutations, a major theme of this chapter. Based on the fundamental affinity of complementary strands of nucleic acids to anneal to their perfect complements, DNA microarrays are, quite simply, exaggerated and miniaturized reverse dot-blots. That is, the "probe" DNA is attached to a solid surface, and the experimental sample or "target" DNA is free in solution. The probe is attached in a repetitive geometric grid pattern (Fig. 26.8); hence the term "array". The ultimate power of the technology lies primarily in the awesome benefits of sheer, brute number—thousands of genes and sequences are screened at one time, in one instantaneous, massive parallel experiment.

To date DNA microarrays have most frequently been utilized in research studies of cellular expression patterns generated by capturing a "snapshot" of cellular mRNA content, which relates directly to gene activity. A comparison of gene expression between any two distinct cell populations provides a rapid means to identify the genotypic components that define the functional difference between the populations. Because numerous genes can be assayed at

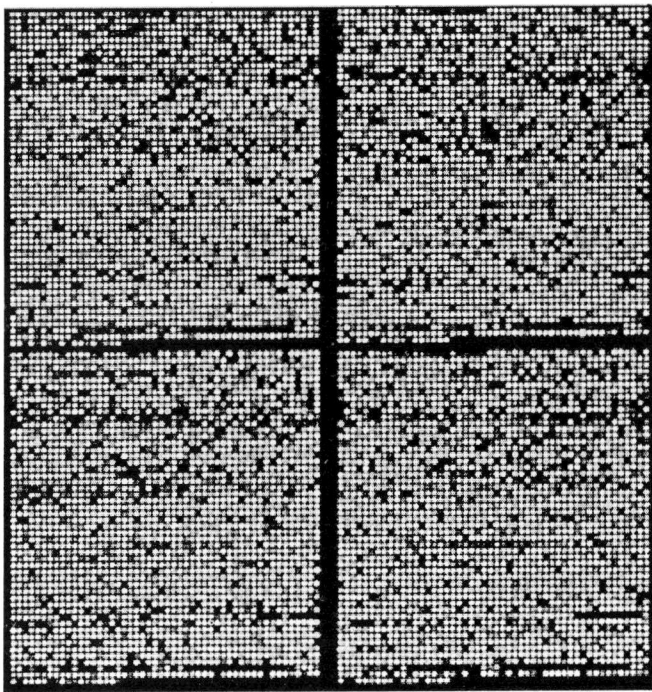

Fig. 26.8. DNA microarray chip, showing the fluorescent results of thousands of individual probe-target hybridizations.

BASIC ARRAY TECHNOLOGY

Several scientific and technological developments have converged to drive the microarray field. In addition to the dramatically increased availability of gene sequence information accruing from the private and public genome sequencing efforts, two concomitant technological advances fueled the microarray revolution: robotic printing techniques on solid supports such as glass, and the adaption of semiconductor and photolithography technology for in situ oligonucleotide probe construction (Fig. 26.9). The former is used to produce arrays principally used in expression studies, while the latter is frequently applied to sequence-based and genotyping analysis, but there is considerable overlap. In another variation, microelectronic chips use an active semiconductor at each test site instead of a passive glass surface for probe attachment. Each site is connected and controlled electronically through a computer. This in essence allows for intelligent and precise assay parameterization, and in a real way brings molecular biology under microelectronic control. Advantages to this platform include improved sensitivity through electronic target concentration and electronically adjustable stringency.

GENOTYPING APPLICATIONS

There are two general approaches to array-based mutation analysis. In the first, a probe panel is created to match all possible known sequences of interest, similar to traditional ASO probe applications. Alternatively, one may interrogate large regions of DNA in a resequencing fashion, which should elucidate all known *and* unknown mutations in the tested region. Array-based sequence analysis methods may be designed to interrogate a single base or, when performed sequentially or in parallel on a large array platform, numerous bases. Most sequence analysis techniques require previous knowledge of a reference sequence so that probes may be constructed relating to this sequence. Another approach, called loss-of-signal analysis, uses only wild type probes on the array. The loss of signal refers to a lack of hybridization when the target has any sequence change that deviates from wild type or other reference. Since the probes are designed to be perfect matches to that sequence only, a homozygous sequence change in the wild-type or reference target yields no signal, and a heterozygous change provides a 50% signal. Because this strategy does not require probes complementary to all of the possible base substitutions at each site, the total number of probes required is reduced. In order to interrogate a string of N bases on one strand for any sequence change, a minimum of 1(N) tiling probes (of any probe length) is needed to overlap the region (for both

one time, their interactions may be analyzed in a more global fashion, closely echoing the normal interplay of physiologic function. This may be likened to watching a football game across the entire field rather than focusing on a single player.

But perhaps the most obvious anticipated application of this technology is in clinical molecular diagnostics, especially in the fields of microbiology, pathology and genetics, where the arrayed probes could represent sequences specific for a spectrum of infectious organisms, malignant tissues or hereditary mutations, respectively. The technology promises to positively impact diagnostic speed, accuracy, comprehensiveness, and ultimately treatment efficacy. For example, of the hundreds of possible mutations responsible for cystic fibrosis or β-thalassemia, it is currently practical to screen for only a few of the most common known mutations, leaving a significant uncertainty to negative test results. A single DNA microarray could potentially contain a full library of sequences complementary to the entire gene and regulatory sequences, which could then be screened for all known and novel mutations, with great sensitivity and specificity. Still, everyday application of the technology has not yet crossed appreciably from the research laboratory to the clinical laboratory, primarily due to considerations of cost, lagging assay development, and robustness of the developed assays.

Cycle 1

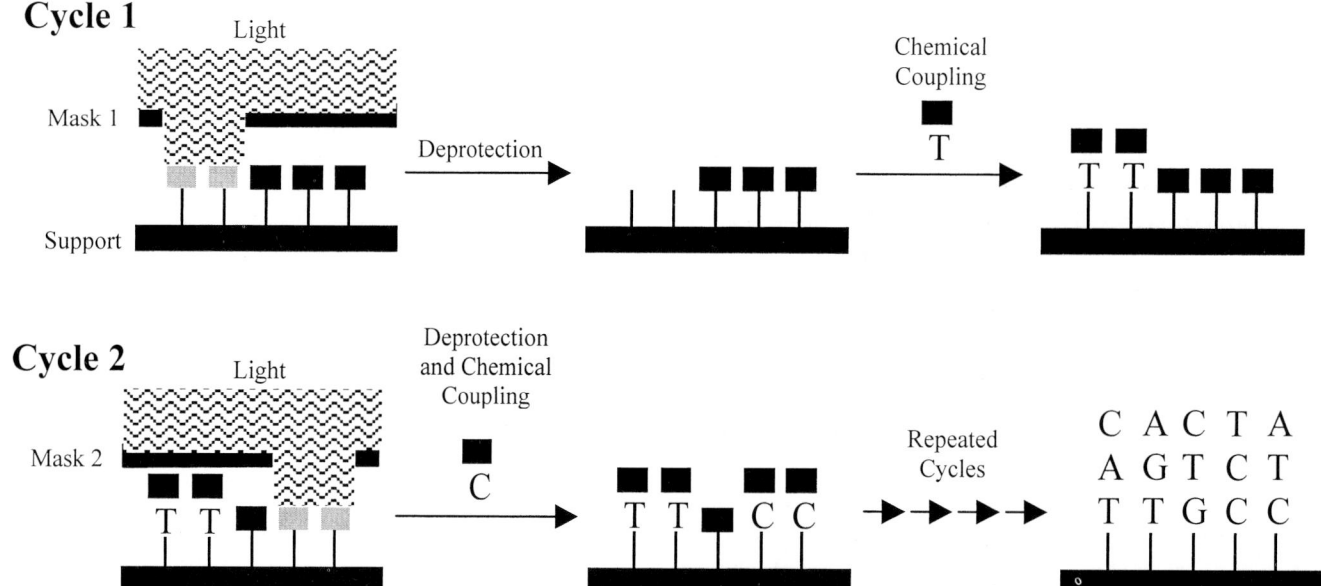

Cycle 2

Fig. 26.9. Construction of a DNA microarray by photolithography and in situ oligonucleotide synthesis. The substrate is first prepared with photolabile protecting groups which can be deprotected when exposed to light. Several masks are used which, at each pass, allow the light to come in contact with the substrate at pre-defined locations. Starting with the 3' nucleotide, an oligonucleotide chain is constructed, adding one base at a time as well as another protecting group. After sequential deprotection and synthesis steps, a precise array of oligonucleotides is constructed. (Adapted from Lipshutz et al., 1999, with permission.)

strands, the number of probes is 2(N)). For example, *BRCA1* has 5.4 kb of coding sequence; to screen both strands of the entire open reading frame, a minimum of 10,800 probes would be required. A disadvantage of this method is that a positive result does not define the nature of the alteration, only that one is present. As such, it is a screening tool, not a specific mutation identifier.

OBSTACLES AND IMPEDIMENTS

One trade-off for embracing microarrays as a platform for genetic testing is currently the small percentage of false negatives that one may find, especially on screening potential heterozygotes for several types of mutations. While the testing palate is greatly increased, so is some element of result uncertainty. Repetitive sequence elements are a particular problem with regard to specificity, and therefore the use of microarrays for analysis of diseases based on triplet repeats remains problematic. Manufacturing obstacles include batch-to-batch feature and array variability, contributing to data dropout and data skewing. Another obstacle is cost. Array cartridges containing the chip and microfluidic stations are complex and expensive as consumables and do not currently provide sufficient user-defined flexibilities. In addition, the complex supporting hardware remains cost-prohibitive for all but the largest commercial and academic laboratories.

Yet despite these hurdles, cautious but strong optimism continues to push the technology forward. The ultimate DNA microarray would incorporate the entire expressed human genome onto a single array, as well as all reasonable gene permutations. With the Human Genome Project approaching its conclusion and array technology speedily maturing, reaching this goal appears to be an inevitability. Another inevitability already in evidence is the application of this platform to other types of analytes, including protein/antibody-based array systems as well as cell and tissue microarrays, which likewise promise to greatly expand the power and scope of genetic testing.

Societal impact of the new genetic technology

The dawn of the twenty-first century has been called the beginning of the age of molecular medicine. Surely there can be no doubt that virtually every patient undergoing diagnosis or treatment in the coming decades will be involved in some sort of molecular genetic procedure. Even if it is on the treatment end (gene therapy), it will have been preceded by a molecular diagnostic procedure, since no patient can become a candidate for gene therapy until his precise molecular defect is known. Also certain is the fact that the diagnostic methods outlined in this chapter will become increasingly automated. Once a DNA chip becomes available as a completely closed system (theoretically) free of complex hands-on manipulations and expert troubleshooting, it could just as easily move into the automated clinical chemistry laboratory as stay in the molecular genetics laboratory. Such a development would not necessarily serve the patients well, however. For even as the technical aspects of DNA tests become easier, their interpretation becomes more complex. Professional organizations have emphasized repeatedly that pre- and post-analytic aspects of genetic tests are just as important as the technical procedures themselves. Even if the technical portion is highly accurate and robust, much harm can ensue if the test was ordered inappropriately or the results information conveyed improperly.

With PCR, microarray and other powerful technologies allowing ever more comprehensive genetic analyses on ever smaller specimens, many complex issues surrounding genetic privacy and informed consent have arisen. Both governmental and professional organizations are attempting to address these concerns through safeguards in the testing process as stipulated in professional practice guidelines and legislation. Especially thorny have been the concerns surrounding predictive genetic testing in presently healthy individuals, since a positive test result carries risks of stigmatization, discrimination, anxiety and depression. For these reasons, most professionals feel specific informed consent and strict confidentiality is prudent for predictive testing. Furthermore, to assure appropriate ordering and results counseling for complex predictive tests, a case can be made that the laboratory accept such orders primarily from genetics professionals or others with specific expertise in the field.

In the United States, more so than in other western countries, risk of insurance discrimination, which has been documented in limited numbers of patients (Billings et al., 1992), is often paramount, influencing many patients to pay out of pocket for expensive tests so that their insurance carrier will not be aware of the result or even the fact that the patient was being tested. Yet this raises other ethical issues such as inequitable access to testing, since only the economically well-off can afford to pay the cost themselves. Sometimes, though, these concerns become so blown out of proportion as to appear slightly irrational. Despite the very real threat, most medical geneticists and genetic coun-

selors would have a difficult time recalling even a single case in their experience of such blatant discrimination as loss of health insurance because of a genetic test result. Furthermore, we (and our patients) must always keep in mind the motivation for the test in the first place. For example, a woman may wish to pay for a predictive BRCA test out of pocket to keep the results secret from the insurance carrier, but if she tests positive and then desires a prophylactic mastectomy or oophorectomy, is she intending to pay for the costs of surgery out of pocket also? Probably not, and yet she cannot expect the insurance company to pay unless it is aware of the indication for surgery, which is the positive test result itself.

What can we expect in the future? A few years from now, will a drop of blood from every newborn, in addition to testing for PKU and other routine newborn screens, be applied to a DNA chip to predict which of hundreds of diseases that child will fall prey to in the course of his lifetime? Aside from the obvious ethical concerns in such a scenario, we should always remain aware of the limitations of molecular genetic testing, no matter how sophisticated the technology. Single genes and mutations rarely act entirely alone, and complex disorders clearly involve tens or perhaps thousands of genes all interacting at the DNA, RNA or protein level and with the outside environment. Thus, no DNA test, no matter how comprehensive, can ever tell the whole story. As the initial phase of the Human Genome Project is completed and we move on to the "post-genomic" or "proteomic" era, we will need to begin to think of genetic disease pathogenesis on a more "three-dimensional" level, taking into view the many interacting gene products in the nucleus and cytoplasm, as opposed to merely the "one-dimensional" string of nucleotides on a strand of DNA. Whether tests of such phenomena, once they arrive, will be part of the domain of the molecular genetics laboratory or will move into a new "proteomics" laboratory section is anyone's guess. But as we await such advances, we can still remain confident that the molecular genetic tests of today, and those added to the menu with each passing month, already offer a tremendous and irreplaceable service to many patients and their families, providing information and choices for their own lives and those of their offspring which had never been available before, in any form, in the entire history of medicine.

REFERENCES

Abbs S, Roberts RG, Mathew CG et al. (1990) Accurate assessment of intragenic recombination frequency within the Duchenne muscular dystrophy gene. Genomics 7:602–606

Akar N, Ozden A, Akar E et al. (1995) Discrimination of HbD Los Angeles (B121 Glu-Gln) and Hb Beograd (B121 Glu-Val) by dual restriction enzyme analysis. Am J Hemat 48:280–281

Almqvist EW, Bloch M, Brinkman R et al. (1999) A worldwide assessment of the frequency of suicide, suicide attempts, or psychiatric hospitalization after predictive testing for Huntington disease. Am J Hum Genet 64:1293–1304

Alter BP (1985) Antenatal diagnosis of thalassemia: a review. Ann NY Acad Sci 445:393–407

American College of Medical Genetics/American Society of Human Genetics Huntington Disease Genetic Testing Working Group (1998) ACMG/ASHG statement: Laboratory guidelines for Huntington disease genetic testing. Am J Hum Genet 62:1243–1247

American College of Medical Genetics (1999a) Genetic Susceptibility to Breast and Ovarian Cancer: Assessment, Counseling and Testing Guidelines—Executive Summary. American College of Medical Genetics and New York State Department of Health, Albany

American College of Medical Genetics (1999b) Standards and Guidelines for Clinical Genetics Laboratories, 2nd edn. Bethesda: American College of Medical Genetics (http://www.faseb.org/genetics/acmg)

Anguiano A, Oates RD, Amos JA et al. (1992) Congenital bilateral absence of the vas deferens: A primarily genital form of cystic fibrosis. JAMA 267:1794–1797

Bakker E, Van Broeckhoven C, Bonten EJ et al. (1987) Germline mosaicism and Duchenne muscular dystrophy mutations. Nature 329:554–556

Barany F (1991) Genetic disease detection and DNA amplification using cloned thermostable ligase. Proc Natl Acad of Sci USA 88:189–193

Beggs AH, Koenig M, Boyce FM et al. (1990) Detection of 98% of DMD/BMD gene deletions by polymerase chain reaction. Hum Genet 86:45–48

Billings PR, Kohn MA, de Cuervas M et al. (1992) Discrimination as a consequence of genetic testing. Am J Hum Genet 50:476–482

Brook JD, McCurrach ME, Harley HG et al. (1992) Molecular basis of myotonic dystrophy: Expansion of a trinucleotide (CTG) repeat at the 3′ end of a transcript encoding a protein kinase family member. Cell 68:799–808

Burger J, Buiting K, Dittrich B et al. (1997) Different mechanisms and recurrence risks of imprinting defects in Angelman syndrome. Am J Hum Genet 61:88–93

Cai SP, Kan YW (1990) Identification of the multiple β-thalassemia mutations by denaturing gradient gel electrophoresis. J Clin Invest 85:550–553

Cai SP, Wall J, Kan YW et al. (1994) Reverse dot blot probes for the screening of β-thalassemia mutations in Asians and American blacks. Hum Mutat 3:59–63

Campuzano V, Montermini L, Molto MD et al. (1996) Friedreich's ataxia: Autosomal recessive disease caused by an intronic GAA triplet repeat expansion. Science 271:1423–1427

Cao A, Galanello R, Rosatelli MC (1998) Prenatal diagnosis and screening of the haemoglobinopathies. Balliees Clin Haematol 11:215–238

Chamberlain JS, Gibbs RA, Ranier JE et al. (1988) Deletion screening of the Duchenne muscular dystrophy locus via multiplex DNA amplification. Nucleic Acids 16:11141–11156

Chang JC, Kan YW (1982) A sensitive new prenatal test for sickle-cell anemia. N Engl J Med 307:30–32

Chehab FF, Kan YW (1990) Detection of sickle cell anaemia mutation by colour DNA amplification. Lancet 335:15–17

Chen T-J, Boles RG, Wong L-J (1999) Detection of mitochondrial DNA mutations by temporal temperature gradient gel electrophoresis. Clin Chem 45:1162–1167

Chong GL, Thibodeau SN (1990) A simple assay for the screening of the cystic fibrosis allele in carriers of the phe 508 deletion mutation. Mayo Clin Proc 65:1072–1076

Clemens PR, Fenwick RG, Chamberlain JS et al. (1991) Carrier detection and prenatal diagnosis in Duchenne and Becker muscular

dystrophy families, using dinucleotide repeat polymorphisms. Am J Hum Genet 49:951–960

Cohn JA, Bornstein JD, Jowell PS (2000) Cystic fibrosis mutations and genetic predisposition to idiopathic chronic pancreatitis. Med Clin North Am 84:621–631

College of American Pathologists (2000) Molecular Pathology: CAP Checklist 12. Chicago: College of American Pathologists (http://www.cap.org)

Coltrera MD, Mathison SM, Goodpaster TA, Gown AM (2000) Abnormal expression of the cystic fibrosis transmembrane regulator in chronic sinusitis in cystic fibrosis and non-cystic fibrosis patients. Ann Otol Rhinol Laryngol 108:576–581

Conner BJ, Reyes AA, Morin C et al. (1983) Detection of sickle cell β^S-globlin allele by hybridization with synthetic oligonucleotides. Proc Natl Acad Sci USA 80:278–282

Couch FJ, DeShano ML, Blackwood MA et al. (1997) BRCA1 mutations in women attending clinics that evaluate the risk of breast cancer. N Engl J Med 336:1409–1415

Crawford DHG, Jazwinska EC, Cullen LM, Powell LW (1998) Expression of HLA-linked hemochromatosis in subjects homozygous or heterozygous for the C282Y mutation. Gastroenterology 114:1003–1008

Cutting GR, Kasch LM, Rosenstein BJ et al. (1990) Two patients with cystic fibrosis, nonsense mutations in each cystic fibrosis gene, and mild pulmonary disease. N Engl J Med 323:1685–1689

Cystic Fibrosis Foundation (1998) Cystic Fibrosis Foundation Patient Registry Annual Data Report

Cystic Fibrosis Genetic Analysis Consortium (1994) Population variations of common cystic fibrosis mutations. Hum Mutat 4:167–177

Cystic Fibrosis Genotype-Phenotype Consortium (1993) Correlation between genotype and phenotype in patients with cystic fibrosis. N Engl J Med 329:1308–1313

Darras BT, Francke U (1988) Normal human genomic restriction-fragment patterns and polymorphisms revealed by hybridization with the entire dystrophin cDNA. Am J Hum Genet 43:612–619

David G, Abbas N, Stevanin G et al. (1997) Cloning of the SCA7 gene reveals a highly unstable CAG repeat expansion. Nat Genet 17:65–70

Decker RA, Peacock ML (1997) Update on the profile of multiple endocrine neoplasia type 2a RET mutations: Practical issues and implications for genetic testing. Cancer 80:557–568

DeMarchi JM, Beaudet AL, Caskey CT, Richards CS (1994) Experience of an academic reference laboratory using automation for analysis of cystic fibrosis mutations. Arch Pathol Lab Med 118:26–32

Di Naro E, Ghezzi F, Vitucci A et al. (2000) Prenatal diagnosis of beta-thalassaemia using fetal erythroblasts enriched from maternal blood by a novel gradient. Mol Hum Reprod 6:571–574

Eichler EE, Richards S, Gibbs RA, Nelson DL (1994) Fine structure of the human FMR1 gene. Hum Mol Genet 3:684–685

Emery AEH, King B (1971) Pregnancy and serum creatine-kinase levels in potential carriers of Duchenne X-linked muscular dystrophy. Lancet 15:1013

Feder JN, Gnirke A, Thomas W et al. (1996) A novel MHC class I-like gene is mutated in patients with hereditary haemochromatosis. Nat Genet 13:399–408

Flint J, Hardin RM, Boyce AL et al. (1998) The population genetics of the haemoglobinopathies. Baillieres Clin Haematol 11:1–51

Forrest SM, Cross GS, Flint T et al. (1988) Further studies of gene deletions that cause Duchenne and Becker muscular dystrophies. Genomics 2:109–114

Frank TS (1999) Laboratory determination of hereditary susceptibility to breast and ovarian cancer. Arch Pathol Lab Med 123:1023–1026

Frank TS, Manley SA, Olopade OI et al. (1998) Sequence analysis of BRCA1 and BRCA2: Correlation of mutation with family history and ovarian cancer risk. J Clin Oncol 16:2417–2425

Garrett CT, Ferreira-Gonzalez A (1996) FDA regulation of analyte-specific reagents (ASRs): Implications for nucleic acid-based molecular testing. Diagn Molec Pathol 5:151–153

Gervais R, Dumur V, Rigot M-M et al. (1993) High frequency of the R117H cystic fibrosis mutation in patients with congenital absence of the vas deferens. N Engl J Med 328:446–447

Geschwind DH, Perlman S, Figueroa CP et al. (1997) The prevalence and wide clinical spectrum of the spinocerebellar ataxia type 2 trinucleotide repeat in patients with autosomal dominant cerebellar ataxia. Am J Hum Genet 60:842–850

Giardello FM, Brensinger JD, Persen GM et al. (1997) The use and interpretation of commercial APC gene testing for familial adenomatous polyposis. N Engl J Med 336:823–827

Gregg JP, Yamane A, Grody WW (1997) The prevalence of the factor V-Leiden mutation in four distinct American ethnic populations. Am J Med Genet 73:334–336

Grody WW (1999) Cystic fibrosis: Molecular diagnosis, population screening, and public policy. Arch Pathol Lab Med 123:1041–1046

Grody WW, Watson MS (1997) Those elusive molecular diagnostics CPT codes. Diagn Molec Pathol 6:131–133

Grody WW, Desnick RJ, Carpenter NJ, Noll WW (1998) Diversity of cystic fibrosis mutation screening practices. Am J Hum Genet 62:1252–1254

Grody WW, Cutting GR, Klinger KW (2001) Laboratory standards and guidelines for population based cystic fibrosis carrier screening. Genet Med 3:149–159

Gryfe R, Di Nicola N, Gallinger S, Redston M (1998) Somatic instability of the APC I1307K allele in colorectal neoplasia. Cancer Res 58:4040–4043

Guru SC, Manickam P, Crabtree JS et al. (1998) Identification and characterization of the multiple endocrine neoplasia type 1 (MEN1) gene. J Intern Med 243:433–439

Halbmayer WM, Kalhs T, Haushofer A et al. (1999) Venous thromboembolism at a young age in a brother and sister with coinheritance of homozygous 20210A/A prothrombin mutation and heterozygous 1691G/A factor V Leiden mutation. Blood Coagul Fibrinolysis 10:297–302

Handyside AH, Lesko JG, Tarin JJ et al. (1992) Birth of a normal girl after in vitro fertilization and preimplantation diagnostic testing for cystic fibrosis. N Engl J Med 327:905–909

Harris H, Scotcher D, Hartley N et al. (1993) Cystic fibrosis carrier testing in early pregnancy by general practitioners. BMJ 306:1580–1583

Highsmith WE, Burch LH, Zhou Z et al. (1994) A novel mutation in the cystic fibrosis gene in patients with pulmonary disease but normal sweat chloride concentrations. N Engl J Med 331:974–980

Hoffman EP, Fischbeck KH, Brown RH et al. (1988) Characterization of dystrophin in muscle-biopsy specimens from patients with Duchenne's or Becker's muscular dystrophy. N Engl J Med 318:1363–1368

Holmes SE, O'Hearn EE, McInnis MG et al. (1999) Expansion of a novel CAG trinucleotide repeat in the 5′ region of PPP2R2B is associated with SCA12. Nat Genet 23:391–392

Hu XY, Burghes AH, Ray PN et al. (1988) Partial gene duplication in Duchenne and Becker muscular dystrophies. J Med Genet 25:369–376

Huisman THJ, Carver MF (1998) The β- and α-thalassemia repository (9th edn, Part 1). Hemoglobin 22:169–195

Huntington's Disease Collaborative Research Group (1993) A novel gene containing a trinucleotide repeat that is expanded and unstable on Huntington's disease chromosome. Cell 72:971–983

Huntington's Disease Society of America (1989) Guidelines for Predictive Testing for Huntington's Disease. New York: HDSA.

Jazwinska EC, Lee SC, Webb SI et al. (1993) Localization of the hemochromatosis gene close to D6S105. Am J Hum Genet 53:347–352

Johnson JP, Vichinsky E, Hurst D et al. (1992) Differentiation of homozygous hemoglobin E from compound heterozygous hemoglobin E-β⁰-thalassemia by hemoglobin E mutation analysis. J Pediatr 120:775–779

Kan YW, Dozy AM (1978) Antenatal diagnosis of sickle-cell anaemia by DNA analysis of amniotic-fluid cells. Lancet 2:910–912

Kang SS, Wong PWK, Susmano A et al. (1991) Thermolabile methylenetetrahydrofolate reductase: An inherited risk factor for coronary artery disease. Am J Hum Genet 48:536–545

Kazazian HH Jr (1990) The thalassemia syndromes: molecular basis and prenatal diagnosis in 1990. Semin Hematol 27:209–228

Kawaguchi Y, Okamoto T, Taniwaki M et al. (1994) CAG expansions in a novel gene for Machado-Joseph disease at chromosome 14q32.1. Nat Genet 8:221–228

Kerem B-S, Rommens JM, Buchanan JA et al. (1989) Identification of the cystic fibrosis gene: Genetic analysis. Science 245:1073–1080

Kiesewetter S, Macek MJ, Davis C et al. (1993) A mutation in CFTR produces different phenotypes depending on chromosomal background. Nat Genet 5:274–277

Knoll JNM, Nicholls RD, Magenis RE et al. (1989) Angelman and Prader-Willi syndromes share a common chromosome 15 deletion but differ in parental origin of the deletion. Am J Med Genet 32:285–290

Kogelnik AM, Lott MY, Brown MD et al. (1996) A human mitochondrial genome database. Nucl Acids Res 24:177–179

Kosaki K, McGinniss MJ, Veraksa AN et al. (1997) Prader-Willi and Angelman syndromes: Diagnosis with a bisulfite-treated methylation-specific PCR method. Am J Med Genet 73:308–313

Kuliev A, Rechitsky S, Verlinsky O et al. (1999) Birth of healthy children after preimplantation diagnosis of thalassemias. J Assist Reprod Genet 16:207–215

Kupferminc MJ, Eldor A, Steinman N et al. (1999) Increased frequency of genetic thrombophilia in women with complications of pregnancy. N Engl J Med 340:9–13

La Spada AR, Wilson EM, Lubahn DB et al. (1991) Androgen receptor gene mutations in X-linked spinal and bulbar muscular atrophy. Nature 352:77–79

Laken SJ, Petersen GM, Gruber SB et al. (1997) Familial colorectal cancer in Ashkenazim due to a hypermutable tract in APC. Nature Genet 17:79–83

Lamberti C, Kruse R, Ruelfs C et al. (1999) Microsatellite instability—a useful diagnostic tool to select patients at high risk for hereditary non-polyposis colorectal cancer: A study in different groups of patients with colorectal cancer. Gut 44:839–43.

Lindor NM, Greene MH, Mayo Familial Cancer Program (1998) The concise handbook of family cancer syndromes. JNCI 90:1039–1071

Lipschutz RJ, Fodor SPA, Gingeras TR, Lockhart DJ (1999) High density synthetic oligonucleotide arrays. Nature Genet 21(Suppl):20–24

Lynch HT, Smyrk T, Lynch J (1997) An update of HNPCC (Lynch syndrome). Cancer Genet Cytogenet 93:84–99

Maggio A, Giambona A, Cai SP et al. (1993) Rapid and simultaneous typing of hemoglobin S, hemoglobin C, and seven Mediterranean β-thalassemia mutations by covalent reverse dot-blot analysis: Application to prenatal diagnosis in Sicily. Blood 81(1):239–242

Mao YP, Cremer M (1989) Detection of Duchenne muscular dystrophy carriers by dosage analysis using the DMD cDNA clone 8. Hum Genet 81:193–195

Merryweather-Clarke, AT, Pointon, JJ, Shearman, JD, Robson, KJ (1997) Global prevalence of putative haemochromatosis mutations. J Med Genet 34:275–278

Monaco AP, Bertelson CJ, Liechti-Gallati S et al. (1988) An explanation for the phenotypic differences between patients bearing partial deletions of the DMD locus. Genomics 2:90–95

NCCLS (2000) Molecular Diagnostic Methods for Genetic Diseases: Approved Guideline. NCCLS Document MM1-A. NCCLS: Wayne, PA.

Nelson DL (1995) The fragile X syndromes. Semin Cell Biol 6:5–11

Nicholls RD (1993) Genomic imprinting and uniparental disomy in Angelman and Prader-Willi syndromes: A review. Am J Hum Genet 46:16–25

Nolin SL, Lewis FA 3rd, Ye LL et al. (1996) Familial transmission of the FMR1 CGG repeat. Am J Hum Genet 59:1252–1261

Orban TI, Csokay B, Olah E (2000) Sequence alterations can mask each other's presence during screening with SSCP or heteroduplex analysis: BRCA genes as examples. BioTechniques 29:94–98

Oron-Karni V, Filon D, Oppenheim A, Rund D (1998) Rapid detection of the common Mediterranean α-globin deletions/rearrangements using PCR. Am J Hematol 58:306–310

Oudet C, Hanauer A, Clemens P et al. (1992) Two hot spots of recombination in the DMD gene correlate with the deletion prone regions. Hum Mol Genet 1:599–603

Park JG, Vasen HF, Park KJ et al. (1999) Suspected hereditary nonpolyposis colorectal cancer: International Collaborative Group on Hereditary Non-Polyposis Colorectal Cancer (ICG-HNPCC) criteria and results of genetic diagnosis. Dis Colon Rectum 42:710–5.

Paulson HL, Fischbeck KH (1996) Trinucleotide repeats in neurogenetic disorders. Annu Rev Neurosci 19:79–107

Peltomaki P, Vasen HF (1997) Mutations predisposing to hereditary nonpolyposis colorectal cancer: Database and results of a collaborative study. The International Collaborative Group on Hereditary Nonpolyposis Colorectal Cancer. Gastroenterology 113:1146–58.

Poort SR, Rosendaal FR, Reitsma PH, Bertina RM (1996) A common genetic variation in the 3′-untranslated region of the prothrombin gene is associated with elevated plasma prothrombin levels and an increase in venous thrombosis. Blood 88:3698–3703

Powell SM, Petersen GM, Krush AJ et al. (1993) Molecular diagnosis of familial adenomatous polyposis. N Engl J Med 329:1982–1987

Press RD (1999) Hereditary hemochromatosis: Impact of molecular and iron-based testing on diagnosis, treatment, and prevention of a common chronic disease. Arch Pathol Lab Med 123:1053–1059

Ridker PM, Hennekens CH, Lindpaintner et al. (1995) Mutation in the gene coding for coagulation factor V and the risk of myocardial infarction, stroke, and venous thrombosis in apparently healthy men. N Engl J Med 332:912–917

Ridker PM, Miletich JP, Hennekens CH, Buring JE (1997a) Ethnic distribution of factor V Leiden in 4047 men and women: Implications for venous thromboembolism screening. JAMA 227:1305–1307

Ridker PM, Hennekens CH, Selhub J et al. (1997b) Interrelation of hyperhomocyst(e)inemia, factor V Leiden, and risk of future venous thromboembolism. Circulation 95:1777–1782

Riordan JR, Rommens JM, Kerem B-S et al. (1989) Identification of the cystic fibrosis gene: Cloning and characterization of complementary DNA. Science 245:1066–1073

Risch N (1997) Haemochromatosis, HFE and genetic complexity. Nat Genet 17:375–376

Roberts RG, Coffey AJ, Bobrow M, Bentley DR (1993) Exon structure of the human dystrophin gene. Genomics 16:536–538

Robson KJ, Merryweather-Clarke AT, Pointon JJ et al. (2000) Diagnosis and management of haemochromatosis since the discovery of the HFE gene: A European experience. Br J Haematol 108:31–3

Rosenberg RN (1995) Spinocerebellar ataxias and ataxins. N Engl J Med 333:1351–1353

Rosendaal FR, Siscovick DS, Schwartz SM et al. (1997) A common prothrombin variant (20210 G to A) increases the risk of myocardial infarction in young women. Blood 90:1747–1750

Rubin EM, Kan YW (1985) A simple sensitive prenatal test for hydrops fetalis caused by α-thalassaemia. Lancet 2:75–77

Ryan D, Nuccie B, Arvan D (1999) Non-PCR-dependent detection of the factor V Leiden mutation from genomic DNA using a homogeneous invader microtiter plate assay. Molec Diagn 4:135–144

Sakamoto N, Chastain PD, Parniewski P et al. (1999) Sticky DNA: Self-association properties of long GAA. TTC repeats in R.R.Y triplex structures from Friedreich's ataxia. Mol Cell 3:465–475

Schapira AHV (1993) Mitochondrial cytopathies. Curr Opin Neurobiol 3:760–767

Sermon K, Seneca S, Vanderfaeillie A et al. (1999) Preimplantation diagnosis for fragile X syndrome based on the detection of the non-expanded paternal and maternal CGG. Prenat Diagn 19:1223–30

Servadio A, Koshy B, Armstrong D et al. (1995) Expression analysis of the ataxin-1 protein in tissues from normal and spinocerebellar ataxia type 1 individuals. Nat Genet 10:94–98

Shattuck-Eidens D, Oliphant A, McClure M et al. (1997) BRCA1 sequence analysis in women at high risk for susceptibility mutations: Risk factor analysis and implications for genetic testing. JAMA 278:1242–1250

Shuber AP, Michalowsky LA, Nass GS et al. (1997) High throughput parallel analysis of hundreds of patient samples for more than 100 mutations in multiple disease genes. Hum Holec Genet 6:337–347

Simon DK, Johns DR (1999) Mitochondrial disorders: Clinical and genetic features. Annu Rev Med 50:111–127

Smeets HJ, Smits AP, Verheij CE et al. (1995) Normal phenotype in two brothers with a full FMR1 mutation. Hum Mol Genet 4:2103–2108

Struewing JP, Hartge P, Wacholder S et al. (1997) The risk of cancer associated with specific mutations of BRCA1 and BRCA2 among Ashkenazi Jews. N Eng J Med 336:1401–8.

Sun X, Evatt B, Griffin JH (1994) Blood coagulation factor Va abnormality associated with resistance to activated protein C in venous thrombophilia. Blood 83:3120–3125

Suzuki A, Yoshida M, Hayashi K et al. (1994) Molecular organization at the glycoprotein-complex-binding site of dystrophin. Three dystrophin-associated proteins bind directly to the carboxy-terminal portion of dystrophin. Eur J Biochem 220:283–292

Tan JAMA, Tay JSH, Lin LI et al. (1994) The amplification refractory mutation system (ARMS): A rapid and direct prenatal diagnostic technique for β-thalassemia in Singapore. Prenatal Diagn 14:1077–1082

Telatar M, Grody WW (2000) Molecular genetic testing for familial Mediterranean fever. Molec Genet Metab 71:256–260

Timchenko LT, Caskey CT (1999) Triplet repeat disorders: Discussion of molecular mechanisms. Cell Mol Life Sci 55:1432–1447

van den Ouweland AMW, van der Est MN, Wesby-van Swaay E et al. (1995) DNA diagnosis of Prader-Willi and Angelman syndromes with the probe PW71 (D15S63). Hum Genet 95:562–567

van Essen AJ, Kneppers AL, van der Hout AH et al. (1997) The clinical and molecular genetic approach to Duchenne and Becker muscular dystrophy: An updated protocol. J Med Genet 34:805–812

Wall J, Cai S, Chehab FF (1995) A 31-mutation assay for cystic fibrosis testing in the clinical molecular diagnosis laboratory. Hum Mutat 5:33–338

Weatherall DJ, Clegg JB (1999) Genetic disorders of hemoglobin. Semin Hematol 36 (suppl 7):24–37

Wevrick R, Francke U (1996) Diagnostic test for the Prader-Willi syndrome by SNRPN expression in blood. Lancet 348:1068–1069

Wilfond BS, Fost N (1990) The cystic fibrosis gene: Medical and social implications for heterozygote detection. JAMA 263:2777–2783

Williams LC, Hegde MR, Nagappan R et al. (2000) Null alleles at the Huntington disease locus: implications for diagnostics and CAG repeat instability. Genet Test 4:55–60

Xu K, Shi ZM, Veeck LL et al. (1999) First unaffected pregnancy using preimplantation genetic diagnosis for sickle cell anemia. JAMA 281:1701–1706

Yamagishi H, Kato S, Hiraishi Y et al. (1996) Identification of carriers of Duchenne/Becker muscular dystrophy by a novel method based on detection of junction fragments in the dystrophin gene. J Med Genet 33:1027–1031

Yazawa I, Nukina N, Hashida H et al. (1995) Abnormal gene product identified in hereditary dentatorubral-pallidoluysian atrophy (DRPLA) brain. Nat Genet 10:99–103

Zhong XY, Holzgreve W, Hahn S (2000) Detection of fetal Rhesus D and sex using fetal DNA from maternal plasma by multiplex polymerase chain reaction. BJOG 107:766–9

Zhuchenko O, Bailey J, Bonnen P et al. (1997) Autosomal dominant cerebellar ataxia (SCA6) associated with small polyglutamine expansions in the α 1A-voltage-dependent calcium channel. Nat Genet 15:62–69

Zielenski J, Rozmahel R, Bozon D et al. (1991) Genomic DNA sequence of the cystic fibrosis transmembrane conductance regulator (CFTR) gene. Genomics 10:214–228

Heterozygote testing and carrier screening

Matthew J. McGinniss
Michael M. Kaback

Introduction

The specific biochemical or genetic abnormality in more than 400 inborn errors of metabolism in man have been determined (Scriver et al., 1995; McKusick 1998). Nearly all inborn errors are transmitted with either autosomal- or X-linked-recessive patterns of inheritance. The ability to identify such conditions in readily available tissues from affected individuals (probands) permits the rapid and accurate diagnosis of such disorders, minimizing the necessity for complicated and, at times, risk-associated diagnostic procedures. Many of these methods have also been applied to permit detection of such disorders in the fetus during early gestation. Such approaches can provide new and vital options in the genetic counseling for many families. And in some instances, the delineation of the underlying metabolic defect has enabled investigators to develop rational and effective therapies for some of these disorders (Desnick, 1990; Morsy et al., 1993; Mountain, 2000).

In addition to the diagnostic and possible therapeutic implications of such discoveries, comparable methodologies have been employed for the detection of heterozygous carriers of many of the recessive traits involved. Accordingly, not only is a striking deficiency of enzymatic activity, gene dosage, or metabolic dysfunction evident in the diagnosis of the homozygous or hemizygous state (the affected male with an X-linked-recessive disorder), but a distinct quantitative decrease of the same function can be demonstrated in the otherwise normal individual carrying the recessive allele. This capability to quantify gene dosage, and thereby to identify carriers of recessive traits, has been reported for many, but not all, of the inborn errors of metabolism where the primary defect is known.

Advances in the applications of molecular genetic techniques have made it possible to identify (either directly or indirectly) heterozygous carriers of an increasing number of mutant alleles. In some instances this may involve direct detection of the mutation (e.g., sickle-cell trait, or carriers of mutations for: β-thalassemia, cystic fibrosis, Tay-Sachs disease, fragile X syndrome). In some conditions where the gene has eluded isolation to date, or where extensive allelic diversity limits direct mutation detection, carrier identification has been achieved with the use of polymorphic genetic markers (restriction fragment length polymorphisms – RFLPs, or short tandem repeats – STRs) segregating in specific families linked very closely to the disease-associated gene (e.g., phenylketonuria (PKU), Duchenne muscular dystrophy (DMD), hemophilia A). In the latter approach, carrier detection through RFLP or STR analysis allows for a statistical probability of carrier (or disease) status to be ascertained. This method requires, however, that comparable linkage determinations be (or have been) carried out on DNA samples from affected members of the same family. In some families, such linkage studies may be totally uninformative while in other families the results of such studies may be only partially informative for carrier identification purposes. The increasing use of the highly informative STRs, or microsatellite markers, has greatly improved the informativeness of linkage testing for carrier detection. Clearly, as more gene loci are isolated, mapped and their nucleotide sequences defined, the applications of these and other sensitive and accurate molecular methods for mutant gene identification will increase.

It is not our intent in this chapter to review all known disorders and their current status regarding carrier detection. Rather, specific disorders will be cited as examples of the issue being discussed. Other chapters in this text will elaborate the fundamental inborn errors associated with such disorders, or deal specifically with issues of prenatal and neonatal screening as well as heterozygote detection. It is also important to make the distinction between heterozygote testing and carrier screening. Heterozygote testing is the use of specific assays to determine the genetic status of individuals already suspected to be at higher risk for an inherited disorder because of a family history or clinical symptoms (Andrews et al., 1994). In contrast, carrier screening is the use of genetic tests to evaluate populations or groups of individuals independent of a family history of a disorder, and without clinical symptoms.

Carrier screening in clinical practice

TO PREVENT ANXIETY IN FAMILY MEMBERS

When a patient is identified with an inborn error of metabolism or the family history reveals such a disorder in a close blood relative, the question of whether to test that individual and other family members for heterozygosity should be considered. In many instances where such tests are available and accurate, this can serve to reduce expressed or hidden anxieties in other family members. Since most of these disorders are individually rare, it is relatively unlikely that other family members need be too fearful of producing affected offspring. For example, taking a maximum risk situation, an American black individual whose brother or sister is a patient with sickle-cell anemia may be concerned about having affected children. Assuming they reproduce with another black person with *no known* sickle-cell anemia in the family – what are the actual risks? The unaffected sib (obviously not SS) of a person with sickle-cell anemia has two chances in three of having sickle trait (if born of the same parents as the patient with sickle-cell anemia). The approximate overall sickle trait frequency in American blacks is about one in ten. Therefore, the likelihood that this person will be at risk for sickle-cell anemia in his or her offspring is: $2/3 \times 1/10 = 1/15$. The likelihood that any given pregnancy will result in a child with sickle-cell anemia is 1/4 of that risk, or one in 60.

TO PREVENT SUBSEQUENT INTRAFAMILIAL CASES OF DISEASE

Although these statistics alone can be somewhat comforting, simple carrier detection studies in the appropriate

persons can put this question out of the realm of "calculation", and definitively establish if one or both individuals are carriers. If both prospective parents are found to be carriers, then comprehensive genetic counseling with a complete discussion of all available options can be initiated including prenatal diagnosis, gamete donation (e.g., sperm or ovum from an established noncarrier donor), preimplantation testing, etc. Where at-risk couples are identified, this can lead to prevention of subsequent intrafamilial cases of disease – a second major reason to consider carrier testing in such families.

MARITAL COUNSELING

A third rationale for carrier screening relates to marital counseling, particularly where consanguinity between prospective parents may exist. Because of religious, moral, or other concerns, individuals might also use information about their carrier status in their decision regarding mate selection. This is the practice in certain Hassidic Jewish communities where strong religious proscriptions against abortion exist (Merz, 1987). Since marriages are "arranged" (often in childhood) and require rabbinical approval, some rabbis have opted for Tay-Sachs disease (TSD) carrier testing among the children or adolescents of their community. Approval for marriage is withheld by the rabbi (to whom solely the results of carrier testing are conveyed) if two carriers are "matched". Alternative "arrangements" are then made without specifying the reason, thus avoiding family or individual stigmatization. While appropriate for individuals of this autocratic socio-religious belief system, generalization of this approach to other individuals or groups is likely to be highly problematic.

ARTIFICIAL INSEMINATION OR OVUM DONATION

Another important consideration for carrier testing is where artificial insemination or ovum donation is being considered by a couple as an alternative reproductive strategy to avoid the birth of a child affected with an autosomal-recessive or X-linked disorder. Potential sperm or ovum donors should be evaluated (where feasible and practical) by appropriate carrier screening tests to avoid what otherwise could be a most unfortunate tragedy. The authors are aware of two children with TSD, conceived by artificial insemination, born to two unrelated families who were attempting to have an unaffected child after they had had a previous child with this fatal condition. In another instance, screening of three medical students as potential sperm donors for a woman who had been previously identified as a TSD heterozygote, showed one of the three to be a TSD carrier also. Of course, he was excluded as a potential donor. Such screening, in addition to a through family history on all potential gamete donors for other relevant issues, can help avert tragedy.

Carrier screening in individuals of defined subpopulation groups

A list of relatively "common" autosomal recessive disorders (Table 27.1) seen in defined subpopulations in the USA is presented with data indicating the respective carrier frequency and newborn disease incidence in those ethnic groups. Gene frequencies and incidence of the disorder may vary considerably in the same ethnic groups in other parts of the world. The fact that selected genetic diseases occur predominantly in certain ethnic, religious, or racial groups is not surprising when one considers the relatively high degree of inbreeding seen in defined subpopulations (McKusick 1998; Ramot 1974). In addition to inbreeding, in some situations, selective environmental factors may have existed at some point in history that provided a biological (reproductive) advantage to carriers of the recessive gene (e.g., relative resistance to malaria in individuals who are heterozygous for sickle cell hemoglobin, β-thalassemia or G6PD deficiency). Because of this selective effect, the gene becomes "enriched" from one generation to the next in that population.

It should be emphasized that while many of these diseases are relatively rare, the frequency of carriers can be quite high. For example, the disease incidence of cystic fibrosis (CF) among caucasians of Northern European ancestry is approximately one in 2500 newborns, yet nearly one in 25 such individuals are carriers of a CF mutation. Similarly, the disease incidence for TSD among Ashkenazi Jewish newborns is about one in 3600, while the carrier rate in this population is approximately one in 30. Because of these population distributions and the availability of relatively simple, accurate, and inexpensive carrier detection methods it is possible to screen individuals in these groups and identify persons and, more critically, couples at risk for homozygous disease in their offspring before affected children are born. With comprehensive genetic counseling, and the important options that prenatal diagnosis can provide, many "at-risk" families, identified through screening such subpopulations, might choose to have only children unaffected with the disorder for which they are found at risk.

For those relatively "common" autosomal disorders which occur within defined ethnic groups, there is usually no known prior history of the disease in either side of the family. Such a positive history may be present in only 20% of instances where a child with such a disorder is diagnosed. For this reason, clinicians should consider carrier screening for all individuals in these subpopulation groups where heterozygote detection is readily available. Certainly, such testing and its implications should be thoroughly discussed with the patients – or they can be referred to appropriate regional agencies for such services. Not only is this considered optimal preventive medicine, but concern has arisen regarding the medicolegal implications of failing to do so (President's Commission 1983; Fost 1993).

TAY-SACHS DISEASE

Perhaps the most effective effort of this nature has been the experience with TSD carrier screening and prenatal diagnosis (Kaback et al., 1993; Kaplan, 1998). From 1970 (when serum carrier detection methods were first described) to 1999, community-based TSD education-screening-counseling programs have been inititated in Jewish communities throughout North America, as well as in Israel, South Africa, Europe, South America, and Australia. More than 1.4 million adults have been screened voluntarily and over 51,000 heterozygotes detected. Most

Table 27.1. Frequency and Incidence for Selected Autosomal-Recessive Disorders in Defined Ethnic Groups in the USA

Disease	Ethnic Group	Gene Frequency	Carrier Frequency	"At-Risk" Couple Frequency	Disease Incidence in Newborns
Sickle cell anemia	Blacks	0.040	0.080	1:150	1:600
Tay-Sachs disease	Ashkenazi Jews	0.016	0.032	1:900	1:3600
β-Thalassemia	Greeks, Italians	0.016	0.032	1:900	1:3600
α-Thalassemia	Southeast Asians and Chinese	0.020	0.040	1:625	1:2500
Cystic fibrosis	Northern Europeans	0.020	0.040	1:625	1:2500
Phenylketonuria	Northern Europeans	0.008	0.016	1:4000	1:16000

[a] Likelihood that both members of a couple are heterozygous for the same recessive allele (assuming nonconsanguinity and that both are of the same ethnic group).

critically, nearly 1400 couples – none of whom had an affected child previously – have been identified as being at risk for this fatal disorder in their offspring. Over 3200 pregnancies at risk for TSD have been monitored by amniocentesis or chorionic villus sampling, and the births of more than 625 affected infants destined to die with this disorder have been prevented. More importantly this approach has been associated with the birth of over 2550 healthy infants. Overall, these efforts have contributed to the more than 90% decline in the incidence of this disorder in Jewish infants throughout North America since 1970 (Desnick and Kaback, 2001).

β-THALASSEMIA

Similar efforts directed at the prevention of β-thalassemia through education, carrier screening, and prenatal diagnosis, have been initiated in several European countries and certain areas of North America. These programs have dramatically reduced the newborn incidence of β-thalassemia in several Mediterranean countries as well as in the Cypriot community in Britain (Modell and Mouzouras 1982; Cao et al., 1984; Kazazian, 1990). In Sardinia, for example, these preventative measures have reduced the incidence of disease by more than 94% of the prescreening levels (Cao et al., 1997).

SICKLE CELL ANEMIA

Screening for sickle cell trait has been initiated in several parts of the world (including the USA). Although the capability to diagnose homozygous sickle cell anemia in early fetal life is well established, through either amniocentesis or chorionic villus sampling, this alternative has not been widely adopted. This may reflect (at least in the USA) some of the complex socio-political issues associated with genetic screening of minority populations (Whitten 1973; Rutkow and Lipton 1974; Fletcher et al., 1985).

CYSTIC FIBROSIS

The cloning of the CF gene in 1989 and subsequent identification of the most common CF mutations has allowed for the direct detection of carriers of 50% to 97% of the 24 most common mutations (The Cystic Fibrosis Genetic Analysis Consortium, 1994). In some parts of the world this has led to widespread CF carrier screening. However, several assemblages (ASHG 1990, 1992; NIH 1990; ACMG 1997) have not yet advocated mass CF carrier screening. This concern is based on the allelic diversity of

CF mutations (over 800 mutations have been identified to date) which limits the sensitivity of carrier detection. In addition, the lack of guidelines for appropriate education of health care providers and consumers, the complex genetic counseling issues involved, the need for appropriate laboratory quality control and proficiency testing, as well as other related issues makes wide-scale screening for CF potentially highly complex. Results of pilot studies (Rowley et al., 1997) suggest that more effective pretest patient education by primary care providers would help avoid some of the adverse outcomes noted such as inadequate informed consent. In 1997, a consensus panel convened by the National Institutes of Health recommended that CF carrier testing be offered to adults with a family history, couples that are planning a pregnancy and to couples that are asking for prenatal testing once an approved infrastructure for education and counseling was in place (NIH Consensus Development Conference Statement, 1997).

Therapeutic implications for heterozygotes

Although in most instances heterozygosity for a recessive trait is of no known health consequence to the individual, there are conditions in which the heterozygous state may impart certain health hazards.

Accordingly, the individuals, knowledge of their carrier status may have therapeutic or preventive health implications for them. For example, persons with AS hemoglobin (sickle-cell trait) should be aware of the possible hazards of exposure to reduced ambient oxygen concentrations (e.g., mountain climbing at high altitude, flying in an unpressurized aircraft above 8000 feet). Also, alerting the anesthetist of the AS trait of their patient prior to gaseous anesthesia could avert inadvertent hypoxia which might be particularly hazardous to such an individual. Heterozygous individuals for type II hypercholesterolemia may be predisposed to premature atherosclerotic degeneration and coronary artery insufficiency. Appropriate therapy (diet, weight control and/or specific medication) may substantially obviate the increased risk for early myocardial infarction in individuals carrying this dominantly expressed disorder. In a similar fashion, persons heterozygous for alpha-1-antitrypsin deficiency (MZ) may be predisposed to chronic obstructive pulmonary disease in early adulthood. Avoidance of tobacco smoke and other noxious inhalants may greatly reduce this risk. Having identified an individual as heterozygous for this mutation, it might be of great practical value for this person to be counseled and to be guided into appropriate job selection and/or environmentally safe areas, as well as informed of the particular importance of not smoking.

Methods and tissues used in carrier identification

Depending upon the genetic nature of the condition, its expression in different organ systems, and the availability of appropriate material for examination, a variety of approaches have been used for heterozygote detection. Table 27.2 lists a series of approaches ranging from physiological studies to direct mutation analysis that are used in carrier detection for different disorders. The disorders listed are representative only of the different categories of methods used and many of these approaches have historical significance only since these have been replaced by more sensitive molecular genetic methods. For example, somatic cell methods assessing the enzymatic (HPRTase) or physiological (^{3}H-hypoxanthine incorporation) properties of clones of skin fibroblast cells were used in the past for carrier detection in

Lesch-Nyhan syndrome. However, molecular genetic techniques (STR linkage analysis and direct mutation detection) have replaced this approach to carrier identification for this disorder (Mansfield et al., 1993a). In both Duchenne muscular dystrophy and hemophilia A, direct mutation detection or linkage analysis has become the method of choice for ascertainment of carrier status in most women (Clemens et al., 1991; Mansfield et al., 1993b; Goodeve, 1998).

MOLECULAR GENETIC TECHNIQUES

A variety of molecular genetic techiques have been used for direct mutation detection in the heterozygote (Table 27.3). In general these are polymerase chain reaction (PCR)-based methods to scan or screen small exon-sized DNA fragments for point mutations or small (e.g., 3–5 base pair) insertions or deletions (Dianzani et al., 1993). Extremely large insertions, deletions, or other rearrangements are best detected with Southern blotting as is the case for the common deletions in α-thalassemia, or the larger premutations and full expansion mutations in fragile X syndrome. In some instances a combination of DNA-based methods may be

Table 27.2. Selected Methods Employed for Carrier Detection in Representative Autosomal- and X-Linked-Recessive Disorders

Approach	Method	Disorder
Structural	Hb electrophoresis	Hemoglobinopathies
Somatic cell	Clonal mosaicism	Lesch-Nyhan syndrome
Immunological	Quantitative immunochemistry	Hemophilias
Statistical	Bayesian pedigree analysis	DMD, Hemophilias
Genetic Linkage	RFLP or STR analysis	DMD, Hemophilia A
Direct mutation analysis	Restriction site alteration	SSA, β-thal, TSD, CF, PKU
	Deletion analysis	DMD, α-thal

PKU, phenylketonuria; TSD, Tay-Sachs disease; CF, cystic fibrosis; DMD, Duchenne muscular dystrophy; β-thal, β-thalassemia; SSA, sickle cell anemia; α-thal, α-thalassemia

Table 27.3. Selected Molecular Genetic Techniques Used for Direct Mutation Detection and Heterozygote Identification

Method	Representative Disorders
Restriction enzyme digestion of PCR products	CF, MCAD deficiency, TSD
Allele-specific oligonucleotide hybridization	CF, β-thalassemia
Southern blotting	α-thal, Hemophilia A, Fragile-X syndrome
Reverse dot blot hybridization	CF
Denaturing gradient gel electrophoresis (DGGE)	Hemophilia A, CF
Single strand conformation polymorphism (SSCP) analysis	Hemophila B
PCR amplification with fluorescent primers	DMD
Direct DNA sequencing of PCR-amplified DNA	β-thalassemia, CF

CF, cystic fibrosis; TSD, Tay-Sachs disease; DMD, Duchenne muscular dystrophy; MCAD, medium chain acyl-CoA dehydrogenase; α-thal, α-thalassemia; β-thal, β-thalassemia

used to optimize carrier detection. For example, carrier identification for fragile X syndrome may involve a combination of Southern blotting and PCR to reliably detect the spectrum of expansion mutations observed within the FMR-1 gene (Snow et al., 1993; Warren and Nelson 1994; ACMG 1994). Finally, advances in technology have led to the ever increasing use of sequencing-based mutation detection. For example, in some laboratories the mutation detection for relatively small genes such as beta-globin has moved from PCR and allele-specific oligonucleotide hybridization to direct sequence based methods using semi-automated capillary electrophoresis systems.

TISSUES USED FOR HETEROZYGOTE DETECTION

Tissues used for heterozygote detection in representative recessive disorders are presented in Table 27.4. In considering carrier detection (either testing an individual or screening a subpopulation) the accessibility of appropriate tissue or material for testing influences the feasibility and cost of such procedures. In some instances, accurate heterozygote identification can be achieved with such readily available tissues such as serum, circulating blood cells, buccal epithelial cells, or tears. In other cases, optimal carrier detection may require cultured skin fibroblasts or even biopsied liver or muscle tissue. Clearly, whether to conduct such studies in individuals related to an affected person, or more generally, will be strongly influenced by such considerations.

DNA-BASED TECHNIQUES

The application of DNA-based techniques in the detection of mutant genes has had great impact on this issue. Since adequate DNA samples are readily obtained from a routine blood sample, the aforementioned reservations are in large part obviated if "DNA methods" can be employed. In some instances, DNA from buccal cells rinsed from the mouth (or even the amount extracted from a single somatic cell) in conjunction with PCR-based methods may provide sufficient material for carrier testing purposes. These PCR-based procedures can be performed more quickly and easily than Southern blot hybridization methods. In addition, PCR methods can be used on small amounts of genomic DNA present on dried blood spots. Accordingly, ease of testing as well as ultimate cost (particularly since such methods are readily automated) should allow for greatly expanded carrier testing for these disorders.

Problems in heterozygote detection

STATISTICAL CONSTRAINTS

The great majority of the inborn errors of metabolism alluded to in this chapter are relatively rare conditions. Although in the aggregate it is estimated that perhaps 1% of all live-born infants will, at some time in life, manifest such a single-gene disorder, there are thousands of such disorders now recognized (McKusick, 1998). This poses critical problems for carrier identification. The only individuals who are obligatory carriers of an autosomal-recessive genetic trait are the biological parents of an affected individual (discounting the 10^{-5} to 10^{-6} possibility of new mutation). Therefore, in the establishment of a carrier identification method, it is critical that a "significant number" of such obligatory heterozygotes be studied (and control

Table 27.4. Tissues Used for Carrier Detection in Representative Recessive Disorders

Tissue	Methods	Disorders
Serum, plasma	Enzyme assay, immunoquantitation, functional assay	TSD, Hemophilias
Erythrocytes	Enzyme assay, electrophoresis	G6PD deficiency, Hemoglobinopathies
Leucocytes	Enzyme assay, histology, functional tests	Gaucher, Batten, CGD
Skin fibroblasts	Enzyme assay, cell cloning	MLD, Hunter
Hair follicles	Enzyme assay/ratio	Lesch-Nyhan, Fabry disease
Tears	Enzyme assay	TSD
Teeth	Vertical banding	Amelogenesis imperfecta-XR
Eyes	Fundoscopy	XR-fundal dystrophies, RP
Liver, muscle biopsy	Enzyme assay, histology	OTC, DMD
DNA from any somatic cell	RFLP/STR linkage, or direct mutation detection	Hemoglobinopathies, CF, DMD, Hemophilias, CF

TSD, Tay-Sachs disease; CGD, chronic granulomatous disease; OTC, ornithine transcarbamylase deficiency; CF, cystic fibrosis; MLD, metachromatic leukodystrophy; DMD, Duchenne muscular dystrophy; RP, retinitis pigmentosa

individuals as well) before statistical validity can be assigned to the testing method. In this regard one must be careful in interpreting research publications in which only small numbers of obligate heterozygotes have been tested and where results suggest that the methods are applicable to carrier detection. Obviously, the larger the samples of obligate carriers and controls studies, and the greater the separation observed in the test results between the two groups, the greater the likelihood for significant applications of the method to heterozygote identification.

It is a very different matter to study persons who the investigator knows must be carriers for a particular trait than individuals who are complete unknowns. Essentially all prior experience with nonmolecular methods used in carrier detection reveals a variable distribution of test results both for carriers and controls. The narrowness of each distribution and the degree of separation between them are critical in assigning a statistical probability that any given test result falls into one or the other distribution.

With molecular methods, however, these constraints are obviated in large part. Certainly, where direct mutation detection is possible, carrier detection is evident without the need for massive numbers in control studies or expansive statistical determinations. With the use of RFLPs or STRs, on the other hand, the proximity of the polymorphic marker to the disease locus is critical to interpretation, since possible meiotic crossover events can confound apparent conclusions drawn by linkage analysis.

WHY VARIABILITY?

One would expect that individuals who are heterozygotes for an autosomal-recessive mutation would reflect 50% of the value (whatever the measurement happens to be) of that found in homozygous normal persons. This is clearly not the case. Not only is there variability of test values in heterozygotes, but considerable variation may also be evident in data obtained from normals. This may reflect the limitations of the methods employed and/or the inherent biological variability of such functions. Other genetic and environmental factors may influence any given biological parameter such that a range of results is seen in carriers and noncarriers. In some instances where, for example, an enzymatic activity measurement is the test employed, there may be levels of activity in heterozygotes distinctly less than 50% of normal. Where the relevant enzyme is composed of multiple subunits — only one of which is under control of the gene in question — random aggregation of normal and abnormal subunits can result in a wide range of activities in the multimeric enzyme. Other mutations may result in only partial reduction in activity of the respective polypeptide. In this instance, the heterozygote may have near-normal activity, or activity of the enzyme in question that overlaps considerably with the range of measurements found in noncarriers.

With X-linked conditions, the carrier female reflects a broad range of test results extending from clearly normal levels to those seen in affected males. This is predominantly a manifestation of the well-known lyonization effect with X chromosome-linked genes. This biological phenomenon makes carrier determination for such X-linked genes particularly difficult. In fact, heterozygous females who carry X-linked recessive genes are mosaic in the expression of most of the genes in question, with a certain proportion of their somatic cells expressing the normal gene and the remainder reflecting the mutant state. Again, the application of molecular methods previously cited (Table 27.3) obviates much of this concern because of their extremely high specificities. The reader is referred to other chapters in this volume concerning specific X-linked disorders for further discussion of carrier-state identification.

OTHER FACTORS INFLUENCING THE CARRIER TEST

In addition to the consideration that other genes in an individual's constitution may modify the expression of a distant specific gene locus, other biological factors may influence gene expression as well. Factors such as age, pregnancy, drugs and medications and certain illnesses might influence the parameter in question, thereby altering the ability to distinguish carriers from non-carriers. Such issues need to be addressed before wide-scale application of a carrier detection method is made.

Genetic heterogeneity

Genetic heterogeneity is an important factor in identifying carriers of mutant genes. Two types of heterogeneity are recognized: genetic heterogeneity and allelic diversity. Genetic heterogeneity can be defined as mutations at two or more genetic loci that produce the same or similar phenotypes (either biochemical or clinical). This is relevant since genetic heterogeneity can present problems for heterozygote detection. For example, forms of Ehlers-Danlos syndrome, a disease of connective tissue, are known to result from alterations at multiple genes inherited with autosomal-dominant, -recessive and X-linked recessive patterns of inheritance. Similarly, the multiple complementation groups in methylmalonic acidemia also indicate genetic heterogeneity for this condition. Many other examples exist as well. Linkage analysis for the purposes of carrier detection and prenatal diagnosis should be used with extreme caution in disorders where evidence exists for genetic heterogeneity.

Allelic diversity

Allelic diversity is the presence of more than one mutation within the same gene that may be associated with highly similar, or very different, biochemical or clinical phenotypes. This has obvious relevance for heterozygote detection. For example, if a standard hemoglobin electrophoresis result (biochemical phenotype) is the only parameter used for sickle cell trait identification, then persons carrying the mutation for hemoglobin-D will be incorrectly identified as carriers of sickle cell trait since the S and D hemoglobins electrophorese similarly under standard conditions. In this instance, of course, the adjunct use of other methods such as hemoglobin solubility studies or sickling on deoxygenation will clarify this possible discrepancy. Similarly, one must be able to differentiate the mutations associated with hemoglobins S and C when performing DNA-based diagnosis of sickle cell trait. Allelic diversity is also an important consideration in disorders such as CF, hemophilia A and β-thalassemia. Direct mutation analysis in these disorders for a set of specific mutations may fail to detect a different disease-causing mutation in a particular family, which may have critical genetic counseling implications for many individuals within that pedigree.

Benign or pseudodeficient mutant alleles

Benign or pseudodeficient mutant alleles are additional examples of allelic diversity with important implications for carrier detection and genetic counseling. These are mutations that mimic the true disease-related carrier state but are not associated with abnormal clinical phenotypes. Such mutations are relatively common in the genes directing the synthesis of various lysosomal hydrolyses (Thomas, 1994). In these disorders, enzyme-based screening tests will fail to distinguish carriers of a disease-causing mutation from carriers of a benign or pseudodeficient allele. For example, in Tay-Sachs disease screening, the enzymatic test employs an artificial substrate in carrier identification. Deficient enzymatic activity is observed both in carriers of pseudodeficient mutations as well as carriers of disease-related mutations (Kaback et al., 1993). These pseudodeficient mutations, however, are not associated with Tay-Sachs disease or any known clinical abnormalities. Two such pseudodeficient alleles are the most common mutations found among the enzyme-defined "carriers" of Tay-Sachs disease in non-Jewish populations. To distinguish true carriers from carriers of pseudodeficient mutations, DNA-based testing is indicated.

Accordingly, DNA testing should be employed after the enzymatic determination of the carrier state in all non-Jewish individuals and all couples that are identified as at-risk (both carriers), regardless of religion. This has obvious implications for accurate genetic counseling and prenatal diagnostic decisions (Kaback et al., 1993). To conduct primary screening with DNA-based testing alone would miss a significant number of carriers and would not be cost effective. Rather, sequential use of gene product and molecular methods in this way optimizes genetic counseling and prenatal diagnostic interpretations, as well as optimizing cost-effectiveness.

Environmental factors

In some instances where nonmolecular methods for carrier detection are employed, certain environmental factors such as drugs, diet, or other agents could affect biological functions and thereby influence their applicability to carrier detection. Iron deficiency can cause hematological changes which mimic the findings of heterozygotes for β-thalassemia. Birth control medications and pregnancy have been shown to result in a relative reduction in serum hexosaminidase A levels, making many of these women appear as carriers for Tay-Sachs disease (Kaback, 1977). These are only two examples where such determinations can be influenced by external factors, resulting in inaccurate carrier identification studies.

Sensitivity and specificity

With all of the above considerations in mind, and having assessed reasonable numbers of obligate heterozygotes and controls with the recommended method(s), significant overlap in the distribution of carriers and noncarriers may still remain. Capabilities of any one laboratory may not be comparable with those of others reflecting, perhaps, differences in preferred methodologies or other inherent variables. Thus the ability to identify all true carriers (sensitivity) is reflected in the false negative frequency of the test employed. The identification of only true carriers (specificity), and not other persons with a false positive test, is also of importance. The greater the overlap in distributions between carrier and noncarrier, the greater the likelihood for either or both types of misclassification.

The advantage of mutation-specific DNA-based testing is that extremely high levels of specificity are achieved. However, since such methods will only identify the specific mutations examined, a decrease in sensitivity is inherent because other mutations in the same gene will not be identified. Since most mutations within a gene affect the gene product, carrier test sensitivities are highest when gene product analysis is the testing method employed. Ideally, carrier screening should be done initially by gene product assay (e.g., enzyme, protein, mRNA) with its high sensitivity. High specificity DNA-based methods can then be employed to confirm abnormal results, to rule out pseudodeficient states, and to identify specific mutations that may have obvious implications for diagnosis or genetic counseling.

With nonmolecular carrier detection methods, even where a defined level of overlap is known to exist, carrier detection studies may still be appropriate. In this context, a test result clearly in the carrier range may indicate, with great likelihood, that the person is heterozygous, while a result in the overlap area would be less definitative and leave the carrier status indeterminate. Similarly, a result at the upper levels of the noncarrier distribution might make the probability of heterozygosity exceedingly small. Where such difficulties exist, carrier screening is (most definitately) best restricted to use only in high-risk individuals (close relatives of probands) rather than in more general or subpopulation screening. Only those approaches in which prior studies have proven the statistical reliability and accuracy of the method and its relative ease of applicability should be candidates for more general use.

Cost and feasibility

Where significant morbidity or cost would be involved in performing carrier detection studies (even where the accuracy is optimal), these issues should be considered and discussed with the individual before proceeding. DNA-based methods, where feasible, can be employed easily with DNA extracted from readily available somatic cells (leukocytes, skin cells, buccal epithelial cells in saliva, etc.) and at reasonable cost.

Age for carrier testing

Heterozygosity for most recessive traits has little if any health consequences for the individual and it is only a matter relevant to reproduction. For this reason, carrier testing is best instituted just prior to, or during, the reproductive age. This has added benefits in that the person's ability to comprehend the meaning of such information is much more likely to be adequate at such an age. Likewise, carrier testing among children or young teenagers should not be undertaken routinely and should be considered only under special circumstances. One's level of maturity and background education may be important factors in obviating any possible stigmatization that carrier identification could entail. A parental request to determine the possible carrier status of their child(ren) need not be a sufficient basis to proceed. Rather, a full discussion with the parents as to the lack of health implications and possible psychosocial hazards of testing youngsters may lead to deferral of testing to a more appropriate time.

Conclusions

From its very outset a number of complex and important social and ethical issues have been identified with genetic screening (Hastings Center, 1972; Bergsma, 1974). Issues such as possible personal, familial, or even more general stigmatization of the identified carrier, – maintenance of utmost confidentiality of test results, rigorous protection of individual privacy, informed consent of the tested individual, are but a few of the more important concerns raised. Clearly, the physician must consider all of these matters in their interaction with the patient where possible genetic testing is anticipated. These issues notwithstanding, heterozygote testing is likely to increase substantially in the future for many of the reasons cited earlier.

Heterozygote detection in the near future will be more efficient and continue to rely heavily upon PCR-based methods including sequencing. The clinical use of highly polymorphic microsatellite, or STR markers (Gyapay et al., 1994), and single nucleotide polymorphisms (SNPs) (Wang et al., 1998) for genotyping in clinical genetics assuredly will increase. Recent advances in molecular genetic research and the Human Genome Project have resulted in the isolation and characterization of literally thousands of human genes (Deloukas et al., 1998). At this time there were over 11,000 entries in the Online Mendelian Inheritance in Man (OMIM) database (OMIM, 2000). Completion of the Human Genome Project in the near future will further accelerate human disease gene identification and mapping and this will lead to additional DNA diagnostic tests. In addition, newer methods may be developed that involve both gene product (e.g., enzyme) and nucleic acid detection schemes using microtitre plates and colorimetric detection schemes. Eventually screening will involve the simultaneous analysis of multiple disease loci by automated methods and the use of so called "DNA chips" containing high density arrays of specific oligonucleotide probes (Caskey, 1993; Fodor, 1993; Brown and Botstein, 1999). With appropriate technical, medical, and educational expertise, the expanded use of these new approaches in the future will serve to reduce the individual, familial and societal burdens associated with many severe, and currently untreatable, hereditary disorders.

Acknowledgements

This work was supported in part by a contract from the Genetic Disease Section, Maternal and Child Health Branch, State of California Department of Health, and by a grant from the National Tay-Sachs and Allied Disorders Association, Incorporated.

REFERENCES

ACMG (American College of Medical Genetics) (1994) Policy statement: Fragile X syndrome: Diagnostic and carrier testing. Am J Med Genet 53:380–381

ACMG (American College of Medical Genetics) (1997) Policy statement: Genetic testing for cystic fibrosis. JAMA 279(14):1068–1069

Andrews LB, Fullarton JE, Holtzman NA, Motulsky AG (eds) (1994) Assessing Genetic Risks Implications for Health and Social Policy. Committee on Assessing Genetic Risks, Institute of Medicine. National Academy Press, Washington, DC

ASHG (American Society of Human Genetics) (1990) The American Society of Human Genetics statement on cystic fibrosis screening. Am J Hum Genet 46:393

ASHG (American Society of Human Genetics). (1992) Statement of the American Society of Human Genetics on cystic fibrosis carrier screening. Am J Hum Genet 51:1443–1444

Bergsma D (ed) (1974) Ethical social and legal dimensions of screening for human genetic disease. Birth Defects: Original Article Series, Vol. X, March of Dimes Birth Defects Foundation

Brown PO, Botstein D (1999) Exploring the new world of the genome with DNA microarrays. Nat Genet 21:33–37

Cao A, Pintus L, Lecca U et al. (1984) Control of homozygous β-thalassemia by carrier screening and antenatal diagnosis in Sardinia. Clin Genet 26:2

Cao A, Saba L, Galanello R, Rosatelli MC (1997) Molecular diagnosis and carrier screening for β-thalassemia. JAMA 278:1273–1277

Caskey CT (1993) Presymptomatic diagnosis: A first step toward genetic health care. Science 262:48–49

Clemens PR, Fenwick RG, Chamberlain JS et al. (1991) Carrier detection and prenatal diagnosis in Duchenne and Becker muscular dystrophy families, using dinucleotide repeat polymorphisms. Am J Hum Genet 49:951–960

Cystic Fibrosis Genetic Analysis Consortium (1994) Population variation of common cystic fibrosis mutations. Human Mutat 4:167–177

Deloukas P, Schuler GD, Gyapay G et al. (1998) A physical map of 30,000 human genes. Science 282:744–746

Desnick RJ (1990) Treatment of inherited Metabolic Diseases. P 2001–10. In Emery and Rimoin (eds): Principles and Practices of Medical Genetics. Volume 2, Churchill Livingstone, Edinburgh

Desnick RJ, Kaback MM (eds) (2001). Tay-Sachs Disease: Deliniation to Prevention. Academic Press, NY

Dianzani I, Camaschella C, Ponzone A, Cotton RGH (1993) Dilemmas and progress in mutation detection. Trends in Genetics 9:403–405

Fletcher JC, Berg K, Tranoy KE (1985) Ethical aspects of medical genetics: A proposal for guidelines in genetic counseling, prenatal diagnosis and screening. Clin Genet 27:199

Fodor SPA, Rava RP, Huang SC et al. (1993) Multiplexed biochemical assays with biological chips. Nature 364:555–556

Fost N (1993) Genetic diagnosis and treatment: Ethical considerations. AJDC 147:1190–1195

Goodeve AC (1998) Review laboratory methods for the genetic diagnosis of bleeding disorders. Clin Lab Haem 20:3–19

Gyapay G, Morrissett J, Vignal A et al. (1994) The 1993–94 Généthon human genetic linkage map. Nat Genet 7 (special issue):246–339

Hastings Center (1972) Ethical and social issues in screening for genetic disease. New Engl J Med 286:1129

Kaback M (ed) (1977) Tay-Sachs Disease: Screening and Prevention. AR Liss, New York

Kaback M, Lim-Steele J, Dabholkar D et al. (1993) Tay-Sachs disease – carrier screening, prenatal diagnosis and the molecular era. JAMA 270(19):2307–2315

Kaplan F (1998) Tay-Sachs disease carrier screening: A model for prevention of genetic disease. Genet Testing 2(4):271–292

Kazazian HH Jr (1990) The thalassemia syndromes: molecular basis and prenatal diagnosis in 1990. Semin Hematol 27(3):209–228

McKusick VA (1998) Mendelian Inheritance in Man, 12th edn. The Johns Hopkins University Press, Baltimore

Mansfield ES, Blasband A, Kronick MN et al. (1993a) Fluorescent approaches to diagnosis of Lesch-Nyhan syndrome and quantitative analysis of carrier status. Molec Cell Probes 7:311–324

Mansfield ES, Robertson JM, Lebo RV et al. (1993b) Duchenne/Becker muscular dystrophy carrier detection using quantitative PCR and fluorescence-based strategies. Am J Med Genet 48:200–208

Merz B (1987) Matchmaking scheme solves Tay-Sachs problem. JAMA 258:2636–2637

Modell B, Mouzouras M (1982) Social consequences of introducing antenatal diagnosis for thalassemia. Birth Defects 18:285

Morsy MA, Mitani K, Clemens P, Caskey CT (1993) Progress toward human gene therapy. JAMA 270:2338–2345

Mountain A (2000) Gene therapy: The first decade. Trends Biotechnol 18(3):119–128

NIH Workshop on Population Screening for the Cystic Fibrosis Gene (1990) Special report: Statement from the National Institutes of Health Workshop on Population Screening for the Cystic Fibrosis Gene. N Engl J Med 323:70

NIH Consensus Development Conference Statement (1997) Genetic testing for cystic fibrosis. Available at: http://odp.od.nih.gov/consensus/cons/106/106_intro.htm Accessed 05 April 2000

Online Mendelian Inheritance in Man, OMIM (TM). McKusick-Nathans Institute for Genetic Medicine, Johns Hopkins University (Baltimore,

MD) and National Center for Biotechnology Information, National Library of Medicine (Bethesda, MD), 2000. World Wide Web URL: http://www.ncbi.nlm.nih.gov/omim/

President's Commission for the Study of Ethical Problems in Medicine and Biomedical Research (1983) Screening and counseling for genetics conditions. US Government Printing Office, Washington, DC

Ramot B (ed) (1974) Genetic Polymorphisms and Diseases in Man. Academic Press, NY

Rowley PT, Loader S, Levenkron JC (1997) Cystic Fibrosis Carrier population screening: A review. Genet Testing 1(1):53–59

Rutkow IM, Lipton JM (1974) Some negative aspects of the state health department's policies related to screening for sickle cell anemia. Am J Public Health 64:217

Scriver CR, Beaudet AL, Sly WS, Valle D (ed) (1995) The Metabolic Basis of Inherited Disease, 7th edn. McGraw-Hill Inc., NY

Snow K, Doud LK, Hagerman R et al. (1993) Analysis of CGG sequence at the FMR-1 locus in fragile X families and in the general population. Am J Hum Genet 53:1217–1228

Thomas GH (1994) Commentary "pseudodeficiencies" of lysosomal hydrolases. Am J Human Genet 54:934–940

Wang DG, Fan J, Siao C et al. (1998) Large-scale identification, mapping, and genotyping of single-nucleotide polymorphisms in the human genome. Science 280:1077–1082

Warren ST, Nelson DL (1994) Advances in molecular analysis of fragile X syndrome. JAMA 271:536–542

Whitten JC (1973) Sickle cell programming: An imperiled promise. New Engl J Med 288:318

Prenatal screening for neural tube defects and aneuploidy

28

David A Aitken
Jennifer A Crossley
Kevin Spencer

Introduction

Prenatal screening for neural tube defects and aneuploidy is an established part of prenatal care in many countries. Most current testing protocols are focused on the second trimester and operate in two stages. The primary screening test identifies women at high risk who can then be offered a specific diagnostic test to confirm or exclude the presence of an affected fetus. In populations where the uptake of screening is high, a combination of maternal serum alpha-fetoprotein testing and ultrasound scanning identifies the majority of pregnancies with open neural tube defects (NTD). Prenatal diagnosis and selective termination of pregnancies affected by NTD combined with a natural decline in prevalence and increasing use of effective primary preventative measures in recent years has reduced the birth incidence of neural tube defects by over 90% in some populations.

For chromosome abnormalities however, in spite of a steady process of evolution and refinement of the biochemical tests upon which most screening is currently based, the impact on the number of affected births has been more modest. Now, a different approach to screening for chromosome abnormalities is emerging. This is based on a combination of biophysical and biochemical measurements in the first trimester and provides the dual benefits of improved sensitivity and specificity and earlier detection of affected pregnancies. Risk assessment, using a combination of ultrasound measurement of fetal nuchal translucency at 11–13 weeks gestation and the analysis of the maternal serum markers free beta human chorionic gonadotrophin and pregnancy associated plasma protein A, can identify 90% of Down's syndrome fetuses. This has implications for the way antenatal care is organized and delivered during the first half of pregnancy.

Neural tube defects

Classification

Anencephaly and spina bifida occur with approximately equal frequency and together constitute 90% of all cases of fetal neural tube defects. Most spina bifida cases and all anencephalic cases are so-called "open" lesions with the neural elements and meninges exposed. However, in 15–20% of spina bifida cases there is a covering of skin over the spinal defect and these "closed" lesions are not detectable by biochemical testing. Encephalocele, where there is herniation of cerebral tissue through a skull defect (usually occipital), and iniencephaly, where spinal and cranial cavities are confluent, are usually closed defects and constitute the remaining 10% of NTD cases.

Frequency and occurrence

A survey of NTD rates in several countries between 1990 and 1994 (World Atlas of Birth Defects, 1998) shows a mean rate of about 12 NTD cases per 10,000 pregnancies but with geographical variation (Table 28.1). Over the last 20 to 30 years there has been a marked decline in the incidence of infants born with NTD in many populations (Davis and Young, 1991; Roberts et al., 1995a). While prenatal diagnosis and selective termination of affected pregnancies has been a major contributor to this reduction, similar trends have been noted in some populations where prenatal screening and diagnosis are not practiced (McDonnell et al., 1999)

763

Table 28.1. Pregnancy prevalance of neural tube defects by type in various populations between 1990 and 1994

| Country | Period | *Crude pregnancy prevalence/10,000 | | | |
		Anencephaly	Spina bifida	Encephalocele	Total
Argentina	1994	9.5	9.1	1.9	20.5
[1]Australia	1994	5.8	8.5	2.9	17.2
Belarus	1994	8.8	17.7	–	26.5
Belgium	1993–4	2.0	4.8	1.6	8.4
Brazil	1994	7.6	8.2	2.5	18.3
Chile	1994	8.5	8.5	1.8	18.8
Czech Republic	1994	3.2	4.0	0.6	7.8
Denmark	1993–4	1.7	3.3	1.7	6.7
[1]France	1993–4	3.5	5.1	1.6	10.2
Eire	1993–4	4.5	3.7	1.3	9.5
[1]Italy	1993–4	2.7	3.4	1.1	7.2
Japan	1994	3.4	3.3	0.7	7.4
Mexico	1994	15.8	16.1	2.9	34.8
Netherlands	1993–4	2.3	3.6	1.0	6.9
Norway	1994	4.1	4.6	0.8	9.5
[1]UK	1993–4	4.8	4.7	1.0	10.5
USA (Atlanta)	1994	1.0	3.8	0.5	5.3
USA (Hawaii)	1994	4.4	4.9	2.9	12.2
[2]USA (California)	1990–4	4.9	4.2	0.8	9.9
Uruguay	1992–3	5.6	3.3	1.4	10.3
Venezuela	1993–4	8.5	10.7	1.1	20.3
Mean rates		4.8	6.2	1.3	12.3

* Includes livebirths, stillbirths and induced abortions. Data from World Atlas of Birth Defects (WHO, 1998).
[1] Data from two or more centers combined.
[2] Feuchtbaum et al. (1999)

and this has been attributed to changing dietary habits of the pregnant population and an increased intake of natural sources of folic acid which is known to have prophylactic effect (Botto et al., 1999). In other populations, little or no decline in pregnancy prevalence has taken place and the reduction in NTD births is almost entirely due to intervention following prenatal diagnosis (Chan et al., 1993; Alembik et al., 1997).

Overall 95% of neural tube defect pregnancies occur spontaneously in women with no family history. However, where a woman has had one previously affected pregnancy the risk of a recurrence is increased to 10-fold the population risk and doubled again for two previously affected pregnancies (and quadrupled for three). A few other cases may be linked to specific teratogens (notably the antiepileptic drug sodium valproate) or may be secondary to chromosomal abnormalities (e.g., trisomy 18) or the autosomal recessive Meckel syndrome and the etiology must be taken into consideration when counseling about the risk of recurrence in any future pregnancy.

Primary prevention

A large multicenter randomized trial has shown that periconceptional folic acid supplementation can prevent the recurrence of many cases of fetal NTD (MRC Vitamin Study, 1991). Other studies reinforce the view that folic acid can also prevent many first occurrences (Milunsky et al., 1989; Berry et al., 1999) and significant falls in the incidence of NTDs would be expected in populations where women were prescribed 0.4 mg of folic acid/day in the perinatal period or where fortification of certain staple foods such as cereals was introduced (Rose and Menutti, 1995).

PRENATAL DIAGNOSIS OF NEURAL TUBE DEFECTS (NTD)

Selective termination of affected pregnancies is a secondary preventative measure which first requires the positive identification of a fetal NTD by a prenatal diagnostic test. Two approaches to diagnosis are available. The first is based on the measurement of alphafetoprotein (AFP) and acetylcholinesterase (AChE) in amniotic fluid. This requires an invasive procedure to obtain amniotic fluid which introduces a risk of procedure related miscarriage estimated to be about 1% (Tabor et al., 1986). Because of the risks associated with amniocentesis it would be highly undesirable to carry out amniocentesis in all pregnancies: the consequence would be the iatrogenic loss of many more normal fetuses than the detection of fetuses with NTD. Thus amniocentesis is appropriate only if the risk of an affected pregnancy is high enough to justify the risks of the procedure, e.g., where there has been a previously affected pregnancy or by selection through serum screening. The second diagnostic approach, using a detailed ultrasound examination of the fetal skull and spine, is non-invasive and in skilled hands has a performance approaching that of amniotic fluid biochemistry. As a result, detailed ultrasonography has largely replaced amniocentesis as the primary diagnostic method for fetal NTD.

PRENATAL DIAGNOSIS BY AMNIOTIC FLUID BIOCHEMISTRY

Alphafetoprotein (AFP) in normal pregnancies

AFP is a fetal protein and its concentration in complex biological solutions can be accurately measured using widely available and highly specific immunoassay methods. AFP levels change with gestation (falling in second trimester amniotic fluid as pregnancy advances) and an accurate estimate of the gestation at which the sample was obtained is therefore essential for interpretation of an amniotic fluid AFP concentration. For this reason AFP concentrations measured in individual samples of amniotic fluid are usually expressed as multiples of the appropriate gestational median (MoM).

Amniotic fluid AFP in pregnancies with open neural tube defects

Where the fetus has an open lesion of the neural tube, the skin barrier is breached and fetal proteins pass into the amniotic fluid at an increased rate, raising their concentrations. Brock and Sutcliffe (1972) first demonstrated elevated levels

of AFP in amniotic fluid from pregnancies with open neural tube defects. The parameters of the association between amniotic fluid AFP concentrations and fetal NTD in the second trimester were defined in a multicenter study of 385 pregnancies with open NTD and over 13,000 unaffected pregnancies (Second Report of the UK Collaborative AFP Study, 1979). The distributions of amniotic fluid AFP levels expressed in MoM in the spina bifida and anencephalic cases showed a small degree of overlap between spina bifida and unaffected pregnancies (Fig. 28.1) and the degree of overlap varied such that the best discrimination between affected and unaffected pregnancies was achieved by setting a sliding scale of cut-off values with gestation (Table 28.2). Overall, a detection rate of 98.2% for anencephaly and 97.6% for open spina bifida was estimated for a false positive rate of 0.48% which reduced to 0.27% when bloodstained samples were excluded. While the precision of these figures may have been influenced by the accuracy of the gestational estimates and doubts over the classification of some of the cases included in the trial, the figures have proved robust in practice and predicted performance has been borne out or exceeded in

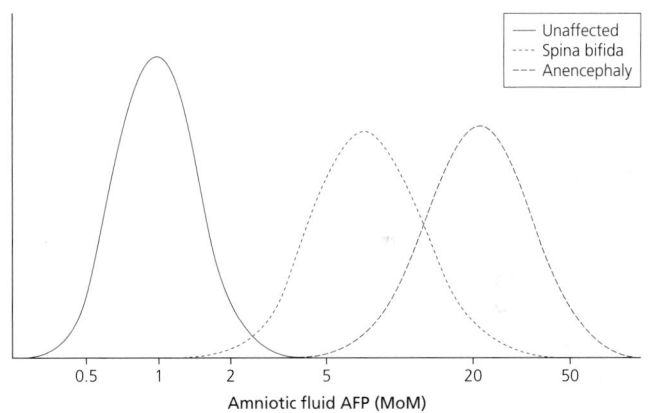

Fig. 28.1 Distribution of amniotic fluid AFP (in MoM) in anencephalic, open spina bifida and unaffected pregnancies.

Table 28.2. Detection rates for open neural tube defects and corresponding false positive rates at specified amniotic fluid AFP cut-off values in multiples of the median (MoM) at different gestations

Gestation (completed weeks)	Cut-off (MoM)	Anencephaly DR (%)		Spina bifida DR (%)		FPR (%)	
		All	*Clear*	*All*	*Clear*	*All*	*Clear*
13–15	2.5	100	100	96	95	0.44	0.31
16–18	3.0	99	97	99	100	0.42	0.24
19–21	3.5	99	97	95	95	0.65	0.30
22–24	4.0	94	96	100	100	1.24	0.30
13–24 combined		98	98	98	98	0.48	0.27

Abbreviations, All—all samples; Clear—bloodstained samples excluded; DR—detection rate FPR—false positive rate.
(Adapted from Second Report of UK Collaborative Study, 1979.)

prospective use (Milunsky et al., 1986). However, not all amniotic fluid AFP levels above the specified gestational cut-off MoM value signal the presence of a pregnancy with an open neural tube defect. Other structural abnormalities of the fetus or complications of pregnancy may result in a raised AFP level in amniotic fluid (and maternal serum) through a variety of mechanisms (Table 28.3).

Occasionally amniotic fluid AFP levels are elevated in the absence of a fetal abnormality. Such false positive results are rare, but of major concern as they may lead to the abortion of unaffected pregnancies. The most common cause of false positive AFP results is contamination of amniotic fluid by fetal blood. Because fetal blood contains on average 100–200 times as much AFP/ml as amniotic fluid at the same gestation even a small amount of fetal blood entering the amniotic fluid will produce a measurable increase in amniotic fluid AFP concentration. Provided the volume of fetal blood contaminating the fluid is small compared to the total volume of the fluid, an estimate of the AFP contribution (in MoM) from the contaminating blood can be made and subtracted from the total AFP level to give a corrected level (Second Report of the UK Collaborative Study, 1979). The additional AFP contribution (in MoM) = the number of fetal red cells per millilitre of amniotic fluid (estimated by the Kleihauer method or by electronic counting and sizing) multiplied by 42×10^{-9}.

Table 28.3. Influence of fetal and pregnancy conditions on amniotic fluid and maternal serum AFP levels in the Second trimester

	Amniotic fluid	Maternal serum
Anencephaly	+++	+++
Open spina bifida	++	++
Closed spina bifida	0	0
Anterior abdominal wall defects	++	++
Teratoma	+++	++
Missed abortion/fetal demise	++	++
Threatened abortion	0	0/+
Fetal infection	0/+	0/+
Congenital nephrosis	+++	++
Duodenal atresia	++	+
Oligohydramnios	++	+
Multiple pregnancy	0	++
Underestimated gestation	–	+
Overestimated gestation	+	–
Lower than average maternal weight	0	+
Higher than average maternal weight	0	–

Abbreviations, + increase; – decrease; 0 no effect.

In the absence of corroborative ultrasound evidence of a specific fetal abnormality, interpretation of a raised amniotic fluid AFP level, particularly in bloodstained samples, may be difficult. The probability that the result indicates an affected pregnancy is heavily dependent upon the indication for amniocentesis. In unselected pregnancies with elevated amniotic fluid AFP results, the odds are still over 3:1 *against* the pregnancy being affected. Table 28.4 shows how these probabilities change according to prior risk and how the odds can be further modified by incorporating the results of acetylcholinesterase (AChE) analysis in amniotic fluid and detailed ultrasound scanning.

Acetylcholinesterase (AChE) in pregnancies with open neural tube defects

The cholinesterases are a group of enzymes with common substrate specificity which can be divided into two types on the basis of their electrophoretic mobility and sensitivity to inhibitors. The non-specific pseudocholinesterases (PChE) are present in serum and amniotic fluid while the acetylcholinesterases (AChE) are not normally present in amniotic fluid but are found in cerebrospinal fluid and as a component of red cell membranes. When samples of amniotic fluid from normal pregnancies are run on polyacrylamide gels and stained to show the site of cholinesterase activity, a single band (PChE) is revealed which can be inhibited by ethopropazine (Lysivane). In pregnancies with open neural tube lesions, cerebrospinal fluid leaks into the amniotic fluid causing the appearance of a second, faster moving AChE band on electrophoresis which can be inhibited by the true cholinesterase inhibitor, BW284C51 (Fig. 28.2) (Smith et al., 1979). The gel electrophoresis test, although qualitative, is a highly effective method of identifying pregnancies with open NTD as it is detecting the presence of a protein (AChE) not normally present in amniotic fluid rather than quantifying a change in concentration. Attempts to distinguish normal and affected pregnancies by measuring PChE and AChE activities are less successful (Aitken et al., 1984). Newer immunoassay methods appear more discriminating (Mehta and Spencer, 1988; Loft et al., 1993), but data on their use is limited.

The performance of the amniotic fluid AChE electrophoresis test has been examined in two large collaborative studies. The first Report of the Collaborative Acetylcholinesterase Study (1981) investigated the value of AChE as a secondary test in 1099 pregnancies which had a high amniotic fluid AFP (> 99.6 percentile) between 13 and 24 weeks of gestation. In 125 of these pregnancies which were not associated with a fetal abnormality or adverse outcome (i.e., false positive AFP results), only eight (6%) had a positive AChE

Table 28.4. Prediction of spina bifida pregnancies by amniotic fluid AFP testing with or without AChE testing and detailed ultrasound (US) scanning according to prior risk.

	NTD present : NTD absent
Prior probability	
1. Average population risk (Table 28.1)	0.12 : 99.88
2. Previously affected pregnancy (10 × 0.12)	1.2 : 98.8
Conditional probability	
3. Elevated maternal serum AFP (≥ 2.5 MoM)	80.0 : 3.0
4. Positive amniotic fluid AFP result, any liquor	91.0 : 0.36
5. Positive amniotic fluid AFP and AChE result	96.0 : 0.14
6. Normal ultrasound scan (unselected pregnancy)	10.0 : 99.0
7. Normal ultrasound scan (high risk pregnancy)	1.0 : 99.9
8. Abnormal ultrasound scan (unselected pregnancy)	85.0 : 0.5
9. Abnormal ultrasound scan (high risk pregnancy)	98.0 : 0.1
Joint probability e.g.	
A. Unselected pregnancy, positive AF AFP i.e. (1) × (4)	1 : 3.3
B. Unselected pregnancy, positive AFP/AChE, normal U/S i.e. (1) × (5) × (6)	1 : 12
C. Unselected pregnancy, elevated MS AFP, abnormal US i.e. (1) × (3) × (9)	32 : 1
D. Previous affected pregnancy, positive AFP/AChE, no U/S i.e. (2) × (5)	8 : 1
E. Previous affected pregnancy, positive AFP/AChE, normal U/S i.e. (2) × (5) × (7)	1 : 12

Best estimates of sensitivity and specificity for ultrasound screening and diagnosis have been used for illustration. Where local performance is accurately known, the appropriate figures should be substituted

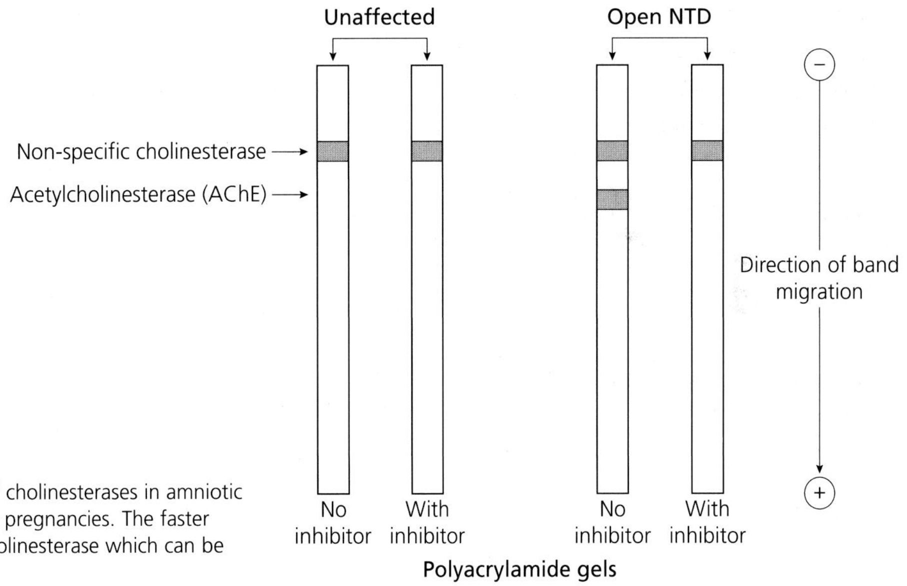

Fig. 28.2 Polyacrylamide gel electrophoresis of cholinesterases in amniotic fluid from normal and open neural tube defect pregnancies. The faster moving, anodal band is neuro-specific acetylcholinesterase which can be selectively inhibited by BW284C51.

gel test (i.e., 2 bands) and seven of these false positive AChE results were associated with bloodstained amniotic fluid. Of the 813 pregnancies in the series with open neural tube defects, 809 (99.5%) had positive amniotic fluid AChE gel results. Thus AChE testing in combination with AFP testing in amniotic fluid produces a major reduction in the false positive rate for virtually no loss in detection.

In the Second Report of the Collaborative Acetylcholinesterase Study (1989) emphasis was placed on estimating the sensitivity and specificity of amniotic fluid AChE testing for cases of open spina bifida. From the analysis of 428 affected pregnancies and over 31,000 unaffected pregnancies at 13–24 weeks of gestation, AChE testing detected a greater percentage of the spina bifida pregnancies than AFP testing using the optimized gestation-specific cut-off AFP MoMs (Table 28.5). Also, corresponding false positive rates were lower for the AChE test. Although the performance of AFP testing in this series was poorer than that predicted by

Table 28.5. Comparison of detection rates for open spina bifida at different gestations by amniotic fluid AFP analysis and amniotic fluid AChE electrophoresis in 428 open spina bifida pregnancies

Gestation (weeks)	AFP Cut-off*	DR (%)	FPR (%)	AChE DR (%)	FPR (%)
13–15	≥ 2·5 MoM	90	0.40	90	0.37
16–18	≥ 3·0 MoM	91	0.36	98	0.31
19–21	≥ 3·5 MoM	89	0.88	100	0.45
22–24	≥ 4·0 MoM	86	0.98	100	0.49

* AFP cut-off as defined in Second Report of UK Collaborative AFP Study (1979)
From Second Report of the Acetylcholinesterase Study, 1989.

earlier studies (Second Report of the UK Collaborative AFP Study, 1979), the best policy was considered to be AFP analysis in all amniotic fluid samples followed by AChE analysis in those with AFP results ≥ 2.0 MoM. This was predicted to give a detection rate of 96% for open spina bifida and a false positive rate of 0.14%. The false positive rate varied according to whether samples were bloodstained (0.12%) or clear (0.06%) and whether the indication for amniocentesis was a raised maternal serum AFP (0.40%). The predictability of combined amniotic fluid AFP and AChE testing for the prenatal diagnosis of NTD is presented in Table 28.4.

Positive AChE results are also encountered in a proportion of other pregnancies with adverse outcome including 63% with exomphalos, 93% with gastroschisis, 29% with Turner syndrome and in 47% ending in miscarriage. However, in cases of autosomal recessive congenital nephrosis syndrome which are associated with high amniotic fluid AFP levels, AChE results are negative, helping to establish the differential diagnosis (Brock et al., 1980).

Amniotic fluid AFP and AChE in the first trimester

Increasing use of early amniocentesis has allowed limited study of amniotic fluid AFP and AChE testing in the first trimester. Successful detection of pregnancies with anencephaly and open spina bifida has been reported by Crandall and Chua (1995) who found elevated AFP levels and positive AChE gel electrophoresis results in 16 cases assessed before 14 weeks of gestation and by Jorgensen et al. (1995) using AFP and AChE immunoassay in two pregnancies with NTD at 10–11 weeks of gestation. However, frequent false positive AChE gel results are found in first trimester amniotic fluid from normal pregnancies (Burton et al., 1989; Muller et al., 1989). This tendency is particularly marked at early gestations and is probably due to the presence of residual AChE activity which persists from before the time of neural tube closure and gradually

disappears towards the end of the first trimester (Eiben et al., 1996a).

Amniotic fluid AFP and AChE in twin pregnancies with NTD

Normal twin pregnancies have amniotic fluid AFP concentrations comparable to those in singleton pregnancies (Second Report of the UK Collaborative AFP Study, 1979). However, AFP concentration may not be identical in neighboring sacs and Drugan et al. (1989) showed that AFP could diffuse between sacs and that this was more likely where there was monochorionic, diamniotic placentation than in twin pregnancies with dichorionic, diamniotic placentation. Aitken (1995) reviewed AFP and AChE results in a series of eight twin pregnancies discordant for open NTD. Elevated AFP levels were associated with the affected fetus and normal AFP levels with the unaffected fetus in six cases which were dichorionic and diamniotic. In two monochorionic, diamniotic pregnancies, elevated AFP levels were found in amniotic fluid from the sacs containing both the affected and unaffected fetuses. In the cases where AChE analysis was carried out, positive results were associated with elevated AFP levels and negative results with normal AFP levels. Thus, amniotic fluid AFP and AChE testing is not reliable in pregnancies where only one twin is affected. Spuriously high AFP levels and positive AChE results are often associated with unaffected fetuses due to diffusion of these proteins across the membranes from the sac with the higher concentration. Detailed ultrasonography is required in twin pregnancies to establish whether one or both twins are affected.

PRENATAL SCREENING AND DIAGNOSIS OF NTD BY ULTRASOUND

Ultrasound screening for NTD

Ultrasonography is an essential part of all screening and diagnostic programmes for NTD. Ultrasound can be used at different levels and the boundary between its role as a method of screening and as a method of diagnosis is blurred. In the UK most pregnant women have a "booking scan" at their first antenatal clinic appointment in the first trimester. In its most basic form the booking scan provides information on the number of viable fetuses, gestational age and the presence of gross abnormalities. As noted above, interpretation of AFP levels in amniotic fluid depends upon an accurate estimate of gestation and this can be derived from an ultrasound measurement of fetal crown-rump length (CRL) before about 12 weeks or bi-parietal diameter of the skull (BPD) after 12 weeks of gestation.

Increasingly however, more detailed anomaly scanning is being carried out in the first trimester, with a systematic search for sonographic features which signal the presence of specific fetal abnormalies. At 10–14 weeks of gestation, anencephaly is readily detectable (Johnson et al., 1997; Chatzipapas et al., 1999). On the other hand, direct ultrasound evidence of spina bifida by visualisation of the spinal defect is difficult to obtain in the first trimester and diagnosis is more usual at later gestations (16–22 weeks). Indirect cranial or cerebellar markers of NTD—the so-called "lemon" and "banana" signs which are prominent in the second trimester (Nicolaides et al., 1986)—may also be useful earlier in pregnancy (Blumenfeld et al., 1993; Sebire et al., 1997a). Apart from NTDs, ultrasound can also identify other types of fetal abnormality, but the timing of the scan is critical. Many abnormalities (e.g., cardiac, renal) can only be visualized successfully in a more mature fetus and in many centers anomaly scanning around 18–22 weeks of gestation is now offered to all pregnant women in addition to the first trimester booking scan.

The performance of ultrasound as a primary screening test for NTD is difficult to estimate as it is subject to local variation determined by such factors as quality of equipment and ultrasound operator training and experience. While detection of anencephaly is consistently high and close to 100%, detection of spina bifida appears more variable. Van den Hof et al. (1990) reported detection of 98% of spina bifida fetuses, Levi et al. (1991) reported 55%, Williamson et al. (1997) 70–84% and Jorgensen et al. (1999) 79.4%. False positive rates for ultrasound screening are generally low, with some studies claiming 100% specificity.

Ultrasound diagnosis of NTD in high risk populations

In pregnancies known to be at high risk of an NTD through family history or a raised serum AFP, detailed ultrasound scanning has largely replaced amniocentesis and

AFP and AChE analysis as a diagnostic test. As most cases of anencephaly are diagnosed by routine first trimester scanning, the residual NTD cases picked up by serum screening at 15–20 weeks of gestation are mainly spina bifida along with some other structural abnormalities such as ventral wall defects. The reliability of ultrasound diagnosis in high risk populations has been documented in numerous studies. For example, Morrow et al. (1991) reported 98% sensitivity and 100% specificity in a series of 50 NTD pregnancies while Lennon and Gray (1999) reported 97% sensitivity and 100% specificity in a series of 68 NTD pregnancies supporting the view that amniocentesis may be avoided within this high risk group unless difficulty is experienced in visualizing the fetal spine or other organs (Nadel et al., 1990; Shields et al., 1996). Apart from avoiding the risk of fetal loss associated with amniocentesis, detailed ultrasound scanning can also provide a differential diagnosis of ventral wall defects and other fetal abnormalities picked up by serum screening.

Ultrasound and amniotic fluid biochemistry combined

Where amniotic fluid is obtained and AFP and AChE analysis carried out, a detailed ultrasound scan can be used to modify the prediction from the amniotic fluid biochemistry results. Where the indication for amniocentesis is a high risk of a NTD because of a previously affected pregnancy, a positive AFP/AChE result will give odds of approximately 8:1 that the pregnancy is affected (Table 28.4) but if a detailed ultrasound scan reveals no obvious abnormality these odds are reduced to 1 chance in 12 that the pregnancy is affected. Where the indication for amniocentesis is some other reason, e.g., chromosomal, AFP and AChE testing will occasionally give positive results, but these are poor predictors of fetal abnormality when the prior risk is low (Table 28.4) and ultrasound scanning is a more specific test (Sepulveda et al., 1995). Several investigators have questioned the value and advisability of carrying out AFP and AChE testing in amniotic fluid samples from pregnancies with a low risk of a fetal NTD (Fisher et al., 1981; Shields et al., 1996).

PRENATAL SCREENING FOR NEURAL TUBE DEFECTS BY MATERNAL SERUM AFP

AFP in maternal serum

AFP reaches the maternal serum by two routes: directly across the placenta and indirectly from the amniotic fluid pool across the chorion and amnion to be taken up by the maternal vasculature of the uterine decidua. In pregnancies where the fetus has an open NTD, maternal serum levels are elevated in most cases and this is a result of increased transfer of AFP across the fetal membranes promoted by the high concentration of AFP in amniotic fluid. In unaffected pregnancies there is a rapid rise in maternal serum AFP concentration through the first and second trimesters peaking at about 32 weeks of gestation. Because of the rising levels with gestation, AFP concentrations in maternal serum are best expressed in MoM and an accurate estimate of gestation is a prerequisite for interpretation of a maternal serum AFP level.

The relationship between maternal serum AFP and fetal neural tube defects was comprehensively examined in a large collaborative study of 301 affected and 18,684 unaffected pregnancies at 10–24 weeks of gestation (Report of the UK Collaborative Study on Alpha-fetoprotein in Relation to Neural Tube Defects, 1977). The results showed that there was a greater overlap of the distributions of AFP in NTD and unaffected pregnancies in maternal serum (Fig. 28.3) than in amniotic fluid (Fig. 28.1) and as a consequence, maternal serum AFP testing has a poorer ability to distinguish between normal and affected pregnancies and cannot be considered diagnostic. Nevertheless, at 16–18 weeks of gestation 88% of anencephalic and 79% of open spina bifida pregnancies included in the study had maternal serum AFP levels ≥ 2.5 MoM for a false positive rate of 3% and it was proposed that this measurement could form the basis of a screening test as a way of selecting women at increased risk for further investigation. The best separation between normal and affected pregnancies is at 17 weeks of gestation but in practice, screening performance is acceptable at 15–20 weeks of gestation, particularly

if ultrasound estimates of gestation based on fetal bi-parietal diameter (BPD) are used. Wald et al. (1980) pointed out that fetuses with spina bifida have smaller BPDs than unaffected fetuses of similar maturity. The consequence is that gestational age, based on ultrasound measurements, is underestimated and the correspondingly lower median AFP value used to calculate an AFP MoM will give a higher result, increasing the likelihood of detection.

Maternal serum AFP should not be used as a marker for NTD before 14 weeks of gestation. Aitken et al. (1993) measured maternal serum AFP in 14 pregnancies with open NTD in which both a first trimester sample and a second trimester sample were collected. None of the samples collected before 14 weeks of gestation had an AFP level above 2.0 MoM but in all cases, the paired second trimester sample had an elevated AFP level. Sebire et al. (1997b) found raised serum AFP (≥ 2.5 MoM) in seven of nine anencephalic pregnancies at 10–14 weeks of gestation while two spina bifida cases had normal serum AFP.

Screening programs for NTD based on maternal serum AFP measurement have evolved since their introduction 25 years ago. The widespread use of ultrasound dating, improvements in the precision of AFP assay methods, and the correction of AFP levels to take account of variables such as maternal weight (Johnson et al., 1990) have contributed to a reduction in variance of the AFP distributions in normal and affected pregnancies reducing the false positive rate determined by fixed AFP MoM cut-offs. This, combined with the replacement of the invasive amniotic fluid AFP/AChE diagnostic test by detailed ultrasound scanning, has allowed the adoption of lower AFP MoM cut-off levels in some program (e.g., 2.0 MoM instead of 2.5 MoM) which results in a useful increase in detection for open spina bifida (to about 85%) at the expense of an increase in follow-up rate (≤ 5%) but without the risk of additional pregnancy losses.

Maternal serum AFP in twin pregnancies

An analysis of maternal serum AFP levels in 1638 normal twin pregnancies gave an average level of 2.14 MoM (Aitken, 1995). In twin pregnancies where one or both fetuses have an open NTD, maternal serum AFP levels are further elevated, but detection rates, particularly for spina bifida, are much poorer than in singleton pregnancies. From data collected by Cuckle et al. (1990a,b) on maternal serum AFP levels in a series of 46 twin pregnancies with NTD, a cut-off level of 5.0 MoM would give a false positive rate of 3% and a detection rate of 83% for anencephaly but only 39% for open spina bifida (Fig. 28.4). A better

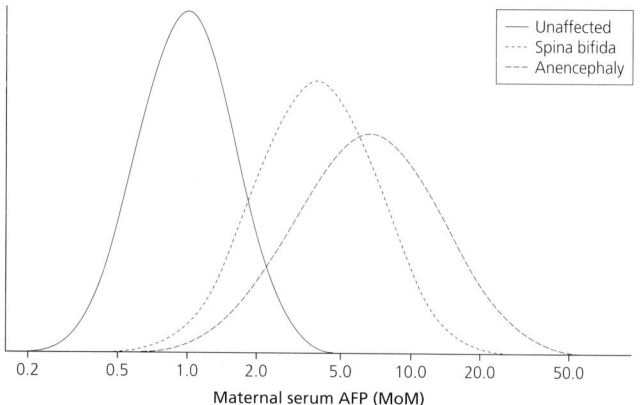

Fig. 28.3 Distribution of maternal serum AFP (in MoM) in anencephalic, open spina bifida and unaffected pregnancies.

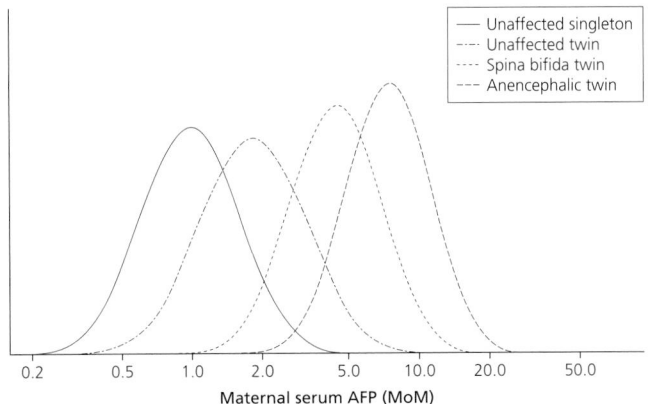

Fig. 28.4 Distribution of maternal serum AFP in normal singleton and twin pregnancies and in anencephalic and open spina bifida twin pregnancies.

strategy would be to use a lower cut-off (3.0–3.5 MoM) and accept a higher follow-up rate (15–20%) of all twin pregnancies for detailed ultrasound scanning. This would increase detection of spina bifida in twin pregnancies to approximately the same level as that in singleton pregnancies obtained using a 2.5 MoM cut-off.

Aneuploidy

Classification, frequency and occurrence

In the absence of prenatal diagnosis, the natural frequency of chromosome abnormalities in newborns has been estimated at a rate of 6/1000 (Hook and Hamerton, 1977). Of these 2/1000 are balanced chromosome rearrangements, 2/1000 are sex chromosome abnormalities and the remaining 2/1000 involve unbalanced rearrangements of the autosomes. Of these unbalanced rearrangements, 1.4/1000 have excess chromosome material in the form of an additional autosome (autosomal trisomies) and the remaining 0.6/1000 are unbalanced structural rearrangements of the autosomes. The most common autosomal abnormality is Down's syndrome (trisomy 21) but an often quoted overall birth frequency of 1 in 800 (Hook and Hamerton, 1977; Hook, 1992) is an underestimate in many pregnant populations due to the increasing median maternal age. The other common autosomal trisomies are Edwards syndrome (trisomy 18) with a birth frequency of 1:6500 and Patau syndrome (trisomy 13) with a birth frequency of 1:12500 (Hook, 1992). These rates were derived from populations which were largely Caucasian, before the advent of prenatal diagnosis.

Maternal age risks

Penrose (1933) first demonstrated the link between advancing maternal age and an increasing risk of having a Down's syndrome child. There have been numerous studies on the rates of Down's syndrome at different maternal ages. Cuckle et al. (1987) compiled data from eight published surveys of Down's syndrome rates in liveborns and provided regressed maternal age risks at individual maternal ages. These risks are in common usage today. However, the use of maternal ages in years plus fractions of years requires that the term "maternal age" in the published equation must be replaced by "age at estimated date of delivery— 0.5" in order to assign the discrete risk per year to the middle of each year class. Hecht and Hook (1996) and Bray et al. (1998) found higher rates than those derived by Cuckle et al. (1987) when the completeness of ascertainment was taken into account when combining data from published studies (Fig. 28.5). Variation in Down syndrome rates between different population groups has been investigated by Carothers et al. (1999) and Hook et al. (1999). An increased rate (about 20%) was reported for mothers of Mexican and Central American origin living in California, but reliable data for most populations is lacking although any real differences are unlikely to be greater than ±25% (Carothers et al., 1999).

Spontaneous fetal loss

The data of Cuckle et al. (1987), Hecht and Hook (1996) and Bray et al. (1998) are estimates of the risks at term, but because of the spontaneous loss of affected fetuses between mid trimester and term, the probability of finding an affected fetus is higher at the time of amniocentesis. Pregnancies affected by autosomal trisomy have a higher rate of spontaneous abortion than unaffected pregnancies. Morris et al. (1999) have combined the results of their own studies with several others and estimate that 43% of Down syndrome pregnancies present at the time of first trimester chorionic villus sampling (CVS) and 23% present at the time of second trimester amniocentesis will end in miscarriage or stillbirth. Trisomy 18 and trisomy 13 have even higher levels of pregnancy loss. Comparing the relative rates of Down syndrome, trisomy 18 and trisomy 13 at CVS (Snijders, 1994; Snijders et al., 1999) and amniocentesis (Ferguson Smith and Yates, 1984) with those found at birth (Hook, 1992), it may be estimated that for the trisomy 18 pregnancies 75% would be lost between CVS and term and 56% between amniocentesis and term and for the trisomy 13 pregnancies the relative rates would

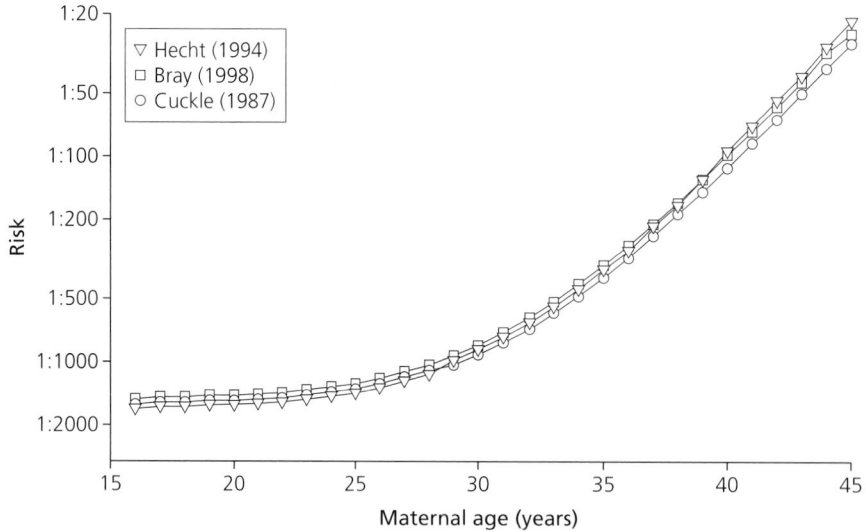

Fig. 28.5 Age-specific risks for Down's syndrome from three different studies.

be 66% and 22%. Since the rates of chromosome abnormalities at amniocentesis and CVS were derived in women aged 35 years and over, these loss rates assume that the rate in younger women is similar to that found in older women, whereas there is evidence to suggest that fetal loss rate increases with advancing maternal age. Trisomy 18 is 8 times less common than Down's syndrome at birth, 5 times less common at amniocentesis, and 3 times less common at first trimester CVS. For trisomy 13 the relative rates vs Down's syndrome are: 15 times less at birth, 16 times less at amniocentesis and 9 times less at first trimester CVS.

Previous affected pregnancy

The risk of an affected pregnancy is increased where a woman has had a previously affected pregnancy. A residual risk of 0.34% at term (0.42% at mid trimester) was estimated by Cuckle and Wald (1990) which is additional to the maternal age risk. The effect is therefore most marked in younger women (Fig. 28.6). For translocation Down's syndrome, the risk of recurrence is at least 1 in 10 if the woman is a carrier of a balanced (14;21) translocation and about 1 in 20 if her partner is a (14;21) translocation carrier (Mikkelsen and Nielsen, 1992). In the rare cases where the

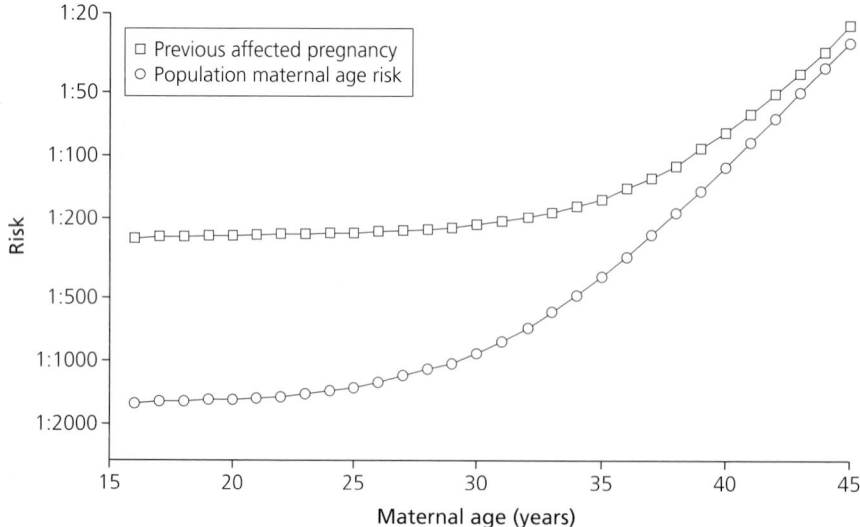

Fig. 28.6 Change in prior risk of Down's syndrome by maternal age in women who have had a previously affected pregnancy.

cause of Down's syndrome is a (21;21) translocation the recurrence rate is 100% for either a female or a male translocation carrier.

Prenatal screening for aneuploidy

MATERNAL AGE SCREENING

From the early 1970s, the association between advancing maternal age and an increased risk of a chromosomally abnormal birth was used to select pregnancies at higher risk of aneuploidy for diagnostic testing by amniocentesis (or latterly chorionic villus sampling) by offering testing to women over a chosen cut-off age, commonly 35 years. However, maternal age alone is an inefficient method of screening for Down's syndrome. In the 1980s only around 30%–35% of the Down's syndrome pregnancies occurred in the approximately 6%–7% of pregnant women who were aged 35 years or over (Fig. 28.7A). The predictive value of maternal age screening in a pregnant population with this age profile is also low, with only one abnormality detected for every 125 diagnostic tests performed, resulting in the possible loss of one normal fetus for each chromosomally abnormal fetus detected. In many populations this method of screening made little impact on the number of Down's syndrome births (Stone et al., 1989), since the uptake of diagnostic testing was low (< 40%) resulting in an average detection rate of around 12–15% (Aitken and Crossley, 1992). Changing population demographics now mean that it is not unusual for 12–15% of a pregnant population to be aged 35 years and over (Fig. 28.7B) and continuing to offer diagnostic testing to this proportion of pregnant women would pose an unacceptable burden on cytogenetic services and result in the iatrogenic loss of many more unaffected fetuses than Down's syndrome fetuses identified. Biochemical screening provides an alternative method of selecting women at increased risk for further testing which allows the follow-up rate to be pre-determined locally.

BIOCHEMICAL SCREENING FOR ANEUPLOIDY

Merkatz et al. (1984) first reported an association between low maternal serum AFP levels and fetal aneuploidy. Many further studies of Down's syndrome and trisomy 18 pregnancies have confirmed significant reductions in AFP concentration in each trisomy (Table 28.6). When AFP concentrations are expressed as MoMs, the distributions in both normal and affected pregnancies are log Gaussian (Fig. 28.8A). Clearly there is no complete separation of AFP levels in unaffected and trisomic pregnancies and Cuckle et al. (1987) proposed the use of a Gaussian model to derive a probability or likelihood that a particular AFP level is associated with an affected pregnancy. This likelihood ratio can then be used as an "odds modifier" to adjust the prior risk based on maternal age. As there is no association between maternal age and maternal serum AFP levels, a combined risk can be obtained by multiplying together the probability of a Down's syndrome pregnancy derived from the woman's age with the probability derived from a serum AFP measurement (in MoM) (Fig. 28.8B). By selecting an appropriate threshold risk (e.g., 1:250) as the decision point for amniocentesis, a fixed proportion of the pregnant population whose combined risks exceed the threshold can be offered amniocentesis. Retrospective studies suggested that an additional 7% of Down's syndrome pregnancies could be detected by AFP/age screening compared to screening by age alone for no increase in

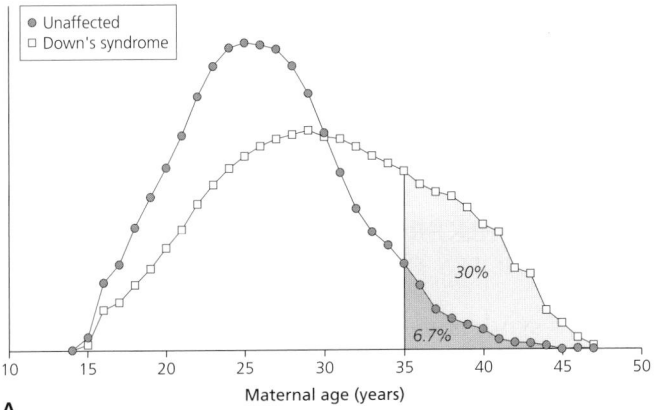

A

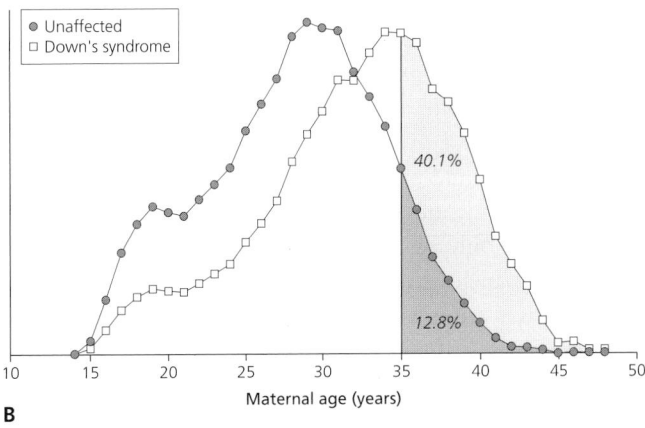

B

Fig. 28.7 Maternal age distribution of unaffected and Down's syndrome pregnancies in the west of Scotland in (A) 1987 and (B) 1999.

Table 28.6. Maternal serum marker median MoM in first and second trimester Down's syndrome and trisomy 18 pregnancies by meta-analysis of published studies

| | Second trimester | | | | First trimester | | | |
| | Down's syndrome | | Trisomy 18 | | Down's syndrome | | Trisomy 18 | |
	n	*Median (MoM)*	*n*	*Median (MoM)*	*n*	*Median (MoM)*	*n*	*Median (MoM)*
AFP	1328	0.75	519	0.65	611	0.80	53	0.91
UE3	733	0.72	263	0.42	210	0.71	–	–
thCG	907	2.06	347	0.32	625	1.33	53	0.38
FβhCG	562	2.20	145	0.33	846	1.98	126	0.27
FαhCG	239	1.43	12	0.86	162	1.00	–	–
Inhibin A	524	1.92	73	0.87	112	1.59	–	–
SP-1	448	1.46	25	1.13	246	0.86	–	–
CA125	187	1.01	–	–	34	1.14	–	–
hPL	81	1.29	12	0.55	–	–	–	–
α inhibin	64	1.63	–	–	112	1.59	–	–
Activin-A	82	1.23	–	–	–	–	–	–
PAPP-A	159	0.97	90	0.11	777	0.45	119	0.20
PALP	70	1.07	18	0.94	–	–	–	–

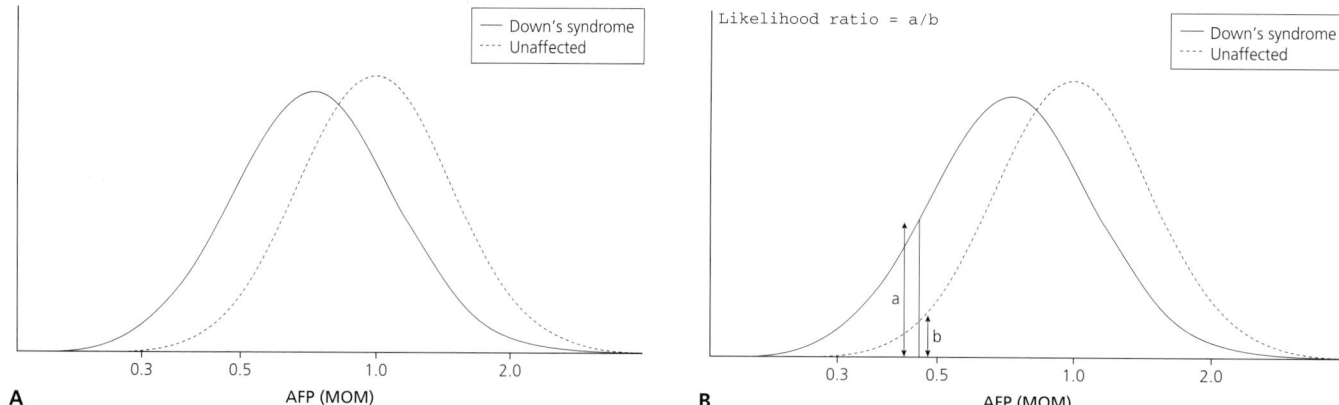

Fig. 28.8 Distribution of maternal serum AFP (in MoM) in unaffected and and Down's syndrome pregnancies (A). Estimation of the likelihood of an affected pregnancy associated with a specific AFP level (B). In this example, an AFP level of 0.45 MoM gives a likelihood ration (a/b) of 4, and therefore a fourfold increase in the risk of a Down's syndrome pregnancy.

the false positive rate (Zeitune et al., 1991) and this has been borne out in practice (Aitken and Crossley, 1995). Using this approach, screening could be offered to women aged 25 years and over and a proportion of women aged over 35 years could avoid invasive testing on the basis of a reduced risk. Although this approach offers an improvement on age-only screening, around 60% of Down's syndrome pregnancies are not detected and detection rates and false positives rates also vary according to maternal age (Zeitune et al., 1991). In an effort to further improve screening performance, a wide range of other serum markers has been investigated for changes in their normal concentrations in chromosomally abnormal pregnancies.

Initially, these studies were largely confined to the second trimester (around 15–20 weeks of gestation) reflecting the stage of sampling for AFP testing for NTDs. Subsequently, marker studies have been extended to the first trimester.

SERUM MARKERS IN ANEUPLOID PREGNANCIES IN THE SECOND TRIMESTER

Down's syndrome

Bogart et al. (1987; 1989) first reported that levels of human chorionic gonadotrophin (hCG) and the free α subunit of hCG (FαhCG) were altered in aneuploid pregnancies at

18–25 weeks of gestation. Numerous subsequent studies using assays which detect either intact (i.e., dimeric) hCG (ihCG) or total hCG (i.e., dimeric + beta subunit hCG; thCG) have confirmed that hCG levels are elevated in Down's syndrome pregnancies in the second trimester (Table 28.6). Less marked but still significant elevations have been found for the FαhCG (Ryall et al., 1992; Spencer 1993a; 1994a; Wald et al., 1994a; 1994b). Macri et al. (1990) and Spencer (1991) reported that maternal serum levels of the free β subunit of hCG (FβhCG) were also elevated in Down's syndrome pregnancies. Meta analysis of published studies of FβhCG levels in over 500 cases indicates that there is a greater shift in the median MoM for FβhCG (2.20) than for dimeric hCG (2.06). The free β subunit of hCG also exists in serum in unstable, nicked form (nFβhCG) which has broken peptide linkages in the region of residues 43–48. Rotmensch et al. (1996) found high levels of nFβhCG (median 4.76 MoM) in a small study of six Down's syndrome and 64 unaffected pregnancies. As with AFP, the distributions of thCG and hCG subunit levels in normal and affected pregnancies are log Gaussian (Fig. 28.9) but with a smaller overlap of normal and affected pregnancies.

Two other placental markers which show significant elevations in Down's syndrome pregnancies are pregnancy specific beta-1 glycoprotein (SP-1) (Graham et al., 1992) and dimeric inhibin A (InhA)(Aitken et al., 1996a; Wald et al., 1996a; Wallace et al., 1996). There have also been reports of changes in the levels of human placental lactogen (hPL) and progesterone (Knight et al., 1989), α inhibin (Van Lith et al., 1992a; Spencer et al., 1993a), placental isoferritin p43 component (Moroz et al., 2000). and total activin A (Lambert-Messerlian et al., 1996; Dalgleish et al., 2001), while pregnancy associated plasma protein A (PAPP-A) (Cuckle et al., 1992), placental alkaline phos-

phatase (PALP) (Aitken et al., 1996b) and cancer antigen 125 (CA125) (Spencer, 1993b; Spencer et al., 1997a) show little change in concentration in Down's syndrome pregnancies in the second trimester (Table 28.6).

Maternal serum unconjugated estriol (UE3) levels, like AFP, are reduced in Down's syndrome pregnancies in the second trimester (Canick et al., 1988; Wald et al., 1988) (Table 28.6). UE3 levels in normal and trisomy 21 pregnancies are a poor fit to both Gaussian and log Gaussian distributions (Crossley et al., 1993). Other markers where significant changes have not been confirmed in Down's syndrome pregnancies are follistatin (Cuckle et al., 1999a), prostate specific antigen (PSA) (Spencer and Carpenter, 1998), and protein S100 (Abraha et al., 1999).

Trisomy 18

Very low levels of thCG and FβhCG have been found in maternal serum from trisomy 18 pregnancies (Bogart et al., 1987; Canick et al., 1990a; Crossley et al., 1991; Spencer et al., 1993b). PAPP-A levels have also been shown to be significantly reduced (Bersinger et al., 1999; Spencer et al., 1999a) while less marked reductions have been reported for AFP and UE3 (Merkatz et al., 1984; Lindenbaum et al., 1987, Norgaard-Pedersen et al., 1990; Crossley et al., 1993). Concentrations of SP-1 (Graham et al., 1992) and inhibin A (Aitken et al., 1996a) are not significantly altered when compared with those found in unaffected pregnancies (Table 28.6).

Other aneuploidies

There is much less information on second trimester maternal serum markers in other types of chromosome abnormality. Apart from those cases of trisomy 13 which have secondary abnormalities, e.g., neural tube defects, trisomy 13 pregnancies tend not to show any marked pattern of change in maternal serum markers in the second trimester. Saller et al. (1999) found UE3 levels to be significantly reduced (0.66 MoM) in 25 cases but no significant change for AFP (1.34 MoM) or hCG (0.89 MoM).

Of the sex chromosome aneuploidies, Turner syndrome (45,X) has been most extensively studied. Here, AFP levels tend to be slightly reduced, UE3 levels markedly reduced and hCG levels either increased or decreased depending on whether hydrops is present or not (Saller et al., 1992). FβhCG levels are also elevated in hydropic cases (Laundon et al., 1996). Lambert-Messerlian et al. (1998; 1999) have found reduced levels of inhibin A (0.64 MoM) and progesterone (0.90 MoM) in Turner syndrome without hydrops

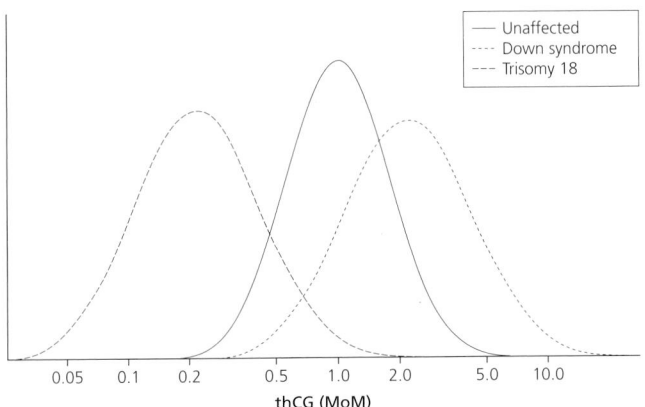

Fig. 28.9 Distribution of thCG (in MoM) in unaffected, Down's syndrome and trisomy 18 pregnancies.

and increased levels (3.91 MoM and 2.11 MoM respectively) in cases where hydrops was present. These data are derived from cases diagnosed prenatally or where there were clinical indications postnatally and therefore they may not reflect the true picture of marker changes in sex chromosomal aneuploidies as many cases are unrecognized at birth.

Triploidy

Triploidy can be classified into two phenotypes based on placental and ultrasound findings (McFadden and Kalousek, 1991; Jauniaux et al., 1996). In Type I the placenta is enlarged and partially multicystic (molar) whereas the fetus is relatively well grown with either proportionate head size or slight microcephaly. Type II, which is the most common, is characterised by a small normal looking placenta and a severely growth restricted fetus with pronounced wasting of the body and sparing of the head. The two phenotypes have been shown to be dependent upon the parental origin of the extra chromosome set. In Type I the additional chromosome set is of paternal origin (diandric) and in Type II it is of maternal origin (digynic) (McFadden et al. 1993; Goshen, 1994; Dietzsch et al., 1995). This different chromosomal origin is also associated with a distinct pattern of marker variation in maternal serum. Type I triploids present with high thCG and high AFP levels in the second trimester while type II have very low levels of thCG and relatively normal AFP (Eiben et al., 1996b)

SERUM MARKERS IN ANEUPLOID PREGNANCIES IN THE FIRST TRIMESTER

Down's syndrome

In the first trimester, a different pattern of change in maternal serum marker levels is observed in trisomic pregnancies. Although AFP levels are reduced in Down's syndrome pregnancies at this stage of gestation, the change is smaller than that observed in the second trimester (Table 28.6). This effect has been noted for several other markers.

Early studies (Cuckle et al., 1988; Bogart et al., 1989; Brock et al., 1990; Aitken et al., 1993) indicated that thCG levels were only modestly raised in trisomy 21 in the first trimester and consequently thCG was a weak marker at this stage. This position has been challenged by Haddow et al. (1998) who suggested that the elevated levels of thCG could be used effectively to screen in the first trimester. A recent large scale study has shown that this is not the case unless screening is carried out at the very end of the first trimester when the levels of thCG in the trisomy 21 cases are increas-

ing to the peak levels seen around 16 weeks (Spencer et al., 2000a). Combining first trimester thCG data from 625 cases gives a median MoM of 1.33 contrasting with a median MoM of 2.06 observed in the second trimester.

Spencer et al. (1992a) reported that levels of FβhCG were elevated in 13 cases of trisomy 21 (median MoM 1.85) in the first trimester and subsequently many other studies have confirmed raised levels. The largest single series to date (Spencer et al., 1999a) containing 210 cases of trisomy 21 had a median MoM of 2.15. Combining FβhCG data from several studies totaling 846 cases gave a median MoM of 1.98, only slightly lower than the levels reported in the second trimester (Table 28.6).

Brambati et al. (1991) were the first to show that levels of pregnancy associated plasma protein A (PAPP-A) were reduced in cases of trisomy 21 in the first trimester and this has subsequently been confirmed in many other studies. Spencer et al. (1999a) have shown that PAPP-A levels are reduced to 0.51 MoM in 210 cases of trisomy 21 and a meta analysis totaling 777 cases gives a median MoM of 0.45 (Table 28.6). However, PAPP-A levels are not markedly altered in Down's syndrome pregnancies in the second trimester and the extent of the median shift in early pregnancy is gestation-related (Berry et al., 1997).

Trisomy 18

Early reports of biochemical markers in the first trimester have suggested that trisomy 18 is associated with a decrease in maternal serum FβhCG (Spencer et al., 1992a) and PAPP-A (Brambati et al., 1993; Spencer et al., 1994a). Since then several reports on small numbers of cases have confirmed these findings. The largest series to date (Tul et al., 1999) of some 50 cases reinforces the view that FβhCG and PAPP-A levels are significantly reduced. Combining data from several sources including the latter study gives a FβhCG median level of 0.27 MoM in a series of 126 cases and a PAPP-A median level of 0.20 MoM in 119 cases (Table 28.6).

When thCG and AFP were examined in the 50 cases reported by Tul et al. (1999) only thCG levels were significantly reduced with a median MoM of 0.38, whilst the AFP median was 0.91MoM (Spencer et al., 2000b). This reduction in thCG in trisomy 18 is less than that observed for FβhCG and shows the same trend as that observed for trisomy 21 in the first trimester.

Trisomy 13

In the first trimester a clear pattern of marker variation in trisomy 13 similar to that in trisomy 18 is now established

(Spencer et al., 2000c). In a study of 42 cases the median MoM Free β-hCG was decreased with a median MoM of 0.51, whilst that for PAPP-A was further reduced with a median MoM of 0.25. Total hCG and AFP have also been studied in the same series (Spencer et al., 2000b) and only the reduced level of thCG was shown to be significant. However this reduction to 0.74 MoM is less marked than that for FβhCG and again supports the view that FβhCG is a more discriminatory marker than thCG. AFP with a median MoM of 0.92 was not significantly reduced.

Sex chromosome aneuploidies

In a study of 46 cases of Turner's syndrome (45,X), the median PAPP-A MoM was significantly lower than that found in controls (0.49 MoM) whilst the median FβhCG MoM was not significantly different (1.11 MoM) (Spencer et al., 2000d). In a series of 13 other sex aneuploidies including cases of 47,XXY; 47,XYY and 47, XXX, the median PAPP-A and FβhCG MoMs were not significantly different (0.88 and 1.07 MoM) from controls. When AFP and thCG were examined the median AFP levels were higher in this group (1.36 MoM) but not different in the Turner's group (1.14 MoM) (Spencer et al., 2000b). Although the median thCG was reduced in the Turner's group (0.80 MoM) and increased in the other sex aneuploidies (1.12 MoM), neither change was significant. As in the second trimester, there is likely to be ascertainment bias in identification of cases of sex chromosome aneuploidy.

Triploidy

Spencer et al. (2000e) have shown that FβhCG levels are elevated (8.04 MoM) in cases with Type I phenotype in the first trimester, as are levels of thCG (4.91 MoM) and AFP (2.76 MoM). PAPP-A on the other hand is mildly decreased (0.75 MoM). In cases of Type II phenotype FβhCG levels are dramatically reduced (0.18 MoM) as are the levels of thCG (0.16 MoM) and PAPP-A (0.06 MoM), whilst AFP is moderately reduced (0.77 MoM) (Spencer et al., 2000e). This effect of raised or lowered hCG is an example of genomic imprinting with the extra paternal set of chromosomes over-expressing hCG (McFadden et al., 1993).

URINE MARKERS

Many circulating pregnancy markers including oestriols, thCG, FαhCG, FβhCG, nicked FβhCG and its terminal degradation product, β-core hCG, are excreted in maternal urine. Cuckle et al. (1994a) first reported substantially ele-

vated urinary β-core hCG (5.34 MoM) in a small study of seven Down's syndrome pregnancies in the second trimester when the levels were corrected against creatinine concentration. Similar results were reported by Canick et al. (1995) and extended by Cuckle et al. (1995) in a larger study of 24 Down's syndrome pregnancies where significant changes were found in the levels of urinary β-core hCG (6.02 MoM) and total estriol (tE) (0.74 MoM) but not FαhCG (1.08 MoM). Low levels of tE but variable changes for β-core hCG and FαhCG were also found in 5 trisomy 18 pregnancies and a group of sex chromosome aneuploides. More modest elevations of β- core hCG (2.35 MoM) were reported by Spencer et al. (1996) in a series of 29 maternal urine samples from Down's syndrome pregnancies. Urinary FβhCG levels were also measured and found to be elevated (2.47 MoM). Lam et al. (1997) reported similar results for β-core hCG (3.44 MoM) in maternal urine from 29 Asian women with Down's syndrome pregnancies. Several other studies of urine samples collected mainly in the second trimester have been reported and summarized by Hsu et al. (1999) and Cole et al. (1999a) who also carried out a prospective study of β-core hCG levels in freshly collected urine samples from 23 women with Down's syndrome pregnancies over a three year period. Markedly elevated β-core hCG levels were found in this study (5.44 MoM) and they proposed that the lower concentrations reported in some other studies may be due to the use of stored/frozen urine samples promoting aggregation of β-core hCG fragments which interferes with the assay of β-core hCG. In a further study of the same sample series, Cole et al. (1999b) used a specially developed immunoassay to measure levels of urinary hyperglycosylated hCG (a form of hCG characterised by a more complex oligosaccharide side chain) and found dramatically elevated levels in trisomy 21 pregnancies (7.8 MoM).

Less marked changes in urinary β-core hCG levels have been reported in aneuploid pregnancies in the first trimester. Spencer et al. (1997b) examined β-core hCG and FβhCG in 22 Down's syndrome pregnancies at 10–14 weeks of gestation. The median β-core hCG level was increased to 2.91 MoM and free β-hCG to 1.81 MoM, but the very wide spread (SD) of the data in controls and cases made both markers poor discriminators of affected pregnancies. In cases of trisomy 18 the levels of both markers were reduced and in trisomy 13 the level of urine FβhCG was elevated while that of β-core hCG was very low. Others have also reported poor discrimination between normal and trisomic pregnancies based on urine β-core analysis in the first trimester (Cuckle et al., 1996; Kornman et al., 1997; ; Macintosh et al., 1997). Recently, Weinans et al. (2000) have reported a median

Table 28.7. Maternal urine marker median MoM in first and second trimester Down's syndrome pregnancies

	n	β-core hCG	n	Total estriol	n	FβhCG
1st trimester	50	2.10	22	0.83	36	1.71
2nd trimester	200	3.88	151	0.62	127	3.16

Table 28.8. Mahalanobis distances for selected first and second trimester markers of trisomy 21

Marker	Mahalanobis distance	
	2nd trimester	1st trimester
Serum		
AFP	0.69	0.23
Unconjugated estriol	1.20	0.68
Intact/total hCG	1.86	0.38
FβhCG	2.04	1.45
Dimeric inhibin A	1.65	0.35
PAPP-A	–	2.08

hyperglycosylated hCG level of 3.6 MoM in eight urine samples from Down's syndrome pregnancies collected at 10–11 weeks gestation. One trisomy 18 and two trisomy 13 cases had levels of 0.3, 0.2 and 0.2 MoM respectively.

A summary of urinary marker medians compiled from published studies in the first and second trimesters is presented in Table 28.7. Although some urinary metabolites of hCG appear to show large median shifts in trisomic pregnancies suggesting that they may be potentially effective markers of Down's syndrome, the spread of values, particularly in the first trimester, are large and questions remain over assay availability, standardization against creatinine and sample stability.

MARKER PREDICTIVE VALUE

The efficacy of a particular screening marker depends not only on the shift of the mean or median level in affected cases, but also on the spread of the values (the standard deviation, SD) in affected and unaffected cases. For two markers with similar SDs, the marker with the greater median shift in affected pregnancies will have better predictive value, while for two markers with similar median shifts, the marker with the smaller spread of values will be more effective. Markers can be graded for effectiveness in screening for Down's syndrome by calculating the Mahalanobis distance which expresses the separation of the affected and unaffected populations as a function of the width of the distributions: (Mean [unaffected] – Mean [affected]/SD [unaffected])^2 where the means and SD are of the $\log_{10}$ distributions (Wright et al., 1993). Table 28.8 shows estimated Mahalanobis distances for some of the screening markers measured in the first and second trimesters. Using this criterion, intact or total hCG, FβhCG and inhibin A are the best markers for second trimester maternal serum screening while FβhCG and PAPP-A can be considered to be suitable markers for use in first trimester screening for aneuploidies. As pioneered with AFP/age screening, each marker could be used individually to provide a separate measure of risk of an affected pregnancy. However, in practice, a much more effective method is to use two or more markers together with maternal age. The

principles of this type of multivariate screening are described by Reynolds and Penney (1990).

MULTIMARKER SCREENING

Second trimester

In practice, the choice of screening markers is influenced by factors other than the median shift (and SD) observed in affected pregnancies. Any association (correlation) between two or more markers used together will reduce their relative contributions to detection. Reported correlation coefficients (r) between pairs of markers tend to vary between different studies, but significant associations have been confirmed between thCG, FβhCG and InhA, and AFP and UE3 and these must be taken into account in the calculation of risk when two or more markers are used together. Also, although AFP is a relatively weak marker for trisomic pregnancies, it is almost always included in second trimester screening protocols because of its value at that stage as a marker for neural tube defects and other structural abnormalities. Other practical issues also influence marker selection such as assay costs, availability, suitability for automation and analyte stability.

The expected screening performance of various marker combinations has been modeled from data obtained in numerous retrospective case control studies of Down's syndrome and trisomy 18 pregnancies. Considerable disparity in estimates of detection and false positive rates has been reported which may be ascribed to a variety of factors including variations in sample size, sample selection, assay methodology, risk calculation methods, estimation of gestational ages, marker distributions and correlations, and corrections for co-variables (Reynolds, 1994). In one study, Wald et al. (1988) predicted a detection rate for Down's syndrome of 61% at a 5% false positive rate based on three markers (AFP, thCG and UE3) in combination with maternal age (the triple test). Crossley et al. (1991) proposed a double test combination of AFP and thCG with maternal age and estimated 57% detection at a 5% false positive rate. Macri et al. (1990) and Spencer (1991) developed double test protocols based on FβhCG, AFP and maternal age and showed that detection rates for Down's syndrome were improved when FβhCG was substituted for thCG. Ryall et al. (1992) proposed a 5 marker test combination (AFP, FαhCG, FβhCG, UE3 and hPL) which was projected to give a 76% detection rate at a 3.9% false positive rate. Much controversy has surrounded the contribution of UE3 to detection of Down's syndrome pregnancies with some groups claiming significant improvements in detection (Cuckle, 1994) and others no benefit (Spencer, 1994b). Recently, test combinations incorporating InhA as a third or fourth marker (Aitken et al., 1996a; Wald et al., 1996a) have been estimated to yield detection rates of over 70% at a 5% false positive rate.

Detection rates for Down's syndrome for various combinations of five different screening markers with maternal age based on parameter sets from one center and gestational estimates by dates and scan have been published (Wald et al., 1997). A better measure of true screening performance might be expected from audit of routine screening programs but here detection rates may be affected by incomplete ascertainment of affected pregnancies (which enhances apparent screening performance) or screening of pregnant populations with atypical age distributions. In the UK where a double test (AFP with either thCG or FβhCG) is most widely used, detection rates for Down's syndrome of 65–70% at a 5% false positive rate have been reported in two large unselected screening populations with complete ascertainement (Spencer and Carpenter, 1993; Crossley et al., 1994). Further experience of screening in these same populations has largely confirmed the initial performance on large numbers of pregnancies. Aitken and Crossley (1997) reported 68% detection of Down's syndrome at a 5.2% false positive rate for AFP/hCG/age in over 100,000 screened pregnancies and Spencer (1999a) reported a 75% detection of Down's syndrome at a 5.1% false positive rate for AFP/FβhCG/age in 67,000 pregnancies. Similar detection rates have been reported for prospective triple marker (AFP/hCG/UE3) testing (Goodburn et al., 1994). Wald et al. (1997) attempted a synthesis of published data from screening programs in prospective use (termed "demonstration projects" although many appear to be reports of screening in routine clinical practice). Although there was considerable variation between individual studies, there appears to be little difference in performance between triple tests which include UE3 and double tests which do not. A detection rate (uncorrected for fetal loss) of 70% at a 5.7% false positive rate was estimated for AFP/hCG/UE3/age

screening by combining data from over 116,000 pregnancies. The corresponding figures for AFP/hCG/age screening were 66% detection at a 4.8% false positive rate in over 110,000 pregnancies. Further improvement in detection seems possible with the inclusion of InhA although prospective data is lacking.

Many routine screening programs also include a separate protocol for trisomy 18 based on multivariate analysis of the reduced marker concentrations generally associated with this aneuploidy. Detection rates comparable with those for Down's syndrome have been reported for various combinations of markers for only a small additional false positive rate. Staples et al. (1991) estimated a 58% detection for a 0.3% false positive rate using UE3, FαhCG, FβhCG, estradiol and human placental lactogen. Spencer et al. (1993b) estimated a 50% detection rate for a 1% false positive rate using AFP and FβhCG while Barkai et al. (1993) estimated 67% detection for a 0.3% false positive rate using AFP/hCG/UE3. Palomaki et al. (1995), in a study of marker levels in 94 affected pregnancies, found UE3 to be the strongest individual predictor of trisomy 18 and estimated a 60% detection rate for a 0.2% false positive rate using an AFP/thCG/UE3/age protocol. Leporrier et al. (1996), using thCG and UE3 and fixed cut-off MoMs for each marker, estimated 48% detection at a 0.8% false positive rate. Further gains in detection could be provided by the addition of PAPP-A analysis (Bersinger et al., 1999; Spencer et al., 1996b), but this is unlikely to be a practical proposition as this marker is not routinely analyzed in the second trimester.

Biochemical screening for aneuploidy has a number of advantages over age-only screening. Sensitivity and specificity are improved resulting in a greater detection of affected pregnancies for fewer invasive diagnostic tests and a consequent reduction in the number of iatrogenic fetal losses. Also a proportion of fetal abnormalities other than Down's syndrome and trisomy 18 are incidentally detected. For example, type I triploids (diandric) are identified by the Down's syndrome screening protocol while type II (digynic) are detected by the trisomy 18 protocol. Difficult counseling issues are raised, however, when cases of Turner syndrome or other conditions with a mild phenotype are found. Other difficulties associated with biochemical screening relate to the variation in detection of affected pregnancies with maternal age, and the anxiety generated by waiting for results. As the starting point for screening is 15 weeks gestation in most programs, the process of screening, counseling of women at increased risk, diagnostic testing and fetal chromosome analysis may often mean a delay of 2–3 weeks before the fetal karyotype is known.

This leads to late intervention in pregnancy where an affected fetus is found and the parents opt for termination. Also, as up to one third of affected pregnancies may be missed by second trimester biochemical screening, further improvements in sensitivity of detection would be desirable.

First trimester

As many markers show a different pattern of variation in cases of aneuploidy in early pregnancy, the second trimester protocols described above are not optimum for use in the first trimester. Also, AFP is an ineffective marker for NTD before 14 weeks gestation and therefore not an automatic selection in first trimester screening protocols. FβhCG and PAPP-A have emerged as the most effective markers for first trimester screening and several retrospective studies have examined the performance of this combination of markers with maternal age at 7–14 weeks gestation. Estimated detection rates for Down's syndrome at a 5% false positive rate of 62% (Wald et al., 1996b), 68% (Krantz et al., 1996), 55% (Berry et al., 1997) and 56% (Forest et al., 1997) have been reported. However, detection rates are affected by the gestation at which samples are obtained. Berry et al. (1997) showed that the median shifts for FβhCG and PAPP-A were not constant across the first and second trimesters by comparing the levels of each marker at different stages in the same pregnancy. In this study, two samples were obtained from each of 45 Down's syndrome pregnancies, one in the first trimester and another in the second trimester. The FβhCG median MoM in the first trimester was 1.99 and in the second trimester 2.79. The corresponding values for PAPP-A were 0.50 MoM and 0.94 MoM. This indicates that the parameters of the distributions vary for FβhCG and PAPP-A at different gestations in the first and second trimesters and that a single unified distribution across 7–14 weeks is not optimum. A large number of cases is required to accurately define the trends for each marker and allow the calculation of gestation-specific medians. This complicates the calculation of risk from biochemical markers in the first trimester.

FIRST TRIMESTER POPULATION DISTRIBUTION PARAMETERS IN TRISOMIES 21, 18 AND 13

Population distribution parameters can be derived in two different ways. The first method is a direct approach in which FβhCG and PAPP-A are measured in maternal serum samples from a large group of affected cases and compared with a much larger group of control unaffected pregnancies

(Wald et al., 1996b; Berry et al., 1997; Haddow et al., 1998; Spencer et al., 1999a). The individual analyte values in both series are converted to MoMs and these values are then $\log_{10}$ transformed and their distributions checked for a gaussian fit. The $\log_{10}$ mean and $\log_{10}$ standard deviation for each analyte in cases and controls can then be calculated and the correlation between each analyte estimated in each series. The second method is to carry out a meta analysis in which data from the literature on all published series is included to derive parameter estimates (Cuckle and van Lith, 1999) and these may then be tailored to an individual center's own population and laboratory conditions using procedures developed for the second trimester (Cuckle, 1995). Although this latter approach enables population parameters to be calculated from larger series of Down's syndrome cases than is possible with most direct measurement series, it is potentially flawed in the first trimester. Firstly it assumes that all of the assays used for each analyte are compatible or that conversion to MoMs removes any assay biases—a fact that is well established to be incorrect in the second trimester for UE3 and AFP (Parvin et al., 1991; Reynolds and John, 1992; Bishop et al., 1994). Also, as noted below, early polyclonal-based PAPP-A assays may detect different forms of PAPP-A and other serum components compared with the specific monoclonal methods now in routine use (Qin et al., 1996) questioning the validity of combining data obtained by different methods. Another problem with the meta analysis approach relates to the fact that the median MoM for both PAPP-A and FβhCG in cases of trisomy 21 changes across the first trimester and therefore grouping data from a wide gestational window will inevitably lead to an error in estimating the performance of the various markers. Although Cuckle and van Lith (1999) have made adjustments to the median MoM to compensate for this variation with PAPP-A they have made no such adjustment for FβhCG and also made no adjustment to the standard deviation. Also, the accuracy of meta analysis is compromised where individual MoM data are extracted from published studies by reading points from a scatter plot—an approach which can lead to some obvious errors.

Direct measurement approaches are also not without problems. The data of Wald et al. (1996b) are derived from 77 cases and 385 controls spread across a wide gestational window (8 to 14 weeks) and takes no account of the gestational variation of either PAPP-A or FβhCG in cases of trisomy 21 (Reynolds et al., 1998). Furthermore the assay used in this study was an earlier polyclonal-monoclonal immunometric assay for PAPP-A known to cross react with other serum components (Pettersson et al., 1993). Similarly the studies of Berry et al. (1997) and Haddow et al. (1998) both used a polyclonal PAPP-A assay and derived parameters from a wide gestational range. Also, Hallahan et al. (1998) have drawn attention to an inconsistency in the distribution parameters given for intact hCG and FβhCG in the study of Haddow et al. (1998). Spencer et al. (1999a) used samples collected in a narrower gestational window (10.5 to 13.5 weeks) and a more specific monoclonal assay for PAPP-A to derive parameters which may be more appropriate for that period of gestation. A comparison of the FβhCG and PAPP-A distribution parameters reported in the above studies is summarized in Table 28.9. From these distribution parameters and an age standardized population distribution it is possible to estimate the Down's syndrome detection rate in each study for a fixed 5% false positive rate (Table 28.10). Better estimates of true screening performance will be possible when a comprehensive analysis of the temporal changes in median analyte levels in Down's syndrome pregnancies across the first and second trimesters is available (see below). However, based on the information currently available, it is unlikely that detection rates will vary by more than 7–10% across the 8 to 14 week window.

As for trisomy 21, population parameters can be estimated for trisomy 18 and trisomy 13 and hence individual risks for trisomy 18 and trisomy 13 can be derived in the first trimester. Only a few studies have been of sufficient size to allow meaningful parameter estimation, including those of Biagiotti et al. (1998) and Tul et al. (1999) for trisomy 18 and that of Spencer et al. (2000c) for trisomy 13. For trisomy 18, Tul et al. (1999) and Biagiotti et al. (1998) estimated that detection rates of around 75% were possible for a 0.5% false positive rate. Detection increases by a further 10% when fetal nuchal translucency thickness is added to the algorithm (Tul et al., 1999). For trisomy 13, detection rates of 69% can be achieved at a 0.5% false positive rate increasing to 90% when fetal nuchal translucency thickness is added to the algorithm (Spencer et al., 2000c).

TEMPORAL CHANGES IN MEDIAN ANALYTE LEVELS ACROSS THE FIRST AND SECOND TRIMESTERS

In the second trimester it is well established that the median MoM FβhCG in cases of trisomy 21 changes across the 14

Table 28.9. Study population and serum FβhCG and PAPP-A parameters in five studies in the first trimester

Statistic	Wald et al., 1996b	Berry et al., 1997	Haddow et al., 1998	Spencer et al., 1999a	Cuckle and van Lith, 1999
Gestation range	8–14	7–14	9–13	10+3–13+6	6–14
Cases	77	54 (52)	48	210	502 (447)
Controls	385	10600 (227)	3169	947	31435 (8623)
Correlation controls	0.1407	−0.223	0.154	0.160	0.111
SD free β controls	0.2833	0.289	0.275	0.249	0.287
MEAN Log$_{10}$ Free β controls	0	−0.003	0	0.004	0
Correlation Down's	0.0648	−0.086	−0.038	0.216	0.130
SD Free β Down's	0.2870	0.306	0.257	0.271	0.290
MEAN Log$_{10}$ Free β Down's	0.2540	0.299	0.311	0.322	0.296
SD PAPP-A controls	0.2659	0.236	0.251	0.237	0.285
MEAN Log$_{10}$ PAPP-A controls	0	−0.011	0	−0.004	0
SD PAPP-A Down's	0.3471	0.481	0.272	0.275	0.326
MEAN Log$_{10}$ PAPP-A Down's	−0.3704	−0.305	−0.370	−0.306	−0.481 to −0.143 at 9 to 13 weeks

Table 28.10. Estimated detection rates for Down's syndrome at a 5% false positive rate for serum markers combined with maternal age in the first trimester

Marker (plus maternal age)	Wald et al., 1996b	Berry et al., 1997	Haddow et al., 1998	Spencer et al., 1999a (Spencer et al., 2000a)	Cuckle and van Lith, 1999
PAPP-A	52%	41%	42%	48%	52%
Free β-hCG	38%	41%	25%	46%	42%
Total hCG	32%		29%	(31%)	
Free β-hCG + PAPP-A	62	55%	60%	67%	65%

to 20 week gestational window (Macri et al., 1990; 1993c; Spencer and Macri, 1992: Spencer et al., 1992b). At the 14 to 16 week period median levels are 18% higher than in the 17 to 19 week period (Spencer et al., 1993c) and such differences lead to 10–15% higher detection rates at 14 to 16 weeks compared with 17 to 19 weeks (Spencer, 1999a). The FβhCG median MoM in a study of 480 cases of trisomy 21 in the second trimester was found to be 2.64 (Macri et al., 1994), this is higher than the average value of 1.98 seen in the first trimester. This suggests that the median MoM in trisomy 21 cases is changing between trimesters and some early evidence for this was also shown by workers (Spencer et al., 1994a; Berry et al., 1997; Spencer 1997a) collecting samples from the same cases in both the first and second trimesters, when similar sized differences were observed. More recently in a large first trimester study over a narrow gestational window of 10.5 to 14 weeks by Spencer et al. (1999a) has confirmed that FβhCG median MoMs do increase in trisomy 21 cases even across this period, with medians of 1.75 at 11 weeks, 2.20 at 12 weeks and 2.25 at 13 weeks. This temporal shift in median is also evident from a meta-analysis of published studies. Very little published data is available prior to 10 weeks but our evidence suggests that FβhCG levels in cases of trisomy 21 fall to normal levels by the 7–8th week. In a series of 53 cases between the sixth and eigth week of gestation the median FβhCG was 1.21 (Berry E, Crossley JA, Aitken DA, Spencer K, 2000, unpublished observations).

In the case of PAPP-A and trisomy 21, in the second trimester levels approach normal by about the 16–17th week, (Cuckle et al., 1992; Knight et al., 1993; Spencer et al., 1994a; Berry et al., 1997) and paired sample analysis on cases between the two trimesters clearly shows the reducing discriminatory power for PAPP-A in the second trimester. In the first trimester the first intimation that the median MoM was also not constant across this period came from Bersinger et al. (1994) who showed a median MoM of 0.47 at 10–11 weeks and 0.85 MoM at 12–13 weeks in a study of 29 cases. In a much larger series of 210 cases, Spencer et al. (1999a) similarly showed a variation across the narrow window of 11 to 13 weeks, with the median MoM of 0.44 at 11 weeks, 0.50 at 12 weeks and 0.69 at 13 weeks. Examination of published literature by meta-analysis based on the median gestation of the study samples confirms this increase in MoM with gestation (Spencer et al., 1999a). Indeed one of the lowest medians reported is the 0.27 MoM of Brambati et al. (1993) which was obtained from a study of samples with a median gestation of eight weeks. This would suggest that better clinical discrimination might be achieved earlier in the first trimester with PAPP-A.

In other aneuploidies, temporal changes in analyte MoMs across the first and second trimester are also evident, but perhaps have less of a clinical impact. For example, in trisomy 18 median PAPP-A levels fall progressively across the first trimester and continue to fall through the second trimester (Spencer et al., 1999b; Tul et al., 1999). In trisomy 13 levels of FβhCG (and presumably thCG) increase from moderately low levels in the first trimester to normal or marginally raised levels in the late second trimester (Spencer et al. 2000c, 2001).

MATERNAL AND PREGNANCY VARIABLES

Effect of co-variables

Numerous factors have been recognized that affect serum marker levels and therefore the risk estimate derived from them. Refinements to multimarker screening programs have been introduced to take account of these factors, allowing a more precise estimate of risk and possible improvements to detection rates as a result of reducing the population variance.

Gestation

All maternal serum marker concentrations vary with gestation. In the second trimester, AFP, UE3 and SP-1 levels rise with advancing gestation, while ihCG, FβhCG and InhA levels fall. As noted above, comparison of levels at different gestations is achieved by conversion of marker concentration to MoM, but the precision of this estimate depends on the accuracy of the gestational estimate, whether derived from an LMP or (preferably) from an ultrasound assessment of fetal maturity. The greatest error associated with inaccurate gestational estimates is found for UE3, which has the greatest rate of change with gestation, and the least error with InhA, which has a relatively flat concentration profile in the second trimester. An overestimated gestation will result in the calculation of lower MoMs for AFP and UE3 (and therefore greater likelihood ratios) and higher MoMs for ihCG, FβhCG and InhA (and therefore greater likelihood ratios) leading to the calculation of a higher than appropriate risk for any combination of these markers. An underestimated gestation will have the opposite effect.

In the first trimester free β-hCG levels rise to a peak at around 64 days with values then declining in an almost linear fashion by about 1 IU/L (1 ng/ml) per day (Berry et al., 1995) to reach plateau levels at around 18 weeks. PAPP-A levels on the other hand show a fairly linear increase in concentration across the first trimester period

(Spencer et al., 1994a). In the first trimester gestational dating errors are probably less likely than in the second trimester since biochemical measurements at this time are normally combined with ultrasound measurement.

Maternal weight

All the maternal serum markers that have been investigated in detail seem to show a tendency for levels to decrease with increasing maternal weight. This is due to the dilution effect of the greater blood volume in heavy women diluting a fixed amount of placental product. Conversely in smaller women the blood volume is less and so the effect is to concentrate the placental product. Correction for maternal weight can be made by dividing either the analyte result in concentration units or in MoM by the expected value for the weight based on a regression curve. In the second trimester this has been done either using a linear regression method (Palomaki et al., 1990) or a reciprocal regression method (Neveux et al., 1996) and the latter has been shown to be more accurate (Kennedy et al., 1999) (Fig. 28.10). It is important however that each center constructs its own weight correction curve since any difference in median weight between populations will introduce inaccuracies. This is particularly important when considering non-Caucasian populations such as Asians or Orientals (Hseih et al., 1995). In the first trimester the reciprocal regression model gives the best fit at the extremes of the distribution. Weight correction equations based on data from 5422 Caucasian women have been published (Spencer et al., 2000 g).

Multiple pregnancy

In common with AFP, other serum markers show increased concentrations in maternal serum from multi-fetal pregnancies in the second trimester. A meta-analysis of published studies gave twin median MoM levels of 2.18 MoM for AFP on 1638 unaffected twin pregnancies, 1.63 MoM for UE3 on 286 pregnancies, 1.89 MoM for ihCG on 559 pregnancies and 2.11 MoM for FβhCG on 645 pregnancies (Aitken, 1995). There are few corresponding data on twin pregnancies affected by Down's syndrome. Spencer et al. (1994b) reported AFP and FβhCG levels in eight sets of dizygous twin pregnancies discordant for Down's syndrome. A twin corrected median MoM of 0.72 MoM was estimated for AFP and 1.54 MoM for FβhCG. Standard deviations of the marker distributions in affected twin pregnancies were similar to those found for affected singleton pregnancies for AFP, but markedly smaller in the case of FβhCG. A detection rate for Down's syndrome of 51% at a 5% false positive rate was estimated using AFP, FβhCG and maternal age. Estimation of an accurate risk of Down's syndrome in a twin pregnancy based on a combination of biochemical markers and maternal age is complicated where chorionicity is unknown. The age related risk of Down's syndrome in monozygous twin pregnancies is approximately equivalent to that of singleton pregnancies of women of the same age, while for dizygous twins the age related risk that either fetus will have Down's syndrome is double that of a singleton pregnancy.

In a series of 159 first trimester twin pregnancies compared with 3466 singleton controls the FβhCG median was 2.1 times higher and the PAPP-A median 1.86 times higher

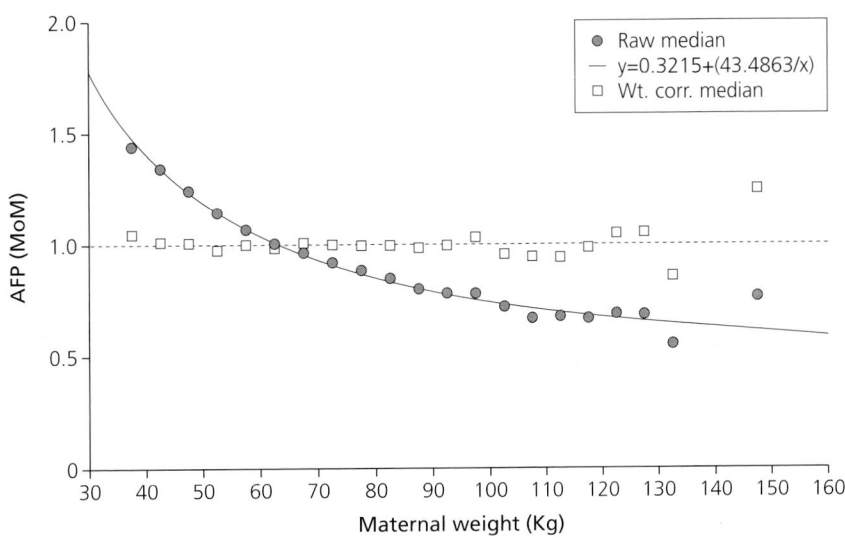

Fig. 28.10 Effect of correction of AFP levels (in MoM) for women of above and below average maternal weight.

than in singletons (Spencer, 2000a). Although screening for twins in the second trimester is considered by some to be problematical because of the significant clinical, technical and ethical challenges posed for the diagnosis and management of such pregnancies, correction methods have been introduced which will produce "pseudo-risks" in such situations (Wald et al., 1991; Spencer et al., 1994b). These are estimated to allow detection of just over 50% of cases in which twins are discordant for trisomy 21. Similar methods have been proposed for correction in the first trimester when detection rates of 52% can be expected in discordant twins (Spencer, 2000a). These methods can also be used alongside nuchal translucency measurements (see later section), when a combination of ultrasound and biochemical measurements can be expected to detect 80% of twins discordant for trisomy 21 (Spencer, 2000a). Such algorithms are already in use in prospective practice (Spencer and Nicolaides, 2000).

Smoking

Maternal smoking during pregnancy is a known health problem associated with significant risks to the fetus. Thomsen et al. (1983) first reported that second trimester maternal serum AFP levels in women who smoked were higher than those in non-smokers. Bernstein et al. (1989) reported that maternal serum levels of hCG and estradiol in early pregnancy were significantly depressed in women who smoked. Cuckle et al. (1990) confirmed these findings noting a 7% increase in AFP, a 5% fall in UE3 and an 11% fall in hCG. This was reinforced by Bartels et al. (1993) who reported a 21% fall in thCG levels and also produced evidence to suggest that this fall in thCG was not dependent on the number of cigarettes smoked. They also found a 3% reduction in UE3 levels. Palomaki et al. (1993) found a 25% reduction in thCG but also reported a weak dose response relationship between nicotine levels and the magnitude of the decrease in hCG levels. The impact of smoking on FβhCG in the second trimester is a reduction in levels in smokers by 14% (Spencer, 1998). Recently, Ferriman et al. (1999) reported that InhA levels are increased by 47% in smokers, suggesting a possible underlying cause for the reductions in thCG and FβhCG levels. When marker levels were investigated in Down's syndrome pregnancies in women who smoked (Cuckle et al., 1990; Spencer, 1998) AFP levels were found to be around 10% higher than in non smokers, UE3 levels were 2% lower, total hCG levels were 27% lower and FβhCG levels were 16% lower than in non smokers. These changes in marker levels in pregnancies affected by Down's syndrome reflect the changes seen in unaffected pregnancies. The consequence is a significantly lower detection rate and a lower false positive rate in women who smoke (Spencer, 1998). However, although correction for smoking would have a significant impact on any one individual's risk, the overall effect on population screening would be only a modest 1–2% improvement in detection rates (Cuckle et al., 1990a,b; Spencer, 1998). These changes in detection rate and false positive rate will also vary from center to center, being dependent on the incidence of smoking in the population, which in turn is significantly influenced by age distribution and socio-economic status.

In the first trimester Brambati et al. (1997) reported a 4% reduction in FβhCG levels in smokers in a series of 740 pregnancies and a 4% reduction in PAPP-A levels. No reduction in FβhCG levels in smokers was apparent amongst a group of 3111 women with unaffected pregnancies (Spencer, 1999b), while for PAPP-A the median weight-corrected level in smokers was significantly reduced to 0.85 MoM. Uncorrected, this 15% reduction was estimated to reduce detection rates for Down's syndrome in smokers from 67% to 61%. Analyte levels have also been examined in women who smoked and had a pregnancy affected by trisomy 21 (Spencer et al., 2000f). FβhCG levels were 13% lower than in non smokers with affected pregnancies and PAPP-A levels were 6% higher although neither change was statistically significant. The implications of this data would be for a decrease in the detection rate and an increase in the false positive rate when screening for trisomy 21 amongst women who smoked.

Suggestions have been made that there is a negative association between Down's syndrome births and maternal cigarette smoking (Klein et al. 1981; Hook and Cross, 1985; Shiono 1986; Christianson and Torfs, 1988). Other studies that were carefully controlled for maternal age (Cuckle et al., 1990; Chen et al., 1999) could not confirm a relationship between maternal smoking and a lower rate of Down's syndrome births. The prevalence of Down's syndrome births increases with advancing maternal age, whereas cigarette smoking decreases with advancing maternal age. Chen et al. (1999) demonstrated that it was important to control for maternal age in individual year increments rather than in broad age bands. In two recent studies, one in the second trimester (Spencer, 1998) and the other in the first trimester (Spencer et al., 2000f), of the effect of maternal smoking on maternal serum markers no deficit of Down's syndrome cases was found in the second trimester study, but in the first trimester there was a reduction of 25% in the Down's syndrome cases amongst smokers. If an association between maternal smoking and Down's syndrome rates is confirmed it would require correction to the a priori age risks in order to provide accurate risks for women who smoke.

Ethnicity

The assessment of the influence of ethnic origin on maternal serum marker levels from published data is often difficult since many earlier studies did not apply maternal weight correction to marker levels. This is an important pre-requisite since average maternal weights in black Afro-Caribbean populations are higher than those in white women while Asian/Oriental women have a much lower maternal weight. When maternal weight is taken into account, there is a significantly higher AFP level (15%), higher thCG level (18%), higher FβhCG level (12%) and lower inhibin A level (8%) in black Afro-Caribbean women in the second trimester than in Caucasians. For UE3 no significant difference has been observed. It is reasonably well established that in Asian and Oriental women, weight corrected second trimester hCG levels (both total and free β) are also higher than in Caucasian women (Hseih et al., 1995; Onda et al., 1996). AFP levels are increased in orientals. Watt et al. (1996) proposed a method of correcting for ethnic origin but a gain of only 0.5% in detection rate could be expected at population level.

In the first trimester a study of Afro-Caribbean and Asian women (Spencer et al., 2000 g) found that weight corrected FβhCG and PAPP-A medians were respectively 21% and 57% higher in Afro-Caribbean women and 4% and 17% higher in Asian women. It was estimated that correcting for ethnicity would increase the overall population detection rate by only 1.4% but the effect at an individual level could be highly significant. For example in a 67 kg, 25-year-old Afro-Caribbean with an uncorrected FβhCG of 2.10 MoM and a PAPP-A of 0.65 MoM, the risk prior to correction would be 1 in 540. After correction the FβhCG MoM becomes 1.73 and the PAPP-A MoM 0.41 with a corrected risk of 1 in 260.

Fetal sex

In the second trimester it is known that the presence of a female fetus results in a 7% higher maternal serum FβhCG MoM and a 3% lower AFP MoM (Spencer, 2000b). These changes lead to a significantly higher false positive rate in women carrying a female fetus and although it has been suggested that this effect would lead to a reduced detection rate in female fetuses affected by trisomy 21 (Bazzett et al., 1998; Ghidini et al., 1998), Spencer et al. (2000b) could find no evidence for any fetal gender bias in detection rates amongst large series of pregnancies. When fetal sex was examined in the first trimester (Spencer et al., 2000h) in both chromosomally normal fetuses and in the presence of fetuses with trisomy 21, FβhCG levels were increased by 15% and 11% respectively in female fetuses. Similarly for PAPP-A levels were increased by 10% and 13% respectively in female fetuses.

In contrast fetal nuchal translucency was 3% to 4% lower in both chromosomally normal and trisomy 21 female fetuses. The consequence of such changes when screening for trisomy 21 will be a reduction in the detection rate in female fetuses of the order of 1–2% (Spencer et al., 2000h).

Gravidity and parity

In the second trimester both maternal serum total hCG and FβhCG have been shown to decrease with an increasing number of pregnancies (gravidity) or an increasing number of previous births (parity) (Haddow et al., 1995; Spencer, 1995). The observed effect (after taking into account an increased maternal weight with increasing number of pregnancies) is quite small—less than 6% between primagravid and multigravid women. Correction for such a small change is not considered worthwhile when screening in the second trimester.

In the first trimester Spencer et al. (2000i) have shown that gravidity and parity is associated with a small but progressive decrease in fetal nuchal translucency and a small but progressive increase in both FβhCG and PAPP-A. None of these changes was statistically significant and correction for this variable was not considered necessary.

Pregnancy complications and adverse outcome

In the second trimester conflicting views have been expressed as to the relationship between biochemical marker levels and the incidence of pregnancy complications and adverse outcomes such as pre-eclampsia, IUGR, low birth weight, pre-term delivery and stillbirth (Spencer, 2000c). It would appear that apart from the association of a raised FβhCG (or thCG) with an increased incidence of pre-eclampsia, an isolated raised FβhCG is not associated with adverse outcome in the second trimester. When this was examined in the first trimester FβhCG levels were not increased in cases developing pre-eclampsia (Ong et al., 2000) and, if anything, values were lower in cases of pregnancy induced hypertension. Low maternal serum PAPP-A was associated with subsequent miscarriage, development of pregnancy induced hypertension and growth restriction. However, the sensitivity and specificity of these tests were low and therefore they are not useful as predictors of subsequent complications of pregnancy (Ong et al., 2000). In contrast Morssink et al. (1998) in a smaller study could find no association between first trimester FβhCG and PAPP-A levels in cases with pre-term delivery or in those with IUGR. Cuckle et al. (1999b) have also shown that low PAPP-A is associated with poor fetal viability, confirming earlier reports (Westergaard et al., 1983).

IDDM

In women with insulin dependent diabetes mellitus (IDDM) second trimester maternal serum marker levels on the whole are reduced, although considerable variation exists in the published literature. This variation is partly due to the fact that maternal weight correction has often not been applied (women with IDDM tend to be around 6 kg heavier) and the possibility that the extent of the reduction is dependent upon the adequacy of diabetic control. Early studies reported marked reductions in AFP levels to around 0.60–0.80 MoM (Wald et al., 1979; 1992; Milunsky et al., 1982). Reese et al. (1987) found a median AFP level of 0.91 MoM which increased to 0.96 MoM when corrected for maternal weight. Canick et al. (1990b) reported a median AFP level of 0.97 MoM and Crossley et al. (1996) found levels of 0.89 MoM (0.98 MoM when corrected for maternal weight). High levels of glycosylated hemoglobin indicate poor control of IDDM during pregnancy and an inverse relationship has been established between the levels of glycosylated hemoglobin and AFP (Reese et al., 1987; Baumgarten and Robinson, 1988; Martin et al., 1990). Although an overall estimate of a 10% reduction for AFP might seem reasonable in IDDM women, genuine differences probably exist between different populations reflecting differences in the level of diabetic control. Ideally, correction factors should be established locally but published data suggests that UE3, thCG, and FβhCG all show reductions of less than 10% (Wald et al., 1992; Palomaki et al., 1994; Wald et al., 1994a,b; Crossley et al., 1996). Dimeric inhibin A on the other hand has been reported raised by 17% in one study (Wallace et al., 1997) but reduced by 12% in another (Wald et al., 1996c).

For first trimester markers, levels of PAPP-A are reduced in IDDM mothers (Pedersen et al., 1998) and in those with pre-existing or gestational diabetes the levels of FβhCG and PAPP-A are reduced by 20% and 25% respectively (Ong et al., 2000). If such reductions are confirmed in other studies correction of both markers will be necessary in diabetic women.

Previous screening results

In women who have an increased Down's syndrome risk in a first pregnancy there is a five-fold greater chance of them also having an increased Down's syndrome risk in a second preg-

nancy (Holding and Cuckle, 1994; Spencer, 1997b). The extent of this is more noticeable in younger women such that at 20 years of age the relative chance is 5-fold, reducing to 1.3-fold at age 40. Such a biological association of serum marker levels between pregnancies suggests that there are additional maternal or genetic factors influencing the levels of these serum markers, other than the physiological factors which in themselves are poorly understood. Correcting for a previous result has been estimated to have only a small (0.2%) impact on false positive rates (Spencer, 1997b), although others consider correction worthwhile (Larsen et al., 1998).

Assisted reproduction

In the second trimester assisted reproduction techniques appear to have an impact on maternal serum marker levels. In women undergoing ovulation induction only, total hCG levels were 9% higher and UE3 8% lower, whilst AFP was not significantly different (Barkai et al., 1996). In women having IVF the various studies are inconsistent. Muller et al. (1993) reported normal hCG levels in 138 IVF pregnancies, whilst Heinonen et al. (1996), Ribbert et al. (1996), Frishman et al. (1997), Lam et al. (1999) and Wald et al. (1999a) reported increases of 52%, 29%, 22%, 22% and 14% respectively. In one study (Barkai et al., 1996) a 7% decrease was reported. For AFP the general consensus is that in IVF pregnancies levels are no different from controls and UE3 levels are reduced by 6–8%. Inhibin A in one small study was not significantly different (Wald et al., 1999a).

In pregnancies conceived by intrauterine insemination the levels of AFP were significantly lower (0.76 MoM) compared with normally conceived pregnancies (1.05 MoM) (Hsu et al., 1999) while the levels of FβhCG were not significantly different. In pregnancies conceived by intracytoplasmic sperm injection (ICSI) the median AFP was also significantly reduced (0.76 v 0.94 MoM) while for thCG the change was not significant (0.88 v 0.94 MoM) (Lam et al., 1999).

In the first trimester FβhCG was increased (14%) in IVF pregnancies whilst PAPP-A was decreased (8%) (Liao et al., 2001). In those having ICSI only PAPP-A was significantly decreased (20%) while in the group having only ovulatory inducing drugs, levels were not significantly different from the controls. The difference in FβhCG and PAPP-A levels in the IVF pregnancies would result in at least a 1% higher false positive rate in this group and correction may be worthwhile (Liao et al., 2001).

An important point to be remembered when estimating risks in IVF pregnancies is that in cases where a donor egg is used the prior risk should be based on the maternal age of the donor rather than the recipient's maternal age.

Vaginal bleeding

The presence of vaginal bleeding in early pregnancy complicates the interpretation of serum screening for Down's syndrome. In one study, AFP levels were significantly increased in cases of vaginal bleeding (by 9%), but the increases in UE3 (5%) and thCG (12%) levels did not reach significance (Cuckle et al., 1994b). Although Cuckle et al. (1994b) proposed a method of correcting for vaginal bleeding which was estimated to increase the detection rate by less than 1%, in practice correction is rarely applied as the magnitude of the marker changes is related to the proximity of the bleed to the time of sampling. Correction is also made more difficult by the fact that vaginal bleeding is more common in older women and that it is also a risk factor for Down's syndrome (Cuckle and Wald, 1990).

ASSAY SPECIFICITY AND SAMPLE STABILITY

FβhCG is present in maternal serum in a milieu of hCG related molecules. Many different forms of hCG exist and include intact hCG (the combined alpha and beta subunits), hyperglycosylated forms of both intact and FβhCG and the various nicked forms of both intact and FβhCG. (Cole, 1994; Cole et al., 1997). The levels of FβhCG for example are 0.5% of the total circulating hCG, thus assays must be very specific and be able to measure the specific free β form against this high background. Since it has been suggested also that nicked FβhCG production in trisomy 21 may account for the improved specificity of FβhCG in the second trimester (Cole, 1994), it may be important that FβhCG assays also measure the nicked and non nicked forms.

Consideration should also be given to sample collection and storage conditions. FβhCG stability at room temperature was originally questioned based on anecdotal evidence of the thermal degradation of intact hCG producing elevated levels of FβhCG. Scientific studies have shown that intact hCG in serum is stable for up to 70 hours at room temperature although FβhCG levels can increase in whole blood after 35 hours at room temperature (Spencer et al., 1993d). Others have shown that these limitations have no impact on screening performance (Cuckle and Jones, 1994; 1995; Muller et al., 1999). Provided samples are in serum form then stability during transport does not become an operational issue. In those situations when shipment of serum is not possible, dried filter paper blood spots provide a reliable alternative with stability in excess of seven days at 37°C (Spencer et al., 1993d; Verloes et al., 1995; Macri et al., 1996).

As noted earlier, assay specificity is also of some concern with respect to PAPP-A which has recently been identified as an insulin-like growth factor (IGF)-dependent protease which cleaves IGF binding protein-4 (Lawrence et al., 1999). In maternal serum PAPP-A exists complexed 2:2 with the preform of eosinophil major basic protein (ProMBP) (Oxvig et al., 1994). ProMBP also can be complexed with angiotensinogen and this new complex can also be complexed with complement 3dg (Christiansen and Norgaard-Pedersen, 1997). Early assays for PAPP-A were either RIAs employing purified and labeled PAPP-A with a short shelf life and questionable specificity or ELISAs employing polyclonal antibodies. The specificity of the polyclonal antibodies has been a source of controversy for some years and a widely used commercial polyclonal antibody (A0230, DAKO) has been shown to cross react with SP1, ProMBP and haptoglobin (Christiansen and Norgaard-Pedersen, 1997) and this could lead to underestimates of the clinical utility of PAPP-A (Qin et al., 1996). More recently assay systems using dual monoclonal antibodies against PAPP-A/ProMBP have been shown to give lower median MoMs in trisomy 21 samples compared with the dual polyclonal assay (Christiansen and Norgaard-Pedersen, 1997; Qin et al., 1997). Now that commercial monoclonal assays are available for PAPP-A (e.g., Brahms (formerly CIS) BioInternational Kryptor; Perkin Elmer Delfia; Johnson & Johnson Amerlex-M) the problem of assay specificity is hopefully resolved.

On the question of stability of PAPP-A little has been published but our own studies have shown that up to five freeze/thaw cycles and storage of samples for up to seven days at room temperature have no effect on measured PAPP-A levels. The only effect noted was that associated with blood collected in EDTA, which complexes the zinc moiety at the center of the PAPP-A protein resulting in a conformational change to the molecule, making it invisible in the monoclonal assay system (Spencer, 1998, unpublished observations).

ULTRASOUND SCREENING FOR FETAL CHROMOSOME ABNORMALITIES IN THE SECOND TRIMESTER

Benacerraf et al. (1985) first reported sonographic evidence of a thickening of the fetal skin or soft tissue in the nuchal area in the second trimester where the fetus had Down's syndrome. This nuchal fold thickness was measured in transverse view of the fetal skull, being the soft tissue thickness behind the occiput which measures between 1 mm and 5 mm at 15–20 weeks gestation in unaffected fetuses. Several studies of nuchal fold measurement as a screening method for Down's syndrome, mainly in high risk populations, have been reported and are reviewed by Benacerraf (1996) and Borrell et al. (1996). Using a cut off of 5 mm or 6 mm detection rates averaged around 40% for a false positive rate of about 2%. Other second trimester sonographic signs have been linked to the presence of fetal Down's syndrome, including short femur length, pyelectasis, echogenic bowel and various structural malformations (Benacerraf, 1996). Although individually, most are weak markers, used together it has been suggested that they may have useful predictive value particularly when combined with maternal age (Vintzileos and Egan, 1995) or maternal serum screening results. Palomaki and Haddow (1995) have criticized this approach due to the uncertainty over false positive rates. Bahado-Singh et al. (1995) found that normal nuchal fold thickness significantly reduced the risk of Down's syndrome in women with positive serum screening results. Nyberg et al. (1995) reported that abnormal sonographic signs increased the risk of Down's syndrome 5.6-fold in screen positive women but half of all cases in the study group were missed by ultrasonography. Normal ultrasonography reduced the risk by approximately half. Recently, Howe et al. (2000) have suggested that a combination of maternal age and mid pregnancy ultrasound scanning may out-perform a combination of maternal age and second trimester serum biochemistry as a screening test for Down's syndrome. The authors identified 36 of 53 (68%) cases of Down's syndrome at a false positive rate of 6.6%. However, of the 53 Down's syndrome pregnancies 36 (68%) were in women aged 35 years or over suggesting some selection bias in the study population. Also, no standardized ultrasound protocol was described, raising concerns expressed previously about control of the false positive rate (Palomaki and Haddow, 1995). Again, if there is no or low correlation between ultrasound markers and biochemical markers, a better approach would be to combine age, ultrasound and biochemical markers in the second trimester.

ULTRASOUND SCREENING FOR CHROMOSOME ABNORMALITIES IN THE FIRST TRIMESTER

A routine ultrasound examination of the fetus in the first trimester has increasingly become an integral part of antenatal care. Apart from confirming fetal viability, the number of fetuses and establishing fetal age, a more detailed examination of the fetus can also reveal chorionicity in twin pregnancies or certain developmental abnormalities such as anencephaly. Ultrasound markers which may be associated with fetal chromosome abnormality at this stage of pregnancy include exomphalos and gastroschisis, fetal heart rate

pattern, reduced crown-rump length (CRL) and increased nuchal translucency (NT).

Fetal heart rate

Studies of heart rate in chromosomally abnormal fetuses have reported conflicting results. In a longitudinal study of one trisomy 21 fetus at 6–9 weeks gestation the heart rate was consistently below the 3rd centile of normal (Schats et al., 1990). In another study of five fetuses at 7–13 weeks the heart rate was always within the normal range (van Lith et al., 1992b). In a study of 17 cases at 10–13 weeks the heart rate was either above the 97th or below the 2.5th centile in 23% of cases (Martinez et al., 1998). Fetal heart rate (FHR) has been comprehensively examined in a series of 472 pregnancies with trisomy 21 and 437 pregnancies with other chromosomal abnormalities between 10–14 weeks of gestation, and compared with 25,000 normal pregnancies (Liao et al., 2000). In trisomy 21, trisomy 13 and Turner syndrome FHR was significantly higher than in controls. In trisomy 18 and triploidy the heart rate was lower and in other sex chromosomal defects it was not significantly different from normal. FHR was above the 95th centile of normal in 10%, 67% and 52% of fetuses with trisomy 21, trisomy 13 and Turner syndrome respectively. The FHR was below the 5th centile in 27% of fetuses with triploidy and 18% of those with trisomy 18. However, the addition of FHR measurement to existing algorithms incorporating fetal nuchal translucency and maternal serum biochemistry is unlikely to yield extra gains in detection.

Nuchal translucency (NT)

In all fetuses there is an ultrasound-translucent area of fluid between the fetal skin and soft tissue overlying the cervical spine. Nicolaides et al. (1992) used the term "nuchal translucency" (NT) to describe this accumulation of fluid which has an average maximum thickness of about 1.4–1.5 mm at 13 weeks of gestation in normal fetuses when measured by ultrasound in the saggital plane (Pajkrt et al., 1995). Studies in high risk pregnancies in the first trimester identified a possible association between an enlarged NT and fetal chromosome abnormalities (Szabo and Gellen 1990; Nicolaides et al. 1992; Shulman et al. 1992). In a series of 1273 high risk pregnancies, 84% of Down's syndrome fetuses and 4.5% of unaffected fetuses were found to have an NT measurement ≥ 2.5 mm (Nicolaides et al., 1994). Other studies have shown that each of the common trisomies (Down's syndrome, trisomy 18 and trisomy 13) and some sex chromosome abnormalities (Turner syndrome) are often associated with an enlarged NT at 10–13 weeks of gestation (Johnson et al., 1993; Pandya et al., 1995a). However, considerable variation in detection rates has been reported (Brambati et al. 1995; Szabo et al., 1995) and the usefulness of NT measurement as a screening test in unselected pregnancies has been questioned (Kornman et al., 1996).

Chitty and Pandya (1997) reviewed the performance of fetal NT measurements for the detection of fetal chromosome abnormalities in several published studies in both selected and routine screening populations. The mean detection rates for Down's syndrome were 77% and 62% respectively and the corresponding false positive rates 6.0% and 4.0% respectively but with wide variation in each population. NT measurements have also been shown to be useful for the detection of fetal abnormality in twin pregnancies (Sebire et al., 1996) where biochemical screening alone is of doubtful value.

Subsequently, in the largest study reported to date (Snijders et al., 1998), NT measurements obtained in 96,127 women attending one of 22 centers in the UK were used to derive risks which were then combined with the mother's age risk to delineate a high risk group. Using an NT/age cut-off risk of 1:300, 82.2% of trisomy 21 pregnancies and 77.9% of pregnancies with other fetal chromosomal abnormalities were identified at an 8.3% false positive rate. At a standardised 5% follow-up rate, 77% of Down's syndrome fetuses were identified. In intervention studies such as this, true detection rates are difficult to measure and the authors have attempted to account for fetal loss between 12 weeks and term although their figures are disputed (Haddow, 1998). There appears to be an increased rate of miscarriage of fetuses with large NT measurements whether chromosomally normal or abnormal (Hyett et al., 1996). Nevertheless, in combination with maternal age, NT measurement in skilled hands appears to be the single most effective marker for Down's syndrome yet identified.

Some of the reported variation between studies undoubtedly relates to the practical problems of measuring NT thickness which is operator dependent. High resolution ultrasound equipment which can measure to the nearest 0.1 mm, with magnification and playback capability and the option of transabdominal or transvaginal transducers assists in the ease of obtaining accurate and reproducible measurements. Specific training in the application of a consistent protocol, an appreciation of factors which may influence NT measurements, e.g., fetal neck position (Whitlow et al., 1998), and a system of quality control based on a review of images (Herman et al., 1998) and an on-going audit of measurements (RCOG, 1997; Crossley et al., 2000), the

results of which are relayed back to the contributors of the data, are essential. Pandya et al. (1995b) proposed the following criteria for NT measurement should be applied in all cases:

- the fetus must be in the saggital plane
- the ultrasound image should be magnified to fill three-quarters of the screen
- care must be taken to distinguish between fetal skin and amnion (aided by waiting for spontaneous fetal movement away from the amnion or by asking the mother to cough or by tapping the abdomen)
- the maximum NT thickness is determined to the nearest 0.1 mm by placing the calipers on the edges of the fetal skin and soft tissue overlying the cervical spine (Fig. 28.11)
- three separate measurements should be obtained.

When this protocol was used to measure NT in 1718 unselected pregnancies in a routine antenatal clinic setting, 63 women (3.6%) had an NT measurement ≥ 2.5 mm, 49 of whom opted for CVS and three of four trisomy 21 pregnancies were detected (Pandya et al., 1995c). These results contrast with those of Roberts et al. (1995b) and Bewley et al. (1995) who attempted NT measurements in 1368 unselected women using their own protocol and rounding measurements to the nearest mm. NT measurements were obtained in 1127 pregnancies (82%) and using a cut-off of ≥ 3.0 mm, 6% of unselected fetuses and one of three trisomy 21 and one of two trisomy 18 fetuses were identified.

In most of the early studies, discrimination between normal and affected pregnancies was based on the use of a simple cut-off NT measurement, commonly 2.5 or 3.0 mm. However, this fails to take account of the change in NT thickness with gestation (Pajkrt et al. 1995; Braithwaite et al. 1996) and NT measurements should be interpreted against gestation using a CRL (or BPD) measurement. As with serum markers, the most effective method of interpreting NT thickness is to convert individual measurements to MoM. Published parameters of the distribution of NT measurements in MoM show that they are $\log_{10}$ normally distributed (Nicolaides et al., 1998). Each individual NT measurement can therefore be converted to a risk (odds ratio) and combined with other risks derived from maternal age or maternal serum marker measurements. This maximizes the value of the NT data as a small NT will give a lower risk just as a large NT will give a higher risk and emphasizes the importance of always obtaining a precise and accurate NT measurement in every pregnancy. Figure 28.12 shows the distribution of NT measurements in MoM in normal and trisomy 21 pregnancies using data

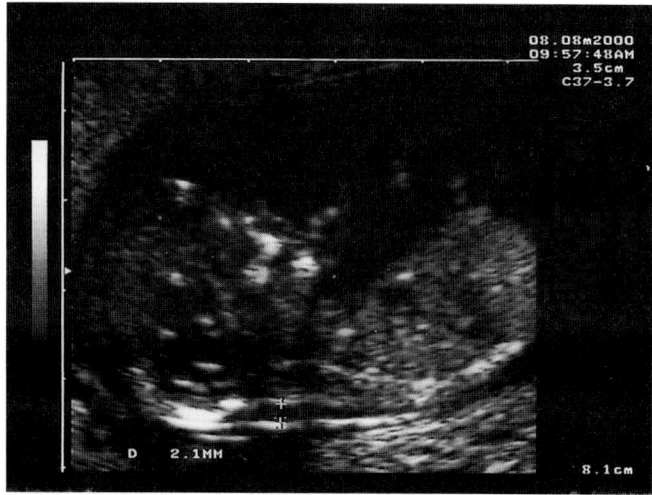

A

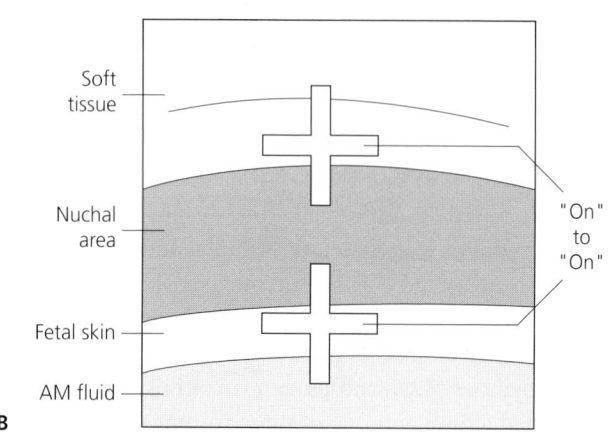

Soft
tissue

Nuchal
area

"On"
to
"On"

Fetal skin

AM fluid

B

Fig. 28.11 A and B. Fetal image, orientation, size and caliper placement for NT measurement.

published by Nicolaides et al. (1998) based on 95,476 normal pregnancies and 326 cases of Down's syndrome. From the parameters of the distributions, the median NT MoM in trisomy 21 pregnancies was 2.02, and the $\log_{10}$ SDs of the distribution in Down's syndrome pregnancies was greater than that in unaffected pregnancies (0.235 vs 0.120). This gives a Mahalanobis distance of 6.46, which is notably larger than that of any of the serum markers in current use (Table 28.8), illustrating the potential discriminatory power of NT. However, it is important to note that not all affected pregnancies will have large NTs, but for those that do e.g., > 5 0 mm) very high odds ratios in favor of an affected pregnancy are derived. The difference in SDs also creates an anomaly on this particular data set such that likelihood ratios decline as MoMs decrease to about 0.8 MoM but thereafter begin to increase again. Thus a lower truncation limit of 0.8 MoM should be used to avoid giving inappropriately high risks for small NT measurements (Crossley and Aitken, 1999).

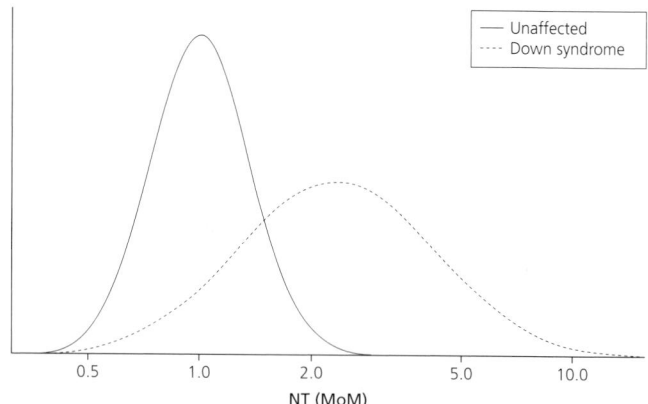

Fig. 28.12 Distribution of NT measurements (in MoM) in unaffected and Down's syndrome pregnancies.

Fetal abnormalities other than chromosomal trisomies are also associated with an enlarged NT. Pandya et al. (1995d) reviewed the outcome of pregnancy in 565 cases with an enlarged NT but a chromosomally normal fetus and found an increased incidence of cardiac, diaphragmatic, renal and ventral wall defects. There was also an increasing risk of miscarriage and perinatal death associated with increasing NT size. Others have also reported increased NT measurements at 10–14 weeks of gestation in fetuses which were later found to have major cardiac defects (Hyett et al., 1997) and fetal echocardiography should be considered in such cases later in pregnancy. Thus, NT is a powerful marker of fetal abnormality which is rapidly being adopted into screening programs. However, its effectiveness as a predictor of aneuploid pregnancies is increased when it is combined with biochemical markers.

Combined ultrasound and biochemical (CUB) screening

Combining ultrasound nuchal translucency and maternal serum biochemistry to produce risks in conjunction with maternal age is simply analogous to the use of three markers in the second trimester described earlier based on the gaussian method of Reynolds and Penney (1990). Spencer et al. (1999a) combined trisomy 21 maternal serum marker population distributions with those established for NT (Nicolaides et al., 1998) based on the large multicenter series described by Snijders et al. (1998). When individual biochemical marker levels were compared against NT there was no significant correlation either in the control group or in the trisomy 21 pregnancies for PAPP-A (r = 0.000 and r = − 0.089, respectively) and FβhCG (r = −0.057 and r = 0.000, respectively). Other combined distribution parameters have been published. Those of Cuckle and van Lith

(1999) use the Nicolaides et al. (1998) NT distribution parameters and the meta-analysis of the serum biochemistry as outlined previously. These parameter sets also assume no correlation between NT and serum markers. The parameter set of Wald and Hackshaw (1997) is based on data from three sources: the biochemical marker data previously discussed (Wald et al., 1996b), NT data extracted from figures from an early study of 86 cases of trisomy 21 (Pandya et al., 1995a) and NT baseline data complied from a separate study of 561 unaffected pregnancies (Schuchter et al., 1998). Distribution parameters have also been derived for biochemical markers and NT for trisomy 18 (Tul et al., 1999) and trisomy 13 (Spencer et al., 2000d).

PREDICTED DETECTION AND FALSE POSITIVE RATES

Using these three different sets of population parameters, predictions have been made on the likely detection rate at a fixed 5% false positive rate using an age standardized population distribution. Wald and Hackshaw (1997) predicted a detection rate of 80%, Cuckle and van Lith (1999) predicted a range between 80–87% depending on the use of specific week median MoMs for PAPP-A. Spencer et al. (1999a), using prospective NT measurements and retrospective analysis of FβhCG and PAPP-A in 210 cases of Down's syndrome, estimated a detection rate of 89%. Table 28.11 shows from the data of Spencer et al. (1999a) how detection rates can be tailored to provide different false positive rates. Other retrospectve studies have reported similar results. De Graaf et al. (1999) estimated 84.6% detection at a 5% false positive rate for FβhCG, PAPP-A, NT and maternal age.

High detection rates for CUB screening have also been reported in prospective non-intervention studies. De Biasio et al. (1999) in a study of 1467 women found 13 cases of trisomy 21 and detected 11 (85%) with a false positive rate of 3.3%. Orlandi et al. (1997) studied 744 women from an advanced maternal age group and found seven cases of trisomy 21 and detected six cases (86%) with a false positive rate of 4.7%. Recently, data from a large multicenter study of over 17,000 unselected pregnancies, shows 82% detection of Down's syndrome pregnancies at a 5% false positive rate when NT, FβhCG, PAPP-A and maternal age are used together (Crossley et al. 2001).

For trisomy 18 the predicted detection rate in one study was 86% at a 0.5% false positive rate (89% at a 1% false positive rate) using combined biochemical markers and NT (Tul et al., 1999). For trisomy 13 the predicted detection rate was 90% at a 0.5% false positive rate (84% at a 0.1% false positive rate) (Spencer et al., 2000c). The multivariate risk algorithm for trisomy 21 incorporating NT, FβhCG, PAPP-A and maternal age would identify 96% of cases of Turner syndrome and 62% of other types of sex chromosomal anomalies (Spencer et al., 2000d). However, many sex chromosomal abnormalities remain unrecognized at birth and beyond and these figures may be an overestimate. Similarly, using a combination of the trisomy 21 risk algorithm and an atypicality approach, over 95% of cases of triploidy would be identified (Spencer et al., 2000e).

PERFORMANCE IN PROSPECTIVE PRACTICE

Prospective intervention CUB screening has been offered in one centre in the UK since early 1998 using a unique approach. The One Stop Clinic for Assessment of Risk for fetal abnormality (OSCAR) is designed to allow the patient, in a one hour visit to the clinic, to have pre-test counseling; phlebotomy; biochemical measurement of FβhCG and PAPP-A; ultrasound assessment of nuchal translucency, crown-rump length and anomaly scan prior to receiving a combined first trimester risk report and post test counseling. The results of the first year of screening over 4000 women showed a detection rate of 86% for trisomy 21 (six out of seven cases), a detection rate of 100% for trisomy 18 and trisomy 13 (nine out of nine cases) and a detection rate of 95% (18 out of 19 cases) for all aneuploidies (Spencer et al., 2000j). Year two figures also show detection of 8 of 9 cases of trisomy 21, and 16 of 17 aneuploides in total with only one case of trisomy 21 missed.

Table 28.11. False positive rates at fixed detection rates for various combinations of serum markers with and without NT

Detection Rate %	Free β-hCG & PAPP-A	NT & free β-hCG	NT & PAPP-A	NT, free β-hCG & PAPP-A
90	23.0	12.0	12.0	6.0
85	16.0	7.0	7.0	3.5
80	11.0	5.0	4.0	2.1
75	8.0	3.0	2.7	1.5
70	6.0	2.2	1.5	1.0

Data from Spencer et al. (1999a)

Krantz et al. (2000) reported the results of CUB screening on 5809 women between 10 weeks and 4 days and 13 weeks and 6 days gestation. A combination of ultrasound NT and biochemical measurements on dried blood spot specimens gave an observed detection for Down's syndrome of 91% at a 7.8% false positive rate. Within the study population, 34% of the women were aged 35 years or over. When the data was modeled on the age distribution of the USA pregnant population, the detection rate was projected to be 91% at a 5% false positive rate.

These reports confirm the superior performance of CUB screening predicted by retrospective studies compared with current second trimester biochemical screening protocols. Apart from the improvement in sensitivity and specificity, the availability of rapid results and earlier diagnosis of affected pregnancies as delivered by the OSCAR approach seems attractive to pregnant women (Spencer et al., 2000j). However, first trimester screening brings many logistical challenges. Women need to be informed about the possibility of CUB screening before they attend for their antenatal appointment. To benefit from the information provided by an NT scan, they must attend within a very narrow gestational window (ideally during the 11th, 12th or 13th week) and, as an accurate assessment of gestation may only become available at that visit, it is inevitable that a proportion of women will come too early or too late for CUB screening. For those attending too early it may be advantagous to collect the blood at that stage so that the serum markers can be measured and the results are available when the woman returns for her NT scan, speeding the provision of the combined risk estimate. For those attending too late, second trimester biochemical screening can be offered as an alternative. Thus, centers offering CUB screening need to retain the ability to provide second trimester biochemical screening as it is likely that there will always be a small proportion of women who will require tests at this stage of pregnancy.

Abandoning the routine second trimester AFP test may lead to an increase in the number of undetected spina bifida pregnancies unless the safeguard of a second trimester anomaly scan is available to all women who have first trimester screening. Where such scanning is not routinely offered to all patients, some centers may consider it worthwhile to continue to offer AFP screening for NTD. As noted above, abnormalities other than aneuploidy (e.g., cardiac defects) are sometimes associated with an enlarged NT measurement in the first trimester and these may be diagnosable by ultrasound later in pregnancy. Therefore, it is important to ensure that all women who have an NT measurement above a certain threshold (e.g., 2.5 MoM),

but have a chromosomaly normal fetus on diagnostic testing or a low risk on CUB screening, are offered a second trimester anomaly scan at around 22 weeks of gestation.

Multistage testing

A danger inherent in the introduction of first trimester NT screening with or without the measurement of FβhCG and PAPP-A is that some women given a normal NT measurement or low CUB risk may, by accident or design, go on to have a second trimester biochemical screening test and possibly additional ultrasound screening. The results from the subsequent test(s) should not be considered in isolation as an accurate estimate of risk requires that the first trimester results must be taken into account. Cuckle and Sehmi (1999) have shown how this may be achieved for a first trimester NT measurement and second trimester biochemical markers (assuming that there is no correlation between the ultrasound and biochemical markers). Calculating the correct risk is more complicated if both first and second trimester biochemical markers are measured. Depending upon the markers tested, there will be some degree of correlation to be taken into account but the necessary data has not been published. Such sequential testing is likely to lead to confusion if women are given different risks at different stages and the probable effect will be an increase in the overall number of diagnostic tests carried out for little gain in detection of affected pregnancies. Wald et al. (1997) pointed out that such an approach was inefficient and recommended that screening should be carried out at one stage in pregnancy only. Subsequently Wald et al. (1999b) proposed a different approach where the information from selected first and second trimester markers is integrated to give a single estimate of risk. Using NT and PAPP-A measurements between 10–13 weeks and thCG, AFP, UE3 and InhA at 15+ weeks of gestation, they estimated that 94% of Down's syndrome pregnancies could be detected at a 5% false positive rate. Although this modeled performance exceeds that found in prospective practice for first trimester CUB screening, the implementation of the integrated screening test as a method of population screening may be difficult in practice. To optimise the effectiveness of this approach women would have to make at least two visits to the antenatal clinic: one in the first trimester to provide blood for PAPP-A and for an NT measurement, and another at 15–16 weeks to provide blood for thCG, AFP, UE3 and InhA measurements. Apart from increasing the cost and inconvenience for patients (and therefore the likelihood that some will default), women will have to endure the additional anxiety associated with a 4–6 week wait for results. As up to 90% of Down's syndrome pregnancies could have been detected by CUB screening four weeks earlier, the majority of women found to have an affected pregnancy by the inegrated test route will have missed out on the benefits of earlier prenatal diagnosis and termination of pregnancy. Also, in some cases a combination of maternal age and a large NT discovered at the first trimester scan visit may produce a risk which is so high that it is unlikely to be modified into the low risk group by subsequent biochemical testing. Under these circumstances reporting of an interim risk based on information available at the time of the NT scan would be of benefit to the patient. The integrated test may, however, find greater acceptance amongst women with pregnancies conceived through IVF or ICSI who are anxious to avoid the risks associated with invasive diagnostic testing.

Summary and conclusions

The introduction of prenatal screening for neural tube defects 25 years ago by measurement of maternal serum AFP changed the pattern of antenatal care for a high proportion of the pregnant population. A visit to the antenatal clinic or physician at 16 weeks gestation became necessary for blood sampling for MSAFP analysis and 3–5% of screened women were recalled because of an elevated MSAFP result for diagnostic amniocentesis or detailed ultrasound examination. Uptake of screening in most programs has remained consistently high, and a major impact on the birth incidence of NTD is apparent as a result of identification and selective termination of affected pregnancies. Ultrasound, initially as a pregnancy dating method and diagnostic procedure, and latterly as a screening method in the first trimester, is an indispensable part of NTD screening programs. The naturally declining prevalence of NTD pregnancies seen in many countries over the last 10–20 years can be accelerated by providing folic acid supplements in the periconceptional period for all women or through fortification of staple foods.

The introduction of biochemical screening for Down's syndrome was initially an add-on to the existing screening infrastructure developed for NTDs with testing confined to the second trimester. The introduction of double marker or triple marker testing and the estimation of a risk that a pregnancy is affected has displaced maternal age as the main method of screening for Down's syndrome in many countries. It allows all women, irrespective of age to have access to prenatal testing but, while overall detection rates are much improved compared with age-only screening, sensitivity is better in older women.

Many practical difficulties and concerns have been recognised over the last 10 years.

Providing adequate information for women contemplating screening is challenging and the complexity of the testing process and interpretation of results make counseling after a high risk result difficult and time consuming. Invasive diagnostic testing is required to confirm the chromosomal constitution of the fetus and this brings the hazard of procedure-related miscarriage and introduces a delay of 2–4 weeks between the finding of a high risk screening result and obtaining a fetal karyotype.

Efforts to address some of these problems have met with mixed success. From the search for new and better markers which would improve the sensitivity of current double and triple second trimester screening protocols, dimeric inhibin A has emerged as the most promising candidate and with some further development of commercially available assays it could become a cost-effective addition to large scale screening programs helping to push detection rates to over 70%. Greater potential, however, appears to lie with screening in the first trimester. The single most effective marker of fetal chromosome abnormalities is the ultrasound measurement of NT which, when combined with maternal age and the serum markers FβhCG and PAPP-A, has the potential to detect 80–90% of Down's syndrome pregnancies at 11–13 weeks gestation. While CUB screening provides a clear improvement over second trimester screening performance, testing has to be carried out within a narrow gestational window, specific training and quality control appear to be essential for satisfactory NT screening performance, and an invasive test is still required to confirm the fetal karyotype. Nevertheless encouraging results have been reported in prospective practice with many women receiving the results from diagnostic CVS before the end of the first trimester. Integrating first trimester NT and PAPP-A testing with second trimester thCG, AFP, UE3 and InhA testing may have the potential to improve sensitivity and specificity further, but this approach delays provision of a result until the second trimester.

These developments offer more effective testing but add to the complexity of screening. As the aim of a screening programme should be to provide universal access for all women to screening based on an informed choice, health professionals must ensure that women are aware of and understand all of the options available to them. This requires training for all staff who need to be fully informed of the range and performance of current tests and the latest developments in screening.

REFERENCES

Abraha HD, Noble PL, Nicolaides KH, Sherwood RA (1999) Maternal serum S100 protein in normal and Down syndrome pregnancies. Prenat Diagn 19:334–346

Aitken DA (1995) Biochemical Screening in Twins. In Ward RH, Whittle M (eds): Multiple Pregnancy. RCOG Press, London, pp. 171–185

Aitken DA, Crossley JA (1992) Screening for chromosome abnormalities. Curr Obstet Gynaecol 2:65–71

Aitken DA, Crossley JA (1995) Prenatal Screening—Biochemical. In Whittle MJ, Connor JM (eds): Prenatal Diagnosis in Obstetric Practice 2nd edn. Blackwell Science, Oxford, pp. 12–29

Aitken DA, Crossley JA (1997) The Glasgow ratio method. In Grudzinskas JG, Ward RHT (eds): Screening for Down's Syndrome in the First Trimester. RCOG Press, London, pp. 67–79

Aitken DA, Morrison NM, Ferguson-Smith MA (1984) Predictive value of amniotic acetylcholinesterase analysis in the diagnosis of fetal abnormality in 3700 pregnancies. Prenat Diagn 4:329–340

Aitken DA, McCaw G, Crossley JA et al. (1993) First trimester screening for fetal chromosome abnormalities and neural tube defects. Prenat Diagn 13:681–689

Aitken DA, Wallace EM, Crossley JA et al. (1996a) Dimeric inhibin A as a marker for Down's syndrome in early pregnancy. N Eng J Med 334:1231–1236

Aitken DA, Syvertsen BS, Crossley JA et al. (1996b) Heat stable and immunoreactive placental alkaline phosphatase in maternal serum from Down's syndrome and trisomy 18 pregnancies. Prenat Diagn 16:1051–1054

Alembik Y, Dott B, Roth MP, Stoll C (1997) Prevalence of neural tube defects in northeastern France, 1979–1994. Impact of prenatal diagnosis. Anales de Genetique 40:69–71

Bahado-Singh RO, Goldstein I, Uerpairojkit B et al. (1995) Normal nuchal thickness in the midtrimester indicates reduced risk of Down syndrome in pregnancies with abnormal triple-screen results. Am J Obstet Gynecol 173:1106–1110

Barkai G, Goldman B, Ries L et al. (1993) Expanding multiple marker screening for Down's syndrome to include Edwards syndrome. Prenat Diagn 13:843–50

Barkai G, Goldman B, Ries L et al. (1996) Down's syndrome screening marker levels following assisted reproduction. Prenat Diagn 16:1111–1114

Bartels I, Hoppe-Sievert B, Bockel B et al. (1993) Adjustment formulae for maternal serum alpha-fetoprotein, human chorionic gonadotropin, and unconjugated oestriol to maternal weight and smoking. Prenat Diagn 13:123–130

Baumgarten A, Robinson J (1988) Prospective study of an inverse relationship between maternal glycosylated hemoglobin and serum alpha-fetoprotein concentrations in pregnant women with diabetes. Am J Obstet Gynecol 159:77–81

Bazzett LB, Yaron Y, O'Brien JW et al. (1998) Fetal gender impact on multiple-marker screening results. Am J Med Genet 76:369–371

Benacerraf BR (1996) The second trimester fetus with Down's syndrome: Detection using sonographic features. Ultrasound Obstet Gynecol 7:147–155

Benacerraf BR, Frigoletto FD, Laboda LA (1985) Sonographic diagnosis of Down syndrome in the second trimester. Am J Obstet Gynecol 153:49–52

Bernstein L, Pike MC, Lobo RA et al. (1989) Cigarette smoking in pregnancy results in marked decrease in maternal hCG and oestradiol levels. Br J Obstet Gynaecol 96:92–96

Berry E, Aitken DA, Crossley JA et al. (1995) Analysis of maternal serum alpha-fetoprotein and free beta human chorionic gonadotrophin in the first trimester: Implications for Down syndrome screening. Prenat Diagn 15:555–565

Berry E, Aitken DA, Crossley JA et al. (1997) Screening for Down's syndrome: Changes in marker levels and detection rates between first and second trimester. Br J Obstet Gynaecol 104:811–817

Berry RJ, Li Z, Erickson JD et al. (1999) Prevention of neural tube defects with folic acid in China. China-U.S. collaborative project for neural tube defect prevention. N Engl J Med 341:1485–1490

Bersinger NA, Brizot ML, Johnson A et al. (1994) First trimester maternal serum pregnancy associated plasma protein A and pregnancy specific beta-1-glycoprotein in fetal trisomies. Br J Obstet Gynaecol 101:970–974

Bersinger NA, Leporrier N, Herrou M, Leymarie P (1999) Maternal serum pregnancy-associated plasma protein A (PAPP-A) but not pregnancy-specific beta1-glycoprotein (SP1) is a useful second-trimester marker for fetal trisomy 18. Prenat Diagn 19:537–41

Bewley S, Roberts LJ, Mackinson AM, Rodeck CH (1995) First trimester fetal nuchal translucency: Problems with screening the general population. 2. Br J Obstet Gynaecol 102:386–388

Biagiotti R, Cariati E, Brizzi L et al. (1998) Maternal serum screening for trisomy 18 in the first trimester of pregnancy. Prenat Diag 18:907–913

Bishop J, Dunstan FDJ, Nix BJ et al. (1994) All MoM's are not equal: Some statistical properties associated with reporting results in the form of multiples of the median. Am J Hum Genet 52:425–430

Blumenfeld Z, Siegler E, Bronshtein M (1993) The early diagnosis of neural tube defects. Prenatal Diagnosis 13:863–871

Bogart MH, Pandian MR, Jones OW (1987) Abnormal maternal serum chorionic gonadotropin levels in pregnancies with fetal chromosome abnormalities. Prenat Diagn 7:623–630

Bogart MH, Golbus MS, Sorg ND, Jones OW (1989) Human chorionic gonadotropin levels in pregnancies with aneuploid fetuses. Prenat Diagn 9:379–384

Borrell A, Costa D, Martinez JM et al. (1996) Early midtrimester fetal nuchal thickness: Effectiveness as a marker of Down syndrome. Am J Obstet Gynecol 175:45–49

Botto LD, Moore CA, Khoury MJ, Erickson JD (1999) Neural-tube defects. N Engl J Med 341:1509–1519

Braithwaite JM, Morris RW, Economides DL (1996) Nuchal translucency measurements: Frequency distribution and changes with gestation in a general population. Br J Obstet Gynaecol 103:1201–1204

Brambati B, Lanzani A, Tului L (1991) Ultrasound and biochemical assessment of first trimester pregnancy. In Chapman M, Grudzinskas JG, Chard T (eds): The Embryo: Normal and Abnormal Development and Growth, Springer-Verlag, NY, pp. 181–194

Brambati B, Macintosh MCM, Teisner B et al. (1993) Low maternal serum levels of pregnancy associated plasma protein A (PAPP-A) in the first trimester in association with abnormal fetal karyotype. Br J Obstet Gynaecol 100:324–326

Brambati B, Cislaghi C, Tului L et al. (1995) First-trimester Down's syndrome screening using nuchal translucency: A prospective study in patients undergoing chorionic villus sampling. Ultrasound Obstet Gynecol 5:9–14

Brambati B, Macri JN, Tului L et al. (1997) First-trimester fetal aneuploidy screening: maternal serum PAPP-A and free β-hCG. In Grudzinskas JG et al. (eds): Screening for Down syndrome in the First Trimester. London, Royal College of Obstet. Gynaecol Press, pp 135–147

Bray I, Wright DE, Davies C, Hook EB (1998) Joint estimation of Down syndrome risk and ascertainment rates: A meta analysis of nine published data sets. Prenatal Diagnosis 18:9–20

Brock DJH, Sutcliffe RG (1972) Alphafetoprotein in the antenatal diagnosis of anencephaly and spina bifida. Lancet ii:197–199

Brock DJH, Hayward C, Seppala M (1980) Distinguishing neural tube defects and congenital nephrosis by amniotic fluid assay. Lancet i:773

Brock DJH, Barron L, Holloway S et al. (1990) First trimester maternal serum biochemical indicators in Down's syndrome. Prenat Diagn 10:245–251

Burton BK, Nelson LH, Pettanati MJ (1989) False positive acetylcholinesterase with early amniocentesis. Obstetrics and Gynecology 74:607–610

Canick JA, Knight GJ, Palomaki GE et al. (1988) Low second trimester maternal serum unconjugated oestriol in pregnancies with Down's syndrome. Br J Obstet Gynaecol 95:330–333

Canick JA, Palomaki GE, Osathanondh R (1990a) Prenatal screening for trisomy 18 in the second trimester. Prenat Diagn. 10:546–548

Canick JA, Panizza DS, Palomaki GE, (1990b) Prenatal screening for Down's syndrome using AFP, UE3 and hCG: Effect of maternal race, insulin dependent diabetes and twin pregnancy. Am J Hum Genet 47:A270

Canick J, Kellner LH, Saller DN et al. (1995) Second trimester levels of maternal urinary gonadotropin peptide in Down syndrome pregnancy. Prenat Diagn 15:752–759

Carothers AD, Hecht CA, Hook EB (1999) International variation in reported livebirth prevalence rates of Down syndrome, adjusted for maternal age. J Med Genet 36:386–393

Chan A, Robertson EF, Haan EA et al. (1993) Prevalence of neural tube defects in South Australia, 1966–91: Effectiveness and impact of prenatal diagnosis. BMJ 307:703–706

Chatzipapas IK, Whitlow BJ, Economides DL (1999) The "Mickey Mouse" sign and the diagnosis of anencephaly in early pregnancy. Ultrasound in Obstet Gynecol 13:196–199

Chen CL, Gilbert TJ, Daling JR (1999) Maternal smoking and Down syndrome: The confounding effect of maternal age. Am J Epidemiol 149:442–446

Chitty LS, Pandya PP (1997) Ultrasound screening for fetal abnormalities in the first trimester. Prenat Diagn 17:1269–1281, Review

Christiansen M, Norgaard-Pedersen B (1997) Maternal serum screening for Down syndrome in first trimester using Schwangerschaftsprotein 1, PAPP-A/proMBP-complex and the proform of eosinophil major basic protein as markers. In Grudzinskas JG, Ward RHT (eds): Screening for Down Syndrome in the First Trimester RCOG Press, London, pp. 148–182

Christianson RE, Torfs CP (1988) Maternal smoking and Down syndrome. Am J Hum Genet 43:545–547

Cole LA (1994) Multiple hCG related molecules. In Grudzinskas JG, Chard T, Chapman M, Cuckle H (eds): Screening for Down's Syndrome. Cambridge University Press, Cambridge, pp. 119–140

Cole LA, Cermik D, Bahado Singh RO (1997) Oligosaccharide variants of hCG-related molecules: Potential screening markers for Down syndrome. Prenat Diagn 17:1188–1190

Cole LA, Rinne KM, Mahajan SM et al. (1999a) Urinary screening tests for fetal Down's syndrome: I. fresh β-core fragment. Prenat Diagn 19:340–350

Cole LA, Shahabi S, Oz UA et al. (1999b) Urinary screening tests for fetal Down syndrome: II. hyperglycosylated hCG. Prenat Diagn 19:351–359

Crandall BF, Chua C (1995) Detecting neural tube defects by amniocentesis between 11 and 15 weeks' gestation. Prenat Diagn 15:339–343

Crossley JA, Aitken DA (1999) Deriving risks of Down's syndrome from nuchal translucency measurements. Ultrasound Obstet Gynecol 14:438

Crossley JA, Aitken DA, Connor JM (1991) Prenatal screening for chromosome abnormalities using maternal serum chorioic gonadotrophin, alphafetoprotein and age. Prenat Diagn 11:88–101

Crossley JA, Aitken DA, Connor JM (1993) Second trimester unconjugated oestriol in maternal serum from chromosomally abnormal pregnancies using an optimised assay. Prenat Diagn 13:271–280

Crossley JA, Aitken DA, Berry E, Connor JM (1994) Impact of a regional screening programme using maternal serum AFP and hCG on the birth incidence of Down's syndrome in the west of Scotland. J Med Screening 1:180–183

Crossley JA, Berry E, Aitken DA, Connor JM (1996) Insulin dependent diabetes and prenatal screening results: Current experience from a regional screening programme. Prenat Diagn 16:1039–1042

Crossley JA, Aitken DA, Cameron AD, Connor JM (2000) Quality assessment of ultrasound nuchal translucency measurements. Eur J Ultrasound 11:S19–20

Crossley JA, Aitken DA, Cameron AD et al. (2001) Combined ultrasound and biochemical (CUB) screening for Down's syndrome in the first trimester: A Scottish multicentre study. Submitted

Cuckle HS (1994) Risk estimation in Down's syndrome screening policy and practice. In Grudzinskas JG, Chard T, Chapman M, Cuckle H (eds): Screening for Down's Syndrome. Cambridge University Press, Cambridge, pp. 31–46

Cuckle H (1995) Improved parameters for risk estimation in Down's syndrome screening. Prenat Diagn 15:1057–1065

Cuckle HS, Jones RG (1994) Maternal serum free beta human chorionic gonadotrophin level: The effect of sample transportation. Ann Clin Biochem 31:97–98

Cuckle HS, Jones RG (1995) Posting maternal blood samples for free beta-human chorionc gonadotrophin testing. Prenat Diagn 15:879–880

Cuckle H, Sehmi I (1999) Calculating correct Down's syndrome risks. Br J Obstet Gynaecol 106:371–372

Cuckle HS, van Lith JMM (1999) Appropriate biochemical parameters in first-trimester screening for Down Syndrome. Prenat Diagn 19:505–12

Cuckle HS, Wald NJ (1990) Screening for Down syndrome. In Lilford RJ (ed): Prenatal Diagnosis and Prognosis. Butterworth-Heinemann, Oxford, pp. 67–92

Cuckle HS, Wald NJ, Thomson SG (1987) Estimating a woman's risk of having a pregnancy associated with Down's syndrome using her age and serum alphafetoprotein level. Br J Obstet Gynaecol 94:387–402

Cuckle HS, Wald NJ, Barkai G et al. (1988) First trimester biochemical screening for Down's syndrome. Lancet ii:851–852

Cuckle HS, Alberman E, Wald NJ et al. (1990a) Maternal smoking habits and Down's syndrome. Prenat Diagn 10:561–7

Cuckle HS, Wald NJ, Stevenson JD et al. (1990b) Maternal serum alphafetoprotein screening for open neural tube defects in twin pregnancies. Prenatal Diagnosis 10:71–77

Cuckle H, Lilford RJ, Teisner B et al. (1992) Pregnancy associated plasma protein A in Down's syndrome. BMJ 305:425

Cuckle HS, Iles RK, Chard T (1994a) Urinary β-core human chorionic gonadotropin: A new approach to Down's syndrome screening. Prenat Diagn 14:953–958

Cuckle H, van Oudgaarden ED, Mason G, Holding S (1994b) Taking account of vaginal bleeding in screening for Down's syndrome. Br J Obstet Gynaecol 101:948–953

Cuckle HS, Iles RK, Sehmi IH et al. (1995) Urinary multiple marker screening for Down's syndrome. Prenat Diagn 15:745–751

Cuckle HS, Canick JA, Kellner LH et al. (1996) Urinary beta-core-hCG screening in the first trimester. Prenat Diagn 16:1057–1059

Cuckle HS, Sehmi I, Jones R, Evans LW (1999a) Maternal serum activin A and follistatin levels in pregnancies with Down syndrome. Prenat Diagn 19:513–516

Cuckle HS, Sehmi IK, Jones RG, Mason G (1999b) Low maternal serum PAPP-A and fetal viability. Prenat Diagn 19:787–790

Dalgliesh GL, Aitken DA, Lyall et al. (2001) Placental and maternal serum inhibin-A and activin-A levels in Down's syndrome pregnancies Placenta 22:227–234

Davis CF, Young DG (1991) The changing incidence of neural tube defects in Scotland. J Pediatr Surg 26:516–518

De Biasio P, Siccardi M, Volpe G et al. (1999) First-trimester screening for Down syndrome using nuchal translucency measurements with free β-hCG and PAPP-A between 10 and 13 weeks of pregnancy—the combined test. Prenat Diagn 19:360–363

De Graaf IM, Pajkrt E, Bilardo CM et al. (1999) Early pregnancy screening of fetal aneuploidy with serum markers and nuchal translucency. Prenat Diagn 19:458–462

Dietzsch E, Ramsay M, Christianson AL et al. (1995) Maternal origin of the extra haploid set of chromosomes in third trimester triploid fetuses. Am J Med Genet 58:360–364

Drugan A, Sokol RJ, Syner FN et al. (1989) Clinical implications of amniotic fluid alpha-fetoprotein in twin pregnancy. J Reprod Med 34:977–980

Dupont A, Vaeth M, Viderbech P (1986) Mortality and life expectancy of Down's syndrome in Denmark. Ment Defic 30:111–120

Eiben B, Goebel R, Hansen S, Hammans W (1996a) Alpha-fetoprotein and AChE in early amniocentesis. Prenatal Diagnosis 16:87–88

Eiben B, Hammans W, Goebel R (1996b) Triploidy, imprinting, and hCG levels in maternal serum screening. Prenat Diagn 16:377–378

Elejalde BR, de Elejalde MM, Acuna JM et al. (1990) Prospective study of amniocentesis performed between weeks 9 and 16 of gestation: Its feasibility, risks, complications and use in early genetic prenatal diagnosis. Am J Med Genet 35:188–196

Ferguson Smith MA, Yates JRW (1984) Maternal age specific rates for chromosome aberrations and factors influencing them: Report of a collaborative study on 52,965 amniocenteses. Prenat Diagn 4:5–44

Ferriman EL, Sehmi IK, Jones R, Cuckle HS (1999) The effect of smoking in pregnancy on maternal serum inhibin A levels. Prenat Diagn 19:372–4

Feuchtbaum LB, Currier RJ, Riggle S et al. (1999) Neural tube defect prevalence in California (1990–1994): Eliciting patterns by type of defect and maternal race/ethnicity. Genet Test 3:265–272

Fisher NL, Luthy DA, Peterson A et al. (1981) Prenatal diagnosis of neural tube defects: Predictive value of AF-AFP in a low-risk population. Am J Med Genet 9:201–209

Forest JC, Masse J, Moutquin JM (1997) Screening for Down syndrome during first trimester: A prospective study using free beta-human chorionic gonadotropin and pregnancy-associated plasma protein A. Clin Biochem 30:333–338

Frishman GN, Canick JA, Hogan JW et al. (1997) Serum triple-marker screening in in vitro fertilization and naturally conceived pregnancies. Obstet Gynecol 90:98–101

Ghidini A, Spong CY, Grier RE et al. (1998) Is maternal serum triple screening a better predictor of Down syndrome in female than in male fetuses? Prenat Diagn 18:123–126

Goldstein H, Neilsen KG (1988) Rates and survival of individuals with trisomy 18 and trisomy 13. Data from a 10 year period in Denmark. Clin Genet 34:366–372

Goodburn SF, Yates JR, Raggatt PR et al. (1994) Second-trimester maternal serum screening using alpha-fetoprotein, human chorionic gonadotrophin, and unconjugated oestriol: experience of a regional programme. Prenat Diagn 14:391–402

Goshen R (1994) The genomic basis of the β subunit of human chorionic gonadotropin diversity in triploidy. Am J Obstet Gynecol 170:700–701

Graham GW, Crossley JA, Aitken DA, Connor JM (1992) Variation in the levels of pregnancy-specific β-1-glycoprotein in maternal serum from chromosomally abnormal pregnancies. Prenat Diagn 12:505–512

Haddow JE (1998) Antenatal screening for Down's syndrome: Where are we and where next? Lancet 352:336–337

Haddow JE, Palomaki GE, Knight GJ (1995) Effect of parity on human chorionic gonadotrophin levels and Down's syndrome screening. J Med Screen 2:28–30

Haddow JE, Palomaki GE, Knight GJ et al. (1998) Screening of maternal serum for fetal Down's syndrome in the first trimester. N Engl J Med 338:955–961

Hallahan T, Krantz D, Khabbaza E et al. (1998) First trimester maternal serum screening for Down syndrome: Intact hCG versus free beta hCG. Am J Hum Genet 63(Suppl):A164

Hecht CA, Hook EB (1996) Rates of Down syndrome at livebirth by one-year maternal age intervals in studies with apparent close to complete ascertainment in populations of European origin: A proposed revised rate schedule for use in genetic and prenatal screening. Am J Med Genet 62:376–385

Heionen S, Ryynanen M, Kirkinen P et al. (1996) Effect of in vitro fertilization on human chorionic gonadotropin serum concentrations and Down's syndrome screening. Fertil Steril 66:398–403

Herman A, Maymon R, Dreazen E et al. (1998) Nuchal translucency audit: A novel image-scoring method. Ultrasound Obstet Gynecol 12:398–403

Holding S, Cuckle H (1994) Maternal serum screening for Down's syndrome taking account of the result in a previous pregnancy. Prenat Diagn 14:321–322

Hook EB (1992) Prevalence, risks and recurrence. In Brock DJH, Rodeck CH, Ferguson-Smith MA (eds): Prenatal Diagnosis and Screening. Churchill Livingstone, Edinburgh, pp. 351–392

Hook EB, Cross PK (1985) Cigarette smoking and Down syndrome. Am J Hum Genet 37:1216–1224

Hook EB, Hamerton JL (1977) The frequency of chromosome abnormalities detected in consecutive newborn studies—differences between studies—results by sex and severity of phenotypic involvement. In Hook EB, Porter IH (eds): Population Cytogenetics, Studies in Humans. Academic Press, NY, pp. 63–79

Hook EB, Carothers AD, Hecht CA (1999) Elevated maternal age-specific rates of Down syndrome liveborn offspring of women of Mexican and Central American origin in California. Prenat Diagn 19:245–251

Howe DT, Gornall R, Wellesley D et al. (2000) Six year survey of screening for Down's syndrome by maternal age and mid-trimester ultrasound scans. BMJ 320:606–610

Hseih TT, Hsu JJ, Chen CP et al. (1995) Down's syndrome screening with AFP and Free Beta hCG: An analysis of the influence of Chinese ethnic origin on screening parameters. Am J Hum Genet 57:A281

Hsu JJ, Spencer K, Aitken DA et al. (1999) Urinary free β hCG, beta care fragment and total oestriol as markers of Down's syndrome in the second trimester of pregnancy. Prenat Diagn 19:146–158

Hsu TY, Ou CY, Hsu JJ et al. (1999) Maternal serum screening for Down syndrome in pregnancies conceived by intra-uterine insemination. Prenat Diagn 19:1012–1014

Hyett JA, Sebire NJ, Snijders RJM, Nicolaides KH (1996) Intrauterine lethality of trisomy 21 fetuses with increased nuchal translucency thickness. Ultrasound Obstet Gynecol 7:101–103

Hyett JA, Perdu M, Sharland GK et al. (1997) Increased nuchal translucency at 10–14 weeks of gestation as a marker for major cardiac defects. Ultrasound Obstet Gynecol 10:242–246

Jauniaux E, Brown R, Rodeck C, Nicolaides KH (1996) Prenatal diagnosis of triploidy during the second trimester of pregnancy. Obstet Gynecol 88:983–989

Johnson AM, Palomali GE, Haddow JE (1990) The effect of adjusting maternal serum alphafetoprotein levels for maternal weight in pregnancies with fetal open spina bifida. A United States collaborative study. Am J Obstet Gynecol 163:9–11

Johnson MP, Johnson A, Holzgreve W et al. (1993) First trimester simple hygroma: cause and outcome. Am J Obstet Gynecol 168:156–161

Johnson SP, Sebire NJ, Snijders RJ et al. (1997) Ultrasound screening for anencephaly at 10–14 weeks of gestation. Ultrasound in Obstet and Gynecol 9:14–16

Jorgensen FS, Sundberg K, Loft AG et al. (1995) Alpha-fetoprotein and acetylcholinesterase activity in first- and early second-trimester amniotic fluid. Prenat Diagn 15:621–625

Jorgensen FS, Valentin L, Salvesen KA et al. (1999) MULTISCAN—a Scandinavian multicentre second trimester obstetric ultrasound and serum screening study. Acta Obstet Gynecolo Scand 78:501–510

Kennedy DM, Edwards VM, Worthington DJ (1999) Evaluation of different weight correction methods for antenatal serum screening using data from two multi-centre programmes. Ann Clin Biochem 36:359–364

Klein J, Stein Z, Susser M, Warburton D (1981) New insights into epidemiology of chromosome disorders; their relevance to the prevention of Down's syndrome. In Miterl (ed.): Frontiers in Knowledge in mental Retardation, Vol 2 Biochemical Aspects. University Park Press, Baltimore, pp. 131–141

Knight GJ, Palomaki GE, Haddow JE et al. (1989) Maternal serum levels of the placental products hCG, hPL, SP1 and progesterone are all elevated in cases of fetal Down syndrome. Am J Hum Genet 45:A263

Knight GJ, Palomaki GE, Haddow JE et al. (1993) Pregnancy associated plasma protein A as a marker of Down syndrome in the second trimester of pregnancy. Prenat Diagn 13:222–223

Kornman LH, Morssink LP, Beekhuis JR et al. (1996) Nuchal translucency cannot be used as a screening test for chromosomal abnormalities in the first trimester of pregnancy in a routine ultrasound practice. Prenat Diagn 16:797–805

Kornman LH, Morssink LP, Wortelboer MJM et al. (1997) Maternal urinary β-core hCG in chromosomally abnormally pregnancies in the first trimester. Prenat Diagn 17:135–139

Krantz DA, Larsen JW, Buchanan PD, Macri JN (1996) First-trimester Down syndrome screening: Free beta-human chorionic gonadotropin and pregnancy-associated plasma protein A. Am J Obstet Gynecol 174:612–616

Krantz DA, Hallahan TW, Orlandi F et al. (2000) First-trimester Down syndrome screening using dried blood biochemistry and nuchal translucency. Obstet Gynecol 96:207–213

Lam YH, Tang MH, Tang LC et al. (1997) Second-trimester maternal urinary gonadotrophin peptide screening for fetal Down syndrome in Asian women. Prenat Diagn 17:1101–1106

Lam YH, Yeung WS, Tang MH et al. (1999) Maternal serum alpha-fetoprotein and human chorionic gonadotrophin in pregnancies conceived after intracytoplasmic sperm injection and conventional in-vitro fertilization. Hum Reprod 14:2120–2123

Lambert-Messerlian GM, Canick JA, Palomaki GE (1996) Maternal serum total activin A in pregnancies affected with fetal Down's syndrome. J Med Screen 3:217

Lambert-Messerlian GM, Saller DN, Tumber MB et al. (1998) Second-trimester maternal serum inhibin A levels in fetal trisomy 18 and Turner syndrome with and without hydrops. Prenat Diagn 18:1061–1067

Lambert-Messerlian GM, Saller DN, Tumber MB et al. (1999) Second-trimester maternal serum progesterone levels in Turner syndrome with and without hydrops and in trisomy 18. Prenat Diagn 19:476–479

Larsen SO, Christiansen M, Norgaard-Oedersen B (1998) Inclusion of serum marker measurements from a previous pregnancy improves Down syndrome screening performance. Prenat Diagn 18:706–712

Laundon CH, Spencer K, Macri JN et al. (1996) Free beta hCG screening of hydropic and non-hydropic Turner syndrome pregnancies. Prenat Diagn 16:853–856

Lawrence JB, Oxvig C, Overgaard MT et al. (1999) The insulin-like growth factor (IGF)-dependent IGF binding protein-4 protease secreted by human fibroblasts is pregnancy-associated plasma protein-A. Procs Natl Acad Sci 96:3149–3153

Lennon CA, Gray DL (1999) Sensitivity and specificity of ultrasound for the detection of neural tube and ventral wall defects in a high-risk population. Obstet Gynecol 94:562–566

Leporrier N, Herrou M, Herlicoviez M, Leymarie P (1996) The usefulness of hCG and unconjugated oestriol in prenatal diagnosis of trisomy 18. Br J Obstet Gynaecol 103:335–338

Levi S, Hyjazi Y, Schaaps JP et al. (1991) Sensitivity and specificity of routine antenatal screening for congenital abnormalities by ultrasound: the Belgium multicentre study. Ultrasound Obstet Gynecol 1:102–110

Liaw AW, Heath V, Kametas N, Spencer K, Nicolaides KM (2001) First trimester screening for trimosy 21 in singleton pregnancies achieved by assisted reproduction. Human Reproduction (In Press)

Liao AW, Snijders R, Geerts L et al. (2000) Fetal heart rate in chromosomally abnormal fetuses. Ultrasound Obstet Gynecol 16:610–613

Lindenbaum RH, Ryynanen M, Holmes-Sieole M et al. (1987) Trisomy 18 and maternal serum and amniotic fluid alpha-fetoprotein. Prenat Diagn 7:511–519

Loft AG, Hogdall E, Larsen SO, Norgaard-Pedersen B (1993) A comparison of amniotic fluid alpha-fetoprotein and acetylcholinesterase in the prenatal diagnosis of open neural tube defects and anterior abdominal wall defects. Prenat Diagn 13:93–109

McDonnell RJ, Johnson Z, Delaney V, Dack P (1999) East Ireland 1980–1994: Epidemiology of neural tube defects. J Epidemiol Comm Health 53:782–788

McFadden DE, Kalousek DK (1991) Two different phenotypes of fetuses with chromosomal triploidy: Correlation with parental origin of the extra haploid set. Am J Med Genet 38:535–538

McFadden DE, Kwong LC, Yam IYL, Langlois S (1993) Parental origin of triploidy in human fetuses: Evidence for genomic imprinting. Hum Genet 92:465–469

Macintosh MCM, Nicolaides KH, Noble P et al. (1997) Urinary β-core hCG: Screening for aneuploides in early pregnancy (11–14 weeks' gestation). Prenat Diagn 17:401–405

Macri JN, Kasturi RV, Krantz DA et al. (1990) Maternal serum Down syndrome screening: Free beta protein is a more effective marker than human chorionic gonadotropin. Am J Obstet Gynecol 163:1248–1253

Macri JN, Spencer K, Anderson R, Cook EJ (1993) Free beta chorionic gonadotropin: A cross reactivity study of two immunometric assays used in prenatal maternal serum screening for Down syndrome. Ann Clin Biochem 30:94–98

Macri JN, Spencer K, Garver K et al. (1994) Maternal serum free beta Down syndrome screening: Results of twelve studies including 480 cases of Down Syndrome. Prenat Diagn 14:97–103

Macri JN, Anderson RW, Krantz DA et al. (1996) Prenatal maternal dried blood screening with alpha-fetoprotein and free β-human chorionic gonadotropin for open neural tube defect and Down syndrome. Am J Obstet Gynecol 174:566–572

Martin AO, Dempsey LM, Minogue J et al. (1990) Maternal serum alpha-fetoprotein levels in pregnancies complicated by diabetes: Implications for screening programs. Am J Obstet Gynecol 163:1209–1216

Martinez JM, Echevarria M, Borell A et al. (1998) Fetal heart rate and nuchal translucency in detecting chromosomal abnormalities other than Down syndrome. Obstet Gynecol 92:68–71

Mehta S, Spencer K (1988) Antenatal diagnosis of neural tube defects using a coated bead immunoassay for acetylcholinesterase in amniotic fluid. Ann Clin Biochem 25:569-576

Merkatz IR, Nitowsky HM, Macri JN, Johnson WE (1984) An association between low maternal serum alpha-fetoprotein and fetal chromosomal abnormalities. Am J Obstet Gynecol 148:886–894

Mikkelsen M, Nielsen KB (1992) Karyotype analysis and chromosome disorders. In Brock DJH, Rodeck CH, Ferguson-Smith MA (eds): Prenatal Diagnosis and Screening. Churchill Livingstone, Edinburgh, pp. 99–125

Milunsky A, Alpert E, Kitzmiller JL et al. (1982) Prenatal diagnosis of neural tube defects. VIII. The importance of serum alpha-fetoprotein screening in diabetic pregnant women. Am J Obstet Gynecol 142:1030–1032

Milunsky A, Jick H, Jick SS et al. (1989) Multivitamin/folic acid supplementation in early pregnancy reduces the prevalence of neural tube defects. J Am Med Assoc 262:2847–2852

Moroz C, Maymon R, Jauniaux E, Traub L, Cuckle H (2000) Screening of trisomies 21 and 18 with maternal serum placental isoferritin p43 component. Prenat Diagn 20:395-399

Morris JK, Wald NJ, Watt HC (1999) Fetal loss in Down's syndrome pregnancies. Prenat Diagn 19:142–145

Morrow RJ, McNay MB, Whittle MJ (1991) Ultrasound detection of neural tube defects in patients with elevated maternal serum alphafetoprotein. Obstet Gynecol 78:1055–1057

Morssink LP, Kornman LH, Hallahan TW et al. (1998) Maternal serum levels of free β-hCG and PAPP-A in the first trimester of pregnancy are not associated with subsequent fetal growth retardation or preterm delivery. Prenat Diagn 18:147–152

MRC Vitamin Study Research Group (1991) Prevention of neural tube defects: Results of the MRC vitamin study. Lancet 338:132–137

Muller F, Oury JF, Boue A (1989) First trimester amniotic fluid acetyl-cholinesterase electrophoresis. Prenat Diagn 9:173–175

Muller F, Aergerter P, Boue A (1993) Prospective maternal serum human chorionic gonadotripin screening for the risk of fetal chromosome anomalies and subsequent fetal and neonatal deaths. Prenatal Diagnosis 13:29-43

Muller F, Doche C, Ngo S et al. (1999) Stability of Free β-subunit in routine practice for trisomy 21 maternal serum screening. Prenat Diagn 19:85–86

Nadel AS, Green JK, Holmes LB et al. (1990) Absence of need for amniocentesis in patients with elevated levels of maternal serum alpha-fetoprotein and normal ultrasonographic examinations. N Engl J Med 323:557–561

Neveux LM, Palomaki GE et al. (1996) Refinements in managing maternal weight adjustment for interpreting prenatal screening results. Prenat Diagn 16:1115–1119

Nicolaides KH, Campbell S, Gabbe SG, Guidette R (1986) Ultrasound screening for spina bifida: Cranial and cerebellar signs. Lancet ii:72–74

Nicolaides KH, Azar G, Byrne D et al. (1992) Fetal nuchal translucency: Ultrasound screening for chromosomal defects in the first trimester of pregnancy. BMJ 304:867–869

Nicolaides KH, Brizot ML, Snijders RJM (1994) Fetal nuchal translucency: Ultrasound screening for fetal trisomy in the first trimester of pregnancy. B J Obstet Gynaecol 101:782–786

Nicolaides KH, Snijders RJM, Cuckle HS (1998) Correct estimation of parameters for ultrasound nuchal translucency screening. Prenat Diagn 519–521

Norgaard-Pedersen B, Larsen SO, Arends J et al. (1990) Maternal serum markers for Down's syndrome. Clin Genet 37:35–43

Nyberg DA, Luthy DA, Cheng EY et al. (1995) Role of prenatal ultrasonography in women with positive screen for Down syndrome on the basis of maternal serum markers. Am J Obstet Gynecol 173:1030–1035

Onda T, Kitagawa M, Takeda O et al. (1996) Triple marker screening in native Japanese women. Prenat Diagn 16:713–717

Ong CYT, Liao AWJ, Spencer K, Nicolaides KH (2000) First trimester maternal serum free β-hCG and PAPP-A as predictors of pregnancy complications. Br J Obstet Gynaecol 107:1265–1270

Orlandi F, Damiani G, Hallahan TW et al. (1997) First-trimester screening for fetal aneuploidy: Biochemistry and nuchal translucency. Ultrasound Obstet Gynecol 10:381–386

Oxvig C, Sand O, Kristensen T et al. (1994) Isolation and characterisation of circulating complex between human pregnancy associated plasma protein-A and proform of eosinophil major basic protein. Biochim Biophys Acta 1201:415–423

Pajkrt E, Bilardo CM, van Lith JM et al. (1995) Nuchal translucency measurement in normal fetuses. Obstet Gynecol 86:994–997

Palomaki GE, Haddow JE (1995) Can the risk for Down syndrome be reliably modified by second-trimester ultrasonography? Am J Obstet Gynecol 173:1639–1640

Palomaki GE, Panizza DS, Canick JA (1990) Screening for Down syndrome using AFP, uE3 and hCG: Effect of maternal weight. Am J Hum Genet 47:245–249

Palomaki GE, Knight GJ, Haddow JE et al. (1993) Cigarette smoking and levels of maternal serum alpha-fetoprotein, unconjugated estriol, and hCG: Impact on Down syndrome screening. Obstet Gynecol 81:675–678

Palomaki GE, Knight GJ, Haddow JE (1994) Human chorionic gonadotropin and unconjugated oestriol measurements in insulin-dependent diabetic pregnant women being screened for fetal Down syndrome. Prenat Diagn 14:65–68

Palomaki GE, Haddow JE, Knight GJ et al. (1995) Risk-based prenatal screening for trisomy 18 using alpha-fetoprotein, unconjugated oestriol and human chorionic gonadotropin. Prenat Diagn 15:713–23

Pandya PP, Snijders RJM, Johnson SP et al. (1995a) Screening for fetal trisomies by maternal age and fetal nuchal translucency thickness at 10 to 14 weeks of gestation. Br J Obstet Gynaecol 102:957–962

Pandya PP, Altman DG, Brizot ML, Nicolaides KH (1995b) Repeatability of measurement of fetal nuchal translucency thickness. Ultrasound Obstet Gynecol 5:334–337

Pandya PP, Goldberg H, Walton B et al. (1995c) The implementation of first-trimester scanning at 10–13 weeks' gestation and the measurement of fetal nuchal translucency thickness in two maternity units. Ultrasound Obstet Gynecol 5:20–25

Pandya PP, Kondylios A, Hilbert L et al. (1995d) Chromosomal defects and outcome in 1015 fetuses with increased nuchal translucency. Ultrasound Obstet Gynecol 5:15–19

Parvin C, Gray D, Kessler G (1991) Influence of assay method differences on multiple of the median distributions: Maternal serum alpha-fetoprotein as an example. Clin Chem 37:637–642

Pedersen JF, Sorensen S, Molsted-Pedersen L (1998) Pregnancy-associated plasma protein A in first trimester of diabetic pregnancy and subsequent fetal growth. Acta Obstet Gynecol Scand 77:932–934

Penrose LS (1933) The relative effects of paternal age and maternal age in mongolism. J Genet 27:219–224

Pettersson K, Norgaard-Pedersen B, Stenman U, Stigbrand T (1993) Optimization of immunometric assays for the measurement of PAPP-A first trimester samples from normal and trisomy 21 pregnancies. In Screening for Down's Syndrome. Royal College Obstet Gynaecol, 24–26 May, Abstract 35

Qin QP, Nguyen TK, Christiansen M et al. (1996) Time resolved immunofluorometric assay of pregnancy-associated plasma protein-A in maternal serum screening for Down's syndrome in first trimester of pregnancy. Clin Chim Acta 253:113–129

Qin QP, Christiansen M, Oxvig C et al. (1997) Double-monoclonal immunofluorometric assays for pregnancy-associated plasma protein A/proeosinophil major basic protein (PAPP-A/proMBP) complex for first-trimester maternal serum screening for Down syndrome. Clin Chem 43:2323–2332

RCOG (1997) Recommendations arising from the 32nd Study Group: Screening for Down syndrome in the first trimester. In Grudzinskas JG, Ward RHT (eds): Screening for Down Syndrome in the first trimester, RCOG Press, London, pp. 353–356

Reese EA, Davis N, Mahoney MJ, Baumgarten A (1987) Maternal serum alpha-fetoprotein in diabetic pregnancy: Correlation with blood glucose control. Lancet ii:275

Report of the Collaborative Acetylcholinesterase Study (1981) Amniotic fluid acetylcholinesterase electrophoresis as a secondary test in the diagnosis of anencephaly and open spina bifida in early pregnancy. Lancet ii:321–324

Report of the UK Collaborative Study on Alpha-fetoprotein in Relation to Neural-tube Defects (1977) Maternal serum alphafetoprotein measurement in antenatal screening for anencephaly and spina bifida in early pregnancy. Lancet I:1323–1332

Reynolds TM (1994) Screening by test combination: A statistical overview. In Grudzinskas JG, Chard T, Chapman M, Cuckle H (eds): Screening for Down's syndrome. Cambridge University Press, Cambridge, pp. 47–71

Reynolds T, John R (1992) A comparison of unconjugated oestriol assay kits shows that expression of results as multiples of the median causes unacceptable variation in calculated Down syndrome risk factors. Clin Chem 38:1888–1893

Reynolds T, Penney M (1990) The mathematical basis of multivariate risk analysis: With special reference to screening for Down syndrome associated pregnancy. Ann Clin Biochem 27:452–458

Reynolds TM, Dunstan F, Nix B et al. (1998) Combining ultrasound and biochemistry in first trimester screening for Down's syndrome. Prenat Diagn 18:511–515

Ribbert LS, Kornman LH, De Wolf BT et al. (1996) Maternal serum screening for fetal Down syndrome in IVF pregnancies. Prenat Diagn 16:35–8

Roberts HE, Moore CA, Cragan JD et al. (1995a) Impact of prenatal diagnosis on the birth prevalence of neural tube defects, Atlanta, 1990–1991. Pediatr 96:880–881

Roberts LJ, Bewley S, Mackinson AM, Rodeck CH (1995b) First trimester fetal nuchal transiuency: Problems with screening the general population. 1. Br J Obstet Gynaecol 102:381–385

Rose NC, Menutti MT (1995) Periconceptional folic acid supplementation as a social intervention. Seminars in Perinatology 19:243–254

Rotmensch S, Liberati M, Kardana A et al. (1996) Nicked free beta-subunit of human chorionic gonadotropin: A potential new marker for Down syndrome screening. Am J Obstet Gynecol 174:609–611

Ryall RG, Staples AJ, Robertson EF, Pollard AC (1992) Improved performance in a prenatal screening programme for Down's syndrome incorporating serum free hCG subunit analyses. Prenat Diagn 12:251–261

Saller DN, Canick JA, Schwartz S, Blitzer MG (1992) Multiple-marker screening in pregnancies with hydropic and nonhydropic Turner syndrome. Am J Obstet Gynecol 167:1021–1024

Saller DN, Canick JA, Blitzer MG et al. (1999) Second trimester maternal serum analyte levels associated with fetal trisomy 13. Prenat Diagn 19:813–816

Schats R, Jansen CAM, Wladimiroff JW (1990) Abnormal embryonic heart rate pattern in early pregnancy associated with Down's syndrome. Hum Reprod 5:877–879

Schuchter K, Wald NJ, Hackshaw AK et al. (1998) The distribution of nuchal translucency at 10–13 weeks of pregnancy. Prenat Diagn 18:281–286

Sebire NJ, Snijders RJM, Hughes K et al. (1996) Screening for trisomy 21 in twin pregnancies by maternal age and fetal nuchal translucency thickness at 10–14 weeks of gestation. Br J Obstet Gynaecol 103:999–1003

Sebire NJ, Noble PL, Thorpe-Beeston JG et al. (1997a) Presence of the "lemon" sign in fetuses with spina bifida at the 10–14 week scan. Ultrasound Obstet Gynecol 10:403–405

Sebire NJ, Spencer K, Noble PL et al. (1997b) Maternal serum alpha-fetoprotein in fetal neural tube and abdominal wall defects at 10 to 14 weeks of gestation. Br J Obstet Gynaecol 104:849–851

Second Report of the Collaborative Acetylcholinesterase Study (1989) Amniotic fluid acetylcholinesterase measurement in the prenatal diagnosis of open neural tube defects. Prenat Diagnosis 9:813–829

Second Report of UK Collaborative Study on Alpha-fetoprotein in Relation to Neural Tube Defects (1979) Amniotic Fluid Alpha-fetoprotein Measurement in Antenatal Diagnosis of Anencephaly and Open Spina Bifida in Early Pregnancy. Lancet ii:651–661

Sepulveda W, Donaldson A, Johnson RD et al. (1995) Are routine alpha-fetoprotein and acetylcholinesterase determinations still necessary at second-trimester amniocentesis? Impact of high-resolution ultrasonography. Obstet Gynecol 85:107–112

Shields LE, Uhrich SB, Komarniski CA et al. (1996) Amniotic fluid alphafetoprotein determination at the time of genetic amniocentesis: has it outlived its usefulness? J Ultrasound in Med 15:735–739

Shiono PH, Klebanoff MA, Berendes HW (1986) Congenital malformations and maternal smoking during pregnancy. Teratology 34:65–71

Shulman LP, Emerson D, Felker R et al. (1992) High frequency of cytogenetic abnormalities with cystic hygroma diagnosed in the first trimester. Obstet Gynecol 80:80–82

Smith AD, Wald NJ, Cuckle HS et al. (1979) Amniotic fluid acetylcholinesterase as a possible diagnostic test for neural tube defects in early pregnancy. Lancet ii:685–688

Snijders RJ, Holzgreve W, Cuckle H, Nicolaides KH (1994) Maternal age-specific risks for trisomies at 9–14 weeks' gestation. Prenat Diagn 14:543–552

Snijders RJM, Noble P, Sebire N et al. (1998) UK multicentre project on assessment of risk of trisomy 21 by maternal age and fetal nuchal translucency thickness at 10–14 weeks of gestation. Lancet 352:343–346

Snijders RJ, Sundberg K, Holzgreve W et al. (1999) Maternal age- and gestation-specific risk for trisomy 21. Ultrasound Obstet Gynecol 13:167–170

Spencer K (1991) Evaluation of an assay of the free beta-subunit of choriogonadotropin and its potential value in screening for Down's syndrome. Clin Chem 37:809–14

Spencer K (1993a) Free alpha subunit of human chorionic gonadotropin in Down syndrome. Am J Obstet Gynecol 168:132–135

Spencer K (1993b) Second-trimester CA 125 and Down's syndrome. Prenat Diagn 13:773–774

Spencer K (1994a) The measurement of hCG subunits in screening for Down's syndrome. In Grudzinskas JG, Chard T, Chapman M, Cuckle H (eds): Screening for Down's Syndrome. Cambridge University Press, Cambridge, pp. 85–100

Spencer K (1994b) Is the measurement of unconjugated oestriol of value in screening for Down's syndrome? In Grudzinskas JG, Chard T, Chapman M, Cuckle H (eds): Screening for Down's Syndrome. Cambridge University Press, Cambridge, pp. 141–161

Spencer K (1995) The influence of gravidity on Down's syndrome screening with free beta hCG. Prenat Diagn 15:87–89

Spencer K (1997a) hCG and its subunits in first trimester Down syndrome screening. In Grudzinskas JG, Ward RHT (eds): Screening for Down Syndrome in the First Trimester RCOG Press, London, pp. 117–131

Spencer K (1997b) Between-pregnancy biological variability of maternal serum alpha-fetoprotein and free beta hCG: Implications for Down syndrome screening in subsequent pregnancies. Prenat Diagn 17:39–45

Spencer K (1998) The influence of smoking on maternal serum AFP and free beta hCG levels and the impact on screening for Down syndrome. Prenat Diagn 18:225–234

Spencer K (1999a) The influence of smoking on maternal serum PAPP-A and free beta hCG levels in the first trimester of pregnancy. Prenat Diag 19:1065–1066

Spencer K (1999b) Second trimester prenatal screening for Down's syndrome using alpha-fetoprotein and free beta hCG: A seven year review. Br J Obstet Gynaecol 106:1287–1293

Spencer K (2000a) Screening for trisomy 21 in twin pregnancies in the first trimester using free β-hCG and PAPP-A, combined with fetal nuchal translucency thickness. Prenat Diagn 20:91–95

Spencer K (2000b) The influence of fetal sex in screening for Down's Syndrome in the second trimester. Prenat Diagn 20:648–51

Spencer K (2000c) Second trimester prenatal screening for Down's Syndrome and the relationship of maternal serum biochemical markers to pregnancy complication with adverse outcome. Prenat Diagn 20:652–656

Spencer K, Carpenter P (1993) Prospective study of prenatal screening for Down's syndrome with free beta human chorionic gonadotrophin BMJ 307:764–769

Spencer K, Carpenter P (1998) Is prostate-specific antigen a marker for pregnancies affected by Down syndrome? Clin Chem 44:2362–2365

Spencer K, Macri JN (1992) Early detection of Down's syndrome using free beta human choriogonadotropin. Ann Clin Biochem 29:349–350

Spencer K, Nicolaides KH (2000) First trimester prenatal diagnosis of trisomy 21 in discordant twins using fetal nuchal translucency thickness and maternal serum free β-hCG and PAPP-A. Prenat Diagn 20:683–684

Spencer K, Macri JN, Aitken DA, Connor JM (1992a) Free beta hCG as a first trimester marker of fetal trisomy. Lancet 339:1480

Spencer K, Coombes EJ, Mallard AS, Milford Ward A (1992b) Free beta human choriogonadotropin in Down syndrome screening: A multicentre study of its role compared with other biochemical markers. Ann Clin Biochem 29:506–518

Spencer K, Wood PJ, Anthony FW (1993a) Elevated levels of maternal serum inhibin immunoreactivity in second trimester pregnancies affected by Down's syndrome Ann Clin Biochem 30:219–220

Spencer K, Mallard AS, Coombes EJ, Macri JN (1993b) Prenatal screening for trisomy 18 with free beta human chorionic gonadotrophin as a marker. BMJ 307:1455–1458

Spencer K, Macri JN, Anderson RW et al. (1993c) Dual analyte immunoassay in neural tube defect and Down's syndrome screening: Results of a multicentre clinical trial. Ann Clin Biochem 30:394–401

Spencer K, Macri JN, Carpenter P et al. (1993d) Stability of intact hCG in serum, liquid whole blood and dried whole blood filter paper spots and its impact on free beta hCG Down's syndrome screening. Clin Chem 39:1064–1068

Spencer K, Aitken DA, Crossley JA et al. (1994a) First trimester biochemistry screening for trisomy 21: The role of free beta hCG, alpha fetoprotein and pregnancy associated plasma protein A. Ann Clin Biochem 31:447–454

Spencer K, Salonen R, Muller F (1994b) Down's syndrome screening in multiple pregnancies using alpha-fetoprotein and free beta hCG. Prenat Diagn 14:537–542

Spencer K, Aitken DA, Macri JN, Buchanan PD (1996) Urine free beta hCG and beta core in pregnancies affected by Down's syndrome. Prenat Diagn 16:605–613

Spencer K, Muller F, Aitken DA (1997a) Amniotic fluid and maternal serum levels of CA125 in pregnancies affected by Down syndrome: A re-evaluation of the role of CA125 in Down syndrome screening. Prenat Diagn. 17:701–706

Spencer K, Noble P, Snijders RJM, Nicolaides KH (1997b) First trimester urine free beta hCG, beta core, and total oestriol in pregnancies affected by Down's Syndrome: Implications for first trimester screening with nuchal translucency and serum free beta hCG. Prenat Diagn 17:525–538

Spencer K, Souter V, Tul N et al. (1999a) A screening program for trisomy 21 at 10–14 weeks using fetal nuchal translucency, maternal serum free β-human chorionic gonadotropin and pregnancy-associated plasma protein-A. Ultrasound Obstet Gynecol 13:231–237

Spencer K, Crossley JA, Green K et al. (1999b) Second trimester levels of pregnancy associated plasma protein-A in cases of trisomy 18. Prenat Diagn 19:1127–1134

Spencer K, Berry E, Crossley JA et al. (2000a) Is maternal serum total hCG a marker of trisomy 21 in the first trimester of pregnancy. Prenat Diagn 20:311–317

Spencer K, Heath V, Flack N et al. (2000b) First trimester maternal serum AFP and Total hCG in aneuploides other than trisomy 21. Prenat Diagn 20:635–639

Spencer K, Ong C, Skentou H et al. (2000c). Screening for Trisomy 13 by fetal nuchal translucency thickness and maternal serum free β-hCG and PAPP-A at 10–14 weeks. Prenat Diagn 20:411–416

Spencer K, Tul N, Nicolaides KH (2000d). Maternal serum free β-hCG and PAPP-A in fetal sex chromosome defects in the first trimester. Prenat Diagn 20:390–394

Spencer K, Liao AWJ, Skentou H et al. (2000e) Screening for triploidy by fetal nuchal translucency and maternal serum free β-hCG and PAPP-A at 10–14 weeks of gestation. Prenat Diagn 20:495–499

Spencer K, Ong CYT, Liao AWJ et al. (2000f) First trimester markers of trisomy 21 and the influence of maternal cigarette smoking status. Prenat Diagn 20:852–853

Spencer K, Ong CYT, Liao AWJ, Nicolaides KH (2000g) The influence of ethnic origin on first trimester biochemical markers of chromosomal abnormalities. Prenat Diagn 20:491–494

Spencer K, Ong CYT, Liao AWJ et al. (2000h) The influence of fetal sex in screening for trisomy 21 by fetal nuchal translucency, maternal serum free β-hCG and PAPP-A at 10–14 weeks of gestation. Prenat Diagn 20:673–675

Spencer K, Ong CY, Liao AW, Nicolaides KH (2000i) The influence of parity and gravidity on first trimester markers of chromosomal abnormality. Prenat Diagn 20:792–794

Spencer K, Spencer CE, Power M et al. (2000j) One stop clinic for assessment of risk for fetal anomalies: A report of the first year of prospective screening for chromosomal anomalies in the first trimester. Br J Obstet Gynaecol 107:1271–1275

Spencer K, Crossley JA, Kennedy D et al. (2001) Second trimester levels of pregnancy associated plasma protein-A, free β hCG and AFP in cases of trisomy 13. Prenat Diagn 20: Submitted

Staples AJ, Robertson EF, Ranieri E et al. (1991) A maternal serum screem for trisomy 18: An extension of maternal serum screening for Down syndrome. Am J Hum Genet 49:1025–1033

Stone DH, Rosenberg K, Womersley J (1989) Recent trends in the prevalence and secondary prevention of Down's syndrome. Paediatr Perinat Epidemiol 3:278–283

Szabo J, Gellen J (1990) Nuchal fluid accumulation in trisomy 21 detected by vaginosonography in first trimester. Lancet 336:1133

Szabo J, Gellen J, Szemere G (1995) First-trimester ultrasound screening for fetal aneuploidies in women over 35 and under 35 years of age. Ultrasound Obstet Gynecol 5:161–163

Tabor A, Philip J, Madsen M et al. (1986) Randomised controlled trial of genetic amniocentesis in 4606 low-risk women. Lancet I:1287–1293

Thomsen SG, Isager-Sally L, Lange AP et al. (1983) Smoking habits and maternal serum alpha-fetoprotein levels during the second trimester of pregnancy. Br J Obstet Gynaecol 90:716–717

Tul N, Spencer K, Noble P et al. (1999) Screening for trisomy 18 by fetal nuchal translucency, maternal serum free β-hCG and PAPP-A at 10–14 weeks of gestation. Prenat Diagn 19:1035–1042

van den Hof MC, Nicolaides KH, Campbell J, Campbell S (1990) Evaluation of the lemon and banana signs in one hundred thirty fetuses with open spina bifida. Am J Obstet Gynecol 162:322–327

van Lith JM, Pratt JJ, Beekhuis JR, Mantingh A (1992a) Second trimester maternal serum immunoreactive inhibin as a marker for fetal Down's syndrome. Prenat Diagn 12:801–806

van Lith JMM, Visser GHA, Mantingh A, Beekhuis JR (1992b) Fetal heart rate in early pregnancy and chromosomal disorders. Br J Obstet Gynaecol 99:741–744

Verloes A, Schoos R, Herens C et al. (1995) A prenatal trisomy 21 screening program using alpha-fetoprotein, human chorionic gonadotropin, and free estriol assays on maternal dried blood. Am J Obstet Gynecol 172:167–174

Vintzileos AM, Egan JFX (1995) Adjusting the risk for trisomy 21 on the basis of second trimester ultrasonography. Am J Obstet Gynecol 172:837–844

Wald NJ, Hackshaw AK (1997) Combining ultrasound and biochemistry in first-trimester screening for Down's Syndrome. Prenat Diagn 17:821–829

Wald NJ, Cuckle HS, Boreham J et al. (1979) Maternal serum alpha-fetoprotein and diabetes mellitus. Br J Obstet Gynaecol 86:101–105

Wald N, Cuckle H, Boreham J, Stirrat G (1980) Small biparietal diameter of fetuses with spina bifida: Implications for antenatal screening. B J Obstet Gynaecol 87:219–221

Wald NJ, Cuckle HS, Densem JW et al. (1988) Maternal serum unconjugated oestriol as an antenatal screening test for Down's syndrome. Br J Obstet Gynaecol 95:334–341

Wald N, Cuckle H, Wu TS, George L (1991) Maternal serum unconjugated oestriol and human chorionic gonadotrophin levels in twin pregnancies: Implications for screening for Down's syndrome. Br J Obstet Gynaecol 98:905–908

Wald NJ, Cuckle HS, Densem JW, Stone RB (1992) Maternal serum unconjugated oestriol and human chorionic gonadotrophin levels in pregnancies with insulin-dependent diabetes: Implications for screening for Down's syndrome. Br J Obstet Gynaecol 99:51–53

Wald NJ, Densem JW, Smith D, Klee GG (1994a) Four marker serum screening for Down's syndrome. Prenat Diagn 14:707–16

Wald NJ, Densem JW, Cheng R, Collishaw S (1994b) Maternal serum free alpha- and free beta-human chorionic gonadotrophin in pregnancies with insulin-dependent diabetes mellitus: implications for screening for Down's syndrome. Prenat Diagn 14:835–837

Wald NJ, Densem JW, George L et al. (1996a) Prenatal screening for Down's syndrome using inhibin-A as a serum marker. Prenat Diagn 16:143–153

Wald NJ, George L, Smith D et al. On behalf of the International Prenatal Screening Research Group (1996b) Serum screening for Down's syndrome between 8 and 14 weeks of pregnancy. Br J Obstet Gynecol 103:407–412

Wald NJ, Watt HC, George L (1996c) Maternal serum inhibin-A in pregnancies with insulin-dependent diabetes mellitus: Implications for screening for Down's syndrome. Prenat Diagn 16:923–926

Wald NJ, Kennard A, Hackshaw A, McGuire A (1997) Antenatal screening for Down's syndrome. J Med Screening 4:181–246

Wald NJ, White N, Morris JK et al. (1999a) Serum markers for Down's syndrome in women who have had in vitro fertilisation: Implications for antenatal screening. Br J Obstet Gynaecol 106:1304–1306

Wald NJ, Watt HC, Hackshaw AK (1999b) Integrated screening for Down's syndrome on the basis of tests performed during the first and second trimesters. N Engl J Med 341:461–467

Wallace EM, Swanston IA, McNeilly AS et al. (1996) Second trimester screening for Down's syndrome using maternal serum dimeric inhibin A. Clin Endocrinol 44:17–21

Wallace EM, Crossley JA, Ritoe SC et al. (1997) Maternal serum inhibin-A in pregnancies complicated by insulin dependent diabetes mellitus. Br J Obstet Gynaecol 104:946–948

Watt HC, Wald NJ, Smith D et al. (1996) Effect of allowing for ethnic group in prenatal screening for Down's syndrome. Prenat Diagn 16:691–698

Weinans MJN, Butler SA, Mantingh A, Cole LA (2000). Urinary hyperglycosylated hCG in first trimester screening for chromosomal abnormalities. Prenat Diagn 20:976–978

Westergaard JG, Sinosich MJ, Bugge M et al. (1983) Pregnancy-associated plasma protein A in the prediction of early pregnancy failure. Am J Obstet Gynecol 145:67–69

Whitlow BJ, Chatzipapas IK, Economides DL (1998) The effect of fetal neck position on nuchal translucency measurement. Br J Obstet Gynaecol 105:872–876

Williamson P, Alberman E, Rodeck C et al. (1997) Antecedent circumstances surrounding neural tube defect births in 1990–1991. The steering committee of the national confidential enquiry into counselling for genetic disorders. B J Obstet Gynaecol 104:51–56

World Atlas of Birth Defects (1998) International Cente for Birth Defects of the International Clearinghouse for Birth Defects Monitoring Systems in Collaboration with EUROCAT, 1st edn. Human Genetics Programme, World Health Organisation 1998, Geneva

Wright D, Reynolds T, Donovan C (1993) Assessment of atypicality: an adjunct to screening for Down syndrome that facilitates detection of other chromosomal defects. Ann Clin Biochem 30:578–583

Zeitune M, Aitken DA, Crossley JA et al. (1991) Estimating the risk of a fetal autosomal trisomy at mid-trimester using maternal serum alphafetoprotein and age: A retrospective study of 142 pregnancies. Prenat Diagn 11:847–857

Techniques for prenatal diagnosis

29

Sherman Elias
Joe Leigh Simpson
Lee P. Shulman

Introduction

Advancing capabilities in the prenatal diagnosis of genetic abnormalities and monitoring fetal growth and development have added an entirely new dimension to genetic counseling (Simpson and Elias, 1994a). Instead of counseling in terms of probabilities alone, in many circumstances it is now possible to determine whether a fetus is affected with a specific genetic disorder in question. This chapter reviews the techniques used for prenatal diagnosis and their safety. Also considered are the new approaches of using first trimester ultrasonography to provide a risk assessment for fetal Down syndrome and isolating fetal cells from maternal blood, a method with potential for noninvasive prenatal diagnosis.

Amniocentesis

TRADITIONAL AMNIOCENTESIS: 15 WEEKS GESTATION AND GREATER

Technique

Amniocentesis, the aspiration of amniotic fluid, has traditionally been performed at and after 15 to 17 weeks gestation (menstrual weeks). At this stage of gestation, the volume of amniotic fluid is approximately 200 ml. The ratio of viable to nonviable cells in the amniotic fluid is relatively high (Fuchs and Riis, 1956), thus allowing timely culture and diagnosis of fetal cytogenetic abnormalities. This allows women the option of pregnancy termination should an abnormality be found.

Amniocentesis is routinely performed in an outpatient facility. An ultrasound examination should be done immediately before the procedure to evaluate fetal number and viability, perform fetal biometric measurements to confirm gestational age, establish placental location, and estimate amniotic fluid volume. In our units, a fetal anatomic survey to screen for major anomalies is standard. In addition, ultrasonography may be useful in discovering maternal gynecologic conditions (e.g., leiomyomata) that could influence the technique and/or timing of the amniocentesis.

Once the preoperative ultrasound examination is completed, a needle insertion site is chosen. We prefer to insert the needle in the midline fundal area of the uterus, but this is not always the site at which the optimal pocket of amniotic fluid is located. Not infrequently, a lower uterine segment or lateral approach is required. If possible, we avoid the placenta; however, transplacental amniocentesis has not been shown to reduce the safety of amniocentesis (Bravo et al., 1995; Marthin et al., 1997; Tharmaratnam et al., 1998). If tapping the optimal pocket of fluid requires traversing the placenta, we select the thinnest portion of the placenta possible through which the needle can be directed. The umbilical cord insertion site should be identified and avoided. The maternal bowel and bladder should also be located, as these should likewise be avoided. A local subcutaneous anesthetic (e.g., 2 to 3 ml of 1% xylocaine) may be used, but we usually find this unnecessary. After the maternal skin is cleaned with an iodine-based solution, sterile drapes are placed around the needle-insertion site to help maintain an aseptic field. We prefer a 22-gauge spinal needle and recommend no larger than a 20-gauge. Ultrasonographic monitoring with continuous visualization of the needle should be performed throughout the procedure. Ultrasound gel (Ultrasonic Scanning Gel, Pharmaceutical Innovations, Newark, NJ) is applied adjacent to the insertion site, and a real-time ultrasound transducer is held in position such that the ultrasound beam is directed parallel to the planned needle track. Needle insertion should be performed with one smooth continuous motion until the needle tip is within the amniotic cavity (Fig. 29.1A,B). Some practitioners locate the needle tip within the subcutaneous fat and assess the distance from tip to amniotic cavity as well as the appropriate needle angle required to successfully enter the amnion and avoid maternal structures and the fetus.

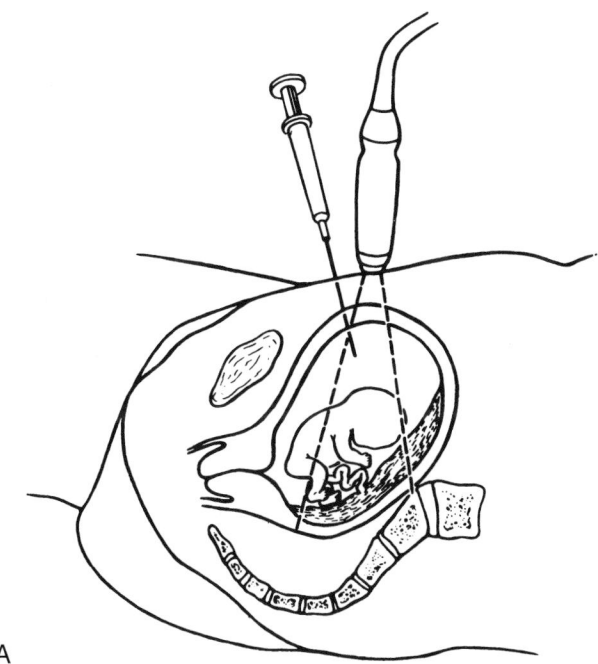

A

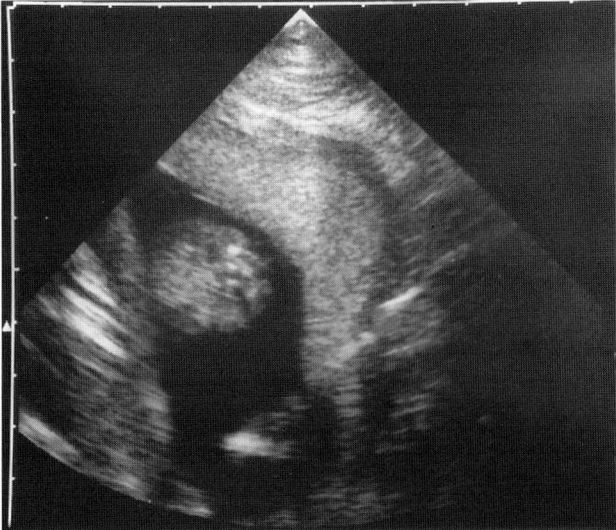

B

Fig. 29.1. (A) Amniocentesis performed concurrently with ultrasound. (From Simpson and Elias, 1994a, with permission.). (B) Ultrasonographic visualization of a transplacental amniocentesis.

The first several milliliters of amniotic fluid are aspirated into a syringe. These first few milliliters are theoretically most likely to contain maternal cells from blood vessels, the abdominal wall, or the myometrium; therefore, this initial sample is usually discarded or set aside for α-fetoprotein (AFP) assay. For a second-trimester amniocentesis performed at 14 to 20 weeks inclusive, 20 to 30 ml amniotic fluid is usually aspirated. Once the amniotic fluid is obtained, the specimen is clearly labeled and transported at ambient temperature to the laboratory.

Amniotic fluid and urine are often indistinguishable in appearance. Analysis of cells derived from maternal urine could obviously lead to erroneous interpretations of fetal status. Inadvertent aspiration of maternal urine is a particular risk when a suprapubic needle insertion site is chosen. If the origin of aspirated fluid is in doubt, tests should be performed to determine its origin. Our group found that the crystalline arborization pattern characteristic of amniotic fluid is observed if the fluid is allowed to dry on an acid-cleaned slide and examined under low power (X 100 magnification) (Elias et al., 1979). This test readily differentiates amniotic fluid from urine. However, only rarely are any tests necessary.

Bloody amniotic fluid is aspirated in perhaps 1% to 2% of amniocenteses. The blood, which is almost always maternal in origin, does not adversely affect amniotic cell growth. Indeed, the performance of a transplacental amniocentesis may increase the risk for a bloody tap; this will not have an adverse affect on the safety or accuracy of the amniocentesis. By contrast, brown or dark red- or wine-colored amniotic fluid is associated with an increased likelihood of poor pregnancy outcome. This color indicates prior intra-amniotic bleeding, with hemoglobin breakdown products accounting for the pigment. Pregnancy loss eventually occurs in about one-third of such cases (Milunsky, 1986). If the abnormally colored fluid is also characterized by an elevated (AFP) level, the outcome is usually unfavorable (fetal death, anencephaly, spontaneous abortion, or fetal abnormality). Green-colored amniotic fluid, presumably due to meconium staining, is apparently not associated with poor pregnancy outcome (Karp and Schiller, 1977; Hess et al., 1986; Isada et al., 1990). By contrast, brown amniotic fluid has been associated with an increased risk of fetal aneuploidy (Isada et al., 1990).

The propriety of administering Rh immunoglobulin (RhIG) to prevent Rh immunization in unsensitized women with Rh-positive fetuses remains controversial. Fetomaternal transfusion by disruption of the fetoplacental circulation logically might have an immunizing effect; however, the magnitude of the risk has not been determined. The task is difficult because one must consider such variables as ABD compatibility, number of needle insertions, placental location, and the amount of fetal blood transfused into the maternal circulation. Early investigators opined that prophylactic RhIG should not be administered following genetic amniocentesis (Golbus et al., 1982), but almost all now advocate its routine use (Henry et al., 1976; Bowman et al., 1978; Hill et al., 1980; Khalil et al., 1984). The dose to be administered is controversial. The American College of Obstetricians and Gynecologists recommends that 300 µg of RhIG be administered for an exposure of 30 ml of fetal blood (ACOG, 1999). In the United Kingdom, the recommended dose of RhIG is 50 µg before 20 weeks gestation and 100 µg thereafter (Turnbull and Mackenzie, 1983). We routinely administer 300 µg of RhIG following genetic amniocentesis, regardless of whether the needle has traversed the placenta.

Following amniocentesis, the fetal heart motion should be documented by ultrasonographic visualization. The patient is observed briefly following the procedure and is instructed to report any vaginal fluid loss or bleeding, uterine cramping, or fever. Reasonably normal activities may be resumed following the procedure; however, we recommend that strenuous exercise (e.g., jogging or aerobic exercises) and coitus be avoided for a day.

Multiple gestations

In multiple gestations, amniocentesis can usually be performed on all fetuses, provided amniotic fluid volume is adequate (Elias et al., 1980a). Following aspiration of amniotic fluid from the first sac, 2 to 3 ml of indigo carmine, diluted 1:10 in bacteriostatic water, is injected prior to needle withdrawal. A second amniocentesis is then performed. The second needle is then inserted into the sac of the second fetus, preferably determined after visualizing the membranes separating the two sacs. Aspiration of clear fluid confirms that the second sac has truly been entered (Fig. 29.2). In experienced hands, amniocentesis is performed successfully in more than 95% of twin pregnancies with ostensibly no increased risks over that of amniocentesis in singleton pregnancies (Elias et al., 1980a; Anderson and Goldberg, 1991). Anderson and Goldberg (1991) observed a postprocedure twin-loss rate of 3.57% up to 28 weeks, a rate interpreted as not increased over the sum of background twin-loss rate plus the loss rate associated with singleton amniocentesis. Triplets and higher-order multiple gestations can be managed similarly by sequentially injecting dye into successive sacs. As long as clear fluid is aspirated, one can be reassured that a new amniotic sac has been

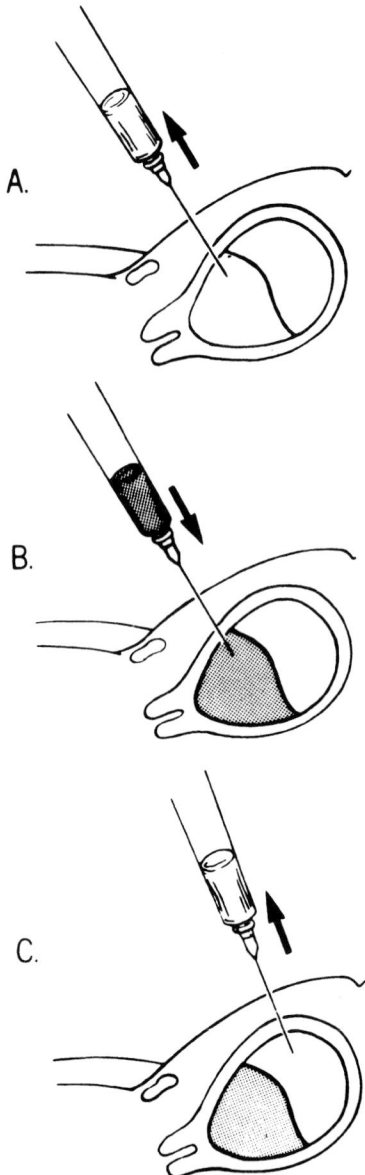

Fig. 29.2. Technique for amniocentesis in twin gestations. (A) Fluid is aspirated from the first amniotic sac. (B) Blue indigo carmine dye is injected into the first amniotic sac. (C) A second tap is made in the ultrasonographically determined location of the second fetus. Clear fluid confirms that the second amniotic sac was successfully aspirated. (From Elias et al., 1980a, with permission.)

entered. However, the overall safety of amniocentesis in triplets and higher-order multiple gestations have not yet been formally determined.

Other techniques for sampling multiple gestations have been reported, including a single puncture technique and an "air-bubble" infusion procedure. Despite the advances in ultrasonography, we have concerns that single-puncture techniques could lead to cross-contamination between sacs, resulting in diagnostic inaccuracies. In addition, we believe it unwise to instill any substance into the amniotic cavity unless the instillation is performed in a strict, aseptic fashion and serves to considerably and consistently improve safety or accuracy. More recently, some operators have not used dye instillation to distinguish separate sacs, instead relying on ultrasonographic visualization alone (Bahado-Singh et al., 1992; Buscaglia et al., 1995; van Vugt et al., 1995). In view of the considerable positive experience with dye instillation techniques over the past 20 years with regard to safety and accuracy, we still prefer the dye instillation procedure described above.

Safety

Any procedure that involves passing a device into an organ, especially the pregnant uterus, carries a risk. Amniocentesis is no exception. Amniocentesis carries potential danger to both mother and fetus. Maternal risks are quite low, with symptomatic amnionitis occurring only rarely. Minor maternal complications such as transient vaginal spotting and minimal amniotic fluid leakage occur in 1% or less of cases, but these are almost always self-limited in nature. Other very rare complications include intra-abdominal organic injury or hemorrhage.

The safety of traditional amniocentesis has been addressed by several large collaborative studies. The U.S. National Institute of Child Health and Human Development (NICHD) (1976) conducted the first major prospective study of genetic amniocentesis that was comprised of 1040 subjects and 992 matched controls. Of the 1040 women undergoing amniocentesis, 950 (91.3%) had the procedure performed for cytogenetic analysis and 90 (8.7%) to evaluate for the possible presence of an inborn error of metabolism. Of all women who underwent amniocentesis, 3.5% experienced fetal loss between the time of the procedure and delivery compared with 3.2% of controls; the slight difference was not statistically significant and disappeared completely when corrected for maternal age. In Canada, a collaborative group conducted a cohort study but did not include a concurrent control group (Simpson et al., 1976; Medical Research Council, 1977). Analysis was based on 1,223 amniocenteses performed during 1020 pregnancies in 900 women. The pregnancy loss rate was 3.2%, a frequency similar to that reported in the US collaborative study.

A later British collaborative study found that the rate of fetal loss following amniocentesis was significantly greater than in controls (2.6% versus 1%) (United Kingdom Medical Research Council, 1978). In the British study, however, one common indication for amniocentesis was elevated maternal serum α-fetoprotein (MSAFP), now recognized itself as a factor associated with fetal loss and adverse perinatal outcome. Analysis after excluding subjects undergoing amniocentesis for that indication lowered the loss rates between subject and control groups to less than 1%, albeit still a significant difference (National Institute of Child Health and Human Development Consensus Conference on Antenatal Diagnosis, 1979).

None of the collaborative studies cited above were conducted with high-quality ultrasonography as defined by today's standards, nor was concurrent ultrasonography universally applied. More relevant recent data are from a Danish randomized controlled study of amniocentesis that involved 4606 women aged 25 to 34 years who were without known risk factors for fetal genetic abnormalities (Tabor et al., 1986). Women with three or more previous spontaneous abortions, diabetes mellitus, multiple gestation, uterine anomalies, or intrauterine contraceptive devices were excluded. Maternal age, social group, smoking history, number of previous induced and spontaneous abortions, stillbirths, livebirths, and low-birthweight infants were comparable in the study and control groups, as was gestational age at time of entry into the study. Amniocentesis was performed under real-time ultrasound guidance with a 20-gauge needle by experienced operators. Follow-up evaluation was available for all but three women. The spontaneous abortion rate after 16 weeks was 1.7% in amniocentesis patients compared with 0.7% in controls (p<0.01), with a 2.6-fold relative risk of spontaneously aborting if the placenta was traversed. Transplacental needle passage is a risk factor that has more recently been shown to not increase the risk for post-procedure loss (see above). The frequency of postural malformations in the infants in the two groups did not differ. However, respiratory distress syndrome was diagnosed more often (relative risk 2.1) in the study group, and more infants were treated for pneumonia (relative risk 2.5). A more recent assessment of the safety of second-trimester amniocentesis can be found in the CEMAT study that compared conventional second-trimester amniocentesis to early amniocentesis (CEMAT 1998). In this multicenter trial performed by experienced operators using concurrent ultrasonography, the total loss rate in the second trimester amniocentesis cohort was 5.9%.

In a study from British Columbia, Baird, et al., (1994) considered the question of whether children delivered of women who had midtrimester amniocentesis can be identified by a population-based database of congenital anomalies and disabilities at a different rate from that of matched controls (i.e., offspring of women who had not undergone amniocentesis). The authors studied 1296 cases (651 males and 645 females) and 3704 matched controls (1867 males and 1837 females) among live births (1972–1983) from the Health Surveillance Registry with data collected to 1990 to allow a follow-up of seven to 18 years. Cases were children of mothers who had midtrimester amniocentesis for advanced maternal age (35 years or older) and whose results were normal for chromosomal disorders and neural tube defects. When possible, three controls per case were matched for age of mother, sex, date of birth, and health from provincial birth records. One hundred twenty-eight (9.9%) of the cases and 308 (8.3%) of the controls were registered (relative risk 1.23); this relative risk was not significantly different from 1. The likelihood of having disabilities was examined for cases as compared to controls, and no difference was found except for an increased ABO isoimmunization associated with amniocentesis. Overall, this study provides reassuring data for patients considering midtrimester amniocentesis with respect to long-term outcome.

In conclusion, we believe it wise to continue to counsel that the risk of pregnancy loss secondary to amniocentesis is 0.5% over baseline, or perhaps slightly less at centers with experienced operators. At our centers, serious maternal complications and fetal injuries are stated to be "remote" risks.

EARLY AMNIOCENTESIS: 14 WEEKS GESTATION OR LESS

With the advent of high-resolution ultrasound equipment, some physicians began offering amniocentesis before 15 weeks gestation. Some programs not offering chorionic villus sampling (CVS) viewed early amniocentesis as an attractive alternative for those women who desired prenatal diagnosis before the time in pregnancy when traditional amniocentesis is performed (i.e., 15 weeks gestation or greater). In other medical centers, early amniocentesis was explored to obviate the inconvenience of patients having to be rescheduled if they came in for CVS, and were determined to be beyond 12 weeks gestation but under 15 weeks gestation.

A number of programs, including our own centers, had reported experiences suggesting early amniocentesis to be a promising technique. In a series of 936 amniocenteses at 12.8 weeks gestation or less reported by Hanson and colleagues (1992), loss rates were 0.7% (7 of 936) within 2 weeks of amniocentesis, with an additional 2.2% before 28 weeks and an additional 0.5% stillbirths or neonatal deaths. Total losses (32 of 936, or 3.4%) were considered comparable with the 2.1 to 3.2% in ultrasonographically normal pregnancies not undergoing a procedure; however, lack of

corrections for maternal age and gestational age render comparisons less than exact. Other series reported include those conducted by Benacerraf, et al., (1988), Elejalde et al., (1990), Penso et al., (1990), Stripparo et al., (1990), Hackett et al., (1991), Assel et al., (1992), Djalali et al., (1992), Henry and Miller (1992), Yang et al., (1993), Eiben et al., (1993), and Kerber and Held (1993). Our group, then at the University of Tennessee, Memphis (Shulman et al., 1994), compared our initial experience with 250 early amniocenteses (14 weeks or less) to that of our first 250 cases of transabdominal CVS (9.5 to 12.9 weeks), finding loss rates for early amniocentesis and transabdominal CVS to be 3.8% and 2.1%, respectively. Our group also reported early amniocentesis in six twin gestations (mean 11.9 weeks; range 10.5 to 13.6 weeks), using a similar dye injection technique as described for traditional amniocentesis (see above) (Shulman et al., 1992a,b). We successfully tapped both amniotic sacs in each of six cases (five requiring two needle insertions, one requiring three needle insertions); all cultures yielded normal cytogenetic results, and all six pregnancies resulted in the delivery of healthy infants.

However, these studies mostly represented observational reports of amniocentesis with most of the procedures being performed at or after 13 weeks gestation. Comparative studies evaluating the safety and efficacy of early amniocentesis have failed to corroborate the generally favorable outcomes reported in the observational studies. Nicolaides et al (1994) reported a comparison of amniocentesis and CVS at 10 to 13 weeks gestation. Early amniocentesis was performed in 731 patients (493 by choice and 238 by randomization) and CVS in 570 (320 by choice and 250 by randomization). Both procedures were performed by transabdominal ultrasound-guided insertion of a 20-gauge needle. The spontaneous loss (intrauterine or neonatal death) was significantly higher after early amniocentesis (total group mean: 5.3%; 95% CI 3.8 to 7.2/randomized subgroup mean: 5.9%; CI 3.3 to 9.7) than after CVS (total group mean, 2.3%, CI 1.2 to 3.9; randomized subgroup: mean, 1.2%, 0.3 to 3.5). Subsequently, Nicolaides and colleagues (Nicolaides et al., 1996) reported further findings of this study. Again, postprocedure loss rates were significantly higher in the total early amniocentesis group (4.9%) and the randomized early amniocentesis sub-group (5.8%) than in the total transabdominal CVS group (2.1%) and the randomized transabdominal CVS sub-group (1.8%). The frequency of talipes equinovarus was higher in the early amniocentesis group, but this difference did not attain statistical significance.

Sundberg and colleagues (1997) performed a similar type of randomized trial comparing early amniocentesis and

CVS. In this study, the rate of talipes equinovarus was significantly increased in the early amniocentesis group, despite the fact that the investigators used a filter system to reduce the amount of fluid removed. This finding led the authors to prematurely terminate their study for safety concerns.

The results of the Canadian Early Amniocentesis versus Mid-Trimester Amniocentesis Trial (CEMAT 1998; Johnson et al., 1999)—a multicenter, randomized trial of early amniocentesis and conventional second-trimester amniocentesis—have been most revealing. This multicenter trial randomized 4374 women into an early amniocentesis cohort (n = 2183) and a conventional mid-trimester amniocentesis cohort (n = 2185). In the early amniocentesis cohort, 1916 women (87.8%) underwent amniocentesis before 13 weeks gestation.

Loss rates were 7.6% for the early amniocentesis cohort and 5.9% for the mid-trimester cohort (p = 0.012). Talipes equinovarus occurred in 1.3% of infants delivered of women in the early amniocentesis group compared to 0.1% in the mid-trimester cohort (p = 0.0001). In addition, postprocedure amniotic fluid leakage occurred more frequently in the early amniocentesis group (3.5%) than in the mid-trimester group (1.7%; p = 0.0007). Failed procedure, multiple needle insertions, and culture failure also occurred more frequently in the early amniocentesis group (CEMAT 1998; Johnson et al., 1999).

In view of these recent studies, the ongoing United States multicenter trial evaluating the safety and efficacy of early amniocentesis with the EATA (Early Amniocentesis-Transabdominal CVS) trial ceased offering early amniocentesis to women less than 14 weeks gestation. These more recent prospective studies strongly suggest that second trimester amniocentesis and first-trimester chorionic villus sampling should remain, for the foreseeable future, as the invasive procedures of choice for the detection of fetal cytogenetic and mendelian abnormalities.

Chorionic villus sampling

Since amniocentesis is most commonly performed in the mid-second trimester (15 to 16 weeks), fetal diagnosis cannot usually be established prior to 17 to 18 weeks gestation. A technique that could be performed during the first trimester would be highly desirable to reduce the psychological stress of awaiting results until mid-pregnancy and to allow a safer method of pregnancy termination, should an abnormality be detected. CVS is such a technique.

Following fertilization, the zygote differentiates first into the blastocyst, which contains an inner cell mass that develops into the fetus and an outer trophoblastic layer that develops into nonfetal structures such as amnion, chorion, and placenta. The genetic complement of the outer cell mass nearly always reflects the genetic constitution of the inner cell mass (i.e., the fetus) because both are derived from the same zygote. It follows that cytogenetic, DNA, or biochemical analysis on trophoblastic cells should provide information comparable with that obtained from cultured amniotic fluid cells. The one major exception is that assays requiring amniotic fluid, specifically AFP, require amniocentesis.

TECHNIQUES FOR CHORIONIC VILLUS SAMPLING

Transcervical chorionic villus sampling

Transcervical CVS is now usually performed at 10 to 12 completed gestational weeks. Absolute contraindications to transcervical CVS include active cervical or vaginal pathology (e.g., herpes, chlamydia or gonorrhea infection) or maternal blood group sensitization. Relative contraindications include leiomyoma obstructing the cervical canal, bleeding from the vagina within two weeks of planned CVS, and a markedly retroverted, retroflexed uterus (Elias et al., 1985). Before CVS, fetal viability and normal fetal growth must be confirmed by ultrasound. The procedure is performed with a device that consists of a plastic cannula enclosing a metal obturator extending just beyond the catheter tip; the diameter of most catheters is approximately 1.5 mm.

At our institutions, CVS is performed in an ultrasound suite. The patient is positioned in the dorsal lithotomy position. The vagina is cleaned with an iodine preparation, and the perineum draped with sterile towels. After insertion of a sterile vaginal speculum, placement of a tenaculum on the anterior lip of the cervix may occasionally be needed to help correct uterine anteflexion or retroflexion. The CVS catheter is introduced transcervically under simultaneous ultrasonographic visualization, with optimal catheter placement being parallel to the long axis of the placenta (Fig. 29.3). The obturator is then withdrawn and the catheter Luer-lock attached to a 20- or 30-ml syringe. Chorionic villi are then aspirated by multiple, rapid aspirations of the syringe plunger to 20- to 30-ml negative pressure. The catheter is withdrawn under continuous maximum negative pressure. An adequate sample is at least 5 mg of villi, but a sample of 10 to 25 mg is preferred.

Following the procedure, fetal heart activity is verified by ultrasonography. Patients are monitored for any untoward

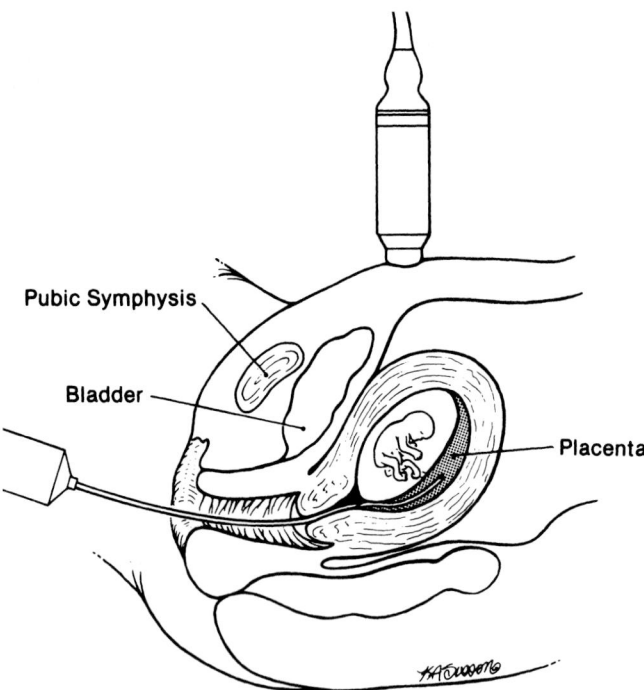

Fig. 29.3. Transcervical chorionic villus sampling. (From Elias and Simpson, 1994, with permission.)

effects for approximately 30 minutes. Unsensitized Rh-negative patients are given Rh1g. Maternal serum AFP screening for fetal neural tube defects is recommended at 16 to 18 weeks gestation.

Transabdominal chorionic villus sampling

Transabdominal CVS can be used to evaluate pregnancies at the same gestational age as transcervical CVS at 10 to 12 weeks; however, this procedure also can be performed later in pregnancy (Holzgreve et al., 1987; Shulman et al., 1990; Podobnik et al., 1997), particularly when fetal abnormalities are visualized at ultrasound and a rapid diagnosis may influence pregnancy management. Placentas especially amenable to the transabdominal approach include those located in the fundus or those located anteriorly in an anteflexed uterus. Transabdominal CVS is also an option in certain circumstances when transcervical sampling is contraindicated (e.g., active herpes or cervical lesions).

Following selection of a needle insertion site based on ultrasound findings, the overlying skin is infiltrated with a local anesthetic, cleaned with an iodine preparation, and draped with sterile towels. As performed at our centers, a 19-gauge spinal needle is inserted percutaneously through the maternal abdominal wall and myometrium under con-

tinuous ultrasound guidance. The tip is then guided into the long axis of the placenta (Fig. 29.4). The needle stylet is withdrawn, and next a syringe housed in an aspiration device (Cameco syringe pistol, Precision Dynamics, San Fernando, CA) is connected to the Luerlock of the needle. Chorionic villi are obtained by repeated (15 to 20) rapid aspirations of the syringe plunger to 20 ml of negative pressure. The needle is then withdrawn under continuous negative pressure. The same postoperative protocol is used as for transcervical CVS.

Most physicians performing transabdominal CVS employ the aforementioned "free-hand" technique. Alternatively, some operators still use a guide-needle or double-needle system device, which punctures the uterine wall once but permits multiple attempts at villus aspiration (Smidt-Jensen and Hahnemann, 1984).

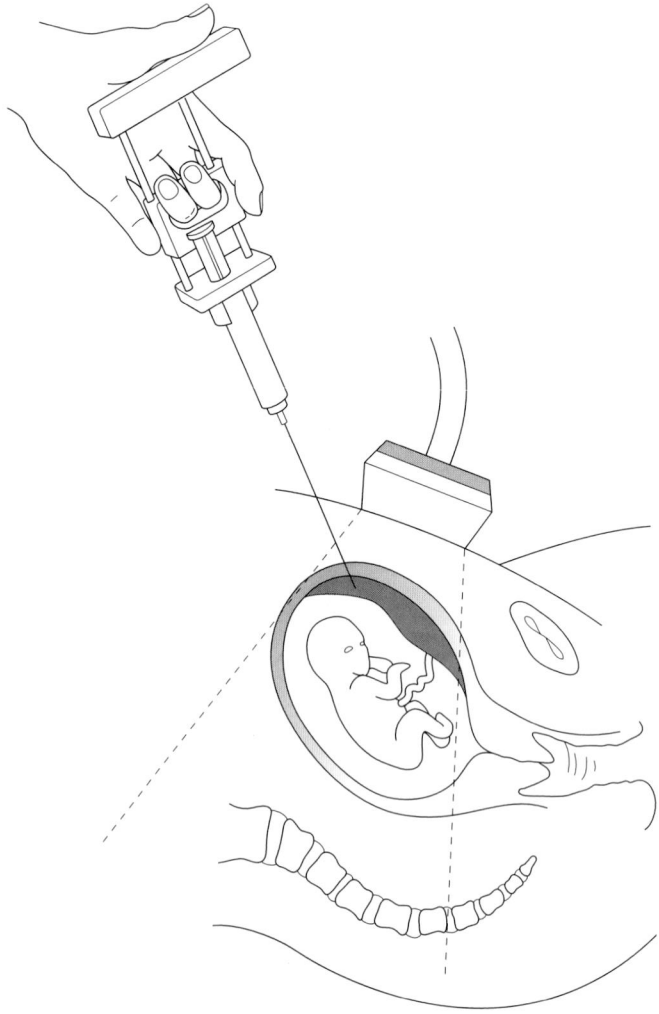

Fig. 29.4. Transabdominal chorionic villus sampling. (From Elias and Simpson, 1994c, with permission.)

Transvaginal chorionic villus sampling

Although not commonly necessary, transvaginal CVS may be the only option in women having a retroverted, retroflexed uterus with a posterior placenta. Patients are prepared in a fashion similar to transcervical CVS. We use a 35-cm 18-gauge aspiration needle to obtain chorionic villi. The wall of the vagina posterior to the cervix is infiltrated with a local anesthetic. Transabdominal ultrasound is used for needle guidance through the vaginal mucosa and myometrium into the placenta. Once within the placenta, the needle stylet is removed, and villi are aspirated in a similar fashion as with transabdominal CVS (Fig. 29.5; Shulman et al., 1993).

SAFETY OF CHORIONIC VILLUS SAMPLING

Pregnancy loss following chorionic villus sampling

The U.S. Cooperative Clinical Comparison of Chorionic Villus Sampling and Amniocentesis study and the Canadian Collaborative CVS-Amniocentesis Trial Group study initially reported the pregnancy loss rate CVS to be 0.8% and 0.6% higher than traditional amniocentesis, respectively (Rhoads et al., 1989; Canadian Collaborative CVS-Amniocentesis Trial Group, 1991). Neither figure was statistically significant. In the U.S. study, 2278 women self-

selected transcervical CVS; 671 women similarly recruited in the first trimester selected amniocentesis. Randomization did not prove possible. The Candian study was randomized, with 1391 subjects assigned to transcervical CVS and 1396 to amniocentesis. Variables shown to influence fetal loss rates adversely included fundal location of the placenta, number of catheter passages, small sample size, and prior bleeding during the current pregnancy (Rhoades et al., 1989; Golbus et al., 1992). Almost all the above invariably reflect technical difficulty. Other obstetric complications (e.g., intrauterine growth restriction [IUGR], placental abruption, premature delivery) did not exceed those in women not undergoing CVS.

Transcervical CVS and transabdominal CVS appear to be equally safe procedures for first-trimester diagnosis. In a later U.S. NICHD collaborative study, in which 1844 patients were randomized to transcervical CVS and 1929 patients randomized to transabdominal CVS, the loss rates of cytogenetically normal pregnancies through 28 weeks were 2.5% and 2.3%, respectively (Jackson et al., 1992). Of note, the overall loss rate (i.e., background plus procedure-related) following CVS decreased by about 0.8% during this 1988–1990 randomization trial, in comparison with rates observed during the transcervical versus amniocentesis self-selection study (1985–1987). This decrease in procedure-related loss rate probably reflects increasing operator experience, as well as availability of both transcervical and transabdominal approaches. In a small Italian randomized trial, Brambati et al., (1990) also found no difference between transabdominal and transcervical CVS. By contrast, in a randomized comparison of amniocentesis, transabdominal CVS, and transcervical CVS in Denmark, Smidt-Jensen et al., (1992) found similar fetal loss rates after transabdominal CVS and amniocentesis, but a significantly increased loss rate associated with transcervical CVS. These results are not surprising, however, since Danish experience with transabdominal CVS is far greater than with transcervical CVS.

The one major study that differs substantively from the U.S., Canadian, and Italian collaborative trials is the Medical Research Council Study (MRC Working Party on the Evaluation of Chorionic Villus Sampling, 1991). In this multicenter randomized comparison between first-trimester CVS performed in whatever fashion deemed suitable by the obstetrician and second-trimester amniocentesis, the ultimate variable measured was completed pregnancies. The 4.4% fewer completed pregnancies in the CVS cohort reflected both unintended and intended pregnancy terminations. The latter, in turn, probably reflected inexperience in cytogenetic interpretation, given some terminations

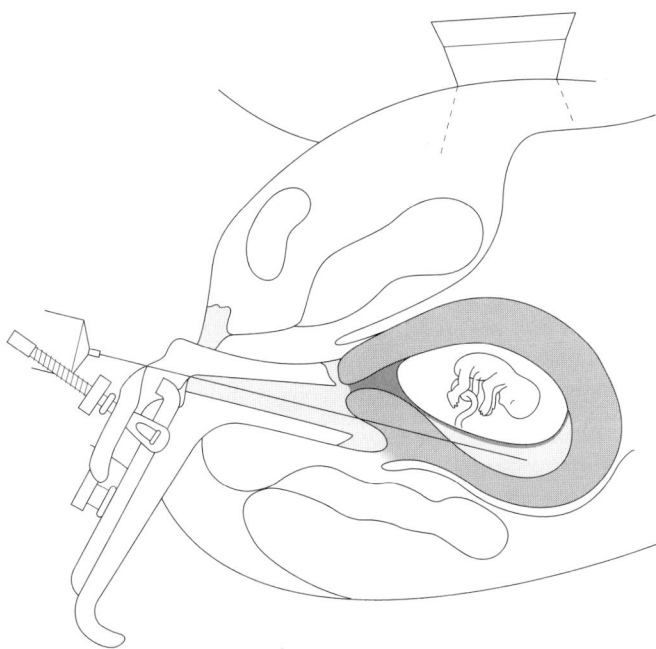

Fig. 29.5. Transvaginal chorionic villus sampling. (From Shulman et al., 1993, with permission).

seemingly arguable in retrospect (i.e., confined placental mosaicism). Experience with CVS by the MRC study operators was also considerably less than in the U.S. operators. For example, the only requirement for participation in the MRC study was 30 "practice" CVS procedures. Some centers also contributed very few cases.

No formal attempts to assess the safety of transvaginal CVS have as yet been attempted. In our own experience (Shulman et al., 1993), as well as that of Sidranski et al., (1990), neither major complications nor obvious excessive fetal loss rates have been observed.

We conclude that clinical judgment and patient individualization in choosing the optimal approach for CVS increases safety. For example, some technically difficult transcervical CVS procedures (e.g., fundal placentas) should be avoided in favor of a technically more straightforward transabdominal approach. The converse is also true.

Chorionic villus sampling in multifetal pregnancy

CVS in multifetal pregnancies has become more widely used with increasing use of fetal reduction resulting from assisted reproductive technologies (ART). Many women requiring ART to become pregnant are also at increased risk for fetal chromosome or mendelian abnormalities. CVS prior to fetal reduction allows for the detection of chromosome or DNA abnormalities, thus allowing for the reduction of only abnormal gestations (Brambati et al., 1995; De Catte et al., 1998; van den Berg et al., 1999).

Few data exist for safety of CVS in multiple gestations. In a major U.S. study involving four centers, the total loss rate of chromosomally normal fetuses (spontaneous abortions, stillborns, neonatal deaths) was 5.0% (Pergament et al., 1992), only slightly higher than the 4.0% observed for singleton pregnancies (Rhoads et al., 1989). We now use CVS in multiple gestations when both placentas can reliably be sampled as determined by ultrasonography. When placental locations preclude the reasonable obtainment of separate and distinct samples, amniocentesis is preferred.

Limb-reduction deformities (LRD)

Evaluation of the safety of CVS has recently shifted focus from concerns about the risk of fetal loss to its being the possible cause for congenital abnormalities. In 1991, Firth and colleagues (1991a, b) reported that five of 289 (1.7%, or 17 in 1000) infants exposed to CVS at 56 to 66 days of gestation (i.e., 42 to 50 days after fertilization) had severe limb-reduction deformities (LRD). Four of the five infants had oromandibular-limb hypogenesis (all transabdominal

CVS); the fifth had a terminal transverse limb reduction alone (transcervical CVS). Subsequently, a number of reports followed, both supporting and refuting such an association (Hsieh et al., 1991; Jackson et al., 1991; Mahoney, 1991; Mastroiacovo and Cavalcanti, 1991; Monni et al., 1991; Scott, 1991). In the United States, Burton et al., (1992) reported a second cluster among 394 infants whose mothers had undergone CVS. Thirteen (3.3%) had major congenital abnormalities, including four with transverse LRD (10 of 1000 or 1%). All four LRDs were transverse distal defects involving hypoplasia or absence of the fingers and toes. Three of these cases followed transcervical sampling, using a device that, in the hands of the reporting physicians, was associated with an 11% fetal loss rate.

Teratogenic mechanisms whereby CVS might cause LRD have been hypothesized (Simpson and Elias, 1994b). These include (1) hypoperfusion due to fetomaternal hemorrhage or pressor substances released by disturbance of villi or the chorion; (2) embolization of chorionic villus material or maternal clots into the fetal circulation; and (3) amniotic puncture and limb entrapment in exocoelic gel.

The potential association of LRD with CVS has been explored through various registries. Based on data from the Italian Multicenter Birth Defects Registry, Mastroiacovo et al., (1992) reported that eight cases of oromandibular-limb hypogenesis complex were entered into the registry from January 1988 through December 1991, four of which had been exposed to CVS, compared to 36 exposed subjects among 8445 controls. There were 166 cases of transverse limb defects alone, four having been exposed to CVS, compared to 36 cases among 8445 controls. A 1994 update of this study, based on 11 CVS-exposed cases, continued to indicate an association with transverse limb defects (Mastroiacovo and Botto, 1994). The highest risk was associated with procedures performed at less than 70 days gestation (OR 23.2; 95% CI 1.31–41.0); a lower, but still increased risk with procedures at 70 to 76 days (OR 17.1; 95% CI 6.7–44.0); over 44 days there were no exposed cases and the risk interpreted as considerably lower. By contrast, analysis of other European registries in aggregate involving more than 600,000 births showed that only four of 336 cases (1.2%) with limb-reduction abnormalities had been exposed to CVS, compared with 78 of 11,883 (0.66%) cases with other malformations (OR 1.8, 95% CI 0.7–5.0) (Dolk et al., 1992).

Firth et al., (1994) summarized LRD in 75 infants exposed to CVS by combining their own cases with those reported in the literature. The median gestational age at CVS ranged from 56 (range 49 to 65) postmenstrual days for the most severe defects to 72 (51 to 98) for the least severe. They concluded that there was a correlation between the severity of the defects and the duration of gestation when CVS was performed.

In 1994, the U.S. Centers for Disease Control (CDC) held an open forum in Atlanta where data were presented from a U.S. multistate case control study in an effort to quantify the risk of LDR associated with CVS (Olney et al., 1995). Case subjects were 131 infants with nonsyndromic limb deficiency from seven population-based birth defects surveillance programs born to women 34 years or older from 1988 through 1992. Controls were 131 infants with other birth defects matched to case subjects by the infant's year of birth, mother's age, race, and state of residence. Overall, the odds ratio for limb deficiency after CVS from eight to 12 weeks gestation was 1.7 (95% CI 0.4 to 6.3). However, when analyzed for specific anatomic subtypes, there was an association for transverse digital deficiency (OR 6.4; 95% CI. 1.1 to 38.6). They concluded that the absolute risk for such defects was approximately 1 in 3000. It should be noted that such transverse digital deficiencies occurred in only seven exposed cases.

Finally, the World Health Organization Committee on Chorionic Villus Sampling recently analyzed data collected through an international voluntary registry (Fishman, 1994; Froster and Jackson, 1996). A total of 77 cases with LRD among 138,996 infants born after CVS was reported from 63 registering centers. Pattern analysis of the types of limb defects and overall frequencies of specific LRD were compared to a background population study from British Columbia (Froster and Baird, 1989). The pattern of defects showed upper limb to be affected in 65%, 13% in the lower limb, and 23% in both upper and lower limbs compared to frequencies in the general population of 68%, 23%, and 9%, respectively. Transverse limb defects occurred in 41% of infants in the cohort exposed to CVS, compared to 43% in the general population and longitudinal limb deficiencies were found in 59% of cases, compared to 57% in the general population. It was concluded that the pattern analysis of the types of limb defects and calculation of overall incidences failed to find a difference between the CVS and background populations.

A more recent review of CVS safety sponsored by the World Health Organization (WHO/PAHO 1999) evaluated the clinical outcomes of 216,381 CVS cases performed worldwide. In this review, a total of 115 LRD were observed with an incidence of 1/1881, similar to the rate of 1/1642 observed in the general population. The distribution of LRD (upper limbs 71.3%, lower limbs 11.3%, both limbs 17.4%) was also similar to that observed in the general population. The authors concluded the data demonstrate that

"...CVS carries no increased risk for fetal loss or congenital malformation, including limb reduction defect ..." compared to conventional mid-trimester amniocentesis.

In summary, CVS is the only established method for first trimester prenatal diagnosis and carries minimal, if any increased risk for adverse pregnancy outcomes when performed by experienced operators. To maximize the safety of CVS, we avoid performing CVS before 10 weeks gestation except in cases of profound risk for fetal abnormalities (e.g., fetal hydrops). We continue to counsel patients about the LRD controversy and inform them that the absolute risk at 10 to 12 weeks is believed to be very low, approximately one in 2000, a rate similar to that observed in the general population (WHO/PAHO 1999). We also stress that this issue be placed in proper perspective and weighed against the substantial advantages that CVS offers first trimester prenatal diagnosis.

Fetal blood sampling

Access to the fetal circulation was initially accomplished by fetoscopy, a method of directly visualizing the fetus, umbilical cord, and chorionic surface of the placenta, using endoscopic instruments (Hobbins and Mahoney, 1974; Elias, 1980). Fetoscopy for this purpose has now been replaced by ultrasound-directed percutaneous umbilical blood sampling (PUBS), also termed cordocentesis or funipuncture.

Fetal blood chromosome analysis has been used to help clarify purported chromosome mosaicism detected in cultured amniotic fluid cells (Gosden et al., 1988) or chorionic villi. Rapid assessment of fetal chromosome complement has been accomplished by "direct" cytogenetic analysis of uncultured nucleated blood cells (Tipton et al., 1990). Short-term fetal lymphocyte cultures can provide a cytogenetic result within 72 hours; direct analysis of spontaneously dividing fetal cells (probably nucleated red blood cells) can provide a karyotype result within 24 hours. This proves particularly useful for patients presenting late in the second trimester, when results from amniocentesis would be available only after pregnancy termination would no longer be available. Also, in cases of fetal structural abnormalities or intrauterine growth retardation (IUGR) presenting in the third trimester, rapid results may prove useful for decision making concerning the mode of delivery (Porreco et al., 1993; Liou et al., 1993a). More recently, fluorescent in situ hybridization (FISH) with chromosome-specific DNA probes has also been used for rapid prenatal diagnosis of aneuploidy using nucleated fetal blood cells from umbilical cord blood, as well as amniotic fluid cells (Bryndorf et al., 2000).

Fetal blood sampling is used in the prenatal evaluation of many fetal hematological abnormalities (Ryan and Rodeck, 1993). Daffos (1989) reported normal hematological values for second-trimester fetuses, and Forestier and colleagues (1987, 1988) reported normal blood chemistry values for second-trimester fetuses. Fetal blood hematocrit can be directly measured to assess hemolysis resulting from Rh or other blood antigen isoimmunization states (Nicolaides et al., 1987). Before this, obstetricians had to rely on indirect evidence of fetal hemolysis, such as maternal antibody titers, past obstetric history, ultrasound findings, and spectrophotometry of bilirubin in amniotic fluid; the need for subsequent transfusions was based on somewhat arbitrary guidelines. Now the decisions about who, when, how much, and how often to transfuse can be made more rationally on the basis of actual fetal blood analyses such as hemoglobin level, hematocrit level, blood group, direct antibody titer, and reticulocyte count. Fetal hemoglobin can be directly evaluated to diagnose sickle cell disease, α- or β-thalassemia or other hemoglobinopathies (Hobbins and Mahoney, 1974), although these disorders are now usually diagnosed by DNA analysis of chorionic villi or amniotic fluid cells. Fetal blood sampling can be used to assess both the quantity of platelets and the quality of function (Donnenfeld et al., 1990). The maternal PLA2 (platelet antigen) alloimmunization PUBS is not only useful for diagnosis, but access to the fetal circulation also allows therapeutic alternatives including in utero platelet transfusion or maternal immunotherapy with gamma-globulin or steroids (Bussel et al., 1988).

Fetal blood has been used for the diagnosis of blood factor abnormalities such as hemophilia A, hemophilia B, or von Willebrand disease (Forestier et al., 1988; Weiner et al., 1989). In addition to hematologic studies, fetal blood samples can be used to diagnose autosomal-recessive or X-linked immunologic deficiencies, including severe combined immunodeficiency (SCID), Chédiak–Higashi syndrome, Wiskott–Aldrich syndrome, and chronic granulomatous disease (Durandy et al., 1982; Holmberg et al., 1983; Diukman et al., 1992).

Recovery of fetal blood permits assessment of viral, bacterial, or parasitic infections of the fetus. Detection of fetal viral or parasitic infection is usually made on the basis of maternal antibody titers or ultrasound-detected fetal structural abnormalities. Serum studies of fetal blood allows for quantification of antibody titers (Daffos et al., 1988; Rodeck and Nicolini, 1988). In addition to antibody studies, PUBS can be used for direct analysis of viral, bacterial, and parasitic infections by culture of fetal blood (Daffos et al., 1988; Hsieh et al., 1989; Peters and Nicolaides, 1990).

Although many of the indications for detecting fetal abnormalities that previously required fetal blood sampling are now performed by amniocentesis or CVS using DNA analysis (Newton 1999; Robert-Gangneux et al., 1999; Bryndorf et al., 2000), the continuing value of fetal blood sampling lies not only with those few remaining diagnostic indications, but also providing the potential for drug therapy. For example, fetal arrhythmias have been treated with direct administration of antiarrhythmic medications and fetal paralysis may be induced to facilitate invasive procedures such as fetal transfusions or for magnetic resonance imaging (MRI) (Moise et al., 1989).

TECHNIQUE

Today the technique most commonly used for fetal blood sampling is ultrasound-directed PUBS. The procedure can be safely undertaken from 18 weeks onward, although successful procedures have been reported as early as 12 weeks (Orlandi et al., 1987; 1990).

PUBS can be performed as an outpatient procedure. Maternal sedation is usually unnecessary, but oral benzodiazepine one or two hours before the procedure may be of benefit to the anxious patient and usually results in a transient decrease in fetal movement that can facilitate the procedure. A preliminary ultrasonographic examination of the fetus is performed to assess fetal viability, placental and umbilical cord location, fetal or placental anomalies, and fetal position. A suitable site for needle insertion is then selected; the skin over this site is anesthetized with 5 ml of 1% xylocaine. A sterile field is established; the skin is cleansed with an iodine-based solution and sterile drapes applied. The ultrasound transducer is placed on the abdomen away from the sterile insertion site, but at a location that permits visualization of the complete path of the needle from skin to fetal blood vessel.

There are several potential sampling sites. Owing to its fixed position, the placental cord root is usually the site of choice whenever it is clearly visible. Alternatively, free loops of cord or the intrahepatic vein are possibilities (Nicolini et al., 1990; Nicolaidis et al., 1991; Ryan and Rodeck, 1993).

Following percutaneous insertion of the spinal needle into the fetal blood vessel under direct ultrasound guidance, a small amount of blood is aspirated. The presence of fetal blood in this initial sample is confirmed using a model ZBI Coulter counter and channelizer to differentiate fetal from maternal blood on the basis of erythrocyte volume.

The amount of blood aspirated for diagnosis depends on the indication for PUBS; rarely is more than 5 ml required.

Upon completion of the fetal blood sampling, the spinal needle is withdrawn and an ultrasound examination is performed to evaluate fetal status. The woman and her fetus are monitored for about 1 hour following PUBS. At our centers, all women at risk of Rh isoimmunization receive 300 μg of Rh immune globulin following the procedure.

SAFETY

Fetal blood sampling appears to be a relatively safe procedure when performed by experienced physicians, albeit carrying more risk than CVS or amniocentesis. Maternal complications are rare but include amnionitis and transplacental hemorrhage (Weiner et al., 1989; Nicolini et al., 1988). Data from large perinatal centers estimate the risk of in utero death or spontaneous abortion to be 3% or less following PUBS (Weiner, 1987; Rodeck and Nicolini, 1988; Daffos, 1989; Hsieh et al., 1989; Ghidini et al., 1993; Wilson et al., 1994; Buscaglia et al., 1996). Collaborative data from 14 North American centers, sampling 1600 patients at varying gestational ages and for a variety of indications, revealed an uncorrected fetal loss rate of 1.6% (Nicolaides et al., 1990).

A more recent assessment of fetal blood sampling loss risk was performed by Antsaklis and colleagues (1998), who reviewed their clinical outcomes based on indication for fetal blood sampling. They divided their cohort into five main indication subgroups and found highly significant differences in procedure-related loss rates between the five groups. The highest loss rates were observed in the two groups characterized by fetal abnormalities and growth restriction, thus demonstrating that indication for fetal blood sampling has a major impact on risk for the procedure. Unfortunately, no studies directly comparing loss rates in control and treated groups have yet been published.

Fetal skin sampling

The prenatal diagnosis of severe hereditary skin diseases (genodermatoses) used to require fetal skin biopsy for ultrastructural or immunohistochemical analysis. Such genodermatoses that have been amenable to diagnosis by fetal skin sampling have included anhidrotic ectodermal dysplasia (Arnold et al., 1984), bullous congenital ichthyosiform dystrophia (epidermolytic hyperkeratosis) (Golbus et al., 1980; Anton-Lamprecht, 1983; Jurkovic and Kurjak, 1989), epi-

dermolysis bullosa dystrophia (Hallopean-Siemens) (Anton-Lamprecht et al., 1981), harlequin ichthyosis (Blanchet-Bardon et al., 1983; Elias et al., 1980c), hypohidrotic ectodermal dysplasia (Gilgenkrantz et al., 1989), epidermolysis bullosa lethalis (Rodeck et al., 1980; Elias et al., 1994), nonbullous ichthyosiform erythroderma (Perry et al., 1987), and Sjögren–Larsson syndrome (Kouseff et al., 1982).

Most of these conditions are now amenable to prenatal diagnosis by DNA analysis of chorionic villi or amniotic fluid cells (Shimizu and Suzumori, 1999). Indeed, one of the more common lethal genodermatoses, Herlitz junctional epidermolysis bullosa, is now amenable to prenatal diagnosis by DNA analysis (Christiano et al., 1997). However, the prenatal diagnosis of harlequin icthyosis still requires fetal skin sampling, although Akiyama and colleagues (1999) have reported that the diagnosis can now be made earlier than 21 to 22 weeks gestation.

On rare occasions, fetal skin sampling is still required and is best performed at 17 to 20 weeks gestation. The procedure was initially performed under direct visualization using fetoscopy, a procedure associated with a total fetal loss rate of 4% to 7% (Elias and Esterly, 1981; Golbus, 1984), or a procedure-related loss rate of perhaps 2%. From a safety standpoint, it seemed reasonable to assume that the smaller the caliber of the instrument introduced into the uterus, the safer the procedure. For this reason, we began to use ultrasound-directed biopsy forceps for fetal skin sampling in the 1980s (Fig. 29.6; Elias et al., 1994). We reported the clinical outcomes of 17 ultrasound-guided fetal skin sampling procedures (Elias et al., 1994). In five cases, a fetal skin disorder was diagnosed, and these pregnancies were terminated. In the remaining 12 cases, all infants were delivered without complications at 37 weeks gestation or later. Despite the use of biopsy forceps that take smaller fetal skin samples than the biopsy forceps used for fetoscopically directed fetal skin sampling, superficial scarring lesions have occasionally been noted.

Fetal muscle sampling

Prenatal diagnosis of Becker-Duchenne muscular dystrophy is usually possible by DNA analysis. However, in a few families, meiotic recombination or homozygosity of multiple restriction fragment length polymorphisms (RFLPs) precludes a DNA-based diagnosis (Evans et al., 1994; Nevo et al., 1999). In these cases, fetal muscle biopsies can be used for immunohistochemical analysis with a fluorescent

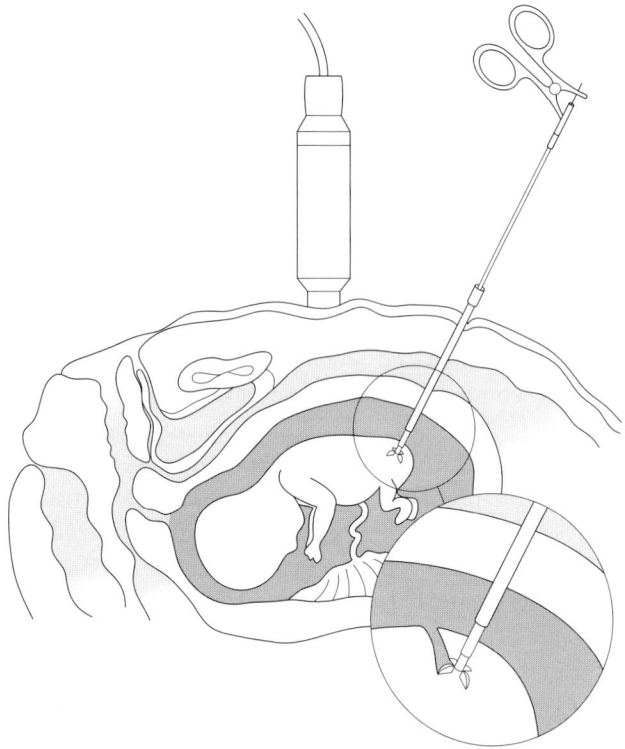

Fig. 29.6. Fetal skin sampling. (From Elias et al., 1994, with permission.)

antidystrophin antibody. Males with Duchenne muscular dystrophy lack dystrophin and with Becker muscular dystrophy lack or demonstrate a variable dystrophin pattern (Evans et al., 1995), whereas muscle biopsies from unaffected male fetuses show normal amounts of dystrophin.

Fetal muscle sampling is usually performed at around 18 weeks gestation using a technique analogous to fetal skin sampling or fetal liver sampling. Muscle biopsies are taken from the gluteal region by directing a Klear Kut (Baxter, Los Angeles, CA) kidney forceps gun toward the fetal buttock. As with fetal skin and liver biopsy procedures, only a small number of fetal muscle sampling procedures have been reported (Gustavii et al., 1983; Evans et al., 1991; 1994). Thus, statements cannot be made concerning the safety of this procedure.

Coelocentesis

Coelocentesis involves the transcervical or transabdominal aspiration of fluid from the extraembryonic coelom. This procedure has been suggested as a possible method for early first-trimester prenatal diagnosis. Jurkovic and colleagues (1989) were successful in aspirating fluid from 48 to 50 (96%) pregnancies between 6 and 10 weeks gestation.

Although the authors were unable to obtain metaphase analyses from these specimens, subsequent work by Cruger and colleagues (1996; 1997) demonstrated success in culturing and karyotyping. In addition, Makrydimas and colleagues (1997) reported successful prenatal detection of β-thalassemia by coelocentesis.

However, Ross and colleagues (1997) reported that short-term pregnancy loss rates associated with coelocentesis were markedly increased. In a comparative study of women undergoing pregnancy termination, 25% of women spontaneously aborted before their termination compared to 5% of women not undergoing coelocentesis ($p < 0.01$). These high loss rates suggest that coelocentesis may not be appropriate as a routine prenatal diagnostic test.

Of interest is the work of Santolaya-Forgas and colleagues. This group has investigated coelecentesis in baboons to determine its potential applicability for fetal therapy. In one series, coelocentesis was performed in 9 baboons; fluid aspiration (1 to 5 cc) was successful in eight cases and seven of the eight pregnancies were continuing 140 days after the procedure (Santolaya-Forgas et al., 1998a). Coelocentesis was subsequently performed in six other baboons; assessment of the extracoelomic fluid osmometry and electrolyte composition in these six samples found that the chorion laeve behaves as a semipermeable membrane at 40 days' gestation (Santolaya-Forgas et al., 1998b), suggesting that it may be useful for maternal-fetal transfer of some substances that could be used for fetal therapy.

Embryoscopy

Embryoscopy is a relatively new and investigational technique that permits direct visualization of the fetus as early as the first trimester (Reece 1992; 1997). Initially, a rigid fiberoptic endoscope was passed transcervically into the extracoelomic cavity, permitting inspection of fetal anatomic structures; fetal blood sampling was also feasible by this method (Reece, 1997). However, improvements and advancements in fiberoptic technology have led to the performance of thin-gauge transabdominal and transcervical embryoscopy (Qunitero et al., 1993), allowing visualization as early as 4 weeks after conception (Reece, 1999).

Initial procedures were performed only on women who had elected pregnancy termination; however, embryoscopy has since been performed on continuing pregnancies (Reece et al., 1997). Ville and colleagues reported a procedure-related loss rate of 12% when the procedure was performed in the first trimester.

Further studies of the safety, accuracy, and applications of this new modality will be needed before embryoscopy is used as a routine prenatal diagnostic tool. However, the ability to access the embryonic circulation may have important application for therapeutic interventions such as drug, gene and cell therapy.

Ultrasonography

Ultrasonography has been one of the most important advances in the practice of obstetrics. At intensities usually produced by diagnostic equipment, ultrasound has not been found to cause any harmful effects on operators, pregnant women, fetuses, or other patients (Stark et al., 1984; Lyons et al., 1988; American Institute of Ultrasound in Medicine, 1993). Indications for ultrasonography during pregnancy are multiple and diverse and include estimation of gestational age by biometric measurements, estimation of fetal growth, bleeding from the vagina, determination of fetal growth, suspected multiple gestation, adjunct to invasive procedure (e.g., CVS or amniocentesis), suspected uterine or adnexal abnormality, suspected fetal demise, and many others (ACOG 1993; 1997).

In the context of prenatal diagnosis, many major, and even some minor, fetal structural anomalies can be detected. It is unrealistic, however, to expect 100% accuracy in detecting fetal anomalies, even with the most expert and thorough scanning. Some anomalies are more readily diagnosed than others. For example, anencephaly and marked hydrocephaly are rarely misdiagnosed, whereas others are more difficult to diagnose and may be overlooked, such as heart defects, facial clefts, diaphragmatic hernias, skeletal abnormalities, and neural tube detects (ACOG 1993; 1997).

Although there is no question that high-resolution ultrasonography is invaluable in detecting fetal anomalies (Sabbagha, 1993; ACOG 1997), accuracy of diagnosis will vary depending on the experience of the sonographer, as well as on equipment, gestational age at time of scanning, and the a priori risk of the abnormality in question (Bernaschek et al., 1996; Dillon and Walton 1997; Queisser-Luft et al., 1998; VanDorsten et al., 1998). As such, the limitations of diagnostic ultrasonography must be recognized. For example, Platt et al., (1992) reviewed the ultrasound findings in 161 fetuses with spina bifida identified in the California MSAFP screening program. Before information regarding elevated MSAFP was made available to the examiner, in 13 of the 161 cases, spina bifida was not initially visualized. Subsequently,

the defect was found in 10 of the 13 fetuses; in the remaining three cases, amniocentesis was declined, and the spina bifida was only diagnosed at birth. In screening for fetal anomalies, data concerning the sensitivity, specificity, and predictive values of diagnostic ultrasound are usually not available (Philip, 1993). It is inappropriate for a given unit to make any claims about diagnostic accuracy unless they have analyzed their own experience.

Controversy persists as to whether ultrasound screening of all obstetric patients to allow prenatal diagnosis of structural birth defects should be routine. The rationale for such a policy would be to allow couples the option of pregnancy termination for lethal or severely handicapping disorders and possibly to improve the chances of survival for infants with life-threatening but treatable conditions by delivery in a tertiary center. These issues have been addressed in a report from the NICHD-sponsored Routine Antenatal Diagnostic Imaging with Ultrasound (RADIUS) study (Crane et al., 1994). Low-risk pregnant women with no indication for ultrasonography were randomly assigned to have either two screening sonograms (15 to 22 weeks and 31 to 35 weeks) or conventional obstetric care with ultrasonography used only on a selective basis as determined by the clinical judgement of the patient's physician. Major congenital anomalies occurred in 2.3% of the 15,281 fetuses and infants. Antenatal ultrasonography detected 35% of the anomalous fetuses in the screened group versus only 11% of the control population (relative detection rate 3.1; 95% CI 2.0 to 5.1). Surprisingly, ultrasonography did not significantly influence the management or outcome of pregnancies complicated by fetuses with congenital malformations. Moreover, ultrasonography screening had no significant impact on survival rates among infants with potentially treatable, life-threatening anomalies despite the opportunity to take precautionary measures such as delivery at a tertiary center. The RADIUS study also provided some insight into the content and limitations of obstetric ultrasound examinations. For example, a four-chamber view of the heart permitted detection of only 43% of fetuses with complex heart disease, and only 30% of fetuses with cleft lip and palate were detected. Finally, it was estimated that a public health policy of routine ultrasonographic screening would increase US health care costs by at least $500 million. This study concluded that "given this extraordinary cost and the lack of measurable benefit, ultrasonographic screening for fetal anomaly detection cannot be justified".

Nonetheless, many groups and centers have reevaluated the RADIUS findings as well as their own experience and have come to the opposite conclusion. DeVore (1994) reported that the RADIUS study demonstrated that second-trimester ultrasonography could be provided in a cost-effective fashion to low-risk women. Skupski and colleagues (1996) reported on their experience with ultrasound in a low-risk population and found that the detection of major and minor malformations had a profoundly positive impact. The Eurofetus Study (Grandjean et al., 1999) combined the ultrasound and clinical outcomes of 61 European centers over a three-year period and found that systematic ultrasound pregnancy detected a large proportion of fetal malformations. Providing ultrasonographic services to all women regardless of risk will continue to be a contentious issue.

New applications of ultrasound may have a considerable impact on our ability to provide prenatal diagnosis. Work in the early 1990s showed that first-trimester ultrasonography could be used to detect fetuses at increased risk for fetal chromosome abnormalities (van Zalen-Sprock et al., 1991; Nicolaides et al., 1992; Shulman et al., 1993). However, further work showed that ultrasound screening, specifically the measurement of the nuchal translucency (Fig. 29.7) could be applied to the screening of high- and low-risk women for fetal chromosome and structural abnormalities (Nicolaides et al., 1992; 1994; Hafner et al., 1998; Snijders et al., 1998). Similar to second-trimester ultrasonography, operator, gestational and mechanical factors can alter diagnostic ultrasonographic outcomes (D'Ottavio et al., 1998; Haddow et al., 1998). The measurement of certain maternal serum markers, including free β-hCG, PAPP-A, AFP, hCG and unconjugated estriol in various combinations, has been shown to provide an adequate, though not optimal, first-trimester screening protocol for fetal Down syndrome (Haddow et al., 1998; Canick and Kellner, 1999).

However, when first-trimester maternal serum marker screening is combined with ultrasonography, the overall sensitivity and specificity of aneuploidy screening has been shown to improve (Benattar, 1999; De Basio et al., 1999). Two multicenter trials are currently underway in the United States that will prospectively assess the efficacy and feasibility of combining ultrasonographic measurement of nuchal translucency and maternal serum markers for first-trimester aneuploidy and structural abnormality screening.

The other new application of ultrasound that may have a considerable effect on prenatal diagnosis is three-dimensional ultrasonography. This investigational technology has been introduced for use in selected centers for only the past two to three years. Reports from individual centers have demonstrated the potential positive impact of three-dimensional ultrasonography on the ability to detect major and minor malformations in all the trimesters of pregnancy (Hata et al., 1998a; Platt et al., 1998), especially with regard to the fetal face (Hata et al., 1998b), heart (Sklansky et al., 1999) and skeleton (Yanagihara and Hata, 2000). Although three-dimensional ultrasonography shows promise in improving our ability to prenatally diagnose fetal abnormalities, further and considerable study will be needed to not only assess the sensitivity and specificity of this technology, but also the feasibility and cost-effectiveness of using this diagnostic tool in high-and low-risk populations.

Isolating fetal cells and DNA from maternal blood

Isolation and analysis of fetal cells in maternal blood now genuinely seem practical (Simpson and Elias, 1994c; Elias and Simpson, 1994b; Elias and Simpson, 1995; Lewis et al., 1996; Bianchi, 1999). Although not yet standard like the diagnostic and screening approaches reviewed above, this is an attractive new approach to noninvasive prenatal screening and diagnosis.

HISTORICAL OVERVIEW

This idea has been considered seriously since Walknowska et al., (1969) found XY metaphases in maternal blood of pregnant women carrying male fetuses. De Grouchy and Trubuchet (1971) also reported male metaphases from pregnant women carrying male fetuses, and other groups followed (Schindler et al., 1972; Takahara et al., 1972; Whang-Peng et al., 1973). Relatively high proportions of fetal cells to maternal cells were claimed, approximately 0.1 to 0.3%. However, several problems were evident. First, not all individuals carrying male fetuses showed XY metaphases, usually explained on the basis that fetal cells are rare events in maternal blood. Second, XY metaphases were also present in some women carrying female fetuses, perhaps explained by the establishment of clones of fetal cells in the

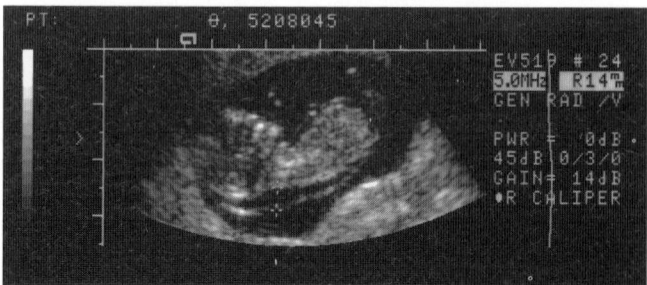

Fig. 29.7. Prominent nuchal translucency (3.9 mm between asterisks) measured in fetus at 10.8 weeks gestation. Fetus found to have 47,XY,+21 complement by CVS.

mother's bone marrow during prior pregnancies. However, the consensus gradually arose that the XY metaphases probably represented cytogenetic misclassifications and the ostensible "Y-chromatin" cells reflected autosomal fluorescence (Sargent et al., 1994).

During the late 1970s, Herzenberg and colleagues applied flow sorting technology to enrich for fetal cells (Herzenberg et al., 1979; Iverson et al., 1981). Their experimental design used HLA-A2-negative women who had an HLA-A2-positive spouse (heterozygote or homozygote). Any A2-positive cells recovered by flow sorting presumably must be fetal in origin, that antigen having been inherited from the father. Analogous to earlier disappointment with karyotyping and initial promise of flow sorting technology had by the mid-1980s proved disappointing to most.

Interest in the hypothesis was rekindled by application of molecular technology. Lo et al., (1989, 1990) showed that fetal cells, or at least fetal DNA, indeed existed in maternal blood. Sensitivity required to make such a statement was achieved by using nested primer polymerase chain reaction (PCR) to amplify for Y sequences. Women carrying a male fetus proved far more likely to show a Y-specific signal than those carrying a female fetus. The original work of Lo et al., (1989; 1990) was performed on unsorted nucleated cells; later our own group (Wachtel et al., 1991) and many others confirmed these results with various separation schemes on sorted and unsorted cells (Bianchi et al., 1990; Mueller et al., 1990; Kao et al., 1992).

FETAL CELLS

Diagnosis of chromosomal abnormalities currently requires fetal interphase cell analysis by FISH with chromosome-specific probes. One must first enrich for the rare fetal cells by targeting a specific cell type. Candidate fetal cell types are trophoblasts, lymphocytes, granulocytes and nucleated red blood cell. Despite some success with all the aforementioned cell types, much of the current work involves evaluation of the nucleated fetal red cell (erythroblast) in the maternal circulation. The fetal nucleated red cell is an attractive candidate because nucleated red blood cells (NRBCs) comprise about 10% of red cells in the 11-week fetus and 0.5% in the 19-week fetus. Nucleated red blood cells do not persist longer than perhaps five days in the adult, and are rare in peripheral adult blood.

Bianchi and co-workers (1990) were the first to focus on NRBCs, flow-sorting for transferrin receptor (CD71) expression and examining by PCR for a Y sequence. After enrichment, Y sequences were found in six of eight pregnancies in which women were carrying male fetuses. Our group was later successful when sorting not only for CD71 but also for cell size, cell granularity and glycophorin-A positivity (Price et al., 1991; Wachtel et al., 1991).

Our group later became the first to detect fetal aneuploidy by maternal blood analysis. Analyzing interphase cells by fluorescent in situ hybridization (FISH) with chromosome-specific probes, we detected trisomy 18 (Price et al., 1991) and trisomy 21 (Elias et al., 1992). By 1993, our experience with 69 maternal blood samples (Simpson and Elias, 1993; Elias and Simpson, 1994a; Simpson and Elias, 1994c) had proved promising, with no false-positive results.

Using an avidin-biotin-based immunoaffinity system, Hall and Williams (1992) estimated that the ratio of fetal nucleated cells to maternal nucleated cells was $1:4.75 \times 10^6$ to 1.6×10^7. Hamada et al., (1993) estimated the ratio of fetal nucleated cells to maternal nucleated cells by performing FISH on unsorted maternal blood using a DNA probe specific for the repetitive Y-DNA sequence DYZ1. Frequencies in successive trimesters were 0.27, 3.52 and 8.56×10^5, respectively. The authors' estimate is $1:1 \times 10^7$ or $1:1 \times 10^8$, based on flow cytometry data. Using quantitative PCR, Bianchi et al., (1997) estimated that a 16 cc maternal blood sample contains perhaps 19 fetal cells. ("DNA equivalents").

Rarity of fetal cells in maternal blood means that detecting aneuploidies requires enrichment for these rare cells. To accomplish this, one utilizes density gradients or protein separation techniques, followed by either flow cytometry (Lewis et al., 1996), or magnetic-activated cell sorting (MACS) (Ganshirt et al., 1994). Flow cytometry has proved most useful in our hands, but the technology is more expensive than MACS (Simpson and Elias, 1995). Wang et al. (2000) compared FACS and MACS and concluded that both techniques have benefits and limitations. FACS had the advantage of higher fetal cell yields, higher purity, higher FISH efficiency and ease in microscope analysis. MACS had the advantage of higher specificity and less cell loss during FISH.

The exception to the consensus reflected above is the work of Wachtel and colleagues, who believe that fetal cells in maternal blood occur more frequently. Their conclusions are based on use of an enrichment technique called charged flow separation. Their approach is said to recover many more fetal cells. At least some of these cells are fetal, and Wachtel's group states that 30% of NRBC in maternal blood are fetal (Wachtel et al., 1998). The group has studied a large sample (225 samples) in a study showing no relationship with recovery of nucleated red blood cells to gestational age (Shulman et al., 1998). However, in very few samples was FISH with chromosome-specific probes studied.

Using nested primer polymerase chain reaction (PCR) for Y-specific DNA, signals can be detected early in pregnancy in the peripheral blood of pregnant women carrying male fetuses. Y-specific signals were detected in 33 and 40 days gestation by Thomas and colleagues (1994). By 6 weeks gestation 18 of 18 pregnancies having a male fetus showed a Y-specific signal in maternal blood. Liou and co-workers (1993b; 1994) found Y sequences indicative of male fetal cells in 19 of 19 pregnancies by 10 to 11 weeks.

A major concern is that fetal cells from a prior pregnancy could persist in the maternal circulation and, hence, lead to diagnostic error. This would especially be troublesome if aneuploid cells were to persist after a chromosomally abnormal live born offspring or spontaneous abortion. It appears that fetal cells disappear after delivery in large part but not completely. One week after gestation, 26 of 28 women delivering males showed XFY and SRY sequences in their blood (Hsieh et al., 1993). By 4 months, only 2 of 23 did. Others have had similar experience, including our group (Elias et al., 1996).

Lo et al., (1999) followed eight women delivered of male fetuses postpartum, obtaining serial blood samples for analysis of Y sequences in maternal *plasma*. All eight women showed fetal DNA sequences, but amounts of fetal DNA fell rapidly postpartum. By two hours levels were undetectable in most women. The mean half-life for circulating DNA was 16.3 minutes.

Bianchi and colleagues (1996) clarified some of the ostensible contradiction by showing that the fetal cells persisting from prior pregnancies are indeed detectable, but not using the same selection criteria employed to isolate cells for prenatal diagnosis. Positive selection for persisting clones is achieved not with CD71 (see below), but by CD38 and CD34. By choosing appropriate selection criteria, clones of fetal cells established in prior pregnancies should not interfere with diagnosis.

Other issues of concern are whether a woman's blood type or Rh status influences the detection of fetal cells in maternal blood. In a study of 1052 women with a mean maternal age of 36.2 years who were carrying male fetuses at a mean gestational age of 14.0 weeks, Elias et al. (2000) found no differences in the cases with any Y signals by FISH by maternal ABO and Rh status. Similarly, maternal race appears to have no effect on fetal cell recovery (Evans et al., 2000).

DETECTING FETAL ABNORMALITIES

In determining the accuracy of detecting chromosomal abnormalities in fetal blood, the initial approach was calcu-

lating the number of pregnancies in which male (XY cells) were correctly detected. However, it seems likely from both clinical evaluation (Price et al., 1991; Simpson and Elias, 1993) as well as quantitative PCR studies (Bianchi et al., 1997) that severalfold more fetal cells are present in the maternal blood in aneuploid pregnancies than in euploid pregnancies. Not all agree with these statements but their supporting data to the contrary are based only on morphologic criteria (NRBCs). Since maternal erythroblasts also increase during pregnancy, we believe studies should utilize FISH with chromosome-specific probes as an unequivocal fetal marker (Fig. 29.8).

In the United States collaborative study funded by the National Institute of Child Health and Human Development, the outcome assessed is numbers of pregnancies in which fetal trisomies are detected per numbers of pregnancies in which fetal trisomies exists. The current detection estimates at least 40% from an ongoing NICHD collaborative study is that of autosomal aneuploidies (trisomy 13,21 and 18) and 50% of sex chromosomal abnormalities can be detected by fetal cell analysis (Elias and Simpson, 1995). Usually 1 to 3 trisomic (and, hence fetal cells) are detected per 20–30 cc specimens. Given that it is believed 1 cc of maternal blood contains a single fetal cell, many fetal cells are being lost. Improved sensitivity would be expected with increased fetal cell recovery and especially better selection criteria.

The rarity of fetal cells in maternal blood could be overcome by fetal cell culture, which if successful could obviously increase the absolute number of fetal cells present. Since maternal stem cells are also present in any given maternal blood samples, techniques designed to stimulate

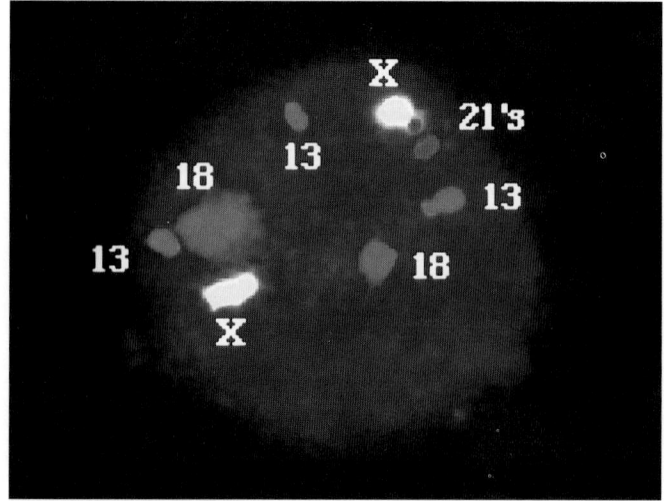

Fig. 29.8. Five color FISH analysis of fetal cell obtained from maternal circulation. Fetus with 47,XX,+13 complement. (See Plate 29.8.)

fetal cells differentially would be desirable. Several groups have reported the successful fetal cells in culture (Lo et al., 1994; Valerio et al., 1996, 1997a,b; Little et al., 1997; Han et al., 1999). However, questions on the reliability of this approach have been raised because of failure to detect fetal specific sequences after culture of maternal blood.

Unlike fetal chromosome abnormalities, detection of fetal mendelian disorders by analysis of fetal cells does not necessarily require enrichment. PCR-based technology alone may suffice, since the DNA may be derived from any type of fetal cell and may represent the detection of an allele different from the maternal complement.

Determining fetal sex is obviously useful in couples at risk for X-linked recessive traits, and can be performed readily. Nested primer analysis for Y-DNA sequences was used initially by Lo et al., (1989; 1990) to establish that fetal cell exist in maternal blood. As already noted, detection rates for fetal sex is approximately 100% by the end of the first trimester (Liou et al., 1993a,b;1994). Primer extension in *situ* techniques can also be employed to detect fetal Y-DNA sequences (Orsetti et al., 1998).

The principle of detecting mendelian disorder by analysis of DNA of the fetal cells present in maternal blood was first shown by Camaschella et al., (1990). DNA was obtained from maternal blood of three pregnancies at risk for α-thalassemia/hemoglobin Lepore$_{Boston}$. Camaschella et al., (1990) used PCR to amplify for hemoglobin Lepore$_{Boston}$-specific DNA in unsorted maternal blood of women whose male partners carried the Lepore$_{Boston}$ mutation. The mutation was correctly identified in two fetuses, and excluded in a third.

Another circumstance permitting detection of a mendelian disorder through analysis of fetal cells in maternal blood arises when the father is heterozygous (Aa) and the mother homozygous (aa) for the autosomal recessive trait. The normal allele, which may or may not be transmitted by the heterozygous father, should be readily detectable. If blood from the homozygous mother reveals DNA of the normal paternal allele (A), the fetus could be deduced as heterozygous. The diagnosis of fetal rhesus (D) by PCR of maternal blood represents such a clinical paradigm. The molecular basis of Rh(D) negative (dd) is usually a gene deletion; "d" representing lack of the DNA sequence that if present encodes "D". RhD isoimmunization occurs only if the mother is Rh negative and the father is homozygous or heterozygous for Rh(D) (Rh positive). If the father is heterozygous, the likelihood is 50% that the fetus would inherit his RhD gene and, hence, be at risk for being affected; the other 50% of pregnancies would not be at risk for Rh-isoimmunization. Nested primers can be constructed such that the CE sequence is concurrently amplified, allowing an "internal control" that assures lack of qualification of D is not the result of primers failing to anneal or absence of cellular DNA in the sample tested. The largest study is that of Lo et al., (1998a) who studied 57 RhD negative women throughout pregnancy. All RhD positive fetuses in the second and third trimester were correctly identified, whereas 10 of 12 in the first trimester were correctly identified.

Until now the discussion has implied that fetal DNA that is to be analyzed is present in the nucleus. Actually, cell-free DNA is also present in maternal plasma and serum (Lo et al., 1997; 1998b). Work on rapid clearance of fetal DNA immediately postpartum involves maternal plasma (Lo et al., 1999). Lo used maternal plasma to derive the data cited on detecting fetal Rh status, and we have shown Rh(D) DNA in maternal serum of Rh negative women (dd) carrying heterozygous (Dd) fetuses (Bischoff et al., 1999).

REFERENCES

Adkison LR, Andrews RH, Vowell NL, Koontz WL (1994) Improved detection of fetal cells from maternal blood with polymerase chain reaction. Am J Obstet Gynecol 170:952–955

Akiyama M, Suzumori K, Shimizu H (1999) Prenatal diagnosis of harlequin icthyosis by the examination of keratinized hair canals and amniotic fluid cells at 19 weeks' estimated gestational age. Prenat Diagn 19:167

American College of Obstetricians and Gynecologists (1993) ACOG Technical Bulletin No. 187. Ultrasonography in Pregnancy. ACOG, Washington, DC

American College of Obstetricians and Gynecologists (1997) ACOG Practice Patterns No. 5: Routine ultrasound in low-risk pregnancy. ACOG, Washington, DC

American College of Obstetricians and Gynecologists (1999) ACOG Practice Bulletin No. 4. Prevention of Rh D Alloimmunization. ACOG, Washington, DC

American Institute of Ultrasound in Medicine (1993) Bioeffects and Safety of diagnostic ultrasound. AIUM, Rockville, MD

Anderson RL, Goldberg JD (1991) Prenatal diagnosis in multiple gestations: 20 years' experience with amniocentesis. Prenatal Diagn 11:263

Anton-Lamprecht I (1983) Genetically induced abnormalities of epidermal differentiation and ultra-structure in ichthyoses and epidermolyses: Pathogenesis, heterogeneity, fetal manifestation and prenatal diagnosis. J Invest Dermatol 81:149S

Anton-Lamprecht I, Ruskolb R, Jovanovic V et al. (1981) Prenatal diagnosis of epidermolysis bullosa dystrophica Hallopean-Siemens with electron microscopy of fetal skin. Lancet 2:1077

Antsaklis A, Daskalakis G, Papantoniou N, Michalas S (1998). Fetal blood sampling – indication-related losses. Prenat Diagn 18:934

Arnold ML, Rauskolb R, Anton-Lamprecht I et al. (1984) Prenatal diagnosis of anhidrotic ectodermal dysplasia. Prenat Diagn 4:85

Assel BG, Lewis SM, Mickerman LH et al. (1992) Single-operator comparison of early and midsecond trimester amniocentesis. Obstet Gynecol 79:940

Bahado-Singh R, Schmitt R, Hobbins JC (1992) New technique for genetic amniocentesis in twins. Obstet Gynecol 79:304

Baird PA, Yee IML, Sadnovnick AD (1994) Population-based study of long-term outcomes after amniocentesis. Lancet 334:1134

Benacerraf B, Green MF, Saltzman DH et al. (1988) Early amniocentesis for prenatal cytogenetic evaluation. Radiology 169:709

Benattar C, Audibert F, Taieb J et al. (1999) Efficiency of ultrasound and biochemical markers for Down's syndrome risk screening. A prospective study. Fetal Diagn Ther 14:112

Benirschke K (1994) Anatomical relationship between fetus and mother. In Simpson JL, Elias S (eds): Fetal Cells in Maternal Blood Prospects for Noninvasive Prenatal Diagnosis. Proc NY Acad Sci 731:9–20

Bernaschek G, Stuempflen I, Deutinger J (1996) The influence of the experience of the investigator on the rate of sonographic diagnosis of fetal malformations in Vienna. Prenat Diagn 16:807

Bianchi DW (1999) Fetal cells in the maternal circulation: Feasibility for prenatal diagnosis. Br J Haemotol 105:574

Bianchi DW, Flint AF, Pizzimenti MF et al. (1990) Isolation of fetal DNA from nucleated erythrocytes in maternal blood. Proc Natl Acad Sci USA 87:3279–3283

Bianchi DW, Klinger KW (1992) Prenatal diagnosis through the analysis of fetal cells in the maternal circulation. p. 759. In Milunsky A (ed): Genetic Disorders and the Fetus. 3rd edn. Johns Hopkins University Press, Baltimore

Bianchi DW, Zickwolf GK, Weil GJ et al. (1996) Male fetal progenitor cells persist in maternal blood for as long as 27 years postpartum. Proc Natl Acad Sci USA 93:705

Bianchi DW, Williams JM, Sullivan LM et al. (1997) PCR quantitation of fetal cells in maternal blood in normal and aneuploid pregnancies. Am J Hum Genet 61:822

Bischoff FZ, Nguyen DD, Marquez D-O et al. (1999) Noninvasive determination of fetal RhD status using fetal DNA in maternal serum. J Soc Gynecol Invest 6:64

Blanchet-Bardon C, Dumez Y, Labée F et al. (1983) Prenatal diagnosis of harlequin fetus, letter. Lancet 1:132

Bowman JM, Chown B, Pollock JM (1978) Rh isoimmunization during pregnancy: antenatal prophylaxis. Can Med Assoc J 118:623

Brambati B, Lanzani A, Tului L (1990) Transabdominal and transcervical chorionic villus sampling: Efficiency and risk evaluation of 2,411 cases. Am J Med Genet 35:160

Brambati B, Tului L, Baldi M et al. (1995) Genetic analysis prior to selective fetal reduction in multiple pregnancy: Technical aspects and clinical outcomes. Hum Reprod 10:818

Bravo RR, Shulman LP, Phillips OP et al. (1995) Transplacental needle passage in early amniocentesis and pregnancy loss. Obstet Gynecol 86:437

Bruch JF, Metezeau D, Garcia-Fonknechten N et al. (1991) Trophoblast-like cells sorted from peripheral maternal blood using flow cytometry: a multiparametric study involving transmission electron microscopy and fetal amplification. Prenat Diagn 11:787–798

Bryndorf T, Lundsteen C, Lamb A et al. (2000) Rapid prenatal diagnosis of chromosome aneuploidies by interphase in situ hybridization: a one-year clinical experience with high-risk and urgent fetal and postnatal samples. Acta Obstet Gynecol Scand 79:8

Burton BK, Schulz CJ, Burd L (1992) Limb anomalies associated with chorionic villus sampling. Obstet Gynecol 79:726

Buscaglia M, Ghisoni L, Belloti M et al. (1995) Genetic amniocentesis in biamniotic twin pregnancies by a single transabdominal insertion of the needle. Prenat Diagn 15:17

Buscaglia M, Ghisoni L, Belloti M et al. (1996) Percutaneous umbilical blood sampling: Indication changes and procedure loss rates in a nine years' experience. Fetal Diagn Ther 11:106–113

Bussel JB, Berkowitz RL, McFarland JG et al. (1988) Antenatal treatment of neonatal alloimmune thrombocytopenia. N Engl J Med 319:1374

Camaschella C, Alfarno A, Gottardi E et al. (1990) Prenatal diagnosis of fetal haemoglobin Lepore Boston disease on maternal peripheral blood. Blood 75:2102–2106

Canadian Collaborative CVS—Amniocentesis Clinical Trial Group (1991) Multicentre randomized clinical trial of chorion villus sampling. Lancet 337:1491

Canick JA, Kellner LH (1999) First trimester screening for aneuploidy: serum biochemical markers. Semin Perinatol 23:359

CEMAT Group (1998) Randomised trial to assess safety and fetal outcome of early and midtrimester amniocentesis. The Canadian early and mid-trimester amniocentesis trial (CEMAT) Group. Lancet 351:242

Christiano AM, Pulkkinen L, McGrath JA, Uitto J (1997) Mutation-based prenatal diagnosis of Herlitz junctional epidermolysis bullosa. Prenat Diagn 17:343

Crandall BF, Hanson FW, Tennant F (1989) Acetylcholinesterase (AChE) electrophoresis and early amniocenteses. Am J Hum Genet 45:A257

Crane JP, LeFevre ML, Winborn RC (1994) A randomized trial of prenatal ultrasonographic screening: Impact on the detection, management, and outcome of anomalous fetuses. Am J Obstet Gynecol 171:392–399

Cruger DG, Bruun-Petersen G, Kolvraa S (1996) Early prenatal diagnosis: Standard cytogenetic analysis of coelomic cells obtained by coelocentesis. Prenat Diagn 16:945

Cruger DG, Bruun-Petersen G, Kolvraa S (1997) Turner's syndrome 45,X found by coelocentesis (letter). Prenat Diagn 17:588

Daffos F (1989) Fetal blood sampling. Annu Rev Med 40:319

Daffos F, Forestier F, Capella-Pavlovsky M et al. (1988) Prenatal management of 746 pregnancies at risk for congenital toxoplasmosis. N Engl J Med 318:271

De Biasio P, Siccardi M, Volpe G et al. (1999) First-trimester screening for down syndrome using nuchal translucency measurement with free beta-hCG and PAPP-A between 10 and 13 weeks of pregnancy—the combined test. Prenat Diagn 19:360

De Catte L, Camus M, Bonduelle M et al. (1998) Prenatal diagnosis by chorionic villus sampling in multiple pregnancies prior to fetal reduction. Am J Perinatol 15:339

deGrouchy J, Trubuchet C (1971) Transfusion foeto-maternelle de lymphocytes sanguins et detection du sexe du foetus. Ann Genet 14:133–137

de la Cruz F, Shifrin H, Elias S (1995) Prenatal diagnosis by use of fetal cells isolated from maternal blood. Am J Obstet Gynecol 173:1354–1355

DeVore GR (1994) The routine antenatal diagnostic imaging with Ultrasound Study: Another perspective. Obstet Gynecol 84:622

Dillon E, Walton SM (1997) The antenatal diagnosis of fetal abnormalities: A 10 year audit of influencing factors. Br J Radiol 70:341

Diukman R, Tanigawara S, Cowan MJ, Golbus MS (1992) Prenatal diagnosis of Chediak-Higashi syndrome. Prenat Diagn 12:1877–1885

Djalali M, Barbi G, Kennerknecht I, Terinde R (1992) Introduction of early amniocentesis to routine prenatal diagnosis. Prenat Diagn 12:661

Dolk H, Beatrand F, Lechat MF (Eurocat) (1992) Chorionic villus sampling and limb abnormalities. Lancet 339:876–877

Donnenfeld AE, Wiseman B, Lavi E et al. (1990) Prenatal diagnosis of thrombocytopenia absent radius syndrome by ultrasound and cordocentesis. Prenat Diagn 10:29

D'Ottavio G, Mandruzzato G, Meir YJ et al. (1998) Comparisons of first and second trimester screening for fetal anomalies. Ann N Y Acad Sci 847:200

Durandy A, Dumez Y, Guy-Grand D et al. (1982) Prenatal diagnosis of severe combined immunodeficiency. J Pediatr 101:995

Eiben B, Goebel R, Rutt G et al. (1993) Early amniocentesis between 12th-14th week of pregnancy. Clinical experience with 1,100 cases. Geburtshilfe Frauenheilkd 53:554

Elejalde BR, de Elejalde MM, Acuña JB (1990) Prospective study of amniocentesis performed between weeks 9 and 16 of gestation: Its feasibility, risks, complications and use in early genetic prenatal diagnosis. Am J Med Genet 35:188

Elias S for the National Institute of Child Health and Human Development Fetal Cell Study (NIFTY) Group (2000). Does a pregnant woman's blood type and/or Rh status influence the detection of Y signals in women carrying male fetuses? Presented at the Society of Gynecologic Investigation, Chicago, Illinois, March 2000

Elias S (1980b) The role of fetoscopy in antenatal diagnosis. Clin Obstet Gynaecol 7:73

Elias S, Esterly NB (1981) Prenatal diagnosis of hereditary skin disorders. Clinical Obstetrics and Gynecology 24:1069–87

Elias S, Simpson JL (1994a) Prenatal diagnosis of aneuploidy using fetal cells isolated from maternal blood: University of Tennessee, Memphis experience. In Simpson JL, Elias S (eds): Fetal Cells in Maternal Blood: Prospects for Noninvasive Prenatal Diagnosis. Vol. 731. New York Academy of Science, NY, p. 80

Elias S, Simpson JL (1994b) Techniques and safety of genetic amniocentesis and chorionic villus sampling. In Sabbagha RE (ed): Diagnostic Ultrasound applied to Obstetrics and Gynecology, 3rd edn. JB Lippincott, Philadelphia, p. 113

Elias S, Simpson JL (1995) Prospects for prenatal diagnosis by isolating fetal cells from maternal blood. Contemp Rev Obstet Gynecol 7:135–139

Elias S, Martin AO, Patel VA et al. (1979) Analysis for amniotic fluid crystallization in second-trimester amniocentesis. Am J Obstet Gynecol 33:401

Elias S, Gerbie AB, Simpson JL et al. (1980a) Genetic amniocentesis in twin gestations. Am J Obstet Gynecol 138:169

Elias S, Mazur M, Sabbagha R et al. (1980b) Prenatal diagnosis of harlequin ichthyosis. Clin Genet 17:275

Elias S, Simpson JL, Martin AO et al. (1985) Chorionic villus sampling for first trimester prenatal diagnosis: Northwestern University Program. Am J Obstet Gynecol 152:204

Elias S, Price J, Dockter M et al. (1992) First trimester prenatal diagnosis of trisomy 21 in fetal cells from maternal blood. Lancet 340:1033

Elias S, Emerson DS, Simpson JL et al. (1994) Ultrasound-directed fetal skin sampling for prenatal diagnosis of genodermatoses. Obstet Gynecol 83:337

Elias S, Lewis DE, Simpson JL et al. (1996) Isolation of fetal nucleated red blood cells from maternal blood: Persistence of cells from prior pregnancy is unlikely to lead to false positive results. J Soc Gyncol Invest 3, 359A

Evans MI, Greg A, Kunkel LM et al. (1991) In utero fetal muscle biopsy for the diagnosis of Duchenne muscular dystrophy. Am J Obstet Gynecol 165:728

Evans MI, Hoffman EP, Cadrin C et al. (1994) Fetal muscle biopsy: Collaborative experience with varied indications. Obstet Gynecol 84:913

Evans MI, Krivchenia EL, Johnson MP et al. (1995) In utero fetal muscle biopsy alters diagnosis and carrier risks in Duchenne and Becker muscular dystrophy. Fetal Diagn Ther 10:71

Evans MI, Elias S, Bianchi D et al. (2000) Racial/ethnic confounders to the detection of Y signals in maternal blood in women carrying male fetuses: The NIFTY study group. J Soc Gynecol Invest 7(S):180A

Firth HV, Boyd PA, Chamberlin P et al. (1991a) Severe limb abnormalities after chorion villus sampling at 55–66 days' gestation. Lancet 337:762

Firth HV, Boyd PA, Chamberlain P et al. (1991b) Limb abnormalities and chorion villus sampling. Lancet 338:51

Firth HV, Boyd PA, Chamberlain P et al. (1994) Analysis of limb reduction defects in babies exposed to chorion villus sampling. Lancet 343:1069

Fishman RHB (1994) WHO on CVS Safety. Lancet 443:1420

Forestier F, Daffos F, Rainaut M et al. (1987) Blood chemistry of normal human fetuses at midtrimester of pregnancy. Pediatr Res 21:579

Forestier F, Cox WL, Daffos F et al. (1988) The assessment of fetal blood samples. Am J Obstet Gyynecol 158:1184

Froster-Ikenius UG, Baird PA (1989) Limb reduction defects in over one million consecutive live births. Teratology 39:127

Froster UG, Jackson L (1996) Limb defects and chorionic villus sampling: Results from an international registry 1992 to 1994. Lancet 347:489–494

Fuchs F, Riis P (1956) Antenatal sex determination. Nature 117:330

Ganshirt-Ahlert D, Börjesson-Stoll R, Burschyk M et al. (1994) Detection of fetal trisomies 21 and 18 from maternal blood using triple gradient and magnetic cell sorting. Am J Reprod Immunol 30:194–201

Ghidini A, Sepulvada W, Lockwood CJ, Romero R (1993) Complications of fetal blood sampling. Am J Obstet Gynecol 168:1339

Gilgenkrantz S, Blanchet-Bardon C, Nazzaro V et al. (1989) Hypohidrotic ectodermal dysplasia: clinical study of a family of 30 over three generations. Hum Genet 81:120

Golbus MS, for the International Fetoscopy Group (1984) Special report: The status of fetoscopy and fetal tissue sampling. Prenat Diagn 4:79

Golbus MS, Sagebiel RW, Filly RA et al. (1980) Prenatal diagnosis of congenital bullous ichthyosiform erythroderma (epidermolytic hyperkeratosis) by fetal skin biopsy. N Engl J Med 302:93

Golbus MS, Stephens JD, Cann HM et al. (1982) Rh-isoimmunization following genetic amniocentesis. Prenat Diagn 2:149

Golbus MS, Simpson JL, Fowler SE et al. (1992) Risk factors associated with transcervical CVS losses. Prenat Diagn 12:373

Gosden C, Nicolaides KH, Rodeck CH (1988) Fetal blood sampling in investigation of chromosome mosaicism in amniotic fluid culture. Lancet 2:613

Grandjean H, Larroque D, Levi S (1999) The performance of routine ultrasonography screening of pregnancies in the Eurofetus Study. Am J Obstet Gynecol 181:446

Gustavii B, Lofberg L, Henrikson KG (1983) Fetal muscle biopsy. Acta Obstet Gynecol Scand 62:369

Hackett GA, Smith JH, Rebello CTH et al. (1991) Early amniocentesis at 11–14 weeks gestation for the diagnosis of fetal chromosomal abnormality – a clinical evaluation. Prenat Diagn 11:311

Haddow JE, Palomaki GE, Knight GJ et al. (1998) Screening of maternal serum for fetal Down's syndrome in the first trimester. N Engl J Med 338:955

Hafner E, Schucher K, Liebhart E, Philipp K (1998) Results of routine fetal nuchal translucency measurement at weeks 10–13 in 4,233 unselected pregnant women. Prenat Diagn 18:29

Hall JM, Williams SJ (1992) Isolation and purification of CD34++ fetal cells from maternal blood. Am J Hum Genet 51:A257

Hamada H, Arinami T, Kubo T et al. (1993) Fetal nucleated cells in maternal peripheral blood: frequency and relationship to gestational age. Hum Genet 91:427

Han J-Y, Je G-H, Kim J-H et al. (1999) Culture of fetal erythroid cells from maternal blood using a two-phase liquid system. Am J Med Genet 87:84

Hanson FW, Tennant F, Hune S, Brookhyser K (1992) Early amniocentesis: Outcome, risks, and technical problems at ≤12.8 weeks. Am J Obstet Gynecol 166:1707

Hata T, Manabe A, Aoki S et al. (1998a) Three-dimensional intrauterine sonography in the early first-trimester of pregnancy: Preliminary study. Hum Reprod 13:740.

Hata T, Yonachara T, Aoki S et al. (1998b) Three-dimensional sonographic visualization of the fetal face. Am J Roentgenol 170:481

Hawes CS, Suskin HA, Kalionis B et al. (1994) Detection of paternally inherited mutations for α-thalassemia in trophoblast isolated from peripheral maternal blood. In Simpson JL, Elias S (eds): Fetal Cells in Maternal Blood: Prospects for Noninvasive Prenatal Diagnosis. Vol. 731. New York Academy of Science, NY, p. 181

Henry GP, Miller WA (1992) Early amniocentesis. J Reprod Med 37:396

Henry G, Wexler P, Robinson A (1976) Rh-immune globulin after amniocentesis for genetic diagnosis. Obstet Gynecol 48:557

Herzenberg LA, Bianchi DW, Schroder J (1979) Fetal cells in the blood of pregnant women: Detection and enrichment by fluorescence-activated cell sorting. Proc Nat Acad Sci USA 76:1453–1455

Hess LW, Anderson RL, Golbus MS (1986) Significance of opaque amniotic fluid at second-trimester amniocentesis. Obstet Gynecol 67:44

Hill LM, Platt LD, Kellogg B (1980) Rh-sensitization after genetic amniocentesis. Obstet Gynecol 56:459

Hobbins JC, Mahoney MJ (1974) In utero diagnosis of hemoglobinopathies: Technique for obtaining fetal blood. N Engl J Med 290:1065

Holmberg L, Gustavii B, Jonsson A (1983) A prenatal study of fetal platelet count and size with application to fetus at risk for Wiskott-Aldrich syndrome. J Pediatr 102:773

Holzgreve W, Miny P, Basarans S et al. (1987) Safety of placental biopsy in the second and third trimester. N Engl J Med 317:1159

Hsieh F-J, Ko TM, Chang FM et al. (1989) Percutaneous ultrasound-guided fetal blood sampling: Experience in the first 100 cases. Taiwan I Hsueh Hui Tsa Chih 88:137

Hsieh F-J, Chen D, Tseng L-H et al. (1991) Limb-reduction defects and chorion villus sampling. Lancet 337:1091–1092

Hsieh TT, Pao CC, Hor JJ et al. (1993) Presence of fetal cells in maternal circulation after delivery. Hum Genet 92:204

Isada NB, Koppitch FC III, Johnson MP et al. (1990) Does the color of amniotic fluid still matter? Fetal Diagn Ther 5:165

Iverson GM, Bianchi DW, Cann HM, Herzenberg LA (1981) Detection and isolation of fetal cells from maternal blood using the fluorescence-activated cell sorter (FACS). Prenat Diagn 1:61–73

Jackson LG, Wapner RJ, Brambai B (1991) Limb abnormalities and chorionic villus sampling. Lancet 337:1423

Jackson LG, Zachary JM, Desnik RJ et al. (1992) A randomized comparison of transcervical and transabdominal chorionic villus sampling. N Engl J Med 327:594

Johnson JM, Wilson RD, Singer J et al. (1999) Technical factors in early amniocetesis predict adverse outcome. Results of the Canadian early (EA) versus mid-trimester (MA) amniocentesis trial. Prenat Diagn 19:732

Jurkovic D, Kurjak A (1989) Prenatina dijagnostika epidermolysis bullosa hereditaria utravuenco vodenum fetalne koze. Lijec Vjesn 111:60

Kao SM, Tang GC, Hsieh TT et al. (1992) Analysis of peripheral blood of pregnant women for the presence of fetal Y chromosome-specific ZFY gene deoxyribonucleic acid sequences. Am J Obstet Gynecol 166:1013–1019

Karp LE, Schiller HS (1977) Meconium staining of amniotic fluid at midtrimester amniocentesis. Obstet Gynecol 50:475

Kennerknecht I, Kramer S, Grab D, Terinde R (1993) Evaluation of amniotic fluid cell filtration: an experimental approach to early amniocentesis. Prenat Diagn 13:247

Kerber S, Held KR (1993) Early genetic amniocentesis-4 years' experience. Prenat Diagn 13:21

Khalil MA, Tabsh MA, Lobherz TB et al. (1984) Risks of prophylactic anti-D immunoglobulin after second-trimester amniocentesis. Am J Obstet Gynecol 149:225

Kouseff BG, Matsuoka LY, Stenn KS et al. (1982) Prenatal diagnosis of Sjögren-Larsson syndrome. Pediatrics 101:998

Lewis DE, Schober W, Murrell S et al. (1996) Rare event selection of fetal nucleated erythrocytes in maternal blood by flow cytometry. Cytometry 23:218–227

Liou JD, Chen CP, Breg WR et al. (1993a) Fetal blood sampling and cytogenetic abnormalities. Prenat Diagn 13:1

Liou JD, Pao CC, Hor JJ, Kao SM (1993b) Fetal cells in the maternal circulation during first trimester in pregnancies. Hum Genet 92:309–311

Liou JD, Hsieh TT, Pao CC (1994) Persistence of cells of fetal origin in maternal circulation of pregnant women. In Simpson JL, Elias S (eds): Fetal Cells in Maternal Blood: Prospects for Noninvasive Prenatal Diagnosis. Vol. 731. New York Academy of Science, NY, p. 237

Little MT, Langlois S, Wilson RD, Lansdorp PM (1997) Frequency of fetal cells in sorted subpopulations of nucleated erythroid and CD34+ hematopoietic progenitor cells from maternal peripheral blood. Blood 89:2347–2358

Lo YMD, Wainscot JS, Gilmer MDG et al. (1989) Prenatal sex determination by DNA amplification from maternal peripheral blood. Lancet 2:1363–1365

Lo YMD, Pate P, Sampietro M et al. (1990) Detection of single-copy fetal DNA sequence from maternal blood. Lancet 335:1463–1464

Lo YMD, Bowell PJ, Selinger M et al. (1993) Prenatal determination of fetal RhD status by analysis of peripheral blood of rhesus negative mothers. Lancet 341:1147–1148

Lo YM, Morey AL, Wainscoat JS et al. (1994) Culture of fetal erythroid cells from maternal peripheral blood. Lancet 344:264

Lo YM, Corbatta N, Chamberlain PF et al. (1997) Presence of fetal DNA in maternal plasma and serum. Lancet 350:458

Lo YM, Hjelm NM, Fidler C et al. (1998a) Prenatal diagnosis of fetal RhD status by molecular analysis of maternal plasma. N Engl J Med 339:1734

Lo YM, Tein MS, Lau TK et al. (1998b) Quantitative analysis of fetal DNA in maternal plasma and serum: implications for noninvasive prenatal diagnosis. Am J Hum Genet 62:768

Lo YM, Zhang J, Leung TN et al. (1999) Rapid clearance of fetal DNA from maternal plasma. Am J Hum Genet 64:218

Lockwood DH, Neu RL (1993) Cytogenetic analysis of 1,375 amniotic fluid specimens from pregnancies with gestational age less than 14 weeks. Prenat Diagn 13:801

Lyons EA, Dyke C, Toms M, Cheang M (1988) In utero exposure to diagnostic ultrasound. A 6-year follow-up. Radiology 166:687–690

Mahoney MJ and USNICHD collaborators (1991) Limb abnormalities and chorionic villus sampling. Lancet 337:1422

Makrydimas G, Georgiou I, Kranas V et al. (1997) Prenatal diagnosis of beta-thalassaemia by coelocentesis. Mol Hum Reprod 3:729

Marthin T, Liedgren S, Hammar M (1997) Transplacental needle passage and other risk-factors associated with second trimester amniocentesis. Acta Obstet Gynecol Scand 76:728

Mastroiacovo P, Botto LD (1994) Chorionic villus sampling and limb deficiencies. Review of case control and cohort studies. p. 71. In Zakut H (ed): Seventh International Conference on Early Prenatal Diagnosis of Genetic Disease, Jerusalem, Israel, May 22–27

Mastroiacovo P, Cavalcanti DP (1991) Limb reduction defects and chorion villus sampling. Lancet 337:1091

Mastroiacova P, Botto LD, Cavalcanti, DP et al. (1992) Limb anomalies following chorionic villus sampling: A registry based case-control study. Am J Med Genet 44:856

Medical Research Council (1977) Diagnosis of Genetic Disease by Amniocentesis During the Second Trimester of Pregnancy. Ottawa, Canada

Milunsky A (1986) The prenatal diagnosis of neural tube and other congenital defects. In Milunsky A (ed): Genetic Disorders and the Fetus. Plenum, NY, p. 453

Moise KJ, Deter RL, Kishorn B et al. (1989) Intravenous pancuronium bromide for fetal neuromuscular blockade during intrauterine transfusion for red cell alloimmunization. Obstet Gynecol 74:905

Monni G, Ibba RM, Lai R et al. (1991) Limb-reduction defects and chorion villus sampling. Lancet 337:1091

MRC Working Party on the Evaluation of Chorionic Villus Sampling (1991) Medical Research Council European trial of chorion villus sampling. Lancet 337:1491

Mueller UW, Hawes CD, Wright AE et al. (1990) Isolation of fetal trophoblast cells from peripheral blood of pregnant women. Lancet 336:197–200

National Institute of Child Health Development National Registry for Amniocentesis Study Group (1976) Midtrimester amniocentesis for prenatal diagnosis: Safety and accuracy. JAMA 236:1471

National Institute of Child Health and Human Development Consensus Conference on Antenatal Diagnosis December (1979) NIH Publication No. 80–1973. Washington, DC

Nevo Y, Shomrat R, Yaron Y et al. (1999) Fetal muscle biopsy as a diagnostic tool in Duchenne muscular dystrophy. Prenat Diagn 19:921

Newton ER (1999) Diagnosis of perinatal TORCH infections. Clin Obstet Gynecol 42:59

Nicolaides KH, Clewel WH, Rodeck CH (1987) Measurement of human fetoplacental blood volume in erythroblastosis fetalis. Am J Obstet Gynecol 157:50

Nicolaides KH, Thorpe-Beeston JG, Noble P (1990) Cordocentesis in assessment and care of the fetus. In Eden RD, Boehm FH (eds): Assessment and Care of the Fetus. Appleton & Lange, Norwalk, CT, p. 291

Nicolaidis P, Nicolini U, Fisk NM et al. (1991) Fetal blood sampling from the intrahepatic vein for rapid karyotyping in the second and third trimesters. Br J Radiol 64:505

Nicolaides KH, Azar G, Byrne D et al. (1992) Fetal nuchal translucency: Ultrasound screening for chromosomal defects in first trimester of pregnancy. BMJ 304:867

Nicolaides KH, Brizot ML, Snijders RJ (1994) Fetal nuchal translucency: Ultrasound screening for fetal trisomy in the first trimester of pregnancy. Br J Obstet Gynaecol 101:782

Nicolaides K, Brizot ML, Patel F, Snijders R (1994) Comparison of chorionic villus sampling and amniocentesis for fetal karyotyping at 10–13 weeks gestation. Lancet 344:435

Nicolaides K, Brizot ML, Patel F, Snijders R (1996) Comparison of chorionic villus sampling and early amniocentesis for karyotyping in 1,492 singleton pregnancies. Fetal Diagn Ther 11:9

Nicolini U, Kochenour NK, Greco P et al. (1988) Consequences of fetomaternal haemorrhage after intrauterine transfusion. BMJ 297:1379

Nicolini U, Nicolaidis P, Fisk NM et al. (1990) Fetal blood sampling from the intrahepatic vein: Analysis of safety and clinical experience with 214 procedures. Obstet Gynecol 76:47

Olney RS, Khoury MJ, Alo CJ et al. (1995) Increased risk transverse digital deficiency after chorionic villus sampling: Results of the United States multistate case-control study, 1988–1992. Teratology 51:20–29

Orlandi F, Damiani G, Jakil C et al. (1987) Clinical results and fetal biochemical data on 140 early second trimester diagnostic cordocentesis. Acta Eur Fertil 18:329

Orlandi F, Damiani G, Jakil C et al. (1990) The risks of early cordocentesis (12–21 weeks): Analysis of 500 procedures. Prenat Diagn 10:425–428

Orsetti B, Lefort G, Boulot P et al. (1998) Fetal cells in maternal blood: the use of primed in situ (PRINS) labelling technique for fetal cell detection and sex assessment. Prenat Diagn 18:1014

Penso CA, Sandstrom MM, Garber MF et al. (1990) Early amniocentesis: Report of 407 cases with neonatal follow-up. Obstet Gynecol 76:1032

Pergament E, Schulman JD, Copeland K et al. (1992) The risk and efficacy of chorionic villus sampling in multiple gestations. Prenat Diagn 12:377

Perry TB, Holbrook KA, Hoff MS et al. (1987) Prenatal diagnosis of congenital non-bullous ichthyos form erythroderm (lamellar ichthyosis). Prenat Diagn 7:145

Peters MT, Nicolaides KH (1990) Cordocentesis for the diagnosis and treatment of human fetal parvovirus infection. Obstet Gynecol 75:501

Philip J (1993) Sensitivity and specificity in ultrasonographic screening. In Simpson JL, Elias S (eds): Essentials of Prenatal Diagnosis. Churchill Livingstone, NY p. 141

Platt LD, Feuchtbaum L, Filly R et al. (1992) The California maternal serum alpha-fetoprotein program: the role of ultrasonography in the detection of spina bifida. Am J Obstet Gynecol 166:1328

Platt LD, Santulli T Jr, Carlson DE et al. (1998) Three-dimensional ultrasonography in obstetrics and gynecology: preliminary experience. Am J Obstet Gynecol 178:1199

Podobnik M, Ciglar S, Singer Z et al. (1997) Transabdominal chorionic villus sampling in the second and third trimesters of high-risk pregnancies. Prenat Diagn 17:125

Porreco RP, Harshbarger B, McGavran L (1993) Rapid cytogenetic assessment of fetal blood samples. Obstet Gynecol 82:242

Price J, Elias S, Wachtel SS et al. (1991) Prenatal diagnosis using fetal cells isolated from maternal blood by multiparameter flow cytometry. Am J Obstet Gynecol 165:1731–1737

Quintero RA, Puder KS, Cotton DB (1993) Embryoscopy and fetoscopy. Obstet Gynecol Clin North Am 20:563

Queisser-Luft A, Stopfkuchen H, Stolz G et al. (1998) Prenatal diagnosis of major malformations: quality control of routine ultrasound examinations based on a five-year study of 20,248 newborn fetuses and infants. Prenat Diagn 18:567

Reece EA (1992) Embryoscopy: new developments in prenatal diagnosis. Curr Opin Obstet Gynecol 4:447

Reece EA (1997) Embryoscopy and early prenatal diagnosis. Obstet Gynecol Clin North Am 24:111

Reece EA (1999) First trimester prenatal diagnosis: embryoscopy and fetoscopy. Semin Perinatol 23:424

Reece EA, Homko CJ, Koch S, Chan L (1997) First-trimester needle embryofetoscopy and prenatal diagnosis. Fetal Diagn Ther 12:136

Rhoads GG, Jackson LG, Schlesselman SE et al. (1989) The safety and efficacy of chorionic villus sampling for early prenatal diagnosis of cytogenetic abnormalities. N Engl J Med 320:609

Robert-Gangneux F, Gavinet MF, Ancelle T et al. (1999) Value of prenatal diagnosis and early postnatal diagnosis of congenital toxoplasmosis: Retrospective study of 110 cases. J Clin Microbiol 37:2893

Rodeck CH, Nicolini U (1988) Fetal blood sampling. Eur J Obstet Gynecol Reprod Biol 28:85

Rodeck CH, Eady RAJ, Gosden CJ (1980). Prenatal diagnosis of epidermolysis bullosa lethalis. Lancet 1:949

Ross JA, Jurkovic D, Nicolaides K (1997) Coelocentesis: A study of short-term safety. Prenat Diagn 17:913

Ryan G, Rodeck CH (1993) Fetal blood sampling. In Simpson JL, Elias S (eds): Essentials of Prenatal Diagnosis. Churchill Livingstone, NY, p. 63

Sabbagha RE (1993) Ultrasound diagnosis of fetal structural anomalies. p. 91. In Simpson JL, Elias S (eds): Essentials of Prenatal Diagnosis. Churchill Livingstone, NY

Santolaya-Forgas J, Vengalil S, Kushwaha A et al. (1998a) Assessment of the risk of fetal loss after the coelocentesis procedure using a baboon model. Fetal Diagn Ther 13:257

Santolaya-Forgas J, Duval J, Prespin C et al. (1998b) Extracoelomic fluid osmometry and electrolyte composition during early gestation in the baboon. Am J Obstet Gynecol 179:1124

Sargent IL, Choo YS, Redman CWG (1994) Isolating and analyzing fetal leukocytes in maternal blood. In Simpson JL, Elias S (eds): Fetal Cells in Maternal Blood: Prospects for Noninvasive Diagnosis. Vol. 731. New York Academy of Science, NY, p. 147

Sbracia M, Scarpellini F, Lalwani S et al. (1994) Possible use of an unusual HLA antigen to select trophoblast cells from the maternal circulation to perform early prenatal diagnosis. p. 170. In Simpson JL, Elias S (eds): Fetal Cells in Maternal Blood: Prospects for Noninvasive Diagnosis. Vol. 731. New York Academy of Science, New York

Schindler AM, Graf E, Martin-Du-Pan R (1972) Prenatal diagnosis of fetal lymphocytes in the maternal blood. Obstet Gynecol 40:340–346

Scott R (1991) Limb abnormalities after chorionic villus sampling. Lancet 337:103

Shimizu H, Suzumori K (1999) Prenatal diagnosis as a test for genodermatoses: Its past, present and future. J Dermatol Sci 19:1

Shulman LP, Tharapel AT, Meyers CM et al. (1990) Direct analysis of cytotrophoblastic cells from second and third trimester placentas: An accurate and very-rapid method-for detecting fetal chromosome abnormalities. Am J Obstet Gynecol 163:1606

Shulman LP, Elias S, Phillips OP et al. (1992a) Early twin amniocentesis prior to 14 weeks gestation. Prenat Diagn 12:625

Shulman LP, Emerson DS, Felker RE et al. (1992b) High frequency of cytogenetic abnormalities in fetuses with cystic hygroma diagnosed in the first trimester. Obstet Gynecol 80:80

Shulman LP, Simpson JL, Elias S et al. (1993) Transvaginal chorionic villus sampling using transabdominal ultrasound guidance: A new technique for first-trimester prenatal diagnosis. Fetal Diagn Ther 8:144

Shulman LP, Elias S, Phillips OP et al. (1994) Amniocentesis performed at 14 weeks gestation or earlier: Comparison with first-trimester chorionic villus sampling. Obstet Gynecol 83:543

Shulman LP, Phillips OP, Tolly E et al. (1998) Frequency of nucleated red blood cells in maternal blood during the different gestational ages. Hum Genet 103:723

Sidransky E, Black SH, Soenksen DM et al. (1990) Transvaginal chorionic villus sampling. Prenat Diagn 10:583

Simpson JL, Elias S (1993) Isolating fetal cells from maternal blood: advances in prenatal diagnosis through molecular technology. JAMA 270:2357–2361

Simpson JL, Elias S (1994a) Prenatal diagnosis of genetic disorders. In Creasy RK, Resnik R (eds): Maternal-Fetal Medicine: Principles and Practice. WB Saunders, Philadelphia, p. 61

Simpson JL, Elias S (1994b) Techniques for prenatal diagnosis of genetic disorders. Reprod Genet 4:197

Simpson JL, Elias S (1994c) Fetal cells in maternal blood: overview and historical perspective. In Simpson JL, Elias S (eds): Fetal Cells in Maternal Blood: Prospects for Noninvasive Prenatal Diagnosis. NY Acad Sci 731:1–8

Simpson JL, Elias S (1995) Isolating fetal cells in the maternal circulation. Hum Reprod Update 1:409–418

Simpson NE, Dellaire L, Miller JR et al. (1976) Prenatal diagnosis of genetic disease in Canada: report of a collaborative study. Can Med Assoc J 15:739

Sklansky MS, Nelson T, Strachan M, Pretorius D (1999) Real-time three-dimensional fetal echocardiography: Initial feasibility study. J Ultrasound Med 18:745

Skupski DW, Newman S, Edersheim T et al. (1996) The impact of routine obstetric ultrasonographic screening in a low-risk population. Am J Obstet Gynecol 175:1142

Smidt-Jensen S, Hahnemann N (1984) Transabdominal fine needle biopsy from chorionic villi in the first trimester. Prenat Diagn 4:163

Smidt-Jensen S, Permin M, Philip J et al. (1992) Randomized comparison of amniocentesis and transabdominal and transcervical chorionic villus sampling. Lancet 340:1237

Snijders RJ, Noble P, Sebire N et al. (1998) UK multicentre project on assessment of risk of trisomy 21 by maternal age and fetal nuchal-translucency thickness at 10–14 weeks of gestation. Fetal Medicine Foundation First Trimester Screening Group. Lancet 352:343

Stark CR, Orleans M, Haverkamp AD, Murphy J (1984) Short- and long-term risks after exposure to diagnostic ultrasound in utero. Obstet Gynecol 63:194–200

Stripparo L, Buscaglia M, Longatti L (1990) Genetic amniocentesis: 505 cases performed before the sixteenth week of gestation. Prenat Diagn 10:359

Sundberg K, Bang J, Smidt-Jensen S et al. (1997) Randomised study of risk of fetal loss related to early amniocentesis versus chorionic villus sampling. Lancet 350:697

Sundberg K, Smidt-Jensen S, Lundsteen C et al. (1993) Filtration and recirculation of early amniotic fluid. Evaluation of cell cultures from 100 diagnostic cases. Prenat Diagn 13:1101

Tabor A, Philip J, Madsen MI et al. (1986) Randomized controlled trial of genetic amniocentesis in 4,606 low-risk women. Lancet 1:1287

Takabayashi H, Kuwabara S, Ukita T, Igarashi T (1994) Fetal nucleated erythrocyte retrieval from maternal blood. p. 45. In Zakut H (ed): Seventh International Conference on Early Prenatal Diagnosis. Monduzzi Editore, Bologna

Takahara H, Kadotani I, Kusumi S, Makino (1972) Some critical aspects of prenatal diagnosis of sex in leukocyte cultures from pregnant women. Proc Jpn Acad 48:603–607

Tharapel AT, Jaswaney V, Dockter M et al. (1989) Can fetal cells in maternal blood be selected through cytogenetic means? Am J Hum Genet, suppl. 45:271

Tharapel AT, Jaswaney VL, Dockter ME et al. (1993) Failure to detect fetal metaphases in lymphocytes flow sorted by maternal-fetal HLA differences. Fetal Diagn Ther 8:95–101

Tharmaratnam S, Sadek S, Streele EK et al. (1998) Transplacental early amniocentesis and pregnancy outcome. Br J Obstet Gynecol 105:228

Thomas MR, Williamson R, Craft I et al. (1994) Y chromosome sequence DNA amplified from peripheral blood in women in early pregnancy. Lancet 343:413

Tipton RE, Tharapel AT, Change HT et al. (1990) Rapid chromosome analysis using spontaneously dividing cells from umbilical cord blood (fetal and neonatal). American Journal of Obstet Gynecol 161:1546

Tse DB, Anderson P, Goldbard S et al. (1994) Characterization of trophoblast-reactive monoclonal antibodies by flow cytometry and their application for fetal cell isolation. p. 162. In Simpson JL, Elias S (eds): Fetal Cells in Maternal Blood: Prospects for Noninvasive Prenatal Diagnosis. Vol. 731. New York Academy of Science, New York

Turnbull AC, MacKenzie IZ (1983) Second-trimester amniocentesis and termination of pregnancy. Br Med Bull 39:315–321

United Kingdom Medical Research Council (1978) Working Party on amniocentesis. An assessment of the hazards of amniocentesis. Br J Obstet Gynaecol, Suppl 21. 85:1

Valerio D, Aiello R, Altieri V et al. (1996) Culture of fetal erythroid progenitor cells from maternal blood for non-invasive prenatal genetic diagnosis. Prenat Diagn 16:1073

Valerio D, Aiello R, Altieri V (1997a) Isolation of fetal erythroid cells from maternal blood based on expression of erythropoietin receptor. Mol Hum Reprod 3:451

Valerio D, Altieri V, Antonucci FR et al. (1997b) Characterization of fetal haematopoietic progenitors circulating in maternal blood of seven aneuploid pregnancies. Prenat Diagn 17:1159

van den Berg C, Braat APG, Van Opstal D et al. (1999) Amniocentesis or chorionic villus sampling in multiple gestations? Experience with 500 cases. Prenat Diagn 19:234

VanDorsten JP, Hulsey TC, Newman RB, Menard MK (1998) Fetal anomaly detection by second-trimester ultrasonography in a tertiary center. Am J Obstet Gynecol 178:742

van Vugt JM, Nieuwint A, van Geijn HP (1995) Single-needle insertion: an alternative technique for early second-trimester genetic twin amniocentesis. Fetal Diagn Ther 10:178

van Zalen-Sprock, van Vugt JMG, Karsdorp et al. (1991) Ultrasound diagnosis of fetal abnormalities and cytogenetic evaluation. Prenat Diagn 11:655

Wachtel SS, Elias S, Price J et al. (1991) Fetal cells in the maternal circulation: Isolation by multiparameter flow cytometry and confirmation by PCR. Hum Reprod 6:1466–1469

Wachtel SS, Sammons D, Twitty G et al. (1998) Charge flow separation: Quantification of nucleated red blood cells in maternal blood during pregnancy. Prenat Diagn 18:455

Walknowska J, Conte FA, Grumback MM (1969) Practical and theoretical implications of fetal/maternal lymphocyte transfer. Lancet 1:119–1122

Wang JY, Zehn DK, Falco VM et al. (2000) Fetal nucleated erythrocyte recovery: Fluorescence activated cell sorting-based positive selection using anti gamma-globulin versus magnetic activated cell sorting using anti-CD45 depletion and anti-gamma globulin positive selection. Cytometry 39:224

Wathen NC, Campbell DJ, Kitau MJ, Chard T (1993) Alphafetoprotein levels in amniotic fluid from 8 to 18 weeks of pregnancy. Br J Obstet Gynaecol 100:380

Watson JD, Craft P (1989) Acetylcholinesterase determination in early amniocentesis. Am J Hum Genet 45:A272

Weiner CP (1987) Cordocentesis for diagnostic indications: Two years experience. Obstet Gynecol 70:664

Weiner CP, Grant SS, Huson J et al. (1989) Effect of diagnostic and therapeutic cordocentesis upon maternal serum alpha fetoprotein concentration. Am J Obstet Gynecol 161:706

Whang-Peng J, Lettin JS, Harris C et al. (1973) The transplacental passage of fetal leukocytes into the maternal blood. Proc Soc Exp Biol Med 142:50–53

Wilson RD, Farquharson DF, Wittmann BK, Shaw D (1994) Cordocentesis: Overall pregnancy loss rate as important as procedure loss rate. Fetal Diagn Ther 9:142

WHO/PAHO Consultation on CVS (1999) Evaluation of chorionic villus sampling safety. Prenat Diagn 19:97

Yanagihara T, Hata T (2000) Three-dimensional sonographic visualization of fetal skeleton in the second trimester of pregnancy. Gynecol Obstet Invest 49:12

Yang CH, Chu-Ho ES, Liucc et al. (1993) Prenatal cytogenetic diagnosis by amniocentesis before 15 weeks gestation. Chung Hua I Hueh Tsa Chih Chinese Med J 52:81

Yeoh SC, Sargent IL, Redman CWG et al. (1991) Detection of fetal cells in maternal blood. Prenat Diagn 11:117–123

Neonatal screening

30

Richard W. Erbe
Harvey L. Levy

Introduction

Genetic screening is a search in a population for persons who possess genotypes that (1) are associated with disease or predispose to disease, (2) may lead to disease in their descendants, or (3) produce other variations not known to be associated with disease (Committee for the Study of Inborn Errors of Metabolism, 1975). The primary focus of this chapter is newborn genetic screening for inborn errors of metabolism. Neonatal screening provides a means of early recognition of disorders in order to initiate treatment where available and to reduce confusion, anxiety and delay associated with late ascertainment. Genetic screening can be a source of epidemiological data regarding birth defects. The nature and number of newborn screening tests vary widely in different localities and may include some or all of the following: (1) cord blood, (2) newborn nursery blood, (3) newborn follow-up blood and/or (4) newborn urine. In addition to tests for classical inborn errors of metabolism, neonatal screening programs in the United States or elsewhere may offer tests for one or more of the following: adenosine deaminase deficiency, α_1-antitrypsin deficiency, congenital adrenal hyperplasia, cystic fibrosis, Duchenne muscular dystrophy, newborn hearing, hemoglobinopathies, hyperlipidemia, hypothyroidism, and toxoplasmosis.

Historical aspects

Genetic screening as we know it dates from the 1960s. As early as 1908, however, Archibald Garrod stated that inborn errors of metabolism could be recognized "... by

some strikingly unusual appearance of surface tissues or of excreta, by the excretion of some substance which responds to a test habitually applied in the routine of clinical work, or by giving rise to obvious morbid symptoms" (Harris, 1963). This observation was first applied on a population-wide basis to phenylketonuria (PKU) but only after two important advances. The first occurred in 1934 when Fölling described the association between PKU and mental retardation (Fölling, 1934). The second occurred when Bickel and coworkers (1954) developed a phenylalanine-restricted diet that was shown to prevent the mental retardation seen regularly in untreated PKU. The remaining challenge was to identify PKU in the presymptomatic newborn infant so that the dietary intervention could be optimally effective. This challenge was met when Guthrie developed a bacterial assay for phenylalanine that required only a few drops of blood, easily obtainable from the heel of newborn infants and dried on filter paper (Guthrie and Susi, 1963). Routine newborn screening for PKU using this method began in Massachusetts in 1962 and, after a successful field trial (MacCready and Hussey, 1964), expanded widely in the United States and abroad. Guthrie subsequently introduced microbiological assays to screen for maple syrup urine disease, homocystinuria, tyrosinemia, histidinemia, galactosemia and other disorders (Guthrie, 1968). Paper chromatographic methods for general newborn screening of blood and urine amino acids were also introduced at this time (Efron et al., 1964; Scriver et al., 1964; Turner and Brown 1967).

The great advantage of Guthrie's newborn screening system resided in the specimen of blood dried on filter paper, now often referred to as the Guthrie specimen or Guthrie card. This specimen is easily collected, readily transported to a central testing laboratory, and can be used

826

Table 30.1. Newborn Metabolic Screening in New England

Test	Metabolite	Primary Disorder	State
MS-MS[a]	Phenylalanine	Phenylketonuria	MA, ME, NH, RI, VT
MS-MS	Leucine	Maple syrup urine disease	MA, ME, NH, RI, VT
MS-MS	Methionine	Homocystinuria	MA, ME, NH, RI, VT
Enzyme assay	Galactose	Galactosemia	MA, ME, NH, RI, VT
Fluoroimmunoassay	T$_4$, TSH	Congenital hypothyroidism	MA, ME, NH, RI, VT
Fluoroimmunoassay	17-OHP	Congenital adrenal hyperplasia	MA, ME, RI
Enzyme assay	Biotinidase	Biotinidase deficiency	
Isoelectric focusing	Hemoglobin	Hemoglobinopathies	MA, ME[b], NH[b], RI, VT
ELISA	IgM	Congenital toxoplasmosis	MA, NH
MS-MS	Multiple metabolites	Organic acid and fatty acid disorders	MA

Tests in this table are performed on dried blood samples obtained from newborns at 1 to 3 days of age.
[a]MS-MS, tandem mass spectroscopy
[b]Testing only on request

in many different tests. In the 1970s, for instance, Dussault et al., (1975) introduced newborn screening for congenital hypothyroidism by developing a radioimmunoassay for thyroxine (T4) that could be applied to the Guthrie specimen. More recently, DNA extracted from the dried blood has been used for molecular testing.

In the 1980s many newborn screening programs added tests for sickle cell diseases (i.e. sickle cell anemia, hemoglobin SC disease, and Sβ-thalassemia) (National Institutes of Health Consensus Conference, 1987). This occurred following demonstration in a large clinical trial that prophylactic treatment with penicillin reduced by 84% the mortality caused by infections with *Streptococcus pneumoniae* that otherwise killed many infants with sickle cell disease (Gaston et al., 1986). In the 1990s, screening for congenital adrenal hyperplasia by immunoassay of 17-hydroxyprogesterone (17-OHP) (Pang and Clark, 1993) and for biotinidase deficiency by assay of biotinidase activity were added. Most recently, programs have expanded further to include screening for cystic fibrosis by immunoassay of trypsinogen (Wilcken et al., 1995) and for many disorders affecting amino acids, organic acids and fatty acid oxidation using the newly introduced technology of tandem mass spectrometry (Levy, 1998; Chace and Naylor, 1999).

Newborn screening for PKU and other inborn errors using dried blood has spread widely throughout the developed world. In the United States, PKU and congenital hypothyroidism are universally screened but coverage of other disorders varies quite widely. Galactosemia and sickle cell disease are screened in almost all states, and maple syrup urine disease is screened in at least 21 states (Tables 30.1 and 30.2). New tests continue to be proposed, with much recent interest focused on those that are DNA-based.

Table 30.2. Disorders Included in Newborn Screening

Disorder	Number of States[a]	Reliably Screened at <24 Hours
PKU	51	Yes
Congenital hypothyroidism	51	Possibly
Sickle cell disease	44	Yes
Galactosemia	44	Yes
Maple syrup urine disease	24	Yes
Homocystinuria	21	No
Biotinidase deficiency	17	Yes
Congenital adrenal hyperplasia	14	Yes
Tyrosinemia	7	No
Cystic fibrosis	3	Possibly
Congenital toxoplasmosis	2	Yes

[a]Includes the District of Columbia.

Newborn metabolic screening

COLLECTION OF SPECIMENS

The newborn Guthrie blood specimen is the only specimen currently used for newborn screening in the United States and, with few exceptions, all other countries. One exception is the Canadian province of Quebec which still collects and tests newborn urine specimens in addition to the newborn blood specimen. In Portugal and a few Latin American countries, cord blood is collected for congenital hypothyroidism screening.

The Guthrie specimen is usually collected in the nursery from the lanced heel of the infant by allowing drops of blood to saturate the filter paper within designated circles. The specimen is air dried in the nursery and then placed in an envelope or a plastic bag for transport to the central testing laboratory. Occasionally, the blood specimen is transferred to the filter paper from a capillary tube or a venous specimen (Lorey and Cunningham, 1994).

The newborn urine specimen in Quebec is collected by the parents when the infant is three weeks old using a kit supplied at the time of nursery discharge. The parent collects the specimen by placing the filter paper between folds of a wet diaper and pressing the diaper to push urine into the specimen card.

ORGANIZATION OF SCREENING

All screening programs in the United States are organized on a state-by-state basis in that the state determines the disorders to be screened. Specimens are sent to the state program, and the follow up is conducted by the program. In most states, the specimen is tested by the state laboratory or in one or more contract laboratories designated by the state. Several regional programs have been formed within which each participating state sends specimens to a testing laboratory within the region yet maintains within the originating state all other elements of the screening program. Whereas services were provided free of charge when first established, most programs now charge a fee for the test alone or with additional charges for program administrative costs, follow up, treatment and/or genetic counseling.

Screening outside the United States has usually been organized similarly to screening in the United States. Nevertheless, there are a few national programs, notably the national screening program in Japan.

BLOOD

Analysis of blood specimens

In the laboratory small discs are punched from the Guthrie filter paper specimen. For the Guthrie-type bacterial inhibition assays, still used in most newborn screening programs, the blood-soaked discs are placed on agar gels that contain both a test strain of bacteria and a chemical compound that inhibits that bacterial strain's growth. The growth inhibitor used is selected to be a structural analogue of the amino acid to be measured in the blood spot. The principle of the assay involves the increasing extent of growth of the test bacteria around the disc in proportion to the increasing concentration of the target amino acid in blood from the disc, the latter competitively reversing the effect of the inhibitor. This allows

for bacterial growth around the disc in a semi-quantitative manner (e.g. in PKU, increased phenylalanine in the blood overcomes the inhibition produced by the β_2-thienylalanine and results in a large bacterial growth around the disc).

Galactosemia is identified by either a metabolite assay for galactose and galactose-1-phosphate or an enzyme assay for galactose-1-phosphate uridyltransferase (GALT) activity. A metabolite assay can identify galactosemia and the two other common galactose metabolic disorders (namely, galactokinase deficiency and uridine diphosphogalactose-4-epimerase deficiency), whereas the enzyme assay is limited to the detection of galactosemia due to GALT activity.

Biotinidase activity is also measured by an enzyme assay in the dried blood specimen. In the semiquantitative assay used in screening (Wolf et al., 1987), biotinidase releases *p*-aminobenzoate from the artificial substrate, biotinyl-*p*-aminobenzoate. Color-developing reagents added subsequently cause samples with biotinidase activity to become purple, while samples lacking biotinidase activity remain clear or straw-colored.

Congenital hypothyroidism, congenital adrenal hyperplasia, and cystic fibrosis are screened by immunoassays for, respectively, thyroxine (T4) and/or thyroid stimulating hormone (TSH), 17-hydroxyprogesterone (17-OHP), and trypsinogen (Levy and Albers, in press). Sickle cell diseases are screened by examination of hemoglobin mobilities using either isoelectric focusing or hemoglobin electrophoresis (Levy and Albers, in press).

Tandem mass spectrometry has been adapted recently for use with the Guthrie specimen and introduced into newborn screening by Neo Gen Screening, a private screening laboratory in Pittsburgh. Use of this method is increasingly widespread in screening programs throughout the world. It allows simultaneous screening for most amino acid disorders as well as for many organic acid and fatty acid oxidation disorders in a single assay (Levy, 1998). The technology employs two mass spectrometers in tandem separated by a collision chamber (Fig. 30.1). The mass of ionized molecules is determined in the first spectrometer and the molecules are identified on the basis of the fragmentation profiles in the second spectrometer (Chace and Naylor, 1999; Rashed et al., 1999). The data are analyzed by means of a computer program and electrically translated into a printout with representative peaks for each metabolite.

Interpretation of the screening results

The majority of positive screening results are not due to a metabolic or other disorder. False positive results occur frequently with the bacterial growth and enzyme activity

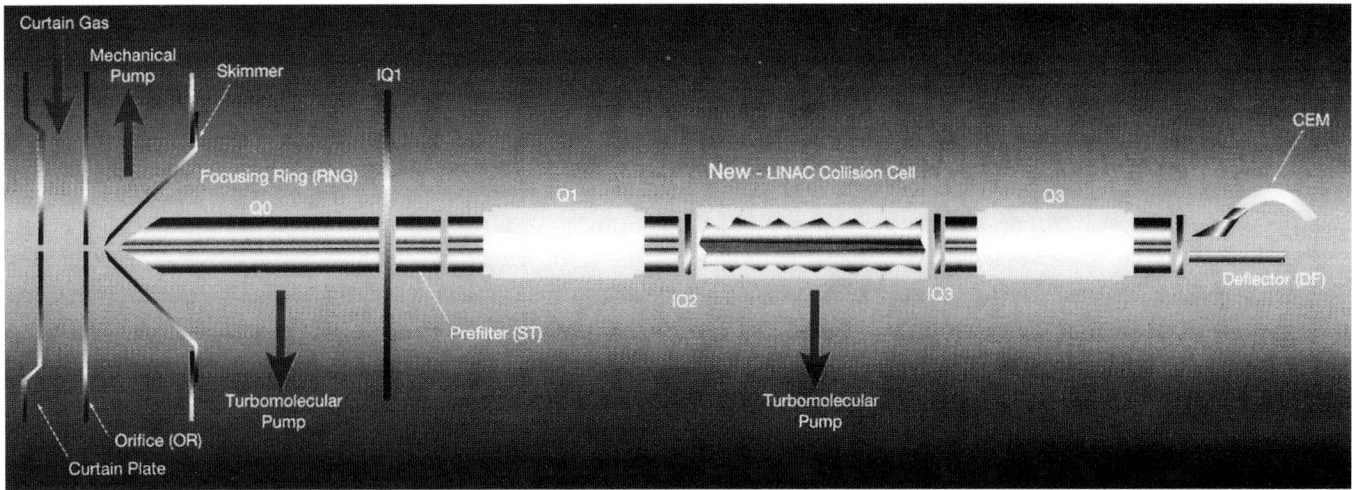

Fig. 30.1. Schematic representation of tandem mass spectrometry (MS-MS). Blood eluted from a disc punched from the Guthrie specimen is subjected to esterification with butanol. After injection and ionization by electrospray, molecules in the blood enter the first MS (Q1) where their masses are determined and they are separated according to ionic (positive and negative) charge. These molecules then enter the collision cell (Q2) where they are fragmented by an inert gas introduced under high pressure. The fragments, either ions or uncharged, pass into the second MS (Q3) where they are separated according to mass and charge and selectively scanned for fragments associated with amino acids (loss of mass 102 from the original ion) and acylcarnitines (ion with mass 85). Computer scanning of the two MSs links the fragment results in the second MS with the parent masses in the first MS. The computer also measures the quantities of each amino acid and acylcarnitine based on the ratio between the masses of the parent molecules and of a known amount of stable isotope for each metabolite injected with each specimen. The results are then electrically displayed and printed out.

assays. False positives frequently result from mild transient elevations in blood of phenylalanine, leucine, methionine and/or tyrosine seen in otherwise normal newborns. Moreover, multiple amino acid elevations are encountered in premature infants receiving hyperalimentation or infants who are very ill, especially in the presence of severe liver dysfunction. Transient deficiencies of galactose-1-phosphate uridyltransferase produce false positive results in galactosemia screening. Transient deficiencies of biotinidase activity, particularly in premature infants, may also be encountered in screening for biotinidase deficiency.

Artifacts also account for many false positive results. Multiple applications of blood to one area of the filter paper or the presence of blood clots can produce "caking" and falsely elevate the apparent concentrations of amino acids in screening assays. Coffee with milk accidentally spilled on filter paper specimens adds lactose to the specimen and produces a false elevation indistinguishable from an increased blood galactose concentration, suggesting galactosemia. Frequent false positive reductions during summer months in blood spot galactose-1-phosphate uridyltransferase activity has been attributed to inactivation of the enzyme by humidity and/or heat (Frazier et al., 1992).

Confirmatory tests

Importantly, an abnormal screening test result, even when present on repeat testing, does not establish a specific diag-

nosis. An abnormality reflected by a positive screening test may have more than one possible genetic or non-genetic cause, and the etiology in each particular case must be ascertained. Confirmation of PKU, galactosemia and other inborn errors of metabolism requires not only additional diagnostic tests but also rigorous clinical diagnostic evaluation before an appropriate plan of management can be formulated. DNA testing for confirmation of diagnosis and identification of mutant alleles is increasingly available for screened disorders. Direct DNA testing for diagnosis and genetic counseling is available for PKU and galactosemia among the "traditional" metabolic disorders, as well as for congenital adrenal hyperplasia, cystic fibrosis and the hemoglobinopathies among the other disorders detectable by neonatal screening. A clear genotype/phenotype relationship has been described in some of the traditional metabolic disorders (e.g., galactosemia) and has been identified in congenital adrenal hyperplasia, cystic fibrosis and the hemoglobinopathies.

Potential problems in newborn screening

Several important potential problems can affect the interpretation of the screening results and should be considered when deciding whether an infant with clinical evidence of disease should have additional metabolic tests and, if so, which tests to order.

False-positive results

Most positive results in newborn screening are transient aberrations not caused by a metabolic disorder or any other pathologic state. In some instances, the transient abnormality is associated with an identifiable temporary influence, such as antibiotic therapy, prematurity or postprandial status, but often no cause is identified. These transient abnormalities are usually of mild degree. The cut-off or threshold level selected for the purpose of suspecting the presence of a metabolic disorder is usually a level that presumably will be exceeded by all affected infants. Inevitably, some unaffected infants will also manifest such levels, producing a range in which affected and unaffected infants will overlap. This means that repeat specimens will be requested from some normal infants.

The proportion of false positive results varies widely among the screening tests. In screening for PKU using the bacterial assay, for example, the ratio of false positive to true positive results is about 10:1. In screening for congenital adrenal hyperplasia, it may be as great as 100:1 because 17-hydroxyprogesterone, the analyte measured, is frequently increased transiently in premature infants (Pang and Clark, 1993). Galactosemia screening also yields a substantial proportion of false-positive results (Levy and Hammersen, 1978).

False-positive results not only produce great anxiety in the parents of infants thus identified, but also add to the expense and workload of newborn screening. Parental anxiety has been studied (Bodegard et al., 1983, Sorenson et al., 1984), and methods for reducing anxiety have been developed. Parents deserve simple and clear explanations of the reasons that the additional specimens are requested (Sorenson et al., 1984). Some newborn screening programs distribute specially prepared written explanations in advance to physicians or include them with requests for follow-up specimens.

A major advantage of new technologies is the potential for reducing false positive results. Tandem mass spectrometry provides a metabolite profile rather than only the single metabolite levels measured by the bacterial assays. In screening for PKU, for instance, it is the ratio of phenylalanine to tyrosine that best distinguishes the infant with PKU from the much larger number of infants with only transient hyperphenylalaninemia. Tandem mass spectrometry readily provides phenylalanine-to-tyrosine ratios (Chace et al., 1998) and ratios of the branched-chain amino acids to alanine that distinguish infants with maple syrup urine disease from those with transient increases in blood leucine concentration (Chace et al., 1995). DNA-based molecular testing as a secondary assay in newborn screening also substantially reduces false positive results in screening for galactosemia and cystic fibrosis (Levy and Albers, in press). In galactosemia, detecting the N314D allele indicating the Duarte variant, a frequent and benign variant, allows a positive initial metabolite screen to be identified as a "false positive" result rather than galactosemia (Urwin et al., 1997). In newborn screening for cystic fibrosis, mutation analysis is especially important for distinguishing the frequent transient increases in the primary screened metabolite, immunoreactive trypsinogen (IRT), from true cystic fibrosis. A secondary molecular assay for ΔF508, the mutant allele present on 70% of cystic fibrosis chromosomes (Gregg et al., 1997), eliminates most of the false positive results (Wilcken et al., 1995).

Early newborn screening

All newborn screening programs require or strongly recommend collection of the Guthrie specimen before the neonate is discharged from the hospital. This essentially guarantees that the newborn will be screened. Traditionally, the specimen would be obtained on the second or third day of life, but the increasing frequency with which newborns are discharged at or before 24 hours of age now means that many neonates are being screened "early" relative to the traditional parameters of newborn metabolic screening. Early discharge has revived concerns about missing affected infants by screening them prior to the time when their metabolic abnormality becomes detectable and has led to the recommendation for collection of a second blood specimen from infants initially tested at or before 24 hours (Editorial, 1994). Most disorders, including PKU, can be identified before 24 hours of age (Jew et al., 1994; DiGeorge, et al., 1982) but usually not much before that age. Biotinidase deficiency and galactosemia can also be detected in Guthrie specimens collected before 24 hours of age since the corresponding enzyme assays are not affected by the timing of specimen collection. In contrast, detection of some disorders is adversely affected by early specimen collection. For homocystinuria due to cystathionine β-synthase deficiency, the elevation of blood methionine concentration used to identify its presence usually does not develop until at least 24 hours of age (Peterschmitt et al., 1999). Detection of congenital hypothyroidism may also be compromised in the early specimen. The current trend is to insist on collection of the initial specimen at discharge regardless of age and to recommend the collection of a second Guthrie specimen at no later than seven days of age from infants discharged "early," that is, prior to 24 hours of age (see Table 30.3).

Table 30.3. Specimen Collection in Newborn Screening

Neonate	Initial Specimen	Repeat Specimen
Normal	≥24 hours	No
	<24 hours	≤7 days
Low birth weight	3 days	No
Transferred	At transfer	Discharge
Transfused	Before transfusion	2 months

Transferred and transfused infants

Failure to collect the newborn screening specimen is not uncommon among infants transferred to a special care nursery, especially when this transfer is to another hospital. Ironically, the transfer may be necessitated by the symptoms of a disease identifiable in routine screening, such as galactosemia (Dennehy et al., 1985) or maple syrup urine disease. To guard against this omission, the initial screening specimen should be collected before transfer and a second screening specimen collected at discharge (Table 30.3).

The infant who receives a blood transfusion is also vulnerable to missed diagnosis in newborn screening. Notably at risk are the diagnoses of galactosemia (Sokol et al., 1989) and sickle cell disease, both of which depend on identifiers in the red blood cell (viz. lack of galactose-1-P uridyltransferase enzyme activity and the presence of hemoglobin S, respectively). Donor erythrocytes in the transfused blood will mask these abnormalities by providing normal red blood cells to the affected infant. The initial screening specimen should be collected prior to any transfusion and a second screening specimen collected at about two months of age when the infant has replaced most of the donor erythrocytes with new red blood cells (Table 30.3).

Missed and uncovered disorders

A common misconception is that all infants with metabolic disorders for which newborn screening is conducted are detected in the screening process. Although the majority are detected, an occasional infant with PKU, congenital hypothyroidism or another screened disorder is missed (McCabe, 1992). The reasons these infants have been missed are debated. Delay in appearance of the identifier (e.g., lack of elevated blood methionine in homocystinuria) is certainly one reason (Peterschmitt et al., 1999), but laboratory error is often the culprit (Holtzman et al., 1986). Despite the presumption of a normal newborn screen or even the presence of a normal newborn screening report, it is important to consider the possibility that an infant with a clinical phenotype compatible with one of the screened

metabolic disorders is indeed affected with the disorder. This can avoid delays in diagnosis and treatment. Evaluation of these patients should include tests for all relevant metabolic disorders, *without excluding* the ones covered by newborn screening.

Misconceptions about newborn screening also extend to the range of coverage for metabolic disorders. Knowledge that newborn screening includes metabolic disorders can be misinterpreted as indicating that *all* metabolic disorders are covered. This misinterpretation can lead to the omission of metabolic testing in a clinically abnormal infant who otherwise would receive these tests, resulting in delays in metabolic diagnosis and therapy.

Disorders and conditions detected by newborn blood screening

The estimated frequencies of metabolic disorders or conditions detectable by newborn blood screening are listed in Table 30.4. The number of states screening for the disorders is shown in Table 30.2. Although detailed descriptions of these disorders are beyond the scope of this chapter, aspects especially pertinent to screening are considered below.

Phenylketonuria and hyperphenylalaninemias

As in many inherited disorders, the detection of a primary abnormality, hyperphenylalaninemia, requires the consideration of a spectrum of possible genetic causes before proper diagnosis and management are possible. The failure to appreciate that several disorders as well as benign metabolic conditions can cause hyperphenylalaninemia was a serious early problem in newborn metabolic screening (Committee for the Study of Inborn Errors of Metabolism 1975; Erbe 1981).

Table 30.4. Frequencies of Some Metabolic Disorders and Conditions Detected by Screening Newborn Blood

Disorder or Condition	Frequency
Hyperphenylalaninemias	
PKU	1:13,000
Other hyperphenylalaninemia	1:20,000
Galactosemia	1:50,000
Biotinidase deficiency	1:72,000
Maple syrup urine disease	1:70,000
Hypermethioninemia (homocystinuria)	1:200,000
Hereditary tyrosinemia	Very low

Frequent causes of hyperphenylalaninemia (Scriver et al., 1995): .

1. Transient hyperphenylalaninemia
2. Persistent non-PKU hyperphenylalaninemia
3. PKU
4. Three disorders causing defective tetrahydrobiopterin synthesis
5. Impaired recycling of tetrahydrobiopterin due to dihydropteridine reductase deficiency.

The phenylalanine concentration in newborn blood is normally less than 120 μM (2 mg/dL). The Guthrie bacterial inhibition assay is considered to be positive when the phenylalanine concentration exceeds 120 μM or 240 μM, depending on which cut-off level is used by the screening laboratory. Positive screening results should be followed promptly by confirmatory tests of blood and urine. Complete amino acid analysis of blood can confirm the elevated phenylalanine and reduced tyrosine concentrations, and rule out the presence of other amino acid abnormalities. Additional blood spots on filter paper should be collected and submitted for measurement of dihydropteridine reductase (DHPR) deficiency. A random specimen of urine should be collected and submitted for pterin analysis. The diagnosis of PKU is generally assigned when: (a) the blood phenylalanine concentrations are 1200 μM (20 mg/dL) or greater in confirmatory follow-up tests while the infant is ingesting a diet normal for age, (b) the tyrosine concentration in blood is no greater than 250 μM (5 mg/dL), and (c) the analyses of DHPR activity in blood and pterins in urine yield normal results. Phenylalanine metabolites, such as phenylpyruvic acid and orthohydroxyphenylacetic acid, may be present but are often absent in neonates with PKU. Mild forms of PKU produce phenylalanine concentrations of 600–1200 μM (10–20 mg/dL). When these criteria are met, a phenylalanine-restricted diet should be instituted promptly in order to prevent the mental retardation seen in untreated PKU.

Classical PKU is due to deficiency of hepatic phenylalanine hydroxylase and must be distinguished from the approximately two percent of hyperphenylalaninemic newborns with defects in tetrahydrobiopterin (BH$_4$) synthesis or recycling. These BH$_4$-deficiency disorders are characterized by hyperphenylalaninemia with progressive neurological deterioration despite dietary phenylalanine restriction (Scriver et al., 1995). Since BH$_4$ is required as a cofactor for phenylalanine hydroxylation, BH$_4$ deficiency results in impaired conversion of phenylalanine to tyrosine. Tyrosine and tryptophan hydroxylases also require BH$_4$, so the conversions of tyrosine to DOPA and tryptophan to 5-hydroxy-

tryptophan are also impaired, thus disrupting synthesis of the neurotransmitters dopamine and serotonin, respectively. A number of patients and families with DHPR deficiency have been collected and studied (Blau et al., 1996), allowing characterization of the heterogeneity and identification of effective therapy. Moreover, the genes for these enzymes have been cloned and several mutations characterized (Scriver et al., 1995).

Since the degrees of hyperphenylalaninemia and the usual clinical manifestations of PKU, DHPR deficiency and the BH$_4$ synthesis deficiencies are similar during the newborn period, accurate diagnosis requires a combination of *in vivo* and *in vitro* tests (Scriver et al., 1995). Although phenylalanine hydroxylase (PAH) activity can be assayed only in the liver, DHPR can be assayed in a filter paper blood specimen (Surplice et al., 1990) as well as in white blood cells, cultured skin fibroblasts and amniotic fluid cells. Urine pterin analysis will distinguish the BH$_4$ synthesis defects on the basis of markedly altered (low) biopterin:neopterin (B:N) ratio. It must be emphasized that all hyperphenylalaninemic subjects identified in newborn screening programs must be appropriately studied to distinguish those with blocks in BH$_4$ generation or conservation who will require more complex therapy from the 97 to 99% of hyperphenylalaninemic newborns who will either respond to phenylalanine-restricted diets or who have mild hyperphenylalaninemia not needing treatment.

Hyperphenylalaninemias not due to PKU or BH$_4$ deficiency are generally associated with lesser elevations of the plasma phenylalanine concentration. Most of these infants have transient hyperphenylalaninemia, which disappears in the first months of life and requires no specific therapy (O'Flynn et al., 1980). In some instances, the hyperphenylalaninemia is accompanied by transient hypertyrosinemia. Other infants, however, will have persistent mild hyperphenylalaninemia. This will be accompanied by a normal tyrosine concentration. Mild hyperphenylalaninemia has been considered benign (Levy et al., 1971; Waisbren et al., 1984). Data have suggested that those with persisting blood phenylalanine levels of 600 μM (10 mg/dL) or greater who have remained untreated have reduced IQs (Costello et al., 1994), but this conclusion has been disputed by another group of investigators (Weglage et al., 1997).

Although most newborns with PKU have plasma phenylalanine concentrations above 360 μM when first tested, occasional phenylketonuric newborns have much milder elevations on initial testing, especially if prior protein intake is low or the infant is discharged early from the nursery. Accordingly, concerns about possible false negative initial

PKU tests have been raised and routine retesting has been recommended in some programs (Meryash et al., 1981). Sepe et al., (1979) surveyed by questionnaire the results of routine follow-up blood screening of infants for PKU in the 13 states that conduct such studies. Some 2,382,300 routine follow-up blood specimens were obtained from infants aged two to six weeks, and eleven of these infants, or 1:217,000, were found to have persistent hyperphenylalaninemia not detected by the initial newborn screening. Seven of these infants had milder forms of hyperphenylalaninemia that did not require treatment, while four had PKU. This analysis of follow-up blood specimens showed that additional cases of PKU were detected at a frequency of 1:596 000 which increased the cost for each PKU case found to $263,000 or 30 times the $8700 cost of identifying an infant with PKU by routine screening. The survey also clearly indicated that incomplete testing poses a problem. Based on the observed compliance rate of only 80% for initial testing, it was estimated that some 640,000 infants each year in the US were not tested at that time and 54 of these would be expected to have PKU.

Maternal PKU can be detected by cord blood or prenatal testing (Levy and Waisbren, 1983). The importance of this condition stems from the occurrence of mental retardation in the non-phenylketonuric offspring of mothers with PKU. Lenke and Levy (1980) collected data on 524 pregnancies in 155 women having PKU or other forms of hyperphenylalaninemia. A slightly higher than expected rate of spontaneous abortion was found but, much more significantly, the 423 live-born offspring showed a marked increase in the frequencies of mental retardation, microcephaly and congenital heart disease. Indeed, of mothers having blood phenylalanine concentrations of 1200 μM (20 mg/dL) or greater, one or more of their children were mentally retarded in 95% of instances. Data from several studies, including the Maternal PKU Collaborative Study, indicate that diet begun before conception with maintenance of good metabolic control throughout pregnancy may be associated with a good outcome (Ghavami et al., 1986; Waisbren et al., 2000).

Galactosemia

At least three disorders of galactose metabolism are detectable in newborn screening. They are appropriate targets for newborn screening because of the need for early intervention. The most frequent of these disorders is classical transferase deficient galactosemia due to deficiency of galactose-1-phosphate uridyltransferase (GALT), an enzyme which is normally present in most tissues, including liver, skin fibroblasts and red blood cells (Segal and Berry, 1995). In this disorder GALT activity is undetectable. The untreated clinical course is characterized in the neonate by failure to thrive, jaundice, hepatomegaly and often death from sepsis, especially due to *E. coli* (Levy et al., 1977). Untreated infants who survive suffer from developmental retardation, cirrhosis and cataracts. Early diagnosis can lead to effective treatment that prevents neonatal death and blunts the later complications. Hence, screening is needed. Moreover, even when the infant is obviously ill, the correct clinical diagnosis of this rare inborn error of metabolism is often not made by the attending physicians.

Several variant forms of GALT deficiency have been described (Segal and Berry, 1995; Segal 1998). In the African-American variant, associated with the S135L (leucine replaces serine at amino acid 135) mutant GALT allele, low but detectable levels of GALT activity are present in liver and intestinal mucosa but not erythrocytes, and the clinical course may be milder. Variants such as Rennes and Indiana may be associated with some or all of the serious clinical abnormalities. The Duarte (D2) variant, associated with the N314D (asparagine replaces aspartate at amino acid 135) mutant allele, is characterized by diminished erythrocyte GALT activity and altered electrophoretic mobility of the enzyme without clinical abnormalities.

The other galactose metabolic disorders are galactokinase deficiency and uridine diphosphate galactose-4-epimerase deficiency. These are much less frequent than transferase deficiency galactosemia. Galactokinase deficiency leads to cataract formation in older untreated patients without other evidence of galactose toxicity, while epimerase deficiency seldom produces clinical abnormalities. Treatment of galactosemia due to either GALT deficiency or galactokinase deficiency aims at rigorous exclusion of galactose from the diet and, if instituted early, is completely effective in preventing or reversing the serious neonatal abnormalities (Segal and Berry, 1995; Segal, 1998). In contrast, even early and continuous dietary galactose restriction in galactosemia appears to have little impact on the risk of abnormal speech, intellectual and neurological functions, and ovarian function which often develop later in the child and adult (Segal, 1998).

Homocystinuria (cystathionine β-synthase deficiency)

The screening of over 30 million newborns by the Guthrie bacterial inhibition assay for methionine has led to the detection of approximately 150 infants with cystathionine β-synthase (CBS) deficient homocystinuria. CBS normally condenses L-homocysteine and L-serine to cystathionine, using pyridoxal-5′-phosphate as a cofactor. CBS deficiency is the most frequently encountered cause of homocystinuria, is inherited in an autosomal recessive pattern and may result in clinical abnormalities that include mental retardation, ectopia lentis, thromboembolism affecting large and small arteries, and skeletal abnormalities. Treatment includes a diet that is restricted in methionine and supplemented with cystine, and, in those patients responsive to pyridoxine, pharmacological doses of the vitamin. Treatment with orally administered betaine has also proved effective in reducing the level of homocysteinemia in many patients (Mudd et al., 1995).

Some cases of CBS deficiency have escaped detection by newborn screening and this has raised concerns about possible slow rises in blood methionine (Levy, 1973). The blood methionine concentration may not exceed normal (1 mg/dL) until after the first week of life in CBS-deficient infants. Lowering the methionine level in screening from the usual 2 mg/dL to 1 mg/dL has resulted in detecting affected infants screened before 48 hours of age who otherwise would have been missed in New England (Peterschmitt et al., 1999). Conversely, later in the neonatal period normal infants may have methionine elevations to 4 mg/dL or greater that are usually transient and related to a high protein diet (Levy, 1973). Other causes of hypermethioninemia include liver disease, tyrosinemia (see below) and, methionine adenosyltransferase deficiency (Mudd et al., 1995; Chamberlin et al., 2000). Homocystinuria and homocysteinemia also result from defects in the metabolism of folates and cobalamins that are required for the transmethylation of homocysteine to methionine (Erbe, 1986; Fenton and Rosenberg, 1995; Rosenblatt, 1995). In these conditions, the concentration of methionine is low or normal, even though the concentrations of homocysteine and related compounds are increased. Consequently, these remethylation disorders escape detection in newborn screening which is limited to detecting increased methionine and not homocyst(e)ine.

Maple syrup urine disease

Identifying increased leucine in newborn screening has allowed detection of some instances of maple syrup urine disease (MSUD). This disorder results from deficient activity of one or more enzymes involved in the oxidative decarboxylation of the α-keto acid derivatives of leucine, isoleucine and valine (Chuang and Shih, 1995). Although apparently healthy at birth, the newborn with MSUD begins to feed poorly by the end of the first week. This is followed by vomiting, lethargy, muscular hypertonicity,

seizures, coma, and death. A distinctive urinary odor resembling maple syrup accompanies the clinical abnormalities. With dramatic severity, the clinical illness can lead to death before the true nature of the disorder is recognized. Levy (1973) has suggested that MSUD may be underdiagnosed because the acute neonatal illness may lead to retention in the hospital and a fatal delay in submission of the appropriate specimens for newborn screening. Attempts at treatment have involved complicated diets which have been partially successful (Chuang and Shih, 1995). Several variants of MSUD with milder clinical and biochemical abnormalities have been described (Chuang and Shih, 1995). A transient elevation (6 mg/dL or greater) of the blood leucine concentration occurs in 0.1 to 0.2% of newborns screened.

Tyrosinemia

While screening for tyrosinemia is formally included in only a few programs, other programs routinely measure tyrosine concentrations in confirmatory testing for hyperphenylalaninemia. In at least 1 to 2% of infants the blood tyrosine concentration exceeds 5 mg/dL at some time during the first three months of life. The frequency is even higher in premature babies (Levy, 1973). This transient tyrosinemia usually disappears spontaneously within a few weeks, and its disappearance can often be promoted by administering vitamin C or with a protein-restricted diet (Mitchell et al., 1995).

Persistent tyrosinemia is caused by at least two inherited disorders. Tyrosinemia I (hereditary tyrosinemia) is an autosomal recessively inherited disorder in which the primary enzyme defect is deficiency of fumarylacetoacetate hydrolase (FAH), the final enzyme in the degradation of tyrosine (Mitchell et al., 1995). The prevalence of this disorder is unusually high in the Quebec province of Canada. The clinical presentations and course are quite variable but the most serious abnormalities are in liver and kidney, the main sites in which toxic tyrosine metabolites accumulate. Tyrosine and methionine metabolism are disturbed, with marked excretion of the p-hydroxyphenyl acids (termed tyrosyluria) and renal tubular defects resulting in hyperphosphaturia, rickets, mellituria, proteinuria and generalized aminoaciduria (Mitchell et al., 1995). The presence of succinylacetone in urine or blood is pathognomonic. Dietary restriction of phenylalanine and tyrosine does not prevent progression of liver disease and approximately one-third of affected individuals develop hepatocellular carcinoma, often in childhood. Liver transplantation was previously the only option for these patients. Lindstedt et al., (1992) introduced treatment with 2-(2-nitro-4-trifluoromethylbenzoyl-)-1,3-cyclohexanedione (NTBC), a potent inhibitor of 4-hydroxyphenylpyruvate dioxygenase, the enzyme catalyzing an early step in tyrosine catabolism. Inhibition of this enzyme reduces the accumulation of toxic metabolities produced more distally in the pathway. NTBC therapy has been helpful in many patients but transplantation of liver or liver and kidney may be needed for patients unresponsive to NTBC and those with hepatic nodules, neurologic crises and hepatic or renal failure (Paradis, 1996; Mohan et al., 1999).

Tyrosinemia type II, also called the Richner-Hanhart syndrome, results from deficiency of hepatic tyrosine aminotransferase and has been reported in fewer than 100 cases (Buist et al., 1985; Mitchell et al., 1995). Blood tyrosine concentrations are 20–50 mg/dL on an unrestricted diet. Mental retardation is present in all cases, but hepatic and renal disease are absent. Other clinical abnormalities include keratitis and palmar hyperkeratosis. Over 1.7 million newborns in six countries were screened without finding a single instance of this disorder, reflecting either its very low frequency or the occurrence of false negatives due to a delayed rise in the blood tyrosine concentration or both (Levy 1973).

Other inherited disorders may lead to an elevation of the blood tyrosine concentration when the infant is ill. Notable among these are transferase deficiency galactosemia and hereditary fructose intolerance due to deficiency of fructose-1,6-biphosphate aldolase in liver, kidney cortex and small intestine. Both of these disorders elevate blood tyrosine concentration by deleterious effects on hepatic metabolism. Since liver disease of any cause can elevate the blood tyrosine concentration, detecting either tyrosinemia or hypermethioninemia may simply signal the presence of liver disease.

Biotinidase deficiency

Biotinidase deficiency can be detected in newborns who, if treated with pharmacological doses of biotin, do not develop the otherwise serious or even fatal abnormalities seen in some untreated patients. Biotinidase deficiency show a wide range of phenotypic severity, and the basis for this variation is incompletely known. Biotin is a water-soluble vitamin that acts as a prosthetic group for four carboxylases required for the catabolism of several branched-chain amino acids, for the first step of gluconeogenesis and for the synthesis of fatty acids (Wolf, 1995). These carboxylases are normally activated by covalent enzymic attachment of biotin. One biotin-containing product of the eventual pro-

teolytic degradation of these carboxylases is known as biocytin. Normally biotinidase hydrolytically releases biotin from biocytin, allowing some of the biotin to be recycled. In biotinidase deficiency the biotin is not released, leading to intracellular deficiency of biotin.

Biotinidase deficiency is inherited in an autosomal recessive pattern (Wolf, 1995). Most symptomatic children have profound biotinidase deficiency. The frequency of the deficiency in newborns has varied between studies but the incidence of the profound deficiency (less than 10% of mean normal serum activity) is estimated at about 1:137,400 and the incidence of partial deficiency at about 1:109,900, for a combined incidence of 1:61,000 (Wolf, 1991). Although some mutant alleles of the biotinidase gene (BTD) have been identified on a research basis (Norrgard et al., 1999), genotype/phenotype correlations are incomplete and confirmation of diagnosis continues to be by assay of biotinidase activity.

Biotinidase deficient persons may become biotin deficient during infancy or early childhood (Wolf, 1995). Signs and symptoms are mainly neurological and cutaneous, and include seizures, feeding and breathing problems, ataxia, hearing loss, hypotonia, developmental delay, skin rash and alopecia. Symptomatic individuals with profound deficiency usually also manifest metabolic acidosis, hyperammonemia and organic aciduria. Metabolic decompensation can terminate in coma and death. Symptomatic children with biotinidase deficiency have consistently responded to treatment with biotin. Importantly, biotinidase deficiency must be differentiated from holocarboxylase deficiency with which it shares many clinical and biochemical features (Wolf, 2000).

URINE

Analysis of urine specimens

Filter paper urine specimens can be analyzed either by unidimensional paper chromatography (Efron et al., 1964), as was formerly done in Massachusetts (Levy et al., 1980) and New South Wales, Australia (Wilcken et al., 1980), or by unidimensional thin-layer chromatography as is still being done in Quebec (Lemieux et al., 1988). In the Massachusetts program two 1/4 inch diameter discs were punched from each filter paper, one analyzed for amino acids by overnight descending chromatography and ninhydrin stain and the other analyzed for methylmalonic acid by ascending chromatography developed with o-dianisidine reagent. Each sheet of chromatography paper accommodated 25 specimens plus appropriate reference standards. The identification, analysis and interpretation of suspected abnormalities have been described in detail (Levy et al., 1980), as have the procedures for follow-up and management.

Confirmatory tests

A variety of confirmatory tests are available depending on the specific disorder or condition suspected. These include spot tests of urine for specific compounds, two-dimensional chromatography electrophoresis and gas chromatography-mass spectrometry. Tests of blood and specific enzyme assays of fluids or cells may also be appropriate.

Frequency of disorders detected by newborn urine screening

Some metabolic disorders and conditions that are not screened by most current methods for analyzing blood specimens are detected by screening newborn urine. Several of these disorders are medically important and can be treated. In other cases, newborn urine screening yields abnormal results but information to assess the natural history, medical significance and management of the disorder is incomplete. Examples of such findings of uncertain significance include cystathioninemia (1:70,000) (Mudd et al., 1995), hyperlysinemia (Phang et al., 1995) and sarcosinemia (1:350,000 in New England, 1:28,000 in Quebec) (Scott, 1995). Several conditions detected are probably benign, including iminoglycinuria (1:12,000) (Chesney, 1995), histidinemia (1:20,000) (Levy et al., 1995), Hartnup disorder (Levy, 1995) (1:25,000) and type I hyperprolinemia (1:200,000) (Phang et al., 1995; see also Table 30.5). Three of the disorders or conditions screened in urine involve defects in renal transport rather than traditional inborn errors of metabolism, viz. cystinuria (Segal and Their, 1995), iminoglycinuria (Chesney, 1995) and

Hartnup aminoaciduria (Levy, 1995). In most other disorders involving aminoaciduria an extrarenal metabolic disturbance leads to accumulation in plasma of one or more amino acids which are filtered in amounts that exceed the reabsorption capacity of the nephron. Blood screening by tandem mass spectrometry now identifies several disorders previously identifiable only by urine screening (e.g., methylmalonic acidemia, citrullinemia, argininosuccinic acidemia).

Other newborn screening

Newborn screening programs in varying numbers of states screen for additional inherited and acquired disorders including congenital adrenal hyperplasia (18 programs), cystic fibrosis (six programs), hemoglobinopathies, hypothyroidism and toxoplasmosis (two programs). Screening for congenital adrenal hyperplasia (CAH) became technically feasible in 1977 when Pang et al., (1977) introduced an immunoassay using Guthrie specimens to measure 17-hydroxyprogesterone (17-OHP) in order to detect CAH due to 21-hydroxylase deficiency, which accounts for over 90% of all cases (New et al., 1995). Nationwide and regional screening programs for CAH were subsequently introduced in several countries (Pang and Clark, 1993). Worldwide incidence of CAH was estimated at 1:15,000 live births, with the salt-wasting form comprising 75% of the total and often causing hypovolemic shock and death in newborns, and the simple-virilizing form, which does not result in spontaneous hypovolemia, comprising 25% (Pang et al., 1988). Initial screening is by immunoassay for 17-OHP, a second screen is performed in some programs, and the cut-off levels among programs, especially as they relate to premature or low-birthweight newborns. Follow up is often by referral to a medical consultant. Neonatal screening aims to prevent deaths from delayed recognition and treatment of the salt-wasting form, to prevent sex misassignment of affected female newborns that can occur with either the salt-wasting or simple-virilizing forms, and possibly to prevent premature epiphyseal closure in children with simple-virilizing CAH (Thilén et al., 1998, Therrell et al., 1998).

The technical feasibility of screening newborns for cystic fibrosis by measuring the serum immunoreactive trypsin in dried blood has been established (Hammond et al., 1987). Moreover, accurate methods are available for the prenatal diagnosis of cystic fibrosis and the identification of carriers by means of direct DNA and linkage analyses. A three base

Table 30.5. Frequencies of Some Metabolic Disorders and Conditions Detected by screening Newborn Urine

Disorder or Condition	Frequency
Cystinuria	1:8,000
Iminoglycinuria	1:12,000
Histidinemia	1:20,000
Hartnup disease	1:25,000
Methylmalonic aciduria	1:50,000
Cystathioninuria	1:70,000
Argininosuccinic aciduria	1:90,000
Hyperglycaemia, nonketotic	1:180,000
Hyperprolinemia	1:200,000

deletion, designated ΔFS08, is found in approximately 70% of the cystic fibrosis chromosomes from patients of northern European ancestry and is present in smaller proportions of cystic fibrosis chromosomes from patients from other populations (The Cystic Fibrosis Genetic Analysis Consortium, 1990). Over 800 additional mutant alleles have been identified, but only a few of these occur in as much as several percent of CF chromosomes, most occurring exclusively in the families in which they were originally identified. Current genotyping strategies allow the identification of the specific mutant alleles in the majority of affected homozygotes and compound heterozygotes, while direct analysis combined with linkage analyses can provide accurate genotyping in nearly all of the remaining families.

Newborn cystic fibrosis screening has been initiated in several countries (Hammond et al., 1987). Both short-and long-term benefits have been claimed. The most convincing evidence of a short-term benefit was the demonstration by Wilcken and Brown that the number of hospital days during the first two years of life required by children with cystic fibrosis identified by screening 400,000 newborns in Australia was lower for the screened patients than in unscreened historical controls (Wilcken and Brown, 1987). As a result of this study, cystic fibrosis has been added to several newborn screening programs (Wilcken, 1993). In other respects, it is not yet established that early diagnosis and treatment will significantly improve the morbidity and mortality of cystic fibrosis. The randomized controlled trial of newborn screening in Wisconsin has suggested improved nutritional status and larger head circumference in children identified early by screening and treated (Farrell et al., 1997). Long-term results, however, have not yet been reported.

Most programs in the United States screen newborns for hemoglobinopathies, particularly those involving sickle hemoglobin. The initial screen is most frequently by means of isoelectric focusing, less often by high performance liquid chromatography (HPLC) or cellulose acetate electrophoresis. Confirmatory testing also uses these methods and programs are increasingly adding genotyping by DNA analysis for this purpose. The early identification of infants with one of the sickling hemoglobinopathies coupled with aggressive follow-up has been shown to result in a significant reduction of mortality during the early years when the risks are especially great (Vichinsky et al., 1988). Moreover, the investigators in the multicenter oral penicillin prophylaxis trial achieved an 84% reduction in the incidence of pneumococcal disease, a major cause of early morbidity and mortality in the sickling disorders, by means of inexpensive and safe treatment with penicillin (Gaston et al., 1986). In addition to the treatment of affected newborns and genetic counseling of their parents, some programs attempt to follow up the parents of carrier newborns in order to identify and counsel those couples in which both are carriers. When ascertained by means of carrier screening in a large program, only a small percentage of those couples whose offspring are at risk for a serious globin disorder have chosen to use prenatal diagnosis (Loader et al., 1991). In contrast, ascertainment of 28 at-risk pregnant women in a large newborn hemoglobinopathy screening program led to amniocentesis in 14 and elective termination of three of the four affected pregnancies (Grover et al., 1986). Screening programs outside major metropolitan areas face the issue of whether to screen all newborns, accepting the additional costs and problems that accompany increasing program size, or to attempt to identify and screen only those newborns considered to be at risk, based on racial or other criteria.

Congenital hypothyroidism screening began in 1974 with the introduction by Dussault (Dussault et al., 1975) of a radioimmunoassay applicable to the newborn filter paper blood specimens. Congenital hypothyroidism screening is now part of many programs and has had the interesting effect of promoting regionalization of screening since the immunoassays used for hypothyroidism are technically more complicated than the tests used for inborn error screening. In this procedure the initial test involves measurement of the newborn blood thyroxine (T_4) concentration. A filter paper disc of dried blood is incubated with labeled T_4 and anti-T_4 antibodies and an inhibitor of thyroxine binding globulin. A low blood T_4 concentration leads to greater labeled T_4 binding by the anti-T_4 antibody and reduced amounts of unbound labeled T_4. Following separation of the bound and unbound fractions, the measurement of activity in each fraction allows estimation of the blood T_4 concentration. The procedure can be automated and the data analysis completed by computer. Commonly the detection of a T_4 value two standard deviations or more below the mean is followed by measurement of the concentration of thyroid stimulating hormone (TSH) by radioimmunoassay using another disc from the blood sample. When both a low T_4 and an elevated TSH concentration are detected, the newborn's parents and physician are advised regarding the need for additional testing and possible treatment (Glorieux et al., 1992). This approach requires TSH testing in 3% of newborns and identifies congenital hypothyroidism in approximately 1:3600–5000 newborns (Rovet and Ehrlich, 2000). Although commonly combined with newborn screening for principally genetic disorders, only a few of the etiologies of congenital hypothyroidism are mendelian (Vassart et al., 1995).

Other disorders considered for screening include α_1-antitrypsin deficiency (Sveger, 1978), Duchenne muscular dystrophy (Lemieux, 1987), adenosine deaminase deficiency (Moore and Meuwissen, 1974), and hyperlipidemia (Wilcken, 1987). Their ultimate place in newborn screening programs remains to be established.

Issues and concerns in screening

Most screening tests are designed to be sensitive in order to minimize false-negative results, but these tests may not be specific and they are seldom diagnostic. Accurate and definitive diagnosis requires additional testing in nearly all instances. Since false negative results do occur with every screening procedure, a negative result from screening should not preclude an appropriate evaluation for a disorder suspected clinically.

Screening programs and procedures should meet a variety of criteria both before they are implemented and continually during their operation (Committee for the Study of Inborn Errors of Metabolism, 1975). These criteria include technical, educational and organizational aspects. A high signal-to-noise ratio is needed to maximize effectiveness and minimize adverse effects. The noise in the system includes the true biological variation of the character being measured in the screened population and the variation within the testing procedure itself. In addition to normal biological variation and transient abnormalities, confusing artifacts are produced by contamination of blood and urine specimens with micro-organisms, drugs used systemically or locally, diaper powder, food supplements and the like. Disentangling these sources of confusion and delay requires great expertise. As noted earlier, positive results in a screening test necessitate repeat testing with follow-up and additional testing, possibly over a period of weeks or months. These can be expensive in terms of personnel, materials and parental anxiety and inconvenience (Sorenson et al., 1984; Fyro and Bodegard, 1987). The rarer the trait being sought by screening, the higher will be the proportion of false positives.

Finally, screening programs should be organized and administered in such a way that they are constantly updated to incorporate the latest technical and medical advances. They must also be responsive to changes in society. After several decades with few fundamental changes in neonatal screening programs, the recent discussions centered on the potential advantages and limitations of screening based on tandem mass spectrometry (MS-MS) has stimulated much debate and discussion. Advocacy groups consisting of professionals, parents of affected children and others have increasingly appealed to screening programs themselves and to state legislatures for the addition of MS-MS screening. Claims have been made that a half dozen or more disorders not detected by other screening methods could be detected by MS-MS. Interest has focused particularly on the rare disorder, glutaric acidemia type 1 (GA1) (Goodman and Frerman, 1995), and medium chain acyl-CoA dehydrogenase deficiency (MCAD), a more common disorder (Roe and Coates, 1995). These two disorders are characterized by abrupt onset of symptoms in early childhood. The initial acute episode in GA1 may result in severe, irreversible neurological abnormalities, and may be fatal in one-quarter to one-third of MCAD cases. Evidence suggests that most newborns affected with these disorders could be identified by MS-MS screening and that prompt metabolic management could prevent the initial acute episode in many or possibly most cases. In both disorders the interval between birth and the first episode is sufficiently long to allow an appropriate metabolic program to be implemented.

The introduction of MS-MS technologies in several of the larger screening programs has stimulated a major reevaluation of newborn metabolic screening after many years of relative constancy. The widespread inclusion of this or other new technologies in screening programs requires that the traditional questions and the issues be addressed. Is the frequency of the disorder detected sufficiently great to justify screening? Are the genetic heterogeneity, expression and natural history of the disorder well characterized? Is an effective treatment available and, if so, must it begin shortly after birth or will it be equally effective if started later? What is the detection rate, and what are the frequencies of false positive and false negative screening test results? Is the screen cost-effective? Discussions and debates regarding the claims, issues and concerns about disorders and conditions to be screened will likely produce major and extensive changes in screening programs over the next few years.

REFERENCES

Bickle H, Gerrard JW, Hickmans EM (1954) Influence of phenylalanine intake an the chemistry and behaviour of a phenylketonuric child. Acta Pediatr 43:64–77

Blau N, Barnes I, Dhondt JL (1996) International database of tetrahydrobiopterin deficiencies. J Inherited Metabolic Diseases 19:8–14

Bodegard G, Fyro K, Larsson A (1983) Psychological reactors in 102 families with a newborn who has a falsely positive secrening test for congenital hypoparathyroidism. Acta Pediatr Scand, suppl. 304

Buist NRM, Kennaway NG, Fellman JH (1985) Tyrosinemia type II: Hepatic cytosol tyrosine aminotransferase deficiency (the "Richner-Hanhart syndrome"). In Bickel H, Wachtel U (eds): Inherited Diseases of Amino Acid Metabolism. George Thieme, Stuttgart, p. 203

Chace DH, Naylor EW (1999) Expansion of newborn screening programs using tandem mass spectrometry. Mental Retardation and Developmental Disability Research Review 5:150–154

Chace DH, Hillman SL, Millington DS et al. (1995) Rapid diagnosis of maple syrup urine disease in blood spots from newborns by tandem mass spectrometry. Clin Chem 41:62–68

Chace DH, Sherwin JE, Hillman SL et al. (1998) Use of phenylalanine-to-tyrosine ratio determined by tandem mass spectrometry to improve newborn screening for phenylketonuria of early discharge specimens collected in the first 24 hours. Clin Chem 44(12):2405–2409

Chamberlin ME, Ubagai T, Mudd SH et al. (2000) Methionine adenosyltransferase I/III deficiency: Novel mutations and clinical variations. Am J Hum Gen 66(2):347–55

Chuang DT, Shih VE (1995) Disorders of branched chain amino acid and keto acid metabolism. In Scriver CR, Beaudet AL, Sly WS, Valle D (eds): The Metabolic and Molecular Bases of Inherited Disease, 7th edn. McGraw-Hill, NY, pp. 1239–1277

Chesney RW (1995) Iminoglycinuria. In Scriver CR, Beaudet AL, Sly WS, Valle D (eds): The Metabolic and Molecular Bases of Inherited Disease, 7th edn. McGraw-Hill, NY, pp. 3643–3653

Committee for the Study of Inborn Errors of Metabolism (1975) Genetic Screening Programs, Principles and Research. National Academy of Sciences, Washington, DC

Costello PM, Beasley MG, Tillotson SL, Smith I (1994) Intelligence in mild atypical phenylketonuria. Eur J Pediatr 153:260–263

Dennehy PH, O'Shea PA, Abuelo DN (1985) A newborn with bilious vomiting and jitteriness. J Pediatr 106:161–166

DiGeorge AM, Rezvani I, Garibaldi LR, Schwartz M (1982) Prospective study of maple-syrup-urine disease for the first four days of life. N Eng J Med 307:1492–1495

Dussault JH, Coulombe P, Laberge C et al. (1975) Preliminary report on a mass screening program for neonatal hypothyroidism. J Pediatr 86:670–674

Editorial (1994) Early discharge from the newborn nursery. A potential threat to effective newborn screening. Screening 3:45–48

Efron ML, Young D, Moser HW, MacCready RA (1964) A simple chromatographic screening test for the detection of disorders of amino acid metabolism. N Engl J Med 270:1378–1383

Erbe RW (1981) Issues in newborn screening. In Bloom AD, James LS (eds): The Fetus and the Newborn (Birth Defects Original Article Series, Vol. 17). Liss, NY, pp. 167–179

Erbe RW (1986) Inborn errors of folate metabolism. In Blakley RL, Whitehead VM (eds): Folates and Pterins. Vol. 3: Nutritional, Pharmacological and Physiological Aspects. Wiley, NY, pp. 413–465

Farrell PM, Kosorok MR, Laxova A et al. (1997) Nutritional benefits of neonatal screening for cystic fibrosis. Wisconsin Cystic Fibrosis Neonatal Screening Study Group. N Engl J Med 337(14):963–369

Fenton WA, Rosenberg LE (1995) Disorders of propionate and methylmalonate metabolism. In Scriver CR, Beaudet AL, Sly WS, Valle D (eds): The Metabolic and Molecular Bases of Inherited Disease, 7th edn. McGraw-Hill, NY, pp. 1423–1449

Fenton WA, Rosenberg LE (1995) Inherited disorders of cobalamin transport and metabolism. In Scriver CR, Beaudet AL, Sly WS, Valle D (eds): The Metabolic and Molecular Bases of Inherited Disease, 7th edn. McGraw-Hill, NY, pp. 3129–3149

Fölling A (1934) Uber Ausscheidung von Phenylbrenztraubensaure in den Harn als Stoffwechselanomalie in Verbindung mit Imbezilliat. Hoppe Seyler Zeitschrift für Physiologische Chemie 227:169–176

Frazier DM, Clemons EH, Kirkman HN (1992) Minimizing false positive diagnoses in newborn screening for galactosemia. Biochem Med Metab Bio 48:199–211

Fyro K, Bodegard G (1987) Four-year follow-up of psychological reactions to false positive screening tests for congenital hypothyroidism. Acta Paediatrica Scandinavica 1987 76(1):107–14

Gaston MH, Verter JI, Woods G et al. (1986) Prophylaxis with oral penicillin in children with sickle cell anemia. A randomized trial. N Eng J Med 314(25):1593–1599

Ghavami M, Levy HL, Erbe RW (1986) Prevention of fetal damage through dietary control of maternal hyperphenylalaninemia. Clin Obstet Gynecol 29:580–585

Glorieux J, Dussault J, Van Vliet G (1992) Intellectual development at age 12 years of children with congenital hypothyroidism diagnosed by neonatal screening. J Pediatr 121(4):581–4

Goodman SI, Frerman FE (1995) Organic acidemias due to defects in lysine oxidation: 2-ketoadipic acidemia and glutaric acidemia. In Scriver CR, Beaudet AL, Sly WS, Valle D (eds): The Metabolic and Molecular Bases of Inherited Disease, 7th edn. McGraw-Hill, NY, pp. 1451–1460

Gregg RG, Simantel A, Farrell PM et al. (1997) Newborn screening for cystic fibrosis in Wisconsin: comparison of biochemical and molecular methods. Pediatr 99(6):819–824

Grover R, Newman S, Wethers D et al. (1986) Newborn screening for hemoglobinopathies: the benefit beyond the target. Am J Public Health 76(10):1236–1237

Guthrie R (1968) Screening for "inborn errors of metabolism" in the newborn infant – a multiple test program. In Bergsma D (ed): Human Genetics. (Birth Defects Original Article Series, Vol. 4 No. 6). National Foundation – March of Dimes, NY, pp. 92–98

Guthrie R, Susi A (1963) A simple phenylalanine method for detecting phenylketonuria in large populations of newborn infants. Pediatr 32:338–343

Hammond K, Naylor E, Wilcken B (1987) Screening for cystic fibrosis. In Therell BL Jr. (ed.): Advances in Neonatal Screening. Excerpta Medica, Amsterdam, pp. 377–382

Harris H (1963) Garrod's Inborn Errors of Metabolism. OUP, London

Holtzman C, Slazyk WE, Cordero JF, Hannon WH (1986) Descriptive epidemiology of missed cases of phenylketonuria and congenital hypothyroidism. Pediatr 78:553–558

Jew K, Kan K, Koch R, Cunningham GC (1994) Validity of screening early collected newborn specimens for phenylketonuria using a fluorometric method. Screening 3:1–9

Kerem B, Rommens JM, Buchanan JA (1989) Identification of the cystic fibrosis gene: genetic analysis. Science 245(4922):1073–1080

Kraus JP, Janosik M, Kozich V et al. (1999) Cystathionine beta-synthase mutations in homocystinuria. Human Mutation 13(5):362–375

Lemieux B (1987) Recommendations regarding neonatal screening for muscular dystrophy In Therell BL Jr. (ed.): Advances in Neonatal Screenings Excerpta Medica, Amsterdam, p. 349

Lemieux B, Auray-Blais C, Giguere R et al. (1988) Newborn urine screening experience with over one million infants in the Quebec network of genetic medicine. J Inherit Metab Dis 11:45–55

Lemna WK, Feldman GL, Kerem B et al. (1990) Mutation analysis for heterozygote detection and the prenatal diagnosis of cystic fibrosis. N Eng J Med 322(5):291–296

Lenke RR, Levy HL (1980) Maternal phenylketonuria and hyperphenylalaninemia: an international survey of the outcome of untreated pregnancies. N Eng J Med 303:1202–1208

Levy HL (1973) Genetic screening. In Harris H, Hirschhorn K (eds): Advances in Human Genetics. Plenum, NY, Vol. 4, p. 1

Levy HL (1995) Hartnup disorder. In Scriver CR, Beaudet AL, Sly WS, Valle D (eds): The Metabolic and Molecular Bases of Inherited Disease, 7th edn. McGraw-Hill, NY, pp. 3629–3642

Levy HL (1998) Newborn screening by tandem mass spectrometry: A new era [editorial]. Clin Chem 44:2401–402

Levy HL, Albers S (in press) Genetic screening of newborns. In Lander E, Lifton R, Page D (eds): Annual Review of Genomics and Human Genetics.

Levy HL, Taylor RG, McInnes RR (1995) Disorders of histidine metabolism. In Scriver CR, Beaudet AL, Sly WS, Valle D (eds): The Metabolic and Molecular Bases of Inherited Disease, 7th edn. McGraw-Hill, NY, pp 1107–1123

Levy HL, Hammersen G (1978) Newborn screening for galactosemia and other galactose metabolic defects. J Ped 92:871–877

Levy HL, Sepe SJ, Shih VE et al. (1977) Sepsis due to Escherichia coli in neonates with galactosemia. N Eng J Med 297:823–825

Levy HL, Shih VE, Karolkewicz V et al. (1971) Persistent mild hyperphenylalaninemia in the untreated state. A prospective study. N Engl J Med 285(8):424–4299

Levy HL, Coulombe JT, Shih VE (1980) Newborn urine screening. In Bickel H, Guthrie R, Hammersen G (eds): Neonatal screening for inborn errors of metabolism. Springer-Verlag, Heidelberg, p. 89

Levy HL, Waisbren SE (1983) Effects of maternal phenylketonuria and hyperphenylalaninemia in the fetus. N Eng J Med 309:1269–1274

Lindstedt S, Holme E, Lock EA et al. (1992) Treatment of hereditary tyrosinaemia type I by inhibition of 4-hydroxyphenyl pyruvate dioxygenase. Lancet 340:813–817

Loader S, Sutera CJ, Segelman SG et al. (1991) Prenatal hemoglobinopathy screening. IV. Follow-up of women at risk for a child with a clinically significant hemoglobinopathy. Am J Hum Genet 49(6):1292–1299

Lorey FW, Cunningham GC (1994) Effect of specimen collection method on newborn screening for PKU. Screening 3:57–65

MacCready RA, Hussey MG (1964) Newborn phenylketonuria detection program in Massachusetts. Am J Public Health 54:2075–2081

McCabe ERB (1992) Neonatal screening for dependents of active-duty military personnel. Pediatr 90:130–131

Meryash DL, Levy HL, Guthrie R et al. (1981) Prospective study of early neonatal screening for phenylketonuria. N Eng J Med 304:294–296

Mitchell GA, Lambert M, Tanguay RM (1995) Hypertyrosinemia. pp. 1077–1106. In Scriver CR, Beaudet AL, Sly WS, Valle D (eds): The Metabolic and Molecular Bases of Inherited Disease, 7th edn. McGraw-Hill, New York, pp. 1077–1106

Mohan N, McKiernan P, Preece MA et al. (1999) Indications and outcome of liver transplantation in tyrosinaemia type 1. Eur J Pediatr 158 Suppl 2:S49–54

Moore EC, Meuwissen HJ (1974) Screening for ADA deficiency. J Pediatr 85:802–804

Mudd SH, Levy HL, Skovby F (1995) Disorders of transsulfuration. In Scriver CR, Beaudet AL, Sly WS, Valle D (eds): The Metabolic and Molecular Bases of Inherited Disease, 7th edn. McGraw-Hill, NY, pp. 1279–1327

National Institutes of Health Consensus Conference (1987) Newborn screening for sickle cell disease and other hemoglobinopathies. J Am Med Assoc 258:1205–1209

New MI, Crawford C, Wilson RC (1995) Genetic disorders of the adrenal gland. In Rimoin DL, Connor JM, Pyeritz RE (eds): Emery and Rimoin's Principles and Practice of Medical Genetics, 3rd edn. Churchill Livingstone, Edinburgh, pp. 1441–1476

Newborn Screening Committee, The Council of Regional Networks for Genetic Services (CORN) (1999) National Newborn Screening Report—1995, CORN, Atlanta

Norrgard KJ, Pomponio RJ, Hymes J, Wolf B (1999) Mutations causing profound biotinidase deficiency in children ascertained by newborn screening in the United States occur at different frequencies than in symptomatic children. Pediatr Research 46(1):20–27

O'Flynn ME, Holtzman NA, Blaskovics M et al. (1980) The diagnosis of phenylketonuria. A report from the collaborative study of children treated for phenylketonuria. Am J Diseases of Children 134:769–774

Pang S, Clark A (1993) Congenital adrenal hyperplasia due to 21-hydroxylase deficiency: Newborn screening and its relationship to the diagnosis and treatment of the disorder. Screening 2:105–139

Pang S, Hotchkiss J, Drash AL et al. (1977) Microfilter paper method for 17 alpha-hydroxyprogesterone radioimmunoassay: Its application for rapid screening for congenital adrenal hyperplasia. J Clin Endocrinol Metab 45(5):1003–1008

Pang SY, Wallace MA, Hofman L et al. (1988) Worldwide experience in newborn screening for classical congenital adrenal hyperplasia due to 21-hydroxylase deficiency. Pediatr 81(6):866–874

Paradis K (1996) Tyrosinemia: The Quebec experience. Clin Invest Med 19(5):311–316

Peterschmitt MJ, Simmons JR, Levy HL (1999) Reduction of false-negative results in screening newborns for homocystinuria. N Eng J Med 341:1572–1576

Phang JM, Yeh GC, Scriver CR (1995) Disorders of proline and hydroxyproline metabolism. In Scriver CR, Beaudet AL, Sly WS, Valle D (eds): The Metabolic and Molecular Bases of Inherited Disease, 7th edn. McGraw-Hill, NY, pp. 1125–1146

Rashed MS, Rahbeeni Z, Ozand PT (1999) Application of electrospray tandem mass spectometry to neonatal screening. Seminars in Perinatology 23(2):183–193

Rashed MS, Ozand PT, Bucknall MP, Little D (1995) Diagnosis of inborn errors of metabolism from blood spots by acylcarnitines and amino acids profiling using automated electrospray tandem mass spectrometry. Pediatr Res 38(3):324–331

Research Group on Ethical, Social and Legal Issues in Genetic Counseling and Genetic Engineering (1972) Ethical and legal issues in screening for genetic disease. N Eng J Med 286:1129–1132

Roe CR, Coates PM (1995) Mitochondrial fatty acid oxidation disorders. In Scriver CR, Beaudet AL, Sly WS, Valle D (eds): The Metabolic and Molecular Bases of Inherited Disease, 7th edn. McGraw-Hill, NY, pp. 1501–1533

Rosenberg LE, Downing SE, Durant JL, Segal S (1966) Cystinuria: biochemical evidence for three genetically distant diseases. J Clin Invest 45:365–371

Rosenblatt DS (1995) Inherited disorders of folate transport and metabolism. In Scriver CR, Beaudet AL, Sly WS, Valle D (eds): The Metabolic and Molecular Bases of Inherited Disease, 7th edn. McGraw-Hill, NY, pp. 3111–3128

Rovet JF, Ehrlich R (2000) Psychoeducational outcome in children with early-treated congenital hypothyroidism. Pediatr 105(3 Pt 1):515–522

Scott CR (1995) Sarcosinemia. In Scriver CR, Beaudet AL, Sly WS, Valle D (eds): The Metabolic and Molecular Bases of Inherited Disease, 7th edn. McGraw-Hill, NY, pp. 1329–1335

Scriver CR, Levy HL (1983) Histidinemia. Part I: Reconciling retrospective and prospective findings. J Inherit Metabolic Disease 6:51–53

Scriver CR, Rosenberg LE (1973) Amino acid metabolism and its disorders. Saunders, New York

Scriver CR, Davies E, Cailen AM (1964) Application of a simple micromethod to the screening of plasma for a variety of aminoacidopathies. Lancet 2:230–232

Scriver CR, Mahon B, Levy HL et al. (1987) The Hartnup phenotype: Mendelian transport disorder, multifactorial disease. Am J Hum Genet 40(5):401–412

Scriver CR, Kaufman S, Eisensmith RC, Woo SLC (1995) The hyperphenylalaninemias. In Scriver CR, Beaudet AL, Sly WS, Valle D (eds): The Metabolic and Molecular Bases of Inherited Disease, 7th edn. McGraw-Hill, N, pp. 1015–1075

Segal S, Berry GT (1995) Disorders of galactose metabolism. In Scriver CR, Beaudet AL, Sly WS, Valle D (eds): The Metabolic and Molecular Bases of Inherited Disease, 7th edn. McGraw-Hill, NY, pp. 967–1000

Segal S (1998) Komrower Lecture. Galactosaemia today: The enigma and the challenge. J Inherited Metabolic Disease 21(5):455–71

Segal S, Their SO (1995) Cystinuria. In Scriver CR, Beaudet AL, Sly WS, Valle D (eds): The Metabolic and Molecular Bases of Inherited Disease, 7th edn. McGraw-Hill, NY, pp. 3581–3601

Sepe SJ, Levy HL, Mount FW (1979) An evaluation of routine follow-up blood screening of infants for phenylketonuria. N Eng J Med 300:606–609

Sokol RJ, McCabe ERB, Kotzer AM, Langendoerfer SI (1989) Diagnosing galactosemia: False negative newborn screening following red blood cell transfusion. J Pediatr Gastroenterology and Nutrition 8:266–268

Sorenson JR, Levy HL, Mangione TW, Sepe SJ (1984) Parental response to repeat testing of infants with "false positive" results in a newborn screening program. Pediatr 73:183–187

Surplice IM, Griffiths PD, Green A, Leeming RJ (1990) Dihydropteridine reductase activity in elevates from dried blood spots: automation of an assay for a national screening service. J Inherited Metabolic Disease 13:169–177

Sveger T (1978) alpha 1-antitrypsin deficiency in early childhood. Pediatr 62(1):22–25

The Cystic Fibrosis Genetic Analysis Consortium (1990) Worldwide survey of the delta F508 mutation—Report from the Cystic Fibrosis Genetic Analysis Consortium. Am J Hum Genet 47(2):354–359

Therrell BL Jr, Berenbaum SA, Manter-Kapanke V (1998) Results of screening 1.9 million Texas newborns for 21-hydroxylase-deficient congenital adrenal hyperplasia. Pediatr 101(4 Pt1):583–590

Thilén A, Nordenstrom A, Hagenfeldt L et al. (1998) Benefits of neonatal screening for congenital adrenal hyperplasia (21-hydroxylase deficiency) in Sweden. Pediatr 101(4):E11 URL: http://www.pediatrics.org/cgi/contents/full/101/4/e11

Turner B, Brown DA (1967) Detection of urinary abnormalities in a well-baby population: results of a survey. Med J Australia 1(11):560–562

Urwin R, Christodoulou J, Wiley V et al. (1997) Evaluation of a second tier to newborn screening for galactosemia: Utility of N314D mutation screening. In International Congress of Inborn Errors of Metabolism, 7th edn. Vienna

Vassart G, Dumont JE, Refetoff S (1995) Thyroid disorders. In Scriver CR, Beaudet AL, Sly WS, Valle D (eds): The Metabolic and Molecular Bases of Inherited Disease, 7th edn. McGraw-Hill, NY, pp. 2883–2928

Vichinsky E, Hurst D, Earles A et al. (1988) Newborn screening for sickle cell disease: Effect on mortality. Pediatr 81:749–755

Waisbren SE, Hanley W, Levy HL et al. (2000) Outcome at age 4 years in offspring of women with maternal phenylketonuria: The Maternal PKU Collaborative Study. J Am Med Assoc 283(6):756–762

Waisbren SE, Schnell R, Levy HL (1984) Intelligence and personality characteristics in adults with untreated atypical phenylketonuria and mild hyperphenylalaninemia. J Pediatr 105:955–958

Waters DL, Wilcken B, Irwing L (1999) Clinical outcomes of newborn screening for cystic fibrosis. Archives of Disease in Childhood Fetal Neonatal Edition 80(1):F1–F7

Weglage J, Ullrich K, Pietsch M (1997) Intellectual, neurologic, and neuropsychologic outcome in untreated subjects with nonphenylketonuria hyperphenylalaninemia. German Collaborative Study on Phenylketonuria. Pediatr Res 42(3):378–84

Wilcken B, Wiley V, Sherry G, Bayliss U (1995) Neonatal screening for cystic fibrosis: a comparison of two strategies for case detection in 1.2 million babies. J Pediatr 127:965–970

Wilcken DEL (1987) Summary of the workshop on hyperlipidemias. In Therrell BL Jr. (ed.): Advances in Neonatal Screening. Excerpta Medica, Amsterdam, pp. 325–327

Wilcken B (1993) Newborn screening for cystic fibrosis: its evolution and a review of the current situation. Screening 2:43–62

Wilcken B, Brown ARD (1987) Screening for cystic fibrosis in New South Wales, Australia: Evaluation of the results of screening 400,000 babies. In Therrell BL Jr. (ed.): Advances in Neonatal Screening. Excerpta Medica, Amsterdam, pp. 385–390

Wilcken B, Chalmers G (1985) Reduced mortality in patients with cystic fibrosis detected by neonatal screening. Lancet 2:1319–1321

Wilcken B, Smith A, Brown DA (1980) Urine screening for aminoacidopathies: Is it beneficial? J Pediatr 97:492–497

Wolf B (1991) Worldwide survey of neonatal screening for biotinidase deficiency. J Inherited Metabolic Disease 14:923–927

Wolf B (1995) Disorders of biotin metabolism. In Scriver CR, Beaudet AL, Sly WS, Valle D (eds): The Metabolic and Molecular Bases of Inherited Disease, 7th edn. McGraw-Hill, NY, pp. 3151–3177

Wolf B (updated 24 March 2000) Biotinidase deficiency. In GeneClinics: Medical Genetics Knowledge Base [database online]. Copyright, University of Washington, Seattle. Available at http://www.geneclinics.org/profiles/[disease name].

Genetic counseling

Ann P. Walker

Historical perspective and philosophy of genetic counseling

THE ORIGINS AND GOALS OF GENETIC COUNSELING

Although Sheldon Reed (1980) is credited with coining the term "genetic counseling" less than a half century ago, this activity has probably been practiced since prehistory when our early ancestors first noticed that people and animals usually resemble their parents. By the time the Talmud was written, the familial basis for hemophilia was well enough understood to know that the brothers of bleeders should not be circumcised. The fact that many cultures have historically forbidden marriages between siblings, or discouraged those between uncles and nieces or between first cousins, shows that they recognized that such unions were more likely to give rise to offspring with problems. In fact, throughout history, most families probably have had their own self-appointed "genetic counselors" who were only too ready to make disparaging predictions about undesirable traits from the *other* side of the family that could crop up in grandchildren. But genetic counseling as we now know it had to wait for a more sophisticated understanding of genetics.

The first real biologic basis for understanding the occurrence of human genetic disease came at the beginning of the twentieth century with the rediscovery of Mendel's work and Garrod's recognition that these principles of inheritance could explain the transmission of alcaptonuria. Up until this time, inheritance had been perceived as a blending of parental features. In fact, for the previous 35 years, Darwin's first cousin, Sir Francis Galton, had been attempting to develop mathematical methods to quantify the respective contributions of "nature and nurture" to human traits such as height or intelligence. These models were also invoked to try to explain more elusive personality or behavioral characteristics. In 1885 Galton introduced the term "eugenics" (derived from the Greek for "well-born"), which he defined as "the study of agencies under social control that may improve or impair racial qualities of future generations, either physically or mentally" (Carr-Saunders, 1929). Coming at a time when considerable social upheaval had resulted from rapid urbanization, industrialization, and immigration, the idea that scientific knowledge could be used to increase desirable social qualities such as intelligence or "law abidingness" and to diminish undesirable ones such as "feeble-mindedness," "pauperism," alcoholism, or "criminality" had great appeal. The distinction between genetic diseases and societal diseases became muddled as numerous organizations devoted to "eugenics" sprang up in over 30 countries.

The eugenic model

By 1910, the eugenics movement had generated a great deal of enthusiasm among respected experimental geneticists like Thomas Hunt Morgan and Charles B. Davenport, and had led to the establishment of institutions like the Eugenics Records Office at Cold Spring Harbor to collect data on genetic traits. Sometimes these agencies also provided consultation so as to discourage families with "undesirable traits" from reproducing. Unfortunately, this eugenic model of genetic counseling persisted for a number of years, until the myriad abuses arising from the eugenics movement—including laws that mandated involuntary sterilization of the mentally retarded or restricted the immigration of certain population groups—caused most scientists to distance themselves from the movement. By the 1930s, "genetic hygiene" had fallen into disrepute, both because it was no longer "politically correct" and because it had relatively little to offer. As Sir Humphry Rolleston, president of the English Eugenics Society, pointed out at a symposium in 1934, "The propaganda of eugenicists [appeared to many] to have outrun the existing knowledge of the laws of human heredity" (Rolleston, 1934).

The medical/preventive model

Initially it was primarily non-medical geneticists, working mostly with plants, *Drosophila*, and mice who began to apply what they were learning to human diseases and to counsel affected families. By the mid-1940's, a handful of "heredity clinics" had been established to provide families with information about the growing number of diseases that were recognized to be clearly inherited. Departments of medical genetics also started to appear in a few universities. In keeping with the new emphasis on preventive medicine, the primary purpose of genetic counseling was felt to be prevention of genetic diseases. Yet, for a variety of reasons, including concern about the recent legacies of the eugenics movement and social Darwinism, and the fact that most of those who were advising patients were research-trained and unaccustomed to participating in families' health care and reproductive decisions, information was generally provided in a neutral manner. This "nondirective" or at least "non-prescriptive" philosophy has remained integral to genetic counseling ever since.

Sheldon Reed (1974) has described genetic counseling as "a type of social work entirely for the benefit of the whole family without direct concern for its effect upon the state or politics." However a mid-1970s study by Sorenson and Culbert (1979) found that only a quarter of the geneticists they surveyed (of whom about 90% were either PhDs or physicians) felt that discussing psychosocial issues was a major obligation. Those geneticists who were more psychosocially oriented were much less likely to endorse prevention of genetic disease or a reduction in its incidence as goals of counseling. However the remaining 75% generally said they steered away from discussing prior values and expectations of the clients and felt that their primary role was to determine and provide accurate information about recurrence risk and disease severity. Nonetheless, virtually all of those studied did agree that lessening client anxiety and guilt and increasing client happiness were appropriate goals of genetic counseling.

The decision-making model

Initially, most who provided genetic counseling subscribed to the philosophy that, given accurate information about risk and burden of disease, clients would generally make "rational" decisions about reproduction, that is, those that would promote societal goals of reducing the incidence of genetic disease and personal goals of reducing pain and suffering. In fact, many early studies of genetic counseling attempted to measure its "success" by determining how well clients retained the information they had been given or by seeing if they had altered their previous reproductive plans. With the 1970s came a general shift in medicine that placed a higher premium on patient autonomy, even if it meant departing from the traditional, somewhat paternalistic, physician-patient relationship. This was mirrored by a subtle shift in the goals of genetic counseling away from encouraging clients to make "rational" decisions, to helping them make their own decisions, whether "rational" or not. Educating clients about the genetic and medical facts of the situation still forms the basis for this type of counseling interaction, but the decision-making model recognizes that clients must process and personalize facts affectively as well as cognitively before they can act on them.

The rationale for this model of genetic counseling is that it requires clients to take responsibility for the consequences of decisions and behavior that are truly their own. By so doing, they increase their sense of control and self-worth (both of which are often assaulted by the occurrence or threat of genetic disease). This model is predicated on the beliefs that people are more likely to be motivated to act on decisions in which they have meaningfully participated, and that they grow and learn about themselves and their relationships by considering the implications of various courses of action. The counselor who creates an atmosphere of respect and understanding in which open discourse can safely occur makes the client feel valued and competent and, in the process, increases his or her own credibility.

Psychotherapeutic genetic counseling model

The psychotherapeutic model of genetic counseling recognizes that there is frequently much more to the genetic counseling interaction than decision-making; that often the real issue is not what to do in the future, but how to cope with what has already occurred. A person's ability to adjust to a disease, or its risk of occurrence/recurrence, involves complex psychosocial factors, such as previous experience with the disorder, personality, motivation, education, values, culture, family and interpersonal dynamics, financial and social resources, and coping styles. Counselors who adopt a psychotherapeutic approach believe that for counseling to succeed, these affective dimensions must be adequately explored throughout the process of providing genetic and medical information. The impact and meaning of virtually identical information about genetic risk and reproductive options is likely to be very different for an individual whose personality has been shaped and world view colored by growing up with a mentally retarded sibling than it will for a couple learning that their newborn has Down syndrome. Neither will be likely to integrate the facts about the diagnosis or the genetic information until their responses are identified, acknowledged, and dealt with.

The use of the term "psychotherapeutic" is as disquieting to many genetics professionals as the use of the term "counseling" is to many clients. Although genetics fellowships and genetic counseling programs validate the importance of psychosocial issues and model behavior that is supposed to encourage addressing them, few geneticists feel adequately prepared in counseling techniques to consider themselves psychotherapists. They are generally more comfortable attending to the medical or genetic aspects of a consultation. Similarly, patients usually come to geneticists seeking information about diagnosis, prognosis, or recurrence, rather than help with the psychological impact of the genetic condition or the decision they are facing. They usually feel that "counseling" or psychotherapy is for people who are dissatisfied with some aspect of themselves or their interpersonal relationships, or worse, who feel "out of control." Since genetic counseling is often suggested at the time when a new diagnosis has assaulted the self-image and generated levels of anxiety, guilt, and depression never before experienced, the referral may be perceived as especially threatening. It may help for the counselor to reassure the client that because the threat or reality of a genetic condition usually generates powerful and frequently unfamiliar responses, exploration of these emotions and their impact is a routine part of the genetic counseling process. However, it is also appropriate to indicate that if issues arise that would be better dealt with by another professional with different types of counseling skills, a referral can be made.

In reality, these various counseling philosophies and orientations are not mutually exclusive, and may need to be used by the same counselor with different clients or at different times in the course of counseling. Nevertheless, an overtly prescriptive or directive eugenic stance is virtually never appropriate, and respect for the autonomy of the individual should remain paramount in any counseling interaction.

DELIVERY OF GENETIC COUNSELING SERVICES

Professional diversity

To some measure, shifts in the approaches to genetic counseling have reflected changes in the disciplinary background and training of those providing the service. The early emphasis on risk assessment and genetic education was consonant with the orientation of biologic researchers. Even in the early 1970s, 85% of PhD. and 57% of MD geneticists, who together represented nine of every ten who were then providing genetic counseling in the United States, said that their primary interest was research (Sorenson and Culbert, 1977). Up until this time virtually all genetics services were affiliated with medical schools, and most recipients of genetic counseling were families at risk for a specific disorder or couples who had had an affected child. By the middle of the decade, screening for sickle cell and Tay-Sachs carriers and the growing availability of prenatal diagnosis had created a new market for genetic counseling among those who had no history of birth defects, but who were at risk solely on the basis of their age or genotype.

While it was becoming apparent that the increased capabilities of medical genetics and the advent of prenatal diagnosis would soon lead to a demand for genetic services that could overwhelm the relatively small number of geneticists and physicians available to provide them, it had also begun to be recognized that there should be more to genetic counseling than diagnosis and interpretation of genetic risk. Psychiatric research had led to a better understanding of the emotional impact of having a handicapped child or a genetic condition, and it was evident that it would be beneficial if genetics, medicine, and psychology could be better integrated. Nurses, social workers, and psychologists began to work with genetics teams, bringing counseling skills and a more psychosocial perspective to patient interactions. The nascent literature in genetic counseling began to reflect this perspective, as did the training of genetics professionals in fellowship and graduate programs. In the United States, a few institutions began educating a new type of master's level professional, initially called a "genetics associate" (now "genetic counselor"), who had not only a solid foundation in medical genetics, but also counseling skills and an awareness of the psychosocial issues surrounding genetic conditions and birth defects. There are currently 31 such programs in the United States, Canada, the United Kingdom and Australia, (National Society of Genetic Counselors, 2001). Twenty-seventeen North American programs are accredited or recognized by the American Board of Genetic Counseling (American Board of Genetic Counseling, 2001). Three additional US programs train masters level clinical nurse specialists in genetics. At least in the United States, master's-level genetic counselors are now responsible for delivering a significant portion of genetic services, usually as part of a team that includes one or more clinical or laboratory geneticists.

Client diversity and access to services

In the mid-1970s the vast majority of clients seeking genetics services were white, educated, and middle to upper class. Today, however, all segments of the population are more aware of genetics and of how to find services. Increasingly, patients refer themselves or request a referral from their provider. Access has been improved as more genetics professionals have been trained and as genetics services have dispersed from universities into private hospitals, commercial laboratories, and satellite clinics. Screening programs such as those for infant metabolic diseases and maternal serum markers have cast a much broader net. People seeking genetics services now come from every social stratum and represent a host of cultures and languages. We are just beginning to learn how the counseling needs of some of these clients may differ from what traditionally has been provided. An exhaustive discussion of genetic issues and the limitations, risks, and benefits of various tests can overwhelm even the most knowledgeable English-speaking family. How does one manage the problem of "information-overload" for a recent immigrant with a grade-school education while still respecting the client's autonomy and avoiding paternalism?

Along with the changes in patient population, higher medical costs and the advent of managed care are demanding that genetics services, like all others, be delivered as efficiently and cost effectively as possible. This means that families must frequently be seen in only one visit and by a single genetics professional. The luxury of the team approach and repeated, lengthy, counseling sessions is rapidly becoming a thing of the past. Furthermore, while technology has brought new reproductive options and a proliferation of testing alternatives, these are not always realistically available to patients who are minimally insured or unable to afford them. Counselors may be caught in a bind if, by giving patients complete information about their choices, they inhumanely dangle unattainable options in front of them.

The approach of this chapter is to discuss how genetic counseling is traditionally provided without the above constraints. As medical care, the capabilities of genetics, and our clients continue to change, genetic counseling will have to adapt to new settings and providers. It is hoped that the essential elements discussed in the following section will be preserved regardless of whether counseling takes place in a single visit of short duration or over a period of years.

Components of genetic counseling

INFORMATION-GATHERING

The (intake interview) really starts at the moment of referral, and the tone that is set can determine the success or failure of counseling. Although demographic and basic historical information can successfully be obtained over the telephone by well-trained administrative personnel, it is helpful to involve a genetics professional early on. With the exception of prenatal diagnosis, genetics services are unfamiliar to most people, and referral for a genetic evaluation can be particularly alarming. It may confirm fears that a family already has regarding a specific diagnosis, like muscular dystrophy, or introduce the possibility of a previously unheard-of and thus especially frightening condition, such as tuberous sclerosis. Furthermore, unlike other types of referrals, a genetics referral raises fears not only for the potentially affected individual, but for other family members—born and unborn. Even an individual who is self-referred may have taken years to work up the courage to call and request testing or counseling. It is critical that the basis for future open communication and trust be established at this point.

The patient's or family's understanding of the reason for referral should be determined at the outset. What has their practitioner shared about his or her concerns? Was a specific diagnosis mentioned? If so, what were they told about the likelihood of this diagnosis or about its implications? How does the family perceive this condition and what, if any, has been their prior experience with it? What have they observed about the person being referred, and do they feel the practitioner's concerns are warranted? Do they have specific expectations of what the genetic evaluation and counseling will entail? Unless there is incontrovertible evidence of a correct diagnosis at the time of referral, it may be beneficial to leave some hope that the genetic evaluation may in fact, reassure them. Correcting initial misinformation (like clarifying that neurofibromatosis was not the "elephant man's" disease) can alleviate unnecessary anxiety. It is also helpful to describe, in broad terms, what the consultation will entail and what types of studies may be necessary. Preparing the family for the fact that it is not always possible to make a diagnosis or determine an etiology will help set realistic expectations.

Adequate assessment at the time of referral can facilitate "triage" and staffing of the case. How anxious is the family? If they are panicked about what they have been told about the possibility of a diagnosis and its potential severity or if there are urgent medical problems that call for immediate evaluation, a visit should clearly be arranged as soon as possible. In other cases, postponing scheduling until results of specific studies or relevant medical records on affected family members can be obtained may make for a much more efficient and productive visit. Issues raised at intake may suggest that the visit should be scheduled when specific team members (e.g., child psychologist, social worker) can attend. If it can be determined that a physical examination will not be needed for risk assessment or counseling (as in the case of a couple requesting information about a deceased infant or multiple miscarriages), it is usually preferable for the visit to take place in an office rather than an examining room. This may be especially important if the genetics visit would otherwise occur in a setting (such as a pediatrics or prenatal diagnosis clinic) that would add to the couple's discomfort because of the previous loss.

Involving a genetics professional during the telephone intake process gives the family a personal contact with whom they can begin to interact before the visit, and helps to "demystify" the referral. This interaction can provide an opportunity to engage the family as an active participant in the counseling process. Giving them responsibility for obtaining records or other tasks may increase their sense of control and their understanding of what information is and is not relevant. Preliminary telephone conversations can also allow for some psychotherapeutic intervention before the appointment. A pitfall of telephone intakes is that, unless it is clearly explained that genetic counseling will not be provided until the visit, the professional can be manipulated into providing more information than is appropriate at this stage. However, with one or more telephone contacts it may be possible to obtain the history, pedigree, and initial psychosocial assessment in advance, so that the clinic visit can be devoted to pursuing pertinent historical and emotional issues, the diagnostic examination, and other aspects of genetic evaluation. Optimally, the professional who has done the initial phone work with the family should be able to brief other team members before clinic, so that they can become aware of relevant medical and psychosocial issues, personalities, and the family's concerns and develop a coherent plan for the visit.

At the initial visit, it is important to explain who the people are who will be seeing the family and what the role of each will be in the evaluation. Describing what will happen, and why, can also help to alleviate anxiety. Ideally this should be done in any medical consultation, but it is especially important in genetics. Not only is the specialty relatively new, but it is often unfamiliar. Few people have the same level of understanding of what may be entailed in evaluating someone for a possible genetic condition as they do for a gallbladder ailment, heart disease, back trouble, or some other more publicly acknowledged condition. Because of the very private and potentially stigmatizing nature of hereditary diseases, even people who have had a genetic evaluation may be reticent to discuss this experience with friends, and so families rarely know what to expect.

Initial telephone contacts will often have been with just one family representative. The first face-to-face contact is likely to involve additional family members—the spouse and child, other siblings, and so on. Asking each about his or her understanding of the reason for the referral and concerns, and verifying with each the relevant parts of the previously obtained history can begin to establish rapport, demonstrate the importance of each member's participation, and provide an opportunity to observe family dynamics. In summarizing the family's stated concerns, one can differentiate the ones that may be able to be addressed by the geneticist from those that should be the province of another professional; and also distinguish the ones that may be able to be answered at the initial visit from those that may have to await further studies.

RISK ASSESSMENT

One of the major purposes in arriving at a diagnosis is to determine genetic risk. Families are usually concerned about why a condition has occurred, if and in whom it might recur, and whether more or less seriously. Early on, such risk assessment was the primary raison d'être for genetic counseling. Even today, geneticists are sometimes much more focused on this aspect of their task than are their patients, and they may go to great ends to refine a risk determination to fractions of a percent. In the case of recessive disorders for which there is accurate and reliable carrier detection, like sickle cell disease, or clearly expressed dominant disorders, like achondroplasia, this exercise is usually fairly straightforward. However, even with well-described mendelian disorders, the water is often muddied by confounding issues like genetic heterogeneity, subtle gene expression, non-penetrance, somatic or gonadal mosaicism, variable and late ages of onset, new mutations, sex limitation, and non-genetic phenocopies. Ironically, locating and characterizing a gene may actually complicate rather than simplify risk assessment because the phenotypic implications of newly recognized mutations and polymorphisms may not be clear. This is now the situation with the myriad changes identified in the cystic fibrosis and breast-ovarian cancer genes, and with the various diseases associated with triplet repeat expansions.

The risks for occurrence and recurrence of chromosomal or presumably multifactorial conditions, when available, are usually based on empirical data. These data are derived from observations of many cases that may actually have varying etiologies, and, while they might be the best risk figures that exist, they may not be accurate for a given family. This may also be true for the chances given for specific complications to occur in variably expressed mendelian disorders. In these types of situation, providing specific risk figures may imply a level of precision that is misleading.

To date, relatively little information exists about recurrence risk and diagnostic implications for disorders caused by newly understood mechanisms like imprinting, uniparental disomy, placental mosaicism, or subtle apparently de novo chromosome deletions, duplications, and translocations. With mitochondrial diseases, heteroplasmy, tissue mosaicism, and the effects of interacting polymorphic nuclear genes may introduce too many variables to make any meaningful prediction about recurrence or severity.

While these uncertainties may make it difficult for the geneticist to arrive at a specific risk figure, it is really the family's perception of risk (rather than the actual risk) that will determine their course of action. Many studies have shown that people perceive chances in a binary fashion: either something will happen or it won't. If a rare condition has already occurred, the fact that it has only a 1% risk of recurring is often meaningless. Families frequently say "If it happened once, it can happen again," or think that since their risk has increased from, for example, 1 in 10,000 before the occurrence to 1 in 100 afterwards, the condition will surely recur.

Risk perceptions are colored not only by having had a condition occur, but by the nature of family's experience with the disorder, and the meaning of its attendant problems. The woman whose high-school years were spent caring for a brother dying with adrenoleukodystrophy will have very different feelings about the disease than the woman whose uncle was diagnosed as an adult. A 2% risk of recurrence of for cleft lip may be unacceptable to a parent for whom physical appearance is very important, while a 50% chance of having a child with a skeletal dysplasia may actually represent the desired outcome to a couple with short stature The same risk figure will also sound different depending on the perception of burden of the outcome; a 35-year-old couple with a history of repeated miscarriages may view a 1/200 procedural risk of amniocentesis as "higher" than their 1/200 chance of having a baby with aneuploidy.

In many cases, families come to counseling with a preconceived notion of what risk they will be given. If the counselor's estimation is significantly different from what they anticipated, their reaction may seem incongruous: "Only 50:50?!", or "As high as 2%?!" The counselor must be careful not to let his or her own perception of the burden of the condition or magnitude of the risk affect how this information is conveyed, and should avoid making qualitative statements that the risk is "high" or "low". On the other hand, risk data must be given in an understandable way. Metaphors that are commonplace in our culture, like "tossing a coin," may be unfamiliar to a recent immigrant from a country in which goods are exchanged by bartering. Percentages and probabilities may be completely arcane to someone whose education ended with grammar school. Even well-educated people often have a difficult time interpreting risk numbers; to many, 1/400 sounds higher than 1/200 because the denominator is bigger. To any of us, 1 in 20 may sound higher than 5%, or vice versa.

It is important to state not only the risk of an untoward outcome, but also the likelihood of a positive one, and also to give the risk in different ways, for example, "There is a 25% (1 in 4) chance that the baby will be affected, but 3 chances in 4 (75%) that it will not have the condition." But simply delivering risk data is not helpful. The counselor needs to explore the clients' impressions of this risk and how each of the possible outcomes would affect them.

INFORMATION-GIVING

Estimating occurrence or recurrence risk and helping clients interpret this information in a way that is meaningful to them is an important part of counseling, but it represents only a small part of the information that must be exchanged. Depending on the situation, clients may be asking about a specific disorder that has already occurred in a family member, or about conditions for which they may be at risk because of a screening result, age, ethnicity, a possible teratogen or mutagen exposure, or maternal disease. They may need to know about available means of diagnosis or carrier detection and the limitations and possible complications of such tests. Usually they will want to understand the genetic or other basis for the condition and to learn who, if anyone, is at risk. They may have concerns about medical management, school progress, or resources available for financial or social support. Or they may need help in adapting to the condition and its impact on their family. Many times, clients do not know the types or extent of information that they can obtain through the counseling, and the counselor may need to guide them by raising issues that are neither medical nor genetic.

Depending on when information is given during the counseling process, families will hear and process it differently. Often, the same information will have to be presented repeatedly and in different ways. Some studies of the efficacy of genetic counseling have found that as few as 20% of clients correctly recollected the counseling information, and others have determined that only half of counseling recipients recalled enough to make an informed choice (Leonard et al. 1972).

In most cases, the genetic aspects of the counseling are not only quite novel, but "concept dense". To educate clients to the point that they can understand the reason the disorder occurred, its chance to recur, or how a genetic test is done may require that they be exposed to more genetics than many primary care physicians have encountered in their medical training. Using diagrams and visual aids that utilize common objects (e.g., switching tops on two differently colored pens to demonstrate a translocation) can make difficult concepts more accessible and will make it easier for clients to explain the genetics to family members. On the other hand, it is important that the "genetics lesson" not overshadow the counseling session.

In giving information about the condition itself, an effort should be made to define all of the medical terminology used and to actually write out key words for the clients to take with them. Terms that are second nature to the geneticist (like "syndrome") may sound like a death sentence to a patient. Even names of conditions that are widely used may be misinterpreted. Once, during an informing interview about an infant with Down syndrome, a mother burst into tears of relief when I explained that the condition was named after the doctor who had first described it; for six weeks she had believed that her baby had a syndrome that "was as low as you could go ... a real 'downer'." Asking the clients to summarize what they have heard or what they recall from previous discussions can be helpful, not only in determining the accuracy of their understanding, but also in assessing what aspects of the information they found most important or most disturbing.

At the conclusion of the genetic evaluation and counseling a letter should be written to the clients summarizing historical data and the test results that were relevant to the diagnosis, as well as the information about etiology, prognosis, or genetic risk that was provided. Such a letter gives the clients a review of the consultation that they can retain as part of their personal medical information and share with other family members, if they wish. Sending the clients a written record also provides another chance to identify any misperceptions that should be corrected, and (when appropriate) can reemphasize the importance of their seeking additional counseling should their family situation or reproductive plans change. It also may provide some measure of medicolegal protection for the geneticist—particularly if there has been discussion about the importance of the counselee's sharing information with other family members who may be at risk.

PSYCHOLOGICAL ASSESSMENT AND COUNSELING

Although information must be incorporated on a cognitive level, it also must be experienced emotionally and personalized before it can be acted upon. As Kessler (1979) points out," ... the psychological responses of clients are not only a normal, but often a necessary step in comprehending, integrating and coping with a medical diagnosis or the content material of genetic counseling." The client's psychological state will determine not only what he is ready to hear but how much he can hear. Therefore, the psychosocial impact as well as the comprehension of information must be continually assessed throughout the counseling process.

There has been much discussion about how psychotherapeutic genetic counseling should be. In reality this is usually determined by the training of the professional involved and his or her level of comfort and competence in working with patients in this way. The clinical situation itself will dictate the utility of a psychotherapeutic approach; for example, extended therapeutic counseling may be very necessary and beneficial for some couples who have elected pregnancy termination after finding a fetal abnormality, but there is usually little need or opportunity for this approach in the preliminary counseling for prenatal diagnosis.

Clients who want genetic counseling are psychologically no different from people in the rest of the population. In coming to us, they are seeking information about genetic issues, not psychotherapy. On the other hand, many unique challenges to the psyche are inherent in the issues raised by genetic counseling, the decisions clients are asked to make, and the threat or occurrence of a genetic disorder or birth defect. Some of these are unlike anything most individuals have ever had to confront. It is incumbent on the provider of genetic counseling to understand the common emotional reactions to these distinct psychic challenges and to be able to differentiate normal and appropriate responses from underlying psychopathology.

A genetic counselor should be able to see most clients through the emotional land mines they can encounter in the course of diagnosis and adjustment to the condition. When issues arise that are beyond the counselor's therapeutic expertise, he or she must be able to recognize this and make an effective referral to the appropriate mental health professional. It is worthwhile cultivating good working relationships with therapists who have demonstrated interest in and sensitivity to the genetic issues. Among these I include clergy, who, in their pastoral counseling, can provide a healing dimension that is lacking in most medical interactions.

HELP WITH DECISION-MAKING

In the course of genetic counseling, clients may need to make decisions about issues as varied as testing options, pregnancy continuation, treatment or placement of a severely impaired child, or reproductive alternatives. To do this, they need to understand this information not only cognitively, but emotionally, and to relate it to their own situation. The counselor may need to help them try different alternatives "on for size," imagining how each would feel with a particular decision and how the possible outcomes of each choice might affect their lives. If the responses of different family members—particularly the husband and wife—are different and would lead to incompatible decisions, the counselor needs to help them resolve the conflict. This can be done by working with them on values clarification. Which of the alternatives is most consonant with what they believe? Which would be most harmful to their relationship (family, status, lifestyle, self-image, etc.)? Sometimes it may help to have each party articulate what he or she perceives as the "best case" and "worst case" outcomes of each decision and why. Specific counseling issues around decisions that clients may confront and responses they may have to particular situations are discussed in the relevant sections below.

ONGOING CLIENT SUPPORT

In most cases, when patients are faced with the possibility or the reality of a birth defect or genetic disease, or of the loss of a wanted pregnancy or child, they find themselves in uncharted territory. The experience is likely to upset their psychological equilibrium in a way that nothing before has ever done. They will discover that our society has not yet developed a collective wisdom to guide them in dealing with the trauma and dilemmas they are encountering, and as a result, they may feel even more isolated and terrified as a result.

Professional support

Genetic counseling can help clients understand their feelings and what is causing them and (in most cases) can provide reassurance that the emotions are appropriate. Many are helped by being forewarned of responses they are likely to have. This "anticipatory guidance" can prepare them for what lies ahead and prevent the additional harm that might occur if they were caught off guard by yet another psychic assault. Professional acceptance, concern, and understanding can provide comfort and reassurance to the client that he or she is not a "bad person" because of what has occurred or what they are thinking. By remaining involved over time, the counselor can encourage behaviors and feelings that increase the client's self-esteem and sense of competence. This involvement can also help clients discover and cultivate other sources of support that they may not have known existed. The goal should be to restore psychological homeostasis and to establish, as much as possible, a healthy acceptance of what may be an ongoing challenge. Providing this type of support does not require extensive training in psychotherapy, but rather, as Kessler (1999) points out, the professional's making the effort to "express kindness, to raise the person's spirits, to give rewards, to bolster self-efficacy, and to teach and encourage the application of coping skills."

Support groups

There now exist a host of organizations that can be an invaluable resource to the professional who cares for families that have a genetic disease or birth defect. These organizations may be regional or international. Some comprise fewer than 20 members, while others have a membership in the millions. Their focus may be as broad as providing support for parents who have lost a child or as narrow as promoting increased understanding of a specific rare chromosome deletion. An organization may provide peer support, advocacy and lobbying, public and professional education, support of research, or all of these. Often its greatest value is in demonstrating to affected families that they are not alone, that others have confronted the same losses, hardships, disappointments, frustrations, and uncertainties they themselves are facing. Local chapters can provide an opportunity for similarly affected individuals or families to become acquainted—either one-on-one, or in meetings that vary from professionally led group therapy to educational presentations by medical specialists and researchers to social or fund-raising events. Many support groups now have Internet web-sites with patient information about the condition, pictures of affected individuals and their families, and even "chat rooms". Since families often will have found their way to these sites before their first genetics visit, the wise counselor will become familiar with the material they contain.

Involvement in a support group or organization can show families that their feelings and reactions have been experienced by others in similar situations, that others have coped, that there can be "light at the end of the tunnel." But referrals need to be made judiciously. The professional should, if at all possible, become familiar with the group and its "players," and know what the families they refer are likely to experience. It can be overwhelming for parents of a newly diagnosed child to be visited by a group member whose enthusiasm and positive outlook on the disorder in question does not "resonate" with the shock and denial that the parents are experiencing. Similarly, the emotional impact of attending a meeting and seeing for the first time a number of affected individuals of varying ages and degrees of severity can create additional anxiety and depression just at a time when some measure of psychological homeostasis was just beginning to return. The person may suddenly have the fact of his new identity (e.g., as the parent of a child with Down syndrome, a young adult with neurofibromatosis, or the spouse of a person with Huntington disease) forcefully driven home. It is helpful for the professional to prepare the patient and family for the fact that they may encounter individuals who have different diagnoses from theirs. One should also reassure them (when appropriate) that certain characteristics they may notice in others (e.g., wheelchair use, mental retardation, congenital heart disease) are not and will not be relevant to their own situation.

While support groups can be valuable resources for patients, involvement with them can also benefit the professional. Such participation is often viewed by families as a show of commitment and emotional support—something that can only increase mutual trust, communication, and respect. Having an opportunity to see the range of physical effects of a disease in people of different ages can provide new insights into the natural history and variability of the condition. Listening to affected individuals and their families talk about challenges and successes with school, work, transportation, insurance, interpersonal relationships, or even mundane aspects of daily life will give the health care provider a more complete awareness of the non-clinical ramifications of the disorder. The geneticist who has a holistic understanding of the disease will be more sensitive to its attendant psychological and social issues and will be better able to provide anticipatory guidance about these, as well as medical complications that may lie ahead. By participating in a support group or serving on its medical advisory board the professional can improve the quality and accuracy of genetic and clinical information the organization provides about the condition—either through their members or with its educational materials. Perhaps less altruistically, support groups can provide the professional with access to subjects for research studies, and sometimes even with funding for these efforts. Information about support groups may be found through local resource directories, hospital social work departments, organizations such as the United Way that give financial help to not-for-profit groups, or from the Genetic Alliance. This last organization also provides technical support for professionals or families who wish to start a group, and it can supply information about such issues as peer support training, incorporation, and fund-raising.

Considerations in specific genetic counseling situations

PRENATAL DIAGNOSIS

How prenatal diagnosis counseling has changed

Initially, much of the growth in demand for genetic counseling services came with the advent of prenatal diagnosis. The most frequent indication for prenatal referral used to be risk for a rare metabolic or chromosomal condition (usually aneuploidy) either because of a previous affected child or advancing maternal age. More recently, screening for neural tube defects and certain trisomies by measuring maternal serum alphafetoprotein, human chorionic gonadotropin, unconjugated estriol and/or inhibin A has become widespread. In addition, the nearly routine use of prenatal ultrasound in the primary care setting now detects not only potential obstetric complications but also unsuspected fetal structural anomalies. This means that many couples who did not embark on a pregnancy knowing of an increased risk are being referred for genetic counseling and are facing unanticipated decisions about prenatal diagnosis. Among these are couples who may initially have declined more definitive prenatal testing because of their personal beliefs, and others who were not entirely aware of the possible ramifications of having a screening blood test. Thus, couples referred for prenatal diagnostic services are much more likely to be in a state of crisis than they were a decade or two ago.

At the same time, the increased volume of prenatal patients and decreased reimbursement for counseling and laboratory services has created pressures on many counselors to diminish the extent of counseling. A 1993 study of genetic counselors in California (Walker, 1993) showed that 58% of them spent less time with their patients than they did 10 years ago, that the time spent in counseling diminished significantly as patient load increased, and that an average of 15 minutes less was spent with prenatal than non-prenatal patients. While the time available for counseling had decreased, many counselors felt that the complexity of information that needed to be discussed had increased, even from what it had been just two years earlier. Fortunately, these counselors also felt that the patients had become more familiar with the issues over time and that most were able to understand the information better. However, this improvement was noted only for English-speaking patients; non-English speaking patients were felt to be significantly less well prepared and equipped to deal with the content material of genetic counseling, even when the interview was conducted by a counselor fluent in the language.

Essential elements of counseling for maternal age and serum marker screening

The likelihood that prenatal patients may be referred in crisis, the increasingly complicated counseling issues, and the stresses of diminished reimbursement and greater patient volume mean that choices often must be made about what is truly important to prenatal genetic counseling. A lengthy counseling session that allows for an extensive discussion of genetics and exploration of psychosocial issues is becoming a luxury that is more difficult to justify. What, then, should be considered essential?

History and pedigree

One of the time-consuming aspects of prenatal counseling is obtaining family and pregnancy history, and some have suggested that the counselor's review of a patient-completed questionnaire should be adequate for this purpose. While this may be so, information gained through constructing at least an abbreviated three-generation pedigree can also be important. Two retrospective analyses of charts from over 2200 patients referred to our center for follow-up of an abnormal maternal serum screening result showed that using both a questionnaire and a pedigree identified additional issues of significance to the pregnancy, to the couple's future reproduction, or to a close family member in over a quarter of patients (Holsinger et al., 1992; Yates, 1999). These issues had not been identified before referral (usually at 17 or more weeks of gestation) and had not been addressed in the primary care setting. In 12% of the cases, the finding changed the patient's management by identifying the need for (1) additional fetal testing that would not otherwise have been offered; (2) parental screening to deter-

mine if additional fetal testing would be appropriate (such as karyotyping for repeated fetal losses, or screening for hemoglobinopathies, Tay-Sachs, and other diseases because of ethnicity); or (3) further evaluation of the mother or alteration of her obstetric care (e.g., because of one patient's own diagnosis of Marfan syndrome and another's family history of intracranial aneurysms). An additional 15% of couples were found to be at increased risk for a fetal anomaly for which no additional diagnosis could be offered, or to need counseling because of a possible teratogenic exposure, or to have a first-degree relative whose history suggested the need for genetic evaluation and counseling.

Discussion of risks

A great deal of the content material of prenatal counseling pertains to risk: the estimated chance that a fetal condition is present, the likelihood that it can be diagnosed with available techniques, the procedural risks, and various background incidences in the general population. Obviously these issues are central to decision-making, and care must be taken not only to ensure that they are understood, but that their emotional impact is addressed. Just the word "risk" elicits a negative response, and while it is difficult to avoid using it, words like "chance" or "likelihood" are more emotionally neutral. Talking about background risks can also be alarming; few people embark on a pregnancy with an awareness that, even without any identifiable risk factors there is a 3% chance that their baby will have a significant abnormality and a 2% chance that they could lose the pregnancy in the second half of gestation. Often the counseling may also involve discussing unfamiliar conditions, such as trisomies other than Down syndrome, for which a couple may not have realized they could also be at higher risk. This generates further anxiety. On the other hand, "older" mothers may perceive that they are at a high risk for any fetal abnormality, and may actually be relieved to learn that their chance of having a baby with a non-chromosomal birth defect is rarely any different from what it was when they were younger.

Helping patients understand how serum screening changes their risk can be especially tricky. Many primary care providers do not have a good understanding of screening tests, and it may be difficult for patients to understand that (in most cases) an "abnormal" test result does not mean a fetal abnormality. Although it may be necessary to use numbers in talking about risk, it is usually more helpful to talk in terms of how their risk factor (be it age, a "triple marker" result, a teratogen exposure, etc.) changes their chances from what it would be without that factor. For instance, it may be easier for a 33-year-old woman whose triple marker screening result has raised her risk for Down syndrome to 1/370 to interpret this figure if she is also told that her chance of having a baby with a chromosome abnormality is now the same as it would be if she were 35. In giving risks, it is also important to emphasize the likelihood that the condition will not be found, or that the complication will not occur.

Discussion of genetic issues and possible diagnoses

Some counselors choose to go into fairly detailed descriptions and show pictures of conditions for which the couple may be at risk, outlining for instance, the genetics and phenotype of Down syndrome or the various potential complications of spina bifida. My bias is that this is time-consuming and unduly anxiety-provoking, given the level of risk that is usually involved in cases of routine maternal age or low maternal serum α-fetoprotein (MSAFP). However, it is important that the patient has a clear understanding of what Down syndrome is—a distinct condition with a specific genetic basis and not, as some perceive, just a general term for mental retardation. Furthermore, since Down syndrome is familiar to most people, it can serve as a point of comparison in discussing other chromosomal disorders, particularly if the counselor takes care to make sure that clients have an appropriate and realistic idea of the condition.

To understand what they are at risk for and how a diagnosis can be made, patients who have increased chance for aneuploidy on the basis of age or serum screening need to know at least the following:

1. The conditions for which they are at risk are caused by changes in the amount of genetic information a baby receives.
2. Genetic information is contained on structures called "chromosomes" that are passed from the parents in the egg or sperm.
3. A change in chromosome number can happen in either the egg or the sperm and is usually present at the time of conception.
4. These accidents occur more often as women get older but can happen at any age and with no family history.
5. Only about half of babies with an abnormal number of chromosomes have Down syndrome.
6. Changes in chromosome number can cause certain other disorders that would be more serious than Down syndrome (i.e., associated with severe mental retardation, multiple malformations, and a greatly shortened life span) or milder conditions that would

not be detectable in many adults (but about which it might be beneficial to know).
7. These disorders can be diagnosed with a high degree of accuracy by studying the chromosomes from a sample of amniotic fluid or chorionic villi.
8. Testing maternal blood will identify some mothers who are carrying a chromosomally abnormal baby (and many who are not), but cannot make a diagnosis.

While this information can be tailored to the clients' sophistication and level of interest, most patients do not need, and indeed do not benefit from, a lengthy genetics explanation or description of chromosomal entities.

In the case of an elevated maternal serum alphafetoprotein result, the essential information to present is more situation-specific and will depend on the counselor's judgment. Many factors, including how high the result is, if ultrasound has previously been used to confirm dates and rule out a multiple gestation, whether this previous scan was done when a major abnormality (like anencephaly) should have been detectable, as well as relevant pregnancy information such as the reliability of the patient's dates and any history of bleeding or threatened abortion, will influence what should be emphasized. Even with a relatively low value (2.5 to 2.9 multiples of the median), about 1/20 patients will have a fetal malformation, demise, or other complication such as oligohydramnios diagnosed at ultrasound (Crandall et al., 1991). When the level is very high (>5 MoM), about 2/3 of patients will be found to have a problem (Crandall et al., 1991). Because the likely abnormalities—neural tube and ventral wall defects and anencephaly—are unfamiliar to most patients, it is important to describe them in general terms. I usually defer using diagrams or discussing chromosomes until specific ultrasound findings suggest that the couple needs more information to understand the implications of the diagnosis or to make a decision about additional testing such as amniocentesis or about pregnancy termination. On the other hand, most patients will have MSAFP levels under 5 MoM, and they can be reassured that the majority of women with results similar to theirs will have no fetal abnormality or pregnancy complication. As with other types of prenatal diagnosis, clients need to be told the chances that a significant abnormality will be missed with ultrasonography alone, or with both ultrasound and amniocentesis. Also, patients need to be cautioned that—unlike maternal age or low α-fetoprotein indications, for which a normal chorionic villus sampling (CVS) or amniocentesis can provide nearly complete reassurance that risk is no longer increased—having a high MSAFP confers a residual risk for an untoward pregnancy outcome even after normal ultrasound and amniocentesis.

Information about testing options

Clearly, a thorough discussion of available means of prenatal diagnosis and the advantages and disadvantages of each is essential to the couple's decision-making. However, the proliferation of prenatal testing options can make this a daunting exercise for both the counselor and the clients. A couple referred early in pregnancy for advanced maternal age may need to choose among CVS, early amniocentesis, "regular" amniocentesis, and one or more serum screening options—with or without ultrasonography. Increasingly, they are also asked to consider carrier screening for CF, hemoglobinopathies, or other conditions more prevalent in their ethnic group. Each of these tests has a different sensitivity and specificity, different attendant risks and limitations, and sometimes a different likelihood of being covered by the patient's health insurance. Some counselors utilize pamphlets, a videotape, or a group presentation to introduce these options. This saves time and gives more opportunity to individualize the subsequent face-to-face discussion.

Even after all the prenatal diagnostic and screening alternatives have been described, patients frequently need the counselor to again compare the options with regard to:

1. Each test's diagnostic accuracy for the condition(s) for which they are at risk.
2. Further testing that might be needed in the case of inconclusive results.
3. The amount of fetal risk or maternal discomfort with each test.
4. Timing for testing and results.
5. Expense

Asking the couple which of these factors is most and least important to them can help them identify the option that is best for them. A reflective summary by the counselor of their decision-making process helps to ensure that they have understood and weighed all the various alternatives and their implications. An example might be: "It sounds as though the most important things for you are to have results of the chromosome study as early as possible and as much reassurance as we can give that the baby does not have any abnormality. You seem to be leaning towards CVS with an AFP blood test a month later and a good ultrasound at about 18 weeks. Am I right in understanding that CVS's slightly higher risk and the very small chance that an amniocentesis might be needed if the results are inconclus-

ive are acceptable to you in exchange for getting results earlier?"

Exploration of feelings about testing and possible outcomes

At the time of referral, some couples may unwaveringly state their desire for a particular mode of prenatal diagnosis and their intentions in case of certain outcomes. Others may remain ambivalent and unsure of what to do about having testing even after extensive counseling. Clients need to understand from the outset that the role of the counselor is to provide information about the tests and to help them make decisions that they are comfortable with. This is particularly important when the issue is follow-up for an abnormal screening result, since the urgency of the referral and the anxiety surrounding it may make patients feel as though they have been thrust into a cascade of events over which they have little control. For some patients, the counselor's nondirective message may not seem to match what they have heard from their primary practitioner. They may indicate that they are there only because their "doctor said I should have this test" or may even fear that their prenatal care will be jeopardized if they do not follow what they perceive is their prenatal provider's recommendation.

It is important that the counseling session not become so focused on the diagnostic methods and the diagnosable conditions that little attention is paid to the reasons for offering testing. Unfortunately, there is still a widespread perception that the sole purpose of prenatal diagnosis is to identify anomalous fetuses so that their birth can be prevented by pregnancy termination. Other valid reasons that should be reviewed with the couple (when appropriate to their situation) include (1) the likelihood that testing will provide reassurance; (2) the fact that knowing more about the baby's condition may change how the pregnancy and delivery are managed; (3) the ability to plan for the baby's treatment in the neonatal period (or in rare cases, prenatally); and (4) the opportunity for the family to adjust, make plans, and marshal resources prior to the baby's birth.

Before a final decision is made about testing, each partner should be asked, separately, if they have considered what they would do in the face of an abnormal outcome. Although this is an uncomfortable question for both counselor and counselee, it does acknowledge that they may not be reassured by testing and could face a painful decision as a result. It also provides an opportunity for patients to ask about the particulars of pregnancy termination if they wish. This is a good time for the counselor to mention that couples do not always end up making decisions they think they would, to normalize the fact that the wait for test results is always difficult, to invite the couple to contact the counselor if they have questions in the interim, and to establish at what time and where they would like to be called with results.

For couples who are undecided about testing and in situations where the two partners are not in accord, it may help to have them describe what they feel would be the impact of several different possible outcomes, for example:

1. They have testing and the baby either appears fine, is affected with a serious condition, or has a relatively mild condition about which they would not otherwise have known.
2. They have testing from which results are inconclusive or ambiguous.
3. They have testing and have a complication that results in pregnancy loss.
4. They do not have testing and have a baby with a problem that could have been diagnosed prenatally.

Additional counseling concerns in other prenatal diagnostic situations

The basic elements of obtaining appropriate history, educating patients about the mechanics, risks, and limitations of testing, and exploring feelings regarding testing options and possible outcomes are common to all prenatal diagnosis counseling, but additional issues may arise when special circumstances surround the pregnancy. Some of these situations are discussed in the following sections.

Previous affected child

When parents are seeking prenatal diagnosis for a condition with which a previous child has been affected, there is bound to be a great deal of ambivalence, particularly if the child is still alive. Having prenatal diagnosis with the intent of aborting a similarly affected fetus may seem to parents to be tantamount to betrayal—denying the positive aspects of the child's existence and implicitly stating "We wouldn't have had you if we had had the choice." Furthermore, anxiety over the possibility of a recurrence can be so overwhelming that emotional investment in the pregnancy is "put on hold" until after the diagnosis is complete. This robs the parents of the excitement and anticipation of the early months of pregnancy and of support from family and friends if they choose to keep the pregnancy private until after the CVS or amniocentesis. It is important to ask the couple whom they have told about the pregnancy and to provide additional emotional support during and after the diagnosis if the couple's

usual social network is not aware of what they are going through. The counselor should be sensitive to the fact that coming to counseling may be especially traumatic if the genetics unit is in the same medical center where the previous child was treated or died and should give the couple a specific opportunity to deal with these reactions.

The family may also have "replacement child" issues. Parents of a child who died in late gestation or in infancy may rush prematurely into a subsequent pregnancy in an attempt to restore the child they lost and to reassure themselves (as well as friends and family) of their potency and fertility. Sometimes this urgency is driven by a sense of "the biological clock ticking", especially if the previous child is (or was) affected with an age-related aneuploidy. When an older child has died he or she may have been idealized to a degree that it is impossible for its potential successor to be welcomed wholeheartedly, causing ambivalence, as well as anxiety about the pregnancy.

The counselor should explore the parents' understanding of the affected child's disorder and clarify which medical problems were related to the condition and how the disorder might differ in another individual. This is especially important when the previous child's condition was compromised by additional complications such as prematurity or a postnatal infection. The previous child may have had multiple anomalies that were associated with a syndrome (e.g., polydactyly, cleft lip and palate, holoprosencephaly, a heart defect, and an omphalocele with trisomy 13). In this case, it is essential that the parents realize that their recurrence risk is for the underlying condition (e.g., the aneuploidy) rather than for a host of individual birth defects.

Affected parent

A delicate situation arises when a couple is referred for counseling and possible prenatal diagnosis of a condition with which one of the parents is affected. It is important to ascertain who has suggested or is seeking the consultation. In some cases, the couple is not concerned about having a similarly affected child, and has come only to placate their prenatal care provider. Unfortunately, such a referral can carry various implicit guilt-provoking and devaluing messages such as "A responsible person wouldn't want to pass on this condition" or "Of course, you wouldn't want to have a child with the same problems you've had." It is well to ask the couple what they think were their practitioner's concerns in suggesting the consultation and how they feel about having been referred.

If the couple has sought counseling on their own, was one of them more interested than the other, and if so why?

What is their perception of the severity and variability of the condition and of the efficacy of currently available treatment? What messages have they gotten from their family, friends, or health care providers about embarking on this pregnancy? Are they interested in the possibility of prenatal diagnosis, and if so, what would they do with the information? Do both the affected and the unaffected parent feel the same way about the possibility of having a child with the condition? If not, which of them is the more unsure? Is guilt being expressed by the affected parent or blame by the unaffected one? Does the affected individual's disease have any implications for parenting (e.g., shortened life span, employability, insurability, ability to cope with the physical demands of child-rearing)? If it is the mother who is affected, are there any concerns about the impact of the pregnancy on her own health? The answers to these questions will speak volumes about the couple's relationship, their family dynamics, and the self-image of the affected individual.

In some cases, adults with genetic conditions or birth defects were treated in childhood but may not have required follow-up. A genetic counseling referral occasioned by pregnancy can provide an opportunity to educate the affected individual and partner about the condition and newer modes of diagnosis or treatment, to address related psychosocial issues, and to refer to social services and support groups when appropriate.

Parental carrier status

Sometimes one or both parents are known to be carrying a recessive gene or chromosome rearrangement that was discovered through genetic screening rather than an affected child. Depending on whether testing was done because of a family history of a specific condition, on the basis of ethnicity, or after repeated fetal losses, the couple's understanding about the potential disorder will vary. In the case of translation carriers and women who carry an X-linked mutation, "responsibility" for the increased fetal risk can be attributed to a single partner, potentially engendering guilt or blame. The carrier parent may also have had one or more family members with the condition, in which case their attitude toward the disorder (and prenatal diagnosis) will be colored by this experience and by their relationship with the affected person. Conversely, parents who are found to be at risk for an autosomal recessive condition (such as Canavan disease or alpha thalassemia) solely because they were screened on the basis of increased ethnic risk may have no experience with the condition. It can require a "leap of faith" for them to believe that they could have a severely affected child when no one they know has ever had such a disorder.

When a translocation has been found after recurrent miscarriages, the couple may be unwilling to have any type of invasive procedure that might jeopardize a "premium" pregnancy that has successfully been carried through the first trimester. They may also perceive (perhaps correctly) that any unbalanced conception would have eliminated itself. Moreover, for many translocations ascertained as a result of miscarriages, little information is available about the phenotype that would be expected if an unbalanced offspring survived to term. This paucity of data makes decision-making about prenatal diagnosis especially difficult.

Possible teratogenic exposures

Exposure to a possible or perceived teratogen is likely to precipitate a real crisis during pregnancy. While this is not strictly a genetic counseling issue, it frequently becomes one, either because the patient is referred for prenatal diagnosis because of the exposure, seeks a second opinion after having been advised (often incorrectly) that the fetus is at greatly increased risk, or mentions the teratogenic agent during counseling for some other indication. In most cases, reassurance can be provided, but it is likely to be believed by the patient only after careful assessment and a thorough explanation of why the exposure is unlikely to have harmed the baby. Points that may be important to emphasize (depending on the patient's situation) include that:

1. An agent that causes birth defects in certain laboratory animals does not necessarily cause problems in humans.
2. The exposure happened at a time that it could not have caused damage in the fetus (i.e., by occurring before implantation or after the susceptible organ system had already formed).
3. The dosage was much too low to have caused damage (e.g., most diagnostic radiographs).
4. An apparently high *relative* risk may not mean a high absolute risk (e.g., even a twenty-fold increase in fetal risk may translate into less than a 1% chance for a specific rare birth defect).
5. The birth defect caused by the agent is of relatively little consequence or remediable (e.g., staining of primary but not secondary teeth with tetracycline exposure).
6. Individual sensitivity to the teratogen may differ depending on maternal and fetal metabolism.
7. There is a small (about 3%) risk of having a baby with a birth defect even with *no* exposures in pregnancy.

Sometimes, the fetal risk may actually be significantly increased due to an exposure, and the patient cannot be reassured. The impact of this information will vary according to what the patient already knows about her risk and how much control she had over the exposure. In certain maternal disease states, such as diabetes or epilepsy, the woman may previously have been admonished not to get pregnant, and thus feel selfish or irresponsible for wanting a child and putting it at risk. The patient who has neglected warnings about specific medications or failed to maintain good diabetic or (in the case of a metabolic disorder like PKU) dietary control may also feel guilty. In many cases, prenatal diagnosis can be provided for certain of the birth defects (such as major cardiac malformations and neural tube defects) for which the maternal condition increases risk. The patient can then be reassured that at least these problems appear not to have occurred, and that the chance of a fetal anomaly is therefore reduced.

Counseling about fetal risk due to chronic alcoholism or drug abuse can be particularly challenging. It is often impossible to determine the actual nature and magnitude of potentially damaging exposures, since the reliability of the history may be questionable. Moreover, since many of the fetal effects of such agents are either unknown or subtle and not amenable to prenatal diagnosis, complete reassurance can rarely be provided as a result of the counseling or testing. In some cases, the patient may have a great deal of ambivalence about the pregnancy and be unable or unwilling to modify her risk-causing behavior. Certain patients may actually hope to be told that the fetal risk is high so that they can justify an abortion decision. For this reason it is especially important to assess the patient's feelings about being pregnant and her plans for the baby. A nonjudgmental counseling stance that acknowledges that fetal damage may already have occurred while emphasizing the benefits of reducing exposures throughout the rest of pregnancy is most appropriate. By maintaining contact as the pregnancy continues and slowly earning the patient's trust, the counselor may be able to make a successful referral for a treatment program, for discussion of adoption, or for services that may help to improve the lifestyle or increase parenting skills.

Abnormal ultrasound findings

With obstetric ultrasound becoming routine in many practices, fetal anomalies are being identified in low-risk pregnancies with increasing frequency. When this happens, the first genetic counseling contact may be after referral for a consultative high-resolution ultrasound. At this point the couple, who had looked forward to their doctor's sonogram providing them with their first baby picture and perhaps a determination of the fetal sex, is in a state of crisis over the unanticipated findings. They may be especially bewildered if their practitioner and the consultative ultrasonographer have given conflicting interpretations of the baby's problems, and may find it hard to believe that such grave prognostic information could derive from a collection of shadowy images.

If the anomaly is found early enough in pregnancy and fetal chromosome studies provide an explanation, the parents can be given specific information to help them make a decision about continuing the pregnancy. However, ultrasound sometimes discovers the abnormality too late for termination to be an option or finds something (e.g., oligohydramnios, incipient hydrocephalus, a cystic kidney) for which the fetal prognosis is unclear. Sometimes repeated assessments may be needed to determine the finding's significance. In these situations, the parents suffer an extended period of uncertainty and anxiety, which may not be resolved until some time after delivery. Scheduling a meeting between the parents and several professionals from appropriate disciplines (e.g., genetics, perinatology, pediatric surgery, neonatal intensive care, social work) who can provide input about the possible implications of the anomalies and the resources that will be available to deal with them can give the parents at least some concrete information and diminish their sense of helplessness.

Surrogacy and assisted reproduction

The proliferation of alternatives for conceiving and bearing a child can lead to unusual genetic counseling situations. To establish a pregnancy, infertile couples and those at risk for genetic diseases may have utilized techniques as routine as artificial insemination with donor sperm or as novel as preimplantation genetic diagnosis. Often a great deal of expense, emotional upheaval and inconvenience has been involved, and the pregnancy may be long awaited or achieved after many disappointments. Given their considerable investment of time, money, and psychic energy, such couples are usually painfully anxious from before the moment of conception (which they can often pinpoint to the hour) until a normal baby is safely home with them and various potential legal pitfalls have been successfully avoided. They may seek, but be very ambivalent about, prenatal diagnosis—on the one hand, wanting every reassurance that the baby is developing normally, while, on the other, being unwilling to do anything to put the pregnancy at risk.

When the couple has utilized ovum or sperm donation, it is important to ascertain the extent of genetic history and screening that was obtained on the donor. If they are unsure about this, the genetic counselor should ask their permission to contact the facility or provider that arranged the donation so that the adequacy of this screening can be documented in the genetics chart. It is also good to ascertain what their policy is on contacting donors in the event that a genetic disorder is found in the fetus or child. I usually obtain a genetic history on both members of the couple—even though one is not the biologic parent—to identify any other issues that could have health implications for either of them or their family members.

Surrogacy presents a more complicated situation since the gestational mother may or may not be the biologic mother. This can have implications in deciding how appropriate it is to offer prenatal diagnosis for maternal age, since presumably it is the age of the mother contributing the egg that will determine the risk for fetal aneuploidy. Moreover, it is not always clear whether it is the contracting couple or the surrogate who is the patient. In some cases, their contract may explicitly state that the surrogate will submit to prenatal diagnosis, even though there is no indication for this other than parental anxiety. This means that the surrogate cannot be entirely autonomous in making her decision about diagnostic procedures or, potentially about pregnancy management if a fetal anomaly is found. Current obstetric guidelines indicate that the gestational mother should have complete autonomy in making decisions about the pregnancy, regardless of whether she is the biologic mother. But even so, the interests of the contracting couple obviously create conflicts and tensions. Although some couples develop a close relationship with their surrogate, it is usually better to have separate genetic counseling sessions, so that both parties feel comfortable in having their questions and concerns addressed. It is especially important to clarify who is to be given the results.

Positive diagnoses and ambiguous findings

Although most couples having prenatal diagnosis can be told they are most likely to receive reassuring news, the counseling should also prepare them for the possibility of an abnormal or inconclusive result. They must also be reminded that because some fetal abnormalities cannot be detected by analysis of amniotic fluid, chorionic villi, serum markers, and/or expert ultrasound, and because complications can occur later in pregnancy, a normal prenatal diagnosis cannot guarantee a normal baby. The anxiety of waiting for results can be miserable, but couples may be

somewhat comforted by knowing what will be going on with their specimen in the interim. The following specific points are worth mentioning:

1. Some cultures normally grow more rapidly than others so there is variability in how long results will take.
2. Their sample will begin to be processed and analyzed as soon as it is at an appropriate stage.
3. There are numerous checks that ensure that specimens are not mixed up.
4. Their results will be reviewed by at least two specialists.
5. The laboratory will notify the counselor (or their doctor, the patient, etc.) as soon as the studies are complete.

The couple should be told how and from whom they will get their results. They also should be asked which of them wants be called and where, and whether they think they will want to know the fetal sex. At our center, the counselor usually gives normal results to the patient by telephone. If at all possible, however, abnormal findings are delivered only face to face. During the pre-diagnosis counseling session, we prepare the couple for this by explaining that we will ask them to come back in if the results are in any way unusual, even if they do not signify a fetal abnormality. This can be presented as a "policy" that has been made because findings are frequently easier to explain in person using pictures and/or because many primary care providers are inexperienced in interpreting genetic studies. It is our preference not to give an abnormal diagnosis over the telephone unless specifically asked. However, when the couple is having prenatal diagnosis to rule out a specific disorder (e.g., an unbalanced chromosome translocation or another condition with which they or a previous child have been affected) they usually ask. We also try not to call if face-to-face counseling cannot be arranged shortly thereafter (i.e., not late on a Friday afternoon or before a holiday unless timing is critical). If couples understand that being asked to return for counseling does not necessarily mean that a fetal abnormality has been found, they are less likely to press for information before they can be given the diagnosis together in the office.

At the informing interview, the counselor should be prepared to discuss not only the implications of the specific findings, but other information (such as available financial and social service resources, or issues surrounding pregnancy termination) that may be relevant to decision-making. When there is a clear diagnosis such as a chromosome abnormality, the features of the condition should be presented as completely and even-handedly as possible. If the fetus appears, by ultrasound, not to have certain anomalies (e.g., a cystic hygroma in 45,X, a major cardiac lesion in trisomy 21), the couple can be reassured that although such a problem *can* be associated with the condition, it apparently has not occurred in their baby. When appropriate, showing pictures that include non-clinical photographs of affected individuals at various ages engaged in characteristic activities can help the couple visualize not only the phenotypic features, but how such a person might (or might not) fit into their lives. It is important to elicit the parents' prior experience (if any) with the condition and to correct misperceptions. Available intervention—surgical, medical, and developmental— should be described, and if affected individuals usually live into adulthood, discussion should include the outlook for independent living, employment, marriage, and family. Some parents may appreciate an offer to meet with a specialist who treats the condition, with a family who has an affected child, or with a representative of a relevant support group. Such referrals should be made carefully, and with an awareness of the personalities and attitudes of both parties.

Especially challenging for both counselors and parents is finding a problem that can be quite variable (e.g., mosaic aneuploidy or a small, low spina bifida), one that may not be evident at birth (e.g., 47,XXX or 47,XXY), or one for which the outcome cannot be predicted with any certainty (e.g., a marker chromosome or an elevated amniotic fluid α-fetoprotein with normal ultrasound and negative acetyl-cholinesterase). A couple who elect to continue such a pregnancy will be left with heightened anxiety and doubts that will persist long after the child is born, and will need a great deal of counseling support over the next several months or even years. If they decide to abort, they should be reminded that while the fetus may appear normal, certain potentially associated problems (e.g., mental retardation, infertility or incontinence) would not be evident. Nonetheless, the couple who makes a decision to end a pregnancy in the face of uncertain information is bound to have persistent fears that they have aborted a normal fetus.

Options and decisions after a fetal abnormality is diagnosed

Unless the couple is quite secure about their course of action, the counselor should specifically discuss the various alternatives and their implications. Other factors besides phenotypic information that may be important in the parents' decision about continuing the pregnancy include:

1. The probability that the fetus might die or be born prematurely.
2. If the fetal diagnosis increases risk to the mother in any way.

3. How the baby's condition might alter pregnancy and delivery management.
4. What decisions about the baby's treatment will need to be made after delivery.
5. What help they can expect in caring for the baby.
6. What options they have in case they decide they *cannot* care for the baby.

With regard to last issue, the possibility of adoption or foster placement can be raised. If the couple has questions about the likelihood that a baby with problems such as theirs would be able to be placed, the counselor should be prepared to put them in touch with an appropriate agency and should offer to communicate directly with the agency about the nature of the fetal diagnosis.

If the couple decides to terminate the pregnancy, they will need information about:

1. What choices they have (if any) about the type of termination.
2. The advantages and disadvantages of each method (e.g., an intact delivery following labor induction might improve the likelihood of establishing or confirming the diagnosis and would allow the couple to view the fetus and release it to a mortuary, but it would mean that the mother would experience labor with possibly unpleasant side effects from medication and would be awake for the delivery).
3. The relative costs of the different abortion methods.
4. The mechanics of scheduling the chosen procedure.

If termination is to be done by induction, the counselor will need to help the couple consider additional issues including whether they wish to see, hold, name, or baptize the fetus, consent for autopsy or other studies, and their preference for disposition of the remains.

Once a couple has made a decision to abort, they usually want the procedure done as soon as possible. It is helpful for the genetics unit and obstetrics to have established a protocol for terminations for fetal anomalies so that patients are treated sensitively and fetuses can be examined and samples obtained as needed. Educating surgical or labor and delivery nurses and house staff about the patient's unusual situation can help ensure that she is segregated as much as possible from other laboring patients and the newborn nursery and that events surrounding the procedure or delivery are handled according to the couple's preferences. If the parents wish to see the fetus, the baby should be presented wrapped in a warmed baby blanket with any anomalies covered until the parents can be prepared for what they will see. It is important to remember that most people have never seen a fetus or markedly pre-term baby and that some fetal characteristics (such as the thin skin and body proportions) at this gestational age can be disarming. The baby's normal features should be pointed out, as well as any that corroborate findings seen on ultrasound or anticipated from chromosome studies.

At our center, parents are told that we routinely take photographs of the fetus for our genetics chart in order to document the abnormalities and provide a record that may be important for future diagnosis. This practice can also be helpful for a parent who is unsure about wanting to see or hold the baby and who may find it more manageable to look at a Polaroid picture before deciding. We tell couples that some parents want one or more pictures for themselves, either at the time of delivery or some months or even years later. For this reason, we take extra photographs with the fetus wrapped to look as normal as possible and others to show the abnormalities. Such photographs can provide parents with a tangible reminder of their baby, as can a lock of hair, or a footprint. Photographs also provide a "fallback" alternative if the parent did not wish to view the fetus at the time of delivery.

Ongoing support following prenatal diagnosis

A pregnancy termination because of a fetal anomaly is psychologically very different from other elective abortions. In the first place, the pregnancy was probably planned and wanted. Second, unless the couple knew they were at increased risk because of a previous disorder or carrier status, they were unlikely to have been prepared for the fetal abnormality. In most cases the problem will not have been diagnosed until well into the second trimester, often at about the time fetal movement was beginning to be felt and usually after friends and family had become aware of the pregnancy. For parents who tried to keep themselves on "emotional hold" because of a pending prenatal diagnosis, the impact of seeing the fetal ultrasound images will often have made it hard to postpone bonding with the baby any longer. The unexpected nature of the diagnosis, the ("taint") of carrying a baby with a birth defect, and strong personal, religious, and societal feelings about abortion may have made it difficult for the parents to call upon their usual sources for emotional support and help with decision-making. If their primary practitioner was also unfamiliar and uncomfortable with the situation, the couple may feel that they were abandoned to face their plight alone.

In addition to the emotional impact of having unexpectedly lost a pregnancy, the parents have suffered an assault to their egos by having produced an "imperfect" child. Many of their responses will be the same as those of parents who have given birth to an abnormal newborn. They may feel unworthy as a marriage partner, and even if the anomaly was not genetic, they will be anxious about their prospects for future reproductive success. At the same time, they will be angry about the unjustness of what has happened to them, and this anger may bewilder them when they unexpectedly find it directed at pregnant strangers, health professionals, each other, or even God. If the decision to terminate was contrary to firmly held personal moral beliefs, the couple's already overwhelming sense of isolation, guilt, and loss is likely to be magnified. Blumberg and his colleagues (1975) showed that couples terminating a pregnancy after prenatal diagnosis suffered depression that was of even greater intensity than that following a stillbirth. In some cases, the termination may revive repressed memories of a previous elective abortion. This can be particularly challenging for the mother, who may feel that she is being punished for her past "sin" or be obsessed with the fact that the previously aborted baby would probably have been normal. If her husband is unaware of this history, she will be completely alone in her self-recriminations.

At the time of the termination and in the weeks immediately following, the counselor can help the couple anticipate some of these reactions and reassure them as to their normalcy. By maintaining periodic telephone contact the geneticist can demonstrate a willingness to be available for questions and "venting" of emotions, reduce the couple's sense of isolation, and monitor the progress of grieving. Many patients report a great sense of relief upon learning that the autopsy or post-procedure chromosome studies have confirmed the abnormality. A return appointment to review the findings and discuss future reproductive risks and interventions can also provide an opportunity to explore how both parents are coping. Times that can be especially difficult for couples who have terminated a pregnancy include the date that delivery would have occurred and the one year anniversary of the abortion. A call from the counselor at these times is often viewed as a real show of emotional support, and can provide another chance for the patient to ask questions and discuss reactions and relationships. Some areas have special support groups for couples who have terminated a pregnancy because of a fetal anomaly. These can be very helpful for some parents and are much more appropriate than groups that focus on infant loss.

The couple who decides to continue a pregnancy in the face of a fetal anomaly can also benefit from ongoing contacts with the counselor. These can provide an opportunity to reinforce the information given at the post-diagnostic session and can reassure the couple that they are not being ignored because the geneticist feels that they made an inappropriate decision in choosing to carry the pregnancy. In fact, it is worthwhile asking the couple if they have told friends and family about the diagnosis, and if so what the reaction has been. Unfortunately, having prenatal diagnosis available sends an implicit societal message that it should be utilized and that a reasonable person would choose not to have a handicapped child if they knew. Parents who are continuing an abnormal pregnancy may need help in responding to inadvertent judgmental comments about their decision.

An advantage of knowing the diagnosis several months in advance of delivery is that some of the grief work can be completed before the baby arrives. During this period, couples are likely to experience many of the same emotions that they would if the diagnosis were made in the newborn period. Until the baby arrives, however, they can only adjust to the loss of the expected child and not to the reality of a child whom they do not yet know. Uncertainties about how the baby will look, what problems it will have, and whether there will be delivery complications can cause great anxiety. At the same time, even when a parent has had no doubts about continuing the pregnancy, he or she may sometimes secretly hope that the baby will die, thereby relieving them of the burden. While it is difficult for a parent to admit to having such alarming and enormously guilt-producing thoughts, the counselor may be able to elicit and deal with them by remarking that even parents who have elected to continue a pregnancy may still be somewhat ambivalent about the baby.

By utilizing the remainder of the pregnancy to familiarize themselves with the condition and to explore resources that will be available, parents can increase their sense of control over what has befallen them. The counselor can help by putting them in touch with families who have a similarly affected child, a support group, an early intervention program, or appropriate social services. While some adjustment to the diagnosis can be accomplished during the latter half of pregnancy, the couple's need for support will not end with the baby's birth. The counselor will be able to capitalize on the relationship and trust that has developed during the prenatal period as the family continues to meet new and different emotional challenges.

INFERTILITY AND FETAL LOSS

Multiple pregnancy loss

A frequent indication for genetic services is repeated miscarriage. Although in many cases couples are sent only for cytogenetic studies, it is worth spending some time in pre-

liminary counseling whenever possible. Previous investigations of the cause of the losses are likely to have focused on obstetric issues, and so a referral for genetic evaluation may add a new and frightening dimension. It is important for the couple to realize that a chromosomal basis for miscarriages will be identified in only about 1 in 20 couples and that such a finding rarely precludes a normal subsequent reproductive outcome. Obtaining a brief family and pregnancy history, particularly if there have been others in the family with increased fetal loss or abnormal liveborns, can help to refine the level of suspicion about a chromosomal etiology and may occasionally identify a different genetic basis for the losses. The couple should be asked what they have already been told about the reasons for the miscarriages and whether any pathology or cytogenetic investigation of the products of conception was done. If appropriate, the possibility of investigating other potential causes of infertility (e.g., thrombophilias, CFTR mutations, etc.) can be raised.

By commenting on how hard it must be to have had repeated disappointments and by asking how the two of them are doing, the counselor can invite discussion of emotional issues surrounding the losses. It is particularly important to specifically include the father in this discussion, since the paternal impact of miscarriage is frequently ignored. Inquiring about the circumstances of the miscarriages and about the reactions of friends and family will often elicit comments about how alone they feel with their loss or how difficult it is for them to respond to unthinking remarks such as "You're young, you'll get pregnant again soon," or "It was good that you miscarried, because there was probably something wrong with it." The counselor can validate the appropriateness of the couple's sorrow by acknowledging that they rightly feel they have lost a baby (and usually more than one baby), not just a pregnancy.

Sometimes, if I sense that the parents are quite sad and frustrated, I will try to normalize feelings they may have had by mentioning that many couples in their situation have told me that they occasionally find themselves resenting the normal pregnancies and children of others, or that they are terrified of initiating another pregnancy, or that they feel they have been avoided by friends and excluded from certain social events like baby showers. Enumerating such characteristic reactions may make it easier for the couple to admit to similar feelings and help reduce their anxiety or guilt about having them. Time spent attending to psychosocial issues before the cytogenetic studies are done can help develop rapport that will be needed in the event a rearrangement is found.

If studies are normal, the couple can be reassured that there is no apparent genetic reason for their miscarriages.

While the possibility exists that some undetermined genetic factor could still be contributing to their losses, relatively few such causes have yet been identified. The couple may view the normal results with relief or with even greater frustration, since they still have no explanation for what is occurring and little information about the likelihood that they will again face disappointment.

When one member of the couple is found to carry a translocation or other chromosome change, a number of issues need to be addressed. Among these are that the rearrangement has no implications for the health of the carrier except in terms of reproductive risk. When it is the father who is found to carry the translocation, he may have more difficulty in dealing with the discovery because until the genetic investigation, "responsibility" for reproductive failure had implicitly been attributed to his partner. Carrier status often jeopardizes a person's self-image. The fact that the chromosome change is present in all the cells of the body, and that there is no remedy for it, may add to the sense of being "damaged". At least with most obstetric causes and other non-genetic reasons for miscarriage, there is some hope that the problem can be corrected.

Another frustrating issue is that the reproductive implications of the translocation may be unclear. Is the couple's increased risk solely for repeated miscarriages, or do they have a chance of having abnormal liveborns? If so, what types of problem might result, and what could be the range of severity? Except in relatively common and well-described rearrangements, such as many of the robertsonian translocations, these questions can rarely be answered satisfactorily. With limited information, the couple faces a quandary in subsequent pregnancies, since they cannot be sure that a chromosomally unbalanced fetus would again miscarry. The uncertainty means that they must consider an invasive diagnostic procedure even if they succeed in getting the pregnancy into the midtrimester.

The last consideration with discovery of a chromosome translocation is the potential risk to other family members. It is usually appropriate to suggest chromosome studies on at least the parents of the carrier to see if siblings and other relatives of reproductive age could be at risk. This puts the newly identified carrier in the awkward position of discussing his or her own evaluation and the reasons for it with family members who may not have been aware of the pregnancy history, and also of raising relatives' anxiety by explaining the potential implications of the finding.

The logistics of testing and insurance considerations can also be problematic for the family. It is not surprising that many carriers are reticent to contact others about their risk, and the counselor may need to facilitate this process by offering to talk with at-risk relatives or by writing an explanatory letter that can be sent by the patient to those who might wish to consider testing. An interesting professional ethical dilemma arises in the situation where, even after extensive counseling, the carrier refuses to notify relatives. If the counselor feels that the risk is high enough that a reasonable person would want this information for reproductive planning, he may need to explain to the patients that warning specific family members is so important that it may be necessary for him to breach confidentiality. In reality, it is rarely necessary (or possible) to do this, and just having this discussion with the patients may motivate them.

Stillbirth or neonatal death

Many of the above issues related to pregnancy loss pertain to genetic counseling for a condition that has resulted in stillbirth or death in the newborn period. Although the parents may hardly have had an opportunity to know the infant, the child they fantasized has been lost—not only because it died, but also because it was not the child they anticipated. When the death was related to one or more malformations, the unfamiliar and alarming nature of these may have seemed repugnant to the parents, making them wish to disavow that they could have created something so unlike them. Such a reaction is bound to engender guilt: "How could a parent not love his child—particularly a sick, helpless baby?" The goals of counseling should be not only to provide information about causation and recurrence risk, but also to demystify the abnormality and to help the couple deal with these complex emotions.

Even if the baby was stillborn, it is important to ask the parents if they named him or her and then to use the name in talking about the baby. This demonstrates that the counselor recognizes the baby's humanity and appreciates the significance of the fact it was the couple's child. I once had a couple tell me six weeks after their baby's neonatal death that I was the only person beside themselves who had ever called their child by name!

As with other types of counseling, asking the parents what they have been told about the baby and what additional things they themselves have noticed is a good place to start. Misperceptions about the baby's features can then be corrected at the outset. In some cases one or both parents may not have seen the baby. If pictures are available, the counselor can offer to show them to the couple, preparing them for what they will see. Sometimes they may want copies of the photographs. When there has been an autopsy, the couple can be given the option of having the geneticist read through it with them. Since the autopsy report may end up in their possession, it is important that they understand the terminology and what was or was not relevant to the baby's diagnosis and cause of death. It is often less scary if malformations or dysmorphic features can be explained in terms of how a normal developmental process either did not finish (such as failure of the lip or neural tube to close), was unable to happen properly because of an underlying genetic abnormality (for instance, in a trisomy), or occurred normally but was later disrupted (e.g., amniotic bands). When appropriate, it is important to clarify that, while the couple may have a risk for recurrence of the condition, they do not have any higher chance of having any of its associated anomalies recur if the condition itself does not.

Since parents of a baby who has died will often have been accused—implicitly or even explicitly—of doing something before or during the pregnancy or of having something in their family that caused the baby's problems, it is essential that such history be obtained sensitively. Depending on the genetic basis of the disorder, the pedigree can assume more or less prominence in the interview. On the other hand, getting a thorough pregnancy history is often critical for pinpointing inappropriate concerns the parents have had about what caused the condition. It may also occasionally be valuable in identifying early clues to the diagnosis or (rarely) to contributing factors. Sometimes the counselor may intuit that there are unarticulated concerns about previous real or imagined misdeeds. One can pursue this hunch with an offhand statement such as "Many parents worry that their baby's problem was caused by doing something like using drugs in high school" (or a fall, stress, previous abortion, etc., as appropriate). This often gives the parent permission to raise the real issue or issues that have been on his or her mind.

In discussing how the family is coping emotionally, the counselor should specifically explore:

1. The reaction of their friends and family to the baby's condition and death.
2. How each of them is dealing with his or her grief.
3. Whether and how experiencing the baby's death has changed their relationship with each other.
4. What they have told their other children about the baby's death.
5. If they have noticed changes in the other children's behavior.
6. Whether supports that have been important to them in the past (friends, family, religious faith) are still helpful.

An extensive discussion of bereavement counseling is beyond the scope of this chapter, but there are many good treatments of this special area of counseling. There is also a growing body of lay literature appropriate for couples who

have had a miscarriage, stillbirth, or neonatal death. Numerous local and international support groups exist for parents who have lost a baby. Social services associated with obstetrics and pediatric units can often be of help in identifying resources for patient referral.

Genetic conditions resulting in infertility or unusual sexual development

Interestingly, despite the fact that surveys done of patients in subfertility clinics have shown that chromosome abnormalities, including rearrangements, are several times more likely to be present than they are in the fertile population, karyotypes are not usually a routine part of the evaluation. For this reason, unlike couples who are found to have a chromosome translocation after fetal losses, the diagnosis of a genetic abnormality in an infertile individual is usually suspected because of his or her phenotype. Often the affected person may not only have been concerned about infertility but also distressed or insecure about his or her diminished, or otherwise unusual, secondary sexual development. This sensitivity about body image makes counseling a teenager or adult for a condition such as Klinefelter or Turner syndrome, or a rarer one like androgen insensitivity or Kallman syndrome particularly delicate.

It is critical that information about the genetic basis for the problem be presented sensitively so as to minimize additional trauma to the sexual identity. For instance, in talking about a condition that affects sexual differentiation it is important to reinforce the gender identification of the affected individual by saying, for example, "Women with androgen insensitivity syndrome ..." or "Men with X/XY mosaicism ...". Whenever it can be done, it is more reassuring to relate the physical features of the condition to normal physiologic or developmental processes. Illustrations of this for three disorders resulting in infertility are given below.

Turner syndrome

In the case of Turner syndrome (except when it is due to 45, X/46,XY mosaicism), points that seem to be helpful to patients include that:

1. Most women have two X chromosomes, but only one is normally active in each cell. Because of this, even though there is only one X, the cells of women with Turner syndrome function normally (except during very early development).
2. Most women's ovaries make eggs during early fetal development and then slowly, over several decades, lose the ability to produce hormones and to maintain and

release eggs. Although eggs are formed in the ovaries of fetuses with Turner syndrome, by birth the ovaries have gone through changes that do not occur in most women until menopause so that infertility is likely.

3. Another result of these early changes is that the ovaries of most women with Turner syndrome don't produce enough female hormones to initiate the changes of puberty.
4. Treatment with growth hormone in childhood and sex hormones in adolescence can increase stature and create a more mature feminine appearance.
5. Unfortunately, while female hormone replacement may create a more mature appearance, it cannot restore fertility. Some women with Turner syndrome have achieved pregnancies using assisted reproductive techniques.

Klinefelter syndrome

Males who are diagnosed with Klinefelter syndrome may actually be relieved to learn that there is a biologic basis for the difficulty they have had in gaining muscle mass, or their gynecomastia, diminished beard growth, or school problems. It is critical that the counseling reassure them about their maleness and the fact that most of these features can be explained by the diminished ability of the testes to produce testosterone. In explaining the karyotype, it is helpful to emphasize that:

1. The fetus develops as a male whenever there is a Y chromosome.
2. The extra X chromosome is inactivated and does not alter the function of cells after birth.
3. Very early in development the XXY chromosome change affects the testes so that they are usually unable to produce sperm or adequate amounts of testosterone.
4. All men produce small amounts of estrogen, and so slight breast development can normally occur in *any* boy as he enters puberty. Usually it goes away as more testosterone is produced. Because boys with Klinefelter syndrome produce less testosterone, the breast prominence may persist, but it can be surgically corrected if desired.
5. Testosterone replacement helps correct the hormone imbalance, and usually improves the self-image by making the physique more masculine and increasing libido.

With both Turner and Klinefelter syndromes, it may help normalize the need for exogenous hormones by comparing the situation to other conditions like diabetes or thyroid deficiency in which people need to take medication because the body is not producing enough of a particular hormone.

Androgen insensitivity syndrome

Clearly, a different approach must be used to explain the karyotype in androgen insensitivity syndrome. Some would argue that an affected individual should not be told about the chromosome result, but I feel that it is better for this finding to be explained in the course of genetic counseling than inadvertently or insensitively divulged when it is later encountered in the patient's medical record. Here it is important to explain that:

1. All embryos start out with gonads that have not yet "decided" whether to become testes or ovaries and thus are initially neither male nor female.
2. The major function of the Y chromosome is to signal these gonads to differentiate, making a substance that prevents development of a uterus, and producing hormones to cause male development.
3. In embryos with androgen insensitivity syndrome the gonad prevents development of a uterus and the upper vagina, but because of a genetic change, the body's cells do not respond to the gonads' other hormonal signals.
4. For this reason the individual develops as a female—both before and after birth.
5. Sexual development and identity is determined not by the presence or absence of a Y chromosome, but by a series of complex biochemical interactions and by how a person grows up thinking about himself or herself.
6. There are numerous reasons why women who are completely feminine—as she is—can be infertile or fail to menstruate.

I think it is preferable to use the term "gonads," rather than testes, and to explain that these will need to be removed because they serve no function (since cells cannot respond to the hormones they produce) and because they have a small but increased chance of developing cancer. Unless there is no vagina, discussing vaginoplasty in terms of "lengthening" rather than "creating" a vagina may be more affirming of the sexual identity. The term "testicular feminization" is emotionally loaded and should be avoided if possible.

DIAGNOSIS IN A CHILD

The infant with a birth defect or a suspected genetic disorder

One of the most painful tasks of genetic counseling is telling parents that their newborn has a birth defect or that it may have a genetic condition. It is also one of the most important tasks to do well. What parents are told may color their perception of the baby from then on. How they are told will be permanently branded in their memories.

In most cases, information about the malformation or the suspicion of a particular diagnosis should be shared with the new parents as soon as possible. It is naive to think that parents will not have noticed a change in expression or behavior among professionals in the delivery room or among those providing postpartum care for the mother. If the baby has been spirited away to intensive care or has not been brought to the couple shortly after birth, they are sure to know that something is amiss. On the other hand, the initial informing should be carefully planned. The professional who gives the information needs to be prepared to remain available and involved over the next days, weeks, or even months, and should try to learn about any significant psychosocial issues (e.g., unplanned pregnancy, prenatal diagnosis declined, drug or alcohol abuse) before meeting with the couple. If at all possible, both parents should be told together, even at the expense of delaying the news for a few hours. It is not fair to rob them of each other's support or to burden one with information the other does not have. If the father is not involved, every effort should be made to find out if there is someone else who can be the mother's emotional mainstay.

The discussion should be arranged to provide as much privacy as possible by reducing the number of professionals to a minimum and by avoiding the situation where another patient is in a nearby bed. If the parents are not fluent in the language, arrangements must be made to have a professional interpreter (not just a bilingual family member) in attendance. The counselor should meet with the translator in advance to review what information will be discussed and how it will be presented and also to ask about any significant cultural considerations.

The interaction may seem more humane to the parents if the counselor and any other professionals are at eye level with them. Asking the baby's name and using it in all subsequent discussions will show that the counselor sees the baby as a person and as their child, rather than the embodiment of a birth defect or syndrome. If the baby is stable and can be brought to the parents, the counselor can demonstrate respect and acceptance in the way he or she handles the baby. Having the infant there can also make it easier to show the parents the specific phenotypic features that have raised concern, or in the case of a visible birth defect, prevent the parents from imaging something worse than the reality.

Asking the couple what they have noticed or been told about the baby is a good point of departure. In most cases,

there is no need for the interview to exceed a half-hour, and information should be limited to what is necessary for them to know at that time. Because of their shock and distress, the parents will retain very little information, and it is premature to discuss causation or recurrence risk. In the case of a congenital malformation, the parents should be told what treatment is planned, when it will be done, and what outcome can be anticipated. When a chromosome abnormality is suspected, the features leading to the suspicion should be described, but it is advisable to indicate that the diagnosis cannot be made solely by a physical examination and will have to await laboratory confirmation. Even when the clinician has little doubt about the diagnosis, it is kinder to leave the couple with some hope until the karyotype is completed, although they should be given an estimate of the level of suspicion if they ask.

It is essential to respond compassionately and without embarrassment to the parents' initial shock and grief. They can be asked if they would like a few minutes to themselves, but the counselor should return shortly thereafter to answer questions they may have. In talking about the possible diagnosis or birth defect, medical jargon and platitudes like "a special child" should be avoided, since they will seem either unintelligible or fatuous. "Lumping terms" such as "children like these" deny the baby's individuality and thus increase the parents' sense of doom and hopelessness. Care should be exercised in making offhand remarks about causation like "an accident of nature," or "a one-in-a million chance" that may later be recollected as an assessment of recurrence risk.

One way to assess the couple's support network and their understanding of what they have been told is to ask them with whom they intend to share the information and what they will tell them. It is also important to ask the couple about their other children (if any), for they are sure to sense the parents' distress and may not only be alarmed about the baby, but fearful that something has happened to their mother. The counselor can help the couple decide how much the other children need to know at this point.

To develop rapport, monitor the couple's reactions, and be available to address questions and concerns, the counselor should make an effort to contact the couple periodically over the next few days. It is critical that they not feel abandoned, and these repeated interactions can help prepare them for the probable confirmation of the diagnosis. During this time, the couple will probably alternate between complete denial—insisting, for example, that dysmorphic features are really familial traits—and showing that they are becoming aware that the baby may actually be affected by asking more about the implications of the diagnosis. These retreats into denial are necessary if the couple is to cope with their anxiety over losing their hoped-for child and their fears about being able to parent a baby with this unfamiliar and threatening condition.

With confirmation of the diagnosis the couple must begin to accept their new reality. This will be accompanied by feelings of responsibility, guilt over real or imagined past misdeeds, anger at the unjustness of the situation, disorientation, and overwhelming sadness. By preparing the couple for these reactions, the counselor can provide reassurance that the emotions are normal and appropriate and that they are not "losing control". They should also be cautioned that the two of them will grieve in different ways and at different times and be admonished to keep the lines of communication open when it seems to one that the other is "uncaring". One of the most devastating blows is that the parents find themselves robbed of the anticipated joy and status of having a new baby while having to adapt to their new identity as the mother or father of a handicapped child.

An occasional couple will be completely unable to accept this identity and the changes in lifestyle, expectations, responsibilities, and prestige that accompany it. In these cases, the possibility of placement, either temporary or permanent, can be raised. For couples who think that institutionalization is their only alternative, it can come as a surprise that this is rarely necessary or appropriate, and that there are families who are willing to adopt a handicapped child, or to provide good short or long-term foster care. They also need to know that a decision to place is (up to a point) reversible. Sometimes, just knowing that they are not "trapped" is enough to allow parents to begin trying to adapt to life with the baby. For couples who place their child, their sense of failure at having produced an "imperfect" child is compounded by their perception that they have also failed in parenting it. They may be guilty because they see themselves as selfish and the adoptive or foster family as unselfish. The counselor should not minimize the couple's feelings, but can remind them of the considerations they took into account in making a decision that they felt was best for them and their child.

For the vast majority of couples who keep their children, repeated counseling sessions can provide a chance for the couple to "flesh out" their understanding of the disorder, to learn about their recurrence risk and reproductive alternatives, and to vent their concerns and frustrations. For many parents, one of the most discouraging features of adjusting to the child's diagnosis is the repetitive and seemingly unending nature of the grief reaction. They may feel that they have finally begun to return to some approximation of normal only to have some unexpected or seemingly

inconsequential event plunge them back into a "slough of despond". Counseling can reinforce that there will be "good days" and "bad days" and remind the couple of the progress they have made. The goal is to restore, as much as possible, their sense of self-worth and to guide the family's return to healthy functioning.

The counselor should specifically inquire about how the child's diagnosis has affected other family members, especially the grandparents and siblings, and about how their relationships with each other and with their friends have changed. It is also important to find out what lifestyle adjustments they have had to make (childcare, employment, recreation) and to help them differentiate between changes they have made because of the child's condition and those that would have been necessary with any new baby. Referrals to an early intervention program or support group can be made when the time seems right. In rare cases, one or both members of the couple will not progress in their grieving process, or maladaptive behavior patterns will emerge. At this point, the possibility of individual, marital, or family counseling with another professional should be raised.

Later diagnosis of a chronic childhood genetic disease

When an older child is found to have a genetic condition, the family will have many of the same concerns about the meaning of the diagnosis as they would in the newborn period. A major difference, however, is that the child is already accepted as an individual and as part of the family constellation. If a child's developmental or health problems have become increasingly apparent over time, much expense and emotional energy may have been devoted to finding a cause, and the family may actually be relieved to have a diagnosis at last. On the other hand, such a diagnosis can bring with it new and distressing information about additional threats that may lie ahead. A youngster who has been thought by the family only to have frequent infections, or to be clumsy and tire easily, may suddenly face a future of potentially grave medical complications when a diagnosis such as cystic fibrosis or muscular dystrophy is made. The family will understandably be thrown into crisis as they try to learn about the condition and initiate treatment amid fears for what lies ahead—emotionally, socially, and financially.

Perhaps even harder for families is having a possible diagnosis raised without warning. For instance this may occur when a pediatrician expresses concern about mild dysmorphism, short stature, delayed development, a suspicious number of café au lait spots, or some other finding in a child whom the family perceives as entirely normal. In terms of the family's shock, denial, and anxiety over the implications of the finding, this situation is not unlike having a genetic diagnosis suspected in a newborn, and warrants the same ongoing counseling involvement.

Impact of the diagnosis and the disease on the family

The pediatrics, mental health, and social work literature is full of discussions about the impact of a chronically ill child on the family, and a distillation of this literature is well beyond the scope of this chapter. Suffice it to say that having a child who requires daily therapy, a special diet, frequent medical visits or hospitalizations, cumbersome hardware, or a great deal of assistance for mobility and self-care places physical, psychic, time, and financial demands that few can imagine on the entire family. The normal siblings may be expected to assume adult-type responsibilities that isolate them from their peers. If their sibling behaves oddly or looks unusual, they may be embarrassed to bring friends home. Activities the family has previously enjoyed together may become impossible, causing sibs (or parents) to resent the affected child for causing this change in lifestyle. It is important to encourage parents to set aside special times where each child gets the mother's or father's undivided attention, and to emphasize that taking care of their own marital relationship is essential. Many couples express concern that having a chronically ill child will precipitate a divorce. They may be reassured to know that most researchers have found the divorce rate not to be significantly different among couples whose child has a disabling condition.

Additional issues relevant to genetic counseling include the fact that diagnosing a genetic disease in a child often has health and reproductive implications for the siblings, who may be carriers, mildly affected, or destined to develop the condition in the future. This may also be true for an affected child's grandparent, aunts or uncles, or cousins. Parents who learn they carry an abnormal gene are likely to feel terribly responsible and guilty for having transmitted it, albeit unknowingly. This is especially true for female carriers of X-linked conditions who had an uncle or brother who was affected with a condition they did not realize was genetic. When, in the course of the child's evaluation, one of the parents is found to be mildly affected, they (or their spouse) may be anxious about implications for their own future health. Furthermore, the mildly affected parent may feel selfish and guilty for worrying about him or herself at a time when it is the child's health that is in jeopardy. The unaffected siblings of the affected child may experience "survivor guilt" or be worried (and afraid to ask) about implications for their own reproductive future. Younger children may even fear that they caused their sibling's illness by something they did or thought. Although many children with chronic genetic diseases or birth defects are cared for in clinics that provide multidisciplinary management, it is worth scheduling a specific genetics visit annually to follow the progress of the condition and to reinforce or update previous genetic counseling information.

ADULT-ONSET GENETIC DISEASES

Two arenas of adult medicine in which genetic counseling has assumed greater importance over the last decade are neurology and cancer. Identifying the causative mutations for a number of neurogenetic disorders, including Huntington disease, familial amyotrophic lateral sclerosis, and myotonic dystrophy, has meant that accurate diagnostic and presymptomatic testing can be done without relying on linkage analysis. The major genes involved in colon and breast-ovarian cancers have also been mapped and cloned, as have a host of others, including those for Von Hippel-Lindau disease, tuberous sclerosis, neurofibromatosis 1 and 2, the multiple endocrine neoplasias, and even rare tumor types like paragangliomas. Although most of these disorders are dominant, the pattern of inheritance may be obscured by new mutation (30% in familial adenomatous polyposis; 50% in NF1), anticipation (most of the trinucleotide repeat expansion disorders) decreased penetrance (nearly all of the cancer syndromes) or sex-limitation (ovarian and prostate cancer). This makes risk assessment and genetic counseling more challenging—particularly with cancers like breast and colon, which are common in the general population and usually result from genetic accidents that accrue during the lifespan rather than from germline mutations. In the next decade, as the scope and variability of pathology for genetic conditions such as hemochromatosis or the thrombophilias is recognized, and as the genetic basis of conditions like Alzheimer's and cardiovascular disease becomes clearer, geneticists are likely to find themselves counseling for conditions that are even more common.

It is the advent of genetic testing for these conditions that is largely responsible for their increased prominence in genetic counseling. In the past, affected individuals were usually cared for by the neurologist, oncologist, cardiologist or other relevant specialist, and often not referred to genetics—despite the hereditary nature of the condition being well known. If family members asked about risk of occurrence or recurrence, information was given on the assumption of straightforward dominant inheritance or (particularly with cancer) based on empiric data. But now, if a genetic test exists, a suspected diagnosis can be confirmed in a symptomatic person (diagnostic testing), or predicted in an asymptomatic one ("predictive" or "presymptomatic" testing). In testing for hereditary cancer syndromes though, finding a mutation neither diagnoses nor predicts the cancer's occurrence, but only indicates cancer predisposition ("predispositional" testing). Certain issues are common to genetic counseling and testing for all of these adult-onset diseases, but the implications of a positive or negative test in each situation can be quite different. Furthermore, with testing for cancer predisposition, the test result may be neither clearly positive nor negative if a mutation of unknown significance is found or if no causative mutation has actually been documented in an affected family member.

Distinctive psychosocial aspects

Genetic counseling for adult-onset disorders differs in that its focus is primarily on implications for the client's own future health, rather than on reproductive risk. Furthermore the client is usually painfully familiar with the condition for which he is at risk by virtue of having observed it in other family members. The disease may actually be a central feature of the family's identity, affecting multiple members and generations and creating a common bond due to the shared risk and burden. Caregivers often know that they themselves may be the next to be stricken. They thus must deal with powerful and complex emotions around two intertwined issues.

A person at risk may refer to himself as a "ticking time bomb" and be constantly on the lookout for any potential symptom. A transient sensation or inconsequential health problem, a normal mood swing or memory lapse that could perhaps signal onset of the disorder can assume enormous significance. In some cases, plans for education, employment, marriage, or reproduction have been altered or put "on hold" because of fears of developing the disease or of needing to become a caretaker for an affected relative. A person at risk may already have concluded that he carries the gene because he shares other traits with the affected parent or because he feels that he has always been "unlucky". Conversely, he may believe that he will be spared, perhaps by virtue of having made certain sacrifices (such as being a caregiver or forgoing a particular career), being very religious, doing good works, etc., by way of "bargaining" with fate. A consequence of predictive or pre-dispositional testing is that these firmly held beliefs about

the future may be overturned. Learning one's true status thus has implications for much more than reproductive decision-making and health care planning. It can change how one is perceived by other family members and indeed, one's own self-concept. There are now many accounts in the literature of at-risk individuals having enormous difficulty after receiving the "good" news that they do not carry a familial mutation.

Counseling considerations and approaches

An at-risk individual may come to counseling alone if he does not want to frighten other family members by showing that he is concerned. Even so, it is important to encourage him to identify someone close who can provide support through the evaluation. If testing is going to be done, it is preferable that this "support person" not be another family member who is also at risk. It may not even be an at-risk individual who seeks counseling, but rather a spouse, parent or child who wants information about the relative's risk. When this happens, the counselor should clarify what the client hopes to gain from counseling, whether the at-risk individual knows (or would approve) that they have come, and if they intend to include him in the process.

In counseling someone at risk for a late-onset familial disorder, various questions should be explored. Why has the client come for genetic evaluation at this time (new information about the "family disorder," a pending life decision, insurance issues, fear that symptoms are beginning, etc.)? Has he come of his own accord or at the instance of his doctor, spouse or partner, or other family member? Has he grown up with surrounded by people with the disease, or has it only recently come to light? How does he perceive the condition, and is this a fair picture? Has his perception been colored by an experience with someone who had a bad surgical outcome, inadequate medication, multiple hospitalizations, poor custodial care, or whose appearance or behavior traumatized him as a child? How old was he when key relatives became ill, and how did the illness affect him and the family? Is he approaching the age when a person with whom he closely identifies was stricken? Are there an unusual number of affected individuals in the family? Have some recently been diagnosed? Does the disease in his family seem unusually mild or severe? If so, might this be because the diagnosis is incorrect, or because the client is unaware of some features of the disease or of people who are in the early stages and mildly affected? How do people in the family deal with the disorder? Is the prevailing attitude positive and matter-of-fact, or do affected individuals view themselves as helpless victims? What are the family's beliefs about the pattern of inheritance or about who will be affected? Does the client think he will or will not get it? Would he want to know, and if so why? Is he aware of factors (like being asymptomatic at an age by which most people show signs of the disease) that may decrease his chances of being a gene carrier? Is he being screened or monitored for symptoms? Has he done anything to try and reduce his chances of becoming affected? What is his understanding of the disease's usual course and available therapies? How much does he know about genetic testing for the condition, and under what circumstances might he utilize it?

Presymptomatic testing

Huntington disease was the first late-onset disease for which presymptomatic genetic testing was offered. For seven years after the gene was mapped, testing was only possible by using linkage analysis. It thus often needed cooperation from several family members. Since 1993 however, it has been possible to directly measure the size of the causative CAG trinucleotide repeat expansion in the Huntington disease gene. This means that direct mutation analysis can now be used for diagnosis or predictive testing in an individual *without* the need to involve the rest of the family. Similar tests can now be done for several other late-onset neurogenetic diseases, such as the spinocerebellar ataxias and Kennedy disease. Causative mutations have also been found that make testing possible for some families with amyotrophic lateral sclerosis or Alzheimer disease. However, since there is currently no intervention to prevent or delay the onset of these disorders, there is no medical benefit to diagnosing them before onset of symptoms. Most people who decide to be tested predictively have a 50% chance of inheriting the disease, and want to resolve the uncertainty.

Although learning whether one carries such a devastating gene can make for more informed life decisions, the change in status from "at-risk" to "not-at-risk" or to "affected-but-when?" may create as many problems as it solves. For these reasons, pretest and posttest counseling for individuals who may want to learn about their status should be provided over time, giving them ample opportunity to explore the implications of having this knowledge and insuring that they have ongoing support whatever the decision or outcome. Most counselors still feel that a team of professionals who can provide not just genetics expertise, but psychotherapy, medical evaluation, and information about treatment and surveillance should ideally be in place where testing for late-onset neurogenetic diseases is offered. This was the model developed in the initial years of Huntington disease testing and the one still used in many academic centers with large neurogenetics clinics. However, since genetic testing for many of these disorders is now done by a number of commercial laboratories, many physicians perceive that presymptomatic genetic testing can be ordered just like any other laboratory study. We have had several patients who were referred for genetic counseling only after a general practitioner or specialist saw them for an unrelated issue and sent blood for predictive testing. I suspect that many other patients are not referred at all unless the result is abnormal. Usually, the patient is in an even greater crisis at this point because he did not have an opportunity to thoroughly consider the implications of testing.

I prefer to see patients considering predictive testing a minimum of three times. Ideally, records on at least one family member should be obtained before the visit to confirm the diagnosis. During the first visit a more complete family history is obtained, and the pedigree constructed. This visit is essential not only for confirming the diagnosis and assessing risk, it also provides a forum for exploring issues around the patient's previous experience with the disease, getting a sense of family dynamics, and assessing the patient's emotional state and social supports.

Among the issues that the at-risk individual should be asked to consider before the testing decision are:

1. What changes they would make in their life, plans or health care if they knew for certain that they would (or would not) develop the disease.
2. Whether the information would affect their reproductive decisions (including possible use of prenatal diagnosis to detect the condition).
3. Possible economic consequences of learning their status.
4. With whom they would share the results of their test and why.
5. How having or sharing this knowledge might change their relationships with these people.
6. How they (and others) would feel if they found out that they were a carrier and that another family member was not (or vice versa).
7. Whether, in balance, they think they would be happier knowing or not knowing.
8. If they feel that this is the best time for them to be tested.

A second visit provides an opportunity to further explore these issues after the patient has had time to reflect more on them. At this visit, it is important to obtain informed consent for testing before getting the blood sample. Although many commercial laboratories no longer require this, some genetics units have created their own "generic" consent form for presymptomatic or predispositional testing. A word-processed form can be easily modified to include the name of the disease, particulars about the test (including which laboratory will be doing it), the test's sensitivity and specificity, and other limitations and liabilities of testing. If the patient did not have a support person at the initial appointment, they should be strongly encouraged to bring one to this visit. This not only gives the counselor a chance to meet this person and assess the quality of support that will be available, but also provides an opportunity to again review information for the support person's benefit. At this visit, I particularly emphasize that having the test done does not commit the patient to getting his results—either when they are complete or at any time in the future.

Usually the third visit is for disclosing test results. I have developed a practice of indicating to the patient at the time blood is drawn that I will call them to schedule an appointment when the studies are complete, but that I will not know their results at the time I make the call. This is so that they will not try to "second guess" the outcome from my tone of voice or force me into disclosing results over the telephone. It also gives the patient another chance to decide not to learn their results and to have them remain sealed in the chart. Most patients feel better knowing that the counselor is not privy to information they themselves do not have. I do recommend, however, opening the results before the disclosure visit, in order to plan for the session, and to make sure that the laboratory report is correct and clear.

There have been some surprising findings from initial studies on the uptake and impact of presymptomatic testing—most of which were for Huntington disease. Among these are that: (1) fewer people than expected from surveys of interest before the test was available have chosen to be tested; (2) some people found *not* to carry the mutation have untoward psychological sequelae; and (3) those who find they carry it usually return to their baseline psychological functioning within a year after getting the news. It has also become evident that testing affects the whole family, not just the person tested. A recent study found that when individuals were tested, some families experienced what they called "changes in membership", including marriage or separation, alterations in reproductive plans, and "disconnections"—particularly of people who tested normal—from the family (Sobel and Cowan, 2000). About half of families they studied experienced changes in patterns of communication among members. The issue of testing sometimes made it possible for the family to talk openly about the disease for the first time, particularly if there had been a "conspiracy of silence" among older family members. In other families, however, communication became more restricted, with persons who tested positive being particularly likely to be isolated. For some families, results also precipitated role changes, as younger family members and those found not to carry the gene realized that they might one day be responsible for caring for the less fortunate ones. People who tested positive, on the other hand, began to examine the care-giving skills of family members who would need to care for them.

These findings point up the need for the counselor to not only assess the patient's psychological state in the weeks and months after giving results, but also to inquire specifically about how relationships within the family have been affected. Unfortunately, follow-up visits are often not covered by third party payors. To my mind, when additional visits are not feasible, the counselor has a responsibility to maintain contact with the patient, at least by telephone, to monitor his and the family's responses to the new information. If the patient has been found to carry the mutation, counseling goals should be to the patient rebuild his self-esteem, find areas of his life where he can exert control, and make decisions and take actions that are necessary because of his changed status.

Predispositional testing

Evaluation of risk for hereditary cancer is a relatively new focus of genetic counseling that has burgeoned as genes responsible for numerous familial cancer syndromes have been identified over the past decade. It is a challenging area, for both risk assessment and testing. First, it must be determined if in fact there is a hereditary basis to cancer in the family, since cancers can occur in several individuals by chance alone rather than by virtue of a shared genetic predisposition. Also, since most cancer syndromes do not have unique pathognomonic features, the "diagnosis" must often be established from the pattern, age of onset, pathology, and particular constellation of tumors occurring in the family. In many cases—particularly when clients are requesting predispositional testing—a physical examination is neither helpful nor necessary. In this situation it is often the counselor who must decide which gene (if any) is appropriate to test. For some cancers (particularly breast/ovarian), the counselor may also need to estimate the chance that a mutation will be found, in order to help the client decide whether it is worthwhile to proceed with expensive testing.

Counseling issues differ depending on who is requesting counseling. Sometimes it is an individual who currently has cancer or who has recovered that comes for evaluation in the hopes of obtaining information to guide treatment decisions or for the benefit of other family members. More frequently however, the person seeking counseling is unaffected and potentially at risk. While many of the same considerations inherent in presymptomatic testing also arise in hereditary cancer counseling and predispositional testing, other aspects are different.

The considerable media attention that has followed discovery of "cancer genes"—particularly those for familial breast/ovarian and colon cancer syndromes—has created unrealistic expectations in both the lay and medical communities. For this reason, it is useful to have the genetic counselor involved at the time of telephone intake in order to determine whether the referral is appropriate and if the patient's goals for the evaluation are realistic. Many potential clients misperceive that they can have a genetic test to tell them if they will get cancer. The counselor's preliminary assessment of family history and brief discussion of the limitations (and costs) of testing can align expectations and identify clients for whom evaluation has a reasonable chance of being productive. Since confirming cases and tumor pathology can be critical to subsequent risk assessment, the client may be asked to track down these records during the initial telephone interaction. This immediately involves the client in the process, and raises issues (like obtaining medical records releases) that may be problematic—thereby providing insight into family dynamics and interrelationships that may need to be considered in counseling.

Genetic testing issues

Unlike many of the late-onset neurogenetic diseases, few cancer syndromes are associated with a unique causative mutation. This means that ideally an affected individual from the family should be tested first to see if a mutation can be documented in the suspected gene. Testing an at-risk individual for a known familial mutation then provides clearer information about risk status. It is important that the client realize, however, that inheriting the mutation (1) does not guarantee that they will ever develop cancer; (2) predict when or where cancer will occur; or (3) indicate that the cancer would be similar to what they may have seen in other family members. Furthermore, for many familial cancers, optimal surveillance and preventive strategies are still not clear. Given these uncertainties, it is essential that pre-test counseling specifically explore what actions the client will take on the basis of test results. Referral to a medical or surgical oncologist may be appropriate at this point if the client is unclear about various options. The counselor should also emphasize that even if test is negative they could still develop cancer for unrelated reasons, and thus need to adhere to the same risk reduc-

tion and screening guidelines as do people with no family history of cancer.

The rapid introduction of commercial testing for cancer predisposition (particularly for breast and ovarian cancer) has meant that results may not provide the hoped-for resolution regarding risk status. A "normal" result should not be completely reassuring to an at-risk person unless a deleterious mutation has already been documented in an affected family member or unless the person comes from a population in which a high proportion of cases are due to a few founder mutations. While failure to find a mutation could indicate that the individual had not inherited the familial risk, it could also mean that gene sequencing missed a deleterious mutation or that the "wrong" gene was tested. Also problematic is identifying a mutation of "unknown significance" that has previously not been described in association with cancer and that would not be expected to clearly affect protein function. Unless this mutation can definitively be shown to segregate with cancer in a number of affected family members (and to be absent in several people who are unaffected at a late age), it has little if any predictive value in an at-risk person. These possible outcomes and how the client would deal with each need to reviewed as part of the consenting process.

With some familial cancers, there is an effective intervention for those found to be mutation carriers. Unfortunately, most of these are surgical and involve removing organs or tissues at risk. However, the benefits of testing are more clear in such situations since learning that one carries a mutation that is highly penetrant (such as one for familial adenomatous polyposis) resolves the uncertainty and means that the carrier can proceed to prophylactic surgery, thereby substantially reducing risk. Conversely, an at-risk person found *not* to carry the mutation can be spared the expensive and sometimes unpleasant surveillance that would otherwise be necessary. In contradistinction to most types of presymptomatic or predispositional testing, it is appropriate to raise the issue of testing minors in the family if the syndrome involves cancers that are likely to arise in childhood and there are options that can significantly reduce the risk of malignancies.

With the majority of familial cancers, however, penetrance is not complete, and so counseling must address not only the chance that an individual has inherited the mutation, but also the likelihood that it will ever lead to cancer. Empiric data are somewhat helpful in this regard, but the client must be cautioned that some of these were derived from high-risk families, and few take into consideration the specific mutation. There are now several published models as well as a computer program (BRCAPRO™) that can estimate the chance that an individual or family carries a BRCA1 or BRCA2 mutation. Some also give a risk of breast or ovarian cancer by specific ages. Caution must be exercised in using these aids, however, since each model is able to take the history of only certain family members into account, and may or may not consider ethnic risk factors. The models thus can give quite different estimates.

LABORATORY SELECTION AND TEST COORDINATING

Genetic counselors are often responsible for identifying the laboratory that will do genetic testing. With testing for chromosomal disorders, this is not usually a problem, since most counselors have a well-established liaison with a cytogenetics laboratory. However, there may be only a handful of laboratories that do a particular molecular (or molecular cytogenetic) test, and the counselor's choice of which to use may affect the success of the evaluation. For this reason it is worth briefly mentioning some considerations in identifying and choosing a laboratory.

An invaluable resource for finding a laboratory to do testing is GeneTests™, an on-line database funded by the National Library of Medicine and the Maternal and Child Health Bureau. The database lists both research and clinical tests. These differ in that the latter are performed in laboratories meeting standards for quality and proficiency established by the Clinical Laboratory Improvement Act/Amendment (CLIA 88, 1992) and thus are qualified to provide results that will be used in patient care. Research tests are usually done as part of a study (e.g., gene mapping or characterization), or when the lab is in the investigational stage of developing a clinical test. Most such testing is conducted under IRB protocols. These protocols usually specify that participants will *not* be given their results.

However, for many diseases, no commercial or clinical test is or is likely to become available, and the only option may be testing through a laboratory doing research on the disorder. If a research laboratory is willing to do a test given that results may be used for decisions about clinical care (e.g., presymptomatic or prenatal diagnosis), the counselor should ask specifically about the lab's previous experience in comparable situations (their success, test sensitivity and specificity) as well as anticipated turn-around time. There should also be a clear understanding about how and to whom results will be transmitted. If a laboratory does *not* have its own consent form, it is prudent for the counselor have a "generic" consent form that can be modified to name the lab doing the test, the disease being tested, and any possible limitations or ambiguities of the test or its results. These issues should be carefully reviewed with the patient and the discussion documented with the signed consent. At the very least, there should be detailed chart notes on what the patient was told about where the testing would be done, and the likelihood that it would be able to provide reliable and useful diagnostic information.

The National Society of Genetic Counselors has published a useful six-page document for gathering information about molecular genetic laboratories (NSGC 1995). It provides helpful guidelines on questions to ask about sample requirements, techniques used in testing, laboratory policies and practices, costs, and billing issues. There is also an excellent review of the "nuts and bolts" of coordinating genetic testing by Uhlmann (1998).

SCREENING AND CARRIER TESTING IN THE ABSENCE OF FAMILY HISTORY

As tests have been developed for conditions common in the general population (e.g., fragile X syndrome) or more prevalent in certain ethnic groups (e.g., Canavan disease, thalassemias) it has been proposed that carrier screening should routinely be offered to pregnant couples or even to the population at large. However, some of these tests have dramatically different sensitivity in different populations (e.g., testing for the common cystic fibrosis mutations detects 97% of Ashkenazi Jewish carriers, but only 30% of those with Asian ancestry [NIH Consensus statement 1997]). Also, for disorders like CF in which hundreds of mutations have been described, the phenotype/genotype correlations associated with all but the most common mutations are poorly understood. Other conditions for which carrier testing can be done, such as Gaucher disease, can be quite variable in their severity. There is little consensus, even among geneticists, about what screening should be offered, at what time, and to whom. Nonetheless, as the tests have become commercially available, they are being requested by anxious patients and practitioners, and are now routinely offered in many prenatal diagnosis centers. It is imperative that genetic counselors take an active part in designing public education materials, establishing "standards of care" and developing public policy regarding the use of these and other genetic tests.

A thorough discussion of all of the conditions for which carrier testing can be done and the indications, costs, limitations and implications of the tests could fill an entire genetic counseling session—overwhelming the patient and diverting the focus from issues more relevant to his or her situation. Moreover, the counselor who becomes little more than a purveyor of repetitive information about genetic tests will not only waste opportunities to do real counseling, but also risk "burn-out". Supplying patients with written materials beforehand gives them time to consider screening and formulate specific questions, making better use of their time with the counselor. Unfortunately, the availability of these numerous tests does potentially increase legal liability. For protection, the chart should document not only that the patient was offered specific tests appropriate to the family history and ethnicity, but also provided written information about other available screening.

COUNSELING THE CULTURALLY AND LINGUISTICALLY DIFFERENT CLIENT

One of the major challenges of genetic counseling comes in working with clients whose language and culture is different from our own. Although less frequently making their way to genetic services by themselves, they may get referred as a result of population-based screening (prenatal, newborn, or hemoglobinopathy) or because a genetic disease or birth defect has occurred in their child. Recent immigrants rarely have had any prior experience with this type of medical interaction. While access to health care may have been good in their country of origin, genetics services are likely to have been less available. Furthermore, even within their newly adopted community, there may be little familiarity with or acknowledgment of genetic services. This is especially likely to be true if birth defects are perceived as very stigmatizing by the culture or if people do not usually use (or at least to admit to using) prenatal diagnosis.

One of the perplexing aspects of genetic counseling for many recently-arrived citizens is its emphasis on respecting patient autonomy. In many cultures, one seeks help from a healer to be advised about what to do to cure a disease or correct a problem. If the clients' primary care physician is from the same culture, he or she may in fact already have told the family what they are expected to do (e.g., to have an amniocentesis). Clients who perceive the genetic counselor's nondirective stance as unauthoritative or indecisive may doubt his or her professional competence. They may also fear that their referring physician will be angry with them or stop seeing them if they do not follow his or her advice. Moreover, trying to elicit the clients' agenda may not be the best way to start a session. They may incorrectly interpret your asking about their understanding of why they have been referred as evidence that you have not prepared for the consultation by becoming familiar with their case. It may be more reassuring if you frame the session by mentioning their physician and by saying what the interview will be about: "Dr X (the referring physician) would like me to talk with you about (his concerns about your child, some tests that we can offer you to find out more about your

baby, etc.)". However, while our attempts at helping clients get what they need from counseling and "make decisions that are best for them" may seem doomed from the start, it is unfair to prejudge that this will be the case.

The importance of good interpreting services cannot be overemphasized. Although sometimes unavoidable, using a family member—especially a child—or expecting one member of a couple to translate for the other really compromises the counseling and can create awkward situations when sensitive information must be obtained or discussed. It is better to cultivate a good relationship with one or more professional medical interpreters who can be available for the extended interactions that counseling requires and who are interested in and can be compassionate about the sometimes delicate topics that arise. By asking the interpreter about relevant cultural issues and practicing with them how to pronounce the patient's name before the patient arrives, and by reviewing with them afterward issues or reactions that came up in the interview, you will demonstrate your respect and interest in their culture and language. Similarly, explaining to them why it is important to obtain certain information, or to explain a genetic concept in just such a way, or to spend time exploring certain emotional issues, will improve the information exchange and make them more understanding of the time counseling takes. A common problem with interpretive services is their limited availability and expense. Some genetics units have trained bilingual and bicultural "genetics aides" to be a permanent part of their staff and even to provide some patient education independently. In our unit, we have had good success with utilizing fluent undergraduate premedical majors who can be available at specific times during the week. In exchange for their work, these students receive independent study credit, have an opportunity to learn some genetics, gain experience in patient care and education, and in many cases, become more aware and appreciative of their own parent culture in the process.

Counselors will increase the effectiveness of their work with clients from another culture if they can learn enough of the language to at least engage in some social conversation with the patient and to monitor the accuracy of translation. Spending time and dining in ethnic areas of the city, asking natives about aspects of their culture, becoming familiar with the geography and religions of the relevant countries, and exploring the anthropology literature that pertains to the culture's health beliefs and behaviors will also increase the counselor's understanding. It is important to keep in mind that immigrants from any country are highly diverse, often representing many ethnic, religious, socioeconomic, or linguistic groups, and varying levels of education and medical sophistication. Stereotyping is a destructive way to begin genetic counseling. However, an awareness of common beliefs about causation of birth defects, cultural attitudes toward mental retardation and physical disability, religious practices surrounding death, and an understanding of family structures and how decisions are made can prepare the counselor for issues that may need to be addressed.

Among things that may need to be modified in genetic counseling is the complexity of the information that is presented. Recent immigrants may not have had the educational background in human anatomy or biology that we take for granted in those who historically have sought genetic counseling. Lengthy descriptions of chromosomal inheritance or complex comparisons of various risks may obscure, rather than illuminate the important issues. Paring the educational content to the minimum that is necessary to make an informed decision may seem paternalistic, but it is less likely to overwhelm a client. It is also important to make sure that the analogies that are used are understandable. Comparing chromosomes to a set of encyclopedias and genes to the paragraphs in them is not helpful to a client who does not read, whether from a different culture or not.

It is essential to address the clients, rather than the interpreter, and to watch them as what was said is being translated. This seems uncomfortable and a little odd at first, but makes it possible to observe reactions and body language. In some cultures, direct eye contact may be considered rude, and it is helpful to take cues from how the interpreter and clients interact. It is also important to know if the conversation should be directed to one member of the couple; sometimes it may diminish the husband's authority if a question is addressed to his wife. In some cultures, decisions are made only after family discussion, or after consultation with an elder or religious leader. The counselor might do well to ask if there are other people with whom the couple will be talking about the matter, or whom they would like to include in a subsequent session.

When a baby has been born with a malformation or other handicap, there may be particular cultural beliefs about its causation. In many cases, clients are embarrassed to admit these concerns. Depending on the culture, it may be helpful to bring up the issue by saying something like "Many people believe that a baby will be born with a malformation if particular things happen during pregnancy, like an eclipse, a curse, or if the mother uses scissors or becomes very upset (whatever the cultural belief related to the malformation may be). Has anyone told you that something you did caused this problem?" Often this will flush out the concern and may also identify who is laying blame. Dealing with the information requires tact however, to diminish guilt over the perceived cause while not denigrating the belief or the person who has made the accusation. Rather than making a doctrinaire statement such as "We know these things don't cause birth defects," it is less judgmental and more sympathetic to say something along the lines of "Every culture finds ways to try and explain things that are hard to understand, or that we can't control." If there is a biologic explanation, it can be offered at that point. If not, it may help to ask the patient if she had any friends that were pregnant at the same time and who had a similar experience. The fact that the other person's baby (presumably) did not have the same problem may give the couple a rational crutch to assuage their guilt and make them less terrified if something similar happens in a subsequent pregnancy. As for any couple, the counselor's statement that it is normal for parents to look for explanations and to blame themselves—even when they have been exemplary in their behavior or care of the pregnancy—may provide some measure of reassurance.

Two useful resources for educating oneself about specific aspects of cultural and ethnic diversity vis à vis genetic counseling are those by Greb (1998) and Fisher (1996). Even if the counselor is awkward in his or her efforts to use another language or to understand another culture, most patients appreciate the attempt. The pain and dilemmas that families experience are universal, although they may handle them in different ways. Showing respect and empathy overcomes cultural barriers and can reward the counselor with glimpses into the wisdom of other societies and with increased human understanding.

Conclusion

As genetic technology becomes ever more sophisticated and options for testing and treatment more numerous, genetic counselors must be vigilant that the counseling aspects of our interaction with patients do not become secondary to the educational aspects. If we neglect the emotional content of the information, we send a message that people should be able to make decisions they can live with just by understanding facts. Nothing could be further from the truth. If it were, genetic counseling could be reduced to a set of videotapes and brochures and group "counseling", as some would have it. We must educate and remind insurers, other professionals, employers, and those who set policy that the implications of genetic information are incredibly complex, and that decisions our patients make affect not only their own lives, but those of future generations. Genetic counseling must be accorded enough time (and reimbursement) that the job can be done properly. When it is, our patients and we both grow as people.

Acknowledgments

I am indebted to Virginia Corson, Cynthia Dolan, Judith Hall, Elsa Reich, and Karen Wcislo for the reflections and ideas that helped this chapter take shape; to Maureen Bocian, Pamela Flodman, Timothy Gawron, Rick Martin, and Joan Scott for their thoughtful comments and careful review of the manuscript for the previous edition; to Diane Baker's suggestions for revisions; and to the many other colleagues who have taught me some of what they have learned over the years. An even greater debt of gratitude is owed, however, to all of the patients who have let me share and learn from their challenges, sorrows, and triumphs.

REFERENCES

American Board of Genetic Counseling (2001) http://www. faseb.org/genetics/abcg/tr-prog1.htm

Blumberg BD, Golbus MS, Hanson KH (1975) The psychological sequellae of abortion performed for a genetic indication. Am J Obstet Gynecol 122:799–808

Carr-Saunders AM (1929) Eugenics. p. 806. In: The Encyclopedia Britannica. 14th edn. Vol. 8. Encyclopedia Britannica Co., London

CLIA88 (1992) Federal/Register 57(40):7001-7288. Public law 100-578, Clinical Laboratory Improvement Amendments of 1988, 42 USC 263a et seg.

Crandall BF, Robinson L, Grau P (1991) Risks associated with an elevated maternal serum α-fetoprotein level. Am J Obstet Gynecol 165:581–585

Fisher NL (1996) Cultural and Ethnic Diversity, a Guide for Genetics Professionals. Johns Hopkins University Press, Baltimore

Greb A (1998) Multiculturalism and the Practice of Genetic Counseling. Ch. 7, p. 171. In Baker DL, Schuette JL, Uhlmann WR (eds): A Guide to Genetic Counseling. Wiley-Liss

Holsinger D, Larabell S, Walker AP (1992) History and pedigree obtained during follow-up for abnormal maternal serum α-fetoprotein identifies additional risk in 25% of patients. Clin Res 40:28A

Kessler S (1979) The psychological foundations of genetic counseling. p. 19. In Kessler S (ed): Genetic Counseling: Psychological Dimensions. Academic Press, New York

Kessler S (1999) Psychological aspects of genetic counseling: XIII. Empathy and decency. J Genet Counsel, 6:333–343

Leonard CO, Chase GA, Childs B (1972) Genetic counseling: a consumer's view. N Engl J Med 287:433–439

National Society of Genetic Counselors (1995) Molecular Genetics Laboratory Questionnaire. NSGC, Wallingford PA

National Society of Genetic Counselors (2001) http://www.hsgc.org

NIH Consensus Statement on Genetic Testing for Cystic Fibrosis. National Institutes of Health 1997, 15(4):8

Reed SC (1974) A short history of genetic counseling. Soc Biol 21:332–339

Reed SC (1980) In the beginning. p. 1. In Counseling in Medical Genetics. 3rd edn Wiley, New York

Rolleston H (1934) Introduction. p. 9. In Blacker CP (ed): The Chances of Morbid Inheritance. William Word, Baltimore

Sobel SK, Cowan DB (2000) Impact of genetic testing for Huntingdan disease on the family system. Am J Med Genet 90:49–59

Sorenson JR, Culbert AJ (1977) Genetic counselors and counseling orientations: unexamined topics in evaluation. p. 138. In Lubs HA, de la Cruz F (eds): Genetic Counseling. Lippincott-Raven, New York

Sorenson JR, Culbert AJ (1979) Professional orientations to contemporary genetic counseling. Birth Defects Orig Art Ser 15:85–102

Uhlmann WR (1998) A Guide to Case Management. Ch. 8, p. 199. In Baker DL, Schuette JL, Uhlmann WR (eds): A Guide to Genetic Counseling. Wiley-Liss

Walker AP (1993) Physician-patient relationship in contemporary genetic counseling. Paper presented at the American Society of Human Genetics, New Orleans, October 6

Yates EE (1999) Identification of additional risk factors prior to prenatal diagnosis in patients referred after positive X-AFP screening. Master's thesis. University of California, Irvine

Gene therapy strategies for the treatment of neurodegenerative and other genetic diseases

32

Edward H. Schuchman
Janet E. Carter
Robert J. Desnick

Introduction

During the past two decades major advances have been made in the elucidation of the molecular pathologies of many genetic diseases (Scriver et al., 1995). For example, the underlying protein defects in more than 700 inborn errors of metabolism have been identified and the specific molecular lesions in the genes encoding these proteins are being described at an ever increasing rate (Antonarakis and McKusick, 2000). Moreover, implementation of biochemical and molecular techniques has made accurate diagnosis, carrier detection and prenatal diagnosis for many of these disorders a reality. Various therapeutic approaches have been undertaken to ameliorate the metabolic abnormalities in genetic disorders, including dietary restriction, use of chelators, cofactor supplementation and, most recently, enzyme replacement and allotransplantation (Table 32.1). The limitations, as well as the encouraging successes, of these strategies have been the subject of many reviews (e.g., Desnick, 1990).

In spite of these major achievements, however, treatment of the neurological complications associated with many of these diseases has remained elusive, particularly for the treatment of neurodegenerative diseases for which no clear etiology has yet been described (e.g., Alzheimer's disease, Parkinson's disease, etc.). The only means to cure these devastating neurological disorders would be to stably express the defective (or other therapeutic genes) in the proper anatomical and cellular sites of pathology in the central nervous system (CNS). Such is the objective of current efforts to develop gene therapy for neurological diseases. This chapter will summarize the principles, current methods and recent advances of gene therapy for genetic diseases with neurodegeneration, with particular emphasis on viral gene transfer methods and cell transplantation strategies for the CNS. A brief discussion of other disease targets also is included.

Table 32.1. Therapeutic Strategies for the Treatment of Genetic Diseases

Metabolic manipulation
 Dietary restriction
 Substrate-depletion techniques
 Chelation-enhanced excretion
 Plasmapheresis/affinity techniques
 Surgical bypass procedures
 Metabolic inhibition
 Product replacement

Gene product therapy
 Cofactor supplementation
 Enzyme induction
 Allotransplantation
 Enzyme replacement therapy

Gene therapy
 Ex vivo correction/transplantation
 In vivo gene delivery

Preventative therapy
 Heterozygote screening
 Genetic counseling
 Prenatal diagnosis

Gene therapy basics

Genes can be transferred into the germ-line or into somatic cells. Germ-line gene therapy involves the insertion of a normal gene into germ cells such that it will correct the genetic defect and be transmitted in a mendelian fashion from generation to generation. In contrast, the goal of somatic gene therapy is the insertion of the therapeutic gene into somatic cells, particularly those with primary disease pathology. In this way only the somatic cells of the patient will be modified, without the possibility of germ-line transmission. The foreign gene must either gain access to the cell nucleus for stable integration into the host chromosome or function in the nucleus as an episomal element, thereby effecting the high-level or tissue-specific expression of the desired gene product.

GERM-LINE GENE THERAPY IN MICE

Although germ-line gene therapy in humans has been prohibited for moral, scientific and practical reasons in most developed countries, such experiments have been permitted in mice and demonstrate the feasibility of inserting functional genes into the germ-line with subsequent cure of the murine disease.

The technique for insertion of a foreign gene or DNA segment (i.e., a transgene) into the mouse germ-line is now commonly performed in laboratories throughout the world and is summarized in Figure 32.1 (for review, see Brinster, 1993). Briefly, one-cell mouse embryos are collected immediately following fertilization. The male pronucleus is visible at this stage and foreign DNA can be inserted into the nucleus by microinjection. Following injection, the embryos are surgically placed into the uterus of a pseudopregnant female mouse. Since only a few injected embryos

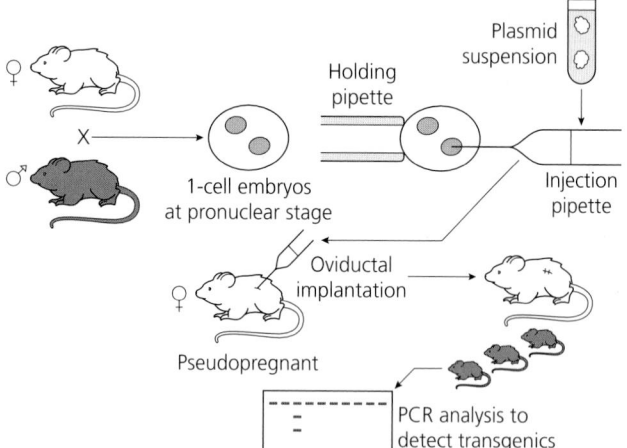

Fig. 32.1. Germ-line gene therapy. DNA can be inserted into the germ-line of mice by microinjection into the pronuclei of single-cell embryos. Gene-modified embryos are then transplanted into the oviducts of pseudopregnant mice, and the offspring are tested to identify those that have the "transgene". These mice can be bred to determine if the transgene has been introduced into the germ-line and to generate homozygous mice carrying the transgene.

will successfully undergo fetal development, 100 or more embryos are usually reimplanted into several pseudopregnant female mice to assure success. After the pups are born, the presence of the transgene can be determined by Southern hybridization analysis or polymerase chain reaction (PCR) using DNA isolated from tail biopsies. These "founder mice" may be chimeric, the foreign gene having only gained access to certain cell types. Those that have the transgene (one to several hundred copies) integrated into their sperm- or egg-producing cells will transmit the gene in a mendelian fashion. Moreover, the integrated genes tend to be expressed with the appropriate tissue specificity. For example, the human β-globin gene, which is normally expressed only in erythrocytes, was expressed only in this cell lineage after transfer into the mouse germ-line (Constantini et al., 1986). Because these mice can express the foreign genes, they are called "transgenic" mice.

The ability to insert foreign genes into the germ-line of mice has provided the opportunity to test the feasibility of gene therapy. Normal genes have been injected into mice with specific genetic defects, and their incorporation into the mouse genome has effectively and dramatically cured the murine disease (Table 32.2). For example, transfer of the rat growth hormone gene into growth hormone-deficient "Dwarf Little" mice resulted in the cure of the growth hormone deficiency and the generation of larger-than-normal mice (Hammer et al., 1984). Similarly, transfer of the human β-globin gene into mice with β-thalassemia (due to a murine β^{maj}-globin gene deletion) resulted in the regulated expression of β-globin molecules in these mice, association of the murine α-globin chains with the human β-globin chains, and correction of the hematopoietic disease (Constantini et al., 1986). These and other early examples illustrated the fact that germ-line gene therapy was feasible, at least in the mouse, and could effectively cure a genetic disease.

SOMATIC CELL GENE THERAPY

Somatic gene therapy involves the insertion of a normal gene into somatic cells such that sufficient quantities of the therapeutic protein will be expressed to correct the metabolic defect. In contrast to germ-line gene therapy, only certain somatic cells of an affected individual are targeted, and there is no transfer of the new genetic material to the treated patients' offspring. As illustrated in Figure 32.2, two approaches can be used to deliver genes to somatic cells. *Ex vivo* gene therapy involves the removal of cells from the patient, the introduction of the therapeutic gene(s) using viral or non-viral vectors, and the autologous trans-

Table 32.2. Correction of Genetic Defects in Transgenic Mice

Murine Disease	Defective Gene	Microinjected Gene	Reference
Growth hormone deficiency Dwarf little mouse (lit)	Growth hormone (deletion)	Rat growth hormone	Hammer et al., (1984)
β-globin Deficiency β-Thalassemia mouse (hbb[th-1])	β-globin (deletion)	Human β-globin	Constantini et al., (1986)
Hypogonadism Hypogonadal mouse (hpg)	18GnRH-GAP[a] (3′ deletion)	Murine GnRH-GAP	Mason et al., (1986)
MBP deficiency[b] shiverer mouse (shi)	MBP (3′ deletion)	Murine MBP	Readhead et al., (1987)
OTC deficiency sparse fur mouse (spf)	OTC (point mutation)	Human OTC	Jones et al., (1990)
β-glucuronidase deficiency MPS VII (gus[MPS])	β-glucuronidase (termination mutation)	Human β-glucuronidase	Kyle et al., (1990)

[a]GnRH-GAP, Gonadotropin releasing hormone and GnRH-Associated Peptide
[b]MBP, myelin basic protein

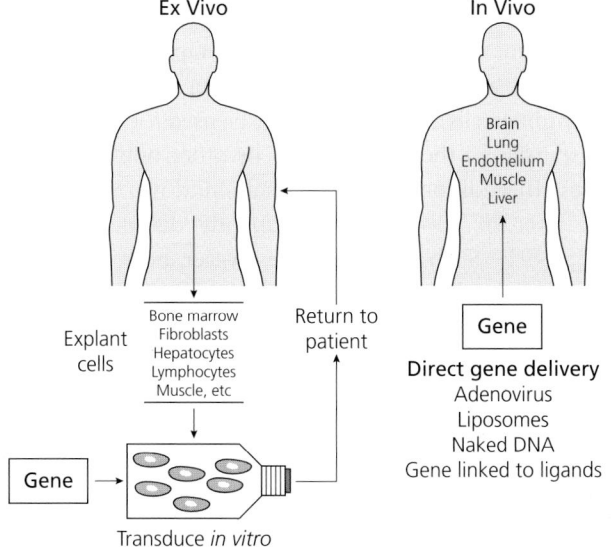

Fig. 32.2. Strategies for somatic cell gene therapy. Somatic cell gene therapy may be accomplished by *ex vivo* or *in vivo* techniques. *Ex vivo* gene therapy requires the removal of target cells from the diseased individual, the introduction of the therapeutic gene into these cells using viral or non-viral vectors, followed by autologous transplantation for gene expression. *In vivo* gene therapy requires techniques for direct gene delivery to the sites of pathology using viral or non-viral vectors.

plantation of the gene-corrected cells into the patient. *In vivo* gene therapy refers to the direct delivery of the therapeutic gene to the target sites of pathology of the diseased individual (e.g., intravenous infusion, stereotaxic injection) without the need for explanting and culturing cells for gene insertion in the laboratory and then performing expensive and potentially dangerous transplantation procedures. Both types of gene therapy procedures will be discussed in this review.

Viral gene delivery systems

Several viruses are currently being used in gene therapy clinical trials or are actively under development as gene transfer vehicles. These include retroviruses (RV), adenovirus (AV), lentiviruses (LV), adeno-associated virus (AAV) and herpes simplex virus (HSV). The genomic structures of these viruses is schematically illustrated in Figure 32.3 and their advantages and limitations are compared in Table 32.3 and discussed below.

RETROVIRAL VECTORS

Retroviruses are uniquely suited for somatic gene transfer because integration into the genome of infected cells is an obligatory and highly efficient part of the viral life cycle and results in transfer of the genetic material to progeny cells. In general, a retroviral envelope glycoprotein binds to a specific cell surface receptor and is internalized and uncoated, releasing the viral RNA genome into the cytoplasm. The viral enzyme, reverse transcriptase, converts the single stranded viral genome into a double stranded DNA copy that forms an "integration complex" with a viral integrase and host cell proteins. The integration complex is transported to the nucleus, where it inserts into host cell DNA and forms a provirus. Transport to the nucleus occurs only with fragmentation of the nuclear membrane at mitosis, hence retroviruses can only transduce dividing cells. The provirus uses host cell machinery to then transcribe and translate the viral genome (Coffin et al., 1997).

Table 32.3. Comparison of Viral Vector Systems

Feature	RV	Ad E1-Deleted	AAV	HSV Amplicon	LV
Size of viral genome	~9.8Kb	~36Kb	~4.7Kb	~152Kb	~7Kb
Insert capacity	<7Kb	7Kb	4.8Kb	15Kb	7Kb
Existence in cell nucleus	Integrated	Episomal	Integrated/ episomal	Episomal	Integrated
Cytotoxicity	No	Yes	No	Yes	No
Transduction efficiency	High	Moderate	High	High	High
Requires dividing cells	Yes	No	No	No Yes/No	

RV = retrovirus; Ad = adenovirus; AAV = adeno-associated virus; HSV = herpes simplex virus; LV = lentivirus

Currently available retroviral vectors for gene therapy represent modified retroviruses in which the genes for replication (*gag, pol* and *env*) have been deleted and replaced by a therapeutic gene of interest. The remaining backbone vector retains genetic information for the long terminal repeats (LTR's), which are necessary for expression of the viral genome and integration of the provirus into the genome of infected cells (Fig. 32.3). Because retroviral vectors are not competent for replication, to produce such vectors the replicating genes are supplied by complementing "packaging cell lines" which constitutively express the *gag, pol* and *env* genes. The vector RNA is transcribed, including the gene of interest, and packaged into viral

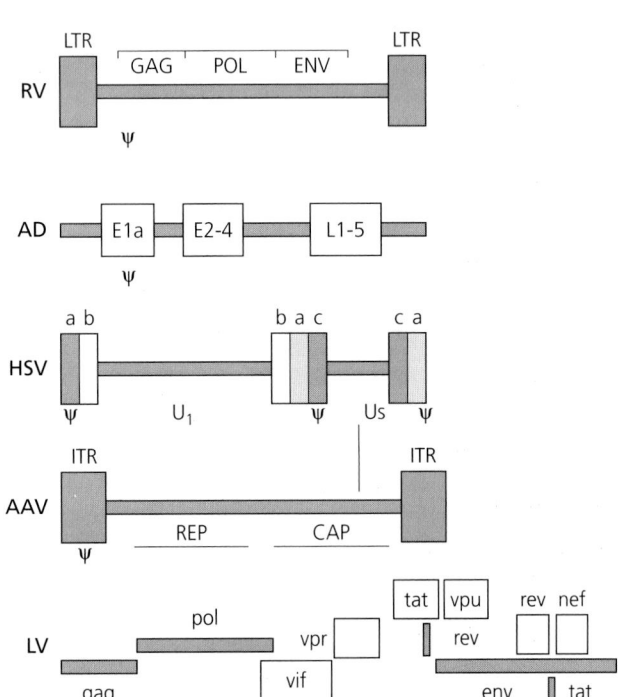

Fig. 32.3. Structures of the five commonly used viruses for gene therapy. The size and basic structure of the five viral genomes is shown. The location of important structural genes and regulatory sequences are shown. ψ indicates the packaging signal. See text for details.

capsids in these cells because it contains an intact encapsidation sequence. However, in the absence of the *gag, pol* and *env* genes, viral particles produced in this way cannot replicate (see Marin et al., 1997 for a more comprehensive overview).

Unfortunately, protypical retroviral vectors based on the Moloney Murine Leukemia Virus (MMLV), which have been widely used for gene transfer to rapidly dividing cells, do not transduce postmitotic neurons of the CNS (or other nondividing cells), and thus cannot be used for direct gene *in vivo* transfer to the mature brain or other non-proliferating tissues. In addition, transcriptional shutdown of the transgene after *in vivo* delivery frequently occurs (Scharfman et al., 1991). Such vectors have, however, been used extensively for the evaluation of *ex vivo* CNS gene therapy in animal model systems, as discussed below.

LENTIVIRAL VECTORS

The limitations in the usefulness of MMLV-based retroviruses led to the investigation of the potential use of another member of the Retroviridiae family, the Lentiviruses. Lentiviruses represent a group of viruses that infect non-proliferating macrophages and lymphocytes and give rise to progressive disease of the immune and nervous systems. Lentiviruses currently used as the basis for gene therapy vectors include Human Immunodeficiency Virus (HIV-1 and -2), Simian Immunodeficiency Virus (SIV), Feline and Equine Infectious Anemia Virus (FIAV/EIAV), Caprine Arthritis encephalitis virus (CAEV), and Bovine Immunodeficiency Virus (BIV). Unlike MMLV, the integration complex of lentivirus contains nuclear localization signals which allow it to be actively transported through the nucleopores to the nucleus, facilitating infection of non-dividing cells (Naldini, 1998). Significant progress in the use of lentiviral vectors as a potential therapeutic vector was made with the discovery of the minimal genetic information required for replication and pathogenesis. This information has allowed development of refined vectors, which eliminate non-essential sequences and thereby improve vector safety (see Federico, 1999 and Klimatatcheva et al., 1999 for comprehensive overviews of HIV vector design). Third generation HIV-1 based vectors and self-inactivating (SIN) vectors represent the most recent advances (Miyoshi et al., 1998; Zufferey et al., 1998).

Contemporary lentiviral vectors are produced using a transient transfection system consisting of three plasmid-based expression constructs; transfer construct, packaging construct and env expression construct. The transfer construct contains cis-acting elements responsible for expression of viral structural proteins; i.e., gag and pol predominantly, and gives rise to the capsid (Fig. 32.3). The envelope construct produces a heterologous envelope glycoprotein, usually vesicular somatitis virus (VSV-G), creating a "pseudo-typed" virus. VSV-G is commonly used as the heterologous coat glycoprotein because of the significant advantage it confers to the vector delivery system. Entry of VSV-G into its target cells occurs by binding to ubiquitous phospholipid components of the cell membrane. This mode of entry confers on VSV-G, and viruses pseudotyped with it, a broad host range including non-mammalian cells (Burns et al., 1993). Current conventional small-scale methods to produce lentiviral vectors depend upon transient transfection of the three plasmids; thus, the infectious titer is subject to great batch-to-batch variability and the resulting volume is limited. Stable packaging cell lines that provide, *in trans*, all of the viral proteins required for viral assembly have therefore been recently constructed.

Clearly, the most urgent issue regarding the safety of lentiviral vectors remains the fact that HIV is a deadly pathogen. The possibility of the appearance of replication-competent virus, albeit remote (Chong and Vile, 1996), has spurred efforts to develop vectors based on other lentiviruses with less potential pathogenicity. Recently, FIV, a non-primate virus thought to have low pathogenic potential in humans, was pseudotyped with VSV-G and used to successfully transduce non-dividing human primary cells *in vitro* (Poeschla et al., 1998). Furthermore, EIAV has also been used to transduce neurons and glial in the adult rat CNS with efficiencies comparable to HIV vectors (Mitrophanous et al., 1999). However, despite these promising results, additional concerns about the use of such non-primate lentivirus vectors for human gene therapy have been raised by reports describing the susceptibility of human peripheral blood lymphocytes to FIV (Johnson and Power, 1999).

Despite the limitations and although, to date, therapeutic evaluations are limited, initial reports of successful transduction and long-term expression in the liver, retina and muscle are encouraging. In addition, in the CNS an HIV-1 vector expressing β-galactosidase demonstrated sustained and efficient transgene expression in rat hippocampus and striatum in the absence of an inflammatory response (Naldini et al., 1996), and suggests that HIV-1 vectors will be useful therapeutic agents for CNS gene delivery (see below).

ADENOVIRAL VECTORS

Adenoviruses are encapsidated double-stranded linear DNA viruses. Commonly used recombinant adenoviruses derive from human serotypes 2 and 5, which have natural tropism for the respiratory tract producing a benign infection. Adenoviral replication can be divided into three phases of gene expression: Intermediate Early (*E1*) and Early (*E2–E4*) genes expressed before viral replication, and Late (*L*) genes expressed after viral replication (Fig. 32.3). *E1a* is the first viral gene expressed after the viral genome enters the nucleus. It activates other viral genes inducing host cells to proliferate and undergo apoptosis.

Recombinant adenoviruses can transduce both quiescent and actively dividing cells, including the main cell types of the CNS (Akli et al., 1993; Davidson et al., 1993; Le Gal de Salle et al., 1993), and is therefore highly attractive for CNS gene transfer. However, high expression of viral proteins causes an immunogenic response which, in turn, can lead to shutdown of transgene expression as a result of destruction of host cells. Despite the ensuing inflammatory response, long-term expression of 2 to 6 months has been observed on stereotactic injection of these vectors into the brain (Byrnes et al., 1996). Efforts are currently directed at trying to eliminate as many adenoviral genes as possible to reduce this inflammatory response to viral proteins. First and second generation vectors have been produced by deletions in the early *E1* gene region. Additional deletions in the *E3* region allow for the insertion of larger transgenes. First generation vectors have been used experimentally with proven success in the CNS. Deletion of *E1* renders the virus replication-incompetent by preventing activation of remaining early and late genes. However, it seems likely that at high multiplicity of infection, the *E1* region becomes dispensable for replication and cellular transactivators with E1-like activity produce E1-independent activation of *E2* such that viral replication proceeds with accumulation of viral gene products. These gene products lead to cytopathic effects on the transduced cells and activation of the immune system (Dai et al., 1995; Byrnes et al., 1995).

Second generation vectors have introduced temperature sensitive mutations into the *E2a* gene. In the liver, such a vector gave rise to transgene expression for up to 70 days but still produced an inflammatory response (Engelhardt et al., 1994). Additional second-generation vectors have been made with larger deletions in *E2a* and *E2b* to ensure that *E2* is not expressed from the vectors in an active form (Gorziglia et al., 1996). Third generation vectors employ deletions in both the *E1* and *E4* gene regions, with retention of only open reading frame (ORF) 6 of the *E4* gene. ORF 6 can complement deletion of the entire *E4* region which in itself is toxic (Armentano et al., 1995). Although the immune response after transfection with *E1/E4* deleted viruses is minimal, such vectors display significantly reduced effectiveness in transgene expression.

Transgene persistence with adenoviral vectors appears dependent on the type of promoter used and the immunogenic nature of the transgene itself (Gao et al., 1996; Dedieu et al., 1997). Defective vectors deleted of all adenoviral genes have also been generated, so called "minimal" or "gutless" vectors (Fisher et al., 1996). These constructs accommodate over 35 kb of foreign sequence, induce tissue-specific transcriptional regulation and high levels of stable expression with significantly reduced toxicity (Kochanek et al., 1996; Scheidner et al., 1998). (See Hermans and Verhaagen, 1998; Barkats et al., 1998 and Smith and Romero, 1999 for more comprehensive overviews of developmental strategies to adapt adenoviral vectors to specific gene therapy applications.) The successful use of adenoviruses for *in vivo* and *ex vivo* approaches in the CNS is considered below.

ADENO-ASSOCIATED VIRAL VECTORS

Adeno-associated virus (AAV) is a non-pathogenic human parvovirus, with a linear single-stranded DNA genome of 4.7 kb which is capable of infecting a wide variety of hosts (Fig. 32.3). Lytic infection normally depends on the presence of a helper virus (Atchison et al., 1965) (Adenovirus or Herpes simplex). In the absence of a helper, the virus integrates into the host cell genome at a specific locus on human chromosome 19 (Kotin et al., 1990). Production of recombinant AAV requires transfection of two plasmids, one carrying the gene of interest inserted between the viral inverted terminal repeats, and one, a helper plasmid containing the replication and capsid genes. Transfection of these two plasmids is followed by super-infection, usually in 293 cells, with helper adenovirus. A by-product of nearly all AAV helper systems is the generation of wild-type AAV-like particles, despite the fact that all packaging systems are designed to prevent this by lack of homology between the wild-type virus and the vector plasmids.

In addition, despite rigorous purification procedures residual adenovirus remains in many AAV preparations and can produce a cytotoxic T lymphocyte response. Alternative approaches to eliminate the use of helper utilize a triple transfection procedure with adenoviral DNA contained in a plasmid vector (Xiao and Samulski, 1998; Ferrari et al., 1997). These constructs produce an increase in AAV without loss of titer and result in Ad-free AAV. Such constructs produced no cytotoxic response and long-term expression in muscle (Monohan et al., 1998). Current efforts are underway to develop packaging cell lines to obviate the need for transfection protocols. Recently, the *in vitro* packaging of AAV as a cell free alternative to transfection and the development of packaging cell lines have been described (Ding et al., 1997). (See Rabinowitz and Samulski, 1998 for more comprehensive review.) AAV has been successfully used to transduce neurons in the brain with persistent transgene expression and in the absence of cytopathic effects. These applications are considered below.

HERPES SIMPLEX VIRAL VECTORS

Herpes simplex virus (HSV) contains a linear double stranded DNA genome of 152 kb and has a natural tropism for epithelial and mucosal cells (Fig. 32.3). However, infectious particles can also enter the sensory neurons which innervate the infection site. Here the virus is retrogradely transported to the cell body to produce one of two types of infection, either lytic of latent. Latency may last for the lifetime of the host but stress, drugs or UV irradiation may induce a lytic infection.

To establish effective HSV delivery systems for gene therapy it is essential to promote the establishment of latency but to remove virally induced cytotoxic functions produced during the early lytic cycle. To date, deletions of immediate early genes expressed during the lytic cycle, *ICP4/ICP27* and a tegument protein, vhs, which is a significant source of cytotoxicity, results in complete block of viral replication, although some viral toxicity remains (Johnson et al., 1992a,b; Johnson et al., 1994).

More promising results have arisen from an alternative approach using defective HSV vectors. These vectors have arisen from the observation that a plasmid containing a transgene and minimal HSV sequences could be amplified and packaged in the presence of a helper virus (Speate and Frenckel, 1982). This plasmid, called an amplicon, allows the production of a defective HSV vector which contains no viral genes, is unable to replicate and contains multiple copies of the transgene per virion. The amplicon can be amplified to high titers to provide high-level gene expression, however, the presence of helper virus is a limiting factor. To disable the helper virus, commonly used methods include temperature sensitive mutations to disable growth at body temperatures. Such defective vectors have been used with promising results for CNS expression of functional genes (see below).

Progress in the development of helper-free packaging systems for HSV has been reported recently with a system involving the use of five cosmids which together represent the HSV genome but from which DNA cleavage and packaging signals have been deleted (Fraefel et al., 1996). Although a significant advance, this system is limited since the preparation is cumbersome and produces only low viral titers.

Clearly, modified viruses carrying foreign genes have been instrumental in the development of gene therapy. However, several disadvantages of these gene delivery systems must be considered. Perhaps most significant is the fact that the repeated injection of viruses, even those modified for gene transfer, is likely to elicit immune responses, thereby limiting their usefulness for in vivo gene delivery. Viruses which do not integrate into the host cell genome, such as AV, are particularly susceptible to this problem since they will require repeated administration for therapeutic effectiveness. In addition, many viruses have cytotoxic and/or oncogenic capabilities. Although the viruses used for gene transfer have been substantially modified to minimize these dangers, the risk remains that they may recombine with endogenous viruses in the recipient cells, leading to the production of replication-competent and potentially dangerous wild-type virus.

For these and other reasons, many investigators have turned towards non-viral gene delivery strategies (see Mahato, 1999; Treco and Selden, 1995 for reviews). While powerful tools in the research laboratory, most non-viral gene transfer methods are inefficient in animal model systems and not useful for CNS gene therapy at the present time. Thus, they will not be included in this review.

Approaches to gene therapy for neurodegenerative diseases

The neuropathological phenotypes seen in common neurodegenerative diseases vary from loss of function in a particular subset of neurons in Parkinson's disease (PD) and Huntington's disease (HD), to global neuronal dysfunction in Alzheimer's Disease (AD). Although this review will focus on gene therapy approaches for these common neurodegenerative diseases, the same methods and approaches which are discussed below could be used to treat many other genetic disorders with neurodegeneration.

IN VIVO APPROACHES

Degeneration of specific subsets of neurons and an associated decline in local specific neurotransmitters is a common feature of AD, PD and HD. The discovery of neurotrophic factors that inhibit neurodegeneration or stimulate regeneration, as well as the isolation of genes involved in the synthesis of neurotransmitter proteins, forms the basis of current in vivo gene strategies in primary neurodegenerative diseases.

Table 32.4 summarizes some of the features required for idealized CNS gene transfer vectors. To date, numerous studies have used HSV, AAV, AV and LV to mediate expression of a reporter gene in the rat brain (Akli et al., 1993; Davidson et al., 1993; Le Gal de Salle et al., 1993; Kaplitt et al., 1991; Kaplitt et al., 1994; Blomer et al., 1997; Naldini et al., 1996; Navarro et al., 1999). With the exception of LV, each of the above vectors also has been used to express tyrosine hydroxylase (TH) in a rodent model of PD by stereotactic intracerebral injection. TH is the enzyme required for conversion of tyrosine to L-Dopa.

For example, multiple injections of an AV expressing TH (Ad-TH) throughout the striatum in a rodent PD model reduced apomorphine-induced turning behavior two weeks after viral injection (Horrelou et al., 1994). In an HSV-TH study, a persistent increase in L-Dopa synthesis was observed at 16 months after multiple injections in the striatum, together with an improvement in behavioral deficits (During et al., 1994). In an AAV-expressing TH vector, transgene expression was detected, predominantly in neurons, at seven months after injection (Kaplitt et al., 1994), and the efficiency of cell transduction in AAV was significantly higher than that observed for AV or HSV.

A further promising approach to the gene therapy of PD is the coincident intrastriatal expression of several enzymes on the biosynthetic pathway for dopamine. For example, a

Table 32.4. Principal Requirements for Ideal CNS Viral Vectors

Able to transduce non-dividing cells
Replication-defective to prevent viral spread and cell damage
Non-toxic viral envelope
No viral gene expression
Absence of immune response
Free from helper virus
Stable integration into host cell genome
Maintenance of transgene expression

bicistronic AAV expressing transgenes for both TH and L-aromatic amino acid decarboxylase stereotactically injected into the striatal cells of dopamine-depleted monkeys, produced elevated levels of dopamine near the injection sites at 2.5 months post-injection (During et al., 1998). A similar approach expressing the same two transgenes, but this time using two separate AAV, produced behavioral recovery in a rodent PD model (Fan et al., 1998). This latter study is significant in that it suggests simultaneous transduction with several vectors is a potentially feasible approach to gene delivery. In a related strategy, separate AAVs encoding TH and GTP cyclohydrolase I, the enzyme necessary to produce the tetrahydrobiopterin cofactor for TH, were injected into denervated rat striatum. Microdialysis assays confirmed an increase synthesis of L-Dopa and metabolites (Mandel et al., 1998).

In a mouse model of mucopolysaccharidosis VII (Sly' syndrome), a neurodegenerative lysosomal storage disorder, sustained production of the missing normal enzyme β-glucuronidase also was achieved in the adult mouse brain using AAV gene transfer. Widespread distribution of the enzyme resulted from only a single treatment and produced reversal of the characteristic lysosomal storage lesions (Skorupa et al., 1999).

An alternative *in vivo* approach to protect degenerating neurons in genetic diseases is to engineer them to produce a trophic factor. Almost all studies on the efficacy of neurotrophic factor expression by viral vectors have been performed with vectors encoding members of the neurotrophin family, particularly, nerve growth factor (NGF) and brain-derived neurotrophic factor (BDNF), together with ciliary neurotrophic factor (CNTF) and glial-derived neurotrophic factor (GDNF). Neurotrophins are a class of structurally related growth factors which promote neuronal survival and differentiation and stimulate neurite outgrowth.

Numerous studies have shown that survival of basal forebrain cholinergic neurons is dependent on neurotrophic factors (Tuszynski et al., 1994). For example, intracerebroventricular infusion of NGF prevents the cholinergic neuronal atrophy and associated memory impairment observed in aged rats. The direct injection of an AV NGF into the basal forebrain in 30 month old rats protected neurons against this atrophy and produced an increase in somal size of the cholinergic neurons (Castel-Barthe et al., 1996). These studies suggest that recombinant AV directing the expression of growth factors can protect neurons against the age-related degenerative process. However, no functional recovery has been demonstrated in experimental animals and the efficacy of this approach for treating AD remains unproven.

In contrast, an AV encoding GDNF has been tested *in vivo* in a rodent model of PD. Injection of the GDNF vector rescued striatal neurons and reduced apomorphine-induced turning at three weeks compared to controls (Choi-Lundberg et al., 1997; Bilang-Bleuel et al., 1997). A similar approach using a recombinant AAV encoding GDNF has replicated these findings (Mandel et al., 1997). In the clinical situation, however, vector delivery prior to the onset of neuropathology (as was carried out in these studies where the rodent model was created by chemical lesioning after vector delivery) is not often possible. In addition, chronic delivery of the vector is likely to be necessary in a growth factor-based therapy. To address the former question, administration of the same AAV-GDNF construct (Mandel et al., 1999), post chemical lesioning in the rat model (i.e., after the onset of progressive striatal degeneration) has also been shown to protect nigral dopamine neurons following a single administration.

A defective HSV has also recently been used to test the hypothesis that apoptotic pathways are involved in the death of dopaminergic neurons in PD. An HSV expressing *Bcl-2* injected into the striatum of the rodent model of PD increased dopaminergic neuron survival as assessed by TH immunostaining. The proto-oncogene *Bcl-2* is a potent inhibitor of cell death. These results demonstrate that death of nigral neurons may be blocked by *Bcl-2* and are consistent with the notion that cell death in this model system is, at least in part, apoptotic (Yamada et al., 1999). This suggests that anti-apoptotic genes may be a target for gene therapy approaches.

Finally, the use of LV in the CNS has, so far, been restricted to expression of reporter genes into rat hippocampus and striatum by intracerebral injection. Prolonged stable expression, up to nine months after a single injection, was observed in the absence of cytotoxicity (Naldini et al., 1996).

EX VIVO APPROACHES

Dramatic advances in isolating cells suitable for neural transplantation pave the way to *ex vivo* gene therapy as a viable therapeutic strategy for CNS disease. It is now possible to isolate and expand, from developing and adult tissues, cells with properties characteristic of early neural multipotent progenitor or stem cells. The tantalizing possibility of using cells with stem cell-like properties as a source of cells for CNS transplantation, neural replacement and brain repair is thus being realized.

Early *ex vivo* approaches to transplantation in neurodegenerative diseases have employed a "survival approach" to amplify dopamine function or to increase expression of growth factors to restore dying neurons in target areas of the corpus striatum. In HD, strategies directed towards preventing degeneration of striatal neurons have a special appeal since potential sufferers can be identified well before the onset of symptoms and neuronal degeneration.

Experiments using heterologous donor tissue in PD have focused mainly on tissue derived from embryonic mesencephalon harvested at the point when the cells start to differentiate to dopaminergic neurons (Brundin et al., 1988). In particular, the use of multiple fetal brains for each graft with the addition of neurotrophic factors has proved a successful strategy to increase graft survival (Takayama et al., 1995). In HD the first study of fetus-to-adult striatal transplantation has recently been performed in three non-demented patients. The patients each received bilateral implantations from multiple fetuses into caudate and putamen in addition to cyclosporin immunosuppression. Magnetic resonance imaging demonstrated good graft survival and growth, and neuropsychological assessment at up to six months post-surgery demonstrated improved cognitive function on some measures (Philpott et al., 1997; Kopyov et al., 1998).

Although promising, ethical controversy over the use of human fetal tissue and serious methodological concerns associated with such techniques, not least the limited number of cells that can be collected from fetal dissections, has restricted their use. Instead, experimental protocols have progressed to attempts to expand cell types which meet the requirements for suitable donor cells with the ultimate aim of generating neural tissue *in vitro*. The ability to generate neural tissue would represent a key milestone in cellular and gene therapy for CNS disorders.

Potential cell types for CNS therapy

A number of potentially useful cell types have attracted attention as sources of donor tissue for transplantation (Table 32.5). No single idealized cell can fit all the requirements for CNS disease, but certain attributes make some cells more suitable for certain replacement functions than others. For example, in the local repair of damaged neurons the ability to integrate and function appropriately at the integration site could be considered a more important feature than migratory capacity. However, long distance migratory capacity is crucial to donor cells required for global CNS disease. In general, ideal candidates for cell transplantation in the CNS should be readily available, capable of rapid expansion in culture, immunologically inert and amenable to stable transfection and long term

Table 32.5. Potential Cell Types For CNS Gene Therapy

Pluripotent cells
Neural stem cells
Embryonic stem cells
Bone marrow stromal cells

Terminally differentiated cells
Skin fibroblasts
Neural cells (e.g., astrocytes)

expression of exogenous genes. Cell types that potentially satisfy these requirements are discussed below.

Non-neuronal cell types

Fibroblasts. As non-neuronal cells, fibroblasts are readily available, and can be easily expanded, transfected and manipulated *in vitro*. Fibroblasts remain *in situ* on transplantation (Morrison et al., 1997), and have been used for local delivery of trophic factors and synthetic enzymes in PD rodent models. For example, retroviral transduction of fibroblasts with brain-derived neurotrophic factor has resulted in reduction in chemically-induced dopaminergic neuronal degeneration (Frim et al., 1994). Similarly, animals implanted with fibroblasts expressing TH show amelioration in lesion-induced dopamine asymmetry for up to eight weeks post-implantation (Fisher et al., 1991). Furthermore, co-introduction of fibroblast growth factor-expressing fibroblasts with fetal dopaminergic neuronal cells, as in the paradigm above, has been shown to potentiate cellular survival and significantly improve behavioral function in a rodent model of PD (Takayama et al., 1995). The rationale for co-grafting is that it serves to enhance survival and function of the graft and decreases reliance on large quantities of fetal cells. Modification of fibroblasts to produce a continuous supply of NGF prevents degeneration of cholinergic neurons and partially reconstitutes spatial memory deficits in both rodent and primate models (Tuszynski et al., 1995; Martinez-Serrano, 1996).

In an adult mouse model of MPS VII (Sly' syndrome), retroviral transduction of transplanted fibroblasts supersecreting high levels of the corrective enzyme β-glucuronidase, resulted in clearance of lysosomal distension in neurons and glial cells in the vicinity of the graft. This demonstrates that corrective enzyme not only reached the diseased cells but also reversed established lesions in the severely diseased adult brain (Taylor and Wolfe, 1997). In a monkey model of HD, intrastriatal implants of polymer-encapsulated hamster kidney fibroblasts, genetically modified to secrete human Ciliary Neurotrophic Factor have been shown to exert a neuroprotective effect on GABAergic striatal neurons following administration of quiniloic acid compared with controls (Emerich et al., 1997).

The advantages of primary cells like fibroblasts are that these cells do not form tumors and the use of autologous cells obviates the need for immunosuppression in hosts. However, such cells have the disadvantage that each batch of transduced cells has to be generated separately, which reduces the reproducibility and degree of control over their properties and eventually, the safety of the engineered material. In addition, it is unclear how long such cells can persist in the CNS following transplantation.

Marrow stromal cells. Another easily available source of cells that satisfy the requirements of donor cells is bone marrow. At least one population of cells in the CNS, the microglia, is bone marrow-derived. Indeed, whole bone marrow cells from male mice systemically infused into female mice have been shown to produce a small but detectable contribution to both microglia and macroglia in the brain, presumably because small numbers of donor cells are capable of crossing the blood brain barrier (Eglitis and Mezey, 1997). However, BMT has been only partially effective in treating CNS defects of genetic diseases (Peters et al., 1996).

In addition to hematopoietic cells, bone marrow contains a subset of cells called marrow stromal cells (MSC's – also known as mesenchymal stem cells, colony-forming fibroblast units), which include stem-like precursors for non-hematopoietic tissues like osteoblasts, chondrocytes, adipocytes and myoblasts. These non-hematopoietic precursors represent hematopoietic support cells important in subsistence, differentiation and growth of hematopoietic stem cells. The potential of adult human MSCs to differentiate to multiple lineages of mesenchymal tissue has recently been confirmed using controlled conditions *in vitro* (Pittenger et al., 1999).

Systemic infusion of MSCs into irradiated three week old mice was followed by the appearance of progeny of the donor cells in a variety of non-hematopoietic tissues, including the brain (Pereira et al., 1998). Direct injection of human MSCs into the brain of albino rats produced 20% engraftment of the infused cells with migration away from the injection sites along known pathways for migration of neural stem cells into successive layers of the brain (Azizi et al., 1998) (see below). Injection of murine MSCs into the lateral ventricle of immune competent neonatal mice produced migration throughout the forebrain and cerebellum with expression of glial fibrillary acidic protein, a marker of differentiation to mature astrocytes (Kopen et al., 1999).

In a combination approach, injection of MSCs, retrovirally transduced with TH and GC, into the striatum of chemically lesioned rats, produced an increase in L-Dopa and a reduction in apomorphine-induced turning behavior. The engrafted cells survived for 87 days but transgene expression ceased by nine days (Schwarz et al., 1999).

These promising results suggest that MSCs may be useful vehicles for transplantation and may provide a realistic option for neurological diseases. One of the advantages to such a system is the readily available source of MSCs from the bone marrow which can be easily expanded. The use of a patient's own bone marrow would circumvent the problem of graft versus host disease.

However, critical issues concerning the types of CNS cells that are derived from the hematopoietic system, whether such cells can acquire the phenotype of mature neural cells, the entry of these cells into the CNS during fetal, neonatal and adult development, and the migration and persistence of the cells within the CNS, remain unanswered at present.

Neuronal cell types

Astrocytes. Among neuronal cell types currently under investigation for gene transfer and cell transplantation, astrocytes are particularly well suited because of their CNS origin, efficient secretory mechanisms, and their role of neuronal support by release of trophic factors. A further potentially useful characteristic of transplanted astrocytes is the ability to migrate along pathways similar to those of neural stem cells (Craig et al., 1996; Mackay, 1997). Human fetal astrocytes have been cultured and successfully transduced with retroviral vectors to express NGF (Lin et al., 1997). Recent studies have also demonstrated that human adult astrocytes isolated from cerebral cortex of patients undergoing surgical resection can be maintained, cryopreserved, expanded as long-term pure primary cultures for up to ten months, and can be efficiently engineered to express transgenes. AV-transduced astrocytes produce human TH in an active form, under the control of a tetracycline based regulatory system, and release L-Dopa (Rider et al., 1999).

These experimental findings confirm that human adult astrocytes can express a transgene of therapeutic interest in a regulatable manner and thus can function as biological "minipumps" for autologous transplantation in neurodegenerative diseases. However, in order to obtain autologous astrocytes invasive procedures must be used, and the immunogenicity of non-autologous cells has not yet been adequately determined.

Immortalized neural stem/progenitor cells. Neural stem/progenitor cells (NSCs) are immature, uncommitted cells that give rise to the array of more specialized cells of the CNS (Mackay, 1997; Morrison et al., 1997; Weiss et al., 1996). Like all stem cells, NSCs are capable of self-renewal and are able to differentiate into cells of all neural lineages. Recognition that neural cells with stem cell properties could be isolated from the developing and adult rodent CNS, could be propagated in culture and re-integrate to stably express foreign genes, has led to the search for analogous human counterparts for gene therapy applications (Synder et al., 1992; Gage et al., 1995).

Once isolated, neural progenitor cells can be rendered immortal, most commonly, by introducing extragenetic information into the cells, usually coding for oncogenic proteins. This acts to halt the progression of development such that the cells remain in a continuous cell cycle (Martinez-Serrano and Bjorklund, 1997). Thus, a homogenous progenitor population can be maintained in a proliferative state in culture to produce a limitless source of donor cells. "Conditionally" immortalized cells contain temperature sensitive alleles of the SV40 large tumor antigen and are thus able to proliferate *in vitro* at "permissive" temperatures, but exit the cell cycle and differentiate at non-permissive temperatures corresponding to mammalian core body temperature (Friederiksen et al., 1998). A remarkable feature of conditionally immortalized progenitors is the ability to integrate and differentiate after implantation into the developing and adult brain. Upon implantation into germinal zones of the brain, such progenitors are able to integrate and migrate over extended distances. The cells also differentiate in a site-specific manner to develop stable phenotypes characteristic of neuronal and glial cells, and establish neuronal connections.

Immortalized neuronal progenitor cell lines from rodents have so far been used successfully to correct metabolic defects in a number of *ex vivo* transduction studies. For example, intracerebroventricular injection of genetically engineered mouse progenitor cells has been used to deliver the missing gene product, β-glucuronidase, throughout the brain in the mouse model of MPS VII. Genetically modified, transplanted progenitors migrated throughout the brain and produced cross-correction of the disease by replacement of the defective enzyme. The widespread neuropathology of lysosomal distention was reduced or disappeared in treated animals (Synder et al., 1995). In a similar manner, immortalized progenitors expressing the β-hexosaminidase α-subunit gene (the genetic defect of Tay-Sachs disease) have been used to correct the diseased cellular phenotype in a human Tay-Sachs fibroblast cell line (Lacorazza et al., 1998). *In vivo*, after grafting to the brains of newborn mice, the cells expressed the enzyme for up to eight weeks, but cross-correction of the metabolic disease and neuropathology has not yet been demonstrated.

In addition to neurons, immortalized cells also represent a source of glial cells. Intracerebroventricular injection at birth of clonal neuronal stem cells resulted in widespread engraftment throughout the brain in a mouse of dysmyelination. Many of the donor cells differentiated into oligodendrocytes and a subgroup myelinated up to 52% of host cell neuronal processes accompanied by a reduction in symptomatic tremors in some animals (Yandava et al., 1999).

These valuable experiments using immortalized rodent progenitor cells confirm that implantation of immortalized neural stem cells can be used to make transgenic proteins available to large brain areas, and therefore may be useful for a variety of diseases characterized by extensive neuronal cell dysfunction. These findings suggest that therapeutic cell replacement in a widely disseminated global manner is a feasible strategy.

Human neural stem cells. That human neural stem cells can function in a manner analogous to their rodent counterparts has been established very recently with the successful isolation of human neural stem cells for the first time from the ventricular zone of the human fetal telencephalon. These cells were expanded, in one study up to 10^7 fold, and reimplanted into the germinal zones of developing and adult mice brains (Flax et al., 1998; Fricker et al., 1999; Vescovi et al., 1999). The human NSCs participated in all aspects of normal development in newborn mice and at all ages, migrated along established pathways to disseminate through the brain, differentiating into regionally appropriate cell types and interspersed with host rodent progenitors.

Neuropoietic cells of the human CNS are generated mainly during embryonic development within the germinal matrix of the ventricular and subventricular zones (VZ and SVZ). The SVZ persists into adulthood in a reduced form as the subependymal zone and represents a proliferative core of the CNS, dubbed "brain-marrow" (Schleffer et al., 1999). Controversial evidence that ependymal cells, too, could be stem cells of the adult brain has been presented recently (Johansson et al., 1999). However, although these cells clearly do show proliferative ability, no capacity for self renewal or multipotential for production of neurons was observed (Chiasson et al., 1999) (see Schleffer et al., 1999 for comprehensive review).

The existence of an additional region for neuropoiesis in the adult human brain has also been confirmed by *in vitro* studies. For example, proliferative stem/progenitor cells, isolated from the adult human hippocampus of surgical biopsy specimens, can generate neuronal and glial progeny

(Kukekov et al., 1999; Erikson, 1998). Manipulation of *in vitro* culture conditions has also been used to induce secretion of TH in neuronal stem cells isolated from mouse embryonic striatum and adult subependyma of the lateral ventricle or from multipotent embryonic forebrain stem cells (Daadi and Weiss, 1999). This development presents the prospect of regulating neurotransmitter phenotypes in such precursor cells for potential therapeutic use. It remains to be seen whether such manipulations can be extended to human neural stem cells. Nevertheless, these findings represent exciting progress in the search for a source of human tissue for repopulating degenerating or damaged brain.

Lineage directed human pluripotent stem cells. One of the potential limitations in introducing neural progenitor cells into the mature CNS may be that the normal adult brain lacks the appropriate environmental signals to realize their broad proliferative potential. In addition, specific neuropathological conditions may alter the balance of required environmental signals, perhaps even producing inappropriate cues which promote apoptotic death of residual populations. This suggests that a more viable alternative to the primary derivation of brain-derived specific stem cells may be to promote lineage commitment of progenitor cells *in vitro* prior to transplantation to the damaged brain. An *in vitro* system in which lineage-directed stem cells could be generated from a founder stem cell population of human pluripotent stem cells would thus be highly valuable.

It is well established that mouse embryonic stem cells are pluripotent and can be propagated in culture and differentiate into multi-lineage phenotypes, including mature neuronal and glial cells (Bain et al., 1995). Until recently, pluripotent stem cells could only be generated from mice. However, in two recent and highly significant reports, isolation and *in vitro* culture of human pluripotent stem cells was demonstrated.

In a similar manner to cultivation of mouse embryonic stem (ES) cells, human ES cell lines were generated from the inner cell mass of blastocysts grown from living embryos donated by participants in an *in vitro* fertilization program, or from the culture of gonadal ridges and mesenteries containing primordial germ cells from non-living fetal issues (Thompson et al., 1998; Shamblott et al., 1998).

Although exciting, it remains uncertain whether expertise from embryonic mouse ES cell lines will be transferable to pluripotent human ES cells. Successful cellular transplantation will require the expansion of the stem cell population to produce millions of cells for transplantation. Mixed cell populations are not suitable for transplantation because of the risk of invoking inappropriate host responses. Further,

if undifferentiated pluripotent stem cells persist there is a risk of initiating teratoma formation. Work is under way towards directing the cells to differentiate into lineage-restricted stem cells, but it is unclear how rapidly such cells could be expanded in culture, how stable the progeny would be over repeated passage, and how pure derived neural cells would be.

Assuming such problems were overcome, it is conceivable that pluripotent human stem cells could thus be primed to differentiate into neural cell populations and serve as tools for cell therapy. This approach may also offer the advantage to genetically manipulate these cells during the culture period. Finally, it is worth noting that grafting of cells might not be the only method of using stem/progenitor cells for neurorepair. In adult rats, intravenous injection of epidermal growth factor into the lateral ventricles was shown to produce a massive expansion of the endogenous subependymal progenitor population with migration into the neocortex and delayed elaboration of oligodendrocytes, astrocytes and neurons (Craig et al., 1996).

Other disease targets for gene therapy

HEMATOPOIETIC DISEASES

The roots of the human gene therapy field lie in the treatment of diseases for which BMT had proven curative and, most specifically, the rare genetic disorder, severe combined immune deficiency due to adenosine deaminase deficiency (Blaese et al., 1995). To date, most investigators have concentrated on retroviral gene transfer into pluripotent hematopoietic stem cells (PHSCs) as the prototype for somatic gene therapy for hematopoietic diseases, although many recent efforts have also focused on the evaluation of new gene transfer systems such as those based on adeno associated- and lenti-viruses (see above). PHSCs can be obtained from the bone marrow or peripheral blood and provide the opportunity to generate a variety of blood elements and hematopoietically-derived cells (e.g., Kupffer cells, osteoclasts, erythrocytes, pulmonary macrophages, etc.) expressing the transferred gene. PHSCs expressing therapeutic genes also may be reintroduced into affected individuals by autologous transplantation (Fig. 32.4), and the transplanted stem cells can migrate from the site of injection and establish a lineage of differentiated cells (e.g., Kupffer cells in the liver, microglia in the brain) which will express the foreign gene product. As noted above, the disease candidates for such therapy include those in which

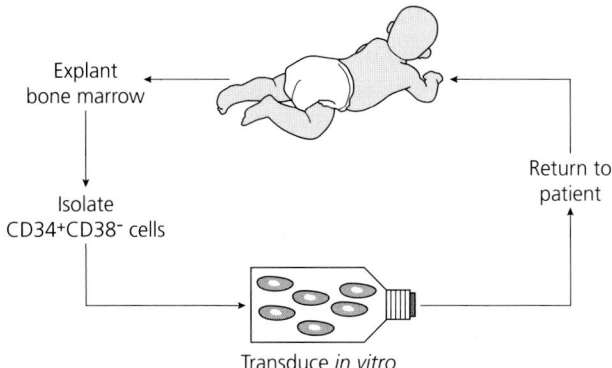

Explant bone marrow

Isolate CD34+CD38- cells

Transduce *in vitro*

Return to patient

Fig. 32.4. Procedure for hematopoietic stem cell gene therapy. Hematopoietic cells can be harvested from the bone marrow or peripheral blood and stem cells can be enriched using anti-CD34 and CD38 antibodies. CD34+/CD38- cells are then cultured in the presence of growth factors (e.g., IL-3, stem cell factor, etc.) in order to stimulate cell division, which is necessary for transduction by retroviral vectors. Meanwhile, the patient is subjected to radiation treatment and/or chemical reagents to destroy his/her remaining immune cells and make "space" for new cells. After retroviral transduction, the genetically-corrected cells are transplanted back into the patient for reconstitution of the immune system and expression of the therapeutic gene product. See text for details.

the primary site of pathology resides within the hematopoietic system and successful allogeneic BMT already has proven therapeutic or curative. Moreover, it has been suggested that the transplantation of stem cells which efficiently secrete a therapeutic protein may also lead to uptake of these proteins by non-hematopoietic target sites of pathology (for review see Lutzko et al., 1999).

Since *ex vivo* gene therapy using hematopoietic stem cells requires that the cells be maintained in culture, research efforts have been directed to develop optimal culture conditions for hematopoietic cell growth. The goal of these studies is to establish conditions which permit the maintenance/proliferation of stem cells such that they can be transduced by gene transfer vectors without the loss of their totipotent capacity. This is particularly important for the oncoretroviral vectors which require cell division for efficient transduction (see above). Initial studies to enhance retroviral transduction of PHSCs focused on the murine system. For example, Bodine et al., (1989) demonstrated that when the hematopoietic growth factors interleukin (IL)-3 and IL-6 were added to the media of cultured murine bone marrow cells, the number of "spleen colony forming units" (CFU-S) increased more than 10-fold over that obtained using standard cell culturing procedures. IL-3 and IL-6 appear to act synergistically to stimulate the division of PHSCs, a prerequisite for the stable integration of the retroviral vector. In the same study, bone marrow cells were infected with a retroviral vector containing the human β-globin gene and reintro-

duced into mice. Six of the 11 mice analyzed showed expression of the human β-globin gene 12 months post-transplantation, demonstrating effective gene transfer into murine PHSCs. Stem cell factor (also known as kit ligand or mast cell growth factor) (Williams et al., 1990; Zsebo et al., 1990) has also often been included in the bone marrow media to promote division of very primitive stem cells.

Concordant with the development of improved stem cell growth conditions, various protocols have been designed to purify murine PHSCs, which normally constitute less than 1% of bone marrow cells. For example, Szilvassy et al., (1989) reported a procedure for the single-step isolation of PHSCs from mice treated with 5-fluorouracil (5-FU). About 25% of the cells obtained in this manner were day 12 CFU-S, and at least 1% were capable of long-term marrow repopulation after transplantation into lethally irradiated mice. These investigators also showed that transplantation of 5 FU-enriched stem cells containing the *neo* gene into irradiated recipients resulted in *neo* expression in lymphoid and myeloid tissues six months post-transplantation. Alternative methods for the enrichment of stem cells also have been developed, such as the use of monoclonal antibodies which recognize stem cell-specific cell surface receptors (Spangrude et al., 1988; van de Rijn et al., 1989).

These and other techniques to enrich and grow murine stem cells have progressed rapidly, and many groups have achieved long-term expression of genes in mice after retroviral transduction of PHSCs and autologous transplantation (for review, see Karlsson, 1991). Moreover, several groups have demonstrated retroviral gene transfer into long-term repopulating marrow cells of larger animal models, such as dogs and non-human primates (Bodine et al., 1990; Kiem et al., 1994; Schuening et al., 1991). However, similar efforts in man have been relatively unsuccessful.

Human cells with "stem cell-like" properties have been isolated from peripheral blood, bone marrow and umbilical cord blood (e.g., Broxmeyer et al., 1992; Eaves et al., 1992) using monoclonal antibodies raised against a cell surface antigen, CD34 (Berenson et al., 1992). CD34 is a heavily glycosylated transmembrane protein whose function remains unknown, despite its universal expression and extensive characterization. CD34+ cell mixtures have been shown to contain totipotent cells and are the current target of most human gene therapy endeavors. In fact, a specialized subset of these cells, refered to as CD34+, HLA DR+, CD38-, are highly enriched for totipotent progenitors. The major advantages of using CD34+ cells for gene therapy as opposed to whole marrow include the smaller quantities of viral supernatants and cytokines needed and the smaller numbers of differentiated cells which would be transplanted.

Despite the identification of CD34+ cells and the development of methods to efficiently isolate them, they account for only 1–4% of mononuclear cells in human bone marrow, peripheral blood or cord blood (Eaves et al., 1992; Broxmeyer et al., 1992; Migliaccio et al., 1992). Moreover, the CD34+ cells isolated from these sources are heterogenous, including both committed and progenitor cells, and specific conditions for optimal retroviral transduction of CD34+ progenitor cells have not been developed.

An alternative method for the isolation of human hematopoeitic stem cells was developed by Berardi et al., (1995), who stimulated the proliferation of bone marrow cells using IL-3 and kit ligand while they were being grown in the presence of 5-FU. Under these conditions, dividing cells were killed, leaving only quiescent cells that could not be stimulated by the cytokines. Such cells, which represented about 1 in 10^5 bone marrow mononuclear cells, had a characteristic stem cell immunophenotype, were highly enriched for long-term culture initiation cells, and produced both myeloid and lymphoid progeny. However, despite the fact that these cells are likely to represent very early progenitors that are capable of long-term reconstitution in transplanted animals, they may be of limited use in retroviral-mediated gene therapy since they do not divide and would be difficult to stably transduce.

As noted above, oncoretroviruses require dividing cells for transduction, while totipotent stem cells are thought to be dormant. Therefore, cytokines are required to stimulate their growth, but this may result in differentiation and loss of totipotency. Thus, protocols differ widely with respect to the concentrations and combinations of cytokines used, the timing of prestimulation and virus exposures, and the presence or absence of stromal cells. Alternatively, vector systems which do not require cell proliferation (such as those using lentiviral vectors) are being actively explored (see Sutton et al., 1998).

Furthermore, little is known about the mechanisms underlying stem cell homing and engraftment following transplantation. Indirect measurements of stem cell homing in mice were initially performed by determining the seeding efficiences of spleen colony forming cells in transplantation studies (Lahiri et al., 1969). More recently, direct labeling of mouse stem cells with fluorescent probes has been achieved and used to monitor stem cell homing and engraftment (Samlowski et al., 1991). However, in these rodent studies the transplant recipients are generally subjected to lethal doses of total body irradiation to kill dividing cells and improve engraftment. Such irradiation treatment has many deleterious effects, including decreased bone growth and disruption of the blood brain barrier

(e.g., Rubin et al., 1994). Thus, alternative strategies must be evaluated. For example, several groups are investigating the use of dominant selectable markers (such as the multiple drug resistance [MDR] protein) to facilitate the *in vivo* selection of transplanted stem cells (for review, see Gottesman and Pastan, 1993). Clearly, to improve the success of hematopoietic stem cell gene therapy in man, the issue of homing and engraftment must be further investigated, animal experiments must be designed to simluate human conditions, and techniques to "scale-up" production of viral supernatants and CD34+ cells must be developed and optimized.

In summary, recent advances in the understanding of hematopoiesis have stimulated new experimental protocols which permit the proliferation and enrichment of murine and human stem cells for the targeting and expression of retrovirally transferred genes. However, the feasibility of stem cell gene therapy has not been fully demonstrated in monkeys or man, and a greater understanding of basic stem cell biology is needed before the successes of the rodent experiments can be duplicated in larger animals.

LIVER DISEASES

Since many inherited diseases result from the deficiency of hepatic-specific enzymes or proteins, the introduction and expression of human genes in hepatic cells has become an active area of investigation. (Fig. 32.5). Among the disease candidates for liver gene therapy are those in which the primary metabolic defect resides in the liver (e.g., familial hypercholesterolemia), as well as other diseases in which the liver may not be the primary site of pathology, but can be used to produce and secrete metabolic products into the circulation which may be therapeutic. Recent progress in this field is considered below.

It is now possible to propagate long-term cultures of hepatocytes that can expand in a clonal fashion and differentiate (Agelli et al., 1997; Bloch et al., 1996). Many studies using animal models indicate that hepatocytes transplanted into the spleen or liver survive, function and participate in the normal liver regenerative process. For example, allogeneic hepatocyte transplantation has been used to prolong survival in anhepatic rats (Arkadopoulos et al., 1998), and in a rat model of Wilson's disease, transplantation of normal hepatocytes before the onset of hepatic disease reduced hepatic copper deposition to 60% of that in untreated animals (Yoshida et al., 1996). In human patients, intrasplenic transplantation of differentiated adult hepatocytes has been used to promote short-term survival while awaiting orthoptic liver transplantation (Strom et al., 1997). Techniques have also

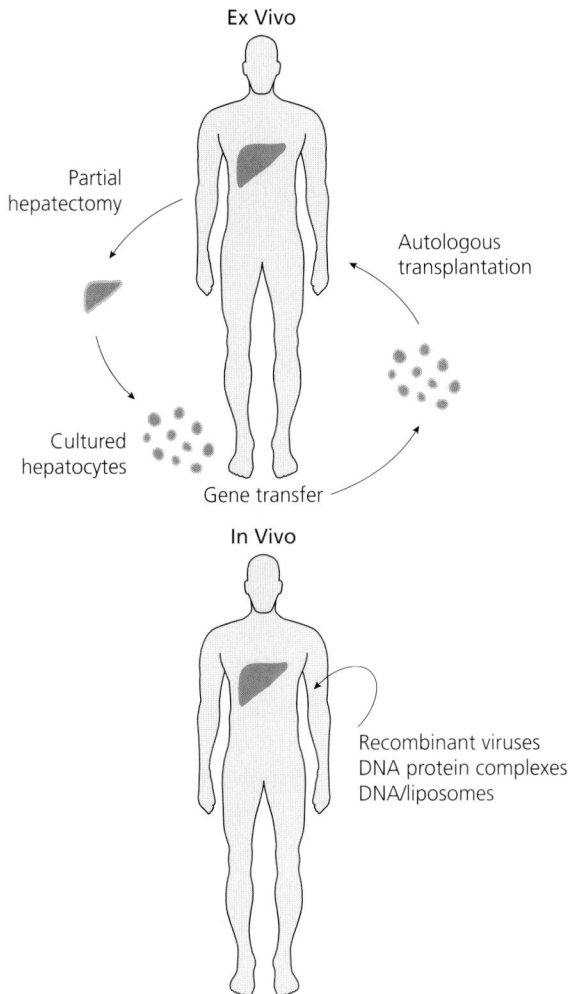

Ex Vivo

Partial hepatectomy

Autologous transplantation

Cultured hepatocytes

Gene transfer

In Vivo

Recombinant viruses
DNA protein complexes
DNA/liposomes

Fig. 32.5. Procedures for liver gene therapy. *Ex vivo* and *in vivo* approaches can be used to deliver and express genes in the liver. Once expressed, the gene products can be used to correct liver cells for primary liver disorders, or can be secreted into the circulation for delivery to other organ systems.

several metabolic diseases in animal model systems. For example, a single intravenous injection of an adenoviral vector encoding the human acid α-glucosidase gene resulted in efficient hepatic transduction, and subsequent systemic distribution to peripheral muscle, with correction of glycogen accumulation in an animal model of glycogen storage disease (Amalfitano et al., 1999). Similarly, a single intraportal injection of a recombinant AAV encoding the canine factor IX cDNA, under the control of a liver-specific promoter, has been used to produce sustained correction of the bleeding diathesis in hemophilia B mice (Wang et al., 1999).

Neonatal transfer of high titer retroviral vectors encoding factor VIII also has been used successfully to treat hemophilia A in a mouse model (Vanden Driessche et al., 1999). The uncharacteristically efficient hepatic gene transfer obtained from retroviral transduction in these experiments was attributed to the rapid growth of mouse hepatocytes and/or targeting to hepatic stem cells in neonatal animals. Recent efforts, in adult animals, have successfully facilitated hepatic transduction with retroviral vectors by employing coincident intramuscular injection of an adenovirus expressing hepatic growth factors (Gao et al., 1999).

Alternative approaches to correcting liver pathology in neonates have included direct intramuscular injection of AAV. *In situ* delivery of an AAV expressing β-glucuronidase resulted in long-term enzyme expression and correction of liver pathology in an experimental mouse model of mucopolysaccharidosis type VII (Daly et al., 1999).

Finally, the ability of lentiviral vectors to transduce non-dividing cells has been harnessed to enhance efficient gene transfer to the liver. Direct intraparenchymal injection of a lentiviral vector expressing a CMV-driven GFP transgene produced sustained expression for more than 22 weeks (Kafri et al., 1997).

Ex vivo liver-directed gene therapy has already proceeded to clinical trials in patients with familial hypercholesterolemia. In this approach, hepatic resection served as a source of hepatocytes that were cultured *in vitro* and transduced with a retrovirus encoding the human LDL receptor. Transplantation into the liver via portal vein cannulation produced transient reduction in serum cholesterol in some patients in the absence of major side effects (Grossman et al., 1995).

As with other organ-based approaches, identification of suitable cell types for *ex vivo* gene therapy remains an important goal. One potentially usefully source may be Oval cells, derived from potential stem cells in the bile ducts. Both *in vitro* and *in vivo* experiments demonstrate that oval cells have the capacity to differentiate into functional hepatocytes

now been established for the cryopreservation of human hepatocytes (Dunn et al., 2000, Jamal et al., 2000), although the shortage of human livers available for hepatocyte isolation limits the clinical usefulness of this procedure.

Recent innovations such as the production of a "reversibly" immortalized human cell line that can be expanded *in vitro* and exhibits the characteristics of differentiated hepatocytes also may provide a viable alternative for *ex vivo* liver gene therapy. Using this approach, intrasplenic transplantation of clonal cells (equivalent to 5% of the total number of hepatocytes) in rodents with liver failure, provided life-saving metabolic support during acute liver failure (Kobayashi et al., 2000).

In vivo gene therapy employing hepatic targeting has also proven a successful strategy for sustained correction of

in situ and can be genetically modified with retroviral vectors (Yashui et al., 1997).

An alternative strategy for the introduction of genetically modified hepatocytes into animals is to entrap such cells in synthetic biodegradable polymer scaffolds that can be permanently transplanted into the peritoneal cavity. Such anchorage-dependent dissociated liver cells tend to reorganize to native structures and proliferate. Using this method, a partial correction of a single liver enzyme defect has been achieved in dogs (Takeda et al., 1995). Efforts are currently under way to enhance long-term survival and engraftment using this approach.

Hepatic cells remain one of the most actively studied and potentially important targets for gene therapy. The proliferative capacity of the liver and the fact that many genetic diseases result from defective function of liver proteins and/or the production of toxic metabolites by the liver makes liver gene therapy an important goal. Although technical obstacles clearly remain to be overcome, it is likely that improved methods will continue to be developed for the genetic transduction of hepatic cells and the reintroduction of such cells into human patients.

Gene therapy—the future

IN UTERO GENE THERAPY

The pathologic abnormalities associated with many genetic diseases often begin in early fetal development, leading to the onset of clinical symptoms soon after birth or during early infancy. Thus, to accomplish effective therapy of these disorders, normal function must be restored as early as possible and, if possible, during the fetal period. This is particularly important for those genetic diseases with CNS involvement, since closure of the BBB during fetal development makes delivery of therapeutic molecules into the brain after birth extremely difficult. Thus, researchers have recently begun to develop and evaluate *in utero* gene delivery strategies for several genetic diseases, particularly those with CNS involvement.

One approach for achieving *in utero* gene therapy is to use genetically corrected pluripotent hematopoietic stem cells for fetal transplantation. Fetal stem cell transplantation has been performed in sheep (Srour et al., 1992; Tan et al., 2000), non-human primates (Roodman et al., 1991; Winkler et al., 1999), mice (Pallavicini et al., 1992; Schneider et al., 1999), and man (Touraine et al., 1991; Flake et al., 1999). Sources of stem cells varied from fetal liver to adult marrow, and the fetal age at the time of transplant spanned the first to third trimester. To date, few attempts at fetal stem cell transplantation have been undertaken in humans (e.g., Touraine et al., 1991). In general, these were unsuccessful, principally because donor cell engraftment was not achieved. Although the experience has been limited, the following facts have been documented or are emerging: 1) direct umbilical cord venipuncture under ultrasonographic guidance is possible in the human fetus as early as 20 weeks of gestation, 2) the source of stem cells is critical for engraftment; at present, fetal liver seems to be the optimal source, 3) successful engraftment appears to depend on transplantation before the fetus achieves immunocompetence, and 4) the proportion of donor to recipient cells is a major factor in determining beneficial response. The frequency of donor cells detected after birth varies from less than 1% to as much as 20% in published reports, and the factors influencing outcome and methods to improve it are not clearly understood.

The most commonly used method in experimental animals for *in utero* gene transfer involves microinjection of normal DNA into the pronuclei of zygotes immediately after fertilization for the generation of transgenic individuals. However, this method accomplishes gene transfer to all cells, including germ-cells, and is not acceptable for humans (see above, "Germ-Line Gene Therapy"). Another intriguing method involves the intravenous injection of DNA constructs into pregnant women for gene transfer into embryos. For example, Tsukamoto et al., (1995) injected cationic liposomes complexed with CAT expression plasmids into pregnant mice and achieved gene transfer and expression in embryos. Efficient gene transfer to embryos was dependent on the formation of a placenta, as attempts to deliver genes earlier in fetal life were unsuccessful. Viral vectors have also been directly injected into early embryos to achieve gene expression (e.g., Jahner et al., 1985), and viral gene delivery may prove useful for the transplacental delivery method described above.

Clearly, *in utero* gene therapy must be carefully evaluated in experimental animals prior to human application. Acceptable methods must accomplish somatic cell gene delivery and expression in the embryos, without the risk of gene delivery to the germ cells. Moreover, considerable effort must be directed to better understand the regulation of gene expression during embryogenesis in order to avoid any deleterious effects of abnormal temporal or spatial gene expression. *In utero* gene therapy remains the only viable approach to treating numerous genetic diseases, particularly those that follow a rapid neurodegenerative course (e.g., Tay-Sachs disease), and will likely remain an important area of research in the foreseeable future.

RIBOZYMES, ANTISENSE RNA AND DOMINANT DISORDERS

Until recently, efforts to develop gene therapy have relied on techniques to introduce and express normal genes into cells containing genetic defects. However, for certain diseases, particular dominantly inherited structural gene defects and certain types of cancer, correction may not only require expression of the normal gene product, but inhibition of the abnormal gene product as well because of a "dominant-negative" phenotype. To accomplish this type of gene therapy, researchers have turned to the use of various RNA strategies, such as antisense RNA and ribozymes (for review, see Altman, 1993; Shippy et al., 1999; Sullenger, 1999).

Ribozymes are RNA enzymes capable of self-cleavage (Altman, 1993). The "enzymatic" domain of such RNAs can be divided into two regions: one serving as the catalytic surface (i.e., the enzyme) and the other as the site of cleavage (i.e., the substrate). These two regions can be independently reconstructed on synthetic oligonucleotides that have primary sequences enabling them to hydrogen bond with each other, permitting cleavage to occur in "trans". Thus, if the sequence of a target RNA is known, an oligonucleotide can be custom-designed to complex with the target and cleave it. The sequence encoding the enzymatic RNA (i.e., ribozyme) may be delivered to the cells using any of the viral or non-viral gene delivery methods discussed above.

Several different types of ribozymes have been engineered. For example, Yu et al., (1993) used the hairpin motif found in tobacco ringspot virus satellite RNA to attack the 5′ leader regulatory sequence encoded by the HIV genome. In contrast, Cantor et al., (1993) used the hammerhead motif found in many viral RNAs to cleave the mRNA coding for the *rex* and *tax* regulatory gene products of bovine leukemia virus. Similarly, Ohkawa et al., (1993) used multiple hammerheads with different flanking sequences to simultaneously attack several targets in HIV RNA. Multi-ribozyme targeting has also been accomplished for the human α-globin gene (Shen et al., 1999). Thus, several approaches can be envisioned for the development of a disease-specific ribozyme, provided the specific disease-causing nucleotide sequence is known.

One question which arises from these studies is whether the observed effect of gene product inhibition is due to site-directed cleavage of the target RNA, or alternatively, antisense RNA effects. In most cases it is likely that both events are occurring and RNA enzyme cleavage events are an addition to whatever level of inhibition is due to antisense effects. The RNA enzyme, in principle, is capable of releasing from the complex after cleavage has occurred for

recycling, an important concept if stable gene therapy is to be accomplished without repeated administration of the RNA. It is also likely that a ribozyme is more stable inside cells than a single-stranded antisense RNA, since the ribozyme rapidly becomes part of a high-order structure that is relatively resistant to cellular nucleases.

Another potential gene therapy application of this technology is the use of ribozymes that catalyze RNA splicing, as opposed to RNA cleavage (Thompson et al., 1995). Such ribozymes could be applied in a gene therapy setting to repair defective genes by replacing a region of an RNA containing a mutation or small rearrangement with a functional piece of RNA. Clearly, improved ribozyme and/or antisense techniques will continue to be developed and have important applications for gene therapy.

GENE REPLACEMENT VERSUS GENE INSERTION

About ten years ago, nearly simultaneous with the first successful retroviral gene transfer experiments, several groups independently demonstrated that cultured mammalian cells possessed the enzymatic machinery to carry out homologous (i.e., site-specific) recombination (for review, see Bollag et al., 1989). Although the frequency of these site-specific insertion events was rare, one important implication of these early findings was that human gene therapy might be accomplished by direct replacement of a defective gene with a normal gene, as opposed to random gene insertion. This possibility offered an important answer to critics who were concerned with the potential risks associated with insertional mutagenesis or abnormal gene activation. Although numerous new and improved gene transfer techniques have been developed during the past decade, the possibility of carrying out direct gene replacement in man remains an elusive and important goal.

Homologous recombination may provide a solution to the correction of dominant diseases and cancers in which expression of the defective gene may interfere with the function of the normal gene product. Such gene replacement techniques also may be useful for certain recessive diseases (i.e., enzyme deficiencies) in which the mutant and normal gene products may form abnormal subunit structures. Clearly, gene replacement, as opposed to gene insertion, remains the long-term goal of most gene therapy efforts. However, increased understanding of the human recombination apparatus is required before the correction of deletions, insertions and base substitutions can become a reality. The development of such technology will represent a defining moment in molecular medicine and herald the emergence of this new technology in the twenty-first century.

Acknowledgements

This review was supported in part by grants from the National Institutes of Health, including research grants (5 R37 DK34045, 5 R01 DK25759, 5 R01 HD28607, 1 P30 HD28822), a grant (5 M01 RR0071) from the National Center for Research Resources for the Mount Sinai General Clinical Research Center, and a grant (1 P30 HD32654) from the National Institutes of Child Health for the Mount Sinai Child Health Research Center, as well as grants (1–578 and 1–1224) from the March of Dimes Birth Defects Foundation. JEC is an MRC Clinician Scientist Fellow.

REFERENCES

Agelli M, Dello Sbarba P et al. (1997) Putative liver progenitor cells: conditions for long-term survival in culture. Histochem J 29:205–217

Akli S, Caillaud C, Vigne E, Stratford-Perricaudet LD et al. (1993) Transfer of a foreign gene into the brain using adenovirus vectors. Nat Genet 3:224–228

Altman S (1993) RNA-enzyme directed gene therapy. Proc Natl Acad Sci USA 90:10898–10900

Amalfitano A, McVie-Wylie AJ, Hu H et al. (1999) Systemic correction of the muscle storage disorder glycogen storage disease type II after hepatic targeting of a modified adenovirus vector encoding human α-glucosidase. Proc Natl Acad Sci USA 96:861–8866

Antonarakis AE, McKusick VA (2000) OMIM passes the 1,000 disease-gene mark. Nat Genet 25:11

Arkadopoulus N, Lilja H, Suh KS et al. (1998) Intrasplenic transplantation of allogenic hepatocytes prolongs survival in anhepatic rats. Hepatology 28:1365–1370

Armentano D, Sookdeo CC, Hehir, KM et al. (1995) Characterization of an adenovirus gene transfer vector containing and E4 deletion. Hum Gene Ther 6:1343–1353

Atchison RW, Casto BC, Hammond WM (1965) Adeno-associated defective virus particles. Science 149:754–756

Azizi SA, Stokes D, Augeli B et al. (1998) Engraftment and migration of human bone marrow stromal cells implanted in the brains of albino rats-similarities to astrocyte grafts. Proc Natl Acd Sci USA 95:3908–3913

Bain G, Kitchens D, Yao M et al. (1995) Embryonic stem cells express neuronal properties in vitro. Dev Biol 168:342–357

Barkats M, Bilang-Bleuel A, Buc-Caron MH et al. (1998) Adenovirus in the brain: recent advances of gene therapy for neurodegenerative diseases. Prog Neurobiol 55:333–341

Berardi AC, Wang A, Levine JD et al. (1995) Functional isolation and characterization of human hematopoietic stem cells. Science 267:104–108

Berenson RJ (1992) Transplantation of CD34+ hematopoietic precursors: clinical rationale. Transpl Proc 24:3032–3034

Bilang-Bleuel A, Revah F, Colin P et al. (1997) Intrastriatal injection of an adenoviral vector expressing glial-derived-neurotrophic factor prevents dopaminergic neuron degeneration and behavioral impairment in a rat model of Parkinson's disease. Proc Natl Acad Sci USA 94:8818–8823

Blaese RM, Culver KW, Miller DW (1995) T-cell directed gene therapy for ADA-SCID. Science 270:475–480

Bloch GD, Locker J, Bowen WC et al. (1996) Population expansion, clonal growth, and specific differentiation of hepatocytes induced by HGF/SF, EGF, TGF in a chemically defined medium. J Cell Biol 132:1133–1149

Blomer U, Naldini L, Kafri T et al. (1997) Highly efficient and sustained gene transfer in adult neurones with lentivirus vector. J Virol 71:6641–6649

Bodine DM, Karlsson S, Nienhuis AW (1989) Combination of interleukins 3 and 6 preserves stem cell function in culture and enhances retrovirus-mediated gene transfer into hematopoietic stem cells. Proc Nat Acad Sci USA 8897–8901

Bollag AJ, Waldman AS, Liskay RM (1989) Homologous recombination in mammalian cells. Ann Rev Genet 23:199–225

Brinster RL (1993) Stem cells and transgenic mice in the study of development. Int J Dev Biol 37:89–99

Broxmeyer HE, Douglas GW, Hangoc G et al. (1992) Human umbilical cord blood as a source of transplantable hematopoietic stem and progenitor cells. Curr Top Microbiol Immunol 177:195–204

Brundin PR, Strecker H, Widner DJ et al. (1988) Human foetal dopamine neurones grafted in a rat model of Parkinson's disease: Immunological aspects, spontaneous and drug-induced behaviour and dopamine release. Exp Brain Res 70:192–208

Burns JC, Friedmann T, Driever W et al. (1993) Vesicular stomatitis virus G glycoprotein pseudotyped retroviral vectors: concentration to very high titre and efficient gene transfer into mammalian and non-mammalian cells. Proc Natl Acad Sci USA 90:8033–8037

Byrnes AP, Wood MJ, Charlton HM (1995) Adenovirus gene transfer causes inflammation in the brain. Neuroscience 16:1015–1024

Byrnes AP, Wood MJ, Charlton HM (1996) Role of T cells in inflammation caused by adenovirus vectors in the brain. Gen Ther 3:644–651

Cantor GH, McElwain TF, Birkebak TA, Palmer GH (1993) Ribozyme cleaves rex/tax mRNA and inhibits bovine leukemia virus expression. Proc Natl Acad Sci USA 90:10932–10936

Castel-Barthe MN, Jazat-Poindessous F, Barneaoud P et al. (1996) Direct intracerebral nerve growth factor gene transfer using a recombinant adenovirus: effects on basal cholinergic forebrain neurones. Neurobiol Dis 3:76–86

Chiasson BJ, Tropepe V, Morshead, CM et al. (1999) Adult mammalian forebrain ependymal and subependymal cells demonstrate proliferative potential but only subependymal cells have neural stem cell characteristics. J Neurosci 19:4462–4471

Choi-Lundberg DL, Lin Q, Chang Y et al. (1997) Dopaminergic neurones protected from degeneration by GDNF gene therapy. Science 255:838–841

Chong H, Vile RG (1996) Replication-competent retrovirus produced by a split-function third generation amphotropic packaging cell line. Gene Ther 3:624–626

Coffin JM, Hughes SH, Varmus HE (1997) Retroviruses. Cold Spring Harbor Laboratory Press, NY

Constantini F, Chad K, Magram J (1986) Correction of murine β-thalassemia by gene transfer into the germ line. Science 233:1192–1194

Craig CG, Tropepe V, Morshead CM et al. (1996) In vivo growth factor expression of endogenous subependymal neural precursor cell populations in the adult rat brain. J Neurosci 2:424–429

Daadi MM, Weiss S (1999) Generation of tyrosine hydroxylase producing neurones from precursors of the embryonic and adult forebrain. J Neurosci 19:4484–4497

Dai Y, Schwartz E, Gu D et al. (1995) Cellular and humeral immune responses to adenoviral vectors containing the factor IX gene: Tolerisation of factor IX and vector antigens allows for long-term expression. Proc Natl Acad Sci USA 92:1403–4105

Daly TM, Okuyama T, Vogler C et al. (1999) Neonatal intramuscular injection with recombinant adeno-associated virus results in prolonged beta-glucuronidase expression *in situ* and correction of liver pathology in MPS VIII mice. Hum Gene Ther 19:85–94

Davidson BL, Allen ED, Kozarsky KF et al. (1993) A model system for *in vivo* transfer into the CNS using an adenoviral vector. Nat Genet 3:219–223

Dedieu J, Vigne E, Torrent C et al. (1997) Long-term gene delivery into the livers of immunocompetent mice with E1/E4 deleted defective adenoviruses. J Virol 71:4626–4637

Desnick RJ (1990) Treatment of inherited metabolic diseases. In Emery AE, Rimoin DL (eds) Principles and Practice of Medical Genetics, Churchill Livingstone, London pp. 2001–2010

Ding L, Lu S, Munshi NC (1997) *In vitro* packaging of an infectious adeno-associated virus. Gene Ther 4:1167–1172

Dunn TB, Kumins NH, Raaofi V et al. (2000) Multiple hepatocyte transplantations in the dalmation dog. Surgery 127:193–199

During MJ, Naegale JR, O'Malley KL et al. (1994) Long-term behavioural recovery in Parkinsonian rats by and HSV vector expressing tyrosine hydroxylase. Science 266:1399–1403

During MJ, Samulski RJ, Elsworth JD et al. (1998) *In vivo* expression of therapeutic human genes for dopamine production in the caudates of MPTP-treated monkeys using an AAV vector. Gene Ther 5:820–837

Eaves CJ, Sutherland HJ, Udomsakdi C et al. (1992) The human hematopoietic stem cell in vitro and in vivo. Blood Cells 18:301–307

Eglitis MA, Mezey E (1997) Haematopoeitic cells differentiate to microglia and macroglia in the brains of adult mice. Proc Natl Acad Sci USA 94:4080–4085

Emerich DF, Winn SR, Hantraye PM et al. (1997) Protective effect of encapsulated cells producing neurotrophic factor CNTF in a monkey model of Huntington's disease. Nature 386:395–399

Engelhardt JF, Ye X, Doranz B et al. (1994) Ablation of E2a in recombinant adenoviruses improves transgene expression and decreases inflammatory response in mouse liver. Proc Natl Acad Sci US 91:6196–6200

Eriksson PS (1998) Neurogenesis in the adult hippocampus. Nat Med 4:113–1317

Fan DS, Ogawa M, Fujimoto KI et al. (1998) Behavioural recovery in 6-hydroxydopamine-lesioned rats by co-transduction of striatum with tyrosine hydroxylase and aromatic Lamino acid decarboxylase genes using two separate AAV vectors. Hum Gen Ther 9:2527–2535

Federico M (1999) Lentiviruses as gene delivery vectors. Curr Opin Biotech 10:448–453

Ferrari FK, Xiao X, McCarty D et al. (1997) New developments in the generation of Adfree high titre rAAV gene therapy vectors. Nat Med 3:1295–1297

Fisher LJ, Jinnah HA, Kale LC et al. (1991) Survival and function of intrastriatally grafted primary fibroblasts genetically modified to produce L-Dopa. Neuron 6:371–380

Fisher KJ, Choi H, Burda J et al. (1996) Recombinant adenovirus deleted of all viral genes for gene therapy of cystic fibrosis. Virology 217:11–22

Flake AW (1999) In utero stem cell transplantation for the treatment of genetic diseases. Schwiz Med Wochenschr 129:1733–1739

Flax JD, Aurora S, Yang C et al. (1998) Engraftable human neural stem cells respond to development cues replace neurones and express foreign genes. Nat Biotech 16:1033–1039

Fraefel C, Song S, Lim F et al. (1996) Helper virus-free transfer of herpes simplex virus type 1 plasmid vectors into neural cells. J Virol 70:7190–7197

Fricker RA, Carpenter MK, Winkler C et al. (1999) Site-specific migration and neuronal differentiation of human neural progenitor cells after transplantation in the adult rat brain. J Neurosci 19:5990–6005

Friederiksen K, Jat PS, Valtz N et al. (1998) Immortalisation of precursor cells from the mammalian CNS. Neuron 1:439–448

Frim DM, Uhler TA, Galpern WR et al. (1994) Implanted fibroblasts genetically engineered to produce brain-derived neurotrophic factor prevent MPTP toxicity to dopaminergic neurones in the rat. Proc Natl Acd Sci USA 91:5104–5108

Gage FH, Coates PW, Palmer TD (1995) Survival and differentiation of adult neuronal progenitor cells transplanted to the adult brain. Proc Natl Acad Sci USA 92:11879–11883

Gao G, Yang Y, Wilsson JM (1996) Biology of adenovirus vectors with E1/E4 deleted for liver-directed gene therapy. J Virol 70:8934–8943

Gao C, Jokerst R, Gondipalli P et al. (1999) Intramuscular injection of an adenoviral vector expressing hepatocyte growth factor facilitates hepatic transduction with a retroviral vector in mice. Hum Gene Ther 10:911–922

Gorziglia MI, Kadan MJ, Yei S et al. (1996) Elimination of both E1 and E2a form adenovirus vectors further improves prospects for *in vivo* gene therapy. J Virol 70:4173–4178

Gottesman MM, Pastan I (1993) Biochemistry of multidrug resistance mediated by the multidrug transporter. Annu Rev Biochemi 62:385–427

Grossman M, Rader DJ, Muller DW et al. (1995) A pilot study of *ex vivo* gene therapy for homozygous familial hypercholesterolaemia. Nat Med 1:1148–1154

Hammer RE, Palmiter RD, Brinster RL (1984) Partial correction of a murine hereditary growth disorder by germ-line incorporation of a new gene. Nature 311:65–6

Hermans WTJMC, Verhaagen J (1998) Viral vectors, tools for gene transfer in the nervous system. Prog Neurobiol 55:399–434

Horrelou P, Vigne E, Castel M et al. (1994) Direct intracerebral gene transfer of an adenoviral vector expressing tyrosine hydroxylase in a rat model of Parkinson's disease. Neuroreport 6:49–53

Jahner D, Haase K, Mulligan R, Jaenisch R (1985) Insertion of the bacterial *gpt* gene into the germ line of mice by retroviral infection. Proc Natl Acad Sci USA 82:6927–6931

Jamal HZ, Weglarz TC, Sandgren EP (2000) Cryopreserved mouse hepatocytes retain their regenerative capacity *in vivo*. Gastroenterology 118:390–394

Johansson CB, Momma S, Clarke DL et al. (1999) Identification of a neural stem cell in the adult mammalian brain. Cell 96:25–34

Johnson PA, Yoshida K, Gage FH, Friedmann T (1992a) Effects of gene transfer into cultured CNS neurons with a herpes simplex virus type 1 vector. Mol Brain Res 12:95–102

Johnson PA, Miyanohara A, Levine F et al. (1992b) Cytotoxicity of a replication-defective mutant of herpes simplex virus type 1. J Virol 66:2952–1956

Johnson PA, Wang MJ, Friedman T (1994) Improved cell survival by the reduction of immediate early gene expression in replication-defective mutants of herpes simplex virus type 1 but not by a mutation in the virion host shut off function. J Virol 68:6347–6362

Johnston J, Power C (1999) Productive infection of human peripheral blood mononuclear cells by FIV: Implications for vector development. J Virol 73:2491–2498

Jones SN, Grompe M, Munir et al. (1990) Ectopic correction of ornithine transfer deficiency in sparse fur mice. J Biol Chem 265:14681–14690

Kafri T, Blomer U, Petersen DA et al. (1997) Sustained expression of genes delivered directly into liver and muscle by lentiviral vectors. Nat Genet 17:314–317

Kaplitt MG, Pfaus JG, Kleopoulos SP et al. (1991) Expression of a functional foreign gene in adult mammalian brain following *in vivo* transfer via a herpes simplex virus type 1. Mol Cell Neurosci 2:320–330

Kaplitt MG, Leone P, Samulski RJ et al. (1994) Long-term expression and phenotypic correction using adeno-associated virus vectors in the mammalian brain. Nat Genet 1994 4:148–154

Karlsson S (1991) Treatment of genetic defects in hematopoietic cell function by gene transfer. Blood 78:2481–2492

Kiem H-P, Darovsky B, von Kalle C et al. (1994) Retrovirus-mediated gene transduction into canine peripheral blood repopulating cells. Blood 83:1467–1473

Klimatatcheva E, Rosenblatt JD, Planelles V (1999) Lentiviral vectors and gene therapy. Fron Biosci 4:481–496

Kobayashi N, Fujiwara T, Westerman KA et al. (2000) Prevention of acute liver failure in rats with reversibly immortalised human hepatocytes. Science 287:1258–1262

Kochanek S, Clemens PR, Mitani K et al. (1996) A new adenoviral vector: replacement for all viral coding sequences with 28 kb of DNA independently expressing both full-length dystrophin and β-galactosidase. Proc Natl Acad Sci 93:5731–5736

Kohn RM, Siniscalco M, Samulski RJ (1990) Site-specific integration by adeno-associated virus. Proc Natl Acad Sci USA 87:2211–2215

Kohn DB, Weinberg KI, Lenarsky C (1995) Gene therapy for neonates with ADA deficiency by transfer of human ADA cDNA into umbilical cord CD34+ cells. Paediatr Res 37:A9

Kohn RM, Siniscalco M, Samulski RJ et al. (1990) Site-specific integration by adeno-associated viruses. Proc Natl Acad Sci USA 87:2211–2215

Kopen GC, Prockop DJ, Phinney DG (1999) Marrow stromal cells migrate throughout forebrain and cerebellum, and they differentiate into astrocytes after injection into neonatal mouse brains. Proc Natl Acad Sci USA 96:10711–10716

Kopyov OV, Jacques S, Lieberman A et al. (1998) Safety of intrastriatal neurotransplantation for Huntington's disease patients. Exp Neurol 149:97–108

Kukekov VG, Laywell ED, Suslov K et al. (1999) Multipotent stem/progenitor cells with similar properties arise from two neurogenic regions of the adult human brain. Exp Neurol 156:333–344

Kyle JW, Birkenmeier EH, Gwynn B et al. (1990) Correction of murine micropolysaccharidosis VII by human β-glucuronidase transgene. Proc Natl Acad Sci USA 87:3914–3918

Lacorazza HF, Flax JD, Snyder EY et al. (1998) Expression of human beta-hexosaminindase alpha-subunit gene the gene defect of Tay-Sachs disease in mouse brains upon the engraftment of transduced progenitor cells. Nat Med 2:424–429

Lahiri SK, Van Putten LM (1969) Distribution and multiplication of colony forming units from bone marrow and spleen after injection in irradiated mice. Cell Tissue Kinet 2:21–28

Le Gal de Salle G, Robert JJ, Berrard S et al. (1993) An adenovirus vector for gene transfer into neurones and glia in the brain. Science 259:988–990

Leinekugel P, Michel S, Conzelmann E et al. (1993) Quantitative correlation of the residual activity of hexosaminindase A and arylsulfatase A and the severity of the resulting lysosomal storage disease. Hum Genet 88:513–523

Lin Q, Cunningham LA, Epstein LG et al. (1997) Human foetal astrocytes as an *ex vivo* gene therapy vehicle for delivering biologically active nerve growth factor. Hum Gene Ther 8:331–339

Lutzko C, Dube ID, Stewart AK (1999) Recent progress in gene transfer into hematopoietic stem cells. Crit Rev Oncol Hematol 30:143–158

Mackay RDG (1997) Stem cells in the central nervous system. Science, 276, 66–71

Mahato RI (1999) Non-viral peptide-based approaches to gene delivery. J Drug Target 7:249–268

Mandel RJ, Spratt SK, Synder RO et al. (1997) Midbrain injection of recombinant adeno-associated virus encoding rat glial cell line-derived neurotrophic factor in a progressive model of 6 hydroxydopamine-induced Parkinson's disease. Proc Natl Acad Sci USA 94:14083–14088

Mandel RJ, Rendahl KG, Spratt SK et al. (1998) Characterisation of intrastriatal recombinant adeno-associated virus-mediated gene transfer of human tyrosine hydroxylase and human GTP-cyclohydrolase I in a rat model of Parkinson's disease. J Neurosci 12:4271–4284

Marin M, Noel D, Piechaczyk M (1997) Towards efficient cell targeting by recombinant retroviruses. Mol Med Today 9:396–403

Martinez-Serrano A, Bjorklund A (1997) Immortalised neural progenitor cells for CNS gene transfer and repair. Trends Neurosci 20:530–538

Martinez-Serrano A, Fischer W, Soderstrom S et al. (1996) Long-term functional recovery from age-induced spatial memory impairments by nerve growth factor gene transfer to the rat basal forebrain. Neurobiol 93:6355–6360

Mason AJ, Pitts SL, Mikolics K et al. (1986) The hypogonadal mouse: reproductive functions restored by gene therapy. Science 234:1372–1378

Migliaccio G, Migliaccio AR, Druzin ML et al. (1992) Long term generation of colony forming cells in liquid culture of CD34+ cord blood cells in the presence of recombinant human stem cell factor. Blood 79:2620–2627

Mitrophanous KA, Yoon S, Rohll JB et al. (1999) Stable gene transfer to the nervous system using a non-primate lentiviral vector. Gen Ther 6:1808–1818

Miyoshi H, Blomer U, Takahashi M et al. (1998) Development of a self-inactivating lentivirus vector. J Virol 728:81150–8157

Monohan PE, Samulski RJ, Tazelaar J et al. (1998) Direct intramuscular injection with recombinant AAV results in sustained expression in a dog model of Haemophilia. Gene Ther 5:40–49

Morrison SJ, Shah NM, Anderson DJ (1997) Regulatory mechanisms in stem cell biology. Cell 88:287–298

Naldini L (1998) Lentiviruses as gene transfer agents for delivery to non-dividing cells. Curr Opin Biotech 9:457–463

Naldini L, Blomer U, Gage FH et al. (1996) Efficient transfer, integration, and long-term expression of the transgene in adult rat brains injected with a lentiviral vector. Proc Natl Acad Sci 93:11382–1188

Navarro V, Millecamps S, Geoffroy M-C et al. (1999) Efficient gene transfer and long-term expression in neurones using a recombinant adenovirus with a neurone-specific promoter. Gene Ther 6:1884–1892

Ohkawa J, Yuyama N, Takebe Y et al. (1993) Importance of independence in ribozyme reactions: Kinetic behavior of trimmed and of simply connected ribozymes with potential activity against human immunodeficiency virus. Proc Natl Acad Sci USA 90:11302–11306

Pallavicini MG, Flake AW, Madden D et al. (1992) Hemopoietic chimerism in rodents transplanted *in utero* with fetal human hemopoietic cells. Transpant Proceed 24:524–543

Pereira R, O'Hara MD, Laptev AV et al. (1998) Marrow stromal cells as a source of progenitor cells from non-haematopoietic tissues in transgenic mice with a phenotype of osteogenesis imperfecta. Proc Natl Acad Sci USA 95:1142–1147

Peters C, Balthazor M, Shapiro EG et al. (1996) Outcome of donor bone marrow transplantation in 40 children with Hurler syndrome. Blood 87:4894–4902

Philpott LM, Kopyov OV, Lee AJ et al. (1997) Neuropsychological functioning following foetal striatal transplantation in Huntington's chorea: three case presentations. Cell Transplant 6:203–212

Pittenger MF, Mackay AM, Beck SC et al. (1999) Multilineage potential of adult mesenchymal stem cells. Science 284:143–147

Poeschla EF, Wong-Staal DJ, Looney L (1998) Efficient transduction of non-dividing human cells by feline leukaemia immunodeficiency virus lentiviral vectors. Nat Med 4:354–347

Polymeropoulus M, Lavedan MH, Leroy E et al. (1997) Mutation in the alpha-synuclein gene identified in families with Parkinson's disease. Science 277:2045–2047

Price DL, Tanzi E, Borchelt DR, Sissodia SS (1998) Alzheimer's disease: genetic studies and transgenic models. Annu Rev Genet 32:461–493

Rabinowitz JE, Samulski J (1998) Adeno-associated virus expression systems for gene transfer. Curr Opin Biotech 9:470–475

Readhead C, Popko B, Takahashi N et al. (1987) Expression of a myelin basic protein gene in trangenic Shiverer mice: correction of dysmyelinating phenotype. Cell 48:703–712

Rider JL, Corti O, Pencalet P et al. (1999) Toward autologous *ex vivo* gene therapy for the central nervous system with human adult astrocytes. Hum Gene Ther 20:271–280

Roodman GD, Kuehl TJ, Vandeberg JL, Muirhead DY (1991) *In utero* bone marrow transplantation of fetal baboons with mismatched adult baboon marrow. Blood Cells 17:367–375

Rubin P, Gash DM, Hansen JT et al. (1994) Disruption of the blood-brain barrier as the primary effect of CNS irradiation. Rad Onc 31:51–60

Samlowski WE, Robertson BA, Draper BK et al. (1991) Effects of supravital fluorochromes used to analyze the *in vivo* homing of murine lymphocytes on cellular function. J Immunol Methods 144:101–115

Scharfman R, Axelrod JH, Verma IM (1991) Long-term *in vivo* expression of retrovirus-mediated gene transfer in mouse fibroblast implants. Proc Natl Acad Sci USA 88:4626–4630

Scheidner G, Morral N, Parjs RJ et al. (1998) Genomic DNA transfer with a high capacity adenovirus vector results in improved gene expression and decreased toxicity. Nat Genet 18:180–183

Schneider H, Adebakin S, Themis M et al. (1999) Therapeutic plasma concentrations of human factor IX in mice after gene delivery into the amniotic cavity: a model for the prenatal treatment of haemophilia B. J Gene Med 1:424–432

Schleffer B, Horn M, Blumcke I et al. (1999) Marrow-mindedness: a perspective on neuropoiesis. Trends Neurosci 22:348–357

Schuening FG, Kawahara K, Miller AD et al. (1991) Retrovirus mediated gene transduction into long term repopulating marrow cells of dogs. Blood 78:2568–2573

Schwartz EJ, Alexander GM, Prockop DJ et al. (1999) Multipotential marrow stromal cells transduced to produce L-DOPA: Engraftment in a rat model of Parkinson's Disease. Hum Gen Ther 10:2539–2549

Scriver CR, Beaudet AL, Sly WS, Valle D (eds) (1995) The Metabolic Basis of Inherited Disease. 8th Ed. McGraw-Hill, New York

Sedivy JM, Dutriaux A (1999) Gene targeting and somatic cell genetics. Trends Gen 15:88–90

Shamblott MJ, Wang S, Bugg EM et al. (1998) Derivation of pluripotent stem cell from cultured human primordial germ cells. Proc Natl Acad Sci USA 95:13726–13731

Shen TJ, Ikonomi P, Smith R et al. (1999) Multi-ribozyme targeting of human alpha-globin gene expression. Blood Cells Mol Dis 25:361–373

Shippy R, Lockner R, Farnsworth M, Hampel A (1999) The hairpin ribozyme. Discovery, mechanism, and development for gene therapy. Mol Biotechnol 12:117–129

Skorupa AF, Fisher KJ, Wilson JM et al. (1999) Sustained production of β-glucuronidase from localised sites after AAV vector gene transfer results in widespread distribution of enzyme and reversal of lysosomal storage lesions in a large volume of brain in Mucopolysaccharidosis VII mice. Exp Neurol 160:17–27

Smith GM, Romero MI (1999) Adenoviral-mediated gene transfer to enhance neuronal survival, growth and regeneration. J Neurosci Res 55:147–157

Synder EY, Deitcher DL, Walsh C et al. (1992) Multipotent cell lines can engraft and participate in the development of mouse cerebellum. Cell 68:1–20

Snyder EY, Taylor RM, Wolfe JH (1995) Neural progenitor cell engraftment corrects lysosomal storage disease throughout the MPS VII mouse brain. Nature 374:367–370

Spangrude GJ, Heimfeld S, Weissman IL (1988) Purification and characterization of mouse hematopoietic stem cells. Science 241:58–62

Speate RR, Frenckel N (1982) The herpes simplex virus amplicon: a new eukaryotic defective virus cloning amplifying vector. Cell 30:295–304

Srour E, Zanjani ED, Brandt JE et al. (1992) Sustained human hematopoiesis in sheep transplanted *in utero* during early gestation with fractionated adult human bone marrow cells. Blood 79:1404–1412

Strom SC, Fisher RA, Thompson MT et al. (1997) Hepatocyte transplantation as a bridge to orthoptic liver transplantation in terminal liver failure. Transplantation 63:559–569

Sullenger BA (1999) RNA repair as a novel approach to genetic therapy. Gene Ther 6:461–462

Sutton RE, Wu HT, Rigg R et al. (1998) Human immunodeficiency virus type 1 vectors efficiently transduce human hematopoietic stem cells. J Virol 72:5781–7588

Szilvassy SJ, Fraser CC, Eaves CJ et al. (1989) Retrovirus-mediated gene transfer to purified hematopoietic stem cells with long-term lympho-myelopoietic repopulating ability. Proc Natl Acad Sci USA 86:8798–8802

Takayama H, Ray J, Ramon HK (1995) Basic fibroblast growth factor increases dopaminergic graft survival and function in a rat model of Parkinson's disease. Nat Med 1:53–58

Takeda T, Kim TH, Lee SK et al. (1995) Hepatocyte transplantation in biodegradable polymer scaffolds using the dalmatian dog model of hyperuricosuria. Transplant Proc 27:635–636

Tan ND, Porada CD, Zhao Y et al. (2000) *In utero* transfer and expression of exogenous genes in sheep. Exp Hematol 28:17–30

Taylor RM, Wolfe JH (1997) Decreased lysosomal storage in the adult MPS VII mouse in the vicinity of retroviral vector-corrected fibroblasts secreting high levels of β-glucuronidase. Nat Med 3:771–774

Thompson JD, Macejak D, Couture L, Stinchomb DT (1995) Ribozymes in gene therapy. Nat Med 1:277–278

Thompson JA, Itskovitz-Edor J, Shapiro AA et al. (1998) Embryonic stem cell lines derived from human blastocysts. Science 282:1145–1147

Touraine JL, Raudrant D, Royo C (1991) *In utero* transplantation of hemopoietic stem cells in humans. Transplant Proceed 23:1706–1708

Treco DA, Selden RF (1995) Non-viral gene therapy. Mol Med Today 1:314–321

Tsukamoto M, Ochiya T, Yoshida S, Sugimura T, Terada M (1995) Gene transfer and expression in progeny after intravenous DNA injection into pregnant mice. Nat Gene 9:243–248

Tuszynski MH, Peterson DA, Ray J, Baird A et al. (1994) Fibroblasts genetically modified to produce nerve growth factor induce robust neuritic ingrowth after grafting to the spinal cord. Exp Neurol 126:1–14

Tuszynski MH, Roberts J, Senut MC et al. (1995) Gene therapy in the adult primate brain: intraparenchymal grafts of cells genetically modified to produce nerve growth factor prevent cholinergic neuronal degeneration. Gen Ther 3:305–314

van de Rijn M, Heimfeld S, Spangrude GJ, Weissman IL (1989) Mouse hematopoietic stem cell antigen Sca-1 is a member of the Ly-6 antigen family. Proc Natl Acad Sci USA 86:4634–4638

Vanden Driessche T, Vanslembrouck V, Goovaerts I et al. (1999) Long-term expression of human coagulation factor VIII and correction of haemophilia A after *in vivo* retroviral gene transfer in factor VIII-deficient mice. Proc Natl Acad Sci USA 96:10379–10384

Vescovi AL, Parati EA, Gritti A et al. (1999) Isolation and cloning of multipotent stem cells from the embryonic human CNS and establishment of transplantable human neural stem cell lines by epigenetic stimulation. Exp Neurol 156:71–83

Wang I, Takabe K, Bidlingmaier SM et al. (1999) Sustained correction of bleeding disorder in haemophilia B mice by gene therapy. Proc Natl Acad Sci USA 96:3906–3910

Weiss S, Reynolds BA, Vescovi AL et al. (1996) Is there a neural stem cell in the mammalian forebrain? Trends Neurosci 19:387–393

Williams DE, Eisenman J, Baird A, Rach C et al. (1990) Identification of a ligand for the C-kit proto-oncogene. Cell 63:167–174

Winkler A, Kiem HP, Shields LE (1999) Gene transfer into fetal baboon hematopoietic progenitor cells. Hum Gene Ther 10:667–677

Wolfe JH, Deshmane SL, Fraser NW (1992) Herpes virus vector transfer and expression of β-glucuronidase in the central and peripheral nervous system of MPS VII mice. Nature Genet 1:379–384

Xiao X, Samulski RJ (1998) Production of high titre recombinant adeno-associated virus vectors in the absence of helper adenovirus. J Virol 72:2224–2232

Yamada M, Oligino T, Mata M et al. (1999) Herpes simplex virus vector mediated expression of Bcl-2 prevent the 6-hydroxydopamine-induced degeneration of neurones in the substantia nigra *in vivo*. Proc Natl Acad Sci USA 96:4978–4083

Yandava B, Billinghurst LL, Synder EY (1999) Global cell replacement is feasible via neural stem cell transplantation: evidence from the dysmelinated shiverer mouse brain. Proc Natl Acad Sci USA 996:7029–2034

Yanez RJ, Porter ACG (1998) Therapeutic gene targeting. Gen Ther 5:149–159

Yashui O, Miura N, Terada K et al. (1997) Isolation of oval cells from Long Evans Cinnamon rats and their transformation into hepatocytes *in vivo* in the rat liver. Hepatology 25:329–334

Yu M, Ojwang J, Yamada O et al. (1993) A hairpin ribozyme inhibits expression of diverse strains of human immunodeficiency virus type 1. Proc Natl Acad Sci USA 90:6340–6344

Zsebo KM, Wypych J, McNiece IK, Lu HS et al. (1990) Identification, purification and biological characterization of hematopoietic stem cell factor from buffalo rat liver conditioned medium. Cell 63:195–201

Zufferey R, Dull T, Mandel RJ et al. (1998) Self-inactivating lentivirus vector for safe and efficient in vivo gene delivery. J Virol 72:9873–9880

Ethical and social issues in clinical genetics

33

Angus Clarke

Introduction

Ethical issues abound in all areas of clinical medicine. These can relate to the medical management of individual patients or to broader social and political issues, such as the access to care for disadvantaged groups within society and the wise deployment of the resources available for health care. Whereas the ethical discussions in some clinical areas focus on "end-of-life" issues, including euthanasia and the withdrawal of futile treatments, in clinical genetics there has been an unusually broad range of contentious topics. Important areas have included "beginning-of-life" issues such as prenatal diagnosis and the selective termination of pregnancies, specifically professional issues such as the role of the clinical geneticist or genetic counselor, and the interrogation of common assumptions and attitudes towards the just treatment of individuals within society.

Two additional factors make any reflection upon ethical issues in the practice of clinical genetics particularly complex. First, there are ethical issues that confront our clients as individuals and families. In most of medicine there are issues that challenge the professional, and there may be complex issues where society has to declare its view—as where regulation or legislation may be needed. In genetics, however, there are numerous occasions where it is our clients who are confronted by the ethical difficulties. Indeed, it is sometimes our role to formulate the issues for our clients to consider. We therefore need to distinguish between the challenges that we face as professionals, those that are faced by society at large and those that are faced by our clients.

Second, our discipline is characterized by the rapid growth of genetic knowledge and, simultaneously, by the rapid development of technologies for applying this new knowledge. The elucidation of the complete DNA sequence of the human genome is but one component of this continuing expansion of the information available both to professionals and to their clients.

It is my aim here to sketch out the principal social and ethical issues that arise in the course of our work in clinical genetics—there being no clear distinction between the social and the ethical in this area, if indeed anywhere. While it may be easier for those not directly involved to view them in a more detached fashion, perhaps as "abstract" issues, ethical difficulties that are experienced by individuals—professionals or clients—are always located in a social context.

On most topics, I will set out the important questions. On some issues, I will assert my opinions or judgments—but I hope it will always be clear where I have done this. In addition to promoting discussion and debate within our profession, I will be particularly pleased if this chapter contributes to the flow of ideas and discussions across the conventional boundaries between health professionals and clients and between health professionals and scholars from such academic disciplines as philosophy and the social sciences. Faced with the challenges that confront us—professionals, clients and society—we can only benefit from the sympathetic understanding and questioning of those with particular skills in these other disciplines.

The historical context

Clinical genetics developed after the Second World War in response to the concerns of families and clinicians about the risk of genetic disease occurring within a family.

Pediatricians were consulted about the risk of recurrence of congenital malformations or childhood genetic disorders and neurologists were consulted about the risk of healthy individuals developing the neurodegenerative or neuromuscular disorders that affected other members of their families. Clinical genetics as we know it arose from the convergence of clinicians tackling these questions and concerns with non-medical scientists interested in human genetics. Human genetics, however, has a longer history than this, which cannot be ignored.

The study of heredity and its influence on human variation, especially on "natural ability", was developed in nineteenth-century Britain by Sir Francis Galton. He regarded intelligence, social virtues (or their lack) and social achievement as primarily genetic and—like many before him—had the goal of improving the genetic constitution of future generations. He coined the term "eugenics" to describe, "the study of agencies under social control that may improve or impair the racial qualities of future generations either physically or mentally". The term soon came to be applied to the social movement promoting the improvement of such qualities. The perennial concern about the moral decay of society, widespread among the older citizens in societies ancient and modern, latched onto theories of heredity in late Victorian Britain as offering solutions to social vices such as alcoholism, pauperism, homelessness and feeble-mindedness. The same set of ideas also reinforced assumptions about the relative evolutionary development of different populations, reassuring the citizens of the major imperial powers that they were justified, indeed destined, to rule over their biologically inferior colonial subjects. Such ideas flourished in literature and the arts, as well as the sciences, and were integral to the mentality of society at large in much of Europe and North America.

The notion that "Biology is Destiny" sometimes has a rather narrow set of connotations—relating to gender—but in its broader sense of a century ago it encapsulates the often tacit, taken-for-granted realities of race and social class as well as of gender. Out of these common social assumptions developed the theories and practices that we now condemn as the eugenic abuses of human genetics. Racist immigration policies were introduced in the USA in the guise of intelligence tests—ensuring the "quality" of immigrants was then acceptable whereas overtly racist legislation was not. Legislation to enable the forced sterilization of those with mental handicap—and a range of other medical and social disorders—was introduced in North America, Sweden, Germany and other countries. Such legislation was not introduced in Britain but the segregation of the sexes in institutions and the involuntary sterilization of many with

mental handicap—especially women—was a widespread practice over many years because the assumptions that led this to appear appropriate, "normal" practice, were so pervasive. Even the horrors of the Nazi campaign of racial hygiene, in which many physicians, anthropologists, geneticists and other scientists actively participated, and the murderous consequences of the related belief in Aryan racial superiority, did not lead to the discontinuation of such practices outside Germany for many years.

It is unhelpful for contemporary geneticists to be perpetually apologizing for the sins committed by their intellectual forebears, but neither can we afford to forget those horrific events that happened so very recently. As the scientific validity of contemporary genetics and its power to impact on society are now much greater than was the case 60 years ago, it is essential that we work hard to identify and make explicit our current taken-for-granted attitudes and our deeply held but often unstated, and perhaps unexamined, convictions. How might these be leading us into errors that we will only recognize too late, once great damage has been done to our profession, to our patients or to society as a whole? This is the hard lesson we should learn from considering the past abuses of human genetics.

Genetic counseling, testing and screening

A crucial distinction, familiar to every practitioner, is the contrast between the clinical genetic services made available in response to the pre-existing concerns of individuals and small family groups, and the population screening programs offered proactively to large groups of the population who have usually not sought the test that is being offered.

In the context of a specific family, the genetics professionals are responding to their particular questions or anxieties—thus, as examples, a) they may be seeking an explanation for a serious developmental problem affecting their child, or b) an individual at risk of a familial neurodegenerative condition or malignancy may wish to know their chance of developing their family's disorder, or c) a couple may wish to know the chance of their future children being affected by an inherited condition that has previously affected other family members. Such a consultation will usually begin with the professional listening to the family's account of their concerns, then performing any relevant clinical assessments or investigations, and then finally providing whatever information is appropriate back to the family. This process may be extended in time—perhaps occupying several consultations separated by weeks or months, especially if the diagnosis is not readily apparent. Great sensitivity is often required to the interactional cues of the client, whether spoken or unspoken, for the professional to respond adequately to their needs. It will often be appropriate to provide emotional support, while skilled counseling will sometimes also be helpful and occasionally more formal psychotherapy will be necessary. In all these cases, however, the professional is responding as best they can to the client's pre-existing concerns.

In the context of population screening, the encounter between professional and client is very different. The professional is actively promoting a specific course of action—that the client/patient should undergo an investigation. The client may never have had any questions or concerns to which the screening test could be understood as a helpful response, so the professionals' suggestion of the screening test may itself generate concerns rather than allaying them, imposing the burden of an unsought decision when one course of action—compliance with the offer of testing—is being heavily recommended in the very act of making the test available at all.

There may well be circumstances in which it is thoroughly appropriate for health services to promote a particular screening test or other health intervention in this way—as with the immunization of infants, the measurement of blood pressure in adults and cervical cytology or mammography in women in the relevant age-groups. In the sphere of reproduction, however, the promotion of screening can be regarded as especially contentious; in this context, individual choice is highly valued. While newborn screening for the remediable disorders, phenylketonuria (PKU) and congenital hypothyroidism, is universally applauded, there is dissent in relation to reproductive genetic screening—including antenatal screening for Down syndrome or congenital malformation, and carrier screening for autosomal recessive diseases. It is unarguable, however, that the context of proactive population screening for genetic disease is very different from that of genetic counseling as a response to pre-existing family concerns. This has important ethical implications for professional practice in these areas.

Goals and outcomes of genetic services

In the bad old eugenic past, the principal aim of reproductive medicine was to improve the biological quality of the next generation. This meant encouraging the gifted and

successful to have more children and discouraging or preventing those with medical or social disadvantages (whether inherited or acquired) from having so many. This would help to overcome what was perceived as the relatively low fertility of the higher social classes and of the "more advanced races". Such concerns about differential fertility still resonate around the globe—they are reflected, in different ways, in contemporary state policies in Singapore and China, and are whipped up from time to time by those politicians in many countries (including European countries) who think they stand to benefit from inter-community strife.

Western society today pays little overt attention to the antiquated concepts of racial hygiene. In the contemporary rhetoric of clinical genetics and genetic counseling, our professional goals are therefore quite different from former ideas of "the health of the people" (i.e., of the race). Respect for the autonomy of the individual takes precedence over measures of impact of genetic services on the population as a whole—such as the incidence of genetic disorders at birth or the number of terminations of pregnancy for specific conditions. To describe our goals in terms of such crude population outcomes would indeed be regarded as frankly eugenic.

There is a context within which such assumptions about the effectiveness of genetic services could be seen as defensible, however, or even laudable. This is the economic frame, in which the primary goal of genetic services would be seen as the reduction of expenditure on caring for those with genetic disease or disability, achieved through a reduction in the birth incidence of conditions for which prenatal or carrier screening has been made available.

Despite the ethically contentious nature of these claims, many studies of prenatal or carrier population screening, including prenatal screening for Down syndrome or carrier screening for cystic fibrosis, do essentially argue for the implementation of such programs on the grounds that screening and the termination of affected pregnancies is less costly than caring for affected individuals. Although many clinicians may regard these arguments as ethically unacceptable, they are still employed. Some of those who use such arguments may have no moral qualms about doing so. Others may value the offer of reproductive choices per se and therefore support the existence of prenatal screening programs while rejecting the monetary, neo-eugenicist arguments. They feel that screening should be available to all pregnant women and that the absence of such a screening program would remove the possibility for many of making important reproductive decisions. This view is considered further below.

Crude monetary arguments are not generally used to justify the provision of family-based clinical genetic and genetic counseling services. Such an analysis might show a net saving to society—because genetic counseling does sometimes have the consequence of reducing the number of infants born with serious (costly) genetic disorders, through parental decisions not to have children or through the selective termination of affected pregnancies—although clinical genetic professionals may refuse to use these arguments to justify their services. Furthermore, the economic analysis would require many assumptions about the future pattern of health and social care provision and about the most appropriate way of discounting the likely future costs of care to be traded against current actual costs of providing the clinical genetics services. Such analyses would therefore be complex and contentious even within a purely economic frame of reference.

How, then, can the outcomes of clinical genetics services be measured to permit a comparison of the worth of different models of clinical genetics services, or their comparison with expenditure on altogether different areas of health service activity? A number of outcome measures have been proposed and employed in research studies, but none so far devised is suitable for the ongoing evaluation of a clinical service.

1. The recall of risk information—concerning the risk of a disease or the risk of its recurrence in a future child—can be assessed after a lapse of months or years, but recall is the result of many psychological processes including the tendency to polarize probabilities towards 0 or 1, i.e., No (it will not happen = 0) or Yes (it is certain to happen = 1). Further, the significance attached to recurrence risks by clients is itself influenced by the way in which the information is framed in the counseling process.
2. Reproductive plans can be assessed before and after genetic counseling—although that is to pre-judge the concerns of the client, many of whom are not specifically seeking information about reproduction. In any case, plans are merely hypothetical and their expression will be heavily dependent upon the context and framing of the question by the professional.
3. Reproductive behaviour could also be measured—but over what time span? What would count as a satisfactory outcome for the assessor? What if this is not the perspective of the clients?
4. Client satisfaction with the service, and levels of anxiety or concern, can be assessed—but may be heavily influenced by the environment in which a service is provided. In addition, the clients may not be aware of how the service they have experienced compares to other services, and their views are likely to be influenced by the information they are given in the clinic—for example, they may be seriously distressed if given an item of "bad news" or they may be resentful if a diagnostic process has failed to identify the cause of some serious disorder in their child.
5. For the same reasons, questionnaire-based measures of healthy physical and mental functioning are unsuitable outcome measures for genetic services, while they may be entirely appropriate for assessing care for osteoarthritis of the hip or for chronic asthma.

The ethical importance of the choice of outcome measure is especially grave in the context of a large population-based health service because the professionals in national health care systems or large insurance-based schemes can be driven to comply with population-based or corporate goals rather more readily and directly than in the context of truly individual health care arranged between the physician and the patient. If a health service decides to reduce the birth incidence of Down syndrome or Duchenne muscular dystrophy, for example, and to judge the performance of health service staff according to their "achievements" in these respects—perhaps with implications for their rates of pay or job security—then it is easy to see how population goals could systematically distort the pattern of health care provided to large numbers of individual patients. This is not an argument for the privatization or fragmentation of health care but for great vigilance in any large health care system; professionals must watch to ensure that their responsibilities are not subverted, perhaps rather subtly, by the imposition of institutional (state or corporate) policies.

I am arguing here that there is no utilitarian calculus that can determine the worth of clinical genetic services in a neutral, detached or objective fashion. There are promising developments, such as a framework for assessing the client's "perceived personal control" (Berkenstadt et al., 1999), but such psychometric outcomes will not amount to a full evaluation of genetic service effectiveness.

Despite these difficulties, there are ways of using research evidence to help decide what services should be made available, and there are ways of assessing the quality of the services that are provided. The decisions about what services to provide will draw upon research evidence about the practical consequences of providing particular, contrasting patterns of service. These decisions are inevitably the product of a political process reflecting the value that society places upon autonomy in the sphere of reproduction and society's concern for the welfare of individuals with genetic disorders and their families. Once the decisions have been made about what services to provide, there are ways of assessing the quality of those services. These include the development of sophisticated approaches to client satisfaction that incorporate the increasingly realistic expectations that clients have of the service as they gain experience of both the disease in their family and the services that are provided to support them.

Non-directiveness in genetic counseling

Respect for client autonomy is one of the core values of the genetic counseling profession. One of the manifestations of this respect for autonomy is the claim that genetic counseling is, or at least should be, "non-directive"—it should not lead the client to make specific choices pre-determined by the counselor or the health care system. In addition to respect for client autonomy, however, there are several other important factors that contribute to the cult of "non-directiveness", and it is necessary to understand these other factors in order to use the concept of non-directiveness in an appropriate fashion.

The claim that genetic counseling is non-directive allows the professional to distance her/himself from emotional involvement in the decision. This may at times be very helpful, in so far as emotional over-involvement can be damaging. The claim that genetic counseling is non-directive can also function well for professionals by ensuring that the legal responsibility for their clients' decisions lies firmly with the clients—an important clarification in these increasingly litigious times. Another function of the claim to be non-directive is that it helps professionals reject suggestions that they may be contaminated by any taint of Nazi eugenics. In all these respects, then, the claim of adherence to the doctrine of non-directiveness may be attractive and helpful to genetic counseling professionals.

There are several other respects, however, in which the concept of "non-directiveness" may be problematic. First, at least some elements of clinical genetic services may inevitably be "directive"—leading clients towards specific decisions and outcomes. This applies particularly to population genetic screening programs, most especially in the context of reproductive genetic screening, where the existence of a screening program must in itself carry the implicit message that screening is worthwhile—indeed, that it is recommended. This can be referred to as "structural" directiveness and does not imply that the individual professionals involved are actively recommending one course of action or another, although they may be doing so, or the screening

program may be so routinized that neither professionals nor clients give active consideration to the issues involved and both parties merely accept screening as standard practice (Barnard, 1985; Clarke, 1991).

Secondly, there are contexts in clinical genetics where it is entirely proper for a professional to recommend a specific course of action to her clients. This may involve the recommendation that a client at risk of a specific disorder should undergo surveillance for complications of that disorder—as with colonoscopy for those at increased risk of bowel cancer, or echocardiography for those with Marfan syndrome. This may involve the recommendation of a predictive genetic test—so that, for example, colonoscopic surveillance for bowel cancer can be targeted to those family members with the high risk, and those who are at population risk can avoid the inconvenience, costs and hazards of unnecessary investigations.

Genetic counseling professionals may also recommend a particular course of action to their clients in relation to the sharing of genetic information within a family. When information about a client's genetic condition could be relevant to other members of the client's family, the professional may very reasonably point this out. It could be relevant to the future health of the client's relatives or to their reproductive decisions. In general, genetic counselors will promote open family communication about any relevant genetic disorder and will indicate the type of problems that can arise if communication is blocked. This is generally acknowledged to be good professional conduct—although it clearly conflicts with "non-directiveness" if that is interpreted in an excessively rigid manner.

There is another sense in which an exaggerated respect for non-directiveness can be unhelpful—when compliance with "non-directiveness" is taken to require that genetic counselors accept without challenge every statement expressed by their clients, even mere preferences that have not been carefully considered. This approach so constrains the counselor that their ability to help the client is severely restricted. Effective counseling, as in scenario decision counseling, helps the client to think through the consequences of any particular decision or course of action that is planned. This inevitably entails the use of authoritative counselor interventions, such as direct questioning to gather information or confrontation of the client with unwelcome information or with the need to consider some previously unanticipated potential consequences of planned action. Not to make use of such interventions would greatly restrict the effectiveness of the genetic counseling. An inappropriate understanding of "non-directiveness" will undermine the authority and effectiveness of the genetic counselor and reflects an inadequate understanding of "counseling" in general, but it is all too easy for such misunderstandings to arise unless professionals monitor their practice with the help of regular supervision (Wolff and Jung, 1995; Kessler, 1997).

Finally, there is the danger that non-directiveness in relation to a complex practical question with extensive moral implications may be felt as abandonment by the client. This has been particularly problematic for those patients recently diagnosed with cancer, who are faced by choices between therapeutic options where the evidence is unclear and difficult to interpret. A detached presentation of the options can then, understandably, be experienced as an emotional withdrawal from the client—as abandonment. In the different context of clinical genetics, the practice of non-directiveness could also be perceived by clients in this way unless the professionals take care to make this concept function on behalf of the clients rather than on behalf of their professional selves.

Any claim that genetic counseling should always be "non-directive", therefore, would be unhelpful—and any claim that it is so would clearly be false. Respect for "non-directiveness" is appropriate but only when it is understood as a rich and complex concept. If this appropriate sense of "non-directiveness" is to be recognized in practice, we will require sensitive tools for the analysis of language in the specific context of genetic counseling—within a sophisticated methodological framework for the understanding of language in its more general social context. Mechanical or formulaic definitions of what constitutes "non-directiveness" will simply be unhelpful.

Predictive genetic testing

Individuals at risk of developing a serious inherited disorder will sometimes wish to find out if they have inherited the relevant gene. For the autosomal dominant neurodegenerative disorders, such as Huntington disease and some of the rare familial forms of early-onset Alzheimer disease, highly accurate predictive testing is possible. Uncertainty as to whether the individual will develop the disease is replaced by uncertainty as to when (and how) it will manifest. In the context of the autosomal dominant familial cancer disorders, testing is also sometimes possible—although there are limitations to the predictive power of these tests, because some individuals with their family's gene mutation, predisposing for example to breast or colon cancer, will be fortunate in escaping the relevant cancer

while others, without the relevant mutation, may nevertheless develop the cancer. Inheritance of the predisposing mutation increases the statistical risk of developing the cancer from the population risk (of more than zero) to a high risk (but still less than 100%). In BRCA1-associated familial breast cancer, the increase in (lifetime) risk may be from approximately 10% to approximately 70%.

The ethical issues that can arise in the course of predictive genetic testing are numerous, and many are considered elsewhere in this chapter. Here, we need to refer to just two particular issues. First, it is instructive to consider what has been learned from the numerous studies performed on the process of predictive genetic counseling and testing. Clients seeking predictive genetic testing and recruited to research studies have been asked to complete psychometric questionnaires; in some studies, they have also been interviewed by a researcher. In general, it has been found that the process of genetic testing for those at risk of a familial disorder has been well tolerated, even when unfavorable results have been generated. Surprising, perhaps counterintuitive, findings have also emerged, however, such as the distress and social dislocation sometimes found in those given a favorable predictive test result. A favorable result can lead to feelings of guilt in young adults with siblings who are already affected or are shown to be at high risk of disease—a form of survivor guilt. Family ties, perhaps strengthened from sharing the impact of the disease, may weaken for those no longer directly involved with the condition. Those who have made important life decisions, perhaps about career, relationships or children, may wish they had acted differently when they find that the basis on which the decisions were made—their genetic risk—has been undermined.

Another finding has been the inadequacy of the understanding of predictive genetic testing to emerge from psychometric assessments of its impact. Any simple interpretation of anxiety as a negative, unhelpful or undesirable response to testing or test results has been challenged by qualitative evidence that such measures of anxiety may reflect an active process of confronting and engaging with the unwelcome facts. So to use evidence of increased anxiety after testing to make a policy decision not to provide such testing services would be completely inappropriate, and some of those in whom the measures of anxiety are increased before receiving the test result may subsequently be in less need of emotional support than others in whom the pre-test measures of anxiety had been lower.

The second issue to consider in relation to predictive testing is the family dimension of predictive tests, sometimes amounting to a conflict of interest between family members. The genetic testing of individuals at 25% prior risk of an autosomal dominant disease provides the most stark examples of such conflicts of interest. What if a young man, whose grandparent has Huntington disease (HD), wants to know if he will develop the disease too? He is wanting to marry and start a family but wishes to clarify his genetic status first. His at-risk parent appears healthy but has made it clear to all concerned that she/he does not want to undergo testing. If the young man is found to carry the HD mutation, then his parent must carry the mutation too. There are ethical issues here for both the young man, his at-risk parent and the genetics professional. In most families, a resolution can be found to the potential conflict if the professionals encourage discussion within the family and are available to discuss the issues with the various parties—a solution through counseling. Occasionally, however, real conflict persists and professionals have to decide whether or not to make testing available to one family member if doing so may have adverse consequences for others. The process of resolving such family disagreements can be particularly difficult when a couple unsure of their genetic situation have a pregnancy and wish to make a decision about prenatal diagnosis—the need for haste in making decisions then adds to the difficulties.

Difficult issues can arise in families with diseases that show marked anticipation—especially myotonic dystrophy. In this case, a diagnostic test (of an infant with possible congenital myotonic dystrophy) is effectively a predictive test when considered from the perspective of the apparently healthy mother who has not yet recognized her minor symptoms. This makes the counseling issues especially difficult if the child is to be given the appropriate diagnosis while the mother—and her parents—are led gently to consider testing for themselves. Similarly complex, transgenerational issues arise in relation to the fragile X syndrome, although testing of the affected child's grandparents is a form of carrier testing rather than predictive testing.

Confidentiality

Respect for confidentiality is one of the oldest principles of medical ethics—at least as old as Hippocrates and certainly older than the contemporary attachment to autonomy. My own view is that confidentiality must continue to be respected at (almost) all costs. In relation to genetics, however, it is subject to challenge on several grounds. First, genetic information might be sought about individuals by their employers or insurance companies or by the state.

Secondly, the fact that we share (almost) all our genes with other members of our families has been used to justify the claim that genetic information about one individual "really" belongs to his/her relatives too—so that genetic privacy, it is argued, need not apply within families.

Third parties

Protecting the individual's right to genetic privacy from third parties, such as employers, insurers and the state, has been robustly defended. While insurance corporations have generally accepted that they should not require genetic testing before making life insurance available to applicants, they have been less ready to concede that prospective clients should be able to have genetic tests performed without passing on that information to the insurance company—as with any other medical information. The counter-argument runs that genetic information is not like other medical information because—if the individual is currently in good health—genetic information about propensity to disease is essentially predictive or risk modifying, and not at all like information about current clinical problems. The danger for the insurance companies is that of "adverse selection" in which their clients will be better informed than they are, and so those at high risk of serious problems may take out more insurance while paying only standard premiums, so that the company—and ultimately its other clients—lose out and higher premiums have to be charged.

In fact, most individuals at high risk of serious genetic disease will have to declare their family history and so the insurance corporation will be aware of their pre-test risks. If they have a favorable test result the company may be informed, but if not then the individual seeking insurance may prefer not to disclose this. The number of adults at high risk of a serious genetic disorder but who are in good health when seeking life insurance is small, however, and the number who are likely to die from the disorder during the term of insurance is smaller, so that the industry is unlikely to suffer much from adverse selection in this context. In relation to health insurance, the potential for adverse selection is probably greater, especially in the context of a predominantly commercial health care sector as in North America. This constitutes an increasingly powerful argument for the organization of health services on a national basis, whether as a single health service (as in the UK) or through a largely private, but regulated, insurance scheme (as in many other European countries and Canada).

Employers may wish to gain access to genetic information about their employees, or potential employees, for several reasons. Genetic information might be used to alter the selection of job applicants or the promotion prospects of staff in post—in favor of those with less likelihood of serious disease developing before retirement age. The scope for genetic screening of the workforce for susceptibility to disease is small because screening tests for susceptibility to the common, complex diseases are simply not available. Screening the workforce for susceptibility to specific occupational disorders is also not feasible at present, but a case has been made for screening some workers for α-1-antitrypsin deficiency because this predisposes individuals to severe, chronic chest disease if their lungs are exposed to cigarette smoke or to dust, as in quarries, building sites and some other workplaces. An argument for caution in genetic testing of a workforce is that the exclusion of susceptible workers from hazardous sites could be used as a cheap substitute for the proper environmental protection that would in fact benefit the whole workforce.

Several countries in Europe and North America have developed national agreements to restrict the gathering and application of genetic information by insurance companies or have introduced legislation to prevent discrimination against those affected by, or at risk of, genetic disease in insurance or employment. Without proper legal protection, there is the fear that individuals at above average risk of specific disorders may become unable to find work or insurance cover. This could lead to the formation of a class of people identified by molecular genetic testing who would be excluded from full participation in society—an underclass reminiscent of Orwell's *1984* or of Nietzsche. This would have especially grave consequences in those societies where health insurance is under commercial control and is linked to employment, because health care would then be denied these individuals in addition to employment, life insurance and mortgages.

Privacy within the family

While conventional medical ethics has insisted upon respecting the confidentiality of patients except in the most extreme and exceptional cases, this view has been challenged in the context of genetic disease. Information about one member of a family can be regarded as information about their relatives too (Somerville and English, 1999). Harm could result, it is argued, if genetic information is not shared with relatives—an individual at risk of a disorder may develop complications that could have been avoided if they had been given foreknowledge of the risk, or a child may be born with a serious disorder when the pregnancy could have been terminated if the parents had been warned of this possibility. To what extent these "harms" could be avoided,

and whether the birth of a child with a genetic condition can be regarded as a "harm", are complex issues that require further analysis—but most of us can at least agree that family members have a moral obligation to pass on potentially relevant genetic information to their relatives, even if we might dispute the legal or professional force of this obligation and contest the notion of genetic harm implicit in this discourse.

The topic of debate then becomes the way in which professionals can best promote the appropriate transmission of information within family networks—accepting that it may be difficult to contact some family members, that others will be distressed by genetic information that may well turn out not to be relevant to them, and that the duty to contact relatives can prove burdensome to our clients. There may be no easy solution to the problems arising from the duty to transmit information. Perhaps a client's niece, at risk of carrying a sex-linked disorder, is getting married next Saturday afternoon and then going on honeymoon for three weeks: what should our client do? (i.e., **when** should he talk with her about the genetic risk?) Perhaps another client has just been told by his physician that his kidney complaint is inherited as an autosomal dominant trait and his (adult) children are at risk—but Sally has just become engaged, Manfred is sitting his university final examinations in two months, Mark's wife is six months pregnant and Maureen has just been admitted to hospital with her second bout of severe depression in two years. Whom should he tell about the polycystic kidney disease? Or our client may suffer from male infertility and find it difficult to discuss this with his wider family, even though they may be carriers of the cystic fibrosis mutations identified in him—or could even themselves be affected. There may be no "right" time to pass on such information, but it usually does need to be transmitted at some point in the not-too-distant future.

One approach is to view these problems from a family systems perspective, and for the genetic counselor to work on managing the situation on behalf of the whole family but through the individuals with whom she already has contact. This counseling-based approach is usually successful, in that the blocks to the flow of important information usually dissolve over time and with sympathetic discussion and support from the genetic counselor. But what should the professional do if an individual persists in refusing to transmit the information or breaks off contact with the genetics team?

There are those who argue that the professionals should then be prepared to pass on information about one family member to others without their consent—although always informing them of this decision in advance of carrying it out. The circumstances in which such a breach of confidence would be justifiable have been considered by several learned bodies (including the American Society of Human Genetics, the Nuffield Council on Bioethics, the Royal College of Physicians) but there is still no consensus either about what to do in specific cases or even about how to resolve these issues.

This could lead us to discuss in detail the various ethical frameworks within which such issues could be addressed, but here we have space merely to outline four approaches to ethical deliberation. One approach would be to reflect on and discuss the competing principles at stake—with the principle of autonomy usually trumping the others in our contemporary, individualistic, western societies. Another approach that is also founded on a positivistic individualism is that of utilitarianism—attempting to weigh up, in a notional calculus, the likely outcomes of particular courses of action, and perhaps considering the concrete particulars of the case in its analysis as a bioethical case discussion (for a critical view, see Chambers, 1999). A third approach is that of "common morality" (Gert et al., 1996), respecting rationality and impartiality in decision making within an open, public framework of moral rules. Finally, a framework that may be less familiar to many readers, but which has a lot to offer, is that of narrative ethics. In this, the professionals do not seek to abstract the issues of principle from the particulars of the case—the context—but to focus on the experience of their clients and encourage them to reflect on the future paths they can envisage taking (Brock, 1995). This approach can draw together a professional ethic derived from MacIntyre's virtue-based morality (Clegg, 2000) with the professional skills of humanistic counseling, making use of narrative approaches to promote the personal growth, development and healing of their clients—and thereby resolving (or dissolving) many of the ethical difficulties that could otherwise persist and become problematic if a confrontational approach is adopted.

Some professionals fear that the development of a formalized framework for breaching confidences will inevitably make such practices a more routine, even an expected or obligatory component of the professional activity of genetic counseling. While it would be inappropriate to announce that there are no circumstances in which a professional could legitimately breach confidences, many problems would be generated by any systematic policy of transmitting confidential genetic information about one individual to their relatives without consent. Professionals could become less inclined to persist with alternative approaches to resolving these communication problems. Clients, aware that confidentiality could be jeopardized by their counselor or clinician, could tend to be less than frank about their disease or their family structure from their first contact with the clinical genetics team. These consequences of altering the rules of professional conduct would be difficult to demonstrate in a tangible, numerical form but would be none the less real for that.

Genetic testing and children

When is it appropriate to carry out genetic tests on children? There are few issues on which there is so much disagreement among health professionals or between professionals and families.

There are circumstances in which all agree that genetic testing is entirely appropriate. Thus, if a child has a clinical disorder that requires a diagnosis and which may be genetic in origin, then genetic testing may be the most appropriate investigation. For example, a young boy with delayed motor and speech development and an elevation of the serum creatine kinase may have Duchenne muscular dystrophy. A molecular genetic investigation—searching for deletions and duplications within the Duchenne muscular dystrophy gene—may well yield a diagnosis and thus may avoid the need for the invasive procedure of muscle biopsy.

Predictive testing for a disorder with onset usually in childhood is another context in which childhood testing can be appropriate. Thus, in the family above, if the boy does have Duchenne muscular dystrophy, it may be thoroughly appropriate to test his younger, apparently healthy, brother. The family are likely to be highly anxious about him—will he develop the same disease?—and it may take months or even years before either the diagnosis becomes apparent or the family is reassured. Some might prefer to wait and watch but most families wish to know one way or the other. Another context in which a child might very reasonably have predictive testing for a genetic disorder, even where the condition might not manifest until adult life, is where the child is at risk of complications for which surveillance can usefully begin in childhood. A few familial cancer syndromes fall into this category.

Predictive testing for disorders that usually have an adult onset and which are untreatable is another matter altogether. To test a child, who is too young to participate in the decision, prevents them from making their own decision later. This may be especially important where, as in Huntington disease (HD), the disorder is untreatable and many at-risk adults choose not to be tested—preferring to live in a state of uncertainty. To carry out a test to resolve the anxieties of the parents would then be quite inappropriate. As well as abrogating the child's future autonomy it also breaches the principle of respect for confidentiality—if tested as an adult, a person has complete control over who else is told about the test result. In addition, there is the possibility that a child's upbringing could be damaged by the result of the genetic testing. Might altered parental expectations of the child's future educational attainments or personal relationships be damaging, and perhaps self-fulfilling? There is no firm evidence on this point, and it would be difficult to gather "evidence" that would resolve this—indeed, what type of evidence would settle this question?—so we have strong grounds for caution without the prospect of readily establishing "the truth". Fortunately, most professional bodies and lay disease support groups share this perspective and would not be prepared to carry out predictive tests for HD or similar disorders on healthy children, at least in Europe and North America. Professionals in other (especially Mediterranean and non-Western) cultures do not all share this perspective, however, and some would be willing to perform predictive tests for HD on even very young children (see chapter by Wertz in Clarke, 1998). The role of the family in less individualistic societies certainly creates a different context to which we should not transfer our culture-bound judgments without great care, although that does not necessarily mean that our value systems have to be discarded in the face of a traditional, authoritarian paternalism just because it is based in a different culture.

Carrier testing in childhood is the most hotly contested issue in relation to the genetic testing of children, and professionals differ in their approaches too. Parents of children with autosomal recessive disorders may wish to know which of their healthy (unaffected) children are genetic carriers. In the context of chromosomal rearrangements, such as balanced translocations, it used to be standard practice to test a whole sibship when the family presented clinically and a similar approach has been adopted by some pediatricians as molecular testing has become possible for mendelian disorders, notably cystic fibrosis. Given that the young children tested for chromosome translocations in the past have not suffered obvious harm, is there any reason why professionals should not comply with parental requests to test young children to determine their carrier status?

One response is to point out that the children themselves will not benefit from the testing until adulthood—the results are not relevant to them until they come to make their own relationship and reproductive decisions in the future. Being identified as a carrier can have subtle effects on an individual's sense of well-being, and we do not know how this could affect a child's developing sense of self.

Carrier testing presents the same challenge to the ethical principles of autonomy and confidentiality as does predictive testing, although there is perhaps rather less at stake because the child's own health is not in question, and there is still the concern that parental expectations could exert an undue influence on future relationships and reproduction. That may apply particularly in the context of sex-linked disorders or chromosome rearrangements, where the child's own future children may be affected irrespective of the genetic constitution of their partner. So there are considerations that weigh in favor of deferring a test until the child can participate in the decision. Furthermore, performing a test in childhood does not ensure that the results will in fact be passed on to the child in a comprehensible and relevant fashion in the future, whether the child does or does not turn out to carry the condition. It is the experience of several studies that genetic carrier test results are not always transmitted to the children tested even by the time they are adolescents or young adults, and there are often misunderstandings about the inheritance of the disorder in the family and about the meaning of the test results (Jolly et al., 1998, in Clarke, 1998; Fanos and Gatti, 1999; Fanos and Mackintosh, 1999; Järvinen, 2000). Carrier testing of the young child, then, is not a complete solution to family concerns, and the offer of genetic counseling is likely to be helpful to the children when older even when the test has been carried out years before.

Discussing these issues with parents who are seeking to have carrier testing for a young child will often lead to an agreement that the family will talk with the child about the genetic issues in the family as she/he grows up. An arrangement can be made with the family either to keep in very occasional contact or to defer future contact until the children decide to seek information and testing for themselves. It cannot be overemphasized that not testing for a condition is not the same as not talking about it! If the family has very strong feelings about testing, wanting the test to go ahead when a child is too young to contribute to the discussion, the counselor can prompt a careful discussion of the issues and an exploration of the parents' expectations from the test, but need not completely block testing if the family are heavily focused on this. Although it may be appropriate to defer testing to allow some further reflection, a complete refusal to perform carrier tests in young children can lead to anger and resentment that may be very unhelpful in the future. It may be better to avoid rigid positions in such a sensitive area and to leave the final decision with the parents.

An approach that can be presented to families as often being the best way forward through the tangled issues and feelings may be the encouragement of discussion and openness within a family but the deferral of testing so as deliberately to leave that decision to the child when she/he is older—in adolescence. This may help these adolescents to arrive at reasonable and responsible decisions, with which they can live more happily in the future.

The final topic to be considered in this section is the handling of requests from a child or adolescent for a predictive or carrier test. The question is whether the legal minor is sufficiently mature to understand the considerations involved in making a decision about testing. Gaining sufficient experience of life to arrive at a wise decision must take time, but it can be argued that living through particular experiences, that have given the child an intimate knowledge of the family's genetic disease, accelerates this process. Living in a family touched by genetic disease may give a child both the need to find out their carrier status and the capacity to make decisions about carrier testing. What might be inappropriate for a minor of the same age in the general population may be very reasonable within a particular family context. There are parallels between children being involved in decisions about genetic testing and the involvement of children with short stature in decisions about leg-lengthening surgery (Alderson, 1993). It is important to recognize that a child can be involved in a decision without necessarily making the decision alone—children can be brought in to the process of making a decision, making a contribution from an earlier stage than has often been appreciated, but this is not an all-or-nothing involvement.

The question as to when children can make their own decisions about genetic testing without parental involvement or even knowledge is separate. An assessment approach has been found helpful in the context of requests from adolescents for predictive testing for Huntington disease (Binedell et al., 1996).

Population genetic screening

The important differences between clinical genetic services made available to individual families and those provided as screening programs to a whole population have been outlined above. There are three ethical aspects to genetic screening programs that need to be considered further here.

First, there is the issue of informed consent. It is always important to ensure that participation in a population screening program is conditional upon informed consent, but it may be difficult to define "informed consent" so that it can be readily operationalized (i.e., readily assessed in a valid and

reliable manner in an evaluation of the screening program). As a minimum, the potential participant needs to recognize that they have been given a choice and to understand what the choice is about. There may be potential disadvantages to participation as well as potential advantages, and this would have to be recognized. Probably the most serious limitations to informed consent for genetic screening arise from the routinization of the offer of testing—its incorporation into standard clinical practice, perhaps with the subtle discouragement of questioning, and the active promotion of testing by committed and enthusiastic staff.

The second issue to be considered here is the decision making process whereby any particular screening program is made available to, or provided for, a population. In a national health care system, this will be decided by the health service—at regional or national level. Under a private insurance scheme, such a decision could be imposed by legislation or determined by commercial factors—the "free" market. What is important from the perspective of ethics is how the decision is made: What evidence is taken into account, being regarded as relevant to the decision? Which interest groups have a say in the decision? On what grounds is the decision made and justified? Are these judgments defensible in open, public debate? This perspective amounts to a procedural ethics, appropriate to the bureaucracies of contemporary government and commerce. From this perspective, it becomes especially important to examine the processes by which such decisions are made in practice, as has been done in the case of two genetic screening and testing programs (Koch and Stemerding, 1994; Nelkin, 1996).

Finally, there is the distinction between maximal and optimal rates of uptake of a screening test. There will often be a tension between the conventional goal of maximizing uptake for a screening test that is considered to be "A Good Thing" and the goal of good clinical practice. A high uptake may be seen as necessary to achieve a maximal efficiency both in the clinic and the laboratory, but a very high uptake may be regarded as evidence of a poor quality of informed consent. There is certainly no point in using scarce resources to provide a screening test that is not wanted by most members of the public, but nor is it adequate to argue that a screening program is worthwhile because it achieves a high rate of uptake. In the context of screening for the health benefit of the individual, it may be assumed that uptake has to be maximized—at least until the marginal cost of promoting further uptake becomes too great—but, especially in the context of reproductive decisions, it may be more helpful to recognize that screening will be valued by some individuals and not by others. It then becomes more appropriate to optimize the uptake of screening rather than maximizing it. This involves making the offer of screening in such a way that those who are likely to find it helpful to participate in screening do so and those who would not find it helpful do not participate. This topic is explored further below.

Newborn screening

The first population screening program to be introduced for genetic disease was the newborn screening program for phenylketonuria (PKU), which transformed the prognosis for affected infants. There is no doubt that this—and the subsequent introduction of screening for congenital hypothyroidism—has been a great success. There is also good evidence that the identification of infants with sickle cell disease, and their prophylactic treatment with penicillin, is to their benefit. What ethical issues arise in these flagship programs, the "acceptable face" of genetic screening?

First, there is the issue of whether newborn screening for these treatable disorders should be mandatory, as it is in some countries and some states of the USA, or whether it should be voluntary—on the basis of assumed or informed parental consent—as elsewhere. The uptake of testing is scarcely influenced in western countries by legal compulsion, and informed parental consent must be the preferred route to implementation on all other grounds, so there seems to be little reason to justify compulsion. Operating on a basis of assumed parental consent does not have the explicit advantages of informed parental consent but may be acceptable in this context, where a degree of routinization is likely in practice even where "informed" consent—which entails the provision of information to parents and their active involvement in the decision—would be preferable. In different health care systems, where primary care might be delivered in a fragmented fashion by multiple, poorly coordinated providers of variable skill and experience, the case for mandatory newborn screening for treatable disorders would be stronger.

The other issues around newborn screening relate to screening for disorders where the child is unlikely to benefit directly from any clinical intervention. There are reasoned arguments both in favour of and against newborn screening for Duchenne muscular dystrophy (DMD), for example, and it is not possible to resolve this issue "in principle", i.e., by reflection in the abstract. This is a good example of a situation where practical experience of both situations is required. For that reason, this is worth discussing at greater length.

There are two principal arguments for screening. First, many families with a boy affected by DMD have noticed a problem in the second or third year of life but they are usually reassured by friends and professionals and it may take several more years before a diagnosis is made. The parents in these families are often bitter about the diagnostic delay and the impact this has had on their treatment of the boy's complaints. They often state that they would like to have known the diagnosis earlier. Second, in some of these families another affected child is born before the elder affected boy has been diagnosed and the family have two (or three) affected sons. If the diagnosis had been made earlier then the parents could have been offered genetic counseling in advance of another pregnancy, perhaps thereby averting the birth of the second affected child. While newborn screening would not have the goal of reducing the birth incidence of DMD, it could have a modest effect in this direction.

Arguments against the program include the distress caused to the family when their relationship with the boy is just beginning—it could spoil the first few years of the child's life, and the family's pleasure in him, without improving the outlook for his health and with the possibility of damage to parent-child relationships.

Practical experience with newborn screening for DMD in Wales, where the program has been running on the basis of informed parental consent for 10 years, has shown that most families are pleased to have the diagnosis early and use this knowledge in practical planning for the future, including for their reproductive decisions. There has, inevitably, been distress at the diagnosis, but most families have been pleased to know about the condition from this early stage. Parental satisfaction with the diagnostic process—adhering to a protocol refined in the early months of the program—has been greater than in a group of families where the diagnosis was made after a clinical presentation with symptoms.

The principal outstanding issue surrounding this program is the adequacy of the informed consent process at entry to screening. The uptake rate of > 90% suggests an element of routinization, which would not be at all appropriate in this context. Alterations to the process of testing—marking this test as different from the therapeutically helpful PKU test—reduce uptake to what may be a more appropriate figure of 75–80%. This emphasizes the influence of structural and social factors on individual decision making about genetic tests.

Newborn screening for other diseases is feasible, as with cystic fibrosis and α-1-antitrypsin deficiency (A1ATD), and is becoming feasible for many inborn errors of metabolism, including medium chain acyl-CoA dehydrogenase deficiency, MCAD. Which of these tests should be made available? The case for introducing newborn screening for CF is strong in that active management of nutrition and infection can commence earlier after newborn screening and it is plausible to suggest that this may improve the long-term prognosis. Experience with screening for A1ATD is limited, but a program in Sweden was discontinued because it seemed to result in parental distress and increased parental smoking, a specific hazard in A1ATD. In relation to MCAD, there could be pressure from enthusiastic medical biochemists to introduce the necessary technology—tandem mass spectrometry—but there is still uncertainty about the natural history of the condition and about the likely balance between the improved prognosis for some of the young children, who are protected from metabolic decompensation, and the imposition of intense medicalization onto those children who would have suffered no ill effects from the condition but may now be admitted to hospital with every minor childhood illness. What is clear is that any process of evaluation of such screening programs must be broad-based—it must examine not only the clinical medical outcomes but also the social impact on the families caught up in screening and the costs imposed on both the health services and the families involved. Those involved in making decisions about the implementation of such screening programs must not just reflect a coalition of vested interest groups—enthusiastic professionals, the manufacturers of the technology and medical administrators interested only in containing health service costs.

Antenatal screening

There are several issues around antenatal screening that need to be discussed, in addition to the issues discussed above about non-directiveness and screening programs in general. First, there is the question of the goals of antenatal screening. Then there are the unanticipated consequences of screening—especially the impact of antenatal screening on women and couples who become caught up in the clinic process but may not have really thought through the issues in advance. Finally, there is the impact of antenatal screening on those affected by the conditions for which screening is made available and which are often subject to the termination of pregnancy.

GOALS

Is the primary purpose of antenatal screening to reduce suffering, to provide choice or to reduce the costs of health

care? Perhaps the best way to address this question is to examine particular screening programs in detail, and test out their rhetoric against their operation in practice. If we do that, what might we find? That is the type of empirical ethics research that is needed in place of yet further cost-benefit analyses which are simply not capable of answering the really important questions.

It is incontestably good to reduce "suffering"—but whose suffering do we mean? Prenatal screening is essentially targeted at Down syndrome and at structural malformations of the fetus; it utilizes maternal serum screening "for" Down syndrome and fetal ultrasound scans "for" malformation and for Down syndrome. Fetal anomaly ultrasound scans can reduce perinatal mortality—but most of this effect consists of bringing forward inevitable neonatal deaths so that they are no longer counted in either perinatal or neonatal mortality figures. Such reclassifications of inevitable deaths need not reflect any improvement in the clinical reality for the mother or family, because a late termination of pregnancy takes the place of a sad but inevitable neonatal death—which might leave the family with fewer regrets and less guilt in a context of greater emotional support.

Neural tube defects (NTDs) certainly can cause physical suffering in the child, although it may be difficult to argue that anencephaly causes the neonate more suffering than a termination of pregnancy, but there is no consensus among adults with NTD about the rights and wrongs of selective termination. Many take a "permissive" view, arguing that screening and termination should not be prohibited, but often maintaining that their lives are worthwhile despite their physical problems and that they are full members of society and must be respected as such. There is a strong tension in this position, discussed further below, between the freedom of pregnant women to make their own reproductive decisions on the one hand and the respect due to our fellow human beings, whatever their physical or intellectual capacities, on the other hand.

While Down syndrome can cause serious physical problems for affected individuals, it is the intellectual limitations and the stigmatizing physical features that are usually thought of as the major problems associated with it. So the suffering to be avoided through selective terminations of pregnancy is as much the suffering likely to be experienced by the parents and the wider family as it is any direct suffering by the child. Such suffering by the parents may have many elements—of sadness and disappointment at the limitations imposed on one's child by their genetic constitution, of irrational but often powerful feelings of guilt, of social stigmatization, of worry about the child's future happiness in society outside the home and concern about their physical frailty or health problems.

The offer of informed reproductive choices is also given as a possible goal of prenatal screening, but this begs many questions. Given that the imposition of decisions about testing and (dis)continuing wanted pregnancies is burdensome, with its own social and emotional costs, which decision-making tasks is it appropriate to impose on every pregnant woman? Who makes this decision and on what grounds? It is not possible to sustain the view that a simple maximization of the number of decisions made is an end in itself. We must examine the context within which these decisions are made.

DECISIONS IN SOCIAL CONTEXT

If the termination of a pregnancy "for" Down syndrome is motivated by the desire to avoid suffering, therefore, it could be argued that there are alternative approaches to this problem that are often not proposed by public health physicians, health economists or genetics professionals. These other approaches may have major advantages over the process of prenatal screening and the termination of wanted pregnancies, with the pain and suffering felt by the pregnant woman and the distress, guilt and depression that so commonly ensue. Society could respond to the challenge of Down syndrome—and mental handicap or intellectual disability more generally—by ensuring that children with such problems are actively welcomed by society and integrated effectively into schooling and work, that parents are provided with a high standard of social support, and that older individuals with Down syndrome are offered adequately sheltered housing near the homes of their friends and families. The decisions made about prenatal screening and the termination of pregnancies might be different if parents were confident that neither they nor their child would experience overt hostility or more subtle forms of stigmatization if their child were to have Down syndrome, and if they could have a realistically optimistic view about the future for their child once they are themselves insolvent, infirm or dead.

This idyllic state of affairs would require major changes in public attitudes and in the provision of health and social services in most societies, but without such developments any promotion of prenatal screening can be understood as (at least implicitly) coercive. Families can feel that they have little real choice about prenatal screening because the support they can expect to receive from society for a baby with special problems and special needs would simply be inadequate. Altering the social context in this broad way, at

the "macro" level, would also be likely to improve "micro" aspects of social functioning—the subtle, intimate hostility sometimes displayed towards individuals with disability and their parents.

In contemporary society, the notion that "reproductive choice" is A Good Thing—good enough to justify the systematic promotion of prenatal genetic screening—is highly questionable. The emphasis on individual choice and autonomy that is so strong in contemporary medical ethics, including ethical discussions of prenatal screening, is really a mirage. To consider ethical issues in the abstract, divorced from the social context of those confronting them, is to inhabit a fantasy. This is not to argue that individual choice is a Bad Thing, or that individuals should be prohibited from utilizing prenatal screening—but the active promotion of screening on the grounds of respecting individual choice is ingenuous if the social framework within which the choice is made available remains unexamined. Such a policy deflects attention away from the processes through which society arrives at decisions about health and social care. These decisions inevitably reflect the interests of different social groups, and to present them as neutral and based solely on objective considerations is actively misleading—making it harder for those with little power and few resources to contribute their views in an effective manner.

ENTRY TO PRENATAL SCREENING

Consent for entry to prenatal screening is often not based on carefully considered and well informed decision-making—as is known from many studies of the antenatal clinic process. Indeed, the way in which the test is offered is often routinized, and this leads to further problems for those women and couples in whom the screening test indicates a possible problem. If they have complied with screening in the expectation that the test will "make sure the baby is alright"—such an ambiguous phrase!—then they can find it very difficult when a real or possible problem is identified. Such women can feel swept along on a diagnostic conveyor belt that often leads to amniocentesis and sometimes towards a termination of pregnancy; it can be very difficult to slow this process sufficiently to permit reflection or to stop the conveyor belt and get off.

Such difficult experiences would be minimized if it were made very clear to all potential screening participants that:

1. The primary purpose of screening is to identify pregnancies in which the fetus has a problem, not to provide reassurance or photographs for the baby album or an emotional glue to "promote bonding".

2. Participation is entirely voluntary.

3. Professionals are likely to raise the question of terminating the pregnancy if the tests do indicate a problem.

4. The reassurance gained through a normal screening test result is never complete.

5. Some test results may be of uncertain significance, being neither completely "normal" nor definitely "abnormal", and would require further investigation and/or consideration before any decision could be made.

6. Services may be available locally to support families who have a child with Down syndrome or spina bifida.

Some pregnancies are terminated in haste when the couple learns about a problem detected on the fetal ultrasound or on fetal chromosome analysis. Then, when the parents learn more about the diagnosis—especially if the child might have enjoyed a very reasonable quality of life—they can bitterly regret their decision. Such problems are less likely to arise when women are informed about the possibility of "gray" results before deciding to go ahead with screening—but it is emotionally difficult and demanding for both staff and pregnant women to confront these issues in every pregnancy. The issues are therefore often evaded until there is a serious decision to be made in a hurry—and those are not the best circumstances in which to make such a decision.

The ethical challenges in this setting are faced by our clients, by society at large and by us professionals.

1. Pregnant women have to decide whether or not to comply with the prenatal screening program on offer. While some will wish to take any available measures to avoid having a child with problems, others will want to welcome their child unconditionally into this world. Yet others may wish to spare their child what they fear might be a life of misery, and would prefer to take any suffering upon themselves—suffering the distress of terminating a wanted pregnancy so as to spare their child from physical suffering or from life in a hostile society.

2. Society has to decide how to support pregnant women and vulnerable children. Should it set out to welcome every infant unconditionally, and to generate confidence in the willingness of society to care lifelong for those with special needs? Or should it adopt a more hard-nosed, instrumentalist approach to its future citizenry by discouraging the birth of those likely to require more than average from its health and social services?

3. Under what circumstances, and with what goals and ethos, are we prepared to make prenatal screening available? To what extent does our compliance with an unsatisfactory system serve to bolster it?

RESEARCH IN PRENATAL SCREENING

It is certainly of crucial ethical importance that our evaluations of prenatal screening programs develop more sophisticated ways of weighing costs and benefits. At present, it is all too easy for a family tragedy to be recorded—for the purposes of clinical audit or health services research—as the successful identification and termination of an abnormal fetus (e.g., with Turner syndrome). At present, most research and audit on prenatal screening avoids the active search for these potentially disastrous outcomes, so the evidence base is systematically distorted. This is not merely an issue of research methodology but a serious ethical issue about the framing of research questions that has received insufficient attention. In this era of "evidence-based medicine", what types of evidence "count" as such? Is evidence to be considered only if it is quantitative? Who makes these decisions?

DISABILITY ISSUES, COST-BENEFIT ANALYSIS AND SEX SELECTION

The persistent focus of research studies investigating population genetic screening programs on crude cost comparisons—the cost to society of either screening and terminating affected pregnancies or of caring for affected individuals—is grossly offensive to many individuals with disability. It may horrify other citizens too, but it is especially offensive to those of us who have the conditions that society seems determined to stamp out on the grounds that affected individuals cost too much to look after. This really does amount to putting a price on a person's head! Such cost-saving arguments—essentially, that it is cheaper to stop your patients being born than to look after them—are totally unacceptable in other medical contexts. Indeed, it is generally accepted that medical care costs money and that society should be prepared to pay for it. The simplistic, narrowly economic approach to prenatal screening reduces human value to a cash price, and reflects a deeply amoral cynicism.

There are other reasons why terminations of pregnancy may be justified, but the widespread use of crude cost calculations to justify prenatal screening "for" Down syndrome suggests that society and the professions have—perhaps by default—decided to promote prenatal screening on those grounds. Such utilitarian attitudes fail to consider the duties we owe other humans, including our future selves when we become unwell or infirm, and fail to recognize the important virtue of human solidarity. Such policies have helped to generate considerable hostility towards genetics within the disability movement. This is most unfortunate because genetics may have a lot to offer society—including those with disabilities—and a rejection of genetics *tout court* could obstruct useful progress on several fronts.

One obstacle to mutual understanding is that "genetics" covers many different activities. The term can be used to describe prenatal screening programs and their apparent contempt for the worth of people with disabilities. It can also be used to describe research into the causes of disability, which may result in a more sophisticated diagnostic taxonomy and give insights into the causation of disabilities—and perhaps eventually lead to the improved treatment of affected individuals. Hostility to one aspect of genetics may carry over to other areas also labeled as "genetics". Furthermore, gene therapy may be many years from widespread application in fields such as the muscular dystrophies, but even a distant prospect of such therapies generates conflicting emotions within affected individuals and their families. On the one hand there can be surges of hope that individuals already born will be helped by such treatments to lead better (healthier, more able, fuller) lives, while waves of resentment can also arise at anyone thinking that therapy would be wanted—this can be taken to imply a lack of respect for the daily achievements of affected individuals, who live their lives creatively and with enjoyment and seek recognition as valued individuals, just as everyone strives to do. Neither the (bio)medical model of disability ("you have a problem with your body and we professionals are doing what we can to fix it") nor the social model ("society is to blame for all the difficulties confronted by individuals with disability") does full justice to the complex relationship between the cause of a disability, its practical manifestations in the life of an affected person, the broader social impact of their disability and the emotional consequences for the individual and those around them.

Those with disabilities may fear that genetics will be used by society to eradicate either their disabilities or the people themselves. Of course the eradication of disabilities is never going to be possible because so many acquire disabilities for nongenetic reasons, but there may still be great resentment that anyone would wish to do so. It is likely that for many years it will remain technically much easier to eradicate people with inherited disabilities prenatally—sometimes, and inappropriately, regarded as a form of disease prevention—than to prevent the loss of these abilities in those with progressive disorders or to restore them to someone who has lost them or never had them. Suspicion of genetics will therefore persist, but it is possible for the disabled and their health professionals to develop a dialogue that slowly breaks down misunderstandings. This is an important activity from which both groups can learn—the professionals can learn more about the experiences and aspirations of the disabled, and the disabled can learn that "genetics" is not a single, monolithic entity that aims to wipe them out but refers to a range of different activities, some of which will help at least to understand the causes of inherited disabilities and may one day provide useful therapies.

One particular disabled community that deserves specific mention here is that of the deaf—those with prelingual deafness who use sign language. This group sees itself as a threatened cultural minority, and genetic research into deafness is perceived by some of this group as a direct threat to their continued existence as a distinct minority culture. This group of the deaf often do not see their deafness as a problem, in contrast to those with later-onset hearing impairments. Is such prelingual deafness, then, a disease? or a disability? or a condition—an innocent trait—like red hair? or a marker of belonging to a specific cultural community?

Finally, mention must be made of fetal sex selection. Many cultures have a preference for sons—this was true until recently of both the ruling and the laboring classes of western societies. The pressure to have sons has powerful socio-economic roots and relates to cultural practices such as the dowry and the need for sons to work in the fields, join the family business or inherit property. In some societies, newborn daughters are sometimes exposed or killed, so that the sex ratio in parts of Asia is substantially distorted. Furthermore, women who have daughters are sometimes abused, assaulted, divorced or murdered—so that the women can be as eager as their menfolk to have a son. In this cultural setting, those who can afford prenatal diagnosis sometimes use it to ensure that a pregnancy does produce a son.

Collusion with requests for fetal sex determination as a means to achieve a son can be regarded in the west as collusion with an offensive, patriarchal system that oppresses woman and is hugely disrespectful to them. British medicine has decided not to permit prenatal diagnosis for such purposes—to do so would be seen as support for a wicked system. This raises two important questions. First, if a woman seeks fetal sex selection out of fear that she will be assaulted or killed if she has a daughter, then is that not at least as powerful a justification for prenatal diagnosis and pregnancy termination as many of the "social" terminations carried out every day? Secondly, if we western professionals adopt this stance because we hold women in such high esteem, what message is conveyed by our collective willing-ness to promote prenatal screening "for" Down syndrome? If the disability movement had a higher profile, would we discontinue that type of prenatal selection too?

Carrier screening

Screening to identify unaffected, healthy carriers of auto-somal recessive diseases in the general population is another form of reproductive genetic screening, and it can be made available in pregnancy—when it may be represented as being "most relevant". Similar issues arise to those in the field of prenatal genetic screening because the simplest outcome measures are the numbers of individuals tested, the number of carriers and of carrier couples identified, the number of pregnancies tested and the number of affected pregnancies terminated. To attempt simply to maximize these figures could lead health professionals to direct their patients into testing, so it is most important that health services do not impose crude testing targets that could encourage unacceptably directive clinical practices.

There are potential benefits from being identified as a carrier—especially the ability to make reproductive deci-sions, such as asking a partner to be tested—but there are disadvantages too. The negative consequences of being identified as a carrier include the emotional impact of this unwelcome information, the burden of future reproductive decisions, possible lingering concerns about one's own health and the potential for stigmatization and discrimin-ation in personal relationships. Granted that there will always be many more individuals identified as carriers than there will be carrier couples who could have an affected child, how does one weigh these minor burdens on many people with the more serious positive and negative effects on carrier couples—who will be given important personal information but will also have the burden of making deci-sions about prenatal testing, and perhaps termination, in their pregnancies?

Given the difficulty in making decisions about what carrier testing services to make available—the principal con-tenders would be screening for cystic fibrosis, the hemo-globin disorders and Tay-Sachs disease—one approach would be to set up pilot schemes and be guided by the interest and response shown by the public. Such pilot schemes have been established in several countries and similar results have been found in most programs. Essentially, the public in general has little interest in carrier screening but will often comply if screening is actively

offered by enthusiastic health professionals. Indeed, the rate of uptake is critically dependent upon the way in which testing is made available—varying from < 10% to > 70%, with higher rates if testing is offered actively and is available on the spot but much lower if a separate appointment is required. It would seem that the mode of offer of the test could be selected to generate whatever rate of uptake of the test was desired. In addition, if screening is made available to women or couples in early pregnancy then the uptake is substantially higher again. How is this to be interpreted—as indicating a real interest in testing? or as compliance with an actively promoted test because of the vulnerability of pregnant women to suggestions that they should have a test "to make sure baby is alright"? Your answer to this question will reflect, or perhaps affect, your attitude to suggestions that cystic fibrosis carrier screening should be introduced widely into the antenatal setting in USA (the NIH Consensus Statement 1998). If you are uncomfortable with this suggestion, you may well ask yourself *cui bono?* How was the NIH consensus arrived at? What evidence was con-sidered, and how was it weighted? What (vested) interests were represented or promoted in the decision-making process?

Further issues arise in antenatal carrier screening as to the precise offer to be made—testing just the pregnant woman, or the couple as individuals or the couple as a unit—because the nature of the offer made reflects the goals of the program and will have implications for how these are perceived.

When testing is actively promoted by the dominant social institutions—as with screening for β-thalassaemia in Cyprus, promoted by the Orthodox Church—it can be very difficult for outsiders to distinguish popular consent from public compliance or, effectively, coercion. Societies certainly differ in the degree to which individuals are willing to comply with decisions made by authority figures within the family or society at large.

The variation in frequency of autosomal recessive dis-eases between populations and ethnic groups means that the frequency of the carrier state varies widely. So a carrier screening program that could be appropriate in one popu-lation may be inappropriate in another. Problems may arise where racial disharmony and discrimination exist in a mixed population, with two (or more) ethnic groups. The promotion of genetic carrier screening could then be used by one ethnic group to stigmatize and discriminate against the other. This indeed occurred in the 1970s in the USA, when screening for sickle cell trait (carrier state) was actively promoted, and led to discrimination against blacks in employment. So the social context within which carrier screening is made available can be a highly charged, political issue—clinicians and scientists should beware.

Other problems in genetic counseling

Several other ethical issues arise in genetic counseling, to which we must refer before passing on to some broader topics. These are cross-cultural issues, the naming of syndromes and the clinician's duty to recontact clients as new information comes to light about their condition.

CROSS-CULTURAL GENETIC COUNSELING

The process of communication in genetic counseling is obviously made much more difficult if the counselor and client do not share a common language in which both can discuss the full range of technical topics and intimate issues that so frequently arise in this context. The use of an interpreter may provide a solution but may also generate its own set of problems. If the interpreter is a member of the family—a young child, perhaps, or the male or female partner of the client—then it may be difficult for the client or the counselor to talk freely, and the counselor may lack confidence that the discussion is being reported fairly to the client. Issues of power between husband and wife may intrude, and the counselor may find it difficult to walk the tightrope between collusion with the more powerful partner and causing him (or her) offence that leads to the complete withdrawal of the family from counseling.

A language barrier is only the most obvious obstacle to communication in genetic counseling. Other cultural issues may arise even more frequently, although they may not always be recognized as such. Religious beliefs may be given as an explanation by the client to the counselor in accounting for their decision not to make use of genetic testing, especially in the context of prenatal diagnosis and a possible termination of pregnancy. Religious traditions, however, do not always give a clear ruling on the "correct" decision for an adherent to make—differences exist within many traditions on such matters, and it may be the cultural assumptions and values surrounding a religion that influence client decisions and understandings more than the details of religious belief per se. Patients' and clients' appeals to "religion" may often be used as a signal by the patient/client that s/he is unwilling to pursue the topic under consideration, having deep-seated objections to the whole process. This signal is usually respected by professionals in a way that the mere expression of an opinion by the client may not otherwise be.

Access to clinical genetic services within multicultural societies may vary between different communities for a number of reasons, including patterns of language use and religion but also broader social and cultural factors. The place of an ethnic minority group in relation to the dominant society may have a crucial role here. Access to all health services may be restricted, and low uptake of genetic services may reflect this as opposed to any specific cultural factor making genetics unacceptable. Access of certain communities in Britain to health care may be restricted by the reluctance of women to be seen by male health professionals (or the reluctance of their menfolk to permit this) but also by the same influences that restrict uptake of health services by others of the same social class but of the dominant "white" majority; these economic and class factors will be especially relevant when recently arrived immigrants are still in the process of establishing themselves economically.

It is important that health professionals do not seize upon either the social or the biological differences between ethnic groups and communities to explain differences in health-related behaviors or in the patterns of disease between the communities without giving very full consideration to other possible factors—such as the material circumstances experienced by the communities. For example, differences in perinatal mortality between groups may reflect differences in socioeconomic class as much as genetic differences or differences in social customs (see chapters in Clarke and Parsons, 1997).

Probably the major cultural factor that is employed to account for differences in the pattern of genetic disease between communities is the practice of customary consanguinity within some communities. In Britain, customary consanguinity is especially prevalent in certain South Asian and Middle Eastern groups, and often more pronounced than is usual in their countries of origin because of the smaller number of potential partners in the relevant community in Britain. While this does increase the risk of autosomal recessive disorders appearing in children born into these communities, it would be all too easy for western health professionals to attribute blame and responsibility for the disorders to the minority culture and its representatives. Such provocative attributions of blame ignore the stabilizing social functions of consanguinity in many communities—this marriage pattern being more widely practiced than exogamy in global terms—and are not likely to promote any useful mutual understanding or change in customs. For communities that place social value on consanguineous marriages but have become concerned because of their high perinatal mortality or the frequency of serious genetic problems in young children, it may be more helpful to explain how the custom of consanguinity can be retained while substantially reducing the risk of genetic problems through promoting marriage between somewhat less closely related individuals. Perinatal mortality may also be tackled by attention to maternal nutrition and the provision of effective antenatal care.

The final problem of cross-cultural genetic counseling to be mentioned here is that of stereotyping. The counselor must not make assumptions about the likely response of an individual to a genetic problem in their family on the basis of how she/he thinks that a client from that community or ethnic group (or social class) would typically respond. Our inevitably patchy understandings of other cultures could all too easily lead us to imagine a spurious homogeneity within these other communities—especially in the case of disadvantaged ethnic minority groups. There is evidence that health professionals are less likely to offer some services to those from minority groups on the grounds that "they" would not want to consider genetic testing or a termination for pregnancy—falling into this trap of inappropriate cultural stereotyping.

THE NAMING OF SYNDROMES

Many families arrive in the genetic clinic with the hope that the condition affecting their child will be diagnosed. The process of labeling, however, can have immense repercussions for the family, which they may not always have foreseen. Attaching a label to the developmental disorder affecting a child is a business to be taken seriously by the family and the professional.

Where a diagnostic label is available, it may have unforeseen negative as well as positive consequences. While it may facilitate access to support services, it may also provide an unwelcome insight into the likely future for their child that a family may not be prepared to confront immediately. There can also be problems even when a diagnosis is not available, as happens quite frequently. The family may then feel bitter and resentful, especially if the lack of a diagnostic label makes it more difficult for them to access appropriate social, educational or health services for their child. Where a diagnostic label can be applied, this too may have adverse consequences if educational provision for the child is altered inappropriately—if the child is treated as the diagnosis and not primarily as an individual. There is also much scope for the self-fulfilling prophecies of low expectations on the part of parent or teacher.

A very real problem for some individuals affected by genetic disorders and their families is the name given to their diagnosis, their syndromes. This applies particularly to the field of dysmorphology. It can be difficult enough for a family to accept that one (or more) of them has a disorder manifest in their physical appearance, without insult being added to injury by the offensive nature of the name given to their condition. While some names are unfortunate but understandable, others are the expression of a brand of medical humor that should not be paraded before the families in our care—it should be relegated to the undergraduate classroom and have no place in clinical practice. Given that families now routinely have access to the internet, they can readily find out all the names given to "their" syndrome, so it is not possible for clinicians to use one name with families and another name for the same condition when talking with their colleagues.

The name "cri du chat" syndrome can be unfortunate when it causes a family to flinch whenever they hear their child's cry—the cry having caused no concern before they were given the name of the condition. This name was coined in good faith as a clinically useful description, and not as a thoughtless witticism, but it does have this unanticipated impact on families. This name, however, need not be used by professionals—5p- syndrome is a good alternative—although I suspect that the more evocative name will linger. There are many other syndrome names, however, especially acronyms, which have surely been devised for their "humorous" effect and with complete disregard for the impact of the name on those affected and on their families. Examples include CATCH 22 syndrome, LEOPARD syndrome, DEFECT syndrome and CRASH syndrome. The giving of a name to a syndrome can be as serious a matter as the giving of a diagnostic label to a child.

Another reason for taking great care in the naming of genetic conditions has been explored by Peter Harper in relation to the eponymous Hallervordern-Spatz disease. These two research neuropathologists made use of the brains of children with neurological and mental disorders who were exterminated in Nazi death camps as part of the German policy of race hygiene, and Hallervordern (at least) was closely and knowingly involved in the work of the death camps. Harper and others have called for this condition to be given a different name.

A final topic to be mentioned under this heading is the process of giving a diagnostic label to a patient or family. This process can be very delicate and information about the diagnosis—even the name itself—may need to be fed slowly to the family as they become ready to accept it. A full and abrupt disclosure of information about a distressing problem in a young child may be unhelpful, especially if the family have not yet recognized the severity of the problem affecting their child, and may block the process of confronting reality. On the other hand, the professional's fear of triggering a strongly emotional reaction should not prevent them from delivering "bad news" when this is necessary. Professionals should keep their practice in this area under review in a supportive process of group or individual supervision.

A DUTY TO RECONTACT?

When a family attends for genetic counseling, the clinician and counselor provide the best answers they can to the family's questions. When new information comes to light some time in the future—especially if it involves treatments or the possibility of prenatal diagnosis—is it reasonable to expect the responsible clinician to recontact the family to pass on this information? If the family is still under review, then no special problem arises—but what if the family has not attended for some years, or follow-up was never planned, or they have changed address? How far does the obligation to recontact such families extend?

A strong duty to recontact could impose such burdens on individual clinicians and counselors, and on clinical genetic services as institutions, that clinical genetics practice could cease to be a viable specialty. There has to be a balance of responsibility, with the physician updating families with whom she/he has ongoing contact but families being obliged to keep the genetics service informed of changes of address and to request occasional review consultations if they think that information may come to light that could be of interest to them.

TENSIONS IN GENETIC COUNSELING

At several points in this chapter, I have expressed the notion that there are ethical tensions inherent in genetic counseling practice, such as that between the reproductive autonomy of pregnant women and the support and respect due to individuals with Down syndrome. Another example is that between the "right" of the adult grandchild at risk of Huntington disease to find out his genetic status as opposed to the right of his at-risk parent *not* to have his/her genetic status determined. This approach—identifying points of tension where ethical principles may be said to conflict—has both rhetorical and heuristic value and can be helpful. It has one major drawback, however, in that it suggests that neither pole of the tension is "correct" and that there will be a middle way to be reached by an appropriate compromise. This thought is itself an ethical danger to be avoided—it could lead to a complete ethical paralysis because any position to be advocated could be (re)presented as being at one pole of a tension, and the desire for

a "middle way" could undermine it. The contemporary, post-modern condition of human life already makes it difficult to sustain and justify any coherent process of ethical reasoning; the use of rhetorical maneuvres to demolish any conclusions emerging from an ethical discussion could easily amount to a form of nihilism.

Pharmacogenetics, commercialization and the common, complex diseases

The promise of "the new genetics" is that an improved understanding of the genetic basis of the major diseases of western society will give new insights into their pathogenesis; this, in turn, will lead to improved, indeed truly rational, therapies. From an understanding of the contribution of genetic variation to disease susceptibility, it will be possible—so goes the implicit promise—to calculate each individual's personal profile of disease susceptibilities and hence define a suitable set of lifestyle measures or preventive medications that will keep the individual in the best possible health. This goal sounds laudable but, as soon as it is examined closely, numerous difficulties and objections appear.

First, there are problems with gathering and analyzing the data that would be required to dissect the genetic basis of the common diseases such as diabetes, hypertension, rheumatoid disease, osteoporosis, cerebrovascular disease, coronary artery disease, Alzheimer disease and the common cancers. While it has proved possible to define gene loci important in a subset of those affected by such conditions—the 5% or so of cases where there is an effectively mendelian predisposition to disease—there has been little progress towards defining the risk-modifying genetic factors of lesser effect. To identify such sequences and their interactions, with each other and with environmental factors, is an enormous and daunting task. Given the realities of human population history, the non-random association of specific sequences with each other and with disease may result from the operation of several different factors other than simple linear processes of disease causation. This will make it highly problematic to establish the causal nature of any associations that are identified, even when they have been replicated in independent studies. Not only are there problems of linkage disequilibrium, but the non-random mating of humans throughout their history and prehistory, for both geographical and cultural reasons, combined with the present rapid mixing of populations, will make it immensely difficult to assess the influence of specific "genetic backgrounds". The dissection of quantitative trait loci in the mouse has only been possible because of the controlled breeding of defined laboratory strains and the close control of environmental variables. The feasibility of both collecting sufficient human data and then conducting an interpretable analysis capable of identifying disease-related polygenic (small effect) molecular variation is small.

Secondly, if molecular variation associated causally with disease susceptibility were identified, it still might not be amenable to effective therapeutic intervention. In the context of genetic disorders, there has been a long lag period between improved understanding of pathogenesis and improved treatments for patients. It would be irresponsible to raise public expectations beyond the point where we have good grounds for confidence that progress in knowledge will lead to progress in therapy.

Thirdly, if molecular variation associated with disease susceptibility (at least in some populations) does become available before improved, more rational therapies, then there may be pressure to apply these results in health care settings. This pressure could easily come from the biotechnology industry, eager to provide a return to their shareholders and anxious because of the lag in therapeutic applications of their prodigious investments. The attempt to create a market for genetic susceptibility testing could be very damaging:

1. It could cause great stress and anxiety, through identifying those at increased risk of disease without offering adequate countermeasures.
2. It could consume limited health care resources without improving health.
3. If marketed direct to the public, it could lead those given increased risks of disease to place inappropriate demands for intervention upon their regular health care providers—posing a threat to these systems.
4. It could distract attention from environmental and lifestyle measures that are already known to be helpful to the whole population (the molding of national food, transport and leisure policies to promote healthy eating and exercise).
5. It could distract attention from the group of individuals at very substantially increased risk of disease, for whom more effective interventions are appropriate and already available (e.g., LDL receptor disorders, HNPCC etc.).
6. It could lead to paradoxical behavioral consequences for those at high and at low risk of disease, as with screening for hypertension and for hypercholesterolemia, through inducing feelings of either fatalistic inevitability or inappropriate invulnerability.

In short, the genetic dissection of the common, complex diseases presents enormous technical and social challenges. The heavy commercial involvement in this research may lead to the inappropriate promotion of consumer demand for genetic susceptibility testing. Such developments must be resisted by those health professionals and scientists who can foresee these problems.

An adequate evaluation of any such susceptibility screening test would include assessments of the clinical, psychological, social and economic consequences of introducing the test—for those given increased as well as decreased risks, and for society as a whole. There will be a temptation to examine only the clinical consequences for those at high risk of disease, and this would be much too narrow an assessment. A full evaluation should preferably be conducted before any such disease susceptibility screening test could be introduced to either a state or a private medical care system, where both types operate in a given country. To apply restrictions to the state health care system but not the private system could undermine the effectiveness of the state system, where such testing does turn out to have a useful clinical role. There is a danger that restrictions on the introduction of clinically helpful susceptibility tests could be exploited as a means of limiting pressures on the health care budget, using appeals to "evidence-based medicine" as a veil.

Perhaps the single most important ethical issue in relation to population screening for susceptibility to disease is the nature of the evidence that would be required to justify and permit screening of this type. Crucially, what evidence would be required? Who makes that decision?

While there are clearly many potential problems with genetic susceptibility screening, not all of which have been discussed here, it must not be forgotten that there could be some useful outcomes of genetic research in the area of the complex disorders. One potentially useful application is the recognition of DNA sequence variation that is causally associated with the risk of disease. Such results—perhaps most likely to come from research in relatively isolated, homogeneous populations—could identify novel links in disease pathogenesis. Such insights could then lead to the development of radically new therapeutic approaches, although it would be many years before any such therapy could be validated for general clinical application, as with any new medicine. More likely, however, and certainly more likely to reach fruition in the shorter term, is the possible use of genetic tests to guide pharmacological therapy.

There are several important clinical entities which may represent a common end-point of rather different pathogenetic processes—including hypertension, depression and epilepsy. It is widely recognized that the selection of the most appropriate therapy for patients with such problems is immensely difficult and is currently a fairly hit-and-miss affair—or, at least, all affected individuals are lumped together for therapeutic trials, which then recognize the medicines most effective in the majority of patients. What might become possible—and this is still only a possibility—is the selection of the most appropriate therapy for each individual given the pattern of the disease-associated molecular genetic variation that has predisposed them to develop the disorder. This tailoring of the treatment to the individual—"Oh, Mr Smith, I would suggest starting on medicine 557 K because your hypertension seems to have been triggered by a sequence on chromosome 13q—and, by the way, you don't have to bother about cutting down on your salt intake because that would make little difference to this type of raised blood pressure"—represents the Holy Grail of therapeutics. We must not expect such developments to work out in the near future, because human biology may simply make this goal unattainable, but it is reasonable to entertain the modest hope that progress in this direction will accumulate over the next few decades. The Holy Grail could be treasure buried beneath a perpetually receding rainbow—but cautious hope is appropriate. Promoting exaggerated expectations, on the other hand, will not be helpful and could be damaging.

Another possible benefit of identifying genetic variation associated with disease susceptibility, where this becomes feasible, could be its application to clinical trials of new therapies. If only those at increased risk of a disease are recruited, it may require fewer trial participants to be followed for fewer years before an effect of the therapy should be apparent. A possible problem here is that this high-risk subgroup, while important in its own right, may not respond to therapies or preventive measures in the same way as the rest of the population, so extrapolation from them may be problematic. Studies correlating DNA sequence variation with adverse drug reactions are also planned and would be an appropriate use of the technology. If individuals susceptible to such adverse drug reactions could be identified, then their suffering and the substantial health care costs associated with iatrogenic disease could both be reduced.

Research in human genetics

At present, research in human genetics is largely non-therapeutic so that the principal issues to be considered are consent, confidentiality and control over the process and application of the research. Many of the issues touched on here are relevant to an appreciation of the debates around the Icelandic healthcare database and its applications in biotechnology-based pharmaceuticals research (see Chadwick 1999; Annas 2000). We will also consider questions relating to the study of human diversity and "race".

CONSENT

At recruitment into a research project, it is important that the participants appreciate that the genetic sample being obtained for study is going to be examined in a research laboratory—the analytic process may not be subject to the same quality control measures as in a regular diagnostic laboratory and the applicability of the results to any health care decisions may not have been established. It may be simplest and cause least confusion if the research studies are thoroughly separated from the clinical services being provided to the patient, although this is not always feasible. It is obligatory, however, to make clear to the participant who is also a patient how, if at all, the research results may alter their prognosis or treatment. If participation will make no difference to their condition or if the results will not be revealed to the participant, then this must be clear at the point of recruitment to the study.

With banked samples of DNA or tissue, it is good practice to return to the sample donor for consent to carry out new investigations for which specific consent had not previously been obtained. This also allows the donor to be given fresh information about the progress of the research. If the donor has died, then it might be appropriate to contact his/her family if information to be generated in the research could have implications for them.

With banked tissue samples that were obtained for diagnostic purposes—perhaps at surgery for the removal of a malignancy—and for which consent for research was not obtained, should researchers have to contact the patient and gain their consent before carrying out the research?—surely Yes, if the investigation might generate information about the patient's genetic constitution, but otherwise perhaps No, if the research is only intended to characterize the tumor tissue. If the patient has died, should the family be asked to give consent before the researchers proceed with their studies?—again, Yes, if the results could be relevant to other members of the family.

It is important to distinguish on the one hand between research investigations carried out on individuals or groups of individuals who have a specific genetic condition or disease, such as a mendelian or chromosomal disorder, and on the other hand those studies of large groups or populations that seek to identify the genetic influences upon the more complex, multifactorial disorders. These population studies either seek to correlate clinical information available at the time of the genetic sample collection with genotypic data generated in the study, or continue to gather clinical information about those who have contributed samples to compare susceptibilities to disease and to drug responses that become apparent over time. There are very substantial differences between these types of research that it is important to clarify at recruitment.

When molecular genetic studies are carried out on individuals with mendelian or chromosomal disorders, this will generate information about the underlying basis of their condition and may provide insight into the pathogenesis or prognosis of their disorder. Although such information should not be used as an inducement to persuade individuals to contribute to research, it may be made available within a suitable clinical framework if that is the wish of the participants. In some studies this may be inappropriate, but it will often be thoroughly reasonable to provide feedback from the study to participants. In population-based research, however, this is much more problematic.

In studies seeking associations between the common, complex diseases and individuals' genotypes, the research—if successful—could provide information that would be relevant to third parties such as insurers or employers as well as to the individuals and their families. This would need to be explained in counseling in advance of recruitment unless either the samples and the relevant clinical information were anonymized or the results of the analysis were provided to participants in the form of general conclusions and not as the particular results applicable to each individual. It is of course impossible to provide individual results when anonymization of the samples and their accompanying clinical information has taken place, but anonymization cannot be performed when clinical information is to be gathered prospectively for use in the analysis. There are good grounds for avoiding the feedback to individual participants in this type of research of their personal results, however, even when it would be a possibility. First, agreement to the principle of being given research results at the end of the project will usually be invalid, because the nature of the result will usually be not at all clear at recruitment. If feedback is left to the discretion of the researchers, when they consider the results to be "relevant" or "important" for the individual, then the inevitable enthusiasm of the researcher is likely to exaggerate the relevance and importance of the results. It would be far more appropriate for the ethics committee approving each population study of a complex disorder to decide at the end of the study—in the light of its findings and of other available research evidence—whether feedback of results to individual participants should be made available. Then participants could be told about the general conclusions of the study and offered access to appropriate counseling and testing (i.e., effectively re-testing) in a clinical environment if they so chose. In this model, participants in anonymized studies would have just the same access to the research findings as participants in the studies with ongoing collection of clinical data.

There are additional ethical problems with obtaining consent for the recruitment of children or incompetent adults. While parents can give valid consent for the recruitment of their children to research, research should in general not be performed on children where it could be conducted adequately on adults. Furthermore, children should be involved in discussions about research to the extent that they can understand the issues and contribute their views. If children withdraw their assent for research then this must be respected—whereas, in contrast, important therapies may be administered against a young child's wishes as long as the parent consents. Particular concerns might be raised by research into the predictive testing of children for later-onset (usually adult-onset) disease for which no useful health intervention is available in childhood. Similar concerns apply to certain newborn screening programs where the natural history of the disorder is unclear, e.g., screening for medium chain acyl-CoA dehydrogenase (MCAD) deficiency in asymptomatic newborns, or where the purpose of recognizing a high-risk subgroup of children would be to recruit them into a trial of possible preventive strategies, e.g., for juvenile-onset diabetes mellitus. In such a case, the goal of recruitment into a trial must be transparent to the consenting parents at the point of entry—otherwise they could agree to participate in screening on the assumption that it would benefit their child and then find that there was no established treatment for a child shown to be at risk.

The important considerations relating to the recruitment of incompetent adults into research are not specific to genetics research and will be passed over here—suffice it to say that any decisions made must take the subject's best interests into account and must not be enforced against their will (i.e., at least the passive assent of the subject is required). The context is very similar to conducting diagnostic investigations on an incompetent adult at the request of a concerned relative, anxious to know if they could have a child affected by the same (so far undiagnosed) disorder.

CONFIDENTIALITY

Medical, personal and demographic information contributed to a research project must of course be kept securely and the privacy of all research participants must be protected. Third parties should not be given personal genetic information about individuals without their specific consent. In studies where the samples and data are anonymized, the protection of genetic privacy is simpler, but elaborate precautions—including encryption and tightly restricted access—may be needed to ensure the confidentiality of subjects in population studies with continuing data collection.

The attachment of research results to patients' medical records without their knowledge is a potentially serious problem—and this danger is one of the reasons for the recommendation that genetic research should be carried out in a different laboratory, and the results recorded in a separate format, to be kept distinct from the individual's regular medical records. Otherwise, a member of staff unaware of the background context could inadvertently pass on research results that are highly sensitive or of uncertain significance, or that the participant had chosen to be told, or staff could act on the results in a clinically inappropriate fashion.

CONTROL AND OWNERSHIP

In most jurisdictions, patients who have donated a sample of blood or tissue for research, or who have had blood or tissue removed as part of their medical care, thereby lose rights in that tissue. Ownership passes to the relevant clinical or research institution. This used not to cause many difficulties, but the commercialization of biotechnology and of biomedical research—with potentially large sums accruing to researchers developing the right molecular technologies, to their institutions and to their investors—has undermined the former "gift relationship" which (in many countries) used to motivate patients and members of the public to give blood and tissue samples for research as well as for blood transfusion services. While individual patients and research subjects are expected to treat their genetic material as a part of their person, and therefore not a commercial resource to be bought, sold or otherwise exploited, the very same genetic material can be treated as property by researchers, institutions and corporations. This contrast is being made explicit in the new generation of consent forms being developed for use in genetics research in Britain, in which patients contributing samples will have to sign away any right to commercial exploitation or benefit in respect of the sample before it will be accepted into research.

Patients and clinicians will generally acknowledge that the practical, clinical application of advances in human molecular genetics to the welfare of individuals with genetic and other diseases requires financial investment and therefore the involvement of biotechnology and pharmaceutical corporations. Many, however, feel revulsion at the way this is working in practice to the advantage of corporations or laboratories who have contributed only to the very last lap of an arduous struggle to identify the genetic basis of the relevant diseases. It offends the sense of justice of many individuals that patients and families with genetic disorders, who have contributed blood or tissue samples to research and often also supported the research by fundraising activities over many years, now find that they—or the health services that care for them—are being charged licence fees for applying the discoveries that "their" research led to.

The question of whether human (or any other organism's) DNA sequences can be patented has roused much passion. Patenting in general is conditional upon three criteria—novelty, an inventive step and an industrial application. Discoveries, therefore, should be clearly distinct from inventions, and so naturally occurring DNA sequences, genes and organisms would seem not to be patentable—but patents that give effective control over certain genetic sequences are being awarded. A landmark legal decision was the granting of a patent on a modified organism—an oil-eating bacterium—by the US Supreme Court in 1980, following which precedent further patents on organisms and DNA sequences have been granted. This heralded—perhaps enabled—the recent spate of investment in biotechnology. A rush for patents on sequences of human DNA has led to a race to complete the sequence of the human genome between an international, publicly-funded collaborative team and a US-based commercial research team. Openness and a collaborative approach among scientists would be preferable to commercial secrecy on any acceptable understanding of the scientific endeavor, even if this would entail slower progress in understanding the mechanisms of the human genome. It seems likely that the new commercial secrecy has distorted the process of research and has slowed the overall pace of scientific progress in this field. Whether a collaborative spirit can be re-established is uncertain, but this must be an important goal for scientists concerned for the ethical conduct of their craft.

HUMAN GENOME DIVERSITY PROJECT, HUMAN (PRE)HISTORY AND "RACE"

One area of human biology that may well be illuminated by genetic research is that of the history of human populations. By defining the human genetic variation present in populations around the globe, the movement of peoples over the millennia may be traced and compared with the understandings reached by other tools such as archeology and comparative linguistics. The making of artefacts and the speaking of languages, however, can be learned—can be transmitted culturally—so that a comparison of the spread of a style of pottery across Europe with molecular data from surviving populations may give an indication of the extent to which the spread of the artefacts reflected the movement of people and how much resulted from the social learning of new customs. One could even imagine tackling classical myths, such as those of the Aeneid: do Romans have Trojan Y chromosomes but Sabine mitochondria?

What problems lurk in this apparently delightful backwater of molecular archeology? One issue is the potential misapplication of molecular results to make "race" a superficially more valid, more concrete concept. While human populations do differ in their physical characteristics, and inevitably their genetic constitutions too, there is no clear demarcation between population groups. We belong to communities socially, and these communities are not biologically distinct entities that correlate with specific genetic differences at the level of the individual. Population genetics describes the variation in gene frequencies between groups in a statistical manner, and its application to individuals is fraught with scientific problems as well as cultural confusion. Even the drawing of geographical boundaries around populations is arbitrary, likely to misrepresent a cline in gene frequency as a biological discontinuity, when the mean frequencies of specific genetic variants in the two constructed groups are found to differ. That is why the term "race" has been discredited in the biological sense, and the term "ethnicity", indicating a social group to which an individual chooses to be affiliated, is used instead in the social sciences.

We must remember that social tensions between ethnic groups, sometimes associated with real differences in biological characteristics, have always been used to justify discrimination against minorities and against neighboring communities or countries. Although scientists may have no such intentions, there is every possibility that genetic studies that focus on the differences between population groups will be systematically misused. Molecular reconstructions of population history are likely to support some popular or traditional "origin myths" and to disconfirm others. How might such evidence be used by those antagonistic to their neighbors? If the myth of a group's distinct origin is supported by a research finding, then discrimination against that group—where it is in the minority—may be strengthened. Where a research finding disputes the oral

or written tradition, then the group may be subject to mockery or abuse. However fascinating, we must be very cautious in pursuing such studies.

The potential application of results from the human genome diversity project to other fields—especially those relating to socially important characteristics, such as intelligence or other valued traits—raises the frightening prospect of major social conflicts and political disputes. The "race and intelligence" debates of the 1970s would appear tame in comparison with what could emerge. There are many problems that can be foreseen as likely consequences of such research, including an increased emphasis on nationalism in politics, higher levels of inter-ethnic conflict within multicultural societies and a greater reluctance of the public or the state to support special educational interventions for children from disadvantaged ethnic minority groups. To pursue the research without attending to the likely social consequences would be irresponsible, and there seems to be no prospect of neutralizing the potential disasters.

One issue that has attracted a lot of discussion is the process through which valid consent for participation in this research could be gained. When dealing with indigenous, aboriginal communities who have had little exposure to external influences, and no science education, it may be effectively impossible for the research team to educate each member of the community to the same understanding of the project and of their rights as in genetics research conducted in a western society. Is there a place for a different type of consent in this setting? Can a community give its consent to participate, through its own processes of discussion, in the light of information from, and discussions with, project representatives? Does each individual still need to give their personal consent—and what would that mean in societies with little concept of individual autonomy? Is there a place for community inducements to participate in research—such as genetic testing for a prevalent disease, or provision of medical care for a defined period?—or would that be improper leverage? What if the project were to identify some important disease resistance factor, which could yield enormous profits when commercially exploited—(how) would the community benefit from this in practice?

Genetics, geneticization and society

Genetics has received increasing levels of public attention over the past decade, and this trend seems set to continue as more findings emerge from the Human Genome Project. Although gratifying to geneticists, there are problems with this focus on genetics—especially when society looks to genetics to explain, and even perhaps intervene to "solve", social problems. The list of social problems for which a gene is being sought is long and strikingly similar to the list of social vices that concerned the eugenics movement 50–100 years ago. This includes homelessness, addiction to drugs and alcohol, learning difficulties, sexual orientation, violence, impulsivity and criminality.

When the phrase "gene for X" is translated into something like scientific language, then the absurdity of some of the public expectations becomes clear. This phrase becomes: "a site in the genome—not necessarily a gene—at which DNA sequence variation is associated with variation in the propensity to develop X as a problem, although this association need not be causal and may only be found in one or a few population groups". The links mediating the social consequences of genetic variation are so long and so complex that, even in principle, it could never be possible to predict these consequences from the molecular causes on a linear model of causality, proceeding from the DNA sequence through cell biology to the behavioral phenotype in its full social context. The genetic sites at which molecular variation correlates with behavioral consequences, for example, if consistent correlations are ever found for any complex phenotype, will not be genes "for" the social problems. Rather, the genes will have distinct biological functions that evolved over millennia and which may be elucidated by the relevant neurosciences. The brain is far too complex an organ for geneticists to be able to make detailed predictions about behavior, although certain statistical associations between molecular variation and the probabilities of specific behaviors may be established.

One arena, in which disputes about the contribution of genetics to behavior may well be argued out in the future, is the legal system. Leaving aside the biological validity of claims that a crime was committed "because" the guilty individual was predisposed to this action by his genetic constitution, there are two possible responses. Either the genetic predisposition can count in mitigation because his responsibility was indeed limited, or the likelihood that the criminal will re-offend should ensure a heavier sentence than usual, perhaps even an indefinite sentence—a form of "preventive detention". A good case can be made for both arguments, and the legal consequences of following either course would be hugely disruptive. Legal systems might be best advised to ignore the evidence presented of a genetic predisposition to criminal behavior except in the most unusual circumstances.

Genetic determinism is the attempt to reduce the whole of biology to the physical sciences, with the behavior of organisms being shaped largely by their genetic constitu-

tion. This is a powerful but destructive concept and in reality is a doomed enterprise. Given the inevitable limitations of the physical sciences in dissecting the functions of the brain, and *a fortiori* our limitations in tackling societal characteristics and problems, how should clinical geneticists respond to the widespread misunderstandings about the relevance of genetics to social issues?

1. We should ensure that we do not inadvertently exacerbate these misunderstandings through the inappropriate use of pseudo-scientific terminology—"genes for X",.

2. We should dissociate ourselves from, and refuse to participate in, research predicated upon such misleading premises or likely to promote such misunderstandings.

3. We should speak out—as individuals or, preferably, collectively—when we see genetics being hijacked and misused by those with damaging social or political motivations, especially if we see that vulnerable and inarticulate groups of our patients are likely to suffer as a result.

4. We should take care not to attribute health problems to genetic causes when social and political factors are likely to be as heavily involved and probably more open to remedy. This could, of course, be to our professional disadvantage—because we might benefit from research funds if the principal cause of a problem is seen as being largely genetic—but this would be dishonest and would, eventually, return to haunt us as our failure to resolve the problem came to be widely recognized.

5. We should combat inappropriate talk about genetics so as to help minimize the harm done to the families in our care by some of the wildly exaggerated expectations current in the media.

The tendency to attribute causation of health or social problems to genetic factors is an example of "geneticization", a term coined by Abby Lippman to describe the more general practice of accounting for observed differences between individuals and populations in terms of underlying genetic differences. This process allows vested political interests to obscure the remediable, environmental causes of social inequalities in health and individual attainment by focusing attention upon the fixed and unalterable genetic constitutions of individuals. This, of course, fits well with a conservative, sociobiological view of human nature, in which social problems are framed as biological inevitabilities determined by our genes. This implicitly leads either to a sense of political apathy and inertia or to the advocacy of technological solutions to problems that would more appropriately be tackled by collective political action. The process of geneticization therefore distracts energy and resources from the social and environmental strategies that could lead to real solutions.

One aspect of genetics research that is particularly alarming—because of the ease with which it could be misapplied, especially in the context of "race" and human diversity—is the genetic dissection of non-disease traits, especially intelligence and personality traits, and including variation in intelligence within the normal range. The apparent rationale for pursuing this research is that it may teach us about mild learning difficulties and about fundamental brain processes involved in learning. Given the barriers to interpreting any associations that may be found between intelligence and molecular variation, however, my judgment is that the more immediate results of such research are likely to be social mayhem than a productive understanding of cognitive processes. The results are likely to be distorted, deliberately, by those intent on mobilizing political support behind racist, or at least nationalist, campaigns.

One final topic to consider here is the "thrifty gene hypothesis"—as an example of geneticization distorting the research agenda. This hypothesis was proposed by James Neel to account for the high frequency of type 2 diabetes mellitus in aboriginal societies undergoing rapid development. A "diabetogenic" genotype would be favored as promoting maximal efficiency in food utilization when food supply is limited. When food becomes abundant, the efficient utilization of food becomes a disadvantage, with type 2 diabetes developing as a consequence. On this understanding, type 2 diabetes will remain prevalent in societies emerging from a harsh subsistence because of their genetic constitution, which will change over some generations as new selective forces operate. The emergence of this hypothesis gave an apparently adequate account for the very high frequencies of type 2 diabetes found in some aboriginal communities; other possible causal factors—including socio-economic factors—received little attention.

Research in a different research paradigm has shown that the risk of developing type 2 diabetes (and other chronic diseases) in adult life is greater for infants born with fetal growth retardation. This research has supported the hypothesis that the fetus is programed by the intrauterine environment to respond throughout postnatal life to nourishment and other environmental factors in a manner reflecting its growth in utero—the Barker hypothesis of the fetal origins of much adult cardiovascular and related morbidity. This challenges the thrifty gene hypothesis, although both could have some validity. How, then, should policy makers respond to evidence that the incidence of type 2 dia-

betes in some aboriginal populations is falling faster than would be expected by selection against a genetic predisposition to diabetes? Public health officials should be delighted, because the post-war improvement in fetal and infant nutrition may now be taking effect—supporting the fetal programing hypothesis. There would be every reason then to hope that attention to the nutrition and general health of the young aboriginal women should prevent this epidemic in future generations.

With hindsight, it can be appreciated that the genetic explanation for an epidemic of morbidity in a deprived ethnic minority population led health professionals to discount further efforts at preventing type 2 diabetes by environmental measures. With hindsight, we can see that at least some of the morbidity could have been avoided by appropriate public health measures in nutrition and antenatal care.

Reproductive technologies and cloning— "reprogenetics"

The two new reproductive technologies to be discussed here are preimplantation genetic diagnosis (PGD) and human reproductive cloning. PGD entails all the procedures of superovulation, oocyte harvesting, sperm collection and in vitro fertilisation (IVF) as in the treatment of infertility—with the strict obligation to use reliable contraception alongside the IVF procedures. The zygotes are allowed to develop to about 6–8 cells, when one or two cells are removed from each morula for analysis—employing either FISH techniques, to look for chromosome anomalies or microdeletions, or polymerase chain reaction methods, to identify specific disease-associated mutations or the number of repeat units in a triplet repeat or a microsatellite sequence. Then, two (or three) embryos without evidence of the family's genetic disorder are implanted into the woman's prepared uterus.

PGD can be the perfect solution for couples with infertility who also have a risk of transmitting a serious genetic disorder to any child they might have. For couples without a fertility problem, but who are concerned about transmitting their genetic disorder to a child and who wish to avoid the procedures of prenatal diagnosis and pregnancy termination, PGD may also appear an attractive option. The process of PGD is inconvenient, however, and it is emotionally and physically draining and expensive.

For those who wish to avoid having a child with their family's genetic disorder, weighing up the potential advantages and disadvantages of PGD against conventional prenatal diagnosis entails weighing up the practical difficulties and costs of PGD against the fear of "needing" a pregnancy termination. Included in this equation may be the welfare of any children the couple already have and disruption to the wider social networks of both partners, including their employment. In discussing this with a couple, it may be helpful to encourage them to assess the strength of their objections to a pregnancy termination—this may clarify their thoughts and feelings.

Objections have been made to PGD because it is a technology that could be applied to choose between embryos on the basis of non-disease traits, including sex. If there are six healthy embryos and two are to be implanted, then it may seem very reasonable to allow the couple to choose the sex of the two embryos. There are good grounds for rejecting fetal sex selection in general, as discussed above, but are there any valid reasons for not permitting a couple in these circumstances to choose between the healthy embryos on the basis of sex or other non-disease traits for which testing might become possible—such as physical or even mental characteristics? If it were permitted for those utilizing PGD because of an infertility problem to select between embryos on the basis of such traits, would the same be permitted for those who had no fertility problem but simply wished to select the characteristics of their child?

PGD can be seen as being located part of the way down the slippery slope to the "designer baby". While the burdensome nature of IVF technology and its costliness make it unlikely that many couples would wish to use it now, testing for non-disease traits may become available and the technology is likely to improve—to be less burdensome—so it is probably worth trying to arrive at a resolution of these problems now. There is no reason why a couple wishing to use such services would consult a clinical geneticist, so in that sense it is not a problem for "us"—but this area of "reprogenetics" lies so close to clinical genetics that we are bound to be affected by these developments.

One temporary resolution is to treat PGD for disease, for sex selection and for selection on the basis of non-disease traits as distinct.

1. PGD for disease presents fewer ethical problems than prenatal diagnosis and selective pregnancy termination and appears a reasonable option for those undergoing infertility treatment or with strong objections to pregnancy termination.
2. PGD for sex selection is disrespectful to women and should not be performed (see the discussion about prenatal diagnosis and sex selection above).
3. PGD for non-disease traits is not available at present because of technical limitations, and testing for socially important characteristics may not become available for many years, if ever. PGD on these grounds would not be part of the work of a clinical geneticist and should probably not be practiced at all. Such a development would be widely understood as the first move towards a brave new world of genetically manipulated children.

The cloning of Dolly the sheep, announced in 1997, attracted acclaim and simultaneously also enormous concern. Human reproductive cloning has not yet been performed, but the world was compelled to acknowledge that it may be technically possible. In the context of clinical genetics, when might our patients seek reproductive cloning? What should our response be if/when such cloning becomes feasible?

Individuals who cannot have their own children because of infertility may find cloning an attractive option. Couples in which one partner has a dominant genetic disorder, or carries a sex-linked disorder or a chromosome rearrangement that could lead to problems with the child, may choose to clone the fertile, healthy or non-carrier partner rather than run the risk of transmitting the condition to an affected child. It is difficult to envisage how the technology, or its public acceptance, will develop—but let us hope that biotechnology will be able to assist in such family scenarios before human cloning becomes available, so that the incentive to work for human reproductive cloning is lessened.

There would be very real concerns about the biological welfare of children born after cloning of an adult human because of cell aging effects, including telomere shortening and the accumulation of mitochondrial and other mutations. They may also suffer from infertility and this could be a special problem for infertile males with Y-chromosome microdeletions. There would also be major concerns about the psychological welfare of cloned adult individuals; the children would find themselves uncannily similar to their mother or father when she/he was a child. The climate of expectations likely to surround these children in at least some families could well cause serious disturbances in their emotional development. If such children are born, however, it will be of the greatest importance to monitor their health and their emotional state, but without excessive intrusion into their family lives.

BIBLIOGRAPHY AND FURTHER READING

GENERAL

Andrews LB, Fullerton JE, Holtzman NA, Motulsky AG (eds) (1994) Assessing Genetic Risks: Implications for Health Policy. National Academy Press Washington, DC

Annas GJ, Elias S (1992) Gene Mapping: Using Law and Ethics as Guides. Oxford University Press, Oxford

Baumiller RC, Comley S, Cunningham G et al. (1996) Code of ethical principles for genetics professionals. Am J Med Genet 65:177–178

Baumiller RC, Comley S, Cunningham G et al. (1996) Code of ethical principles for genetics professionals: An explication. Am J Med Genet 65:179–183

Bosk CL (1992) All God's Mistakes: Genetic Counseling in a Pediatric Hospital. University of Chicago Press, Chicago

British Medical Association (1998) Human Genetics: Choice and responsibility. Oxford University Press, Oxford

Brock SC (1995) Narrative and medical genetics: On ethics and therapeutics. Qualitative Health Research 5:150–168

Burley J (ed) (1998) The Genetic Revolution and Human Rights. The Oxford Amnesty Lectures. Oxford University Press, Oxford

Carson RA, Rothstein MA (eds) (1999) Behavioral Genetics. Johns Hopkins University Press,

Chambers T (1999) The Fiction of Bioethics (Cases as Literary Texts). Routledge, NY

Clarke A (ed) (1994) Genetic Counselling: Practice and Principles. Routledge, London

Clarke A (ed) (1998) Genetic Testing of Children. Bios Scientific Publishers, Oxford

Clarke A, Parsons EP (eds) (1997) Culture, Kinship and Genes. Macmillan, London

Clegg J (2000) Beyond ethical individualism. J Intellectual Disability Research 44:1–11

Duster T (1990) Backdoor to Eugenics. Routledge, London

Gert B, Berger EM, Cahill GF et al. (1996) Morality and the New Genetics. A Guide for Students and Health Care Providers. Jones and Bartlett, Sudbury, Mass

Harper PS, Clarke AJ (1997) Genetics, Society and Clinical Practice. Bios Scientific Publishers, Oxford

Kitcher P (1996) The Lives to Come: the Genetic Revolution and Human Possibilities. Penguin Books, London

Lewontin RC (1991) The Doctrine of DNA: Biology as Ideology. Penguin Books, London

Maclean A (1993) The Elimination of Morality. Reflections on Utilitarianism and Bioethics. Routledge, London

Marteau TM, Richards MPM (eds) (1996) The Troubled Helix: Social and Psychological Implications of the New Human Genetics. Cambridge University Press, Cambridge

Nelkin D, Lindee MS (1995) The DNA Mystique: The Gene as a Cultural Icon. WH Freeman, NY

Nuffield Council on Bioethics (1993) Genetic Screening: Ethical Issues. Nuffield Council on Bioethics, London

Nuffield Council on Bioethics (1998) Mental disorders and genetics: the ethical context. Nuffield Council on Bioethics, London

Rifkin J (1998) The Biotech Century. The coming age of genetic commerce. Victor Gollancz, London

Rose S (1997) Lifelines. Biology, Freedom, Determinism Penguin Books, London

Rothman BK (1988) The Tentative Pregnancy. Pandora, London

Royal College of Physicians' Committees on Clinical Genetics and on Ethical Issues in Medicine (1991) Ethical Issues in Clinical Genetics. Royal College of Physicians of London, London

Sarkar S (1998) Genetics and Reductionism. Cambridge University Press, Cambridge

Thompson AK, Chadwick RF (1999) Genetic Information: Acquisition, Access and Control. Kluwer Academic/Plenum, New York

Wilkie T (1993) Perilous Knowledge: the Human Genome Project and its Implications. Faber and Faber, London

Williamson R, Savulescu J (eds) (1999) Journal of Medical Ethics 25 (2):75–214

CARRIER SCREENING

Bekker H, Modell M, Denniss G et al. (1993) Uptake of cystic fibrosis testing in primary care: Supply push or demand pull? BMJ 306:1584–1586

Evers-Kiebooms G, Denayer L, Welkenhuysen M et al. (1994) A stigmatising effect of the carrier status for cystic fibrosis? Clin Genet 46:336–343

Fanos JH, Johnson JP (1995) Perception of carrier status by cystic fibrosis siblings. Am J Hum Genet 57:431–438

Fanos JH, Johnson JP (1995) Barriers to carrier testing for adult cystic fibrosis sibs: The importance of not knowing. Am J Med Genet 59:85–91

Loeben GL, Marteau TM, Wilfond BS (1998) Mixed messages: Presentation of information in cystic fibrosis-screening pamphlets. Am J Hum Genet 63:1181–1189

Marteau TM, van Duijn M, Ellis I (1992) Effects of genetic screening on perceptions of health. J Med Genet 29:24–26

Marteau TM, Michie S, Miedzybrodzka ZH, Allanson A (1999) Incorrect recall of residual risk three years after carrier screening for cystic fibrosis: A comparison of two-step and couple screening. Am J Obstet & Gynecol 181:165–169

National Institutes of Health (1997) NIH consensus statement: Genetic testing for cystic fibrosis. NIH Consensus Statement: volume 15 (4)

Zeesman S, Clow CL, Cartier L, Scriver CR (1984) A private view of heterozygosity: Eight-year follow-up study on carriers of the Tay-Sachs gene detected by high school screening in Montreal. Am J Med Genet 18:769–778

CONFIDENTIALITY: PRIVACY WITHIN THE FAMILY

American Society of Human Genetics (1998) ASHG statement: Professional disclosure of familial genetic information. Am J Hum Genet 62:474–483

Manjoney DM, McKegney FP (1978) Individual and family coping with polycystic kidney disease: The harvest of denial. Intl J Psychiatry in Medicine 9:19–31

Somerville A, English V (1999) Genetic privacy: Orthodoxy or oxymoron? J Med Ethics 25:144–150

Wilcke JTR, Seersholm N, Kok-Jensen A, Dirksen A (1999) Transmitting genetic risk information in families: Attitudes about disclosing the identity of relatives. Am J Hum Genet 65:902–909

(For discussion see also Nuffield Council 1993 Royal College of Physicians 1991, BMA 1998 and Clarke—chapter 10, pp 149–164, in Harper and Clarke, 1997 (see under "General".)

CONFIDENTIALITY: THIRD PARTIES

Geller LN, Alper JS, Billings PR et al. (1996) Individual, family and societal dimensions of genetic discrimination. Science and Engineering Ethics 2:71–88

Light DW (1992) The practice and ethics of risk-related health insurance. J Am Med Assoc 267:2503–2508

Rothenberg K, Fuller B, Rothstein M et al. (1997) Genetic information and the workplace: legislative approaches and challenges. Science 275:1755–1757

Zick CD, Smith KR, Mayer RN, Botkin JR (2000) Genetic testing, adverse selection and the demand for life insurance. Am J Med Genet 93:29–39

CROSS-CULTURAL ISSUES

Clarke A, Parsons EP (eds) (1997) Culture, Kinship and Genes Macmillan, London

Hepper F (1999) "A woman's heaven is at her husband's feet"? The dilemmas for a community learning disability team posed by the arranged marriage of a Bangladeshi client with intellectual disability. J Intellect Disability Research 43:558–561

DISABILITY

Asch A (1999) Prenatal diagnosis and selective abortion: A challenge to practice and policy. Am J Public Health 89:1649–1657

Diesfeld K (1999) International ethical safeguards: Genetics and people with learning disabilities. Disability & Society 14:21–36

Middleton A, Hewison J, Mueller RF (1998) Attitudes of deaf adults toward genetic testing for hereditary deafness. Am J Hum Genet 63:1175–1180

Parens E, Asch A (1999) The disability rights critique of prenatal genetic testing. Special Supplement to the Hastings Center Report, Sept/Oct 1999 S1-S21

Shakespeare T (1998) Eugenics, genetics and disability equality. Disability and Society 13:665–682

DUTY TO RECONTACT

Fitzpatrick JL, Hahn C, Costa T, Huggins MJ (1999) The duty to recontact: Attitudes of genetics service providers. Am J Hum Genet 64:852–860

Sharpe NF (2000) The duty to recontact: Benefit and harm. Am J Hum Genet 65:1201–1204

GENES, GENETICIZATION AND SOCIETY

Beckwith J (1997) The responsibility of scientists in the genetics and race controversies. In Smith E, Sapp W (eds): Plain Talk About The Human Genome Project. Tuskegee University, Tuskegee, pp 83-94

Carson RA, Rothstein MA (eds.) (1999) Behavioural Genetics. Johns Hopkins University Press,

Conrad P (1999) A mirage of genes. Sociology of Health & Illness 21:228–241

Hattersley AT, Tooke JE (1999) The fetal insulin hypothesis: An alternative explanation of the association of low birthweight with diabetes and vascular disease. Lancet 353:1789–1792

Koch L, Stemerding D (1994) The sociology of entrenchment: A cystic fibrosis test for everyone? Soc Sci Med 39:1211–1220

Lippman A (1993) Worrying—and worrying about—the geneticization of reproduction and health. In Basen G, Eichler M, Lippman A, eds.: Misconceptions. Voyageur Publishing, Quebec, Vol 1, pp 39–65

McDermott R (1998) Ethics, epidemiology and the thrifty gene: Biological determinism as a health hazard. Soc Sci Med 47:1189–1195

Nelkin D (1996) The social dynamics of genetic testing: The case of fragile-X. Med Anthrop Quart 10:537–550

Nazroo JY (1998) Genetic, cultural or socio-economic vulnerability? Explaining ethnic inequalities in health. Sociology of Health & Illness 20:710–730

Rollo CD (1994) Phenotypes. Chapman and Hall,

Salthe S (1993) Development and Evolution. Bradford Books, MIT Press,

GENETIC TESTING OF CHILDREN

Alderson P (1993) Children's consent to surgery. Open University Press, Buckingham

Binedell J, Soldan JR, Scourfield J, Harper PS (1996) Huntington's disease predictive testing: The case for an assessment approach to requests from adolescents. J Med Genet 33:912–918

Clarke A (1997) Chapter 2, pp 15–29, in Harper and Clarke, 1997 (see under "General")

Clarke A (ed) (1998) Genetic Testing of Children. Bios Scientific Publishers, Oxford

Clinical Genetic Society (1994) Report of the Working Party on the Genetic Testing of Children. J Med Genet 31:785–797

Fanos JH, Gatti RA (1999) A mark on the arm: Myths of carrier status in sibs of individuals with ataxia-telangiectasia. Am J Med Genet 86:338–346

Fanos JH, Mackintosh M-A (1999) Never again joy without sorrow: The effect on parents of a child with ataxia-tèlangiectasia. Am J Med Genet 87:413–419

Harper PS, Clarke A (1990) Should we test children for "adult" genetic diseases? Lancet 335:1205–1206

Järvinen O (2000) Genetic carrier testing in childhood. A retrospective study of psychosocial consequences, attitudes, and comprehension of the test results. Doctoral thesis, University of Helsinki

Wertz DC, Fanos JH, Reilly PR (1994) Genetic testing for children and adolescents: Who decides? J Am Med Assoc 272:875–881

GOALS AND OUTCOMES OF GENETIC SERVICES

Berkenstadt M, Shiloh S, Barkai G et al. (1999) Perceived personal control (PPC): A new concept in measuring outcome of genetic counselling. Am J Med Genet 82:53–59

Clarke A (1997) Chapter 12, pp 165–178, in Harper and Clarke, 1997 (see under "General")

Fryer AE, Cheese IAF Lister (on behalf of the College's Clinical Genetics Committee) (1998) Clinical genetic services: Activity, outcome, effectiveness and quality. Royal College of Physicians of London, London

Kessler S (1989) Psychological aspects of genetic counselling VI. A critical review of the literature dealing with education and reproduction. Am J Med Genet 34:340–353

Michie S, Marteau TM, Bobrow M (1997) Genetic counselling: The psychological impact of meeting patients' expectations. J Med Genet 34:237–241

Shiloh S, Sagi M (1989) Effect of framing on the perception of genetic risk recurrence risks. Am J Med Genet 33:130–135

HISTORICAL CONTEXT

Kevles D (1986) In the Name of Eugenics. Knopf, and Harmondsworth, NY

Mazumdar PMH (1992) Eugenics, Human Genetics and Human Failings. The Eugenics Society, its Sources and its Critics in Britain. Routledge, London

Müller-Hill B (1988) Murderous Science. Oxford University Press, Oxford
Proctor RN (1988) Racial Hygiene. Medicine under the Nazis. Cambridge, Mass and Harvard University Press,

HUMAN GENOME DIVERSITY, HUMAN (PRE)HISTORY AND "RACE"

Beckwith J (1997) The responsibility of scientists in the genetics and race controversies. In Smith E, Sapp W (eds.): Plain Talk About The Human Genome Project. Tuskegee University, Tuskegee, pp. 83–94

Foster MW, Sharp RR, Freeman WL et al. (1999) The role of community review in evaluating the risks of human genetic variation research. Am J Hum Genet 64:1719–1727

Juengst ET (1998) Group identity and human diversity: Keeping biology straight from culture. Am J Hum Genet 63:673–677

Lock M (1994) Interrogating the human genome diversity project. Soc Sci Med 39:603–606

Schibeci R, Barns I, Shaw R, Davison A (1999) Genetic medicine: An experiment in community-expert interaction. J Med Ethics 25:335–339

Weijer C, Goldsand G, Emanuel EJ (1999) Protecting communities in research: current guidelines and limits of extrapolation. Nat Genet 23:275–280

NAMING OF SYNDROMES

Armstrong D, Michie S, Marteau TM (1998) Revealed identity: A study of the process of genetic counselling. Soc Sci Med 47:1653–1658

Harper PS (1997) The naming of enetic syndromes and unethical activities. The case of Hallervordern and Spatz. Chapter 16, pp 221–225 in Harper and Clarke, 1997 (see under "General")

Schrander-Stumpel CTRM (1998) What's in a name? Am J Med Genet 79:228

Zola IK (1993) Self, identity and the naming question: Reflections on the language of disability. Soc Sci Med 36:167–173

NON-DIRECTIVENESS IN GENETIC COUNSELING

Barnard D (1985) Unsung questions of medical ethics. Soc Sci Med 21:243–249

Clarke A (1991) Is non-directive genetic counselling possible? Lancet 338:998–1001

Clarke A (1997) Chapter 13, pp 179–200 in Harper and Clarke, 1997 (see under "General")

Elwyn G, Gray J, Clarke A (2000) Shared decision making and non-directiveness in genetic counselling. J Med Genet 37:135–138

Kessler S (1997) Psychological aspects of genetic counselling XI Nondirectiveness revisited. Am J Med Genet 72:164–171

Wolff G, Jung C (1995) Nondirectiveness and genetic counselling. J Genet Counseling 4:3–25

(See also Gert et al. 1996, under "General").

PHARMACOGENETICS AND GENETIC SUSCEPTIBILITY SCREENING

Clarke A (1997) The genetic dissection of multifactorial disease. Chapter 7, pp 93–106 in Harper and Clarke, 1997 (see under General)

Lerman C, Gold K, Audrain J et al. (1997) Incorporating biomarkers of exposure and genetic susceptibility into smoking cessation treatment: Effects on smoking-related cognitions, emotions and behaviour change. Health Psychology 16:87–99

Roses AD (2000) Pharmacogenetics and future drug development and delivery. Lancet 355:1358–1361

Senior V, Marteau TM, Peters TJ (1999) Will genetic testing for predisposition for disease result in fatalism? A qualitative study of parents' responses to neonatal screening for familial hypercholesterolaemia. Soc Sci Med 48:1857–1860

Welch HG, Burke W (1998) Uncertainties in genetic testing for chronic disease. JAMA 280:1525–1527

Wolf CR, Smith G, Smith RL (2000) Pharmacogenetics. BMJ 320:987–990

PREDICTIVE GENETIC TESTING

Binedell J, Soldan J, Harper PS (1998) Predictive testing for Huntington's disease II Qualitative findings from a study of uptake in South Wales. Clinical Genetics 54:489–496

Codori A-M, Brandt J (1994) Psychological costs and benefits of predictive testing for Huntington's disease. Am J Med Genet (Neuropsychiatric Genetics) 54:174–184

DudokdeWit AC, Tibben A, Duivenvoorden HJ et al. and the Rotterdam/Leiden Genetics Workgroup (1998) Distress in individuals facing predictive DNA testing for autosomal dominant late-onset disorders: comparing questionnaire results with in-depth interviews. Am J Med Genet 75:62–74

Grosfeld FJM, Lips CJM, Beemer FA et al. (2000) Distress in MEN2 family members and partners prior to DNA test disclosure. Am J Med Genet 91:1–7

Harper PS (1997) chapter 3, pp 31–48 in Harper and Clarke, 1997 (see under "General")

Huggins M, Bloch M, Wiggins S et al. (1992) Predictive testing for Huntington disease in Canada: adverse effects and unexpected results in those receiving a decreased risk. Am J Med Genet 42:508–515

Sobel SK, Cowan DB (2000) Impact of genetic testing for Huntington disease on the family system. Am J Med Genet 90:49–59

PRENATAL GENETIC SCREENING

Abramsky L, Chapple J (eds) (1994) Prenatal Diagnosis: the Human Side. Chapman and Hall, London

Bernhardt BA, Geller G, Doksum T et al. (1998) Prenatal genetic testing: Content of discussions between obstetric providers and pregnant women. Obstet Gynecol 91:648–655

Browner CH, Preloran HM, Cox SJ (1999) Ethnicity, bioethics and prenatal diagnosis: The amniocentesis decisions of Mexican-origin women and their partners. Am J Public Health 89:1658–1666

Chitty LS, Barnes CA, Berry C (1996) Continuing with pregnancy after a diagnosis of lethal abnormality: Experience of five couples and recommendations for management. BMJ 313:478–480

Green J (1990) Calming or Harming: A critical review of psychological effects of fetal diagnosis on pregnant women. Galton Institute Occasional Papers, Second Series, No. 2. Galton Institute, London

Lippman A (1991) Prenatal genetic testing. Constructing needs and reinforcing inequities. Am J Law & Medicine 17:15–50. Reprinted in Clarke (ed) 1994 (see under "General")

Press N, Browner CH (1997) Why women say yes to prenatal diagnosis. Soc Sci Med 45:979–989

Rapp R (1988) Chromosomes and communication: The discourse of genetic counselling. Med Anthrop Quart (new series) 2:143–157

Rothman BK (1988) The Tentative Pregnancy. Pandora, London

REPRODUCTIVE TECHNOLOGIES AND CLONING

Baird PA (1999) Cloning of animals and humans: What should the policy response be? Perspectives in Biology and Medicine 42:179–194

Pergament E, Bonnicksen A (1994) Preimplantation genetics: A case for prospective action. Am J Med Genet 52:151–157

Shenfield F (ed) (1998) Societal, medical and ethical implications of cloning. Proceedings of a workshop held at the Royal Society, London, November 1997. European Communities, Luxembourg

Wellcome Trust's Medicine In Society Programme (1998) Public Perspectives on Human Cloning. Wellcome Trust, London

RESEARCH IN HUMAN GENETICS

American College of Medical Genetics (1995) Statement on storage and use of genetic materials. Am J Hum Genet 57:1499–1500

American Society of Human Genetics (1996) Statement on informed consent for genetic research. Am J Hum Genet 59:471–474

Annas GJ (2000) The Icelandic healthcare database and informed consent. New Eng J Med 342:1827–1833

Chadwick R (1999) The Icelandic database—do modern times need modern sagas? BMJ 319:441–444

Clayton EW, Steinberg KK, Khoury MJ (1995) Consensus statement: Informed consent for genetic research on stored tissue samples. JAMA 274:1786–1792

Knoppers BM (1999) Status, sale and patenting of human genetic material: An international survey. Nat Genet 22:23–26

Marshal E (1997) Whose DNA is it anyway? Science 278:564–567

Wilcox AJ, Taylor JA, Sharp RR, London SJ (1999) Genetic determinism and the overprotection of human subjects. Nat Genet 21:362

Legal issues in genetic medicine

Philip Reilly

34

Introduction

From a medical perspective, genetic data may be characterized in two ways: information that has diagnostic or predictive value about one's health or the health of one's children or relatives, and information that determines identity or biologic relationship. Advances in our understanding of the human genome are having and will continue to have a major impact in both arenas. After providing some general comments on the broad impact of genetics on society, I shall focus on the legal issues raised by its impact on the practice of medicine.

With increasing frequency, advances in clinical genetic testing are permitting physicians to discern critical facts about health that are relevant to the patient and, by inference, to one or more relatives. Thus, genetic diagnostic testing challenges clinicians to reconsider one of the cornerstones of medicine: the principle of confidentiality. As genetic testing becomes routine in medicine, it is likely to reshape the contours of doctor-patient confidentiality. For example, the rules governing disclosures to third parties may eventually be amended to accommodate a clinician's need to make limited disclosures to third parties.

The decision to offer genetic testing to an individual may have serious implications for the manner in which others perceive that individual. During the 1990s a sustained discourse emerged concerning the need to be vigilant in preventing genetic discrimination, defined here as actions taken by a social institution such as an insurance company, an employer or a school, in response to genetic information that harms an individual's interests. In the United States during the 1990s fears about genetic discrimination stimulated much legislation. At the close of 1999 about 30 states

had laws that generally prohibit health insurers from using genetic information in underwriting (Hall, 1999). At the federal level, the Health Insurance Portability and Accountability Act (1996) prohibits group health insurers from denying access to coverage on the basis of genetic information. In the United Kingdom a report to the Parliament (Science and Technology Select Committee, 1995) addressed concerns of genetic discrimination. Probably because health care in the United Kingdom is provided through a National Health Service, the public there has not been as concerned as have citizens in the United States about this issue. A few states have sought to regulate the use of genetic information in life and other kinds of insurance, with little impact.

For the foreseeable future advances in carrier screening and prenatal diagnosis will outpace the introduction of new therapies. For that reason elective abortion will remain an important option in obstetrics. In that regard the political struggle to limit or overturn Roe v. Wade (1973), the United States Supreme Court opinion that held that the constitutional right to privacy included a woman's right to terminate a pregnancy, is relevant. Although political efforts in the United States to reverse the holding in Roe v. Wade will not succeed, in many states there are those who persist in attempting to pass laws that interpret that decision as narrowly as possible. As most of these bills focus on requiring teenagers to inform parents about their decision to seek an abortion or (more recently) on banning certain techniques used in performing late abortions, they do not much effect women who are seeking termination on genetic grounds. Far more problematic is the fact that many states will not fund elective abortions for poor people.

Progress in developing somatic cell gene therapy, which looked so promising in the early 1990s, has been slower than some have anticipated. The death of Jesse Gelsinger while participating in a gene therapy experiment at the University of Pennsylvania in 1999 had a major impact at NIH on the regulatory approach to such research. Reports of other deaths and injuries during the course of gene therapy trials virtually guarantees that institutional Review Boards (IRBs) will intensely scrutinize and monitor gene therapy research over the next few years. Late in the 1990s, before the unfortunate events just noted, a few scientists were asserting that germ-line gene therapy might not be so far in the future. That possibility has now receded and there is little basis to anticipate that regulatory bodies will permit experiments with humans in that field in the next decade.

Advances in molecular biology have revolutionized the approach to drug development in the pharmaceutical industry and to crop deployment in agriculture. But the public reaction to genetically modified food, especially in Europe, has been dramatically negative (Grove-White et al., 1997). Although the United States Department of Agriculture approved its first genetically engineered food (a tomato with a transgene that affected ripening and provided a much longer shelf life) in 1994 and favorably reviewed more than 50 other products in the ensuing five years, the public outcry that developed in 1999 ensures that there will be much more thorough review of new products and new rules that require foods containing genetically engineered components to be so labeled. The reaction to the large-scale application of genetic engineering to our food recalls the public controversy over environmental release of genetically engineered bacteria that was a hot political topic in the United States in the mid-1970s (Berg et al., 1974). This concern will ultimately be resolved in the legislatures, the courts, and the marketplace. The debate over the safety of such products is tangential to medicolegal concerns arising out of genetic screening, genetic testing, genetic counseling, and genetic research, but it is well for the clinical geneticist to remain familiar with them.

The results of genetic testing may greatly alter the reproductive plans of an individual or a couple. In addition to avoidance of pregnancy, prenatal diagnosis and selective abortion and artificial insemination by donor, in vitro fertilization, and surrogate motherhood are options that some couples burdened with substantial genetic risks in childbearing now consider. Preimplantation embryo genetic testing is gradually emerging as an alternative to prenatal testing and selective abortion (Grifo et al., 1994). However, this technology is not yet perfected, and there have been several lawsuits filed after the birth of a child with a genetic disorder to parents who were told that an unaffected embryo had been placed in the woman. These

technologies have raised a host of ethical and legal questions that are beyond the scope of this chapter, but about which there is ample literature. Among the most prominent are reports issued by a committee in Australia (Victoria, 1984), the Warnock Commission Report (United Kingdom, 1984), the Ontario Law Reform Commission Report (1985) produced in Canada (Elias and Annas, 1987) and the report of the Ethics Committee of the American Fertility Society (1990).

Particularly because of the work done by the Home Office in the United Kingdom, DNA-based testing has had a dramatic impact on the forensic sciences. It has altered the investigation of crimes of violence, it has fostered the rise of DNA felon data banks (McEwen and Reilly, 1994), and it has virtually ended once common paternity litigation. In the United States in 1990 only one state had a law requiring that samples be taken from certain convicted felons for (non-DNA based) identity typing and storage. In 2000 every state in the United States had enacted a DNA felon data banking law and all were using or planning to use a set of probes developed by the Federal Bureau of Investigation. While this topic is beyond the scope of this chapter, it should be noted that DNA felon data banking may significantly improve our ability to apprehend violent offenders and to exonerate quickly the wrongfully accused (Sheck et al., 1999). Also, the rapid resolution of paternity disputes can improve the economic well being of hundreds of thousands of children by enhancing the efficiency with which the social welfare system forces fathers to support their offspring.

Who should have access to genetic information?

The most important ethical and legal issue that arises from our growing power to read the genetic code is summarized in two closely related questions: 1) who should have access to genetic information? and 2) for what purposes may such information be used? The responses that a society develops will reflect the underlying dimensions of the individual's right of privacy which varies widely around the globe. In the United States, the United Kingdom, Canada, the European Community, and Australia, societal discussion of the need to develop rules on the acquisition, storage, and control of genetic information is well advanced (Nuffield Council on Bioethics, 1993). Many private and public bodies, ranging from the World Health Organization (Wertz et al., 1995) to local church groups, have published relevant guidelines. In the late 1990s there was global discussion concerning the decision by the government of Iceland to enact a law that gave exclusive access in the nation's health data base to DeCode Genetics, Inc, an Icelandic biotech company (Jonatansson, 2000). The debate helped crystallize privacy issues.

With the emergence of efforts to deliver genetic information and provide genetic services over the internet, there will be a need for new standards concerning technical support to physicians and counseling patients. Although the law of electronic medical privacy is in its infancy, it is likely that current prohibitions concerning the practice of medicine across state lines in cyberspace will disappear.

Although there has been much interest in regulating the uses of genetic information, until recently there has been relatively little effort to regulate the development and deployment of genetic tests. In the United States in 2000, genetic tests that are performed using manufactured kits are subject to approval by the Food and Drug Administration (FDA). However, most DNA based tests are performed by labs with reagents that are prepared in house. Under the so-called "home brew" exception, such tests currently are not subjected to FDA review (Malinowski and Blatt, 1997). the Secretary's Advisory Committee on Genetic Testing (2000) will issue a report that will strongly advocate for increased pre-market oversight of the development of genetic tests. Whether the report will generate statutory or regulatory change is less certain. At the state level only New York and California are likely to demonstrate any sustained interest in regulating the deployment of genetic tests.

Depending on the particular context, spouses, parents, children, siblings, and other relatives may have an interest in knowing genetic facts about an individual. For example, when a physician determines that a child is suffering from an X-linked genetic disorder, that information may be extremely important to the reproductive planning of the child's maternal aunts. Should the child's parents refuse to communicate with relatives, are there circumstances that would justify the decision by the physician to warn relatives? The common law expectation that the physician-patient encounter will be conducted in confidence offers some guidance about how to regulate the flow of genetic information within families, but novel questions will challenge established rules and lead to nuanced exceptions.

Informed consent

The decision-making process that precedes genetic testing is governed by the doctrine of informed consent, derived from case law and medical literature that developed largely in the United States since the 1960s (President's Commission for the Study of Ethical Problems in Medicine and Biomedical and Behavioral Research, 1983). The term *informed consent* first appeared in the case law in 1957 (Salgo v. Leland Stanford Jr. Univ. Bd. of Trustees), and the concept was developed at length three years later by the Supreme Court of Kansas (Natanson v. Kline, 1960). Over the years the courts have steadily enlarged the duty of the physician to make material disclosures of fact to enable the patient to make an informed choice (Canterbury v. Spence, 1972; Cobbs v. Grant, 1972).

In the context of genetic testing the physician should, at a minimum, inform the individual about the nature and purpose of the test, any significant risks associated with it, the potential consequences of deciding not to be tested, and foreseeable problems that may arise from undergoing the procedure or learning the result (Canterbury v. Spence, 1972). The individual should also be informed that test results could discern that assumed biologic relationships are incorrect (e.g., non-paternity or undisclosed adoption). It may eventually become a standard practice to inform persons that the presymptomatic diagnosis of disease or recognition of increased risk for a serious disorder could compromise access to health and life insurance and restrict employment opportunities (Billings et al., 1992). It is also appropriate, if relevant, to determine whether an individual has any objection to the subsequent use of a tissue sample for research purposes and whether or not he or she wishes to be contacted about potentially relevant results derived from such research (Reilly et al., 1997).

The question of when one individual may consent to genetic testing on behalf of another will become more important as predictive genetic testing proliferates. There is a well-established body of case law concerning the determination of competency (essentially, a judicial decision that turns on the evaluation of expert testimony concerning the intellectual and emotional capacity of the individual who is the subject of the proceeding) among impaired adults, which is key to the decision about whether or not to appoint a guardian.

In Europe and the United States there is a general societal consensus that parents are the appropriate decision makers for the health needs of their children. As the United States Supreme Court wrote, "The law's concept of the family rests on a presumption that parents possess what a child lacks in maturity, experience, and capacity or judgment required for making life's difficult decisions" (Parham v. J.R., 1979). In regard to predictive genetic testing in children, even where there is no clear clinical benefit, the presumption should be that the parents are acting in the best interests of the child. However, should a physician be firmly convinced that genetic testing is more likely to harm than help the child, he should consider dissuading the parents, and he certainly has the right to refuse to order the test. For example, most clinicians will not order a test for Huntington disease in non-symptomatic, at risk persons under the age of 18 (Hugging et al., 1990). The majority view is that testing should be deferred (if clinically possible) until the child reaches an age when he or she can make the decision (Wertz et al., 1994).

In both the United States and Europe there is a definite trend to recognize the right of adolescents to seek medical testing and treatment. In the United Kingdom the Family Law Reform Act of 1969 specifically permits persons 16 years of age to consent to medical treatment. A case decided in the House of Lords in 1986 (Nuffield Council on Bioethics, 1993) recognized that even younger persons had the right to consent to treatment if they had the capacity to understand the alternatives placed before them.

Confidentiality

There is a strong presumption in clinical practice that medical information should be regarded as confidential. Nonetheless, many states have laws that require disclosure by physicians in a variety of circumstances, usually in connection with highly contagious diseases. Except for a few statutes relating to the reporting of birth defects and the results of sickle cell anemia testing, these laws were not written with consideration of the familial nature of genetic information. If individuals think that they have been harmed by the disclosure of genetic information, they could sue for breach of an implied promise of confidentiality.

Physicians and genetic counselors frequently acquire genetic information from one patient that may be important to other family members. Is there a right, or even an obligation, to disseminate such information to a patient's relatives despite the general presumption of confidentiality over the objection of the prebend? Disclosure of genetic data within families does not typically expose patients to the type or degree of harm that the common law of privacy evolved to protect, and the potential benefit of the information to a relative may be substantial. Nevertheless, in some situations families may be sundered by the emotional impact of information derived from a genetic test. Obviously, any warning to third parties should be undertaken with care. Probably the most common problem will arise when a patient refuses to alert relatives to a risk that

may be directly inferred from the results of a genetic test. The inadvertent discovery of nonpaternity or the acknowledgment of nonpaternity or secret adoption may also trigger difficult disclosure issues.

Although it is fading in clinical importance, linkage testing, when it is necessary, is a cooperative effort. When a key relative refuses to undergo testing he or she may, in effect, block other family members from learning whether they are likely or unlikely to be at risk. Do those who wish to be tested have any recourse? Currently, there is no legal right to compel a reluctant relative to undergo testing. Even if the disease in question is a life-threatening disorder for which preventive therapy is available, it is unlikely that a court would order a person to provide a blood sample for testing to benefit a relative.

What are the dimensions of a physician's rights and obligations when he or she becomes aware of data that could be important to the health or reproductive plans of a patient's relatives? May a physician ever communicate information to other relatives without the consent of his patient? Are there circumstances when he ought to do so? In the United States two blue ribbon panels have considered this question: the Committee for the Study of Inborn Errors of Metabolism (1975) convened by the National Academy of Sciences concluded that the privacy right was paramount and that there were no circumstances under which it should be subordinated to other interests, however compelling. Eight years later, the President's Commission for the Study of Ethical Problems in Medicine and Biomedical and Behavioral Sciences (1983) took a different position. It concluded that:

> A professional's ethical duty of confidentiality to an immediate patient or client can be overridden only if several conditions are satisfied: (1) reasonable efforts to elicit voluntary consent to disclosure have failed, (2) there is a high probability both that harm will occur if the information is withheld and that the disclosed information will actually be used to avert harm, (3) the harm that identifiable individuals would suffer would be serious, and (4) appropriate precautions are taken to ensure that only the genetic information needed for diagnosis and/or treatment of the disease in question is disclosed.

A report by a committee convened by the Institute of Medicine (Andrews et al., 1994) reiterated this view. In the United Kingdom the Nuffield Council on Bioethics (1993) also concluded that there are circumstances in which it is appropriate for a physician to override a patient's request not to share genetic data with other family members. As yet there have been no lawsuits arising out of a decision by a physician to warn relatives of a patient, despite the patient's express instructions not to alert them.

Physicians who believe that certain information should be shared with specific relatives should so inform persons before testing. The physician who believes that he or she has a moral obligation to warn other at-risk relatives should seek written authority to do so. He or she may then contact those relatives and ask them if they wish to be informed of the implications of a test result derived from another family member (Reilly, 1997).

The inadvertent discovery of nonpaternity poses a vexing dilemma which geneticists have been wrestling with for years. There is an informal consensus as to the appropriate course of action. In typical cases involving children with autosomal recessive disorders, the counselor meets alone with the woman to report the finding of probable non-paternity and to note that a child conceived with her husband is not likely to develop the disorder that afflicts the existing child. The woman usually acknowledges the non-paternity. In the past, this information was not shared with the husband. The rationale is that the geneticist owes a higher allegiance to protecting the integrity of the family than to being absolutely truthful with each family member. Although it may be true that disclosing to the husband might do more harm than good, this deception is not easily defended on legal grounds. If the husband presses the physician as to why a subsequent pregnancy is not at risk, the clinician should tell the truth.

Adoption poses special issues in genetic testing largely because the curtain of secrecy that has traditionally been drawn between the child and his or her biologic parents confounds the effort to share key facts. Imagine that three years after a young woman has given her infant son up for adoption it is discovered that he has Duchenne muscular dystrophy. Does the child's pediatrician have a right to attempt to alert the biologic mother to the potential risks in future pregnancies? Does that physician have a duty to warn her? Alternatively, if, 10 years after she has given her son for adoption, a birth mother develops a late-onset, dominantly inherited genetic disease, does the mother or her physician (assuming he is aware of the adopted child) have an ethical obligation to warn the boy or his adoptive parents of the risks? Although there is currently a movement to eliminate some of the legal obstacles, it remains difficult to acquire or transmit relevant medical or genetic information between the birth child and the parent through the adoption curtain. It will be necessary to develop a means to acquire family histories from the biologic parents, evaluate genetic data as it emerges, and have an effective means to transmit information when there is a compelling reason to do so. This can best be accomplished by influencing the content of adoption laws and educating the staff of appropriate social agencies (American Society of Human Genetics Social Issues Committee, 1991; American Society of Human Genetics and the American College of Medical Genetics Social, Ethical and Legal Issues Committee, 2000). The decision by a governmental agency or private service to withhold information about a child's risk for a serious genetic disorder from the adopting parents could provoke a successful lawsuit.

A dilemma arises when an identical adult twin seeks predictive testing, but his or her cotwin does not. How should the physician respond to a request for testing that will diagnose not one, but two individuals? Does he have an ethical obligation to ask the cotwin to assent to testing? May the disinclined cotwin veto the interests of the other? If the physician tests the twin who has requested the service, has he violated the privacy interest of the other? No. A physician who learns that his patient is an identical twin may wish to advise him or her to inform the cotwin about plans for testing, but his ethical obligation extends no further. The adult patient is an autonomous being with the right to discover medical data about himself.

Are there circumstances in which a clinician *must* disclose genetic data to a patient's relatives? The recognition of a possible obligation to breach confidentiality to protect third parties derives in part from a California case holding that a psychotherapist had a duty to warn a woman that the therapist's patient had threatened her life when the therapist had reason to believe that the threat would be carried out (Tarasoff v. Regents of the University of California, 1976). While this case suggests that there may be duty to warn a person about important facts that may affect health, the risk that one may someday parent a child with a genetic disease is not, in my view, analogous to the risk of an immediate, directed threat of violence. Of perhaps greater relevance is an opinion of the Supreme Court of Tennessee (Bradshaw v. Daniel, 1993) that held that a physician had a legal duty to warn the wife of one of his patients of the risk to her created by the diagnosis of Rocky Mountain spotted fever in her husband. The finding of an obligation to warn was anchored in the severity of the risk and the immediacy of the danger, both of which are more compelling than in most genetic scenarios.

In the United States two courts have considered the dimensions of the physician's duty to warn about the familial implications of a genetic diagnosis. The Florida Supreme Court held that physicians have a duty to inform patients about risks to relatives (Pate v. Threkel, 1996). A New Jersey court held that physicians have a duty to warn the relatives known to be at risk (Safer v. Estate of Pack, 1996).

Of course these two decisions do not necessarily signal an evolving legal standard.

Liability for failure to inform about a genetic test

Most of the litigation concerning genetic information has focused on whether or not a physician owed a duty to warn a patient that she was at increased risk for having a child with a serious genetic disorder. This litigation has led to the recognition of two novel causes of action known as *wrongful birth* and *wrongful life*. The notion of wrongful life arose originally in a discussion of whether a child should have legal recourse against his parents for the stigmatization of illegitimacy (Tedeschi, 1966); the concept of wrongful birth was developed from about 1975 to 1985 as a number of court decisions (Jacobs v. Theimer, 1975; Becker v. Schwartz, 1978) and law review articles explored the topic (Capon, 1979).

In the United States the vast majority of states will not permit children with birth defects or genetic disorders to bring wrongful life lawsuits against physicians that are based on an alleged failure of the physician to warn parents about a risk to childbearing that subsequently occurred (Cow v. Forum Group, Inc., 1991). On the other hand, most states will permit the parents of children with birth defects or genetic disorders to bring wrongful birth lawsuits on the theory that the physician's failure to warn deprived them of an opportunity to avert the birth of an affected child (Show, 1984). This distinction grew out of juridical concerns about the law of damages. The plaintiff in a wrongful life suit must argue that, but for the disclosure that a physician failed to make, he or she would not have been born. This requires the jury to measure the value of an impaired life (due to a serious genetic or congenital disorder) against nonexistence, a charge that many judges found impossible to deliver. Wrongful birth lawsuits, those brought by the parents of the child with the disorder, usually focus on the failure to inform. If a jury decides that such a duty exists, that the physician breached it, and that an injury occurred, then it must decide the damages. Virtually all jurisdictions that recognize wrongful birth claims permit the jury to calculate the special costs of raising a child with the particular disorder, some permit additional damages to be awarded to the parents for the related loss of economic productivity (for example, because a parent must stop work in order to care for the child), and a few permit damages to be awarded for emotional harm (Andrews, 1987).

The majority of wrongful birth actions are filed against obstetricians, not clinical geneticists. The critical question in such cases is to determine whether or not in the context of the facts the physician had a duty to alert a couple or a woman to a particular risk. The relevant body of case law permits some general statements. There is a duty to take a family history that includes questions concerning genetic disorders and developmental disabilities, to follow up with appropriate tests or referrals, and, where necessary, to alert the patient about unusual reproductive risks (Holder, 1978). Although case law varies from state to state, it is well established that a physician caring for a pregnant woman who will be 35 at delivery has a duty to warn her of the age-associated risk of carrying a fetus with Down syndrome (Becker v. Schwartz, 1978). Although there is little case law directly on point, courts are likely to recognize a duty to warn individuals of risks of bearing children with genetic diseases that are associated with ethnicity or race. Presumably, this includes warnings about Tay-Sachs disease to Ashkenazi Jews, sickle cell disease to persons of African descent, and β-thalassemia to Mediterranean peoples. Lawsuits alleging failure to warn about these disorders have been filed, but very few have reached the appellate courts, the level at which policy is set.

There has been much discussion about the duty to inform persons of northern European ancestry, but who have no family history of the disease, about carrier testing for cystic fibrosis. During the early 1990s the majority view was that despite the high prevalence of CF alleles, there should not be a duty to inform such persons about their 1 in 25 chance of being a carrier and their 1 in 2,500 chance of parenting an affected child. However, the publication in 1997 by a group convened under the auspices of NIH of a statement recommending that physicians should inform young white adults about the availability of a screening test signal the beginning of a change of practice.

In the United States a number of lawsuits have been filed that allege failure to offer MSAFP testing to a woman who later gave birth to a child with a neural tube defect. In California, where physicians are required by law to inform women about this screening test, several cases have led to large settlements. The standard of care for offering a test for Fragile X syndrome is also becoming the subject of some litigation. Given the availability, reliability, and moderate cost of the DNA-based test, it is possible that a jury would decide that by the mid-1990s the workup of a young boy with an undiagnosed developmental disability should include Fragile X testing and that failure to offer this test could lead to liability of the pediatrician and/or geneticist associated with the birth of another affected child in the family (American College of Medical Genetics, 1994b).

The availability of ever more genetic tests, some intended to diagnose only mild to moderately severe disorders, will eventually force the courts to define the limits of the duty to warn. It is likely that actions for wrongful birth will be limited to situations where the physician knew or should have known that the parents faced a significantly increased risk of bearing a child with a serious disease for which a test is available and that manifests at birth or in childhood. Physicians should always alert patients to risks associated with invasive procedures like amniocentesis and chorionic villus sampling (Centers for Disease Control and Prevention, 1995).

The maturation of clinical genetics as a medical specialty will eventually change standards of practice. The formal recognition of such experts suggests a duty among non-specialists to refer difficult cases and presumes a higher standard of performance among the specialists. This comes just as the explosion of genetic knowledge is likely to create an acute shortage of trained personnel. Given the paucity of board-certified geneticists and the fact that current training programs cannot satisfy the demand for genetic counselors and clinical geneticists, there is a pressing need to develop new approaches to training in this field. In particular, recognition by third party payers that genetic counselors should be reimbursed for their work would be helpful.

The proliferation of academic and commercial genetic testing laboratories has renewed concerns about maintaining high standards of laboratory practice (Andrews et al., 1994). The American College of Medical Genetics (1994a) has strongly supported the development of comprehensive, rigorous guidelines for clinical genetics laboratories. The report of the aforementioned Secretary's Advisory Committee on Genetic Testing (2000) may stimulate greater federal oversight of genetic testing laboratories. Should there be significant growth of commercial DNA banking, it too is likely to become the subject of regulatory oversight.

An overriding concern for testing laboratories and DNA banking facilities is the security of the information and the tissue or DNA samples. In the United States no single federal or state law or regulation comprehensively addresses this concern. In the United Kingdom the Data Protection Act of 1984 has been interpreted to apply to genetic information stored in a computer (Nuffield Council of Bioethics, 1993). Diagnostic laboratories and any other entity involved in storing DNA for clinical purposes should develop and adhere to appropriate written protocols for this activity (McEwen and Reilly, 1995).

Our growing power to discern a genetic cause for birth defects is likely to influence some lawsuits filed by the parents of children with disabilities who claim that the injuries were caused by the negligence of the obstetrician or were due to an environmental toxin. In some cases, a thorough evaluation by a clinical geneticist will demonstrate unequivocally that the child was not injured during delivery, but instead has a condition that was present from conception. Unfortunately, courts will not always appreciate the importance of the genetic evidence (Martinez v. Botsford General Hospital, 1995)

Genetic screening

Beginning in 1962 with the first law to mandate newborn screening for phenylketonuria (PKU), there has been a steady growth of state-operated, population-based, newborn screening in the western world. In the United States every state participates in newborn screening, most as mandated by state law (Andrews, 1985). The programs were originally aimed at identifying children with treatable inborn errors of metabolism, but now include screening for sickle cell anemia and congenital adrenal hyperplasia, two disorders where early diagnosis can be life-saving (Council of Regional Networks for Genetic Services, 1992).

Screening statutes and regulations typically mandate testing, but some states exempt children whose parents object on religious grounds. Only the Wyoming law specifically requires that there be informed consent (Clayton, 1992), but a few other states, notably Maryland, conduct newborn screening only if the parent has consented (Maryland Ann. Code, 1986). A report from the Institute of Medicine concluded that newborn screening can be safely and efficiently conducted on a voluntary basis. It also recommended that new tests be added to the current menu only when pilot studies have confirmed their potential benefit (Committee on Assessing Genetic Risks, 1994).

Mandatory newborn screening programs have not been constitutionally challenged, but they would probably be upheld based on the state's police power – the same power that justifies vaccination and disease reporting requirements. The courts might recognize a limited right to refuse newborn screening under the First Amendment, which protects freedom of religious belief, and in accord with the long-recognized right of parents to make decisions about rearing their children without unnecessary state interference. The likelihood that a child who is not screened will actually be affected with one of the relevant disorders (assuming there is not a positive family history) is extremely low (although rising as the number of disorders screened increases) and the risk associated with a refusal of screening is less than the risks inherent in many other decisions about children that parents routinely make on behalf of children (Clayton, 1992).

The scope of newborn screening is – under the influence of technological advance – changing rapidly. The availability of tandem mass spectrometry (TMS) as a highly efficient, low cost method of detecting infants with organic acidemias and other rare biochemical disorders led to the decision in Massachusetts early in 1999 to add medium chain acyl-coA dehydrogenase (MCAD) deficiency to the list of disorders for which testing is mandatory. Massachusetts also launched a pilot program (for which parental agreement is required) that uses TMS to screen for an additional group of disorders. In addition to Massachusetts, Pennsylvania and Washington DC have added TMS to their screening programs, and several other states, including California and New York, are planning to do so. At least one company is seeking to use TMS to sell a broad array of newborn tests. When Massachusetts issued regulations to block efforts by the company to transact business it sued for restraint of trade, but lost at trial and on appeal. The outcome suggests that state public health departments will for a time be able to delay the evolution of a private market in newborn screening. On the other hand the disparity created by the uneven deployment of TMS by state and regional screening programs could invite lawsuits by parents of children who are born with disorders in states that have not yet expanded their programs and are thus diagnosed much later than otherwise, often when they are in a metabolic crisis.

Carrier screening is intended to identify otherwise healthy persons who may, depending upon whom they marry, be at high risk for having children with a severe genetic disorder. In the United States, population-based screening programs have been undertaken to identify carriers for sickle cell anemia and Tay-Sachs disease. Since its start in the mid-1970s Tay-Sachs screening has been community-based, conducted without legislative mandate, and highly utilized by the Ashkenazi Jewish population. In contrast, sickle cell screening programs were often implemented by law. Between 1970 and 1972 twelve states and the District of Columbia enacted statutes that mandated carrier screening of black persons, usually by tying it to entry into the public schools or to obtaining a marriage license. Most state laws failed to offer pretest education or to provide access to genetic counseling. Concerns about genetic discrimination provoked a strong outcry from the black community (Reilly, 1975).

Voluntary mass screening for β-thalassemia has been conducted in Sardinia, Cyprus, and Greece. In 1975 geneticists

in Sardinia initiated a voluntary screening program that was heavily endorsed by prominent social institutions, which developed into perhaps the world's largest eugenics program. By 1991 more than 167,000 people had been tested and about 90% of carrier couples had been identified. The vast majority of at-risk couples have chosen prenatal diagnosis, and most women have aborted affected fetuses. In 15 years the number of children born with β-thalassemia in Sardinia has declined by 90% (Cao, 1991).

The cloning of the cystic fibrosis gene in 1989 sparked debate over the criteria that should be met before mass carrier screening for this common allele could be offered. In England several population-based cystic fibrosis screening programs were introduced regionally, and a large, voluntary effort was deployed quickly in Denmark. During the 1990s scores of labs in Europe launched CF carrier testing. An effort is underway there to systematize uptake of the technology. In the United States there is general agreement that population-based cystic fibrosis screening effort must be voluntary, preceded by adequate education, and anchored to the availability of competent genetic counseling (National Institutes of Health, 1990). In 1997 a group convened by NIH recommended that young adults should be informed about the availability of CF carrier testing regardless of the family history, but that has not yet become standard practice.

Prenatal genetic screening is widely practiced in the United States, Europe and elsewhere. During the 1970s obstetricians acquired sufficient experience with amniocentesis and there were such significant advances in fetal karyotyping that by about 1978 it had become standard of care to inform women who would be 35 or older at delivery about the age-associated risk of carrying a fetus with Down syndrome. The age of 35 was chosen based on studies showing that among women 34 and under who underwent amniocentesis the risk of miscarriage after the procedure was greater than the risk of bearing a child with Down syndrome. The requirement that women be informed about this risk is not imposed by statute; it reflects clinical consensus and court decisions.

The rapid growth of screening to identify women at increased risk for carrying fetuses with neural tube defects has been significantly influenced by public health, and in the United States, by legal considerations. Screening programs that measure the concentration of α-fetoprotein (AFP) in maternal serum (MS) to identify women at increased risk of having a child with anencephaly or spina bifida were first used in England and Wales in the 1970s (UK Collaborative Study, 1977). During the 1970s and 1980s live births of children with neural tube defects in

England and Wales declined by about 95% (Wald and Kennard, 1996). In the United States concerns that the test generated too many false positives, that some laboratories would perform it inaccurately, and that adequate counseling would not be available to assist women in understanding the results led the FDA to delay licensure of the reagents until 1983. In 1986 California enacted a law that requires physicians to inform women about the availability and purpose of MSAFP screening, but through 1993 only the District of Columbia had enacted a similar rule. About 70% of women in California choose to be tested (Cunningham and Kizer, 1990).

During the late 1980s in the United States MSAFP screening grew rapidly. This was partly the result of reports on successful screening experiences, but a bulletin published by the legal department of the American College of Obstetricians and Gynecologists that warned physicians of a liability risk if they did not inform their patients about the test also had a substantial impact (American College of Obstetricians and Gynecologists, 1985). The rapid growth of MSAFP testing stimulated the American Society of Human Genetics to develop a policy statement on laboratory practices (American Society of Human Genetics, 1987). California controls test quality in part by permitting only a few laboratories within the state to provide the service. Elsewhere most MSAFP tests are performed by commercial laboratories operating under standard state public health and federal Clinical Laboratory Improvement Act (CLIA) licenses.

The newest population-based prenatal screening program emerged due to the discovery in 1984 that low levels of α-fetoprotein suggest increased risk for carrying a fetus with Down syndrome (Merkatz et al., 1984). The subsequent development of a "triple marker" test (which also measures human chorionic gonadotropin and unconjugated estriol in maternal serum) led to a new approach to screening to detect fetuses with Down syndrome. Although the test could only detect about 65% of all cases of Down syndrome if it were used in every pregnancy regardless of the woman's age, and despite the significant number of false-positive results, in the United States more than half of all pregnant women are screened. In the late 1990s some labs added a fourth marker (Inhibin-A) because it appeared to improve the detection rate by 5 to 10%. There are as yet no reported legal decisions that hold that physicians have a legal duty to inform women about a test that can (independent of age) assess risk for bearing a child with Down syndrome.

The test could be used to refine the age-related risk of carrying a fetus with Down syndrome among women 35 and older. If clinicians and consumers agreed to use the results to decide whether to seek fetal karyotyping, the number of amniocenteses could be reduced and the yield (defined here as the percentage of fetal karyotypes that detect an abnormality) increased (Haddow et al., 1994). To implement such a change of practice, relevant clinical communities would have to publish unequivocal guidelines to protect the practicing physician who changes his recommendations as to whom is a candidate for amniocentesis.

Genetic testing and insurance

There is growing concern that genetic data acquired to assist in the resolution of a clinical problem or in the course of screening might be used in a manner that could harm the economic or social interests of the individual or his or her relatives (Gostin, 1991). The origins of this concern can be traced to the eugenics movement that flourished in the 1920s and 1930s during which many states in the United States and some European nations enacted involuntary sterilization laws targeting institutionalized persons. United States immigration law from 1921 until 1968 favored entry by immigrants from northern and western Europe over eastern and southern Europe, a pattern rationalized in part by eugenic beliefs (Reilly, 1991).

During the early 1970s in the United States some persons who participated in sickle cell screening programs and who were found to be carriers suffered employment discrimination. For a short time a few life insurance companies placed persons with sickle cell trait outside the normal risk pool (Reilly, 1977). This led several states to enact legislation that specifically forbade the use of sickle cell testing to determine insurability and employability. Concern about genetic discrimination (originally defined as discrimination against an otherwise healthy person on the basis of information concerning his genotype) as a consequence of screening and testing has grown among geneticists since the mid-1980s (Billings et al., 1992). The possibility that genetic data could be used to deny individuals access to health insurance was a major topic throughout the 1990s (NIH-DOE Working Group on Ethical, Legal and Social Implications of Human Genome Research, 1993). During the mid to late 1990s more than a dozen bills targeting this issue were introduced before Congress (Colby, 1998). Concern about the threat that genetic information could affect access to health insurance elicited commentary from President Clinton on several occasions (Clinton, 1997).

Efforts to prevent discriminatory behavior by insurers are not new. Virtually all states have laws prohibiting "unfair discrimination", statutes that require that like individuals be treated alike (McEwen and Reilly, 1992). Such laws are too general, however, to address the problem of genetic discrimination. Since 1990 legislative interest in preventing genetic discrimination has grown sharply.

In the early 1990s California enacted laws that forbid denial of access to health insurance because an individual carries an allele that could result in the birth of a child with a serious genetic disorder. Maryland forbids both life and health insurers from charging higher premiums due to the presence of "any genetic trait that is harmless within itself". During the mid-1990s there was a dramatic increase in bills before state legislatures intended to curb the use by insurers of genetic risk data in health insurance underwriting. The trend continued throughout the 1990s, and by 1999 at least 30 states had adopted laws that forbade any use of genetic data by group health insurers (Hall, 1999). However, the only available studies of them suggest that they have had no discernible impact – probably because they address a problem that is substantially more theoretical than real (Hall and Rich, 2000).

For more than a decade there has been periodic discussion of the value of employer-based genetic screening as a means of averting occupational disease in genetically susceptible individuals. In 1992 Wisconsin enacted a law that prohibits the use of genetic test information in employment decisions (McEwen and Reilly, 1992). As there are few tests that would disclose relevant information, there has been relatively little activity in this arena. A few employers have screened to detect persons with sickle cell anemia and there has been discussion about screening to identify persons with glucose-6-phosphate dehydrogenase (G6PD) deficiency. A cotton textile plant in Jutland (Denmark) has screened workers to identify persons who carry an allele for a-1-antitrypsin deficiency. Two surveys of the largest corporations in the United States have indicated that a small minority would consider screening should appropriate tests become available (Office of Technology Assessment, 1990). There does not appear to be much employer interest in occupationally based genetic screening in the United Kingdom (Nuffield Council on Bioethics, 1993). Nevertheless, by 1999 at least 19 states in the United States had enacted laws that forbid employers from using genetic information in decisions about hiring or promotion (Yesley, 1999). On February 8, 2000 President Clinton issued an Executive Order banning genetic discrimination in decisions about hiring in the federal workplace (Gillis, 2000).

In the 1980s several companies with manufacturing processes that expose workers to high concentrations of lead (a known teratogen) refused to employ women of childbearing age unless they could prove that they were incapable of having children. These "fetal exclusion" policies were intended to protect the employer from being sued by an employee who bears a child with birth defects or developmental disabilities that were arguably caused by a exposure to a toxin in the work place (Annas, 1991). In 1985 women employees at Johnson Controls, Inc. sued their employer, arguing that conditioning employment on proof of infertility violated Title VII of the Civil Rights Act of 1964 as amended by the Pregnancy Discrimination Act of 1978. Six years later the United States Supreme Court, reversing the lower courts, held that employers could not ban non-pregnant women from a workplace simply because they were exposed to chemicals that could cause birth defects should they become pregnant and continue to work (International Union, UAW v. Johnson Controls, Inc., 1991).

The Americans With Disabilities Act (1990) forbids employers from discriminating against disabled persons who, with reasonable accommodation, can do the job for which they have applied. The law recognizes three definitions of disability of which the most relevant is the third, which defines a person as being disabled (and therefore subject to the protection of the Act) if he or she is merely *perceived* as being disabled. The third definition has provoked debate as to whether persons who have undergone genetic testing and are found to be highly likely to develop a single gene disorder or who are found to be at greatly increased risk for cancer or heart disease could claim the protection of the law. The Equal Employment Opportunity Commission has interpreted the ADA as extending protection to otherwise healthy persons who carry a mutation that puts them at high risk for a serious, genetically influenced disease (Equal Employment Opportunity Commission, 1995). However, several decisions by the United States Supreme Court in 1999 regarding the scope of coverage afforded by the ADA, while not directly addressing genetically based risks, suggest that the stance taken by the EEOC would not survive constitutional attack.

For individuals who are affected with a serious, chronic, illness or at high risk for such a disorder, or who have dependents who are or may be at increased risk for becoming seriously ill, until recently there were in the United States significant potential costs associated with changing group health plans (Office of Technology Assessment, 1992). This problem, known as "job lock", is a consequence of "preexisting condition" clauses. A person enrolling in a new plan who has a chronic disorder or who has a dependent with a chronic disorder faces a period ranging from 30 days to nine months during which the problem for which coverage is most needed is not protected by the health plan. This lack of coverage can constitute a risk of such magnitude that persons will not change jobs. The Health Insurance Portability and Accountability Act (1996) specifically insulates persons who are enrolled in group health plans and who are known to be at a genetically based increased risk for disease from being labeled as having a "pre-existing condition".

In 1991 Montana became the first state to bar insurers from refusing to consider applications for life or disability insurance from persons with a "specific chromosomal or single gene condition". It also requires that any rejection of an application for insurance and any rating decision be justified by the medical history of the applicant, not fear of potential illness.

By its very nature the marketplace for life insurance discriminates among its applicants. Not all people are alike; they differ by gender, age, occupation, avocation, health history, family history, and a host of other factors. Based on decades of statistical analysis, life insurers know that among certain classes of persons the likelihood of dying in a given period is greater than among others. This statistical knowledge provides the foundation for underwriting, the decision about how to price the cost of a particular policy for a particular individual. The premium represents the price of entry for the policyholder to the pool of purchasers to which he or she in essence has been assigned.

The American Council of Life Insurance has asserted that genetic testing is not essentially different from other kinds of medical information, but that it is not yet sufficiently developed for disorders such as heart disease and cancer, the illnesses that are their overriding concern, to be of value in underwriting in the near future (Pokorski, 1989). The Council has acknowledged that when good DNA based predictive tests are developed, they may choose to use them. It recognized that predictive tests do not provide absolute answers and that underwriters must interpret them in the context of other parameters such as "age, gender, current health status, occupation, and health enhancing factors such as exercise and avoidance of tobacco and excessive amounts of alcohol".

A task force convened by the American Council of Life Insurance (ACLI) and the Health Insurance Association of America (HIAA) concluded that public's concern about insurer use of genetic tests turn on the larger public policy issues about providing universal access to health care. The task force recommended that the insurance industry should continue to propose methods to cover the uninsured, including state implementation of small group reforms and the creation of high-risk pools. But it also concluded that the industry should "aggressively defend the need to have access to and to consider any relevant health information for underwriting purposes, including genetic information" (Report of the ACLI-HIAA Task Force on Genetic Testing, 1991)

Genetic testing to determine whether an individual with a positive family history is at increased risk, for example, for breast cancer or colon cancer could soon become of interest to life insurance underwriting. Unless there is a dramatic change in the way that the life insurance industry is regulated, insurers will have the right to review an applicant's family history, evaluate test results that are in the medical record, and require that applicants be tested. This does not mean they will act irresponsibly. In 1997 the Association of British Insurers (ABI) voluntarily agreed not to use genetic testing in underwriting modestly sized life insurance policies tied to home mortgages (Association of British Insurers, 1997).

During the next decade, we are likely to see the policy questions raised by genetic testing played out on several stages. Surely, there will be litigation brought pursuant to the ADA and relevant state statutes to expand the definition of disability to include healthy persons at risk for genetic disease. Escalating fears about the interest that insurers and employers have in genetic data will foster ever more state legislation. In response various insurance and trade associations will issue reassuring policy statements while keeping a watchful eye on and lobbying against some state bills. An organization such as the National Conference of Commissioners on Uniform State Laws could play an important role by drafting comprehensive model legislation that defines rules for disclosure of medical data in non-medical contexts. The better solution is to develop a comprehensive statute that protects that privacy of all medical data. Such legislation is (perennially) before the U.S. Congress.

Regulation of human genetic research

Accelerating efforts to find the alleles that cause or increase the risk for human diseases led the Office for Protection from Research Risks (OPRR) of the National Institutes of Health to issue guidelines for use by local Institutional Review Boards in their assessment of grant applications that would involve genetic testing of human subjects. Although they are advisory in nature, the OPRR guidelines shape the conduct of research and have substantial regulatory weight. They stress that the decision to participate in human genetic research requires an informed consent, that subjects must have access to adequate genetic counseling, and that participants must be told that should they enter and then withdraw from a study, the researcher is not required to purge existing data or destroy cell lines or DNA derived from them. The OPRR has instructed local Institutional Review Boards that in gathering family histories investigators may seek information that is routinely available from other public sources (such as names and addresses), but may not seek non-public information such as about illnesses or adoptions, a position that could impede data gathering (Office for Protection from Research Risks, 1993).

During the mid to late 1990s advances in human genetics triggered a policy debate over the relationship between human subjects and researchers that touched on a number of issues that were not directly addressed when the relevant federal regulations were drafted in the late 1970s. In part due to the influence of concerns about genetic discrimination in health care, there emerged an argument that participation in gene mapping research involved more than "minimal risk" (defined in the federal rules as the risk associated with everyday life activities) (Clayton et al., 1995). Earley and Strong (1995) suggested that for some research projects it might be worthwhile to seek a Federal Certificate of Confidentiality which, if issued, insulates research date even from the reach of a judicial subpoena. Others cautioned that genetic research could result in the inadvertent discovery of nonpaternity or undisclosed adoption, findings that would create disclosure dilemmas for researchers. There also emerged uncertainty as to the scope of the researchers' ethical obligation to inform subjects about findings of potential relevance in regard to risk for disease (Reilly et al., 1997). The debate over the ownership and future use of the DNA obtained during the research was especially heated. In 1993 the OPRR asserted that subjects could not be coerced to waive a right such as a potential economic interest in their tissue. Those working in industry responded that without the certainty that they could obtain patent protection on and economic control over their work, they could not conduct commercial research. A decision by the California Supreme Court (Moore v. Regents of the University of California, 1990), the only case law on point, supports the economic interests of the research community so long as the subject is informed of and consents to the uses of his tissue. None of the aforementioned issues has been resolved, but there is a general trend to address them in the consent process and document them in the consent form that is signed by the individual who chooses to participate in the research.

Much genetic research is conducted on special populations, many of which have in the past have been (and may

still be) the object of discrimination by members of a dominant society. In the late 1990s some proposed that genetic research constituted a special risk to such groups and that consent should be sought from the *group* itself (via its designated leaders) before researchers could claim the right to recruit individuals to participate (Foster et al., 1998; Foster et al., 1999). Still a minority view and not without its critics (Reilly, 1998), this argument nevertheless appears to be gaining adherents.

A major issue in the oversight of human subjects research in the United States is that a growing fraction of it is conducted in the private sector in settings that are technically not subject to the federal regulations. In 1997 Senator John Glenn introduced a bill to extend the rules to cover all human subject research regardless of its source of funding, but it garnered little attention. In 1998 and 1999 several reports by various agencies within the United States government were published that expressed serious reservations about the ability of the existing system of Institutional Review Boards to protect human subjects. The death in 1999 of a young man during gene therapy research at the University of Pennsylvania (along with decisions by OPRR to suspend research at several well known universities) helped to focus much public attention on the protection of human subjects. It appears likely that there will soon be significant revisions in the system for oversight of research involving human subjects, and it will not be surprising if gene therapy is singled out for special attention.

In the United States experiments in which recombinant DNA is introduced into cells of a human subject with the intent of modifying the genome are regulated by the NIH Guidelines for Research Involving Recombinant DNA Molecules (49 Federal Register 46266 1990), and its subsequent amendments. Every human gene therapy protocol must be reviewed by the local Institutional Review Board. In addition, federally funded experiments involving recombinant DNA must be approved by the Recombinant DNA Advisory Committee (RAC) at the NIH. In Canada the Medical Research Council Standing Committee on Ethics in Experimentation has taken a similar approach, one that requires both local and national review (Prior, 1992).

Somatic cell gene therapy, probably the most thoroughly anticipated clinical research in the history of medicine, does not raise novel legal issues. It has been fully reviewed by several national commissions (President's Commission for the Study of Ethical Problems in Medicine and Biomedical and Behavioral Research, 1982), and Congress has held hearings about it. The civic, religious, scientific and medical groups that have studied the topic have concluded that this therapy does not present unique ethical problems (Office of

Technology Assessment, 1984). Commentators in Canada and the European Medical Research Councils have concluded that it is not fundamentally different from other medical therapies (News Report, 1988; Knoppers and LeBris, 1993).

Unlike somatic cell therapy, in which the impact of the intervention is limited to an individual patient, germ-line therapy – the manipulation of the genome in cells that are the progenitors of egg or sperm cells – affects the patient's descendants. This fact coupled with the concern that genetic engineering may some day permit germ-line enhancement (the introduction of genes intended to increase the likelihood of having a child with desired traits rather than to avert disease) has provoked much concern. Religious and civic groups have urged a ban on such genetic manipulations, and the RAC has stated that it would not approve proposals to do research intended to further this goal in humans. The Parliamentary Assembly of the Council of Europe has recommended that the Committee of Ministers provide for explicit recognition in the European Convention on Human Rights of the right to a genetic inheritance which has not been artificially interfered with, unless it is in accord with principles that are compatible with respect for other human rights, language that would permit interventions to prevent disease (Knoppers, 1991). The European Medical Research Councils of Austria, Denmark, Finland, France, The Netherlands, Norway, Spain, Sweden, Switzerland, United Kingdom and West Germany have declared that "Germ-line therapy for the introduction of heritable genetic modification is not acceptable" (News Report, 1988). The United Nations Educational, Scientific, and Cultural Organization (UNESCO) has issued a "Universal Declaration on the Human Genome and Human Rights" (UNESCO, 1997) that opposes such research.

The report that researchers had successfully used somatic cell nuclear transfer technology to clone a sheep named Dolly (Wilmut et al., 1997) initiated a worldwide debate over the appropriate response to the possibility of cloning humans. The overwhelming sentiment was that the technology should never be used for this purpose. Many international bodies adopted resolutions condemning human cloning, and several nations in Europe enacted laws that criminalized efforts to clone humans. A number of states in the United States considered similar laws that (because of imprecision in drafting) if enacted would have forbidden any experiments that replicated DNA molecules. At the request of President Clinton, the National Bioethics Advisory Commission (1997) quickly produced a superb analysis of the issue that did much to stabilize discourse.

While it is likely that at some point in the future we will be able to create humans by cloning and it is impossible to prevent the technology from ever being used, it is highly unlikely that it will ever be legally permissible or ethically defended.

Rapid advances in the ability to identify, isolate and clone stem cells from early human embryos (Thompson et al., 1998) triggered an intense debate over the morality of that research, one that is caught in the web of the intractable debate over abortion (National Bioethics Advisory Commission, 1999). Interpreting the relevant federal rules that ban fetal research, the NIH in 1999 decided that it would not fund efforts to obtain human tissue for stem cell research (usually, frozen human embryos originally created to overcome infertility), but that it would fund work on the use of stem cells in a variety of arenas including as novel therapeutic agents in degenerative disorders like Parkinson disease (Robertson, 1999).

Genes and patents

During the 1990s human genetics was dominated by the Human Genome Project. The decade saw an explosive growth in the number of biotechnology companies with a core business strategy that centered on the creation of intellectual property as a result of massive DNA sequencing efforts. The complex history of efforts to patent human DNA sequence is beyond the scope of this chapter. However, it may be helpful to note that the general trend in patent policy in regard to genomics is clear. Expressed sequence tags (ESTs) are not patentable. However, even though they exist in nature, newly published cDNA sequences are potentially patentable, under the rationale that they do not naturally exist in a useful form. Sequence variations that are linked to other knowledge (such as the correlation of a single nucleotide polymorphism with increased risk for a particular disease) are patentable (Rai, 1999).

During the late 1990s some geneticists and consumer groups began to raise concerns that they were being denied access to a test for a rare disorder because a university-based lab was charging an unreasonable licensing fee. While such issues may arise periodically, it is likely that in the vast majority of cases market forces will influence those who control intellectual property to price access to it in a reasonable way. Despite the debate over patenting genes, I do not foresee new restrictions in the United States on the right to patent DNA sequences for defined purposes.

Intellectual property is the cornerstone of biotechnology; without it access to capital for research would vanish.

Conclusion

We have entered an era in which our rapidly growing understanding of the role that genes play in complex disorders such as heart disease, cancer, and mental illness promises to bring about a paradigmatic shift in how we understand, avert, and treat disease and bring genetics to the center of medicine. The potential clinical benefits that may be derived from genetic information are vast. But the growth of genetic testing also means that family members, insurers, employers, school systems, and the state might be able to acquire ever more genetic information about individuals. We must guard against the possibility that genetic information could be misused. The means to accomplish this will almost certainly be legislation that subordinates the interests of third parties in the data to the individual's right to privacy.

REFERENCES

American College of Medical Genetics (1994a) Standards and Guidelines. Clinical Genetics Laboratories, Bethesda, MD

American College of Medical Genetics (1994b) Policy statement: Fragile X syndrome: Diagnostic and carrier testing. Bethesda, MD

American College of Medical Genetics/American Society of Human Genetics Working Group (1995) Statement on use of apolipoprotein E testing for Alzheimer Disease. JAMA 274:1627–29

American College of Obstetricians and Gynecologists (1985) Professional Liability Implication of AFP Tests: Department of Professional Liability Alert. American College of Obstetricians and Gynecologists, Washington, DC

American Society of Human Genetics (1987) Policy statement for maternal serum alpha-fetoprotein screening programs and quality control for laboratories performing maternal serum and amniotic fluid alpha-fetoprotein assays. Am J Hum Genet 40:75–82

American Society of Human Genetics Social Issues Committee (1991) Report on genetics and adoption: Points to consider. Am J Hum Genet 48:1009–1010

American Society of Human Genetics Social Issues Committee and the American College of Medical Genetics Social, Ethical, and Legal Issues Committee (2000) Genetic testing and adoption. Am J Hum Genet 66:761–67

American Society of Human Genetics Social Issues Subcommittee on Familial Disclosure (1998) Professional disclosure of familial genetic information. Am J Hum Genet 62:474–83

Americans With Disabilities Act (1990) Pub. L. No. 101–336, 104 Stat. 377, 42 USC 12101–12213

Andrews LB (1985) State Laws and Regulations Governing Newborn Screening. American Bar Association, Chicago

Andrews LB (1987) Medical Genetics: A Legal Frontier. American Bar Foundation, Chicago

Andrews L, Fullarton J, Holtzman N, Motulsky A (eds) (1994) Assessing Genetic Risks: Implications for Health and Social Policy. National Academy Press, Washington, DC

Annas GJ (1991) Fetal protection and employment discrimination: the Johnson Controls case. N Engl J Med 325:740–743

Annas GJ, Glanz LH, Roche PA (1995) The Genetic Privacy Act and Commentary. Health Law Department, Boston University School of Public Health, Boston

Association of British Insurers (1997) Genetic testing: ABI code of practice. London (www.abi.org.uk)

Becker v. Schwartz (1978) 46 N.Y.2d 401, 386 N.E.2d 807, 413 N. Y. S. 895

Berg P, Baltimore DS, Boyer HW (1974) Potential biohazards of recombinant DNA molecules. Science 1985:303–305

Billings PR, Kohn MA, de Cuevas M et al. (1992) Discrimination as a consequence of genetic testing. Am J Hum Genet 50:476–82

Bradshaw v. Daniel (1993) No. 02–5–01–9206 cv 00035 Supreme Court of Tennessee

Canterbury v. Spence (1972) 464 F. 2d 772 D.C. Circuit

Cao A (1991) Antenatal diagnosis of β-thalassemia in Sardinia. pp. 72–79. In Bankowski Z, Capon A M (eds): Genetics, Ethics and Human Values. Proceedings of the XXIVth CIOMS Conference. Geneva CIOMS

Capon AM (1979) Tort liability and genetic counseling. Columbia Law Rev 79:618–704

Centers for Disease Control and Prevention (1995) Chorionic villous sampling and amniocentesis: Recommendations for prenatal counseling. Morbidity and Mortality Weekly Report, Atlanta

Clayton EW (1992) Screening and treatment of newborns. Houston Law Rev 29:85–148

Clayton E, Steinberg K, Khoury M et al. (1995) Informed consent for genetic research on stored tissue samples. JAMA 274:1786–92

Clinton W (1997) Science in the 21st century. Science 276:1971

Cobbs v. Grant (1972) 8 Cal. 3rd 229, 502 P.2d 1, 104 Cal. Rptr. 505

Colby JA (1998) An analysis of genetic discrimination legislation proposed by the 105th congress. Am J Law & Med 24;443–480

Committee for the Study of Inborn Errors of Metabolism (1975) Genetic Screening: Programs, Principles, and Research. National Academy of Sciences, Washington, DC

Council of Regional Networks for Genetic Services (CORN) (1992) Newborn Screening Report. New York CORN Central Office

Cow v. Forum Group, Inc. (1991) 575 NE 2d 630–7 (Indiana)

Cunningham GC, Kizer KW (1990) Maternal serum alpha-fetoprotein screening activities of state health agencies: a survey. Am J Hum Genet 47:899–903

Earley CL and Strong LC (1995) Certificate of confidentiality: A valuable tool for protecting genetic data. Am J Hum Genet 57:727–31

Elias S, Annas G (1987) Reproductive Genetics and the Law. Year Book Medical Publishers, Chicago

Equal Employment Opportunity Commission (1995) Compliance Manual. Section 902–45 Government Printing Office, Washington, DC

Ethics Committee of the American Fertility Society (1990) Ethical Consideration of the New Reproductive Technologies. Fertil Steril 53 (Suppl 2)

Foster MW, Bernstein D, and Carter TH (1998) A model agreement for genetic research in socially identifiable populations. Am J Hum Genet 63:696–702

Foster MW, Sharp RR, Freeman WL et al. (1999) The role of community review in evaluating the risks of human genetic variation research. Am J Hum Genet 64:1719–27

Gillis J (2000) Clinton targets misuse of gene data. Washington Post 2/8 p9

Goldgar D, Reilly PR (1995) A common BRCA1 mutation in the Ashkenazim. Nat Genet 11:113–114

Gostin L (1991) Genetic discrimination: The use of genetically based diagnostic and prognostic tests by employers and insurers. Am J Law Med 17:109–144

Grifo JA, Tang YX, Santiago M et al. (1994) Healthy deliveries from biopsied human embryos. Hum Repro 9:912–916

Grove-White R, Macnaghten P, Mayer S, and Wynne B (1997) Uncertain world: genetically modified organisms, food and public attitudes in Britain. Centre for the Study of Environmental Change. Lancaster University, Lancaster, UK. csec@lancaster.ac.uk

Haddow JE, Palomaki GE, Knight GJ et al. (1994) Reducing the need for amniocentesis in women 35 years of age or older with serum markers for screening. N Engl J Med 330:1115–1118

Hall MA (1999) Legal rules and industry norms: The impact of laws restricting health insurers' use of genetic information. Jurimetrics 40:93–122

Hall MA and Rich SS (2000) The impact on genetic discrimination of laws restricting health insurers' use of genetic information. Am J Hum Genet 66:293–308

Health Insurance Portability and Accountability Act of 1996. Pub L No 110:104–91, Stat 1936

Holder AR (1977) Legal Issues in Pediatrics and Adolescent Medicine. Wiley, New York

Holder AR (1978) Medical Malpractice Law, 2nd edn. Wiley, NY

Hugging M, Block M, Kanani S et al. (1990) Ethical and legal dilemmas arising during predictive testing for adult-onset disease: The experience of Huntington disease. Am J Hum Genet 47:4–12

International Union UAW v. Johnson Controls, Inc. (1991) 111 S. Ct. 1196

Jacobs v. Theimer (1975) 519 SW 2d 846 (Texas)

Jonantansson H (2000) Iceland's health sector database: a significant head start in the search for the biological grail or an irreversible error? Am J Law & Med 26(1):31–68

Knoppers BM (1991) Human Dignity and Genetic Heritage. Ottawa Law Reform Commission of Canada

Knoppers BM, Le Bris S (1993) Ethical and legal concerns: reproductive technologies 1990–1993. Curr Opinion Obstet Gynecol 5:630–635

McEwen JE, Reilly PR (1992) State legislative efforts to regulate the use and potential misuse of genetic information. Am J Hum Genet 51:637–647

McEwen JE, Reilly PR (1994) A review of state legislation on DNA forensic databanking. Am J Hum Genet 54:941–958

McEwen JE, Reilly PR (1995) A survey of DNA diagnostic laboratories regarding DNA banking. Am J Hum Genet 56:1477–1486

Malinowski MJ and Blatt RJR (1997) Commercialization of genetic testing services: the FDA, market forces, and biological tarot cards. Tulane L Rev 71(4) 1211–1312.

Martinez v. Botsford General Hospital (1995) Mich. Ct. App.

Maryland Ann. Code Art. (1986) 48A §223 (a) (3);223(b)(4)

Merkatz JR, Nitowsky HM, Macri JN (1984) An association between low maternal serum α-fetoprotein and fetal chromosomal abnormalities. Am J Obstet Gynecol 148:886

Moore v. Regents of University of California (1990) 793 P.2d 479

Natanson v. Kline (1960) 186 Kan. 393, 350 P.2d 1093, opinion on denial of motion for rehearing, 187 Kan. 186, 354 P.2d 670

National Bioethics Advisory Commission (1997) Cloning Human Beings. Rockville, MD

National Bioethics Advisory Commission (1999) Ethical Issues in Human Stem Cell Research. Rockville, MD

National Institutes of Health (1990) Statement from the workshop on population screening for the cystic fibrosis gene. N Engl J Med 323:70–71

News Report (1988) Gene therapy in man: recommendations of the European research councils. Lancet 1:1271–1272

NIH-DOE Working Group on Ethical, Legal, and Social Implications of Human Genome Research (1993) Genetic information and health insurance. Bethesda NIH Publication No. 93–3686

Nuffield Council on Bioethics (1993) Genetic Screening: Ethical Issues. Nuffield Foundation, London

Office for Protection from Research Risks (1993) Protecting Human Research Subjects: Institutional Review Board Guidebook. U.S. Government Printing Office, Washington, DC

Office of Technology Assessment (1984) Human Gene Therapy. U.S. Government Printing Office, Washington, DC

Office of Technology Assessment (1990) Genetic Screening and Monitoring in the Workplace. OTA-BA 455. U.S. Government Printing Office, Washington, DC

Office of Technology Assessment (1992) Genetic Tests and Health Insurance: Results of a Survey: Background Paper. U.S. Government Printing Office, Washington, DC

Ontario, Law Reform Commission (1985) Report on Human Artificial Reproduction and Related Matters. Ministry of the Attorney General, Toronto

Parham v. J.R. (1979) 442 US 584

Pate v. Threkel (1996) 661 So. 2d 278

Pokorski RJ (1989) Principles of insurance and risk classification. In: Report of the Genetic Testing Committee to the Medical Section of the American Council of Life Insurance, Hilton Head, S.C. June 10, p. 46

Pokorski RJ (1998) A test for the life insurance industry. Nature 391:935–6.

President's Commission for the Study of Ethical Problems in Medicine and Biomedical and Behavioral research (1982) Splicing Life. U.S. Government Printing Office, Washington, DC

President's Commission for the Study of Ethical Problems in Medicine and Biomedical and Behavioral Research (1983) Screening and Counseling for Genetic Conditions. U.S. Government Printing Office, Washington, DC

Prior L (1992) Somatic and germ line gene therapy: Current status and prospects. In Technologies of Sex Selection and Prenatal Diagnosis. Vol. 14: Research Studies. Ontario Royal Commission on New Reproductive Technologies, pp. 233–263

Rai AK (1999) Intellectual property rights in biotechnology – addressing new technology. Wake Forest Law Rev 34:791–33

Reilly PR (1975) Genetic screening legislation. In Hirschhorn K and Harris H (eds): Adv Hum Genet V. Plenum, NY 319–376

Reilly PR (1977) Genetics, Law and Social Policy. Harvard University Press, Cambridge, MA

Reilly PR (1991) The Surgical Solution. Johns Hopkins University, Baltimore

Reilly PR (1997) Genetic information in families: Rethinking confidentiality. Microb & Comp Genom 2:7–18

Reilly PR (1998) Rethinking risks to human subjects in genetic research. Am J Hum Genet 63:682–85

Reilly PR, Boshar M, and Holtzman SH (1997) Ethical issues in genetic research; disclosure and informed consent. Nat Genet 15:16–20

Report of the ACLI-HIAA Task Force on Genetic Testing (1991) The American Council of Life Insurance and the Health Insurance Association of America, Washington, DC

Robertson J (1999) Ethics and policy in embryonic stem cell research. Kennedy Inst of Ethics J 9(2):109–36

Roe v. Wade (1973) 410 U.S. 113

Safer v. Estate of Pack (1996) 677 A2d 1188 (NJ Super A.D.)

Salgo v. Leland (1957) Stanford Jr. Univ. Bd. of Trustees, 154 Cal. App. 2d 560, 317 P.2d 170

Science and Technology Select Committee (1995) Human Genetics: The Science and Its Consequences. Her Majesty's Stationery Office, London

Secretary's Advisory Committee on Genetic Testing (2000) A public consultation on oversight of genetic tests. NIH www4.od.nih.gov/oba/sacgt.htm

Sheck B, Neufeld P and Dwyer J (1999) Actual Innocence. Doubleday, NY

Show MW (1984) To be or not to be? That is the question. Am J Hum Genet 35:1–9

Tarasoff v. Regents of the University of California (1976) 17 Cal. 3d 425, 551 d P.2334, 131 Cal. Rptr. 14

Tedeschi I (1966) On tort liability for wrongful life. Israel Law Rev 1:513–549

Thomson JA, Itskovitz-Elder J, Shapiro S (1998) Embryonic stem cell lines derived from human blastocysts. Science 282:1145–47

U.K. Collaborative Study of Alpha-Fetoprotein in Relation to Neural Tube Defects (1977) Maternal serum alpha-fetoprotein measurement in antenatal screening for anencephaly and spina bifida in early pregnancy. Lancet 1:1323–332

United Kingdom, Department of Health and Social Security (1984) Report of the Committee of Inquiry into Human Fertilization and Embryology. Her Majesty's Stationery Office, London

United Nations Educational, Scientific and Cultural Organization (1997) Universal declaration on the human genome and human rights.

Victoria, Australia, Committee to Consider the Social, Ethical, and Legal Issues Arising from In Vitro Fertilization (1984) Report on the Disposition of Embryo Produced by In Vitro Fertilization. F.D. Atkinson, Government Printer, Melbourne

Wald N and Kennard A (1996) Prenatal screening for neural tube defects and Down syndrome. In Emery and Rimoin DL (eds): Principles and Practice of Medical Genetics, 3rd edn., pp. 545–62

Walters L (1986) The ethics of human gene therapy. Nature 320:225–227

Wertz D, Fanos JH, Reilly PR (1994) Genetic testing for children and adolescents – who decides? JAMA 272:875–881

Wertz DC, Fletcher JC, and Berg K (1995) Guidelines on ethical issues in medical genetics and the provision of genetic services. WHO, Geneva

Wilmut I, Schnieke AE, McWhir J et al. (1997) Viable offspring derived from fetal and adult mammalian cells. Nature 385:810–13

Yesley MS (1999) Genetic difference in the workplace. Jurimetrics 40:129–42

APPROACHES TO CLINICAL PROBLEMS

The genetic basis of female infertility

35

Lawrence C. Layman

Introduction

Most of the genes involved in human fertility remain unknown at the present time, but with the completion of the Human Genome Mapping Project within the next several years, we can expect an accelerated rate of discovery. Genes that affect development and function of the hypothalamic-pituitary-gonadal axis have been demonstrated to cause infertility. Similarly, genes that affect uterine and vaginal development and function could impair fertility. Although many of the genetic causes of infertility affect both males and females, only those disorders affecting female fertility will be discussed. Those causes of female infertility have been categorized according to the primary location of the observed defect–hypothalamus, pituitary, gonad, uterus/vagina (Fig. 35.1).

Infertility

Infertility is most commonly defined as the absence of pregnancy for one year of unprotected intercourse. Causes of infertility include male (40%) or female (40%) factor, or both male and female factors (20%) (Speroff, 1999) For any given individual or couple, more than one factor may be present. Known female factors include fallopian tubal obstruction and/or adhesions, ovulation disorders, and endometriosis, while male disorders include reduced sperm parameters (decreased concentration, motility, and/or morphology) due to testicular, obstructive, and endocrine causes. The present chapter will focus on the genetic causes of infertility in patients presenting with a female phenotype,

regardless of karyotype. For a discussion of male factor infertility, see Chapter 36.

Although most patients with infertility display normal pubertal development with evidence of estrogen production, most of the gene mutations causing infertility also result in anovulatory cycles or amenorrhea. In women with amenorrhea, it must first be determined if estrogen is being produced, and this is usually done by administering progesterone, which should induce a withdrawal bleed. (Layman and Reindollar, 1994; Layman, 1999a). If no menstrual period is induced, serum levels of serum gonadotropins follicle stimulating hormone (FSH) and luteinizing hormone (LH) are obtained to rule out ovarian failure (Fig. 35.1). If gonadotropins are elevated on several separate occasions, ovarian failure is present, and a karyotype should be obtained to exclude chromosomal causes including 45,X cell line, a partial X chromosome deletion, or a translocation (see below) (Layman 1994; 1999a). This is particularly true for the woman with delayed puberty and primary amenorrhea, where the frequency of karyotypic abnormalities exceeds 50% (Table 35.1) (Reindollar, 1981; 1986). When amenorrhea occurs after a normal onset of puberty and menses, the probability of chromosomal abnormalities is decreased, but should be considered.

However, if gonadotropins are low or normal in the face of low estrogen (which is inappropriate), the cause is hypothalamic or pituitary (discussed below). An MRI is recommended to exclude a pituitary tumor, usually a prolactinoma, but occasionally a craniopharyngioma in adolescence. If the MRI is negative, a hypothalamic cause is most likely, particularly if there are no signs or symptoms of pituitary failure of TSH, ACTH, GH, or prolactin. A family history of extreme short stature suggests the possibility of inherited forms of pituitary failure. Single gene mutations

947

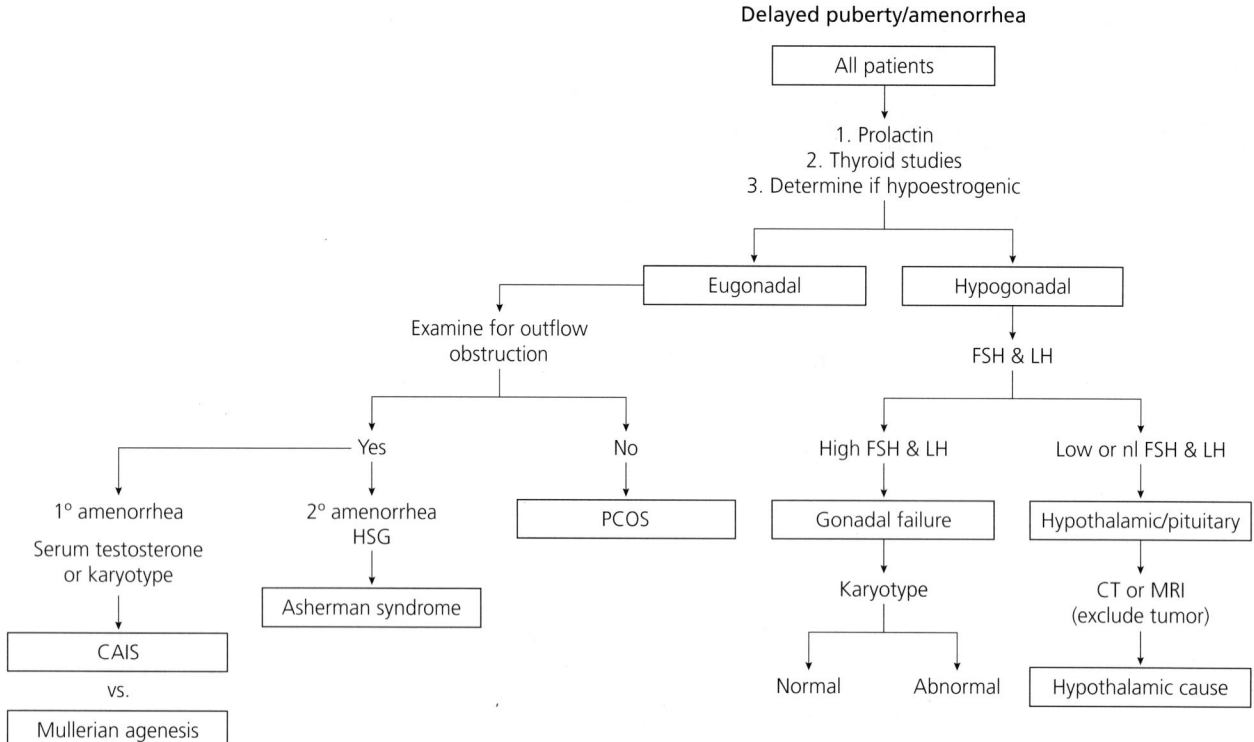

Delayed puberty/amenorrhea

Fig. 35.1. An evaluation of primary with delayed puberty and secondary amenorrhea is shown. Outflow obstruction can occur with both primary amenorrhea (developmental causes such as vaginal agenesis) and secondary amenorrhea (adhesions from prior uterine curettage–Asherman syndrome). CAIS = complete androgen insensitivity syndrome; PCOS = polycystic ovary syndrome.

Table 35.1. The Prevalence of diagnostic categories of primary amenorrhea and secondary amenorrhea.

	Primary amenorrhea[a]	Secondary amenorrhea[b]
I. Hypogonadism		
A. Hypergonadotropic	43%	11%
1. Abnormal karyotype	27%	0.5%
2. Normal karyotype	16%	10%
B. Hypogonadotropic	31%	42%
1. Reversible	19%	39%
2. Irreversible	12%	3%
II. Eugonadism	26%	46%
1. Ovulation disorder	8%	7%
2. Outflow obstruction	18%	18%

[a]From Reindollar, 1981; [b] from Reindollar, 1986.

of hypothalamic and pituitary genes have been described (Layman and Reindollar, 1994; Layman, 1999a).

If there is evidence of normal estrogen production, then anovulation or obstruction of the outflow tract (uterus and/or vagina) must be excluded. Thyroid stimulating hormone and prolactin levels are usually ordered in an amenorrheic or anovulatory patient, regardless of whether the patient demonstrates endogenous estrogen production, in order to exclude primary hypothyroidism and hyperprolactinemia. At the time of this writing, only two disorders of outflow tract obstruction are caused by a single gene defect.

Hypothalamic causes of female infertility

Identified gene mutations affecting hypothalamic development and/or function are summarized in Table 35.2.

THE *KAL* GENE

Kallmann syndrome is an X-linked recessive form of human hypogonadotropic hypogonadism accompanied by anosmia (Fig. 35.1; Table 35.2). The causative *KAL* gene was independently characterized by two different groups of investigators, who mapped and cloned the gene from the pseudoautosomal region of Xp (Franco et al., 1991; Legouis et al., 1991). The KAL protein anosmin appears to provide a scaffold for GnRH neurons and olfactory nerves to migrate from the olfactory placode across the cribriform plate to synapse with mitral cells of the olfactory bulb. With deficient or impaired anosmin, GnRH and olfactory neurons fail to

Table 35.2. Gene mutations affecting hypothalamic function in females

Gene	Localization	Phenotype	Inheritance
KAL	Xp22.3	HH and anosmia	X-linked recessive
AHC	Xp21	Adrenal hypoplasia congenita & HH	X-linked recessive
Leptin	7q31.3	Obesity, HH	Autosomal recessive
Leptin receptor	1p31	Obesity, HH	Autosomal recessive

synapse normally, so Kallmann syndrome results (Francs et al., 1991; Legouis et al., 1991). All of the mutations described to date affect only males, so this will not be discussed further, except to state that the expression patterns of *KAL* correlate very well with the phenotype of the clinical syndrome (HH, anosmia, renal agenesis, clefting, neurologic abnormalities) (Hardelin et al., 1993; Rugarli et al., 1993).

THE DSS REGION AND THE *AHC* (*DAX1*) GENE

Another X-linked cause of human HH is adrenal hypoplasia congenita (AHC)/HH due to mutations of the *AHC* gene. Males present with adrenal failure in infancy or childhood due to a deficient formation of the permanent zone of the adrenal gland. Children who are adequately treated with steroid replacement fail to undergo puberty due to HH, which may be accompanied by cryptorchidism (Muscatelli et al., 1994; Zanaria et al., 1994; Guo et al., 1995). The observation that AHC may also sometimes be accompanied by Duchenne muscular dystrophy and glycerol kinase deficiency suggested a contiguous gene deletion syndrome on Xp21.

AHC was cloned from the dosage sensitive sex reversal (DSS) region of human chromosome Xp21. The DSS region is the portion of Xp21, which when duplicated, produces undermasculinization (observed as feminization) of 46,XY males (Bardoni et al., 1994). *AHC* contains two exons that code for a 470 amino acid protein, DAX1 (*DSS-AHC* critical region of the *X* chromosome, gene *1*). DAX1 has no known ligand (an orphan receptor) which belongs to the steroid hormone superfamily, and is a transcription factor required for normal development of the pituitary gonadotropes and adrenal cortex. Greater than 50 different mutations, both deletions and point mutations, in *AHC* have been reported in AHC patients, which have almost been completely in males (Zhang et al., 1998). Of interest is the observation of a homozygous *AHC* mutation in a female affected with IHH (without adrenal failure) within a family with two males with adrenal hypoplasia congenita (Merke et al., 1999). Her homozygosity was thought to be due to a gene conversion event.

DAX1 appears to regulate gonadotropin secretion at both hypothalamic and pituitary sites within the neuro-endocrine axis (Habiby et al., 1996). There is also evidence that DAX1 inhibits transcription of another important steroid receptor, SF-1, which is expressed in the same tissues (Achermann et al., 1999). The interaction between these two factors is probably important in initiation of sexual development.

Initial studies suggested that DAX1 might be an ovarian determinant gene because it was localized within a region of chromosome Xp (the DSS region), which when duplicated, is associated with sex reversal (feminization) of 46,XY males (Bardoni et al., 1994). Recent studies, however, do not support its role as an ovarian determinant gene, but rather a gene important in spermatogenesis. Yu et al. (1998) recently described a targeted knockout of the mouse homologue of *AHC* (the *Ahch* gene) using the Cre-loxP system (since standard neomycin selection marker cassettes failed to produce undifferentiated embryonic stem cells). Surprisingly, ovarian development and function were normal similar to wild-type mice, however, degeneration of testicular germinal epithelium occurred independent of gonadotropin and testosterone abnormalities (Yu et al., 1998). These data demonstrate the importance of *Ahch* as a spermatogenesis gene, not as an ovarian determinant gene.

THE LEPTIN GENE

The identification of the leptin deficient *ob/ob* mice due to mutations in the leptin gene indicated that similar mutations in the human gene might be present in obese, hypogonadal individuals. The first human leptin mutation was demonstrated in a family with two obese prepubertal children with exceedingly low leptin levels (Montague et al., 1997). However, since none of the probands were pubertal-age, the effects of the gene mutation upon reproduction were not able to be assessed. However, another leptin mutation was identified in a consanguineous family containing three affected obese individuals (Strobel et al., 1998). Of the two affected individuals who were young adults, both had delayed puberty. In this family, a 14-year-old female presented with primary amenorrhea and a 22-year-old male had irreversible pubertal delay, low testosterone, low gonadotropins, but a normal response to exogenous hCG and to exogenous GnRH.

Both affected individuals were homozygous for Arg105Trp missense mutation failed to result in any secreted leptin into the media from transfected COS-1 cells. The phenotype of humans with leptin gene mutations is similar to the *ob/ob* mice as they manifest extreme obesity, hyperinsulinemia, and hypogonadism, but unlike the mice, the patients did not have hyperglycemia, and hypercortisolemia, and stunted height (Strobel et al., 1998). The prevalence of human leptin mutations is unknown, but is likely to be uncommon since leptin mutations are uncommon in obesity. However, extremely obese, hypogonadotropic patients should be considered for leptin gene testing.

THE LEPTIN RECEPTOR GENE

Leptin resistant *db/db* mice were found to have mutations of the leptin receptor gene, and recently, similar mutations have also been identified in humans. Leptin resistance was observed in a family of affected females with obesity, hypogonadotropic hypogonadism, and elevated serum levels of leptin (Clement et al., 1998). A homozygous point mutation (G to A) was identified in the splice donor site just downstream to exon 16, which resulted in exon skipping during splicing. The resulting truncated receptor lacked both the transmembrane and intracellular domains of the protein. In addition to HH, this patient also had a mild diminution of GH and TSH secretion.

Pituitary causes of female infertility

Identified gene mutations affecting pituitary development, function or both are summarized in Table 35.3.

THE GONADOTROPIN RELEASING HORMONE RECEPTOR (GNRHR) GENE

GnRH constitutes a pivotal neuroendocrine regulator of reproductive function, and was considered to be the most likely candidate for mutations in IHH. Although a naturally occurring partial GnRH gene deletion was characterized in the hypogonadal mouse (Mason et al., 1986), no human GnRH gene deletions have been identified to date (Layman, 1999b). However, since patients with IHH have a variability in their response to GnRH, the GnRH receptor (GnRHR) became a plausible candidate for mutations. The GnRHR belongs to the G protein coupled receptor class of receptors, which contain an extracellular domain for ligand binding, a seven-transmembrane domain, three extracellular loops, three intracellular loops, and an intracellular carboxy-terminal tail (Fig. 35.2).

Until recently, gene mutations in humans with HH were X-linked recessive and confined to males. Mutations in the GnRHR gene were the first identifiable cause of autosomal recessive HH (Table 35.3) (de Roux et al., 1997; Layman et al., 1998a,b). Both males and females have been described, with either completely delayed puberty and sterility (Layman et al., 1998a,b) or with partial pubertal development and sterility (de Roux et al., 1997). Because it is the trophic

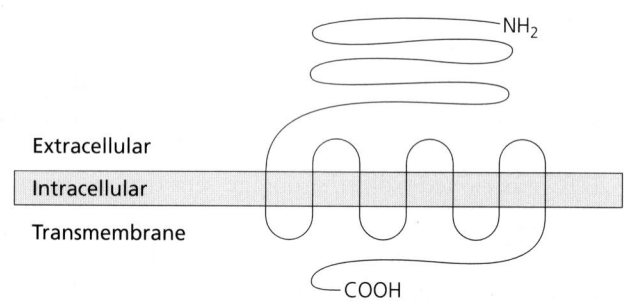

Fig. 35.2. The basic structure of a G-protein coupled receptor is shown. The GnRHR, LH/hCGR, and FSHR share this basic structure. In general, mutations of the extracellular domain reduce ligand binding, while those at other locations affect signal transduction.

Table 35.3. Gene mutations affecting pituitary function in females

Gene	Localization	Phenotype	Inheritance
GNRHR	4q21.2	HH	Autosomal recessive
HESX1	3p21.1-21.2	Septo-optic dysplasia	Autosomal recessive
LHβ	19q13.3	Isolated LH deficiency	Autosomal recessive
FSHβ	11p13	Isolated FSH deficiency	Autosomal recessive
PROP1	5q	Short stature, hypothyroid, HH	Autosomal recessive
HESX1	3p21.1-21.2	Septo-optic dysplasia	Autosomal recessive

stimulus that is deficient, i.e., gonadotropins, sterility here refers only to the untreated state. If gonadotropins are provided, fertility may be achieved.

Females with GnRHR gene mutations may present with absent breast development, no menstrual periods, low estradiol, low FSH and LH, and they lack CNS tumors which could impinge upon GnRH neurons (Layman et al., 1997). Other affected females have had normal breast development and one or two menstrual periods before becoming irreversibly amenorrheic and proband was a male who presented at age 22 with hypogonadism and no evidence of anosmia (de Roux et al., 1997). The administration of exogenous GnRH results in either an absent, blunted, or nearly normal gonadotropin response, demonstrating the heterogeneity of the disorder (Layman et al., 1997). The reported mutations have all been missense mutations that affect either ligand binding, signal transduction or both (de Roux et al., 1997; 1999; Layman et al., 1997; Caron et al., 1999). One woman received a prolonged treatment with subcutaneous GnRH given at physiologic intervals (every 90 minutes), but failed to ovulate, while her affected sister had two ovulatory cycles with gonadotropins (Layman et al., 1997). These findings suggested the possibility of GnRH resistance.

The prevalence of GnRHR gene mutations is unknown, but in a small study of 46 unrelated IHH probands (32 males and 14 females) screened for GnRHR gene mutations by GC-clamped denaturing gradient gel electrophoresis, only 2.2% (1 of 46) total IHH patients, and 7.1% (1 of 14) of patients in which an affected female was present (Layman et al., 1997).

THE LUTEINIZING HORMONE-BETA/HUMAN CHORIONIC GONADOTROPIN-BETA (LHβ/HCGβ) GENES

The pituitary glycoprotein hormones consist of a common α-subunit encoded by a single gene and a specific β-subunit (LH, hCG, FSH, and TSH). No human α-subunit mutations have been described yet, but the phenotype would be expected to include hypogonadotropic hypogonadism and hypothyroidism due to gonadotropin and TSH deficiency, similar to the α-subunit knockout mouse. In the homozygous knockout mice, neonatal gonads appeared normal, but adult gonads had a prepubertal appearance, suggesting that gonadotropins are not necessary for prenatal sexual differentiation (Kendall et al., 1995).

The LHβ/hCGβ gene complex consists of six hCGβ and one LHβ genes, which are highly polymorphic (Weiss et al., 1992). However, the only one known human mutation in the LHβ gene to date was found in a male with pubertal delay, small testes, oligospermia, and deficient testosterone, with elevated immunoreactive, but reduced biologically active LH levels. Merke and Colleagues (1999) studied a family in which two males had a nonsense mutation of codon 172 of the DAX1 gene as the cause of congenital adrenal hypoplasia with gonadotropic hypogonadism. Their mother was heterozygous for this mutation as was their maternal grandfather, both of whom were asymptomatic. The results of mutational analysis of DNA from urinary sediment were similar to those in leukocyte DNA. A maternal aunt, who had isolated hypogonadotropic hypogonadism, was homozygous for the mutation. This homozygosity was thought to have resulted from gene conversion, the non-reciprocal transfer of DNA from one parental allele to the other. This is a novel suggestion for manifestations in heterozygous females. No mutations of the LHβ/hCGβ gene complex were identified in couples with unexplained infertility or in women with recurrent abortion (Layman et al., 1997). Although not yet described, females with LHβ gene mutations would be expected to exhibit normal puberty with anovulation.

THE FOLLICLE STIMULATING HORMONE-BETA (FSHβ) GENE

Mutations in the FSHβ gene have been described in several males and females (Matthews et al., 1993; Layman et al., 1997; Lindstedt et al., 1998; Phillip et al., 1998). All mutations (missense, nonsense, or 2 bp deletion) in females have been identified in exon 3, and those studied in vitro result in low immunoreactive and low bioactive FSH levels (Matthews et al., 1993; Layman et al., 1997). Most females display a complete absence of pubertal development, completely lacking breasts and never having any menses. Estradiol levels are menopausal, FSH is very low or undetectable, and LH levels are elevated (Matthews et al., 1993; Layman et al., 1997). Isolated FSH deficiency is inherited in an autosomal recessive fashion.

Although females with isolated FSH deficiency have elevated levels of LH, they do not exhibit hyperandrogenism or hirsutism (Layman et al., 1997). This finding was not expected since women with polycystic ovary syndrome (PCOS), defined as chronic hyperandrogenic anovulation (with or without polycystic appearing ovaries on ultrasound), have elevated LH levels and hyperandrogenism. These findings question the two-gonadotropin two-cell hypothesis, which states that LH stimulates ovarian thecal cells to produce androgens, which serve as precursors for estrogens in the granulosa cell where FSH induces aromatization to estrogen (Layman et al., 1997). The fact that isolated FSH deficiency is associated with low androgens suggests that FSH plays an important role in ovarian androgen production, perhaps by increasing LH receptors, or by inducing 17-hydroxylase activity (an androgen dependent enzyme), inhibin, or growth factors. Ovarian follicles typically show primordial, primary, and antral follicles, and normal fertility may be restored with FSH treatment (Matthews et al., 1993; Layman et al., 1997).

THE *PROP1* GENE

Mutations in pituitary transcription factors have the potential to cause hypogonadotropic hypogonadism with or without deficiencies of other pituitary hormones. *PROP1* appears to be important for the early pituitary development since mutations of *PROP1* have been shown to cause combined pituitary hormone deficiency (Wu et al., 1998). *PROP1*-deficient patients have an autosomal recessive form of GH, TSH, prolactin, and gonadotropin deficiency. They display extremely short stature secondary to deficient TSH and GH levels. Affected individuals from several different families demonstrated a failure of the pituitary to respond normally to GHRH, TRH, and GnRH stimulation (Wu et al., 1998). A variety of mutations have been identified including missense mutations and small deletions. Mutations of the mouse homolog (*Prop1*) cause a similar phenotype in the Ames dwarf mouse.

It has been suggested that milder mutations of *PROP1* might be expected to cause gonadotropin deficiency, sparing GH, TSH, and ACTH. However, in a large study of 175 patients with idiopathic hypogonadotropic hypogonadism (IHH), no *PROP1* mutations were identified by denaturing gradient gel electrophoresis of GC-clamped PCR products, suggesting that *PROP1* mutations rarely result in this phenotype.

THE *HESX1* GENE

Several homeobox genes were hypothesized to be excellent candidate genes for human idiopathic hypogonadotropic hypogonadism (IHH). *EMX2* mutations result in schizencephaly (a defect in the cerebrum in which hemispheres are physically separated by clefts), and because it also expressed in the olfactory bulbs and kidneys, it represents a reasonable candidate gene for IHH, but no mutations have been identified to date (Taylor et al., 1999).

However, an Arg53Cys missense mutation in *HESX1* was identified in one family with affected individuals with septo-optic dysplasia, a disorder characterized by panhypo-

pituitarism, optic nerve atrophy, and other midline CNS abnormalities such as agenesis of the corpus callosum and septum pellucidum (Table 35.3) (Dattani et al., 1998). The mutation occurred in the homeodomain and reduced DNA binding, an important function of this transcription factor. *Hesx1*, the mouse homologue of *HESX1*, is expressed in the early forebrain. Later, *Hesx1* expression is restricted to Rathke's pouch, which ultimately becomes the anterior pituitary gland. Although the phenotype is not described in detail in this report, HH is a common feature of septo-optic dysplasia (Datteni et al., 1998).

Ovarian causes of female infertility

Identified gene mutations affecting ovarian development and/or function are summarized in Table 35.4. It should be noted that although hypergonadotropic hypogonadism has been reported in myotonic dystrophy, the incidence in affected females is very low, so it will not be discussed (Layman, 1997).

X-CHROMOSOME DISORDERS ASSOCIATED WITH OVARIAN CAUSES OF INFERTILITY

1 Whole X chromosome deletions

Women completely lacking an X chromosome include patients with a pure 45,X karyotype, but also include those with another cell line, such as 46,XY, 46,XX, 47,XXX, or 46,X iXq. About 90% of these patients with a single 45,X cell line with or without another cell line, present with primary amenorrhea, the complete lack of pubertal development with absent breast development. Typically, patients with 45,X cell line have ovarian failure with irreversibly elevated levels of gonadotropins FSH and LH and low levels of estradiol. Only about 10–15% of women with a 45,X cell line experience pubertal development with menstruation, although regular ovulatory cycles do not last very long as ovarian failure ensues (Layman and Reindoller, 1994; Layman, 1997).

Because of these endocrinologic deficiencies, very few 45,X women become pregnant spontaneously, since donor oocyte in vitro fertilization (IVF) is usually necessary for most 45,X patients. However, at least 138 pregnancies (without IVF) have been reported in 62 women with a 45,X cell line, most of whom have a second cell line (Kaneko et al., 1990). No patients with a 46,XY cell line have achieved pregnancy without IVF. In patients with complete X chromosome deletions, fetal wastage is

Table 35.4. Gene mutations/chromosomal abnormalities affecting gonadal function in females

Gene	Localization	Phenotype	Inheritance
Whole Del X	45,X (with or without other cell line)	Short stature & ovarian failure	Sporadic
Partial Del X	Xp & Xq	Variable: delayed puberty/infertility	X-linked dominant
t(X-A)	Variable	Variable; delayed puberty/infertility	Sporadic or X-linked dominant
DIAPH2	Xq21	Ovarian failure	Disruption in X-autosome translocation
FMR1	Xq27.3	Fragile X; ovarian failure	X-linked dominant
SRY	Yp11.3	Swyer syndrome	Sporadic, Y linked
FSHR	2p21p16	Primary amenorrhea (F); Oligospermia (M)	Autosomal recessive
LHR	2p21	Anovulation (F) Undermasculinization (M)	Autosomal recessive
CYP17	10q24.3	17-hydroxylase deficiency	Autosomal recessive
CYP19	15q21.1	Aromatase deficiency	Autosomal recessive
AIRE	21q22.3	APECED	Autosomal recessive
FTZF1 (SF1)	9q33	Adrenal failure/sex reversal (M)	Autosomal recessive
GALT	9p13	Galactosemia (with ovarian failure)	Autosomal recessive

common, as 26% had spontaneous abortions, and another 6% had stillborns. In addition, about 18% had a chromosomal abnormality or significant congenital anomaly. When just the liveborn are evaluated, 23/102 (23%) had chromosomal or congenital anomalies (Kareko et al., 1990). Important to note is the 4% risk that a woman with a 45,X cell line will have a child with Down syndrome. Although advanced maternal age must be considered in situations of increased aneuploidy, this is an unlikely factor in 45,X patients since most will have experienced gonadal failure before age 35. Ten percent of pregnant women with a 45,X cell line will have a sex chromosome aneuploid female with ovarian failure with reported karyotypes in their offspring including 45,X (3%), 45,X/46,XX (4%), 45,X/46,XY (1%), and 45,X/46,XX/47,XXX (2%) (Kaneko et al., 1990).

The molecular basis of 45,X gonadal dysgenesis or Turner syndrome remains unknown. It is likely that it is due to haploinsufficiency of multiple genes on the X chromosome which affect ovarian function and stature (Layman, 1997; Simpson and Rajkovic, 1999). Depending upon the severity, other phenotypic effects, such as shield chest, widely spaced nipples, webbed neck, multiple nevi, may or may not be present (Layman, 1997; Simpson and Rajkovic, 1999). The most constant feature is short stature, and a statural determinant gene has been identified in short patients with X deletions. Recently, a gene from the pseudoautosomal region of the X chromosome (with a pseudogene on the Y chromosome) was found to be a statural determinant gene, and the authors suggested it might be involved in the short stature of Turner syndrome (Rao et al., 1997). The pseudo-

autosomal homeobox containing osteogenic (*PHOG*) gene, also known as the short stature homeobox (*SHOX*) gene, is a transcription factor expressed primarily in osteogenic cells.

One patient of 91 males and females with idiopathic short stature (and none of 300 controls) was found to harbor a nonsense mutation (Arg195X) in *SHOX* (Rao et al., 1997). A different nonsense mutation (Tyr199X) was observed in a three-generation family with Leri-Weill Dyschondrosteosis, a skeletal dysplasia with disproportionate short stature, mesomelic limbs, and the Madelung deformity (sometimes seen in Turner syndrome) (Shears et al., 1998). A *SHOX* deletion on both X chromosomes has also been characterized in a female child with Langer mesomelic dysplasia, whose mother had a hemizygous deletion (Belin et al., 1998). Although deletions of *SHOX* have been postulated to cause the short stature of Turner syndrome, there are no studies of Turner patients documenting mutations in this gene.

2 X-chromosome deletions

Deletions of part of the X chromosome have been reported in a large number of patients, most of whom all the only case in the family. In general, deletions affecting Xp11 result in ovarian failure in about half of women, and menstrual function in the other half (Fig. 35.3); (Simpson and Rajkovic, 1999). Even in those with normal menstruation, fertility is rare. When the deletion on the X chromosome is more distal, such as the p21 region, patients usually have a less severe phenotype with normal menarche, although they

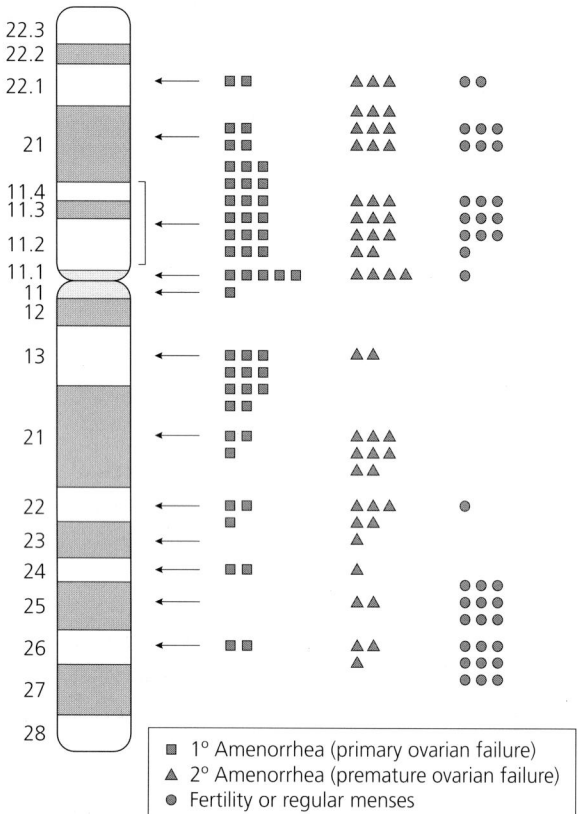

22.3
22.2
22.1

21

11.4
11.3
11.2
11.1
11
12

13

21

22
23
24
25
26
27
28

■ 1° Amenorrhea (primary ovarian failure)
▲ 2° Amenorrhea (premature ovarian failure)
● Fertility or regular menses

Fig. 35.3. The X chromosome is shown with the locations of different deletions and their corresponding phenotype. (From Simpson and Rajkovic, 1999.) Ovarian differentiation and ganadal failure. Am J Genet 89:186–200. ©1999 Reprinted by permission of Wiley-Liss Inc., a subsidiary of John Wiley Sons, Inc.

commonly manifest secondary amenorrhea or infertility. Most women with Xp deletions are short, regardless of their ovarian function, indicating that statural determinant genes likely lie within these regions (Simpson and Rajkovic, 1999). Several familial Xp deletions have also been reported (reviewed in Simpson and Rajkovic, 1999).

Deletions involving the q arm of X generally result in ovarian failure if they involve the proposed critical region (the critical region hypothesis), i.e., Xq13-q26. Although nearly all patients with deletions within this region do have gonadal failure, exceptions do occur. Similar to short arm deletions, proximal (Xq13) deletions are usually more severe, manifesting absent thelarche, primary amenorrhea, and hypergonadotropic hypogonadism. At the more distal end of the long arm, menarche may occur, with or without ovarian failure (Fig. 35.3). Patients with apparently the same breakpoints determined by karyotype may have different breakpoints at the molecular level, thereby contributing to the discrepancy in genotype/phenotype correlations in patients with X chromosome deletions.

There have been reports of familial X chromosome deletions in which gonadal failure in females occurs (reviewed in Simpson and Rajkovic, 1999 and Layman, 1997). Krauss and Colleagues (1987) reported a family with three women having normal puberty, pregnancy (in two women), and subsequent premature ovarian failure from ages 24–37. These three women and a fourth family member with normal puberty and irregular menses were found to have an interstitial deletion of Xq21.3-q27 by molecular analysis, which was thought to be a terminal deletion by cytogenetic studies. Heights of the proband (POF at age 24) and her sister with irregular menses and the same deletion were 155 cm (61 inches) and 152.5 cm (60 inches), respectively (others were not provided). The disorder appears to be inherited in an X-linked dominant fashion in this family since the phenotype was expressed when females had a single X chromosome with the interstitial deletion. Several other cases of molecular analysis of familial X chromosome deletions have been described. These studies of Xp and Xq deletions suggest that a number of ovarian determinant genes reside on the X chromosome (Layman, 1997; Simpson and Rajkovic, 1999).

One possible explanation for gonadal failure in women with partial X chromosome deletions is the loss of a putative ovarian determinant gene(s) necessary to be present in two copies during ovarian development. With an X chromosome deletion, the dosage of a normal gene is decreased and gonadal failure could ensue since reactivation of the previously inactivated X chromosome occurs during oogenesis. (Layman, 1997; Simpson and Rajkovic, 1999). Since many of these patients had normal puberty, but subsequently developed gonadal failure, deleted ovarian determinant genes probably increase follicular atresia, but not to the extent of that observed in patients with a 45,X cell line. It is also possible that the Xq deletion might affect mitosis or meiosis. If oocytes are unable to complete meiosis, enhanced follicular atresia could occur (Layman, 1999a,b).

3   X chromosome-autosome translocations

In contrast to most autosomal translocations, X-autosome translocations may affect reproductive capacity depending upon the location of break points of the X chromosome. In a balanced X-autosome translocation, when one X is normal (Xn), and the other is an X-autosome-translocation (Xt) chromosome, X-inactivation usually is not random, so that Xn is inactivated. If the translocated chromosome were inactivated (associated with *XIST* expression), the autosome would also be inactivated (Layman, 1997). Since monosomy of an autosome is lethal, the normal X chromosome must be inactivated to secure normalcy. In an unbalanced translocation involving the X chromosome, Xn is normally active while the X-autosome translocated product Xt containing *XIST* is inactivated in some cells.

X-autosome translocations are extremely rare, being estimated to occur in about 1/30,000 live births. This low frequency in the population is due to the observation that nearly all males and half of the females with X-autosome translocations are sterile (Layman, 1997). In females, the phenotype of a balanced X-autosome translocation depends upon the position of the breakpoint and the functional status of the Xt chromosome. Those patients with an active Xt (and inactive Xn) comprise about three quarters of those reviewed by Schmidt and Du Sart (1992). In the remaining one-fourth, Xt was subjected to inactivation in some cells. In females where Xt is active in all cells and the breakpoint does not interrupt any functional gene, approximately half have a normal phenotype and half have ovarian failure (Schmidt and Du Sart 1992). Although some exceptions exist, in general, those with ovarian failure have breakpoints within the Xq13-q26 region, while those with normal gonadal function do not have breakpoints outside this range.

For females with an active Xt in all cells (and inactivated Xn), when the breakpoints interrupt important genes on either the X chromosome or the autosome, a single gene disorder may occasionally result, such as the X-linked recessive diseases Duchenne muscular dystrophy or Hunter syndrome. These types of translocations have been useful for mapping disease-producing genes, since the breakpoint signals where the candidate gene is localized. In the one-fourth of balanced X-autosome translocations, Xt is inactivated in a proportion of cells, which generally produces multiple anomalies and mental retardation (Schmidt and Du Sart, 1992). In only 3 of 122 (2.5%) cases was the same X-autosome translocation identified in other family members (Xp11.22). None of these probands with the X-A translocation had gonadal failure, so transmission of a balanced X-autosome translocation is extremely unlikely.

The location of the X chromosome breakpoints involved in the translocation is evenly distributed when different studies are combined, although regions Xq24 and Xq25 were underrepresented in one study (Schmidt and Du Sart, 1992). The most common autosomes involved in X-autosome translocations include chromosomes 15, 21, and 22. The pericentromeric regions of these acrocentric autosomes are particularly predisposed to pairing with the X chromosome. It has been hypothesized that translocations involving the X chromosome cause ovarian failure by a position effect (the order of important ovarian determinant gene(s) is altered) or by the deletion of ovarian determinant genes.

Alternatively, the translocation could impair the normal activity of the X chromosome in meiosis or mitosis, which could also render the oocytes dysfunctional predisposing them to accelerated atresia, as discussed for X chromosome deletions.

Single gene disorders causing ovarian infertility

THE DIAPHANOUS GENE

As discussed under X chromosome deletions and translocations, multiple ovarian determinant genes are likely to reside throughout the X chromosome. In a woman with POF who had a balanced X;12 translocation, t(X;12)(q21;p1.3), the last intron of the diaphanous 2 (*DIAPH2*) gene was found to be disrupted (Bione et al., 1998). *DIAHP2* disruption was proposed to be the etiologic event since this gene has high homology to the DIA gene of Drosophila, which is expressed in the testes and ovary, and results in sterility when mutations occur (Bione et al., 1998). However, the importance of this gene remains to be determined, as no point mutations have yet been described and other females with deletions of Xq21 may not have *DIAPH2* disruption (Simpson and Rajkovic, 1999).

THE *FMR1* GENE

Fragile X syndrome is an X-linked dominant disorder with incomplete penetrance characterized by mental deficiency, macroorchidism, and large ears and jaws in affected males. The mental deficiency may be subtle and be manifested as autistic behavior. At the location of the fragile site on the long arm (Xq27) of the X chromosome resides the *FRMR1* gene, which contains a triplet repeat of CGG base pairs (bp) normally in the range of 6–50 bp. Affected males have an expansion of these repeated sequences to greater or equal to 200 repeats, while carrier females are said to possess a premutation allele of 50–200 repeats. Interestingly, some females with premutation alleles may be affected with mild degrees of mental deficiency or learning disability.

Although males with fragile X syndrome have macroorchidism as a feature and normal testicular histology, premature ovarian failure has been observed more frequently in carrier females (see Layman, 1997). Conversely, *FMR1* premutations have been identified frequently in women with idiopathic premature ovarian failure, with 6/147 (4%) of women having premutations, including four familial and two sporadic cases. Similar to the findings of other investigators, no women in this large study had full mutations in *FMR1* (Murray et al., 1998). Although there is not general agreement upon the association of POF and *FMR1* mutations, it has been hypothesized that premutations of *FMR1* might affect ovarian development or function, or both.

THE *SRY* GENE

Most individuals with 46,XY gonadal dysgenesis (Swyer syndrome) have sexual infantilism, a normal vagina and uterus, and streak gonads with the propensity for gonadoblastoma with or without an accompanying germ cell tumor (Cameron and Sinclair, 1997; McElreavey and Fellous, 1999). Since the gonad is dysgenetic, Mullerian inhibiting substance (MIS) is deficient, explaining the presence of a uterus. Testosterone, is also deficient resulting in undermasculinization of 46,XY males. Most cases are isolated and have been presumed to be caused by mutations in *SRY* (sex determining region on the Y chromosome), a single exon gene encoding a transcription factor with a conserved HMG (high mobility group) domain. However, only about 15% of such patients possess *SRY* mutations suggesting that other etiologies must be present in these patients (Cameron and Sinclair, 1997; McElreavey and Fellows, 1999).

THE FOLLICLE STIMULATING HORMONE RECEPTOR (*FSHR*) GENE

The FSHR is a heptohelical G-protein coupled receptor located on the membrane surface of ovarian granulosa cells (Fig. 35.2). Several *FSHR* mutations have been described in humans, and they result in a clinical syndrome of FSH resistance (Aittomaki et al., 1995; 1996; Beau et al., 1998). Females usually present with primary amenorrhea, and about half have breast development, while the other half completely lack thelarche (Aittomaki et al., 1995; 1996). One case has also been described in which the female had normal breast development and menarche, but ceased menstruating within a few years of menarche (Beau et al., 1998). Serum FSH and LH are typically elevated, and estradiol levels are low-normal to normal. Ovarian follicles range from primordial to mature, indicating that the defect is not quite as severe as that of the FSHβ ligand. These patients usually have irreversible hypergonadotropic hypogonadism, and require donor oocyte in vitro fertilization for treatment.

The Finnish mutation, a missense Ala189Val mutation of exon 7, results in a protein with normal binding affinity, but markedly decreased capacity (Aittomaki et al., 1995), while the other two mutations (found as a compound heterozygote

in the one patient) affect binding or signal transduction (Beau et al., 1998). The Finnish mutation is extremely rare outside Finland, and there is very little data concerning the prevalence of *FSHR* mutations in women with hypergonadotropic amenorrhea (Jiang et al., 1998; Layman et al., 1998a,b).

THE LUTEINIZING HORMONE/HUMAN CHORIONIC GONADOTROPIN RECEPTOR (LH/HCGR) GENE

The LH/hCGR is also a G-protein coupled receptor expressed in the thecal cells of the ovary and the Leydig cells of the testis (Fig. 35.2). The phenotype of patients with LH/hCGR gene mutations depends upon the karyotype. Genetic females with LH/hCGR gene mutations have normal puberty, with full breast development and menarche (Toledo et al., 1996). However, they become anovulatory with usually elevated, but occasionally normal, LH and FSH levels. They do not have testes; therefore they have a normal vagina and uterus. Genetic males with inactivating LH/hCGR mutations also usually present as phenotypic females but have delayed puberty with absent breast development and normal appearing external genitalia, but with a blind vaginal pouch (Kremer et al., 1995; Latronico et al., 1996). Since the testes is normal and produces MIS, no uterus or upper two-thirds of the vagina is present. The external genitalia phenotype, however, ranges from normal-appearing female to sexual ambiguity to bilaterally descended testes (Kremer et al., 1995; Latronico et al., 1996). Serum gonadotropins are both usually elevated, suggesting a gonadal etiology for the LH resistance. The testes are small and devoid of Leydig cells.

Inactivating mutations of the LH/hCGR gene are inherited in an autosomal recessive fashion (Latronico et al., 1996), in contrast to activating mutations of the LH/hCGR, which cause autosomal dominant familial male precocious puberty (Shenker et al., 1993).

THE *CYP17* GENE

CYP17 encoding for the cytochrome P450 enzyme with at least two functions, a 17-hydroxylase activity (converting progesterone to 17-hydroxyprogesterone and pregnenolone to 17-hydroxypregnenolone) and a 17–20 desmolase activity (converting 17-hydroxypregnenolone to dehydroepiandrosterone (DHEA) and 17-hydroxyprogesterone to androstenedione). With *CYP17* mutations, an autosomal recessive deficiency in the production of androgens, progestins, and estrogens results (Simpson and Kakjovic, 1999). Cortisol is also deficient since it is derived from 17-hydroxyprogesterone; however, mineralocorticoids such as 11-deoxycorticosterone (DOC) and corticosterone may be elevated, with associated hypertension and hypokalemic alkalosis.

The phenotype in 46,XX females includes delayed puberty with absent breast development, primary amenorrhea, and elevated gonadotropins (Yanase et al., 1991). The vagina, uterus, and ovaries are present, but they are hypoestrogenic. 46,XY males have a similar phenotype except that they will not have a uterus or upper vagina since MIS is produced from their normal testes. Some males with partial deficiency may have sexual ambiguity. A variety of mutations in CYP17 have been identified, consisting predominantly of deletions and insertions (Yanase et al., 1991).

THE *CYP19* GENE AROMATASE

Mutations in CYP19 encoding the cytochrome P450 enzyme aromatase, cause autosomal recessive aromatase deficiency. Females with aromatase deficiency are unable to convert androgens testosterone and androstenedione to estradiol and estrone, respectively (Simpson and Rakjovic, 1999). Females are born with sexual ambiguity with clitoromegaly, but since they have ovaries, they do not have labioscrotal gonads (Ito et al., 1993; Simpson and Rakjovic, 1999). When these children approach the time of puberty, FSH rises, and multicystic ovaries develop (Ito et al., 1993). However, the increased FSH cannot elicit the production of ovarian estrogen and no breast development or menses occur. LH levels are also usually elevated in these patients.

An interesting feature of aromatase deficiency is that the heterozygous mother carrying an affected female fetus can also develop hyperandrogenism and hirsutism (Shozu et al., 1991). This is because the fetal placenta (derived from the fetus, having the same genotype as the fetus) cannot convert androgens to estrogens. Normally, the placenta is quite capable of aromatase production, which helps protect the mother from hyperandrogenism.

THE AUTOIMMUNE REGULATORY (*AIRE*) GENE

The autoimmune polyglandular syndrome type 1, also known as autoimmune polyendocrinopathy-candidiasis-ectodermal dystrophy (APECED) is an autosomal recessive disorder in which multisystem autoimmune disease is observed. APECED is more common in the Finnish population and in Iranian Jews. Moniliasis (60%) is a common initial presenting feature, but can occur at anytime. Hypoparathyroidism (80%) and adrenal failure (70%) represent the most frequent endocrine manifestations, but

ovarian failure (60%) and testicular failure (14%) may also occur with sufficient frequency (Layman, 1997).

Mutations in AIRE (autoimmune regulator) a transcriptional factor with two PHD-type zinc-finger motifs, have been identified in patients with APECED (Consortium, 1997; Nagamine et al., 1997). The identification and characterization of AIRE mutations represented the first report of a single gene defect causing systemic autoimmune disease in humans (Consortium, 1997; Nagamine et al., 1997). Approximately 80% of mutations in the Finnish patients consist of a single nonsense mutation (Arg257X) (Nagamine et al., 1997), while a 13 bp deletion accounts for more than half of mutations in North American patients (Heino et al., 1999), and a single nonsense mutation (Arg139X) occurred in about 80% of Sardinian AIRE alleles (Rosatelli et al., 1998). Currently, it is unclear whether certain mutations increase the likelihood of ovarian failure vs other endocrinopathies.

THE *FTZF1* GENE

FTZF1 encodes for steroidogenic factor 1 (SF1) protein, a transcription factor important in steroidogenesis in the gonad and adrenal glands. Similar to targeted disruption of the homologous gene in the mouse, a mutation in FTZF1 caused undermasculinization of a 46,XY male (Achermann et al., 1999). The patient presented as a phenotypic female with adrenal failure in neonatal life, who later was studied before puberty at age 10. Her baseline serum levels of gonadotropins increased in response to exogenous GnRH, but the testosterone did not increase to hCG administration suggesting defective gonadal function. At laparotomy, the proband had a normal uterus and bilateral streak gonads. Estrogen replacement induced normal breast development, and combination estrogen and progesterone induced normal withdrawal periods (Achermann et al., 1999).

Upon DNA sequencing of FTZF1, a heterozygous 2 bp point mutation in the proximal box of the first zinc finger was identified, which upon in vitro analysis, eliminates SF1 from binding to DNA (Achermann et al., 1999). To date, this is the only case described in humans. The phenotype in genetic females would be expected to consist of adrenal failure, delayed puberty with absent breast development and primary amenorrhea, with elevated gonadotropins.

THE *GALT* (GALACTOSE-1-PHOSPHATE URIDYLTRANSFERASE) GENE

Galactosemia is an autosomal recessive disorder in which galactose cannot be properly metabolized to glucose. The phenotype typically consists of failure to thrive, nausea, and vomiting, cataracts, hepatomegaly, mental retardation, speech abnormalities, and hemolytic anemia. If treated by a galactose-free diet, the prognosis for liver function and mental capacity is improved, but not to the level expected (Gitzelmann and Steinmann, 1984). Although several enzymes are involved in the process, galactosemia caused by mutations in *GALT* have been shown to have a sex-specific effect upon reproduction in that females, but not males, develop gonadal failure. This enzyme is responsible for the conversion of galactose-1-phosphate and UDP-glucose to UDP-galactose and glucose-1-phosphate.

In a study by Kaufman et al. (1979), 12/18 (67%) of women with galactosemia had premature ovarian failure, while none of eight men had testicular failure. Females had normal pubertal development, but half presented with primary amenorrhea, while the other half had secondary amenorrhea. However, gonadotropins were elevated in both groups. The exact cause of the ovarian failure is unknown, but could represent a detrimental metabolic defect during development caused by galactose-1-phosphate, abnormal glycosylation of gonadotropin glycoproteins or their receptors. More than 150 *GALT* mutations have been described, many of which are missense mutations. Heterozygotes do not develop gonadal failure as homozygotes do. Of interest, the *GALT* knockout mouse has a less severe phenotype, and no effect upon gonadal development and function (Leslie et al., 1996).

Uterine/vaginal genetic causes of infertility

THE HUMAN ANDROGEN RECEPTOR GENE

The human androgen receptor (hAR) belongs to the steroid superfamily of nuclear hormone receptors, and is encoded by an 8 exon gene. The protein has an amino-terminus, a DNA binding domain, and a carboxyterminal androgen binding domain. 46,XY males with complete androgen insensitivity syndrome (CAIS) due to mutations in the hAR present as phenotypic females with normal breast development, minimal axillary and pubic hair, and a blind vaginal pouch (Gottlieb

et al., 1999). The phenotype results from the absence of normal androgen interaction with its receptor at the target level. Since testes are normal, MIS is produced, which inhibits the formation of the uterus and upper vagina. The vagina appears as a blind vaginal pouch and no cervix is identified. The testes, which may be intra-abdominal or inguinal, are capable of making testosterone, and normal adult male levels are produced (300–1100 ng/dL). Incomplete forms of AIS have also been described, but these will not be discussed here since they cause sexual ambiguity in males.

More than 300 different mutations, most commonly missense mutations, in the hAR gene have been reported to cause AIS. Interestingly, nearly all of the exon 1 mutations cause CAIS or incomplete AIS, and most of these produce a premature stop codon (Gottlieb et al., 1999). However, most of the mutations causing AIS occur in exons 2–8, despite the fact that exon 1 encodes for more than half of the protein (Gottlieb et al., 1999).

THE *HOXA13* GENE

To date, only one single gene disorder has been shown to affect uterine development in genetic females. A nonsense mutation in the *HOXA13* homeobox gene has been identified in women with the hand-foot-genital syndrome (Mortlock and Innis, 1997). The mutation truncates 20 amino acids from the mature protein and is predicted to reduce the ability of the protein to bind DNA (Mortlock and Innis, 1997). Patients with this autosomal dominant disorder typically have small hands and feet, along with a double uterus. The specific hand anomalies include short first metacarpals, short middle phalanges of the fifth fingers, small distal phalanges of the thumbs, and delayed ossification or fusion of wrist bones. The great toe demonstrates a short first metatarsal and a small pointed distal phalanx. Uterine anomalies typically include bicornuate or didelphic abnormalities of midline Mullerian fusion (Mortlock and Innis, 1997). Urinary anomalies, such as displaced urethral or ureteral openings are also associated with hand-foot-genital syndrome. Males may have varying degrees of hypospadius. Although congenital absence of euterus and vagina seems like another potential phenotype of *HOXA13* mutations, none have been described in these patients to date.

Table 35.5. Gene mutations abnormalities affecting uterine development in females

Gene	Localization	Phenotype	Inheritance
hAR	Xq11q12	Androgen insensitivity syndrome (M)	X-linked recessive
HOXA13		Hand-foot-uterus syndrome	Autosomal dominant

Conclusion

At the present time, there is little information regarding the genetic basis of human female fertility. A relatively small number of mutations in genes affecting hypothalamic, pituitary, gonadal, and uterine/vaginal development and func-

tion have been characterized. Most of the disorders described are rare, and there have been very few studies on the prevalence of these mutations in infertile patients. When the genome mapping project is completed, we can expect an exponential increase in the number of gene mutations in newly identified genes.

REFERENCES

Achermann JC, Ito M, Ito M et al. (1999) A mutation in the gene encoding steroidogenic factor-1 causes XY sex reversal and adrenal failure in humans. Nat Genet 22:125–126

Aittomaki K, Lucena JLD, Pakarinen P et al. (1995) Mutation in the follicle-stimulating hormone receptor gene causes hereditary hypergonadotropic hypogonadism. Cell 82:959–968

Aittomaki K, Herva R, Stenman U-H et al. (1996) Clinical features of primary ovarian failure caused by a point mutation in the follicle stimulating hormone receptor gene. J Clin Endocrinol Metab 81:3722–3726

Bardoni B, Zanaria E, Guioli S et al. (1994) A dosage sensitive locus at chromosome Xp21 is involved in male to female sex reversal. Nat Genet 7:497–501

Beau I, Touraine P, Meduri G et al. (1998) A novel phenotype related to partial loss of function mutations of the follicle stimulating hormone receptor. J Clin Invest 102:1352–1359

Belin V, Cusin V, Viot G et al. (1998) SHOX mutations in dyschondrosteosis (Leri-Weill syndrome). Nat Genet 19:67–69

Bione S, Sala C, Manzini C et al. (1998) A human homologue of the Drosophila melanogaster diaphenous gene is disrupted in a patient with premature ovarian failure: Evidence for conserved function in oogenesis and implications for human sterility. Am J Hum Genet 62:533–541

Cameron R, Sinclair AH (1997) Mutations in SRY and SOX9: Testis-determining genes. Hum Mutat 9:388–395

Caron P, Chauvin S, Christin-Maitre S et al. (1999) Resistance of hypogonadotropic patients with mutated GnRH receptor genes to pulsatile GnRH administration. J Clin Endocrinol Metab 84:990–996

Clement K, Vaisse C, Lahlou N et al. (1998) A mutation in the human leptin receptor gene causes obesity and pituitary dysfunction. Nature 392:398–401

Consortium F-GA (1997) An autoimmune disease, APECED, caused by mutations in a novel gene featuring two PHD-type zinc-finger domains. Nat Genet 17:399–403

Dattani MT, Martinez-Barbera J-P, Thomas PQ et al. (1998) Mutations in the homeobox gene HESX1/Hesx1 associated with septo-optic dysplasia in human and mouse. Nat Genet 19:125–133

de Roux N, Young J, Misrahi M et al. (1997) A family with hypogonadotrophic hypogonadism and mutations in the gonadotropin-releasing hormone receptor. N Engl J Med 337:1597–1602

de Roux N, Young J, Brailly-Tabard S et al. (1999) The same molecular defects of the gonadotropin-releasing hormone determine a variable degree of hypogonadism in affected kindred. J Clin Endocrinol Metab 84:567–572

Franco B, Guioli S, Pragliola A et al. (1991) A gene deleted in Kallmann's syndrome shares homology with neural cell adhesion and axonal path-finding molecules. Nature 353:529–536

Gitzelmann R, Steinmann B (1984) Galactosemia how does long-term treatment change the outcome? Enzyme 32:37–46

Gottlieb B, Pinsky L, Beitel LK, Trifiro M (1999) Androgen insensitivity. Am J Med Genet 89:210–217

Guo W, Mason JS, Stone CG et al. (1995) Diagnosis of X-linked adrenal hypoplasia congenita by mutation analysis of the DAX1 gene. JAMA 274:324–330

Habiby RL, Boepple P, Nachtigall L et al. (1996) Adrenal hypoplasia congenita with hypogonadotropic hypogonadism: Evidence that DAX-1 mutations lead to combined hypothlamic and pituitary defects in gonadotropin production. J Clin Invest 98:1055–1062

Hardelin JP, Levilliers J, Blanchard S et al. (1993) Heterogeneity in the mutations responsible for X chromosome-linked Kallmann syndrome. Hum Mol Genet 2:373–377

Heino M, Scott HS, Chen Q et al. (1999) Mutation analysis of North American APS-1 patients. Hum Mutat 13:69–74

Ito Y, Fisher CR, Conte FA et al. (1993) Molecular basis of aromatase deficiency in an adult female with sexual infantilism and polycystic ovaries. Proc Natl Acad Sci USA 90:11673–11677

Jiang M, Aittomaki K, Nilsson C et al. (1998) The frequency of an inactivating point mutation (^{566}C–T) of the human follicle-stimulating hormone receptor gene in four populations using allele-specific hybridization and time-resolved fluorometry. J Clin Endocrinol Metab 83:4338–4343

Kaneko N, Kawagoe S, Hiroi M (1990) Turner's syndrome–review of the literature with reference to a successful pregnancy outcome. Gynecol Obstet Invest 29:81–87

Kaufman FR, Kogut MD, Donnell GN et al. (1979) Hypergonadotropic hypogonadism in female patients with galactosemia. N Engl J Med 304:994–998

Kendall SK, Samuelson LC, Saunders TL et al. (1995) Targeted disruption of the pituitary glycoprotein hormone alpha-subunit produces hypogonadal and hypothyroid mice. Genes Develop 9:2007–2019

Krauss CM, Turksoy RN, Atkins L et al. (1987) Familial premature ovarian failure due to interstital deletions of the long arm of the X chromosome. N Engl J Med 317:125–131

Kremer H, Kraaij R, Toledo SPA et al. (1995) Male pseudohermaphroditism due to a homozygous missense mutation of the luteinizing hormone receptor gene. Nat Genet 9:160–164

Latronico AC, Anasti J, Arnhold IJP et al. (1996) Brief report: testicular and ovarian resistance to luteinizing hormone caused by inactivating mutations of the luteinizing hormone-receptor gene. N Engl J Med 334:507–512

Layman LC (1997) Familial ovarian failure. In Lobo RA, (ed): Perimenopause. NY, ch. 6, Springer-Verlag, pp. 46–77

Layman LC (1999a) Genetic aspects of amenorrhea. Contemp Obstet Gynecol 44:27–40

Layman LC (1999b) The genetics of human hypogonadotropic hypogonadism. Am J Med Genet 89:240–248

Layman LC, Reindollar RH (1994) The diagnosis and treatment of pubertal disorders. Adolesc Med: State of the art reviews 5:37–55

Layman LC, Edwards JL, Osborne WE et al. (1997) Human chorionic gonadotropin-b sequences in women with disorders of HCG production. Mol Hum Reprod 3:315–320

Layman LC, Lee EJ, Peak DB et al. (1997) Delayed puberty and hypogonadism caused by a mutation in the follicle stimulating hormone β-subunit gene. N Engl J Med 337:607–611

Layman LC, Peak DB, Xie J et al. (1997) Mutation analysis of the gonadotropin releasing hormone receptor gene in idiopathic hypogonadotropic hypogonadism. Fertil Steril 68:1079–1085

Layman LC, Amde S, Cohen DP et al. (1998) The Finnish follicle stimulating hormone receptor (FSHR) gene mutation in women with 46,XX ovarian failure is rare in the United States. Fertil Steril 69:300–302

Layman LC, Cohen DP, Jin M et al. (1998) Mutations in the gonadotropin-releasing hormone receptor gene cause hypogonadotropic hypogonadism. Nat Genet 18:14–15

Legouis R, Hardelin J, Levilliers J et al. (1991) The candidate gene for the X-linked Kallmann syndrome encodes a protein related to adhesion molecules. Cell 67:423–435

Leslie ND, Yager KL, McNamara PD, Segal S (1996) A mouse model of galactose-1-phosphate uridyl transferase deficiency. Biochem Mol Med 59:7–12

Lindstedt G, Nystrom E, Matthews C et al. (1998) Follitropin (FSH) deficiency in an infertile male due to FSHbeta gene mutation. A syndrome of normal puberty and virilization but underdeveloped testicles with azoospermia, low FSH but high lutropin and normal serum testosterone concentrations. Clin Chem Lab Med 36:663–665

McElreavey K, Fellous M (1999) Sex determination and the Y chromosome. Am J Med Genet 89:176–185

Mason AJ, Hayflick JS, Zoeller T et al. (1986) A deletion truncating the gonadotropin-releasing hormone gene is responsible for hypogonadism in the hpg mouse. Science 234:1366–1371

Matthews CH, Borgato S, Beck-Peccoz P et al. (1993) Primary amenorrhea and infertility due to a mutation in the β-subunit of follicle-stimulating hormone. Nat Genet 5:83–86

Merke DP, Tajima T, Baron J, Cutler GB, Jr (1999) Hypogonadotropic hypogonadism in a female caused by an X-linked recessive mutation in the DAX1 gene. N Eng J Med 340:1248–1252

Montague CT, Farooqi S, Whitehead FP et al. (1997) Congenital leptin deficiency is associated with severe early-onset obesity in humans. Nature 387:903–908

Mortlock DP, Innis JW (1997) Mutation of HOXA13 in hand-foot-genital syndrome. Nat Genet 15:179–181

Murray A, Webb J, Grimley S et al. (1998) Studies of FRAXA and FRAXE in women with premature ovarian failure. J Med Genet 35:637–640

Muscatelli F, Strom TM, Walker AP et al. (1994) Mutations in the DAX-1 gene give rise to both X-linked adrenal hypoplasia congenita and hypogonadotropic hypogonadism. Nature 372:672–676

Nagamine K, Peterson P, Scott HS et al. (1997) Positional cloning of the APECED gene. Nat Genet 17:393–398

Phillip M, Arbelle JE, Segev Y, Parvari R (1998) Male hypogonadism due to a mutation in the gene for the b-subunit of follicle stimulating hormone. N Engl J Med 338:1729–1732

Rao E, Weiss B, Fukami M et al. (1997) Pseudoautosomal deletions encompassing a novel homeobox gene cause growth failure in idiopathic short stature and Turner syndrome. Nat Genet 16:54–63

Reindollar RH, Byrd JR, McDonough PG (1981) Delayed sexual development: A study of 252 patients. Am J Obstet Gynecol 140:371–380

Reindollar RH, Novak M, Tho SPT, McDonough PG (1986) Adult-onset amenorrhea: A study of 262 patients. Am J Obstet Gynecol 155:531–543

Rosatelli MC, Meloni A, Meloni A et al. (1998) A common mutation in Sardinian autoimmune polyendocrinopathy-candiasis-ectodermal dystrophy patients. Hum Genet 103:428–434

Rugarli EI, Lutz B, Kuratani SC et al. (1993) Expression pattern of the Kallmann syndrome gene in the olfactory system suggests a role in neuronal targeting. Nat Genet 4:19–26

Schmidt M, Du Sart D (1992) Functional disomies of the X chromosome influence: The cell selection and hence the X inactivation pattern in females with balanced X-autosome translocations: A review of 122 cases. Am J Med Genet 42:161–169

Shears DJ, Vassal HJ, Goodman FR et al. (1998) Mutation and deletion of the pseudoautosomal gene SHOX cause Leri-Weill dyschondrosteosis. Nat Genet 19:70–73

Shenker A, Laue L, Kosugi S et al. (1993) A constitutively acting mutation of the luteinizing hormone receptor in familial male precocious puberty. Nature 365:652–654

Shozu M, Akasofu K, Harada T, Kubota Y (1991) A new cause of female pseudohermaphroditism: placental aromatase deficiency. J Clin Endocrinol Metab 72:560–566

Simpson JL, Rajkovic A (1999) Ovarian differentiation and gonadal failure. Am J Med Genet 89:186–200

Speroff L. (1999) Women's healthcare in the 21st century. Maturitas 32:1–9

Strobel A, Issad T, Camoin L et al. (1998) A leptin missense mutation associated with hypogonadism and morbid obesity. Nat Genet 18:213–215

Taylor H, Block K, Olive D et al. (1999) Absence of EMX2 gene mutations in Kallmann syndrome. Fertil Steril 72:910–914

Toledo SPA, Brunner HG, Kraaij R et al. (1996) An inactivating mutation of the luteinizing hormone receptor causes amenorrhea in a 46,XX female. J Clin Endocrinol Metab 81:3850–3854

Weiss J, Axelrod L, Whitcomb RW et al. (1992) Hypogonadism caused by a single amino acid substitution in the β subunit of luteinizing hormone. N Engl J Med 326:179–183

Wu W, Cogan JD, Pfaffle RW et al. (1998) Mutations in PROP1 cause familial combined pituitary hormone deficiency. Nat Genet 18:147–149

Yanase T, Simpson ER, Waterman MR (1991) 17-Alpha-hydroxylase/17,20-lyase deficiency: From clinical investigation to molecular definition. Endocr Rev 12:91–108

Yu RN, Ito M, Saunders TL et al. (1998) Role of Ahch in gonadal development and gametogenesis. Nat Genet 20:353–357

Zanaria E, Muscatelli F, Bardoni B et al. (1994) An unusual member of the nuclear hormone receptor superfamily responsible for X-linked adrenal hypoplasia congenita. Nature 372:635–641

Zhang Y-H, Guo W, Wagner RL et al. (1998) DAX1 mutations provide insight into structure-function relationships in steroidogenic tissue development. Am J Hum Genet 62:855–864

Male infertility

Willy Lissens
Inge Liebaers
André Van Steirteghem

Introduction

Infertility and subfertility are estimated to affect approximately one in seven couples worldwide (Greenhall and Vessey, 1990). A male factor is the only, or an important contributory cause, in about half of these involuntary childless couples. Many different factors have been recognized as being involved in the etiology of male infertility and it has been shown, especially over the last decade, that genetic disorders account for a significant fraction of cases. It is to these genetic aspects of male infertility that this chapter is devoted.

Recombinant DNA technology has dramatically increased our knowledge of many biological processes in the last twenty years, including those leading to normal fertility in males. As evidence of how complex these processes are likely to be, many genetic defects interrupt the normal process, and consequently lead to infertility. In addition, the development of artificial reproductive technology (ART) has opened new perspectives for many couples suffering from infertility in the male. The introduction of intracytoplasmic sperm injection (ICSI) at the beginning of the 1990s, especially, gave rise to new possibilities for the alleviation of longstanding severe andrological infertility (Palermo et al., 1993; Van Steirteghem et al., 1993). In contrast to conventional *in vitro* fertilization (IVF), ICSI with sperm of poor quality is associated with considerably better fertilization rates and produces more embryos capable of implantation in the uterus. Moreover, couples who would not usually have been accepted for conventional IVF because of poor semen concentration, motility or morphology can now be helped since ICSI involves the injection of a single spermatozoon directly into the oocyte (Fig. 36.1 a–d). While concern has been expressed about the safety of the ICSI procedure itself, which

sometimes involves recovering spermatozoa or elongated spermatids from the epididymis or the testis, another source of concern has been the possible transmission of genetic disease (Bonduelle et al., 1999). Many couples, formerly unable to have their own genetic children, can now be treated successfully, but will thereby transmit infertility or genetic disease to their children if the infertility is linked to genetic factors. These factors can be transmitted as autosomal recessive, autosomal dominant, X-linked and Y-linked traits.

The World Health Organization (WHO) has proposed a standardized approach to the investigation and diagnosis of the infertile couple (Rowe et al., 1993). The recommendations provide the clinician with clear guidelines and a logical sequence of steps to reach quickly an accurate diagnosis of the underlying cause of infertility. For the male partner, the WHO manual defines 16 diagnostic categories covering the whole spectrum of causes including, among others, acquired and idiopathic ones. Since the aim of this chapter is to review what is known of the different genetic aspects of male infertility, a classification as proposed by the WHO could not be followed. After an overview of genes involved in early sexual development of the male, and of known defects in these genes leading to sex reversal, sexual ambiguity and/or infertility, we describe what is known of monogenic and chromosomal causes of infertility. In some instances the genetic defects occur in infertile but otherwise healthy males while in others the infertility is associated with additional minor or major clinical symptoms (Table 36.1).

Early sexual differentiation and sex reversal

In early fetal life, sexual development of male and female mammals is indistinguishable. The reproductive system

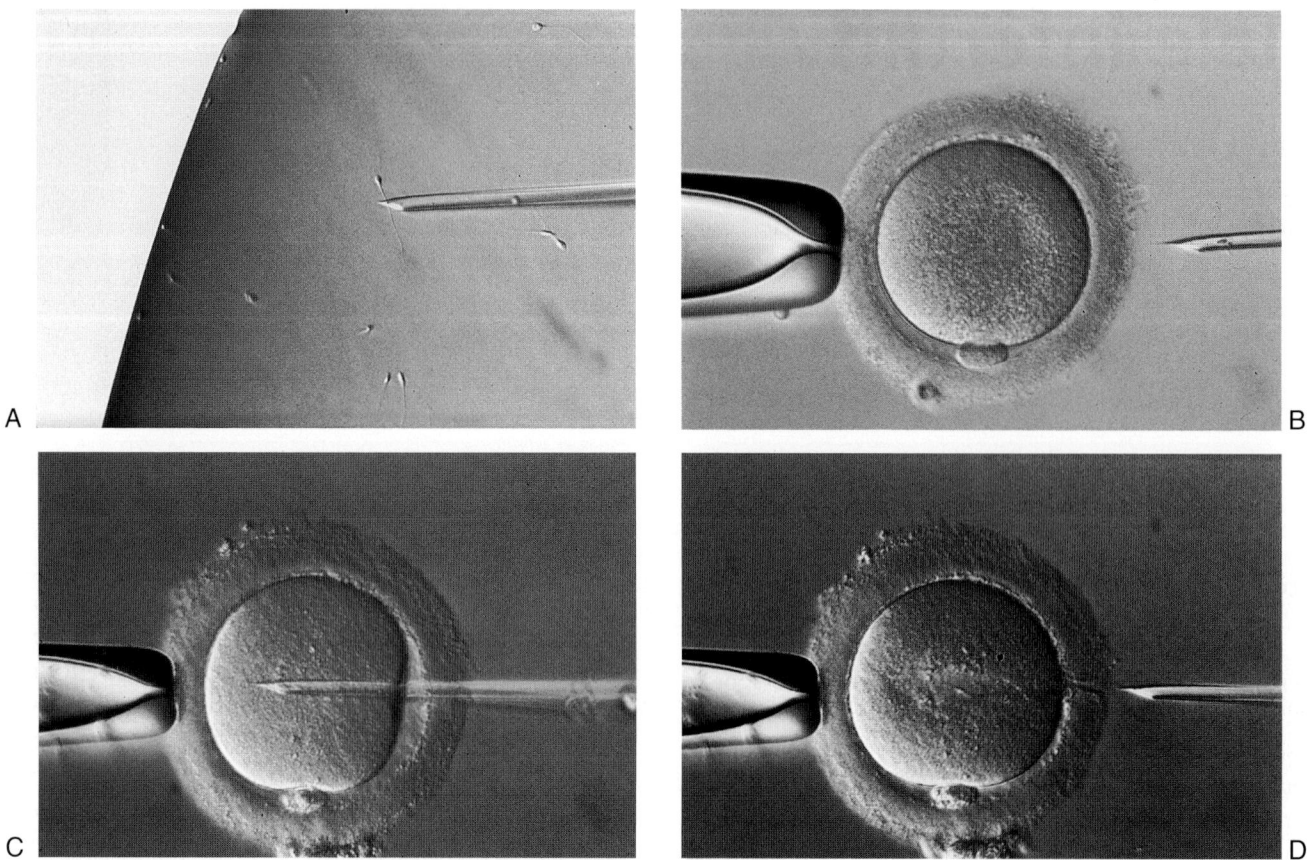

Fig. 36.1. Different steps in the ICSI procedure. **(A)** The injection pipette presses the tail of the spermatozoon against the bottom of the Petri dish until it stops moving. The spermatozoon is then aspirated, tail first, into the injection pipette. **(B)** The metaphase II oocyte is immobilized by slight negative pressure exerted on the holding pipette at 9 o'clock. The polar body is held at 6 o'clock **(C)** The micropipette containing a single spermatozoon is pushed through the zona pellucida and the oolemma into the ooplasm at 3 o'clock. **(D)** The injection pipette is withdrawn gently and the injected oocyte is released from the holding pipette.

consists of an indifferent bipotential gonad and two adjacent primitive ducts, the Müllerian and Wolffian ducts, precursors of the oviducts, uterus and upper vagina, and epididymis, vas deferens, seminal vesicles and ejaculatory ducts, respectively (Bogan and Page, 1994; Ramkissoon and Goodfellow, 1996; McElreavey and Fellous, 1997; Roberts et al., 1999). Differentiation into male or female will depend in the first place on the content of the sex chromosomes at fertilization (**genetic sex**). While an oocyte will always contribute an X chromosome to the embryo, a spermatozoon may contribute an X or a Y chromosome and this determines the genetic sex (female in the presence of two X chromosomes and male in the presence of an X and a Y chromosome). Male gonadal differentiation starts with the expression of the SRY (*s*ex-determining *r*egion Y; OMIM *480000) gene located on the short arm of the Y chromosome (**gonadal sex**). SRY is a single-exon gene that codes for a protein containing a DNA-binding motif called high-mobility group (HMG) (Sinclair et al., 1990). The protein is able to bind DNA and to produce a dramatic bend in the target DNA, thereby probably facilitating transcription of other genes in the sex-determining cascade (Haqq et al., 1994). However, direct target genes of SRY remain unknown. The expression of SRY in cells of the supporting cell precursor lineage induces their differentiation into Sertoli cells, which express anti-Müllerian hormone (AMH or Müllerian inhibiting substance, MIS). AMH is involved in the regression of the Müllerian duct and the production of testosterone in the Leydig cells which are thought to differentiate as a result of factors produced by Sertoli cells. The production of testosterone induces the formation of the internal male genitalia such as the epididymis, vas deferens, seminal vesicles and ejaculatory duct; the synthesis of dihydrotestosterone from testosterone results in the formation of the prostate, the urethra and the external genitalia (**phenotypic sex**). In a later stage of development, Leydig cells produce insulin-like hormone 3 (InsL3) that is required for descent of the testes (Zimmermann et al., 1998; 1999).

Table 36.1. Male Infertility: Clinical and Genetic Characteristics

Condition	Frequency	Physical Examination	Hormones	Sperm Characteristics	Karyotype	Cause	Gene	Locus	Infertility Treatment	OMIM
XX-Sex reversal	1:20000	male phenotype, hypogonadism, gonadal dysgenesis	↑ FSH, LH; ↓ T; ↑ estrogens	azoospermia	46,XX	X–Y recombination in 80% ? in 20%	SRY –	Yp11.3 –	AID AID	480000 Y-L
XY-Sex reversal	rare	female phenotype, gonadal dysgenesis		–	46,XY	SRY mutations in 20%, other causes in 80%	SRY ?	Yp11.3 –	oocyte donation	–
Numerical sex chromosomal aberrations	1:500 males	male phenotype, hypogonadism male phenotype	↑ FSH, LH; ↓ T; ↑ estrogens normal	azoospermia OAT OAT or NS	47,XXY, mosaics 47,XYY	NN NN	– –	– –	AID or ICSI + PGD AID or ICSI + PGD	– –
Chromosomal translocations	1:1000 males	male phenotype	–	OAT or NS	t(R) t(r)	NN NN	–	–		–
Persistent Müllerian Duct Syndrome (PMDS)	rare	male phenotype, cryptorchidism, pseudohermaphroditism, gonadal dysgenesis	normal	azoospermia	46,XY	Anti Müllerian Hormone deficiency Anti Müllerian Hormone type II receptor deficiency Anti Müllerian Hormone type I receptor deficiency postulated	AMH AMH II-receptor AMH I-receptor	19q13 12q13 NN	AID AID AID	261550 600957 AR 261550 600956 AR 261550 NN
Testosterone synthesis defects	rare	male phenotype, pseudohermaphroditism	↓ T	–	46,XY	CYP17 deficiency HSD3B2 deficiency HSD17B3 deficiency	CYP17 HSD3B2 HSD17B3	10q24.3 1p13.1 9q22	AID?	202110 AR 201810 AR 264300 AR
5α-reductase deficiency (Pseudovaginal perineoscrotal hypospadias)	rare	sex ambiguity, pseudohermaphroditism	↓ DHT, T/DHT ↑, T normal	OAT azoospermia	46,XY	5α-reductase 2 deficiency	SRD5A2	2p23	surgery + hormone substitution AID?	264600 AR male limited
Androgen resistance (Testicular feminization Complete/incomplete)	1:60000	female phenotype or sex ambiguity, pseudohermaphroditism, gonadal dysgenesis	T normal or ↑, E2 ↑, LH ↑, FSH normal or ↑	azoospermia	46,XY	androgen receptor deficiency complete/incomplete	AR point mutations	Xq11–q12	surgery towards male or female	300068 X-L

continued

Table 36.1. Male Infertility: Clinical and Genetic Characteristics (*contd*)

Condition	Frequency	Physical Examination	Hormones	Sperm Characteristics	Karyotype	Cause	Gene	Locus	Infertility Treatment	OMIM
Kennedy disease (SBMA)	1:50000	male phenotype, spinal bulbar and muscular atrophy (gynecomastia)	↑ LH, FSH T subnormal in 1/3	azoospermia oligospermia	46,XY	androgen receptor deficiency	AR "CAG expansion"	Xq11-q12	AID or ICSI/PGD	313200 X-L
Luteinizing hormone deficiency	rare	male phenotype, hypogonadism	FSH normal T↓ LH↓	azoospermia	46,XY	luteinizing hormone deficiency	β-subunit of LH point mutation	19q13.32	Hormonal substitution	152780 AR
Luteinizing hormone receptor defect	rare	female phenotype, pseudohermaphroditism	↓T ↑LH FSH normal	No germ cells	46,XY	LH receptor	LH receptor inactivating mutations	2p21	AID?	152790 AR
	rare	male phenotype, precocious puberty	↑T	?	46,XY	LH receptor	LH receptor activating mutations	2p21	AID?	176410 AD male limited
Idiopathic Hypogonadotropic Hypogonadism (IHH)	?	male phenotype, pubertal delay, hypogonadism	FSH, LH↓ T↓ No response to GnRH test	azoospermia (AT?)	46,XY	GnRH deficiency	GnRH	–		146110 AR
	rare					GnRH receptor mutation	GnRH receptor	4q21.2		138850 AR
Kallmann syndrome	1:10000	male phenotype, pubertal delay, anosmia	FSH, LH↓ T↓ No response to GnRH test	azoospermia	46,XY	abnormal neuronal migration	KAL-1	Xp22.3	hormonal substitution	308700 XL
		males & females					NN	NN		147950 AD
		males & females					NN	NN		144200 AR
Bardet-Biedl syndrome	1:100000	male phenotype, MCA/MR, hypogonadism	normal FSH, LH and T	NN	46,XY	NN	NN NN NN NN NN MKKS deficiency	11q13 (BBS1) 16q21 (BBS2) 3p12 (BBS3) 15q22.3-q23 (BBS4) 2q31 (BBS5) 20p12 (BBS6)	–	209901 AR 209900 AR 6001151 AR 600374 AR 603650 AR 605231 AR
Prader–Willi syndrome	1:10000	male phenotype, MR, obesity, hypogonadism	T, LH, FSH subnormal	NN	46,XY	paternal deletion (70%) maternal disomy (29%) imprinting defect (1%)	NN	15q11-q13	–	176270

Table 36.1. (contd)

Condition	Frequency	Physical Examination	Hormones	Sperm Characteristics	Karyotype	Cause	Gene	Locus	Infertility Treatment	OMIM
Noonan syndrome	1:5000	male fenotype, MCA	normal	azoospermia oligospermia	46,XY	NN	NN other NN	12q-24 other NN	Correction cryptorchidism?	163950 AD
Myotonic dystrophy (Steinert disease)	1:8000	male phenotype, myotonia, …	LH and FSH ↑ T ↓ or normal	OAT	46, XY	CTG expansion	DMPK	19p13.3	ICSI + PGD	160900 AD
CF	1:2500	male phenotype, pulmonary gastrointestinal problems, CBAVD	normal	azoospermia (obstructive)	46, XY	bilateral absence of vas deferens	CFTR	7q31.2	TESE, ICSI (+ PGD)	219700 AR
CBAVD		male phenotype	normal	azoospermia (obstructive)	46,XY	bilateral absence of vas deferens	CFTR	7q31.2	TESE, ICSI (+ PGD)	277180 AR
Primary ciliary dyskinesia	NN	male phenotype	normal	asthenozoospermia	46,XY	dynein deficiency		9p21-p13 other	ICSI	242620 AR
Yq microdeletion	1:400? males	male phenotype	normal	azoospermia OAT	46,XY	XY disturbed abnormal spermatogenesis	RBM family DAZ family other	Yq11	ICSI (+ PGD) or AID	400006 Y-L 400003 Y-L Y-L

Abbreviations

T testosterone; AID artificial insemination with donorsperm; FSH follicle stimulating hormone; LH luteinizing hormone; OAT oligoasthenoteratospermia; NS normospermia; t(R) robertsonian translocation of chromosomes; t(r) reciprocal translocation of chromosomes; NN not known.

Y-L Y-linked; X-L X-linked; AR autosomal recessive; AD autosomal dominant; DHT dihydrotestosterone; GnRH gonadotropin releasing hormone; MCA multiple congenital anomalies; MR mental retardation; ICSI intracytoplasmic sperm injection; PGD preimplantation genetic diagnosis.

Sex reversal due to the presence of SRY in XX individuals or the presence of mutant SRY in XY individuals can occur (Ferguson-Smith and Goodfellow, 1995) (OMIM 278850 and *306100). In about 80% of 46,XX males, sex reversal is due to the presence of the SRY gene on one of the X chromosomes. This unusual localization of the SRY gene results from recombination during male meiosis between homologous sequences near the pseudoautosomal region of the X and Y chromosomes (Weil et al., 1994; Wang et al., 1995; Schiebel et al., 1997). The prevalence of 46,XX male sex reversals is around 1/20,000 in the general population; the patients have small testes and are infertile. In 20% of 46,XY females (phenotypic females with XY gonadal dysgenesis resulting in streak gonads) mutations are present in the HMG motif of the SRY gene that probably destroy the DNA-binding capacity of the protein. The absence of SRY in 20% of 46,XX males and of SRY mutations in the majority of 46,XY females indicates that in many cases sex reversal must result from mutations in other genes involved in sexual development (see further).

In genetically normal females, the lack of SRY production (due to absence of a Y chromosome), and consequently of MIS and testosterone, allows development of the Müllerian duct and the degeneration of the Wolffian duct. Female sexual development could thus be considered the default pathway in sexual differentiation, although this idea is probably an oversimplification in view of recent experimental evidence.

Several other genes and gene products have been shown to be involved in early sexual development. Two zinc-finger-containing proteins, steroidogenic factor 1 (SF1) and Wilms tumor 1 (WT1), seem to play an important role in the commitment and maintenance of the indifferent gonad. SF1 is also involved in the regulation of the synthesis of MIS and testosterone and is important for the development of the hypothalamic-pituitary-gonadal axis (Teixeira and Donahoe, 1996). So far, one heterozygous mutation in the SF1 gene (FTZF1; OMIM *184757) has been described in humans that results in XY sex reversal and adrenal failure (Achermann et al., 1999). WT1 is essential for gonadal and kidney development. WT1 mutations are associated with childhood kidney tumors and three syndromes involving genital and/or gonadal abnormalities (Little and Wells, 1997): the contiguous gene syndrome WAGR (Wilms tumor, aniridia, genitourinary anomalies and mental retardation; OMIM #194072), Denys-Drash syndrome (Wilms tumor with congenital nephrotic syndrome and genital and gonadal abnormalities, often XY pseudohermaphroditism; OMIM #194080) and Frasier syndrome (progressive glomerulopathy and male pseudohermaphroditism; OMIM

#136680). Four isoforms of the WT1 protein exist and these result from alternative splicing of the WT1 gene: presence or absence of 17 amino acids corresponding to alternative splicing of exon 5 and presence or absence of 3 amino acids (lysine-threonine-serine, KTS) between zinc fingers 3 and 4 due to an alternative splice donor site at the 3′ end of exon 9 (WT1 + KTS and WT1 − KTS isoforms). WAGR results from heterozygous loss of WT1, while in Denys-Drash syndrome (heterozygous) dominant-negative mutations probably lower effective WT1 levels to less than 50% by dimerization of wild type and mutant WT1 (Mueller, 1994). Heterozygous mutations disrupting the exon 9 alternative splice donor site resulting in lower levels of the WT1 + KTS isoform (about 1:2 as opposed to 2:1 for normal) are probably the major cause of Frasier syndrome (Barbaux et al., 1997; Klamt et al., 1998). However, mutations not affecting the WTS +/− KTS isoforms have also been described in two patients with Frasier syndrome (Kohsaka et al., 1999).

Another gene, SOX9 (SRY-like HMG box), is expressed before SRY induction but is strongly up-regulated in XY genital ridges at the time of SRY expression and is repressed in XX genital ridges (Foster et al., 1994, Wagner et al., 1994). Besides its role in sex determination, SOX9 is a regulator of chondrogenesis, through the activation of the type II collagen gene COL2A1 (Bell et al., 1997). Expression of SOX9 in several non-skeletal tissues may indicate that it also plays a role in these tissues (Bi et al., 1999). Nevertheless, heterozygous mutations in SOX9 cause campomelic dysplasia, a dwarfism syndrome, which is associated in 75% of cases with an autosomal (SOX9 maps to 17q24.3-q25.1) form of XY sex reversal (OMIM *114290). In one genetic female, XX sex reversal due to an extra copy (three instead of two) of the SOX9 gene has also been described, indicating that an extra dose of SOX9 is sufficient to initiate testis differentiation in the absence of SRY (Huang et al., 1999). Duplication of DAX-1 (Dosage-sensitive sex – Adrenal hypoplasia congenita critical region on the X, gene), an X-linked (Xp21.2-p21.3) gene encoding an orphan nuclear receptor, causes dosage-sensitive sex reversal (DSS) in genetic males (Muscatelli et al., 1994; Zanaria et al., 1994) (OMIM *300200). Deletion or mutation of DAX-1 is associated with primary adrenal insufficiency and often with hypogonadotropic hypogonadism. The gene is transcribed in genital ridges of males and females at the time SRY expression starts in males, but expression is soon switched off in males while it continues in females.

Recent experiments, especially in the mouse, allow us to build a picture of early sexual differentiation in mammals. The WT1 − KTS isoform and SF1 synergyze to promote

AMH production, and DAX-1 antagonizes this synergy probably through a direct interaction with SF1 (Nachtigal et al., 1998; Kim et al., 1999). DAX-1 has also been shown to be an antagonist of SRY (Swain et al., 1998), which might explain the sex reversal seen in human genetic males with *DAX-1* duplication. At normal concentrations of DAX-1, SRY could function as an inhibitor of *DAX-1* expression in the male gonad, thereby allowing continued expression of *SOX9*. Recently, a signaling molecule Wnt-4 has been shown to be essential for the development of the female reproductive system and for repression of the male reproductive system in females (Vainio et al., 1999).

Besides the genes described above, other regions of the genome mapped to 1p, 9p and 10q, have been associated with primary sex reversal in genetic males (Bennett et al., 1993; Wilkie et al., 1993; Wieacker et al., 1996; Suzuki et al., 1998). Of special interest here are deletions of 9p, since two genes with sequence similarity to genes involved in the regulation of sexual development in nematodes and insects have been isolated recently (Raymond et al., 1998; 1999). Genetic males with large 9p deletions show phenotypes including mental retardation and craniofacial abnormalities often in association with partial or complete sex reversal. This broad range of phenotypes probably results from a contiguous gene syndrome involving several different genes (Flejter et al., 1998; Guioli et al., 1998; Veitia et al., 1998). By studying different patients with deletion breakpoints ranging from 9p21 to 9p24, a minimal critical sex-reversing region was defined in 9p24.3. From this region, two genes have been isolated that show homology to the *mab-3* gene of *C. elegans*, which is required for male sexual differentiation, and the sex regulator doublesex (*dsx*) gene of Drosophila. *Mab-3* and *dsx* encode proteins with a novel DNA-binding motif that is also present in the 2 genes isolated from the 9p24.3 region: *DMRT1* and *DMRT2* (*D*oublesex and *M*ab-3 *r*elated *t*ranscription factor 1 and 2). The precise function of *DMRT1* and *DMRT2* is not yet known and their position in the early sexual differentiation pathway remains to be determined. Nevertheless, XY sex reversal linked to 9p deletion seems to be due to hemizygosity of both *DMRT1* (OMIM *602424) and *DMRT2*. Variability in the sexual phenotypes of 9p deleted patients might depend on a sensitive threshold for the activity of the *DMRT1* and *DMRT2* genes, in the same way as has been described for *SOX9*, *WT1* and *DAX-1*.

Primordial germ cells (PGCs) are the precursors of spermatozoa and oocytes. PGCs migrate from the extraembryonic mesoderm at the base of the allantois through the dorsal mesentery into the coelomic epithelium covering the genital ridges that are composed of somatic cells derived from the mesonephros. In the early developing testis, PGCs (prespermatogonia) aggregate with differentiated Sertoli cells to form solid cell cords. The rate of mitotic proliferation of the prespermatogia thus enclosed into testicular cords at the time of testicular differentiation will decrease and finally stop at birth. Proliferation will resume some time before puberty, before spermatogenesis is started. A stem-cell population of mitotically dividing spermatogonia will be maintained throughout adult life. Spermatogenesis starts when some spermatogonia enter meiotic prophase (spermatocyte stage). The haploid post-meiotic spermatids become round spermatids, elongating spermatids and finally spermatozoa. The regulatory mechanisms underlying mitotic arrest and resumption of mitotic proliferation, and the initiation of meiosis are not well understood. However, many gene products underlying these processes as well as the processes leading to mature spermatozoa capable of fertilizing an oocyte are involved, and upon deficiency, can lead to male infertility. Genetic factors known to impair spermatogenesis in the human male are discussed below.

Chromosome anomalies

More than 40 years ago it was first recognized that male infertility is associated with an increased frequency of chromosome anomalies. In a cohort of 91 azoospermic or severely oligozoospermic males, 10 patients with Klinefelter syndrome showed the presence of an extra X chromosome (Ferguson-Smith et al., 1957) and the karyotype of these males was later shown to be 47,XXY (Jacobs and Strong, 1959). Since then, many surveys have been conducted to determine the chromosomal contribution to male infertility. In a review by Van Assche et al. (1996), the cytogenetic results of seven relevant studies of infertile men (including males with azoospermia and oligozoospermia) were collected. The frequency of chromosomal aberrations in almost 8 000 infertile males was compared to a large group of newborn children. In the infertile group the frequency of sex chromosome abnormalities was 27 times greater (3.8% versus 0.14%) and five times greater for autosomes (1.3% versus 0.25%) with a combined greater frequency of 13 times (5.1% versus 0.38%). On pooling data from five surveys of oligozoospermic men and six studies of azoospermic men, frequencies of chromosome abnormalities of 4.6% and 13.7% were obtained respectively. Although the frequency of chromosomal abnormalities differs among individual studies as a result of varying inclusion criteria, some general conclusions can be drawn: the frequency of constitutional chromosome abnormalities increases as the number of spermatozoa in the ejaculate decreases. Moreover, the frequency of sex chromosome abnormalities is highest in the group of males with non-obstructive azoospermia, while autosomal structural aberrations predominate in patients with oligozoospermia.

In the group of numerical sex chromosome aberrations, patients with Klinefelter syndrome (47,XXY or mosaics 46,XY/47,XXY) are the most frequent. These patients present with small firm testes with hyalinisation of seminiferous tubules, hypergonadotrophic hypogonadism with or without gynecomastia and azoospermia or extremely severe oligozoospermia. The reason for the infertility in these males has not been determined but is probably associated with a dosage effect resulting from the extra X chromosome. At present, assisted reproduction techniques such as ICSI using seminal or testicular spermatozoa have enabled some patients with Klinefelter syndrome to fertilize oocytes and father children (Staessen et al., 1996; Tournaye et al., 1996). Patients with a 47,XYY karyotype are also observed more frequently among infertile men (0.26%) than in the series of newborn males (0.07%). However, their spermatogenic picture can range from one of severe impairment to apparent normality. The frequency of Y chromosome structural rearrangements and the condition of 46,XX maleness are found to be higher in infertile males than in newborn infants. Since these aberrations cause spermatogenic failure, they are seen more often in azoospermic males.

Robertsonian translocations are by far the most frequent structural autosomal rearrangement found in infertile men. In the review by Van Assche et al. (1996), 0.7% of the infertile males present this aberration. This is 8.5 times higher than the frequency reported in the newborn studies that these authors used. A correlation exists between the increased frequency of the XY bivalent and the Robertsonian trivalent association, present during the pachytene stage of meiosis, and the extent of germ cell impairment (Johannisson et al., 1993).

Pooling the data from the different series of infertile males, 0.5% reciprocal translocations were observed as opposed to 0.1% in the newborn children (Fig. 36.2). The correlation between reciprocal translocations with involvement of the chromosomes 3, 4, 5, 6, 7, 9, 11, 13, 14, 15, 16, 17, 19, 20, 21, 22 and the impairment of sperm production is well known (Chandley et al., 1986; Gabriel-Robez et al., 1986; Guichaoua et al., 1991; 1992; Gabriel-Robez and Rumpler, 1996). Observations at the pachytene stage of meiosis revealed a high frequency of centromeric contacts, especially with chain configurations,

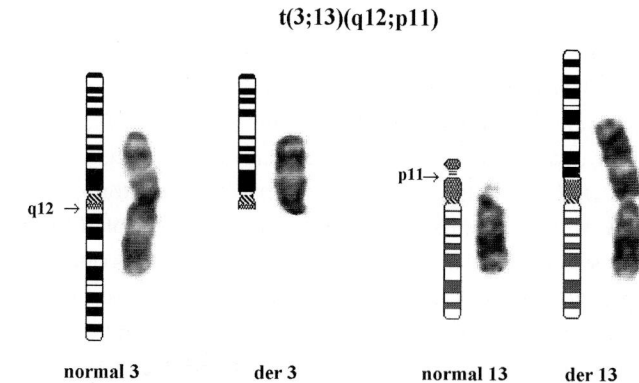

t(3;13)(q12;p11)

normal 3   der 3   normal 13   der 13

Fig. 36.2. Partial somatic karyotype, with G-banding, of a male with severe OAT. The patient is carrier of a balanced reciprocal translocation t(3;13)(q12;p11).

between the translocation quadrivalent and the XY bivalent. Such contacts were not seen to any important extent among fertile translocation carriers.

Hormonal defects

PERSISTENT MÜLLERIAN DUCT SYNDROME

Persistent Müllerian duct syndrome (PMDS; OMIM #261550) is characterized by a lack of reduction of the Müllerian duct in otherwise normally virilized males. PMDS leads to an uncommon (less than 200 cases described) autosomal recessive form of male pseudohermaphroditism with cryptorchidism (and associated azoospermia) and/or inguinal hernia as the most prominent clinical features. In the absence of longstanding cryptorchidism, the testes usually contain germ cells (Josso et al., 1997).

In normal males, regression of the Müllerian duct is conducted by the action of the anti-Müllerian hormone (AMH) and two receptors necessary for AMH ligand binding (AMH type II receptor) and signal transduction (AMH type I receptor) (Teixeira and Donahoe, 1996). So far mutations leading to PMDS have been identified in *AMH* (19q13) and in the AMH type II receptor (*AMHR2*, chromosome 12q13) (Knebelmann et al., 1991; Carré-Eusèbe et al., 1992; Imbeaud et al., 1994; 1995; 1996). Depending on the affected gene, either normal quantities of AMH are present in the testis (*AMHR2* mutations; OMIM *600956) or no AMH is produced (*AMH* mutations; OMIM *600957). However, some PMDS patients have no mutations in either of these two genes, indicating that still other genes are involved in PMDS. The type I

AMH receptor would be a likely candidate but mutations in this receptor have not yet been identified.

DEFECTS IN THE SYNTHESIS OF ANDROGENS AND THE ANDROGEN RECEPTOR

Androgen action consists of the interaction, in target cells, of the major circulating androgens, testosterone and dihydrotestosterone, with the androgen receptor (AR; OMIM #313700). The activation of the AR results in its translation to the nucleus where the protein binds to androgen responsive elements (AREs) in the promoter regions of androgen-responsive genes, thereby regulating the expression of these target genes. Androgen action is impaired when defects either in the synthesis of the androgens or in the AR itself are present. Since androgen action is necessary in males for the differentiation of the indifferent gonad into male urogenital structures, impaired or deficient androgen action will lead to a broad range in abnormalities of male phenotypic development.

Testosterone synthesis occurs in Leydig cells starting from cholesterol. The genes of all four enzymes involved are localized on the autosomes and mutations in three of these genes have been identified in genetic males with pseudohermaphroditism. Dihydrotestosterone is synthesized in extraglandular tissues from testosterone by the enzyme 5α-reductase 2. The gene encoding this enzyme is also autosomal. Deficiency of the enzyme due to mutations in both autosmal copies leads, as for deficiency in enzymes in testosterone synthesis, to male pseudohermaphroditism (Mendonça et al., 1996; Sinnecker et al., 1996) (OMIM *264600).

Defects in the AR lead to androgen resistance syndromes (prevalence around 1/60,000 male births) that have been shown to present with a broad spectrum of clinical manifestations in genetic males (Quigley et al., 1995; Hiort et al., 1998) (OMIM #300068). The phenotypes of affected patients range from complete or incomplete testicular feminization (female phenotype) through genital ambiguity to undervirilized infertile males. The gene for the AR is on the long arm of the X chromosome (AR, Xq11-q12) and disorders of the AR are transmitted as an X-linked disease (Chang et al., 1988; Lubahn et al., 1988). So far more than 300 mutations have been identified and most of these impair the DNA-binding and hormone-binding capacities of the receptor (Gottlieb et al., 1999). Nevertheless, mutations are found in all regions of the gene. In most instances, identical mutations lead to similar phenotypes but several exceptions have been described.

Expansion of a CAG trinucleotide repeat, coding for a polyglutamine tract, in the transactivation domain of the AR has been associated with Kennedy disease or X-linked spinal bulbar muscular atrophy (SBMA; OMIM #313200) (La Spada et al., 1991). SBMA is a neurodegenerative disease associated with testicular atrophy and oligozoospermia or azoospermia (Kennedy et al., 1968). In normal individuals, the CAG repeat is polymorphic and ranges from 10–36 repeats; in SBMA patients the number is increased to 40–62 repeats and disease severity correlates well with the number of repeats (Igarashi et al., 1992). The elongation of the polyglutamine tract in the receptor has been shown to impair the transactivation capacity of the receptor and to cause a toxic gain of function that is possibly fundamental to the neuronal degeneration seen in SBMA patients (MacLean et al., 1995).

The broad range of phenotypes seen in genetic males with defects in the AR might imply that infertile but otherwise normal phenotypic males might also have defects in the AR. These defects may be mild in relation to the phenotypic sex but may for instance impair spermatogenesis. Several studies have recently been conducted to test this hypothesis in infertile males with impaired spermatogenesis of unknown etiology. Although a very low frequency of possible pathogenic mutations were found, mutations in the AR do not seem to be an important cause of idiopathic male infertility. The length of the polyglutamine tract has also been studied in a similar population of patients. A possible association of infertility with the number of repeats towards the upper limit of normal has been suggested in some studies but has not been confirmed by others. More studies are certainly required to confirm or disapprove this hypothesis. Furthermore, it is not yet clear how small increases in the number of CAG repeats seen in infertile patients, but with numbers still in the control range, might influence action of the AR and be impaired in the pathogenesis of oligozoospermia/azoospermia and infertility (Tincello et al., 1997; Tut et al., 1997; Wang et al., 1998; Dowsing et al., 1999).

LUTEINIZING HORMONE AND LUTEINIZING HORMONE RECEPTOR

The gonadotropins, luteinizing hormone (LH), follicle stimulating hormone (FSH) and human chorionic gonadotropin (hCG), consist of a common α-subunit and a hormone-specific β-subunit. So far, mutations in the α-subunit have not been described, but on the basis of a knockout mouse model, the phenotype would probably include hypogonadotropic hypogonadism, and hypothyroidism due to thyroid stimulating hormone (TSH) deficiency (Kendall et al., 1995).

The important role of LH in the maintenance of Leydig cell function is demonstrated by the description of a single patient with the same mutation in both alleles of the β-subunit LH gene (LH-β; OMIM *152780). This patient presented with hypogonadism (small, bilaterally descended testes) and pubertal delay (Weiss et al., 1992). Immunoreactive LH was higher than normal, but bioactive LH was lower, explaining the delayed puberty. A testicular biopsy revealed spermatogenic arrest and a complete absence of Leydig cells, indicating the absolute requirement of LH in Leydig cell formation. Molecular analysis of his LH-β gene demonstrated the presence in both alleles of an arginine substitution for a glutamine. The patient's parents and maternal grandparents were first cousins. His mother and three of her infertile brothers were carriers of the same mutation. It could not be determined whether the infertility in these three males was related to heterozygosity for the LH-β mutation or to an unrelated cause. In any case, the patient's father had no history of infertility and he must have been an obligate carrier, but this could not be proven experimentally since DNA was not available for study. LH-β deficiency is probably a very rare cause of autosomal recessive hypogonadism since no other patients have been described.

The gonadotropins LH and hCG bind to the same receptor, the LH/hCG receptor (LH receptor; OMIM #152790). Both inactivating and activating mutations have been described for this receptor (Latronico and Segaloff, 1999). Inactivating mutations were first reported in two siblings with 46,XY karyotype who presented with female external genitalia and primary amenorrhea (around 40 years of age) (Kremer et al., 1995). Histology of the gonads showed the presence of testes with normal Sertoli cells but with Leydig cell hypoplasia. Autosomal recessive inheritance was demonstrated by the presence of a homozygous substitution of proline for alanine at amino acid position 593 of the LH receptor. In this family, ligand binding (hCG) of the receptor was normal but cAMP production was absent. Several other patients of male genetic sex with inactivating mutations in the LH receptor have since been described, and the mutations impair either signal transduction, ligand binding, or both (Laue et al., 1995; Latronico et al., 1996). The presence of testes and associated structures in these patients indicates that while the initiation of testosterone production is independent of Leydig cells, LH and LH receptor are necessary for the proliferation and maturation of Leydig cells at a later fetal stage. Inactivating mutations in the LH receptor in females do not result in an abnormal female sex phenotype but probably result in primary amenorrhea (Toledo et al., 1996).

Activating mutations in the LH receptor lead to a constitutively activated receptor without stimulation by a gonadotropin ligand (Latronico and Segaloff, 1999; Layman, 1999). These mutations are associated with familial male-limited precocious puberty, an autosomal dominant condition in which puberty begins between 1–4 years of age (OMIM #176410). The constitutively activated LH receptor does not induce puberty in females, probably because LH and FSH are both required for the activation of ovarian steroidogenesis.

HYPOGONADOTROPIC HYPOGONADISM

Idiopathic hypogonadotropic hypogonadism and Kallmann syndrome

Patients with idiopathic hypogonadotropic hypogonadism (IHH) have reduced or defective secretion of gonadotropin-releasing hormone (GnRH), which manifests as pubertal delay, and low levels of gonadotropins (OMIM 146110). IHH in association with the inability to smell (anosmia) is known as Kallmann syndrome (Rugarli and Ballabio, 1993). IHH and Kallmann syndrome both present as sporadic and inherited cases, with autosomal recessive, autosomal dominant and X-linked recessive inheritance. The distinction between IHH and Kallmann syndrome is not always obvious because GnRH deficiency with and without anosmia often occurs in different members of the same family. The exogenous administration of gonadotropins or GnRH is usually effective in inducing pubertal development and fertility.

An autosomal recessive mouse model for IHH exists and results from a partial deletion of the GnRH gene (GNRH1) (Mason et al., 1986). Although this gene is a likely candidate for IHH in humans, mutations in the human GnRH gene have not yet been identified. However, a low proportion of autosomal recessive IHH can be attributed to mutations in the GnRH receptor gene (GNRHR, chromosome 4q21.2) (de Roux et al., 1997; Layman et al., 1998) (OMIM *138850). In both families described, affected patients were compound heterozygotes of missense mutations affecting ligand binding or signal transduction capacities of the receptor. In one family, there was incomplete GnRH deficiency with some signs of pubertal development while in the other family complete IHH with delayed puberty was observed, a difference probably due to intragenic heterogeneity.

The incidence of Kallmann syndrome is about 1 in 10,000 males with a five to seven times lower frequency in females. Because of the overrepresentation of males with Kallmann syndrome, a predominant X-linked recessive form was suspected. An X-linked gene (KAL1) from the pseudoautosomal region (Xp22.3) was indeed isolated and shown to be responsible for X-linked Kallmann syndrome

(OMIM *308700) by the demonstration of the presence of deletions and point mutations in affected males (Franco et al., 1991; Legouis et al., 1991). The KAL1 protein shows similarities with neural adhesion molecules and proteins involved in neuronal migration and axonal pathfinding; it interferes with the migration of GnRH neurons and olfactory nerves to their position in the hypothalamus (Rugarli, 1999). Although this dual function of the KAL1 protein may explain its involvement in both IHH and anosmia, only approximately 50% of X-linked families present with mutations in *KAL1*. In sporadic patients with Kallmann's syndrome or IHH, this frequency is even lower (5%). So far, autosomal genes involved in Kallmann syndrome have not been identified (OMIM *147950; OMIM *244200).

Bardet–Biedl syndrome

Bardet–Biedl syndrome is characterized by obesity, polydactyly, mental retardation, renal anomalies, retinal pigmentary dystrophy and hypogenitalism (Beales et al., 1999; Green et al., 1989). Additional characteristics include deafness, diabetes mellitus, dental anomalies and small stature. In females, vaginal atresia and delayed puberty are observed. In males, hypogenitalism includes cryptorchidism, micropenis and various degrees of hypospadias.

Bardet–Biedl syndrome is inherited as an autosomal recessive disease with an incidence of less than one in 100,000 live births. The condition is genetically very heterogeneous. So far, one gene, called MKKS, involved in the developmental anomaly syndrome of McKusick-Kaufman (MKKS) has also been implicated in Bardet-Biedl syndrome (BBS6 at chromosome 20p12; OMIM #605231) (Katsanis et al., 2000; Slavonitek et al., 2000). The MKKS protein shows similarities to the chaperonins, a protein family involved in protein processing, but its actual function is still unknown. At least five other candidate loci have been identified, at 11q13 (BBS1; OMIM *209901), 16q21 (BBS2; OMIM *209900), 3p12 (BBS3; OMIM *600151), 15q22.3-q23 (BBS4; OMIM *600374) and 2q31 (BBS5; OMIM *603650) (Beales et al., 1997; Bruford et al., 1997; Carmi et al., 1995a,b; Kwitek-Black et al., 1993; Leppert et al., 1994; Sheffield et al., 1994; Young et al., 1999). The syndrome seems to be associated with the BBS1 locus in most of the families (36–55%).

Prader–Willi syndrome (see also Ch. 32)

Prader–Willi syndrome (PWS; OMIM #176270) is a neurobehavioral disease that affects both males and females and is characterized by infantile hypotonia, developmental delay and mental retardation, obesity and hypogonadism (Cassidy, 1997). In males, the hypogonadism manifests as cryptorchidism and scrotal hypoplasia. The prevalence of PWS is from 1/10,000 to 1/15,000.

PWS is caused by a disturbance in the parent-of-origin pattern of inheritance at chromosome region 15q11-q13 (imprinting) and results from the absence of expressed paternal genes from this imprinted region (Horsthemke et al., 1997). Imprinting refers to the differential expression of genes depending on the parental origin of a chromosomal region thereby making this genetic region functionally nonequivalent in the presence of both a maternal and a paternal contribution (Feil and Khosla, 1999). Several genes at 15q11-q13 are expressed only from the paternal chromosome and PWS results from paternal interstitial deletion of the region (about 70% of patients), maternal disomy (29%) or a defect in the imprinting mechanism (1%). The mechanism underlying imprinting is not well understood but parent-of-origin specific DNA methylation is important in the regulation of the expression of imprinted genes.

Other monogenic defects

OBSTRUCTIVE AZOOSPERMIA: CONGENITAL BILATERAL ABSENCE OF THE VAS DEFERENS

Congenital bilateral absence of the vas deferens (CBAVD; OMIM #277180) is characterized by the absence of the scrotal vasa, which results in a blockade of the transport of the spermatozoa from the testis or the epididymis to the distal genital tract. This form of obstructive azoospermia is responsible for 1 to 2% of male infertility and for up to 6% of all obstructive azoospermias (Dubin and Amelar, 1971). CBAVD is also present in most males with cystic fibrosis (CF; OMIM #219700), the commonest autosomal recessive disease in populations of Caucasian origin (Zielenski and Tsui, 1995). The hallmarks of CF are chronic pulmonary obstruction and infection and pancreatic dysfunction (see Ch. 32). CF occurs with a frequency of about one in 2500 live births (carrier frequency one in 25) and is caused by mutations in the cystic fibrosis transmembrane conductance regulator (*CFTR*) gene, which codes for a protein involved in chloride conduction across epithelial cell membranes (Kerem et al., 1989; Riordan et al., 1989; Rommens et al., 1989). One mutation, a three base pair deletion in exon 10 of *CFTR* that leads to the deletion of a phenylalanine at amino acid position 508 of the protein, ΔF508, is responsible for the majority of defects found in CF: it accounts for

66% of almost 44,000 CF chromosomes (Cystic Fibrosis Genetic Analysis Consortium, 1994). Another 20 to 30 mutations have been found to occur on 50 or more chromosomes. So far, over 800 mutations have been identified in *CFTR* of CF patients and most of these occur with a low frequency or are even unique to single CF families. A wide variation in disease presentation exists in CF patients (Kerem and Kerem, 1996). Patients with the severest form of CF have mutations in both alleles of *CFTR* that leave no residual CFTR activity (severe mutations). Patients with milder presentations have a severe mutation in one allele and a mild mutation, leaving some residual CFTR activity, or they have 2 mild mutations.

The similarity between infertility in CF males and in males with CBAVD without other clinical characteristics of CF led to the hypothesis that isolated CBAVD is an incomplete form of CF (Holsclaw et al., 1971). This hypothesis was confirmed for the majority of males with CBAVD (about 80%) since a high frequency of *CFTR* mutations was indeed found in these patients (Dumur et al., 1990; 1995; 1996; Anguiano et al., 1992; Oates and Amos, 1994; Mercier et al., 1995; Lissens et al., 1996; Lissens and Liebaers, 1997). As expected, none of these patients have two severe mutations, but have either a severe and a mild mutation or two mild mutations (De Braekeleer and Férec, 1996). Many of these mutations are unique to CBAVD and are not found in CF patients. Moreover, a splice site variant in intron 8 (the 5T variant) of *CFTR* appears to occur at a much higher frequency in CBAVD than in the general population (21% versus 5%) (Chillon et al., 1995). The 5T variant results in a high degree of exon 9 skipping on transcription of *CFTR* which leads to the production of a nonfunctional CFTR protein. The splicing efficiency of the 5T variant is variable among different individuals and different tissues of the same individual but is consistently lower in epididymal epithelium and vas deferens than in other tissues (Rave-Harel et al., 1997; Teng et al., 1997; Cuppens et al., 1998; Larriba et al., 1998). For all of these reasons, the 5T variant has been classified as a mutation associated with CBAVD but with incomplete penetrance. In addition, the splicing efficiency of the 5T variant is further influenced by other polymorphisms in *CFTR* (Cuppens et al., 1998).

In about 20% of patients, CBAVD does not seem to represent a mild form of CF (Dumur et al., 1995). These patients have CBAVD-associated urinary tract malformations and *CFTR* mutations are found in this situation at a frequency no higher than the general population. The etiology of this form of CBAVD remains unknown but is probably caused by damage to the Wolffian duct before it splits into a reproductive and an ureteral part at about 7 weeks of gestation. This can be deduced from the fact that the ureteral ducts are not affected in CF patients and in CF-associated CBAVD patients. In these patients, CFTR dysfunction probably leads to damage, either through a morphogenetic defect or through a progressive obstruction by excessive mucus secretion, of the genital ducts after splitting of the Wolffian duct (Patrizio and Zielenski, 1996).

The condition of congenital unilateral absence of the vas deferens (CUAVD) also seems to be a mild form of CF when contralateral genitourinary anomalies are present (Casals et al., 1995; Mickle et al., 1995; Schlegel et al., 1996). This is not the case when anatomically complete and patent vasa are present on the side of the palpable vas. These patients often present with renal abnormalities at the ipsilateral side of the absent vas.

Young syndrome (OMIM 279000) is characterized by obstructive azoospermia in combination with chronic sinopulmonary disease. No increased frequency of *CFTR* mutations is found in these patients, indicating that Young syndrome is not related to CF (Friedman et al., 1995; Le Lannou et al., 1995). Young syndrome might be related to childhood mercury poisoning and thus be an acquired disease (Hendry et al., 1993).

Involvement of the CF gene in other conditions of male infertility has recently been suggested (Jarvi et al., 1995; van der Ven et al., 1996; Meschede et al., 1997). An increased frequency of *CFTR* mutations was indeed described in patients with obstructive azoospermia (non-CBAVD) and in patients with reduced sperm quality and quantity. However, these data need to be confirmed in a larger population.

PRIMARY CILIARY DYSKINESIA

Primary ciliary dyskinesia (PCD, also known as immotile cilia syndrome; OMIM #242650) is a genetically heterogeneous group of disorders resulting from the absence of mucociliary clearance of the airways and other ciliated structures due to severe or complete immotility of the cilia (Afzelius, 1998). The major clinical features are chronic respiratory tract disease, rhinitis and sinusitis. Most males are also infertile because of immotility or poor mobility of spermatozoa as a consequence of structural and functional abnormalities in the central part of the sperm flagella. About half of the patients with PCD also display situs inversus, a condition known as Kartagener syndrome (OMIM *244400). The prevalence of PCD is around 1/25,000 and that of Kartagener syndrome 1/50,000. The mode of inheritance is autosomal recessive in the majority of cases.

Cilia are complex structures containing at least 130 different polypeptide species, and the diagnosis of PCD can be made only by electron microscopy to identify the defective components. The main defect found in PCD is an absence of dynein arms, the structures necessary for the generation of movement of cilia and sperm tails. At the molecular level, a first human gene related to the *Chlamydomonas reinhardii* dynein gene IC78 has been shown to be defective in one family with PCD (Pennarun et al., 1999). The patient was a compound heterozygote for 2 truncating mutations, one- and four-base pair insertions in the gene; the unrelated parents were carriers. In another 5 families studied by the same authors, the condition of PCD was not linked to this gene. However, the same gene was recently shown to be responsible for a small fraction of patients with Kartagener syndrome since three of 34 patients (9%) were compound heterozygotes for defects in this gene (Guichard et al., 2001)

NOONAN SYNDROME (see Ch. 32)

Noonan syndrome (OMIM *163950) is characterized by short stature, congenital heart defects (most often pulmonary valve stenosis or hypertrophic cardiomyopathy) and a typical facial dysmorphism with posteriorly rotated ears. About half of male patients with Noonan syndrome have azoospermia or oligozoospermia resulting from bilateral cryptorchidism. Affected females and males with normally descended testes are fertile (Elsawi et al., 1994).

The incidence of Noonan syndrome is estimated at 1/1000 to 1/5000 live births. Half of the cases show an autosomal dominant pattern of inheritance while the other half occur as a result of new mutations (sporadic cases). Some cases of Noonan syndrome have been found in association with neurofibromatosis type 1 (chromosome 17q11) and with deletion 22q11 syndromes (Ahlbom et al., 1995; Robin et al., 1995; Bahuau et al., 1996; Colley et al., 1996; Donnai et al., 1996; Digilio et al., 1996). This association is probably purely coincidental, since a first gene for Noonan syndrome has been localized to the long arm of chromosome 12 at q22-qter (Jamieson et al., 1994; Legius et al., 1998). Not all families show linkage to this locus, so that genetic heterogeneity of the condition is probable (Jamieson et al., 1994).

MYOTONIC DYSTROPHY (see Chap. 32)

Myotonic dystrophy (DM; OMIM *160900) is an autosomal dominant disease caused by a trinucleotide (CTG) repeat expansion in *DMPK* at 19p13.3 (Aslanidis et al., 1992; Brook et al., 1992; Fu et al., 1992; Mahadevan et al., 1992). It is the commonest form of adult muscular dystrophy (prevalence 1/7000 to 1/8000 births) characterized by myotonia and muscle weakness and wasting. Additional anomalies include cardiac conduction disturbances, cataracts and progressive testicular tubular atrophy in 60 to 80% of males.

The number of CTG repeats in the 3′ untranslated region of *DMPK* is polymorphic in normal individuals and ranges from five to 35. Genes with 50 to 80 repeats are unstable and are likely to expand in the number of repeats on transmission to the offspring. The severity and time of onset of the disease will in general be related to the number of repeats, a phenomenon called anticipation (Ashizawa et al., 1992a; 1992b; Hunter et al., 1992). In its severest form, a few thousand repeats are present. A second locus for myotonic dystrophy has been described recently in one five-generation family (Ranum et al., 1998). This form of DM (OMIM *602668) is clinically very similar to classic DM and the gene has been mapped to chromosome 3q.

Microdeletions of the Y chromosomes and male infertility

The presence on the Y chromosome of genes necessary for spermatogenesis was first suggested by a cytogenetic study of azoospermic males in 1976 (Tiepolo and Zuffardi, 1976). In 6 of these males, deletions were found in part of the non-fluorescent (euchromatic) region at band q11 and these deletions were not present in the fertile fathers and brothers of the patients. On the basis of the association of cytogenetic detectable deletions and azoospermia, the presence of a gene encoding an azoospermia factor (*AZF*) in the distal region of the Y chromosome was suggested. In more recent years, it has turned out that the proposed existence of a single *AZF* was an oversimplification and that, instead, the presence of several putative Y-linked spermatogenesis genes or gene families are involved.

The Y chromosome can be divided into three parts based on cytogenetic criteria: the euchromatic parts on the short (Yp11) and on the long (Yp11) arm and the heterochromatic part on the long arm (Yp12). The heterochromatic part consists primarily of repetitive DNA sequences of variable length in normal fertile males. By using DNA from patients with various deletions, the Y chromosome has further been divided into 7 regions with intervals 1–4 comprising the short arm and the centromere and intervals 5–7 the long arm (Foote et al., 1992; Vollrath et al., 1992). These intervals have been further subdivided, especially by the use of sequence-tagged sites (STSs), which are known sequences of genomic DNA that can be amplified by the polymerase chain reaction (PCR). Many investigators have taken advantage of this fine mapping of the Y chromosome to detect deletions and to define the extent of these deletions in males with azoospermia or oligozoospermia (reviewed in McElreavey and Krausz, 1999; Roberts, 1998; Vogt, 1998). Since in many cases these deletions are not detectable by cytogenetic analysis, they are termed microdeletions. On the basis of non-overlapping deletions in patients with non-obstructive azoospermia or oligozoospermia, the original *AZF* region has been subdivided into *AZFa*, *AZFb* and *AZFc* (Vogt et al., 1996). A possible fourth *AZF* region, *AZFd*, localized between *AZFb* and *AZFc*, has been suggested recently (Kent-First et al., 1999). Deletions of the Y chromosome appear to be associated with a wide range of histopathologies ranging from Sertoli-cell-only syndrome (SCOS or complete absence of germ cells), through spermatogenic arrest (maturation arrest) to severe hypospermatogenesis. Although a strict classification is not possible, Vogt et al. (1996) suggested that *AZFa* deletions result in a complete absence of germ cells, *AZFb* deletions mostly exhibit maturation arrest at the spermatocyte stage while *AZFc* deletions show a more variable phenotype ranging from SCOS to severe oligozoospermia with all germ-cell types present. *AZFd* deletions have been associated with mild oligozoospermia or normal cell counts with abnormal sperm morphology. Nevertheless, this classification should be used with caution since the phenotype might change over time, as described by Girardi et al. (1997) in a patient carrying an *AZFc* deletion, who initial by had severe oligozoospermia but azoospermia on follow-up. Fertility in two patient with an *AZFc* deletion has also been described (Chang et al., 1999; Saut et al., 2000). In these families, the father and their respectively four and three naturally conceived sons all carried an apparently identical deletion in *AZFc*. The father were not aware of a fertility problem.

As mentioned before, many clinical studies looking for microdeletions of the Y chromosome have been conducted. From these studies it can be concluded that deletions are found mainly in patients with azoospermia or severe oligozoospermia and that most deletions affect either *AZFc* or *AZFb* together with *AZFc* (Figs 36.3 and 4). *AZFa* deletions occur with a frequency of less than 5%. Strikingly, the frequency of deletions can vary enormously among studies: 1 to 55% of deletions have been found (mean around 8%). The reasons for this extreme variability are not known, although some indicative factors can be found. First, patient selection criteria are likely to be important. Some studies include only patients with non-obstructive azoospermia or severe oligozoospermia (sperm count less than ficve million) of idiopathic origin while others include patients with known causes of infertility or with oligozoospermia (sperm counts up to 20 million). In many cases, testis histopathology is not available so that patients are classified on the basis of sperm counts and not on the basis of defec-

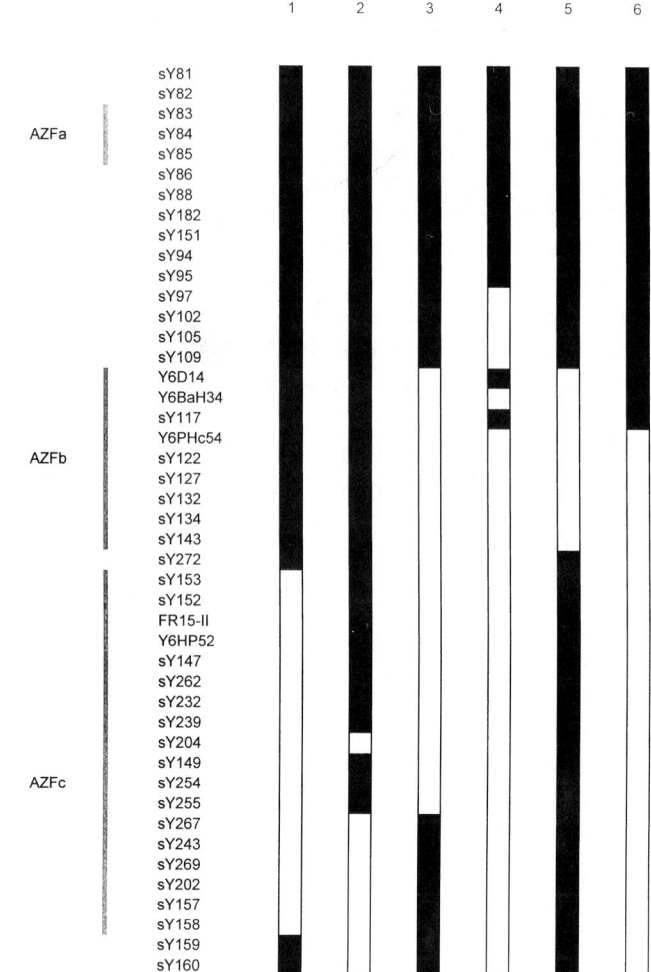

Fig. 36.3. Schematic overview of the Yq11 microdeletions detected in 13 patients. Almost 300 cytogenetically normal males with azoospermia, cryptozoospermia (sperm count less than 0.1×10^6/ml) or extreme oligozoospermia (sperm count $0.1–5 \times 10^6$/ml), including some patients with varicocele or a history of cryptorchidism, were studied for the presence of 27 sequence-tagged sites (STS) of Yq11 and *SRY* by using five multiplex PCR reactions. Additional PCR markers were studied in those patients showing absence of one or more of the 27 markers studied. Eight patients showed a similar deletion pattern (represented by pattern 1) in *AZFc*, while other patterns were seen in five patients (patterns 2–6). Open/closed boxes: absence/presence of STS. Part of the results shown here has been published (Van Landuyt et al., 2000).

tive spermatogenesis. Second, a large variation in the number of STSs used to detect microdeletions is observed. In some instances, the use of a limited number of STSs might leave some microdeletions undetected. Third, problems related to the technology used might be involved. Finally, the possibilities of ethnic, geographical or environmental influences cannot be excluded.

In the last few years, several genes have been isolated from the *AZFb* and *AZFc* regions (Ma et al., 1993; Reijo et al., 1995; Lahn and Page, 1997). A first gene family,

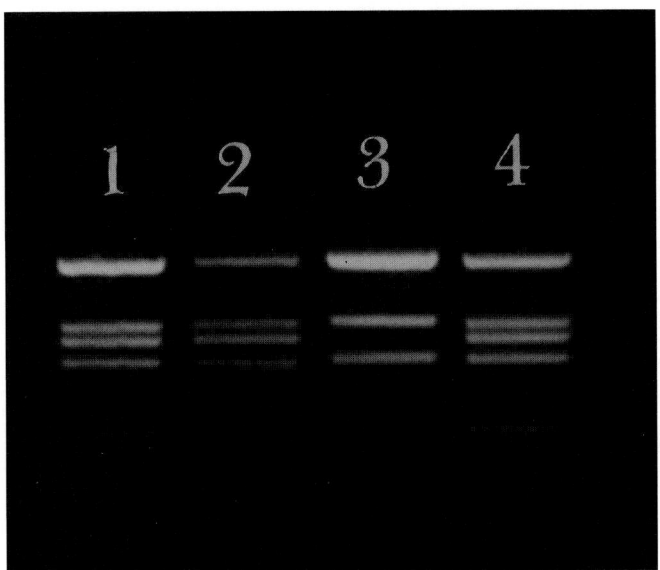

Fig. 36.4. Example of one of five multiplex PCRs used to obtain results represented in Figure 36.3. The STS used are, from top to bottom, sY14 (*SRY*), sY95, sY127, sY109 and sY149. Lanes 1–3 represent the results in three of the infertile patients, lane 4 shows a positive control (normal fertile male). No bands are visible in the negative control (female DNA) in the lane to the left of lane 1. Patients 2 and 3 both lack a signal for STS sY149 (*AZFc*), while patient 3 also lacks sY127 (*AZFb*). Additional studies showed deletion patterns 1 and 3 for patients 2 and 3, respectively (see Figure 36.3).

called *RBMY* (RNA binding motif), consists of 30 to 50 genes and pseudogenes spread over the euchromatic region of the Y chromosome. These genes contain an RNA recognition motif (RRM) and an internal repeated sequence typical of proteins interacting with RNA or single-stranded DNA. RBM is a member of the heterogeneous nuclear ribonucleoprotein G (hnRNPG) family of proteins that encodes proteins involved in pre-mRNA processing and transport (Weighardt et al., 1996), but in contrast to other family members it is expressed only in the testis. The functional copies of RBMY have recently been localized to the *AZFb* region (Elliott et al., 1997). Another multicopy family of genes has been isolated from the *AZFc* region: the *DAZ* (*d*eleted in *az*oospermia)/*SPGY* (*sp*ermatogenesis *g*ene on the *Y*) family. This gene family, with an estimated seven to 10 copies on the Y chromosome, also codes for RNA binding proteins. A functional homologue of *DAZ/SPGY* is present on chromosome 3p24 (*DAZL1* for DAZ like 1); in other mammals, except primates, only an autosomal single-copy gene of *DAZ/SPGY* exists. *DAZ/SPGY* and *DAZL1* are expressed only in the testis in males, but the autosomal *DAZL1* gene is also expressed in prenatal and postnatal germ cells in females. The *DAZ/SPGY* family resembles a gene termed *boule* in Drosophila that results, when absent, in azoospermia in male flies (Eberhart et al.,

1996). In contrast to RBMY, which is a nuclear protein, DAZ/SPGY protein is localized in the cytoplasm. Therefore, it is unlikely that the protein has a function in transcription or RNA splicing, but it might be involved in translational control of mRNAs. Recently, another 12 genes were isolated from the long arm of the Y chromosome, some showing expression only in the testis while others are expressed ubiquitously and have functional homologues on the X chromosome (Lahn and Page, 1997; 1999). The functions of these genes and resulting proteins have not been studied so far and their possible role in spermatogenesis remains to be uncovered. Many of the Y-specific genes are also present in multicopies and, according to their localization, are also supposed to be deleted in most patients with *AZFb* and *AZFc* deletions.

Three functional genes have recently been localized to the *AZFa* region (*USP9Y*, formerly known as *DFFRY*, and *DBY*) and its vicinity (*UTY*) (Lahn and Page, 1997; Brown et al., 1998). Patients with deletion of the entire *AZFa* region have lost functional copies of *USP9Y* and *DBY* genes and no testicular germ cells are present. In contrast, patients lacking *USP9Y* but not *DBY* function have hypospermatogenesis with the presence of pre-meiotic and meiotic germ cells in most seminiferous tubules and small numbers of post-meiotic cells in a few tubules (Sun et al., 1999). Both *USP9Y* and *DBY* are ubiquitously expressed and have functional homologues on the X chromosome. Their role in spermatogenesis remains to be determined.

Other genes associated with male infertility

Several other genetic syndromes have, in varying degrees, been associated with male infertility. A few examples of these are Aarskog-Scott syndrome (X-linked recessive; cryptorchidism and sperm acrosome defects; OMIM *305400), Beckwith–Wiedemann syndrome (imprinting defect at chromosome 11p15.5; cryptorchidism; OMIM #130650), adrenomyeloneuropathy (X-linked recessive; azoospermia or oligozoospermia; OMIM *300100) and autoimmune polyglandular syndrome type 1 (APECED, autosomal recessive; hypogonadism in 10–20% of males; OMIM *240300). For all of these, genes or candidate genes underlying the clinical phenotype have been isolated (Mosser et al., 1993; Elliot and Maher, 1994; Pasteris et al., 1994; Hatada et al., 1996; Meschede et al., 1996; Nagamine et al., 1997; Ward, 1997). For others such as chromosome 1 deletion q44 (Sertoli-cell-only syndrome) and contiguous gene syndrome associated with X-linked myotubular myopathy type 1 (ambiguous genitalia; OMIM #309219), only a rough positioning of genes involved in genital development and male infertility is available (Hu et al., 1996; Laporte et al., 1997; Hathout et al., 1998). For still others, such as mitochondrial DNA deletions, only a possible involvement in male infertility is surmised (Kao et al., 1995; Johns et al., 1997; 1998; Lestienne et al., 1997; Reynier et al., 1997; 1998).

It seems reasonable to presume that many more genes involved in the process of normal reproductive functioning in males will be identified in the future. Besides learning from associations of genetic disease and male infertility in the human, an important contribution might come from the study of genes involved in reproduction in animals. As already shown in the previous sections, this approach can be used to identify the human gene homologs, to study their precise function in man and to assess them at the molecular level as possible candidates in human male infertility. A few recent examples of this approach are the studies of the involvement of transcription factors and RNA-binding proteins in spermatogenesis and male infertility (Engelkamp and van Heyningen, 1996; Venables and Eperon, 1999) and the identification of genes or candidate genes for complex infertility conditions such as cryptorchidism (Kolon et al., 1999; Zimmermann et al., 1999) and globozoospermia (Xu et al., 1999).

Conclusions

The data presented in this chapter show that an increasing number of genetic causes has been associated with male reproductive dysfunction. In many cases genes and gene products have been isolated and have been shown to be implicated, when defective, in male infertility. For some other causes of male infertility, a genetic basis has been recognized but the genetic defect has either only been localized to a chromosomal region or remains as yet unmapped.

Today the clinician confronted with male infertility can, by performing a complete personal and family history, a thorough physical examination and a number of complementary investigations, reach a causal diagnosis in an increasing number of patients. The physical examination distinguishes among a normal male phenotype, a male phenotype with hypogonadism, and a male phenotype with extragenital symptoms such as obesity, mental retardation, neuromuscular defects and other dysmorphic signs. The basal complementary investigations should include a sperm analysis, an analysis of hormone concentrations (gonadotropins, steroids, ...) and a karyotype. In addition a search for microdeletions at the Yq11 locus should be included in case of non-obstructive azoospermia or OAT with concentrations below 5 or 10.10^6 spermatozoa/ml. In case of obstructive azoospermia due to bilateral absence of the vas deferens (without kidney anomalies), analysis of *CFTR* should be performed. Furthermore specific tests can be done according to the presence of specific symptoms such as in myotonic dystrophy or Kennedy disease. To improve knowledge, the researcher may, in collaboration with the clinician, perform other investigations such as testis biopsies for morphological and molecular studies, chromosomal segregation studies in gametes, functional or positional cloning studies in families to isolate novel genes and mutations.

In exceptional cases, hormone treatment may reverse infertility. More often, no causal treatment is available. However, the development of artificial reproductive technology, especially ICSI, now offers new perspectives for reproduction. The risk of transmitting genetic disease, infertility or both to the offspring is often high in such cases. The identification of a genetic defect is therefore very important for these couples opting for ICSI, so that appropriate genetic counseling can be offered. In many cases preimplantation genetic diagnosis in combination with ICSI will offer a means to prevent the transmission of genetic disease.

REFERENCES

Achermann JC, Ito M, Ito M et al. (1999) A mutation in the gene encoding steroidogenic factor-1 causes XY sex reversal and adrenal failure in humans. Nat Genet 22:125–126

Afzelius BA (1998) Immotile cilia syndrome: Past, present, and prospects for the future. Thorax 53:894–897

Ahlbom BE, Dahl N, Zetterqvist P, Annerén G (1995) Noonan syndrome with café-au-lait spots and multiple lentigines syndrome are not linked to the neurofibromatosis type 1 locus. Clin Genet 48:85–89

Anguiano A, Oates RD, Amos JA et al. (1992) Congenital bilateral absence of the vas deferens. A primarily genital form of cystic fibrosis. J Am Med Assoc 267:1794–1797

Ashizawa T, Dubel JR, Dunne PW et al. (1992a) Anticipation in myotonic dystrophy. Neurology 42:1877–1883

Ashizawa T, Dunne CJ, Dubel JR et al. (1992b) Anticipation in myotonic dystrophy. Neurology 42:1871–1877

Aslanidis C, Jansen G, Amemiya C et al. (1992) Cloning of the essential myotonic dystrophy region and mapping of the putative defect. Nature 355:548–551

Bahuau M, Flintoff W, Assouline B et al. (1996) Exclusion of allelism of Noonan syndrome and neurofibromatosis-type 1 in a large family with Noonan syndrome-neurofibromatosis association. Am J Med Genet 66:347–355

Barbaux S, Niaudet P, Gubler M-C et al. (1997) Donor splice-site mutations in WT1 are responsible for Frasier syndrome. Nat Genet 17:467–470

Beales PL, Warner AM, Hitman GA (1997) Bardet-Biedl syndrome: A molecular and phenotypic study of 18 families. J Med Genet 34:92–98

Beales PL, Elcioglu N, Woolf AS et al. (1999) New criteria for improved diagnosis of Bardet-Biedl syndrome: Results of a population survey. J Med Genet 36:437–446

Bell DM, Leung KKH, Wheatley SC et al. (1997) SOX9 directly regulates the type-II collagen gene. Nat Genet 16:174–178

Bi W, Min Deng J, Zhang Z et al. (1999) Sox9 is required for cartilage formation. Nat Genet 22:85–89

Bogan JS, Page DC (1994) Ovary? Testis? – A mammalian dilemma. Cell 76:603–607

Bonduelle M, Camus M, De Vos A et al. (1999) Seven years of intracytoplasmic sperm injection and follow-up of 1987 subsequent children. In Diedrich K, Felberbaum R (eds): ART in the year 2000. Oxford University Press, Oxford, UK. Hum Reprod 14(suppl 1):243–264

Brook DJ, McCurrach ME, Harley HG et al. (1992) Molecular basis of myotonic dystrophy: expansion of a trinucleotide (CTG) repeat at the 3′ end of a transcript encoding a protein kinase family member. Cell 68:799–808

Brown GM, Furlong RA, Sargent CA et al. (1998) Characterisation of the coding sequence and fine mapping of the human DFFRY gene and comparative expression analysis and mapping to the Sxr^b interval of the mouse Y chromosome of the Dffry gene. Hum Mol Genet 7:97–107

Bruford EA, Riise R, Teague PW et al. (1997) Linkage mapping in 29 Bardet-Biedl syndrome families confirms loci in chromosomal regions 11q13, 15q22.3-q23 and 16q21. Genomics 41:93–99

Carmi R, Elbedour K, Stone EM, Sheffield VC (1995a) Phenotypic differences among patients with Bardet-Biedl syndrome linked to three different chromosome loci. Am J Med Genet 59:199–203

Carmi R, Rokhlina T, Kwitek-Black A et al. (1995b) Use of a DNA pooling strategy to identify a human obesity syndrome locus on chromosome 15. Hum Mol Genet 4:9–13

Carré-Eusèbe D, Imbeaud S, Harbison M et al. (1992) Variants of the anti-Müllerian hormone gene in a compound heterozygote with the persistent Müllerian duct syndrome and his family. Hum Genet 90:389–394

Casals T, Bassas L, Ruiz-Romero et al. (1995) Extensive analysis of 40 infertile patients with congenital absence of the vas deferens: in 50% of cases only one CFTR allele could be detected. Hum Genet 95:205–211

Cassidy SB (1997) Prader–Willi syndrome. J Med Genet 34:917–923

Chandley AC, Speed RM, McBeath S, Hargreave TB (1986) A human 9;20 reciprocal translocation associated with male infertility and analysed at prophase and metaphase I of meiosis. Cytogenet and Cell Genet 41:145–153

Chang C, Kokontis J, Liao S (1988) Molecular cloning of human and rat complementary DNA encoding androgen receptors. Science 240:324–326

Chang PL, Sauer MV, Brown S (1999) Y chromosome microdeletion in a father and his four infertile sons. Hum Reprod 14:2689–2694

Chillon M, Casals T, Mercier B et al. (1995) Mutations in the cystic fibrosis gene in patients with congenital absence of the vas deferens. N Eng J Med 332:1475–1480

Colley A, Donnai D, Evans DGR (1996) Neurofibromatosis/Noonan phenotype: a variable feature of type 1 neurofibromatosis. Clin Genet 49:59–64

Cuppens H, Lin W, Jaspers M et al. (1998) Polyvariant mutant cystic fibrosis conductance regulator genes. The polymorphic (TG)m locus explains the partial penetrance of the T5 polymorphism as a disease mutation. J Clin Investigation 101:487–496

Cystic Fibrosis Genetic Analysis Consortium (1994) Population variation of common cystic fibrosis mutations. Hum Mutation 4:167–177

De Braekeleer M, Férec C (1996) Mutations in the cystic fibrosis gene in men with congenital bilateral absence of the vas deferens. Mol Hum Reproduction 2:669–677

de Roux N, Young J, Misrahi M et al. (1997) A family with hypogonadotropic hypogonadism and mutations in the gonadotropin-releasing hormone receptor. N Eng J Med 337:1597–1602

Digilio MC, Marino B, Giannotti A, Dallapiccola B (1996) Exclusion of 22q11 deletion in Noonan syndrome with tetralogy of Fallot. Am J Med Genet 62:413–414

Dowsing AT, Yong EL, Clark M et al. (1999) Linkage between male infertility and trinucleotide repeat expansion in the androgen-receptor gene. Lancet 44:640–643

Dubin L, Amelar RD (1971) Etiologic factors in 1294 consecutive cases of male infertility. Fertility and Sterility 22:469–474

Dumur V, Gervais R, Rigot J-M et al. (1990) Abnormal distribution of CF ΔF508 allele in azoospermic men with congenital aplasia of epididymis and vas deferens. Lancet 336:512

Dumur V, Gervais R, Rigot J-M et al. (1995) Congenital bilateral absence of the vas deferens in absence of cystic fibrosis. Lancet 345:200–201

Dumur V, Gervais R, Rigot J-M et al. (1996) Congenital bilateral absence of vas deferens (CBAVD) and cystic fibrosis transmembrane regulator (CFTR): correlation between genotype and phenotype. Hum Genet 97:7–10

Eberhart CH, Maines JZ, Wasserman SA (1996) Meiotic cell cycle requirement for a fly homologue of human deleted in azoospermia. Nature 381:783–785

Elliot M, Maher ER (1994) Beckwith–Wiedemann syndrome. J Med Genet 31:560–564

Elliott DJ, Millar MR, Oghene K et al. (1997) Expression of RBM in the nuclei of human germ cells is dependent on a critical region of the Y chromosome long arm. Proc Natl Acad Sci USA 94:3848–3853

Elsawi MM, Pryor JP, Klufio G et al. (1994) Genital tract function in men with Noonan syndrome. J Med Genet 31:468–470

Engelkamp D, van Heyningen V (1996) Transcription factors in disease. Cur Opin in Genet Dev 6:334–342

Feil R, Khosla S (1999) Genomic imprinting in mammals. Trends Genet 15:431–435

Ferguson-Smith MA, Goodfellow PN (1995) SRY and primary sex-reversal syndromes. In Scriver CR, Beaudet AL, Sly WS, Valle D (eds): The Metabolic and Molecular Bases of Inherited Disease. McGraw-Hill, NY, ch. 17, p. 739–748

Ferguson-Smith MA, Lennox B, Mack WS, Stewart JSS (1957) Klinefelter's syndrome. Frequency and testicular morphology in relation to nuclear sex. Lancet ii:167–169

Flejter WL, Fergestad J, Gorski J et al. (1998) A gene involved in XY sex reversal is located on chromosome 9, distal to marker D9S1779. Am J Hum Genet 63:794–802

Foote S, Vollrath D, Hilton A, Page DC (1992) The human Y chromosome: Overlapping DNA clones spanning the euchromatic region. Science 258:60–66

Foster JW, Dominguez-Steglich MA, Guioli S et al. (1994) Campomelic dysplasia and autosomal sex-reversal caused by mutations in an SRY-related gene. Nature 372:525–530

Franco B, Guioli S, Pragliola A et al. (1991) A gene deleted in Kallmann's syndrome shares homology with neural cell adhesion and axonal path-finding molecules. Nature 353:529–536

Friedman KJ, Teichtahl H, de Kretser DM et al. (1995) Screening Young syndrome patients for CFTR mutations. Am J Respir Crit Care Med 152:1353–1357

Fu H-Y, Pizzuti A, Fenwick RG et al. (1992) An unstable triplet repeat in a gene related to myotonic muscular dystrophy. Science 255:1256–1258

Gabriel-Robez O, Ratompoirina C, Dutrillaux B et al. (1986) Meiotic association between the XY chromosomes and the autosomal quadrivalent of a reciprocal translocation in two infertile men, 46,XY,t(19;22) and 46,XY,t(17;21). Cytogenet Cell Genet 43:154–160

Gabriel-Robez O, Rumpler Y (1996) The meiotic pairing behaviour in human spermatocytes carrier of chromosome anomalies and their repercussions on reproductive fitness. II Robertsonian and reciprocal translocations. A European collaborative study. Ann Génét 39:17–25

Girardi SK, Mielnik A, Schlegel PN (1997) Submicroscopic deletions in the Y chromosome of infertile men. Hum Reprod 12:1635–1641

Guichaoua MR, de Lanversin A, Cataldo C et al. (1991) Three dimensional reconstruction of human pachytene spermatocyte nuclei of a 17;21 reciprocal translocation carrier: study of XY-autosome relationships. Hum Genet 87:709–715

Guichaoua MR, Speed RM, Luciani JM et al. (1992) Infertility in human males with autosomal translocations. Cytogenet Cell Genet 60:96–101

Gottlieb B, Beitel LK, Lumbroso R et al. (1999) Update of the androgen receptor gene mutations database. Hum Mutat 14:103–114

Green JS, Parfrey PS, Harnett JD et al. (1989) The cardinal manifestations of Bardet–Biedl syndrome, a form of Laurence–Moon–Bardet–Biedl syndrome. N Eng J Med 321:1002–1009

Greenhall E, Vessey M (1990) The prevalence of subfertility: our view of the current confusion and a report of two new studies. Fertil Steril 54:978–983

Guichard C, Harricane M-C, Lafitte J-J et al. (2001) Axonemal dynein intermediate-chain gene (DNAI1) mutations result in situs inversus and primary ciliary dyskinesia (Kartagener syndrome). Am J Hum Genet 68:1030–1035

Guioli S, Schmitt K, Critcher R et al. (1998) Molecular analysis of 9p deletions associated with XY sex reversal: refining the localization of a sex-determining gene to the tip of the chromosome. Am J Hum Genet 63:905–908

Haqq CM, King C-Y, Ukiyama E et al. (1994) Molecular basis of mammalian sexual determination: activation of Müllerian inhibiting substance gene expression by SRY. Science 266:1494–1500

Hatada I, Ohashi H, Fukushima Y et al. (1996) An imprinted gene p57KIP2 is mutated in Beckwith-Wiedemann syndrome. Nat Genet 14:171–173

Hathout EB, Thompson K, Baum M, Dumars KW (1998) Association of terminal chromosome 1 deletion with Sertoli cell-only syndrome. Am J Med Genet 80:396–398

Hendry WF, A'Hern RP, Cole PJ (1993) Was Young's syndrome caused by exposure to mercury in childhood? BMJ 307:1579–1582

Hiort O, Holterhuis P-M, Nitsche EM (1998) Physiology and pathophysiology of androgen action. Baillière's Clin Endocrinol Metab 12:115–132

Holsclaw DS, Lober B, Jockin H, Schwachman H (1971) Genital abnormalities in male patients with cystic fibrosis. J Urol 106:568–574

Horsthemke B, Dittrich B, Buiting K (1997) Imprinting mutations on human chromosome 15. Hum Mutation 10:329–337

Hu L-J, Laporte J, Kress W et al. (1996) Deletions in Xq28 in two boys with myotubular myopathy and abnormal genital development define a new contiguous gene syndrome in a 430 kb region. Hum Mol Genet 5:139–143

Huang B, Wang S, Ning Y et al. (1999) Autosomal XX sex reversal caused by duplication of SOX9. Am J Med Genet 87:349–353

Hunter A, Tsilfidis C, Mettler G et al. (1992) The correlation of age of onset with CTG trinucleotide repeat amplification in myotonic dystrophy. J Med Genet 29:774–779

Igarashi S, Tanno Y, Onodera O et al. (1992) Strong correlation between the number of CAG repeats in androgen receptor genes and the clinical onset features of spinal and bulbar atrophy. Neurology 42:2300–2302

Imbeaud S, Carré-Eusèbe D, Rey R et al. (1994) Molecular genetics of the persistent Müllerian duct syndrome: a study of 19 families. Hum Mol Genet 3:125–131

Imbeaud S, Faure E, Lamarre J et al. (1995) Insensitivity to anti-Müllerian hormone due to a mutation in the human anti-Müllerian hormone receptor. Nat Genet 11:382–388

Imbeaud S, Belville C, Messika-Zeitoun L et al. (1996) A 27 base-pair deletion of the anti-Müllerian type II receptor gene is the most common cause of the persistent Müllerian duct syndrome. Hum Mol Genet 5:1269–1277

Jacobs PA, Strong JA (1959) A case of human intersexuality having a possible XXY sexdetermining mechanism. Nature 183:302–303

Jamieson CR, van der Burgt I, Brady AF et al. (1994) Mapping a gene for Noonan syndrome to the long arm of chromosome 12. Nat Genet 8:357–360

Jarvi K, Zielenski J, Wilschanski M et al. (1995) Cystic fibrosis transmembrane conductance regulator and obstructive azoospermia. Lancet 345:1578

Johannisson R, Schwinger E, Wolff HH et al. (1993) The effect of 13;14 Robertsonian translocation on germ-cell differentiation in infertile males. Cytogenet Cell Genet 63:151–155

Johns JC, Cook ID, Barratt C (1997) Mitochondrial mutations and male infertility. Nat Med 3:124–125

Josso N, Picard J-Y, Imbeaud S et al. (1997) Clinical aspects and molecular genetics of the persistent Müllerian duct syndrome. Clin Endocrinol 47:137–144

Kao SH, Chao HT, Wei YH (1995) Mitochondrial deoxyribonucleic acid 4977-bp deletion is associated with diminished fertility and motility of human sperm. Biol Reprod 52:729–736

Kao SH, Chao HT, Wei YH (1998) Multiple deletions of mitochondrial DNA are associated with the decline of motility and fertility of human spermatozoa. Molec Hum Repro 4:657–666

Katsanis N, Beales PL, Woods MO et al., (2000) Mutations in the MKKS cause obesity, retinal dystrophy and renal malformations associated with Bardet-Biedl syndrome. Nat Genet 26:67–70

Kendall SK, Samuelson LC, Saunders TL (1995) Targeted disruption of the pituitary glycoprotein hormone alpha-subunit produces hypogonadal and hypothyroid mice. Genes Dev 9:2007–2019

Kennedy WR, Alter M, Sung JH (1968) Progressive proximal spinal and bulbar muscular atrophy of late onset: a sex-linked recessive trait. Neurology 18:671–680

Kent-First M, Muallem A, Shultz J et al. (1999) Defining regions of the Y-chromosome responsible for male infertility and identification of a fourth AZF region (AZFd) by Y-chromosome microdeletion detection. Mol Reprod Dev 53:27–41

Kerem B, Kerem E (1996) The molecular basis for disease variability in cystic fibrosis. Eur J Hum Genet 4:65–73

Kerem B, Rommens JM, Buchanan JA et al. (1989) Identification of the cystic fibrosis gene: genetic analysis. Science 245:1073–1080

Kolon TF, Wiener JS, Lewitton M et al. (1999) Analysis of homeobox gene HOXA10 mutations in cryptorchidism. J Urol 161:275–280

Kremer H, Kraaij R, Toleda SPA et al. (1995) Male pseudohermaphroditism due to a homozygous missense mutation in the luteinizing hormone receptor gene. Nat Genet 9:160–164

Kwitek-Black AE, Carmi R, Duyck GM et al. (1993) Linkage of Bardet–Biedl syndrome on chromosome 16q and evidence for non-allelic genetic heterogeneity. Nat Genet 5:392–396

Lahn BT, Page DC (1997) Functional coherence of the human Y chromosome. Science 278:675–680

Lahn BT, Page DC (1999) Retroposition of autosomal mRNA yielded testis-specific gene family on human Y chromosome. Nat Genet 21:429–433

Kim J, Prawitt D, Bardeesy N et al. (1999) The Wilms' tumor suppressor gene (wt1) product regulates Dax-1 gene expression during gonadal differentiation. Mol Cell Biol 19:2289–2299

Klamt B, Koziell A, Poulat F et al. (1998) Frasier syndrome is caused by defective alternative splicing of WT1 leading to an altered ratio of WT1 +/– KTS splice isoforms. Hum Mol Genet 7:709–714

Knebelmann B, Boussin L, Guerrier D et al. (1991) Anti-Müllerian hormone Bruxelles: a nonsense mutation associated with the persistent Müllerian duct syndrome. Proc Natl Acad Sci USA 88:3767–3771

Kohsaka T, Tagawa M, Takekoshi Y et al. (1999) Exon 9 mutations in the WT1 gene, without influencing KTS splice isoforms, are also responsible for Frasier syndrome. Hum Mutat 14:466–470

Laporte J, Kioschis P, Hu L-J et al. (1997) Cloning and characterization of an alternatively spliced gene in proximal Xq28 deleted in 2 patients with intersexual genitalia and myotubular myopathy. Genomics 41:458–462

Larriba S, Bassas L, Gimenez J et al. (1998) Testicular CFTR splice variants in patients with congenital absence of the vas deferens. Hum Mol Genet 7:1739–1744

La Spada AR, Wilson EM, Lubahn DB et al. (1991) Androgen receptor gene mutations in X-linked spinal and bulbar muscular atrophy. Nature 352:77–79

Latronico AC, Segaloff DL (1999) Naturally occurring mutations of the luteinizing-hormone receptor: lessons learned about reproductive physiology and G protein-coupled receptors. Am J Hum Genet 65:949–958

Latronico AC, Anasti J, Arnhold IJP et al. (1996) Testicular and ovarian resistance to luteinizing hormone caused by inactivating mutations of the luteinizing hormone-receptor gene. N Eng J Med 334:507–512

Laue L, Wu S-M, Kudo M et al. (1995) A nonsense mutation of the human luteinizing hormone receptor gene in Leydig cell hypoplasia. Hum Mol Genet 4:1429–1433

Layman LC (1999) Mutations in human gonadotropin genes and their physiologic significance in puberty and reproduction. Fertility and Sterility 71:201–218

Layman LC, Cohen DP, Jin M et al. (1998) Mutations in gonadotropin-releasing hormone receptor gene cause hypogonadotropic hypogonadism. Nat Genet 18:14–15

Legius E, Schollen E, Matthijs G, Fryns J-P (1998) Fine mapping of Noonan/cardio-facio cutaneous syndrome in a large family. Eur J Hum Genet 6:32–37

Legouis R, Hardelin J, Levilliers J et al. (1991) The candidate gene for the X-linked Kallmann syndrome encodes a protein related to adhesion molecules. Cell 67:423–435

Le Lannou D, Jézéquel P, Blayau M et al. (1995) Obstructive azoospermia with agenesis of the vas deferens or with bronchiectasia (Young's syndrome): A genetic approach. Hum Reprod 10:338–341

Leppert M, Baird L, Anderson KI et al. (1994) Bardet–Biedl syndrome is linked to DNA markers on chromosome 11q and is genetically heterogeneous. Nat Genet 7:108–112

Lestienne P, Reynier P, Chrétien MF et al. (1997) Oligoasthenospermia associated with multiple mitochondrial DNA rearrangements. Mol Hum Reprod 3:811–814

Lissens W, Liebaers I (1997) The genetics of male infertility in relation to cystic fibrosis. Baillière's Clin Obstet Gynaecol 11:797–817

Lissens W, Mercier B, Tournaye H et al. (1996) Cystic fibrosis and infertility caused by congenital bilateral absence of the vas deferens and related clinical entities. Hum Reprod 11(suppl 4):55–80

Little M, Wells C (1997) A clinical overview of WT1 gene mutations. Hum Mutation 9:209–225

Lubahn DB, Joseph DR, Sullivan PM et al. (1988) Cloning of human androgen receptor complementary DNA and localization to the X-chromosome. Science 240:327–330

Ma K, Inglis JD, Sharkey A et al. (1993) A Y chromosome gene family with RNA-binding protein homology: candidates for the azoospermia factor AZF controlling human spermatogenesis. Cell 75:1287–1295

McElreavey K, Fellous M (1997) Sex-determining genes. Trends Endocrinol Metab 9:342–345

McElreavey K, Krausz C (1999) Male infertility and the Y chromosome. Am J Hum Genet 64:928–933

MacLean HE, Choi W-T, Rekaris G et al. (1995) Abnormal androgen receptor binding affinity in subjects with Kennedy's disease (spinal and bulbar muscular atrophy) J Clin Endocrinol Metab 80:508–516

Mahadevan M, Tsilfidid C, Sabourin L et al. (1992) Myotonic dystrophy mutation: An unstable CTG repeat in the 3″ untranslated region of the gene. Science 255:1253–1255

Mason AJ, Hayflick JS, Zoeller T et al. (1986) A deletion truncating the gonadotropin-releasing hormone gene is responsible for hypogonadism in the hpg mouse. Science 234:1366–1371

Mercier B, Verlingue C, Lissens W et al. (1995) Is congenital bilateral absence of the vas deferens a primary form of cystic fibrosis? Analysis of the CFTR gene in 67 patients. Am J Hum Genet 56:272–277

Meschede D, Rolf C, Neugebauer D-C et al. (1996) Sperm acrosome defects in a patient with Aarskog-Scott syndrome. Am J Med Genet 66:340–342

Meschede D, Dworniczak B, Behre HM et al. (1997) CFTR gene mutations in men with bilateral ejaculatory-duct obstruction and anomalies of the seminal vesicles. Am J Hum Genet 61:1200–1202

Mickle J, Milunsky A, Amos JA, Oates RD (1995) Congenital unilateral absence of the vas deferens: a heterogeneous disorder with two distinct subpopulations based upon aetiology and mutational status of the cystic fibrosis gene. Hum Reprod 10:1728–1735

Mosser J, Douar AM, Sarde CO et al. (1993) Putative X-linked adrenoleukodystrophy gene shares unexpected homology with ABC transporters. Nature 361:726–730

Mueller RF (1994) The Denys–Drash syndrome. J Med Genet 31:471–477

Muscatelli F, Strom TM, Walker AP et al. (1994) Mutations in the DAX-1 gene give rise to both X-linked adrenal hypoplasia congenita and hypogonadotropic hypogonadism. Nature 372:672–676

Nachtigal MW, Hirokawa Y, Enyeart-VanHouten DL et al. (1998) Wilms' tumor 1 and Dax-1 modulate the orphan nuclear receptor SF-1 in sex-specific gene expression. Cell 93:445–454

Nagamine K, Peterson P, Scott HS et al. (1997) Positional cloning of the APECED gene. Nat Genet 17:393–403

Oates RD, Amos JA (1994) The genetic basis of congenital bilateral absence of the vas deferens and cystic fibrosis. J Androl 15:1–9

Palermo G, Joris H, Devroey P, Van Steirteghem AC (1992) Pregnancies after intracytoplasmic injection of a single spermatozoon into an oocyte. Lancet 340:17–18

Pasteris NG, Cadle A, Logie LJ (1994) Isolation and characterization of the faciogenital dysplasia (Aarskog-Scott syndrome) gene: A putative rho/rac guanine nucleotide exchange factor. Cell 79:669–678

Patrizio P, Zielenski J (1996) Congenital absence of the vas deferens: a mild form of cystic fibrosis. Mol Med Today 1:24–31

Pennarun G, Escudier E, Chapelin C et al. (1999) Loss-of-function mutations in a human gene related to Chlamydomonas reinhardtii dynein IC78 result in primary ciliary dyskinesia. Am J Hum Genet 65:1508–1519

Quigley CA, De Bellis A, Marschke KB et al. (1995) Androgen receptor defects: historical, clinical and molecular perspectives. Endocrine Reviews 16:271–321

Ramkissoon Y, Goodfellow P (1996) Early steps in mammalian sex determination. Curr Opin Genet Dev 6:316–321

Ranum LPW, Rasmussen PF, Benzow KA et al. (1998) Genetic mapping of a second myotonic dystrophy locus. Nat Genet 19:196–198

Rave-Harel N, Kerem E, Nissim-Rafinia M et al. (1997) The molecular basis of partial penetrance of splicing mutations in cystic fibrosis. Am J Hum Genet 60:87–94

Raymond CS, Shamu CE, Shen MM et al. (1998) Evidence for evolutionary conservation of sex-determining genes. Nature 391:691–695

Raymond CS, Parker ED, Kettlewell JR et al. (1999) A region of human chromosome 9p required for testis development contains two genes related to known sexual regulators. Hum Mol Genet 8:989–996

Reijo R, Lee T-Y, Salo P et al. (1995) Diverse spermatogenic defects in humans caused by Y chromosome deletions encompassing a novel RNA-binding protein gene. Nat Genet 10:383–393

Reynier P, Chrétien MF, Penisson-Besnier I et al. (1997) Male infertility associated with multiple mitochondrial DNA rearrangements. Compte Rendu de l'Académie 320:629–636

Reynier P, Chrétien MF, Savanger F et al. (1998) Long PCR of human gamete mtDNA suggests defective mitochondrial maintenance in spermatozoa and supports the bottleneck theory for oocytes. Biochem Biophys Res Commun 252:373–377

Riordan JR, Rommens JM, Kerem B et al. (1989) Identification of the cystic fibrosis gene: cloning and characterization of complementary DNA. Science 245:1066–1073

Roberts KP (1998) Y-chromosome deletions and male infertility: state of the art and clinical implications. J Andrology 19:255–259

Roberts LM, Shen J, Ingraham HA (1999) New solutions to an ancient riddle: defining the differences between Adam and Eve. Am J Hum Genet 65:933–942

Robin NH, Sellinger B, McDonald-McGinn D et al. (1995) Classical Noonan syndrome is not associated with deletions of 22q11. Am J Med Genet 56:94–96

Rommens JM, Iannuzzi MC, Kerem B et al. (1989) Identification of the cystic fibrosis gene: Chromosome walking and jumping. Science 245:1059–1065

Rowe PJ, Comhaire FH, Hargreave TB, Mellows HJ (1993) WHO Manual for the Standardized Investigation and Diagnosis of the Infertile Couple. Cambridge University Press, NY

Rugarli EI (1999) Kallmann syndrome and the link between olfactory and reproductive development. Am J Hum Genet 65:943–948

Rugarli EI, Ballabio A (1993) Kallmann syndrome. From genetics to neurobiology. J Am Med Assoc 270:2713–2716

Saut N, Terriou P, Navarro A et al. (2000) The human Y chromosome genes BPY2, CDY1 and DAZ are not essential for sustained fertility. Mol Hum Reprod 6:789–793

Schiebel K, Winkelmann M, Mertz A et al. (1997) Abnormal XY interchange between a novel isolated protein kinase gene, PRKY, and its homologue, PRKX, accounts for one third of all (Y+)XX males and (Y–)XY females. Hum Mol Genet 6:1985–1989

Schlegel PN, Shin D, Goldstein M (1996) Urogenital anomalies in men with congenital absence of the vas deferens. J Urology 155:1644–1648

Sheffield VC, Carmi R, Kwitek-Black A et al. (1994) Identification of a Bardet–Biedl syndrome locus on chromosome 3 and evaluation of an efficient approach to homozygosity mapping. Hum Molec Genet 3:1331–1335

Sinclair AH, Berta P, Palmer MS et al. (1990) A gene from the human sex-determining region encodes a protein with homology to a conserved DNA-binding motif. Nature 346:240–244

Slavotinek AM, Stone EM, Mykytyn K et al. (2000) Mutations in MKKS cause Bardet-Biedl syndrome. Nat Genet 26:15–16

Staessen C, Coonen E, Van Assche E et al. (1996) Preimplantation diagnosis for X and Y normality in embryos from three Klinefelter patients. Hum Reprod 11:1650–1653

Sun C, Skaletsky H, Birren B et al. (1999) An azoospermic man with a de novo point mutation in the Y-chromosomal gene USP9Y. Nat Genet 23:429–432

Suzuki Y, Sasagawa I, Nakada T, Onmura Y (1998) Bilateral cryptorchidism associated with terminal deletion of 10 q. Urol Int 61:186–187

Swain A, Narvaez V, Burgoyne P et al. (1998) Dax1 antagonizes Sry action in mammalian sex determination. Nature 391:761–767

Teixeira J, Donahoe PK (1996) Molecular biology of MIS and its receptors. J Androl 17:336–341

Teng H, Jorissen M, Van Poppel H et al. (1997) Increased proportion of exon 9 alternatively spliced CFTR transcripts in vas deferens compared with nasal epithelial cells. Hum Mol Genet 6:85–90

Tiepolo L, Zuffardi O (1976) Localization of factors controlling spermatogenesis in the nonfluorescent position of the human Y chromosome long arm. Hum Genet 34:119–124

Tincello DG, Saunders, PTK, Hargreave TB (1997) Preliminary investigations on androgen receptor gene mutations in infertile men. Mol Hum Reprod 3:941–943

Toledo SPA, Brunner HG, Kraaij R et al. (1996) An inactivating mutation of the luteinizing hormone receptor causes amenorrhea in a 46,XX female. J Clin Endocrinol Metab 81:3850–3854

Tournaye H, Staessen C, Liebaers I et al. (1996) Testicular sperm recovery in nine 47,XXY Klinefelter patients. Hum Repro 11:1644–1649

Tut TG, Ghadessy FJ, Trifiro MA (1997) Long polyglutamine tracts in the androgen receptor are associated with reduced transactivation, impaired sperm production, and male infertility. J Clin Endocrinol Metab 82:3777–3782

Vainio S, Heikkilä M, Kispert A et al. (1999) Female development in mammals is regulated by Wnt-4 signalling. Nature 397:405–409

Van Assche E, Bonduelle M, Tournaye H et al. (1996) Cytogenetics of infertile men. Hum Reprod 11 (suppl 4):1–26

van der Ven K, Messer L, van der Ven H et al. (1996) Cystic fibrosis mutation screening in healthy men with reduced sperm quality. Hum Repro 11:513–517

Van Landuyt L, Lissens W, Stouffs K et al. (2000) Validation of a simple Yq deletion screening programme in an ICSI candidate population. Mol Hum Reprod 6:291–297

Van Steirteghem AC, Nagy Z, Joris H et al. (1993) High fertilization and implantation rates after intracytoplasmic sperm injection. Hum Reprod 8:1061–1066

Veitia RA, Nunes M, Quintana-Murci L et al. (1998) Swyer syndrome and 46,XY partial gonadal dysgenesis associated with 9p deletions in the absence of monosomy-9p syndrome. Am J Hum Genet 63:901–905

Venables JP, Eperon IC (1999) The roles of RNA-binding proteins in spermatogenesis and male infertility. Curr Opin Genet Dev 9:346–354

Vogt PH (1998) Human chromosome deletions in Yq11, AZF candidate genes and male infertility: History and update. Mol Hum Reprod 4:739–744

Vogt PH, Edelmann A, Kirsch S et al. (1996) Human Y chromosome azoospermia factors (AZF) mapped to different subregions in Yq11. Hum Mol Genet 5:933–943

Vollrath D, Foote S, Hilton A et al. (1992) The human Y chromosome: a 43-interval map based on naturally occurring deletions. Science 258:52–59

Wagner T, Wirth J, Meyer J et al. (1994) Autosomal sex reversal and campomelic dysplasia are caused by mutations in and around the SRY-related gene SOX9. Cell 79:1110–1120

Wang Q, Ghadessy FJ, Yong EL (1998) Analysis of the transactivation domain of the androgen receptor in patients with male infertility. Clin Genet 54:185–192

Wang I, Weil D, Levilliers J et al. (1995) Prevalence and molecular analysis of two hot spots of recombination leading to XX maleness. Genomics 28:52–58

Weighardt F, Biamonti G, Riva S (1996) The roles of heterogeneous nuclear ribonucleoproteins (hnRNP) in RNA metabolism. Bioessays 18:747–756

Weil D, Wang I, Dietrich A (1994) Highly homologous loci on the X and Y chromosomes are hot-spots for ectopic recombination resulting in XX maleness. Nat Genet 7:414–419

Weiss J, Axelrod L, Whitcomb RW et al. (1992) Hypogonadism caused by a single amino acid substitution in the β subunit of luteinizing hormone. N Eng J Med 326:179–183

Wieacker P, Missbach D, Jakubiczka S (1996) Sex reversal in a child with the karyotype 46,XY, dup (1) (p22.3p32.3). Clin Genet 49:271–273

Xu X, Toselli PA, Russell LD, Seldin DC (1999) Globozoospermia in mice lacking the casein kinase II α' catalytic subunit. Nat Genet 23:118–121

Young T-L, Penney L, Woods MO et al. (1999) A fifth locus for Bardet-Biedl syndrome maps to chromosome 2q31. Am J Hum Genet 64:900–904

Zanaria E, Muscatelli F, Bardoni B et al. (1994) An unusual member of the nuclear hormone receptor superfamily responsible for X-linked adrenal hypoplasia congenita. Nature 372:635–641

Zielenski J, Tsui L-C (1995) Cystic fibrosis: Genotypic and phenotypic variations. Annu Rev Genet 29:777–807

Zimmermann S, Schwärzler A, Buth S et al. (1998) Transcription of the Leydig insulin-like gene is mediated by steroidogenic factor-1. Molec Endocrin 12:706–713

Zimmermann S, Steding G, Emmen JMA et al. (1999) Targeted disruption of the Insl3 gene causes bilateral cryptorchidism. Mol Endocrinol 13:681–691

Fetal loss

Rhona Schreck
Neil Silverman

37

Introduction

Pregnancy loss can be defined as the unexpected and unplanned spontaneous loss of a pregnancy before the fetus is capable of extrauterine survival. In the United States and Australia, the term spontaneous abortion is used for pregnancy loss up to 20 weeks gestation, after which time the loss is defined as either an intrauterine fetal death (IUFD) or a premature delivery. Various studies on spontaneous abortion estimate the frequency of pregnancy loss to be between 10% and 50% of all pregnancies (Simpson and Mills, 1986; Wilcox et al., 1988), depending on differences in methods for estimating the fetal loss rate (such as evaluation of beta human chorionic gonadotropin (β-HCG) in early gestation, versus evaluation of clinically recognized pregnancies). Numerous different factors have been suggested to contribute to fetal loss, although good supporting data are limited for many of them. These factors can be grouped under specific classes, such as chromosomal, genetic, maternal (anatomic features and other maternal disease), endocrinologic, immunologic, disorders of coagulation, and exogenous, although some factors span these categories.

Definitions of terms

Spontaneous abortion is subdefined further based on pathologic findings and gestational age at abortion (Table 37.1). The term biochemical pregnancy is used to describe the presence of the β-subunit of human chorionic gonadotropin (β-HCG) in maternal blood seven to 10 days after ovulation without subsequent disruption of the menstrual cycle. A biochemical pregnancy implies failure of the implantation process at one of three critical stages. First, the embryo must appose itself to the endometrium such that the trophoblast beneath the inner cell mass is oriented toward the endometrial implantation site. The second stage occurs when the blastocyst forms microvilli, which interdigitate with the endometrial cells to initiate the adhesion process. Finally, hyperplasia of the trophoblast allows for penetration into the endometrium; the trophoblast becomes the placenta, and the inner cell mass becomes the fetus. If either implantation or differentiation of the inner cell mass fail to proceed normally, menstruation will most likely occur at the expected time.

Preclinical abortion (prior to six menstrual weeks gestation), occurs when the conceptus fails to implant or aborts

Table 37.1. Terms to describe various stages of pregnancy loss

Term	Description
Biochemical pregnancy	Positive maternal β-HCG within 10 days of ovulation without further evidence of pregnancy
Preclinical abortion	Abortion prior to 6 menstrual weeks due to failed implantation or disruption following implantation
Blighted ovum or anembryonic pregnancy	Empty gestational sac usually diagnosed at 5–7 weeks
Missed abortion	Disorganized fetal parts without cardiac activity retained in uterus beyond the time of fetal death
Intrauterine fetal death	Fetal demise after 20 weeks gestation but before the onset of labor

shortly after implantation. Even among investigations that include strict protocols for early β-HCG assays, preclinical abortion rates differ between studies, most likely due to the timing of the initial assay, the definition of pregnancy (based on β-HCG values), and the cross-reactivity of β-HCG assays with luteinizing hormone (LH).

Clinically recognized abortion rates are well established to be between 10% and 15% with the majority of these occurring in the first trimester of pregnancy (Yerushalmy et al., 1956; Warburton and Fraser, 1964; Leridon, 1977). Overall, 45% of clinically recognized spontaneous losses occur between seven and 11 menstrual weeks (Stevenson et al., 1959). The majority of spontaneous abortions occur in pregnancies with incomplete fetal development; however, abnormal development does not always end in spontaneous abortion, as is evident from the 3% to 4% population incidence of sporadic congenital anomalies. If the underlying cause of abortion occurs early and is severe, embryogenesis is disrupted, and ultrasound at six to eight weeks will demonstrate an empty sac classified as a blighted ovum or anembryonic pregnancy. The term missed abortion is used when the fetus has died, but is retained in the uterus, usually for several weeks. With a missed abortion, ultrasound reveals disorganized fetal parts without cardiac activity. Pathologic examination demonstrates a disorganized embryo, 1 to 10 mm in length, usually attached directly to the amion or chorion.

Failure of continued fetal growth and development beyond six to seven weeks is usually followed by vaginal bleeding at seven to 10 weeks gestation. The pregnancy is classified as an inevitable abortion when uterine contractions cause dilation of the cervix leading to either a complete abortion (all products of conception are expelled and the cervix subsequently closes), or an incomplete abortion (only a portion of the products of conception are passed through the cervix).

An ectopic pregnancy is a gestation that implants outside of the endometrial cavity. Because ectopic pregnancy poses imminent risks to the mother's health and future reproductive potential, prompt intervention is indicated. The majority (95%) of ectopic pregnancies implant within various segments of the fallopian tube, with less frequent implantation occurring in the abdomen, ovary, and the uterine cervix. The natural history of ectopic pregnancies include (1) embryonic death due to poor blood supply, (2) continued growth of the pregnancy leading to tubal rupture; or, rarely, (3) progressive fetal growth in the parietal peritoneum associated with a viable infant, more commonly termed an "abdominal" pregnancy.

Cytogenetic abnormalities

The most common cause of miscarriage is the presence of an abnormal chromosome complement. Although the frequency of chromosomal abnormalities in newborn surveys is in the range of 0.5% to 0.7%, it has been estimated that the rate at conception is many fold higher (Jacobs et al., 1974; Hamerton et al., 1975). Indeed 25–71% of preimplantation embryos obtained following *in vitro* fertilization demonstrate chromosome abnormalities (Papadopoulos et al., 1989). The 40-fold reduction in the frequency of chromosome abnormalities between conception and delivery is due to the selective loss of chromosomally abnormal fetuses during gestation.

It is well documented that chromosome abnormalities account for at least 50% of all spontaneous losses and about 60% of first trimester losses. (Warburton et al., 1980; Boue et al., 1985). Even these numbers may underestimate reality. More recent studies, with cultured chorionic villi, as opposed to suspected fetal tissue, found an abnormality rate of 69.4% (Ohno et al., 1991). In these authors' laboratory, it has been observed that 95% of the chromosomally normal abortus cultures have a 46,XX normal female karyotype, suggesting that many of the "normal results" actually represent maternal cell contamination. This idea is supported by another study, which used PCR and fluorescent in situ hybridization to investigate archival samples from "normal female abortuses", and found 29% of them contained Y-chromosome specific DNA (Bell et al., 1999). Thus, "normal" results may be over represented, and it is likely that the vast majority of spontaneous losses are to due an imbalance of genetic material as the result of chromosome abnormalities in the fetus.

Among spontaneous abortions due to chromosome disorders, autosomal trisomies are the most frequently recognized abnormality, accounting for more than 50% of cytogenetically abnormal abortuses. All autosomal trisomies have been documented with the exception of trisomy 1. The failure to detect trisomy 1 is most likely due to its early lethality, leading to embryonic death before implantation. It is well established that maternal age is strongly associated with the presence of a trisomic embryo, most likely as a result of maternal nondisjunction. Warburton's series demonstrates that for trisomies in general, the mean maternal age increases with decreasing size of the autosome, which is trisomic (Warburton et al., 1991). For example, in trisomies 2–6, the mean maternal age at the time of abortion is 26.8 years, while for trisomy 22 it is 33.5 years. The majority of autosomal trisomies are lost between eight and 14 weeks (mean: 12.4 weeks) gestation; these are not known to be associated with a significantly increased risk for recurrence in future pregnancies (Morton et al., 1987; Warburton, 1987). The only possible exceptions are spontaneous abortions involving trisomies 13, 18, or 21, which may conservatively be regarded as implicating the same recurrence risk as would be estimated if the pregnancy resulted in a term delivery. It is feasible that a proportion of this increased risk may be due to low-level parental mosaicism for these trisomies. Increasing maternal age is one risk factor for spontaneous loss, nondisjunction and aneuploidy. Maternal age also shows a direct correlation with the presence of abnormal karyotypes, specifically trisomy, in abortus material (Cowchock et al., 1993) leading to the suggestion that the majority of oocytes in woman aged 40 and above may be aneuploid (Hassold and Chiu, 1985). Thus, it is likely that the overwhelming majority of spontaneous losses in older woman can be attributed to chromosome abnormalities.

The most common trisomy (30% of all trisomies) seen in first trimester abortion specimens is trisomy 16, which is associated with only minimal embryonic development. Full trisomy 16 has not been reported in liveborn infants or in second trimester amniotic fluid specimens, indicating the severe lethality of this condition. Despite the nonviability of trisomy 16, the mean gestational age for abortion (11.7 weeks) is not significantly different from the mean age at abortion for other nonviable trisomies (12.1 weeks) or from the mean age for viable trisomies (13.1 weeks). Trisomy 16 in placental tissue (detected by CVS), even when associated with a chromosomally normal fetus, is associated with intrauterine growth retardation (Kalousek, 1993). Mosaic trisomy 16 has been reported in amniotic fluid specimens with and without uniparental disomy, and associated with distinctive dysmorphic features (Garber et al., 1994; Hsu et al., 1998). Other commonly observed trisomies in abortus material include trisomy 15 and trisomy 22.

Although trisomies are very common, autosomal monosomy is almost never seen and probably results in preimplantation lethality. However, approximately 20% of all first trimester losses are a result of X chromosome monosomy, which typically leads to abortion at 12 to 14 weeks gestation and is associated with only minimal fetal development. In contrast to liveborns with Turner syndrome, the vast majority of X chromosome monosomy abortus specimens have a pure 45,X karyotype (Boue and Gallano, 1984). The lethality of this condition is further demonstrated by the finding that 75% of 45,X fetuses detected by amniocentesis abort spontaneously following the diagnosis (Hook, 1983). Unlike many trisomies, monosomy X is inversely associated with maternal age, possibly because this aneuploidy is usually associated with paternal nodisjunction (Warburton et al., 1980; Chandley, 1981). Molecular analysis of monosomy X

cases demonstrate that this condition frequently (75%) occurs as a result of the loss of the paternal X or Y chromosome (Hassold et al., 1988). Mean gestational age at abortion is 13.1 weeks with the products of conception exhibiting normal female genitalia, and the placenta demonstrating subchorial thromboses. Cystic hygroma, edema, and coarctation of the aorta are common characteristics in monosomy X fetuses that survive into the second trimester. However, intact first trimester aborted embryos do not demonstrate these features, suggesting that their abnormal development begins at least as late as the end of the first trimester. Unlike monosomy X, the 47,XXX, 47,XXY, and 47,XYY chromosome complements are only rarely seen in abortus specimens (0.2%) and often survive to term.

Triploidy accounts for another 15% of cytogenetically abnormal abortuses, and is associated with a disproportionately large sac on ultrasound evaluation, and with syndactyly, hydrocephaly, cardiac defects, and hypoplastic kidneys on pathologic examination. Triploidy most frequently (66%) results from dispermy producing a 69,XXX or 69,XXY karyotype (Kajii and Nikawa, 1977; Jacobs et al., 1978; Zaragoza, 2000), although there is molecular evidence for some resulting from diploid sperm. More rarely, triploidy results from two maternal and one paternal set of chromosomes, due to complete nondisjunction at maternal meiosis I or II and retention of a polar body. For clinically recognized triploid losses, the gestational age at abortion is broadly distributed from seven to 17 weeks. Nonclassic, or partial hydatidiform moles are often triploid and show evidence of fetal parts as well as trophoblastic hyperplasia and hydatidiform changes of some villi (Jacobs et al., 1982; Szulman, 1984). The complete form of hydatidiform mole is associated with a 46,XX karyotype, with duplication of the paternal haploid complement resulting in homozygosity at all loci. Complete moles are rare, and are characterized by extensive hyperplasia of the trophoblast with hydropic chorionic villi, and without evidence of a fetus. Complete moles are associated with malignant or residual trophoblastic disease and should be followed for evidence of malignant sequelae.

Tetraploidy, due to failure of postconceptional cell cleavage at the first mitotic division, is observed in about 5% of karyotyped abortus specimens. The resulting cell, with 92 chromosomes, always has an XXXX or XXYY sex chromosome complement. Abortion usually occurs at 10 to 14 menstrual weeks, although embryonic development ceases much earlier (Warburton et al., 1991). Rarely, tetraploidy may be associated with a live birth (Golbus et al., 1976; Shiono et al., 1988), but is also seem in cultured chorionic villi and amniocytes from normal pregnancies.

Only about 2% of karyotyped spontaneous abortion specimens are characterized by unbalanced structural chromosome abnormalities, about half of these being de novo. Of special interest is the group with inherited cytogenetic abnormalities as these families are at a greatly increased risk of repeated pregnancy loss (see the section below).

Recurrent abortion

Spontaneous abortion is a frequent enough event that, merely by chance, some couples would be expected to experience repeated pregnancy loss. Indeed, if the risk of pregnancy loss is 15% in any given pregnancy, the likelihood of three consecutive pregnancy losses, which is the classic gynecologic definition of habitual abortion, would be 0.34% (34/1000). However, about 1.0% to 2% of couples experience three or more consecutive spontaneous pregnancy losses (Drugan et al., 1990; Regan, 1991, Brigham, 1999), suggesting some underlying operative mechanism. Empirical data show that a history of pregnancy loss increases the risk of miscarriage at subsequent pregnancies (Warburton and Fraser, 1964; Risch, et al., 1988; Clifford et al., 1997), with the risk increasing from 12% without any prior history, to 24% after one loss, 32% after three losses and to 53% after six or more losses. Even though the chance of a successful pregnancy for such couples is generally better than 60% (Regan, 1991; Brigham et al., 1999), many seek medical help to identify the cause involved, in the hopes of determining a strategy to alleviate the problem. Factors that seem to influence the recurrence risk include loss of a chromosomally normal fetus (Ogasawara et al., 2000), loss after the first trimester, history of preterm deliveries, infertility problems (Warburton and Strobino 1987), and maternal age (Risch, et al., 1988; Clifford et al., 1997; Nybo Anderson et al., 2000a,b). In a Danish study of all reported pregnancies between 1978 and 1992, (Nybo Anderson et al., 2000) the overall rate of spontaneous pregnancy loss was reported to be 13.5%, with the rate in woman aged 20–24 years being only 8.9%, while the rate of loss at age 42 was 50%, with nearly 75% of pregnancies in woman 45 years of age and older resulting in a spontaneous loss. A similar, but not as steep, increase was reported in combined US and Canadian data, with a doubling of the spontaneous loss rate in women over 40 years of age (Risch, 1988), while the rate of about 50% in women over 40 was confirmed in another study (Clifford et al., 1997). Ironically, as a woman's age at each subsequent pregnancy is more advanced, failure to achieve successful pregnancies, and the delay involved, can contribute to the risk of loss.

Traditionally, anatomic defects in the mother (associated with second trimester loss) or luteal phase inadequacies (first trimester losses) have been suggested as the most common causes for recurrent losses, although there are inadequate data on the frequencies of these conditions in the normal population to establish a clear relationship. The anatomic defects most frequently reported to be involved are uterine abnormalities, specifically variations of failure of Mullerian development, resulting in bicornuate, septate, or didelphic uteri. Structural defects of the uterus have been reported in 15% to 30% of women who habitually abort as compared to 0.5 to 2% of normal controls (Stirrat, 1990; Makino, 1994), and sonohysterography of women with at least two prior losses revealed interuterine abnormalities in 50% (Keltz, 1997), suggesting a causal relationship. Surgical correction of uterine abnormalities may be a reasonable option if other causes of recurrent pregnancy loss have been excluded. While no controlled trials have studied this approach, approximately 70–85% of patients with histories of recurrent loss, who underwent surgical correction of either a septate or bicornuate uterus, delivered viable infants in their subsequent pregnancies (DeCherney et al., 1986, March and Israel, 1987). However, there is no compelling evidence that uterine myomas affect either spontaneous abortion or preterm delivery rates (Exacoustos and Rosati, 1993). An "incompetent" cervix has been observed in 13% to 20% of patients experiencing repeated loss, but without good data from a control population (McDonald, 1987). This condition, when diagnosed, is amenable to treatment by cerclage. The recognition of a treatable anatomic abnormality usually precludes the search for other causes.

Maternal endocrine problems have been suggested to be associated with recurrent pregnancy loss. Progesterone produced by the corpus luteum is essential for implantation and subsequent pregnancy maintenance until the placenta is functional at about eight weeks of gestation. While a progesterone deficit in the luteal phase (luteal phase defect or LPD) has been considered by some investigators to be responsible for 20–40% of early trimester losses (Daya et al., 1988; Check, 1994), there are no published studies that include concurrently tested controls. The diagnosis of LPD is commonly made empirically, but requires the presence of a histologically out-of-phase endometrial biopsy, ideally in two of three consecutive menstrual cycles. Uncontrolled studies have reported that patients with recurrent losses and LPD are more likely to achieve pregnancy when treated with supplemental progesterone, though this is not a uniform finding (Ogasawara, 1997) and a meta-analysis of controlled trials found progesterone therapy to be no better than placebo (Goldstein et al., 1989). In patients whose endometrial biopsies or serum hormone results show evidence of reduced progesterone, hormone therapy may lower the loss rate, although not all investigations support this. Additionally, ultrasound examination has revealed polycystic ovaries in 44% to 56% of women with at least three spontaneous pregnancy losses, as compared with 20% of controls (P = .06) (Johnson and Pearce, 1990; Clifford, 1994). Polycystic ovaries are associated with elevated basal concentrations of lutenizing hormone (Johnson and Pearce, 1990). Pituitary suppression with bromocriptine has been reported to reduce the risk of miscarriage in women with this condition.

Both genetic and immunologic factors have been identified as causes of repeated pregnancy loss. Genetic factors can include both single gene defects as well as parental chromosome abnormalities. Although chromosome defects are the most common cause of first trimester pregnancy loss, chromosome abnormalities only account for a relatively small proportion of couples with recurrent losses. Fetuses with double trisomies, associated with two nondisjunctional events, do occur in women in the oldest age groups (Kline and Stein, 1987). There is evidence from other species of genes that predispose to nondisjunction and aneuploidy (Sandler and Lindsley, 1974). Some studies have shown a repeating pattern of either normal or abnormal chromosome studies in abortus material from women, with successive losses either showing both normal (85%) or abnormal (65%) outcomes (Maier, 1987). The risk of subsequent pregnancy loss was higher if the previous loss had been cytogenetically normal (Warburton and Strobino, 1987), suggesting that other factors were responsible for the recurrent loss.

Numerous studies have shown that about 5.5% of couples experiencing three or more losses have one partner who carries a balanced chromosomal rearrangement, in comparison to less than 0.55% of the general population (Sant-Cassia and Cooke, 1981; Stoll, 1981; Husslein et al., 1982; Michels et al., 1982; Osztovics et al., 1982; Diedrich et al., 1983; Lippman-Hand and Vekemans, 1983; Neri, 1983; Schwartz and Palmer, 1983; Fryns et al., 1984; Pantzar et al., 1984; Soh et al., 1984; Toth et al., 1984; Sachs et al., 1985; Bourrouillou et al., 1986; Castle and Bernstein, 1988; Fortuny et al., 1988; Portnoi et al., 1988; Cammarata et al., 1989; Makino et al., 1990; Fryns and Van Buggenhout, 1998). These rearrangements are detected about twice as often in the female partner with a history of pregnancy loss (Lippman-Hand and Vekemans,

1983; Simpson and Bombard, 1987). Rearrangements in males may more often be associated with infertility (Maier, 1987). History of an abnormal offspring is about fourfold more likely if it is the mother who carries the rearrangement (Simpson et al., 1981; Boue and Gallano, 1984). The most commonly observed rearrangements are either reciprocal or Robertsonian translocations (Neri et al., 1983), which predispose to genetically unbalanced gametes because of the dispersion of tetrads during meiosis resulting in nonviable fetuses. Fryns and Van Buggenhout (1998) reported that of the chromosome abnormalities observed in couples with two or more pregnancy losses, two-thirds were balanced autosomal translocations, with the incidence of such translocations in this group being 30 times higher than in the general population. Prospective studies of couples identified as balanced translocation carriers indicate that as many as 80% of their pregnancies end in abortion, while 16% lead to the birth of a healthy newborn. Their risk of giving birth to an abnormal child with chromosome imbalance is relatively low (approximately 4–6%) (Neri et al., 1983), particularly when the parental rearrangement has been ascertained through a history of miscarriage rather than through the birth of an abnormal child (Boue and Gallano, 1984). However, only one-third of these losses result from an unbalanced fetal karyotype related to the rearrangement in the parent, suggesting that translocation carriers may be at increased risk for other types of aneuploidy (Warburton and Strobino, 1987). The high rate of loss, but low rate of viable abnormals (Petrosky and Borgaonkar, 1984), needs to be considered when counseling ongoing pregnancies and when evaluating the risks of prenatal diagnosis in these patients. The specific chromosomes involved in the translocation also influence these statistics. For instance, carriers of Robertsonian translocations involving both copies of chromosome 21 (e.g., 45,XX, der (21;21) (q10; q10) will lose half of their pregnancies as a result of monosomy 21, while all of their liveborn children will have Down syndrome.

Chromosomal inversions have been identified in about 0.3% of recurrent aborters (Maier, 1987) and carry a 4% to 8% risk for an abnormal liveborn infant (Boue and Gallano, 1984). This risk is highly dependent on the type of inversion, as paracentric inversions almost always result in nonviable gametes (with acentric or dicentric chromosomes), in distinction to pericentric inversions. The larger the inverted segment, the smaller the amount of duplicated or deleted material in the unbalanced gametes, as only the material outside of the inversion loop formed during meiosis is subject to alterations in the amount of euchromatin. The commonly reported human inversions, [inv(9) (p12q13) and inv(2)(p11q12)] are unlikely to be associated with either pregnancy loss or abnormal offspring, as the inversion loop created by this inversion contains heterochromatin, in which crossing-over is suppressed.

Anecdotal evidence and occasional reports (Diedrich et al., 1983; Hecht et al., 1984; Holzgreve et al., 1984; Wu et al., 1992; Sachs et al., 1985) from cytogenetics laboratories suggest that the finding of low-level sex chromosome mosaicism is more common among phenotypically normal individuals being karyotyped for a history of recurrent abortion than those being evaluated for other indications, although not all studies support this idea (Reinisch et al., 1981). In our own laboratory, attempts to confirm the finding of low-level mosaicism in such patients with repeat lymphocyte cultures or skin fibroblast cultures has usually produced normal results (Wu et al., 1992). Whether the observation of sex chromosome mosaicism represents an artifact of culture, an age-related phenomenon, or an indication of ovarian dysfunction as seen in Turner syndrome is still speculative. In the absence of a large-scale study to evaluate the relative frequency of a low percentage of 45,X and/or 47,XXX cells in habitual aborters and matched controls, the biologic importance of these observations cannot be discerned. However, evidence for sex chromosome aneuploidy has also been observed in evaluation of sperm chromosome complements (Rubio et al., 1999) with about 0.8–1% of sperm from men with a history of pregnancy loss showing sex chromosome disomy as opposed to 0.4% of controls.

The presence of inherited disorders with low viability within a family can also be associated with repeated pregnancy loss. This is frequently the case for X-linked dominant disorders (Table 37.2) such as incontinentia pigmenti, Rett syndrome, or Aicardi syndrome, where male fetuses are not viable, and only females survive. Skewing of X chromosome inactivation (> 90% of cells showing the same active X as opposed to the 50% expected by chance) has been observed in women with a history of recurrent spontaneous abortion (Lanasa et al., 1999a,b; Sangha et al., 1999) supposedly resulting from the presence of one X chromosome carrying a deleterious mutation. After random X-inactivation, a selective disadvantage would eliminate these cells producing a cell population with "nonrandom" or skewed X-inactivation. In two separate studies, women with recurrent spontaneous loss showed skewing of X-inactivation in 14–18% as compared to 1.5–5% of control women (Lanasa et al., 1999a; Sangha et al., 1999). Skewing of X-inactivation in one family helped identify a deletion in the factor VIII gene. All woman with the deleted X showed "preferential inactivation" of that X chromosome as well as a statistically significant increase in spontaneous abortions

Table 37.2. Single gene disorders associated with pregnancy loss

Disorder	Mode of Inheritance
Aicardi syndrome	X-linked dominant
Chondrodysplasia punctata	X-linked dominant
Focal dermal hypoplasia	X-linked dominant
Incontinenti pigmenti	X-linked dominant
Orofaciodigital syndrome	X-linked dominant
Osteogenesis imperfecta	Autosomal recessive
Rett syndrome	X-linked dominant
Thalassemia major	Autosomal recessive
Wildervanck syndrome	X-linked dominant or polygenic, sex-limited

(Pegoraro et al., 1997). In addition, genetic diseases producing nonimmune hydrops, as well as those associated with connective tissue disorders (see Chs 149-151), hemoglobin anomalies (see Chs 68-72) and kidney disorders (see Chs 59-63) can be associated with perinatal death (Mueller et al., 1983).

The presence of autoimmune antibodies with or without other stigmata of autoimmune disease, has been ascertained as a risk factor for recurrent pregnancy loss. Elevated levels of both antiphospholipid antibodies (lupus anticoagulant) and anticardiolipin antibodies have been reported in women with a history of pregnancy loss (Parke et al., 1986; Love and Santoro, 1990; Blumenfeld et al., 1991; Brown, 1991; Creagh et al., 1991). Both of these classes of antibodies lead to a higher incidence of thrombotic events (lupus anticoagulant interferes with the conversion of promthrombin to thrombin) causing placental thrombosis and infarction (Brown, 1991). Thus while the presence of these antibodies can lead to pregnancy loss in any trimester, most of the losses occur later in pregnancy (Love and Santoro, 1990).

A unique syndrome, antiphospholipid syndrome (OMIM 107320), involving the presence of a spectrum of antibodies directed against cellular phospholipid components, arterial and venous thrombosis, recurrent pregnancy loss, and immune thrombocytopenia in the absence of rheumatic connective tissue disease has been described and can show a familial aggregation (Parke et al., 1986; Mackie et al., 1987; Matthey et al., 1989) with most likely dominant or codominant inheritance (Goel et al., 1999). Antiphospholipid antibodies were detectable in 16% of patients with three or more pregnancy losses as compared with 7% of normal controls, and only 3% of women who had never reported a pregnancy (Parke et al., 1986). Creagh et al. (1991) reported the incidence of women with lupus anticoagulant or anticardiolipin as 7/35 and 6/35, respectively, in a group with more than two losses, as compared to 1/31 and 0/31 in a group with two or fewer losses. However, low-positive IgG fractions of antiphospholipid antibodies or isolated IgM fractions do not make a diagnosis of the antiphospholipid syndrome. Women with prior fetal losses and high levels of anticardiolipin IgG antibodies appear to be at the highest risk of fetal loss in subsequent pregnancies and may benefit the most from preventive therapies (Branch et al., 1992; Rai et al., 1997). An elevation of antinuclear antibodies occurred in the sera of a woman with previous pregnancy loss, even when the loss had been explained by other causes (anatomic or luteal phase defects; (Creagh et al., 1991). However, anti-nuclear antibodies alone appear to be non-specific markers in women with pregnancy loss, with other investigators demonstrating no difference in the proportion of positive anti-nuclear antibody tests between women with recurrent losses and appropriate controls (Cowchock et al., 1986; Maier and Parke, 1989). Takakuma (1997) observed that the incidence of chromosomally abnormal abortuses was lower in women with elevated anticardiolipin antibodies (20% as compared to 60% in controls), suggesting that some of their losses were caused by other events. Whether some of these autoimmune antibodies are generated in response to fetal demise in susceptible women, rather than being the cause of the pregnancy loss, has been cause for speculation. However, immunoglobulin isolated from women with elevated anticardiolipin levels can induce abortion in pregnant mice (Stirrat, 1990), suggesting that the antibodies themselves are the underlying etiology of the loss. In addition, several studies have shown the efficacy of corticosteroids, heparin, aspirin, and immunoglobulin therapy in preventing pregnancy loss in women with autoimmune antibodies (Stirrat, 1990; Blumenfeld et al., 1991; Festin et al., 1997; Cowchock, 1998; Greaves, 1999; Wechsles et al., 1999).

The role of autoimmune antibodies as the cause or result of the pregnancy loss has been influenced by studies of the effect of thrombophila on pregnancy loss rates (Table 37.3). Several causes of inherited thrombophilia, and the associated thrombosis of placental vessels, have been proposed to influence pregnancy loss (Preston et al., 1996; Bonnar, 1998; Blumenfield and Brenner, 1999). Factor XII deficiency was reported in 9.4% of woman with recurrent losses as opposed to 0% of controls in one study (Gris, 1999) and has been associated with recurrent pregnancy loss by other groups (Braulke et al., 1993; Yamada et al., 2000). Mutations in the genes for both factor V and prothrombin have also been associated with unexplained late fetal loss and other thrombosis-related pregnancy complications in recent studies (Kupferminc et al., 1999; Martinelli et al., 2000). factor V

Table 37.3. Factors that contribute to vascular problems in the placenta

Autoantibodies	anti-cardiolipin lupus anticoagulant antiphospholipid syndrome systemic lupus erythematosus
Clotting factors	factor V Leiden factor XII protein C prothrombin
Metabolic problems	hyperhomocyst(e)inemia methylenetetrahydrofolate reductase deficiency
Other	45,X karyotype

Leiden mutations and the associated resistance to activated protein C have been found to be more prevalent in women with a history of pregnancy loss in several studies (Grandone, 1997; Ridker et al., 1998; Kupferminc et al., 1999; Meinardi et al., 1999; Souza, 1999; Tormene, 1999; Foka et al., 2000; Gerhardt, 2000; Younis, 2000) with an incidence of 7–44% in those with losses as compared to 1.6–6% of controls. Studies on mice, made deficient for factor V through gene targeting, show that half of the embryos die during the first half of gestation, probably as a result of abnormalities in yolk-sac vasculature (Cui et al., 1996). Factor V deficiency is also associated with pre-eclampsia, abruptio placentae, fetal growth retardation, late pregnancy loss and stillbirth. Therapy with heparin and low-dose aspirin treatment has been proposed as a treatment (Bonnar, 1998). Currently, testing for both the factor V Leiden mutation and the prothrombin gene mutation has been incorporated into pregnancy loss evaluation at our center.

An additional hereditary thrombophilic tendency implicated in recurrent pregnancy loss has been hyperhomocysteinemia, which has also been associated with other thrombotic morbidities, such as adult myocardial infarction (Steegers-Theunissen et al., 1992; Quere, 1998; Ray, 1999; Nelen, 2000a,b). Some recent reports have shown an association between a homozygous C->T polymorphism at nucleotide 677 in the gene coding for methyenetetrahydrofolate reductase which leads to a thermolabile variant of the enzyme and low levels of serum folate, hyperhomocysteinemia and early pregnancy loss (Quere, 1998; Lissak, 1999; Durnwald, et al., 2000). The combination of serum folate deficiency and hyperhomocysteinemia has been reported to result in defective chorionic villus vascularization (Nelen, 2000a,b) and would be amenable to treatment with relatively high doses of folic acid (5 mg/day) along with pyridoxine supplementation (Quere, 1998). Testing for the methyenetetrahydrofolate reductase (MTHFR) mutation is also a component of pregnancy loss assessment at our center.

The sharing of HLA antigens between partners, or more specifically the lack of differences in their major histocompatibility complexes, was proposed to prevent the formation of blocking antibodies that would protect the fetus from rejection by the mother and lead to fetal loss. This theory led to an immunotherapy that utilized lymphocytes or sperm from the partner in an attempt to alter the maternal humoral immune system (Makino, 1994). However, an extensive study of the highly inbred Hutterite community, which has a high degree of sharing of HLA alleles, did not show an increase in the miscarriage rate in that community (Ober et al., 1985). Moreover, recent reports, including two large meta-analyses, have shown that such immunotherapy approaches do not significantly reduce the risk of pregnancy loss (Fraser et al., 1993; Jeng et al., 1995; Ober et al., 1999; Scott, 2000).

Some women, who experience repeated losses, do so because of underlying maternal diseases. Any disease that can potentially decrease uterine-placental blood flow profoundly may be implicated in causing a fetal demise. These would include maternal hypertension, systemic lupus erythematosus, insulin-dependent diabetes mellitus, sickle cell disease, renal disease with hypertension, severe maternal trauma, and cocaine use. There has been some suggestion that mild thyroid disorders are associated with pregnancy loss (Vaquero et al., 2000). Other studies have shown an association between the presence of anti-thyroid antibodies in euthyroid women with recurrent pregnancy loss (Bussen and Steck, 1997; Lazarus and Kokandi, 2000). Women, who were themselves exposed to diethylstilbestrol *in utero*, also show an increased incidence of spontaneous abortion, ectopic pregnancies and preterm births, presumably as a result of congenital tubal or uterine abnormalities induced by their exposure during development (Kaufman et al., 2000).

During pregnancy and the postpartum period, systemic lupus erythematosus (SLE) is associated with a series of remissions and exacerbations with a 20% to 40% risk of exacerbation (Tincani et al., 1992). If the disease is in remission at the time of conception, the fetal survival rate is good (about 85%) (Hayslett, 1992; Georgiou et al., 2000), but still below that seen in unaffected women. However, if SLE is active during the pregnancy, the fetal survival rate decreases to 50% to 75% due to complications of placental thrombosis and hypertension (Petri and Allbritton, 1993) associated with lupus flares. Several rheumatic connective tissue diseases produce circulating antibodies, such as Ro (SS-A), and La (SS-B) that lead in utero to complete heart block (Buyon and Winchester, 1990). A good review of the less common autoimmune diseases in pregnancy was provided by Giacoia and Azubuike (1991).

In non-pregnant women, type 1 diabetes often is used to include all insulin-dependent diabetes, while type 2 implies non-insulin-dependent disease. In pregnancy, the classification is based on whether or not a woman has had diabetes before pregnancy. Pregestational diabetes is then subdivided into alphabetical classes (B-D and F,R,H) depending on the age of onset, duration of the disease, or both and whether any diabetic vascular complications occurred. Gestational diabetics have diabetes only during pregnancy and are classed as A-1 if controlled with diet only, and A-2 if insulin is needed (ACOG, 1986a). Metabolic control of diabetes prior to conception and during the first trimester dramatically influences both the risk of spontaneous abortion and the incidence of major congenital anomalies (Dorman et al., 1999; Greene, 1999). The perinatal mortality rate of 3.9% in well-controlled diabetic women has been stable for over 15 years (Martin et al., 1987). Poorly controlled diabetes is associated with an increased perinatal death rate. Excluding lethal fetal anomalies, the maternal complications of ketoacidosis, pregnancy induced hypertension (PIH), pyelonephritis, or neglect increase the perinatal mortality rate to as high as 17% (Diamond et al., 1987). In a study by Garner and colleagues (1990) preeclampsia was diagnosed in about 10% of diabetic women with a 6% perinatal mortality rate. In the same study, 4% of non-diabetics developed preeclampsia, with a 0.3% perinatal mortality rate. Major congenital anomalies are increased threefold in diabetic pregnancies, but it appears that excellent pre-pregnancy control can markedly reduce the incidence of malformations (Reece et al., 1988; Greene, 1999). Early detection, excellent control, fetal surveillance, and blood pressure monitoring are key factors in lowering the perinatal mortality rate associated with maternal diabetes.

Exogenous factors and pregnancy loss

The use of certain teratogenic agents during human pregnancy is known to produce abnormalities of form or function, including fetal wastage in exposed fetuses. The pathogenetic mechanisms leading to fetal death may occur through the disturbance of one or more developmental processes. These include hypoplasia or hyperplasia of developing tissues, failure of cell differentiation or interaction, or mechanical disruption of cells. Often, the end result of teratogenic action is an organ with too few cells.

Subsequently, the organ system may fail to develop fully because of a lack of critical mass required for differentiation. Pregnancy loss due to teratogenetic agents is often difficult to prove conclusively, and many relatively safe agents have been incorrectly implicated from anecdotal experience.

The majority of known teratogens are not associated with an outcome as severe as fetal death. Table 37.4 lists agents that include pregnancy loss as part of their related effects. Certain classes of drugs, such as folic acid antagonists (aminopterin and methotrexate) are well-documented abortofacients and have been specifically studied in terms of the timing and dose required for subsequent fetal wastage (Feldkamp and Carey, 1993). Because certain vaccines (measles, mumps, smallpox) are associated with a small increase in pregnancy loss, primary care providers should inquire as to the possibility of pregnancy before administering vaccines in this category.

Antineoplastic agents in general raise serious concerns regarding the mutagenic, teratogenic, and abortifacient effects on the human embryo. With the exception of aminopterin and methotrexate (Feldkamp and Carey, 1993), these agents have not been sufficiently studied to determine whether a clear risk for pregnancy loss exists. However, in a case-control study, 124 nurses exposed to cyclophosphamide, doxorubicin, or vincristine had a significantly higher fetal loss rate than unexposed nurses (odds ratios: 2.66, 3.96, and 2.46, respectively) (Selevan et al., 1985). Although investigators have questioned this observation (Chabner, 1986; Kalter, 1986), the documented risks for congenital anomalies, as well as the potential for inducing abortions, warrant careful precautions among pharmacy and nursing personnel to avoid these agents.

Infections are a rare, but occasional cause of fetal loss. Mumps and measles, when acquired during pregnancy, have been associated with increased rates of spontaneous abortion, though not prematurity, stillbirth, or congenital malformations (Schwartz, 1950; Siegel, 1973; Eberhart-Phillips et al., 1993). Other maternal infections, such as parvovirus B19 and syphilis, can result in second or third trimester fetal death (Ricci et al., 1989; Sanghi et al., 1997) because of the sequelae of overwhelming fetal infection. Other infectious diseases may produce a substantially increased risk of structural fetal abnormalities, such as rubella and varicella (Freij et al., 1988; Enders et al., 1994) or developmental abnormalities, such as cytomegalovirus (Hagay et al., 1996) without intrinsically increasing risk of fetal loss.

Battering is the most common form of maternal trauma that occurs in pregnancy. It is believed to be the most underreported crime in the United States, but recent studies indicate that 4% to 8% of women are hit at least once during pregnancy. One-fourth of these women report being struck in the abdomen (Berenson et al., 1994). Repetitive severe blows to the gravid uterus can result in direct trauma to the fetus or in partial separation of the placenta and preterm labor (Morey et al., 1981; Berenson et al., 1994). Car accidents are also common in pregnancy. Use of seat belts has decreased the fetal loss rate significantly and all health workers should encourage their use. Trauma that causes maternal death usually results in fetal death unless the fetus is delivered within 4 minutes of maternal cardiac arrest (Katz et al., 1986).

Multiple gestations

Several lines of evidence, including early ultrasound and chorionic villus sampling (CVS), suggest that twinning in human pregnancies may be much more common than the rate seen at delivery, with the difference being due to pregnancy loss, sometimes referred to as the "vanishing twin phenomenon" (Jackson and Benirschke, 1989; Landy and Keith, 1998). An ultrasound review of 1000 first trimester pregnancies revealed evidence of 329 twin pregnancies, of which 21.2% showed one twin to "vanish" (Landy et al., 1986). Multiple gestations may constitute more than 12% of natural pregnancies at conception with only 14% of these surviving to term (2% as twin pregnancies and the rest as singleton births) (Boklage, 1990). Falik-Borenstein and colleagues (1994) described chimerism detected during CVS with both a 46,XX normal female karyotype and a

Table 37.4. Teratogenic agents associated with fetal wastage in human pregnancy

Anticoagulants	coumarin derivatives
Anticonvulsants	paramethadione trimethadione
Antineoplastic agents	aminopterin methotrexate
Sedatives	ethyl alcohol
Illicit drugs	cocaine
Vaccines	measles mumps smallpox
Vitamin retinoids	etretinate isotretinate
Gastrointestinal agents	misoprostol

47,XY,+9 trisomy 9 male karyotype, and only a singleton pregnancy seen by ultrasound. The pregnancy resulted in a normal female birth, although there were abnormal male cells in the term placenta. The male co-twin was assumed to have suffered an early demise as a result of the chromosome abnormality.

A measure of the risk for fetal death associated with abnormal multiple gestation pregnancies was demonstrated in a large study in which the reported perinatal mortality rates for twin A and twin B were 58.8 and 64.1, respectively, compared with 10.4 per 100 births for singleton controls (Spellacy et al., 1990). The increased risk was due to the complications of maternal hypertension, placental abruption, and the increased rate of congenital anomalies in twins.

Second and third trimester fetal loss

HYPERTENSION

Fetal life is dependent on a normal functioning placenta, therefore severe impairment in fetal perfusion from the placental bed can eventually result in fetal demise. The American College of Obstetrics and Gynecology defines pregnancy-induced hypertension (PIH) as blood pressure greater than 140/90 mm Hg that develops as a consequence of pregnancy and regresses postpartum. Three subclassifications of PIH are (1) hypertension without proteinuria, (2) preeclampsia characterized by hypertension, proteinuria, and/or edema, and (3) eclampsia characterized by preeclampsia that evolves into convulsions. Preexisting hypertension is separated into two large groups: coincidental hypertension, a chronic underlying hypertension that exists before pregnancy and persists after pregnancy, and a,b, pregnancy-aggravated hypertension, an underlying hypertension that becomes more severe during pregnancy in the form of preeclampsia or eclampsia (ACOG, 1996). Pregnancy-aggravated hypertension and severe preeclampsia/eclampsia are associated with increased perinatal mortality (Lenox et al., 1990). Isolated essential hypertension does not increase the fetal mortality rate (Sibai et al., 1993), but hypertension as a complication of another disease process is associated with increased fetal wastage.

Both animal and human studies demonstrate that hypertension of any cause results in a two- to threefold decrease in uteroplacental perfusion, most likely due to abnormal histologic changes in the placenta (Browne and Veall, 1953).

The risk of intrauterine growth retardation or restriction (IUGR) is markedly increased in the presence of maternal hypertension. More specifically, absent end-diastolic flow demonstrated by Doppler velocimetry in the presence of maternal hypertension, intrauterine growth restriction, or both has been associated with a high risk for perinatal death (Pattinson et al., 1994). It is important to emphasize that each patient must be individually evaluated to improve fetal salvage and maternal morbidity.

RENAL DISEASE

The perinatal loss rate is not increased in women with mildly impaired renal function (serum creatinine < 1.4 mg/dl). In women with moderate disease (creatinine of 1.5 to 3.0 mg/dl), the perinatal mortality rate is about 10%, but one-third of these mothers have a marked increase in hypertension with the associated risks previously outlined (Davison, 1985). Women with severe renal insufficiency on dialysis (serum creatinine > 3.0 mg/dl) are usually anovulatory, but if they do become pregnant the perinatal mortality rate is as high as 50% (Hou, 1994). The deaths usually result from severe hypertension associated with IUGR and placental separation. Davison (1985) reviewed the outcomes in 3382 pregnancies in 2409 women who had renal transplants, 80% of which were cadaveric; 35% of the pregnancies resulted in spontaneous and elective abortion, and of the remaining 65% continuing pregnancies, 90% had a successful outcome. In a similar study, Hou (1989) reported only a 5% perinatal mortality rate in continuing pregnancies, and a 30% preeclampsia rate, which accounted for much of the loss. The optimal factors for a good outcome were: good health without severe hypertension for two years after transplant; no signs of graft rejection; and no persistent proteinuria.

CARCINOMA

Cancer occurs in 0.07% to 0.1% of all pregnancies (Zemlickis et al., 1992). The most common malignancies include those of the breast, cervix, thyroid, ovary, and colon, and leukemia, lymphoma, and melanoma. Pregnancy outcome appears to be extremely good in women with hematologic malignancies (Zuazu et al., 1991). Malignant melanoma can, though very rarely, metastasize to the placenta and the fetus, but in general does not result in fetal death (Wong and Strassner, 1990). Breast cancer, which complicates 1 in 3000 pregnancies, does not seem to be influenced by pregnancy (Parente et al., 1988). Although 1 in 30 cases of cervical cancer occurs during pregnancy, fetal mortality is uncommon (Koren et al., 1990).

FETAL ABNORMALITIES

There are many abnormalities that result in stillbirth. Most of these fetuses do not die before delivery, but cannot survive outside of the uterus because of a small thorax or a severe neurologic impairment that inhibits normal breathing. These abnormalities would include many skeletal dysplasias (see Ch. 152), Fraser cryptophalmos syndrome, males with incontinentia pigmenti, Meckel-Gruber syndrome, megacystic-microcolon hypoperistalsis syndrome, Neu-Laxova syndrome, Walker-Warburg syndrome, Zellweger syndrome, large irreparable diaphragmatic hernias, and anencephaly and other severe neural tube defects (Schauer et al., 1992). Anomalies in the fetus that cause *in utero* death in the late second and third trimesters often present as nonimmune hydrops fetalis.

NONIMMUNE HYDROPS FETALIS

Nonimmune hydrops fetalis (NIHF) is a fetus with two or more fluid-filled spaces, including skin edema, pleural effusions, ascites, or pericardial effusion. NIHF is not a diagnosis, but a descriptor of the effect of an underlying disease process. More than 150 different disease states can potentially result in NIHF, the more common conditions include those listed in Table 37.5 (Meizner et al., 1990; Newbould et al., 1991; Poeschmann et al., 1991). The most recognizable causes of NIHF are fetal cardiac malformations such as hypoplastic right ventricle, Ebstein anomaly, abnormal tricuspid valve and pulmonary atresia that results in right-sided cardiac failure. Left-sided lesions can result in hydrops, but do so rarely and very late in pregnancy (Ruiz et al., 1990). Homozygous α-thalassemia results in the failure to produce normal hemoglobin F or any adult hemoglobin. Maternal viral (e.g., parvovirus B19) and bacterial pathogens may be passively transmitted to the fetus where hydrops develop and then due to severe anemia. Rh and other blood group incompatibilities result in immune hydrops fetalis. Blood group incompatibilities and parvovirus infection may be successfully treated with in utero fetal transfusions.

Abnormal uterine environment

Abnormalities in the environment of the fetus that may cause demise include oligohydramnios from preterm rupture of

Table 37.5. Leading causes of nonimmune hydrops fetalis

System	Disorder
Cardiovascular	Malformation Supreventricular tachycardia Complete heart block Myocarditis Rhabdomyoma Teratoma Subendocardial fibroelastosis
Aneuploidy	Trisomy 13 Trisomy 18 Trisomy 21 45,X Triploidy Other
Placental	Twin-twin transfusion Chorioangioma
Hematologic/metabolic	α- Thalassemia Fetomaternal hemorrhage Gaucher's disease GM1 gangliosidosis type I Mucolipidosis type I Niemann-Pick disease
Infectious pathogens	Cytomegalovirus Parvovirus B19 Toxoplasmosis Syphilis
Respiratory tract	Cystic adenomatoid malformation Pulmonary sequestration
Skeletal dysplasia	Achondrogenesis Osteogenesis imperfecta
Other	Sacroccygeal teratoma/vascular teratomas Urogenital tract malformation-perforation Bowel perforation

membranes, uteroplacental insufficiency from maternal diseases, aneuploidy, intrauterine growth restriction, postmaturity, and renal aplasia (Peirpert and Donnenfield, 1991). Prostaglandin synthetase inhibitors (indomethecin) and angiotensin converting enzyme inhibitors (enalapril) have also been implicated in oligohydramnios (De Wit et al., 1988; Cunniff et al., 1990). Polyhydramnios is defined as an amniotic fluid index of more than 24 cm and is often associated with a wide range of fetal abnormalities, but may be present in the case of spontaneous fetal death without any identifiable abnormality or aneuploidy (Carlson et al., 1990; Alessandri et al., 1992). Placental abruption or vasa previa can lead to fetal death from acute blood loss (Clark, 1999).

Summary

The single most common reason for pregnancy loss, is the presence of a chromosome abnormality in the fetus, particularly if the loss occurs early in the pregnancy and there is no history of prior losses. As these are the result of random events, little follow-up may be indicated, other than the reminder that as women ages, her risk will increase. However, a thorough workup, indicated when there has been a recurrence or there is significant maternal concern, would include a careful maternal history with attention to diseases known to be associated with demise, maternal viral studies and/or bacterial cultures, dysmorphic examination of the fetus, photographs, autopsy, chromosome studies when possible and radiographic studies (Curry and Honore, 1990). The coordinated efforts of the medical geneticist, fetal dysmorphologist, perinatologist, obstetrician, pathologist and genetic counselor can often uncover the cause of this unfortunate event. In the case of maternal disease, this information can allow the mother to receive optimal preconceptual care to enhance the outcome of a subsequent pregnancy. If a fetal abnormality or the uterine environment was the cause of the pregnancy loss, or there is no identified etiology, careful antenatal monitoring will often avert another tragic outcome.

REFERENCES

American College of Obstetricians and Gynecologists (ACOG) (1986a) Classification of diabetes in pregnancy. Technical Bulletin 92

American College of Obstetricians and Gynecologists (1986b) Management of preeclampsia. Technical Bulletin 92

Alessandri LM, Stanley FJ, Garner JB et al. (1992) A case-control study of unexplained antepartum stillbiths. Br J Obstet Gynecol 99:711–718

Bell KA, Van Deerlin PG, Haddad BR, Feinberg RF (1999) Cytogenetic diagnosis of "normal 46,XX" karyotypes in spontaneous abortions frequently may be misleading. Fertil Steril 71(2):334–41

Berenson AB, Wiemann CM, Wilkinson GS et al. (1994) Perinatal morbidity associated with violence experienced by pregnant women. Am J Obstet Gynecol 170:1760–1769

Blumenfeld Z, Brenner B (1999) Thrombophilia-associated pregnancy wastage. Fertil Steril 72:765–74

Blumenfeld Z, Weiner Z, Lorber M (1991) Anticardiolipin antibodies in patients with recurrent pregnancy wastage. Obstet Gynecol 78:584–589

Boklage CE (1990) Survival probability of human conceptions from fertilization to term. Int J Fertil 35:75

Bonnar J, Green R, Norris L (1998) Inherited thrombophilia and pregnancy: The obstetric perspective. Semin Thromb Hemost. 24 Suppl 1:49–53

Boue A, Gallano P (1984) A collaborative study of the segregation of inherited chromosomal structural rearrangements in 1356 prenatal diagnosis. Prenat Diagn 4:45–67

Boue A, Boue J, Gropp A (1985) Cytogenetics of pregnancy wastage. In: Harris H, Hirschorn K (eds). Adv Hum Genet 14

Bourrouillou G, Colombies P, Dastugue N (1986) Chromosome studies in 2136 couples with spontaneous abortions. Hum Genet 74:399–401

Branch DW, Dudley DS, Scott JR, Silver RM (1992) Antiphospholipid antibodies and fetal loss. New Engl J Med 326:952–954

Braulke I, Pruggmayer M, Melloh P et al. (1993) Factor XII (Hageman) deficiency in women with habitual abortion: New subpopulation of recurrent aborters? Fertil Steril 59:98–101

Brigham SA, Conlon C, Farquharson RG (1999) A longitudinal study of pregnancy outcome following idiopathic recurrent miscarriage. Hum Reprod 14:2868–71

Brown H (1991) Antiphospholipid antibodies and recurrent pregnancy loss. Clin Obstet Gynecol 34:17–26

Browne JCM, Veall N (1953) The maternal placental blood flow in normotensive and hypertensive women. J Obstet Gynecol Br Empire 60:141–147

Bussen SS, Steck T (1997) Thyroid antibodies and their relation to antithrombin antibodies, anticardiolipin antibodies and lupus anticoagulant in recurrent spontaneous abortions (antithyroid, anticardiolipin and antithrombin autoantibodies and lupus anticoagulant in habitual aborters). Eur J Obstet Gynecol Reprod Biol 74:139–43

Buyon JP, Winchester R (1990) Congenital complete heart block. Arthritis Rheum 33:608

Cammarata M, Corsello G, Marino M et al. (1989) Genetic factors of recurrent abortions. Acta Eur Fertil 20:367–70

Carlson DE, Platt LD, Medearis AL, Horenstein J (1990) Quantifiable polyhydramnios: Diagnosis and management. Obstet Gynecol 75:989–993

Castle D, Bernstein R (1988) Cytogenetic analysis of 688 couples experiencing multiple spontaneous abortions. Am J Med Genet 29:549–56

Chabner BA (1986) Antineoplastic drugs and spontaneous abortion in nurses. N Engl J Med 314:1049–1050

Chandley AC (1981) The origin of chromosome aberrations in man and their potential for survival and reproduction in the adult human population. Ann Genet 24:5

Check JH (1994) The role of progesterone in suppository implantation and preventing early pregnancy loss. In Barnea ER, Cheek JH, Grudzinskas JG, Marvo T (eds): Implantation and Early Pregnancy in Humans. Pathenon, London

Clark SL (1999) Placenta previa and abruptio placentae. In Creasy RK, Resnik R (eds): Maternal-fetal Medicine, 4th edn. W.B. Saunders, Philadelphia, pp:616–31

Clifford K, Rai R, Watson H, Regan L (1994) An informative protocol for the investigation of recurrent miscarriage: Preliminary experience of 500 consecutive cases. Hum Reprod 9:1328–32

Clifford K, Rai R, Regan L (1997) Future pregnancy outcome in unexplained recurrent first trimester miscarriage. Hum Reprod 12:387–9

Cnattingius S, Forman MR, Berendes HW, Isotalo L (1992) Delayed childbearing and risk of adverse perinatal outcome. JAMA 268:886

Cowchock FS, Smith JB, Gocial B (1986) Antibodies to phospholipids and nuclear antigens in patients with repeated aborters. Am J Obstet Gynecol 155:1002–1010

Cowchock FS, Gibas Z, Jackson LG (1993) Chromosome errors as a cause of spontaneous abortion: The relative importance of maternal age and obstetric history. Fertil Steril 59:1011–4

Cowchock S (1998) Treatment of antiphospholipid syndrome in pregnancy. Lupus. 7 Suppl 2:S95–7

Creagh MD, Malis RG, Cooper SM et al. (1991) Screening in lupus anticoagulant and anticardiolipin antibodies in women with fetal loss. J Clin Pathol 44:45–47

Cui J, O'Shea KS, Purkayastha A et al. (1996) Fatal haemorrhage and incomplete block to embryogenesis in mice lacking coagulation factor V. Nature 384:66–8

Cunniff C, Jones KL, Phillipson J et al. (1990) Oligohydramnios sequence and renal tubular malformation associated with maternal enalapril use. Am J Obstet Gynecol 162:187–189

Curry CJ, Honore LH (1990) A protocol for the investigation of pregnancy loss. Clin Perinatol 17:723–742

Davison JM (1985) The effect of pregnancy on kidney function in renal allograft recipients. Kidney Int. 27(1):74–9

Daya S, Ward S, Burrows E (1988) Progesterone profiles in luteal phase defect cycles and outcome of progesterone treatment in patients with recurrent spontaneous abortion. Am J Obstet Gynecol 158:225–32

De Wit W, Van Mourik I, Weisenhaan PF (1988) Prolonged maternal indomethacin therapy associated with oligohydramnios. Br J Obstet Gynecol 95:303

DeCherney AH, Russell JB, Graebe RA, Polan ML (1986) Resectoscopic management of mullerian fusion defects. Fertil Steril 45:726–8

Diamond MP, Salyer SL, Vaughn WK et al. (1987) Reassessment of White's classification and Pedersen's prognostically bad signs of diabetic pregnancies in insulin-dependent diabetic pregnancies. Am J Obstet Gynecol 156:599

Diedrich U, Hansmann I, Janke D et al. (1983) Chromosome anomalies in 136 couples with a history of recurrent abortions. Hum Genet 65:48–52

Dorman JS, Burke JP, McCarthy BJ et al. (1999) Temporal trends in spontaneous abortion associated with Type 1 diabetes. Diabetes Res Clin Pract 43:41–7

Drugan A, Koppitch FC, Williams JC et al. (1990) Prenatal genetic diagnosis following recurrent early pregnancy loss. Obstet Gynecol 75:381–384

Durnwald CP, Flora R, Agamanolis D et al. (2000) Hereditary thrombophilia as a cause of fetal loss. Obstet Gynecol 95(4 Suppl 1):S11–S12

Eberhart-Phillips JE, Frederick PD, Baron RC, Mascola L (1993) Measles in pregnancy: A descriptive study of 58 cases. Obstet Gynecol 82:797–801

Enders G, Miller E, Cradock-Watson J et al. (1994) Consequences of varicella and herpes zoster in pregnancy: Prospective study of 1739 cases. Lancet 343:1548–51

Exacoustos C, Rosati P (1993) Ultrasound diagnosis of uterine myomas and complications in pregnancy. Obstet Gynecol 82:97–101

Falik-Borenstein Z, Korenberg J, Schreck RR (1994) Confined placental chimerison: Prenatal and postnatal cytogenetic and molecular analysis, and pregnancy outcome. Am J Med Genet 50:51–56

Feldkamp M, Carey J (1993) Clinical teratology counseling and consultation case report: Low-dose methotrexate exposure in the early weeks of pregnancy. Teratology 47:533–539

Festin MR, Limson GM, Maruo T (1997) Autoimmune causes of recurrent pregnancy loss. Kobe J Med Sci 43:143–57

Foka ZJ, Lambropoulos AF, Saravelos H et al. (2000) Factor V leiden and prothrombin G20210A mutations, but not methylenetetrahydrofolate reductase C677T, are associated with recurrent miscarriages. Hum Reprod 15:458–62

Fortuny A, Carrio A, Soler A et al. (1988) Detection of balanced chromosome rearrangements in 445 couples with repeated abortion and cytogenetic prenatal testing in carriers. Fertil Steril 49:774–9

Fraser EJ, Grimes DA, Schulz KF (1993) Immunization as therapy for recurrent spontaneous abortion: A review and meta-analysis. Obstet Gynecol 82:854–9

Freij BJ, South MA, Sever JL (1988) Maternal rubella and the congenital rubella syndrome. Clin Perinatol 15:247–57

Fryns JP, Van Buggenhout G (1998) Structural chromosome rearrangements in couples with recurrent fetal wastage. Eur J Obstet Gynecol Reprod Biol 81:171–6

Fryns JP, Kleczkowska A, Kubien E et al. (1984) Cytogenetic survey in couples with recurrent fetal wastage. Hum Genet 65:336–354

Garber A, Carlson D, Schreck R et al. (1994) Prenatal diagnosis and dysmorphic features in mosaic trisomy 16. Prenat Diagn 14:257–266

Garner PR, D'Alton ME, Dudley DK et al. (1990) Preeclampsia in diabetic pregnancies. Obstet Gynecol 163:505

Georgiou PE, Politi EN, Katsimbri P et al. (2000) Outcome of lupus pregnancy: a controlled study. Rheumatology 39:1014–9

Gerhardt A, Scharf RE, Beckmann MW et al. (2000) Prothrombin and factor V mutations in women with a history of thrombosis during pregnancy and the puerperium N Engl J Med 342:374–80

Giacoia GP, Azubuike K (1991) Autoimmune diseases in pregnancy: Their effect on the fetus and newborn. Obstet Gynecol Surv 46:723–732

Goel N, Ortel TL, Bali D et al. (1999) Familial antiphospholipid antibody syndrome: Criteria for disease and evidence for autosomal dominant inheritance. Arthritis Rheum 42:318–27

Golbus MS, Bachman R, Wiltse S, Hall BD (1976) Tetraploidy in a newborn infant. J Med Genet 13:329–332

Goldstein P, Berrier J, Rosen S et al. (1989) A meta-analysis of randomized control trials of progestational agents in pregnancy. Br J Obstet Gynaecol 96:265–74

Grandone E, Margaglione M, Colaizzo D et al. (1997) Factor V Leiden is associated with repeated and recurrent unexplained fetal losses. Thromb Haemost 77:822–4

Greene MF (1999) Spontaneous abortions and major malformations in women with diabetes mellitus. Semin Reprod Endocrinol 17:127–36

Greaves M (1999) Antiphospholipid antibodies and thrombosis. Lancet 1999 353:1348–53

Gris JC, Quere I, Monpeyroux F et al. (1999) Case-control study of the frequency of thrombophilic disorders in couples with late foetal loss and no thrombotic antecedent–the Nimes Obstetricians and Haematologists Study5 (NOHA5). Thromb Haemost 81:891–9

Hagay ZJ, Biran G, Ornoy A, Reece EA (1996) Congenital cytomegalovirus infection: a long-standing problem still seeking a solution. Am J Obstet Gynecol 174:241–5

Hamerton JL, Canning N, Ray M et al. (1975) A cytogenetic survey of 14,069 newborn infants: I. Incidence of chromosome abnormalities. Clin Genet 8:223

Hassold TJ (1980) A cytogenetic study of repeated spontaneous abortions. Am J Hum Genet 32:723–30

Hassold T, Chiu D (1985) Maternal age-specific rates of numerical chromosome abnormalities with special reference to trisomy. Hum Genet 70:11–7

Hassold T, Warburton D, Kline J, Stein Z (1984) The relationship of maternal age and trisomy among trisomic spontaneous abortions. Am J Hum Genet 36:1349–56

Hassold T, Benhan F, Leppert M (1988) Cytogenetic and molecular analysis of sex-chromosome monosomy. Am J Hum Genet 42:534–541

Hayslett JP (1992) The effect of systemic lupus erythematosus on pregnancy and pregnancy outcome. Am J Reprod Immunol 28:199–204

Hecht F, Hecht BK, Berger CS (1984) Aneuploidy in recurrent spontaneous abortions: The tendency to parental nondisjunction. Clin Genet 26:43–45

Higgs DR, Vickers MA, Wilkie AOM et al. (1989) A review of the molecular genetics of the human a-globin gene cluster. Blood 73:1081

Holzgreve W, Schonberg SA, Douglas RG, Golbus MS (1984) X-chromosome hyperploidy in couples with multiple spontaneous abortions. Obstet Gynecol 63:237–240

Hook EB (1983) Chromosome abnormalities and spontaneous fetal death following amniocentesis: Further data and associations with maternal age. Am J Hum Genet 35:110–116

Hou S (1989) Pregnancy in organ transplant recipients. Med Clin North Am 73:667

Hou SH (1994) Frequency and outcome of pregnancy in women on dialysis. Am J Kidney Dis 23:60–63

Hsu WT, Shehepin D, Mao R et al. (1998) A new clinical entity-Mosaic trisomy 16 ascertained through amniocentesis. Amer J Med Genet 80:473–480

Husslein P, Huber J, Wagenbichler P, Schnedl W (1982) Chromosome abnormalities in 150 couples with multiple spontaneous abortions. Fertil Steril 37:379–83

Ian F, Martin R, Heath P, Mountain KR (1987) Pregnancy in women with diabetes mellitus. Med J Aust 146:187–190

Jackson J, Benirschke K (1989) The recognition and significance of the vanishing twin. J Am Board Fam Pract 2:58–63

Jacobs PA, Melville M, Ratcliffe S et al. (1974) A cytogenetic survey of 11,680 newborn infants. Am Hum Genet 37:359

Jacobs PA, Angell RR, Buchanan JM et al. (1978) The origin of human triploids. Am Hum Genet 42:49

Jacobs PA, Hunt PA, Matsura JS (1982) Complete and partial hydatidiform moles in Hawaii: cytogenetics, morphology and epidemiology. Br J Obstet Gynecol 89:258

Jeng GT, Scott JR, Burmeister LF (1995) A comparison of meta-analytic results using literature vs individual patient data. Paternal cell immunization for recurrent miscarriage. JAMA 274:830–6

Johnson P, Pearce JM (1990) Recurrent spontaneous abortion and polycystic ovary disease: Comparison of two regimas to induce ovulation BMJ 300:154–156

Kajii T, Nikawa N (1977) Origin of triploidy and tetraploidy in man: Cases with chromosome markers. Cytogenet Cell Genet 18:109

Kalousek DK, Langlois S, Barrett I et al. (1993) Uniparental disomy for chromosome 16 in humans. Am J Hum Genet 52:8–16

Kalter H (1986) Antineoplastic drugs and spontaneous abortion in nurses. N Engl J Med 314:1048–1049

Katz VL, Doters DJ, Droegemueller W (1986) Perimortem cesarean delivery. Obstet Gynecol 68:571

Kaufman RH, Adam E, Hatch EE et al. (2000) Continued follow-up of pregnancy outcomes in diethylstilbestrol-exposed offspring. Obstet Gynecol 96:483–9

Keltz MD, Olive DL, Kim AH, Arici A (1997) Sonohysterography for screening in recurrent pregnancy loss. Fertil Steril 67:670–4

Kline J, Stein Z (1987) Epidemiology of chromosomal abnormalities in spontaneous abortion: Prevalence, manifestation and determinant. In Bennett MJ, Edmonds DK (eds): Spontaneous and Recurrent Abortion. Blackwell: Oxford

Koren G, Weiner L, Lishner M et al. (1990) Cancer in pregnancy: Identification of unanswered questions on maternal and fetal risks. Obstet Gynecol Surv 45:509

Kupferminc MJ, Eldor A, Steinman N et al. (1999) Increased frequency of genetic thrombophilia in women with complications of pregnancy. N Engl J Med 340:9–13

Lanasa MC, Hogge WA, Kubik C et al. (1999a) Highly skewed X-chromosome inactivation is associated with idiopathic recurrent spontaneous abortion. Am J Hum Genet 65:252–54

Lanasa MC, Hogge WA, Hoffman EP (1999b) The X chromosome and recurrent spontaneous abortion: the significance of transmanifesting carriers. Am J Hum Genet 64:934–38

Landy HJ, Keith LG (1998) The vanishing twin: A review. Hum Reprod Update 4:177–83

Landy HJ, Weiner S, Corson SL, Batzer FR, Bolognese RJ (1986) The "vanishing twin": Ultrasonographic assessment of fetal disappearance in the first trimester. Am J Obstet Gynecol 155:14–9

Lazarus JH, Kokandi A (2000) Thyroid disease in relation to pregnancy: A decade of change. Clin Endocrinol 53:265–78

Lenox JW, Uguru V, Cibils LA (1990) Effects of hypertension on pregnancy monitoring and results. Am J Obstet Gynecol 163:1173–1179

Leridon H (1977) Human Fertility. University of Chicago Press, Chicago

Lippman-Hand A, Vekemans M (1983) Balanced translocations among couples with two or more spontaneous abortions: Are males and females equally likely to be carriers. Hum Genet 63:252–257

Lissak A, Sharon A, Fruchter O et al. (1999) Polymorphism for mutation of cytosine to thymine at location 677 in the methylenetetrahydrofolate reductase gene isassociated with recurrent early fetal loss. Am J Obstet Gynecol 181:126–30

Love PE, Santoro SA (1990) Antiphospholipid antibodies: Anticardiolipin and the lupus anticoagulant in systemic lupus erythematosus and in non-SLE Disorders. Ann Intern Med 112:682–698

McDonald IA (1987) Cervical incompetence as a cause of spontaneous abortion. In Bennett MJ, Edmonds DK (eds): Spontaneous and Recurrent Abortion. Blackwell, Oxford

Mackie IJ, Colaco CM, Machin SJ (1987) Familial lupus anticoagulants. Br J Haemetol 67:359–363

Maier DB (1987) Genetic and infectious causes of habitual abortion. In Gondas B, Riddick DH, (eds): Pathology of Infertility. Thieme, NY

Maier DB, Parke A (1989) Subclinical autoimmunity in recurrent aborters. Fertil Steril 51:280–5

Makino T, Tabuchi T, Nakada K et al. (1990) Chromosomal analysis in Japanese couples with repeated spontaneous abortions. Int J Fertil 35:266–70

Makino V (1994) Early pregnancy loss and possible etiologic factors. In Barnea ER, Cheek JH, Grudzinskas JG, Marvo T (eds): Implantations and Early Pregnancy in Humans. Pathenon: London

March CM, Israel R (1987) Hysteroscopic management of recurrent abortion caused by septate uterus. Am J Obstet Gynecol 156:834–42

Martin FR, Health P, Mountain KR (1987) Pregnancy in women with diabetes. Med J Aust 146:187

Martinelli I, Taioli E, Cetin I et al. (2000) Mutations in coagulation factors in women with unexplained late fetal loss. N Engl J Med 343:1015–8

Matthey F, Walshe K, Mackie IJ, Machin SJ (1989) Familial occurrence of the antiphospholipid syndrome. J Clin Pathol 42:495–497

Meinardi JR, Middeldorp S, de Kam PJ et al. (1999) Increased risk for fetal loss in carriers of the factor V Leiden mutation. Ann Intern Med 130:736–9

Meizner I, Levy A, Carmi R, Robinson C (1990) Niemann-Pick disease associated with nonimmune hydrops fetalis. Am J Obstet Gynecol 163:128–129

Michels VV, Medrano C, Venne VL, Riccardi VM (1982) Chromosome translocations in couples with multiple spontaneous abortion. Am J Hum Genet 34:507–513

Morey MA, Begleiter ML, Harris DJ (1981) Profile of a battered fetus. Lancet 2:1294

Morton NE, Chiu D, Holland C et al. (1987) Chromosome anomalies as predictors of recurrence risk for spontaneous abortion. Am J Med Genet 28:353–360

Mueller RF, Sybert VP, Johnson J et al. (1983) Evaluation of a protocol for post-mortem examination of stillbirths. N Engl J Med 309:586–590

Nelen WL, Blom HJ, Steegers EA et al. (2000) Homocysteine and folate levels as risk factors for recurrent early pregnancy loss. Obstet Gynecol 95:519–24

Nelen WL, Bulten J, Steegers EA et al. (2000) Maternal homocysteine and chorionic vascularization in recurrent early pregnancy loss. Hum Reprod 15:954–60

Neri G, Serra A, Campana M, Tedeschi B (1983) Reproductive risks for translocation carriers: Cytogenetic study and analysis of pregnancy outcome in 58 families. Am J Med Genet 16:535–561

Newbould MJ, Armstrong GR, Barson AJ (1991) Endocardial fibroelastosis in infants with hydrops fetalis. J Clin Pathol 44:576–579

Nybo Andersen AM, Wohlfahrt J, Christens P et al. (2000) Maternal age and fetal loss: Population based register linkage study. BMJ 320:1708–12

Ober CL, Hauck WW, Kostyu DD et al. (1985) Adverse effects of human leukocyte antigen-DR sharing on fertility: A cohort study in a human isolate. Fertil Steril 44:227–32

Ober C, Karrison T, Odem RR et al. (1999) Mononuclear-cell immunisation in prevention of recurrent miscarriages: A randomised trial. Lancet 354:365–9

Ogasawara M, Kajiura S, Katano K et al. (1997) Are serum progesterone levels predictive of recurrent miscarriage in future pregnancies? Fertil Steril 68:806–9

Ogasawara M, Aoki K, Katano K et al. (1998) Activated partial thromboplastin time is a predictive parameter for further miscarriages in cases of recurrent fetal loss. Fertil Steril 70:1081–4

Ogasawara M, Aoki K, Okada S, Suzumori K (2000) Embryonic karyotype of abortuses in relation to the number of previous miscarriages. Fertil Steril 73:300–4

Ohno M, Maeda T, Matsunobu A (1991) A cytogenetic study of spontaneous abortions with direct analysis of chorionic villi. Obstet Gynecol 77(3):394–8

Osztovics MK, Toth SP, Wessely JA (1982) Cytogenetic investigations in 418 couples with recurrent fetal wastage. Ann Genet 25:232–236

Pantzar JT, Allanson JE, Kalousek DK, Poland BJ (1984) Cytogenetic findings in 318 couples with repeated spontaneous abortion: A review of experience in British Columbia. Am J Med Genet 17:615–20

Papadopoulos G, Templeton AA, Fisk N, Randall J (1989) The frequency of chromosome anomalies in human preimplantation embryos after in-vitro fertilization. Hum Reprod 4:91–8

Parke A, Maier D, Hakim C et al. (1986) Subclinical autoimmune disease and recurrent spontaneous abortion. J Rheumatol 13:1178–1180

Parente JT, Amsel M, Lerner R et al. (1988) Breast cancer associated with pregnancy. Obstet Gynecol 71:861

Pattinson RC, Norman K, Odendaal HJ (1994) The role of Doppler velocimetry in the management of high risk pregnancies. Br J Obstet Gynecol 101:114–120

Pegoraro E, Whitaker J, Mowery-Rushton P et al. (1997) Familial skewed X inactivation: A molecular trait associated with high spontaneous-abortion rate maps to Xq28. Am J Hum Genet 61:160–70

Peirpert JF, Donnenfeld AE (1991) Oligohydramnios: A review. Obstet Gynecol Surv 46:325–335

Petrosky DL, Borgaonkar DS (1984) Segregation analysis in reciprocal translocation carriers. Am J Med Genet 19:137–159

Petri M, Allbritton J (1993) Fetal outcome of lupus pregnancy: A retrospective case-control study of the Hopkins Lupus Cohort. J Rheumatol 20:650–656

Phung Thi Tho, Byrd JR, McDonough PG (1979) Etiologies and subsequent reproductive performance of 100 couples with recurrent abortion. Fertil Steril 32:389–95

Plachot M, Junc AM, Mandelbaum J et al. (1987) Chromosome investigations in early life: human preimplantation embryos. Hum Reprod 2:29–35

Poeschmann RP, Verheijen RHM, Van Dongen PWJ (1991) Differential diagnosis and causes of nonimmunological hydrops fetalis: A review. Obstet Gynecol Surv 46:223–231

Portnoi MF, Joye N, van den Akker J et al. (1988) Karyotypes of 1142 couples with recurrent abortion. Obstet Gynecol 72:31–4

Preston FE, Rosendaal FR, Walker ID et al. (1996) Increased fetal loss in women with heritable thrombophilia. Lancet 348:913–6

Quere I, Bellet H, Hoffet M et al. (1998) A woman with five consecutive fetal deaths: Case report and retrospective analysis of hyperhomocysteinemia prevalencein 100 consecutive women with recurrent miscarriages. Fertil Steril 69:152–4

Rai RS, Clifford K, Cohen H, Regan L (1995) High prospective fetal loss rate in untreated pregnancies of women with recurrent miscarriage and antiphospholipid Hum Reprod 10:3301–4

Rai R, Cohen H, Dave M, Regan L (1997) Randomised controlled trial of aspirin and aspirin plus heparin in pregnant women with recurrent miscarriage associated with phospholipid antibodies (or antiphospholipid antibodies) BMJ 314:253–7

Rai R, Backos M, Rushworth F, Regan L (2000) Polycystic ovaries and recurrent miscarriage–a reappraisal. Hum Reprod 15:612–5

Rai R, Backos M, Baxter N, Chilcott I, Regan L (2000) Recurrent miscarriage–an aspirin a day? Hum Reprod 15:2220–3

Ray JG, Laskin CA (1999) Folic acid and homocyst(e)ine metabolic defects and the risk of placental abruption, pre-eclampsia and spontaneous pregnancy loss: A systematic review. Placenta 20:519–29

Reece EA, Gabrielli S, Abdall AM (1988) The prevention of diabetes-associated birth defects. Semin Perinatol 12:292

Regan L (1991) Recurrent miscarriage. BMJ 302:543–544

Reinisch LC, Silvery KL, Dumms KW (1981) Sex chromosome mosaicism in couples with repeated fetal loss. Am J Hum Genet 33:117–A

Ricci JM, Fojaco RM, O'Sullivan MJ (1989) Congenital syphilis: The University of Miami/Jackson Memorial Medical Center experience, 1986–1988. Obstet Gynecol 74:687–93

Ridker PM, Miletich JP, Buring JE et al. (1998) Factor V Leiden mutation as a risk factor for recurrent pregnancy loss. Ann Intern Med 128:1000–3

Risch HA, Weiss NS, Clarke EA, Miller AB (1988) Risk factors for spontaneous abortion and its recurrence. Am J Epidemiol 128:420–30

Rubio C, Simon C, Blanco J et al. (1999) Implications of sperm chromosome abnormalities in recurrent miscarriage. J Assist Reprod Genet 16:253–8

Ruiz VA, Suarez MMP, Lopez FP et al. (1990) Nonimmunologic hydrops fetalis: an etiopathogenetic approach through the postmortem study of 59 patients. Am J Med Genet 35:274–279

Sachs ES, Jahoda MG, Van Hemel JO, Hoogeboom AJ, Sandkuyl LA (1985) Chromosome studies of 500 couples with two or more abortions. Obstet Gynecol 65:375–8

Sandler L, Lindsley DL (1974) Some observations on the study of the genetic control of meiosis in Drosophila melanogaster. Genetics 78:289–297

Sangha KK, Stephenson MD, Brown CJ, Robinson WP (1999) Extremely skewed X-chromosome inactivation is increased in women with recurrent spontaneous abortion. Am J Hum Genet 65:913–17

Sanghi A, Morgan-Capner P, Hesketh L, Elstein M (1997) Zoonotic and viral infection in fetal loss after 12 weeks. Br J Obstet Gynaecol 104:942–5

Sant-Cassia LJ, Cooke P (1981) Chromosomal analysis of couples with repeated spontaneous abortions. Br J Obstet Gynecol 88:52–8

Schauer GM, Kalousek DK, Magee JF (1992) Genetic causes of stillbirth. Semin Perinatol 16:341–351

Schwartz A (1950) Mumps in pregnancy. Am J Obstet Gynecol 60:875–6

Schwartz S, Palmer CG (1983) Chromosomal findings in 164 couples with repeated spontaneous abortions with special consideration to prior reproductive history. Hum Genet 63:28–34

Scott JR (2000) Immunotherapy for recurrent miscarriage. Cochrane Database Syst Rev 2000:CD000112

Selevan SG, Lindbohm ML, Hornung RW, Hemminki K (1985) A study of occupational exposure to antineoplastic drugs and fetal loss in nurses. N Engl J Med 313:1173–1178

Shiono H, Azumi J, Fukiwara M et al. (1988) Tetraploidy in a 15-month old girl. Am J Med Genet 29:543–547

Sibai BM, Ramadan MK, Usta I et al. (1993) Maternal morbidity and mortality in 442 pregnancies with hemolysis, elevated liver enzymes, and low platelets (HELLP syndrome). Am J Obstet Gynecol 69:1471–1474

Siegel M (1973) Congenital malformations following chickenpox, measles, mumps, and hepatitis. Results of a cohort study. JAMA 226:1521–4

Simpson JL, Bombard A (1987) Chromosomal abnormalities in spontaneous abortion: frequency, pathology and genetic counseling. In Bennett MJ, Edmonds DK (eds): Spontaneous and Recurrent Abortion. Blackwell, Oxford

Simpson JL, Mills JL (1986) Methodologic problems in determining fetal loss rates. In Brambati B, Simoni G, Fabro S (eds): Chorionic Villus Sampling. Marcel Deckker, NY

Simpson JL, Elias S, Martin AO (1981) Parental chromosomal rearrangements associated with repetitive spontaneous abortion. Fertil Steril 36:584–590

Smythe JF, Copel JA, Kleinman CS (1992) Outcome of prenatally detected cardiac malformations. Am J Cardiol 69:1471–1474

Soh K, Yajima A, Ozawa N et al. (1984) Chromosome analysis in couples with recurrent abortions. Tohoku J Exp Med 144:151–63

Souza SS, Ferriani RA, Pontes AG, Zago MA, Franco RF (1999) Factor V leiden and factor II G20210A mutations in patients with recurrent abortion. Hum Reprod 14:2448–50

Spellacy WN, Handler A, Ferre CD (1990) A case-control study of 1253 twin pregnancies from a 1982–1987 perinatal data base. Obstet Gynecol 75:168–171

Steegers-Theunissen RP, Boers GH, Blom HJ et al. (1992) Hyperhomocysteinaemia and recurrent spontaneous abortion or abruptio placentae. Lancet 339:1122–3

Stern JJ, Dorfmann AD, Gutierrez-Najar AJ, Cerrillo M, Coulam CB (1996) Frequency of abnormal karyotypes among abortuses from women with and without a history of recurrent spontaneous abortion. Fertil Steril 65:250–3

Stevenson AC, Dudgeon MY, McClure HI (1959) Observations on the result of pregnancies in women residents in Belfast: II. Abortions, hydatidiform moles, and ectopic pregnancies. Am Hum Genet 23:395

Stirrat GM (1990) Recurrent miscarriage. II: Clinical associations, causes and management. Lancet 336:728–33

Stoll C (1981) Cytogenetic findings in 122 couples with recurrent abortions. Hum Genet 57:101–3

Szulman AE (1984) Syndromes of hydatidiform moles: Partial versus complete. J Reprod Med 29:788

Takakuwa K, Asano K, Arakawa M et al. (1997) Chromosome analysis of aborted conceptuses of recurrent aborters positive for anticardiolipin antibody. Fertil Steril 68:54–8

Tincani A, Faden D, Tarantini M et al. (1992) Systemic lupus erythematosus and pregnancy: A prospective study. Clin Exp Rheumatol 10:439–436

Tormene D, Simioni P, Prandoni P et al. (1999) The risk of fetal loss in family members of probands with factor V Leiden mutation. Thromb Haemost 82:1237–9

Toth A, Gaal M, Bosze P, Laszlo J (1984) Chromosome abnormalities in 118 couples with recurrent spontaneous abortions. Gynecol Obstet Invest 18:72–7

Vaquero E, Lazzarin N, De Carolis C et al. (2000) Mild thyroid abnormalities and recurrent spontaneous abortion: Diagnostic and therapeutical approach. Am J Reprod Immunol 43:204–8

Warburton D, Fraser FC (1964) Spontaneous abortion risks in man: Data from reproductive histories collected in a medical genetics unit. Am J Hum Genet 16:1–24

Warburton D, Strobino B (1987) Recurrent spontaneous abortion. In Bennett MJ, Edmonds DK (eds): Spontaneous and Recurrent Abortion. Blackwell, Oxford

Warburton D, Stein Z, Kline J, Susser M (1980) Chromosome abnormalities in spontaneous abortions: Data from the New York city study. In Porter JH, Hook EB (eds): Human Embryonic and Fetal Death. Academic Press, NY

Warburton D, Kline J, Stein Z et al. (1987) Does the karyotype of a spontaneous abortion predict the karyotype of a subsequent abortion? Evidence from 273 women with two karyotyped spontaneous abortions. Am J Hum Genet 41:465–483

Warburton D, Byrne J, Canki N (1991) Chromosome anomalies and prenatal development: an atlas. Oxford Monogroms in Medical Genetics, Vol 24

Wechsler B, Huong Du LT, Piette JC (1999) Is there a role for antithrombotic therapy in the prevention of pregnancy loss? Haemostasis 29 Suppl S1:112–20

Wilcox AJ, Weinberg CR, O'Connor JF et al. (1988) Incidence of early loss of pregnancy. N Engl J Med 319:189–94

Wong DJ, Strassner HT (1990) Melanoma in pregnancy. Clin Obstet Gynecol 33:782–791

Wu D, Schreck RR (1992) Sex chromosome aneuploidy is more common in patients with multiple SAB's, abstracted. Applied Cytogenet 18:25

Yamada H, Kato EH, Ebina Y et al. (2000) Factor XII deficiency in women with recurrent miscarriage. Gynecol Obstet Invest 49:80–3

Yerushalmy J, Bierman JM, Kemp DH et al. (1956) Longitudinal studies of pregnancy on the island of Kauai, Territory of Hawaii. Am J Obstet Gynecol 71:80–96

Younis JS, Brenner B, Ohel G et al. (2000) Activated protein C resistance and factor V Leiden mutation can be associated with first- as well as second-trimester recurrent pregnancy loss. Am J Reprod Immunol 43:31–5

Zaragoza MV, Surti U, Redline RW et al. (2000) Parental origin and phenotype of triploidy in spontaneous abortions: Predominance of diandry and association with the partial hydatidiform Mole. Am J Hum Genet 66:1807–1820

Zemlickis D, Lishner M, Degendorfer P et al. (1992) Fetal outcome after in utero exposure to cancer chemotherapy. Arch Intern Med 152:573–576

Zuazu J, Julia A, Sierra J et al. (1991) Pregnancy outcome in hematologic malignancies. Cancer 67:703–709

A clinical approach to the dysmorphic child

38

Kenneth L. Jones
Marilyn C. Jones

Introduction

The purpose of this chapter is to present a clinical approach to the child with structural defects. The approach is predicated upon the concept that the nature of the structural defects presents clues to the time of onset, mechanism of injury, and probable etiology of the problem, all of which determine the direction of the evaluation. It presumes that the dysmorphic child represents an experiment in human development, which, if interpreted correctly, can provide answers regarding the etiology of various structural defects, as well as permit insights into mechanisms of normal and abnormal morphogenesis. The method upon which this approach is based has been most articulately set forth by Sir Arthur Conan Doyle's fictional character Sherlock Holmes, who showed "how much an observant man might learn by accurate and systematic examination of all that came within his way". This chapter adapts this method to the evaluation of the child with structural defects. By sharpening the faculties of observation, the clinician can narrow systematically the diagnostic possibilities so that the laboratory and the literature can be consulted in a rational fashion to arrive at an accurate diagnosis. Texts by Gorlin, Cohen and Levin (1990) and Jones (1997) are particularly useful. In recent years computerized databases on CD ROM have become useful adjuncts to diagnosis (Winter and Baraister, 1999; Bankier, 2000).

Prenatal versus postnatal onset of developmental problems

A method of approach to children with structural defects is set forth diagrammatically in Figure 38.1. Although the lines of distinction between these two categories are becoming increasingly blurred, a history and physical exam-

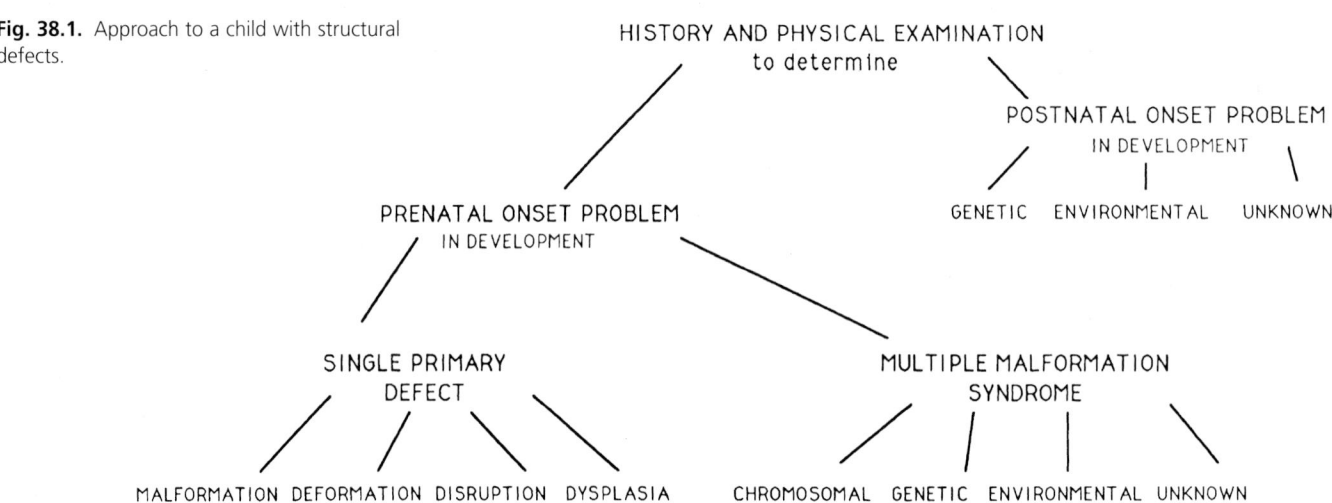

Fig. 38.1. Approach to a child with structural defects.

998

ination usually make it possible to determine if the structural abnormality is of prenatal or postnatal onset. In this chapter, "prenatal onset" designates structural abnormalities that are present at birth, and "postnatal onset" designates structures that have previously developed and differentiated normally. Although the genetic alteration responsible for many of the disorders included under postnatal-onset structural defects is present at the time of conception, the structural manifestations of that genetic alteration do not become obvious until postnatal life. On the basis of this distinction a more rational approach to the problem can be developed, since this determination narrows considerably the diagnostic probabilities and, it is hoped, permits a more judicious selection of adjunctive laboratory tests.

Generally speaking, prenatal-onset problems in development are a consequence of genetic or chromosomal alterations that cause programing problems in the development and/or differentiation of structure or are the result of factors unique to the pregnancy itself, such as environmental agents, abnormalities of placentation, or mechanical constraint. Although always evident at birth, most prenatal-onset problems remain static or improve postnatally without evidence of neurologic deterioration. By contrast, postnatal-onset problems in development usually result in deterioration in structure or function that has previously been normal. Deterioration may reflect postnatal accumulation of a toxic metabolic product (as in phenylketonuria), progressive storage of a metabolite (as in Hurler syndrome), deteriorating energy production (as in mitochondrial myopathies), or ongoing infection (as in deafness from cytomegalovirus). Children with postnatal problems usually appear to have thrived *in utero*. The structural and functional consequences of the problem manifest after the newborn period.

Certain historical information can be particularly helpful in determining onset of the problem. Structural defects of prenatal onset are frequently associated with the following abnormalities noted by the mother during pregnancy and at the time of delivery, while, by contrast, with postnatal-onset structural defects, the pregnancy and delivery usually are normal.

Alterations of pregnancy associated with prenatal onset of developmental problems are as follows:

1. *Alterations in gestational timing (prematurity or postmaturity).* As discussed in several other chapters, the majority of conceptuses do not survive to be born at 40 weeks gestation. Much of this loss occurs in the very early part of pregnancy and is the result of gross

chromosomal abnormities and/or malformation. Numerous studies have documented an increased frequency of chromosomal and genetic abnormalities in losses from the second and third trimesters. Premature delivery may reflect late fetal wastage rather than maternal disease. Postmaturity rarely occurs today because of improved fetal monitoring techniques. In years before the widespread use of ultrasound, anencephaly typically presented in pregnancies that were post-dates since the fetal pituitary-adrenal axis is involved in the triggering of labor.

2. *Alterations in onset of fetal activity, nature of fetal activity, or both.* Although it is clear that fetal activity begins much earlier, it is usually not felt by the mother until about 18 weeks of gestation. Fetal activity increases in amount and intensity from that time, reaches a maximum between the 29th and 38th weeks and then decreases somewhat until delivery (Sadovsky and Yaffe, 1973). Discussion with mothers who have given birth to babies with structural defects suggests that certain structural defects are often associated with delayed onset and/or decreased intensity of fetal activity. Moreover, fetal movement may be localized to one particular quadrant of the abdomen, for example, when the defect represents deformation due to intrauterine compression in a previously normally formed structure. Other examples are defects in brain development and meningomyelocele, conditions in which the decreased fetal activity is secondary to neurologic impairment.

3. *Abnormalities in amount of amniotic fluid, for example, polyhydramnios or oligohydramnios.* During the latter part of gestation, amniotic fluid is maintained in equilibrium by fetal urination and fetal swallowing. Polyhydramnios occurs when the fetus has difficulty swallowing amniotic fluid, for example, early problems in central nervous system development or upper gastrointestinal obstruction. Oligohydramnios is usually present following chronic leakage of amniotic fluid or whenever fetal urinary excretion is decreased, for example, renal agenesis, infantile polycystic kidney disease, or urethral obstruction.

Alterations noted at delivery associated with prenatal onset of developmental problems are as follows:

1. *Increased incidence of breech presentation.* Breech presentation occurs in 3.1% of normal deliveries at 40 weeks gestation (Berendes et al., 1965). However, it occurs much more frequently in some disorders that adversely affect the form and/or function of the fetus.

Defects of form include structural abnormalities such as hydrocephalus, which would be less compatible with the vertex position because of the large head, and joint dislocations, which may limit the capacity of the fetus to alter its position. Defects of function include some conditions associated with neuromuscular dysfunction, for example, the trisomy 18 syndrome and Smith–Lemli–Opitz syndrome associated with hypertonia and the Prader–Willi syndrome and Zellweger syndrome associated with hypotonia. Braun et al. (1975) documented an increased incidence of breech presentation in 11 recognized patterns of malformation, selected because each showed a problem in fetal morphogenesis and/or function.

2. *Prenatal onset growth deficiency*. Drillen (1970) studied the incidence of malformations, mental retardation, and/or neurologic defects in 180 one-year-old children whose birth weight was 2000 g or less and who were small for gestational age. She documented an increased incidence of prenatal onset malformations as weight-for-gestational age decreased. In addition, she showed a marked increase in suspected mental and neurologic defects in those small-for-gestational-age children who had some structural anomaly.

3. *Difficulty with neonatal adaptation*. Children with prenatal-onset structural defects frequently have problems with neonatal respiratory adaptation, probably secondary to malformations of brain structure. Therefore, one should always be cautious when attributing mental retardation to a perinatal insult in a child who has associated prenatal-onset structural malformations. Mental retardation in such patients may well be related to a problem in brain development of prenatal onset. The most helpful way to determine whether a structural defect is of prenatal or postnatal onset is a careful physical examination (Aase, 1990). In the vast majority of situations the nature of the problem will determine the direction the diagnostic evaluation should take.

Prenatal onset problems in development

Once a given problem has been determined to be of prenatal onset, a distinction should be made between those that are single primary defects in development and those that are multiple malformation syndromes. Although the concepts are not totally analogous, separation of prenatal problems into these two categories permits some practical generaliz-

ations that can be extremely helpful in counseling about recurrence risk.

Conceptually, "single primary defect in development" is an anatomic or morphogenetic designation. In most cases, the defect involves only a single structure, and the child is otherwise completely normal. Table 38.1 sets forth the seven most common single primary defects in development. For most of them, the specific etiology is unknown, making definitive recurrence risk counseling difficult. However, from a practical standpoint, most single primary defects are explained on the basis of multifactorial inheritance, which is thought to carry a recurrence risk for first-degree relatives of between 2% and 5%. Thus, recognition that a child's structural defect represents a single primary defect in development usually enables the clinician to suggest recurrence risk percentages between 2% and 5% for unaffected parents with one affected child.

The multifactorial model is a theoretical construct that was developed to explain the observed 2% to 5% recurrence risk for many common single defects, such as cleft lip with or without cleft palate. The model stipulates that expression of a given characteristic represents the interaction between genetic susceptibility to a given biologic error and a threshold beyond which a given characteristic is expressed (see Chs 3 and 12). Susceptibility is depicted as a normal distribution in the population. The threshold may be manipulated by environmental factors, which may either increase or decrease the likelihood that a defect will be evident. The extent to which multifactorial inheritance contributes to the etiology of some of the less common single defects in development is at present unclear. The fact that single primary defects are etiologically heterogeneous implies that some will have a clearly environmental etiology, while others will result from dominantly or recessively inherited single altered genes. Craniosynostosis secondary to in utero constraint (Graham et al., 1979) is an example of the former, and postaxial polydactyly (Castilla et al., 1973) illustrates the latter. Before multifactorial risk figures are used for

Table 38.1. Common Single Primary Defects in Development

Malformation
Cleft lip +/– cleft palate
Cleft palate
Cardiac septal defects
Defect in neural tube closure
Deformation
Congenital hip dislocation
Talipes equinovarus
Dysplasia
Pyloric stenosis

counseling, references such as *Mendelian Inheritance in Man* (McKusick, 1998) should be consulted to determine if other risk figures have been reported.

In contrast to the anatomic concept of the single primary defect in development, the designation "multiple malformation syndrome" indicates that the observed structural defects all have the same cause. The defects themselves usually include a number of anatomically unrelated errors in morphogenesis. Multiple malformation syndromes are caused by gross chromosomal abnormalities, chromosomal microdeletions, teratogens, and single gene defects usually inherited in mendelian patterns. Recurrence risk depends upon an accurate diagnosis and ranges from zero in cases that represent fresh gene mutations or are caused by one-time teratogen exposures to 100% for the unusual case of a child with the Down syndrome in which one parent is a balanced 21/21 translocation carrier. To review, recognition that a child has a prenatal onset single primary defect in development suggests a 2% to 5% risk; recognition that a child has a multiple malformation syndrome is not helpful with respect to recurrence risk counseling unless a specific diagnosis can be made.

SINGLE PRIMARY DEFECT IN DEVELOPMENT

Single primary defects can be subcategorized, as shown in Table 38.1, according to the nature of the error in morphogenesis that has produced the observed structural defect (Spranger et al., 1982). Thus single primary defects involve either malformation, deformation, disruption, or dysplasia of developing structure. A malformation implies a primary structural defect arising from a localized error in morphogenesis. A deformation should be thought of as an alteration, usually through compression, in shape and/or structure of a part that has differentiated normally; the term disruption is used for a structural defect resulting from destruction of a previously normally formed part. The term dysplasia refers to an abnormal organization of cells and the structural consequences. Dysplasias may be localized or generalized. Localized dysplasias (e.g., hemangiomas) are generally single primary defects in development. However, generalized dysplasias such as connective tissue disorders usually present as multiple malformation syndromes in that a variety of structures are involved because of the widespread distribution of the dysplastic tissue.

Table 38.1 sets forth the most common single primary defects in development. Four are malformations, the result of a localized error in morphogenesis. Two (congenital hip dislocation and talipes equinovarus) are the result of intrauterine molding and thus represent deformation of previously normally formed structures. One (pyloric stenosis) is a dysplasia resulting from abnormal muscular hypertrophy at the gastric outlet. Each of these seven anomalies occurs with a frequency of 0.5 to 1 per 1000 in liveborn infants. The major reason for separating single defects in development into malformation, deformation, disruption and dysplasia is to gain information that can be helpful relative to prognosis. Of the deformations noted at birth, 90% will correct spontaneously; of those that do not, the vast majority can be corrected with early postural interventions, such as casting or bracing. Conversely, spontaneous correction of both malformations and disruptions almost never occurs, and, when correction is possible, surgery is virtually always necessary. Since dysplasias involve abnormal organization and localized deregulation of growth in affected structures, many change over time with involution occurring in some and malignant transformation taking place in others.

MALFORMATIONS

Most children with a localized malformation in development, such as a cardiac septal defect or cleft lip and palate are otherwise completely normal. Following appropriate reconstruction, prognosis is excellent. In those cases in which mendelian inheritance has not been previously documented, multifactorial recurrence risk figures (2% to 5%) can be given to unaffected parents. If the malformation in development involves a structure that is not amenable to surgical correction, such as the brain, the long-term prognosis may be poor. The environmental factors that modify the threshold for expression of most malformations are for the most part unknown. For neural tube malformations, however, folic acid supplementation before conception reduces the risk for recurrence (MRC Vitamin Study Research Group, 1991).

DEFORMATIONS

Most deformations involve the musculoskeletal system and are believed to be caused by intrauterine molding (Dunn, 1976). The pressure required to produce such molding may be intrinsic (e.g., neuromuscular imbalance within the fetus), or may be extrinsic (e.g., fetal crowding). In either case, the ability of the fetus to kick is impaired, resulting in decreased fetal movement, an important factor in the development of a normal musculoskeletal system. This is particularly true with respect to joint development because motion is essential for normal development of the joints. In addition, because of fetal plasticity, marked positional deformation of any body part can occur when the fetus is unable to change position and thus alter the direction along which potentially deforming extrinsic forces are being directed.

Intrinsically derived prenatal-onset deformations

Disorders involving muscle degeneration, such as the Steinert myotonic dystrophy disease, and disorders involving motor neurons, such as Werdnig–Hoffmann disease, are uncommon causes of positional deformations. Early defects in development of the central nervous system are more common causes and should be seriously considered whenever a structural defect is thought to be an intrinsically derived prenatal-onset deformation.

Extrinsically derived prenatal-onset deformations

Fetal crowding, the common pathway in extrinsically derived postural deformations, is usually due to a decreased volume of amniotic fluid, a situation that occurs normally during the later weeks of gestation when the fetus in undergoing extremely rapid growth (Cunningham et al., 1993). However, it also occurs abnormally when fetal urinary output is diminished and in cases of chronic leakage of amniotic fluid (Thomas and Smith, 1974). Other extrinsic factors associated with the development of deformations include breech presentation and the shape of the amniotic cavity. When a fetus is held in the breech position, the legs may be trapped between the body and the uterine wall. In that position, the fetus is unable to kick optimally and therefore is immobilized and more susceptible to molding and deformation. Breech presentation is associated with a tenfold increase in the incidence of deformations (Dunn, 1976). The shape of the amniotic cavity, which has a profound influence on the shape of the fetus that lies within it, is influenced by many factors, among which are the following: uterine shape; volume of amniotic fluid; size and shape of the fetus; presence of more than one fetus; site of placental implantation; presence of uterine tumors; shape of the abdominal cavity, which is influenced by the pelvis, sacral promontory; and neighboring abdominal organs; and tightness of the abdominal musculature (Graham, 1988).

The various forms of talipes and congenital hip dislocation are the most frequently observed congenital postural deformities. Most children with these deformations are otherwise completely normal, and their prognosis is excellent. Correction usually occurs spontaneously. However, recognition that a structural defect represents a deforma-

tion does not always imply fetal crowding and should lead to careful consideration of other etiologic possibilities that might have far greater importance to the child. For example, since decreased fetal movement can be secondary to serious neurologic abnormalities, multiple joint contractures should always alert the clinician to the possibility of a malformation in central nervous system development. Although the most common deformational single primary defects – congenital hip dislocation and talipes – have a 2% to 5% recurrence risk, most deformations are the result of physiologic crowding and have virtually no recurrence risk. Deformations that are due to pathologic crowding (e.g., uterine tumors or malformation) have a much higher recurrence risk unless the factors leading to crowding are altered before subsequent pregnancies. Deformations that are the result of an underlying malformation (e.g., renal agenesis) have a recurrence risk similar to that for the underlying malformation.

DISRUPTIVE DEFECTS

Disruptive defects occur when there is destruction of a previously normally formed part. There are at least two basic mechanisms known to produce disruption. One involves entanglement followed by renting, amputation, or both of a normally developed structure, usually a digit, arm, or leg, by strands of amnion floating within amniotic fluid ("amniotic bands") (Higginbottom et al., 1979).

The second mechanism through which disruption occurs involves the interruption of blood supply to a developing part, leading to infarction, necrosis, and resorption of structures distal to the insult. If interruption of blood supply occurs early in gestation, the disruptive defect seen at term usually involves atresia or absence of a particular part. If the infarction occurs later, necrosis is more likely to be present. Examples of disruptive single primary defects for which infarctive mechanisms have been implicated include non-duodenal intestinal atresia (Louw, 1966), gastroschisis (Hoyme et al., 1981), porencephaly (Lemire et al., 1975), and transverse limb reduction defects (Hoyme et al., 1982). The extent to which disruption of developing structures plays a role in dysmorphogenesis is unknown.

Because disruptions do not involve programing errors intrinsic to the fetus, genetic factors play a minor role in their pathogenesis. Thus, most disruptive defects are sporadic events in otherwise normal families. Cocaine is an environmental agent whose mechanism of action is vascular disruption. Multiple disruptive defects have been seen in the offspring of women who abuse this agent in pregnancy (Hoyme et al., 1990). The prognosis for a disruptive defect is determined entirely by the extent and location of the tissue loss. Thus a child with a limb amputation has an excellent prognosis for normal function but a child with porencephaly does not.

DYSPLASIA

The causes of the vast majority of localized dysplasias are unknown. Since many generalized dysplasias are the result of abnormal genes, it is possible that localized dysplasias will reflect somatic mutation in specific tissues. This hypothesis is consistent with the observation that empirical recurrence risks for localized dysplasias are low. The process of dysplasia appears to involve deregulation of growth; hence most dysplasias change over time. Capillary hemangiomas become involuted; the bathing trunk nevus illustrated in Figure 38.5 carries a risk for malignant transformation. Knowledge of the natural history of a lesion is critical in the long-term follow-up of children with localized dysplasias.

SEQUENCE

"Sequence" describes the pattern of multiple anomalies that occurs when a single primary defect in early morphogenesis produces multiple abnormalities through a cascading process of secondary and tertiary errors in morphogenesis. When evaluating a child with multiple anomalies, it is extremely important from the standpoint of recurrence risk counseling to differentiate between multiple anomalies secondary to a single localized error in morphogenesis (a sequence) and a multiple malformation syndrome. In a sequence, recurrence risk counseling for the multiple anomalies depends entirely upon the recurrence risk for the initiating, localized error. The words malformation, deformation, disruption, and dysplasia sequence are used if the nature of the initiating error in morphogenesis is known.

The patient depicted in Figure 38.2 has mandibular hypoplasia, glossoptosis, and cleft palate, an example of multiple anomalies secondary to a single localized error in morphogenesis. The primary defect in this case is mandibular hypoplasia, a malformation. Since the tongue is relatively large for the oral cavity, it drops back (glossoptosis), blocking closure of the posterior palatal shelves, resulting in a U-shaped cleft palate. This condition has previously been referred to as the Pierre Robin syndrome. However, since both the glossoptosis and cleft palate are secondary to mandibular hypoplasia, the disorder is now referred to as the Robin malformation sequence. Recognition that all of the observed defects are due to a single localized error in

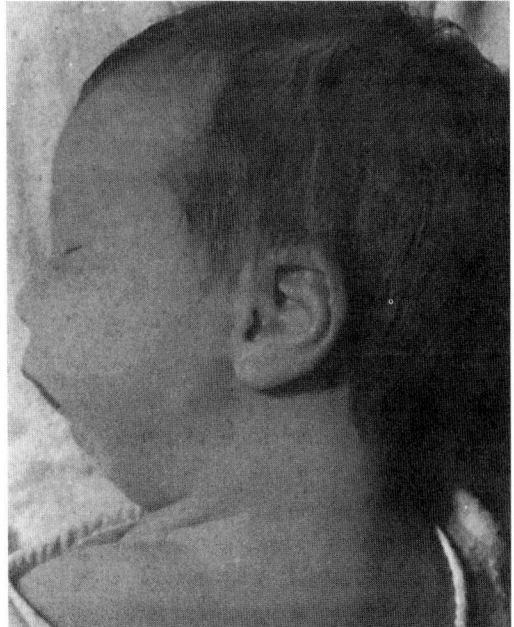

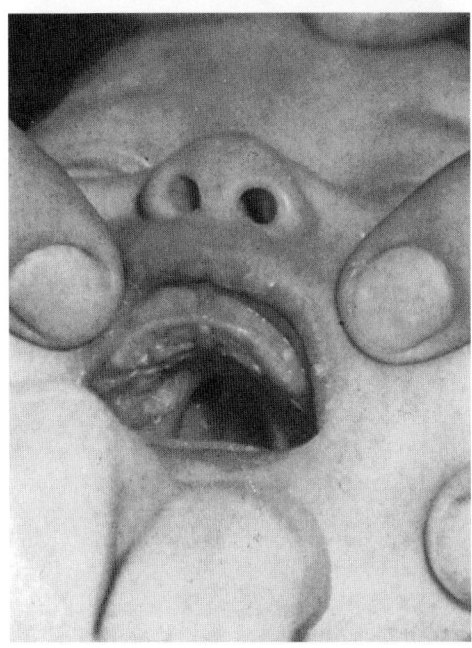

Fig. 38.2. Infant with the Robin malformation sequence. **(A)** Micrognathia. **(B)** U-shaped palatal cleft.

morphogenesis (mandibular hypoplasia) permits recurrence risk counseling based upon the etiology of the single defect. The patient depicted in Figure 38.3 has bathrocephaly, torticollis, facial asymmetry, a dislocated right hip, and valgus anomalies of both feet. All of the structural defects are the result of compression of developing fetal parts. The pattern of abnormalities in this patient is referred to as the breech deformation sequence. Intrauterine crowding in this situation was the result of a large infant with a birth length of

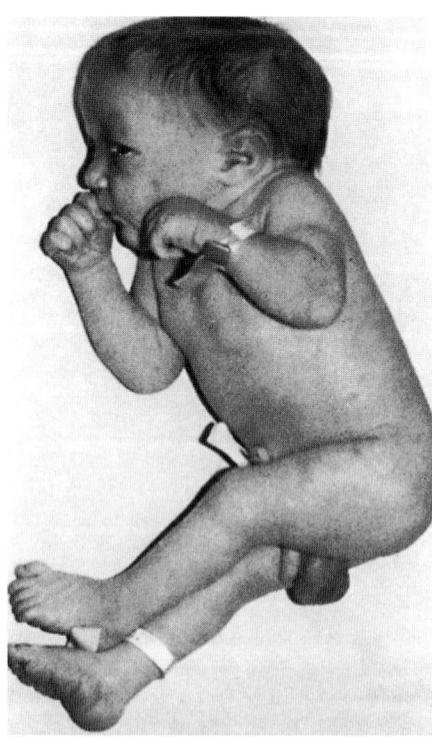

Fig. 38.3. Newborn infant with breech deformation sequence. Note the deformed cranial shape and positional deformities at the hips and feet.

54 cm, birth weight of 3.9 kg, and head circumference of 36 cm, delivered from a breech position to a small, primagravida mother. Recurrence risk is therefore negligible. Recognition of the deformational nature of the abnormalities is helpful with respect to prognosis. All of the problems should resolve spontaneously or with postural therapy.

The patient depicted in Figure 38.4 has the amnion rupture sequence. All of the craniofacial and limb defects are secondary to multiple fibrous strands of amnion extending from the placental insertion of the umbilical cord to the surface of the amnion-denuded chorion or floating freely within the chorionic sac. These strands of amnion, which result from disruption of the normally formed membrane, cause secondary defects through any one or more of the following mechanisms. Malformations occur if a strand of amnion interferes with the normal sequence of embryologic development. For example, a strand of amnion could interrupt fusion of the facial processes so that a cleft lip would result. Disruptions, on the other hand, are secondary to tearing apart of structures that have previously developed normally. As such, an amniotic band might act to cleave areas in the developing craniofacies along a line not conforming to the normal planes of facial closure. Deformations due to fetal

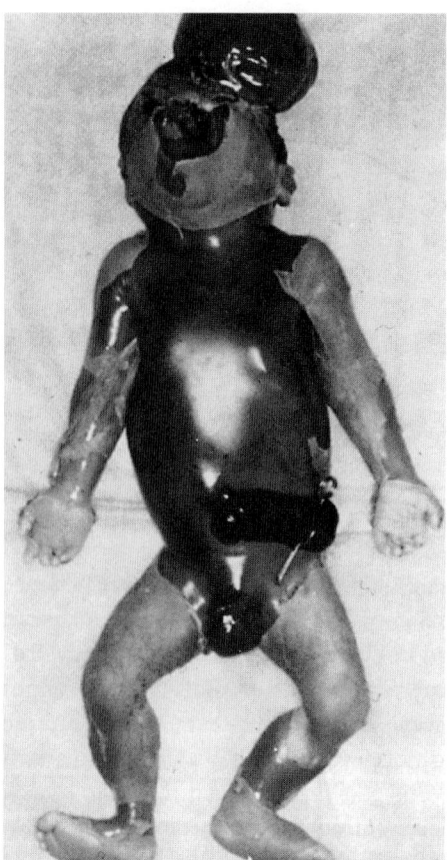

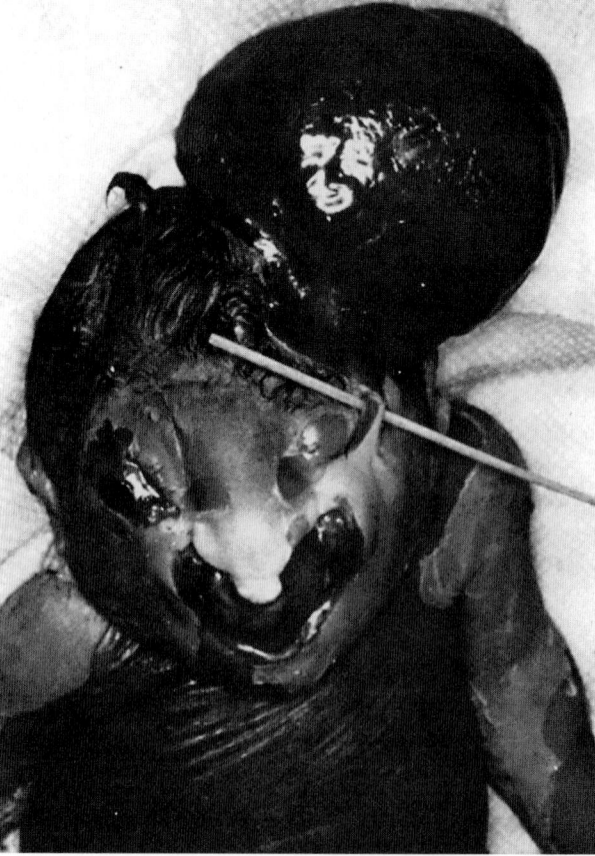

Fig. 38.4. Infant with amniotic band disruption sequence. Note the asymmetrical encephalocele, severe disruption of facial development, and digital anomalies.

compression occur secondary to oligohydramnios, tethering of a fetal part, or both. The former situation may result from rupture of both amnion and chorion, leading to chronic leakage of amniotic fluid. Tethering occurs when the fetus or one of its parts becomes immobilized by the constraining effect of an amniotic band such that it is unable to change position and thus alters the direction along which potentially deforming forces are being directed.

When used in conjunction with the word "sequence", malformation, deformation, disruption, and dysplasia describe only the initiating error in morphogenesis of the sequence. The nature of the individual secondary defects that ensue from the initiating event depend upon the manner in which the initiating error alters subsequent morphogenesis. In the case of the amnion rupture sequence, the initiating event, disruption, can lead to multiple structural defects through three of the mechanisms listed above.

The child depicted in Figure 38.5 has a neurocutaneous melanosis sequence. In this dysplasia sequence, melanocytic hamartosis of the skin occurs in conjunction with similar

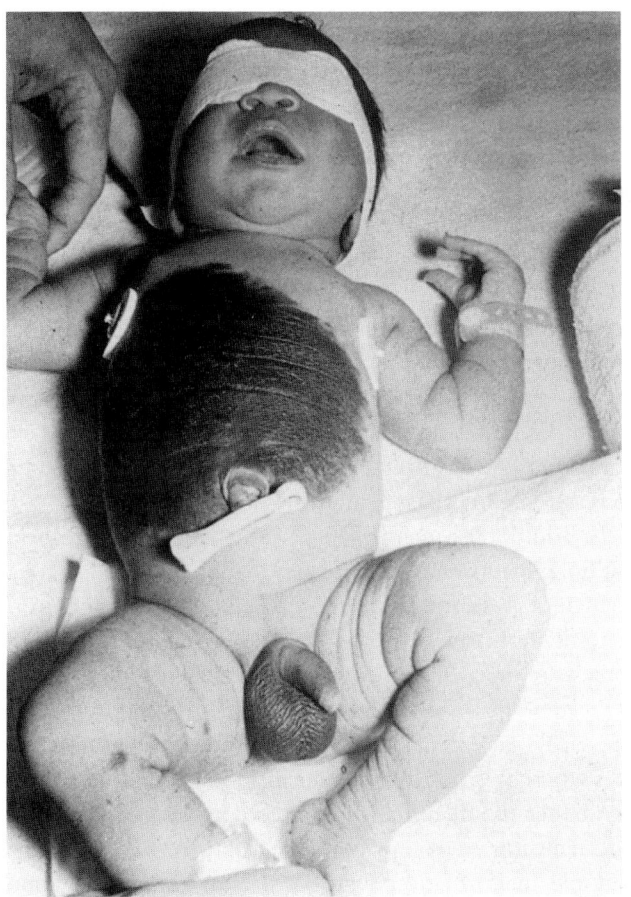

Fig. 38.5. Infant with neurocutaneous melanosis. Note the bathing trunk nevus. This infant also had seizures, presumably from melanocytic infiltration of the pia and arachnoid.

changes in the pia and arachnoid. Affected individuals are at risk for malignant degeneration within the hamartoses and are also at risk for neurologic sequelae, including seizures and mental retardation. Although the etiology of this sporadic condition is unknown, the single defect in development is presumed to involve melanoblastic precursors migrating from the neural crest.

Finally, a sequence, like any other single defect in development, can occur by itself in an otherwise normal individual or may be one feature in a multiple malformation syndrome. Stickler syndrome, cerebrocostomandibular syndrome, and spondyloepiphyseal dysplasia congenita are examples of multiple malformation syndromes in which the Robin malformation sequence represents one feature. In this situation, recurrence risk counseling is based on the etiology of the overall condition.

MULTIPLE MALFORMATION SYNDROMES

The category of multiple malformation syndromes includes patients in whom a primary developmental anomaly of two or more systems has occurred, all of which are thought to be due to a common etiology. Other than Down syndrome, which has an incidence of 1:660, and XXY syndrome (1:500 males), few of these disorders occur more frequently than 1 in 3000 live births.

As shown in Figure 38.1, multiple malformation syndromes can be categorized on the basis of etiology.

CHROMOSOMAL ABNORMALITIES

The ability to perform chromosomal studies has led to the recognition of a number of multiple malformation syndromes due to chromosomal abnormalities. Two excellent references delineate the features of the most common of these (Schinzel, 1984; Borgaonkar, 1997). Certain generalizations are important to consider when deciding whether or not a chromosome study should be performed. First, since chromosomes are present in most cells of the body, a chromosome aberration may be expected to affect adversely many parts of the body. Consequently, a person with only an incurved fifth finger and a heart defect is very unlikely to have those features on the basis of a chromosome problem. Second, some sex-chromosome disorders (e.g., XXX, XXY, and XYY) have few, if any, defects recognizable at birth. In addition, as more experience is gained with chromosomal abnormalities involving very small deletions and duplications, it becomes increasingly clear that prenatal growth deficiency and mental retardation should not be the only requirements for chromosome studies.

The most common disorder associated with a chromosomal abnormality is the Down syndrome (21 trisomy). The principal features of the disorder (flat facies with upward slant to the palpebral fissures, hypotonicity and small ears) are usually present at birth, making a clinical diagnosis possible in the newborn period. Ear length is measured by the maximum distance from the superior aspect to the inferior aspect of the ear. Aase and colleagues (1973) documented decreased ear length as a consistent feature in newborn infants with the Down syndrome. In their series no full-term white infant with the Down syndrome had an ear length greater than 3.4 cm (mean 3 cm), and no normal full-term white infant had an ear length less than 3.2 cm (mean 3.8 cm).

A routine G-banded chromosome study is the only widely available screening test that can be done to define the etiology of an unrecognized, prenatal-onset multiple malformation syndrome. In certain circumstances, further investigation for cytogenetic abnormalities may be warranted. High-resolution chromosome analysis should be considered in children with unexplained developmental delay, prenatal growth deficiency or both who also have multiple minor malformations. In a study of 2245 patients presenting with malformations and developmental delay, 1.1% were found to have chromosome abnormalities on high-resolution analysis that would have been missed, standard methodology (Mascarello and Hubbard, 1991).

Another technique that may be useful in diagnosis is fluorescent in situ hybridization (FISH) analysis (see Chapter 26). Since the probes used to perform FISH are specific to defined areas of the genome, FISH analysis is usually not a screening technique, but rather is best applied when (1) there is high clinical suspicion of a recognized pattern of malformation for which FISH analysis is available, and (2) the high resolution studies are normal (i.e., Prader–Willi syndrome or Williams syndrome, see below).

New techniques are being developed to screen for balanced and unbalanced rearrangements using either FISH probes or microsatellited DNA markers specific to the subtelomeric regions of chromosomes (Nature Genetics, 1996; Knight et al., 1997; Slavotinek et al., 1999). These regions have a high concentration of genes; however, subtle rearrangements are difficult to detect using G-banding. The DNA methodology has the disadvantage of requiring parental samples; however, a pilot study of 27 subjects with mental retardation and dysmorphic features who were cytogenetically normal on G-banded analysis detected two previously unrecognized alterations (Slavotinek et al., 1999). The literature is replete with single cases of subtle chromosome anomalies detected by FISH. As the methodology improves, subtelomeric analysis may become a more widespread second-line screening test.

Recurrence risk counseling for chromosome abnormalities depends on the nature of the cytogenetic abnormality identified. Risk is usually low in aneuploidy; however, the risk for certain trisomies (21, 18, XXX and XXY) may increase with increasing maternal age. In case of an unbalanced translocation, parental karyotypes are warranted before specific risks are cited. In cases of *de novo* abnormalities, the risk is usually low except for the rare circumstance of gonadal mosaicism in a parent.

DISORDERS WITH KNOWN GENETIC ETIOLOGY

A single mutant allele or a pair of mutant alleles have been implicated as the cause of some recognizable multiple malformation syndromes of prenatal onset. Correct diagnosis in most of these disorders depends on clinical recognition, since in the vast majority of cases there is no testing available for the abnormal gene. A family history of a similarly affected individual can be extremely helpful. However, in many patients with multiple malformation syndromes of genetic etiology, the occurrence is sporadic and thus represents a fresh gene mutation. In such situations all family members do not have the malformation. Diagnosis depends entirely on evaluation of the patient's phenotype. The type of laboratory evaluation that may be helpful as an adjunct to clinical recognition is usually an extension of the physical examination, for example, radiographic assessment of bony structure or tissue histopathology. As the genetic basis for many single gene disorders is elucidated, diagnosis by mutation analysis may become routine. To date, however, transfer of mutation detection from the research to the clinical laboratory has been extremely slow. Thus most diagnosis rests on clinical assessment.

In addition to mendelian patterns of inheritance, some multiple malformation syndromes may arise as a consequence of dosage imbalance of a gene. At some loci in the genome, only one copy of a gene is active even though two copies are normally present. Inactivation of one member of a gene pair involves the process of imprinting (see Ch. 130). Parent of origin effects are evident at imprinted sites where it is possible in a normal individual to document that either the maternally inherited copy of the gene or the paternally inherited copy of the gene is active. Prenatal-onset multiple malformation syndromes may occur if an abnormality in the imprinting process causes both the maternal and paternal genes to be active at a specific locus or if an affected individual inherits two copies of a gene from one parent and none from the other. The latter situation is termed uniparental disomy. Both of these mechanisms have been implicated in cases of the Beckwith–Wiedemann syndrome. In addition, loss of the normally active allele has been documented to produce phenotypic effects in certain multiple malformation syndromes in which the genetic locus for the condition appears to be imprinted. The extent to which these mechanisms play a role in the etiology of genetically determined multiple malformation syndromes is at present unknown.

DISORDERS CAUSED BY TERATOGENS

Disorders caused by teratogens include multiple malformation syndromes due to the effect of specific infections, drugs or chemical agents with which the embryo or fetus has come into contact. These disorders take on special importance because they represent the only group of dysmorphologic conditions in which prevention before conception may be feasible. This is particularly true in the case of drugs and chemicals if the mother is aware that the agent in question can affect her baby. It is difficult, on the other hand, for a pregnant woman to avoid contact with all infectious agents. Immunization of at-risk individuals with new vaccines may assist in prevention of birth defects caused by specific viral infections (e.g., varicella-zoster virus).

A careful history of drug intake and chemical exposure should be obtained from the parents of all children with multiple malformation syndromes. This is particularly true when the etiology of the disorder is unknown. Two excellent references in determining the teratogenic potential of any environmental factor with which the mother has had contact are available (Briggs et al., 1998; Shepard, 1998). In addition, several online databases are available through subscription including Reprotox (2000) and Teris (2000) (which includes Shepard, 1988).

Although a specific and easily distinguishable phenotype does not exist for each of the infectious agents that are commonly associated with altered fetal development, intrauterine infection can frequently be suspected, based on the overall pattern of malformation. Any small-for-gestational-age patient with microcephaly or hydrocephalus, ocular findings including microphthalmia, chorioretinitis, cataracts and/or glaucoma, hepatosplenomegaly and thrombocytopenia, and who is developmentally delayed should be suspected of having had an intrauterine infection. It should be emphasized that each of these intrauterine infections has a wide spectrum, from fetal death, to the severely affected newborn infant with multiple malformations, to the child with no malformation disabilities. The latter situation is illustrated by a study by Hanshaw and coworkers (1976) indicating a significant increase in school failure and deafness after clinically inapparent congenital cytomegalovirus infection.

RECOGNIZED PATTERNS

There are some well-recognized multiple malformation syndromes in which virtually all cases have been sporadic and, until recently, the etiology unknown. The de Lange syndrome, Williams syndrome, and Rubenstein–Taybi syndrome are three of the most common disorders included in this category. Each occurs with a frequency of more than 1 per 10,000. Experience with many children with each of these disorders has provided a vast amount of information that can be extremely helpful to parents in understanding their child's behavior and to educators in planning an appropriate curriculum. For example, a specific behavioral phenotype has been delineated for de Lange syndrome (Johnson et al., 1976). Awareness by parents that the child's aberrant behavior is "normal" for de Lange syndrome rather than "their fault" can be extremely helpful in relieving anxiety and guilt. For the Williams syndrome, Bennett and colleagues (1970) demonstrated a characteristic psychological profile that indicates delayed motor and perceptual development with relatively good verbal performance and sociability. It is hoped that knowledge of a child's particular strengths and weaknesses will allow educators to develop a curriculum that will give children with specific disorders a better chance to reach their potential.

Within the last few years, the etiology of some of the conditions in this category has become clear. The de Lange syndrome has been transmitted vertically within a family suggesting that the condition, in fact, has a genetic etiology with autosomal dominant inheritance (Robinson et al., 1985). The observation that the overwhelming majority of cases occur sporadically within families reflects the fact that the condition is usually a reproductive lethal.

Williams syndrome has been documented to be the result of a submicroscopic deletion of chromosomal material on chromosome 7q11.23 in an area encompassing the elastin gene (Ewart et al., 1993). Although technically disorders caused by submicroscopic chromosomal deletion could be considered chromosomal malformation syndromes, we prefer to consider them recognized patterns for the purposes of this approach, since neither a routine nor high-resolution karyotype will necessarily detect the chromosomal abnormality. Although chromosomal microdeletion syndromes may be vertically transmitted in a pattern consistent with dominant inheritance, the physical and functional effects of the condition are usually such as to preclude transmission. The practical risk for recurrence for unaffected parents is low, but not zero. The major exception to this statement currently is the 22q11 microdeletion syndrome discussed in detail in Chapter 48.

Rubenstein–Taybi syndrome is produced by functional loss of one copy of the gene encoding the transcriptional coactivator CREB-binding protein on chromosome 16p13.3 (Petrij et al., 1995). Microdeletions of this region, first thought to be causal in the majority of cases (Breuning et al., 1993), actually account for only 11% of affected cases and produce a more severe phenotype than point mutations in the gene which account for the majority of cases (Wallerstein, 1997). Rubenstein–Taybi syndrome is typical of a growing number of recognized patterns of malformation in which different genetic mechanism may produce the same phenotype.

Postnatal-onset problems in development

Most children with postnatal-onset malformation problems are normal at birth, having appeared to thrive *in utero*. Neurologic problems frequently begin within the first week of life, and deterioration is often rapid. A specific pattern of malformation usually does not occur; structural abnormalities are usually the result of neurologic deterioration, storage of metabolites, or progressive loss of function in a specific tissue. In disorders with a known metabolic aberration, other manifestations of the metabolic defect such as cataracts, sparse hair, coarse facies, unusual skin pigmentation, and hepatosplenomegaly are frequently present. As set forth in Figure 38.1, these disorders can be categorized on the basis of etiology.

GENETIC

Metabolic

Most metabolic conditions are the result of a specific enzyme deficiency. Because of the possibility that early institution of dietary therapy may help to prevent mental retardation, these disorders are of particular interest and newborn screening is offered for some of these conditions throughout the United States. Since the placenta is able to compensate for the metabolic deficiency, affected infants are normal at birth (e.g., aminoacidurias and organic acidurias). Most of these conditions have an autosomal recessive mode of inheritance. Their incidence is extremely low. Phenylketonuria (1:14, 000) is the most common and represented, in its untreated state, about 1% of most institutionalized populations surveyed before newborn screening programs were instituted. A second group of metabolic conditions produces a phenotype through abnormal accumulation or storage of material in various tissues in the body. Although the placenta does not compensate for the enzymatic deficiency, the phenotype does not manifest until a period of time has passed during which accumulation of metabolites occurs (e.g., glycogen storage diseases and mucopolysaccharidoses). Consequently, there is usually a postnatal presentation.

Central nervous system degenerative states

A metabolic defect will probably be found for most of these disorders. However, at present, although the clinical features and mode of inheritance have been delineated, the biochemical abnormality is unknown; diagnosis relies on histopathology. The incidence of these conditions is extremely low, representing 0.9% of the 1378 mentally retarded individuals at the Walter E. Fernald State School (Holmes et al., 1972).

Myopathies and connective tissue disorders

Myopathies and connective tissue disorders represent a group of conditions in which structures deteriorate with wear and tear over time – hence the postnatal presentation. A diagnosis may be suspected by the communality of the involved tissue (i.e., wound healing problems and ligamentous laxity for connective tissue disorders or cardiomyopathy and weakness for muscle disorders).

ENVIRONMENTAL FACTORS

Trauma, infection, hypoxia, and metabolic derangements can result in severe neurologic impairment. Progressive joint immobility, abnormal positioning, and paralysis secondary to central nervous system deterioration are the most frequent structural anomalies resulting from this type of injury. Deafness and cataract may also be seen.

Summary

A clinical approach to children with structural defects has been set forth. It is based upon the concept that the diagnostic evaluation should be directed by the nature of the structural defects. The ultimate goal of this approach is a specific overall diagnosis. In such cases, appropriate recurrence risk counseling for the parents, accurate prognostication relative to the child's future development, and an appropriate plan to help the child reach his potential usually are possible. When an overall diagnosis is lacking, the most that can be expected is a better understanding of the nature and onset of the problem. That in itself can often be helpful to parents and to all others dealing with children who have structural defects.

REFERENCES

Aase JM (1990) Diagnostic Dysmorphology. Plenum, NY

Aase JM, Wilson AC, Smith DW (1973) Small ears in Down's syndrome: a helpful diagnostic aid. J Pediatr 82:845–847

Bankier A (2000) POSSUM CD ROM Version 5.2. The Murdoch Institute for Research in to Birth Defects, Melbourne Australia URL http://www.possum.net.au

Bennett FC, LaVeck B, Sells CJ (1970) The Williams elfin facies syndrome: the psychological profile as an aid in syndrome identification. Pediatr 61:303–305

Berendes HW, Weiss W, Dentschberger J, Jackson E (1965) Factors associated with breech delivery. Am J Public Health 55:708–719

Borgaonkar DS (1997) Chromosomal Variation in Man: A Catalog of Chromosomal Variants and Anomalies. 8th edn. Wiley-Liss, NY

Braun FHT, Jones KL, Smith DW (1975) Breech presentation as an indicator of fetal abnormality. J Pediatr 86:419–421

Breuning MH, Dauwerse HG, Fugazza G et al. (1993) Rubinstein-Taybi syndrome caused by submicroscopic deletions within 16p13.3 Am J Hum Genet 52:249–254

Briggs GG, Yaffe SJ, Freeman RK (1998) Drugs in Pregnancy and Lactation: A Reference Guide to Fetal and Neonatal Risk, 5th edn. Williams & Wilkins, Baltimore

Castilla E, Paz J, Mutchinick O et al. (1973) Polydactyly: A genetic study in South America. Am J Hum Genet 25:405–412

Cunningham FG, MacDonald PC, Gant NF et al. (1993) William's Obstetrics. p. 184. Appleton & Lange, E Norwalk, Connecticut

Doyle AC. n.d. The Complete Sherlock Holmes. Doubleday, Garden City, NY, p. 23

Drillen CM (1970) The small-for-date infant: Etiology and prognosis. Pediatr Clin N Am 17:9–24

Dunn PM (1976) Congenital postural deformities. Br Med Bull 32:71–76

Ewart AK, Morris CA, Atkinson D et al. (1993) Hemizygosity at the elastin locus in a developmental disorder, Williams syndrome. Nature Genet 5:11–16

Gorlin RJ, Cohen MM, Levin LS (1990) Syndromes of the Head and Neck. 3rd edn. OUP, NY

Graham JM (1988) Smith's Recognizable Pattern of Human Deformation, 2nd edn. WB Saunders, Philadelphia

Graham JM, deSaxe M, Smith DW (1979) Sagittal craniostenosis: Fetal head constraint as one possible cause. J Pediatr 95:747–750

Hanshaw JB, Scheiner AP, Moxley AW et al. (1976) School failure and deafness after silent congenital cytomegalovirus infection. N Engl J Med 295:468–470

Hanson JW, Smith DW (1975) U-shaped palatal defect in the Robin anomalad: developmental and clinical relevance. J Pediatr 87:30–33

Higginbottom MC, Jones KL, Hall BD, Smith DW (1979) The amniotic band disruption complex: Timing of amniotic rupture and variable spectra of conseqeunt defects. J Pediatr 95:544–549

Holmes LB, Mack C, Moger HW et al. (1972) Mental Retardation: An Atlas of Diseases with Associated Physical Abnormalities. Macmillan, NY

Hoyme HE, Higginbottom MC, Jones KL (1981) The vascular pathogenesis of gastroschisis: Intrauterine interruption of the omphalomesenteric artery. J Pediatr 98:228–231

Hoyme HE, Jones KL, Van Allen MI et al. (1982) Vascular pathogenesis of transverse limb reduction defects. J Pediatr 101:839–843

Hoyme HE, Jones KL, Dixon SD et al. (1990) Prenatal cocaine exposure and fetal vascular disruption. Pediatr 85:743–747

Johnson HQ, Ekman P, Friesen W et al. (1976) A behavioral phenotype in the de Lange syndrome. Pediatr Res 10:843–850

Jones KL (1997) Smith's Recognizable Patterns of Human Malformation, 5th edn. WB Saunders, Philadelphia

Knight SJ, Horsley SW, Regan R et al. (1997) Development and clinical application of an innovative fluorescence in situ hybridization technique which detects submicroscopic rearrangements involving telomeres. Euro J Hum Genet 5:1–8

Lemire RJ, Loeser JD, Leech RW, Alvord EC (1975) Normal and Abnormal Development of the Human Nervous System. Harper/Collins, NY, p. 251

Louw JH (1966) Jejunoileal atresia and stenosis. J Pediatr Surg 1:8–23

Mascarello JT, Hubbard (1991) Routine use of methods for improved G-banded resolution in a population of patients with malformations and developmental delay. Am J Med Genet 38:37–42

McKusick VA (1998) Mendelian Inheritance in Man. Catalogs of Human Genes and Genetic Disorders, 12th edn. Johns Hopkins University Press, Baltimore http://www.ncbi.nlm.nih.gov/Omim/

MRC Vitamin Study Research Group (1991) Prevention of neural tube defects: results of the Medical Research Council Vitamin Study. Lancet 338:131–137

1996 A complete set of human telomeric probes and their clinical application. National Institutes of Health and Institute of Molecular Medicine collaboration. Nature Genet 14:86–89

Petrij F, Giles RH, Dauwerse HG et al. (1995) Rubenstein-Taybi syndrome caused by mutation in the transcriptional co-activator CBP. Nature 376:348–351

Reprotox system (2000) URL http://www.micromedex.com/products/pd-reportox.htm

Robinson LK, Wolfsberg E, Jones KL (1985) Brachmann-de Lange syndrome: evidence for autosomal dominant inheritance. Am J Med Genet 22:109–115

Sadovsky E, Yaffe H (1973) Daily fetal movement recording and fetal prognosis. Obstet Gynaecol 41:845–850

Schinzel A (1984) Catalog of Unbalanced Chromosome Aberrations in Man. Walter de Gruyter, Berlin

Shepard TH (1998) A Catalog of Teratogeneic Agents, 9th edn. Johns Hopkins University Press, Baltimore

Slavotinek A, Rosenberg M, Knight S et al. (1999) Screening for submicroscopic chromosome rearrangements in children with idiopathic mental retardation using microsatellite markers for the chromosome telomeres. J Med Genet 36:405–411

Spranger J, Benirschke K, Hall JG et al. (1982) Errors of morphogenesis: concepts and terms. J Pediatr 100:160–165

Teris (2000) URL http://depts.washington.edu/~terisweb/

Thomas IT, Smith DW (1974) Oligohydramnios, cause of the nonrenal features of Potter's syndrome, including pulmonary hypoplasia. J Pediatr 84:811–814

Wallerstein R, Anderson CE, Hay B et al. (1997) Submicroscopic deletions at 16p13.3 in Rubenstein-Taybi syndrome: Frequency and clinical manifestations in a North American population. J Med Genet 34:203–206

Winter RM, Baraister M (1999) London Dysmorphology Database CD ROM. Version 2.2. Oxford Medical Databases, OUP, Oxford

Clinical teratology

J. M. Friedman
James W. Hanson

Introduction

Pregnant patients who are undergoing genetic evaluation or prenatal diagnosis often have concerns about possible adverse effects of non-genetic factors, such as exposures to drugs or occupational agents. Less than one-third of families seen in most genetics clinics have conditions that are principally genetic in origin, and the differential diagnosis often includes disorders that have a predominant non-genetic cause. Accordingly, it is incumbent upon practitioners of clinical genetics to be aware of the nonheritable sources of human variability, their potential interactions with genetic factors, and their implications for human health, growth, and development.

Teratology is the branch of medical science devoted to study of the environmental contribution to abnormal prenatal growth and development. Teratological effects include both structural congenital anomalies, growth disturbances and functional deficits such as behavioral and cognitive abnormalities that may not be apparent until some time after birth. The term "teratogen" has been used to denote an agent that can cause abnormalities of form, function or both in an exposed fetus, but this usage is somewhat misleading. It implies that any given agent either is or is not teratogenic and that clinical teratology consists merely of memorizing a list of "human teratogens". In reality, teratogenicity is a property of an *exposure* taken as whole, which involves not only the physical and chemical nature of the agent but also the dose, route, and gestational timing involved. The occurrence of other, concurrent exposures as well as the biological susceptibility of the mother and embryo or fetus are also factors that can determine whether a given exposure produces damage in a particular instance.

Although interest in teratogenic effects is recorded in surviving fragments of tablets from ancient Middle Eastern cultures, much of the information available in this field before 1950 can hardly be classified as more than folklore (Warkany, 1977). Despite the pioneering studies of Warkany and Nelson (1940) and others, the rekindling of serious scientific and medical interest in teratology awaited the successive tragedies of thalidomide and the rubella pandemics in the early 1960s.

The succeeding decades have seen a significant growth of basic, clinical, and epidemiologic investigation into problems of teratogenesis. Regulatory agencies have erected barriers against the introduction of teratogenic exposures into our environment. Furthermore, the past two decades have seen the development of teratogen information services (Hanson, 1987; Koren and Pastuszak, 1994; Koren et al., 1998). These services, supported by computer-based information resources such as *TERIS* (Friedman and Polifka, 2000) (http://depts.washington.edu/~terisweb/teris/index.html) and *REPROTOX* (Scialli et al., 1995; (http://www.reprotox.org), have improved the access of health care providers and the general public to available information and have fostered a systematic approach to risk assessment and risk management. Unfortunately, the mechanisms by which most teratogenic exposures produce their pathogenic effects are still unknown, significant gaps remain in public health barriers, and our goal of primary prevention through the avoidance of hazardous prenatal exposures remains substantially unrealized.

While considerable debate still rages regarding the relative contribution of teratogenic exposures to the total load of birth defects in our population, it is increasingly clear that genetic factors per se cannot account for many such abnormalities. With this realization has come a renewed emphasis on the prevention of teratogenic exposures. A few generalizations have emerged that help us to characterize and recognize teratogenic exposures.

Characterization of teratogenic exposures

Teratogenic exposures may act by a relatively limited number of pathogenetic processes (Brent et al., 1993; Finnell, 1999) that may produce cellular death, alter tissue growth (hyperplasia, hypoplasia, or asynchronous growth), or interfere with cellular differentiation or other basic morphogenetic processes, including mechanical ones. Some agents may also act by destroying ("disrupting") normally developing structures. Furthermore, similar general effects may be produced by a number of teratogenic exposures. For instance, many exposures may stunt growth (though possibly by different mechanisms), resulting in a neonate who is small for gestational age. Thus, certain characteristics are common to a wide range of teratogenic exposures and may be used as general indicators of potential teratogenicity. Such indicators that a teratogenic effect may have occurred include:

1. Infertility or fetal wastage
2. Prenatal-onset growth deficiency
3. Alterations of morphogenesis
4. Alterations of central nervous system performance

Exposures that produce one or more of these effects should be considered likely to be teratogenic. Fetal wastage and prenatal-onset growth deficiency seem to be particularly common indicators of teratogenicity.

These general indicators of teratogenic activity reflect disturbances of basic processes occurring in many tissues. Such processes affect critical events in growing cells and developing organisms, and commonly are manifest in more than one tissue or organ in the developing embryo or fetus at any one time. It is not surprising, therefore, to find that teratogenic exposures commonly have the capability of producing abnormalities in more than one tissue or organ system and that teratogenic exposures tend to produce characteristic patterns of abnormal growth and morphogenesis. For this reason, while individual abnormalities of morphogenesis are usually not specific for a particular teratogenic exposure, certain patterns of abnormal growth and development may be distinctive.

Agents are teratogenic only under certain conditions of exposure. This is why classifying some agents as "teratogens" and others as "non-teratogens" is misleading (Scialli,

1997). One critical factor is the developmental stage of the embryo at the time of exposure. The most sensitive period for an exposure to alter embryonic development appears to be from roughly two weeks after conception to the fourth or fifth week after conception. Exposures occurring later than this time may produce problems of cell depletion and could therefore be related to such effects as growth retardation. Data from animal experiments suggest that earlier adverse exposures usually are either lethal to the embryo or produce no demonstrable effects on morphogenesis, although malformations can be produced by exposure of rodents to some mutagens between conception and the time of implantation (Rutledge, 1997). Agents that lead to fetal constraint and consequent deformations are likely to have their most significant effect in the third trimester of pregnancy, during the phase of most rapid fetal growth. Exposures, such as those to infectious agents, that produce cell death or tissue necrosis may cause disruption at any stage of gestation.

Thalidomide and angiotensin-converting enzyme (ACE) inhibitors provide especially vivid illustrations of the importance of timing to teratogenesisis. The pattern of limb reduction defects, facial hemangioma, microtia, ocular abnormalities, renal malformations, and congenital heart disease that characterizes the thalidomide embryopathy only occurs in children whose mothers are treated between 27 and 40 days of gestation (Lenz and Knapp, 1962). In contrast, maternal treatment with the ACE inhibitors captopril and enalapril only produces fetal renal failure and oligohydramnios during the latter stages of pregnancy (Barr, 1994; Mastrobattista, 1997). These effects appear to result from exquisite sensitivity of the fetus to the pharmacological hypotensive action of ACE inhibitors during the second and third trimester of gestation (Barr, 1994).

Dose is a critical feature of any teratogenic exposure. Teratogenic effects occur only when the dose exceeds a certain threshold (Brent, 1995a). Exposures to agents that are generally considered to be safe may have adverse effects on the embryo or fetus if given in doses high enough to produce maternal toxicity This is an especially important consideration in exposures associated with suicide attempts, drugs of abuse (e.g., toluene inhalation) or agents encountered occupationally. Chronic exposure is usually of more concern than a single exposure, given similar doses.

The route of exposure is also of importance—there is unlikely to be a risk associated with any agent when the exposure occurs by a route that does not permit systemic absorption. This is the case with many dermal exposures. Exposure to methylene blue illustrates the importance of dose to teratogenicity. Several studies have found a strong association between the occurrence of intestinal atresia and the instillation of methylene blue into the amniotic sac during midtrimester genetic amniocentesis in twin pregnancies (Cragan, 1999). The risk of intestinal atresia in an infant born after this procedure is about 20% (van der Pol et al., 1992). Neither oral nor topical administration of methylene blue to the mother has been associated with a similar teratogenic risk.

Some agents, such as ionizing radiation, have direct access to the embryo whereas others do not reach the embryo until after extensive metabolism by the mother. The teratogenicity of agents that are metabolized by the mother may depend on whether teratogenic metabolites reach the embryo or fetus in sufficient quantities to produce adverse effects. This, in turn, depends on a number of factors including route of entry, physical properties of the agent, maternal dose, and amount of systemic absorption.

Another factor that influences teratogenicity is the chemical and/or physical nature of the agent itself. Some agents are inherently more risky than others. Maternal thalidomide treatment during embryogenesis is the classic example of an exposure that usually presents little direct risk to the mother but has strong developmental toxicity. There are only a few other examples of exposures that exhibit such selective developmental toxicity.

The teratogenicity of an exposure is also influenced by both the maternal and fetal genotypes, which may result in differences in cell sensitivity, placental transport, metabolism, receptor binding, and distribution. These differences explain why only some of the children of women who have exposures that are similar with respect to agent, dose and gestational timing exhibit adverse effects. The importance of the genetic susceptibility of the fetus to teratogenesis is clearly illustrated by the higher rate of concordance for fetal alcohol syndrome among monozygotic twins than dizygotic twins of mothers who heavily abuse alcohol during pregnancy (Streissguth and Dehaene, 1993).

Together, these factors probably account for most variation encountered among patients adversely affected by prenatal exposures. It must be recognized that the teratogenic potential of an exposure is commonly expressed over a wide spectrum when all exposed individuals are considered. That is to say, when dealing with affected individuals, variability of effect is the rule, not the exception.

These generalizations lead to the following conclusions:

1. Teratogenic exposures are most easily recognized (that is, the effects are most specific) at the severe end of the spectrum where a clear-cut pattern of abnormalities of growth and development often emerges.

2. As such patterns are clear only at the severe end of the spectrum, "milder" or partial effects, including single major abnormalities of morphogenesis, may be more frequent among exposed individuals and less specific to individual teratogenic exposures. Such effects may sometimes be viewed as being "consistent with a prenatal teratogenic exposure" even though they are not specific.

3. Certain general features of teratogenic exposures may be sought in screening for potentially hazardous agents, and the use of agents displaying some of these characteristics would be most prudently avoided during pregnancy.

4. All of the above features should be taken into account for complete clinical characterization of the effects of a teratogenic exposure and in order to interpret this information in a meaningful way to patients. A checklist of the types of information needed for the clinical characterization of a teratogenic exposure is presented in Table 39.1. Table 39.2 presents a list of features used to characterize effects that may occur in the child as the result of such exposures. Much more information on each of these points is needed for virtually every known or suspected teratogenic exposure.

Table 39.1. Characterization of teratogenic exposures

Agent
  Nature of the chemical, physical, or infectious agent
  Inherent developmental toxicity
  Capacity to produce other kinds of toxicity in the mother

Dosage to embryo or fetus
  Single, repeated, or chronic exposure
  Duration of exposure
  Maternal dose
  Maternal route of exposure
  Maternal absorption
  Maternal metabolism and clearance
  Placental transfer

Period of pregnancy
  Between conception and onset of embryogenesis
  Embryogenesis
  Fetal period

Other factors
  Genetic susceptibility of mother
  Genetic susceptibility of the fetus
  Other concurrent exposures
  Maternal illness or other condition associated with exposure
  Availability of tests to quantify the magnitude of maternal exposure

Table 39.2. Characterization of teratogenic effects

General effects
   Alterations of morphogenesis
   Alterations of CNS function
   Other functional impairments
   Death of the conceptus, embryo, or fetus
   Prenatal-onset growth deficiency
   Carcinogenesis

Specific effects
   Recognizable syndrome
   Other distinctive features

Magnitude of risk
   Absolute
   Relative

Prenatal diagnosis
   Detailed ultrasound examination
   Amniocentesis or other invasive method
   Availability
   Reliability
   Utility

Risk assessment and counseling for teratogenic effects

Clinical geneticists and genetic counselors need to consider the possibility of teratogenic effects in three clinical settings. The first is during the evaluation of a patient, usually a child, in whom the medical history and/or physical findings suggest the possibility of a teratogenic effect. Both a high index of suspicion and considerable skepticism are required in such cases. Careful review of the prenatal history for the nature and circumstances of any potentially teratogenic exposure is essential, and the child should be examined for major and minor abnormalities known to be associated with such exposures. Except in the case of some infectious agents, laboratory confirmation of the diagnosis is not possible, and recognition of a teratogenic cause may require the skills of an expert dysmorphologist (Aase, 1990; Jones, 1997; Graham et al., 1999). In many instances, a firm diagnosis can only be made by exclusion of alternative explanations for any abnormalities identified and long-term follow-up of the patient.

Concern is often voiced that informing couples of the adverse effects of a drug or other potential teratogenic exposure on a child with birth defects may create serious psychological problems, particularly in situations that involve maternal drug abuse, such as excessive consumption of ethanol. However, only through such a frank approach will there be an opportunity to provide optimal care for the affected child and the potential for prevention of similar problems in future children. It is clear, however, that the sharing of such information may indeed produce psychological problems. Under these circumstances long-term support for affected families through community agencies and health care mechanisms is extremely important.

A second setting in which the geneticist or genetic counselor must consider a teratogenic effect is when a patient who is not currently pregnant but wishes to have children is concerned about possible teratogenic effects of a current or future medical treatment or occupational exposure. The most certain way to prevent birth defects from teratogenic exposures is exclusion of the exposure from the prenatal environment. The approach in this instance involves determining whether the exposure is of concern and, if so, whether it can be avoided, replaced by a safer alternative, completed prior to pregnancy, or deferred until the pregnancy is over. Although this is not always possible, increased attention should be paid by physicians to patient education to help avoid unnecessary exposures to potentially teratogenic agents during pregnancy, particularly during the first trimester. When a woman of reproductive age requires drug therapy, the prescribing physician's discussion of risks and benefits should include the potential for teratogenic risks. Failure to inform a pregnant patient or potentially pregnant patient of hazards relating to medical treatment or procedures may place the physician in legal jeopardy.

Sometimes it is impossible or unwise for a woman to avoid a potentially teratogenic exposure, e.g., when failure to use a potentially teratogenic treatment poses a greater risk to the woman than the treatment does even if she is pregnant. When it is not possible or prudent to avoid such treatment, it may still be possible to minimize the magnitude of the exposure or to avoid it during the most sensitive period of fetal development. In the final analysis, decisions regarding the use of potentially teratogenic treatments during pregnancy are best left to an informed couple, supported through a comprehensive pregnancy risk assessment, risk communication, and management process by a sensitive and knowledgeable physician.

A third circumstance in which a geneticist or genetic counselor must consider a teratogenic effect is when a patient is concerned about the possible adverse effect of a previous or ongoing exposure during her current pregnancy. For example, a patient may have abused alcohol or "recreational drugs" before she realized that she was pregnant, or she may have become pregnant while taking a particular medication that she has now stopped. In this case, any benefits of the exposure are no longer relevant, and the patient's concern may be whether she should terminate the pregnancy, consider prenatal diagnosis, or accept the additional risk (if any) and continue the pregnancy. Providing appropriate teratogen risk counseling in such situations requires careful evaluation of the patient, her fetus and the exposure, as well as review of the relevant scientific literature.

EVALUATING THE PATIENT AND HER EXPOSURE

In order to provide a context for the counseling, the counselor should review the patient's general medical, obstetrical, and family history. The purpose of teratogenic risk assessment is to determine whether a pregnant woman's exposure increases her risk of having a child with congenital anomalies above the risk that she would have if she were unexposed. The "background" risk of serious congenital anomalies usually quoted is 3–5% for the general population, but the risk for a particular woman may be much greater because of her age, family history, medical condition, or other exposures. It is common for the risk of congenital anomalies associated with these other factors to equal or exceed the risk associated with a particular exposure of concern to the patient.

The dose, route, duration, and timing for each exposure of concern should be determined as precisely as possible. For example, one can usually obtain the name, amount, frequency, and length of time that a medication was taken. This is much more informative than just knowing what was prescribed. In some cases, blood levels of a drug or occupational chemical to which the patient was exposed can be used to define the exposure very precisely. In other instances, measurements of a chemical or its metabolite in the urine or an occupational hygiene assessment can help to quantify an exposure of particular concern. One should always establish the reason the exposure occurred (e.g., medical treatment of a particular disease) and whether the woman experienced any toxic effects as a result of the exposure. If toxic effects did occur, they should be described as fully as possible. The evaluation should also include information about any relevant occupational exposures and the patient's use of other medications, alcohol, tobacco and other "recreational" drugs.

ASSESSING THE SCIENTIFIC LITERATURE

Characterization of human teratogenic exposures requires careful interpretation of data obtained from several kinds of studies (Brent et al., 1993; Koren et al., 1998; Polifka and Friedman, 1999). Fortunately, the problem of collecting and analyzing the available data has been greatly simplified for families and physicians by the advent of teratogen information services (Hanson, 1987; Koren and Pastuszak, 1994) and clinical teratology knowledgebases (Scialli et al., 1995; Friedman and Polifka, 2000).

For many exposures, the only kind of teratological studies available are those done in laboratory animals. Such studies are valuable because they provide a means of identifying exposures with teratogenic potential before humans have been harmed. Unfortunately, however, it is usually impossible to extrapolate findings directly from animal experiments to a clinical situation involving an individual pregnant woman except in a very general way. Comparisons between species are confounded by differences in placentation, pharmacodynamics, embryonic development, and other factors that may influence the likelihood of teratogenic effects. In addition, the doses and routes of exposure used in animal teratology experiments often are not comparable to those that are likely to occur in humans.

Teratogenic exposures typically produce qualitatively distinct patterns of congenital anomalies in affected children. Almost all exposures that are currently known to be teratogenic in humans were initially identified in case reports and clinical series on the basis of such characteristic patterns of anomalies. The evidence of a causal relationship can be compelling when a highly characteristic pattern of congenital anomalies is recognized in children whose mothers experienced similar well-defined exposures at similar times in pregnancy, especially if both the pattern of anomalies and the exposure are otherwise rare. Unfortunately, however, case reports and clinical series cannot provide quantitative estimates of the strength or statistical significance of a teratogenic effect. Properly-conducted epidemiological studies are needed to determine the magnitude of a teratogenic risk.

Epidemiological studies must also be interpreted with caution. These investigations may be subject to biases of ascertainment or recall, and the maternal disease or situation that occasioned the exposure rather than the agent itself may be responsible for an observed association. Moreover, the usefulness of many birth defects epidemiology studies is limited by failure to consider the etiologic heterogeneity of human congenital abnormalities or the fact that most teratogenic exposures produce a characteristic pattern of congenital anomalies and not a single malformation in an otherwise normal child.

A statistically significant association in an epidemiological study is not sufficient to establish causality without other evidence to support such a conclusion. It is critically important that observed associations make biological sense. A chemical exposure cannot be teratogenic unless it is systemically absorbed by the mother and it or its metabolic products reach susceptible sites in the embryo or placenta.

Exposures that produce congenital anomalies do so only during times in which the involved structures in the embryo or fetus exhibit appropriate sensitivity. In most cases, exposure to a greater quantity of the agent can be expected to increase the likelihood of abnormalities. The existence of a reasonable pathogenic mechanism for the observed effect may provide further support for a causal inference.

TERATOGEN RISK COUNSELING

Providing teratogen risk counseling involves more than just identifying and estimating the magnitude of risk. The information must be communicated to the patient in a way that allows her to make informed decisions about the management of her pregnancy. The approach varies from patient to patient and depends on many factors, including the patient's cultural and social background, her understanding of the counselor's language, her level of general and scientific knowledge, and her commitment to the pregnancy. The uncertainty that usually exists complicates teratogen counseling and requires that information be provided as risks, which are difficult for many people to understand. Counselors need to be aware of the information and misinformation patients bring with them to the counseling session and how it affects their perception of risk (Koren et al., 1989). Finally, the importance most women place on having healthy children and the emotional circumstances that often surround teratogen risk counseling require that the counselor have considerable clinical skill as well as a thorough knowledge of clinical teratology.

Categories of teratogenic exposures

Teratogenic exposures may be conveniently grouped into four major categories on the basis of the kind of agent involved: infectious agents, physical agents, drug and chemical agents, and maternal metabolic factors. Since our current information on specific agents is incomplete, in this chapter we present only general summaries for several of the more important teratogenic exposures in each group. The reader is cautioned that considerable disagreement still exists over the role of many of these exposures in the production of human birth defects. Thus, the following discussion should be used as a guide, and standard medical references and the current literature should be consulted for a more thorough consideration of any particular agent. One should *not* use the information included in this chapter for counseling pregnant patients regarding the teratogenic

potential of particular exposures without consulting up-to-date information resources such as *TERIS* (http://depts.washington.edu/~terisweb/teris/index.html) or *REPROTOX* (http://www.reprotox.org) that are designed for this purpose.

Infectious agents

For many years clinicians have been aware of infectious agents that may attack the fetus in utero. Recognized effects on the fetus include death, intrauterine growth retardation, congenital defects, and mental retardation. The pathogenesis of these abnormalities can generally be ascribed to direct fetal infection, which may be associated with inflammation of fetal tissues and cellular death. Many, if not all, of these defects represent the "disruption" pathogenetic category (see Ch. 38).

Certain signs and symptoms characterize prenatal infections of the fetus and can therefore be used as indicators of a potential infectious etiology for a child's congenital abnormalities. Direct invasion of the nervous system may result in microcephaly, often associated with cerebral calcifications, mental retardation, disorders of movement and muscle tone (sometimes mischaracterized as "cerebral palsy", see Ch. 40), seizures, and central auditory and visual deficits. As the eye represents a direct developmental extension of the central nervous system, it is not surprising to find it frequently involved with such defects as chorioretinitis, cataracts, and microphthalmia. Furthermore, as the central nervous system controls limb movement, contractures and other fetal positional limb deformations are sometimes encountered in cases where severe central nervous system damage has occurred. However, other limb anomalies such as major intercalary limb reduction malformations, polydactyly, and syndactyly are not typically associated with teratogenic infections. Other general abnormalities associated with prenatal infections include prematurity, low birth weight for gestational age, and failure to thrive. Affected infants may exhibit evidence of widespread sepsis such as pneumonitis, hepatitis with hepatosplenomegaly and jaundice, and bleeding disorders manifested by petechiae and purpura. Chronic skin rashes and certain categories of congenital heart disease, such as stenotic vascular anomalies and defects due to disturbed blood flow, may also be associated with congenital infections (Klein and Remington, 1995).

Ophthalmologic examination and imaging studies in the infant may reveal additional signs of congenital infection. Serological studies in the mother and infant may be helpful, but "TORCH" screening alone is usually insufficient in newborns in whom a congenital infection is suspected because not all transplacental infections are included in this test and its sensitivity and specificity are limited. Specialized serological studies, culture of the organism, PCR for the organism's DNA, or other more specific approaches are usually necessary to diagnose a congenital infection in an affected infant with certainty (Klein and Remington, 1995).

VIRUSES

Rubella

Abnormalities associated with prenatal infection with rubella vary substantially in frequency, severity, and type according to the month of gestation in which the infection occurred (Cooper et al., 1995; Webster, 1998). From 40–85% of infants born to women with serologically-proven rubella infection during the first trimester of pregnancy have features of congenital rubella infection in early infancy. The incidence of severely affected children drops off rapidly with maternal rubella infection after the first trimester of pregnancy, but later-appearing manifestations, such as hearing loss, delayed intellectual development, and diabetes, are encountered in offspring of women infected later in pregnancy.

Rubella infection of the embryo may lead to miscarriage. Infants who are born after first-trimester rubella virus infection may display a wide variety of birth defects and health problems, including intrauterine growth retardation, subsequent failure to thrive, and congenital anomalies (Fig. 39.1). Ocular defects such as cataracts, pigmentary retinopathy, microphthalmia, and glaucoma are often present. Various cardiovascular anomalies, including patent ductus arteriosus, valvular and peripheral pulmonary arterial stenoses, atrial and ventricular septal defects, and possibly, other vascular stenotic lesions and tetralogy of Fallot, may occur. Myocardial damage, presumably stemming from myocarditis, has also been observed. Central nervous system abnormalities may include microcephaly, mental retardation, hypotonia, and convulsions. Signs of acute meningo-encephalitis or progressive panencephalitis may occur, and senorineural deafness or other sensory or functional disturbances often are present. Signs and symptoms of widespread systemic infection are common and may include hepatosplenomegaly, jaundice, thrombocytopenia, anemia, irregularities of ossification of the long bones, and delayed ossification of the calvarium. Affected children may also exhibit pneumonitis, a chronic rubelliform rash, generalized

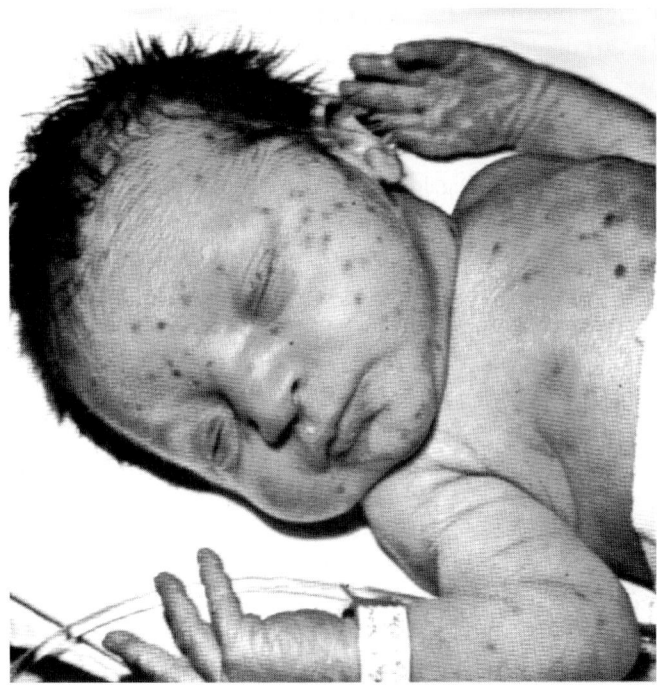

Fig. 39.1. A child with rubella embryopathy. Note the "blueberry muffin" petechial rash. (Photograph courtesy of Susan Reef, MD, National Congenital Rubella Syndrome Registry, Centers for Disease Control and Prevention.)

adenopathy, chronic diarrhea, diabetes mellitus, or thyroid disease. A variety of immune defects, such as thymic hypoplasia and hypogammaglobulinemia, may occur, often in association with recurrent or persistent infections. It is particularly important to note that the hearing and other neurologic deficits and endocrine disturbances may not be noted in the neonatal period but rather become apparent only after several months or years of age (Cooper et al., 1995).

Intrauterine diagnosis of fetal rubella infection can be accomplished by immunologic or molecular methods in the second trimester of pregnancy, but these methods cannot distinguish fetuses that will have rubella embryopathy from those that will have asymptomatic infections at birth (Valente and Sever, 1994; Jacquemard et al., 1995). Some manifestations of rubella embryopathy, such as cardiac defects or fetal growth retardation, can sometimes be identified prenatally by detailed ultrasound examination.

Prevention of congenital rubella syndrome is possible through routine immunization of children with rubella vaccine (Cooper et al., 1995). Although use of attenuated live rubella vaccines in pregnant women is contraindicated, inadvertent immunization of women with such vaccines early in pregnancy has not been associated with an increased risk to the fetus (Best, 1991).

Cytomegalovirus

Congenital cytomegalovirus infection has assumed a position of increasing importance in recent years as a recognized cause of perinatal morbidity and mortality. Indeed, in periods when rubella is not epidemic, cytogemalovirus may represent the most common congenital infectious cause of mental retardation and other central nervous system disorders, including deafness (Daniel, et al., 1995; Stagno, 1995).

Congenital cytomegalovirus infection is common, but most infected infants are asymptomatic. Between 0.2% and 2.2% of newborn infants are congenitally infected, but only about 10% of these infants exhibit serious manifestations at birth (Daniel et al., 1995; Stagno, 1995). The risk of symptomatic involvement is highest in the children of women who had a primary cytomegalovirus infection during the first six months of gestation. Previous maternal infection and the presence of antibodies in the mother's blood do not prevent fetal infection, although such antibodies appear to reduce the risk of symptomatic disease.

The classical picture of severe congenital cytomegalovirus infection includes central nervous system manifestations such as microcephaly, typically associated with diffuse periventricular calcifications reflecting an extensive encephalitis (Daniel, 1995; Stagno, 1995; Demmler, 1996). Less frequently, hydrocephalus may develop secondary to obstruction of the flow of cerobrospinal fluid. These central nervous system abnormalities are associated with functional disturbances, including mental retardation, spasticity, hypotonia, seizures, and strabismus. Ocular involvement is common with chorioretinitis, optic atrophy, microphthalmia, cataracts, retinal necrosis, calcifications and anomalies of the anterior chamber and optic disc, all of which may produce severe visual impairment. Hepatitis with resultant hepatosplenomegaly and jaundice may occur, and bone marrow disturbances may result in thrombocytopenia, with a generalized petechial rash or hemolytic anemia. Non-CNS malformations do not appear to be unusually frequent among infants with congenital cytomegalovirus infections.

Although most infants infected in utero with cytomegalovirus do not display clinical symptoms in the neonatal period, 10–15% of these children develop neurodevelopmental handicaps as a result of their infection later in life. Senosorineural hearing loss is most common. Other manifestations may include mental retardation, movement and coordination disorders, behavioral disturbances, and chorioretinitis (Daniel, 1995; Stagno, 1995; Demmler, 1996).

There is presently no effective vaccine against cytomegalovirus infection. Furthermore, since naturally acquired infection does not completely protect against subsequent maternal or fetal infection, it is not clear that immunization would be worthwhile. Thus, primary prevention consists mainly of avoiding cytomegalovirus exposures during pregnancy, a not-inconsiderable feat in view of the ubiquity of these organisms.

Detailed ultrasound examination can be used for prenatal diagnosis of fetal ventriculomegaly, cerebral calcification, and some other serious manifestations of fetal cytomegalovirus infection in the second or third trimester of pregnancy (Nelson and Demmler, 1997; Brown and Abernathy, 1998). Invasive testing can be used to demonstrate fetal infection but does not distinguish symptomatic from asymptomatic involvement of the fetus. Such invasive testing is most informative when there is evidence of fetal disease on ultrasound examination.

Varicella-zoster virus

Although varicella infections and zosteriform eruptions during pregnancy are relatively infrequent, a congenital varicella syndrome has been recognized since 1947 (Laforet and Lynch). The risk for the fetus to display significant teratogenic effects when the mother contracts varicella during pregnancy is small—2% or less, depending on gestational age (Enders et al., 1994; Jones et al., 1994; Pastuszak et al., 1994). The most susceptible period of pregnancy for such effects is between 13 and 20 weeks gestation (Enders et al., 1994). The risk of fetal damage related to maternal zoster during pregnancy appears to be much lower than with maternal varicella (Enders et al., 1994; Gershon, 1995).

Children infected with varicella-zoster virus in utero may display growth deficiency and microcephaly with cortical atrophy, often resulting in convulsions and mental retardation. Other neurologic sequelae may include peripheral nerve palsies, muscle weakness, and paralysis or muscular atrophy. Secondary positional limb deformities may occur, and ocular involvement—microphthalmia, cataracts, and chorioretinitis—may be seen. Limb anomalies may include distal phalangeal hypoplasia or hypoplasia of an entire limb, possibly secondary to denervation. Cutaneous abnormalities—scars, vesicles, epidermal hypoplasia, and other bizarre craniofacial or limb anomalies, possibly secondary to in utero ulceration—may be present. Respiratory distress, pneumonitis, repeated infections and hearing deficiency have occasionally been reported (Enders et al., 1994; Gershon, 1995).

Some manifestations of varicella embryopathy can be detected prenatally by ultrasound examination (Ghidini and

Lynch, 1994; Chapman, 1998), but affected fetuses cannot always be identified. No reliable means has been established for prenatal diagnosis of varicella embryopathy by amniocentesis or chorionic villus sampling (Gershon, 1995).

Varicella infection of children or adults usually confers long-term immunity to chickenpox, although reactivation of a latent varicella-zoster virus infection may occur, producing zoster. Passive immunization with varicella-zoster immune globulin (VZIG) within 96 hours of exposure is recommended for pregnant women who have been in close contact with someone with varicella or zoster and who are seronegative or have no history of having had chickenpox themselves (Gershon, 1995; Holmes et al., 1996). Passive immunization of a pregnant woman who has already developed clinical manifestations of chickenpox seems unlikely to prevent transmission of varicella-zoster virus to the fetus.

Limited information is currently available concerning possible risks to the fetus arising from maternal immunization during pregnancy with live attenuated varicella virus vaccine. A registry to collect outcome data from unintentionally exposed pregnancies has been initiated by the manufacturer with assistance from the Centers for Disease Control and Prevention (Anonymous, 1996). Preliminary analysis of data from this registry shows no indication of an adverse effect on the fetus, but the data are insufficient to rule out an effect similar in magnitude to that seen with natural maternal chicken pox during pregnancy. Secondary transmission of vaccine virus may occur.

Human immunodeficiency virus (HIV; AIDS)

Rates of HIV transmission from mother to fetus range from 14–25% in most studies from the United States and Europe in which maternal antiretroviral treatment was not given during pregnancy (Rodriguez et al., 1997; Minkoff, 1998). Maternal antiretroviral treatment late in pregnancy decreases the rate of vertical transmission of HIV by about two-thirds (Anonymous, 1998; Burns and Mofenson 1999). The safety of antiretroviral treatment early in pregnancy with respect to teratogenesis has not been established.

Congenital HIV infections usually follow one of two courses in untreated children (Scarlatti, 1996; Wiznia et al., 1996; Burns and Mofenson, 1999). Most have a slow progression that resembles AIDS in adults, but 10–25% of congenitally infected infants become symptomatic in the first year of life, suffer rapid progression, and die very early. Affected infants may exhibit failure to thrive, interstitial pneumonia, recurrent bacterial and other infections, chronic diarrhea, and generalized lymphadenopathy (Wiznia et al., 1996; Rodriguez et al., 1997). Growth retardation is common, and microcephaly, developmental delay, progressive encephalopathy, and other neurological abnormalities are often seen. Malformations do not appear to be unusually frequent among the children of HIV-infected women (Mueller and Pizzo, 1995; Brocklehurst and French, 1998).

Parvovirus B19

Parvovirus infection causes fifth disease (erythema infectiosum) in children. Infections in adults may produce a rash or arthropathy but are often asymptomatic. Fetal infection with parvovirus B19 can cause severe anemia, hydrops, and death (Torok, 1995; Levy et al., 1997; Markenson and Yancey, 1998; Rodis et al., 1998). Many infected fetuses that develop hydrops die, but the hydrops may spontaneously resolve. Less-severely affected fetuses may have meconium peritonitis, isolated ascites, increased nuchal thickness, or pleural or pericardial effusions.

Transplacental parvovirus B19 infection occurs in $\frac{1}{4}$ to $\frac{1}{2}$ of cases of maternal primary infection during pregnancy, but in most instances there is no apparent adverse effect on the fetus (Torok, 1995; Miller et al., 1998a). The excess fetal loss attributable to parvovirus B19 infection during the first 20 weeks of gestation is estimated to be between 2–9% in various studies. The risk of fetal death is lower with maternal infection later in pregnancy.

Persistent congenital anemia has been observed in infants born after intrauterine parvovirus B19 infection (Brown et al., 1994). Myocarditis, myositis, arthrogryposis, and ocular and central nervous system anomalies have also been reported after documented intrauterine parvovirus B19 infection (Rodis et al., 1998; Torok, 1995), but such observations are rare. No measurable increase in the frequency of malformations or neurological abnormalities was found among the infants of women who had parvovirus B19 infections during pregnancy in most studies (Miller et al, 1998a; Rodis et al., 1998).

Testing for specific IgM antibody in serum is the standard means of diagnosing parvovirus B19 infection and of distinguishing primary and secondary infection in a pregnant woman (Brown et al., 1994b; Torok, 1995; Markenson and Yancey, 1998; Rodis, 1999). Prenatal diagnosis of affected fetuses is often possible by ultrasonography and maternal serum α-fetoprotein and human chorionic gonadotropin screening (Torok, 1995; Markenson and Yancey, 1998). Detection of viral DNA in amniotic fluid or fetal blood is useful in documenting fetal infection with parvovirus B19 (Torok, 1995; Levy et al., 1997; Markenson and Yancey, 1998). Intrauterine transfusion may be beneficial in some cases of fetal hydrops associated with parvovirus B19 infection (Levy et al., 1997; Markenson and Yancey, 1998; Rodis, 1999).

Other possible teratogenic viral infections

Herpes simplex virus infections are very common, and once they occur, are persistent and recurrent. Transplacental fetal infection with herpes simplex virus is, fortunately, rare, but the effects on the fetus can be devastating (Whitley and Arvin, 1995). They may include chorioretinitis, microcephaly, various disruptive structural lesions of the brain, growth retardation and typical skin lesions. Disseminated infection with death in the neonatal period may occur; surviving children may be mentally retarded. This severe herpes simplex embryopathy must be distinguished from neonatal herpes simplex infection acquired during or immediately after delivery, a much more frequent and better recognized entity (Whitley and Arvin, 1995; Jacobs, 1988).

Transplacental infection with lymphocytic choriomeningitis virus is an uncommon occurrence that is often asymptomatic in the mother. Fetal infection has been associated with abortion and with hydrocephalus and chorioretinitis in surviving infants (Arvin and Maldonado, 1995).

Concerns have been raised about possible teratogenic effects of several other viruses, including influenza virus, Ebstein-Barr virus, measles virus, mumps virus, and various enteroviruses (Remington and Klein, 1995). Most of these viruses have been associated with miscarriage in epidemiological studies, but evidence that these agents infect the embryo or fetus and cause serious disruptive lesions is lacking or very limited and controversial. It can be anticipated that future studies will clarify these questions and identify other teratogenic viral infections.

BACTERIA

Although a host of bacterial agents may infect the fetus antenatally, only syphilis is thought to have a significant teratogenic potential. Nevertheless, many intraamnionic bacterial infections can have devastating fetal consequences. Furthermore, as discussed later, high sustained fever associated with such infections may itself cause damage. The clinical signs and symptoms, which could be used as indicators of a possible prenatal bacterial infection, are very similar to those for the various viral agents described previously.

Congenital heart defects were more frequent than expected in an area where Lyme disease is endemic in one study (Williams et al., 1995), but no association between congenital heart defects and maternal Lyme disease during pregnancy was found in a more recent large case-control study (Strobino et al., 1999). Prompt antibiotic treatment is recommended for women who develop Lyme disease during pregnancy (Gardner, 1995; Silver, 1997).

Syphilis

Congenital syphilis is certainly the oldest if not the most venerable of the known prenatal teratogenic infections, having been recognized now for more than five hundred years. Presently available information indicates that the clinical manifestations of prenatal syphilis are related to both the time of gestation in which the fetal infection occurs and the duration of the untreated infection in the mother prior to pregnancy (Ingall et al., 1995). Although little direct information is available to confirm such a conclusion, it has been generally believed that infection of the fetus usually does not occur before the fourth month of pregnancy. The frequency of congenital syphilis in the child of a woman who has untreated primary or secondary syphilis during pregnancy is 40–50%. Many such pregnancies are delivered prematurely, and many of the infants are stillborn or die in the perinatal period. Syphilitic infections later in pregnancy result in lower risks to the fetus, with approximately 70% of late syphilitic infections resulting in the birth of normal healthy infants and only 10% showing signs of congenital syphilis. Fetal growth retardation may occur, and a wide variety of congenital problems may result.

The manifestations in the fetus may be overlooked in the newborn infant, and structural congenital anomalies are not frequent. Signs of syphilis in the child have been grouped into those that present within the first two years of life (early congenital syphilis) and those that appear later. Infants with early congenital syphilis are often hydropic, have a relatively large placenta and may display widespread evidence of hematogenous infection such as hepatosplenomegaly, jaundice, generalized lymphadenitis, anemia, thrombocytopenia, and leukemoid reactions. Rhinitis and various other cutaneous and mucosal rashes and lesions—including vesicular or bullous eruptions, maculopapular rashes that may desquamate, mucous patches, petechial lesions, edema, and condylomata lata—may occur in up to 60% of patients. Osteitis is frequent and may mimic an Erb's palsy or present as an irritable infant. Syphilitic nephrosis may appear during the second or third month of life, and other evidence of generalized infection such as bronchopneumonia, failure to thrive, or malabsorption may be encountered. Nervous system manifestations such as meningitis, cranial nerve palsies, intracerebral vascular lesions, and progressive hydrocephalus are frequent. Convulsions and hemiplegia may also occur.

There may be a generalized chorioretinitis and uveitis, and optic atrophy, glaucoma, and chancres of the eyelid may be seen (Ingall et al., 1995).

Later manifestations of congenital syphilis, commonly occurring beyond the age of two years, are also widespread. The most characteristic features are Hutchinson teeth (peg-shaped and notched permanent upper central incisors), mulberry molars, interstitial keratitis, and sensorineural deafness. Frontal bossing is also a frequent, but not specific, finding. Poor maxillary growth and saddle nose deformity are frequent craniofacial manifestations, and deep linear facial scars, particularly around body orifices (rhagades) are typical late cutaneous manifestations. Late neurological features include mental retardation, hydrocephalus, convulsions, cranial nerve palsies and optic atrophy (Ingall et al., 1995).

Prompt treatment of mother and infant is extremely important in congenital syphilis, particularly if the infant is symptomatic. Penicillin is the drug of choice.

PARASITES

Although several parasitic agents are known to cross the placenta and infect the fetus, only toxoplasmosis has been clearly shown to produce congenital anomalies. Malaria may rarely produce central nervous system damage (Remington and Klein, 1995).

Toxoplasmosis

Congenital toxoplasmosis has been recognized for several decades. The major risk to the fetus arises from primary toxoplasmosis infections during pregnancy. The frequency and severity of fetal effects are strongly related to the stage of gestation in which the exposure occurs. The risk of transmission with primary maternal infection increases from about 1% around the time of conception to more than 90% near term. Most fetal infections do not cause permanent damage, but clinical manifestations of the disease are more likely and more severe with infections earlier in pregnancy. The highest risk for having a baby with severe manifestations is estimated to be 10–40% with maternal infection between 10 and 24 weeks of gestation (Remington et al., 1995; Lynfield and Guerina, 1997). Many more infants, especially those whose mothers acquire *Toxoplasma* infection in the second or third trimester of pregnancy, have mild or subclinical involvement, but these infants may develop chorioretinitis or neurological abnormalities later in childhood if not treated after birth (Remington et al., 1995).

As with other prenatal infections, congenital toxoplasmosis includes a wide range of manifestations (Remington et al., 1995; Boyer, 1996). It is often overlooked in the newborn period because of the subtlety of its manifestations. Clinically-apparent disease is commonly associated with central nervous system abnormalities. These may include microcephaly, hydrocephaly, intracranial calcification, mental retardation and seizures. In addition, chorioretinitis, microphthalmia, glaucoma, and cataracts are frequent. Other signs of generalized sepsis may occur with hepatitis, resulting in hepatomegaly and jaundice, and thrombocytopenia, resulting in anemia. Pneumonitis, diarrhea, skin rash, lymphadenopathy and other signs of generalized infection may be present. Even if the features are more subtle in the neonatal period, long term follow-up has revealed a high percentage of mental retardation, convulsions, spasticity, visual impairment, and deafness in children with serious toxoplasmosis infections. *Toxoplasma* infection during pregnancy can also cause miscarriage.

Diagnosis of primary maternal infection by *Toxoplasma* is usually based on serological studies. Prenatal diagnosis by amniocentesis, chorionic villus sampling, or fetal blood sampling can be used to demonstrate most, but not all, fetal infections in pregnant women with primary *Toxoplasma* infections (Abboud et al., 1997; Fricker-Hidalgo et al., 1997; Beazley and Egerman, 1998). Ultrasound examination is useful in identifying hydrocephalus, hydrops, and other severe manifestations of fetal infection but is not a reliable means of determining whether transmission of *Toxoplasma* to the fetus has occurred. Prompt treatment of the infant is important when congenital toxoplasmosis is diagnosed at birth (Remington et al., 1995; Lynfield and Guerina, 1997). Treatment of the mother is often recommended when maternal *Toxoplasma* infection is documented early in pregnancy (Boyer, 1996; Alger, 1997; Wallon et al., 1997).

Screening of pregnant women remains controversial and is not generally recommend in North America or the United Kingdom (Boyer, 1996; Alger, 1997; Wallon et al., 1999). The only satisfactory preventive measure is avoidance of *Toxoplasma* infection during pregnancy by avoiding ingestion of infected foods and contact with the oocysts. Generally, this means avoiding handling or eating raw meat (especially red meat) and eggs, and avoiding exposure to materials such as cat feces that may contain the oocysts.

Physical agents

A wide variety of physical agents are potentially teratogenic for the fetus (Brent, 1999a). Among these, the most important are ionizing radiation, mechanical factors, and possibly heat. Although public concern continues, present evidence does not support any causal relationship between birth defects in humans and commonly-encountered low-energy exposures to sound waves, ultrasound examination, microwaves, or computer terminals (Bentur, 1994; Brent 1999a, b; Robert, 1996, 1999; Ziskin, 1999).

IONIZING RADIATION

A considerable amount of attention has been directed to the possibility of adverse effects from high-energy radiation on fetal growth and development. In particular, episodes such as the Chernobyl nuclear power reactor accident have unrealistically heightened concern over the role high-energy radiation plays in human malformations (Castronovo, 1999; Dolk and Nichols, 1999). A careful examination of available information must address three related concerns: teratogenesis, mutagenesis, and carcinogenesis. Although most exposures to high-energy radiation during pregnancy are avoidable, some exposures in both medical facilities and in the workplace continue to occur. In some instances, valid medical indications exist for deliberate exposure of a pregnant woman to ionizing radiation. In such cases, as with the use of any potentially teratogenic agent during pregnancy, risk/benefit comparisons must be carefully made and a decision reached by the patient and her physician after careful discussion and consideration. When exposure of a pregnant woman to ionizing radiation is necessary, the dosage to the fetus should be minimized.

Teratogenesis

Concern over possible teratogenic effects of high-energy radiation came both from studies with experimental animals and epidemiologic studies of the offspring of survivors of nuclear explosions at the end of World War II. These experiences suggest that very high doses of high-energy radiation (>200 cGy) can produce prenatal-onset growth retardation, central nervous system damage, including microcephaly, and ocular defects (Brent, 1999a). Other abnormalities produced by large doses of high-energy radiation appear to be exceedingly rare in humans, if they exist at all. Furthermore, both the rate and fractionation of the radiation dosage are extremely important considerations, as slow dosage rates or division of the dose over a period of days markedly reduces the effects of the total dosage. Thus, it would appear that under ordinary circumstances, only therapeutic levels of radiation delivered to the region of the developing embryo during the first months of pregnancy have a demonstrable risk of significant anomalies for the fetus (Brent, 1999a).

Much lower doses of radiation, as might occur from intravenous pyelography, gastrointestinal tract examination, CT scanning or other diagnostic studies are, of course, far more frequent in the population. Exposure of a pregnant woman to such low radiation doses at any time during gestation produces an extremely low or negligible risk for malformations in the offspring (Bentur, 1994; Brent, 1999a). This is not to imply that radiographic exposures may be conducted with total impunity during pregnancy. Even an extremely low risk should be avoided unless there is an important benefit expected.

Mutagenesis

The mutagenic effect of high-energy radiation is well known. Present evidence suggests that there may be no threshold for this effect. Thus, even low-dose natural exposures to radiation contribute to the total population load of mutations. By the same token then, radiation exposures even at diagnostic levels may have potential mutational implications for an exposed fetus (Brent, 1999a). It is estimated that 1 cGy of radiation to a particular gene locus in a particular cell produces a risk of mutation on the order of 10^{-7}. This would suggest that a germ cell exposed to 1 cGy of radiation may have on the order of 1 chance in 1000 to have undergone a mutation of some type. However, as most such mutations are probably lethal, the chance for fertilization of that cell to result in an individual with a genetic disorder is probably substantially less.

Ordinarily the radiation-exposed fetus would itself not suffer from a genetic disorder produced in this fashion. Rather, potential offspring of that fetus in subsequent generations might manifest the disorder. By implication then, gonadal irradiation at any time during life before conception may have some small risk of a significant mutation in the offspring. The load of such mutations presumably increases throughout a person's lifetime but in the aggregate is still a very small absolute risk under ordinary circumstances.

Carcinogenesis

Concern over the carcinogenic potential of prenatal radiation may be a slightly more realistic concern (Boice and Miller, 1999). However, the magnitude of the risk is again substantially lower than is ordinarily understood by the lay public. Studies of leukemogenesis stemming from prenatal exposures to X-irradiation suggest that the relative risk from common low-dose exposures is no greater than 1.5 and may be substantially less for an exposed fetus to develop leukemia. In other words, the absolute risk at worst may rise from 1 chance in 3000 to 1 chance in 2000 for such an exposed individual to develop leukemia.

Summary

Common environmental exposures to high-energy radiation through diagnostic X-ray examination or other similar low-dose exposures produce only very low risks to the fetus or offspring of an individual (Bentur, 1994; Brent, 1999a). Although such exposures should be avoided whenever possible as a matter of prudence, inadvertent exposures or exposures for valid medical indications should not be a major source of concern.

HEAT

Possible sources of fetal hyperthermia include high fever of whatever origin and other factors that produce substantial elevation in the body temperature, such as excessive use of a steam bath or hot tub. Studies in laboratory animals strongly suggest that hyperthermia may be teratogenic at critical stages of neural tube development (Edwards et al., 1995; Graham et al., 1998). The situation is less clear for humans, but most studies are limited by poor documentation of the degree and duration of fever or other form of hyperthermia that occurred during pregnancy. In addition, fever usually accompanies serious infections, and such infections or their treatment may also have teratogenic potential in some instances. Nevertheless, an increased frequency of neural tube defects has been found in association with high fever during the period of neural tube closure in some studies (Chambers et al., 1998; Graham et al., 1998; Shaw et al, 1998). A number of anecdotal cases of neuromigrational errors, Moebius syndrome, and neurogenic arthrogryposis have also been reported in the offspring of women having hyperthermic events during the first or second trimester of pregnancy (Graham et al., 1998). The risk associated with substantial hyperthermia during pregnancy has not been clearly defined and probably depends on the severity, duration, and gestational timing of the fever or other exposure. It would seem prudent to avoid extreme prolonged hyperthermic exposures whenever possible during pregnancy.

Serial detailed ultrasound examination is useful for prenatal diagnosis of some kinds of severe central nervous system damage following such episodes, and maternal serum α-fetoprotein screening for neural tube defects is indicated if the exposure occurred between four and six weeks after the last normal menstrual period. Infants born after such exposures should be carefully examined and followed for possible central nervous system abnormalities.

MECHANICAL FACTORS

Although the effects of fetal constraint on fetal growth have been recognized for some years, relatively little attention has been paid to the effects of in utero mechanical factors on fetal morphogenesis. Fetal growth or movement may be constrained by a variety of mechanical factors, for example, uterine malformation, large uterine myomas, oligohydramnios (whether of maternal of fetal origin), intraamniotic fibrous bands, or multifetal gestation.

It is relatively easy to understand how fetal constraint could result in the category of anomalies known as *deformations*. Such anomalies are the result of mechanical forces that entrap and physically compress structures of the developing fetus (Smith and Graham, 1988). Included in this category are plagiocephaly and such positional limb deformities as clubfoot, dislocated hips, and perhaps arthrogryposis, particularly in predisposed fetuses. Such anomalies could theoretically be produced at any time during prenatal life and would seem particularly likely to occur if the degree of constraint is severe or if the fetus is predisposed because of neurologic impairment. All of these fetal anomalies are etiologically heterogenous, and similar defects may result from mechanisms other than constraint.

Recognition of factors such as uterine malformation, oligohydramnios or multifetal gestation, that predispose to fetal constraint should alert the physician to the possibility of adverse consequences to the fetus or newborn. These anomalies are often effectively treated by taking advantage of the relatively normal growth potential of the "deformed" tissues through casting or other essentially mechanical forms of therapy.

By the same token, recognition of deformations in the newborn infant should alert the physician to the possibility of fetal constraint in utero. For instance, features of severe in utero compression are a common part of the so-called Potter sequence as a consequence of oligohydramnios, whether of fetal (renal hypoplasia) or nonfetal (premature rupture of the fetal membranes with amniotic fluid leakage) origin. The presence of deformations should alert the practitioner to the possibility of other disturbances of fetal growth that may commonly be associated, e.g., club foot and pulmonary hypoplasia with consequent respiratory distress resulting from oligohydramnios.

Evidence that the mechanical trauma associated with early prenatal diagnosis by chorionic villus sampling (CVS) or amniocentesis may occasionally cause fetal anomalies is of particular concern to medical geneticists. CVS prior to 10–11 weeks gestation, i.e., during or shortly after formation of the limbs in the embryo, has been associated with an increased risk of limb reduction defects and oromandibular-limb hypogenesis syndrome (Botto et al., 1996; Firth, 1997). The risk appears to be greater and the defects more severe with earlier procedures. It is unclear whether or not an increased risk for fetal limb defects exists with later CVS procedures; if so, the risk is very small (Firth, 1997; Jenkins and Wapner, 1999). There is also some evidence that cavernous hemangiomas, intestinal atresia, gastroschisis, and club foot are more common than expected among children born to women who had CVS (Stoler et al., 1999), but further study is needed to define these risks more clearly and to determine whether they also depend on the gestational age at which the procedure is done.

Two randomized controlled trials of early amniocentesis found a small but significantly increased frequency of talipes equinovarus among infants born to women who had undergone the procedure at $11–12^6/_7$ weeks gestation (Sundberg et al., 1997; CEMAT Group, 1998; Farrell et al., 1999). The risk was much greater when amniotic fluid leakage occurred following early amniocentesis. Talipes equinovarus does not appear to be more frequent than expected among the children of women who have undergone amniocentesis after 15 weeks gestation.

Drug and chemical agents

Since the thalidomide disaster, increasing attention has been focused on the role of drug and chemical agents in the environment to which pregnant women might be exposed. Unfortunately, not only has there been a proliferation of both therapeutic agents and environmental chemicals during the past four decades, it has also become increasingly clear that self-medication by pregnant women using a variety of over-the-counter, herbal, and traditional medicines is a common practice. In addition, many pregnancies are unplanned, and inadvertent chemical and drug exposures are frequent. Finally, women may have medical conditions for which treatment is necessary regardless of pregnancy.

For all of these reasons, health professionals who care for pregnant women often must deal with their concerns about possible teratogenic effects of drug and other chemical exposures. Far too little is known about the teratogenic potential of most drug and chemical exposures. Several major categories of agents are considered here: environ-mental chemicals, nonprescription drugs, and prescription drugs.

The pathogenetic mechanisms by which most drug and chemical agents produce birth defects are just beginning to be understood. These mechanisms probably include derangements of cellular growth, controlled cell death (apotosis), cell signaling and other basic morphogenetic processes. In addition, some agents can kill cells and destroy tissue directly, leading to defects of the disruption category. It is also possible that some agents act by interfering with nervous system function, thereby enhancing the liability to deformation-type fetal anomalies.

ENVIRONMENTAL CHEMICALS

Recognition of the pollution of our environment by an ever-proliferating group of compounds has caused serious concern regarding the potential impact on the developing fetus. Relatively little is known about the teratogenic potential of many of these exposures in humans. Fortunately, however, efforts to limit exposures for the public at large and for occupationally-exposed adults often provide a measure of protection for the fetus as well. Nevertheless, organic mercurial compounds provide testimony to the teratogenic potential that environmental exposures can have.

Organic mercury compounds

Ingestion by a pregnant woman of food that is heavily contaminated with methylated mercury compounds can cause severe damage to the developing central nervous system of her fetus (Choi, 1989; Harada, 1995). Clusters of affected infants have been observed after maternal consumption of methylmercury-contaminated fish in Minamata, Japan, and of grain treated with methylmercury fungicides in Iraq. The frequent outcome of such pregnancies is children with severe central nervous system damage and microcephaly, resulting in a static encephalopathy that presents as "cerebral palsy." Maternal neurotoxicity often occurs in these cases as well, but the fetus appears to be more sensitive than the adult to this effect. Malformations do not appear to be unusually frequent in affected infants.

Other environmental chemicals

Women who used cooking oil that was heavily contaminated with PCBs during pregnancy had infants with intra-uterine growth retardation and a transient dark-brown staining of the skin ("cola-colored babies") (Schantz, 1996; Jacobson and Jacobson, 1997). Developmental delay was also observed in these children. Subsequent studies of infants whose mothers consumed PCBs in much smaller amounts during pregnancy have produced inconsistent findings.

Although there has been considerable concern about maternal exposures to other environmental contaminants, there is no compelling evidence of teratogenic effects of such exposures in humans. Adequate studies are often difficult to perform because of uncertainty about the magnitude of individual exposures and the causal heterogeneity of birth defects in humans. Avoiding toxic exposures during pregnancy as much as possible is certainly a prudent precaution.

"RECREATIONAL" DRUGS

Among the host of drugs that individuals in our society habitually use and abuse, alcohol and tobacco clearly stand out as the most important public health problems for both adults and the developing embryo or fetus. Adverse effects on the offspring have also been associated with maternal abuse of cocaine and some other "recreational" drugs during pregnancy.

Ethyl alcohol

Ethanol leads the list of abused drugs in the United States and in many other parts of the world. Thus, it is perhaps surprising that recognition of the adverse effects of this agent on fetal growth and development did not occur sooner. Historical reviews suggest that such a possibility was indeed recognized by at least some individuals for hundreds if not thousands of years (Warner and Rosett, 1975). However, the studies of Smith and Jones (Jones et al., 1973; Hanson et al., 1976) and others (Ouellette et al., 1977; Streissguth, 1977; Clarren and Smith, 1978) during the 1970s led to general acceptance of the teratogenic potential of maternal alcohol abuse during pregnancy. Pathogenesis, treatment, and prevention of alcohol-related birth defects are now subjects of intensive investigation, and recognition of the fetal alcohol syndrome has resulted in important changes in public policy and social norms regarding drinking by pregnant women (Stratton et al., 1995)

It is now clear that prenatal exposure to ethanol can result in a wide spectrum of effects on the embryo and fetus. The frequency and severity of these anomalies appears to be dose-related and ranges from apparently unaffected children to severely affected children with the fetal alcohol syndrome. Severe fetal alcohol syndrome occurs among infants born to chronically alcoholic women, but there is

considerable disagreement about the amount of ethanol necessary to cause milder degrees fetal damage (Mills and Graubard, 1987; Stratton et al., 1995). Some evidence suggests that consumption of as little as two drinks per day in early pregnancy, or periodic binge drinking (e.g., five or more drinks on a single occasion) in early pregnancy, may be associated with recognizable (though milder) abnormalities in a significant percentage of exposed newborns (Streissguth, 1992; Gladstone et al., 1996; Jacobson et al., 1998). Studies of binge drinking in a primate model support concern about this pattern of drinking (Clarren et al., 1988; 1992).

Full clinically-recognizable fetal alcohol syndrome occurs in about 6% of children of women who drink heavily during pregnancy (Day and Richardson, 1991). Less severe alcohol-related birth defects and neurocognitive deficits occur in a much larger proportion of these children, but the estimated frequency varies widely in different studies. The risk of full fetal alcohol syndrome is much higher for alcoholic women who have already had an affected child (Abel, 1988).

The fetal alcohol syndrome is characterized by a distinctive facial appearance, prenatal-onset growth deficiency, developmental delay and mental retardation, and an increased frequency of major congenital anomalies. Children with this syndrome display a rather flat midface with narrow palpebral fissures, a low nasal bridge, short upturned nose, and long smooth philtrum with a narrow vermilion border of the upper lip (Fig. 39.2). Presenting as small-for-gestational-age babies in the neonatal period, they continue to grow poorly and often are admitted to the hospital for evaluation of "failure to thrive." They may be described as jittery or tremulous babies, a feature that often results in confusion with drug withdrawal symptoms. However, these necrologic abnormalities persist and in addition to developmental delay and mental retardation, such children are often poorly coordinated, tremulous, and sometimes hyperactive in later life. A wide variety of congenital anomalies has been associated with this syndrome, including cleft palate, cardiac malformations (especially atrial and ventricular septal defects), microphthalmia, joint anomalies, and a variety of dermal and skeletal abnormalities (Ginsburg et al., 1991; Coles, 1992). Neuropathologic examination often shows abnormalities of neuronal migration, occasionally associated with microcephaly, hydrocephaly, absence of the corpus callosum, and other midline anomalies, as well as cerebellar abnormalities (Roebuck et al., 1998). In addition, maternal alcohol use during pregnancy has been associated with an increased risk of acute myeloid leukemia and other malignant neoplasms in the offspring (Kiess et al., 1984; Severson et al., 1993; Shu et al., 1996).

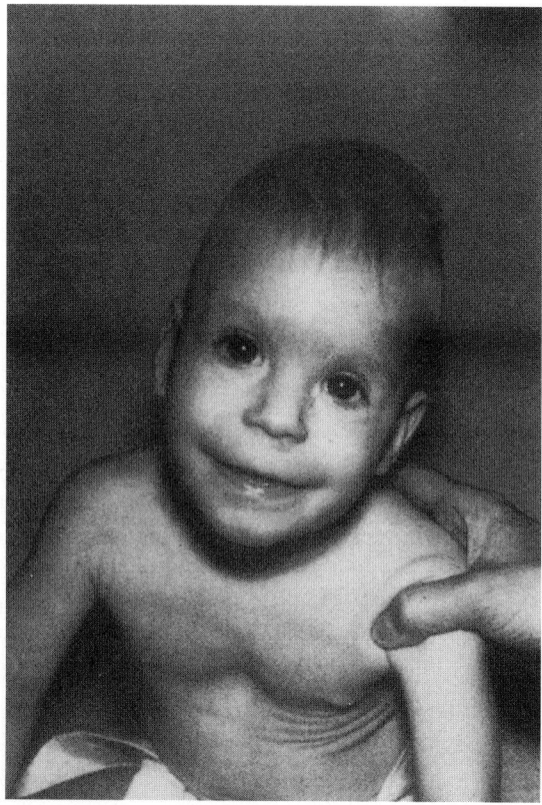
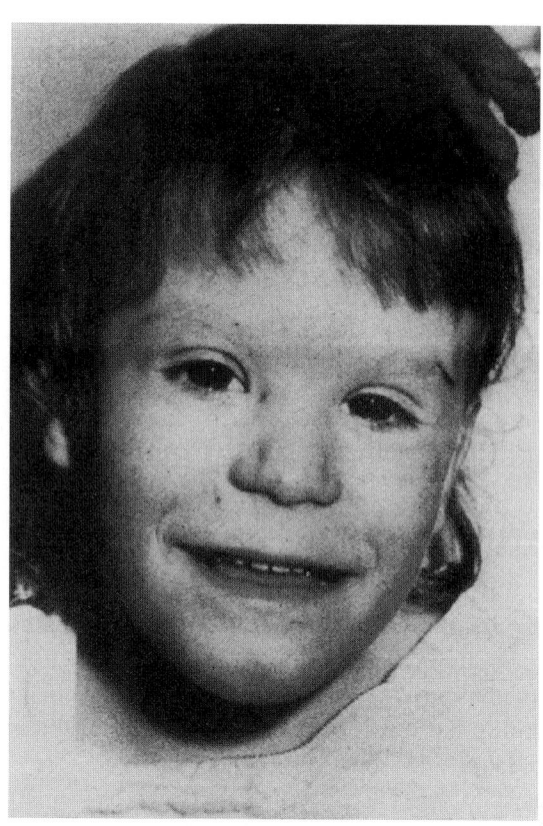

A   B

Fig. 39.2. Facial features of the fetal alcohol syndrome in a child (A) at 16 months of age (B) at four years of age. Note narrow palpebral fissures, midfacial hypoplasia and long philtrum with narrow vermilion border. (From Hanson et al., 1976, with permission.)

Epidemiologic studies suggest that prenatal damage from maternal alcohol abuse may be one of the most frequent recognizable causes of mental deficiency in the United States (Sampson et al., 1997). Disabilities due to prenatal alcohol abuse are an important public health problem (Sampson et al., 1997; Fast et al., 1999)—particularly distressing because virtually all such exposures are avoidable. The increase in ethanol abuse by children and adolescents suggest that this problem may well become more prevalent in the near future. Pregnant women, or women who might become pregnant, should avoid ethanol as much as possible—the safest amount being none at all.

Tobacco smoking

Maternal smoking during pregnancy interferes with fetal growth in a significant fashion (Werler, 1997). Birth weight, length and head circumference tend to be decreased in exposed babies. This growth deficiency is dose-related and reversible in early childhood (Lassen and Oei, 1998).

Women who smoke heavily during pregnancy also have higher than expected rates of spontaneous abortion, late fetal death, neonatal death, and prematurity (Werler, 1997; Greenhouse and Stillman, 1998). Slightly lower measured intelligence levels and increased frequencies of hyperactivity have been reported in these children (Lassen and Oei, 1998). Maternal smoking during pregnancy has also been associated with a small increase in some birth defects, especially cleft lip and palate and cleft palate alone (Werler, 1997; Wyszynski et al, 1997). The risk appears to be greater among a subset of infants who have genetic variants that predispose to orofacial clefting (Shaw et al., 1996; Romitti et al., 1999).

The common association between smoking and concomitant alcohol and other drug abuse raises concern about potential interactive effects between tobacco and other potentially teratogenic exposures. Pregnant women should be advised to avoid smoking. Smokers who are unable to stop should be advised to cut down the amount of smoking as much as possible, as this would appear to improve fetal outcome.

Cocaine

The extensive medical literature on the effects of maternal cocaine use in pregnancy is difficult to interpret (LaGasse et al., 1999; Tronick and Beeghly, 1999). Most studies are bedeviled by confounding factors, deficiencies in design, and poor documentation of the frequency, timing, and dosage of the mothers' use of cocaine, other illicit drugs, and alcohol. Moreover, there appears to be a systematic publication bias in favor of studies that show an association and against those that do not find an association between maternal cocaine use and untoward pregnancy outcomes.

Vascular disruptions occur with increased frequency in infants whose mothers abused cocaine during pregnancy, especially in the second or third trimester. Involvement of the central nervous system has been reported most often (Frank et al., 1998). Other congenital anomalies thought to result from vascular disruption—segmental intestinal atresia, gastroschisis, sirenomelia, limb-body wall complex, and limb reduction defects—have also been associated with maternal abuse of cocaine during pregnancy in some studies (Delaney-Black et al., 1994). Associations with other kinds of congenital anomalies have been reported as well, but the findings are inconsistent. Cocaine's vasoconstrictive and hypertensive actions probably account for the increased frequency of placental abruption observed among pregnant women who abuse this drug (Frank et al., 1996; Hulse et al., 1997).

Prenatal growth retardation has consistently been noted among infants whose mothers abused cocaine during pregnancy, but the effect appears to be due at least in part to concomitant exposure to alcohol or cigarette smoking (Frank et al., 1996; Hulse et al., 1997). By school age the growth of these children is indistinguishable from controls.

Many studies have demonstrated a subtle pattern of neonatal behavioral abnormalities among infants born to women who used cocaine during pregnancy (Frank et al., 1998; Chiriboga, 1998; Held et al., 1999). This pattern has been characterized as affecting "the four A's of infancy": attention, arousal, affect, and action. Studies in older children have been inconsistent, and interpretation is confounded by other differences that distinguish mothers who abuse cocaine during pregnancy from other women (Chiriboga, 1998; Tronick and Beeghly, 1999).

Toluene abuse

Maternal abuse of toluene by inhalation during pregnancy can produce a characteristic toluene embryopathy in the offspring (Wilkins-Haug, 1997; Jones and Balster, 1998). Affected children exhibit central nervous system dysfunction, developmental delay, attention deficit disorder, microcephaly, growth deficiency, short palpebral fissures, deep-set eyes, microagnathia, abnormal auricles, and small fingernails. The features resemble fetal alcohol syndrome.

Toluene embryopathy is associated with maternal inhalation of toluene in acute doses that may be 10–100 times greater than the occupational limit, which is averaged over a workday. Adverse fetal effects are unlikely with maternal exposure to less than the occupational threshold limit value of toluene during pregnancy, but it is prudent to avoid such exposure if possible.

Other drugs of abuse

Although many conflicting claims have been made regarding prenatal use of recreational drugs such as opiates, amphetamines, and LSD and other hallucinogens, there is little objective evidence that clearly implicates maternal abuse of such drugs as a cause of birth defects (Behnke and Eyler, 1993). Maternal drug abuse during pregnancy is associated with fetal growth retardation, increased perinatal mortality, and neonatal behavioral abnormalities, including drug withdrawal (Woods, 1996; Wagner et al., 1998). Children of women who abuse such drugs during pregnancy are clearly at increased risk for adverse outcomes, but it is difficult to determine whether these are effects of the drugs themselves or of social problems, infectious diseases, poor nutrition, or abuse of alcohol or cocaine, all of which often accompany drug abuse (Eyler and Behnke, 1999; LaGasse et al., 1999). For many reasons, including potential hazards to the fetus associated with all of these factors, pregnant women should not abuse drugs.

Caffeine

While caffeine is teratogenic in high doses in some species, no convincing evidence linking this substance to human congenital anomalies has emerged (Nehlig and Debry, 1994; Golding, 1995). Associations between maternal coffee drinking during pregnancy and miscarriage or poor fetal growth have been repeatedly observed in epidemiological studies, but these studies are often confounded by cigarette smoking and other factors (Golding, 1995; Fernandes et al., 1998). If moderate coffee drinking by pregnant women does adversely influence fetal growth or the rate of miscarriage, the effect is small. Nevertheless, it is sensible for pregnant women to avoid excessive caffeine intake (Eskenazi, 1999).

NONPRESCRIPTION DRUGS

Many over-the-counter preparations are widely used for the treatment of viral illnesses, allergies, headache, aches and pains, sleep disturbances, anxiety, and gastrointestinal discomfort. Little formal evaluation has been conducted of the potential reproductive toxicity of most over-the-counter drugs. It seems prudent in the absence of specific information to avoid these medications whenever possible, particularly in the earliest parts of pregnancy.

Salicylates and other antiinflammatories

Although aspirin and other salicylate compounds are believed to be among the safest and most effective drugs in the marketplace, excessive use may be associated with an increased risk of fetal hemorrhages, and limited evidence suggests that chronic aspirin consumption may interfere with fetal growth (Shepard, 1995; Schardein, 2000a). No evidence of an effect on intelligence has been identified (Klebanoff and Berendes, 1988).

Malformations do not appear to be associated with the prenatal use of salicylates, but use of these agents in the latter stages of pregnancy may interfere with closure of the ductus arteriosus. Similar concerns exist for other nonsteroidal anti-inflammatory agents (Briggs et al., 1995). More information on these agents is needed before definitive conclusions can be reached.

PRESCRIPTION DRUGS

Numerous prescription medications are potentially teratogenic when used at conventional therapeutic doses. Some other drugs can be used safely during pregnancy, and in some instances such treatment is highly beneficial to both the mother and the fetus. Unfortunately, however, available data are insufficient to determine whether maternal treatment with most prescription drugs during pregnancy poses a substantial teratogenic risk. Postmarketing studies of prescription drugs for potential teratogenicity need to be greatly expanded to permit more adequate counseling of pregnant women. In the absence of specific information strongly supporting the safety of treatment with a particular agent during pregnancy, prudence dictates that such treatment be avoided whenever possible. All women of reproductive age who are given prescription drugs should be counseled regarding potential teratogenic effects, because many exposures occur when women become pregnant unintentionally or before they recognize that they are pregnant.

Thalidomide

The most dramatic epidemic of drug-induced birth defects ever recognized occurred in the early 1960s when thalido-mide was sold in several countries, but not the United States, as an over-the-counter sedative preparation. The dramatic events that followed are now a matter of historical record. For many years after the recognition of thalidomide embryopathy, the drug was not marketed in most countries. However, discovery of thalidomide's immunomodulatory action led to its use in a variety of neoplasms and immuno-lopathological disorders, including AIDS. In 1998, the United States Food and Drug Administration approved prescription use of thalidomide for erythema nodosum leprosum, a complication of leprosy, under strict controls. It is not yet clear how successful these controls will be in preventing unintentional thalidomide treatment during pregnancy. Substantial concern surrounds the use of thalidomide for other indications, so called "off-label" use, in view of the growing numbers of prescriptions reported by the manufacturer.

Over 10,000 babies were damaged by this drug between 1958 and 1963. The association between maternal drug use and birth defects was independently noted by Widukind Lenz (1962) and William McBride (1961). Subsequent studies indicated that the susceptible period for the embryo ranged between days 20 and 35 after conception (Lenz and Knapp, 1962). The thalidomide embryopathy includes a very unusual and characteristic pattern of congenital anomalies (Smithells and Newman, 1992). The manifestations depend primarily on the stage of embryonic development at which exposure occurred. Typical anomalies are phocomelia and other limb reduction malformations, anomalies of the external ear, ocular anomalies and cardiovascular malformations ranging from septal defects to complex conotruncal defects. Involvement of the central nervous system and other organ systems may occur but is less common.

Anticancer agents

As the therapeutic efficacy of antineoplastic agents is dependent on their ability to kill cells, particularly undifferentiated cell lines, all such agents should be regarded as potentially teratogenic. The folic acid antagonists and several of the alkylating agents, in particular, have caused concern (Schardein, 2000b).

Folic acid antagonists (aminopterin and methotrexate)

An unusual and characteristic pattern of congenital anomalies has been reported in more than 20 children whose mothers took one of the folic acid antagonists, aminopterin or methotrexate, during pregnancy. In addition to its use as an antineoplastic agent, methotrexate is employed in the therapy of rheumatoid arthritis and other immunopathic diseases (Kremer, 1998) and as part of a medical regimen to induce abortion (Grimes, 1997).

Children with aminopterin or methotrexate embryopathy have distinctive craniofacial anomalies with abnormal head shape and ocular hypertelorism, shallow orbits, mild midfacial hypoplasia, micrognathia, cleft palate, and facial asymmetry (Warkany, 1978; Schardein, 2000b). Malformations of the auricles, skin tags, and numerous skeletal anomalies, especially vertebral segmentation abnormalities with anomalous ribs, abnormalities of ossification of sacral structures, ectrodactyly, syndactyly, longitudinal limb reduction malformations, and positional limb deformities are common. Central nervous system abnormalities may occur and developmental delay is the rule in childhood, but affected adults may have normal or only mildly reduced intelligence. Women who are treated with methotrexate or aminopterin in pregnancy have increased rates of miscarriage, early intrauterine growth retardation, stillbirth, and neonatal death.

The risk of a teratogenic effect after first-trimester maternal treatment with methotrexate is probably dose-related, and much lower doses of the drug are used to treat immunopathic diseases than neoplasia. Most babies born to women treated with low-dose methotrexate during pregnancy appear normal at birth (Feldkamp and Carey, 1993), but typical folic acid embryopathy has been reported even with low-dose treatment (Buckley et al., 1997; Wiebe and Sipila, 1994). This may reflect a particular genetic susceptibility.

Other antineoplastic agents

Maternal treatment early in pregnancy with alkylating agents—busulfan, chlorambucil, cyclophosphamide, and nitrogen mustard—have been anecdotally associated with a variety of fetal anomalies (Schardein, 2000b), including severe intrauterine growth retardation, microphthalmia, cleft palate, genitourinary anomalies, and limb-reduction defects. The risk for such exposure to produce malformations has not been clearly defined. Early pregnancy appears to be a particularly hazardous time for the use of alkylating agents.

Treatment with high doses of most other anticancer agents is teratogenic in laboratory animals (Schardein, 2000b). Unlike most kinds of drug therapy, cancer chemotherapy is often given at the maximum dose tolerated by the mother, i.e., the doses are near or within the range of maternal toxicity. Under such conditions, treatment may carry a substantial risk of teratogenic effects, especially when it occurs during the first trimester and with several drugs at once. Apparently normal children have been born to women who underwent cancer chemotherapy during the first trimester or later in pregnancy (Aviles et al., 1991; Buekers and Lallas, 1998), and the risk of teratogenic effects in a particular case depends on the agent or combination of agents, dose, route, and gestational timing in a complex way that is unique for almost every woman.

In general, the risk of miscarriage and congenital anomalies appears to be increased with many kinds of cancer chemotherapy during the first trimester of pregnancy, and the risks of premature delivery and of fetal death, growth retardation, and myelosuppression may be increased with treatment later in pregnancy (Buekers and Lallas, 1998). Women who are undergoing cancer chemotherapy should be advised to avoid pregnancy during the period of treatment. Patients who require such treatment during pregnancy should receive appropriate counseling regarding the risk of congenital anomalies in exposed offspring.

Warfarin anticoagulants (Coumadin®)

A very uncommon and striking pattern of congenital anomalies has been reported in more than 50 children whose mothers were treated with coumarin derivatives during pregnancy (Fig. 39.3) (Barbour, 1997; Bates and Ginsberg, 1997). Affected children typically have abnormal facial features with severe nasal hypoplasia, which may also affect the ethmoid complex, resulting in choanal atresia. Microcephaly is common and optic atrophy has been repeatedly observed. Radiographic studies often reveal a lag in skeletal maturation with stippling of epiphyseal growth centers. Prenatal-onset growth deficiency with subsequent failure to thrive, developmental delay, mental deficiency, and other neurologic abnormalities are frequent features. Other serious congenital anomalies are less frequent.

The period of greatest concern for the production of fetal facial and skeletal anomalies extends from six to nine weeks after conception. Beyond nine weeks of age, ocular defects and central nervous system malformations may be produced. Children with these abnormalities often have a poor outcome. However, survivors not suffering from mental retardation usually do relatively well except for the various craniofacial cosmetic abnormalities. Children with similar defects have been described who have a genetic disorder of vitamin K-dependent coagulation factors (and whose mothers did not take coumarin derivatives during pregnancy) (Pauli et al., 1987; Menger et al., 1997). Further study of these children may help to clarify the pathogenic mechanism of the coumarin embryopathy.

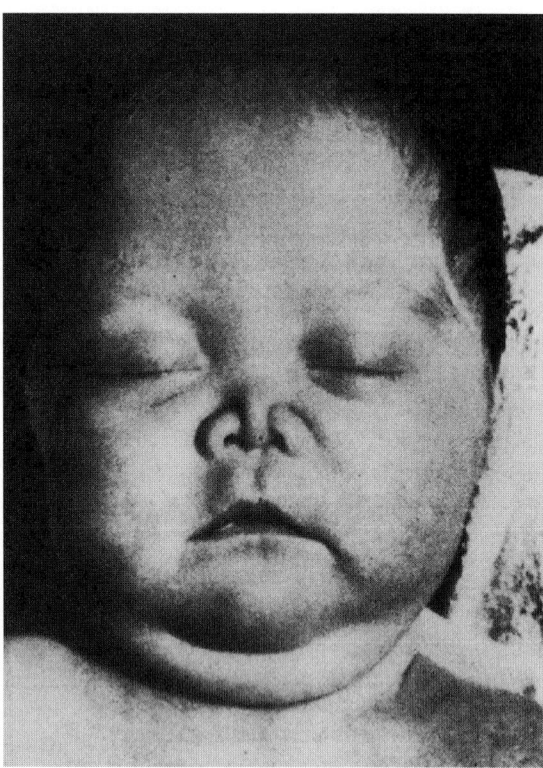

Fig. 39.3. Fetal warfarin syndrome, note severe nasal hypoplasia. (From Pauli et al., 1976, with permission.)

The frequency of coumarin embryopathy among infants of women who are treated with this drug throughout pregnancy has not been clearly established but is in the range of 5%. Miscarriage appears to occur more often than expected when the mother is treated with coumarin derivatives early in pregnancy. Stillbirth and fetal, placental, and neonatal hemorrhage are substantially more frequent when the mother is treated with coumarin anticoagulants late in pregnancy (Oakley, 1995).

Antibiotics

With the exception of a few anecdotal reports of anomalies thought most likely to be coincidental, available studies have not revealed an increased risk to the fetus associated with prenatal treatment with most antibiotics, including penicillins, sulfas, cephalosporins, and related agents (Dashe and Gilstrap, 1997; Schardein, 2000c; 2000d). Exceptions to this generalization are treatment with tetracyclines, aminoglycosides, high-dose quinine, or high-dose fluconazole. Most newer antibacterial and antiviral agents have not been adequately evaluated with regard to their teratogenic potential.

Tetracyclines

Maternal treatment with tetracyclines during the second and third trimesters of pregnancy produces staining of the infant's primary teeth (Cohlan, 1977). The risk for malformations does not appear to be increased among the children of women who were treated with tetracyclines during pregnancy.

Aminoglycosides

Several cases of sensorineural deafness, sometimes with accompanying vestibular dysfunction, have been reported in children whose mothers were treated during pregnancy with streptomycin (Warkany, 1979). Asymptomatic abnormalities of auditory or vestibular function have been observed in up to 10% of such children, but symptomatic disturbances of eighth cranial nerve function are much less common (Donald et al., 1991). Studies have not been reported regarding the relationship, if any, of aminoglycoside-induced fetal ototoxicity to the A1555G mutation of the mitochondrial 12s ribosomal RNA gene associated with such ototoxicity in adults (Prezant et al., 1993).

Quinine and related antimalarials

Maternal use of very high doses of quinine in an attempt to induce abortion have been associated in case reports and clinical series with deafness and optic nerve abnormalities in the offspring (Dannenberg et al., 1983). A causal association seems possible because quinine treatment, especially in large doses, may cause auditory and visual damage in adults. Such abnormalities do not appear to be unusually common among the children of pregnant women who are given much lower doses of quinine to treat malaria or usual prophylactic or therapeutic doses of chloroquine (Roubenoff et al., 1988).

Fluconazole

Four children have been described with a very unusual pattern of congenital anomalies whose mothers were treated for coccidioidomycosis meningitis during the first trimester of pregnancy with daily high-dose fluconazole (Lee et al., 1992; Pursley et al., 1996; Aleck and Bartley, 1997). The features in these infants include brachycephaly, abnormal calvarial development, cleft palate, arthrogryposis, and congenital heart disease. The pattern of anomalies resembles the Antley-Bixler syndrome, an autosomal recessive condition, and two of the affected children were sibs. Nevertheless, the occurrence of a similar rare pattern of congenital anomalies in four children whose mothers received the same, very unusual treatment during pregnancy suggests a causal relationship. A teratogenic effect is unlikely with the much lower doses of fluconazole used to treat vaginal candidiasis.

Anticonvulsants

Because seizures affect 0.5% to 1.0% of pregnant women, the potential teratogenicity of anticonvulsants has been a source of substantial ongoing concern for several decades. Although there was confusion in the past about the relative contribution of the underlying convulsive disorder and that of the medications used to treat it, a growing body of data has helped to illuminate this issue (Dansky and Finnell, 1991; Lindhout and Omtzigt, 1992; Kaneko et al., 1992; Yerby, 1994; Zahn et al., 1998; Schardein, 2000e). A consensus has emerged that women with seizures treated with anticonvulsant medications during pregnancy are at an increased risk for fetal abnormalities. The overall magnitude of this risk is two to three times that of the normal population. The risk is higher in women who require treatment with multiple anticonvulsants than in those who are adequately treated with a single medicine (Czeizel et al., 1992; Lindhout and Omtzigt, 1992; Janz, 1994; Kaneko et al., 1999). The observation of characteristic patterns of abnormal fetal growth and development associated with maternal treatment with some anticonvulsants during pregnancy supports the concept of a unique role for anticonvulsants in the pathogenesis of these birth defects.

It seems prudent to suggest that all epileptic women be cautioned before beginning pregnancy about the potential adverse outcomes for their offspring. In some instances, a trial off drug therapy before conceiving may be warranted. In other cases, where it is deemed unsafe to remove a woman from such drug therapy, she should be placed on the least number of anticonvulsant agents and the lowest dosages compatible with adequate seizure control, and the potential hazards of anticonvulsant therapy to her offspring should be discussed in detail. Women of childbearing age who take anticonvulsant medications should also take 0.4–5 mg/day of supplemental folic acid (Committee on Educational Bulletins of the American College of Obstetricians and Gynecologists, 1997; Rochester and Kirchner, 1997; Morrell, 1998; Zahn et al., 1998; Champel et al., 1999). Taking such supplements is very unlikely to cause harm and may reduce the risk of neural tube defects and other congenital anomalies in the children, although this benefit has not yet been demonstrated specifically among epileptic women who take anticonvulsants during pregnancy.

Maternal serum α-fetoprotein measurement and detailed ultrasound examination are useful for prenatal diagnosis of fetal neural tube defects associated with maternal use of valproic acid or carbamazepine during pregnancy (Delgado-Escueta and Janz, 1992; Committee on Educational Bulletins of the American College of Obstetricians and Gynecologists, 1997; Rochester and Kirchner, 1997). Some other serious malformations have also been diagnosed prenatally in fetuses of women treated with anticonvulsant medications during pregnancy, but the subtle dysmorphic syndromes and functional deficits that occur more frequently in these children cannot usually be identified before birth.

Many of the same major malformations and a similar pattern of minor anomalies, sometimes called the "fetal anticonvulsant syndrome", have been reported among children of epileptic women treated with a variety of anticonvulsant medications (Gaily and Granstrom, 1992; Janz, 1994; Nulman et al., 1997). Some investigators attribute these similarities to underlying genetic predispositions involved in the pathogenesis of maternal epilepsy, while other researchers interpret the similarities as indicating common teratogenic mechanisms of various maternal anticonvulsive treatments. The discussion below emphasizes these similarities as well as some serious malformations that are only associated with maternal use of particular drugs during pregnancy.

Trimethadione

Trimethadione is the only oxazolidine anticonvulsant that is still used clinically. It is prescribed infrequently, usually for the treatment of petit mal epilepsy—an uncommon seizure disorder among women of reproductive age. There is little justification for the use of this particularly toxic drug in pregnant women. Nevertheless, trimethadione is important because it was the first maternal anticonvulsant treatment found to produce a unique pattern of abnormalities of growth and development in infants exposed prenatally (Goldman and Yaffe, 1978; Dansky and Finnell, 1991). Moreover, maternal trimethadione treatment during pregnancy, especially when used in combination with other drugs, appears to cause serious birth defects in an unusually large proportion of exposed pregnancies (Nakane et al., 1990; Czeizel et al., 1992)

The anomalies observed include a characteristic facial appearance with flattening of the midface, short upturned nose, synophrys with upslant of the eyebrows in a V-like configuration, and auricular anomalies, particularly overfolded cup-like helices. In addition, prenatal-onset growth deficiency and an increased frequency of abnormalities of central nervous system performance, including mental deficiency and delayed speech development, occur. Major congenital anomalies, particularly cleft palate, cardiovascular malformations (such as septal defects, tetralogy of Fallot, and transposition of the great vessels), urogenital malformations, and limb defects, appear to be more frequent than expected in these children. Several affected children have had tracheoesophageal malformations, and a few have had malformations of the brain and nervous system.

Hydantoin anticonvulsants

Although concern about a possible role of hydantoin anticonvulsants in the production of birth defects was voiced more than 25 years ago, there is still disagreement about the extent to which these congenital anomalies are an effect of the maternal epilepsy or genetic factors that caused it or of the maternal phenytoin treatment during pregnancy (Kelly, 1984; Friis, 1989; Gaily and Granstrom, 1992; Janz, 1994; Holmes et al., 1994; Nulman, 1997). About 10% of infants born to epileptic women treated with phenytoin during pregnancy have a recognizable pattern of minor anomalies known as the fetal hydantoin syndrome (Kelly, 1984; Hanson, 1986), while an additional 30% show lesser degrees of alteration. The abnormalities found in these children include a characteristic facial appearance with midface hypoplasia, low nasal bridge, ocular hypertelorism, and an accentuated cupid's bow of the upper lip (Fig. 39.4). Prenatal-onset growth deficiency, including poor growth for weight, length, and head circumference, is occasionally seen. Increased frequencies of distal digital hypoplasia and of major malformations, particularly clefts of the lip and palate and cardiovascular anomalies, have been noted (Hanson, 1986; Friis, 1989). In addition, small but significant reductions in cognitive function have been observed among the children of epileptic women treated with phenytoin during pregnancy (Vanoverloop et al., 1992; Scolnik et al., 1994). Genetic differences in maternal or fetal metabolism appear to be important risk factors for congenital anomalies among the children of epileptic women treated with phenytoin during pregnancy (Strickler et al., 1985; Buehler et al., 1990, 1994; Dean et al., 1999).

Children whose mothers were treated with phenytoin during pregnancy also have a higher than expected risk of developing neuroblastoma (Stage et al., 1998). Fortunately, such neoplasia is rare in childhood, and tumors are uncommon even in children whose mothers took phenytoin during pregnancy.

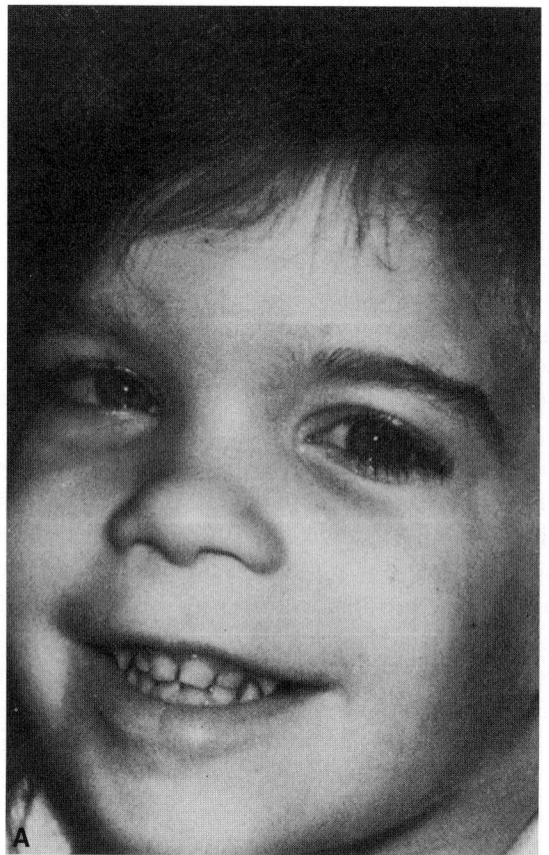

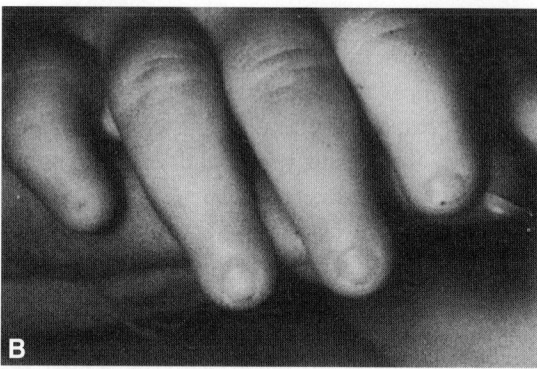

Fig. 39.4. Features of the fetal hydantoin syndrome. (A) Facial, (B) Digital. Note the ocular hypertelorism, ptosis and strabismus, short nose with low bridge and accentuated "cupid's bow" of lip. Distal phalangeal and nail hypoplasia are common digital anomalies. (From Hanson, 1986, with permission.)

Valproic acid

The risk of spina bifida is increased to about 2% among the children of epileptic women treated with valproic acid during the first trimester of pregnancy (Robert, 1988; Omtzigt et al., 1992). The increased risk for spina bifida is not associated with an increased risk for anencephaly, suggesting that the pathogenetic mechanism may not be related to neural tube closure but rather to factors that affect canalization posterior to the caudal neuropore.

A characteristic pattern of craniofacial and other anomalies has been observed in up to half of children born to epileptic women treated with valproic acid during pregnancy (Ardinger et al., 1988; Thisted and Ebbesen, 1993; Clayton-Smith and Donnai, 1995). Features of this "fetal valproate syndrome" include abnormalities of the calvaria with metopic ridging, trigonocephaly, narrow bifrontal diameter, relative deficiency of the outer orbital region, midfacial hypoplasia, short upturned nose with a broad flat bridge, and long flat philtrum with a thin vermilion border of the upper lip. Cleft lip or palate or both, congenital heart disease, radial ray defects, and other malformations have been seen occasionally. Inherited variations in maternal drug metabolism may increase the susceptibility of certain pregnancies to these adverse effects (Dean et al., 1999).

Carbamazepine

A fetal anticonvulsant syndrome has also been observed among the children of epileptic women who were treated with carbamazepine during pregnancy (Jones et al., 1989; Ornoy and Cohen, 1996). Frequent features include minor craniofacial anomalies, fingernail hypoplasia, and delayed growth and development. Spina bifida occurs in about 1% of children whose mothers took carbamazepine while they were pregnant (Kaneko et al., 1992; Omtzigt et al., 1993; Samren et al., 1997). The frequency of other major malformations among the children of epileptic women treated with carbamazepine during pregnancy appears to be similar to that observed in children of women treated with other anticonvulsants (Samren et al., 1997; Kaneko et al., 1999).

Other anticonvulsant agents

Phenobarbital is not often used as an anticonvulsant in adults, but primidone, which is partially metabolized to phenobarbital, is sometimes used. In most studies, the frequency of congenital anomalies among children of epileptic women treated with these drugs during pregnancy is similar to that observed with other anticonvulsants (Bertollini et al., 1987; Dansky and Finnell, 1991; Samren et al., 1997; Kaneko et al., 1999). A distinctive pattern of minor dysmorphic features and poor growth, i.e., a "fetal anticonvulsant syndrome" occurs in some children whose mothers were treated for epilepsy with either phenobarbital or primidone during pregnancy (Hoyme, 1990; Koch et al., 1992).

Insufficient data are available to determine the risk of congenital anomalies in the children of pregnant women treated with the succinimide anticonvulsants, ethosuximide or methsuximide. In the last several years, felbamate, gabapentin, and lamotrigine have also been used to treat seizure disorders. Insufficient information is available to determine whether the risk of birth defects in children of women who are treated with these newer drugs during pregnancy is higher, lower, or similar to that of children whose mothers took conventional anticonvulsants during gestation. There is some evidence that maternal use of lamotrigine during pregnancy may be associated with an increased risk of neural tube defects in the offspring (Mackay et al., 1997), but this has not yet been established.

Endocrine agents

A number of reports have suggested possible teratogenic effects of treatment with agents used for endocrine disorders. These drugs are often taken by women of reproductive age.

Male sex hormone agents

Maternal treatment with androgens during pregnancy can cause masculinization of the external genitalia of female fetuses (Schardein, 2000f). The effect appears to be dose-related. Similar masculinization of female fetuses may occur after maternal treatment with large doses of anabolic steroids such as danazol that have androgenic and antiestrogenic activity (Brunskill, 1992). No clear evidence of other teratogenic effects of androgens has been reported.

Female sex hormone agents

Agents with female sex hormone-like activity, especially various synthetic progestins and estrogens, have received considerable attention because of their widespread use in contraceptive agents and for other medical purposes that could result in fetal exposures.

Diethylstibestrol. Diethylstilbestrol (DES) was widely used in the 1950s as a treatment for threatened abortion and for estrogen replacement during pregnancy. The daughters of women who received such treatment during pregnancy have a greatly increased risk of gross structural anomalies of the uterus and vagina and of developing vaginal adenosis and clear cell adenocarcinoma of the vagina or cervix (Giusti et al., 1995; Mittendorf, 1995). At least one-third to one-half of women who were exposed in utero to diethylstilbestrol have gross or histological abnormalities of genital tract, but the absolute risk of developing vaginal malignancy is, fortunately, quite small. Ectopic pregnancy, miscarriage, and premature delivery also occur with increased frequency among "DES daughters". The sons of women who were treated with DES during pregnancy have higher than expected frequencies of epididymal cysts, hypoplastic testes, and cryptorchidism, but fertility and sexual function are usually not impaired (Giusti et al., 1995; Mittendorf, 1995).

Estrogens and progestins. Other estrogens have not been clearly associated with similar risks. Early reports of feminization of male fetuses after maternal treatment with other estrogens during pregnancy have not been substantiated.

Maternal treatment during pregnancy with high doses of androgenic progestins is associated with an increased risk of masculinization of the external genitalia in female fetuses. The degree of masculinization depends upon the time of treatment and is unlikely to occur after the twelfth week of gestation. The magnitude of this risk is no more than 1% with high doses and is less with lower doses. Maternal treatment with high doses of norethindrone are particularly likely to produce such abnormalities (Schardein, 2000f). Despite reports associating maternal progestin use during pregnancy with various other malformations in the offspring, no consistent pattern of abnormalities has emerged, and epidemiologic studies have failed to confirm such associations.

Combinations of estrogens and lower-dose progestins in the form of contraceptive agents have also been alleged to produce fetal anomalies. Studies claiming a relationship between maternal use of these agents and various congenital anomalies have been reported, but the results have generally not been reproducible (Brent et al., 1993; Schardein, 2000f). A woman who has inadvertently become pregnant while taking an oral contraceptive can be reassured that her use of birth control pills is very unlikely to have harmed the fetus.

Other endocrine-active agents

Clomiphene. Induction of ovulation with clomiphene has been associated with an increased risk of neural tube defects in some studies, but most investigations do not show such an association (Greenland and Ackerman, 1995; Schardein, 2000f). The effects of treatment with these agents may be confounded in some studies with the effects of underlying maternal disorders that led to the need for therapy.

An association between clomiphene use and multifetal gestation has been clearly established (Cittadini and Palermo, 1992; Venn et al., 1994). Six to thirteen percent of treated pregnancies result in multiple births, in which the risk for premature delivery and positional limb deformations may be increased. Similar risks apply to other treatments that induce multiple gestation.

Corticosteroids. Although maternal treatment with adrenal corticosteroids is teratogenic in some animal species, most epidemiologic studies do not support such an association in humans. Any risk to the fetus associated with maternal use of these drugs during pregnancy appear to be extremely low (Rayburn, 1992; Kallen, 1998).

Antithyroid agents. Maternal treatment during pregnancy with antithyroid agents such as radioactive iodine (^{131}I), propylthiouracil, or methimazole is associated with an increased risk of hypothyroidism and consequent mental retardation in the offspring (Schardein, 2000g). In addition, it appears that maternal treatment with methimazole or the related thioamide, carbimazole, during pregnancy can occasionally cause cutis aplasia of the scalp or, rarely, a methimazole embryopathy in the fetus (Greenberg, 1987; Clementi et al., 1999). The features of this unusual pattern of anomalies include developmental delay, cloanal atresia, esophageal atresia, absent or hypoplastic nipples, and scalp defects.

Iodides have the potential for producing neonatal goiter and hypothyroidism, particularly when taken by a pregnant woman after the first trimester (Schardein, 2000h). Fetal goiter can also be produced by maternal treatment with other medications, such as amiodarone, that contain large amounts of iodine (Cox and Gardner, 1993; Grosso et al., 1998).

Retinoids and vitamin A

Preformed retinoids, including retinol, retinaldehyde, and retinoic acid, possess vitamin A activity directly. They are contained in substantial amounts in some foods, especially liver. Isotretinoin, etretinate, and acitretin are synthetic retinoid congeners that are used orally and topically to treat a variety of skin disorders. Absorption of the topical forms is usually quite limited. β-Carotene and related carotenoids, which are contained in many orange or dark green leafy vegetables, can be metabolized by the body to vitamin A.

Although information linking vitamin A to birth defects has been available in laboratory animals since the 1950s, the relevance of these observations to human beings remained uncertain until a characteristic pattern of birth defects was recognized in children whose mothers had been treated with isotretinoin during pregnancy (Lammer, 1985). A growing body of studies has subsequently demonstrated the teratogenic potential of oral therapy with isotretinoin or etretinate, and anecdotal evidence suggests that acetretin and preformed vitamin A itself in high doses may have similar potential (Coberly et al., 1996; Miller et al., 1998b; Schardein, 2000i). Concern about the teratogenic potential of preformed vitamin A in doses as low as 10,000 IU per day has been raised (Rothman et al., 1995) but appears to unfounded (Miller et al., 1998b; Wiegand et al., 1998). An exact threshold dose for the teratogenic risk associated with use of preformed vitamin A in pregnancy has not been determined but is likely to be greater than 30,000 IU per day. Ingestion of β-carotene, even in high doses, has not been associated with a teratogenic risk (Polifka et al., 1996).

The characteristic retinoid embryopathy has been most clearly delineated in children of women who were treated with isotretinoin during the first trimester of pregnancy (Lammer, 1985; Schardein, 2000i). Typical craniofacial anomalies include microcephaly, facial asymmetry with midfacial hypoplasia (Fig. 39.5A), microphthalmia, cleft palate, micrognathia, and microtia (Fig. 39.5B) or anotia. Central nervous system abnormalities, such as hydrocephaly or posterior fossa cysts, and cardiovascular malformations, especially conotruncal defects, are common. Thymic hypoplasia and genitourinary anomalies, including hypoplastic kidneys and hydroureter, are also frequent. Children with isotretinoin embryopathy who survive often have developmental delay, cortical blindness, or facial nerve palsies (Adams and Lammer, 1993).

Dosage and timing are major factors, the highest risk period being with maternal treatment between two and five weeks after conception. However, it should be noted that both etretinate and retinol have half-lives of weeks to months, leading both to longer risk periods after discontinuation of use and to the possibility of substantial bioaccumulation (Lammer, 1988). The half-life of isotretinoin is much shorter—less than one day.

Despite a program designed by the manufacturer to prevent use of isotretinoin in pregnancy, recent reviews confirm that substantial numbers of fetal exposures continue to occur (Mitchell, 1995; Anonymous, 2000). Women who are pregnant or may become pregnant should not be treated systemically with isotretinoin or related drugs. Pregnant women should not take more than the recommended dietary allowance of preformed vitamin A (Teratology Society, 1991; Miller et al., 1998b). Vitamin supplements containing β-carotene are preferable to those containing preformed vitamin A for women of reproductive age.

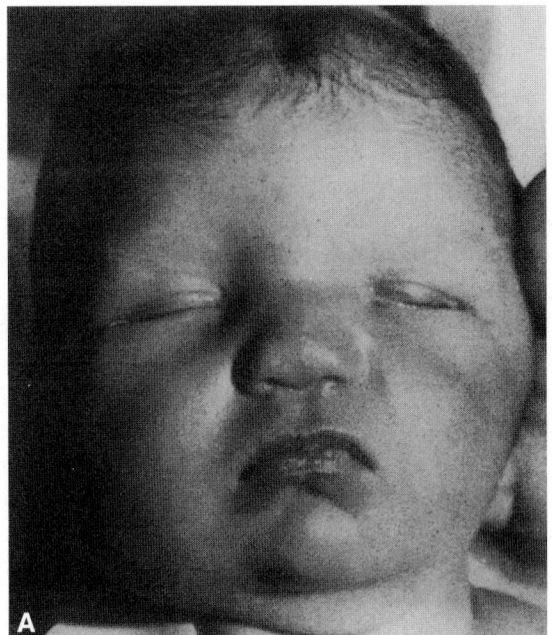

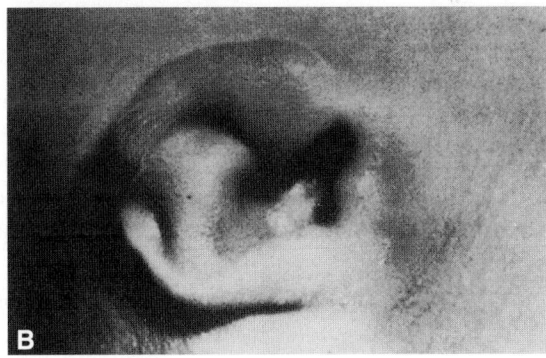

Fig. 39.5. Fetal retinoid syndrome. (A) Dysmorphic facial features. (B) Microtia. (Fig. A from Lammer 1987, with permission; Fig. B from Fernhoff and Lammer, 1984, with permission.)

Other drugs

Lithium

Children of women who are treated with lithium during pregnancy appear to have an increased risk of Ebstein's anomaly of the heart, although epidemiological studies indicate that this risk is likely to be small (Cohen et al., 1994; Moore, 1995). Fetal echocardiography should be offered to women who are treated with lithium during the first trimester of pregnancy for prenatal diagnosis of fetal cardiac disease.

Treatment of severe depression in pregnant women and those of reproductive age presents a clinical dilemma. The small but serious teratogenic risk associated with lithium use may need to be balanced against a substantial risk to the mother's health if treatment is stopped or with possible maternal or fetal risks associated with alternative treatments (Cohen and Rosenbaum, 1998; Llewellyn et al., 1998).

Selective seratonin reuptake inhibitors

Selective seratonin reuptake inhibitors, SSRIs, are very widely used as antidepressants. These drugs are also given to treat obsessive compulsive disorder, panic disorders, and other psychiatric illnesses. Most studies have not found any association between maternal treatment with an SSRI during pregnancy and the risk of congenital anomalies in the infant (Loebstein and Koren, 1997; Wisner et al., 1999), but available data are insufficient to rule out a small increase in risk. Transient behavioral alterations and other abnormalities of neonatal adaptation may occur in infants whose mothers are treated with an SSRI near the time of delivery.

Misoprostol

Misoprostol is prostaglandin analogue that is used in the prevention and treatment of peptic ulcer disease. The drug has recently been licensed by the US. Food and Drug Administration, in combination with mifepristone, to induce abortion. Associations have been observed between unsuccessful maternal use of misoprostol to induce abortion in the first trimester of pregnancy and the occurrence of Moebius syndrome, terminal transverse limb reduction defects, arthrogryposis, and brain defects such as holoprosencephaly and hydrocephalus in the offspring (Pastuszak et al., 1998; Orioli and Castilla, 2000). Vascular disruption is a biologically plausible explanation for these associations (Brent, 1993). The risks for severe anomalies among fetuses surviving attempted therapeutic abortion with mifepristone and misoprostol should be explained to women contemplating such treatment. These risks contribute to the recommendation that pregnancies which continue in spite of attempted medical abortion be surgically terminated.

Penicillamine

Several infants whose mothers were treated with penicillamine during pregnancy have been reported with an unusual syndrome of abnormal connective tissue similar to cutis laxa (see Ch. 151) (Domingo, 1998). Limited data from clinical series suggest that such abnormalities are uncommon among these children. Nevertheless, a causal relationship seems likely, given the fact that similar skin lesions occur as a rare complication of chronic penicillamine therapy in adults and that such treatment is known to affect crosslinking of elastin and collagen.

Angiotensin coverting enzyme inhibitors

Neonatal renal failure and hypotension as well as fetal anuria resulting in oligohydramnios, joint contractures, pulmonary hypoplasia and death, have been observed repeatedly after maternal treatment with captopril, enalapril or lisinopril during pregnancy (Sedman et al., 1995; Buttar, 1997). Several cases of neonatal hypocalvaria and other skeletal anomalies have also been noted after maternal treatment during pregnancy with one of these angiotensin converting enzyme (ACE) inhibitors (Sedman et al., 1995). Accurate risk estimates are not available, but the effects appear to result from hypersensitivity of the fetus to the pharmacologic action of ACE inhibitors during the latter half of pregnancy (Barr, 1994; Buttar, 1997). There is no evidence suggesting that maternal ACE inhibitor therapy early in pregnancy is likely to harm the fetus, but women who conceive while taking one of these drugs should be switched during the first trimester to an antihypertensive agent of a different class if treatment continues to be necessary.

Indomethacin and other prostaglandin synthethesis inhibitors

Maternal treatment with indomethocin late in pregnancy has been associated with decreased fetal urinary output and oligohydramnios, as well as with premature closure of the ductus arteriosus in the fetus and consequent persistent pulmonary hypertension in the infant (Lione and Scialli, 1995; Norton, 1997). These effects appear to result from transplacental pharmacological activity of this prostaglandin synthesis inhibitor. Maternal treatment late in pregnancy with other inhibitors of prostaglandin synthesis, such as ketoprofen and sulindac, may have similar action on the fetal ductus arteriousus and kidneys (Ostensen, 1998). There is no indication that maternal treatment with these drugs early, but not later, in pregnancy poses a substantial teratogenic risk.

Methylene blue

Up to 20% of twins born after genetic amniocentesis in which methylene blue is used as a marker develop small bowel atresia (Cragan, 1999). The affected twin is the one whose amniotic sac was injected with the dye, and the risk appears to be greater with higher doses. The risk of fetal death is also increased after injection of methylene blue during genetic amniocentesis (Kidd et al., 1996). It is important to note that these risks are only associated with intra-amniotic instillation of methylene blue, not with oral or topical use by the mother during pregnancy.

HMG-CoA reductase inhibitors

Treatment with HMG-CoA reductase inhibitors such as lovastatin and simvastatin is contraindicated during pregnancy because of unlikely benefit to the mother and concern about the potential teratogenicity of reducing cholesterol synthesis. However, limited available data provide no indication that women who conceive while taking these medicines have a greatly increased risk of birth defects in their children (Manson et al., 1996).

Bendectin® (Diclectin®)

A fixed combination of pyridoxine (vitamin B_6) and doxylamine (an antihistamine), marketed in the past as Bendectin® and more recently as Diclectin®, is used in the treatment of nausea and vomiting of pregnancy. This medication was removed from the market by its manufacturer and was unavailable for many years in the United States because of excessive litigation alleging that Bendectin® caused a variety of serious birth defects in children whose mothers took it early in pregnancy. However, extensive epidemiological studies provide no indication that maternal use of this medication during pregnancy increases the risk of congenital anomalies above the rate expected in the general population (McKeigue, 1994; Brent, 1995b).

Maternal metabolic and genetic factors

Although not strictly environmental, factors that alter maternal metabolism or otherwise affect a woman's reproductive potential can be considered to alter the intrauterine fetal environment. Thus, an additional category of potential teratogenic factors are maternal metabolic and genetic factors. Of particular importance in this category are diabetes mellitus, maternal phenylketonuria, and maternal nutritional disturbances, especially folic acid intake.

MATERNAL METABOLIC DISORDERS: DIABETES MELLITUS

The principal maternal metabolic disorder that raises concern for the developing fetus is type I diabetes mellitus. The risk of congenital anomalies in infants of women who have insulin-dependent diabetes is 2–3 times greater than that in the general population (Becerra et al., 1990; Garner, 1995; Ryan, 1998). A variety of congenital anomalies is associated with maternal diabetes, but congenital heart defects and neural tube defects are most common. Preconceptional and early postconceptional folic acid supplementation is, there-

fore, especially important for women with type 1 diabetes, and pregnant diabetic women should be offered prenatal diagnosis by detailed ultrasound examination, fetal echocardiography, and serum α-fetoprotein measurement.

Caudal regression, focal femoral hypoplasia, and holoprosencephy are also more frequent than expected among the children of women with type 1 diabetes mellitus but are, fortunately, uncommon even among this group. Diabetic pregnancies are at increased risk of spontaneous abortion, abnormal fetal growth, neonatal hypoglycemia, and various obstetrical complications (Garner, 1995; Greene, 1999). Risks for congenital anomalies and adverse neonatal outcomes can be minimized by very good control of maternal diabetes from the time of conception and throughout pregnancy (Ryan, 1998; Greene, 1999; Wiznitzer and Reece, 1999).

There is controversy over whether women with gestational diabetes also are at increased risk to have children with malformations. When maternal diabetes does not develop until after the first trimester of pregnancy, an effect on embryogenesis would seem unlikely. However, some women with gestational diabetes have unusually high blood glucose levels at the time of diagnosis and may actually have pre-existing abnormalities of glucose metabolism. The infants of such women may be more likely to have malformations of the types seen in children of mothers with pre-existing type 1 diabetes (Ryan, 1998; Kjos and Buchanan, 1999; Schaefer-Graf et al., 2000).

MATERNAL GENETIC DISORDERS

Maternal genetic disorders may present hazards to the developing fetus through a direct alteration of the intrauterine environment, a physical or chemical effect, or an interaction between an affected mother and affected fetus. Relatively few disorders of these types have been defined. However, maternal phenylketonuria deserves special comment.

Phenylketonuria

Children of women with PKU who are not adequately treated during pregnancy are mentally retarded and microcephalic in 75–90% of cases and may also have prenatal growth retardation and congenital heart disease (Levy and Ghavami, 1996; Rouse et al., 2000). Their appearance is reminiscent of fetal alcohol syndrome (Lipson et al., 1984). These children, who are usually heterozygous but do not have PKU themselves, are damaged during gestation by exposure to very high levels of phenylalanine, phenylpyruvic acid, and other potentially toxic metabolities in the maternal blood.

Effective treatment of the mother beginning before conception and continuing throughout pregnancy reduces the risk substantially (Rouse et al., 1997, 2000; Platt et al., 2000). It is extremely important to ensure that all female phenylketonuric children receive this information before and during the advent of their reproductive years. Unfortunately, adult women with undiagnosed phenylketonuria have occasionally been identified after they have become pregnant (Hanley et al., 1999). A few of these women have near-normal intelligence; others have milder degrees of intellectual deficit than is commonly associated with classical phenylketonuria. Some present with major psychotic disorders. Such women may come to attention only through the birth of an abnormal child. Thus, maternal screening for phenylketonuria subsequent to the birth of a child with the above-described abnormalities is one way of preventing the birth of additional affected children.

Nutritional disturbances

The recognition that many malformations, including most neural tube defects, can be prevented by maternal folic acid supplementation prior to and during pregnancy has provided an unparalleled opportunity for the prevention of birth defects. Dietary supplementation with folic acid before and after conception may reduce the overall risk of birth defects by 40% (Czeizel, 1998; Lewis et al., 1998). Not all malformations are affected equally—neural tube defects may be reduced by as much as 85% (Czeizel and Dudas, 1992; Berry et al., 1999; Botto et al., 1999), but the reductions in orofacial clefts, cardiac malformations, and renal anomalies are smaller (Czeizel, 1998; Lewis et al., 1998). The mechanism of prevention is not understood, but certain genetic variants (e.g., in folate metabolism) may put some patients at greater risk than others for such birth defects when folic acid supplementation is not provided (Bailey and Gregory, 1999; Botto et al., 1999).

All women of childbearing age should take 0.4 mg of supplemental folic acid daily (Centers for Disease Control and Prevention, 1992; Bailey, 1998; Locksmith and Duff, 1998). Larger doses of folic acid are sometimes recommended for women who are at increased risk to have a child with a neural tube defect. As compliance with regimens requiring daily vitamin supplements is problematical, some authorities are urging that the level of folic acid fortification in the food supply be increased (Oakley, 1997; Bentley et al, 1999; Botto et al., 1999).

Paternal exposures

Concern is often voiced about the potential role of paternal exposures to toxic agents in the pathogenesis of birth defects (Olshan and Mattison, 1994). However, it seems unlikely that such paternal exposures could produce birth defects in a subsequent child except by germ cell mutation. Although this possibility certainly exists for many agents to which fathers might potentially be exposed, the overall risk for mutation would presumably apply to many different genetic loci, each at a relatively low frequency. Thus, one would not expect to see any consistent pattern of abnormalities among the offspring of an exposed male. Rather, a low-frequency increase in a variety of disorders resulting from new autosomal dominant mutations would be anticipated.

No paternal exposure to any chemical or physical agent, including a number of known mutagens, has been convincingly shown to increase the risk of birth defects in subsequently-conceived children (Rudiger, 1991; Shelby, 1994). It is certainly possible, indeed likely, that germ cell mutations do occur but that their contribution to the burden of birth defects is too small to measure in comparison to the background risk of congenital anomalies. Paternal mutagenic exposures may contribute to infertility or early miscarriage and may be of importance from a population perspective, especially when considered over many generations. However, an individual couple who are concerned about exposure of the father to a potentially teratogenic or mutagenic agent can be reassured that such exposures probably present minimal risk to the fetus if they occur before conception and none at all if they occur postconceptionally.

Summary

In conclusion, a wide variety of potentially teratogenic exposures may be encountered during pregnancy. Insufficient evidence is available for the complete characterization of most such agents and further information in this area is badly needed. In the interim, emphasis should be placed on the avoidance of potentially hazardous agents unless benefits to the mother or infant from the proposed exposure clearly outweigh hazards to the fetus. Well-informed women, supported by knowledgeable and sensitive health care providers, form one of the strongest lines of defense for the fetus against potentially hazardous exposures.

REFERENCES

Aase Jon M (1990) Diagnostic Dysmorphology: Plenum Medical Book Co. N Y

Abboud P, Villena I, Chemla C, et al. (1997) Screening for congenital toxoplasmosis: Pregnancy outcome after antenatal diagnosis in a series of 211 cases. J Gynecol Obstet Biol Reprod 26:40–46

Abel EL (1988) Fetal alcohol syndrome in families. Neurotoxicol Teratol 10:1–2

Adams J, Lammer EJ (1993) Neurobehavioral teratology of isotretinoin. Reprod Toxicol 7:175–177

Aleck KA, Bartley DL (1997) Multiple malformation syndrome following fluconazole use in pregnancy: Report of an additional patient. Am J Med Genet 72:253–256

Alger LS (1997) Toxoplasmosis and parvovirus B19. Infect Dis Clin North Am 11:55–75

Anonymous (1996) Establishment of VARIVAX Pregnancy Registry. JAMA 275:1073

Anonymous (1998) Public Health Service task force recommendations for the use of antiretroviral drugs in pregnant women infected with HIV-1 for maternal health and for reducing perinatal HIV-1 transmission in the United States. MMWR 47:1–30

Anonymous (2000) Accutane-exposed pregnancies—California, 1999. MMWR Morb Mortal Wkly Rep. 49:28–31

Ardinger HH, Atkin JF, Blackston RD et al. (1988) Verification of the fetal valproate syndrome phenotype. Am J Med Genet 29:171–185

Arvin AM, Maldonado YA (1995) Other viral infections of the fetus and newborn. In Remington JS, Klein JO (eds): Infectious Diseases of the Fetus and Newborn Infant. 4th edn. WB Saunders, Philadelphia, pp. 745–756.

Aviles A, Diaz-Maqueo JC, Talavera A et al. (1991) Growth and development of children of mothers treated with chemotherapy during pregnancy: Current status of 43 children. Am J Hematol 36:243–248

Bailey LB (1998) Dietary reference intakes for folate: The debut of dietary folate equivalents. Nutr Rev 56:294–299

Bailey LB, Gregory JF 3rd (1999) Polymorphisms of methylenetetrahydrofolate reductase and other enzymes: Metabolic significance, risks and impact on folate requirement. J Nutr 29:919–922

Barbour LA (1997) Current concepts of anticoagulant therapy in pregnancy. Obstet Gynecol Clin North Am 24:499–521

Barr M (1994) Teratogen update: angiotensin-converting enzyme inhibitors. Teratology 50:339–409

Bates SM, Ginsberg JS (1997) Anticoagulants in pregnancy: Fetal effects. Baillieres Clin Obstet Gynaecol 11:479–488

Beazley DM, Egerman RS (1998) Toxoplasmosis. Semin Perinatol 22:332–338

Becerra JE, Khoury MJ, Cordero JF, Erickson JD (1990) Diabetes mellitus during pregnancy and the risks for specific birth defects: A population-based case-control study. Pediatrics 85:1–9

Behnke M, Eyler FD (1993) The consequences of prenatal substance use for the developing fetus, newborn, and young child. Int J Addict 28:1341–1391

Bentley JR, Ferrini RL, Hill LL (1999) American College of Preventive Medicine public policy statement. Folic acid fortification of grain products in the U.S. to prevent neural tube defects. Am J Prev Med 16:264–267

Bentur Y (1994) Ionizing and nonionizing radiation in pregnancy. In Koren G (ed): Maternal-Fetal Toxicology: A Clinician's Guide, 2nd edn. Marcel Dekker, N Y, pp. 515–572.

Berry RJ, Li Z, Erickson JD et al. (1999) Prevention of neural-tube defects with folic acid in China. China-U.S. Collaborative Project for Neural Tube Defect Prevention. N Engl J Med 341:1485–1490

Bertollini R, Kallen B, Mastroiacovo P, Robert E (1987) Anticonvulsant drugs in monotherapy. Effect on the fetus. Eur J Epidemiol 3:164–171

Best JM (1991) Rubella vaccines: Past, present, and future. Epidemiol Infect 107:17–30

Boice JD Jr, Miller RW (1999) Childhood and adult cancer after intrauterine exposure to ionizing radiation. Teratology 59:227–233

Botto LD, Olney RS, Mastroiacovo P et al. (1996) Chorionic villus sampling and transverse digital deficiencies: Evidence for anatomic and gestational-age specificity of the digital deficiencies in two studies. Am J Med Genet 62:173–178

Botto LD, Moore CA, Khoury MJ, Erickson JD (1999) Neural-tube defects. N Engl J Med 341:1509–1519

Boyer KM (1996) Diagnosis and treatment of congenital toxoplasmosis. Adv Pediatr Infect Dis 11:449–467

Brent RL (1986) Evaluating the potential teratogenicity of environmental agents. Clin Perinatol 13:615–648

Brent RL (1993) Congenital malformation case reports: The editor's and reviewer's dilemma. Am J Med Genet 47:872–874

Brent RL (1995a) The application of the principles of toxicology and teratology in evaluating the risks of new drugs for treatment of drug addiction in women of reproductive age. NIDA Res Monogr 149:130–184

Brent RL (1995b) Bendectin: Review of the medical literature of a comprehensively studied human nonteratogen and the most prevalent tortogen-litigen. Reprod Toxicol 9:

Brent RL (1999a) Utilization of developmental basic science principles in the evaluation of reproductive risks from pre-and postconception environmental radiation exposures. Teratology 59:182–204

Brent RL (1999b) Reproductive and teratologic effects of low-frequency electromagnetic fields: A review of in vivo and in vitro studies using animal models. Teratology 59:261–86

Brent RL, Beckman DA, Landel CP (1993) Clinical teratology. Curr Opin Pediatr 5:201–211

Briggs GG, Freeman RK, Yaffe SJ (1995) Chlorhexidine, diclofenac, etodolac, fluorescein sodium, flurbiprofen, mefanimic acid, nabumetone, oxaprozin, sulindac. Update: Drugs pregnancy and lactation 8:11–20

Brocklehurst P, French R (1998) The association between maternal HIV infection and perinatal outcome: A systematic review of the literature and meta-analysis. Br J Obstet Gynaecol 105:836–848

Brown HL, Abernathy MP (1998) Cytomegalovirus infection. Semin Perinatol 22:260–266

Brown KE, Young NS, Liu JM (1994) Molecular, cellular and clinical aspects of parvovirus B19 infection. Crit Rev Oncol Hematol 16:1–31

Brunskill PJ (1992) The effects of fetal exposure to danazol. Br J Obstet Gynaecol 99:212–215

Buckley LM, Bullaboy CA, Leichtman L, Marquez M (1997) Multiple congenital anomalies associated with weekly low-dose methotrexate treatment of the mother. Arthritis Rheum 40:971–973

Buehler BA, Delimont D, van Waes M, Finnell RH (1990) Prenatal prediction of risk of the fetal hydantoin syndrome. N Engl J Med 322:1567–1572

Buehler BA, Rao V, Finnell RH (1994) Biochemical and molecular teratology of fetal hydantoin syndrome. Neurol Clin. 12:741–748

Buekers TE, Lallas TA (1998) Chemotherapy in pregnancy. Obstet Gynecol Clin North Am 25:323–329

Burns DN, Mofenson LM (1999) Paediatric HIV-1 infection. Lancet 354 Suppl 2:SII1–6

Buttar HS (1997) An overview of the influence of ACE inhibitors on fetal-placental circulation and perinatal development. Mol Cell Biochem 176:61–71

Castronovo FP Jr (1999) Teratogen update: Radiation and Chernobyl. Teratology 60:100–106

CEMAT Group (1998) Randomised trial to assess safety and fetal outcome of early and midtrimester amniocentesis. The Canadian Early and Mid-trimester Amniocentesis Trial (CEMAT) Group. Lancet 351:242–247

Centers for Disease Control and Prevention (1992) Recommendations for the use of folic acid to reduce the number of cases of spina bifida and other neural tube defects. MMWR 41:1–7

Chambers CD, Johnson KA, Dick LM et al. (1998) Maternal fever and birth outcome: a prospective study. Teratology 58:251–257

Champel V, Radal M, Moulin-Vallez M et al. (1999) Should folic acid be given to women treated with valproic acid and/or carbamazepine? Folic acid and pregnancy in epilepsy. Rev Neurol (Paris) 155:220–224

Chapman S (1998) Varicella in pregnancy. Semin Perinatol 22:339–346

Chiriboga CA (1998) Neurological correlates of fetal cocaine exposure. Ann NY Acad Sci 846:109–125

Choi BH (1989) The effects of methylmercury on the developing brain. Prog Neurobiol 32:447–470

Cittadini E, Palermo R (1992) Outcomes of induced conception. Acta Eur Fertil 23:111–116

Clarren SK, Smith DW (1978) The fetal alcohol syndrome: A review of the world literature. N Engl J Med 298:1063–1067

Clarren SK, Astley SJ, Bowden DM (1988) Physical anomalies and developmental delays in nonhuman primate infants exposed to weekly doses of ethanol during gestation. Teratology 37:561–569

Clarren SK, Astley SJ, Gunderson VM, Spellman D (1992) Cognitive and behavioral deficits in nonhuman primates associated with very early embryonic binge exposures to ethanol. J Pediatr 121:789–796

Clayton-Smith J, Donnai D (1995) Fetal valproate syndrome. J Med Genet 32:724–727

Clementi M, Di Gianantonio E, Pelo E et al. (1999) Methimazole embryopathy: Delineation of the phenotype. Am J Med Genet 83:43–46

Coberly S, Lammer E, Alashari M (1996) Retinoic acid embryopathy: Case report and review of literature. Pediatr Pathol Lab Med 16:823–36

Cohen LS, Friedman JM, Jefferson JW et al. (1994) A reevaluation of risk of in utero exposure to lithium. JAMA 271:146–150

Cohen LS, Rosenbaum JF (1998) Psychotropic drug use during pregnancy: Weighing the risks. J Clin Psychiatry 59 Suppl 2:18–28

Cohlan SQ (1977) Tetracycline staining of teeth. Teratology 15:127–130

Coles CD (1992) Prenatal alcohol exposure and human development. In Miller MW (ed): Development of the Central Nervous System: Effects of Alcohol and Opiates, Wiley-Liss, N Y, pp. 9–36

Committee on Educational Bulletins of the American College of Obstetricians and Gynecologists (1997) ACOG educational bulletin: Seizure disorders in pregnancy. Number 231, December 1996. Int J Gynaecol Obstet 56:279–286

Cooper LZ, Preblud SR, Alford CA (1995) Rubella. In Remington JS, Klein JO (eds): Infectious Diseases of the Fetus and Newborn Infant, 4th edn. WB Saunders, Philadelphia, pp. 268–311

Cox JL, Gardner MJ (1993) Treatment of cardiac arrhythmias during pregnancy. Prog Cardiovasc Dis 36:137–178

Cragan JD (1999) Teratogen update: Methylene blue. Teratology 60:42–48

Czeizel AE (1998) Periconceptional folic acid containing multivitamin supplementation. Eur J Obstet Gynecol Reprod Bio 78:151–161

Czeizel AE, Dudas I (1992) Prevention of the first occurrence of neural-tube defects by periconceptional vitamin supplementation. N Engl J Med 327:1832–1835

Czeizel AE, Bod M, Halasz P (1992) Evaluation of anticonvulsant drugs during pregnancy in a population-based Hungarian study. Eur J Epidemiol 8:122–127

Daniel Y, Gull I, Peyser MR, Lessing JB (1995) Congenital cytomegalovirus infection. Eur J Obstet Gyencol Reprod Biol 63:7–16

Dannenberg AL, Dorfman SF, Johnson J (1983) Use of quinine for self-induced abortion. South Med J 76:846–849

Dansky LV, Finnell RH (1991) Parental epilepsy, anticonvulsant drugs and reproductive outcome: Epidemiologic and experimental findings spanning three decades. 2: Human studies. Reprod Toxicol 5:301–335

Dashe JS, Gilstrap LC (1997) Antibiotic use in pregnancy. Obstet Gynecol Clin North Am 24:617–629

Day NL, Richardson GA (1991) Prenatal alcohol exposure: A continuum of effects. Semin Perinatol 15:271–279

Dean JC, Moore SJ, Osborne A et al. (1999) Fetal anticonvulsant syndrome and mutation in the maternal MTHFR gene. Clin Genet 56:216–220

Delaney-Black V, Covington C, Sokol RJ (1994) Maternal cocaine consumption: Birth outcome and child development. Fetal Matern Med Rev 6:119–134

Delgado-Escueta AV, Janz D (1992) Consensus guidelines: Preconception counseling, management, and care of the pregnant woman with epilepsy. Neurology 42(4 Suppl 5):149–160

Demmler GJ (1996) Congenital cytomegalovirus infection and disease. Adv Pediatr Infect Dis 11:135–162

Dolk H, Nichols R (1999) Evaluation of the impact of Chernobyl on the prevalence of congenital anomalies in 16 regions of Europe. EUROCAT Working Group. Int J Epidemiol 28:941–948

Domingo JL (1998) Developmental toxicity of metal chelating agents. Reprod Toxicol 12:499–510

Donald PR, Doherty E, Van Zyl FJ (1991) Hearing loss in the child following streptomycin administration during pregnancy. Cent Afr J Med 37:268–271

Edwards MJ, Shiota K, Smith MSR, Walsh DA (1995) Hyperthermia and birth defects. Reprod Toxicol 9:411–425

Enders G, Biber M (1990) Parvovirus B19 infections in pregnancy. Behring Inst Mitt 85:74–78

Enders G, Miller E, Craddock-Watson J et al. (1994) Consequences of varicella and herpes zoster in pregnancy: prospective study of 1739 cases. Lancet 343:1548–1551

Eskenazi B (1999) Caffeine—filtering the facts. N Engl J Med 341:1688–1689

Eyler FD, Behnke M (1999) Early development of infants exposed to drugs prenatally. Clin Perinatol. 26:107–50

Farrell SA, Summers AM, Dallaire L et al. (1999) Club foot, an adverse outcome of early amniocentesis: Disruption or deformation? J Med Genet 36:843–846

Fast DK, Conry J, Loock CA (1999) Identifying fetal alcohol syndrome among youth in the criminal justice system. J Dev Behav Pediatr 20:370–372

Feldkamp M, Carey JC (1993) Clinical teratology counseling and consultation case report: Low dose methotrexate exposure in early weeks of pregnancy. Teratology 47:533–539

Fernandes O, Sabharwal M, Smiley T et al. (1998) Moderate to heavy caffeine consumption during pregnancy and relationship to spontaneous abortion and abnormal fetal growth: a meta-analysis. Reprod Toxicol 12:435–444

Feruhoff PM, Lammer EJ (1984) Craniofacial features of igotretinoin embryopathy. J Pediatr 595–597

Finnell RH (1999) Teratology: General considerations and principles. J Allergy Clin Immunol 103(2, Part 2):S337–S342

Firth H (1997) Chorion villus sampling and limb deficiency—cause or coincidence? Prenat Diagn 17:1313–1330

Frank DA, Bresnahan K, Zuckerman BS (1996) Maternal cocaine use: Impact on child health and development. Curr Probl Pediatr 26:52–70

Frank DA, Augustyn M, Zuckerman BS (1998) Neonatal neurobehavioral and neuroanatomic correlates of prenatal cocaine exposure. Problems of dose and confounding. Ann NY Acad Sci 846:40–50

Fricker-Hidalgo H, Pelloux H, Muet F, et al. (1997) Prenatal diagnosis of congenital toxoplasmosis: Comparative value of fetal blood and amniotic fluid using serological techniques and cultures. Prenat Diagn 17:831–835

Friedman JM, Polifka JE (2000) Teratogenic Effects of Drugs: A Resource for Clinicians (TERIS) 2nd edn. Johns Hopkins University Press, Baltimore

Friis ML (1989) Facial clefts and congenital heart defects in children of parents with epilepsy: Genetic and environmental etiologic factors. Acta Neurol Scand 79:433–459

Gaily E, Granstrom ML (1992) Minor anomalies in children of mothers with epilepsy. Neurology 42(4 Suppl 5):128–131

Gardner T (1995) Lyme Disease. In Remington JS, Klein JO (eds) Infectious Diseases of the Fetus and Newborn Infant, 4th edn. Philadelphia, WB Saunders, pp. 447–528

Garner P (1995) Type I diabetes mellitus and pregnancy. Lancet 346:157–161

Gershon AA (1995) Chickenpox, measles and mumps. In Remington JS, Klein JO (eds): Infectious Disease of the Fetus and Newborn Infant, 4th edn. WB Saunders, Philadelphia, pp. 566–590

Ghidini A, Lynch L (1994) Management strategies for congenital infections. Mt Sinai J Med 61:376–388

Ginsburg KA, Blacker CM, Abel EL, Sokol RJ (1991) Fetal alcohol exposure and adverse pregnancy outcomes. Contrib Gynecol Obstet 18:115–129

Giusti RM, Iwamoto K, Hatch EE (1995) Diethylstibestrol revisited: A review of the long-term health effects. Ann Intern Med 122:778–788

Gladstone J, Nulman I, Koren G (1996) Reproductive risks of binge drinking during pregnancy. Reprod Toxicol 10:3–13

Golding J (1995) Reproduction and caffeine consumption—a literature review. Early Hum Dev 43:1–14

Goldman AS, Yaffe SJ (1978) Fetal trimethadione syndrome. Teratology 17:103–105

Graham JM Jr, Edwards MJ, Edwards MJ (1998) Teratogen update: Gestational effects of maternal hyperthermia due to febrile illnesses and resultant patterns of defects in humans. Teratology 58:209–221

Graham JM Jr, Jones KL, Brent RL (1999) Contribution of clinical teratologists and geneticists to the evaluation of the etiology of congenital malformations alleged to be caused by environmental agents: ionizing radiation, electromagnetic fields, microwaves, radionuclides, and ultrasound. Teratology 59:307–313

Greenberg F (1987) Choanal atresia and athelia: Methimazole teratogenicity or a new syndrome? Am J Med Genet 28:931–934

Greene MF (1999) Spontaneous abortions and major malformations in women with diabetes mellitus. Semin Reprod Endocrinol 17:127–136

Greenhouse SJ, Stillman RJ (1998) Cigarette smoking and reproduction. Effects on fecundity and early pregnancy outcomes. Infertil Reprod Med Clin North Am 9:699–723

Greenland S, Ackerman DL (1995) Clomiphene citrate and neural tube defects: A pooled analysis of controlled epidemiologic studies and recommendations for future studies. Fertil Steril 64:936–941

Grimes DA (1997) Medical abortion in early pregnancy: A review of the evidence. Obstet Gynecol 89:790–796

Grosso S, Berardi R, Cioni M, Morgese G (1998) Transient neonatal hypothyroidism after gestational exposure to amiodarone: A follow-up of two cases. J Endocrinol Invest 21:699–702

Hanley WB, Platt LD, Bachman RP et al. (1999) Undiagnosed maternal phenylketonuria: The need for prenatal selective screening or case finding. Am J Obstet Gynecol 180:986–994

Hanson JW (1979) Anticonvulsants and the fetus: the fetal hydantoin syndrome and related problems. In Wada JA (ed): Epilepsy: Neurotransmitter, Behavior and Pregnancy. Canadian League Against Epilepsy and Western Institute on Epilepsy, Vancouver, BC

Hanson JW (1986) Teratogen update: Fetal hydantoin effects. Teratology 33:349–53

Hanson JW (1987) Teratogen information services: Developmental, clinical, and public health aspects. Banbury Report 26: Developmental Toxicology: Mechanisms and Risk, Cold Spring Harbor Laboratory

Hanson JW, Jones KL, Smith DW (1976) Fetal alcohol syndrome: Experience with 41 patients. JAMA 235:1458–1460

Harada M (1995) Minamata disease: methylmercury poisoning in Japan caused by environmental pollution. Crit Rev Toxicol 25:1–24

Held JR, Riggs ML, Dorman C (1999) The effect of prenatal cocaine exposure on neurobehavioral outcome: A meta-analysis. Neurotoxicol Teratol 21:619–625

Holmes LB, Harvey EA, Brown KS (1994) Anticonvulsant teratogenesis: I. A study design for newborn infants. Teratology 49:202–207

Holmes SJ, Reef S, Hadler SC et al. (1996) Prevention of varicella: Recommendations of the Advisory Committee on Immunization Practices (ACIP). MMWR 45:1–36

Hoyme HE (1990) Teratogenically induced fetal anomalies. Clin Perinatol 17:547–567

Hulse GK, English DR, Milne E et al. (1997) Maternal cocaine use and low birth weight newborns: A meta-analysis. Addiction 92:1561–1570

Ingall D, Sanchez PJ, Musher DM (1995) Syphilis. In Remington JS, Klein JO (eds): Infectious diseases of the fetus and newborn infant, 4th edn. WB Saunders, Philadelphia, pp. 529–564

Jacobs RF (1988) Neonatal herpes simplex virus infections. Semin Perinatol 22:64–71

Jacobson JL, Jacobson SW (1997) Teratogen update: Polychlorinated biphenyls. Teratology 55:338–347

Jacobson JL, Jacobson SW, Sokol RJ, Ager JW Jr (1998) Relation to maternal age and pattern of pregnancy drinking to functional significant cognitive deficit in infancy. Alcohol Clin Exp Res 22:345–351

Jacquemard F, Hohlfeld P, Mirlesse V et al. (1995) Prenatal diagnosis of fetal infections. In Remington JS, Klein JO (eds): Infectious Diseases of the Fetus and Newborn Infant, 4th edn. WB Saunders, Philadelphia, pp. 99–107

Janz D (1994) Are antiepileptic drugs harmful when taken during pregnancy? J Perinat Med 22:367–377

Jenkins TM, Wapner RJ (1999) First trimester prenatal diagnosis: Chorionic villus sampling. Semin Perinatol 23:403–413

Jones HE, Balster RL (1998) Inhalant abuse in pregnancy. Obstet Gynecol Clin North Am 25:153–167

Jones KL (1997) Smith's Recognizable Patterns of Human Malformations, 5th edn., W.B. Saunders Philadelphia

Jones KL, Lacro RV, Johnson KA, Adams J (1989) Pattern of malformations in the children of women treated with carbamazepine during pregnancy. N Engl J Med 320:1661–1666

Jones KL, Johnson KA, Chambers TA (1994) Offspring of women infected with varicella during pregnancy: A prospective study. Teratology 49:29–32

Jones KL, Smith DW, Ulleland N, Streissguth AP (1973) Pattern of malformation in offspring of chronic alcoholic mothers. Lancet 1:1267–1271

Kallen B (1998) The teratogenicity of antirheumatic drugs—what is the evidence? Scand J Rheumatol Suppl 107:119–124

Kaneko S, Battino D, Andermann E et al. (1999) Congenital malformations due to antiepileptic drugs. Epilepsy Res 33:145–158

Kaneko S, Otani K, Kondo T et al. (1992) Malformation in infants of mothers with epilepsy receiving antiepileptic drugs. Neurology 42(4 Suppl 5):68–74

Kelly TE (1984) Teratogenicity of anticonvulsant drugs. I: Review of the literature. Am J Med Genet 19:413–434

Kidd SA, Lancaster PA et al. (1996) Fetal death after exposure to methylene blue dye during mid-trimester amniocentesis in twin pregnancy. Prenat Diagn 16:39–47

Kiess W, Linderkamp O, Hadorn H-B, Haas R (1984) Fetal alcohol syndrome and malignant disease. Eur J Pediatr 143:160–161

Kjos SL, Buchanan TA (1999) Gestational diabetes mellitus. N Engl J Med 341:1749–1756

Klebanoff MA, Berendes HW (1988) Aspirin exposure during the first 20 weeks of gestation and IQ at four years of age. Teratology 37:249–255

Klein JO, Remington JS (1995) Current concepts of infections of the fetus and newborn infant. Remington JS, Klein JO (eds): Infectious Diseases of the Fetus and Newborn Infant, 4th edn. WB Saunders, Philadelphia, pp. 1–19.

Koch S, Losche G, Jager-Roman E et al. (1992) Major and minor birth malformations and antiepileptic drugs. Neurology 42(4 Suppl 5):83–88

Koren G, Bologa M, Long D et al. (1989) Perception of teratogenic risk by pregnant women exposed to drugs and chemicals during the first trimester. Am J Obstet Gynecol. 160(5 Pt 1):1190–1194

Koren G, Pastuszak A (1994) Teratogen Information Services. In Koren G (ed): Maternal-Fetal Toxicology: A Clinician's Guide. 2nd edn. Marcel Dekker, N Y, pp. 683–705

Koren G, Pastuszak A, Ito S (1998) Drugs in pregnancy. N Engl J Med 338:1128–1137

Kremer JM (1998) Methotrexate and emerging therapies. Rheum Dis Clin North Am 24:651–658

Laforet EG, Lynch CL (1947) Multiple congenital defects following maternal varicella. N Engl J Med 236:534–537

LaGasse LL, Seifer R, Lester BM (1999) Interpreting research on prenatal substance exposure in the context of multiple confounding factors. Clin Perinatol 26:39–54

Lammer EJ (1985) Retinoic acid embryopathy. N Engl J Med 313:837–841

Lammer EJ (1987) Patterns of malformation among fetuses and infants exposed to retinoic acid (Isotretinoin). Banbury Report 26: Developmental Toxicology: Mechanisms and Action. Cold Spring Harbor Laboratory, pp. 213–255

Lammer EJ (1988) Embryopathy in infant conceived one year after termination of maternal etretinate. Lancet 2:1080–1081

Lammer EJ, Hayes A, Schunior A (1987) Risk for major malformation among human fetuses exposed to isotretinoin (13-cis-retinoic acid), abstracted. Teratology 35:68

Lassen K, Oei TPS (1998) Effects of maternal cigarette smoking during pregnancy on long-term physical and cognitive parameters of child development. Addict Behav 23:635–653

Lee BE, Feinberg M, Abraham JJ, Murthy ARK (1992) Congenital malformations in an infant born to a woman treated with fluconazole. Pediatr Infect Dis J 11:1062–1064

Lenz W (1962) Thalidomide and congenital abnormalities. Lancet 1:45–46

Lenz W, Knapp K (1962) Thalidomide embryopathy. Arch Environ Health 5:100–105

Levy HL, Ghavami M (1996) Maternal phenylketonuria: A metabolic teratogen. Teratology 53:176–184

Levy R, Weissman A, Blomberg G, Hagay ZJ (1997) Infection by parvovirus B19 during pregnancy: A review. Obstet Gynecol Surv 52:254–259

Lewis DP, Van Dyke DC, Stumbo PJ, Berg MJ (1998) Drug and environmental factors associated with adverse pregnancy outcomes. Part II: Improvement with folic acid. Ann Pharmacother 32:947–961

Lindhout D, Omtzigt JG (1992) Pregnancy and the risk of teratogenicity. Epilepsia 33 (Suppl 4):S41–48

Lione A, Scialli AR (1995) The developmental toxicity of indomethacin and sulindac. Reprod Toxicol 9:7–20

Lipson A, Beuhler B, Bartley J et al. (1984) Maternal hyperphenylalaninemia fetal effects. J Pediatr 104:216–220

Llewellyn A, Stowe ZN, Strader JR Jr (1998) The use of lithium and management of women with bipolar disorder during pregnancy and lactation. J Clin Psychiatry 59 Suppl 6:57–65

Locksmith GJ, Duff P (1998) Preventing neural tube defects: The importance of periconceptional folic acid supplements. Obstet Gynecol 91:1027–1034

Loebstein R, Koren G (1997) Pregnancy outcome and neurodevelopment of children exposed in utero to psychoactive drugs: The Motherisk experience. J Psychiatry Neurosci 22:192–196

Lynfield R, Guerina NG (1997) Toxoplasmosis. Pediatr Rev 18:75–83

Mackay FJ, Wilton LV, Pearce GL et al. (1997) Safety of long-term lamotrigine in epilepsy Epilepsia 38:881–886

Manson JM, Freyssinges C, Ducrocq MB, Stephenson WP (1996) Postmarketing surveillance of lovastatin and simvastatin exposure during pregnancy. Reprod Toxicol 10:439–446

Markenson GR, Yancey MK (1998) Parvovirus B19 infections in pregnancy. Semin Perinatol 22:309–317

Mastrobattista JM (1997) Angiotensin converting enzyme inhibitors in pregnancy. Semin Perinatol 21:124–134

McBride WG (1961) Thalidomide and congenital abnormalities. Lancet 2:1358

McKeigue PM, Lamm SH, Linn S, Kutcher JS (1994) Bendectin and birth defects: I. A meta-analysis of the epidemiologic studies. Teratology 50:27–37, 1994

Menger H, Lin AE, Toriello HV et al. (1997) Vitamin K deficiency embryopathy: A phenocopy of the warfarin embryopathy due to a disorder of embryonic vitamin K metabolism. Am J Med Genet 72:129–134

Miller E, Fairley CK, Cohen BJ, Seng C (1998a) Immediate and long term outcome of human parvovirus B19 infection in pregnancy. Br J Obstet Gynaecol 105:174–178

Miller RK, Hendrickx AG, Mills JL et al. (1998b) Periconceptional vitamin A use: How much is teratogenic? Reprod Toxicol 12:75–88

Mills JL, Graubard BI (1987) Is moderate drinking during pregnancy associated with an increased risk for malformations? Pediatrics 80:309–314

Minkoff HL (1998) Human immunodeficiency virus infection in pregnancy. Semin Perinatol 22:293–308

Mitchell AA, Van Bennekom CM, Louik C (1995) A pregnancy-prevention program in women of childbearing age receiving isotretinoin. N Engl J Med 333:101–106

Mittendorf R (1995) Teratogen update: Carcinogenesis and teratogenesis associated with exposure to diethylstilbestrol (DES) in utero. Teratology 51:435–445

Mofenson LM (1996) The role of antiretroviral therapy in the management of HIV infection in women. Clin Obstet Gynecol 39:361–385

Moore JA (1995) An assessment of lithium using the IEHR Evaluative Process for Assessing Human Developmental and Reproductive Toxicity of Agents. IEHR Expert Scientific Committee. Reprod Toxicol 9:175–210

Morrell MJ (1998) Guidelines for the care of women with epilepsy. Neurology 51(Suppl 4):S21–27

Mueller BU, Pizzo PA (1995) Acquired immunodeficiency syndrome in the infant. In Remington JS, Klein JO (eds): Infectious Diseases of the Fetus and Newborn Infant, 4th edn. WB Saunders, Philadelphia, pp. 377–403.

Nehlig A, Debry G (1994) Potential teratogenic and neurodevelopmental consequences of coffee and caffeine exposure: A review on human and animal data. Neurotoxicol Teratol 16:531–543

Nelson CT, Demmler GJ (1997) Cytomegalovirus infection in the pregnant mother, fetus, and newborn infant. Clin Perinatol 24:151–160

Norton ME (1997) Teratogen update: Fetal effects of indomethacin administration during pregnancy. Teratology 56:282–292

Nulman I, Scolnik D, Chitayat D et al. (1997) Findings in children exposed in utero to phenytoin and carbamazepine monotherapy: Independent effects of epilepsy and medications. Am J Med Genet 68:18–24

Oakley CM (1995) Clinical perspective. Anticoagulation and pregnancy. Eur Heart J 16:1317–1319

Oakley GP Jr (1997) Let's increase folic acid fortification and include vitamin B-12. Am J Clin Nutr 65:1889–1890

Olshan AF, Mattison DR (eds) (1994) Male-mediated developmental toxicity. Plenum Press, N Y

Omtzigt JGC, Los FJ, Grobbee DE et al. (1992) The risk of spine bifida aperta after first-trimester exposure to valproate in a prenatal cohort. Neurology 42 (Suppl 5):119–125

Omtzigt JGC, Los FJ, Meijer JWA, Lindhout D (1993) The 10, 11-epoxide-10, 11-diol pathway of carbamazepine in maternal serum, urine, and amniotic fluid: Effect of dose, comedication, and relation to outcome of pregnancy. Ther Drug Monit 15:1–10

Orioli IM, Castilla EE (2000) Epidemiological assessment of misoprostol teratogenicity. BJOG 107:519–523

Ornoy A, Cohen E (1996) Outcome of children born to epileptic mothers treated with carbamazepine during pregnancy. Arch Dis Child 75:517–520

Ostensen M (1998) Nonsteroidal anti-inflammatory drugs during pregnancy. Scand J Rheumatol Suppl 107:128–132

Ouellete EM, Rosett HC, Rosman NP, Weiner L (1977) Adverse effects on offspring of maternal alcohol abuse during pregnancy. N Engl J Med 297:528–530

Pastuszak A, Levy M, Schick RN et al. (1994) Outcome after maternal varicella infection in the first 20 weeks of pregnancy. N Engl J Med 330:901–905

Pastuszak AL, Schuler L, Speck-Martins CE et al. (1998) Use of misoprostol during pregnancy and Mobius' syndrome in infants. N Engl J Med 338:1881–1885

Pauli RM, Lian JB, Mosher DF et al. (1987) Association of congenital deficiency of multiple vitamin K-dependent coagulation factors and the phenotype of the warfarin embryopathy: clues to the mechanism of teratogenicity of coumarin derivatives. Am J Hum Genet 41:566–583

Pauli RM, Madden JD, Kranzler KJ et al. (1976) Warfarin therapy initiated during pregnancy and phenotypic chondrodysplasia punctata. J Pediatr 506–508

Platt LD, Koch R, Hanley WB et al. (2000) The international study of pregnancy outcome in women with maternal phenylketonuria: Report of a 12-year study. Am J Obstet Gynecol 182:326–333

Polifka JE, Dolan CR, Donlan MA, Friedman JM (1996) Clinical teratology counseling and consultation report: High dose beta-carotene use during early pregnancy. Teratology 54:103–107

Polifka JE, Friedman JM (1999) Clinical teratology: Identifying teratogenic risks in humans. Clin Genet 56:409–420

Prezant TR, Agapian JV, Bohlman MC et al. (1993) Mitochondrial ribosomal RNA mutation associated with both antibiotic-induced and non-syndromic deafness. Nat Genet 4:289–294

Pursley TJ, Blomquist IK, Abraham J et al. (1996) Fluconazole-induced congenital anomalies in three infants. Clin Infect Dis 22:336–340

Rayburn WF (1992) Glucocorticoid therapy for rheumatic diseases: maternal, fetal, and breast-feeding considerations. Am J Reprod Immunol 28:138–140

Remington JS, Klein JO (1995) Infectious Diseases of the Fetus and Newborn Infant, 4th edn. WB Saunders, Philadelphia, pp. 140–267.

Remington JS, McLeod R, Desmonts G (1995) Toxoplasmosis. In Remington JS, Klein JO (eds): Infectious Diseases of the Fetus and Newborn Infant. 4th edn. WB Saunders, Philadelphia.

Robert E (1988) Valproic acid as a human teratogen. Congen Anom 28(Suppl):S71–S80

Robert E (1996) Teratogen update: Electromagnetic fields. Teratology 54:305–13

Robert E (1999) Intrauterine effects of electromagnetic fields—(low frequency, mid-frequency RF, and microwave): Review of epidemiologic studies. Teratology 59:292–8

Rochester JA, Kirchner JT (1997) Epilepsy in pregnancy. Am Fam Physician 56:1631–1636, 1638

Rodis JF: Parvovirus infection (1999) Clin Obstet Gynecol 42:107–120

Rodis JF, Rodner C, Hansen AA et al. (1998) Long-term outcome of children following maternal human parvovirus B19 infection. Obstet Gynecol 91:125–128

Rodriguez EM, Diaz C, Fowler MG (1997) The clinical management of children perinatally exposed to HIV. Primary Care 24:643–666

Roebuck TM, Mattson SN, Riley EP (1998) A review of the neuroanatomical findings in children with fetal alcohol syndrome or prenatal exposure to alcohol. Alcohol Clin Exp Res 22:339–344

Romitti PA, Lidral AC, Munger RG et al. (1999) Candidate genes for nonsyndromic cleft lip and palate and maternal cigarette smoking and alcohol consumption: Evaluation of genotype-environment interactions from a population-based case-control study of orofacial clefts. Teratology 59:39–50

Rothman KJ, Moore LL, Singer MR et al. (1995) Teratogenicity of high vitamin A intake. N Engl J Med 333:1369–1373

Roubenoff R, Hoyt J, Petri M et al. (1988) Effects of antiinflammatory and immunosuppressive drugs on pregnancy and fertility. Semin Arthritis Rheum 18:88–110

Rouse B, Azen C, Koch R et al. (1997) Maternal Phenylketonuria Collaborative Study (MPKUCS) offspring: Facial anomalies, malformations, and early neurological sequelae. Am J Med Genet 69:89–95

Rouse B, Matalon R, Koch R et al. (2000) Maternal phenylketonuria syndrome: Congenital heart defects, microcephaly, and developmental outcomes. J Pediatr 136:57–61

Rudiger HW (1991) Clinical, genetic and regulatory consequences of exposure to mutagens. Ann Genet 34:173–178

Rutledge JC (1997) Developmental toxicity induced during early stages of mammalian embryogenesis. Mutat Res 396:113–127

Ryan EA (1998) Pregnancy in diabetes. Med Clin North Am 82:823–845

Sampson PD, Streissguth AP, Bookstein FL et al. (1997) Incidence of fetal alcohol syndrome and prevalence of alcohol-related neurodevelopmental disorder. Teratology 56:317–26

Samren EB, van Duijn CM, Koch S et al. (1997) Maternal use of antiepileptic drugs and the risk of major congenital malformations: a joint European prospective study of human teratogenesis associated with maternal epilepsy. Epilepsia 38:981–990

Scarlatti G (1996) Paediatric HIV infection. Lancet 348:963–868

Schaefer-Graf UM, Buchanan TA, Xiang A et al. (2000) Patterns of congenital anomalies and relationship to initial maternal fasting glucose levels in pregnancies complicated by type 2 and gestational diabetes. Am J Obstet Gynecol 182:313–320

Schantz SL (1996) Developmental neurotoxicity of PCBs in humans: What do we know and where do we go from here? Neurotoxicol Teratol 18:217–227; discussion 229–276

Schardein JL (2000a) Agents used for pain. In Chemically Induced Birth Defects, 3rd edn. Marcel Dekker, N Y, pp. 139–166

Schardein JL (2000b) Cancer chemotherapeutic agents. In Chemically Induced Birth Defects, 3rd edn. Marcel Dekker, N Y, pp. 559–611

Schardein JL (2000c) Antimicrobial agents. In Chemically Induced Birth Defects, 3rd edn. Marcel Dekker, N Y, pp. 379–434

Schardein JL (2000d) Antiparasitical drugs. In Chemically Induced Birth Defects, 3rd edn. Marcel Dekker, N Y, pp. 435–452

Schardein JL (2000e) Anticonvulsants. In Chemically Induced Birth Defects, 3rd edn. Marcel Dekker, N Y, pp. 179–235

Schardein JL (2000f) Hormones and hormonal antagonists. In Chemically Induced Birth Defects, 3rd edn. Marcel Dekker, N Y, pp. 281–357

Schardein JL (2000g) Thyroid-acting agents. In Chemically Induced Birth Defects, 3rd edn. Marcel Dekker, N Y, pp. 463–473

Schardein JL (2000h) Drugs used in respiratory and allergic disorders. In Chemically Induced Birth Defects, 3rd edn. Marcel Dekker, N Y, pp. 359–377

Schardein JL (2000i) Foods, nutrients, and dietary factors. In Chemically Induced Birth Defects, 3rd edn. Marcel Dekker, N Y, pp. 653–691.

Scialli AR (1997) Identifying teratogens: the tyranny of lists. Reprod Toxicol 11:555–559

Scialli AR, Lione A, Boyle Padgett GK (1995) Reproductive effects of chemical, physical and biologic agents: REPROTOX. Johns Hopkins University Press, Baltimore

Scolnik D, Nulman I, Rovet J et al. (1994) Neurodevelopment of children exposed in utero to phenytoin and carbamazepine monotherapy. JAMA 271:767–770

Sedman AB, Kershaw DB, Bunchman TE (1995) Recognition and management of angiotensin converting enzyme inhibitor fetopathy. Pediatr Nephrol 9:382–385

Severson RK, Buckley JD, Woods WG et al. (1993) Cigarette smoking and alcohol consumption by parents of children with acute myeloid leukemia: An analysis within morphological subgroups—A report from the Childrens Cancer Group. Cancer Epidemiol Biomarkers Prev 2:433–439

Shaw GM, Todoroff K, Velie EM, Lammer EJ (1998) Maternal illness, including fever and medication use as risk factors for neural tube defects. Teratology 57:1–7

Shaw GM, Wasserman CR, Lammer EJ et al. (1996) Orofacial clefts, parental cigarette smoking, and transforming growth factor-alpha gene variants. Am J Hum Genet 58:551–561

Shelby MD (1994) Human germ cell mutagens. Environ Mol Mutagen 23 Suppl 24:30–34

Shepard TH (1995) Catalog of Teratogenic Agents, 8th edn. Johns Hopkins University Press, Baltimore

Shu X-O, Ross JA, Pendergrass TW et al. (1996) Parental alcohol consumption, cigarette smoking, and risk of infant leukemia: A Children's Cancer Group study. J Natl Cancer Inst 88:24–31

Silver HM (1997) Lyme disease during pregnancy. Infect Dis Clin North Am 11:93–97

Smith DW, Graham JM Jr (1988) Recognizable Patterns of Human Deformation, 2nd edn. WB Saunders, Philadelphia

Smithells RW, Newman CGH (1992) Recognition of thalidomide defects. J Med Genet 29:716–723

Stage D, Sasco AJ, Little J (1998) Antenatal therapeutic drug exposure and fetal/neonatal tumours: Review of 89 cases. Paediatr Perinat Epidemiol 12:84–117

Stagno S (1995) Cytomegalovirus. In Remington JS, Klein JO (eds): Infectious Diseases of the Fetus and Newborn Infant, 4th edn. WB Saunders, Philadelphia, pp. 312–353

Stoler JM, McGuirk CK, Lieberman E et al. (1999) Malformations reported in chorionic villus sampling exposed children: A review and analytic synthesis of the literature. Genetics in Medicine 1:315–322

Stratton K, Howe C, Battaglia F (1995) Fetal Alcohol Syndrome: Diagnosis, Epidemiology, Prevention, and Treatment. Institute of Medicine, National Academy Press, Washington, DC

Streissguth AP (1977) Maternal drinking and the outcome of pregnancy: Implications for child mental health. Am J Orthopsychiatry 47:422–431

Streissguth AP (1992) Fetal alcohol syndrome and fetal alcohol effects: A clinical perspective of later developmental consequences. In Zagon IS, Slotkin TA (eds): Maternal Substance Abuse and the Developing Nervous System, Academic Press, San Diego, California, pp. 5–25

Streissguth AP, Dehaene P (1993) Fetal alcohol syndrome in twins of alcoholic mothers: concordance of diagnosis and IQ. Am J Med Genet 47:857–861

Strickler SM, Miller MA, Andermann E et al. (1985) Genetic predisposition to phenytoin-induced birth defects. Lancet 2:746–749

Strobino B, Abid S, Gewitz M (1999) Maternal Lyme disease and congenital heart disease: A case-control study in an endemic area. Am J Obstet Gynecol 180:711–716

Sundberg K, Bang J, Smidt-Jensen S et al. (1997) Randomised study of risk of fetal loss related to early amniocentesis versus chorionic villus sampling. Lancet 350:697–703

Teratology Society (1991) Recommendations for isotretinoin use in women of childbearing potential. Teratology 44:1–6

Thisted E, Ebbesen F (1993) Malformations, withdrawal manifestations, and hypoglycaemia after exposure to valproate in utero. Arch Dis Child 69(3 Spec No):288–291

Torok TJ (1995) Human parvovirus B19. In Remington JS, Klein JO (eds): Infectious Diseases of the Fetus and Newborn Infant, 4th edn. WB Saunders Co, Philadelphia, pp. 668–702

Tronick EZ, Beeghly M (1999) Prenatal cocaine exposure, child development, and the compromising effects of cumulative risk. Clin Perinatol 26:151–171

Valente P, Sever JL (1994) In utero diagnosis of congenital infections by direct fetal sampling. Isr J Med Sci 30:414–420

van der Pol JG, Wolf H, Boer K et al. (1992) Jejunal atresia related to the use of methylene blue in genetic amniocentesis in twins. Br J Obstet Gynaecol 99:141–143

Vanoverloop D, Schnell RR, Harvey EA, Holmes LB (1992) The effects of prenatal exposure to phenytoin and other anticonvulsants on intellectual function at 4 to 8 years of age. Neurotoxicol Teratol 14:329–335

Venn A, Lumley J (1994) Clomiphene citrate and pregnancy outcome. Aust N Z J Obstet Gynaecol 34:56–66

Wagner CL, Katikaneni LD, Cox TH, Ryan RM (1998) The impact of prenatal drug exposure on the neonate. Obstet Gynecol Clin North Am 25:169–194

Wallon M, Liou C, Garner P, Peyron F (1999) Congenital toxoplasmosis: Systematic review of evidence of efficacy of treatment in pregnancy. Br Med J 318:1511–1514

Warkany J (1978) Aminopterin and methotrexate: Folic acid deficiency. Teratology 17:353–358

Warkany J (1977) History of teratology. In Wilson JG, Fraser FC (eds): Handbook of Teratology. Vol. 1. Plenum, N Y, pp. 3–45

Warkany J (1979) Teratogen update: Antituberculous drugs. Teratology 20:133–138

Warkany J, Nelson CR (1940) Appearance of skeletal abnormalities in the offspring of rats reared on a deficient diet. Science 92:383–384

Warner RH, Rosett HL (1975) The effects of drinking on offspring: An historical survey of the American and British literature. J Stud Alcohol 36:1395–1420

Webster WS (1998) Teratogen Update: Congenital rubella. Teratology 58:13–23

Werler MM (1997) Teratogen update: Smoking and reproductive outcomes. Teratology 55:382–388

Whitley RJ, Arvin AM (1995) Herpes simplex virus infections. In Remington JS, Klein JO (eds): Infectious Diseases of the Fetus and Newborn Infant, 4th edn. WB Saunders, Philadelphia, pp. 354–376.

Wiebe VJ, Sipila PEH (1994) Pharmacology of antineoplastic agents in pregnancy. Crit Rev Oncol Hematol 16:75–112

Wiegand UW, Hartmann S, Hummler H (1998) Safety of vitamin A: Recent results. Int J Vitam Nutr Res 68:411–416

Wilkins-Haug L (1997) Teratogen update: Toluene. Teratology 55:145–151

Williams CL, Strobino B, Weinstein A et al. (1995) Maternal Lyme disease and congenital malformations: A cord blood serosurvey in endemic and control areas. Paediatr Perinat Epidemiol 9:320–330

Wisner KL, Gelenberg AJ, Leonard H et al. (1999) Pharmacologic treatment of depression during pregnancy. JAMA 282:1264–1269

Wiznia AA, Lambert G, Pavlakis S (1996) Pediatric HIV infection. Med Clin North Am 80:1309–1336

Wiznitzer A, Reece EA (1999) Assessment and management of pregnancy complicated by pregestational diabetes mellitus. Pediatr Ann 28:605–613

Woods JR Jr (1996) Adverse consequences of prenatal illicit drug exposure. Curr Opin Obstet Gynecol 8:403–411

Wyszynski DF, Duffy DL, Beaty TH (1997) Maternal cigarette smoking and oral clefts: A meta-analysis. Cleft Palate Craniofac J 34:206–210

Yerby MS (1994) Pregnancy, teratogenesis, and epilepsy. Neurol Clin 12:749–771

Zahn CA, Morrell MJ, Collins SD et al. (1998) Management issues for women with epilepsy: A review of the literature. Neurology 51:949–956

Ziskin MC (1999) Intrauterine effects of ultrasound: Human epidemiology. Teratology 59:252–60

ADDITIONAL READING

Briggs GG, Freeman RK, Yaffe SJ (1998) Drugs in Pregnancy and Lactation, 5th edn. Williams & Wilkins, Baltimore

Friedman JM, Polifka JE (2000) Teratogenic Effects of Drugs: A Resource for Clinicians (TERIS), 2nd edn. Johns Hopkins University Press, Baltimore

Jones KL (1997) Smith's Recognizable Patterns of Human Malformations, 5th edn. W.B. Saunders, Philadelphia

Koren G (1994) Maternal-Fetal Toxicology: A Clinician's Guide, 2nd edn. Marcel Dekker, N Y

Remington JS, Klein JO (eds) (2000) Infectious Diseases of the Fetus and Newborn Infant, 5th edn. W.B. Saunders, Philadelphia

Scialli AR, Lione A, Boyle Padgett GK (1995) Reproductive Effects of Chemical, Physical and Biologic Agents: REPROTOX. Johns Hopkins University Press, Baltimore

Shepard, Thomas H (1998) Catalog of Teratogenic Agents, 9th edn. Johns Hopkins University Press, Baltimore

Abnormal mental development

Gerald V. Raymond

40

Introduction

The formation of the nervous system is a complex process that begins early in embryogenesis and continues through intrauterine development and into the postnatal period. Alterations in the development of the nervous system result in alterations of function. While it is traditional to think of alterations in mental development as limited to disorders of intelligence or cognition, nearly all aspects of what makes us human are functions of higher cerebral development. Alterations in function can result in mental retardation, cerebral palsy, autism, and other developmental delays and these disorders have significant impact on the individual, their families, and society.

That there is a significant genetic component and that alterations in this development is an important clinical genetic problem is self-evident. In fact, the recognition of genetic causes of these disorders and in appropriate circumstances, their treatment as in PKU and other inborn errors, has been one of the major triumphs of genetic medicine of the last century.

This chapter will discuss the approach to genetic evaluation of the child with disordered development of the nervous system and will include mental retardation, cerebral palsy and autism. As will become apparent, they often coexist in the same individual and the genetic evaluation of these conditions does not significantly differ.

Definitions and epidemiology

MENTAL RETARDATION

Mental retardation is a serious and lifelong disability that places heavy demands on society and the health system (Hunter et al., 1980; McQueen et al., 1987). It is not a specific medical diagnosis, but rather as with all of the entities to be discussed here, a symptom. There have been multiple definitions proposed over the years with differing levels of acceptance (King et al., 1997). Mental retardation is generally accepted as having three components: (1) significantly abnormal intellectual performance – generally determined by a test of intelligence; (2) onset during development before the age of 18; and, (3) impairment of the ability to adapt to the environment (Batshaw, 1993).

The standard intelligence test centers on an average intelligence quotient (IQ) of 100 with a standard deviation of approximately 15; therefore, significantly subnormal intelligence is more than two SD below the mean or an IQ of 70 or less (Batshaw, 1993). The severity of the mental retardation can be divided into mild (50–70) or severe (<50). Severe mental retardation was formerly divided into moderate, severe, and profound, a system still used by many. Most epidemiologic studies rely on the simpler split into two groups, which will be the system used in this chapter (Roeleveld et al., 1997).

Published prevalence rates have varied from two through 85 per 1000. According to the World Health Organization, the rate of total mental retardation in industrialized nations is close to 3%, whereas in the United States the rate is said to be between 1 to 3% (King et al., 1997), and the Scandinavian countries have found a much lower rate of less than 1% (Gustavson et al., 1977; Hagberg et al., 1983).

A recent survey using the Metropolitan Atlanta Developmental Disabilities Study determined the overall prevalence to be 12.0 per 1000 in 10-year-olds (Murphy et al., 1995). The rate for mild mental retardation was 8.4/1000 compared to 3.6/1000 for severe mental retardation. The prevalence was higher in black children than in white children (prevalence odds ratio (POR) of 2.7), and in boys than in girls (POR = 1.4). In this study, not all individuals with mental retardation, especially in the mild range, were identified since case ascertainment was predominantly through the school system. Not unexpectedly, they found an increased incidence of other developmental disabilities, such as cerebral palsy and epilepsy, among the subjects. The rates were 12% in children with mild mental retardation and 45% in children with severe mental retardation (Murphy et al., 1995).

Most prevalence studies have focused on individuals requiring services, represented by the number of cases recorded by the authorities. However, the true prevalence rate is actually the number of individuals in the population with mental retardation whether or not they ever require services (Roeleveld et al., 1997; Murphy et al., 1995). Rates will vary depending on the study design, assessment criteria used, and method of identifying cases as well as the true rate in the studied population. Prevalence is age-dependent with the peak prevalence usually noted around 10 years of age, which reflects the fact that individuals with milder mental retardation will not come to attention until school age and that there are individuals who may be far along in school before their limitations are noted (Roeleveld et al., 1997).

A review by Roeleveld et al. (1997) highlighted these variables as the critical problems in all prevalence studies. They arrived at a relatively constant value of 3.8 per 1000 for severe mental retardation. While generally held to not vary depending on age, this was not the case for most of the studies presented. Most children with severe mental retardation do come to attention in the first years of life, but the highest prevalence is still among school age children. The prevalence of severe mental retardation declines with age, probably secondary to increased mortality and loss of contact with social services as they approach adulthood. The prevalence figures for mild mental retardation were higher than those for severely retarded and the variation in rates were significantly larger. Since these data were obtained from multiple studies, it is not clear the variation represents real differences among populations or differences in ascertainment. An overall rate of 29.8 per 1000 was obtained. The majority of individuals with mental re-

tardation fell into the mild range with a male predominance of 1.6–1.9:1 (Roeleveld et al., 1997).

A higher prevalence of mild mental retardation in lower socioeconomic classes has been found in many studies, and there is less class distinction in severe mental retardation. Because of this, it has been proposed that some individuals with mild mental retardation actually suffer from social disadvantage and the low IQ reflects an artefact. However, this influence has not been clear and there is increasing evidence of genetic influences even in lower socioeconomic classes (Blomquist et al., 1981; Costeff et al., 1983; Gillerot et al., 1989; Rutter et al., 1996; Satcher, 1995; Stromme and Hagberg, 2000; Yeargin-Allsopp et al., 1995).

The etiology of mental retardation includes genetic, infectious, and perinatal events. In almost all series, there remains a substantial number of individuals for whom no definite cause is found. More individuals with severe mental retardation will have a specific cause-identified than will individuals with mild mental retardation. This is reflected both in cases examined pathologically and by the increased genetic recurrence risk for severe mental retardation (Tables 40.1, 40.2).

CEREBRAL PALSY

Cerebral palsy (CP) is a heterogeneous collection of clinical presentations that are characterized by abnormal motor actions and postural mechanisms. The term does not imply causation (Miller and Clark, 1998). The symptoms and signs are by definition due to nonprogressive abnormalities of the developing brain. In other words, the pathologic appearance of lesions and their clinical expression may change with time as the brain matures, but there is no ongoing pathologic process. Voluntary movements that in an unaffected individual are complex, coordinated and varied become limited, stereotypic and uncoordinated. Cerebral palsy may coexist with other manifestations of brain injury including mental retardation, seizures, visual and hearing impairment, and other behavior abnormalities (Murphy et al., 1993; Boyle et al., 1996).

Cerebral palsy is typically classified according to the type and distribution of the motor abnormalities – hemiplegia, spastic diplegia, tetraplegia, dyskinetic or dystonic, ataxic, atonic/hypotonic, and mixed. Rarely is the presentation pure, and often clinical distinction between types may be difficult. Hemiplegia is a unilateral motor disturbance that is usually spastic. Bilateral spastic cerebral palsy involves both sides of the body. When limited to the legs, it is referred to as diplegia, and when it significantly involves the arms, quadriplegia or tetraplegia. Dyskinetic CP goes by a

Table 40.1. Etiology of Severe Mental Retardation

Category	Uppsala N=122	Hertfordshire n=146	Akershus N=79
Clearly genetic			
Chromosome abnormality	36	32.9	22
Down syndrome	32	32.2	
Other chromosome disorder	4	0.7	
Single gene disorder	5	14.4	27
Multiple congenital anomaly	20	13.0	9
CNS malformations	2	7.6	9
Perinatal or unidentified prenatal cause	16		8
Infectious disease	7	2.8	
Postnatal injury excluding infection	1	1.4	5
Infantile Psychosis	2		
Unclassified	12	12.3	18
Total	~100	~100	~100

Comparison of three regional surveys (Uppsala, Hertfordshire, and Akershus) expressed as percentage of total cases in each survey. Because multiple congenital anomalies or CNS malformations may be secondary to genetic or environmental causes, they are reported separately. Note that the percentage of patients with Down syndrome in the institutional group is low since the facility served individuals with severe or complex disabilities (Gustavson et al., 1977; Laxova et al., 1977; Stromme and Hagberg, 2000).

Table 40.2. Causes of mild mental retardation

Causes	Blomquist et al. (1981, 1983) 171 children	Hagberg et al. (1981) 126 children	Bundey et al. (1989) 439 children
Chromosomal			
Down syndrome	11	2	25
Fragile X	5	Not tested	7
Other	2	3	2
Single gene disorder	10	4	5
Malformation/syndrome	2	13	
Acquired			
Prenatal	19	8	
Perinatal	12	15	12 (combined pre- and perinatal)
Postnatal	8	4	14
Psychosis	3	2	0
Unclassified	99 (58%)	75 (60%)	364 (83%)

variety of other names including dystonic, extrapyramidal, and choreathetoid. The underlying abnormality is the inability to coordinate and organize voluntary movements with superimposed adventitial ones. Ataxic CP is characterized by signs that are generally felt to reflect cerebellar involvement. These include tremor, titubation, and wide, fluctuating movements of the limbs. Children with ataxic CP are usually hypotonic. The atonic or hypotonic category is reserved for individuals with a decrease in muscle tone beyond the first years of life. Many children in the first year or two of life who will ultimately develop another form of

CP will appear hypotonic with limited motor movements (Aicardi, 1998; Miller and Clark, 1998).

The prevalence of CP is about 2.5 per 1000 live births (Murphy et al., 1993). In full term infants the cause is usually of prenatal origin. Intrapartum events play only a limited role and may be influenced by preexisting conditions (Illingworth, 1985). Contrary to general perception, intrapartum asphyxia accounts for only 10–20% of CP (Holm, 1982; Freeman and Nelson, 1988; Shields and Schifrin, 1988). Other risk factors include prematurity, birth weight <1500 g, infection, and teratogens (Nelson and Ellenberg, 1986). In terms of genetic causes, children with cerebral dysgenesis and neuronal migration defects as well as children with major malformations are at increased risk for developing CP.

AUTISM

Autism is a behaviorally defined syndrome characterized by atypical social interaction, disordered verbal and nonverbal communication, restricted areas of interest, limited imaginative play, and a need for sameness. Many terms have been used to describe this presentation and include infantile autism, pervasive developmental disorder, childhood schizophrenia, and autistic psychoses. Varying definitions exist for autism and include those published in the DSM-IV (American Psychiatric Association, 1994) and the ICD-10 (WHO, 1993). Under the DSM-IV, several related childhood developmental disorders share these features: autistic disorder, Asperger disorder, childhood disintegrative disorder, pervasive developmental disorder (PDD-NOS (not otherwise specified), and atypical autism. The overarching term autistic spectrum is now often used because of the variability in the specific definitions (Filipek et al., 1999).

Children with infantile autism may have normal initial development, but then can undergo regression of language and social abilities between 15 to 21 months. It is estimated that 10–50% of children with autism will have a loss of previously acquired language (Tuchman and Rapin, 1997).

"Childhood disintegrative disorder", a separate DSM-IV diagnosis, refers to a specific group of children with early normal development until two years of age followed by rapid regression resulting in autism. This regression typically occurs between the ages of 36 to 48 months, later than that seen in autistic disorder. The hallmark signs include the loss of previously normal language, social, play, or motor skill and is marked by the onset of the restrictive repetitive behaviors typical for autism. Whether this disorder with the later regression is separate from the other forms of autistic spectrum disorder is uncertain, but the resultant symptoms in childhood disintegrative disorder are usually more severe than autistic disorder or pervasive developmental disorder (Volkmar, 1992).

Asperger syndrome is classically defined as individuals with milder autistic behavior and normal IQ. The DSM-IV criteria state that there should be no clinically important language delay, although the specific limits are unspecified. However, language is not normal and is often concrete and literal. Additionally, affected individuals have social deficits with restrictive, repetitive interests and are unable to form friendships with resultant social isolation.

Estimates of the prevalence of autism have varied greatly. This variation over time can be explained by differing definitions, study methods, and population. Prevalence was originally described as 4–5 per 10,000 (Lotter, 1966), but using a broader clinical phenotype others have reported a much higher incidence of 10–20 per 10,000 (Filipek et al., 1999). A recent investigation by the Centers for Disease Control and Prevention in Brick Township, New Jersey found a prevalence rate for autism of 4.0 per 1000 children and a rate of 6.7 for the autistic spectrum disorder. These prevalence rates are significantly higher and have raised alarms about increasing occurrence of this disorder, but at this time this awaits reconfirmation and further study.

The overall ratio of males to females with autism has been generally reported as 2:1 to 4:1 (Lotter, 1966; Wing and Gould, 1979; Volkmar et al., 1993). The male to female ratio appears to vary with intelligence ranging from 2:1 when associated with severe mental retardation to 4:1 with average IQ (Bryson, 1996; Ehlers and Gillberg et al., 1993; Wing and Gould, 1979). Most studies have found the incidence of co-existing mental retardation between 60–80% and epilepsy is seen in up to 25% of children.

Genetic evaluation of the child with developmental delay

NORMAL DEVELOPMENT AND ASSESSMENT

As emphasized in the opening section, function follows development of the neuronal substrate. It is important to realize how complex the brain becomes in gestation and how rapidly it continues to change postnatally. Development of the brain and functional ability occur in a sequential and orderly fashion; temporal norms are referred to as developmental milestones (Table 40.3).

The infant at birth is predominantly governed by reflex activity. The CNS has little myelination. The earliest motor activities, represented by automated reactions at the level of the brainstem and spinal cord, become suppressed during the first three to six months of life and are not continuous with later motor skills. This is one of the reasons that the predictive value of gross motor development is limited. Even children with severe mental retardation may have a relatively normal sequence of gross motor acquisition. The assessment of gross motor function does serve a role, however, in that abnormalities should alert the clinician to look at other areas of neurodevelopment and may be diagnostic for CP (Capute and Accardo, 1996).

Table 40.3. Developmental Milestones

Age (months)	Gross motor	Visual motor/Adaptive	Language
1	Raises head slightly from prone	Regards face Follows to midline	Alerts to sound Smile
4	Head and chest up in prone Rolls prone to supine	Grasps with both hands Midline play	Orients to voice Cooing Laughs
6	Sits unsupported	Reaches with either hand and transfers	Babbles
9	Pivots while sitting Pulls to stand Cruises	Overhand pincer grasp Finger-feeds	Imitates sounds
12	Cruising or walking independently	Pincer grasp Throws objects Cooperates with dressing	One step commands One word Comes when called
18	Running Throws objects	Uses a spoon Drinks from a cup	2 word phrases by 21 months
24	Goes up stairs	Undresses Uses fork	50 or more words Points to 6 body parts Follows 2-step commands
36	Pedals a tricycle	Dresses self Toilet trained	3 or more word sentences States full name

Ultimate intelligence correlates best with the progressive integration of visual and motor function and language development. Social and adaptive aspects of development come later as the child develops awareness of self and independence. Useful screens and measures of early development include the Denver Developmental Screening Test (DDST-revised), Bayley Scores of Infant Development, Cattell Infant Scales, Peabody Picture Vocabulary Test – revised (PPVT-R), and the Stanford Binet test of intelligence (King et al., 1997).

Global delay or delays in all the areas of development – gross and fine motor, language, social, and visual perception – even at early age, is suggestive of mental retardation. One specific area of delay, for example language, should not prompt prematurely diagnosing mental retardation, but should suggest further, specific evaluations. Other deviations from the normal route of development, even precocity, must also be addressed. Failing single items or achieving single milestones should never be viewed in isolation nor should the developmental quotient scores derived from individual areas of development be over-interpreted. Single findings should not elicit a diagnosis, but point to the need for further study and assist in diagnosis (Capute and Accardo, 1996).

GENETIC EVALUATION

The clinical assessment including prenatal and birth history, family pedigree, and a physical and neurological examin-

ation by the clinician emphasizing assessment of growth, major and minor anomalies, and development are the mainstays of a clinical genetic evaluation.

Certain approaches increase the yield in the evaluation of an individual with developmental delay. Serial examinations increase the rate of diagnosis (Majnemer and Shevell, 1995; Curry et al., 1997; Daily et al, 2000; Hunter, 2000; Shevell et al, 2000) because of the evolution of a specific recognizable physical or behavioral phenotype. In other cases, it is the result of new or more specific diagnostic methods. Testing focused on diagnosis should be performed sequentially when possible. The frequency of reevaluation varies depending on the severity, complexity, and age at presentation. The use of algorithms or standardized forms rarely can augment clinical expertise (Newell and Green, 1987; Battaglia et al., 1999).

The review of the family medical history should pay attention to the presence of individuals with mental retardation, autism, psychiatric disorders, learning problems, and congenital abnormalities. It is essential to obtain as much clinical documentation as possible on the patient and, where appropriate, on other family members. Diagnostic formulations on relatives may or may not be valid, and clinical documentation is essential.

The developmental assessment will be based partially on history and partially on the examination of the individual. In most situations the recall of developmental milestones by parents will be accurate. The reliance on events reported by the family will depend to some extent on the degree of delay, familiarity with normal milestones, and intactness of the family. There are many assessment scales put forward that rely heavily on specific milestones that may or may not be remembered. Memory will depend to an extent on time from acquisition (age at assessment) and number of children in the family. It is extraordinarily useful to review videos, home movies, or photographs of the child at various ages.

Physical examination

The examination of the individual with alterations of mental abilities will as any other genetic examination need to be as complete as necessary. One should determine present and previous growth, perform a general examination paying particular attention to other congenital abnormalities, and assess neurologic function.

Head circumference

Head circumference is an important sign of brain growth. The head circumference at birth can be very helpful for determining the timing of injury. Since head growth occurs rapidly in the third trimester, a second trimester prenatal ultrasound may have been normal, so head circumference at birth is very important. Microcephaly at birth is referred to as primary microcephaly and needs to be assessed for genetic causation. Unfortunately, many disorders can give rise to primary microcephaly, so it is rarely diagnostic. There are genetic causes of secondary microcephaly, but the majority are environmental. Important genetic causes of secondary microcephaly include Rett syndrome and certain inborn errors of metabolism e.g. sulfite oxidase deficiency, homocystinuria, and other disorders that can lead to loss of neuronal tissue.

The converse, macrocephaly is also important. Macrocephaly in a strict sense only refers to the size of the head and should not be confused with megalencephaly, an enlarged brain. Macrocephaly is most often due to hydrocephalus or an external fluid collection. When it is due to true enlargement of the brain, it is useful to distinguish between nonprogressive and progressive. Nonprogressive congenital megalencephaly may be seen in fragile X syndrome, Sotos syndrome, neurofibromatosis, tuberous sclerosis, and others. The progressive disorders include glutaric aciduria type 1, Alexander disease, Canavan disease, and Tay-Sachs disease (Lyon et al., 1996).

Ophthalmologic/eye abnormalities

The eye is embryologically very closely associated with cerebral development and the presence of structural eye abnormalities should always be noted. The presence of colobomas of the lids, iris, or retina may assist diagnosis. Microophthalmia may be noted in trisomy 13, 18, other chromosomal abnormalities, the Walker-Warburg lissencephaly syndrome, Frasier cryptophthalmos, and Aicardi syndrome. Cataracts are seen in certain genetic disorders as well as congenital infections. The telengiectasia of ataxia telengiectasia, aniridia of aniridia-Wilms tumor syndrome (WAGR), Lisch nodules in neurofibromatosis or ectopia lentis of homocystinuria may be viewed in the anterior eye. Retinal abnormalities are seen in Aicardi syndrome, peroxisome assembly disorders, Lebers amaurosis, as well as other progressive disorders. Optic atrophy and macular abnormalities may either be congenital or acquired. Eye movement abnormalities associated with other alterations in mental development usually indicate congenital blindness, but may also represent structural or functional abnormalities of the centers that control eye movements and may be seen in the newborn period in the X-linked Pelizaeus-Merzbacher syndrome and the autosomal recessive Joubert syndrome, or later in onset neuronal ceroid lipofuscinosis, peroxisomal diseases, Niemann-Pick syndrome. These are merely examples and the interested reader should refer to the section on ophthalmologic disorders (Chapters 132–139) or other reviews of genetic eye abnormalities (Birch, 1999; Cassidy and Taylor, 1999, Kerrison, 1999; Perrault et al., 1999; Traboulsi, 1995; Traboulsi, 1998; Traboulsi, 1999; Yen et al., 1999).

Hearing

The evaluation of hearing is particularly important in evaluating the child with developmental delay. Early language development is dependent on functional hearing. While hopefully rare and an event of the past, reports of deaf individuals being mistakenly labeled as mentally retarded exist. Deafness and mental retardation do coexist, examples being peroxisome assembly disorders, mitochondrial diseases, and the Cockayne syndrome, and should prompt further appropriate evaluation.

Abnormalities of the skin, hair, and skeletal/joints

Abnormalities of the ectoderm may assist in diagnosis and are required for diagnosis of several disorders (Lyon et al., 1996). Adenoma sebaceum, shagreen patches, or cafe au lait patches may be indicative of tuberous sclerosis, neurofibromatosis or other neurocutaneous disorders. Detection may be assisted by illuminating the skin with UV rays (e.g., a Woods lamp). Abnormalities of pigmentation may be generalized or patchy – the latter indicating possible chromosomal mosaicism. Other specific skin lesions include the angiokeratoma seen in fucosidosis, ichthyosis in multiple sulfatase deficiency and the Sjögren-Larsson syndrome, and photosensitive skin in xeroderma pigmentosa and Cockayne syndrome. Alopecia or thin hair are seen in a number of conditions including certain microcephaly syndrome. Hair whorls and other abnormalities of pattern may indicate underlying abnormalities of the brain. Abnormalities of the texture of the hair can be seen in Menkes disease, arginosuccinic aciduria, trichothiodystrophy, and giant axonal neuropathy.

Neurologic assessment

The brain is the organ responsible for cognition, language, motor activity, social interaction, and adaptive abilities and so it should really come as no surprise that in the evaluation of abnormalities of that function, a neurologic examination is highly recommended. The basic parts of the neurologic assessment should include the mental status, cranial nerve function, motor examination including tone, muscle strength, and mass; sensory examination, coordination, station and gait, and reflexes. The exam is age and state dependent; the sleeping infant has a different exam than an awake, hungry one. It has been appropriately pointed out that much can be learned from simply observing the child at play and interact with others and this opportunity should never be ignored (Aicardi, 1998).

The degree of mental impairment should be determined by appropriate psychometric assessment and the choice of tests and their interpretation is one area that is appropriately left with the professional psychologist.

Diagnostic tests

CHROMOSOME ANALYSIS

Chromosome abnormalities are the single most common cause found in series of unselected patients with mental retardation. The percentage of clinically relevant chromosome abnormalities found in the literature surveys is difficult to assess accurately since sites of ascertainment (clinic, institution, special schools), severity of mental handicap, and the presence of congenital anomalies as well as the type of cytogenetic study varies. Rates range from 4–28% in surveys of severe mental retardation with slightly lower rates for mild mental retardation (Table 40.4). Unless it is specifically excluded, the most common abnormality found is trisomy 21 or Down syndrome (see Ch. 44). The relevance of certain sex chromosome abnormalities and abnor-

malities found in studies prior to the availability of banding is uncertain.

Chromosomal abnormalities are also seen in individuals with autism. In one series of 233 individuals with autism in Utah, 5% had a major chromosomal abnormality (Gillberg, 1998). While nearly all chromosomes have been implicated in autism, the most common abnormality is that involving the long arm of chromosome 15 (15q11-13) occurring in 1–4% of consecutive cases meeting criteria for autistic disorder (Cook et al., 1997; Schroer et al., 1998). These are usually maternally derived duplications either pseudodicentric 15 (inverted duplication 15) or other markers involving 15q11-13. These patients are in general moderate to profoundly retarded although there have been reports of more mildly affected individuals (Bundey et al., 1994). In patients with IQ >35, interstitial duplications of 15q11-13 were found in more than 1% of patients and at a greater frequency than fragile X (Pericak-Vance et al., 1997; Gillberg, 1998; Schroer et al., 1998; Weidmer-Mikhail et al., 1998; Filipek et al., 1999).

Does a mentally retarded child without other physical features require cytogenetic assessment? Curry et al. (1996) showed that of those individuals with undiagnosed developmental delay in a genetics clinic, 16 out of 150 (11%) had chromosomal abnormalities. Four of these 16 were labeled as nondysmorphic by a clinical geneticist. Two had Klinefelter syndrome 47,XXY, one with tetrasomy 15q, and one with an unidentified marker found in a mosaic state in his mother. In addition as will be discussed, there is an increasing role for more advanced techniques in individuals with idiopathic mental retardation. There are patients who have been identified as having microdeletions who do not have unusual or characteristic features (Flint et al., 1995; Doheny et al., 1997).

Fluorescent in situ hybridization (FISH), the use of fluorescently tagged DNA, has proven invaluable in diagnosing and delineating the range of microdeletion or contiguous gene syndromes. It is certainly indicated in those patients with clear features of a known contiguous gene syndrome and should be combined with a standard banded karyotype. The yield of targeted FISH for microdeletions is naturally going to depend on the clinical indication, but in unselected cytogenetic series varied from 10–20% (Curry et al., 1997).

Every child with mental retardation without a clear diagnosis should have cytogenetic analysis at the 500 band level. In patients with asymmetry or pigmentary abnormalities, single or multiple biopsies for a fibroblast karyotype should be performed to examine for somatic mosaicism. Even in those with known syndromic causes, it may still be warranted

Table 40.4. Chromosomal Studies in Series of Individuals with Mental Retardation

Study	Source	Year	Number who received chromosome study	% Abnormal	Number with autosome abnormality	Down syndrome n(%)	Other autosome abnormality	Sex chromosome abnormality	FraX
Gustavson et al (1977)	Severe MR Uppsala Sweden	1959–1970	122	36	43	39	4		
Laxova et al (1977)	Severe MR Hertfordshire	1965–1967	146 children out of 46.960 total	~33	49	47	2		
Hagberg et al (1981)	Mild MR Gothenburg, Sweden	1966–1970	91[a]	4.4	3	2	1	1	
Hunter et al (1980)	Institutionalized Severe MR Manitoba	1975–1978	406[a]		55	48	6	1	
Rasmussen et al (1982)	Registered MR Aarhus, Denmark	1976	1905	18.8	326	281	45	33	
Bundey et al (1989)	Mild MR Special Schools Coventry, England	1984–1985	439[a]	10.7	26	25	1	1	20
Fryns et al. (1986)	Severe MR Institutional Belgium	1985	173	15.1	26	22	4		2/40
Wuu et al (1991)	Mentally retarded school children Taiwan	1988–1990	1323	MMR 7.87 SMR 17.51	116	64	52	9	
Hou et al (1998)	Identified MR in Taiwan 11,892	1991–1996	4372	43.2	1854	1557 (82.4)	297[b]	Not reported	233

MMR – mild mental retardation
SMR – severe mental retardation
[a]not all karyotyped
[b]includes 98 contiguous gene syndromes

due to findings of cytogenetic rearrangements. An important question remains of how many children with a "presumed known" diagnosis should be studied especially those with evidence of perinatal hypoxic-ischemia, since there is a role for prenatal or genetic causes in some of these cases.

There are several techniques presently becoming available that promise to add significantly to the evaluation of individuals with alteration of mental development. Using various strategies, 1–23% of cases of idiopathic mental retardation have been explained by deletions of the subtelomeric region (Anderlid et al., 1999; Joyce et al., 1999; Knight et al., 1999; Lamb et al., 1999; Slavotinek et al., 1999; Viot et al., 1998; Vorsanova et al., 1998). While it is generally agreed that there is a need for fast, reliable screening sets for the subtelomeric regions (Knight and Flint, 2000), it is not certain what the yield of these tests over standard karyotype will be and as yet there are no screening methods for duplications.

Uniparental disomy (UPD), the inheritance of both chromosomes or segments of a chromosome from a single parent rather than its usual biparental inheritance, has been demonstrated to involve chromosomes including 7, 14, 16, 20, and others (Chudoba et al., 1999; Fokstuen et al., 1999; Hall, 1999; Hordijk et al., 1999; Kotzot et al, 2000; Martin et al., 1999; Mergenthaler et al, 2000; Ralph et al., 1999). The role of imprinting involving chromosome 15 has been especially important in explaining the discrepant syndromes, Prader-Willi and Angelman and UPD has been shown to be an important cause of both conditions (Hall, 1999; Lalande et al., 1999). Techniques have been developed to rapidly screen for biparental inheritance (Buchholz et al., 1998; Dittrich et al., 1992; Glenn et al, 2000; Kubota et al., 1996; Muralidhar et al., 1998). However, Flint et al. (1995) did not find any instances of UPD in their evaluation of 99 individuals with idiopathic mental retardation and concluded that UPD accounted for idiopathic mental retardation in less than 5% of their population.

Fragile X

About 40% of X-linked mental retardation is attributable to the fragile X syndrome (FRAXA) (see Ch. 103). Two to six percent of males in residential and community programs have fragile X. Population prevalence ranges from 1:1000 to 1:6000 males and mental retardation has been noted in half of the females with a full mutation (Rousseau et al., 1991; Turner et al., 1992; Turner et al., 1996; Youings et al, 2000). In a study of boys attending special schools in Wessex in southern England, Youings et al (2000) found a prevalence of full mutation of FRAXA in males of 1 in 5530 and 1 in 23,423 for FRAXE, another fragile site located on the X chromosome believed to be associated with a milder phenotype.

The gene for the fragile X syndrome has been isolated (*FMR1*) and mutational analysis is standardized (Rousseau et al., 1991, Yu et al., 1991). Laboratory testing of the fragile X requires molecular analysis of *FMR1*. This permits differentiation of a normal complement of CGG repeats (less than 50), premutations (50–230), and full mutations (>230 repeats). The rarer deletions and point mutations of the *FMR1* must be considered as a cause of the phenotype when no abnormality of repeat number is found. Cytogenetic analysis is still indicated for other fragile sites (FRAXE) and since numerical and structural alterations are still as common, a banded karyotype is also indicated (Curry et al., 1997).

A variety of scoring systems have been proposed to assist with determining which males with mental retardation to test (Arvio et al., 1997; Butler et al., 1991; Giangreco et al., 1996; Jain et al., 1998). Most of them contain behavioral features, mental retardation, physical features including an elongated face, large testes, and large ears, and whether or not there is a family history. Since the laboratory confirmation of fragile X is relatively inexpensive and has implications for the patient and family assessment, it has been proposed that it be performed in all males and females with unexplained mental retardation (Curry et al., 1997).

NEUROIMAGING

Neuroimaging is performed to examine for structural abnormalities of the brain. However, computerized tomography (CT) has been shown to have little value in the routine assessment of children with severe mental retardation and autism. Lingam and associates (1982) examined 76 children with severe mental retardation: 72% had normal scans, 20% had cerebral atrophy, and 8% had a specific abnormality (agenesis of the corpus callosum, arachnoid cyst, and communicating hydrocephalus). It was felt that none of the findings had any positive genetic implications. Moeschler et al. (1981) demonstrated only one abnormality out of 23 scans (incidence of 4.3%) and again it did not assist in making the diagnosis. This is to be contrasted with the use of magnetic resonance imaging (MRI) which shows a high rate of abnormality when used in specific populations (Gabrielli et al., 1990; Sugimoto et al., 1993; Tamraz et al., 1987).

Magnetic resonance imaging is, in general, superior to CT. It is a more complete study of the brain since it images better the cranial base and the posterior fossa, allows evaluation of myelin, and has improved detection of subtle abnormalities – such as heterotopia, mild atrophy, and abnormalities of the corpus callosum. MRI does not directly visualize calcium and therefore cannot image bone directly or intracerebral calcifications. CT is therefore necessary in cases of suspected craniosynostosis or where there is a suspicion for calcification.

In most circumstances, some form of neuroimaging will be indicated. In the evaluation of children suspected of having a metabolic disorder, the areas of involvement and nature of the signal abnormality may be diagnostic (Brismar and Ozand, 1994; Forsting, 1999; Hirano and Pavlakis, 1994; Kohlschutter, 1994; Nyhan et al., 1999; Valk and van der Knaap, 1991; van der Knaap et al., 1996). It is also important in the individual with definite abnormalities in head growth, loss of skills, neurologic signs, or seizures. The value is less clear in an individual with either mental retardation or autism without any of the above. In known conditions such as Down syndrome or fragile X where the individual does not have any other neurologic signs, neuroimaging should be restricted to research questions only.

Newer techniques used to analyze other chemical constituents of the brain will have an increasing role in the future of assessing patients. Magnetic resonance spectroscopy (MRS), positron emission tomography (PET) and single photon emission computer tomography (SPECT) all demonstrate specific abnormalities in individuals with mental retardation, cerebral palsy, and autism (Deb, 1997; Deb and Thompson, 1998; Hoon et al., 1997; Jenkins and Kraft, 1999; O'Tuama and Treves, 1993; Santosh, 2000; Shevell et al., 1999).

METABOLIC TESTING

The prevalence of identified metabolic disease in the disorders under discussion is reportedly low although it is not known if this is true or rather reflects the difficulty in identifying a specific defect in a myriad of possibilities. Focused testing is clearly indicated in a wide variety of clinical situations ranging from neonatal hypotonia to loss of developmental milestones, and may encompass assessment of acid/base, plasma and urine amino acids, organic acids, thyroid studies, lysosomal enzyme analysis, carnitine determinations, and peroxisomal studies (Table 40.5). It is important to emphasize that often standard studies may give important diagnostic clues and are relatively inexpensive. These studies include a full hematologic panel, electrolytes, chemistry studies with special attention to creatinine kinase and uric acid, and urinanalysis especially for reducing substances.

In the list of the commonly treatable conditions (hypothyroidism, phenylketonuria, galactosemia, homocystinuria), most children will have been screened in the newborn period. It is important, however, to recognize that tested conditions vary from country to country and even among states of the USA, and a subset of the population may not deliver in hospital and partake of newborn screening.

Table 40.5. Biochemical Disorders that may Give Rise to Abnormal Mental Development

Mental Retardation
 Phenylketonuria
 Galactosemia
 Mucopolysaccharidosis
 Glycoprotein disorders
  Alpha-mannosidosis
  Fucosidosis
 Mitochondrial disease
  Pyruvate dehydrogenase deficiency
 Peroxisomal assembly disorders

Cerebral Palsy
 Arginase deficiency
 Sjögren-Larsson syndrome (fatty aldehyde dehydrogenase deficiency)
 Lesch-Nyhan syndrome
 Pyruvate dehydrogenase deficiency
 Hyperornithemia-hyperammonemia-homocitullinuria (HHH syndrome; ornithine translocase deficiency)

Autistic spectrum
 Adenylosuccinate lyase
 Phenylketonuria

OTHER STUDIES

As emphasized above, all children with mental retardation, autism, and cerebral palsy require a complete audiologic evaluation. A specific opthalmologic evaluation for diagnosis will depend on findings and concerns, but is generally indicated in the health care of any child. The examination of other tissue types or organ systems will depend on the situation – the routine examination of fibroblasts, skeletal X-rays, echocardiography, ultrasound examination of the kidneys, and others is not warranted.

Electroencephalogram (EEG) is appropriate in patients suspected to have seizures and is probably indicated in children who have regression of language abilities to evaluate for the nongenetic Landau-Kleffner syndrome or acquired epileptic aphasia. Whether it is justified in all children with autism is presently evolving (Tuchman, 1994; Rapin, 1995). EEG is not recommended in children with non-specified mental retardation or cerebral palsy. It does not assist with a genetic diagnosis. In many instances the test will be normal, but may also be abnormal, unnecessarily raising anxiety when there is no clinical indication to treat.

Specific clinical situations

STRUCTURAL BRAIN LESIONS

Structural brain abnormalities have been demonstrated in 34–98% of severely retarded individuals in postmortem studies (Cole et al., 1994; Crome, 1960; Freytag and Lindenberg, 1967; Warkany, 1971). Neuroimaging now gives us important information on the structure of the brain and congenital brain abnormalities are now routinely diagnosed during life and specifically at an early enough age to give parents important information about recurrence risk. The clinical signs of these malformations may include abnormalities of head size, abnormalities in skull shape, other dysmorphic features, delays in development, cerebral palsy, and seizures. The degree of structural changes are time-related so that earlier events lead to disorders of telencephalon development – holoprosencephaly, followed by disorders of migration giving rise to abnormalities of gyral formation with resultant lissencephaly (literally smooth brain), to the later occurrence of polymicrogyria. The specific brain abnormality will determine the specificity of the lesion and the recurrence risk. There are now known to be several genetic loci which will give rise to holoprosencephaly, lissencephaly, and several genetic/nongenetic causes of polymicrogyria. It is to be emphasized that not all examples will affect the cortical gray matter – abnormalities of the vermis will be seen in Joubert syndrome, agenesis of the corpus callosum in Aicardi syndrome, and tubers in tuberous sclerosis, enlargement of the ventricular system, abnormal signal of the white matter. Beside structural or developmental gene abnormalities, there are also biochemical abnormalities which can result in malformations. Some examples of both groups are provided in Table 40.6 and 40.7.

MICROCEPHALY

Microcephaly is an abnormality of head growth and is indicated by a decreased head circumference. The importance of this measurement cannot be overemphasized. When not secondary to craniosynostosis (an important, treatable cause not to be ignored), this single measure is an important indication of brain size. While many authors state that the head circumference must be 3 SD below the mean, the majority of clinicians use −2 SD. There is nothing inherently wrong with one definition versus the other, but decreased specificity will result in a slightly increased frequency of individuals and subsequently more individuals who are normal in the group. There are also clear differences between the sexes, age – both gestational and postnatal, and probably also between different ethnic groups (Nellhaus, 1968; Nellhaus, 1971; Raymond and Holmes, 1994).

Microcephaly vera ("true" microcephaly) represents an entity that is often genetic. It is characterized by extreme microcephaly without other abnormalities. Penrose (1972) suggested that autosomal recessive microcephaly had a characteristic phenotype consisting of a receding forehead, large ears, short stature, and a shuffling gait, and that spasticity and seizures were not common. Others have not found this to be the case and have emphasized that concordance for these features is poor (Adler, 1961; Powdermaker, 1930; Tolmie et al., 1987). That this is still a genetically heterogeneous group is reflected by other modes of inheritance both autosomal dominant and X-linked and that certain population groups have been determined to have either metabolic abnormalities or differing genetic localizations. It has been reported that the autosomal dominant form of microcephaly is usually free of neurologic signs and profound microcephaly rare (Haslam and Smith, 1979) and affected individuals may be only mildly retarded or intellectually normal (Crowe and Dickerman, 1986; Leung, 1987).

The empiric recurrence risk for microcephaly with mental retardation ranges widely from 6% (Herbst and Baird, 1982) to 20% (Opitz and Holt, 1990)(see Table 40.8). Tolmie and

Table 40.6. Cerebral Malformations

Malformation	Chromosome Localization	Gene	Recurrence Risk in Sibs
Holoprosencephaly			13–14% (Odent et al., 1998)
HPE1	21q22.3		
HPE2	2p21	SIX3	
HPE3	7q36	SHH	
HPE4	18p11.3	TGIF	
Lissencephaly			
Miller-Dieker (MDS)	17p13.3 deletion	LIS1	Parent – balanced translocation 12% MDS (Pollin et al., 1999)
			Parents normal – 5%
Isolated Lissencephaly	17p13.3 (no chromosomal deletion)	LIS1	5% empiric If mutation found 1% based on germline mosaicism
X-linked lissencephaly in males Subcortical laminar heterotopia in females	Xq22.3-q23	LISX doublecortin	50% for male and female although clinical variability in females
Walker-Warburg (Type II)	9q31		
Schizencephaly	10q26.1	EMX2	Mainly sporadic, one documented instance of presumed germline mosaicism (Faiella et al., 1997)
Hydrocephalus			4% (Varadi et al., 1988)
Hydrocephalus with aqueductal stenosis in males	Xq28	L1CAM HSAS1	6–25%

Table 40.7. Biochemical Disorders that can Cause Cerebral Malformations

Nonketotic hyperglycinemia

Pyruvate dehydrogenase deficiency

Pyruvate carboxylase deficiency

Zellweger syndrome

Glutaric acidemia type II

Smith-Lemli-Opitz syndrome

Table 40.8. Studies of Recurrence Risk of Microcephaly

Reference	Sib recurrence risk (%)
Brandon et al. (1959)	6
Bundey and Carter (1974)	0
Bundey and Griffiths (1977)	13
Opitz et al. (1978)	20
Bartley and Hall (1978)	11
Herbst and Baird (1982)	5.9
Tolmie et al. (1987)	19

associates (1987) reported their experience with microcephaly as the major finding – all children had at least one determination of head circumference less than 3 SD. They only included individuals who had been born after counseling for the first affected child which excluded 2 recurrences which were determined only after the second occurrence. Using these criteria, they determined an empiric recurrence risk of 19%.

Prenatal diagnosis of microcephaly before the third trimester is difficult. In two prospectively followed cases in the report of Tolmie et al. (1987), head growth was determined to slow, but was not diagnostic until the third trimester. This is not surprising since much of head and body growth occurs in the third trimester making a determination of this specific growth failure challenging.

MOTOR ABNORMALITIES (CEREBRAL PALSY)

There is clearly the opinion that CP or static motor abnormalites are rarely genetic. This would appear to be born out in several large series that have examined for the recurrence risk of cerebral palsy. Asher and Schonell (1950) in their survey of CP in Birmingham found only one affected sib in 349 families. Gustavson et al. (1969) in a study of CP in Sweden found 30 families out of 3150 in which there were affected sibs with normal parents. Bundey and Griffiths (1977) found a risk of about 1 in 9 for sibs of children with symmetrical spasticity and suggested that about half of such children have a recessive condition. What these series fail to account for are newly recognized entities and the fact that many metabolic or structural disorders are then excluded from the lists of CP. Unfortunately the converse is not known, how many structural, metabolic, and other genetic disorders are not uncovered in the rolls of cerebral palsy clinics. It is also not certain epidemiologically how many children are not completely characterized/defined – i.e., children who may receive the diagnosis of profound mental retardation, but never receive a static motor diagnosis as well. The list of conditions that can result in motor abnormalities is quite extensive and includes the structural abnormalites as well as metabolic processes (see Tables 40.6 and 40.7).

Certain subtypes of CP are stated to be at more risk for recurrence. Estimates are that one-third to one-half of all cases of congenital ataxia with mental retardation are genetic (Gustavson et al., 1969; Miller, 1988; Yannet, 1944). Several investigators have demonstrated a higher recurrence risk for spastic cerebral palsy if the spasticity was symmetrical (Böök, 1953; Bundey and Griffiths, 1977; Penrose, 1938; Yannet, 1944).

Athetoid CP is generally stated to be environmental except in rare instances – Lesch-Nyhan with hyperuricemia and self-mutilation as well as reports of other X-linked forms (Adler, 1961; Baar and Gabriel, 1966; Bundey and Carter, 1974). Athetoid CP may be secondary to genetic or metabolic disorders and that there may be a characteristic appearance on MRI (Hoon et al., 1997).

Children who suffer a hemorrhage in the newborn period which would be expected to result in motor and other neurologic sequella may have an underlying genetic coagulopathy (Harum et al., 1999a; Harum et al., 1999b) as the cause of their acquired hemorrhage.

BEHAVIORAL ABNORMALITIES

A behavioral phenotype refers to the specific and characteristic behavioral repertoire exhibited by patients with a genetic or chromosomal disorder (Flint, 1996; Flint, 1998). There are conditions that are more easily diagnosed by the recognition of their resultant behaviors than by any specific physical features. This is an expanding field and further experience with certain manifestations will produce new insights.

Several disorders are noted for their incidence of autism and include fragile X, dup 15q, and adenylosuccinase deficiency. Self-mutilation, a dramatic symptom, has been seen in Lesch-Nyhan, Smith-Magenis, and Prader-Willi syndromes, but can also be seen in other individuals with congenital neuropathies, mental retardation, and autism. Characteristic hand wringing and breathing abnormalities are typical for the Rett syndrome. Similar breathing abnormalities outside of metabolic derangement are seen in Joubert syndrome and in the oral-facial-digital syndrome, Type VI. Angelman syndrome is notable for laughing and giggling and Prader-Willi for hyperphagia and food-driven behaviors. The Williams syndrome is notable for its preservation of language and social openness.

Flint (1998) has pointed out that the whole category of behavioral abnormalities raises a number of conceptual and methodologic issues. The strictness of the behavioral phenotype is a problem of expression. For example, Lesch-Nyhan is so characterized by self-mutilation that if the behavior is absent, the diagnosis is often called into question (Christie et al., 1982; Anderson et al., 1994), but other conditions may not always demonstrate a specific behavioral phenotype as completely. The second issue is demonstrating that a particular behavior is part of a behavioral phenotype, as illustrated by fragile X and autism. The sample size needed to establish an association at a statistically significant level is difficult to obtain and will likely be impossible for a rare syndrome. As an example, fragile X accounts for 5% of autism (Bailey et al., 1993; Bailey et al., 1998) while in the general population, autism occurs at the lower rate of approximately four per 10,000. While autism occurs at a higher incidence in fragile X, demonstrating a direct connection that fragile X results in autism has been difficult. As an alternative, it has been proposed that mental retardation, a nonspecific consequence of FRAXA, predisposes to autism (Fisch, 1992).

Finally, there are unusual behaviors for which no validated measures exist. For example, Smith Magenis (del 17p11.2) can result in an unusual forms of self injury, such as biting, pulling out toe and fingernails, inserting foreign bodies into various orifices and no rating scales exist for such severe behaviors (Flint, 1998).

PROGRESSIVE CONDITIONS

While this chapter deals mainly with static conditions, identifying progressive deterioration is extremely important. Many clearly degenerative conditions will initially only demonstrate protean symptoms and may present at nearly any age – infancy to the progressive selective neuronal degenerations of Huntington and Alzheimer disease in the elderly. There are also genetic disorders that will appear initially to be a static condition, but which can progress. These disorders can range from the peroxisome assembly disorders such as neonatal adrenoleukodystrophy, associated with blindness, deafness, and a leukodystrophy on the backdrop of a child with hypotonia and developmental delay, through the progressive Alzheimer-like dementia that can appear at a young age in Down syndrome.

The clinical clues to a progressive condition may be obvious or may be subtle and nonspecific. It is apparent that the child who has previously reached some milestone, clearly mastered it, and is now losing that ability has a degenerative condition. The greater difficulty is with the child who is not attaining milestones at the appropriate ages and who appears to have some preexisting condition. The child with skills that plateau presents a special problem. In some cases this will be the opening sign of deterioration, but in many more circumstances it will be shown to be a static process whose severity was underappreciated.

Regression of developmental milestones should always prompt an appropriate and thorough assessment, for it is only by determining the cause that possible treatment may be sought, prognosis broadly applied, and possible prenatal diagnosis in subsequent pregnancies made in appropriate circumstances.

The diagnosis of a progressive neurologic condition rests on the presentation – areas involved as determined by symptoms, signs, and neuroradiologic findings, age at onset, family history, and associated areas of involvement, such as hepatomegaly, retinal involvement, skeletal abnormalities. Algorithms and other devices for diagnosis have been proposed, but are rarely exhaustive or uniformly appropriate, cannot account for variations, and should only be relied upon for general guidance. There are several sources that are appropriate to consult in evaluating an individual with a suspected progressive condition (Dyken, 1996; Lyon et al., 1996; Dyken and Krawiecki et al., 1983).

Genetic recurrence risks for undiagnosed causes of mental retardation and autism

One of the main reasons to determine a diagnosis is to obtain recurrent risk figures. When a genetic diagnosis can be made, it will provide important iformation for the individual and their family.

However, even after appropriate evaluation, some individuals with either mental retardation or autism will not have either a diagnosis or a cause. Nonspecific mental retardation or autism refers to the patient with a normal head circumference, no recognizable dysmorphic syndrome, and no other neurologic signs who has been appropriately evaluated. The recurrence risks of CP have already been discussed.

Risks for siblings

Data on recurrences of severe mental retardation in sibs are provided by the British Columbia survey of many patients (Herbst and Baird, 1982) as well as other smaller studies (Bundey et al., 1985). In the study by Herbst and Baird (1982), the risks to sibs ranged from 11.7% for brothers of severely retarded males to 1.8% for sisters of moderately retarded males, with an overall risk of $4.4 \pm 0.6\%$ for sibs (Table 40.9). The sex of the index case influences the recurrence risk with a higher risks for brothers of a male index case and a much lower risk for sisters of a male index case. This sex difference is secondary to X-linked mental retardation, both fragile X as well as other X-linked mental retardation syndromes. The level of mental retardation did not significantly change the recurrence risk for all sibs. However, the brothers of male index patients again had a significantly increased risk at the moderate and severe mental retardation level. This was not apparent at the mild and profound level where there were no significant differences in risk. This was similar to the results of Turner et al. (1971), but differed from that of Bundey et al. (1989) who found a very high recurrence risk of one in four to one in five for mild mental retardation. The recurrence risk after two affected sibs with nonspecific MR is increased to $12 \pm 7\%$ (Herbst and Baird, 1982).

Recurrence risks for sons of unaffected sisters of probands

Risks for sisters' sons depend upon the risks of a mentally retarded boy having an X-linked condition and for the proband's mother being a carrier. Herbst and Miller (1980) considered this question in regard to non-specific mental retardation by analyzing the British Columbia Health

Table 40.9. Sib Recurrence Risks for Severe Nonspecific Mental Retardation

Study	Brothers	Sisters	All Sibs
Male Index Case			
Herbst and Baird, 1982	1 in 12	1 in 33	1 in 18
Bundey et al., 1985	1 in 10	1 in 20	1 in 13
Female Index Case			
Herbst and Baird, 1982	1 in 22	1 in 17	1 in 19

Table 40.10. Approximate Risks for X-linked Inheritance of Nonspecific Mental Retardation in Those Families in Which the Fragile X has Been Excluded

Patient	Risk of boy being a new mutation for X-linked disease	Risk of boy with a carrier mother	Risk for sister being a carrier
Isolated male	1/20	1/20	1/40
Two similarly affected brothers but no other affected relative	0	1/3	1/6

surveillance registry for children with nonspecific mental retardation born between 1950 to 1969. They determined the excess of affected brother-brother pairs over affected sister-sister pairs, on the assumption that all such sibships were examples of X-linked inheritance. There were 35 sibships with two or more affected sisters and 107 sibships with two or more affected brothers, giving an excess of 72 sibships with presumed X-linked mental retardation, and therefore 72 carrier mothers. It was then estimated how many more carrier mothers there should be who either had one or no affected sons and an adjustment of 1/3 was made for new mutations in males. From these figures they estimated the total number of all boys with X-linked mental retardation who might be expected to be born during the study period and they found this number approximated the observed excess of males over females with nonspecific mental retardation. The estimate of the proportion of males with X-linked mental retardation was 27% of whom approximately one-third had an affected brother. The assumption was then made, based on data from other studies, that about one-half of such males would have the fragile X syndrome.

These figures can then be used to estimate genetic counseling risk figures for sisters. Approximately 27% of males with nonspecific mental retardation will have an X-linked condition which will be the fragile X syndrome in half of cases. So 13.5% of males will have the other forms of X-linked mental retardation. Approximately 1/3 will be new mutations, 1/3 will have an affected brother, 1/3 will have a carrier mother but no affected brother. Therefore, of isolated males without the fragile X syndrome about 9% will have another form of X-linked mental retardation.

If one now considers sibships with two or more affected males, about 1/3 will have autosomal recessive disease (based on the British Columbia data of 107 all male sibships to 35 all female sibships), about 1/3 will have the fragile X syndrome, and about 1/3 another X-linked mental retardation syndrome with affected males on the maternal side in about half the cases. Therefore if there are two brothers with a similar type of nonspecific mental retardation, without affected uncles or cousins and who test negative for fragile X their overall chance of having an X-linked form of mental retardation 1 in 3. The family risks are set out in Table 40.10.

Risks for offspring

Risks are assessed in relation to offspring of mildly retarded adults since very few severely retarded adults become parents. Risks are provided by Reed and Reed (1965) with the overall risks for mental retardation in offspring being 1 in 7 (14%); the risks were higher for the offspring of retarded females, in this series close to 20% (see Table 40.11), which most likely reflects the presence of fragile X and the other causes of X-linked mental retardation.

RECURRENCE RISK FOR AUTISM

Studies on the recurrence risk of autism have been limited by differences in definitions and criteria used in ascertainment. The recurrence risk of autism is estimated to be between 3% and 7% across several studies (Bolton et al., 1994; Jorde et al., 1990; Piven et al., 1990; Szatmari et al., 1993). Baird and August (1985) found 3 (5.9%) of 51 siblings of 29 probands. Ritvo et al. (1989) performed an epidemiologic study of autism in Utah, and found 20 (9.7%) of families with more than one child with autism. The overall recurrence risk was 8.6%, but varied with the sex of the firstborn autistic child becoming 7.0% if the proband was male and 14.5% if female. The sibling risk for autism was 4.5% (Ritvo et al., 1989). This recurrence risk is substantially higher for having a second child on the autistic spectrum, 1 in 20 to 1 in 10, as compared with 1 in 500–1000 for the general population.

Table 40.11. Offspring of Mentally Retarded Adults

Parent	IQ Range in Offspring		
	<50	50–70	>70
Mentally retarded male with normal or unknown partner	3/341 (1%)	28/341 (8%)	310/341 (91%)
Mentally retarded female with normal or unknown partner	16/313 (5%)	44/313 (14%)	253/313 (81%)

Conclusion

The genetic evaluation of the child with abnormal mental development continues to be an important problem in genetic medicine. Improved techniques of both genetic analysis and neuroimaging, enhance the ability to diagnose the individual with mental retardation or other developmental delays. When undertaking the initial evaluation, the goals of the evaluation should be discussed with the family. In most situations, diagnosis will not significantly alter care of the child, but may assist families in understanding the condition, its prognosis and recurrence risks, and allow them access to prenatal diagnosis. It is important to emphasize that even in modern series, a significant percentage of cases will not have a clear cause of the delays and this should also be stated to the family. Empiric recurrence risks continue to be essential in the counseling of families in which a definite cause cannot be determined.

Acknowledgement

This chapter is dedicated to the memory of Dr Sarah Bundey. Dr Bundey, who was the previous author of this chapter, made many important contributions to the field of genetics and especially in the area of mental retardation and developmental delay. Her work continues to provide important information on the incidence and recurrence risks of a variety of problems in development which ultimately served the patient and family.

REFERENCES

Adler E (1961) Familial cerebral palsy. J Chronic Disease 13:207–214

Aicardi J (1998) Diseases of the Nervous System in Childhood, 2nd edn. Mac Keith Press, London

American Psychiatric Association (1994) Diagnostic and Statistical Manual of Mental Disorder, 4th edn. Washington, D.C.

Anderlid B, Anneren G, Blennow E, Nordenskjold M (1999) Subtelomeric rearrangements detected by FISH in patients with idiopathic mental retardation. Am J Hum Genet 65:A67

Anderson LT, Ernst M (1994) Self-injury in Lesch-Nyhan disease. J Autism and Developmental Disorders 24:67–81

Arvio M, Peippo M, Simola KO (1997) Applicability of a checklist for clinical screening of the fragile X syndrome. Clinic Genet 52:211–215

Asher P, Schonell FE (1950) A survey of 400 cases of cerebral palsy in childhood. Archives of Disease in Childhood 25:360–379

Baar HS, Gabriel AM (1966) Sex-linked spastic paraplegia. Am J Mental Deficiency 71(1):13–18

Bailey A, Bolton P, Butler L et al. (1993) Prevalence of the fragile X anomaly amongst autistic twins and singletons. J Child Psychology and Psychiatry 34:673–688

Bailey DBJ, Mesibov GB, Hatton DD et al. (1998) Autistic behavior in young boys with fragile X syndrome. J Autism and Developmental Disorders 28:499–508

Bamforth F, Bamforth S, Poskitt K et al. (1988) Abnormalities of corpus callosum in patients with inherited metabolic diseases [letter]. Lancet 2:451

Bartley JA, Hall BD (1978) Mental retardation and multiple congenital anomalies of unknown etiology: Frequency of occurrence in similarly affected sibs of the proband. Birth Defects Original Article Series 14(6B):127–137

Batshaw ML (1993) Mental retardation. Pediatric Clinics of North America 40:507–521

Battaglia A, Bianchini E, Carey JC (1999) Diagnostic yield of the comprehensive assessment of developmental delay/mental retardation in an institute of child neuropsychiatry. Am J Med Genet 82:60–66

Birch DG (1999) Retinal degeneration in retinitis pigmentosa and neuronal ceroid lipofuscinosis: An overview. Molec Genet and Metabolism 66:356–366

Blomquist HK, Gustavson KH, Holmgren G (1981) Mild mental retardation in children in a northern Swedish county. J Mental Deficiency Research 25:169–186

Blomquist HK, Gustavson KH, Holmgren G et al. (1983) Fragile X syndrome in mildly mentally retarded children in a northern Swedish county. A prevalence study. Clin Genet 24:393–398

Bolton P, Macdonald H, Pickles A et al. (1994) A case-control family history study of autism. J Child Psychology and Psychiatry 35:877–900

Böök JA (1953) A genetic and neuropsychiatric investigation of a north-Swedish population. Part II. Mental deficiency and convulsive disorders. Acta Genetica et Statistica Medica 4:345–414

Boyle CA, Yeargin-Allsopp M, Doernberg NS et al. (1996) Prevalence of selected developmental disabilities in children 3–10 years of age: the Metropolitan Atlanta Developmental Disabilities Surveillance Program, 1991. Morbidity Mortality Weekly Report CDC Surveillance Summary 45:1–14

Brandon MWG, Kirman BH, Williams CE (1959) Microcephaly. J Mental Science 105:721–747

Brismar J, Ozand PT (1994) CT and MR of the brain in disorders of the propionate and methylmalonate metabolism. AJNR American Journal of Neuroradiology 15:1459–1473

Bryson SE (1996) Brief report: Epidemiology of autism. J Autism and Developmental Disorders 26:165–167

Buchholz T, Jackson J, Robson L, Smith A (1998) Evaluation of methylation analysis for diagnostic testing in 258 referrals suspected of Prader-Willi or Angelman syndromes. Hum Genet 103:535–539

Bundey S, Carter CO (1974) Recurrence risks in severe undiagnosed mental deficiency. J Mental Deficiency Research 18:115–134

Bundey S, Griffiths MI (1977) Recurrence risks in families of children with symmetrical spasticity. Developmental Medicine and Child Neurology 19:179–191

Bundey S, Hardy C, Vickers S et al. (1994) Duplication of the 15q11-13 region in a patient with autism, epilepsy and ataxia. Developmental Medicine and Child Neurology 36:736–742

Bundey S, Webb TP, Thake A, Todd J (1985) A community study of severe mental retardation in the West Midlands and the importance of the fragile X chromosome in its aetiology. J Med Genet 22:258–266

Bundey S, Thake A, Todd J (1989) The recurrence risks for mild idiopathic mental retardation. J Med Genet 26:260–266

Butler MG, Mangrum T, Gupta R, Singh DN (1991) A 15-item checklist for screening mentally retarded males for the fragile X syndrome. Clin Genet 39:347–354

Capute AJ, Accardo PJ (1996) The infant neurodevelopmental assessment: a clinical interpretive manual for CAT-CLAMS in the first two years of life, part 1. Current Problems in Pediatrics 26:238–257

Cassidy L, Taylor D (1999) Congenital cataract and multisystem disorders. Eye 13:464–473

Christie R, Bay C, Kaufman IA et al. (1982) Lesch-Nyhan disease: Clinical experience with nineteen patients. Developmental Medicine and Child Neurology 24:293–306

Chudoba I, Franke Y, Senger G et al. (1999) Maternal UPD 20 in a hyperactive child with severe growth retardation. Euro J Hum Genet 7:533–540

Cole G, Neal JW, Fraser WI, Cowie VA (1994) Autopsy findings in patients with mental handicap. J Intellectual Disability Research 38:9–26

Cook EH, Jr, Lindgren V, Leventhal BL et al. (1997) Autism or atypical autism in maternally but not paternally derived proximal 15q duplication. Am J Hum Gene 60:928–934

Costeff H, Cohen BE, Weller LE (1983) Biological factors in mild mental retardation. Developmental Medicine and Child Neurology 25:580–587

Crome L (1960) The brain and mental retardation. BMJ 1:897–904

Crowe CA, Dickerman LH (1986) A genetic association between microcephaly and lymphedema. Am J Med Genet 24:131–135

Curry CJ, Sandhu A, Frutos L and Wells R (1996) Diagnostic yield of genetic evaluations in developmental delay/mental retardation. Clinical Research 44:130A

Curry CJ, Stevenson RE, Aughton D et al. (1997) Evaluation of mental retardation: recommendations of a Consensus Conference: American College of Medical Genetics. Am J Med Genet 72:468–477

Daily DK, Ardinger HH, Holmes GE (2000) Identification and evaluation of mental retardation. American Family Physician 61:1059–67, 1070

Deb S (1997) Structural neuroimaging in learning disability. B J Psychiat 171:417–419

Deb S, Thompson B (1998) Neuroimaging in autism. BJ Psychiat 173:299–302

Dittrich B, Robinson WP, Knoblauch H et al. (1992) Molecular diagnosis of the Prader-Willi and Angelman syndromes by detection of parent-of-origin specific DNA methylation in 15q11-13. Hum Genet 90:313–315

Dobyns WB (1989) Agenesis of the corpus callosum and gyral malformations are frequent manifestations of nonketotic hyperglycinemia. Neurology 39:817–820

Doheny KF, McDermid HE, Harum K et al. (1997) Cryptic terminal rearrangement of chromosome 22q13.32 detected by FISH in two unrelated patients. J Med Genet 34:640–644

Dyken P, Krawiecki N (1983) Neurodegenerative diseases of infancy and childhood. Annals of Neurology 13:351–364

Dyken PR (1996) Neurodegenerative diseases in pediatric neurology. Introduction. Seminars of Pediatric Neurology 3:257–259

Ehlers S, Gillberg C (1993) The epidemiology of Asperger syndrome. A total population study. J Child Psychology and Psychiatry 34:1327–1350

Faiella A, Brunelli S, Granata T et al. (1997) A number of schizencephaly patients including 2 brothers are heterozygous for germline mutations in the homeobox gene EMX2. Euro J Hum Genet 5:186–190

Filipek PA, Accardo PJ, Baranek GT et al. (1999) The screening and diagnosis of autistic spectrum disorders. J Autism and Developmental Disorders 29:439–484

Fisch GS (1992) Is autism associated with the fragile X syndrome? Am J Med Genet 43:47–55

Flint J (1996) Annotation: behavioural phenotypes: a window onto the biology of behaviour. J Child Psychology and Psychiatry 37:355–367

Flint J (1998) Behavioral phenotypes: Conceptual and methodological issues. Am J Med Genet 81:235–240

Flint J, Wilkie AO, Buckle VJ et al. (1995) The detection of subtelomeric chromosomal rearrangements in idiopathic mental retardation. Nat Genet 9:132–140

Fokstuen S, Ginsburg C, Zachmann M, Schinzel A (1999) Maternal uniparental disomy 14 as a cause of intrauterine growth retardation and early onset of puberty. J Pediatr 134:689–695

Forsting M (1999) MR imaging of the brain: Metabolic and toxic white matter diseases. Euro Radiology 9:1061–1065

Freeman JM, Nelson KB (1988) Intrapartum asphyxia and cerebral palsy. Pediatr 82:240–249

Freytag E, Lindenberg R (1967) Neuropathologic findings in patients of a hospital for the mentally deficient. A survey of 359 cases. Johns Hopkins Medical Journal 121:379–392

Fryns JP, Kleczkowska A, Dereymaeker A et al. (1986) A genetic-diagnostic survey in an institutionalized population of 173 severely mentally retarded patients. Clin Genet 30:315–323

Gabrielli O, Salvolini U, Coppa GV et al. (1990) Magnetic resonance imaging in the malformative syndromes with mental retardation. Pediatric Radiology 21:16–19

Giangreco CA, Steele MW, Aston CE et al. (1996) A simplified six-item checklist for screening for fragile X syndrome in the pediatric population. J Pediatr 129:611–614

Gillberg C (1998) Chromosomal disorders and autism. J Autism and Developmental Disorders 28:415–425

Gillerot Y, Koulischer L, Yasse B, Wetzburger C (1989) The geneticist and the so-called "socio cultural" familial mental retardation. Journal de Genetique Humaine 37:103–112

Glenn CC, Deng G, Michaelis RC et al. (2000) DNA methylation analysis with respect to prenatal diagnosis of the Angelman and Prader-Willi syndromes and imprinting. Prenatal Diagnosis 20:300–306

Gustavson KH, Hagberg B, Sanner G (1969) Identical syndromes of cerebral palsy in the same family. Acta Paediatrica Scandinavia 58(4):330–340

Gustavson KH, Hagberg B, Hagberg G, Sars K (1977) Severe mental retardation in a Swedish county. II. Etiologic and pathogenetic aspects of children born 1959–1970. Neuropadiatrie 8:293–304

Hagberg B, Hagberg G, Lewerth A, Lindberg U (1981) Mild mental retardation in Swedish school children. II. Etiologic and pathogenetic aspects. Acta Paediatrica Scandinavia 70:445–452

Hagberg B, Kyllerman M (1983) Epidemiology of mental retardation – a Swedish survey. Brain Development 5:441–449

Hall JG (1999) Human diseases and genomic imprinting. Results and Problems in Cell Differentiation 25:119–32:119–132

Harum KH, Hoon AH, Jr., Kato GJ et al. (1999) Homozygous factor-V mutation as a genetic cause of perinatal thrombosis and cerebral palsy. Developmental Medicine and Child Neurology 41(11):777–780

Harum KH, Hoon AH, Jr., Casella JF (1999) Factor-V Leiden: a risk factor for cerebral palsy. Developmental Medicine and Child Neurology 41(11):781–785

Haslam RH, Smith DW (1979) Autosomal dominant microcephaly. J Pediatr 95:701–705

Herbst DS, Baird PA (1982) Sib risks for nonspecific mental retardation in British Columbia. Am J Med Genet 13:197–208

Herbst DS, Miller JR (1980) Nonspecific X-linked mental retardation II: The frequency in British Columbia. Am J Med Genet 7:461–469

Hirano M, Pavlakis SG (1994) Mitochondrial myopathy, encephalopathy, lactic acidosis, and strokelike episodes (MELAS): Current concepts. J Child Neurology 9:4–13

Holm VA (1982) The causes of cerebral palsy. A contemporary perspective. JAMA 247(10):1473–1477

Hoon AH, Jr., Reinhardt EM, Kelley RI et al. (1997) Brain magnetic resonance imaging in suspected extrapyramidal cerebral palsy: Observations in distinguishing genetic-metabolic from acquired causes. J Pediatr 131:240–245

Hordijk R, Wierenga H, Scheffer H et al. (1999) Maternal uniparental disomy for chromosome 14 in a boy with a normal karyotype. J Med Genet 36:782–785

Hou JW, Wang TR, Chuang SM (1998) An epidemiological and aetiological study of children with intellectual disability in Taiwan. J Intellectual Disabilities Research 42:137–143

Hughes I, Newton R (1992) Genetic aspects of cerebral palsy. Developmental Medicine and Child Neurology 34:80–86

Hunter AG (2000) Outcome of the routine assessment of patients with mental retardation in a genetics clinic. Am J Med Genet 90:60–68

Hunter AG, Evans JA, Thompson DR, Ramsay S (1980) A study of institutionalized mentally retarded patients in Manitoba. I: Classification and preventability. Developmental Medicine and Child Neurology 22:145–162

Illingworth RS (1985) A paediatrician asks – why is it called birth injury. B J Obstet and Gynaecol 92(2):122–130

Jain U, Verma IC, Kapoor AK (1998) Prevalence of fragile X(A) syndrome in mentally retarded children at a genetics referral centre in Delhi, India. Indian Journal of Medical Research 108:12–6:12–16

Jenkins BG, Kraft E (1999) Magnetic resonance spectroscopy in toxic encephalopathy and neurodegeneration. Current Opinion in Neurology 12:753–760

Jones MB, Szatmari P (1988) Stoppage rules and genetic studies of autism. J Autism and Developmental Disorders 18:31–40

Jorde LB, Mason-Brothers A, Waldmann R et al. (1990) The UCLA-University of Utah epidemiologic survey of autism: genealogical analysis of familial aggregation. Am J Med Genet 36:85–88

Joyce CA, Hart HH, Fisher AM and Browne CE (1999) Use of subtelomeric FISH probes to detect abnormalities in patients with idiopathic mental retardation and characterize rearrangements at the limit of cytogenetic resolution. J Med Genet 36(suppl):S16

Kaveggia EG, Durkin MV, Pendleton E and Opitz JM (1975) Diagnostic/genetic studies of 1224 patients with severe mental retardation. Warsaw, Polish Medical Publishers. Proc 3rd Congress of the Inter Assoc for the Scientific Study of Mental Deficiency, pp 82–93

Kerrison JB (1999) New genetic, pathophysiologic, and therapeutic issues in nystagmus. Current Opinions in Ophthalmology 10:411–419

King BH, State MW, Shah B et al. (1997) Mental retardation: A review of the past 10 years. Part I. J American Academy of Child and Adolescent Psychiatry 36:1656–1663

Knight SJ, Flint J (2000) Perfect endings: a review of subtelomeric probes and their use in clinical diagnosis. J Med Genet 37:401–409

Knight SJ, Regan R, Nicod A et al. (1999) Subtle chromosomal rearrangements in children with unexplained mental retardation [see comments]. Lancet 354:1676–1681

Kohlschutter A (1994) Neuroradiological and neurophysiological indices for neurometabolic disorders. Euro J Pediatr 153:S90–S93

Kotzot D, Balmer D, Baumer A et al. (2000) Maternal uniparental disomy 7 – review and further delineation of the phenotype. Euro J Pediat 159:247–256

Kubota T, Sutcliffe JS, Aradhya S et al. (1996) Validation studies of SNRPN methylation as a diagnostic test for Prader-Willi syndrome. Am J Med Genet 66:77–80

Lalande M, Minassian BA, DeLorey TM, Olsen RW (1999) Parental imprinting and Angelman syndrome. Advance in Neurology 79:421–9:421–429

Lamb AN, Lytle CH, Aylsworth AS et al. (1999) Low proportion of subtelomeric rearrangements in a population of patients with mental retardation and dysmorphic features. Am J Hum Genet 65:A169

Laxova R, Ridler MA, Bowen-Bravery M (1977) An etiological survey of the severely retarded Hertfordshire children who were born between January 1, 1965 and December 31, 1967. Am J Med Genet 1:75–86

Lequin MH, Barkovich AJ (1999) Current concepts of cerebral malformation syndromes. Current Opinions in Pediatrics 11:492–496

Leung AK (1987) Dominantly inherited syndrome of microcephaly and congenital lymphedema with normal intelligence [letter]. Am J Med Genet 26:231

Lingam S, Read S, Holland IM et al. (1982) Value of computerised tomography in children with non-specific mental subnormally. Archives of Disease in Children 57:381–383

Lotter V (1966) Epidemiology of autistic conditions in young children. I. Prevalence. Social Psychiatry 1:124–137

Lyon G, Adams RD, Kolodny EH (1996) Neurology of Hereditary Metabolic Diseases of Children, 2nd edn. McGraw-Hill, NY

McQueen PC, Spence MW, Garner JB et al. (1987) Prevalence of major mental retardation and associated disabilities in the Canadian Maritime Provinces. Am J Mental Deficiency 91:460–466

Majnemer A, Shevell MI (1995) Diagnostic yield of the neurologic assessment of the developmentally delayed child. J Pediatr 127:193–199

Martin RA, Sabol DW, Rogan PK (1999) Maternal uniparental disomy of chromosome 14 confined to an interstitial segment (14q23-14q24.2). J Med Genet 36:633–636

Mergenthaler S, Wollmann HA, Burger B et al. (2000) Formation of uniparental disomy 7 delineated from new cases and a UPD7 case after trisomy 7 rescue. Presentation of own results and review of the literature. Annales Genetique 43:15–21

Miller G (1988) Ataxic cerebral palsy and genetic predisposition. Archives of Diseases in Children 63(10):1260–1261

Miller G, Clark GD (1998) The Cerebral Palsies. Causes, Consequences, and Management. Buterworth-Heinemann, Boston

Moeschler JB, Bennett FC, Cromwell LD (1981) Use of the CT scan in the medical evaluation of the mentally retarded child. J Pediatr 98:63–65

Muralidhar B, Butler MG (1998) Methylation PCR analysis of Prader-Willi syndrome, Angelman syndrome, and control subjects. Am J Med Genet 80:263–265

Murphy CC, Yeargin-Allsopp M, Decoufle P, Drews CD (1993) Prevalence of cerebral palsy among ten-year-old children in metropolitan Atlanta, 1985 through 1987. J Pediatr 123:S13–S20

Murphy CC, Yeargin-Allsopp M, Decoufle P, Drews CD (1995) The administrative prevalence of mental retardation in 10-year-old children in metropolitan Atlanta, 1985 through 1987. Am J Public Health 85:319–323

Nellhaus G (1968) Head circumference from birth to eighteen years. Practical composite international and interracial graphs. Pediatr 41:106–114

Nellhaus G (1971) Head circumference in black and white and Indian (New Delhi) children. Pediatr 48:494–495

Nelson KB, Ellenberg JH (1986) Antecedents of cerebral palsy. Multivariate analysis of risk. N Eng J Med 315:81–86

Newell SJ, Green SH (1987) Diagnostic classification of the aetiology of mental retardation in children. B M J 294:163–166

Nyhan WL, Bay C, Beyer EW, Mazi M (1999) Neurologic nonmetabolic presentation of propionic acidemia. Archives of Neurology 56:1143–1147

O'Tuama LA, Treves ST (1993) Brain single-photon emission computed tomography for behavior disorders in children. Seminars in Nuclear Medicine 23:255–264

Odent S, Le Marec B, Munnich A et al. (1998) Segregation analysis in nonsyndromic holoprosencephaly. Am J Med Genet 77:139–143

Opitz JM, Holt MC (1990) Microcephaly: general considerations and aids to nosology. J Craniofacial Genetics and Developmental Biology 10:175–204

Opitz JM, Kaveggia EG, Durkin-Stamm MV, Pendleton E (1978) Diagnostic/genetic studies in severe mental retardation. Birth Defects Original Articles Series 14:1–38

Penrose LS (1938) A clinical and genetic study of 1288 cases of mental defect. Spec. Rep.Ser.med.Res.Coun.Lond. 229:42

Penrose LS (1972) The Biology of Mental Defect, 4th edn. Sidgwick and Jackson, London

Pericak-Vance MA, Wolpert CM, Menold MM et al. (1997) Linkage evidence supports the involvement of chromosome 15 in autistic disorder. Am J Hum Genet 61:A40

Perrault I, Rozet JM, Gerber S (1999) Leber congenital amaurosis. Molec Genet Metabolism 68:200–208

Piven J, Gayle J, Chase GA et al. (1990) A family history study of neuropsychiatric disorders in the adult siblings of autistic individuals. J Am Acad of Child and Adolescent Psychiatry 29:177–183

Pollin TI, Dobyns WB, Crowe CA et al. (1999) Risk of abnormal pregnancy outcome in carriers of balanced reciprocal translocations involving the Miller-Dieker syndrome (MDS) critical region in chromosome 17p13.3. Am J Med Genet 85:369–375

Powdermaker F (1930) Familial congenital spastic diplegia. Am J Diseases in Children 39:148–156

Ralph A, Scott F, Tiernan C et al. (1999) Maternal uniparental isodisomy for chromosome 14 detected prenatally. Prenatal Diagnosis 19:681–684

Rapin I (1995) Autistic regression and disintegrative disorder: how important the role of epilepsy? Seminar in Pediatric Neurology 2:278–285

Rasmussen K, Nielsen J, Dahl G (1982) The prevalence of chromosome abnormalities among mentally retarded persons in a geographically delimited area of Denmark. Clin Genet 22:244–255

Raymond GV, Holmes LB (1994) Head circumferences standards in neonates. J Child Neurology 9:63–66

Reed EW, Reed SC (1965) Mental retardation: a family study. WB Saunders, Philadelphia

Ritvo ER, Jorde LB, Mason-Brothers A et al. (1989) The UCLA-University of Utah epidemiologic survey of autism: recurrence risk estimates and genetic counseling. Am J Psychiatry 146:1032–1036

Roeleveld N, Zielhuis GA, Gabreels F (1997) The prevalence of mental retardation: a critical review of recent literature. Developmental Medicine and Child Neurology 39:125–132

Rousseau F, Heitz D, Biancalana V et al. (1991) Direct diagnosis by DNA analysis of the fragile X syndrome of mental retardation. N Eng J Med 325:1673–1681

Rutter M, Simonoff E, Plomin R (1996) Genetic influences on mild mental retardation: concepts, findings and research implications. J Biosocial Science 28:509–526

Santosh PJ (2000) Neuroimaging in child and adolescent psychiatric disorders. Archives of Disease in Children 82:412–419

Satcher D (1995) The sociodemographic correlates of mental retardation. Am J Public Health 85:304–306

Schroer RJ, Phelan MC, Michaelis RC et al. (1998) Autism and maternally derived aberrations of chromosome 15q. Am J Med Genet 76:327–336

Shevell MI, Ashwal S, Novotny E (1999) Proton magnetic resonance spectroscopy: clinical applications in children with nervous system diseases. Seminars in Pediatric Neurology 6:68–77

Shevell MI, Majnemer A, Rosenbaum P et al. (2000) Etiologic yield of subspecialists' evaluation of young children with global developmental delay. Journal of Pediatrics 136:593–598

Shields JR, Schifrin BS (1988) Perinatal antecedents of cerebral palsy. Obstet Gynecol 71:899–905

Slavotinek A, Rosenberg M, Knight S et al. (1999) Screening for submicroscopic chromosome rearrangements in children with idiopathic mental retardation using microsatellite markers for the chromosome telomeres. J Med Genet 36:405–411

Stromme P, Hagberg G (2000) Aetiology in severe and mild mental retardation: a population-based study of Norwegian children. Developmental Medicine and Child Neurology 42:76–86

Sugimoto T, Yasuhara A, Nishida N et al. (1993) MRI of the head in the evaluation of microcephaly. Neuropediatr 24:4–7

Szatmari P, Jones MB, Tuff L et al. (1993) Lack of cognitive impairment in first-degree relatives of children with pervasive developmental disorders. J Am Acad of Child and Adolescent Psychiatry 32:1264–1273

Tamraz JC, Rethore MO, Iba-Zizen MT et al. (1987) Contribution of magnetic resonance imaging to the knowledge of CNS malformations related to chromosomal aberrations. Hum Genet 76:265–273

Tint GS, Irons M, Elias ER et al. (1994) Defective cholesterol biosynthesis associated with the Smith-Lemli-Opitz syndrome. N Eng J Med 330:107–113

Tolmie JL, McNay M, Stephenson JB et al. (1987) Microcephaly: genetic counselling and antenatal diagnosis after the birth of an affected child. Am J Med Genet 27:583–594

Traboulsi EI (1995) Practice guidelines for the patient with suspected ocular nonretinal genetic disorder. Seminars in Ophthalmology 10:318–322

Traboulsi EI (1998) Ocular malformations and developmental genes. Journal of AAPOS 2:317–323

Traboulsi EI (1999) Genetic Diseases of the Eye. OUP, Oxford

Tuchman RF (1994) Epilepsy, language, and behavior: clinical models in childhood. J Child Neurology 9:95–102

Tuchman RF, Rapin I (1997) Regression in pervasive developmental disorders: seizures and epileptiform electroencephalogram correlates. Pediatr 99:560–566

Turner G, Collins E, Turner B (1971) Recurrence risk of mental retardation in sibs. Medical Journal of Australia 1:1165–1166

Turner G, Robinson H, Laing S et al. (1992) Population screening for fragile X Lancet 339:1210–1213

Turner G, Webb T, Wake S, Robinson H (1996) Prevalence of fragile X syndrome. Am J Med Genet 64:196–197

Valk J, van der Knaap MS (1991) White matter disorders. Curr Opin Neurol Neurosurg 4:843–851

van der Knaap MS, Jakobs C, Valk J (1996) Magnetic resonance imaging in lactic acidosis. Journal of Inherited Metabolic Diseases 19:535–547

Varadi V, Toth Z, Torok O, Papp Z (1988) Heterogeneity and recurrence risk for congenital hydrocephalus (ventriculomegaly): a prospective study. Am J Med Genet 29:305–310

Viot G, Gosset P, Fert S et al. (1998) Cryptic subtelomeric rearrangements detected by FISH in mentally retarded and dysmorphic patients. Am J Hum Genet 63:A10

Volkmar FR (1992) Childhood disintegrative disorder: Issues for DSM-IV. J Autism and Developmental Disorders 22:625–642

Volkmar FR, Szatmari P, Sparrow SS (1993) Sex differences in pervasive developmental disorders. J Autism and Developmental Disorders 23:579–591

Vorsanova SG, Koloti D, Sharaonin VO et al. (1998) FISH analysis of microaberrations at telomeric and subtelomeric regions in chromosomes of children with mental retardation. Am J Hum Genet 65:A154

Warkany J (1971) Congenital Malformations. Year Book Medical Publishers, Chicago

Webb TP, Bundey S, Thake A, Todd J (1986) The frequency of the fragile X chromosome among schoolchildren in Coventry. J Med Genet 23:396–399

Weidmer-Mikhail E, Sheldon S, Ghaziuddin M (1998) Chromosomes in autism and related pervasive developmental disorders: A cytogenetic study. J Intellectual Disability Research 42:8–12

Wing L, Gould J (1979) Severe impairments of social interaction and associated abnormalities in children: Epidemiology and classification. J Autism and Developmental Disorders 9:11–29

World Health Organization (1993) The ICD-10 Classification of mental and behavioral disorders: Diagnostic criteria for research. World Health Organization, Geneva

Wuu KD, Chiu PC, Li SY et al. (1991) Chromosomal and biochemical screening on mentally retarded school children in Taiwan. Japanese Hum Genet 36:267–274

Yannet H (1944) The etiology of congenital cerebral palsy. J Pediatr 24:38

Yeargin-Allsopp M, Drews CD, Decoufle P, Murphy CC (1995) Mild mental retardation in black and white children in metropolitan Atlanta: a case-control study. Am J Public Health 85:324–328

Yen MT, Lam BL (1999) Update on hereditary optic neuropathy. Seminars in Ophthalmology 14:74–80

Youings SA, Murray A, Dennis N et al. (2000) FRAXA and FRAXE: the results of a five year survey. J Med Genet 37:415–421

Yu S, Pritchard M, Kremer E (1991) Fragile X genotype characterized by an unstable region of DNA. Science 252:1179–1181

Abnormal body size and proportion

41

John M. Graham, Jr
David L. Rimoin

Introduction

Normal stature varies widely among ethnic groups, and also varies within each ethnic group, approximating a normal distribution. "Short stature" or "tall stature" are, therefore, relative terms and related to a person's ethnic, familial, and nutritional background. Before beginning a complex diagnostic evaluation or contemplating growth-promoting or growth-limiting therapy, one must be able to differentiate between pathologic, short, or tall stature, as well as normal variants within each end of the normal range. This can be done by utilizing standard growth curves. However, growth curves must be appropriate for the individual's genetic and ethnic background. In addition, allowances must be made for parental height, nutritional background, and the impact of chronic disease before an individual can be declared pathologically short or tall (Tanner et al., 1970; Harvey et al., 1979). One must also rule out constitutional delay or acceleration of maturation by correlating bone age and height. This normal variation in the timing of growth accounts for a large proportion of children referred for variations in growth.

Pathologic short stature

When it is established that a person is truly short for his or her genetic background, and does not simply have constitutional delay, the exact cause of the pathologic short stature must be delineated. If possible, it is essential that a specific diagnosis be made because there are literally hundreds of causes of short stature that have differing prognoses, complications, and responses to treatments. A specific diagnosis is essential to provide accurate genetic counseling (Smith, 1977; Hall, 1985; Rimoin et al., 1986).

The first step in the clinical evaluation of short stature is to determine whether the body habitus is proportionate or disproportionate (Fig. 41.1). Children with disproportionate short stature usually have a skeletal dysplasia, while those with proportionate short stature may have a more generalized disorder (i.e., malnutrition, chronic disease, psychosocial dwarfism, endocrine disorder, genetic syndrome, or a chromosomal or teratogenic disorder. Exceptions to this rule occur, and disproportionate dwarfism occurs in cases of severe cretinism, while proportionate shortening may occur in persons with osteogenesis imperfecta.

A mildly disproportionate body habitus may not be apparent on casual examination, and anthropometric measurements, such as sitting height, upper/lower segment ratio, and/or arm span must be made before a relatively mild skeletal dysplasia (e.g., hypochondroplasia) can be excluded. Once a person with short stature is found to be proportionate, it is helpful to determine whether the growth deficiency was of prenatal or postnatal onset. Prenatal-onset growth deficiency usually implicates a fetal environmental insult or a generalized cellular genetic defect. Late fetal insults are more likely to demonstrate catch-up growth postnatally, when compared with environmental factors which have an early impact in fetal life (Smith et al., 1976; Smith, 1977; Graham, 2002). On the other hand, postnatal onset of proportionate growth deficiency usually implicates a postnatal environmental insult, such as infection, chronic disease, malnutrition, or an endocrine, psychological, or malabsorption disorder. These generalizations hold true whether or not the cause of the short stature is a single-system disorder, such as growth hormone

1066

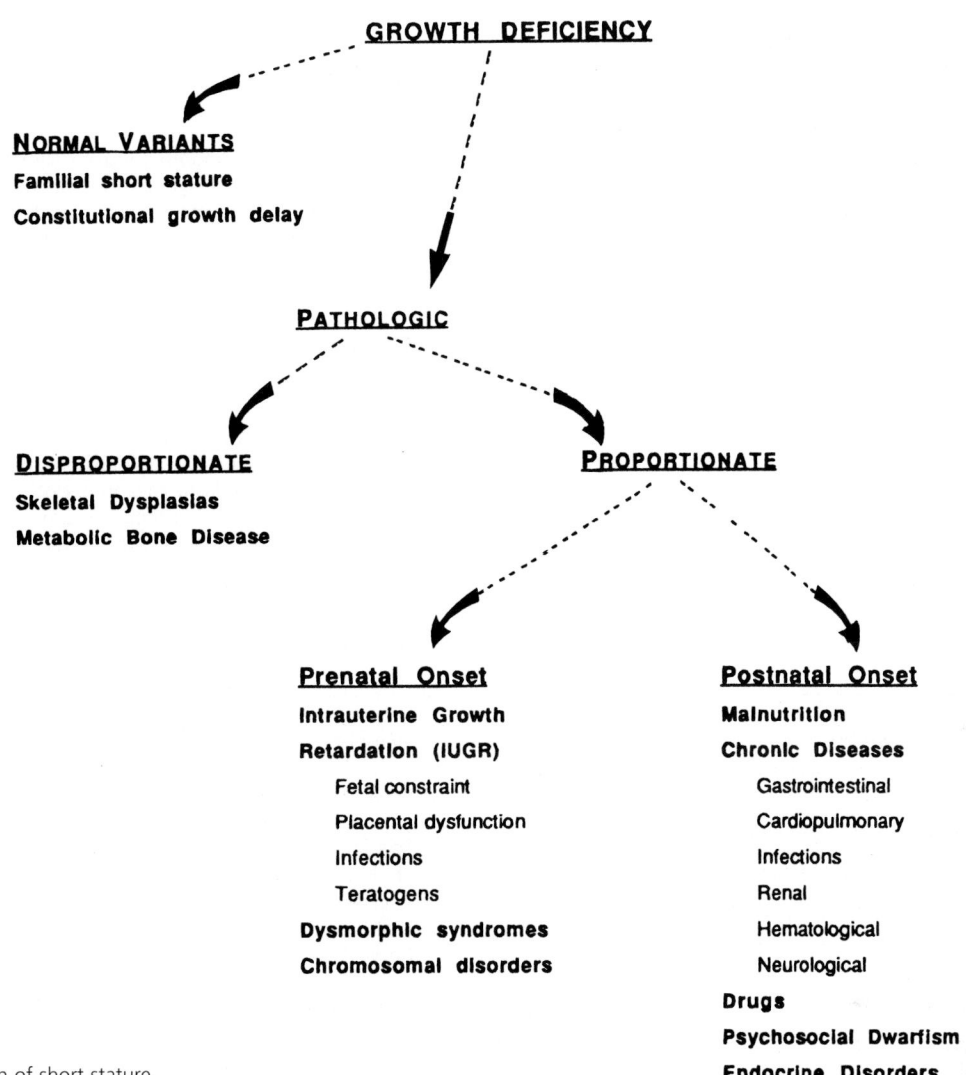

GROWTH DEFICIENCY

NORMAL VARIANTS
Familial short stature
Constitutional growth delay

PATHOLOGIC

DISPROPORTIONATE
Skeletal Dysplasias
Metabolic Bone Disease

PROPORTIONATE

Prenatal Onset
Intrauterine Growth
Retardation (IUGR)
    Fetal constraint
    Placental dysfunction
    Infections
    Teratogens
Dysmorphic syndromes
Chromosomal disorders

Postnatal Onset
Malnutrition
Chronic Diseases
    Gastrointestinal
    Cardiopulmonary
    Infections
    Renal
    Hematological
    Neurological
Drugs
Psychosocial Dwarfism
Endocrine Disorders

Fig. 41.1. Classification of short stature.

deficiency or diabetes mellitus, or the short stature is associated with other abnormalities in a complex syndrome.

Proportionate short stature of prenatal onset

Prenatal growth deficiency or intrauterine growth retardation (IUGR) can be due to numerous causes, both genetic and acquired. Practice guidelines for infants born with IUGR has been presented by Alkalay et al. (1998). Mechanical late gestational constraint has been emphasized as the most common cause of prenatal growth deficiency (Graham, 2002). Most commonly, such small babies are born to small mothers with fathers of normal size, and they readily catch up into the normal range within the first few months of postnatal life. Late fetal causes of growth deficiency, such as preeclampsia or

placental insufficiency, usually show prompt resolution with postnatal catch-up growth. However, disorders that adversely affect growth from early fetal life, such as chronic maternal hypertension, maternal diabetes mellitus with vascular changes, and heavy maternal smoking may not show catch-up growth during the first six months of postnatal life. These latter conditions may be the result of diminished maternal blood flow to the placenta. There are a wide variety of fetal malformation syndromes caused by single gene disorders, chromosomal disorders, teratogens, or in utero infections, where fetal hypoplasia is part of the overall disorder (Jones, 1997; Smith, 1977) (Table 41.1). These babies would not be expected to show catch-up growth and some of these disorders can be associated with a high degree of perinatal lethality.

Though etiologically heterogeneous, small size at birth may be associated with significant functional implications.

Table 41.1. Prenatal-onset growth deficiency disorders

Disorder	Inheritance	Key clinical findings
Teratogenic disorders		
Fetal alcohol effects		Microcephaly, thin smooth philtrum, short palpebral fissures
Fetal hydantoin effects		Ocular hypertelorism, hypoplastic nails, short nose
Fetal trimethadione effects		Arched eyebrows, cupped helix, heart defects
Fetal warfarin effects		Hypoplastic nose, stippled epiphyses, short limbs
Fetal rubella effects		Deafness, cataracts, patent ductus arteriosus
Fetal varicella effects		Cicatricial skin defects, limb hypoplasia, mental deficiency, seizures
Maternal phenyketonuria effects		Microcephaly, cardiac defects, mental deficiency
Chromosome abnormalities		
Trisomy 18		Clenched hands, short sterum, low arch dermal patterns
Trisomy 13		Scalp defects, polydactyly, holoprosencephaly facies
Triploidy		3–4 Syndactyly, dysplastic cavarium, cystic placenta
4p-syndrome		Ocular hypertelorism, hypospadias, preauricular pits
5p-syndrome		Catlike cry, microcephaly, down-slanted palpebral fissures
13q-syndrome		Central nervous system defects, short thumbs, anal anomalies
18p-syndrome		Ptosis, protruding ears, mental deficiency
18q-syndrome		Prominent antihelix, midface hypoplasia, long palms
45, X Turner syndrome		Lymphoedema hands and feet, webbed neck, broad chest with wide-set nipples
Proportionate syndromes		
Brachmann-de Lange syndrome	Sporadic, autosomal dominant @ 3q26.3	Synophrys, thin down-turned upper lip, micromelia
Rubinstein-Taybi syndrome	Sporadic, autosomal dominant @ 16p13.3	Broad thumbs and halluces, down-slanted palpebral fissures, prominent nasal septum
Russell-Silver syndrome	Sporadic heterogeneous	Triangular face, normal-sized cranium, incurved 5th fingers
Dubowitz syndrome	Autosomal recessive	Shallow supraorbital ridges, ptosis and blepharophimosis, eczema
Bloom syndrome	Autosomal recessive	Malar erythema/telangiectasia, malar hypoplasia, microcephaly
Fanconi pancytopenia syndrome	Autosomal recessive	Radial hypoplasia, hyperpigmentation, pancytopenia
De Sanctis-Cacchione syndrome	Autosomal recessive	Xeroderma pigmentosa, hypogonadism, microcephaly
Johansen-Blizzard syndrome	Autosomal recessive	Hypoplastic alae nasi, scalp defects, sensorineural deafness
Leprechaunism syndrome	Autosomal recessive	Adipose deficiency, thick lips, islet cell hyperplasia
Seckel syndrome	Autosomal recessive	Microcephaly, prominent nose, micrognathia
Hallermann-Streiff syndrome	Sporadic	Microphthalmia, small pinched nose, hypotrichosis
Smith-Lemli-Opitz syndrome	Autosomal recessive	Ptosis, syndactyly of 2nd and 3rd toes, hypospadias
Williams syndrome	Sporadic, autosomal dominant 7q11.2	Prominent lips, periorbital fullness, supravalvular aortic stenosis
Noonan syndrome	Autosomal dominant	Webbed neck, pectus excavatum, pulmonary stenosis
Aarskog syndrome	X-linked	Ocular hypertelorism, brachydactyly, shawl scrotum
Robinow syndrome	Autosomal dominant and autosomal recessive	Broad forehead with flat facial profile, short forearms, hypoplastic genitalia
Opitz syndrome	Autosomal dominant	Ocular hypertelorism, hypospadias, swallowing difficulties
Coffin-Sirus syndrome	Probably autosomal dominant	Hypoplastic 5th digits and nails, coarse face, hirsutism with sparse scalp hair
Disproportionate syndromes		
Achondrogenesis (A & B)	Autosomal recessive	Very short limbs, low nasal bridge, incomplete ossification of spine
Achondrogenesis II/ hypochondrogenesis	Autosomal dominant	Short limbs, poor ossification of spine, metaphyseal abnormalities
Spondyloepiphyseal dysplasia congenita	Autosomal dominant	Short trunk, delayed epiphyseal mineralization, myopia
Ellis-van Creveld syndrome	Autosomal recessive	Short distal limbs, polydactyly, nail hypoplasia auricular cartilage

continued

Table 41.1. Prenatal-onset growth deficiency disorders (*continued*)

Disorder	Inheritance	Key clinical findings
Kniest dysplasia	Autosomal dominant	Flat facies, thick joints, platyspondyly with comel clefts, cleft palate myopia
Cerebrocostomandibular syndrome	Autosomal recessive	Bell-shaped small thorax, rib gaps, micrognathia
Jarcho-Levin syndrome	Autosomal recessive	Short thorax with diminished ribs, vertebral segmentation defects, comptodactyly/syndactyly
Atelosteogenesis syndromes	Sporadic	Very short proximal limbs, depressed nasal bridge, cleft palate
Short rib-polydactyly syndrome	Autosomal recessive	Short limbs, short horizontal ribs, polydactyly
Thanatophoric dysplasia	Autosomal dominant	Hypotonia with large cranium, short limbs, telephone receiver femus
Camptomelic dysplasia	Autosomal dominant	Anteriorly bowed tibias with skin dimples, XY sex reversal, flat facies
Rhiaomelic chondrodysplasia punctata	Autosomal recessive	Short humeri and femurs, coronal cleft in vertebrae, punctate epiphyseal mineralization

Longterm follow-up of over 1000 adults who were born small for gestational age (SGA) at term with no congenital abnormalities demonstrated small but significant deficits in academic achievement, with teachers less likely to rate them in the top 15th percentile of the class at age 16 years, and more likely to recommend special education (Strauss, 2000). At age 26 years, those who had been born SGA were less likely to have professional or managerial jobs, with significantly lower levels of weekly income. Those born SGA with a small head size had substantially lower rates of professional attainment than those born SGA who had a normal head size at age five years. Also, adults born SGA had significant adult height deficits of approximately 5 cm (Strauss, 2000).

Syndromic disorders

When the onset of growth deficiency is prenatal, one must differentiate between the numerous forms of intrauterine growth retardation (Hall, 1985; Graham, 2002; Jones, 1997). This is a very heterogeneous group of disorders with multiple causes ranging from placental insufficiency, to teratogenic exposure, to specific genetic and chromosomal syndromes. Although in most cases the causes are obscure, a specific diagnosis of a recognizable syndrome usually can be made. This may be done on the basis of associated clinical findings, such as the characteristic facial features of Brachmann-de Lange syndrome, Rubinstein-Taybi syndrome, Russell-Silver syndrome, Johansen-Blizzard syndrome, leprechaunism, Seckel syndrome, Hallerman-Streiff syndrome, Smith-Lemli-Opitz syndrome, Williams syndrome, Noonan syndrome, Aarskog syndrome, and Coffin-Sirus syndrome; or the limb malformations that may be the distinctive parts of the Brachmann-de Lange syndrome, Rubinstein-Taybi syndrome, Silver-Russell syndrome, Fanconi-pancytopenia syndrome, Aarskog syndrome, and Robinow syndrome (Table 41.1 and Figs 41.2 and 41.3). Thus, the clinical evaluation and analysis of dysmorphic features present in each case often permits reaching a conclusive diagnosis. In certain syndromes, diagnosis can be confirmed with specific laboratory studies, such as chromosomal analysis for sister chromatid exchanges in the Bloom syndrome, analysis of chromosome breakage in the Fanconi-pancytopenia syndrome, assessment of DNA repair in the Cockayne and xeroderma pigmentosa syndromes, use of fluorescent *in situ* hybridization (FISH) probes in Williams syndrome, and insulin receptor studies in leprechaunism.

Many of these syndromes are inherited as autosomal-recessive traits, such as Bloom syndrome, Seckel syndrome, Donahue syndrome, and Dubowitz syndrome, whereas others usually occur sporadically, such as Hallerman-Streiff syndrome, Rubinstein-Taybi syndrome, Russell-Silver syndrome, Brachmann-de Lange syndrome, and Williams syndrome. Such disorders may be due to a new mutation or a submicroscopic chromosomal deletion, e.g., Rubinstein-Taybi syndrome, which is mapped to 16p13.3, and Williams syndrome at 7q11.2. The development of FISH probes for such disorders should help to facilitate an early clinical diagnosis, and establishing a diagnosis is essential for accurate prognosis and genetic counseling.

Chromosomal disorders

With the exception of sex chromosome excess, trisomy 21, and trisomy 8 mosaicism, most chromosomal disorders

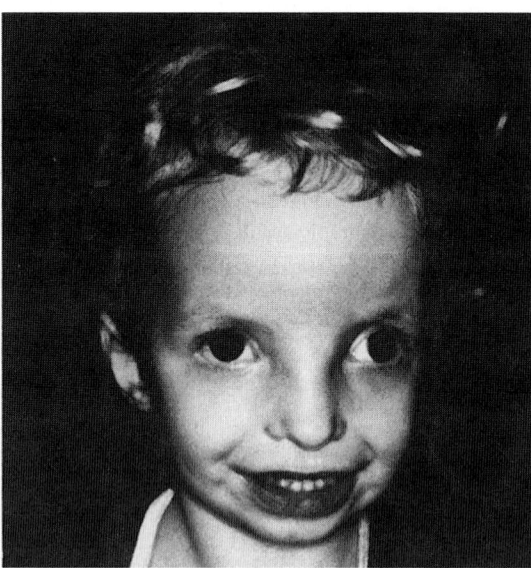
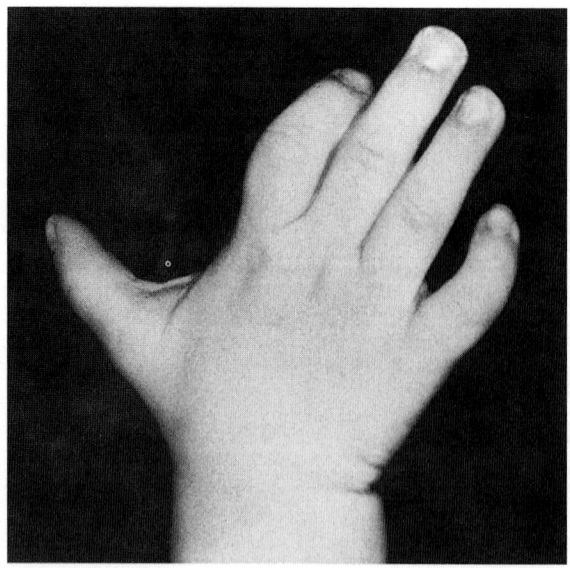

Fig. 41.2. This three-year-old child with Russell-Silver syndrome had delayed motor development, prenatal growth deficiency that persisted postnatally, triangular face shape, and inturning of his fifth finger. In addition, he demonstrated a liability toward fasting hypoglycemia, mild skeletal asymmetry, and a deficit of adipose tissue with blue (thin) sclerae. (From Graham, 1983, with permission.)

result in some degree of intrauterine growth retardation. In those syndromes compatible with survival beyond infancy, such as Turner syndrome and a variety of autosomal partial deletion or duplication syndromes, there is continued diminished growth throughout childhood and a blunted pubertal growth spurt as well. As the number of recognized chromosomal disorders increases due to new technologies, such as FISH techniques, it has become important to make an accurate clinical diagnosis to focus the laboratory's attention on specific chromosomal regions. A patient with intrauterine growth retardation, developmental delay, and dysmorphic features who does not manifest a recognizable syndrome should always undergo a high-resolution cytogenetic evaluation.

In patients with a syndrome suggestive of a specific chromosomal deletion syndrome (e.g., 18q-syndrome or 4p-syndrome (Figs 41.4 and 41.5), it may be necessary to repeat chromosome studies with newer techniques or to use FISH probes, if previous studies were done before such high-resolution techniques were available. Some chromosomal syndromes may only be detectable in skin fibroblast samples (e.g., diploid/triploid mixoploidy or tetrasomy 12p) (Graham et al., 1981; Hersh et al., 1983). It is also important to remember that some girls with Turner syndrome, especially those with mosaicism, express few phenotypic features prepubertally, except for short stature. Thus, chromosomal studies should be done on all girls who are projected to be short for their family background, with relatively normal body proportions, and for whom another diagnosis has not been made.

Several chromosomal deletion syndromes have also been found to be associated with growth hormone deficiency (Rimoin et al., 1986), indicating the locations of genes or chromosomal regions that result in short stature. Since the growth hormone gene is on the long arm of chromosome 17, it is not surprising that deletion of this part of chromosome 17 will result in growth hormone deficiency. Leprechaunism (Donohue syndrome) has been linked to mutations in the insulin receptor gene on 19p13, resulting in insulin resistance and IUGR, since insulin is a major fetal growth factor. For some of the more common chromosome disorders (e.g., Turner syndrome and Down syndrome), syndrome-specific growth curves are available to aid in following these patients (Saul, 1988), and these curves are quite useful for detecting when secondary hormonal problems might be present.

Growth deficiency in Turner syndrome has been attributed to haploinsufficiency of the SHOX gene at Xpter-p22.32 (Rao et al., 1997), and maternal uniparental disomy has been identified in approximately 10% of patients with Russell-Silver syndrome (Price et al., 1999).

Teratogens

A variety of teratogenic exposures are associated with intrauterine growth retardation, including alcohol, cigarettes, and anticonvulsants (Table 41.1). Although maternal smoking may result in otherwise normal small-for-dates babies, most

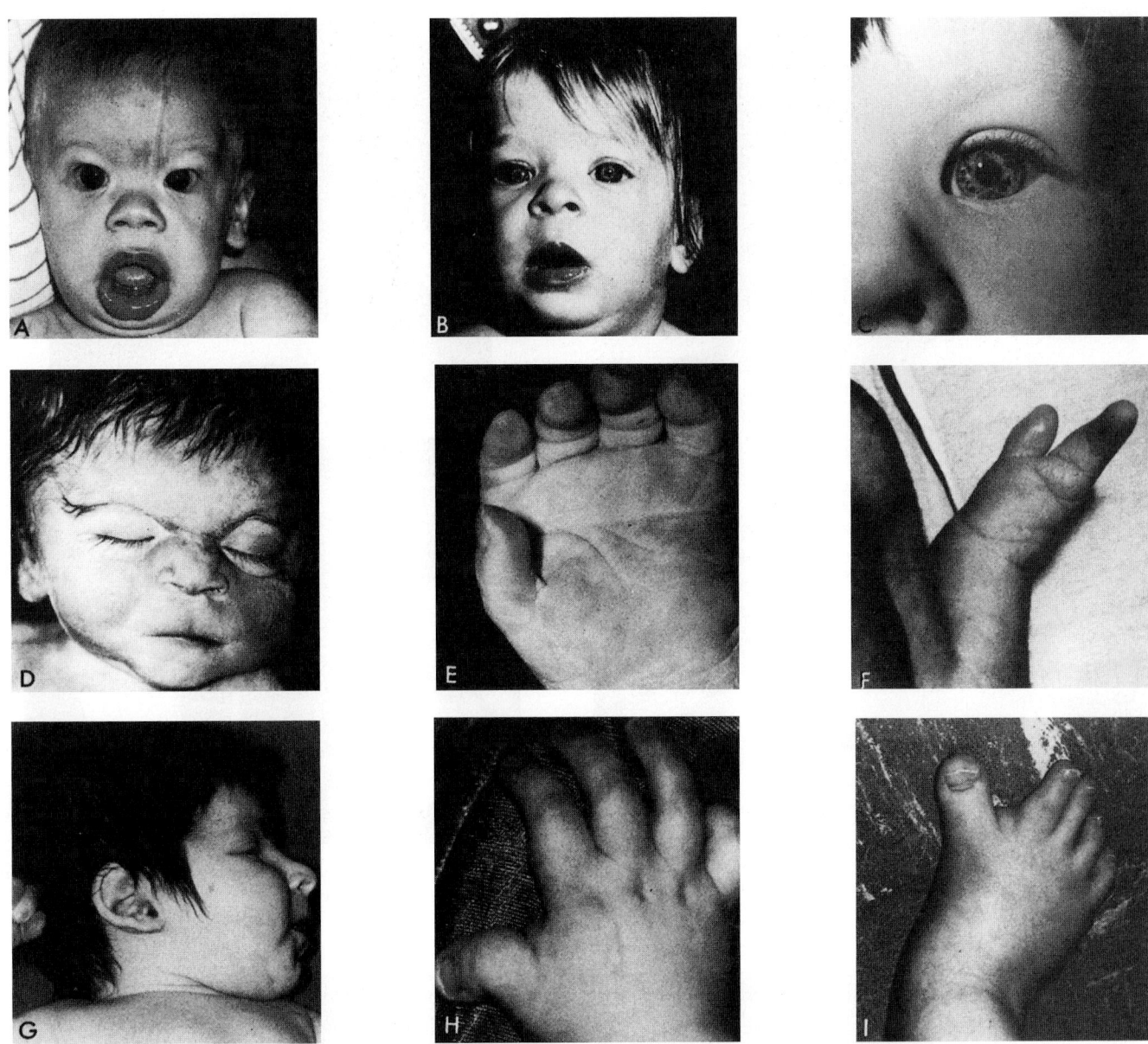

Fig. 41.3. Three different sporadic syndromes now localized to specific chromosomal regions: (A–C) Williams syndrome at 17q11.2; (D–F) Brachmann-de Lange syndrome at 3q26.3, and (G–I) Rubinstein-Taybi syndrome at 16p13.3. Each is associated with relatively proportionate short stature and varying degrees of mental deficiency. (A–C) These two young children with Williams syndrome demonstrate the facial features characteristic of this disorder (Laskari et al., 1999). The nose is short with a flat nasal bridge and anteverted nares, giving rise to the impression of an elongated philtrum. The lips appear full, with a tendency toward an open mouth. The iris reveals a stellate pattern (C). (D–F) The facial features shown here are typical of the Brachmann-de Lange syndrome: microbrachycephaly, marked facial hirsutism, synophrys, a short nose with anteverted nares, and thin lips with a characteristic midline notch and downturned angles of the mouth. Limb deficiency in this condition can range from brachydactyly with micromelia (E) to oligodactyly, which usually affects the ulnar aspects of the hand to a greater extent (F). (G–I) This infant with Rubinstein-Taybi syndrome shows the characteristic beaked nose with a nasal septum that extends below the alae nasi. He is relatively hirsute, with broadening and flattening of the distal thumb. The thumb (H) and great toe (I) also tend to deviate to one side, as shown here in the hands and feet of an older child with the Rubinstein-Taybi syndrome. (From Graham, 1983, with permission.)

other teratogens result in well-characterized teratogenic syndromes. It must be stressed, however, that the clinical variability in these teratogenic syndromes is great, and it is the exceptional case that has all of the features of a teratogenic syndrome. Therefore, a careful history of maternal drug and teratogen ingestion must be taken for all children who demonstrate intrauterine growth retardation. The most frequent teratogenic cause of growth deficiency is fetal alcohol syndrome (Sampson et al., 1997) (Fig. 41.6). Maternal disease that can result in the accumulation of toxic

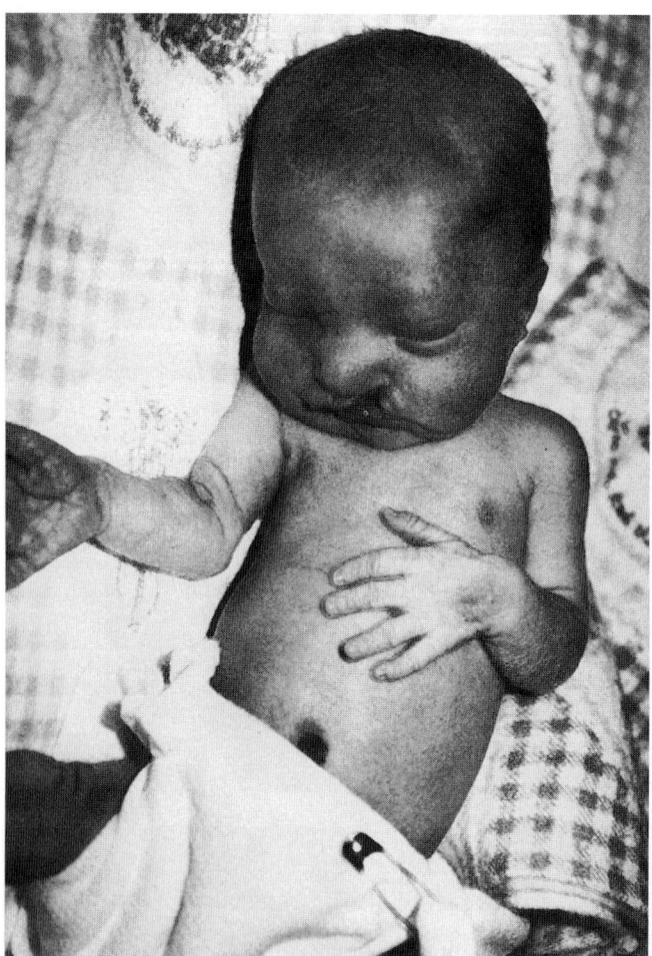

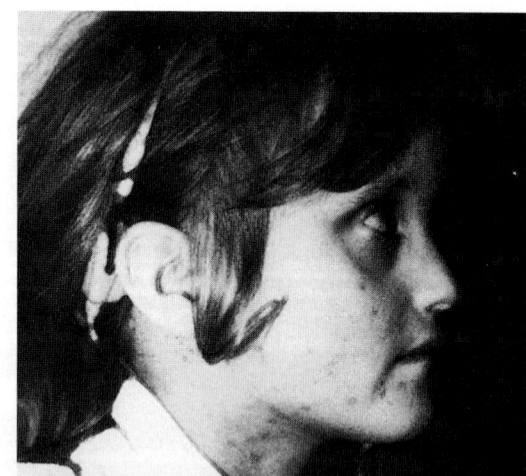

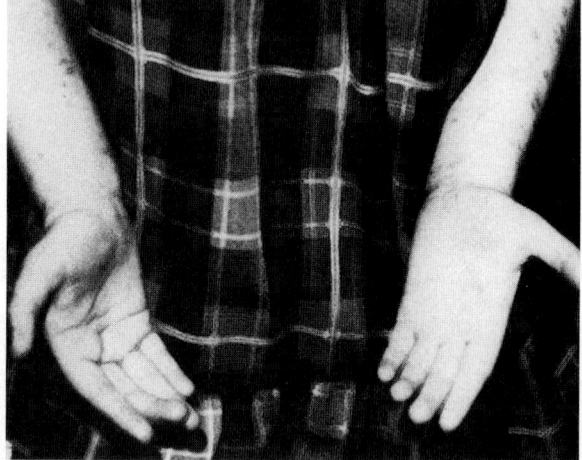

Fig. 41.4. Patient with 4p-syndrome. Note ocular hypertelorism with cleft lip. Also present were hypospadius and preauricular pits with intrauterine growth deficiency.

Fig. 41.5. Patient with 18q-syndrome. Note long palms, tapered fingers, mid-face deficiency, conductive hearing loss, and prominent antitragus.

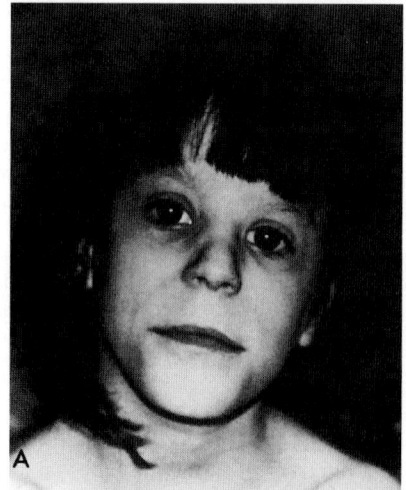

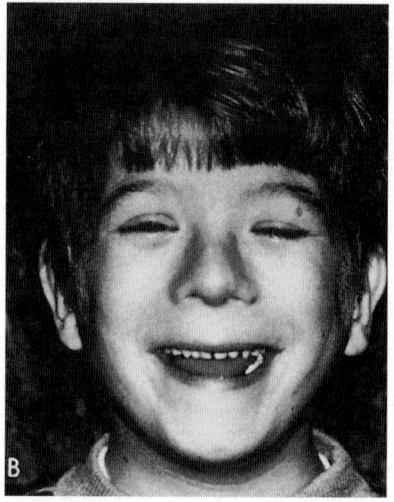

Fig. 41.6. (A) Fetal alcohol effects. This eight-year-old girl is mildly retarded and growth-deficient, with facial features typical of fetal alcohol syndrome (short palpebral fissures, short nose with flat nasal bridge, and thin lips with a smooth philtrum). (B) This eight-year-old boy shows similar facial features, is mildly retarded and growth-deficient. He weighed 2 kg at birth after a term gestation in a gravida 5, para 4, abortus 1, 28-year-old woman who drank one-fifth of hard liquor every one to two days during the first four months of pregnancy. (From Graham, 1983, with permission.)

substances that cross the placenta also result in teratogenic effects on the fetus. This is clearly evident in the maternal phenylketonuria syndrome (Jones, 1997). Intrauterine infections with rubella, syphilis, toxoplasmosis, and cytomegalic inclusion disease can produce prenatal growth retardation that result in postnatal proportionate short stature. Affected neonates may show systemic manifestations, including microcephaly, chorioretinitis, heptosplenomegaly, petechiae, and seizures. The diagnosis should be suspected perinataly, so that appropriate studies can be done to document the diagnosis.

Proportionate short stature of postnatal onset

Persons with postnatal-onset proportionate short stature usually have some kind of postnatal environmental insult, such as a chronic disease or an endocrine disorder, all of which may be associated with decreased insulinlike growth factor (IGF) or peripheral unresponsiveness to its action (Rimoin et al., 1986). There may be direct suppression of hepatic IGF synthesis, deficient HGH secretion with secondarily reduced IGF production, inability to respond to growth hormone (GH) stimulation of IGF, circulating IGF inhibitors, or peripheral unresponsiveness to the actions of IGF. These children usually have a bone age commensurate with, or even more severely retarded than, their height age, depending upon the state of their gonadal and thyroid systems. An accurate diagnosis is especially important for persons with this group of disorders because many of them will respond to specific therapeutic measures.

Psychosocial dwarfism

In certain children, emotional disturbances may result in pronounced growth retardation (Powell et al., 1967). Although these children usually come from homes where marital discord, separation, alcoholism, and social upheaval are found, they can also be seen in well-to-do and seemingly well-adjusted families. There is usually a poor plasma GH response to growth hormone stimulation tests, and levels of circulating IGF are low. Bone age maturation is usually greatly delayed. When removed from their adverse environment, these children usually show a striking catch-up in their bone age, and GH and IGF levels return to normal. Psychosocial dwarfism is thought to represent functional hypopituitarism in which psychic factors have produced a pituitary insufficiency through hypothalamic

suppression. This condition appears to be relatively common, but it usually occurs in only one member of a family.

Malnutrition

Chronic malnutrition retards growth and is associated with reduced synthesis of IGF (Phillips and Vassilopoulou-Sellin, 1980a,b). The absence of an adequate substrate for growth may contribute to growth failure in malnutrition as well. Malnutrition resulting from malabsorption may also result in growth retardation (Kaplan, 1982). Several cases of otherwise asymptomatic celiac disease and proportionate growth retardation have been reported. Small-bowel biopsies are sometimes helpful in the workup of such children in whom other causes of growth retardation have been excluded.

Chronic disease

Many chronic childhood diseases are associated with growth failure. Chronic liver disease, renal disease, celiac disease, regional enteritis, infectious disease, diabetes mellitis, hemoglobinopathies, asthma, congenital heart disease, and many others fit into this category. Often, reduced growth may be the dominant clinical feature. Low insulinlike growth factor (IGF) levels are usually found and, in addition, many patients are in a state of negative nitrogen balance. After cure or control of the basic disease, there is usually significant catch-up growth and some may ultimately reach a near-normal final adult stature, depending on the duration and severity of the disease, the age at the onset of the disorder, and its therapy.

Drug administration

In addition to various intrinsic causes of reduced human growth hormone secretion, certain medications used in treating hyperactivity, such as methylphenidate hydrochloride (Ritalin) and dextroamphetamine may alter the normal regulation of GH secretion (Aarskog et al., 1977; Roche et al, 1979). Children often show a lower than expected growth rate during the first few years after treatment commences, but tolerance to the growth suppression may develop later. Similarly, glucocorticoids used in treating certain diseases, such as asthma, nephrotic syndrome, juvenile rheumatoid arthritis, and leukemia may significantly retard growth. The growth-suppressing effects of steroids may be seen with relatively small doses that are often thought to be harmless, such as prolonged use of topical ointments, nasal spray, or eyedrops containing these compounds. The long-term effects of these and other drugs, on final adult height, have not been well established.

Endocrine disorders

Many disturbances in the endocrine system can impair growth. Thyroid hormone deficiency can result in either proportionate or disproportionate short stature, depending on the degree of secondary epiphyseal dysplasia. Cushing's disease can lead to proportionate short stature similar to that seen with the exogenous administration of steroids. Excess androgen secretion, as in the adrenogenital syndrome, can lead to accelerated growth with advanced bone age in early childhood, but significant adult short stature results from premature closure of epiphyses. The prototype of endocrine short stature is GH deficiency. Growth hormone-related causes of short stature can result from many interruptions in the hypothalamic-pituitary-peripheral tissue axis. The various types of pituitary dwarfism can be classified on the basis of the level of the defect, whether genetic or acquired. If genetic, is it associated with an obvious developmental or degenerative disease of the hypothalamus? If pituitary, is the deficiency monotropic (isolated growth hormone deficiency) or is it multitropic? In the cases due to a defect in growth hormone action, is IGF generation normal or defective ?. The most common causes of acquired pituitary insufficiency are birth trauma, cranial irradiation for neoplasia, craniopharyngioma with the expanding tumor mass compromising pituitary function, and hemosiderosis following chronic transfusion therapy. In addition, trauma, surgical damage, infection, and sarcoidosis can also lead to pituitary insufficiency.

Developmental anomalies and genetic syndromes associated with hypopituitarism

A number of developmental anomalies or genetic syndromes affecting the hypothalamus and pituitary may result in HGH deficiency with or without other trophic hormone deficiencies. Many of these syndromes are associated with facial or optic anomalies. In certain disorders, such as congenital absence of the pituitary, empty sella syndrome, transsphenoidal encephalocele, and two rare syndromes associated with unusual or large sella turcica, lateral skull radiographs may be sufficient to suspect the intracranial anomaly. In other disorders, however, such as holoprosencephaly and septooptic dysplasia, computed tomography scans or magnetic resonance imaging of the brain and hypothalamus may be necessary to detect the malformations. Therefore, any HGH-deficient child with malformations of the face or eyes should have imaging of the brain and sella turcica to rule out a malformation affecting the hypothalamus or pituitary gland.

There are a number of genetic syndromes not associated with known developmental malformations of the hypothalamus or pituitary, which have pituitary insufficiency as a common component. Children with Pallister-Hall syndrome (hypothalamic hamartoma or hamartoblastoma, polydactyly, anal or renal anomalies, and facial changes) may present with hypopituitarism (Biesecker and Graham, 1996), and this disorder is caused by mutations in the transcription factor gene GL13 (Kang et al., 1997). In other disorders, such as histiocytosis X and hemochromatosis, the hormonal deficiencies are due to a degenerative disease of the hypothalamus and pituitary. In most of these syndromes, however, the pathogenesis of the pituitary insufficiency is unknown. Both sickle cell anemia and thalassemia are associated with delayed growth and sexual development that result in adult short stature. In the thalassemias, this is apparently due to posttransfusion therapy, resulting in hemosiderosis that affects the pituitary. In persons with sickle cell anemia the exact cause of the short stature is unknown.

Growth hormone deficiency unassociated with developmental anomalies or multisystem genetic syndromes

The most common form of growth hormone deficiency is the "idiopathic-type" (i.e., one where no organic lesions exist). This heterogeneous group of disorders can be classified on the basis of whether only growth hormone is deficient, if there are multitropic hormone deficiencies, and if it is genetic or acquired. In addition, these disorders must be distinguished from the various forms of IGF or growth hormone resistance. Prenatal problems, such as breech or forceps deliveries, early vaginal bleeding, or prolonged or unusually short labors, frequently occur in persons with acquired hypopituitarism, as do signs of intrapartum fetal stress or anoxia. It has been suggested that these perinatal insults lead to the hypopituitarism in the nongenetic forms of this disease. The many genetic forms of growth hormone deficiency or resistance are discussed in Chapter **80**.

Disproportionate short stature

If a disproportionate body habitus is found on physical examination, the patient is likely to have a form of skeletal dysplasia. This is a heterogeneous group of heritable disorders affecting connective tissue in which the predominant clinical feature is dwarfism. Well over 100 distinct disorders have now been recognized, and it is important to make an accurate diagnosis so that a specific prognosis and proper genetic counseling can be provided. Furthermore, each of these disorders is associated with a variety of skeletal and nonskeletal complications, so that an accurate diagnosis will help one to develop a realistic treatment plan. These osteochondrodysplasias and dyosostoses are discussed in detail in Chapters **152** and **155, respectively**.

As illustrated in Fig. 41.1, the diagnostic workup for short stature should be approached rationally, before determining the mode of therapy. Disproportionate short stature may require an entirely different therapeutic approach than what is used for proportionate short stature. Likewise, prenatal-onset disorders must be separated from postnatal-onset disorders, and each category of growth deficiency will manifest different responses to specific treatments. In general, prenatal-onset growth deficiency that persists postnatally is generally assumed to be due to a genetic, syndromal, cytogenetic, or teratogenic disorder that results in generalized hypoplasia or dysproportionate skeletal hypoplasia. Growth deficiency that is secondary to chronic disease, endocrine insufficiency, nutritional insufficiency, or psychosocial deprivation responds best to treatment of the primary disease state. Recurrence risk counseling must also be individualized based on the underlying diagnosis. As the human genome becomes completely mapped and sequenced, future diagnostic and therapeutic modalities will change dramatically.

Pathologic overgrowth

The array of pathologic conditions which can result in overgrowth is much more restricted than the numerous conditions that have a negative impact on growth. There are a number of growth factors that function at various times during development and impact the growth of specific tissues in either a generalized or localized way. Similarly, other factors function to suppress growth. Thus, overgrowth disorders result in either localized or generalized effects on growth.

As with short stature, the pathologic determination of overgrowth should be made in relation to family and ethnic background. Once a careful assessment has been made and pathologic overgrowth is indicated, every effort should be made to reach an accurate diagnosis in order to provide adequate medical management and genetic counseling. The vast majority of prenatal syndromic overgrowth disorders persists postnatally, and, in some cases, mental deficiency, risk for tumor development or both, are important associated features. The risk for tumor development involves embryonal neoplasms, perhaps related to overexpression of growth factors, or lack of suppressing factors. A comprehensive review and classification system for overgrowth disorders has been presented by Cohen (1989) and updated (Cohen, 1999), and the diagnosis and treatment of these disorders has also been reviewed by Sotos (1996; 1997). The early history of the study of overgrowth, beginning in the eighteenth century, has been reviewed by Beckwith (1998).

Generalized overgrowth disorders

The optimum birthweight for the lowest perinatal mortality and morbidity is 3500 to 4000 g (Kessner, 1973), with 5.3% of newborns exceeding 4000 g, and 0.4% to 0.9% exceeding 4500 g (Horger et al., 1975). Factors related to large fetal weight include genetic predispositions; excessive maternal weight gain, obesity, and diabetes; postmaturity; and multiparity (Spellacy et al., 1985). Although many macrosomic infants demonstrate proportionate overgrowth, infants of diabetic mothers are often disproportionately overgrown with increased weight-to-length ratios. Some infants with anasarca are macrosomic primarily due to increased extracellular fluid volumes. True somatic overgrowth is often accompanied by increased placental size, as is commonly seen in Beckwith-Wiedemann syndrome (Weng et al., 1995).

At the cellular level, the onset of most prenatal overgrowth results from (1) excessive cellular proliferation (hyperplasia); (2) excessive cellular size (hypertrophy); (3) an increase in the interstitium (e.g., anasarca); or (4) a combination of these factors (Cohen, 1999). Overgrowth conditions can be subdivided between normal variants, such as familial tall statue or familial rapid maturation, prenatal-onset growth excess, or postnatal-onset growth excess (Fig. 41.7), however, primary growth excess results from intrinsic cellular hyperplasia, while secondary growth excess is due to humorally mediated factors outside the skeletal system (Cohen, 1989).

Among pathologic overgrowth disorders, most prenatal-onset growth excess is of the primary type, such as is seen with Beckwith-Wiedemann syndrome or Sotos syndrome. Secondary growth excess of prenatal-onset is usually not syndromic. The best examples include diabetic macrosomia and congenital nesidioblastosis (a diffuse abnormality of the pancreas with extensive and often disorganized formation of new islets of Langerhans, overproduction of insulin, and consequent severe neonatal hypoglycemia requiring pancreatectomy). Based on recurrence in siblings born to unaffected parents, this disorder is thought to manifest autosomal recessive inheritance (Schwartz et al., 1979).

Postnatal-onset growth excess is usually secondary, involving overproduction of estrogens or androgens (precocious puberty), overproduction of growth hormone (acromegaly), or overproduction of thyroid hormone. A few primary excess growth disorders manifest the majority of their overgrowth in the postnatal period (e.g., XYY syndrome, XXY syndrome, fragile X syndrome, and Marfan syndrome). These disorders are discussed more fully in Chapters **103** and **149**.

Other overgrowth disorders

There are only a few disorders that result in regional overgrowth (e.g., familial macrocephaly, congenital hemihyperplasia, cutis marmorata telangiectasia congenita, Klippel-Trenaunay-Weber syndrome, Maffuci syndrome, Ollier syndrome, Patterson-David syndrome, and Proteus

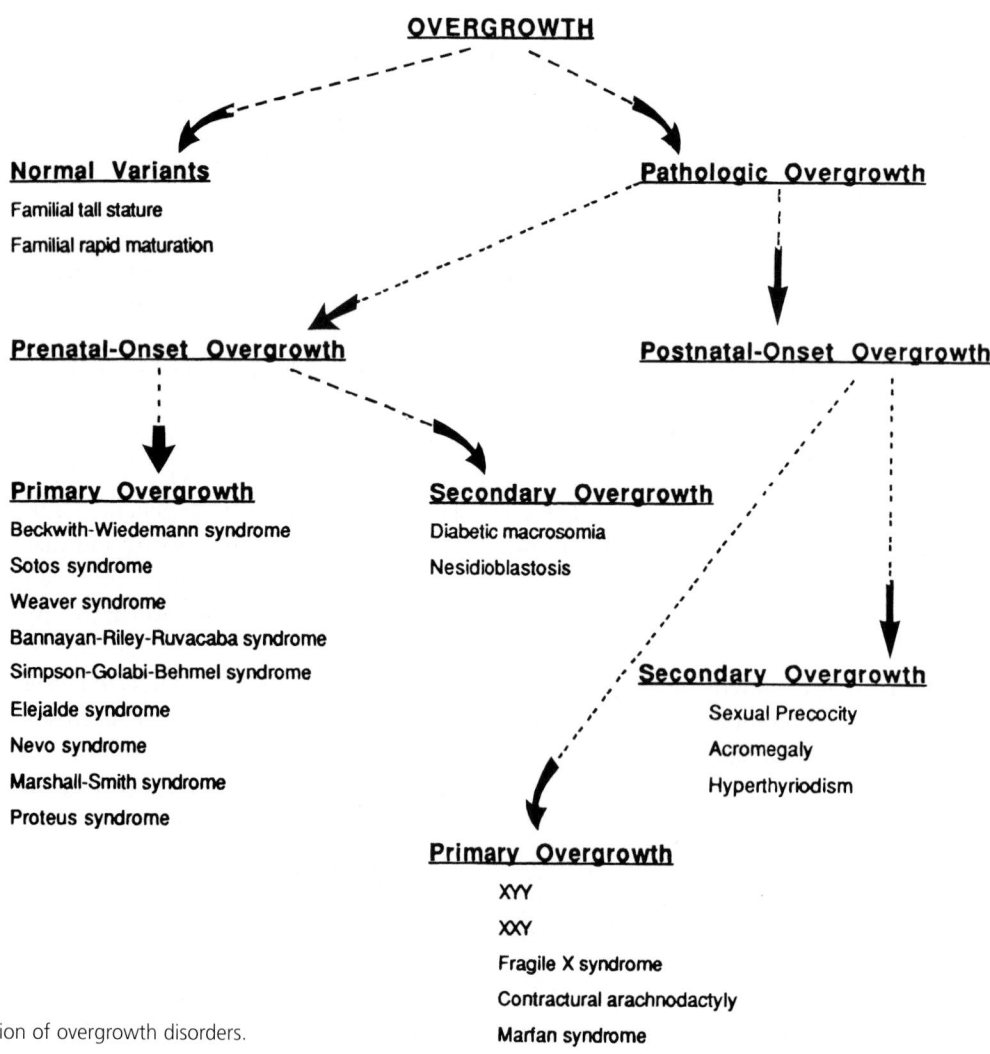

Fig. 41.7. Classification of overgrowth disorders.

syndrome). Parameter-specific overgrowth disorders contrast with generalized overgrowth disorders in that usually only a single growth parameter (e.g., weight) is affected. Examples of such disorders include those associated with obesity (e.g., Prader-Willi syndrome, Cohen syndrome, Borjesson-Forssman-Lehman syndrome, or familial idiopathic obesity), or with accelerated skeletal maturation (e.g., Marshall-Smith syndrome or Berardinelli lipodystrophy).

Prenatal overgrowth syndromes

The major diagnostic features for some of the prenatal-onset overgrowth syndromes are listed in Table 41.2.

Because of their importance and frequency, five of these disorders are discussed in more detail below.

BECKWITH-WIEDEMANN SYNDROME

Beckwith-Wiedemann syndrome is the most common congenital overgrowth syndrome, with a frequency of 1 case per 13,700 births (Weng et al., 1995; Cohen, 1999). It is associated with abdominal wall defects, macroglossia, prenatal-onset overgrowth, neonatal hypoglycemia, and visceromegaly. Other distinctive features include earlobe creases and pits, facial nevus flammeus, and infraorbital creases (Fig. 41.8). Large size at birth is associated with placental overgrowth, long umbilical cord, and polyhydramnios, which often results in premature delivery and

Table 41.2. Prenatal-onset overgrowth syndromes

Syndrome	Inheritance	Key clinical findings
Beckwith-Wiedemann	Autosomal dominant, sporadic	Macroglossia, infraorbital creases, ear lobe creases, and pits, abdominal wall defects, neonatal hypoglycemia, visceromegaly, risk for abdominal neoplasms, hemihypertrophy, polyhydramnios, large placenta
Perlman	Autosomal dominant	Hypotonia, mental retardation, serration of upper alveolar ridge, nephromegaly, bilateral cortical hamartomas and nephroblastomatosis
Sotos	Sporadic	Macrocephaly, dolichocephaly, downslanting palpebral fissures, hypertelorism, prognathism, high narrow palate, premature eruption of teeth, large hands and feer, kyphoscoliosis, mental deficiency
Weaver	Sporadic	Mental retardation, hypertonia, hoarse voice, macrocephaly, round face, ocular hypertelorism, down-slanting palpebral fissures, long philtrum, large ears, micrognathia, camptodactyly, thin deep-set nails, prominent fingertip pads
Bannayan-Riley-Ruvalcaba	Autosomal dominant	Delayed gross motor development, hypotonia, speech delay, mental deficiency, macrocephaly, prominent schwalbe lines, prominent corneal nerves, pseudo-papilledema, mesodermal hamartomas, pigmented macules penis, and lipid storge myopathy
Simpson-Golabi-Behmel	X-linked recessive	Macrocephaly, ocular hypertelorism, short broad nose, large mouth, macroglossia, variable mental retardation, hypotonia, postaxial polydactyly of hands, nail hypoplasia, partial cutaneous syndactyly, cryptorchidism, supernumerary nipples, cardia defects, gastrointestinal defects, large cystic kidneys
Elejalde	Autosomal recessive	Craniosynostosis, gross edema, short limbs, postaxial polydactyly, redundant neck skin, cystic renal dysplasia, congenital heart defect, spleen anomaly micromelia
Nevo	Autosomal recessive	Large, low-set malformed ears, cryptorchidism, accelerated osseous maturation, dolichocephaly, large extremities, clumsiness and retarded motor and speech development, generalized edema, hypotonia, contractures of the feet, wrist drop, clinodactyly
Marshall-Smith	Sporadic	Accelerated linear growth, skeletal maturation, postnatal failure to thrive, hypotonia, developmental delay, structural brain anomalies, respiratory tract anomalies, recurrent pneumonia, pulmonary hypertension, dolichocephaly, coarse eyebrows, shallow orbits, blue sclerae, upturned nose, low nasal bridge, small mandibular ramus, hypertrichosis, umbilical hernia, choanal atresia, omphalocele
Proteus	Sporadic	Regional overgrowth of hand and/or feet, asymmetry of limbs, plantar hyperplasia, hemangiomas, lipomas, lymphangiomas, varicosities, verucous epidermal nevi, macrocephaly, cranial hypertoses, long bone overgrowth, variable moderate mental deficiency

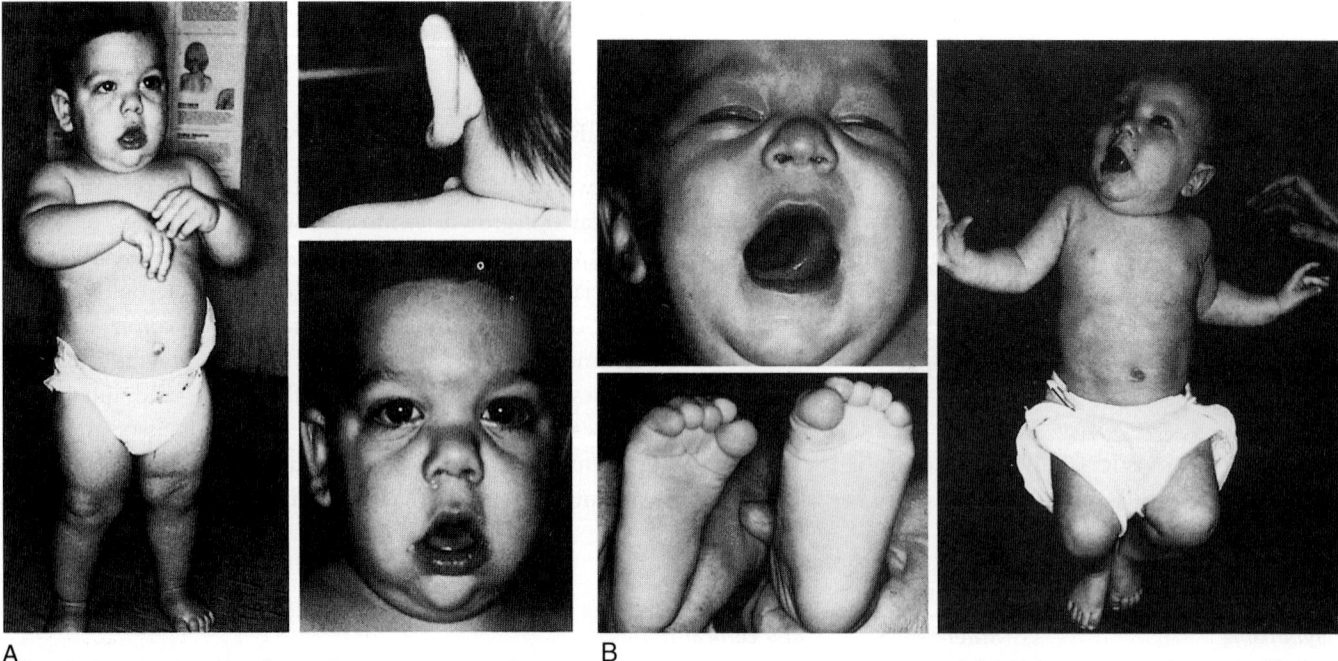

A   B

Fig. 41.8. (A) This 15 ½-month-old boy was born weighing 4700 g with macroglossia, umbilical hernia, glabellar nevus flammeous, prominent infraorbital creases and posterior ear pit superiorly. Other children on the side of mother's siblings were born weighing over 4500 g with large tongues. (B) This 4 ½-month-old female was born with hemihyperplasia of the left side of the body, including the tongue. The overgrowth also involved the left kidney, in relation to the size of the right kidney. Family history was negative for others with signs of Beckwith-Wiedemann syndrome.

contributes to a 21% perinatal mortality (Weng et al., 1995). The large size-for-age continues through early childhood and is associated with accelerated osseous maturation, but overgrowth is usually no longer evident by adulthood. Prompt recognition of this disorder is important because of the dangers associated with hypoglycemia and prematurity in overgrown neonates, and associated risk for embryonal neoplasms, affecting abdominal organs (primarily nephroblastoma, adrenocortical carcinoma, and hepatoblastoma). Intelligence is usually normal in the absence of complications related to prematurity and/or neonatal hypoglycemia.

Beckwith-Wiedemann syndrome is caused by genetic alterations in chromosomal region 11p15, an area which is subject to imprinting. In addition to the major fetal growth factor, insulin-like growth factor type 2 (IGF2), there are a number of genes in this region which may play roles in enhancing and suppressing growth, and imbalance of these gene functions may lead to fetal overgrowth. For example, IGF2 is a paternally active growth-enhancing gene with imprinting of the maternal allele, while H19 appears to be a maternally active growth-suppressor gene, with imprinting of the paternal allele. Cohen (1994) indicates that Beckwith-Wiedemann syndrome can arise in at least three different ways: (1) familial cases with genetic linkage to 11p15 (with 5% of cases demonstrating mutations in p57^{KIP2}); (2) cases with karyotypic abnormalities (2% of cases), due to either

paternal duplications of 11p15 (Fig. 41.9), or to maternal translocations or inversions with breakpoints in 11p15; and (3) sporadic cases (85% of cases). Familial cases (15% of cases) are inherited in an autosomal dominant fashion with incomplete penetrance, and most are born to female carriers.

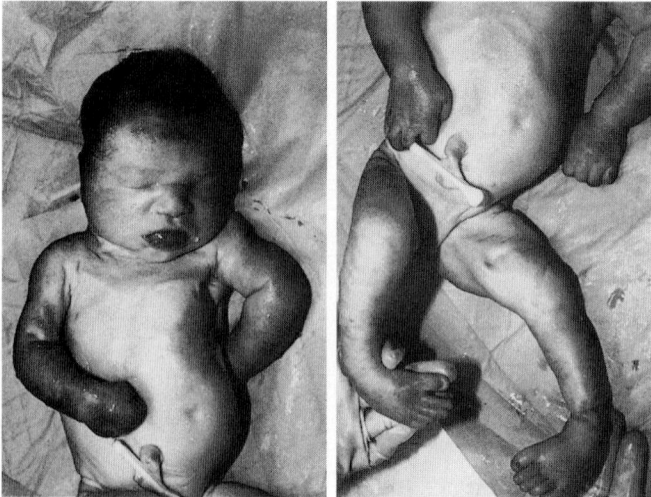

Fig. 41.9. Paternal duplication of 11p15 with prenatal-onset overgrowth, macroglossia, and other features representing a combination of Beckwith-Wiedemann syndrome and 18q- deletion syndrome. The father had a balanced 11p:18q chromosomal translocation, while this fetus had an unbalanced translocation resulting in partial trisomy 11p and partial monosomy 18q.

Sporadic cases can arise through *de novo* germline or somatic mutations. Among cases with normal chromosomes, paternal uniparental disomy is present in 10–20% of cases, and somatic mosaicism for partial paternal isodisomy occurs in some cases of hemihypoplasia (Henry et al., 1993; Li et al., 1998). About half of the sporadic cases show biallelic expression of IGF2 (Weksberg et al., 1993; Li et al., 1998). Cohen (1994) noted that hemihyperplasia rarely occurs in familial cases, and hemihyperplasia and neoplasms seem to occur more frequently in sporadic cases, possibly due to an imbalance in the biallelic expression of IGF-2 and H19. Paternal trisomy or uniparental disomy for 11p15 could lead to an excess of expressed paternal alleles, while relaxation of the maternal imprint for 11p15 might give rise to biallelic expression of IGF-2 and/or suppression of H19. Other genes of interest in the 11p15 region include KVLQT1, HASH2, and INS, but overexpression of IGF2 appears to be most common pathogenetic mechanism for the prenatal overgrowth.

Because of the risk of tumor development in Beckwith-Wiedemann syndrome and in some common types of congenital hemihypertrophy, Clericuzio (1993) proposed the following screening protocol: (1) baseline abdominal CT at age six months (or at time of initial diagnosis); (2) abdominal ultrasound every three months until age seven years, then every six months until skeletal growth completion; (3) abdominal palpation and urinalysis every three months until age seven years, then every six months until skeletal growth completion; and (4) serum α-fetoprotein determination at time of initial diagnosis, then annually. Patients with hemihyperplasia may need more frequent determinations because of their increased risk for hepatoblastoma.

CEREBRAL GIGANTISM (SOTOS SYNDROME)

Cerebral gigantism is associated with prenatal-onset overgrowth and affects length more than weight. Initially, there is rapid linear growth accompanied by advanced osseous maturation and large hands and feet. The head is large and dolichocephalic with frontoparietal balding, down-slanted palpebral fissures, prognathism with pointed chin, and premature eruption of teeth (Fig. 41.9). Commonly, there is developmental delay affecting the development of both motor and speech functions, with associated clumsiness, and EEG abnormalities. On cranial imaging, dilatation of cerebral ventricles is common (63% of cases), especially prominent occipital horns (75%); other abnormalities include absent corpus callosum, prominent cortical sulci, cavum septum pellucidum, and cavum velum interpositi (Schaefer et al., 1997). Opitz et al (1998) reviewed this syn-drome, along with Weaver syndrome, and noted it was a relatively frequent overgrowth syndrome that occurred 10 times more frequently than Weaver syndrome. A slightly increased risk for malignancy may exist, but the sites and types of neoplasia vary considerably, and no formal screening protocol, other than periodic clinical evaluation, has been suggested (Hersh et al., 1992). Most cases appear to be sporadic occurrences in otherwise normal families, with associated increased paternal age, and autosomal dominant inheritance has been suggested in some cases, with the affected parents showing primarily mild mental retardation, long facies and large hands and feet, but without tall stature (Cole and Hughes, 1994; Opitz et al., 1998).

WEAVER SYNDROME

In Weaver syndrome overgrowth is usually evident at birth, with most affected individuals at or above the 97th centile by age 1 year for length and weight (Weaver et al., 1974). Overgrowth continues throughout life, with adult height and weight above the 97th centile, and markedly accelerated osseous maturation during childhood. Most affected individuals are mentally deficient. Their distinctive features include hypertonia, hoarse low-pitched cry, macrocephaly, round face, ocular hypertelorism, down-slanting palpebral fissures, long philtrum, large ears, micrognathia, campto-dactyly, clinodactyly, broad thumbs, prominent fingertip pads, and limited elbow and knee extension (Fig. 41.10). Most cases appear to be sporadic occurrences in otherwise normal families, with parent-to-child transmission noted in five instances (Opitz et al., 1998).

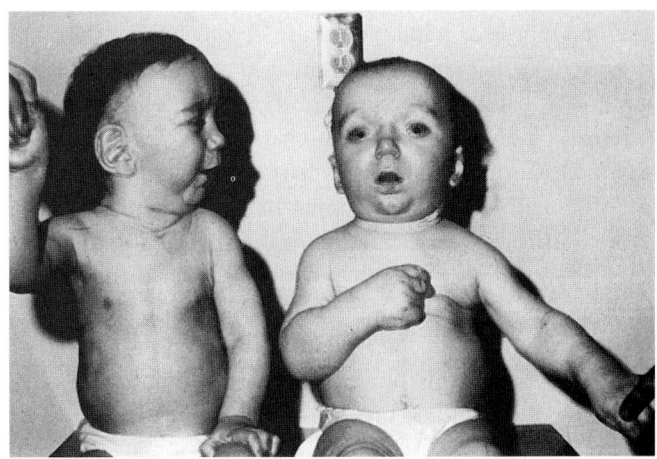

Fig. 41.10. Two unrelated boys with Weaver syndrome at ages 18 months and 11 months. (From Weaver et al. (1974) A new overgrowth syndrome with accelerated skeletal maturation, unusual facies, and conptodactyly. J Pediatr 84:547–552. © 1974.)

BANNAYAN-RILEY-RUVALCABA SYNDROME

This disorder was initially reported in 1960 by Riley and Smith as the association of macrocephaly, pseudo-papilledema, and multiple hemangiomas. Bannayan (1971) described the association of macrocephaly with multiple lipomas and hemangiomas, and Zonana and colleagues (1976) confirmed these findings as a clinical entity. In 1980, Ruvalcaba and colleagues reported two males with macrocephaly, intestinal polyposis, and pigmented spotting of the penis (initially interpreted as new features of Sotos syndrome, illustration the phenotypic overlap between these two disorders). This disorder was further delineated by DiLiberti and associates (1984) who documented an associated lipid storage myopathy. In 1988, Dvir and coworkers suggested that each of these conditions represented different combinations of the same autosomal dominant syndrome that consisted of mesodermal hamartomas, macrocephaly, and pseudopapilledema. Cohen (1989) suggested combining the names of the first authors of these three original reports to reflect the coalescence of the syndromes, fusing them into one clinical entity, the Bannayan-Riley-Ruvalcaba syndrome, consisting of macrocephaly, vascular malformations, lipomas, hamartomatous intestinal polyps, pigmented penile macules, and Hashimoto's thyroiditis.

At birth, length and weight are usually greater than the 97th centile, but growth tends to normalize by midchildhood with the final height within the normal adult range. Bone age is usually consistent with chronological age, and macrocephaly persists into adulthood with normal ventricular size. Delayed gross motor development may be associated with a lipid storage myopathy which appears to respond to treatment with carnitine. This autosomal dominant syndrome is caused by mutations in the PTEN gene, a tumor-suppressor gene which also results in Cowden syndrome (a hamartomatous disorder that results in cobblestone-like papules of the gingiva, facial trichilemmomas, intestinal polyps, and carcinoma of the breast andlor thyroid). Germline mutations have been identified in 81% of Cowden syndrome families and in about 57% of Bannayan-Riley-Ruvalcaba syndrome families, though a hot spot for Cowden syndrome mutations occurs in the PTPase core motif (43%), but mutations for both disorders appear to occur throughout the gene (Cohen, 1999; Marsh et al., 1999). Even though these two disorders are allelic, their phenotypes commonly breed true (Cohen, 1999).

SIMPSON-GOLABI-BEHMEL SYNDROME

This distinctive X-linked syndrome, with partial expression in female carriers, was initially confused with Beckwith-Wiedemann syndrome in earlier reports (Hughes-Benzi et al., 1992) due to striking prenatal-onset overgrowth that persists into adulthood (Fig. 41.11). Distinctive features include congenital macrocephaly, mental deficiency, ocular hypertelorism with short broad nose, cleft palate, wide mouth, central groove of the lower lip, supernumerary nipples, pectus excavatum, rib and vertebral abnormalities, hypotonia, postaxial polydactyly of the hands, nail hypoplasia (especially involving the index fingers), partial cutaneous syndactyly, cryptorchidism, heart defects, and large cystic kidneys (Neri et al., 1998). Features in common with Beckwith-Wiedemann syndrome include prenatal overgrowth, macroglossia, ear lobe creases and pits, umbilical hernia, intestinal malrotation, and hypoglycemia from

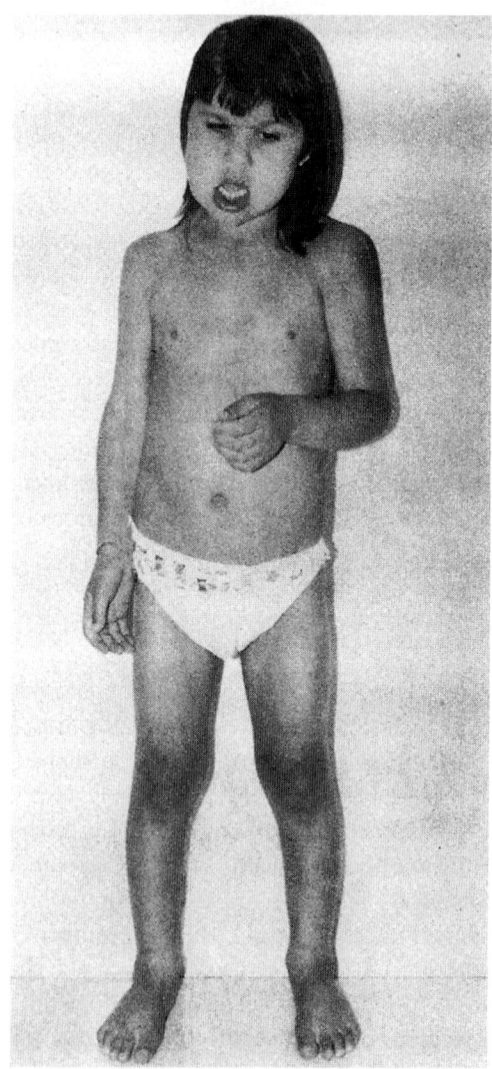

Fig. 41.11. Affected female carrier with Simpson-Golabi-Behmel syndrome, initially misdiagnosed with Beckwith-Wiedemann syndrome, was later diagnosed properly after fetal demise of subsequent male sibling with postaxial polydactyly of the hands.

excessive islets of Langerhans. Infant mortality is approximately 50%, occurring primarily from cardiorespiratory causes. This disorder results from mutations in the cell surface heparan sulfate proteoglycan glipican gene GPL3, which appears to play a role in controlling the growth of mesodermal tissues and binds to IGF2, whereby it helps to modulate its action (Neri et al., 1998; Cohen, 1999).

A few other important and distinctive prenatal-onset overgrowth syndromes are described in Table 41.2. Further analysis and study of these interesting syndromes should help shed light on the normal processes of human growth and morphogenesis.

Acknowledgements

We appreciate the generous support of SHARE's Child Disability Center and the Steven Spielberg Pediatric Research Center. In addition, this work was supported by the UCLA Intercampus Training Program Grant #GM08243 from the National Institutes of Health, and Grant #P01 HD22657 from the U.S. Department of Health and Human Services, Public Health Service.

REFERENCES

Aarskog D, Ferang FO, Klore H et al. (1977) The effect of the stimulant drugs, dextroamphetamine and methylphenidate on secretion of growth hormone in hyperactive children. J Pediatr 90:136–139

Alkalay AL, Graham JM Jr, Pomerance JJ (1998) Evaluation of neonates born with intrauterine growth retardation: Review and practice guidelines. J Perinatol 18:142–151

Bannayan GA (1971) Lipomatosis, angiomatosis and macroencephaly: a previously underscribed congenital syndrome. Arch Pathol 92:1–5

Beckwith JB (1998) Vignettes from the history of overgrowth and related syndromes. Am J Med Genet 79:238–248

Biesecker LB, Graham JM Jr (1996) Syndrome of the month: Pallister-Hall syndrome. J Med Genet 33:585–589

Clericuzio CL (1993) Clinical phenotypes and Wilms tumor. Med Pediatr Oncol 21:182–187

Cohen MM Jr (1989) A comprehensive and critical assessment of overgrowth and overgrowth syndromes. Advan Hum Gene 18:181–303

Cohen MM Jr (1994) Wiedemann-Beckwith syndrome, imprinting, IGF2, and H19: Implications for hemihyperplasia, associated neoplasms, and overgrowth. Am J Med Genet 52:233–234

Cohen MM Jr (1999) Overgrowth syndromes: An update. Advan Pediatr 46:441–491

Cole TRP, Hughes HE (1994) Sotos syndrome: A study of the diagnostic criteria and natural history. J Med Genet 31:20–32

DiLiberti JH, D'Agostino AN, Ruvalcaba RHA, Schimshock JR (1984) A new lipid storage myopathy observed in individuals with the Ruvalcaba-Myhre-Smith syndrome. Am J Med Genet 18:163–167

Dvir M, Beer S, Aladjem M (1988) Heredofamilial syndrome of mesodermal hamartomas, macrocephaly, and pseudopapilledema. Pediatrics 81:287–290

Edwards MJ, Park J, Wurster-Hill DH, Graham JM Jr (1994) Mixoploidy in humans: two surviving cases of diploid tetraploid mixoploidy and comparison with diploid triploid mixoploidy. Am J Med Genet 52:324–330

Graham JM Jr (1983) In Congenital Anomalies: Developmental Behavioral Pediatrics. W B Saunders: Philadelphia, p. 378

Graham JM Jr (2002) In: Smith's Recognizable Patterns of Human Deformation. W B Saunders, Philadelphia

Graham JM Jr, Hoehn H, Lin MS and Smith DW (1981) Diploid-triploid mixoploidy: Clinical and cytogenetic features. Pediatrics 68:23–28

Hall BD (1985) A diagnostic approach to genetic causes of short stature. Alabama J Med Sci 22:431–435

Harvey MAS, Smith DW, Skinner AL (1979) Infant growth standards in relation to parental stature. Clin Pediatr 18:602–603, 611–613

Henry I, Puech A, Riesewijk A et al. (1993) Somatic mosaicism for partial paternal isodisomy in Wiedemann-Beckwith syndrome: A post-fertilization event. Eur J Hum Genet 1:19–29

Hersh JH, Graham JM Jr, Destrempes BS, Greenstein RM (1983) Teschler-Nicola Killian syndrome: A case report. J Clin Dysmorphol 1:20–24

Hersh JH, Cole TRP, Bloom AS et al. (1992) Risk of malignancy in Sotos syndrome. J Pediatr 120:572–574

Horger EO, Facog M, Miller C, Conner ED (1975) Relation of large birthweight to maternal diabetes mellitus. Obstetr Gynecol 45:150–154

Hughes-Benzie RM, Hunter AGW, Allanson JE, Mackenzie AE (1992) Simpson-Golabi-Behmel syndrome associated with renal dysplasia and embryonal tumor: Localization of the gene to Xqcen-q21. Am J Med Genet 43:428–435

Jones KL (1997) In Smith's Recognizable Patterns of Human Malformation. WB Saunders, Philadelphia

Kang S, Graham JM Jr, Olney AH, Biesecker LG (1997) GL13 frameshift mutations cause autosomal dominant Pallister-Hall syndrome. Nature Genet 15:266–268

Kaplan SA (1982) In Clinical Pediatric and Adolescent Endocrinology. WB Saunders, Philadelphia

Kessner DM (1973) Infant death: An analysis by maternal risk and health care. Proc Acad Sci USA 70:90–195

Laskari A, Smith AK, Graham JM Jr (1999) Williams-Behrens Syndrome: An update and review for the primary pediatrician. Clin Pediatr 38:189–208

Li M, Squire J, Weksberg R (1998) Molecular genetics Wiedemann-Beckwith syndrome. Am J Med Genet 79:253–259

Marsh DJ, Kum JB, Lunetta KL et al. (1999) PTEN mutation spectrum and genotype-phenotype correlations in Bannayan-Riley-Ruvalcaba syndrome suggest a single entity with Cowden syndrome. Hum Mol Genet 8:1461–1472

Neri G, Gurrieri F, Zanni G et al. (1998) Clinical and molecular aspects of the Simpson-Golabi-Behmel syndrome. Am J Med Genet 79:279–283

Opitz JM, Weaver DW, Reynolds JF Jr (1998) The syndromes of Sotos and Weaver: Reports and review. Am J Med Genet 79:294–304

Phillips LS, Vassilopoulou-Sellin P (1980a) Somatromedins: Part 1 (medical progress). N Engl J Med 302:371–80

Phillips LS, Vassilopoulou-Sellin P (1980b) Somatromedins: Part 2 (medical progress). N Engl J Med 302:438–446

Powell GF, Brasel JA, Blizzard RM (1967) Emotional deprivation and growth retardation simulating idiopathic hypopituitarism: 1. Clinical evaluation of the syndrome. N Engl J Med 276:1271–1278

Price SM, Stanhope R, Garrett C, Preece MA, Trembath RC (1999) The spectrum of Silver-Russell syndrome: A clinical and molecular genetic study and new diagnostic criteria. J Med Genet 36:837–842

Rao E, Weiss B, Fukami M et al. (1997) Pseudoautosomal deletions encompassing a novel homeobox gene cause growth failure in idiopathic short stature and Turner syndrome. Nature Genet 16:54–63

Riley HD, Smith WR (1960) Macrocephaly, pseudopapilledema and multiple hemangiomata. Pediatrics 26:293–300

Rimoin DL, Borochowitz Z, Horton WA (1986) Short stature: Physiology and pathology (medical progress). West J Med 144(6):710–721

Roche AF, Lipman RS, Overall JE et al. (1979) The effects of stimulant medications on the growth of hyperkinetic children. Pediatrics 63:847–850

Ruvalcaba RHA, Myhre S, Smith DW (1980) Sotos syndrome with intestinal polyposis and pigmentary changes of the genitalia. Clin Genet 18:413–416

Sampson PD, Streissguth AP, Bookstein FL et al. (1997) The incidence of fetal alcohol syndrome and the prevalence of alcohol-related neurodevelopmental disorder. Teratology 56:317–325

Saul RA, Stevenson RE, Rogers RC et al. (1988) Growth references from conception to adulthood. Proceed Greenwood Genet Center, Supplement No. 1

Schaefer GB, Bodensteiner JB, Buehler BA et al. (1997) The neuroimaging findings in Sotos syndrome. Am J Med Genet 68:462–465

Schwartz SS, Rich BH, Lucky AW et al. (1979) Familial nesidioblastosis: Severe neonatal hypoglycemia in two families. J Pediatr 95:44–53

Smith DW, Truog W, Rogers JE et al. (1976) Shifting linear growth during infancy: illustration of genetic factors in growth from fetal life through infancy. J Pediatr 89:225–230

Smith DW (1977) In Growth and Its Disorders. WB Saunders, Philadelphia

Sotos JF (1996) Overgrowth. Clin Pediatr 35:517–529, 579–590, 637–648

Sotos JF (1997) Overgrowth. Clin Pediatr 36:39–49, 91–103, 157–170

Spellacy WN, Miller S, Winegar A, Peterson PQ (1985) Macrosomia-maternal characteristics and infant complications. Obstetr Gynecol 66:158–161

Strauss RS (2000) Adult functional outcome of those born small for gestational age: Twenty-six-year follow-up of the 1970 British birth cohort. J Am Med Assoc 283:625–632

Tanner JM, Goldstein H, Whitehouse RH (1970) Standards for children's heights at ages 2–9 years allowing for heights of parents. Arch Disabled Children 45:755–762

Weaver DD, Graham CB, Thomas IT, Smith DW (1974) A new overgrowth syndrome with accelerated skeletal maturation, unusual facies, and comptodactyly. J Pediatr 84:547–552

Weksberg R, Shen DR, Fei YL et al. (1993) Disruption of insulin-like growth factor 2 imprinting in Beckwith-Wiedemann syndrome. Nature Genet 5:143–150

Weng EY, Mortier GR, Graham JM Jr (1995) Beckwith-Wiedemann syndrome: An update and review for the primary pediatrician. Clin Pediatr 34:317–326

Zonana J, Rimoin DL, Davis DC (1976) Macrocephaly with multiple lipomas and hemangiomas. J Pediatr 89:600–603

Susceptibility and response to infection

Michael F. Murray
James Versalovic

Introduction

Microbial infection likely represents primary driving force of natural selection in humans, particularly in the last five thousand years (Haldane, 1949). In the spirit of his day, Haldane (1957) suggested that "the abolition of infectious diseases, which is now a possibility, and may be a reality in fifty years, should lead not only to an immediate improvement in human physique, but to a progressive improvement through many centuries". Since that time, we have learned a great deal more about genetic susceptibility to infection, and the selective pressure of microbes on humans. It has also become clear that despite the optimism associated with the antibiotic revolution of the mid-twentieth century, both new (e.g., human immunodeficiency virus) and old infections (e.g., malaria) are continuing to exert substantial selective pressure on human populations (Marshall, 2000). Although infectious diseases will likely persist due to microbial and host evolution, a detailed understanding of host genetic susceptibility and response to infection will facilitate improvements in existing therapies and the development of new therapies.

In this chapter, the discussion of genetics and infection does not focus exclusively on the immune system. While primary immune defects represent an important set of genetic disorders, and they are reviewed in Chapters 77 through 79, this chapter will examine the wide range of genetic polymorphisms that alter susceptibility to infection and associated complications. The organizing principle of the chapter is the location of the gene product in the context of the cell. Cell surface proteins, intracellular proteins, and extracellular proteins represent the designated categories. The first set of genes, the human leukocyte antigen (HLA) genes, display a high degree of polymorphism and serve as a model for human genes in an apparent state of co-evolution with infecting microbes.

Cell surface proteins

HUMAN LEUKOCYTE ANTIGEN GENES (HLA)

The HLA genes, which are encoded in the short arm of chromosome 6 (6p21.3), have been implicated as a modulating influence in a large number of infections (see Table 42.1). The HLA system, which is part of the human major histocompatibility complex (MHC), has been concisely reviewed elsewhere (Klein and Sato, 2000a, 2000b). MHC proteins, encoded by class Ia genes including HLA-A, HLA-B, and HLA-C, are expressed on most nucleated cells. The class II genes, also known as HLA-D, are designated with a three-letter code (e.g., HLA-DRB), which indicates class (D), family (M, O, P, Q, or R), and chain (A or B). Proteins encoded by class II genes are expressed on leukocytes (both B and T), macrophages, dendritic cells, and thymus cells. In both classes, numbers are assigned to each allele; this nomenclature is different for sequence-defined and for serologically-defined variants. An asterisk followed by a number indicates a genotypic variant (e.g., HLA-A*0101), while a number without an asterisk represents a serologic variant (e.g., HLA-A1) (Bodmer et al., 1999). An online HLA sequence database is available at http://www.ebi.ac.uk/imgt/hla (Robinson et al., 2000).

The class II molecules are heterodimers, which allows for alpha/beta matching within and between families (e.g., DRA and DQB), and results in approximately 12different class

Table 42.1 HLA Class Ia and Class II associated diseases

Microbe	Type of Organism	Disease(s)	Class	References
Human T-lymphotropic virus-1 (HTLV-1)	RNA Virus	Myelopathy	Ia	Jeffery
Human immunodeficiency virus-1 (HIV-1)	RNA Virus	AIDS	Ia and II	Kaslow Carrington MacDonald
Hepatitis C virus	RNA Virus	Viremia Mixed Cryoglobulinemia	II Ia and II	McKierna Lenzi
Dengue virus	RNA Virus	Hemorrhagic fever Shock	Ia	Paradoa
Puumala Hantavirus	RNA Virus	Renal Disease	Ia and II	Mustone
Ross River virus	RNA Virus	Arthritis	II	Fraser
Measles	RNA Virus	Subacute sclerosing panencephalitis	Ia	Kahana
Hepatitis B virus	DNA Virus	Viremia	II	Thurz
Herpes simplex virus 2 (HSV-2)	DNA Virus	Genital ulcers	Ia	Lekstrom-Hines
Epstein Barr virus	DNA Virus	Nasopharyngeal Cancer	Ia and II	Wu
Cytomegalovirus	DNA Virus	Retinitis	Ia and II	Schrier
Human herpes virus 8 (HHV-8)	DNA Virus	Kaposi Sarcoma	Ia	Prince
Human papilloma virus	DNA Virus	Cervical Cancer	Ia and II	Apple Krul
Mycobacterium tuberculosis	Bacteria	Tuberculosis	II	Goldfeld Meyer
Mycobacterium leprae	Bacteria	Leprosy	II	Meyer
Mycobacterium avium	Bacteria	Bacteremia Pneumonitis	II Ia and II	LaBlanc Kubo
Chlamydia trachomatis	Bacteria	Trachoma Fallopian tube scarring	Ia II	Conway Cohen
Haemophilus influenzae	Bacteria	Meningitis and Bacteremia	Ia	Tejani
Helicobacter pylori	Bacteria	Atrophic Gastritis	II	Sakai
Borrelia burgdorferi	Bacteria	Lyme Arthritis	II	Gross
Streptococcus pyogenes	Bacteria	Rheumatic Fever	II	Visentainer
Plasmodium falciparum	Protozoa	Malaria	Ia and II	Hill 1
Trypanosoma cruzi	Protozoa	Chagas Disease	Ia	Llop 1
Toxoplasma gondi	Protozoa	Congenital hydrocephalus	II	Mack
Leishmania spp.	Protozoa	Mucocutaneous ulceration	II	Petzl-Erler
Giardia lamblia	Protozoa	Gastroenteritis	II	el-Gananyni
Schistosomiasis spp.	Helminth	Hepatic fibrosis	II	Hirayama
Echinococcus spp.	Helminth	Liver abscess	II	Eiermann
Brugia spp.	Helminth	Elephantiasis	Ia and II	Yazdanbaknsh
Onchocerca volvulus	Helminth	River blindness	II	Meyer
Paracoccidiodes spp.	Fungus	Mycosis	Ia	Lacerda
Fronsecaea pedrosoi	Fungus	Chromoblastomycosis	Ia	Tsuneto
Trichosporon spp.	Fungus	Hypersensitivity pneumonitis	II	Ando
Cryptococcus neoformans	Fungus	Meningitis	Ia	Van Dam

Table 42.2 Non-HLA microbe-gene susceptibility associations

Microbe	Gene/Gene Product	Associated Susceptibility
HIV-1	FUT 2	Heterosexually acquired infection
	CCR5	Infection and progression to AIDS
	CCR2	Progression to AIDS
	CX$_3$CR1	Progression to AIDS
	NRAMP1	Progression to AIDS
	SDF1-3'A	Progression to AIDS
Parvovirus B19	P^K synthase	Infection
Hepatitis B Virus	VDR	Persistent infection
H. influenzae	FUT 2	Invasive infection
S. pneumoniae	FUT 2	Invasive infection
N. meningitidis	FUT 2	Invasive infection
Pseudomonas aeruginosa	CFTR	Pulmonary infection
Salmonella spp.	CFTR	Gastrointestinal infection
	IFNGR	Systemic infection
V. cholerae	Blood group O	Gastrointestinal infection
E. coli	GALT	Bacteremia
H. pylori	Lewis Ag	Gastric infection
	IL 1β	Gastric carcinoma
Mycobacterium spp.	VDR	Symptomatic infection
	IFNGR	Systemic infection
	IL 12RB1	Systemic infection
	NRAMP 1	Symptomatic infection
	IL1β	Pleural tuberculosis
	TNF2	Symptomatic infection
	MBP	Pulmonary tuberculosis
P. falciparum	Blood group A	Severe infection
	α Hgb	Severe infection
	βHgb	Severe infection
	G6PD	Severe infection
	TNF2	Cerebral malaria
P. vivax	DARC	Infection
Leishmania spp.	TNF2	Mucocutaneous infection

II antigens available on the cell surfaces of heterozygotes (Lechler et al., 1995). Heterozygotes also express six different class Ia antigens. Due to codominant expression, homozygotes likely express half as many different surface antigens as heterozygotes. Recombination within the MHC region allows for individuals who are homozygous for one locus or for an entire haplotype. Thus, there is a range of expressed HLA types within human populations.

HLAs are pivotal in the processing and presentation of microbial antigens to the human immune system. Inefficiency or failure of peptide presentation can result in disadvantages for the host when combating infection. Twenty-one highly polymorphic HLA genes with greater than 1000 recognized HLA alleles have been described (Robinson et al., 2000). This diversity is as yet unmatched elsewhere in the human genome. Infections may represent a driving force of HLA genetic diversity. Proposed mechanisms of infection-driven diversity include: overdominant selection (or heterozygous advantage) and frequency dependent selection (Parham and Ohta, 1996). The overdominant selection hypothesis holds that the *individual* with the most available HLA types will be best suited to handle the largest variety of microbial antigens. The frequency dependent selection hypothesis suggests that in a *population*, the selective force of the microbe on the host will favor uncommon HLAs to which the microbe has not yet adapted. Both mechanisms favor diversity and they are not mutually exclusive processes.

The overdominant selection hypothesis has been supported both in principle (Hughes and Nei, 1988), and with empirical data of specific infectious diseases. Heterozygous advantage has been demonstrated in three chronic viral infections: human papillomavirus, hepatitis B virus, and

HIV-1 (Gregoire et al., 1994; Thurz et al., 1997; Carrington et al., 1999a). On the other hand, though not predicted by those seeking to explain HLA diversity, homozygous advantage has also been demonstrated (Hill et al., 1991; Burt et al, 1994). Homozygous advantage in the context of a specific infection can be explained by increased numbers of a "preferred" HLA protein capable of peptide presentation specific microbial antigens.

Frequency dependent selection can be invoked to explain variations in the frequency of HLA-B53 in Africa. This HLA is associated with protection against severe malaria in studies performed in Gambia (Hill et al., 1991). While population frequencies in black South Africans are only about 2%, this class Ia antigen reaches frequencies of up to 40% in malaria-prone regions of West Africa. HLA-B53 is extremely rare or altogether absent in most non-African populations. Malaria appears to have acted as a directional selective force on local populations for 10,000 years. Plasmodial infections may have increased the frequency of HLA-B53 to levels greater than expected by genetic drift, as observed currently in West Africa (Howard, 1991).

Co-evolution of humans and microbes is an important concept in the study of HLA and infection. An African study of malaria peptides and HLA-B35 found evidence for bi-directional effects of human and parasitic alleles (Gilbert et al., 1998). Although observations such as this are still relatively rare, the opportunity for important observations in this area will grow with acquisition of human and microbial sequence data. For example, the use of a HIV1 sequence database together with knowledge of HLA peptide constraints and epidemiological data on HLA influence on outcomes, has allowed one group to correlate protective HLA types with their anticipated capacity to bind the observed range of motifs in the highly mutable HIV1 (Nelson et al., 1997).

Specific HLA alleles have been associated with cancers linked with chronic viral infections. HLA associations have been reported for several viral infections, including hepatitis B virus (HBV), hepatitis C virus (HCV), human papillomavirus (HPV) and Epstein-Barr virus (EBV). Hepatocellular carcinoma is associated with persistent viremia in both HBV and HCV, and while there is little direct evidence at this point for HLA associations with hepatocellular carcinoma, HLA associations have been reported with persistent viremia in chronic HBV or HCV infection (Ahn et al., 2000; McKiernan et al., 2000). HPV is a primary etiologic factor in the development of cervical carcinoma (Walboomers and Meijer, 1997), and HLA associations have been documented in cervical dysplasia and cervical carcinoma (Krul et al., 1999). Undifferentiated nasopharyngeal carcinoma is tightly linked with chronic EBV infection and has been associated with specific HLA antigens (Wu et al., 1989).

The exclusive application of serology-based (phenotypic) rather than sequence-defined (genotypic) HLAs represents a significant limitation with earlier HLA association studies. HLA genotyping emerged in the 1990s and yielded relatively greater specificity in HLA association studies. HLA antigens defined by serotyping represent phenotypes that have been useful with particular rheumatologic disease associations (e.g., HLA-B27 and ankylosing spondylitis, see Ch. 75), but relatively non-specific results obtained by such studies may be confounding. An example of the relative specificity of HLA genotyping and its ability to clarify otherwise contradictory data was demonstrated in the case of HLA-DR1 and HIV-1 infection. One group reported DR1 to be protective (Kaplan et al., 1990), while another group's data suggested that DR1 increased risk for progression (Mann et al., 1988). In a third report, it was found that HLA-DRB1*0101 was associated with a risk for progression, and HLA-DRB1*0102 appeared to be protective against progression; both of these alleles are serologically grouped as HLA-DR1 (Kroner et al., 1995). It can be expected that most studies will use genotypically defined alleles alone or in combination with serologically defined groups in the future.

Linkage disequilibrium among HLA and non-HLA genes within the MHC region may confound results obtained in the study of HLA and infection. HLA haplotypes, such as the "8.1 haplotype" [A1, B8, DR3] (Price et al., 1999), have been associated with several infectious diseases; the association of the 8.1 haplotype with HIV-1 (McNeil et al., 1996; Kaslow et al., 1990), HCV (Lenzi et al., 1998), or HSV (Lekstrom-Hines et al., 1999) infection may be due to individual HLA loci, the combination of HLA loci, or the non-HLA genes carried with the MHC. Non-HLA effector genes closely linked with HLA loci include tumor necrosis factor (TNF), transporters associated with antigen processing (TAP), and complement component genes.

The prevalence and cumulative effects of multiple infections, each with a different selective influence and occurring within the same human population must be considered when studying the role of HLA antigens in infection. Most studies have attempted to evaluate the influence of a single microbe with the HLAs of a discrete human population. However, human populations are subject to numerous microbial infections that occur sequentially and concomitantly during a lifetime. This multipronged attack may favor HLA diversity, although it makes isolating the effects of one infection from another in a given population challenging. Insight may be gained into this situation by re-examining the interaction between HLA and two infections: one that exerts strong directional selection and one that does not exert obvious selective pressure. In the study referred to previously, HLA protection from malaria was associated with both Class Ia and Class II antigens (Hill et al., 1991). Howard (1991) predicted that increases of specific HLA frequencies in response to malaria would ultimately result in either a counter-response from *Plasmodium falciparum* or the opportunity for another pathogen to "take advantage". Three years later, the DQB1*0501 allele, which together with HLA-B53 had been associated with protection against severe malaria, was linked with susceptibility to generalized *Onchocerca volvulus* infection (Meyer et al., 1994). This chronic helminthic infection, which causes "river blindness" late in life, has no recognized effects on reproductive fitness, while malaria (fatal in 1% of local children prior to their fifth birthday) has a major effect on reproductive fitness. The price of 10,000 years of selection for HLAs protective against malaria appears to be susceptibility to *Onchocerca* infection.

Several HLA class and loci associations have been repeatedly reported with specific bacterial and viral infections. Tuberculosis studies performed in multiple countries since 1989 have consistently found Class II, in particular DRB1, associations with infectious outcomes (Meyer et al., 1998). Class I associations have consistently been significant in HIV-1 outcomes (Carrington et al., 1999a).

In summary, the study of HLA-microbe interactions continues to be a complex task of studying two moving targets, i.e., the highly polymorphic human MHC region and continuously evolving microbial pathogens. Published studies have been limited by numerous variables but a greater understanding of the complex relationship between HLA and infection is emerging. Despite reports of HLA antigens functioning as co-receptors for viral entry (Haan et al., 2000), most available evidence suggests that the variability in infectious disease outcomes associated with specific HLA alleles is due to qualitative differences in the microbial peptide presentation to the immune system. Unfavorable outcomes are generally attributed to inefficient peptide presentation; however, it has been suggested that overly efficient HLA peptide presentation may lead to an excessive inflammatory reaction and poor outcomes (Carter et al., 1992). The role of HLA in host susceptibility to infection continues to be defined, and though some reported associations may ultimately prove to be due to genes linked to the MHC other than HLA, two principles have emerged: (1) HLA and microbial populations co-

evolve, and consequently (2) multiple alleles at specific loci appear to be linked to outcomes in different populations.

THE ABH ANTIGEN AND FUCOSYLTRANSFERASE GENES

Genes coding for five different glycosyltransferases determine classical "blood group" type, "secretor" status, and Lewis antigens. Alpha 1–3-N-actylgalactosaminyltransferase (transferase A) and alpha 1–3-galactosyltransferase (transferase B) genes are located in the long arm of chromosome 9 (9q34). These transferases act upon the "H" antigen to form the oligosaccharide blood group antigens "A" and "B". In the absence of transferase activity the unmodified "H" antigen defines the "O" phenotype. The enzymatic activity of fucosyltransferase 1 (FUT 1) provides the oligosaccharide substrate for either transferase by creating the H antigen. ABH antigens types are co-dominant in their expression (Spitalnik and Spitalnik, 2000). ABH antigens have a wide distribution in addition to erythrocytes, including vascular endothelial cells, and intestinal, cervical, urothelial, and mammary epithelial cells. These antigens can also be found in the body fluids of persons with inherited FUT 2 activity—i.e., positive "secretor" status (Spitalnik and Spitalnik, 2000). The non-erythrocytic distribution of antigens may account for many reported infectious disease associations.

The genes encoding FUT 1 and FUT 2 lie in the long arm of chromosome 19 (19q13.3). Individuals with the nonsecretor phenotype are homozygous for mutations associated with non-functional FUT 2 enzyme, thereby giving secretor status an autosomal recessive inheritance pattern. In an American study, homozygous alleles for a nonsense mutation were found at codon 143 of FUT 2 in 20% of persons tested (Kelly et al., 1995), while different mutations resulting in a non-functional enzyme have been found in other populations (Kudo et al., 1996). Secretor status is associated with FUT 2 activity and results in secreted ABH antigens in saliva, plasma, urine, milk, and feces.

Since the first reported associations of ABO blood groups to disease states, numerous attempts have linked infectious diseases with specific ABH antigens and secretor status, and this extensive literature has been reviewed elsewhere (Berger et al., 1989; Rios and Bianco, 2000). ABH antigens and secretor status influence susceptibility to infectious diseases, in most cases, by acting at mucosal sites of microbial exposure. The mucosal sites involved include the oropharyngeal, respiratory, gastrointestinal, and genitourinary tracts. Three common agents of bacterial meningitis, gain access to the central nervous system via the upper respiratory tract mucosa and are linked to nonsecretor status (Blackwell et al., 1986a; 1986b). An association between the presence of the O blood group and cholera susceptibility has been demonstrated in multiple studies (Glass et al., 1985; Swerdlow et al., 1994). In a Senegalese population, women who were exposed to HIV-1 positive heterosexual partners appeared to be at increased risk of infection if they were secretors, suggesting that the presence of ABH antigens in vaginal secretions increased the risk of HIV-1 transmission (Ali et al., 2000). The association of blood group A with malaria was recently described (Fischer and Boone, 1998), providing an apparent link between an erythrocyte antigen and intraerythrocytic infection by *Plasmodium falciparum*.

A third fucosyltransferase gene at locus 19q13.3 (i.e., FUT 3) determines the expression of Lewis antigen. Although the results have been debated, studies have linked Lewis antigen status to *Helicobacter pylori* infection in the gastric antrum (Boren et al., 1993) and Gram negative urinary tract infections. Expression of particular Lewis antigens by gastric epithelial cells may enhance colonization and infection by *H. pylori*.

DUFFY ANTIGEN RECEPTOR FOR CHEMOKINES (DARC)

Chromosome 1q22–23 includes the loci encoding the glycoprotein duffy antigen receptor for chemokines (DARC). This antigen has had several other names in the literature, including Duffy antigen, FY antigen, and glycoprotein D (GPD). DARC binds IL-8 (interleukin 8), MGSA (melanoma growth stimulatory factor), RANTES (regulated upon activation, normally T-cell expressed and secreted), and MCP-1 (monocyte chemotactic peptide 1) (Horuk et al., 1993). Vascular endothelial cell expression of DARC may underly its primary chemokine receptor function (Peiper et al., 1995).

DARC was first described in a patient named Duffy with alloantibodies against this glycoprotein (Cutbush et al., 1950). Subsequently it was discovered that three common alleles exist in USA populations, i.e., FY*A, FY*B, and FY*O (also known as Duffy null or FY*B^ES). These co-dominant alleles lead to four serologic red blood cell phenotypes i.e. Fy (a+b–), Fy (a–b+), Fy (a+b+) and Fy (a–b–). The Fy (a–b–) phenotype, which is genotypically homozygous for the FY*O allele, is common in African-Americans and West Africans (Pogo and Chaudhuri, 2000). The coding sequence for FY*B and FY*O is identical (Chaudhuri et al., 1995). A single point mutation in the FY*B 5′UTR leads to disruption of the GATA binding site for erythroid transcription factor

(Tournamille et al., 1995). Hence, FY*O is the "erythroid silent" allele (FY*B^ES) but is present in a typical distribution on non-erythroid cells.

Plasmodium vivax, the second most common cause of human malaria, is incapable of establishing infection in individuals homozygous for FY*O (Miller et al., 1976). Thus, the FY*O allele is an example of a human polymorphism that prevents a specific microbial infection. In a remarkable demonstration of the bi-directional selective pressure in human-microbial populations, the region of West Africa where FY*O predominates is free of *P. vivax* infection, thereby making this region unique within its latitude (Hadley and Peiper, 1997).

P^K SYNTHASE

Erythrocyte P antigens have been characterized by serologic studies to yield at least five surface antigenic variants. P antigens are present in multiple cell types, including lymphocytes in which the P antigen comprises part of the CD77 molecule (Spitalnik and Spitalnik, 1995). The P null (or p) phenotype is quite rare in the general population. However, in northern Sweden there is a carrier rate of up to 2% for the null phenotype in some population groups (Nordstrom and Cedergren, 1989). Persons who are homozygous for a point mutation in the P^K synthase gene in chromosome 22q13.2 are phenotypically P null (Steffensen et al., 2000). These individuals lack active P^K synthase, the specific galactosyltransferase activity required to convert lactosylceramide to globotriaosylceramide (Steffensen et al., 2000).

Parvovirus B19 is a ubiquitous human pathogen, infecting most individuals around the world with a seroprevalence of up to 90% in some adult populations (Cohen and Buckley, 1988). It causes a range of diseases including erythema infectiosum, hydrops fetalis and transient aplastic anemia (Brown and Young, 1997). Since P antigen is the erythrocyte receptor for human parvovirus B19, P null individuals are uniquely resistant to parvovirus B19 infection (Brown et al., 1994). However, this rare phenotype does not appear to afford a significant selective advantage and it is believed that the elevated P null frequencies in northern Sweden result from founder effect and genetic drift (Cedergren, 1973).

CYSTIC FIBROSIS TRANSMEMBRANE CONDUCTANCE REGULATOR (CFTR)

The cystic fibrosis transmembrane conductance regulator (CFTR) functions as a cytoplasmic membrane chloride channel and ion transport regulatory protein. The CFTR gene has been localized in chromosome 7q31. Cystic fibrosis (CF) is an autosomal recessive disease associated with inheritance of mutant CFTR in either homogyzous or compound heterozygote fashion (see Chap. 55).

CFTR mutations result in defects in the internalization and clearing of *Pseudomonas aeruginosa* in the respiratory tract. In the absence of normal clearing by the respiratory epithelial cells, *Pseudomonas aeruginosa* infection occurs in 75–90% of patients with cystic fibrosis (CF). Notably, *Pseudomonas* strains in the respiratory tract of CF patients adapt to this host alteration by transitioning from isolates with smooth lipopolysaccharide (LPS) and no extracellular mucoid exopolysaccharide to isolates with rough LPS and mucoid hyperexpression. The microbial advantage gained by this adaptation has not been fully elucidated (Pier, 2000). Wild type CFTR also serves as a receptor for *Salmonella typhi* on gastrointestinal epithelial cells (Pier et al., 1998). Mutant CFTR results in diminished translocation of *S. typhi* across the mucosal barrier; this diminished invasiveness of *Salmonella* is postulated to represent the heterozygous advantage of the carrier state, which allowed the carrier frequency of mutated CFTR to reach 4% in some Caucasian populations. A recent study also suggested that cases of chronic sinusitis may be associated with mutations in the CFTR gene (Wang et al., 2000).

INTERFERON GAMMA RECEPTOR (IFNγR)

The interferon gamma receptor (IFNγR) is expressed in all nucleated cells as a tetramer composed of two IFNγR1 subunits and two IFNγR2 subunits (Dorman and Holland, 2000). IFNγR1 maps to 6q23–24 and IFNγR2 maps to 21q22.1–22.2.

Mutations associated with *Salmonella* and mycobacterial infections have been reported in both subunits, although IFNγR1 mutations appear to be more common. Three cases with IFNγR2 were associated with three different homozygous mutations. A total of 34 cases of IFNγR1 have been reported, 15 of which involved individuals with homozygous mutations. The remaining 19 cases however are attributed to a mutational hotspot leading to a single mutant allele and resulting in recurrent infections with a dominant inheritance pattern (Jouanguy et al., 1999).

INTERLEUKIN 12 RECEPTOR, BETA-1 (IL12Rβ1)

The cell surface receptor for interleukin 12 (IL12) is a heterodimer composed of beta 1 (β1) and beta 2 (β2) chains. The β1 receptor is encoded at chromosome 19p13.1, and the β2 gene is in 1p31.2. Co-expression of both functional subunits is required for IL12 binding.

Homozygous mutations in the IL12Rβ1 gene have been associated with *Salmonella* and *Mycobacterium* infections in seven published cases (Altare et al., 1998a; de Jong et al., 1998). Six different mutations were demonstrated in the IL12Rβ1 gene of six different patients (Dorman and Holland, 2000). One child who died at eight years of age without sequence analysis was presumed homozygous for the same mutation as his brother. The six patients included in the sequence analysis had intermittent infections but were apparently free of adverse consequences. (Altare et al., 1998b).

CHEMOKINE RECEPTOR 5 (CCR5)

Chemokine receptor 5 (CCR5) serves as a natural receptor for β-chemokines including RANTES, MIP1-α, and MIP1-β. CCR5 also acts as a viral coreceptor for macrophage tropic (M-tropic) strains of HIV-1 (Deng et al., 1996; Dragic et al., 1996). This receptor is encoded in 3p21 and its gene product is present on the cell surface.

Intragenic deletions in the chemokine coreceptor 5 (CCR5) gene may explain why multiply exposed individuals may be resistant to HIV-1 infection, and a subset of HIV-infected persons may progress slowly to AIDS and death, relative to the average infected individual. A 32 base pair deletion (nucleotides 794 to 825) in the CCR5 gene (CCR5-Δ 32) (Dean et al., 1996) confers resistance to HIV-1 infection in the homozygous state (Liu et al., 1996) and slower progression to AIDS in the heterozygous state (Samson et al., 1996). Meta-analysis revealed a consistently lower serum viral load associated with the presence of the CCR5-Δ 32 mutation (Ionnidis et al., 1998). In one study of 334 men in Amsterdam, wild type CCR5 was associated with an increased relative risk for HIV-1 disease progression (by a factor of 2.5) compared to heterozygous CCR5-Δ 32 (de Roda Husman et al., 1997).

A survey involving 4166 individuals suggested that CCR5-Δ 32 was absent in African, American Indian, and East Asian populations while present in 0–14% of Eurasian groups. Stephens and colleagues (1998) estimated that the CCR5-Δ 32 mutation arose approximately 700 years ago (range 275–1875). It has been suggested that a strong positive selective pressure, such as an infection via the CCR5 coreceptor, drove a recently increased gene frequency. Since HIV-1 is estimated to have infected human populations during the last 70 years (Korber et al., 2000), CCR5-Δ 32 is postulated to provide protection against at least one other as yet unidentified microbe.

Two other protective polymorphisms and one deleterious polymorphism have been associated with CCR5 and HIV-1 infection. Homozygous individuals with a point mutation at position −502 relative to the transcription initiation site had delayed onset (3.8 years) of AIDS when compared to individuals with wild type CCR5 (McDermott et al., 1998). This variant was very common (43–68%) compared to either CCR5-Δ 32 or to the third protective variant, known as the m303 mutation. While m303 occurred in less than 2% of individuals in the surveyed population, it was discovered in a multiply exposed HIV-1-negative individual. The compound heterozygous state with m303 and CCR5-Δ 32 in one patient conferred complete in vitro resistance to HIV-1 (Quillent et al., 1998). In contrast, Martin and colleagues (1998) have attributed rapid HIV-1 disease progression (i.e., development of AIDS in less than or equal to 3.5 years) to homozygosity for a polymorphism in the CCR5 promoter region (CCR5P1). Homozygosity of CCR5P1 occurred in 12.7% of Caucasian Americans and 6.7% of African Americans.

CHEMOKINE RECEPTOR 2 (CCR2)

Chemokine receptor 2 (CCR2) is encoded at gene locus 3p21, in close proximity to CCR5. A point mutation causing the neutral substitution of isoleucine for valine (V641) has been studied as a potential AIDS susceptibility polymorphism. CCR2-V641 was present in 10% of Caucasian Americans, 15% of African Americans, 17% of Hispanic Americans and 25% of Asian Americans in one large study (Smith et al., 1997). Wild type CCR2 is in strong linkage disequilibrium with CCR5-Δ 32, which facilitates examination of distinct effects of each two polymorphism (Smith et al., 1997). CCR2-V641 is not associated with differences in HIV infectivity, but it is associated with a 2–4 year delay in the onset of AIDS in HIV infected persons (Smith et al., 1997).

CCR2 is unlikely to be a primary cellular coreceptor for HIV-1 when compared to CCR5 and CXCR4. Evidence suggests that the CCR2-V641 mutation could inhibit HIV-1 indirectly, through the desensitization of CCR5 and CXCR4 receptors to their normal ligand responses (Lee et al., 1998). However, the worldwide presence of exceptionally strong linkage disequilibrium between CCR2-V641 and a CCR5 promoter polymorphism (CCR5–59635T), and the fact that V641 encodes a neutral amino acid change in a transmembrane domain, has led to speculation that CCR2-V641 could be a marker for a different biologically significant mutation (Carrington et al., 1999b).

CHEMOKINE RECEPTOR CX₃CR1

The chemokine receptor CX_3CR1 is a leukocyte chemotactic and adhesion receptor for the chemokine fractalkine (Bazan et al., 1997). The gene for this receptor lies in the short arm of chromosome 3 (3p21). In addition to being a receptor for fractalkine, this cell surface molecule also acts as a co-receptor for HIV-1. HIV-1 infected patients homozygous for a polymorphic allele including two point mutations (V2491 and T280M) were statistically more likely to have rapid progression of disease relative to those with the wild type gene (Faure et al., 2000). Although this allele had a frequency of 13.5% in the uninfected French population studied, and ranged from 12.6% to 19.8% in three infected cohorts examined, the polymorphism was not detected in the non-Caucasian populations tested (Faure et al., 2000).

TOLL LIKE RECEPTORS (TLR)

At least nine different human toll like receptors (TLRs) have been described and they are homologous with the *Drosophila* toll protein (Du et al., 2000). These receptors appear to function as endotoxin sensors. Two missense mutations in *TLR4* have been associated with a blunted response to inhaled bacterial lipopolysaccharide (LPS), and these mutations may affect sensitivity to bacterial antigens in the environment (Arbour et al., 2000). In another study, polymorphisms in *TLR2* were examined and a missense mutation was found in 9% of patients with staphylococcal sepsis (Arg 753Gln), compared to less than 3% of normal controls (Lorenz et al., 2000). The emerging data since the description of the first human TLR in 1997 suggest that these receptors are important in the human response to microbial infection (Medzhitov et al., 1997).

Intracellular proteins

ALPHA HEMOGLOBIN (αHB)

Four functional alpha hemoglobin (αHgb) genes are present per diploid erythroblast, with two tandem αHgb genes at each 16p 13.3 locus. The protein product αHgb combines with βHgb to form the functional $\alpha_2\beta_2$ tetramer of adult hemoglobin. "thalassemia" is used to describe inherited defects in globin synthesis; α-thalassemia is secondary to αHgb mutations (see Ch. 68). Greater than thirty different α-thalassemia inducing mutations exist (Krawczak et al., 2000). Persons with α-thalassemia trait have three functional genes and an essentially normal hematologic phenotype, while persons with a mild hypochromic anemia generally have two functional copies.

Before the mid-1980s, it was difficult to dissect the interactions of α-thalassemia and infection from the effects of the β-hemoglobinopathies. Flint and colleagues studied human populations in the Southwest Pacific nations of Papua New Guinea and Melanesia, who have α-thalassemia and no β-thalassemia or sickle cell disease. This study suggested that the level of malaria endemicity correlated with the gene frequency of α-thalassemia, and argued that a selective pressure was being exerted by malaria in favor of α-thalassemia (Flint et al., 1986). Further study has now demonstrated that the α-thalassemia trait is associated with a reduced risk of severe malaria (0.66) with an even greater reduced risk associated with α-thalassemia itself (0.40) (Allen et al., 1997). There was also a reduced risk for other serious infections associated with α-thalassemia and trait in this study, although the reason for this association is not apparent (Allen et al., 1997).

BETA HEMOGLOBIN (βHgB)

Two functional genes encode wild type beta hemoglobin [βHgb], one at each 11p15 locus. This difference in gene copy number distinguishes the hemoglobinopathies associated with βHgb from the α-hemoglobinopathies which stem from mutations in any of the four functional αHgb loci. In addition to β-thalassemias associated with defects in βHgb synthesis, there are important structural β-hemaglobinopathies (Clarke and Higgins, 2000).

Sickle hemoglobin (HgbS) is encoded by a βHgb allele with a point mutation on the sixth codon. In a series of scientific discoveries spanning 1949 to 1977, this structural hemoglobinopathy was first described as "a molecular disease" based on hemoglobin electrophoresis differences (Pauling et al., 1949), then as a single amino acid substitution linked disease (Ingram, 1957), and finally as a single nucleotide polymorphism (SNP)-linked disease (Marotta et al., 1977). The A to T change which codes for the known glutamic acid to valine substitution, constituted the first host microbial resistance trait and the first human disease linked to a SNP.

In countries with endemic malaria, HgbS demonstrates the principle of balanced polymorphism since the heterozygous state (i.e., sickle cell trait) is associated with a reduced risk of severe malaria. Either homozygous state confers a disadvantage: HgbS/HgbS causing sickle cell anemia and βHgb/βHgb risking severe morbidity or even mortality due to malaria. Heterozygous advantage may be responsible for

the success of the five different HgbS alleles occurring as separate mutational events in five different human populations (Pagnier et al., 1984; Zago et al., 2000). In addition to its multiple clinical manifestations, sickle cell anemia is associated with an increased susceptibility to a number of infectious complications including parvovirus-induced aplastic crisis, and bacterial infections with encapsulated bacterial pathogens such as *Streptococcus*, *Haemophilus*, and *Salmonella* organisms (Overturf, 1999).

Unlike HgbS, β-thalassemia is associated with a variety of genetic alterations including SNPs, substitutions, deletions, insertions, and rearrangements. The shared features of these various mutations are quantitative defects in βHgb synthesis. The heterogeneous group of mutations which lead to β-thalassemia occur in a manner which suggests that β thalassemia affords protection against malaria (Flint et al., 1993).

VITAMIN D RECEPTOR (VDR)

The vitamin D receptor (VDR) is an intracellular protein which is believed to act as a transcriptional regulatory factor (Haussler et al., 1988). This receptor binds to 1,25 dihydroxyvitamin D3. The VDR gene maps to 12q12-q14, and contains a total of 11 exons including eight protein coding exons. Along with their role in calcium metabolism, vitamin D and VDR are also involved in the immunoregulatory functions of monocytes and activated lymphocytes.

The VDR allele containing a T to C substitution at codon 352 may confer susceptibility to several important infectious diseases. Although this "silent" polymorphism does not alter the protein's amino acid sequence, it is associated with increased mRNA quantities (Morrison et al., 1994). Mutant alleles containing the C substitution are labeled as "t" genotype, while "T" genotype represents the wild type allele. Homozygotes for "t" (i.e., tt) appear to have decreased risk for chronic hepatitis B, and decreased active tuberculosis (Bellamy et al., 1999; Wilkinson et al., 2000). Heterozygotes for Tt appear less likely to develop leprosy (Roy et al., 1999). Whether this single nucleotide polymorphism is causally related or simply linked to the causative mutation is not yet fully elucidated (Morrison et al, 1994).

GLUCOSE-6-PHOSPHATE DEHYDROGENASE (G6PD)

The gene encoding glucose-6-phosphate dehydrogenase (G6PD) is located in chromosome Xq28. This enzyme is believed to be essential to cellular function, and quantitative variations in enzyme function appear to be clinically significant in mature erythrocytes. The phenomenon of X-linked inactivation in females was uncovered in the study of G6PD-deficiency; this results in heterozygous females having two cellular populations: G6PD-deficient and G6PD-nondeficient cells (Gartler and Riggs, 1983). At least 95 different mutations have been associated with G6PD deficiency (Krawczak et al., 2000), and these sequence changes account for the observed range of enzyme activities (from mild to severe deficiency). The known mutations are almost entirely point mutations, although four small in-frame deletions (of 3 or 6 base pairs) have been reported. It appears that a mutation which would result in a completely non-functional enzyme would be lethal (Pandolfi et al., 1995).

In the 1960s when the increased population prevalence of G6PD-deficiency in malarious zones was noted, it was suggested that like sickle cell disease and thalassemia, G6PD-deficiency likely offers a survival advantage in malaria. Epidemiologic support for his hypothesis in 1995 suggested that both female heterozygotes and male hemizygotes have a 46–58% reduced risk for severe malaria (Ruwende et al., 1995). While many mechanisms of selective advantage have been proposed, recent data suggests that early phagocytosis of *Plasmodium falciparum*-infected erythrocytes occurs. Phagocytosis is induced by parasite-associated erythrocyte membrane damage more readily in G6PD-deficient cells (Cappadoro et al., 1998).

A selective disadvantage to of G6PD deficiency has been proposed to explain the lack of allelic fixation in sub-Saharan African populations (Ruwende et al., 1995). The disadvantage is not clear, but an increased incidence of bacterial sepsis in neonates may be a contributing factor (Abu-Osba et al., 1989).

GALACTOSE-1-PHOSPHATE URIDYLTRANSFERASE (GALT)

The galactose-1-phosphate uridyltransferase (GALT) gene is located in chromosome 9 (9p13). GALT deficiency represents an autosomal recessive inborn error of metabolism that has been associated with greater than 100 different mutant genotypes (Krawczak et al., 2000). This metabolic disorder is discussed in detail in Chapter 95, but warrants mention here due to the association of neonatal gram negative sepsis with this disorder (Levy et al., 1977). Although a comprehensive understanding of the pathogenesis of this bacteremic state is not available, impaired neutrophil function in neonates attributed to increased galactose is likely to be a significant contributing factor (Kobayashi et al., 1983).

NATURAL RESISTANCE ASSOCIATED MICROPHAGE PROTEIN 1 [NRAMP 1]

NRAMP 1 is a human macrophage membrane protein which is recruited to the phagosomal membrane after phagocytosis, and apparently acts as a divalent cation transporter (Jabado et al., 2000). The human gene and its protein product were sought following identification of the murine homologue in which a point mutation was associated with increased susceptibility to intracellular parasites (Vidal et al., 1993). *NRAMP 1* is located in chromosome 2q35 (Cellier et al., 1994) and is expressed exclusively in immune phagocytes (Canonne-Hergaux et al., 1999).

Eleven NRAMP 1 polymorphisms have been identified (Gao et al., 2000), including four mutations that have been associated with increased susceptibility to active tuberculosis (Bellamy et al., 1998; Gao et al., 2000; Ryu et al., 2000). Data suggests that NRAMP 1 plays a role in the development of lepromatous leprosy (Abel et al., 1998) and HIV-1 infection (Marquet et al., 1999), as well as idiopathic conditions such as sarcoidosis (Maliarik et al., 2000) and autoimmune diseases (Searle and Blackwell, 1999).

Extracellular proteins

Relative levels of expression or activity of secreted immunoactive proteins have been associated with enhanced susceptibility to infection and associated complications. Polymorphisms in cytokine genes will be emphasized since multiple mutations affecting relative levels of cytokine expression have been associated with various infectious diseases. Cytokine genes have been mapped to several different chromosomes in the human genome. Relative imbalances of pro-inflammatory and immunomodulatory cytokines in the immune network may play prominent roles in host susceptibility to infection and disease outcome in vivo (Mosmann and Coffman, 1989; Kelso, 1998). Interestingly, increased levels of both pro-inflammatory or immunomodulatory cytokines appear to increase susceptibility to severe or persistent infections. Pro-inflammatory cytokines such as interleukin-1 (IL-1) or tumor necrosis factor (TNF) are important effector molecules of the immune response but also contribute to disease pathogenesis when expressed at high levels during infection. Elevated levels of immunomodulatory cytokines such as interleukin-4 (IL-4) or interleukin-10 (IL-10) may contribute to the pathogenesis of acute and chronic infections. Relative predispositions for the development of autoimmune or infectious disease may depend on relative levels of pro-inflammatory or immunomodulatory cytokines.

INTERLEUKIN-1

Pro-inflammatory cytokines such as IL-1 or TNF drive T-helper lymphocyte 1 (Th1) responses and stimulate the synthesis of T cell proliferative cytokines such as interleukin-2 (IL-2) (Mosmann and Coffman, 1989). Interleukin-1 is synthesized as a precursor and proteolytic cleavage is required for synthesis of functional IL-1β (Cerretti et al., 1992). Genetic determinants in virulent pathogens may alter production of active IL-1β. Virulent clones of *Streptococcus pyogenes* encode a cysteine protease that cleaves human IL-1, promoting formation of active IL-1β (Kapur et al., 1993). Polymorphisms in the human IL-1 gene have been associated with altered levels of expression of functional IL-1 in response to infectious agents. Induction of IL-1β mRNA by *M. tuberculosis* was elevated in subjects with the IL-1β (+3953) A1-haplotype (Wilkinson et al., 1999). This pro-inflammatory haplotype, when combined with a particular haplotype associated with reduced levels of interleukin-1 receptor antagonist (IL-1Ra), was more common in patients with pleural tuberculosis. Promoter polymorphisms that enhance production of functional IL-1β have also been associated with hypochlorhydria induced by gastric infection with *Helicobacter pylori* and the associated development of gastric carcinoma (El-Omar et al., 2000).

TUMOR NECROSIS FACTOR

TNF-α is a potent pro-inflammatory cytokine produced by monocytes/macrophages and T and B lymphocytes (Vassalli, 1992). The TNFA and TNFB genes lie in the class III region of the human MHC complex in chromosome 6, approximately 250 kilobases centromeric of the HLA-B locus and 850 kilobases telomeric of HLA-DR. Polymorphisms within TNF genes may contribute to the association of MHC alleles with specific autoimmune and infectious diseases. Specific TNFA promoter polymorphisms have been associated with altered expression of TNFα. Substitutions (G-A) at either positions −308 or −238 have been characterized as rare alleles in the human TNFA promoter region. The −308 allele (*TNF2*) is part of an extended MHC haplotype and studies have indicated that carriage of *TNF2* is associated with worse outcomes in cerebral malaria (McGuire et al., 1994) and leishmaniasis (Cabrera et al., 1995). The G-A substitution at position −308 (TNF2) allele results in a much stronger transcriptional activator and increased levels of TNFα expression (Wilson et al., 1997). Presumably, increased levels of TNFα may contribute to disease severity and morbidity in systemic infections. Increased levels of plasma TNFα were present in Gambian children with cerebral malaria and the highest TNFα levels were noted in fatal cases (Kwiatkowski et al., 1990). Excessive levels of the potent cytokine TNFα may predispose to greater disease morbidity and fatal outcome. Gambian children homozygous for the *TNF2* allele were at significantly increased risk for death or severe neurologic sequelae due to cerebral malaria (McGuire et al., 1994). In contrast to cerebral malaria, severe malarial anemia was associated with the TNF −238A allele (*TNFA-A*) after stratification for HLA haplotype (McGuire et al., 1999). The *TNF2* allele was also associated with development of mucocutaneous leishmaniasis (Cabrera et al., 1995) and lepromatous leprosy (Roy et al., 1997).

Both the TNFA and TNFB loci have been implicated in the development of severe sepsis due to multiple infectious agents. *TNF2*, containing a TNFα promoter polymorphism (Mira et al., 1999), and *TNFB2*, with an intronic substitution in the TNFβ gene (Stuber et al., 1996; Majetschak et al., 1999), have been independently associated with severe sepsis. Interestingly, both the *TNF2* and *TNFB2* alleles are associated with elevated TNFα levels in peripheral blood (Majetschak et al., 1999; Mira et al., 1999). The *TNF2* allele has also been independently associated with the development of autoimmune diseases such as ankylosing spondylitis (McGarry et al., 1999). Adequate expression of TNFα is likely essential for surmounting infectious challenges, but overexpression of this potent pro-inflammatory agent may result in deleterious consequences for the host. The greater than expected prevalence of *TNF2* in western Africa suggests a protective role for *TNF2* during exposure to infectious or environmental challenges (McGuire et al., 1994). Family studies of patients with fatal meningococcal disease indicate that increased levels of TNFα may be important in acute infection as reduced TNFα levels were associated with fatal outcomes (Westendorp et al., 1997b).

INTERLEUKIN-10

Immunomodulatory cytokines such as IL-4, IL-10, and transforming growth factor-β (TGF-β) counteract effects of pro-inflammatory cytokines such as IL-1 and TNF in the cytokine network. The human IL-10 gene has been mapped to chromosome 1q31–1q32 and its 5′ regulatory region has been characterized (Eskdale et al., 1997). Multiple cytokine response elements have been mapped and represent target sites for TNF, interferon-gamma (IFN-γ), and IL-6 (Eskdale et al., 1997) upstream of the IL-10 coding sequence.

Lipopolysaccharides (LPS) of gram-negative bacteria (Hessle et al., 2000) and viral pathogens such as Epstein-Barr virus (EBV) (Andersson, 1996) induce expression of human IL-10 from mononuclear cells. Microbial pathogens may induce the expression of human cytokines and specific polymorphisms in regulatory sequences may influence the course of infection with specific pathogens.

Elevated levels of IL-10 production appear to increase susceptibility to chronic infectious diseases, whereas diminished levels of IL-10 may increase the risk of autoimmune disease. Family studies previously linked elevated systemic IL-10 levels with fatal outcome due to meningococcal infection (Westendrop et al., 1997a). IL-10 promoter polymorphisms affecting levels of gene expression have been associated with human autoimmune and infectious diseases. Nucleotide substitution polymorphisms at positions −854 and −627 were identified in a population of healthy individuals but seem to lack effects on IL-10 expression (Eskdale et al., 1997). Other nucleotide substitutions in the promoter region of human IL-10 at positions −592, −819, and −1082 have been identified and yield different IL-10 haplotypes. These haplotypes GCC, ACC, and ATA have been linked with high, intermediate, and low IL-10 production, respectively (Edwards-Smith et al., 1999). The GCC haplotype, linked with high levels of IL-10, has been associated with poor treatment response to interferon-α (IFN-α) in patients with chronic hepatitis C virus (HCV) infection (Edwards-Smith et al., 1999). Consistent with these findings, elevated levels of serum IL-10 were observed in patients with chronic HCV infection (Cacciarelli et al., 1996; Piazzolla et al., 2000) and Epstein-Barr virus (EBV) (Andersson, 1996) infections. One study has suggested that the −1082 allele 1 associated with elevated IL-10 production protects against EBV infection although promoter haplotypes were not studied (Helminen et al., 1999). In contrast, the ATA IL-10 promoter haplotype associated with low IL-10 production has been linked with autoimmune diseases such as juvenile rheumatoid arthritis (JRA) (Crawley et al., 1999) and systemic lupus erythematosus (SLE) with neuropsychiatric manifestations (Rood et al., 1999). The JRA phenotype may represent an exaggerated response to infectious agents due to relative deficiencies in immunomodulatory agents such as IL-10.

TRANSFORMING GROWTH FACTOR-β AND INTERLEUKIN-4

Transforming growth factor-β (TGF-β) and interleukin-4 (Il-4) represent potent immunomodulatory cytokines active in various organs and tissues. TGF-β knockout mice develop systemic inflammatory disease in various organs (Christ et al., 1994), indicating the ubiquitous importance of TGF-β as an important immunomodulatory agent. Multiple TGF-β gene polymorphisms have been identified in the promoter region, 5′ untranslated region, and the signal sequence (Awad et al., 1998). A signal sequence polymorphism at position +915 (codon 25) resulting in the homozygous arginine/arginine genotype has been associated with high levels of TGF-β production in stimulated lymphocytes from patients (Awad et al., 1998). Pulmonary fibrosis and HCV-associated hepatic fibrosis (Powell et al., 2000) have been linked with fibrogenic TGF-β overproduction due to the arginine/arginine signal sequence genotype. IL-4 is a pleiotropic cytokine that regulates Th2 lymphocyte subset development and IgE production (Paul and O'Hara, 1987; Mosmann and Coffman, 1989). IL-4 downregulates HIV-1 coreceptor CCR5 expression and upregulates CXCR4 expression, stimulating the phenotypic switch from non-syncytium induction (NSI) to syncytium induction (SI). An IL-4 promoter polymorphism (−589T) associated with increased expression of IL-4 has been correlated with acquisition of the SI phenotype in HIV-1-infected individuals (Nakayama et al., 2000) and its associated poor prognosis.

MANNOSE BINDING PROTEIN

Collectins are proteins secreted by the innate immune system to facilitate opsonization and phagocytosis of extracellular microbial pathogens (Holmskov, 2000). Mannose binding protein (MBP; mannose binding lectin) is a serum collectin secreted by hepatocytes, binding surface mannans on bacterial cell surfaces. MBP recruits macrophages, facilitating phagocytosis by opsonization and activates the classical complement pathway via MBP-associated serine proteases (MASPs) independent of C1. Mutations in several MBP codons affecting opsonization have been associated with severe infections (Summerfield et al., 1995) including pulmonary tuberculosis (Selvaraj et al., 1999). Severe systemic infections including septicemia were associated with homozygous codon 54 (exon 1) mutations (Summerfield et al., 1997). Codon 52 missense mutations in the MBP gene were associated with chronic hepatitis B virus (HBV) infection in Caucasian individuals (Thomas et al., 1996). As with IL-10, specific MBP promoter polymorphisms have been correlated with altered levels of MBP expression and implicated in susceptibility to infection (Crosdale et al., 2000; Juliger et al., 2000). Chinese individuals with rheumatoid arthritis (RA) had significantly reduced levels of serum MBP (Ip et al., 2000). Lower levels of serum MBP were correlated with codon 54 mutations and promoter polymorphisms associated with reduced MBP expression (Ip et al., 2000). RA patients with erosive and prominent extraarticular disease had the lowest serum MBP levels (Ip et al., 2000). Reduced MBP levels may result in exaggerated inflammatory responses due to diminished microbial clearance, contributing to chronic inflammation in RA.

CHEMOKINES

Chemokines are small proteins expressed by various cell types that chemoattract and activate immune cells and bind to transmembrane G-protein-coupled receptors (Rossi and Zlotnik, 2000; Baggiolini and Loetscher, 2000). RANTES and stromal cell-derived growth factor 1 (SDF1) represent important soluble chemokine mediators of the immune response (Schroder et al., 1994). RANTES is a C-C chemokine produced by cytotoxic CD8+ T lymphocytes with anti-HIV-1 suppressive effects. Specific promoter sequences have been characterized as LPS-responsive elements lying upstream of the murine RANTES gene (Shin et al., 1994). Although not identified to date in humans, point mutations in the LPS-response elements may abrogate the immediate-early transcriptional activation of RANTES in macrophages stimulated by the presence of LPS. Upregulation of C-C chemokine expression has been associated with allergic inflammation and atopic diseases. A proximal promoter mutation upstream of the human RANTES gene has been identified, resulting in enhanced transcriptional activation and expression of RANTES (Nickel et al., 2000). This mutant allele with an additional GATA transcription factor binding site has been associated with atopic dermatitis (Nickel et al., 2000), although a role for this mutant allele in infection remains speculative.

SDF1 is a CXC chemokine that binds exclusively to the CXC chemokine factor receptor 4 (CXCR4) and is essential for embryogenesis and lymphopoeisis (Nagasawa et al., 1996). CXCR4 acts as a coreceptor for HIV-1 (Feng et al., 1996). SDF1 protects individuals against HIV-1 infection by competing with gp120 for binding to CXCR4 and by downregulation of the receptor (Amara et al., 1997). A polymorphism in the 3′ untranslated region of the human SDF1 gene has been linked with nonprogression or delayed progression to acquired immunodeficiency syndrome (AIDS) during HIV-1 infection (Winkler et al., 1998). The homozygous state, SDF1-3′A/3′A, delayed the onset of AIDS in large study (>2800 patients), and the SDF1–3′A allele complemented CCR5 and CCR2 mutations in delaying the onset of AIDS. In contrast, Magierowska et al. (1999) observed that long-term nonprogression in HIV-1-infected individuals was associated with the combined presence of the CCR5-(del) 32 and homozygous wild type SDF1.

REFERENCES

Abel L, Sanchez FO, Oberti J et al. (1998) Susceptibility to leprosy is linked to the human NRAMP1 gene. J Infect Dis 177:133–45

Abu-Osba YK, Mallouh AA, Hann RW (1989) Incidence and causes of sepsis in glucose-6-phosphate dehydrogenase-deficient newborn infants. J Pediatr 114:748–52

Ahn SH, Han KH, Park JY et al. (2000) Association between hepatitis B virus infection and HLA-DR type in Korea. Hepatology 31:1371–3

Ali S, Niang MA, N'Doye I et al. (2000) Secretor polymorphism and human immunodeficiency virus infection in Senegalese women. J Infect Dis 181:737–9

Allen SJ, O'Donnell A, Alexander ND et al. (1997) Alpha+-Thalassemia protects children against disease caused by other infections as well as malaria. Proc Natl Acad Sci USA 94:14736–41

Altare F, Lammas D, Revy P et al. (1998a) Inherited interleukin 12 deficiency in a child with bacille Calmette-Guerin and *Salmonella enteritidis* disseminated infection. J Clin Invest 102:2035–40

Altare F, Jouanguy E, Lamhamedi S et al. (1998b) Mendelian susceptibility to mycobacterial infection in man. Curr Opin Immunol 10:413–7

Amara A, Gall SL, Schwartz O et al. (1997) HIV coreceptor downregulation as antiviral principle: SDF-1 alpha-dependent internalization of the chemokine receptor CXCR4 contributes to inhibition of HIV replication. J Exp Med 186:139–46

Andersson J (1996) Clinical and immunological considerations in Epstein-Barr virus-associated diseases. Scand J Infect Dis Suppl 100:72–82

Ando M, Hirayama K, Soda K et al. (1989) HLA-DQw3 in Japanese summer-type hypersensitivity pneumonitis induced by *Trichosporon cutaneum*. Am Rev Respir Dis 140:948–50

Apple RJ, Erlich HA, Klitz W et al. (1994) HLA DR-DQ associations with cervical carcinoma show papillomavirus-type specificity. Nat Genet 6:157–62

Arbour NC, Lorenz E, Schutte BC et al. (2000) TLR4 mutations are associated with endotoxin hyporesponsiveness in humans. Nat Genet 25:187–91

Baggiolini M, Loetscher P (2000) Chemokines in inflammation and immunity. Immunol Today 21:418–20

Bazan JF, Bacon KB, Hardiman G et al. (1997) A new class of membrane-bound chemokine with a CX3C motif. Nature 385:640–4

Bellamy R, Ruwende C, Corrah T et al. (1998) Variations in the NRAMP1 gene and susceptibility to tuberculosis in West Africans. N Engl J Med 338:640–4

Bellamy R, Ruwende C, Corrah T et al. (1999) Tuberculosis and chronic hepatitis B virus infection in Africans and variation in the vitamin D receptor gene. J Infect Dis 179:721–4

Berger SA, Young NA, Edberg SC (1989) Relationship between infectious diseases and human blood type. Eur J Clin Microbiol Infect Dis 8:681–9

Blackwell CC, Jonsdottir K, Hanson M et al. (1986a) Non-secretion of ABO antigens predisposing to infection by *Neisseria meningitidis* and *Streptococcus pneumoniae*. Lancet 2:284–5

Blackwell CC, Jonsdottir K, Hanson MF, Weir DM (1986b) Non-secretion of ABO blood group antigens predisposing to infection by *Haemophilus influenzae*. Lancet 2:687

Bodmer JG, Marsh SG, Albert ED et al. (1999) Nomenclature for factors of the HLA System, 1998. Hum Immunol 60:361–95

Boren T, Falk P, Roth KA et al. (1993) Attachment of *Helicobacter pylori* to human gastric epithelium mediated by blood group antigens. Science 262:1892–5

Brown KE, Young NS (1997) Parvovirus B19 in human disease. Annu Rev Med 48:59–67

Brown KE, Hibbs JR, Gallinella G et al. (1994) Resistance to parvovirus B19 infection due to lack of virus receptor (erythrocyte P antigen). N Engl J Med 330:1192–6

Burt RD, Vaughan TL, Nisperos B et al. (1994) A protective association between the HLA-A2 antigen and nasopharyngeal carcinoma in US Caucasians. Int J Cancer 56:465–7

Cabrera M, Shaw MA, Sharples C et al. (1995) Polymorphism in tumor necrosis factor genes associated with mucocutaneous leishmaniasis. J Exp Med 182:1259–64

Cacciarelli TV, Martinez OM, Gish RG et al. (1996) Immunoregulatory cytokines in chronic hepatitis C virus infection: pre- and posttreatment with interferon alfa. Hepatology 24:6–9

Canonne-Hergaux F, Gruenheid S, Govoni G, Gros P (1999) The NRAMP 1 protein and its role in resistance to infection and macrophage function. Proc Assoc Am Physicians 111:283–9

Cappadoro M, Giribaldi G, O'Brien E et al. (1998) Early phagocytosis of glucose-6-phosphate dehydrogenase (G6PD)—deficient erythrocytes parasitized by *Plasmodium falciparum* may explain malaria protection in G6PD deficiency. Blood 92:2527–34

Carrington M, Nelson GW, Martin MP et al. (1999a) HLA and HIV-1: heterozygote advantage and B*35-Cw*04 disadvantage. Science 283:1748–52

Carrington M, Dean M, Martin MP and O'Brien SJ (1999b) Genetics of HIV-1 infection: Chemokine receptor CCR5 polymorphism and its consequences. Hum Mol Genet 8:1939–45

Carter R, Schofield L, Mendis K (1992) HLA Effects in Malaria: Increased parasite-killing immunity or reduced immunopathology. Parasitology Today 8:41–42

Cedergren B (1973) Population studies in northern Sweden. IV. Frequency of the blood type p. Hereditas 73:27–30

Cellier M, Govoni G, Vidal S et al. (1994) Human natural resistance-associated macrophage protein: cDNA cloning, chromosomal mapping, genomic organization, and tissue-specific expression. J Exp Med 180:1741–52

Cerretti DP, Kozlosky CJ, Mosley B et al. (1992) Molecular cloning of the interleukin-1 beta converting enzyme. Science 256:97–100

Chaudhuri A, Polyakova J, Zbrzezna V, Pogo AO (1995) The coding sequence of Duffy blood group gene in humans and simians: Restriction fragment length polymorphism, antibody and malarial parasite specificities, and expression in nonerythroid tissues in Duffy-negative individuals. Blood 85:615–21

Christ M, McCartney-Francis NL, Kulkarni AB et al. (1994) Immune dysregulation in TGF-beta 1-deficient mice. J Immunol 153:1936–46

Clarke GM, Higgins TN (2000) Laboratory investigation of hemoglobinopathies and thalassemias: Review and update. Clin Chem 46:1284–90

Cohen BJ, Buckley MM (1988) The prevalence of antibody to human Parvovirus B19 in England and Wales. J Med Microbiol 25:151–3

Cohen CR, Sinei SS, Bukusi EA et al. (2000) Human leukocyte antigen class II DQ alleles associated with *Chlamydia trachomatis* tubal infertility. Obstet Gynecol 95:72–7

Conway DJ, Holland MJ, Campbell AE et al. (1996) HLA class I and II polymorphisms and trachomatous scarring in a *Chlamydia trachomatis*-endemic population. J Infect Dis 174:643–6

Crawley E, Kay R, Sillibourne J et al. (1999) Polymorphic haplotypes of the interleukin-10 5′ flanking region determine variable interleukin-10 transcription and are associated with particular phenotypes of juvenile rheumatoid arthritis. Arthritis Rheum 42:1101–8

Crosdale DJ, Ollier WE, Thomson W et al. (2000) Mannose binding lectin (MBL) genotype distributions with relation to serum levels in UK Caucasoids. Eur J Immunogenet 27:111–7

Cutbush M, Mollison PL, Parkin DM (1950) A new human blood group. Nature 165:188

de Jong R, Altare F, Haagen IA et al. (1998) Severe mycobacterial and *Salmonella* infections in interleukin-12 receptor-deficient patients. Science 280:1435–8

de Roda Husman AM, Koot M, Cornelissen M et al. (1997) Association between CCR5 genotype and the clinical course of HIV-1 infection. Ann Intern Med 127:882–90

Dean M, Carrington M, Winkler C et al. (1996) Genetic restriction of HIV-1 infection and progression to AIDS by a deletion allele of the CKR5 structural gene. Hemophilia Growth and Development Study, Multicenter AIDS Cohort Study, Multicenter Hemophilia Cohort Study, San Francisco City Cohort, ALIVE Study. Science 273:1856–62

Deng H, Liu R, Ellmeier W et al. (1996) Identification of a major co-receptor for primary isolates of HIV-1. Nature 381:661–6

Du X, Poltorak A, Wei Y, Beutler B (2000) Three novel mammalian toll-like receptors: Gene structure, expression, and evolution. Eur Cytokine Netw 11:362–71

Dragic T, Litwin V, Allaway GP et al. (1996) HIV-1 entry into CD4+ cells is mediated by the chemokine receptor CC-CKR-5. Nature 381:667–73

Edwards-Smith CJ, Jonsson JR, Purdie DM et al. (1999) Interleukin-10 promoter polymorphism predicts initial response of chronic hepatitis C to interferon alfa. Hepatology 30:526–30

Eiermann TH, Bettens F, Tiberghien P et al. (1998) HLA and alveolar echinococcosis. Tissue Antigens 52:124–9

el-Ganayni GA, Attia RA, Motawea SM (1994) The relation between ABO blood groups, HLA typing and giardiasis in children. J Egypt Soc Parasitol 24:407–12

El-Omar EM, Carrington M, Chow WH et al. (2000) Interleukin-1 polymorphisms associated with increased risk of gastric cancer. Nature 404:398–402

Eskdale J, Kube D, Tesch H, Gallagher G (1997) Mapping of the human IL10 gene and further characterization of the 5′ flanking sequence. Immunogenetics 46:120–8

Faure S, Meyer L, Costagliola D et al. (2000) Rapid progression to AIDS in HIV+ individuals with a structural variant of the chemokine receptor CX3CR1. Science 287:2274–7

Feng Y, Broder CC, Kennedy PE, Berger EA (1996) HIV-1 entry cofactor: Functional cDNA cloning of a seven-transmembrane, G protein-coupled receptor. Science 272:872–7

Fischer PR, Boone P (1998) Short report: Severe malaria associated with blood group. Am J Trop Med Hyg 58:122–3

Flint J, Hill AV, Bowden DK et al. (1986) High frequencies of alpha-thalassaemia are the result of natural selection by malaria. Nature 321:744–50

Flint J, Harding RM, Clegg JB, Boyce AJ (1993) Why are some genetic diseases common? Distinguishing selection from other processes by molecular analysis of globin gene variants. Hum Genet 91:91–117

Fraser JR, Tait B, Aaskov JG, Cunningham AL (1980) Possible genetic determinants in epidemic polyarthritis caused by Ross River virus infection. Aust N Z J Med 10:597–603

Gao PS, Fujishima S, Mao XQ et al. (2000) Genetic variants of NRAMP1 and active tuberculosis in Japanese populations. International Tuberculosis Genetics Team. Clin Genet 58:74–6

Gartler SM, Riggs AD (1983) Mammalian X-chromosome inactivation. Annu Rev Genet 17:155–90

Gilbert SC, Plebanski M, Gupta S et al. (1998) Association of malaria parasite population structure, HLA, and immunological antagonism. Science 279:1173–7

Glass RI, Holmgren J, Haley CE et al. (1985) Predisposition for cholera of individuals with O blood group. Possible evolutionary significance. Am J Epidemiol 121:791–6

Goldfeld AE, Delgado JC, Thim S et al. (1998) Association of an HLA-DQ allele with clinical tuberculosis. JAMA 279:226–8

Gregoire L, Lawrence WD, Kukuruga D et al. (1994) Association between HLA-DQB1 alleles and risk for cervical cancer in African-American women. Int J Cancer 57:504–7

Gross DM, Forsthuber T, Tary-Lehmann M et al. (1998) Identification of LFA-1 as a candidate autoantigen in treatment-resistant Lyme arthritis. Science 281:703–6

Haan KM, Kwok WW, Longnecker R, Speck P (2000) Epstein-Barr virus entry utilizing HLA-DP or HLA-DQ as a coreceptor. J Virol 74:2451–4

Hadley TJ, Peiper SC (1997) From malaria to chemokine receptor: The emerging physiologic role of the Duffy blood group antigen. Blood 89:3077–91

Haldane JBS (1949) Disease and evolution. La Ricerca Scientifica 19 (Suppl.):68

Haldane JBS (1957) Natural selection in man. Acta genet. 6:321–332

Haussler MR, Mangelsdorf DJ, Komm BS et al. (1988) Molecular biology of the vitamin D hormone. Recent Prog Horm Res 44:263–305

Helminen M, Lahdenpohja N, Hurme M (1999) Polymorphism of the interleukin-10 gene is associated with susceptibility to Epstein-Barr virus infection. J Infect Dis 180:496–9

Hessle C, Andersson B, Wold AE (2000) Gram-positive bacteria are potent inducers of monocytic interleukin-12 (IL-12) while gram-negative bacteria preferentially stimulate IL-10 production. Infect Immun 68:3581–6

Hill AV, Allsopp CE, Kwiatkowski D et al. (1991) Common West African HLA antigens are associated with protection from severe malaria. Nature 352:595–600

Hirayama K, Chen H, Kikuchi M et al. (1999) HLA-DR-DQ alleles and HLA-DP alleles are independently associated with susceptibility to different stages of post-schistosomal hepatic fibrosis in the Chinese population. Tissue Antigens 53:269–74

Holmskov UL (1999) Collectins and collectin receptors in innate immunity. APMIS Suppl 100:1–59

Horuk R, Chitnis CE, Darbonne WC et al. (1993) A receptor for the malarial parasite *Plasmodium vivax*: The erythrocyte chemokine receptor. Science 261:1182–4

Howard JC (1991) Immunology. Disease and evolution. Nature 352:565–7

Hughes AL, Nei M (1988) Pattern of nucleotide substitution at major histocompatibility complex class I loci reveals overdominant selection. Nature 335:167–70

Ingram VM (1957) Gene mutations in human haemoglobin: The chemical difference between normal and sickle cell haemoglobin. Nature 180:326–328

Ioannidis JP, O'Brien TR, Rosenberg PS et al. (1998) Genetic effects on HIV disease progression. Nat Med 4:536

Ip WK, Lau YL, Chan SY et al. (2000) Mannose-binding lectin and rheumatoid arthritis in southern Chinese. Arthritis Rheum 43:1679–87

Jabado N, Jankowski A, Dougaparsad S et al. (2000) Natural resistance to intracellular infections. Natural resistance-associated macrophage protein 1 (nramp 1) functions as a ph-dependent manganese transporter at the phagosomal membrane. J Exp Med 192:1237–48

Jeffery KJ, Usuku K, Hall SE et al. (1999) HLA alleles determine human T-lymphotropic virus-I (HTLV-I) proviral load and the risk of HTLV-I-associated myelopathy. Proc Natl Acad Sci USA 96:3848–53

Jouanguy E, Lamhamedi-Cherradi S, Lammas D et al. (1999) A human IFNGR1 small deletion hotspot associated with dominant susceptibility to mycobacterial infection. Nat Genet 21:370–8

Juliger S, Luckner D, Mordmuller B et al. (2000) Promoter variants of the human mannose-binding lectin gene show different binding. Biochem Biophys Res Commun 275:617–22

Kahana E, Brautbar C (1991) HLA antigens in subacute sclerosing panencephalitis patients in Israel. Acta Neurol Scand 83:367–9

Kaplan C, Muller JY, Doinel C et al. (1990) HLA-associated susceptibility to acquired immune deficiency syndrome in HIV-1-seropositive subjects. Hum Hered 40:290–8

Kapur V, Majesky MW, Li LL et al. (1993) Cleavage of interleukin 1 beta (IL-1 beta) precursor to produce active IL-1 beta by a conserved extracellular cysteine protease from *Streptococcus pyogenes*. Proc Natl Acad Sci USA 90:7676–80

Kaslow RA, Duquesnoy R, VanRaden M et al. (1990) A1, Cw7, B8, DR3 HLA antigen combination associated with rapid decline of T-helper lymphocytes in HIV-1 infection. A report from the Multicenter AIDS Cohort Study. Lancet 335:927–30

Kaslow RA, Carrington M, Apple R et al. (1996) Influence of combinations of human major histocompatibility complex genes on the course of HIV-1 infection. Nat Med 2:405–11

Kelly RJ, Rouquier S, Giorgi D et al. (1995) Sequence and expression of a candidate for the human secretor blood group alpha(1,2)fucosyltransferase gene (FUT2). Homozygosity for an enzyme-inactivating nonsense mutation commonly correlates with the non-secretor phenotype. J Biol Chem 270:4640–9

Kelso A (1998) Cytokines: Principles and prospects. Immunol Cell Biol 76:300–17

Klein J, Sato A (2000a) The HLA system: First of two parts. N Engl J Med 343:702–709

Klein J, Sato A (2000b) The HLA system: Second of two parts. N Engl J Med 343:782–786

Kobayashi RH, Kettelhut BV, Kobayashi AL (1983) Galactose inhibition of neonatal neutrophil function. Pediatr Infect Dis 2:442–5

Korber B, Muldoon M, Theiler J et al. (2000) Timing the ancestor of the HIV-1 pandemic strains. Science 288:1789–96

Krawczak M, Ball EV, Fenton I et al. (2000) Human gene mutation database-a biomedical information and research resource. Hum Mutat 15:45–51

Kroner BL, Goedert JJ, Blattner WA et al. (1995) Concordance of human leukocyte antigen haplotype-sharing, CD4 decline and AIDS in hemophilic siblings. Multicenter Hemophilia Cohort and Hemophilia Growth and Development Studies. Aids 9:275–80

Krul EJ, Schipper RF, Schreuder GM et al. (1999) HLA and susceptibility to cervical neoplasia. Hum Immunol 60:337–42

Kubo K, Yamazaki Y, Hanaoka M et al. (2000) Analysis of HLA antigens in *Mycobacterium avium*-intracellulare pulmonary infection. Am J Respir Crit Care Med 161:1368–71

Kudo T, Iwasaki H, Nishihara S et al. (1996) Molecular genetic analysis of the human Lewis histo-blood group system. II. Secretor gene inactivation by a novel single missense mutation A385T in Japanese nonsecretor individuals. J Biol Chem 271:9830–7

Kwiatkowski D, Hill AV, Sambou I et al. (1990) TNF concentration in fatal cerebral, non-fatal cerebral, and uncomplicated *Plasmodium falciparum* malaria. Lancet 336:1201–4

Lacerda GB, Arce-Gomez B, Telles Filho FQ (1988) Increased frequency of HLA-B40 in patients with paracoccidioidomycosis. J Med Vet Mycol 26:253–6

LeBlanc SB, Naik EG, Jacobson L, Kaslow RA (2000) Association of DRB1*1501 with disseminated *Mycobacterium avium* complex infection in North American AIDS patients. Tissue Antigens 55:17–23

Lechler RI, Simpson E, Bach FH (1995). *In* FH Bach and H. Auchincloss (eds.): *Transplant Immunology* Wiley-Liss, N Y pp. 1–34

Lee B, Doranz BJ, Rana S et al. (1998) Influence of the CCR2-V64I polymorphism on human immunodeficiency virus type 1 coreceptor activity and on chemokine receptor function of CCR2b, CCR3, CCR5, and CXCR4. J Virol 72:7450–8

Lekstrom-Himes JA, Hohman P, Warren T et al. (1999) Association of major histocompatibility complex determinants with the development of symptomatic and asymptomatic genital herpes simplex virus type 2 infections. J Infect Dis 179:1077–85

Lenzi M, Frisoni M, Mantovani V et al. (1998) Haplotype HLA-B8-DR3 confers susceptibility to hepatitis C virus-related mixed cryoglobulinemia. Blood 91:2062–6

Levy HL, Sepe SJ, Shih VE et al. (1977) Sepsis due to Escherichia coli in neonates with galactosemia. N Engl J Med 297:823–5

Liu R, Paxton WA, Choe S et al. (1996) Homozygous defect in HIV-1 coreceptor accounts for resistance of some multiply-exposed individuals to HIV-1 infection. Cell 86:367–77

Llop E, Rothhammer F, Acuna M, Apt W (1988) HLA antigens in cardiomyopathic Chilean chagasics. Am J Hum Genet 43:770–3

Lorenz E, Mira JP, Cornish KL et al. (2000) A novel polymorphism in the toll-like receptor 2 gene and its potential association with staphylococcal infection. Infect Immun 68:6398–401

MacDonald KS, Fowke KR, Kimani J et al. (2000) Influence of HLA supertypes on susceptibility and resistance to human immunodeficiency virus type 1 infection. J Infect Dis 181:1581–9

Mack DG, Johnson JJ, Roberts F et al. (1999) HLA-class II genes modify outcome of Toxoplasma gondii infection. Int J Parasitol 29:1351–8

Magierowska M, Theodorou I, Debre P et al. (1999) Combined genotypes of CCR5, CCR2, SDF1, and HLA genes can predict the long-term nonprogressor status in human immunodeficiency virus-1-infected individuals. Blood 93:936–41

Majetschak M, Flohe S, Obertacke U et al. (1999) Relation of a TNF gene polymorphism to severe sepsis in trauma patients. Ann Surg 230:207–14

Maliarik MJ, Chen KM, Sheffer RG et al. (2000) The natural resistance-associated macrophage protein gene in African Americans with sarcoidosis. Am J Respir Cell Mol Biol 22:672–5

Mann DL, Murray C, Yarchoan R et al. (1988) HLA antigen frequencies in HIV-1 seropositive disease-free individuals and patients with AIDS. J Acquir Immune Defic Syndr 1:13–7

Marotta CA, Wilson JT, Forget BG, Weissman SM (1977) Human beta-globin messenger RNA. III. Nucleotide sequences derived from complementary DNA. J Biol Chem 252:5040–53

Marquet S, Sanchez FO, Arias M et al. (1999) Variants of the human NRAMP1 gene and altered human immunodeficiency virus infection susceptibility. J Infect Dis 180:1521–5

Marshall E (2000) A renewed assault on an old and deadly foe. Science 290:428–430

Martin MP, Dean M, Smith MW et al. (1998) Genetic acceleration of AIDS progression by a promoter variant of CCR5. Science 282:1907–11

McDermott DH, Zimmerman PA, Guignard F et al. (1998) CCR5 promoter polymorphism and HIV-1 disease progression. Multicenter AIDS Cohort Study (MACS). Lancet 352:866–70

McGarry F, Walker R, Sturrock R, Field M (1999) The –308.1 polymorphism in the promoter region of the tumor necrosis factor gene is associated with ankylosing spondylitis independent of HLA-B27. J Rheumatol 26:1110–6

McGuire W, Hill AV, Allsopp CE et al. (1994) Variation in the TNF-alpha promoter region associated with susceptibility to cerebral malaria. Nature 371:508–10

McGuire W, Knight JC, Hill AV et al. (1999) Severe malarial anemia and cerebral malaria are associated with different tumor necrosis factor promoter alleles. J Infect Dis 179:287–90

McKiernan SM, Hagan R, Curry M et al. (2000) The MHC is a major determinant of viral status, but not fibrotic stage, in individuals infected with hepatitis C. Gastroenterology 118:1124–30

McNeil AJ, Yap PL, Gore SM et al. (1996) Association of HLA types A1-B8-DR3 and B27 with rapid and slow progression of HIV disease. QJM 89:177–85

Medzhitov R, Preston-Hurlburt P, janeway CA Jr (1997) A human homologue of the Drosophila Toll protein signals activation of adaptive immunity. Nature 388:394–7

Meyer CG, Gallin M, Erttmann KD et al. (1994) HLA-D alleles associated with generalized disease, localized disease, and putative immunity in Onchocerca volvulus infection. Proc Natl Acad Sci USA 91:7515–9

Meyer CG, May J, Stark K (1998) Human leukocyte antigens in tuberculosis and leprosy. Trends Microbiol 6:148–54

Miller LH, Mason SJ, Clyde DF, McGinniss MH (1976) The resistance factor to Plasmodium vivax in blacks. The Duffy-blood-group genotype, FyFy. N Engl J Med 295:302–4

Mira JP, Cariou A, Grall et al. (1999) Association of TNF2, a TNF-alpha promoter polymorphism, with septic shock susceptibility and mortality: A multicenter study. Jama 282:561–8

Morrison NA, Qi JC, Tokita A et al. (1994) Prediction of bone density from vitamin D receptor alleles. Nature 367:284–7

Mosmann TR, Coffman RL (1989) TH1 and TH2 cells: Different patterns of lymphokine secretion lead to different functional properties. Annu Rev Immunol 7:145–73

Mustonen J, Partanen J, Kanerva M et al. (1998) Association of HLA B27 with benign clinical course of nephropathia epidemica caused by Puumala Hantavirus. Scand J Immunol 47:277–9

Nagasawa T, Hirota S, Tachibana K et al. (1996) Defects of B-cell lymphopoiesis and bone-marrow myelopoiesis in mice lacking the CXC chemokine PBSF/SDF-1. Nature 382:635–8

Nakayama EE, Hoshino Y, Xin X et al. (2000) Polymorphism in the interleukin-4 promoter affects acquisition of human immunodeficiency virus type 1 syncytium-inducing phenotype. J Virol 74:5452–9

Nelson GW, Kaslow R, Mann DL (1997) Frequency of HLA allele-specific peptide motifs in HIV-1 proteins correlates with the allele's association with relative rates of disease progression after HIV-1 infection. Proc Natl Acad Sci USA 94:9802–7

Nickel RG, Casolaro V, Wahn U et al. (2000) Atopic dermatitis is associated with a functional mutation in the promoter of the C-C chemokine RANTES. J Immunol 164:1612–6

Nordstrom S, Cedergren B (1989) Genetic genealogical studies of 20 north Swedish families with the rare blood group p. Hum Hered 39:20–5

Overturf GD (1999) Infections and immunizations of children with sickle cell disease. Adv Pediatr Infect Dis 14:191–218

Pagnier J, Mears JG, Dunda-Belkhodja O et al. (1984) Evidence for the multicentric origin of the sickle cell hemoglobin gene in Africa. Proc Natl Acad Sci USA 81:1771–3

Pandolfi PP, Sonati F, Rivi R et al. (1995) Targeted disruption of the housekeeping gene encoding glucose 6-phosphate dehydrogenase (G6PD): G6PD is dispensable for pentose synthesis but essential for defense against oxidative stress. EMBO J 14:5209–15

Paradoa Perez ML, Trujillo Y, Basanta P (1987) Association of dengue hemorrhagic fever with the HLA system. Haematologia 20:83–7

Parham P, Ohta T (1996) Population biology of antigen presentation by MHC class I molecules. Science 272:67–74

Paul WE, O'Hara J (1987) B-cell stimulatory factor-1/interleukin 4. Annu Rev Immunol 5:429–59

Pauling L, Itano HA, Singer SJ, Wells IC (1949) Sickle cell anemia, a molecular disease. Science 110:543–8

Peiper SC, Wang ZX, Neote K et al. (1995) The Duffy antigen/receptor for chemokines (DARC) is expressed in endothelial cells of Duffy negative individuals who lack the erythrocyte receptor. J Exp Med 181:1311–7

Petzl-Erler ML, Belich MP, Queiroz-Telles F (1991) Association of mucosal leishmaniasis with HLA. Hum Immunol 32:254–60

Piazzolla G, Tortorella C, Schiraldi O, Antonaci S (2000) Relationship between interferon-gamma, interleukin-10, and interleukin-12 production in chronic hepatitis C and in vitro effects of interferon-alpha. J Clin Immunol 20:54–61

Pier GB (2000) Role of the cystic fibrosis transmembrane conductance regulator in innate immunity to *Pseudomonas aeruginosa* infections. Proc Natl Acad Sci USA 97:8822–8

Pier GB, Grout M, Zaidi T et al. (1998) *Salmonella typhi* uses CFTR to enter intestinal epithelial cells. Nature 393:79–82

Pogo AO, Chaudhuri A (2000) The Duffy protein: A malarial and chemokine receptor. Semin Hematol 37:122–9

Powell EE, Edwards-Smith CJ, Hay JL et al. (2000) Host genetic factors influence disease progression in chronic hepatitis C. Hepatology 31:828–33

Price P, Witt C, Allcock R et al. (1999) The genetic basis for the association of the 8.1 ancestral haplotype (A1, B8, DR3) with multiple immunopathological diseases. Immunol Rev 167:257–74

Prince HE, Schroff RW, Ayoub G et al. (1984) HLA studies in acquired immune deficiency syndrome patients with Kaposi's sarcoma. J Clin Immunol 4:242–5

Quillent C, Oberlin E, Braun J et al. (1998) HIV-1-resistance phenotype conferred by combination of two separate inherited mutations of CCR5 gene. Lancet 351:14–8

Rios M, Bianco C (2000) The role of blood group antigens in infectious diseases. Semin Hematol 37:177–85

Robinson J, Malik A, Parham P et al. (2000) IMGT/HLA database—a sequence database for the human major histocompatibility complex. Tissue Antigens 55:280–7

Rood MJ, Keijsers V, van der Linden MW et al. (1999) Neuropsychiatric systemic lupus erythematosus is associated with imbalance in interleukin 10 promoter haplotypes. Ann Rheum Dis 58:85–9

Rossi D, Zlotnik A (2000) The biology of chemokines and their receptors. Annu Rev Immunol 18:217–42

Roy S, McGuire W, Mascie-Taylor CG et al. (1997) Tumor necrosis factor promoter polymorphism and susceptibility to lepromatous leprosy. J Infect Dis 176:530–2

Roy S, Frodsham A, Saha B et al. (1999) Association of vitamin D receptor genotype with leprosy type. J Infect Dis 179:187–91

Ruwende C, Khoo SC, Snow RW et al. (1995) Natural selection of hemi- and heterozygotes for G6PD deficiency in Africa by resistance to severe malaria. Nature 376:246–9

Ryu S, Park YK, Bai GH et al. (2000) 3′UTR polymorphisms in the NRAMP1 gene are associated with susceptibility to tuberculosis in Koreans. Int J Tuberc Lung Dis 4:577–80

Sakai T, Aoyama N, Satonaka K et al. (1999) HLA-DQB1 locus and the development of atrophic gastritis with *Helicobacter pylori* infection. J Gastroenterol 34:24–7

Samson M, Libert F, Doranz BJ et al. (1996) Resistance to HIV-1 infection in caucasian individuals bearing mutant alleles of the CCR-5 chemokine receptor gene. Nature 382:722–5

Schrier RD, Freeman WR, Wiley CA, McCutchan JA (1994) CMV-specific immune responses and HLA phenotypes of AIDS patients who develop CMV retinitis. HNRC Group. HIV Neurobehavioral Research Center. Adv Neuroimmunol 4:327–36

Schroder JM, Kameyoshi Y, Christophers E (1994) RANTES, a novel eosinophil-chemotactic cytokine. Ann N Y Acad Sci 725:91–103

Searle S, Blackwell JM (1999) Evidence for a functional repeat polymorphism in the promoter of the human NRAMP1 gene that correlates with autoimmune versus infectious disease susceptibility. J Med Genet 36:295–9

Selvaraj P, Narayanan PR, Reetha AM (1999) Association of functional mutant homozygotes of the mannose binding protein gene with susceptibility to pulmonary tuberculosis in India. Tuber Lung Dis 79:221–7

Shin HS, Drysdale BE, Shin ML et al. (1994) Definition of a lipopolysaccharide-responsive element in the 5′-flanking regions of MuRantes and crg-2. Mol Cell Biol 14:2914–25

Smith MW, Dean M, Carrington M et al. (1997) Contrasting genetic influence of CCR2 and CCR5 variants on HIV-1 infection and disease progression. Hemophilia Growth and Development Study (HGDS), Multicenter AIDS Cohort Study (MACS), Multicenter Hemophilia Cohort Study (MHCS), San Francisco City Cohort (SFCC), ALIVE Study. Science 277:959–65

Spitalnik PF, Spitalnik SL (1995) The P blood group system: Biochemical, serological, and clinical aspects. Transfus Med Rev 9:110–22

Spitalnik PF, Spitalnik SL (2000) In Hoffman (ed.): Hematology, Basic Principles and Practices

Steffensen R, Carlier K, Wiels J et al. (2000) Cloning and expression of the histo-blood group Pk UDP-galactose: Ga1beta-4G1cbeta 1-cer alpha 1, 4-galactosyltransferase. Molecular genetic basis of the p phenotype. J Biol Chem 275:16723–9

Stephens JC, Reich DE, Goldstein DB et al. (1998) Dating the origin of the CCR5-Delta32 AIDS-resistance allele by the coalescence of haplotypes. Am J Hum Genet 62:1507–15

Stuber F, Petersen M, Bokelmann F, Schade U (1996) A genomic polymorphism within the tumor necrosis factor locus influences plasma tumor necrosis factor-alpha concentrations and outcome of patients with severe sepsis. Crit Care Med 24:381–4

Summerfield JA, Ryder S, Sumiya M et al. (1995) Mannose binding protein gene mutations associated with unusual and severe infections in adults. Lancet 345:886–9

Summerfield JA, Sumiya M, Levin M, Turner MW (1997) Association of mutations in mannose binding protein gene with childhood infection in consecutive hospital series. Bmj 314:1229–32

Swerdlow DL, Mintz ED, Rodriguez M et al. (1994) Severe life-threatening cholera associated with blood group O in Peru: Implications for the Latin American epidemic. J Infect Dis 170:468–72

Tejani A, Mahadevan R, Dobias B et al. (1981) Occurrence of HLA types in H. influenzae type B disease. Tissue Antigens 17:205–11

Thomas HC, Foster GR, Sumiya et al. (1996) Mutation of gene of mannose-binding protein associated with chronic hepatitis B viral infection. Lancet 348:1417–9

Thursz MR, Thomas HC, Greenwood BM, Hill AV (1997) Heterozygote advantage for HLA class-II type in hepatitis B virus infection. Nat Genet 17:11–2

Tournamille C, Colin Y, Cartron JP, Le Van Kim C (1995) Disruption of a GATA motif in the Duffy gene promoter abolishes erythroid gene expression in Duffy-negative individuals. Nat Genet 10:224–8

Van Dam MG, Seaton RA, Hamilton AJ (1998) Analysis of HLA association in susceptibility to infection with *Cryptococcus neoformans* var. gattii in a Papua New Guinean population. Med Mycol 36:185–8

Vassalli P (1992) The pathophysiology of tumor necrosis factors. Annu Rev Immunol 10:411–52

Vidal SM, Malo D, Vogan K et al. (1993) Natural resistance to infection with intracellular parasites: Isolation of a candidate for Bcg. Cell 73:469–85

Visentainer JE, Pereira FC, Dalalio MM et al. (2000) Association of HLA-DR7 with rheumatic fever in the Brazilian population. J Rheumatol 27:1518–20

Walboomers JM, Meijer CJ (1997) Do HPV-negative cervical carcinomas exist? J Pathol 181:253–4

Wang X, Moylan B, Leopold DA et al. (2000) Mutation in the gene responsible for cystic fibrosis and predisposition to chronic rhinosinusitis in the general population. Jama 284:1814–9

Westendorp RG, Langermans JA, Huizinga et al. (1997a) Genetic influence on cytokine production in meningococcal disease. Lancet 349:1912–3

Westendorp RG, Langermans JA, Huizinga TW et al. (1997b) Genetic influence on cytokine production and fatal meningococcal disease. Lancet 349:170–3

Wilkinson RJ, Patel P, Llewelyn M et al. (1999) Influence of polymorphism in the genes for the interleukin (IL)-1 receptor antagonist and IL-1 beta on tuberculosis. J Exp Med 189:1863–74

Wilkinson RJ, Llewelyn M, Toossi Z et al. (2000) Influence of vitamin D deficiency and vitamin D receptor polymorphisms on tuberculosis among Gujarati Asians in west London: A case-control study. Lancet 355:618–21

Wilson AG, Symons JA, McDowell TL et al. (1997) Effects of a polymorphism in the human tumor necrosis factor alpha promoter on transcriptional activation. Proc Natl Acad Sci USA 94:3195–9

Winkler C, Modi W, Smith MW et al. (1998) Genetic restriction of AIDS pathogenesis by an SDF-1 chemokine gene variant. ALIVE Study, Hemophilia Growth and Development Study (HGDS), Multicenter AIDS Cohort Study (MACS), Multicenter Hemophilia Cohort Study (MHCS), San Francisco City Cohort (SFCC). Science 279:389–93

Wu SB, Hwang SJ, Chang AS et al. (1989) Human leukocyte antigen (HLA) frequency among patients with nasopharyngeal carcinoma in Taiwan. Anticancer Res 9:1649–53

Yazdanbakhsh M, Sartono E, Kruize YC et al. (1995) HLA and elephantiasis in lymphatic filariasis. Hum Immunol 44:58–61

Zago MA, Silva WA, Jr, Dalle B et al. (2000) Atypical beta(s) haplotypes are generated by diverse genetic mechanisms. Am J Hematol 63:79–84

Transplantation genetics

43

Massimo Trucco
Wilma B. Bias

Introduction

The idea of replacing a diseased, or damaged part of the body of an individual, the *recipient*, with the same part provided by another healthy individual, the *donor*, has always been present in the human mind. Greek mythology is full of examples of chimeras – imaginary animals composed of parts coming from individuals of different species. If, on the one hand, chimeras can represent an artistic version of a successful xenotransplantation intervention (i.e., a transplant between individuals of different species), on the other hand, picturesque examples of dreamed allotransplantation (i.e., a transplant between two genetically different individuals of the same species) are also available (Rossini et al., 1999).

The most elegant representation of this mental concept is perhaps the famous painting of Fra Angelico (1387–1455), an altar piece in the San Marco Church in Florence, Italy (Fig. 43.1). The painter here represented the miracle performed by Saints Cosmas and Damian in Constantinople as narrated in a third century legend. According to the legend, these twin brothers, one a physician and the other a surgeon, replaced the cancerous leg of a white church sacristan with a healthy limb from a recently deceased Moor. The story is told that the sacristan walked around for the rest of his life with one white leg and one black leg (Klein, 1986; Silverstein, 1988; Rossini et al., 1999).

There is, however, evidence that transplantation surgery was actually successfully performed more than 2,000 years ago by ancient Hindu vaidya (Majno, 1975; Rossini et al., 1999). The reported clinical interventions that involved the reconstruction of the nose using pedicle flap grafts from the patient's own forehead, were similar in approach to the one more clearly described by the historian Calinzio who, in 1503, wrote in praise of the surgeon Branca who reconstructed the nose of a gentleman using skin removed from his slave (Wright, 1898). Calinzio added that "for a time the new nose functioned well", then "suddenly grew cold", "turned blue", and "eventually fell off". Since the slave died on the same day, the slave's demise was blamed for the loss of the engrafted nose. Today we know that the difference between these successful and unsuccessful transplants is that the first was an autologous transplant, the other an allotransplant. While Branca's patient actually suffered a typical graft rejection, the physician, Gaspare Tagliacozzi, was instead successful when, one hundred years later (1597), he tried to reproduce the vaidya's results by performing similar reconstructive rhinoplasty using skin flaps from the patient's arm (Silverstein, 1988; Rossini et al., 1999).

The beginning of the 20th century brought a fresh look to the transplantation problem. In 1912, George Schöne clearly summarized conclusions he gathered from different transplant attempts mostly performed in animals. The "Laws of transplantation" were so defined: (1) autografts generally succeed; (3) allografts usually fail; (2) xenografts invariably fail. "Blood relationship" was proposed as the biological barrier that separates donor from recipient: the closer the relationship, the more likely the graft will be accepted (Silverstein, 1988; Rossini et al., 1999).

The scientific basis of this postulated blood relationship was defined twenty-five years later by Peter Gorer, an expert on tumor resistance in mice (Gorer, 1937). Gorer was interested in explaining why tumors that could often be transplanted from one mouse to another, failed to grow when transplanted in another strain of recipient mice. To determine what was different between the acceptor strain

1101

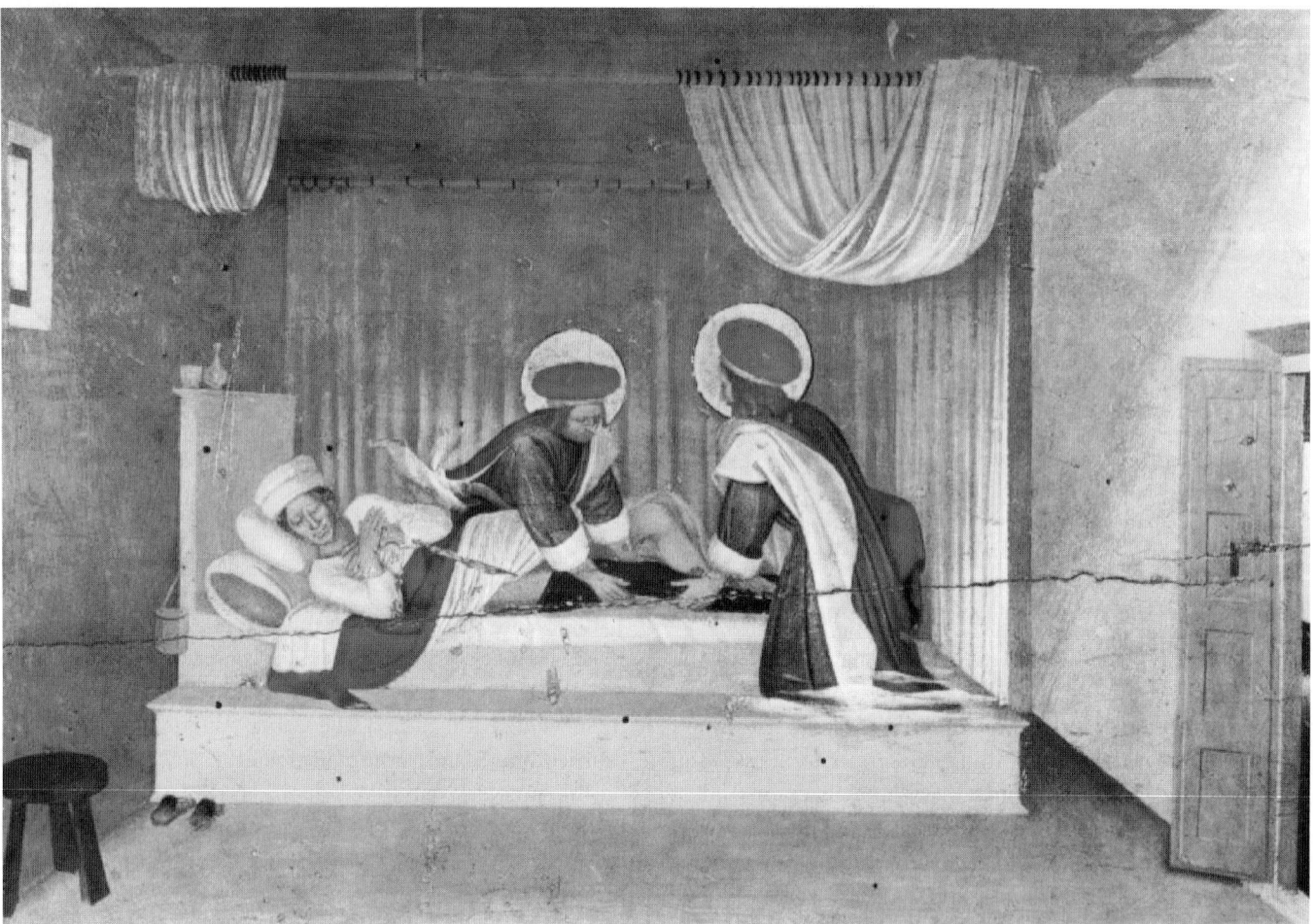

Fig. 43.1. The miracle of Cosmas and Damian as portrayed by Fra Angelico in his painting conserved in the museum of San Marco Church in Florence, Italy. (See Plate 43.1.)

versus the rejecting strain, Gorer performed tumor transplants in F_1, F_2, and backcross progeny of the three inbred strains of mice. The permissive trait was attributed to two independent genetic loci. On the basis of his knowledge of the blood groups, Gorer also attempted to distinguish the tumor-susceptible from the tumor-resistant animals on the basis of mouse erythrocyte agglutination driven by human serum. The successful experiments also proved that, like for the ABO system, agglutination behaved as a simple mendelian dominant trait. Furthermore, rabbit anti-mouse erythrocyte sera were sufficient to define three mouse red blood cell antigens. The detection in the serum of the mice of anti-type II antigen antibodies coincided with rejection propensity (Gorer, 1938). It was on this basis that Gorer joined forces with George Snell at the Jackson Laboratory in Bar Harbor, ME, where they expanded the studies to Snell's "congenic" inbred mouse strains (Snell, 1948). Congenic strains are genetically identical except at a single chromosomal locus. Using congenic strains of the mice,

Gorer and Snell were able to determine that engrafted tumors were most likely able to "take" when the recipient mouse was of the same strain as the donor (Gorer et al., 1948). More importantly, they also realized that survival of donor tissue was not limited to tumors, but applied to any graft including skin. Also, donor-specific antibodies first noted by Gorer in the graft rejecting recipient were induced not only by tumor grafting, but also by any other tissue graft or blood transfusion (reviewed in Klein, 1986). By appropriate genetic crosses and backcrosses among their congenic inbred strains, Snell and Gorer identified a number of genetically independent loci controlling these immune responses, which they designated H for histocompatibility (i.e., compatibility between different tissues), followed by an arabic numeral in the order of discovery. The locus designated H-2 appeared to be more immunogenic than the others and corresponded to Gorer's original type II antigen. This locus became known with time as the murine major histocompatibility gene complex (MHC).

The MHC can be considered the molecular embodiment of Schöne's "blood relationship" (Rossini et al., 1999).

Sir Peter Medawar tried to apply these concepts to help World War II burned soldiers with skin grafts (Medwar, 1944; 1958). He also came to the conclusion that while autografts succeed, allografts fail after an initial period of survival. A second allograft from the same donor did not experience the latent period of the first; rather, it rejected in an accelerated fashion. The survival of a second graft from a different donor was instead similar to that of the original graft, rejecting only after a latent period. Since the accelerated rejection could also be induced by injecting the recipient with donor leukocytes prior to engraftment, he concluded that "destruction of the foreign epidermis was brought about by a mechanism of active immunization". Specific antigens analogous to those of the ABO blood groups were supposed to be shared by skin and leukocytes and were responsible for the rejection response. Medawar's conclusions constituted the theoretical basis to postulate that immunosuppression might overcome the laws of transplantation.

In 1954, the first successful kidney transplant was performed between monozygotic twins for which immunosuppression was not necessary (Merrill et al., 1956). In 1959, the same team used an efficient immunosuppressive regimen to perform the first kidney graft between unrelated individuals (Merrill, 1978). The graft survived for 20 years.

The observations that antibodies against transplantation antigens could be generated as the result of an immune response against transfused blood components suggested the possibility of identifying human histocompatibility antigens by serologic methods. The first human histocompatibility antiserum was produced by Jean Dausset in 1958, by deliberate immunization of one blood donor with leukocytes from another (Dausset, 1958). This antiserum agglutinated the white blood cells of about 60% of his French donor panel. Concurrently, Payne and Rolfs showed that the sera of multiparous women often contained leuko-agglutinins (Payne and Rolfs, 1958). This important finding promised readily available sources of reagent antisera with which to characterize human leukocyte antigens (HLA).

The physiologic function of MHC molecules

The interpretation of the genetics of histocompatibility initially was, as presented, based upon experiments in which the histocompatibility antigens were only seen as the factors limiting tissue transplantation by promoting graft rejection.

Later the physiologic function of the MHC molecules was fully elucidated (Bjorkman et al., 1987a).

Although with different efficiency, macrophages, monocytes, dendritic cells, and mature B cells are all able to phagocytose foreign molecules, thus capturing "non-self" proteins invading the body and enzymatically cleaving them into peptides. This function is called "processing" of the antigenic protein. The peptides generated as the result of antigen processing are then protected from further cleavage and brought to the cell surface by MHC molecules able to accommodate the peptides in their antigen-combining site. The function of this site, the so-called peptide binding groove, was clearly determined once the interpretation of the crystal structure of the HLA molecule was completed (Bjorkman et al., 1987b). The HLA/peptide complex is then exposed at the cell surface (i.e., "presented") to a T lymphocyte that recognizes and engages it by its T-cell receptor (TCR) molecule. The antigen presenting cell (APC) activates T lymphocytes, causing them to divide and secrete specific factors (Davis and Bjorkman, 1988). The signal from the engaged TCR to the inside of the cell is transmitted by a chain of molecules, the CD3 complex, that ultimately activates the enzymes necessary to stimulate cell division, lymphokine receptor upregulation and lymphokine production (Jorgensen et al., 1992; Weiss, 1993) (Fig. 43.2). Lymphokines are secreted cellular hormones that can inhibit or stimulate other cells to become activated.

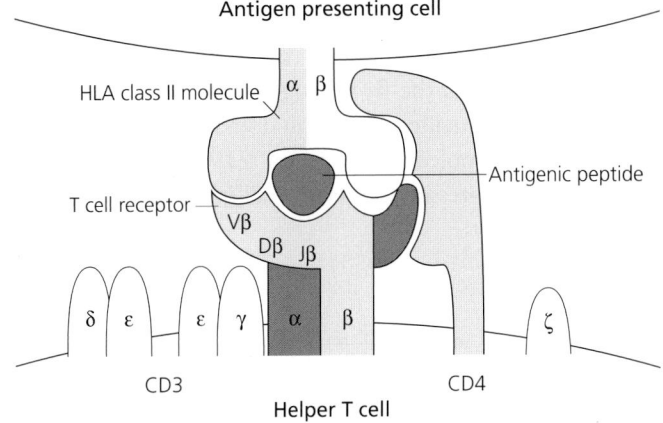

Fig. 43.2. The HLA class II molecule, expressed at the surface of an antigen presenting cell (APC), interacts with the processed antigenic peptide, lodged in the Bjorkman's groove of the molecule. The T helper cell recognizes the complex HLA molecule/antigenic peptide with its α/β T cell receptor (TCR). The accessary molecule CD4 stabilizes the binding of the TCR with the HLA molecule. CD4 provides antigen-mediated specific T cell activation functions. The CD3 complex composed of δ, ε, and γ molecules, transfers the signal of the successfully engaged TCR into the cytoplasm of the T cell. (Modified from Conrad and Trucco, *Diabetes/Metabolism Reviews*, 10:309–338, 1994 © John Wiley & Sons Limited. Reproduced with permission.)

T-cells producing "helper" factors are known as T-helper cells (Th). Based upon preferential secretion of certain lymphokines, Th cells are conventionally divided into Th_1 and Th_2 subgroups (Romagnani, 1992). Th_2 cells primarily promote activation of B lymphocytes and subsequent antibody production via secretion of interleukins 4, 5, 6 and 10 (Tony and Parker, 1985). Th_1 cells, which preferentially secrete interleukin 2, interferon γ, and TNF-β, help other T cells, already committed to the cytotoxic T-cell lineage, to proliferate (Mosmann et al., 1986). These cytotoxic T cells (Tc) destroy cells that are infected or altered by the same foreign antigen to which the Th initially reacted.

Th cells can easily be recognized and distinguished from Tc cells by differences in co-receptor expression and MHC-restriction. CD4 and CD8 are T-cell co-receptor molecules that stabilize the TCR/antigenic peptide/MHC molecule complex while recognition is taking place (Fig. 43.2). In general, CD4+ T-cells preferentially recognize MHC class II molecules (see below) that have bound peptides derived from internalized, exogenous proteins, whereas CD8+ T-cells react with MHC class I molecules (see below) complexed with cell-derived endogenous peptides.

The structure of human histocompatibility molecules

HLA molecules are grouped into two classes based on their structure, function, and cellular expression. Class I (HLA-A, -B, and -C molecules) are characterized by a heavy (43 kD) α chain with three domains ($α_1$, $α_2$ and $α_3$) (Fig. 43.3) that dimerizes with the $β_2$ microglobulin, a short (12 kD) protein, which provides the fourth domain necessary to stabilize the HLA molecule (Grey et al., 1973). Class I molecules are co-expressed on nearly all nucleated cells and

platelets, and are anchored via the transmembrane portion and the short cytoplasmic tail of the α chain only. Class II molecules (HLA-DR,-DQ and -DP) consist of α (34 kD) and β (29 kD) chains, each with two domains. Class II molecules are anchored by both chains, each of which can communicate across the membrane with cytoplasmic structures (Fig. 43.3). These molecules are expressed primarily on B lymphocytes, macrophages, dendritic cells, activated T cells and endothelial cells.

The two outermost domains of each molecule (α1 and α2 in class 1; α1 and β1 in class II) fold together to form the cleft in which the antigenic peptide can find appropriate lodging (Fig. 43.4). These first external domains are approximately 90 amino acids, or 270 base pairs in length. The antigen-combining site (also know as the Bjorkman's groove) is comprised of a β-pleated sheet with eight antiparallel strands forming the floor of the groove, and sides assuming the shape of α helices (Fig. 43.5). The amino acid residues forming this cleft are very polymorphic and are particularly immunologically-relevant in the α helical regions. As the protein folds into the tertiary structure, some of the hypervariable regions assume a location pointing into the cleft, i.e., an optimal position for interaction with the processed antigen. Other hypervariable segments are instead located on the external part of the molecule and constitute the determinants potentially involved with TCR recognition. These same hypervariable regions form the molecular basis of alloreactivity in tissue transplantation, i.e., donor differences in these amino acids are recognized as "foreign" by the recipient who immunologically reacts against them. These same, antigenically relevant differences are the human leukocyte antigens originally recognized by Dausset and Payne.

The HLA class I and class II molecules constitute the most highly polymorphic genetic system in humans. A

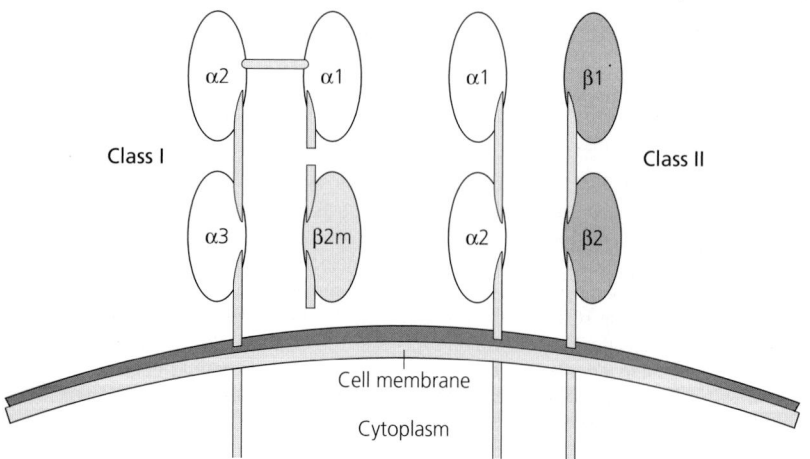

Fig. 43.3. The secondary structure of the HLA class I molecule with the α1, α2, and α3 domains (i.e., amino acid sequences that show similarities and are present more than once in the same polypeptide) of the α chain completed by the β2-microglobulin, is here compared with the structure of the class II molecule with its α1 and α2 domains of the α chain. Domains β1 and β2 are characteristic of the class II β-chain only. Both class I and class II heterodimers form, at their most external end, a peptide combining site composed of the α1 and α2 domains for class I, and α1 and β1 domains for class II molecules. (Modified from Rosner, Martell, Trucco, *Bone Marrow Transplantation*, Chapter 2.2.1.1, 2000.)

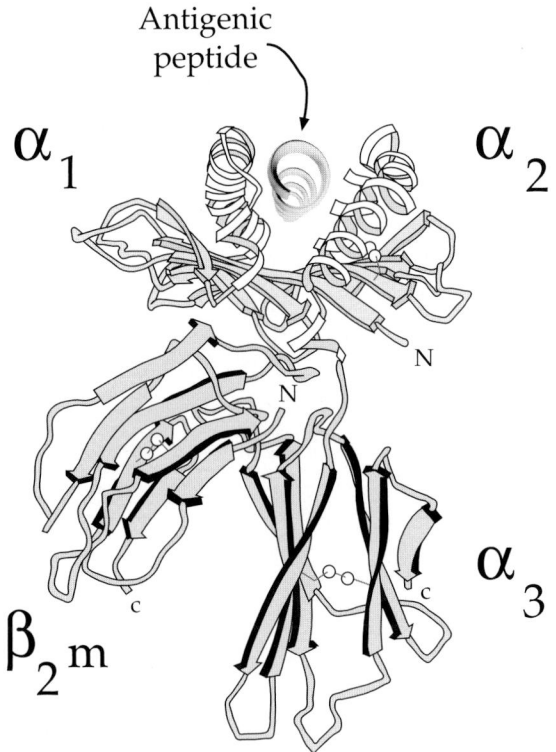

Fig. 43.4. The resolution of the structure of crystallized HLA-A2 class I molecule. The molecule, shown here from the side, has its most external domains (α_1 and α_2) able to form the antigen combining site in which the processed antigenic peptide is lodged. In this position the complex HLA molecule/antigenic peptide is recognized by the T cell via its receptor molecule (Modified from Faas and Trucco, *Diabetes Mellitus: A Fundamental and Clinical Text*, Ch. 34, pp. 326–333, 1996 © Lippincott Williams & Wilkins.)

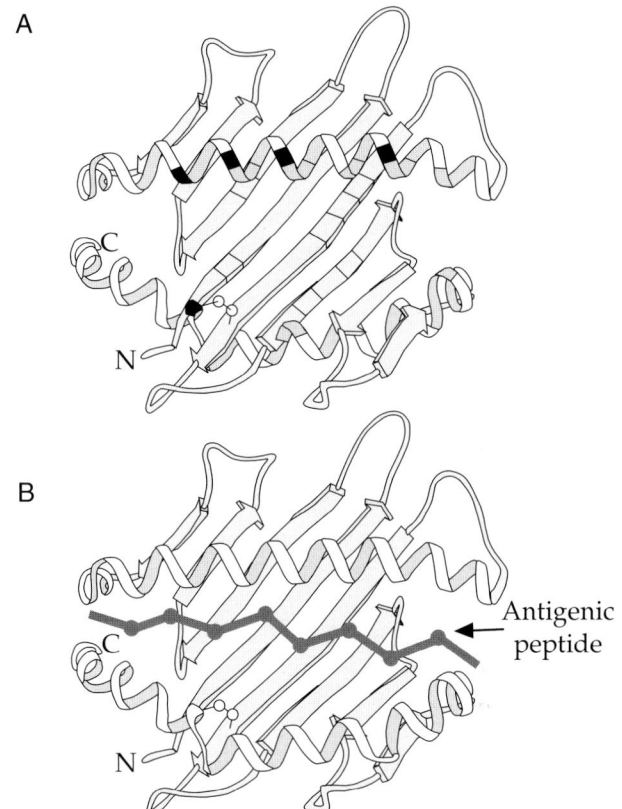

Fig. 43.5. The antigen combining site in which the antigenic peptide can find appropriate lodging. In **A**, the HLA molecule is seen from the top. The polymorphic regions are indicated in different nuances of color from grey to black. In **B**, a schematic, 9 amino acid-long peptide is shown present in the groove of the molecule. The antigenic peptides found in HLA class I molecule grooves are normally of this same size, while the antigenic peptides most frequently found associated with HLA class II molecules are longer than 9 amino acids and can vary considerably in size. (Modified from Trucco, *Diabetes Care*, 15:705–715, 1992.)

stable, inherited polymorphism gives rise to alternative forms of the protein, the *alleles*. Nearly all the HLA molecules have various alleles, with the numbers identified consistently rising (Marsh, 1999).

The molecular basis for the HLA polymorphic alleles resides in nucleotide sequence differences present in the coding regions of the HLA genes. Polymorphisms cluster into three or four discrete hypervariable regions, which become more evident when their amino acid sequences are aligned (Fig. 43.6). These nucleic acid sequence differences account for amino acid differences among the various HLA molecules. While most HLA alleles occur in all ethnic groups, they may vary in frequency from group to group.

The chromosomal organization of the HLA complex

The genes encoding HLA class I and class II molecules are located in a 4000 kilobases (kb) long DNA segment present on the short arm of chromosome 6. This DNA segment can be subdivided into three major regions which encode: class I molecules (2000 kb), class III molecules (1000 kb) and class II molecules (1000 kb) (Campbell and Trowsdale, 1993). The organization of the genes included in the HLA complex is shown in Fig. 43.7. The physical location, the *locus*, of each HLA gene determines its order on the chromosome, while the nomenclature instead recapitulates the chronological characterization of the genes at the various loci. The A locus is the most distant from the centromere and was the first to be characterized. The characterization of the B locus immediately followed that of the A locus; however, A and B are geographically separated by the C locus, which was the last to be characterized. The first class II locus was characterized by cellular tests after C and was then called D. Subsequently, by absorbing out anti-class I antibodies, sera able to recognize the same alleles defined by

```
               1                                    10                                   20                                  30
DQB1*0501   AGA GAC TCT CCC GAG GAT TTC GTG TAC CAG TTT AAG GGC CTG TGC TAC TTC ACC AAC GGG ACG GAG CGC GTG CGG GGT GTG ACC AGA CAC ATC TAT AAC CGA
DQB1*0502   --- --- --- --- --- --- --- --- --- --- --- --- --- --- --- --- --- --- --- --- --- --- --- --- --- --- --- --- --- --- --- --- --- ---
DQB1*05031  --- --- --- --- --- --- --- --- --- --- --- --- --- --- --- --- --- --- --- --- --- --- --- --- --- --- --- --- --- --- --- --- --- ---
DQB1*05032  *** *** *** *** *** *** *** *** *** *** *** *** *** *** *** *** *** *** *** *** *** *** *** *** *** *** **- --- --- --- --- --- --- ---
DQB1*0504   *** *** *** *** *** *** *** *** --- --- --- --- --- --- --- --- --- --- --- --- --- --- --- --- --- --- --- --- --- T-- --- --- --- ---
DQB1*06011  --- --- C-- --- --- --- --- --- CT- --- --- --- -C- A-- --- --- --- --- --- --T --- --- --- --- -T TA- --- --- T-- --- --- --- ---
DQB1*06012  *** *** *** *** *** *** *** *** *** *** *** -C- A-- --- --- --- --- --- --- --- --- --- --- -T TA- --- --- T-- --- --- --- ---
DQB1*0602   --- --- --- --- --- -T- --- --- --- A-- --- --- --- --- --- --- --- --- --- --- --- -T CT- --- --- T-- --- --- --- ---
DQB1*0603   --- --- --- --- --- --- --- --- --- A-- --- --- --- --- --- --- --- --- --- --- --- -T CT- --A --- --- --- ---
DQB1*0604   --- --- --- --- --- --- --- --- --- A-- --- --- --- --- --- --- --- --- --- --- --- -T CT- --A --- --- --- ---
DQB1*06051  --- --- --- --- --- --- --- --- --- A-- --- --- --- --- --- --- --- --- --- --- --- -T CT- --A --- --- --- ---
DQB1*06052  *** *** *** *** *** *** *** *** *** *** *** *** *** *** *** *** *** *** *** *** *-- --- -T CT- --A --- --- T-- --- --- --- ---
DQB1*0606   *** *** *** *** *** *** *** *** *** *** *** *** *** *** *** *** *** *** *** *** *-- --- -T CT- --A --- --- --- ---
DQB1*0607   *** *** *** *** *** *** *** *** --- A-- --- --- --- --- --- --- --- --- --- --- --- -T CT- --A --- --- --- ---
DQB1*0608   *** *** *** *** *** *** *** *** --- A-- --- --- --- --- --- --- --- --- --- --- --- -T CT- --A --- --- --- ---
DQB1*0609   *** *** *** *** --- A-- --- --- --- --- --- --- --- --- --- --- --- --- -T CT- --A --- --- T-- --- --- --- ---
DQB1*0201   --- --- --- --- --- --- --- --- --- --- --- --- --- --- --- --- --A --- --- --- --- -T CT- --- -G- --- AG- --- --- --- ---
DQB1*0202   --- --- --- --- --- --- --- --- --- --- --- --- --- --- --- --- --A --- --- --- --- -T CT- --- -G- --- AG- --- --- --- ---
DQB1*0301   --- --- --- --- --- --- --- --- -C- A-- --- --- --- --- --- --- --- --- --- --- --- -T TA- --- --- T-- --- --- --- ---
DQB1*0302   --- --- --- --- --- --- --- --- --- A-- --- --- --- --- --- --- --- --- --- --- --- -T CT- --- --- T-- --- --- --- ---
DQB1*03032  --- --- --- --- --- --- --- --- --- A-- --- --- --- --- --- --- --- --- --- --- --- -T CT- --- --- T-- --- --- --- ---
DQB1*0304   --- --- --- --- --- --- --- --- -C- A-- --- --- --- --- --- --- --- --- --- --- --- -T TA- --- --- T-- --- --- --- ---
DQB1*0305   *** *** *** *** --- A-- --- --- --- --- --- --- --- --- --- --- --C --- --- --- --- T-- --- --- --- ---
DQB1*0401   --- --- --- --- --- --- -T- --- --- A-- --- --- --- --- --- --- --- --- --C --- -T- --- --- T-- --- --- --- ---
DQB1*0402   --- --- --- --- --- --- -T- --- --- A-- --- --- --- --- --- --- --- --- --C --- --- --- --- T-- --- --- --- ---

               40                                   50                                   60
DQB1*0501   GAG GAG TAC GTG CGC TTC GAC AGC GAC GTG GGG GTG TAC CGG GCA GTG ACG CCG CAG GGG CGG CCT GTT GCC GAG TAC TGG AAC AGC CAG AAG GAA GTC CTG
DQB1*0502   --- --- --- --- --- --- --- --- --- --- --- --- --- --- --G --- --- --- --- --- AGC --- --- --- --- --- --- --- --- --- --- ---
DQB1*05031  --- --- --- --- --- --- --- --- --- --T --- --G --- --- --- --- --- --AC --- --- --- --- --- --- --- --- --- --- --- ---
DQB1*05032  --- --- --- --- --- --- --- --- --- --T --- --G --- --- --- --- --- --A- --- --- --- --- --- --- --- --- --- --- --- ---
DQB1*0504   --A --- --- --- --- --- --- --- --- --- --G --- --- --- --- --- AGC --- --- --- --- --- --- --- --C A-- ---
DQB1*06011  --- --- G-- --- --- --- --- --- --T --- --G --- --- --C --- --- -AC --- --- --- --- --- --- --- --- --C A-- ---
DQB1*06012  --- --- G-- --- --- --- --- --- --T --- --G --- --- --C --- --- -AC --- --- --- --- --- --- --- --- --C A-- ---
DQB1*0602   --- --- --- -C- --- --- --- --- --- --C --G --- --- --- --- --- -A- --- --- --- --- --- --- --- ---
DQB1*0603   --- --- --- -C- --- --- --- --- --- --C --G --- --- --- --- --- -A- --- --- --- --- --- --- --- ---
DQB1*0604   --- --- --- -C- --- --- --- --- --- --- --G --- --- --- --- --- --- --- --- --- --- --- --- ---
DQB1*06051  --- --- --- -C- --- --- --- --- --- --- --G --- --- --- --- --- --- --- --- --- --- --- --- ---
DQB1*06052  --- --- --- -C- --- --- --- --- --- --- --G --- --- --- --- --- --C --- --- --- --- --- --- ---
DQB1*0606   --- --- --- -C- --- --- --- --- --- --- --G --- --- --- --- --- --- --- --- --- --- --- --- ---
DQB1*0607   --- --- --- -C- --- --- --- --- --- --C --G --- --- --- --- --- -A- --- --- --- --- --- --- --- ---
DQB1*0608   --- --- --- -C- --- --- --- --- --- --C --G --- --- --- --- --- -A- --- --- --- --- --- --- --- ---
DQB1*0609   --- --- --- -C- --- --- --- --- --- --- --G --- --- --- --- --- --- --- --- --- --- --- --- ---
DQB1*0201   --A --- AT- --- --- --- --- --- --- -A- -T- --- --G --- --- -T- -T- --- -T- --- --CC --- --- --- --- --C A-- ---
DQB1*0202   --A --- AT- --- --- --- --- --- --- -A- -T- --- --G --- --- -T- -T- --- -T- --- --CC --- --- --- --- --C A-- ---
DQB1*0301   --- --- --- -CA --- --- --- --- --- -A- --- --G --- --- --- --T --- -C- --- -AC --- --- --- ---
DQB1*0302   --- --- --- -CA --- --- --- --- --- --T --- --G --- --- --- --T --- -C- --- --CC --- --- --- ---
DQB1*03032  --- --- --- -CA --- --- --- --- --- --T --- --G --- --- --- --T --- -C- --- -AC --- --- --- ---
DQB1*0304   --- --- --- -CA --- --- --- --- -A- --- --- --G --- --- --- --T --- -C- --- --CC --- --- --- ---
DQB1*0305   --- --- --- -C- --- --- --- --- --- --- --G --- --- --- --- --T --- -C- --- --CC --- --- --- ---
DQB1*0401   --- --- --- -C- --- --- --- --- --- --T --- --G --- --- --- --T --- -T- -AC --- --- --T --- --C A-- ---
DQB1*0402   --- --- --- -C- --- --- --- --- --- --T --- --G --- --- --- --T --- -T- -AC --- --- --T --- --C A-- ---

               70                                   80                                   90                               100
DQB1*0501   GAG GGG GCC CGG GCG TCG GTG GAC AGG GTG TGC AGA CAC AAC TAC GAG GTG GCG TAC CGC GGG ATC CTG CAG AGG AGA GTG GAG CCC ACA GTG ACC ATC TCC
DQB1*0502   --- --- --- --- --- --- --- --- --A --- --- --- --- --- --- --- --- --- --- --- --- --- --- --- --- --- --- --- --- --- --- --- ---
DQB1*05031  --- --- --- --- --- --- --- --- --A --- --- --- --- --- --- --- --- --- --- --- --- --- --- --- --- --- --- --- --- --- --- --- ---
DQB1*05032  --- *** *** *** *** *** *** *** *** *** *** *** *** *** *** *** *** *** *** *** *** *** *** *** *** *** *** *** *** *** *** *** *** ***
DQB1*0504   --- --- --- --- --- --- --- --- -** *** *** *** *** *** *** *** *** *** *** *** *** *** *** *** *** *** *** *** *** *** *** *** ***
DQB1*06011  --- A-- A-- --A GA- T-- -C- *** *** *** *** *** *** *** *** -T- --- T-- --- --- --- --- --- --- --- --- --- --- --- ***
DQB1*06012  --- A-- A-- --A GA- T-- -C- *** *** *** *** *** *** *** *** --- --- --- --- --- --- --- --- --- --- ***
DQB1*0602   --- A-- A-- --- GA- T-- -C- --- --- --- --- --- --- --- -T- --- T-- --- --- --- --- --- ---
DQB1*0603   --- A-- A-- --- GA- T-- -C- --- --- --- --- --- --- --- -T- --- T-- --- --- --- --- --- ---
DQB1*0604   --- A-- A-- --- GA- T-- -C- --- --- --- --- --- --- --- --G --- --- --- --- --- --- ---
DQB1*06051  --- A-- A-- --- GA- T-- -C- --- --- --- --- --- --- --- --G --- --- --- --- --- --- ---
DQB1*06052  --- A-- A-- --- GA- T-- -C- *** *** *** *** *** *** *** *** *** *** *** *** *** *** *** *** *** *** *** *** *** *** ***
DQB1*0606   --- A-- A-- --- G-- --- --- --- *** *** *** *** *** *** *** *** *** *** *** *** *** *** *** *** *** *** *** *** *** ***
DQB1*0607   --- A-- A-- --- GA- T-- -C- --- -** *** *** *** *** *** *** *** *** *** *** *** *** *** *** *** *** *** *** ***
DQB1*0608   --- --- A-- --- GA- T-- -C- --- -** *** *** *** *** *** *** *** *** *** *** *** *** *** *** *** *** *** *** ***
DQB1*0609   --- A-- A-- --- GA- T-- -C- --- --- -** *** *** *** *** *** *** *** *** *** *** *** *** *** ***
DQB1*0201   --- A-- AAA --- G-- --- --- --- C-- T-- -A- CT- --- AC- -C- T-- --- C-- C-- --- --- --- --- ---
DQB1*0202   --- A-- AAA --- G-- --- --- --- C-- T-- -A- CT- --- AC- -C- T-- --- C-- C-- --- --- --- --- ---
DQB1*0301   --- A-- A-- --- GA- T-- -C- --- C-- T-- -A- CT- --- AC- -C- T-- --- C-- C-- --- --- --- --- ---
DQB1*0302   --- A-- A-- --- GA- T-- -C- --- C-- T-- -A- CT- --- AC- -C- T-- --- C-- C-- --- --- --- --- ---
DQB1*03032  --- A-- A-- --- GA- T-- -C- --- C-- T-- -A- CT- --- AC- -C- T-- --- C-- C-- --- --- --- --- ---
DQB1*0304   --- A-- A-- --- GA- T-- -C- --- C-- T-- -A- CT- --- AC- -C- T-- --- C-- C-- --- --- --- --- ---
DQB1*0305   --- A-- A-- --- GA- T-- -C- --- C-- T-- -A- CT- --- AC- -C- T-- --- C-- C-- --- --- --- --- ---
DQB1*0401   --- -A- -A- --- --- --- -CC --A --- C-- T-- -A- CT- --- AC- -C- T-- --- C-- C-- --- --- --- --- ---
DQB1*0402   --- -A- -A- --- --- --- -CC --A --- C-- T-- -A- CT- --- AC- -C- T-- --- C-- C-- --- --- --- --- ---
```

Fig. 43.6. In the case of HLA class II molecules, the most polymorphic (i.e., hypervariable) regions between allelic chains are encoded by nucleotides contained in the second exon of the gene. The nucleotides in the sequences are here grouped three-by-three to reflect the amino acid composition of the most external domain of the molecule, i.e., the first 90 amino acids. In this example, allelic nucleotide sequences of the HLA-DQB1 gene are shown. (Modified from Morel et al, Proc Nat Acad Sci USA 85:8111–8115, 1988.)

mixed lymphocyte reaction (MLR) were also obtained. The alleles recognized by these anti-class II antibodies were then defined as D related, and eventually became known as DR alleles. Class II loci DQ and DP were characterized after DR in this chronological order and actually are in the same physical order on chromosome 6, closer to the centromere than class I loci with DP as the most centromeric (Fig. 43.7). The class I and class II regions are physically separated on the chromosome by genes encoding MHC class III molecules. Class III genes encode components of the complement cascade, C2, Bf, C4A, C4B, the functional steroid hydroxy-lase gene CYP21, a CYP21 pseudogene, and the genes for tumor necrosis factors (TNF-α and TNF-β) that are not relevant in the context of histocompatibility.

The class I genes present at the A, B and C loci encode molecules that can present antigenic peptides efficiently

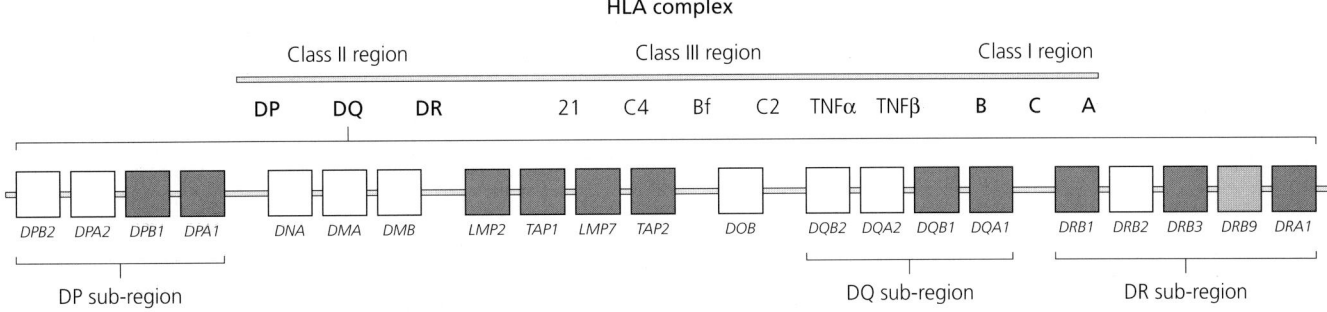

HLA complex

Class II region   Class III region   Class I region

DP   DQ   DR   21   C4   Bf   C2   TNFα   TNFβ   B   C   A

DPB2 DPA2 DPB1 DPA1   DNA DMA DMB   LMP2 TAP1 LMP7 TAP2   DOB   DQB2 DQA2 DQB1 DQA1   DRB1 DRB2 DRB3 DRB9 DRA1

DP sub-region   DQ sub-region   DR sub-region

Fig. 43.7. The HLA complex present on human chromosome 6, can be subdivided into 3 regions: class I, class III, and class II. The class II region is closest to the centromere of the chromosome and is conventionally subdivided into 3 additional sub-regions, DR, DQ, and DP. In black are the genes that encode functional molecules; in white are genes that are not functioning, i.e., pseudogenes, or that might encode proteins not yet characterized. The DRA1 gene encodes a non-polymorphic α chain able to pair with the products of each of the functional DRB genes. In this example, a DR3 haplotype is shown. DRB1 gene encodes for the DR3 allele, DRB2 is a pseudogene, and DRB3 encodes for the so-called DR52 molecule, which is always found associated with DR3. The DRB9 gene has not been well studied yet but seems to be able to encode for a non-functionally stable protein chain. (Modified from Luppi, Rossiello, Faas, Trucco, J Mol Med, 73:381–393, 1995 © Springer-Verlag New York Inc.)

once paired with the β_2 microglobulin, which is actually encoded on chromosome 15. The class I region also contains non-functional genes (i.e. pseudogenes HLA-H, -J, -K, and -L) and genes that are potentially functional, but whose gene products are not yet known like HLA-E and -F. HLA-G, a protein preferentially expressed at the surface of cytotrophoblasts at the maternal-fetal interface of the placenta, has been shown by Pazmany et al. (1996) to sufficiently protect otherwise susceptible target cells from lysis promoted by activated natural killer (NK) cells. In addition to the ones at the DR, DQ and DP loci, the class II region includes genes encoding proteins involved in antigen processing and in peptide transport from the cytoplasm to the cell surface (Campbell and Trowsdale, 1993). Besides the large multifunctional protease (LMP) and transporter associated with antigen processing (TAP) encoding genes, others (i.e., the α chain encoding genes DMA and DNA, or the β chain encoding genes DOB and DMB) are present in this region for which a physiologic function still awaits determination.

The class II are heterodimers, i.e., molecules consisting of two MHC-encoded polypeptide chains: the α, (encoded by "A" genes), non-covalently bound to the β (encoded by "B" genes) (Fig. 43.3). For DQ molecules, only the DQA1 and DQB1 gene products are known to be expressed as functional DQ α/β heterodimers. The DQA2 and DQB2 genes are pseudogenes (Fig. 43.7). Likewise, only the DPA1 and DPB1 genes encode the chains of functional DP molecules. In contrast, more than one type of DR molecule can be encoded by the same chromosome and all are co-expressed at the surface of the same cell. Different DRB genes are present in different numbers and in different combinations on chromosome 6 in different individuals

(Fig. 43.7 and 43.8). Each type of DRβ-chain pairs with the single non-polymorphic α chain encoded by the DRA1 gene (Fig. 43.7) (Dupont and Yang, 1994).

Each individual has one maternal and one paternal chromosome 6 and consequently one maternal and one paternal allele at any HLA locus. If the maternal allele and the paternal allele differ, as they often do, the person is said to be *heterozygous* at that HLA locus. If the inherited maternal and paternal alleles happen to be the same, the person is *homozygous* at that locus. As the maternal and paternal alleles are expressed codominantly, each cell of an individual will express two sets of each HLA molecule, e.g., 2 HLA-A molecules, 2 HLA B-molecules, etc. The combined expression of both sets of molecules constitute the HLA *phenotype* of the cells of an individual. The *genotype* of an individual is instead constituted by two (i.e., one paternal and one maternal) sets of arrays of closely linked genes, many with multiple alleles, inherited as a unit.

In 1967, Ceppellini coined the term *haplotype* to define each genetic unit inherited from one or the other parent. An HLA haplotype includes the class I, III and II genes present on one chromosome 6 of an individual. The HLA genotype of an individual is composed of one paternal and one maternal HLA haplotype. Each HLA haplotype is transmitted from the parent to the child in mendelian fashion so that each child shares one haplotype with each parent (Fig. 43.9). Within a family, one can find siblings that share two haplotypes (i.e., they are HLA *identical*), one haplotype (i.e., they are HLA *haploidentical*), or no haplotypes (i.e., they are HLA *different*) with the probability of 25%, 50% and 25%, respectively. Recombination may occur during parental gametogenesis by crossing over during meiosis. However, due to the relative proximity of

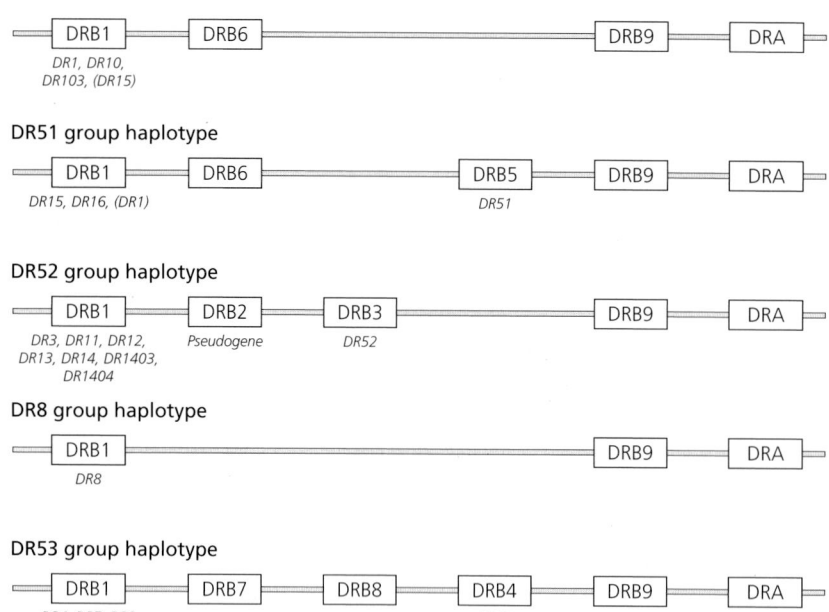

Fig. 43.8. DRB genes are present in different numbers and in different combinations on the chromosome 6 of different individuals. While DRB1 encodes the serologically best defined DR alleles, DRB3, 4 and 5 encode three molecules (DR52, 53 and 51, respectively) always associated with certain DRB1 alleles like DR3, DR4 and DR1, respectively. Thus, DR51, 52 and 53 are not allelic forms at a certain locus, like the DRB1 alleles, but are different protein products, each encoded by its own genes at different loci, and each only present in certain haplotypes. (Modified from Rosner, Martell, Trucco, *Bone Marrow Transplantation*, Ch. 2.2.1.1 2000.)

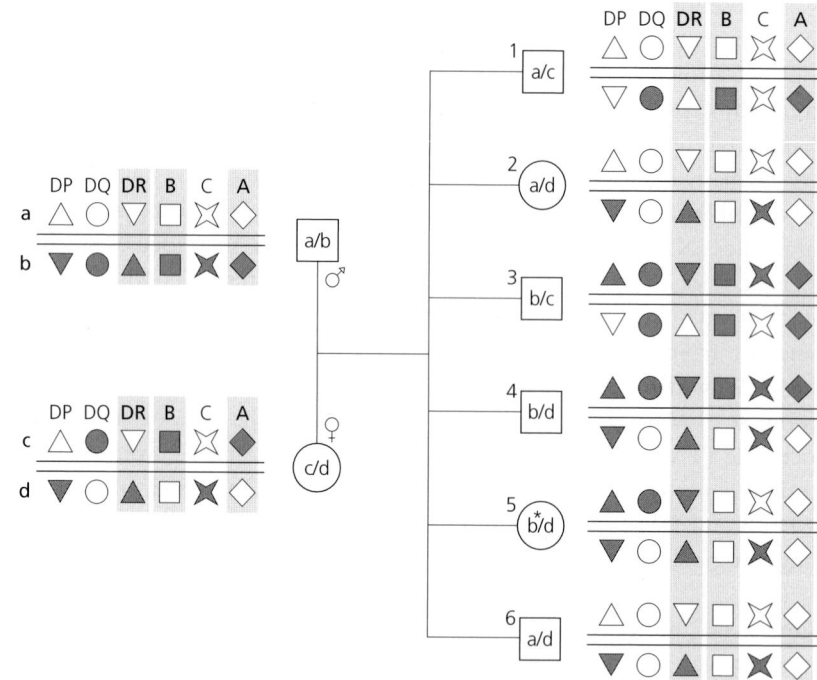

Fig. 43.9. HLA typing determines the HLA *phenotype* of an individual. Segregation analysis of the HLA phenotypes on at least the two parents and a child or on 3 HLA-different members of the same family enables determination of the four *haplotypes* (normally called **a, b, c** and **d**) present in the family, or the *genotype* of each individual. Consequently the definition of individuals as *heterozygous* or *homozygous* at certain loci (e.g., sibling 1 is homozygous at DP, DR and C, both alleles are white; but heterozygous at DQ, B and A loci, 1 white and 1 black allele), together with the recognition of individuals who share one haplotype only (e.g., siblings 1, 2 and 6 share the "a" haplotype, and are HLA *haploidentical*) or two haplotypes (e.g., siblings 2 and 6 share the "a" and the "d" haplotypes and are HLA *identical*), or none (e.g., siblings 2 and 3 and are HLA *different*) becomes possible, as well. A bone marrow transplant always offers the best chance of success if it is performed between HLA identical siblings. "Six antigen matching" refers to the situation in which two individuals share both alleles at the locus A, B and DR (grey background) and to the unique situation in which national sharing of kidneys is considered mandatory. In this simplistic example, father and mother are phenotypically the same since they are sharing the alleles at the A, B and DR loci and constitute a 6 antigen matching pair, although they are not HLA "identical", like siblings 2 and 6, since their haplotypes are actually different. Although it is considered a very rare event, it is possible to find individuals, represented here by sibling 5, in which a crossing over between class I and class II gene regions, involving the paternal and maternal haplotypes of the father, cause an a-b recombination flagged here with an asterisk: b*. (Modified from Rosner, Martell, Trucco *Bone Marrow Transplantation*, Chap. 2.2.1.1 2000.)

the HLA genes, recombination events between loci within a region, or even between regions, though possible, are quite rare. In addition, the selective pressure seems to maintain the genes of each established HLA haplotype together, i.e., in *linkage disequilibrium* (Bodmer, 1972). With linkage disequilibrium we define the non-random association of the alleles of linked loci present in one haplotype. For example, among Caucasoids, the most frequent HLA-A and HLA-B haplotype, if we disregard all other loci in the complex, encodes HLA-A1; B8 molecules. This combination occurs in about 10% of the population. However, the allele frequencies are 0.142 and 0.096, respectively. If the population were in Hardy-Weinberg equilibrium, i.e., non-influenced by external forces and then in a situation which occurs when the genes considered are independently segregating through successive generations, the HLA-A1; B8 haplotype frequency would be $0.142 \times 0.096 = 0.014$, or about one-tenth the observed frequency. Linkage disequilibrium, Δ, can be determined by calculating the difference between the observed haplotype frequency and the expected frequency. At equilibrium, $\Delta = 0$. As a logical consequence, an HLA haplotype composed in part of the paternal and in part by the maternal genes (i.e., a *recombinant* haplotype) is quite difficult to find.

On one hand, recombination is a very rare event across a few generations. On the other hand, it is considered the most efficient mechanism of HLA gene evolution. During the course of evolution, a primitive HLA gene duplicated and mutated; yet, by chance or because of selective advantage, the ancestral complex remained linked. Once gene duplication had occurred, reciprocal recombination was available to generate new haplotype arrangements. Sequence analyses suggest that both intrallelic and intergenic recombinational events were major contributors to HLA diversity. Some of these events have been likened to the one-way "gene conversion" process, first described in yeast, in which a segment of nucleotides from a "donor" gene is translocated or inserted into another gene.

One proposed example of an HLA interallelic conversion is the specificity DRB1*1304 reported by Lee and coworkers (1990). The nucleotide sequence of this allele is identical to that of DRB1*1102 except for codons 57, 58, and an intervening sequence that DRB1*1304 shares with DRB1*0801, *0803, and *0405. These authors suggested that one of the three latter alleles donated codons 57, 58, and the intervening sequence to *1102, which led to serologic reactivity with antisera to DR13.

A possible example of intergenic conversion is HLA-B46. This allele, which is relatively common in Orientals, appears to have derived from the donation of a cluster of nucleotides from HLA-Cw1 into HLA-B62. The donated Cw1 nucleotides resulted in a lack of serologic reactivity with anti-B62 or any other B locus antisera, but an acquisition of reactivity to anti-Cw3 (Zemmour et al., 1992). HLA-B46 haplotypes typically carry the Cw1 gene. If the B46+ cell is heterozygous at the HLA-C locus, it will type for three HLA-C alleles, Cw1, Cw3 and the allele carried on the alternate haplotype.

By convention, the paternal haplotypes are designated as *a* and *b* and the maternal haplotypes as *c* and *d*. Children in a family are designated as genotypes ac, bc, ad, or bd. If a = HLA-A1; B8; C7; DR3; DQ2; DP4 while *b* = A2; B7; C7; DR2; DQ6; DP1, and *c* = A3; B65; C3; DR7; DQ2; DP2, or *d* = A11; B35; C4; DR1; DQ1; DP4, the phenotype of a child b/d will be A2,11;B7,35;C4,7; DR1,2;DQ1,6; DP1,4, and the recombinant haplotype resulting from a crossing over that took place somewhere in between class I and class II regions of the father's paternal (*a*) and maternal (*b*) haplotypes, will be b* A1;B8;C7;DR2;DQ6;DP1 as described in Fig. 43.9 in simplified terms. Family studies are therefore recommended, both to confirm the alleles present in each of the patient's haplotypes, and to rule out the possibility of recombination. Only a family study and the analysis of allele segregation can positively elucidate the genotype of an individual.

Minor histocompatibility systems

Determining the HLA phenotype of an individual is the goal of histocompatibility testing (i.e., tissue typing) to determine who is a suitable donor for a particular recipient. It can be achieved using serologic and/or molecular techniques (see below). Generally a sibling HLA-identical to the recipient constitutes the first choice as a donor, although transplants from haploidentical donors are more frequently being performed today. In fact, although bone marrow transplantation (BMT) between genetically HLA identical siblings has the highest chance of success, with the declining birthrate in the US and Western Europe, the likelihood of finding a genotypically-identical sibling has dwindled. An estimated 65–75% of individuals requiring BMT will not have a suitable donor in their family (Kernan et al., 1993).

To overcome this problem, alternative sources of hematopoietic stem cells from phenotypically HLA-matched, unrelated donors have been sought, and utilized with much success. The National Marrow Donor Program (NMDP) has facilitated unrelated marrow transplants throughout the world, using HLA-matched marrow from donors which were chosen among the volunteers listed in the NMDP registry (Kernan et al., 1993; Mori et al., 1997; Yancey et al., 1997; Murata, 1998; Walker, 1999). Places such as the Placental Blood Center in New York are also having success with transplants using umbilical cord blood instead of bone marrow cells from HLA-matched and partially mismatched unrelated donors (Kurtzberg et al., 1996).

Unlike related donors who match at all loci within the haplotypes they share, unrelated donors can match at some, but not all loci. Therefore, precise HLA typing at the various loci becomes essential.

Although to date, clinical experience in transplanting bone marrow from unrelated donors has proven that relatively long-term survival is achievable, the high risks of graft failure and serious, acute graft-versus-host-disease (GVHD) remain major obstacles when compared to transplants between related donors. One plausible explanation for the increased incidence of severe GVHD among allogeneic combinations of donor and recipient is that, unlike genotypically-identical HLA-matched siblings who are "identical by descent" for HLA and other poorly characterized MHC or non-MHC (i.e., minor) histocompatibility antigens (Goulmy et al., 1996), the phenotypically HLA-matched unrelated donors may not be matched for a subset of antigens that can still contribute to alloreactivity. Furthermore, recent advances in HLA typing by DNA analysis have revealed additional polymorphisms only evident at the genetic level. These differences may have so far still undetermined functional and clinical relevance. The failure to identify these differences using older techniques suggests that unrelated donor/recipient pairs thought to be phenotypically-matched actually were somewhat mismatched (Nademanee et al., 1995).

All instances of graft rejection and most instances of GVHD in MHC-identical transplants can be attributed to non-MHC systems. The preponderance of evidence of their impact on human transplantation comes primarily from BMT. Approximately 60% of patients who receive bone marrow from an HLA-identical sibling will have some evidence of GVHD, and in about 20% it will be severe. In the mouse, the number of minor histocompatibility (mH) loci has been estimated to be more than 100, about 40 of which have been identified by skin graft experiments and genetic segregation analysis. It appears that the alleles of a particular locus vary in antigenic strength (as determined by mean survival time of skin grafts), and that the effects of different loci are additive (reviewed in Klein, 1975). This is probably true in humans because, in general, GVHD increases in

severity with decreasing degree of relatedness even with HLA identity.

Cytotoxic T lymphocytes (CTL) have been observed from patients with graft rejection following HLA-identical BMT for aplastic anemia, in multiply transfused patients and in multiparous women (Parkman et al., 1976; Zier et al., 1983; Tekolf and Shaw, 1983). In some human and mouse CTL studies the reactions have shown MHC class I restriction, including H-Y, a minor antigen encoded by a gene on the Y chromosome (Bevan, 1975; Goulmy, 1988; Voogt et al., 1988). Class II restriction of proliferating T cells reactive to mH antigens following HLA-identical BMT has been reported by Reinsmoen and coworkers (1984) and van Els and coworkers (1992). The MHC restriction of T cell responses to these antigens suggests that they are naturally processed peptides of intracellular proteins which, presumably, associate with MHC antigen-binding sites for presentation to T cell receptors (Rotzschke et al., 1990). However, not all responses to mH antigens appear to be MHC restricted. For example, as early as 1957, Snell and colleagues showed that a B10.LP (H-2b) mouse preimmunized with tissue from C57BR (H-2k) rejected a C57BL/10 (H-2b) tumor. All B10.LP mice that were not preimmunized succumbed to the tumor. The tumor donor strain differed from the host only at the H-3 locus, whereas the C57BR strain differs from B10LP at the H-2 complex as well as H-3 and other minor loci. Confirmation that responses to mH are not always restricted was later provided by Murasko (1978) who showed that BALB/c (H-2d) mice preimmunized against B10.D2 (H-2d) rejected C57BL/10 (H-2b) skin grafts in an accelerated manner. The interpretation was that the accelerated rejection was against mH antigens, since the preimmunizing strain was H-2 identical to the recipient, whereas the skin donor was not. Inasmuch as the mH loci probably encode a very heterogeneous group of molecules whose structures and primary functions are unknown, it is not surprising that both restriction and non-restriction have been observed.

In humans, there is indirect evidence of the presence of an HLA-linked mH gene. The first report of this minor locus came from Eisvoogel and colleagues (1972), who observed weak mixed lymphocyte reactivity between siblings, one of whom was a recombinant between HLA-A and HLA-B. This locus, which appeared to map near HLA-A, was designated MLR weak (MLRw). Later, Hsu and coworkers (1981) reported a similar location for genes controlling in vitro cellular responses to the synthetic polypeptides (T,G)-A–L and (H,G)-A–L. Family studies suggested that the gene, or genes, lie distal to HLA-A. Then, in 1989, in an analysis of 142 HLA-identical sibling donor bone marrow transplants, Hopkins and colleagues implicated this, or a similar locus, in the etiology of GVHD. These patients were selected from a total of 323 because they were informative for polymorphisms of clotting factor 13 (F13A), which maps distal to HLA-A, and the red cell enzyme glyoxalase-1 (GLO), which maps proximal to the HLA-D region. No double recombinants between these two loci were observed. Of 68 GLO-informative donor-recipient pairs, 22 were GLO mismatched, that is, one of each pair was a DR/GLO recombinant. There was no significant difference in acute GVHD between the DQ/GLO recombinant and nonrecombinant groups (32% vs 48%). Of 33 pairs informative for F13A, 18 had a donor or recipient recombinant. Among this HLA-A/F13A recombinant group, 67% of the patients had acute GVHD in contrast to 33% of patients in the nonrecombinant group, providing statistical significance to the difference. A relative risk of acute GVHD attributable to this putative immune response gene that maps near but distal to HLA-A is 4.0. This, or another, HLA-linked mH locus was described by Vinci and associates (1994) who obtained a cytotoxic T-cell line from a patient who rejected bone marrow from an HLA-identical sibling. The cells lysed EBV-transformed B cells of the donor and some, but not all, unrelated subjects who shared HLA-B44 with the patient. An EBV-transformed line of the patient's pretransplant B cells were not lysed by the cytotoxic cells.

Neither transplantation nor transfusions elicit much demonstrable antibody production to mH antigens. For this reason, in vitro cellular assays, especially the generation of CTL, has been the method of choice for studying mH antigens in both mouse and man. However, Bias and coworkers (1980) found 31 unique non-MHC lymphocytotoxic antibodies in the sera of multitransfused kidney transplant patients who rejected HLA-identical organs, multitransfused bone marrow transplant candidates whose sera reacted with cells of HLA-identical siblings, and in multiparous women. These sera were tested against cells from 60 families with an average of seven children each. Analysis of reaction patterns revealed that the reacting antigens segregated independently of the MHC.

It is important to note that GVHD, unrelated to histoincompatibility, often occurs in syngeneic or autologous BMT (reviewed in Santos et al., 1985). It appears that the development of the immune system following bone marrow transplantation is similar to normal ontology. It has been shown in animal studies that syngeneic GVHD can be induced by neonatal thymectomy, thymic irradiation prior to engraftment, ciclosporine treatment for six weeks after engraftment followed by withdrawal of the drug, or various other treatments. It appears that these treatments cause a failure of the developing immune system to discriminate self from nonself, resulting in the generation of autoreactive cells, indicating that tolerance to self-antigens is controlled by regulatory T cells. Syngeneic or autologous GVHD is similar to chronic GVHD, a complex of reactions resulting from an imbalance of immunoregulatory cells. In acute GVHD, immunologic recovery occurs when the non-specific regulatory T cells are able to control autoreactivity. Chronic GVHD appears to be an extension of acute GVHD in which the immune dysregulation continues, resulting in clinical manifestations characteristic of certain autoimmune diseases such as scleroderma.

Serologic methods for HLA typing

Tissue typing for transplantation refers to determination of the class I and class II specificities (i.e., the HLA phenotype) of both the potential donor(s) and the recipient. Finding the best donor for a kidney transplant generally means finding a "six-antigen match" by looking at each of the 2 alleles at HLA-A, -B and -DR loci (Figure 43.9). For bone marrow transplant, however, HLA-C and -DQ are also typed and often considered.

Until recent years, the most frequently used HLA typing method has been the microlymphocytotoxicity assay (Takasugi et al., 1971). This technique utilizes as target cells a suspension of pure and viable lymphocytes which have been separated from whole peripheral blood using density gradient separation. The lymphocytes are incubated with a panel of alloreactive antisera and a source of complement (C'), usually rabbit serum. The anti-HLA antibodies present in the various sera are quite specific for the individual structural determinants that characterize the polymorphism of the HLA antigens. When a specific antigen-antibody complex is formed, C' activation results in cell lysis. Following addition of a vital dye, the percentage of dead versus live cells can be visualized by phase contrast microscopy. A positive reaction is scored when at least half of the cells are killed. The HLA type is assigned by interpreting the patterns of reactivity of dozens of sera whose specificities are known. Most antisera are obtained from donors who have been exposed by transfusion or multiple pregnancies to cells bearing foreign HLA molecules. As first proven by Rose Payne, multiparous women become immunized against the alleles encoded by the paternal HLA haplotype when blood from the fetus enters the mother's bloodstream at delivery (Payne et al., 1967; Ceppellini et al., 1971).

Originally, it was the responsibility of the individual tissue typing laboratory to procure, test, and maintain quality control of the antisera used in testing. The pioneering HLA investigators soon realized, however, the need for standardizing their own reagents. This was achieved by organizing international workshops which have been held every three to four years since 1963. These international workshops originally aimed at sharing and consequently standardizing alloantisera, target cells or cell lines, and technical procedures, soon became the forum for recognition of new loci, the definition of new alleles, the adoption of the standard methods, the acceptance and then the utilization of a common nomenclature.

Today, sera can be obtained locally or through national or international serum exchange programs. Commercial trays with well-characterized sera are most widely used. All accredited histocompatibility laboratories are required to adhere to rigorous standards regarding reagents, protocols, and quality assurance set forth by the American Society for Histocompatibility and Immunogenetics (ASHI). In addition, most laboratories participate in several proficiency testing programs administered by such agencies as the College of American Pathologists (CAP).

However, even with all the refinement and standardization promoted through the years, many problems still confound the results obtainable by serologic methods. As mentioned, serology is encumbered by the requirement for relatively pure populations of viable lymphocytes. This has the greatest impact on class II typing, as HLA-DR and -DQ molecules are expressed most abundantly on B lymphocytes and less significantly on activated T cells and macrophages which, all together, comprise at best 20% of the peripheral blood lymphocyte population. Therefore, a relatively large quantity of blood (30 ml) from each individual must be processed in order to obtain enough class II positive cells to allow a complete HLA typing. This may constitute a problem when the individual to be HLA typed is a child. Also, if the cells are not essentially 100% viable at the beginning of the test procedure as a consequence of disease, chemotherapy, or the assumption of other drugs, the subsequent isolation procedures (e.g., spinning the blood through a Ficoll-Hypaque gradient, collecting cells at the serum/Ficoll interface, and separating B from T cell subpopulations to facilitate the typing of class II and class I alleles, respectively) may further damage them. This cell damage can generate a background of dead cells that, when the cytotoxic reaction is read, will make the results of the specific killing mediated by the antisera and C' indistinguishable from the negative controls. Also, serology cannot be used to HLA type a patient recently treated with anti-

CD3 antibodies, like OKT3, since these antibodies are cytotoxic in the presence of C' and per se cause cell death limiting the specificity of the assay. Finally, the C' itself can be a source of variability in these tests, as it can by itself be slightly cytotoxic.

In many leukemias (e.g., chronic myelogenous leukemia) and other disorders, insufficient numbers of B-cells and/or reduced antigen expression can completely preclude class II testing. Although Epstein-Barr (EB) virus transformation (Bodmer et al., 1977), and a variety of other procedures, have been developed in attempts to procure sufficient numbers of B-cells for testing, they can be labor-intensive, time-consuming, and expensive, besides often being quite unproductive (Trucco et al., 1979). A major drawback to EB-virus transformation is that the blastoid nature of the transformed B-cells makes them overly sensitive to C' activity. Although complement pre-adsorption with each cell-line to be tested can avoid this problem, such treatment is impractical for a general clinical use.

Also, cross-reactivity (i.e., lack of specificity) of alloantisera still remains an unsolved problem for serological typing. The HLA types defined by serologic methods are often not directly correlated to single alleles. Certain groups of class I antigens belong to cross-reactive groups (CREGs) that share distinct immunogenic epitopes referred to as *public*, or broad specificities (Klein, 1971). All the cells sharing a public epitope react with the same antiserum. Further, the antisera used for class II typing are not naturally class-II specific. These sera are frequently "contaminated" with class I antibodies, which may cause false positive reactions. The donor's immune system is exposed simultaneously to the two classes of molecules both present on the immunizing cells. While extensive absorption with platelets (which express class I, but not class II proteins) can provide a relatively pure preparation of anti-class II antibodies, these antisera have generally lower titers and are in shorter supply than anti-class I antisera.

The need for ongoing screening programs to replenish sera is further complicated in that two donors (e.g., two polygranidae) will never have exactly the same specificity. Also, only 200 ml of blood can legally be collected postpartum, and even serum obtained from the same donor, following subsequent pregnancies, can differ with respect to titer or range of reactivity. Accurate serologic HLA typing largely depends upon experience and extensive knowledge of protocols and reagents of specialized HLA laboratory personnel.

In 1977, the development of mouse anti-human monoclonal antibodies was seen as the best alternative source to increase specificity and have an unlimited supply of standardized reagents (Trucco et al., 1978). Their use, however, is not yet widespread due to the limited number of "private" specificities recognized by the mouse which reacts preferentially against "public" specificities. Trays containing only monoclonal antibodies that allow a relatively informative typing recently became commercially available.

Despite its limitations, the microlymphocytotoxicity test remains the most popular test for clinical use to provide class I and class II typing at a moderate level of resolution in one working day. A drastic improvement in the analysis of percentages of reactive antibodies (PRA) has, however, improved the results of transplant (kidney, in particular) interventions, eliminating the negative conditions frequently found associated with fulminant or hyperacute rejections. The use of the flow cytometer to determine the presence in the recipient serum of anti-T and anti-B cell antibodies that are not reactive against the major histocompatibility antigens, drastically improved the one-year survival.

Cellular methods for HLA typing

Other alleles, including those at HLA-C, -DQ, -DP and perhaps at other loci, are not strongly immunogenic and therefore do not elicit antibodies in large quantity or with high affinity. Reasons could be that these molecules are shed quite rapidly from the cell surface, are in a very limited quantity per single cell, or their critical amino acid differences point into the Bjorkman's groove instead of outside. They may, however, be clinically-relevant and detectable by alloreactive T-cells.

As previously mentioned, the first cellular approach successfully used for recognition of HLA class II alleles was the so-called mixed lymphocyte culture (MLC) or mixed lymphocyte reaction (MLR). To perform this test, lymphocytes from two individuals are co-incubated for several days in tissue culture. If the two individuals are disparate for a class II allele or a non-MHC minor histocompatibility antigen undetectable by serology, both cell types undergo lymphoblastogenesis, synthesize DNA and proliferate. In the presence of ^{3}H-thymidine, the degree of newly synthesized DNA can be estimated. Cells that are HLA-identical are non-reactive in MLC and the incorporation of ^{3}H-thymidine equals the negative controls.

In 1969, in order to separately monitor the response of the recipient (host-versus-graft) and the donor (graft-versus-host), Fritz Bach proposed to perform two separate unidirectional MLRs (Bach et al., 1969). The cells chosen as *stimulators* are irradiated to inhibit DNA synthesis and ^{3}H-thymidine incorporation. The non-irradiated *responders* are instead still able to incorporate the thymidine. Every MLC typing test is set up as a complicated matrix of many one-way reactions. In general, three unrelated HLA-mismatched individuals are used as positive controls of the maximum proliferative ability of the responder cells. Every cell should be tested as both stimulator and responder. In addition, autologous controls (i.e., each individual's cells incubated with its own irradiated cells) are used to normalize the response of each cell type to its stimulators. The results are expressed as a relative response (RR) or as a stimulation index (SI). Ideally, when two individuals are HLA-identical, the proliferative responses are less that 20% of the positive controls (Meo et al., 1973).

The MLC test has been used most widely in bone marrow transplantation and was developed primarily to help select the most compatible (i.e., least stimulatory) donor when several compatible family members are available (Bach et al., 1969). It is best used for confirmation of genotypic identity in siblings, especially in cases in which a complete haplotype could not be determined, such as when one parent is unavailable for testing or one appears to be serologically homozygous for DR or DQ.

Although the MLC is a cellular crossmatch predominantly triggered by class II alleles, it does not define an individual HLA type. One reason could be that DR is thought to have dominance over DQ, perhaps because the expression at the cell surface of the former is 10 times higher than the one of the latter. The role of DP, with 100 times fewer molecules than DR expressed on a single cell, remains controversial. This is the reason cellular specificities recognized by MLC testing were originally designated as HLA-Dw ("D" because these specificities were considered to be encoded by a different locus than A, B and C; "w" because they were still to be officially recognized in the context of an international workshop). HLA-Dw antigens were in reality immunogenic combinations of HLA-DR, -DQ and/or -DP determinants recognized as such by alloreactive T cells, but not necessarily by alloantisera. When, by absorbing the antisera with platelets to remove anti-class I antibodies and using purified B cells as cytotoxicity test targets, the HLA-Dw determinants were also recognized by certain antisera. They were then defined as D-related serological specificities and eventually DR alleles.

A variation of this test can be performed in which the lymphocytes to be tested are used as responders in an MLC test in which a panel of HLA homozygous cells are used as irradiated stimulators. These homozygous typing cells (HTC) are able to define the HLA-Dw specificities but are quite difficult and costly to procure. Inasmuch as the majority of HTC are Epstein Barr virus transformed cell lines, the results of the testing is frequently difficult to interpret. Other available cellular tests are the primed lymphocyte test (PLT) frequently used to identify DP alleles better, and the cell-mediated lympholysis (CML) test which primarily reflects the stimulatory and effector functions of cytotoxic T lymphocytes (CTLs) in culture (Dormoy et al., 1992; Yamamoto et al., 1994). Although proven extremely useful for research purposes, these tests are too complex and the results too difficult to standardize to be included in routine typing procedures.

Until recent years, the convention was to use HLA-A, -B and -DR serology (i.e., 6 antigens matching) to select a donor, with the MLC as the final arbiter of donor-recipient compatibility. In addition, a pre-transplant crossmatch of patient's serum against donor lymphocytes (i.e., PRA determination) is generally done to ensure that there is no recipient presensitization to donor HLA antigens, which could prevent engraftment. However, the MLC lacks sensitivity and specificity, in particular, when used for patients with hematologic disorders. Spontaneous proliferation of malignant blast cells in culture and/or poor HLA antigen expression, can contribute to false positives or false negatives, respectively. The MLC is technically difficult and as many as 40% of the tests are uninterpretable. Furthermore, it does not have good predictive value for either rejection or GVHD. Therefore, despite being the only functional test for assessing class II histocompatibility, the National Marrow Donor Program (NMDP) no longer requires it before performing a bone marrow transplant (Mickelson et al., 1993).

Molecular methods for HLA typing

The practical limitations of both serologic and cellular assays, as well as their inability to resolve clinically-relevant subtypes, prompted the rapid development of molecular biologic techniques for HLA typing. Molecular techniques can precisely define differences missed by serologic typing and/or those suggested by an incompatible MLC.

In the 1980s, molecular biology technologies, such as gene cloning and sequencing, became simple to perform. This facilitated the isolation and characterization of the HLA genes at different loci from hundreds of individuals. By comparing sequence variations from person to person, the nature and locations of the polymorphism of the HLA complex were revealed (Fig. 43.6).

The first attempts to perform molecular HLA typing was based on restriction fragment length polymorphism (RFLP) analysis (Turco et al., 1990). RFLP testing uses a specific DNA probe to recognize the presence of a certain HLA gene on a set of DNA fragments. These fragments are generated by digesting genomic DNA with commercially-prepared bacterial restriction endonucleases (i.e., restriction enzymes) which recognize short, specific nucleotide sequences. The resulting array of restriction fragments are separated on agarose gels by electrophoresis, transferred by capillary action to a nitrocellulose or nylon membrane (Southern blotting), and sequentially hybridized with radiolabelled DNA probes specific for each HLA locus. After repetitive washings, the radioactive probes specifically hybridized to their DNA fragment are revealed by exposing the membranes to X-ray film. The positive fragments differ in size and number from one individual to another, thus creating a polymorphism useful for typing. Although by RFLP it was possible to generate results more precisely and completely than serological typing (Cascino et al., 1986; Carlsson et al., 1987), in some laboratories, the use of radioactivity was problematic and high quality Southern blots could not be achieved. Also, the turn around time for even a small number of tests was very long, thus precluding the use of these DNA tests in a clinical setting.

The Xth International Histocompatibility Workshop was organized with the specific aim of transferring RFLP technology to laboratories specialized in HLA serology. All participant laboratories received a common set of HTC lines and a panel of DNA probes. Although the proceeds of this workshop, published in 1987, were useful in establishing standards for RFLP analysis of class II loci, and the collective data obtained revealed strong associations between certain DR and DQ alleles and the RFLPs (Trucco and Ball, 1987), the results were not definitive, largely due to strong homology and cross-reactivity between different alleles and even different loci. These obvious limiting aspects did not preclude, however, their application to fulfill specific aims, like the characterization of HLA-DQ alleles that confer susceptibility to type 1 diabetes (Trucco et al., 1989), or the comparison between serologic and molecular typing in promoting kidney graft survival (Hsia et al., 1993; Tong et al., 1993). As other techniques which directly analyze HLA polymorphism were being developed, RFLP analysis was, however, quickly deemed unsuitable for general clinical use.

The introduction of polymerase chain reaction (PCR) (Mullis and Faloona, 1987; Saiki et al., 1988) revolutionized HLA molecular typing. PCR is a powerful and versatile technique for generating millions of copies of specific genomic DNA fragments from minute amounts of starting material once the nucleotide sequence of a certain gene is known. Amplification is accomplished automatically in a DNA thermal cycler by incubating nanogram quantities of DNA, isolated from any possible source in solution with buffer, free deoxynucleotide triphosphates (dNTPs), specific oligonucleotide primers and thermostable DNA polymerase. The most common of analyses are performed by dot blotting a few microliters of the amplified DNA onto replicate nylon membranes. Each membrane is then hybridized with a different sequence-specific oligonucleotide probe (SSOP) labelled with a reporter moiety. After washing away the unbound excess, the retention of specific probe can be visualized by a variety of methods, the most common of which is chemiluminescence (Fig. 43.10A). This approach allowed typing of hundreds of samples with a relatively small number of probes to determine, for example, that variants of sequences involving codon 57 of the second exon of the HLA-DQB1 gene were reliable markers for insulin-dependent diabetes mellitus susceptibility (Todd et al., 1987; Morel et al., 1988).

As the extremely large sequence diversity of the class II gene second exon was revealed, the possibility of using this technique for complete HLA class II typing seemed difficult, yet feasible. This daunting task was promoted and organized by the XIth International Histocompatibility Workshop which provided standardized conditions and a battery of probes to each of its participant laboratories (Bodmer, 1992).

The advantages of this technique, often referred to as "oligotyping" are many (Fig. 43.10A). The requirement for viable, purified lymphocytes expressing HLA antigens is eliminated. Reagents can be standardized and synthesized in unlimited quantities. Functionally-relevant subtypes and polymorphisms as small as one nucleotide substitution can be precisely defined, as stringency conditions for hybridization can be perfected for each probe. However, to provide a high resolution HLA typing, up to seven separate PCR amplifications may need to be done for DRB and DQB1 typing alone. A complete set of results, no matter how large or small the set, requires 4–5 days to be finalized.

Therefore, this technique is not well-suited for routine clinical applications in which a relatively small number of samples should be tested as quickly as possible.

A different format referred to as the "reverse dot blot" has proven advantageous in reducing the amount of technical manipulation, and in improving turn-around time (Saiki et al., 1989; Rudert and Trucco, 1992). Reverse dot blots feature a pre-made membrane to which the entire battery of probes has been fixed. The DNA to be tested incorporates the reporter moiety during amplification, and is then hybridized against the probes present on the membrane. Advantages include labelling one or few DNA samples per donor instead of many probes, performing an entire test with only one membrane, and obtaining results in one working day.

The canonical size of specific oligonucleotides normally used as probes is about 20 nucleotides, a minimal size for discriminating all difference of one nucleotide. For the reverse dot blot, the direct attachment of probes this size is inefficient, and involves formations of chemical bonds to portions of the probe, resulting in reduced hybridization capability. These difficulties have been solved by enzymatically adding a large number of thymidine nucleotides to the

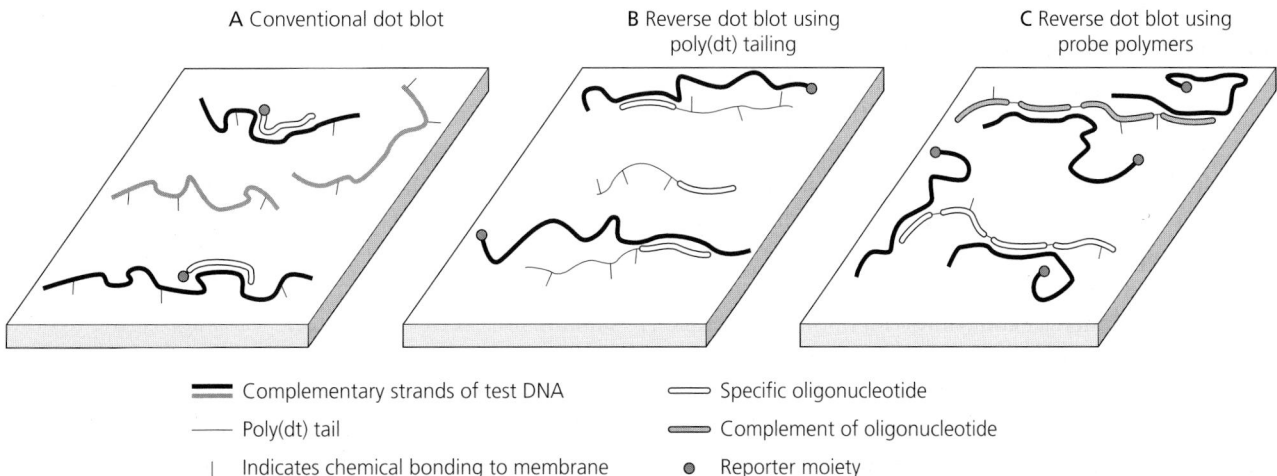

| A Conventional dot blot | B Reverse dot blot using poly(dt) tailing | C Reverse dot blot using probe polymers |

Complementary strands of test DNA

Poly(dt) tail

Indicates chemical bonding to membrane

Specific oligonucleotide

Complement of oligonucleotide

Reporter moiety

Fig. 43.10. "Conventional" dot blot used in SSOP typing A is compared with reverse dot blot after poly DT tailing of the various probes B, and with reverse dot blot of polymeric probes C. (Modified from Rudert and Trucco, *Histocompatibility Testing 1991*, pp. 352–356, 1992 By permission of Oxford University Press.)

end of the probe (poly dT tailing) (Saiki et al., 1989b). The increased length facilitates binding efficiency, and favors formation of chemical bonds in the poly dT tails, thus leaving the sequence specific parts of the probe available for hybridization (Fig. 43.10B). This approach is being used in some commercial kits for HLA typing.

A new method developed in our laboratory (Rudert and Trucco, 1992) uses a different approach to bind nucleotide probes to the membrane. Long polymers, usually greater than 25 repeats of the specific nucleotide sequence are synthesized and bound to the membrane with high efficiency (Rudert and Trucco, 1990). Although chemical bonds between the membrane and the DNA will prevent the hybridization to some sequences, the result is that many more specific sequences remain available for hybridization. Another important advantage of this method is that both complementary strands of probe sequence are bound to the membrane, i.e., the probes are double-stranded. This allows both strands of amplified DNA to hybridize to the probe, further increasing the sensitivity of this assay (Fig. 43.10C). Finally, a large quantity of polymers of the same size can be generated from those cloned into plasmid vectors. This level of reproducibility is not obtainable with poly dT tailing, and would enhance standardization of this technique.

Other "reverse" techniques involve fixing probes to 96-well plastic trays with either colorimetric or fluorescent detection (Chia et al., 1993; Giorda et al., 1993).

More recently, a new technique based on the use of sequence-specific primer (SSP) pairs and PCR has been proven more suitable for clinical use. SSP consists of a battery of primer pairs, each capable of only amplifying a specific gene segment. The numerous PCR products obtained are then loaded onto an agarose gel. Following electrophoresis and staining, the presence of the specifically amplified DNA segments can be visualized on a UV light-box so to allow correct allele definition. The presence of determined bands combinations allow the attribution of each allele. SSP offers the possibility of obtaining moderate-high resolution HLA typing in a few hours. Techniques for DRB molecular typing using 32 sequence-specific pairs of primers (Olerup and Zetterquist, 1992) and DQB typing using 14 primer pairs (Olerup et al., 1993) have been published. Several commercial companies offer SSP testing kits.

Both SSP and SSOP methodologies have also been applied to class I typing, which is proving to be a much more formidable task due to the high degree of widespread polymorphism compared to the class II genes, and complications presented by the presence of pseudogenes. One method for SSP typing (Browning et al., 1993) uses nine coding-strand and seven non-coding strand primers in

various combinations to generate HLA-A specific amplification products. The specificity of PCR priming is increased by taking advantage of the amplification refractory mutation system (ARMS), in which non-specific reactions are inhibited by introducing a nucleotide mismatch near the 3′ end of the primer (Newton et al., 1989). Fifteen HLA-A group specificities can be successfully characterized using this method which appears to be comparable to routine serology with respect to identification and resolution of HLA-A specificities. Subtypes of each group can be more specifically resolved using additional primer pairs (Krausa et al., 1993). Low resolution typing of the HLA-B alleles has also been described (Sadler et al., 1994) using a similar approach. Twenty-four PCRs using 34 primers are sufficient to determine the majority of, but not all, serologically-defined specificities at the B locus. ARMS-PCR has also been used to detect alleles at the HLA-C locus (Bunce and Welsh, 1994).

The SSP approach is especially amenable for use in clinical laboratories that do not have a great deal of molecular biology experience, as the equipment and special techniques required are minimal. From DNA extraction to allele identification, reliable and easily interpretable results can be generated in less than four hours; thus, SSP typing is an especially attractive alternative to serology for clinical laboratories. However for laboratories performing large-scale molecular typing, the SSP method may be too labor-intensive.

To answer to these limiting aspects, we devised a strategy that combines the high throughput advantages of SSOP with the speed, high resolution and relative ease of SSP analysis. To this end, we have applied a method (Holland et al., 1991) that permits amplification *and* direct detection of specific target DNA to the SSP approach. Our method does not require post-amplification hybridization or gel analysis steps (Faas et al., 1996), rather it takes advantage of the 5′ to 3′ exonuclease activity of the Taq polymerase normally used in PCR amplifications. An oligonucleotide probe, labelled at the 5′ end with a "reporter" fluorescent dye and at the 3′ end with a "quencher" fluorescent dye, is pre-mixed in each PCR with the allele-specific primers. The annealing of the probe to one of the PCR template strands during the course of amplification generates a substrate suitable for exonuclease attack. Cleavage of the hybridized probe releases the reporter from the quenching residue, enabling its detection by an increase in sample fluorescence (Fig. 43.11). The fluorescence signal is read directly from the PCR mixture using a luminescence spectrometer. The sequence-specific priming and exonuclease released fluorescence (SSPERF) assay is a highly specific, sensitive and rapid method already successfully tested for the detection of

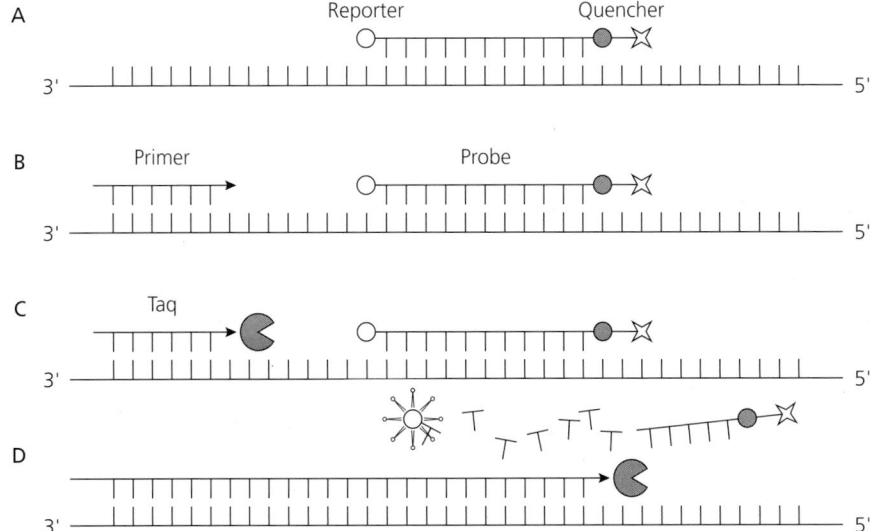

Fig. 43.11. Sequence-specific priming and exonuclease-released fluorescence (SSPERF) method. In A, hybridization of a doubly-labeled fluorogenic probe to the target DNA sequence. The reporter (○) and the quencher (●) dyes portions are indicated. The 3′ phosphate added to inhibit the primer function of the probe is indicated with a star (★). In B, the annealing of the primer to the DNA template follows the annealing of the probe to it since its size is shorter than the one of the probe. In C, Taq polymerase catalyzes the extension of the primer. In D, Taq polymerase exerts its exonuclease function once it encounters the double-stranded template formed by the probe hybridizing to one of the strands of the DNA to be amplified. The cleavage of the probe physically separates the reporter from the quencher dye, promoting an increase in reporter fluorescence. (From Faas, Menon, Braun, Rudert, Trucco, *Tissue Antigens* 48:97–112. © 1996 Munks-goard International Publishers Ltd, Copenhagen.)

HLA-A, B, DQB1, DQA1 and DRB alleles (Faas et al., 1996; Rudert et al., 1997; Menon et al., 1997).

Although the preparation and purification of fluorescent probes is more time-consuming than the simple synthesis and labelling of conventional fluorescent or radioactive probes for SSOP-based typing, the probes, once validated in the assay, can be generated in large-scale (1–10μM) syntheses that will provide sufficient reagents for at least 200,000 reactions (Rudert et al., 1997). The doubly-labelled probes, together with SSP primers, buffer, dNTPS and $MgCl_2$ can be aliquotted and stored indefinitely at −20°C in PCR strip tubes. Subsequent use would involve manual addition of extracted DNA and Taq polymerase to each tube. The rest is automated. A machine that serves both as a DNA thermocycler and spectrometer is commercially available.

The time has come, however, to convert all the suitable methods for molecular HLA typing to microchip technology. Microarray technology can accommodate thousands of perfectly distributed DNA spots on a microscope glass slide where hybridization can take place, saving reagent quantities, avoiding time consuming manipulations, and providing automatically read results (Guo et al., 1999).

Clinical significance of HLA molecular typing

A possible criticism of DNA typing is that it gives "too much" information. Although it has been hypothesized that even one nucleotide difference, and hence one amino acid disparity, can result in increased risk of alloreactivity *in vivo* (Fleischauer et al., 1990), many nucleotide substitutions do not cause amino acid changes. Given the huge number of detectable alleles at the various loci, it would be important to determine which mismatches are allowable and which ones are instead non-permissive for a positive clinical outcome.

A number of studies have been done to determine the clinical impact of HLA matching in unrelated bone marrow transplants. Many reports have shown that the incidence of both acute GVHD and rejection are significantly higher among patients transplanted with phenotypically-matched bone marrow cells from unrelated donors compared with cells from genotypically identical siblings (Anasetti et al., 1989; Beatty et al., 1993), in particular when serologic techniques were used for HLA typing (Santamaria et al., 1994). Further, the incidence and severity tend to increase with increasing HLA mismatch, except in very young patients, in whom a one HLA locus mismatch can be tolerated (Davies et al., 1995).

It must be also considered, however, that bone marrow transplant is a case apart in general tissue transplantation since drastic immunosuppressive regimens cannot be applied as they are for any other type of organ to be transplanted. For solid organs, immunosuppressive therapy is necessary to prevent graft rejection even when donor and recipient are HLA-identical siblings. It is the effectiveness of the immunosuppressive therapy that permits the survival, often for many years, of allogeneic grafts, many of which are poorly HLA matched. There is an abundance of data that show little or no difference between well-matched and poorly matched grafts as measured by one-year survival (Starzl et al., 1993a). These considerations added to the need for transplantation in a relatively short amount of time for the most severely diseased patients, and to the limited number of donor organs available, has led many to propose that organ allocation should be governed primarily by criteria other than HLA matching (Starzl et al., 1993b). This discussion is particularly "hot" these days (Stolberg, 1999a,b,c). However, if we consider a longer time of transplanted organ survival, we can see how HLA matching of donors and recipients may actually have a relevant effect. In 1992, Terasaki and colleagues developed logarithmic plots predicting 10-year rates of graft survival and rates of loss in organ half-life. They compared these predictions with actual graft survival of transplants done from 1975 to 1980. Their half-life actuarial estimate of 16,320 first cadaveric kidney grafts from the United Network for Organ Sharing (UNOS) registry was 10.3 years. From the 1975–1980 actual 10-year survival data, they calculated a half-life of 24.0 years when the donor was an HLA-identical sibling, 11.8 with a parental donor, and 7.9 with a cadaveric donor. When the cadaveric donor grafts were evaluated by HLA matching, the half-life was 19.7 for no A, B, DR mismatch (or 6 antigens match), and 7.5 years for complete mismatches. However, the estimated half-life was similar for one, two, three, four, and five mismatches. All other variables analyzed did not make any difference, including race, sex, original disease, and other non-histocompatibility factors. Based on their conclusion that "HLA matching is the single most important factor that can improve nationwide 10-year graft survival rates," the equitable system of organ allocation approved by UNOS was the following: the priority system adopted for non-renal patients included the length of time a patient has been on the waiting list, the severity of his or her illness, and the proximity of the available organ to the patient. For kidney allocation, the degree of HLA matching and the degree of HLA presensitization (i.e., PRA values or presence of antibodies against donor HLA specificities) were added to the above criteria (Wujciak and Opelz, 1997). UNOS has also mandated national sharing of perfect HLA matches, irrespective of other criteria. The probability for a kidney patient to find a perfect match anywhere is, however, no more than 5%.

The results recently presented by Opelz and collaborators (1997 and 1998) relative to the cumulative results from various European transplant centers seem to confirm the appropriateness of these criteria. Starzl, Terasaki and collaborators (Starzl et al., 1997) using more recently updated results obtained from UNOS registry have also proven the importance of perfect HLA matching for kidney transplants, although the negative effect of mismatches seems to be the same for more than 1 or all the six alleles

and limited to a small percentage even in a ten-year survival analysis (Fig. 43.12). This is the reason why all kidney patients are still typed for HLA and ABO blood groups before entry on the waiting list and their sera screened for anti-HLA antibodies.

DNA methodologies for HLA typing have shown that unrelated donors who appeared HLA-identical by serology are indeed not matched at the DNA level, and that DNA-matched pairs survive much better. More recent studies using DNA methods for both class I and class II typing have shown that molecular matching may reduce the risks of acute GVHD and patient mortality (Speiser et al., 1996).

The likelihood of finding a matched donor in the registries also depends on whether the patient has a common or rare HLA genotype. Not only are some alleles more common or rare within a particular ethnic or racial group, but because of linkage disequilibrium, certain alleles can give rise to different haplotypes within different populations. NMDP is making an extraordinary effort to enroll in its registry and HLA type by DNA different minority groups so as to increase the likelihood that minority patients requiring any type of transplant, particularly of kidney or bone marrow, can find a more suitable HLA-matched donor.

Even considering all the possible genotypically-identical sibs as donors and the large number of potential donors enrolled in the NMDP registry, a substantial number of patients will not be able to find an HLA-matched donor. Also, as new loci and alleles are discovered that potentially must be matched, the odds of finding a complete match will decrease even further. Therefore, the most important charge for those involved in bone marrow transplantation is a more precise definition of HLA mismatches that are clinically permissible versus those that are functionally significant with respect to rejection, GVHD and overall patient mortality.

The transplantation of organs other than bone marrow or kidney affords, a completely different scenario. Patients are routinely transplanted on the basis of their clinical condition and undergo transplant as soon as an organ becomes available. The HLA typing is generally performed *a posteriori* and the presence of reacting antibodies in the recipient only used to modify the immunosuppressive regimen. The possibility to successfully transplant the liver across the histocompatibility barriers seems to be due to the intrinsic characteristics of human organs (Yagihashi et al., 1992). The liver is able to absorb a large quantity of antibodies without having its function impaired, and the quantity of immunocompetent cells present in the liver at the moment of the transplant is considered by some the possible reason

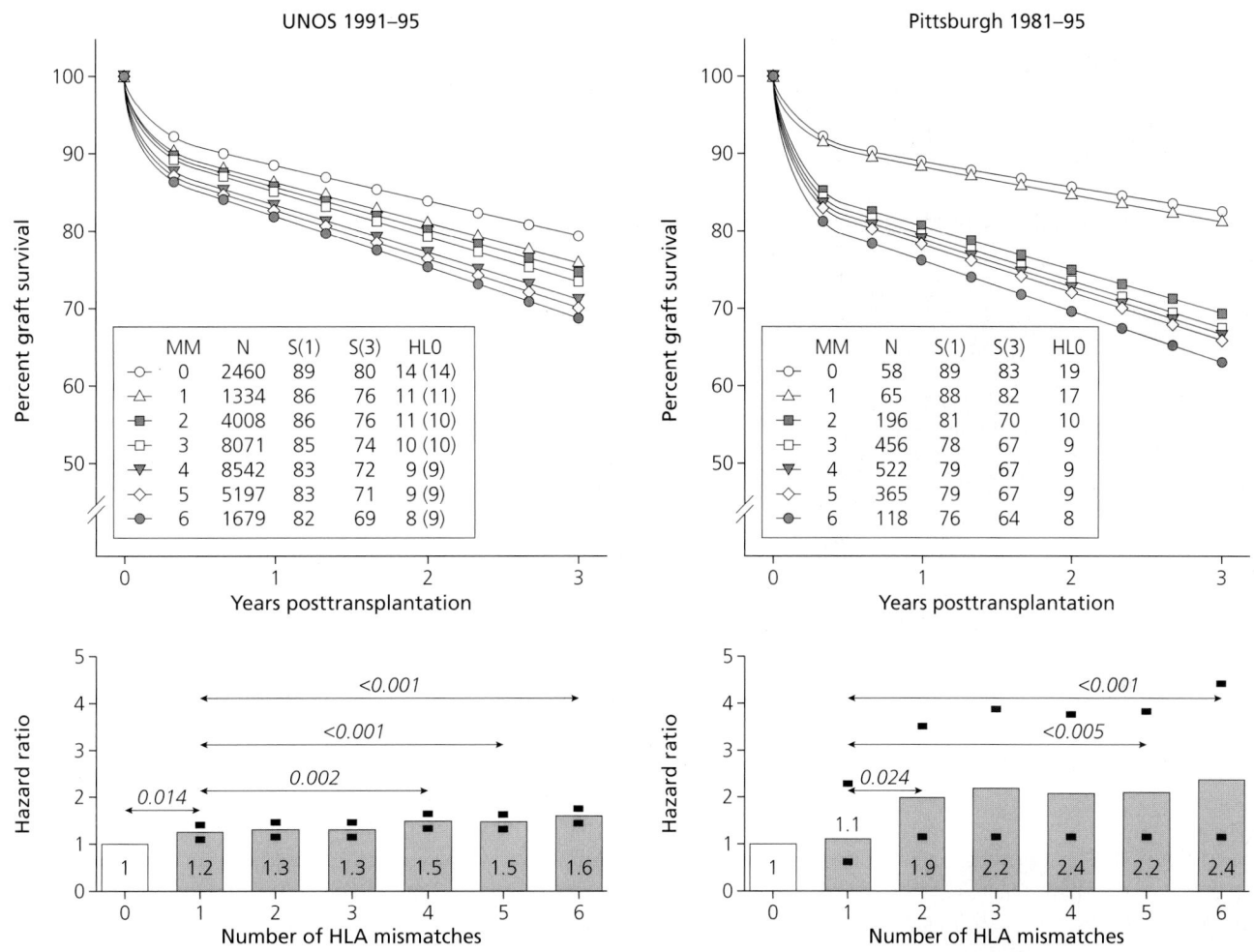

Fig. 43.12. Survival percentages of kidney transplants subdivided by 0 to 6 HLA antigen mismatches (MM): (From Starzl et al, HLA and cross-reactive antigen group matching for cadaver kidney allocation. *Transplantation*, 64:983–987, 1997. © Lippincott Williams & Wilkins.)

for the liver's tolerogenic power. Under the protective umbrella of immunosuppression, immunocompetent stem cells present in the liver are able to migrate into the recipient body where they are not strongly confronted by a drug-impaired immune system of the recipient. In this peculiar context, the immune system of the recipient may become "accustomed" to the presence of immunocompetent cells of the donor so that both systems harmoniously survive in the transplanted individual. This exceptional situation known as *immunologic chimerism* (Fig. 43.13), can offer the invaluable advantage of generating a donor-specific type of tolerance in the recipient that *ipso facto* becomes able to host the foreign tissue without the need of a massive and, in general, particularly dangerous immunosuppressive regimen. These types of considerations were actually supported by the finding of immunocompetent cells of donor origin in the tissues (e.g., skin) or in the blood of patients who received a liver transplant 30 years before (Starzl et al.,

1992a,b; 1993b,c). In different proportions, a certain degree of immunologic chimerism, or a "microchimerism", was also found in kidney and heart transplant patients years after transplantation (Starzl et al., 1993). The enthusiasm produced by these incontrovertible findings promoted the implementation of therapeutic protocols aimed at favoring the establishment of immunologic chimerism. One protocol suggested the augmentation of immunocompetent cells obtainable by co-transplanting with a solid organ not generally rich in these cells (like the heart or the kidney) bone marrow cells from the same donor (Fontes et al., 1994). Although this therapeutical intervention did not cause any appreciable harm to the recipient, the benefits associated with the procedure were not easy to define in terms of graft survival. Quality of cells, quantity of cells, time of administration, and prolongation of chimeric status were all considered variables that supported the suspicion of improved results, but did not offer any unquestionable and tangible

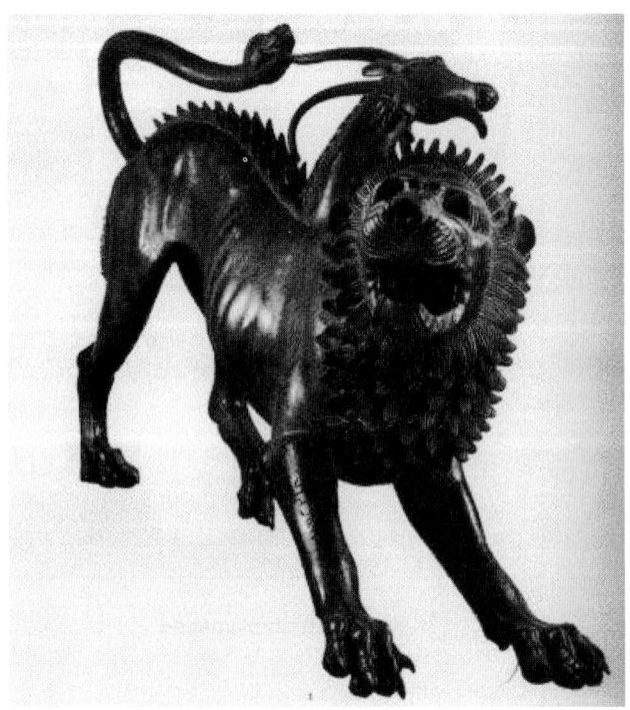

A

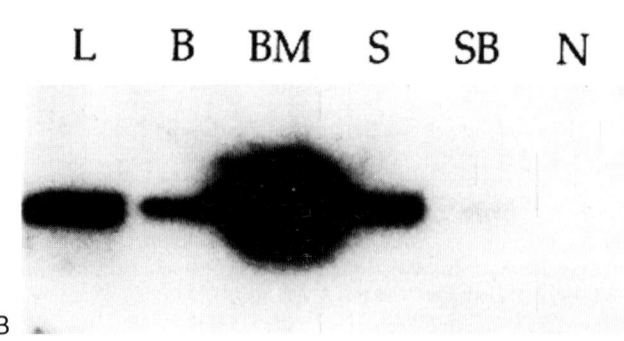

L   B   BM   S   SB   N

B

Fig. 43.13. Artistic representation of a chimera from the Greek mythology and evidence of an immunologic chimera in a patient with Gaucher's disease. In A, Khimaira, also spelled in the Latin Chimera, was a powerful beast with the head of a male lion, the body of a goat, and as a tail, a serpent. The legend states that she was slain by Bellerophon with a golden arrow, while he rode on the back of Pegasus, a horse with wings. The Chimera of Arezzo is conserved at the Archaeologic Museum in Florence, Italy. In B, Genomic DNA was extracted from the recipient's tissues and amplified with HLA-DR beta-chain "generic" oligonucleotide primers to determine the subgroup of the donor's alleles. "Specific" primers were then used to amplify the alleles selectively. The alleles were identified by hybridizing the amplified DNA to radiolabeled allele-specific probes. HLA-DR1 was only present in the donor. After HLA-DR1-specific amplification of DNA from the liver (L), blood (B), bone marrow (BM), skin (S), and small bowel (SB) of the recipient, the DNA was separated by electrophoresis on an agarose gel and then analyzed by Southern blotting. The denatured DNA present on the nylon membrane was hybridized to a labeled HLA-DR1 (donor)-specific oligonucleotide probe. For liver DNA, the quantity analyzed was reduced to 1 percent of the other samples. Although lower in intensity, the signal from donor DNA in the small bowel was clearly positive in the original film, although this can be seen here only faintly. The negative control was a reaction run without DNA (last lane; N=Negative control). (From Starzl et al, N Engl J Med 328:745–749, 1993 © 1993 Massachusetts Medical Society. All rights reserved.)

parameters to quantitate this sense of improvement (Schlitt et al., 1993a,b; Rudert et al., 1994; Suberbiele et al., 1994; Hisanga et al., 1996; Wood and Sachs, 1996).

A more drastic but also theoretically valid alternative is the one originally proposed by Ildstad and Sachs (1984), and more recently revamped (Bracy et al., 1998), that considers the radiologic ablation of the recipient bone marrow followed by the transplant of mature-T-cell-free mixture of recipient and donor bone marrow cells. In the mouse, the simultaneous presence of the two immunologic systems, even from individuals with different histocompatibility phenotypes, allows the immunologic reconstitution of the recipient by both types of cells together. The established chimerism is in this case quite stronger in percentage of donor versus recipient cells than the one obtainable by bone marrow augmentation. Once proven durable, this chimerism permits the acceptance of any organ coming from the same donor. This approach has even been proposed to set the basis for possible xenotransplantation (Bracy et al., 1998). However, the risks involved in treating the recipient with a potentially lethal preparative regimen have so far precluded any application of this type of protocol in humans, but may constitute a very valuable tool in the future.

While all of these approaches are designed to bypass the limitations imposed by genotypic differences between donor and recipient, a somewhat revolutionary alternative has recently been offered. Pluripotent stem cells can be found in different tissues of an individual, and they are able to replace differentiated cells of different organs. For example, stem cells isolated from the bone marrow were able to replace malfunctioning myocytes in a mouse model of Duchenne muscular dystrophy (Gussoni et al., 1999). Furthermore, stem cells isolated from muscle tissue and possessing a slightly different phenotype than the bone marrow precursors, were not only able to replace diseased myocytes, but also replace the bone marrow precursors in a syngeneic recipient. Apart from ethical considerations that pertain to this type of experimentation, the stem cell avenue seems to be the most promising and exciting approach to autologous, as well as allogeneic, transplantations.

Conclusion

The data presented clearly show that HLA matching does not and cannot influence solid organ distribution. However, these analyses support the wisdom of the UNOS Board of Directors to mandate national sharing of the serologically perfectly matched HLA cadaveric donor kidneys in the rare cases where they occur. HLA matching for other solid organ grafts is even more problematic because the patients needing livers or thoracic organs are generally critically ill and cannot tolerate extensive waiting periods. The recent success in transplanting a single lobe of the lung or liver from alive or cadaveric donors into one or more recipients, respectively, may expand these limited chances. On average only about 30% of candidates for bone marrow transplantation will have an HLA-identical sibling or other related donor. Leukemia is the most common indication for BMT. Survival and cure rates for acute nonlymphocytic leukemics are almost as great following autologous BMT as for HLA-identical sib BMT. This is not the case for acute lymphocytic leukemia patients, however. Unfortunately, those patients with uncommon HLA phenotypes will not survive a lengthy search for an unrelated donor. At the present time few patients with chronic lymphocytic leukemia are considered candidates for bone marrow transplant; therefore, the NMDP and other registries of unrelated donors benefit primarily patients with chronic myelogenous leukemia (CML). Thus far, the outcome of unrelated transplants for CML has been poor because of HLA mismatching not detected by serologic and cellular assays. It is anticipated that improvement will be seen now that typing by DNA-based methods for class II are in place. Once this is accomplished, the next major effort for the future will be to identify which minor differences between variants can be tolerated with little or no risk of rejection or GVHD, or which tolerogenic protocol can offer safe but effective means to allow transplants across HLA boundaries or even across different species without the need for massive immunosuppression.

REFERENCES

Anasetti C, Amos D, Beatty PG et al. (1989) Effect of HLA compatibility on engraftment of bone marrow transplants in patients with leukemia or lymphoma. N Eng J Med 320:197–204

Bach FH, Albertini RJ, Amos DB et al. (1969) Mixed leukocyte culture studies in families with known HL-A genotypes. Transplantation Proc 1:339–341

Beatty PG, Anasetti C, Hansen JA et al. (1993) Marrow transplantation from unrelated donors for treatment of hematologic malignancies: Effect of mismatching for one HLA locus. Blood 81:249–253

Bevan MJ (1975) The major histocompatibility complex determines susceptibility to cytotoxic T cells directed against minor histocompatibility antigens. J Exper Med 142:1349–1364

Bias WB, Pollard K, Pardo S (1980) Preliminary studies of 31 antisera that identify non-HLA histocompatibility antigens. In Gale RP, Fox CF (eds): Biology of Bone Marrow Transplantation. Academic Press, NY, pp. 553–562

Bjorkman P, Saper M, Samraoui W et al. (1987a) Structure of the human class I histocompatibility antigen, HLA-A2. Nature 329:506–512

Bjorkman P, Saper M, Samraoui B et al. (1987b) The foreign antigen binding site and T cell recognition regions of class I histocompatibility antigens. Nature 329:512–518

Bodmer WF (1972) Population genetics of the HL-A system: Retrospect and prospect. In Dausset J, Colombani J (eds): Munksgaard, Copenhagen, p. 611

Bodmer WF (1992) HLA 1991. In Tsugi K, Aizawa M, Sasazuki T (eds): HLA 1991: Proceedings of the Eleventh International Histocompatibility Workshop and Conference. Oxford Science, UK, p 7

Bodmer J, Yound D, Jones E et al. (1977) Serological characterization of human Ia antigens using B cell lymphoid lines. Transplantation Proc 9:121–126

Bracy JL, Sachs DH, Iacomini J (1998) Inhibition of xenoreactive natural antibody production by retroviral gene therapy. Science 281:1845–1847

Browning MJ, Krausa P, Rowan A et al. (1993) Tissue typing the HLA-A locus from genomic DNA by sequence-specific PCR: Comparison of HLA genotype and surface expression on colorectal tumor cell lines. Proc Nat Ac Sci USA 90:2842–2845

Bunce M, Welsh KI (1994) Rapid DNA typing for HLA-C using sequence-specific primers (PCR-SSP): Identification of serological and non-serologically defined HLA-C alleles including several new alleles. Tissue Antigens 43:7–17

Campbell RD, Trowsdale J (1993) Map of the human MHC. Immunology Today 14:349–352

Carlsson B, Wallin J, Bohme J, Moller E (1987) HLA-DR-DQ haplotypes defined by restriction fragment length analysis: Correlation to serology. Hum Immunology 20:95–113

Cascino I, Rosenshire S, Turco E et al. (1986) Relationship between DQ alpha and DQ beta RFLP and serologically defined class II HLA antigens. J Immunogenet 13:387–400

Ceppellini R, Curtoni ES, Mattiuz PL et al. (1967) Genetics of leukocyte antigens: a family study of segregation and linkage. In Curtoni ES, Mattiuz PL, Tosi R (eds): Histocompatibility Testing Munksgaard, Copenhagen pp. 149–187

Ceppellini R, Connard GD, Coppo F et al. (1971) Transplantation antigens: Introductory symposium. Mixed leukocyte cultures and HL-A antigens. I. Reactivity of young fetuses, newborns and mothers at delivery. Transplantation Proc 3:58–63

Chia D, Terasaki P, Chan H et al. (1993) Direct detection of PCR products for HLA class II typing. Tissue Antigens 42:146–149

Dausset J (1958) Iso-leuco-anticorps. Acta Haematology 20:156–166

Davies SM, Shu XO, Blazar BR et al. (1995) Unrelated donor bone marrow transplantation:influence of HLA A and B incompatibility on outcome. Blood 86:1636–1642

Davis MM, Bjorkman PJ (1988) T-cell antigen receptor genes and T-cell recognition. Nature 334:395–402

Dormoy A, Urlacher A, Tongio MM (1992) Complexity of the HLA-DP region: RFLP analysis versus PLT typing and oligotyping. Hum Immunology 34:39–46

Dupont B, Yang SY (1994) Histocompatibility. In Forman S, Blume K, Thomas ED (eds): Bone Marrow Transplantation. Blackwell Science Publishing, chapter 4, pp. 22–40

Eisvoogel VP, van Rood JJ, du Toit ED, Schelekens PTA (1972) Position of a locus determining mixed lymphocyte reaction distinct from the known HLA loci. Euro Immunology 2:413–418

Faas SJ, Menon R, Braun ER et al. (1996) Sequence-specific priming and exonuclease-released fluorescence detection of HLA-DQB1 alleles. Tissue Antigens 48:97–112

Fleischhauer K, Kernan NA, O'Reilly R et al. (1990). Bone marrow-allograft rejection by T lymphocytes recognizing a single amino acid difference in HLA-B44. N Eng J Med 323:1818–1822

Fontes P, Rao A, Demetris AJ et al. (1994) Bone marrow augmentation of donor-cell chimerism in kidney, liver, heart, and pancreas islet transplantation. Lancet 344:151–155

Giorda R, Lampasona V, Kocova M, Trucco M (1993) Non-radioisotopic typing of human leukocyte antigen class II genes on microplates. Bio Techniques 15:918–925

Gorer PA (1937) The genetic and antigenic basis of tumor transplantation. J Pathology Bacteriology 44:691–697

Gorer PA (1938) The antigenic basis of tumor transplantation. J Pathology and Bacteriological Pathology 47:231–252

Gorer PA, Lyman S, Snell GD (1948) Studies of the genetic and antigenic basis of tumor transplantation: linkage between a histocompatibility gene and "fused" in mice. Proc R Soc Lond Ser B 135:499–505

Goulmy E (1988) Minor histocompatibility antigens in man and their role in transplantation. Transplantation Reviews 2:29–53

Goulmy E, Schipper R, Pool J et al. (1996) Mismatches of minor histocompatibility antigens between HLA-identical donors and recipients and the development of graft-versus-host disease after bone marrow transplantation. N Eng J Med 334:281–285

Grey HM, Kubo RT, Colon SM et al. (1973) The small subunit of HLA antigens is beta-2 microglobulin. J Experimental Medicine 138:1608–1612

Guo Z, Hood L, Peterdorf EW (1999) Oligonucleotide arrays for high resolution HLA typine. Reviews in Immunogenetics 1:220–230

Gussoni E, Soneoka Y, Strickland C et al. (1999) Dystrophin expression in the *mdx* mouse restored by stem cell transplantation. Nature 401:390–394

Hisanaga M, Hundrieser J, Boker K et al. (1996) Development, stability and clinical correlations of allogeneic microchimerism after solid organ transplantation. Transplantation 61:40–45

Holland PM, Abramson RD, Waton R, Gelfand DH (1991) Detection of specific polymerase chain reaction product by utilizing the 5′ to 3′ exonuclease activity of Thermus aquaticus DNA polymerase. Proc Nat Ac Sci 88:7276–7280

Hopkins KA, Vogelsang GB, Delaney NL et al. (1989) Implication of a gene distal to HLA-A in the etiology of graft-versus-host disease. Transplantation Proc 21:2971–2973

Hsia S, Tong JY, Parris GL et al. (1993) Molecular compatibility and renal graft survival: the HLA DRB1 genotyping. Transplantation 55:395–399

Hsu SH, Chan MM, Bias WB (1981) Genetic control of MHC linked immune responses to synthetic polypeptides in man. Proc Nat Ac Sc USA 78:440–444

Ildstad ST, Sachs DH (1984) Reconstitution with syngeneic plus allogeneic or xenogeneic bone marrow leads to specific acceptance of allografts or xenografts. Nature 307:168–170

Jorgensen PAR, Ehrich EW, Davis MM (1992) Molecular components of T-cell recognition. Annual Reviews in Immunology 10:835, 1992

Krausa P, Bodmer JG, Browning MJ (1993) Defining the common subtypes of HLA A9, A10, A28 and A19 by use of ARMS/PCR. Tissue Antigens 42:91–99

Kernan NA, Bartsch G, Ash RC et al. (1993) Analysis of 462 transplantations from unrelated donors facilitated by the National Marrow Donor Program. N Eng J Med 328:593–602

Klein J (1971) Private and public antigens of the mouse H-2 system. Nature 229:635–637

Klein J (1975) Biology of the Mouse H-2 Complex. Springer-Verlag, NY

Klein J (1986) Natural history of the Major Histocompatibility Complex. Wiley-Interscience, NY

Kurtzberg J, Laughlin M, Graham ML et al. (1996) Placental blood as a source of hematopoietic stem cells for transplantation into unrelated recipients. N Eng J Med 335:157–166

Lee KW, Johnson AH, Hurley CK (1990) Two divergent routes of evolution gave rise to the DRw13 haplotypes. J Immunology 145:3119–3125

Majno G (1975) The Healing Hand. Man and Wound in the Ancient World. Harvard University Press, Cambridge, MA, pp. 261–312

Marsh SG (1999) Nomenclature for factors of the HLA system, update March 1999. WHO Nomenclature Committee for factors of the HLA system. Human Immunology 60:627

Medawar PB (1944) The behavior and fate of skin autografts and skin homografts in rabbits. J Anat 78:176–280

Medawar PB (1958) The homograft reaction. Proc Roy Soc Lond Ser B 148:145–166

Menon R, Rudert WA, Faas SJ et al. (1997) HLA-A molecular typing by SSPERF. Molecular Diagnosis 2:99–111

Meo T, Vives J, Miggiano V, Shreffler D (1973) A major role for the lr-1 region of the mouse H-2 complex in the mixed leukocyte reaction. Transplantation Proc 5:377–381

Merrill JP, Murray JE, Harrison JH et al. (1956) Successful homotransplantation of the human kidney between identical twins. JAMA 160:277–282

Merrill JP (1978) Transplantation immunology 1957–1975. Annals of Immunology 129:347–352

Mickelson EM, Bartsch GE, Hansen JA, Dupont B (1993) The MLC assay as a test for HLA-D region compatibility between patients and unrelated donors: Results of a National Marrow Donor Program involving multiple centers. Tissue Antigens 42:465–472

Morel P, Dorman J, Todd J et al. (1988) Aspartic acid at position 57 of the HLA DQ-beta chain protects against type I diabetes: A family study. Proc Nat Ac Sci USA 85:8111–8115

Mori M, Beatty PG, Graves M et al. (1997) HLA gene and haplotype frequencies in the North American population: The National Marrow Donor Program Donor Registry. Transplantation 64:1017–1027

Mosmann TR, Cherwinski H, Bond MW et al. (1986) Two types of murine helper T cell clones. I. Definition according to profiles of lymphokine activities and secreted proteins. Journal of Immunology 136:2348–2357

Mullis KB, Faloona FA (1987) Specific synthesis of DNA *in vitro* via a polymerase-catalyzed chain reaction. In Diego RW (ed): Methods in Enzymology, Academic Press, San Diego, CA, p. 335

Murasko DM (1978) Apparent lack of H-2 restriction of allograft rejection. Journal of Immunology 121:958–961

Murata M, Haneda M, Nishida T et al. (1998) Unrelated donor bone marrow transplantation in Japanese patients facilitated by the National Marrow Donor Program of the United States. Transplantation Proc 30:150–152

Nademanee A, Schmidt GM, Parker P et al. (1995) The outcome of matched unrelated donor bone marrow transplantation in patients with hematologic malignancies using molecular typing for donor selection and graft-versus-host disease prophylaxis regimen of cyclosporine, methotrexate, and prednisone. Blood 86:1228–1234

Newton CR, Graham A, Heptinstall LE et al. (1989) Analysis of any point mutation in DNA. The amplification refractory mutation system (ARMS). Nucleic Acids Research 17:2503–2516

Olerup O, Zetterquist H (1992) HLA-DR typing by PCR amplification with sequence-specific primers (PCR-SSP) in 2 hours: An alternative to serological DR typing in clinical practice including donor-recipient matching in cadaveric transplantation. Tissue Antigens 39:225–235

Olerup O, Aldener A, Fogdell A (1993) HLA-DQB1 and -DQA1 typing by PCR amplification with sequence-specific primers (PCR-SSP) in 2 hours. Tissue Antigens 41:119–134

Opelz G (1997) Impact of HLA compatibility on survival of kidney transplants from unrelated live donors. Transplantation 64:1473–1475

Opelz G (1998) HLA compatibility and kidney grafts from unrelated live donors. Collaborative Transplant Study. Transplantation Proc 30:704–705

Parkman R, Rosen FS, Rappeport J et al. (1976) Detection of genetically determined histocompatibility antigen differences between HLA identical and MLC nonreactive siblings. Transplantation 21:110–116

Payne R, Rolfs MR (1958) Fetomaternal leukocyte incompatibility. J Clin Invest 37:1756–1763

Payne R, Bodmer WF, Troup GM, Walford RL (1967) Serologic activities and specificities of eleven human leukocyte antisera produced by planned immunization. Transplantation 5:597–605

Pazmany L, Mandelboim O, Vales-Gomez M et al. (1996) Protection from natural killer cell-mediated lysis by HLA-G expression on target cells. Science 274:792–795

Reinsmoen NL, Kersey JH, Bach FH (1984) Detection of HLA restricted anti-minor histocompatibility antigens reactive cells from skin GVHD lesions. Human Immunology 11:249–257

Romagnani S (1992) Induction of Th21 and Th2 responses: A key role for the "natural" immune respone? Immunology Today 13:379–381

Rossini A, Greiner D, Mordes J (1999) Induction of immunologic tolerance for transplantation. Physiology Reviews 79:99–141

Rotzschke O, Falk K, Wallny HJ et al. (1990) Characterization of naturally occurring minor histocompatibility peptides including H-4 and H-Y. Science 249:283–287

Rudert WA, Trucco M (1990) DNA polymers of protein binding sequences generated by PCR. Nucleic Acid Research 18:6460

Rudert WA, Trucco M (1992) Rapid detection of sequence variations using polymers of specific oligonucleotides. Nucleic Acid Research 20:1146

Rudert WA, Kocova M, Rao A, Trucco M (1994) Fine quantitation by competitive PCR of circulating donor cells in post-transplant chimeric recipients. Transplantation 58:964–965

Rudert WA, Braun ER, Faas SJ et al. (1997) Strategies for synthesis of double-labeled fluorescent oligonucleotide probes for 5′ nuclease assay. Bio Techniques 22:1140–1145

Sadler AM, Petronzelli F, Krausa P et al. (1994) Low-resolution DNA typing for HLA-B using sequence-specific primers in allele-or group-specific ARMS/PCR. Tissue Antigens 44:148–154

Saiki RK, Gelfand OH, Stoffel S et al. (1988) Primer-directed enzymatic amplificiation of DNA with a thermostable DNA polymerase. Science 239:487–491

Saiki RK, Walsh PS, Levenson CH, Erlich HA (1989) Genetic analysis of amplified DNA with immobilized sequence-specific oligonulceotide probes. Proc Nat Ac Sci USA 86:6230–6234

Santamaria P, Reinsmoen NL, Lindstrom AL et al. (1994) Frequent HLA class I and DP sequence mismatches in serologically (HLA-A, HLA-B, HLA-DR) and molecularly (HLA-DRB1, HLA-DQA1, HLA-DQB1) HLA-identical unrelated bone marrow transplant pairs. Blood 83:280–287

Santos GW, Hess AD, Vogelsang GB (1985) Graft-versus-host reactions and disease. Immunology Reviews 88:169–192

Schlitt HJ, Raddatz G, Steinhoff G et al. (1993) Passenger lymphocytes in human liver allografts and their potential role after transplantation. Transplantation 56:951–955

Schlitt HJ, Hundrieser J, Ringe B, Pichlmayr R (1994) Donor-type microchimerism associated with graft rejection eight years after liver transplantation (letter). N Eng J Med 330:646–647

Schlitt HJ, Hundrieser J, Hisanaga M et al. (1994) Patterns of donor-type microchimerism after heart transplantation. Lancet 343:1469–1471

Silverstein AM (1988) A History of Immunology. Academic Press, San Diego, CA, p 1–422

Snell GD (1948) Methods for the study of histocompatibility genes. J Genet 49:87–103

Snell GD, Wheeler N, Aaron M (1957) A new method of typing inbred strains of mice for histocompatibility antigens. Transplant Bull 4:18–21

Speiser DE, Tiercy J-M, Rufer N et al. (1996) High resolution HLA matching associated with decreased mortality after unrelated bone marrow transplantation. Blood 87:4455–4462

Starzl TE, Demetris AJ, Murase N et al. (1992a) Cell migration, chimerism, and graft acceptance. Lancet 339:1579–1582

Starzl TE, Demetris AJ, Trucco M et al. (1992b) Systemic chimerism in human female recipients of male livers. Lancet 340:876–877

Starzl TE, Demetris AJ, Trucco M et al. (1993) Chimerism after liver tranplantation for type IV glycogen storage disease and type I Gaucher's disease. N Eng J Med 328:745–749

Starzl TE, Demetris AJ, Trucco M et al. (1993a) Cell migration and chimerism after whole organ transplantation: The basis of graft acceptance. Hepatology 17:1127–1152

Starzl TE, Trucco M, Rao A, Demetris A (1993b) The role of HLA typing in clinical kidney transplants: 30 years later. The blind-folding of HLA matching (editorial). Clinic Transplants 7:423–425

Starzl TE, Eliasziw M, Gjerston D et al. (1997) HLA and cross-reactive antigen group matching for cadaver kidney allocation. Transplantation 64:983–991

Stolberg SG (1999a) Agreement on plan to revamp organ distribution. New York Times, November 12

Stolberg SG (1999b) Deal to revamp organ allocation is at risk. New York Times, November 19

Stolberg SG (1999c) Iowa turf war over transplants mirrors feuds across the nation. New York Times, December 29

Suberbiele C, Caillat-Zucman S, Legendre C et al. (1994) Peripheral microchimerism in long-term cadveric-kidney allograft recipients. Lancet 343:1468–1469

Takasugi M, Sengar DP, Terasaki PI (1971) Microassays in transplantation immunology. American Journal of Medical Technology 37:470–472

Tekolf WA, Shaw S (1983) In vitro generation of cytotoxic cells specific for human minor histocompatibility antigens by lymphocytes from a normal donor potentially primed during pregnancy. J Ex Med 157:2172–2177

Terasaki PI, Cecka JM, Gjertson DW et al. (1992) A ten-year prediction for kidney transplant survival. In Terasaki PI, Cecka JM (eds): Clinical Transplants. UCLA Tissue Typing Laboratory, Los Angeles, pp. 501–512

Todd JA, Bell JI, McDevitt HO (1987) HLA-DQ-beta gene contributes to susceptibility and resistance to insulin-dependent diabetes mellitus. Nature 329:559–604

Tong JY, Hsia S, Parris GL et al. (1993) Molecular compatibility and renal graft survival: the HLA DQB1 genotyping. Transplantation 55:390–395

Tony HP, Parker DC (1985) Major histocompatibility complex-restricted, polyclonal B cell responses resulting from helper T cell recognition of anti-immunoglobulin presented by small B lymphocytes. J Ex Med 161:223–241

Trucco M, Stocker JW, and Ceppellini R (1978) Monoclonal antibodies against human lymphocyte antigens. Nature 273:666–668

Trucco M, Garotta G, Stocker JW and Ceppellini R (1979) Murine monoclonal antibodies against HLA structures. Immunological Reviews 47:219–252

Trucco M, Ball E (1987) RFLP analysis of DQ-beta chain gene: Workshop report. In Histocompatibility Testing 1987. Vol. 1:1989:860

Trucco G, Fritsch R, Giorda R, Trucco M (1989) Rapid detection of IDDM susceptibility, using amino acid 57 of the HLA-DQ beta chain as a marker. Diabetes 38:1617–1622

Turco E, Fritsch R and Trucco M (1990) Use of immunologic techniques in gene analysis. In Herberman R, Mercer DW (eds): Immunodiagnosis of Cancer, 2nd edn, 53:205

van Els CACM, D'Amaro J, Pool J et al. (1992) Immunogenetics of human minor histocompatibility antigens: their polymorphism and immunodominance. Immunogenet 35:161–165

Vinci G, Masset M, Semana G, Vernant JP (1994) A human minor histocompatibility antigen which appears to segregate with the major histocompatibility complex. Transplantation 58:361–367

Voogt PJ, Goulmy E, Veenhof WFJ et al. (1988) Cellularly defined minor histocompatibility antigens are differentially expressed on human hematopoietic progenitor cells. J Ex Med 168:2337–2347

Walker T (1999) The national marrow donor program. Minnesota Med 82:26–28

Weiss A (1993) T cell antigen receptor signal transduction: a tale of tails and cytoplasmic protein-tyrosine kinases. Cell 73:209–212

Wood K, Sachs DH (1996) Chimerism and transplantation tolerance: cause and effect. Immunol Today 17:584–588

Wright J (1898) The nose and throat in medical history. Published privately

Wujciak T, Opelz G (1997) Matchability as an important factor for kidney allocation according to the HLA match. Transplantation Proceedings 29:1403–1405

Yagihashi A, Kobayashi M, Noguchi K et al. (1992) HLA matching effect in liver transplantation. Transplantation Proceedings 24:2432–2433

Yamamoto M, Sugihara K, Ohtsuki F et al. (1994) Generation of self HLA-DR-specific CD3+CD4-CD8+ cytotoxic T cells in chronic graft-versus-host disease. Bone Marrow Transplantation 14:525–533

Yancey AK, Coppo P, Kawanishi Y (1997) Progress in availability of donors of color: The National Marrow Donor Program. Transplantation Proc 29:3760–3765

Zemmour J, Gumperz JE, Hildebrand WH et al. (1992) The molecular basis for reactivity of anti-Cw1 and anti-Cw3 alloantisera with HLA-B46 haplotypes. Tissue Antigens 39:249–257

Zier KS, Elkins WL, Pierson GR, Leo MM (1983) The use of cytotoxic T cell lines to detect the segregation of a human minor alloantigen within families. Hum Immunol 7:117–129

APPROACHES TO SPECIFIC DISORDERS

- Chromosomal disorders
- Cardiovascular disorders
- Respiratory disorders
- Renal disorders
- Gastrointestinal disorders
- Hematologic disorders
- Immunologic disorders
- Endocrinologic disorders
- Metabolic disorders
- Mental and behavioral disorders
- Neurologic disorders
- Neuromuscular disorders
- Ophthalmologic disorders
- Deafness
- Craniofacial disorders
- Dermatologic disorders
- Connective tissue disorders
- Skeletal disorders

Chromosomal disorders

Down syndrome and other autosomal trisomies

44

John L. Tolmie

Introduction

This chapter discusses the common autosomal trisomy syndromes that affect livebirths, namely trisomy for chromosome 21, 18, and 13. It also considers genetic counseling aspects of other autosomal trisomies and mosaic autosomal trisomies that present following prenatal cytogenetic diagnosis.

Concerning trisomy 21 Down syndrome, in the past five years most articles published in the medical literature have dealt with aspects of prenatal screening for trisomy 21. This topic is now reviewed in Chapter 28. The year 2000 has seen publication of the DNA sequence of chromosome 21, followed by the determination of DNA sequences of the other human chromosomes. This huge advance was preceded by excellent progress in the detailed early maps of chromosome 21 and the development of trisomy 16 mouse models for Down syndrome. Chromosome 21 DNA sequence data and creation of mice models to investigate Down syndrome phenotype and molecular genetics bode well for the future research. Progress in understanding how autosomal trisomies arise, the mechanisms of chromosome nondisjunction, has been slower, although the important role of chromosome recombination has become clearer.

Autosomal trisomies: rates and survival

RATES IN SPONTANEOUS ABORTIONS AND PRENATAL DIAGNOSIS

Although the cumulative birth rates of trisomy 21, 18, and 13 are considerably less than 1 in 100, in large series of spontaneously aborted pregnancies that have been karyo-typed, autosomal trisomy was identified in 20% of cases and comprised the most common type of chromosomal abnormality (Hassold and Jacobs, 1984; Warburton et al., 1991). Trisomy for every chromosome except chromosome 1 has been reported although trisomy 1 has only ever been found in an early embryo after in vitro fertilization (Watt et al., 1987). Even double autosomal trisomies occur at appreciable frequency in spontaneous abortions (Reddy, 1997) although much less commonly in newborns (Hecht et al., 1969), underlining the predominant embryonic lethal effect of autosomal aneuploidy. Liveborn, affected infants trisomic for chromosome 21, 18, or 13 constitute a tiny minority of all trisomic conceptions, the vast majority of which are nonviable.

Cytogenetic surveys of human gametes have revealed 10% of spermatozoa and 25% of mature oocytes are chromosomally abnormal (Martin et al., 1987; Pellestor, 1991). Aneuploidy accounts for at least 90% of the abnormalities present in oocytes but structural chromosomal aberrations are relatively more common in sperm (Baumgartner et al., 1999). Studies that have examined the karyotype of morphologically normal embryos have found the rate of chromosomal abnormality is correspondingly high, at about 20% (Angell et al., 1988; Plachot et al., 1988). Among untransferred, morphologically poor-quality embryos from an in vitro fertilization program, where cytogenetic analysis was possible, this indicated that 36% of the embryos were aneuploid (Pellestor et al., 1994). Other groups have obtained similar results with newer techniques such as multiple-probe (X, Y, 16, 18) fluorescence in situ hybridization: Munne et al. (1995) found numeric aberrations in 23% and 42%, respectively, of normally and abnormally developing embryos, an observation that is relevant to women undergoing in vitro fertilization since aneuploidy increases with advancing maternal age.

For the three common autosomal trisomies, livebirth rates may be compared with rates observed at amniocentesis and chorionic villus sampling (Fig. 44.1). Hook (1992) calculated that only about 25% of trisomy 21 conceptions, 5% of trisomy 18 conceptions, and 2.5% of trisomy 13 conceptions survive to birth. Most intrauterine deaths occur in early pregnancy and Morris et al. (1999a,b) estimated that the trisomy 21 spontaneous loss rate was 43% after identification at first trimester chorionic villus sampling (CVS) and 23% after identification at second trimester amniocentesis. The methodological difficulties with studies of spontaneous fetal loss rates have been discussed (Cuckle 1999; Snijders, 1999; Morris and Wald, 2000).

Curiously, there are different sex ratios in autosomal aneuploidies. In prenatal life, the Down syndrome M/F ratio is increased at 1.28 whereas in trisomies 18 and 13 the ratio is reduced. In trisomy 18 the ratio (0.65) is even more reduced at term (Ferguson-Smith, 1962), and in trisomy 21, the ratio at birth (1.2) is still greater than the ratio in chromosomally normal infants (1.05). However, in trisomy 21 mosaicism the ratio at birth is less than 1. The origins of these sex ratio differences are unclear (Mutton et al., 1996; Carothers et al., 1999b; Hook et al., 1999).

LIVEBIRTH RATES

Smith and Berg (1976) were able to amass data from 32 previous studies of Down syndrome that, in total, indicated the birth rate was 1 in 700. Summarizing data from 10 independent studies in which newborn infants were unselectively screened for chromosomal abnormalities, Bond and Chandley (1983) concluded that trisomy 21, 18, and 13 had respective incidences in livebirths of 1 in 800, 1 in 10,000, and 1 in 21,000. Hook (1992) reviewed these data and included additional studies to calculate that trisomy 21, 18, and 13 occurs in 1 in 826, 1 in 6666 and 1 in 12,500 live births, respectively.

The maternal-age specific livebirth rates for trisomy 21 are very important in prenatal screening programmes. Hook (2000) noted that recent data from the England and Wales Down Syndrome Register (Huang et al., 1998) gives higher observed rates than the rates predicted by Cuckle et al. (1987) and it is the latter that are currently used in computer programs to calculate risks for Down syndrome in prenatal diagnosis. Many studies have given adjusted Down syndrome rates in different populations, some have been combined, but analyses and comparisons are hampered by differences in accuracy, reporting and methodo-

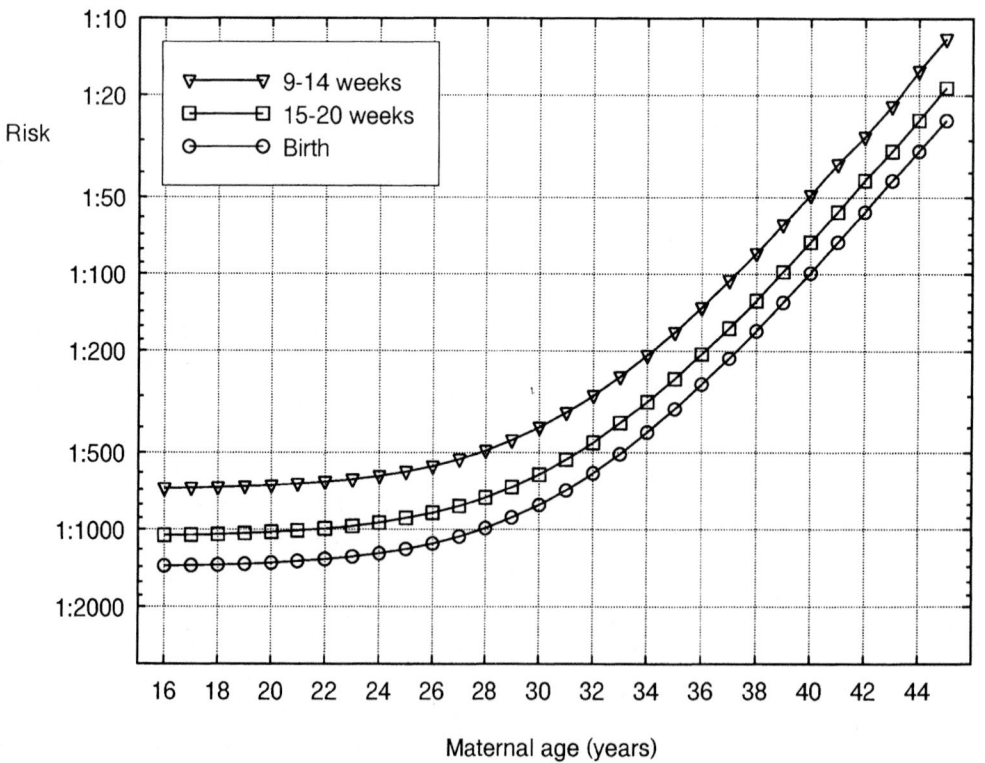

Fig. 44.1. Graphic representation of the odds of viable autosomal trisomy (chromosomes 13, 18, and 21) present at birth, at 15 to 20 weeks gestation and at 9 to 14 weeks gestation. Odds derived from data of Cuckle et al. (1987); Hook et al. (1988), and Snijders et al. (1994), with calculations made as in Zeitune et al. (1991).

logy (Hecht and Hook, 1994; 1996). Thus, Carothers et al. (1999a) examined technical aspects and offered advice on presentation and analysis of data.

Clusters of Down syndrome births have been described but these are difficult to investigate and sophisticated computer techniques have been described (Hook and Carothers, 1997). A remarkable cluster of Down syndrome infants was born to mothers who attended one school in the Irish Republic. This was investigated by Dean et al. (2000) who concluded that chance was the most likely explanation. In England and Wales there was no evidence of space/time clustering in Down syndrome at the level of the district health authority (Morris et al., 1998), and in published studies from different populations there is no evidence of seasonality (Stolwijk et al., 1997).

SURVIVAL OF INFANTS AND ADULTS WITH AUTOSOMAL TRISOMY

Postnatal mortality associated with trisomy 18 and 13 is high and the median survival times of infants with trisomy 13 and 18 are both under one week (Wyllie et al., 1994; Embleton et al., 1996). Fewer than 5% of trisomy 18 and 13 infants survive to one year of age (Goldstein and Nielsen, 1988; Root and Carey, 1994). By contrast, trisomy 21 survival data indicates that over 85% of infants survive to one year of age, 80% survive to age 10 years and more than 50% can expect to live longer than 50 years (Baird and Sadovnick, 1989; Bell et al., 1989; Mikkelsen et al., 1990). Thus, there is greatly improved life expectancy for infants with Down syndrome, but trisomy 13 and 18 remain lethal disorders in infancy.

In Down syndrome, congenital heart disease, often in combination with respiratory tract infections, has been a major cause of mortality in early childhood. Improved survival largely reflects the higher proportion of infants with heart disease who now survive to adulthood, although the combination of cardiac and non-cardiac congenital abnormalities, especially gastrointestinal abnormalities, is still a major cause of death (Baird and Sadovnick, 1988; Frid et al., 1999). Leukemia, the malignancy most widely associated with Down syndrome, accounts for fewer than 10% of deaths (Scholl et al., 1982).

In the context of prenatal counseling, mortality statistics are an important part of the description of Down syndrome natural history (Noble, 1998), but when discussing a live-born infant's prognosis, parents are generally told long survival is the rule. The low but not negligible possibility of long survival in trisomy 13 and 18 should also be mentioned to parents after-prenatal or postnatal cytogenetic diagnosis, especially if no major malformations are detected. Otherwise, parents may have great difficulty caring for a profoundly handicapped infant to whom no hope of life had previously been given.

Trisomy 21 Down syndrome

The English physician, John Langdon Haydon Down, wrote in 1866 the clinical description of the condition that was subsequently given his name (Down, 1866). Down was a distinguished physician who was ahead of his time in describing patients with other genetic or part-genetic disorders, including pseudohypertrophic muscular dystrophy, Prader-Willi syndrome, and Asperger syndrome (his writings are reprinted by the McKeith Press in their series Classics in Developmental Medicine [Down, 1990]). Although, in naming the condition mongolian idiocy, Down incorrectly speculated that affected individuals had reverted to an earlier phylogenetic type, he differed from many of his contemporaries in recognizing the "unity of the human species" and he ardently opposed apologists for racial subjugation and slavery. The terms "mongol", "mongoloid" and "mongolism" were widely adopted at the time but are now long-abandoned, being replaced by Down syndrome and trisomy 21.

A milestone in Down syndrome research was Shuttleworth's study of 350 affected individuals, which led him to conclude that either advanced maternal age per se or maternal reproductive exhaustion brought about by repeated pregnancies, were causative factors that accounted for the association he observed between increased maternal age and birth of an affected infant (Shuttleworth, 1909). The observation that children with Down syndrome tend to be born at the end of large sibships had been made in the nineteenth century by Fraser and Mitchell, but it was Jenkins and Penrose who, independently, established in the 1930s that there is a relationship between the chance of a Down syndrome birth and increased maternal age, as opposed to maternal parity or advanced paternal age. In contrast with these early advances in understanding the epidemiology of Down syndrome, unproductive speculations were being made in the nineteenth and early twentieth centuries about the cause of Down syndrome, with maternal syphilis, tuberculosis, hypothyroidism, alcoholism, fetal endocrine dysfunction, ovum degeneration, and maternal emotional trauma during gestation all implicated at one time or another. However, the ophthalmologist Waardenburg and the American pediatrician, Bleyer, did suggest a chromosomal cause for Down syndrome more than 25 years prior to the demonstration of the extra acrocentric chromosome in 1959. Ursula Mittwoch observed 24 chromosomes in a meiotic preparation from a testicular biopsy derived from a Down syndrome individual, but this was in the early 1950s when the normal diploid number was thought to be 48. Thus, Lejeune et al. (1959) are credited with the discovery of the chromosomal basis of Down syndrome some three years after Tijo and Levan (1956) established that the normal diploid number was 46. In 1960, Polani et al. (1960) discovered translocation Down syndrome in the daughter of a 21-year-old mother who was selected for study because the investigators had reasoned that some individuals may be affected through a separate, maternal age-independent chromosomal mechanism. The following year, Clarke et al. (1961) reported mosaic Down syndrome, having found both normal diploid and trisomy 21 cells in skin and blood derived from a two-year-old girl with physical stigmata of Down syndrome but near-normal intelligence.

DOWN SYNDROME PHENOTYPE

Down syndrome is usually diagnosed at birth. No single phenotypic feature is pathognomonic but the combination of dysmorphisms is recognizable and specific. Although clinical diagnosis of Down syndrome is readily made, chromosome analysis is necessary in each case for confirmation of the diagnosis and also to assess the genetic implications for the family.

Fetus with Down syndrome

Although the first trimester fetus with trisomy 13 or trisomy 18 has growth restriction as evidenced by reduced crown-rump length, this early effect is not evident in Down syndrome (Bahado-Singh et al., 1997). Also, pictures reveal that the major postnatal clinical clue, the facial appearance, cannot be relied on (Fig. 44.2). Instead, at fetal autopsy, a simian crease, clinodactyly, septal heart defects, and small size collectively form the best indicators of trisomy 21 (Stephens and Shepherd, 1980). Post-mortem radiographic studies of Down syndrome fetuses have identified three key radiological markers for trisomy 21: brachycephaly, absence of nasal bone ossification, and hypoplasia of the middle phalanx of the fifth finger. An increased iliac angle may be added to this list (Zook et al., 1999). These features can also be identified by antenatal ultrasound (Stempfle et al., 1999), but the main ultrasound marker of trisomy 21 is fetal nuchal translucency and this has been incorporated into antenatal risk calculation in some screening programs (Nicolaides et

al., 1992a; Chitty and Pandya, 1997) (see Ch. 28). Other ultrasound-detectable markers and malformations, such as isolated atrioventricular canal defect, in the hands of some experts, have high enough sensitivity and specificity to be usefully incorporated into screening and risk assessment (Vautier-Rit et al., 2000; Winter et al., 2000). But many sonographic signs of Down syndrome have questionable utility. For example, Vergani et al. (2000) undertook a critical reappraisal of sonographic fetal femur length and concluded this measurement is not a reliable sonographic predictor of Down syndrome. In France, where high resolution ultrasound examinations are routine, the sensitivity of ultrasound diagnosis was 25% (Stoll et al., 1998a). In the UK, even if positive ultrasound signs are identified, subsequent antenatal management is quite variable and there is scope for its improvement (Mclachlan et al., 2000).

Infant Down syndrome

A plethora of clinical signs have been described in affected newborns, but facial recognition typically precedes systematic examination. The rounded head, a third fontanelle, the appearance of the eyes especially on crying, an apparently large tongue in a small mouth, a short neck and single palmar creases may all be appreciated at birth (Fig. 44.3). Brachycephaly, upslanting palpebral fissures, epicanthic folds, flattened nasal root and midfacial hypoplasia, small dysplastic pinnae, protruding tongue, brachymesophalangy and clinodactyly of the fifth digit, and a wide gap between the first and second toes are non-specific signs frequently documented in infants with trisomy 21. Yet, experienced or inexperienced clinicians may rightly or wrongly suspect the diagnosis in newborn infants with only hypotonia and subtle facial or limb dysmorphism. In such cases, if chromosome analysis is ordered, it is important to inform the parents, otherwise difficulties arise if the parents are unaware that a chromosome test result is pending. Where abandonment of Down syndrome babies at birth occurs (10% to 60% of cases), an important factor is the advice which is given to the parents in the neonatal period (Dumaret et al., 1996).

The presence of a characteristic heart defect or a leukemoid blood picture may be helpful adjuncts to diagnosis in newborns, whereas extreme prematurity or the presence of an uncommon malformation such as omphalocoele may be a hindrance (Khoury et al., 1988; Reddy et al., 1994). Clinical diagnosis in the rare cytogenetic varieties of Down syndrome including trisomy 21 mosaicism may be straightforward or simply impossible. Experience from South Africa has also indicated that delayed diagnosis is commonplace in black neonates in whom clinical features of Down

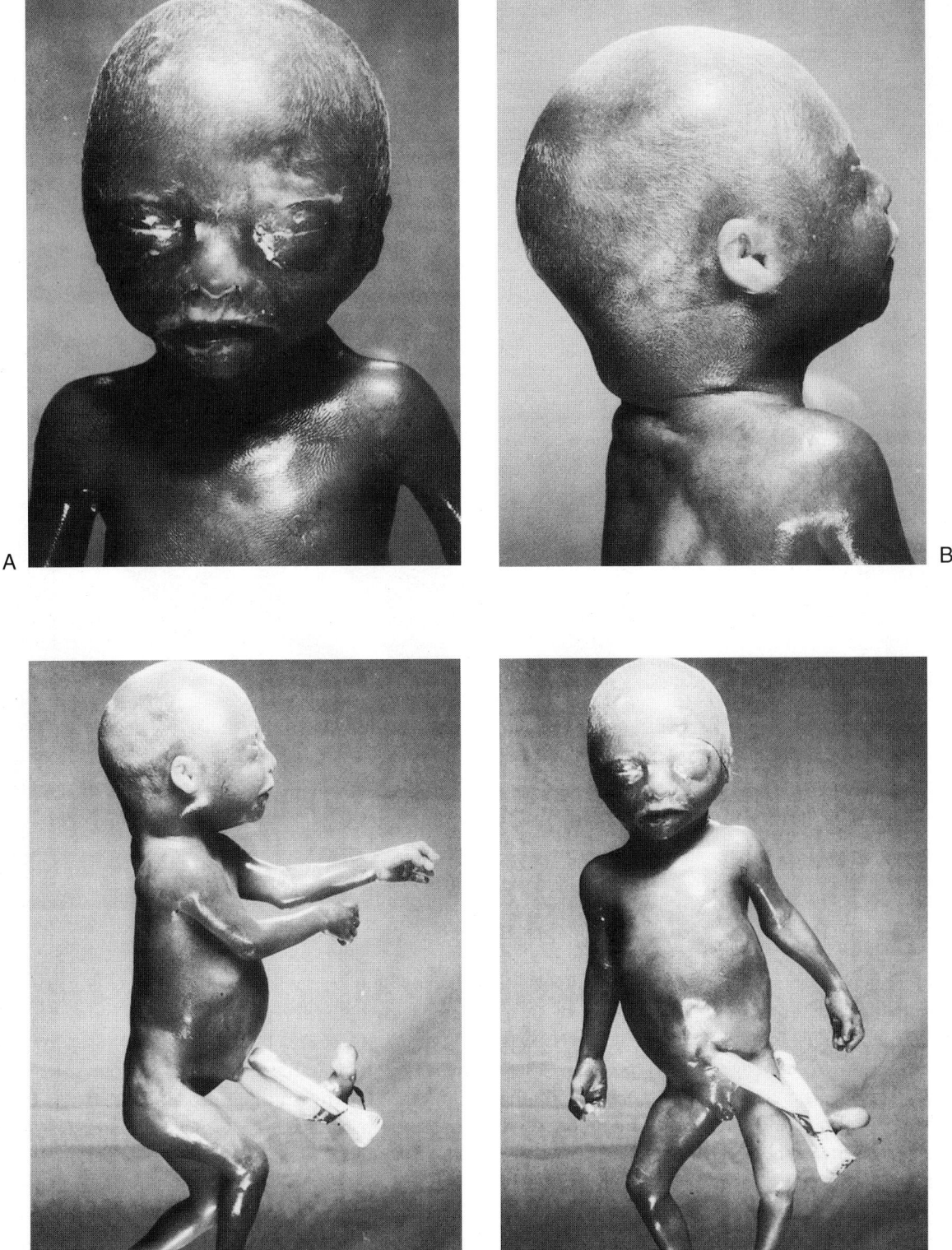

Fig. 44.2. A–D Facial features of Down syndrome are not evident in midtrimister, nor is limb shortening but note apparent nuchal thickening.

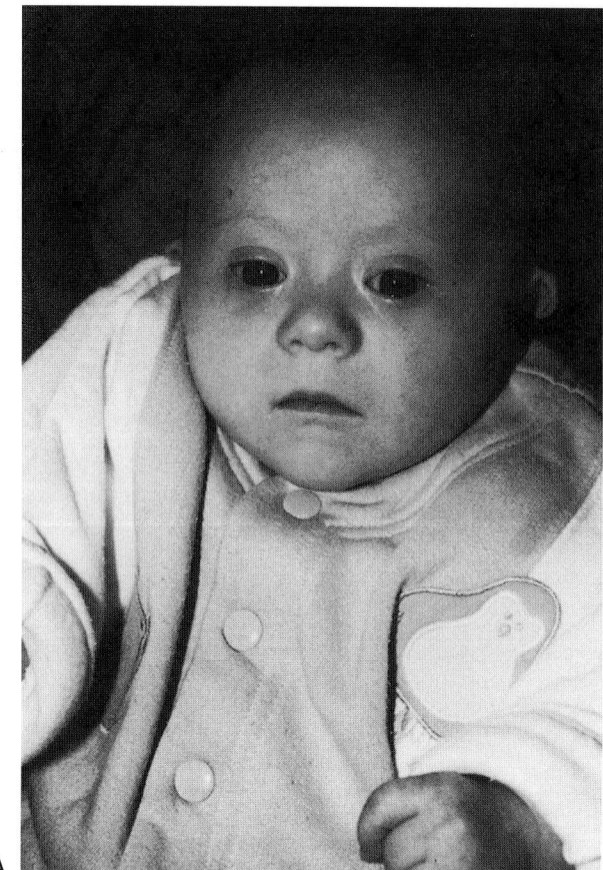

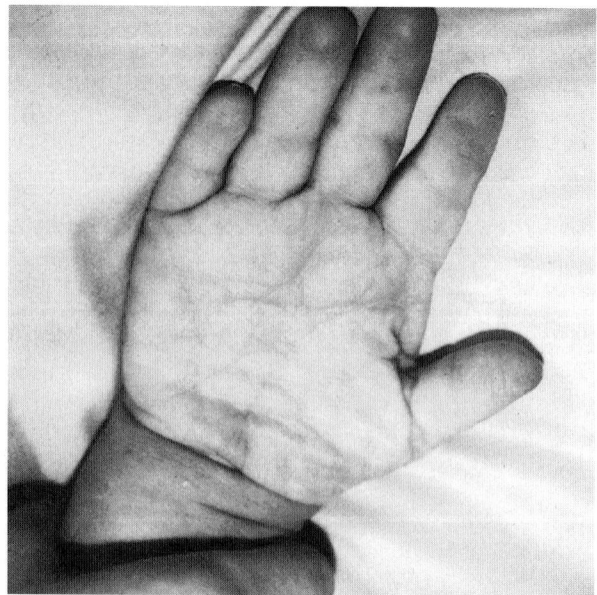

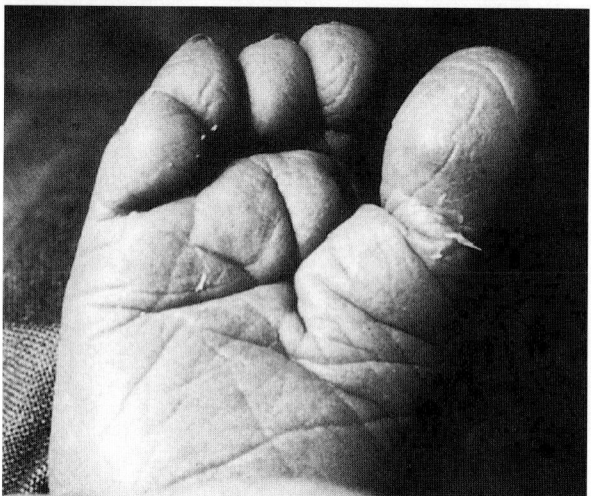

Fig. 44.3. A–C Down syndrome appearance and distal limb signs in infancy: a single palmar crease and brachymesophalangy V; a "sandal gap" and deep crease between the first and second toes.

syndrome are often difficult to recognize (Christianson, 1997). Detailed clinical diagnostic protocols have been published (Rex and Preus, 1982; Epstein et al., 1991) and in children under two years of age, the 10 most discriminating clinical signs of trisomy 21 are brachycephaly, oblique palpebral fissure, nystagmus, flat nasal bridge or root, narrow palate, folded ear, short broad neck, incurved fifth finger, sandal gap between great toe and second toe, and hypotonia (Jackson et al., 1976).

Adult with Down syndrome

The clinical diagnosis of Down syndrome has often been illustrated with the most obvious signs such as upslanting palpebral fissures, Brushfield spots on the iris, thickened,

everted and cracked lips, a fissured tongue, small rounded ears with underdeveloped lobes, short broad neck, short stature and obesity (Figs. 44.4 and 44.5). However, this is just as often unrepresentative and an attractive, smart appearance with normal body weight for height may confuse many would-be diagnosticians. Facial features change with age in trisomy 21; the nasal root becomes more prominent, epicanthic folds become less prominent, and increased growth of the lower face occurs with aging, just as it does in chromosomally normal individuals.

Mosaic Trisomy 21 Down Syndrome

About 2% to 4% of affected individuals have a mixture of normal diploid and trisomy 21 cells. Clearly, if a low pro-

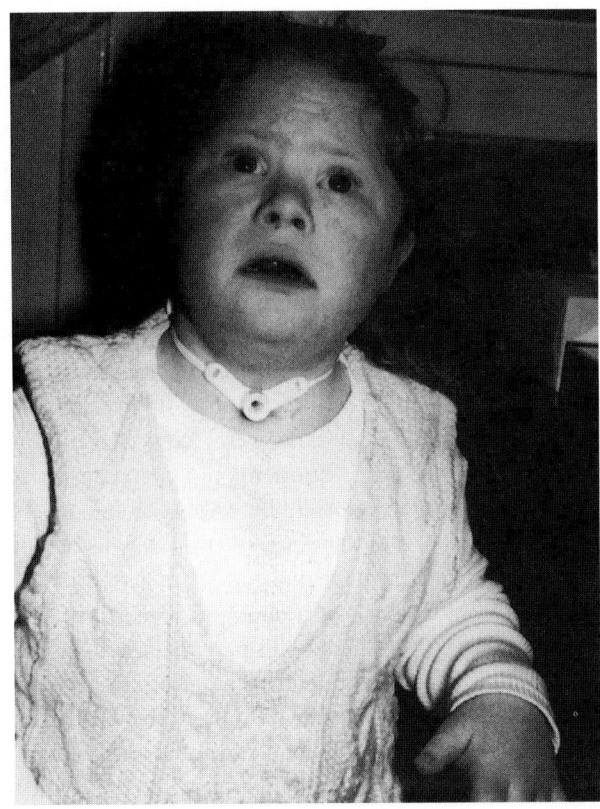

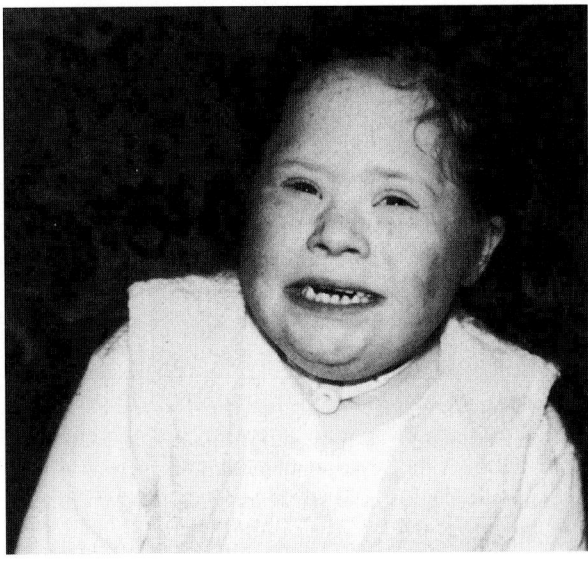

B

Fig. 44.4. (A–B) Six-year-old, tracheostomy-dependent child with trisomy 21 who previously underwent surgical repair of atrioventricular canal defect and a vascular ring. Note how a change in the facial expression may aid recognition of Down syndrome. (See Shapiro et al, 2000, for discussion of tracheal stenosis and congenital heart disease in Down syndrome.)

A

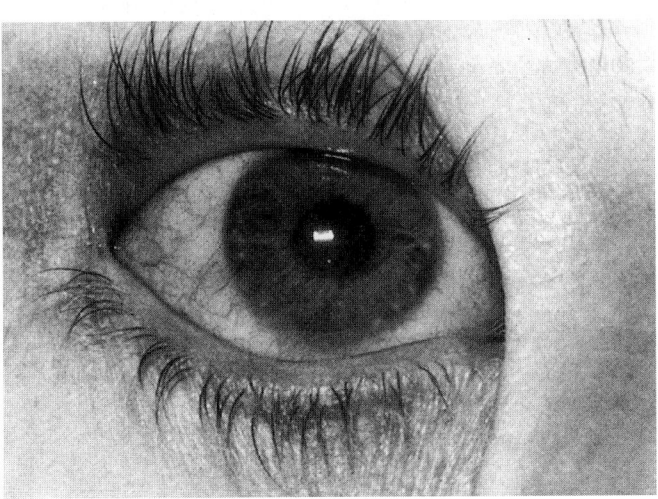

Fig. 44.5. Epicanthic fold and Brushfield spots on the iris of a 20-year-old man with trisomy 21.

portion of abnormal cells are present, or if the proportions vary markedly in samples from different tissues, it may be very difficult to detect mosaicism, even when the phenotype suggests Down syndrome.

Like full trisomy 21, mosaic trisomy 21 (and other autosomal mosaic aneuploidies) is detected more often in prenatal life (Hsu et al., 1997; Wallerstein et al., 2000).

Presumably, factors that affect the survival of the mosaic pregnancy include the percentage of chromosomally abnormal cells, whether or not severe fetal malformation is present, and the mother's age, with decreased survival expected as this advances (Kratzer et al., 1992; Mutton et al., 1996).

Clarke et al. (1961) first reported chromosomal mosaicism in a two-year-old girl who was selected for detailed study because she had physical features of Down syndrome but superior intellectual development compared with a trisomic case. In Clarke's case, 13% of cells from blood leukocyte cultures were trisomy 21 and 34% of cells examined from fibroblast cultures were trisomy 21, the remaining cells being karyotypically normal. In general, there is a tendency for the proportion of trisomic cells to be higher in fibroblasts and in early life, so the measured proportions in one individual are not necessarily constant with time (Taysi et al., 1970; Percy et al., 1993).

On average, signs of Down syndrome in trisomy 21 mosaicism are less prominent compared with full trisomy 21 (Smith and Berg, 1976), but in individual cases the proportion of abnormal cells in one or two tissue samples may give a false indication of the severity or mildness of the phenotype (Kohn et al., 1970). Poor correlation between mental development and the proportion of trisomic cells in blood or skin has an important implication for genetic counseling: following prenatal or postnatal diagnosis of mosaic trisomy 21, it is hazardous to predict the phenotype based upon the proportion of abnormal cells. However, there are data to indicate that after diagnosis of mosaicism in amniocytes, abnormal pregnancy outcome does, to an extent, correlate with finding trisomy 21 cells in a fetal blood sample and with ultrasonographically detected abnormalities (Wallerstein et al., 2000). Also, from anecdotal reports of cases with low-grade mosaicism and no malformation, hope for a better prognosis in such cases is not unreasonable (Moreira et al., 2000). Indeed, phenotypically normal or near normal mosaic trisomy 21 parents are known in whom the cytogenetic diagnosis was made serendipitously or after the birth of trisomy 21 siblings (Smith et al., 1962; Casati et al., 1992).

Down syndrome development, personality, and learning difficulties

A large body of detailed literature reports changes in the brain in Down syndrome (Wisniewski, 1990; Cairns, 1999). This occurs at all levels, visible changes in magnetic resonance images, neuropathological changes, and neurochemical changes. For example, there are cortical development anomalies that occur during the emergence of lamination (Golden and Hyman, 1994); there is poor dendritic maturation and atrophy with early reappearance of beta-amyloid and overexpression of membrane proteins in the brain (Takashima et al., 1994); earlier amyloid plaque formation preceded by increased amounts of soluble amyloid beta peptide 42 (Teller et al., 1996); there is an increased tendency for cortical neurones to undergo apoptosis in cell culture (Busciglio and Yankner 1995); there is a different pattern of ramified microglial cell development (Wierba-Bobrowicz et al., 1999). But for parents, though, the crucial question is what kind of development can be expected?

Although a typical stereotype might be the floppy, sociable but undemanding infant who turns into a placid, affectionate, good-natured, music-loving, moderately intellectually disabled adult, people who get to know Down syndrome individuals well know this to be false (Wishart and Johnston, 1990; Carr, 1995). In fact, Down syndrome individuals are just as different from each other as their chromosomally normal peers: some are happy, others are sad, some are flighty and impulsive, others are careful and steady. Just like the general population, a minority exhibit deviant behaviors or suffer more serious conditions such as autism spectrum disorders (Pueschel et al., 1991b; Kent

et al., 1999). Interestingly, there is evidence that adults with Down syndrome exhibit fewer maladaptive behaviors (Collacott et al., 1998).

The definitive work on the development of children with Down syndrome has been carried out by Janet Carr, a psychologist who recruited all 54 babies with Down syndrome who were born in a region of south east England in 1964 (Carr, 1995). A control for each case was also recruited and a remarkable 21 year, longitudinal study ensued. The total population size was small but there was great variation between cases and it emerged that Down syndrome children, like other children, mostly grow up in happy families. Ages at which different skills were acquired varied greatly, and higher intelligence quotients did correlate with earlier development. Transcripts of interviews and conversations with patents and their families conveyed details of family life and relationships, which, nowadays, are also topics for discussion in popular magazines and on the Internet.

In discussing prognosis with parents, it may be said that, generally, in Down syndrome early social and emotional development is mildly delayed during the first year, while language and motor delay becomes more apparent in the second year of life. Central hypotonia is present to some degree in nearly every infant and there is some evidence associating severe hypotonia in infancy with more severe retardation in motor and mental development in later childhood (Gath and Gumley, 1984). Developmental milestones, such as sitting independently, walking, being toilet trained, and using words with meaning, are usually but not always delayed, and the range of delays in different children is wide (Carr, 1995).

Studies employing psychometric tests to assess cognitive development have found that children with Down syndrome generally score in the IQ range 20 to 85. In other words, children at the top end of the range achieve scores in the lower normal range, whereas children at the bottom end fall into the range of scores commonly associated with severe mental impairment (Carr, 1995). There is also evidence of decline in measured intelligence quotients from peak values gained in the first years of life. In the clinic, it is often more helpful to point out that there is a pattern of stops and starts in the developmental progress of children with Down syndrome. Pauses in development define alternating periods of progress and plateaus in cognitive, adaptive, and linguistic spheres. This pattern was studied in detail by Gibson (1966), who carried out multiple regression analysis of early developmental markers in more than 300 Down syndrome individuals. Gibson found that during the first four years, there was early acceleration followed by a short plateau when the median developmental age was about 17 months. Between five years and eight or nine years, acceleration occurred, terminating at a median mental age of 31 months. From eight to 11 years, there was stability, followed by a third period of developmental progress terminating on a plateau by age 12 or 13 years, when development was assessed to be equivalent to a median mental age of 40 months. Given advances in education theory and practice, better averages might be expected today. Parents who press for a candid assessment of their infant's prognosis may be told that, very roughly, most children with Down syndrome attain overall learning abilities equivalent to those of an unaffected child aged six to eight years. However, it is very important to emphasize that some affected infants do considerably better.

Aspects of learning, speech and language development and auditory short term memory, all show different patterns of development in Down syndrome (see detailed studies by Caselli et al., 1998; Chapman et al., 1998; 2000). As far as language is concerned, Down syndrome children appear to have special difficulties that place them behind chromosomally normal children of equivalent mental age or children with mental retardation of unknown etiology (Kernan, 1990). The reason for this is not clear: volumetric MRI studies have shown no correlation between performance on speech and language tests, and size of the superior temporal gyrus or planum temporale, parts of the brain concerned with language (Frangou et al., 1997). Some evidence suggests that within language, social communication is less behind, whereas grammatical syntactic difficulties are severe (Fowler, 1990). Though the wide range of individual abilities renders early prediction of potential unreliable, parents may be reassured the vast majority of Down syndrome children learn to speak.

In summary, longitudinal studies indicate that children with Down syndrome go through stages of development but simple slowing of the normal process is not the problem. The extra chromosome 21 disrupts learning and renders acquired skills unstable (Wishart, 1993). Temperament characteristics of children with Down syndrome do differ, but whether a behavioral phenotype can be defined (e.g., see Chapman and Hesketh, 2000) is more controversial.

Down syndrome: growth

At birth, infants with Down syndrome show mild growth retardation, with mean birthweight, length, and head circumference (OFC) lying between the 10th and 15th centiles calculated for chromosomally normal infants (Cronk, 1978; Clementi et al., 1990). Growth velocity in infancy is near-normal, but after the first year it reduces, so that by three years of age, height approaches −3 SD. Growth velocity tends not to fall any further after three years; a study from Sicily of nearly 400 affected children aged up to 14 years found that height, weight, and OFC were seldom less than −3 SD (Piro et al., 1990). Growth charts for children with Down syndrome are available (Cronk et al., 1988; Toledo et al., 1999) but measurements, including body mass index, should probably also be plotted on standard charts since there are reservations about Down syndrome charts that may have been created with growth data from some trisomy 21 individuals with specific growth abnormalities.

Puberty usually occurs normally in Down syndrome although some individuals have hormonal evidence of hypogonadism (Hsiang et al., 1987; Arnell et al., 1996). The pubertal growth spurt is diminished and final height is usually within the range 140 to 160 cm. Hormone studies have shown reduced levels of insulin-like growth factor-1 in children and adolescents (Annerén et al., 1990), but not in adults with Down syndrome (Hestnes et al., 1992). There has been doubt as to whether normal levels of growth hormone are present in some cases (Castells et al., 1992). In recent years, growth hormone therapy has been used to increase growth velocity in children, including Down syndrome children, who have short stature without evidence of growth hormone deficiency. Children with Down syndrome who are not growth hormone deficient do show height response to growth hormone therapy (Annerén et al., 1993; Torrado et al., 1994) but the effect on final height is not yet clear. One trial of growth hormone injections commencing from age six to nine months had no effect on craniofacial development or morphology (Carlstedt et al., 1999) but the need for long term studies of growth hormone therapy has been emphasized repeatedly. At present, blanket prescription of growth hormone treatment is not recommended in the absence of proven growth hormone deficiency (Annerén et al., 1999). In the United States, the Lawson Wilkins Pediatric Endocrine Society (1993) highlighted dubious claims of possible benefits from treatment and recent results from Sweden showed no evidence of behavioral and cognitive improvements in treated young children (Annerén et al., 1999).

From early childhood onward, Down syndrome individuals have a tendency to be overweight. In the United States, by nine years of age, the average child with Down syndrome is above the 95th percentile of the National Center for Health Statistics weight-for-height growth chart (Cronk et al., 1988; Luke et al., 1994). In adult life, obesity is a frequent problem (Rubin et al., 1998). A study of 58 Down syndrome individuals living in the community found that 96% of females and 71% of males were above the acceptable weight range, compared with normal population figures of 32% and 40%, respectively (Bell and Bhate, 1992). Clearly, prevention of obesity is preferable to radical or ineffectual dieting to combat an established weight problem, but evidence suggests that obesity in Down syndrome is not due simply to increased food intake and deceased energy expenditure. It is encouraging that a program of athletics training led to improvement in measurements of strength, speed and endurance in Down syndrome subjects with an added benefit being a "tendency to a more athletic morphotype" (Peran et al., 1997). Scheduled training in the company of peers would be in keeping with the notion that lifestyle factors such as friendship and social opportunities are important to oppose any biological influences the extra chromosome may have on the resting metabolic rate in Down syndrome children (Luke et al., 1994; Fujiura et al., 1997). Nevertheless, although common sense indicates benefits from exercise and good eating habits are best established in childhood, obesity will still be a problem for many Down syndrome individuals.

Down syndrome: congenital heart disease

Congenital heart defects comprise the most frequently occurring major malformation in Down syndrome but their reported incidence, with estimates ranging from 16% to 62%, has varied because of the selected nature of many case series. A study of fetuses aborted after cytogenetic prenatal diagnosis revealed a major heart defect in 45%, not including patent ductus arteriosus and some types of atrial septal defect which are expected to close after birth (Rehder, 1981). A similar incidence (42%) was observed in a study from Northern Ireland that prospectively screened with echocardiography all Down syndrome infants born during a two-year period (Tubman et al., 1991). Given this high incidence, the important practical point is that all newborn infants with Down syndrome undergo echocardiographic examination by age six weeks since clinical, radiographic and ECG examinations combined only detect 70% of lesions (Tubman et al., 1991; Wren et al., 1999).

A frequently observed lesion (approximately 40% of all lesions) is atrioventricular canal defect, which comprises an atrial septal defect with abnormality of the atrioventricular valves and ventricular septum. Isolated ventricular septal defect, secundum atrial septal defects, and patent ductus arteriosus are the next most common lesions (representing more than 40% of the total), while tetralogy of Fallot and other complex lesions make up the remainder. In fetal life, atrioventricular canal defects may be visualized by sonographic examination (an abnormal four-chamber view) and since about 50% of fetuses with isolated canal defect have trisomy 21 (Delisle et al., 1999), identification of this malformation constitutes an indication to offer fetal chromosome examination. However, in routine obstetric practice, fetal anomaly scans often miss atrioventricular canal defects and other heart lesions that are present in Down syndrome (Stoll et al., 1998b; Allan, 1999).

Medical and surgical treatments of heart defect in children with Down syndrome are not fundamentally different from the treatments used in the care of chromosomally normal children (Schneider et al., 1989). Current data on the survival of Down syndrome children with congenital heart disease show great improvement in recent years, from 15% overall mortality rate for infants undergoing major cardiac surgical procedures to, at one institution, an insignificant difference between the mortality rates in children with Down syndrome and children with normal chromosomes (Baciewicz et al., 1989). In another study only complete atrioventricular septal defect had higher perioperative and late mortality in Down syndrome versus controls (Reller and Morris, 1998). Untreated, atrioventricular septal defects are associated with high mortality in infancy, and young adult survivors may have profound morbidity and gross impairment of quality of life due to pulmonary hypertension and right heart failure. Thus, early surgical intervention is necessary to relieve symptoms of cardiac failure and minimize the likelihood of pulmonary vascular disease (Frontera-Izquierdo and Cabezuelo-Huerta, 1990; Amark and Sunnegardh, 1999). Results of early surgical repair of atrioventricular canal defect show an 80% or greater survival to age 15 years, but some children still develop irreversible pulmonary vascular disease that has its onset in infancy (Suzuki et al., 2000), and optimal medical management remains very important (Bull et al., 1985).

Why pulmonary hypertension should be so frequent in Down syndrome is unclear (Clapp et al., 1990). Suggested precipitating factors include abnormal development of lung parenchyma with diminished numbers of alveoli and pulmonary hypoplasia (Cooney and Thurlbeck, 1982); thinning of the medial layer of small pulmonary arteries (Yamaki et al., 1983); other anatomic variations such as maxillary hypoplasia, macroglossia, hypertrophy of the tonsils and adenoids; and sleep apnea with or without upper airway obstruction (Wilson et al., 1979; Loughlin et al., 1981; Levine and Simpser, 1982; Southall et al., 1987). Of these possible causes, obstructive airway disease, causing sleep disturbance and hypoxemia, can sometimes have a surgical remedy (Strome, 1986).

When cardiac mortality was higher in infancy, past surveys revealed that adults with Down syndrome had less severe types of congenital heart defects than affected young children. Valvular heart disease, such as aortic regurgitation and mitral valve prolapse, was relatively common and sometimes asymptomatic (Goldhaber et al., 1986; 1987), so a routine echocardiographic examination has been recommended for all young adults. However, the availability of improved treatments for children with major cardiac lesions and good community-based medical care for affected adults will result in increased prevalence of serious symptomatic heart disease. Curiously, several reports have indicated a decreased prevalence of coronary artery disease in adults with trisomy 21 (Yla-Herttuala et al., 1989). This is not well established, however, and Pueschel et al. (1992) found no evidence that trisomy 21 individuals have lipid and lipoprotein profiles associated with reduced risk of atherosclerosis.

In the United Kingdom, a recent survey discovered surprisingly few referrals of Down syndrome individuals for heart and heart-lung transplantation. This was the subject of a British Medical Journal editorial (Leonard et al., 2000a) and subsequent correspondence from readers of the article (gathered together in the electronic edition at http://bmj.com) made it perfectly clear that Down syndrome patients are equally deserving of optimal medical and surgical care.

Down syndrome: oral health

Good oral health is especially important in individuals with congenital heart disease and it is long known that Down syndrome children often have poor condition teeth and gums. Thus, Hennequin et al. (1999) performed a service for those who care for Down syndrome individuals by reviewing the literature on oral health problems. A subsequent survey of over 200 Down syndrome individuals and their families revealed a high prevalence of problems that fall into two main areas.

Firstly, the main oral functions, breathing, sucking, chewing and swallowing are delayed and remain impaired in later childhood. Weak sucking, fatigue during feeding, coughing and spluttering due to uncoordinated breathing and swallowing are all frequent in infancy. Abnormally positioned anterior mandible, tooth grinding and tongue thrusting combine to impair chewing and this often contributes to poor dietary fibre intake and constipation.

Secondly, periodontal disease in trisomy 21 is related to oral hygiene problems and in the French study, some 50% of young Down syndrome children and 23% of older children were unable to clean their teeth (Hennequin et al., 1999). Bleeding gums and halitosis were frequent. But, since the periodontal disease in trisomy 21 is early in its onset, severe and resistant to plaque control measures, poor

oral hygiene is not the only contributory factor. Whether poorly defined immune deficiencies associated with Down syndrome such as imbalance in the proportions of T cell subpopulations contribute to the increased susceptibility to infection (Murphy and Epstein, 1992), remains unproven (Cichon et al., 1998; Amano et al., 2000).

In any event, researchers agree that the oral health of Down syndrome individuals could be improved by provision of improved dental services from an early age with related services including dietetics and speech therapy also being readily available.

Down syndrome: gastrointestinal complications

Two major gastrointestinal malformations associated with Down syndrome are duodenal atresia and Hirschsprung disease. Between 2% and 15% of infants with Down syndrome have duodenal atresia, and 20% to 30% of children with duodenal atresia have trisomy 21 (Fonkalsrud et al., 1969). About 2% of patients with Down syndrome have Hirschsprung disease, and 10% to 15% of patients with Hirschsprung disease have trisomy 21 (Harrison et al., 1987; Canniano et al., 1990). A small number of trisomy 21 infants have both duodenal atresia and Hirschsprung disease. In these cases, the dual pathology may cause a considerable diagnostic problem because the presenting features of duodenal atresia overshadow signs of Hirschsprung disease (Surana et al., 1994). Clinicians should therefore have a low threshold for investigating and excluding Hirschsprung disease as the cause of persistent constipation following surgery for duodenal atresia. Surgical management of gastrointestinal tract atresia in trisomy 21 carries a higher mortality in infants with additional malformations (Beasley et al., 1997). A major problem in managing Hirschsprung disease in infants with trisomy 21 is an increased risk of enterocolitis (Canniano et al., 1990).

Other congenital intestinal abnormalities that probably or possibly occur more frequently in trisomy 21 infants include omphalocele, duodenal bands, annular pancreas, ileal and jejunal atresias and microcolon (Källén et al., 1996). Imperforate anus without fistula is an associated malformation that has a good prognosis (Torres et al., 1998). Achalasia was identified recently as an uncommon problem in trisomy 21 children and adults (Zarate et al., 1999).

Celiac disease also has a recognized association with Down syndrome and screening for subclinical varieties of this condition with IgG and IgA antigliadin antibody determinations has been recommended, whether or not the Down syndrome child has gastrointestinal symptoms (Gale et al., 1997; Zachor et al., 2000. A gene locus for trisomy

21 associated celiac disease susceptibility is being sought, but so far without success (Morris et al., 2000).

The most frequent and persistent gastrointestinal complaint is constipation. In infancy this may be caused by anal stenosis (Spahis and Wilson, 1999) or Hirschsprung disease (Quin et al., 1994). But many older children and adults are affected in the absence of gastrointestinal tract abnormality. In such cases the origins of constipation are complex and may date from early life when hypotonia, delayed introduction of solid foods and other dietary factors probably combined to disturb the establishment of a regular bowel habit.

Down syndrome: hearing loss

The small dysmorphic pinna is a well-recognized clinical pointer to the diagnosis of Down syndrome (Mazzoni et al., 1994), and other diverse malformations affect middle and inner ear structures (reviewed by Rogers and Coleman, 1992). Therefore, there is no shortage of mechanisms by which hearing may be impaired in Down syndrome individuals. Several studies have found that unilateral or bilateral hearing loss is present in 40% to 75% of children and adults (Brooks et al., 1972; Keiser et al., 1981; Roizen et al., 1993). Hearing loss may be conductive, sensorineural, or mixed, and of mild, moderate, or severe degree. It may occur at any age, so lifelong surveillance by testers with expertise in working with people with learning disability is required. Observer-based testing is often difficult in Down syndrome (Werner et al., 1996). Full audiological assessments should be carried out between six months and one year and older children may have annual assessments dropping to two yearly intervals in adults as presbyacusis is frequently evident in Down syndrome individuals by the second decade (Buchanan, 1990).

Middle ear disease is the commonest cause of hearing loss. A high frequency of upper respiratory infections is reported in Down syndrome but these coughs and colds are not necessarily causing the repeated episodes of acute otitis media that precede development of effusion within the middle ear. Symptoms and signs of acute otitis media may be difficult to recognize and detect in Down syndrome children because the external auditory meatus and canal are frequently narrow, occluded by wax and difficult to examine. In general, more than 50% of cases of otitis media with effusion (glue ear) resolve spontaneously within eight weeks, but 5% result in bilateral hearing loss persisting for one year (De Melker, 1993). Glue ear is thus a common cause of hearing loss in Down syndrome, so screening for this complication followed by appropriate treatment is important (Mandel et al., 1987; Thomsen et al., 1989). Debate surrounds the choice and effectiveness of both medical therapies (antibiotics, oral corticosteroids, and decongestants) and surgical treatments including adenoidectomy, myringotomy, and the placement of ventilatory tubes (grommets). In chromosomally normal children, surgical procedures for glue ear have been subject to scrutiny following recognition that, in England at least, such operations were the commonest reason for elective surgery in all children, despite controversy surrounding the effectiveness of different procedures. Treatment of Down syndrome children with grommet insertion may be especially prone to failure. Selikowitz (1993a) found no improvement in hearing six to nine weeks after operation in 40% of ears. Yet in one series of Down syndrome children, 28% had grommets inserted by the time the cohort reached a mean age of nine years and two months (Turner et al., 1990). An Australian review reported that 51% of school age children with Down syndrome had had grommets inserted (Selikowitz, 1992). The recognition that most episodes of glue ear are self-limiting, and that permanent resolution of symptoms or significant improvement in hearing deficits may not follow from even the most aggressive treatment plans is important (Iino et al., 1999). Moreover, surgical treatment carries a small risk (although standard positioning for ear surgery in the child with no radiological abnormality of the neck is safe [Todd et al., 2000]). It is also not clear that improved hearing is followed by amelioration of language, cognitive, and behavioral problems. Thus, there should be measured enthusiasm for surgical treatments for hearing-impaired Down syndrome individuals and conservative management is preferred for all but the most severe cases of glue ear (Iino et al., 1999).

Down syndrome: ophthalmic disorders

Apart from the minor ocular features in children and adults with Down syndrome such as epicanthic folds, upward-slanting palpebral fissures, and Brushfield spots on the iris, there is a high prevalence of anomalies, such as congenital cataract, glaucoma, strabismus, keratoconus, and major refractive errors, which are important to detect and manage.

In a study of 77 children with Down syndrome (all cared for at home and referred to a Down syndrome clinic in a teaching hospital), 61% had ophthalmic disorders that warranted monitoring and treatment (Roizen et al., 1994). Also, prior pediatric physical examination had failed to detect treatable abnormalities, including refractive errors, strabismus, cataracts, and nystagmus, which were subsequently detected by an ophthalmologist in 16 children.

Since the percentage of children with ophthalmic disorders, especially refractive disorders, nearly doubles from the first year of life to about 70% in the five to 12-year-old group, annual examinations are recommended in the first five years after initial examination in infancy to exclude congenital cataract (Courage et al., 1994; Wong and Ho, 1997; Tsiaras et al., 1999). Teller visual acuity cards (Teller et al., 1986) are good for rapidly and accurately assessing acuity in Down syndrome infants, whose acuities become more impaired compared with their chromosomally normal peers, as they get older (Courage et al., 1994).

Other ophthalmic complications include tear film alteration with dry spots and frequent anterior segment infections (Filippelo et al., 1997). In adults, there is a high incidence of latent nystagmus that is also best identified by specialist ophthalmic examination techniques (Averbuch-Heller et al., 1999).

Leukemia, solid tumors and Down syndrome

A remarkable longitudinal study, based upon the Danish cytogenetic register, found that in Down syndrome there is a decreased chance of solid tumors in adults and in children, including neuroblastoma and Wilms tumor (Hasle et al., 2000). This discovery is of course in stark contrast to the well-known increased risk of leukemia in Down syndrome children. The reasons for solid tumor resistance and leukemia susceptibility are unknown (Zipursky, 2000).

A 10-year retrospective study by the Children's Cancer Study Group found that about 2% of children with acute lymphoblastic leukemia (ALL) and 2% of patients with acute nonlymphoblastic leukemia (ANLL), had Down syndrome (Robinson et al., 1984). The UK Medical Research Council Trial, UKALL X (Chessells et al., 1995) recruited more than 90% of eligible cases of ALL, 1% of whom had Down syndrome. Overall, the rate of leukemia in Down syndrome is estimated to be about 1 in 150 and some 20 times greater than the rate in the general population (reviewed by Fong and Brodeur, 1987; Zipursky et al., 1992). Trisomy 21 is also one of the most frequent acquired chromosomal abnormalities in leukemia (Mittelman et al., 1990). Acquired non-Down syndrome trisomy 21 cases tend to be older than Down syndrome cases, a finding consistent with an earlier peak age for leukemia in Down syndrome.

At birth, transient myeloproliferative disorder associated with splenic enlargement and liver fibrosis is not uncommon (Miyauchi et al., 1992). This disorder comprises clonal proliferation of immature myeloid cells and although spontaneous resolution in the first year of life is usual, a minority of affected children subsequently develop acute megakaryoblastic leukemia or acute nonlymphoblastic leukemia (Wong et al., 1988; Zipursky et al., 1997). Disomic homozygosity in the pericentromeric region of 21q has been found in trisomy 21 individuals with transient abnormal myelopoiesis and/or ANLL-M7 leukemia (Niikawa et al., 1991; Shen et al., 1995; Dagna-Bricarelli et al., 1997; Cavani et al., 1998). It has been proposed that this region may house a gene encoding a product with tumor suppressor or growth control functions (Niikawa et al., 1991; Ohta et al., 1996).

Comparison of clinical and laboratory characteristics and treatment outcomes of Down syndrome and non-Down syndrome cases of ALL demonstrated that Down syndrome children are less tolerant of intensive treatment regimens, particularly methotrexate therapy (Kalwinsky et al., 1990; Ragab et al., 1991), giving them a poorer outcome in most trials (Chessells et al., 1995). By contrast, Down syndrome children with acute myeloid leukemia (AML) can respond better to intensive therapy than non-Down syndrome patients, and may not need to have bone marrow transplantation in first remission (Ravindranath et al., 1992; Craze et al., 1999). Therefore, an important general message is that although certain drug and radiation toxicities are more common and severe in leukemics with Down syndrome, the results of intensive therapies are impressive and more Down syndrome individuals are being entered into leukemia trials than previously (Dordelmann et al., 1998; Lange et al., 1998).

The immune system and Down syndrome

Immune system disturbances are commonly observed in Down syndrome individuals including an increased frequency of autoimmune disorders, altered proportions of peripheral blood lymphoid subsets, and an increased susceptibility to infection. However, most Down syndrome individuals do not have immunological disease (Mikkelsen et al., 1990; Cuadrado and Barrena 1996), and detailed investigation of antibody-mediated immunity and cell-mediated immunity in Down syndrome has not identified critical immunodeficiencies. Abnormalities that are documented include many lesser immune system defects, often inconstantly present and of uncertain clinical significance, such as leukopenia and macrocytosis (Roizen and Amarose, 1993), which may date from prenatal life to old age (Ugazio et al., 1990; Thilaganathan et al., 1993). These immunological alterations are often age-related changes and may be one feature of a general, early onset senescence in Down syndrome (Cuadrado and Barrena, 1996; Holland, 2000). Complex and sometimes conflicting descriptions of in vivo or in vitro immunological impairments usually makes interpretation of clinical relevances difficult. The next sections briefly outlines reported immunologic abnormalities and implications for care of Down syndrome individuals.

Cell-mediated immunity

Many abnormalities are observed, but clinical implications are difficult to discern. The thymus in Down syndrome is smaller than in chromosomally normal control individuals. Thymus histologic abnormalities include reduced cortical area, thymocyte depletion, loss of corticomedullary demarcation, enlarged cystic Hassal's corpuscles, and evidence of defective expansion of T-cell precursors (discussed by Larocca et al., 1990). Whereas the total number of circulating T lymphocytes is normal or slightly reduced, the distribution of different T-cell subsets may differ from the distribution in controls (Philip et al., 1986). Some changes may be age-related observations such as the appearance of functionally defective natural killer (NK) cells (Cossarizza et al., 1991) or depletion of T lymphocytes, especially in males (Park et al., 2000). Some but not all reports demonstrate low phytohemagglutinin responsiveness in older Down syndrome individuals compared with chromosomally normal controls, which may or may not correlate with reduced interleukin-2 (IL-2) production and, consequently, reduced proliferative response to antigens and mitogens (Ugazio et al., 1990). Studies suggest evidence of diminished cell surface expression of the alpha, beta-chains of the T-cell receptor in Down syndrome thymocytes (the T-cell receptor being necessary for antigen specific recognition [Marrack and Kappler, 1987]), as well as low levels of expression of the CD3 antigen (Murphy et al., 1990; Musiani et al., 1990). Thus, Ugazio et al. (1990) suggested that reduced expansion of T-cell precursors may play an important role in Down syndrome immunodeficiency leading to an incomplete cell repertoire and abnormality of cell-mediated immune response. The defective proliferative response of T lymphocytes has been further investigated and Scotese et al. (1998) concluded T cell activation deficiency is characterized by partial signal transduction through a TCR/CD3 complex, and associated with a selective failure of ZAP-70 tyrosine phosphorylation.

Humoral immunodeficiencies

Humoral immunodeficiencies are generally agreed to be less striking than cell-mediated deficiencies in Down syndrome, but interpretation is difficult because of the variety of reported changes (reviewed by Levin, 1987). There are no major abnormalities of the B-lymphocytes, and serum immunoglobulin levels are not grossly deranged, although there is a tendency for high IgG and low IgM levels after early childhood. The antibody response to various viral protein antigens is inconsistent in Down syndrome subjects, and some studies find reduced response, for example, to influenza virus, but other studies find no such differences. However, there is no doubt that the prevalence of hepatitis B surface antigen (HBsAg) is higher in Down syndrome individuals, whether they are in institutional care or living with their family at home (Madden et al., 1976; Renner et al., 1985). Down syndrome individuals do respond to hepatitis B vaccination, albeit to a lesser degree (Avanzini et al., 1990), so vaccination is indicated to avoid the high risk of becoming an HBsAg carrier. Hepatitis B carriers with Down syndrome were, in one study, at increased risk of developing autoimmune thyroid disease compared with hepatitis B carriers without Down syndrome (May et al., 1996).

Nonspecific immunity

While the number of polymorphonuclear phagocytes is normal, decreased neutrophil chemotaxis, deficient leukocyte opsonization and phagocytosis, decreased leukocyte bactericidal activity, and low leukocyte chemiluminescence activity after phagocytic activation have all been reported in Down syndrome individuals (see Licastro et al., 1990). The gene encoding copper-zinc superoxide dismutase (SOD-1) is located on chromosome 21 and enzymatic activity shows a gene dosage effect leading to 150% activity in Down syndrome individuals. It is speculated that increased SOD-1 leads to low levels of superoxide anions and reduced destruction of organisms which require superoxide radicals for efficient killing. Low serum zinc levels have also been proposed as a possible reason for impaired chemotaxis observed in Down syndrome individuals, since that mineral has a role in promoting chemotaxis as well as being a cofactor in T-cell responsiveness (Locktich et al., 1987; Ugazio et al., 1990). However, Down syndrome individuals do not usually develop clinical signs associated with zinc deficiency and, from published trials (e.g., Licastro et al., 1994), almost all of which are open without controls, the case for convincing clinical benefit from zinc therapy is not proven.

Thyroid disorders and autoimmunity

Hypothyroidism and Down syndrome are strongly associated at all ages (Loudon et al., 1985; Pueschel and Pezullo, 1985;

Kennedy et al., 1992; Karlsson et al., 1999). About one-third of Down syndrome individuals have thyroid autoantibodies, discovery of which often predates diagnosis of hypothyroidism in adults, but not so often in children. In a survey of 106 Down syndrome adults, more than 30% had raised microsomal autoantibodies, but only 5% were hypothyroid, with a further 4% having elevated mildly elevated TSH with normal T3 and T4 levels (Dinani and Carpenter, 1990). In Down syndrome children, a longitudinal study of thyroid function in 107 children who attended a developmental clinic concluded that a high proportion of thyroid dysfunction is compensated and transient, possibly related to inappropriate secretion of thyroid-stimulating hormone (TSH) or thyroid gland insensitivity to TSH, rather than to autoimmune thyroiditis (Selikowitz, 1993b).

Neither thyroid dysfunction nor thyroid autoantibodies have correlated with particular HLA alleles, as might have been expected in the case of an autoimmune disorder (Zori et al., 1990). It is also peculiar that individuals with X chromosome aneuploidy, Klinefelter syndrome and Turner syndrome, seem to have an increased chance of developing thyroid disease (Kelnar, 1989). Presumably this may indicate nonspecific influence of either sex chromosomal or autosomal aneuploidy on immunity and the thyroid gland.

In practice, the high frequency of thyroid dysfunction and the difficulty recognizing clinical signs of hypothyroidism in Down syndrome individuals (lethargy, decreased growth, increased weight, depression, dementia [which is reversible]) has led to proposals of screening protocols. Newborn infants must be screened for congenital hypothyroidism which, along with transient elevation of TSH, occurs at increased frequency (Fort et al., 1984). Older children and adults should have regular checks including thyroid antibodies, thyroxine and TSH estimations, since thyroid disease may develop at any age (Murdoch et al., 1977). The optimal frequency of checks is not clear but annual screening is easier to schedule and in children this is conveniently performed through school-based dried blood spot analysis (Noble et al., 2000). Abnormal thyroid function tests often require careful consideration before treatment is commenced. For example, elevated TSH with normal T4/T3 levels have been reported in association with growth retardation in young children (Sharav et al., 1988), but this was not confirmed by Selikowitz (1993b), and there was no evidence of benefit from short-term T4 treatment for Down syndrome individuals with compensated hypothyroidism (Tirosh et al., 1989).

Data on the frequency of other autoimmune disorders in Down syndrome individuals are puzzling. Celiac disease and insulin dependent diabetes mellitus (IDDM) are more common (Anwar et al., 1998; Pueschel et al., 1999) as are

alopecia and vitiligo (Brown et al., 1977; Shield et al., 1999; Tazi-Ahnini et al., 2000). Thyroid disease plus IDDM has higher prevalence in children with Down syndrome (Griffin et al., 1997), but other conditions such as systemic lupus erythematosus are rarer (Suwa et al., 2000). One of the strongest autoimmune disease associations is between Down syndrome and a poly- or pauciarticular arthropathy which resembles juvenile rheumatoid arthritis and which affects about 1% of trisomy 21 individuals (Yancey et al., 1984; Olson et al., 1990). Symptoms respond to treatment with nonsteroidal anti-inflammatory drugs but remission of the disease may not occur. Rarer types of arthropathy such as psoriatic arthropathy (Tudor, 1976; Jorgensen et al., 1995) or gout (Dacre and Huskisson, 1988; Kamantani et al., 1996) have also been reported.

Down syndrome: epilepsy

Epileptic seizures are present in at least 5% to 10% of individuals with Down syndrome (Stafstrom et al., 1991; Johannsen et al., 1996). Seizures are therefore commoner than in chromosomally normal individuals, but they occur less frequently in Down syndrome than in other types of mental retardation. The prevalence of seizures in Down syndrome is also age dependent (Veall, 1974), with peaks in infancy and late adult life when they are associated with the onset and progression of dementia (Pueschel et al., 1991a; Stafstrom et al., 1991). In childhood, different seizure types have been reported, including tonic-clonic seizures, myoclonic epilepsy and reflex anoxic seizures. Clinical aspects and biologic mechanisms are reviewed by Stafstrom (1993). The most important practical point is that the diagnosis of fits, faints and epilepsy in Down syndrome children and adults is primarily clinical and crucially dependent on reliable history and accurate observation. The electroencephalogram (EEG) is not a primary diagnostic tool and, if used as such, will lead to misdiagnosis and inappropriate treatment. However, EEG studies are often essential to clarify the type of epilepsy following positive clinical diagnosis and to manage certain epilepsies such as the epileptic encephalopathy associated with infantile spasms (Stephenson and King, 1989). Treatment of different seizure disorders in Down syndrome should follow the same principles and practice applicable to epilepsy treatments prescribed for chromosomally normal individuals.

One particular seizure type, infantile spasms, merits special mention because subtle expression of this seizure may delay diagnosis in Down syndrome infants (Stephenson, 1990). Also, the poor prognosis attributed to infantile spasms affecting chromosomally normal infants does not necessarily apply;

seemingly fewer trisomy 21 infants with spasms suffer developmental regression or go on to develop other types of epilepsy that are difficult to control with anticonvulsants (Stafstrom and Konkol, 1994; Silva et al., 1996).

Febrile seizures are infrequently reported in Down syndrome children, but this does not mean that they occur infrequently; for example, Romano et al. (1990) recorded febrile seizures in six out of 15 Down syndrome individuals with different types of seizure.

Down syndrome: Alzheimer disease

The brains of adults with Down syndrome who are over 40 years old virtually all have neuropathologic changes similar to those seen in Alzheimer disease; the relationship between neuropathologic changes and the development of dementia in Down syndrome individuals is complex as the number of adults with Down syndrome who develop cognitive impairments is lower than that expected from the neuropathological studies (see Dalton and Wisniewski, 1990; Oliver et al., 1998; Petronis, 1999; Sadowski et al., 1999). Clinical diagnosis of dementia is difficult in Down syndrome (Burt et al., 1998; Deb and Breganza, 1999) and studies have suggested that the prevalence of dementia has been overestimated (e.g., Devenny et al., 1992, 1996). A prospective study indicated overall prevalence of Alzheimer disease of 8% by age 49 years rising to more than 75% among those over 60 years of age (Lai and Williams, 1989). By comparison, among chromosomally normal individuals, the prevalence of Alzheimer disease is about 20% between ages 75 and 85 years, and 45% for individuals over 85 years of age. Males with Down syndrome are more likely to dement (Schupf et al., 1998) and there is some blood biochemical and cytological evidence to support the notion that Down syndrome adults "age" and lose skills at a faster rate than other individuals with conditions such as unexplained mental retardation, cerebral palsy, and epilepsy (Zigman et al., 1987; Nakamura and Tanaka, 1998).

Although the symptoms and signs of Alzheimer disease are similar in Down syndrome and non-Down syndrome individuals—personality change, gait disturbance, loss of daily living skills, epilepsy, and incontinence, diagnosis in Down syndrome is more difficult. Functional decline is also a feature of depression or hypothyroidism (or both) in adults with Down syndrome and these are important treatable conditions to rule out in each case (Geldmacher et al., 1997).

The average interval between onset of dementia and death is 3.2 years (Lai and Williams, 1989). Cranial computed tomography (CT) scans show atrophic changes, with variable widening of cerebrospinal fluid (CSF) spaces and, after 50 years of age, occasional marked enlargement of the temporal horns (LeMay and Alverez, 1990). Magnetic resonance images show the atrophic process in greater detail (Pearlson et al., 1998). Postmortem examination findings, extensively documented in the literature for many years, are senile plaques containing beta-amyloid, neurofibrillary tangles, and amyloid angiopathy. Modern, detailed case studies also reveal additional findings such as neuronal sprouting, that may have significance for future understanding (Ohara et al., 1999).

Initial genetic linkage studies suggested a locus for early-onset, familial Alzheimer disease on chromosome 21 (St George-Hyslop et al., 1987). Subsequently, some mutations in the beta-amyloid precursor protein gene (APP) on chromosome 21 were found to co-segregate with dementia in a proportion of families with early-onset familial Alzheimer disease (other mutations within this gene are associated with different neurologic phenotypes especially cerebro-arterial amyloidosis OMIM 104760). Relationships between dementia, beta-amyloid, and Down syndrome have been the subject of many studies (see Petronis, 1999) and animal models promise to increase understanding (Kola and Hertzog, 1997). In the meantime, conventional genetic association studies with demented and non-demented Down syndrome individuals have mostly indicated that specific apolipoprotein genotypes confer similar risk effects in Down syndrome dementia and non-Down syndrome dementia: apolipoprotein ε4 allele carriers have increased risk of dementia and, possibly, homozygous ε2 individuals have decreased risk (Schupf et al., 1998; Lai et al., 1999; Rubinsztein et al., 1999; Deb et al., 2000). A presenilin (chromosome 14) gene polymorphism in Down syndrome probands and their parents was examined by Petersen et al. (2000) who found some evidence of a rather complex association between an intron 8 polymorphism in the mothers' presenilin-1 gene, the stage of the meiotic error leading to trisomy 21 and the mothers' apolipoprotein E genotype.

The unknown basis of the association between Down syndrome and Alzheimer disease has also been the subject of epidemiologic studies. The EURODEM collaborative reanalysis of published case-control studies investigated the frequency of Down syndrome births in the families of individuals with Alzheimer disease and the frequency of Alzheimer disease in relatives of Down syndrome individuals. The study revealed that there is 2.7 times greater risk of developing Alzheimer disease if the subject has a first-degree relative with Down syndrome (van Duijn et al., 1991). A subsequent case-control study (Schupf et al., 1994), designed in the knowledge that an age-related, maternal nondisjunction event provides the usual source of the extra chromosome in Down syndrome, found an increased risk of dementia among mothers of Down syndrome probands compared with control mothers (risk ratio 2.6, 95% confidence limits 0.9 to 7.3). Moreover, the increased risk was five times greater among mothers aged under 35 at the birth of the Down syndrome infant and was not increased at all among mothers who were over 35 years at the proband's birth. The authors of this study hypothesized that there is shared genetic susceptibility to Down syndrome and Alzheimer disease, and Petronis (1999) suggested aberrant meiotic recombination in chromosome 21 may play a role, similar to observations in trinucleotide repeat expansion diseases. As Petronis (1999) comments, the aberrant meiotic recombination hypothesis lends itself to experimental testing.

The similarity between the neuropathology of Down syndrome and Alzheimer's dementia led Scinto et al. (1994) to investigate whether Down syndrome-associated hypersensitivity to drugs that block the neurotransmitter acetylcholine is also present in individuals with a clinical diagnosis of Alzheimer disease. Remarkably, 18 out of 19 patients with probable Alzheimer disease had hypersensitivity to the mydriatic effect of locally instilled tropicamide. Evidence of functional and neuropathological similarity between Alzheimer disease and dementia associated with Down syndrome suggests that adults with trisomy 21 might benefit from acetylcholinesterase inhibitors that have, in clinical trials, conferred benefits to mildly and moderately affected Alzheimer disease patients (Wilcock et al., 2000).

Down syndrome: rare neurologic problems

Among the rare neurologic problems that may be more frequent or underdiagnosed in Down syndrome are congenital malformations such as severe microcephaly and holoprosencephaly (Martinez-Frias, 1989), cerebrovascular disorders including moya-moya disease (Vicari and Albertini, 1991; Leno et al., 1998; Dai et al., 2000); multiinfarct dementia (Collacott et al., 1994); and intracerebral hemorrhage with cerebral amyloid angiopathy (Donahue et al., 1998). Late-onset mania has been reported (Cooper et al., 1994) but Down syndrome individuals generally suffer less bipolar affective disease compared with both intellectually impaired and nonimpaired chromosomally normal individuals (Craddock and Owen, 1994). Of individuals with Down syndrome and psychiatric disease, males tend to be more disturbed than females (Lund, 1988) and Haveman et al. (1994) noted that increased psychiatric morbidity in elderly people with Down syndrome often corresponded with physicians' diagnosis of "dementia".

Down syndrome: atlantoaxial subluxation and instability and other orthopedic problems

Nomenclature is not always consistent: atlantoaxial subluxation is widely regarded as a serious, infrequent complication of Down syndrome that causes neurologic symptoms and signs of spinal cord compression. In contrast, atlantoaxial instability is defined radiologically as an atlantoaxial gap of greater than 4 mm (Locke et al., 1966) and this is frequently observed without any symptoms or clinical signs in lateral-view radiographs of the cervical region in full flexion and extension. Instability does not predict increased risk of cord compression (Davidson, 1988; Selby et al., 1991; Cremers et al., 1993; Morton et al., 1995). Moreover, the measurement of instability has limited intraobserver reproducibility and interobserver reliability (Wellborn et al., 2000).

Peuschel (1998) took issue with the revised recommendations of the American Academy of Pediatrics who, in 1995, withdrew an older recommendation that radiological screening should be employed to detect atlantoaxial instability in Down syndrome (Atlantoaxial Instability in Down syndrome, 1995). The American Academy's view that lateral X-rays have no predictive value and should not be routinely used has been endorsed by the medical advisors of the British Down Syndrome Association. In practice, whether or not radiographs are performed and whether or not physical activities are restricted, a few Down syndrome individuals will develop symptoms and signs of spinal cord compression and early diagnosis is vital. In practice, neck flexion and extension radiographs are often carried out before a first anesthetic is given or prior to commencing a contact sport such as judo or trampolining (Chapman, 1995). Of course, after any accidental injury, but especially a road traffic accident, great care is required in case there has been cervical spine injury.

Ferguson et al. (1997) studied 84 patients with Down syndrome who underwent flexion-extension lateral X rays of the C1-C2 articulation for the purpose of dividing the group into subluxators and nonsubluxators. Seventeen patients (20%) were defined as subluxators, and five of the subluxaters had positive neurologic findings. However, 18 (27%) of the nonsubluxators had similar positive neurologic findings. Ferguson et al. concluded that positive neurologic findings and an abnormal atlanto-dens interval are not alone adequate criteria to judge need for surgical stabilization of the C1-C2 articulation in patients with Down syndrome.

Worrying symptoms and signs of cord compression are sudden or gradual onset of neck pain, change in bowel or bladder function, clumsy hand movements, torticollis, sudden preference for sitting, poor balance, decreased walking, increased tendon reflexes, ankle clonus, upgoing plantar response, and spasticity. Such signs may occur at any age, even in young children (Tseng and Cheng, 1998) and they demand urgent neurologic evaluation since surgical treatment of craniovertebral junction abnormalities can produce good or excellent results (Taggard et al., 2000).

Degenerative cervical spine abnormalities may also be more frequent among Down syndrome individuals and there are anecdotal accounts of delayed diagnosis of serious cervical spondyloarthritic myelopathy in patients in their fifth decade (Bosma et al., 1999; Frost et al., 1999). Cervical spine degeneration occurs in karyotypically normal individuals at the C4, C5, and C6 vertebral levels especially. In Down syndrome, the changes are distributed in various cervical interspaces but may be comparatively more frequent at the C2 and C3 vertebral levels (Tangerud et al., 1990).

Osteoporosis is probably underdiagnosed in Down syndrome adults. Reduced bone mineral density has been demonstrated in adults living at home (Angelopoulou et al., 1999) and histologically proven osteoporosis was found in a previously mobile 49-year-old adult male who died of pulmonary embolus six days after surgical repair of fractured femoral neck (Grimwood et al., 2000).

CONTROVERSIAL TREATMENTS FOR DOWN SYNDROME

A balanced review of controversial therapies for Down syndrome is given by Rogers and Coleman (1992). Plastic surgery has been performed on Down syndrome children to uplift the flat nasal profile, remove epicanthic folds, alter palpebral fissure angle, and reduce tongue size. Assessing the role of surgical alteration to Down syndrome facial attributes is not straightforward. Certain operations may be justified on the basis of oral or facial pathology that merits similar treatment in the chromosomally normal child. Other operations, for example, to reduce the size of an ulcerated, protruding tongue, may have a medical goal that is inextricably entwined with a cosmetic advantage. Yet other procedures may not have a conventional medical goal but are justified by the argument that it is easier to change the appearance of a child with Down syndrome than to remove the misconceptions and prejudices of others which that appearance engenders. Ethical issues are to the fore (Aylott 1999; Jones, 2000) and, interestingly, there is evidence that cosmetic surgery is favored more by people who

are less involved on a day-to-day basis with Down syndrome children (Saviolo-Negrin and Cristante, 1992).

Treatment with vitamin and mineral supplements is less dramatic than plastic surgery but may be no less contentious. Nowadays, many healthy individuals supplement a normal, balanced diet with a variety of vitamins and trace elements. As a commercial enterprise, vitamin supplementation is a large and highly profitable business which is heavily advertised on television and in the press. Generally, across-the-counter supplements taken at recommended dosages do no harm but some alternative treatments including megavitamin therapies can produce dangerous side effects (Bidder et al., 1989). The scientific evidence for the use of nutritional supplements in Down syndrome was the subject of an excellent review by Ani et al. (2000). In summary, although there is some evidence to implicate increased oxidative stress in the pathology of Down syndrome (e.g., see Odetti et al., 1998), Ani et al. (2000) stated there is no consistent or rigorous proof that any form of nutritional supplement improves the outcome in Down syndrome. Well-conducted clinical trials are required to investigate effects of antioxidant therapy. The same may be said of the new class of psychoactive drugs such as piracetam (Holmes, 1999) which are claimed to enhance cognition.

CYTOGENETICS OF DOWN SYNDROME

Trisomy 21

Mikkelsen et al. (1980) investigated the origin of trisomy 21 using cytogenetic methods and discovered that most nondisjunction errors occurred during the first meiotic division in the mother. Hassold and Sherman (2000) reviewed their own studies and those of others who have used chromosome 21 DNA polymorphisms to prove that approximately 90% of trisomy 21 cases result from a maternal meiosis nondisjunction error, 75% of which occur at maternal meiosis 1. In the 8% of cases in which the extra chromosome is paternal in origin, meiosis 1 and meiosis 2 nondisjunction events are equally frequent. Chromosome fluorescence in situ hybridization (FISH) studies carried out on the sperm of fathers who had trisomy 21 conceptions of paternal origin, showed no increase in the incidence of disomy 21 sperm above the frequency of 0.15%, present in non-trisomy 21 fathers (Hixon et al., 1998). Whether such cases are relatively more frequent in pregnancies sampled at mid gestation, as Muller et al. (2000) found, remains to be confirmed.

Hassold and Sherman (2000) also reviewed evidence they and others have gathered on the genetic recombination and human nondisjunction. The risk of maternal meiosis 1 error is increased when the chromosome 21 bivalent is either achiasmate (a very rare observation in normal female meiosis) or when a single cross over is observed in distal 21q. Such "distal-only" exchanges seem to be less efficient at segregating the chromosomes than proximally placed crossovers. But a surprising finding was made by Lamb et al. (1997) who discovered that in trisomy 21 of maternal meiosis 2 origin, an exchange near the centromere increases the chance of nondisjunction. Lamb et al. (1997) suggested that this may be explained if maternal meiosis 2 errors are more apparent rather than real, and such errors really originate at meiosis 1 by chromosome entanglement due to proximal exchange, or by premature separation of sister chromatids at meiosis 1 with migration together due to chance at meiosis 2. Certainly, the maternal age effect operates for maternal meiosis 1 and maternal meiosis 2 errors.

Evidence on the role of genetic recombination in other human chromosome nondisjunctions varies: achiasmate bivalents are responsible for most paternally derived cases of 47,XXY, some maternal meiosis 1 sex chromosome trisomy, but not for trisomy 16 (Hassold and Sherman, 2000). The distal placed exchanges are important in trisomies 16 and 21 but not in other trisomies. The main origin of trisomy 18 cases appears to be maternal meiosis 2 errors (Fisher et al., 1995) and no significant effect of recombination has been observed (Bugge et al., 1998).

Compared with the maternal age effect, other maternal factors have a much weaker or unsubstantiated influence on the chance of a trisomy 21 conceptus. For example, an increased risk occurs with a diminished oocyte pool and earlier menopause (Kline et al., 2000); reduced ovarian complement, whether due to congenital absence or surgical removal (Freeman et al., 2000); the presence of certain methylenetetrahydrofolate reductase gene polymorphisms in the mother (Botto and Yang, 2000; Hobbs et al., 2000); the accumulation of spontaneous mitochondrial DNA deletion mutations that diminish the supply of energy to cells surrounding the oocyte (Schon et al., 2000).

Hook (1992) has provided a concise summary of evidence on other factors, such as exposure to certain chemicals, drugs, or irradiation, which have been implicated but not confirmed in the causation of trisomy 21. There has been debate about the effect of the 1986 nuclear accident at Chernobyl on the incidence of Down syndrome in parts of Europe, but no firm conclusion was reached (Boice and Linet, 1994; Sperling et al., 1994; Verger, 1997; Stoll et al., 1998c). Maternal glucose intolerance or gestational diabetes mellitus have been considered risk factors for trisomy

21 (Milunsky, 1976; Narchi and Kulayat, 1997), and the influence of maternal smoking is unproven (Chen et al., 1999) although certain malformations in Down syndrome may be more common if the mother smokes (Torfs and Christianson, 1999).

Whether a general, chromosome nonspecific, tendency to nondisjunction exists is unresolved. Such a phenomenon might account for case reports describing predisposition to suffer different trisomies in successive pregnancies (e.g., FitzPatrick and Boyd, 1986). Prenatal diagnosis data also suggest a slightly increased tendency for mothers who had a pregnancy with trisomy 21 to have greater chance of recurrence of any other trisomy, as well as trisomy 21, although the overall increase in risk for any autosomal trisomy does not exceed by more than 1% the maternal age-specific risk for all chromosomal abnormalities at that age (Stene et al., 1984). The existence of a recessive gene mutation which might underlie a predisposition to general or chromosome specific mitotic nondisjunction in the zygote was postulated by Alfi et al. (1980), who observed an increased frequency of parental consanguinity among the parents of their patients with Down syndrome. Subsequent studies (Cereijo and Martinez–Frias, 1993; Zlotogora, 1997; Sayee and Thomas, 1998) failed to confirm a higher incidence of close consanguinity among parents of individuals with Down syndrome. Nevertheless, the suggestion lingers and there are observations in some populations that are compatible with the hypothesis that lesser degrees of kinship between father and mother of Down syndrome cases may operate to prevent spontaneous loss of trisomy 21 conceptions (Roberts et al., 1991; de Braekeleer et al., 1994).

Trisomy 21 mosaicism

Richards (1974) analyzed maternal ages at the time of mosaic Down syndrome births and estimated that in a minority of phenotypically diagnosed cases, the extra chromosome arose through a mitotic nondisjunction. Molecular methods have since confirmed that only about 2% of all cases with trisomy 21 arise from a mitotic error in somatic cells of the zygote (Antonarakis et al., 1993a; Sherman et al., 1994; Zaragoza et al., 1994). While the trisomic cell line generated by mitotic nondisjunction survives, its reciprocal product, the 45, –21 cell line dies, leaving the embryo with euploid and trisomy 21 cells.

Mosaic trisomy 21 is more often caused by a maternal meiotic error; Pangalos et al. (1994) found this in 10 out of 17 cases, with a mean maternal age of 31.4 years. A mitotic error was a likely mechanism in the remaining cases, which had a lower mean maternal age of 27.4 years. The meiotic origin of most cases of mosaic Down syndrome means that couples who have had an affected child or fetus should be given the same genetic counseling advice that follows diagnosis of full trisomy 21. While this may overestimate the risk in some families, it avoids surprise in other families where mosaic trisomy 21 with origins in full trisomy, is followed a by a full trisomy 21 pregnancy (Bruyere et al., 2000).

Translocation Down syndrome

In about 5% of all cases of Down syndrome, the extra chromosome 21 is fused with another large or small acrocentric chromosome (13, 14, and 15 are D-group acrocentrics; 21 and 22 are G-group acrocentrics). The fusion, sometimes described as a whole arm exchange, is called a Robertsonian translocation in recognition of Robertson's contribution from his studies on insect cytogenetics early last century. Usually, the Robertsonian chromosome is dicentric although true monocentric chromosomes resulting from centromere fusion do occur. Some dicentrics appear monocentric because one centromere is suppressed. Nonhomologous Robertsonian translocations, involving fusion of two different acrocentrics, are much more frequent than homologous Robertsonian translocations.

There are no clinical differences between individuals with trisomy 21 Down syndrome and those with Robertsonian translocation Down syndrome. To describe the rearranged chromosomes Gardner and Sutherland (1996) employed a clear, shortened nomenclature that is mostly followed here. In cases with D;21 translocations, about one third are inherited from one parent who has the balanced translocation karyotype, for example, 45,XX, rob (14q21q). Among inherited cases, in more than 90% of instances, the mother is the carrier parent. Only about 7% of affected individuals with G;21 Robertsonian translocations have a carrier parent and, once again, the mother is usually the carrier (Hook, 1981). All de novo Robertsonian (14q21q) trisomies studied have had their origins in maternal germ cells (Petersen et al., 1991; Shaffer et al., 1992), and the mean maternal age (29.2 years) is only slightly raised above the population mean maternal age (27 years).

The majority of homologous Robertsonian translocations are not centric fusion or whole arm exchange chromosomes, rather, they are isochromosomes from fusion of sister chromatids, leading to homozygosity, at a very early postzygotic mitosis (see Grasso et al., 1989; Shaffer et al., 1993). It is argued that isochromosomes can arise postconception in somatic tissues of trisomic conceptuses (Robinson et al., 1994). In the minority of cases proved to be true homologous Robertsonian (21;21) chromosomes, the abnormal chromosome arises from fusion, in the mother, of paternal and maternal homologs so that heterozygosity is maintained (Antonarakis et al., 1990; Shaffer et al., 1993).

Down syndrome with a normal karyotype

Rarely, features of the Down syndrome phenotype are present in individuals with normal chromosomes (see Epstein et al., 1991; Ayme and Philip, 1997). Possible explanations for apparent phenotype-karyotype discrepancy include undetected mosaicism for trisomy 21 and cryptic imbalance of chromosome 21 that can now be revealed by chromosome 21 FISH (Bartsch et al., 1997; Garcia-Heras et al., 1999). Simple misdiagnosis can occur: infants with Zellweger syndrome, Smith–Magenis syndrome or tetrasomy 12p may bear some resemblances to Down syndrome, but not usually for long.

MOLECULAR GENETICS

Chromosome 21 was the first human chromosome to have its DNA sequence reported (Hattori et al., 2000). Analysis revealed 127 known genes, 98 predicted genes and 59 pseudogenes. Compared with chromosome 22, chromosome 21 is gene-poor having half the number of genes of the former. It is thought that the low number of genes on chromosome 21 contributes to the increased chance of survival in this autosomal aneuploid syndrome compared with other trisomies.

Identification of cases with clinical features of Down syndrome in association with duplication of specific regions of chromosome 21 (e.g., see Nadal et al., 2001) has resulted in the designation of a "Down syndrome critical region" at 21q22 to qter. The role of the extra copy of genes in this region in determining the Down syndrome phenotype is unknown at present, but it seems unlikely that all phenotypic effects are attributable to critical gene dosage (see Kurnit et al., 1987; and Delabar et al., 1993; Korenberg et al., 1994; Pritchard and Kola, 1999). While genes such as DSCR1, through its evolutionary conservation, interaction with transcription regulators and its expression pattern in Down syndrome fetal tissues, are prime candidates for involvement in the molecular pathology of Down syndrome (Fuentes et al., 2000), until the functions of all the genes on chromosome 21 are understood, the molecular pathology of Down syndrome remains largely speculative.

Studies may now be designed in mouse models of Down syndrome. The trisomy 16 mouse has three copies of the

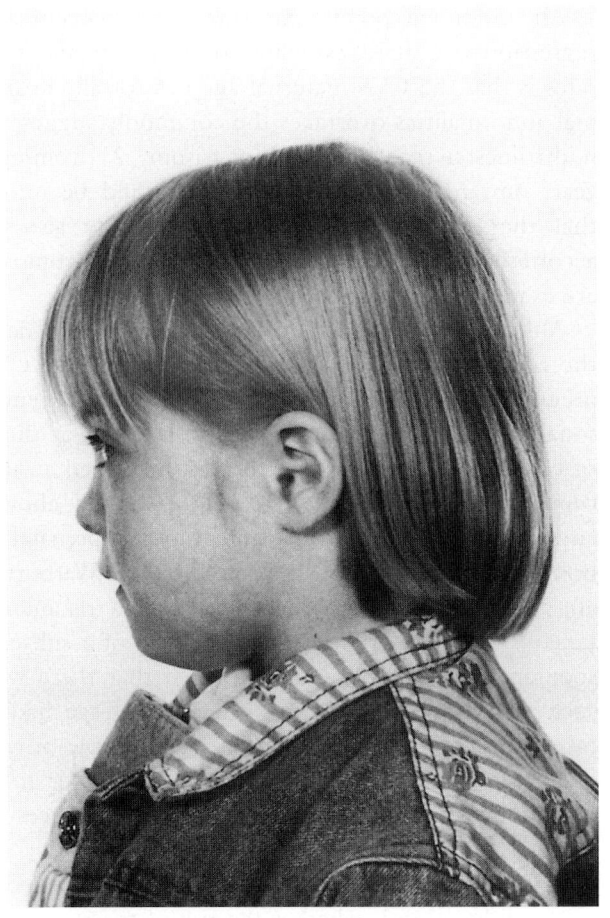 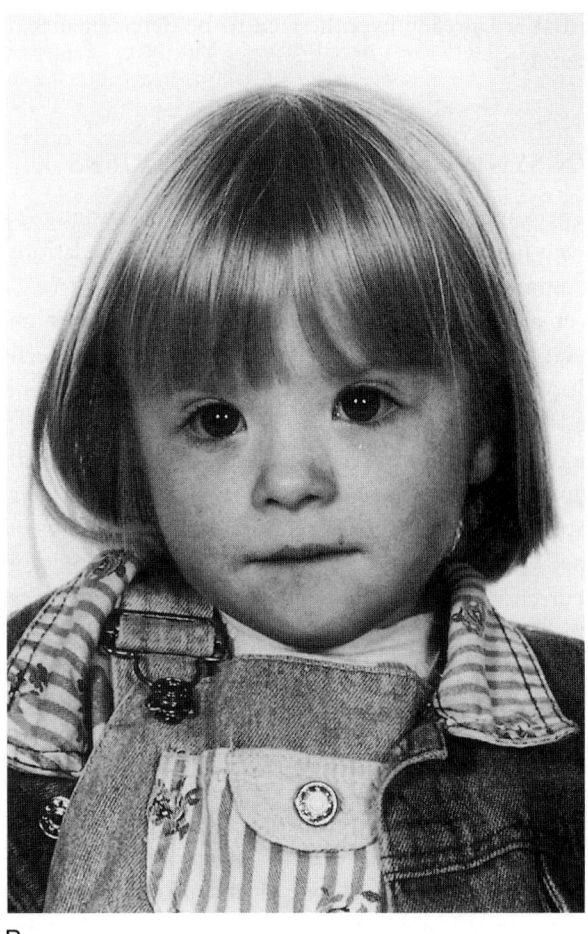

A

B

Fig. 44.6. (A & B) Down syndrome was diagnosed in the newborn period but the phenotype was due to an unbalanced translocation, leading to triplication of 21q21 → qter and deletion of distal Xp. The abnormal X chromosome is preferentially inactivated, accounting for minimal phenotypic expression of Down syndrome features in this bright four-year-old child with short stature.

distal segment of mouse chromosome 16, syntenic with human chromosome 21. Trisomy 16 mice display a number of phenotypes including deficits in learning and memory (Reeves et al., 1995; Sago et al., 2000), and their underlying neocortical abnormalities are being analysed (e.g., see Haydar et al., 2000). Investigation of the Down syndrome phenotype may now occur at neurochemical and neuroanatomical levels. For example, it is known that deficits in the cholinergic system characterize Down syndrome and Alzheimer disease; in the trisomy 16 mouse, cerebral cortical astroglia are less able to support cholinergic function in neurones (Nelson et al., 1997) and loss of cholinergic function occurs with cognitive decline (Granholm et al., 2000). Another observation is Down syndrome individuals have disproportionate reduction in the size of the cerebellum, and reduction in the cerebellar granule cell density is visible in both the trisomic mouse and in Down syndrome (Baxter et al., 2000).

The influence of chromosome 21 genes on complex traits such as learning can also be studied in panels of transgenic mice that carry defined segments of the genome—in vivo libraries (Smith and Rubin, 1997). The human homologue of the Drosophila minibrain gene, MNBH, and human SIM2 gene, homologous to Drosophila singleminded (sim) gene, both map in the Down syndrome "critical region" of chromosome 21 at 21q22. These genes have important roles in central nervous system development and learning in Drosophila. Their roles in Down syndrome are being analyzed in different ways including examination of expression patterns and studies of behavior in trisomy 16 and transgenic mice (Smith and Rubin, 1997; Chrast et al., 1999; Ema et al., 1999). Another approach to understanding Down syndrome is the creation of animal models with gain-of-function or loss-of-function mutations in genes that are not presupposed to be candidates for the trisomy 21 phenotype, as well as genes such as MNBH and

Sim2, that are already hypothesized to be determinants of the phenotype.

DOWN SYNDROME RECURRENCE RISKS

Prevalence and recurrence risk estimates for trisomy 21 have been made at different times in different populations. These estimates have been compared and combined (e.g., Stene et al., 1984; Cuckle et al., 1987; Halliday et al., 1995; Hook et al., 1988; Hook and Cross, 1989; Hecht and Hook, 1994;1996; Snijders et al., 1994a; Hecht and Hook, 1996; Carothers et al., 1999a; Uehara et al., 1999). Although data are now very detailed, when dealing with individuals at the antenatal clinic, it is apparent that numerical expressions of low probability may cause confusion (e.g., see Quagliarini et al., 1998) and small differences in the recurrence risk figures quoted by clinicians may exacerbate this. In the clinic, therefore, it is often helpful to give a rounded risk estimate supplemented with a contextual description.

Trisomy 21 recurrence risk

Data on the chance of recurrence of trisomy 21 in children of mothers who had one liveborn affected infant were summarized by Hook (1992): when the mother was younger (less than 30 years), the recurrence risk was 1.4%, and when she was 30 years or older, the risk was 0.5%. These risks were based on quite small numbers of cases. Hook (1992) also analyzed data on the mid-trimester risk of recurrence diagnosed through amniocentesis. These data indicate that for genetic counseling purposes the chance of recurrence of Down syndrome can be rounded to 1% greater than the maternal age-specific risk at that age. Clearly, this represents a significant increase over the maternal age risk in mothers under 35 years of age, but for mothers over 35 years, the increase over the maternal age risk is less apparent. Hook (1992) points out that women older than 35 years who had their first affected pregnancy under age 30 are more likely to have greater underlying predisposition to recurrence compared with older mothers who had their first affected pregnancy after age 35 years. Preimplantation genetic diagnosis is now being used to enhance the chance of a chromosomally normal child being born to couples who have increased risk of Down syndrome occurrence and recurrence (e.g., see Conn et al., 1999) and, as expected, older recipients of donor embryos do not have an increased risk of aneuploidy (Kornafel and Sauer, 1994).

An additional point concerning recurrence risk and regression-smoothed estimates of maternal age specific rates is that the CVS maternal age risk for all chromosomal abnormalities overtakes the commonly suggested 1% mid-trimester recurrence risk of trisomy 21 from age 36 years onward. Thus, older women should be informed that the risk of chromosomal abnormality also varies according to the stage in gestation when chromosomes are examined.

Although there are no substantive published data on the risk of recurrence measured at the time of CVS in pregnancies subsequent to a first occurrence, it seems reasonable to anticipate that the recurrence risk at the time of CVS will be greater than the risk measured at amniocentesis. The recurrence risk data discussed above are largely derived from rates at mid-trimester prenatal diagnosis following birth of an affected infant. Warburton et al. (1987) asked whether the karyotype of a trisomic spontaneous abortion predicts the karyotype of a subsequent spontaneous abortion and discovered that there was no such trend after information on maternal age had been taken into account. Nevertheless, reasonable advice to couples assumes a trisomy 21 spontaneous or induced abortion has the same recurrence risk consequences as the livebirth of an affected infant.

An issue arising from evidence for general predisposition to nondisjunction is whether the risk of trisomy for chromosomes other than chromosome 21 is increased after prenatal diagnosis or birth of a trisomy 21 fetus or child. Conversely, does the risk of trisomy 21 increase after prenatal diagnosis or birth of a child with any other maternal age-related autosomal aneuploidy? While Warburton et al. (1987) found in the case of spontaneous abortions the risk is insignificantly low, Hook (1992) re-examined published and unpublished data before suggesting the risk of trisomies other than trisomy 21 is slightly increased for women with a previous trisomy 21 infant. Again, reasonable advice is that young women who have had a child or fetus with trisomy 21 or any other viable autosomal trisomy have 1% risk of viable autosomal aneuploidy affecting a future pregnancy and older mothers have a recurrence risk of 1% plus their maternal age risk.

The frequency of trisomy 21 and most mosaic trisomy 21 increases with advancing maternal age, but the frequency of translocation Down syndrome is independent of maternal age. Hook (1982) provided data on the likelihood of the different cytogenetic types of Down syndrome in affected individuals with unknown karyotype based on the mother's age at their birth. In summary, the probability of translocation Down syndrome is very low when the mother is over

35 years and no greater than 10% at the youngest maternal age. Therefore, chromosome analysis carried out on a parent with a positive family history of Down syndrome rarely discloses a balanced Robertsonian translocation, but it remains important to offer blood chromosome analysis to blood relatives of patients when the karyotype of the proband is unknown. When the proband has confirmed trisomy 21, relatives other than the proband's parents may be advised they are not at appreciably increased risk of having a trisomy 21 child.

Translocation Down syndrome

Following the diagnosis of translocation Down syndrome, karyotyping the parents of the affected child or fetus is the first stage in assessing the chance of recurrence in a future pregnancy. If both parents have normal blood chromosomes, the translocation is presumed to have arisen as a result of a new mutation (de novo) and is unlikely to recur. However, Steinberg et al. (1984) and Hall (1985) and others have documented cases in which a parent of a Down syndrome child with a de novo isochromosome (21q) was found on re-examination to be a low-grade mosaic or to have a more complex karyotype. Steinberg et al. (1984) concluded that the recurrence risk for Down syndrome due to

apparently de novo chromosome 21 rearrangements could be between 2% and 3%. Thus, it is appropriate to offer prenatal cytogenetic diagnosis to cytogenetically normal parents who had a fetus or child with Down syndrome due to a de novo structural abnormality.

Where one parent is shown to carry a balanced Robertsonian translocation that has given rise to a child affected by Down syndrome, the risk of recurrence depends on the sex of the carrier parent, as well as the particular chromosomes involved in the translocation (Table 44.1). Most importantly, if the mother is a rob(14q21q) carrier, the risk of recurrence at amniocentesis is 15% (closer to 10% at term due to fetal demise after 16 weeks gestation), compared with a much lower risk of less than 5%, or even less than 1%, if the father is the translocation carrier. Although data are scanty, the same risks and sex difference most probably apply for the rarer rob(13q21q), rob (15q21q) and rob(21q22q) heterozygotes. When chromosome 15 is involved in a Robertsonian translocation, there is a further complication, namely the possibility of an abnormal phenotype due to uniparental disomy, this is discussed below. The highest risk of recurrence, virtually 100%, applies when one parent carries a homologous rob(21q21q) translocation. Most such cases are isochromosomes. The same 100% risk applies for rob(13q13q), rob (15q15q) and rob (22q22q)

Table 44.1. Risks of chromosome abnormality at amniocentesis when one parent carries a balanced, non-homologous Robertsonian translocation (Boué and Gallano, 1984; Hook, 1992).

Robertsonian translocation	No. of fetuses tested	Unbalanced (%)	95% Confidence interval
(13q14q) all	230	0	0–1.3%
maternal	157	0	0–1.9%
paternal	73	0	0–4%
(13q15q) all	15	0	0–18.1%
(13q21q) all	31	2 (6%)	0–11.2%
maternal	20	2 (10%)	0–16.8%
paternal	11	0	0–23.8%
(13q22q)	3	1 (33%)	0.8–90.6%
maternal	1	0	0–95%
paternal	2	1 (50%)	1.3–98.7%
(14q21q)	188	21 (11%)	7.1–16.3%
maternal	137	21 (15%)	9.8–22.4%
paternal	51	0	0–7.0%
(15q21q)	14	1 (7%)	0.2–33.9%
maternal	9	1 (11%)	0.3–48.3%
paternal	5	0	0–45.1%
(21q22q)	22	3 (14%)	2.9–34.9%
maternal	19	3 (16%)	3.4–39.6%
paternal	3	0	0–63.2%

In summary, if chromosome 21 is involved, the risk of Down syndrome approaches 15% for a female carrier and is less than 5% for a male carrier. If chromosome 13 is involved, the risk of Patau syndrome is less than 1% for male and female carriers. Gardner and Sutherland's monograph (1996) provides excellent, detailed discussion of chromosome imbalance recurrence risks.

carrier parents, although the vast majority of unbalanced conceptions will not develop or miscarry early in pregnancy.

Two Down syndrome pregnancies

Up to 3% of couples may have a much greater risk of recurrence of either trisomy 21 or translocation Down syndrome due to the presence of mosaicism in one parent (Harris et al., 1982; Uchida and Freeman, 1985; Cozzi et al., 1999). For example, Sachs et al. (1990) detected mosaicism in two parents who had three pregnancies and four pregnancies, respectively, affected by trisomy 21. One of these parents had 47% trisomy 21 cells present in cultures derived from an ovarian biopsy. A third couple, who had normal chromosomes, had three pregnancies with (21;21) translocation Down syndrome. Sachs et al. (1990) concluded that after two pregnancies with trisomy 21 or translocation 21 Down syndrome, gonadal mosaicism should be considered as the cause of an elevated recurrence risk. The actual figure is unknown but in some families it may approach 50%.

Gonadal mosaicism is very difficult to detect. Molecular techniques were used by James et al. (1998) to demonstrate novel chromosome 21 alleles in the trisomic offspring of one young mother—evidence that the mother had been conceived as a trisomy with three different chromosomes 21. FISH in lymphocytes (Shi et al., 2000) may also be used to detect low level somatic mosaicism, as seen in an unusual case of a clinically normal father and his mosaic son who also had no features of Down syndrome (Casati et al., 1992). The same authors reviewed other such cases with and without features of Down syndrome and proposed a genetically determined predisposition to mitotic nondisjunction, noting the work of Fitzgerald et al. (1986), who recorded premature centromere division of chromosome 21, presumed to give rise to repeated primary nondisjunction in subjects with Down syndrome offspring.

Rarely, women with trisomy 21 may become pregnant and in this situation the risk of trisomy 21 in the offspring is close to 50% (Bovicelli et al., 1982). Fertility in males with trisomy 21 is exceptional, but there are at least two well-documented reports of an affected male fathering an unaffected child (Bobrow et al., 1992; Zühlke et al., 1994).

Trisomy 18—Edwards syndrome

Trisomy 18, or Edwards syndrome (Edwards et al., 1960), was described one year after trisomy 21 but, unlike Down

syndrome, there was little or no appreciation of the clinical syndrome prior to the discovery of the additional E group chromosome.

The birth frequency of trisomy 18 is approximately 1 in 6000 (Bond and Chandley 1983; Young et al., 1986; Goldstein and Nielsen, 1988; Carothers et al., 1999b). At birth, the sex ratio (M/F) is 0.65, significantly less than unity (Ferguson-Smith, 1962; Weber, 1967), and this is also the case during gestation but the difference then is less marked, suggesting decreased in utero survival in males with trisomy 18 (Carothers et al., 1999b).

Well-documented clinicopathologic data on trisomy 18 have been supplemented by data on the prenatal phenotype of fetuses with trisomy 18 diagnosed through ultrasound scanning. Inevitably, clinical data on the phenotype does vary with the mode of case ascertainment.

TRISOMY 18 PHENOTYPE

Fetus with trisomy 18

In cytogenetic surveys of spontaneous abortions, trisomy 18 is less common than trisomy 21 (Warburton et al., 1991). However, among fetuses karyotyped after ultrasound diagnosis of fetal malformation and/or growth retardation, trisomy 18 is the commonest cytogenetic disorder, occurring about 50% more frequently than trisomy 21 (Eydoux et al., 1989; Nicolaides et al., 1992b). Thus, while trisomy 21 is difficult to diagnose by prenatal ultrasound scanning, trisomy 18 (and trisomy 13) are readily diagnosed by virtue of ultrasonographically detectable major malformations in association with growth retardation, oligohydramnios or polyhydramnios (Fig. 44.7). (Twining, 1995). As discussed at the beginning of this chapter, intrauterine mortality associated with trisomy 18 is high, and Hook (1992) calculated that only 2.5% of all trisomy 18 conceptions survive to be liveborn with about 30% of those alive at midtrimester amniocentesis surviving to term.

Diagnosis may be made in the first trimester during screening for trisomy 21 by a combination of maternal age and fetal nuchal translucency thickness (NT) at 10–14 weeks (Nicolaides et al., 1992a). In a multicentre study of 91,091 singleton pregnancies, there were 106 fetuses with trisomy 18 (a remarkably high trisomy 18 rate of 1 in 859, reflecting the selected nature of the population) and 83% were identified by NT screening (Sherod et al., 1997). Trisomy 18 may also be detected in early gestation through its strong association with fetal hand abnormalities (Lam and Tang, 1998; Shields et al., 1998) and ultrasound findings in the cranium including choroid plexus cysts, minimal

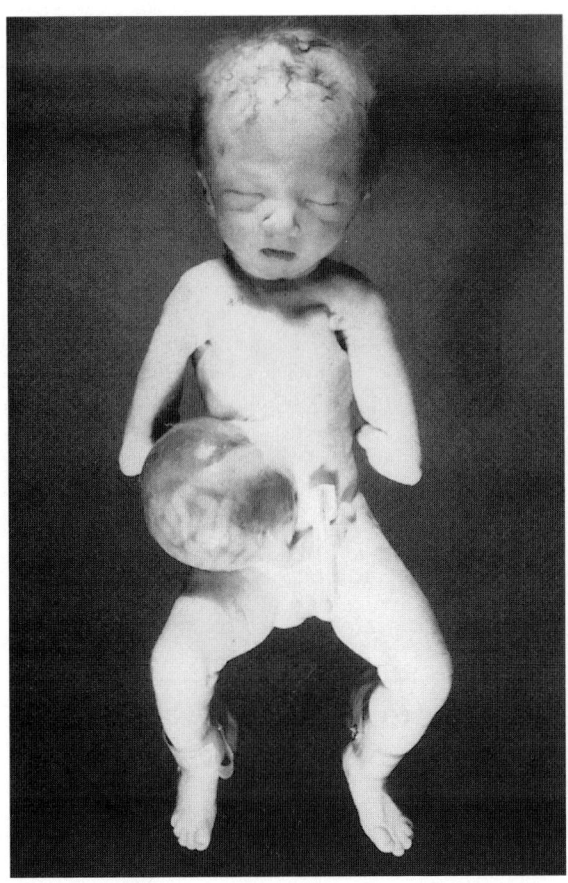

Fig. 44.7. Exomphalos and limb defects associated with trisomy 18. See Beccerra et al. (1992) for review of limb defects in trisomy 18.

central nervous system malformations, an abnormal nuchal skin fold, ventricular septal defect, outflow tract abnormalities of the heart, and right-to-left chamber disproportion of the heart) and one interaction between markers (right-to-left chamber disproportion and outflow tract abnormalities) contributed most to the identification of 93% of fetuses with trisomy 18, with a false-positive rate of 8.9%. Noncardiovascular markers (choroid plexus cysts, central nervous system malformations, and abnormal nuchal skin fold) identified 77% of fetuses with trisomy 18, with a false-positive rate of 3.9%. Conversely, normal anatomy can be used to reduce but not abolish the risk of trisomy 18 using a Bayesian approach (Nadel et al., 1995).

Phenotype in infancy

Mean birthweight is reduced, characteristically lying within the range 1.5 to 2.5 kg at or near term (Young et al., 1986; Baty et al., 1994a). The placenta of the trisomy 18 infant is also small (Hecht, 1963). Notably, over 50% of trisomy 18 infants, mostly undiagnosed, are delivered by cesarean section, the main reasons being IUGR and/or fetal distress in labor (Embleton et al., 1996; Saller et al., 1996). At birth, the typical affected neonate has a small, narrow head, open metopic suture, and prominent occiput. Pinnae have unusual morphology, are positioned low on the skull, and are often posteriorly rotated. The mouth is small and micrognathia is present (Fig. 44.8). A short sternum is often hidden by ECG pads, but congenital heart disease with dysmorphism of the hands and feet can be diagnostic—flexed and overlapping digits such that the index finger overlaps the third and the fifth finger overlaps the fourth, small nails, prominence of the heels with convexity of the soles (rocker-bottom feet), and short, dorsiflexed great toes with a slight degree of second and third toe syndactyly. A preponderance of low arch fingerprint patterns (six or more) is a helpful sign but one that is hard to elicit in the neonate.

Phenotype and management of the child with trisomy 18

Information is based on a relatively small number of reported cases with prolonged survival (e.g., Surana et al., 1972; Smith and Dulk, 1980; Karayalcin et al., 1981; Robinson and McQuorquodale, 1981; Mehta et al., 1986; Smith et al., 1989), as well as the questionnaire responses of parents and case record reviews (Baty et al., 1994a; 1994b).

After cytogenetic confirmation of trisomy 18, parents may be told that median survival is less than one week

cerebral ventricular dilation and enlarged cysterna magna (Chen et al., 1998). As with Down syndrome, the value of minor fetal markers of trisomy 18 depends on the frequency of these signs in low-risk populations. Such data are not always available, but in the well-studied case of choroid plexus cysts, Walkinshaw (2000) concluded that the prevalence of such cysts in the general population at mid-gestation is about 1% and the chance of trisomy 18 affecting the fetus is about 1 in 80 if choroid plexus cysts are the only ultrasonographic marker. The chance of trisomy 18 rises sharply if additional abnormalities are present. In practice, any combination of ultrasonographically detectable major malformations (heart defects, exomphalos, myelomeningocele, obstructive uropathy, polyhydramnios due to esophageal atresia, clenched fists, or radial limb defects) with intrauterine growth retardation (IUGR), with or without an abnormal maternal serum biochemical screen result suggests trisomy 18 (Merkatz et al., 1984; Ozturk et al., 1990; Donaldson et al., 1999; Quereshi et al., 2000).

The strong relationship between trisomy 18 and abnormal anatomy was evident in 97% of 30 fetuses with trisomy 18 (DeVore, 2000). Six markers (choroid plexus cysts,

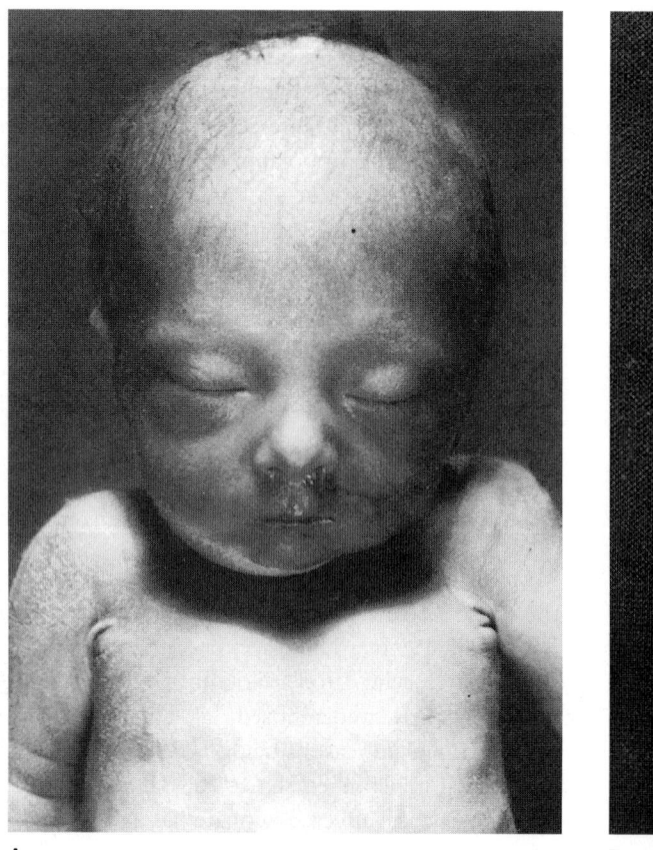 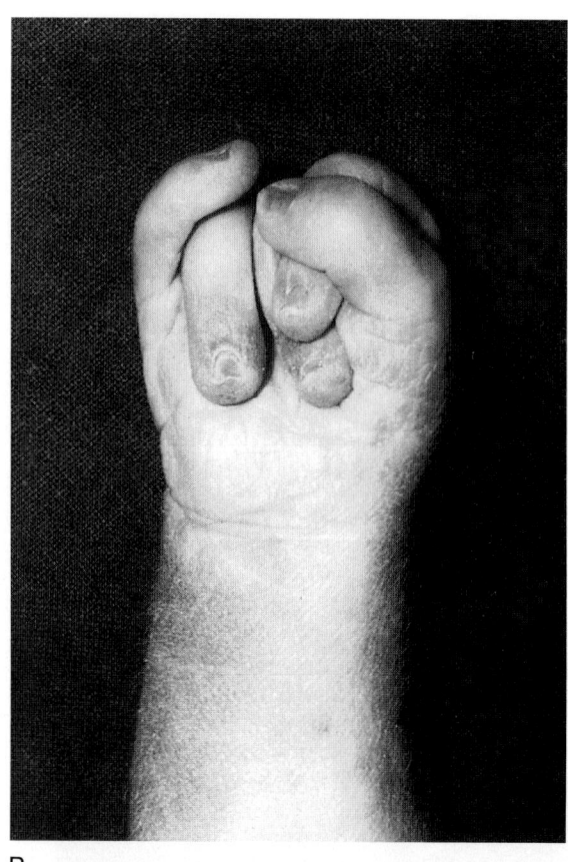

A   B

Fig. 44.8. (A & B) Microstomia, micrognathia, and characteristic positioning of the digits in a deceased infant with trisomy 18.

(Embleton et al., 1996) and 90% of babies die by six months. Of equal importance, up to 5% are still alive at age one year (Root and Carey, 1994). Once the prognosis has been explained to the parents, a joint decision is usually made to eschew aggressive therapies aimed at prolonging life (Anon, 1992; Bos et al., 1992). Couples may prefer to care for their critically ill infant at home, an ideal arrangement provided good, medical, psychological, and social support are available.

Congenital heart disease or cardiopulmonary arrest are frequently stated to be the cause of death in trisomy 18, but this may be an oversimplification, with ill-defined CNS abnormalities and respiratory system problems also contributing (Baty et al., 1994a). Ventricular septal defects, present in about two-thirds of cases, are large and unlikely to undergo spontaneous closure. Double outlet right ventricle is common (Rogers et al., 1965). Polyvalvular disease may not be clinically important, but cyanosis combined with right ventricular enlargement usually portends early demise (Musewe et al., 1990). Whether the patient undergoes surgical treatment for congenital heart disease or for any other major malformation depends upon parents'

wishes and available medico-surgical resources. Cardiac surgery and other major operations are not usually performed in the United Kingdom and Europe, except when the chromosomal diagnosis is masked by a malformation that demands urgent treatment, for example extrahepatic biliary atresia (Ikeda et al., 1999). However, in the United States a questionnaire survey of parents ascertained through a family support group did discover that surviving infants with trisomy 18 (and 13) had approximately two operations in the first year after birth (Baty et al., 1994a). One trisomy 18 infant underwent successful repair of an aortic coarctation at four months but died on cardiopulmonary bypass at age 14 months after operative treatment for double outlet right ventricle.

In survivors, profound physical and mental retardation is inevitable and overall development in full trisomy 18 usually does not progress beyond that of a six-month-old, chromosomally normal infant (Fig. 44.9). Functional visual impairments are severe (Holmes and Coates, 1994) and ear malformation is frequent (Chrobok and Simakova, 1997). Somatic growth is very poor in childhood but growth curves are available (Baty et al., 1994a). Some dysmor-

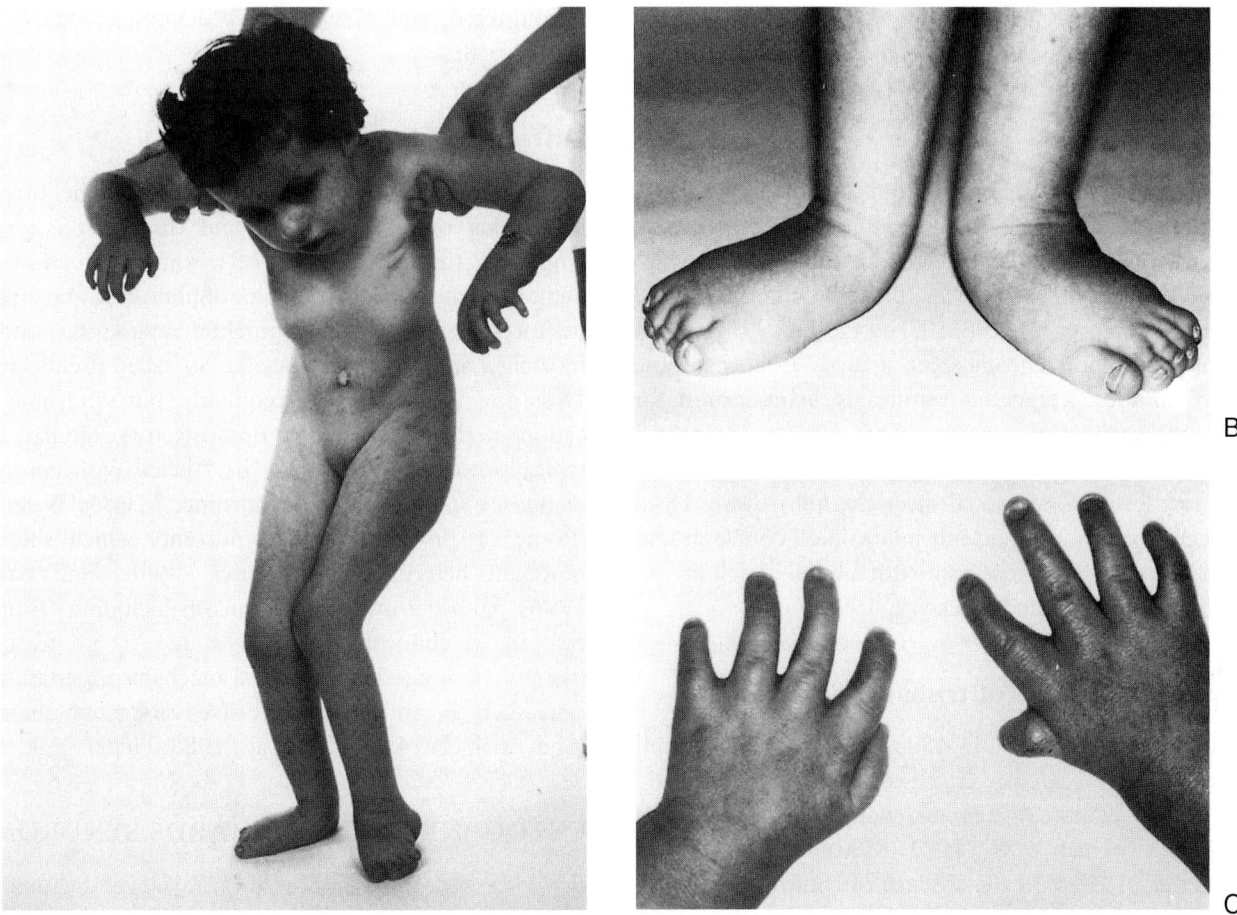

Fig. 44.9. Profound mental and physical handicaps present in a nine-year-old girl with trisomy 18.

phisms such as overlapping fingers and prominent occiput may become less apparent, while other skeletal abnormalities such as severe kyphoscoliosis or a tendency to spontaneous fracture of long bones emerge (Ries et al., 1990). A wide spectrum of clinical features is possible and one 19-month-old girl had alopecia and absence of finger prints on both hands (Shim et al., 1993). Among surviving infants, major congenital malformations are less likely to be present, but infection causes considerable morbidity and mortality (Van Dyke and Allen, 1990). Immune system defects may predispose to infection but these defects are most likely multifaceted, similar to the situation in Down syndrome. By analysis of cordocentesis samples from eight trisomy 18 fetuses at 20 to 36 weeks gestation, Makrydimas et al. (1994) found that the mean T-cell and NK cell counts were significantly lower compared with values in chromosomally normal pregnancies, although the mean B-cell count was not significantly different. Various malignant tumors, including Wilms tumor (Karaylcin et al., 1981), neurogenic tumor (Robinson and McQuorquodale, 1981), and hepatoblastoma (Dasouki and Barr, 1987; Teraguchi et al.,

1997; Bove et al., 1996), have been reported in trisomy 18 survivors.

Longevity is limited by the medical effects of major malformation and nonspecific factors such as requirement for nasogastric tube feeding, which is known to decrease survival of infants with profound handicap arising for any reason. In individual cases, there may be difficult management problems posed by complications such as progressive scoliosis causing respiratory dysfunction (Ries et al., 1990). Van Dyke and Allen (1990) discuss psychological and medical considerations that are prominent when supporting the family with a trisomy 18 child.

Mosaic trisomy 18

The clinical phenotype displayed by individual cases of trisomy 18 mosaicism may range from that of full trisomy 18 syndrome in cases with a small proportion of chromosomally normal cells (Greve et al., 1993), through a milder, nonspecific dysmorphic phenotype (Sarigol and Rogers, 1994), perhaps with a history of female subfertility (Uehara et al., 1996; Satge et al., 1996), to normal or near-normal phenotype in cases ascertained serendipitously (Kohn and Shohat, 1987; Gersdorf et al., 1990; Butler, 1994; Lim and Su, 1998). In some cases the phenotype is atypical to the extent that the low proportion of trisomy 18 cells may be non-contributory (Shashi et al., 1996; Plessis et al., 1997). Nonspecific clinical signs of underlying tissue mosaicism, such as asymmetry of body proportions and linear skin pigmentary abnormalities following Blaschko's lines, may be present (Chemke et al., 1983; Ukita et al., 1997) and in such cases if blood chromosome analysis is normal, the presence of these cutaneous features is an indication for cytogenetic analysis of skin fibroblast cultures. Interphase FISH of peripheral lymphocytes may also be useful in identifying low level mosaicism. Conversely, full trisomy 18 in blood cells with an unexpectedly mild clinical course should suggest chromosome mosaicism with a euploid cell line in other tissues (Dennis and Cockwell, 1992).

Pathologic diagnosis of trisomy 18

Pathologic features of trisomy 18 have been detailed, tabulated, and reviewed extensively (Lewis, 1964; Warkany et al., 1966; Terplan et al., 1970; Hodes et al., 1978; Matsuoka et al., 1983; Moerman et al., 1982; Kinoshita et al., 1989; Gorlin et al., 1990). In the absence of confirmatory cytogenetic diagnosis, a trisomy 18 clinical score based upon 52 individually weighted features of the syndrome can provide objective support for a tentative diagnosis (Marion et al., 1988). Where tissue has been retained, chromosome FISH is possible on macerated and autolysed formalin-fixed tissue, to retrospectively diagnose trisomy (Isaksen et al., 2000).

Broadly, the clinical and pathologic diagnosis relies on observation of characteristic external dysmorphic features in the presence of nonspecific internal malformations such as reduced brain size with or without gyral abnormalities, cerebellar abnormalities, myelomeningocoele, hydrocephalus, corpus callosum defects, neuronal heterotopias, or cardiac ventricular septal defect. Ocular malformations, such as microphthalmos, cataract, optic nerve hypoplasia, and colobomatous malformation, are less common than in trisomy 13 (Calderone et al., 1983; Pe'er and Braun, 1986), but a striking, rare finding is ankyloblepharon filiforme adnatum (Evans et al., 1990). Abnormal low placement of the external ear and dysmorphism affecting the pinna are constant findings, while mental aplasia and inner ear malformation are documented in some cases (Wright et al., 1985). Abdominal wall defect, esophageal atresia, diaphragmatic hernia, and imperforate anus are regularly encountered, and Meckel's diverticulum is almost invariably present.

Differential diagnosis

Early reports of infants with trisomy 18 phenotype but normal karyotype (e.g., Hook and Yunis, 1965) served to emphasize that clinical signs of trisomy 18 such as prominent occiput, small ears, blepharophimosis, distal limb contractures, profound developmental retardation, and high mortality, are not totally specific. So-called pseudo-trisomy 18 is now diagnosed less frequently, but syndrome delineation in this area remains unsatisfactory. Similar, karyotypically normal infants may be labeled with eponymous diagnoses such as Fryn's syndrome, Marden-Walker syndrome or Bowen-Conradi syndrome, which themselves represent heterogeneous entities (Winter and Baraitser, 1996). Unusual multiple mosaicism including trisomy 18 cells in an abnormal infant with few or no features of trisomy 18 suggests an unusual mechanism or rare condition such as autosomal recessive variegated aneuploidy (Shih et al., 1974; Tolmie et al., 1988; Flejter et al., 1998).

CYTOGENETICS OF EDWARDS SYNDROME

Edwards syndrome is almost always associated with an extra free chromosome 18, and very few cases are associated with translocations or other chromosome 18 structural abnormalities (Schinzel, 1984). Trisomy 18 is a maternal age-related autosomal trisomy with the rate at prenatal diagnosis or birth rising until 43 years and then leveling off, possibly due to greater difficulty experienced by the older mother in maintaining a trisomy 18 fetus (Ferguson-Smith and Yates, 1984).

Molecular genetic studies employing polymorphic DNA markers indicated that the extra chromosome in trisomy 18 is of maternal origin in more than 90% of cases and maternal meiosis 2 errors predominate (Fisher et al., 1995; Eggerman et al., 1996; Ramesh and Verma, 1996). This is unlike trisomy 21 which results from maternal meiosis 1 errors.

The relationship between chromosome recombination and the meiotic error was studied by Bugge et al. (1998). In the few maternal meiosis 1 trisomy 18 cases, there was a low frequency of recombination in proximal 18p and medial 18q, with 30% of cases being nullichiasmate. Chromosome 18 maternal meiosis 2 nondisjunction did not show a significant relationship with recombination and did not fit the entanglement model that predicts increased recombination near the centromere, in contradistinction to chromosome 21 meiosis 2 errors which showed the predicted increase in recombination proximally (discussed earlier). They concluded that observations made about recombination and the meiotic error in chromosome nondisjunction are chromosome specific, and a model of susceptible chiasma distributions interacting with age-dependent deterioration of the meiotic mechanism may not apply to all chromosome meiotic nondisjunctions.

Among a small number of cases with a paternally derived extra chromosome 18, most have arisen from a post-fertilization mitotic error (Kondoh et al., 1988; Kupke and Müller, 1989; Fisher et al., 1993; 1995; Ya-Gang et al., 1993). The frequency of sperm cells disomic for chromosome 18 averages about 0.4%, which is not significantly different from the disomy frequency for other chromosomes (Guttenbach et al., 1994; Griffin et al., 1995).

Phenotype-karyotype correlations in trisomy 18 are difficult due to paucity of reports of individuals with pure, partial duplications of segments of chromosome 18q. Also, a wide spectrum of clinical abnormalities exists among those cases recorded in the literature (Turleau et al., 1980; Matsuoka et al., 1981; Muecke et al., 1982). In the past, clinical case studies employing conventional cytogenetic techniques have shown that chromosome 18 short arm is unlikely to have a phenotypic effect, in view of the lack of abnormalities present in individuals with trisomy for 18p (Turleau et al., 1980; Wolff et al., 1991). Detailed review of phenotypes attributed to different triplicated chromosome 18q regions led Wilson et al. (1990) to conclude that genetic interaction among individual triplicated loci most likely determines the trisomic phenotype; important regions are 18q11 → q12.1 and 18q21 → qter. Mewar et al. (1993) excluded the region 18q11 from being a critical determinant of the Edwards syndrome phenotype. Boghasian-Sell et al. (1994) studied six patients, four of whom were mildly affected by duplications of the distal half of 18q (18q21.1 → qter), while the remaining two patients were more like full trisomy 18 patients and carried duplication of most of 18q (18q12.1 → qter). The last named authors also concluded that no single region on 18q is sufficient to produce the trisomy 18 phenotype, proximal and distal regions of 18q are both important and severe mental retardation is associated with 18q12.3 → q21.1 duplication.

Little is known about the role of specific segments of chromosome 18. One candidate that has been studied is transthyretin (TTR), which is localized to 18q11 → 12.1. TTR protein (prealbumin) is expressed in visceral yolk sac and various fetal organs; its function is the transport of thyroxine and retinol (Sparkes et al., 1987). Mutations within TTR cause familial amyloidotic polyneuropathy (Ferlini et al., 1992). Although the gene is conserved in mammalian species, mice with null mutations do not suffer malformations but do have reduced levels of thyroxine and retinol in plasma (Episkopou et al., 1993). Overexpression of TTR in trisomy 18 is measurable in fetal liver and intestine at 20 to 23 weeks gestation, but not at 10 to 14 weeks gestation (Loughna et al., 1995).

RECURRENCE RISK

Data on the recurrence risk after the birth of one fetus or infant with trisomy 18 is scanty. Hecht et al. (1964) pointed out an increased risk of Down syndrome in families in which the index case had trisomy 18. Forty-four such index cases had 104 siblings, three of whom had Down syndrome. In a Japaneses study, 170 pregnancies followed a trisomy 18 offspring and there were no recurrences (Uehara et al., 1999).

Certainly, trisomy 18 is a maternal age-related trisomy, and there are several anecdotal reports of women who have either had two trisomy 18 pregnancies or successive pregnancies with trisomy 18 and trisomy 13 or trisomy 21 (reviewed by Baty et al., 1994a) or even trisomy for 13, 18, and 21 (FitzPatrick and Boyd, 1989). As each of these three autosomal aneuploidies is associated with advanced maternal age, it is difficult to disentangle this effect from any other association that the aneuploidies may have with each other. Whether there is such a phenomenon as general predisposition to autosomal nondisjunction and aneuploidy was discussed in relation to trisomy 21 recurrence. Following an analysis of available data, Hook (1992) concluded that there is evidence of general predisposition to aneuploidy in some women, therefore, it is reasonable to add 1% to the maternal age-specific risk of trisomy 21 when estimating the chance of recurrence of viable autosomal trisomy (trisomy 18, 13, or 21) after an index case with trisomy 18. Prenatal cytogenetic diagnosis may be offered to provide reassurance.

If Edwards syndrome phenotype results from a chromosome 18 balanced structural rearrangement present in one parent, the risk of recurrence will almost always be significantly higher, but a more precise risk estimate will depend on the type of rearrangement and the pattern of its segregation in the extended family tree, if this is known (Gardner and Sutherland, 1996).

Trisomy 13—Patau syndrome

Patau et al. (1960) reported trisomy 13 syndrome in a Lancet paper adjacent to the original description of trisomy

18 (Edwards et al., 1960). The initial case was noted to have an extra D-group acrocentric chromosome and microcephaly, anophthalmia or microphthalmia, bilateral cleft lip and palate, and polydactyly. Notably, she was still alive at age 13 months. The trisomy 13 phenotype is thus striking and was almost certainly the subject of detailed case reports in earlier centuries (Warkany, 1971; Oostra et al., 1998).

TRISOMY 13 PHENOTYPE

Fetus with Patau syndrome

Patau syndrome is commoner among spontaneous abortions, making up 8% of abortuses with any autosomal trisomy in the series reported by Jacobs et al. (1987). Growth retardation may be detected early with reduced crown rump length (Bahado-Singh et al., 1997). Some major malformations, such as exomphalos, may be evident at the end of the first trimester (Snijders et al., 1995), but malformations are mostly diagnosed in the second trimester (see below). Abramsky and Chapple (1993) found that approximately 50% of cases of trisomy 13 were prenatally diagnosed by a combination of maternal age and serum screening, and routine ultrasound screening. By comparison, about 66% of trisomy 18 cases and 33% of Down syndrome cases were prenatally diagnosed. Recently, Snijders et al. (1999) found that 80% of trisomy 13 fetuses could be detected at 10–14 weeks gestation using the protocol of a combined maternal age/nuchal thickness, first trimester, screening programme for trisomy 21.

In mid-trimester, detailed fetal ultrasound examination will readily visualize major brain, facial, heart, renal, and limb malformations caused by the extra chromosome 13 (Twining, 1995; Lehman et al., 1995) (Figs. 44.10 and 44.11). Holoprosencephaly especially is associated with trisomy 13 and is present in about 66% of cases. Conversely, in one series of fetuses with holoprosencephaly, 40% had trisomy 13 (Greene et al., 1987). Synophthalmia or anophthalmia, nasal malformation and facial clefting are also diagnosed by ultrasound examination (Fig. 44.11), as are the congenital heart defect, renal abnormalities (hydronephrosis, cystic changes, hypoplasia) and post axial polydactyly.

Postnatal phenotype and management of child with Patau syndrome

A history of pre-eclampsia may be a clue (Boyd et al., 1987; 1995; Heydanus et al., 1995) and the placenta may be abnormal or show changes like those of a partial mole (Jauniaux et al., 1998) but clinical diagnosis of trisomy 13

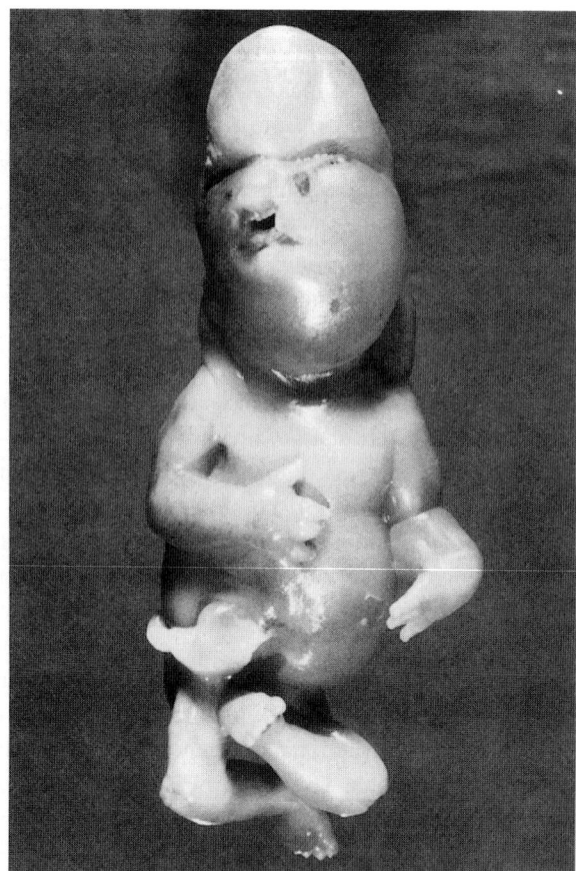

Fig. 44.10. Fetus with trisomy 13. Abnormalities diagnosed by ultrasound include hydropic appearance, nuchal cystic change, and bilateral cleft lip and palate.

is usually straightforward. The mean birthweight is reduced at 2.6 kg. Polydactyly plus any combination of microcephaly, ocular malformation, cleft lip and palate, heart defect, or renal abnormality are typical. If clinical examination reveals only one major malformation and no polydactyly, then scalp defects, present in nearly 50% of cases, are diagnostically helpful (Fig. 44.12). Polydactyly is always postaxial, and may affect fingers or toes and be bilateral or unilateral.

The immediate management of newborn infants with trisomy 13 and subsequent management of children with trisomy 13 raises similar problems to those discussed above in relation to management of infants and children with trisomy 18. Parents may ask for a guide to the likelihood of prolonged survival; most studies find median survival is less than one week (Wyllie et al., 1994), more than 80% of affected infants die during the first month, but about 3% are alive at six months (Goldstein and Nielsen, 1988). If major congenital heart and renal defects are present, prolonged survival is less likely, but it should be noted that infants with severe alobar holoprosencephaly may survive well into

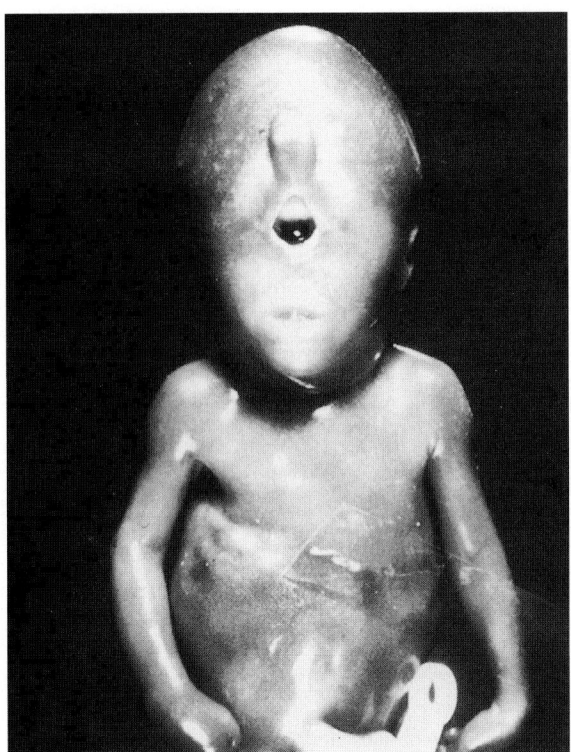

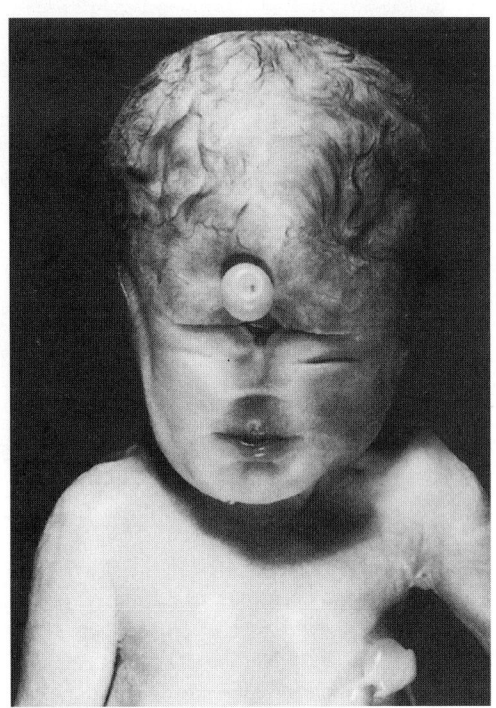

Fig. 44.11. Synophthalmia and proboscis in trisomy 13 fetus (A) and infant (B). In both cases, there was underlying alobar holoprosencephaly.

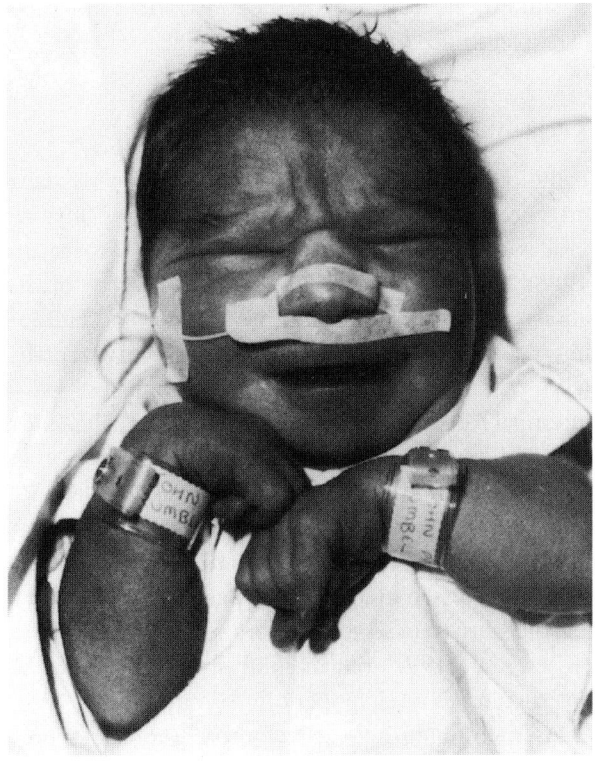

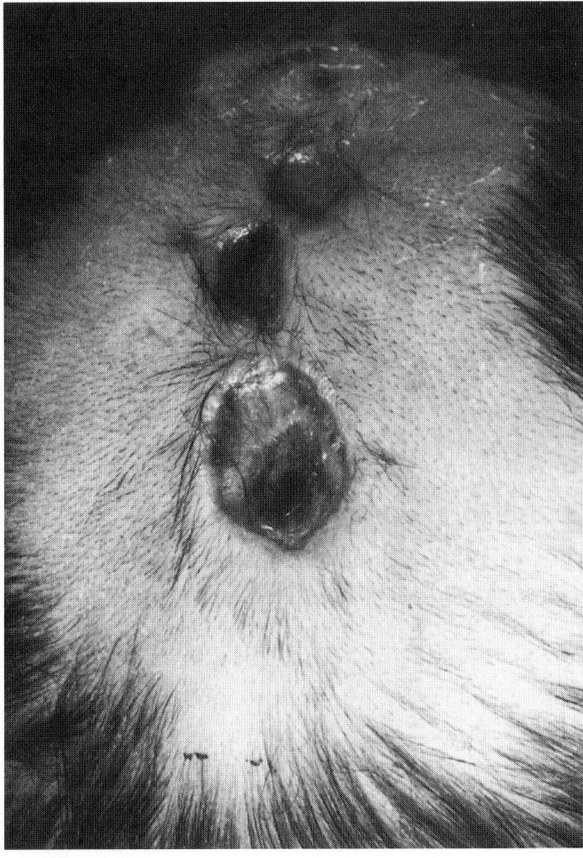

Fig. 44.12. Microphthalmos and scalp defects present in trisomy 13.

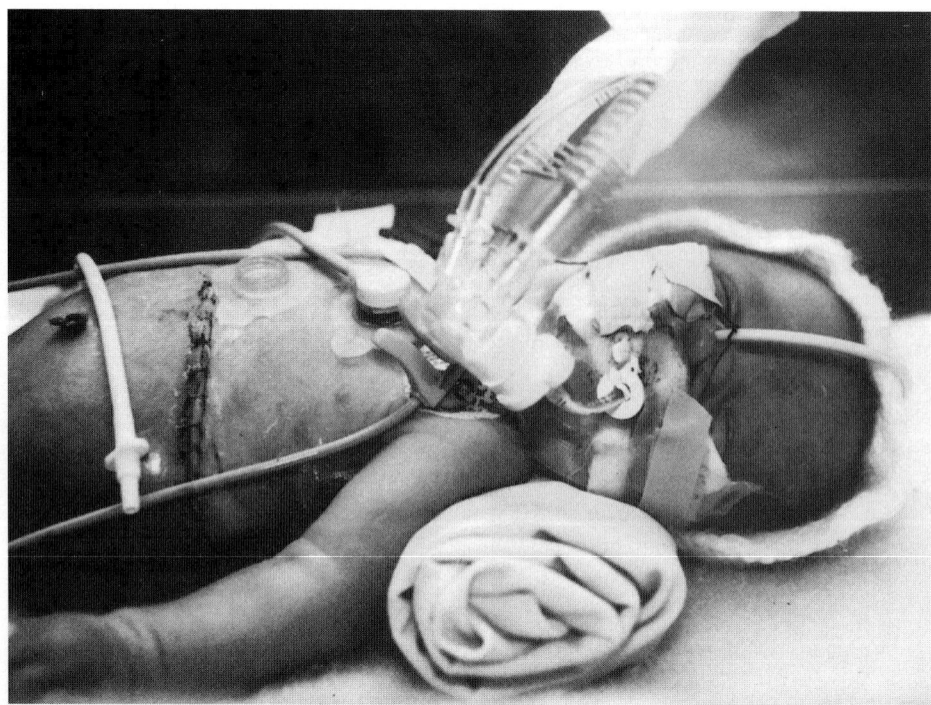

Fig. 44.13. Delayed diagnosis of trisomy 13 after surgical repair of esphageal atresia. Note the obvious difficulties in examining the infant.

infancy. Several individuals with trisomy 13 but no life-threatening malformations have survived into adulthood but physical and mental retardation is profound, with development arrested at the six-month level or less (Mankinen and Sears 1976; Cowen et al., 1979; Redheendran et al., 1981; Boraz, 1987; Singh, 1990; Zoll et al., 1993). Trisomy 13 individuals are often blind and deaf. Severe epilepsy, feeding difficulties, and difficult behaviors (e.g., self-mutilation) have all been reported, although some parents have also reported developmental responses, which, in chromosomally normal children, emerge in later infancy (Baty et al., 1994b). Wilms tumor has been reported in a four-year-old child (Sweeney and Pelegano, 2000).

Trisomy 13 mosaicism

Like trisomy 18 mosaicism, there is great variation in the phenotype of cases. If the cytogenetic diagnosis is made in prenatal life and no fetal malformation is visible, then there is a chance of a normal outcome (Delatycki et al., 1998; Eubanks et al., 1998). Such cases have a low proportion of trisomic cells. If a fetal malformation is identified through ultrasound examination, it is likely to be due to the mosaic chromosome result.

As far as clinical diagnosis of trisomy mosaicism is concerned, phylloid hypomelanosis, a type of "pigmentary mosaicism characterized by congenital hypochromic macules resembling a floral ornament with various elements such as round or oval patches, macules resembling the asymmetrical leaves of a begonia, or oblong lesions" (Happle, 2000), may be a very specific sign.

Pathology of trisomy 13

Pathologic findings associated with trisomy 13 have been presented in detail (Warkany et al., 1966; Taylor, 1968; Hodes et al., 1978; Koole et al., 1986; Moerman et al., 1988; Fujinaga et al., 1990) and the pattern of malformations can be used to diagnose or rule out trisomy 13. Typical internal anomalies are atrial and ventricular septal defects with patent ductus arteriosus, exomphalos, incomplete intestinal rotation or malrotation with unattached mesentery, enlarged lobulated kidneys with cystic change in the cortex and medulla, accessory spleen, and abnormal liver lobation. Good markers of trisomy 13 are microscopic pancreatic dysplasia (Moerman et al., 1988) and supranormal spleen and kidney weights in midgestation (Barr, 1994). As with trisomy 18, there are changes in the morphology of the axial skeleton (Kjaer et al., 1997) but in contrast to trisomy 18, Meckel's diverticulum is rarely present in trisomy 13.

As mentioned above, holoprosencephaly is present in about 66% of cases with the face frequently, but not always, "predicting" the brain as evidenced by synophthalmia or hypotelorism and premaxillary agenesis. Most frequently, the cerebral malformation comprises a monoventricular cerebrum without corpus callosum, septum pellucidum, or fornices. Posterior fossa intracranial abnormalities with cerebellar malformation and heterotopias, microscopic abnormalities with pyramidal tract hypoplasia, and neural tube defects have also been described (Moerman et al., 1988). Cortical dysplasia may be evident with MRI (Nuri Sener, 1996) and detailed Golgi studies have revealed a variety of structural abnormalities (Marin Padilla, 1974), but the conclusion is that the neuropathological features of trisomy 13 (and other chromosomal syndromes) are neither constant nor obligatory (Gullotta et al., 1981).

Differential diagnosis

Young and Madders (1987) described a karyotypically normal, stillborn male infant with holoprosencephaly, premaxillary agenesis, microphthalmos, congenital heart defect, and postaxial polydactyly. Subsequently, it became clear that an autosomal recessive disorder, sometimes reported as pseudotrisomy 13 syndrome, may be mistaken for trisomy 13 (Amor and Woods, 2000). In cases in which cytogenetic studies are normal or not performed, parental consanguinity should raise suspicion of this diagnosis. Other syndromes such as Meckel, hydrolethalus, Pallister-Hall, and Smith-Lemli-Opitz type 2 are monogenic conditions that should be considered in the differential diagnosis of holoprosencephaly, heart defect, and polydactyly without karyotypic evidence of trisomy 13 (Hennekam et al., 1991).

Cytogenetics of Patau syndrome

Magenis et al. (1968) discovered that the distribution of the age of mothers at the birth of trisomy 13 infants was bimodal, consistent with trisomy 13 arising from two distinct mechanisms: the presence of an extra chromosome 13 being a maternal age-dependent phenomenon, while Patau syndrome associated with a rob(D;D) translocation is independent of the mother's age. The same bimodality was observed by Jacobs et al. (1987), who studied trisomy 13 in spontaneous abortions. This study also found no evidence for a reduction in the frequency of cases born to mothers over the age of 40 years, contrary to amniocentesis data (Ferguson-Smith and Yates, 1984; Hook et al., 1984), or another study of spontaneous abortions (Risch et al., 1986). With, in one study, reduced mean maternal age for trisomy 13 compared with trisomy 21, there is some indirect evidence that older women may be less able to sustain a trisomy 13 pregnancy (Drugan et al., 1999).

About 75% of spontaneous abortuses and the same proportion of liveborn infants with Patau syndrome have trisomy 13. Cytogenetic and DNA marker studies by Hassold et al. (1987), Robinson et al. (1996) and others, have revealed that the extra chromosome in free trisomy 13 is maternally derived in about 90% of cases. There is evidence of genetic recombination in the majority of cases of free trisomy 13, making lack of chiasmata an unlikely reason for chromosome nondisjunction.

About a quarter of cases with Patau syndrome have a Robertsonian translocation, usually rob(13q14q). This is the most common structural chromosome rearrangement being carried by about 1 in 1500 individuals and it is estimated that the rate of unbalanced rob(13q14q) translocations is 1 per 25,000 livebirths (Hook, 1981). Female carriers of rob(13q14q) are fertile; male carriers of this translocation are usually fertile, but they have an increased chance of abnormal spermatogenesis and infertility (Plymate et al., 1976). Cytogenetic analyses of sperm from rob(13q14q) translocation carriers have revealed about 25% of sperm are chromosomally unbalanced (Martin, 1988; Escudero et al., 2000). Analysis of sperm from a rob(13q15q) translocation carrier also revealed a high (10%) frequency of unbalanced sperm (Pellestor, 1990). However, the observed risks of chromosomally abnormal progeny in the offspring of male Robertsonian translocation carriers are very low (Table 44.1).

Studies of the rob(13q14q) have demonstrated that the chromosomes are dicentric with the chromosome 14 breakpoint within the p11 region and the chromosome 13p breakpoint between the pTRI-6 satellite sequence and ribosomal DNA (Shaffer et al., 1993; Han et al., 1994). Among rob(13q14q) translocations, equal proportions are de novo and inherited. In cases of de novo rob(13q14q) Patau syndrome, the translocation may be formed in either parent, but note that the extra chromosome 13 may still be derived from a maternal meiotic nondisjunction event (Robinson et al., 1996).

Other translocations such as rob(13q15q) and rob(13q13q) comprise a minority of all cases with translocation Patau syndrome. As expected, the majority of rob(13q13q) cases arise de novo and just as with the isochromosome (21q), some (13q13q) rearrangements are isochromosomes arising from prezygotic fusion of long arm sister chromatids, but other mechanisms for the origin of these unusual rearrangements have been discovered, such as somatic translocation between maternal and paternal homologs (Robinson et al., 1996). Very rarely, a rob(13q15q) translocation has been identified in one parent of an infant with Patau syndrome (Mori et al., 1985).

RECURRENCE RISKS

Trisomy 13

Data on the risk of recurrence after diagnosis of trisomy 13 in a fetus or child are scanty. In a questionnaire and telephone survey of families with trisomy 18 and 13 children, Baty et al. (1994a) found that for trisomy 13 and 18 probands combined, there was only one aneuploid sibling. That case was a prior fetus with trisomy 18. Otherwise, among more than 200 siblings of trisomy 13 and 18 index cases, there were no recurrences. Uehara et al. (1999) also found there were no recurrences in the offspring of 46 women who had had a trisomy 13 pregnancy. There is anecdotal evidence from case reports (see above in discussions of trisomy 21 and 18 recurrence risks) and evidence summarized by Hook (1992), that some women have a general predisposition to autosomal aneuploidy, having conceived infants and fetuses with trisomy 13, 18, and 21 in successive pregnancies. In such cases it also possible that the maternal age effect is responsible but, similar to the situation for trisomy 18, the young mother of a fetus or infant with trisomy 13 may be offered a 1% recurrence risk for any viable autosomal trisomy being present in midtrimester, and older mothers may be given appropriate maternal age specific risk for trisomy 21 plus 1%. Cytogenetic prenatal diagnosis is customarily offered.

Robertsonian translocation Patau syndrome

If one parent is known to carry rob(13q14q), a low (1%) risk for fetus or infant with Patau syndrome is given, largely based on data from the European Collaborative Amniocentesis Study (Boué and Gallano, 1984), which found no unbalanced offspring in 230 pregnancies among rob(13q14q) translocation carriers. Every genetic center is aware of one or more infants with Patau syndrome who were born to rob(13q14q) carriers (Daniel et al., 1989), so the risk is not zero. For Patau syndrome that may be due to any other nonhomologous Robertsonian rearrangement, the risks are similarly low (Table 44.1). When chromosome 15 is involved in a Robertsonian translocation, there is a further complication, namely the possibility of an abnormal phenotype due to uniparental disomy and this is discussed below.

Autosomal trisomy mosaicism, prenatal diagnosis and uniparental disomy

Mosaicism for autosomal trisomies occurs more frequently in spontaeous abortions and amniotic fluid samples than in newborns. In 1978 Warburton et al., pointed out this could be due to underestimation of mosaicism in live births or due to mosaicism that is restricted to extraembryonic tissue. When parents are informed of the coexistence in a prenatal diagnosis sample of aneuploid and normal diploid cells, they wish to know whether chromosomally abnormal cells are present in the fetus and, if they are present, whether these cells will harm the fetus. The responses to these key questions are often unsatisfactory, as the very nature of chromosome mosaicism is such that exact proportions of aneuploid cells in all the body organs are indeterminable. Although cytogenetic tests cannot totally exclude significant chromosome mosaicism, and the clinical phenotype autosomal mosaicism produces is highly unpredictable, most prenatally detected mosaicism does not harm the fetus (Hsu et al., 1997; Smith et al., 1999; Wallerstein et al., 2000). In practice, a pragmatic approach to chromosome mosaicism draws on experience in prenatal cytogenetics and knowledge of the literature. Before discussing commoner autosomal trisomy mosaicism problems, it is helpful to consider some general aspects of prenatally detected mosaicism.

Mosaicism in amniotic fluid

When chromosomally abnormal cells are present in the fetus, true mosaicism exists. In contrast, pseudomosaicism arises from an in vitro cultural artifact. Rarely, true mosaicism can be misreported as pseudomosaicism, or it can be missed completely. Protocols for analysis of amniotic fluid samples are designed to be practical, have maximum detection rates for cytogenetically abnormal fetuses and minimize the chance of false negative and false positive diagnoses. Hsu et al. (1992) built upon a staged classification of mosaicism advocated by Worton and Stern (1984). Stage III mosaicism is most important, since it most likely represents abnormal cells in the fetus and is defined as one or more cells with an identical karyotypic abnormality present in at least two independent primary cultures. By contrast, stage 1 mosaicism, defined as a single abnormal cell, and stage II mosaicism, defined as a clone of identical abnormal cells in a single flask or colony, very rarely reflect true fetal mosaicism.

Hsu and colleagues (Hsu et al., 1992; Hsu and Benn, 1999; Wallerstein et al., 2000) have gathered data on amniotic fluid chromosome mosaicism that informs clinical decisions about further investigation and assessment of the risk of fetal abnormality.

Common trisomy mosaicism is mosaicism for chromosomes, 13, 18, 20, 21, and accounts for 70% of autosomal trisomy mosaicism. Wallerstein et al. (2000) studied cases of common trisomy mosaics that were ascertained without prior knowledge of fetal malformation being present. These cases were then examined at birth or at termination and categorized as normal or abnormal. As expected in a collaborative study, the intensity of efforts made to confirm the prenatal chromosome findings varied, but there were higher mosaicism confirmation rates in pregnancies with abnormal versus normal outcome. Over 300 cases were included and the risk of an abnormal outcome did, in general, increase as the proportion of trisomy cells amongst amniocytes increased. The risk of an abnormal outcome was in the range of 40% to 55% for trisomy 13, 18 and 21. However, in trisomy 20 mosaicism there was a lower risk of an abnormal outcome (8.2%) and for this chromosome the cytogenetic confirmation rates were similar in cases with and without an abnormal outcome (47% and 40% respectively). As far as further prenatal investigation of cases was concerned, in a small number of cases of trisomy 13, 18 or 21, detecting mosaicism in a fetal blood sample increased the risk of abnormal outcome but, in general, when the first amniotic fluid sample result was adequate from the technical viewpoint, repeat chromosome tests did not add information. In summary, true mosaicism at amniocentesis for trisomy 13, 18 or 21 has a high risk for an abnormal outcome at termination or at birth. Detailed fetal ultrasound examination was recommended to seek evidence of malformation, but a normal result would not be totally reassuring since there would still be an unquantifiable concern about long-term cognitive development in such cases.

· *Rare trisomy mosaicism* is defined as mosaicism for autosomes apart from 13, 18, 20 and 21. Based on examination of 151 prenatally diagnosed cases, who were again evaluated at birth or at termination, Hsu and colleagues (Hsu et al., 1997; Hsu and Benn, 1999) concluded the risk of fetal abnormality varied with the chromosome involved. In the 1997 study, the chromosomes with the highest risks attached to autosomal trisomy mosaicism were 2, 16, and 22 where the risk was at least 60%; a high risk of 40–59% was found for chromosomes 5, 9, 14, and 15; a moderately high risk of 20–39% was found for 12; and moderate risks of up to 19 per cent were attached to chromosomes 7, and 8; a low risk was attached to chromosome 17 mosaicism; and due to lack of cases, an undetermined risk was applied to the remaining autosomal trisomy mosaics. As additional data is gathered, these risks may be modified (Hsu and Benn, 1999). At first reading, it is slightly surprising that rare trisomy mosaics could have as high or even higher risks of clinical abnormality than the common trisomy mosaics. It seems possible that the rare trisomy mosaics, if born alive or

stillborn, go undiagnosed because we fail to analyse chromosomes in tissues other than blood as often as we should: in rare trisomy mosaicism, blood lymphocytes are more likely to be cytogenetically normal. In the report of Hsu et al. (1997) it was important that the cytogenetic confirmation rate was highest in abnormal pregnancies, and that comparison of the phenotypes of prenatally and postnatally diagnosed abnormal cases showed some concordance. Hsu et al emphasized that to maximize the confirmation rate (85% was the highest achieved) both fibroblasts and placental tissues should be studied. Except for 46/47, +8 and 46/47, +9, fetal blood sampling is of limited value for prenatal diagnosis of rare trisomy mosaicism. DNA studies for uniparental disomy were suggested for certain chromosomes with imprinting effects, such as chromosomes 7, 11, 14, and especially 15. Most importantly, since the majority of abnormalities noted could be visualized by prenatal ultrasound, a detailed scan should be performed in all cases.

Even if ultrasound examination is normal, problems remain in individual cases. An example from the "low risk" group is the case report of trisomy 17 mosaicism (Shaffer et al., 1996). This child had mental retardation, seizures, hearing loss, growth retardation, microcephaly, and minor anomalies that would not be diagnosed by antenatal ultrasound. Peripheral blood lymphocyte chromosomes were normal, so fetal blood analysis would not have helped, but trisomy 17 cells were present in skin fibroblasts 18% of cells analyzed at age three years and 80% at 8 years. Molecular analysis demonstrated the extra chromosome 17 in the skin was of paternal origin but since three alleles were never seen in the trisomic cell line, the extra chromosome probably arose after conception.

Mosaicism in chorionic villus sampling

The various technical procedures adopted by different laboratories to process and analyze cells from chorionic villus sampling (CVS) reduce the general applicability of the robust, staged, definition of mosaicism that has been possible for amniotic fluid studies. However, the experience derived from a series of collaborative studies from Europe, the United States, the United Kingdom, and Canada (Vejerslev and Mikkelsen, 1989; Ledbetter et al., 1992; Teshima et al., 1992; Association of Clinical Cytogeneticists [ACC] 1994; Smith et al., 1999) has led to empirically-based distinction between clinically significant mosaicism and clinically insignificant mosaicism.

Couples who are about to undergo CVS may be told that diagnostic pitfalls due to chromosome mosaicism are quantified in a false-negative rate of 0.04% and a false-positive rate of 1% to 2% (Simoni and Sirchia, 1994). An important point is 15% to 20% of mosaic cases show complete discordance between the karyotype from the direct preparation and that from cultured cells, and this would have resulted in a false positive or false negative result if only one technique had been employed (Smith et al., 1999). More reliable cytogenetic results are obtained on cells obtained from long term cultures, with their origins in the extra-embryonic mesoderm that has closer lineage to the fetus proper.

In cases with common mosaic autosomal aneuploidies, the ACC Study (1994) concluded that mosaic trisomy 13, 18, and 21 in CVS were all "unreliable" indicators of the fetal karyotype, and that further cytogenetic studies employing a different method of prenatal diagnosis, such as amniocentesis, were warranted. In the ACC follow-up study (Smith et al., 1999), many mosaic trisomy 13, 18, and 21 cases were associated with normal outcomes but a significant proportion (12 out of 34 cases) were cytogenet-

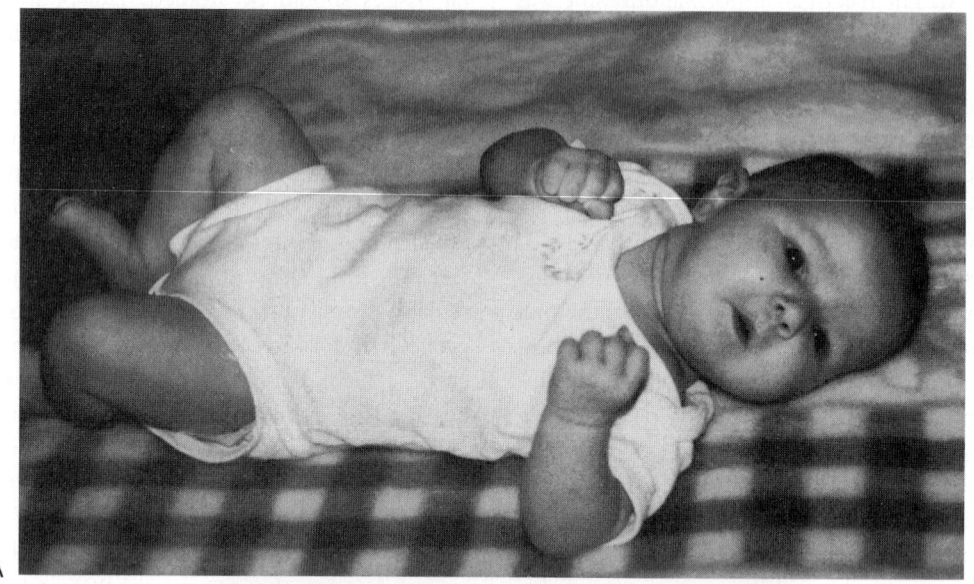

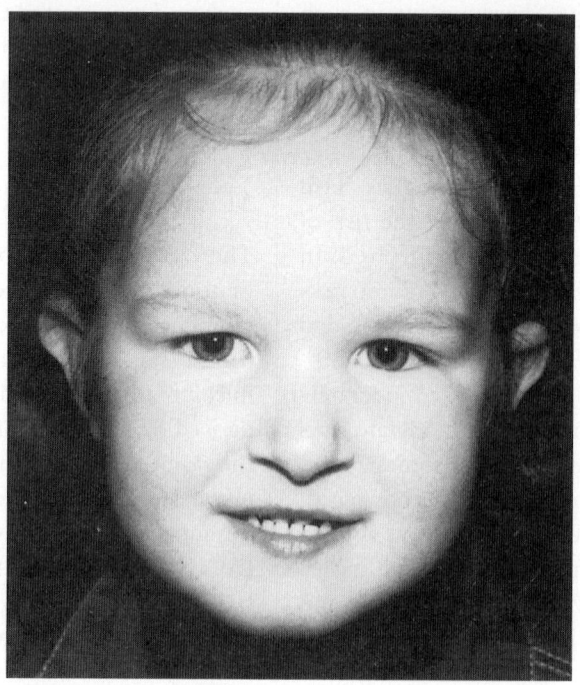

Fig. 44.14. (A & B) Trisomy 13 mosaicism (5% to 10% trisomy 13 cells in blood and skin samples in a normal child at ages two months and five years. Chromosomes were initially checked in the newborn period simply because there was a single umbilical artery.

ically confirmed. In the case of mosaic (and nonmosaic) autosomal trisomies for chromosomes other than 13, 18, and 21, detected at CVS, Smith et al., concluded that the cytogenetic findings are unlikely to be representative of the fetal karyotype and unless fetal abnormalities are visualized by ultrasound scanning, the risk of fetal abnormality is low. This conclusion should be given to parents who may wish to consider whether to undergo further invasive procedures for additional cytogenetic tests.

Nevertheless, there are always complicated cases in clinical practice and this is where knowledge of the literature can help. For example, the issues raised by confirmation of a mosaic trisomy 21 result restricted to the long-term culture of chorionic villi and to one amniotic fluid culture were discussed in relation to diagnosis of mosaic Down syndrome confirmed by cordocentesis and by post-abortion fibroblast culture by Beverstock et al. (1998). In another case, false negative diagnosis of trisomy 18 pseudomosaicism was reported in amniocytes and this provides a salutary reminder that such an uncommon event does occur (van Ravenswaaij-Arts et al., 1997).

Confined mosaicism

The reasons why autosomal trisomy mosaicism in CVS is an unreliable indicator of the fetal karyotype are better understood. If chromosome mosaicism is present in the blastocyst, which first appears approximately one week after conception, and before the development of the embryo proper, it will probably be present in both placental and fetal tissue. On the other hand, if chromosome mosaicism arises at later stage in gestation, the abnormal cells may be confined to the placenta or, less commonly, to the fetus. At an incidence of 2% in CVS, confined placental mosaicism is about seven times more common than mosaicism in amniocytes.

Confined placental mosaicism may arise if a diploid zygote gains a trisomic cell line through mitotic non disjunction, or a trisomic zygote acquires a diploid cell line. Confirmation of the diagnosis of confined placental mosaicism requires cytogenetic follow-up studies on the fetus or infant as well as on the placenta and membranes. Detailed classification schemes categorize five types of confined mosaicism (see Bianchi et al., 1993) but since confined placental mosaicism is more often presumed to be present from the cytogenetic findings in the initial chorionic villus sample, perhaps followed by a confirmatory normal result in amniotic fluid or fetal blood, a practical scheme was presented by Kalousek and Vekemans (1996).

Type I: Mosaicism in the direct cytotrophoblast preparation (chorionic ectoderm, reflects mosaicism in the placenta),

but not in cultured chorionic stroma cells (extraembryonic mesenchyme with closer lineage to the fetus)

Type II: Mosaicism in cultured chorionic stroma cells but not in direct cytotrophoblast preparation

Type III: Mosaicism in direct cytotrophoblast preparation and in cultured chorionic stroma cells

As discussed above, the collaborative studies indicated that mosaicism in direct *and* cultured CVS does not necessarily reflect mosaicism in the fetus (a false positive result). Conversely, the fetus can be mosaic despite normal results in direct and cultured CVS (a true false-negative result). After a mosaic CVS result, the chance that chromosomally abnormal cells will be detected in the fetus may be no more than 10% overall (Fryburg et al., 1993; Wang et al., 1994; Phillips et al., 1996; Goldberg and Wohlferd, 1997). Mosaicism confined to the placenta may still be harmful to the fetus, though. Kalousek and Dill (1983) first suggested that chromosomal abnormalities in the placenta causes growth retardation of a chromosomally normal fetus. Confined placental mosaicism may also increase the chance of spontaneous abortion (Wapner et al., 1992). Conversely, a diploid cell line in the placenta may help ensure viability of a fetus with nonmosaic trisomy 13 or 18 (Kalousek et al., 1989). Overall, the results of follow-up studies point to a low risk of adverse pregnancy outcome with confined placental mosaicism causing IUGR in about 10% of cases (Fryburg et al., 1993; Roland et al., 1994; Wolstenholme et al., 1994).

Mosaicism, trisomy and uniparental disomy

Uniparental disomy occurs if both members of a pair of homologous chromosomes are derived from one parent and there is no contribution from the other parent (Engel, 1980). Uniparental disomy (UPD) can result from several different mechanisms but the best known is loss of an extra chromosome in a trisomic conceptus leading to a diploid cell line. UPD is clinically important since it may cause disease or malformation through several different mechanisms. For example, a genomic imprinting effect was identified following experimental work in mice; in effect, this means some regions of the genome must show particular patterns of expression and non-expression of maternally and paternally derived genes during gametogenesis and in the preimplantation embryo for normal development to occur (Kotzot, 1999; Pfeifer, 2000). UPD could prevent this occurring. Another mechanism for disease in UPD is if both homologs are derived from a single parental chromosome and are genetically identical; this is termed uniparental isodisomy and it may lead to homozygosity for a recessive gene mutation. In uniparental heterodisomy both parental homologs are represented and heterozygosity is maintained.

Relationships between autosomal trisomy, confined mosaicism and UPD were explored by Robinson et al. (1997) in 101 cases of confined placental mosaicism. A somatic (postmeiotic) origin of the trisomy was observed in the majority of cases with confined placental mosaicism for trisomy 2, 7, 8, 10, and 12. Most cases of confined placental mosaicism involving trisomy 9, 16, and 22 were meiotic in origin and had higher levels of autosomal trisomy in CVS, moreover, fetal UPD was common in these cases. Fetal maternal UPD was found in nearly 20% of informative confined placental mosaicism cases, including trisomy 2, 7, 16, and 22. Growth retardation in the fetus correlated with meiotic origin of the trisomy, the presence of fetal UPD, and the level of trisomy in trophoblast but not with the level of trisomy in CVS or term chorion. The authors concluded that molecular determination of origin is a useful predictor of pregnancy outcome, whereas the level of trisomy observed in cultured CVS is not. In addition, UPD for some chromosomes may affect prenatal, but not postnatal, development, possibly indicating that imprinting effects for these chromosomes are confined to placental tissues.

In total, genomic imprinting effects are uncommon. Only nine imprinted human genes, mostly considered to have controlling roles in aspects of placental growth and embryonic development, were listed by Bartolomei and Tilghman (1997). The most frequent diseases that result from imprinting abnormalities are Prader-Willi syndrome due to maternal UPD in proximal 15q, and Angelman syndrome due to paternal UPD in the same chromosomal region (Robinson et al., 2000). The existence of normal phenotypes in many patients with UPD for most chromosomes constitutes evidence against an imprinting effect on these chromosomes. Nevertheless, if UPD is detected antenatally, difficult genetic counseling problems may ensue for other mechanisms, such as undiagnosed trisomy mosaicism or homozygosity for a recessive gene mutation may cause disease. Slater et al. (2000) discussed the difficulties presented by antenatal detection of UPD of chromosome 9 and residual trisomy mosaicism. In this case the baby was born and at one year of age was developing normally albeit with minor facial dysmorphism and skeletal abnormalities, and had 8% trisomy 9 mosaicism in peripheral blood lymphocytes.

In summary, the associations between UPD and disease are quite rare (Engel and De Lozier-Blanchet, 1991; Kalousek and Barrett, 1994; Shaffer et al., 1998). Typically, UPD cases come to attention with clinical abnormalities

but the abnormal phenotypes may have resulted from any one of several mechanisms—genomic imprinting effects, autosomal trisomy mosaicism, or homozygosity for recessive genes in uniparental isodisomy.

Uniparental disomy and Robertsonian translocations

Phenotypically abnormal individuals with balanced, non-homologous Robertsonian translocations and acrocentric isochromosomes are known (Groupe de Cytogeneticiens Francais, 1989; Temple et al., 1991; Robinson et al., 1994). Different mechanisms might explain this unexpected observation, such as homozygosity for a recessive disorder in cases with isodisomy (Pentao et al., 1992) or an unrelated cryptic chromosome abnormality (Bonthron et al., 1993).

Berend et al. (2000) carried out a prospective study of the risk of UPD in a total of 174 prenatally identified acrocentric rearrangements, that is Robertsonian translocations and isochromosomes. Only one case of UPD 13 was identified in 168 nonhomologous Robertsonian rearrangements (risk estimate 0.6%), but four out of six homologous acrocentric rearrangements showed UPD. Normal phenotypes have been observed in both maternal and paternal UPD of chromosome 13, maternal and paternal UPD of chromosome 21, and maternal UPD of chromosome 22. The risk of an abnormal phenotype specifically relates to maternal and paternal UPD of chromosome 15 and, possibly, chromosome 14. Thus, if a chromosome 15 Robertsonian translocation is discovered prenatally, molecular analysis to rule out UPD is indicated, and in the case of homologous acrocentric rearrangements, the low clinical risk of UPD relates to isodisomy and the possibility of homozygosity for a recessive gene mutation.

AUTOSOMAL TRISOMY MOSAICISM: TRISOMY 8, 16, AND 20 MOSAICISM

Trisomy 8 and 8 mosaicism

Mosaicism for trisomy 8 occurs much more frequently than full trisomy 8 syndrome, and the majority of apparent trisomy 8 cases exhibit mosaicism in at least one somatic tissue (Schinzel, 1984). In contrast with other autosomal trisomy mosaics (21, 13, or 18) that commonly arise from chromosome loss in a trisomic zygote (Zaragoza et al., 1994), trisomy 8 mosaicism arises more frequently from somatic gain of one chromosome 8 in the early development of a normal diploid zygote (Robinson et al., 1995). In a collaborative study on 26 probands with trisomy 8 and mosaic trisomy 8, twenty cases (13 maternal, 7 paternal) were probably due to postzygotic mitotic duplication (Karadima et al., 1998).

The birth frequency of trisomy 8 mosaicism is low—only one case was discovered in a Danish survey of more than 30,000 unselected consecutive newborn infants (Nielsen and Wohlert, 1991), but only about 5 to 10 cells are analyzed in such surveys. Nevertheless, mosaic trisomy 8 is one of the commoner cytogenetic abnormalities among spontaneous abortions comprising 12% of autosomal trisomies in one major series (Warburton et al., 1991). Trisomy 8 mosaicism occurs in up to 1 in 12,000 amniotic fluid samples (Hsu and Perlis, 1984), and the authoritative review of mosaic trisomy 8 syndrome was based on more than 100 published cases (Schinzel, 1984).

As with the other mosaic autosomal trisomies, identification of a typical postnatal phenotype is difficult because of great variability in clinical expression; for example, a 19-year-old girl who presented with primary amenorrhoea due to gonadal dysgenesis had mosaic trisomy 8 and 21 (Sulewski et al., 1980). Mosaic trisomy 8 is not necessarily associated with even mild handicap (e.g., Chandley et al., 1980; Finley et al., 1993), but among cases who present with phenotypic abnormalities, a recognizable clinical syndrome does emerge (Schinzel, 1984). Birthweight is normal. Typical clinical presentation is in early childhood with developmental delay and dysmorphism. The facies may have a myopathic appearance with open mouth and everted lower lip (Fig. 44.15A). Radiographic studies have indicated disturbed vertical growth of the face in some cases (Beemer et al., 1984). Cleft palate, pronounced anterior open bite, complete reserved unilateral buccal cross-bite, slightly increased width of alveolar processes, and gingival enlargement were recorded in a case in which orofacial complications were studied in detail (Henderson and Crawford, 1996). Corneal opacities may be diagnostically helpful (Frangoulis and Taylor, 1983). Commonly reported bone and joint abnormalities include vertebral abnormalities, hypoplastic patellae, and restricted movement at both large and small joints. Radiologic features were reviewed by Silengo et al. (1979). Cardiovascular malformations are infrequent, but hydronephrosis may be common. The lack of life-threatening major malformations means that survival in trisomy 8 mosaicism does not appear to be significantly reduced.

Two aspects of the trisomy 8 phenotype merit special attention. First, deep plantar and palmar grooves are well-recognized findings among other less striking dermatoglyphic abnormalities (Rodewald et al., 1977) (Fig. 44.15B,C).

Secondly, in cases in which neuroimaging studies are performed, agenesis of the corpus callosum is frequently identified. Indeed, on the basis of phenotype-karyotype correlation in individuals with different duplicated regions of chromosome 8, it was suggested that there is a gene important for corpus callosum development located in the region 8p21 → pter (Digilio et al., 1994). However, neither deep palmar and plantar furrows nor agenesis of the corpus callosum are specific for trisomy 8 mosaicism: deep plantar grooves are often present in boys with fragile X syndrome; corpus callosum abnormalities may be associated with many different chromosomal, mendelian, and nongenetic disorders.

Within the context of prenatal diagnosis, Wang et al. (1994) had four cases of trisomy 8 mosaicism in cultured tissue from 4000 consecutive CVS cases. Follow-up studies in amniocytes did not reveal a trisomic cell line. A false-negative amniocentesis result has also been recorded in trisomy 8 mosaicism (Schneider et al., 1994). An important point is the need for longer term follow up information in prenatally diagnosed cases (Camurri et al., 1991). Trisomy 8 mosaicism is not associated with major congenital malformations, so the phenotype is not readily recognized in a fetus or at birth. Nevertheless, since a characteristic clinical syndrome with mental retardation is evident in later childhood, prenatal diagnosis of trisomy 8 mosaicism is usually followed by pregnancy termination without visible fetal abnormality being present (Hsu et al., 1997). An exception was the follow-up study reported by Klein et al. (1994): a 37-year-old woman had normal direct cytogenetic analysis of CVS material, trisomy 8 mosaicism in CVS cultures, but normal diploid cells after amniocentesis. In peripheral blood samples taken after the birth of a normal infant, very low-level mosaicism for trisomy 8 (less than 5% trisomic cells) was detected. Clinical examination confirmed normality at 2.5 years of age.

Trisomy 16 mosaicism

Nonmosaic trisomy 16 is by far the commonest autosomal trisomy found among first trimester and early second trimester spontaneous abortions, and in such cases there is highly abnormal or minimal or no embryonic development (Warburton et al., 1991). Trisomy 16 and mosaic trisomy 16 has been the subject of excellent, recent reviews (Wolstenholme, 1995; Benn 1998). The estimated incidence of trisomy 16 in the first trimester is 15 per 1000 recognized pregnancies. About 90% of trisomy 16 pregnancies are lost by 12 weeks gestation, but 10% survive, mostly

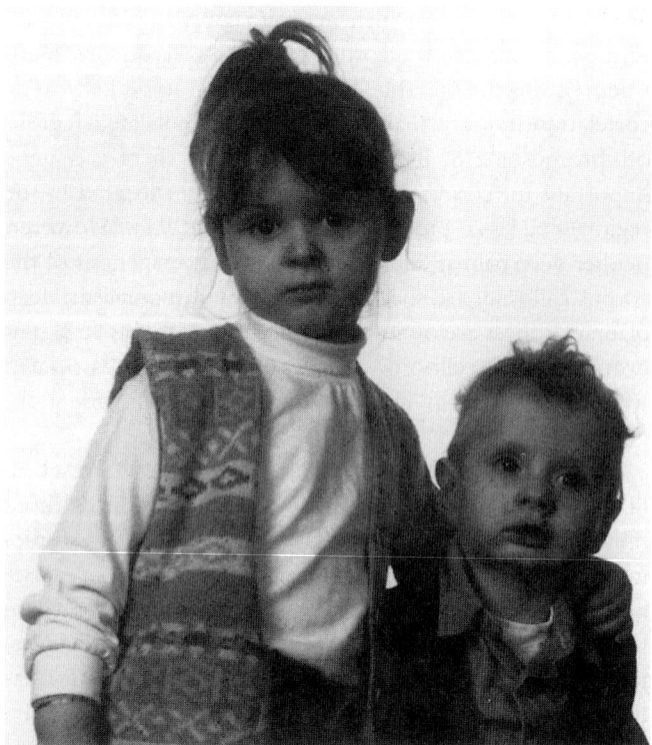

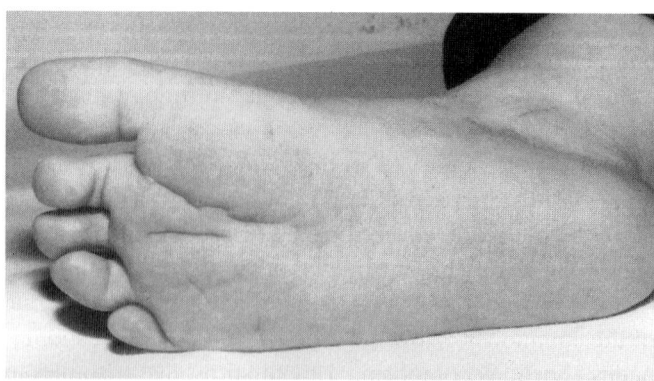

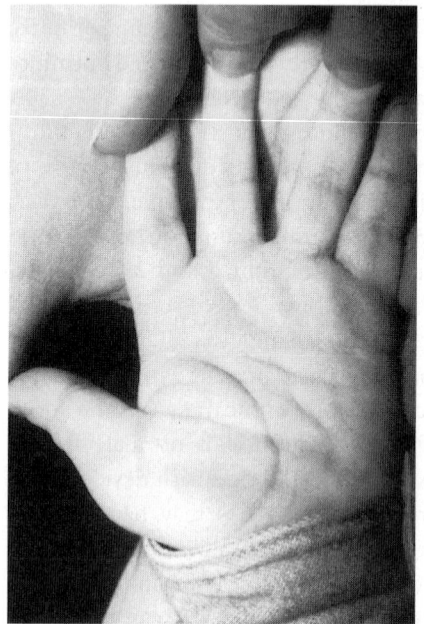

Fig. 44.15. (A) Two-year-old boy with trisomy 8 mosaicism detected in fibroblasts, and his unaffected sister. Deep palmar and plantar creases with agenesis of the corpus callosum (B & C) prompted fibroblast chromosome analysis although the blood lymphocyte karyotype was normal.

having spontaneously reduced to disomy 16 in fetal tissues. Reduction to disomy gives rise to confined placental mosaicism and may result in fetal UPD. There is now good evidence that high levels of trisomy 16 cells within placental tissue can cause pathological changes therein and retard fetal growth, leading to miscarriage (Kalousek et al., 1993; Astner et al., 1998). Trisomy 16 cells have also been detected in the fetus, albeit uncommonly, almost always in fibroblasts (Garber et al., 1994; Pletcher et al., 1994; Benn, 1998; Stavropoulos et al., 1998). It is well-established that mosaicism in amniotic fluid is a much better indicator of mosaicism in the fetus than mosaicism in CVS and, through elevated maternal serum HCG and alphafetoprotein levels, such true mosaic cases may be detected in screening programs for Down syndrome and spina bifida.

An analysis of the phenotype in trisomy 16 mosaicism showed there was much variation (Benn, 1998) but heart defects, hernias, hypospadias and imperforate anus seem to be more common (Fig. 44.16). Additional evidence for a recognizable phenotype due to chromosome 16 trisomy mosaicism, as opposed to UPD 16, is that these abnormalities are also present in cases of nonmosaic partial duplications of chromosome 16. But a variety of atypical and even mild abnormalities were present in other cases. In both severely and mildly affected fetuses, trisomy 16 cells were most often conspicuous by their absence, even in skin fibroblasts. Benn (1998) suggested the term "occult mosaicism" should be used to describe the situation where the presence of an abnormal cell line is suspected on clinical grounds but cannot be proven by cytogenetics. Recently, skewed X chromosome inactivation has been identified in clinically abnormal mosaic trisomy 16 cases and it is postulated that this reflects a failure to eliminate trisomic cells from all fetal tissues (Lau et al., 1997; Peñaherrera et al., 2001).

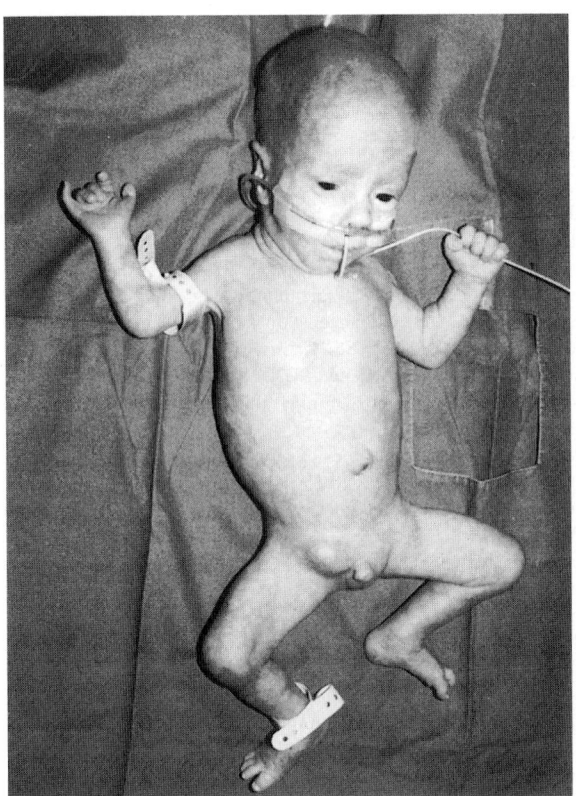

Fig. 44.16. Uniparental disomy of chromosome 16. Trisomy 16 mosaicism in placental tissue and complex congenital heart disease were diagnosed prenatally, but no trisomy 16 cells were detected in this infant, who had growth retardation and dysmorphism and who died at age three months. (From Whiteford et al, 1995, with permission.)

The net result is that parents cannot be absolutely reassured following detection of mosaic trisomy 16 in amniocytes from a fetus without visible malformation. Further tests such as DNA analysis to look for UPD may be offered but are not expected to provide a definitive answer as to the future health of the fetus. Detailed ultrasonographic examination of the fetus may, at least, rule out placental abnormalities, growth retardation and major congenital malformation.

Trisomy 20 mosaicism

Trisomy 20 mosaicism is diagnosed in about 1 in every 6000 amniotic fluid samples examined (Worton and Stern, 1984). Previously, this prenatal diagnosis has resulted in parents receiving a cautious or guarded prognosis for normal physical and intellectual development in a liveborn infant. Therefore, it was not surprising that pregnancies were terminated after prenatal diagnosis of trisomy 20 mosaicism and a diverse array of insignificant, and some apparently significant developmental abnormalities were reported in the fetuses with and without trisomy 20 cells identified postmortem. However,

since trisomy 20 mosaicism is not detected in postnatal life among children with handicaps, some geneticists took the view that this cytogenetic abnormality did not have clinical significance, and more optimistic prenatal counseling was followed by the birth of normal infants with normal blood and skin karyotypes. Subsequently, however, trisomy 20 cells were isolated from normal children born after positive prenatal diagnosis (Hsu et al., 1991; Brothman et al., 1992), as well as from abortuses and infants with abnormalities. The trisomic cells tend to be in highest proportions in the gastrointestinal and renal tracts.

The net result is that from 144 cases of trisomy 20 mosaicism, 91% were associated with a grossly normal phenotype, and the remainder did not have any particular pattern of abnormalities that could be said to constitute a clinical cytogenetic syndrome (Hsu, 1992). Recently, low level (10%) trisomy 20 cells were identified in fetal blood obtained after midtrimester termination of pregnancy in a woman referred for amniocentesis because of the suspicious ultrasound findings of short femurs and nuchal thickening. Molecular analysis revealed the origin of the extra chromosome 20 was due to mitotic non-disjunction in the zygote (Micale et al., 1996). Generally, however, fetal blood sampling is unhelpful as the trisomic cells are not identified, and even if they were, their clinical significance would most likely still be uncertain.

Conclusion

Once mosaicism has been discovered and reported to the parents, great anxiety ensues that is not necessarily allayed by normal cytogenetic or ultrasound findings in subsequent analyses or tests. Genetic counseling is often difficult—parents are informed that there is an abnormality in the prenatal chromosome test result, but do not worry, the fetus is probably unaffected, although we cannot be absolutely sure. Also, whereas the genetic counselor may be able to accept that, in a statistical sense, the prenatal finding of trisomy 7 mosaicism or trisomy 15 mosaicism is unlikely to have clinical consequences given normal appearances on ultrasound examination, the couple at the clinic may find this harder to believe, especially after becoming acquainted with one or two case reports describing exceptions to the rule. In practice, some couples terminate their pregnancy after prenatal diagnosis of chromosome mosaicism, and a greater number of couples elect to continue. The reasons for these different actions may be related to the style of genetic counseling received (Marteau et al., 1994) or may be personal to the couple concerned. Whatever the explanation, further investigation of the counseling process is warranted.

REFERENCES

Abramsky L, Chapple J (1993) Room for improvement? Detecting autosomal trisomies without serum screening. Public Health 107:349–354

Alfi OS, Chang R, Azen SP (1980) Evidence for genetic control of non-disjunction in man. Am J Hum Genet 32:477–483

Allan LD, (1999) Atrioventricular septal defect in the fetus. Am J Obstet Gynecol 181:1250–1253

Amano A, Kishima T, Kimura S et al. (2000) Periodontopathic bacteria in children with Down syndrome. J Periodontol 71:249–255

Amark K, Sunnegardh J (1999) The effect of changing attitudes to Down's syndrome in the management of complete atrioventricular septal defects. Arch Dis Child 81:151–154

Amor DJ, Woods CG (2000) Pseudotrisomy 13 syndrome in siblings. Clin Dysmorphol 9:115–118

Angell RR, Hillier SG, West JD et al. (1988) Chromosome anomalies in early human embryos. J Reprod & Fert Suppl 36:73–81

Angelopoulou N, Souftas V, Sakadamis A, Mandroukas, K (1999) Bone mineral density in adults with Down's syndrome. Eur Radiol 9:648–651

Ani C, Grantham-McGregor S, Muller D (2000) Nutritional supplementation in Down syndrome: Theoretical considerations and current status. Dev Med Child Neurol 42:207–213

Annerén G, Gustavson K-H, Sara V et al. (1990) Growth-retardation in Down syndrome in relation to insulin-like growth factors and growth hormone. Am J Med Genet Suppl 7:59–62

Annerén G, Gustafsson J, Sara VR et al. (1993) Normalised growth velocity in children with Down's syndrome during growth hormone therapy. J Intell Disabil Res 37:381–387

Annerén G, Tuvemo T, Carlsson-Skwirut C et al. (1999) Growth hormone treatment in young children with Down's syndrome: Effects on growth and psychomotor development. Arch Dis Child 80:334–338

Anon (1992) Clinical management of trisomy 18. Lancet 339:904

Antonanarakis SE, Avramopoulos D, Blouin J-L et al. (1993a) Mitotic errors in somatic cells cause trisomy 21 in about 4.5% of cases and are not associated with advanced maternal age. Nature Genet 3:146–150

Antonarakis SE, Blouin JL, Maher J et al. CC (1993b) Maternal uniparental disomy for human chromosome 14, due to loss of a chromosome 14 from somatic cells with t (13;14) trisomy 14. Am J Hum Genet 52:1145–52

Anwar AJ, Walker JD, Frier BM (1998) Type 1 diabetes mellitus and Down's syndrome: Prevalence, management and diabetic complications. Diabet Med 15:160–163

Arnell H, Gustafsson J, Ivarsson SA, Anneren G (1996) Growth and pubertal development in Down syndrome. Acta Paediatr 85:1102–1106

Association of Clinical Cytogeneticists Working Party on Chorionic Villi in Prenatal Diagnosis (1994) Cytogenetic analysis of chorionic villi for prenatal diagnosis: an ACC collaborative study of U.K.data. Prenat Diagn 14:363–379

Astner A, Schwinger E, Caliebe A, Jonat W, Gembruch U (1998) Sonographically detected fetal and placental abnormalities associated with trisomy 16 confined to the placenta. A case report and review of the literature. Prenat Diagn 18:1308–1305

Avanzini M, Monafo V, de Amici M et al. (1990) Humoral immunodeficiencies in Down syndrome: Serum IgG subclass and antibody response to hepatitis vaccine. Am J Med Genet Suppl 7:231–233

Averbuch-Heller L, Dell'Osso LF, Jacobs JB, Remler BF (1999) Latent and congenital nystagmus in Down syndrome. J Neuroophthalmol 19:166–172

Aylott J (1999) Should children with Down's syndrome have cosmetic surgery? Br J Nurs 8:33–38

Ayme S, Philip N (1997) Apparently new syndrome of congenital cataracts, sensorineural deafness, Down syndrome like facial appearance, short stature and mental retardation. Am J Med Genet 70:333–335

Baciewicz FA, Melvin WS, Basilius D et al. (1989) Congenital heart disease in Down syndrome patients: A decade of surgical experience. Thorac Cardiovasc Surg 37:369–371

Bahado-Singh RO, Lynch L, Deren O et al. (1997) First-trimester growth restriction and fetal aneuploidy: The effect of type of aneuploidy and gestational age. Am J Obstet Gynecol 176:976–980

Baird PA, Sadovnick AD (1988) Causes of death to age 30 in Down syndrome. Am J Hum Genet 43:239–248

Baird PA, Sadovnick AD (1989) Life tables for Down syndrome. Hum Genet 82:291–292

Barr MJ (1994) Growth profiles of human autosomal trisomies at midgestation. Teratology 50:395–398

Bartolomei MS, Tilghman SM (1997) Genomic imprinting in mammals. Annu Rev Genet 31:493–525

Bartsch O, Hinkel GK, Petersen MB et al. (1997) A large family with subtelomeric translocation t(18; 21) (q23;q22.1) and molecular breakpoint in the Down syndrome critical region. Hum Genet 100:669–675

Baty BJ, Blackburn BL, Carey JC (1994a) Natural history of trisomy 18 and trisomy 13: 1 Growth, physical assessment, medical histories, survival, and recurrence risk. Am J Med Genet 49:175–188

Baty BJ, Jorde LJ, Blackburn BL et al. (1994b) The natural history of trisomy 18 and trisomy 13. 2 Psychomotor development. Am J Med Genet 49:189–194

Baumgartner A, Van Hummelen P, Lowe XR et al. (1999) Numerical and structural chromosomal abnormalities detected in human sperm with a combination of multicolor FISH assays. Environ Mol Mutagen 33:49–58

Baxter LL, Moran TH, Richtsmeier JT et al. (2000) Discovery and genetic localization of Down syndrome cerebellar phenotypes using the Ts65Dn mouse. Hum Mol Genet 9:195–202

Beasley SW, Allen M, Myers N (1997) The effects of Down syndrome and other chromosomal abnormalities on survival and management in oesophageal atresia. Pediatr Surg Int 12:550–551

Beatty BG, Qi S, Pienkowska M (1999) Chromosomal localization of phospholipase A2 activating protein, an Ets2 target gene, to 9p21. Genomics 62:529–532

Beccerra M, Moya F, Lacassie Y et al. (1992) Clinico-pathological conference: a preterm infant with multiple congenital abnormalities. Am J Med Genet 44:503–507

Beemer FA, Van Doorne JM, Gorlin RJ et al. (1984) Roentgencephalometric measurements in trisomy 8 mosaicism. Report of three cases. J Craniofac Genet Dev Biol 4:233–241

Bell AJ, Bhate MS (1992) Prevalence of overweight and obesity in Down's syndrome and other mentally handicapped adults living in the community. J Intellect Disabil Res 36:359–364

Benn P (1998) Trisomy 16 and trisomy 16 mosaicism: a review. Am J Med Genet 79:121–133

Berend SA, Horwitz J, McCaskill C, Shaffer LG (2000) Identification of uniparental disomy following prenatal detection of Robertsonian translocations and isochromosomes. Am J Hum Genet 66:1787–1793

Beverstock GC, Hansson K, Helderman-van den Enden AT et al. (1998) A near false-negative finding of mosaic trisomy 21—a cautionary tale. Prenat Diagn 18:742–746

Bidder RT, Gray P, Newcombe RG et al. (1989) The effects of multivitamins and minerals on children with Down syndrome. Dev Med Child Neurol 31:532–537

Bobrow M, Barby T, Hajianpour A et al. (1992) Fertility in a male with trisomy 21. J Med Genet 29:141

Boghosian-Sell L, Mewar R, Harrison W et al. (1994) Molecular mapping of the Edwards syndrome phenotype to two noncontiguous regions on chromosome 18. Am J Hum Genet 55:476–483

Boice J, Linet M (1994) Chernobyl, childhood cancer, and chromosome 21. BMJ 309:139–140

Bond DJ, Chandley AC (1983) Aneuploidy. Oxford University Press,

Bonthron DT, Smith SJL, Fantes J et al. (1993) De novo microdeletion on an inherited Robersonian translocation chromosome: A cause for dysmorphism in the apparently balanced translocation carrier. Am J Hum Genet 53:629–637

Boraz RA (1987) Trisomy 13 syndrome: A rare case of long term survival. J Pedodont 11:288–294

Bos AP, Broers CJM, Hazebroek FWJ et al. (1992) Avoidance of emergency surgery in newborn infants with trisomy 18. Lancet 339:913–915

Bosma GP, van Buchem MA, Voormolen JH et al. (1999) Cervical spondylarthrotic myelopathy with early onset in Down's syndrome: Five cases and a review of the literature. J Intellect Disabil Res 43:283–288

Botto LD, Yang Q (2000) 5, 10-Methylenetetrahydrofolate reductase gene variants and congenital anomalies: A HuGE review. Am J Epidemiol 151:862–877

Boué A, Gallano P (1984) A collaborative study of the segregation of inherited chromosome structural rearrangements in 1346 prenatal diagnoses. Prenat Diagn (special issue) 4:45–67

Bove KE, Soukup S, Ballard ET, Ryckman F (1996) Hepatoblastoma in a child with trisomy 18: Cytogenetics, liver anomalies, and literature review. Pediatr Pathol Lab Med 16:253–262

Bovicelli L, Orsini LF, Rizzo N et al. (1982) Reproduction in Down's syndrome. Obstet Gynaecol 59 (suppl 6):13s–17s

Boyd PA, Lindenbaum RH, Redman C (1987) Pre-eclampsia and trisomy 13: A possible association. Lancet 11:425–427

Boyd PA, Maher EJ, Lindenbaum RH et al. (1995) Maternal 3; 13 chromosome insertion, with severe pre-eclampsia. Clin Genet 47:17–21

Brooks DN, Wooley A, Kanjilal D (1972) Hearing loss and middle ear disorders in patients with Down's syndrome (Mongolism) J Ment Defic Res 16:21

Brothman AR, Rehberg K, Storto PD et al. (1992) Confirmation of true mosaic trisomy 20 in a phenotypically normal liveborn male. Clin Genet 42:47–49

Brown AC, Olkowski ZL, Mclaren JR et al. (1977) Alopecia areata and vitiligo associated with Down's syndrome (mongolism). Arch Dermatol 113:1296

Bruyere H, Rupps R, Kuchinka BD et al. (2000) Recurrent trisomy 21 in a couple with a child presenting trisomy 21 mosaicism and maternal uniparental disomy for chromosome 21 in the euploid cell line. Am J Med Genet 94:35–41

Buchanan LH (1990) Early onset of presbyacusis in Down syndrome. Scand Audiol 19:103–110

Bugge M, Collins A, Petersen MB et al. (1998) Non-disjunction of chromosome 18. Hum Mol Genet 7:661–669

Bull C, Rigby ML, Shinebourne EA (1985) Should management of complete atrioventricular canal defect be influenced by coexistent Down syndrome? Lancet 1:1147–1149

Burt DB, Loveland KA, Primeaux-Hart S et al. (1998) Dementia in adults with Down syndrome: Diagnostic challenges. Am J Ment Retard 103:130–145

Busciglio J, Yankner BA (1995) Apoptosis and increased generation of reactive oxygen species in Down's syndrome neurons in vitro. Nature 378:776–779

Butler MG (1994) Trisomy 18 mosaicism in a 24yr old white woman with normal intelligence and skeletal abnormalities. Am J Med Genet 53:92–93

Cairns NJ (1999) Neuropathology. J Neural Transm Suppl 57:61–74

Calderone JP et al. (1983) Intraocular pathology of trisomy 18 (Edwards syndrome): Report of a case and review of the literature. Br J Ophthalmol 67:162–169

Camurri L, Chiesi A et al. (1991) A three-year follow-up on a child with low level trisomy 8 mosaicism which was diagnosed prenatally. Prenat Diag 11:59–62

Canniano DA, Teitelbaum DH, Qualman SJ (1990) Management of Hirschsprung's disease in children with trisomy 21. Am J Surg 159:402–404

Carlstedt K, Anneren G, Huggare J et al. (1999) The effect of growth hormone therapy on craniofacial growth and dental maturity in children with Down syndrome. J Craniofac Genet Dev Biol 19:20–23

Carothers AD, Hecht CA, Hook EB (1999a) International variation in reported livebirth prevalence rates of Down syndrome, adjusted for maternal age. J Med Genet 36:386–393

Carothers AD, Boyd E, Lowther G et al. (1999b) Trends in prenatal diagnosis of Down syndrome and other autosomal trisomies in Scotland 1990 to 1994, with associated cytogenetic and epidemiological findings. Genet Epidemiol 16:179–190

Carr J (1988) Six weeks to twenty-one years old. A longitudinal study of children with Down syndrome and their families. J Child Psychol & Psych 29:407–431

Carr J (1995) Down's Syndrome: Children Growing Up. Cambridge University Press, Cambridge

Casati A, Giorga R, Lanza A et al. (1992) Trisomy 21 mosaicism in two subjects from two generations. Ann Genet 35:245–250

Caselli MC, Vicari S, Longobardi E et al. (1998) Gestures and words in early development of children with Down syndrome. J Speech Lang Hear Res 41:1125–1135

Castells S, Torrado C, Bastian W et al. (1992) Growth hormone deficiency in Down's syndrome children. J Intellect Disabil Res 36:29–43

Cavani S, Perfumo C, Argusti A (1998) Cytogenetic and molecular study of 32 Down syndrome families: potential leukaemia predisposing role of the most proximal segment of chromosome 21q. Br J Haematol 103:213–216

Cereijo AI, Martinez-Frias ML (1993) Consanguineous marriages amongst parents of patients with Down syndrome. Clin Genet 44:221–222

Chandley AC, Hargreave TB, Fletcher JM et al. (1980) Trisomy 8: report of a mosaic human male with near-normal pheonotype and normal IQ ascertained through infertility. Hum Genet 55:31

Chapman S (1995) Commentary on "Atlantoaxial instability instability in Down's syndrome: A five year follow up study." Arch Dis Child 72:118–119

Chapman RS, Hesketh LJ (2000) Behavioral phenotype of individuals with Down syndrome. Ment Retard Dev Disabil Res Rev 6:84–95

Chapman RS, Seung HK, Schwartz SE, Kay-Raining BE (1998) Language skills of children and adolescents with Down syndrome: II. Production deficits. J Speech Lang Hear Res 41:861–873

Chapman RS, Seung HK, Schwartz SE, Bird EK (2000) Predicting language production in children and adolescents with Down syndrome: The role of comprehension. J Speech Lang Hear Res 43:340–350

Chemke J, Rappaport S, Etrog R (1983) Aberrant melanoblast migration associated with trisomy 18 mosaicism. J Med Genet 20:135–137

Chen CP, Hung TH, Jan SW, Jeng CJ (1998) Enlarged cisterna magna in the third trimester as a clue to fetal trisomy 18. Fetal Diagn Ther 13:29–34

Chen CL, Gilbert TJ, Daling JR (1999) Maternal smoking and Down syndrome: The confounding effect of maternal age. Am J Epidemiol 149:442–446

Chessells JM, Bailey C, Richards SM (1995) Intensification of treatment and survival in all children with lymphoblastic leukaemia: Results of the UK Medical Research Council trial UKALL X. Lancet 345:143–148

Chitty LS and Pandya PP (1997) Ultrasound screening for fetal abnormalities in the first trimester. Prenat Diagn 17:1269–1281

Chrast R, Scott HS, Madani R et al. (2000) Mice trisomic for a bacterial artificial chromosome with the single-minded 2 gene (Sim2) show phenotypes similar to some of those present in the partial trisomy 16 mouse models of Down syndrome. Hum Mol Genet 9:1853–1864

Christianson AL (1997) Down syndrome in black South African infants and children—clinical features and delayed diagnosis. S Afr Med J 87:992–995

Chrobok V, Simakova E (1997) Temporal bone findings in trisomy 18 and 21 syndromes. Eur Arch Otorhinolaryngol 254:15–18

Cichon P, Crawford L, Grimm WD (1998) Early-onset periodontitis associated with Down's syndrome—clinical interventional study. Ann Periodontol 3:370–380

Clapp SK, Perry BL, Farooki ZQ et al. (1990) Down's syndrome complete atrioventricular canal and pulmonary obstructive disease. J Thorac Cardiovasc Surg 100:115–121

Clarke CM, Edwards JH, Smallpiece V (1961) 21 trisomy/normal mosaicism in an intelligent child with mongoloid characteristics. Lancet 1:1028–1030

Clementi M, Calzolari E, Turolla L et al. (1990) Neonatal growth patterns in a population of consecutively born Down syndrome children. Am J Med Genet Suppl 7:71–74

Collacott RA, Cooper S-A, Ismail IA (1994) Multi-infarct dementia in Down's syndrome. J Intellect Disabil Res 38:203–208

Collacott RA, Cooper SA, Branford D, McGrother C (1998) Behaviour phenotype for Down's syndrome. Br J Psychiatry 172:85–89

Committee on Sports Medicine and Fitness. American Academy of Pediatrics (1995) Atlantoaxial instability in Down syndrome. Pediatrics 96:151–4

Conn CM, Cozzi J, Harper JC et al. (1999) Preimplantation genetic diagnosis for couples at high risk of Down syndrome pregnancy owing to parental translocation or mosaicism. J Med Genet 36:45–50

Cooney TP, Thurlbeck WM (1982) Pulmonary hypoplasia in Down's syndrome. N Engl J Med 307:1170–1182

Cooper SA, Collacott RA, Hauck A (1994) Late-onset mania in Down syndrome. J Intellect Disabil Res 38:73–78

Cossarizza A, Ortolani C, Forti E et al. (1991) Age-related expansion of functionally inefficient cells with markers of natural killer activity in Down's syndrome. Blood 77:1263–1270

Courage ML, Adams RJ, Reyno S, Kwa P-G (1994) Visual acuity in children with Down syndrome. Dev Med Child Neurol 36:586–593

Cowen JM, Walker S, Harris F (1979) Trisomy 13 and extended survival. J Med Genet 16:155

Cozzi J, Conn CM, Harper J et al. (1999) A trisomic germ cell line and precocious chromatid segregation leads to recurrent trisomy 21 conception. Hum Genet 104:23–28

Craddock N, Owen M (1994) Inverse relationship between Down syndrome and bipolar affective disorder. J Intellect Disabil Res 38:73–78

Craze JL, Harrison G, Wheatley K et al. (1999) Improved outcome of acute myeloid leukaemia in Down's syndrome. Arch Dis Child 81:32–37

Cremers MJA, Ramos L, Bol E et al. (1993) Radiological assessment of the atlantoaxial distance in Down's syndrome. Arch Dis Child 69:347–350

Cronk C (1978) Growth of children with Down syndrome. Birth to age 3 years. Pediatrics 61:564–568

Cronk C, Crocker AC, Pueschel SM et al. (1988) Growth charts for children with Down syndrome: 1 month to 18 years of age. Pediatrics 81:102–110

Cuadrado E, Barrena MJ (1996) Immune dysfunction in Down's syndrome: Primary immune deficiency or early senescence of the immune system? Clin Immunol Immunopathol 78:209–214

Cuckle H (1999) Down syndrome fetal loss rate in early pregnancy. Prenat Diagn 19:1177–1179

Cuckle HS, Wald NJ, Thompson SG (1987) Estimating a woman's risk of having a pregnancy associated with Down's syndrome using her age and serum alpha-fetoprotein level. Brit J Obstet Gynaecol 94:387–402

Dacre JE, Huskisson EC (1988) Arthritis in Down's syndrome. Ann Rheum Dis 47:254–255

Dai AI, Shaikh ZA, Cohen ME (2000) Early-onset Moyamoya syndrome in a patient with Down syndrome: Case report and review of the literature. J Child Neurol 15:696–699

Dalton A, Wisniewski H (1990) Down syndrome and dementia of Alzheimer disease. Int Rev Psychiatry 2:41–50

Daniel A, Hook EB, Wulf G (1989) Risks of unbalanced progeny at amniocentesis to carriers of chromosome rearrangements: Data from United States and Canadian laboratories. Am J Med Genet 33:14–53

Dasouki M, Barr M (1987) Trisomy 18 and hepatic neoplasia. Am J Med Genet 27:203–205

Davidson RG (1988) Atlantoaxial instability in individuals with Down syndrome: A fresh look at the evidence. Pediatrics 81:857–865

de Braekeleer M, Landry T, Cholette A (1994) Consanguinity and kinship in Saguenay Lac-Saint-Jean (Québec) Ann Génét 37:86–88

De Melker R (1993) Treating persistent glue ear in children (editorial) BMJ 306:5–6

Dean G, Nevin NC, Mikkelsen M et al. (2000) Investigation of a cluster of children with Down's syndrome born to mothers who had attended a school in Dundalk, Ireland. Occup Environ Med 57: 793–804

Deb S, Braganza J (1999) Comparison of rating scales for the diagnosis of dementia in adults with Down's syndrome. J Intellect Disabil Res 43:400–407

Deb S, Braganza J, Norton N et al. (2000) APOE epsilon 4 influences the manifestation of Alzheimer's disease in adults with Down's syndrome. Br J Psychiatry 176:468–472

Delabar J, Theophile D, Rahmani Z et al. (1993) Molecular mapping of 24 features of Down syndrome on chromosome 21. Eur J Hum Genet 1:114–124

Delatycki M, Gardner RJ (1997) Three cases of trisomy 13 mosaicism and a review of the literature. Clin Genet 51:403–407

Delatycki MB, Pertile MD, Gardner RJ (1998) Trisomy 13 mosaicism at prenatal diagnosis: dilemmas in interpretation. Prenat Diagn 18:45–50

Delisle MF, Sandor GG, Tessier F, Farquharson DF (1999) Outcome of fetuses diagnosed with atrioventricular septal defect. Obstet Gynecol 94:763–767

Dennis NR, Cockwell A (1992) Clinical management of trisomy 18. Lancet 339:1235

Devenny DA, Hill AL, Patxot O et al. (1992) Aging in higher functioning adults with Down syndrome: An interim report in a longitudinal study. J Intellect Disabil Res 36:41–250

Devenny DA, Silverman WP, Hill AL et al. (1996) Normal ageing in adults with Down's syndrome: A longitudinal study. J Intellect Disabil Res 40:208–221

DeVore GR (2000) Second trimester ultrasonography may identify 77 to 97% of fetuses with trisomy 18. J Ultrasound Med 19:565–576

Digilio MC, Giannotti A, Floridia G (1994) Trisomy 8 syndrome due to isodicentric 8p chromosomes: Regional assignment of a presumptive gene involved in corpus callosum development. J Med Genet 31:238–241

Dinani S, Carpenter S (1990) Down's syndrome and thyroid disorder. J Ment Def Res 34:187–193

Donahue JE, Khurana JS, Adelman LS (1998) Intracerebral hemorrhage in two patients with Down's syndrome and cerebral amyloid angiopathy. Acta Neuropathol (Berl.) 95:213–216

Donaldson SJ, Wright CA, de Ravel TJ (1999) Trisomy 18 with total cranio-rachischisis and thoraco-abdominoschisis. Prenat Diagn 19:580–582

Donnenfeld AE, Scott S, Henscider-Kimmel M, Dampier CD (1994) Prenatally diagnosed non-immune hydrops caused by congenital transient leukemia. Prenat Diagn 14:721–724

Dordelmann M, Schrappe M, Reiter A et al. (1998) Down's syndrome in childhood acute lymphoblastic leukemia: Clinical characteristics and treatment outcome in four consecutive BFM trials. Berlin-Frankfurt-Munster Group. Leukemia 12:645–651

Down JL (1866) Observations on an ethnic classification of idiots. London Hospital Reports 3:259–262

Down JL (republished in 1990) On some of the mental affections of childhood and youth. MacKeith Press, Blackwell, Oxford

Drugan A, Yaron Y, Zamir R et al. (1999) Differential effect of advanced maternal age on prenatal diagnosis of trisomies 13, 18 and 21. Fetal Diagn Ther 14:181–184

Dumaret AC, Donnelly A, Rosset DJ (1996) Announcing the trisomy 21 diagnosis and care of the infant in the maternity ward: Counseling offered to the parents. J Gynecol Obstet Biol Reprod (Paris) 25:629–635

Edwards JH, Harnden DG, Cameron AH et al. (1960) A new trisomic syndrome. Lancet 1:787

Eggermann T, Nothen MM, Eiben B et al. (1996) Trisomy of human chromosome 18: Molecular studies on parental origin and cell stage of nondisjunction. Hum Genet 97:218–223

Ema M, Ikegami S, Hosoya T et al. (1999) Mild impairment of learning and memory in mice overexpressing the mSim2 gene located on chromosome 16: an animal model of Down's syndrome. Hum Mol Genet 8:1409–1415

Embleton ND, Wyllie JP, Wright MJ et al. (1996) Natural history of trisomy 18. Arch Dis Child Fetal Neonatal Ed 75:F38–F41

Engel E (1980) A new genetic concept: Uniparental disomy and its potential effect. Am J Genet 6:137–43

Engel E, De Lozier-Blanchet CD (1991) Uniparental disomy, isodisomy and imprinting: Probable effects in man and strategies for their detection. Am J Med Genet 40:432–439

Episkopou V, Maeda S, Nishiguchi S et al. (1993) Disruption of the transthyretin gene results in mice with depressed levels of plasma retinol and thyroid hormone. Proc Natl Acad Sci USA 90:2375–2379

Epstein CJ, Korenberg JR, Anneren G et al. (1991) Protocols to establish Genotype-Phenotype correlations in Down syndrome. Am J Hum Genet 49:207–305

Escudero T, Lee M, Carrel D et al. (2000) Analysis of chromosome abnormalities in sperm and embryos from two 45, XY, t (13; 14) (q10; q10) carriers. Prenat Diagn 20:599–602

Eubanks SR, Kuller JA, Amjadi D, Powell CM (1998) Prenatal diagnosis of mosaic trisomy 13: A case report. Prenat Diagn 18:971–974

Evans DGR, Evans ID, Donnai D et al. (1990) Anklyoblepharon filiforme adnatum in trisomy 18 Edwards syndrome. J Med Genet 27:720–721

Eydoux P, Choiset A, Le Porrier N et al. (1989) Chromosomal prenatal diagnosis: Study of 936 cases of intrauterine abnormalities after ultrasound assessment. Prenat Diagn 9:255–269

Ferguson RL, Putney ME, Allen BLJ (1997) Comparison of neurologic deficits with atlanto-dens intervals in patients with Down syndrome. J Spinal Disord 10:246–252

Ferguson-Smith MA (1962) Abnormal sex ratios in the autosomal trisomy syndromes. Lancet 2:357–358

Ferguson-Smith MA, Yates JRW (1984) Maternal age specific rates for chromosome aberrations and factors influencing them: Report fo a collaborative European study on 52965 amniocentesis. Prenat Diag 4:5–44

Ferlini A, Fini S, Salvi F et al. (1992) Molecular strategies in genetic diagnosis of transthyretin-related hereditary amyloidosis. FASEB J 6:2864–2866

Filippello M, Cascone G, Zagami A, Scimone G (1997) Impression cytology in Down's syndrome. Br J Ophthalmol 81:683–685

Finley MJ, Neale MC, Corey LA et al. (1993) Common fragile site expression in lymphocytes from an individual mosaic for trisomy 8. Am J Med Genet 45:570–571

Fisher JM, Harvey JF, Lindenbaum RH et al. (1993) Molecular studies of trisomy 18. Am J Hum Genet 52:1139–1144

Fisher JM, Harvey JF, Morton NE et al. (1995) Trisomy 18: studies of the parent and cell division of origin and the effect of abberrant recombination on nondisjunction. Am J Hum Genet 56:669–683

Fitzgerald PH, Archer SA, Morris CM (1986) Evidence for the repeated primary non-disjunction of chromosome 21 as a result of premature centromere division (PCD). Hum Genet 72:58–62

FitzPatrick DR, Boyd E (1989) Recurrence of trisomy 18 and trisomy 13 after trisomy 21. Hum Genet 82:301

Flejter WL, Issa B, Sullivan BA et al. (1998) Variegated aneuploidy in two siblings: Phenotype, genotype, CENP-E analysis, and literature review. Am J Med Genet 75:45–51

Fong C-T, Brodeur GM (1987) Down's syndrome and leukemia: Epidemiology, genetics, cytogenetics and mechanisms of leukemogenesis. Cancer Genet Cytogenet 28:55–76

Fonkalsrud EW, de Lorimier AA, Hays DM (1969) Congenital atresia and stenosis of the duodenum. Pediatrics 43:79–83

Fort P, Lifshitz F, Bellisario R et al. (1984) Abnormalities of thyroid function in infants with Down syndrome J Pediatr 104:545–549

Fowler A (1990) Language abilities in children with Down syndrome: Evidence for a specific syntactical delay. p. 302. In Cicchetti D, Beeghly M (eds): Children with Down syndrome. Cambridge University Press, Cambridge

Frangou S, Aylward E, Warren A et al. (1997) Small planum temporale volume in Down's syndrome: A volumetric MRI study. Am J Psychiatry 154:1424–1429

Frangoulis M, Taylor D (1983) Corneal opacities—a diagnostic feature of the trisomy 8 mosaic syndrome. Br J Ophthalmol 67:619–622

Freeman SB, Yang Q, Allran K et al. (2000) Women with a reduced ovarian complement may have an increased risk for a child with Down syndrome. Am J Hum Genet 66:1680–1683

Frid C, Drott P, Lundell B et al. (1999) Mortality in Down's syndrome in relation to congenital malformations. J Intellect Disabil Res 43:234–241

Frontera-Izquierdo P, Cabezuelo-Huerto G (1990) Natural and modified history of complete atrioventricular septal defect—a 17 year study. Arch Dis Child 65:964–967

Frost M, Huffer WE, Sze CI et al. (1999) Cervical spine abnormalities in Down Syndrome. Clin Neuropathol 18:250–259

Fryburg JS, Dimaio MS, Yang-Fen TL et al. (1993) Follow-up of pregnancies complicated by placental mosaicism diagnosed by chorionic villus sampling. Prenat Diagn 13:481–494

Fuentes JJ, Genesca L, Kingsbury TJ et al. (2000) DSCR1, overexpressed in Down syndrome, is an inhibitor of calcineurin-mediated signaling pathways. Hum Mol Genet 9:1681–1690

Fujinaga M, Shephard TH, Fitzsimmons J (1990) Trisomy 13 in the fetus. Teratology 41:233–238

Fujiura GT, Fitzsimons N, Marks B, Chicoine B (1997) Predictors of BMI among adults with Down syndrome: The social context of health promotion. Res Dev Disabil 18:261–274

Garber A, Carlson D, Schreck R et al. (1994) Prenatal diagnosis and dysmorphic findings in mosaic trisomy 16. Prenat Diagn 14:257–266

Garcia-Heras J, Rao PN (1999) A brief review of cryptic duplications of 21q as an emerging cause of Down syndrome: Practical considerations for accurate detection. Clin Genet 55:207–211

Gardner RJM, Sutherland GR (1996) Chromosome Abnormalities and Genetic Counselling, 2nd. Oxford University Press, Oxford

Gath A, Gumley D (1984) Down's syndrome and the family: Follow up of children first seen in infancy. Dev Med Child Neurol 26:500

Geldmacher DS, Lerner AJ, Voci JM et al. (1997) Treatment of functional decline in adults with Down syndrome using selective serotonin-reuptake inhibitor drugs. J Geriatr Psychiatry Neurol 10:99–104

Gersdorf E, Utermann B, Utermann G (1990) Trisomy 18 mosaicism in an adult woman with normal intelligence and a history of miscarriage. Hum Genet 84:298–299

Gibson D (1966) Early developmental staging as a prophesy index in Down syndrome. Am J Ment Defic 70:825–828

Goldberg JD, Wohlferd MM (1997) Incidence and outcome of chromosomal mosaicism found at the time of chorionic villus sampling. Am J Obstet Gynecol 176:1349–1352

Golden JA, Hyman BT (1994) Development of the superior temporal neocortex is anomalous in trisomy 21 J Neuropathol Exp Neurol 53:513–520

Goldhaber SZ, Rubin IL, Brown W (1986) Valvular heart disease (aortic regurgitation and mitral valve prolapse) amongst institutionalised adults with Down's syndrome. Am J Cardiol 57:278–281

Goldhaber SZ, Brown WD, St John Sutton MG (1987) High frequency of mitral valve prolapse and aortic regurgitation among asymptomatic adults with Down's syndrome. JAMA 258:1793–1795

Goldstein H, Nielsen KG (1988) Rates and survival of individuals with trisomy 13 and trisomy 18. Clin Genet 34:366–372

Gordon LS (1990) Cardiac conditions. In Van Dyke DC, Lang DJ, Heide F, (eds): Clinical Perspectives in the Management of Down Syndrome. Springer-Verlag, NY p. 55.

Gorlin RJ, Cohen MM, Levin LS (1990) Syndromes of the Head and Neck. Oxford University Press, Oxford

Granholm AC, Sanders LA, Crnic LS (2000) Loss of cholinergic phenotype in basal forebrain coincides with cognitive decline in a mouse model of Down's syndrome. Exp Neurol 161:647–663

Grasso M, Giovannucci ML, Pierluigi M et al. (1989) Isochromosome not translocation in trisomy 21q21q. Hum Genet 84:63–65

Greene MF, Benacerraf BR, Frigoletto FD (1987) Reliable criteria for prenatal sonographic diagnosis of alobar holoprosencephaly. Am J Obs Gyn 156:687–689

Greve G, Waaler PE, Rosendahl K (1993) Low frequency of mosaicism of normal cells in a 16-year-old girl with trisomy 18. Clin Genet 43:83–87

Griffin DK, Abruzzo MA, Millie EA et al. (1995) Non-disjunction in human sperm: Evidence for an effect of increasing paternal age. Hum Mol Genet 4:2227–2232

Griffin ME, Fulcher T, Nikookam K et al. (1997) Down's syndrome, IDDM, and hypothyroidism. Diabetes Care 20:1202–1203

Grimwood JS, Kumar A, Bickerstaff DR, Suvarna SK (2000) Histological assessment of vertebral bone in a Down's syndrome adult with osteoporosis [letter]. Histopathology 36:279–280

Groupe de Cytogeneticiens Français (1989) Robertsonian translocations and abnormal phenotypes. Ann Génét 32:5–9

Gullotta F, Rehder H, Gropp A (1981) Descriptive neuropathology of chromosomal disorders in man. Hum Genet 57:337–44

Guttenbach M, Schakowski R, Schmid M (1994) Incidence of chromosome 18 disomy in human sperm nuclei as detected by nonisotopic in situ hybridization. Hum Genet 93:421–423

Hall BD (1985) Recurrence risk in de novo 21q21q translocation Down syndrome. Am J Med Genet 22:417–418

Halliday JL, Watson LF, Lumley J et al. (1995) New estimates of Down syndrome risks at chorionic villus sampling, amniocentesis, and livebirth in women of advanced maternal age from a uniquely defined population. Prenat Diagn 15:455–465

Han J-Y, Choo KHA, Shaffer LG (1994) Molecular cytogenetic characterisation of 17 rob(13q14q) Robertsonian translocations by FISH, narrowing the region containing the breakpoints. Am J Hum Genet 55:960–967

Happle R (2000) Phylloid hypomelanosis is closely related to mosaic trisomy 13. Eur J Dermatol 10:511–512

Hardy J (1992) Framing Beta amyloid. Nat Genet 1:233–234

Harris DJ, Begleiter ML, Chamberlain J et al. (1982) Parental trisomy 21 mosaicism. Am J Hum Genet 34:125–133

Harrison MW, Deitz DM, Campbell JR, Campbell JT (1987) Diagnosis and management of Hirschsprung's disease: A 25 year perspective. Am J Surg 152:49–56

Hassold TJ, Jacobs PA (1984) Trisomy in man. Annu Rev Genet 18:69–97

Hassold T, Sherman S (2000) Down syndrome: Genetic recombination and the origin of the extra chromosome 21. Clin Genet 57:95–100

Hasle H, Clemmensen IH, Mikkelsen M (2000) Risks of leukaemia and solid tumours in individuals with Down's syndrome. Lancet 355:165–169

Hassold T, Warburton D, Kline J, Stein Z (1984) The relationship of maternal age and trisomy among trisomic spontaneous abortions Am J Hum Genet 36:1349–1356

Hassold T, Jacobs PA, Leppert M, Sheldon M (1987) Cytogenetic and molecular studies of trisomy 13. J Med Genet 24:725–732

Hattori M, Fujiyama A, Taylor TD et al. (2000) The DNA sequence of human chromosome 21. The chromosome 21 mapping and sequencing consortium. Nature 405:311–319

Haveman MJ, Maaskant MA, van Schrojenstein HM (1994) Mental health problems in elderly people with and without Down syndrome. J Intellect Disabil Res 38:341–355

Haydar TF, Nowakowski RS, Yarowsky PJ, Krueger BK (2000) Role of founder cell deficit and delayed neuronogenesis in microencephaly of the trisomy 16 mouse. J Neurosci 20:4156–4164

Hecht F (1963) The placenta in trisomy 18 syndrome. Obstet Gynec 22:147

Hecht CA, Hook EB (1994) The imprecision in rates of Down syndrome by 1-year maternal age intervals: A critical analysis of rates used in biochemical screening. Prenat Diagn 14:729–738

Hecht CA, Hook EB (1996) Rates of Down syndrome at livebirth by one-year maternal age intervals in studies with apparent close to complete ascertainment in populations of European origin: A proposed revised rate schedule for use in genetic and prenatal screening. Am J Med Genet 62:376–385

Hecht F, Bryant JS, Motulsky AG et al. (1964) The nonrandomness of chromosome abnormalities: Association of trisomy 18 and Down's syndrome. N Eng J Med 271:1081–1086

Hecht F, Nievaard JE, Duncanson N (1969) Double aneuploidy: The frequency of XXY in males with Down's syndrome. Am J Hum Genet 21:352–359

Henderson NJ, Crawford PJ (1996) The oro-facial manifestations of trisomy 8 mosaicism: A case report. Int J Paediatr Dent 6:129–132

Hennekam RCM, Van Noort G, De La Fuente AA (1991) Familial holoprosencephaly, heart defects, and polydactyly. Am J Med Genet 41:258–262

Hennequin M, Faulks D, Veyrune JL, Bourdiol P (1999) Significance of oral health in persons with Down syndrome: A literature review. Dev Med Child Neurol 41:275–283

Hestnes A, Stovner LJ, Husoy O et al. (1992) Somatomedin C (insulin-like growth factor 1) in adults with Down's syndrome. J Ment Def Res 35:204–208

Heydanus R, Defoort P, Dhont M (1995) Pre-eclampsia and trisomy 13. Eur J Obstet Gynecol Reprod Biol 60:201–202

Hixon M, Millie E, Judis LA et al. (1998) FISH studies of the sperm of fathers of paternally derived cases of trisomy 21: No evidence for an increase in aneuploidy. Hum Genet 103:654–657

Hobbs CA, Sherman SL, Yi P et al. (2000) Polymorphisms in genes involved in folate metabolism as maternal risk factors for Down syndrome. Am J Hum Genet 67:623–630

Hodes ME, Cole J, Palmer LG et al. (1978) Clinical experience with trisomies 18 and 13. J Med Genet 15:48–60

Holmes LB (1999) Concern about Piracetam treatment for children with Down syndrome. Pediatrics 103:1078–1079

Holmes JM, Coates CM (1994) Assessment of visual acuity in children with trisomy 18. Ophthalmic Genet 15:115–120

Hook EB (1981) Unbalanced Robertsonian translocations associated with Down's syndrome or Patau's syndrome: Chromosome subtype, proportion inherited, mutation rates, and sex ratio. Hum Genet 59:235–239

Hook EB (1982) Epidemiology of Down syndrome. In Pueschel SM, Rynders JE (eds): Down Syndrome. Advances in Biomedical and Behavioural Sciences. Ware Press, Cambridge, MA, p. 11

Hook EB (1992) Chromosome abnormalities: Prevalence, risks and recurrence. In Brock DH, Rodeck CH, Ferguson-Smith MA (eds): Prenatal Diagnosis and Screening. Churchill Livingstone, Edinburgh, p. 351

Hook EB (2000) Maternal age-specific rates of Down syndrome used in serum screening are biased low [letter]. Prenat Diagn 20:169

Hook EB, Carothers AD (1997) Use of computer simulation to evaluate a putative cluster of genetic or teratologic outcomes: Adjustment for "multiple hypotheses" and application to a reported excess of Down's syndrome. Genet Epidemiol 14:133–145

Hook EB, Cross PK (1989) Maternal age-specific rates of chromosome abnormalities at chorionic villus study: A revision. Am J Med Genet 45:474–477

Hook EB, Yunis JJ (1965) Trisomy 18 syndrome in a patient with a normal karyotype. JAMA 193:840–843

Hook EB, Cross PK, Regal RR (1984) The frequency of 47, +21, 47, +18, and 47+13 at the uppermost extremes of maternal ages: Results on 56,094 fetuses studied prenatally and comparisons with data on livebirths. Hum Genet 68:211–220

Hook EB, Cross PK, Jackson L et al. (1988) Maternal age specific rates of 47, +21 and other cytogenetic abnormalities diagnosed in the first trimester pf pregnancy in chorionic villus biopsy specimens: Comparison to rates expected from observations at amniocentesis. Am J Hum Genet 42:797–807

Hook EB, Cross PK, Mutton DE (1999) Female predominance (low sex ratio) in 47, +21 mosaics Am J Med Genet 84:316–319

Hsiang YH, "Berkovitz GD, Bland GL et al. (1987) Gonadal function in patients with Down syndrome. Am J Med Genet 27:449–458

Hsu LYF, Perlis TE (1984) US survey on chromosome mosaicism. Prenat Diagn Spec issue 4:97–130

Hsu LYF, Kaffe S, Perlis TE (1991) A revisit of trisomy 20 mosaicism in prenatal diagnosis—an overview of 103 cases. Prenat Diagn 11:7–15

Hsu LYF, Kaffe S, Jenkins E et al. (1992) Proposed guidelines for diagnosis of chromosome mosaicism in amniocytes based on data derived from chromosome mosaicism and pseudomosaicism studies. Prenat Diagn 12:555–573

Hsu LY, Yu, MT, Neu RL et al. (1997) Rare trisomy mosaicism diagnosed in amniocytes, involving an autosome other than chromosomes 13, 18, 20, and 21: karyotype/phenotype correlations. Prenat Diagn 17:201–242

Huang T, Watt H, Wald N et al. (1998) Birth prevalence of Down's syndrome in England and Wales 1990 to 1997 [letter]. J Med Screen 5:213–214

Huether CA, Martin RL, Stoppelman SM et al. (1996) Sex ratios in fetuses and liveborn infants with autosomal aneuploidy. Am J Med Genet 63:492–500

Iannello RC, Crack PJ, de Haan JB, Kola I (1999) Oxidative stress and neural dysfunction in Down syndrome. J Neural Transm Suppl 57:257–67

Iino Y, Imamura Y, Harigai S, Tanaka Y (1999) Efficacy of tympanostomy tube insertion for otitis media with effusion in children with Down syndrome. Int J Pediatr Otorhinolaryngol 49:43–149

Ikeda S, Sera Y, Yoshida M et al. (1999) Extrahepatic biliary atresia associated with trisomy 18. Pediatr Surg Int 15:137–138

Isaksen CV, Ytterhus B, Skarsvag S (2000) Detection of trisomy 18 on formalin-fixed and paraffin-embedded material by fluorescence in situ hybridization. Pediatr Dev Pathol 3:249–255.

Jackson JF, North ER, Thomas JG (1976) Clinical diagnosis of Down's syndrome. Clin Genet 9:483–487

Jacobs PA, Hassold TJ, Henry A et al. (1987) Trisomy 13 ascertained in a survey of spontaneous abortions. J Med Genet 24:721–724

James RS, Ellis K, Pettay D, Jacobs PA (1988) Cytogenetic and molecular study of four couples with multiple trisomy 21 pregnancies. Eur J Hum Genet 6:207–212

Jauniaux E, Halder A, Partington C (1998) A case of partial mole associated with trisomy 13. Ultrasound Obstet Gynecol 11:62–64

Jenkins EC, Schupf N, Genovese M et al. (1997) Increased low-level chromosome 21 mosaicism in older individuals with Down syndrome. Am J Med Genet 68:147–151

Johannsen P, Christensen JE, Goldstein H et al. (1996) Epilepsy in Down syndrome—prevalence in three age groups. Seizure 5:121–125

Jones RB (2000) Parental consent to cosmetic facial surgery in Down's syndrome. J Med Ethics 26:101–102

Jorgensen C, Bologna C, Sany J (1995) Vasculitis and psoriatic arthritis associated with Down's syndrome. Clin Exp Rheumatol 13:749–751

Källén B, Mastroiacovo P, Robert E (1996) Major congenital malformations in Down syndrome. Am J Med Genet 65:160–166

Kalousek DK (2000) Pathogenesis of chromosomal mosaicism and its effect on early human development. Am J Med Genet 91:39–45

Kalousek DK, Barrett I (1994) Genomic imprinting related to prenatal diagnosis. Prenat Diagn 14:1191–1201

Kalousek DK, Dill FJ (1983) Chromosome mosaicism confined to the placenta in human conceptions. Science 221:665–667

Kalousek DK, Vekemans M (1996) Confined placental mosaicism. J Med Genet 33: 529–533

Kalousek DK, Barrett IJ, McGillvray BC (1989) Placental mosaicism and intrauterine survival of trisomy 13 and 18. Am J Hum Genet 44:338–343

Kalousek DK, Langlois S, Barrett I et al. (1993) Uniparental disomy for chromosome 16 in humans. Am J Hum Genet 52:8–16

Kalwinsky DK, Raimondi SC, Bunin NJ et al. (1990) Clinical and biological characteristics of acute lymphocytic leukemia in children with Down syndrome. Am J Med Genet 7:267–271

Kamatani N, Yamaanaka H, Totokawa S et al. (1996) Down syndrome with coexistent gout: Report of six patients and possible reasons for scarcity of descriptions of this association. Ann Rheum Dis 55:649–650

Karadima G, Bugge M, Nicolaidis P et al. (1998) Origin of nondisjunction in trisomy 8 and trisomy 8 mosaicism. Eur J Hum Genet 6:432–438

Karayalcin G, Shanske A, Honigman R (1981) Wilms' tumor in a 13 year old girl with trisomy 18. Am J Dis Child 135:665–667

Karlsson B, Gustafsson J, Hedov G et al. (1998) Thyroid dysfunction in Down's syndrome: Relation to age and thyroid autoimmunity. Arch Dis Child 79:242–245

Keiser H, Montague J, Wold D et al. (1981) Hearing loss of Down syndrome adults. Am J Ment Defic 86:467–472

Kelnar CJH (1989) Thyroid disturbances in cytogenetic disease. Dev Med Child Neurol 31:400–404

Kennedy RL, Jones TH, Cuckle HS (1992) Down's syndrome and the thyroid Clin Endocrinol (Oxf) 37:471–476

Kent L, Evans J, Paul M, Sharp M (1999) Comorbidity of autistic spectrum disorders in children with Down syndrome. Dev Med Child Neurol 41:153–158

Kernan KT (1990) Comprehension of syntactically indicated sequence by Down's syndrome and other mentally retarded adults. J Ment Defic Res 34:168–178

Khoury MJ, Cordero JF, Rasmussen S (1988) Ectopia cordis, midline defects and chromosome abnormalities: an epidemiological perspective. Am J Med Genet 30:811–817

Kilpatrick LM, Kola I, Salamonsen LA (1999) Transcription factors Ets1, Ets2, and Elf1 exhibit differential localization in human endometrium across the menstrual cycle and alternate isoforms in cultured endometrial cells Biol Reprod 61:120–126

Kinoshita M, Nakamura Y, Nakano R et al. (1989) Thirty-one autopsy cases of trisomy 18: Clinical features and pathological findings. Pediatr Pathol 9:445–457

Kjaer I, Keeling JW, Fischer HB (1997) Pattern of malformations in the axial skeleton in human trisomy 13 fetuses. Am J Med Genet 70:421–426

Klein J, Graham JM, Platt LD et al. (1994) Trisomy 8 mosaicism in chorionic villus sampling: Case report and counselling issues. Prenat Diagn 14:451–454

Kline J, Kinney A, Levin B, Warburton D (2000) Trisomic pregnancy and earlier age at menopause. Am J Hum Genet 67:395–404

Kohn G, Shohat M (1987) Trisomy 18 mosaicism in an adult with normal intelligence Am J Med Genet 26:298–299

Kohn G, Taysi K, Atkins TE et al. (1970) Mosaic mongolism I Clinical studies. J Pediatr 76:874–879

Kola I, Hertzog PJ (1997) Animal models in the study of the biological function of genes on human chromosome 21 and their role in the pathophysiology of Down syndrome. Hum Mol Genet 6:1713–1727

Kola I, Hertzog PJ (1998) Down syndrome and mouse models. Curr Opin Genet Dev 8:316–321

Kola I, Hertzog PJ (1999) The "gene dosage effect" hypothesis versus the "amplified developmental instability" hypothesis in Down syndrome. J Neural Transm Suppl 57:293–303

Kondoh T, Tonoki H, Matsumoto T et al. (1988) Origin of the extra chromosome in trisomy 18. Hum Genet 79:377–378

Koole FD, Velzeboer CM, van der Harten JJ (1986) Ocular abnormalities in Patau syndrome (chromosome 13 trisomy syndrome). Ophthalm Pediatr Genet 11:15–21

Korenberg JR, Chen X-N, Schipper R et al. (1994) Down syndrome phenotypes: The consequences of chromosomal imbalance. Proc Natl Acad Sci USA 91:4997–5001

Kornafel KL, Sauer MV (1994) Increased rates of aneuploidy in older women. Increased rates of aneuploidy do not occur in gestations of older embryo recipients. Hum Reprod 9:1981–1982

Kotzot D (1999) Abnormal phenotypes in uniparental disomy (UPD): fundamental aspects and a critical review with bibliography of UPD other than 15 Am J Med Genet 82:265–274

Kratzer WM, Golbus MS, Schonberg SA et al. (1992) Cytogenetic evidence for enhanced selective miscarriage of trisomy 21 pregnancies with advancing maternal age. Am J Med Genet 44:657–663

Kupke KG, Müller U (1989) Parental origin of the extra chromosome in trisomy 18. Am J Hum Genet 45:599–605

Kurnit DM, Layton WM, Matthysse S (1987) Genetics, chance and morphogenesis. Am J Hum Genet 41:979–995

Lai F, Williams RS (1989) A prospective study of Alzheimer disease in Down syndrome. Arch Neurol 46:849–853

Lai F, Kammann E, Rebeck GW et al. (1999) APOE genotype and gender effects on Alzheimer disease in 100 adults with Down syndrome. Neurology 53:331–336

Lam YH, Tang MH (1999) Sonographic features of fetal trisomy 18 at 13 and 14 weeks: four case reports. Ultrasound Obstet Gynecol 13:366–369

Larocca LM, Lauriola L, Ranelletti FO et al. (1990) Morphological and immunohistochemical study of Down syndrome thymus. Am J Med Genet, suppl 7:225–230

Lau AW, Brown CJ, Penaherrera M et al. (1997) Skewed X-chromosome inactivation is common in fetuses or newborns associated with confined placental mosaicism. Am J Hum Genet 61:1353–1361

Lawson Wilkins Pediatric Endocrine Society (1993) Growth hormone for children with Down syndrome. J Pediatr 123:742–743

Ledbetter DH, Zachary JM, Simpson JL et al. (1992) Cytogenetic results from the US collaborative study of CVS. Prenat Diagn 12:313–347

Lehman CD, Nyberg DA, Winter TC et al. (1995) Trisomy 13 syndrome: prenatal US findings in a review of 33 cases. Radiology 194:217–222

Lejeune J, Gauthier M, Turpin R (1959) Les chromosomes humains en culture des tissus. C R Acad Sci 248:602–603

LeMay M, Alvarez R (1990) The relationship between enlargement of the temporal horns of the lateral ventricles and dementia in ageing patients with Down syndrome. Neuroradiology 32:104–107

Leno C, Mateo I, Cid C et al. (1998) Autoimmunity in Down's syndrome: Another possible mechanism of Moyamoya disease. [letter] Stroke 29: 868–869

Leonard H, Eastham K, Dark J (2000) Heart and heart-lung transplantation in Down's syndrome. The lack of supportive evidence means each case must be carefully assessed [editorial] BMJ 320:816–817

Leonard S, Bower C, Petterson B, Leonard H (2000) Survival of infants born with Down's syndrome: 1980–96 Paediatr Perinat Epidemiol 14:163–171

Levine OR, Simpser M (1982) Alveolar hypoventilation and cor pulmonale associated with chronic airway obstruction in infants with Down syndrome. Clin Pediatr 21:25–29

Lewis AJ (1964) The pathology of 18 trisomy. J Pediatr 65:92–101

Licastro F, Melotti C, Parente R et al. (1990) Derangement of non-specific immunity 1 Down syndrome subjects: Low leukocyte chemiluminescence activity after phagocytic activation. Am J Med Genet suppl 7:242–246

Licastro F, Chiricolo M, Mocchegiani E et al. (1994) Oral zinc supplementation in Down syndrome subjects decreased infections and normalised some humoral and cellular immune parameters. J Intellect Disabil Res 38:149–162

Lim AS, Su LC (1998) Mosaic trisomy 18 male with normal intelligence who fathered a normal baby girl. [letter] Am J Med Genet 76:365–366

Locke GR, Gardner JI, Van Epps EF (1966) Atlas-dens interval (ADI) in children. A survey based on 200 normal cervical spines. AJR 97:135–140

Locktich G, Singh V, Puterman LM et al. (1987) Age-related changes in humoral and cell-mediated immunity in Down syndrome children living at home. Pediatr Res 22:536–540

Loudon MM, Day RE, Duke EM (1985) Thyroid disease in Down's syndrome. Arch Dis Child 60:1149–1151

Loughlin GN, Wyne JW, Victorica BE (1981) Sleep apnea as a possible cause of pulmonary hypertension in Down syndrome. J Pediatr 98:435–437

Loughna S, Bennett P, Moore G (1995) Molecular analysis of the expression of transthyretin in intestine and liver from trisomy 18 fetuses. Hum Genet 95:89–95

Luke A, Roizen NJ, Sutton M, Schoeller DA (1994) Energy expenditure in children with Down syndrome: correcting metabolic rate of movement. J Pediatr 125:829–838

Lund J (1988) Psychiatric aspects of Down syndrome. Acta Psychiatr Scand 78:369–374

McGrother CW, Marshall B (1990) Recent trends in incidence morbidity and survival in Down's syndrome. J Ment Defic Res 34:49–57

Maclachlan N, Iskaros J, Chitty L (2000) Ultrasound markers of fetal chromosomal abnormality: A survey of policies and practices in UK maternity ultrasound departments. Ultrasound Obstet Gynecol 15:387–90

McLaughlin F, Ludbrook VJ, Kola I et al. (1999) Characterisation of the tumour necrosis factor (TNF)–(alpha) response elements in the human ICAM-2 promoter. J Cell Sci 112:4695–4703

Madden DL, Matthew EB, Dietzman DE et al. (1976) Hepatitis and Down's syndrome. Am J Ment Defic 80:401–406

Magenis ER, Hecht F, Milham S (1968) Trisomy-13 (D) syndrome: Studies on parental age, sex ratio and survival. J Pediatr 73:222–228

Makrydimas G, Plachouras N, Thilaganathan B, Nicolaides KH (1994) Abnormal immunological development in fetuses with trisomy 18. Prenat Diagn 14:239–241

Mandel EM, Rockette HE, Bluestone CD et al. (1987) Efficacy of amoxycillin with and without decongestant—antihistamine for otitis media with effusion in children. N Engl J Med 316:432–437

Mankinen CB, Sears JW (1976) Trisomy 13 in a female over 5 years of age. J Med Genet 13:157–161

Marin Padilla M (1974) Structural organization of the cerebral cortex (motor area) in human chromosomal aberrations: A Golgi study of D (13–15) trisomy, Patau syndrome. Brain Res 66:375–391

Marion RW, Chitayat D, Hutcheon RG (1988) Trisomy 18 score: A reliable diagnostic test for trisomy 18. J Pediatr 113:45–48

Marrack P, Kappler J (1987) The T cell receptor. Science 238:1073–1079

Marteau T, Drake H, Bobrow M (1994) Counselling following diagnosis of a fetal abnormality: The differing approaches of obstetricians, clinical geneticists, and genetic nurses. J Med Genet 31:864–867

Martin RH (1988) Cytogenetic analysis of sperm from a male heterozygous for a 13; 14 Robertsonian translocation. Hum Genet 80:357–361

Martin RH, Rademaker AW, Hildebrand K (1987) Variation in the frequency and type of sperm chromosomal abnormalities among normal men. Hum Genet 77:108–114

Martinez-Frias ML (1989) Association of holoprosencephaly and Down syndrome. Am J Med Genet 32:435

Matsuoka R, Matsuyama S, Yamamoto Y et al. (1981) Trisomy 18q: A case report and review of karyotype phenotype correlations. Hum Genet 57:78–82

Matsuoka R, Misugi K, Goto A et al. (1983) Congenital heart anomalies in the trisomy 18 syndrome with reference to congenital polyvalvular disease. Am J Med Genet 14:657–668

May P, Kawanishi H (1996) Chronic hepatitis B infection and autoimmune thyroiditis in Down syndrome. J Clin Gastroenterol 23:181–184

Mazzoni DS, Ackley RS, Nash DJ (1994) Abnormal pinna type and hearing loss correlations in Down's syndrome. J Intellect Disabil Res 38:549–560

Mehta L, Shannon RS, Duckett DP, Young ID (1986) Trisomy 18 in a 13 year old girl. J Med Genet 23:256–278

Merkatz IR, Nitowsky HM, Macri JN et al. (1984) An association between low maternal serum alphafetoprotein and fetal chromosomal abnormalities. Am J Obstet Gynecol 148:886

Mewar R, Kline AD, Harrison W et al. (1993) Clinical and molecular evaluation of four patients with partial duplications of the long arm of chromosome 18. Am J Hum Genet 53:1629–1278

Micale MA, Wolff DJ, Dickerman LH et al. (1996) Cytogenetic and molecular genetic characterization of trisomy 20 mosaicism in fetal blood and tissues. Prenat Diagn 16:893–897

Mikkelsen M, Poulsen H, Grinsted J, Lange A (1980) Non-disjunction in trisomy 21: Study of chromosomal heteromorphisms in 110 families. Ann Hum Genet 44:17–28

Mikkelsen M, Poulsen H, Nielsen KG (1990) Incidence, survival and mortality in Down syndrome in Denmark. Am J Med Genet suppl 7:75–78

Milunsky A (1970) Glucose intolerance in the parents of children with Down's syndrome. Am J Ment Defic 74:475–478

Mittelman F, Heim S, Mandahl N (1990) Trisomy 21 in neoplastic cells. Am J Med Genet, suppl 7:262–266

Miyauchi J, Ito Y, Kawano T et al. (1992) Unusual diffuse liver disease accompanying transient myeloproliferative disorder in Down's syndrome: a report of four autopsy cases and proposal of a hypothesis. Blood 80:1521–1527

Moerman P, Fryns J-P, Goddeeris P et al. (1982) Spectrum of clinical and autopsy findings in trisomy 18 syndrome. J Genet Hum 30:17–38

Moerman P, Fryns JP, van der Steen K et al. (1988) The pathology of trisomy 13 syndrome. Hum Genet 80:349–356

Moreira LMdeA, San Juan A, Pereira PS, de Souza CS (2000) A case of mosaic trisomy 21 with Down's syndrome signs and normal intellectual development. J Intellect Disabil Res 44:91–96

Mori MA, Huertras H, Pinel I et al. (1985) Trisomy 13 in the child of two carriers of a 13/15 translocation. Am J Med Genet 20:17–20

Morris J, Wald N (2000) Down syndrome fetal loss rate in early pregnancy. Prenat Diagn 20:685–686

Morris JK, Alberman E, Mutton D (1998) Is there evidence of clustering in Down syndrome? Int J Epidemiol 27:495–498

Morris JK, Wald NJ, Watt HC (1999a) Fetal loss in Down syndrome pregnancy. Prenat Diagn 19:142–145

Morris MA, Yiannakou JY, King AL et al. (1999b) Coeliac disease and Down syndrome: Associations not due to genetic linkage on chromosome 21. Scand J Gastroenterol 35:177–180

Morton RE, Ali Khan M, Murray-Leslie C et al. (1995) Atlantoaxial instability in Down's syndrome: A five year follow-up study. Arch Dis Child 72:115–118

Muecke J, Trautmann U, Sandig K-R et al. (1982) The crucial band for phenotype of trisomy 18. Hum Genet 60:205

Muller F, Rebiffe M, Taillandier A et al. (2000) Parental origin of the extra chromosome in prenatally diagnosed fetal trisomy 21. Hum Genet 106:340–344

Munne S, Sultan KM, Weier HU et al. (1995) Assessment of numeric abnormalities of X, Y, 18, and 16 chromosomes in preimplantation human embryos before transfer. Am J Obstet Gynecol 172:1191–1199

Murdoch JC, Ratcliffe WA, McLarty DG et al. (1977) Thyroid function in adults with Down syndrome. J Clin Endocrinol Metab 44:53–458

Murphy M, Lempert M, Epstein L (1990) Decreased level of T cell receptor expression by Down syndrome (trisomy 21) thymocytes. Am J Med Genet suppl 7:234–237

Musewe NN, Alexander DJ, Teshima I et al. (1990) Echocardiographic evaluation of the spectrum of cardiac anomalies associated with trisomy 13 and trisomy 18. J Am Coll Cardiol 15:673–677

Musiani P, Valitutti S, Castellino F et al. (1990) Intrathymic deficient expansion of T cell precursors in Down syndrome. Am J Med Genet suppl 7:219–224

Mutton D, Alberman E, Hook EB (1996) Cytogenetic and epidemiological findings in Down syndrome, England and Wales 1989 to 1993. National Down Syndrome Cytogenetic Register and the Association of Clinical Cytogeneticists. J Med Genet 33:387–394

Nadal M, Vigo CG, Melaragno MI et al. (2001) Clinical and cytogenetic characterisation of a patient with down syndrome resulting from a 22q22→22qter duplication. J Med Genet 38:73–76

Nadel AS, Bromley B, Frigoletto FD Jr, Eenacerraf BR (1995) Can the presumed risk of autosomal trisomy be decreased in fetuses of older women following a normal sonogram? J Ultrasound Med 14:297–302

Nakamura E, Tanaka S (1998) Biological ages of adult men and women with Down's syndrome and its changes with aging. Mech Ageing Dev 105:89–103

Narchi H, Kulaylat N (1997) High incidence of Down's syndrome in infants of diabetic mothers. Arch Dis Child 77:242–244

Nelson PG, Fitzgerald S, Rapoport SI et al. (1997) Cerebral cortical astroglia from the trisomy 16 mouse, a model for Down syndrome, produce neuronal cholinergic deficits in cell culture. Proc Natl Acad Sci USA 94:12644–12648

Nicolaides KH, Azar G, Byrne D (1992a) Fetal nuchal translucency: Ultrasound screening for chromosome defects in the first trimester of pregnancy. BMJ 304:704–707

Nicolaides KH, Snijders RJM, Gosden CM et al. (1992b) Ultrasonographically detectable markers of fetal chromosomal abnormalities. Lancet 340:704–707

Nielsen J, Wohlert M (1991) Chromosome abnormalities found among 34, 910 newborn children; results from a 13-year incidence study in Aarhus, Denmark. Hum Genet 87:81–83

Niikawa N, Deng H-X, Abe K et al. (1991) Possible mapping of the gene for transient myeloproliferative syndrome at 21q11.2. Hum Genet 87:561–566

Noble J (1998) Natural history of Down's syndrome: A brief review for those involved in antenatal screening. J Med Screen 5:172–177

Noble SE, Leyland K, Findlay CA et al. (2000) School based screening for hypothyroidism in Down's syndrome by dried blood spot TSH measurement. Arch Dis Child 82:27–31

Nuri Sener R (1996) Bilateral, perisylvian and rolandic cortical dysplasia in trisomy 13 syndrome. J Neuroradiol 23:231–233

Odetti P, Angelini G, Dapino D et al. (1998) Early glycoxidation damage in brains from Down's syndrome. Biochem Biophys Res Commun 243:849–851

Ohara S, Tsukada M, Ikeda S (1999) On the occurrence of neuronal sprouting in the frontal cortex of a patient with Down's syndrome. Acta Neuropathol (Berl) 97:85–90

Oliver C, Crayton L, Holland A et al. (1998) A four year prospective study of age-related cognitive change in adults with Down's syndrome. Psychol Med 28:1365–1377

Olson JC, Bender JC, Levinson JE et al. (1990) Arthropathy of Down syndrome. Pediatrics 86:931–936

Oostra RJ, Baljet B, Dijkstra PF, Hennekam RC (1998) Congenital anomalies in the teratological collection of Museum Vrolik in Amsterdam, The Netherlands I: Syndromes with multiple congenital anomalies. Am J Med Genet 77:100–115

Ozturk M, Milunsky A, Brambati B et al. (1990) Abnormal maternal serum levels of human chorionic gonadotrophin free subunits in trisomy 18. Am J Med Genet 36:480–483

Pangalos C, Avramopoulos D, Blouin J-L et al. (1994) Understanding the mechanism(s) of mosaic trisomy 21 by using DNA polymorphism analysis. Am J Hum Genet 54:473–481

Park E, Alberti J, Mehta P et al. (2000) Partial impairment of immune functions in peripheral blood leukocytes from aged men with Down's syndrome. Clin Immunol 95:62–69

Patau K, Smith DW, Therman E et al. (1960) Multiple congenital anomaly caused by an extra autosome. Lancet 1:790–793

Pearlson GD, Breiter SN, Aylward EH et al. (1998) MRI brain changes in subjects with Down syndrome with and without dementia. Dev Med Child Neurol 40:326–334

Pe'er J, Braun JT (1986) Ocular pathology in trisomy 18 (Edwards syndrome). Ophthalmologica 192:176–178

Pellestor F (1990) Analysis of meiotic segregation in a man heterozygons for a 13; 15 Robertsonian translocation and review of the literature. Hum Genet 85:49–54

Pellestor F (1991) Differential distribution of aneuploidy in human gametes according to their sex. Hum Reprod 6:1252–1258

Pellestor F, Dufour M-C, Arnal F, Humeau C (1994) Direct assessment of the rate of chromosomal abnormalities in grade IV human embryos produced by in-vitro fertilization procedure. Hum Reprod 9:292–302

Pentao L, Lewis RA, Ledbetter DH et al. (1992) Maternal uniparental isodisomy of chromosome 14: An association with autosomal recessive rod monochromacy. Am J Hum Genet 50:690–699

Peñaherrera MS, Barrett IJ, Brown CJ et al. (2001) An association between skewed X chromosome inactivation and abnormal outcome in mosaic trisomy 16 confined predominantly to the placenta. Clin Genet 58:436–446

Peran S, Gil JL, Ruiz F, Fernandez-Pastor V (1997) Development of physical response after athletics training in adolescents with Down's syndrome. Scand Med Sci Sports 7:283–288

Percy ME, Markovic VD, Dalton AJ et al. (1993) Age-associated chromosome 21 loss in Down syndrome: Possible relevance to moasaicism and Alzheimer disease. Am J Med Genet 45:584–588

Petersen MB, Adelsburger PA, Schinzel AA et al. (1991) Down syndrome due to de novo Robertsonian translocation t(14;21): DNA polymorphism analysis suggests that the origin of the extra 21 is maternal. Am J Hum Genet 49:529–536

Petersen MB, Karadima G, Samaritaki M et al. (2000) Association between presenilin-1 polymorphism and maternal meiosis II errors in down syndrome. Am J Med Genet 93:366–372

Petronis A (1999) Alzheimer's disease and Down syndrome: From meiosis to dementia? Exp Neurol 158:403–413

Pfeifer K (2000) Mechanisms of genomic imprinting. Am J Hum Genet 67:777–787

Philip R, Berger AC, McManus NH et al. (1986) Abnormalities of the in vitro cellular and humoural response to tetanus and influenza antigens with concomitant numerical alterations in lymphocyte subsets in Down syndrome. J Immunol 136:1661–1667

Phillips OP, Tharapel AT, Lerner JL et al. (1996) Risk of fetal mosaicism when placental mosaicism is diagnosed by chorionic villus sampling. Am J Obstet Gynecol 174:850–855

Piro E, Pennino C, Cammarata M et al. (1990) Growth charts of Down syndrome in Sicily Evaluation of 382 children 0–14 years of age. Am J Med Genet, suppl 7:66–70

Plachot M, de Grouchy J, Junca AM et al. (1988) Chromosome analysis of human oocytes and embryos: Does delayed fertilization increase chromosome imbalance? Hum Reprod 3:627–635

Plessis G, Le Treust M, Lemaire F et al. (1997) Trisomy 18 mosaicism in a mildly retarded boy with postnatal overgrowth. Ann Genet 40:235–237

Pletcher BA, Sanz MM, Schlessel JS et al. (1994) Postnatal confirmation of prenatally diagnosed trisomy 16 mosaicism in two phenotypically abnormal liveborns. Prenat Diagn 14:933–940

Plymate SR, Brenner J, Paulsen CA (1976) The association of D-group chromosomal translocations and defective spermatogenesis. Fertil Steril 27:139–144

Polani PE, Briggs JH, Ford CE et al. (1960) A mongol girl with 46 chromosomes Lancet 1:721

Pritchard MA, Kola I (1999) The "gene dosage effect" hypothesis versus the "amplified developmental instability" hypothesis in Down syndrome J Neural Transm Suppl 57:293–303

Pueschel SM (1990) Clinical aspects of Down syndrome from infancy to adulthood. Am J Med Genet, suppl 7:52–56

Pueschel SM (1998) Should children with Down syndrome be screened for atlantoaxial instability? Arch Pediatr Adolesc Med 152:123–125

Pueschel SM, Pezzullo JC (1985) Thyroid dysfunction in Down syndrome. Am J Dis Child 139:636–639

Pueschel SM, Louis S, McKnight P (1991a) Seizure disorders in Down syndrome. Arch Neurol 48:318–320

Pueschel SM, Bernier JC, Pezzullo JC (1991b) Behavioural observations in children with Down's syndrome. J Ment Defic Res 35:502–511

Pueschel SM, Craig WY, Haddow JE (1992) Lipids and lipoproteins in persons with Down syndrome. J Intellect Disabil Res 36:365–369

Pueschel SM, Romano C, Failla P et al. (1999) A prevalence study of celiac disease in persons with Down syndrome residing in the United States of America. Acta Paediatr 88:953–956

Quagliarini D, Betti S, Brambati B, Nicolini U (1998) Coping with serum screening for Down syndrome when the result is given as a numeric value. Prenat Diagn 18:816–821

Quinn FM, Surana R, Puri P (1994) The influence of trisomy 21 on outcome in children with Hirschsprung's disease. J Pediatr Surg 29:781–783

Qureshi F, Jacques SM, Feldman B et al. (2000) Fetal obstructive uropathy in trisomy syndromes. Fetal Diagn Ther 15:342–347

Ragab AH, Abel-Mageed A, Shuster JJ et al. (1991) Clinical characteristics and treatment outcome of children with acute lymphatic leukemia and Down syndrome. Cancer 67:1057–1063

Ramesh KH, Verma RS (1996) Parental origin of the extra chromosome 18 in Edwards syndrome. Ann Genet 39:110–112

Ravindranath Y, Abella E, Krischer JP et al. (1992) Acute myeloid leukemia (AML) in Down's syndrome is highly responsive to chemotherapy: Experience on pediatric oncology group AML study 8498. Blood 80:2210–2214

Reddy KS (1997) Double trisomy in spontaneous abortions. Hum Genet 101:339–345

Redheendran R, Neu RL, Bannerman RM (1981) Long survival in trisomy-13-syndrome: 21 cases including prolonged survival in two patients 11 and 19 years old. Am J Med Genet 8:167–172

Reeves RH (2000) Recounting a genetic story. Nature 405:283–284

Reeves RH, Irving NG, Moran TH et al. (1995) A mouse model for Down syndrome exhibits learning and behaviour deficits. Nat Genet 11:177–184

Rehder H (1981) Pathology of trisomy 21—with particular reference to persistent common atrioventricular canal of the heart. In Burgio GR, Fraccaro M, Tiepolo L, Wolf U (eds): Trisomy 21. Springer-Verlag, Berlin, p 57

Reller MD, Morris CD (1998) Is Down syndrome a risk factor for poor outcome after repair of congenital heart defects? J Pediatr 132:738–741

Renner F, Andrie M, Horak W et al. (1985) Hepatitis A and B in non-institutionalised mentally retarded patients. Hepatogastroenterology 32:175–177

Rex AP, Preus M (1982) A diagnostic index for Down syndrome. J Pediatr 100:903–906

Richards BW (1974) Investigation of 142 mosaic mongols and mosaic parents of mongols: Cytogenetic analysis and maternal age at birth. J Ment Defic Res 18:199–208

Ries MD, Ray S, Winter RB, Bowen JR (1990) Scoliosis in trisomy 18. Spine 15:1281–1284

Risch N, Stein Z, Kline J et al. (1986) The relationship between maternal age and chromosome size in autosomal trisomy. Am J Hum Genet 39:68–78

Roberts DF, Roberts MJ, Johnston AW (1991) Genetic epidemiology of Down's syndrome in Shetland. Hum Genet 87:57–60

Robinson LL, Nesbit ME, Sather HN et al. (1984) Down's syndrome and acute leukemia in children: A 10-year retrospective study from the Childrens' Cancer Study Group. J Pediatr 105:235–242

Robinson MG, McQuorquodale MM (1981) Trisomy 18 and neurogenic neoplasia. J Pediatr 99:428–429

Robinson WP, Bernasconi F, Basaran S et al. (1994) A somatic origin of homologous Robertsonian translocations and isochromosomes. Am J Hum Genet 54:290–302

Robinson WP, Bernasconi F, Dutly G et al. (1996) Molecular studies of translocations and trisomy involving chromosome 13 Am J Med Genet 61:158–163

Robinson WP, Barrett IJ, Bernard L et al. (1997) Meiotic origin of trisomy in confined placental mosaicism is correlated with presence of fetal uniparental disomy, high levels of trisomy in trophoblast, and increased risk of fetal intrauterine growth restriction. Am J Hum Genet 60:917–927

Robinson WP, Christian SL, Kuchinka BD et al. (2000) Somatic segregation errors predominantly contribute to the gain or loss of a paternal chromosome leading to uniparental disomy for chromosome 15. Clin Genet 57:349–358

Rodewald A, Zankl H, Wischerath H, Borkowsky-Fehr B (1977) Dermatoglyphic patterns in trisomy 8 syndrome. Clin Genet 12:28–38

Rogers PT, Coleman M (1992) Medical Care in Down Syndrome. Marcel Dekker, New York

Rogers TR, Hagstrom JWC, Engle MA (1965) Origin of both great vessels from the right ventricle associated with the trisomy 18 syndrome. Circulation 32:802–807

Roizen NJ, Amarose AP (1993) Hematologic abnormalities in children with Down syndrome. Am J Med Genet 46:510–512

Roizen NJ, Wolters C, Nicol T et al. (1993) Hearing loss in children with Down syndrome. J Pediatr (suppl) 123:S9–S12

Roizen NJ, Mets BM, Blondis TA (1994) Ophthalmic disorders in children with Down syndrome. Dev Med Child Neurol 36:594–600

Roland B, Lynch L, Berkowitz G, Zinberg R (1994) Confined placental mosaicism in CVS and pregnancy outcome. Prenat Diagn 14:589–593

Romano C, Tine A, Fazio G et al. (1990) Seizures in patients with trisomy 21 Am J Med Genet (suppl) 7:298–300

Root S, Carey JC (1994) Survival in trisomy 18. Am J Med Genet 49:170–174

Rubin SS, Rimmer JH, Chicoine B et al. (1998) Overweight prevalence in persons with Down syndrome. Ment Retard 36:175–181

Rubinsztein DC, Hon J, Stevens F et al. (1999) Apo E genotypes and risk of dementia in Down syndrome. Am J Med Genet 88:344–347

Sachs EJS, Jahoda MGJ, Pijpers L et al. (1990) Trisomy 21 mosaicisms in gonads with unexpectedly high recurrence risks. Am J Med Genet suppl 7:186–188

Sadowski M, Wisniewski HM, Tarnawski M (1999) Entorhinal cortex of aged subjects with Down's syndrome shows severe neuronal loss caused by neurofibrillary pathology. Acta Neuropathol (Berl) 97:156–164

Sago H, Carlson EJ, Smith DJ et al. (2000) Genetic dissection of region associated with behavioral abnormalities in mouse models for Down syndrome. Pediatr Res 48:606–613

St George Hyslop PH, Tanzi R, Polinsky RJ et al. (1987) The genetic defect causing familial Alzheimer's disease maps on chromosome 21. Science 235:885–890

Saller DNJ, Oyer CE, Star J, Canick JA (1996) A normative study of obstetric complications associated with fetal trisomy 18. J Perinatol 16:117–120

Sarigol SS, Rogers DG (1994) Trisomy 18 mosaicism in a thirteen-year-old girl with normal intelligence, delayed pubertal development, and growth failure. Am J Med Genet 50:94–95

Satge D, Geneix A, Goburdhun J et al. (1996) A history of miscarriages and mild prognathism as possible mode of presentation of mosaic trisomy 18 in women. Clin Genet 50:470–473

Saviola-Negrin N, Cristante F (1992) Teacher's attitudes towards plastic surgery in children with Down's syndrome. J Intellect Disabil Res 36:143–155

Sayee R, Thomas IM (1998) Consanguinity, non-disjunction, parental age and Down's syndrome. J Indian Med Assoc 96:335–337

Schinzel A (1984) Catalogue of Unbalanced Chromosome Aberrations in Man. Walter de Gruyter, Berlin

Schinzel AA, Basaran S, Bernasconi F et al. (1994) Maternal uniparental disomy 22 has no impact on the phenotype. Am J Hum Genet 54:21–24

Schneider DS, Zahka KG, Clark EB, Neill CA (1989) Patterns of cardiac care in infants with Down syndrome. Am J Dis Child 143:363–365

Schneider VM, Klein-Vogler U, Tomiuk J et al. (1994) Pitfall: amniocentesis fails to detect mosaic trisomy 8 in a male newborn. Prenat Diagn 14:651–652

Scholl T, Stein Z, Hansen H (1982) Leukaemia and other cancers, anomalies and infections as causes of death in Down syndrome in the United States during 1976. Dev Med Child Neurol 24:817–829

Schon EA, Kim SH, Ferreira JC et al. (2000) Chromosomal non-disjunction in human oocytes: is there a mitochondrial connection? Hum Reprod Suppl 2:160–172

Schupf N, Kapell D, Lee JH et al. (1994) Increased risk of Alzheimer's disease in mothers of adults with Down's syndrome. Lancet 344:353–356

Schupf N, Kapell D, Nightingale B et al. (1998) Earlier onset of Alzheimer's disease in men with Down syndrome. Neurology 50: 991–995

Scinto LFM, Daffner KR, Dressler D et al. (1994) A potential noninvasive neurobiological test for Alzheimer's disease. Science 266:1051–1054

Scotese I, Gaetaniello L, Matarese G et al. (1998) T cell activation deficiency associated with an aberrant pattern of protein tyrosine phosphorylation after CD3 perturbation in Down's syndrome. Pediatr Res 44:252–258

Selby KA, Newton RW, Gupta S et al. (1991) Clinical predictors and radiological reliability in atlantoaxial subluxation in Down's syndrome. Arch Dis Child 66:876–878

Selikowitz M (1992) Health problems and health checks in school-aged children with Down syndrome. J Paed Child Health 28:383–386

Selikowitz M (1993a) Short-term efficacy of tympanostomy tubes for secretory otitis media in children with Down syndrome. Dev Med Child Neurol 35:511–515

Selikowitz M (1993b) A five year longitudinal study of thyroid function in children with Down syndrome. Dev Med Child Neurol 35:396–401

Shaffer LG, Jackson-Cook CK, Stasiowski BA et al. (1992) Parental origin determination in 30 de novo Robertsonian translocations. Am J Med Genet 43:957–963

Shaffer LG, McCaskill C, Haller V et al. (1993) Further characterisation of 19 cases of rea(21q21q) and delineation as isochromosomes or Robertsonian translocations in Down syndrome. Am J Med Genet 47:957–963

Shaffer LG, McCaskill C, Han J-Y et al. (1994) Molecular characterisation of de novo secondary trisomy 13. Am J Hum Genet 55:968–974

Shaffer LG, McCaskill C, Hersh JH et al. (1996) A clinical and molecular study of mosaicism for trisomy 17. Hum Genet 97:69–72

Shaffer LG, McCaskill C, Adkins K, Hassold TJ (1998) Systematic search for uniparental disomy in early fetal losses: the results and a review of the literature Am J Med Genet 79:366–372

Shapiro NL, Huang RY, Sangwan S et al. (2000) Tracheal stenosis and congenital heart disease in patients with Down syndrome: Diagnostic approach and surgical options. Int J Pediatr Otorhinolaryngol 54:137–142

Sharav T, Collins RM, Baab PJ (1988) Growth studies in infants and children with down syndrome and elevated levels of thyrotrophin. Am J Dis Child 142:1302–1306

Shashi V, Golden WL, von Kap-Herr C, Wilson WG (1996) Constellation of congenital abnormalities in an infant: A new syndrome or tissue-specific mosaicism for trisomy 18? Am J Med Genet 62:38–41

Shen JJ, Williams BJ, Zipursky A et al. (1995) Cytogenetic and molecular studies of Down syndrome individuals with leukemia. Am J Hum Genet 56:915–925

Sherman SL, Petersen MB, Freeman SB et al. (1994) Non-disjunction of chromosome 21 in maternal meiosis 1 Evidence for a maternal age-dependent mechanism involving reduced recombination. Hum Mol Genet 3:1529–1535

Sherod C, Sebire NJ, Soares W et al. (1997) Prenatal diagnosis of trisomy 18 at the 10–14-week ultrasound scan. Ultrasound Obstet Gynecol 10:387–390

Shi Q, Adler ID, Zhang J et al. (2000) Incidence of mosaic cell lines in vivo and malsegregation of chromosome 21 in lymphocytes in vitro of trisomy 21 patients: detection by fluorescence in situ hybridization on binucleated lymphocytes Hum Genet 106:29–35

Shield JP, Wadsworth EJ, Hassold TJ et al. (1999) Is disomic homozygosity at the APECED locus the cause of increased autoimmunity in Down's syndrome? Arch Dis Child 81:147–150

Shields LE, Carpenter LA, Smith KM, Nghiem HV (1998) Ultrasonographic diagnosis of trisomy 18: is it practical in the early second trimester? J Ultrasound Med 17:327–331

Shih L, Hsu LY, Sujansky E, Kushnick T (1974) Trisomy 18 mosaicism in two siblings. Clin Genet 5:420–427

Shim DT, Kim YK, Whang KU et al. (1993) Atypical dermatoglyphics in trisomy 18 (Edwards syndrome). Ann Dermatol 5:30–33

Shuttleworth GE (1909) Mongolian idiocy. BMJ 2:661

Silengo MC, Davi GF, Franceschini P (1979) Radiologic features in trisomy 8. Pediatr Radiol 8:116–118

Simoni G, Sirchia SM (1994) Confined placental mosaicism. Prenat Diagn 14:1185–1189

Singh KST (1990) Trisomy 13 (Patau's syndrome): A rare case of survival into adulthood. J Ment Defic Res 34:91–93

Silva ML, Cieuta C, Guerrini R et al. (1996) Early clinical and EEG features of infantile spasms in Down syndrome. Epilepsia 37:977–982

Slater HR, Ralph A, Daniel A et al. (2000) A case of maternal uniparental disomy of chromosome 9 diagnosed prenatally and the related problem of residual trisomy. Prenat Diagn 20:930–932

Smith A, Dulk GMD (1980) Follow up of case of advanced survival and trisomy 18. J Ment Defic Res 24:157–158

Smith A, Field B, Learoyd BM (1989) Trisomy 18 at 21 years. Am J Med Genet 34:338–339

Smith DJ, Rubin EM (1997) Functional screening and complex traits: human 21q222 sequences affecting learning in mice. Hum Mol Genet 6:1729–1733

Smith DW, Therman EM, Patau KA et al. (1962) Mosaicism in the mother of two mongoloids. Am J Dis Child 104:534

Smith GF, Berg JM (1976) Down's Anomaly. 2nd edn. Churchill Livingstone: Edinburgh

Smith K, Lowther G, Maher E et al. (1999) The predictive value of findings of the common aneuploidies, trisomies 13, 18 and 21, and numerical sex chromosome abnormalities at CVS: experience from the ACC UK Collaborative Study Association of Clinical Cytogeneticists Prenatal Diagnosis Working Party. Prenat Diagn 19:817–826

Snijders R (1999) Fetal loss in Down syndrome pregnancies. Prenat Diagn 19:1180

Snijders RJ, Holzgreve W, Cuckle H et al. (1994) Maternal age-specific risks for trisomies at 9–14 weeks' gestation. Prenat Diagn 14:543–552

Snijders RJ, Brizot ML, Faria M, Nicolaides KH (1995) Fetal exomphalos at 11 to 14 weeks of gestation J Ultrasound Med 14:569–574

Snijders RJ, Sebire NJ, Nayar R, Souka A, Nicolaides KH (1999) Increased nuchal translucency in trisomy 13 fetuses at 10–14 weeks of gestation. Am J Med Genet 86:205–207

Spahis JK, Wilson GN (1999) Down syndrome: Perinatal complications and counseling experiences in 216 patients. Am J Med Genet 89:96–99

Southall DP, Stebbens VA, Mirza R et al. (1987) Upper airway obstruction with hypoxaemia and sleep disturbance in Down syndrome. Dev Med Child Neurol 29:734–732

Sparkes RS, Sasaki H, Mohandas T et al. (1987) Assignment of the prealbumin (PALB) gene (familial amyloidotic polyneuropathy) to human chromosome region 18q11.2–q12.1. Hum Genet 75:151–154

Sperling K, Pelz O, Wegner R-D et al. (1994) A significant increase of trisomy 21 in Berlin nine months after the Chernobyl accident: temporal correlation or causal relation? BMJ 309:158–162

Stafstrom CE (1993) Epilepsy in Down syndrome: Clinical aspects and possible mechanisms. Am J Ment Retard suppl 98:12–26

Stafstrom CE, Konkol RJ (1994) Infantile spasms in children with Down syndrome. Dev Med Child Neurol 36:576–585

Stafstrom CE, Patxot OF, Gilmore HE, Wisniewski KE (1991) Seizures in children with Down syndrome: Etiology, characteristics and outcome. Dev Med Child Neurol 33:191–200

Stavropoulos DJ, Bick D, Kalousek DK (1998) Molecular genetic detection of confined gonadal mosaicism in a conceptus with trisomy 16 placental mosaicism. Am J Hum Genet 63:1912–1914

Steinberg C, Zackai EH, Eunpu DL (1984) Recurrence rate for de novo translocation Down syndrome: A study of 112 families. Am J Med Genet 17:523–530

Stempfle N, Huten Y, Fredouille C et al. (1999) Skeletal abnormalities in fetuses with Down's syndrome: A radiographic post-mortem study. Pediatr Radiol 29:682–688

Stene J, Stene E, Mikkelsen M (1984) Risk for chromosome abnormality at amniocentesis following a child with a non-inherited chromosome aberration. Prenat Diagn 4:81–95

Stephens TD, Shepherd TH (1980) The Down syndrome in the fetus. Teratology 22:37–41

Stephenson JBP (1990) Fits and Faints. Clinics in Developmental Medicine No. 109, MacKeith Press, London

Stephenson JBP, King MD (1989) Handbook of Neurological Investigations in Children. Wright, London

Stoll C, Alembik Y, Dott B (1998a) Impact of routine fetal ultrasonographic screening on the prevalence of Down syndrome in non aged mothers. Ann Genet 41:27–30

Stoll C, Alembik Y, Dott B et al. (1998b) Evaluation of prenatal diagnosis of congenital heart disease. Prenat Diagn 18:801–807

Stoll C, Alembik Y, Dott B, Roth MP (1998c) Study of Down syndrome in 238, 942 consecutive births. Ann Genet 41:44–51

Stolwijk AM, Jongbloet PH, Zielhuis GA, Gabreels FJ (1997) Seasonal variation in the prevalence of Down syndrome at birth: A review J Epidemiol Community Health 51:350–353

Strome M (1986) Obstructive sleep apnea in Down syndrome children: A surgical approach. Laryngoscope 96:1340–1342

Sulewski JM, Thao,phuong Dang, Ward S, Ladda RL (1980) Gonadal dysgenesis in a 46,XY female mosaic for double autosomal trisomies 8 and 21. J Med Genet 17:321–323

Surana RB, Bain HW, Conen PE (1972) 18-trisomy in a 15 year old girl. Am J Dis Child 123:75–77

Surana R, Quinn FJM, Puri P (1994) Hirschsprung's disease in association with trisomy 21 and duodenal obstruction. Pediatr Surg 9:366–367

Suwa A, Hirakata M, Satoh S et al. (2000) Systemic lupus erythematosus associated with Down syndrome. Clin Exp Rheumatol 18:650–651

Suzuki K, Yamaki S, Mimori S et al. (2000) Pulmonary vascular disease in Down's syndrome with complete atrioventricular septal defect Am J Cardiol 86:434–437

Sweeney H, Pelegano J (2000) Wilms tumor in a child with trisomy 13. J Pediatr Hematol Oncol 22:171–172

Taggard DA, Menezes AH, Ryken TC (2000) Treatment of Down syndrome-associated craniovertebral junction abnormalities. J Neurosurg 93 (2 Suppl):205–213

Takashima S, Iida K, Mito T, Arima M (1994) Dendritic and histochemical development and ageing in patients with Down's syndrome. J Intellect Disabil Res 38:265–273

Tangerud A, Hestnes A, Sand T et al. (1990) Degenerative changes in the cervical spine in Down's syndrome. J Ment Defic Res 34:179–185

Taylor AJ (1968) Autosomal trisomy syndromes: A detailed study of 27 cases of Edwards syndrome and 27 cases of Patau's syndrome. J Med Genet 5:227–241

Taysi K, Kohn G, Mellman WJ (1970) Mosaic mongolism 2. Cytogenetic studies. J Pediatr 76:880–885

Tazi-Ahnini R, di Giovine FS, McDonagh AJ et al. (2000) Structure and polymorphism of the human gene for the interferon-induced p78 protein (MX1): evidence of association with alopecia areata in the Down syndrome region. Hum Genet 106:639–645

Teller DY, McDonald M, Preston K et al. (1986) Assessment of visual acuity in infants and children: The acuity card procedure. Dev Med Child Neurol 28:779–789

Teller JK, Russo C, DeBusk LM et al. (1996) Presence of soluble amyloid beta peptide precedes plaque formation in Down's syndrome. Nature Medicine 2:93–95

Temple IK, Cockwell A, Hassold T et al. (1991) Maternal uniparental disomy for chromosome 14. J Med Genet 28:511–514

Teraguchi M, Nogi S, Ikemoto Y et al. (1997) Multiple hepatoblastomas associated with trisomy 18 in a 3-year-old girl Pediatr Hematol Oncol 14:463–467

Terplan KL, Lopez EC, Robinson HB (1970) Histologic structural anomalies in the brain in trisomy 18 syndrome. Am J Dis Child 119:228–235

Teshima IE, Kalousek DK, Vekmans MJJ et al. (1992) Canadian multicentre randomised clinical trial of chorion villus sampling and amniocentesis Annex 6: Chromosome mosaicism in CVS and amniocentesis samples. Prenat Diagn 12:443–459

Thilaganathan B, Tsakonas D, Nicolaides K (1993) Abnormal immunological development in Down's syndrome. Br J Obstet Gynaecol 100:60–62

Thomsen J, Sederberg-Olsen J, Balle V et al. (1989) Antibiotic treatment of children with secretory ototis media. Arch Otolaryngol Head Neck Surg 115:447–451

Tijo HJ, Levan A (1956) The chromosome number of man. Hereditas 42:1–6

Tirosh E, Taub Y, Scher A et al. (1989) Short term efficacy of thyroid hormone supplementation for patients with Down syndrome and low-borderline thyroid function. Am J Ment Retard 93:652–656

Todd NW, Holt PJ, Allen AT (2000) Safety of neck rotation for ear surgery in children with Down syndrome. Laryngoscope 110:1442–1445

Toledo C, Alembik Y, Aguirre JA, Stoll C (1999) Growth curves of children with Down syndrome. Ann Genet 42:81–90

Tolmie JL, Boyd E, Batstone P et al. (1988) Siblings with chromosome mosaicism, microcephaly, and growth retardation: The phenotypic expression of a human mitotic mutant? Hum Genet 88:197–200

Torfs CP, Christianson RE (1999) Maternal risk factors and major associated defects in infants with Down syndrome. Epidemiology 10:264–270

Torrado C, Bastien W, Wisniewski KE et al. (1994) Treatment of children with Down syndrome and growth retardation with recombinant human growth hormone. J Pediatr 119:478–483

Torres R, Levitt MA, Tovilla JM et al. (1998) Anorectal malformations and Down's syndrome. J Pediatr Surg 33:194–197

Tseng SH, Cheng Y (1998) Occiput-cervical fusion for symptomatic atlantoaxial subluxation in a 32-month-old child with Down syndrome: A case report. Spinal Cord 36:520–522

Tsiaras WG, Pueschel S, Keller C et al. (1999) Amblyopia and visual acuity in children with Down's syndrome. Br J Ophthalmol 83:1112–1114

Tubman TRJ, Shields MD, Craig BG et al. (1991) Congenital heart disease in Down's syndrome: Two year prospective early screening study. BMJ 302:1425–1427

Tudor RB (1976) Psoriatic arthritis in a child with Down Syndrome. Arthritis Rheum 19:561

Turleau C, Chavin-Colin F, Narbouton R et al. (1980) Trisomy 18q- Trisomy mapping of chromosome 18 revisited. Clin Genet 18:20–26

Turner S, Sloper P, Cunningham C, Knussen C (1990) Health problems in children with Down syndrome. Child Care Health Dev 16:83–97

Twining P (1995) Ultrasound diagnosis of chromosomal disease. Reed GB, Claireaux AE, Cockburn F (eds) In Disease of the Fetus and Newborn,. 2nd edn. Chapman & Hall: London, 939–953

Uchida IA, Freeman VCP (1985) Trisomy 21 Down syndrome. Parental mosaicism. Hum Genet 70:246–248

Uehara S, Obara Y, Obara T et al. (1996) Trisomy 18 mosaicism associated with secondary amenorrhea: Ratios of mosaicism in different samples and complications. Clin Genet 49:91–94

Uehara S, Yaegashi N, Maeda T et al. (1999) Risk of recurrence of fetal chromosomal aberrations: analysis of trisomy 21, trisomy 18, trisomy 13, and 45, X in 1,076 Japanese mothers. J Obstet Gynaecol Res 25:373–379

Ugazio AG, Maccario R, Notarangelo LD et al. (1990) Immunology of Down syndrome: A review. Am J Med Genet suppl 7:204–217

Ukita M, Hasegawa M, Nakahori T (1997) Trisomy 18 mosaicism in a woman with normal intelligence, pigmentary dysplasia, and an 18 trisomic daughter. Am J Med Genet 68:240–241

van Duijin, Clayton D, Chandra V et al. (1991) Familial aggregation of Alzheimer's disease and related disorders: A collaborative reanalysis of case-control studies. Int J Epidemiol 20 (suppl 2):S13–S20

van Ravenswaaij-Arts CM, Tuerlings JH, Van Heyst AF et al. (1997) Misinterpretation of trisomy 18 as a pseudomosaicism at third-trimester amniocentesis of a child with a mosaic 46,XY/47,XY, +3/48,XXY, +18 karyotype. Prenat Diagn 17:375–379

Van Dyke DC, Allen M (1990) Clinical management considerations in long term survivors with trisomy 18. Pediatrics 85:753–759

Vautier-Rit S, Subtil D, Vaast P et al. (2000) Actual value of Down syndrome's echographic signs in the second trimester of pregnancy: Review of literature. J Gynecol Obstet Biol Reprod (Paris) 29:445–453

Veall RM (1974) The prevalence of epilepsy amongst mongols related to age. J Ment Defic Res 18:99–106

Vejerslev LO, Mikkelsen N (1989) The European collaborative study on mosaicism in chorionic villus sampling data from 1986 to 1987. Prenat Diagn 9:575–588

Vergani P, Locatelli A, Piccoli MG et al. (2000) Critical reappraisal of the utility of sonographic fetal femur length in the prediction of trisomy 21. Prenat Diagn 20:210–214

Verger P (1997) Down syndrome and ionizing radiation. Health Phys 73:882–893

Vicari S, Albertini G (1991) Moyamoya disease in Down's syndrome: A report of two cases. J Ment Defic Res 35:392–397

Walkinshaw S (2000) Choroid plexus cysts: Are we there yet? Prenat Diagn 20:657–662

Wallerstein R, Yu MT, Neu RL et al. (2000) Common trisomy mosaicism diagnosed in amniocytes involving chromosomes 13, 18, 20 and 21: Karyotype-phenotype correlations. Prenat Diagn 20:103–122

Wang BT, Peng W, Cheng K-T et al. (1994) Chorionic villi sampling: Laboratory experience with 4,000 consecutive cases. Am J Med Genet 53:307–316

Wapner RJ, Simpson JL, Golbus MS et al. (1992) Chorionic mosaicism: Association with fetal loss but not with adverse perinatal outcome. Prenat Diagn 12:347–355

Warburton D, Yu CY, Kline J, Stein Z (1978) Mosaic autosomal trisomy in cultures from spontaneous abortions. Am J Hum Genet 30:606–619

Warburton D, Kline J, Stein Z et al. (1987) Does the karyotype of a spontaneous abortion predict the karyotype of a subsequent abortion? Evidence from 273 women with two karyotyped spontaneous abortions. Am J Hum Genet 41:465–483

Warburton D, Byrne J, Canki N (1991) Chromosome Anomalies and Prenatal Development: An Atlas. Oxford University Press, NY

Warkany J (1971) Congenital Malformations. Notes and Comments. Year Book, Chicago

Warkany J, Passarge E, Smith LB (1966) Congenital malformation in autosomal trisomy syndromes. Am J Dis Child 112:502–517

Watt JL, Templeton AA, Messinis I et al. (1987) Trisomy 1 in an eight cell human pre-embryo. J Med Genet 24:60–64

Weber WW (1967) Survival and the sex ratio in trisomy 17–18. Am J Hum Genet 19:369–377

Wellborn CC, Sturm PF, Hatch RS et al. (2000) Intraobserver reproducibility and interobserver reliability of cervical spine measurements. J Pediatr Orthop 20:66–70

Werner LA, Mancl LR, Folsom RC (1996) Preliminary observations on the development of auditory sensitivity in infants with Down syndrome. Ear Hear 17:455–468

Whiteford MW, Coutts J, Al-Roomi L et al. (1995) Uniparental isodisomy for chromosome 16 in a growth-retarded infant with congenital heart disease. Prenat Diagn 15:579–584

Wierzba-Bobrowicz T, Lewandowska E, Schmidt-Sidor B Gwiazda E (1999) The comparison of microglia maturation in CNS of normal human fetuses and fetuses with Down's syndrome. Folia Neuropathol 37:227–234

Wilcock GK, Lilienfeld S, Gaens E (2000) Efficacy and safety of galantamine in patients with mild to moderate Alzheimer's disease: Multicentre randomised controlled trial. BMJ 321:1445–1449

Wilson SK, Hutchins GM, Neill CA (1979) Hypertensive pulmonary vascular disease in Down syndrome. J Pediatr 95:722

Wilson WG, Shires MA, Willson KA et al. (1983) Trisomy 18/trisomy 13 mosaicism in an adult with profound mental retardation and multiple malformations. Am J Med Genet 16:131–136

Winter RM, Baraitser M (1996) The London Dysmorphology Database. Oxford University Press, Oxford

Winter TC, Uhrich SB, Souter VL, Nyberg DA (2000) The "genetic sonogram": Comparison of the index scoring system with the age-adjusted US risk assessment. Radiology 215:775–782

Wishart JG (1993) The development of learning difficulties in children with Down's syndrome. J Intellect Disabil Res 37:389–403

Wishart JG, Johnston FH (1990) The effects of experience on attribution of a stereotyped personality to children with Down syndrome. J Ment Defic Res 34:409–420

Wisniewski KE (1990) Down syndrome children often have brain with maturation delay, retardation of growth, and cortical dysgenesis. Am J Med Genet, suppl 7:274–281

Wolff DJ, Raffel LJ, Ferré MM et al. (1991) Prenatal ascertainment of an inherited dup(18p) associated with an apparently normal phenotype. Am J Med Genet 41:319–321

Wolstenholme J (1995) An audit of trisomy 16 in man. Prenat Diagn 15:109–121

Wolstenholme J, Rooney DE, Davidson EV et al. (1994) Confined placental mosaicism, IUGR, and adverse pregnancy outcome: A controlled retrospective collaborative survey. Prenat Diagn 14:345–361

Wong KY, Jones MM, Srivastava AK et al. (1988) Transient myeloproliferative disorder and acute nonlymphoblastic leukemia in Down syndrome. J Pediatr 112:18–22

Wong V, Ho D (1997) Ocular abnormalities in Down syndrome: an analysis of 140 Chinese children. Pediatr Neurol 16:311–314

Worton RG, Stern R (1984) A Canadian collaborative study of mosaicism in amniotic fluid cell cultures. Prenat Diagn spec issue 4:131–144

Wren C, Richmond S, Donaldson L (1999) Presentation of congenital heart disease in infancy: Implications for routine examination. Arch Dis Child Fetal Neonatal Ed 80:F49–F53

Wright CG, Brown OE, Meyerhoff WL et al. (1985) Inner ear anomalies in two cases of trisomy 18. Am J Otolaryngol 6:392–404

Wyllie JP, Wright MJ, Burn J, Hunter S (1994) Natural history of trisomy 13. Arch Dis Child 71:343–345

Ya-Gang X, Robinson WP, Spiegal R et al. (1993) Parental origin of the extra chromosome in trisomy 18. Clin Genet 44:57–61

Yamaki S, Horiuchi T, Sekino Y (1983) Quantative analysis of pulmonary vascular disease in simple cardiac anomalies with the Down syndrome. Am J Cardiol 51:1502–1506

Yancey CL, Zmijewski C, Athreya BH, Doughty RA (1984) Arthropathy of Down's syndrome. Arthritis Rheum 27:929–934

Yla-Herttuala S, Luoma J, Nikkari T et al. (1989) Down's syndrome and atherosclerosis. Atherosclerosis 76:269–272

Young ID, Madders DJ (1987) Unknown syndrome: Holoprosencephaly, congenital heart defects and polydactyly. J Med Genet 24:714–715

Young ID, Cook JP, Mehta L (1986) Changing demography of trisomy 18. Arch Dis Child 61:1035–1036

Zachor DA, Mroczek-Musulman E, Brown P (2000) Prevalence of celiac disease in Down syndrome in the United States. J Pediatr Gastroenterol Nutr 31:275–279

Zaragoza M, Jacobs PA, James RS et al. (1994) Nondisjunction of human acrocentric chromosomes: Studies of 432 fetuses and liveborns. Hum Genet 94:411–417

Zarate N, Mearin F, Gil-Vernet JM et al. (1999) Achalasia and Down's syndrome: Coincidental association or something else? Am J Gastroenterol 94:1674–1677

Zeitune M, Aitken DA, Crossley JA et al. (1991) Estimating the risk of fetal autosomal trisomy at mid-trimester using maternal serum alphafetoprotein and age: a retrospective study of 142 pregnancies. Prenat Diagn 11:847–857

Zigman WB, Schupf N, Lubin R, Silverman WP (1987) Premature regression of adults with Down syndrome. Am J Ment Defic 92:161–168

Zipursky A (2000) Susceptibility to leukemia and resistance to solid tumors in Down syndrome. Pediatr Res 47:704 (required?)

Zipursky A, Brown E, Christensen H et al. (1997) Leukemia and/or myeloproliferative syndrome in neonates with Down syndrome. Semin Perinatol 21:97–101

Zhou J, NG AY, Tymms MJ et al. (1998) A novel transcription factor, ELF5, belongs to the ELF subfamily of ETS genes and maps to human chromosome 11p13-15, a region subject to LOH and rearrangement in human carcinoma cell lines. Oncogene 17:2719–2732

Zlotogora J (1997) Genetic disorders among Palestinian Arabs: 1. Effects of consanguinity. Am J Med Genet 68:472–475

Zoll B, Wolf J, Lensing-Hebben D et al. (1993) Trisomy 13 with an 11 year survival. Clin Genet 43:46–50

Zook PD, Winter TC, Nyberg DA (1999) Iliac angle as a marker for Down syndrome in second-trimester fetuses: CT measurement. Radiology 447:447–451

Zori RT, Schatz DA, Ostrer H et al. (1990) Relationship of autoimmunity to thyroid dysfunction in children and adults with Down syndrome. Am J Med Genet, suppl 7:238–241

Zühlke C, Thies U, Braukle I et al. (1994) Down syndrome and male fertility: PCR-derived fingerprinting, serological and andrological investigations. Clin Genet 46:324–326

Sex chromosome abnormalities

Judith E. Allanson
Gail E. Graham

45

Introduction

The X and Y chromosomes are structurally quite distinct
and are subject to different forms of genetic regulation.
They are thought to have descended from a common progenitor, with the Y chromosome becoming depleted of
genes. A number of genes retain copies on both the X and
Y chromosomes, many being present in two pseudoautosomal regions, at the termini of the short and long arms of
the sex chromosomes. Pairing at meiosis facilitates
exchange of information at both pseudoautosomal regions.

In somatic cells of normal females one X chromosome is
inactivated. The Barr body, a chromatin mass visible in
interphase, represents the late-replicating inactive X. The
number of Barr bodies is always one less than the total
number of X chromosomes per cell. Inactivation is believed
to occur early in embryonic life and to be complete by the
end of the first week of development. There is random inactivation of the maternally and paternally derived X chromosomes in any one female somatic cell. Inactivation is
permanent and clonal. These features are the basis of the
Lyon hypothesis (Lyon, 1962).

Three consequences of X inactivation are dosage compensation, variability of expression in heterozygotes, and
mosaicism. X inactivation transcriptionally silences most but
not all of the genes on one of the two Xs in females. Some
genes, particularly those in the pseudoautosomal regions,
escape inactivation and are expressed from both active and
inactive X chromosomes. The number and distribution of
these genes are the subject of considerable research. A recent
study reported that a third of genes on the X short arm may
escape inactivation while only 5% of those genes on the X
long arm do so, suggesting that imbalance involving the X

short arm might be predicted to have more significant consequences (Carrel et al., 1999). The clinical significance of
genes that escape inactivation is uncertain; however, these
genes may explain clinical features in sex chromosome aneuploidy as gene products may be either under- or overexpressed in relation to normal females and males.

Because inactivation is random, but established at a stage
of embryonic development when the embryo has 16 to 64
cells, females with one X carrying an altered gene, such as
Duchenne muscular dystrophy or hemophilia A, have a
varying proportion of cells in which the altered allele is
active. Consequently they exhibit variable phenotypes. The
range can be extreme, from a normal female to one in
whom there are significant and potentially severe clinical
manifestations of the disorder. In addition, females have
two populations of cells, in which one or the other X chromosome is the active one; in other words they are mosaic
with respect to their X-linked genes.

The process of inactivation is incompletely understood.
This process is under the control of the X inactivation
centre, located at Xq13. *XIST*, a gene which is transcribed
exclusively from the inactive X, is both necessary and sufficient for initiation and propagation of X inactivation, and
does so by coating the inactive X, perhaps boosted by chromosomal domains which each have a signal sequence. It is
not clear whether *XIST* plays a role in maintenance of inactivation, which likely occurs through differential methylation (reviewed by Lyon, 1998).

There are exceptions to random inactivation. In almost all
individuals with structural abnormalities of the X chromosome, the structurally abnormal X is inactivated, mediating
against unbalanced cells and their effect on phenotype. This
preferential inactivation means X structural anomalies are
better tolerated than autosomal equivalents and are thus more

frequently observed. Non-random inactivation is also the rule in X;autosome translocations. If the translocation is balanced, the normal X is preferentially inactivated, and the two parts of the translocated chromosome remain active, reflecting selection against a situation which would silence autosomal genes. In an unbalanced translocation, only the product carrying the X inactivation centre is present and this chromosome is invariably inactivated, the normal X being always active. These non-random events minimize the likelihood of clinical consequences of a particular chromosomal defect.

Sex chromosome abnormalities include monosomy X, polysomy of X and/or Y, structural changes in the X and Y chromosomes, and mosaicism. Early data on the health and developmental prognosis of these individuals was extremely biased by the method of ascertainment. Studies of unselected newborns, followed long-term, have provided a more accurate natural history emphasizing how many aspects of these phenotypes fall within the range of "normal".

The parental origin of non-disjunction of the sex chromosomes has been studied. In XXY males, the origin of the extra X is equally likely to be maternal or paternal; in XXX females, the extra X is maternal in over 90% of cases; in monosomy X, the paternal X is lost in 80% of individuals. Recent data have suggested that a parent of origin effect (imprinting) is demonstrated in these latter cases. When the retained X is paternal, there is evidence of superior verbal and higher-order executive function skills, which mediate social interactions. These females with Turner syndrome are likely to be better adjusted (Skuse et al., 1997).

The risk of polysomy X rises with increasing maternal age, while mothers of offspring with monosomy X are predominantly younger than average. A sex chromosome abnormality will be diagnosed in about 1 in 250 amniocenteses performed on women 35 years of age and older. These abnormalities may be more common in chorionic villous sampling (CVS). This rate is higher than that found at term, suggesting that there is significant loss of these fetuses in the latter half of pregnancy (Ferguson-Smith and Yates, 1984). Since the advent of widespread maternal serum screening with alphafetoprotein, estriol and human chorionic gonadotrophin, it has been recognized that abnormal analytes may be detected in the presence of sex chromosome aneuploidy, particularly 45,X (Kaffe and Hsu, 1992).

Turner syndrome

Turner syndrome, also known as Ullrich-Turner or Bonnevie-Ullrich-Turner syndrome, was described by Turner in 1938, although the chromosome abnormality was not recognized until 1959 (Ford et al., 1959). A myriad of features have been described including short stature, gonadal dysgenesis, and in utero lymphedema which may cause a variety of differences including neck webbing, congenital heart defects, dysplastic nails and subtle facial dysmorphism (Figs. 45.1 and 45.2). No single feature is pathognomonic or universally present.

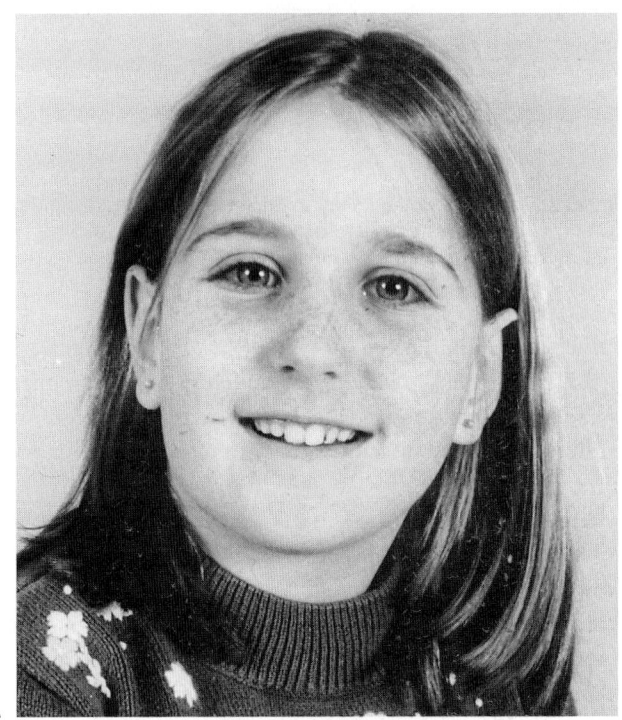

A

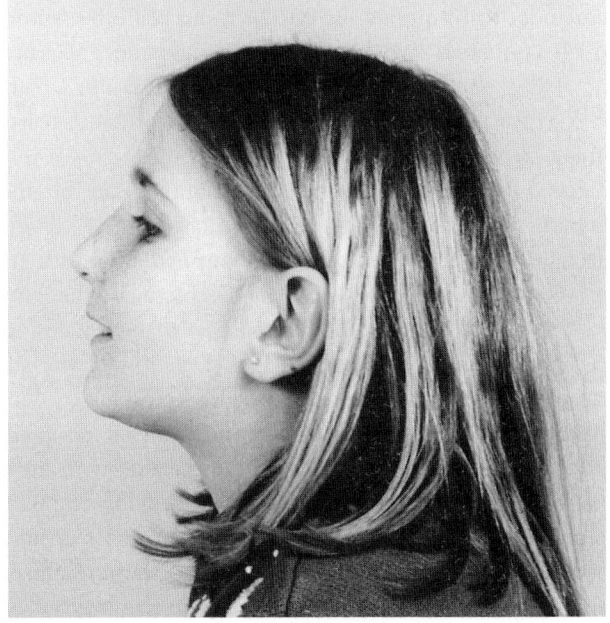

B

Fig. 45.1a and b. A young woman with Turner syndrome, showing unremarkable facial appearance.

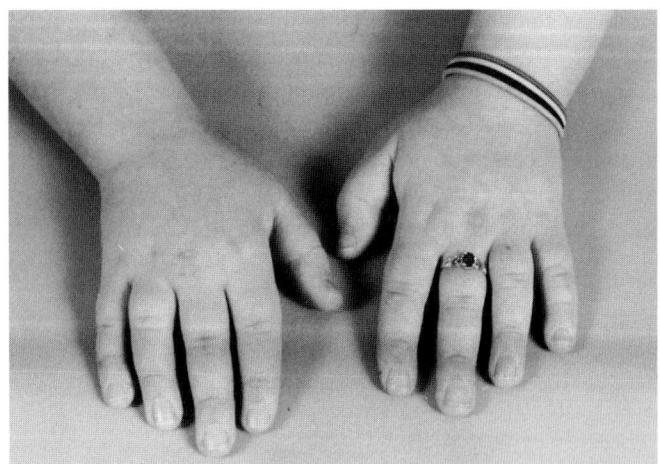

Fig. 45.2. The hands of the female in Figure 45.1, demonstrating short fourth metacarpals bilaterally (the dimple overlying the fourth metacarpophalangeal joint is proximally placed).

Turner syndrome occurs in 1/2500 to 1/3000 female live births, but is found much more frequently among pregnancy losses. It is hypothesized that the 45,X conceptuses that survive to live birth must be mosaic for a cell line with normal chromosomes.

Absence of a second normal sex chromosome is diagnostic of Turner syndrome. The cytogenetic alteration may be deletion of part or all of an X or Y chromosome. In a large series (Sybert, 2001) 45,X was found in half of the females diagnosed with Turner syndrome. Five to 10% had an isochromosome of the X long arm (duplication of the long arm, with loss of the short arm) – 46,X,i(Xq). Most of the remainder were mosaic for one or more cell lines, some of which contained two normal X chromosomes. Mosaicism for two abnormal cell lines can also be found. 45,X/46,X,i(Xq) will generally lead to physical features similar to those in isolated 45,X.

Some karyotype-phenotype correlations can be made (Sybert, unpublished data). Individuals with 45,X more often demonstrate congenital lymphedema and neck webbing. Females with 45,X/46,XX mosaicism are more likely to have spontaneous menarche than females with 45,X, isochromosomes or ring (X). Deletion of the short arm of the second copy of the X or homologous sequences on the Y leads to short stature and gonadal dysgenesis, although terminal deletions may be associated with normal ovarian function. Deletion of interstitial or telomeric material on the long arm of the second X chromosome programs short stature and primary or secondary ovarian failure. A ring or marker X chromosome of variable size may be associated with a more severe phenotype and an increased chance of mental retardation. 45X/46,XX mosaicism, when

diagnosed at birth, will generally show phenotypic similarity to 45,X. However, when prenatal diagnosis demonstrates 45,X/46, XX or 45,X/46, XY, in the absence of ultrasound anomalies, the liveborn is more likely to be phenotypically normal. The presence of Y chromosomal material, in whole or in part, confers a risk for gonadoblastoma. There are no clinical guidelines regarding the extent to which a search for Y material should be conducted. Studies using H-Y antigen and fluorescent in situ hybridization have suggested that up to 8% of females will be positive (Muller and Skakkeback, 1990). Many clinicians would only choose to pursue this testing if there is evidence of masculinization or mosaicism for an unidentified ring or marker (Sybert, personal communication). It is very important to remember that despite these karyotype-phenotype correlations, predictions in any one individual with Turner syndrome are imprecise.

ETIOLOGY AND PATHOGENESIS

Loss of all or part of a second sex chromosome may occur during spermatogenesis, oogenesis, or as a consequence of postzygotic non-disjunction. There does not seem to be a link with advanced maternal age, nor an increased risk for recurrence once a couple have had a child with Turner syndrome. Considerable research has focused on the particular genes on the X and Y chromosomes which lead to the Turner syndrome phenotype. Deletion of the *SHOX* gene in the pseudoautosomal region of the X and Y short arms is believed to be responsible for short stature (Rao et al., 1997). Deletion of the *SRY* gene, or testis-determining factor, on the short arm of the Y chromosome will lead to the features of Turner syndrome. Those individuals with a ring (X) and more severe phenotype may lack the X chromosome locus which controls X inactivation (*XIST*) located at Xq13.2. Lack of inactivation could lead to overexpression of X chromosomal material which, in the presence of a large ring chromosome, could have significant clinical consequences (Turner et al., 2000).

DIFFERENTIAL DIAGNOSIS

Many of the physical features of Turner syndrome are a consequence of in utero lymphedema, as mentioned earlier. Very similar features can be found in Noonan syndrome, a single gene disorder that affects males and females, in which short stature and congenital heart defects (usually right sided or cardiomyopathy) are also present. The differential diagnosis of short stature is large. Turner syndrome is one of the most common conditions and should always be excluded with this presentation. The third cardinal feature of Turner syndrome is gonadal dysgenesis. Other causes of primary or premature ovarian failure such as galactosemia and carriage of the fragile (X) gene should be excluded.

GROWTH

Birth weight is usually below the mean but within the normal range (Lindsten and Fraccaro, 1969; Sybert, personal communication). Mean birth length, at term, is at the fifth centile (Sybert, 2001). Growth velocity is reduced even in infancy, although the impact is gradual with diagnosis of short stature often delayed until five to ten years of age. Frequently, it is lack of the pubertal growth spurt that brings the female to medical attention. Studies of the efficacy of growth hormone treatment have been carried out since the mid 1980s. As a result, growth hormone treatment has become standard, even though, in general, females with Turner syndrome make sufficient quantities of growth hormone. Gain in final adult height is extremely variable, and may depend on age at start of treatment, duration of therapy and dosage (Plotnick et al., 1998). Families should be fully informed about the modest gains in height expected from treatment with growth hormone to be balanced against the burden of injections and monitoring. Human growth hormone does not appear to have negative sequelae, and should be initiated at age four or at the time of diagnosis, whichever comes first. Most adult females will remain small in comparison with their peers. They may also be overweight, likely as a result of excess caloric intake over expenditure, rather than a metabolic derangement; however, hypothyroidism should be excluded.

GONADAL FUNCTION AND FERTILITY

Gonadal dysgenesis is a cardinal feature of Turner syndrome and only 10% of women will have spontaneous puberty and fertility. These women are more likely to have mosaicism with a chromosomally normal cell line, or to have a terminal deletion of the short arm of the X chromosome. Many will subsequently experience premature ovarian failure. Many girls with Turner syndrome will show signs of adrenarche with some pubic and axillary hair development; however, the majority will require hormone replacement to fully develop secondary sexual characteristics and to have cyclical ovarian bleeding. In teenage years, FSH, LH and estradiol levels can provide guidance regarding hormonal supplementation. Ovarian hormone therapy should be initiated at around age 14, unless the individual is receiving growth hormone and has completed growth early. Hormone replacement therapy will decrease the complication of

primary or premature ovarian failure, particularly osteoporosis and heart disease. There is no recommended regimen but, in general, the lowest effective dose should be used and, in the first year, continuous dosage or cycling can be prescribed. After this time, unopposed estrogen should not be given and cycling with a progestational agent is recommended on a monthly basis, at least until the usual age of menopause. After this age, the approach to the "postmenopausal" woman with Turner syndrome does not differ from the general population.

Women with Turner syndrome who have become pregnant have demonstrated an increased risk of miscarriage, and of non-disjunction leading to chromosomal trisomy, particularly trisomy 21 (3%) and sex chromosome aneuploidy (20%) (Tarani et al., 1998). Twinning may also be more common. In women who are infertile, pregnancy, using gamete intrafallopian transfer (GIFT) techniques and donor eggs, has been successful. Normal sexual functioning can be expected, although dyspareunia may occur because of a small vagina or atrophic vaginal lining (Sybert, 1995). Dyspareunia may respond to vaginal dilation, hormone replacement therapy or lubrication, depending on the cause.

INTELLIGENCE, PERSONALITY AND BEHAVIOR

Most females with Turner syndrome have normal intellectual functioning. Verbal IQ exceeds performance IQ, and specific learning deficits are common, particularly visual-spatial functioning, right-left discrimination, processing speed and sequencing. These may lead to problems in mathematics, direction-finding and driving (Ross et al., 1995). In some females, additional difficulties occur because of short attention span and hyperactivity. About one in ten females with Turner syndrome will have significant delays requiring special education. The risk for intellectual handicap is greatest when the karyotype reveals a marker or ring chromosome (Sybert, 1995). When school difficulties are appreciated a full developmental assessment should be carried out and an individualized education program prepared.

Many girls with Turner syndrome display immature behavior in comparison to their peers, and experience particular isolation in adolescence. They are at an older age than their peers when they begin dating, leave home and marry (Pavlidis et al., 1995). Adults also have fewer social contacts, but most do not perceive this as a problem and express satisfaction with employment and social life (Pavlidis et al., 1995). The risk of psychiatric disease, including major reactive depression, affective disorder, eating disorders, substance abuse and obsessive-compulsive disorder, is approximately 10%, which is unlikely to be increased above the risk in the general population (Sybert, 2001).

CARDIOVASCULAR SYSTEM

Coarctation is the most common congenital heart defect, and bicuspid aortic valve is found frequently. Up to 45% of women with Turner syndrome will have a congenital cardiac anomaly (Sybert, 1998). The natural history of these defects and their treatment regimens do not differ from the general population. Hypertension is frequently found in Turner syndrome, and becomes more common with increasing age and with obesity. The likelihood of lipid abnormalities, myocardial infarction and atherosclerosis does not appear to be elevated (Sybert, 2001). There has been some concern that acquired heart defects, specifically aortic dissection, may be more common in Turner syndrome. Coarctation of the aorta, bicuspid aortic valve, and hypertension are all risk factors for aortic dissection. There seems little evidence of an increased risk for dissection in the absence of these risk factors (Lin et al., 1998).

Echocardiography should be arranged when the diagnosis of Turner syndrome is made. The frequency with which it should be carried out thereafter is under debate (American Academy of Pediatrics Committee on Genetics 1995; Sybert, 1998; Lin et al., 1998).

LYMPHATIC SYSTEM

Lymphatic abnormalities are a common feature of Turner syndrome and frequently manifest in utero with lymphedema and even hydrops. Lymphatic hypoplasia and delayed connection between the jugular veins and lymphatic channels are two of the causes postulated. Several physical features are found as a consequence, including redundant neck skin, which, over time, will change to broad or webbed neck, puffy hands and feet, dysplastic finger and toe nails, protuberant ears, ptosis, and shield-shaped chest (Fig. 45.3). Some studies suggest a correlation between the in utero presence of edema and the development of a structural defect of the heart (Clark, 1984; Lacro et al., 1988). Treatment of congenital edema is rarely necessary as it will generally resolve spontaneously.

ENDOCRINE SYSTEM

Hypothyroidism occurs in five to 10% of girls in mid to late childhood and may exacerbate growth retardation (Sybert,

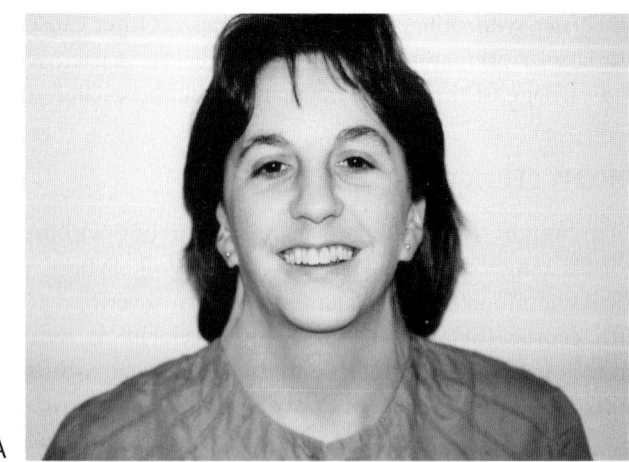

A

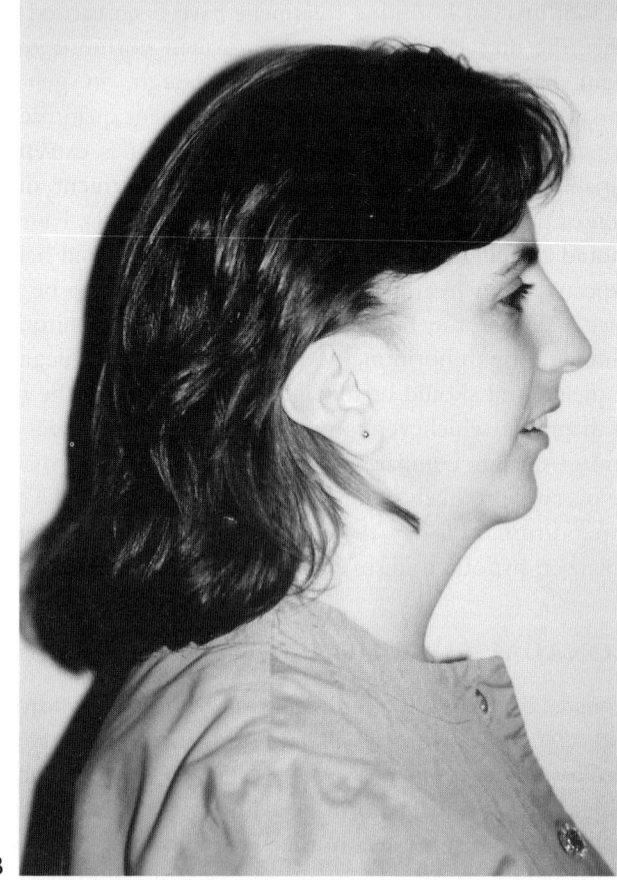

B

Fig. 45.3a and b. An adult female with Turner syndrome. Note the broad webbed neck, and lowset mildly posteriorly rotated ears which are a characteristic shape.

1995). It is also described in up to a third of adult women with Turner syndrome. Insulin resistance and diabetes are said to be more common in Turner syndrome although meta-analysis does not provide clear evidence of this (Sybert, personal communication).

RENAL SYSTEM

Structural anomalies of the renal tract occur in up to 40% of people with Turner syndrome (Lippe, 1998). Renal agenesis, horseshoe kidney, duplicated collecting system, obstructed outflow and aberrant vasculature are all described. Although vesicoureteric reflux and recurrent infection may be severe, dysfunction is rare. Renal ultrasound should be performed at diagnosis.

45,X/46,XY mosaicism

Substantial variation in the phenotype associated with 45,X/46,XY mosaicism exists, and much depends on whether diagnosis is made postnatally, or, fortuitously, prenatally. In the latter circumstance, 90 to 95% of babies, at delivery, have a normal male phenotype (Chang et al., 1990; Telvi et al., 1999). These boys have an increased risk of abnormal gonadal histology. Few prospective data are available on pubertal development, fertility, risk of testicular failure and likelihood of gonadoblastoma. When this diagnosis is made prenatally, detailed ultrasound evaluation will help to identify the minority with ambiguous genitalia and thus facilitate counseling regarding natural history and prognosis (Lazebnik et al., 1996). There does not appear to be a correlation between phenotype and the proportion of cells with 45,X in lymphocyte or fibroblast studies.

When diagnosis of 45,X/46,XY is made postnatally it is generally because of an abnormal phenotype, however there are rare normal males. The most common presentation is Turner syndrome. These females with a Y bearing cell line have an increased risk of gonadoblastoma. Less frequently, this karyotype is found in the investigation of male pseudohermaphroditism or mixed gonadal dysgenesis, with hypospadias, cryptorchidism, rudimentary phallus, urogenital sinus or, rarely, true hermaphroditism (Telvi et al., 1999). Associated mental retardation has been described but is unusual. Some apparently normal males, with normal genitalia, have been ascertained because of infertility, with abnormal sperm number or morphology. Studies of these males have documented an increased risk of sex chromosome and autosomal aneuploidy in sperm (Newberg et al., 1998).

X;Y translocations

X;Y translocations in humans are the result of abnormal male meiotic recombination. Translocations involving the X and Y chromosomes generally involve breakpoints in Xp22 and Yq11, producing partial monosomy of Xp with the addition of Yq material. The normal two-copy complement of Xcen-Xq11, a putative Turner syndrome critical interval, is present. SRY is most often absent, so the individual with this translocation is usually a woman with normal intelligence and fertility but short stature. The latter feature likely reflects the absence of the SHOX gene in the pseudoautosomal regions of Xp and Yp, but this can rarely be offset by the presence of GCY, a growth-promoting locus on Yq. Like women with Turner syndrome, women with t(X;Y) may have demonstrable growth hormone deficiency and may benefit from growth hormone administration. A smaller percentage of women with breakpoints proximal to Xp22 have gonadal dysgenesis, infertility and variable Turner stigmata in addition to short stature.

Less often, the translocation breakpoint is in Yq and the product retains the SRY gene, but important coding regions of the Y long arm may be deleted. The phenotype is highly variable and these males may have hypogonadism, infertility, dysmorphism and a degree of cognitive impairment. When the Y chromosome translocation breakpoint is more distal and only heterochromatic long arm material appears to be lost, there may still be submicroscopic loss of euchromatin that can have important clinical consequences. This possibility should be addressed by molecular methods.

Klinefelter syndrome

Klinefelter syndrome is the most common sex chromosome aneuploidy, occuring in all racial groups with an estimated incidence of 1/500 to 1/1000 male births. This condition is characterized by the addition of at least one extra X chromosome to a 46, XY male karyotype. Klinefelter syndrome usually refers to male patients with infertility and/or hypogonadism with a 47, XXY karyotype. Males with variable numbers of X and Y chromosomes have also been described, including 48, XXXY, 49, XXXXY, and mosaicism for 47, XXY. In addition, 46, XX males with Y sequences due to an X-Y interchange at paternal spermatogenesis, may manifest the Klinefelter phenotype. These variant forms of Klinefelter syndrome may modify the phenotype and have a different prognosis and management.

Klinefelter syndrome was initially described in a series of nine men with infertility, gynecomastia, and high urinary gonadotrophins (Klinefelter et al., 1942). These features are not present in newborns and children and some geneticists reserve the use of the term Klinefelter syndrome for the untreated adult phenotype, preferring 47,XXY in other circumstances. Pre-pubertal boys with 47,XXY appear normal, and it is unusual for the diagnosis to be made prior to this time. Most males will typically be identified through an evaluation for delayed puberty, infertility or gynecomastia in adolescence or adulthood. Infrequently, diagnosis will be made during an evaluation of developmental delay or behavioural problems in childhood or adolescence, or by prenatal diagnosis. The characteristic physical features of eunuchoid body habitus, sparse facial and body hair, gynecomastia, small testes and azoospermia are found in only a small proportion of men with 47,XXY.

ETIOLOGY

Non-mosaic 47,XXY occurs because of non-disjunction of the sex chromosomes during the first or second meiotic division of gametogenesis in either parent. The extra X chromosome is contributed slightly more frequently by the mother (56%) than the father (Harvey et al., 1990). When the origin is maternal, an error in meiosis one is more likely. There is a small association with advanced maternal age (Carothers and Filippi, 1988).

GROWTH AND PHYSICAL DEVELOPMENT

The newborn with 47,XXY has no significant dysmorphism. Height, weight and head circumference are in the normal range. Height velocity is increased by age five, and by adolescence most males will be in the tallest quartile (Robinson et al., 1990). Head circumference remains average, and the face may be long and slender with prominence of the lower jaw.

GONADAL FUNCTION AND FERTILITY

Gynecomastia is found in 15 to 30% of adolescent and adult males with 47,XXY, although some experts report a higher frequency after careful examination (Paulsen and Plymate, 1992). The pathogenesis is unclear but may be related to increased conversion of testosterone to estradiol. Muscle mass is quite variable, however muscle strength is usually reduced, a finding also noted pre-puberty. Facial, axillary and body hair all increase during puberty, but this usually occurs to a lesser degree than males with a normal chromosomal constitution. Untreated males may shave only once a week.

The sexual development of 47,XXY males is normal in infancy and childhood, when penile length, testicular volume, testosterone and gonadotrophin levels are normal (Robinson et al., 1990). The onset of puberty is no different than in the general male population and stimulates a normal elevation of testosterone that begins to plateau at around age 14. By mid- to late-adolescence most males with 47,XXY are hypergonadotrophic with normal to low testosterone levels (Salbenblatt et al., 1985). As these endocrine alterations progress, testicular growth is arrested, testes are small and firm, with progressive hyalinization and fibrosis of the seminiferous tubules. Leydig cells decrease in number, and become hyperplastic with reduced capacity to synthesize testosterone. Relatively low levels of testosterone put adults with 47,XXY at risk for osteoporosis (Horowitz et al., 1992).

Since adolescents and adults with 47,XXY are generally unable to produce normal quantities of testosterone, supplemental testosterone is used to raise and subsequently maintain levels within the normal range. This is usually considered in mid-adolescence. Testosterone levels should be closely monitored during the initiation process, since excess dosage may increase aggression. Supplementation allows support of androgen-dependent processes, including facial and body hair and muscle mass development, energy, drive, and libido. It may promote an improved sense of well-being, with less fatigue, more alertness, and an improved ability to concentrate. Supplementation will reduce the rate of bone resorption and increase calcium absorption to promote bone mineralization and reduce the risk of osteoporosis.

Historically, intramuscular injections have been the most common method of replacement, with injections every 10 to 14 days. This source clearly does not mimic normal physiologic production, and may lead to fluctuations in mood and physical functioning. Transdermal patches provide more appropriate bioavailability, and newer, non-scrotal, patches do not increase levels of dihydrotestosterone. They rarely cause acne, edema or local skin reactions and are preferred by most males. Development of alternative formulations of testosterone are encouraging. Implantable pellets, sublingual tablets, gels and long-lasting injections are currently under investigation.

Sexual functioning in 47,XXY is normal (Yoshida et al., 1997) but the ejaculate shows either oligospermia or azoospermia, with resultant infertility. A few 47,XXY fertile males have been reported, but these men likely are mosaic for a normal 46,XY cell line. Some men with 47,XXY have been shown to have a few sperm in their testes despite absence in ejaculate. For these men, testicular sperm extraction and ICSI (intracytoplasmic sperm injection) holds the promise of biological fatherhood (Harari et al., 1995). Genetic counseling should be provided prior to these advanced reproductive techniques being carried out, since there appears to be an increased risk for chromosome anomaly in the offspring (Kruse et al., 1998). Thus this technique is generally combined with prenatal or preimplantation diagnosis.

INTELLIGENCE, PERSONALITY AND BEHAVIOR

The developmental progress of most infants with 47,XXY is unremarkable; however, mild delays in motor and language milestones can be found, and expressive verbal skills often lag behind non-verbal skills. Language deficits include reduced processing speeds, word retrieval and fluency. By school entry, mild sensorimotor integration problems may be evident with hypotonia, apraxia, and coordination difficulties. Reading skills, which are highly dependent on other verbal abilities, are most problematic, although specific remediation in this area will generally allow continued academic progress in a regular classroom. Fine motor skills are often well-developed. The proportion of boys with diminished cognitive and learning abilities may increase towards adolescence (Stewart et al., 1990). Despite these trends, meta-analysis of six studies demonstrated a performance IQ equivalent to control males while verbal IQ was reduced (Netley, 1986), emphasizing that cognitive difficulties are largely verbal.

Evidence of delayed development should prompt a detailed assessment with standard interventions if deficits are identified. Special education support in reading, math, and comprehension may be needed (Robinson, 1990).

Many boys with 47,XXY are shy, unassertive and immature. Their difficulties in verbal performance may contribute to reduced peer interactions. Sensorimotor integrative problems may lead to reduced success in physical achievements which add to immaturity and isolation. In adolescence, boys with 47,XXY may be more passive and less confident (Theilgaard, 1984). Some experience serious emotional and behavioral difficulties. Psychiatric problems are rare, but clinical depression and bipolar disorder have been described. Depression, loss of interest, decline in school performance or suspected substance abuse should lead to individual counseling.

Every attempt should be made by parents and teachers to facilitate successful experiences and build self-esteem and self-confidence. Improved behavioral adaptation can be linked to a nurturing and supportive family life (Bender et al., 1987). Most boys progress towards independence from their families but tend to emancipate later than their peers. While educational achievements tend to lag behind those of siblings, some men with 47,XXY complete college and pursue professional careers. Work performance and adult adaptation are poorly studied. In general these men are gainfully employed. Many marry, although perhaps less often than their siblings. The incidence of psychiatric difficulty is increased in adults, but does not appear to be greater than that identified in adolescents (Bender et al., 1999).

MALIGNANCY

The risk of neoplasia in Klinefelter syndrome is no greater than in the general population. However, an association with extra-gonadal, primarily mediastinal, germ cell tumours and breast cancer has been documented (Hasle et al., 1995; Hultborn et al., 1997). Persistent unexplained respiratory symptoms should lead to a high index of suspicion. Regular self and clinical breast examination is recommended.

CARDIOVASCULAR SYSTEM

Men with Klinefelter syndrome have an increased incidence of vascular insufficiency, leg ulceration, deep vein thrombosis and pulmonary embolism (Veraart et al., 1995). The underlying cause of leg ulcers may be androgen deficiency or vascular abnormality. Mitral valve prolapse may also be more common in men with Klinefelter syndrome (Fricke et al., 1984). Aortic valve disease and subarachnoid hemorrhage may be more frequent than in the population as a whole, leading to a higher mortality rate (Price et al., 1985). High cholesterol levels are also found in untreated males, and should therefore be monitored in conjunction with testosterone assays.

IMMUNE SYSTEM

Adults with Klinefelter syndrome have a slightly increased risk of several auto-immune disorders, including systemic lupus erythematosis, thyroid disease, rheumatoid arthritis, Sjögren syndrome and diabetes mellitus. Although treatment of these disorders would usually be the same as that in the general population, a specific response to testosterone treatment may be found.

47,XYY karyotype

47,XYY is present in approximately one in 1000 newborn boys. This sex chromosome aneuploidy is not characterized by distinct physical features and, since there does not appear to be a recognizable pattern of neurodevelopmental or behavioral characteristics, the use of the term "syndrome" may be inappropriate. Males with an extra Y chromosome are phenotypically normal, and the vast majority never come to medical attention. This seems to be reflected in the paucity of recent clinical literature on individuals with this karyotype. There are relatively small numbers of controlled prospective studies, so knowledge of the medical and psychological profiles of boys with this chromosome constitution remains subject to both ascertainment and reporting biases.

ETIOLOGY

The additional Y chromosome is derived from paternal meiosis II non-disjunction or post-zygotic mitotic non-disjunction (Robinson and Jacobs, 1999). 47,XYY is therefore not associated with increased maternal or paternal age. Not surprisingly, the incidence of 47,XYY at amniocentesis is similar to that at birth, indicating that few of these fetuses are lost in the second and third trimesters of pregnancy.

GROWTH AND PHYSICAL DEVELOPMENT

The length and weight of newborns with an extra Y chromosome are indistinguishable from others and there are few, if any, clinical differences to suggest the karyotype (Fryns, 1998). There have been reports that the presence of the extra Y chromosome is more often associated with renal malformations and Potter sequence (Rudnick-Schoneborn et al., 1996), but no increase in any major anomaly has been seen in large studies with unbiased ascertainment. There are rare reports of radioulnar synostosis in boys with 47,XYY (Franceschini et al., 2000), though this finding is more consistently associated with the presence of more than two Y chromosomes (48, XYYY and 49, XYYYY) or with mosaic karyotypes that include multiple Y chromosomes. While an increased frequency of minor anomalies such as clinodactyly, inguinal hernia, and pectus carinatum has also been suggested, no consistent clinical picture has emerged. Similarly, no distinction in growth or appearance can be made between infants with 47,XYY and those with 46,XY karyotypes.

Accelerated linear growth may be present as early as the preschool years, and most adult males with 47,XYY are tall, reaching the 75th centile by adolescence. Gron et al. (1997) also documented larger craniofacial dimensions in these males than were present in controls.

GONADAL FUNCTION AND FERTILITY

Pubertal development, testicular histology and spermatogenesis have been repeatedly reported as normal. There is no indication that the sexual orientation of boys and men with 47,XYY is any different than it is in those with a 46,XY karyotype and many XYY men have fathered chromosomally normal children. It has generally been observed that reproductive risks for males with 47,XYY are no higher than for euploid males, despite the fact that in-situ hybridisation studies demonstrate a variably higher rate of spermatozoa with XY and chromosome 13 disomy in the former group (Martin et al., 1999). These observations, based on the analysis of more than 10,000 sperm in 47,XYY and control men, reach a very high degree of statistical significance. However, the absolute frequencies of XY and disomy 13-bearing sperm from 47,XYY men remain low at 0.55% and 0.40%, respectively. It appears that the extra Y chromosome in 47,XYY men is eliminated in the majority of cells during spermatogenesis and that the increased rate of sperm aneuploidy is small enough to have had little clinical effect. In many of the case reports describing aneuploid offspring born to men with 47,XYY, the aneuploidy has been of maternal origin, and in other reports an ascertainment bias is likely (Grass et al., 1984). In a number of instances, smaller than normal testes, decreased spermatogenesis, spermatogenic arrest, subfertility, and sterility have also occurred. In these relatively unusual situations, the problem may not always be related to the presence of an extra Y chromosome.

INTELLIGENCE, PERSONALITY AND BEHAVIOR

The commonest indications for karyotyping in boys with 47,XYY are developmental delay and/or behavioral difficulties. Some population-based studies have demonstrated that intellectual abilities tend to be lower on average than those of siblings and matched controls, and that boys with an extra Y chromosome are more likely to require educational help. However, Linden et al. (1996) report a full-scale average IQ of 105 (range 65–129) among 39 boys identified at birth and followed prospectively. Interestingly, boys with Klinefelter syndrome, as well as females with 47,XXX, have significantly smaller whole brain volumes on MRI than age- and sex-matched controls, while this difference is not seen in males with 47,XYY (Warwick et al., 1999). There are also case reports describing pervasive developmental delay in a few boys with 47,XYY but these may be the result of ascertainment bias. Since the vast majority of boys with an extra Y chromosome do not have pervasive developmental delay, Nicolson et al. (1998) speculate that the extra Y chromosome might set the stage for aberrant brain development. Pervasive developmental delay could then develop in a small number of these boys when a sufficient number of additional predisposing factors, such as a family history of learning or social difficulties, are present.

During school age, learning disabilities requiring educational intervention may be present in up to 50%, and are as responsive to therapy as they are in children with normal chromosomes. Expressive and receptive language difficulties and reading disorders are common. Hyperactivity, distractibility, and temper tantrums have been present in some boys, and may affect their school performance. Aggression is not frequently observed. Psychological studies have suggested that certain personality traits, such as infantilism, lack of emotional control, increased impulsiveness after emotional stimulation and a weak concept of self are so characteristic that men with 47,XYY can be recognized by psychological tests alone (Noel et al., 1974). Such findings are largely contradicted by prospective studies in which males with 47,XYY are behaviorally indistinguishable from controls. There may be a weak predisposition to behavioral problems in the setting of a stressful environment, as adolescents and young adults with 47,XYY from dysfunctional families seem to be less well adjusted than their siblings. This is not true in those whose environments have been more supportive. An important bias is that any psychosocial difficulties experienced by an individual with 47,XYY are likely to be attributed to his karyotype when they could well be caused or influenced by a myriad of environmental factors.

The karyotype XYY has probably aroused more public interest than any other chromosome abnormality, since the extra Y chromosome was demonstrated in tall, mentally retarded criminals. Prospective studies of XYY males detected at birth are now starting to yield data on adults. Gotz et al. (1999) identified 16 newborns with 47,XYY and 13 newborns with Klinefelter syndrome by population screening over a twelve-year period ending in 1979. Twenty years later, these men were compared to 45 controls with normal karyotypes and normal intelligence for rates of antisocial behavior and criminal convictions. The males with 47,XYY demonstrated a significantly higher frequency of criminal convictions and antisocial behavior in adolescence and adulthood than did controls, but multiple regression analysis suggested that these differences were mediated through lowered intelligence. The same observations were not seen in the Klinefelter group, but the small number of subjects precluded any firm conclusions.

There is some suggestion, therefore, that the extra Y chromosome leads to a slightly, but only slightly, increased risk of social maladjustment. There is little information on adaptation in an unselected group of XYY adults.

However, it would seem that the above-noted cognitive and psychological characteristics combined with environmental stressors may increase their risk for problems with the law.

HEALTH

Severe facial acne has occasionally been reported. There is poor evidence for a purported increase in varicose veins, electroencephalographic, or electrocardiographic abnormalities. Several reports of hematologic malignancies in boys and men with 47,XYY appear to be coincidental and due to the routine inclusion of a karyotype in the diagnostic work-up (Oguma et al., 1996; Sandlund et al., 1997).

Structural abnormalities of the Y chromosome

The length of the human Y chromosome shows considerable inter-individual variation. This trait is stable and inherited, father and son generally having identical Y chromosomes. When a structural abnormality is diagnosed in utero, comparison with the paternal Y chromosome is essential for interpretation and the possibility of non-paternity must always be considered. Structural abnormalities of the Y chromosome cannot usually be well-delineated by routine karyotyping, so molecular and in situ hybridization studies are generally recommended.

Yp DELETIONS

Individuals who have neither molecular nor cytogenetic evidence of the testis-determining factor (*SRY*), located on Yp just proximal to the pseudoautosomal region, are not usually masculinized. De novo deletions of Y p11 are therefore associated with a female Turner syndrome phenotype and often include lymphedema, streak gonads, infertility and a significant risk for gonadoblastoma. They differ from Turner syndrome by the absence of short stature (Hsu, 1994).

Yq DELETIONS

Deletions of the long arm are thought to be the result of intrachromosomal recombination involving highly repetitive DNA sequences unique to the Y chromosome. These deletions do not involve the *SRY* locus and do not affect testicular determination; hence they produce phenotypic males. Some such patients have normal or near-normal sized testes with histologic evidence of absent spermatogenesis or spermatogenic arrest, while others have more pronounced testicular maldevelopment, additional signs of hypogonadism and short stature. Studies of deletions have suggested that proximal Yq11 contains genes controlling stature, while distal Yq11 contains genes controlling spermatogenesis. The existence of a locus for stature on the long arm of the Y chromosome is supported by observations that XY males are taller than XX males, XY females are taller than XX females and XYY males are taller than XY males. This locus has been termed *GCY* for "growth control Y".

Cytogenetically-visible deletions of the long arm of the Y chromosome have been recognized in some males with non-obstructive azoospermia for over two decades. More recently PCR and FISH techniques have identified submicroscopic deletions in a larger percentage of these men, and three different non-overlapping Yq microdeletion regions known as azoospermia factors (AZFa, AZFb and AZFc) have been demonstrated (Krausz et al., 1999). The incidence of Yq deletion among azoospermic males varies from zero to 55.5%, the latter figure pertaining to the narrowly defined idiopathic Sertoli cell-only syndrome (SCOS), in which there is a complete absence of germ cells on testicular biopsy (Foresta et al., 1998). The world-wide frequency of Y chromosome microdeletions in azoospermic males is approximately 13% and does not appear to be influenced by ethnic or geographic factors (Oliva et al., 1998). The majority of these microdeletions include the *DAZ* (deleted in azoospermia) gene in the AZFc region of Yq11, while most of the remainder appear to involve the *RBM-1* gene in AZFb or, rarely, the *DFFRY* gene in AZFa (Ferlin et al., 1999). Two of these three genes are RNA binding proteins, but their role in spermatogenesis is unclear. There are additional candidate genes in these regions that may prove to be important.

A smaller and more variable percentage of males with fairly severe oligospermia and low reproductive capacities also have Yq microdeletions. There is speculation that males with mild or moderate oligospermia may be mosaic for such deletions. Interestingly, one Yq microdeletion that encompassed the *DAZ* gene was transmitted in natural conceptions from a father to his four infertile sons (Chang et al., 1999). At the time of ascertainment, this man was 63 and oligospermic, but he conceived his children between the ages of 25 and 38 years. This family demonstrates that Y chromosome microdeletions are subject to variable expressivity and do not necessarily imply a life-long history of infertility. Approximately 5% of oligospermic males participating in intracytoplasmic sperm injection (ICSI) programs have non-mosaic Y chromosome microdeletions, and the

advent of this technique for the treatment of male infertility has enabled the father to son transmission of these deletions (Page et al., 1999). It has therefore been recommended that all males with reduced or absent sperm counts seeking assisted reproductive technologies be screened for Y chromosome deletions.

DICENTRIC Yp

Dicentric Yp is among the most common Y chromosome rearrangements, and is often associated with the mosaic karyotype 45,X/46,X,dic(Yp). The dicentric Y chromosome may be created during male gametogenesis, the observed mosaicism presumably reflecting post-zygotic instability. It may also result from a very early post-conceptional mitotic event. Not surprisingly, the phenotype is highly variable and includes females with genital ambiguity and/or Turner stigmata, males with Turner stigmata and males that are phenotypically normal. The degree of 45,X mosaicism seems to correlate loosely with the probability of a female Turner syndrome phenotype but this may also depend on the tissue distribution of *SRY*-containing cells. Cytogenetic studies to estimate the proportion of cells containing the dicentric Y chromosome may be misleading because of inherent dicentric instability. It appears that the majority of dicentrics contain two copies of most of the functional euchromatin with breakpoints close to or within the heterochromatic region. However, only limited genotype:phenotype correlations can be derived from molecular studies to determine the amount of Yq between the two centromeres. *SRY* is usually present, but the mosaic nature of the Y-bearing cell line seems to reduce its ability to produce a male phenotype. The presence of Y material is known to predispose to gonadoblastoma, so gonadectomy is recommended for these individuals. Occasionally males with this karyotype are fertile, presumably due to the presence of one or more Y-linked genes controlling spermatogenesis. More frequently, however, phenotypic males are deleted for important regions of the Y chromosome long arm and consequently have short stature and azoospermia. Very rarely, microcephaly and mental retardation have been reported.

DICENTRIC Yq

Dicentric Yq is less common than dicentric Yp and it is also generally associated with 45,X mosaicism. The recombinant chromosome loses a variable amount of Yp, so that some of these individuals are males and others are females. Once again, the presence of *SRY* in a proportion of cells does not guarantee a male phenotype (Teraoka et al., 1998).

Isochromosome Yq is rare and when present usually results in females with little or no masculinization.

RING Y

Rings and very small Y-derived marker chromosomes can best be characterised with the use of molecular and in situ hybridization techniques. Many of the rings represent complex Y chromosome rearrangements, some have multiple centromeres and all are generally unstable. The phenotype varies widely depending to some degree on the extent of Y chromosome rearrangement and deletion, but generally an 45,X cell line is also present and there is overlap with the dicentric spectrum described above.

PERICENTRIC INVERSIONS OF THE Y

Pericentric inversions of the Y are heritable and have no phenotypic effects. One form leading to an almost metacentric Y chromosome is common in India and probably represents an ancient mutation. The paternal Y chromosome should be checked when the condition is diagnosed prenatally.

47,XXX karyotype

The 47,XXX karyotype occurs in approximately 1 in 1000–1200 female newborns. Unlike Turner syndrome, this is essentially the same incidence found at amniocentesis (Ferguson-Smith and Yates, 1984), suggesting that prenatal loss after mid-gestation is rare.

ETIOLOGY

In a study of 50 females with 47,XXX, 90% of the time the extra X chromosome was maternally-derived (MacDonald et al., 1994). Molecular studies indicated that 64% of these were the result of meiosis I non-disjunction, 18% the result of meiosis II non-disjunction and 16% the result of post-zygotic non-disjunction. In another 37 women with 47,XXX karyotypes, 93.5% resulted from maternal non-disjunction with increasing maternal age being present in meiosis I but not in meiosis II.

GROWTH AND PHYSICAL DEVELOPMENT

Females with X chromosome trisomy cannot be identified by the presence of physical differences at any age. The mean birth weights are somewhat lower than those of 46,XX girls. Many girls with 47,XXX will reach the 80th percentile during adolescence. The greater height seems to be attributable to increased growth of the lower segment relative to the trunk. Variability is great and stature is also influenced by parental heights in the usual multifactorial fashion. Relative microcephaly is present with an average head circumference at the 25th to 35th percentile. Those who have been followed prospectively from birth have a higher incidence of minor anomalies such as epicanthic folds, ear anomalies, and clinodactyly than females with a euploid karyotype.

GONADAL FUNCTION AND FERTILITY

The vast majority of adult women with an extra X chromosome go through puberty in the usual fashion, are no different with regard to their sexual orientation and lead a normal sexual life. Most also have normal reproductive capacities and bear children without sex chromosome aneuploidy. While precocious puberty, early-onset menarche and primary or secondary amenorrhea, including premature ovarian failure, have also been reported, prospective studies have not found them to be more common in women with triple X than they are in the general population. The incidence of sex chromosome aneuploidy in the offspring of women with 47,XXX does not appear to be substantially increased.

INTELLIGENCE, PERSONALITY AND BEHAVIOR

Neuromotor deficits with an increased tendency for delays in the acquisition of gross motor skills are frequently present and usually mild, but may result in poor coordination, and reduced athleticism. To a somewhat greater extent than other individuals with sex chromosome abnormalities, females with 47,XXX karyotypes are often delayed in the acquisition of language and academic skills. IQ is usually 10 to 15 points below that of siblings, but mental retardation (IQ <70) is rare. The average IQ in the prospectively followed group of 46 females is about 85 with a broad range (64–120). Verbal IQ is significantly less than performance IQ, with deficits in both expressive and receptive language being present in approximately 50%. A total of 70% have learning disabilities that require some form of educational intervention. A study of 11 adolescent girls with 47,XXX found, in addition to a reduced mean full-scale IQ, impaired scores on individual tests of attention, concept formation, mental flexibility, spatial thinking, verbal fluency and basic academic skills compared with controls (Bender et al., 1993). Retention and retrieval of previously learned information did not differ from controls. As might be expected based on their lower average IQ, these 11 adolescent girls with 47,XXX found the academic demands of high school particularly problematic. Nine of them required remedial placements and less than half completed their high school degrees (Bender et al., 1995). From a social point of view, these girls were immature, passive and prone to aberrant behavior and depression. One of the 11, however, attended college and remained free of psychologic dysfunction, while an additional two overcame significant psychological and behavioral problems to have good outcomes.

A study examining the transition from adolescence to adulthood in these 11 young women with 47,XXX and nine female sibling controls found the former group to be less well-adapted, experience more stress, have more work, leisure and relationship problems, and demonstrate more psychopathology (Harmon et al., 1998). Psychological dysfunction was not wholly attributable to lowered intelligence, though the latter did appear to exert an influence. Nevertheless, most of the group experienced mild disturbances and functioned reasonably well. The authors concluded that previously reported outcomes of antisocial behavior and severe psychopathology, including schizophrenia, are rare in women with 47,XXX and that the variability in behavioral phenotype is much larger than was originally appreciated.

RENAL SYSTEM

Urogenital malformations, including cloacal exstrophy, Mullerian anomalies, renal anomalies and lower mesodermal defects (single umbilical artery, sacral vertebral fusions and anal agenesis) have been reported in a small number of individuals (Lin et al., 1993), but an increased association with 47,XXX has not been substantiated by prospective studies. Routine investigation of the urogenital tract in females who are incidentally found to carry an extra X chromosome is probably unwarranted.

X chromosome mosaicism

45,X/47,XXX,45,X/46,XX/47,XXX and 46,XX/47,XXX mosaicisms are the product of nondisjunction in the first mitotic division of a 46,XX zygote. The increased frequency with which these mosaic diagnoses are made prenatally indicates that many mosaic individuals are not identified postnatally.

The majority of these women have been described in the obstetrical literature, indicating that they do not, for the most part, have physical stigmata of Turner syndrome that bring them to earlier attention. A study examining growth in approximately 50 women with triple mosaicism found a direct correlation between height standard deviation scores and the proportion of 46,XX cells in peripheral lymphocytes, and an indirect correlation between these scores and the proportion of 45,X cells (Partsch et al., 1994). The 47,XXX cell line did not seem to have a significant influence on stature. The interpretation of studies relying on one tissue in mosaic patients must be cautious, however, since the frequency of the cell lines in other tissues remains unknown. In vivo selection for the euploid cell line may occur over time.

Spontaneous pubertal development and menarche occur in many girls with these mosaic karyotypes. Premature ovarian failure or recurrent miscarriages have been observed in some women, but the majority have chromosomally and phenotypically normal pregnancy outcomes.

Adolescent women with this karyotype generally have neuropsychological profiles that are indistinguishable from controls and developmental or learning problems are the exception rather than the rule.

Sex chromosome tetrasomy and pentasomy (polysomy)

While 45,X, 47,XXX, 47,XXY and 47,XYY collectively occur with an incidence of approximately 1 in 400 newborns, sex chromosome polysomies are much rarer events. Unfortunately, their rarity precludes prospective studies that would present an unbiased picture. These individuals all have been identified clinically. The additional sex chromosomes seem to produce a lowering of IQ and an increase in somatic malformations.

MALE

48,XXXY and 49,XXXXY

The most significant effects of additional X chromosomes on phenotype are a reduction in intellectual functioning and an increase in somatic manifestations. None of these polysomic situations is common, except 49,XXXXY. Here, tall stature is less common than in 47,XXY; IQ is between 20 and 60; facial appearance is coarse; and gonadal hypoplasia and skeletal anomalies such as radioulnar synostosis are common. 48,XXXY is somewhat less common and is associated with severe cognitive and behavioral problems. IQ is lower than in 47,XXY, but reduced to a lesser extent than 49,XXXXY.

48,XYYY and 49,XYYYY

Males with poly-Y karyotypes containing three Y chromosomes (48,XYYY) are usually identified by tall stature and aberrant behavior (impulsivity and low frustration tolerance), with low-normal or subnormal intelligence, developmental delay, abnormal dentition, radioulnar synostosis and hypergonadotropic hypogonadism. Normal-appearing external genitalia seem to be the rule, but testicular biopsies have demonstrated variable abnormalities and azoospermia is common. Recurrent respiratory infections, inguinal hernias and additional abnormalities of the humerus, radius and ulna have also been reported. Minor anomalies include brachydactyly, clinodactyly and single transverse palmar creases. The phenotype is, however, inconsistent.

Males with four Y chromosomes are even fewer in number than those with 48,XYYY. In addition to the features outlined above, case reports suggest that these males are ascertained at birth because of the presence of craniofacial dysmorphism, including trigonocephaly, hypertelorism, upslanting palpebral fissures, epicanthic folds, low-set ears and micrognathia or prognathia. These boys are not uniformly tall and appear to have a more severe degree of intellectual deficits, hypotonia, motor delay and speech delay than their counterparts with three Y chromosomes. Little is known about the extent of phenotypic variability.

FEMALE

48,XXXX

More than 40 women with a 48,XXXX karyotype have been described. These individuals are often tall with an average height of 169 cm (Bender et al., 1995). Otherwise there are no consistent clinical features. Epicanthic folds, hypertelorism, nystagmus, radioulnar synostosis and clinodactyly are often reported. Genitalia are generally normal, but secondary sex characteristics may be incompletely developed. In one series, half of the adult women with this karyotype had normal menarche and menopause (Linden et al., 1995). With one exception, mental retardation has been consistently reported, with an average IQ of 60, but a range from 30 to 75. There is no characteristic behavioral phenotype. The mechanism of origin seems to be successive maternal meiosis I and II non-disjunction in most instances (Deng et al., 1991; Martini et al., 1993).

49,XXXXX

The penta-X karyotype is less common than 48,XXXX and none of the case reports describe a girl older than sixteen. All of these individuals demonstrate a more markedly abnormal physical and developmental phenotype than is seen in girls with quadruple-X karyotypes. Unlike other sex chromosome polysomies, girls with 49,XXXXX often demonstrate intrauterine and postnatal growth retardation, so they are more likely to be short than tall. The phenotype consists of microcephaly and coarse facial features, including hypertelorism, epicanthic folds, up-slanting palpebral fissures, a depressed and/or broad nasal bridge and a short broad neck. Congenital heart defects, particularly ventricular septal defect and patent ductus arteriosus, radioulnar synostosis, generalized joint laxity with multiple dislocations and talipes equinovarus have also been reported. Minor anomalies include single transverse palmar creases and clinodactyly. Puberty is delayed, secondary sex characteristics are incompletely developed and several girls have been noted to have small uteri. Fertility remains unknown. Mental retardation has been universal with an average IQ of 50 and no distinct behavioral profile.

Prenatal diagnosis of sex chromosome abnormalities

As more couples are availing themselves of chorionic villus sampling or amniocentesis for both fetal and maternal indications, sex chromosome aneuploidy is an increasingly common prenatal finding. Most geneticists and obstetricians would agree that these counseling sessions are more complex and challenging than those for autosomal trisomies, in which the phenotypes are generally less subtle from a physical, developmental and prognostic point of view. The goal of counseling is to present the couple with accurate information that empowers them to make an informed decision about the pregnancy that is best for them and their families. The counselor can be faced with at least two different scenarios. When there has been a sonographic identification of major fetal anomalies such as hydrops, the couple will have received some information prior to the prenatal diagnostic procedure. In this scenario, they generally arrive for counseling with a highly variable degree of understanding that there are physical problems with the baby that may be the result of a chromosome abnormality. On the contrary, when prenatal diagnosis has been performed because of advanced maternal age or the presence of "soft" markers for autosomal trisomies, the finding of sex chromosome aneuploidy is often incidental and completely unanticipated.

Irrespective of the particular situation, the general principles of prenatal counseling apply. The couple is often aware of "an abnormality" on arrival at the counselor's door. For most couples the term "chromosome abnormality" is synonymous with "Down syndrome", since this is the most common type of aneuploidy in liveborn children and the only one with which they may have personal experience. They are usually in a state of extreme distress that is exacerbated by fear of what they are about to be told. A compassionate acknowledgement of this at the outset is often helpful and should be followed by a brief attempt to elicit what details the couple already knows. The counselor should then proceed as quickly as possible to a discussion of the particular chromosome finding and it's implications, allowing the couple to dictate the agenda with their questions. Management options, which generally include continuing or ending the pregnancy, should be approached in a non-judgmental and non-directive manner. As in any counseling situation, empathic verbal and body language are extremely important. The counselor must be prepared to respond compassionately to expressions of grief and to repeat the information as often as necessary.

Of the more common sex chromosome aneuploidies (45,X, 47,XXX, 47,XXY and 47,XYY), only Turner syndrome and related mosaic karyotypes are often associated with major congenital anomalies and an increased risk of pregnancy loss. Turner syndrome counseling will depend to a great extent on the mode of ascertainment. If the indication for prenatal diagnosis is fetal hydrops on a midtrimester ultrasound examination, there is a very high probability of intrauterine death. Since the majority of 45,X losses occur in the first trimester, this is not true of a fetus with 45,X and normal sonographic findings who is incidentally ascertained by second trimester amniocentesis for advanced maternal age. Obviously, the content and emphasis of the counseling session will be dramatically different in these two situations.

In general, however, counseling for common sex chromosome aneuploidies should include a thorough discussion of the highly variable spectrum of physical findings, which may be cosmetically significant in 45,X and 47,XXY, but are essentially restricted to taller than average stature in 47,XXX and 47,XYY. The involvement of sex chromosomes suggests to many couples a fundamental difference in the gender of their child. The counselor should volunteer the fact that the extra or missing chromosome usually precludes fertility in Klinefelter and Turner syndromes, but has no impact on sexual orientation and the capacity for normal sexual function. The mention of hypogonadism in Turner and Klinefelter syndromes must be accompanied by a review of available treatments, including cosmetic surgery for breast enlargement in 45,X, and for gynecomastia and testicular enlargement in 47,XXY. Hormone replacement therapy is a mainstay of treatment in both conditions and growth hormone therapy is an option in the former. Under some circumstances, a referral to a pediatric endocrinologist during the pregnancy is appropriate and helpful with regard to decision-making. The couple should also be made aware of the availability of alternative parenting options (in vitro fertilization with donor egg or sperm, intracytoplasmic sperm injection, adoption) for the adult individual with Turner or Klinefelter syndrome.

Perhaps most importantly, the counselor must thoroughly review the intellectual, psychological and behavioral observations summarized above and make absolutely clear the difference between distinct learning disabilities (which are often present and amenable to educational support) and mental retardation (which is almost always absent and implies a degree of permanent disability). For 47,XXX and 47,XYY, emphasis should be placed on the fact that most of these children would have gone through life undetected, particularly in a stable environment. The importance of a supportive home environment cannot be over-emphasized, as children with sex chromosome aneuploidy from stable and nurturing families have no more psychologic disorders than do their siblings (Linden et al., 1996). Abramsky and Chapple (1997) recognized that the label of a "chromosome abnormality" may lead to a worse perception of the phenotype (and an increased likelihood of pregnancy termination) than would otherwise be the case. How many couples, they wondered, would consider termination of a euploid pregnancy if they were told the child's IQ would be normal but 10–15 points lower than that of his or her siblings? They also draw attention to the fact that background rates of learning disability, developmental delay and psychologic difficulties in chromosomally normal children should be quoted to enable the couple to put the implications for children with sex chromosome aneuploidy in context. There is no such thing as a "perfect" child.

In a retrospective review of 169 pregnancies in which 45,X, 47,XXX, 47,XXY and 47,XYY were diagnosed between 1971 and 1997, 32% of couples chose to continue their pregnancies (Christian et al., 2000). Of those who had normal ultrasound examinations, 60% ended their pregnancies; the equivalent figure in pregnancies with abnormal ultrasound examinations was 82%. Half of the latter pregnancies were ended on the basis of ultrasound findings alone, as many of them consisted of 45,X-associated fetal hydrops or cystic hygroma, both of which are known to predict a poor prognosis. Among pregnancies with a normal ultrasound examination, those with a diagnosis of 47,XXX and 47,XYY were continued significantly more often than those with a diagnosis of 45,X and 47,XXY. Fifty percent of sonographically normal pregnancies with mosaic findings were continued, compared with 35% of pregnancies with non-mosaic karyotypes. The method of prenatal diagnosis as well as the marital status, education and profession of parents did not exert a significant influence on decision-making. There was a significant difference in parental decision-making over the course of the study, likely related to the lack of adult outcome data prior to 1990. None of the couples continued their pregnancies between 1976 and 1979, in contrast to a 46% continuation rate between 1995 and 1997. Recent studies have reported continuation rates as high as 60–70%. Interestingly, follow-up of a small number of these children suggests that they are developmentally ahead of children with sex chromosome aneuploidies that were diagnosed by newborn screening. The fact that these parents made a conscious decision to continue their pregnancies, possibly combined with the advantage of early anticipatory intervention, appears to have had a positive effect on outcome.

REFERENCES

Abramsky L, Chapple J (1997) 47,XXY (Klinefelter Syndrome) and 47,XYY: Estimated rates of and indication for postnatal diagnosis with implications for prenatal counselling. Prenat Diagn 17:363–8

American Academy of Pediatrics Committee on Genetics (1995) Health supervision for children with Turner syndrome. Pediatrics 96:1166–1173

Bender BG, Linden MG, Robinson A (1987) Environment and developmental risk in children with sex chromosome abnormalities. J Acad Child Psych 26:499–503

Bender BG, Linden MG, Robinson A (1993) Neuropsychological impairment in 42 adolescents with sex chromosome abnormalities. Am J Med Genet 48:169–73

Bender BG, Harmon RJ, Linden MG, Robinson A (1995) Psychosocial adaptation of 39 adolescents with sex chromosome abnormalities. Pediatr 96:302–308

Bender BG, Harmon RJ, Linden MG et al. (1999) Psychological competence of unselected young adults with sex chromosome abnormalities. Am J Med Genet 88:200–206

Carothers AD, Filippi G (1988) Klinefelter's syndrome in Sardinia and Scotland. Comparative studies of parental age and other aetiological factors in 47, XXY. Hum Genet 81:71–75

Carrel L, Cottle A, Willard HF (1999) X inactivation profile of the X chromosome: survey of the first 125 genes. Am J Hum Genet 65 A2

Chang HJ, Clark RD, Bachman H (1990) The phenotype of 45, X/46, XY mosaicism: an analysis of 92 prenatally diagnosed cases. Am J Hum Genet 46:156–167

Chang PL, Sauer MV, Brown S (1999) Y chromosome microdeletion in a father and his four infertile sons. Hum Repro 14:2689–2694

Clark EB (1984) Neck web and congenital heart defects: a pathogenic association in 45, XO Turner syndrome? Teratology 29:355–361

Christian SM, Koehn D, Pillay R et al. (2000) Parental decisions following prenatal diagnosis of sex chromosome aneuploidy: A trend over time. Prenatal Diag 20:37–40

Deng H-X, Abe K, Kondo I et al. (1991) Parental origin and mechanism of formation of polysomy X: an XXXXX case and four XXXXY cases determined with RFLPs. Hum Genet 86:541–44

Ferguson-Smith MA, Yates JRW (1984) Maternal age specific rates for chromosome aberrations and factors influencing them: report of a collaborative study on 52 965 amniocenteses. Prenatal Diag 4:5–44

Ferlin A, Moro E, Garolla A, Foresta C (1999) Human male infertility and Y chromosome deletions: role of the AZF-candidate genes *DAZ*, *RBM* and *DFFRY*. Hum Reprod 14:1710–16

Ford CE, Jones KW, Polani PE et al. (1959) A sex-chromosome anomaly in a case of gonadal dysgenesis (Turner's syndrome). Lancet I:711–712

Foresta C, Ferlin A, Garolla A et al. (1998) High frequency of well-defined Y-chromosome deletions in idiopathic Sertoli cell-only syndrome. Hum Reprod 13:302–307

Franceschini P, Lictata D, Guala A et al. (2000) Radioulnar synostosis and XYY syndrome. Clin Dysmorphology 9:77

Fricke GR, Mattern HJ, Schweikert HU, Schwanitz G (1984) Klinefelter's syndrome and mitral valve prolapse, an echocardiographic study in twenty-two patients. Biomed Pharmacotherapy 38:88–97

Fryns JP (1998) Mental status and psychosocial functioning in XYY males. Prenatal Diag 18:303–304

Gotz MJ, Johnstone EC, Ratcliffe SG (1999) Criminality and antisocial behaviour in unselected men with sex chromosome abnormalities. Psychol Med 29:953–62

Grass F, McCombs J, Scott CI et al. (1984) Reproduction in XYY males: two new cases and implications for genetic counseling. Am J Med Genet 19:553–560

Gron M, Pietila K, Alvesalo L (1997) The craniofacial complex in 47,XYY males. Arch Oral Biol 42:579–86

Harari O, Bourne H, Baker G et al. (1995) High fertilization rate with intracytoplasmic sperm injection in mosaic Klinefelter's syndrome. Fertil Steril 63:182–184

Harmon RJ, Bender BG, Linden MG, Robinson A (1998) Transition from adolescence to early adulthood: Adaptation and psychiatric status of women with 47,XXX. J Am Acad Child Adol Psych 37:286–91

Harvey J, Jacobs PA, Hassold T, Pettay D (1990) The parental origin of 47,XXY males. Birth Defects Original Article Series 26:289–296

Hasle H, Mellemgaard A, Nielsen J, Hansen J (1995) Cancer incidence in men with Klinefelter syndrome. Brit J Cancer 71:416–420

Horowitz M, Wishart JM, O'Loughlin PD et al. (1992) Osteoporosis and Klinefelter's syndrome. Clin Endocrin 36:113–118

Hsu LYF (1994) Phenotype/karyotype correlations of y chromosome aneuploidy with emphasis on structural aberrations in postnatally diagnosed cases. Am J Med Genet 53:108–140

Hultborn R, Hanson C, Kopf I et al. (1997) Prevalence of Klinefelter's syndrome in male breast cancer patients. Anticancer Research 17:4293–4297

Joseph M, Cantu ES, Pai GS et al. (1996) Xp pseudoautosomal gene haploinsufficiency and linear growth deficiency in three girls with chromosome Xp22;Yq11 translocation. J Med Genet 33:906–11

Kaffe S, Hsu LYF (1992) Maternal serum alpha-fetoprotein screening and fetal chromosome anomalies: Is lowering maternal age for amniocentesis preferable? Am J Med Genet 42:801–806

Klinefelter HF Jr, Reifenstein EC Jr, Albright F (1942) Syndrome characterized by gynecomastia, aspermatogenesis with a-Leydigism and increased excretion of follicle-stimulating hormone. J Clin Endocrin Metabolism 2:615–627

Krausz C, Quintana-Murci L, Barbaux S et al. (1999) A high frequency of Y chromosome deletions in males with non-idiopathic infertility. J Clin Endocrin Metabolism 84:3606–3612

Kruse R, Guttenbach M, Schartmann B et al. (1998) Genetic counselling in a patient with XXY/XXXY/XY mosaic Klinefelter's syndrome: estimate of sex chromosome aberrations in sperm before intracytoplasmic sperm injection. Fertility and Sterility 69:482–485

Lacro RV, Jones KL, Benirschke K (1988) Coarctation of the aorta in Turner syndrome: A pathogenetic study of fetuses with nuchal cystic hygromas, hydrops fetalis, and female genitalia. Pediatr 81:445–451

Lazebnik N, Filkins KA, Jackson CL et al. (1996) 45,X/46,XY mosaicism: the role of ultrasound in prenatal diagnosis and counselling. Ultrasound in Obstetr and Gynec 8:325–328

Lin HJ, Ndiforchu F, Patell S (1993) Exstrophy of the cloaca in a 47,XXX child: Review of genitourinary malformations in triple-X patients. Am J Med Genet 45:761–3

Lin A, Lippe B, Rosenfeld R (1998) Further delineation of aortic dilation, dissection, and rupture in patients with Turner syndrome. Pediatrics 102(1). URL: http://www.pediatrics.org/cgi/content/full/102/1/el2

Linden MG, Bender BG, Robinson A (1995) Sex chromosome tetrasomy and pentasomy. Pediatrics 96:672–82

Linden MG, Bender BG, Robinson A (1996) Intrauterine diagnosis of sex chromosome aneuploidy. Obstetr and Gynec 87:468–75

Lindsten J, Fraccaro M (1969) Turner's syndrome. In Rashad MN, Morton (eds): Genital anomalies. CC Thomas, Springfield, IL, pp396–456

Lippe B, Geffner ME, Dietrich RB et al. (1998) Renal malformations in patients with Turner syndrome: imaging in 141 patients. Pediatr 82:852–856

Lyon MF (1962) Sex chromatin and gene action in the mammalian X-chromosome. Am J Hum Genet 14:135–148

Lyon MF (1998) X-chromatin inactivation spreads itself: Effects in autosomes. Am J Hum Genet 63:17–19

MacDonald M, Hassold T, Harvey J et al. (1994) The origin of 47,XXY and 47,XXX aneuploidy: Heterogeneous mechanisms and role of aberrant recombination. Hum Mol Genet 8:1365–71

Martin RH, McInnes B, Rademaker AW (1999) Analysis of aneuploidy for chromosomes 13, 21, X and Y by multicolour fluorescence in situ hybridization (FISH) in a 47,XYY male. Zygote 7:131–4

Martini G, Carillo G, Catizone F et al. (1993) On the parental origin of the X's in a prenatally diagnosed 49,XXXXX syndrome. Prenatal Diag 13:763–66

Muller J, Skakkeback NE (1990) Gonadal malignancy in individuals with sex chromosome anomalies. Birth Defects Original Article Series 26:247–257

Netley C (1986) Summary overview of behavioural development in individuals with neonatally identified X and Y aneuploidy. In Ratcliffe SG, Paul N (eds): Prospective studies on children with sex chromosome aneuploidy. Birth Defects Original Article Series 22:293–306

Newberg MT, Francisco RG, Pang MG et al. (1998) Cytogenetics of somatic cells and sperm from a 46,XY/45,X mosaic male with moderate oligoasthenoteratozoospermia. Fertil Steril 69:146–148

Nicolson R, Bhalerao S, Sloman L (1998) 47,XYY karyotypes and pervasive developmental disorders. Can J Psychiat 43:619–622

Noel B, Dupont JP, Revil O et al. (1974) The XYY syndrome: reality or myth? Clin Genet 5:387–394

Oliva R, Margarit E, Ballesca, J-L et al. (1998) Prevalence of Y chromosome microdeletions in oligospermic and azoospermic candidates for intracytoplasmic sperm injection. Fertility and Sterility 70:506–509

Oguma N, Shigeta C, Kamada N (1996) XYY male and hematologic malignancy. Cancer Genet Cytogenet 90:179–181

Page DC, Silber S, Brown LG (1999) Men with infertility caused by AZFc delection can produce sons by intracytoplasmic sperm injection, but are likely to transmit the deletion and infertility. Hum Reprod 14:1722–26

Partsch C-J, Pankau R, Sippell WG, Tolksdorf M (1994) Normal growth and normalization of hypergonadotrophic hypogonadism in atypical Turner syndrome (45,X/46,XX/47,XXX). Correlation of body height with distribution of cell lines. Eur J Pediatr 153:451–55

Paulsen CA, Plymate SR (1992) Klinefelter's syndrome. In King RA, Rotter J, Motulsky AH (eds): The Genetic basis of Common Diseases. Oxford University Press, New York, pp. 876–894

Pavlidis K, McCauley E, Sybert VP (1995) Psychosocial and sexual functioning in women with Turner syndrome. Clin Genet 47:85–89

Plotnick L, Attie KM, Blethen SL, Sy JP (1998) Growth hormone treatment of girls with Turner syndrome: The National Cooperative Growth Study experience. Pediatrics 102:479–481

Price WH, Clayton JF, Wilson J et al. (1985) Causes of death in X chromatin positive males (Klinefelter's syndrome). J Epidem Commun Health 39:330–336

Rao E, Weiss B, Fukami M et al. (1997) Pseudoautosomal deletions encompassing a novel homeobox gene cause growth failure in idiopathic short stature and Turner syndrome. Nature Genet 16:54–63

Robinson A, Bender BG, Linden MG (1990) Summary of clinical findings in children and adults with sex chromosome anomalies. Birth Defects Original Article Series 26:225–228

Robinson DO, Jacobs PA (1999) The origin of the extra Y chromosome in males with a 47,XYY karyotype. Hum Molec Genet 8:2205–2209

Ross JL, Stefanatos G, Roeltgen D et al. (1995) Ullrich-Turner syndrome: neurodeveopmental changes from childhood through adolescence. Am J Med Genet 58:74–82

Rudnick-Schoneborn S, Schuler HM, Schwanitz G et al. (1996) Further arguments for non-fortuitous association of Potter sequence with XYY males. Annals Genetique 39:43–6

Salbenblatt JA, Bender BG, Puck MH et al. (1985) Pituitary-gonadal function in Klinefelter syndrome before and during puberty. Pediatric research 19:82–86

Sandlund JT, Krance R, Pui CH et al. (1997) XYY syndrome in children with acute lymphoblastic leukemia. Med Pediatr Oncology 28:6–8

Skuse DH, James RS, Bishop DVM et al. (1997) Evidence from Turner's syndrome of an imprinted X-linked locus affecting cognitive function. Nature 387:705–708

Spranger S, Kirsch S, Mertz A et al. (1997) Molecular studies of an X;Y translocation chromosome in a women with deletion of the pseudoautosomal region but normal height. Clin Genet 51:346–50

Stewart DA, Bailey JD, Netley CT, Park E (1990) Growth, development, and behavioural outcome from mid-adolescence to adulthood in subjects with chromosome aneuploidy: The Toronto study. Birth Defects Original Article Series 26:131–188

Sybert VP (1995) The adult patient with Turner syndrome. In Albertsson-Wikland K and Ranke MB (eds): Turner Syndrome in a Lifespan Perspective: Research and Clinical Aspects. NY, Elsevier, pp. 205–218

Sybert VP (1998) Cardiovascular malformations and complications in Turner syndrome. Pediatrics 101(1). URL:http://www.pediatrics.org/cgi/content/full/101/1/e11

Sybert VP (2001) Turner syndrome. In Cassidy SB, Allanson JE (eds) Management of Genetic Syndromes, pp. 459–484. Wiley & Co, New York

Tarani L, Lampariello S, Raguso G et al. (1998) Pregnancy in patients with Turner's syndrome: six new cases and review of the literature. Gynecol Endocrinol 12:83–87

Telvi L, Lebbar A, Del Pino O et al. (1999) 45,X/46,XY mosaicism: Report of 27 cases. Pediatr 104:304–308

Teraoka M, Narahara K, Yokoyama Y et al. (1998) 45,X/46,X,idic(Yq) mosaicism: Clinical, cytogenetic and molecular studies in four individuals. Am J Med Genet 78:424–8

Theilgaard A (1984) A psychological study of the personalities of XYY – and XXY – men. Acta Psych Scand Suppl 315:1–133

Turner HH (1938) A syndrome of infantilism, congenital webbed neck, and cubitus valgus. Endocrinolgy 23:566–574

Turner C, Dennis NR, Skuse D, Jacob PA (2000) Seven ring (X) chromosomes lacking the XIST locus, six with an unexpectedly mild phenotype. Hum Genet 106:93–100

Veraart JC, Hamulyak K, Neumann HA (1995) Leg ulcers and Klinefelter's syndrome. Arch Dermatol 131:958–959

Yoshida A, Miura K, Nagao K et al. (1997) Sexual function and clinical features of patients with Klinefelter's syndrome with the chief complaint of male infertility. Int J Androl 20:80–85

Warwick MM, Doody GA, Lawrie SM et al. (1999) Volumetric magnetic resonance imaging study of the brain in subjects with sex chromosome aneuploidies. J Neurol Neurosurg Psych 66:628–632

Deletions and other structural abnormalities of the autosomes

46

Nancy B. Spinner
Beverly S. Emanuel

Introduction

The human genome is composed of 3×10^9 base pairs of DNA, which codes for an estimated 30,000 to 40,000 structural genes (International Human Genome Sequencing Consortium, 2001). Approximately 10–15% of the DNA codes for genes (transcripts and their regulatory sequences), while the remainder consists of repeated sequences and sequences of unknown function. The DNA is packaged into 23 pairs of chromosomes; 22 pairs of non-sex chromosomes (autosomes) and one pair of sex chromosomes: XX in females and XY in males. When examined at metaphase at the 550 band stage (standard cytogenetic analysis), an "average" chromosomal band contains approximately 5×10^6 DNA base pairs that could code for as many as 100–200 genes. Therefore, patients with cytogenetically visible chromosomal abnormalities involving gains or losses of a single band or part of a band have abnormal dosage for numerous genes. Given this, it is not surprising that almost all individuals with a cytogenetically detectable chromosomal imbalance demonstrate some phenotypic abnormality.

Structural constitutional chromosomal anomalies are usually a consequence of chromosome breakage that has occurred during meiosis. In the simplest case, a single break occurs within a chromosome arm. This does not affect the centromere, and results in a shorter chromosome plus an acentric fragment (i.e., lacking a centromere). Chromosomal fragments lacking a centromere are unstable through mitosis and fragments are usually lost during a subsequent cell division. Therefore, the result of the breakage event is a shorter (deleted) chromosome.

If two chromosomal breaks occur within a single cell, repair enzymes can rejoin the broken ends resulting in a new configuration of the chromosomal material. Chromosomes can apparently break at any point and the broken ends can be re-joined to form a wide variety of new combinations. Rarely, the breakage occurs within a critical disease-causing gene, resulting in a recognizable phenotype and allowing the precise localization of the disease locus. Very few site specific constitutional rearrangements have been observed to occur in multiple unrelated individuals. In addition to disruption of a single gene, the consequences of chromosomal rearrangements include the following: loss of genetic material (deletion); gain of genetic material (duplication); or reunion of the disrupted chromosomal segments in an abnormal configuration accompanied by no loss or gain (balanced translocation, inversion). Alterations in the normal banding pattern after these rearrangements often permit their detection on standard cytogenetic analysis. There is an extensive literature regarding structural abnormalities of the chromosomes (Schinzel, 1984; 1994). Clinically, the most numerous structural rearrangements are translocations and deletions. Duplications, inversions, ring chromosomes and isochromosomes are observed less frequently.

In this chapter we review the most frequently observed translocations, deletions and duplications to provide access to information on the most common of the myriad of cytogenetic abnormalities. In addition, we present some of the more rare disorders which provide new insights into the mechanisms of cytogenetic disease.

The information presented in this chapter has been obtained through a combined cytogenetic and molecular cytogenetic approach. However, it should be noted that the field of molecular cytogenetics is continuing to grow at a very rapid pace, fueled in part by the fruits of the Human Genome Project. There are an increasing number of probes available for molecular cytogenetics, which will be used to continue to refine the critical regions for many of the clinical phenotypes discussed in this chapter. In addition, new techniques such as comparative genomic hybridization (CGH) (Kallioniemi et al., 1992), M-FISH (Uhrig et al., 1999) and spectral karyotyping (SKY) (Schrock et al., 1996) are beginning to make their way into clinical laboratories. We anticipate that the next decade will be one of vastly increased understanding of the mechanisms of genomic rearrangements. The fruits of the human genome project will provide increased understanding of the clinical consequences of deletions and duplications of specific chromosomal regions.

Translocations

CYTOGENETICALLY BALANCED TRANSLOCATIONS

Homologous chromosomes are chromosomes that have very similar nucleotide sequences and pair with each other during meiosis, (e.g., the two 1's in a human cell; one maternally inherited and one paternally inherited are homologues). A translocation results from exchange of chromosomal segments between non-homologous chromosomes. If the transfer of genetic information between the two chromosomes appears to be complete, and is not associated with a loss of material, the translocation is reciprocal and balanced. Robertsonian translocations (discussed below) are a special case, being technically associated with a loss of genetic material, but generally not associated with phenotypic abnormalities. Translocations can be inherited (familial) or de novo (newly occurring).

Balanced translocations occur in approximately 1 in 500 individuals (Van Dyke et al., 1983; Hook et al. 1984). The majority of balanced translocation carriers do not have any associated clinical problems except decreased fertility and the risk of abnormalities to their offspring as a result of malsegregation of the translocation (discussed below). However, there is evidence that the frequency of apparently balanced translocation, particularly *de novo* rearrangements, is higher in the mentally retarded population than it is in the newborn population (Fryns et al., 1986, Jacobs, 1974, Funderburk et al., 1977). To estimate the frequency of abnormalities among carriers of reciprocal translocations, Warburton analyzed data on 163 children with de novo reciprocal translocations that had been ascertained at amniocentesis. Six percent were found to have a significant congenital anomaly (Warburton et al., 1991). Clearly, some apparently balanced translocations are not benign. In some cases, balanced translocation carriers manifest features of a recognizable, dominant genetic disease. It has been demonstrated that this occurs because the breakpoint on one of the involved chromosomes disrupts the disease locus. There are several autosomal dominant and X-linked diseases which, in rare cases, have been caused by balanced translocation. These include Duchenne muscular dystrophy (Ray et al., 1985), neurofibromatosis 1 (Wallace et al., 1990), supravalvular aortic stenosis (Morris et al., 1993), aniridia (Davis et al., 1988) and Alagille syndrome (Spinner et al., 1994) among others. Another explanation for the association of congenital anomalies and apparently balanced reciprocal translocations is that the presence of a balanced rearrangement in a parent may be a pre-disposing factor for uniparental disomy in offspring. This is discussed in some detail in a later section of this chapter.

CYTOGENETICALLY CRYPTIC TRANSLOCATIONS

Cryptic translocations are those which involve exchange of segments that are either so small or which are cytogenetically so similar in appearance that they would not be identified reliably by G-band analysis at the 400–550 band stage of cytogenetic resolution. Most often they involve the exchange of telomeres (ends) of chromosomes. Many cryptic translocations have been identified because a patient presented with a phenotype suggestive of a deletion or duplication syndrome in the presence of apparently normal chromosomes. They are usually identified by molecular or molecular cytogenetic techniques after initial cytogenetic studies reveal an apparently normal karyotype (Ledbetter, 1992). Studies have been carried out to investigate the frequency of cryptic rearrangements in series of patients with normal karyotypes. Flint et al. (1995) found cryptic rearrangements in 3/99 individuals with idiopathic mental retardation. They searched for evidence of abnormal inheritance of 28 highly polymorphic probes located near chromosome ends. Using a combination of molecular and molecular cytogenetic techniques they identified cryptic chromosome rearrangements in three individuals (Flint et al., 1995). In another study, 2/20 individuals with mental retardation and dysmorphic features, with a normal karyotype, were found to have cryptic rearrangements using a multiplex FISH assay (Uhrig et al., 1999). Multiplex FISH (M-FISH) is a technique that permits visualization of each of the 24 different human chromosomes in a unique color using a combination of probes. There are numerous examples in the literature of cryptic translocations in patients with features of well-studied clinical syndromes including Wolf-Hirschhorn (Altherr et al., 1991), cri-du-chat (Overhauser et al., 1989), Miller-Dieker syndrome (Kuwano et al., 1991) and Down syndrome (Scott et al., 1995). Some of these cases are discussed in more detail later in this chapter.

ROBERTSONIAN TRANSLOCATIONS

These are a specific class of translocation in which two acrocentric chromosomes fuse at their centric ends (Robertson, 1916). In humans, 13,14,15,21, and 22 are acrocentric chromosomes and there are numerous examples of Robertsonian translocations involving each of them. Because chromosomal translocation is assessed by counting the number of centromeres in a metaphase spread, individuals with a Robertsonian translocation have 45 chromosomes. The small reciprocal product which contains the remnants of the short arms of the two fused chromosomes is usually lost. The short arms of all of the acrocentric chromosomes contain numerous duplicated copies of the genes which code for ribosomal RNA. Therefore, the loss of the short arms of two acrocentric chromosomes is not deleterious and individuals with this type of rearrangement are generally phenotypically normal. Certain Robertsonian translocation carriers may, however, be at increased risk for having children with abnormalities either due to mal-segregation of the translocation chromosome, or as a consequence of their increased risk for having offspring with uniparental disomy.

Consequences of and counseling for reciprocal translocations

Carriers of balanced translocations are subject to increased risk of abnormal chromosomal segregation during meiosis. The consequences include infertility, multiple pregnancy losses and liveborn abnormal offspring with multiple congenital malformations as a result of chromosomal imbalance.

During meiosis, homologous chromosomes pair to form a synaptonemal complex. When there is a balanced translocation, all four homologues (the two involved and the two non-involved chromosomes) pair to produce a quadrivalent configuration (Fig. 46.1). Normal gamete formation relies upon the segregation of alternating centromeres into two daughter cells (i.e. chromosome A with C and B with D). Thus, alternate segregation produces either a normal gamete (AC), or a gamete containing both partners of the balanced translocation (BD). However, if adjacent centromeres segregate together, A with D and B with C (adja-

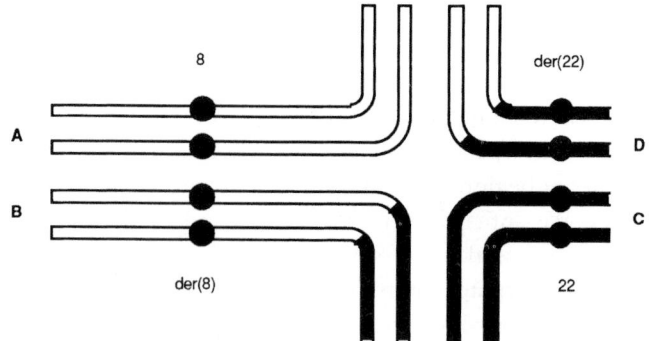

Fig. 46.1. Pachytene diagram of a hypothetical translocation between chromosomes 8q and 22q. The normal chromosome 8 is labeled as A, the der(8) as B, the normal 22 as C and the der(22) as D. As indicated in the text, segregation of A with C or B with D produces a balanced complement in daughter cells whereas A with B or D; or C with B or D produces an unbalanced complement.

cent I) or A with B and C with D (adjacent II), this results in production of chromosomally unbalanced gametes. If a gamete containing abnormal adjacent segregants is fertilized by a normal gamete from the non-translocation carrier parent, this results in a zygote with partial trisomy (duplication) and partial monosomy (deletion) for the relevant portions of the involved chromosomes. In some cases the imbalance is so severe that it results in miscarriage before a pregnancy is recognized. Clinically, these early pregnancy losses can present as infertility. For couples in which one partner has a balanced translocation, these abnormal segregations lead to recurrent miscarriages, stillborn offspring or liveborn offspring with multiple congenital abnormalities occur. Pregnancy outcome is related to the size and genetic composition of the rearranged portions of the chromosomes.

Most balanced rearrangements are unique (i.e., they are only observed within a given pedigree) so it is not easy to provide precise risk figures for each of the outcomes. Studies of segregation outcomes, for many balanced translocations, suggest that the risk to a balanced translocation carrier for producing a chromosomally abnormal offspring varies according to the manner in which the translocation was initially ascertained.

If an individual was ascertained because of the birth of a chromosomally abnormal live born child, then it is known that at least one of the unbalanced karyotypes is compatible with life, such that the risk for a subsequent abnormal child is high (5% to 30% by empirical data) with a significant risk for miscarriage or stillbirth (Neri et al., 1983; Daniel et al., 1986; Hook and Cross 1987). In the cases where the balanced carriers were ascertained in an unbiased fashion (for example, newborn screening studies) the risk for a chromosomally unbalanced child is lower (1–5%) with a significant risk for miscarriage or stillbirth (Ferguson-Smith, 1983). Clearly, in this latter group there are many reciprocal translocations whose unbalanced products result in a phenotype that is severe enough to be incompatible with life.

Counseling for Robertsonian translocations

As with reciprocal translocation carriers, there is a risk to carriers of Robertsonian translocations for producing unbalanced offspring. Clinically, the most significant is for carriers of a Robertsonian translocation that involves chromosome 21. These individuals are at risk for producing a child with Down syndrome. Female carriers have about a 15% risk for a liveborn child with Down syndrome and male carriers have a much lower risk (about 1–2%) (Ferguson-Smith, 1983). Four percent of Down syndrome patients have 46 chromosomes, one of which is a Robertsonian translocation involving chromosome 21. The translocation is familial (inherited) in 25% of these patients and de novo in 75% (Gardner and Sutherland, 1989). Theoretically, carriers of Robertsonian translocations involving chromosome 13 could produce offspring with trisomy 13 (Patau's syndrome), but this is rarely observed. Robertsonian translocation carriers are at increased risk for spontaneous abortions (Neri et al., 1983) and there has been an association observed between Robertsonian translocations and male infertility (Luciani et al., 1987).

Robertsonian translocations between homologous chromosomes (e.g., 21;21 or 13;13) pose unique problems, since carriers of these are rearrangements cannot produce any normal gametes.

Robertsonian translocations, uniparental disomy and disease

Uniparental disomy (UPD) is the inheritance of a pair of chromosomes (or a portion of a pair) from only one parent (Engel, 1980). UPD is sometimes associated with clinical abnormalities and this can occur by two mechanisms. The first is the inheritance of two copies of one homologue from a parent (parental *iso*disomy) on which there is a mutant allele for a recessive disorder. Duplication of a single deleterious recessive allele will cause the disease, even though only one parent is a disease carrier. Uniparental disomy is most easily identified by the study of polymorphic loci, which reveals failure to inherit an allele from one parent, and a pattern consistent with the presence of two alleles from the other parent. This has been observed for cystic fibrosis (Spence et al., 1988; Voss et al., 1989) and Bloom syndrome (Woodage et al., 1994) and has been hypothesized to account for disease

in a patient with spinal muscular atrophy (Brzustowicz et al., 1994). The second mechanism, is the uniparental inheritance of a region of the genome containing an imprinted gene. Imprinted genes are differentially expressed depending on whether they are inherited from the male or female parent (Hall, 1990). In this case, the two uniparental chromosomes can represent both homologues (parental *hetero*disomy, refers to the presence of both homologues from one parent) or there can be uniparental *iso*disomy. The best studied examples of this phenomenon in humans are the Prader-Willi and Angelman syndromes. Both of these disorders can be associated with loss of genetic material from 15q11q13 by deletion. *Maternal* uniparental disomy for 15q11q13 leads to the Prader-Willi syndrome, while *paternal* uniparental disomy for this same region leads to Angelman syndrome, a clinically distinct syndrome (Malcolm et al., 1991; Nicholls et al., 1989a, b). In other words, absence of paternally derived sequences from 15q11q13 causes Prader-Willi syndrome, whether the loss is the result of deletion of the paternally derived chromosome, or failure to inherit a paternal chromosome with concomitant duplication of the maternal chromosome. Likewise, absence of maternally derived sequences from 15q11q13 by either mechanism causes Angelman syndrome. Another disorder in which uniparental disomy plays a significant and consistent role is the Silver-Russell syndrome. In this disorder, characterized by pre- and postnatal growth retardation, triangular facies, and facial limb or truncal asymmetry, maternal uniparental disomy for chromosome 7 is seen in about 10% of cases (Kotzot et al., 1995). In this case, there is evidence that the phenotype is due to an imprinted gene, as there are no consistently isodisomic areas found in five patients with this disorder (Preece et al., 1999). It was also demonstrated that duplication of maternal genes within 7p11.2–p13 is associated with this disorder. Therefore, Silver-Russell syndrome appears to be caused by extra copies of maternal genes rather than by loss of a paternally imprinted gene (Monk et al., 2000).

An association has been observed between uniparental disomy and inherited or de novo Robertsonian translocations. Malsegregation of familial Robertsonian translocations has resulted in uniparental disomy for one of the chromosomes involved in the translocation in multiple cases (UPD for chromosome 13; Slater et al., 1994; UPD for chromosome 14: Temple et al., 1991; Wang et al. 1991; UPD for chromosome 15: Smith et al., 1993). Uniparental disomy has also been observed in association with *de novo* Robertsonian translocations (chromosome 14: Antonarakis et al., 1993; Healey et al., 1994; chromosome 15: Freeman et al., 1993; chromosome 21: Blouin et al., 1993; chromosome 22: Schinzel et al., 1994).

Among the acrocentric chromosomes, UPD for chromosomes 13, 21 or 22 does not appear to be associated with phenotypic abnormalities, while UPD for chromosome 15 is associated with Prader-Willi or Angelman syndromes and UPD for chromosome 14 has been associated with multiple abnormalities.

Knowledge of the frequency of uniparental disomy in normal individuals and in individuals with abnormal phenotypes is incomplete. A survey undertaken to determine the frequency of uniparental disomy among 18 first trimester spontaneous abortions revealed that all demonstrated biparental inheritance for each of the chromosomes (Shaffer et al., 1998).

t(11;22) SYNDROME (Fig. 46.2)

The t(11;22)(q23;q11.2) is the only recurrent, non-Robertsonian, constitutional translocation seen in humans (Fraccaro, et al., 1980; Zackai and Emanuel, 1980; Iselius et al., 1983). Several hundred families with this rearrangement have been described. The translocation appears to be independent of environmental factors and is estimated to have a low rate of mutation based on the paucity of de novo cases.

Clinical presentation and cytogenetics

Carriers of the constitutional t(11;22) are phenotypically normal, but come to attention subsequent to the birth of abnormal offspring with the der(22) as a supernumerary chromosome [47, XX or XY, +der(22)t(11;22)] or upon being treated for infertility. It has been observed that in multiple unrelated families the breakpoints on both chromosomes 11 and 22 are tightly clustered (Edelmann et al. 1999; Shaikh et al., 1999). Further, similar breakpoints in several families have been identified within AT-rich repeat regions on chromosomes 11q23 and 22q11, suggestive of genomic instability as the mechanism mediating the rearrangement (Kurahashi et al., 2000).

Only one type of unbalanced karyotype is seen in association with this translocation, 47, XX(Y), +der(22)t(11;22)(q11.2;q23). Presumably, unbalanced karyotypes with 46 chromosomes and the der(11) or the der(22) are non viable. The syndrome associated with the presence of a supernumerary chromosome in the proband is designated the supernumerary der(22)t(11;22) syndrome (+der(22) syndrome). (The phenotype of individuals with the der(22) is discussed later in this chapter along with other examples of segmental duplication.) The minimal overall recurrence risk for producing unbalanced offspring is estimated to be 2%. The risk could be as high as 5.6%, if one includes the non-karyotyped stillborn children who were reported as malformed (Iselius, 1983). The abortion frequency is 27%. There is apparently no difference in the risk to male versus female carriers but there appears to be an excess of female balanced carriers among the phenotypically normal offspring of females with the t(11;22).

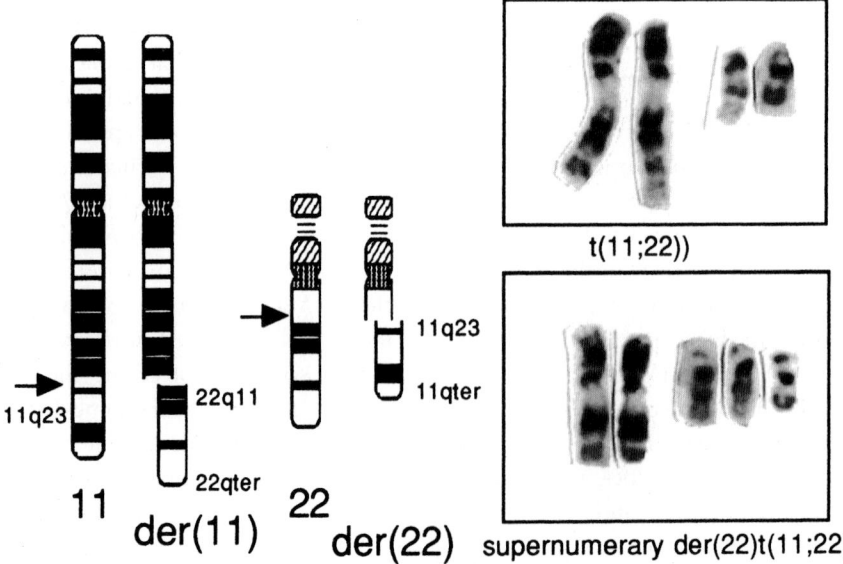

Fig. 46.2. Ideogram and partial karyotype demonstrating the reciprocal t(11;22). The upper box indicates the partial karyotype for chromosomes 11 and 22 of a balanced carrier, with the derivative chromosome of each pair on the right. The lower box shows the composition of an unbalanced proband with the supernumerary der(22). (This figure and all subsequent cytogenetic figures were prepared with the help of Tammy Grov).

Deletion

Loss, or deletion of a chromosomal segment results in an individual having only one copy of a portion of the genome. This leads to hemizygosity or haploinsuffiency for several or many loci. A deletion may be terminal (at the end of the chromosome) or it may be interstitial (within the chromosome). The clinical consequences depend on the size of the deleted segment and the number and function of the genes that it contains. Deletions can either occur de novo or they can be inherited from a parent with a deletion. Alternatively they can occur as a result of malsegregation of a parental balanced translocation. Such translocation-mediated deletions are generally accompanied by partial trisomy of another chromosomal region, resulting in partial duplication accompanying the deletion. There have been isolated reports of deletions of many regions of the genome. However, there are several regions that have been found to be deleted in multiple patients so that a clinical syndrome has been clearly established. The best known of these are the 4p- (Wolf-Hirschhorn) and 5p- (cri-du-chat) syndromes.

In addition to deletions which are easily detected cytogenetically because of their size, high resolution banding and molecular cytogenetic techniques have led to the identification of deletions that are too small to be seen in standard metaphase chromosome preparations. These combined molecular and cytogenetic analyses have led to the identification of small deletions in a percentage of patients with a number of clinically recognizable syndromes. Prader-Willi, Angelman, DiGeorge, velo-cardio-facial, and Miller-Dieker syndromes are the best studied of these disorders. The proportion of patients who demonstrate visible cytogenetic deletions ranges from about 20–30% for DiGeorge and velo-cardio-facial syndromes to over 50% for Prader-Willi, Angelman and Miller-Dieker syndromes. These disorders have been referred to as "contiguous gene deletion syndromes" (Schmickel, 1986). It has been presumed that the commonly deleted chromosomal regions associated with each of the respective syndromes contains numerous genes. It is hypothesized that clinical features result from deletion of several different genes that happen to lie in proximity to one another in the same chromosomal region. While only a proportion of patients with these disorders demonstrate cytogenetically visible deletions, molecular-cytogenetic studies frequently reveal sub-microscopic deletions.

Other disorders have been thought to demonstrate features of contiguous gene deletion syndromes. These include the Langer-Gideon (8q deletions) and WAGR (Wilms tumor, anirida, genital abnormalities and retardation) (11p deletions) syndromes (Schmickel 1986), Alagille syndrome (20p deletions) (Schnittger et al., 1989), Rubinstein-Taybi syndrome (16p deletions) (Breuning et al., 1993), Williams syndrome (7q deletions) (Ewart et al., 1993), and Smith-Magenis syndrome (17p deletions) (Smith et al., 1986). Clinically, these disorders are characterized by abnormalities in multiple systems and each of them has been associated with cytogenetic or molecular deletions in a percentage of patients. In recent years, a few of these disorders have been shown to be caused by the loss of a single gene (e.g., Alagille and Rubenstein-Taybi syndromes). Even for these disorders thought to be caused by loss of multiple genes, it is unlikely that all of the genes that map within the consistently deleted segment in these disorders play an important role in the causation of the major features of the phenotype. Thus, it might be more appropriate to refer to these disorders as microdeletion syndromes or as segmentally aneusomic disorders. Segmental aneusomy refers to a condition in which numerous contiguous genes could have abnormal dosage as a result of a cytogenetic abnormality (or imprinting effect) amongst which a smaller number of genes contribute to the cardinal features of the phenotype. Some of these disorders might in actuality be caused by a single gene which will ultimately be determined when all the genes in the commonly deleted region are identified and analyzed.

One of the most challenging tasks in human clinical cytogenetics is the identification of cytogenetically undetectable microdeletions in association with phenotypic features of known deletion syndromes. Analysis of small deletions of human chromosomes is best approached by using fluorescence in situ hybridization and hybridizing with probes that are targeted to the critical region responsible for the syndrome.

WOLF-HIRSCHHORN SYNDROME (4p-)

Partial monosomy of the short arm of chromosome 4 is associated with a clinically distinct syndrome characterized by recognizable facial dysmorphism in combination with marked growth retardation of pre-natal onset and severe mental deficiency (Hirschhorn et al., 1965; Wolf et al., 1965; Lurie et al., 1980 and Wilson et al., 1981). The true incidence of this syndrome is not known. It was estimated as 1 in 50,000 by Goodman and Gorlin (1983) and in a study of 27,472 newborns at a large maternity hospital in Japan, 1 patient was identified (Higurashi et al., 1990). This could be an underestimate as it does not account for patients with submicroscopic deletions.

Clinical presentation

The distinctive face has been called the "Greek helmet" facies, characterized by frontal bossing with a high frontal hairline; prominent glabella, ocular hypertelorism; proptosis due to hypoplasia of the orbital ridges; slanted palpebral fissures and epicanthal folds; a broad and beaked nose with a large, prominent bridge and shallow septum (Fig. 46.3). Strabismus is common. Ears are low-set, large, and simple, commonly with pre-auricular pits or tags. The mouth is downturned, with a short upper lip and philtrum; micrognathia is present. Closure defects are common including cleft lip and/or palate in about 15% of patients, coloboma of the iris, cardiac septal defects (present in more than 50% of patients and a leading cause of mortality); and genital anomalies such as hypospadias, scrotal hypoplasia, cryptorchidism or testicular hypoplasia.

Mental deficiency is usually severe, with IQs below 20. Seizures are frequent and usually begin within the first two years of life. Postnatal mortality is high, with at least one-third of patients dying during the first year of life. Heart disease and a high susceptibility to infection are frequently the cause of death.

Cytogenetics

The Wolf-Hirschhorn syndrome (WHS) is caused by partial deletion of the short arm of chromosome 4 (4p-). The critical region for development of this disorder is located within band 4p16.3 (Gandelman et al., 1992) (Fig. 46.4).

Approximately 85–90% of cases result from de novo deletions and 10–15% result from translocations (Lurie et al., 1980). The size of the deleted region can very greatly between patients, although such variations do not apparently result in significant differences in phenotype, suggesting that there are relatively few genes responsible for the major characteristics of this syndrome (Wilson et al., 1981).

Molecular cytogenetics

A number of patients have been described with very subtle translocations and deletions. In many of these cases, cytogenetic studies were normal, but a small deletion within 4p16 was detectable by molecular analysis. Sub-microscopic deletions have been detected by Southern blotting (Altherr et al., 1991), PCR (Altherr et al., 1992) and fluorescence in situ hybridization (FISH) (Gandelman et al., 1992). Many clinical cytogenetics laboratories are currently offering molecular cytogenetic diagnosis of this disorder using FISH. Definitive phenotypic features of the Wolf-Hirschhorn syndrome, in the presence of normal chromosomes, warrant molecular investigation of the patient. If a submicroscopic deletion is detected, analysis of parental chromosomes by molecular cytogenetic techniques is of primary importance, because one of the parents could carry a cryptic translocation. If this is the case, prenatal diagnosis for future pregnancies could be offered.

Analysis of the deletions seen in patients with WHS has lead to the identification of a 165 kb critical region within

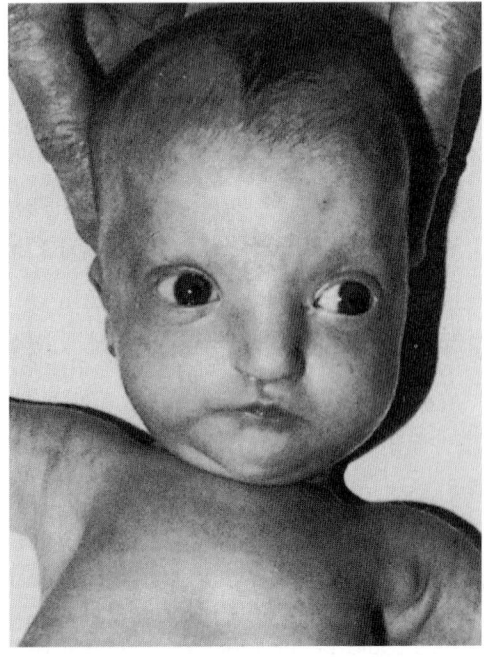
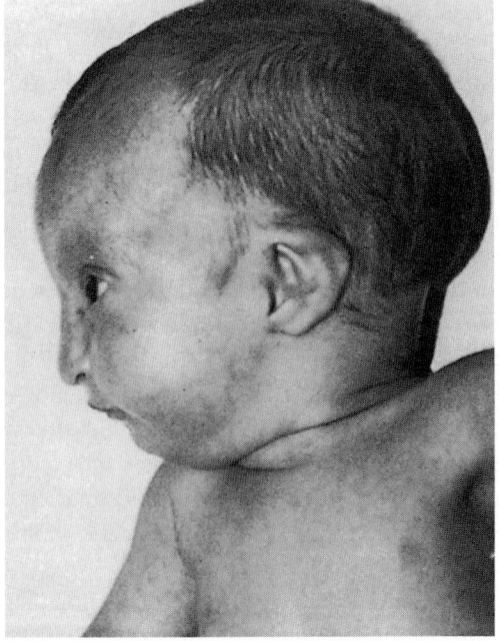

Fig. 46.3. Patient with 4p monosomy.

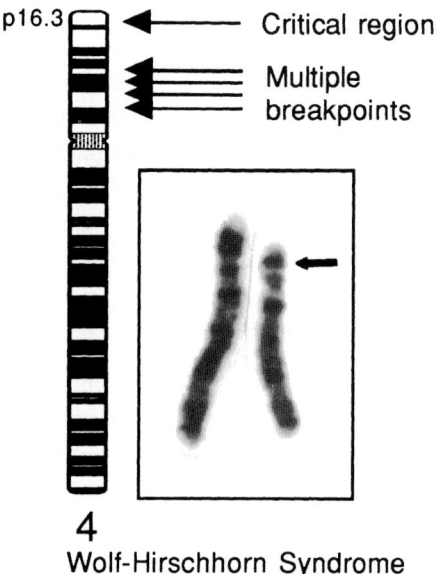

4
Wolf-Hirschhorn Syndrome

p16.3 ← Critical region
← Multiple
breakpoints

Fig. 46.4. Ideogram and partial karyotype of chromosome 4 showing the critical region and various reported breakpoints in a patient with Wolf-Hirschhorn syndrome.

4p16.3 (Wright et al., 1998). At least nine independent transcription units (putative genes) have been identified within this region. Characterization of these genes is currently underway with the ultimate goal of determining which of the genes in this region contribute to the phenotype when present in only one copy (Wright et al., 1999; Stec et al., 1998).

Submicroscopic deletions of 4p16.3 have also been found in patients with the Pitt-Rogers-Danks syndrome. This disorder demonstrates phenotypic overlap with Wolf-Hirschhorn syndrome and it has been proposed that Pitt-Rogers-Danks may represent a milder form of the Wolf-Hirschhorn syndrome (Clemens et al., 1996; Lindeman-Kusse et al., 1996). The Pitt-Rogers-Danks syndrome is characterized by pre- and postnatal growth retardation, microcephaly, ocular proptosis, mid face hypoplasia, short and flat philtrum, wide mouth and history of seizures (Pitt et al., 1984). The original chromosome studies on patients with this disorder were interpreted as normal, but subsequent molecular cytogenetic analysis revealed submicroscopic deletions involving 4p16.3. The critical regions for the deletions in WHS and the Pitt-Rogers-Danks syndromes have been shown to be overlapping (Wright et al., 1998).

CRI-DU-CHAT SYNDROME (5p-)

Partial deletion of the short arm of chromosome 5 results in the cri-du-chat syndrome. The syndrome is named because it is associated with a laryngeal defect, which causes

a distinctive cry resembling the mewing of a cat. The incidence has been reported to range from 1 in 15,000 to 1 in 50,000 newborns (Niebuhr 1978a; Higurashi et al., 1990). These figures could be underestimates as they do not take into account patients with smaller chromosomal deletions (discussed below).

Clinical presentation

Patients present in the newborn period with the characteristic cry and craniofacial dysmorphism consisting of microcephaly, a round (moon-like) face, hypertelorism, epicanthal folds and broad nasal bridge (Niebuhr, 1978a,b) (Fig. 46.5). Most patients demonstrate muscular hypotonia and strabismus is common. About one-third of patients demonstrate variable types of heart disease.

The cat-like cry disappears over the first year and development is severely delayed. Head control is attained at about one year, sitting occurs at two years and walking begins at four years. Speech development is particularly slow. Many

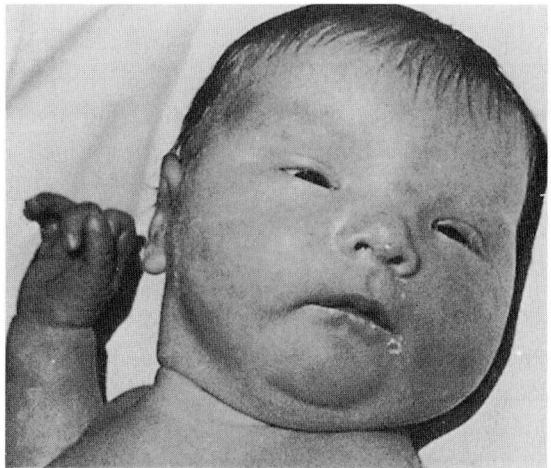

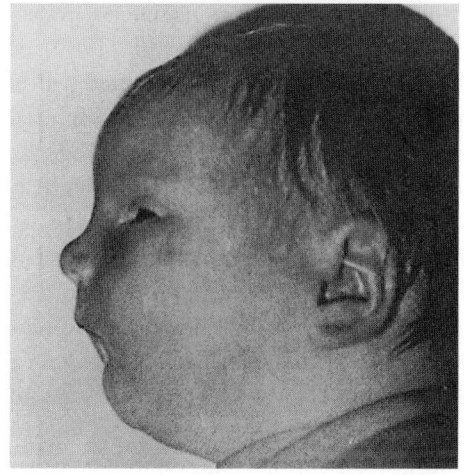

Fig. 46.5. Patient with cri-du-chat syndrome (5p monosomy).

patients with this disorder survive into adulthood and there is a report of a mentally retarded woman with the cri-du-chat syndrome who delivered a similarly affected daughter. Both individuals had an interstitial deletion of 5p (Martinez et al., 1993). Mental retardation is usually severe with IQs below 50 in infants and below 20 in adults. In a recent study of 50 individuals with an age range of one to 31 years (90% of patients below the age of 16), development was studied using the Vineland Adaptive Behavior Scales test. The range of IQs was from 20 to 75, with a mean of 35. Eighteen of the 50 individuals scored at the bottom of the scale (20). The previously reported trend of lower IQs in older patients was also seen in this study (Marinesc et al., 1999). It has been reported that early intensive programs of special education have been beneficial, resulting in social and psychomotor development at the level of five to six year old normal child (Wilkins et al., 1980).

Cytogenetics

As with the Wolf-Hirschhorn syndrome, 85–90% of cases result from de novo deletions, with 10–15% resulting from the malsegregation of a balanced translocation in one of the parents (Niebuhr, 1978b). The extent of deletion of 5p in patients with features of the cri-du-chat syndrome varies widely, but critical chromosomal regions for specific features of the syndrome have been identified (Fig. 46.6). The cat-cry phenotype maps within 5p15.3, while the facial features map proximally, within 5p15.2 (Gersh et al., 1995). There does not appear to be a consistent correlation between the size of the deletion and the level of developmental delay (Marinescu et al., 1999). Cri-du-chat patients with cryptic translocations have been reported. These have been found in individuals with features of the cri-du-chat syndrome, whose chromosomes appeared normal. Using molecular cytogenetic techniques, cryptic rearrangements involving 5p15 have been identified. Overhauser et al. (1989) described a family with three individuals who presented with features of the cri-du-chat syndrome (cat-like cry, microcephaly, epicanthic folds and failure to thrive). While cytogenetic studies revealed normal karyotypes, molecular studies demonstrated hemizygosity for multiple loci distal to 5p14. Five individuals within the family were identified as being balanced carriers of a translocation involving 5p14 and another region of the genome. Bernstein et al. (1993) reported identification of a cryptic translocation involving chromosomes 5 and 7 in the mother of an infant with the cri-du-chat syndrome. As for Wolf-Hirschhorn Syndrome, patients with features of cri-du-chat and normal chromosomes warrant further molecular analysis of the 5p15 critical region. Based on molecular

mapping studies, the critical region for cri-du-chat clinical features in combination with mental retardation spans approximately 4–5 Mb, and few genes have been identified within this region. The few identified genes are currently under study to determine the role they play in this disorder (Medina et al., 2000).

18p MONOSOMY

Clinical presentation

The pattern of abnormalities seen in patients with deletion of 18p may not be striking at birth, but becomes more evident by three years of age. Newborns have mild to moderate growth retardation (mean birth weight at the 5–10 centile). Affected neonates demonstrate brachycephaly, a broad face with ptosis of the upper lids, strabismus, hypertelorism, a broad nose, downturned corners of the mouth, micrognathia with a wide mouth and large protruding ears (Fig. 46.7). Teeth are irregularly set and are particularly prone to caries (Lurie and Lazjuk, 1972). Holoprosencephaly in varying severity is present in at least 10% of patients. Heart defects, primarily septal defects are seen in under 10% of patients. IQs range from 25 to 75 with an average of 45 to 50. Speech is particularly delayed and many patients do not speak before seven years. Prognosis is poor for patients with holoprosencephaly, but patients without this defect do not have a shortened life expectancy (Schinzel, 1984). There are reports of patients who have reproduced (Uchida et al. 1965).

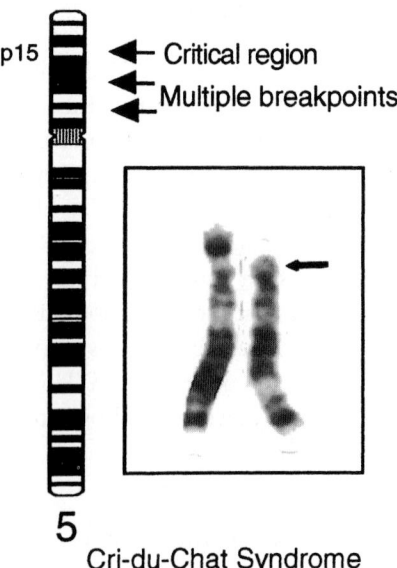

Fig. 46.6. Ideogram and partial karyotype of chromosome 5 showing the critical region and various reported breakpoints in patients with cri-du-chat syndrome.

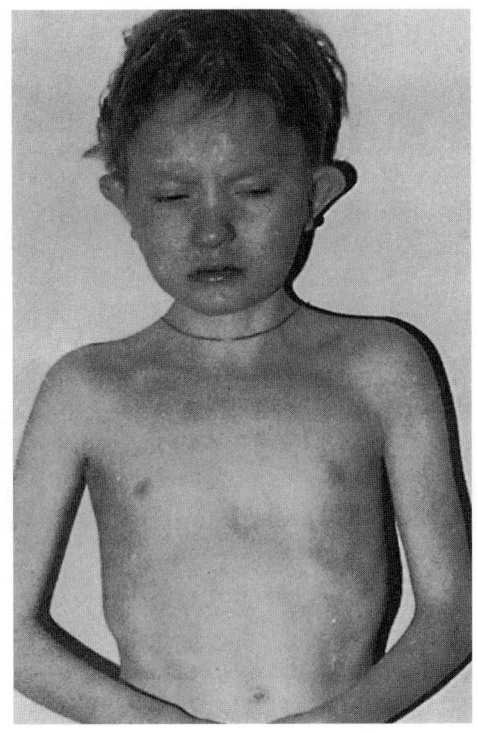
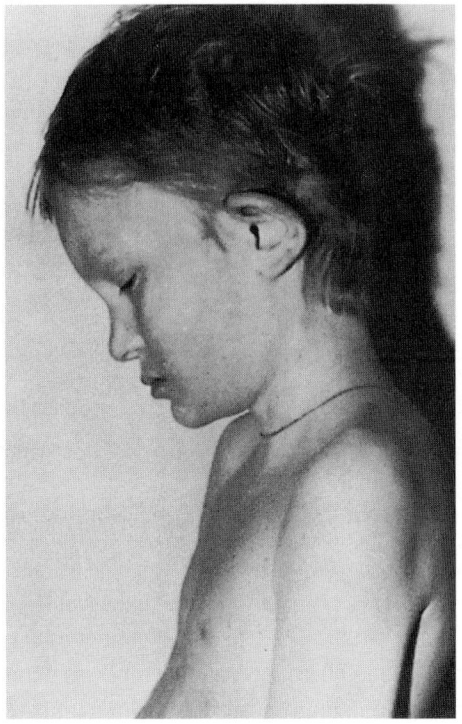

Fig. 46.7. Patient with 18p monosomy.

Cytogenetics

Most 18p- patients have a cytogenetically detectable deletion of almost the entire short arm of chromosome 18 (Fig 46.8). This deletion occurs de novo in about 85% of patients, with the remainder of 18p- individuals resulting from the segregation of familial rearrangements. With the availability of FISH probes for analysis of human subtelomeric regions, smaller deletions have been reported. Some have been the result of cryptic translocations involving other chromosome subtelomeric regions (Horsley et al., 1998).

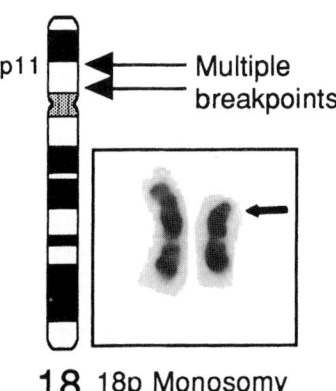

Fig. 46.8. Ideogram and partial karyotype of chromosome 18 showing the breakpoints in patients with 18p.

18q MONOSOMY

Clinical features

Partial deletion of the long arm of chromosome 18 leads to a recognizable syndrome distinguished by growth deficiency, facial dysmorphia, microcephaly, genitourinary malformations, necrologic abnormalities, developmental delay and mental retardation. Facial dysmorphia consists of mid face hypoplasia, deeply set eyes, short nose, and a "carp" mouth (large, open mouth with corners slanting downward, short upper lip, absent Cupid's bow) (Fig. 46.9). Ears are characteristic with prominent antitragus and antihelix. Atresia of the external auditory canal can be present and hearing loss has been noted. Fingers are long, thin and tapered with protuberant fingertips and toes are irregularly implanted and overriding. Both sexes demonstrate abnormal genitalia, with cryptorchidism and hypospadias in males and hypoplasia of the labia minora in females. Growth hormone insufficiency is a common cause of growth failure in 18q- individuals.

Necrologic findings have been found to include hypotonia, poor coordination, choreoathetotic movements and spinal muscular atrophy. Mental retardation is generally present, but varies from mild to severe. Patients have been reported with only learning disabilities (Weiss et al., 1991) although half of the patients have an IQ between 30 and 50. Life expectancy is apparently normal and many affected

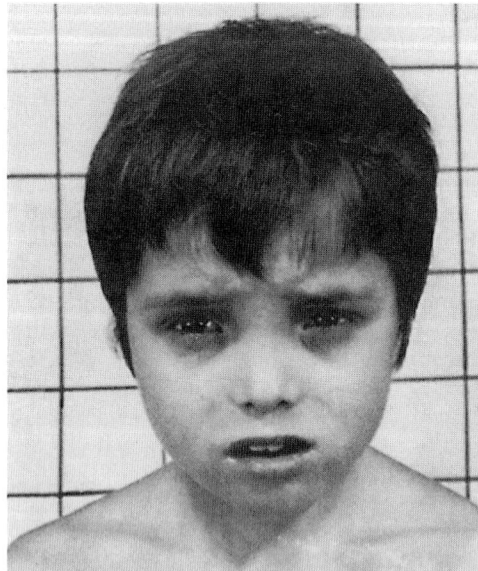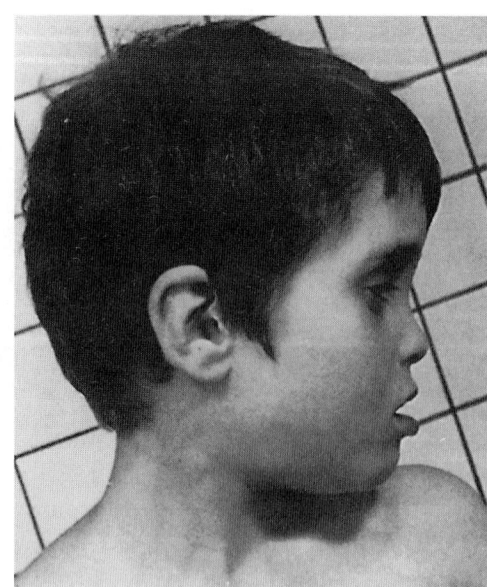

Fig. 46.9. Patient with 18q partial monosomy.

adults have been described. There are multiple reports of this chromosomal abnormality being transmitted from parent to child (Subrt and Pokorny, 1970; Fryns et al., 1979).

Cytogenetics

The breakpoint of the deletions on the long arm of chromosome 18 have been found to vary between 18q21 and 18q23 (Fig. 46.10). Seventy-five percent of patients have a de novo deletion, with the remainder resulting from familial rearrangements. Eighty-five percent of de novo deletions are paternal in origin with no evidence for a paternal age effect (Cody et al, 1997). Further, some of the deletions are interstitial deletions that retain the distal end of 18q or more complex cryptic rearrangements. These findings indicate that detailed cytogenetic characterization of the

deletion is relevant to phenotypic characterization and assignment of appropriate recurrence risks (Brkanac et al., 1998). In a molecular analysis of 7 patients with 18q deletions, Kline et al. (1993) demonstrated that the four individuals with the largest deletions demonstrated full blown features of the 18q- syndrome, with two of the four being more severely affected. Recent analysis of 42 subjects indicate that large deletions are associated with significantly decreased head circumference and the presence of anomalous or proximally placed thumbs (Cody et al., 1999). As a group, the smaller deletions produced milder phenotypes, but the smallest deletion did not have the mildest phenotype. Possible explanations for this might include differences in the precise genes that are missing from deletion to deletion, or variation in alleles on the normal chromosome 18 which may modify the effect of deletion on one chromosome. Further molecular definition and identification of the genes involved in deletions with different phenotypic effects will eventually lead to better understanding of the genotype-phenotype relationships in this region. Toward that end, a 2 Mb region has been delineated in the patients with growth hormone insufficiency (Cody et al., 1997). This region contains the genes for myelin basic protein and the galanin receptor, both of which are candidates for the growth hormone insufficiency phenotype.

CHROMOSOME 15 MICRODELETION SYNDROMES

There are two distinct disorders associated with small interstitial deletions of proximal chromosome 15q. These are

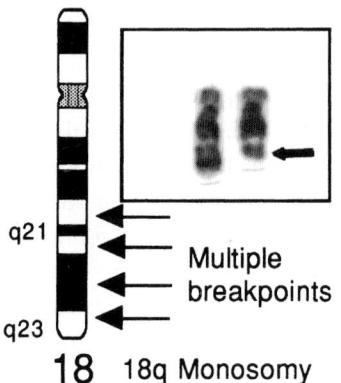

Fig. 46.10. Ideogram and partial karyotype of chromosome 18 showing breakpoints reported in patients with 18q.

the Prader-Willi and Angelman syndromes. The deleted regions in these two clinically distinct conditions are often overlapping, although it has been determined that Prader-Willi syndrome results when the deletion is on the paternally inherited chromosome, while Angelman syndrome results from deletion on the maternally derived chromosome. This unusual finding demonstrates the importance of imprinting in the etiology of human disease. Recent work has greatly refined the regions involved in the deletions in these two disorders, and demonstrated that there is unusual heterogeneity in the mechanisms leading to loss of maternally imprinted genes that cause Angelman syndrome, and loss of paternally imprinted genes causing Prader-Willi syndrome. These mechanisms include deletion, uniparental disomy, gene mutation and imprinting center defects, and will be discussed in more depth below.

PRADER-WILLI SYNDROME

Clinical presentation

Prader-Willi syndrome (PWS) is characterized by severe muscular hypotonia, poor suck and hypogonadism in the neonatal period. Decreased fetal activity has been documented and serves as a prenatal indication to pursue cytogenetic and molecular studies in the neonatal period. During the second year poor feeding is succeeded by hyperphagia leading to obesity (Fig. 46.11). PWS patients gain weight even when subjected to restricted diets. Patients have mild to moderate mental retardation, behavioral disorders and characteristic facial features including almond shaped eyes, narrow bitemporal diameter, upslanting palpebral fissures and strabismus. Additional clinical features include short stature, small hands and feet and in about 75% of patients, fair hair and skin color as compared to other family members. Adults frequently suffer from diabetes and cardiac disease, secondary to weight gain. Prader-Willi syndrome occurs with an estimated incidence of 1 in 10,000 to 1 in 20,000 live births (Cassidy, 1997).

Genetics and cytogenetics

The molecular mechanisms underlying the PWS are complex and consist of 1) chromosomal deletions (~70–75%); 2) maternal uniparental disomy (UPD) for chromosome 15 (20–25%), 3) abnormalities of imprinting (2–4%); and 4) balanced translocations involving 15q11q13 (<1%). A cytogenetic cause of Prader-Willi syndrome was first suggested by the finding of a few patients with translocations involving proximal 15q. These observations prompted high resolution

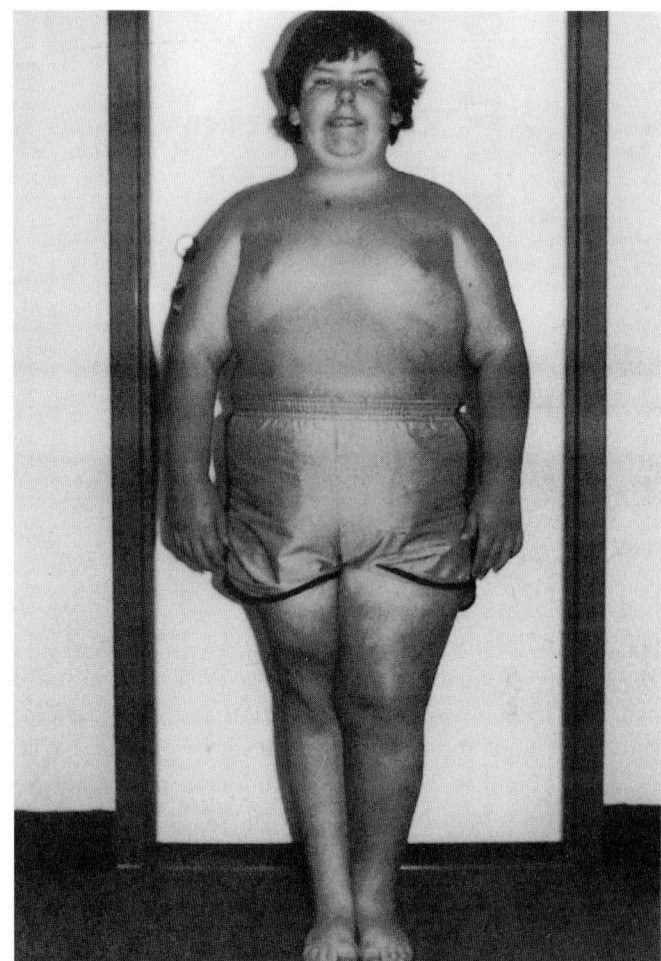

Fig. 46.11. Prader-Willi syndrome. An 11-year-old boy with typical facial appearance (narrow bifrontal diameter, almond-shaped eyes, and triangular mouth), small hands and feet, and characteristic obesity. (From Butler, 1990, with permission.)

cytogenetic studies of five Prader-Willi patients that demonstrated interstitial deletion of 15q11q13 in four out of the five (Ledbetter et al., 1981). Greater than 50–60% of patients have been found to have a cytogenetically visible deletion of 15q11q13 (Ledbetter et al., 1982; Butler et al., 1986) (Fig. 46.12). The majority are sporadic, de novo deletions, although there are a few patients with deletion secondary to familial translocation (Smeets et al., 1992). Molecular studies of patients with normal chromosomes has demonstrated that an additional 15% have a microdeletion of sequences from 15q11q13. In all Prader-Willi syndrome patients studied, the deletion of chromosome 15 occurs on the paternally inherited chromosome (Butler et al., 1986; Nicholls et al., 1989a, 1989b; Robinson et al., 1991). This unusual finding led to studies of the parental origin of chromosome 15q11q13 in chromosomally normal Prader-Willi syndrome patients. These studies demonstrated that a number of patients had

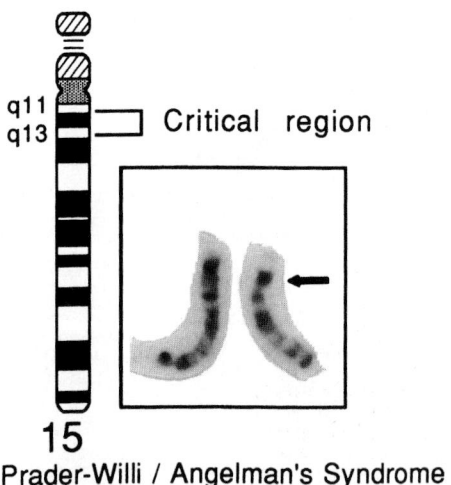

Critical region

15

Prader-Willi / Angelman's Syndrome

Fig. 46.12. Ideogram and partial karyotype of chromosome 15 demonstrating the interstitial deletion of chromosome 15 reported in patients with Prader-Willi and Angelman syndromes.

uniparental disomy for chromosome 15 (Mascari et al., 1992). Approximately 25% of Prader-Willi patients have maternal UPD. In addition to deletion and maternal uniparental disomy, there are other rare causes of Prader-Willi syndrome found in 2–5% of patients. These include abnormalities in the imprinting process, such that all paternally inherited genes are present, but the pattern of methylation and hence imprinting is abnormal (Ohta et al., 1999). Finally, a few patients have been identified who have apparently balanced translocations with no evidence for deletion (Schulze et al., 1996; Kuslich et al., 1999).

The combined data suggest that loss of the paternal 15q11q13 region, whether by deletion or maternal UPD, causes Prader-Willi syndrome. The common deletions in PWS encompass a 4 MB region, containing a number of paternally imprinted genes (Lee and Wevrick, 2000). While *SNRPN* (*s*mall *n*uclear *r*ibonucleoprotein *p*olypeptide N) has been a leading candidate for the PWS disease gene, it is not sufficient to cause the disease based on patients with interruption of *SNRPN* who do not demonstrate the full phenotype (Schulze et al., 1996). It is most likely that PWS is caused by loss of more than one gene. Besides *SNRPN*, there are 10 paternally expressed transcripts that have been identified in the critical region including a zinc finger gene (*ZNF127*), *NECDIN* (a gene shown to be involved in neural differentiation) and *IPW* (an RNA transcript not known to encode a protein) (Lee and Wevrick, 2000).

Diagnosis of PWS can be carried out by a combination of molecular and/or cytogenetic studies. Parent specific imprinting can be detected at the DNA level by examination of the methylation pattern of specific regions of DNA. This fact has been exploited to develop diagnostic assays for PWS.

DNA-based testing to detect maternal or paternal patterns of methylation will currently detect 99% of PWS patients (i.e., those due to deletion, UPD or imprinting center mutations). If a maternal only pattern of methylation is revealed, the diagnosis of PWS can be confirmed, but further studies are needed to determine the molecular class of the mutation (deletion, UPD or imprinting center mutation). FISH, using the *SNRPN* probe, is most commonly used to detect deletions and standard cytogenetic analysis is necessary to rule out a translocation. UPD can be confirmed by analysis of the inheritance of chromosome 15 markers.

Recurrence risks for PWS vary with the molecular mechanism identified. Recurrence is low in the case of de novo deletions and uniparental disomy. However, multiple familial cases have been identified in which there is an imprinting center defect (Ohta et al., 1999) or balanced chromosomal rearrangement (Hulten et al., 1991, Smeets et al., 1992).

ANGELMAN SYNDROME

Clinical Presentation

Features of Angelman syndrome include severe motor and intellectual retardation, a puppet-like ataxic gait, hypotonia, epilepsy, absence of speech, microcephaly and unusual facies consisting of a large mandible and open mouth expression with the tongue revealed (Fig.46.13). Patients are reported to have a happy disposition and demonstrate excessive, inappropriate laughter. There are characteristic EEG changes and abnormal choroidal pigmentation. The combination of excessive laughter and jerky movements led to the term "happy puppet syndrome", which has fallen out of favor. Its frequency of occurrence is estimated at 1 in 15,000.

Cytogenetics and molecular genetics

Like the Prader-Willi syndrome, the genetic etiology of Angelman syndrome is very complex. Approximately 60% of patients with Angelman syndrome have a cytogenetically detectable deletion of 15q11q13 that is similar to that seen in association with the Prader-Willi syndrome (Fig. 46.12). Another 10–15% have a normal karyotype, but a submicroscopic deletion is detectable by FISH (Hamabe et al., 1991). At the molecular level, the PWS and AS deletions are distinct, although closely linked. The deletions in Angelman patients have been found to be exclusively of maternal origin and consistent with this, 3–5% of patients have been found to have paternal uniparental disomy. In 1994, the *UBE3A* gene (E6–AP ubiquitin-protein ligase) was mapped to 15q11q13 within the deletion critical

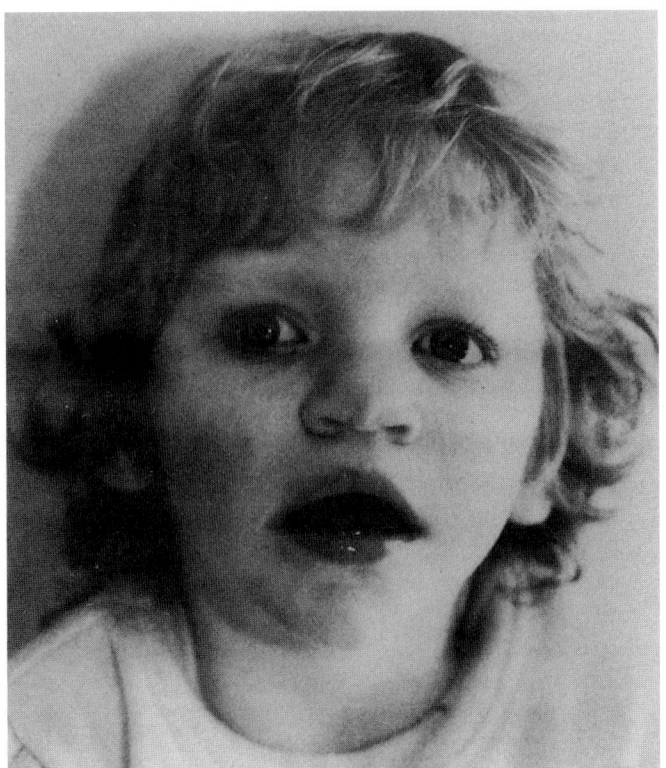

Fig. 46.13. Angelman syndrome. A 29-month-old girl with characteristic facial features apparent hypertelorism, prominent nasal tip, anteverted nares, large mouth, and prognathism. (Courtesy of Elaine Zackai, MD, and Donna McDonald-McGinn, MS, The Children's Hospital of Philadelphia, PA.)

region for Angelman syndrome. Initial studies of gene expression in lymphoblastoid and fibroblast cell lines indicated that the gene is not imprinted in these tissues, and *UBE3A* was therefore not considered a good candidate gene for Angelman syndrome (Nakao et al., 1994). However, further studies demonstrated that *UBE3A* is imprinted in some parts of the brain and, therefore, maternally inherited mutations would be expected to result in phenotypic abnormalities, consistent with findings in Angelman syndrome. Subsequent studies have shown that 4–6% of Angelman patients have mutations in *UBE3A*, and these mutations have been found to account for a significant proportion of familial cases (Jiang et al., 1999). The *UBE3A* gene functions to catalyze the transfer of ubiquitin to substrates which are then targeted for degradation by the proteasome. This is the first member of the ubiquitination pathway to be implicated in a genetic disease; however, the mechanism by which loss of function of *UBE3A* leads to Angelman syndrome is not understood. As in the Prader-Willi syndrome, there is also a class of Angelman patients (4–6%) who have imprinting mutations. That is, there is a defect in the imprinting center such that the affected chro-

mosome is incapable of becoming appropriately imprinted. Failure to assume a maternal imprint results in lack of expression of genes that are only active when maternally expressed. In some cases, these mutations are caused by small deletions and, in other cases, the precise defect has not been identified (Jiang et al., 1999). In addition to all of the mechanisms of mutation leading to Angelman syndrome discussed above, there are still 10–14% of patients in whom no molecular defect has yet been found.

The most straightforward diagnostic test for Angelman syndrome is analysis of methylation status which can detect all cases except those caused by mutations in the *UBE3A* gene. If methylation analysis is shown to be abnormal, the molecular class of the abnormality can be determined in order to provide accurate counseling information (low recurrence for large deletions and UPD, higher for small deletions that affect the imprinting center). If methylation studies are normal, point mutations in the UBE3A gene can be investigated by mutation analysis.

THE CHROMOSOME 22 MICRODELETION SYNDROMES

Deletions of the proximal long arm of chromosome 22 are associated with two well-studied clinical syndromes, the DiGeorge syndrome and the velo-cardio-facial syndrome (Driscoll et al., 1992a,b). These two syndromes are distinct, but have a number of overlapping features. In addition, the same 22q11.2 deletion is also associated with conotruncal anomaly-face syndrome (Burn et al., 1993). Conotruncal anomaly face syndrome (CAFS) has striking similarities to DGS and VCFS and is characterized by the presence of conotruncal cardiac defects in association with a characteristic facial appearance. Cardiac defects are common to all three syndromes and studies have shown that there is a subgroup of patients identified at birth with conotruncal cardiac defects who also demonstrate deletions of 22q (Goldmuntz et al., 1993)

DIGEORGE SYNDROME

Clinical presentation

DiGeorge syndrome is characterized by the absence or hypoplasia of the thymus, and the parathyroid glands, cardiac malformations and dysmorphic facial features. Affected organs are derived from the embryonic third and fourth pharyngeal pouches and the syndrome is presumably a developmental defect of these structures. It is characterized by a variation in the severity of symptoms and a wide spectrum of involvement.

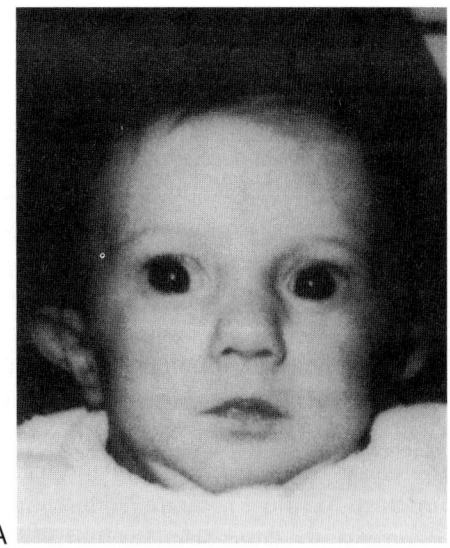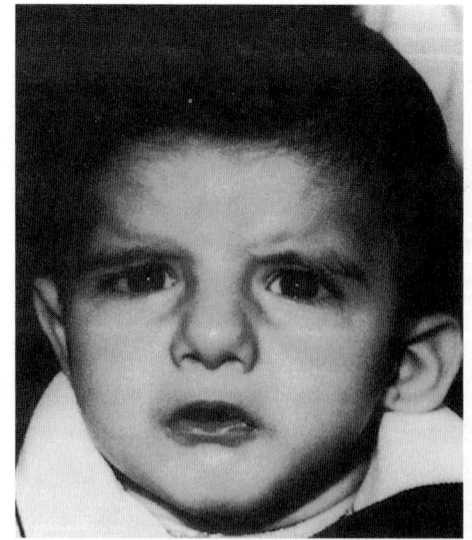

Fig. 46.14. DiGeorge syndrome. Two patients showing characteristic facies. (A) A three-month-old girl with a bulbous nasal tip, small mouth, and protuberant ears. (B) A six-month-old boy with a bulbous nasal tip, small mouth, and protuberant ears. (Courtesy of Elaine Zackai, MD. and Donna McDonald-McGinn, MS., The Children's Hospital of Philadelphia, PA.)

Absence or hypoplasia of the parathyroid glands may lead to hypocalcemia which presents as neonatal tetany or seizures. Hypoplasia of the thymus causes susceptibility to infection due to a deficit of T cells. The cardiac malformations include tetralogy of Fallot, interrupted aortic arch type B, truncus arteriosus, conoventricular septal defect, right sided aortic arch and aberrant right subclavian artery. Craniofacial dysmorphia can include: micrognathia, cleft palate, bifid uvula, low set ears and hypertelorism with short palpebral fissures (Fig. 46.14). Defects in other organ systems have been reported (DiGeorge, 1965; Robinson, 1975; Conley et al., 1979; Greenberg et al., 1988).

Genetics and cytogenetics

The etiology of DGS was originally presumed to be heterogeneous with reported cases demonstrating autosomal dominant, autosomal recessive, X-linked and chromosomal modes of inheritance (Lammer and Opitz, 1986). Today, it is accepted that the vast majority of DGS patients have a microdeletion of 22q11.2 (Fig. 46.15). Approximately 15–20% of patients with DGS have visible chromosomal abnormalities (Greenberg et al., 1988). The majority of these cytogenetically abnormal cases involve chromosome 22. These are either unbalanced translocations with monosomy 22pter→q11 (Back et al., 1980; Bowen et al. 1986; de la Chapelle et al. 1981; Faed et al. 1987; Kelley et al. 1982; Greenberg et al. 1984; 1988) or interstitial deletions, del(22)(q11.21q11.23) (Augusseau et al., 1986; Driscoll et al., 1992C; 1989;Greenberg et al.

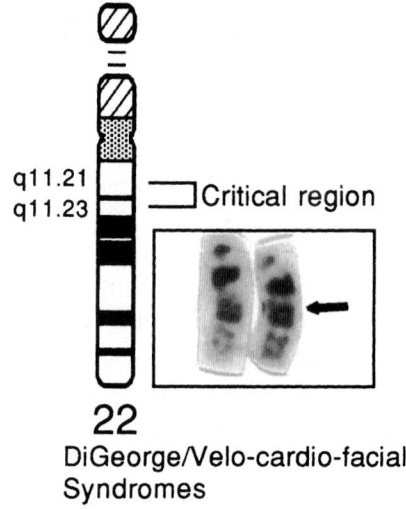

Fig. 46.15. Ideogram and partial karyotype of chromosome 22 demonstrating the interstitial deletion seen in patients with DiGeorge and velocardiofacial syndromes.

1988; Mascarello et al., Wilson et al., 1992a,b). Even with high resolution banding techniques, translocation-mediated or interstitial deletions are only observed in less than 25% of cases. However, since the DGS chromosomal region (DGCR) lies within 22q11.21–q11.23, DNA markers from within the commonly deleted region can be utilized for molecular diagnosis. Using molecular techniques (most often FISH or alternatively DNA dosage), deletions of 22q11 can be demonstrated in approximately 90% of patients (Driscoll et al, 1992a; Wilson et al., 1992a).

Although the majority of cases of DGS are now attributable to a 22q11 deletion, other chromosome defects have been seen in association with DGS, including 10p13 monosomy, and deletion of 18q21.33 (Greenberg et al., 1988, Monaco et al., 1991)

Additionally, there is evidence that teratogens and maternal diabetes are potential causes of DGS, especially in individuals without a 22q11 deletion. Wilson et al. (1993) reported on two infants with DGS and renal agenesis born to women with insulin dependent diabetes. In both cases, cytogenetic and molecular studies failed to detect a deletion within the DiGeorge chromosomal region (DGCR) in 22q11.2.

The cytogenetic management of a patient with DGS should include a standard karyotype to exclude all visible structural rearrangements followed by fluorescence in situ hybridization (FISH) with probes from within the most consistently deleted portion of the DGCR to detect submicroscopic deletions. In the case of a deletion-positive proband, parents should be screened to determine their carrier status.

VELOCARDIOFACIAL SYNDROME

Clinical presentation

Velocardiofacial syndrome (VCFS) is an autosomal dominant disorder in which patients manifest cleft palate, cardiac defects, speech and learning disabilities and a typical facial appearance (Fig 46.16) (Shprintzen et al., 1978; 1981; Williams et al., 1985). Some VCFS patients have phenotypic findings which overlap with features of DGS such as neonatal hypocalcemia and decreased lymphoid tissue (Shprintzen et al., 1985; Williams et al., 1985). Manifestations of DGS in some patients with VCFS suggested that DGS and VCFS might share a common pathogenesis. It is now known that the majority of patients with VCFS have deletions of 22q11 which completely overlap with the deletions of 22q11 seen in DGS (Driscoll et al., 1992b). Thus, VCFS and DGS are presumed to be different manifestations of the same disorder. The major clinical features in patients with VCFS include cleft palate or velo-pharyngeal insufficiency (VPI), cardiac defects, learning disabilities and a characteristic facial appearance. Patients diagnosed with VCFS associated with a 22q11 deletion demonstrate extreme phenotypic variability. Intrafamilial variability has also been observed. Since the disorder and the microdeletion segregate in an autosomal dominant mode, one should pay particular attention to the presence of minor features such as facial dysmorphia and mild cognitive impairment in the parents of deletion-positive probands. It is recommended that parents of deletion-positive children be

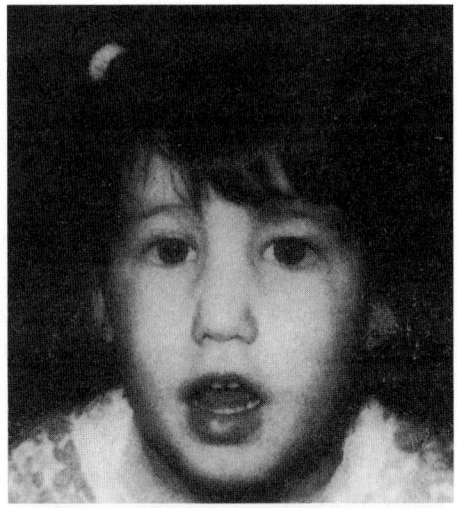

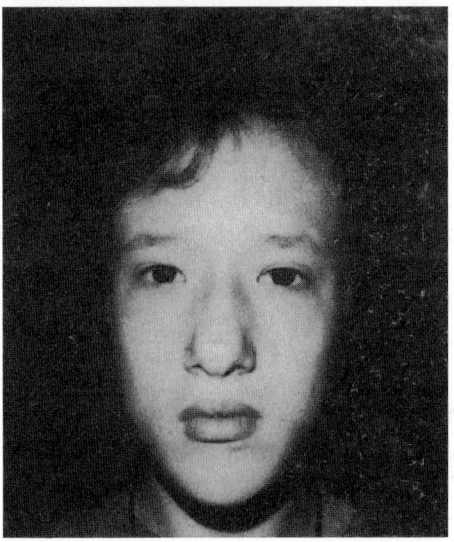

Fig. 46.16. Velocardiofacial syndrome. (A) A girl at two years eight months and (B) a girl at 12 years 10 months both of whom have characteristic bulbous nasal tip and mid face hypoplasia. (Courtesy of Elaine Zackai, MD and Donna McDonald-McGinn, MS, The Children's Hospital of Philadelphia, PA.)

examined by a clinical geneticist and be tested to ascertain their carrier status with regard to a 22q11 deletion.

Cytogenetics

Cytogenetic studies using high resolution banding techniques have detected interstitial deletions in 20% of VCFS patients (Driscoll et al., 1992b) (Fig. 46.15). Molecular studies including FISH with chromosome 22 probes previously shown to be deleted in DGS have shown that over 80% of patients with VCFS have deletions of 22q11 (Driscoll et al., 1992a). In addition, it has been shown that the autosomal dominant inheritance of this disease is the result of acquiring a deletion-bearing chromosome from an affected parent (Driscoll et al., 1992b).

Conotruncal anomaly face syndrome

Conotruncal anomaly face syndrome (CAFS) has striking similarities to DGS and VCFS and is characterized by the presence of conotruncal cardiac defects in association with a characteristic facial appearance. The facial features include ocular hypertelorism, lateral displacement of the inner canthi, flat nasal bridge, small mouth, narrow palpebral fissures, bloated eyelids, and malformed ears. This syndrome has been well characterized in a population of Japanese patients. The finding of 22q11 deletions in CAFS patients confirmed an earlier suggestion that CAFS and VCFS are the same entity.

Conotruncal cardiac defects

Conotruncal cardiac malformations occur with an increased frequency in patients with DGS and VCFS. Interrupted aortic arch type B (IAA), truncus arteriosis (TA), and tetralogy of Fallot (TOF) are the predominant cardiac lesions observed in DGS patients while TOF and ventricular septal defects (VSD) are common in VCFS. Goldmuntz et al. (1993) have shown that 20–30% percent of newborns and infants with apparently non-syndromic conotruncal cardiac defects have microdeletions of 22q11. Deletions of 22q11 have been described in cases of familial CHD as well. Careful examination of these individuals may identify subtle dysmorphic facial features or learning disabilities which are more suggestive of the diagnosis of VCFS; however, some of these features may not be apparent until a child reaches school age. Individuals with a 22q11 deletion have a 50% risk of transmitting the deletion-bearing chromosome to his or her offspring. Antenatal detection of the deletion using FISH has been successfully performed on cultured amniocytes and chorionic villi obtained from at risk pregnancies. However, as there is a wide range of phenotypic features seen in association with the 22q11 deletion, one cannot predict the phenotypic outcome based on the results of molecular-cytogenetic studies.

MILLER-DIEKER SYNDROME

Deletion of the distal end of the short arm of chromosome 17 is associated with a distinct syndrome of facial dysmorphia in combination with lissencephaly (Dobyns et al., 1991). Some patients with isolated lissencephaly, in the absence of other dysmorphic features have also been found to have deletions of this region of the genome (Ledbetter et al., 1992).

Clinical presentation

Miller-Dieker syndrome is characterized by type I lissencephaly (smooth brain, absent gyri and smooth cortical

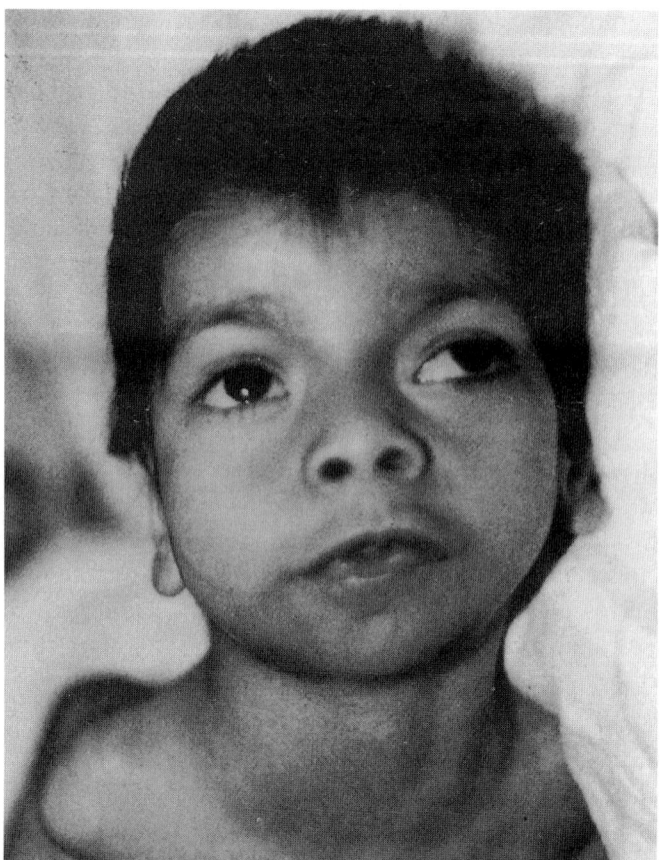

Fig. 46.17. Miller-Dieker syndrome. A 30-month-old girl with characteristic facial features, including bitemporal hollowing, short upturned nose, small jaw, and thin vermilion border. (Courtesy of William Dobyns, M.D., University of Minnesota Medical School, Minneapolis, MN.)

surface) and distinctive facial features including bitemporal hollowing, mid face hypoplasia, a small jaw, short nose with upturned nares, and a protuberant upper lip with thin vermilion border (Fig. 46.17). Patients also demonstrate severe postnatal growth retardation and seizures (Dieker et al., 1969; Jones et al., 1980; Miller, 1963). Polyhydramnios is common during pregnancy, probably due to poor fetal swallowing movements. All patients have profound mental retardation, diminished spontaneous movements, prominent opisthotonus and limb spasticity. In one study of 26 patients, six of the 26 had died by the age of four years (Dobyns et al., 1991).

Genetics and cytogenetics

The occurrence of several families in which there were multiple affected siblings initially suggested that Miller-Dieker syndrome was a recessive condition. It has now been shown that most of the known familial cases are due to a parental balanced translocation or pericentric inversion (Greenberg et al.,

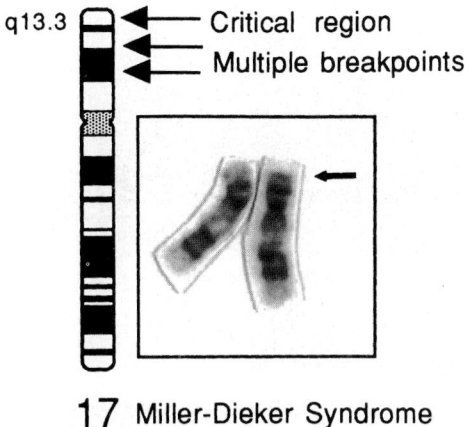

q13.3

Critical region
Multiple breakpoints

17 Miller-Dieker Syndrome

Fig. 46.18. Ideogram and partial karyotype of chromosome 17 demonstrating a deletion in a patient with Miller-Dieker syndrome. (Chromosomes courtesy of Mary C. Phelan, Ph.D., Greenwood Genetic Center, Greenwood, SC.)

1986; Stratton et al. 1994). MDS is associated with a microdeletion of chromosome 17p13.3 which is visible by high-resolution cytogenetic methods in about 50% of cases (Dobyns et al., 1991) (Fig. 46.18). The size of the deletion in these patients is variable, ranging from the majority of band 17p13 to a small region within 17p13.3. There is no apparent difference in clinical manifestation among patients with different size deletions, suggesting that perhaps only one or a small number of genes within band 17p13.3 is responsible for the phenotype. Microdeletions of 17p13.3 have been detected in many patients with apparently normal chromosomes and features of Miller-Dieker syndrome. Using cytogenetic and molecular techniques, deletions of 17p13 are detectable in about 90% of Miller-Dieker syndrome patients and in about 15% of patients with isolated lissencephaly (Kuwano et al., 1991; Ledbetter et al., 1992). Studies to define the smallest region of overlap of patients identified a critical 350 kb region and a gene called *LIS1* (lissencephaly-1) that maps to this region. This gene is deleted in all patients studied. The deduced amino acid sequence shows homology to beta subunits of heterotrimeric G proteins, suggesting that this gene may be involved in a signal transduction pathway that is crucial for cerebral development. It has been proposed that *LIS-1* is the gene for lissencephaly and the associated dysmorphic facial features seen in Miller-Dieker syndrome patients (Reiner et al., 1993).

LANGER-GIEDION SYNDROME (TRICHO-RHINO-PHALANGEAL SYNDROME TYPE II)

The Langer-Giedion syndrome (TRPS II) is a well-defined clinical entity that is characterized by multiple cartilaginous exostoses in combination with the clinical features of TRPS type I (see below). Cytogenetically visible aberrations of chromosome band 8q24.1 (which include deletions, translocations or insertions) can occur in both syndromes, but large deletions accompanied by mental retardation are more common in type II (Langer-Giedion). TRPS I patients with a normal karyotype and a submicroscopic deletion have recently been described, suggesting that on rare occasions, microdeletion can be the etiology for TRPS I (Lüdecke et al., 1999; Nardmann et al., 1997). The presence of maternal and paternal deletions suggests that there is no preferential parent of origin for TRPS-associated deletions. Mutations in TRPSI patients have been detected in the *TRPSI* gene which is predicted to be a novel transcription factor with zinc-finger motifs (Momeni et al., 2000).

CLINICAL FEATURES

Langer-Giedion syndrome is characterized by sparse scalp hair, large and laterally protruding ears, bushy eyebrows that are sometimes thinning laterally, broad nasal bridge and bulbous nose, an elongated upper lip, and thin upper vermilion border (Fig. 46.19). Malocclusion, mandibular retrognathia and dental abnormalities are common. There is frequently marked laxity of the skin in infancy and early childhood which diminshes with age. Brittle nails and multiple nevi are seen frequently. Patients have winged scapulae and short stature of postnatal onset. Multiple cartilaginous exostoses are a defining feature of the disorder (Fig. 46.19). The exostoses may appear in the first year, but may not develop until the fifth year, and they usually increase in size and number until skeletal maturation. There is considerable variability of intelligence and while mild to moderate retardation has been seen in many patients, it does not appear to be a constant feature of the disorder (Langer et al, 1984).

CYTOGENETICS

In 1980, Buhler et al. reported a girl with a terminal deletion of chromosome 8q (del(8)(q24)) with features of Langer-Giedion syndrome (Fig. 46.20). Since that time, deletions or other rearrangements involving 8q24 have been identified in a high percentage of patients (Lüdecke et al., 1991). Patients with TRPS type I have also been found to have deletions of 8q24, although their deletions are generally smaller than those of the Langer-Giedion patients. There is evidence that the presence of mental retardation may correlate with the size of the cytogenetic deletions. Recent work by Lüdecke et al. have demonstrated that there are at

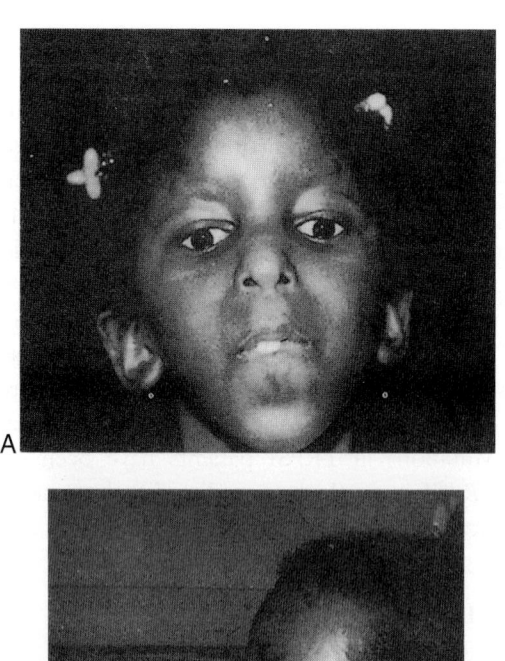

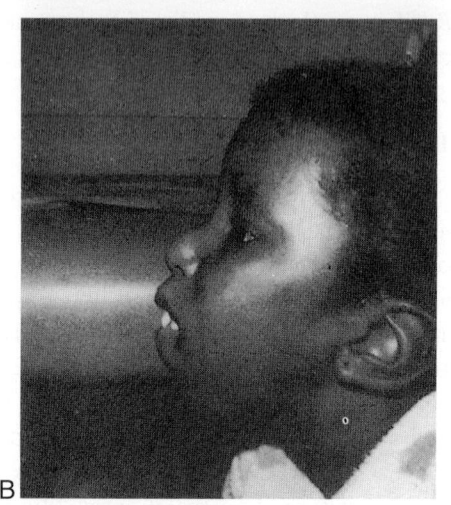

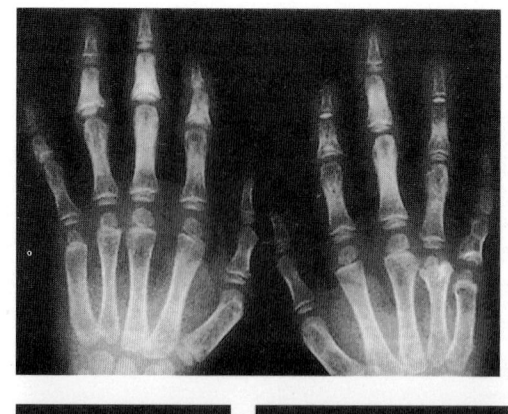

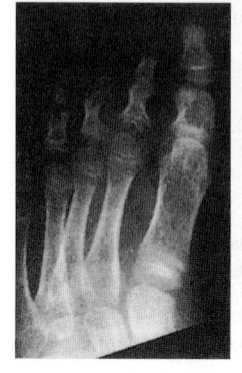
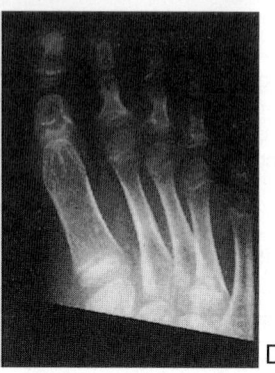

Fig. 46.19. Langer-Giedion syndrome. Left: Frontal (*a*) and lateral (*b*) view of the face of a six-year-old patient. Characteristic facial features include "pear-shaped" nose, thick lips, and prominent ears.
Right: Radiograph of both hands (A) and feet (B) of the patient showing multiple abnormal cone-shaped epiphyses and multiple small exostoses in the hands and feet. (From Ramos, 1992, with permission.)

least two separate genes within 8q24, deletion of which seem to give rise to the Langer-Giedion phenotype. One of these genes (*TRPS*) is deleted in all TRPS type I patients, and the

second (*EXT*) gives rise to the multiple cartilaginous exostoses. They therefore hypothesize that the Langer-Giedion syndrome is a true contiguous gene deletion syndrome and not due to pleiotropic effects of mutations in a single gene (Lüdecke et al., 1995).

WILLIAMS SYNDROME

Williams syndrome is characterized by cardiovascular abnormalities, most commonly supravalvular aortic stenosis; hypertension, intermittent hypercalcemia, growth retardation, dysmorphic facial features, and mental retardation with a unique, outgoing personality. Renal abnormalities have been reported including structural abnormalities, renal artery stenosis and problems secondary to hypercalcemia (Pober et al., 1997). The frequency of the disorder is estimated at 1 in 20,000 to 1 in 50,000 (Greenberg, 1990). A high percentage of patients have a microdeletion of the long arm of chromosome 7 which involves the elastin gene. Cytogenetically visible deletions of chromosome 7 have been reported, but these are rare.

q24.1   □ Critical region

8 Langer-Giedion Syndrome

Fig. 46.20. Ideogram and partial karyotype of chromosome 8 demonstrating the common deletion in patients with Langer-Giedion syndrome.

Clinical presentation

Patients may present at birth with congenital heart disease (supravalvular aortic stenosis is seen in 50% of patients and peripheral pulmonary stenosis in 27%), but the syndromic nature of the disorder often goes unrecognized in the newborn period (Morris et al., 1988). Failure to thrive is a common feature during infancy. The characteristic facial features include a broad forehead, medial eyebrow flare, periorbital fullness, strabismus, stellate iris pattern, flat nasal bridge, malar flattening, full cheeks and lips, a long smooth philtrum, pointed chin and wide mouth (Fig. 46.21). The face is reported to become more coarse with age (Burn, 1986). Mental retardation is a consistent feature with a range from severe to borderline. In one study, 13% of 46 patients had severe MR with IQ less than 49, 78% had mild/moderate mental retardation, and 9% had a border-line IQ (<75) (Perez Jurado et al., 1996). Patients have been shown to demonstrate a highly characteristic pattern of cognitive skills; performance is higher on tasks requiring auditory input and verbal output than on tasks requiring complex visual analysis for receiving information and visual motor expression (Morris et al., 1988). This deficit in the ability to visualize objects as a set of parts (which is crucial to the ability to draw the object) is termed visual-motor integration. This feature of the Williams syndrome has been found to be associated with deletion of LIM-kinase 1, one of the genes in the Williams syndrome critical region (see below) (Frangiskakis et al., 1996).

Genetics and cytogenetics

Williams syndrome is usually a sporadic disorder. In 1993, autosomal dominant supravalvular aortic stenosis was demonstrated to be caused by disruption of the elastin gene on the long arm of chromosome 7. The knowledge that SVAS is a consistent feature of Williams syndrome led to the hypothesis that Williams syndrome may be a contiguous gene disorder and that the vascular and connective tissue abnormalities are caused by deletion of one elastin allele, with the other features being caused by additional adjacent genes. Hemizygosity for elastin was demonstrated in familial and sporadic Williams syndrome (Ewart et al., 1993). Further studies have demonstrated that deletion of the elastin gene occurs in about 90% of Williams syndrome patients (Nickerson et al., 1995) (Fig. 46.22). The commonly deleted region in patients with Williams syndrome is about 1.5 megabases in size and includes elastin (associated with supravalvular aortic stenosis), LIM-kinase 1 (associated

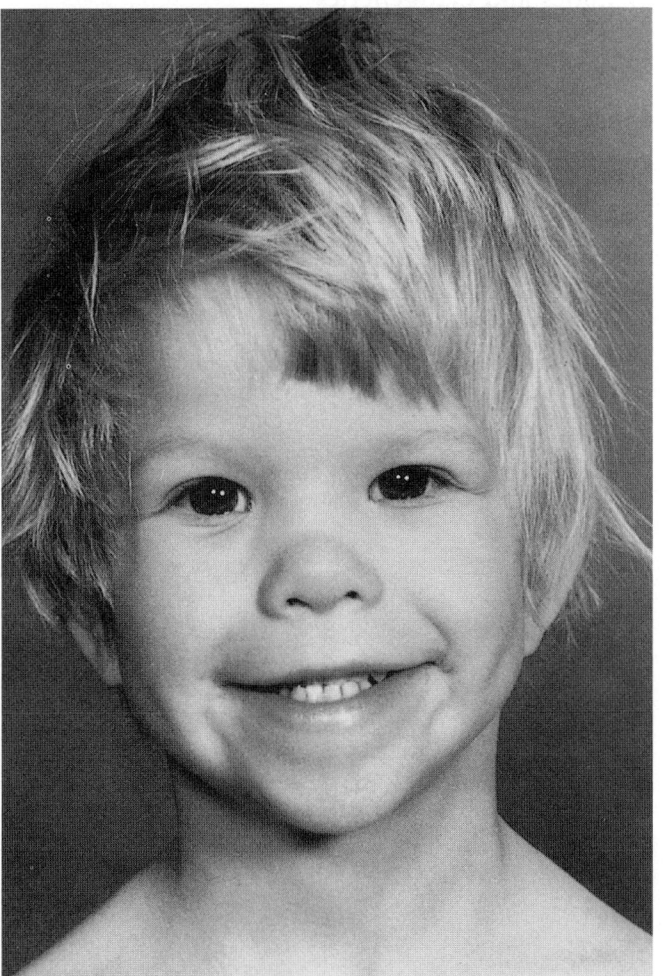

Fig. 46.21. William syndrome. Female proband at 2 years of age demonstrating characteristic facial features of William syndrome (periorbital fullness, full nasal tip, full lips with decreased cupid's bow, full cheeks with prominent nasolabial fold). (Courtesy of Paige Kaplan, MD.)

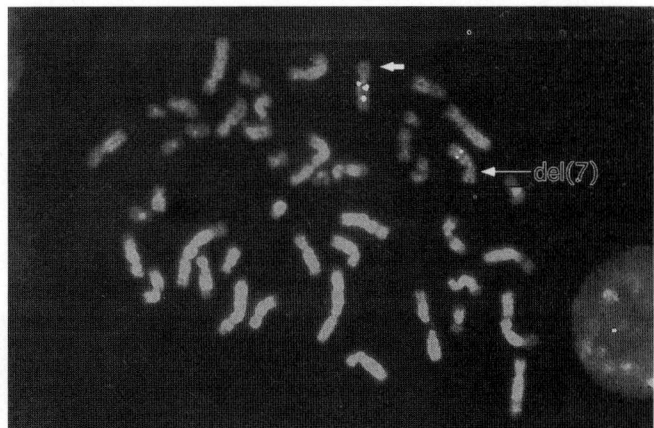

Fig. 46.22. The deletion of chromosome 7 in patients with William syndrome is generally not detectable by gene banding, but can easily by detected by FISH. The Williams syndrome critical region probe (180 kb) contains markers *ELN*, *LIMK1* and D7S613 (red signal). A chromosome 7 control probe that maps to 7q31 (green signal) is also shown.

with impaired visual motor integration), syntaxin 1A (hypothesized to be associated with attention deficit and hyperactivity seen in some patients with Williams syndrome) and other less well studied genes (Meng et al., 1998). Delineation of the contribution of haploinsufficiency of each of the genes in the Williams syndrome critical region will undoubtedly occur over the next few years.

ALAGILLE SYNDROME (SYNDROMIC BILE DUCT PAUCITY, ARTERIOHEPATIC DYSPLASIA)

Bile duct paucity, in combination with heart defects, skeletal anomalies, ocular abnormalities and characteristic facies are the features of Alagille syndrome. Approximately 5% of patients have been described with cytogenetic deletions of chromosome 20p (Krantz et al., 1997). In 1997 deletions were used as the basis of a positional cloning study and Jagged 1 (*JAG1*) was identified within the deletion critical region. JAGI is a cell surface ligand for the Notch transmembrane receptor. This ligand receptor pair functions in the evolutionarily conserved Notch signaling pathway, which is involved in regulation of cell fate during development (Artavanis-Tsakonas et al., 1995). AGS patients were subsequently identified who had mutations in *JAG1* as the cause of Alagille syndrome (Li et al., 1997; Oda et al., 1997). The syndrome has a frequency of about 1 in 50–1 in 100,000 (Krantz et al., 1999).

Clinical presentation

Alagille syndrome is characterized by bile duct paucity in association with other clinical features including cholestasis,

cardiac defect (most frequently pulmonary artery stenoses at various sites in the proximal and distal tree), musculoskeletal abnormality (most commonly butterfly vertebrae), ocular findings (most commonly posterior embryotoxon) and a characteristic facial appearance (Fig. 46.23). Additional defects may include growth retardation, long bone abnormalities and renal disease (Alagille et al., 1975; 1987). Patients with Alagille syndrome may present with jaundice and cholestasis in the first three months of life although clinical manifestations are highly variable. Some patients demonstrate progressive pruritus, cirrhosis or liver failure, resulting in liver transplantation while others have few or no symptoms and remain undiagnosed as adults. Most patients present with hepatic manifestations; however, mortality from cardiac disease equals that from liver failure (Emerick et al., 1999).

Genetics and cytogenetics

Examination of a few multi-generation families initially suggested autosomal dominant inheritance with reduced penetrance and variable expressivity (Watson and Miller, 1973; LaBrecque et al., 1982; Shulman et al., 1984). Since 1986 the disease was mapped to the short arm of chromosome 20 based on identification of Alagille patients with cytogenetically visible deletions with the shortest region of overlap at 20p11.23–p12 (Byrne et al. 1986; Krantz et al., 1997) (Fig. 46.24). There has been one report of a mother and child who both were affected and demonstrated a deletion of 20p11.23–p12.2 (Anad et al., 1990). In this case, the mother had typical facies, heart defect and embryotoxon, but no hepatic involvement, while her son had liver disease, heart disease, renal dysplasia, and abnormal facies. An apparently

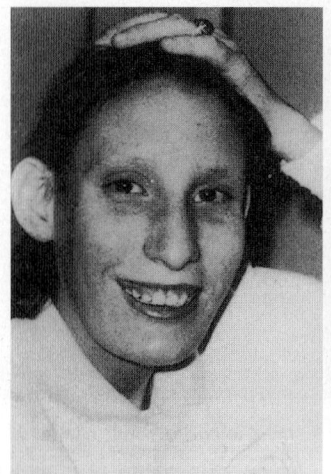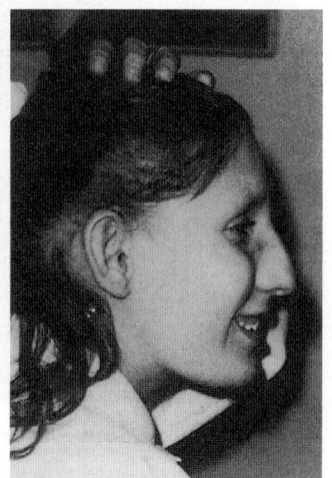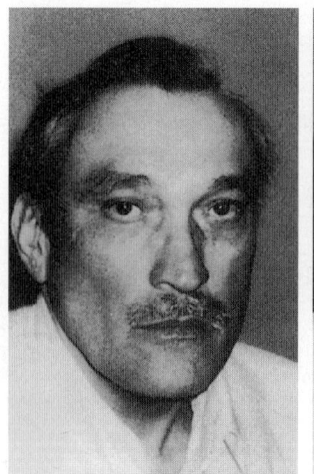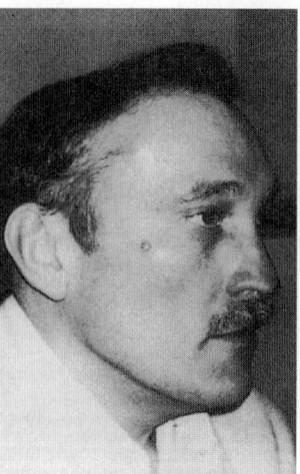

Fig. 46.23. Alagille syndrome. (A) A 15-year-old girl. (B) Her subclinically affected father. Characteristic facial features in both individuals include prominent forehead, triangular facies, deep-set eyes, and anteriorly pointed chin. (From Spinner et al., 1994, with permission.)

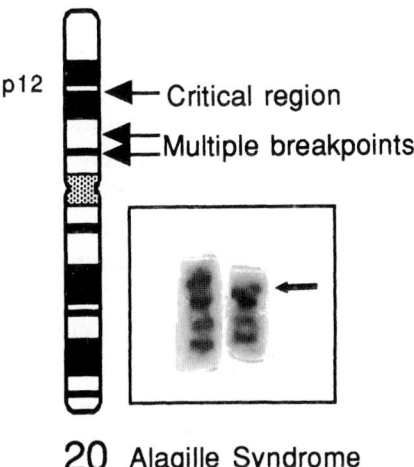

Fig. 46.24. Ideogram and partial karyotype of chromosome 20 demonstrating a deletion in a patient with Alagille syndrome.

balanced translocation with a breakpoint at 20p12 was demonstrated to segregate with Alagille syndrome in one family with two affected sisters and a sub-clinically affected father. Subsequent molecular analysis of this family demonstrated a deletion at the translocation breakpoint (Spinner et al., 1994; Krantz et al., 1997).

In 1997 two groups identified *JAG1* as the AGS disease gene based on its localization within the deletion critical region and the finding that non-deleted patients had mutations that segregated with the disease in families (Li et al., 1997; Oda et al., 1997). *JAG1* is one of two Jagged genes (*JAG1* and *JAG2*) identified in humans and these genes code for proteins that are cell surface ligands for the Notch transmembrane receptors. These receptor-ligand pairs are components of the highly conserved Notch signaling pathway, which is involved in cell fate determination (Artavanis-Tsakonas et al., 1999).

Overall, approximately 5% of Alagille syndrome patients have total gene deletions of *JAG1*, and another 60–65% have been found to have mutations that lead to production of an abnormal and presumably non-functional protein (Krantz et al., 1998; Crosnier et al., 1999; Spinner et al., 2001).

SMITH-MAGENIS SYNDROME

Smith-Magenis syndrome was first described in 1986 and patients have a constellation of features including facial dysmorphism, short stature, cleft palate, behavioral problems and mental retardation. The syndrome is associated with cytogenetically detectable interstitial deletion of the short arm of 17p (Smith et al., 1986; Stratton et al., 1986). The birth incidence is estimated at 1 in 25,000.

Clinical presentation

The phenotype includes brachycephaly, mid facial hypoplasia with a broad flat mid face, broad nasal bridge, prognathism, hoarse voice, and speech delay, cognitive delay, psychomotor and growth retardation, and behavioral problems (Greenberg et al., 1996). The brows are heavy with excess lateral extension of the eyebrows. The nose has a depressed root and, in the young child, a scooped nasal bridge (Fig. 46.25). Hearing loss is seen in ~50% of cases and hyperactivity, and behavioral problems are present in most. Two-thirds of the patients demonstrate self-injurious behavior including pulling out fingernails and toenails and insertion of foreign bodies into body orifices as well as head banging. Ocular abnormalities are frequent and include high myopia, retinal detachments, iris anomalies, microcornea, strabismus and cataracts (Smith et al., 1986; Stratton et al., 1986; Greenberg et al., 1991; Finucane et al., 1993; Smith et al., 1998).

The patients demonstrate normal nerve conduction velocities, despite the fact that signs suggestive of peripheral neuropathy (e.g., decreased or absent deep tendon reflexes, pes planus or pes cavus, decreased sensitivity to pain, and decreased leg muscle mass) are found in 75% of patients (Greenberg et al., 1996). Notable symptoms of sleep

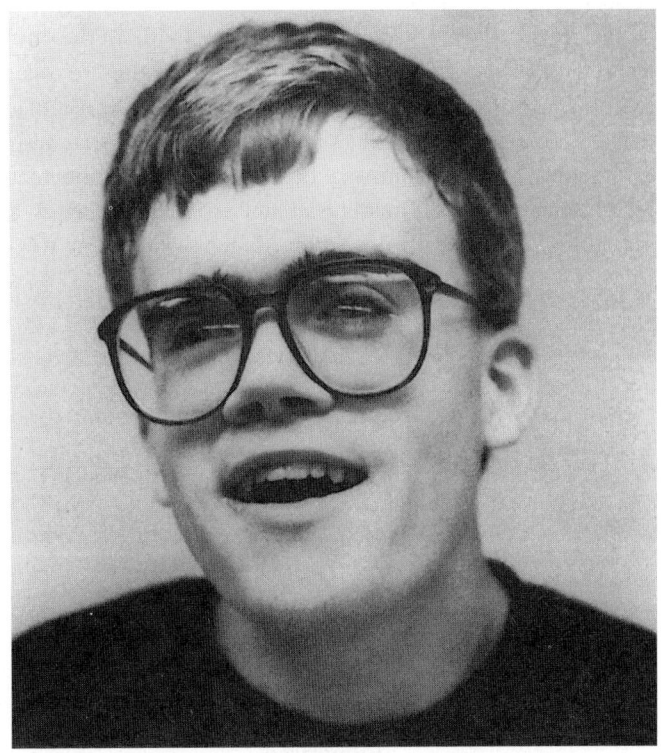

Fig. 46.25. Smith-Magenis syndrome. A 20-year-old male with characteristic features including brachycephaly, midfacial hypoplasia, prognathism, and myopia. (From Finucane et al., 1993, with permission.)

disturbance (difficulty falling asleep, difficulty staying asleep, and frequent awakening during the night) have been observed in a significant number of patients (Smith et al., 1998). In 57% of patients abnormalities in REM sleep has been demonstrated by polysonography (Greenberg et al., 1996; Smith et al., 1998). Patients with Smith-Magenis syndrome manifest unusual hand- or arm-clasping behavior (self-hugging) which appears to be part of a complex upper body tic which is exacerbated by happiness, excitement or over stimulation (Finucane et al., 1994).

CYTOGENETICS AND MOLECULAR CYTOGENETICS

In the majority of patients, the syndrome is related to a cytogenetically visible, de novo, interstitial deletion of a portion of 17p11.2 [del(17)(p11.2p11.2)] (Smith et al., 1986; Stratton et al., 1986) (Fig. 46.26). One patient with complete deletion of band 17p11.2 was more severely affected with facial malformations, cleft palate, and major anomalies of the cardiac, skeletal and genitourinary systems. Parent of origin studies on 15 patients demonstrated nine paternal and six maternal deletions. The apparent random parental origin suggested that genomic imprinting does not play a role in expression of the SMS clinical phenotype (Greenberg et al., 1991).

Progress has been made in molecular mapping of the critical region of this disorder. Using probes from the proximal region of 17p Moncla et al. (1993) generated a molecular map of the deleted region in three patients with cytogenetically visible deletions and they defined a critical region that included two 17p11.2 markers. These markers will allow a search for patients with the Smith-Magenis phenotype who

do not have visible deletions. More recently, it has been demonstrated that recombination between copies of a repeat gene cluster (*SMS-REP*) in 17p which flanks the deletion is responsible for this microdeletion disorder (Chen et al., 1997). Interestingly, duplication of a more telomeric region of 17p adjacent to the region missing in Smith-Magenis syndrome causes Charcot-Marie-Tooth Disease (type 1A). CMT1A is a dominant disorder characterized clinically by distal muscle atrophy and weakness and electrophysiologically by decreased nerve conduction velocities. The disease was initially linked to 17p11.2-p12 and it has been shown that patients with cytogenetically identifiable duplications of 17p demonstrate abnormal nerve conduction velocities consistent with a diagnosis of CMT1A (Chance et al., 1992; Lupski et al., 1992).

Duplication

SUPERNUMERARY CHROMOSOMES

Small supernumerary chromosomes are seen in approximately 0.06% of the population (Sachs et al., 1987). These small chromosomes are sometimes referred to as "marker" chromosomes. Marker chromosomes are defined as abnormal chromosomes that cannot be fully characterized based on standard cytogenetic analyses because of their paucity of banding landmarks. These markers are known to be heterogeneous with respect to size and composition and some are associated with mental retardation and other abnormalities, while others seem to have no recognizable phenotypic effects.

Numerous studies have used fluorescence in situ hybridization to identify the chromosomal origin of marker chromosomes. In many cases, use of chromosome specific pericentromeric alphoid satellite probes have indicated the chromosomal origin of the markers (Callen et al., 1992; Blennow et al., 1995). Correlation between phenotype and the chromosomal origin is being made to permit a distinction between those markers that carry a high risk for phenotypic abnormality and those markers with a low risk. The risk for phenotypic abnormality is correlated with whether the marker is de novo or familial (with the risk being higher for de novo markers), and with the chromosomal origin of the marker. Once a marker has been identified by standard cytogenetics, further characterization is carried out by fluorescence in situ hybridization (FISH). However, this technique requires selection of which chromosome specific probes should be tested. Initial cytogenetic analysis usually

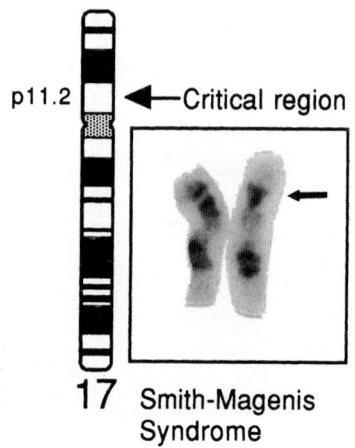

Fig. 46.26. Ideogram and partial karyotype of chromosome 17 showing the commonly deleted region in patients with Smith-Magenis syndrome.

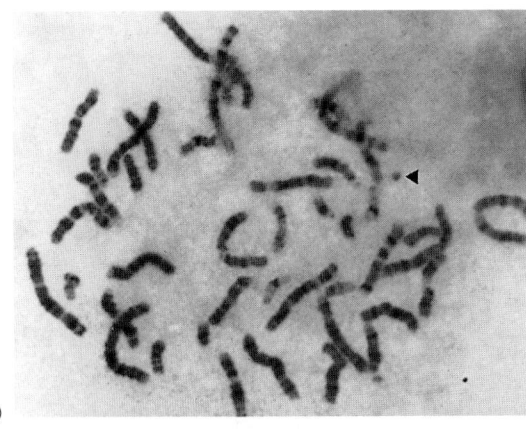
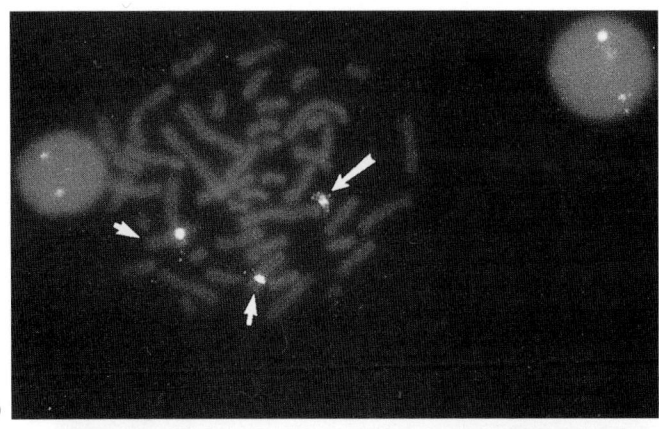

(A)   (B)

Fig. 46.27. (A) Photograph of G-banded metaphase from a patient with a small supernumerary marker chromosome (*arrowhead*). (B) Pohotomicrograph of a metaphase after fluorescence in situ hybridization using a biotin-labeled α-satellite probe for the pericentrometric region of chromosome 8. *Large arrow* indicates the brightly fluorescent marker chromosome. The two normal 8s (*smaller arrows*) also give a positive signal. (From Spinner NB, Rehberg-Grace K, Owens NL et al. (1995) Mosaicism for a chromosome 8 derived marker chromosome in a patient with manifestations of trisomy 8 mosaicism. Am J Med Genet 56:22–24, with permission.) (See Plate 46.27.)

provides some guidance with the most useful classification being separation of satellited and non satellited markers. In some cases, the marker chromosomes are large enough and have some banding characteristics which allow the cytogeneticist to make educated guesses about their origin. Other markers are very small and have no cytogenetic landmarks. If these markers are identified postnatally, it may be possible to use clinical information about the proband to suggest which chromosome is involved and this can be tested with chromosome specific alpha satellite probes (Spinner et al., 1995a) (Fig. 46.27). In a study of 50 marker chromosomes, Blennow et al. identified 37 markers that were of acrocentric origin (25 from chromosome 15), 5 isochromosomes for 18p, one isochromosome for 12p (Pallister-Killian), and one each derived from chromosomes 4, 7, 8, 9, 19, 20. In this section, we describe five syndromes associated with relatively well studied supernumerary chromosomes i.e., the (inv dup(15), the "cat eye" marker, the i(18p), the der(22)t(11;22) and the i(12p) associated with Pallister-Killian syndrome.

INVERTED DUP(15)

Clinical presentation

Inv dup(15)'s account for approximately 40% of marker chromosomes. They have been reported in normal individuals (Stetten et al., 1981; Knight et al., 1984) individuals with mental retardation and other anomalies (inv dup(15) syndrome) (Schreck et al., 1977; Wisniewski et al., 1979,) and in a few patients with Prader-Willi and Angelman syndromes (Fujita et al., 1980; Ledbetter et al., 1982; Mattei et al.,

1984). However, molecular cytogenetic studies have shown that the inv dup(15's) seen in normal individuals and in PWS and AS patients are smaller than those seen in patients with mental retardation (Robinson et al., 1993; Cheng et al., 1994; Spinner et al., 1995b). It appears that in patients with Prader-Willi or Angelman syndromes and an inv dup(15) chromosome, the inv dup(15) most likely has no relationship to the etiology of the syndrome. In 4/4 patients studied, another cause for PWS or AS (deletion of 15q11q13 or UPD 15) was found (discussed in more detail below).

Most reported cases of inv dup(15) have been identified in patients studied because of mental retardation. These patients are generally non-dysmorphic, although facial features have been described as coarse and various minor dysmorphic features have been described (Fig. 46.28) (Schinzel, 1984). Affected individuals demonstrate developmental delay from an early age and other associated features include psychomotor retardation, seizures, hyperactivity and behavioral disturbances, including violent behavior (Wisneiwski et al., 1979; Maraschio et al., 1988; Lazarus et al., 1991; Crolla et al, 1995). Autistic features have been reported in multiple patients. (Cheng et al., 1994; Leana-Cox et al., 1994; Crolla et al., 1995). Lifespan does not appear to be reduced although there have been a few reports of progressive loss of function (Zannotti et al., 1980).

CYTOGENETICS AND MOLECULAR CYTOGENETICS

Inv dup(15) chromosomes are dicentric and bisatellited and consist of two copies of the p arm, centromere and proximal long arm of chromosome 15 which are fused at the

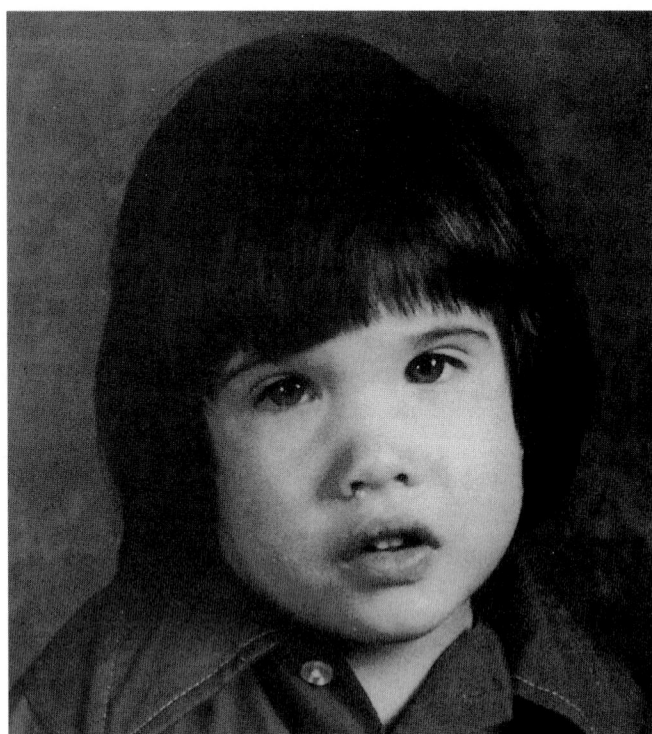

Fig. 46.28. Inverted dup(15) syndrome. Male proband at three and a half years of age with a "large" inv dup(15) (inv dup(15) syndrome). Minor dysmorphic features include coarse facies and bilateral epicanthal folds. (Courtesy of Brenda Finucane, MS, Elwyn Inc., Elwyn, PA.)

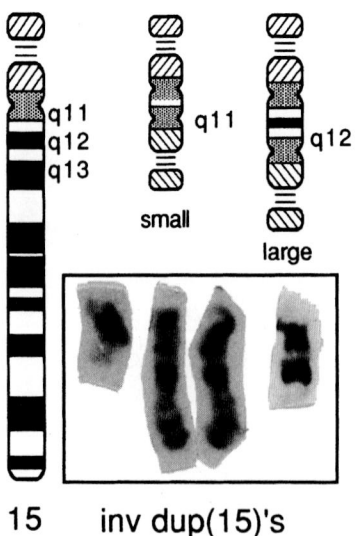

Fig. 46.29. Ideogram and partial karyotype of chromosome 15 showing two different sizes of inverted duplication 15 chromosomes. As described in the text, the smaller inverted dup (left) does not appear to cause phenotypic abnormalities, while the larger inverted dup(15) (right) is associated with an abnormal phenotype.

proximal long arm (Fig. 46.29). Various techniques have been useful in demonstrating that a bisatellited chromsome derives from chromosome 15. Before the introduction of molecular cytogenetic techniques, chromosomes were stained with Distamycin-DAPI, which produces a brightly fluorescent signal on chromosome 15p, but not on any of the other acrocentric chromosomes. Therefore, any acrocentric that was positive for a signal with Distamycin-DAPI could be identified as deriving from chromosome 15. Variation in the size of the inv dup(15's) has been observed, but this has been difficult to quantify based on standard cytogenetics.

Fluorescence in situ hybridization provides an improved means of identifying the origin and composition of marker chromosomes. Probes are available that map to the pericentromeric region of most human chromosomes and use of a chromosome 15 pericentromeric (alpha satellite) probe can confirm the identity of an inv dup(15). Studies have focused on the molecular characterization of inv dup(15's) from the three classes of individuals in whom these markers are found (normal individuals, individuals with the "inv dup(15) syndrome" and patients with Prader-Willi or Angelman syndrome) (Robinson et al., 1993; Cheng et al., 1994; Leana-Cox et al., 1994; Spinner et al., 1995b, Mignon et al., 1996).

These studies have demonstrated a correlation between the amount of material present on the inv dup(15) and phenotype. Normal individuals have been found to have relatively smaller inv dup(15's) with duplication of only the most proximal centromeric loci. Individuals with mental retardation and other features of the inv dup(15) syndrome had larger markers, with duplication of a number of more distal loci (Cheng et al., 1994; Leana-Cox et al., 1994; Crolla et al., 1995). The situation with Prader-Willi and Angelman patients who have inv dup(15's) is more complex. In all cases studied, the inv dup(15)'s were found to be relatively small, with duplication of only the most proximal markers, however; all patients demonstrated either uniparental disomy for chromosome 15 or deletion of loci from 15q11q13 (on one of the cytogenetically normal appearing 15's) which was believed to be the cause of their disease. Therefore, the inv dup(15)'s were not considered to be related to the phenotype (Robinson et al., 1993; Spinner et al., 1995b). These studies have raised the possibility that patients with inv dup(15's) may be at increased risk for uniparental disomy of chromosome 15 or deletion of proximal 15q11q13.

The fact that these inv dup(15) chromosomes are relatively common among markers, suggests a pre-disposing mechanism inherent in the sequence of the proximal region of chromosome 15. Studies to delineate the breakpoints of a series of inv dup(15's) have demonstrated that there are two common regions in which the breakage occurs. These regions are known to contain a large number of low copy repeat sequences, and it has been proposed that illegitimate recombination between these repeats may be involved as a mechanism in the formation of structural anomalies involving 15q11q13 (Wandstrat et al., 1998).

CAT EYE SYNDROME

Clinical presentation

The name for the condition is derived from the "cat eye-like" appearance of the pupil which results from coloboma of the iris, one of the features of the syndrome (Fig. 46.30). Other features include imperforate anus, preauricular tags or fistulas, heart malformations, urinary tract anomalies, and mild to moderate mental retardation. Some patients have been of normal intelligence, but emotionally disturbed. Inferior iris coloboma occurs in less than half of cases. Preauricular skin tags and/or pits constitute the most consistent feature. Renal malformations, congenital heart defects, and anal atresia with fistula, are frequent. There is a high variability of clinical features noted.

Cytogenetics

The characteristic chromosomal change is the presence of a small extra acrocentric marker chromosome, derived from chromosome 22, which is often bisatellited (Fig. 46.31). Schinzel et al. (1991) recommended that the designation "cat eye syndrome" be reserved for cases with little or no mental retardation and with trisomy or tetrasomy of 22pter-22q11.

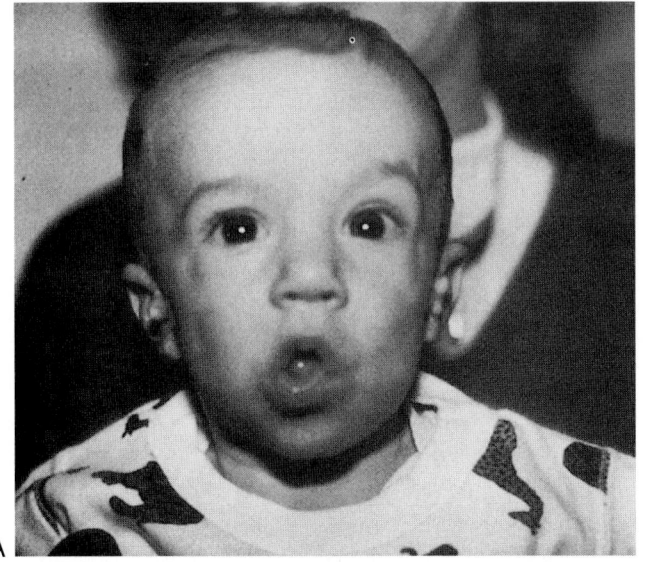

A

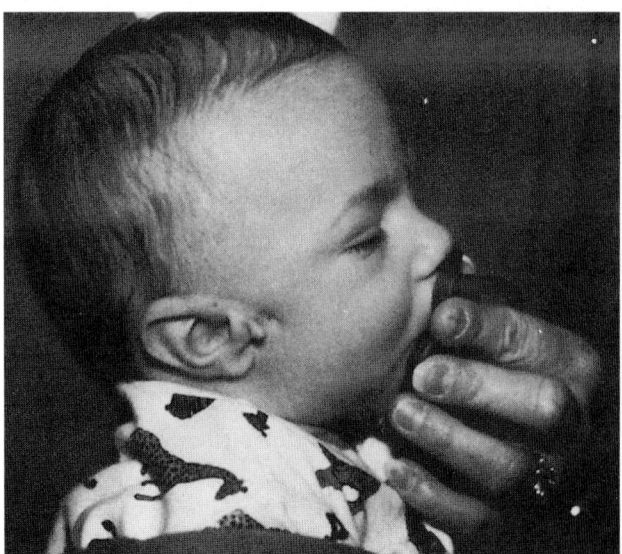

B

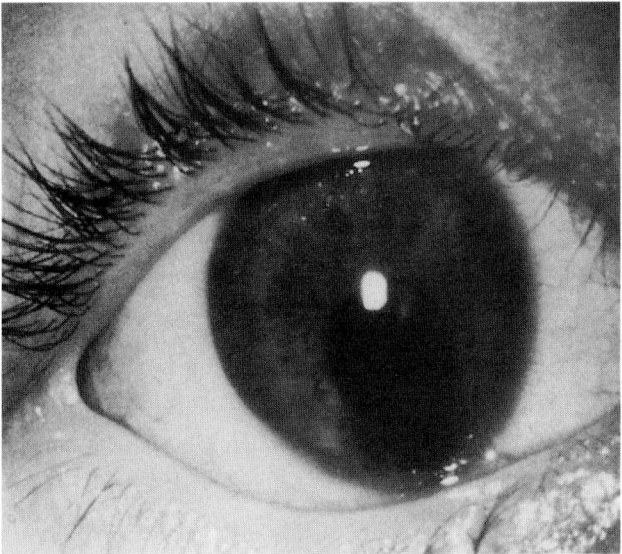

C

Fig. 46.30 Cat eye syndrome. (A) Frontal and (B) lateral view of the face of a male infant with a supernumerary "cat eye" chromosome. Note the ear pits and tags. This patient does not have an iris coloboma, which is seen in less than 50% of patients. (C) Iris coloboma from another patient with cat eye syndrome (Figures 5A and B courtesy of Elaine Zackai, M.D. and Donna McDonald-McGinn, MS, The Children's Hospital of Philadelphia, PA and Figure C courtesy of R. Ellen Magenis, MD, Oregon Health Sciences University, Portland, OR.)

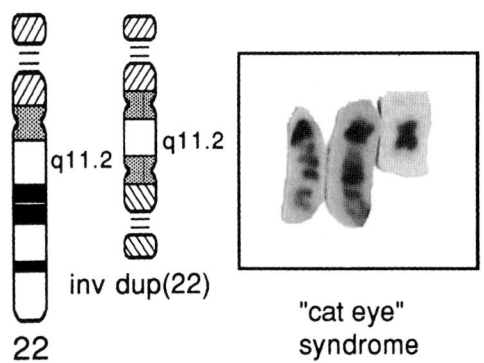

Fig. 46.31. Ideogram and partial karyotype of chromosome 22 and an inverted dup(22) or cat eye chromosome.

Using a DNA probe that had been previously localized to 22q11 by in situ hybridization, McDermid et al. (1986) using DNA dosage analysis showed that patients with cat eye syndrome and a supernumerary chromosome had four copies of the probe. The cat eye syndrome marker chromosomes are variable in size and can be asymmetric with regard to the region duplicated (Mears et al., 1994). Three types of CES chromosomes have been identified. They are classified based on the location of the breakpoints required to generate them. The smaller CES chromosomes are always symmetrical and classified as Type I CES chromosomes. The larger type II CES chromosomes are either symmetric or asymmetric type. Since the phenotype associated with the larger duplicated chromosome is no more severe than that of the smaller cat eye chromosome, sizing the duplicated segment has little prognostic value (McTaggart et al., 1998). The critical region has been further defined to include markers D22S9, D22S43 and *ATP6E* based upon molecular characterization of a familial ring chromosome (Mears et al., 1995). There have been numerous examples of transmission of the marker from parent to child with variability in the phenotype (Schinzel et al, 1981; Mears et al., 1994).

ISOCHROMOSOME 18p

Clinical presentation

Patients with i(18p) demonstrate a recognizable phenotype characterized by low birth weight, microcephaly, hypotonia, camptodactyly or adducted thumbs and a typical facial appearance. There is hypotonia and feeding difficulties in the first year and spasticity develops by the second year. Mental retardation in the moderate to severe range is present in all individuals studied. Some patients (about 50%) suffer from seizures. Facial dysmorphism includes dolicocephaly, a round face with small, low set ears, short

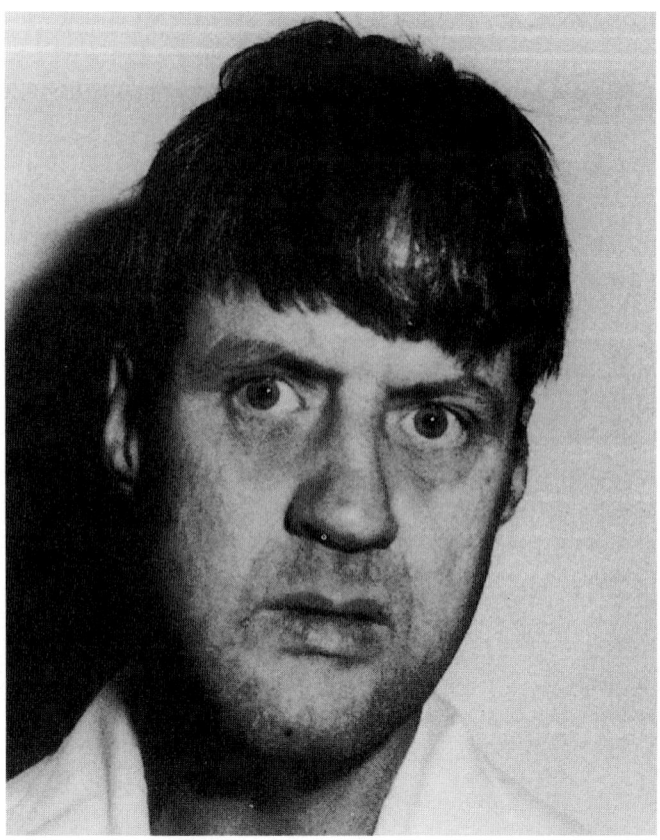

Fig. 46.32. i(18p) syndrome. A 44-year-old man with characteristic facial features: prognathism, long philtrum, and small mouth. (Courtesy of Mary C. Phelan, PhD, Greenwood Genetic Center, Greenwood, SC.)

palpebral fissures and small mouth; although, with increasing age, prognathism develops and the mouth and nose become more normal in size (Batista et al, 1983; Rivera et al., 1984; Callen et al., 1990) (Fig. 46.32)

Cytogenetics

The marker chromosome is a small, metacentric marker, which can usually be identified as an i(18p) on the basis of its size and banding pattern (Fig. 46.33). Callen et al. (1990) studied nine patients with marker chromosomes thought to be an i(18p) based on banding and confirmed their origin from chromosome 18 using a chromosome 18 alpha satellite probe in combination with a probe mapping to 18p11.3. The 18p11.3 probe was present on both arms of the marker as expected for an isochromosome (Callen et al., 1990). This marker chromosome usually occurs de novo, however a few familial cases have been reported Takeda et al., 1989; Abeliovich et al., 1993). In most, but not all cases studied, the marker was maternally derived (Eggerman et al., 1996; 1997).

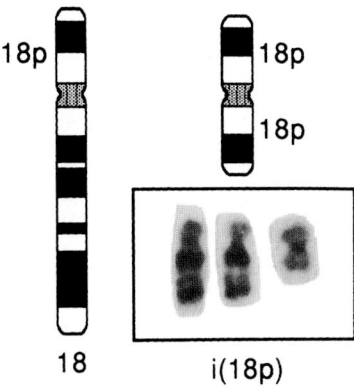

Fig. 46.33. Ideogram and partial karyotype from a patient with an isochromosome 18p.

SUPERNUMERARY DER(22)t(11;22) SYNDROME

Clinical presentation

As discussed in an earlier section of this chapter, patients with the +der(22) t(11;22) syndrome have a distinctive phenotype which consists of severe mental retardation, preauricular tag or sinus (Fig. 46.34), ear anomaly, cleft or high arched palate, micrognathia, heart defects (Lin et al., 1986) and genital abnormalities in the male. The vast majority of instances of this syndrome occur as the result of 3:1 meiotic malsegregation of the translocation (Shaikh et al., 1999). The mechanisms leading to 3:1 as opposed to 2:2 segregation, have yet to be definitely determined (Lindenbaum and Bobrow, 1975; Lindenbaum, 1990). However, results of recent studies of meiosis in a male translocation carrier have suggested that this pattern is due to selection against the other aberrant karyotypes after fertilization rather than preferential 3:1 meiotic segregation (Armstrong et al., 2000).

PALLISTER-KILLIAN SYNDROME

The Pallister-Killian syndrome is a relatively rare disorder characterized by multiple dysmorphic features and severe mental retardation. It is relatively rare but warrants mention because it is an excellent example of tissue specific mosaicism. The cytogenetic abnormality is not generally observed in peripheral blood lymphocytes and therefore the diagnosis could be missed if the proper tissue is not obtained for study.

Clinical presentation

Patients with Pallister-Killian syndrome have a very coarse face with pigmentary skin anomalies, localized alopecia, profound

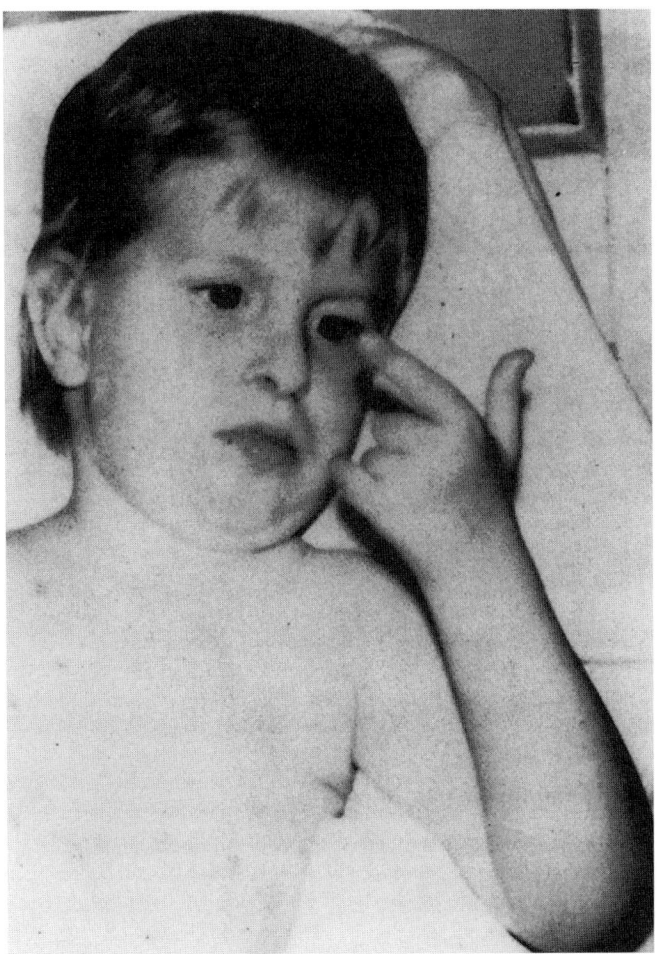

Fig. 46.34. Supernumerary der(22) syndrome. Affected patient at age five and a half years. Features in this patient consistent with the diagnosis include prominent forehead, cleft palate, preauricular sinus and skin tags, a short broad flat nose, long prominent philtrum, and microretrognathia. (From Emanuel et al., 1976, with permission.)

mental retardation and seizures. In infancy the hair is sparse, particularly in the frontal area. patients have a prominent, high forehead, hypertelorism, epicanthal folds, flat nasal bridge, large mouth with downturned corners and abnormal ears. The neck is often short and webbed, with excess nuchal skin (Fig. 46.35). There is a relatively high incidence of diaphragmatic defects and supernumerary nipples. Affected newborns are profoundly hypotonic. Adults with the disorders demonstrate severe mental retardation, epilepsy, coarse facies and macroglossia (Pallister et al., 1977; Killian et al., 1981; Schinzel, 1991; Reynolds et al., 1987).

Cytogenetics

In most Pallister-Killian patients studied, lymphocyte chromosomes are found to be normal but fibroblasts show an extra, small metacentric chromosome. The supernumerary

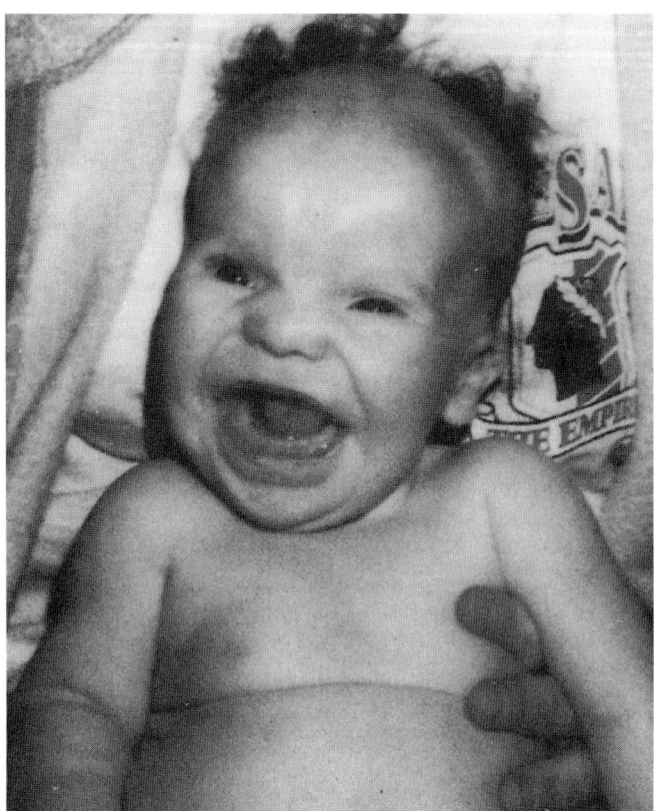

Fig. 46.35. Pallister-Killian (tetrasomy 12p) syndrome. As three and a half month-old female with sparse scalp hair, eyebrows, and lashes; long philtrum; large mouth with downturned corners; and thin upper lip. (Courtesy of Elaine Zackai, MD and Donna McDonald, McGinn, MS, The Children's Hospital of Philadelphia, PA.)

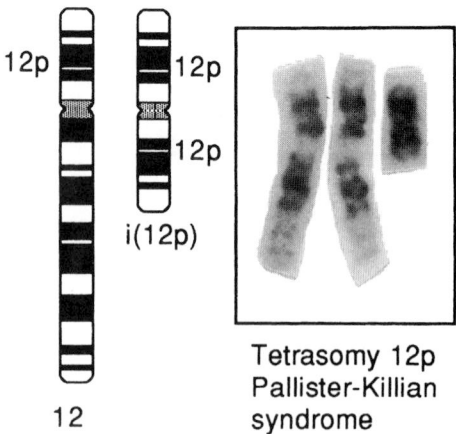

Tetrasomy 12p
Pallister-Killian
syndrome

Fig. 46.36. Ideogram and partial karyotype of chromosome 12 demonstrating the isochromosome 12p found in mosaic form in fibroblasts, epithelial cells, and bone marrow of patients with the Pallister-Killian syndrome. This supernumerary chromosome is rarely identified in peripheral blood lymphocytes.

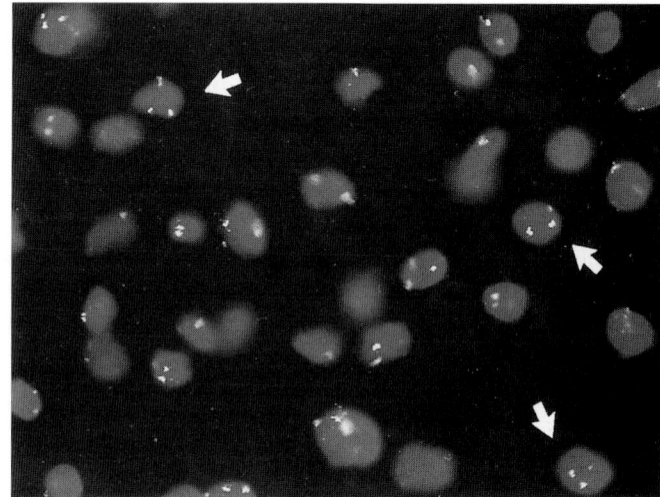

Fig. 46.37. Photomicrograph of interphase cells from the buccal mucosa of a patient with Pallister-Killian syndrome after fluorescent in situ hybridization, using an α-satellite probe from the pericentromeric region of chromosome 12. Note that some cells in the field (*arrows*) have three signals, consistent with the presence of the isochromosome 12p. (See Plate 46.37.)

chromosome has been demonstrated to be an isochromosome for the short arm of chromosome 12 (i(12p)) (Peltomaki et al., 1987) (Fig. 46.36). The i(12p) has been demonstrated in a high percentage of cells on direct bone marrow analysis, in a lower, but significant percentage of cells from cultured bone marrow and it has been seen in fibroblasts from skin, lung, and testes. The percentage of cells containing the supernumerary i(12p) has varied widely among patients studied. This disorder demonstrates tissue specific mosaicism, since the abnormal chromosome is apparently limited to certain tissues. It can be hypothesized that the four copies of 12p are toxic to lymphocytes and therefore there is selection in favor of the cells that have lost the supernumerary chromosome. The percentage of fibroblasts containing the marker has been observed to decrease over time (Ward et al., 1988; Wenger et al., 1990; Schubert et al., 1997). The marker can be inherited from either parent, although of six cases reported, it was maternal in five(Struthers et al., 1999).

Using interphase FISH, the marker has been identified in buccal smear preparations (Ohashi et al., 1993) (Fig. 46.37).

This technique is relatively simple, requiring a slide of cells that have been scraped from the buccal mucosa and fixed onto a microscope slide. Fluorescence in situ hybridization can then be carried out on this sample and in the presence of the isochromosome three signals will be seen, one each from the two normal 12's and one from the isochromosome. This has important diagnostic value as it eliminates the need for a tissue biopsy.

The consistently mosaic nature of this chromosome abnormality can make prenatal diagnosis difficult. Prenatal findings on ultrasound that indicate a risk of the Pallister-Killian syndrome include broad neck, short limbs, abnormal hands or feet, diaphragmatic hernia and hydramnios. The frequency of the i(12p) has been found to be higher in amniotic fluid than in choronic villi or cord blood. It has also been found to be higher on FISH studies, indicating that tissues with a high mitotic index may selectively lose the marker (Chiesa et al., 1998). A prudent approach to diagnosis of this abnormality would therefore include amniocentesis with both standard cytogenetics and FISH studies, with possible follow up by cordocentesis in the event of a severe ultrasound abnormality and a negative result.

REFERENCES

Abeliovic D, Dagon J, Levy A et al. (1993) Isochramosome 18p is a mother and her child. Am J Med Genet 46:392–393

Alagille D, Odièvre M, Gautier M, Dommergues JP (1975) Hepatic ductular hypoplasia associated with characteristic facies, vertebral malformations, retarded physical, mental and sexual development, and cardiac murmur. J Pediatr 86:63–71

Alagille D, Estrada A, Hadchouel M et al. (1987) Syndromic paucity of interlobular bile ducts (Alagille syndrome or arteriohepatic dysplasia): Review of 80 cases. J Pediatr 110:195–200

Altherr MR, Bengtsson U, Elder FFB et al. (1991) Molecular confirmation of Wolf-Hirschhorn syndrome with a subtle translocation of chromosome 4. Am J Hum Genet 49:1235–1242

Anad F, Burn J, Matthews D et al. (1990) Alagille syndrome and deletion of 20p. J Med Genet 27:729–737

Antonarakis SE, Blouin J, Maher J et al. (1993) Maternal uniparental disomy for human chromosome 14 due to loss of a chromosome 14 from somatic cells with t(13;14) Trisomy-14. am J Hum Genet 52:1145–1152

Armstrong SJ, Goldman ASH, Speed RM, Hultén MA (2000) Meiotic studies of a human male carrier of the common translocation, t(11;22), suggests postzygotic selection rather than preferential 3:1 MI segregation as the cause of liveborn offspring with an unbalanced translocation. Am J Hum Genet 67:601–609

Artavanis-Tsakonas S, Rand MD, Lake RJ (1999) Notch signaling: Cell fate control and signal integration in development. Science 284:770–776

Augusseau S, Jouk S, Jalbert P, Prieru M (1986) DiGeorge syndrome and 22q11 rearrangements. Hum Genet 74:206

Back E, Stier R, Bohsen N et al. (1980) Partial monosomy 22pter->q11 in a newborn with the clinical features of trisomy 13 syndrome. Ann Genet (Paris) 23:244–48

Batista DAS, Vianna-Morgante AM, Richieri-Costa A (1983) Tetrasomy 18p: tentative delineation of a syndrome. J Med Genet 20:144–147

Bernstein R, Bocian ME, Cain MF et al. (1993) Identification of cryptic t(5;7) reciprocal translocation by fluorescent in situ hybridization. Am J Med Genet 46:77–82

Blennow E, Nielsen KB, Telenius H et al. (1995) Fifty probands with extra structurally abnormal chromosomes characterized by fluorescence in situ hybridization. Am J Med Genet 55:85–94

Blouin J-L, Avramopoulos D, Pangalos C, Antonarakis SE (1993) Normal phenotype with paternal uniparental isodisomy for chromosome 21. Am J Hum Genet 53:1074–1078

Bowen P, Pabst H, Berry D et al. (1986) Thymic deficiency in an infant with a chromosome t(18;22)(q12.2;p11.2)pat arrangement. Clin Genet 29:174–77

Breuning MH, Dauwerse HG, Fugazza G et al. (1993) Rubinstein-Taybi syndrome caused by submicroscopic deletions within 16p13.3. Am J Hum Genet 52:249–254

Brkanac Z, Cody JD, Leach RJ, DuPont BR (1998) Identification of cryptic rearrangements in patients with 18q- deletion syndrome. Am J Hum Genet 62:1500–6

Brzustowicz LM, Allitto BA, Matseoane D et al. (1994) Paternal isodisomy for chromosome 5 in a child with spinal muscular atrophy. Am J Hum Genet 54:482–488

Buhler EM, Buhler UK, Stalder GR (1980) Chromosome deletion and multiple cartilaginous exostoses. Eur J Pediatr 133:163–166

Burn J (1986) Williams syndrome. Syndrome of the Month. J Med Genet 23:389–395

Burn J, Takao A, Wilson D et al. (1993) Conotruncal anomaly face syndrome is associated with a deletion within chromosome 22. J Med Genet 30:822–824

Butler MG, Meany FJ, Palmer CG (1986) Clinical and cytogenetic survey of 39 individuals with prader-Labhart-Willi syndrome. Am J Med Genet 23:793–809

Byrne JLB, Harrod MJE, Friedman JM, Howard-Peebles PN (1986) Del(20p) with manifestations of arteriohepatic dysplasia. Am J Med Genet 24:673–678

Callen DF, Freemantle CJ, Ringenbergs ML et al. (1990) The isochromosome 18p syndrome: Confirmation of cytogenetic diagnosis in nine cases by in sigu hybridization. Am J Hum Genet 47:493–498

Callen DF, Eyre H, Yip M-Y et al. (1992) Molecular cytogenetic and clinical studies of 42 patients with marker chromosomes. Am J Med Genet 43:709–715

Cassidy SB (1997) Prader-Willi syndrome. J Med. Genet 34:917–923

Chance PF, Bird TD, Matsunami N et al. (1992) Trisomy 17p associated with Charcot Marie Tooth Neuropathy 1A phenotype: Evidence for gene dosage as a mechanism in CMT 1A. Neurology 42:2295–2299

Chen KS, Manian P, Koeuth T et al. (1997) Homologous recombination of a flanking repeat gene cluster is a mechanism for a common contiguous gene deletion syndrome. Nat Genet 17:154–63

Cheng SD, Spinner NB, Zackai EH, Knoll JHM (1994) Cytogenetic and molecular characterication of inverted duplicated chromosomes 15 from 11 patients. Am J Hum Genet 55:753–759

Chiesa J, Hoffet M, Rausseow O et al. (1998) Pallister-Killian syndrome [i(12p)]: First pre-natal diagnosis using cordocentesis in the second trimester confirmed by in situ hybridization. Clin Genet 54:294–303

Clemens M, Martsolf JT, Rogers JG et al. (1996) Pitt-Rogers-Danks syndrome: the result of a 4p microdeletion

Cody JD, Hale DE, Brkanac Z et al. (1997a) Growth hormone insufficiency associated with haploinsufficiency at 18q23. Am J Med Genet 1997 71:420–5

Cody JD, Pierce JF, Brkanac Z et al. (1997b) Preferential loss of the paternal alleles in the 18q- syndrome. Am J Med Genet 69:280–6

Cody JD, Ghidoni PD, DuPont BR et al. (1999) Congenital anomalies and anthropometry of 42 individuals with deletions of chromosome 18q. Am J Med Genet 85:455–62

Conley ME, Beckwith JB, Mancer JFK, Tenchkhoff L (1979) The spectrum of the DiGeorge syndrome. J Pediatr 94:883

Crolla JA, Harvey JF, Sitch FL, Dennis NR (1995) Supernumerary marker 15 chromosomes: a clinical, molecular and FISH approach to diagnosis and prognosis. Hum Genet 95:161–170

Crosnier C, Driancourt C, Raynaud N et al. (1999) Analysis of mutations of the *Jagged1* gene in patients with Alagille syndrome: Evidence for most cases being sporadic. Gastroenterology 116:1141–1148

Daniel A, Boue A, Gallano P (1986) Prospective risk in reciprocal translocation heterozygotes at amniocentesis as determined by potential chromosome imbalance sizes. Data of the European collaborative prenatal diagnosis centers. Prenatal Diagn 6:315–350

Davis LM, Stallard R, Thomas GH et al. (1988) Two anonymous DNA segments distinguish the Wilms' tumor and aniridia loci. Science 241:840–842

de la Chapella A, Herva R, Koivisto M, Aula P (1981) A deletion in chromosome 22 can cause DiGeorge syndrome. Hum Genet 57:253–256

Dieker H, Edwards RH, Zu Rhien et al. (1969) The Lissencephaly syndrome. Birth Defects 5:53

DiGeorge AM (1965) Discussions on a new concept of the cellular basis of immunology. J Pediatr 67:907

Dittrich B, Robinson WP, Knoblauch H et al. (1992) Molecular diagnosis of the Prader-Willi and Angleman syndromes by detection of parent-of-origin specific DNA methylation in 15q11q13. Hum Genet 90:313–315

Dobyns WB, Curry CJR, Hoyme HE et al. (1991) Clinical and molecular diagnosis of Miler-Dieker syndrome. Am J Hum Genet 48:584–594

Donnai D (1996) Editorial comment: Pitt-Rogers-Danks syndrome and Wolf-Hirschhorn syndrome. Am J Med Genet 66:101–103

Driscoll DA, Budarf ML, Emanuel B (1992a) A genetic etiology for DiGeorge syndrome: Consistent deletions and microdeletions of 22q11. Am J Hum Genet 50:924–933

Driscoll DA, Spinner NB, Budarf ML et al. (1992b) Deletions and microdeletions of 22q11.2 in velo-cardio-facial syndrome. Am J Med Genet 44:261–268

Driscoll DJ, Waters MF, Williams CA et al. (1992c) A DNA methylation imprint, determined by the sex of the parent, distinguishes the Angelman and Prader-Willi Syndromes. Genomics 13:917–924

Edelmann L et al. (1999) A common breakpoint on 11q23 in carriers of the constitutional t(11;22) translocation. Am J Hum Genet 65:1608–16

Eggermann T, Engels H, Moskalonek B et al. (1996) Teterasomy 18p de novo: identification by FISH with conventional and microdissection probes and analysis of parental origin and formation by short sequence repeat typing. Hum Genet 97:568–572

Eggerman T, Engels H, Apacik C et al. (1997) Tetrasomy 18p caused by paternal meiotic nondisjunction. Eur J Hum Genet. 5:175–177

Emerick KM, Rand EB, Goldmuntz E et al. (1999) Features of Alagille syndrome in 92 patients: frequency and relation to prognosis. Hepatology 29:822–829

Engel E (1980) A new genetic concept: Uniparental disomy and its potential effect, isodisomy. Am J Med Genet 6:137–143

Ewart AK, Morris CA, Atkinson D et al. (1993) Hemizygosity at the elastin locus in a developental disorder, Williams syndrome. Nat Genet 5:11–16

Faed MJW, Robertson J, Swanson Beck J et al. (1987) Features of DiGeorge syndrome in a child with 45,XX,–3,–22,+der(3),t(3;22)(p25;q11). J Med Genet 25:224–34

Ferguson-Smith MA (1983) Prenatal chromosome analysis and its impact on the birth incidence of chromosome disorders. Br Med Bulletin 39:355–364

Finucane BM, Jaeger E, Kurtz MB et al. (1993) Eye abnormalities in the Smith-Magenis syndrome. Am J Med Genet 45:443–446

Finucane BM, Konar D, Haas-Givler et al. (1994) The spasmodic upper body squeeze: a characteristic behavior in Smith-Magenis syndrome. Dev Med and Child Neurol 36:70–83

Flint J, Wilkie AOM, Buckle VJ et al. (1995) The detection of subtelmomeric chromosomal rearrangements in idiopathic mental retardation. Nature Genet 9:132–139

Fraccaro M, Lindsten J, Ford CE, Iselius L (1980) The 11q;22q translocation: A European collaborative analysis of 43 cases. Hum Genet 56:21–51

Frangiskakis JM, Ewart AK, Morris CA (1996) LIM-kinasel hemizygosity implicated in impaired visuospatial constructive cognition. Cell 86:59–69

Freeman SB, May KM, Pettay D et al. (1993) Paternal uniparental disomy in a child with a balanced 15;15 translocation and Angelman syndrome. Am J Med Genet 45:625–630

Fryns JP, Logghe N, van Eygen M, van den Berghe H (1979) 18q-syndrome in mother and daughter. Eur J Pediatr 130:189–192

Fryns JP, Kleczkowska A, Kubien E, Van den Berge H (1986) Excess of mental retardation and/or congenital malformation in reciprocal translocations in man. Hum Genet 72:1–8

Fujita H, Sakamoto Y, Hamamoto Y (1980) An extra idic (15p)(q11) chromosome in Prader-Willi syndrome. Hum Genet 55:409–411

Funderburk SJ, Spence MA, Sparkes RS (1977) Mental retardation associated with "balanced" chromosome rearrangements. Am J Hum Genet 29:136–141

Gandelman K-Y, Gibson L, Meyn MS, Yang-Feng TL (1992) Molecular definition of the smallest region of deletion overlap in the Wolf-Hirschhorn syndrome. Am J Hum Genet 51:571–578

Garcia-Heras J, Rao PN (1999) A brief review of cryptic duplications of 21q as an emerging cause of Down syndrome: Practical considerations for accurate detection. Clin Genet 55:207–211

Gardner RJM and Sutherland GR (1989) Chromosomal Abnormalities and Genetic Counseling. Oxford University Press, N Y, Oxford

Gersh M, Goodart SA, Pasztor LM et al. (1995) Evidence for a distinct region causing a cat-like cry in patients with 5p deletions. Am J Hum Genet 56:1404–1410

Goldmuntz E, Driscoll D, Budarf ML et al. (1993) Microdeletions of chromosomal region 22q11 in patients with congenital cardiac defects. J Med Genet 20:807–812

Goodman RM, Gorlin RJ (1983) The Malformed Infant and Child. Oxford University Press, N Y

Greenberg F (1990) Williams syndrome professional symposium. Am J Med Genet Suppl 6:85–88

Greenberg F, Crowder WE, Paschall V et al. (1984) Familial DiGeorge syndrome and asociated partial monosomy of chriomosome 22. Hum Genet 65:317–19

Greenberg F, Stratton RF, Lockhart LH et al. (1986) Familial Miller-Dieker syndrome associated with pericentric inversion of chromosome 17. Am J Med Genet 23:853

Greenberg F, Elder FFB, Hafner P et al. (1988) Cytogenetic findings in a prospective series of patients with DiGeorge Anomaly Am J Hum Genet 43:605–611

Greenberg F, Guzzetta V, Montes de Oca-Luna R et al. (1991) Molecular analysis of the Smith-Magenis syndrome: A possible contiguous gene syndrome associated with del(17)(p11.2). Am J Hum Genet 49:1207–1218

Greenberg F, Lewis RA, Potocki L et al. (1996) Multi-disciplinary clinical study of Smith-Magenis syndrome. Am J Med Genet 62:247–54

Hall JG (1990) Genomic imprinting: Review and relevance to human diseases. Am J Hum Genet 46:857–873

Hamabe J, Kuroki Y, Imaizumi K et al. (1991) DNA deletion and its parental origin in origin in Angelman syndrome patients. Am J Med Genet 41:64–68

Healey S, Powell F, Battersby M et al. (1994) Distinct phenotype in maternal uniparental disomy of chromosome 14. Am J Med Genet 51:147–149

Higurashi M, Oda M, Iijima K et al. (1990) Livebirth prevalence and follow up of malformation syndromes in 27,472 newborns. Brain Dev 12:770–773

Hirschhorn K, Cooper HL, Firschein IL (1965) Deletion of short arms of chromosome 4–5 in a child with defects of midline fusion. Humangenetik 1:479–482

Hook EB and Cross P (1987) Rates of mutant and inherited structural cytogenetic abnormalities detected by amniocentesis: Results on about 63,000 fetuses. Ann Hum Genet 51:27–55

Hook EB, Schreinemachers DM, Willey AM, Cross PK (1984) Inherited structural cytogenetic abnormalities detected incidentally in fetuses diagnosed prenatally: Frequency, parental-age associations, sex-ratio trends, and comparisons with rates of mutants. Am J Hum Genet 36:422–443

Horsley SW, Knight SJ, Nixon J et al. (1998) Del(18p) shown to be a cryptic translocation using a multiprobe FISH assay for subtelomeric chromosome rearrangements. J Med Genet 35(9):722–726

Hulten M, Armstrong S, Challinor P et al. (1991) Genomic imprinting in an Angelman and Prader-Willi translocation family (Letter) Lancet 338:638–639

International Human Genome Sequencing Consortium (2001) Initial sequencing and analysis of the human genome. Nature 409:860–921

Iselius L, Lindsten J, Aurias A et al. (1983) The 11q;22q translocation: A collaborative study of 20 new cases and analysis of 110 families. Hum Genet 64:343–355

Jacobs PA (1974) Correlation between euploid structural chromosomal rearrangements and mental subnormality in humans. Nature 249:164–165

Jiang Y-h, Lev-Lehman E, Bressler J et al. (1999) Neurogenetics '99 Genetics of Angelman syndrome. Am J Hum Genet 65:1–6

Jones KL, Gilber EF, Kaveggia EG, Opitz JM (1980) The Miller-Dieker syndrome. Pediatrics 66:277

Kallioniemi A, Kallioniemi O-P, Sudar D et al. (1992) Comparative genomic hybridization for molecular cytogenetic analysis of solid tumors. Science 258:818–821

Kelley RI, Zackai EH, Emanuel BS et al. (1982) The association of the DiGeorge anomalad with partial monosomy of chromosome 22. J Pediatr 101:197–200

Kline AD, White ME, Wapner R et al. (1993) Molecular analysis of the 18q-phenotype. Am J Hum Genet 52:895–906

Killian W, Teschler-Nicola M (1981) Case report 72: Mental retardation, unusual facial appearance, abnormal hair. Syndrome Identification 7:6–7

Knight LA, Lipson M, Mann J, Bachman R (1984) Mosaic inversion duplication of chromosome 15 without phenotypic effect: occurrence in a father and daughter. Am J Med Genet 17:649–654

Kotzot D, Schmitt S, Bernasconi F et al. (1995) Uniparental disomy 7 in Silver-Russell syndrome and primordial growth retardation. Hum Mol Genet 4:583–587

Krantz ID, Colliton RP, Genin A et al. (1998) Spectrum and frequency of Jaggedl (JAG1) mutations in Alagille syndrome patients and their families. Am J Hum Genet 62:1361–1369

Krantz ID, Rand EB, Genin A et al. (1997) Deletions of 20p12 in Alagille syndrome: Frequency and molecular characterization. Am J Med Genet 70:80–86

Krantz ID, Piccoli DA, Spinner NB (1999) Alagille syndrome: Clinical and Molecular Genetics. Current Opinions in Pediatrics 11:558–564

Kurahashi H, Shaikh TH, Hu P et al. (2000) Regions of genomic instability on 22q11 and 11q23 as the etiology for the recurrent constitutional t(11;22). Hum Mol Genet, In Press

Kuslich CD, Kobori JA, Mohapatra G et al. (1999) Prader-Willi syndrome is caused by disruption of the SNRPN gene. Am J Hum Genet 64:70–76

Kuwano A, Ledbetter SA, Dobyns WB et al. (1991) Detection of deletions and cryptic translocations in Miller-Dieker syndrome by *in situ* hybridization. Am J Hum Genet 49:707–714

LaBrecque DR, Mitros FA, Nathan RJ et al. (1982) Four generations of arteriohepatic dysplasia. Hepatology 2:467–474

Lammer EJ, Opitz JM (1986) The DiGeorge anomaly as a developmental field defect. Am J Med Genet Suppl 2:113–127

Langer LO, Krassikoff N, Laxova R et al. (1984) The Tricho-Rhino-Phalangela syndrome with exostoses (or Langer-Giedion Syndrome):

Four additional patients without mental retardation and review of the literature. Am J Med Genet 19:81–111

Lazarus AL, Moore KE, Spinner NB (1991) Recurrent neuroleptic malignant syndrome associated with inv dup(15) and mental retardation. Clin Genet 39:65–67

Leana-Cox J, Jenkins L, Palmer CG, et al. (1994) Molecular cytogenetic analysis of inv dup(15) chromosomes, using probes specific for the Prader-Willi/Angelman syndrome region: Clinical implications. Am J Hum Genet 54:748–756

Ledbetter DH (1992) Minireview: Cryptic translocations and telomere integrity. Am J Hum Genet 51:451–456

Ledbetter DH, Riccardi VM, Airhart SD et al. (1981) Deletions of chromosome 15 as a cause of the Prader-Willi syndrome. New Engl J Med 304:325–329

Ledbetter DH, Mascarello JT, Riccardi VM et al. (1982) Chromosome 15 abnormalities and the Prader-Willi syndrome: A follow up report of 40 cases. Am J Hum Genet 34:278–285

Ledbetter SA, Kuwano A, Dobyns WB, Ledbetter DH (1992) Microdeletions of chromosome 17p13 as a cause of isolated lissencephaly. Am J Hum Genet 50:182–189

Lee S, Wevrick R (2000) Identification of novel imprinted transcripts in the Prader-Willi syndrome and Angelman syndrome deletion region: Further evidence for regional imprinting controi. Am J Hum Genet 66:848–858

Legius E, Fryns J-P, Eyskens B et al. (1990) Alagille syndrome (arteriohepatic dysplasia) and del(20)(p11.2). Am J Med Genet 35:432–535

Li L, Krantz ID, Deng Y et al. (1997) Alagille syndrome is caused by mutations in human Jagged1, which encodes a ligand for Notch1. Nature Genet 16:243–251

Lin AE, Bernar J, Chin A et al. (1986) Congenital heart disease in supernumerary der(22), t(11;22) syndrome. Clin Genet 29:269–275

Lindeman-Kusse MC, Van Haeringen VA, Hoorweg-Nijman JJG and Brunner HG (1996). Am J Med Genet 66:104–112

Lindenbaum RH (1990) Unusual segregation of constitutional 11q;22q translocation may be explained by crossover in interchange segment followed by 3:1 segregation at meiosis I. Hum Genet 85:143

Lindenbaum RH, Bobrow (1975) Reciprocal translocations in man: 3:1 meiotic disjunction resulting in 4- or-45 chromsome offspring. J Med Genet 12:29–43

Lubinsky M, Zellweger H, Greenswag L et al. (1987) Familial Prader-Willi syndrome with normal chromosomes Am J Med Genet 28:37–43

Luciani JM, Guichaoua MR, Delafontaine D et al. (1987) Pachytene analysis in a 17;21 reciprocal translocation carrier: Role of the acrocentric chromosomes in male sterility. Hum Genet 77:246–250

Lüdecke HJ, Johnson C, Wagner MJ et al. (1991) Molecular definition of the shortest region of deleion overlap in the Langer-Giedion syndrome. Am J Hum Genet 49:1197–1206

Lüdecke HJ, Wagner MJ, Nardmann J et al. (1995) Molecular dissection of a contiguous gene syndrome: Localization of the genes involved in the Langer-Giedion syndrome. Hum Molec Genet 4:31–36

Lüdecke HJ, Schmidt O, Nardmann J et al. (1999) Genes and chromosomal breakpoints in the Langer-Giedion syndrome region on human chromosome 8. Hum Genet 105:619–628

Lupski JR, Wise CA, Kuwano A et al. (1992) Gene dosage is a mechanism for Charcot-Marie-Tooth disease type 1A. Nature Genet 1:29–33

Lurie IW and Lazjuk GI (1972) Partial monosomies 18. Review of cytogenetical and phenotypical variants. Humangenetik 15:203–222

Lurie IW, Lazjuk GI, Ussova YI et al. (1980) The Wolf-Hirschhorn syndrome I. Genetics. Clin Genet 17:375–384

McDermid HE, Duncan AMV, Brasch KR et al. (1986) Characterization of the supernumerary chromosome in cat eye syndrome. Science 232:646–48

McTaggart KE, Budarf ML, Driscoll DA et al. (1998) Cat eye syndrome chromosome breakpoint clustering: Identification of two intervals also associated with 22q11 deletion syndrome breakpoints. Cytogenet. Cell Genet. 81:222–228

Malcolm S, Clayton-Smith J, Nichols M et al. (1991) Uniparental paternal disomy in Angelman's syndrome. Lancet 1:694–697

Maraschio P, Cuoco C, Gimelli G (1988) Origin and clinical significance of inv dup(15). In Daniels A (ed): The cytogenetics of Mammalian Autosomal Rearrangements. Liss, N Y, pp. 615–634

Marinescu RC, Johnson EI, Dykens EM et al. (1999) No relationship between the size of the deletion and the level of developmental delay in Cri-Du-Chat syndrome. Am J Med Genet 86:66–70

Martinez JE, Tuck-Muller CM, Superneau D, Wertelecki W (1993) Fertility and the cri-du-chat syndrome Clin Genet 43:212–214

Mascarello JT, Bastian JF, Jones MC (1989) Interstitial deletion of chromosome 22 in a patient with the DiGeorge malformation sequence. Am J Med Genet 32:112–114

Mascari MJ, Gottlieb W, Rogan PK et al. (1992) The frequency of uniparental disomy in Prader-Wilii syndrome: Implications for molecular diagnosis. New Engl J Med 326:1599–1607

Mattei MG, Souiah N, Mattei JF (1984) Chromosome 15 anomalies and the Prader-Willi syndrome: Cytogenetic analysis. Hum Genet 66:313–334

Mears AJ, Duncan AMV, Budarf ML et al. (1994) Molecular characterization of the marker chromosome associated with cat eye syndrome. Am J Hum Genet 55:134–142

Mears AJ, el-Shanti H, Murray JC et al. (1995) Minute supernumerary ring chromosome 22 associated with cat eye syndrome: Further delineation of the critical region. Am J Hum Genet 57:667–73

Medina M, Marinescu RC, Overhauser J et al. (2000) Hemizygosity of delta-catenin (CTNND2) is associated with severe mental retarded in cri-du-chat syndrome. Genomics 63:157–164

Meng X, Lu X, Li Z et al. (1998) Complete physical map of the common deletion region in Williams syndrome and identification and characterization of three novel genes. Hum Genet 103:590–599

Miller JG (1963) Lissencephaly in 2 siblings. Neurology 13:841–850

Mignon C, Malzac P, Moncla A et al. (1996) Clinical heterogeneity in 16 patients with inv dup 15 chromosome: Cytogenetic and molecular studies, search for an imprinting effect. Eur J Hum Genet 4:88–100

Momeni P, Glockner G, Schmidt O et al. (2000) Mutations in a new gene, encoding a zinc-finger protein, cause tricho-rhino-phalangeal syndrome type I. Nat Genet. 24:71–74

Monaco G, Pignata C, Rossi E et al. (1991) DiGeorge anomaly associated with 10p deletion. Am J Med Genet 39:215–216

Moncla A, Piras L, Arbex OF et al. (1993) Physical mapping of microdeletions of the chromosome 17 short arm associated with Smith-Magenis syndrome. Hum Genet 90:657–660

Monk D, Wakeling EL, Proud V et al. (2000) Duplication of 7p11.2-p13, including GRB10, in Silver-Russell syndrome. Am J Hum Genel 66:36–46

Morris CA, Demsey SU, Leonard CO et al. (1988) Natural history of Williams syndrome: Physical characteristics. J Peds 113:318–326

Morris CA, Loker J, Ensing G, Stock AD (1993) Supravalvular aortic stenosis cosegregates with a familial 6;7 translocation which disrupts the elastin gene. Am J Med Genet 46:737–744

Nakao M, Sutcliffe JS, Durschi B et al. (1994) Imprinting analysis of three genes in the Prader-Willi/Angelman region: SNRPN, E6-associated protein and PAR-2 (D15S225E). Hum Mol Genet: 309–315

Nardmann J, Tranebjaerg L, Horsthemke B, Ludecke HJ (1999) The tricho-rhino-phalangeal syndromes: Frequency and parental origin of 8q deletions. Hum Genet 99:638–43

Neri G, Serra A, Campana M, Tedeschi B (1983) Reproductive risks for translocation carriers: Cytogenetic study and analysis of pregnancy outcome in 58 families. Am J Med Genet 16:535–561

Nicholls RD (1993) Genomic imprinting and uniparental disomy in Angelman and Prader-Willi syndromes: A review. Am J Med Genet 46:16–25

Nicholls RD (1994) Invited Editorial. New insights reveal complex mechanisms involved in genomic imprinting. Am J Hum Genet 54:733–740

Nicholls RD, Knoll JHM, Glatt K et al. (1989a) Restriction fragment length polymorphisms within proximal 15q and their use in molecular cytogenetics and the Prader-Willi syndrome. Am J Med Genet 33:66–77

Nicholls RD, Knoll JH, Butler MG et al. (1989b) Genetic imprinting suggested by maternal uniparental heterodisomy in nondeletion Prader-Willi syndrome. Nature 342:281–285

Nickerson E, Greenberg F, Keating MT et al. (1995) Deletions of the elastin gene at 7q11.23 occur in approximately 90% of patients with Williams Syndrome. Am J Hum Genet 56:1156–1161

Niebuhr E (1978a) The cri-du-chat syndrome, epidemiology, cytogenetics, and clinical features. Hum Genet 44:227–275

Niebuhr E (1978b) Cytologic observations in 35 individuals with a 5p-karyotype. Hum Genet 42:146–156

Oda T, Elkahlous AG, Pike BL et al. (1997) Mutations in the human Jagged I gene are responsible for Alagille syndrome. (1997) Nature Genet 16:235–242

Ohashi H, Ishikiriyama S, Fukushima Y (1993) New diagnostic method for Pallister-Killian syndrome: Detection of i(12p) in interphase nuclei of buccal mucosa by fluorescence in situ hybridization. Am J Med Genet 45:123–128

Ohta T, Gray TA, Rogan PK et al. (1999) Imprinting mutation mechanisms in Prader-Willi syndrome. Am J Hum Genet 64:397–413

Orstavik KH, Tangsrud SE, Kiil R et al. (1992) Prader-Willi syndrome in a brother and sister without cytogenetic or detectable molecular genetic abnormality at chromosome 15q11q13. Am J Med Genet 44:534–538

Overhauser J, Beaudet AL, Wasmuth JJ (1986) A fine structure physical map of the short arm of chromosome 5. Am J Hum Genet 39:562–572

Overhauser J, Bengtsson U, McMahon J et al. (1989) Prenatal diagnosis and carrier detection of a cryptic translocation by using DNA markers from the short arm of chromosome 5. Am J Hum Genet 45:296–303

Overhauser J, Huang X, Gersh M et al. (1994) Molecular and phenotypic mapping of the short arm of chromosome 5:sublicalization of the critical region for the cri-du-chat syndrome. Hum Molec Genet 3:247–252

Pallister PD, Meisner LF, Elejalde BR et al. (1977) The Pallister mosaic syndrome. In Bergsma D, Lowry RB (eds): New Syndromes. N Y: Alan R. Liss, Inc. for the National Foundation-March of Dimes. Birth Defects: OAS XIII(3B):103–110

Peltomaki R, Knuutila S, Ritvanen A, Chapelle A de la (1987) Pallister-Killian syndrome: Cytogenetic and molecular studies. Clin Genet 31:399–405

Perez Jurado LA, Peoples R, Kaplan P et al. (1996) Molecular definition of the chromosome 7 deletion in Williams syndrome and parent-of-origin effects on growth. Am J Hum Genet 59:781–792

Piccoli DA, Witzleben CL (1991) Disorders of the intrahepatic bile ducts. In Walker DA, Durie PR, Hamilton JR et al. (eds) Gastrointestinal Disease: Pathophysiology, Diagnosis, Management, 3rd edn. BC Decker, Inc, Philadelphia, PA, pp 1124–1140

Pitt DB, Roger JG, Danks DM (1984) Mental retardation, unusual face, and intrauterine growth retardation: a new recessive syndrome? Am J Med Genel 19:307–313

Pober BR, Lacro RV, Rice C et al. (1997) Renal findings in 40 individuals with Williams syndrome Am J Med Genet 46:271–274

Preece MA, Abu-Amero SN, Ali Z et al. (1999) An analysis of the distribution of hetero and isodisomic regions of chromosome 7 in five MUPD Silver-Russell syndrome probands. Med Genel 36:457–460.

Rand EB, Spinner NB, Piccoli DA et al. (1995) Molecular analysis of 24 Alagille syndrome families identifies a single submicroscopic deletion and further localizes the Alagille region within 20p12. Am J Hum Genet 57:1068–1073

Ray PN, Belfall B, Duff C, et al. (1985) Cloning of the breakpoint of an X;21 translocation associated with Duchenne muscular dystrophy. Nature 318:672–675

Reiner O, Carrozzo R, Shen Y et al. (1993) Isolation of a Miller-Dieker lissencephaly gene containing G protein B subunit-like repeats. Nature 364:717–721

Reynolds JF, Daniel A, Kelly TE et al. (1987) Isochromosome 12p mosaicism (Pallister mosaic aneuploid or Pallester-Killian syndrome): report of 11 cases. Am J Med Genet 27:257–274

Rivera H, Moller M, Hernandez A et al. (1984) Tetrasomy 18p: a distinctive syndrome. Ann Genet 27:187–189

Robertson W (1916) Chromosome studies. I. Taxonomic relationships shown in the chromosomes of Tettigidae and Acrididae. V-shaped chromosomes and their significance in Acrididae, Locutididae and Gryllidae: Chromosomes and variation. J Morphol 27:179

Robinson WP, Bottani A, Yagang X et al. (1991) Molecular, cytogenetic and clinical investigations of Prader-Willi syndrome patients. Am J Hum Genet 49:1219–1234

Robinson WP, Wagstaff J, Bernasconi F et al. (1993) Uniparental disomy explains the occurrence of the Angelman or Prader-Willi syndrome in patients with an additional small inv dup(15) chromosome. J Med Genet 1993 30:756–760

Sachs ES, Van Hemel JO, Den Hollander JC, Jahoda MGJ (1987) Marker chromosomes in a series of 10,000 prenatal diagnoses. Cytogenetic and follow up studies Prenat Diag 7:81–89

Schinzel A (1984) Catalog of unbalanced Chromosome Aberrations in Man, Walter de Gruyter, Berlin

Schinzel A (1991) Tetrasomy 12p (Pallister-Killian syndrome). J Med Genet 54:294–302

Schinzel A (1994) Human Cytogenetics Database. Oxford Medical Database Series. Oxford University Press.

Schinzel A, Schmid W, Fraccaro M et al. (1981) Dicentric small marker chromosome probably derived from a no.: 22 (tetrasomy 22pterq11) associated with a characteristic phenotype. Hum Genet 57:148–158

Schinzel AA, Basaran S, Bernasconi F et al. (1994) Maternal uniparental disomy 22 has no impact on the phenotype. Am J Hum Genet 54:211–24

Schmickel RD (1986) Contiguous gene syndromes: A component of recognizable syndromes. J Pediatr 109:231–241

Schnittger S, Hofers C, Heidemann P et al. (1989) Molecular and cytogenetic analysis of an intersitital 20p deletion associated with syndromic intrahepatic ductular hypoplasia (Alagille syndrome). Hum Genet 83:239–244

Schreck RR, Breg WR, Erlanger BF, Miller OJ (1977) Preferential derivation of abnormal human G-group like chromosomes from chromosome 15. Hum. Genet 36:1–12

Schrock E, du Manoir S, Veldman T et al. (1996) Multicolor spectral karyotyping of human chromosomes. Science 273:494–7

Schubert R, Viersbach R, Eggermann T et al. (1997) Report of two new cases of Pallister-Killian syndrome confirmed by FISH: Tissue-specific mosaicism and loss of i(12p) by in vitro selection. Am J Med Genet 72:106–110

Schulze A, Hansen C, Skakkebaek NE et al. (1996) Exclusion of the SNRPN as a major determinant of Prader-Willi syndrome by a translocation breakpoint. Nature Genet 12:452–454

Scott JA, Wenger SL, Steele MW, Chakravarti A (1995) Down syndrome consequent to a cryptic maternal 12p;21q translocation. Am J Med Genet 56:67–71

Shaikh TH, Budarf ML, Celle L et al. (1999) Clustered 11q23 and 22q11 breakpoints and 3:1 meiotic malsegregation in multiple unrelated t(11;22) families. Am J Hum Genet. 65:1595–1607

Shprintzen RJ, Goldberg RB, Lewin ML et al. (1978) A new syndrome involving cleft palate, cardiac anomalies, typical facies and learning disabilities: velo-cardio-facial syndrome. Cleft Palate J. 15:56

Shprintzen RJ, Goldberg RB, Young D, Wolford L (1981) The velo-cardio-facial syndrome: A clinical and genetic analysis. Pediatr 67:167–172

Shprintzen RJ, Wang F, Goldberg R, Marion R (1985) The expanded velo-cardio-facial syndrome: additional features of the most common clefting syndrome Am J Hum Genet 37:A77

Shulman SA, Hyams JS, Gunta R et al. (1984) Arteriohepatic dysplasia (Alagille Syndrome): Extreme variability among affected family members. Am J Med Genet 19:325–332

Slater H, Shaw JH, Dawson G et al. (1994) Maternal uniparental disomy of chromosome 13 in a phenotypically normal child. J Med Genet 31:644–646

Smeets DFCM, Hamel BCJ, Nelen MR et al. (1992) Prader-Willi syndrome and Angelman syndrome in cousins from a family with a translocation between chromosomes 6 and 15. New Engl J Med 326:807–811

Smith ACM, McGavran L, Robinson J et al. (1986) Interstitial deletion of (17)(p11.2p11.2) in nine patients. Am J Med Genet 24:393–414

Smith A, Robson L, Neuman A et al. (1993) Flurescence in situ hybridisation and molecular studies used in the characterisation of a Roberstonian translocation t(13q15q) in Prader-Willi syndrome. Clin Genet 43:5–8

Smith AC, Dykens E, Greenberg F (1998) Sleep disturbance in Smith-Magenis syndrome (del 17 p11.2). Am J Med Genet 81:186–91

Spence JE Perciaccante RG, Grieg GM et al. (1988) Uniarental disomy as a mechanism for human genetic disease. Am J Hum Genet 42:217–226

Spinner NB, Rand EB, Fortina P et al. (1994) Cytologically balanced t(2;20) in a two-generation family with Alagille syndrome: cytogenetic and molecular studies. Am J Hum Genet 55:238–243

Spinner NB, Rehberg-Grace K, Owens NL et al. (1995a) Mosaicism for a chromosome 8 derived minute marker chromosome in a patient with manifestations of trisomy 8 mosaicism. Am J Med Genet 56:22–24

Spinner NB, Zackai E, Cheng S-D, Knoll JHM (1995b) Supernumerary inv dup(15) in a patient with Angelman syndrome and a deletion of 15q11q13. Am J Med Genet 57:61–65

Spinner NB, Colliton RP, Crosnier C, Krantz ID, Hadchouel M, Heunier-Rotival H (2001) Mutation Update: Jagged/ Mutations in Alagille Syndrome. Human Mutat 17:18–33

Stetten G, Sroka-Zacaek B, Corson VL (1981) Prenatal detection of an accessory chromosome identified as an inversion duplication (15). Hum Genet 57:357–359

Stratton RF, Dobyns WB, Greenberg F et al. (1986) Interstitial deletion of (17)(p11.2p11.2) Report of six additional patients with new chromosome deletion syndrome. Am J Med Genet 24:421–432

Stratton RF, Dobyns WB, Airhart SD, Ledbetter DH (1994) New chromosome syndrome: Miller-Dieker syndrome and monosomy 17p13. Hum Genet 67:193

Struthers JL, Cuthbert CD, Khalifa MM (1999) Parental origin of the isochromosome 12p in Pallister-Killian syndrome: Molecular analysis of one patient and review of the reported cases. Am J Med Genet 84:111–115

Subrt I and Pokorny J (1970) Familial occurrence of 18q-. Humangenetik 10:181–187

Sutcliffe JS, Nakao M, Christian S et al. (1994) Deletions of a differentially methylated CpG island at the SNRPN gene define a putative imrprinting control region. Nature Genet 8:52–58

Takeda K, Okamura T, Hasegawa T (1989) Sibs with tetrasomy 18p born to a mother with trisomy 18p. J Med Genet 26:195–197

Taylor KM, Wolfinger HL, Brown MG et al. (1975) Origin of a small metacentric chromosome: familial and cytogenic evidence. Clin Genel 8:364–369

Teebi AS, Krishna Murthy DS, Ismail EAR, Redha AA (1992) Alagille syndrome with de novo del(20(p11.2). Am J Med Genet 42:35–38

Temple IK, Cockwell A, Hassold T et al. (1991) Maternal uniparental disomy for chromosome 14. J Med Genet 28:511–514

Uchida IA, McRae KN, Wang HC, Ray M (1965) Familial short arm deficiency of chromosome 18 concomitant with arhinencephaly and alopecia congenita. Am J Hum Genet 17:410–419

Uhrig S, Schuffenhaver S, Fauth C et al. (1999) Multiplex-FISH for pre- and postnatal diagnostic applications. Am J Hum Genet 65:448–462

Van Dyke DL, Weiss L, Roberson JR, Babu VR (1983) The frequency and mutation rate of balanced autosomal rearrangements in man estimated from prenatal genetic studies for advanced maternal age. Am J Hum Genet 35:301–308

Voss R, Ben-Simon E, Avital A et al. (1989) Isodisomy of chromosome 7 in a patient with cystic fibrosis: Could uniparental disomy be common in humans? Am J Hum Genet 45:373–380

Wagstaff J, Knoll HJM, Glatt KA et al. (1992) Maternal but not paternal transmission of 15q11-q13 linked nondeletion Angelman syndrome leads to phenotype expression. Nature Genet 1:291–294

Wallace MR, Marchuk DA, Andersen LB et al. (1990) Type 1 neurofibromatosis gene: Identification of a large transcript disrupted in three NF1 patients. Science 249:181–186

Wandstrat AE, Leana-Cox J, Jenkins L, Schwartz S (1998) Molecular cytogenetic evidence for a common breakpoint in the largest inverted duplications of chromosome 15. Am J Hum Genet 62:925–936

Wang J-CC, Passage MB, Yen PH (1991) Uniparental heterodisomy for chromosome 14 in a phenotypically abnormal familial balanced 13/14 Robertsonian translocation carrier. Am J Hum Genet 48:1069–1074

Warburton D (1991) De Novo Balanced chromosome rearrangements and extra marker chromosomes identified at prenatal diagnosis: clinical significance and distribution of breakpoints. Am J Hum Genet 49:995–1013

Ward BE, Hayden MW, Robinson A (1988) Isochromosome 12p mosaicism (Pallister-Killian Syndrome): Newborn diagnosis by direct bone marrow analysis. Am J Med Genet 31:835–839

Watson GH and Miller V (1973) Arteriohepatic dysplasia, familial pulmonary arterial stenosis with neonatal liver disease. Arch Dis Childhood 48:459–466

Weiss BJ, Kamholz J, Ritter A et al. (1991) Segmental spinal muscular atrophy and dermatological findings in a patient with chromosome 18q deletion. Annals Neurol 30:419–423

Wenger SL, Boone LY, Steele MW (1990) Mosaicism in Pallister i(12p) syndrome. Am J Med Genet 35:523–525

Wilkins LE, Brown JA, Wolf B (1980) Psychomotor development in 65 home-reared children with cri-du-chat syndrome. J Pediatr 97:401–405

Wilson DI, Cross IE, Goodship JA et al. (1992a) A prospective cytogenetic study of 36 cases of DiGeorge syndrome. Am J Hum Genet 51:957–963

Wilson DI, Goodship JA, Burn J et al. (1992b) Deletions within chromosome 22q11 in familial congenital heart disease. Lancet 340:573–575

Williams MA, Shprintzen RJ, Goldberg RB (1985) Male to male transmission of the velo-cardio-facial syndrome: A case report and review of 60 cases. Craniofacial Genet 5:175–180

Wilson MG, Towner JW, Coffin GS et al. (1981) Genetic and clinical studies in 13 patients with the Wolf-Hirschhorn syndrome [del(4p)]. Hum Genet 59:297–307

Wilson TA, Blethen SL, Vallone A et al. (1993) Di George anormaly with renal agenesis in infants of mothers with diabetes. AM J Med Genel 47:1078–1082

Wisniewski L, Hassold T, Heffelfinger J, Higgins JV (1979) Cytogenetic and clinical studies in five cases of inv dup(15). Hum Genet 50:259–270

Wolf U, Reinwein H, Porsch R et al. (1965) Defizienz an den kurzen Armen eines Chromosomes Nr. 4. Humangenetik 1:397–413

Woodage T, Prasad M, Dixon JW et al. (1994) Bloom syndrome and maternal uniparental disomy for chromosome 15. Am J Hum Genet 55:74–80

Wright TJ, Clemens M, Quarrell O, Altherr MR (1998) Wolf-Hirschhorn and Pitt-Rogers-Danks Syndromes caused by overlapping 4p deletions. Am J Med Genet 75:345–350

Zackai EH, Emanuel BS (1980) Site specific reciprocal translocation, t(11;22)(q23;q11) in several unrelated families with 3:1 meiotic disjunction. Am J Med Genet 7:507–521

Zhang F, Deleuze JF, Aurias A et al. (1990) Interstitial deletion of the short arm of chromosome 20 in arteriohepatic dysplasia (Alagille syndrome). J Pediatr 116:73–77

Zannoti M, Preto A, Giovanardi PR, Dallapiccola B (1980) Extra dicentric 15pter→21/22 chromosomes in five unrelated patients with a distinct syndrome of progressive psychomotor retardation, seizures, hyper-reactivity and dermatoglyphic abnormalities. J Ment Defic Res 24:235–242

Cardiovascular disorders

Congenital heart disease

47

John Burn
Judith Goodship

Introduction

Heart malformations are the most common form of birth defect, affecting about 7 in 1000 newborns. Despite this, they have received relatively little attention from geneticists. The wide availability of pre- and postnatal diagnostic echocardiography, coupled with the greatly improved life expectancy thanks to surgical advances, such that adults with major congenital heart defects are becoming parents, have increased awareness of genetic predisposition among pediatric cardiologists and their patients. The greater sophistication of cytogenetic and molecular genetic techniques and an increased willingness among geneticists to address complex traits has resulted in a similar growth in interest among geneticists. The approach in this chapter is to focus on practical presentation and incorporate theoretical and research aspects where relevant.

As with all birth defects, chromosomal aneuploidy should be suspected in any newborn with congenital heart disease. The association of heart disease with a specific pattern dysmorphic features may suggest a syndrome. Maternal history will identify those associated with the known teratogens. Clinical examination will identify those liable to be associated with a chromosomal deletion not apparent to routine karyotype analysis. A combination of family history and dysmorphic features can identify a further group of heart defects associated with monogenic syndromes. In a small proportion of isolated heart defects, the pedigree is sufficient to recognize monogenic inheritance. The rest must be addressed in the clinic using empirical data from traditional family studies. In the future we may anticipate a greater focus in counseling based on molecular testing for genes that predispose a person to heart defects. The likely success of this approach will depend on the relative contribution of genetic *versus* nongenetic factors and the likely number of genes involved in an individual.

Embryology and terminology

The complexity of cardiovascular embryology and the equally complex terminology that describes anomalies have been a deterrent to geneticists. The heart becomes recognizable when the cardiogenic ridges unite in the midline at four weeks post-fertilization. The resultant cardiac tube grows rapidly, bulging forward in the midline. The tube is pulsatile and begins to produce a circulation before valve development. It has an inlet or atrium, a central dilatation (ventricle) and an outlet portion—the bulbus cordis—leading to the single outlet artery—the truncus arteriosus. Differential growth of the right and left sides of the tube causes it to bend to the right (Fig. 47.1). The heart is unique in being an essential organ from the earliest stages of development. It must remain operational as it converts from a simple tube to a four-chamber, valved organ.

Venous blood entering the heart from below through the future inferior vena cava is oxygenated by the placenta. Most of the blood is routed through to the left hand side of the atrium and forms the left-sided stream of blood that supplies the rapidly growing brain. Deoxygenated blood from the head and upper body forms most of the right-sided flow. Provided the bend is at the correct angle, the two streams of blood retain their laminar flow as they pass through the ventricle to the outflow tract. Preservation of laminar flow allows normal septal growth, while correct positioning of the endocardial cushions allows them to

1239

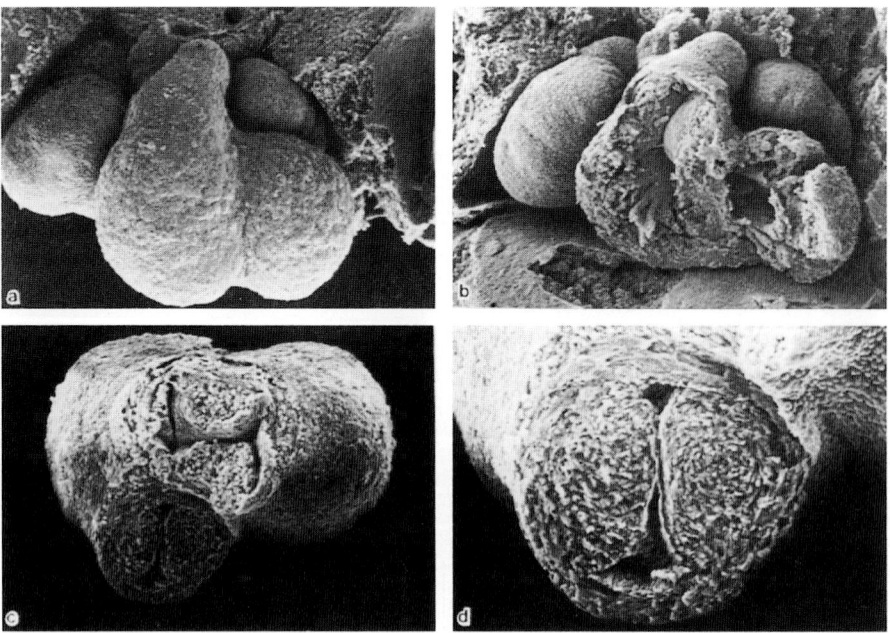

Fig. 47.1 Scanning electron micrograph of the early heart tube of the mouse, showing the normal curve to the right allowing the ventricle and bulbus cordis to lie beside each other and allow the expansion to form the "left" and "right" ventricles. The sections show the cushions that septate the inlet to and outlet from the ventricles. (Courtesy of Kathy Sulik, MD.)

meet appropriately. The septum primum separates the left and right atria. To allow fetal circulation, a hole forms in the middle, which is covered by an infolding of the wall. The right-to-left flow in the fetus separates the two septa and allows blood to cross. After birth, pulmonary flow raises the pressure in the left atrium and presses the two septa together, closing the communication. If the hole – the fossa ovalis – is too big, or the septum secundum too small, a hole persists, known as a secundum atrial septal defect (ASD). The venous return to the heart enters a sinus venosus in early heart development. As organogenesis proceeds, this chamber becomes incorporated into the posterior wall of the atria. If this process is incomplete, a gap persists in the atrial septum, the much rarer sinus venosus ASD.

The superior and inferior endocardial cushions grow toward each other and septate the opening between the atrium and ventricle. Valves form in the two openings – the mitral valve on the left and tricuspid valve on the right. Failure of this process causes the development of a single-valve structure with a septal defect above and below it. The atrioventricular septal defect (AVSD) is a severe heart defect with specific clinical features and genetic associations. In the American literature the term AV canal defect is favored. The valve apparatus may become attached to the lower edge of the septum primum above it, resulting in blood flow only between the ventricles, an inlet ventricular

septal defect (VSD). More commonly, the valve structure tethers to the upper edge of the ventricular septum leaving only a hole between the atria, an ostium primum ASD. From a genetic viewpoint, AVSD, inlet VSD, and ostium primum ASD are synonymous and must be distinguished from the much more common secundum ASD and other types of VSD. The atria develop on the left and right sides of the heart and are thus truly lateralized structures. The two ventricles, on the other hand, develop from the single ventricle and bulbus cordis. The heart loop rotates the central tubular structure to cause them to lie in a left-right orientation. The ventricles are not, therefore, lateralized in the sense that they derive from the left and right sides of the early embryo. Blood enters the outflow tract from the bulbus cordis, which is part of the future right ventricle. It reaches this part of the heart from the future left ventricle through the opening between the ventricle and bulbus cordis. As the two ventricles bulge away caudally, the relative size of this opening becomes less. It is eventually closed off during septation of the outflow tract to form the small membranous part of the ventricular septum. Failure of this process results in the common and relatively minor membranous ventricular septal defect (VSD). Most of the wall between the ventricles comprises the myocardium, which becomes part of the pump chamber. Much of the surface is trabeculated, giving it a web-like appearance. The right ventricle is distinguished from the left by the coarser structure of the trabeculae. The programed cell death involved in this process is a likely factor in the appearance of holes through the wall, allowing blood to cross from left to right after birth. These muscular VSDs often close spontaneously as hypertrophy of the surrounding muscle obstructs the flow. Membranous VSDs are sometimes closed secondarily by valve tissue from the tricuspid valve. In genetic counseling terms, these resolving heart murmurs are significant. Failure of equal and appropriate growth of the two ventricles may result from abnormal heart looping, abnormal inlet orifices, or obstruction of the outlet vessels. The most serious is failure of growth of the left ventricle, known as hypoplastic left heart. A more specific defect of development of the right ventricular muscular wall results in a distended saclike right ventricle with various names, including *right* ventricular dysplasia and Uhl anomaly.

The outflow tract is septated by cells migrating in from the neural crest. Since these cells also form many other structures, including the face, outflow tract defects are often seen in a variety of syndromes. Complete failure of septation results in a common arterial trunk or, as it is more commonly known, persistent truncus arteriosus. The septation of the outflow tract continues to generate intense debate among embryologists, but there is, in effect, a spiral separation that produces the aorta on the left and the pulmonary artery on the right. The plane of the septum is rotated further from the heart so that the pulmonary artery lies anterior to the aorta. The effect of growth is to move the aorta back into an indented or wedged position so that when the septum extends down onto the margin of the ventricular septum the aorta becomes connected to the left ventricle, leaving the pulmonary artery as the sole outlet of the right. If this process is incomplete or distorted, the aorta overrides the upper margin of the ventricular septum; the membranous septum remains incomplete, and the outlet of the right ventricle is narrowed. These malformations combine to cause hypertrophy of the right ventricle. The combination of an aorta overriding a VSD with right ventricular outflow tract (RVOT) obstruction and RV hypertrophy constitute the tetralogy of Fallot. If the process if further distorted, the aorta lies predominantly over the right ventricle and the term DORV (double outlet right ventricle) is applied. This anomaly may also form part of the spectrum that results in an abnormal plane of the outflow septum such that the anterior vessel becomes connected to the left ventricle and the morphologic aorta to the right ventricle. Transposition of the great arteries (TGA) is thus distinct from most outflow defects in that it results from a malformation of the septum rather than a neural crest migration anomaly. This distinction is reflected in the syndrome associations and recurrence risks.

Malformations involving the major vessels connected to the heart are generally included with heart defects in discussions of cause and recurrence risk. Systemic venous drainage is rarely of major genetic importance, although absence of the last segment of the inferior vena cava and its replacement by an azygous connection to the superior vena cava is a valuable diagnostic sign of lack of a morphologic right atrium in left isomerism sequence. Abnormality of pulmonary venous drainage is of much greater significance. Four pulmonary veins rendezvous with an outgrowth from the back of the left atrium. The coalescence incorporates into the posterior wall, producing four separate orifices. If one or more of the orifices are displaced, the term anomalous pulmonary venous drainage is applied, which may be partial, involving up to three vessels, or complete, when it is known as total anomalous venous drainage (TAPVD). Displacement to the right on the posterior atrial wall is one cause of a sinus venosus ASD. In the absence of a morphologic left atrium in cases of disturbed laterality, the pulmonary veins find an outlet to one of the neighboring venous structures, such as the superior vena cava or to the hepatic veins below the diaphragm.

The aorta is assembled from several embryologic origins. The ascending aorta is from the original midline outflow tract, while the arch is the persistent left fourth aortic arch. The aortic arches begin as a symmetrical branching structure in the branchial arches and are distinguished by an elastic tunica media of neural crest origin. The most serious malformation is the absence of the aortic arch, which results in a descending aorta connected to the heart only through the ductus arteriosus. Interrupted aortic arch is often seen in association with anomalies involving the branchial arch and hence neural crest derivatives.

The ductus arteriosus (arterial duct) connects the right ventricular outflow to the descending aorta. It is usually called the sixth aortic arch, but it is morphologically distinct and has evolved to have an oxygen-sensitive lining, which allows it to constrict and occlude after birth, allowing the pulmonary circulation to open. It often stays open after birth, particularly in preterm infants in whom the duct is not mature. The persistent ductus arteriosus (PDA) is, therefore, one of the most common anomalies of the cardiovascular system in postnatal life, but an essential physiologic structure in utero.

This brief overview has focused on anomalies relevant to a group of major defects that are serious after birth but compatible with intrauterine survival. The dependence of the embryo and fetus on a functional circulation means that any defect that compromises intrauterine function is lost at an early stage.

Chromosomal defects and heart malformation

The previous section illustrates the complexity of heart development, which requires precise timing and migration to achieve correct function. It is hardly surprising that cardiovascular embryology involves a large number of genes; indeed, most chromosome defects are associated with an increased incidence of heart defects. In most cases of aneuploidy there is no specific type of heart defect, and counseling is based on the underlying karyotype. As a general rule, chromosome analysis should be performed in any infant presenting with a heart defect associated with other malformations, or dysmorphic features, or both. If the defect is suspected at or before birth, there are usually sufficient mitotic cells in cord blood to allow a rapid analysis. More often, there is time to perform standard analysis, particularly now that widespread use of prostaglandin inhibitors to keep the duct open and maintain circulation has made the need to intervene immediately less common. An exception is that transposition of the great arteries with an intact septum requires immediate action to prevent death. It is rarely associated with chromosomal defects.

ANEUPLOIDY (see also Ch. 28)

The term aneuploidy means "not good set". It has two meanings in the literature. Some writers use the term to denote any abnormality of the chromosomes. Cytogeneticists tend to apply the term to numerical departures from the norm: monosomies, trisomies, and tetrasomies. The three most common trisomies are worthy of detailed discussion, together with the only common examples of monosomy (Turner syndrome) and tetrasomies, (cat eye syndrome and Pallister-Killian syndrome).

Trisomy 21 (Down syndrome) (see also Ch. 44)

Trisomy 21 remains the most important association between major chromosome defects and heart malformation. Before the introduction of widespread maternal serum screening for Down syndrome, 5% of heart defects in newborn infants were accounted for by trisomy 21 cases. In addition to this numerical importance, there is a specific association of great interest in the molecular studies of heart defects; about 40% of children with Down syndrome have heart defects, and of these, almost half have the otherwise rare AVSD. On the basis of quantitative Southern blot analysis and fluorescent in situ hybridization (FISH) studies in cases of partial duplication, Korenberg and colleagues

(1990a; 1990b, 1992; Barlow et al., 2001) have localized the critical region for the Down phenotype to the telomeric segment of the chromosome beyond 21q22.12. Mouse chromosome 16 has a large segment of homology with human trisomy 21; the trisomy 16 mouse has heart defects that closely resemble those seen in trisomy 21. The most telomeric segment, including most of band 22.3, does not share homology with the mouse chromosome 16. The gene or genes responsible for the AVSD in Down syndrome likely reside in a 6.63 Mb segment of which 21q22.2 forms the middle third (Korenberg and Kurnit, 1995). A gene which continues to attract great interest is the col6A1 gene (Davies et al, 1995). Haplotype analysis within this gene in Down syndrome families revealed a nonrandom distribution, suggesting that the contribution from the disjoining parent may be a determinant of CHD risk in Down syndrome babies.

Collagen VI is a candidate gene because it maps to human chromosome 21, but a major argument against this gene is that it does not map to chromosome 16 in the mouse (MacDonald et al, 1991). The growth and/or adhesion of the endocardial cushions or the cellular structures in their immediate vicinity, is highly likely to be implicated in the disease process. Identification of genes expressed in the cushion region that are chromosome 21-specific should greatly reduce the number of genes of interest. Elaborate analysis of heart cDNA libraries may be necessary, since the relevant gene may be more widely expressed. Kurnit and colleagues (1985) put forward the hypothesis that there was a failure to form the atrioventricular septum because the overexpression of a gene involved in cell adhesion led to premature cessation of growth.

From the clinical perspective, the geneticist is often consulted when a neonate presents with features of Down syndrome (see Ch. 44). While the major features are well-recognized and documented, it is not unusual for doubt to persist until the karyotype is available. In these circumstances, examination of the dermatoglyphic pattern is of great help in making a diagnosis (Fig. 47.2). Routine examination should detect single palmar creases (common in the general population), loss of a flexion crease on the fifth digit, and a wide first-toe cleft. Closer examination requires magnification. At the bedside, the best approach is to use an otoscope without an earpiece. On the fingertips the presence of at least eight ulnar loops are typical of Down syndrome. Bilateral ulnar loops on the index fingers are least often seen in the normal population. Other findings typical of Down syndrome are displacement of the axial triradius toward the palm and a simple arch (instead of a whorl) on the feet over the first metatarsal head. If all these

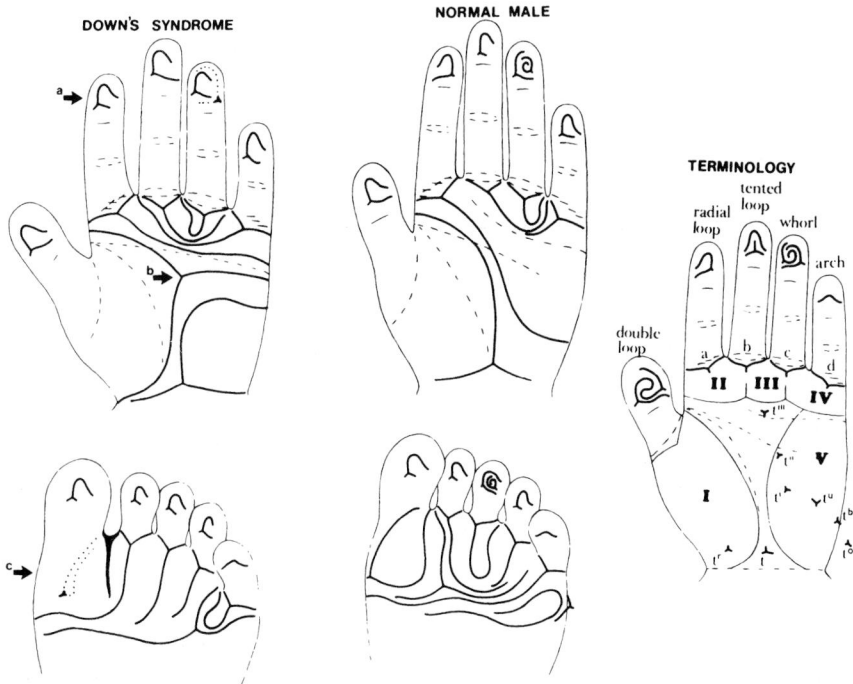

Fig. 47.2 Dermatoglyphics in Down syndrome. The dotted lines illustrate the palmar creases. The continuous lines illustrate the fine ridge patterns. Examination is possible with the naked eye, but is easier with an auroscope without earpiece or ophthalmoscope using a plus 20 lens. To support a diagnosis of trisomy 21, first check with naked eye for absence of the distal flexion crease on the fifth finger and single "simian" palmar creases. Then, with a lens, examine the index finger of the right hand for an ulna loop (a) which occurs in over 90% of children with trisomy 21. If time permits examine the other fingers. There should be 8–10 ulnar loops whereas normally there are less than 7. Next follow the ridge pattern from the thenar eminence across the palm to identify the triradius where it meets the ridge pattern from the wrist, and that from the hypothenar eminence. The triradius should be distally placed (b). Finally, check the pattern over the head of the first metatarsal. There should be a tibial arch—the ridge pattern crosses to the medial border without forming a triradius. (From Pedro Saldana-Garcia, with permission.)

dermatoglyphic features are present in a child whose dysmorphic features suggest trisomy 21, the diagnosis is secure. If the facial features and dermatoglyphics are conflicting, mosaicism or another syndrome that can cause early confusion, such as Zellweger syndrome, should be considered.

Trisomy 18 (Edwards syndrome)

Figure 47.3 illustrates the typical apparance of an infant with trisomy 18 or Edwards syndrome, the second most common autosomal aneuploidy after Down syndrome. This is an important bedside diagnosis, because the prognosis is so poor; a positive diagnosis may influence medical management. In addition to the prominent occiput, low-set ears, micrognathia, and small palpebral fissures, particular diagnostic clues are the short sternum, typical finger clenching with the second and fifth fingers overlapping third and fourth fingers, and a predominance of simple arches on the fingers. Heart defects are a recognized association and are often quoted as the cause of early demise. Embleton and colleagues (1996) reviewed all cases of

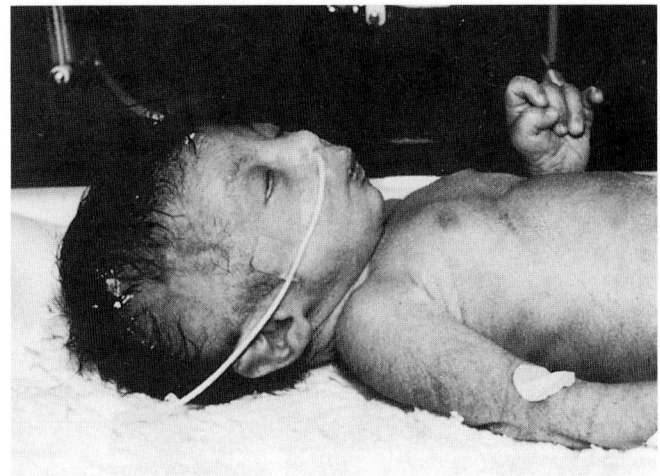

Fig. 47.3. Trisomy 18 (Edwards syndrome). Note the small jaw, small palpebral fissure, short stemum and typical hand posture with the outer fingers overlapping the third and fourth.

trisomy 18 over a six-year period in northern England and identified 66 babies and fetuses among 282,583 births, giving a prevalence at 18 weeks gestation of 1 in 8333 and a birth prevalence of 1 in 4274, figures in keeping with reports from Denmark and Utah (Goldstein and Nielsen, 1988; Root and Carey, 1994). Postmortem examination, echocardiography, or both was carried out in 25 babies of which 21 had a heart defect. Of the remaining nine liveborn neonates, six had no heart murmur or heart failure, and two had murmurs without failure but died of apnea. Of the 21 heart defects, seven were VSDs, five were AVSDs, two were double outlet right ventricles, and three were hypoplastic left hearts. In only five was the heart defect considered the cause of death, yet all babies in the series had died by the end of the first year. The spectrum was similar to that reported in a postmortem series.

Trisomy 13 (Patau syndrome)

The birth incidence of trisomy 13 is about 1 in 7000. The majority die as neonates. Survival beyond the first year of life is exceptional (Wyllie et al., 1994). The characteristic clinical features are postaxial polydactyly, cleft lip and palate (often bilateral and severe) and hypotelorism associated with holoprosencephaly (Fig. 47.4). There is a high incidence of cardiac defects, in particular atrial and ventricular septal defects. Disturbance of cardiac position, including dextrocardia, is common (Schinzel, 1983), suggesting a role for a gene or genes on chromosome 13 in laterality development.

Tetrasomy 22p (cat eye syndrome)

Tetrasomy 22p individuals typically show a marker chromosome, an isochromosome of 22p. The marker may be lost

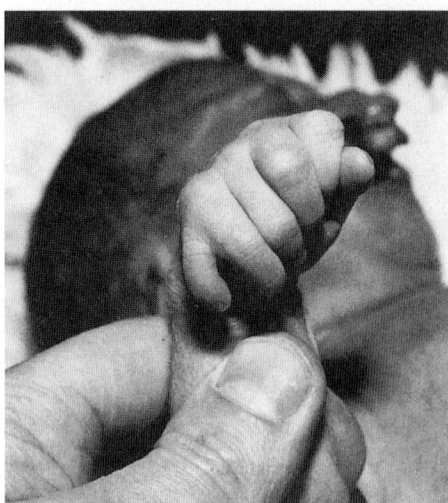

Fig. 47.4. Postaxial polydactyly with or without facial clefting make trisomy 13 a strong possibility. Facial clefts are often midline, tending towards holoprosencephaly. Heart defects including dextrocardia are relatively common.

from the blood and other tissues with age (McDermid et al., 1986). The syndrome is characterized by a variable pattern of anomalies, including learning disability, ear tags, imperforate anus, and iris colobomata. The last of these is no more consistent than the others, which makes the title "cat eye syndrome" misleading. The child shown in Figure 47.5 did not have the iris defect but did have the other features and was noted to have clinical features of heart failure when seen in the genetic clinic despite an absence of heart murmurs. The strong association of tetrasomy 22p with total anomalous pulmonary venous drainage prompted referral for echocardiography. TAPVD was found and treated, but not before irreversible lung damage due to pulmonary hypertension had resulted. The strong association

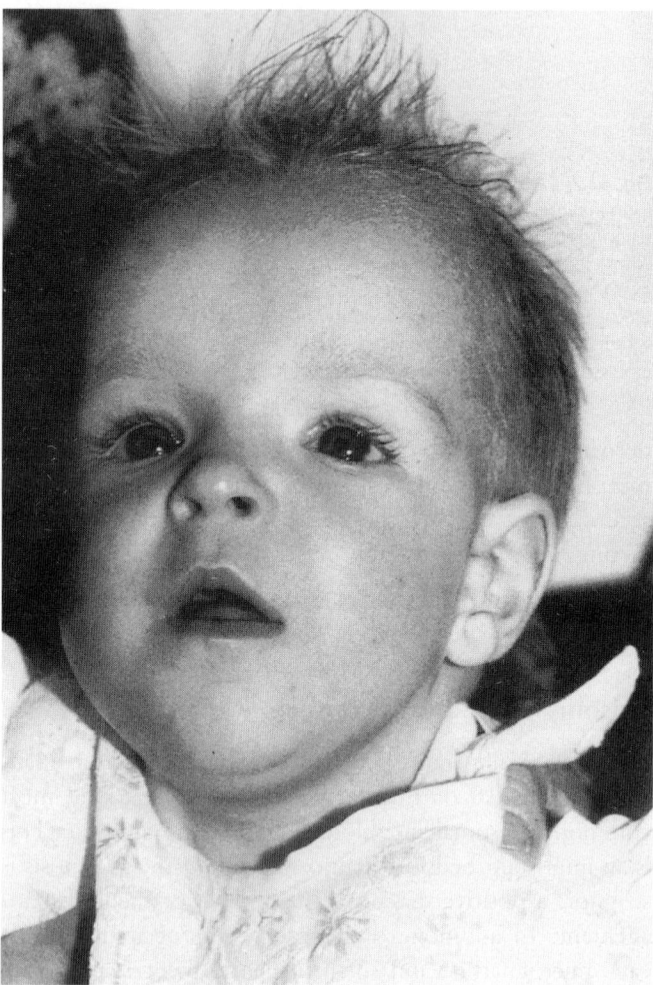

Fig. 47.5. Tetrasomy 22p usually results from the presence of an additional marker chromosome made up of two 22 short arms attached end-to-end. The popular name cat eye syndrome refers to the presence of iris coloboma. As this child shows, the ocular anomaly is not consistent. Fleshy ear tags and anal anomalies are seen. There is an association with TAPVD, which was overlooked in this child until pulmonary hypertension had developed.

of TAPVD with tetrasomy 22p is another clue to the location of key genes in heart development.

Tetrasomy 12p (Pallister-Killian syndrome)

Pallister-Killian syndrome is an important aneuploidy to remember when dealing with infants with congenital heart defects because there is always mosaicism. Blood karyotyping almost always gives a normal result, and the marker 12p isochromosome is only found if a skin biopsy is taken. Severe developmental delay, coarse facies (Fig. 47.6), and parietal alopecia should prompt a skin biopsy. Other clinical features of note are a tendency to seizures, hypertelorism, small mandible in infants becoming prominent in the adult, diaphragmatic hernias, and supernumerary nipples. About a

quarter of children with tetrasomy 12p have heart defects, VSD being the most common. Other common defects include coarctation of the aorta, PDA, ASD, and aortic stenosis (Reynolds et al., 1987).

45, X Turner syndrome

The only viable human monosomy, 45,X, is attributed to Turner, although it was first described by Ullrich eight years earlier. Absence of the second sex chromosome results in short stature, gonadal dysgenesis, and a variable dysmorphic appearance with neck webbing (pterygium colli), a "shark" mouth and occasionally down-slanting palpebral fissures and low-set ears (Fig. 47.7). The prevalence of cardiovascular malformation varies with the method of ascertainment. Based on studies of aborted fetuses, it is estimated that up to 99% of 45,X fetuses are lost as early miscarriages. At least some of these losses have a cardiovascular basis, particularly hypoplastic left heart. The birth incidence is at least 1 in 1850 live female births (Nielsen and Wohlert, 1991). Earlier estimates were discrepant because of the varying phenotype and age at presentation. Simpson (1976) reviewed reports of heart defects associated with Turner syndrome in published studies based on gonadal dysgenesis, amenorrhea, or population studies.

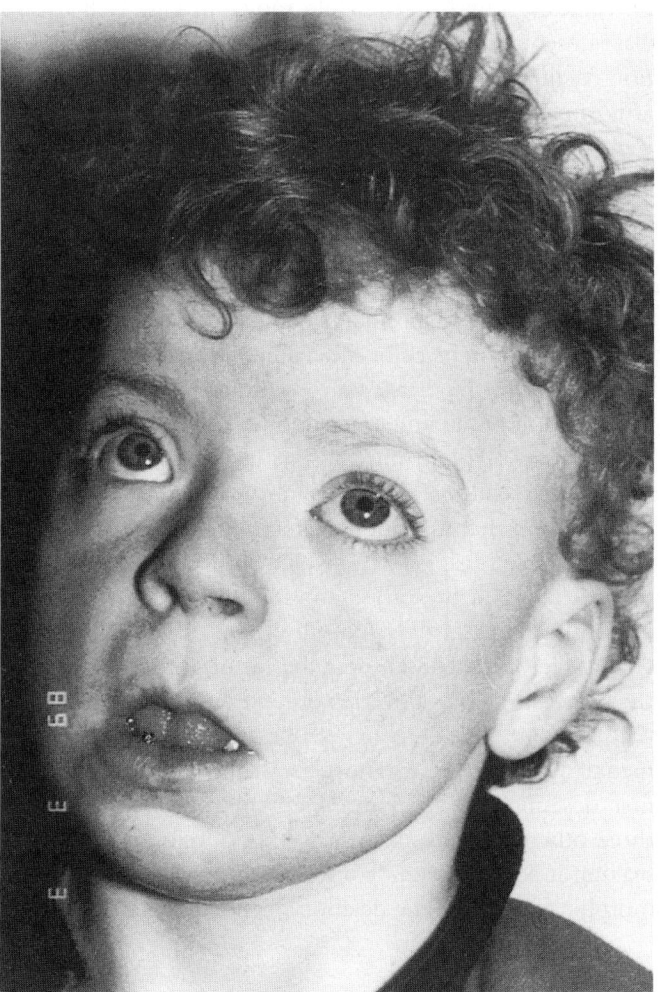

Fig. 47.6. Pallister Killian syndrome. The most striking early feature is the thinning of the hair over the temples. Diagnosis depends on skin biopsy since only children with a mosaic chromosome pattern survive to term.

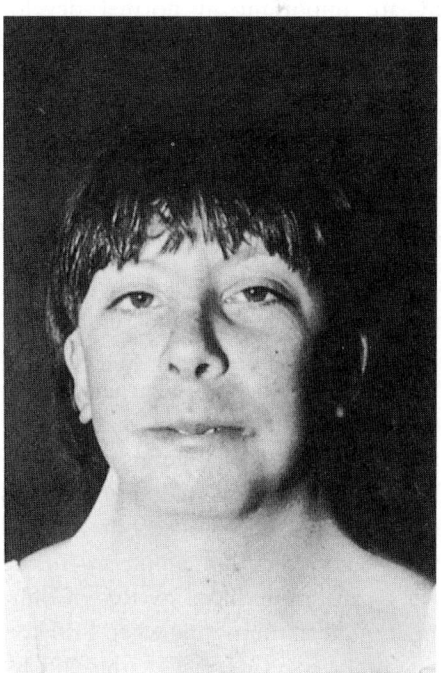

Fig. 47.7. Turner syndrome. The typical facial appearance with neck webbing in a girl with a 45, X karyotype.

Among 228 pooled cases, 22 cases (10%) of heart defect were listed, though details of cardiovascular status were provided in only 119, for a potential prevalence of 16%. Miller and colleagues (Muller et al., 1983) identified 80 girls with 45,X in a pediatric endocrinology clinic, 13 of whom had aortic coarctation, the most common defect in all series. In 35 girls not known to have a heart defect, echocardiography revealed bicuspid aortic valve in 12, mitral valve prolapse in two, and idiopathic aortic root dilatation in two. Conversely, heart defects are rarer in women presenting with Turner syndrome in gynecology clinics. There is likely to be an association between dysmorphic features such as neck webbing and heart defects, which would result in a greater prevalence of heart defects in cases diagnosed earlier. As a general guide it would be reasonable to deduce that 10% of all girls with Turner syndrome have a clinically evident heart defect and that a further 10% will display pathology at echocardiography.

Studies of parental origin of the chromosomal loss reveals evidence of imprinting. Chu and colleagues (1994) found nine out of 43 girls who had retained the maternal X had heart defects as opposed to only one out of 20 girls with a retained paternal X. With pooled data from three previous studies, there were 34 of 90 cases of heart malformation where the mother's X chromosome was retained and only four of 38 where the father's X chromosome was retained. Unrecognized mosaicism could explain the results, but it seems more likely that a gene or genes on the paternal X are important in normal development of the aorta or its surrounding structures. There was a similar parent of origin effect on the presence of neck webbing, supporting the belief that these malformations may have a common pathogenesis (Clark, 1984).

CHROMOSOME DELETION SYNDROMES

A tradition has developed for calling phenotypes associated with deletions detectable by standard cytogenetic techniques "deletion syndromes", and those detected more recently by using FISH or molecular analysis "microdeletion syndromes". When a syndrome is attributed to loss of adjacent genes the term "contiguous gene syndrome" is applied. These are pointless and misleading distinctions. For example, Wolf-Hirshhorn syndrome due to 4p– was first described before Giemsa staining was introduced, yet the phenotype can be produced by loss of only the most distal segment of the chromosome when FISH or allele loss studies are employed. Conversely, the 22q11 deletion described below is sometimes detectable on a standard karyotype, but the true prevalence of the deletion became evident only when FISH techniques were introduced. The two factors that determine the size of the deletion appear to be the propensity of different segments for deletion and, more important to the terminology, the number of genes in the vicinity that produce a phenotype when hemizygous. The fact that loss of most of the short arm of chromosome 4 produces essentially the same syndrome as loss of the terminal band suggests that there are few, if any, genes on 4p that produce a dominant loss of function phenotype. In short, deletion syndromes, however they are demonstrated, define the position of loss of function dominant genes.

Wolf-Hirshhorn syndrome

The Wolf-Hirshhorn syndrome is an important phenotype because it relies heavily on the clinician to recognize the pattern so that the cytogeneticist can focus on the terminal segment of 4p. Wolf-Hirshhorn syndrome was diagnosed on clinical grounds in the child shown in Fig. 47.8A, who was subsequently shown to have an unbalanced translocation resulting in loss of the telomeric segment of the short arm of chromosome 4. The father carried a balanced 4;10 translocation, which had led to the birth and early demise of a previous child with the same phenotype. The heart malformations are frequent but not specific to the syndrome. Prognosis is poor, although the cardiovascular problems are rarely a major factor in survival. Much is made of the Greek helmet profile, likening the bridge of the nose to the metal nosepiece of the helmets worn by early Greek soldiers. More important to recognition of the face is the combination of sagging everted lower eyelids, a short nose, and very short philtrum, causing the mouth to be carp-shaped. The child in Fig. 47.8B also had 4p- due to a 4;10 translocation that was not detected on Giemsa banding but was easily seen using FISH, which showed the chromosomal exchange in the carrier mother was similarly detected (Goodship et al., 1992). Wright et al. (1997) reduced the critical region to 165 kb near the tip of 4p on the basis of the shortest region of overlap of reported deletions. Within that segment, Stec et al. (1998) described a novel developmental gene WHSC1. The gene shares the SET domain first described in a *Drosophila* dysmorphy gene and has three other domains characteristic of developmental genes making it a good candidate for the cardiac and other dysmorphic features of the deletion phenotype.

Williams syndrome

The discovery of the deletion underlying Williams syndrome is a dramatic example of the recent advances in what

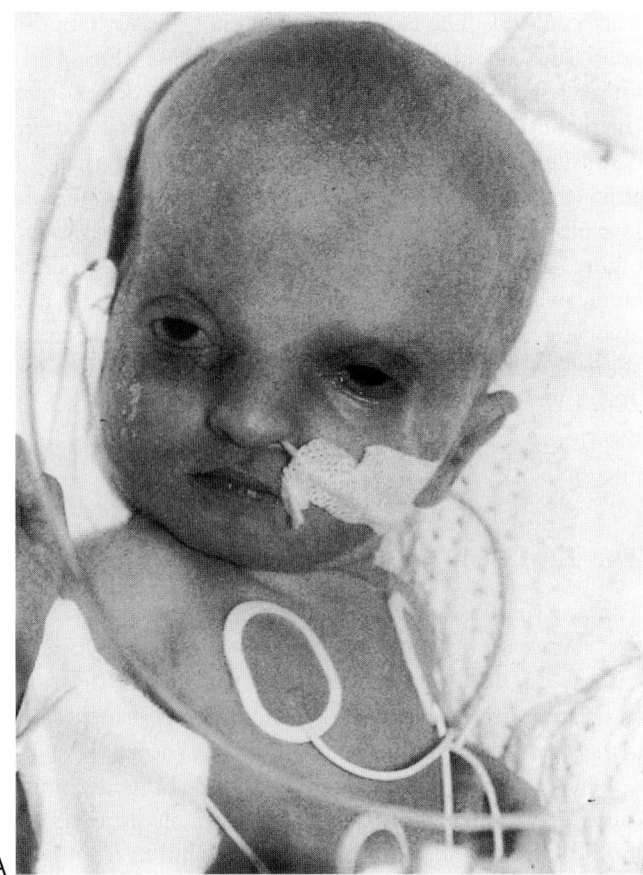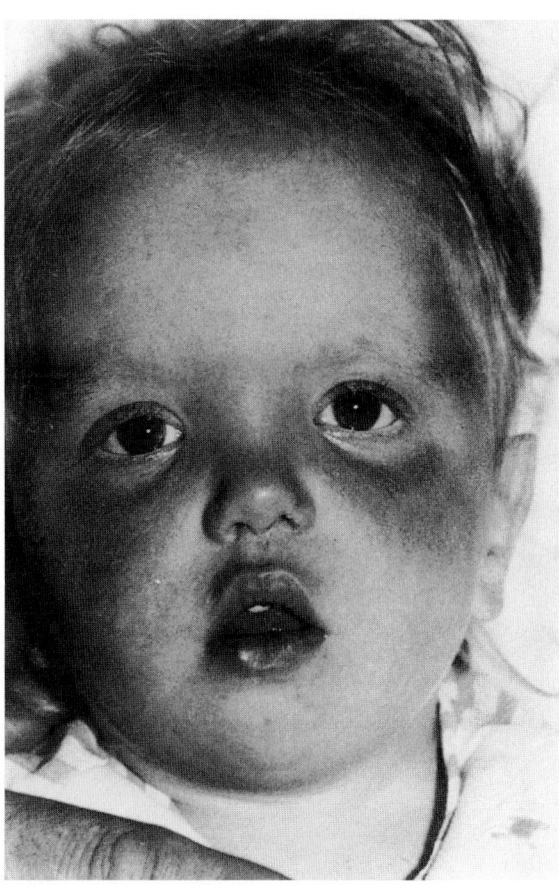

A   B

Fig. 47.8. (A) The typical facial appearance of a child with Wolf-Hirschhorn syndrome due to deletion of the terminal region of 4p. Note the "Greek helmet" appearance of the nasal bridge and the sagging lower eyelids and short upper lip. (B) Another child with much more subtle features of 4p-, diagnosis of which depended on FISH using probes for the terminal band of 4p. The mother carried a balanced 4;10 translocation. (From Goodship et al., 1992, with permission.)

might be called molecular dysmorphology. Williams syndrome, or Williams-Beuren syndrome, is characterized by learning disability with a "cocktail party manner", so called because of a readiness to converse in a friendly outgoing fashion but with little content. The dysmorphic features are easily recognized by the trained eye (Fig. 47.9); malar flattening, periorbital fullness, heavy sagging cheeks, short nose, poorly developed Cupid's bow on the upper lip and everted lower lip. The cardinal cardiovascular malformation in this syndrome is supravalvular aortic stenosis (SVAS). Less well recognized and more difficult to detect are peripheral pulmonary artery stenoses, which produce murmurs over the lung fields. The striking association with SVAS, which had been described as an isolated dominant trait in many families, prompted the speculation that Williams syndrome would turn out to be a deletion involving the gene responsible for SVAS (Burn, 1986). The identification of a balanced translocation associated with SVAS provided the clue. Curran and associates (1993) showed first that dominant SVAS mapped to chromosome 7 at a translocation

break point (Ewart et al., 1993a) and subsequently that most Williams syndrome cases could be shown to have a deletion of this region of chromosome 7 (Ewart et al., 1993b). Elastin was shown to be the causative gene in isolated SVAS by the demonstration of loss of function mutations (Ewart et al., 1994). Osborne et al. (1996) characterised a 500 kb region in 7q11.23 deleted in a series of 30 patients with Williams syndrome. A total of nine transcribed segments were identified including the previously recognised genes *ELN*, for tropoelastin, *LIMK1* and *RFC2*.

Alagille syndrome

Alagille syndrome is characterized by hypoplasia of the intrahepatic bile ducts, leading to a variable degree of cholestasis, which may present with neonatal jaundice or become apparent later in life (Alagille et al., 1987). Up to 90% of affected individuals have single or multiple areas of peripheral pulmonary artery stenosis. In about one-third, a variety of other intra and extra-cardiac malformations are seen (Mueller and

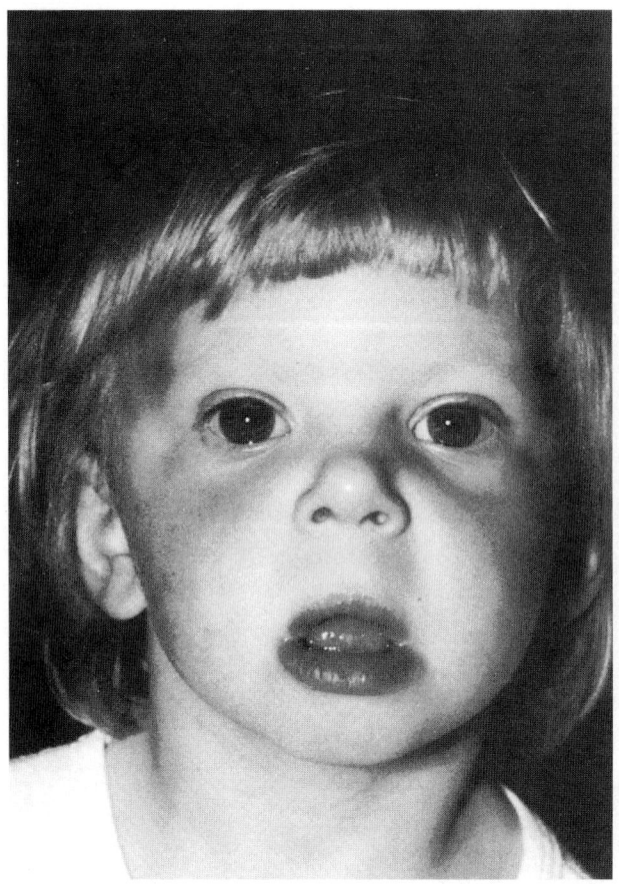

Emslie, 1995). The face is mildly dysmorphic with a prominent forehead, deep-set eyes, and thin nose (Fig. 47.10). Other typical clinical features include skeletal defects (particularly butterfly vertebrae) and anterior chamber eye defects, confusingly called posterior embryotoxon. Externally, the striking feature is a pale ring around the iris known as arcus juvenilis (Li et al., 1997). The mother and child shown in Figure 47.10 were the first example of a two-generation family with a demonstrable deletion (Anad et al., 1990) involving 20p11–2. This deletion is demonstrable in only about 10% of cases. The critical region was found to be at 20p11.2–20p12 (Hol et al., 1995). Subsequent studies have shown that loss of the *JAGGED1* gene is responsible for the phenotype.

The 22q11 phenotype

The most important development in our understanding of the causes of heart malformation since the discovery of trisomy 21 has been the discovery that 22q11 deletion is associated with a wide spectrum of heart malformations and is the most common autosomal deletion known.

The recognition that deletion of 22q11 is a common cause of varied malformations and clinical disorders took more than a decade to achieve. The evolution from "small print" to "mainstream" involved a convergence of two lines of study: clinicians described a series of interrelated, but apparently distinct, syndromes over two decades, while the geneticists reported cytogenetic and later molecular genetic

Fig. 47.9. Williams syndrome. The typical facial appearance resulting from deletion of the elastin gene and neighbouring areas. Note the periorbital fullness, malar flattening, sagging cheeks and full everted lower lip. A stellate iris pattern is often seen. (From Burn, 1986, with permission.)

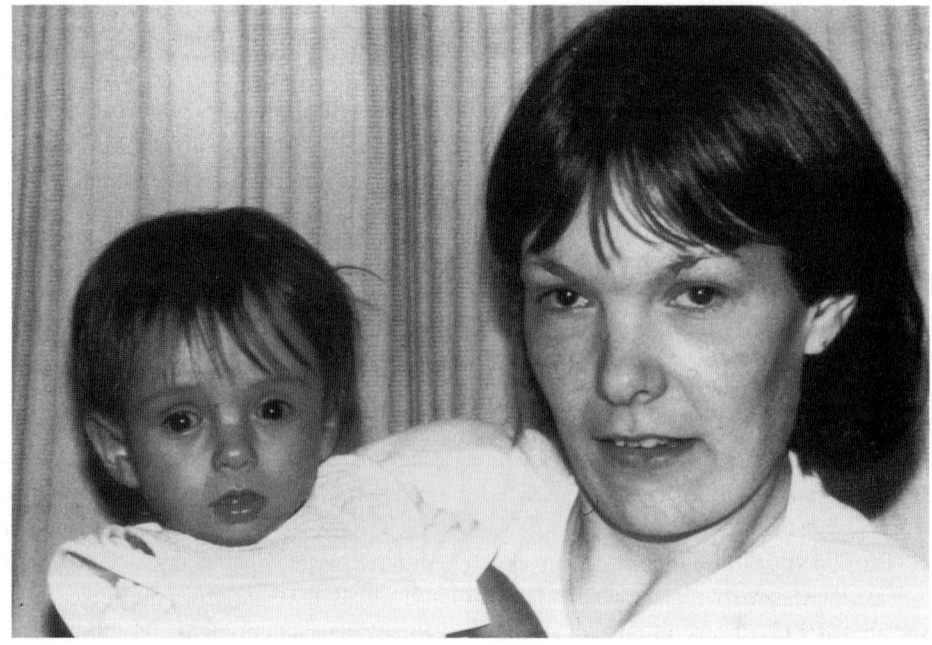

Fig. 47.10. Alagille syndrome, in mother and child due to a deletion of chromosome 20p. (From Arad et al., 1990, with permission.)

analyses and noted the clinical consequences of these genetic disturbances and their relationship to published syndromes.

DiGeorge syndrome and the immunology perspective

Cooper and colleagues (1965) recorded the observation by DiGeorge in 1965 that absence of the thymus might be associated with hypocalcemia due to parathyroid hypoplasia. Although Lobdell (1959) had made this observation in 1959, the passing note and the subsequent expansion by DiGeorge (1968) established the eponym. With the additional reports came the realization that cardiac malformation, particularly defects of the outflow tract, were a key feature of the syndrome (Freedom et al., 1972). Dysmorphic facial features were noted: a small mouth, a square nasal tip with pinched nares, abnormalities of the pinnae with impaired pattern of folding and reduction in vertical diameter, and short palpebral fissures with variable slant of the eyes. Figure 47.11A illustrates the typical features in a neonate. We have reviewed the dysmorphic features (Wilson et al., 1993a,b); variable features include both sensorineural and conductive hearing loss, cleft palate, and, rarely, lip, facial palsy, renal anomalies, and hypothyroidism. Hypocalcemia may be symptomatic and present with seizure activity, but responds promptly to replacement therapy and becomes less apparent with age. The immune deficit also resolves with time and is often less overt than in the original cases. The tendency of the thymic shadow to become smaller in stressed infants makes recognition of true thymic hypoplasia more difficult with radiography. Reduced white blood cell counts may not be present in children with DiGeorge syndrome, while, conversely, sick infants may have a reduced white blood cell count but a normal thymus. In order to demonstrate thymic hypoplasia with confidence, it is necessary to assess the number of T lymphocytes that are recorded as CD4 positive cells. In the sick neonate it should be assumed that cellular immunity is compromised until proven otherwise, and any transfusion should involve irradiated blood to avoid graft versus host disease.

Shprintzen (velocardiofacial) syndrome and the craniofacial clinic perspective

The group led by Shprintzen has played a pivotal role in elucidation of the phenotypes associated with 22q11 deletion. Using the descriptive title velocardiofacial syndrome (VCFS), their reports began with a description of 12 cases of hypernasal speech due to cleft palate, cardiac anomalies,

and characteristic facial appearance (Shprintzen and Mea, 1978; 1981). The craniofacial emphasis of the referral pattern is reflected in the proportion of cases of the syndrome with cleft palate (98%), pharyngeal hypotonia (90%), retrognathia (80%), and malar flatness (70%) (Goldberg et al., 1993). The later presentation as patients in the craniofacial clinic can account for the recognition of learning disability and short stature as frequent features. They reported mental retardation in 40% of cases. An important observation is the frequency of psychiatric disorders: 13 of their patients had suffered a variety of problems, including manic depressive psychosis, general anxiety disorder, and paranoia. Given the age distribution of the patients, it is possible that neuropsychiatric complications may be a bigger problem as the cohort is followed through to adulthood. Conversely, there is a strong likelihood that, as more mild cases are identified, the proportion of cases with these severe features will decrease.

Takao (conotruncal anomaly face) syndrome and pediatric cardiology perspective

The Japanese group led by Takao (1980) was the first to recognize the major contribution of the phenotype to the patient population with outflow tract defects. The term "conotruncal anomaly face" correctly describes the presenting features but has not found widespread use partly because it is a difficult term to use with patients in a Western clinical practice, and in part because terms based on embryologic assumptions of cause are not ideal.

Radford (1985; 1988) also recognized the association of dysmorphic facies with outflow tract defects, (Burn, 1989) particularly truncus arteriosus and tetralogy of Fallot. The overlap between the differing phenotypes and the likelihood of a common pathogenesis was emphasized soon thereafter.

Strong syndrome and the "familial" perspective

Strong (1968) reported on a family with right-sided aortic arch, mental deficiency, and facial dysmorphism. This report was the first to draw together the wide spectrum of clinical features in what was almost certainly the same phenotype. It is of interest that these patients had hypernasal speech and the mother had a psychotic illness. Several authors, for example, Greenberg and colleagues (1984), have described familial DiGeorge syndrome.

Setting aside the discussion of terminology, these familial cases in more than one generation pointed to a mendelian inheritance pattern due to either a single-gene defect or

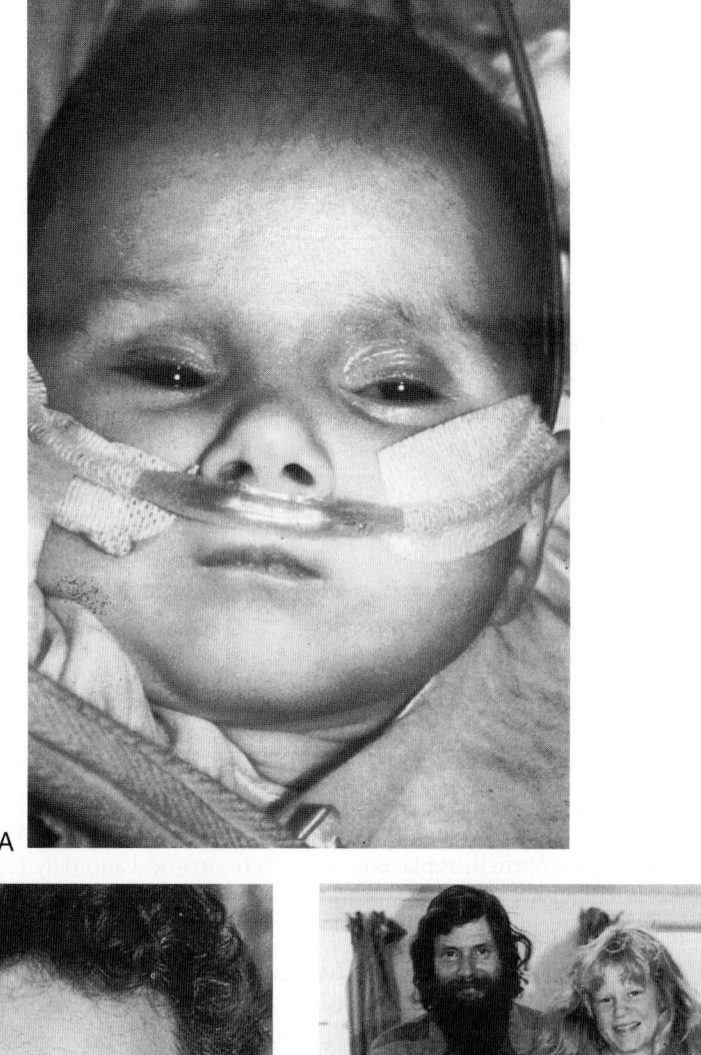

A

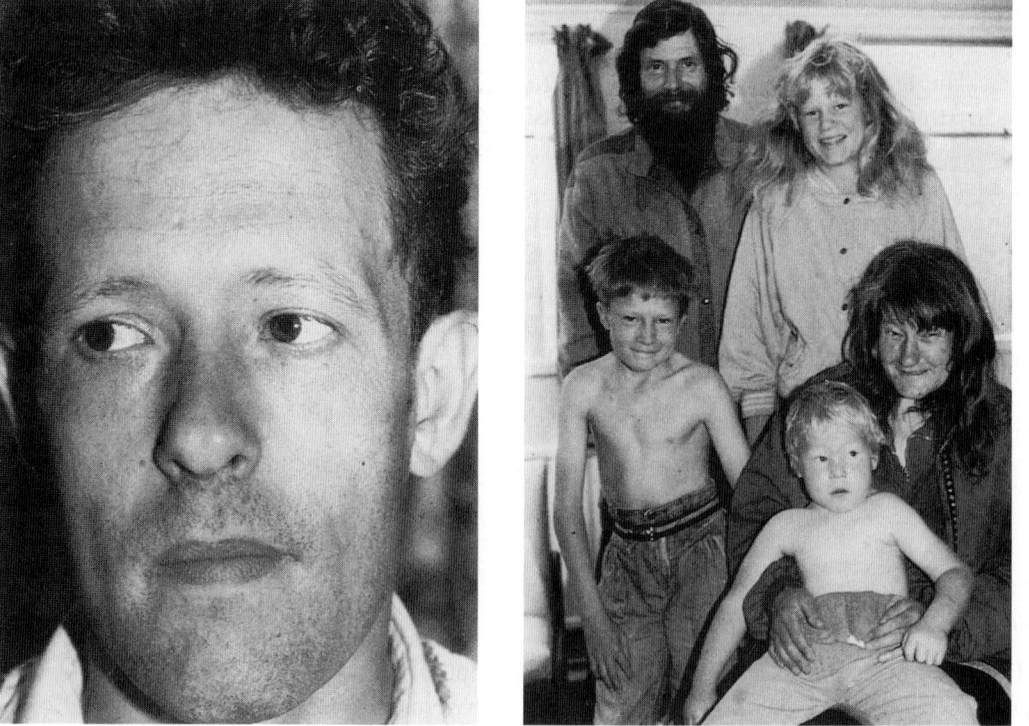

B   C

Fig. 47.11. (A) DiGeorge syndrome-typical neonatal features. (From Wilson et al., 1991, with permission) (B) A father with CATCH phenotype with minimal problems, both of whose children had severe heart defects. (C) A mother with CATCH phenotype without a heart defect but with typical facial features. Both boys had a heart defect. (From Wilson et al., 1993a,b, with permission.)

microdeletion. This proved to be the case with the surprising discovery that complete deletion was the rule, and this could be identified using the new technique of FISH.

Other syndromes

A number of other syndromes have been shown to be associated in some cases with 22q11 deletion; Noonan syndrome (Wilson et al., 1993a), Opitz syndrome (McDonald-McGinn et al., 1995), CHARGE syndrome (Emanuel et al., 1992) and Cayler (asymmetric crying face) syndrome (Giannotti et al., 1994) are described below.

The 22q11 Genotype

De la Chapelle and associates (1981) reported a familial 20:22 translocation associated in its unbalanced form with features of DiGeorge syndrome. Subsequent reports beginning with Kelley and colleagues (1982), confirmed that the 22 deletion was the cause. As case reports accumulated it became apparent that 22q11 deletion was often associated with DiGeorge syndrome, but the latter continued to be regarded as a field defect likely to have multiple causes linked by disturbance of the migratory neural crest. The association of the syndrome with an apparently balanced translocation through 22q11 suggested that a small segment of the deleted area might be critical to the clinical phenotype (Augusseau et al., 1986). While the systematic study by Greenberg and colleagues (1988) established the importance of 22q11 deletion but was also somewhat misleading; the available cytogenetic technology limited the resolution such that a minority of cases had a visible 22 deletion. Cases were found with deletion of chromosome 10p13 and involving chromosome 18. The chromosome 10 connection has been supported by other reports but it may be assumed that defects on other chromosomes are rarely important, given the dramatic developments with improved resolution of the 22 deletions by FISH.

FISH revealed a 22q11 deletion in 90% of cases of DiGeorge syndrome, over 75% of Shprintzen syndrome (Driscoll et al., 1992; 1993; Scambler et al., 1992; Kelly et al., 1993), and in similar proportions of the conotruncal anomaly face syndrome or Takao syndrome (Burn et al., 1993a,b). In almost all cases, a segment of chromosome extending over 2 Mb is lost. (Ryan et al., 1997; Jerome and Papaioannou, 2001)

There are about 20 genes in the deleted segment most commonly lost. A number of these have been implicated in the neural crest migration defect implicated in the phenotypes resulting from 22q11 deletion. An early candidate was *TUPLE1* (Halford et al., 1993), later renamed *HIRA*, which has a role in development of the outflow tract of the heart (Farrell et al., 1999). It shows an expression pattern which predicts a neural crest role. Most recently, mice homozygous for a deletion of *TBX1*, a transcription factor, have been shown to manifest the CATCH phenotype (Jerome and Papaioannou, 2001). Lindsay et al. (2001) in parallel experiments also demonstrated the pivotal role of *TBX1* using an elegant transgenic mouse approach. Having engineered a deletion (*df1*) of the mouse chromosome 16 area syntenic to 22q11.2, they narrowed the critical area to 200kb, including *Tbx1*. Gene targeting of *Tbx1* reproduced the aortic arch abnormalities in a *Tbx1/df1* compound heterozygote. Heterozygous mice were normal. This may reflect a greater developmental sensitivity in humans or, more likely, that several of the genes in the critical region including *TBX1*, *HIRA*, *UFD1L* (Yamagishi et al., 1999) and *CRKL* (Guris et al., 2001) are implicated. It remains unclear whether several genes must be haploinsufficient to cause a clinical phenotype or whether a single locus predominates. Of the 14 coding sequences identified in the critical region to date (Roberts et al., 1990; Adam et al., 1991; Halford et al., 1993; Kelly et al., 1994; Budarf et al., 1995a; 1995b, Demczuk et al., 1995; Kurahashi et al., 1995; Lamour et al., 1995; Wadey et al., 1995), the most interesting remains *Tuple 1* (Halford et al., 1993).

A working hypothesis is that people with a 22q11.2 deletion have impairment of several steps in one or more neural crest migration pathways which, collectively, lead to a sufficient impairment of delivery of cells to the end destination, delay in migration, or capacity to differentiate that a clinical syndrome results. Heterozygosity at a single locus cannot do sufficient damage to produce the full phenotype. This interpretation would explain the fact that cases have occurred with a smaller 22q11 deletion and these cases do not have an overlapping span. It would also accommodate the failure of several groups, including our own, to identify loss of function mutations in the individual genes in the critical region. The final proof will come from compound heterozygotes for the different mouse models produced to date.

In the early stage of the laboratory study, the family of the infant illustrated in Figure 47.11 became the focus of attention. This important family comprised four sibs, two of whom had undergone surgical correction of heart defects before the birth of the girl with DiGeorge syndrome. One had had a coarctation of the aorta and the other a ventricular septal defect. All three were found to have a deletion inherited from the mother (Wilson et al., 1991). The mother (Fig. 47.11C) had the same dysmorphic features as the children with short narrow up-slanting palpebral fissures, a bulbous nasal tip with narrow base and thin lips. This family lent support to the hypothesis that familial outflow tract defects might result from 22q11 deletion in the absence of other features of the syndromes.

We carried out deletion analysis in a series of families where there had been more than one case of heart malformation with at least one case involving the outflow. In five of the nine families, 22q11 deletion was apparent (Wilson et al., 1992). This finding made 22q11 deletion of primary importance in the genetic management of families with children affected by heart defects; any child with an outflow tract defect and dysmorphic features became eligible for deletion analysis.

Goldmutz and colleagues (1993) found five cases among 17 patients with isolated outflow tract defects. In our series, deletion is particularly likely in type B interrupted aortic arch and truncus arteriosus but is rarely associated with transposition of the great arteries. In the northern region of England, detailed analysis of all significant heart defects over five years revealed a steady annual rate of around 200 cases among 40,000 births. Among 1993 births, 10 affected children had been found by spring 1994. This suggests that 22q11 deletion can account for 5% of all heart defects and has a minimum prevalence of around 1 in 4000. One of the affected infants born in 1993 died at the time of catheterization. The father, shown in Figure 47.11B, was found to carry the deletion. He had mild learning disability in childhood but had suffered no major physical problem. His heart was normal on echocardiography. His wife was pregnant at the time of diagnosis. The couple chose prenatal diagnosis, which revealed a deletion in the fetus. Subsequent fetal echocardiography revealed a complex outflow tract malformation with pulmonary atresia, and the parents decided to terminate the pregnancy.

In 1997, our group led a European consortium that assembled data on 558 cases of 22q11 deletion (Ryan et al., 1997). Twenty-eight per cent of the cases where parents had been tested had inherited deletions with a marked excess of maternally inherited deletions. Eight per cent had died, over half within a month of birth primarily due to severe congenital heart defects, though a contribution from immune deficiency is likely in many. Clinically diagnosed immune deficiency was uncommon. When measured, calcium was low in 60% of cases, and 75% had a clinically significant heart defect. Among 409 patients with a heart defect, 355 fell into the five diagnostic categories tetralogy of Fallot, ventricular septal defect, interrupted aortic arch, pulmonary atresia ventricular septal defect and truncus arteriosus.

Other points of relevance to counseling were short stature, renal malformation and learning disabilities, each reported in about a third of cases, though some degree of learning impairment is probably present in up to 75%.

PHENOTYPE/GENOTYPE CORRELATION: THE CATCH PHENOTYPE

In our review of DiGeorge syndrome (Wilson et al., 1993b) we suggested that a useful acronym would be CATCH22: *c*ardiac defect, *a*bnormal facies, *T*-cell deficit, *c*left palate, *h*ypocalcemia due to *22*q11 deletion. There is obvious attachment to existing eponyms and it is reasonable to retain these. DiGeorge anomaly has been associated with other chromosomal and teratogenic causes, for example, while Shprintzen syndrome has become well-established in the literature. One solution is to accept that CATCH22 embraces several phenotypes. In particular, patients presenting with the neonatal phenotype with severe T-cell deficiency and hypocalcemia may be described as DiGeorge syndrome, those presenting with clefting and nasal speech fit the Shprintzen phenotype, and those presenting with a predominantly cardiac phenotype may be called Takao syndrome in preference to conotruncal anomaly face syndrome.

In some communities, catch 22 is used to denote a "no win" situation after the famous novel of that name by James Heller. Clinicians must judge how their patients will react to these various labels. Whichever name is used, it must be remembered that any label is likely to be distressing to an unprepared family. The term "syndrome" is now often associated in the lay mind with Down syndrome and connotes severe mental handicap. Reference to chromosome deletions and to some of the reviews might lead the professional to a similar conclusion. In practice, it is likely that most carriers of 22q11 deletion are able to function intellectually within the broad range of normal. With these points in mind, we have suggested recently (Burn, 1999) that the term CATCH22 be dropped, either in favour of VCFS or CATCH phenotype. The acronym should be adjusted to:

*C*ardiac, *A*bnormality/abnormal facies, *T*-cell deficit due to thymic hypoplasia, *C*left palate/palatal dysfunction, *H*ypocalcemia.

If the CATCH phenotype presents in infancy with immune problems, it is likely to be called "DiGeorge syndrome". If the problems of nasal speech and palate problems are the major presenting problem in an older child the terms "velo-cardiofacial" (VCFS) or "Shprintzen syndrome" may be used. If the main presenting feature is a heart defect, together with a facial resemblance to other children with the same pattern of problems, the terms, "Takao syndrome" may be used. CATCH phenotype may be used as an overarching collective term for all three or it may be used as an alternative for all syndromic cases where a 22 deletion has been shown to be present. This avoids the complexity for the family of offering different syndrome labels to family members with the same underlying cause.

Whatever descriptive terms are used, the convergence of these many lines of phenotypic and genotypic research has brought us to the point that all children with an outflow tract defect and dysmorphic features should have a deletion analysis. It is highly likely that the prevalence studies now underway will confirm that all children with significant defects of the outflow tract of the heart or the palate should be tested in view of the possibility of recurrence in a more severe form.

Other chromosome segments associated with heart malformation

Brewer et al. (1998) performed a meta-analysis of reports of chromosome deletion and identified several areas frequently associated with particular heart defects. Important associations, other than those listed above, include deletion of distal 11q in hypoplastic heart. Such cases are associated with trigonocephaly and attract the eponym Jacobsen syndrome. Another association worthy of note is 8p deletion with atrioventricular septal defect.

Other major "cardiac" syndromes

The frequency of heart defects and the complexity of heart formation result in cardiovascular malformation being described in a large number of syndromes. Appendix 47.1 contains an analysis of over 370 syndromes which may be seen among children with cardiac malformation. This table draws heavily on the Oxford Medical Database (Winter and Baraitser), published by Oxford University Press, which is available in CD-ROM form and is strongly recommended as a reference source for anyone confronted by the need to diagnose dysmorphic syndromes. A few of those listed are worthy of particular mention.

NOONAN SYNDROME

One of the best recognized syndromes in the pediatric cardiology clinic is Noonan syndrome. Earliest descriptions have been traced back over a century, but the syndrome derives its name from the report by Noonan and Ehmke in 1963 of nine children with valvar pulmonary stenosis, short stature, mild learning difficulties, and dysmorphic appearance. The variable phenotype is illustrated by the mother and two daughters in Figure 47.12. Collectively, they have the full picture, yet neither has the complete pattern.

In infancy the striking features are the hyperteloric, down-slanting eyes with low-set posteriorly rotated ears and low posterior hairline. Later the face becomes more triangular and rather coarse in appearance. In adulthood the eyes are less prominent and the nose has a thinner bridge and pinched root with wide base; the neck becomes longer accentuating the prominent trapezius and/or neck webbing, which caused original confusion with Turner syndrome in the literature.

Other important features are the feeding difficulties of infancy, pectus excavatum/carinatum with wide-spaced nipples, cryptorchidism, a predisposition to lymphatic dysplasia and bleeding diathesis, and a high frequency of naevi and cafe-au-lait spots.

Two-thirds of children with Noonan syndrome have a heart defect with valvar pulmonary stenosis in 50%. Often the valve is dysplastic making balloon dilatation more difficult. Among a variety of other defects reported the most frequent are atrial septal defect, asymmetric septal hypertrophy, and persistent ductus arteriosus. Ventricular septal defect occurs in about 5%. The electrocardiograph typically shows left axis deviation with a wide QRS complex, giant Q waves and a negative pattern in the left precordial leads.

There is a phenotypic overlap with a number of syndromes, particularly LEOPARD syndrome, Costello syndrome, Watson syndrome (cafe-au-lait spots, pulmonary stenosis, learning difficulty) and neurofibromatosis type 1. The syndrome is genetically heterogeneous. Tassabehji and associates (1993) demonstrated a tandem duplication of an exon in the *NF1* gene (neurofibromin) in a family with features of Noonan and Watson syndromes. Linkage mapping has shown there to be a gene on the long arm of chromosome 12 that can produce the dominant Noonan phenotype, but haplotype studies in smaller families show that not all cases map to this area (Jamieson et al., 1994).

HOLT-ORAM SYNDROME

Holt-Oram syndrome is the best recognized of the heart-hand syndromes. The characteristic anomalies are underdevelopment of the shoulder girdle with triphalangeal thumb and atrial septal defect (Newbury-Ecob et al., 1996) (Fig. 47.13). The limb defects can vary from phocomelia to

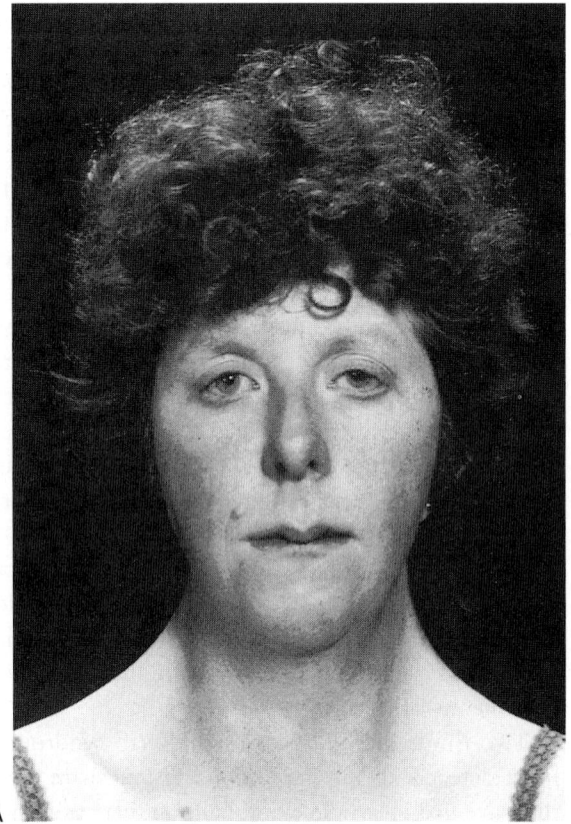
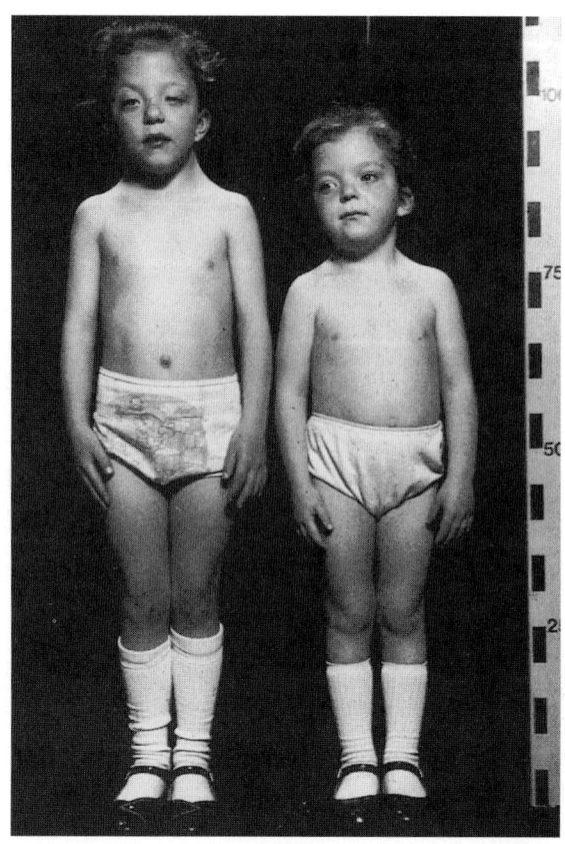

Fig. 47.12. Noonan syndrome mother and two daughters. Mother shared neck webbing with her older daughter who also had ptosis and learning disability. The younger child had pulmonary stenosis, ASD and short stature.

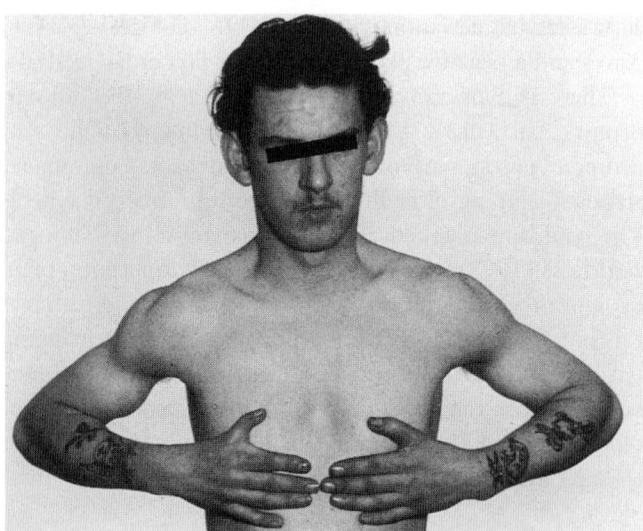

Fig. 47.13. Holt-Oram syndrome. Typical hypoplasia of both thumbs.

minor anomalies of joint movement at the thumb, elbow, or shoulder. About half of gene carriers have a secundum ASD with occasional reports including VSD, AVSD, and truncus arteriosus. Genetic studies have shown this autoso-

mal dominant trait to be heterogeneous. Some families map to 12q21.3-q22 (Bonnet et al., 1994), but Terrett and associates (1994) found two clinically indistinguishable families which did not show linkage. The causative gene defect involves loss of function of *TBX5*, another of the 12 or so transcription factors characterized by the presence of the T box domain, a DNA-binding motif (Basson et al., 1999).

ELLIS VAN CREVELD SYNDROME

Ellis van Creveld is an extremely rare autosomal recessive syndrome characterized by a short rib/polydactyly skeletal dysplasia (Fig. 47.14), natal teeth, oral frenulae, and other features of an ectodermal dysplasia and what the original authors called congenital morbus cordis. About 60% of affected individuals have a heart malformation. Apart from certain inbred populations, notably the Old-Order Amish in the United States and the aboriginal population of western Australia (Goldblatt et al., 1992), the birth prevalence is less than 1 in 200,000. The syndrome deserves particular mention because of the nature of the heart defect; the most common defect involves failure of the primum

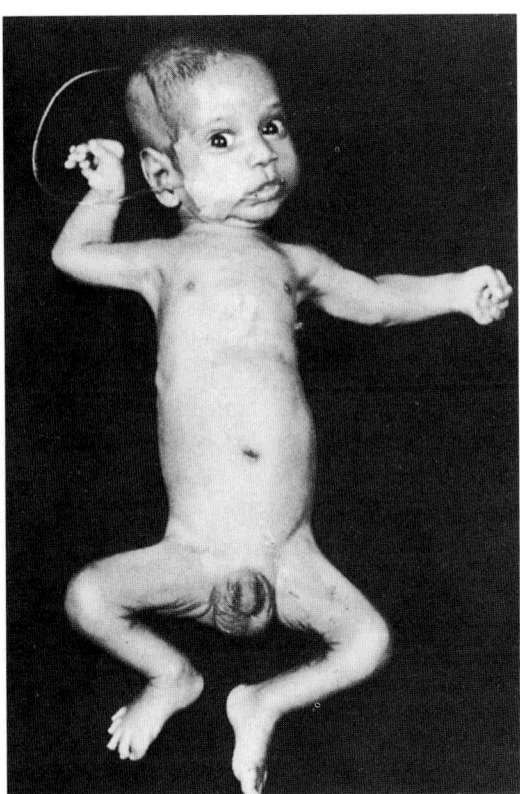

Fig. 47.14. Ellis van Creveld syndrome.

atrial septum. In some cases, this is associated with abnormality of the AV valves, and, rarely, there is a complete AVSD. In some children there is a common atrium, suggesting that the gene plays a key role in formation of the primum septum rather than the endocardial cushions.

Our group led an international consortium which identified the causative gene on chromosome 4p16. The gene, designated *EVC*, encodes a 992 amino acid residue protein of uncertain function (Ruiz-Perez et al., 2000). Pathological mutations were identified in seven pedigrees. Of interest in the search for additive genes relevant to non-syndromic heart defects was a missense mutation in another family, a father and daughter, both of whom had the typical heart defect and polydactyly but normal stature.

Heart malformation and metabolic disorders

The inborn errors of metabolism, such as the mucopolysaccharidoses, (see Ch. 98), develop cardiac involvement as a postnatal event, particularly involving valve dysfunction due to deposition of storage material and, most dramatically in type 2 glycogenosis or Pompe disease, with accumulation of material in the cardiac muscle. More recently, it has become

apparent that some metabolic defects are not corrected by the maternal influence and can produce congenital malformations that may include the heart. Two are worthy of mention, since simple diagnostic biochemical tests exist making prenatal diagnosis available.

ZELLWEGER SYNDROME

Zellweger or cerebrohepatorenal syndrome was originally described as a lethal multiple malformation syndrome of infancy characterized by profound hypotonia, a marked paucity of facial movement, open anterior fontanelle, hypoplastic supraorbital ridges, and a broad nasal bridge (Fig. 47.15). Hepatomegaly, renal cortical cysts, deafness, cataracts, and calcific stippling of the patellae complete the typical phenotype (Opitz et al., 1969). Following the discovery of peroxisomal defect in a child with this syndrome, it has become apparent that this pattern represents one end of a clinical spectrum that may result from at least ten genetic defects in peroxisomal assembly or the function of the single matrix enzymes including *PEX1* on chromosome 7q (Fitzpatrick, 1996). Severe cerebral dysfunction results from premature arrest of migrating neuroblasts. Thymic hypoplasia and outflow tract cardiac malformations occur (Heymanns, 1984).

SMITH-LEMLI-OPITZ SYNDROME

Smith-Lemli-Opitz (SLO) syndrome is characterized by severe learning disability, failure to thrive, cleft palate, hypospadias in males, and 2/3 syndactyly. The facies are dysmorphic with bitemporal narrowing and anteverted nares (Fig. 47.16). Heart malformations are common (Wallace et al., 1994; Kelley et al., 1995; Lin et al., 1995)

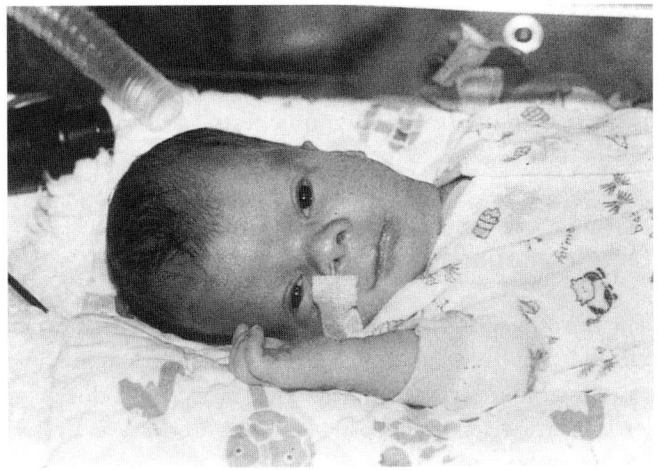

Fig. 47.15. Zellweger syndrome.

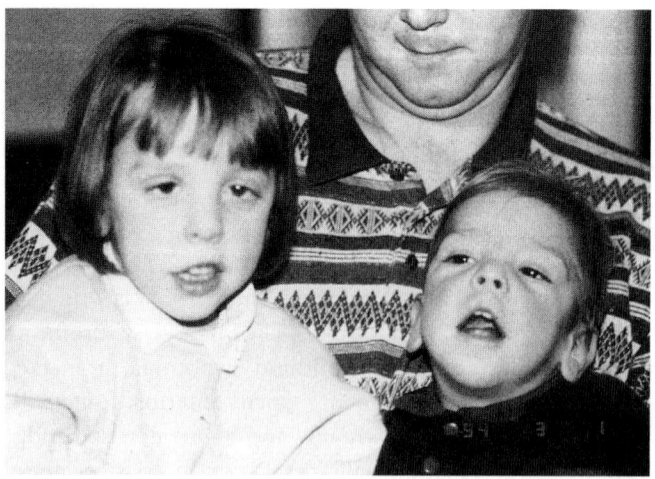

Fig. 47.16. Smith-Lemli-Opitz syndrome.

affecting almost half of cases. Lin's group (1995) found 16 of 68 patients with SLO to have AVSD and a further three to have primum ASD, and one a common atrium. Five of the series had anomalous pulmonary venous drainage, a significant overrepresentation compared to the distribution of types of heart defects in the general population. Our group coordinated a review of all UK cases; 86 patients with the clinical diagnosis revealed 49 with the classic metabolic defect. A marked excess of males was attributed to the difficulty of making the diagnosis in females. Of 18 proven cases with a heart defect, six were AVSDs.

The discovery that affected individuals have hypocholesterolemia and markedly elevated levels of 7-dehydrocholesterol due to a defect in the 7-dehydrocholesterol reductase gene showed that another multiple malformation syndrome had a metabolic basis (Tint et al., 1994). How and why a defect in the cholesterol biosynthesis pathway should have such an adverse effect on, for example, the septation of the ventricular inlet, remains to be established, but from the practical perspective, the possibility of SLO syndrome must be considered in a dysmorphic infant with a heart defect in view of the recessive mode of inheritance and the availability of pre- and postnatal diagnostic tests.

Genes responsible for congenital heart malformations as mongenic traits

The investigation of deletion syndromes and traditional mapping have identified the location of genes, and in some cases their identity, which, when defective can produce isolated heart defects. The classic examples are *ELN* as a cause of supravalvar aortic stenosis and *JAG1* leading to peripheral pulmonary artery stenosis. Mapping studies and candidate gene analysis led to the discovery of *Zic3* as a cause of X-linked laterality syndrome (see below), and the same approach yielded *TFAP2B* as the cause of autosomal dominant PDA (Satoda et al., 2000). Mapping studies point to a locus at 4q12–13 (Bleyl et al., 1995) responsible for total anomalous pulmonary venous drainage and another at 1p31–21 (Sheffield et al., 1997) causes one form of autosomal dominant AVSD.

Animal models, particularly zebra fish and mouse, will continue to generate candidate genes for heart malformation in ever increasing numbers. It should not be assumed that the role of the gene in humans will be the same. The extreme example of this is provided by *NKX2.5*. This homologue of the *Drosophila* gene *Tinman*, a gene so named because without it the fly has no heart, is responsible for an autosomal dominant cardiac syndrome characterized by ASD with atrioventricular conduction defects (OMIM 108900). About 18% of cases manifest a VSD instead (Schott et al., 1998; Benson, 1999). Mutations leading to loss of function and upregulation seem to produce the same phenotype. The propensity to sudden death in these patients makes it of clinical importance to recognize this phenotype. *NKX2.5*, also known as *CSX*, is a cardiac transcription factor containing a homeobox domain.

Environmental causes and the teratogen syndromes

The search for specific environmental associations has scored notable successes. This began with congenital rubella, which has now receded as a cause of heart defects in European populations where inoculation is widespread but will continue to cause heart defects in other populations. In Britain, as recently as the mid-1970s the average notification was 64 cases per annum, of which 39% had multiple malformations. This gave a rate of 3.27 in 100,000, although this was almost certainly a major underestimate due to failure of diagnosis in many cases. Table 47.1 lists several well-recognized teratogenic situations. In practical terms, maternal diabetes and alcohol abuse remain the most important external threats to normal heart development, but it is important to take a history of drug ingestion before offering recurrence risks. This is important when the consultation is with an affected individual, since recognition of a teratogenic cause enables the counselor to give a very small recurrence risk. This assumes, of course, that it is possible to remove the cause in the next pregnancy. The most important teratogenic influences involve chronic maternal disease and maternal medication or drug abuse.

Table 47.1. Some common teratogens

Teratogenic influence	Risk of heart defect (%)	Commonest type[a]
Maternal rubella	35	Persistent ductus arteriosus, peripheral pulmonary artery stenosis, septal defects
Maternal diabetes	3–5	VSD, coarctation, transposition of the great arteries
Maternal phenylketonuria	25–50	Tetralogy of Fallot
Systematic lupus erythematosus	20–40	Complete heart block
Maternal alcohol abuse	25–30	Septal defects
Hydantoin	2–3	Pulmonary and aortic stenosis, coarctation of aorta, PDA
Trimethadione	15–30	Tetralogy of Fallot, TGA, hypoplastic left heart
Thalidomide	<5	Tetralogy of Fallot, septal defects, truncus arteriosus
Lithium		Ebstein's anomaly, tircuspid atresia, ASD
Retinoic acid	10–20	Conotruncal heart defects

[a] See the text for abbreviations

MATERNAL DIABETES

Fetuses born to mothers with diabetes mellitus are at increased risk of heart malformation, either isolated or in association with other features of diabetic embryopathy. In particular, exposed fetuses are at increased risk of defective development of the caudal end of the spinal column, variously called caudal regression or sacral agenesis. In milder cases, the pattern of femoral hypoplasia-unusual facies syndrome results (Burn et al., 1984). Williamson (1970) found heart defects in 20% of children with the skeletal features of diabetic embryopathy. Rowland (1973) reported a 4% risk of heart defects in the offspring of diabetic mothers. Subsequent studies that took account of glycemic control found rates of heart malformation little different from the general population risk when mothers maintained good control (Jovanovic et al., 1981; Watkins, 1982). The Baltimore-Washington Infant Study, a population-based, case-control study of heart malformation found 1.5% of mothers to have overt diabetes and 4.2% to have gestational diabetes in their series of 2259 cases compared to rates of 0.5% and 3% among controls. The highest odds ratio was for double-outlet right ventricle (OR 21.33 CI 3.34–136.26) and truncus arteriosus (OR 12.81 CI 1.43–114.64). Splitt and Goodship, (1997) reported a strong association of left isomerism sequence with maternal diabetes. Slavotinek et al. (1996) reported three babies with disturbed laterality born to mothers with diabetes, one of which had the rare combination of left isomerism with asplenia.

The basis for the pattern of malformations seen is unclear though it is likely that some embryologic pathways are particularly susceptible to disruption by disturbance of glucose homeostasis and that some mother/fetus pairs are genetically more susceptible to disturbed development.

MATERNAL DRUG INGESTION

Alcohol

Alcohol is the non-therapeutic drug most frequently ingested by pregnant women. Alcohol induces heart defects in some exposed fetuses; VSD is most common, but ASD, tetralogy of Fallot, and other defects can also occur. Fetal alcohol syndrome produces a typical phenotype (Fig. 47.17). The overall incidence of the fetal alcohol syndrome in the general population may be 0.1–3.3 per 1000 (Smith, 1982) with

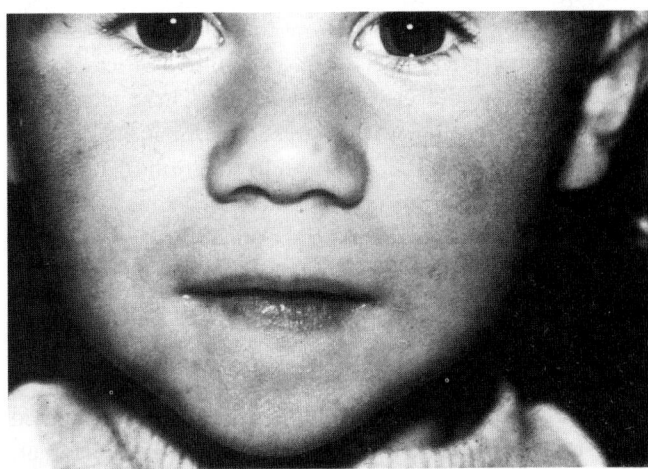

Fig. 47.17. Fetal alcohol syndrome. Short palpebral fissures and poorly developed philtral piers on the top lip can be seen. The child also had a VSD, short stature, and learning disability.

cardiovascular defects present in 29% to 70% of affected infants (Fang et al., 1987). Heavy alcohol drinkers, defined as women consuming a daily average equivalent of 45 ml or more absolute alcohol, had offspring with a higher incidence of major anomalies compared to more moderate drinkers. A "safe" level of alcohol intake during pregnancy has not been established.

Lithium

Lithium, used in the treatment of bipolar disease was first recognized as a teratogen because of the increased number of babies born with Ebstein anomaly, a relatively rare defect of the tricuspid valve. In one study of 143 infants exposed in utero, 13 (9%) had malformations, including ten with congenital cardiovascular defects; four had Ebstein anomaly plus other cardiac malformations (Weinberg and Goldfield, 1975). Data from the Swedish registry revealed four exposed infants with CHDs when 0.2 were expected, but none had Ebstein anomaly (Kallen, 1987). More recent studies have failed to confirm this high risk. Four case-control studies of Ebstein's anomaly covering a total of 227 cases failed to identify a single mother on lithium. Two cohort studies gave risk ratios for cardiac defects of 7.7 and 1.2 with wide confidence limits (Cohen et al., 1994).

MATERNAL PHENYLKETONURIA

With successful treatment for phenylketonuria (PKU) through dietary modification, a small but significant number of homozygous females of normal intellect have reached childbearing age (Walter, 1995). Most relinquish the unpleasant diet in adolescence and may enter pregnancy with high blood levels of phenylalanine. Among 524 offspring of non treated PKU mothers, Lenke and Levy (1980) found microcephaly in two-thirds of cases and congenital heart defects in one-quarter. There is a dose-response relationship with fewer malformations as the maternal blood levels fall. Only reintroduction of a phenylalanine-free diet before conception ensured a malformation rate no different from the general population.

FOLIC ACID SUPPLEMENTATION

Folic acid supplementation reduces by over half the number of neural tube defects in offspring. A less well recognized effect is a probable reduction in conotruncal heart malformations. For example, O'Malley et al. (1996) reported a 40% reduction in the prevalence of conotruncal heart defects in supplemented pregnancies. It will be interesting

to see if the C677T polymorphism in the methylene tetrahydrofolate reductase gene, which reduces bioavailable folate in homozygotes, is associated with an increased risk of heart malformation. There are early reports of a fall in the number of neural tube defects in the USA following the decision to supplement flour in 1998. The effect on heart malformation rates will be awaited with great interest.

Genes versus environment

Heart malformations outnumber all other major structural defects combined. As Figure 47.18 illustrates, there is remarkable similarity in reported birth rates in different centers. Most differences may be attributed to ascertainment differences. In the New England study, children presenting to referral centers in the first year of life were included. In the Baltimore-Washington Infant Study any first-year diagnoses were included. The availability of echocardiography increased early diagnosis. In both studies there was very little variation from year to year. In the other studies, heart defects diagnosed clinically gave a variable overall estimate of 6 to 8 per 1000 with an underlying steady rate of 4 per 1000 in those diagnosed by catheter, operation, or autopsy. A recent publication of a thorough study of all heart defects in Northern Ireland in the period 1974 to 1978 with at least five-year follow-up identified 972 cases of heart malformation with an annual rate varying from 6.0 to 8.59 in 1000 and a mean of 7.34 in 1000. Abu Harb and collaborators (1994) used the malformation register in northern England to arrive at an annual figure of just over 5 per 1000 births presenting to the regional

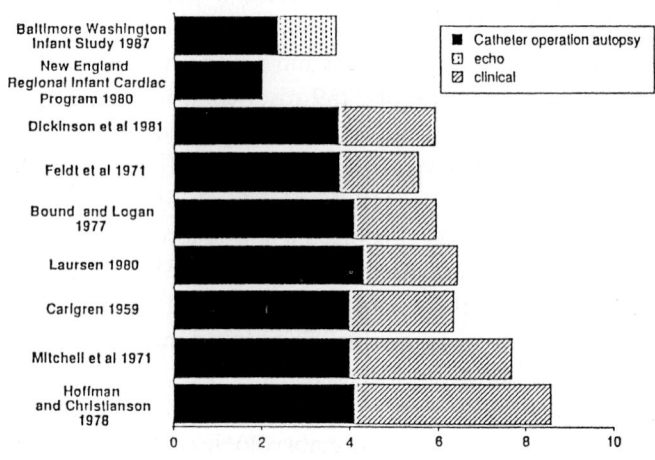

Fig. 47.18. Heart malformations.

cardiology service from all sources. The overall message from these studies is that heart defects are remarkably constant in time and place, which tends to argue against "hidden teratogens" as a major cause of heart defects. Despite this, many authors have favored a major environmental contribution on the basis of twin studies.

The "twin method" provides an estimate of genetic contribution to a disorder by comparing concordance rates in monozygotic (MZ) and dizygotic (DZ) twins; since the former share all their genes, any trait with a genetic component should be more likely to affect both members of the pair than in DZ twins where they share only half their genes. An underlying assumption is that twins are biologically comparable to singletons. This may be true of DZ twins but cannot be assumed in MZ twins, who are exposed to major and unique intrauterine influences. MZ twins are "a malformation to whom nature was kind". Galton in his original work avoided the issue by focusing on disorders perceived to be of postnatal origin. Price (1950) first enumerated the ways in which the influences of the twinning process might disturb early development and concluded that application of the twin method to malformations would result in an underestimate of genetic contribution. This did not deter several authors stating that heart defects are not genetic because they usually affect only one member of MZ twin pairs.

McKeown and Record in 1960 noted an apparent excess of heart defects in like-sex twins. Leck (1960) and Campbell (1961) raised the possibility that the twinning process itself might result in a heart defect in one of the pair. Most subsequent hospital series contained an excess of MZ pairs, and heart defects were more numerous among like-sex pairs in population studies. All reports were open to criticism on one or more of four counts: proof of zygosity, method of ascertainment, reliability of cardiac diagnosis, and sample size. In 1984, Burn and Corney reported a series of 195 twin pairs ascertained by complete case review in Newcastle and Great Ormond Street, London. Exclusion of uncertain diagnoses, monogenic and chromosomal syndromes, conjoined pairs, and PDA left 155 pairs. Exclusion of PDA was based on the high incidence of this disorder in premature babies; twins are more likely to be born "too small or too soon". Zygosity was established in 130, using physical examination and blood polymorphism analysis. A total of 65 of 130 (50%) were MZ, a highly significant excess over the general British population where only 35% of twins are MZ. Even taking account of the unknown zygosity cases did not alter the conclusion that there were either too many MZ or too few DZ twin pairs presenting with a heart defect in one or both of the pair. A subsequent

investigation of twin individuals identified through an unlimited ascertainment using existing British twin/malformation registers confirmed the MZ twin excess. Using data from Liverpool, Birmingham, and Aberdeen it was possible to study all heart defects in a population of over 20,000 individual twins. Again, only established diagnoses other than PDA were included. In Aberdeen the records of the perinatal mortality survey were combined with a cross-reference of the twins register and cardiac register to identify 43 children with heart murmurs. Only 13 of these qualified for inclusion as proven structural defects in a population of 1449 twins giving an overall twin rate of 8.97 in 1000. The incidence among singletons in the same time period was 6.0 in 1000 (AGM Campbell, personal communication).

In Liverpool, the incidence of heart defects in singletons in the period 1960–1969 was just under 6 per 1000 (Kenna et al., 1975). Among all twins recorded in Liverpool, the prevalence of confirmed heart defects was 11.09 in 1000. In Birmingham only inpatient heart defects were recorded; the singleton and twin heart defect rates were 3.69 and 5.03 in 1000, respectively. The excess was confined to like-sex twins pointing to an excess in MZ twins.

A second study in Birmingham looked at births in two maternity units between 1960 and 1965 with zygosity analysis: 13 out of 228 MZ twins had heart defects compared to four out of 628 DZ twin individuals. Combined with the data from Aberdeen where routine zygosity studies were undertaken, these data prove conclusively that MZ twin individuals are at increased risk; the combined data shown in Figure 47.19 give a prevalence of 17.2 in 1000 compared to a singleton figure of 6.0 in 1000.

These findings confirm the theoretical criticism of the twin method in relation to malformations. Heritability estimates are liable to major error if the twinning process itself is associated with the disorder under study. A variety of mechanisms have been invoked to account for excess malformations among twins (discussed further below). The likelihood is that any of the possible mechanisms would cause a defect in only one of a pair, increasing the number of discordant pairs. Figure 47.20 shows the effects of removing the presumed excess of discordant MZ twin pairs. The ratio of concordant pairs in MZ compared to DZ twins is almost doubled and with it the twin heritability estimate is increased to 60%. In practice, the wide variation in heritability estimates emphasizes the unreliability of the twin approach and the likelihood that genetic contribution is greater than twin studies have suggested.

A variety of mechanisms can be invoked to account for the MZ twin excess. Early effects of a reduced cell mass and, later in pregnancy, the adverse effects of shared circulation

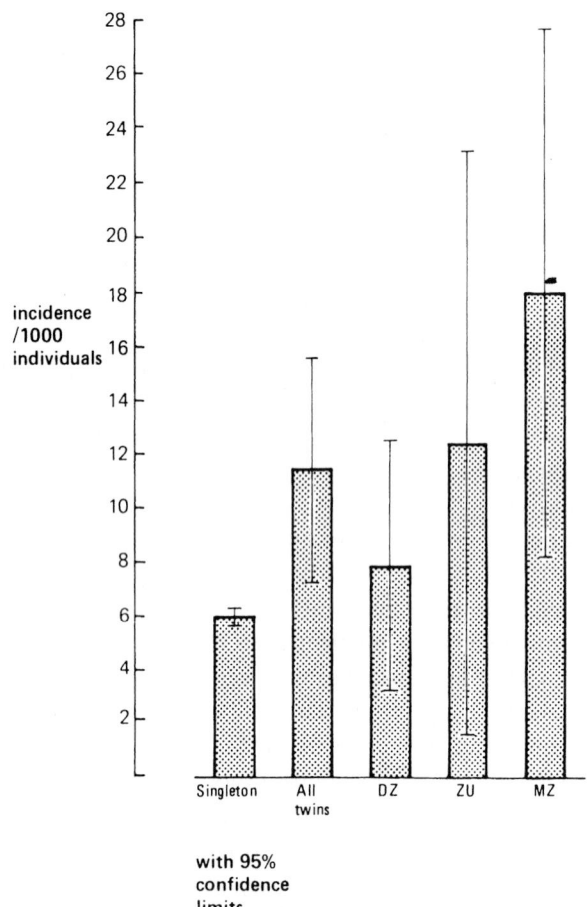

with 95%
confidence
limits

Fig. 47.19. Incidence of heart defects in twins (and higher multiples) compared to singletons with 95% confidence internal. (From Burn, 1988, with permission.)

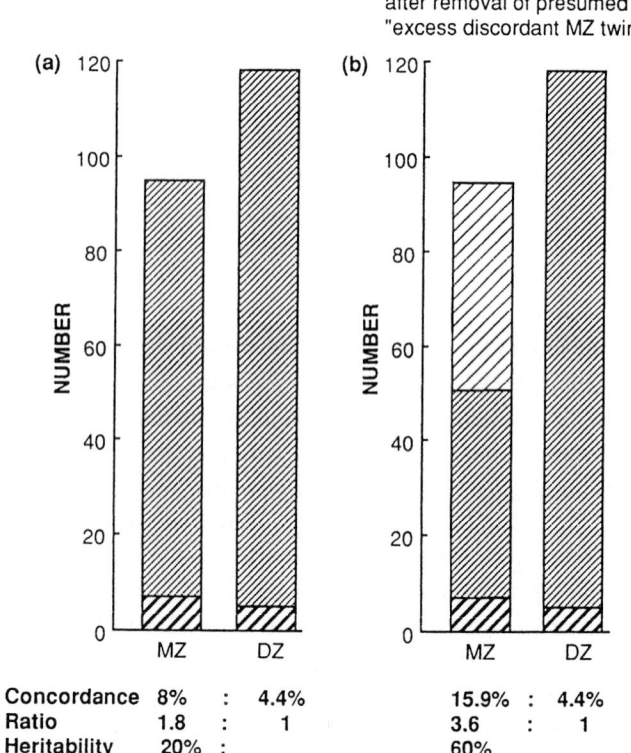

	Concordance		Ratio		Heritability	
(a)	8% : 4.4%		1.8 : 1		20% :	
(b)	15.9% : 4.4%		3.6 : 1		60%	

Fig. 47.20. Twin concordance for heart malformation. MZ:DZ ratio. Discordant; one of the pair affected (fine crosshatch). Concordant; both affected (heavy crosshatch).

are mechanisms liable to account for some of the excess heart defects in MZ twins. A more potent factor is the potential for disturbance of laterality. This is seen most clearly in conjoined twins where there have been several reports of right isomerism in the right half of some pairs joined side to side (Rossi et al., 1987). There is general evidence of a left lead in determination of the left-right gradient (Corballis and Morgan, 1978). From this it may be deduced that in the conjoined pairs, separation of the right side of the early embryo from the left results in the left half producing an embryo with normal situs while the right half, having lost its point of reference is at risk of a major disturbance of laterality, with right isomerism as its most extreme manifestation (Burn, 1991). The monoamniotic twins shown in Figure 47.21A had conjoined cords. Their mother, a midwife, had noted that they were mirror-imaged for tooth eruption and thumb-sucking. Their hair whorls were mirror-imaged with the right half having a crown deflected to the right of the midline and the other a deflec-

tion to the left. The "right half" of this twin pair had tetralogy of Fallot. Figure 47.21B shows MZ twins who both have the CATCH phenotype but only the twin on the right suffered tetrology of Fallot. His brother had a normal heart (Goodship et al., 1995).

Disturbance of laterality and the heart

The association of laterality disturbance and heart defects in twins draws attention to an embryonic mechanism of major importance in cardiac development. There is evidence in family studies and mouse models of a variety of monogenic causes for disturbance of laterality. The left-right axis is defined from the beginning of embryonic development with the formation of the dorso ventral and rostral/daudal axes. Creation of an asymmetric organism requires breaking of symmetry and maintenance of the asymmetry. In humans, the curvature of the heart tube to the right, the dextral heart loop, is the first evidence of asymmetry but clearly at the cellular level the left-right gradient was estab-

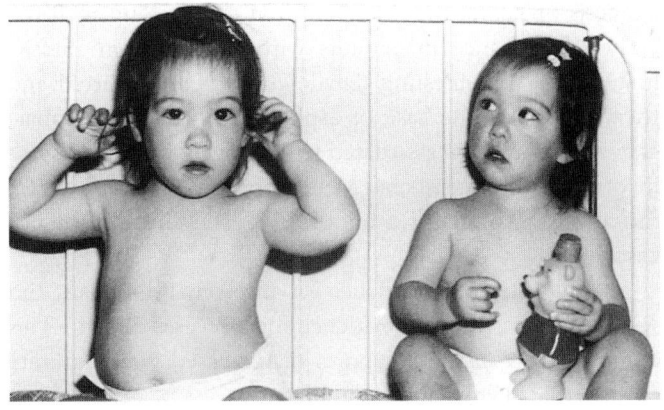

A

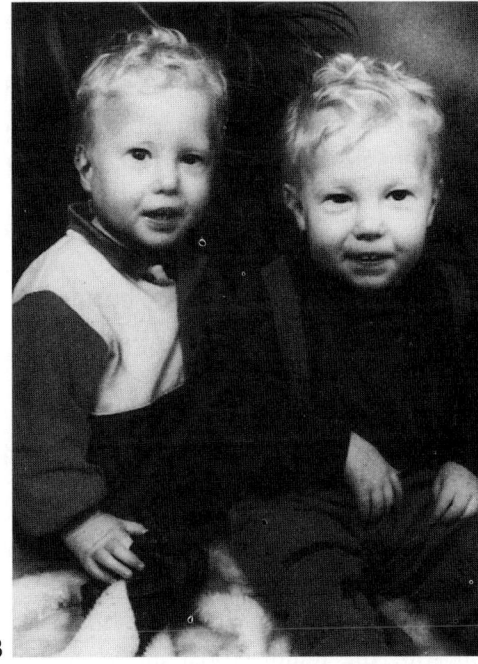

B

Fig. 47.21. (A) Monoamniotic twins discordant for Fallot's tetralogy. The morphologic "left half" developed normally. (B) MZ twins with CATCH phenotype.

lished earlier. If the gradient is reversed but all other processes are normal, complete situs inversus results. The heart should be normal, apart from being on the right (dextrocardia), though heart defects are present in 3% to 9% of cases (Merklin and Varano, 1995). This is presumed to be due to the reversal being less than perfect for even minor disturbance of laterality is liable to alter the shape and flow characteristics of the heart tube with resultant abnormality of connections and septation. When there is incomplete reversal with lateralization being different in internal organs, the terms visceral heterotaxy and situs ambuguus are used interchangeably.

The patterns of malformation can be divided into those with and without primary ciliary dyskinesia (PCD). The association of PCD with situs inversus, nasal polyps and bronchiectasis is known by the eponym Kartagener syndrome (OMIM No. 244400). The ciliary anomaly obeys the predictions of autosomal recessive inheritance while the bronchiectasis has become a rarity with more effective therapy. Situs inversus occurs in about half of affected homozygotes suggesting that determination of situs is a chance phenomenon in such individuals. Heart defects occur in about 10% of affected individuals indicating less than complete reversal of laterality in these individuals. This is a heterogeneous disorder. Histologically cilia typically lack dynein arms. The ciliary axoneme comprises over 100 polypeptides while dynein itself is a complex protein with several subunits. Mutations have been found in axonemal dynein intermediate chain gene 1 (*DNAI1*) (Guichard et al., 2001). The human arthologue of *lrd*, the gene defective in the *iv* mouse, is on chromosome 7 and a mutation has been identified in this gene in a child known to have paternal uniparental disomy of chromosome 7 and primary ciliary dyskinesisa (Bartoloni et al., 2000).

ISOMERISM SEQUENCE

Laterality defects without cilial anomalies are a major factor in the etiology of heart defects, particularly those at the more severe end of the clinical spectrum. In isomeric children the body displays pathological symmetry. In right isomerism, typically the individual has bilateral right atrial appendages, bilateral short eparterial bronchi and bilateral "right" trilobed lungs. Left isomerism is characterized by left atrial appendages, bilateral long hyparterial bronchi and bilateral bilobed lungs. In right isomerism the spleen, which arises from the left side of the dorsal mesogastrium, is usually absent. In left isomerism multiple spleens often develop. The terms asplenia/polysplenia syndrome and Ivemark syndrome (Ivemark, 1955) are often used but a more precise descriptive term of the underlying disorder is isomerism sequence (Burn, 1991).

There are no population-based studies of isomerism sequence but asplenia was found to affect 1 in 22,000 births in Canada (Webber et al., 1992). In a retrospective study of children undergoing catheterization, 1 in 24,000 children in a Caucasian population had evidence of laterality sequence including isomerism sequence, accounting for at least 1% of all heart defects (Gatrad et al., 1984). Both right and left isomerism sequence are associated with a wide spectrum of heart defects shown in Table 47.2. Some anomalies are attributable to the direction of lateralization.

Table 47.2. Frequency of common heart lesions found in patients with isomerism sequence[a]

Principal heart defects	Left isomerism (%)	Right isomerism (%)
Interruption of IVC with azygos continuation	75	7
Total anomalous pulmonary venous connection	0	35
Common atrium	47	67
Single ventricle	30	70
Atrioventricular septal defect	68	93
Double outlet right ventricle	7	47
Pulmonary stenosis/atresia	48	78

[a] *The table refers to the mean of the percentages given in references 1, 2 and 3 for right isomerism (Ho et al., 1991; Chiu et al., 1988; Sapire et al., 1986) and 1, 3 and 4 for left isomerism (Ho et al., 1991; Sapire et al., 1986; Sharma et al., 1987). isomerism sequence, accounting for at least 1% of all heart defects (Gatrad et al., 1984).*

For example, in left isomerism there is a failure of development of the suprarenal portion of the inferior vena cava in the absence of a morphological right atrium. Blood reaches the heart *via* an azygos connection to the superior vena cava. In right isomerism, lack of a morphological left atrium is associated with anomalous pulmonary venous connection in 35% of cases. Disturbances of atrioventricular connection and separation and conotruncal anomalies occur in both types of isomerism, though right isomerism is associated with more severe defects overall. Absence of a spleen adds to morbidity and mortality due to predisposition to infection. It is important to recognize asplenia by a search for Howell Jolly bodies in the blood and abdominal ultrasound with antibiotic pophylaxis if the spleen is absent.

In the last five years a large number of genes in the pathway by which the left–right axis is established have been identified. Mutation screening has been undertaken in some of these in patients with laterality disturbance and heterozygous mutations found in lefty 1, nodal activin receptor 2b and cryptic, in a minority of patients (Kosaki et al., 1999; Casey and Hackett, 2000). When parental samples have been available it has been noted that the changes have been inherited from a phenotypically normal parent. Whilst it is likely that the changes contribute to the phenotype this is difficult to prove. The changes could be dominant with low penetrance or require a second event, either a mutation in a second gene in the pathway or an environmental factor.

Only one of the genes in the pathway was identified through investigation of a family with laterality disturbance, *ZIC3* (Gebbia et al., 1997). Midline defects such as sacral agenesis or neural tube defects often occur along with laterality disturbance in patients with mutations in this X-linked gene. Manifesting females have been reported and there has been one case of a phenotypically normal male carrying a mutation associated with congenital heart disease in other family members (Mégarbané et al., 2001). *ZIC3* mutations account for a minority of laterality disturbance cases.

In addition to the evidence for autosomal dominant and X-linked forms there is evidence for a recessive form. This comes from consistent reports of increased consanguinity (Burn et al., 1986) and a significant excess of cases among inbred groups (Gatrad et al., 1984).

A careful family history and pregnancy history are essential before counseling. In one study half of the cases of left isomerism occurred in the offspring of women with diabetes (Splitt et al., 1999) and undoubtedly the incidence of laterality disturbance is increased in the offspring of diabetic women. In the absence of significant previous family history, consanguinity or maternal diabetes, an empiric recurrence risk of 5–10% for future pregnancies seems appropriate based on the prospective study of over 1000 mothers referred for echocardiography because of a previous child with a heart defect (Allan et al., 1986).

Counseling and isolated heart malformations

Isolated heart malformations are usually sporadic, but occasionally particular defects can be shown to be inherited as a simple mendelian trait (Yao et al., 1968). In the past, a preoccupation with the multifactorial model together with misinterpretation of twin data led to the general statement that risks to sibs and offspring would be similar and would be small. Observational data have not supported these assumptions. A starting point for analysis of empirical data on heart defects in sibs and offspring has been the polygenic threshold model. The possibility that several genes might act additively was originally introduced to allow Mendel's laws to be applied to graded characters. A number of expectations of a polygenic trait allow observational data to be tested against this model:

1. Risk to first-degree relatives equates to the square-root of the population incidence.
2. Risk to sibs and offspring should be about equal.
3. Risk for more distant relatives declines rapidly.
4. Risk increases when there are multiple affected family members.

5. Risk increases with the severity of the disorder.
6. Risk is greater among relatives of the more rarely affected sex.

Persistent ductus arteriosus is associated with preterm delivery and, more rarely, results from exposure to rubella. These two obvious causes have tended to obscure the underlying genetic predisposition to PDA, study of which provides an elegant demonstration of a polygenic trait. The possibility of a genetic predisposition in isolated PDA was first raised by the repeated observation of two or more affected individuals in the same family (Carleton et al., 1958). Systematic analyses based on family studies in the term infant began with Record and McKeown (1953) and Anderson (1954). Their combined data revealed five, or possibly six, cases of PDA among 269 later-born sibs, a recurrence risk of 1 in 50. Anderson further noted that among his uncomplicated cases, only 27% were male. A number of subsequent studies have confirmed that these early estimates were essentially correct (Polani and Campbell, 1960; Wilkins, 1969; Ando et al., 1977; Nora and Nora, 1978). One other study stands out for its size, precision, and attention to detail. Zetterqvist (1972) examined the records of 479 patients who underwent ligation of the arterial duct in one of three Swedish centers between 1941 and 1965. He selected those born before 1945 who were of Swedish origin, and who had reproduced. He was able to trace 435 of the 479 eligible for study and examine their families. The ratio of males:females was 1:3. Among 663 siblings, 17 had congenital heart disease. One had Down syndrome and an atrioventricular septal defect and one had preductal aortic coarctation. The rest had persistence of the arterial duct giving a recurrence risk of 15 in 663 or 2.3 ($\pm$ 0.6)%.

Among 490 offspring, 18 had congenital heart disease; three of these did not have a persistently patent duct and were probably random associations. The remaining 15 had persistence of the duct, giving a recurrence risk of 3.7% among offspring. As this is substantially higher than the sib risk, the effect of single dominant genes was considered possible. This was confirmed when Zetterqvist identified two families with a total of six children of whom three had a PDA. All three children had features of a generalized connective tissue disorder. Excluding these two "syndromic" families, 12 offspring of 484 families had PDA. This is 2.5 ($\pm$ 0.7)%—the same risk as was seen in sibs. Zetterqvist looked for evidence of a major environmental contribution, but found none. Birth rank, parental age, and seasonal incidence showed no significant associations. Earlier authors had an excess of females in the third quarter of the year. A

similar trend was present in the Swedish data but did not reach significant levels. It remains possible that a few cases result from some insult such as fever, cold medications, or viral infection affecting women who become pregnant in midwinter. The lack of statistical significance suggests that such an environmental contribution is small.

Zetterqvist's report suggests that PDA is a polygenic threshold trait. The recurrence risk is the same for sibs and offspring. The risk in first-degree relatives is the same as the square root of the population incidence. Carlgren (1959) found the incidence of PDA in a comparable group of 116,419 Swedish children to be 6 in 10,000. The square-root of this figure is 2.4%.

Cousins share only one-eighth of their alleles in common as opposed to sibs and offspring who share one-half. When a disorder depends on "negative" alleles being present at several gene loci, it is to be expected that the likelihood of this happening is much smaller in cousins (or third-degree relatives) than in first-degree relatives. Therefore, the occurrence of a polygenic disorder in one member of a family should be reflected in a high recurrence risk in first, but not in second- and third-degree relatives. Zetterqvist found only 0.6% of the latter group to be affected with PDA.

It was also possible to assess the effect of "severity" on recurrence risks. At operation, the surgeons measured routinely the widest diameter of the duct. Zetterqvist had 71 probands with a wide duct. They had seven affected children among a total of 146 (4.8% $\pm$ (1.7)). The probands in the "narrow" and "moderate" categories had five affected children among 271 or 1.8 ($\pm$ 0.9)%. This is in keeping with the fifth category in the above list; greater severity implies a greater genetic predisposition, which is reflected in the higher risk to relatives: 20 children were born to probands who themselves had affected sibs; two of these offspring were affected, which is comparable to the 10% recurrence risk used generally in counseling families with two sibs affected by a polygenic trait. The risk of recurrence rises with more affected family members.

The "Carter effect" states that when there is a sex difference in a polygenic trait the recurrence risk is greater in the relatives of the more rarely affected sex. This is based on the assumption that the more rarely affected sex is, on average, further from the "threshold" and so requires a greater genetic disadvantage before the "disease" occurs. The excess of deleterious genes is reflected in a higher incidence of the disorder among close relatives. Since persistence of the arterial duct is two to three times as common among females, the recurrence risk should be greater among the relatives of male probands. In the Zetterqvist study, male probands had 100 children of whom three had a duct (3.0 (± 1.7%)), while female probands had nine affected among 384 offspring (2.3 (± 0.8%)). The difference is in the predicted direction, but is not statistically significant.

Persistent patency of the arterial duct provides an excellent example of a multifactorial or polygenic threshold trait. One environmental insult, rubella, produces persistence of the duct regardless of genetic makeup. With the other important environmental factors, (altitude and preterm delivery) there is the possibility that genetic predisposition determines which individuals "cross the line". Apart from these categories, there is little evidence of other significant environmental "variance", or contribution to the number of cases born. The family studies, on the other hand, reveal PDA to comply very well with the six "polygenic predictions". The greatest risk would be to the daughter of a man who himself had been found to have a widely patent duct. In Zetterqvist's series there were 16 daughters of such men, of whom two were affected.

The animal models of Patterson et al.(1971) provide biologic support for a "graded character". In breeding experiments with collies, he found some to have an arterial duct and others to have ductal diverticula in which the duct had closed at the extreme pulmonary end, but remained patent over the rest of its length. As in humans, those with a PDA varied in severity from a narrow channel to a diameter equal to that of the aorta. Crossing an affected dog with an unrelated collie resulted in 22% offspring crossing the diverticulum threshold and a small number having an open duct. When affected dogs were back-crossed with unaffected first-degree relatives, there was a much higher incidence of duct anomaly among offspring, which suggests that the population curve for liability was shifted further across the threshold. The worst situation resulted from mating between two affected collies; only 16% of the offspring had normal closure of the duct. Patterson and his colleagues extended their work to histologic examination of abnormal ducts. In cases of ductal diverticulum, they found, instead of the normal muscular media with a few elastic fibers, that the segment of duct adjacent to the aorta had an elastic aorta-like media while normal duct wall was present at the pulmonary end. In cases of persistently patent ducts this "aortification" extended along the whole length.

Zetterqvist reported two families in which an apparent autosomal dominant single gene defect, involving connective tissue structure, seemed to be the cause of patency of the duct. Burman (1961) reported a female infant whose father was affected. PDA was diagnosed in two of the father's sibs and their mother died at 48 years of age from "dropsy", with features compatible with PDA. Davidson

(1992) described a large dominant PDA pedigree with nine affected members. A single dominant gene seemed likely in this family. As yet, such families may only be recognized in retrospect, when multiple family members are affected (Satoda et al., 2000). This was one of the families shown to have Char syndrome with a mutation in *TFAP2B*, which encodes a transcription factor (Satoda et al., 2000)

EMPIRICAL RISKS FOR SIBLING OF CHILDREN WITH HEART DEFECTS

Table 47.3 reviews the major traditional studies of recurrence risk in sibs of children with heart defects. The general principle that sibling risks fall into the 2% to 5% range so often used by genetic counselors is apparent. Most of the studies did not distinguish between sibs born before and after the proband, which may have distorted figures, since families who have had a child with a heart defect are likely to be somewhat less likely to try for further children. Nevertheless, the counseling figures shown are sufficient in practical terms, since the advances in fetal echocardiography and postnatal care of affected children have improved to the point where it is reasonable to counsel in terms of the risk of recurrence being small.

EMPIRICAL RISKS FOR OFFSPRING

In early studies of recurrence risks in the offspring of adults born with major heart defects, the limited available literature suggested a recurrence risk in offspring of 3% to 5%, comparable to sibs and compatible with the multifactorial model. In 1982, Whittemore and colleagues reported a study that was not in keeping with a polygenic predisposition; they found 60 children with heart defects among 372 children born to mothers with heart malformations of various types, a recurrence risk of 16%. Emanuel and colleagues (1983) found five (10%) out of 52 children born to individuals with atrioventricular septal defects to have a major heart defect. Rose and associates (1985) studied the families of adults with coarctation of the aorta, aortic stenosis, ASD, and dextrocardia. In the first three categories, offspring recurrence was seen in 9/90 (10%), 11/96 (11%), and 22/194 (11%), respectively. These higher offspring risks are now widely quoted, but the possibility of selection bias cannot be excluded. The study by Whittemore and collaborators related to women who responded to an invitation to be followed in subsequent pregnancy but no estimate of the participation rate was obtained. In the study of Emanuel and colleagues the families of 60 probands from an initial cohort of 123 were included, giving a

Table 47.3. Recurrence risks in sibs

Malformation	Probands	Affected sibs	Total sibs	% affected	Counseling figure	Reference
Situs inversus	240	28	1271	2.2	3	Torgersen, 1950
Isomerism sequence	60	3	63	4.75	5	Rose et al, 1975
	98	2(4)	109	2.0 (4.1)		Burn et al., 1984
						Allan et al., 1986
Tricuspid atresia	33	0 (1)	92	0 (0.9)	1	Fuhrmann, 1968
	52	0 (1)	98	0 (0.1)		Nora and Nora, 1983
Mitral atresia		0 (2)	110	0(2)	2	Child and Dennis, 1977
Transposition of great arteries	184	6(22)	442	1.4(5.0)	2	Fuhrmann, 1968
	153	3	171	1.8		Ando et al., 1977
	45	2		1.4		Sanchez- Cascos, 1978
Truncus arteriosus	43	1	86	1.2	1	Nora and Nora, 1983
Pulmonary atresia secundum ASD	36	0(1)	80	1.3	1	Nora and Nora, 1983
		9(10)	279	3.2(3.7)	3	Nora et al., 1967
		13	1110	1.2		Ando et al., 1977
	172	11	380	2.9		Nora and Nora, 1983
	191	6	645	1.0		Zetterqvist, 1972
	135	11	335	3.3		Sanchez-Cascos, 1978
		7	190	3.7		Williamson, 1969
AVSD	73	4	151	2.6	2	Nora and Nora, 1983
	92	4	229	1.7		Emanuel et al., 1968
	80	2	103	1.9		Ando et al., 1977
	51	14 1st degree relatives		8.7		Sanchez-Cascos, 1978
Ebstein's anomaly	47	1	105	1	1	Nora and Nora, 1983
VSD	180	6	359	1.7	3	Campbell, 1965
	1241	18	1237	1.5		Ando et al., 1977
	214	345	12	1.7		Sanchez-Cascos, 1978
	161	3	672	0.9		Dennis and Warren, 1981
	306	28	61	4.2		Nora and Nora, 1983
		2		3.3		Czeizel and Meszaros, 1981
Pulmonary stenosis	125	6	282	2.1	2	Campbell, 1962
	123	3	99	1.5		Ando et al., 1977
	101	1	208	0.5		Dennis and Warren, 1981
	166	10	375	2.7		Nora and Nora, 1983
Tetralogy of Fallot	100	4	189	2.1	2	Boon et al., 1972
	196	6	380	1.6		Ando et al., 1977
	113	4	327	1.2		Sanchez-Cascos, 1978
	61	0	100	0		Dennis and Warren, 1981
	180	11	366	3.0		Nora and Nora, 1983
Aortic stenosis	126	10	246	4.1	3	Zoethout et al., 1964
	29	2	41	4.9		Ando et al., 1977
	155	8	361	2.2		Nora and Nora, 1983
Coarctation of aorta	109	1	252	0.4	2	Campbell and Polani, 1961
	94	5	283	1.8		Zetterqvist, 1972
	100	1	112	0.5		Boon and Roberts, 1976
	131	5	281	1.8		Nora and Nora, 1983
PDA	241	3	198	1.5	2.5	Wilkins, 1969
	435	15	663	2.3		Zetterqvist, 1972
	295	8	408	2.0		Ando et al., 1977
	220	18	516	3.5		Nora and Nora, 1983

participation rate of just below 50%, and families of an additional 30 probands from an unspecified total were included. Again, the participation rate in the study of Rose and colleagues was low (219 of a total of 507 who were alive and had children; 43%), in part because the investigators were restricted to a two-year period in which to contact the study subjects and because ascertainment was restricted to the state in which the hospital was based. This may have resulted in an excess of families with affected children who were more likely to remain close to the specialist center. A further difficulty when comparing different studies is the choice of heart defect. Czeizel and colleagues (1982) followed up adult survivors regardless of heart defect and found an overall recurrence risk of 4%. A study that differs dramatically from the study by Whittemore and colleagues is the report by Zellers and colleagues (1990) based on 395 patients with tetralogy of Fallot. They identified three affected children among 253 offspring; all three were girls and their defects were VSD, truncus arteriosus, and tetralogy of Fallot. In two of the three cases the father was the affected parent. The authors recognized that their study had important methodologic weaknesses; they relied on postal questionnaires and only 58% were returned. They were unable to examine the offspring, and thus some defects may have been overlooked. Despite a mean age of 38 years among the respondents, they identified only 127 parents. Not only did their recurrence risk of 1.2% fall well below that found by Whittemore and others, the risk of recurrence in their group was greater if the father was affected. This is in contrast to the other literature. For example, Nora and Nora (1987) drew attention to the greater recurrence risk in the offspring of affected mothers in almost all reports published up to that time. Table 47.4 summarizes this literature.

The British Heart Foundation Offspring Study (Burn et al., 1998) identified 1094 individuals from the pediatric records of the Hospital for Sick Children, Great Ormond Street, Guy's Hospital, National Heart Hospital, and the cardiac units in Newcastle, Southampton, Leeds, and Liverpool. The available cohort was reduced to 943 by exclusion of 108 patients who had died, 31 who had emigrated, and 12 who were found to be mentally retarded; 62 cases could not be traced through available channels, 29 refused to participate, and 158 were traced but failed to respond. Interviews with 694 individuals (74% of the available cohort) were recorded. A total of 32 heart defects were recorded among 1436 sibs (2.2%). There was no significant difference in recurrence rate in sibs of affected males or females (Table 47.4). There were 17 heart malformations among 380 offspring (4.5%), which is significantly greater than the sib risk. Normality of the other offspring was based on parental report in 19% and medical report in the remainder. Table 47.5 shows the abnormal offspring as a proportion of total offspring in relation to the nature of the malformation in the proband and the sex of the proband. As most of the categories of disturbed situs and connection were small, these are grouped together. There were four recorded cases of heart defect among the 179 offspring of males. A case was excluded where a child born to another partner was said to have died in childhood but where no

Table 47.4. Recurrence rates in offspring of males and females with heart defects

Authors	Defect	% offspring affected		Ratio F:M
		Male	Female	
Williamson, 1969	Atrial septal defect	0	11.1	
Taussig, 1971	Tetralogy of Fallot	0	3.1	
Zetterqvist, 1972	Atrial septal defect Persistent ductus arteriosus Coarctation	1.6	3.1	1.94
Dennis and Warren, 1981	Pulmonary valve stenosis Pulmonary infundibular stenosis Ventricular septal defect	3.0	2.9	0.97
Czeizel et al., 1982	Mixed	1.4	5.1	3.64
Emanuel et al., 1983	Atrioventricular septal defect	0	13.9	
Rose et al., 1985	Aortic stenosis Atrial septal defect Coarctation	7.3	13.0	1.78
Nora and Nora, 1987	Mixed	2.4	5.5	2.29

Table 47.5. The british offspring study. Affected and total offspring according to proband sex and malformations

	Proband No.	Offspring				
		Of Males		Of Females		
		Aff/Total	%	Aff/Total	%	
Anom. pulmonary venous drainage	38	0/14	–	1/20	5.0	
Transposition great arteries	97	0/10	–	0/3	–	
Abnormal situs and other abnormal connections	90	1/14	7.1	2/13	15.4	
AV septal defects	85	1/12	8.3	4/38	10.5	
Tetralogy of Fallot	384	2/129	1.6	6/127	4.7	
Totals		**Males**	**%**	**Females**	**%**	
Heart defects		4/179	2.2	13/201	6.5*	
All major malformations		4/179	2.2	16/201		

Contrast M:F* p = 0.10. (From Burn et al. 1998)

record of any illness or the death could be found. One case included in this group was a boy with the typical electrocardiographic changes seen in AVSD, the disorder in his father. Echocardiography revealed trivial mitral regurgitation but no septal defect. Included in the recurrences among the offspring of females with tetralogy of Fallot is a case of TAPVC associated with a marker chromosome of maternal origin, that is tetrasomy 22 or cat eye syndrome; the mother was of normal intelligence but had colobomata; a second affected pregnancy was terminated, but the heart was said to have been normal and was not included. The two recurrences among the 13 offspring of mothers in the "abnormal situs or connection" group were born to one woman with double outlet left ventricle.

The numbers in each category are small, but in all groups the recurrence rate is greater in the offspring of females. This reaches statistical significance when all heart defects are grouped together ($p = 0.038$). All three cases of major malformation other than heart defects were born to affected mothers. The excess of all malformations in the offspring of females is highly significant ($p = 0.01$). A significant excess of miscarriages were recorded where the mother was affected compared to the male group (45:15; $p = 0.0009$).

Recurrence risk ratios were analyzed using a computer modeling method developed by Farrall and Holder (1992) based on the work of Risch (1990) reported after exclusions, data from 290 offspring, 861 siblings, 2364 second degree and 4230 third degree relatives were used in modeling. The best fit model for Fallot's tetralogy was one of three loci acting in a multiplicative mode. AVSD, on the other hand was compatible with a heterogeneous monogenic model, i.e., most cases probably result from a defect in a single gene but different genes cause the problem in different families.

Future developments

Chromosome analysis including FISH for small deletions such as 22q11 deletion, a history of diabetes and alcohol abuse, and a check for one of the 370 plus dysmorphic syndromes that feature a heart defect can account for perhaps a quarter of all heart defects. The remainder are likely to result from the interaction of several genes with or without external triggers and chance factors in early development. Completion of the Human Genome Project and the availability of comprehensive sets of single nucleotide polymorphisms amenable to high throughput analysis open the way to complex trait analysis. The large scale mutagenesis screens in zebra fish and mouse and the dissection of key developmental pathways such as neural crest migration and laterality determination will yield a large number of candidate genes. The future will involve a large-scale collaborative effort to bring together the necessary clinical resources to permit evaluation of the contribution of these genes. The coming decade may bring congenital heart disease closer to being a solved problem in terms of cause. Prevention will have to wait much longer.

REFERENCES

Abu-Harb M, Hey E, Wren C (1994) Death in infancy from unrecognised congenital heart disease. Arch Dis Child 71:3–7

Adam LR, Davison EV, Malcolm AJ et al. (1991) Cytogenetic analysis of a congenital fibrosarcoma. Cancer Genet Cytogenet 52:37–41

Alagille D, Estrada A et al. (1987) Syndromic paucity of interlobular bile ducts Alagille syndrome or arteriohepatic dysplasia: Review of 80 cases. J Pediatr 110:195–200

Allan LD, Crawford DC, Chita SK et al. (1986) Familial recurrence of congenital heart disease in a prospective series of mothers referred for fetal echocardiography. Am J Cardiol 58:334–337

Alonso S, Pierpont ME, Radtke W et al. (1995) Heterotaxia syndrome and autosomal dominant inheritance. Am J Med Genet 56:12–15

Anad F, Burn J, Matthews D, Cross I, Davison BCC, Mueller R et al. (1990) Alagille syndrome and deletion of 20p. J Med Genet 27:729–737

Anderson RC (1954) Causative factors underlying congenital heart malformations. Pediatrics 14:143–152

Ando M, Takao A, Mori K (1977) Genetic and environmental factors in congenital heart disease. In Inouye E, Nishimura H (eds): Gene-Environmental Interaction in Common Diseases. University Park Press, Baltimore, pp. 71–88

Augusseau S, Jouk S, Jalbert P, Prieur M (1986) DiGeorge syndrome and 22q11 rearrangements. Hum Genet 74:206

Bamford RN, de la Cruz J, Roessler E et al. (2000) Mutations in the EGF-CFC gene, CRYPTIC cause human left-right axis abnormalities and transposition of the great arteries. Am J Hum Genet 67

Bamford RN, Roessler E, Burdine RD et al. (2000) Loss of function mutations in the EGF-CFC gene CFC1 are associated with human left-right laterality defects. Nature Genetics 26:501505–501

Bartoloni L, Pan Y, Rossier C et al. (2000) The DNAH11 axonemal heavy chain dynein type 11; gene is mutated in one form of primary ciliary dyskinesia. Am J Hum Genet 67:27

Bleyl S, Nelson L, Odelberg SJ et al. (1995) A gene for familial total anomalous pulmonary venous return maps to chromosome 4p13-q12. Am J Hum Genet 56:408–415

Bonnet D, Pelet A, Legeai-Mallet L, Sidi D, Mathieu M, Parent P et al. (1994) A gene for Holt-Oram syndrome maps to the distal long arm of chromosome 12. Nature Genet 6:405–408

Boon AR, Roberts DF (1976) A family study of coarctation of the aorta. J Med Genet 13:420–433

Boon AR, Farmer MB, Roberts DF (1972) A family study of Fallot's tetralogy. J Med Genet 9:179–192

Boughman JA, Berg KA, Astemborski JA et al. (1987) Familial risks of congenital heart defect assessed in a population-based epidemiologic study. Am J Med Genet 26:839–849

Bound JR, Logan WF (1977) Incidence of congenital heart disease in Blackpool 1947–1971. Br Heart J 39:445–450

Brewer C, Holloway S, Zawalnyski P, Schinzel A, FitzPatrick D (1998) A chromosomal deletion map of human malformations. Am J Hum Genet 63:1153–9

Britz-Cunningham SH, Shah MM, Zuppan CW, Fletcher WH (1995) Mutations of the *Connexin43* gap-junction in patients with heart malformations and defects of laterality. N Engl J Med 332:1323–1329

Budarf ML, Collins J, Gong W et al. (1995a) Cloning a balanced translocation associated with DiGeorge syndrome and identification of a disrupted candidate gene. Nature Genet 10:269–278

Budarf ML, Konkle BA, Ludlow LB et al. (1995b) Identification of a patient with Bernard-Soulier syndrome and a deletion in the DiGeorge/velo-cardio-facial chromosomal region in 22q11.2. Hum Mol Genet 4:763–766

Burman D (1961) Familial patent ductus arteriosus. Br Heart J 23:603–604

Burn J (1986) Williams syndrome. J Med Genet 23:389–395

Burn J (1989) The face and immune system in tetralogy of Fallot (editorial). Int J Cardiol 22:237–239

Burn J (1991) Disturbance of morphological laterality in humans. In: Bock GR, Marsh J (eds): Biological asymmetry and handedness. Chichester: Wiley, 282–299

Burn J (1999) Closing time for CATCH 22. J Med Genet **36**,737–738

Burn J, Corney G (1984) Congenital heart defects and twinning. Acta Genet Med Gemellol 33:61–69

Burn J, Winter RM, Baraitser M, Hall CM, Fixsen J (1984) Femoral hypoplasia-unusual facies syndrome. J Med Genet 21:331–340

Burn J, Coffey R, Allan LD et al. (1986) Isomerism: A genetic analysis. In Doyle EF, Engle MA, Gersony WM, Rashkind WJ, Talner NS, (eds): Paediatric Cardiology. NY, Springer Verlag, pp. 1126–1128

Burn J, Takao A, Wilson D, Cross I, Momma K, Wadey R et al. (1993) Conotruncal anomaly face syndrome is associated with a deletion within chromosome 22q11. J Med Genet 30:822–824

Burn J, Brennan P, Holloway S et al. (1998) Recurrence risks in offspring of adults with major heart defects: results from first cohort of British collaborative study. Lancet 351:311–316

Burns MA, McLeod R, Linton LR, Butler MG (1993) Metacarpophalangeal pattern profile analysis in Williams syndrome. Am J Med Genet 47:471–474

Campbell M (1961) Twins and congenital heart disease. Acta Genet Med Gemellol 10:443–455

Campbell M (1962) Factors in the aetiology of pulmonary stenosis. Br Heart J 24:625–632

Campbell M (1965) Malformation of the heart. BMJ ii:895–904

Campbell M, Polani P (1961) The aetiology of coarctation of the aorta. Lancet i:463–468

Capdevila J, Vogan K, Tabin CJ, Beomonte JCI (2000) Mechanisms of left-right determination in vertebrates. Cell 101:9–21

Carleton RA, Abelman WH, Hancock EW (1958) Familial occurrence of congenital heart disease: Report of three families and review of the literature. N Engl J Med 26:1237–1245

Carlgren LE (1959) The incidence of congenital heart disease in children born in Gothenburg 1941–1950. Br Heart J 1959; 21:40–50

Casey B, Hackett BP (2000) Left-right axis malformations in man and mouse. Current Opinion in Genetics and Development 10:257–261

Casey B, Devoto M, Jones KL, Ballabio A (1993) Mapping a gene for familial situs abnormalities to human chromosome Xq24–q27.1. Nature Genet 5:403–407

Child AH, Dennis NR (1977) The genetics of congenital heart disease. Birth Defects 13:85–89

Chitayat D, McIntosh N, Fouron JC (1992) Pulmonary artresia with intact ventricular septum and hypoplastic right heart in sibs: A single gene disorder? Am J Med Genet 42:304–306

Chiu I, How S, Wang J et al. (1988) Clinical implications of atrial isomerism. Br Heart J 60:72–77

Chu C, Donaldson MDC (1994) Possible role of imprinting in the Turner phenotype. J Med Genet 31,840–842

Clark EB (1984) Neck web and congenital heart defects: A pathogenic association in 45 X-O Turner syndrome. Teratology 29:355–361

Cohen LS et al. (1994) A re-evaluation of risk of in utero exposure to lithium J Am Med Assoc 27:146–150

Colley A, Thakker Y, Ward H, Donnai D (1992) Unbalanced 13;18 translocation and Williams syndrome. J Med Genet 29:63–65

Cooper MD, Peterson RDA, Good RA (1965) A new concept of the cellular basis of immunity. J Pediatr 67:907–908

Corballis MC, Morgan MJ (1978) On the biological basis of human laterality: Evidence of a maturational left to right gradient. Behav Brain Sci 2:261–269

Cotter PD, Kaffe S, McCurdy LD, Jhaveri M, Wilner JP, Hirschhorn K (1997) Paternal uniparental disomy for chromosome 14: A case report and review. Am J Med Genet 70:74–79

Cousineau AJ, Lauer RM, Pierpont ME et al. (1994) Linkage analysis of autosomal dominant atrioventricular canal defects: Exclusion of chromosome 21. Hum Genet 93:103–108

Cunniff C, Kratz LE, Moser A, Natowicz MR, Kelley RI (1997) Clinical and biochemical spectrum of patients with RSH/Smith-Lemli-Opitz syndrome and abnormal cholesterol metabolism. Am J Med Genet 68:263–269

Curran ME, Atkinson DL, Ewart AK et al. (1993) The elastin gene is disrupted by a translocation associated with supravavular aortic stenosis. Cell 73:159–168

Czeizel A, Meszaros M (1981) Two family studies of children with ventricular septal defect. Eur J Pediatr 13:81–85

Czeizel A, Pornoi A, Peterffy E, Tarcal E (1982) Studies of children of parents operated on for congenital cardio-vascular malformations. Br Heart J 47:290–293

Danos MC, Yost HJ (1995) Linkage of cardiac left-right asymmetry and dorsal anterior development in Xenopus. Development 121:1467–1474

Davidson HR (1992) A large family with patent ductus arteriosus and an unusual face. J Med Genet 30:503–505

Davies GE, Howard CM, Farrer MJ et al. (1995) Genetic variation in the COL6A1 region is associated with congenital heart defects in trisomy 21 Down's syndrome. Ann Hum Genet 59:253–269

De Biase L, Di Commo V, Ballerini L et al. (1986) Prevalence of left-sided obstructive lesions in patients with atrioventricular canal without Down's syndrome. J Thorac Cardiovasc Surg 91:467–472

De la Chapelle A, Herva R, Koivisto M, Aula P (1981) A deletion in chromosome 22 can cause Digeorge syndrome. Hum Genet 57:253–256

Demczuk S, Aledo R, Zucman J et al. (1995) Cloning of a balanced translocation breakpoint in the DiGeorge syndrome critical region and isolation of a novel potential adhesion receptor gene in its vicinity. Hum Mol Genet 4:551–558

Dennis NR, Warren J (1981) Risks to the offspring of patients with some common congenital heart defects. J Med Genet 18:8–16

Dickinson DF, Arnold R, Wilkinson JL (1981) Congenital heart disease among 160,480 liveborn children in Liverpool 1960 to 1969. Implications for surgical treatment. Br Heart J 46:55–62

DiGeorge AM (1968) Congenital absence of the thymus and its immunologic consequences: Concurrence with congenital hypothyroidism. Birth Defects 4:116–121

Digilio MC, Marino B, Gianotti A, Dallapiccola B (1996) Search for 22q11 deletion in non-syndromatic conotruncal cardiac defects. Eur J Pediatr 155:619–624

Driscoll DA, Spinner NB, Budarf ML et al. (1992) Deletions and microdeletions of 22q11.2 in velo-cardio-facial syndrome. Am J Med Genet 44:261–268

Driscoll DA, Salvin J, Sellinger B et al. (1993) Prevalence of 22q11 microdeletions in DiGeorge and velocardiofacial syndromes: Implications for genetic counselling and prenatal diagnosis. J Med Genet 30:813–817

Emanuel R, Nichols J, Anders JM et al. (1968) Atrioventricular defects: A study of 92 families. Br Heart J 30:645–653

Emanuel R, Somerville J, Inns A, Withers R (1983) Evidence of congenital heart disease in the offspring of parents with atrioventricular defects. Br Heart J 49:144–147

Emanuel BS, Budarf ML, Sellinger B et al. (1992) Detection of microdeletions of 22q11.2 with fluorescence in situ hybridization

FISH: Diagnosis of DiGeorge syndrome DGS, velo-cardio-facial VCF syndrome, CHARGE association and conotruncal cardiac malformations, abstracted. Am J Hum Genet 51:A3

Embleton ND, Wyllie JP, Wright MJ, Burn J, Hunter AS (1996) Natural history of trisomy 18. Arch Dis Child 751:F38–F41

Epstein CJ (1988) Mouse models for Down's syndrome and Alzheimer's disease. Le Foundation pur l'étude de système nerveux. 5:127–134

Epstein CJ, Cox DR, Epstein LB (1985) Mouse trisomy 16: An animal model of human trisomy 21 Down syndrome. Ann NY Acad Sci 450:157–168

Ewart AK, Morris CA, Atkinson D et al. (1993a) Hemizygosity at the elastin locus in a developmental disorder, Williams syndrome. Nature Genet 5:11–16

Ewart AK, Morris CA, Ensing GJ et al. (1993b) A human vascular disorder, supravalvular aortic stenosis, maps to chromosome 7. Proc Natl Acad Sci 90:3226–3230

Ewart AK, Jin W, Atkinson D et al. (1994) Supravalvular aortic stenosis associated with a deletion disrupting the elastin gene. J Clin Invest 93:1071–1077

Fang T, Bruyere HJJ, Kargas SA et al. (1987) Ethyl alcohol-induced cardiovascular malformations in the chick embryo. Teratology 35:95–103

Farrell MJ et al. (1999) HIRA, a DiGeorge syndrome candidate gene is required for cardiac outflow tract septation. Circ Res 84:127–135

Feldt RH, Avasthey P, Yoshimasu F et al. (1971) Incidence of congenital heart disease in children born to residents of Olmsted County, Minnesota. 1950–1969. Mayo Clin Proc 46:794–799

Fitzpatrick DR (1996) Zellweger syndrome and associated phenotypes. J Med Genet 33:863–868

Freedom RM, Rosen FS, Nadas AS (1972) Congenital cardiovascular disease and anomalies of the third and fourth pharyngeal pouch. Circulation 46:165–172

Fuhrmann W (1968) A family study of transposition of the great vessels and in tricuspid atresia. Humangenetik 6:148–157

Gassman M, Casagranda F, Orioli D et al. (1995) Aberrant neural and cardiac development in mice lacking erB4 neuregulin receptor. Nature 378:390–394

Gatrad AR, Read AP, Watson GH (1984) Consanguinity and complex cardiac anomalies with situs ambiguus. Arch Dis Child 59:242–245

Giannotti A, Digilio MC, Marino B et al. (1994) Cayler cardiofacial syndrome and del 22q11: Part of the CATCH22 phenotype. Am J Med Genet 53:303–304

Goldberg R, Motzkin B, Marion R, Scambler PJ, Shprintzen RJ (1993) Velo-cardio-facial syndrome: A review of 120 patients. Am J Med Genet 45:313–319

Goldblatt J, Minutillo C, Pemberton PJ, Hurst J (1992) Ellis van Creveld syndrome in a Western Australian aboriginal community. Postaxial polydactyly as a heterozygous manifestation. Med J Aust 157:271–272

Goldmuntz E, Driscoll D, Budarf ML et al. (1993) Microdeleions of chromosomal 22q11 in patients with congenital conotruncal cardiac defects. J Med Genet 30:807–812

Goldstein HI, Nielsen KB (1988) Rates and survival of individuals with trisomy 13 and 18. Data from a 10-year period in Denmark. Clin Genet 34:366–372

Goodship J, Curtis A, Cross J et al. (1992) A submicroscopic translocation, 14;10;, responsible for recurrent Wolf-Hirschhorn syndrome identified by allele loss and fluorescent in situ hybridisation. J Med Genet 29:451–454

Goodship J, Cross I, Scambler P, Burn J (1995) Monozygotic twins with chromosome 22q11 deletion and discordant phenotype. J Med Genet 32:746–748

Greenberg F, Crowder WE, Paschall V et al. (1984) Familial DiGeorge syndrome and associated partial monosomy of chromosome 22. Hum Genet 65:317–319

Greenberg F, Elder FFB, Haffner P et al. (1988) Cytogenetic findings in a prospective series of patients with DiGeorge anomaly. Am J Hum Genet 43:605–611

Guris DL, Fanles J, Taro D et al. (2001) Nice lacking the homologue of the human 22q11.2 gene cell phenocapy neurochristepathe of DiGeorge syndrome. Nature Genet 27:293–298

Guichard C, Harricane M-C, Lafitte J-J et al. (2001) Axonemal dynein intermediate-chain gene DNA11; mutations result in situs inversus and primary ciliary dyskinesia Kartagener syndrome. Am J Hum Genet 68:1030–1035

Halford S, Wadey R, Roberts C et al. (1993) Isolation of a putative transcriptional regulator from the region of 22q11 deleted in Di George syndrome, Shprintzen syndrome and familial congenital heart disease. Hum Mol Genet 2:2099–2107

Hanna J (1994) Congenital heart disease in Northern Ireland. J Med Genet 31:858

Heymanns HSA (1984) Cerebrohepatorenal Zellweger; syndrome: Clinical and biochemical consequences of peroxisomal dysfunction. University of Amsterdam,

Hoffman JE, Christianson R (1978) Congenital heart disease in a cohort of 19,502 births with long-term follow-up. Am J Cardiol 42:641–647

Hol FA, Hamel BCJ, Guerds MPA et al. (1995) Localization of Alagille syndrome to 20p11.2-p12 by linkage analysis of a three generation family. Hum Genet 95:687–690

Ho SY, Cook A, Anderson RH et al. (1991) Isomerism of the atrial appendages in the fetus. Pediatr Pathol 11:589–608

Hurst JA, Hall CM, Baraitser M (1995) Holt-Oram syndrome. Donnai D, Winter RM (eds): In Congenital Malformation Syndromes. Chapman & Hall, London, pp. 317–324

Ivemark BI (1955) Implications of agenesis of the spleen on the pathogenesis of cono-truncus anomalies in childhood. Acta Paediatr Scand 44:1–110

Jamieson RC, van der Burgt I, Brady AF, van Reen M, Elsawi MM, Hol F et al. (1994) Mapping a gene for Noonan syndrome to the long arm of chromosome 12. Nature Genet 8:357–360

Jerome, LA, Papaioannou VE (2001) DiGeorge syndrome phenotype in mice mutant for the T-box gene, Tbxl. Nature Genet 27:286–291

Jovanovic L, Druzin M, Peterson CM (1981) Effect of euglycemia on the outcome of pregnancy in insulin-dependent diabetic women as compared with normal control subjects. Am J Med 71:921–927

Kallen B (1987) Search for teratogenic risks with the aid of malformation registries. Teratology 35:47–52

Kelley RI, Zackai EH, Emanuel BS et al. (1982) The association of the DiGeorge anomalad with partial monosomy of chromosome 22. J Pediatr 101:197–200

Kelly D, Goldberg R, Wilson D et al. (1993) Confirmation that the velo-cardio-facial syndrome is associated with haplo-insufficiency of genes at chromosome 22q11. Am J Med Genet 45:308–312

Kelly MD, Essex DW, Shapiro SS et al. (1994) Complementary DNA cloning of the alternatively expressed endothelial cell glycoprotein lbβ (GPIbβ); and localization of the GPIbβ gene to chromosome 22. J Clin Invest 93:2417–2424

Kenna AP, Smithells RW, Fielding DW (1975) Congenital heart disease in Liverpool 1960–9. Q J Med 44:17–44

Korenberg JR, Kurnit DM (1995) In Clark EB, Markwald RR, Takao A (eds): Developmental mechanisms of Heart Disease. Futura, NY

Korenberg JR, Kawashima H, Pulst S et al. (1990a) Molecular definition of a region of chromosome 21 that causes features of the Down Syndrome phenotype. Am J Hum Genet 47:236–246

Korenberg JR, Kawashima H, Pulst SM et al. (1990b) Down syndrome: toward a molecular definition of the phenotype. Am J Med Genet 7:91–97

Korenberg JR, Bradley C, Disteche CM (1992) Down syndrome: Molecular mapping of the congenital heart disease and duodenal stenosis. Am J Hum Genet 50:294–302

Konkol RJ (1992) Is there a cocaine baby syndrome? Editorial. J Child Neurol 146:748–752

Kosaki R, Marinella G, Kenjiro K et al. (1999a) Left-right axis malformations associated with mutations in ACVR2B, the gene for human activin receptor type IIB. Am J Med Genet 82:70–76

Kosaki K, Bassi MT, Kosaki R et al (1999b) Characterization and mutation analysis of human LEFTY A and LEFTY B, hamologues of murine genes implicated in left -right aixs development. Am J Hum Genet 64:712–717

Kousseff BG, Gallardo LA, Mueller OT (1992) Unusual clinical presentation associated with uniparental disomy of chromosome 10 in a child presymptomatic for multiple endocrine neoplasia type 2A Abstract. Am J Hum Genet 51:A219

Kurahashi H, Akagi K, Inazawa J et al. (1995) Isolation and characterization of a novel gene deleted in DiGeorge syndrome. Hum Mol Genet 4:541–549

Kurihari Y, Kurihara H, Oda H et al. (1995) Aortic arch malformations and ventricular septal defect in mice deficient in endothelin-1. J Clin Invest 96:293–300

Kurnit DM, Aldridge JF, Matsuoka R, Matthysse S (1985) Increased adhesiveness of trisomy 21 cells and atrioventricular canal malformations in Down syndrome: A stochastic model. Am J Med Genet 20:385–399

Lammer EJ, Chen DT, Hoar RM et al. (1985) Retinoic acid embryopathy. N Engl J Med 313:837–841

Lamour V, Lécluse Y, Desmaze C et al. (1995) A human homolog of the S. cerevisiae HIR1 and HIR2 transcriptional repressors cloned from the DiGeorge syndrome critical region. Hum Mol Genet 4:791–799

Laursen HB (1980) Some epidemiological aspects of congenital heart disease in Denmark. Acta Pediatr Scand 69:619–624

Layton WM (1978) Heart malformations in mice homozygous for a gene causing situs inversus. Birth Defects 14:277–293

Lee KF, Simon H, Chen H et al. (1995) Requirement for neuregulin crB2 in neural and cardiac development. Nature 378:394–398

Lenke RR, Levy HL (1980) Maternal phenylketonuria and hyperphenylalaninemia: An international survey of the outcome of untreated and treated pregnancies. N Engl J Med 1202–1208

Li L, Krantz ID, Deng Y, Genin A, Banta AB, Collins CC et al. (1997) Alagille syndrome is caused by mutations in human. Jagged1, which encodes a ligand for Notchl. Nature Genet 16:243–251

Lin AE, Ardinger HH, Ardinger RH Jr, Cunniff C, Kelley RI (1997) Cardiovascular malformations in Smith-Lemli-Opitz syndrome. Am J Med Genet 68:270–278

Lindsay EA, Vitelli F, Su H, Morishima M, Huynh T, Pramparo TV, Ogunrinu G, Sutherland HF et al. (2001) Tbxl haploinsufficiency in the DiGeorge syndrome region causes aortic arch defects in mice. Nature 410:97–101

Lobdell DH (1959) Congenital absence of the parathyroid glands. Arch Pathol 67:412–418

McDermid HE, Duncan AM, Brasch KR et al. (1986) Molecular analysis of the supernumerary chromosome in cat eye syndrome. Science 232:646–648

MacDonald G, Chu ML, Cox DR (1991) Fine structure physical mapping of the region of mouse chromosome 10 homologous to human chromsome 21. Genomics 11:317–323

McDonald-McGinn DM, Driscoll DA, Bason L et al. (1995) Autosomal dominant "Opitz" GBBB syndrome due to a 22q11.2 deletion. Am J Med Genet 59:103–113

McIntosh N, Chitayat D, Bardanis M, Fouron JC (1992) Ebstein anomaly: Report of a familial occurence and prenatal diagnosis. Am J Med Genet 42:307–309

McKeown T, Record RG (1960) Malformations in a population observed for five years after birth. Ciba Found Symp 0:2–21

Marino B, Reale A, Giannotti A et al. (1992) Nonrandom association of atrioventricular canal and del 8p; syndrome. Am J Med Genet 42:424–427

Mégarbané A, Salem N, Stephan E et al. (2001) X-linked transposition of the great arteries. Incomplete penetrance in a male with a nonsense mutation in: ZIC3. Eur J Hum Genet 8:704–708

Merklin RJ, Varano NR (1995) Situs inversus and cardiac defects: A study of 111 cases of reversed asymmetry. J Thorac Cardiovasc Surg 45:334–342

Merscher S, Funke B, Epstein JA, Heyer J, Puech A, Lu MM et al. (2001) TBX1 is responsible for cardiovascular defects in velo-cardio-facial/DiGeorge syndrome. Cell 104:619

Meyer D, Birchmeier C (1995) Multiple essential functions of neuregulin in development. Nature 378:386–390

Miller MJ, Geffner IH, Lippe BM et al. (1983) Echocardiography reveals a high incidence of bicuspid aortic valve in Turner syndrome. J Pediatr 102:47–50

Mitchell SC, Sellmann AH, Westphal MC, Park J (1971) Etiologic correlates in a study of congenital heart disease in 56,109 births. Am J Cardiol 28:653–657

Monteleone PL, Fagan LF (1969) Possible X linked congenital heart disease. Circulation 39:611–614

Morris CA, Thomas IT, Greenberg F (1993) Williams syndrome: Autosomal dominant inheritance. Am J Med Genet 47:478–481

Mueller RF, Emslie FV (1995) The Alagille syndrome arteriohepatic dysplasia. In Donnai D, Winter RM (eds): Congenital Malformation Syndromes. Chapman & Hall, London, pp. 569–580

Musowo NN, Alexander DJ, Teshima LI et al. (1990) Echocardiographic evaluation of the spectrum of cardiac anomalies associated with trisomy 13 and 18. JACC 15:673–677

Narayan D, Desai T, Banks A et al. (1994) Localization of the human cytoplasmic dynein heavy chain DNECL; to 14qter by fluorescence in situ hybridization. Genomics 22:660–661

Newbury-Ecob RA, Leanage R, Raeburn JA, Young ID (1996) Holt-Oram syndrome: A clinical genetic study. J Med Genet 33:300–307

Nielsen J, Wohlert M (1991) Chromosome abnormalities found among 34910 newborn children: Results from a 13-year incidence study in Aårhus, Denmark. Human Genet 87:81–83

Nora JJ, Nora AH (1978) The evolution of specific genetic and environmental counseling in congenital heart disease. Circulation 57:205

Nora JJ, Nora AH (1983) Genetic epidemiology of congenital heart diseases. Prog Med Genet 5:91–137

Nora JJ, Nora AH (1987) Maternal transmission of congenital heart diseases: New recurrence risk figures and the questions of cytoplasmic inheritance and vulnerability to teratogens. Am J Cardiol 59:459–463

Nora JJ, McNamarra DG, Clarke Fraser F (1967) Hereditary factors in atrial septal defect. Circulation 35:448–456

O'Malley CD, Shaw GM, Wassermann CR, Lammer EJ (1996) Epidemiologic characteristics of conotruncal heart defects in California, 1987–1988. Teratology 53:374–377

Opitz JM, ZuRhein GM, Vitale L, Shahidi NT, Howe JJ, Chou SM et al. (1969) The Zellweger syndrome cerebrohepatorenal syndrome. Birth Defects 2:144–160

Patterson DF, Pyle RL, Buchanan JW (1971) Hereditary patent ductus arteriosus and its sequelae in the dog. Circ Res 29:1–13

Penman Splitt M, Burn J, Goodship J (1995) Connexin43 mutations in sporadic and familial defects of laterality, letter. N Engl J Med 333:941

Polani PE, Campbell M (1960) Factors in the causation of persistent ductus arteriosus. Ann Hum Genet 24:343–357

Price B (1950) Primary biases in twin studies. Am J Hum Genet 2:293–352

Radford DJ (1985) Truncus arteriosus and facial dysmorphism. Aust Paediatr J 21:131–133

Radford DJ (1988) Spectrum of DiGeorge syndrome in patients with truncus arteriosus: Expanded DiGeorge syndrome. Pediatr Cardiol 9:95–101

Rahmani Z, Blouin JL, Creau-Goldberg N, Critical role of the D21S55 region on chromosome 21 in the pathogenesis of Down syndrome. Proc Natl Acad Sci USA 86:5958–5962

Record RG, McKeown T (1953) Observations relating to the aetiology of patent ductus arteriosus. Br Heart J 15:376–386

Reynolds JF, Daniel A, Kelly TE et al. (1987) Isochromosome 12p mosaicism pallister mosaic aneuploidy or Pallister-Killian syndrome. Am J Med Genet 27:257–274

Rezaee M, Isokawa K, Halligan N (1993) Identification of an extracellular 130 kDa protein involved in early cardiac morphogenesis. J Biol Chem 268:14404–14411

Roberts DF, Lanchbury J, Papiha SS (1990) Genetic variation in north-east England. Ann Hum Biol 17:265–276

Root S, Carey JC (1994) Survival in trisomy 18. Am J Med Genet 492:170–174

Rose V, Izukawa T, Moes CAF (1975) Syndromes of asplenia and polysplenia: A review of cardiac and noncardiac malformations in 60 cases with special reference to diagnosis and prognosis. Br Heart J 37:840–852

Rose V, Gold RJM, Lindsay G, Allen M (1985) A possible increase in the incidence of congenital heart defects among the offspring of affected parents. J Am Coll Cardiol 6:376–382

Rossi MB, Burn J, Ho SY et al. (1987) Conjoined twins, right atrial isomerism, and the sequential segmental analysis. Br Heart J 58:518–524

Rossiter JP, Hofman KJ, Kelley RI (1995) Smith-Lemli-Opitz Syndrome: Prenatal diagnosis by quantification of cholesterol precursors in amniotic fluid. Am J Med Genet 56:272–275

Rowland TW, Hubell JP, Nadas AS (1973) Congenital heart disease in infants of diabetic mothers. J Pediatr 83:815–820

Ruiz-Perez VL et al (2000) Mutations in a new gene in Ellis-van Creveld syndrome and Weyers acrodental dyostosis. Nat Genet 24:283–286

Ryan AK, Goodship JA, Wilson DI, Philip N, Levy A, Siedel H et al. (1997) Spectrum of clinical features associated with interstitial chromosome 22q11 deletions: A European collaborative study. J Med Genet 34:798–804

Saga Y, Yagi T, Ikawa Y et al. (1992) Mice develop normally without tenascin. Genes Dev 6:1821–1831

Sanchez-Cascos A (1978) The recurrence risk in congenital heart disease. Eur J Cardiol 7:197–210

Sapire DW, Ho SY, Anderson RH et al. (1986) Diagnosis and significance of atrial isomerism. Am J Cardiol 58:342–346

Satoda M, Zhao F, Diaz GA et al. (2000) Mutations in TFAP2B cause Char syndrome, a familial form of patent ductus arteriosus. Nature Genet 25:42–46

Scambler PJ, Kelly D, Lindsay E, Williamson R, Goldberg R, Shprintzen R et al. (1992) Velo-cardio-facial syndrome associated with chromsome 22 deletions encompassing the DiGeorge locus. Lancet 339:1138–1139

Schinzel A (1983) Catalogue of Unbalanced Chromosome Aberrations in Man. Walter de Gruyter, Berlin

Schinzel A, Savoldelli G, Briner J, Sigg P, Massini C (1983) Antley-Bixler syndrome in sisters: A term newborn and a prenatally diagnosed fetus. Am J Med Genet 14:139–147

Schott JJ, Benson DW, Basson CT, Pease W, Silberbach GM, Moak JP et al. (1998) Congenital heart disease caused by mutations in the transcription factor NKX2–5. Science 281:108–111

Sharma S, Devine W, Anderson RH, Zuberbuhler J (1987) Identification and analysis of left atrial isomerism. Am J Cardiol 60:1157–1160

Sheffield VC, Pierpont ME, Nishimura D, Beck JS, Burns TL, Berg MA et al. (1997) Identification of a complex congenital heart defect susceptibility locus by using DNA pooling and shared segment analysis. Hum Mol Genet 61:117–121

Shprintzen RJ, Mea GRL (1978) A new syndrome involving cleft palate, cardiac anomalies, typical facies and learning disabilties: Velo-cardio-facial syndrome. Cleft Palate J 15:56–62

Shprintzen RJ, Goldberg RB, Young D, Wolford L (1981) The velo-cardio-facial syndrome: A clinical and genetic analysis. Pediatrics 67:167–171

Shull MM, Ormsby I, Kier AB et al. (1992) Targeted disruption of the mouse transforming growth factor β1 gene results in multifocal inflammatory disease. Nature 359:693–699

Simpson JL (1976) Gonadal dysgenesis in disorders of sexual differentiation etiology and clinical delineation. Academic Press, NY

Sinet PM, Rahmani Z, Theophile D et al. (1991) Molecular definition of 7 minimal regions on chromosome 21 involved in the pathogenesis of 23 features of Down syndrome. Cytogenet Cell Genet 58:2040

Slavotinek A, Clayton-Smith J, Super M (1997) Familial patent ductus arteriosus: A further case of CHAR syndrome. Am J Med Genet 712:229–232

Smith DW (1982) Recognizable Patterns of Human Malformation. WB, Saunders, Philadelphia

Splitt MP, Goodship JA (1997) Another case of maternal uniparental disomy chromosome 14 syndrome. Am J Med Genet 722:239–240

Splitt M, Wright C, Sen D, Goodship J (1999) Left-isomerism sequence and maternal type-1 diabetes. The Lancet 354:305–306

Stec I, Wright JT, Van Ommen GJB, De Boer PAJ, van Haeringen A, Moorman AFM et al. (1998) WHSCI, a 90 kb SET domain-containing gene, expressed in early development and homologous to a Drosophila dysmorphy gene maps in the Wolf-Hirschhorn syndrome critical region and is fused to IgH in t4;14; multiple myeloma. Hum Mol Genet 77:1071–1082

Strong WB (1968) Familial syndrome of right-sided aortic arch, mental deficiency, and facial dysmorphism. J Pediatr 73:882–888

Takao A, Ando M, Cho K, Kinouchi A, Murakami Y (1980) Etiological categorization of common congenital heart disease. In Van Praagh R, Takao A (eds): Etiology and Morphogenesis of Congenital Heart Disease, pp.252–269

Tassabehji M, Strachan T, Sharland M, Colley A, Donnai D, Harris R et al. (1993) Tandem duplication within a neurofibromatosis type 1 NFI; gene exon in a family with features of Watson syndrome and Noonan syndrome. Am J Hum Genet 53:90–95

Taussig HB, Kallman CH, Nagel D et al. (1975) Long term observations on the Blalock-Taussig VIII, 20 to 28 year follow-up on patients with a tetralogy of Fallot. Johns Hopkins Med J 37:13–19

Terrett JA, Newbury-Ecob R, Cross GS, Fenton I, Raeburn JA, Young ID et al. (1994) Holt-Oram syndrome is a genetically heterogeneous disease with one locus mapping to human chromosome 12. Nature Genet 6:401–404

Threadgill DW, Dlugosz AA, Hansen LA et al. (1995) Targeted disruption of mouse EGF receptor: Effect of genetic background on mutant phenotype. Science 69:230–234

Torgersen J (1950) Situs inversus, asymmetry and twinning. Am J Med Genet 2:361–370

Van Praagh E, Truman T, Firpo A et al. (1989) Cardiac malformations in trisomy 18. A study of 41 postmortem cases. JACC 13:1586–1597

Wadey R, Daw S, Taylor C et al. (1995) Isolation of a gene encoding an integral membrane protein from the vicinity of a balanced breakpoint associated with DiGeorge syndrome. Hum Mol Genet 4:1027–1033

Wallace M, Zori RT, Alley T, Whidden E, Gray BA, Williams CA (1994) Smith-Lemli-Opitz syndrome in a female with a de novo, balanced translocation involving 7q32: Probable disruption of an SLOS gene. Am J Med Genet 50:368–374

Walter JH (1995) Late effects of phenylketonuria. Arch Dis Child 73:485–486

Watkins PJ (1982) Congenital malformations and blood glucose control in diabetic pregnancy. Br Med J 1357–1358

Webber SA, Sandor GGS, Patterson MWH et al. (1992) Prognosis in asplenia syndrome: A population based review. Cardiol Young 2:129–135

Weinberg MR, Goldfield MD (1975) Cardiovascular malformations with lithium use during pregnancy. Am J Psychiatry 132:529–531

Whittemore R, Hobbins EJ, Engle MA (1982) Pregnancy and its outcome in women with and without surgical treatment of congenital heart disease. Am J Cardiol 50:361–370

Wilkins JL (1969) Risks to offspring of patients with patent ductus arteriosus. J Med Genet 6:1–4

Williamson DAJ (1970) A syndrome of congenital spinal anomalies in infants of diabetic mothers. Dev Med Child Neurol 12:145–152

Williamson EM (1969) A family study of atrial septal defect. J Med Genet 6:255–261

Wilson DI, Cross IE, Goodship JA et al. (1991) DiGeorge syndrome with isolated aortic coarctation and isolated ventricular septal defect in three sibs with a 22q11 deletion of maternal origin. Br Heart J 66:308–312

Wilson DI, Goodship JA, Burn J et al. (1992) Deletions within chromosome 22q11 in familial congenital heart disease. Lancet 340:573–575

Wilson DI, Bennett Britton S, McKeown C et al. (1993a) Noonan's and DiGeorge syndromes with monosomy 22q11. Arch Dis Child 68:187–189

Wilson DI, Burn J, Scambler P, Goodship J (1993b) DiGeorge syndrome: Part of CATCH 22. J Med Genet 30:852–856

Wright TJ, Ricke DO, Denison K, Abmayr S, Cotter PD, Hirschhorn K et al. (1997) A transcript map of the newly defined 165 kb Wolf-Hirschhorn syndrome critical region. Hum Mol Genet 62:317–324

Wyllie JP, Wright MJ, Burn J, Hunter S (1994) Natural history of trisomy 13. Arch Dis Child 71:343–345

Yamagishi H, Garg V, Matsuoko R et al. (1999) A molecular pathway revealing a genetic basis for human cardiac and craniofacial defects. Science 283:1158–1161

Yao J, Thompson MW, Trusler GA, Trimble AS (1968) Familial atrial septal defect of the primum type: A report of four cases in one sibship. Can Med Assoc J 98:218–219

Yokoyama T, Copeland NG, Jenkins NA et al. (1993) Reversal of left-right asymmetry: A situs inversus mutation. Science 260:679–682

Zellers TM, Driscoll DJ, Michels VV (1990) Prevalence of significant congenital heart defects in children of parents with Fallot's tetralogy. Am J Cardiol 65:523–526

Zetterqvist P (1972) A Clinical and Genetic Study of Congenital Heart Defects. University of Uppsala, Sweden

Zoethout HE, Bonham Carter RE, Carter CO (1964) A family study of aortic stenosis. J Med Genet 1:2–9

Appendix 47.1
Syndromes Associated with
Cardiac Malformation

Syndrome name	Clinical features	Etiology	Cardiac defects	Key reference
Aase syndrome	Triphalangeal thumbs, radial hypoplasia, narrow shoulders, late closure of anterior fontanelle, hypoplastic anemia, mild short stature, variable hepatosplenomegaly. Overlaps with Diamond Blackfan syndrome.	Unclear; probable autosomal dominant.	Ventricular septal defect most common anomaly. Common arterial trunk described.	Hing and Dowton, 1993.
Aase-Smith syndrome	Dandy Walker cerebral malformation, multiple joint contractures, poorly formed flexion creases, cleft palate, ptosis.	Autosomal dominant.	Muscular ventricular septal defects and cardiac hypertrophy reported.	Patton et al., 1985.
Achard syndrome	Arachnodactyly, brachycephaly, micrognathia, dislocation of lens, joint laxity, normal body proportions, normal stature.	Unknown; all cases have been sporadic.	Ventricular septal defects.	Duncan, 1975.
Acrocallosal syndrome	Hallux duplication, postaxial polydactyly of fingers and toes, syndactyly, mental retardation (agenesis of corpus callosum), growth retardation, high forehead, prominent occiput, hypertelorism, downslanting eyes, short nose, occasional cleft palate.	Autosomal recessive.	Ventricular septal defect, atrial septum defect, tetralogy of Fallot, dysplastic pulmonary valve, dextroposition of aorta.	Courtens et al., 1997.
Acromicric dysplasia	Short slature, brachydactyly chondrodysplasia, blepharophimosis, anteverted nares.	All cases sporadic.	Atrial septal defect, ventricular septal defect.	Hennekam et al., 1996.
Adams syndrome (tachycardia, hypertension, microphthalmos, hyperglycinuria)	Paroxysmal tachycardia, hypertension and seizures with microphthalmos, cataracts and renal stones due to hyperglycinuria.	Affected sibs; previous generation had eye and renal defects only. May be two disorders co-existing.	Paroxysmal tachycardia.	Adams and Nance, 1967.

continued

Appendix 47.1 (*continued*)

Syndrome name	Clinical features	Etiology	Cardiac defects	Key reference
Adams-Oliver syndrome	Scalp defects, terminal transverse defects, cutis marmorata. Probable mechanism: early vascular disruption sequence.	Autosomal dominant.	Tetralogy of Fallot, ventricular septal defect, atrial septal defect; coarctation of aorta, pulmonary stenosis, aortic valve stenosis, mitral valve prolapse reported.	Zapata et al., 1995.
Aglossia-situs inversus	Tongue hypoplasia, small mandible, situs inversus.	Uncertain.	Dextrocardia.	Dunham and Austin, 1990.
Agnathia-holoprosencephaly (agnathia malformation complex)	Absent mandible, extremely low-set ears, sometimes synotia, microstomia, holoprosencephaly, cyclopia, anal atresia, horse-shoe kidneys.	Autosomal recessive or unrecognized chromosome defect.	Situs inversus most common anomaly, tetralogy of Fallot. Ventricular septal defect and various other defects reported.	Porteous et al., 1993.
Alagille Syndrome (arteriohepatic dysplasia)	Intrahepatic cholestasis (95%), defects of the arterior chamber of the eye (80%), mainly posterior embryotoxon, abnormal facies (90%), vertebral anomalies (70%).	Autosomal dominant; defects in JAG1 gene at 20p12.	Peripheral pulmonary stenosis. Tetralogy of Fallot and various other defects reported.	Krantz et al., 1997. Oda et al., 1997. Li et al., 1997.
Aldolase A deficiency	Hemolytic anemia, learning disability, microcephaly, flat face, ptosis, epicanthic folds, telangiectasia eyelids, small penis.	Autosomal recessive.	Unspecified heart defect.	Hurst et al., 1987.
Alkaptonuria syndrome (ochronosis)	Deposition of homogentisic acid, pigmentation sclerae, cartilage, late arthritis.	Autosomal recessive; defects in the HGO gene at 3q21 lead to deficiency in homogentisate 1,2-dioxygenase.	Accelerated cardiovascular disease, aortic stenosis, calcified aortic valve disease.	Fernandez-Canon et al., 1996.
Alstrom syndrome	Retinitis pigmentosa, cataracts, sensorineural deafness, obesity, diabetes mellitus, short stature, hypogonadism, hepatic dysfunction, acanthosis nigricans.	Autosomal recessive; gene mapped to 2p.	Dilated cardiomyopathy.	Marshall et al., 1997. Collin et al., 1997.
Anophthalmia, dextrocardia, skeletal anomalies	Bilateral anophthalmia, large ears with fleshy lobes, melatarsus adductus, fusion defects of T5-T6, 13 pairs of ribs.	Uncertain, with parents being of second cousins.	Cardiac situs inversus/dextrocardia.	Aughton, 1990.
Antley-Bixler syndrome	Coronal, lambdoid suture synostosis, frontal bossing, severe midface hypoplasia, proptosis, choanal stenosis, bowed femora and ulnae, vaginal atresia, renal anomalies.	Probable autosomal recessive. Possible FGFR2 association.	Atrial septal defect.	Crisponi et al., 1997.

continued

Appendix 47.1 (*continued*)

Syndrome name	Clinical features	Etiology	Cardiac defects	Key reference
Apert syndrome	Severe craniosynostosis, flat face, hypertelorism, syndactyly (mitten hands), occasional cleft palate, deafness, mental retardation, renal and genitourinary anomalies.	Autosomal dominant; defects in FGFR2 gene at 10q. Almost all have a mutation in exon 7.	Ventricular septal defect, atrial septal defect, persistent arterial duct, coarctation, various other defects.	Lajeunie et al., 1999.
Aplasia cutis, retinal folds, brain anomalies	Scalp defects, absent fingers with nails attached to the metacarpals, periventricular and thalamic calcification, ventricular dilatation and cerebral atrophy, agenesis of corpus callosum, broad bulbous nose, small chin, long philtrum.	Autosomal recessive, with affected brother and sister reported.	Ventricular septal defect.	Orstavik et al., 1995.
Apple peel congenital intestinal atresia	Duodenal or high jejunal atresia associated with an absence of the small bowel mesentery and occlusion of the superior mesenteric artery, 15% other defects including, imperforate anus, biliary atresia, microphthalmia, ureteropelvic junction obstruction.	Autosomal recessive. Can be a feature of cystic fibrosis.	Atrial septal defect.	Seashore et al., 1987.
Astley-Kendall syndrome (short-limbed dwarfism with extensive stippling)	Lethal, short limbed dwarfism, flared metaphyses, spicule like projection from long bone ends, transverse defects of long bones, absent calcification of skull vault, stippling of spine bones.	Sporadic.	Dextrocardia.	Astley and Kendall, 1980.
Asymmetric crying face syndrome (Cayler syndrome)	Hypoplasia or absence of depressor angularis oris on one side. Genito-urinary, musculo-skeletal, respiratory, cervicofacial defects. Intestinal and central nervous system anomalies, neuroblastoma.	Sporadic; ? part of the CATCH phenotype (22q11 deletions in some patients)	Atrial septal defects, patent ductus arteriosus, ventricular septal defects. Various other defects reported.	Rauch et al., 1998.
Asymmetric crying facies, microcephaly	Microcephaly, asymmetric crying facies, mental retardation, failure to thrive.	Uncertain. ? Autosomal dominant	Atrial septum defect, coarctation/interrupted aorta, patent ductus arteriosus, ventricular septal defect.	Silengo et al., 1986.
Atkin syndrome (oculo-cerebro-acral syndrome)	Hypertelorism, cleft lip, micrognathia, Dandy Walker cyst, renal anomalies, malformed ears, ectrodactyly, cloudy cornea, microphthalmia.	Single case report.	Atrial septal defect, ventricular septal defect, persistent arterial duct, dysplastic pulmonary valve.	Atkin and Patil, 1984.

continued

Appendix 47.1 (*continued*)

Syndrome name	Clinical features	Etiology	Cardiac defects	Key reference
Atrial septal defect with atrioventricular conduction defects	Sudden death in some patients.	Autosomal dominant; defect in *CSX* at 5q34.	Atrial septal defect secundum type, other malformations reported, atrioventricular block.	Schott et al., 1998.
Atrial septal defect-lymphedema	Lymphedema, hydroceles of the testes, prominent forehead, epicanthal folds, upslanting palpebral fissures, wide nasal bridge, horizontal cleft of the chin, hydrops fetalis, accessory spleen, omphalocele.	Autosomal recessive.	Atrial septum defect, patent ductus arteriosus.	Irons et al., 1996.
Axial mesodermal dysplasia syndrome (caudal regression sequence with Goldenhar syndrome)	Hemifacial microsomia, microtia, renal anomalies (agenesis, ectopia, hydronephrosis), absent uterus, anal stenosis, hemivertebrae, fusion of vertebrae, absent sacrum.	Unknown; usually sporadic.	Dextrocardia, patent ductus arteriosus.	Bini et al., 1996.
Baller-Gerold syndrome (craniosynostosis radial aplasia)	Craniosynostosis, radial aplasia, missing thumbs, anal anomalies, skeletal defects, central nervous system defects, urogenital defects.	Autosomal recessive. Possibly due to defects in *TWIST*.	Ventricular septal defect, tetralogy of Fallot. Subaortic stenosis, pulmonary artesia reported.	Gripp et al., 1999.
Baraitser-Winter syndrome	Severe learning disability, iris colobomata, ptosis, epicanthic folds, short stature, cryptorchidism.	Autosomal recessive.	Ventricular septal defect.	Baraitser and Winter, 1988.
Bardet-Biedl syndrome	Mental retardation, ulnar polydactyly, obesity, retinal dystrophy, hypogenitalism, kidney disease, occasional short stature, hearing loss, vaginal atresia.	Autosomal recessive; 4 gene loci mapped at 11q13 (BBS1), 16q21 (BBS2), 3p12 (BBS3), 15q22 (BBS4).	Rare congenital defects, atrial septal defect, bicuspid aortic valve, pulmonary stenosis, acquired heart disease including dilated or hypertrophic cardiomyopathy.	Elbedour et al., 1994. Beales et al., 1997. Young et al., 1999.
Barrow syndome	Short-limbed dwarfism (rhizomelic), undescended testes, severe micrognathia, sloping forehead, prominent nasal bridge, facial hemangloma.	Single case.	Single ventricle, truncus arteriosus.	Barrow and Fitzsimmons, 1984.
Barth syndrome (X-linked cardioskeletal myopathy)	Neutropenia, peripheral myopathy, abnormal mitochondria, growth retardation, premature death. Heart disease may be isolated.	X linked; mutations in *TAZ* at Xq28.	Dilated cardiomyopathy, endocardial fibroelastosis.	Orstavik et al, 1998.

continued

Appendix 47.1 (*continued*)

Syndrome name	Clinical features	Etiology	Cardiac defects	Key reference
Beals syndrome (congenital contractural arachnodactyly)	Long slim limbs, arachnodactyly, large joint contractures, camptodactyly, "crumpled" ears, kyphoscoliosis, hypoplasia of calf muscles, occasional myopia, keratoconus and ectopia lentis, osteopenia.	Autosomal dominant; mutations in *FBN2* at 5q.	Mainly mitral valve prolapse and regurgitation, occasional aortic root dilatation, ventricular septal defect, atrial septal defect, persistent arterial duct, aortic arch anomalies.	Putman et al., 1995.
Beckwith-Wiedemann syndrome	Macroglossia, overgrowth, exomphalos, visceromegaly, ear creases, hypoglycemia, renal anomalies, hemihypertrophy.	Autosomal dominant, parental rearrangements of 11p15, loss of imprinting of *IGF2*. defect in p57 gene, replicated in mice over-expressing *IGF2*.	Cardiomegaly, variety of malformations include septal defects, common arterial trunk.	Sun et al., 1997.
Beemer-Robinow syndrome	Hydrocephalus, increased bone density, bulbous nose, low-set ears, down-slanting palpebral fissures, ambiguous genitalia, thin ribs and fibulae, peroxisomal dysfunction.	Recessive; 2 brothers in one family, one sporadic male case.	Double outlet right ventricle, tetralogy of Fallot.	Robinow and Beemer, 1990.
Berardinelli syndrome (generalized congenital lipodystrophy, Seip syndrome)	Generalized lipoatrophy, hepatomegaly, hyperlipidemia, acanthosis nigricans, organomegaly, tall stature, non-ketotic insulin-resistant diabetes mellitus.	Autosomal recessive.	Hypertrophic cardiomyopathy, multiple peripheral pulmonary artery stenosis.	Uzun et al., 1997.
Bindewald syndrome	Severe failure to thrive, microcephaly, large protruding ears, a hairy forehead, down-slanting of palpebral fissures, high-arched palate, micrognathia.	Autosomal recessive, with four sibs of consanguineous parents described.	Atrial septum defect, anomalous venous return, tetralogy of Fallot, patent ductus arteriosus, pulmonary stenosis, ventricular septum defect, transposition of great vessels.	Bindewald et al., 1994.
Bonneau syndrome (polysyndactyly with cardiac defects)	Polysyndactyly, hypertelorism, hallux duplication, large nares, low-set ears.	Probable autosomal recessive.	Septal defects, double inlet ventricle, discordant ventriculoarterial connexion.	Rajab, 1997.
Bonnemann-Meinecke syndrome	Hydrocephalus, cerebellar hypoplasia, cortical defects.	Autosomal recessive.	Tetralogy of Fallot, situs inversus, atrial septal defect.	Bonnemann and Meinecke, 1996.
Bowen syndrome	Developmental delay, glaucoma, corneal opacities, depressed nasal bridge, omphalocele, camptodactyly.	Autosomal recessive.	Ventricular septal defect.	Billette de Villemeur et al., 1992.

continued

Appendix 47.1 (*continued*)

Syndrome name	Clinical features	Etiology	Cardiac defects	Key reference
Brachydactyly type E with atrial septal defect (ASD) syndrome	Brachydactyly type E, synostosis of terminal phalanges, small extra bones in lower limbs.	Autosomal dominant. May be part of a contiguous gene syndrome at 2q37.	Atrial septal defect, pulmonary stenosis, tricuspid atresia, ventricular septal defect, mitral atresia.	Wilson et al, 1995.
Burn-McKeown syndrome	Choanal atresia, cardiac defect, dysmorphic facies, deafness, external ear anomalies, eye defect, occasionally cleft lip.	Autosomal recessive.	Atrial septal defect, ventricular septal defect.	Burn et al., 1992.
Camptodactyly-arthritis-pericarditis syndrome	Camptodactyly, infant onset progressive contractures and polyarthritis.	Autosomal recessive; gene mapped to 1q25-q31. Defects found in *CACP*	Pericarditis, mitral valve prolapse in one patient.	Marcelino et al., 1999.
Camptomelic dysplasia syndrome	Polyhydramnios, anterior bowed tibiae and femur, hypotonia, small scapulae, poor ossification of pubis, cleft palate, micrognathia, flat nasal bridge, sex reversal in males, small thorax, respiratory distress, early death.	Autosomal dominant; defects in *SOX9* at 17q.	Mainly ventricular and septal defects; tetralogy of Fallot. Aortic stenosis and persistent arterial duct also reported.	Meyer et al., 1997.
Cantrell pentalogy syndrome	Anterior body wall defect, short or bifid sternum, diaphragmatic pericardium defect, anterior diaphragm deficiency.	Sporadic. Some cases linked to Xq26.1.	Atrial septal defect, ventricular septal defect, aortic stenosis, double outlet right ventricle, truncus arteriosus, total anomalous pulmonary venous drainage, ectopic heart, transposition of great arteries, tetralogy of Fallot.	Parvari et al., 1996.
Carbohydrate-deficient glycoprotein syndrome, type 1A (Jaeken syndrome)	Early signs include hypotonia, developmental delay, enlarged dysfunctional liver, progressive ataxia with cerebellar atrophy, microcephaly, pigmentary retinopathy. Later signs include neuropathic muscle wasting, hypogonadism.	Autosomal recessive; defects in phosphomannamutase gene (*PMM2*) at 16p13.	Non-restrictive pericarditis, hypertrophic cardiomyopathy.	Imtiaz et al, 2000.
Carbohydrate-deficient glycoprotein syndrome, type II	Severe developmental delay, hypotonia, seizures, kyphoscoliosis, sparse fine hair, minor dysmorphic features with large dysplastic pinnae and beaked nasal profile.	Autosomal recessive; defect in N-acetyl glucosaminyltransferase II gene at 14q21.	Ventricular septal defect.	Tan et al., 1996.

continued

Appendix 47.1 (*continued*)

Syndrome name	Clinical features	Etiology	Cardiac defects	Key reference
Cardio-auditory syndrome of Sanchez-Cascos	Severe sensorineural deafness, excess whorls on fingertips.	Autosomal recessive.	Cardiac hypertrophy.	Sanchez-Cascos et al, 1969.
Cardio-facio-cutaneous syndrome	Noonan like, large head with bitemperal restriction, coarse facies, sparse curly hair, hyperkeratosis, icthyosis, short stature, mental retardation. Overlap with Noonan and Costello syndromes.	Sporadic; ?autosomal dominant, ?allelic to Noonan syndrome (gene mapped to 12q24 in one family with both phenotypes).	Mainly pulmonary stenosis, atrial septal defect, hypertrophic cardiomyopathy, other defects including ventricular septal defect.	Legius et al., 1998.
Carpenter syndrome.	Pre-axial polydactyly of feet, brachysyndactyly, craniosynostosis (acrocephaly), mental retardation, high forehead, mid face hypoplasia, ptosis, hypogenitalism, obesity, possible cerebral malformations.	Autosomal recessive.	Ventricular septal defect, persistent arterial duct, atrial septal defect, pulmonary stenosis, tetralogy of Fallot.	Cohen et al., 1987.
CATCH syndrome (acronym)	Cardiac abnormality, thymic hypoplasia, cleft palate, hypocalcemia (see also DiGeorge syndrome, velo-cardio-facial syndrome and Takao syndrome).	22q11 deletion; dominantly inherited in 10–15%. Heart defect attributed to loss of *Tbx1*.	Outflow tract defects, mainly tetralogy of Fallot, ventricular septal defect, interrupted aortic arch, pulmonary atresia, truncus arteriosus.	Ryan et al, 1997. Thomas and Graham, 1997.
Catel-Manzke syndrome (digitopalatal syndrome)	Pierre Robin sequence, short, flexed ulnar-deviated index finger with accessary proximal phalanx, occasional hypoplastic/absent thumb or radius, vertebral anomalies, joint laxity, mental retardation.	?X-linked, ? autosomal recessive.	Mainly ventricular septal defect, atrial septal defect, tetralogy of Fallot, transposition of great arteries, coarctation, hypoplastic aortic arch.	Kant et al, 1998.
Cerebellar hypoplasia-lymphedema-neuronal migration defect	Cerebellar hypoplasia, hydro/macrocephaly, lissencephaly, seizures, Dandy Walker malformation, severe learning disability.	Autosomal recessive.	Ventricular septal defect.	Dobyns et al., 1996.
Cerebro-costo-mandibular syndrome	Severe micrognathia, cleft palate, Pierre Robin sequence, gaps in posterior ribs, respiratory distress, mental retardation, growth retardation; occasional tracheomalacia, cerebral anomalies.	Uncertain; autosomal recessive and autosomal dominant transmission reported.	Ventricular septal defect reported in one patient.	Plötz et al., 1996.

continued

Appendix 47.1 (*continued*)

Syndrome name	Clinical features	Etiology	Cardiac defects	Key reference
Cerebro-facio-thoracic dysplasia	Mental retardation, narrow forehead, bushy eyebrows, synophrys, triangular-shaped mouth with down-turned corners, brachycephaly, marked maxillary hypoplasia, hemivertebrae, bifid or bridged ribs.	Autosomal recessive, with 2 sisters and 1 brother of second-cousin parents reported.	Atrial septal defect.	Guion-Almeida et al., 1996.
Char syndrome	Patulous lips, short philtrum, large forehead, flared eyebrows, flat nasal bridge, hypertelorism, short flattened nose, clinodactyly of 5th finger; occasional ptosis, delay, limited movements of interphalangeal joints.	Autosomal dominant. Neural crest defect due to defect in *TFAP2B*.	Patent ductus arteriosus.	Satoda et al, 2000.
CHARGE association (acronym)	Colobomata (iris and/or retina), heart defects, atresia choanae, retardation of growth and development and/or CNS anomalies, genitalia hypoplasia in males, ears cup-shaped and deaf.	Unknown; all cases sporadic.	Tetralogy of Fallot, patent ductus arteriosus, ventricular, atrial and atrioventricular septal defects, aortic arch anomalies, hypoplastic left heart, double outlet right ventricle.	Tellier et al., 1996; 1998.
CHILD syndrome (acronym)	Congenital hemidysplasia, ichthyosiform nevus, limb defects, occasional visceral hypoplasia, CNS lesions and mental retardation.	X-linked dominant with lethality in males.	Defect of septation with abnormal valves and/or common arterial trunk, Shone's complex, ventricular septal defect.	Happle et al., 1996.
Chondrodysplasia punctata Conradi-Hunermann type (CDPX2)	Asymmetric shortening of limbs, stippled epiphysis, contractures, patchy skin changes, sparse hair, flat facies.	X-linked dominant; due to *EBP* at Xp11.2 defect in cholesterol biosynthesis.	Heart defects described occasionally.	Braverman et al., 1999
Chondrodysplasia punctata rhizomelic type	Short proximal limbs, stippled epiphysis, coronal cleft of vertebrae, contractures, flat face, full cheeks, cataracts, ichthyosis, early death, retardation in survivors.	Autosomal recessive; defects in *PEX7* at 6q2 (type 1) or in *DHAP-AT* (type 2).	Various heart defects.	Subramani, 1997. Motley et al., 1997.
Chromosome 16 maternal disomy	Variable features depend on level of mosaicism. Asymmetry, hypertelorism, small hands and feet, 5th finger clinodactyly, microcephaly, hypospadias, scoliosis.	Sporadic.	Atrial septal defect, atrio-ventricular septal defect, ventricular septal defect.	Kalousek et al., 1993.

continued

Appendix 47.1 (*continued*)

Syndrome name	Clinical features	Etiology	Cardiac defects	Key reference
Coffin-Siris syndrome	Growth deficiency, mental retardation, microcephaly, coarse facies, wide mouth, sparse scalp hair, hirsutism, deficient terminal phalanges, hypoplastic nails.	Possible autosomal recessive.	Atrial septal defect, persistent arterial duct, tetralogy of Fallot, pulmonary stenosis, persistent left superior vena cava.	Swillen et al., 1995.
Cohen syndrome	Truncal obesity, mental retardation, hypotonia, microcephaly, delayed puberty, joint laxity, long narrow hands and feet, down-slanting eyes, short philtrum, prominent upper central incisors, occasional chorioretinal dystrophy, neutropenia.	Autosomal recessive; gene mapped to 8q.	Mitral valve prolapse, ventricular septal defect; aortic dilatation. Transient neonatal cardiomyopathy reported.	Kolehmainen et al., 1997.
Congenital short gut-mairotation-dysmotility of the small bowel	Short bowel, malrotation, pyloric stenosis, frontal bossinig, hypertelorism and telecanthus, thrombocytopenia.	X-linked inheritance; ?contiguous gene defect.	Persistent arterial duct.	FitzPatrick et al., 1997.
Conotruncal anomaly face syndrome (Takao syndrome). Part of the CATCH phenotype	Small mouth, short philtrum, micrognathia, hypertelorism, short palpebral fissures, dysplastic ears, nasal voice, occasional cleft palate, mild retardation.	Dominant due to 22q11 deletion.	Common arterial trunk, tetralogy of Fallot with major aortico pulmonary artery collaterals.	Ryan et al., 1997.
Conradi-Hünermann syndrome (chondrodysplasia punctata)	Hydramnios and early death in some, punctate epiphyseal calcification, limb asymmetry, scoliosis, contractures, flat facies, cataracts (20%), dry skin and alopecia (20%).	Variable autosomal dominant.	Heart defects an occasional feature.	Hyndman et al., 1976.
Cornel syndrome	At least two generations with ptosis and coarctation associated with speech delay, probably due to sensorineural hearing loss.	Autosomal dominant.	Coarctation, interrupted aorta.	Cornel et al., 1987.
Cornelia de Lange syndrome	Mental retardation, growth failure, microbrachycephaly, hirsutism, synophrys, neat eyebrows, short up-turned nose, long philtrum, thin upper lip, variable upper limb reduction defects, gastroesophageal reflux, occasional diaphragmatic hernia.	Autosomal dominant; genes possibly mapped to 3q26.	Mainly ventricular septal defect, pulmonary stenosis, other possible defects including tetralogy of Fallot, persistent arterial duct, coarctation.	Tsukahara et al., 1998.
Costello syndrome	Polyhydramnios, mental retardation, post-natal growth failure, coarse face, thick lips, excess of skin on neck, hands and feet, deep palmar and plantar crease, papillomata, sparse curly hair, acanthosisnigricans.	Probable autosomal dominant.	Hypertrophic cardiomyopathy, dysrhythmia, ventricular septal defect, atrial septal defect, pulmonary stenosis, mitral valve defects.	Siwik et al., 1998. Philip and Sigaudy, 1998.

continued

Appendix 47.1 (*continued*)

Syndrome name	Clinical features	Etiology	Cardiac defects	Key reference
Cranioectodermal dysplasia (Sensenbrenner syndrome)	Dolichocephaly, sparse hair, epicathic folds, hypodontia, short limbs, brachydactyly, narrow thorax, sagittal suture synostosis, renal failure, retinal dystrophy.	Autosomal recessive.	Divided left atrium and bicuspid aortic valve reported in one patient.	Savill et al., 1997.
Cri du chat syndrome (5p-)	Growth deficiency, cat-like cry. Developmental delay, microcephaly, round face, hypertelorism.	Sporadic; translocation in 10–15% of families.	Variable.	Niebuhr, 1978.
Cutis laxa (dominant form)	Lax skin, prematurely aged appearance, beaked nose, occasional hoarse voice, joint dislocations, hernias.	Autosomal dominant; defects in *ELN* at 7q11.	Rarely, pulmonary artery stenosis, mitral valve prolapse, toluosity and dilatation of carotid arteries and aorta, dilatation of sinuses of Valsalva, coarctation of aorta.	Tassabehji et al., 1998.
Cutis laxa syndrome (recessive form)	Lax skin, permaturely aged appearance, everted lower eyelids, hooked nose, long upper lip, bladder and colon diverticulae, vaginal and rectal prolapse, hernias, severe emphysema.	Autosomal recessive.	Cor pulmonale, aortic root dilatation, pulmonary artery stenosis, dilated and tortuous carotid, cerebral and pulmonary arteries.	Van Maldergem et al., 1988.
Desmosterolosis	Macrocephaly, hypoplastic nasal bridge, cleft palate, gingival nodules, rhizomelic limb shortening, defect in cholesterol biosynthesis.	Autosomal recessive; deficiency of 3-beta-hydroxysterol-delta-24-reductase.	Anomalous pulmonary venous return.	FitzPatrick et al., 1998.
DiGeorge syndrome	Thymic a/hypoplasia or dysfunction, hypocalcemia (hypoparathyroidism), low set ears, micrognathia, short palpebral fissues, telecanthus, short philtrum, small mouth, occasional renal abnormalities.	22q11 deletion; autosomal dominantly inherited in about 10% cases, some cases due to 10p or 4p deletions or maternal diabetes.	Outflow defects-interrupted aorta, common arterial trunk, tetralogy of Fallot.	Ryan et al., 1997;
Distichlasis-lymphedema syndrome	Extra row of eyelashes, late onset lymphedema; occasional cleft palate, micrognathia, pterygium colli, ptosis, Arnold-Chiari malformation, urinary tract malformations, spinal extradural cysts, vertebral anomalies, double uterus.	Autosomal dominant; linked to 16q.	Ventricular septal defect, patent ductus arteriosus, tetralogy of Fallot, peripheral pulmonary stenosis, arrhythmia, conduction defects.	Mangion et al., 1999.

continued

Appendix 47.1 (*continued*)

Syndrome name	Clinical features	Etiology	Cardiac defects	Key reference
Donnai-Barrow syndrome	Diaphragmatic hernia, exomphalos, agenesis corpus callosum, deafness.	Autosomal recessive.	Double outlet right ventricle.	Donnai and Barrow, 1993.
DOOR syndrome (acronym)	Deafness, onychodystrophy, onycholysis, mental retardation, triphalangeic 1st digits, poor/absent nails, ptosis, short broad nose, hydronephrosis, epilepsy.	Autosomal recessive.	Atrial septal defect, ventricular septal defect.	Thornton et al., 1994.
Down syndrome (trisomy 21)	Hypotonia, developmental delay, upslanting palbebral fissures, speckling of iris, epicanthric folds, brachycephaly, short metacarpals and phalanges, single palmar crease.	Sporadic; associated with increased maternal age; 5% unbalanced Robertsonian translocation.	Cardiac defect in 40%; atrioventricular septal defect, ventricular septal defect, atrial septal defect, persistent arterial duct, tetralogy of Fallot.	Wells et al., 1994.
Early amnion rupture syndrome (includes ADAM complex, limb body wall complex)	Major structural defects of head, limbs and/or body wall, associated with amniotic bands and short umbilical cord.	Presumed to be due to amnion rupture; severe end of spectrum of amniotic band disruption.	Mainly common atrium/primitive ventricle, other defects including truncus arteriosus, ventricular septal defect, atrial septal defect, ectopia cordis.	Moerman et al., 1992. Bamforth, 1992.
Ebstein anomaly-skeletal abnormalities	Camptodactyly/clinodactyly. Limited elbow flexion, edema.	Autosomal dominant.	Ebstein anomaly.	Balaji et al., 1991.
Ectopia cordis–cleft lip and palate	Cleft lip/palate/mandible. Asternia.	Sporadic; ? due to early amnion rupture.	Ectopia cordis.	Gorlin et al., 1990.
Edwards syndrome (trisomy 18)	Developmental delay, growth failure, hypertonia, prominent occiput, small palpebral fissure, clenched hands with overlapping fingers, omphalocele, spina bifida, radial defect.	Sporadic.	Ventricular septal defect, valvular anomalies, atrial septal defect, persistent arterial duct, double outlet right ventricle, tetralogy of Fallot.	Embleton et al., 1996.
Ehlers-Danlos syndrome type IV (arterial or Sack-Barabas type)	Most severe form, skin easily bruised and prematurely aged skin with prominent veins and keloid scars but only slight increase in elasticity, tendency to bowel rupture.	Autosomal recessive and dominant forms; defects in *COL3A1* at 2q31.	Aneurysms and spontaneous rupture of large and medium-sized arteries, mitral valve prolapse.	Pope et al., 1999;
Ellis-van Creveld syndrome (chondroectodermal dysplasia)	Short stature, postaxial polydactyly, limb meso/acromelic shortening, short ribs, small chest, oral frenulae, natal teeth, nail dysplasia, genu valgum, small trident pelvis, occasional Dandy Walker malformation.	Autosomal recessive; EVC protein gene mapped to 4p16 with unknown function.	50% have heart defects, typically common atrium, large atrial septal defect ostium primum type, atrioventricular septal defect; hypoplastic left heart reported.	Ruiz-Perez et al., 2000.

continued

Appendix 47.1 (*continued*)

Syndrome name	Clinical features	Etiology	Cardiac defects	Key reference
Ellis-van Creveld syndrome (chondroectodermal dysplasia)	Short stature, postaxial polydactyly, limb meso/acromelic shortening, short ribs, small chest, oral frenulae, natal teeth, nail dysplasia, genu valgum, small trident pelvis, occasional Dandy Walker malformation.	Autosomal recessive; EVC protein gene mapped to 4p16 with unknown function.	50% have heart defects, typically common atrium, large atrial septal defect ostium primum type, atrioventricular septal defect; hypoplastic left heart reported.	Ruiz-Perez et al., 2000.
Fabry disease	Acroparesthesia, abdominal pains, angiokeratomas, corneal opacities, renal failure.	X-linked; defect in alpha-galactosidase A gene at Xq22.	Hypertrophic cardiomyotrophy, mitral valve prolapse, arrhythmias, myocardial ischemia, cerebrovascular diseases.	Desnick et al, 1995.
Facio-auriculo-vertebral spectrum (Goldenhar syndrome, hemifacial microsomia, oculo-auriculo-vertebral dysplasia)	Hemifacial microsomia, epibulbar dermoid, preauricular tags, deafness, colobomata of eyelids, small jaw, cleft palate, vertebral anomalies, microtia.	Sporadic; occasional autosomal dominant or recessive.	Mainly ventricular septal defects, tetralogy of Fallot, other defects including atrial septal defect, coarctation, transposition of great arteries.	Kumar et al., 1993.
Faciocardiomelic dysplasia	Hypoplastic or absent radius, ulna, tibia, fibula and thumb bilaterally, talipes, camptodactyly, webbed neck, hypoplastic or absent tongue, hypertelorism.	Autosomal recessive.	Hypoplastic left heart. Common arterial trunk.	Cantu et al., 1975.
Facio-cardio-renal syndrome (Eastman-Bixler syndrome)	Horseshoe kidney, mental retardation, malar hypoplasia, broad nose, short smooth philtrum, prominent mandible, prominent low-set ears; occasional cleft palate.	Single report; 3 sibs.	Conduction defects, endocardial fibroelastosis.	Eastman and Bixler, 1977.
Fanconi anemia	Pancytopenia, leukemia, short stature, cafe au lait spots, absent/hypoplastic thumb, small genitalia, microcephaly, renal abnormalities, mental retardation, small eyes, hearing loss, occasional CNS, gastrointestinal abnormalities.	Autosomal recessive; defect mainly in *FAA* at 16q24 or *FAC* at 9q22, unidentified *FAD* gene mapped to 3p2, at least 5 other genes, B,E,F,G,H.	Cardiac defects in 1 in 6 of various types.	Giampietro et al., 1997. Joenje et al., 1997.
Farag syndrome (hypertelorism and tetralogy of Fallot)	Mental retardation, hypertelorism, hypospadias, narrow palebral fissures, flat nasal bridge, posteriorly rotated ears.	? Autosomal recessive.	Tetralogy of Fallot, patent foramen ovale, pulmonary atresia, persistent arterial duct.	Farag and Teebi, 1990.

continued

Appendix 47.1 (*continued*)

Syndrome name	Clinical features	Etiology	Cardiac defects	Key reference
Femoral hypoplasia-unusual facies syndrome	Short bowed femora, long philtrum radio-ulnar synostosis, cleft palate.	2/3 sporadic; 1/3 maternal diabetes.	Heart defects mainly ventricular septal defects (in maternal diabetic cases only).	Burn et al., 1984.
Fetal alcohol syndrome	Short stature, prenatal onset, short palpebral fissures, hairy forehead, smooth philtrum, thin upper lip, hypoplastic terminal phalanges, hypotonia, mental retardation.	Maternal alcohol disruption.	Typically septal defects 1/3 of classic cases. Tetralogy of Fallot, atrial septal defect.	Sandor et al., 1981.
Fetal aminopterin syndrome	Growth deficiency, microcephaly, hypoplastic facial bones, broad nasal bridge, upsweep of hair, short forearm, talipes.	Folate antagonist.	Right-sided heart defects in some.	Shaw and Steinback, 1968.
Fetal cytomegalovirus syndrome	Hepatosplenomegaly, thrombocytopenia, anemia, microcephaly, calcification in brain, chorioretinitis, deafness.	Viral disruption.	Occasional mitral or pulmonary valve stenosis, atrial septal defect.	Ko et al., 2000.
Fetal hydantoin syndrome	Growth deficiency, microcephaly, mild retardation, broad depressed nasal bridge, hypoplastic nails.	Drug disruption.	Aortic and pulmonary valve stenosis coarctation, patent arterial duct, septal defects.	Meadow, 1991.
Fetal thalidomide	Limb reduction, microphthalmia, coloboma, microtia, cleft lip/palate, facial palsy, hypoplastic kidneys, cryptorchidism, duodenal stenosis, anal stenosis, sacral agenesis.	Intrauterine exposure to thalidomide.	Ventricular septal defect, pulmonary stenosis, patent arterial duct, conotruncal anomalies.	Smithells and Newman, 1992.
Fetal valproate syndrome	Metopic ridging bifrontal narrowing, epicanthus, broad flat nasal bridge, short upturned nose, long-flat philtrum, occasional neural tube defects, cleft lip/palate, radial defects, tracheomalacia, genitourinary malformations, distal phalangeal hypoplasia.	Drug disruption.	Ventricular septal defect, atrial septal defect, patent ductus arteriosus, coarctation, hypoplastic left heart, aortic stenosis, peripheral pulmonary stenosis.	Clayton-Smith et al., 1995.
Fetal vitamin A syndrome	Mental retardation, anotia/microtia, hypertelorism, micrognathia, hydrocephalus and other CNS malformation, thymic hypoplasia.	Drug disruption.	Common arterial trunk, transposition of the great vessels, atrial septal defect, ventricular septal defect, tetralogy of Fallot.	Lammer et al., 1985.

continued

Appendix 47.1 (*continued*)

Syndrome name	Clinical features	Etiology	Cardiac defects	Key reference
Fetal warfarin syndrome	Chondrodysplasia punctata with short limbs and stippled epiphyses. Hypoplastic nasal bridge and/or alae nasae. Occasional eye and cerebral defects.	Drug disruption.	Pulmonary stenosis and persistent arterial duct described.	Hall et al., 1980.
FG syndrome (Opitz Kaveggia syndrome)	Postnatal growth failure, hypotonia, severe constipation, anal anomalies, large forehead with developmental delay, agenesis of corpus callosum.	X-linked recessive; probably heterogeneous.	Mainly ventricular septal defects; pulmonary stenosis; hypoplastic left heart reported.	Opitz et al., 1988. Romano et al., 1994. Zwambom-Hanssen et al., 1995.
Floating-Harbor syndrome	Short stature, delayed bone age, broad nose, unusual speech, mental retardation.	Uncertain.	Pulmonary stenosis.	Lazebnik et al., 1996.
Forney syndrome	Proportionate short stature, conductive deafness, vertebral fusion, carpo-tarsal synostosis, skin pigmentation.	Autosomal dominant.	Mitral incompetence.	Forney et al., 1966.
Fournier syndrome (pulmonic stenosis and congenital nephrosis)	Congenital nephrotic syndrome.	? Autosomal recessive.	Pulmonary stenosis.	Fournier et al., 1963.
Fragile X syndrome	Severe learning disability, long face, large ears, enlarged testes.	X-linked recessive; FMR1 gene.	Mitral valve prolapse.	Crabbe et al., 1993. de Vries et al., 1998.
Fraser syndrome	Cryptophthalmos, renal agenesis, atresia stenosis larynx and vagina, syndactyly, heart defect.	Autosomal recessive.	Various defects described.	Burn and Marwood, 1982.
Frontonasal dysplasia with heart defect	Hypertelorism, broad nasal root, median nasal cleft, short stature, microcephaly.	Sporadic.	Tetralogy of Fallot, aortic stenosis.	De Moor et al., 1987. Meinecke and Blunck, 1989.
Fucosidosis	Progressive mental and motor deterioration, coarse face, hepatomegaly, thick skin, angiokeratoma, growth failure, stiff joints, umbilical hernia, recurrent infections.	Autosomal recessive; defect in alpha-fucosidase gene at 1p34.	Cardiomyopathy.	Williams et al., 1991.
Gastrocutaneous syndrome	Peptic ulcer hiatus hernia, lentigines/cafe au lait patches, hypertelorism, myopia.	Autosomal dominant.	Single pedigree; 10 affected, 1 of whom had mitral valve prolapse, and 1 peripheral pulmonary stenosis.	Halal et al., 1982.
Gay syndrome	Laryngeal web, short stature.	Autosomal dominant.	Ventricular septal defect.	Gay, 1981.

continued

Appendix 47.1 (*continued*)

Syndrome name	Clinical features	Etiology	Cardiac defects	Key reference
Geleophysic syndrome	Short stature, small hands and feet, short broad tubular bones, joint contractures, up-slanting eyes, short up-turned nose, thin lip, smooth philtrum, hepatosplenomelaly, premature death.	Autosomal recessive.	Glycoprotein deposit in all cardiac valves causing stenosis and incompetence.	Pontz et al., 1996. Shohat et al., 1990.
Glycogen storage disease type IIA (Pompe disease)	Severe hypotonia, hyperglosia, muscle weakness, hepatomegaly.	Autosomal recessive; defect in acid alpha-glucosidase gene at 17q23.	Progressive cardiac hypertrophy.	Hirschhorn, 1995.
Glycogen storage disease type IV (Brancher deficiency)	Cirrhosis in infancy, rapidly progressive myopathy, failure to thrive, early death.	Autosomal recessive; defect in *GBE* at 3p12.	Cardiomyopathy.	Bao et al., 1996.
Glycogen storage disease type V (McArdle disease)	Muscle cramp, rapid fatigue and myoglobinuria on exercise, progressive muscle wasting.	Autosomal recessive; defect in *PYGM* at 11q13.	Congestive failure due to increased blood flow on exercise and ? involvement of myocardium.	Chen and Burchell, 1995.
Golabi Ito syndrome	Mental retardation, microcephaly, protruding ears, hypertelorism, brittle dry hair, narrow palate, macrodontia, cutis marmorata.	X-linked recessive.	Atrial septal defect.	Golabi et al., 1984.
Goltz syndrome	Focal dermal hypoplasia, oligodactyly, hypoplastic teeth, micropthalmos, coloboma, alopecia, mental retardation, osteopathia-striata.	Almost all sporadic and female. Possibly X-linked dominant with early lethality in males.	Rare; pulmonary stenosis, atrial septal defect, persistent arterial duct.	Goltz, 1992.
Gorlin syndrome (basal cell nevus syndrome)	Macrocephaly, frontal bossing, prognathism, multiple basal cell carcinomas after puberty, palmar/plantar pits, multiple odontogenic keratocyst of jaw, rib anomalies, occasional falx calcification, mild mental retardation, ovarian fibromas.	Autosomal dominant; defect in *patched* gene at 9q22.	Cardiac fibromas.	Kimonis et al., 1997.
Gorlin-Chaudhry-Moss syndrome	Craniofacial dystosis, hypertrichosis, genital hypoplasia, dental defects, small eyes, lid defects, short stature, dysplastic ears, conductive deafness, hypoplastic distal phalangx.	? Autosomal recessive.	Persistent arterial duct.	Ippel et al., 1992.

continued

Appendix 47.1 (*continued*)

Syndrome name	Clinical features	Etiology	Cardiac defects	Key reference
Hajdu-Cheney syndrome	Acroosteolysis in late childhood, skull deformities, basilar impression, distinctive facies, osteoporosis, joint laxity, kyphoscoliosis, short stature, early loss of teeth, hearing loss, occasional hydrocephalus, cystic renal disease, cleft palate.	Autosomal dominant.	Mainly persistent arterial duct, ventricular septal defect, mitral incompetence and aortic stenosis.	Crifasi et al., 1997.
Hallerman-Streiff syndrome	Microphthalmia, cataract, small jaw, frontal prominence, thin pointed nose, dental anomalies, hypotrichosis, skin atrophy, short stature, occasional retardation.	Almost always sporadic.	Occasional, tetralogy of Fallot, pulmonary stenosis, ventricular septal defect, atrial septal defect, persistent arterial duct.	Cohen, 1991. Imaizumi et al., 1994.
Hay-Wells syndrome (AEC syndrome)	Ankyloblepharon, ectodermal dysplasia, cleft lip and/or palate; hypodontia, dystrophic nails, wiry sparse hair, scalp dermatitis or erosion.	Autosomal dominant.	Occasional ventricular septal defect or persistent arterial duct.	Hay and Wells, 1976. Greene et al., 1987.
Heart-hand II syndrome	Hypoplastic or absent ulna, narrow sloping shoulders, short metacarpals, broad short thumbs, short 4th and 5th fingers, anterior displacement of lower end of ulna.	ECG abnormality.	Atrial tachycardia and fibrillation.	Temtamy and McKusick, 1978.
Heart-hand III syndrome	Brachydactyly, hypoplastic phalanges, extra ossicle in index fingers.	Autosomal dominant.	Intraventricular conduction defect, sick sinus syndrome.	Ruiz de la Fuente and Prieto, 1980.
Heart-hand IV syndrome	Proportionate short stature, torticollis, small genitalia, pre- and postaxial polydactyly, synostosis of metacarpals.	Possible autosomal dominant.	Common atrium, pulmonary stenosis, ventricular septal defect, anomalous systemic venous drainage.	Martinez et al., 1981.
Heart-hand V syndrome (ventricular extrasystoles, perodactyly and Robin sequence)	Syncopes, micrognathia, glossoptosis, overt or submucous cleft palate, hypoplasia/agenesis of distal phalanges of hands and feet.	Autosomal dominant.	Ventricular extrasystoles occurring as bigeminy or multifocal tachycardia.	Stoll et al., 1992. Toriello, 1992.
Hennekam syndrome	Early onset lymphedema, intestinal lymphangiectasia, growth retardation, mental retardation, seizures, flat mid-face, flat nasal bridge, epicanthus, hypertelorism, ears anomalies, teeth anomalies, renourinary malformations, deafness, skeletal anomalies	Autosomal recessive.	Ventricular septal defect.	Angle and Hersh, 1997.

continued

Appendix 47.1 (*continued*)

Syndrome name	Clinical features	Etiology	Cardiac defects	Key reference
Hereditary hemorrhagic telangiectasia	Pinpoint spider and nodular telanglectasia, lips, face, mucous membranes and occasionally on viscera, recurrent epistaxis.	Autosomal dominant; heretogeneous, mutations in endoglin gene at 9q3 (*HHT1*), ALK1 gene at 12q13 (*HHT2*), other unidentified genes at different loci.	Arteriovenous fistulas, cavernous hemangiomata, cerebral vascular anomalies.	Johnson et al, 1996.
Ho syndrome	Small jaw, cleft palate, pre-axial polydactyly, hip dislocation, hypoplastic/absent tibia, talipes, persistent fontanelle, wormian bones.	Single case; ? due to multiple drug exposures.	Ventricular septal defect, aberrant subclavian artery.	Ho et al., 1975.
Hollister syndrome	Brachydactyly with long thumb, narrow shoulders, slight shortness of limbs, stiff joints.	Autosomal dominant.	Pulmonary stenosis, ? conduction defect, first-degree heart block.	Hollister and Hollister, 1981.
Holmes-Schimke syndrome	Microcephaly, mental retardation, seizures, micropenis, mild hypotelorism, depressed nasal bridge, coarse facies, rib abnormalities.	Single report; 2 brothers.	Hypoplastic aortic arch, atrial septal defect, ventricular septal defect.	Holmes and Schinke, 1989; 1993.
Holt-Oram syndrome	Triphalangeal or hypoplastic to absent or bifid thumb, variable hypoplasia of first metacarpal, radius or whole limb, narrow shoulders.	Autosomal dominant; mutations in *TBX5* at 12q21.	Mainly atrial septal defect, isolated ECG abnormality, other defects including ventricular septal defect, aortic stenosis, tetralogy of Fallot.	Li et al., 1997.
Holzgreve syndrome	Renal agenesis, meso-post-axial polydactyly, cleft lip/palate. Overlap with Thomas syndrome.	Sporadic.	Hypoplastic left heart, atretic aortic arch, atrioventricular septal defect, ventricular septal defect, atrial septal defect.	Meinecke et al., 1993.
Homocystinuria	Lens dislocation, mild retardation, seizures, psychiatric disturbance, Marfanoid habitus, osteoporosis, malar flush.	Autosomal recessive; defects in at 21q22. *CBS*	Vascular thrombosis.	Welch and Loscalzo, 1998.
Humero-spinal dysostosis	Coronal clefts of vertebrae, bifid distal humerus, dislocated elbow, rhizomelia upper limbs, talipes equinovarus.	Uncertain; maternal half-sibs affected and one sporadic case.	Thickened mitral valve; possible ventricular septal defect in one case.	Hall, 1997.
Hunter syndrome (mucopolysaccharidosis II)	Coarse facies, growth deficiency, stiff joints, clear corneas, hepatosplenomegaly, progressive deafness, mental retardation.	X-linked recessive; defect in iduronate sulfatase gene at Xq27–28.	Heart failure due to valve stenosis and incompetence, coronary artery narrowing, myocardial disease.	Neufeld and Muenzer, 1995.

continued

Appendix 47.1 (*continued*)

Syndrome name	Clinical features	Etiology	Cardiac defects	Key reference
Hurler syndrome (mucopolysaccharidosis IH)	Coarse facies, dysotosis multiplex, hepatosplenomegaly, corneal clouding, deafness, mental retardation, macroglossia, premature death.	Autosomal recessive; defect in *IDUA* gene at 4p16.	Cardiomyopathy, valve incompetence and stenosis, coronary artery disease.	Neufeld and Muenzer, 1995.
Hurst syndrome	Microcephaly, short stature, choanal stenosis, mental retardation, epicanthic folds, small nose, long philtrum, thin upper lip.	? Autosomal recessive.	Atrioventricular septal defect, ventricular septal defect.	Hurst et al., 1989.
Hydrolethalus syndrome	Hydrocephalus, hydramnios, lethality, CNS malformation, polydactyly, micrognathia, occipitoschisis, cleft lip and palate, laryngotracheal stenosis.	Autosomal recessive; mapped to 11q24.	Atrioventricular septal defect, ventricular septal defect and other defects.	Visapaa et al., 1999.
Hypertelorism-microtia-clefting (HMC) syndrome	Hypertelorism, cleft lip/palate, small dysplastic ears, broad nasal root, mental retardation, ectopic kidneys, short stature.	Autosomal recessive.	Atrial septal defect, atrioventricular septal defect.	Verloes, 1994.
Hypertrichosis-osteochondrodysplasia	Congenital hypertrichosis, macrosomy, osteopenia, narrow chest, broad ribs, platyspondyly.	? Autosomal recessive.	All 4 cardiomegaly, 1 had patent arterial duct, 1 had aortic stenosis.	Cantu et al., 1982.
Hypertrichosis-osteodysplasia-cardiomyopathy	Hypertrichosis, macrosomia, macrocephaly, coarse face, osteopenia, narrow chest, broad ribs, platyspondyly, mild mental retardation.	? Autosomal recessive.	Cardiomegaly, pericardial effusion, patent arterial duct, aortic stenosis.	Garcia-Cruz et al., 1997.
Idiopathic infantile arterial calcification	Cerebral arterial disease, deposition of hydroxyapatite due to defect in elastic lamina, early death.	? Autosomal recessive.	Coronary arterial disease.	Bellah et al., 1992. Pao et al., 1998.
Ieshima syndrome	Hypotonia, failure to thrive, hypertelorism, arched eyebrows, small nose, microtia, micrognathia, cleft palate, microcephaly, mental retardation, deafness, small penis, cryptorchidism.	? Autosomal recessive.	Persistent arterial duct, pulmonary hypertension.	Ieshima et al, 1986.
Infantile Refsum disease	Hypotonia, deafness, retinopathy, demyelinating neuropathy, liver fibrosis.	Autosomal recessive.	Conduction defects.	FitzPatrick, 1996.

continued

Appendix 47.1 (*continued*)

Syndrome name	Clinical features	Etiology	Cardiac defects	Key reference
Isomerism sequence	Right—typically 2 right atria, bronchi and lungs, absent spleen; left—typically 2 left atria, bronchi and lungs, multiple spleens; both—central liver, mal-rotation of gut.	Probably heterogeneous; incomplete penetrance, recessive in some cases.	Disturbance of embryonic septation and connexion, worse in right, abnormal venous connection, systemic in left, pulmonary in right.	Burn, 1991.
Jarcho-Levin syndrome (spondylothoracic dysplasia)	Severe short stature, short trunk, fan-like ribs, hemi-vertebrae, hydronephrosis, imperforate anus.	Autosomal recessive; defect of *DLL3* gene at 19q13, part of Notch signaling pathway.	Atrio-ventricular septal defect, coarctation/interrupted aorta, pulmonary stenosis, ventricular defect.	Bulman et al, 2000.
Jennings syndrome	Prominent forehead, crumpled ears, small palpebral fissures, jaw, and genitalia, moderate retardation and seizures.	Single report; 2 brothers.	Endocardial fibroelastosis.	Jennings et al, 1980.
Jervell-Lange-Nielson syndrome	Sensorineural deafness, syncope, sudden death, occasional seizures.	Autosomal recessive; hetero-geneous, homozygous defects in *KVLQT1* at 11p15, in *KCNE1* at 21q11.	Long QT interval, arrhythmia.	Tyson et al, 1997.
Jeune thoracic dysplasia	Severe rib shortening, short-limbed dwarfism, respiratory insufficiency, pelvis anomalies, polydactyly, cone-shaped epiphysis, occasional cystic kidney disease, retinal dystrophy, hepatic and pancreatic fibrosis.	Autosomal recessive.	Congestive heart failure, cor pulmonale, cardiomyopathy and congenital heart defects uncommon.	Tahernia and Stamps, 1977. Turkel et al., 1985.
Johannson-Blizzard syndrome	Failure to thrive, pancreatic insufficiency, hypothyroidism, aplasia cutis congenita, abnormal hair, hypoplastic alae nasi, mental retardation, sensorineural deafness.	Probably autosomal recessive.	Atrial septal defect, ventricular septal defect, pulmonary stenosis, transposition of the great arteries, situs inversus.	Hurst and Baraitser, 1989.
Johnson-McMillan syndrome	Alopecia, anosmia, conductive deafness, microtia and/or atresia of external auditory canal, hypogonadatrophic hypogonadism, occasional mental retardation, cleft palate.	Autosomal dominant.	Ventricular septal defect, complex heart defect.	Bankier and Rose, 1994.
Jones-Waldman syndrome	Prominent forehead, proptosed eyes, broad nasal tip, preauricular pits, short stature, clinodactyly, cryptorchidism.	Autosomal dominant.	Tetralogy of Fallot.	Schuler et al., 1994.

continued

Appendix 47.1 (*continued*)

Syndrome name	Clinical features	Etiology	Cardiac defects	Key reference
Kabuki syndrome (Niikawa-Kuroki syndrome)	Mental retardation, short stature, characteristic face with tented eyebrows and everted lower lids, long palpebral fissures, prominent ears, finger pads. Occasional skeletal and visceral malformations including cleft palate, vetebral anomalies and renal anomalies.	Probable autosomal dominant.	Ventricular septal defect, atrial septal defect, coarctation and aortic valve anomalies, mitral valve prolapse, transposition of the great arteries; other defects reported.	Hughes and Davies, 1994.
Kartagener syndrome	Cilial dyskinesia due to absent dynein arms, bronchiectasis, conductive deafness.	Autosomal recessive; half of homozygotes have situs inversus. Defect reported in axonal dynein intermediate chain 1 (DNAI1)	Mirror-image arrangement rarely associated with major defects (? overlap with isomerism sequence).	Guichard et al., 2001
Kashani syndrome	Obstructive uropathy, ureteral reflux, hydronephrosis.	Single report; 2 sisters.	Diffuse hypoplasia of pulmonary arteries, mild hypoplasia of ascending aorta.	Kashani et al., 1984.
Kaufman syndrome	Duplication of ureters, vertebral fusion, hemi-vertebrae, anal stenosis, cleft lip and palate.	Probably autosomal recessive.	Hypoplastic left heart. coarctation of aorta. venticular septal defect, atrial septal defect, patent ductus arteriosus.	Kaufman, 1974.
Kaufman-McKusick syndrome	Postaxial polydactyly, hydrometrocolpos, vaginal atresia, anal atresia/stenosis, hydronephrosis, Hirschsprung disease.	Autosomal recessive; gene mapped at 20p12.	Atrioventricular septal defect, single atrium, ventricular septal defect.	Cantani et al., 1987. Lurie and Wulfsberg, 1994. Stone et al., 1998.
Kawashima syndrome (isotretinoin embryopathy-like syndrome)	Hypertelorism, dysplastic ears, preauricular tags, sensorineural deafness, broad nasal tip, micrognathia.	Single report; 3 sibs.	Interrupted aortic arch, atrial septal defect, ventricular septal defect, aortic stenosis.	Kawashima, 1987.
Kearns-Sayre syndrome	Mitochondrial myopathy, opthalmoplegia, retinitis pigmentosa, ptosis, optic atrophy, short stature, deafness, endocrine and neurologic dysfunction.	Mitochondrial DNA deletions/duplications.	Conduction defects, cardiomyopathy.	Alaike et al., 1997. Fromenty et al., 1997.
Keutel syndrome	Calcification of ear cartilage, larynx and trachea, brachytelephalangy, mid-face hypoplasia, mixed deafness, short stature, infection-prone, mental retardation.	Autosomal recessive.	Multiple peripheral pulmonary artery stenoses, ventricular septal defect.	Teebi et al., 1998.
Klippel-Feil syndrome	Short neck, low hairline, abnormal cervical vertebrae, deafness, Sprengel shoulder, cleft palate, renal agenesis in some.	Most sporadic; may be dominant in some cases.	Variety of defects, usually ventricular septal defects.	Nagib, 1985.

continued

Appendix 47.1 (*continued*)

Syndrome name	Clinical features	Etiology	Cardiac defects	Key reference
Klippel-Trenaunay-Weber syndrome	Asymmetric limb hypertrophy, cutaneous hemangiomata, mild retardation in case of facial involvement, thromboembolic episodes.	Sporadic.	Arteriovenous fistula, cavernous hemangiomata, varicose veins.	Viljoen, 1988.
Kousseff syndrome	Sacral meningocoele, renal agenesis, low set posteriorly rotated ears, retrognathia, short neck, low posterior hairline.	Autosomal recessive.	Tetralogy of Fallot, truncus arteriosus, pulmonary stenosis/atresia, ventricular septal defect.	Toriello et al., 1985.
Lambert syndrome	Mild retardation, preauricular tags/pits, dysplastic ears, talipes, macrostomia, hypospadias, inguinal herniae, biliary atresia.	? Autosomal recessive.	Ventricular septal defect.	Lambert et al., 1990.
Larsen syndrome	Multiple joint dislocations, club-foot deformities, spatulate thumb, flat face, depressed nasal bridge, cleft palate, short stature, abnormal segmentation of vertebrae, accessory carpal bones.	Autosomal dominant; one gene mapped to 3p, possible autosomal recessive forms.	Aortic root dilatation, valvular anomalies of arterial duct, septal defects, pulmonary stenosis, endocardial fibroelastosis.	Vujic et al., 1995.
Laterality sequence (includes situs ambiguous heterotaxy, poly-/asplenia, Ivemark syndrome, isomerism sequence.	Asplenia/polysplenia, disturbance of visceral lateralization, right/left atrial and branchial isomerism.	Heterogeneous; mostly sporadic, some autosomal recessive and some dominant with imcomplete penetrance.	Complex defects including total anomalous pulmonary venous drainage, common atrium, atrioventricular septal defect, transposition of the great arteries, pulmonary atresia, interrupted inferior vena cava.	Hashmi et al., 1998.
Laurence syndrome	Hirschsprung's disease, post-axial polydactyly of hands, bifid big toes.	Probable recessive.	Ventricular septal defect, atrial septal defect, mitral stenosis, coarctation of aorta.	Nowaczyk et al., 1997.
Lenz microphthalmia	Mental retardation, micropthalmlia, microcephaly, skeletal, digital, genitourinary anomalies, occasional cleft lip/palate.	X-linked recessive.	Unspecified heart defects usually occur.	Traboulsi et al., 1988.
LEOPARD syndrome (acronym) (multiple lentigines syndrome)	Multiple lentigines, ECG anomalies, ocular hypertelorism, pulmonary stenosis, abnormal genitalia, retardation, deafness; occasional learning difficulties; overlap with Noonan syndrome and neurofibromatosis.	Autosomal dominant.	Pulmonary stenosis, dysplastic pulmonary valve, hypertrophic cardiomyopathy, electrocardiographic abnormalities; subaortic stenosis and patent ductus arteriosus reported.	Coppin and Temple, 1997.

continued

Appendix 47.1 (*continued*)

Syndrome name	Clinical features	Etiology	Cardiac defects	Key reference
Levin syndrome	Colobomata of retina, weakness of depressor angularis. ?Overlap with CHARGE association.	Both of a pair of monozygotic twins,? genetic, ? twinning disruption.	Hypoplastic aortic arch.	Levin et al., 1973.
Linear sebaceous nevus syndrome	Linear pigmented nevus, moderate retardation, hydrocephaly, cloudy cornea, coloboma, renal tumours, seizures.	Sporadic.	Coarctation of aorta, ventricular septal defect. Others less often.	Zaremba, 1978.
Linear sebaceous nevus syndrome	Linear verrucous pigmented lesions, mental retardation, seizures, CNS malformations, skeletal, ocular anomalies.	Sporadic.	Ventricular septal defect, coarctation, pulmonary stenosis, persistent arterial duct, hypoplastic left heart.	Grebe et al., 1993.
Lin-Gettig syndrome	Sagittal craniosynostosis, agenesis corpus callosum, developmental delay, camptodactyly blepharophimosis/ptosis, hypoplastic genitalia.	2 brothers; ? recessive.	Ventricular septal defect.	Lin and Gettig, 1990.
Lowry-MacLean syndrome	Severe learning disability, microcephaly, craniosynostosis, cleft palate, eventration of the diaphragm, hypospadias.	Uncertain.	Atrial septal defect, ventricular septal defect, pulmonary stenosis.	Kousseff et al., 1994.
Lujan Fryns syndrome (X-linked mental retardation with Marfanoid habitus)	Mental retardation, slender habitus, long thin hands and feet, long narrow face, sharp nose, high-arched palate, hypernasal voice, behavior problems.	X-linked recessive.	Atrial septal defect in only one patient.	Lacombe et al., 1993.
Lymphedema with cardiac anomalies (Irons syndrome)	Congenital lymphedema of lower limbs, hydrocele, prominent forehead, epicanthus, flat wide nasal bridge, hydrops, omphalocele.	Single report; 3 sibs.	Atrial septal defect.	Irons et al., 1996.
Maffuci syndrome	Enchondromatosis, multiple cutaneous hemangiomata.	Sporadic.	Cavernous hemangiomata.	Lewis and Ketcham, 1973.
Malouf syndrome	Ovarian dysgenesis, hypergonadotrophic hypogonadism, ptosis.	Probably autosomal recessive.	Cardiomyopathy.	Malouf et al., 1985.
Mandibulofacial dysostosis	Short stature, microcephaly, downslanting palpebral fissures, low-set protruding ears, hearing loss, cryptorchidism.	X-linked recessive.	Subvalvar pulmonary stenosis.	Toriello et al., 1985.

continued

Appendix 47.1 (*continued*)

Syndrome name	Clinical features	Etiology	Cardiac defects	Key reference
Marden Walker syndrome	Blepharophimosis, multiple congenital joint contractures, delayed development, growth retardation, decreased muscle mass, immobile face, micrognathia, kyphoscoliosis.	Autosomal recessive.	Dextrocardia, abnormal vena cavae connection, septal defects, cardiomyopathy.	Ramer et al., 1993.
Marfan syndrome	Tall and slim, long limbs, arachnodactyly, chest deformity, scoliosis, joint laxity, high palate, myopla, lens subluxation, herniae, skin striae, pneumothorax, dural ectasia.	Autosomal dominant; defect in the *FBN1* at 15q21.	Dilatation of ascending aorta, aortic dissection, mitral regurgitation, mitral valve prolapse.	Gray and Davies, 1996.
Marfanoid hypermobility syndrome	Disproportionate tall stature, arachnodactyly, joint dislocation hyperelastosis	Probable collagen defect; ? autosomal dominant	Aortic and mitral valve incompetence	Walker et al., 1969.
Maroteaux-Lamy syndrome (Mucopolysaccharidosis VI)	Growth failure, coarse face, joint contracture, chest deformity, corneal clouding, hearing loss, hepatosplenomegaly.	Autosomal recessive; defect in arylsulfatase B gene at 5q1.	Valve stenosis and incompetence, cardiomyopathy reported.	Neufeld and Muenzer, 1995.
Marshall-Smith syndrome	Increased length, advanced bone age, failure to thrive, developmental delay, prominent forehead and eyes, early death.	Sporadic.	Atrial septal defect, persistent arterial duct.	Williams et al, 1997.
Maternal diabetes disruption syndrome	Variety of malformations, sacral agenesis (caudal regression), femoral hypoplasia, cleft palate, vertebral anomalies.	(? Poorly treated) maternal diabetes.	Up to 5%—defects include ventricular septal defects and complete transposition.	Rowland et al, 1973. Ferencz et al, 1990.
Maternal phenylketonuria disruption syndrome	Microcephaly, mental retardation, intrauterine growth retardation, occasional cleft palate, microphthalmos.	Disruption by high phenylalanine levels *in utero*.	25% of cases—variety of defects include septal defects and outflow obstructions.	Levy and Ghavami, 1996.
McDonough syndrome	Mental retardation, large nose, bat ears, diastasis recti, kyphoscoliosis, simian crease.	? Autosomal recessive.	Aortic stenosis, pulmonary stenosis, atrial septal defect, ventricular septal defect.	Garcia-Sagredo et al, 1984.
Meckel syndrome	Occipital encephalocele, microcephaly, cystic renal dysplasia, post-axial axial polydactyly, microphthalmia, cleft lip/palate, hepatic fibrosis/cysts, other CNS abnormalities including Dandy Walker malformation.	Autosomal recessive; heterogeneous, one gene mapped to 17q22.	Various defects reported, mainly septal defects.	Salonen, 1984. Salonen and Paavola, 1998.
Megacystis-microcolon-intestinal hypoperistalsis	Megacystis/megaureter/hydronephrosis; microcolon/dilated small bowel.	Autosomal recessive.	Rhabdomyoma, truncus arteriosus, complex heart defects reported.	Anneren et al, 1991.

continued

Appendix 47.1 (*continued*)

Syndrome name	Clinical features	Etiology	Cardiac defects	Key reference
Microcephaly-cardiomyopathy	Microcephaly, mental retardation, cup-shaped ears, clinodactyly, narrow thorax.	? Autosomal recessive.	Cardiomyopathy.	Winship et al., 1991.
Microphthalmia-microtia-truncus arteriosus	Microphthalmia, microtia, joint contractures, middle finger camptodactyly.	Multiple sibs. ? Recessive.	Truncus arteriosus.	Digilio et al., 1997.
Mietens syndrome (Mietens-Weber syndrome)	Corneal opacity, nystagmus, flexion contracture of elbow, dislocation of redius, short/absent radi and ulna, growth failure, narrowed nose.	Autosomal recessive.	Vascular aneurysms.	Mietens and Weber, 1966.
Miller syndrome (postaxial acrofacial dysostosis; Genee-Wiedemann syndrome)	Postaxial reduction defect, malar hypoplasia, downslanting eyes, ectropion, eyelid coloboma, micrognathia, cleft lip/palate, dysplastic ears, hearing loss.	Probably autosomal recessive.	Ventricular septal defect, atrial septal defect.	Neumann et al., 1996.
Miller-Dieker lissencephaly syndrome	Lissencephaly type I, severe redardation, seizures, growth failure, tall furrowed forehead, bitemporal narrowing, short upturned nose, prominent upper lip.	Autosomal dominant; deletions at 17p13.3 in > 90% causing haploinsufficiency for genes, including *LIS-1*	Variety of defects, including tetralogy of Fallot, ventricular septal defect, pulmonary stenosis, persistent arterial duct.	Dobyns et al., 1991; 1993. Pilz and Quarrell, 1996.
Morquio syndrome (muco-polysaccharidosis IV)	Mild coarse face, dwarfism, short trunk, severe kyphoscoliosis, genu valgum, odontoid hypoplasia, corneal clouding, hearing loss, hepatomegaly.	Autosomal recessive; defects in *GALNS* at 16q24 (type A) or in *GLB1* at 3p21 (type B).	Aortic and mitral valve stenosis and incompetence.	Neufeld and Muenzer, 1995. Northover et al., 1996.
Mucke syndrome	Congenital lymphedema, down slanting palpebral fissures, long philtrum, retrognathia.	Single report; 2 brothers.	Coarctation of aorta, persistent arterial duct.	Mucke et al., 1986.
Mucolipidosis II (I cell disease)	Coarse psychomotor retardation, short stature, poor weight gain, coarse face, thick alveolar ridges, joint stiffness, kyphoscoliosis, hepatomegaly, macroglossia, early death.	Autosomal recessive; deficiency of GlcNAc-P transferase; gene mapped to 4q2.	Aortic valvar thickening and incompetence; cardiomegaly.	Kornfeld and Sly, 1995.
Mucolipidosis type III (Pseudo-Hurler polydystrophy)	Mild coarse face, mild mental retardation, corneal clouding, short stature, joint stiffness, scoliosis.	Autosomal recessive; deficiency of enzyme GNPTA; gene mapped to 4q2.	Aortic valve incompetence.	Kornfeld and Sly, 1995.

continued

Appendix 47.1 (*continued*)

Syndrome name	Clinical features	Etiology	Cardiac defects	Key reference
Mulibrey nanism	Severe short stature, triangular face, large skull, J-shaped sella tunica, yellowish retinal dots, hepatomegaly, muscle wasting, nevus flammeus.	Autosomal recessive; gene mapped to 17q2.	Constrictive pericarditis.	Avela et al., 1997.
MURCS syndrome	Mullerian duct/renal aplasia, cervicothoracic somite dysplasia (MURCS), absent uterus, vaginal atresia, short stature.	Sporadic.	Anomalous venous return, conduction defects, cardiac situs inversus/dextrocardia, ventricular septal defect.	Braun-Quentin et al, 1996.
Mutchinick syndrome	Mental retardation, microcephaly, speech disorders, short stature, hypertelorism, down-slanting eyes, large simple ears, broad straight nose.	Probably autosomal recessive.	Atrial septal defect, pulmonary stenosis, right bundle block.	Doerfler et al., 1997.
Myhre syndrome	Mental retardation, short stature, joint limitation, muscular hypertrophy, short digits, blepharophimosis, short philtrum, prognathism, hearing loss (maybe the same as GOMBO syndrome).	? Autosomal recessive.	Atrial septal defect, left ventricular hypertrophy.	Bottani and Verloes, 1995.
Myotonic dystrophy	Myotonia, cataract, ptosis, small testes, frontal balding, muscle weakness.	Autosomal dominant.	Conduction defects, rhabdomyoma.	Forsberg et al., 1990.
Nager acrofacial dysostosis	Acrofacial dysostosis resembling Treacher Collins syndrome combined with predominantly radial limb defects.	Evidence for both autosomal dominant and recessive inheritance in different families.	Tetralogy of Fallot, ventricular septal defect.	Thompson et al., 1985.
Najjar syndrome (cardiogenital syndrome)	Hypospadias, small penis, small testis, cyptorchidism, mental retardation.	Recessive; 3 brothers in one family, 2 in 2 others —? autosomal, ? X-linked.	Congestive cardiomyopathy.	Thomas et al., 1993.
NAME syndrome (acronym) (LAMB syndrome, Carney syndrome)	Nevi, atrial myxoma, myxoid neurofibromata (mucinosis of the skin), ephelides (endocrine overactivity); malignant endocrine tumors.	Autosomal dominant; gene mapped to 2p16.	Atrial myxomata.	Nwokoro et al., 1997.
Nathalie syndrome	Sensorineural deafness, cataract, muscular atrophy, osteochondrosis, growth retardation, hypoplastic breasts.	Autosomal recessive.	Short PR intervals and QRS ventricular extrasytoles.	Cremers et al., 1975.
Naxos disease (palmoplantar keratosis with cardiac anomalies)	Palmoplantar keratosis, dense, rough bristly hair, brachydactyly.	Autosomal recessive; gene mapped to 17q21.	Ventricular arrhythmias, endomyocardial fibrodysplasia, Ebstein anomaly.	Coonar et al., 1998.

continued

Appendix 47.1 (*continued*)

Syndrome name	Clinical features	Etiology	Cardiac defects	Key reference
Necrotizing myopathy-cataract-cardiomyopathy	Hypotonia, cataracts, cerebral/corpus callosum atrophy, necrotizing myopathy, mental retardation.	Probably autosomal recessive.	Cardiomyopathy.	Lyon et al., 1990.
Neish-Roberts syndrome	Wide forehead, bifid nasal tip, micrognathia, camptodactyly, non-obstructive hydronephrosis, absent septum pellucidum.	2 affected sibs.	Hypoplastic left heart, aortic hypoplasia.	Neish and Roberts, 1992.
Neurofibromatosis type I	Cafe au lait patches, lisch nodules, peripheral neurofibromas, macrocephaly, CNS tumors including optic glioma, pheochromocytoma, malignant tumors, scoliosis, pseudoarthrosis, mild mental retardation.	Autosomal dominant; defect in neurofibromin gene at 17q11.	Hypertension, renal artery, internal carotid artery, aortic stenosis, aneurysms, heart congestions, heart neurofibromas, occasional pulmonary valve stenosis, neurofibromata of heart.	Femer, 1998.
Noonan syndrome	Short stature, short webbed neck, pectus excavatum/carinatum, hypertelorism, down-slanting eyes, low-set ears, mild mental retardation, cryptorchidism.	Autosomal dominant; heterogeneous one gene mapped to 12q22.	Pulmonary valve stenosis, atrial septal defect, hypertrophic cardiomyopathy, ventricular septal defect.	Brady et al., 1997.
Noonan-like/Multiple giant cell lesion	Short stature, low/normal intelligence, hypertelorism, posteriorly rotated ears, giant cell lesions of bones, joints and soft tissues.	Sporadic.	Pulmonary stenosis.	Cohen and Gorlin, 1991.
Noonan-neurofibromatosis syndrome	Noonan phenotype associated with manifestation of neurofibromatosis.	Autosomal dominant; mechanism still unknown.	Pulmonary stenosis, multiple other defects described.	Carey, 1998.
Oculo-facio-cardio-dental syndrome	Congenital cataract, microphthalmia, radiculomegaly, oligodontia, persistent primary teeth, long face, high nasal bridge, notched alae nasi; occasional cleft palate, hearing loss, mental retardation.	? X-linked dominant.	Atrial septal defect, ventricular septal defect, mitral valve prolapse.	Obwegeser and Gorlin, 1997.
Ohdo syndrome	Mental retardation, blepharophimosis, ptosis, hypoplastic teeth, dysplastic ears, characteristic nose, small mouth, hearing loss.	? Autosomal dominant.	Ventricular septal defect, atrial septal defect, persistent arterial duct, pulmonary stenosis.	Mhanni et al., 1998.

continued

Appendix 47.1 (*continued*)

Syndrome name	Clinical features	Etiology	Cardiac defects	Key reference
Omodysplasia	Rhizomelic limb shortening, particularly of the humeri, dislocation of radial heads, club-like femurs, characteristic facies with small nose with round tip, depressed nasal bridge, and long philtrum.	Autosomal recessive and dominant.	Mitral stenosis.	Baxova et al., 1994.
Omphalocele-extrophy of bladder-imperforate anus-spinal defects (OEIS)	Omphalocele, everted bladder, abnormal or absent genitalia, segmentation defects of lumbar spine and sacrum.	Sporadic.	Atrioventricular canal defect, persistent left superior vena cava, aberrant right subclavian artery.	Kant et al., 1997.
Onat syndrome (subaortic stenosis and myopia)	Proportionate short stature, upturned nose, anteverted nares, hoarse voice, kyphosis inguinal hernia, obstructive lung disease.	Possible autosomal recessive.	Aortic stenosis.	Onat et al., 1984.
Opitz G/BBB syndrome (Opitz-Frias syndrome)	Hypertelorism, cleft lip and palate, dysphagia, laryngotracheal cleft, hypospadias, imperforate anus, developmental delay.	X-linked; defects in the *MID1* at Xp22.3, autosomal dominant forms map to 22q11.	Patent ductus arteriosus, ventricular septal defect, tetralogy of Fallot, atrial septal defect, coarctation of aorta, complex heart defects.	Quaderi et al., 1997.
Oral-cardiac-digital syndrome	Hypertelorism, oral hamartomata, malocclusion, postaxial polydactyly, hydrometrocolpos.	Autosomal recessive.	Aortic incompetence, atrioventricular septal defect. coarctation/interrupted aorta.	Orstavik et al., 1992.
Oral-facial-digital (OFD) syndrome, type IV (Mohr-Majewski syndrome)	Midline cleft upper lip, multiple frenulae, harmatomas of tongue, absent tibiae, pre-/postaxial polydactyly of feet, postaxial polydactyly of hands, cerebral atrophy.	Autosomal recessive.	Tetralogy of Fallot, atrioventricular septal defect, anomalous venous return.	Toriello et al., 1997.
Oro-facial-digital syndrome type II (Mohr syndrome)	Midline cleft lip, lobulated tongue, hamartomata, encephalocele, pre-/postaxial polydactyly.	Autosomal recessive.	Atrioventricular septal defect, interrupted aorta, atrial septal defect.	Baraitser, 1986.
Oro-facial-digital syndrome type VI (Varadi-Papp syndrome)	Bifid big toes, central polydactyly of hands, Y-shaped third metacarpal, cleft lip/palate, oral frenulae, lingual nodules, cerebellar defects, growth and mental retardation.	Autosomal recessive.	Aortic stenosis, atrioventricular septal defect, and coarctation reported.	Munke et al., 1990.

continued

Appendix 47.1 (*continued*)

Syndrome name	Clinical features	Etiology	Cardiac defects	Key reference
Osteogenesis imperfecta (4 clinical types)	Multiple fractures, osteopenia, wormian bones, and/or soft deformed cranium, and/or blue sclerae, and/or abnormal tooth enamel, progressive hearing loss.	Autosomal dominant; defects in *COL1A1* at 17q or *COL1A2* at 7q.	Aortic root dilatation, mitral valve prolapse, mitral chordal rupture, aortic regurgitation.	Byers, 1993. Hortop et al., 1986.
Osteogenesis imperfecta-microcephaly-cataracts	Multiple fractures, broad bones, cataracts, low set ears, microcephaly, cerebral atrophy, joint laxity.	Single report; 3 sibs, ? autosomal recessive.	1 small left ventricle, 1 ventricular septal defect.	Buyse and Bull, 1978.
Oto-Palato-Digital syndrome type II.	Hypertelorism, downslanting eyes, micrognathia, cleft palate, long bone bowing, flexed overlapping fingers, fanned toes, short 1st metacarpal; occasional polydactyly, small or absent fibula, omphalocele.	X-linked recessive.	Ventricular septal defect, atrial septal defect, aortic stenosis, patent ductus arteriosus.	Robertson et al., 1997.
Pailister-Hall syndrome	Hypothalamic hamartoblastoma, central-/postaxial polydactyly, imperforate anus, brachytelephalangism, dysplastic nails, larynx anomalies, pituitary dysfunction, renal anomalies, abnormal facies.	Autosomal dominant; defect in *GLI3* gene at 7p13.	Pulmonary stenosis, coarction, aterial septal defect, ventricular septal defect, all described.	Kang et al., 1997.
Pallister-Killian syndrome	Severe mental retardation, seizures, short stature, coarse face, frontal bossing, temporal balding, upturned nose, full cheeks, droopy mouth, depigmented skin areas, diaphragmatic hernia, supernumerary nipples.	Mosaic 12p tetrasomy.	Mainly ventricular septal defect, coarctation, atrial septal defect, persistent arterial duct, aortic stenosis reported.	Schinzel, 1991.
Palmer-Pagon syndrome	Hydrocephalus, urinary reflux, low insertion umbilical cord, flat nasal bridge, bulbous nasal tip.	2 brothers; ? recessive.	Tetralogy of Fallot, anomalous venous return, atrial septal defect, persistent arterial duct.	Palmer and Pagon, 1993.
Pancreatic hypoplasia-congenital congenital heart defect.	Pancreatic hypoplasia leading to diabetes mellitus.	Autosomal dominant.	Tetralogy of Fallot, transposition of the great arteries, atrial septal defect, persistent arterial duct.	Yorifuji et al., 1994.

continued

Appendix 47.1 (*continued*)

Syndrome name	Clinical features	Etiology	Cardiac defects	Key reference
Patau syndrome (Trisomy 13)	Mental retardation, incomplete development of forebrain, polydactyly, microcephaly, microphthalmia, cleft lip, cleft palate, deafness, cryptorchidism, scalp defects.	Sporadic.	Heart defect in 80%; ventricular septal defect, patent arterial duct, atrial septal defect.	Wyllie et al., 1994.
Pena-Shokeir syndrome	Multiple ankyloses, pulmonary hypoplasia, intra-uterine growth retardation, hypertelorism, micrognathia, short neck, low set ears.	Some recessive (10–15%). Some due to maternal anti-acetylcholine receptor antibodies.	Many occasionally described, including atrial septal defect, coarctation and hypoplastic heart.	Brueton et al., 2000.
Percin syndrome	Skin syndactyly of the fingers and toes, cleft lip.	Autosomal dominant, with a father and two daughters reported.	Atrial septum defect, tetralogy of Fallot.	Percin et al., 1995.
Peters anomaly-congenital heart defect	Peters anomaly of eye with sclerocornea, glaucoma, iris dysplasia.	Sporadic.	Tetralogy of Fallot, duplicated/right aortic arch, dextrocardia, ventricular septal defect.	Chen and D'Souza, 1990.
Peters-plus syndrome (Krause-Kivlin syndrome)	Peters anomaly, short stature, short limbs, brachydactyly, round face, thin lip, long philtrum, mental retardation, occasional cleft lip/palate, renal abnormalies.	Autosomal recessive.	Atrial septal defect, ventricular septal defect, pulmonary stenosis, subvalvular aortic stenosis.	Hennekam et al., 1993. Thompson et al., 1993.
Pfeiffer type cardiocranial syndrome	Sagittal craniostenosis, growth retardation, joint contractures, mental retardation, occasional renal anomalies, limited mouth opening.	? Autosomal recessive.	Atrial septal defect, tetralogy of Fallot, ventricular septal defect, persistent arterial duct, pulmonary stenosis.	Digilio et al., 1997.
Pfeiffer-Singer-Zschiesche syndrome	Saggital craniosynostosis, failure to thrive, joint contractures, developmental delay, hypertelorism, micrognathia, low-set ears, submucous cleft palate, hypoplastic kidneys, abnormal ribs.	Uncertain. ? autosomal recessive.	Atrial septal defect, ventricular septum defect, patent ductus arteriosus, tetralogy of Fallot, peripheral pulmonary stenosis, and an azygous vein.	Willamson-Kruse and Biesecker, 1995.
PHAVER syndrome	Pterygia, heart defects, autosomal recessive inheritance, vertebral defects, ear anomalies and radial defects.	Autosomal recessive.	Ventricular septum defect, atrial septum defect, hypoplastic aortic arch, double outlet right ventricle, pulmonary atresia.	Powell et al., 1993.
Poland syndrome	Unilateral terminal limb, reduction defect, ipsilateral absent sternal head of pectoralis major, microcephaly, renal agenesis, diaphragmatic hernia.	Usually sporadic.	Dextrocardia, stenosis of left subclavian artery.	Bamforth et al., 1992.

continued

Appendix 47.1 (*continued*)

Syndrome name	Clinical features	Etiology	Cardiac defects	Key reference
Polydactyly postaxial with dental and vertebral anomalies	Postaxial polydactyly, hypoplasia and fusion vertebral bodies, teeth large, of reduced number with defective enamel, broad toes, submucous cleft.	Autosomal recessive.	Right ventricular outflow murmurs in 2, in 1 a common arterial trunk giving rise to 2 pulmonary arteries.	Rogers et al., 1977.
Progeria syndrome (Hutchinson-Gilford syndrome)	Premature aging leading to growth failure, loss of subcutaneous fat, hair and teeth, atrophic skin.	Mostly sporadic; autosomal dominant mutations, possible autosomal recessive forms.	Coronary artery disease, general atherosclerosis, congestive heart failure, cerebrovascular accident.	Badame 1989.
Prune belly-pulmonary stenosis-deafness-mental retardation	Prune belly syndrome, sensorineural deafness, mental retardation, hydronephrosis.	Autosomal recessive.	Pulmonary stenosis.	Lockhart et al., 1979.
Pseudo-Hurler polydystrophy (mucolipidosis III)	Coarse face, corneal opacities, mild retardation, stiff joints, short stature, lysosomal enzymes high in serum, low in fibroblasts.	Autosomal recessive.	Aortic regurgitation due to valve involvement.	Kelly et al., 1975.
Pseudoxanthoma elasticum	Flexural cutaneous yellowish papular lesions, mild skin redundancy, retinal angioid streaks, chorioretinopathy.	Autosomal dominant and recessive forms; both due to, *ABCC6*, at 16p13.	Angina, claudication, hypertension, cerebrovascular accidents, possible mitral valve prolapse, restrictive cardiomyopathy.	Ringpfeil et al., 2000.
Rabenhorst syndrome (cardio-acro-facial syndrome)	Narrow face, micrognathia, prominent narrow nasal bridge, small mouth, hand and feet anomalies.	Probable autosomal dominant (father and daughter).	Ventricular septal defect, pulmonary stenosis.	Grosse, 1974.
Reardon syndrome	Rhizomelic limb shortening, flared metaphyses, flared iliac wings, narrow thorax, coronal clefts of vertebrae.	Probably autosomal recessive.	Hypoplastic right ventricle, pulmonary atresia, atrial septal defect, ventricular septal defect.	Reardon et al., 1990.
Refsum disease	Retinal pigmentary degeneration, chronic polyneuropathy, ataxia, occasional sensorineural deafness, ichthyosis.	Autosomal recessive; defect in *PAHX* (or *PHYH*) gene at 10p.	ECG abnormalities: ST, T wave changes, conduction defects; congestive cardiomyopathy.	Steinberg, 1995. Mihalik et al., 1997. Jansen et al.,1997.
Renal-hepatic-pancreatic dysplasia	Cystic renal dysplasia, pancreas cystofibrosis, biliary dysgenesis and hepatic fibrosis, occasional a-/poly splenia, situs inversus.	Some autosomal recessive.	Hypoplastic left ventricle, transposition of great arteries, patent foramen ovale, persistent arterial duct.	Crawfurd, 1978. Lurie et al., 1991.
Rett syndrome	Regression from 6 months, loss of social and motor skills, hand wringing, gait ataxia, epilepsy, late spasticity.	X-linked dominant. Mutations in methyl-CpG-binding protein-2 (MECP2) at Xq28	Long QT and T wave abnormalities. ? Sudden death.	Amir et al., 1999

continued

Appendix 47.1 (*continued*)

Syndrome name	Clinical features	Etiology	Cardiac defects	Key reference
Ritscher-Schinzel syndrome (3C syndrome)	Dandy Walker malformation or variant, macrocephaly, large fontanelles, hypertelorism, downslanting eyes, mental retardation, hypotonia, growth delay; occasional coloboma.	Autosomal recessive.	Ventricular septal defect, atrial septal defect, atrioventricular septal defect, tetralogy of Fallot; other various defects reported.	Lurie and Ferencz, 1996. Kosaki et al., 1997. Orstavik et al., 1998.
Roberts syndrome (pseudothalidomide (SC) syndrome)	Variable reduction limb defects, growth delay, cleft lip and palate, hypertelonism, delay, renal defects, neonatal death, premature centromere separation.	Autosomal recessive.	Patent ductus arteriosus, ventricular septal defect, atrial septal defect; aortic and pulmonary valve stenosis, coarctation, aortic arch-atresia reported.	Van den Berg and Francke, 1993.
Robin sequence Pierre-Robin syndrome	Micrognathia, posterior horse-shoe-shaped cleft palate, posterior displacement of tongue (small jaw displaces tongue which prevents palate closure).	Most are sporadic.	Heart defects strongly associated	Hanson and Smith, 1975.
Robin sequence-Persistence of left superior vena cava	Robin sequence, talipes equinovarus.	X-linked.	Left sided superior vena cava, atrial septal defect.	Gorlin et al., 1970.
Robinow syndrome	Short-limbed dwarfism, "fetal" face, broad forehead, hypertelorism, small up-turned nose, wide mouth, thick gums, micropenis, hemi-vertebrae.	Heterogeneous; autosomal dominant and recessive forms described.	Heart defects, including tetralogy of Fallot are described.	Robinow, 1993. Atalay et al., 1993. Sabry et al., 1997.
Romano-Ward syndrome (long QT syndrome)	Recurrent syncope, sudden death.	Autosomal dominant; heterozygous mutations in *KVLQT1* at 11p15, *HERG* at 7q3, *SCN5A* 3p2, or *KCNE1* at 21q22, 1 unidentified gene at 4q2	Prolonged QT interval, ventricular arrhythmias.	Burn et al., 1997. Moss et al., 1991. Zareba et al., 1998.
Rommen syndrome	Mental retardation, failure to thrive, microcephaly, hypotonia, seizures, down slanting palpebralfissures, prominent ears.	Single report, 2 brothers.	Tetralogy of Fallot.	Rommen et al., 1983.
Rubinstein-Taybi syndrome	Developmental delay, broad deviated thumbs and great toes, short stature, microcephaly, downslanting eyes, beaked nose with nasal septum extending below nasal alae.	Autosomal dominant; mutations in *CBP* at 16p13. About 10% have a deletion.	38%, mainly ventricular septal defect, persistent arterial duct, aortic valve anomalies, coarctation.	Stevens and Bhakta, 1995.

continued

Appendix 47.1 (*continued*)

Syndrome name	Clinical features	Etiology	Cardiac defects	Key reference
Ruvalcaba syndrome	Mental retardation, microcephaly, short stature, hooked nose, downslanting eyes, small mouth and alae nasi, short fingers, cone-shaped epiphysis, osteochondritis of spine, occasional craniosynostosis.	Autosomal dominant.	Atrial septal defect, pulmonary stenosis.	Bialer et al., 1989.
Saethre-Chotzen syndrome	Coronal synostosis, brachycephaly, low frontal hairline, facial asymmetry, ptosis, broad great toes, skin syndactyly, prominent ear crus, variable development delay.	Autosomal dominant; defects in *Twist* at 7p21 or in *FGFR2* or *FGFR3*	Occasional heart defect described.	Paznekas et al., 1998.
Sanfilippo syndrome (mucopolysaccharidosis type III)	Intellectual deterioration, behavior problems, mild coarse face, hirsutism, mild dysostosis multiplex.	Autosomal recessive; gene defects in *HSS* at 17q25 (type A), *NAGLU* at 17q21 (B), *GNS* at 12q14 (D), acetylCoA alpha-glucosaminide acetyl-transferase(C).	Mitral valve thickening leading to incompetence.	Zhao et al., 1996.
Scheie syndrome (mucopolysaccharidosis type I S)	Broad mouth, full lips, big jaw, cloudy corneas, stiff joints, occasional hepatomegaly and hearing loss, carpal tunnel syndrome.	Autosomal recessive; defect in *IDUA* at 4p16.	Aortic valve stenosis and incompetence	Neufeld and Muenzen, 1995.
Schinzel-Giedion syndrome	Mental retardation, severe midface hypoplasia, patent ductus, hirsutism, hydronephrosis, genital anomalies, skeletal anomalies, choanal stenosis, brain malformations, sacrococcygeal tumors.	Probably autosomal recessive.	Mainly atrial septal defect, persistent arterial duct, valve anomalies reported.	Elliott et al., 1996.
Short rib-polydactyly syndrome type 1 (Saldino-Noonan)	Hydrops, neonatal death, short ribs, ulnar polydactyly, short tubular bones, metaphyseal irregularities, rounded scapulae, vertebral and pelvis anomalies; possible renal, intestinal, genitourinary malformations, sex-reversal in males.	Autosomal recessive.	Variety of heart defects including transposition of great arteries, coarctation, ventricular septal defect.	Martinez-Frias et al., 1993.
Short rib-polydactyly syndrome type 2 (Majewski)	Hydrops, neonatal death, short ribs, pre/postaxial polydactyly, midline cleft upper lip, short ovoid tibia; possible intestinal, renourinary, cerebral malformations, ambiguous genitalia, cleft palate.	Autosomal recessive.	Atrioventricular septal defect, coarctation/interrupted aorta, ventricular septal defect.	Digilio et al., 1997.

continued

Appendix 47.1 (*continued*)

Syndrome name	Clinical features	Etiology	Cardiac defects	Key reference
Short rib-polydactyly syndrome type 3 (Verma-Naumoff)	Hydrops, neonatal death, short ribs, ulnar polydactyly, short tubular bones, metaphyseal irregularities, shortened cranial base, vertebral and pelvis anomalies; possible renal, intestinal, genito-urinary malformations, sex reversal in males.	Autosomal recessive.	Dextocardia/situs inversus, hypoplastic left heart, patent ductus arteriosus, ventricular septal defect.	Bernstein et al., 1985.
Short rib-polydactyly syndrome type 4 (Beemer-Langer syndrome)	Hydrops, short ribs, short tubular bones, bowed radii and ulnae, variable polydactyly, median cleft lip; possible renal, genital and cerebral malformations, omphalocele and cleft palate; neonatal death.	Autosomal recessive.	Aortic arch atresia, coarctation, transposition of great arteries, ventricular septal defect, atrial septal defect, patent ductus arteriosus.	Lurie, 1994. Chen et al., 1994.
SHORT syndrome	Short stature, hyperextensible joints, ocular depression, rieger anomaly (anterior chamber of the eye), teeth delayed.	Autosomal recessive.	Hypoplastic left heart, heart tumors.	Sorge et al., 1996.
Shprintzen-Goldberg syndrome	Craniosynostosis, exomphalos, maxillary & mandibular hypoplasia, abdominal hernias, arachnodactyly. camptodactyly, learning disability, marfanoid physique.	Sporadic cases. Mutations in *FBN1* (same gene as for Marfan syndrome)	Mitral incompetance.	Megarban and Hokayem,1998.
Shwachman syndrome	Exocrine pancreatic insufficiency, failure to thrive, bone marrow dysfunction, pancytopenia, short-limbed drawfism with metaphyseal changes, occasional ichthyotic rash, mental retardation.	Autosomal recessive.	Cardiac failure due to myocardial lesions, endocardial fibrosis reported.	Mack et al., 1996.
Simpson-Golabi-Behmel syndrome	Pre- and post-natal overgrowth, coarse facies, hypertelorism, broad nose, wide mouth, macroglossia, prominent jaw, broad hands, cleft/high palate, extra nipples, occasional hypoplastic finger nails, polydactyly, hernias, renal tract abnormalities, mild mental retardation, embryonal tumors, sudden death.	X-linked; defect in glypican 3 gene at Xq26.	Conduction defects, tachyarrhythmia, malformations mainly ventricular septal defect, atrial septal defect, pulmonary stenosis.	Pilia et al., 1996.

continued

Appendix 47.1 (*continued*)

Syndrome name	Clinical features	Etiology	Cardiac defects	Key reference
Singleton-Merten syndrome	Dental dysplasia, osteoporosis, expanded medullary cavities of hand bonds, occasional short stature.	Autosomal dominant (variable expression).	Progressive calcification of aortic arch and aortic valve, high mortality.	Feigenbaum et al., 1988.
Sinus node disease and myopia	Degenerative myopia with atrophy of choroid and pigmentary epithelium.	?Autosomal dominant (father, son and daughter).	Sick sinus syndrome.	Onat, 1986.
Smith-Lemli-Opitz syndrome (includes types I and II)	Mental retardation, failure to thrive, feeding difficulties, premature death, microcephaly, micrognathia, ptosis, anteverted nostrils, 2/3 syndactyly of toes, broad alveolar ridges, short stature, genital anomalies; occassional polydactyly, cleft palate, various other visceral malformations, cataract.	Autosomal recessive; defect in the 7-dehydrocholesterol reductase gene at 11q12–15.	Mainly atrioventricular canal, atrial septal defect, patent ductus arteriosus, ventricular septal defect, anomalous pulmonary venous return, coarctation, aortic stenosis, hypoplastic left heart, tetralogy of Fallot reported.	Ryan et al., 1998. Wassif et al., 1998.
Smith-Magenis syndrome	Severe developmental delay and self destructive behavior, disturbed sleep pattern, short and plump, brachydactyly, deaf, scoliosis, renal anomalies.	Microdeletion 17p11.2.	37% cardiac defects, atrioventricular septal defects, atrial septal defect, aortic stenosis, pulmonary stenosis, ventricular septal defect.	Greenberg et al., 1996.
Sonoda syndrome	Short stature, developmental delay, round face, depressed nasal bridge, small mouth.	Autosomal recessive.	Pulmonary stenosis, ventricular septal defect, hypospadias.	Sonoda et al., 1988.
Sotos (cerebral gigantism) syndrome	Pre- and postnatal overgrowth, macrocephaly, prominent forehead, down slanting palpebral fissures, pointed chin, mental retardation.	Mostly sporadic; occasional autosomal dominant.	Atrial septal defect, ventricular septal defect, patent arterial duct. Tricuspid/pulmonary atresia.	Noreau et al., 1998.
Spinal muscular atrophy with contractures and congenital heart disease	Spinal muscular atrophy, arhinencephaly.	Autosomal recessive.	Atrial septal defect, valvular aortic stenosis.	Moller et al., 1990.
Spondyloepimetaphyseal dysplasia with joint laxity	Short stature, joint laxity, kyphoscoliosis, dislocation of radial heads, talipes, spatulate terminal phalanges, oval face, long upper lip, prominent eyes, blue sclerae, soft hyperelastic skin, occasional cleft palate, dislocation of hip.	Autosomal recessive.	Mitral valve incompetence, ventricular septal defect, atrial septal defect.	Beighton et al., 1994.
Sturge-Weber syndrome	Facial capillary hemangioma, glaucoma, epilepsy, retardation, intracranial calcification.	Sporadic.	Leptomeningeal angioma.	Griffiths, 1996.

continued

Appendix 47.1 (*continued*)

Syndrome name	Clinical features	Etiology	Cardiac defects	Key reference
ter Haar syndrome	Prominent eyes, congenital glaucoma, prominent forehead, micrognathia, brachycephaly, hypertelorism, wide fontanelle, brachydactyly, metaphyseal flaring, bowed tibiae and radii, irregular ribs.	Probably autosomal recessive.	Double outlet right ventricle, persistent arterial duct, ventricular septal defect, mitral valve prolapse.	Wallerstein et al., 1997.
Thakker-Donnai syndrome	Hypertelorism, down slanting palpebral fissures, broad nasal bridge, hydrocephalus, agenesis of corpus callosum, vertebral anomalies, diaphragmatic hernia, anal atresia.	Autosomal recessive.	Transposition of great arteries, tetralogy of Fallot, ventricular septal defect.	Thakker and Donnai, 1991.
Thanatophoric dysplasia	Severe short-limbed dwarfism, narrowed chest, neonatal death, macrocephaly, depressed nasal bridge, curved short femurs, metaphyseal flaring, H-shaped flattened vertebrae, brain anomalies; occasional cloverleaf skull.	Autosomal dominant; defect in *FGFR3* at 4p16.	Atrial septal defect, persistent ductus arteriosus, 1 case of great artery "abnormality".	Wilcox et al., 1998.
Thiamine-responsive megaloblastic anemia syndrome (Rogers syndrome)	Sensorineural hearing loss, diabetes, thiamine responsive megaloblastic anemia, decreased activity of ketoglutarate dehydrogenase.	Autosomal recessive; gene mapped to 1q23. Probable defect in thiamine transporter protein.	Ventricular septal defects, atrioventricular septal defect, situs inversus.	Neufeld et al., 1997.
Thomas syndrome	Renal hypoplasia, dysplasia, agenesis, cleft lip/palate (resembles Holzgreve syndrome).	Autosomal recessive.	Hypoplastic left heart sequence, common atrium, truncus arteriosus, persistent arterial duct, tetralogy of Fallot, ventricular septal defect, coarctation, hypertrophic cardiomyopathy.	Zlotogora et al., 1996.
Thoracoabdominal syndrome	Diaphragmatic hernia, hypoplastic lungs, ventral hernia (including female carriers).	X-linked dominant, gene mapped to Xq25–q26.	Hypoplastic pulmonary artery, transposition of great arteries, persistent arterial duct, total anomalous pulmonary drainage, hypoplastic left heart, ventricular septal defect.	Parvari et al., 1996.

continued

Appendix 47.1 (*continued*)

Syndrome name	Clinical features	Etiology	Cardiac defects	Key reference
Thrombocytopenia-absent radius (TAR) syndrome	Bilateral absent radius, ulnar hypoplasia, thumbs present, occasionally (7%) mentally retarded, squint, small jaw.	Autosomal recessive.	33% have congenital heart defect including tetralogy of Fallot and atrial septal defect.	Hall, 1987.
Toriello-Carey syndrome	Agenesis corpus callosum, short palpabal fissures, telecanthus, micrognathia, cleft palate, brachydactyly, hypotonia, learning disability.	Autosomal recessive.	Atrial septal defect, persistent arterial duct, cardiomyopathy, pulmonary stenosis.	Lacombe et al., 1992.
Townes-Brocks syndrome	Triphalangeal thumbs, imperforate anus, overfolded ear helices, sensorineural deafness, pes planus, preauricular tags, renal agenesis.	Autosomal dominant. Probable gene is *SALL1*, a transcription factor at 16q12.1.	Truncus arteriosus, ventricular septal defect.	Powell and Michaelis, 1999.
Treacher-Collins syndrome (mandibulofacial dystosis)	Mandibular and malar hypoplasia, malformed ears, deafness, down-slanting eyes, lower eyelid colobomata, cleft palate.	Autosomal dominant; defect in *TCOF1* on 5q leading to haplo-insufficiency.	Unspecified heart defects seen on occasion.	Dixon, 1995, 1996. Gladwin et al., 1996.
Trigonocephaly C syndrome (Opitz C syndrome)	Mental retardation, metopic ridge, broad alveolar ridges, up-slanting eyes, epicanthus, forehead hemangioma, up-turned nose, loose skin, joint, kidney, genital and brain anomalies.	Autosomal recessive.	Variety of defects including persistent arterial duct, ventricular septal defect, tetralogy of Fallot.	Glickstein et al., 1995.
Tuberous sclerosis	Depigmented skin patches, adenoma sebaceum, periungual fibromas, renal tumor, dental pits, mental retardation, seizures, cerebral lesions, occasional polycystic kidney disease.	Autosomal dominant; defects in hamartin gene at 9q34 (*TSC1*), or in tuberin gene at 16q13 (*TSC2*).	Cardiac rhabdomyomas, Wolff-Parkinson-White syndrome.	Van Slegtenhorst et al., 1997.
Turner syndrome	Short stature, gonadal dysgenesis, broad chest, widely spaced nipples, webbed neck, congenital lymphedema, renal anomalies.	Sporadic. 45X	Coarctation of the aorta, aortic valve anomalies, partial anomalous pulmonary venous drainage, ascending aortic aneurysm.	Gotzsche and Krag-Olsen, 1994.
VACTERL syndrome	Acronym–vertebral anomalies, anal atresia, cardiac defects, tracheo-esophageal fistula, renal anomalies, limb reduction defects (radial).	Sporadic? early generally disruption of development. 1 report of associated mitochondrial mutation.	Variety of defects: ventricular septal defects most common.	Damian et al., 1996.

continued

Appendix 47.1 (*continued*)

Syndrome name	Clinical features	Etiology	Cardiac defects	Key reference
Van Allen-Myhre syndrome	Exomphalos, absent anterior diaphragm, absent sacrum, limb defects, microphthalmia, skin defects.	Probable autosomal recessive.	Ectopia cordis, primum atrial septal defect.	Van Allen and Myhre, 1991.
Van Bever syndrome	Limited supination of forearms due to subluxated radial heads, scoliosis, carpal fusions.	Autosomal dominant.	Septal defects, mitral valve prolapse, conduction defects.	Van Bever et al., 1998.
Varadi syndrome	Bifid big toes, ulnar polydactyly, cleft lip/palate, lingual nodules, growth and mental retardation.	Autosomal recessive.	Aortic stenosis described.	Varadi et al., 1980.
Velo-cardio-facial syndrome (Shprintzen syndrome)	Cleft palate, nasal voice, narrow almond shaped palpebral fissues, bulbous nasal tip, small open mouth, micrognathia, short stature, slender fingers, mild retardation, occasional renal abnormalities, psychiatric disturbance.	22q11 deletion; dominantly inherited in-10% cases.	Ventricular septal defect, tetralogy of Fallot, pulmonary atresia.	Ryan et al., 1997.
Ventricular extrasystoles–plus (heart hand II)	Short stature, microcephaly, mental retardation, patchy skin pigmentation, hypertelorism, premature loss of teeth.	Possible autosomal dominant.	Multifocal ventricular ectopic beats.	Char et al., 1975.
Verloove-Vanhorick syndrome	Cleft lip and palate, micrognathia, short femori and humeri. Absent metacarpal/metatarsal, syndactyly, horseshoe kidney, cryptorchidism.	Autosomal recessive.	Common arterial trunk.	Verloove et al., 1981.
Von Hippel-Lindau syndrome	Retinal angiomata, cerebellar hemangioblastoma, spinal hemangioma, cysts of pancreas, liver and/or kidneys, phaeochromocystoma, renal carcinoma.	Autosomal dominant, defect in *VHL* at 3p2.	Vascular abnormalities, hypertension associated with hypernephroma or phaechromocytoma.	Maddock et al., 1996.
Waardenburg syndrome	White forelock, sensorineural deafness, heterochromia of iris, telecanthus, occasional cleft palate and Hirschsprung disease.	Autosomal dominant; heterogeneous, defects in *PAX3* at 2q35 (WS1,3), in *MITF* at 3p1 (15% of WS2), *EDN3* at 20q13, *EDNRB* at 13q22, *SOX 10* at 22q13 (WS4).	Occasional heart defect of various type.	Read and Newton, 1997.
Watson syndrome	Cafe au lait patches, axillary freckling, mental retardation, short stature.	Autosomal dominant; allelic to NF-1.	Pulmonary stenosis.	Upadhyaya et al., 1992.

continued

Appendix 47.1 (*continued*)

Syndrome name	Clinical features	Etiology	Cardiac defects	Key reference
Webbed neck-facial dysmorphism-congenital heart disease	Short stature, macrocephaly, short webbed neck, incurved little finger, pectus carinatum or excavatum, down-slanting palpebral fissures, arched eyebrows, hypoplastic supraorbital ridges, large nose, low-set ears, mental retardation.	Autosomal recessive.	Atrial septal defect, ventricular septum defect.	Al-Gazali et al., 1996.
Weill-Marchesani syndrome	Short stature, brachydactyly, myopia, glaucoma, dislocated and/or spherical lenses, joint stiffness.	Heterogeneous; autosomal recessive forms, autosomal dominant forms with one gene mapped to 15q21.	Cases of infundibular pulmonary stenosis, ventricular septal defect, persistent arterial duct and subvalvular aortic stenosis described.	Wirtz et al., 1996.
Werner syndrome	Arrest of growth at puberty, cataracts, premature graying and balding, muscle wasting, diabetes mellitus, hypogonadism, soft tissue calcification, atrophic skin.	Autosomal recessive; defect in WRN gene at 8p1, a helicase involved in DNA unwinding and repair and chromosome segregation.	Premature arteriosclerosis leading to congestive heart failure, valvular sclerosis.	Yu et al., 1996.
White forelock with multiple abnormalities	White forelock, hypertelorism, blue sclerae, epicanthic folds, high palate, prominent philtrum, clinodactyly, joint hyperlaxity. Resembles Kabuki syndrome.	Single report, 2 brothers.	Atrial septal defect.	Goodman et al., 1980.
Wiedemann-Rautenstrauch (neonatal progeria) syndrome.	Low birth weight, aged appearance from birth, pinched features, development delay, sparse hair, lack of subcutaneous fat apart from pads over buttocks.	Autosomal recessive.	Atrial septal defect, ventricular septal defect.	Hagadorn et al., 1990.
Williams syndrome	Mild/moderate mental retardation, friendly personality, infantile hypercalcemia, stellate iris, full cheeks, wide mouth, thick lips, malar flattening, periorbital fullness, hyperacusis.	Probable contiguous gene syndrome due to dominantly inherited deletion of 7q11 encompassing *ELN* and LIMK1	Supravalvular aortic stenosis, peripheral pulmonary artery stenosis.	Wu et al., 1998.
Wolf-Hirschhorn syndrome	Growth deficiency, severe mental retardation, microcephaly, seizures, hypertelorism, prominent glabella, highly arched eyebrows, proptosis, strabismus, cleft lip/palate, agenesis of corpus callosum, talipes, hypospadias, cryptorchidism.	Sporadic; *de novo* deletion in a 165 kb critical region translocations in 10–15 % cases.	Ventricular septal defect, atrial septal defect.	Stec et al., 1998.

continued

Appendix 47.1 (*continued*)

Syndrome name	Clinical features	Etiology	Cardiac defects	Key reference
Woodhouse syndrome	Hypogonadism, sparse hair and eyebrows, diabetes mellitus, mental retardation, deafness, failure of female sexual maturation, short stature.	Autosomal recessive.	Variable ST depression and T wave abnormalities.	Woodhouse and Sakati, 1983.
X-linked laterality sequence	Laterality anomaly, poly-/asplenia, spina bifida, cerebral malformations, sacral agenesis.	X-linked; defect in gene *Zic3* at Xq26.	Complex defects including total anomalous pulmonary venous drainage, common atrium, atrioventricular septal defect, transposition of the great arteries, pulmonary atresia, interrupted inferior vena cava.	Gebbia et al., 1997.
Young-Madders syndrome	Holoprosencephaly, microphthalmos, cryptorchidism, post-axial polydactyly, choanal stenosis.	Uncertain, ? Recessive.	Dextrocardia, atrial septal defect, ventricular septal defect, atrioventricular septal defect.	Hennekam et al., 1991.
Young-Simpson syndrome	Microcephaly, blepharophimosis, low set posteriorly rotated ears, micrognathia, hypothyroidism.	Uncertain. Possibly autosomal recessive.	Atrioventricular septal defect, atrial and ventricular septal defect.	Bonthron et al., 1993.
Yunis-Varon syndrome	Dolichocephaly, wide anterior fontanelles, sparse hair, dysmorphic, thin lips, short philtrum, micrognathia, absent thumbs, hypoplastic clavicles.	Autosomal recessive.	Tetralogy of Fallot, cardiomyopathy.	Ades et al., 1993.
Zellweger syndrome	Severe hypotonia and retardation, large fontanelle, high forehead, up-slanting eyes, epicanthic folds, hypoplastic supra-orbital ridges, seizures, hepatomegaly, stippled epiphyses, renal cysts, deafness, retinal dysfunction.	Autosomal recessive; hetero-geneous, defects in several different genes involved in peroxisome biogenesis, mainly *PEX1* at 7q2.	Persistent arterial duct, ventricular septal defect, various anomalies of aorta.	Reuber et al., 1997.

Heart defects and mental retardation/abnormal face (major)

Syndrome name

Acrocallosal syndrome	Hurler syndrome
Alagille syndrome arteriohepatic dysplasia	Hydrolethalus
Asymmetric crying face syndrome	LEOPARD syndrome
Beckwith-Wiedemann syndrome	Manzke syndrome, digitopalatal syndrome
Campomelic dysplasia syndrome	Maternal phenylketonuria disruption syndrome

continued

Heart defects and mental retardation/abnormal face (major) (continued)

Syndrome name

Cardio facio cutaneous syndrome	Meckel syndrome
Carpenter syndrome	Miller Dieker syndrome, lissencephaly syndrome
CATCH syndrome (DiGeorge syndrome)	Mulibrey Nanism syndrome
CHARGE syndrome	Noonan syndrome
Cohen syndrome	Noonan-neurofibromatosis syndrome
Conotruncal anomaly face syndrome	Patau's syndrome
Costello syndrome	Pompe's disease, glycogen storage disease type IIA
Cri du chat syndrome (5p-)	Pseudo-Hurler polydystrophy, mucolipidosis III
De Lange syndrome	Rubinstein-Taybi syndrome
Down syndrome	Smith-Lemli-Opitz syndrome
Edward's syndrome (Trisomy 18)	Smith-Magenis syndrome
Fetal alcohol syndrome	Sotos (cerebral gigantism) syndrome
Fetal hydantoin syndrome	Turner syndrome
Fragile X syndrome	Velo-cardio-facial syndrome, Shprintzen syndrome
Goldenhar syndrome	Williams syndrome
Goltz syndrome	Wolf-Hirschhorn syndrome
Heart-hand IV syndrome	Zellweger syndrome, cerebrohepatorenal syndrome
Hunter syndrome	

Heart defects and mental retardation/abnormal face (minor)

Syndrome name

Aase Smith syndrome	Cardiomyopathy, mental retardation autophagic myopathy
Acrofacial dysostosis (Miller) syndrome	Cerebellar hypoplasia-lymphedema-neuronal migration defect
Acromicric dysplasia syndrome	Cerebro-costo-mandibular syndrome
Adams-Oliver syndrome	Cerebro-facio-thoracic dysplasia
Aglossia-situs inversus	Char syndrome
Agnathia-holoprosencephaly agnathia	Chromosome 16 maternal disomy
Malformation C	Coffin Siris syndrome
Aldolase A deficiency	Collins syndrome
Alstrom syndrome	Congenital hypothyroidism
Antley-Bixler syndrome	Conradi Hunerman syndrome
Apert syndrome	Conradi syndrome
Atkin syndrome (oculo cerebro acral syndrome)	Cranioectodermal dysplasia syndrome
Atrial septal defect–lymphedema	C-trigonocephaly syndrome (Opitz C syndrome)
Auralcephalosyndactyly syndrome	Cutis laxa syndrome (recessive form)
Baller Gerold syndrome	DOOR syndrome (acronym)
Baraitser-Winter syndrome	Early amnion rupture syndrome
Barrow syndrome	Faciocardiomelic syndrome
Basal cell nevus syndrome	Facio-cardio-renal syndrome
Behmel syndrome	Fanconi syndrome
Beighton type spondyloepimetaphyseal dysplasia	Femoral hypoplasia–unusual facies syndrome
Berardinelli syndrome (generalized lipodystrophy)	Fetal aminopterin syndrome
Bindewald syndrome	Fetal thalidomide syndrome
Bonneau syndrome	Fetal toxoplasmosis syndrome
Bonnemann-Meinecke syndrome	Fetal trimethadione syndrome
Bowen syndrome	Fetal valproate syndrome
Burn McKeown syndrome	Fetal vitamin A syndrome
Carbohydrate deficient glycoprotein syndrome, type 1A	Fetal warfarin syndrome
(Jaeken syndrome)	FG syndrome (Opitz Kaveggia syndrome)
Carbohydrate deficient glycoprotein syndrome, type II	Fraser syndrome
Frontonasal dysplasia	Neish-Roberts syndrome
Frontonasal dysplasia with tetralogy of Fallot	Neurofibromatosis syndrome
Fryns syndrome	Oculo-facio-cardio-dental syndrome
Fucosidosis	Ohdo syndrome
Gastrocutaneous syndrome	Onat syndrome
Geleophysic syndrome	Opitz G/BBB syndrome
Golabi Ito syndrome	Oral-cardiac-digital syndrome
Goodman syndrome	Oral-cardiac-digital syndrome type II (Mohr syndrome)

continued

Heart defects and mental retardation/abnormal face (minor) (continued)

Syndrome Name

Gorlin-Chaudhary-Moss syndrome
Grix syndrome
Hadju-Cheney syndrome
Hallerman-Streiff syndrome
Hay-Wells syndrome
Hemifacial microsomia radial defects
Hennekam syndrome
Holmes Schimke syndrome
Homocystinuria
Horst syndrome
Hypertelorism-microtia-clefting
Hypertrichosis-osteochondrodysplasia Ieshima syndrome
Jennings syndrome
Johnson-Blizzard syndrome
Johnson syndrome
Jones syndrome
Kakubi make-up syndrome
Kawashima syndrome
Killian Pallister syndrome
Klippel-Feil syndrome
Klippel-Trenaunay-Weber syndrome
Kousseff syndrome
Krause Kivlin syndrome
Lambert syndrome
Laurence-Moon-Biedl syndrome
Lebenthal syndrome
Lenz microthalamia syndrome
Limb reduction ichthyosis syndrome
Linear sebaceous nevus syndrome
Lin-Gettig syndrome (spondylothoracic dysplasia)
Lowry-MacLean syndrome
Lujan syndrome
Lyon syndrome
Majewski syndrome short rib-polydactyly syndrome I
Mandibulofacial dystosis
Marden Walker syndrome
Maroteaux-Lamy syndrome
Marshall-Smith syndrome
Maternal diabetes disruption syndrome
McDonough syndrome
Microcephaly-cardiomyopathy
Mietens syndrome
Morquio syndrome, mucopolysaccharidosis
Mucke syndrome
Mucolipidosis II (I cell disease)
Mutchinick syndrome
Myotonic dystrophy syndrome
Najjar syndrome

Osteogenesis imperfecta
Osteogenesis imperfecta-microcephaly-cataracts
Pallister-Hall syndrome
Palmer Pagon syndrome
Pena-Shokeir syndrome
Percin syndrome
Pfeiffer-Singer-Zschiesche syndrome
Rabenhorst syndrome, cardio-acro-facial syndrome
Ritscher-Schinzel syndrome
Robin sequence–persistence of left superior vena cava
Robin sequence, Pierre Robin syndrome
Robinow syndrome
Rogers syndrome
Rutledge syndrome
Ruvalcaba syndrome
Saethre-Chotzen syndrome
Saito syndrome
Sanfilippo syndrome, mucopolysaccharidosis
Type III
Scheie syndrome, mucopolysaccaridosis IS
Schinzel-Giedion syndrome
Shprintzen-Goldberg syndrome
Simpson-Golabi-Behmel syndrome
Singleton-Merten syndrome
Sonada syndrome
Spinal muscular atrophy with contractures and congenital heart disease
Steinfield syndrome
Strong syndrome
Sturge Weber syndrome
Tamari Goodman syndrome
Thakker-Donnai syndrome
Thanatrophoric dysplasia syndrome
Thrombocytopenia-absent radius (TAR) syndrome
Toriello-Carey syndrome
Trigonocephaly C syndrome opitz C syndrome
Tuberous sclerosis syndrome
Varadi syndrome
Waadenburg syndrome
Watson syndrome
Webbed neck-facial dysmorphism-congenital heart disease
Werner syndrome
Wiedemann-Rautenstrauch (neonatal progeria) syndrome
Woodhouse syndrome
Young-Madders syndrome
Young-Simpson syndrome
Yunis-Varon syndrome
Zellweger syndrome Cerebrohepatorenal syndrome

Heart defects and limb reduction defects (major)

Syndrome name

Adams-Oliver syndrome
De Lange syndrome
Early amnion rupture syndrome
Fanconi syndrome
Goltz syndrome
Holt-Oram syndrome

Maternal diabetes disruption syndrome
Poland syndrome
Roberts syndrome, pseudothalidomide (SC) syndrome
Thrombocytopenia-absent radius (TAR) syndrome
VACTERL syndrome

Heart defects and limb reduction defects (minor)

Syndrome name

Acrofacial dysostosis (Miller syndrome)	Heart-hand III syndrome
Aplasia cutis, retinal folds, brain anomalies	Hemifacial microsomia radial defects
Atkin syndrome (Oculo cerebro acral syndrome)	Hollister syndrome
Baller Gerold syndrome	Keutel syndrome
Brachydactyly type E with ASD syndrome	Krause Kivlin syndrome
Coffin Siris syndrome	Limb reduction ichthyosis syndrome
Faciocardiomelic syndrome	Nagar acrofacial dysostosis
Fetal alcohol syndrome	Pena-Shokeir syndrome
Fetal aminopterin syndrome	PHAVER syndrome
Fetal hydantoin syndrome	Protonotarios syndrome
Fetal thalidomide	Saito syndrome
Fetal valproate syndrome	Shokeir syndrome
Fetal vitamin A syndrome	Steinfield syndrome
Hajdu-Cheney syndrome	ter Haar syndrome
Heart-hand II syndrome	Treacher Collins syndrome, mandibulofacial dystosis

Heart defects and polydactyly (major)

Syndrome name

Carpenter syndrome	Meckel syndrome
Ellis van Creveld syndrome	Orofacial digital syndrome Type II (Mohr syndrome)
Heart-hand IV syndrome	Saldino Noonan syndrome, short rib polydactyly I
Hydrolethalus syndrome	

Heart defects and polydactyly (minor)

Syndrome name

Acrocallosal syndrome	Majewski syndrome, short rib-polydactyly syndrome I
Anocerebrodigital syndrome, CNS hamartoblastoma syndrome	Mohr-Majewski syndrome
Basal cell nevus syndrome	Oral-cardiac-digital syndrome
Bonneau syndrome	Oral-facial-digital (OFD) syndrome type IV
C-trigonocephaly syndrome (Opitz C syndrome)	Pallister-Hall syndrome
Forney syndrome	Rogers syndrome
Hemifacial Microsomia radial defects	Schinzel-Giedion syndrome
Ho syndrome	Short rib polydactyly syndrome III
Holzgreve syndrome	Short rib polydactyly type II (Majewski)
Jeune thoracic dysplasia	Simpson-Golabi-Behmel syndrome
Kaufman-McKusick syndrome	Single atrium–polydactyly
Laurence syndrome	Smith-Lemli-Opitz syndrome
Laurence-Moon-Biedl syndrome	Varadi syndrome
	Young-Madders syndrome

Heart defects and other skeletal defects (major)

Syndrome name

Beighton type spondyloepimetaphyseal dysplasia	Jarcho-Levin syndrome (spondylothoracic dysplasia)
Campomelic dysplasia syndrome	Manzke syndrome, digitopalatal syndrome
Cardio facio cutaneous syndrome	Marfan syndrome
Carpenter syndrome	Maternal diabetes disruption syndrome
Ellis-van Creveld syndrome	Mulibrey Nanism syndrome
Goldenhar syndrome	Noonan syndrome
Homocystinuria	Rubinstein-Taybi syndrome

Heart defects and other skeletal defects (minor)

Syndrome name

Aase Smith syndrome	Kaufman syndrome
Aase syndrome	Klippel-Feil syndrome
Achard syndrome	Klippel-Trenaunay-Weber syndrome

continued

Heart defects and other skeletal defects (minor) (continued)

Syndrome name

Acrofacial dysostosis (Miller) syndrome	Jeune thoracic dysplasia
Acromicric dysplasia syndrome	Kozlowski syndrome
Adams-Oliver syndrome	Larsen syndrome
Alagille syndrome, arteriohepatic dysplasia	Lujan syndrome
Alkaptonuria syndrome	Majewski syndrome, short rib polydactyly syndrome I
Alstrom syndrome	Marden Walker syndrome
Antley-Bixley syndrome	Marfanoid hypermobility syndrome
Apert syndrome	Martinez syndrome
Astley Kendall syndrome	McDonough syndrome
Auralcephalosyndactyly syndrome	Microcephaly-cardiomyopathy
Barrow syndrome	Mietens syndrome
Barth syndrome, X-linked cardioskeletal myopathy	Morquio syndrome, mucopolysaccharidosis
Basal cell nevus syndrome	Mucolipidosis II (I cell disease)
Beal syndrome	Myhre syndrome
Beemer-Robinow syndrome	Noonan-like/multiple giant cell lesion
Brachydactyly type E with ASD syndrome	Omodysplasia
Camptodactyly-arthritis-pericarditis syndrome	Onat syndrome
Cerebro-costo-mandibular syndrome	Osteogenesis imperfecta-microcephaly-cataracts
Conradi Hunerman syndrome	Pfeiffer-Singer-Zschiesche syndrome
Conradi syndrome	Pseudo-Hurler polydystrophy, mucolipidosis III
Cranioectodermal dysplasia syndrome	Reardon syndrome
C-trigoncephaly syndrome (Opitz C syndrome)	Ritscher-Schinzel syndrome
Desmosterolosis	Robin sequence—persistence of left superior vena cava
Early amnion rupture syndrome	Robinow syndrome
Ebsteins anomaly-skeletal abnormalities	Ruvalcaba syndrome
Ectopia cordis-cleft lip and palate	Saethre-Chotzen syndrome
Femoral hypoplasia–unusual facies syndrome	Scheie syndrome, mucopolysaccharidosis IS
Fetal thalidomide	Schinzel-Giedion syndrome
Fetal vitamin A syndrome	Schwachman syndrome
Fetal warfarin syndrome	Short rib syndrome, Beemer-Langer type
Forney syndrome	Short rib polydactyly syndrome III
Fucosidosis	Short rib-polydactyly type 2 (majewski)
Gay syndrome	Singleton-Merten syndrome
Geleophysic syndrome	Tamari Goodman syndrome
Gorlin-Chaudhary-Moss syndrome	Ter Haar syndrome
Grix syndrome	Thanatophoric dysplasia syndrome
Hajdu-Cheney syndrome	Van Bever syndrome
Holmes Schimke syndrome	Verloove-Vanhorick syndrome
Hunter syndrome	Weil Marchesani syndrome
Hurler syndrome	Yunis-Varon syndrome
Hypertrichosis-osteochondrodysplasia	Zellweger syndrome cerebrohepatorenal syndrome

Heart defect and deafness/ear abnormalities (major)

Syndrome name

Beckwith-Wiedemann syndrome	Noonan syndrome
CHARGE syndrome	Patau's syndrome
DiGeorge syndrome	Townes-Brocks syndrome
Goldenhar syndrome	Treacher Collins syndrome, mandibulofacial dystosis
Jervell-Lange-Nielsen syndrome	Velo-cardio-facial syndrome, shprintzen syndrome
LEOPARD syndrome (acronym)	Waardenburg syndrome

Heart defect and deafness/ear abnormalities (minor)

Syndrome name

Acrofacial dysostosis (Miller) syndrome	Jennings syndrome
Agnathia-holoprosencephaly agnathia	Johanson-Blizzard syndrome
Malformation C	Johnson syndrome

continued

Heart Defect and Deafness/Ear Abnormalities (Minor) (continued)

Syndrome Name

Alstrom syndrome
Antley-Bixler syndrome
Apert syndrome
Atkin syndrome (oculo cerebro acral syndrome)
Auralcephalosyndactyly syndrome
Axial mesodermal dysplasia syndrome
Baller Gerold syndrome
Beal syndrome
Cardio-auditory syndrome of Sanchez-Cascos
Diabetes; ketoglutarate dehydrogenase deficiency;
DOOR syndrome (acronym)
Fanconi syndrome
Farag syndrome
Fetal cytomegalovirus syndrome
Fetal thalidomide
Fetal trimethadione syndrome
Fetal vitamin A syndrome
Forney syndrome
Fraser syndrome
Golabi Ito syndrome
Gorlin-Chaudhary-Moss syndrome
Hajdu-Cheney syndrome
Hemifacial microsomia radial defects
Hunter syndrome
Hurler syndrome

Hypertelorism–microtia–clefting Ieshima syndrome
Jones syndrome
Kartagener syndrome
Kawashima syndrome
Kearns-Sayre syndrome
Keutel syndrome
Klippel-Feil syndrome
Kousseff syndrome
Lenz microthalmia syndrome
Lujan syndrome
Maroteaux-Lamy syndrome
McDonough syndrome
Medium chain Acyl Co-A dehydrogenase deficiency
Microcephaly-cardiomyopathy
Microphthalmia-microtia-truncus arteriosus
Morquio syndrome, mucopolysaccharidosis
Mutchinick syndrome
Nathalie syndrome
Osteogenesis imperfecta
Osteogenesis imperfecta-microcephaly-cataracts
Prune belly-pulmonary stenosis–deafness–mental retardation
Roberts syndrome, pseudothalidomide (SC) syndrome
Scheie syndrome, mucopolysaccharidosis IS
Smith-Magenis syndrome
Woodhouse syndrome

Heart defects and eye defects (major)

Syndrome name

Alagille syndrome arteriohepatic dysplasia
CHARGE syndrome
Cohen syndrome
Fraser syndrome
Goldenhar syndrome
Goltz syndrome
Homocystinuria

Hurler syndrome
Laurence-Moon-Biedl syndrome
Marfan syndrome
Patau's syndrome
Scheie syndrome, mucopolysaccharidosis IS
SHORT syndrome
Waardenburg syndrome

Heart defect and eye defects (minor)

Syndrome name

Achard syndrome
Acrofacial dysostosis (Miller) syndrome
ADAMS syndrome
Agnathia-holoprosencephaly agnathia
Malformation C
Alkaptonuria syndrome
Alstrom syndrome
Anophthalmia, dextrocardia, skeletal anomalies
Antley-Bixler syndrome
Atkin syndrome (oculo cerebro acral syndrome)
Baraitser-Winter syndrome
Beal syndrome
Berardinelli syndrome (generalized lipodystrophy)
Bowen syndrome
Burn McKeown syndrome
Conradi Hunerman syndrome
Conradi syndrome
Cranioectodermal dysplasia (Sensenbrenner syndrome)
De Lange syndrome

Hay-Wells syndrome
Kearns-Sayre syndrome
Klippel-Trenaunay-Weber syndrome
Krause Kivlin syndrome
Lenz microthalmia syndrome
Levin syndrome
Linear sebaceous nevus syndrome
Lyon syndrome
Maroteaux-Lamy syndrome
Maternal phenylketonuria disruption syndrome
Meckel syndrome
Medium chain Acyl Co-A dehydrogenase deficiency
Microphthalmia-microtia-truncus arteriosus IV
Mietens syndrome
Morquio syndrome, mucopolysaccharidosis
Mulibrey nanism syndrome
Myotonic dystrophy syndrome
Nathalie syndrome
Neurofibromatosis syndrome

continued

Heart defect and eye defects (minor) (continued)

Syndrome Name

Fabry's disease	Noonan-like/multiple giant cell lesion
Fanconi syndrome	Oculo-facio-cardio-dental syndrome
Fetal cytomegalovirus syndrome	Ohdo syndrome
Fetal thalidomide	Onat syndrome
Fetal toxoplasmosis syndrome	Osteogenesis imperfecta
Fetal vitamin A syndrome	Osteogenesis imperfecta-microcephaly-cataracts
Fetal warfarin syndrome	Peters' anomaly-congenital heart defect
Fryns syndrome	Pseudo-Hurler polydystrophy, mucolipidosis III
Gastrocutaneous syndrome	Von Hippel-Lindau syndrome
Goodman syndrome	Waardenburg syndrome
Gorlin-Chaudhary-Moss syndrome	Weil Marchesani syndrome
Hajdu-Cheney syndrome	Werner syndrome
Hallerman-Streiff syndrome	Young-Madders syndrome

Heart defects and gastrointestinal/genitourinary anomalies (major)

Syndrome name

Beckwith-Wiedemann syndrome	LEOPARD syndrome (acronym)
Campomelic dysplasia syndrome	Maternal diabetes disruption syndrome
Cantrell pentalogy syndrome	MURCS syndrome
CHARGE syndrome	Noonan syndrome
Edwards syndrome (trisomy 18)	Rubinstein-Taybi syndrome
Fraser syndrome	Smith-Lemli-Opitz syndrome
Isomerism sequence	Towne-Brocks syndrome
Laterality sequence (includes situs ambiguous	VACTERL syndrome
heterotaxy, asplenia/polysplenia, Ivemark syndrome)	Zellweger syndrome, cerebrohepatorenal syndrome

Heart defects and gastrointestinal/genitourinary anomalies (minor)

Syndrome name

Alstrom syndrome	Antley-Bixler syndrome
Anocerebrodigital syndrome, CNS hamartoblastoma syndrome	Apert syndrome
Atkin syndrome	Apple peel congenital intestinal artresia
Atrial septal defect-lymphedema	Asymmetric crying face syndrome
Axial mesodermal dysplasia syndrome	Klippel-Feil syndrome
Beemer-Robinow syndrome	Kousseff syndrome
Chromosome 16 maternal disomy	Krause Kivlin syndrome
Cohen syndrome	Lambert syndrome
Congenital short gut malrotation-dysmotility of the small bowel	Laurence syndrome
De Lange syndrome	Laurence-Moon-Biedl syndrome
Diabetes; ketoglutarate dehydrogenase deficiency	Lenz microthalmia syndrome
Donnai-Barrow syndrome	Linear sebaceous naevus syndrome
Ehlers-Danlos syndrome type IV	Majewski syndrome, short rib-polydactyly syndrome
Fabry's disease	Malouf syndrome
Facio-cardio-renal syndrome	Marfan syndrome
Fanconi syndrome	Meckel syndrome
Farag syndrome	Megacystis-microcolon-intestinal hypoperistalsis
Fetal hydantoin syndrome	Najjar syndrome
Fetal thalidomide	NAME (Nevi-atrial myxoma-myxoid
Fetal trimethadione syndrome	Neurofibromata-epiphelides) syndrome
FG syndrome (Opitz Kaveggia syndrome)	Neish-Roberts syndrome
Fournier syndrome	Omphalocele-extrophy of bladder—imperforate anus—spinal
Fucosidosis	defects (OEIS)
Gastrocutaneous syndrome	Opitz G/BBB syndrome
Gorlin-Chaudhary-Moss syndrome	Pallister-Hall syndrome
Harris syndrome	Pancreatic hypoplasia-congenital heart defect
Heart-hand IV syndrome	Poland syndrome
Hemifacial microsomia radial defects	Renal-hepatic-pancreatic dysplasia
Holmes Schimke syndrome	Robinow syndrome

continued

Heart defects and gastrointestinal/genitourinary anomalies (minor) (continued)

Syndrome name

Holzgreve syndrome	Sacks syndrome
Hydrolethalus syndrome	Saito syndrome
Hypertelorism-microtia-clefting Ieshima syndrome	Schinzel-Giedion syndrome
Jarcho-Levin syndrome (spondylothoracic dysplasia)	Schwachman syndrome
Jennings syndrome	Short rib-polydactyly type 2 (Majewski)
Jeune thoracic dysplasia	Smith-Magenis syndrome
Johnson syndrome	Steinfeld syndrome
Jones syndrome	Thakker-Donnai syndrome
Kashani syndrome	Thomas syndrome
Kaufman syndrome	Thoracoabdominal syndrome
Kaufman-McKusick syndrome	VACTERL syndrome
Kearns-Sayre syndrome	Verloove-Vanhorick syndrome
Rutledge syndrome	Von-Hippel-Lindau syndrome
Ruvalcaba syndrome	Woodhouse syndrome

Heart defects and organomegaly (major)

Syndrome name

Alagille syndrome, arteriohepatic dysplasia	Hurler syndrome
Beckwith-Wiedemann syndrome	Maroteaux-Lamy syndrome
Berardinelli syndrome (generalized lipodystrophy)	Pompex's disease, glycogen storage disease
Glycogen storage disease type IV	Type IIA
Hunter syndrome	Zellweger syndrome, cerebrohepatorenal syndrome

Heart defects and organomegaly (minor)

Syndrome name

Aase syndrome	Klippel-Trenaunay-Weber syndrome
Carbohydrate deficient glycoprotein syndrome	Long chain Acyl Co-A dehydrogenase deficiency
Type IA (Jaeken syndrome)	Medium chain Acyl Co-A dehydrogenase deficiency
Fetal cytomegalovirus syndrome	Morquio syndrome, mucopolysaaccharidosis IV
Fetal toxoplasmosis syndrome	Noonan syndrome
Fucosidosis	Scheie syndrome, mucopolysaaccharidosis IS
Geleophysic syndrome	

Syndromes involving cardiomyopathy (major)

Syndrome name

Duchenne muscular dystrophy syndrome	Najjar syndrome
Emery-Dreifuss muscular dystrophy	Noonan syndrome
Friedreich's ataxia	Oral-cardiac-digital syndrome type II (Mohr syndrome)
Glycogen storage disease type IV	Pompe's disease, glycogen storage disease type IIA
LEOPARD syndrome (acronym)	Sacks syndrome

Syndromes involving cardiomyopathy (minor)

Syndrome name

Alstrom syndrome	Kearns-Sayre syndrome
Barth syndrome X-linked cardioskeletal myopathy	Keutel syndrome
Berardinelli syndrome (generalized lipodystrophy)	Long chain Acyl Co-A dyhydrogenase deficiency
Carbohydrate deficient glycoprotein syndrome	Maroteaux-Lamy syndrome
Type 1A (Jaeken syndrome)	McArdle's disease, glycogen storage disease type V
Cardiomyopathy, mental retardation autophagic myopathy	Medium chain Acyl Co-A dyhydrogenase deficiency
Congenital hypothyroidism	Nemaline myopathy syndrome
Costello syndrome	Refsum disease, phytonic acid storage disease
Fetal toxoplasmosis syndrome	Rigid spine syndrome
Fucosidosis	Spinal muscular atrophy syndrome
Hurler syndrome	Tuberous sclerosis syndrome
Jeune thoracic dysplasia	

Syndromes involving conduction defects (major)

Syndrome name

Heart-hand III syndrome	LEOPARD syndrome
Jervell-Lange-Nielson syndrome	Romano Ward syndrome

Syndromes involving conduction defects (minor)

Syndrome name

ADAM syndrome	Myotonic dystrophy syndrome
Behmel syndrome	Nathalie syndrome
Cardiomyopathy, mental retardation, autophagic myopathy	Onat syndrome
Facio-cardio-renal syndrome	Protonotarios (Naxos) syndrome
Heart-hand II syndrome	Refsum disease, phytanic acid storage disease
Hollister syndrome	Rett syndrome
Holt-Oram syndrome	Simpson-Golabi-Behmel syndrome
Infantile Refsum disease	Van Bever syndrome
	Woodhouse syndrome

Syndromes involving vascular defects (major)

Syndrome name

Cutis laxa	Marfan syndrome
Ehlers-Danlos syndrome type IV (arterial or Sack type)	Osler's hereditary hemorrhagic telangiectasia
Fabry's disease	Progeria syndrome, hutchinson-Gilford syndrome
Homocystinuria	Pseudoxanthoma elasticum syndrome
Isomerism sequence	Von Hippel-Landau syndrome
Klippel-Trenaunay-Weber syndrome	Williams syndrome

Syndromes involving vascular defects (minor)

Syndrome name

Alkaptonuria syndrome	Idiopathic arterial calcification syndrome
Berardinelli syndrome (generalized lipodystrophy)	Lymphedema with cardiac anomalies (Irons syndrome)
Cutis laxa syndrome (recessive form)	Mucolipidosis II (I cell disease)
Hennekam syndrome	Singleton-Merten syndrome
Holt-Oram syndrome	Sturge Weber syndrome
Hunter syndrome	Werner syndrome

REFERENCES

Adams CW, Nance WE. Persistent tachycardia, paroxysmal hypertension, and seizures: association with hyperglycinuria, dominantly inherited microphtalmia, and cataracts. JAMA 1967; 202:525–530.

Ades LC, Morris LL, Richardson M et al. Congenital heart malformation in Yunis-Varon syndrome. J Med Genet 1993; 30:788–792.

Al-Gazali LI, Farndon PA, Burn J, Flannery DB, Davison C, Mueller RF. Schinzel-Giedion syndrome. In: Donnai D, Winter RM, editors. Congenital Malformation Syndromes. London: Chapman and Hall, 1995: 481–492.

Alaike M, Kawai H, Yokoi K, Kunishige M, Mine H, Nishjda Y et al. Cadiac dysfunction in patients with chronic progressive external ophthalmoplegia. Clinical Cardiology 1997; 20(3):239–243.

Amir RE, Van der Veyver IB, etal. Rett syndrome is caused by mutations in x-linked MECPZ encoding methyl CpG-binding Protein 2. Nat Gent 23, 185–188. 1999.

Angle B, Hersh JH. Expamsion of the phenotype inHennekam syndrome: a case with new manifestations. Am J Med Genet 1997; 71(2):211–214.

Anneren G, Meurling S, Olsen L. Megacystis-microcolon-intestinal hypoperistalsis syndrome (MMIHS), an autosomal recessive disorder: clinical reports and review of the literature. Am J Med Genet 1991; 41:251–254.

Astley R, Kendall AC. A bone dysplasia for diagnosis. Ann Radiol (Paris) 1980; 23:121.

Atkin JF, Patil S. Apparently new oculo-cerebro-acral syndrome. Am J Med Genet 1984; 19:585–587.

Aughton DJ. Clinical anophthalmia, dextrocardia and skeletal anomalies in an infant born to consanguineous parents. Am J Med Genet 1990; 37:178–181.

Avela K, Lipsanen-Nyman M, Perheentupa J, Wallgren-Pettersson C, Marchand S, Faure S et al. Assignment of the mulibrey nanism gene to 17q by linkage and linkage-disequilibrium analysis. Am J Hum Genet 1997; 60(4):869–902.

Badame AJ. Progeria [Review]. Arch Dermatol 1989; 125:540–544.

Balaji S, Dennis NR, Keeton BR. Familial Ebstein's anomaly: a report of six cases in two generations associated with mild skeletal abnormalities. Br Heart J 1991; 66:26–28.

Bamforth JS, Fabian C, Machin G, Honore L. Poland anomaly with a limb body wall disruption defect: case report and review. Am J Med Genet 1992; 43:780–784.

Bankier A, Rose CM. Johnson-McMillin syndrome: report of another family. [Letter]. Am J Med Genet 1994;(52):493.

Bao Y, Kishnani P, Wu JY, Chen YT. Hepatic and neuromuscular forms of glycogen storage disease type IV caused by mutations in the same glycogen-branching enzyme gene. J Clin Invest 1996; 97(4):941–8.

Baraitser M. Syndrome of the month: the orofaciodigital (OFD) syndromes. J Med Genet 1986; 23:116–119.

Baraitser M, Winter RM. Iris coloboma, ptosis, hypertelorism and mental retardation: a new syndrome. J Med Genet 1988; 25:41–43.

Barrow M, Fitzsimmons JS. A new syndrome: Short limbs, abnormal facial appearance and congenital heart defect. Am J Med Genet 1984; 18:431–433.

Baxova A, Maroteaux P, Barosova J, Netriova I. Parental consanguinity in two sibs with omodysplasia. Am J Med Genet 1994; 49:263–265.

Beighton P. Spondyloepimetaphyseal dysplasia with joint laxity (SEMDJL) [Review]. J Med Genet 1994; 31:136–140.

Bernstein R, Isdale J, Pinto M, Du Toit Zaaijman J, Jenkins T. Short rib-polydactyly syndrome: a single or heterogeneous entity? A re-evaluation prompted by four new cases. J Med Genet 1985; 22(1):46–53.

Bialer MG. Apparent Ruvalcaba syndrome with genitourinary abnormalities. [Review]. Am J Med Genet 1989; 33(3):314–7.

Billette de Villemeur T, Bijaoui G, Beauvais P, Richardet JM. Bowen syndrome: congenital glaucoma, flexion contracture of the fingers and facial dysmorphism without peroxial abnormalities (Letter). Eur J Pediatr 1992; 151:146–147.

Bindewald B, Ulmer H, Muller U. Fallot complex, severe mental and growth retardation: a new autosomal recessive syndrome? Am J Med Genet 1994; 50:173–176.

Bini R, Danti DA, Materassi M, Pela I. Report of a new case of axial mesodermal dysplasia complex. Clin Genet 1996; 50(5):407–410.

Bonnemann CG, Meinecke P. Bilateral porencephaly, cerebellar hypoplasia, and internal malformations: two siblings representing a probably new autosomal recessive entity. Am J Med Genet 1996; 63:428–433.

Bonthron DT, Barlow KM, Burt AM, Barr DGD. Parental consanguinity in the blepharophimoses, heart defect, hypothyroidism, mental retardation syndrome (Young-Simpson syndrome). J Med Genet 1993; 30:255–256.

Bottani A, Verloes A. Myhre-GOMBO syndrome: possible lumping of two 'old' new syndromes [letter]. Am J Med Genet 1995; 59(4):523–4.

Brady AF, Jamieson CR, van der Burgt I, Crosby A, van Reen M, Kremer H et al. Further delineation of the critical region for Noonan syndrome on the long arm of chromosome 12. Eur J Hum Genet 1997; 5(5):336–7.

Braun-Quentin C, Biles C, Bowling B, Kotzot D. MURCS association: case report and reviw. J Med Genet 1996; 33:618–620.

Braverman N LPMFOCeal. Mutations in the gene encoding 3 beta-hydroxysteroid-delta 8, delta 7–isomerase cause X-linked dominant Conradi-Hunermann syndrome. Nature Genet 1999; 22:291–294.

Brueton L, Huson S, Cox P, Shirley I, Et al. Asymptomatic maternal myasthenia as a cause of the Pena-Shokeir phenotype. Am J Med Genet 2000; 92:1–6.

Bulman M, Kusami K, Frayling T, McKeown C, Et al. Mutations in the human delta homologue, DLL3, cause axial skeletal defects in spondylocostal dysostosis. Nat Genet 2000; 24:438–441.

Burn J. Disturbance of morphological laterality in humans. In: Bock GR, Marsh J, editors. Biological asymmetry and handedness. Chichester: Wiley, 1991: 282–299.

Burn J, Coffey R, Allan LD, Robinson P, Pembrey ME, Macartney FJ. Isomerism: a genetic analysis. In: Doyle EF, Engle MA, Gersony WM, Rashkind WJ, Talner NS, editors. Paediatric Cardiology. New York: Springer Verlag, 1986: 1126–1128.

Burn J, Martin N. Two retarded male cousins with odd facies, hypotonia and severe constipation: possible examples of the X linked FG syndrome. J Med Genet 1983; 20:97–99.

Burn J, Marwood RP. Fraser syndrome presenting as bilateral renal agenesis in three sibs. J Med Genet 1982; 19(5):360–361.

Burn J, Winter RM. Femoral hypoplasia-unusual facies syndrome. Journal of Medical Genetics 19, 370. 1982.

Burn J, Winter RM, Baraitser M, Hall CM, Fixsen J. Femoral hypoplasia-unusual facies syndrome. J Med Genet 1984; 21:331–340.

Buyse M, Bull MJ. A syndrome of osteogenesis imperfecta, microcephaly and cataracts. Birth Defects 1978; XIV(6):95–98.

Cantu JM, Garcia-Cruz D, Sanchez-Corona J, Hernandez A, Nazara Z. A distinct osteochondrodysplasia with hypertrichosis - individualisation of a probable autosomal recessive entity. Hum Genet 1982; 60(1):36–41.

Cantu JM, Hernandez A, Ramirez J, Bernal M, Rubio G, Urrusti J et al. Lethal faciocardiomelic dysplasia: a new autosomal recessive disorder. Birth Defects 1975; 11(5):91–98.

Carey JC. Neurofibromatosis-Noonan syndrome [editorial]. [Review]. Am J Med Genet 1998; 75(3):263–4.

Char F, Douglas JE, Dungan WT. Familial multiforme ventricular extrasystoles with short stature, hyperpigmentation and microcephaly - a new syndrome. Birth Defects 1975; 11(5):63–69.

Chen H, Mirkin D, Yang S. De novo 17q paracentric inversion mosaicism in a patient with Beemer-Langer type short rib-polydactyly syndrome with special consideration to the classification of short-rib polydactyly syndromes. Am J Med Genet 1994; 53:165–171.

Chen SC, D'Souza N. Familial tetralogy of Fallot and glaucoma. Am J Med Genet 1990; 37:40–41.

Chen Y-T, Burchell A. Glycogen storage diseases. In: Scriver CR, Beaudet AL, Sly WS, Valle D, editors. The metabolic and molecular bases of inherited disease. New York: McGraw-Hill, 1995: 935–965.

Clayton-Smith J, Donnai D. Fetal valproate syndrome. J Med Genet 1995; 32:724–727.

Coffin GS, Siris E. The Coffin-Siris syndrome. Am J Dis Child 1985; 139:12.

Cohen DM, Green JG, Miller J, Gorlin RJ, Reed JA. Acrocephalopolysyndactyly type II–Carpenter syndrome: clinical spectrum and an attempt at unification with Goodman and Summitsyndromes. Am J Med Genet 1987; 28(2):311–324.

Cohen MM, Gorlin RJ. Noonan-like/multiple giant cell lesion syndrome. Am J Med Genet 1991; 40:159–166.

Collin GB, Marshall JD, Cardon LR, Nishina PM. Homozygosity mapping at Alstrom syndrome to chromosome 2p. Hum Mol Genet 1997; 6(2):213–219.

Coonar AS, Protonotarios N, Tsatsopoulou A, Needham EW, Houlston RS, Cliff S et al. Gene for arrhythmogenic right ventricular cardiomyopathy with diffuse nonepidermolytic palmoplantar keratoderma and woolly hair (Naxos disease) maps to 17q21. Circulation 1998; 97(20):2049–58.

Coppin BD, Temple IK. Multiple lentigines syndrome (LEOPARD syndrome or progressive cardiomyopathic lentiginosis). J Med Genet 1997; 34:582–586.

Cornel G, Sharratt GP, Virmani S, Rosales T, Lacson A. Familial coarctatio f the aortic arch with bilateral ptosis: a new syndrome? J Pediatr Surg 1987; 22:724–726.

Courtens W, Vamos E, Christophe C, Schinzel A. Acrocallosal syndrome in an Algerian boy born to consanguineous parents: review of the literature and further delineation of the syndrome. Am J Med Genet 1997; 69(1):17–22.

Cremers CWRJ, Ter Haar BGA, Van Rens TJG. The Nathalie syndrome. A new hereditary syndrome. Clin Genet 1975; 8:330–340.

Crifasi PA, Patterson MC, Bonde D, Michels VV. Severe Hajdu-Cheney syndrome with upper airway obstruction. [Review]. Am J Med Genet 1997; 70(3):261–6.

Crisponi G, Porcu A, Piu ME. Antley-Bixler syndrome:,case report and review of the literature. Clin Dysmorph 1997; 61(1):61–68.

Damian MS, Seibel P, Schachenmayr W, Et al. VACTERL with the mitochondrial np 3243 point mutation. Am J Med Genet 1996; 65:213–217.

De Vries BBA. The fragile syndrome. J Med Genet 1998;(35):579–589.

Desnick RJ, Iannou YA, Eng CM. alpha-Galactosidase A deficiency: Fabry disease. In: Scriver CR, Beaudet AL, Sly WS, Walle D, editors. The metabolic and molecular basis of inherited disease. New York: McGraw-Hill, 1995: 2741–84.

Digilio MC, Marino B, Borzaga U, Giannotti A, Dallapiccola B. Infrafamilial variability of Pfeiffer-type cardiocranial syndrome. Am J Med Genet 1997; 73(4):480–483.

Digilio MC, Marino B, Giannotti A, Dallapiccola B. Conotruncal heart defect/microphthalmia syndrome: delineation of an autosomal recessive syndrome. J Med Genet 1997; 34:927–929.

Digilio MC, Marino B, Giannotti A, Dallapiccola B. Single atrium, atrioventricular canal defect is the congenital heart disease connecting short rib-polydactyly and oral-facial-digital syndromes. Am J Med Genet 1997; 68(1):110–112.

Dixon MJ. Treacher Collins syndrome. Hum Mol Genet 1996; 5(Spec No.):1391–6.

Dobyns WB, Patton MA, Stratton RF, Mastrobattista JM, Blanton SH, Northrup H. Cobblestone lissencephaly with normal eyes and muscle. Neuropediatrics 1996; 27:70–75.

Doerfler W, Wieczorek D, Gillessen-Kaesbach G, Albrecht B, Passarge E. Three brothers with mental and physical retardation, hydrocephalus, microcephaly, internal malformations, speech disorder, and facial anomalies: Mutchinick syndrome. [Review]. Am J Med Genet 1997; 73(2):210–6.

Donnai D, Barrow M. Diaphragmatic hernia, exomphalos, absent corpus callosum, hypertelorism, myopia, and sensorineural deafness: a newly recognised autosomal recessive disorder? Am J Med Genet 1993; 47:679–682.

Duncan PA. The Achard syndrome. Birth Defects: Original Article Series 1975; 11(6):69–73.

Dunham ME, Austin TL. Congenital aglossia and situs inversus (review). Int J Pediatr Otorhinolaryngology 1990; 19:163–168.

Eastman JR, Bixler D. Facio-cardio-renal syndrome: A newly delineated recessive disorder. Clin Genet 1977; 11:424–430.

Elliott AM. Schinzel-Giedion syndrome: further delineation of the phenotype. [Review]. Clin Dysmorph 1996; 5(2):135–42.

Embleton ND, Wyllie JP, Wright MJ, Burn J, Hunter AS. Natural history of Trisomy 18. Arch Dis Child 1996; 75(1):F38–F41.

Farag TI, Teebi AS. Autosomal recessive inheritance of a syndrome of hypertelorism, hypospadias and tetralogy of Fallot. Am J Med Genet 1990; 35:516–518.

Feigenbaum A, Kumar A, Weksberg R. Singleton-Merten (S-M) syndrome: autosomal dominant transmission with variable expression. Am J Hum Genet 1988;(43):48.

Ferencz C, Rubin JD, McCarter RJ, Clark EB. Maternal diabetes and cardiovascular malformations: predominance of doublt outlet right ventricle and truncus arteriosus. Teratology 1990; 41:319–326.

Fernandez-Canon JM, Granadino B, Beltran-Valero de Bernabe D, Renedo M, Fernandez-Ruiz E, Penlava MA et al. The molecular basis of alkaptonuria. Nature Genet 1996; 14(1):19–24.

Ferner RE. Clinical aspects of neurofibromatosis. In: Upadhyaya M, Cooper DN, editors. Neurofibromatosis type 1. From genotype to phenotype. Bioscientific Publishers, 1998: 21–38.

Fitzpatrick DR. Zellweger syndrome and associated phenotypes. [Review]. J Med Genet 1996; 33(10):863–868.

Fitzpatrick DR, Keeling JW, Evans MJ, Kan AE, Et al. Clinical phenotype of desmosterolosis. Am J Med Genet 1998; 75:145–152.

Fitzpatrick DR, Strain L, Thomas AE, Barr DGD, Todd A, Smith NM et al. Neurogenic chorinic idiopathic intestinal pseudo-obstruction, patent ductus arteriosis, and thrombocytopenia segregating as an X-linked recessive disorder. J Med Genet 1997; 34:666–669.

Forney WR, Robinson SJ, Pascoe DJ. Congenital heart disease, deafness and skeletal malformations: a new syndrome? J Pediatr 1966; 68:14–26.

Forsberg H, Olofsson B-O, Eriksson A, Andersson S. Cardiac involvement in congenital myotonic dystrophy. Br Heart J 1990; 63:119–121.

Fournier A, Paget M, Pauli A, Devin P. Syndromes nephrotiques familiaux: syndrome nephrotique associe a une cardiopathie congenitale chez quatre soeurs. Pediatrie 1963; 18:677–685.

Garcia-Cruz D, Sanchez-Corona J, Nazara Z, Garcia-Cruz MO, Figuera LE, Castaneda V et al. Congenital hypertrichosis, osteochondrodysplasia, and cardiomegaly: further delineation of a new genetic syndrome. Am J Med Genet 1997; 69(2):138–51.

Garcia-Sagredo JM, Lozano C, Ferrando P, San Roman C. Mentally retarded siblings with congenital heart defect, peculiar facies and cryptorchidism in the male: possible McDonough syndrome with coincidental (X;20) translocation. Clin Genet 1984; 26:117–124.

Gay I, Feinmesser R, Cohen T. Laryngeal web, congenital heart disease and low stature: A syndrome? Arch Otolaryngol 1981; 107:510–512.

Gebbia M, Ferrara GB, Pilia G, Aylsworth AS, Penman Splitt M, Bird IM et al. X-linked situs abnormalities result from mutations in ZIC3. Nature Genet 1997; 17(3):305–309.

Giampietro PF, Verlander PC, Davis JG, Auerbach AD. Diagnosis of Fanconi anemia in patients without congenital malformations: an international Fanconi Anemia Registry Study. Am J Med Genet 1997; 68(1):58–61.

Gladwin AJ, Dixon J, Loftus SKea. Treacher Collins syndrome may rsult from insertions, deletions or splicing mutations which introduce a termination codon into the gene. Hum Molec Genet 1996; 5:1533–1538.

Glickstein J, Karasik J, Caride DG, Marion RW. "C" Trigonocephaly Syndrome: Report of a child with agenesis of the corpus callosum and tetralogy of Fallot, and review. Am J Med Genet 1995; 56:215–218.

Golabi M, Ito M, Hall BD. A new X-linked multiple congenital anomalies/mental retardation syndrome. Am J Med Genet 1984; 27:367–374.

Goltz RW. Focal dermal hypoplasia syndrome. An updated [editorial; comment]. Arch Dermatol 1992; 128(8):1108–11.

Goodman RM, Yahav Y, Frand M, Barzilay Z, Nisan E, Hertz M. A new white forelock (poliosis) syndrome with multiple congenital malformations in two sibs. Clin Genet 1980; 17:437–442.

Gorlin RJ, Cervenka J, Anderson RC. Robin's syndrome: a probaly X-linked recessive subvariety exhibiting persistence of left superior vena cava and atrial septal defect. Am J Dis Child 1970; 119:176–178.

Gorlin RJ, Cohen MMJr, Levin LS. Syndromes of the Head and Neck. Oxford: Oxford University Press, 1990.

Gotzsche CO, Krag-Olsen B, Nielson J, Sorenson KE, Kristensen BO. Prevalence of cardiovascular malformations and association karyotypes in Turners syndrome. Arch Dis Childhood 1994; 71(5):433–436.

Gray JR, Davies SJ. Marfan syndrome. J Med Genet 1996; 33:403–408.

Grebe TA, Rimsza ME, Richter SF, Hansen RC, Hoyme HE. Further delineation of the epidermal nevus syndrome: two cases with new findings and literature review. Am J Med Genet 1993; 47(1):24–30.

Greenberg F, Lewis RA, Potocki L, Glaze D, Parke J, Killian JM et al. Multi-disciplinary clinical study of Smith-Magenis syndrome (deletion 17p11.2). Am J Med Genet 1996; 62:247–254.

Greene SL, Michels VV, Doyle JA. Variable expression in ankyloblepharon-ectodermal defects-cleft lip and palate syndrome. Am J Med Genet 1987; 27(1):207–12.

Griffiths PD. Sturge-Weber syndrome revisited: the role of neuroradiology. [Review]. Neuropediatrics 1996; 27(6):284–94.

Gripp KW, Stolle CA, Celle L, Et al. TWIST gene mutation in a patient with radial aplasia and craniosynostosis: further evidence for heterogeneity of Baller-Gerold. Am J Med Genet 1999; 82:170–176.

Grosse FR. The Rabenhorst syndrome - a cardio-acro-fascial syndrome. Z Kinderheilkd 1974; 117:109–114.

Guichard C, Harricane M-C LJ-J, Et al. Axonemal Ðynein intermediate-chain gene DNAI1: mutations result in situs inversus and primary ciliary dyskinesia Kartagener syndrome. American Journal of Human Genetics 68, 1030–1035. 2001.

Guion-Almeida ML, Richieri-Costa A. Cerebrofaciothoracic syndrome. Am J Med Genet 1996; 61:152–153.

Hagadorn JI, Wilson WG, Hogge WA, Et al. Neonatal progeroid syndrome: more than one disease?. Am J Med Genet 1990; 35:91–94.

Halal F, Gervais MH, Baillargeon J, Lesage R. Gastro-cutaneous syndrome: Peptic ulcer/hiatal hernia, multiple lentigines/cafe-au-lait spots, hypertelorism and myopia. Am J Med Genet 1982; 11:161–176.

Hall BB. Humero-spinal dystosis: report of the fourth case with emphasis on generalised skeletal involvement, abnormal craniofacial features, and mitral valve thickening. Journal of Pediatric Opthalmology 1997; 6:11–14.

Hall JG. Syndrome of the month: thrombocytopenia and absent radius (TAR) syndrome. J Med Genet 1987; 24:79–83.

Hall JG, Pauli RM, Wilson KM. Maternal and fetal sequelae of anticoagulation during pregnancy. The American Journal of Medicine 1980; 68:122–140.

Hansen JW, Smith DW. U-shaped palatal defect in the Robin anomalad: Developmental and clinical relevance. J Pediatr 1975; 87:30–33.

Happle R, Effendy I, Megahed M, Orlow SJ, Kuster W. CHILD syndrome in a boy. Am J Med Genet 1996; 62(2):192–4.

Hashmi A, Abu-Sulaiman R, McCrindle BW, Smallhorn JF, Williams WG, Freedom RM. Management and outcomes of right atrial isomerism: a 26 year experience. Journal of American College of Cardiology 1998; 31(5):1120–6.

Hennekam RC, Tilanus M, Hamel BC, Voshart-van Heeren H, Mariman EC, van Beersum SE et al. Deletion at chromosome 16p13.3 as a cause of Rubinstein-Taybi syndrome: clinical aspects. Am J Hum Genet 1993; 52(2):255–262.

Hennekam RC, van Bever Y, Oorthuys JW. Acromicric dysplasia and geleophysic dysplasia: similarities and differences. Eur J Pediatr 1996; 155(4):311–314.

Hennekam RCM, Van Noort G, De La Fuente AA. Familial holoprosencephaly, heart defects, and polydactyly. Am J Med Genet 1991; 41:258–262.

Hing AV, Dowton SB. Aase syndrome: novel radiographic features. Am J Med Genet 1993; 45(4):413–415.

Hirschhorn R. Glycogen storage disease type II: Acid alpha-glucosidase (Acid Maltase) deficiency. In: Scriver CR, Beaudet AL, Sly WS, Valle D, editors. The Metabolic and Molecular Base of Inherited Disease. New York: McGraw-Hill, 1995: 2443–64.

Ho C-K, Kaufman RL, McAlister WH. Congenital malformations: Cleft palate, congenital heart disease, absent tibiae and polydactyly. Am J Dis Child 1975; 129:714–716.

Hollister DW, Hollister WG. The 'long thumb' brachydactyly syndrome. Am J Med Genet 1981; 8:6–16.

Holmes GE, Schimke RN, Goertz K, Et al. Continuation of a case report (Letter). J Med Genet 1993; 30:445.

Hortop J, Tsipouras P, Hanley JA, Maron BJ, Shapiro JR. Cardiovascular involvement in osteogenesis imperfecta. Circulation 1986; 73(1):54–61.

Hughes HE, Davies SJ. Coarctation of the aorta in Kabuki syndrome. Arch Dis Child 1994; 70(6):512–514.

Hurst JA, Baraitser M. Johanson-Blizzard syndrome. J Med Genet 1989; 26:45–48.

Hurst JA, Baraitser M, Winter RM. A syndrome of mental retardation, short staure, hemolytic anemia, delayed puberty, and abnnormal facial appearance: similarities to a report of aldolase A deficiency. Am J Med Genet 1987; 28:965–970.

Hurst JA, Berry AC, Tettenborn MA. Unknown syndrome: congenital heart disease, choanal stenosis, short stature, developmental delay, and dysmorphic facial features in a brother and sister. J Med Genet 1989; 26:407–409.

Hyndman WB, Alexander DS, Mackie KW. Chondrodystrophia calcificans congenita (the Conradi-Hunermann syndrome). Clin Pediatr 1976; 15:317–321.

Ieshima A, Koeda T, Inagaki M. Peculiar face, deafness, cleft palate, male pseudohermaphroditism, and growth and psychomotor retardation: a new autosomal recessive syndrome? Clin Genet 1986; 30:136–141.

Imaizumi K, Makita Y, Masuno M, Kuroki Y. Congenital heart defect in a patient with the Hallermann-Streiff syndrome [letter; comment]. Am J Med Genet 1994; 53(4):386–7.

Imtiaz F, Worthington V, Champion M, Et al. Genotypes and phenotypes of patients in the UK with carbohydrate-deficient glycoprotein syndrome type 1. J Inherit Metab Dis 2000; 23:162–174.

Ippel PF, Gorlin RJ, Lenz W, van Doorne JM, Bijlsma JB. Craniofacial dysostosis, hypertrichosis, genital hypoplasia, ocular, dental, and digital defects: confirmation of the Gorlin-Chaudhry-Moss syndrome. Am J Med Genet 1992; 44(4):518–22.

Irons MB, Bianchi DW, Geggel RL, Marx GR, Bhan I. Possible new autosomal recessive syndrome of lymphedema, hydroceles, atrial septal defect, and characteristic facial changes. Am J Med 1996; 66:69–71.

Jansen GA, Mihalik SJ, Watkins PA, Moser HW, Et al. Phytanoyl-CoA hydroxylase is not only deficient in classical Refsum disease but also in rhizomelic chondrodysplasia punctata. J Inherit Metab Dis 1997; 20:444–446.

Jennings MT, Hall JG, Kukolich M. Endocardial fibroelastosis, neurologic dysfunction and unusual facial appearance in two brothers coincidentally associated with dominantly inherited macrocephaly. Am J Med Genet 1980; 5:271–276.

Joenje H, Oostra AB, Wijker M, di Summa FM, van Berkel CG, Rooimans MA et al. Evidence for at least eight Fanconi anemia genes. Am J Med Genet 1998; 61(4):940–944.

Johnson DW, Berg JN, Baldwin MA, Gallione CJ, Marondel I, Yoon SJ et al. Mutations in the activin receptor-like kinase 1 gene in hereditary haemorrhagic telangiectasia type 2. Nature Genet 1996; 13(2):189–95.

Journeau P, Lajeunie E, Renier D, Et al. Syndactyly in Apert syndrome. Utility of a prognostic classification. Annales de Chirurgie de la Main et du Membre Superieur 1999; 18:13–19.

Kalousek DK, Langlois S, Barrett I, Yam I, Wilson DR, Howard-Peebles PN et al. Uniparental Disomy for Chromosome 16 in humans. Am J Hum Genet 1993; 52:8–16.

Kang S, Graham JM, Jr., Olney AH, Biesecker LG. GLI3 frameshift mutations cause autosomal dominant Pallister-Hall syndrome. Nature Genet 1997; 15(3):266–8.

Kant SG.Polinkovsky A.Mundlos S., Et al. Acromesomelic dysplasia Maroteaux type maps to human chromosome 9. Am J Hum Genet 1998; 63:155–162.

Kant SG, Bartelings MM, Kibbelaar RE, Van Haeringen A. Severe cardiac defect in a patient with the OEIS complex. Clin Dysmorph 1997; 6:371–374.

Kashani IA, Strom CM, Utley JE, Marin-Garcia J, Higgins CB. Hypoplastic pulmonary arteries and aorta with obstructive uropathy in 2 siblings. Journal of Vascular Diseases 1984; 35:252–256.

Kaufman RL, McAlister WH, Ho C-K, Et al. The association of severe obstructive left heart lesions, vertebral and renal anomalies: a second family (family studies in congenital heart disease VI). BDOAS 1974; 10(7):93–104.

Kawashima H, Ohno I, Ueno Y, Nakaya S, Kato E, Taniguchi N. Syndrome of microtia and aortic arch anomalies resembling isotretinoin embryopathy. J Pediatr 1987; 111:738–740.

Kelly TE, Thomas GH, Taylor JrHA, Et al. Mucolipidosis III (Pseudo-Hurler polydystrophy): clinical and laboratory studies in a series of 12 patients. Johns Hopkins Medical Bulletin 1975; 137:156–175.

Kimonis VE, Goldstein AM, Pastakia B, Yang ML, Kase R, DiGiovanna JJ et al. Clinical manifestation in 105 persons with nevoid basal cell carcinoma syndrome. [Review]. Am J Med Genet 1997; 69(3):299–308.

Ko CY, Rusin LC, Schoetz DJ, Moreau L, Coller JA, Murray JJ et al. Does Better Functional Result Equate with Better Quality of Life?

Implications for Surgical Treatment in Familial Adenomatous Polyposis. Dis Colon Rectum 2000; 43(6):829–835.

Kolemainen J, Norio R, Kivitie-Kallio S, Tahvanainen E, De la Chapelle A, Lehesjoki AE. Refined mapping of the Cohen syndrome gene by linkage disequilibrium. Eur J Hum Genet 1997; 5(4):206–213.

Kornfeld S, Sly WS. I-Cell disease and pseudo-Hurler polydystrophy: Disorder of lysosomal enzyme phosphorylation and localization. In: Scriver CR, Beaudet AL, Sly WS, Valle D, editors. The Metabolic and Molecular Basis of Inherited Disease. New York: McGraw-Hill, 1995: 2495–2508.

Koussseff BG. Sacral meningocele with conotruncal heart defects: a possible autosomal recessive trait. Pediatr 1984; 74:395–398.

Krantz ID, Piccoli DA, Spinner NB. Alagille syndrome. J Med Genet 1997; 34:152–157.

Krantz ID, Rand EB, Genin A, Hunt P, Jones M, Louis AA et al. Deletions in 20p12 in Alagille syndrome: Frequency and molecular characterization. Am J Med Genet 1997; 70:80–86.

Kumar A, Friedman JM, Taylor GP, Patterson MW. Pattern of cardiac malformation in oculoauriculovertebral spectrum. Am J Med Genet 1993; 46(4):423–6.

Lacombe D, Creusot G, Battin J. New case of Toriello-Carey syndrome. Am J Med Genet 1992; 42(374):376.

Lacombe D, Donneau D, Verloes A, Couet D, Koulischer L, Battin J. Lujan-Fryns syndrome (X-linked mental retardation with marfanoid habitus): report of three cases and review. Genetic Counseling 1993; 4(3):193–8.

Lambert JC, Saint-Paul MC, Bastiani F, Et al. Branchial dysplasia, mental deficiency, club feet, and inguinal herniae: report of two further cases associated with paucity of the interlobular bile ducts. J Med Genet 1990; 27:330–332.

Lammer EJ, Chen DT, Hoar RM, Et al. Retinoic acid embryopathy. N Engl J Med 1985; 313:837–841.

Lazebnik N, McPherson E, Rittmeyer LJ, Mulvihull JJ. The floating harbor syndrome with cardiac septal defect (review). Am J Med Genet 1996; 66:300–302.

Legius E, Schollen E, Matthijs G, Fryns J-P. Fine mapping of Noonan/cardio-facio cutaneous syndrome in a large family. Eur J Hum Genet 1998;(6):32–37.

Levin DL, Muster AJ, Newfield EA, Paul MH. Concordant aortic arch anomalies in monozygotic twins. J Pediatr 1973; 83:459–461.

Levy HL, Ghavami M. Maternal phenylketouria: a metabolic teratogen. [Review]. Teratology 1996; 53(3):176–84.

Lewis RJ, Ketcham AS. Maffucci's syndrome: functional and neoplastic significance. J Bone and Joint Surg 1973; 55:1465–1479.

Li L, Krantz ID, Deng Y, Genin A, Banta AB, Collins CC et al. Alagille syndrome is caused by mutations in human *Jagged1*, which encodes a ligand for Notch1. Nature Genet 1997; 16:243–251.

Li QY, Newbury-Ecob RA, Terrett JA, Wilson DI, Curtis ARJ, Yi CH et al. Holt-Oram syndrome is caused by mutations in *TBX5*, a member of the *Brachyury (T)* gene family. Nature Genet 1997; 15(1):21–29.

Lin AE, Gettig E. New syndrome: craniosyntosis, agnesis of the corpus callosum, severe mental retardation, distinctive facies, camptodactyly, and hypogonadism. Am J Med Genet 1990; 35:582–585.

Lockhart JL, Reeve HR, Bredael JJ, Krueger RP. Siblings with prune belly syndrome and associated pulmonic stenosis, mental retardation and deafness. Urology 1979; 14:140–142.

Lurie IW. Further delineation of the Beemer-Langer syndrome using concordance rates in affected sibs. Am J Med Genet 1994; 50:313–317.

Lurie IW, Kirillova IA, Novikova IV, Burakovski IV. Renal-hepatic-pancreatic dysplasia and its variants. Genetic Counseling 1991; 2:17–20.

Lyon G, Arita F, Le Galloudec E, Vallee L, Mission JP, Ferriere G. A disorder of axonal development, necrotizing myopathy, cardiomyopathy and cataracts: a new familial disease. Ann Neurol 1990; 27:193–199.

Mack DR, Forstner CG, Wilschanski M, Freedman MH, Durie PR. Shwachman syndrome: exocrine pancreatic dysfunction and variable phenotypic expression. Gastroentrology 1996; 111(6):1593–602.

Maddock IR, Moran A, Maher ER, Teare MD, Norman A, Payne SJ et al. A genetic register for von Hippel-Lindau disease. J Med Genet 1996; 33(2):120–7.

Malouf J, Alam S, Kary H, Mufarrij A, Der Kaloustian VM. Hypergonadotropic Hypogonadism with Congestive Cardiomyopathy: An Autosomal-Recessive Disorder? Am J Med Genet 1985; 20:483–489.

Mangion J.Rahman N.Mansour S.Brice G., Et al. A gene for lymphedema-distichiasis maps to 16q24.3. Am J Hum Genet 2001; 65:427–432.

Marcelino J, Carpten JD, Suwaira WMA, etal. CACP, encoding a secreted proteoglycan is mutated in camptodactyly-arthropathy-coxa vara-pericarditis syndrome. Nat Gent 1999; 23:319–322.

Marshall JD, Ludman MD, Shea SE, Salisbury SR, Willi SM, LaRoche RG et al. Genealogy, natural history, and phenotype of Alstrom syndrome in a large Acadian kindred and three additional families. Am J Med Genet 1997; 73(2):150–161.

Martinez-Frias ML, Bermejo E, Urioste M, Huertas H, Arroyo I. Lethal short rib-polydactyly syndromes: further evidence for their overlapping in a continuous spectrum. J Med Genet 1993; 30(11):937–941.

Martinez y Martinez R, Corona-Rivera E, Jimenez-Martinez M, Ocampo-Campos R, Garcia-Maravilla S. A new probably autosomal recessive cardiomelic dysplasia with mesoaxial hexadactyly. J Med Genet 1981; 18(2):151–154.

Meadow R. Anticonvulsants in pregnancy. Arch Dis Child 1991; 66:62–65.

Megarbane A, Hokayem N. Craniosynostosis and marfanoid habitus without mental retardation: report of a third case. Am J Med Genet 1998; 77:170–171.

Meinecke P, Blunck W. Frontonasal dysplasia, congenital heart defect, and short staure: a further observation. J Med Genet 1989; 86(6):408–409.

Meinecke P, Ziegenrucker W, Peters A. Potter sequence due to renal aplasia and postaxial hexadactyly, a distinct entity? [Review]. Genetic conseling 1993; 4(2):127–30.

Meyer RA, Cohen MF, Recalde S, Zakany J, Bell SM, Scott WJ, Jr. et al. Developmental regulation and asymmetric expression of the gene encoding Cx43 gap junctions in the mouse limb bud. Dev Genet 1997; 21(4):290–300.

Mietens C, Weber H. A syndrome characterised by corneal opacity, nystagmus, flexion contracture of the elbows, growth failure, and mental retardation. J Pediatr 1966; 69:624–629.

Mihalik SJ, Morrell JC, Kim D, Saint-Paul MC. Identification of PAHX, a refsum disease gene. Nat Gent 1997; 17:185–189.

Moerman P, Fryns JP, Vandenberghe K, Lauweryns JM. Constrictive amniotic bands, amniotic adhesions, and limb-body wall complex: discrete disruption sequences with pathogenetic overlap. Am J Med Genet 1992; 42(4):470–9.

Moller P, Moe N, Saugstad OD, Et al. Spinal muscular atrophy type I combnined with atrial septal defect in three sibs. Clin Genet 1990; 38:81–83.

Motley AM, Hettema EH, Hogenhout EM, Et al. Rhizomelic chondrodysplasia punctata is a peroxisomal protein targetting disease caused by a non-functional PTS2 receptor. Nat Gent 1997; 15:377–380.

Mucke J, Hoepffner W, Scheerschmidt G, Gornig H, Beyreiss K. Early onset lymphoedema, recessive form - a new form of genetic lymphoedema syndrome. Eur J Pediatr 1986; 145:195–198.

Munke M, McDonald DM, Cronister A, Stewart JM, Gorlin RJ, Zackai EH. Oral-facial-digital syndrome type VI (Varadi syndrome): further clinical delineation [see comments]. Am J Med Genet 1990; 35(3):360–9.

Nagib MG, Maxwell RE, Chou SN. Klippel-Feil syndrome in children: clinical features and management. Child's Nervous System 1985; 1:255–263.

Neish AS, Roberts DJ. Hypoplastic left heart, neuromegaly, and distinctive facies in two siblings. Am J Hum Genet 1992; 50:153.

Neufeld EF, Muenzer J. The mucopolysaccharidoses. In: Scriver CR, Beaudet AL, Sly WS, Valle D, editors. The Metabolic and Molecular Bases of Inherited Disease. New York: McGraw-Hill, 1995: 2465–2494.

Neufeld EJ, Mandel H, Raz T, Yandava CN, Szargel R, Stagg A et al. Localization of the gene for thiamine-responsive megaloblastic anemia dyndrome, on the long arm of chromosome 1, by homozygosity mapping. Am J Hum Genet 1997; 61(6):1335–1341.

Neumann L, Pelz J, Kunze J. A new observation of two cases of acrofacial dysostosis type Genee-Wiedemann in a family – remarks on the mode of inheritance: report on two sibs. Am J Med Genet 1996; 64(4):556–62.

Niebuhr E. The cri du chat syndrome: epidemiology, cytogenetics, and clinical features. Hum Genet 1978; 44:227–275.

Noreau DR, Al-Ata J, Jutras L, Teebi AS. Congenital heart defects in Sotos syndrome. Am J Med Genet 1998; 79(4):327–328.

Northover H, Cowie RA, Wraith JE. Mucopolysaccharidosis type IVA (Morquio syndrome): a clinical review. [Review]. J Inher Metab Dis 1996; 19(3):357–65.

Nowaczyk MJM, James AG, Superina R, Siegel-Bartelt J. Hirschprung disease, postaxial polydactyly, and atrial septal defect. Am J Med Genet 1997; 68:74–75.

Nwokoro NA, Korytkowski MT, Rose S, Gorin MB, Penles Stadler MP, Witchel SF et al. Spectrum of malignancy and premalignancy in Carney syndrome. Am J Med Genet 1997; 73:369–377.

Obwegeser HL, Gorlin RJ. Oculo-facio-cardio-dental (OFCD) syndrome. Clin Dysmorph 1997; 6:281–283.

Oda T, Elkahloun AG, Pike BL, Okajima K, Krantz ID, Genin A et al. Mutations in the human Jagged1 gene are responsible for Alagille syndrome. Nature Genet 1997; 16:235–242.

Onat A. Familial sinus node disease and degenerative myopia - a new hereditary syndrome? Hum Genet 1986; 72:182–184.

Onat A, Onat T, Domanic N. Discrete subaortic stenosis as part of a short stature syndrome. Hum Genet 1984; 65:331–335.

Orstavik KH, Bechensteen AG, Fugelseth D, Orderud W. Sibs with Ritscher-Schinzel (3C) syndrome and anal malformations. Am J Med Genet 1998; 75(3):300–303.

Orstavik KH, Lindemann R, Solberg LA, Et al. Congenital heart defects, hamartomas of the tongue and polysyndactyly in a sister and brother. Clin Genet 1992; 42:19–21.

Palmer SE, Pagon RA. Familial hydrocephalus with a low-insertion umbilicus. Clin Dysmorph 1993; 2:351–359.

Pao DG, DeAngelis GA, Lovell MA, Hagspiel KD. Idiopathic arterial calcification of infancy: sonographic and magnetic resonance findings with pathologic correlation. Rediatric Radiology 1998; 28(4):256–9.

Parvari R, Carmi R, Weissenback J, Pilia G, Mumm S, Weinstein Y. Refined genetic mapping of X-linked thoracoabdominal syndrome. Am J Med Genet 1996; 61:401–402.

Parvari R, Mumm S, Galil A, Manor E, Bar-David Y, Carmi R. Deletion of 8.5 Mb, including the FMR1 gene, in a male with the fragile X syndrome phenotype and overgrowth. Am J Med Genet 1999; 83(4):302–307.

Patton MA, Sharma A, Winter RM. The Aase-Smith syndrome. Clin Genet 1985; 28(6):521–525.

Paznekas WA, Cunningham ML, Howard TD, Korf BR, Lipson MH, Grix AW et al. Genetic heterogenity of Saethre-Chotzen syndrome, due to TWIST and FGFR mutations. Am J Hum Genet 1998; 62(6):1370–80.

Percin EF, Duzcan F, Kafali G, Sezgin I. A new syndrome with cardiac malformation, cleft lip-palate, microcephaly and digital anomalies? Clin Genet 1995; 48:264–267.

Philip N, Sigaudy S. Costello syndrome. J Med Genet 1998;(35):238–40.

Pilia G, Hughes-Benzie RM, MacKenzie A, Baybayan P, Chen EY, Huber R et al. Mutations in GPC3, a glypican gene, cause the Simpson-Golabi-Behmel overgrowth syndrome. Nature Genet 1996; 12(3):241–7.

Pilz DT, Quarrell OW. Syndromes with lissencephaly/ [Review]. J Med Genet 1996; 33(4):319–23.

Plotz FB, Van Essen AJ, Bosschaart AN, Bos AP. Cerebro-costo-mandibular syndrome [published erratum appears in Am J Med Genet 1996 Aug 23;64(3):527]. [Review][20refs]. Am J Med Genet 1996; 62(3):286–292.

Pontz BF, Stoss H, Henschke F, Freisinger P, Karbowski A, Spranger J. Clinical and ultrastructural findings in three patients with geleophysic dysplasia. Am J Med Genet 1996; 63(1):50–54.

Pope FM, Burrows NP. Ehlers-Danlos syndrome has varied molecular mechanisms. J Med Genet 1997; 34(5):400–410.

Porteous MEM, Wright C, Smith D, Burn J. Agnathia-holoprosencephaly; a new recessive syndrome ? Clin Dysmorph 1993; 2:161–164.

Powell CM, Michaelis R. Townes-Brocks syndrome (review). J Med Genet 1999; 36:89–93.

Powell SM, Petersen GM, Krush AJ, Booker S, Jen J, Giardiello FM et al. Molecular diagnosis of familial adenomatous polyposis. N Engl J Med 1993; 329:1982–1987.

Putnam EA, Zhang H, Ramirez F, Milewicz DM. Fibrillin-2 (FBN2) mutations result in the Marfan-like disorder, congenital contractural arachnodactyly. Nature Genet 1995; 11(4):456–58.

Quaderi NA, Schweiger S, Gaudenz K, Franco B, Rugarli EI, Berger W et al. Opitz G/BBB syndrome, a defect of midline development, is due to mutations in a new RING finger gene on Xp22. Nature Genet 1997; 17:285–291.

Rajab A. Bonneau syndrome: a further case report. Clin Dysmorph 1997; 6:85–88.

Ramer JC, Frankel CA, Ladda RL. Marden-Walker phenotype:spectrum of variability in three infants. [Review]. Am J Med Genet 1993; 45(3):285–91.

Rasmussen M, Stromme P. Congenital ptosis and blepharophimosis in a mentally retarded girl: a new case of Ohdo syndrome? [Review]. Clin Dysmorph 1998; 7(1):61–3.

Rauch A, Hofbeck M, Bahring S, Leipold G, Trautmann U, Singer H et al. Monozygotic twins concordant for Cayler syndrome. Am J Med Genet 1998; 75(1):113–117.

Read AP, Newton VE. Waardenburg syndrome. J Med Genet 1997; 34(8):656–65.

Reardon W, Hurst J, Farag TI, Hall C, Baraitser M. Two brothers with heart defects and limb shortening: case reports and review. J Med Genet 1990; 27:746–751.

Reuber BE, Germain-Lee E, Collins CS, Morrell JC, Ameritunga R, Moser HW et al. Mutations in PEX1 are the most common cause of peroxisome biogenesis disorders. Nature Genet 1997; 17(4):445–8.

Ringpfeil F, Lebwohl MG, Christiano AM, Uitto J. Pseudoxanthoma elasticum: mutations in the MRP6 gene encoding a transmembrane ATP-binding cassette (ABC) transporter. Proceedings of the National Academy of Sciences of the USA 2000; 97:6001–6006.

Robertson EJ. Development - Left-right asymmetry. Science 1997; 275(5304):1280.

Robinow M, Beemer FA. New syndrome (Letter). Am J Med Genet 1990; 36:375.

Rogers JG, Levin LS, Dorst JP, Temtamy SA. A postaxial polydactyly-dental-vertebral syndrome. J Pediatr 1977; 90:230–235.

Rommen I, Mueller RF, Sybert VP. Developmental delay, growth deficiency, congenital heart defect and multiple craniofacial anomalies. J Clin Dysmorph 1983; 1(4):10–13.

Ruiz-Perez VL, Ide SE, Strom TM, Lorenz B, Wilson D, Woods K et al. Mutations in a new gene in Ellis-van Creveld syndrome and Weyers acrodental dysostosis. Nature Genet 2000; 24:283–286.

Ruiz de la Fuente S, Prieto F. Heart-Hand syndrome III. Hum Genet 1980; 55:43–47.

Ryan AK, Bartlett K, Clayton P, Eaton S, Mills K, Collins J et al. Smith Lemli Opitz syndrome: a variable phenotype caused by 7 dehydro cholesterol reductase deficiency. Journal of Medical Genetics 34[Supplement 1], S23. 1997.

Ryan AK, Bartlett K, Clayton P, Eaton S, Mills K, Donnai D et al. Smith-Lemli-Opitz syndrome: a variable clinical and biochemical phenotype. J Med Genet 1998; 35:558–565.

Ryan AK, Goodship JA, Wilson DI, Philip N, Levy A, Siedel H et al. Spectrum of clinical features associated with interstitial chromosome 22q11 deletions: A European collaborative study. J Med Genet 1997; 34:798–804.

Ryan SG, Chance PF, Zou C-H, Spinner NB, Golden JA, Smietana S. Epilepsy and mental retardation limited to females: an X-linked dominant disorder with male sparing. Nature Genet 1997; 17:92–95.

Sabry MA, Ismail EA, al-Naggar RL, al-Torki NA, Farah S, Al-Awadi SA et al. Unusual traits associated with Robinow syndrome. J Med Genet 1997; 34(9):736–40.

Salonen R, Paavola P. Meckel syndrome. J Med Genet 1998;(35):497–501.

Sanchez Cascos A, Sanchez Harguindey L, DeRabago P. Cardioauditory syndromes: cardiac and genetic study of 511 deaf-mute children. Br Heart J 1969; 31:26–33.

Sandor GGS, Smith DF, MacLeod PM. Cardiac Malformations in the Fetal Alcohol Syndrome. J Pediatr 1981; 98:771–773.

Satoda MZFDGABJGJDHRPMEM&GBD. Mutations in TFAP2B cause Char syndrome, a familial form of patent ductus arteriosus. Nature Genet 2000; 25:42–46.

Savill GA, Young ID, Cunningham RJ, Ansell ID, Evans JH. Chronic tubulo-intestinal nephropathy in children with cranioectodermal dysplasia. Pediatr Nephrol 1997; 11(2):215–217.

Schinzel A. Tetrasomy 12p. J Med Genet 1991; 28(2):122–125.

Schott JJ, Benson DW, Basson CT, Pease W, Silberbach GM, Moak JP et al. Congenital heart disease caused by mutations in the transcription factor NKX2–5. Science 1998; 281(5373):108–111.

Schuler L, Puga ACS, Scwartz IVD, Netto C. Jones-Waldman syndrome: another report? (Letter). Am J Med Genet 1994; 51:83.

Seashore JH, Et a. Familial apple peel jejunal artresia. Paediatrics 1987; 80:540–544.

Shaw EB, Steinback HL. Aminopterin-induced fetal malformation. Am J Dis Child 1968; 115:477–482.

Silengo MC, Bell GL, Biagioli M, Et a. Asymmetric crying facies with microcephaly and mental retardation. An autosomal dominant syndrome with variable expressivity. Clin Genet 1986; 30:481–484.

Siwik ES, Zahka KG, Wiesner GL, Limwongse C. Cardiac disease in Costello syndrome. Pediatr 1998; 101(4 pt 1):706–709.

Smithells RW, Newman CG. Recognition of thalidomide defects. J Med Genet 1992; 29(10):716–723.

Sonoda T, Ohdo S, Madokoro H, Ohba K. A new recognisable syndrome in three sibs with congenital heart disease, round face with depressed nasal bridge, short stature and developmental retardation. Med Genet 1988; 25:711–713.

Sorge G, Ruggieri M, Polizzi A, Scuderi A, Di Pietro M. SHORT syndrome: a new case with probable autosomal dominant inheritance. Am J Med Genet 1994; 83:786–788.

Stec I, Wright JT, Van Ommen GJB, De Boer PAJ, Van Haeringen A, Moorman AFM et al. WHSC1, a 90 kb SET domain-containing gene, expressed in early development and homologous to a Drosophila dysmorphy gene maps in the Wolf-Hirschhorn syndrome critical region and is fused to IgH in t(4;14) multiple myeloma. Hum Mol Genet 1998; 7(7):1071–1082.

Stevens CA, Bhakta MG. Cardiac abnormalities in the Rubinstein-Taybi syndrome. Am J Med Genet 1995; 59(3):346–348.

Stoll C, Kieny JR, Dott B, Alembik Y, Finck S. Ventricular extrasystoles with syncopal episodes, perodactyly, and Robin sequence in three generations: a new inherited MCA syndrome? Am J Med Genet 1992;(42):480–486.

Stone DL, Agarwala R, Schaffer AA, Weber JL, Vaske D, Oda T et al. Genetic and physical mapping of the McKusick-Kaufman syndrome. Hum Mol Genet 1998; 7(3):475–481.

Subramani S. PEX gene on the rise. [news]. Nature Genet 1997; 15(4):331–333.

Sun FL, Dean WL, Kelsey G, Allen ND, Reik W. Transactivation of Igf2 in a mouse model of Beckwith-Wiedemann syndrome. Nature 1999; 389:809–815.

Swillen A, Glorieux N, Peeters M, Fryns JP. The Coffin-Siris syndrome: data on mental development, language, behaviour and social skills in 12 children. Clin Genet 1995; 48:177–182.

Tan J, Dunn J, Jaeken J, Schachter H. Mutations in th MGAT2 gene controlling complex N-glycan synthesis cause carbohydrate-deficient glycoprotein syndrome type II, an autosomal recessive disease with defective brain development. Am J Hum Genet 1996; 59:810–817.

Tassabehji M, Metcalfe K, Hurst J, Ashcroft GS, Kielty C, Wilmot C et al. An elastin gene mutation producing abnormal tropoelastin and abnormal elastic fibres in a patient with autosomal dominant cutis laxa. Hum Mol Genet 1998; 7(6):1021–1028.

Teebi AS, Lambert DM, Kaye GM, Al Fifi S, Tewfik TL, Azouz EM. Keutel syndrome: further characterization and review. Am J Med Genet 1998; 78(2):182–187.

Tellier AL, Cormier-Daire V, Abadie V, Et al. CHARGE syndrome: report of 47 cases and review. Am J Med Genet 1998; 76:402–409.

Tellier AL, Loyonnet S, Cormier-Daire V, Et al. Increased paternal age in CHARGE association. Clin Genet 1996; 50:548–550.

Temtamy S, McKusick VA. Heart-Hand syndrome II (Tabatznik syndrome). Birth Defects 1978; XIV(3):241–244.

Thakker Y, Donnai D. A new recessive syndrome of unusual facies and multiple structural abnormalities. J Med Genet 1991; 28:633–635.

Thomas JA, Graham JM, Jr. Chromosome 22q11 deletion syndrome: an update and review for the primary pediatrician. [Review]. Clin Pediatr 1997; 36(5):253–66.

Thompson EM, Winter RM, Baraister M. Kivlin syndrome and Peters'-Plus syndrome: are they the same disorder? Clin Dysmorph 1993; 2(4):301–16.

Thornton CM, Magee AC, Thomas PS, Et a. Congenital heart disease and urinary tract anomalies in two siblings with DOOR syndrome. Pediatr Pathol 1994; 14:797–803.

Toriello HV. New syndrome: heart-hand syndrome V. Dysmorph Clin Genet 1992;(6):41.

Toriello HV, Higgins JV, Abrahamson J, Et al. X-linked syndrome of branchial arch and other defects. Am J Med Genet 1985; 21:137–142.

Traboulsi EI, Lenz W, Gonzales-Ramos M, Siegel J, Macrae WG, Maumenee IH. The Lenz microphthalmia syndrome. [Review]. Am J Ophthalmol 1988; 105(1):40–45.

Tsukahara M, Okamoto N, Ohashi H, Kuwajima K, Kondo I, agai T et al. Brachmann-de Lange syndrome and congenital heart disease. Am J Med Genet 1998; 75:441–442.

Turkel SB, Diehl EJ, Richmond JA. Necropsy findings in neonatal asphyxiating thoracic dystrophy. J Med Genet 1985; 22(2):112–118.

Tyson J, Tranebjaerg L, Bellman S, Wren C, Taylor JF, Bathers J et al. IsK and KvLQT1: mutation in either of the two subunits of the slow compnent of the delayed rectifier potassium channel can cause Jervell and Lange-Nielsen syndrome. Hum Mol Genet 1997; 6(12):2179–85.

Upadhyaya M, Shen M, Cherryson A, Farnham J, Maynard J, Huson SM et al. Analysis of mutations at the neurofibromatosis 1 (NF1) locus. Hum Mol Genet 1992; 1(9):735–40.

Uzun O, Blackburn ME, Gibbs JL. Congenital total lipodystrophy and peripheral pulmonary artery stenosis. Arch Dis Child 1997; 76(5):456–457.

Van Allen MI, Myhre S. New multiple congenital anomalies syndrome in a stillborn infant of consanguinous paremts and a prediabetic pregnancy. Am J Med Genet 1991; 38:523–528.

van Bever Y, Dijkstra PF, Hennekam RCM. Autosomal dominant familial radial luxation, carpal fusion and scapular dysplasia with variable heart defects. Am J Med Genet 1998; 65:213–217.

Van Den Berg DJ, Francke U. Roberts syndrome: a review of 100 cases and a new rating system for severity. Am J Med Genet 1993; 47(7):1104–1123.

Van Maldergem L, Vamos E, Liebaers I, Petit P, Vandevelde G, Simonis-Blumenfrucht A et al. Severe congenital cutis laxa with pulmonary emphysema: a family with three affected sibs. Am J Med Genet 1988; 31(2):455–64.

van Slegtenhorst M, de Hoogt R, Hermans C, Nellist M, Janssen B, Verhoef S et al. Identification of the tuberous sclerosis gene TSC1 on chromosome 9q34. Science 1997; 277(5327):805–8.

Varadi V, Szabo l, Papp Z. Syndrome of polydactyly, cleft lip/palate or lingual lump, and psychomotor retardation in endogamic gypsies. J Med Genet 1980; 17(2):119–22.

Verloes A. Hypertelorism-microtia-clefting (HMC) syndrome. Genetic Counseling 1994; 5(3):283–7.

Verloove-Vanhorick SP, Brubakk AM, Ruys JH. Extensive congenital malformations in two siblings. Maternal pre-diabetes or a new syndrome? A case report. Acta Paediatr Scand 1981; 70:767–769.

Viljoen D. Pseudoxanthoma elasticum (Gronblad-Strandberg syndrome). J Med Genet 1988; 25(7):488–490.

Visapaa I, Salonen R, Varilo T, Paavola P, Peltonen L. Assignment of the locus for hydrolethalus syndrome to a highly restricted region on 11q23–25. Am J Hum Genet 1997; 65:1086–1095.

Vujic M, Hallstensson K, Wahlstrom J, Lundberg A, Langmaack C, Martinson T. Localization of a gene for autosomal dominant Larsen syndrome to chromosome region 3p21.1 - 14.1 in the proximity of, but distinct from, the COL7A1 locus. Am J Hum Genet 1995; 57(5):1104–13.

Walker BA, Beighton PH, Murdock JL. The Marfanoid hypermobility syndrome. Ann Intern Med 1969; 71:349–352.

Wallerstein R, Scott CIJ, Nicholson L. Extended survival in a new case of ter Haar syndrome: further delineation of the syndrome. Am J Med Genet 1997; 70(3):267–72.

Wassif CA, Maslen C, Kachilele-Linjewile S, Lin D, Linck LM, Connor WE et al. Mutations in the human sterol Delta7–reductase gene at 11q12–13 causes Smith Lemli Opitz syndrome. Am J Hum Genet 1998; 63:55–62.

Webster WS, Brown-Woodman PDC. Cocaine as a cause of congenital malformations of vascular origin: experimental evidence in the rat. Teratology 1990; 41:689–697.

Welch GN, Loscalzo J. Homocystinuria and atherothrombosis. [Review]. N Engl J Med 1998; 338(15):1042–50.

Wells GL, Barker SE, Finley SC, Colvin EV, Finley WH. Congenital heart disease in infants with Down's syndrome. South Med J 1994; 87(7):724–7.

Wilcox WR, Tavormina PL, Krakow D, Kitoh H, Lachman RS, Wasmuth JJ et al. Molecular, radiologic, and histopathologic correlations in thanatophoric dysplasia. Am J Med Genet 1998; 78(3):274–81.

Williams DK, Carlton DR, Green SH, Pearman K, Cole TRP. Marshall-Smith syndrome: the expanding phenotype. J Med Genet 1997; 34:842–845.

Williams PJ, Gatti R, Darby JK, Et al. Fucosidosis revisited: a review of 77 patients. Am J Med Genet 1991; 38:111–131.

Williamson-Kruse L, Biesecker LG. Pfeiffer type cardiocranial syndrome: a third case report. J Med Genet 1995; 32:901–903.

Wilson LC, Leverton K, Oude Luttikhuis MEM, Oley CA, Flint J, Wolstenholme J et al. Brachydactyly and mental retardation: an Albright hereditary osteodystrophy-like syndrome localized to 2q37. Am J Hum Genet 1995; 56:400–407.

Winship IM, Viljoen DL, Leary PM, De Moor MM. Microcephaly-cardiomyopathy: a new autosomal recessive phenotype? J Med Genet 1991; 28:619–621.

Wirtz MK, Samples JR, Kramer PLea. Weill-Marchesani syndrome - possible linkage of the autosomal dominant form to 15q21.1. Am J Med Genet 1996; 65:68–75.

Woodhouse NJ, Sakati NA. A syndrome of hypogonadism, alopecia, diabetes mellitus, mental retardation, deafness, and ECG abnormalities. J Med Genet 1983; 20(3):216–219.

Wu YQ, Sutton VR, Nickerson E, Lupski JR, Potocki L, Korenberg JR et al. Delineation of the common critical region in Williams syndrome and clinical correlation of growth, heart defects, ethnicity, and parental origin. Am J Med Genet 1998; 78(1):82–9.

Wyllie JP, Wright MJ, Burn J, Hunter S. Natural history of trisomy 13. Arch Dis Child 1994; 71:343–345.

Yorifuji T, Matsumura M, Okuno T, Et al. Hereditary pancreatic hypoplasia, diabetes mellitus, and congenital heatr disease: a new syndrome? J Med Genet 1994; 31:331–333.

Young TL, Penney L, Woods MO, Et al. A fifth locus for Bardet-Biedl syndrome maps to chromosome 2q31. Am J Hum Genet 1999; 64:900–904.

Yu CE, Oshima J, Fu YH, Wijsman EM, Hisama F, Alisch R et al. Positional cloning of the Werner's syndrome gene [see comments]. Science 1996; 272(5259):258–62.

Zapata HH, Sletten LJ, Pierpont MEM. Congenital cardiac malformations in Adams-Oliver syndrome. Clin Genet 1995; 47(2):80–84.

Zareba W, Moss AJ, Schwartz PJ, Vincent GM, Robinson JL, Priori SG et al. Influence of the genotype on the clinical course of the Long-QT syndrome. N Engl J Med 1998; 339(14):960–5.

Zaremba J. Jadassohn's naevus phakomatosis: A study based on a review of thirty seven cases. J Mental Deficiency Research 1978; 22:103–123.

Zhao HG, Li HH, Bach G, Schmidtchen A, Neufeld EF. The molecular basis of Sanfilippo syndrome type B. Proc Natl Sci U S A 1996; 93(12):6101–5.

Zlotogora J, Ariel I, Ornoy A, Yagel S, Eidelman AI. Thomas syndrome: potter sequence with cleft lip/palate and cardiac anomalies [see comments]. Am J Med Genet 1996; 62(3):224–6.

Zwamborn-Hanssen AM, Schrander-Stumpel CT, Smeets E, Decock P, Fryns JP. FG syndrome: the trias mental retardation, hypotonia and constipation reviewed. Genetic Counseling 1995; 6(4):313–319.

Common genetic determinants of coagulation and fibrinolysis

48

Angela M. Carter
Peter J. Grant

Introduction

Thrombotic disorders are a major cause of morbidity and mortality in the western hemisphere. These disorders can be classified into those affecting the venous system, characterized by fibrin rich thrombi, and those affecting the arterial system, characterized by platelet rich thrombi superimposed upon atheromatous plaque. Elucidating the mechanisms involved in the development and progression of these disorders has been a major health care initiative for many years. It has become clear that for both venous and arterial thrombotic disorders, abnormalities of hemostasis play a key role.

The hemostatic system maintains a delicate balance between the processes of coagulation and anticoagulation, platelet activation and platelet inhibition, and activation/inhibition of fibrinolysis in order to maintain vascular patency. Activation of the coagulation cascade and activ-

ation of platelets occurs in rapid response to endothelial cell injury leading to thrombin generation, platelet deposition and fibrin formation (Fig. 48.1). Activation of the anticoagulant pathway by interaction of thrombin with membrane bound thrombomodulin and activation of protein C inhibits further thrombin generation and serves to localize coagulation at the site of vascular injury and prevent widespread systemic coagulation. Finally the fibrinolytic system helps to maintain vascular patency by lysis of the fibrin matrix.

Any perturbation of these processes may give rise to either deficiencies in platelet adhesion and fibrin formation leading to bleeding disorders (these tend to be rare familial defects and are not within the scope of this chapter), or to excessive platelet adhesion and fibrin deposition giving rise to thrombosis. Perturbation of hemostasis may arise through a variety of environmental and genetic influences and ultimately the duration of exposure and the accumulation of risk factors will determine the overall risk for thrombosis.

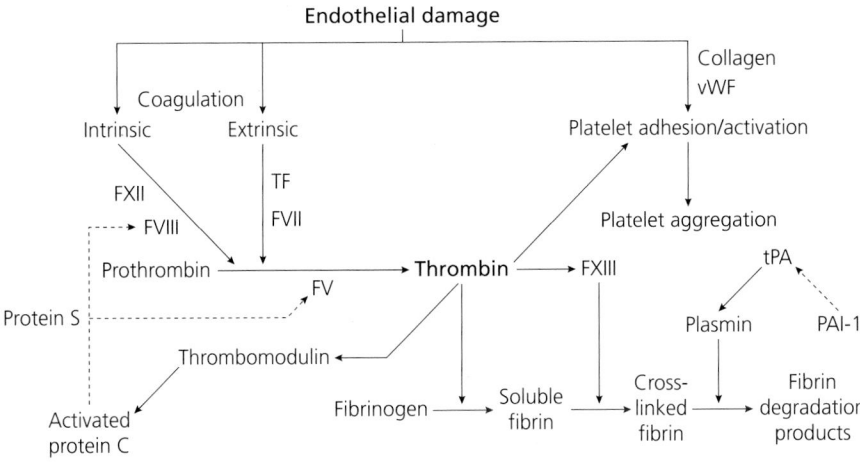

Fig. 48.1. Schematic representation of activation of the coagulation cascade and platelet adhesion following endothelial damage. Activation of the coagulation cascade (both intrinsic and extrinsic) and adhesion of platelets to exposed collagen and von Willebrand factor and subsequent activation occurs in rapid response to endothelial cell injury leading to thrombin generation, platelet deposition and fibrin formation. Activation of the anticoagulant pathway by interaction of thrombin with membrane bound thrombomodulin and activation of protein C inhibits further thrombin generation and serves to localize coagulation at the site of vascular injury and prevent widespread systemic coagulation. Finally the fibrinolytic system helps to maintain vascular patency by lysis of the fibrin matrix.

1327

Risk factors for thrombosis

VENOUS THROMBOSIS

The contribution of genetic factors to the pathogenesis of venous thrombosis is indicated by a strong family history in many individuals presenting with premature thrombosis. Commonly, deficiencies in the anticoagulant proteins, protein C, protein S and antithrombin were identified in these subjects, which highlighted the importance of abnormalities of hemostasis, and anticoagulant pathways in particular, in the pathogenesis of venous thrombosis (Egberg, 1965; Dahlback et al., 1993; Bertina et al., 1994). The contribution of genetic factors to the pathogenesis of venous thrombosis is most apparent in young subjects in whom spontaneous thrombosis may occur without obvious environmental stimuli such as surgery, pregnancy or malignancy. Additionally thrombosis often occurs in sites that are unusual in the general population such as the portal, subclavian and inferior vena caval vessels.

ARTERIAL THROMBOSIS

It is clear that, as with venous thrombosis, the development of arterial thrombosis involves complex interactions between environmental and genetic factors. In comparison to the venous circulation, the arterial system is a high flow, high pressure system in which the development of atherosclerotic plaques on the vessel wall is followed by plaque instability and rupture, which precipitates the acute thrombotic event. A number of large prospective and case-control studies have addressed the question as to whether changes in plasma levels of components of the hemostatic system are related to the pathogenesis of cardiovascular disorders. These have demonstrated associations of several coagulation and fibrinolytic factors, including fibrinogen, factor VII, von Willebrand factor, PAI-1 and tPA with atherothrombotic events (Hamsten et al., 1987; Jansson et al., 1991; Meade et al., 1986; Ridker et al., 1994; Wilhelmsen et al., 1984). It is apparent that whatever the predisposing factors, activation of coagulation is intimately involved in both the progression of atherosclerosis and the manifestation of acute thrombosis. As with venous thrombosis, the contribution of genetic factors has been indicated by the clustering of cardiovascular diseases within families, however, due to the complex pathogenesis of CAD (coronary artery disease), elucidating the genetic factors contributing to the disease process has proved to be more complicated.

Candidate genes for thrombosis

Disturbances of hemostasis are central to the pathogenesis of both venous and arterial thrombosis and the genes encoding the proteins involved in coagulation/anticoagulation, platelet activation/inhibition, and activation/inhibition of fibrinolysis can be considered to be candidates for both arterial and venous thrombosis. Sequence variation within a gene may have several possible consequences. For instance, variation within the 5′ gene regulatory domains may create or destroy binding sites for transcription factors that could result in altered expression of the gene and ultimately plasma levels of the respective protein. Similarly, variation within the 3′-untranslated region of the resultant mRNA may give rise to alterations in mRNA stability or protein translation thereby influencing plasma levels of the protein. Variation within the coding region of a gene can result in amino acid substitutions (missense mutations) which may alter the structure of the protein and its function.

STRATEGIES FOR THE DETECTION OF SEQUENCE VARIATION WITHIN GENES

Several methods have been developed to identify novel polymorphisms in candidate genes. These include single strand conformation polymorphism (SSCP) analysis, chemical mismatch analysis, denaturing gradient gel electrophoresis analysis and Cleavase fragment length polymorphism analysis (Brow et al., 1996; Hayashi et al., 1992; Newton and Graham, 1994). Due to the relative complexity of a number of these methods, the most commonly used is SSCP, which is a relatively straightforward method. It relies on the fact that under non-denaturing conditions, single-stranded DNA has a folded structure due to the formation of intra-strand interactions, and this is highly sequence specific (Orita et al., 1989). More recently an automated system for detection of polymorphisms has been developed based on high performance liquid chromatography, known as temperature modulated heteroduplex analysis. This system has the advantage of analyzing larger fragments (up to 500 bp), without the loss of sensitivity, and is a more rapid and sensitive method for polymorphism detection than SSCP (O'Donovan et al., 1998). For all methods of detection, the characterization of the sequence variation is carried out by DNA sequencing.

COMMON MUTATIONS OF GENES ENCODING HEMOSTATIC FACTORS

Over the past 15 years the search for common sequence variations (population prevalence of 1% or greater) within the genes encoding the various hemostatic factors has accelerated and many polymorphisms have been identified. The aim of the present chapter is to summarize the polymorphisms in the genes encoding key elements of coagulation and fibrinolysis. We will present the data regarding associations of these polymorphisms with levels of the respective protein and with protein function where these studies have been carried out. Finally, where appropriate, any associations with thrombotic disease will be indicated, although for a comprehensive overview of hemostatic gene polymorphisms in relation to thrombotic disease the reader is directed to a recent review of the subject (Lane and Grant, 2000).

Coagulation factors

FACTOR XII

Factor XII is a serine protease which is involved in several hemostatic processes including the activation of the intrinsic coagulation cascade and the contact system of fibrinolysis (Levi et al., 1991). Subjects with inherited deficiencies of factor XII are predisposed to thromboembolic complications and this observation has clouded views on the physiological importance of FXII. Elevated levels of activated FXII have been associated with the extent of coronary stenosis and a history of MI, suggesting that FXIIa may be indicative of a hypercoagulable state (Kohler et al., 1998a). In support of this, FXIIa correlates with cholesterol, triglyceride, FVII clotting activity, BMI, tPA, PAI-1 and insulin (Miller et al., 1997; Kohler et al., 1998a). There is considerable inter-individual and racial variation in plasma levels of FXII and Kanaji et al. (1998) have identified a common polymorphism (46 C/T) in the 5'-untranslated region of the FXII gene four bases upstream of the translation initiation ATG codon that is associated with significant differences in plasma FXII levels. In addition, the 46 C/T genotype distributions of Oriental and Caucasian subjects are significantly different with T allele frequencies of 73% and 20% respectively. Kohler et al. (1999a) confirmed an association of 46 C/T and plasma levels of activated FXII, with genotype accounting for 18% of the inter-individual variation in levels. The presence of the 46 T allele creates an ATG codon 5 bp upstream from the original ATG codon

and *in vitro* transcription/translation analyses suggest that the T allele results in decreased translation efficiency of FXII (Kanaji et al., 1998). Despite the association of 46 C/T with FXII levels and the previous association of FXIIa with extent of coronary stenosis and history of MI, there was no corresponding association of genotype with stenosis or MI (Kohler et al., 1999a). Since FXII deficiency is associated with venous thromboembolic complications, further work is required to determine whether 46 C/T is associated with this disorder.

FACTOR VIII

Elevated plasma FVIII levels have been associated with increased risk for vascular disease (Koster et al., 1995). Evidence of a genetic contribution to plasma FVIII levels comes from the observation of an association with ABO blood group and clustering of FVIII levels in families (Orstavik et al., 1989). However, to date no common polymorphisms have been identified within the FVIII gene which are associated with elevated plasma FVIII (Mansvelt et al., 1998).

FACTOR VII

Factor VII is a vitamin K-dependent coagulation factor circulating as an inactive zymogen. In the Northwick Park Heart Study, elevated levels of FVII coagulant activity were associated with fatal (but not non-fatal) coronary events (Meade et al., 1986). However, this association has not been substantially confirmed by other large studies (Lane et al., 1996; Smith et al., 1997). There are 6 common polymorphisms so far identified within the FVII gene (Green et al., 1991; Marchetti et al., 1993; Pollak et al., 1996; van't Hooft et al., 1999), four of which occur within the 5' gene regulatory region: -122 T/C, -401 G/T, -402 G/A and a decanucleotide insertion at position -323. In addition, a single base mutation (A/G) within the coding region gives rise to the missense mutation Arg353Gln, and finally a polymorphism within the hypervariable region 4 of intron 7 gives rise to 3 different alleles H5, H6 and H7. The 10 bp insertion and the Arg353Gln are in strong linkage disequilibrium and account for approximately 20% of the inter-individual variation in plasma factor VII. Possession of Gln353 is associated with lower plasma levels of FVIIC and antigen and it has been demonstrated that Gln353 is less efficiently secreted than Arg353 *in vitro* (Hunault et al., 1997). The -401 G/T and -402 G/A together account for approximately 30% of the variation in plasma FVII levels, with -401G and -402A alleles associated with increased transcriptional activity *in vitro* and elevated plasma FVII levels (van't Hooft et al., 1999). The 10 bp insertion and the -122 T/C show no difference in nuclear binding profile or transcriptional activity, suggesting that they are unlikely to be functional polymorphisms (van't Hooft et al., 1999). In relation to disease, the association of these polymorphisms with coronary artery disease remains controversial, with most studies showing no association; this issue has been discussed in detail elsewhere (Lane and Grant, 2000).

TISSUE FACTOR PATHWAY INHIBITOR

Tissue factor pathway inhibitor (TFPI) is a heparin-releasable inhibitor of tissue factor dependent coagulation and functions by formation of a quaternary FXa/TFPI/FVIIIa/TF complex (Lindahl et al., 1992). A number of polymorphisms in the gene encoding TFPI have been recently described including the -399 C/T and Val264Met polymorphisms. Despite being located in a putative AP-1 binding domain of the TFPI 5′ regulatory region, there was no association of the -399 C/T with plasma TFPI (Miyata et al., 1998). However, the Val264Met polymorphism has been associated with both baseline and heparin releasable TFPI, with lower levels in those possessing Met264 (Moatti et al., 1999). No association of these polymorphisms with venous or arterial thrombosis was found (Miyata et al., 1998; Moatti et al., 1999).

FACTOR V

Factor V plays central roles in coagulation and anticoagulation. Activated FV is a cofactor in the conversion of prothrombin to thrombin whereas zymogen factor V is thought to act as a cofactor in the activated protein C inhibition of FVa and FVIIIa along with protein S (Shen and Dahlbakc, 1994; Thorelli et al., 1998). Resistance to activated protein C (APCR) is strongly associated with venous thromboembolism (Koster et al., 1993) and a missense polymorphism of the factor V gene (Arg506Gln, Factor V Leiden) accounts for the majority (but not all) of the observed APCR (Bertina et al., 1994). The Gln506 variant of FVa is less readily inactivated by APC and Gln506 is also less effective as a co-factor for the inactivation of FVIIIa, hence leading to a hypercoagulable state (reviewed by Lane and Grant, 2000). A number of other polymorphisms of the FV gene have been identified, one of which (A4070G) gives rise to His1299Arg. A haplotype including nine of the FV polymorphisms always associates with Arg1299 and the haplotype has been referred to as HR2. This haplotype is associated with reduced plasma FV levels (Bernardi et al.,

1997) and APCR even in the presence of Gln506. In addition to the association of Gln506 and HR2 with APCR both polymorphisms are associated with venous thromboembolism, with a doubling of the risk for thrombosis in carriers of Gln506 in the presence HR2 (Faioni et al., 1999).

PROTEIN C

As indicated above, protein C is a major anticoagulant factor and deficiency is associated with venous thromboembolism. Three common polymorphisms in the 5′ regulatory region of the protein C gene have been identified: -1654 C/T, -1641 A/G and -1476 A/T and these polymorphisms are in close linkage disequilibrium (Spek et al., 1994). The five most frequent genotype combinations are CC/GG/TT, CT/AG/AT, CC/AG/AT, CT/AA/AA, TT/AA/AA. There is a significant association with protein C activity levels with the lowest levels observed in CC/GG/TT individuals and the highest levels in TT/AA/AA with intermediate levels in the other genotype groups (Spek et al., 1995; Aich et al., 1999). In addition, in the Leiden Thrombophilia Study, CC/GG/TT was associated with an increased risk for venous thrombosis compared with TT/AA/AA (Spek et al., 1995).

PROTEIN S

Protein S is a cofactor to activated protein C in the inactivation of factors Va and VIIIa. As with protein C, deficiency of protein S is associated with venous thrombosis. Two common polymorphisms of the protein S gene have been described; the 2148 A/G (Pro626) and the 2698 C/A located 520 bp from the termination codon, in the 3′-untranslated region (Diepstraten et al., 1991; Mustafa et al., 1996). These polymorphisms are significantly associated with plasma levels of total protein S antigen, the highest levels in those of AA/AA genotype and the lowest in those of GG/CC genotype (Leroy-Matheron et al., 1999). The mechanism(s) by which the 2148 A/G and 2698 C/A polymorphisms influence plasma levels is unknown at present. No associations of these polymorphisms with venous thrombosis or cardiovascular disease have been reported.

THROMBOMODULIN

Thrombomodulin acts as a receptor for thrombin on the endothelial cell surface and converts thrombin from a coagulant into an anticoagulant capable of activating protein C.

An inverse association of thrombomodulin and risk of coronary heart disease was reported in the ARIC study (Salomaa et al., 1999). A number of polymorphisms of the thrombomodulin gene have been recently identified, including three promoter polymorphisms -133 C/A, -33 G/A and GG -9/-10 AT (Ireland et al., 1997; LeFlem et al., 1999), and two missense polymorphisms, Ala25Thr and Ala455Val (Norland et al., 1997; van der Velden et al., 1991). Associations of the -133 C/A, GG -9/-10 AT, Ala25Thr and Ala455Val polymorphisms with plasma thrombomodulin or in vitro expression systems have yet to be reported. The -33 G/A polymorphism has been reported to confer a weak decrease in promoter activity in a luciferase reporter gene assay. Due to the relatively low incidence of these polymorphisms, reported associations with vascular disease have been contradictory in studies with insufficient power to detect a difference (Lane and Grant, 2000).

ENDOTHELIAL CELL PROTEIN C/ ACTIVATED PROTEIN C RECEPTOR

Endothelial cell protein C/activated protein C receptor (EPCR) is now considered to be a component of the protein C anticoagulant pathway and serves to localize protein C at the endothelial cell surface where it can interact with thrombomodulin bound thrombin. A single 23 bp insertion polymorphism in exon 3 of the EPCR gene has been reported, which gives rise to a STOP codon six codons downstream of the insertion point resulting in a truncated protein missing part of exon 3 and all of exon 4 (Merati et al., 1999). Despite the low frequency of this polymorphism, an association with venous thrombosis, but not MI, was reported. Further studies are required to determine the influence of this polymorphism on receptor expression and function.

VON WILLEBRAND FACTOR

Elevated levels of plasma von Willebrand factor (vWF) have been associated with increased risk for cardiovascular disease (Folsom et al., 1993; Catto et al., 1997). The contribution of genetic factors in determining plasma levels of vWF are indicated by the association of plasma vWF with ABO blood group, with the lowest levels observed in those of blood group O (Orstavik et al., 1989). A number of common polymorphisms of the von Willebrand Factor gene have been identified, including 4 polymorphisms within the 5′ gene regulatory region: -1793 C/G, -1234 C/T, -1185 A/G, -1051 G/A (Heywood et al., 1997; Keightley et al., 1999). There have been differences in binding of nuclear

proteins reported for the -1234 C/T and − 1051 G/A polymorphisms and the -1234 C/T, -1185 A/G and -1051 G/A polymorphisms are in strong linkage disequilibrium with 2 major haplotypes, haplotype 1: -1234C/-1185A/ -1051G; and haplotype 2: -1234T/-1185G/-1051A. These haplotypes are associated with plasma vWF levels in subjects of blood group O, with the highest levels observed in subjects homozygous for haplotype 1 and lowest in those homozygous for haplotype 2 (Keightley et al., 1999). The association of these polymorphisms with vascular disease is yet to be fully investigated.

PROTHROMBIN

The conversion of prothrombin to thrombin is the final step in the common coagulation pathway leading to the conversion of fibrinogen to fibrin and the activation of platelets. A polymorphism in the 3′-untranslated region of the gene, G20210A, has been identified which occurs at the last base of the prothrombin mRNA before the poly(A) addition site (Poort et al., 1996). This polymorphism is associated with plasma levels of prothrombin, with the highest levels observed in those homozygous for the 20210A allele (Poort et al., 1996; Zawadski et al., 1998). The mechanism by which the 20210A allele gives rise to elevated plasma prothrombin is at present unclear, although its proximity to the poly(A) addition site suggests a possible influence on polyadenylation efficiency. Alternatively, it may influence mRNA stability since mRNA stability motifs are commonly located within the 3′-untranslated region, however, given the stability of prothrombin mRNA this may be a less likely explanation (Carter et al., 1999). The 20210A allele has been related to venous thromboembolism in a number of studies and the association with VTE in the Leiden Thrombophilia Study was accounted for entirely by its association with plasma prothrombin level (Poort et al., 1996).

FIBRINOGEN

Fibrinogen is a large and complex protein comprised of pairs of three non-identical polypeptides, referred to as the α, β and γ chains, and each of these chains is encoded by a separate gene. In studies of heritability, the contribution of genetic factors to plasma levels of fibrinogen have been estimated to be in the region of 50% (Hamsten et al., 1987; Friedlander et al., 1995). Fibrinogen levels have been consistently associated with cardiovascular disease (Wilhelmsen et al., 1984; Meade et al., 1986). There are a number of polymorphisms within the fibrinogen gene cluster

(Behague et al., 1996) and several studies have investigated their relationship with circulating levels of fibrinogen, with particular interest in the β fibrinogen gene promoter region due to its apparent rate-limiting influence on fibrinogen secretion (Yu et al., 1984). A number of polymorphisms have been studied with respect to plasma fibrinogen level, in particular the -455 G/A β-fibrinogen polymorphism. Elevated plasma fibrinogen has been fairly consistently reported to be higher in subjects possessing the -455 A allele compared with subjects homozygous for the -455 G allele (Behague et al., 1996). Despite the association of these polymorphisms with fibrinogen levels, the reports of genotype associations with disease have been inconsistent, as summarized in Table 48.1. There are a number of excellent review articles addressing these issues and since little new information has been reported in recent years the reader is directed to the following articles for further information (Humphries et al., 1999; Lane and Grant, 2000).

In terms of polymorphisms within the coding region of fibrinogen, only 2 missense mutations, the β-fibrinogen Arg448Lys and α fibrinogen Thr312Ala polymorphisms, have been reported to date (Baumann and Henschen, 1993). The Arg448Lys is in strong linkage disequilibrium with the promoter polymorphisms, is associated with variation in plasma fibrinogen levels and no reports of structural differences between the two variants have been reported to date. Of more interest is the Thr312Ala polymorphism, which occurs within a region of α-fibrinogen important in a number of FXIII-dependent processes,

including α-fibrin/α-fibrin and α-fibrin/α_2-antiplasmin cross-linking (amino acid residues Aα 328 and Aα 303 respectively) (Kimura and Aoki, 1986; Muszbek et al., 1996). The region of α-fibrinogen encompassing this polymorphism (residues Aα 242–424) is also important in promoting the dissociation of the FXIII A and B subunit dimers thereby enhancing activation of FXIII itself (Credo et al., 1981). Thr312Ala is not in linkage disequilibrium with the β-fibrinogen polymorphisms, shows no association with plasma fibrinogen levels but has been related to more rigid and less porous fibrin gel structures (Curran et al., 1998). In addition we have shown associations of the 312Ala allele with post-stroke mortality in subjects with artrial fibrillation (Carter et al., 1999) and with pulmonary embolism (Carter et al, 2000) supporting the possibility that Thr312Ala influences clot stability, although the exact mechanism(s) remains unclear at present.

FACTOR XIII

FXIII is a transglutaminase that plays a crucial role in fibrin clot formation by cross-linking adjacent γ and α chains of polymerised fibrin thereby ensuring the structural integrity of the clot (Ichinose, 1994). In addition, FXIIIa-dependent cross-linking of α_2-antiplasmin to α-fibrin renders the clot more resistant to lysis by plasmin. Deficiency of FXIII is associated with severe bleeding but there is little information regarding elevated plasma FXIII and vascular disease. Results from animal studies, however, indicate that factor

Table 48.1. Fibrinogen gene polymorphisms: associations with fibrinogen levels and disease. A number of studies have determined the association of β fibrinogen gene polymorphisms with plasma fibrinogen level and with cardiovascular disease. Although associations with plasma fibrinogen have been fairly consistent, associations with disease have been contradictory as indicated.

Genotype	Genotype/Phenotype	Phenotype/Disease	Genotype/Disease	Study (controls/cases)
Bcl I	–level	+PAD	+PAD	EAS (126/121) Fowkes et al., 1992
-455 G/A	+level	+PAD/+CAD	+PAD/–CAD	EAS (423/88/195) Lee et al., 1999
-455 G/A	–level	+CAD	–CAD	(0/545) Wang et al., 1997
-455 G/A	+level	+CAD/+MI	–CAD/–MI	(0/923/224/222) Gardemann et al., 1997
-455 G/A	+level	–CAD progression	+/–CAD progression	REGRESS (0/339/343) de Maat et al., 1998
Bcl I	+level	+CAD	–MI +CAD	ECTIM (567/668) Behague et al., 1996
-455 G/A	+level	+IHD	–IHD	CCHS (9127/470) Tybjaerg-Hansen et al., 1997
-455 G/A	+level	–MI	–MI	EARS (1106/585) Humphries et al., 1995
Bcl I	+level	+MI	+MI	GISSI 2 (173/102) Zito et al., 1997
-148 C/T	–level	+carotid atheroma	+carotid atheroma	ASPS (399/0) Schmidt et al., 1998

CAD = coronary artery disease
PAD = peripheral artery disease
IHD = ischaemic heart disease
MI = myocardial infarction
+ indicates significant association, –indicates no association

XIII is a major determinant of endogenous and exogenous fibrinolysis and suggest associations with MI and pulmonary embolism (Shebuski et al., 1996; Reed and Houng, 1999). A number of common polymorphisms of the FXIII gene have been identified, including four missense polymorphisms, Val34Leu, Pro564Leu, Val650Ile and Glu651Gln (Suzuki et al., 1994; Suzuki et al., 1996). There is no association of these polymorphisms with plasma FXIII A subunit antigen or FXIII B subunit antigen. However, Val34Leu and Pro564Leu are significantly associated with FXIII cross-linking activity (Fig. 48.2), with enhanced activity associated with possession of Leu34 and Pro564. However, after accounting for Val34Leu genotype the association of Pro564Leu with FXIII activity was weak (Kohler et al., 1999b). Val34Leu, which occurs in close proximity to the thrombin cleavage site, is the only one of these polymorphisms that has been consistently associated with vascular disease, with significant inverse associations of Leu34 with

MI, venous thromboembolism and cerebral infarction, as summarised in Table 48.2. These clinical findings appear at variance to the *in vitro* finding of an increase in FXIII activity associated with the Leu34 allele, which might have been expected to confer an increased risk for thrombosis (Anwar et al., 1999; Kangsadalampai and Board, 1998; Kohler et al., 1998c). Recent results from our group have indicated that the Leu34 allele is activated at a lower concentration of thrombin than the Val34 allele. In addition, the Leu34 allele is associated with differences in cross-linked fibrin structure (Ariëns et al, 2000). The exact mechanism(s) giving rise to the apparent protective effect of Leu34 is the subject of ongoing investigation.

Fibrinolysis

TISSUE-TYPE PLASMINOGEN ACTIVATOR

Tissue-type plasminogen activator (tPA) is an endothelial cell-derived activator of the fibrinolytic system that is considered to be protective against thrombotic disorders, a view supported by the clinical use of recombinant tPA following acute myocardial infarction. In contradistinction, however, elevated plasma levels of tPA have been associated with an increased risk of myocardial infarction in a number of prospective and case-control studies (Jansson et al., 1993; Ridker et al., 1994; Thompson et al., 1995). The reason for this paradoxical observation is unclear but may reflect the association of tPA with plasma PAI-1 or other risk factors for vascular disease. However, the role of elevated levels of tPA in the pathogenesis of cardiovascular disease remains unclear at present.

A number of polymorphisms in the tPA gene occur including a common Alu insertion/deletion in intron 8 (Ludwig et al., 1992). There is no evidence of association of this polymorphism with arterial or venous tPA levels,

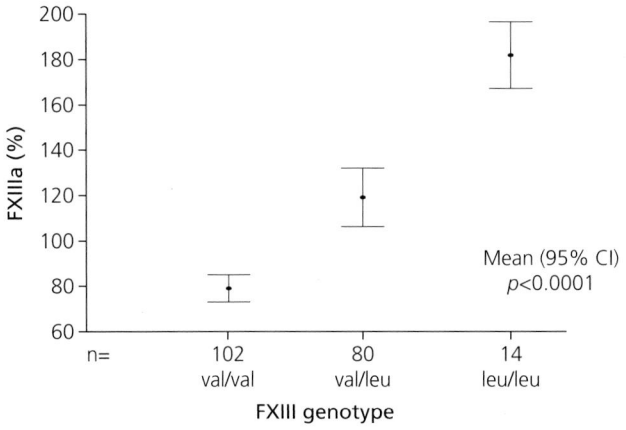

Fig. 48.2. FXIII Val34Leu genotype is a major determinant of plasma FXIIIa cross-linking activity. FXIII cross-linking activity was determined by a 5-biotinamido pentylamine incorporation assay and results expressed as a percentage of pooled normal plasma (Ariëns et al., 1999). Subjects homozygous for the Leu34 allele demonstrated the highest activity and subjects homozygous for the Val34 allele the lowest, with intermediate activity in heterozygous subjects.

Table 48.2. The FXIII-Val34Leu polymorphism and thrombosis. A number of studies have confirmed that possession of the Leu34 allele confers a relative protection from vascular disease compared with the Val34 allele.

Disease	Odds Ratio	Reference
Myocardial infarction	0.67 (0.54–0.85)	Kohler et al., 1998a,b,c
Myocardial infarction	0.59 (0.38–0.93)	Wartiovaara et al., 1999
Myocardial infarction	0.60 (0.4–0.9)	Franco et al 2000
Myocardial infarction	0.46 (0.27–0.79)	Barbosa et al 2000
Venous thromboembolism	0.63 (0.38–0.82)	Catto et al., 1999
Venous thromboembolism	0.16 (0.05–0.50)	Franco et al., 1999
Cerebral infarction	0.58 (0.44–0.75)	Elbaz et al 2000

however an association with local basal tPA release rate determined by a modified perfused forearm model has been described (Jern et al., 1999). Higher release rates were observed in subjects homozygous for the insertion allele compared with those possessing the deletion allele. The insertion allele of this polymorphism has also been associated with MI in the Rotterdam Study (van der Bom et al., 1995), although this association has not been confirmed in other studies (reviewed by Lane and Grant, 2000).

PLASMINOGEN ACTIVATOR INHIBITOR-1

Plasminogen activator inhibitor-1 (PAI-1) is a serine protease inhibitor that is the major circulating inhibitor of tPA. Elevated PAI-1 has been consistently associated with cardiovascular disease (Margaglione et al., 1994; Thogersen et al., 1998) and high PAI-1 levels are found in atherosclerotic plaques (Sobel et al., 1998). In addition PAI-1 clusters with a number of features of the insulin resistance syndrome (Mansfield et al., 1997), which is itself strongly associated with cardiovascular events. Several common polymorphisms of the PAI-1 gene have been identified, including the 4G/5G insertion/deletion at -675, a CA dinucleotide repeat within intron 3 and a 3' *Hind* III RFLP. The only consistent associations with plasma PAI-1 have been observed for the -675 4G/5G polymorphism, with approximately 25% higher levels in those homozygous for the 4G compared to the 5G allele (Eriksson et al., 1995; Ye et al., 1995; Ossei-Gerning et al., 1997). *In vitro* studies have confirmed higher rates of transcription associated with the 4G allele and a difference in binding of nuclear factors has been identified, with the 4G allele apparently binding an enhancer whereas the 5G allele binds both an enhancer and a repressor resulting in decreased transcription of the 5G allele relative to the 4G allele (Dawson et al., 1993). As with many gene-disease association studies, there have been a number of studies demonstrating associations with disease and an almost equal number refuting these associations, (Grant, 1997; Lane and Grant, 2000).

Platelet receptors

PLATELET $\alpha_{IIb}\beta_3$ RECEPTOR

The platelet $\alpha_{IIb}\beta_3$ (glycoprotein IIb/IIIa) receptor is a member of the integrin family of cell adhesion molecules (Bennett, 1996) and activation of $\alpha_{IIb}\beta_3$ is the final common mediator of platelet aggregation. Aggregation arises as a result of fibrinogen or vWF binding to activated $\alpha_{IIb}\beta_3$ receptors on adjacent platelets. Deficiency of $\alpha_{IIb}\beta_3$ (Glanzmann thrombasthenia) is associated with bleeding tendency. The importance of $\alpha_{IIb}\beta_3$ in the pathogenesis of cardiovascular disease has been highlighted by the effective clinical use of anti-$\alpha_{IIb}\beta_3$ agents in the secondary prevention of coronary occlusion following high-risk coronary interventions (Moliterno and Topol, 1997; Tcheng, 1997).

A number of polymorphisms of the genes encoding α_{IIb} and β_3 have been identified (Nurden, 1995). For β_3 these include 3 polymorphisms in the 5' gene regulatory region, -468 G/A, -425 A/C and -400 A/C and 2 missense polymorphisms Leu33Pro (HPA-1, Pl^A) and Arg489Gln (HPA-9). For α_{IIb} these include Ile843Ser (HPA-3) and the 10480 C/G polymorphism in intron 21 (Negrier et al., 1998). The Leu33Pro polymorphism has been the most extensively studied of these polymorphisms to date. It has not been demonstrated to influence the platelet $\alpha_{IIb}\beta_3$ receptor expression, however the Pro33 allele is associated with enhanced platelet fibrinogen binding in response to ADP, with a lower threshold for ADP stimulated fibrinogen binding for the Pro33 compared with the Leu33 allele (Feng et al., 1999; Michelson et al, 2000). In addition, Chinese hamster ovary and human kidney embryonal 293 cells which over-expressed Leu33 and Pro33 variants of human $\alpha_{IIb}\beta_3$ demonstrated increased binding of the Pro33 variant on immobilised fibrinogen, which was unrelated to surface receptor expression. This was associated with enhanced cell spreading, a greater extent of polymerized actin, increased pp125^{FAK} phosphorylation and increased fibrin clot retraction for cells expressing the Pro33 variant compared with the wild-type (Vijayan et al, 2000).

Little is known regarding the functional consequences of the other polymorphisms mentioned in terms of receptor expression, ligand binding or outside-in signaling. A number of studies have investigated the association of Leu33Pro and Ile843Ser with vascular disease. Results have been largely conflicting with positive and negative associations with MI, coronary stent occlusion and stroke. These issues have been addressed in recent comprehensive reviews by Bray (1999) and Goldschmidt-Clermont (1999).

PLATELET GLYCOPROTEIN Ib-IX-V RECEPTOR

The platelet GPIb-IX-V receptor, encoded by 4 separate genes, is involved in the shear dependent adhesion of platelets to vWF exposed at sites of vascular injury. Deficiency of GPIb-IX-V (Bernard Soulier syndrome) is associated with bleeding tendency. A number of polymorphisms of the genes encoding the GPIb-IX-V receptor have been described (Nurden, 1995), the most extensively studied in relation to vascular disease are located in the GPIbα gene including the -5 T/C, a 39 base pair variable number tandem repeat (VNTR) polymorphism and a missense polymorphism Thr145Met (HPA-2) (Corral et al., 1998). The VNTR polymorphism results in one to four copies of a 13 amino acid repeat sequence within the macroglycopeptide region of the protein. It has been postulated that this might result in extension of the vWF binding region (located at the amino terminal of glycoprotein Ibα) further into the circulation, thereby influencing platelet adhesion at sites of vascular injury (Lopez et al., 1992). There are no data to support this hypothesis at present nor do any studies address receptor expression or function with regard to the Thr145Met polymorphism. For the more recently described -5 C/T polymorphism, *in vitro* expression experiments have demonstrated increased expression of the C compared with the T variant. In addition, the C variant is associated with increased platelet surface expression of GPIb-IX-V, with expression dependent on gene dosage (Afshar-Khargan et al., 1999). There have been few reports relating these polymorphisms to vascular disease and the results are again conflicting (Corral et al, 2000; Lane and Grant, 2000).

PLATELET α₂β₁ RECEPTOR

The platelet α₂β₁ (glycoprotein Ia–IIa) receptor is also a member of the integrin family of cell adhesion molecules and acts as a receptor for collagen. There is considerable inter-individual variation in the surface expression of this receptor, which is reflected in a wide variation in response to collagen (Kuniki et al., 1993). A number of polymorphisms in the genes encoding this receptor have been identified including Lys505Glu (HPA-5), and the silent coding region polymorphisms 807 C/T (Phe224) and 873 G/A (Thr246) (Kuniki et al., 1997). The 807 C/T and 873 G/A polymorphisms are in linkage disequilibrium and both are associated with platelet α₂β₁ receptor density. The 807 C and 873 G alleles were associated with lower receptor density than the 807 T and 873 A alleles (Kuniki et al., 1997) and receptor density was correlated with the rate of platelet adhesion to type I collagen even under conditions of high shear (Kritzig et al., 1998). Possession of the 807 T allele has been associated with premature MI (Santoso et al., 1999) and stroke (Carlsson et al., 1999), although the association with MI was not confirmed in a large case-control study (Croft et al., 1999). In contrast there was an increased incidence of the 807 C allele in patients with Type

I von Willebrand disease, suggesting an association with bleeding (Di Paola et al., 1999).

Gene/environment and gene/gene interactions

In the previous sections we have described in excess of 50 common polymorphisms in the genes encoding various components of the hemostatic system. For many of these polymorphisms there is evidence of associations with protein expression or function, and for some of these there is also evidence of associations with vascular disease. In many cases, however, these associations are inconsistent, particularly with respect to disease. This highlights the emerging complexity of genotype/phenotype associations. The epidemiology of myocardial infarction has demonstrated a fluctuating prevalence this century, and migrant studies clearly demonstrate acquisition of risk at a level associated with the destination of migrant populations. These observations indicate the impossibility of common causes of myocardial infarction being related simply to inter-individual variations in genotype and highlight the importance of understanding of the role of gene/environment interactions in the pathogenesis of this disease.

For many hemostatic proteins there is considerable inter-individual variation in levels, and both genetic and environmental factors contribute to the overall determination of an individual's steady state level of both circulating and membrane bound proteins. Therefore, to study the influence of common polymorphisms of hemostatic protein genes on associated levels of proteins or protein function in population studies without due consideration of the potential confounding effect of environmental and other genetic influences is fraught with difficulty. Similarly, investigating the influence of a polymorphism in an isolated *in vitro* system will not account for the complexity of the coagulation and fibrinolytic cascades and the numerous positive and negative feedback mechanism regulating these processes, which may act to compensate for differences in protein levels or function *in vivo*. To highlight some of these points, next we describe a few recent examples of gene/environment and gene/gene interactions.

Interactions of the β-fibrinogen -455 G/A polimorphism in determining plasma fibrinogen level

Fibrinogen levels are elevated in smokers compared with non-smokers and also in the presence of an acute phase reaction. Interactions of the -455 G/A polymorphism with smoking in the determination of fibrinogen levels have been described, with a greater association of this polymorphism with fibrinogen levels being observed in smokers compared with non-smokers (Behague et al., 1996; Green et al., 1993). In addition, -455 G/A has also been associated with a differential elevation of fibrinogen levels in response to a two-day period of strenuous exercise in Army recruits, with the greatest acute-phase rise in fibrinogen levels observed in subjects prossessing the A allele (Montgomery et al., 1996). Similarly, Gardemann et al. (1997) reported a more pronounced difference in levels of fibrinogen between those homozygous for the G allele and those homozyguous for the A allele in subjects with evidence of an acute phase reaction compared to those without such evidence.

Interactions of the PAI-1 4G/5G polymorphism in determining plasma PAI-1 level

Plasma PAI-1 levels are significantly correlated with plasma triglyceride level and a 4G/5G genotype specific response to triglyceride has been reported (Mansfield et al., 1995; Panhaloo et al., 1995). The highest levels of PAI-1 were observed in subjects with 4G/4G genotype and high plasma triglyceride levels. A triglyceride responsive region has since been identified within the PAI-1 5′ region adjacent to the 4G/5G site (Eriksson et al., 1998). An interaction between 4G/5G and an exercise-induced decrease in PAI-1 has also been reported, with a significant reduction (36%) in PAI-1 observed only in those of 4G/4G genotype (Vaisanen et al., 1999). This was suggested to be related to an exercise induced decrease in triglyceride, which would be reflected in a more profound effect on PAI-1 in the triglyceride responsive 4G/4G genotype.

Interactions of the FV ARG506GLN polymorphism in determining risk for venous thrombosis

The risk associated with Arg506Gln in conjunction with one or more other risk factors for venous thrombosis have been determined and significant interactions of Arg506Gln with smoking, oral contraceptive use, the prothrombin G20210A polymorphism and other rarer inherited disorders of protein C and protein S have been identified (Vandenbroucke et al., 1994; van Boven et al., 1996; Rosing et al., 1997). In most cases the risk associated with FV Arg506GIn is synergistic (as opposed to additive) with the risk conferred by the other

factors. Interactions such as this may have serious clinical implications with regard to therapy. For instance, whilst in those subjects with FV 506Gln alone, no long-term prophylactic treatment may be deemed necessary after an acute thrombotic event, given a multiplicity of risk the impetus for long-term pharmacological intervention might be greatly enhanced.

Interactions of the FXIIIVAL34LEU polymorphism in determining risk for vascular disease

Interactions between the FXIIIVal34Leu, PAI-1 4G/5G genotype and insulin resistance have been identified. Patients with a history of MI had higher plasma levels of PAI-1 and an increased prevalence of the PAI-1 4G/5G genotype in those who possessed the FXIIILeu34 allele compared with those homozygous for the FXIIIVal34 allele (Kohler et al., 1998b). These findings suggested that the FXIIILeu34 allele is protective against MI unless there is coexistent suppression of fibrinolysis occurring in association with underlying insulin resistance. In addition, a significant interaction between FXIIIVal34Leu and the α-fibrinogen Thr312Ala polymorphism has been identified in relation to pulmonary embolism, with the apparent protective effect of FXIIILeu34 being lost in the presence of the α-fibrinogen Ala312 allele (Carter et al, 2000).

Conclusion

The development of molecular epidemiology as a scientific discipline, coupled with the relative accessibility of molecular technology, has transformed the scientific landscape over the last 15 years. In the field of thrombosis and hemostasis this has rejuvenated the study of coagulation in relation to thrombotic disorders and in certain cases, such as Factor V Leiden, produced significant advances in understanding. We have now identified a large number of relatively common polymorphisms in genes coding for proteins that are considered important in thrombotic processes. In several cases, there is clear and consistent evidence of circulating levels of the expressed protein being related to sequence variation(s) of the gene encoding the protein in question. This would appear to open the way to providing evidence of relationships between genetic variation and clinical disease. Problems do remain in this area, however, as evidenced by the real difficulty in obtaining consistent relationships between genotype and clinical phenotype, most notably in relation to arterial disease.

It is important to be aware of the complex processes that underpin the development of atherothrombotic disorders. It is virtually certain that atheroma formation alone is governed by hundreds of genes interacting with a variety of environmental and metabolic factors. The study of plaque rupture is in its infancy, mainly due to the difficulty in identifying an unstable plaque, but there are again many potential candidates that could be extrapolated from histological changes in an unstable plaque. Thrombosis is the final insult in a coronary artery that leads to vessel occlusion and tissue death, yet even despite its clear importance, the study of genetics is relatively new and has focused on a small number of candidate genes. All of this indicates that in the final analysis there may be many hundreds of candidates that are involved in these processes, and the number of potential genotype combinations is probably greater than the number of individuals on the planet. Add into this the fact that most genotypes have a relatively small influence on levels of the protein and it is little wonder that difficulty is being experienced in elucidating genetic responsibility for this disease.

Part of the reason for some of this confusion lies in the fact that we seem to have forgotten some basic facts about the disorders being studied. For example, epidemiology indicates quite clearly that migrants attain the cardiovascular risk of the country to which they migrate rather than retaining that of their country of origin. In western communities the prevalence of myocardial infarction increased dramatically at the turn of the 19th century; increased to a maximum in the 1970s and has thereafter decreased. All this tells us that genotpe is not directly responsible for the present epidemic of vascular disease, but rather that environmental influences remain dominant. Any theory of vascular disease must encompass what we know clinically. Our patients with myocardial infarction statistically will be overweight, diabetic, hypertensive, hypercholesterolemic, exercise-negative smokers. The answer to the genetics of myocardial infarction will probably lie in the interaction between genes and risk factors such as these. Rather than searching for genes that directly cause heart disease, which is the basis of association studies, we should be looking for protective or neutral genotypes that are converted to being pathogenic by environmental influences. If accepted, this argument suggests more time should be spent on old fashioned coagulation biochemistry, but focusing on how genotype affects biochemical reactions.

The knowledge accrued thus far, and outlined in this chapter, represents the first tentative steps towards achieving clinically useful information about disease processes. Future studies directed at understanding the pharmacogenetics of vascular disease will eventually enable the interruption of these processes by the development of new generations of therapeutics, with the possibility of altering the course of this common disorder.

REFERENCES

Afshar-Khargan V, Li CQ, Khoshnevis-Asi M, López JA (1999) Kozak sequence polymorphism of the glycoprotein (GP) Ibα gene is a major determinant of the plasma membrane levels of the platelet GP Ib-IX-V complex. Blood 94:186–191

Aich M, Nicaud V, Alhenc-Gelas M et al. (1999) Complex association of protein C gene promoter polymorphism with circulating protein C levels and thrombotic risk. Arterioscler Thromb Vasc Biol 19:1573–1576

Anwar R, Gallivan L, Edmonds SD, Markham AF (1999) Genotype/phenotype correlations for coagulation factor XIII: Specific normal polymorphisms are associated with high or low factor XIII specific activity. Blood 93:897–905

Ariëns RAS, Kohler HP, Mansfield MW, Grant PJ (1999) Subunit antigen and activity levels of blood coagulation factor XIII in healthy individuals. Relation to sex, age, smoking and hypertension. Arterioscler Thromb Vasc Biol 19:2012–2016

Ariëns RAS, Philippou H, Nagaswami C et al. (2000) The factor XIII Val34Leu polymorphism accelerates thrombin activation of factor XIII and affects crosslinked fibrin structure. Blood (in press)

Baumann RE, Henschen AH (1993) Human fibrinogen polymorphic site analysis by restriction endonuclease digestion and allele-specific polymerase chain reaction amplification: identification of polymorphisms at positions Aα312 and Bβ448. Blood 82:2117–2124

Behague I, Poirier O, Nicaud V et al. (1996) Beta fibrinogen gene polymorphisms are associated with plasma fibrinogen and coronary artery disease in patients with myocardial infarction. The ECTIM Study. Etude Cas-Temoins sur l'Infarctus du Myocarde. Circulation 93:440–449

Bennett JS (1996) Structural biology of glycoprotein IIb-IIIa. Trends Cardiovasc Med 6:31–37

Bernardi F, Faioni EM, Castoldi E et al. (1997) A factor V genetic component differing from factor V R506Q contributes to the activated protein C resistance phenotype. Blood 90:1552–1557

Bertina RM, Koeleman BP, Koster T et al. (1994) Mutation in blood coagulation factor V associated with resistance to activated protein C. Nature 369:64–67

Bray PF (1999) Integrin polymorphisms as risk factors for thrombosis. Thromb Haemost 82:337–344

Brow MA, Oldenburg MC, Lyamichev V et al. (1996) Differentiation of bacterial 16S rRNA genes and intergenic regions and *Mycobacterium tuberculosis kat* G genes by structure-specific endonuclease cleavage. J Clin Microbiol 34:3129–3137

Carlsson L, Santoso S, Spitzer C et al. (1999) The α2 gene coding sequence T$_{807}$/A$_{873}$ of the platelet collagen receptor integrin α2β1 might be a genetic risk factor for the development stroke in younger patients. Blood 93:3583–3586

Carter AM, Catto AJ, Grant PJ (1999a) The association of the α-fibrinogen Thr312Ala polymorphism with post-stroke mortality in subjects with atrial fibrillation. Circulation 99:2423–2426

Carter AM, Maurer FG, Medcalf RL (1999b) The relationship between the prothrombin G20210A polymorphism and prothrombin mRNA stability. Thromb Haemost Supplement 403 (abstract)

Carter AM, Catto AJ, Kohler HP et al. (2000) α-Fibrinogen Thr312Ala polymorphism and Venous Thromboembolism. Blood (in press)

Catto AJ, Carter AM, Barrett J et al. (1997) von Willebrand Factor and Factor VIII:C in acute cerebrovascular disease: relationship to stroke subtype and mortality. Thromb Haemost 77:1104–1108

Catto AJ, Kohler HP, Coore J et al. (1999) Association of a common polymorphism in the factor XIII gene with venous thrombosis. Blood 93:906–908

Corral J, González-Conejero R, Lozano ML et al. (1998) New alleles of the platelet glycoprotein Ibα gene. Br J Haematol 103:997–1003

Corral J, Lozano ML, González-Conejero R et al. (2000) A common polymorphism flanking the ATG initiator codon of GPIb alpha does not affect expression and is not a major risk factor for arterial thrombosis. Thromb Haemost 83:23–28

Credo RB, Curtis CG, Lorand L (1981) α-chain domain of fibrinogen controls generation of fibrinoligase (coagulation factor XIIIa). Calcium ion regulatory aspects. Biochemistry 20:3770–3778

Croft SA, Hampton KK, Sorrell JA et al. (1999) The GpIa C807T dimorphism associated with platelet collagen receptor density is not a risk factor for myocardial infarction. Br J Haematol 106:771–776

Curran JM, Evans A, Arveiler D et al. (1998) The α fibrinogen T/A312 polymorphism in the ECTIM study. Thromb Haemost 79:1057–1058

Dahlback B, Carlsson M, Svensson PJ (1993) Familial thrombophilia due to a previously unrecognized mechanism characterized by poor anticoagulant response to activated protein C: Prediction of a cofactor to activated protein C. Proc Natl Acad Sci USA 90:1004–1008

Dawson SJ, Wiman B, Hamsten A et al. (1993) The two allele sequences of a common polymorphism in the promoter of the plasminogen activator inhibitor-1 (PAI-1) gene respond differently to interleukin-1 in HepG2 cells. J Biol Chem 268:10739–10745

de Maat MP, Kastelein JJ, Jukema JW et al. (1998) -455G/A polymorphism of the beta-fibrinogen gene is associated with the progression of coronary atherosclerosis in symptomatic men: proposed role for an acute-phase reaction pattern of fibrinogen. REGRESS group. Arterioscler Thromb Vasc Biol 18:265–71

Di Paola J, Federici AB, Mannucci PM et al. (1999) Low platelet α2β1 levels in type I von Willebrand disease correlate with impaired platelet function in a high shear stress system. Blood 93:3578–3582

Diepstraten CM, Ploos van Amstel JK, Reitsma PH, Bertina RM (1991) A CCA/CCG neutral polymorphism in the codon for Pro 626 in the human protein S alpha (PROS1). Nuc Acids Res 19:5091

Egeberg O (1965) Inherited antithrombin III deficiency causing thrombophilia. Thromb Diath Haem 13:516

Elbaz A, Poirier O, Canaple S, Chédru F, Cambien F, Amarenco P, on behalf of the GÉNIC investigators (2000) The association between the Val34Leu polymorphism in the factor XIII gene and brain infarction. Blood 95:586–591

Eriksson P, Kallin B, van't Hooft FM, PB, Hamsten A (1995) Allele-specific increase in basal transcription of the plasminogen-activator inhibitor 1 gene is associated with myocardial infarction. Proc Natl Acad Sci USA 92:1851–1855

Eriksson P, Nilsson L, Karpe F, Hamsten A (1998) Very-low-density lipoprotein response element in the promoter region of the human plasminogen activator inhibitor-1 gene implicated in the impaired fibrinolysis of hypertriglyceridemia. Arterioscler Thromb Vasc Biol 18:20–26

Faioni EM, Franchi F, Bucciarelli P et al. (1999) Coinheritance of the HR2 haplotype in the factor V gene confers an increased risk of venous thromboembolism to carriers of factor V R506Q (Factor V Leiden). Blood 94:3062–3066

Feng D, Lindpaintner K, Larson MG et al. (1999) Increased platelet aggregability associated with platelet GPIIIa PlA2 polymorphism: the Framingham Offspring Study. Arterioscler Thromb Vasc Biol 19:1142–1147

Folsom AR, Wu KK, Shahar E, Davis CE (1993) Association of hemostatic variables with prevalent cardiovascular disease and asymptomatic carotid artery atherosclerosis. The Atherosclerosis Risk in Communities (ARIC) Study Investigators. Arterioscler Thromb 13:1829–1836

Fowkes FG, Connor JM, Smith FB et al. (1992) Fibrinogen genotype and risk of peripheral atherosclerosis. Lancet 339:693–696

Franco RF, Reitsma PH, Lourenco D et al. (1999) Factor XIII Val34Leu is a genetic factor involved in the aetiology of venous thrombosis. Thromb Haemost 81:676–679

Franco RF, Pazin-Filho A, Tavella MH et al. (2000) Factor XIII val34leu and the risk of myocardial infarction. Haematologica 85:67–71

Friedlander Y, Elkana Y, Sinnreich R, Kark JD (1995) Genetic and environmental sources of fibrinogen variability in Israeli families: the Kibbutzim Family Study. Am J Hum Genet 56:1194–1206

Gardemann A, Schwartz O, Haberbosch W et al. (1997) Positive association of the β fibrinogen H1/H2 gene variation to basal fibrinogen levels and to the increase in fibrinogen concentration during acute phase reaction but not to coronary artery disease and myocardial infarction. Thromb Haemost 77:1120–1126

Goldschmidt-Clermont PJ, Roos CM, Cooke GE (1999) Platelet PlA2 polymorphism and thromboembolic events: from inherited risk to pharmacogenetics. J Thromb Thrombol 8:89–103

Grant PJ (1997) Polymorphisms of coagulation/fibrinolysis genes: gene environment interactions and vascular risk. Prostaglandins Leukot Essent Fatty Acids 57:473–477

Green F, Kelleher C, Wilkes H et al. (1991) A common genetic polymorphism associated with lower coagulation factor VII levels in healthy individuals. Arterioscler Thromb 11:540–546

Green F, Hamsten A, Blomback M, Humphries S (1993) The role of β-fibrinogen genotype in determining plasma fibrinogen levels in young survivors of myocardial infarction and healthy controls from Sweden. Thromb Haemost 70:915–920

Hamsten A, De Faire U, Walldius G (1987) Plasminogen activatory inhibitor in plasma: Risk factor for recurrent myocardial infarction. Lancet 2:3–9

Hamsten A, Iselius L, De Faire U, Blomback M (1987) Genetic and cultural inheritance of plasma fibrinogen concentration. Lancet 2:988–990

Hayashi K (1992) PCR-SSCP: a method for detection of mutations. Genet Anal Tech Appl 9:73–79

Heywood DM, Ossei-Gerning, Grant PJ (1997) Two novel polymorphisms of the von Willebrand factor gene promoter and association with ischaemic heart disease. (abstract).Thromb Haemost Supplement 375

Humphries SE, Ye S, Talmud PJ et al. (1995) European Atherosclerosis Research Study: Genotype at the fibrinogen locus (G-455-A β-gene) is associated with differences in plasma fibrinogen levels in young men and women from different regions in Europe. Evidence for gender-genotype-environment interaction. Arterioscler Thromb Vasc Biol 15:96–104

Humphries SE, Luong LA, Montgomery HE et al. (1999) Gene-environment interaction in the determination of levels of plasma fibrinogen. Thromb Haemost 82:818–825

Hunault M, Arbini AA, Lopaciuk S et al. (1997) The Arg353GIn polymorphism reduces the level of coagulation factor VII. In vivo and in vitro studies. Arterioscler Thromb Vasc Biol 17:2825–2829

Ichinose A (1994) The physiology and biochemistry of factor XIII. In Bloom AL, Forbes CD, Thomas DP, Tuddenham EGD (eds): Haemostasis and Thrombosis, 3rd edn. Churchill Livingstone, Edinburgh, p. 531

Ireland H, Kunz G, Kyriakoulis K et al. (1997) Thrombomodulin gene mutations associated with myocardial infarction. Circulation 96:15–18

Jansson JK, Nilsson TK, Johnson O (1991) von Willebrand factor in plasma: a novel risk factor for recurrent myocardial infarction and death. Br Heart J 66:351–355

Jansson JH, Olofsson BO, Nilsson TK (1993) Predictive value of tissue plasminogen activator mass concentration on long-term mortality in patients with coronary artery disease. Circulation 88:2030–2034

Jern C, Ladenvall P, Wall U, Jern S (1999) Gene polymorphism of t-PA is associated with forearm vascular release rate of t-PA. Arterioscler Thromb Vasc Biol 19:454–459

Kanaji T, Okamura T, Osaki K et al. (1998) A common genetic polymorphism (46 C to T substitution) in the 5′-untranslated region of the coagulation factor XII gene is associated with low translation efficiency and decrease in plasma factor XII level. Blood 91:2010–2014

Kangsadalampai S, Board PG (1998) The Val34Leu polymorphism in the A subunit of coagulation Factor XIII contributes to the large normal range in activity and demonstrates that the activation peptide plays a role in catalytic activity. Blood 92:2766–2770

Keightley AM, Lam YM, Brady JN et al. (1999) Variation at the von Willebrand factor (vWF) gene locus is associated with plasma vWF:Ag levels: identification of three novel single nucleotide polymorphisms in the vWF gene promoter. Blood 93:4277–4283

Kimura S, Aoki N (1986) Cross-linking site in fibrinogen for α_2-plasmin inhibitor. J Biol Chem 261:15591–15595

Kohler HP, Carter AM, Stickland MH, Grant PJ (1998a) Levels of activated FXII in survivors of myocardial infarction. Association with circulating risk factors and extent of coronary artery disease. Thromb Haemost 79:14–19

Kohler HP, Stickland MH, Ossei-Gerning N, Carter et al. (1998b) Association of a common polymorphism in the factor XIII gene with myocardial infarction. Thromb Haemost 79:8–13

Kohler HP, Ariëns RAS, Whitaker P, Grant PJ (1998c) A common coding polymorphism in the Factor XIII A subunit gene (FXIIIVal34Leu) affects cross linking activity. Thromb Haemost 80:704

Kohler HP, Futers TS, Grant PJ (1999a) FXII (46C->T) polymorphism and in vivo generation of FXII activity – gene frequencies and relationship in patients with coronary artery disease. Thromb Haemost 81:745–747

Kohler HP, Futers TS, Grant PJ (1999b) Prevalence of three common polymorphisms in the A-subunit gene of factor XIII in patients with coronary artery disease. Thromb Haemost 81:511–515

Koster T, Rosendaal FR, de Ronde H et al. (1993) Venous thrombosis due to poor anticoagulant response to activated protein C: Leiden Thrombophilia Study. Lancet 342:1503–1506

Koster T, Blann AD, Briet E et al. (1995) Role of clotting factor VIII in effect of von Willebrand factor on occurrence of deep vein thrombosis. Lancet 345:152–155

Kritzig M, Savage B, Nugent DJ et al. (1998) Nucleotide polymorphisms in the α_2 gene define multiple alleles which are associated with differences in platelet $\alpha_2\beta_1$. Blood 92:2382–2388

Kunicki TJ, Orchekowski R, Annis D, Honda Y (1993) Variability of integrin $\alpha 2\ \beta 1$ activity on human platelets. Blood 82:2693–2703

Kuniki TJ, Kritzig M, Annis DS, Nugent DJ (1997) Hereditary variation in platelet integrin $\alpha_2\beta_1$ density is associated with two silent polymorphisms in the α_2 gene coding sequence. Blood 89:1939–1943

Lane A, Green F, Scarabin PY et al. (1996) Factor VII Arg/Gln353 polymorphism determines factor VII coagulant activity in patients with myocardial infarction (MI) and control subjects in Belfast and in France but is not a strong indication of MI risk in the ECTIM study. Atherosclerosis 119:119–127

Lane DA, Grant PJ (2000) Role of hemostatic gene polymorphisms in venous and arterial thrombotic disease. Blood 95:1517–1532

Lee AJ, Fowkes FG, Lowe GD et al. (1999) Fibrinogen, factor VII and PAI-1 genotypes and the risk of coronary and peripheral atherosclerosis: Edinburgh Artery Study. Thromb Haemost 81:553–560

LeFlem L, Picard V, Emmerich J et al. (1999) Mutations in the promoter region of thrombomodulin and venous thromboembolic disease. Arterioscler Thromb Vasc Biol 1999 19:1098–1104

Leroy-Matheron C, Duchemin J, Levent M, Gouault-Heilmann M (1999) Genetic modulation of plasma protein S levels by two frequent dimorphisms in the PROS1 gene. Thromb Haemost 82:1088–1092

Levi M, Hack CE, de Boer JP et al. (1991) Reduction of contact activation related-fibrinolytic activity in factor XII deficient patients. J Clin Invest 88:1155–1160

Lindahl AK, Sandset PM, Abildgaard U (1992) The present status of tissue factor pathway inhibitor. Blood Coag Fib 3:439–449

Lopez JA, Ludwig EH, McCarthy BJ (1992) Polymorphism of human glycoprotein Ib alpha results from a variable number of tandem repeats of a 13-amino acid sequence in the mucin-like macroglycopeptide region. Structure/function implications. J Biol Chem 267:10055–10061

Ludwig M, Wihn K-D, Scheuning W-D, Olek K (1992) Allelic dimorphism in the human tissue-type plasminogen activator (tPA) gene as a result of an Alu insertion/deletion event. Hum Genet 88:388–392

Mansfield MW, Stickland MH, Grant PJ (1995) Plasminogen activator inhibitor-1 promoter polymorphism and coronary artery disease in non-insulin dependent diabetes. Thromb Haemost 74:1032–1034

Mansfield MW, Stickland MH, Grant PJ (1997) PAI-1 concentrations in first degree relatives of patients with non-insulin-dependent diabetes mellitus: Metabolic and Genetic Associations. Thromb Haemost 77:357–361

Mansvelt EPG, Laffan M, McVey JH, Tuddenham EGD (1998) Analysis of the F8 gene in individuals with high plasma factor VIII:C levels and associated venous thrombosis. Thromb Haemost 80:561–565

Marchetti G, Patracchini P, Papaschini M et al. (1993) A polymorphism in the 5′ region of coagulation factor VII gene (F7) caused by an inserted decanucleotide. Hum Genet 90:575–576

Margaglione M, Di Minno G, Grandone E et al. (1994) Abnormally high circulation levels of tissue plasminogen activator and plasminogen activator inhibitor-1 in patients with a history of ischemic stroke. Arterioscler Thromb 14:1741–1745

Meade TW, Mellows S, Brozovic M et al. (1986) Haemostatic function and ischaemic heart disease: principal results of the Northwick Park Heart Study. Lancet 2:533–537

Merati G, Biguzzi F, Oganesyan N et al. (1999) A 23bp insertion in the endothelial protein C receptor (EPCR) gene in patients with myocardial infarction and deep vein thrombosis. (abstract) Thromb Haemost Supplement 507

Michelson AD, Furman MI, Goldschmidt-Clermont P et al. (2000) Platelet GP IIIa Pl^A polymorphisms display different sensitivities to agonists. Circulation 101:1013–1018

Miller GJ, Esnouf MP, Burgess AI et al. (1997) Risk of coronary heart disease and activation of FXII in middle aged men. Arterioscler Thromb Vasc Biol 17:2103–2106

Miyata T, Sakata T, Kumeda K et al. (1998) C-399T polymorphism in the promoter region of human tissue factor pathway inhibitor (TFPI) gene does not change the plasma TFPI antigen level and does not cause venous thrombosis. Thromb Haemost 80:345–346

Moatti D, Seknadji P, Galand C et al. (1999) Polymorphisms of the tissue factor pathway inhibitor (TFPI) gene in patients with acute coronary syndromes and in healthy subjects: impact of the V264M substitution on plasma levels of TFPI. Arterioscler Thromb Vasc Biol 19:862–869

Moliterno DJ, Topol EJ (1997) Conjunctive use of platelet glycoprotein IIb/IIIa antagonists and thrombolytic therapy for acute myocardial infarction. Thromb Haemost 78:214–219

Montgomery HE, Clarkson P, Nwose OM et al. (1996) The acute rise in plasma fibrinogen concentration with exercise is influenced by the G-453-A polymorphism of the beta-fibrinogen gene. Arterioscler Thromb Vasc Biol 16:386–391

Mustafa S, Pabinger I, Mannhalter C (1996) Two new frequent dimorphisms in the protein S (PROS1) gene. Thromb Haemost 76:393–396

Muszbek L, Adany R, Mikkola H (1996) Novel aspects of blood coagulation factor XIII. I. Structure, distribution, activation, and function. Crit Rev Clin Lab Sci 33:357–421

Negrier C, Grenier C, Attali O et al. (1998) Identification of new and known polymorphisms in glycoprotein IIb and IIIa genes by denaturing gradient gel elecrophoresis. Platelets 9:374–380

Newton CR, Graham A (1994) Characterizing unknown mutations. In Graham JM, Billington D (eds): PCR. BIOS Scientific Publishers, Oxford, pp. 113–122

Norlund L, Holm J, Zoller B, Ohlin AK (1997) A common thrombomodulin amino acid dimorphism is associated with myocardial infarction. Thromb Haemost 77:248–251

Nurden AT (1995) Polymorphisms of human platelet membrane glycoproteins: structure and clinical significance. Thromb Haemost 74:345–351

O'Donovan MC, Oefner PJ, Roberts SC et al. (1998) Blind analysis of denaturing high-performance liquid chromatography as a tool for mutation detection. Genomics 52:44–49

Orita M, Suzuki Y, Sekiya T, Hayashi K (1989) Rapid and sensitive detection of point mutations and DNA polymorphisms using the polymerase chain reaction. Genomics 5:874–879

Orstavik KH, Kornstad L, Reisner H, Berg K (1989) Possible effect of secretor locus on plasma concentration of factor VIII and von Willebrand factor. Blood 73:990–993

Ossei-Gerning N, Mansfield MW, Stickland MH et al. (1997) Plasminogen activator inhibitor-1 (PAI-1) promoter 4G/5G genotype and levels in relation to a history of myocardial infarction in patients characterised by coronary angiography. Arterioscler Thromb Vasc Biol 17:33–37

Panahloo A, Mohamed-Ali V, Lane A et al. (1995) Determinants of plasminogen activator inhibitor-1 activity in treated NIDDM and its relation to a polymorphism in the plasminogen activator inhibitor-1 gene. Diabetes 44:37–42

Pollak ES, Hung HL, Godin W et al. (1996) Functional characterization of the human factor VII 5′ flanking region. J Biol Chem 271:1738–1747

Poort SR, Rosendaal FR, Reitsma PH, Bertina RM (1996) A common genetic variation in the 3′-untranslated region of the prothrombin gene is associated with elevated plasma prothrombin levels and an increase in venous thrombosis. Blood 88:3698–3703

Reed GL, Houng AK (1999) The contribution of activated Factor XIII to fibrinolytic resistance in experimental pulmonary embolus. Circulation 99:299–304

Ridker PM, Hennekens CH, Stampfer MJ et al. (1994) Prospective study of endogenous tissue plasminogen activator and risk of stroke. Lancet 343:940–943

Rosing J, Tans G, Nicolaes GAF et al. (1997) Oral contraceptives and venous thrombosis: different sensitivities to activated protein C in women using second- and third-generation oral contraceptives. Br J Haematol 97:233–238

Salomaa V, Matei C, Aleksic N et al. (1999) Soluble thrombomodulin as a predictor of incident coronary heart disease and symptomless carotid artery atherosclerosis in the Atherosclerosis Risk in Communities (ARIC) Study: a case-cohort study. Lancet 353:1729–1734

Santoso S, Kunicki TJ, Kroll H et al. (1999) Association of the platelet glycoprotein Ia C807T gene polymorphism with nonfatal myocardial infarction in younger patients. Blood 93:2449–2453

Schmidt H, Schmidt R, Niederkorn K et al. (1998) Beta-fibrinogen gene polymorphism (C148→T) is associated with carotid atherosclerosis: results of the Austrian Stroke Prevention Study. Arterioscler Thromb Vasc Biol 18:487–92

Shebuski RJ, Sitko GR, Claremon DA et al. (1990) Inhibition of factor FXIIIa in a canine model of coronary thrombosis: Effect of reperfusion and acute reocclusion after recombinant tissue-type plasminogen activator. Blood 75:1455–1459

Shen L, Dahlback B (1994) Factor V and protein S as synergistic cofactors to activated protein C in degradation of factor VIIIa. J Biol Chem 269:18735–18738

Smith FB, Lee AJ, Fowkes FGR et al. (1997) Hemostatic factors as predictors of ischemic heart disease and stroke in the Edinburgh Artery Study. Arterioscler Thromb Vasc Biol 17:3321–3325

Sobel BE, Woodcock-Mitchell J, Schneider DJ et al. (1998) Increased plasminogen activator inhibitor type 1 in coronary artery atherectomy specimens from type 2 diabetic compared with non-diabetic patients. A potential factor predisposing to thrombosis and its persistence. Circulation 97:2213–2221

Spek CA, Poort SR, Bertina RM, Reitsma PH (1994) Determination of the allelic and haplotype frequencies of three polymorphisms in the promoter region of the human protein C gene. Blood Coag Fib 5:309–311

Spek CA, Koster T, Rosendaal FR et al. (1995) Genotypic variation in the promoter region of the protein C gene is associated with plasma protein C levels and thrombotic risk. Arterioscler Thromb Vasc Biol 15:214–8

Suzuki K, Iwata M, Ito S et al. (1994) Molecular basis for subtype differences of the "a" subunit of coagulation factor XIII with description of the genesis of the subtypes. Hum Genet 94:129–135

Suzuki K, Henke J, Iwata M et al. (1996) Novel polymorphisms and haplotypes in the human coagulation factor XIII A-subunit gene. Hum Genet 98:393–395

Tcheng JE (1997) Platelet glycoprotein IIb/IIIa integrin blockade: recent clinical trials in interventional cardiology. Thromb Haemost 78:205–209

Thogersen AM, Jansson JH, Boman K et al. (1998) High plasminogen activator inhibitor and tissue plasminogen activator levels in plasma precede a first acute myocardial infarction in both men and women. Evidence for the fibrinolytic system as an independent primary risk factor. Circulation 98:2241–2247

Thompson SG, Kienast J, Pyke SDN et al. (1995) Hemostatic factors and the risk of myocardial infarction or sudden death in patients with angina pectoris. N Engl J Med 332:635–641

Thorelli E, Kaufman RJ, Dahlback B (1998) The C-terminal region of the factor V B-domain is crucial for the anticoagulant activity of factor V. J Biol Chem 273:16140–16145

Tybjaerg-Hansen A, Agerholm-Larsen B, Humphries SE et al. (1997) A common mutation (G-455→A) in the beta-fibrinogen promoter is an independent predictor of plasma fibrinogen, but not of ischaemic heart disease. A study of 9,127 individuals based on the Copenhagen City Heart Study. J Clin Invest 99:3034–9

Vaisanen SB, Humphries SE, Lunong L-A et al. (1999) Regular exercise, plasminogen activator inhibitor-1 (PAI-1) activity and the 4G/5G promoter polymorphism in the PAI-1 gene. Thromb Haemost 82:1117–1120

Van Boven HH, Reitsma PH, Rosendaal FR et al. (1996) Factor V Leiden (FV R506Q) in families with inherited antithrombin deficiency. Thromb Haemost 75:417–421

Van der Bom JG, de Knijff P, Haverkate F et al. (1995) Tissue plasminogen activator and the risk of myocardial infarction: the Rotterdam Study. Circulation 95:2623–2627

Van der Velden PA, Krommenhoekvanes T, Allart CF et al. (1991) A frequent thrombomodulin amino acid diamorphism is not associated with thrombophilia. Thromb Haemost 65:511–513

Vandenbroucke JP, Koster T, Briet E et al. (1994) Increased risk of venous thrombosis in oral-contraceptive users who are carriers of factor V Leiden mutation. Lancet 344:1453–1457

van't Hooft FM, Silverira A, Tornvall P et al. (1999) Two common functional polymorphisms in the promoter region of coagulation factor VII gene determining plasma factor VII activity and mass concentration. Blood 93:3432–3441

Vijayan KV, Goldschmidt-Clermont P, Ross C, Bray PF (2000) The PI^{A2} polymorphism of integrin β3 enhances outside in signalling and adhesive functions. J Clin Invest 105:793–802

Wang XL, Wang J, McCredie RM, Wilcken DE (1997) Polymorphisms of factor V, factor VII, and fibrinogen genes. Relevance to severity of coronary artery disease. Arterioscler Thromb Vasc Biol 17:246–251

Wartiovaara U, Perola M, Mikkola H et al. (1999) Association of FXIII Val34Leu with decreased risk of myocardial infarction in Finnish males. Atherosclerosis 142:295–300

Wilhelmsen L, Svardsudd K, Korsan-Bengtsen K et al. (1984) Fibrinogen as a risk factor for stroke and myocardial infarction. N Engl J Med 311:501–505

Ye S, Green FR, Scarabin PY et al. (1995) The 4G/5G genetic polymorphism in the promoter of the plasminogen activator inhibitor-1 (PAI-1) gene is associated with differences in plasma PAI-1 activity but not with risk of myocardial infarction in the ECTIM study. Thromb Haemost 74:837–841

Yu S, Sher B, Kudryk B, Redman CM (1984) Fibrinogen precursors. Order of assembly of fibrinogen chains. J Biol Chem 259:10574–10581

Zawadski C, Gaveriaux V, Trillot N et al. (1998) Homozygous G20210A transition in the prothrombin gene associated severe venous thrombotic disease: Two cases in a French family. Thromb Haemost 80:1027–1028

Zito F, Di Castelnuovo A, Amore C et al. (1997) Bcl I polymorphism in the fibrinogen beta-chain gene is associated with the risk of familial myocardial infarction by increasing plasma fibrinogen levels. A case-control study in a sample of GISSI-2 patients. Arterioscler Thromb Vasc Biol 17:3489–94 1997

Cardiomyopathies

49

Hans–Peter Vosberg
William J. McKenna

Introduction

The term "cardiomyopathy" was introduced by Brigden (1957) to distinguish between myocardial disease of unknown cause and the more commonly recognized myocardial abnormalities arising from systemic hypertension, coronary artery and valvular disease. Case reports of probable primary cardiomyopathies were communicated more than a century ago in Paris in the 1860s (Hallopeau, 1869; Liouville, 1869) and, later, in Germany (Krehl, 1895; Schmincke, 1907).

The first systematic characterization in the field of primary myocardial disease was presented by the British forensic pathologist D Teare (1958). He reported nine cases of asymmetric septal hypertrophy, first identified at necropsy. All of the patients had died suddenly; three were first-degree relatives from one family. A complete clinical account of this family was published by Hollman and colleagues (1960); the cause of disease in this sibship (a β-myosin heavy-chain mutation) was determined much later (Watkins et al., 1992a;b).

The classification of cardiomyopathies can be attributed to proposals made by Goodwin and his collaborators in the 1960s and 70s which were later confirmed by a WHO/ISFC Task Force (1980). This scheme has recently been refined and extended by considering the advances, in particular of the past decade, in knowledge of the etiology and pathogenesis of these cardiac disorders (Richardson et al., 1996). Cardiomyopathies have now been defined as "diseases of the myocardium associated with cardiac dysfunction". Four different classes are distinguished, hypertrophic cardiomyopathy (HCM), dilated cardiomyopathy (DCM), restrictive cardiomyopathy (RCM) and arrhythmogenic right ventricular cardiomyopathy (ARVC). Two additional categories comprise "unclassified" and "specific cardiomyopathies". The first of these categories includes cases which do not readily fit into any group, such as fibroelastosis, systolic dysfunction with minimal dilation, or diseases presenting with features of more than one type of cardiomyopathy. The second category covers heart muscle disease associated with specific cardiac or systemic disorders. Ischemia, valvular defects, hypertension, metabolic disorders, general system disease, toxins and other conditions may cause "secondary" cardiomyopathy. Secondary cardiomyopathies are classified by the primary condition responsible for cardiac dysfunction, e.g., valvular, ischemic, metabolic or hypertensive cardiomyopathy (see Richardson et al., 1996, and also earlier discussions by Keren and Popp, 1992).

This chapter is predominantly focused on hypertrophic and dilated cardiomyopathies. The reason for this bias is the enormous increase in knowledge of etiology and pathogenesis, in particular of HCM. This disease, which is as a rule a familial condition, has been intensively studied in recent years. Following the lead of the Seidman group and their collaborators in Boston, the molecular genetic basis of this disease has been determined with major contributions from many laboratories worldwide. In addition, progress has been made in understanding cellular and molecular mechanisms presumably involved in the clinical manifestation of HCM-related cardiac dysfunction. Clinical features, the current molecular genetic knowledge and the functional studies which led to the designation of HCM as a "disease of the cardiac sarcomere", are discussed in detail.

Dilated cardiomyopathy is a more heterogeneous condition than hypertrophic cardiomyopathy. DCM probably comprises a number of different disease entities that, in their later stages, are clinically similar, but etiologically distinct.

1342

The commonly accepted recognition of familial disease with apparent autosomal dominant inheritance applies to at least 25% or more of cases of DCM. Our knowledge of genetic causes is growing, albeit slowly, and will eventually allow genetic classification and phenotypic distinction of an increasing number of these disorders.

RCM is defined by restrictive filling and reduced ventricular volume with normal or near-normal systolic function and wall thickness. As a primary condition it is extremely rare and is more often observed in connection with myocardial fibrosis accompanying HCM or DCM, or as a consequence of endocardial fibroelastosis (which may be inherited). Thus, RCM is probably in most cases a "specific cardiomyopathy" rather than a primary muscle disease of the heart and the evidence does not suggest a familial or genetic basis.

Arrhythmogenic right ventricular cardiomyopathy (ARVC) was not included in the original Goodwin scheme. It has increasingly been recognized over the past two decades. The condition is characterized by fibro-fatty replacement of right ventricular myocardium. It appears to be familial in the majority of cases with autosomal dominant inheritance. Recessive families from the island of Naxos have also been reported and a disease causing gene has been identified (McKoy et al., 2000). Growing awareness of this disorder may lead to new insights soon. The few known data will be discussed in a separate section.

This contribution is an update of a text printed in a previous edition of this series (Vosberg and McKenna, 1996). Genetics is the *leitmotiv*, but clinical aspects will be considered in particular with a special emphasis on new developments in the management of these diseases. Nevertheless for additional discussion, pertinent review articles—some of them which have been superceded, but still informative—are also recommended (Maron et al., 1987a, 1987b; Abelmann and Lorell, 1989; Goodwin, 1992; Keren and Popp, 1992; Kelly and Strauss, 1994; Dec and Fuster, 1994; McKenna and Watkins, 1995; Wigle et al., 1995; Watkins et al., 1996; Spirito et al., 1997, Bonne et al., 1998; McKenna, 2001; Pyeritz, 2001).

Hypertrophic cardiomyopathy

CLINICAL FEATURES

Diagnosis

Hypertrophic cardiomyopathy is characterized by a hypertrophied and nondilated left and/or right ventricle in the absence of an alternative cardiac or systemic cause. Thus, the diagnosis requires the exclusion of other conditions that might induce ventricular hypertrophy, for example, systemic hypertension or aortic stenosis. However, the presence of an alternative condition does not exclude a primary cardiomyopathy. Patients may suffer from two diseases. A summary of the properties of HCM is presented in Table 49.1. The diagnosis is usually based on the demonstration of unexplained hypertrophy detected by two-dimensional echocardiography (discussed below in the subsection Imaging). When unequivocal clinical and electrocardiographic features of the disease are present, or when more subtle features of the disease are associated with a positive family history, echocardiography serves to confirm the diagnosis. If typical features are lacking and history is inconclusive, the clinician must rely on echocardiographic findings for a diagnosis.

Failure to detect hypertrophy in the young in affected families does not exclude the disease. Hypertrophy may not become apparent until adolescent growth is completed

Table 49.1. Clinical and genetic properties of HCM (OMIM 192600)

Clinical presentation	Onset of symptoms variable Many asymptomatic Varying degrees of clinical severity Sudden death common initial presentation in the young
Diagnosis	Based on symptoms and family history, ECG, 2-D echocardiography and nuclear magnetic resonance imaging
Pathology	Asymmetric hypertrophy Myocardial hypertrophy Interstitial fibrosis Altered intramural vessel walls
Pathophysiology	Systolic hypercontractility Diastolic dysfunction Outflow obstruction
Genetics	Usually familial, autosomal dominant Sporadic disease uncommon Sarcomeric contractile gene mutations Eight genes confirmed, β-myosin heavy chain most frequently affected
Pathogenesis	Stepwise process with long latency (about two decades), slow progression of compensatory biological changes in the myocardium
Prognosis	Variable, slow progression of symptoms and severity, course of disease often benign High risk of sudden death in a subpopulation of mutation gene carriers

Abbreviation: *OMIM, entry number in the reference list of* Online Mendelian Inheritance in Man (www.ncbi.nlm.nih.gov/OMIM).

(Maron et al., 1986a). Subsequent reassessments at regular intervals are indicated. Incomplete penetrance of HCM may occasionally mask the disease even in adults. De novo manifestation of HCM beyond the age of 30 is however uncommon and to date appears to be associated with a particular gene abnormality.

Diagnostic problems may arise in highly trained athletes and in patients with mild hypertension. In these cases it can be difficult to assign ventricular hypertrophy to a defined cause and to discriminate between pathologic and physiologic responses. Highly trained sportsmen normally have an increase in muscle mass corresponding to an upward shift of about 3 mm in the bellshaped distribution of left ventricular wall thickness (Shapiro et al., 1985; Pellicia et al., 1991). Echocardiographic features that favor the diagnosis of HCM rather than secondary hypertrophy include left ventricular hypertrophy larger than 15 mm, small left ventricular cavity dimensions, features of an outflow tract gradient and abnormalities of diastolic function.

Natural history

The natural history of HCM is one of slow progression of symptoms, gradual deterioration of left ventricular function, and a significant incidence of sudden death (Frank and Braunwald, 1968; McKenna and Goodwin, 1981). Dyspnea, chest pain, impairment of exercise tolerance, and syncopal episodes are the commonest initial complaints in adults (McKenna et al., 1981b). In children and adolescents sudden death remains a common initial manifestation of the disease. Symptomatic presentation may be at any age. Occasionally, HCM is found at autopsy in a stillborn or presents during infancy with cardiac failure that is usually fatal (Maron et al., 1982b).

About 50% of adults present with symptoms, and in the other half diagnosis is made during family screening or following the incidental detection of an abnormality on physical, ECG, or echocardiographic examination (Maron et al., 1976; Fiddler et al., 1978; McKenna et al., 1981b). About half of the patients with symptoms experience dyspnea (Braunwald et al., 1964; McKenna and Goodwin, 1981).

Slow progression of symptoms is typically associated with an increase in end-diastolic volume and a gradual reduction in left ventricular systolic performance. These events are usually accompanied by increasing myocardial wall thinning, presumably as a consequence of myocyte necrosis and fibrosis (Spirito et al., 1987). In such patients, end-diastolic volume increases, but even in the end stages it rarely exceeds normal limits; these patients resemble those who have DCM mainly in the degree of impairment of systolic

performance. Other patients who experience severe symptomatic deterioration may present with a clinical picture resembling that of restrictive cardiomyopathy (see the section Restrictive and Infiltrative Cardiomyopathy later in this chapter). Atria can be grossly enlarged and signs of right heart failure may be prominent.

Atrial fibrillation develops in 10% to 15% of patients and is considered to indicate a poor prognosis (Glancy et al., 1970; Wigle et al., 1985; Olivotto et al., 1999) though in the largest study of atrial fibrillation patients five-year survival was similar to age matched patients who remained in sinus rhythm (Robinson et al., 1990). Sustained ventricular tachycardia is uncommon but 20–25% of adults with HCM will have episodes of nonsustained ventricular tachycardia detected during 24 hour ECG (Holter monitoring). Both atrial and ventricular arrhythmias are related to age and disease progression.

Sudden death, which may occur at any age, is the most dreaded complication of HCM (McKenna and Goodwin, 1981). Data from tertiary referral centers indicate that the annual mortality from sudden death in adults is about 1%. In children and adolescents it is about 2% (Spirito et al., 1997). Mortality is greater in those who have recurrent syncope or a strong family history of sudden deaths from HCM (Maron et al., 1976; 1978b; Fiddler et al., 1978; McKenna and Deanfield, 1984). Although the mortality figures from nonreferral hospitals are lower, the risk of sudden death is still present (Spirito et al., 1989). Autopsy studies have shown that undiagnosed hypertrophic cardiomyopathy is the most common cause of sudden death in the young and in competitive athletes (Maron et al., 1980a, 1982a; Maron, 1998; Corrado et al., 1990).

In summary, HCM has a wide spectrum of clinical presentation, ranging from severe cardiac failure or sudden death at a young age to an incidental finding at any age.

Physical examination

In the majority of patients with HCM, the physical examination is unremarkable. Abnormalities such as a rapid upstroke arterial pulse, a palpable atrial beat or prominent ventricular impulse may be subtle and difficult to be distinguished from normal. An ejection murmur caused by left ventricular outflow tract obstruction is present in approximately 20–25% of patients. The intensity of this murmur can be increased by physiologic and pharmacologic maneuvers that lower afterload or venous return (amyl nitrite, standing, Valsalva maneuver) and decreased by measures that enhance afterload and venous return (squatting, phenylephrine). Such patients usually also have co-existant mitral regurgitation which may be difficult to distinguish by auscultation, but which can be readily assessed by echo/Doppler evaluation.

For further information, see common textbooks of cardiology (Julian et al, 1996; Braunwald et al., 2001).

INVESTIGATIONS

Imaging

Two-dimensional echocardiography, including Doppler interrogation, has largely replaced chest radiography and invasive catheterization in routine diagnostic and morphologic or functional cardiac assessment in HCM (Maron et al., 1984). Echocardiography was introduced in diagnosis of HCM three decades ago (Shah et al., 1971; Abbasi et al., 1972; Henry et al., 1973). Left ventricular hypertrophy may be symmetric or asymmetric and localized to the spectrum or the free wall, but usually involves the septum and free wall with relative sparing of the posterior wall. To be diagnostic, thickness measurements should exceed two standard devi-

ations for sex-, age-, and size-matched populations because myocardial mass increases with both age and body size. In practice, in an adult of normal size, the presence of a left ventricular myocardial segment of 15 mm or more is usually considered to be diagnostic (Maron et al., 1981a; 1981b; Shapiro and McKenna, 1983). About one third of patients also have hypertrophy of the right ventricular free wall; the severity of right ventricular hypertrophy is strongly related to the severity of left ventricular hypertrophy (McKenna et al., 1988b). Isolated right ventricular hypertrophy has not been described.

Apical hypertrophy seems to be common in Japan (Yamaguchi et al., 1979), but it is also seen elsewhere (Shapiro and McKenna, 1983; Chikamori et al., 1988). Typically, left ventricular end-systolic and end-diastolic dimensions are reduced, and the left atrial dimension is increased, while indices of systolic function, such as ejection fraction and velocity of fiber shortening, are normal or increased. Right ventricular cavity dimensions are usually normal. The left ventricular outflow tract is narrowed, when there is gross upper septal hypertrophy. An example

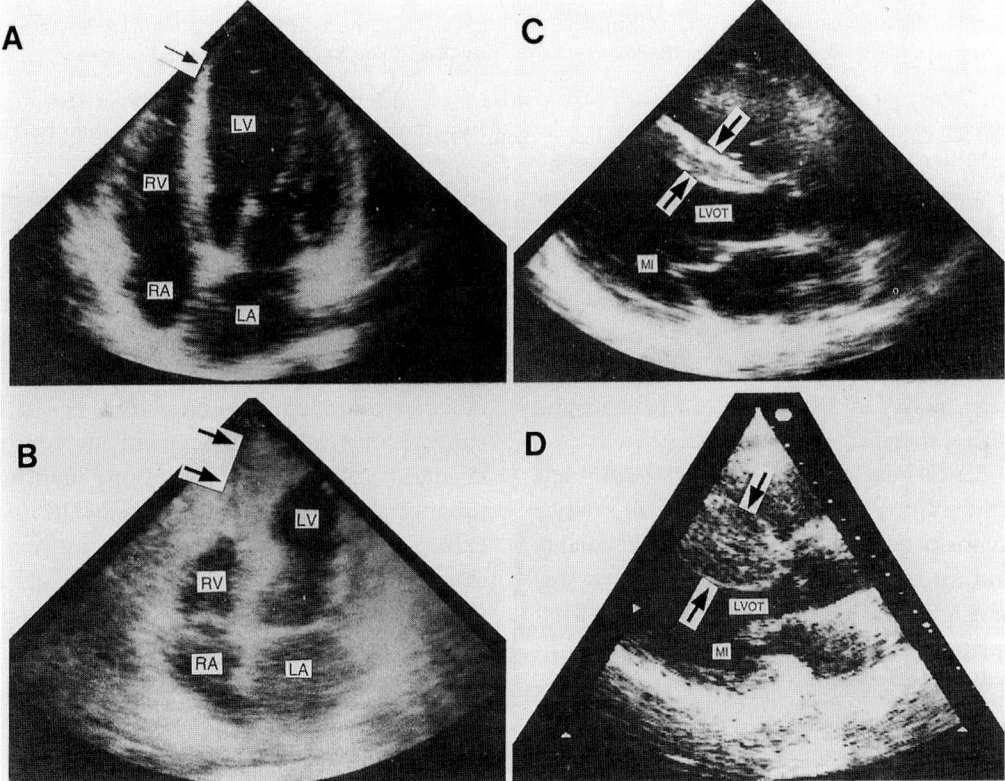

Fig. 49.1. Hypertrophic cardiac muscle investigated by two-dimensional echocardiography. (A) Four-chamber-view of a normal heart. The arrow points to the barely visible apical region. (B) Four-chamber-view of a severe hypertrophy in the apex region (arrows). (C) Normal left ventricle in the long-axis-view with a septum of normal thickness (arrows), normal dimensions of the LVOT (left ventricular outflow tract). The mitral valve is closed. (D) Left ventricle with massive hypertrophy in the long-axis-view. Wall thickness is about 25 mm (see the arrows from either side). The outflow tract is obstructed. LV left ventricle, LA left atrium, RV right ventricle, RA right atrium, MI mitral valve. (From Vosberg and Haberbosch, 1998, with permission.)

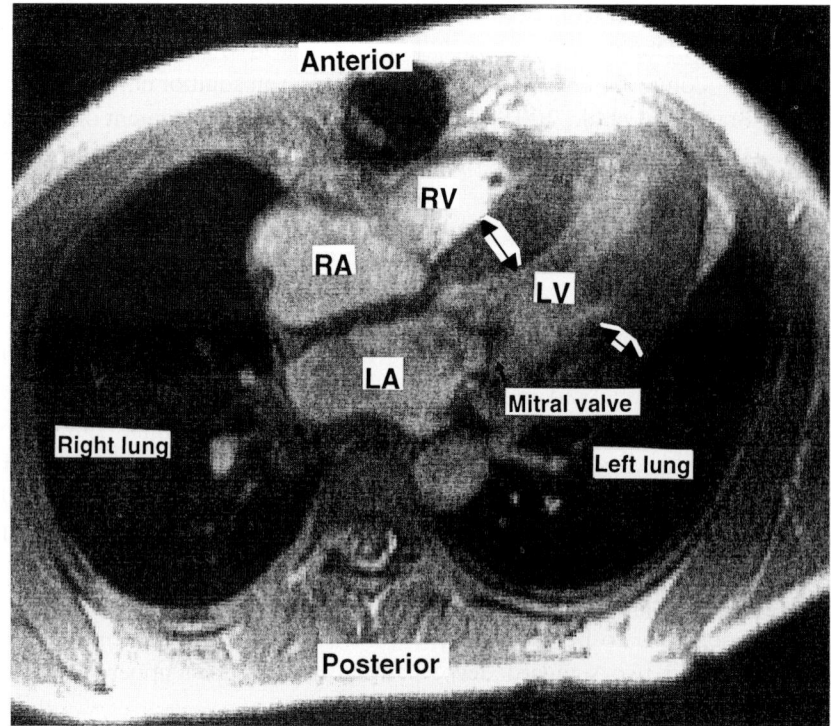

Fig. 49.3. Magnetic resonance imaging of a hypertrophic heart in a HCM patient. The picture shows all four chambers in end-diastolic phase of ventricular activity. The two double arrows indicate the extent of the thickness of the septum (> 20 mm) and the lateral left-ventricular wall. The hypertrophy is associated in this case with an outflow tract obstruction that is not visible at this slice. RA, right atrium; LA, left atrium; RV, right ventricle, LV, left ventricle. The black arrow points to the closed mitral valve. (Courtesy Dr Bachmann, Bad Nauheim.)

of septal hypertrophy assessed by echocardiography is presented in Figure 49.1. Color and continuous-wave Doppler scanning provide a measurement of left ventricular outflow tract gradients that correlate well with those measured invasively. When the calculated outflow tract gradient is higher than 30 mmHg, systolic anterior motion of the mitral valve is usually present (Doi et al., 1980; Gilbert et al., 1980; Pollick et al., 1984). Limitations of 2D echo in HCM include poor image quality in 10% to 20% of patients and difficulties in imaging the apex of the ventricles.

Magnetic resonance imaging (MRI) will not routinely replace echocardiography, but it offers an alternative imaging modality for patients in whom echo image quality is substandard and for those in whom apical HCM is suspected on the basis of ECG abnormalities. A typical MRI cross-section depicting the four chambers of the heart is shown in Figure 49.2.

Electrocardiography

The 12-lead ECG remains a valuable diagnostic tool. Recent family studies reveal that ECG changes often precede echocardiographic left ventricular hypertrophy in adolescents, and in some adults who do not have marked hypertrophy, ECG abnormalities may be the predominant expression of the disease.

The 12-lead ECG is abnormal in 90% to 95% of patients who fulfill diagnostic echocardiographic criteria (Braunwald et al., 1964; Savage et al., 1978). At the time of diagnosis, 10% of patients are in atrial fibrillation, 20% have left axis deviation, while 10% have either right or left bundle branch block (Savage et al., 1978; McKenna et al., 1981a). The latter may develop as an immediate or late complication of surgical myectomy. ST-segment depression and T-wave changes are the most common abnormalities and are usually associated with increased QRS voltage (Savage et al., 1978). Occasionally, giant negative T waves are seen (Yamaguchi et al., 1979; Alfonso et al., 1990). Isolated voltage criteria for left ventricular hypertrophy are unusual. About 20% of patients have abnormal Q waves. Preexcitation of the ventricle, a hallmark of the Wolff-Parkinson-White (WPW) syndrome, is occasionally seen. The coexistence of HCM with WPW syndrome appears to be more common than expected by chance alone. There are now at least 10 families (unpublished) in which the disease causing gene has been mapped to a locus on chromosome 7 suggesting that at least in these families the WPW and the HCM have a common genetic determinant.

P-wave abnormalities of left, right or biatrial overload are common, reflecting the difficulties faced by the atria in emptying their contents into poorly relaxing, stiff ventricles. As there are so many electrophysiologic abnormalities, there is no ECG typical of HCM. A useful rule is to consider the diagnosis whenever the ECG is abnormal, particularly in younger patients (Fig. 49.3).

Holter monitoring is useful to confirm suspected arrhythmia and to detect occult arrhythmia which may be of clinical or prognostic significance. For example, nonsustained ventricular tachcardia is a marker of increased risk of sudden death. Short episodes of supraventricular tachycardia and paroxysmal atrial fibrillation are detected in 30% to 35% of patients. Sustained supraventricular arrhythmias (> 30 seconds) are poorly tolerated unless the ventricular response is controlled; they carry an increased risk of embolism (Robinson et al., 1990). The incidence of supraventricular arrhythmias relates directly to age and is associated with increased atrial dimensions and increased filling pressures.

Exercise electrocardiography provides useful functional and prognostic information. Measurement of exercise cap-acity, ideally performed with simultaneous respiratory gas analysis, provides an objective endpoint to assess symptom severity and guide management. During exercise, ST-segment changes of 2 mm from baseline are documented in 25% of patients and associated with symptoms of angina.

Continuous measurement of the blood pressure during exercise reveals that approximately one-third of patients have abnormal blood pressure response with either flat (failure to increase by at least 20 mmHg) or hypotensive responses (drops of 15 mmHg) from peak recordings (Frenneaux et al., 1990; Counihan et al., 1993). In most patients these changes are asymptomatic, but they are associated with premature sudden death and are a marker of the high risk young patients (aged < 40 years) (Olivotto et al., 1999; Sadoul et al., 1999).

Hemodynamics and electrophysiology

Catheterization is not necessary for diagnosis. It may be indicated for measurements of filling pressures in patients with refractory symptoms or mitral regurgitation, and for coronary arteriography in middle-aged or older patients (> 40 y) with refractory chest pain or marked ST-segment changes during exercise (details in Wigle et al., 1985). Electrophysiologic studies are occasionally necessary to exclude an accessory pathway or guide management of symptomatic arrhythmia. The initial enthusiasm for ventricular tachycardia stimulation studies in the evaluation of high risk individuals has not been confirmed and is not recommended (Slade et al., 1996).

PATHOLOGY

Morphology and histology

The heart shows characteristic macroscopic and microscopic alterations in HCM. Hypertrophy is usually symmetric in the right ventricle (McKenna et al., 1988b), but in the left ventricle may be symmetric or asymmetric, involving the septum, free wall, or posterior wall; occasionally it is restricted to the distal ventricle. A patch of endocardial thickening just below the aortic valve, resulting from contact with the anterior mitral leaflet, is often found in patients with reduced left ventricular dimensions, particularly that of the outflow tract (Maron and Epstein, 1980; Maron et al., 1981a; 1981b; Shapiro and McKenna, 1983).

The histologic findings in HCM are distinctive (Davies, 1984). Within areas of affected myocardium interstitial fibrosis is seen together with gross disorganization of the muscle bundles, resulting in a characteristic whorled array.

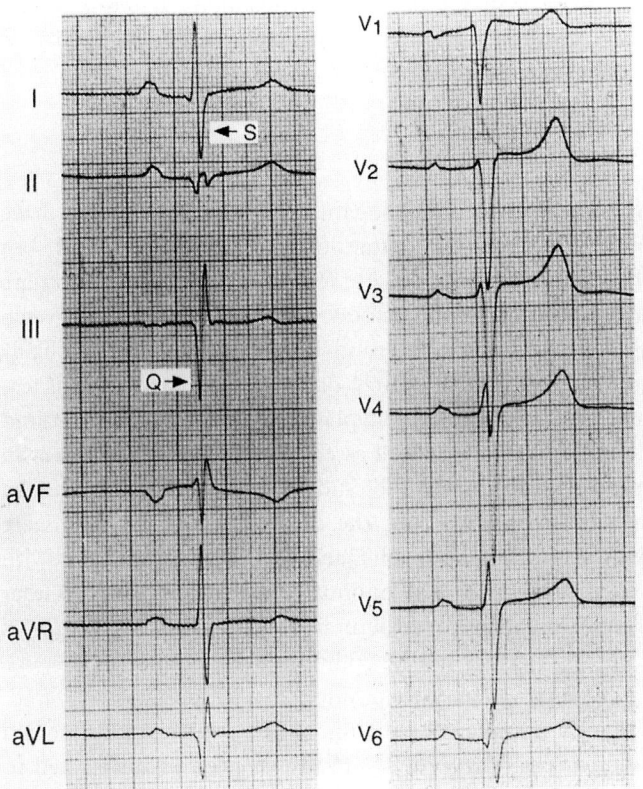

Fig. 49.2. Abnormal ECG in a patient (30 years old) with a severe obstructive HCM and marked septal hypertrophy. The following changes are seen: deep S wave in lead I and deep Q wave in lead III. Deep Q waves in leads II and aVF and deep S waves in leads V2–V5. (Courtesy Prof Döhlemann, Munich.)

In Figure 49.4 the typical disarray is depicted with loss of regular cell-to-cell orientation of muscle cells. Electron-microscopic studies reveal that the contractile myofilaments have lost their normal parallel alignment (Ferrans et al., 1972). Myocardial cells are wide, short, and often bizarre in shape. Foci of disorganized cells are often interspersed among areas of hypertrophied muscle cells that are otherwise normal in appearance.

These alterations are usually diagnostic, but they are not entirely specific. Some disarray may also be found in normal subjects at the junction of the septum with the anterior and posterior walls of the left ventricle (Becker and Caruso, 1982). Fiber disarray may also be seen in some cases of congenital malformations of the heart (Bulkley et al., 1977). Although the specificity of microscopic changes may be debatable, the diagnosis at autopsy is usually not difficult to

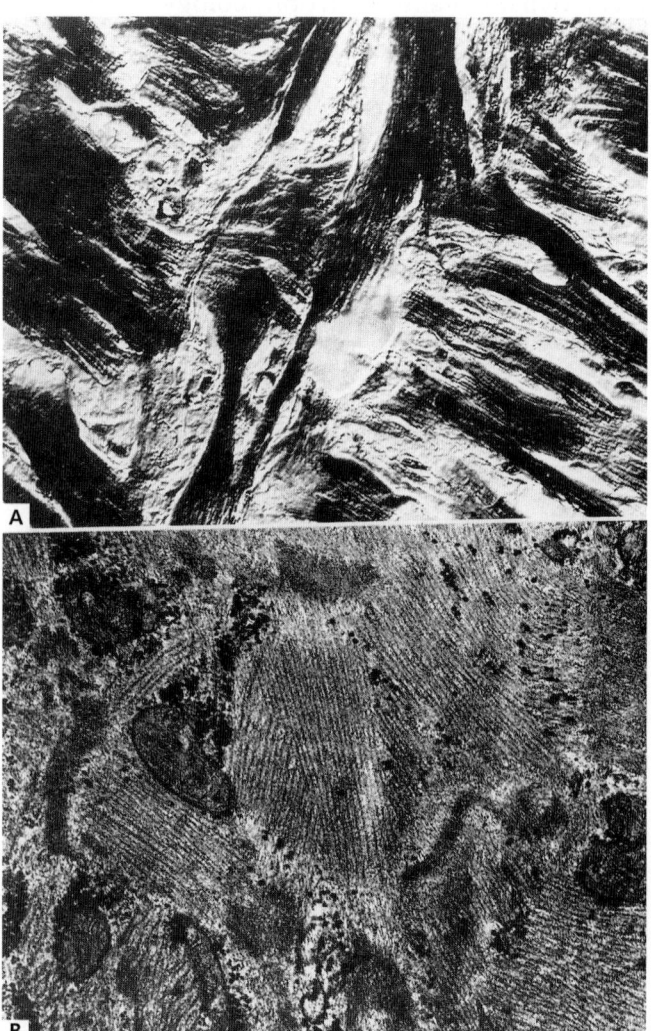

Fig. 49.4. Cellular and filamentous disarray in hypertrophic myocardium. (A) Polyrization light microscopy of cardiac tissue (600 ×). (B) Electron microscopy of myofilaments (43.000 ×). (From Mall, 1988, with permission.)

make (Davies, 1984). Occasionally, myocyte disarray with the other histologic features of HCM is detected in the absence of increased myocardial mass in individuals with familial disease who have died suddenly or have complications resulting from diastolic abnormalities (McKenna et al., 1990). In addition to hypertrophy and cellular disorganization fibrous tissue formation may be found at autopsy in the left ventricular myocardium. This ranges from patchy interstitial fibrosis to extensive and visible scars that may even be transmural (Roberts and Ferrans, 1975; St John Sutton et al., 1980; Maron et al., 1987a). The causes for these changes in cardiac tissue are not known. In addition, small intramural coronary arteries are abnormal in about 40% to 80% of patients with HCM studied at autopsy (James and Marshall, 1975; Maron et al., 1986b; Davies and McKenna, 1995). The walls of these intramural vessels are thickened, and frequently the lumina appear to be narrowed. The pathogenesis of "small vessel disease" (Maron et al., 1987a) is unexplained. It may contribute to myocardial ischemia and necrosis observed in some patients. It should be noted, however, that these alterations are not unique to HCM. They are also found in patients with other cardiac or systemic diseases, for example, systemic hypertension, aortic valvular stenosis, dilated cardiomyopathy, or coronary heart disease.

Pathophysiology

Molecular genetic investigations of the past decade have unraveled numerous mutations associated with HCM, but the mechanisms responsible for myocardial dysfunction are still insufficiently understood. Morphological changes such as disarray, hypertrophy and interstitial fibrosis very likely contribute either separately or cooperatively to clinical features of HCM including hyperdynamic systolic and impaired diastolic function, as well as electrical instability which is in many cases responsible for sudden cardiac death (McKenna et al., 1990). However, the observation of severe disease with marked hypertrophy and minimal disarray, or with extensive disarray and minimal hypertrophy suggests that the relationship of structural and functional changes is complex and may not be common to all mutations.

Hyperdynamic systolic function resulting in early, rapid, and near-complete emptying of the ventricle (Braunwald et al., 1964; Maron et al., 1981a) is presumably related to increased muscle mass, to concomitant changes in ventricular geometry or to alterations of cross-bridge cycling between thick and thin myofilaments. Some time ago it was also suggested that altered handling of calcium by the myocardium is also involved in pathogenesis (Goodwin and

Krikler, 1976; Kaltenbach et al., 1976; Lorell, 1985; Pearce et al., 1985; Wagner et al., 1989).

Hemodynamic dysfunction results from pressure gradients between the outflow tract and the left ventricular cavity either at rest (in 20% of patients) or with provocative maneuvers that increase myocardial contractility or reduce ventricular volume (McKenna et al., 1981b). The mechanisms leading to these gradients are not entirely clear. The discussion in the literature has been controversial. Whereas some authors have maintained that gradients occur in conjunction with hyperdynamic emptying of the left ventricle (Criley et al., 1965; Criley and Siegel, 1986), others have linked the process of outflow tract gradient formation to the development of Venturi forces and systolic anterior motion of the mitral valve (Pollick et al., 1984; Wigle et al., 1986). Regardless, it is generally accepted that those patients who have a gradient at rest are a distinct subset with respect to ease of diagnosis and management options (see the section on Management).

Diastolic abnormalities are common, although less obvious (Sanderson et al., 1978; Sutton et al., 1978; Hanrath et al., 1980; Bonow et al., 1981). The period during which the heart is isovolumic in end-systole and early diastole is prolonged, filling is slow, and the contribution from atrial systolic contraction may be increased. Occasionally, there is early rapid filling with restrictive physiology that resembles the situation in patients with constrictive pericarditis or endocardial fibrosis. Diastolic abnormalities may result in congestive heart failure despite preservation of ventricular systolic function.

The lack of distensibility of the heart may be related to increased interstitial fibrosis or to molecular events controlling the kinetics of contraction. Abnormal handling of calcium and distorted patterns of electromechanical activation with regional asynchrony, possibly influenced by ischemia are also possible (Abelmann and Lorell, 1989; Wagner et al., 1989). In most cases it is not possible to identify the predominant pathophysiologic mechanism of altered diastolic function; most patients have myocardial hypertrophy, evidence suggestive of ischemia and architectural abnormalities, including myocardial disarray and fibrosis.

About 50% of HCM patients suffer from dyspnea. This symptom, usually associated with reduced exercise capacity, is thought to be a consequence of elevated ventricular pressures during diastole, resulting from impaired ventricular relaxation, filling and compliance. Other mechanisms such as control of muscle energetics and central perception of breathlessness may also be important (Frenneaux et al., 1989).

Chest pain may be exertional, atypical, or both, in similar proportions of patients (McKenna et al., 1981a; Cannon et al., 1985). Atypical pain may be precipitated by emotional or physical stress or occur post prandially and may persist long after the stress has been removed. The origin of chest pain is not clear, but is probably related to ischemia (Maron et al., 1986b).

Syncopal episodes occur in 15% to 25% of patients with HCM, but triggering mechanism is not usually determined despite investigations. Occult tachyarrhythmia or conduction disease and altered vascular responses may contribute to complications (McKenna et al., 1981a; Loogen et al., 1983). Rarely, patients may present with symptoms attributable to left or right heart failure with paroxysmal nocturnal dyspnea, cough, ascites, or peripheral edema.

CLINICAL GENETICS

Familial versus sporadic

A report by W Evans on familial cardiomegaly which appeared in the British Heart Journal (1949) is one of the earliest publications about inherited cardiomyopathy. Numerous cases of familial HCM reported in the 1950s and 1960s all suggested autosomal dominant inheritance (Brigden, 1957; Teare, 1958; Brent et al., 1960; Hollman et al., 1960; Paré et al., 1961; Wigle et al., 1962; Braunwald et al., 1964; Horlick et al., 1966; Maurice et al., 1966; Meerschwam, 1972; for a complete record see Emanuel and Withers, 1992).

A particularly impressive account of a single family was published in 1961 by P Paré and colleagues. This pedigree included five generations, with 30 patients who could be traced to an emigrant from France to Quebec in the later years of the seventeenth century (Fig. 49.5). The disease transmitted in this family was, three centuries later, the first case of hypertrophic cardiomyopathy for which a molecular cause was determined.

In another single family reported by Horlick and colleagues (1966), 10 persons in four generations were judged to be affected. Braunwald and colleagues (1964) reported a study of 64 patients with multiple cases in 11 families. Retrospective clinical inheritance analyses were done in a series of investigations over several years (Clark et al., 1973; van Dorp et al., 1976; Maron et al., 1976, 1984; ten Cate et al., 1979). These authors estimated that about 50% of cases were familial (Maron et al., 1987a). A similar proportion of familial disease was found by Greaves and associates (1987). HCM is clearly autosomal dominant in most cases.

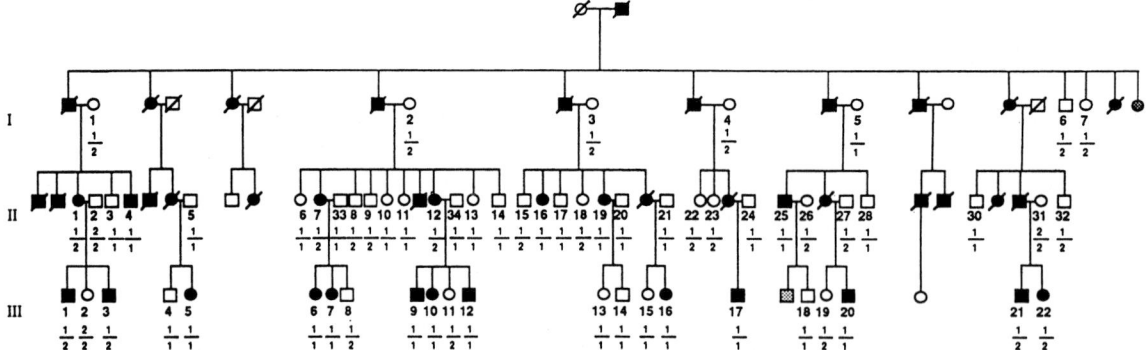

Fig. 49.5. Pedigree of the family that was later shown to carry a mutation in codon 403 of the β-myosin heavy chain gene (MYH7). The allele numbers 1 and 2 refer to an intragenic restriction fragment length polymorphism (RFLP) in intron 24 of the β-MHC gene. All patients have the same allele no. 1. Females, circles; males, squares; filled, patients; slashed, deceased persons; stippled, not available for study. (From Solomon et al., 1990a, with permission.)

Penetrance of familial HCM is age-related. In adults it is in many cases complete; however, expression of the phenotype is different for different genes and mutations within these genes. Clinical manifestations typically develop during periods of growth. Even adult populations, however, may show incomplete penetrance, as obligate gene carriers without clinical manifestations are occasionally recognized. Variable expression regarding morphology and clinical severity in families—even in monozygotic twins (Reid et al., 1989)—suggests that expression of the phenotype is determined by environmental and possibly multiple "modifying genes" that contribute to the control of cardiovascular functions (see below).

How common is the true sporadic (noninherited) variety of the disease? The retrospective clinical studies that estimate 50% sporadic disease include many instances where relatives could not be studied and sporadic HCM was assumed. Prospective pedigree analyses suggest that familial disease is present in approximately 90% of cases. Clinical and morphological features were very similar in familial and sporadic disease. Recent data showing that de novo mutations occur (see below) makes it seem likely that HCM is in most cases a genetic disease.

Epidemiology

HCM has been reported in Western, Asian and African populations. Information on the prevalence of this disease is, however, incomplete. Data are available only for European and North American regions. For the northern parts of the United Kingdom a clinical prevalence of 3.2 per 100,000 population has been documented (Bennett et al., 1987). In Iceland, in a pathologic postmortem survey, 33/100,000 were counted (Bjarnason and Hallgrimsson, 1980). In a study by the Mayo Clinic for the residents in Olmsted

County, Minnesota, a prevalence ratio of 20/100,000 was found (Codd et al., 1989). If these numbers are representative, 1 person in about 5000 could be affected. This estimate is undoubtedly conservative because an unknown fraction of mildly affected individuals and families would have been missed with the diagnostic criteria that were applied. Spirito and colleagues (1989) reported that HCM patients in an outpatient population were much less severely affected compared with patients investigated in referral institutions. The condition is probably more common than suggested by the numbers obtained in referral-based institutions. Selection biases and the difficulty of identifying all cases of affected first-degree relatives are likely to obscure the real (higher) frequencies.

A high prevalence of cardiac hypertrophy of about 1 in 500 was reported recently (Maron et al., 1995). This study was based on echocardiographic analyses of men and women between 23 and 35 years of age selected from the general population. Of 4111 individuals, seven fulfilled diagnostic criteria for HCM. An additional five had left ventricular hypertrophy, which was interpreted to be the consequence of systemic hypertension. The true prevalence of unexplained left ventricular hypertrophy in young adults is probably in the range of 1 in 500. These figures are based on the analysis of phenotypes, not on genotypes or mutations, they seem, however, to represent a well-considered assessment of disease prevalence and indicate that in young adults HCM is more common than previously recognized.

ETIOLOGY

Linkage studies

The search for genetic defects causing HCM was originally based on linkage analysis and positional cloning (see Ch. 8).

Early reports suggested linkage of HCM with the HLA region on chromosome 6 (Matsumori et al., 1979; 1981; Kishimoto et al., 1983). This proposal, however, was never confirmed (Gardin et al., 1982; Haugland et al., 1986; Zezulka et al., 1986; Solomon et al., 1990a). Instead, nine or possibly ten different loci for genetically distinct forms of HCM have been reported since then. These loci are found on nine different chromosomes (Fig. 49.6). Within the exception of one locus on chromosome 7 the genes and their products are known. All HCM proteins are involved in force production or in the control of force production by the myofilaments of cardiac muscle. The genes code for β-myosin heavy chain (MYH7, on chromosome 14, designated β-MHC or β-myosin HC hereafter), cardiac troponin T (TNNT2, chromosome 1, or cTnT), cardiac troponin I (TNNI3, chromosome 19, or cTnI), titin (TTN, chromo-some 2), α-tropomyosin (TMSA, chromosome 15, or α-TM), essential myosin light chain (MYL3, chromosome 3, or ELC), regulatory myosin light chain (MYL2, chromosome 12, or RLC), cardiac α-actin (ACTC, chromosome 15) and for myosin binding protein-C (MYBPC3, chromosome 11, or MyBP-C). The heavy chain of β-myosin and cardiac actin directly participate in myosin-actin cross-bridge formation, while the other proteins are either structural components of the sarcomere or proteins involved in the control of cardiac contractility (Bagshaw, 1993; Jontes, 1995; Holmes, 1996). The steps that led to the identification of these genes are outlined below.

Figure 49.7 summarizes schematically the thin and thick filament associations of the nine different sarcomeric proteins (titin included) which have been implicated in HCM.

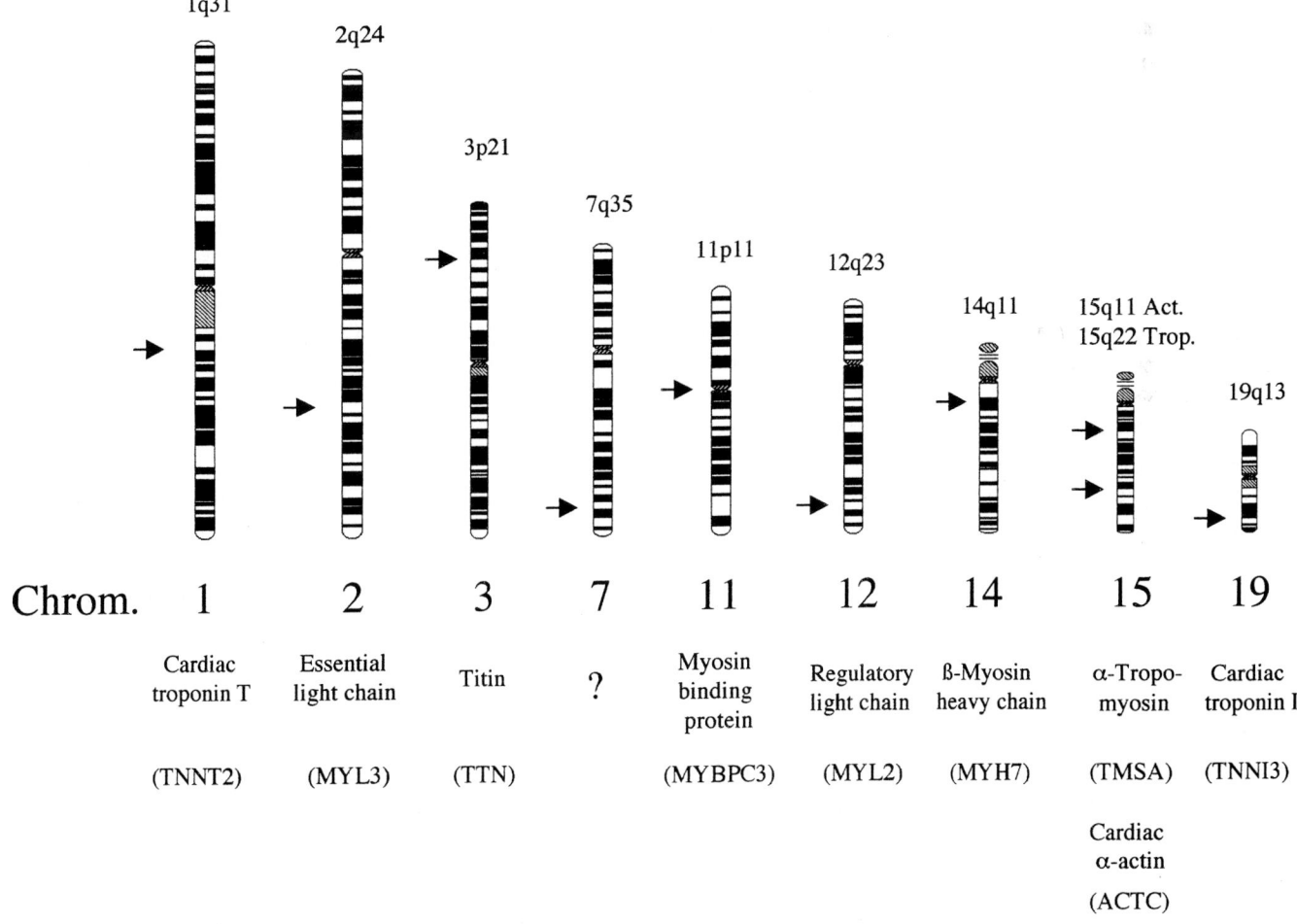

Fig. 49.6. Genomic localization of mutated HCM genes. Eight loci have been confirmed by pedigree analysis. One locus (titin) on chromosome 2 should be considered provisional. A locus on chromosome 7 has been determined by linkage; the gene is, however, not known. The chromosomal positions are indicated on top and by the arrows. The genetic acronyms are written in brackets. It should be noted that in three HCM genes (*MYH7*, *ACTC* and *TNNT2*) mutations have been identified which cause DCM rather than HCM (Olson et al., 1998; Kamisago et al., 2000).

Sarcomeric genes contributing to HCM

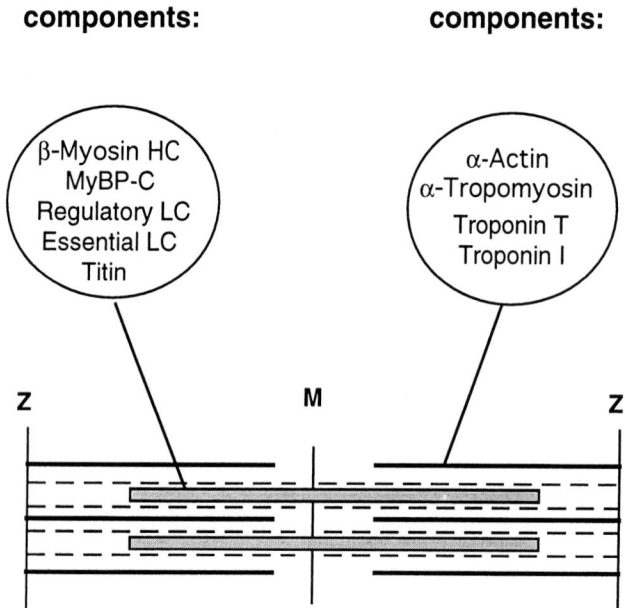

Thick filament components:

β-Myosin HC
MyBP-C
Regulatory LC
Essential LC
Titin

Thin filament components:

α-Actin
α-Tropomyosin
Troponin T
Troponin I

Z   M   Z

Fig. 49.7. HCM gene products are associated with thick and thin filaments in the sarcomere. Z, Z-discs limiting the length of the sarcomeres, M, M-line. The broken lines indicate titin molecules which extend from the M-line to the Z-discs.

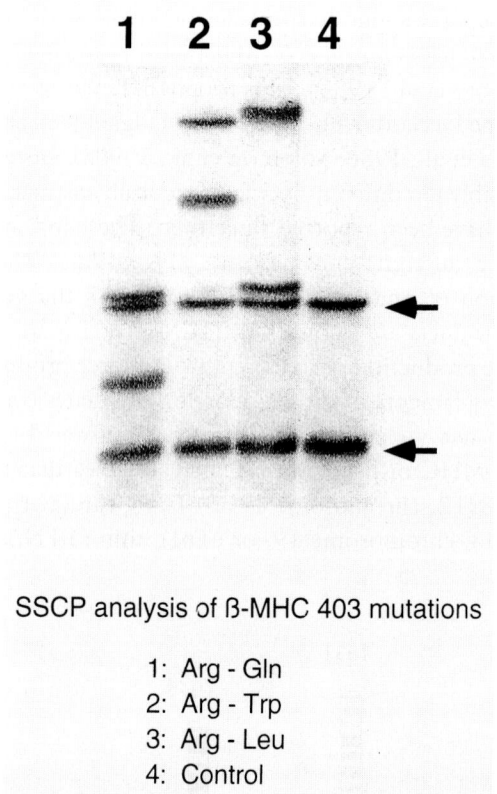

1 2 3 4

SSCP analysis of ß-MHC 403 mutations

1: Arg - Gln
2: Arg - Trp
3: Arg - Leu
4: Control

Fig. 49.8. SSCP analysis of three different mutations of codon 403 in exon 13 of the β-MHC gene (see also Fig. 49.12). Genomic DNA regions of patients were amplified by the polymerase chain reaction (PCR) over a length of 165 basepairs. DNA single strands were obtained by melting double strands and migrated in a nondenaturing polyacrylamide gel for 15 hrs at 400 V. DNA strands were visualized by silver staining. Lane 1: a C→T transition (Arg→Trp); lane 2: a G→T transversion (Arg→Leu), lane 3: a G→A transition (Arg→Gln). Lane 4: wildtype DNA. Wildtype DNA bands are clearly visible in all samples (see the arrows). (Courtesy Dr Weist, Bad Nauheim.)

Methods for testing of candidate genes

Since HCM is associated with mutations in nine genes that may be responsible for 75% of all index cases, the identification of genetic changes will increasingly rely on direct analysis of candidate genes rather than on linkage studies or locus-related haplotyping (which serves as an "abridged" linkage analysis in small families). Although linkage analysis remains to be an important procedure for the study of causes of HCM, five of the nine known genes have been identified by direct candidate gene analysis (the genes for the myosin light chains, cTnI, cardiac actin, and titin).

The identification of a mutation is no problem at all if in a family with a known cause a potential carrier has to be confirmed or excluded. A number of convenient methods are available, such as single strand conformation polymorphism (SSCP) (Orita et al., 1989), chemical cleavage of heteroduplexes (Cotton et al., 1988), oligonucleotide ligation (Landegren et al., 1988), reverse dot blot hybridization or the current chip hybridization techniques, which are based on reverse hybridization (Cronin et al., 1996). The discriminating power of the SSCP technique is demonstrated in Figure 49.8 where three amplified DNA regions have been separated that differ by only one basepair in

codon 403 of the β-myosin HC (exon 13). Direct sequencing or direct cycle sequencing of DNA is an important "reference method" for the ultimate confirmation of sequence changes in genes. Restriction analysis is, where appropriate, a method easy to perform, since it is sensitive, specific and inexpensive. For rapid high throughput screening of large numbers of samples the new technique of pyrosequencing (Ronaghi et al., 1998) seems to offer some advantages, since it is fast, robust and also relatively inexpensive. Reference handbooks or protocol collections, which provide necessary technical information, are available (see Dracopoli et al., 1994 and continuous updates in "Current Protocols in Human Genetics").

If a new, previously unknown mutation has to be searched for, methods with reasonable or high efficiency are either SSCP (with some limits in sensitivity) or the heteroduplex recognition based on denaturing high performance liquid

Table 49.2. Analysis of HCM mutations in candidate genes

Method	Experimental features	Advantages	Disadvantages
A Screening for new mutations			
SSCP	Altered mobility of ssDNA	Easy to perform	Limited rate of detection
CCM/ECM	Chemical/enzymatic cleavage of DNA/DNA heteroduplex	High rate of detection	Laborious
DHPLC	Altered mobility of DNA/DNA heteroduplex	Fast, sensitive	Expensive
Cycle sequencing	Direct sequencing of PCR products, electrophoresis	Detects exact position	Time-consuming
Chip sequencing	Hybridization of PCR products to high-density probe arrays	High-throughput	Restricted availability
B Detection of known mutations			
Restriction site analysis	Digestion of PCR products	Easy to perform	Low-throughput
Reverse dot blot (DNA chips)	Hybridization of PCR products to low-density probe arrays	High-throughput, no electrophoresis	Experimental, not generally available
Pyrosequencing	Oligo-base sequencing of PCR products, online detection	High-throughput, no electrophoresis	Simple, but expensive

Abbreviations: CCM, chemical cleavage of mismatch; ECM, enzymatic cleavage of mismatch; DHPLC, denaturing high-performance liquid chromatography; SSCP, single-strand conformation polymorphism; ssDNA, single-stranded DNA.

chromatography (also known as Wave technique) (Underhill et al., 1997; Liu et al., 1998). Occasionally it is required to clone and sequence genomic DNA if alleles are not easily resolved from each other, e.g., if deletions or insertions are involved and if expensive equipment is not available. The TOPO cloning procedure is a convenient and very efficient method for this purpose (Shuman, 1994). A list of frequently used or appropriate methods for mutation detection is presented in Table 49.2.

MUTATIONS IN HYPERTROPHIC CARDIOMYOPATHY

β-Myosin heavy chain gene

The first mutation responsible for HCM was found in a French-Canadian pedigree originally studied in the early sixties (Paré et al., 1961). Nearly 30 years later, 78 members of this family were reexamined. Sixty-four were siblings, parents, or offspring of an affected person (Jarcho et al., 1989) (see Fig. 49.5). Children of unaffected parents were not included. On the basis of previous clinical investigations or postmortem examinations, 24 deceased members had HCM; 20 died prematurely (< 45 years) of a disease-related complication. HCM was diagnosed in 20 living family members. These clinical and electrocardiographic features were typical, showing left ventricular hypertrophy. The mean maximal thickness of the left ventricular wall was 22 mm (the maximum was 34 mm), 40% had right ventricular hyper-

trophy in addition, and most had enlargement of the left atrium. Two members were considered to be affected despite the absence of echocardiographic left ventricular hypertrophy. Fifty-eight members were clinically unaffected.

The assignment of a disease region was based on linkage of the disease locus to restriction fragment length polymorphisms (RFLP) (see Ch. 8). A marker locus on chromosome 14 (designated D14S26, located on the long arm close to the centromere) (Cox et al., 1990) was determined to be linked to the HCM disease locus (Fig. 49.9). A maximal multipoint lod score was calculated as 9.37, with no recombination between marker loci and the presumed disease gene, suggesting that in this family the probability of linkage of the HCM locus to the D14S26 marker was greater than 10^9:1 (Jarcho et al., 1989).

The next step was the determination of a candidate gene within the region tagged by D14S26. The cardiac α- and β-myosin heavy-chain genes were known to be located on the long arm of chromosome 14 next to the centromere (Saez et al., 1987; Matsuoka et al., 1989; Solomon et al., 1990a). These two subtypes of the myosin heavy chains belong to a multiprotein family of about eight members, all functioning in striated (i.e., skeletal and cardiac) muscle (Weiss et al., 1999). The corresponding genes are clustered on chromosomes 17 (skeletal muscle) and 14 (cardiac muscle) (Saez et al., 1987). The α-isoform is expressed at high levels in atrial cardiocytes, while the β-isoform is primarily ventricular and is also present in the myofibers of slow skeletal muscles (Sinha et al., 1982; Lompré et al., 1984; Lichter et al., 1986).

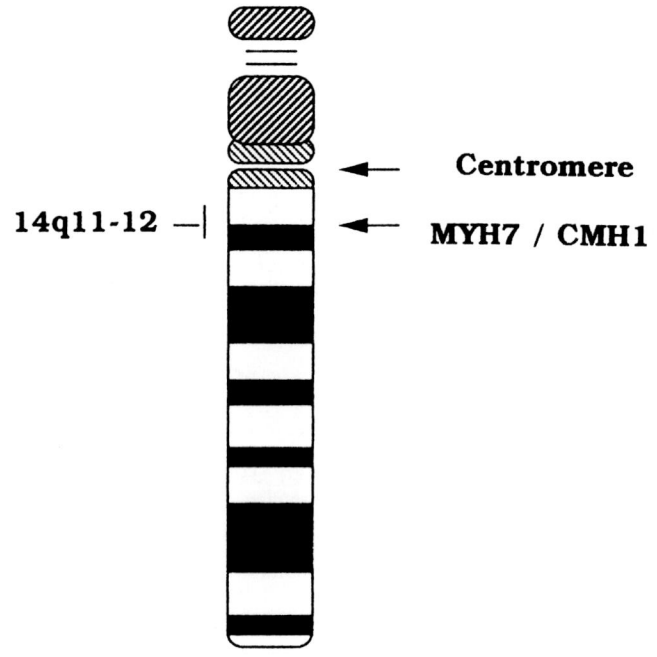

Chromosome 14

Fig. 49.9. Map position of the cardiac myosin heavy chain gene cluster (α- and β-myosin HC) in the vicinity of the centromere of chromosome 14. The myosin gene cluster is labeled *MYH7*. Its position has also been designated CMH1 ("cardiac myopathy, hypertrophic, disease locus no. 1").

A known RFLP within intron 28 of *MYH7* (Siewertsen et al., 1990) was applied to reassess linkage of the disease to the myosin heavy-chain locus. A two-point lod score of 4.62 (with no recombination) was consistent with the suggestion that cardiac myosin heavy-chain genes were probable candidates.

Evidence favoring the hypothesis that myosin heavy-chain genes are disease genes was obtained from another HCM family where a genomic rearrangement was detected in the myosin gene cluster on chromosome 14 (Tanigawa et al., 1990). This rearrangement was presumably the result of a meiotic unequal crossing-over between the α- and β-myosin HC genes. These two highly homologous genes are closely spaced on chromosome 14 (about 5 kb apart). The hybrid α/β-myosin heavy-chain allele was informative because in this family it was found only in patients, not in unaffected individuals, and also not in any of 200 unrelated persons. It turned out later, however, that the rearranged allele was a linked genomic marker rather than the disease gene. This conclusion was based on the observation that the affected members also carried a missense mutation in the nonrearranged *MYH7* on the same chromosome. The identification of unrelated patients who had the same missense mutation, but not the hybrid α/β-allele, made it unlikely that the rearrangement contributed to the phenotype (Watkins et al., 1992b). But this marker was extremely useful because it prompted the molecular examination of *MYH7* for mutations (Geisterfer-Lowrance et al., 1990).

By sequencing cloned genomic DNA from HCM patients of the French-Canadian family, a G→A transition was determined in codon 403 located in exon 13 of *MYH7* (Geisterfer-Lowrance et al., 1990). The change of a CGG triplet to CAG resulted in the replacement of an arginine by a glutamine in position 403 of the protein molecule (Fig. 49.10). This was the first mutation known to cause HCM. To date, missense mutations in *MYH7* have been detected as the most frequent cause of HCM, with about 35% of all cases traced to this gene. The genomic structure of the β-myosin gene (Jaenicke et al., 1990; Liew et al., 1990) is shown in Fig. 49.11. The gene is about 24 kb long and comprises 40 exons, 38 of which are translated into protein.

More than 68 different missense mutations in *MYH7* have been detected (not all have been published and some

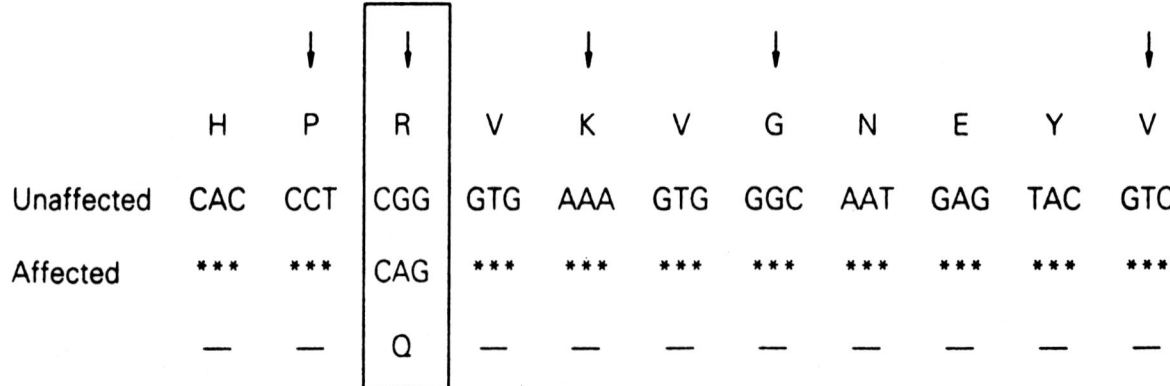

Fig. 49.10. The missense mutation in position 403 of exon 13 of the β-myosin heavy chain gene. DNA and protein sequence flanking codon 403 are shown. The disease involves an arginine (R) to glutamine (Q) exchange. The arrows point to amino acid residues highly conserved in the evolution of myosin heavy chains.

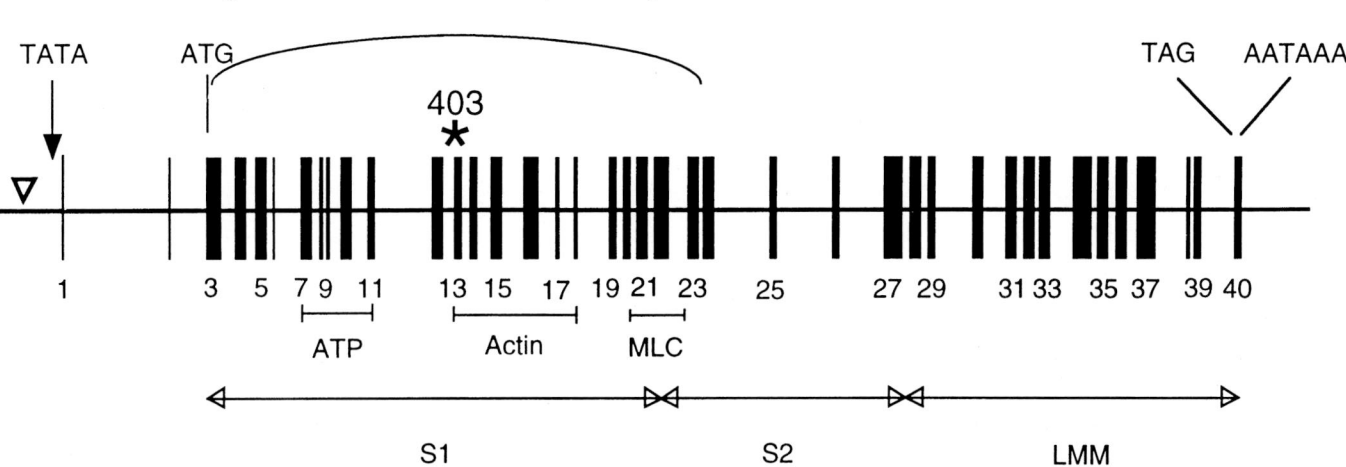

Fig. 49.11. The β-myosin heavy chain gene. The numbered thick bars are exons, thin lines in between are introns. TATA, AATAAA, ATG, and TAG are start and stop signals for transcription and translation, respectively. Protein regions within the heavy chain molecule responsible for ATP binding, cross-bridge formation with actin and internal flexibility of the otherwise filamentous rod (hinge) are labeled. S1, S2 and LMM are proteolytically defined subdomains of the heavy chain molecule. The arrow points to the codon position 403 in exon 13, which is the single most frequently involved mutational site in this gene.

only in the form of an abstract) (Table 49.3). With one exception they are all located in the globular head or in the head rod junction of the β-myosin molecule. One missense mutation has been detected to date in the rod (in codon 1205, a Glu→Lys exchange), located in the "hinge" between the S2 and the LMM domain of the rod. The apparently low prevalence of mutations in this domain suggests that altered rod structures are not viable.

The most frequent base exchanges are G→A transitions, in the majority of cases involving a CpG dinucleotide. The single most frequently lost amino acid is arginine (20/70). This amino acid has a highly degenerate genetic code with four of six codons comprising a CpG dinucleotide. This preference suggests that oxidative deamination of methylated cytosine residues may at least in part be responsible for the mutational events (Coulondre et al., 1978; Youssoufian et al., 1988; Green et al., 1990; Rideout et al., 1990). The validity of this suggestion was convincingly confirmed by recent experimental results demonstrating directly the instability of methylated cytosins, in this case in the cTnT gene (D'Cruz et al., 2000).

Several mutations have been reported repeatedly, for example those in position 403 (Arg→Gln), 606 (Val→Met) or 719 (Arg→Gln). Others have thus far been unique to particular pedigrees. The chance to find a new ("private") mutation in a family not previously genotyped may be as high as 50%. Haplotype analysis in families sharing identical mutations led to the conclusion of independent mutational events rather than of founder effects (Watkins et al.,

1993b). Founder constellations have been described, but they are uncommon (Moolman-Smook et al., 1999). This implies that many mutations were of relatively recent origin. In conjunction with the identification of de novo mutations (Watkins et al., 1992b; Greve et al., 1994; Jeschke et al., 1998), a relatively high mutation rate of this gene can be assumed. Exact numbers, however, have not been determined.

The single most frequently mutated site is codon 403, which was the location of the first known HCM mutation. In studies of at least eight unrelated families the CGG→CAG transition, or Arg→Gln exchange, has been observed. In addition, a G→T transversion and a C→T transition have been detected in this codon (Dausse et al., 1993; Moolman et al., 1993) suggesting a hotspot of mutation (Fig. 49.12). Some other codons (e.g., 143, 719, 741 and 870) have also been characterized with more than one amino acid replacement.

Double mutations have been reported twice. On one occasion an established disease-related mutation in codon 719 (in this case a de novo mutation) was identified in a child that later died from a cardiac arrest (at the age of nine years). No other member in this family was carrier of this mutation. The change occured in the paternal allele (paternity was confirmed). A missense mutation (in codon 349$^{Met→Thr}$) transmitted by the mother was presumably a silent genetic variant. The child, however, died from severe HCM. It carried both mutations. It was therefore conceivable that the non-penetrant variant was a confounding

Table 49.3. Mutations in the β-myosin heavy chain gene (*MYH7*)

A Nucleotide substitutions (missense / nonsense)

No	Exon/ codon	Nucleotide change	Amino acid change	Change in charge	Reference
1.	3/26	GCG → GTG	Ala → Val	no	Marian et al., 1992
2.	3/54	CGA → TGA	Arg → Stop	n.a.[1]	Nishi et al., 1995
3.	3/59	GTC → ATC	Val → Ile	no	Harada et al., 1992
4.	5/124	ACC → ATC	Thr → Ile	no	Rayment et al., 1995
5.	5/143	CGG → CAG	Arg → Gln	yes	Weist and Vosberg, 1995
6.	5/143	CGG → TGG	Arg → Trp	yes	Koyanagi et al., 1996
7.	5/162	TAT → TGT	Tyr → Cys	no	Cuda et al., 1993b
8.	7/187	AAC → AAG	Asn → Lys	yes	Marian and Roberts, 1995a
9.	7/190	AGG → ACG	Arg → Thr	yes	Bundgaard et al., 1994
10.	8/222	CAG → AAG	Gln → Lys	yes	Rayment et al., 1995
11.	8/232	AAT → AGT	Asn → Ser	no	Bundgaard et al., 1999
12.	8/244	n.r.[2]	Phe → Leu	no	Rayment et al., 1995
13.	9/246	AAA → CAA	Lys → Gln	yes	Rottbauer et al., 1996
14.	9/249	CGA → CAA	Arg → Gln	yes	Rosenzweig et al., 1991
15.	9/256	GGA → GAA	Gly → Glu	yes	Fananapazir et al., 1993
16.	9/259	GCA → GAA	Ala → Glu	yes	Vosberg et al., 1999
17.	9/263	ATA → ACA	Ile → Thr	no	Tesson et al., 1998
18.	11/326	GCT → CCT	Ala → Pro	no	Coviello et al., 1997b
19.	12/349	ATG → ACG	Met → Thr	no	Jeschke et al., 1998
20.	13/383	AAG → AAT	Lys → Asn	yes	Kuang et al., 1996
21.	13/390	CTG → GTG	Leu → Val	no	Andersen et al., 1998a
22.	13/403	CGG → CAG	Arg → Gln	yes	Geisterfer-Lowrance et al., 1990
23.	13/403	CGG → CTG	Arg → Leu	yes	Dausse et al., 1993
24.	13/403	CGG → TGG	Arg → Trp	yes	Dausse et al., 1993
25.	14/450	AAG → GAG	Lys → Glu	yes	Arbustini et al., 1998
26.	14/453	CGC → TGC	Arg → Cys	yes	Watkins et al., 1992b
27.	15/483	GAG → AAG	Glu → Lys	yes	Richard et al., 1999
28.	15/499	GAG → AAG	Glu → Lys	yes	Moolman-Smook et al., 1999
29.	15/513	TTT → TGT	Phe → Cys	no	Anan et al., 1994
30.	16/584	GGC → CGC	Gly → Arg	yes	Watkins et al., 1992b
31.	15/587	GAC → GTC	Asp → Val	yes	Marian and Roberts, 1995b
32.	16/606	GTG → ATG	Val → Met	no	Watkins et al., 1992b
33.	16/606	GTG → TTG	Val → Leu	no	Andersen et al., 1998
34.	16/615	AAG → AAC	Lys → Asn	yes	Nishi et al., 1992
35.	16/624	TAT → AAT	Tyr → Asn	no	Ohsuzu et al., 1997
36.	18/663	CGC → TGC	Arg → Cys	yes	Coviello et al., 1997b
37.	18/663	CGC → CAC	Arg → His	yes	Rayment et al., 1995
38.	19/694	CGC → TGC	Arg → Cys	yes	Andersen et al., 1999
39.	19/696	AAT → AGT	Asn → Ser	no	Jaaskelainen et al., 1998
40.	19/712	CGC → CTC	Arg → Leu	yes	Sakthivel et al., 2000
41.	19/716	GGG → AGG	Gly → Arg	yes	Anan et al., 1994
42.	19/719	CGG → CAG	Arg → Gln	yes	Consevage et al., 1994
43.	20/723	CGC → TGC	Arg → Cys	yes	Watkins et al., 1992c
44.	19/719	CGG → TGG	Arg → Trp	yes	Anan et al., 1994
45.	20/731	CCT → CTT	Pro → Leu	no	Toyo-oka et al., 1994
46.	20/736	ATT → ATG	Ile → Met	no	Harada et al., 1992
47.	20/741	GGG → CGG	Gly → Arg	yes	Fananapazir et al., 1993
48.	20/741	GGG → TGG	Gly → Trp	no	Arai et al., 1995
49.	20/741	GGG → AGG	Gly → Arg	yes	Fananapazir et al., 1993
50.	20/741	GGG → GCG	Gly → Ala	yes	Fananapazir et al., 1993
51	21/778	GAC → GGC	Asp → Gly	yes	Harada et al., 1993
52	21/797	GCC → ACC	Ala → Thr	no	Moolman et al., 1995
53.	22/846	GAG → AAG	Glu → Lys	yes	Coviello et al., 1997b
54.	22/846	GAG → CAG	Glu → Gln	yes	Andersen et al., 1998
55.	22/869	CGC → TGC	Arg → Cys	yes	Anan et al., 1998
56.	22/869	CGC → GGC	Arg → Gly	yes	Richard et al., 2000

continued

Table 49.3. Mutations in the β-myosin heavy chain gene (*MYH7*) (continued)

A Nucleotide substitutions (missense / nonsense)

No	Exon/codon	Nucleotide change	Amino acid change	Change in charge	Reference
57.	22/870	CGC → CAC	Arg → His	yes	Rayment et al., 1995
58.	23/908	CTG → GTG	Leu → Val	no	Fananapazir et al., 1993
59.	23/924	GAG → AAG	Glu → Lys	yes	Watkins et al., 1992c
60.	23/930	GAG → AAG	Glu → Lys	yes	Mares et al., 1993
61.	23/935	GAG → AAG	Glu → Lys	yes	Nishi et al., 1994
62.	23/949	GAG → AAG	Glu → Lys	yes	Watkins et al., 1992b
63.	27/1205	GAG → AAG	Glu → Lys	yes	Vosberg et al., 1999
B Small deletions					
66.	3/10	del[3] 3 bp	ΔGly10	no	Nakajima-Tamaguchi et al., 1995
67.	23/927	del 3 bp	ΔLys927	yes	Waldmüller et al., 1999
68.	23/930	del[3] 3 bp	ΔGlu930	yes	Tesson et al., 1998
C Gross deletions					
69.	40/1931–35	deletion ≈ 2,5 kb	del 5 aa[4] at the C-terminus	n.a.[1]	Marian et al., 1992
D Insertion/deletion					
70.	13/395, 404	ins[5]G/del[3]G	[395–404][6]	n.a.[1]	Cuda et al., 1996

Footnotes: 1) n.a., not applicable; 2) n.r., base exchange not reported; 3) del, deletion; 4) aa, amino acids; 5) ins, insertion; 6) altered reading frame between insertion and deletion. The mutation in exon 9/codon 246 may cause HCM and DCM (see Rottbauer et al., 1996).

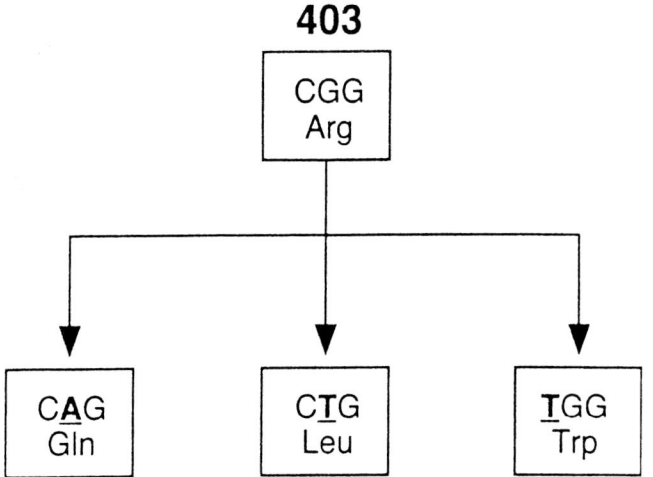

Fig. 49.12. Hot spot of mutation in codon 403 of the β-myosin gene: three different nucleotide exchanges have been identified in this codon. They are discriminated by DNA sequencing, restriction enzyme cleavage or SSCP analysis (see also Fig. 49.8).

second genetic factor contributing to the clinical result of the 719 mutation (Jeschke et al., 1998). In another familial case, a composite genotype was reported with one mutation in the β-myosin gene (in codon 483[Glu→Lys]), and a second one in the MyBP-C gene (a nonsense mutation in codon 1096, Glu→stop). Since these genes do not map to the same chromosome, they did not cosegregate in the affected family. Both genes are typical HCM genes. Those

probands who had inherited both mutations suffered more severely than carriers of only one of the mutations (Richard et al., 1999). Thus, pathogenic effects of separate HCM genes may be additive. Finally, two reports have been communicated about the consequences of homozygous mutations in β-myosin. In one case a missense mutation in codon 935 caused a mild phenotype in the heterozygous state, but it was lethal for those who had inherited both mutated alleles from their heterozygous parents (Nishi et al., 1994). The second case resulted from a β-myosin missense mutation in codon 869 (Arg→Gly). Two children of heterozygous parents were affected. Whereas the parents were only mildly affected, the children exhibited a severe form of HCM, again suggesting that if two mutations are present they have a confounding effect on the phenotype (Richard et al., 2000).

Two major rearrangements or deletions in *MYH7* have been reported that do not involve single amino acid replacements and presumably are not related to disease: (1) the α/β-hybrid allele discussed above; (2) a 2.4-kb deletion removing the terminal exon 40, the 3′ untranslated region, including the polyadenylation signal (required for correct transcriptional termination) and part of the intergenic region between the α- and the β-myosin gene (Marian et al., 1992). This deletion did not cosegregate with the disease. In addition, a nonsense mutation in codon 54 (exon 3) was not associated with a disease phenotype (Nishi et al., 1995).

MYH7 mutations have been reported worldwide. However, ethnic and regional differences in the relative frequencies may exist. It was reported from a Finnish study that the prevalence of myosin mutations in this country is probably much lower than in other regions. In contrast, α-tropomyosin mutations (in codon 175, Asp→Asn), usually regarded to be rare, seem to be frequent in Finland (Jääskelainen et al., 1998).

Two missense mutations have been identified recently that are associated with DCM rather than HCM (Ser532Pro and Phe764Leu) (Kamisago et al., 2000).

α-Tropomyosin gene

The heterogeneity of the clinical presentations and features of HCM led investigators to speculate that this disorder may have different causes (Maron et al., 1987a; 1987b; Davies, 1990; McKenna et al., 1990). The first convincing evidence in favor of heterogeneous causes was the observation that not all HCM families could be linked to the β-myosin heavy chain gene on chromosome 14 (Solomon et al., 1990b; Epstein et al., 1992a; Schwartz et al., 1992).

A second locus encoding the gene for the muscle protein α-tropomyosin (*TMSA*) was identified on chromosome 15 in two families of German origin. The patients in one of them had a relatively mild disease phenotype, the majority of gene carriers being asymptomatic. Such a finding is uncommon in patients with HCM caused by mutations in *MHY7*. In a second family with an α-tropomyosin mutation the disease was more severe with premature sudden death and only 2 of 8 gene carriers being asymptomatic (Thierfelder et al., 1993; 1994).

Linkage analyses were performed with 120 polymorphic microsatellites (Litt and Luty, 1989; Weber and May, 1989). Approximately 50% of the genome was excluded before a disease locus could be assigned to a region recognized by a microsatellite polymorphism (designated D15S108) on chromosome 15q2. Multipoint linkage calculations based on neighboring marker sequences yielded a peak lod score of 4.16. A second, smaller family with a more severe form of the disease resulted in a lod score of 2.28 (at a recombination frequency = 0) for the chromosome 15q2 locus. A comparison of the lod score values by the HOMOG program (see Ch. 8 indicated that in both families the same gene was involved) (Thierfelder et al., 1993).

The identification of the chromosome 15 locus was not associated with a strong candidate gene. The cardiac actin gene was a conceivable candidate (Gunning et al., 1984); however, it was soon ruled out by linkage analysis. Instead, the identification of the α-tropomyosin gene was mediated by genomic map information obtained from the mouse, in which the α-tropomyosin gene was assigned to chromosome 9 within a region syntenic with part of human chromosome 15 (Schleef et al., 1993). Since the sequence of the human α-tropomyosin gene was not known, respective DNA clones and polymorphic microsatellites therein were isolated to establish linkage of the disease to this gene in the two families. With linkage reconfirmed, the tropomyosin gene was screened by PCR amplification of individual exons and direct sequencing. In the two families two different missense mutations in exon 5 were identified, one in codon 175 (Asp → Asn) and one in codon 180 (Glu → Gly). The two mutations were closely spaced in the same domain of the protein conserved in rat, mouse, and frog. Since they were both accompanied by a change in electrical charge a severe cardiac dysfunction was presumed (see the discussion below) (Thierfelder et al., 1994). The known mutations in the α-tropomyosin gene are listed in Table 49.4. The most frequent mutation in this gene is the Asp →Asn exchange in codon 175. Figure 49.13 is a schematic view of the *TMSA* gene.

Cardiac troponin T gene

With the identification of mutations in cardiac myosin and tropomyosin genes, other genes coding for contractile filament components were implicated as candidates for HCM. The two α-tropomyosin mutations in codon 175 and 180 were in a region of the molecule known to interact with troponin T in a calcium-dependent manner (White et al., 1987; Zot and Potter, 1987). Thus, the gene coding for a heart-specific troponin T (*TNNT2*) was a plausible candidate.

Table 49.4. Mutations in the α-tropomyosin gene (*TMSA*)

No.	Exon/codon	Nucleotide change	Amino acid change	Reference
1.	2/63	GCT → GTT	Ala → Val	Yamauchi-Takihara et al., 1996
2.	2/70	AAG → ACG	Lys → Thr	Yamauchi-Takihara et al., 1996
3.	5/175	GAC → AAC	Asp → Asn	Thierfelder et al., 1994
4.	5/180	GAG → GGG	Glu → Gly	Thierfelder et al., 1994

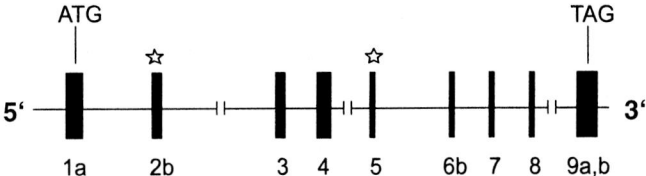

Fig. 49.13. Genomic structure of the α-tropomyosin gene on chromosome 15. The gene has 15 exons, 9 of which are spliced to yield the α-TM mRNA in cardiac and skeletal muscle. Asterisks delineate exons in which mutations have been found. ATG, TAG translational start and stop signals.

To test this assumption, the previously unknown genomic location of this gene was mapped to chromosome 1q31 (Watkins et al., 1993a). The linkage of this gene to HCM in a family unlinked to the chromosome 14 and 15 loci was confirmed in a family of 42 members. A lod score of 6.66 (in the absence of recombination) indicated odds of 5×10^6 to 1 in favor of linkage to *TNNT2*.

To date, 15 different *TNNT2* mutations have been identified; 13 of them are missense, one is a deletion of an entire codon (codon 160), and one is a splice site mutation. The latter mutation (in intron 15) changes the processing pattern of troponin T mRNA (Watkins et al., 1995a) (Table 49.5). A scheme of the cardiac troponin T gene (adapted from Farza et al., 1998) depicting the known mutations is shown in Figure 49.14. The identification of the troponin T

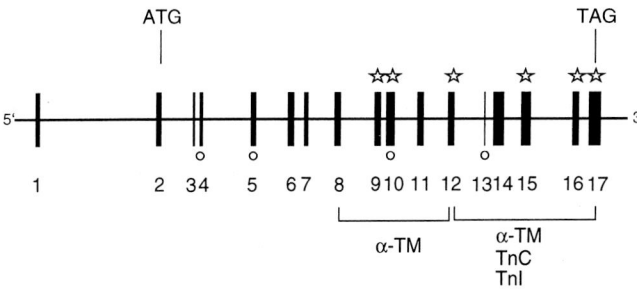

Fig. 49.14. Genomic structure of the cardiac troponin T gene based on recently published information (Farza et al., 1998). Asterisks denote exons containing mutations. Open circles indicate alternatively spliced exons. Internal and C-terminal regions of the protein interacting with other thin filament components are indicated: α-TM is α-tropomyosin, TnC and TnI are subunits of the trimeric troponin complex. ATG and TAG, translational start and stop signals.

Table 49.5. Mutations in the cardiac troponin T gene (*TNNT2*)

A. Nucleotide substitutions (missense/nonsense)

No.	Exon[1]/codon	Nucleotide change	Amino acid change	Reference
1.	8/79	ATC → AAC	Ile → Asn	Watkins et al., 1995a
2.	9/92	CGG → CAG	Arg → Gln	Watkins et al., 1995a
3.	9/92	CGG → CTG	Arg → Leu	Forissier et al., 1996
4.	9/92	CGG → TGG	Arg → Trp	Moolman et al., 1997
5.	9/94	CGC → CTC	Arg → Leu	Varnava et al., 1999
6.	9/104	GCG → GTG	Ala → Val	Nakajima-Taniguchi et al., 1997
7.	9/110	TTT → ATT	Phe → Ile	Watkins et al., 1995a
8.	10/130	n.r.[2]	Arg → Cys	Nakata et al., 1996
9.	11/163	GAG → AAG	Glu → Lys	Watkins et al., 1995a
10.	11/179	TCC → TTC	Ser → Phe	Ho et al., 2000
11.	14/244	GAG → GAT	Glu → Asp	Watkins et al., 1995a
12.	16/278	CGC → TGC	Arg → Cys	Watkins et al., 1995a
13.	16/278	CGC → CCC	Arg → Pro	Erdmann et al., 1998

B. Nucleotide substitutions in intron (splicing mutation)

No.	Position in the gene	Nucleotide change	mRNA change	Reference
14.	Intron 15, ds[3]	G → A, +1[4]	Loss of exon 15	Thierfelder et al., 1994

C. Small deletion

No	Exon/codon	Nucleotide change	Amino acid change	Reference
15.	11/160	del[5] 3 bp	ΔGlu	Watkins et al., 1995a

Footnotes: [1] No final agreement has been reached about exon annotations. Numbers given in this Table are as they are used in notation databases and in the general literature. They account for those exons present in the mRNA encoding the adult cardiac troponin T with cognate rat mRNA taken as the reference (Jun et al., 1992). The respective human gene contains four exons which are differentially spliced. Not all of them are included in adult mRNA (see Forisser et al., 1996; Farza et al., 1998). [2] [3] ds, splice donor site; [4] +1, located in intron 15, 3′ to splice donor site; [5] del,

gene is instructive because it allows exploitation of existing biochemical knowledge about the cooperation between components of the thin filament of cardiac muscle.

Troponin T mutations are relatively frequent causes of HCM. It has been estimated that they contribute to about 15% of all cases. Mutations are usually heterozygous. One case of a homozygous mutation in codon 179 (Ser→Phe) with a severe phenotype has been described (Ho et al., 2000). The parents in the family (third degree cousins) were both heterozygous carriers with mild symptoms. One of their sons had inherited both mutated alleles. He suffered from a severe form of HCM and died suddenly at the age of 17 years. Two of his siblings (genetically unassessed) had died suddenly, both at a young age (15 and 12 years). While the heterozygous carriers were either asymptomatic or only mildly affected, the doubling of the gene dose was apparently lethal. This constellation is reminiscent of two reports discussed above showing that mutations in the β-myosin gene were less severe in the heterozygous than in the homozygous state (Nishi et al., 1994; Richard et al., 2000). One recently discovered mutation, a deletion of codon 210 (ΔLys210), is responsible for a DCM, not for HCM (Kamisago et al., 2000).

Cardiac troponin I gene

After the troponin T and α-tropomyosin genes had been identified as disease genes, it was obvious to expect that mutations in other thin filament components may also contribute to HCM. Likely candidates were troponin I and C, with subunit C being a Ca++-dependent trigger of cross-bridge cycling and subunit I inhibiting this process in the absence of Ca++. A direct search for mutations in the gene for cardiac troponin I (on chromosome 19) in 184 patients resulted in the identification of five missense mutations and one codon deletion. (Kimura et al., 1997). All mutations, missense mutations and one deletion (Table 49.6) were located in the two C-terminal exons. The gene is schematically shown in Figure 49.15. For one of these mutations, the Lys183 deletion, a clinical investigation on 25 patients from seven families was performed. The most conspicuous features were high phenotypic penetrance of the mutation and a relatively high rate of premature sudden death in four of the seven families. Other clinical features and outcomes were variable. Systolic dysfunction was frequent in adults (> 40 years) and some patients developed a dilated cardiomyopathy. Wall thickness values were on the average low to moderate (Kokado et al., 2000). This is the first report on the clinical consequences of a *TnI* mutation. A conclusion about severity and risks related to mutations in this gene can not as yet be drawn.

At present no mutation has been detected in the cardiac troponin C gene.

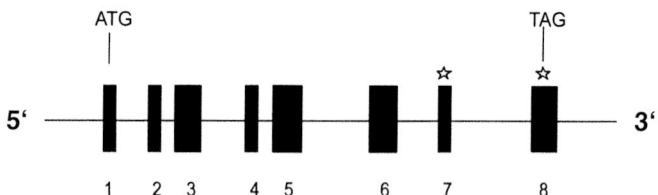

Fig. 49.15. Genomic structure of the cardiac troponin I gene. Asterisks point to exons containing mutations. ATG and TAG, translational start and stop signals.

Table 49.6. Mutations in the cardiac troponin I gene (*TNNI3*)

A. Nucleotide substitutions (missense / nonsense)

No.	Exon/codon	Nucleotide change	Amino acid change	Reference
1.	5/58	AAG → AAT	Lys → Asn	Kimura et al., 1997
2.	7/145	CGG → CAG	Arg → Gln	Kimura et al., 1997
3.	7/145	CGG → GGG	Arg → Gly	Kimura et al., 1997
4.	7/162	CGG → TGG	Arg → Trp	Kimura et al., 1997
5.	8/203	GGC → AGC	Gly → Ser	Kimura et al., 1997
6.	8/206	AAA → CAA	Lys → Gln	Kimura et al., 1997

B. Small deletion

No.	Position in the gene	Nucleotide change	Amino acid change	Reference
7.	7/183	del AAG	Δ Lys	Kimura et al., 1997

C. Large deletion

No.		Nucleotide change	Amino acid change	Reference
8.	Exon 8	Deletion of 33 bp in exon 8, incl. the stop codon	Loss of 8 amino acids at the C-terminus	Mörner et al., 2000

Cardiac myosin binding protein C gene

Myosin binding proteins were originally discovered as co-purifying contaminants in myosin preparations. Three isoforms encoded by three genes are present in slow-skeletal, fast-skeletal and cardiac muscle, respectively. Structurally they belong to the intracellular immunoglobulin superfamily. They have a modular structure composed of 8 Ig1-like and 3 fibronectin-like domains (Fig. 49.16). The cardiac protein (≈ 137 kDa) interacts with myosin and titin (Furst et al., 1992). The respective binding sites are located at the C-terminus of MyBP-C. The function of this protein is not completely understood. It may be involved in thick filament assembly and maintainance. In addition, it has been implicated in phosphorylation reactions which possibly modulate cardiac contraction (Gautel et al., 1995; Kunst et al., 2000).

The gene for the cardiac isoform of MyBP-C (Fig. 49.16) is located on chromosome 11. It was identified as a HCM disease gene through linkage analysis in a French family unlinked to chromosomes 1, 14 or 15 (Carrier et al., 1993). Two-point lod scores for two marker loci on chromosome 11 (D11S905 and D11S986) were high enough (3.81 and 4.98) to suggest a previously unknown HCM

gene. Since *MyBP-C* gene had been independently mapped to the same region (Gautel et al., 1995) it was considered to be a candidate for HCM. A mutation in intron 20 cosegregated with the disease in two families. The mutation created a cryptic splice site associated with loss of exon 21 due to aberrant splicing of mRNA. The predicted consequence was a truncated protein (Bonne et al., 1995). At the same time two families were reported with two different mutations, an internal duplication of 18 bp and a splice site mutation in a region known to interact with myosin and titin (Watkins et al., 1995b). These three mutations were an early indication of an unusual feature of the MyBP-C gene: almost two-thirds of the known mutations induce major structural changes in the protein either due to translational frameshifts resulting from insertions, deletions or rearrangements, or due to point mutations which affect normal splicing, resulting in both cases in a premature stop of protein synthesis (see Table 49.7). Since these changes are accompanied by a loss of myosin and titin binding sites, functions related to contraction should be affected. Filament structure may also suffer. The prevalence of *MyBP-C* mutations is high. It has been estimated that this gene is responsible for about 15% of all cases of HCM.

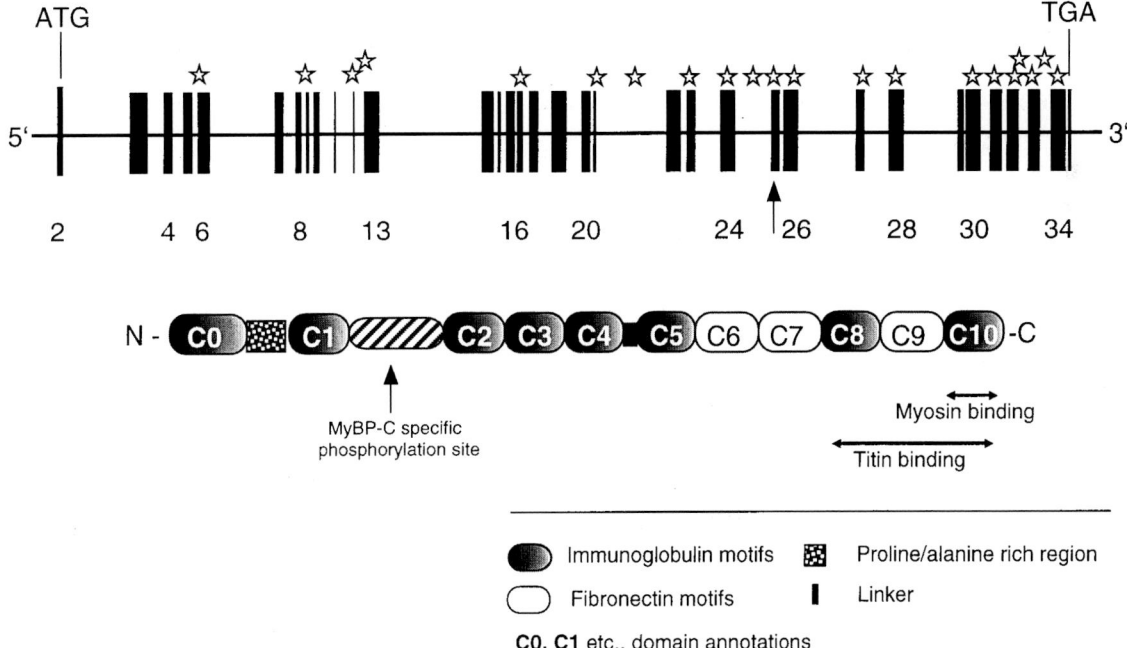

Fig. 49.16. Genomic structure of the cardiac myosin binding protein-C gene and a schematic view of the modular domain structure of the protein. Asterisks, exons and introns in which mutations have been found. The arrow points to a single base insertion in exon 24 which has been repeatedly seen in independent studies. About two thirds of the mutations induce reading frame shifts and premature translational stops in the mRNA due to deletions, insertions, duplications or mutations which affect normal splicing. The predicted result is truncated proteins of variable lengths. The protein has a modular structure consisting of immunoglobulin and fibronectin-like domains. In addition, a unique phosphorylation site (for three phosphates) exists between the domains C1 and C2. The C-terminus binds to myosin filaments and to titin. The N-terminal region around the phosphorylation site reacts with the S2 domain of myosin. MyBP-C acts in the dephosphorylated state presumably as a modulator of contraction (Kunst et al., 2000). Asterisks, positions of known mutations. ATG and TGA, translational start and stop signals. A key to the structural motifs is included in the lower part of the figure.

Table 49.7. Mutations in the myosin binding protein-C gene (*MYBPC3*)

A. Nucleotide substitutions (missense / nonsense)

No.	Exon/codon	Nucleotide change	Amino acid change	Reference
1.	6/258	GAG → AAG	Glu → Lys	Niimura et al., 1998
2.	12/451	GAG → CAG	Glu → Gln	Niimura et al., 1998
3.	17/495	CGG → CAG	Arg → Gln	Niimura et al., 1998
4.	17/502	CGG → CAG	Arg → Gln	Niimura et al., 1998
5.	17/542	GAA → CAA	Glu → Gln	Carrier et al., 1997
6.	21/654	CGC → CAC	Arg → His	Moolman-Smook et al., 1998
7.	23/755	AAC → AAA	Asn → Lys	Yu et al., 1998
8.	27/896	GTG → ATG	Val → Met	Moolman-Smook et al., 1999
9.	27/969	CAA → TAA	Gln → Stop	Yu et al., 1998
10.	31/1096	GAA → TAA	Glu → Stop	Richard et al., 1999

B. Nucleotide substitutions in introns (splicing mutations)

No.	Intron. ds[1], as[2]	Relative location[3]	Nucleotide change	Reference
11.	8/ds	+5	G → A	Carrier et al., 1997
12.	8/ds	+1	G → A	Niimura et al., 1998
13.	12/as	−2	A → G	Niimura et al., 1998
14.	21/as	−2	A → G	Bonne et al., 1995
15.	24/as	−26	A → G	Carrier et al., 1997
16.	24/ds	+1	G → A	Carrier et al., 1997
17.	24/ds	+1	G → T	Niimura et al., 1998
18.	31/ds	+5	G → C	Watkins et al., 1995b
19.	32/ds	+1	G → A	Rottbauer et al., 1997
20.	33/ds	+1	G → A	Niimura et al., 1998

C. Small deletions

No	Exon, codon	Deletion	Reference
21.	23/698	Deletion of 1 bp in codon 699 (ΔC)	Niimura et al., 1998
22.	24/755	Deletion of 1 bp in codon 756 (ΔC)	Moolmann-Smook et al., 1999
23.	26/845–846	Deletion of 5 bp in codon 845–46 (ΔGCGTC)	Carrier et al., 1997
24.	28/954	Deletion of 2 bp in codon 955 (ΔCT)	Niimura et al., 1998

D. Small insertions

No	Exon, codon	Insertion	Reference
25.	25/791	1 bp (G)	Niimura et al., 1998
26.	30/1042	2 bp (AA)	Niimura et al., 1998
27.	33/1253	18 bp (GGGGGCATCTATGTCTGC) between codon 1253 and 1254	Watkins et al., 1995b

E. Small insertion/deletion

No	Exon/codon	Insertion/deletion	Reference
28.	34/1220	Duplication of 12 bp (codon 1215–1218) and insertion in codon 1220, deletion of 4 bp (ACCT) in codon 1220 and 1221	Carrier et al., 1997

Footnotes: [1]ds, splice donor site;[2] as, splice acceptor site;[3] relative location: + indicates a base position 3′ to a splice donor site, and—is a position 5′ to a splice acceptor site both within intron regions.

Cardiac actin gene

The cardiac actin gene has been implicated in the pathogenesis of dilated cardiomyopathy in two unrelated families (Olson et al., 1998) (see below in section DCM). A mutation in the same gene was later also identified in HCM patients of one Danish family (Mogensen et al., 1999). This mutation, Ala295Ser, is localized on the surface of actin in proximity to a putative myosin-binding site (Kabsch et al., 1990; Rayment et al., 1993a,b) suggesting that cross-bridge formation and force generation in cardiocytes may be affected. A scheme of the gene is presented in Figure 49.17. (The 3-dimensional structure of actin is shown in the section DCM in Figure 49.30). The two DCM muta-

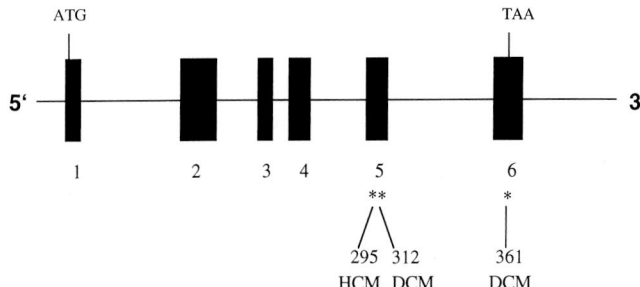

Fig. 49.17. The genomic structure of the cardiac actin gene. Three missense mutations have been identified in exon 5 and 6. Only one mutation (in codon 295) has been implicated in HCM, the two other mutations in codons 312 and 361 are associated with DCM. ATG and TAA, translational start and stop signals.

tions in positions 312 and 361, in contrast, have been implicated in an altered attachment of thin filaments to Z bands of sarcomeres. The two types of actin-related cardiac diseases may tentatively be associated with different mechanisms of pathogenesis: HCM to impaired motor functions (or "force production") and DCM to changes in the structural or cytoskeletal components of cardiocytes (involved in "force transmission"). Whether this or some other mechanism is responsible remains to be shown. Mutations in the cardiac actin gene are apparently rare in both HCM and DCM patients (Takai et al., 1999).

The genes for essential and regulatory myosin light chains

Two types of myosin light chains are involved in contraction, the "essential" light chain (ELC, molecular weight

about 15 kDa) and the "regulatory" light chain (RLC, molecular weight about 20 kDa). They form a complex with myosin heavy chains by binding to a region separating the globular head and the filamentous tail of myosin (see Fig. 49.18). Conceivably, light chains act by stabilizing the single α-helix connecting head and rod against bending stress and protecting the hypothetical "lever arm" of myosin possibly involved in driving the myosin head along actin filaments (Holmes, 1997). A direct interaction of light chains with actin in thin filaments has also been suggested (Morano et al., 1995). Light chains play an essential role in muscle contraction. It was demonstrated in vitro using muscle fiber preparations that the absence of light chains does not affect the ATPase function of myosin; however, the speed of fiber shortening during contraction is markedly decreased (Lowey et al., 1993). *Dictyostelium* myosin heavy chains from which the light chain binding regions were deleted moved more slowly than intact myosin as shown by in vitro motility assays (Ueyada et al., 1993). In agreement with the notion of light chains controlling velocity was the observation that an additional "essential" light chain binding domain was associated with increased speed of in vitro motility of myosin (Ueyada et al., 1996). The consequence of a loss of a light chain binding domain on in vivo function of the myocardium was reported recently from studies of transgenic mice: these animals under the influence of an appropriately mutated myosin transgene developed hypertrophy and other morphological changes similar to those in human HCM and, in vitro, decreased Ca²⁺-sensitivity of force development and

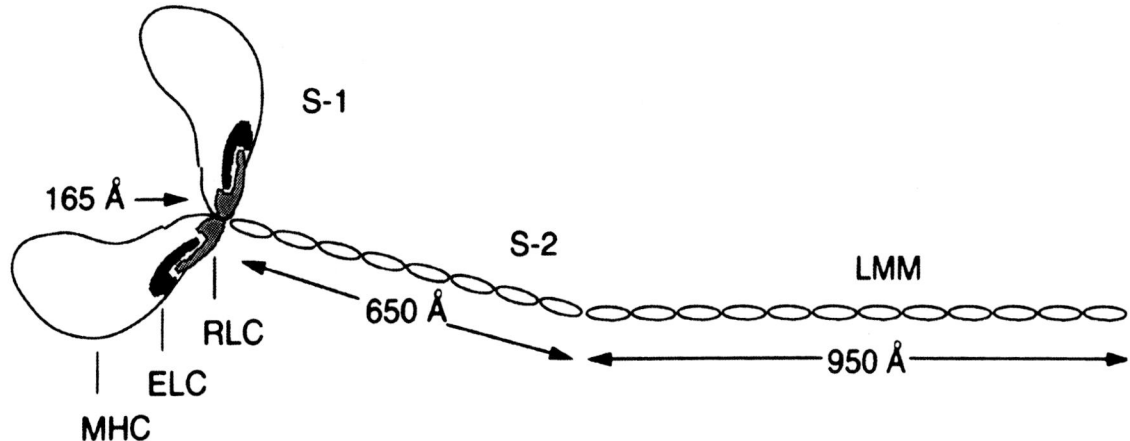

Fig. 49.18. Schematic drawing of a sarcomeric myosin heavy chain molecule. The protomeric myosin is a filamentous hexameric molecule (length ≈160 nm). It consists of two usually identical heavy chain molecules (≈220 kDa) and two pairwise identical light chains (between 16 and 20 kDa). The N-terminal region, about 45% of the total mass, forms the globular head (or S1 region), which is connected by a α-helical neck to the filamentous rod. The S1 domain is the motor unit of myosin. It carries the ATP binding site and interacts reversibly with actin filaments. The light chains bind to the neck by stabilizing the neck (see also Fig 49.21). The rod is subdivided into two domains, S2 and LMM, connected by a flexible hinge. The rods participate in thick filament assembly. MHC, myosin heavy chain, ELC, essential light chain, RLC, regulatory light chain. S1, S2 and LMM designate regions of the protein obtained by mild proteolytic cleavage.

Table 49.8. Mutations in cardiac myosin light chain genes (*MYL2/RLC* and *MYL3/ELC*)

A. MYL2: nucleotide substitutions (missense)

No.	Exon/codon	Nucleotide change	Amino acid change	Reference
1.	2/13	GCC → ACC	Ala → Thr	Poetter et al., 1996
2.	2/18	TTC → CTC	Phe → Leu	Flavigny et al., 1998
3.	2/22	GAA → AAA	Glu → Lys	Poetter et al., 1996
4.	3/58	CGA → CAA	Arg → Gln	Flavigny et al., 1998
5.	5/94	CCG → CGG	Pro → Arg	Poetter et al., 1996

B. MYL3: nucleotide substitutions (missense)

No.	Exon/codon	Nucleotide change	Amino acid change	Reference
1.	4/149	ATG → GTG	Met → Val	Poetter et al., 1996
2.	4/154	CGC → CAC	Arg → His	Poetter et al., 1996

impaired relaxation (Welikson et al., 1999). These results demonstrate that a deficiency related to light chains can have pathological consequences that resemble those known from patients. (A deletion mutation has not been seen in patients.)

The genes for *MYL3/ELC* and *MYL2/RLC* are located on chromosome 3 (ELC) and 12 (RLC) (Fodor et al., 1989; Macera et al., 1992). By screening these genes in several hundred unrelated index patients five missense mutations have been identified (Table 49.8). In the inital report an unusual phenotype with predominantly mild hypertrophy and midventricular obstruction was noted (Poetter et al., 1996). This phenomenon was, however, not observed in a second report on RLC mutations by others (Flavigny et al., 1998). Mutation in light chain genes are apparently rare, they may account for < 1% of all causes of HCM.

Titin gene

Titin is a giant protein (molecular weight ≈ 2.5×10^3 kDa) that plays a key role in muscle assembly and resting tension (Trinick, 1994; Labeit and Kolmerer, 1995). It is expressed in cardiac and skeletal muscle cells. Within sarcomeres single titin molecules span the distance from Z-disk to M-line interacting with the myosin rods and with myosin binding protein-C. In the Z-disk titin is anchored through interaction of tandem protein motifs with α-actinin (Sorimochi et al., 1997). The cDNA and part of the genomic structure of the gene (exons 1 to 16) are known (Labeit and Kolmerer, 1995; Satoh et al., 1999). The gene is located on chromosome 2q31. A contribution of this gene to the prevalence of HCM may be postulated; however, linkage of HCM to this chromosome—in contrast to DCM—has not been detected.

By SSCP screening of exons 2 to 16 in 82 index patients with no mutations in other known HCM genes, a single proband was identified with a heterozygous missense mutation in codon 740 (CGC → CTC, Arg → Leu, in exon 14) (Satoh et al., 1999). This change was located in a domain involved in the interaction of titin with α-actinin. Hence, a disease association was proposed. Since, however, cosegregation of the mutation with the disease was not shown (there were no affected relatives of the proband available for study) this conclusion should be considered provisional. The exchange could also be a silent genetic variant.

An unidentified locus on chromosome 7

A fifth disease locus has been mapped to chromosome 7q3 in a large Irish family in which the phenotype includes HCM, premature conduction disease and the Wolff-Parkinson-White syndrome (WPW), which results from an anomalous atrioventricular conduction pathway that can produce ventricular preexcitation and paroxysmal tachycardia (see Ch. 50). An association between these conditions was suggested in one of the earliest accounts of hypertrophic cardiomyopathy (Braunwald et al., 1960). In the Irish pedigree, 25 patients affected by HCM or WPW or both were analyzed. Linkage to 10 polymorphic loci on chromosome 7 was assessed with a maximum two-point lod score of 7.80 (locus D7S505; recombination frequency = 0) (MacRae et al., 1995). The causative gene remains to be identified.

Note added to the current state of knowledge

The currently known mutations identified in seven of eight (or possibly nine) HCM genes are documented in Tables 49.3 to 49.8 in this section. Actin and titin mutations have not been included. Since reports on new mutations are constantly communicated, these tables will be outdated soon. Mutation databases accessible through the World Wide Web have been implemented in recent years and are continuously updated (see Fung et al., 1999). For hypertrophic cardiomyopathy an online service is available at: http://www.angis.org.au/Databases/Heart. Additional service is offered through Online Mendelian Inheritance in Man (OMIM), http://www.ncbi.nlm.nih.gov/OMIM, and the Human Gene Mutation Database at http://archive.uwcm.ac.uk/uwcm/mg/hgmd (in Cardiff, UK).

Evidence that sarcomeric genes are directly responsible for hypertrophic cardiomyopathy

The nine genes shown or suggested to cause HCM code for proteins directly or indirectly involved in contraction of heart muscle. Although noncontractile proteins cannot *a priori* be excluded as candidates at loci (e.g., that on chromosome 7) for which the genes are not yet known, it seems reasonable to speculate that genes encoding other components of the sarcomere are probably responsible for related varieties of this disorder (Thierfelder et al., 1994).

The conclusion that the identified genes are themselves causative of disease rests on the following arguments:

1. The disease is a cardiac disease, and the mutated genes code for essential cardiac functions.
2. The mutations have been found only within HCM families and not as genetic polymorphisms in the general population. A few polymorphisms or genetic variants have been reported (missense mutations) which do not cosegregate with the disease in affected families (Greve et al., 1994; Nishi et al., 1995; Watkins et al., 1995a; Jeschke et al., 1998).
3. Within affected families all patients are carriers of these mutations. Probands who are gene carriers without having symptoms are direct descendents of patients. In these cases the diagnosis is considered to be preclinical.
4. The mutations are frequently located in evolutionarily conserved protein regions (exemplified in Fig. 49.10 depicting the 403 mutation of β-myosin).
5. Since most of the mutational amino acid exchanges induce an altered electrochemical charge in the protein, they can be expected to have a major impact on the protein structure and function.
6. It has been shown that homozygosity for a missense mutation was associated with a more severe phenotype than in heterozygotes: two sons of a Japanese couple died prematurely from sudden death and cardiac failure, respectively. The clinically asymptomatic patients were first cousins and both heterozygous (Nishi et al., 1994).

7. Molecular genetic evidence has shown that de novo mutations in MYH7 are transmitted together with the disease (Watkins et al., 1992c; Greve et al., 1994). A similar result has been obtained with the α-tropomyosin gene (Watkins et al., 1995a).
8. In vitro analysis of β-myosin heavy chains and other contractile proteins isolated from skeletal and cardiac muscle tissue samples or synthesized using DNA expression cloning has demonstrated that proteins with HCM related mutations are functionally impaired with respect to contraction, force development or ATPase activity.
9. Finally, gene-targeted and transgenic animal models involving mutated HCM genes have been developed (predominantly mice, in a few experiments rats and rabbits also) which reproduce various cardiac dysfunctions similar to those seen in patients.

FUNCTIONAL CONSEQUENCES OF HCM-RELATED MUTATIONS

Genetic mechanisms

In general, mutations may affect function by two different mechanisms. One is related to gene dosage or concentration of a given protein in the cell. If an allele is missing due to a deletion in genomic DNA or if a mutation prevents the expression of the affected gene (null/functional null mutation causing haploinsufficiency), the cell depends on the remaining intact allele. The decreased concentration of a gene product may cause dysfunction. In *Drosophila melanogaster*, a heterozygous null mutation in either an actin gene or the single muscle myosin heavy-chain gene results in a flightless phenotype (Beall et al., 1989). This observation may be relevant to the interpretation of cardiac troponin T mutations in humans where an altered splice donor site might create a functional null mutation (Thierfelder et al., 1994). A decreased amount of troponin T could lead to a disordered thin filament. Other examples of conceivable haploinsufficiency are certain splicing defects in the gene encoding myosin binding protein-C (Rottbauer et al., 1997; Moolman et al., 2000). In these cases cardiac tissue was available for analysis. The predicted truncated proteins were undetectable in the affected myocardium. Under in vivo conditions the situation might, however, be more complex. A null mutation in the human β-myosin heavy-chain gene (a nonsense or stop mutation in codon 54) did not seem to induce a disease phenotype (Nishi et al., 1994; 1995).

The second type of mutational effect results from a dominant-negative mechanism. The incorporation of wild-type and mutated proteins into multisubunit structures such as thick filaments might induce a distorted function even if the normal product is present in excess. The difficulties may begin with filament assembly and could extend to enzymatic functions and force development. In *Caenorhabditis elegans*, as little as 2% of an altered myosin heavy chain (designated unc54) can produce a dominant mutant phenotype (Bejsovic and Andersen, 1990). Since all nine of the known HCM causing sarcomeric proteins participate in the formation of complex multimeric structures, the dominant-negative concept appears most appropriate to explain cardiac dysfunction in HCM patients. The finding of mutated β-myosin mRNA and protein in cardiac tissue of patients lends support to this concept (Perryman et al., 1992; Yu et al., 1993; Cuda et al., 1997). Although dominant-negative effects are a priori more likely to cause functional changes in affected hearts, haploinsufficiency may in exceptional cases also be responsible for disease development.

General considerations

Dysfunction resulting from mutations in sarcomeric proteins would be expected to operate at different levels of cardiac activity. The basic level is related to the function of proteins and myofilaments as well as the intracellular morphology of cardiac muscle cells. Altered contraction may at some later stage affect growth behavior of these cells, their correct alignment within the myocardial tissue and their interaction with other tissue components (extracellular matrix, fibroblasts, small intramural vessels). Altered functional properties and structural changes in hypertrophied tissue are presumably together responsible for the promotion of symptoms and other clinical features. Symptoms may depend on both primary contractile dysfunction and slowly progressing secondary changes in the myocardium.

The analysis of the morphology of the heart and of cardiac performance in patients is essentially restricted to clinical investigation by echocardiography, MRI and some other techniques which all monitor only gross changes of heart morphology and function. In a few exceptional cases myocardial biopsy samples or surgical specimens were available for study of biochemical or contractile properties. Some investigations relied on mutated β-myosin isolated from human skeletal muscle. That is feasible because β-myosin in humans (as in other large mammals) is expressed not only in the ventricles of the heart, but also in slow-twitch skeletal muscle, e.g., m. soleus. For most functional studies, though, one has to rely on model systems. One such system was based on recombinant methods including biosynthesis of proteins in pro- or eucaryotic cells.

Alternatively, appropriately mutated cDNAs were transfected into a variety of cultured cells (cardiocytes, muscle and nonmuscle cells) to study properties of the products of these cDNAs (force development, calcium-control of contraction, filament assembly). The most advanced studies were done, as will be discussed, with transgenic or gene-targeted animals, predominantly mice, and recently rats and rabbits also.

Following these routes, significant progress has been achieved in recent years in the functional analysis of mutated myofibrillar proteins, including single myosin molecules, as well as of cardiac function in living mice in situ and in extracorporal whole organ preparations ("working hearts"). Most efforts have been concentrated on the β-myosin heavy chain, but mutated cardiac troponin T has also been studied. A few data have been obtained by studying α-tropomyosin and myosin binding protein-C. A single in vitro study was conducted with a mutated essential myosin light chain. Transgenic mice as hosts of mutated light chain genes have been generated twice.

Normal cardiac sarcomeres

The mutations associated with HCM are either in those proteins which directly contribute to motility and force development (actin, myosin heavy chain) or in actin and myosin associated components which have accessory or control function (myosin light chains, myosin binding protein-C, tropomyosin and the subunits of the troponin complex). Actin and myosin assemble into long cylindrical structures, the thin (actin) and thick (myosin) filaments, which reversibly associate depending on ATP binding and hydrolysis to produce transient cross-bridges between the actin binding domains of the myosin heads and the myosin binding regions of actin subunits in the thin filament. Sarcomere shortening is caused by sliding of myosin past actin filaments. These are arranged in a polar fashion with "minus ends" pointing to the sarcomere center (the M line) and "plus ends" attached to the Z bands which define the structural limits at both ends of the sarcomere (length $\approx 2,5\ \mu m$). Myosin heads slide towards the plus ends of the actin filaments.

The single most frequently affected protein is the ventricular β-isoform of myosin heavy chain. This protein is 1,935 amino acids long. The protomeric myosin unit has a molecular mass of about 500 kDa. It consists of two identical heavy chains (in cardiocytes either type α or β, each about 220 kDa) and four small light chains, two essential light chains and two regulatory light chains, respectively. The heavy chains are highly asymmetric with a globular head at the N-terminus and a long filamentous tail. The head containing the ATP binding site and the crossbridge region extends from amino acid 1 to 838. The junction between head and rod is the region where light chains form complexes with heavy chains. The filamentous tail comprising more than half of the molecule extends to the C-terminus. In the native hexameric myosin molecule the two helical tails are wound around each other forming a coiled coil. Individual myosins assemble to form multimeric thick filaments. This assembly is apparently controled by the C-termini of the myosin hexamer. Figure 49.18 depicts a simplified scheme of the myosin emphasizing its highly asymmetric structure.

Two types of light chains, the essential and the regulatory (phosphorylatable) myosin light chains (ELC/16 kDa; RLC/20 kDa), bind to the neck region linking the globular head to the filamentous tail of myosin. The function of light chains is presumably to stabilize the long α-helical neck between head and tail. This region acts presumably as an intramolecular "lever arm" of myosin which may have a central function in the myosin-actin sliding process (Holmes, 1997).

Myosin binding protein-C (the former "C-protein" of muscle, 137 kDa) binds to the C-terminus of myosin heavy chain and also to titin (a giant protein spanning the entire distance between two Z-discs and functioning as a structural organizer of the sarcomere). Myosin binding protein-C may—as mentioned—modulate the activity of the myosin head through phosporylation, presumably depending on a β-adrenergic signaling pathway (Gautel et al., 1995; Kunst et al., 2000).

Tropomyosin (46 kDa) is in its native state composed of two identical subunits. It has a filamentous shape and is attached to the actin filament. It is one of the factors bound to the thin filament involved in the calcium-dependent initiation of the cross-bridge cycle.

The troponin complex consists of three heterologous subunits associated with thin filaments in regular intervals (molecular mass of the trimer ~ 80 kDa). The subunits are denoted C, I and T. Subunit C (structurally related to calmodulin, an ubiquitous calcium-binding protein) is the key component which upon binding of calcium enables myosin to approach actin. Not all of the molecular steps involved in this regulation are known.

HCM-related mutations have been identified in these proteins with the exception of troponin C. Whether one reported missense mutation in titin is significant in functional terms (Satoh et al., 1999) has to be confirmed. A scheme of a section of the sarcomere with its main protein components is shown in Figure 49.19.

Contraction is initiated by a sudden rise in cytosolic calcium which enters the cytoplasm through special "Ca^{2+} release channels" in the sarcoplasmic reticulum in response to changing action potentials in the cytoplasmic membrane. The Ca^{2+} dependence is mediated by the calcium-binding subunit C of the troponin complex. It is generally believed

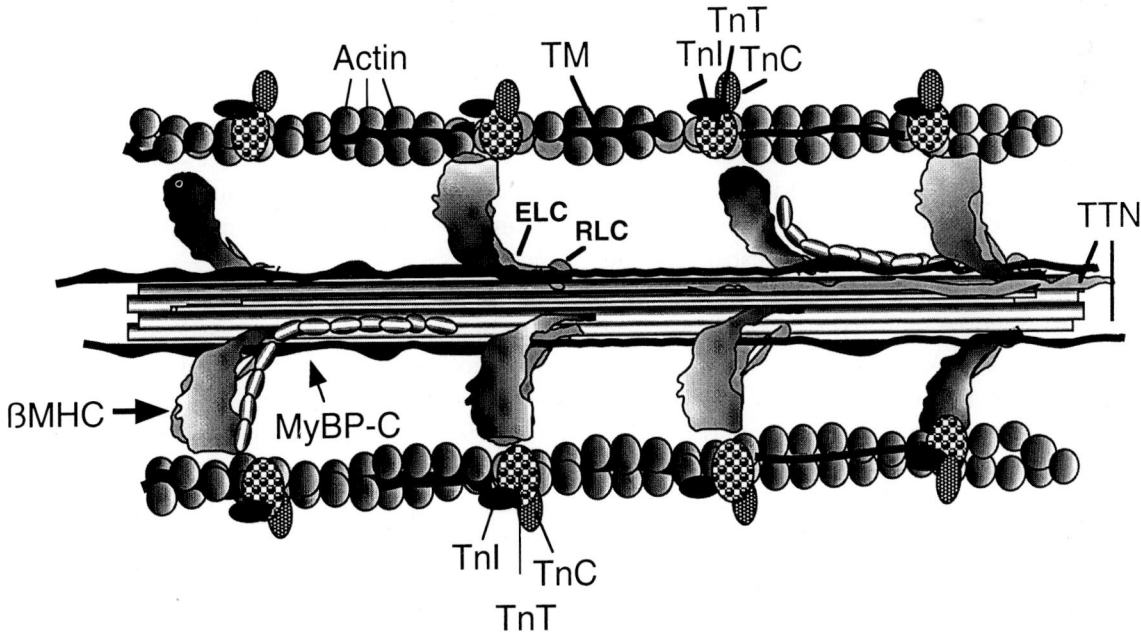

Fig. 49.19. An artificial sketch of the sarcomere. Thick filaments (central part) are flanked by thin filaments (top and bottom). Titin is considered to function as a filament organizer which is also provided with internal elasticity. The interaction of the N-terminal region of myosin binding protein-C with the S2 domain of myosin is not shown. The stoichiometry of myosin HC molecules to MyBP-C molecules is about 8 to 1. The proteins associated with the thin actin filaments are involved in the Ca++ control of contraction. The sarcomeric components are designated by their common abbreviations.

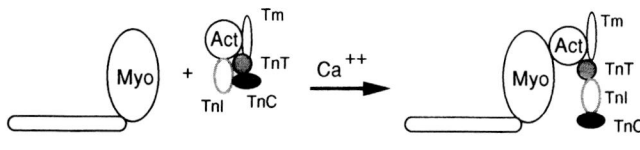

OFF - state   **ON - state**

Fig. 49.20. A scheme of cross-bridge cycling with emphasis on the role of calcium. The ON state: Ca⁺⁺ binding to troponin C allows actin and myosin filaments to assiciate transiently. The OFF state: dissociation of Ca⁺⁺ (and concomitant replacement of ADP by ATP in the S1 head, not shown) leads to separation of actin and myosin.

that Ca^{2+}-binding by subunit C is responsible for a reorientation of the troponin I and T subunits on the actin filaments with subunit T in turn cross-reacting with tropomyosin. The Ca^{2+}-troponin-tropomyosin system may Ca^{2+} prevents myosin from binding to actin, whereas in the presence of Ca^{2+} myosin and actin are free to form cross-bridges. The role of ATP in this reaction is twofold. First, it enables myosin by binding to a specific site in the head to dissociate from actin, and secondly, it provides the energy for the force generating "power stroke" which requires ATP hydrolysis and release of inorganic phosphate from the myosin head. Subsequent replacement of ADP by a new ATP molecule prepares the system for another cycle. A scheme of this cycle is shown in Figure 49.20.

Mutations in the β-myosin heavy chain

Amino acid replacements may be either conservative or nonconservative depending on the assignment of respective residues to one of the four main classes of amino acids (hydrophobic, neutral polar, positively charged and negatively charged). Conservative replacements are generally assumed to be less disruptive for the protein structure and function than nonconservative changes. A change in charge is therefore considered to have a major impact on the stability of a protein. Most of the known β-myosin heavy chain mutations are accompanied by a change in charge (39 of 68, see Table 49.3). While the consequences of such changes are unknown, suggestions have been made that a change in charge of the β-myosin molecule has in general a more detrimental effect on cardiac functions than electrochemically neutral exchanges. Truly conservative replacements have been observed only in a minority of cases (e.g., in positions 124, 232, 606, 870, and 908). While final conclusions are premature, at least some observations may be taken to suggest that mutations associated with changes in charge predispose to a more severe disease

than neutral mutations without such change (Anan et al., 1994).

The positions of the mutations within the myosin molecule may be of critical importance for pathogenic mechanisms. Altered positions are restricted to the globular head or the head-rod junction. Within this domain they occur over a wide range. The three-dimensional structure of the head of chicken-fast skeletal muscle myosin has been reported (Rayment et al., 1993a; 1993b). Since myosins of striated muscle, including human cardiac muscle, are highly conserved in evolution, the chicken data can be used for the interpretation of homologous proteins. The diagram shown in Figure 49.21 indicates the location within the molecule of active sites for ATP binding and for the interaction with actin. (This scheme is a modification of the version published by Rayment et al., 1993a.) Only a minority of the mutation sites listed in Table 49.3 are localized close to the sites controlling these activities. The corresponding amino acid residues are in positions 232, 244, 249, 256, and 403. Mutated residues 232 (Asn-Ser), 249 (Arg-Gln) and 256 (Gly-Glu) could be part of the ATP binding site; and the residue 403 (Arg-Gln/Trp/Leu) is part of the region directly involved in cross-bridge formation with actin filaments (Rayment et al., 1993a; 1993b; Schröder et al., 1993). One might expect that mutations in the active center of myosin (the ATP binding pocket) are deleterious, or even nonviable. However, at least four mutations are located at the base of this pocket: Thr124Leu, Asn187Lys, Asn232Ser and Phe244Leu.

A theoretical attempt has been made to relate mutational positions to distinct functional effects (Rayment et al., 1995). It is not clear, however, whether knowledge of structure is sufficient to predict altered function in detail. Conceivably, many of the mutations could from a distance disturb proper folding affecting more than one property of myosin.

The first reports of abnormal function of mutated β-myosin heavy chains were based on measurements of in vitro motility of β-myosins containing amino acid replacements in position 403 (Arg-Gln) and 908 (Leu-Val) (Cuda et al., 1993a). These myosins were isolated from slow fibers of skeletal muscle (m. soleus) biopsies. A decrease in motility was seen with both mutations. The effect of a 403 mutation (80% decrease) was more pronounced than that of a 908 mutation (60% decrease). In vitro motility studies describe an experimental situation that is not directly comparable to physiologic events in vertebrate skeletal or cardiac muscle. It is not coupled to mechanical work (as it is in muscle), and the myosin molecules are not assembled in a manner comparable to native thick filaments.

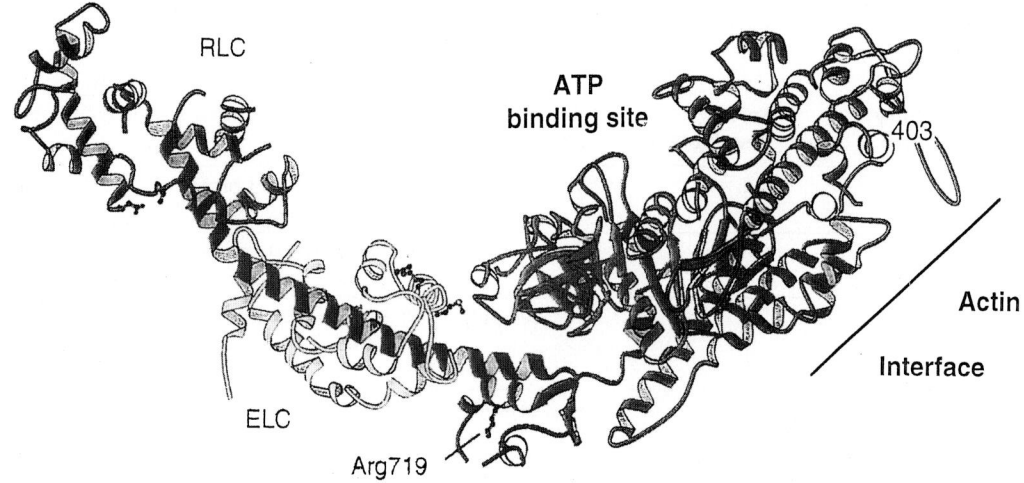

Fig. 49.21. Three-dimensional representation of the myosin S1 structure. This scheme is based on the X-ray analysis of the chicken-fast skeletal muscle myosin (Rayment et al., 1993a). Due to the high degree of evolutionary conservation of myosins across species it applies with minor modifications to human cardiac myosin also. The ATP binding site (a cleft in the S1 head) and the actin binding interface are indicated. The two light chains, ELC (yellow) and RLC (purple) that bind to the α-helical neck are shown. The colors refer to the tryptic fragments of myosin: red 50 kDa, green 25 kDa and blue 20 kDa. The positions of two missense mutations, which are both associated with a severe course of HCM, are indicated: 403[Arg-Gln] and 719[Arg-Gln]. From Poetter et al. (1996). Nature Genetics, 13:63–69. © 1996 Nature Publishing Group. (See Plate 49.21.)

Altered in vitro motility was also tested with a recombinant rat α-myosin heavy chain mutated in the equivalent position 403 and consisting of a fragment comprising the globular head and part of the tail (S2) (Sweeney et al., 1994) (Fig. 49.22). Again, the mutation induced a reduction in the sliding speed of actin filaments. In addition, the actin dependent ATPase activity of this myosin was found to be lower than that of wild-type molecules. In another investigation of slow muscle, single fibers with altered contractile properties were demonstrated, such as a decreased isometric force generation and a depressed velocity of shortening (with β-myosins mutated in position 403[Arg-Gln] and 741[Gly-Arg]). The properties of a mutation in position 256 (Gly-Glu) were indistinguishable from normal (Lankford et al., 1995).

Mutated β-myosin heavy chains were also obtained as an artificial biosynthetic protein synthesized in insect cells transfected with recombinant baculovirus (Sata and Ikebe, 1996). Alternatively, various cDNAs were used to transiently transfect cells of different origin to study properties of muscle proteins within these cells. Thus, filament assembly was found to be impaired either in nonmuscle cells (COS cells) transfected with rat α-myosin heavy chain cDNA which carried site-directed mutations otherwise found in β-myosin heavy chains (Straceski et al., 1994) or in feline cardiac myocytes infected with recombinant adenovirus particles harboring cDNA coding for mutated human β-myosin heavy chains (Marian et al., 1995). However, in other experiments with HCM-related mutations transfected into cardiocytes no effect on filament integrity was observed (Becker et al., 1997).

Table 49.9 summarizes results obtained with mutated β-myosins heavy chains and in one case with a mutated myosin light chain. Parameters tested were in vitro motility (unloaded sliding) of actin filaments along immobilized myosin molecules, the development of force and power output, and actin-activated Mg^{++}-ATPase of myosin. Most

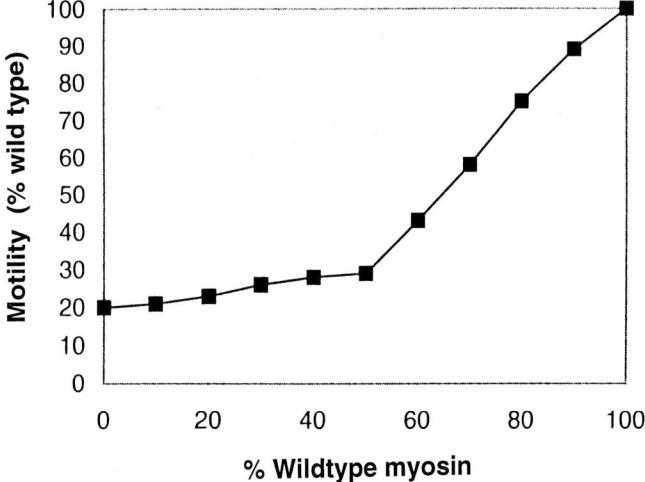

Fig. 49.22. Functional in vitro analysis of recombinant mutated myosin. α-Myosin fragments (rat) containing the S1 and S2 region were mutagenized in position 403 (Arg-Gln) and synthesized in insect cells. The functional test was in vitro motility of actin filaments which were propelled by membrane fixed myosin molecules. Mixtures of wildtype and mutated α-myosin fragments in variable relative proportions were tested. In the absence of wildtype myosin actin motility was reduced to 20% of normal values. Up to a ratio of 50% the mutant myosin was dominant over wildtype. Only if wildtype myosin exceeded 50% did the speed increase in relation to the wildtype content. (From Sweeney et al., 1994, modified.)

Table 49.9. Contraction parameters of mutated β-myosin heavy chains and essential myosin light chain

Mutation	Contraction parameters				
	Motility in vitro	**Force development**	**Actin-activated ATPase**	**Origin of myosin tested**	**References**
β-MHC 249[Arg-Gln]	n.d.	n.d.	V_{max} ↓	Recombinant protein from insect cells	Sata and Ikebe, 1996
β-MHC 256[Gly-Glu]	↓	normal	n.d.	Slow twitch muscle fiber Cuda, Sata and Lankford: v.i.	Lankford et al., 1995 Cuda et al., 1993a
β-MHC 403[Arg-Gln]	severely ↓	↓	V_{max} severely ↓	Sweeney: recomb. α-myosin (rat) from insect cells	Sweeney et al., 1994 Lankford et al., 1995 Sata and Ikebe, 1996
β-MHC 453[Arg-Cys]	↓	n.d.	V_{max} severely ↓	Recombinant protein from insect cells	Sata and Ikebe, 1996
β-MHC 606[Val-Met]	almost normal	n.d.	V_{max} normal	Recombinant protein from insect cells	Sata and Ikebe, 1996
β-MHC 741[Gly-Arg]	normal	↓	n.d.	Slow twitch muscle fiber	Lankford et al., 1995
β-MHC 908[Leu-Val]	↓	n.d.	n.d.	Slow twitch muscle fiber	Cuda et al., 1993a
ELC 149[Met-Val]	↑	n.d.	n.d.	Cardiac muscle biopsy	Poetter et al., 1996

In one experiment (Sweeney et al., 1994) α-myosin of rat was synthesized in insect cells. It comprised the head domain and the S2 region of the tail (HMM fragment). For experimental details see the above references.

of the mutations studied exhibited reduced function with respect to the three parameters tested. Thus, mutations in ventricular myosin heavy chain is associated with loss of function, or in a few cases in this series of experiments with normal properties. However, one mutation in the essential myosin light chain (codon 149[Met-Val]) showed increased motility. The same result was obtained with a myosin HC mutated in codon 741[Gly-Arg], which is located close to the binding site of the essential light chain (Poetter et al., 1996). These observations are not easily explained, but they were early indications that disease mechanisms may not only be explained in terms of "loss of function", but presumably also in terms of "gain of function". (A similar "gain of function" result was obtained even prior to this experiment in an in vitro study of a mutated troponin T, see below.)

At least for some mutations the extent of functional change (loss of function) has tentatively been related to the apparent clinical severity of the disease. The paradigm for this kind of relation is the Arg-Gln missense mutation in codon 403, which is associated with severe disease and premature cardiac death and which exhibits a significant loss of function in these studies. It should be added that the in vitro reduction of sliding speed of the mutation (60% to 80%) was similar in extent regardless of whether the myosin was extracted from skeletal or cardiac muscle cells (Cuda et al., 1997). A point of concern, however, is the discrepancy between these results and data which were obtained in

studies with gene-targeted mice carrying the 403[Arg-Gln] mutation in their adult ventricular myosin isoform (which is α in mice and β in humans). In these mice the 403 exchange caused a "gain of function" rather than a loss, as will be discussed below.

β-Myosin mutations tested in animal models

To investigate mutation-dependent effects on cardiac structure and performance in vivo, a number of animal models have been created by introducing either extra copies of mutated genes or cDNAs under the expression control of cardiac specific promoters, or by using gene-targeting methods aimed at modifying one of two mouse myosin heavy chain alleles. A synopsis of various animal models involving HCM-related mutated genes is presented in Table 49.10.

The targeted modification of a single gene has the advantage of being close to the human condition characterized by a heterozygous genotype with one mutated and one normal allele. The most advanced model for the study of functional changes was a gene-targeted mouse carrying the 403[Arg-Gln] mutation in the ventricular myosin heavy chain (Geisterfer-Lowrance et al., 1996). In mice the fast α-isoform of myosin heavy chain is expressed in the adult heart, rather than the slow β-isoform which is the predominant motor protein in adult human ventricles. (This gene-targeted mouse is designated "403 mouse" hereafter.)

Table 49.10. HCM disease mutations in gene-targeted/transgenic animals

Genetic model	Similarities to human HCM	Differences from human HCM	Comments	References
I. Experiments with mice				
Myosin heavy chain: Targeted mutation in codon 403 (Arg → Gln) of the murine αMHC gene.	Diastolic dysfunction; some hypertrophy, disarray, outflow tract pressure gradients, hypercontraction.	Gender differences; massive atrial dilatation; no sudden death; homozygous lethal.	Use of homologous recombination. Males more severely affected. Mutation is associated with "gain of function" of myosin activities. Intracavity pressure gradients. Decreased free energy of ATP hydrolysis.	Geisterfer-Lowrance et al., 1996 Spindler et al., 1998 Fatkin et al., 1999 Blanchard et al., 1999 Georgakopoulos et al., 1999 Tyska et al., 2000
Myosin heavy chain: Transgenic mouse αMHC mutated in codon 403 (Arg → Gln) plus deletion of the actin binding domain.	Hypertrophy, disarray, increased collagen content, abnormally small coronary vessels.	Genotype: Two normal alleles plus mutated transgene copies. Gender differences; no sudden death.	Rat αMHC promotor and modified coding sequence; females show more extensive hypertrophy. No artrial dilation.	Vikstrom et al., 1996
Myosin light chain: Transgenic mouse with human ELC gene mutated in codon 149 (Met → Val).	Midcavity hypertrophy in the left ventricles of mice similar to morphological changes seen in patients.	Genotype: Two normal alleles plus copies of mutated transgenes.	The human ELC promoter was used. Studies were focussed on distorted stretch activation response of papillary muscles prior to the onset of hypertrophy.	Vemuri et al., 1999
Myosin light chain: Transgenic mouse with mutated human mutations in ELC and RLC genes (ELC: codon 149, Met → Val, RLC: codon 22, Glu → Lys). Transgenes were of mouse origin, mutations were human.	Myocyte disarray and impaired relaxation.	The mutated cDNA was of mouse origin. No midcavity obstruction as reported for the human disease and for transgenic mice (as reported by Vemuri et al., 1999)	Rat αMHC promoter.	Sanbe et al., 2000
Cardiac troponin T: Transgenic cTnT with truncation of exons 15 and 16.	Myocellular disorganization. Diastolic dysfunction.	Genotype: Two normal alleles plus mutated transgene copies. Homozygous lethal; decreased ventricular mass (loss of cardiocytes); no hypertrophy; no sudden death.	c-Myc tag; rat αMHC promotor (allows expression in the atria).	Tardiff et al., 1998
Cardiac troponin T: Transgenic cTnT with missense in codon 92 (Arg → Gln)	Diastolic dysfunction; impaired relaxation; disarray, increased collagen content. Either hypercontraction or normal systolic function.	Genotype: Two normal endogenous alleles plus mutated transgene copies. No hypertrophy; no sudden death. Left ventricle smaller than in controls. Decreased left ventricular ejection. Abnormal systolic function in some animals.	Promoter control: mouse cTnT or rat αMHC. Variable levels of expression. Induction of ANF and βMHC genes in the left ventricle.	Oberst et al., 1998 Lim et al., 2000a Tardiff et al., 1999

(continued)

Table 49.10. HCM disease mutations in gene-targeted/transgenic animals (*continued*)

Genetic model	Similarities to human HCM	Differences from human HCM	Comments	References
I. Experiments with mice (continued)				
α-Tropomyosin: Transgenic αTM with missense mutation in codon 175 (Asp-Asn)	Mild myocellular disorganization and hypertrophy. Severely impaired relaxation and contractility. Trend to formation of thrombi in left atrium.	Genotype: Normal alleles plus mutated transgene copies. No hypertrophy. No sudden death. Mild increase in fibrosis and disarray.	Rat αMHC promotor; modified αTM cDNA from mouse. Altered function in vitro: enhanced calcium sensitivity of force development.	Muthuchamy et al., 1999
Myosin binding protein-C: Transgenic MyBP-C cDNA with C-terminal truncations. (A) Short cDNA, lacking the myosin and titin binding domain, break in protein domain C5. (B) Long cDNA, lacking the myosin binding domain only, break between domain C9 and the terminal domain C10.	Reduced power output. Structural changes in the heart (disarray).	Genotype: Two normal alleles plus mutated transgene copies. No hypertrophy; no sudden death.	c-myc tag: mouse αMHC promotor; cDNA of mouse origin. In vitro increase in calcium sensitivity of force development and decreased contractile power output. Short cDNA: stably expressed, but not assembled into sarcomeres. Long cDNA: low level of expression.	Yang et al., 1998 Yang et al., 1999
Myosin binding protein-C: Targeted replacement of myosin- and titin-binding domain by novel amino acid residues.	Hypertrophy of cardiac myocytes, disarray, fibrosis, diastolic and systolic dysfunction.	Targeted animals were bred to homozygosity. Pathology was indicative of ventricular dilatation and dilated cardiomyopathy rather than of hypertrophic cardiomyopathy.	Two different truncations were tested, both starting in exon 30 (or in the C9 domain of the protein) and both lacking ~200 residues. Changes were analogous to a known cause of human HCM. The genotype in humans is heterozygous.	McConnell et al., 1999
α-**Tropomyosin:** Targeted ablation (knockout) of the gene.	None. Heterozygous mice had no phenotype. Reduced gene dosage had no effect.	A heterozygous null mutation of a TM gene has not been reported.	Homozygous null mutations were not viable.	Blanchard et al., 1997
II. Experiments with rats				
Cardiac troponin T: Deletion of exon 16 and deletion of exon 15 and 16 (two models).	Systolic and diastolic dysfunction without cardiac hypertrophy. Sudden death and ventricular fibrillation. Myocardial dissaray.	Overexpression of the transgenes. The wildtype cTnT caused moderate myocardial hypertrophy.	Sudden death and fibrillation after 6 months of daily physical exercise.	Frey et al., 2000
III. Experiments with rabbits				
Myosin heavy chain: Transgenic βMHC of mouse origin with missense mutation in codon 403 (Arg-Gln).	Substantial disarray, increased septal hypertrophy, interstitial fibrosis. Premature death frequent (including occasional sudden death).	The genotype: Two normal alleles plus a variable number of mutated transgenes.	Promotor: Murine βMHC.	Marian et al., 1999

Conventional transgenic animals (mostly mice, in a few cases rats and rabbits) that carry the normal complement of wildtype alleles in addition to variable numbers of randomly inserted transgenes have also been generated.

The 403 mouse was generated by introducing an appropriately mutated α-myosin heavy chain gene fragment into embryonic stem cells. These cells were then transferred into blastocysts to establish lines carrying the mutation in their germline (Hasty et al., 1991). The procedure by which the mutated gene was obtained is schematically depicted in Fig. 49.23. Structural changes in the hearts of the heterozygous mice were similar to alterations recognized in human HCM: myocyte disarray, hypertrophy and fibrosis, all increasing with age. Male mice were more severely affected than their female counterparts (Geisterfer-Lowrance et al., 1996).

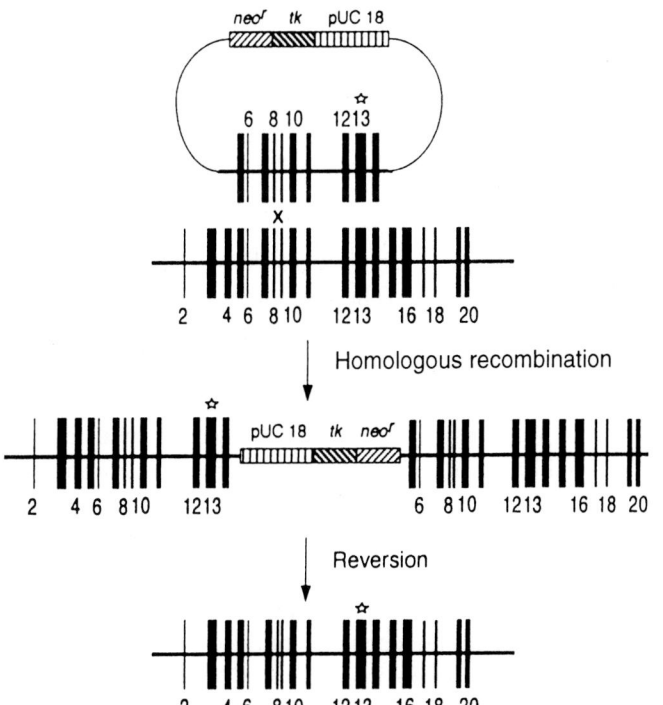

Fig. 49.23. Gene-targeted modification of the α-myosin heavy chain of the mouse (replacement of Arg 403 by Gln). This scheme illustrates the principle of the recombination procedure. In the first step ("homologous recombination") a plasmid carrying part of the α-myosin gene including the mutated codon 403 (asterisk in exon 13) was integrated into the genome of an mouse embryonic stem cell (ES). Recombinant ES cells were selected for the integrated neomycin resistence gene (neo'). In a second step ("reversion") cells were selected for the absence of the tk (thymidine kinase) gene. (The procedure is also called "hit and run" method.) Cells in which the partial gene duplication had been corrected by means of intramolecular crossing-over without losing the 403 mutation were expanded and introduced into blastocysts of mice. Resulting chimeric founders were bred to heterozygous homogeneity of the 403 mutation. (The latter part of the experiment is not shown here. For details see Geisterfer-Lowrance et al., 1996; Hasty et al., 1991.)

Homozygous mice with two mutated alleles were not viable, they died seven days after birth. The neonatal lethality of homozygous 403 mice is caused by a rapidly progressive cardiomyopathy characterized by loss of myocytes and severe cardiac dysfunction. These changes become obvious between days four and six after birth. They are associated with wall thinning, dilatation of the left ventricle and systolic failure (Fatkin et al., 1999). The cardiac performance of viable heterozygous 403 mice has meanwhile been investigated in considerable depth. Results were obtained *in vivo* and *in vitro*, in part by using newly developed methods to assess mouse cardiac dimensions and blood flow by high frequency (45 MHz) echocardiography, the energetic status of magnetic resonance spectroscopy in organ preparations, the in situ investigation of pressure-volume relationships, as well as by studying muscle strips and single myosin molecules.

Hearts of young 403 mice (six weeks old) analysed in vivo had altered contraction kinetics before morphologic or histologic abnormalities of the myocardium became apparent. Systolic pressure rise was accelerated, while pressure drop and chamber filling were delayed. Fibrosis and disarray were seen in older mice (20 weeks), which also showed hyperdynamic contraction, increased end-systolic chamber stiffness and outflow tract gradients (Georgakopoulos et al., 1999). Cardiac performance analysed in isolated, isovolumic heart preparations and studied under conditions of regulated pacing (i.e., at a constant heart rate) was altered in the following respects: diastolic function was impaired as indicated by a decreased rate of relaxation and an increased end-diastolic pressure; measurements of cardiac energetics by ^{31}P nuclear magnetic resonance spectroscopy exhibited lower phosphocreatine and increased inorganic phosphate contents resulting in a decrease of the value calculated for the free energy obtained from ATP hydrolysis (see Fig. 49.24). The ^{31}P-spectrum observed with isolated hearts of 403 mice closely resembled the ^{31}P NMR spectra reported from in vivo investigations of HCM patients (Jung et al., 1998). (No attempt had been made, however, to determine the mutations responsible for the disease of these patients.) In mice, the impaired relaxation and the decrease in free energy release were augmented with increasing calcium concentration as was shown in a "working heart" whole organ preparation (Fig. 49.25). Thus, under conditions of an increased contractile performance the functional deficits were enhanced. This result was corroborated by the finding that 403 hearts led to a marked decrease in heart rate (by 40%) as compared to wildtype hearts (Spindler et al., 1998).

Furthermore, measurements of cross-bridge kinetics in skinned left ventricular papillary muscle strips from 403

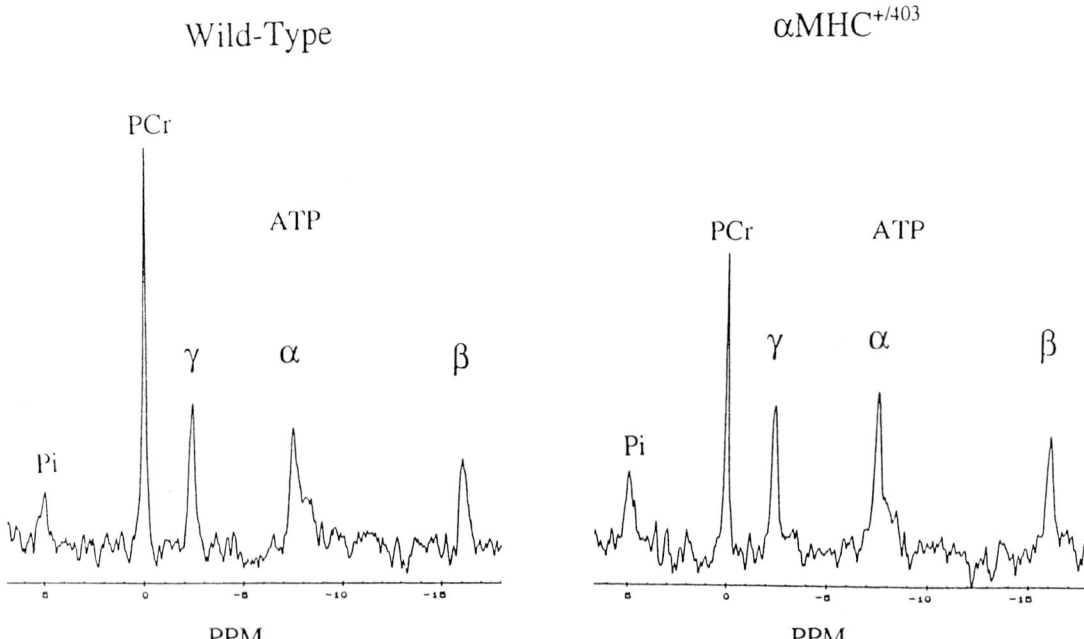

Wild-Type   αMHC$^{+/403}$

PPM   PPM

Fig. 49.24. ^{31}P NMR spectra obtained with isolated hearts from wildtype mice and from heterozygous 403 mice. Wildtype spectra are left, 403 myosin spectra are right. The major resonances refer to inorganic phosphate (P$_i$), phosphocreatin (PCr) and to the γ-, α- and β-phosphates of ATP. The area under each peak is proportional to the number of molecules in the heart. The hearts of 403 mice have similar ATP contents as wildtype hearts, but smaller PCr and larger P$_i$ areas. (From Spindler et al., 1998, with permission.)

hearts showed increased dynamic stiffness in resting strips (at low, non stimulatory calcium concentrations, pCa 8, that is 10^{-8} moles Ca^{2+} per liter) and reduced power output under conditions of maximal stimulation (calcium: pCa 5). These results were consistent with the assumption that the 403$^{Arg-Gln}$ mutation reduces the strong binding affinity of myosin for actin. Myosin heads may attach in a preforce state (preceding the power stroke) that favors activation of thin filaments if calcium is low, but it reduces tension and force production if calcium is high. Thus under conditions of submaximal activity, relaxation may be impaired due to an increased myosin-actin ON rate which in turn should result in increased stiffness. (A reduced OFF rate would probably lead to a similar effect.) Maximal activation at high calcium may be associated with reduced force due to depressed cross-bridge kinetics. A conceivably important implication for the human disease is that—in addition to morphological changes such as fibrosis and disarray—the activation status of the myocardium, e.g., increased stiffness at rest, reduced power output with heavy exercise, may contribute to the compromised function of the diseased myocardium (Blanchard et al., 1999).

An intriguing further extension of these studies was achieved by analyzing the in vitro performance of isolated myosin as purified from cardiac tissue of homozygous neonatal 403 mice. Since these animals die within seven days of birth, hearts—and control hearts—had to be prepared within this time. The mutant myosin was shown to have a 2.3-fold higher actin-activated Mg^{++}-ATPase activity, 2.2-fold greater average force generation and a 1.6-fold faster actin filament sliding in the motility assay. In addition, the analysis of single myosin molecules in an optical trap (Guilford et al., 1997) showed that the mutation has a marked effect on the average step size (or displacement amplitude) during single cross-bridge cycles. The data was interpreted in terms of normal two-headed single myosin molecules being able to coordinate the activity of their two heads, whereas homogeneously mutated myosin molecules operate in an uncoordinated fashion (Tysta et al, 2000).

The difference between mutated and wildtype myosins in force development was measured using myosin populations, not single molecules. On the level of single molecules the force development (the unitary force developed by a single molecule in a single cycle) was equal in both myosin species. This suggested that kinetic differences, e.g., an increased rate of ADP release from myosin, may be accompanied by an accelerated rate of recruiting myosin heads for the cross-bridge cycle. A likely consequence would be that at any one time during muscle contraction more mutated myosin heads are engangend in contraction than wildtype heads which would lead to a relative increase in force development and shortening velocity. This "gain in function"

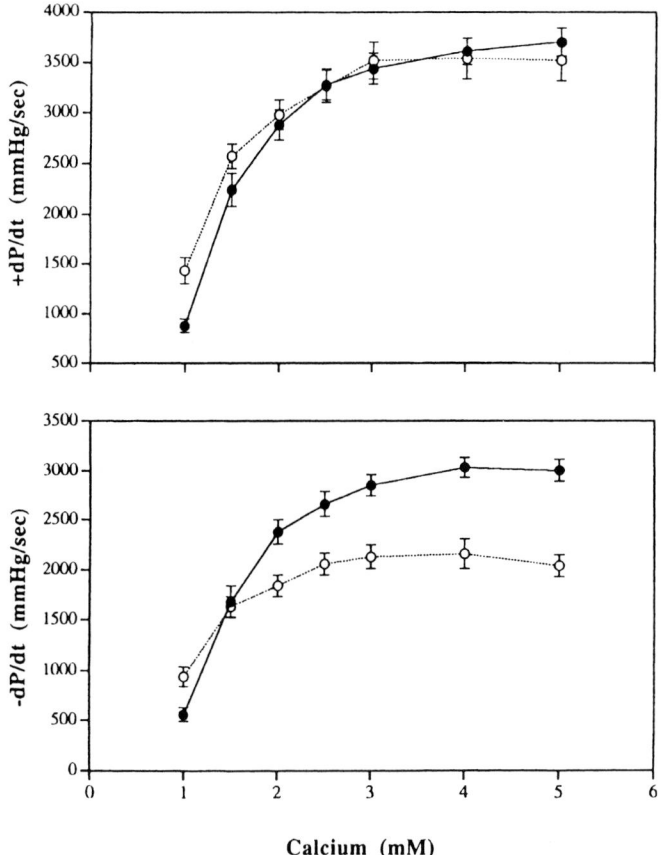

Fig. 49.25. Systolic and diastolic activity of isolated hearts of wildtype and 403 mice. In this experiment the increase in blood pressure (+dP/dt) during systole as an indicator of contraction and the decrease in blood pressure (–dP/dt) during diastole as an indicator of relaxation was measured as a function of the Ca++ concentration in the perfusing medium. In a low Ca++ concentration the systolic pressure rise was increased in 403 hearts as compared to wildtype hearts (hypercontraction), but at higher Ca++ concentrations the difference disappeared. In diastole the increase of Ca++ was associated with a marked decrease in the rate of relaxation of 403 hearts. Filled circles, wild-type hearts; open circles, 403 hearts. (From Spindler et al., 1998, with permission.)

has a price, that is an increased energy demand in terms of ATP hydrolysis. The lack of ATP would affect not only the muscle filaments, but other ATP-dependent functions in the cell also. Compensatory mechanisms for the relief of stress and energy demand may then be the triggers of secondary events leading to structural and metabolic perturbations and ultimately to disease.

The critical step in this process seems to be the altered interaction between myosin and actin, because in the absence of actin, mutated and wildtype myosins have the same ATPase activity. It is interesting to note that the enhanced ATPase activity can be induced in smooth muscle myosin (chicken gizzard) by replacing the amino acid that corresponds to 403[Arg] in human β-myosin (Yamashita et al., 1997). It seems therefore not very likely that the effects seen with

mouse α-myosin are due to an intrinsic property of that particular myosin. They may rather reflect a change of general importance for myosin function. (For further details and discussion, see Tyska et al., 2000.)

The results obtained with 403 mice cause two major questions. First, how should the discrepancies be explained that obviously exist between different studies that do not converge with respect to gain or loss of function caused by the 403[Arg-Gln] mutation. The second question is, what are the implications of the data obtained with these mice for the understanding of the human disease.

The "gain of function" results discussed above are in contrast to results of earlier experiments by others using either recombinant myosin or myosin extracted from slow skeletal muscle (Cuda et al., 1993a; Sweeney et al., 1994; Sata and Ikebe, 1996; Fujita et al., 1998; Roopnarine et al., 1998). The general tendency was "loss of function". In some experiments myosin fragments (heavy meromyosin) have been used. The systems applied for expressing myosin posed difficulties and might have been compromised. Further, different types of actin (regulated and unregulated) might have contributed to different outcomes in motility studies. Finally, although α- and β-myosin are remarkably similar (McNally et al., 1989), minor variations in relevant regions of these proteins may contribute to major functional differences. Thus, it cannot be excluded that the same mutation in the two cardiac isoforms have different consequences for their function. Taken together, the discrepancies are not fully explained. Further studies are required.

With respect to the human condition one had to assume that no critical differences exist between murine fast α-myosin and slow β-myosin. With this presumption the well-known ventricular hypercontraction in human hearts could be explained. That property would then suggest that the hypertrophic response in individuals expressing this mutation is not due to depressed force or reduced kinetics of contraction (which would constitute a loss of function), but instead due to a chronically increased energy demand by the contractile system and other cellular systems too. Hypertrophy and other changes would be indicative of compensatory or adaptive measures of the heart to reduce wall stress and energy consumption per unit cardiac muscle mass (Moss and Pereira, 2000). These changes presumably develop slowly and may be accompanied with altered gene expression profiles in different parts of the myocardium. Secondary changes in the handling of calcium may in addition be involved. Calcium is not only a regulator of muscle contraction, but also of other cytoplasmic and nuclear activities, e.g., signal transduction and control of gene expression (see the discussion below about the presumed role of calcineurin).

These results have been obtained with a single HCM-related mutation in myosin ($403^{Arg-Gln}$). It is open to question whether this concept applies only to myosin mutations or to other genes and mutations, too. Since not all of the known HCM mutations are associated with marked hypertrophy and since penetrance and expressivity may vary considerably, it is conceivable or even likely that different mechanisms are responsible for the ultimate phenotype. For instance, mutations in the gene encoding cardiac troponin T may cause premature sudden cardiac death with mild or absent clinical left ventricular hypertrophy. This kind of HCM may be caused by a specific mechanism that does not apply to other kinds of the disorder.

In addition to the targeted 403 α-myosin mutation, experiments with partial deletions of internal sequences of rat α-MHC have been done using conventional transgene protocols (DNA injection into zygotes of mice). In the first experiment the actin binding domain was deleted (over a length of 58 amino acids). A further mutation in the same DNA was a $403^{Arg-Gln}$ exchange (Vikstrom et al., 1996) (see Table 49.10). In a second experiment 65 amino acids had been removed from the site that interacts with the regulatory light chain (RLC) (Welikson et al., 1999) (see Table 49.12). The host animals in both experiments exhibited structural changes in the heart that closely resembled those recognized in patients (hypertrophy, disarray). The loss of the RLC binding site was associated with decreased Ca^{2+} sensitivity of force development and impaired relaxation in skinned cardiac muscle fibers. Although these deletions do not reflect mutational changes identified in patients, they suggest that different kinds of changes in the ventricular α- or β-MHC gene have similar phenotypic consequences.

The fact that fast α- and slow β-MHC have different kinetics in Mg-ATPase activity and in cross-bridge formation (Sugiura et al., 1998a;b) is cause of persistent concern whether data obtained in mice reliably explain human disease mechanisms. An animal model closer to the human heart would in principle be preferable. Rabbits might be suitable targets. They are not as easily bred as mice, but the larger mammals have the advantage to express β-myosin and not α-myosin in their ventricles. Human and rabbit β-myosin are about 98% homologous (Kavinsky et al., 1984; Jaenicke et al., 1990). One such experiment with rabbits has been reported. The transgene used was human β-myosin with the 403 mutation (Marian et al., 1999). The cardiac phenotype observed resembled the typical human HCM pathology regarding left ventricular hypertrophy with increased septal thickness, disarray and fibrosis and

premature death. Thus, to choose the rabbit as a model may be preferable, although the investigations with this animal are slower and more expensive than experiments with mice. The single published report indicates a success rate for the transgenic manipulation of about 4%: four surviving rabbits, two wildtype and two mutation carriers, were obtained from 95 recipient foster mothers.

Mutations in α-tropomyosin

Mutations in this gene are uncommon. Impaired contractile properties have been demonstrated in a number of reports on two of four known mutations, $175^{Asp-Asn}$ and $180^{Glu-Gly}$. Thin filaments (containing F-actin from rabbit skeletal muscle) were reconstituted with human cardiac troponin and recombinant α-tropomyosin. The latter protein synthesized in *E. coli* cells was equipped with a modification at the N-terminus to compensate for the lack of acetylation upon synthesis in bacterial cells. They exhibited in vitro an increased Ca^{2+} sensitivity of motility, that is, at a given Ca^{2+} concentration in a range between pCa 6 and 6.6 a larger fraction of filaments was moving with mutated α-tropomyosin than with the respective wildtype protein. The effect was more pronounced with the $180^{Glu-Gly}$ mutation than with the $175^{Asp-Asn}$ exchange. Other parameters tested (velocity, isometric force development) showed no difference (Bing et al., 2000). An increased Ca^{2+} sensitivity may be interpreted as a "gain of function" which was also seen in other experiments with mutated tropomyosins. Thus, isometric force produced by human skeletal muscle containing 50% α-tropomyosin ($175^{Asp-Asn}$) showed a small increase in Ca^{2+} sensitivity with no change in maximal force (Bottinelli et al., 1998). Likewise, in experiments with material from transgenic mice carrying $175^{Asp-Asn}$ α-tropomyosin an increased Ca^{2+} sensitivity of skinned cardiac muscle fibers was observed. These animals exhibited in addition severe impairment of cardiac contractility and relaxation (Muthuchamy et al., 1999). Finally, transfection of cardiac myocytes with adenovirus vectors carrying mutant α-tropomyosin led to an increase in Ca^{2+} sensitivity of isometric tension with the $180^{Asp-Asn}$ mutation (but not with the $175^{Asp-Asn}$ mutation) (Michele et al., 1999).

In addition to those changes related to Ca^{2+} sensitivity, altered affinity of mutated α-tropomyosin to F-actin (measured by consedimentation) was also observed. Whereas no change was seen with $180^{Asp-Asn}$ α-tropomyosin, the affinity of $175^{Asp-Asn}$ α-tropomyosin was about two fold weaker, irrespective of the presence of troponin T. The affinity to troponin was unaffected (Golitsina et al., 1997). Thus, composite and pleiotropic effects might result in a distorted equilibrium of ON- and OFF-states of the cross bridge cycle. The physiological consequences of an increased Ca^{2+} sensitivity of contraction would be a somewhat slower and incomplete relaxation during diastole (as was discussed above in the context of properties of 403 mice).

Not all of the observations are fully explained. In one of the studies with mutated α-tropomyosin (Bing et al., 1997) a difference between the in vitro properties of human mutant and wildtype protein became apparent only in the presence of heterologous troponin T (rabbit, skeletal muscle TnT), but not in the presence of homologous troponin T (human, cardiac TnT). This result indicates that observations made in vitro are sometimes not easily interpreted.

Further studies of α-tropomyosin-related dysfunction were done using genetically manipulated mice. One report was focussed on the targeted inactivation ("knockout") of the α-tropomyosin gene (Blanchard et al., 1997), and a second investigation was aimed at the characterization of the consequences of an Asp-Asn exchange in amino acid position 175 of this protein (Muthuchamy et al., 1999). Homozygous knockout mice were not viable. They died before birth. Heterozygous knockouts mice had an essen-

tially normal phenotype. α-Tropomyosin mRNA was reduced to 50%, but the protein content was normal, suggesting that haploinsufficiency is not a major mechanism of disease promotion presumably due to control processes compensating for a reduced gene dosage.

The 175[Asp-Asn] mutation in transgenic mice was found to be associated with a severe impairment of contraction and relaxation. Hearts of these animals were hypodynamic. The maximum rate of contraction (+dP/dt = increase in systolic pressure over time, as measured in isolated perfused heart preparations) was reduced, as was the rate of relaxation (–dP/dt). The latter result may be explained by a marked increase in Ca^{2+} sensitivity of force development (Fig. 49.26). This observation is in agreement with a number of reports about changes induced by other HCM-related mutations in myosin heavy chain and troponin T. Increased Ca^{2+} sensitivity of force development may be a common feature in the early stage of HCM pathogenesis.

Mutations in cardiac troponin T

Dysfunction related to mutated cardiac troponin T have been analysed in numerous in vitro studies and to some

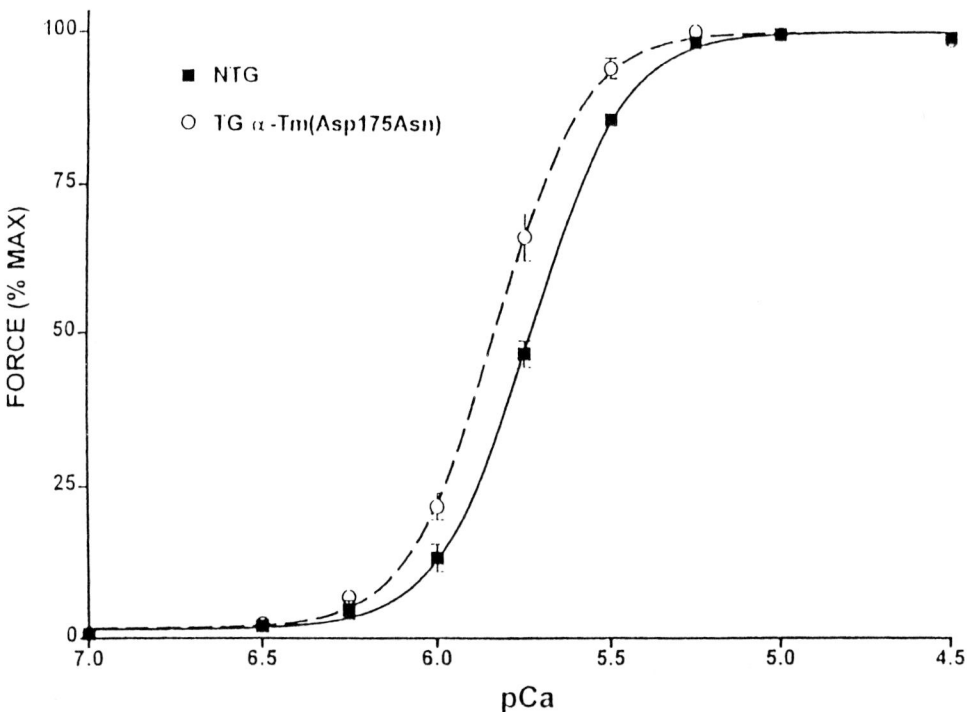

Fig. 49.26. Ca^{2+}-force relationship in skinned cardiac fibers isolated from transgenic mice carrying a mutated α-tropomyosin gene (175[Asp-Asn]). Force development as a function of increasing Ca^{++} concentrations was studied in fiber bundles prepared from transgenic mouse hearts and from hearts of wildtype mice. A shift to the left was seen in the bundles of transgenic mice with the mutated tropomyosin indicating increased sensitivity of contraction to Ca^{++} as a consequence of the mutation. Filled squares and open circles represent fibers from nontransgenic controls and from transgenic animals, respectively. From Muthuchamy et al., 1999.

degree also in transgenic mice. The results obtained by different investigators are complex and not in all respects in agreement. The in vitro experiments were predominantly focussed on myofibrillar Mg^{2+}-ATPase activity, on velocity of sliding (motility) and on force development. The test systems included permeabilized (skinned) rabbit or porcine cardiac muscle fibers and cDNA transfer into skeletal muscle myoblasts from quail (committed, but undifferentiated muscle stem cells which in culture develop into contractile myotubes). Cultured adult cardiac myocytes were also used.

Eight different HCM-related troponin T mutations have been studied: $79^{Ile\text{-}Asn}$, $92^{Arg\text{-}Gln}$, $110^{Phe\text{-}Ile}$, $163^{Glu\text{-}Lys}$, $244^{Glu\text{-}Asp}$, $278^{Arg\text{-}Cys}$, a deletion of 160^{Glu} ($\Delta E160$) and a deletion of the exons 15 and 16, due to a splicing mutation in intron 15 ($\Delta Ex15$–16) associated with a loss of exon 15 and 16 in the transcript. These exons encode the C-terminus of troponin T which in vivo interacts with tropomyosin. The results show both enhanced and decreased properties, or "gain" and "loss of function". The first observation suggesting a somewhat unexpected gain of function was made in a study of a $91^{Ile\text{-}Asn}$ mutation introduced into rat cardiac troponin T. This mutation corresponds to the $79^{Ile\text{-}Asn}$ mutation of human cardiac troponin T (Lin et al., 1996). The amino acid exchange had no effect on troponin T binding to α-tropomyosin, troponin T-induced binding of α-tropomyosin to actin, the cooperative binding of myosin to thin filaments and the Ca^{++} regulation of actin-activated Mg^{2+}-ATPase. However, the maximal in vitro migration speed of thin filaments complexed with mutated troponin T was faster by 50% as compared to wild-type troponin T. The reason for this change is not known. It has been hypothesized by the authors that the increased motility might be due to an "acceleration effect" restricted to the regulatory "unit" of thin filaments (consisting of seven actin monomers plus regulatory proteins) (Lin et al., 1996). But a change in the kinetics of actin-myosin cross-bridge formation, or more specifically an enhanced detachment rate of actin and myosin may also be considered.

The same mutation was also studied by others (Morimoto et al., 1998; Sweeney et al., 1998; Rust et al., 1999; Yanaga et al., 1999; Szczesna et al., 2000) and the increased motility was confirmed. For both $79^{Ile\text{-}Asn}$ and $92^{Arg\text{-}Gln}$. Another functional change of the $92^{Arg\text{-}Gln}$ mutation was an enhanced shortening velocity of transfected myotubes in the absence of load (Sweeney et al., 1998). The agreement between different investigators was, however, not perfect for all functional parameters tested, in particular regarding the Ca^{2+} sensitivity of force development. A decreased sensitivity was measured by some investigators for the mutations $79^{Ile\text{-}Asn}$, $92^{Arg\text{-}Gln}$ and $\Delta Ex15$–16

(Watkins et al., 1996; Sweeney et al., 1998; Rust et al., 1999). In contrast, enhanced sensitivity has been reported by others (Morimoto et al., 1998; Nakaura et al., 1999; Yanaga et al., 1999). Discordant results have also been obtained for maximum force associated with the $79^{Ile\text{-}Asn}$ mutation of troponin T, which was either reduced (Sweeney et al., 1998; Tobacman et al., 1999) or normal (Morimoto et al., 1998; Rust et al., 1999). Not all of the properties of the eight troponin T mutations have been studied by more than one investigator. Some of the reported data should therefore be considered provisional. Gain of function effects have been assessed—in addition to in vitro motility or Ca^{2+} sensitivity of force development—for the maximal rate of myofibrillar Mg^{2+}-ATPase with two mutations, $110^{Phe\text{-}Ile}$ and $244^{Glu\text{-}Asp}$ (Yanaga et al., 1999). The myofibrillar Ca^{2+} sensitivity measured at half-maximal Ca^{2+} concentration was increased with $79^{Ile\text{-}Asn}$ and $92^{Arg\text{-}Gln}$, most notably at low pH values (pH 7.0 and 6.5) (Yanaga et al., 1999). Since the myocardium is never operating under conditions of maximal rate of Mg^{2+}-ATPase, some of the proposed functional changes may not have a major effect in normal life. Others, e.g., pH-dependent parameters, may be ineffective under normal conditions, but not under stress conditions, e.g., ischemia or acidosis.

Loss of function was reported for maximal force with the mutations $79^{Ile\text{-}Asn}$, $\Delta E160$ and $\Delta Ex15$–16 (Watkins et al., 1996; Sweeney et al., 1998; Tobacman et al., 1999). Marked sarcomeric disarray was observed in quail myotubes expressing the $\Delta Ex15$–16 mutation (Watkins et al., 1996) and in transgenic mice carrying the same mutation (Tardiff et al., 1998).

Table 49.11 summarizes the in vitro data obtained for different functional parameters associated with specific mutations in cardiac troponin T.

In addition, troponin T-related dysfunctions have also been investigated in transgenic mice. Two mutations have been analyzed, $92^{Arg\text{-}Gln}$ and $\Delta Ex15$–16. Major results obtained with mice carrying the $92^{Arg\text{-}Gln}$ mutation were impaired diastolic function as deduced from decreased early diastolic filling of the left ventricle (Oberst et al., 1998), and reduced systolic function with a diminished left ventricular ejection fraction (from 53% of ventricular volume down to 39%) in another study (Lim et al., 2000a,b). Furthermore, hearts of $92^{Arg\text{-}Gln}$ mice were found to induce the expression of the genes encoding atrial natriuretic factor and β-myosin HC, indicating the reactivation of a prenatal gene expression program. Impaired relaxation and diastolic dysfunction were demonstrated with isolated cardiocytes and whole heart preparations of these animals. Mitochondria in the cardiac tissue were found to be abnor-

Table 49.11. Functional consequences of cardiac troponin T mutations

Function tested	Mutation						
	79^{Ile-Asn}	92^{Arg-Gln}	110^{Phe-Ile}	Δ160^{Glu}	244^{Glu-Asp}	278^{Arg-Cys}	ΔEx15–16
Sliding speed	↑	↑	n.d.[1]	normal or ↓	↑	n.d.	↑
Maximal force	↓ or normal	normal	n.d.	↓	n.d.	n.d.	↓
Maximal rate of myofibrillar ATPase	normal	normal	↑	n.d.	↑	normal	n.d.
Ca²⁺ sensitivity of force	↑ or ↓	↓	↑	↑	n.d.	↑	↓ or ↑
Myofibrillar Ca²⁺ sensitivity	↑	↑	normal	n.d.	normal	n.d.	n.d.
Disorganized sarcomeres	none or mild	none or mild	n.d.	mild	n.d.	n.d.	severe

The data was adapted from the following sources: Lin et al., 1996; Watkins et al., 1996; Tobacman et al., 1999; Rust et al., 1999, Morimoto et al., 1998; Nakaura et al., 1999; Yanaga et al., 1999 and Szczesna et al., 2000. Arrows up indicate increased and arrows down decreased activities as compared to wildtype controls. The decreased calcium sensitivity with ΔEx15–16 was observed after transient transfection of quail myotubes (Watkins et al., 1996). In all other experiments reconstituted skinned cardiac muscle fibers were used. Data obtained with mutation in codon 163 (Glu-Lys) is not included. This mutation caused almost no change in calcium sensitivity of force, but an elevated actin-activated ATPase (Szczesna et al., 2000). Footnote: n.d., not determined.

mal, with respect to both number (which was increased) and gross changes in morphology. Disarray and fibrosis were frequent, but not observed in all animals. A notable result was hypercontractility in isolated hearts, even in those that did not show disarray or interstitial collagen deposition (Tardiff et al., 1999). The second mutation tested in mice was the ΔEx15–16 C-terminal troponin T truncation. Animals that expressed >10% of their total cardiac troponin T in the truncated form were not viable and died within 24 h of birth. Expression at lower levels was associated with small hearts (possibly indicating loss of cardiocytes), diastolic and mild systolic dysfunction and disarray. Cultured cardiocytes from these mice demonstrated an unusual hypersensitivity to Ca²⁺. If Ca²⁺ was added to the medium, cells responded with hypercontracture and death (Tardiff et al., 1998) (see Table 49.10).

Recently a transgenic rat expressing a truncated troponin T has been described which mimics certain aspects of human troponin T disease (Frey et al., 2000), e.g., sudden death occurred (after long term physical training) in some of the animals tested. A conspicuous feature was the absence of left ventricular hypertrophy, a feature that is typically seen in those human cases caused by cTnT mutations.

Mutations in myosin binding protein-C

Mutations in this gene are not infrequent. The penetrance of HCM caused by MyBP-C is late in onset, but once disease expression occurs clinical manifestations and risk of complications are similar to the spectrum of disease seen with beta myosin heavy chain (Watkins et al., 1992b; Charron et al., 1997; Niimura et al., 1998; Moolman et al.,

2000). A striking genetic feature is the high frequency of deletions, insertions and mutations in sequences involved in mRNA splicing (see Table 49.7). Hence, truncations of the protein at the C-terminus resulting from frameshifts in the mRNA have been predicted for a considerable number of mutations (for review, see Bonne et al., 1998). However, attempts to demonstrate the occurrence of a truncated MyBP-C in affected cardiac tissue of patients have failed on two different occasions (Rottbauer et al., 1997; Moolman et al., 2000). It is therefore undecided whether a dominant-negative effect on cardiac sarcomeres or lack of protein is responsible for the phenotype.

A few experiments have been initiated to elucidate structural and functional consequences of mutations in this gene. The only in vitro analysis reported to date utilized transient transfection of fetal rat cardiocytes with different cDNAs encoding truncated versions of MyBP-C. Regions of variable length extending from internal positions to the C-terminus were missing in these constructs. All mutations had previously been identified in patients. The major result of this study was, briefly, the demonstration of a diffuse localization of truncated MyBP-C in most of the cells tested and a disrupted sarcomere structure in roughly half of the cells. In contrast, full length protein carrying a missense mutation in position 542 (out of a total of 1273 amino acid residues) was found to be incorporated in a regular fashion without alteration of the sarcomere structure in most of the cells. The main conclusion was that truncated MyBP-C presumably acts via a dominant-negative mechanism (Flavigny et al., 1999).

Sarcomere organization was also investigated in two transgenic mouse models of HCM-related truncated

MyBP-C. In one experiment the titin and myosin domains at the C-terminus were missing, whereas a smaller truncation restricted to the myosin binding site was tested in the second experiment. In the first mouse model loss of the long binding domain was associated with stable expression of the transgene. Its product, though, was not efficiently incorporated into sarcomeres. Rather, extensive disarray and sarcomere dysgenesis were obvious. In functional assays muscle fibers from these hearts showed reduced power output and a slightly increased Ca^{2+} sensitivity of force development indicative of subtle changes in cardiac performance in addition to structural disorganization (Yang et al., 1998). In the second experiment which focussed on the myosin binding site with the retained titin binding domain, a surprisingly low expression (ca. 10%) of the transgene was detected in cardiac tissue. However, significant structural changes of cardiac tissue were nevertheless visible (Yang et al., 1999). Some unexplained mechanism responsible for variable expression of different MyBP-C mutations may be involved.

An alternative attempt to create a disease model was the generation of a targeted modification of the MyBP-C gene in mice obtained by the insertion of either of two foreign DNA sequences into exon 30 of the gene: loxP and a neomycin gene flanked by two loxP sequences, respectively (McConnell et al., 1999). The result was in both cases deficient splicing of precursor mRNA in the region of exon 30 and subsequent loss of the C-terminal titin and myosin binding sites of MyBP-C. Mice homozygous for the altered MyBP-C alleles were viable, expressed reduced levels of the truncated protein and exhibited surprisingly normal sarcomere structures. However, right after birth they developed progressive ventricular dilatation, myocyte hypertrophy, disarray and fibrosis. In addition, the analysis of cardiac function in homozygous neonatal and adult mice by echocardiography demonstrated reduced systolic contractility and impaired diastolic function. These results suggest that MyBP-C does not play a major role in myofilament assembly or development of sarcomeres, but that it is required for long-term maintainance of sarcomere function and cardiac morphology. A concept, however, to explain the mechanism of the human condition (which is heterozygous and not homozygous) does not present itself easily from these observations. These targeted mice demonstrate that a mutation in a sarcomeric protein may cause ventricular dilatation rather than hypertrophy—which may require a revision of the previous view that mutations in force producing, i.e., sarcomeric, components of the myocardium are always associated with HCM and not with DCM. (See also the discussion on causes of DCM below.)

Transgenic mice with a mutation in the human essential light chain gene ELC

A transgenic mouse has been generated carrying copies of the human ventricular ELC gene with a missense mutation in codon 149 (Met-Val) (Poetter et al., 1996; Vemuri et al., 1999). This mouse exhibited—similar to one report of the human phenotype—ventricular hypertrophy restricted to the midcavity region, or more specifically to the papillary muscles. The investigators of this model focused on stretch-activation responses of fibers from papillary muscles. Stretch activation refers to the ability of muscle fibers to develop a sequence of tension pulses upon stretching, with a first strong pulse followed by a delayed (and much weaker) second one. Oscillating high frequency stretch-activation responses have been identified long ago in insect flight muscles (Pringle, 1949), but they have also been implicated (with lower frequencies) in mammalian cardiac and skeletal muscle activities (Kawai et al., 1993, and references in Vemuri et al., 1999). These responses conceivably help to optimize heart muscle activity by augmenting power per heart beat—provided their time course matches the heart rate. Papillary muscle strips of transgenic mice carrying mutated ELC exhibited a distorted (shortened) time delay between the two pulses of tension development. This finding suggests an altered synchrony between heart rate and stretch response, which in turn may result in a chronically suboptimal power output of affected muscle. Hypertrophy restricted to papillary muscles indicates that these muscles depend on rate-synchronized stretch-activation more than the bulk of the working myocardium (Vemuri et al., 1999). In a similar experiment with transgenic mice also carrying light chain mutations the very special papillary muscle phenotype was not reproduced (Sanbe et al., 2000). That result, however, does not exclude a contribution of a distorted stretch-activation response to the disease in humans.

Cardiomyopathic phenotypes in mice as response to the manipulation of various nonsarcomeric genes

In recent years a growing number of reports has been communicated documenting that cardiac morphology and performance of mice can be altered in a more or less predicted manner by the introduction of transgenes or by gene-targeting of endogenous genes which—in the majority of cases—do not code for sarcomeric proteins. These experiments were not intended to re-model a human "sarcomeric disease", but they were focussed on studying altered signaling pathways and other functions in cells and tissues. The methods used were injection of genes into zygotes of mice or targeted knockout of endogenous genes. The analysis of altered structures and functions in these animals may provide clues to an improved understanding of various disease mechanisms.

It is beyond the scope of this contribution to discuss these experiments in detail. They are only indirectly related to the pathology of cardiomyopathies. They are mentioned here because they may ultimately help to understand mechanisms which are involved in the pathogenesis of HCM and also of other cardiomyopathies. A summary of some relevant experiments is included in a tabulated form with a brief description of the salient features of 13 distinct investigations which share as a common result altered myocardial structure and function (Table 49.12). In a few cases genes coding for sarcomeric proteins were also studied. For further discussion of these and similar experiments in mice see the DCM section below.

Calcium handling in cardiac disease

Long before mutations in sarcomeric protein genes became known as causes of HCM, it was suspected by some that calcium may play a role in the pathogenesis of this disorder (Goodwin and Krikler, 1976; Kaltenbach et al., 1976; Wagner et al., 1989). Reasons in favor of this notion were the well-established diastolic dysfunction of the myocardium in HCM and also the successful use of calcium channel antagonists in the treatment of patients. Impaired relaxation could be due to an excess of calcium in the myocardial cytoplasm or to an altered calcium sensitivity of proteins regulating contraction. In both cases the lowering of calcium influx into the myocardial cell by inhibiting calcium channels in the membrane may conceivably be beneficial.

A specific contribution of calcium to the hypertrophic phenotype was recently corroborated by transgenic mice experiments showing that the activation of calcineurin, a cytoplasmic calcium-dependent phosphatase, is accompanied by increased myocardial cell size and reactivation of fetal cardiac genes (Molkentin et al., 1998). The mode of action of this process involves dephosphorylation of the transcription factor NF-AT3, which in its phosphorylated (inactive) state is present in the cytoplasm and which upon dephosphorylation translocates into the nucleus. There it interacts with the cardiac zinc finger protein GATA4 (and possibly with other nuclear factors) resulting in the activation of cardiac gene transcription. Independent evidence of calcineurin potentially being involved in progression of HCM is the observation that in transgenic mice overexpressing this phosphatase, cardiac hypertrophy can be prevented by administering cyclosporin or FK506. Both compounds are known to inhibit calcineurin.

Further support in favor of a pathogenic process which includes in a late stage non-contractile calcium mediated events came from experiments with transgenic mice that developed cardiomyopathy in response to aberrant expression of either tropomodulin (an actin-capping protein), or of ventricular myosin light chain 2 (applied in a form that could not be phosphorylated) or of fetal β-tropomyosin. The effect of tropomodulin was ventricular dilatation rather than hypertrophy. Interestingly, both dilatation and hypertrophy in these model studies were prevented by the application of cyclosporin. Moreover, in a different model of cardiac disease—pressure overload hypertrophy in rats—the calcineurin inhibition was also effective in preventing cardiac hypertrophy (Sussman et al., 1998). The same authors have reported more recently that in two transgenic mouse models overexpressing calcineurin or tropomodulin even reversal of existing hypertrophy was achieved by calcineurin inhition (Lim et al., 2000b).

In these experiments different pathological manifestations were targeted: hypertrophic and dilated cardiomyopathy as well as myocardial damage *resulting* from pressure overload. Since in these cases the phenotype was prevented or reverted by cyclosporin (or FK506), one might consider calcium-related events to constitute a "final common pathway" of cardiomyopathies, or even cardiac disease in general (Towbin, 1998). In addition, these results may be taken to discuss the possibility that calcineurin inhibition may offer a new route to the treatment of human cardiac disease (Sussman et al., 1998). (Cyclosporin itself, however, due to its known suppression of the immune system, its renal toxicity and its ability to promote cancer, is not a candidate substance for the treatment of patients.) For the time being, the attractive concept of a "final common pathway" as well as the notion of a potential benefit of calcineurin inhibition for therapy require further investigation. One reason to ask for careful analysis is the observation that not all kinds of cardiac hypertrophy in mice respond positively to the application of cyclosporin or FK 506, a functionally related drug. For instance, hypertrophy induced by increased afterload following aortic banding is refractive to cyclosporin (Ding et al., 1999; Zhang et al., 1999). It seems that more than only one mechanism is responsible for increased cardiac growth activities.

FUNCTIONAL CONSEQUENCES—A SUMMARY

Numerous studies both in vitro and in vivo have been performed to determine nature and extent of myocardial dysfunction caused by mutated sarcomeric proteins.

Table 49.12. Complex mouse models of impaired cardiac function associated with hypertrophy or dilatation

Genetic model	Features of the experiments and comments	References
Myosin heavy chain: Transgenic murine αMHC with light chain binding domain deleted (internal truncation of 64 amino acids).	Mice with this cardiac transgene (tagged with a *c-myc* epitope and under the control of the rat αMHC promoter) are exposed to changes known from human pathology: hypertrophy, disarray, abnormal small coronary vessels and valvular disease. No atrial dilatation and no sudden death were reported from these mice.	Welikson et al., 1999
Lack of **dystrophin** and **myoD** in *mdx* mice.	In *mdx* mice with a deficient dystrophin cardiac disease does not occur. A lack of muscle specific transcription factor *myoD* in these mice (*mdx:myoD*$^{-/-}$) causes, however, severe cardiomyopathy. These results suggest functional cross-connections between skeletal and cardiac muscle.	Megeney et al., 1999
SV40 T antigen ts58 transgenesis targeted to the myocardium.	The temperature-sensitive tumor antigen (TA) gene A58, a viral oncogene, was used to enhance the proliferative capacity of cardiac and skeletal muscle cells. Expression was targeted to heart/muscle cells by the rat β-MHC promoter. The phenotype of a subset of mice was indicative of cardiac and skeletal myopathy. In the heart: fibrosis, loss of cross striation, enlarged nuclei. In muscle: variable fiber size and fiber degeneration.	De Leon et al., 1994
Gene-targeted mice with **phospholamban** deficiency.	Phospholamban (PLB) deficient (homozygous knockout) mice were tested by echocardiography for changes in cardiac performance. Results indicated increased rates of relaxation and contraction. Left ventricular dimensions were normal. However, PLB-deficient mice did not respond to isoproterenol.	Hoit et al., 1995; 1997
Oncogenic **ras** transgenesis targeted to the myocardium.	The activated ras oncogene targeted to the heart by the ventricular myosin light chain 2 promoter (MLC2v) caused increased left ventricular wall thickness. Other features: marked disarray, variable degrees of fibrosis, increase of natriuretic peptides ANP and BNP, and decreased survival in juvenile off-spring of parents selected by echocardiography for enhanced phenotype.	Gottshall et al., 1997
Transgenes affecting calcium-dependent regulations in cardiac cells: **calcineurin, tropomodulin.**	Transgenic mice carrying overexpressed calcium-insensitive calcineurin or tropomudulin develop cardiac hypertrophy, dilatation and heart failure. Hypertrophy in young mice is reversible by cyclosporin A treatment. The nuclear transcription factor NFAT3, normally regulated by calcineurin dephosphorylation, is not affected by cyclosporin A in transgenic mice with a constitutively active NFAT3.	Sussman et al., 1998 Lim et al., 2000b
Lack of **guanylyl cyclase A** gene (GCA).	Targeted mutation in the GCA gene, bred to homozygosity (GCA –/–). GCA is a membrane-bound receptor for atrial natriuretic peptide that contains an intracellular guanylyl cyclase domain. The mutation causes salt resistant hypertension and cardiac hypertrophy. The animals were used to assess the use of MRI for monitoring cardiac hypertrophy in mice.	Lopez et al., 1995 Franco et al., 1998
Protein kinase C, β isoform (PKC-β), transgenes under control of tetracycline.	A modified tetracycline repressor was used to condition the expression of transgeneic PKC-β, targeted to the heart. In adult animals expression was associated with mild progressive ventricular hypertrophy (more marked in males) and impaired diastolic relaxation. Transgene expression during pregnancy caused changes in the calcium regulation of cardiac myocytes (increased calcium transient duration and decreased transient amplitude) and sudden death in newborns.	Bowman et al., 1997
Oncogenic **ras** gene selectively expressed in ventricular cardiocytes under control of ventricle-specific MLC-2v promotor.	Mice homozygous for the transgene exhibited cardiac hypertrophy and functional changes as known from human hypertrophic cardiomyopathy, e.g., impaired relaxation. **Ras** seems to bee sufficient to the hypertrophic response.	Hunter et al., 1995
Transgenic mice carrying a peptide **inhibitor** of β-adrenergic receptor kinase 1 (**BARKct**) mated to a mouse model of cardiac failure (MLP$^{-/-}$)	MLP$^{-/-}$ Mice exhibited chamber dilatation and reduced myocardial function. Mice expressing in addition βARKct had normal chamber morphology and function indicating that inhibition of β-adrenergic receptor phosphorylation is benefical.	Rockman et al., 1998

continued

Table 49.12. Complex mouse models of impaired cardiac function associated with hypertrophy or dilatation (*continued*)

Genetic model	Features of the experiments and comments	References
DNA encoding **ELC1v** (adult ventricular essential light chain 1)	Cardiac overexpression of ELC1v to test the limits of transgene concepts. Moderate overexpression (16 fold) was correlated with no change in cardiac morphology, where an extensive overexpression (up to 50 fold) was associated with atrial hypertrophy, ventricular dilatation and cardiomyopathy. (For related results see also Gulick et al., 1997.)	James et al., 1999
A knockout inactivation of the **gp130 cytokine receptor** gene (through CreloxP recombination) with knockout restricted to ventricles.	gp130 (a cytokine) is a "survival factor" controlling adaptation of myocardial tissue under stress conditions, e.g., pressure overload. Lack of gp 130 receptor is associated with dilated cardiomyopathy and induction of apoptosis.	Hirota et al., 1999
Overexpression of skeletal muscle **β-tropomyosin** in hearts of transgenic mice.	Replacement of cardiac α- by β-tropomyosin in cardiocytes induces: reduced rate of contraction and relaxation, unchanged extent of shortening, increased Ca^{++} sensitivity of force development and ATPase rate. Less maximal tension with cross-bridge turnover unaffected. Reduced activity level conceivably due to differences in electrochemical charge between α- by β-tropomyosin.	Wolska et al., 1999

However, a comprehensive concept of molecular, cellular and cardiac tissue-related mechanisms responsible for HCM does not yet exist. The lack of definite knowledge has various reasons. First, nine genes with more than 140 different mutations have been ascertained as causing HCM. It is not clear whether all mutations in these genes are equivalent or not with respect to dysfunctional mechanisms. In addition, little is known about the role of inherited polymorphisms in nonsarcomeric genes involved in the regulation of cardiac function ("modifying genes"). It had been observed long ago that penetrance and phenotype of HCM differ even within families. Thus, it seems plausible that more than one mechanism contributes to the manifestation of the disease.

The apparent discrepancies in the results reported by different researchers may in part be explained by differences in sample composition of the materials tested or by the complexities of test systems involved (molecules of different origin, transfected cells, animals with different genetic background). Transgenic animals have been introduced into these studies in order to create models for the human disease. Certain features such as disarray, fibrosis, ventricular hypercontraction and diastolic dysfunction, could be reconstructed. However, one has to accept that cardiac physiology and biology of mice or other animals and humans differ in many respects. It is therefore still undecided to what degree results obtained in studies of transgenic hearts serve as a useful tool to advance the identification of mechanisms causing human disease.

Nevertheless, a few conclusions about HCM disease mechanisms seem justified. In Fig. 49.28 we resort to a hypothetical scheme by Marian (2000) designed to delineate pathogenesis of HCM. An essential ingredient of that scheme is the long latency of disease expression during which time biological changes are taking place. The beginning—incorporation of mutated proteins into sarcomeres, or in a few cases lack of protein—goes in most cases unnoticed by the person at risk, but exposes the myocardium to a continuous stress that is increasingly associated with functional deficits, compensatory changes in myocytes and other alterations which affect the overall performance of the heart. Upregulation of stress-responsive factors such as TGF-β1, IGF-1 and endothelin 1 may contribute to secondary abnormalities which in turn are responsible for the pathological phenotype of HCM (Hasegawa et al., 1996; Li et al., 1997).

The scheme of Fig. 49.28 implies that "low contractility" (loss of function) is a key trigger of downstream events that eventually lead to clinical HCM. This may apply to some of the known mutations, but not necessarily to all of them. It cannot be excluded or even seems likely on the basis of existing evidence—in particular that obtained with the 403[Arg-Gln] mice discussed above—that at least in some inherited cases the primary change is "increased contractility" (gain of function) associated with an augmented energy requirement. This alteration may be responsible for subsequent secondary structural and functional changes that ultimately lead to disease. Mild changes in the concentration and handling of calcium may also affect disease progression either by sensitizing or desensitizing contractile parameters or by reshaping normal gene expression patterns. As indicated hypothetically in Marian's scheme, upregulation of stress-responsive factors may ultimately play a major role in

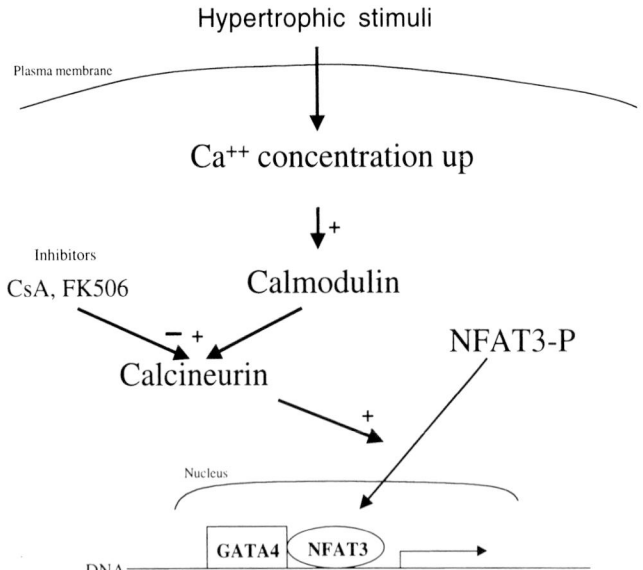

Fig. 49.27. A hypothesis: how hypertrophy may be linked to the activity of calcineurin. Under conditions of elevated intracellular calcium (or increased Ca++ sensitivity?) calmodulin regulates calcineurin (a phosphatase), which is in turn involved in the activation of the transcription factor NFAT3. This factor, when inactive, is a phosphorylated cytoplasmic protein. Upon dephosphorylation it translocates into the nucleus where it interacts with other transcription factors such as GATA4, resulting in the activation of genes, among them presumably some which promote growth. Cyclosporin and FK506 are known inhibitors of calcineurin and of certain types of cardiac hypertrophy in experimental animals. It is not clear whether all types of growth induction, i.e., induction in response to altered genetic conditions versus induction due to stimulation by hormones, react in the same way by activating calcineurin and the regulatory cascade depending on it. (Adapted from Molkentin et al., 1998.)

pathogenesis. However, details need to be investigated further.

MANAGEMENT OF HCM

There have been major advances in the understanding of the molecular genetic basis of HCM. Progress in therapy, particularly in symptomatic treatment, however, has been relatively modest. Pharmacologic treatment modulates cardiac contractility and chronotropic response and suppresses arrhythmias. In patients with left ventricular outflow tract obstruction, gradient reduction with surgical myotomy/myectomy, non-surgical septal reduction and dual chamber pacing are available. Improved knowledge of etiology and pathogenesis of HCM could conceivably help to improve therapy. In particular, if the disease is recognized in a preclinical state it may be possible to intervene before irreversible structural and functional changes in the heart muscle (hypertrophy, disarray, fibrosis) occurs.

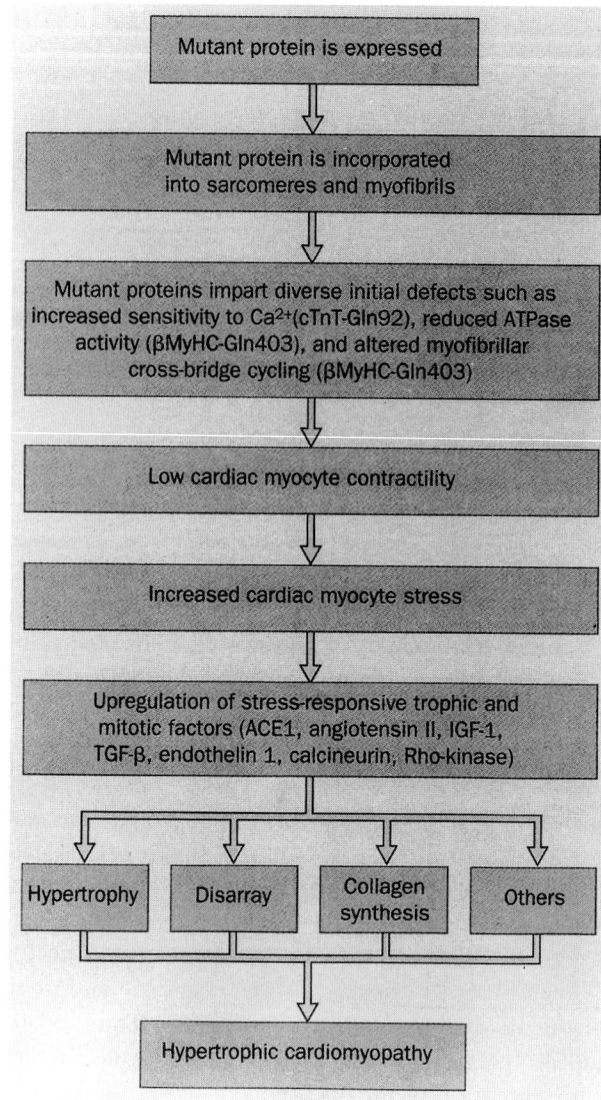

Fig. 49.28. A conceivable scheme of HCM disease development. This proposal was taken from the literature. It illustrates how HCM may develop in carriers of cardiac sarcomeric mutations. The early stages are characterized by a long latency period with no overt functional deficiencies or symptoms. These appear as a rule in young adults or even later. It is not clear whether myocardial contractility is decreased (as suggested by this scheme, or increased (as it may be deduced from a number of recent experiments). Different mutations may have divergent consequences. The major point in this proposal is the gradually increasing impact secondary responses have in the pathogenesis and the development of symptoms. (From Marian, 2000, with permission.)

However, it has yet to be proved whether preventive measures of this kind will be available.

Prognosis, indicators of risk, genotyping

The identification of high-risk patients and the prevention of sudden death are major challenges in the management of

Table 49.13. β-Myosin heavy chain missense mutations: correlation with survival

Good prognosis	232/–	256/+	513/–	606/–	908/–
Intermediate prognosis	249/+				
Poor prognosis	403/+	453/+	719/+		

The numbers refer to the positions of the amino acids in mutated β-myosin heavy chain molecules (see Table 49.3). A plus sign refers to a change in charge as a consequence of the mutation, a minus sign refers to a neutral mutation. For further details see text.

Table 49.14. Risk markers for sudden death

Unexplained syncope (within previous 12 months)

Family history of 2 or more cases of premature sudden death (< 40 years)

Severe and diffuse LVH[1] (≤ 30 mm wall thickness)

Nonsustained ventricular tachycardia[2] on Holter

Abnormal exercise blood pressure response[3]

Footnotes: [1]*LVH, left ventricular hypertrophy;* [2]*tachycardia of ≥ 3 beats at ≥ 120 bpm;* [3]*response during maximal upright exercise (see: Electrocardiography)*

patients with HCM. All patients should undergo risk assessment for sudden death regardless of their symptomatic status or the apparent severity of disease on 2D echo evaluation. In addition to diagnostic ECG and echo this should include careful history to determine the occurrence and circumstances of syncopal episodes, pedigree evaluation to assess potentially disease-related premature deaths, 24–48 hour Holter monitoring and measurement of blood pressure responses during maximal upright exercise testing. The presence of several features which reflect the genetic background and underlying hemodynamic and electrical stability are associated with increased risk of sudden death. (Maron et al., 1981c; McKenna et al., 1981b; McKenna and Deanfield, 1984; McKenna, 1987; Sadoul et al., 1999) (see Table 49.13). In a middle-aged or older adult the presence of any of these risk markers in isolation confers a relative risk of approximately two which in general is insufficient to warrant prophylactic treatment. In contrast, in a child adolescent or young adult (< 25 years) the presence, in isolation of unexplained recurrent or exertional syncope, of nonsustained ventricular tachycardia on Holter or severe and diffuse left ventricular hypertrophy of > 3 cm is of sufficient prognostic significance to consider prophylactic treatment with amiodarone and/or an implantable cardioverter defibrillator as appropriate (see below). When two or more risk factors are present the annual sudden death mortality is 1% to 2% (depending on age and on the combination of factors and their severity), sufficient to recommend prophylactic treatment (details of risk factor stratification in McKenna, 1989; McKenna and Camm, 1989; Maron et al., 1990; 2000; Elliott et al., 2001).

Preliminary evidence suggests that knowledge of the molecular genetic abnormalities may aid risk factor stratification. A number of observations concerned with this problem have been reported. They are all based on the retrospective evaluation of family histories with specific emphasis on life expectancies and severity of the clinical phenotype caused by known mutations (Rosenzweig et al., 1991; Epstein et al., 1992b; Watkins et al., 1992b; 1995a; Anan et al., 1994; Dufour et al., 1994; Fananapazir and

Epstein, 1994). The life expectancy of gene carriers has been assessed for 14 mutations in families large enough for a statistical evaluation (10 mutations in the β-myosin heavy chain gene and 4 in the cardiac troponin T gene).

Life expectancy was evaluated by calculating survival curves (according to Kaplan and Meier, 1958). Premature death frequencies observed in families with identified mutations in the two genes is depicted in Figure 49.29. Regarding β-myosin (Fig. 49.29A) one mutation (606, no change in charge) was benign, one was interpreted as intermediate (249), and three were malignant (403, 453, 719), with premature death being frequent. The intermediate and malignant mutations were all accompanied by a change in charge of the mutant protein, while 4 of 5 of the mutations evaluated with a benign prognosis had a neutral exchange (Table 49.13).

Fig. 49.29B depicts the survival plots of families with cardiac troponin T mutations. Two were missense mutations in positions 79 (Ile-Asn) and 92 (Arg-Gln), both inducing a change in charge, and a deletion of codon 160 (loss of a negatively charged glutamic acid residue) (Watkins et al., 1995a). A splice donor site mutation, which leads to a truncated version of troponin T, is also characterized by a malignant phenotype with a high incidence of sudden death.

These results indicate that a correlation may exist between the mutation and the prognosis of familial HCM caused by altered β-myosin heavy-chain and cardiac troponin T genes. The number of families studied, however, is still small. In addition, discordant observations have been communicated for identical mutations in codon 606 (Val-Met) (Fananapazir and Epstein, 1994), though on occasion these apparent discrepancies have been explained by the discovery of additional potential disease causing mutations following systematic evaluation of the entire DNA of eight recognized gene abnormalities (Blair et al., 2001). Studies of more families are required to determine whether genotyping will aid identification of high-risk families and individuals.

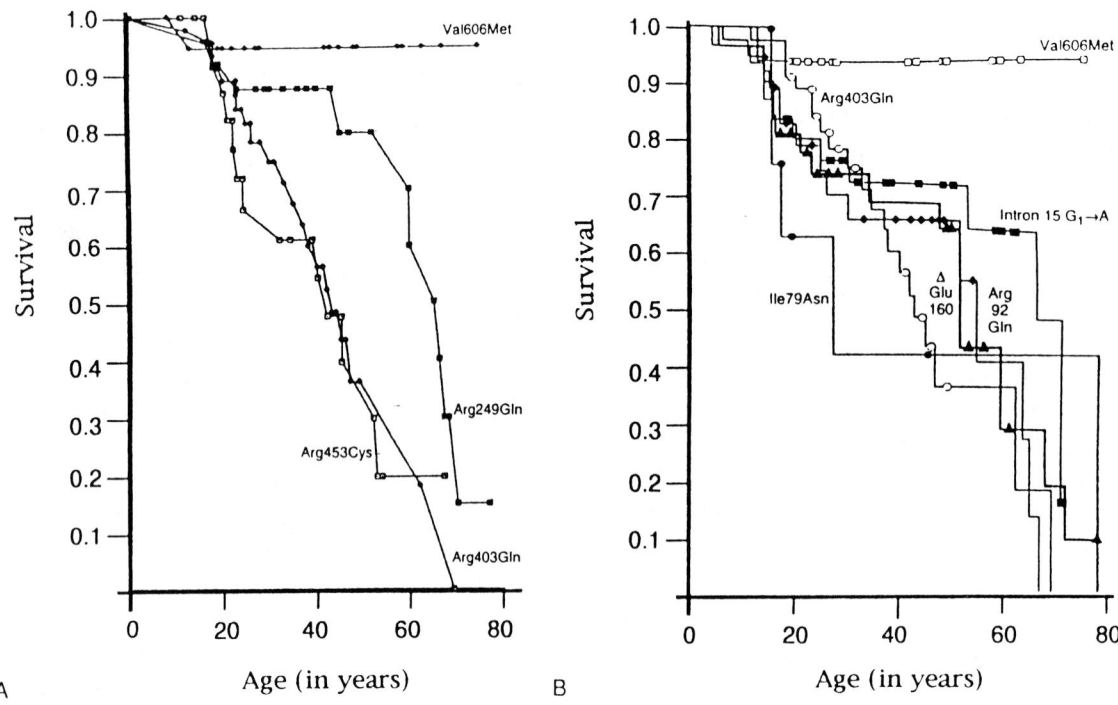

Fig. 49.29. (A) Survival curves of patients with missense mutations in the β-myosin heavy chain gene. Survival data is plotted as Kaplan–Meier product limit curves (Kaplan and Meier, 1958). Curves are shown for patients of families with each of four mutations indicated in the figure. (B) Survival of patients with hypertrophic cardiomyopathy caused by mutations in the troponin T gene, which is similar to that in patients with the "malignant" β-myosin heavy chain mutations in codon 403. Also shown are the effects of the benign β-myosin heavy chain mutation in codon 606. (Modified from Watkins et al., 1992c; 1995a, with permission.)

Pharmacology

The major goals of drug therapy are the relief of symptoms and the prevention of complications. The standard pharmacologic treatment involves β-blockade or calcium channel blockade, usually with verapamil or diltiazem. These compounds have well-established effects against chest pain and dyspnea and offer several advantages. They improve angina pectoris by decreasing myocardial oxygen consumption, and they blunt the heart rate response during exercise providing increased time for chamber filling in patients who suffer from poor relaxation and filling (Frank et al., 1978; Alvares and Goodwin, 1982). These drugs have, in addition, a negative inotropic effect, reducing hyperdynamic systolic function and left ventricular gradients (Goodwin et al., 1964; Goodwin, 1973; Rosing et al., 1979).

Beta-blockers and calcium antagonists are usually well tolerated. Beta-blockers have few serious side effects, but are not always effective. Verapamil and diltiazem may occasionally be responsible for conduction problems or precipitate acute pulmonary edema in patients with unrecognized preexisting conduction disease or raised filling pressures. Beta-blockers should be tried first, and if they are ineffective, verapamil or diltiazem can be tried. Results with diltiazem and verapamil are comparable (Suwa et al., 1984).

The use of nifedipine cannot be recommended because of the marked lowering of systemic vascular resistance, rarely a desirable endpoint in patients with HCM (Betocchi et al., 1985).

Arrhythmia and prevention of sudden death

Both supraventricular and ventricular arrhythmias are common (Savage et al., 1979). The development of established atrial fibrillation can usually be attenuated by the use of low-dose amiodarone, and this agent is particularly effective in the prevention of paroxysmal episodes. Supraventricular arrhythmias predispose to embolic complications and the threshold for the introduction of anticoagulation should be low, particularly in patients with grossly enlarged atria. Symptomatic ventricular arrhythmias are uncommon and can usually be managed with conventional antiarrhythmia treatment (drugs, implantable defibrillator).

The application of therapy to prevent sudden death is predicated on the ability to identify the high-risk cohort and within this group to identify likely mechanisms or determinants of sudden death (McKenna, 1987). In approximately one-third of high-risk patients a probable mechanism/determinant of sudden death, to which treatment can be targeted, is identified during risk stratification. Therapeutic measures include:

1. Paroxysmal atrial fibrillation: amiodarone
2. Ventricular arrhythmias: amiodarone/ICD
3. Ischemia: high-dose verapamil
4. Occult conduction disease: pacemaker
5. Accelerated atrioventricular conduction: ablation
6. Severe left ventricular obstruction (>100 mmHg): myectomy

In adults with nonsustained ventricular tachycardia, low-dose amiodarone has been associated with improved prognosis (McKenna et al., 1985; Stewart and McKenna, 1994). In other high-risk patients where a specific mechanism has not been identified, such as those with recurrent syncope or out-of-hospital ventricular fibrillation, and in cases of multiple sudden deaths in families, treatment remains empirical. An implantable cardioverter defibrillator provides the greatest margin of safety and is recommended. The experience of a recently published retrospective registry revealed appropriate annual discharge rates of 5% in patients with one or more risk factors (Maron et al., 2000). Although randomized clinical trials are lacking, the available evidence suggests that risk stratification and appropriate treatment will be effective in preventing sudden death.

Myectomy and DDD pacing for symptoms

The majority of patients with left ventricular outflow tract gradients do not have significant symptomatic or functional limitation or they respond to pharmacological suppression of myocardial contractility with β-adrenergic blockers, disopyramide, or both. A minority of patients, however, are refractory to these medications or develop side effects (Goodwin, 1973; Epstein and Rosing, 1981; Harris et al., 1983; Hopf and Kaltenbach, 1990; Wigle et al., 1995). In this group, ventricular myotomy/myectomy or the replacement of the mitral valve provides a well-established surgical option that can be anticipated to improve symptoms in 75% to 80% (Morrow et al., 1968; Cooley et al., 1973; Gill et al., 1982; Beahrs et al., 1983; Schulte et al., 1993). Perioperative mortality and morbidity varies (Morrow et al., 1975; Maron et al., 1978a; Beahrs et al., 1983; McIntosh and Maron, 1988), but major centers with the most experience all show mortality rates of less than 2% (Seiler et al., 1991; Schulte et al., 1993). The influence of surgery on prognosis has not been assessed. The immediate surgical goal is to remove the intraventricular pressure gradient, and, when successful, this also results in a lowering of left ventricular filling pressures. Numerous surgical approaches have been proposed. Currently, most sur-

geons use a transaortic approach for access to remove septal tissue, thereby increasing the outflow tract dimension and eliminating systolic anterior motion of the mitral valve. Mitral valve replacement should be reserved for the minority of patients with significant mitral regurgitation associated with abnormalities of the mitral valve that would not be anticipated to be relieved by myectomy.

Two additional therapeutic options are now available as alternatives to surgery for patients who are refractory to drugs. Dual chamber pacing aims to alter the sequence of electrical activation, such that contraction at the apex will occur well in advance of septal activation, so that the stroke volume can be ejected before the development of systolic anterior motion of the mitral valve (McDonald et al., 1988; Fananapazir et al., 1992; Kappenberger, 1995). Earlier anecdotal observations which suggested that a cohort of patients will benefit from pacemaker implantation (Fananapazir et al., 1992a; Jeanrenaud et al., 1992; Cannon et al., 1994; Slade et al., 1994), have been confirmed in randomized trials (Nishimura et al., 1997; Kappenberger et al., 1999; Maron et al., 1999). Overall, however, the magnitude of gradient reduction with pacing is modest (50%–60%), interpretation of symptomatic improvement is confounded by a significant placebo effect (an important outcome of the trials) and objective measures of exercise capacity are usually unchanged. Clinical experience indicates that a small cohort will benefit from DDD pacing though patient selection remains a problem. One of the trials suggested that elderly patients with milder and less diffuse hypertrophy did best.

Non-surgical septal reduction with the percutaneous injection of alcohol down a catheter positioned in the relevant septal artery is a novel and potentially useful approach to reducing septal thickness, left ventricular contractility and outflow tract obstruction. (Knight et al., 1997; Kuhn et al., 1997; Faber et al., 2000). It may not be practical to perform randomized trials versus surgery. Careful observational studies, however, indicate that experienced teams can achieve symptomatic and objective exercise improvement in association with analagous gradient reduction to that achieved with myectomy. The procedure requires diligence with contrast injection to ensure that alcohol is delivered only to the desired area of the septum and not more distally to papillary muscles or other myocardial segments. Other concerns include the long-term effects on myocardial systolic performance and arrhythmia risk. The availability of different therapeutic options for the treatment of left ventricular obstruction has increased awareness concerning the importance of mitral and papillary muscle anatomy as well as the distribution of hypertrophy as determinants of successful gradient reduction procedures.

Clinical application of genetic knowledge: counseling and prenatal and preclinical diagnosis

What is the potential for the new genetic knowledge to influence management of HCM? The condition is usually inherited, and the eight identified disease genes, which can be screened directly, probably account for 60% to 70% of HCM. The most frequently used protocols are summarized in Table 49.2 (see the section Etiology). Also, a preclinical diagnosis in children and adolescents is now possible.

In families with adverse prognosis or in those patients whose familial background cannot be ascertained for whatever reason, a preclinical diagnosis and knowledge of whether the mutation is associated with good, intermediate, or poor prognosis would provide the basis for a management strategy in the young. Those affected with a mutation associated with intermediate or poor prognosis would then undergo risk-factor stratification, with the aim of selecting appropriate therapy to prevent sudden death (see above). Application of preclinical diagnosis would not be warranted where there have been no sudden deaths in families of sufficient size to be confident that the young did not carry a "malignant" mutation.

The disadvantages associated with preclinical diagnosis have been well-reported (Clarke and Harper, 1992; Harper and Clarke, 1993; 1995). Although unproven, it is anticipated that, with appropriate counseling including the recommendation to avoid competitive sport and the introduction of appropriate therapy, the improved survival rate would outweigh the negative psychological and other effects associated with early diagnosis.

The role for prenatal diagnosis is small and might be limited to those families with a known mutation clearly associated with very adverse prognosis. Similarly, in vitro fertilization (Verlinsky et al., 1994) must be limited to the very small cohort of very high-risk families. The application of molecular genetic information for the purpose of genetic or preclinical counseling is in its infancy and will require careful evaluation (McLatchie et al., 1993; Ryan et al., 1995; Vosberg et al., 2000).

Dilated cardiomyopathy

DEFINITION AND PREVALENCE

Dilated cardiomyopathy (DCM) is defined as a myocardial disorder characterized by dilatation and impaired contractile performance of the left or both ventricles (Goodwin and Oakley, 1972; Dec and Fuster, 1994). It may be idiopathic, familial/genetic, viral and/or immune, alcohol/toxic, or associated with recognized cardiovascular disease where the degree of myocardial dysfunction is not explained by the abnormal loading conditions or the extent of ischemic damage. For the purposes of this discussion toxic causes and cardiomyopathy associated with other cardiovascular disease will not be considered.

DCM typically affects young men and frequently presents with advanced heart failure. It is seen worldwide. Epidemiologic information is available for Europe and North America where the prevalence is 36 per 100,000, with an annual incidence of 5 to 8 per 100,000 (Codd et al., 1989). It is probable that these figures are underestimates, since DCM has a long preclinical phase during which patients are asymptomatic, and in many cases the disorder may remain unrecognized altogether (Gillum, 1986; Codd et al., 1989).

A summary of typical properties of DCM is presented in Table 49.15

Clinical features

Patients normally present between 20 and 50 years of age, but children and the elderly may also be affected. The most common manifestation is heart failure, which is often advanced (New York Heart Association functional class III or IV). Symptoms include diminished exercise capacity, exertional dyspnea, and paroxsymal nocturnal dyspnea/ orthop-

Table 49.15. Clinical and genetic properties of DCM (OMIM 115200)

Clinical presentation	Age of onset between 20 and 50 Heart failure frequent (NYHA III and IV)
Diagnosis	2-D echocardiography most useful Nuclear magnetic resonance imaging Symptoms of left ventricular dysfunction Conduction abnormalities frequent
Pathology	Dilatation of both ventricles Increase in heart weight Hypertrophy and degeneration of myocytes Coronary arteries unaffected
Pathogenesis	Heterogeneous factors and processes involved Viral infections and immune responses
Genetics	Mendelian inheritance in ~25% of patients Usually autosomal dominant, rarely X-linked 8 autosomal DCM loci with unknown genes 5 genes known: lamin A/C, β-myosin HC, actin, tafazzin (X-linked), dystrophin (X-linked)
Prognosis	Poor, with 30–50% 5-year mortality

Abbreviations: *OMIM, entry number in the reference list of* Online Mendelian Inheritance in Man (www.ncbi.nlm.nih.gov/). *NYHA, indicator for different degrees of severity of cardiac insufficiency according to the New York Heart Association (class IV is the most severe category).*

nea. Chest pain, occasionally indistinguishable from angina pectoris, is also reported as an initial symptom. Sometimes cardiomegaly or ECG abnormalities are detected as incidental findings in asymptomatic patients. Atrial fibrillation and ventricular arrhythmias are common and in cases of advanced heart failure systemic or pulmonary emboli may be the initial presentation. Rarely, syncope or sudden death may be seen as the initial manifestation, usually in association with histologic or immunohistochemical evidence of inflammation.

Diagnosis

The diagnosis of dilated cardiomyopathy requires exclusion of all potentially reversible causes of left ventricular dysfunction, particularly excess alcohol consumption, coronary heart disease, and systemic hypertension (Keeling and McKenna, 1994; Dec and Fuster, 1995; Keeling et al., 1995). Assessment for diagnosis and management should include physical examination, chest radiography, 12-lead electrocardiography, and two-dimensional echocardiography/Doppler (Shah, 1988). Typical findings include left ventricular dilatation, normal or reduced septal and free-wall thickness, and global hypokinesis (Shah, 1988). Abnormal ventricular contractility is an essential component of DCM, and, in the absence of familial disease, a decreased ejection fraction (< 45%) is generally required for diagnosis (Johnson and Palacios, 1982; Manolio et al., 1992). Radioisotope or magnetic resonance imaging may be useful when echocardiography does not provide adequate images. Coronary artery disease needs to be excluded by history, exercise electrocardiography, and where appropriate, coronary arteriography. It is not necessary to perform cardiac catheterization on a routine basis for diagnosis; myocardial biopsy should be performed if expertise is available to assess the presence of viral genome and immunohistochemical evidence of inflammation. For the diagnosis of DCM within families, see below in Clinical genetics.

Pathology

The major pathologic finding is increased heart weight with dilatation of both ventricles (Roberts et al., 1987; Ferrans, 1989) (Table 49.15). Secondary dilatation of valvular annuli is frequently observed. Microscopic features include hypertrophy and degeneration of myocytes, varying degrees of interstitial fibrosis, and, occasionally, small clusters of lymphocytes (Tazelaar and Billingham, 1986).

The pathogenesis of DCM has not been determined in humans. Most probably multiple factors contribute to this syndrome. An enteroviral trigger (Coxsackie virus type B)

(Cambridge et al., 1979; Bowles et al., 1986; Kandolf, 1988; Muir et al., 1989), with autoimmune-mediated damage (Maisch et al., 1983; Caforio et al., 1990; 1992) in the genetically predisposed individual (Mestroni et al., 1990; Michels et al., 1992; Zachara et al., 1993) has been proposed. This hypothesis arises from experience in various murine models of viral and immune-mediated myocarditis/dilated cardiomyopathy (Wolfgram et al., 1986; Neu et al., 1987).

Pathophysiology

The natural history is not well understood because the disease is frequently asymptomatic until myocardial impairment is well advanced. The rate of progression of asymptomatic left ventricular dysfunction to overt heart failure is unknown. Symptomatic patients have, in general, a poor prognosis. Survival data from tertiary referral centers show mortality rates of about 50% in five years (Dec and Fuster, 1994). The improved survival rates in some studies may be due to earlier detection of disease (Manolio et al., 1992; Sugrue et al., 1992).

The clinical course of DCM is unpredictable. Some patients experience an extended period of clinical stability. Occasionally the improvement of ventricular function is independent of the initial degree of dysfunction. The majority of those presenting with advanced disease improve with initiation of treatment, but then gradually deteriorate over 3–5 years. The natural history in those in whom the diagnosis is made early is not well defined. The great variation in natural history may be explained in part by the difficulties in making a reliable diagnosis at an early stage of the disease.

Clinical genetics

Familial occurrence of DCM has been documented in a number of published pedigrees. The reports from retrospective studies are consistent with autosomal dominant or X-linked transmission. Whether autosomal recessive causes contribute to the prevalence, is open to debate. Since these studies were based on retrospective assessments and/or selective screening for families suspected to have familial disease, they were unable to determine the prevalence of familial DCM. A number of prospective studies from different countries provide evidence that familial disease is diagnosed in at least 25% and possibly up to 35% of probands.

In a study at the Mayo Clinic (Michels et al., 1992) the families of 59 consecutive unrelated DCM patients were screened for affected relatives. DCM was diagnosed in 18 of 325 relatives (5.5%) from 12 families with a familial prevalence of 20% (12/59). This study demonstrated the potential importance of family evaluation; 83% of the affected relatives were asymptomatic and would have been missed by reliance on proband history alone. The mode of transmission was consistent with autosomal dominant inheritance in all cases. In the U.K. prospective study the families of 40 consecutive patients with DCM were evaluated and high ascertainment was achieved (Keeling et al., 1995). Of 236 relatives from 10 families, 25 (10.6%) were identified as affected with a familial prevalence of 25% (10/40). The pedigrees of three typical DCM families described by Keeling and colleagues (1995) are shown in Figure 49.30. Segregation of familial DCM is most consistent with autosomal dominant transmission though recessive transmission cannot be excluded (see family FJ in Fig. 49.30).

In another prospective study 35% of probands had evidence of familial DCM. This study was based on 445 consecutive patients and their families (Grünig et al., 1998). The authors of this investigation discriminated between different phenotypes suggesting that distinct, predominantly unknown genes are responsible for separate types of disease:

A rare form of DCM is X-linked and associated with elevated total serum creatine kinase (CK) activity; this type of DCM is known to be caused by mutations in the dystrophin gene which is otherwise responsible for Duchenne/Becker muscular dystrophy. However, skeletal muscle disease was not obvious in these patients.

Juvenile DCM with rapid progression in males and milder courses with late onset in females without skeletal involvement (CK normal).

DCM with segmental left ventricular functional impairment (hypokinesia). Symptoms which were mild remained stable over a period of up to 10 years.

DCM with progressive conduction disease leading to A-V block documented before left ventricular dysfunction became apparent, usually in the fifth or sixth decade.

Finally, in one family DCM was associated with sensorineural hearing loss. The mode of transmission was likely to be autosomal dominant. A genomic locus for DCM and associated sensorineural hearing loss has recently been identified on chromosome 6q (Schönberger et al., 2000).

The experience from prospective studies confirms that segregation analysis is in the majority of cases consistent with autosomal dominant transmission. X-chromosomal inheritance has been documented, but it is rare. An unequivocal autosomal recessive mode for primary DCM has, as yet, not been documented.

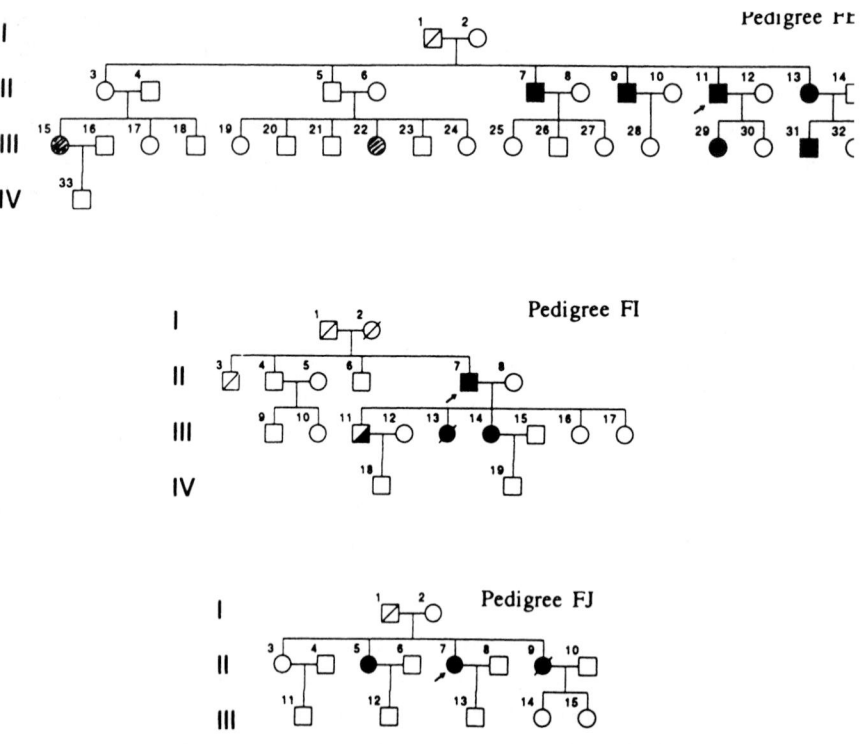

Fig. 49.30. Pedigrees of three families with inherited dilated cardiomyopathy. Incomplete penetrance is likely in family FE (left ventricular enlargement in III, 1 and III, 8). Family FI: Dominant inheritance is evident; LV enlargement in III, 3. A recessive mode of transmission cannot be excluded in family FJ, but seems unlikely considering the sudden cardiac death of I, 1 (at the age of 57). The arrows point to index patients. Symbols are as in Figure 49.5. SD, sudden death. (Adapted from Keeling et al., 1995, with permission.)

A typical aspect of familial DCM is its variable, frequently age-dependent penetrance. In a series of family investigations in Italy penetrance was estimated to be 10% for young (below 20 years), 34% in those age 20–30 years, 60% in those aged 30–40 years and 90% for affected family members older than 40 years (Mestroni et al., 1994). These observations underscore the difficulties of clinical assessment in young individuals who may be carriers of the genetic trait but show none of the diagnostic features. The current figures of the frequency of genetic transmission may be underestimated, since according to current knowledge no clinical or pathologic feature distinguishes between familial and non-familial disease. In addition, as was shown for hypertrophic cardiomyopathy, it is possible that sporadic cases without family history may be caused by de novo mutations in a parental germline cell with the potential to be transmitted to progeny (Watkins et al., 1992c). Incomplete penetrance in small families or insufficient family evaluation may also contribute to the failure to detect inheritance of the condition.

To diagnose familial cases reliably, guidelines have been developed by a European working group for the study of DCM in families (Mestroni et al., 1999). This proposal is based on the distinction between major and minor criteria of DCM. It has been recommended that the diagnosis of familial DCM is fulfilled in a first-degree relative of a proband in the presence of one major criterion, or left-ventricular dilatation plus one minor criterion, or three minor criteria.

Major criteria are:

a reduced ejection fraction of the left ventricle (< 45% of the normal value), fractional shortening (< 25%) or both; and
an increased left ventricular end-diastolic diameter corresponding to > 117% of the predicted value corrected for age and body surface area (Manolio et al., 1992).

Minor criteria are:

unexplained supraventricular or ventricular arrhythmia;
mild left ventricular dilatation (> 112% of the predicted value);
an intermediate impairment of left ventricular dysfunction;
unexplained conduction defects;
segmental wall motion abnormalities in the absence of intraventricular conduction defect, or ischemic heart disease;
unexplained sudden death or stroke before 50 years of age of a first-degree relative.

Recognition of the broader DCM related phenotype may help to guide the identification of affected members in families at risk. Once disease-related mutations in DCM genes in single families become known, a DNA analysis would provide the "gold standard" for the assessment of the carriers even in a preclinical, asymptomatic state.

Molecular genetics

Although complete knowledge of the causes of DCM does not exist, some progress has been made in recent years. Eleven autosomal disease loci have been identified or suggested in DCM families either by linkage analysis or by direct investigation of candidate genes (for locus assignments and references see Fig. 49.31 and Table 49.16). The candidate genes which have been invoked to contribute to DCM code for cardiac actin on chromosome 15q11 (Olson et al., 1998), desmin on chromosome 2q35 (Li et al., 1999) and lamin A/C in chromosome 1q1–q21 (Fatkin et al., 1999). In addition, two genes on the X-chromosome coding for dystrophin (Xp21) and protein G4.5 (also called taffazin, with unknown function, at Xq28) are responsible for rare X-linked recessive forms of DCM. Thus, according to current knowledge 13 different genomic loci may be associated with DCM. It is assumed that this number is not final. A mutation in the metavinculin gene has been claimed to cause a recessive form of DCM (Maeda et al., 1997). (Metavinculin is an actin binding protein involved in anchoring filamentous actin in intercalated discs of cardiomyocytes). This claim requires further study. Also, whether desmin mutations are bona fide disease causing mutations remains to be confirmed.

The first family with an identified autosomal DCM locus (on chromosome 1p1–q1) (Kass et al., 1994) was a seven-generation pedigree with 23 affected members with DCM and conduction disease. The disease gene region is that of the lamin A/C locus, which was recently shown to be frequently involved in DCM in conjunction with conduction disease (Fatkin et al., 1999). (A lamin mutation has, however, not been detected in the family investigated by Kass and co-workers.) Two different DCM genes may exist in this region. An alternative explanation would be a mutation affecting the expression of the gene rather than the structure of the lamin A/C.

An interesting type of autosomal dominant syndromic DCM has been mapped in two families to 6q23–q24 (Schönberger et al., 2000). In this case DCM is associated with sensorineural hearing loss. The syndromic phenotype exhibited age-related penetrance. The hearing loss developed during childhood/adolescence; cardiac symptoms

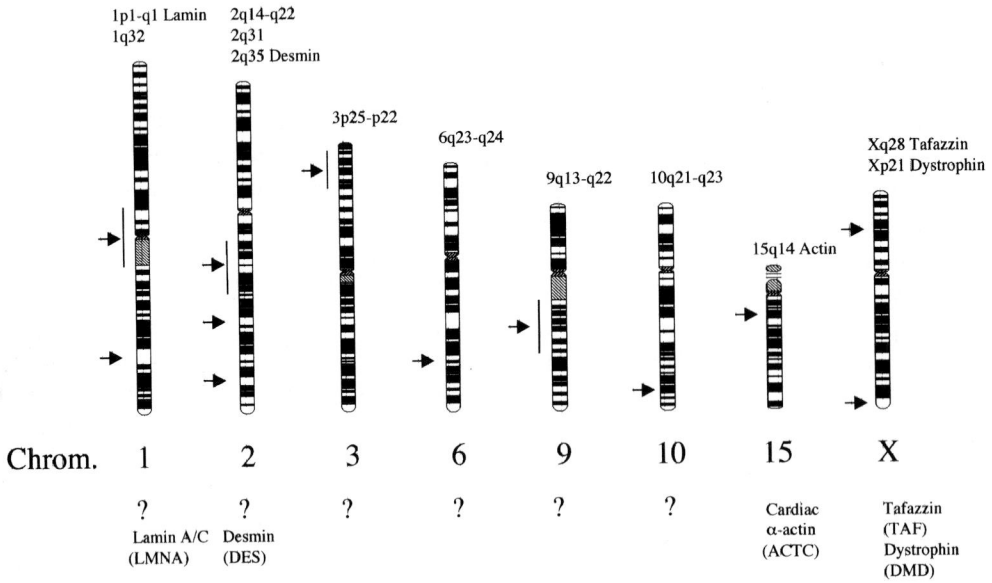

Fig. 49.31. Genomic localization of DCM genes. At least 12 DCM loci have been determined, most of them by linkage without knowledge of the genes involved. In a few cases the disease can be traced to a gene. Extensive information (5 families) is available about lamin A/C mutations and also about dystrophin mutations. (In this case DCM may be regarded as "polymorphic" to DMD/BMD.) Of major interest is the recent detection of DCM mutations in genes that otherwise are typical HCM genes: β-myosin HC and cardiac troponin T (Kamisago et al., 2000). Chromosome 1 is depicted here, for chromosome 14 see Figure 49.6.

Table 49.16. Dilated cardiomyopathy: genomic Loci

Chromosomal localization	Gene	OMIM[1]	Comments	Reference
1p1–q21	Lamin A/C	115200	Five families with DCM and conduction disease[2]	Fatkin et al., 1999
1q32	unknown	601494	One family. Early onset and high penetrance	Durand et al., 1995
2q14–2q22	unknown	604288	One DCM family with DCM and conduction disease	Jung et al., 1999
2q31	unknown	604145	One family with early onset DCM	Siu et al., 1999
2q35	Desmin	604765	Two patients from one DCM family with a desmin mutation. (No linkage)	Li et al., 1999
3p25–p22	unknown	601154	One family with DCM impaired conduction	Olson and Keating, 1996
6q23	unknown	602067	One family. DCM associated with impaired conduction and muscle disease	Messina et al., 1997
6q23–q24	unknown	n.a.	Two families. This disease is associated with hearing loss	Schönberger et al, 2000
9q13–q22	unknown	600884	Three families linked to this locus	Krajinovic et al., 1995
10q21–q23	unknown	601493	A mutation in the metavinculin gene (at 10q22) was reported in addition (Maeda et al., 1997)	Bowles et al., 1996
15q14	Cardiac actin	102540	Two small families. One additional mutation causes HCM (No linkage)	Olson et al., 1998
Xq28	Tafazzin	302060	This disease is known as Barth syndrome: cardioskeletal myopathy with neutropenia and abnormal mitochondria (Barth et al, 1983)	Bione et al., 1996
Xp21	Dystrophin	310200	Duchenne/Becker muscular dystrophy here with no or very mild effects on skeletal muscle. Altogether five families reported separately	Muntoni et al., 1993

Footnotes: [1]OMIM, entry number in the reference list of Online Mendelian Inheritance in Man (www.ncbi.nlm.nhi.gov/omim); [2] In the first family linked to this locus (Kass et al., 1994) no mutation in the lamin A/C gene was detected.

were unusual before 40 years of age, but then progressed rapidly. All affected patients required transplantation or died in their fifties or sixties. A deafness gene, DFNA10 (O'Neill et al., 1996) maps near the DCM locus. Although cardiac disease was not reported in several large families with inherited deafness, it cannot be excluded that a different mutation in the same gene or a defect in a contiguous gene could account for the cardiac defect in these families. Furthermore, another DCM locus has also been mapped to 6q23 (Messina et al., 1997). Since, however, hearing loss has not been observed in these individuals, and since they have symptoms of skeletal myopathy which has not been experienced in the hearing loss families, the causes of the diseases linked to these closely spaced loci are probably not allelic. It is noted that inherited hypertrophic cardiomyopathy in combination with hearing loss has been traced at least once to a mutation in a mitochondrial tRNA gene (tRNA lys) (Santorelli et al., 1996).

Cardiac actin mutations have been demonstrated in two small families by direct screening of this gene (located on chromosome 15q4). The mutations were found in exons 5 and 6. In codon 312 (exon 5) a G→A transition caused an Arg →His amino acid exchange, and in codon 361 (exon 6) an A→G transition was responsible for a Glu→Gly exchange. The mutations cosegregated with the disease; however, the families were small. The main argument against the assumption of these mutations being neutral polymorphisms was their absence in a large cohort of healthy individuals. Considering the generally high degree of evolutionary sequence conservation of actins, the chance that these mutations are functionally relevant is a priori high. The intramolecular regions (located in domain 1 and 3 of actin) affected by these changes are not primarily involved in cross-bridge formation with myosin, but most likely in the interaction of thin filaments with α-actinin in Z-disks. Defective attachment of filamentous actin to anchoring polypeptides may relate mutation 312 to force transmission rather than to force production (see Kabsch et al., 1990). The 3-dimensional structure of actin is shown in Fig. 49.32.

As was discussed in the section on Hypertrophic cardiomyopathy a third substitution in the cardiac actin gene (Ala→Ser in codon 295) has been found close to the positions of the above mutations (Mogensen et al., 1999). In this case the position of the change in the protein, although part of domain 3, does not preclude an effect on myosin binding and, hence, cross-bridge cycling. (Kabsch et al., 1990; Rayment et al., 1993). The divergent phenotypic consequences of two amino acid exchanges in close proximity within the same protein (in codons 312 and 295) are remarkable, but unexplained. It remains to be seen whether the

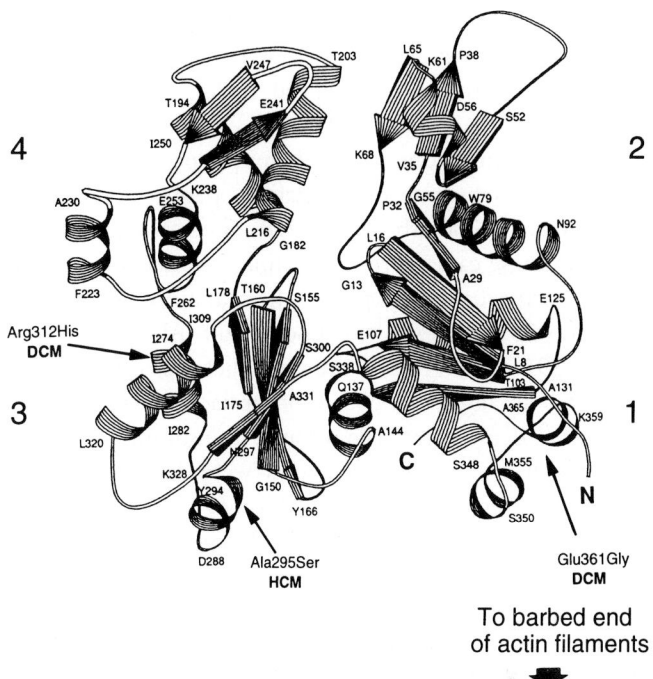

Fig. 49.32. Schematic representation of the three-dimensional structure of actin (rabbit skeletal muscle). The molecule consists of two domains that are further subdivided into two subdomains. The positions of the mutations associated with DCM (two missense mutations in codon 312 and 361) or HCM (one missense mutation in codon 295) are indicated. The main myosin HC interface involved in cross-bridge cycling is subdomain 2. (From Kabsch et al., 1990, modified with permission.)

current popular distinction between force production mutations causing HCM, and force transmission mutations causing DCM is useful to discriminate between different types of cardiomyopathy. The notion of an impaired α-actinin binding of actin mutated in the DCM-related position 312 would render the vast majority of actin protomers of the thin filaments functionally neutral, since only a few subunits at the barbed ends of the actin polymers would cause dysfunction. But it cannot be excluded that the change to which only few subunits contribute is disease relevant.

The desmin mutation associated with DCM was found in one of 44 consecutive probands investigated for changes in the desmin gene by PCR amplification of exons and subsequent direct sequencing of DNA. Desmin is a component of intermediate filaments in skeletal and myocardial cells. A missense mutation, resulting from a C→G transversion causing an Ile451Met exchange in exon 8, was identified in two symptomatic patients (father and son) and in two asymptomatic carriers (sisters). Two deceased obligate carriers from a previous generation and three first-degree cousins who had died prematurely could not be studied. The mutation was located in the C-terminal tail region of desmin and is presumably responsible for a significant change in three-dimensional conformation of its immediate environment (Li et al., 1999). The desmin tail region does not contribute to the α-helical rod. Its functional role is not known.

Missense mutations in the desmin gene have also been recognized as a cause of skeletal myopathies with cardiac involvement (Goldfarb et al., 1998). The cardiac manifestations in these cases were conduction disorders of the heart and restrictive cardiomyopathy. The mutations were located in codon 337 (Ala→Pro), in codon 360 (Ala→Pro) and in codon 392 (Asn→Ile). Compound heterozygosity associated with an aggressive course of cardiac and skeletal myopathy was demonstrated in a family transmitting the latter two mutations. These exchanges were localized in rod forming subregions of desmin. This may again demonstrate that mutations—here in different domains of the rod-like desmin—are associated with different disease manifestations.

A particularly striking example of variable and phenotypically distinguishable position effects of mutations within one protein is lamin A/C. The gene (designated *LMNA*) is located on chromosome 1p1–q21 (Fatkin et al., 1999) (Fig. 49.33). Lamin A/C is an asymmetrical protein (MW ~65.000) consisting of a central α-helical rod domain flanked by globular N-terminal head and C-terminal tail domains. Lamins contribute to the formation of nuclear lamina, a meshwork of intermediate filaments that line the inner surface of nuclear membranes in eucaryotic cells. The α-helical rods are involved in coiled coil-dimerization. The meshwork forms through interactions between charged side chains on the surface of the dimers. Three types of lamins exist, A, B and C. They are encoded by two genes, one for lamin B and one for lamin A/C. Lamins A

and C are predominantly expressed in differentiated cells. These two isoforms result from differential splicing in exon 10 close to the C-terminus (see Fig. 49.33). Lamin A is slightly longer (by 74 amino acids) than lamin C. Homozygous lamin A/C knockout mice are viable; however, they suffer from severe muscular dystrophy in their adult life (Sullivan et al., 1999). Lamin A/C mutations in man cause a broad spectrum of disease.

Four different (partially overlapping) manifestations of lamin A/C mutations have been described in humans. These are dilated cardiomyopathy in conjunction with conduction disease (Fatkin et al., 1999), autosomal dominant or recessive Emery-Dreifuss muscular dystrophy (Bonne et al., 1999; Raffaele Di Barletta et al., 2000), a subtype of limb-girdle muscular dystrophy, and familial partial lipodystrophy (Shackleton et al., 2000). Emery-Dreifuss muscular dystrophy is characterized by early onset contractures, progressive dystrophy in humeroperoneal muscles and cardiomyopathy with conduction block. A related muscle disease is limb-girdle muscular dystrophy with impaired atrioventricular conduction (Muchir et al., 2000). Partial lipodystrophy is a disorder of adipose tissue associated with absence or reduction of subcutaneous fat at the time of puberty. Variable degrees of hyperlipidemia may also be seen. A common denominator of these diseases is the lamin A/C gene with mutations causing substitutions in different parts of the protein. About 25 different mutations have been identified in families and patients affected by these four different disorders. A consistent correlation between mutated positions in the gene and phenotypic consequences is not obvious. A possible exception are mutations leading to lipodystrophy. They are clustered close to the

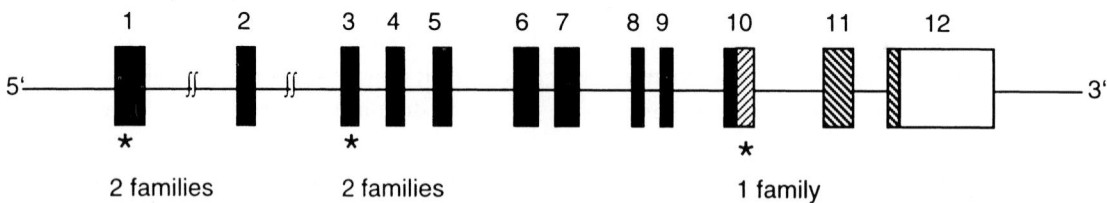

The mutations:

exon 1: 60[Arg-Gly] and 85[Leu-Arg]
exon 3: 195[Asn-Lys] and 203[Glu-Gly]

exon 10: 571[Arg-Ser] (in isoform C only)

Fig. 49.33. Lamin A/C mutations associated with DCM. Mutations in this gene have been implicated in four different, but partially overlapping clinical manifestations, among them DCM and Emery-Dreifuss muscular dystrophy. Lamin A/C is a nuclear protein with unknown function. The gene shown here encodes two isoforms A and C, which arise through alternative splicing in exons 10 to 12. Exons 1 to 10 (5′ half) are common to both isoforms. Lamin A results from skipping the second half of exon 10 but includes exon 11 and 12. Lamin C contains the entire exon 10.4 families have mutations in the region shared by both isoforms, one family has a mutation in the small C-terminal stretch, which is specific for the C isoform. The mechanisms by which mutations in this gene cause cardiac or other diseases are not known.

C-terminus of the protein. This region may be involved in the maintainance of adipocytes. But other mutations in the same region of the gene are determinants of cardiac or skeletal muscle manifestations. To explain the pathogenesis of these heterogeneous phenotypes in terms of distinct position effects will be a formidable task.

Two DCM loci have been determined on the X-chromosome, one in position Xq28 close to the end of the long arm, and the other one at Xp21. The latter region comprises the locus of the dystrophin gene responsible for the X-linked recessive muscular dystrophy of the Duchenne or Becker type (DMD, BMD) (Ahn and Kunkel, 1993). Dystrophin is a large filamentous component of myofibers closely associated with the inner membrane of all muscle fibers (see Ch. 110). It is expressed in skeletal muscle, heart, brain, and also in other organs. Mutations in this gene cause progressive and ultimately lethal wasting of skeletal muscle. Cardiac dysfunction is frequently involved, but normally not as the dominant manifestation. Occasionally, however, mutations in the dystrophin gene are associated with dilated cardiomyopathy rather than skeletal muscle dystrophy. It appears that certain mutations preferentially affect cardiac but not skeletal muscle functions.

An X-linked, dystrophin-related phenotype restricted to cardiac muscle was initially reported over a decade ago (Berko and Swift, 1987). Later, the investigation of an unusual course of a Becker type dystrophy with prominent cardiac symptoms led to the identification of an in-frame deletion spanning exons 2–7 of the dystrophin gene resulting in a truncated protein (Gold et al., 1992). In a subsequent study of a cardiac disorder with chamber dilatation a truncation of the 5′ end of the dystrophin gene was suggested (Towbin et al., 1993). Finally, in two reports of

Italian families with X-linked DCM a deletion of muscle-specific exon 1 presumably including part of the dystrophin promoter region and a mutation affecting correct splicing of exon 1 were documented (Muntoni et al., 1993; Milasin et al., 1996).

The reasons for the different phenotypic consequences of these mutations are not fully understood. The association of changes in dystrophin 5′ gene regions with cardiac manifestations led to the suggestion that ablation of certain parts of the dystrophin promoter (or of the muscle specific exon 1) may affect the heart, but not skeletal muscle. At least five distinct promoters with separate cell type specificities have been identified (Ahn and Kunkel, 1993). Two of them, a brain specific promoter (PB) and a skeletal muscle specific promoter (PM), are located at the 5′ end of the gene, where they precede two respective exons, exon 1 b and exon 1 m. Exon 1 b is expressed in brain-mRNA, whereas exon 1 m is muscle-specific. Fig. 49.34 summarizes results of the first completely analysed case of a DCM associated with a mutation in the 5′ region of the dystrophin gene (Muntoni et al., 1993). A long deletion (≈ 100 kb) including PM and exon 1 m, but not PB can substitute as a promoter in skeletal muscle but not in cardiac muscle (Milasin et al., 1996). Altered promoter activities may not be the only explanation, since mutations (deletions) in a mutational hot spot region around exons 48 and 49 also seem to affect the heart preferably (see references in Ferlini et al., 1999). The mechanism in these cases is not known. It may be hypothesized that loss of a central protein domain has specific consequences in the heart, or that loss of intron sequences with regulatory capacity are accompanied by cardiac dysfunction. Mild disease seems to be characteristic for cases associated with these central deletions.

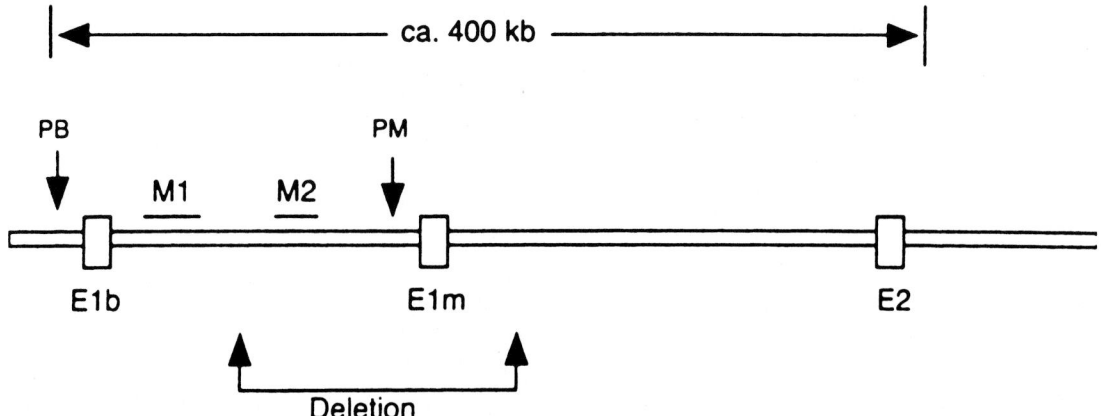

Fig. 49.34. The 5′ region of the dystrophin gene with a promoter deletion. This scheme depicts the 5′ region of the dystrophin gene where two promoter sequences, PB (brain) and PM (skeletal muscle), direct transcription in a tissue specific fashion. In an Italian family with X-linked DCM a deletion was found (approximate size about 100 kb) associated with loss of PM and the first muscle specific exon (E1m). PB and its adjacent brain specific exon E1b were retained (Muntoni et al., 1993). M1 and M2 were informative microsatellite marker sequences used in the mapping of the deletion.

Another mutation has been identified in exon 29—generating a stop codon associated with skipping of that exon—which is also cardiac specific with no or little effect on skeletal muscle (Franz et al., 2000). This mutation has been shown to distort the stability of the membraneous sarcoglycan complex which connects the intracellular cytoskeleton, of which dystrophin forms part, to the extracellular matrix of the myocardium.

An interesting observation pointing to the role of dystrophin as a major structural component of cardiocytes has been communicated recently from in vitro studies of a protease encoded by the cardiotropic virus Coxsackie B3 (Badorff et al., 1999). This protease selectively cleaves dystrophin and hence may disrupt the cytoskeleton of cardiocytes. This result could explain why virus infections contribute to cardiac disease, cardiac failure and dilatation. Viral myocarditis is not an inherited disease; however, certain aspects of its pathogenesis may help to unravel the mechanism possibly involved in disease development of X-linked inherited DCM.

The rare finding of a Duchenne/Becker genotype with a DCM phenotype led—together with other arguments—to the notion that DCM may ultimately result from a distorted myocardial cytoskeleton, or in a more general sense, from dysfunctional force transmission between cells. In contrast, the primary deficiency in HCM may be dysfunctional force production in sarcomeres resulting from mutations in proteins of the contractile apparatus.

The second X-linked locus associated with DCM is in the region Xq28. In this case DCM is part of a syndrome described over two decades ago, called Barth syndrome. It consists of early onset DCM, myopathy, lack of neutrophil leucocytes and abnormal mitochondria (Barth et al., 1983). The gene—designated G4.5—is known including mutations which cosegregate with the disease in affected families (D'Adamo et al., 1997). Its product, named *taffazin*, has been derived from DNA sequences. The function of this protein is, however, not known.

ANIMAL MODELS OF DCM

Animal models serve a double function in research related to cardiomyopathies. Pertinent analysis includes both carriers of randomly induced or spontaneous mutations and transgenic or gene-targeted animals. To be useful the model phenotypes have to mimic human disease. Of increasing importance is the genetic manipulation of experimental animals, usually mice, to investigate functions thought to contribute to pathogenisis. One option is the "reconstruction" of causes as has been successfully achieved with the

murine carrier of a 403 Arg-Gln myosin heavy chain mutation responsible for HCM in humans (Geisterfer-Lowrance et al., 1996). The second option is the targeted alteration of functions that are tested for their ability to change a phenotype in a way that improves understanding of disease mechanisms. Since the analysis of DCM mutations is still in its infancy (with the exception of actin and lamin A/C mutations, and changes in some candidate genes, which require confirmation), animal models of DCM are restricted to random mutations or to targeted manipulations of functions supposed to contribute to a DCM-like phenotype.

Syrian hamsters and dogs

Syrian hamsters inheriting cardiomyopathy and muscular dystrophy as an autosomal recessive trait have been known for a long time (see the references in Sakamoto et al., 1997; Büchner et al., 1978). The cardiac manifestation is either hypertrophic or dilated cardiomyopathy. The cause has been determined recently: both DCM and HCM hamsters carry a 27.4 kb deletion comprising the 5′ end of the gene encoding δ-sarcoglycan (this is one of four different sarcoglycan subunits). The loss includes the major transcription initiation site of this gene. δ-Sarcoglycan participates in the formation of the sarcolemmal dystrophin-associated glycoprotein complex, which links the intracellular cytoskeleton to the extracellular matrix (Sakamoto et al., 1997). Use of a cryptic promoter upstream of the deletion allows some transcription, but the resulting mRNA is for unknown reasons unable to trigger synthesis of δ-sarcoglycan. Lack of this protein disrupts the dystrophin-associated glycoprotein complex and causes muscle wasting and cardiac dysfunction. It seems noteworthy that hamster lines exposing either HCM or DCM were derived from a common cardiomyopathic founder line, BI01.50 (Jasmin and Eu, 1979). HCM- and DCM-hamsters have the same deletion in the δ-sarcoglycan gene. To explain the difference the suggestion was made that DCM hamsters have a second, modifying mutation responsible for the "dilated" phenotype (Sakamoto et al., 1997).

In humans mutations in any of the four sarcoglycan genes cause autosomal recessive limb-girdle muscular dystrophy (Perloff et al., 1966, Merlini et al., 2000). Cardiac abnormalities documented by electro- or echocardiography have been described in up to 30% of cases with severe muscular dystrophy. But myocardial involvement was usually mild (Fadic et al., 1996, Melacini et al., 1999). In functional terms, the DCM hamster resembles the human X-linked dystrophin-related DCM more than the limb-girdle muscular dystrophy. The fact that loss of δ-sarcoglycan also causes HCM rather than DCM, is unexplained.

An intriguing case of severe animal DCM has recently been reported from dog breeding. A recessive mutation occured in Portuguese Water dogs and was lethal in the homozygous state. Untreated affected pups died suddenly. Dilatation of the left ventricle and disrupted sarcomeres were reminiscent of the human condition. The causes are not known. Since, however, the animals responded positively to dietary taurin supplementation, the primary cause may be a metabolic dysfunction rather than a primary deficiency of sarcomeric force production or force transmission (Alroy et al., 2000).

Transgenic and gene-targeted mice

A number of reports have been published in recent years suggesting that a broad spectrum of functions contributes to a DCM-like phenotype (see Table 49.12). The homozygous knockout mice lacking the muscle LIM-protein (MLP) (Arber et al., 1997) are instructive. This protein is involved in myogenesis during development. It disappears later from adult muscle, but it persists in the myocardium. There it presumably acts as a "scaffold protein", which contributes to the stability of the actin-based cytoskeleton. The absence of this protein results in abnormally soft cardiac tissue and in disarray of myofibrils and disordered gap junctions between cells. Cardiac muscle develops compensatory hypertrophy before dilatation prevails. Lifespan is drastically reduced in most homozygous MLP-deficient animals.

Since MLP mutations have not been identified in patients (the human MLP gene maps to chromosome 11p15), these animals do not truly mimic human disease. However, MLP-deficient mice offer an opportunity to study the pathogenesis of dilatation and cardiac failure in molecular terms. An interesting aspect of this model is the dual function of MLP, which is both a structural protein contributing to mechanical strength of the myocardium and a (presumed) regulatory factor that may be involved in the control of gene expression. The assumption of MLP being a regulatory factor is based on the presence of two LIM zinc fingers, the so-called LIM motif, otherwise present in diverse proteins including LIM kinases and LIM homeodomain proteins (for review see Dawid et al., 1995). These proteins control cell differentiation and related events depending on complex gene regulation. Lack of MLP may result not only in mechanical weakness but also in altered patterns of gene expression.

Ca++ handling by the sarcoplasmic reticulum is another factor that might contribute to the manifestations of DCM.

The cardiac Ca++-ATPase, SERCA2a, which during diastole actively transports Ca++ into the sarcoplasmic reticulum, is controlled by phospholamban (PLB) as inhibitor. (Phospholamban is itself regulated by phosphorylation; phosphorylated PLB is inactive as inhibitor.) Ablation of PLB by genetic manipulation rescued in a dominant fashion the contractility of ventricular muscle cells in a mouse devoid of muscle LIM protein (MLP) (Minamisawa et al., 1999). These observations suggested that the SERCA2a-PLB interaction may be a target for therapeutic intervention in heart failure patients.

A likely contribution of altered myocyte survival (apoptosis) to the DCM phenotype was discussed earlier on theoretical grounds (MacLellan and Schneider, 1997). In a mouse with a knockout loss of the gene for gp130, a membrane bound cytokine receptor controlling viability of cells, rapid onset of DCM and massive induction of apoptosis was observed if the animals were exposed to aortic pressure overload (Hirota et al., 1999).

A DCM-like phenotype has also been described as a consequence of an experimentally induced dysfunction of oxygen peroxide metabolism. The targeted inactivation (knockout) of the gene coding for superoxide dismutase (SOD) in mice was associated with pathological changes reminiscent of DCM (ventricular chamber dilatation and impaired systolic function) (Li et al., 1995). Conceivably, the pathogenic mechanism involves loss of mitochondria or mitochondrial function due to an accumulation of oxygen radicals.

Another component triggering a DCM-phenotype is cardiac specific overexpression of tumor necrosis factor (Kubota et al., 1997). Finally, disruption of the smooth muscle MHC gene in the homozygous state also causes gross dilatation of the left ventricle (Morano et al., 2000). These and other changes that can be explained by the lack of smooth muscle functions apparently develop in utero and the animals die early after birth.

Ablation of the murine cardiac actin gene with concomitant expression of non-muscle γ-actin in heart muscle (Kumar et al., 1997) exhibits features of both HCM and DCM. These hearts exhibited hypertrophy and diastolic dysfunction, with additional dilatation and impaired systolic function. Thus, this genetic construct was able to partially rescue the missing cardiac actin function, but at the price of a diminished force generation and of abnormal force transmission.

Finally, a different kind of experimental DCM was observed in genetically targeted mice bred to homozygosity for myosin-binding protein-C mutations (McConnell et al., 1999). The mutation involved a truncation in MyBP-C, analogous to a change found in patients (who are, however, heterozygous). The animals with no normal gene product had ventricular dysfunction, which at birth induced compensatory hypertrophy and a pattern of altered gene expression as typically seen in other models of dilated cardiomyopathy: increased synthesis of α-skeletal actin and brain natriuretic protein (BNP) mRNAs, as well as altered myosin isoform expression in the myocardium. Echocardiography and cardiac catheterization demonstrated the DCM phenotype.

These observations, which cover a fairly broad range of cardiac functions, suggest that DCM may be the common endpoint of different mutations and pathways, contributing to both myocardial structure and the control of metabolic or signaling processes. In rare cases even sarcomeric proteins (which otherwise cause HCM) may be responsible for DCM, at least in animals.

It has been a popular topic among those interested in cardiomyopathies that HCM and DCM are different disease categories with different and, at least conceptually, mutually exclusive causes. According to this scheme HCM is a disease triggered by mutations in sarcomeric genes, and DCM is a disease with less well defined, but in any event different causes. Now there seem to be overlaps that suggest that definitions should be flexible to allow for exceptions. It has been reported recently that human DCM can also be caused by mutations in sarcomeric genes. Two mutations in β-myosin and one in cardiac troponin T cause DCM, and not HCM, as one might have expected (Kamisago et al., 2000). These mutations are two missense mutations in β-myosin (Ser532Pro and Phe764Leu) and a triplet deletion in the cardiac troponin T gene: ΔLys210. In the light of these new results one might look again at actin mutations, which are either associated with DCM or with HCM. They may have been a precedent for the new findings. It appears that not only the mutated gene determines the history of the disease, but additional and unknown factors also. Model studies with these mutations may be attractive because they could produce information about the early steps involved in dilatation rather than in growth.

SUMMARY

There is a common, albeit provisional understanding that DCM is a disease resulting from impaired functions of the myocardial cytoskeleton. The points in favor of this concept are:

DCM related mutations in cardiac actin are in positions not involved in force production, but probably in anchoring thin filaments to Z-bands of the sarcomeres.

Desmin mutations presumably affect the stability of intermediate filaments in cardiac and skeletal muscle. Phenotypes may depend on the type of mutation. Distinct mutations may preferentially affect the myocardium, others the myocardium and skeletal muscle.

Certain mutations in dystrophin cause DCM rather than skeletal muscle dystrophy which is otherwise the prevailing feature of DMD/BMD. Dystrophin contributes to cellular stability and integrity by connecting cardiocytes to the extracellular matrix.

Proteolytic cleavage of dystrophin in Coxsackie virus-infected myocardium may be involved in the pathogenesis of cardiac failure.

δ-Sarcoglycan mutations in cardiomyopathic hamsters underline the importance of mechanical stability of cardiac muscle cells.

Knockout mice suffering from a lack of the cytoskeletal muscle-LIM-protein (MLP) have a severe form of DCM.

These observations are suggestive of cellular/cytoskeletal instability being a major aspect in the pathogenesis of DCM. It should be noted, however, that for the majority of the genomic loci involved in the human DCM the genes have not as yet been identified.

MANAGEMENT OF DCM

Treatment is aimed at relieving symptoms, retarding disease progression, preventing complications, and improving survival. Management is not specific for DCM versus other causes of heart failure with the exception of the need for pedigree evaluation and genetic counseling. Supportive measures include weight control, moderation in alcohol consumption, and maintenance of physical activity with appropriate levels of submaximal exercise. Sodium intake should be restricted in patients with congestive symptoms. Treatment should include ACE inhibitors and possibly digitalis glycosides; those with congestive symptoms should also have diuretics. The use of low dose spironolactone is recommended. In the RALES study, which enrolled over 1600 patients approximately half of whom had DCM, sprironolactone 25 mg daily significantly reduced the number of sudden deaths as well as those due to progressive heart failure (Pitt et al., 1999). The risk of thromboembolic complication appears high, and anticoagulation should be considered in those with severe chamber dilatation, sustained arrhythmia, or both (Fuster et al., 1981; Johnson and Palacios, 1982; Diaz et al.,

1987). The judicious use of β-blocking drugs (Waagstein et al., 1989; Hjalmarson and Waagstein, 1991) has been associated with clinical improvement and increased survival (Dec and Fuster, 1994; Packer et al., 1996; Anonymous, 1999). Ventricular arrhythmias are common and are markers of disease severity. Non-sustained ventricular tachycardia during ECG monitoring is seen in approximately 20% of asymptomatic or mildly symptomatic patients and in up to 70% of severely symptomatic patients. The prognostic significance of ventricular tachycardia, however, is controversial. Its presence early in the course of disease when left ventricular function is relatively preserved is probably an independent marker of sudden death risk, whereas in general, markers of haemodynamic severity (e.g., ejection fraction, left ventricular end diastolic dimension, filling pressures) are more predictive of disease related mortality and sudden death (Dec and Fuster, 1994). Antiarrhythmic therapy with drugs (Cleland et al., 1987; Hamer et al., 1989) and/or implantable cardioverter/defibrillator (Knight et al., 1999) should be reserved for those with sustained symptomatic arrhythmias (Packer et al., 1996). The absence of a clear risk profile for sudden death precludes recommendations for primary prevention, though the use of an implantable defibrillator appears to be beneficial in DCM patients with unexplained syncope (Knight et al., 1999). It is known that many patients with DCM have a chronic inflammatory myocardial process (Caforio et al., 1990; Kuhl et al., 1994). The results from trials involving immunosuppression have been disappointing (Latham et al., 1989; Parillo et al., 1989; Mason et al., 1995). These trials, however, have been few, with small numbers of patients, and immunologic characterization has been incomplete (McKenna and Davies, 1995). It is probable that some patients with DCM would benefit from immunosuppression at particular stages of the disease process. The algorithm for the identification of such individuals remains to be established.

Non-pharmacological treatment of advanced heart failure includes surgical left ventricular remodeling procedures, mitral valve surgery in selected patients with severe mitral regurgitation, the use of left ventricular assist devices and biventricular pacing. Remodelling the ventricle in DCM remains an experiment, but the improvement in symptoms and exercise capacity associated with greater synchronization of left and right ventricular activation by biventricular pacing offers a useful therapeutic option in patients with marked inhomogeneity of ventricular activiation (i.e., QRS > 150 ms).

DCM is still the principal indication for heart transplantation in both adults and children (Kaye, 1992; Mudge et al., 1993). The presence of legitimate pharmacological options and the improvements in symptoms and prognosis associated with modern drug therapy have lessened reliance on transplant in DCM.

In summary, although some progress has been made regarding the genetic etiology of DCM, the full extent of causes is still undetermined and even less is known about pathogenic mechanisms. Disease specific management of DCM targeting pathogenetic mechanisms remains a major challenge.

Genetic counseling

Recognition that there is a familial basis to DCM in a significant proportion of patients raises issues of risk to offspring and other relatives. Probands should be evaluated for the cardiac (including conduction disease) and neuromuscular manifestations of the disease phenotype. Similar evaluation of first-degree relatives is recommended. The presence of impaired myocardial performance with either conduction disease and/or neuromuscular abnormalities in a proband is highly likely to be associated with familial disease. In contrast, only a third of probands with left ventricular dilatation and impaired systolic function who do not have other manifestations of the broader DCM phenotype will exhibit evidence of familial disease. The fact that age-related penetrance extends into the middle decades limits the practical significance of a normal finding in a first-degree relative, particularly in the young. Precise algorithms for serial evaluation remain to be established. Once a relative is shown to have a normal ECG and echo, reevaluation at five yearly intervals is pragmatic and probably sufficient unless cardiac symptoms develop. Preliminary evidence suggests that when the DCM phenotype is limited to impaired myocardial function, disease is slowly progressive over decades. Ultimately, the identification of disease-causing genes will provide a molecular diagnosis to identify those at risk of DCM. Whether preliminary work examining serial markers of immune activation (organ specific myosin antibody, raised CRP) and tissue damage (raised CK-MB, troponin T) will identify disease predisposition and early disease remains to be determined. Potential benefits of a preclinical diagnosis include evaluation of treatment to prevent or attenuate disease development, surveillance and early treatment to reduce arrhythmia, embolic and sudden death risk, and lifestyle advice concerning career, competitive sport and alcohol consumption. The clinical and psychosocial impact of a preclinical diagnosis, however, will require evaluation when and if it becomes a practical possibility.

Arrhythmogenic right ventricular cardiomyopathy

Arrhythmogenic right ventricular cardiomyopathy (ARVC) is a heart muscle disorder characterized pathologically by fibrofatty replacement of the right ventricular myocardium (Fontaine et al., 1982; Marcus et al., 1982; Thiene et al., 1988). The disease was previously called right ventricular "dysplasia" (Frank et al., 1978). It is a progressive disorder. Early on, segmental right ventricular disease is usual, but evolution to more diffuse right ventricular involvement, with or without left ventricular abnormalities, and the development of cardiac failure are recognized. The clinical manifestations of the disease (which may be subtle) include structural and functional abnormalities of the right ventricle, electrocardiographic depolarization and repolarization changes, and presentation with arrhythmias of right ventricular origin or sudden death (Fontaine et al., 1998). Data from prospective pedigree studies are limited. However, autosomal dominant transmission was reported in the early series (Marcus et al., 1982; Ruder et al., 1985).

The true prevalence of ARVC is not known. Retrospective pathological series suggest that it is second only to HCM as a cause of sudden death in apparently healthy young athletes. A study from Italy revealed it to be the commonest cause of sudden death in the Veneto area (Corrado et al., 1990). The prevalence for this region was estimated to be about 1:5000 (Thiene et al., 1997). The available evidence suggests that the lack of general awareness about ARVC and the difficulties in making an accurate diagnosis results in it being under-recognized clinically and at post mortem evaluation. Thus, the disease may be much more common than current figures suggest.

The diagnosis of ARVC is often problematic. Definitive diagnosis is based on the histologic demonstration of transmural fibrofatty replacement of right ventricular myocardium at either biopsy, surgery or necropsy. A tissue diagnosis is often impractical and diagnosis is based on the clinical presentation with arrhythmias of right ventricular origin and on structural, functional and electrocardiographic abnormalities of the right ventricle that reflect the pathological changes. Criteria for diagnosis are based on classification of clinical features into major and minor criteria (McKenna et al., 1994). These criteria remain to be validated prospectively in relation to clinical outcome.

Presentation in the young is usually with symptoms of arrhythmia (sustained palpitation, syncope or sudden death). Typically the arrhythmias respond to pharmacologic therapy with beta-blockers and amiodarone. A major role for catheter ablation and arrhythmia surgery is limited in large part because of disease progression. If arrhythmia can be suppressed, survival is usually good, although in later stages the hemodynamic consequences of right heart failure with atrial arrhythmias and congestive symptoms will require therapy to treat heart failure and and prevent atrial emboli (anticoagulants). Progressive, severe left ventricular dysfunction occurs but is uncommon. Primary prevention with an implantable cardioverter defibrillator is limited by the absence of a clear risk profile of the high-risk patient.

Genetic causes of the dominant forms of ARVC are not known. Linkage studies in families have identified chromosomal loci at 14q23 (Rampazzo et al., 1994), 1q42 (Rampazzo et al., 1995)(ARVD2, possibly related to ryanodine receptor deficiencies), 14q12 (Severini et al., 1996), 2q32 (Rampazzo et al., 1997) and 2p23 (Ahmad et al., 1998) (Fig. 49.35). Recently mutations have been identified in the cardiac ryanodine receptor gene in four families (previously mapped to the ARVD2 locus) (Tiso et al., 2001). The phenotype in affected individuals was characterized by presentation with polymorphic ventricular tachycardia without significant structural heart disease and it is uncertain whether the families reported are part of the spectrum of ARVC. Indeed, other reports also identify ryanodine receptor mutations in patients with polymorphic ventricular tachycardia in the absence of ARVC features (Laitinen et al., 2001; Priori et al., 2001).

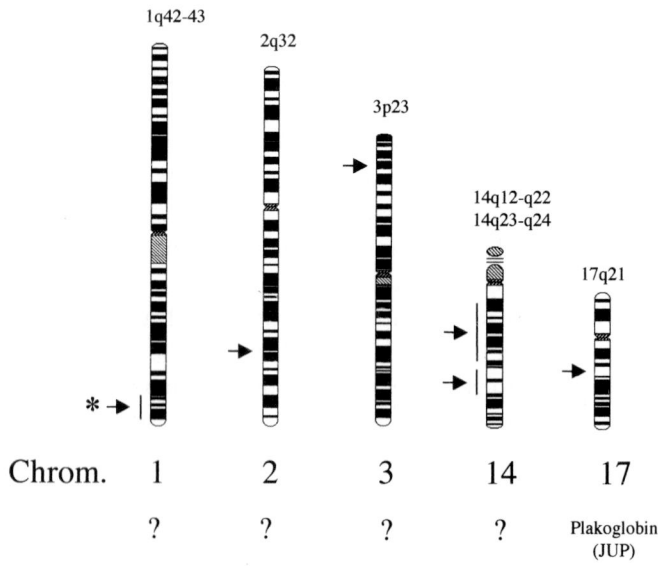

Fig. 49.35. Genomic loci linked to ARVC. Six loci have been identified by linkage analysis. A gene with a disease-related mutation has been identified for the rare syndromic recessive Naxos disease. The locus on chromosome 1 (asterisk) has previously been designated ARVC2 (or ARVD2) locus (Rampazzo et al., 1995). Whether diseases mapped to this locus fulfill conventional ARVC criteria requires further study.

Recently, an autosomal recessive ARVC has also been reported (Coonar et al., 1998; McKoy et al., 2000). It was previously designated Naxos disease (named after the Greek island of Naxos where the first families with this disorder were diagnosed). Naxos disease is a syndrome of ARVC, non-epidermolytic palmoplantar keratoderma and woolly hair (Protonotarios et al., 1986). The recessive form of ARVC is similar to autosomal dominant ARVC with respect to age and mode of clinical presentation, distribution of right and left ventricular involvement, electrocardiographic abnormalities and morphological and histological features (McKoy et al., 2000). This disorder was mapped to chromosome 17q21 (Coonar et al., 1998). After refining the region of homozygosity to a locus containing the gene for plakoglobin as a candidate, a homozygous deletion mutation (loss of two basepairs) was identified that cosegregated with the Naxos disease syndrome (McKoy et al., 2000). The deletion caused a shift in the reading frame and a premature stop in the cognate mRNA. The associated truncation of the protein was demonstrated by immunoblotting protein of palmar punch biopsies (Fig. 49.36). Heterozygous carriers of the deletion were clinically unaffected.

Plakoglobin is a member of the armadillo protein family and a constituent cytoplasmic protein in adherens and desmosomal junctions. It is involved in cell adhesive and signaling functions. Mice with homozygous null mutations exhibit heart and skin abnormalities analogous to Naxos disease (Bierkamp et al., 1996; Ruiz et al., 1996). The mutation in a protein, which is an important constituent of the cytoskeleton and also involved in cell signaling processes, has implications for autosomal dominant forms of ARVC and possibly for other types of cardiomyopathies. The fact that families with both ARVC and DCM are recognized, and that Naxos ARVC like DCM may be seen as a disease of the cardiac cytoskeleton, suggests common pathogenetic mechanisms for these true cardiomyopathies.

RESTRICTIVE AND INFILTRATIVE CARDIOMYOPATHY

The revised classification of cardiomyopathies by the WHO/ISCF Task Force (Richardson et al., 1996) assigns the restrictive cardiomyopathy (RCM) to the category of "diseases of the myocardium associated with cardiac dysfunction". RCM

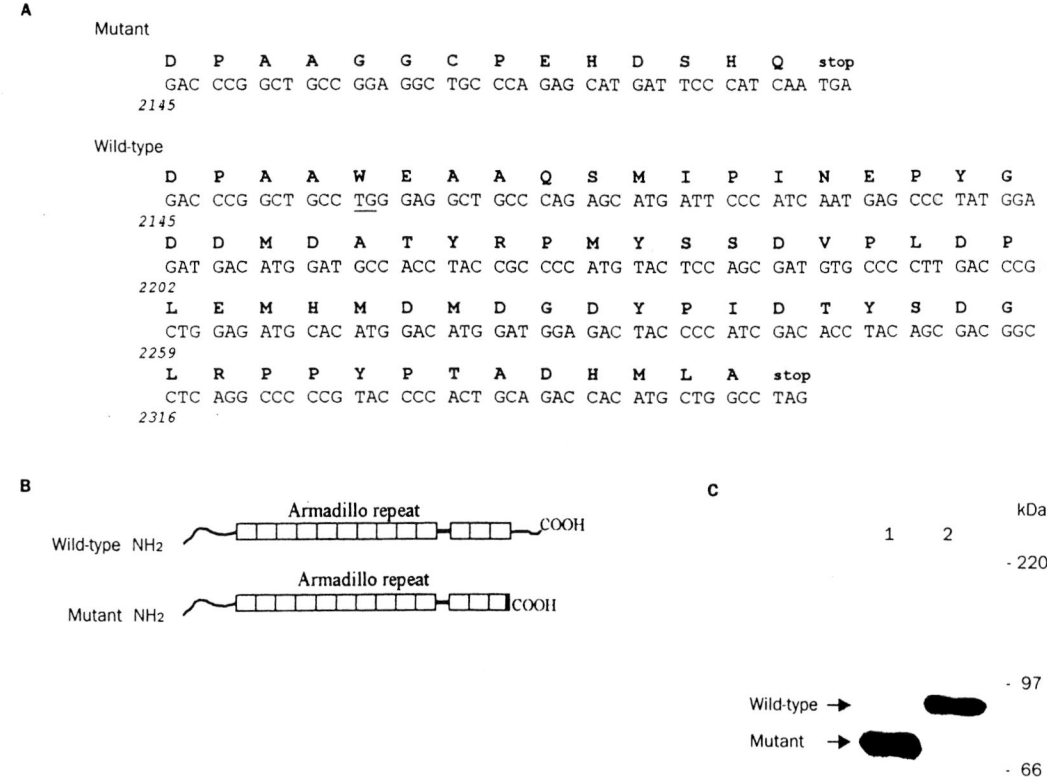

Fig. 49.36. Mutation in the plakoglobin gene causing recessive ARVC (Naxos disease). Features of this syndromic disease are cardiomyopathy with palmoplantar keratoderma and woolly hair (which served to recognize patients). (A) A homozygous 2 base pair deletion (TG, underlined) in the plakoglobin gene was identified in 19 patients. The result was a frameshift and premature termination of translation at the 3' end of the gene. (B) Structural consequence of the mutation is loss of the C-terminus. (C) Electrophoretic demonstration of the truncated protein expressed in a biopsy sample of the left ventricle of a patient. Plakoglobin is a cell-cell adhesion protein. Dysfunction presumably results in loss of myocyte integrity.

is usually the consequence of a nonmyocardial pathologic process and not a primary myocardial disease. It may be idiopathic or associated with other diseases, such as infiltrative disorders and endomyocardial disease with or without eosinophilia. Primary RCM is extremely rare in the Western world. The hallmark of the condition (be it primary or secondary) is abnormal diastolic function, characterized by restrictive filling and reduced diastolic volume of either or both ventricles. Systolic function and myocardial wall thickness are normal or near-normal. A few reports indicate that RCM can be inherited, albeit rarely, as a primary cardiac disease (Aroney et al., 1988; Fitzpatrick et al., 1990). Endomyocardial fibroelastosis has been observed in primary genetic forms as well as in sporadic cases. It is characterized by fibrotic thickening of the endocardium, with gross impairment of diastolic function. Clinical symptoms are failure to thrive, tachypnea, and tachycardia. Cardiac decompensation is the most serious complication. There is no effective therapy, with the possible exception of cardiac transplantation. Histologic analysis shows extensive deposition of extracellular matrix components such as collagen and elastic fibers in the endocardium.

Genetic studies of families with endomyocardial fibroelastosis have revealed that X-linked inheritance is the most frequent pattern of transmission (Hodgson et al., 1987). In addition, a few reports have suggested that autosomal recessive inheritance may also occur (Hallidie-Smith and Olsen, 1968; Opitz, 1982). Fibroelastosis can be found at autopsy in patients with autosomal dominant DCM (Ross et al., 1978). It is not known whether in these cases the endocardial changes are primary, representing a separate mendelian disease, or whether they are a symptom of the underlying cardiomyopathy.

Inherited fibroelastosis has also been described as part of a congenital syndrome of which the major symptoms are kidney malformation, mental retardation, characteristic facies and heart defects, among them fibrotic depositions in the endocardium (Eastman and Bixler, 1977; Nevin et al., 1991).

The structural and functional effects of infiltrative disorders are variable, but often provide a secondary form of RCM (Table 49.17). For further details and discussion of systemic and metabolic diseases affecting the heart, informative summaries by Kelly and Strauss (1994) and Pyeritz (2001) are recommended.

NEUROMUSCULAR DISORDERS WITH CARDIOMYOPATHY AS A SECONDARY FEATURE

Several neuromuscular disorders, in particular those primarily affecting muscle functions, are associated with heart

Table 49.17. Genetic disorders associated with restrictive cardiomyopathy

	OMIM
A. Familial restrictive cardiomyopathy	115210
B. Primary endocardial fibroelastosis:	
Familial endocardial fibroelastosis	226000, 305300
Facio-cardio-renal syndrome	227280
C. Diseases associated with myocardial infiltration:	
Transthyretin amyloidosis	176300
Gaucher disease type I	230800
Fabry disease	301500
Glycogen storage disease II	232300
Glycogen storage disease III	232400
Hemosiderosis	235500
Mucopolysaccharidosis type I	252800
Mucopolysaccharidosis type II	309900

Abbreviation: OMIM, entry number in the reference list of Online Mendelian Inheritance in Man (www.ncbi.nlm.nih.gov/)

muscle disease. Most prominent among them are the X-chromosomal Duchenne/Becker muscular dystrophy, the X-chromosomal and autosomal Emery-Dreifuss muscular dystrophies, the autosomal dominant myotonic dystrophy, the autosomal recessive Friedreich ataxia and the autosomal dominant Noonan syndrome. Of major interest are also diseases with mutations in the mitochondrial DNA (Kearns-Sayre syndrome). Salient cardiac features of these diseases are listed in Table 49.18.

Duchenne/Becker muscular dystrophy is characterized by progressive muscle weakness and wasting. Cardiomyopathy and heart failure are frequent in the Duchenne type dystrophy, but uncommon in the Becker type. In rare cases the disease is restricted to the heart with DCM being the main manifestation, as discussed above.

The diseases listed in Table 49.18 have been characterized in depth in separate chapters in this volume. For further detail we therefore refer to these chapters: Duchenne/Becker muscular dystrophy—Ch. 123; Myotonic dystrophy—Ch. 120. Mitochondrial diseases (Kearns-Sayre syndrome) are subjects of Ch. 11.

Conclusions and future developments

Significant progress has been achieved in the past five years, in particular in the analysis of the genetics of HCM and to a lesser degree of DCM and ARVC. Regarding HCM,

Table 49.18. Neuromuscular disorders associated with cardiac disease

Condition	Cardiac pathology	OMIM	Transmission	Genomic position	Genetic defect
Duchenne/Becker muscle dystrophy	Replacement fibrosis with fatty infiltration, degeneration of Purkinje fibers, conduction defects, DMD: CM uncommon, but CHF is observed; BMD: CM and CHF are common	310200	XR	Xp21	Dystrophin
Emery-Dreifuss muscle dystrophy	Atrophy of cardiac fibers, myocardial fibrosis, atrial fibrillation, SD not uncommon	310300	XR and AD	Xp28 and 1q11	"Emerin" and lamin A/C
Myotonic dystrophy	Diffuse myocardial changes, conduction defects, cardiac death frequent	169900	AD	19q31	cAMP-dependent protein kinase
Friedreich ataxia	Concentric hypertrophy, conduction defects, cardiac death frequent	160900	AR	9q13	"Frataxin", located in the mitochondrial membrane
Noonan syndrome	Variable cardiovascular defects, predisposition to hypertrophic cardiomyopathy	163950	AD	chrom. 12?	not known
Kearns-Sayre syndrome	AV block conduction defects	530000	mitochondrial	mitoch. DNA	Duplications, deletions in mitoch. DNA

DMD and BMD, muscular dystrophy type Duchenne and Becker; OMIM, entry number in the reference list of Online Mendelian Inheritance in Man (www.ncbi.nlm.nih.gov/); CM, cardiomyopathy; CHF, congestive heart failure; AV block, atrioventricular conduction block; SD, sudden death; AR, autosomal recessive; AD, autosomal dominant; XR, X-linked recessive.

mutations in eight genes (possibly nine, if titin is included) have been confirmed as causes of disease. More than 160 mutations have been detected within these genes and the list is constantly growing. Clinical information has not been communicated in all cases, but neutral inherited variants are apparently rare. There is no doubt that the majority of the mutations cause disease. The mutations are randomly distributed within the genes, but a few hot spots have been delineated. Most prominent among them is the codon 403 hot spot in the β-myosin heavy chain, which was the first HCM mutation discovered more than a decade ago (Geisterfer-Lowrance et al., 1990). CpG dimers are prefered mutational target sites as was convincingly shown by direct experimentation (D'Cruz et al., 2000). Although not all the genes known to cause HCM have been analyzed in depth in different centers, there is little doubt that three genes are responsible for roughly 50% of all cases: β-myosin HC, MyBP-C and cardiac troponin T. The five remaining genes are apparently less frequently involved. However, these numbers are provisional.

The concept of HCM as a "disease of the sarcomere" (Thierfelder et al., 1994) has been corroborated. The HCM phenotype is ultimately the consequence of a dysfunction in myocardial muscle contraction or "force production". A considerable amount of data has been ana-lyzed by studying, in particular, the properties of the hearts of gene-targeted mice carrying the 403 missense mutation in the ventricular isoform of myosin heavy chain (which is α in mouse and β in man). Salient features of these hearts, their myofilaments and single myosin molecules included: hypercontraction, increased Ca^{2+} sensitivity of force development, a decrease of free energy from ATP hydrolysis and lack of coordination in the action of the two "heads" of native myosin molecules (all results from the Seidman group in Boston). The fact that 30% to 40% of disease remain unexplained does, however, suggest that not all HCM is a "disease of the sarcomere". The HCM phenotype may also develop as a consequence of defects in energy metabolism and mitochondrial function. The importance of mitochondrial disease and related abnormalities in energy production as causes of HCM remains to be determined.

Inherited DCM, in contrast, has conceptually been treated by different authors as a disease resulting from a deficiency of the cytoskeleton and/or its structural links to the extracellular matrix. This was interpreted as a functional defect in "force transmission". There are some data in support of this notion, e.g., the (rare) contribution of dystrophin to the DCM phenotype without effect on skeletal muscle (Ferlini et al., 1999), the pathological role of sarcoglycan mutations (most clearly in hamster, see Sakamoto et al., 1997), the presumed consequences of desmin mutations (Li et al., 1999), and some others. However, it is not clear whether general conclusions about the "primary" pathogenesis of DCM can be drawn. For most of the linked DCM loci the genes are not known. But more importantly, mutations in cardiac actin (Olson et al., 1998), in β-myosin and in cardiac troponin T (Kamisago et al., 2000) provide evidence that DCM—in presumably rare cases—can be traced to deficient "force production" rather than to "force transmission". It seems that occasionally a dysfunction in the motor unit is "translated" in a second step into a gradually increasing disruption of the myocardial cell and tissue architecture. It would be interesting to know whether other sarcomeric proteins (e.g., titin?) are able to trigger DCM, as well as HCM.

A reasonable conclusion at this time may be that HCM has a clearly defined set of causes that direct the pathologic development towards growth and other secondary changes characteristic of HCM. In contrast, DCM might not be linked to one specific set of causes. Disparate primary defects, various dysfunctions or loss of structural integrity, are conceivably able to independently initiate pathways that result in dilatation and not in growth. The original pathogenic change may be in the cytoskeleton, or in mitochondria, possibly also in enzymes involved in unscheduled or aberrant cleavage of proteins required for normal function (Margossian et al., 1992; Badorff et al., 1999), in mutated nuclear proteins (Fatkin et al., 1999), or—as it is now known—in altered motor proteins. One may conclude that HCM is a disease with a fairly well defined etiology, whereas DCM is the final common pathway of different underlying pathologic processes. Observations in animals carrying mutations or studies of certain transgenic mouse models seem to support the conclusion that DCM is the result of heterogeneous causes. But clearly, more information is required to identify and separate causes and effects in the development of this disease. The same is true for ARVC.

Very little is known about the impact of modifying genes on penetrance and expression of cardiomyopathies. For HCM, for some cases of DCM and for one case of ARVC, causes have been traced to single gene mutations. The well known phenotypic variability documented even within families is still a puzzling phenomenon. It appears that the disorder resulting from a single (mendelian) mutation is, in addition, subject to multifactorial (polygenic or environmental) modulation, which may either result in enhanced or in mitigated expression of symptoms. The analysis of the contribution of modifying genes is still in its infancy. Although a considerable number of association studies have been communicated (which we did not comment in detail), strong conclusions cannot be drawn.

Advances in the clinical management have been achieved in risk stratification for sudden death and preventive measures, most notably ICD implantation. Pharmacologic therapy of HCM in the absence of controlled clinical studies still depends to a large degree on experience and careful monitoring of patients by the cardiologist.

The increasing experience and success of percutaneous alcohol ablation of hypertrophied myocardial tissue to treat outflow tract obstruction suggests that this technique will have a major therapeutic role to play, particularly once appropriate patient selection is better defined.

The clinical management of DCM and ARVC has not changed significantly. The main goal is the relief of symptoms and the early recognition of major risks.

A point of growing interest (and concern by others) is the impact genetic knowledge has on clinical practice. At this time the discussion is largely restricted to HCM, since little is known about causes of other cardiomyopathies. Cardiologists want to know what kind of mutation they are confronted with, be it to obtain knowledge of a (rare) "malignant" mutation before complications develop or simply to confirm the diagnosis. Geneticists want to use genetic information to counsel patients and families. It is obvious that for counseling it is useful or even necessary to have knowledge of causes, in particular in families with a history of severe disease and premature sudden death. If mutations are known, preclinical diagnosis is possible that affords either the exclusion or the confirmation of carrier status. In the long run with further improvement of management the identification of a mutation may have a beneficial effect by the timely implementation of preventive measures or by advice regarding lifestyle to avoid particular risks. To foster the cooperation between geneticists and cardiologists, the establishment of patient and family registers is mandatory. These registers should permit systematic assessment of penetrance and outcome within families and single patients in relation to a specific mutation. This should aid counseling clinical risk assessment. Some regional registers exist or are in preparation, but cooperation between regional centers is lacking.

In summary, the potential of molecular genetics has been used in recent years to broaden the scope of knowledge about causes of cardiomyopathies and also about pathogenic mechanisms to a significant extent. Further advances will be required to bring this knowledge to completion with particular emphasis on myocardial events and changes responsible for the risk of sudden death and other aspects of the clinical phenotype.

REFERENCES

Abbasi AS, MacAlpin RN, Eber LM, Pearce ML (1972) Echocardiographic diagnosis of idiopathic hypertrophic cardiomyopathy without outflow obstruction. Circulation 46:897–904

Abelmann WH, Lorell BH (1989) The challenge of cardiomyopathy. Coll Cardiol 13:1219–1239

Ahmad F, Li DX, Karibe A et al. (1998) Localization of a gene responsible for arrhythmogenic right ventricular dysplasia to chromosome 3p23. Circulation 98:2791–2795

Ahn AH, Kunkel LM (1993) The structural and functional diversity of dystrophin. Nature Genet 3:283–291

Alfonso F, Nihoyannopoulos P, Stewart J et al. (1990) Clinical significance of giant negative T waves in hypertrophic cardiomyopathy. J Am Coll Cardiol 15:965–971

Alroy J, Rush JE, Freeman L et al. (2000) Inherited infantile dilated cardiomyopathy in dogs: Genetic, clinical, biochemical, and morphologic findings. Am J Med Genet 95:57–66

Alvares RF, Goodwin JF (1982) Non-invasive assessment of diastolic function in hypertrophic cardiomyopathy on and off beta adrenergic blocking drugs. Br Heart J 48:204–212

Anan R, Greve G, Thierfelder L et al. (1994) Prognostic implications of novel β-cardiac myosin heavy chain gene mutations that cause familial hypertrophic cardiomyopathy. J Clin Invest 93:280–285

Anan R, Shono H, Kisanuki A et al. (1998) Patients with familial hypertrophic cardiomyopathy caused by a Phe 110Ile missense mutation in the cardiac troponin T gene have variable cardiac morphologies and a favorable prognosis. Circulation 98:391–397

Andersen PS et al. (1998) Beta myosin heavy chain mutations in Danish patients suffering from hypertrophic cardiomyopathy. Am J Pathol 153:1651

Andersen PS, Havndrup O, Bundgaard H et al. (1999) Adult-onset familial hypertrophic cardiomyopathy caused by a novel mutation, R694C, in the MYH7 gene. Clin Genet 56:244–246

Anonymous (1999) Effect of metoprolol CR/XL in chronic heart failure: Metoprolol CR/XL Randomised Intervention Trial in Congestive Heart Failure (MERIT-HF). Lancet. 353:2001–2007

Arai S, Matsuoka R, Hirayama K et al. (1995) Missense mutation of the beta-cardiac myosin heavy chain gene in hypertrophic cardiomyopathy. Am J Med Genet 58:267–276

Arber S, Hunter J, Ross J et al. (1997) MLP-deficient mice exhibit a disruption of cardiac cytoarchitectural organization, dilated cardiomyopathy, and heart failure. Cell 88:393–403

Arbustini E, Fasani R, Morbini P et al. (1998) Coexistence of mitochondrial DNA and β myosin heavy chain mutations in hypertrophic cardiomyopathy with late congestive heart failure. Heart 80:548–558

Aroney C, Bett N, Radford D (1988) Familial restrictive cardiomyopathy. Aust NZ J Med 18:877–878

Badorff C, Lee GH, Lamphear BJ et al. (1999) Enteroviral protease 2A cleaves dystrophin: Evidence of cytoskeletal disruption in an acquired cardiomyopathy. Nature Med 5:320–326

Bagshaw CR (1993) Muscle Contraction. Chapman and Hall, London

Barth PG, Scholte JA, Berden JA (1983) An X-linked mitochondrial disease affecting cardiac muscle, skeletal muscle and neutrophil leucocytes. J Neurol Sci 62:327–355

Beahrs MM, Tajik AJ, Seward JB et al. (1983) Hypertrophic obstructive cardiomyopathy: Ten to 21-year follow-up after partial septal myectomy. Am J Cardiol 51:1160–1166

Beall CJ, Sepanski AM, Fyrberg EA (1989) Genetic dissection of Drosophila myofibril formation: Effects of actin and myosin heavy chain null alleles. Genes Dev 3:131–140

Becker AE, Caruso G (1982) Myocardial disarray: A critical review. Br Heart J 47:527–538

Becker KD, Gottshall KR, Hickey R et al. (1997) Point mutations in human β cardiac myosin heavy chain have differential effects on sarcomeric structure and assembly: An ATP binding site change disrupts both thick and thin filaments, whereas hypertrophic cardiomyopathy mutations display normal assembly. J Cell Biol 137:131–140

Bejsovic A, Anderson P (1990) Functions of the myosin ATP and actin binding sites are required for C. elegans thick filament assembly. Cell 60:133–140

Berko BAM, Swift M (1987) X-linked dilated cardiomyopathy. N Engl J Med 316:1186–1191

Bennett CP, Burn J, Moore G (1987) Prevalence of hypertrophic cardiomyopathy in the Northern region of England. J Med Genet 94:243

Betocchi S, Cannon RO, Watson RM et al. (1985) Effects of sublingual nifedipine on hemodynamics and systolic and diastolic function in patients with hypertrophic cardiomyopathy. Circulation 72:1001–1007

Bierkamp C, Mclaughlin KJ, Schwarz H et al. (1996) Embryonic heart and skin defects in mice lacking plakoglobin. Developmental Biology 180:780–785

Bing W, Redwood CS, Purcell IF et al. (1997) Effects of two hypertrophic cardiomyopathy mutations in alpha-tropomyosin. Asp 175 Asn and Glu 180 Gly, on Ca2+ regulation of thin filament motility. Biochem Biophys Res Com 236:760–764

Bing W, Knott A, Redwood C et al. (2000) Effect of hypertrophic cardiomyopathy mutations in human cardiac muscle alpha-tropomyosin (Asp 175Asn and Glu180Gly) on the regulatory properties of human cardiac troponin determined by in vitro motility assay. J Mol Cell Cardiol 32:1489–1498

Bione S, D'Adamo P, Maestrini E et al. (1996) A novel X-linked gene, GA.5, is responsible for Barth syndrome. Nature Genet 12:385–389

Bjarnason I, Hallgrimsson J (1980) Hypertrophic cardiomyopathy: an autopsy study of the years 1966–78. Icel Med J 66:205–209

Blair E, Price SJ, Baty CJ (2001) Mutations in cis can confound genotype-phenotype correlations in hypertrophic cardiomyopathy. J Med Genet, in press

Blanchard EM, Izuka K, Christe M et al. (1997) Targeted ablation of the murine alpha-tropomyosin gene. Circ Res 81:1005–1010

Blanchard E, Seidman C, Seidman JG et al. (1999) Altered crossbridge kinetics in the alphaMHC403/+ mouse model of familial hypertrophic cardiomyopathy. Circ Res 84:475–583

Bonne G, Carrier L, Bercovici J et al. (1995) A splice acceptor site mutation in the cardiac myosin binding protein-C gene is associated with familial hypertrophic cardiomyopathy. Nature Genet 11:438–440

Bonne G, Carrier L, Richard P et al. (1998) Familial hypertrophic cardiomyopathy. From Mutations to functional defects. Circ Res 83:580–593

Bonne G, Di Barletta MR, Varnous S et al. (1999) Mutations in the gene encoding lamin A/C cause autosomal dominant Emery-Dreifuss muscular dystrophy. Nature Genet 21:285–288

Bonow RO, Rosing DR, Bacharach SL et al. (1981) Effects of verapamil on left ventricular systolic function and diastolic filling in patients with hypertrophic cardiomyopathy. Circulation 64:787–796

Bottinelli R, Coviello DA, Redwood CS et al. (1998) A mutant tropomyosin that causes hypertrophic cardiomyopathy is expressed in vivo and associated with an increased calcium sensitivity. Circ00 Res 82:106–115

Bowles NE, Richardson PJ, Olsen EG, Archard LC (1986) Detection of Coxsackie-B-virus-specific RNA sequences in myocardial biopsy samples from patients with myocarditis and dilated cardiomyopathy. Lancet I:1120–1123

Bowles KR, Gajarski R, Porter P et al. (1996) Gene mapping of familial autosomal dominant dilated cardiomyopathy to chromosome 10q21–23. J Clin Invest 98:1355–1360

Bowman JC, Steinberg SF, Jiang T et al. (1997) Expression of protein kinase C beta in the heart causes hypertrophy in adult mice and sudden death in neonates. J Clin Invest 100:2189–2195

Braunwald E, Morrow A, Cornell W et al. (1960) Idiopathic hypertrophic subaortic stenosis. Clinical, hemodynamic and angiographic manifestation. Am J Med 29:924–945

Braunwald E, Lambrew CT, Rockoff SD (1964) Idiopathic hypertrophic subaortic stenosis: I. A description of the disease based upon an analysis of 64 patients. Circulation 29–30:3–119

Braunwald E, Zipes DP, Libby P (eds) (2001) Heart Disease, 6th edition. Saunders, Philadelphia

Brent LB, Aburano A, Fisher DL (1960) Familial muscular subaortic stenosis, an unrecognised form of "idiopathic heart disease," with clinical and autopsy finding. Circulation 21:167–180

Brigden W (1957) Uncommon myocardial diseases: The non-coronary cardiomyopathies. Lancet 2:1179–1184

Büchner F, Onishi S, Wada A (1978) Cardiomyopathy associated with Systemic Myopathy. Genetic Defect of Actomyosin Influencing Muscular Structure and Function. Urban & Schwarzenberg, Baltimore

Bulkley BH, Weisfeldt ML, Hutchins GM (1977) Asymmetric septal hypertrophy and myocardial fiber disarray: Features of normal, developing, and malformed hearts. Circulation 56:292–298

Bundgaard H, Havndrup O, Anderson PS et al. (1999) Familial hypertrophic cardiomyopathy associated with a novel missense mutation affecting the ATP-binding region of the cerdiac beta-mayosin heavy chain. J Mol Cell Cardiol 31:745–750

Caforio ALP, Stewart JP, Bonifacio E et al. (1990) Inappropriate major histocompatibility complex expression on cardiac tissue in dilated cardiomyopathy: Relevance for autoimmunity? J Autoimmun 3:187–200

Caforio ALP, Grazzini M, Mann JM et al. (1992) Identification of the α and β cardiac myosin heavy chain isoforms as major autoantigens in dilated cardiomyopathy. Circulation 85:1734–1742

Cambridge G, MacArthur CG, Waterson AP et al. (1979) Antibodies to Coxsackie B viruses in congestive cardiomyopathy. Br Heart J 41:692–696

Cannon RO, Rosing DR, Maron BJ et al. (1985) Myocardial ischemia in patients with hypertrophic cardiomyopathy: Contribution of inadequate vasodilator reserve and elevated left ventricular filling pressures. Circulation 71:234–243

Cannon RO, Tripodi D, Dilsizian V et al. (1994) Results of permanent dual-chamber pacing in symptomatic nonobstructive hypertrophic cardiomyopathy. J Cardiol 73:571–575

Carrier L, Hengstenberg C, Beckmann JS et al. (1993) Mapping of a novel gene for familial hypertrophic cardiomyopathy to chromosome 11. Nature Genet 4:311–313

Carrier L, Bonne G, Bährend E et al. (1997) Organization and sequence of human cardiac myosin binding C gene (MYBPC3) and identification of mutations predicted to produce truncated protein in familial hypertrophic cardiomyopathy. Circ Res 80:427–434

Charron P, Dubourg O, Desnos M et al. (1997) Diagnostic value of electrocardiography and echocardiography for familial hypertrophic cardiomyopathy in a genotyped adult population. Circulation 96:214–219

Chikamori T, Doi Y, Odawara H et al. (1988) Clinical pictures and prognosis of mitral valve prolapse in the middle-aged and old-aged patients. J Cardiol 18:113–8, discussion 119–120

Clark CE, Henry WL, Epstein SE (1973) Familial prevalence and genetic transmission of idiopathic hypertrophic subaortic stenosis. N Engl J Med 289:709–714

Clarke A, Harper P (1992) Genetic testing for hypertrophic cardiomyopathy. N Engl J Med 327:1175–1176

Cleland JGF, Dargie HJ, Findlay IN, Wilson JT (1987) Clinical, hemodynamic, and antiarrhythmic effects of long term treatment with amiodarone of patients in heart failure. Br Heart J 57:436–445

Codd MB, Sugrue DD, Gersh BJ, Melton LJ III (1989) Epidemiology of idiopathic dilated and hypertrophic cardiomyopathy: A population based study in Olmsted County, Minnesota, 1975–1984. Circulation 80:564–572

Consevage MW, Salada GC, Baylen GB et al. (1994) A new missense mutation, Arg719Gln, in the β-cardiac heavy chain myosin gene of patients with hypertrophic cardiomyopathy. Hum Mol Genet 3:1025–1026

Cooley DA, Leachman RD, Wukasch DC (1973) Diffuse muscular subaortic stenosis: Surgical treatment. Am J Cardiol 31:1–6

Coonar AS, Protonotarios N, Tstsopoulou A et al. (1998) Gene for arrhythmogenic right ventricular cardiomyopathy with diffuse nonepidermolytic palmoplantar keratoderma and woolly hair (Naxos disease) maps to 17q21. Circulation 97:2049–2058

Corrado D, Thiene G, Nava A et al. (1990) Sudden death in young competitive athletes: Clinicopathologic correlations in 22 cases. Am J Med 89:588–596

Cotton RG, Rodrigues NR, Campbell RD et al. (1988) Reactivity of cytosine and thymine in single-base-pair mismatches with hydroxiylamine and osmium tetroxide and ist application to the study of mutations. Proc Natl Acad Sci USA 85:4397–4401

Coulondre C, Miller JH, Farabaugh PJ, Gilbert W (1978) Molecular basis of base substitution hotspots in Escherichia coli. Nature 274:775–780

Counihan PJ, Fei I, Bashir Y et al. (1993) Assessment of heart rate variability in hypertrophic cardiomyopathy. Association with clinical and prognostic feature. Circulation 88:1682–1690

Coviello DA, Maron BJ, Spirito P et al. (1997a) Clinical features of hypertrophic cardiomyopathy causes by mutation of a "hot spot" in the alpha-tropomyosin gene. J Am Coll Cardiol 29:635–640

Coviello DA et al. (1997b) Molecular and funchoral analysis of mutant sarcomeric genes responsible for familial hypertrophic cardiomyopathy. Am J Hum Genet 61:A329

Cox DW, Nakamura Y, Gedde-Dahl T Jr (1990) Report of the committee on the genetic constitution of chromosome 14. Cytogenet Cell Genet 55:183–188

Criley JM, Siegel RJ (1986) Obstruction is unimportant in the pathophysiology of hypertrophic cardiomyopathy. Postgrad Med J 62:515–529

Criley JM, Lewis KB, White RI, Ross RS (1965) Pressure gradients without obstruction: A new concept of "hypertrophic subaortic stenosis." Circulation 32:881–887

Cronin MT, Fucini RV, Kim SM et al. (1996) Cystic fibrosis mutation detection by hybridization to light-generated DNA probe arrays. Hum Mut 7:244–255

Cuda G, Fananapazir L, Zhu W et al. (1993a) Skeletal muscle expression and abnormal function of β-myosin in hypertrophic cardiomyopathy. J Clin Invest 91:2861–2865

Cuda G, Sellers J, Epstein ND et al. (1993b) In vitro motility activity of β-cardiac myosin depends on the nature of the β-myosin heavy chain gene mutation in hypertrophic cardiomyopathy, abstracted. Circulation 88:1–343

Cuda G, Perrotti N, Perticon F et al. (1996) A previously undescribed de novo insertion-deletion mutation in the β-myosin heavy chain gene in a kindred with familial hypertrophic cardiomyopathy. Heart 76:451–452

Cuda G, Fananapazir L, Epstein ND et al. (1997) The in vitro motility activity of beta-cardiac myosin depends on the nature of the beta-myosin heavy chain gene mutation in hyper2trophic cardiomyopathy. J Muscle Res Cell Motility 18:275–283

D'Adamo P, Fassone L, Gedeon A et al. (1997) The X-linked gene G4.5 is responsible for different infantile dilated cardiomyopathies. Am J Hum Genet 61:862–867

Dausse E, Komajda M, Fetler L et al. (1993) Familial hypertrophic cardiomyopathy: Microsatellite haplotyping and identification of a hot spot for mutations in the β-myosin heavy chain gene. J Clin Invest 92:2807–2813

Davies MJ (1984) The current status of myocardial disarray in hypertrophic cardiomyopathy. Br Heart J 51:361–363

Davies MJ (1990) Hypertrophic cardiomyopathy: One disease or several? Editorial. Br Heart J 63:263–264

Davies MJ, McKenna WJ (1995) Hypertrophic cardiomyopathy: Pathology and pathogenesis. Histopathology 26:493–500

Dawid IB, Toyama R, Taira M (1995) LIM domain proteins. Comptes Rendus de l'Academie des Sciences–Serie Iii, Sciences de la Vie 318:295–306

D'Cruz LG, Baboonian C, Phillimore H et al. (2000) Cytosine methylation confers instability on the cardiac troponin T gene in hypertrophic cardiomyopathy. J Med Genet 37:0–5

De Leon JR, Fegeroff HJ, Dickson DW et al. (1994) Cardiac and skeletal myopathy in β-myosin heavy-chain simian virus 40 tsA59 transgenic mice. Proc Nat Acad Sci USA 91:519–523

Dec GW, Fuster V (1994) Idiopathic dilated cardiomyopathy. N Engl J Med 331:1564–1575

Diaz RA, Obasohan A, Oakley CM (1987) Prediction of outcome in dilated cardiomyopathy. Br Heart J 58:393–399

Ding B, Price RL, Borg TK et al. (1999) Pressure overload induces severe hypertrophy in mice treated with cyclosporine, an inhibitor of calcineurin. Circ Res 84:729–734

Doi YL, McKenna WJ, Gehrke J et al. (1980) M mode echocardiography in hypertrophic cardiomyopathy: Diagnostic criteria and prediction of obstruction. Am J Cardiol 45:6–14

Dracopoli NC, Haines JL, Korf BR et al. (1994) In Current Protocols in Human Genetics. Section 7: Searching Candidate Genes for Mutations. Wiley, N Y

Dufour C, Dausse E, Fetler L et al. (1994) Identification of a mutation near a functional site of the β-cardiac myosin heavy chain gene in a family with hypertrophic cardiomyopathy. J Cell Mol Cardiol 26:1241–1247

Durand JB, Bachinski LL, Bieling LC et al. (1995) Localization of a gene responsible for familial dilated cardiomyopathy to chromosome 1q32. Circulation. 92:3387–3389

Eastman JR, Bixler D (1977) Facio-cardial-renal syndrome: A newly delineated recessive disorder. Clin Genet 11:424–430

Elliott PM, Brecker SJ, McKenna WJ (2000) Left ventricular opacification during selective intracoronary injection of echocardiographic contrast in patients with hypertrophic cardiomyopathy. Heart 83:E7

Elliott PM, Gimeno Blanes JR, Mahon NG et al. (2001) Relation between the severity of left ventricular hypertrophy and prognosis in patients with hypertrophic cardiomyopathy. Lancet 357:420–423

Emanuel R, Withers R (1992) The cardiomyopathies. In Emery AEH, Rimoin DL (eds): General Principles and Practice of Medical Genetics. Churchill Livingstone, Edinburgh, pp. 1263–1272

Epstein SE, Rosing DR (1981) Verapamil: Its potential for causing serious complications in patients with hypertrophic cardiomyopathy. Circulation 64:437–441

Epstein ND, Cohn GM, Cyran F, Fananapazir L (1992b) Differences in clinical expression of hypertrophic cardiomyopathy associated with two distinct mutations in the β-myosin heavy chain gene. A $908^{leu-val}$ mutation and a $403^{nrg-gln}$ mutation. Circulation 86:345–352

Epstein ND, Fananapazir L, Lin HJ et al. (1992a) Evidence of genetic heterogeneity in five kindreds with familial hypertrophic cardiomyopathy. Circulation 85:635–647

Erdmann J et al. (1998) A new mutation (Arg-278-Pro) in the cardiac troponin T gene (TNNT2) was identified in one patient with hypertrophic cardiomyopathy (HCM). Circulation (Suppl) 98:I–245 (Abstract 1273)

Evans W (1949) Familial cardiomegaly. Br Heart J 11:68–82

Faber L, Meissner A, Ziemssen P, Seggewiss H (2000) Percutaneous transluminal septal myocardial ablation for hypertrophic obstructive cardiomyopathy: long term follow up of the first series of 25 patients. Heart 83:295–256.

Fadic R, Sunada Y, Waclawik AJ et al. (1996) Deficiency of a dystrophin-associated glycoprotein (adhalin) in a patient with muscular dystrophy and cardiomyopathy. N Engl J Med 334:362–366

Fananapazir L, Epstein ND (1994) Genotype-phenotype correlations in hypertrophic cardiomyopathy: Insights provided by comparisons of kindreds with distinct and identical beta-myosin heavy chain gene mutations. Circulation 89:499–502

Fananapazir L, Cannon RO, Tripodi D, Panza JA (1992) Impact of dual-chamber permanent pacing in patients with obstructive hypertrophic cardiomyopathy with symptoms refractory to verapamil and β-adrenergic blocker therapy. Circulation 85:2149–2161

Fananapazir L, Dalakas MC, Cyran F et al. (1993) Missense mutations in the β-myosin heavy chain gene cause central core disease in hypertrophic cardiomyopathy. Proc Nat Acad Sci USA 90:3993–3997

Farza H, Townsend PT, Carrier L et al. (1998) Genomic organisation, alternative splicing and polymorphisms of the human cardiac troponin T gene. J Mol Cell Cardiol 30:1247–1253

Fatkin D, Christe ME, Aristizabal O et al. (1999) Neonatal cardiomyopathy in mice homozygous for the Arg403Gln mutation in the alpha cardiac myosin heavy chain gene. J Clin Invest 103:147–153

Ferlini A, Galie N, Merlini L et al. (1998) A novel Alu-like element rearranged in the dystrophin gene causes a splicing mutation in a family with X-linked dilated cardiomyopathy. Am J Hum Genet 63:436–446

Ferlini A, Sewry C, Melis MA et al. (1999) X-linked dilated cardiomyopathy and the dystrophin gene. Neuromuscular Disorders 9:339–346

Ferrans VJ (1989) Pathologic anatomy of the dilated cardiomyopathies. Am J Cardiol 64 Suppl:9C–11C

Ferrans VJ, Morrow AG, Roberts WC (1972) Myocardial ultrastructure in idiopathic hypertrophic subaortic stenosis. A study of operatively excised left ventricular outflow tract muscle in 14 patients. Circulation 45:769–792

Fiddler GI, Tajik AJ, Weidman W et al. (1978) Idiopathic hypertrophic subaortic stenosis in the young. Am J Cardiol 42:793–799

Fitzpatrick AP, Shapiro LM, Rickards AF, Poole-Wilson P (1990) Familial restrictive cardiomyopathy with atrioventricular block and skeletal myopathy. Br Heart J 63:114–118

Flavigny J, Richard P, Isnard R (1998) Identification of two novel mutations in the ventricular regulatory myosin light chain gene (MYL2) associated with familial and classical forms of hypertrophic cardiomyopathy. J Mol Med 76:208–214

Flavigny J, Souchet M, Sebillon P et al. (1999) COOH-terminal truncated cardiac myosin-binding protein C mutants resulting from familial hypertrophic cardiomyopthy mutations exhibit altered expression and/or incorporation in fetal rat cardiomyocytes. J Mol Biol 294:443–456

Fodor WL, Darras B, Sehareseyon J et al. (1989) Human ventricular/slow twitch myosin alkali light chain gene characterization, sequence, and chromosomal location. J Biol Chem 264:2143–2149

Fontaine G, Frank R, Chomette G et al. (1982) Recurrent ventricular tachycardia caused by right ventricular dysplasia. Association with left ventricular anomalies. Archives des Maladies du Coeur et des Vaisseaux. 75:1222

Fontaine G, Fontaliran F, Frank R (1998) Arrhythmogenic right ventricular cardiomyopathies: clinical forms and main differential diagnoses. Circulation. 97:1532–1535

Forissier JF, Carrier L, Farza H et al. (1996) Codon 102 of the cardiac troponin T gene is a putative hot spot for mutations in familial hypertrophic cardiomyopathy. Circulation 94:3069–3073

Franco F, Dubois SK, Peshock RM et al. (1998) Magnetic resonance imaging accurately estimates LV mass in a transgenic mouse model of cardiac hypertrophy. Am J Physiol 274:H679–683

Frank R, Fontaine G, Vedel J et al. (1978) Electrocardiologie de quatre cas de dysplasie ventriuculaire droite arythmogène. Arch Mal Coeur Vaiss 71:963–972

Frank S, Braunwald E (1968) Idiopathic hypertrophic subaortic stenosis. Clinical analysis of 126 patients with emphasis on the natural history. Circulation 37:759–788

Franz WM, Müller M, Müller OJ et al. (2000) Association of nonsense mutation of dystrophin gene with disruption of sarcoglycan complex in X-linked dilated cardiomyopathy. Lancet 355:1781–1785

Frenneaux MP, Porter A, Caforio AL et al. (1989) Determinants of exercise capacity in hypertrophic cardiomyopathy. J Am Coll Cardiol 13:1521–1526

Frenneaux MP, Counihan PJ, Caforio AL et al. (1990) Abnormal blood pressure response during exercise in hypertrophic cardiomyopathy. Circulation 82:1995–2002

Frey N, Franz WM, Gloeckner K et al. (2000) Transgenic rat hearts expressing a human cardiac troponin T deletion reveal diastolic dysfunction and ventricular arrhythmias. Cardiovas Res 47:254–264

Fujita H, Sugiura S, Momomura S et al. (1998) Functional characterization of Dictyostelium discoideum mutant myosins equivalent to human familial hypertrophic cardiomyopathy. Adv Exper Med Biol 453:131–137

Fung DC, Yu B, Littlejohn T et al. (1999) Trent RJ. An online locus-specific mutation database for familial hypertrophic cardiomyopathy. Hum Mut 14:326–332

Furst DO, Vinkemeyer U, Weber K (1992) Mammalian skeletal muscle C-Protein: Purification from bovine muscle, binding to titin and the characterization of full length cDNA. J Cell Sci 102:769–778

Fuster V, Gersh BJ, Giuliani ER et al. (1981) The natural history of idiopathic dilated cardiomyopathy. Am J Cardiol 47:525–531

Gardin JM, Gottdiener JS, Radvany R et al. (1982) HLA linkage versus association in hypertrophic cardiomyopathy. Evidence for the absence of an association in a heterogenous Caucasian population. Chest 81:466–472

Gautel M, Zuffardi O, Freiburg A, Labeit S (1995) Phosphorylation switches specific for the cardiac isoform of myosin binding protein C: A modulator of cardiac contraction? EMBO J 14:1952–1960

Geisterfer-Lowrance AA, Kass S, Tanigawa G et al. (1990) A molecular basis for familial hypertrophic cardiomyopathy: A β cardiac myosin heavy chain gene missense mutation. Cell 62:999–1006

Geisterfer-Lowrance AA, Christe M, Conner DA et al. (1996) A mouse model of familial hypertrophic cardiomyopathy. Science 272:731–734

Georgakopoulos D, Christe ME, Giewat M et al. (1999) The pathogenesis of familial hypertrophic cardiomyopathy: Early and evolving effects from an alpha-cardiac myosin heavy chain missense mutation. Nature Med 5:327–330

Gilbert BW, Pollick C, Adelman AG, Wigle ED (1980) Hypertrophic cardiomyopathy: Subclassification by M mode echocardiography. Am J Cardiol 45:861–872

Gill CC, Duda AM, Kitazume H et al. (1982) Idiopathic hypertrophic subaortic stenosis and coronary atherosclerosis: Results of coronary artery bypass alone and myectomy combined with coronary artery bypass. J Thorac Cardiovasc Surg 84:856–860

Gillum RF (1986) Idiopathic cardiomyopathy in the United States 1970–1982. Am Heart J 111:752–755

Glancy DL, O'Brien KP, Gold HK, Epstein SE (1970) Atrial fibrillation in patients with idiopathic hypertrophic subaortic stenosis. Br Heart J 32:652–659

Gold R, Kress W, Meurers B et al. (1992) Becker muscular dystrophy: Detection of unusual disease courses by combined approach to dystrophin analysis. Muscle Nerve 15:214–218

Goldfarb LG, Park KY, Cervenakova L et al. (1998) Missense mutation in desmin associated with familial and skeletal myopathy. Nature Genet 19:402–403

Golitsina N, An Y, Greenfield NJ et al. (1997) Effects of two familial hypertrophic cardiomyopathy-causing mutations on alpha-tropomyosin structure and function. Biochemistry 36:4637–4642

Goodwin JF (1973) Treatment of cardiomyopathies. Am J Cardiol 32:341–351

Goodwin JF (1992) Cardiomyopathies and specific heart muscle diseases: Definitions, terminology, classification and new and old approaches. Postgrad Med J 68:S3–S6

Goodwin JF, Oakley CM (1972) The cardiomyopathies. Br Heart J 34:545–552

Goodwin JF, Krikler DM (1976) Arrhythmia as a cause of sudden death in hypertrophic cardiomyopathy. Lancet 2:937–940

Goodwin JF, Shah PM, Oakley CM et al. (1964) The clinical pharmacology of hypertrophic obstructive cardiomyopathy. Ciba Found Symp 99:189–199

Gottshall KR, Hunter JJ, Tanaka N et al. (1997) Ras-dependent pathways induce obstructive hypertrophy in echo-selected transgenic mice. Proc Nat Acad Sci USA 94:4710–4715

Greaves SC, Roche AHG, Neutze JM et al. (1987) Inheritance of hypertrophic cardiomyopathy: A cross sectional and M-mode echocardiographic study of 50 families. Br Heart J 58:259–266

Green PM, Montandon AJ, Bentley DR et al. (1990) The incidence and distribution of CpG–TpG transitions in the coagulation factor IX gene: A fresh look at CpG mutational hotspots. Nucleic Acids Res 18:3227–3231

Greve G, Bachinski L, Friedman DL et al. (1994) Isolation of a de novo mutant myocardial β-MHC protein in a pedigree with hypertrophic cardiomyopathy. Hum Mol Genet 3:2073–2075

Gulick J, Hewett TE, Klevitsky R. et al. (1997) Transgenic remodeling of the regulatory light chains in the mammalian hearts. Circ Res 80:655–664

Grünig E, Tasman JA, Kucherer H et al. (1998) Frequency and phenotypes of familial dilated cardiomyopathy. J Am Coll Cardiol 31:186–194

Guilford WH, Dupuis DE, Kennedy G et al. (1997) Smooth muscle and skeletal muscle myosins produce similar unitary forces and displacements in the laser trap. Biophys J 72:1006–1021

Gunning P, Ponte P, Kedes L et al. (1984) Chromosomal location of the co-expressed human skeletal and cardiac actin genes. Proc Nat Acad Sci USA 81:1813–1817

Hallidie-Smith KA, Olsen EGJ (1968) Endocardial fibroelastosis, mitral incompetence, and coarctation of abdominal aorta: A report of 3 sibs. Br Heart J 30:850–858

Hallopeau L (1869) Retrecissement ventriculo-aortique. Gaz Med Paris 24:683–684

Hamer AWF, Arkles LB, Johns JA (1989) Beneficial effects of low dose amiodarone in patients with congestive cardiac failure: A placebo-controlled trial. J Am Coll Cardiol 14:1768–1774

Hanrath P, Mathey DG, Siegert R, Bleifeld W (1980) Left ventricular relaxation and filling pattern in different forms of left ventricular hypertrophy: An echocardiographic study. Am J Cardiol 45:15–23

Harada H, Kimura A, Nishi H et al. (1992) Genetic analysis of hypertrophic cardiomyopathy, abstracted. Circulation 86:I–591

Harada H, Kimura A, Nishi H et al. (1993) A missense mutation of cardiac β-myosin heavy chain gene linked to familial hypertrophic cardiomyopathy in affected Japanese families. Biochem Biophys Res Commun 194:791–798

Harper PS, Clarke AJ (1993) Screening for hypertrophic cardiomyopathy. Br Med J 306:859–860

Harper PS, Clarke A (1995) Testing may be unhelpful. Br Med J 310:857–858

Harris L, McKenna WJ, Rowland E et al. (1983) Side effects of long-term amiodarone therapy. Circulation 67:45–51

Hasegawa K, Fujiwara H, Koshiji M. et al. (1996) Endothelin-1 and its receptor in hypertrophic cardiomyopathy. Hypertension 27:259–264

Hasty P, Ramirez-Solis R, Krumlauf R et al. (1991) Introduction of a subtle mutation into the Hox-2.6 locus in embryonic stem cells. Nature 350:243–246

Haugland H, Ohm OJ, Roman H, Thorsby E (1986) Hypertrophic cardiomyopathy in three generations of a large Norwegian family: A clinical, echocardiographic, and genetic study. Br Heart J 55:168–175

Henry WL, Clark CE, Epstein SE (1973) Asymmetric septal hypertrophy: Echocardiographic identification of the pathognomonic anatomic abnormality of IHSS. Circulation 47:225–233

Hirota H, Chen J, Betz UA et al. (1999) Loss of a gp130 cardiac muscle cell survival pathway is a critical event in the onset of heart failure during biomechanical stress. Cell 97:189–198

Hjalmarson A, Waagstein F (1991) New therapeutic strategies in chronic heart failure: Challenge of long-term beta-blockade. Eur Heart J 12:63–69

Ho CY (2000) Homozygous mutation in cardiac troponin T. Implications for HCM. Circulation 102:1950–1955

Hodgson S, Child A, Dyson M (1987) Endocardial fibroelastosis: Possible X-linked inheritance. J Med Genet 24:210–214

Hoit BD, Khoury SF, Kranias EG et al. (1995) In vivo echocardiographic detection of enhanced left ventricular function in gene-targeted mice with phopholamban deficiency. Circ Res 77:632–637

Hoit BD, Khan ZU, Pawloski-Dahm CM et al. (1997) In vivo determination of left ventricular wall stress-shortening relationship in normal mice. Am J Physiol 272:H1047–1052

Hollman A, Goodwin JF, Teare D, Renwick JW (1960) A family with obstructive cardiomyopathy (asymmetrical hypertrophy). Br Heart J 22:449–456

Holmes KC (1996) Muscle proteins—their actions and interactions. Curr Opinion Struct Biol 6:781–789

Holmes KC (1997) The swinging lever-arm hypothesis of muscle contraction. Curr Bio 7:R112–R118

Hopf R, Kaltenbach M (1990) Management of hypertrophic cardiomyopathy. Ann Rev Med 41:75–83

Horlick L, Petkovich NJ, Bolton CF (1966) Idiopathic hypertrophic subvalvular stenosis. Am J Cardiol 25:70–77

Hunter JJ, Tanaka N, Rockman HA et al. (1995) Ventricular expression of a MLC-2v-ras fusion gene induces cardiac hypertrophy and selective diastolic dysfunction in transgenic mice. J Biol Chem 270:23173–23178

Jääskelainen P, Soranta M, Miettinen R et al. (1998) The cardiac beta-myosin heavy chain gene is not the predominant gene for hypertrophic cardiomyopathy in the Finnish population. J Am Coll Cardiol 32:1709–1716

Jaenicke T, Diederich KW, Haas W et al. (1990) The complete sequence of the human β-myosin heavy chain gene and a comparative analysis of its product. Genomics 8:194–206

James J, Osinska H, Hewett TE et al. (1999) Transgenic over-expression of a motor protein at high levels results in severe cardiac pathology. Transgen Res 8:9–22

James TN, Marshall TK (1975) De subitaneis mortibus. XII. Asymmetrical hypertrophy of the heart. Circulation 51:1149–1166

Jarcho JA, McKenna W, Paré JAP et al. (1989) Mapping a gene for familial hypertrophic cardiomyopathy to chromosome 14q1. N Engl J Med 321:1372–1378

Jasmin G, Eu HY (1979) Cardiomyopathy of hamster dystrophy. Ann NY Acad Sci 317:46–58

Jeanrenaud X, Goy J-J, Kappenberger L (1992) Effects of dual chamber pacing in hypertrophic obstructive cardiomyopathy. Lancet 339:1318–1323

Jeschke B, Uhl K, Weist B et al. (1998) A high risk phenotype of hypertrophic cardiomyopathy associated with a compound genotype of two mutated β-myosin heavy chain genes. Hum Genet 102:299–304

Johnson RA, Palacios I (1982) Dilated cardiomyopathy of the adult. N Engl J Med 307:1051–1058, 1119–1126

Jontes JD (1995) Theories of muscle contraction. J Struct Biol 115:119–143

Julian DG, Camm AJ, Fox KM et al. (1996) Diseases of the Heart, 2nd edn. Saunders, London

Jung M, Poepping I, Perrot A et al. (1999) Investigation of a family with autosomal dominant dilated cardiomyopathy defines a novel locus on chromosome 2q14-q22. Am J Hum Genet 65:1068–1077

Jung WI, Sieverding I, Breuer J et al. (1998) 31P NMR spectroscopy detects metabolic abnormalities in asymptomatic patients with hypertrophic cardiomyopathy. Circulation 97:2536–2542

Kabsch W, Mannherz HG, Suck D et al. (1990) Atomic structure of the actin:DNase I complex. Nature 347:37–44

Kaltenbach M, Hopf R, Keller M (1976) Calciumantagonistische Therapie bei hypertrophisch-obstruktiver Kardiomyopathie. Dtsche Med Wochenschr 101:1284–1287

Kamisago M, Sharma SD, DePalma SR (2000) Mutations in sarcomere protein genes as a cause of dilated cardiomyopathy. N Engl J Med 343:1688–1696

Kandolf R (1988) The impact of recombinant DNA technology on the study of enterovirus Coxsackie Viruses: A General Update. In Bendinelli M, Friedman H (eds): Heart Disease. Plenum, N Y pp. 293–318

Kaplan EL, Meier P (1958) Nonparametric estimation from incomplete observations. J Am Stat Assoc 53:457–481

Kappenberger L (1995) Pacing for obstructive hypertrophic cardiomyopathy. Commentary. Br Heart J 73:107

Kappenberger L (1999) Pacing in hypertrophic cardiomyopathy. Eur Heart J 20:169–170

Kass S, MacRae C, Graber HL et al. (1994) A gene defect that causes conduction system disease and dilated cardiomyopathy maps to chromosome 1p1–1q1. Nature Genet 7:546–551

Kavinsky CJ, Umeda PK, Levin JE et al. (1984) Analysis of cloned mRNA sequences encoding subfragment 2 and part of subfragment 1 of alpha- and beta-myosin heavy chains of rabbit heart. J Biol Chem 259:2775–2781

Kaye M (1992) The Registry of the international society for heart and lung transplantation: Ninth Official Report–1992. J Heart Lung Transplant 11:599–606

Kawai M, Saeki Y, Zhao Y (1993) Crossbridge scheme and the kinetic constants of elementary steps deduced from chemically skinned papillary and trabecular muscles of the ferret. Circ Res 73:35–50

Keeling PJ, McKenna WJ (1994) Clinical genetics of dilated cardiomyopathy. Herz 19:91–96

Keeling PJ, Gang Y, Smith G et al. (1995) Familial dilated cardiomyopathy in the United Kingdom. Br Heart J 73:417–421

Kelly DP, Strauss AW (1994) Inherited cardiomyopathies. N Engl J Med 330:913–919

Keren A, Popp RL (1992) Assignment of patients into the classification of cardiomyopathies. Circulation 86:1622–1633

Kimura A, Harada H, Park JE et al. (1997) Mutations in the cardiac troponin I gene associated with hypertrophic cardiomyopathy. Nat Genet 16:379–382

Kishimoto C, Kaburagi T, Takayama S et al. (1983) Two forms of hypertrophic cardiomyopathy distinguished by inheritance of HLA haplotypes and left ventricular outflow tract obstruction. Am Heart J 105:988–994

Knight C, Kurbaan AS, Seggewiss H et al. (1997) Nonsurgical septal reduction for hypertrophic obstructive cardiomyopathy: Outcome in the first serires of patients. Circulation 95:2075

Knight BP, Goyal R, Pelosi F et al. (1999) Outcome of patients with nonischemic dilated cardiomyopathy and unexplained syncope treated with an implantable defibrillator. J Am Coll Cardiol 33:1964–1970

Kokado H, Shimizu M, Yoshio H et al. (2000) Clinical features of hypertrophic cardiomyopathy caused by a Lys183 deletion mutation in the cardiac troponin I gene. Circulation 102:663–669

Koyanagi T, Harada H, Nishi H et al. (1996) Structural and functional aspects of cardiac β-myosin heavy chain gene mutations in hypertrophic cardiomyopathy. Circulation 94:1–110

Krajinovic M, Pinamonti B, Sinagra G et al. (1995) Linkage of familial dilated: Cardiomyopathy to chromosome 9. Am J Hum Genet 57:846–852

Krehl L (1895) Beitrag zur Kenntnis der idiopathischen Herzmuskelerkrankungen. Dtsches Arch Klin Med 48:414–431

Kuang SQ, Yu JD, Lu L et al. (1996) Identification of a novel missense mutation in the cardiac β myosin heavy chain gene in a Chinese patient with sporadic hypertrophic cardiomyopathy. J Mol Cell Cardiol 28:1879–1883

Kubota T, McTierman CF, Frye CS et al. (1997) Dilated cardiomyopathy in transgenic mice with cardiac-specific overexpression of tumor necrosis factor-alpha. Circ Res 81:627–635

Kuhl U, Noutsias M, Seeberg B et al. (1994) Chronic inflammation in the myocardium of patients with clinically suspected dilated cardiomyopathy. J Cardiac Failure 1:13–25

Kuhn H, Gietzen F, Leuner C et al. (1997) Induction of subaortic septal ischaemia to reduce obstruction in hypertrophic obstructive cardiomyopathy. Studies to develop a new catheter-based concept of treatment. Eur Heart J 18:846–851

Kumar A et al. (1997) Rescue of cardiac alpha-actin-deficient mice by enteric smooth muscle gamma-actin. Proc Natl Acad Sci. USA. 94:4406–4411

Kunst G, Kress KR, Gruen M et al. (2000) Myosin binding protein C, a phosphorylation-dependent force regulator in muscle that controls the attachment of myosin heads by its interaction with myosin S2. Circ Res. 86:51–58

Labeit S, Kolmerer B (1995) Titins: Giant proteins in charge of muscle ultrastructure and elasticity. Science 270:293–296

Laitinen PJ, Brown KM, Piippo K et al. (2001) Mutations of the cardiac ryanodine receptor (RyR2) gene in familial polymorphic ventricular tachycardia. Circulation 103:485–490

Landegren U, Kaiser R, Sanders J et al. (1988) A ligase-mediated gene detection technique. Science 241:1077–1080

Lankford EB, Epstein ND, Fananapazir L, Sweeney HL (1995) Abnormal contractile properties of muscle fibers expressing β-myosin heavy chain gene mutations in patients with hypertrophic cardiomyopathy. J Clin Invest 95:1409–1414

Latham RD, Mulrow JP, Virmani R et al. (1989) Recently diagnosed idiopathic dilated cardiomyopathy: Incidence of myocarditis and efficacy of prednisone therapy. Am Heart J 117:876–882

Li D, Tapscoft T, Gonzales O et al. (1999) Desmin mutation responsible for idiopathic dilated cardiomyopathy. Circulation 100:461–464

Li Y, Huang TT, Carlson EJ et al. (1995) Dilated cardiomyopathy and neonatal lethality in mutant mice lacking manganese superoxide dismutase. Nature Genet 11:376–381

Lichter P, Umeda PK, Levin JE, Vosberg HP (1986) Partial characterization of the human β-myosin heavy-chain which is expressed in heart and skeletal muscle. Eur J Biochem 160:419–426

Liew CC, Sole MJ, Yamauchi-Takihara K et al. (1990) Complete sequence and organization of the human cardiac β-myosin heavy chain gene. Nucleic Acids Res 18:3647–3651

Lim DS, Oberst L, McCluggage et al. (2000a) Decreased left ventricular ejection fraction in transgenic mice expressing mutant cardiac troponin T-Q92, responsible for human hypertrophic cardiomyopathy. J Mol Cell Cardiol 32:365–374

Lim HW, De Windt LJ, Mante J et al. (2000b) Reversal of cardiac hypertrophy in transgenic disease models by calcineurin inhibition. J Mol Cell Cardiol 32:697–709

Lin D, Bobkova A, Homsher E et al. (1996) Altered cardiac troponin T in vitro function in the presence of a mutation implicated in familial hypertrophic cardiomyopathy. J Clin Invest 97:2.842–2848

Liouville H (1869) Retrecissment cardiaque sous aortique. Gaz Med Paris 24:161

Litt M, Luty JA (1989) A hypervariable microsatellite revealed by in vitro amplification of a dinucleotide repeat within the cardiac muscle actin gene. Am J Hum Genet 44:397–401

Liu W, Smith DI, Rechtzigel KJ et al. (1998) Denaturing high performance liquid chromatography (DHPLC) used in the detection of germline and somatic mutations. Nucleic Acids Res 26:1396–1400

Lompré A-M, Nadal-Ginard B, Mahdavi V (1984) Expression of the cardiac ventricular alpha- and beta-myosin heavy chain genes is developmentally and hormonally regulated. J Biol Chem 259:6437–6446

Loogen F, Kuhn H, Gietzen F et al. (1983) Clinical course and prognosis of patients with typical and atypical hypertrophic obstructive and with hypertrophic non-obstructive cardiomyopathy. Eur Heart J 4:145–153

Lopez MJ, Wong SK, Kishimoto I et al. (1995) Salt-resistant hypertension in mice lacking the guanylyl cyclase-A receptor for atrial natriuretic peptide. Nature 378:65–68

Lorell BH (1985) Use of calcium channel blockers in hypertrophic cardiomyopathy. Am J Med 78:43–54

Lowey S, Waller GS, Trybus KM (1993) Skeletal muscle myosinlight chains are exxential for physiological. Nature 365:454–456

Macera MJ, Szabo P, Wadgaonkar R et al. (1992) Localization of the gene coding for ventricular myosin regulatory light chain (MYL2) to human chromosome 12q23–q24.3. Genomics 13:829–831

MacRae CA, Ghaisas N, Kass S et al. (1995) Familial hypertrophic cardiomyopathy with Wolff-Parkinson-White syndrome maps to a locus on chromosome 7q3. J Clin Invest 96:1216–1220

Maeda M, Holder E, Lowes B et al. (1997) Dilated cardiomyopathy associated with deficiency of the cytoskeletal protein. Circulation 95:17–20

Maisch B, Deeg P, Liebau G, Kochsiek K (1983) Diagnostic relevance of humoral and cytotoxic immune reactions in primary and secondary dilated cardiomyopathy. Am J Cardiol 52:1072–1078

Mall G (1988) Kardiomyopathie aus der Sicht des Pathologen. Therapiewoche 38:1175–1184

Manolio TA, Baughman KL, Rodeheffer R et al. (1992) Prevalence and etiology of idiopathic dilated cardiomyopathy (summary of a national heart, lung, and blood institute workshop). Am J Cardiol 69:1458–1466

Marcus FI, Fontaine GH, Guiraudon G et al. (1982) Right ventricular dysplasia: A report of 24 adult cases. Circulation 65:384–398

Mares A, Greve G, Tapscott T, Roberts R (1993) Screening and identification of known and novel mutations in hypertrophic cardiomyopathy based on scanning with chemical cleavage. Circulation 88:I–572

Margossian SS, White HD, Caulfield JB et al. (1992) Light chain 2 profile and activity of human ventricular myosin during dilated cardiomyopathy: Identification of a causal agent for impaired myocardial function. Circulation 85:1720–1733

Marian AJ (2000) Pathogenesis of diverse clinical and pathological phenotypes in hypertrophic cardiomyopathy. Lancet 355:58–60

Marian AJ, Roberts R (1995a) Recent advances in the molecular genetics of hypertrophic cardiomyopathy. Circulation 92:1336–1347

Marian AJ, Roberts R (1995b) Molecular genetics of hypertrophic cardiomyopathy. Annu Rev Med 46:213–222

Marian AJ, Yu Q-T, Mares A et al. (1992) Detection of a new mutation in the β-myosin heavy chain gene in an individual with hypertrophic cardiomyopathy. J Clin Invest 90:2156–2165

Marian AJ, Yu Q-T, Mann DL et al. (1995) Expression of a mutation causing hypertrophic cardiomyopathy disrupts sarcomere assembly in adult feline cardiac myocytes. Circ Res 77:98–106

Marian AJ, Wu Y, Lim DS et al. (1999) A transgenic rabbit model for human hypertrophic cardiomyopathy. J Clini Invest 104:1683–1692

Maron BJ (1998) Cardiovascular risks to young persons on the athletic field. Ann Int Med 129:79–86

Maron BJ, Epstein SE (1980) Hypertrophic cardiomyopathy. Recent observations regarding the specificity of three hallmarks of the disease: Asymmetric septal hypertrophy, septal disorganization and systolic anterior motion of the anterior mitral leaflet. Am J Cardiol 45:141–154

Maron BJ, Henry WL, Clark CE et al. (1976) Asymmetric septal hypertrophy in childhood. Circulation 53:9–19

Maron BJ, Merrill WH, Freier PA et al. (1978a) Long-term clinical course and symptomatic status of patients after operation for hypertrophic subaortic stenosis. Circulation 57:1205–1213

Maron BJ, Lipson LC, Roberts WC et al. (1978b) "Malignant" hypertrophic cardiomyopathy: Identification of a subgroup of families with unusually frequent premature death. Am J Cardiol 41:1133–1140

Maron BJ, Roberts WC, McAllister HA et al. (1980) Sudden death in young athletes. Circulation 62:218–229

Maron BJ, Gottdiener JS, Bonow RO, Epstein SE (1981a) Hypertrophic cardiomyopathy with unusual locations of left ventricular hypertrophy undetectable by M-mode echocardiography: Identification by wide-angle two-dimensional echocardiography. Circulation 63:409–418

Maron BJ, Gottdiener JS, Epstein SE (1981b) Patterns and significance of distribution of left ventricular hypertrophy in hypertrophic cardiomyopathy: A wide angle, two dimensional echocardiographic study of 125 patients. Am J Cardiol 48:418–428

Maron BJ, Savage DD, Wolfson JK, Epstein SE (1981c) Prognostic significance of 24 hour ambulatory electrocardiographic monitoring in patients with hypertrophic cardiomyopathy: A prospective study. Am J Cardiol 48:252–257

Maron BJ, Roberts WC, Epstein SE (1982a) Sudden death in hypertrophic cardiomyopathy: A profile of 78 patients. Circulation 65:1388–1394

Maron BJ, Tajik AJ, Ruttenberg HD et al. (1982b) Hypertrophic cardiomyopathy in infants: Clinical features and natural history. Circulation 65:7–17

Maron BJ, Nichols PF III, Pickle LW et al. (1984) Patterns of inheritance in hypertrophic cardiomyopathy: Assessment by M-mode and two dimensional echocardiography. Am J Cardiol 53:1087–1094

Maron BJ, Spirito P, Wesley Y, Arce J (1986a) Development and progression of left ventricular hypertrophy in children with hypertrophic cardiomyopathy. N Engl J Med 315:610–614

Maron BJ, Wolfson JK, Epstein SE, Roberts WC (1986b) Intramural ("small vessel") coronary artery disease in hypertrophic cardiomyopathy. J Am Coll Cardiol 8:545–557

Maron BJ, Bonow RO, Cannon RO et al. (1987a) Hypertrophic cardiomyopathy: Interrelations of clinical manifestations, pathophysiology, and therapy (Part I). N Engl J Med 316:780–789

Maron BJ, Bonow RO, Cannon RO et al. (1987b) Hypertrophic cardiomyopathy: Interrelations of clinical manifestations, pathophysiology, and therapy (Part II). N Engl J Med 316:844–852

Maron BJ, Kragel AH, Roberts WC (1990) Sudden death in hypertrophic cardiomyopathy with normal left ventricular mass. Br Heart J 63:308–310

Maron BJ, Gardin JM, Flack JM et al. (1995) Prevalence of hypertrophic cardiomyopathy in a general population of young adults: Echocardiographic analysis of 4111 subjects in the CARDIA study. Circulation 92:785–789

Maron BJ, Nishimura RA, McKenna WJ et al. (1999) Assessment of permanent dual-chamber pacing as a treatment for drug-refractory symptomatic patients with obstructive hypertrophic cardiomyopathy. A randomized, double-blind, crossover study (M-PATHY). Circulation 99:2927–2933

Maron BJ, Shen WK, Link MS et al. (2000) Efficacy of implantable cardioverter-defibrillators for the prevention of sudden death in patients with hypertrophic cardiomyopathy. N Engl J Med 342:365–373

Mason JW, O'Connell JB, Herskowitz A et al. (1995) A clinical trial of immunosuppressive therapy for myocarditis. N Engl J Med 333:269–275

Matsumori A, Hirose K, Wakabayashi A et al. (1979) HLA and hypertrophic cardiomyopathy. Am Heart J 97:428–431

Matsumori A, Kawai C, Wakabayashi A et al. (1981) HLA-DRW4 antigen linkage in patients with hypertrophic obstructive cardiomyopathy. Am Heart J 101:14–16

Matsuoka R, Yoshida MC, Kanda N et al. (1989) Human cardiac myosin heavy chain gene mapped within chromosome region 14q11.2-q13. Am J Med Genet 32:279–284

Maurice P, Ben-Ismail M, Penther PH et al. (1966) Les myocardiopathies obstructive. I. Etude clinique et radiologique. Arch Mal Coeurs Vaiss 59:375–390

McConnel BK, Jones KA, Fatkin D et al. (1999) Dilated cardiomyopathy in homozygous myosin-binding protein-C mutant mice. J Clin Invest 104:1235–1244

McDonald K, McWilliams E, O'Keefee B, Maurer B (1988) Functional assessment of patients treated with permanent dual chamber pacing as a primary treatment for hypertrophic cardiomyopathy. Eur Heart J 9:893–899

McIntosh CL, Maron BJ (1988) Current operative treatment of obstructive cardiomyopathy. Circulation 78:487–495

McKenna WJ (1987) Sudden death in hypertrophic cardiomyopathy: Identification of the "high risk" patient. In Brugada P, Wellens HJJ (eds): Cardiac Arrhythmias: Where to Go From Here? Futura Publishing, Munt Kisco, NY, pp. 352–365

McKenna WJ (1989) Hypertrophic cardiomyopathy. In Julian DG, Camm AJ, Fox KM et al. (eds): Diseases of the Heart. Bailliere-Tindall, London, pp. 933–950

McKenna WJ (2001) The Cardiomyopathies: Hypertrophic, Dilated, Restrictive and Right Ventricular. In Warrell Da, Cox TM, Firth JD and Benz EJ (eds): Oxford Textbook of Medicine, 4th edn. Oxford University Press.

McKenna WJ, Goodwin JF (1981) The natural history of hypertrophic cardiomyopathy. Curr Probl Cardiol 6:1–26

McKenna WJ, Deanfield JE (1984) Hypertrophic cardiomyopathy: An important cause of sudden death. Arch Dis Child 59:971–975

McKenna WJ, Camm AJ (1989) Sudden death in hypertrophic cardiomyopathy: Assessment of patients at high risk. Circulation 80:1489–1492

McKenna WJ, Davies JF (1995) Immunosuppression for myocarditis, editorial. N Engl J Med 333:312–313

McKenna WJ, Watkins H (1995) Hypertrophic cardiomyopathy. In Scriver CR, Beaudet AL, Sly WS, Valle D (eds): The Metabolic and Molecular Basis of Inherited Disease. McGraw-Hill, NY, p. 4253

McKenna WJ, England D, Doi YL et al. (1981a) Arrhythmia in hypertrophic cardiomyopathy. I: Influence on prognosis. Br Heart J 46:168–172

McKenna W, Deanfield J, Faruqui A et al. (1981b) Prognosis in hypertrophic cardiomyopathy: Role of age and clinical, electrocardiographic and hemodynamic features. Am J Cardiol 47:532–538

McKenna WJ, Oakley CM, Krikler DM, Goodwin JF (1985) Improved survival with amiodarone in patients with hypertrophic cardiomyopathy and ventricular tachycardia. Br Heart J 53:412–416

McKenna WJ, Kleinebenne A, Nihoyannopoulos P, Foale R (1988b) Echocardiographic measurement of right ventricular wall thickness in hypertrophic cardiomyopathy: Relation to clinical and prognostic features. J Am Coll Cardiol 11:351–358

McKenna WJ, Stewart JT, Nihoyannopoulos P et al. (1990) Hypertrophic cardiomyopathy without hypertrophy: Two families with myocardial disarray in the absence of increased myocardial mass. Br Heart J 63:287–290

McKenna WJ, Thiene G, Nava A et al. (1994) Diagnosis of arrhythmogenic right ventricular dysplasia/cardiomyopathy. Br Heart J 71:215–218

McKenna WJ, Spirito P, Desnos M et al. (1997) Experience from clinical genetics in hypertrophic cardiomyopathy: proposal for new diagnostic criteria in adult members of affected families. Heart 77:130–132

McKoy G, Protonotarios N, Crosby A et al. (2000) Identification of a deletion in plakoglobin in arrhythmogenic right ventricular cardiomyopathy with palmoplanatar keratoderma and woolly hair (Naxos disease). Lancet 355:2119–2124

McLatchie GR, Pedoe DS, McKenna WJ et al. (1993) Screening for hypertrophic cardiomyopathy. Br Med J 306:860

McLellan WR, Schneider MD (1997) Death by design. Programmed cell death in cardiovascular biology and disease. Circ Res 81:137–144

McNally EM, Kraft R, Bravo-Zehnder M et al. (1989) Full-length rat alpha and beta cardiac myosin heavy chain sequences. Comparisons suggest a molecular basis for functional differences. J Mol Biol 210:665–671

Meerschwam IS (1972) Hypertrophic obstructive cardiomyopathy. Nederlands Tijdschrift voor Geneeskunde 116:607–612

Megeney LA, Kablar B, Perry RL et al. (1999) Severe cardiomyopathy in mice lacking dystrophin and MyoD. Proc Nat Acad Sci USA 96:220–225

Melacini P, Fanin M, Duggan DJ et al. (1999) Heart involvement in muscular dystrophies due to sarcoglycan gene mutations. Muscle & Nerve 22:473–479

Merlini L, Kaplan JC, Navarro C et al. (2000) Homogeneous phenotype of the gypsy limb-girdle MD with the gamma-sarcoglycan C283Y mutation. Neurology 54:1075–1079

Messina DN, Speer MC, Pericak-Vance MA et al. (1997) Linkage of familial dilated cardiomyopathy with conduction defect and muscular dystrophy to chromosome 6q23. Am J Hum Genet 61:909–917

Mestroni L, Miani D, Di LA et al. (1990) Clinical and pathologic study of familial dilated cardiomyopathy. Am J Cardiol 65:1449–1453

Mestroni L, Krajinovic M, Severini GM et al. (1994) Familial dilated cardiomyopathy. Br Heart J 72:35–41

Mestroni L, Maisch B, McKenna WJ et al. (1999) Guidelines for the study of familial dilated cardiomyopathies. Eur Heart J 20:93–102

Michele DE, Albayya FP, Metzger JM (1999) Direct, convergent hypersensitivity of calcium-activated force generation produced by hypertrophic cardiomyopathy mutant alpha-tropomyosins in adult cardiac myocytes. Nature Med 5:1413–1417

Michels VV, Moll PP, Miller FA et al. (1992) The frequency of familial dilated cardiomyopathy in a series of patients with idiopathic dilated cardiomyopathy. N Engl J Med 326:77–82

Milasin J, Muntoni F, Severine GM et al. (1996) A point mutation in the 5' splice site of the dystrophin gene first intron responsible for X-linked dilated cardiomyopathy. Hum Mol Genet 5:73–79

Minamisawa S, Hoshijima M, Chu G et al. (1999) Chronic phospholamban-sarcoplasmic reticulum calcium ATPase interaction is the critical calcium cycling defect in dilated cardiomyopathy. Cell 99:313–322

Mogensen J, Klausen IC, Pedersen AK et al. (1999) α-Cardiac actin is a novel disease gene in familial hypertrophic cardiomyopathy. J Clin Invest 103:R39–R43

Molkentin JD, Lu JR, Antos CL et al. (1998) A calcineurin-dependent transcriptional pathway for cardiac hypertrophy. Cell 93:215–228

Moolman JA, Reith S, Uhl K et al. (2000) A newly created splice donor site in exon 25 of the MyBP-C gene is responsible for inherited hypertrophic cardiomyopathy with incomplete disease penetrance. Circulation 101:1396–1402

Moolman JC, Brink PA, Corfield VA (1993) Identification of a new missense mutation at Arg403, a CpG mutation hotspot, in exon 13 of the β-myosin heavy chain gene in hypertrophic cardiomyopathy. Hum Mol Genet 2:1731–1732

Moolman JC, Brink PA, Corfield VA (1995) Identification of a novel Ala797Thr mutation in exon 21 of the beta-myosin heavy chain gene in hypertrophic cardiomyopathy. Hum Mut 6:197–198

Moolman JC, Corfield VA, Posen B et al. (1997) Sudden death due to troponin T mutations. J Am Coll Cardiol 29:549–555

Moolman-Smook JC, Mayosi B, Brink P et al. (1998) Identification of a new missense mutation in MyBP-C associated with hypertrophic cardiomyopathy. J Med Genet 35:253–254

Moolman-Smook JC, De Lange WJ, Bruwer EC et al. (1999) The origins of hypertrophic cardiomyopathy-causing mutations in two

South African subpopulations: A unique profile of both independent and founder events. Am J Hum Genet 65:1308–1320

Morano I, Ritter O, Bonz A et al. (1995) Myosin light chain-actin interaction regulates cardiac contractility. Circ Res 76:720–725

Morano I, Chai GX, Baltas LG et al. (2000) Smooth-muscle contraction without smooth muscle myosin. Nature Cell Bio Vol 2:371–375

Morimoto S, Yanaga F, Minakami R et al. (1998) Ca2+-sensitizing effects of the mutations at Ile-79 and Arg-92 of troponin T in hypertrophic cardiomyopathy. Am J Physiol 275:C200–207

Mörner S, Richard P, Kazzam E et al. (2000) Deletion in the cardiac troponin I gene in a family from northern Sweden with hypertrophic cardiomyopathy. J Mol Cell Cardiol 32:521–525

Morrow AG, Fogarty TJ, Hannah H III, Braunwald E (1968) Operative treatment in idiopathic hypertrophic subaortic stenosis: Techniques and the results of preoperative and postoperative and hemodynamic assessments. Circulation 37:589–596

Morrow AG, Reitz BA, Epstein SE et al. (1975) Operative treatment in idiopathic hypertrophic subaortic stenosis: techniques and the results of pre- and postoperative assessments in 83 patients. Circulation 57:1205–1213

Moss RL, Periera JS (2000) Enhanced myosin function due to a point mutation causing a familial hypertrophic cardiomyopathy. Circ Res 86:720–722

Muchir A, Bonne G, van der Kooi AJ et al. (2000) Identification of mutations in the gene encoding lamins A/C in autosomal dominant limb girdle muscular dystrophy with atrioventricular conduction disturbances (LGMD1B). Hum Mol Genet 9:1453–1459

Mudge GH, Goldstein S, Addonizio LJ et al. (1993) Twenty-fourth Bethesda Conference: Cardiac transplantation: Task Force 3: recipient guidelines/prioritization. J Am Coll Cardiol 22:21–31

Muir P, Nicholson F, Tilzey AJ et al. (1989) Chronic relapsing pericarditis and dilated cardiomyopathy: Serological evidence of persistent enterovirus infection. Lancet I:804–807

Muntoni F, Cau M, Ganau A et al. (1993) Brief report: Deletion of the dystrophin muscle-promoter region associated with X-linked dilated cardiomyopathy. N Engl J Med 329:921–925

Muthuchamy M, Pieples K, Rethinasamy P et al. (1999) Mouse model of a familial hypertrophic cardiomyopathy mutation in α-tropomyosin manifests cardiac dysfunction. Circ Res 85:47–56

Nakajima-Taniguchi C, Matsui H, Nagata S et al. (1995) Novel missense mutation in alpha-tropomyosin gene found in Japanese patients with hypertrophic cardiomyopathy. J Mol Cell Cardiol 27:2053–2058

Nakajima-Taniguchi C, Matsui H, Fujio Y et al. (1997) Novel missense mutation in cardiac troponin T gene found in Japanese patient with hypertrophic cardiomyopathy. J Mol Cell Cardiol 29:839–843

Nakata M, Nishi H, Iwami G et al. (1966) Different clinical manifestations of hypertrophic cardiomyopathy between patients with cardiac beta-maosin heavy chain gene and cardiac troponin T gene mutations, abstracted. Circulation 9:I–110

Nakaura H, Morimoto S, Yanaga F et al. (1999) Functional changes in troponin T by a splice donor site mutation that causes hypertrophic cardiomyopathy. Ame J Physiol 277:C225–232

Neu N, Craig SW, Rose NR et al. (1987) Coxsackie virus induced myocarditis in mice: Cardiac myosin autoantibodies do not cross-react with the virus. Clin Exp Immunol 69:566–574

Nevin NC, Hill AE, Carson DJ (1991) Facio-cardio-renal (Eastman-Bixler) syndrome. Am J Med Genet 40:31–33

Niimura H, Bachinski LL, Sangwatanaroj S et al. (1998) Mutations in the gene for cardiac myosin-binding protein C and late-onset familial hypertrophic cardiomyopathy. N Eng J Med 4:1248–1256

Nishi H, Kimura A, Harada H et al. (1992) Novel missense mutation in cardiac β-myosin heavy chain gene found in a Japanese patient with familial hypertrophic cardiomyopathy. Biochem Biophys Com 188:379–387

Nishi H, Kimura A, Harada H et al. (1994) Possible gene dose effect of a mutant cardiac β-myosin heavy chain gene on the clinical expression of familial hypertrophic cardiomyopathy. Biochem Biophy Res Com 200:549–556

Nishi H, Kimura A, Harada H et al. (1995) A myosin missense mutation, not a null allele, causes familial hypertrophic cardiomyopathy. Circulation 91:2911–2915

Nishimura RA, Trusty JM, Hayes DL et al. (1997) Dual-chamber pacing for hypertrophic cardiomyopathy: a randomized, double-blind, crossover trial. J Am Coll Cardiol 29:435–441

Oberst L, Zhao G, Park JT et al. (1998) Dominant-negative effect of a mutant cardiac troponin T on cardiac structure and function in transgenic mice. J Clin Invest 102:1498–1505

Ohsuzu F, Katsushika S, Akanuma M et al. (1997) Hypertrophic obstructive cardiomyopathy due to a novel T-to-A transition at codon 624 in the beta-myosin heavy chain (beta-MHC) gene possibly related to the sudden death. Int J Cardiol 62:203–209

Olivotto I, Cecchi F, Santoro G et al. (1999) Atrial fibrillation is an important determinant of outcome in patients with hypertrophic cardiomyopathy. Circulation 1000:176 (abstract)

Olson TM, Keating MT (1996) Mapping a cardiomyopathy locus to chromosome 3p22-p25. J Clin Invest 97:528–532

Olson TM, Michels W, Thibodeau SN et al. (1998) Actin mutations in dilated cardiomyopathy, a heritable form of heart failure. Science 280:750–752

O'Neill ME, Marietta J, Nishimura D et al. (1996) A gene for autosomal dominant late-onset progressive non-syndromic hearing loss, DFNA10, maps to chromosome 6. Hum Mol Genet 5:853–856

Opitz JM (1982) The developmental field concept in clinical genetics. J Pediatrics 101:805–809

Orita M, Suzuki Y, Sekiya T, Hayashi K (1989) A rapid and sensitive detection of point mutations and DNA polymorphisms using the polymerase chain reaction. Genomics 5:874–879

Packer M, Bristow MR, Cohn JN et al. (1996) The effect of carvedilol on morbidity and mortality in patients with chronic heart failure. U.S. Carvedilol Heart Failure Study Group. N Engl J Med 334:1349–1355

Paré JAP, Fraser RG, Pirozynski WJ et al. (1961) Hereditary cardiovascular dysplasia: A form of familial cardiomyopathy. Am J Med 31:37–62

Parrillo JE, Cunnion RE, Epstein SE et al. (1989) A prospective, randomized, controlled trial of prednisone for dilated cardiomyopathy. N Engl J Med 321:1061–1068

Pearce PC, Hawkey C, Symons C, Olsen EG (1985) Role of calcium in the induction of cardiac hypertrophy and myofibrillar disarray: Experimental studies of possible cause of hypertrophic cardiomyopathy. Br Heart J 54:420–427

Pelliccia A, Maron BJ, Spataro A et al. (1991) The upper limit of physiologic cardiac hypertrophy in highly trained elite athletes. N Engl J Med 324:295–301

Perloff JK, de Leon AC Jr, O'Doherty D (1966) The cardiomyopathy of progressive muscular dystrophy. Circulation 33:625–648

Perryman MB, Yu Q, Marlan AJ et al. (1992) Expression of missense mutation in the messenger RNA for β-myosin heavy chain in myocardial tissue in hypertrophic cardiomyopathy. J Clin Invest 90:271–277

Pitt B, Zannad F, Remme WJ et al. (1999) The effect of spironolactone on morbidity and mortality in patients with severe heart failure. Randomized Aldactone Evaluation Study Investigators. N Engl J Med 341:709–717

Poetter K, Jiang H, Hassanzadeh S et al. (1996) Mutations in either the essential or regulatory light chains of myosin are associated with a rare myopathy in human heart and skeletal muscle. Nat Genet 13:63–69

Pollick C, Rakowski H, Wigle ED (1984) Muscular subaortic stenosis: the quantitative relationship between systolic anterior motion and the pressure gradient. Circulation 69:43–49

Pringle JWS (1949) The excitation and contraction of the flight muscles of insects. J Physiol 108:226–234

Priori SG, Napolitano C, Tiso N et al. (2001) Mutations in the Cardiac Ryanodine Receptor Gene (hyRy2) underline carecholaminergic polymorphic ventricular Tachycardia. Circulation 103:196–200

Protonotarios N, Tsatsopoulou A, Patsourakos P et al. (1986) Cardiac abnormalities in familial palmoplantar keratosis. Br Heart J 56:321–326

Pyeritz RE (2001) Genetics and cardiovascular disease. In Braunwald E, Zipes DP, Libby P (eds): Heart Disease, 6th edn. WP Saunders, Philadelphia, pp. 1977–2018

Raffaele Di Barletta M, Ricci E, Galluzzi G et al. (2000) Different mutations in the LMNA gene cause autosomal dominant and autosomal recessive Emery-Dreifuss muscular dystrophy. Am J Hum Gen 66:1407–1412

Rampazzo A, Nava A, Danieli GA et al. (1994) The gene for arrhythmogenic right ventricular cardiomyopathy maps to chromosome 14q23–q24. Hum Mol Genet 3:959–962

Rampazzo A, Nava A, Erne P et al. (1995) A new locus for arrhythmogenic right ventricular cardiomyopathy (ARVD2) maps to chromosome 1q42–q43. Hum Mol Genet 4:2151–2154

Rampazzo A, Nava A, Miorin M et al. (1997) ARVD4, a new locus for arrhythmogenic right ventricular cardiomyopathy, maps to chromosome 2 long arm. Genomics 45:259–263

Rayment I, Rypniewski WR, Schmidt-Bäse K et al. (1993a) Three-dimensional structure of myosin subfragment-1: A molecular motor. Science 261:50–58

Rayment I, Holden HM, Whittaker M et al. (1993b) Structure of the actin-myosin complex and its implications for muscle contraction. Science 261:58–65

Rayment I, Holden HM, Sellers J et al. (1995) Structural interpretation of the mutations in the β-cardiac myosin that have been implicated in familial hypertrophic cardiomyopathy. Proc Natl Acad Sci 92:3864–3868

Reid JM, Houston AB, Lundmark E (1989) Hypertrophic cardiomyopathy in identical twins. B Heart J 62:384–388

Richard P, Ismard R, Carrier L et al. (1999) Double heterozygosity for mutations in the beta-myosin heavy chain and in the cardiac myosin binding protein C genes in a family with hypertrophic cardiomyopathy. J Med Genet 36:542–545

Richard P, Charron P, Leclercq C et al. (2000) Homozygotes for a R869G mutation in the beta-myosin heavy chain gene have a severe form of familial hypertrophic cardiomyopathy. J Mol Cell Cardiol 32:1575–1583

Richardson P, McKenna W, Bristow M et al. (1996) Report of the 1995 World Health Organization/International Society and Federation of Cardiology Task Force on the definition and classification of cardiomyopathies. Circulation 93:841–842

Rideout WM, Coetzee GA, Olumi AF, Jones PA (1990) 5-Methylcytosin as an endogenous mutagen in the human LDL receptor and p53 genes. Science 249:1288–1290

Roberts WC, Ferrans VJ (1975) Pathologic anatomy of the cardiomyopathies: Idiopathic dilated and hypertrophic types, infiltrative types, and endomyocaridal disease with and without eosinophilia. Hum Pathol 6:287–342

Roberts WC, Siegel RJ, McManus BM (1987) Idiopathic dilated cardiomyopathy: Analysis of 152 necropsy patients. Am J Cardiol 60:1340–1355

Robinson K, Frenneaux MP, Stockins B et al. (1990) Atrial fibrillation in hypertrophic cardiomyopathy: A longitudinal survey. J Am Coll Cardiol 15:1279–1285

Rockman HA, Chien KR, Choi DJ et al. (1998) Expression of a beta-adrenergic receptor kinase 1 inhibitor prevents the development of myocardial failure in gene-targeted mice. Proc Natl Acad Sci USA 95:7000–7005

Ronaghi M, Uhlen M, Nyren P (1998) A sequencing method based on real-time pyrophosphate. Science 281:363, 365

Roopnarine O, Leinwand LA et al. (1998) Functional analysis of myosin mutations that cause familial hypertrophic cardiomyopathy. Biophys J 75:3023–3030

Rosenzweig A, Watkins H, Hwang DS et al. (1991) Preclinical diagnosis of familial hypertrophic cardiomyopathy by genetic analysis of blood lymphocytes. N Engl J Med 325:1753–1760

Rosing DR, Kent KM, Borer JS et al. (1979) Verapamil therapy: A new approach to the pharmacologic treatment of hypertrophic cardiomyopathy. I. Hemodynamic effects. Circulation 60:1201–1207

Ross RS, Bulkley BH, Hutchins GM et al. (1978) Idiopathic familial myocardiopathy in three generations: A clinical and pathological study. Am Heart J 96:170–178

Rottbauer W, Grünig E, Brown BD et al. (1996) A novel β-myosin heavy chain mutation in a large family suffering from dilated and hypertrophic cardiomyopathy. Circulation 94:I–162–163

Rottbauer W, Gautel M, Zehelein J et al. (1997) Novel splice donor site mutation in the cardiac myosin-binding protein-C gene in familial hypertrophic cardiomyopathy. Characterization of cardiac transcript and protein. J Clin Invest 100:475–482

Ruder MA, Winston SA, Davis JC et al. (1985) Arrhythmogenic right ventricular dysplasia in a family. Am J Cardiol 59:799–800

Ruiz P, Brinkmann V, Ledermann B et al. (1996) Targeted mutation of plakoglobin in mice reveals essential functions of desmosomes in the embryonic heart. J Cell Biol 135:215–225

Rust EM, Albayya FP, Metzger JM (1999) Identification of a contractile deficit in adult cardiac myocytes expressing hypertrophic cardiomyopathy-associated mutant troponin T proteins. J Clin Invest 103:1459–1467

Ryan MP, French J, Al-Mahdawi S et al. (1995) Genetic testing for familial hypertrophic cardiomyopathy in newborn infants. Br Med J 310:856–857

Sadoul N, de Chillou C, Aliot E et al. (1999) Evaluation of the risk of sudden death in hypertrophic cardiomyopathy. Archives des Maladies du Coeur et des Vaisseaux. 92 Spec No 1:65–73

Saez LJ, Gianola KM, McNally EM et al. (1987) Human cardiac myosin heavy chain genes and their linkage in the genome. Nucleic Acids Res 15:5443–5459

St John Sutton MG, Lie JT, Anderson KR et al. (1980) Histopathological specificity of hypertrophic obstructive cardiomyopathy: Myocardial fibre disarray and myocardial fibrosis. Br Heart J 44:433–443

Sakamoto A, Ono K, Abe M et al. (1997) Both hypertrophic and dilated cardiomyopathies are caused by mutation of the same gene, α-sarcoglycan, in hamster: An animal model of disrupted dystrophin-associated glycoprotein complex. Proc NatAcad Sci USA 94:13873–13878

Sakthivel S, Joseph PK, Tharakan JM et al. (2000) A novel missense mutation (R712L) adjacent to the "active thiol" region of the cardiac beta-myosin heavy chain gene causing hypertrophic cardiomyopathy in an Indian family. Hum Mut 15:298–299

Sanbe A, Nelson D, Gulick J et al. (2000) In vivo analysis of an essential myosin light chain mutation linked to familial hypertrophic cardiomyopathy. Circ Res 87:296–302

Sanderson JE, Traill TA, Sutton MG et al. (1978) Left ventricular relaxation and filling in hypertrophic cardiomyopathy: An echocardiographic study. Br Heart J 40:596–601

Santorelli FM, Mak SC, El-Schahawi M et al. (1996) Maternally inherited cardiomyopathy and hearing loss associated with a novel mutation in the mitochondrial tRNA (Lys) gene (G8363A). Am J Hum Gen 58:933–939

Sata M, Ikebe M (1996) Functional analysis of the mutations in the human cardiac β-myosin that are responsible for familial hypertrophic cardiomyopathy. J Clin Invest 98:2.866–2873

Satoh M, Takahashi M, Sakamoto T et al. (1999) Structural analysis of the titin gene in hypertrophic cardiomyopathy: Identification of a novel disease gene. Biochem Biophys Res Com 262:411–417

Savage DD, Seides SF, Clark CE et al. (1978) Electrocardiographic findings in patients with obstructive and nonobstructive hypertrophic cardiomyopathy. Circulation 58:402–408

Savage DD, Seides SF, Maron BJ et al. (1979) Prevalence of arrhythmias during 24-hour electrocardiographic monitoring and exercise testing in patients with obstructive and nonobstructive hypertrophic cardiomyopathy. Circulation 59:866–875

Schleef M, Werner K, Satzger U et al. (1993) Chromosomal location and genomic cloning of the mouse α-tropomyosin gene Tpm-1. Genomics 17:519–521

Schmincke A (1907) Uber linksseitige muskulöse Conusstenosen. Dtsche Med Wochenschr 33:2082–2083

Schönberger J, Levy H, Grünig E et al. (2000) Dilated cardiomyopathy and sensorineural hearing loss. Circulation 101:1812–1818

Schröder RR, Manstein D, Jahn W et al. (1993) Three-dimensional atomic model of F-actin decorated with Dictyostelium myosin S1. Nature 364:171–174

Schulte HD, Bircks WH, Loesse B et al. (1993) Prognosis of patients with hypertrophic obstructive cardiomyopathy after transaortic myectomy. Late results up to twenty-five years. J Thor Cardiovasc Surg 106:709–717

Schwartz K, Beckmann J, Dufour C et al. (1992) Exclusion of cardiac myosin heavy chain and actin gene involvement in hypertrophic cardiomyopathy of several French families. Circulation Res 71:3–8

Seiler C, Hess OM, Schoenbeck M et al. (1991) Long-term follow-up of medical versus surgical therapy for hypertrophic cardiomyopathy: A retrospective study. J Am Coll Cardiol 17:634–642

Severini GM, Krajinovic M, Pinamonti B et al. (1996) A new locus for arrhythmogenic right ventricular dysplasia on the long arm of chromosome 14. Genomics 31:193–200

Shackleton S, Lloyd DJ, Jackson SNJ et al. (2000) LMNA, encoding lamin A/C, is mutated in partial lipodystrophy. Nature Gen 24:153–156

Shah PM (1988) Echocardiography in congestive or dilated cardiomyopathy. J Am Soc Echocardiogr 1:20–30

Shah PM, Gramiak R, Adelman AG, Wigle ED (1971) Role of echocardiography in diagnostic and hemodynamic assessment of hypertrophic subaortic stenosis. Circulation 44:891–898

Shapiro LM, McKenna WJ (1983) Distribution of left ventricular hypertrophy in hypertrophic cardiomyopathy: A two-dimensional echocardiographic study. J Am Coll Cardiol 2:437–444

Shapiro LM, Kleinebenne A, McKenna WJ (1985) The distribution of left ventricular hypertrophy in hypertrophic cardiomyopathy: Comparison to athletes and hypertensives. Eur Heart J 6:967–974

Shuman S (1994) Novel approach to molecular cloning and polynucleotide synthesis using vaccinia DNA topoisomerase. J Biol Chem 269:32678–32684

Siewertsen MA, Vosberg HP, Cox DW (1990) A polymorphism of the MYH7 gene. Nucleic Acids Res 18:6173

Sinha AM, Umeda PK, Kavinsky CJ et al. (1982) Molecular cloning of mRNA sequences for cardiac alpha- and beta-form myosin heavy chains: expression in ventricles of normal, hypothyroid, and thyrotoxic rabbits. Proc Nat Acad Sci USA 79:5847–5851

Siu BL, Niimura H, Osborne JA et al. (1999) Familial dilated cardiomyopathy locus maps to chromosome 2q31. Circulation 99:1022–1026

Slade AKB, Keeling PJ, Prased K et al. (1994) Hypertrophic cardiomyopathy: Pacing and defibrillator therapy, J Am Coll Cardiol 24:484A

Slade AK, Sadoul N, Shapiro L. et al (1996) DDD pacing in hypertrophic cardiomyopathy: a multicentre clinical experience. Heart 75:44–49

Solomon SD, Geisterfer-Lowrance AAT, Vosberg HP et al. (1990a) A locus for familial hypertrophic cardiomyopathy is closely linked to cardiac myosin heavy chain genes, CRI-L436 and CRI-L329 on chromosome 14 at q11–q12. Am J Hum Genet 47:389–394

Solomon SD, Jarcho JA, McKenna W et al. (1990b) Familial hypertrophic cardiomyopathy is a genetically heterogeneous disease. J Clin Invest 86:993–999

Sorimachi H, Freiburg A, Kolmerer B et al. (1997) Tissue-specific expression and alpha-actinin binding properties of the Z-disc titin:

implications for the nature of vertebrate Z-discs. J Mol Biol 270:688–695

Spindler M, Saupe KW, Christe ME et al. (1998) Diastolic dysfunction and altered energetics in the alphaMHC403/+ mouse model of familial hypertrophic cardiomyopathy. J Clin Invest 101:1775–1783

Spirito P, Maron BJ, Bonow RO, Epstein SE (1987) Occurrence and significance of progressive left ventricular wall thinning and relative cavity dilatation in hypertrophic cardiomyopathy. Am J Cardiol 60:123–129

Spirito P, Chiarella F, Carratino L et al. (1989) Clinical course and prognosis of hypertrophic cardiomyopathy in an outpatient population. N Engl J Med 320:749–755

Spirito P, Seidman CE, McKenna WJ et al. (1997) The management of hypertrophic cardiomyopathy. N Engl J Med 336:775–785

Stewart JT, McKenna WJ (1994) Management of arrhythmias in hypertrophic cardiomyopathy. Cardiovasc Drugs Ther 8:95–99

Straceski AJ, Geisterfer-Lowrance AAT, Seidman CE et al. (1994) Functional analysis of myosin missense mutations in familial hypertrophic cardiomyopathy. Proc Nat Acad Sci USA 91:589–593

Sugiura S, Kobayakawa N, Fujita H et al. (1998) Comparison of unitary displacements and forces between 2 cardiac myosin isoforms by the optical trap technique: Molecular basis for cardiac adaptation. Circ Res 82:1029–1034

Sugiura S, Kobayakawa N, Fujita H et al. (1998) Distinct kinetic properties of cardiac myosin isoforms revealed by in vitro studies. Adv Experim Med Biol 453:125–130

Sugrue DD, Rodeheffer RJ, Codd MB et al. (1992) The clinical course of idiopathic dilated cardiomyopathy: A population based study. Ann Intern Med 117:117–123

Sullivan T, Escalante-Alcalde D, Bhatt H et al. (1999) Loss of A-type lamin expression compromises nuclear envelope intergrity leading to muscular dystrophy. J Cell Biol 147:913–920

Sussman MA, Lim HW, Gude N et al. (1998) Prevention of cardiac hypertrophy in mice by calcineurin inhibition. Science 281:1690–1693

Sutton MG, Tajik AJ, Gibson DG et al. (1978) Echocardiographic assessment of left ventricular filling and septal and posterior wall dynamics in idiopathic hypertrophic subaortic stenosis. Circulation 57:512–520

Suwa M, Hirota Y, Kawamura K (1984) Improvement in left ventricular diastolic function during intravenous and oral diltiazem therapy in patients with hypertrophic cardiomyopathy: An echocardiographic study. Am J Cardiol 54:1047–1053

Sweeney HL, Straceski AJ, Leinwand LA et al. (1994) Heterologous expression of a cardiomyopathic myosin that is defective in its actin interaction. J Biol Chem 269:1603–1605

Sweeny HL, Feng HS, Yang Z et al. (1998) Functional analyses of troponin T mutations that cause hypertrophic cardiomyopaathy: insights into disease pathogenesis and troponin function. Proc Nat Acad Sci USA 95:14406–14410

Szczesna D, Zhang Ren, Zhao J et al. (2000) Altered regulation of cardiac muscle contraction by troponin T mutations that cause familial hypertrophic cardiomyopathy. J Biol Chem 275:624–630

Takai E, Akita H, Shiga N et al. (1999) Mutational analysis of the cardiac actin gene in familial and sporadic dilated cardiomyopathy. Am J Med Genet 86:325–327

Tanigawa G, Jarcho JA, Kass S et al. (1990) A molecular basis for familial hypertrophic cardiomyopathy: An α/β cardiac myosin heavy chain hybrid gene. Cell 62:991–998

Tardiff JC, Factor SM, Tompkins BD et al. (1998) A truncated cardiac troponin T molecule in transgenic mice suggests multiple cellular mechanisms for familial hypertrophic cardiomyopathy. J Clin Invest 101:2800–2811

Tardiff JC, Hewett TE, Palmer BM et al. (1999) Cardiac troponin T mutations result in allele-specific phenotypes in a mouse model for hypertrophic cardiomyopathy. J Clin Invest 104:469–481

Tazelaar HD, Billingham ME (1986) Leukocytic infiltrates in idiopathic dilated cardiomyopathy: A source of confusion with active myocarditis. Am J Surg Pathol 10:405–412

Teare D (1958) Asymmetrical hypertrophy of the heart in young adults. Br Heart J 20:1–8

ten Cate FJ, Hugenholtz PG, van Dorp WG, Roelandt J (1979) Prevalence of diagnostic abnormalities in patients with genetically transmitted asymmetric septal hypertrophy. Am J Cardiol 43:731–737

Tesson F, Richard P, Charron P et al. (1998) Genotype-phenotype analysis in four families with mutations in beta-myosin heavy chain gene responsible for familial hypertrophic cardiomyopathy. Hum Mut 12:385–392

Thiene G, Nava A, Corrado D et al. (1988) Right ventricular cardiomyopathy and sudden death in young people. N Engl J Med 318:129–133

Thiene G, Basso C, Danieli GA et al. (1997) Arrhythmogenic right ventricular cardiomyopathy. A still uncrecognized clinical entitity. Trends Cardiocvasc Med 7:84–90

Thierfelder L, MacRae C, Watkins H et al. (1993) A familial hypertrophic cardiomyopathy locus maps to chromosome 15q2. Proc Natl Acad Sci USA 90:6270–6274

Thierfelder L, Watkins H, MacRae C et al. (1994) α-Tropomyosin and cardiac troponin T mutations cause familial hypertrophic cardiomyopathy: A disease of the sarcomere. Cell 77:701–712

Tiso N, Stephan DA, Nava A et al. (2001) Identification of mutations in the cardiac ryanodine receptor gene in families affected with arrhythmogenic right ventricular cardiomyopathy type 2 (ARVD2). Hum Mol Genet 10:189–194

Tobacman LS, Lins D, Butters C et al. (1999) Functional consequences of troponin T mutations found in hypertrophic cardiomyopathy. J Biol Chem 274:28363–28370

Towbin JA (1998) The role of cytoskeletal Proteins in cardiomyopathies. Curr Opin Cell Biol 10:131–139

Towbin JA, Hejtmancik JF, Brink P (1993) X-linked dilated cardiomyopathy: Molecular genetic evidence of linkage to the Duchenne muscular dystrophy (dystrophin) gene at the Xp21 locus. Circulation 87:1854–1865

Toyo-oka T et al. (1994) A novel mutation for myosin heavy chain gene from cardiac β to foetal skeletal type in a family with HCM, DCM and sudden death. EJH (Abstract)

Trinick J (1994) Titin and nebulin: protein rulers in muscle? Trends Biochem Sci 19:405–409

Tyska MJ, Hayes E, Giewat M et al. (2000) Single-molecule mechanics of R403Q cardiac myosin isolated from the mouse model of famillial hypertrophic cardiomyopathy. Circ Res 86:737–744

Underhill PA, Jin L, Lin AA et al. (1997) Detection of numerous Y chromosome biallelic polymorphisms by denaturing high-performance liquid chromatography. Gen Res 7:996–1005

Uyeda TQ, Spudich JA (1993) A functional recombinant myosin II lacking a regulatory light chain-binding site. Science 262:1867–1870

Uyeda TQ, Abramson PD, Spudich JA (1996) The neck region of the myosin motor domain acts as a lever arm to generate movement. Proc Natl Acad Sci USA 93:4459–4464

van Dorp WG, ten Cate FJ, Vletter WB et al. (1976) Familial prevalence of asymmetric septal hypertrophy. Eur J Cardiol 4:349–357

Varnava A, Baboonian C, Davison F et al. (1999) A new mutation of the cardiac troponin T gene causing familial hypertrophic cardiomyopathy without left ventricular hypertrophy. Heart 82:621–624

Vemuri R, Lankford EB, Poetter K et al. (1999) The stretch-activation response may be critical to the proper functioning of the mammalian heart. Proc Nat Acad Sci USA 96:1048–1053

Verlinsky Y, Handyside A, Grifo J et al. (1994) Preimplantation diagnosis of genetic and chromosomal disorders. J Ass Reprod Genet 11:236–243

Vikstrom KL, Factor SM, Leinwand LA (1996) Mice expressing mutant myosin heavy chains are a model for familial hypertrophic cardiomyopathy. Mol Med 2:556–567

Vosberg HP (2000) Genetic counselling for hypertrophic cardiomyopathy: are we ready for it? Curr Control Trials Cardiovasc Med 1:41–44

Vosberg HP, McKenna WJ (1996) Cardiomyopathies. In Rimoin DL, Connor JM, Pyeritz RE (eds): Principles and Practice of Medical Genetics, 3rd edn. Churchill Livingstone, NY, pp. 843–877

Vosberg HP, Haberbosch W (1998) Kardiomyopathien–Genetische Ursachen und Pathogenese. In Ganten D, Ruckpaul K (eds): Handbuch der Molekularen Medizin Band 3. Springer Verlag Berlin, pp. 61–110

Vosberg HP, Weist B, Uhl K et al. (1999) Molecular diagnosis of causes of dominantly inherited hypertrophic cardiomyopathies. In Schumacher G, Sauer U (eds): Genetics of Cardiopathies. Wiss. Verl.-Ges, Stuttgart, 233–247

Waagstein F, Caidahl K, Wallentin I et al. (1989) Long-term beta-blockade in dilated cardiomyopathy: Effects of short- and long-term metoprolol treatment followed by withdrawal and readministration of metoprolol. Circulation 80:551–563

Wagner JA, Sax FL, Weisman HF et al. (1989) Calcium-antagonist receptors in the atrial tissue of patients with hypertrophic cardiomyopathy. N Engl J Med 320:755–761

Waldmüller S, Sakthivel S, Vosberg HP (1999) Eine Myosin "rod"-Mutation ist assoziiert mit einer schweren hypertrophischen Kardiomyopathie. Zeitschr für Kardiologie 88:E927

Watkins H, Seidman CE, MacRae C et al. (1992a) Progress in familial hypertrophic cardiomyopathy: Molecular genetic analyses in the original family studied by Teare. Br Heart J 67:34–38

Watkins H, Rosenzweig A, Hwang DS et al. (1992b) Characteristics and prognostic implications of myosin missense mutations in familial hypertrophic cardiomyopathy. N Engl J Med 326:1108–1114

Watkins H, Thierfelder L, Hwang DS et al. (1992c) Sporadic hypertrophic cardiomyopathy due to de novo myosin mutations. J Clin Invest 90:1666–1671

Watkins H, MacRae C, Thierfelder L et al. (1993a) A disease locus for familial hypertrophic cardiomyopathy maps to chromosome 1q3. Nature Genet 3:333–337

Watkins H, Thierfelder L, Anan R et al. (1993b) Independent origin of identical beta cardiac myosin heavy chain mutations in hypertrophic cardiomyopathy. Am J Hum Genet 53:1180–1185

Watkins H, McKenna WJ, Thierfelder L et al. (1995a) Mutations in genes for cardiac troponin T and α-tropomyosin in hypertrophic cardiomyopathy. N Engl J Med 332:1058–1064

Watkins H, Conner D, Thierfelder L et al. (1995b) Mutations in the cardiac myosin binding protein-C gene on chromosome 11 cause familial hypertrophic cardiomyopathy. Nature Genet 11:434–437

Watkins H, Seidman CE, Seidman JG et al. (1996) Expression and functional assessment of a truncated cardiac troponin T that cause hypertrophic cardiomyopathy. Evidence for a dominant negative action. J Clin Invest 98:2456–2461

Weber JL, May PE (1989) Abundant class of human DNA polymorphisms which can be typed using the polymerase chain reaction. Am J Hum Genet 44:388–396

Weiss A, Schiaffino S, Leinwand LA (1999) Comparative sequence analysis of the complete human sarcomeric myosin heavy chain family: implications for functional diversity. J Mol Biol 290:61–75

Weist B, Vosberg HP (1995) Identification of a new FHC mutation in the human β-MHC gene, abstracted. J Mol Cell Cardiol 26:119

Welikson RE, Buck SH, Ratel JR et al. (1999) Cardiac myosin heavy chains lacking the light chain binding domain cause hypertrophic cardiomyopathy in mice. Am J Physiol 276:H2148–H2158

White SP, Cohen C, Phillips GN (1987) Structure of cocrystals of tropomyosin and troponin. Nature 325:826–828

WHO/ISFC (1980) Report of the WHO/ISFC Task Force on the definition and classification of cardiomyopathies. Br Heart J 44:672–673

Wigle ED, Heimbecker RO, Gunton RW (1962) Idiopathic ventricular septal hypertrophy causing muscular subaortic stenosis. Circulation 26:325–340

Wigle ED, Sasson Z, Henderson MA et al. (1985) Hypertrophic cardiomyopathy: the importance of the site and the extent of hypertrophy: A review. Prog Cardiovasc Dis 28:1–83

Wigle ED, Henderson M, Rakowski H, Wilansky S (1986) Muscular (hypertrophic) subaortic stenosis (hypertrophic obstructive cardiomyopathy): the evidence for true obstruction to left ventricular outflow. Postgrad Med J 62:531–536

Wigle ED, Rakowski H, Kimball BP, Williams WG (1995) Hypertrophic cardiomyopathy. Clinical spectrum and treatment. Circulation 92:1680–1692

Wolfgram LJ, Beisel KW, Herskowitz A, Rose NR (1986) Variations in the susceptibility to coxsackie virus B3-induced myocarditis among different strains of mice. J Immunol 136:1846–1852

Wolska BM, Keller RS, Evans CC et al. (1999) Correlation between Myofilament response to Ca^{2+} and altered dynamics of contraction and relaxation in transgenic cardiac cells that express β-Tropomyosin. Circ Res 84:745–751

Yamaguchi H, Ishimura T, Nishiyama S et al. (1979) Hypertrophic nonobstructive cardiomyopathy with giant negative T waves (apical hypertrophy): Ventriculographic and echocardiographic features in 30 patients. Am J Cardiol 44:401–412

Yamaguchi-Takihara K, Nakajima-Taniguchi C, Matsui H et al. (1996) Clinical implications of hypertrophic cardiomyopathy associated with mutations in the α-tropomyosin gene. Heart 76:63–65

Yamashita H, Lowey S, Trybus KM (1997) Functional consequences of myosin heavy chain mutation implicated in familial hypertrophic cardiomyopathy. Biophys J 72:A339

Yanaga F, Morimoto S, Ohtsuki I (1999) Ca2+ sensitization and potentiation of the maximum level of myofibrillar ATPase activity caused by mutations of troponin T found in familial hypertrophic cardiomyopathy. J Biol Chem 274:8806–8812

Yang O, Sanbe A, Osinska H et al. (1998) A mouse model of myosin binding protein C human familial hypertrophic cardiomyopathy. J Clin Invest 102:1292–1300

Yang O, Sanbe A, Osinska H et al. (1999) In vivo modeling of myosin binding protein C familial hypertrophic cardiomyopathy. Circ Res 85:841–847

Yamashita H, Lowey S, Trybus KM (1997) Functional consequences of myosin heavy chain mutations implicated in familial hypertrophic cardiomyopathy. Biophys J 72:A339

Youssoufian H, Antonarakis SE, Bell W et al. (1988) Nonsense and missense mutations in hemophilia A: Estimate of the relative mutation rate at CG dinucleotides. Am J Hum Genet 42:718–725

Yu B, French JA, Carrier L et al. (1998) Molecular pathology of familial hypertrophic cardiomyopathy caused by mutations in the cardiac myosin binding protein C gene. J Med Genet 35:205–10

Yu QT, Ifegwu J, Marian AJ et al. (1993) Hypertrophic cardiomyopathy mutation is expressed in messenger RNA of skeletal as well as cardiac muscle. Circulation 87:406–412

Zachara E, Cafario ALP, Carboni GP et al. (1993) Familial aggregation of idiopathic dilated cardiomyopathy: Clinical features and pedigree analysis in 14 families. Br Heart J 69:129–135

Zhang W, Kowal RC, Rusnak F et al. (1999) Failure of calcineurin inhibitors to prevent pressure-overload left ventricular hypertrophy in rats. Circ Res 84:722–728

Zezulka A, MacKintosh P, Jobson S et al. (1986) Human lymphocyte antigens in hypertrophic cardiomyopathy. Int J Cardiol 12:193–202

Zot AS, Potter JD (1987) Structural aspects of troponin-tropomyosin regulation of skeletal muscle contraction. Annu Rev Biophys Biophys Chem 16:535–559

Familial dysrhythmias and conduction disorders

Jeffrey A. Towbin

Introduction

Dysrhythmias typically are thought to occur due to primary or secondary abnormalities in cardiac electrophysiology. These abnormalities can include primary alterations in myocardial conduction and repolarization or those occurring as a result of structural heart disease. A significant portion of the individuals found to have abnormalities of rhythm and conduction are now known to have specific genetic mutations. Familial inheritance of dysrhythmias and conduction disorders indicates that genetic factors play an integral role in development of these abnormalities. Understanding the underlying genetic defects responsible for these disorders has provided insights to pathogenesis and promises to impact the therapeutic strategies used in clinical management. Over the course of the past decade, our understanding of the genetic abnormalities in hypertrophic cardiomyopathy, long QT syndrome and Brugada syndrome has led to general concepts of cardiovascular disease. In this chapter, the clinical features and management of familial dysrhythmias and conduction disorders will be discussed and the current understanding of the genetic abnormalities associated with these disorders will be reviewed.

Specific cardiac dysrhythmias

The entire cardiac electrical system can be affected by genetic abnormalities, leading to atrial and ventricular tachydysrhythmias, sinus node dysfunction (SND), or atrioventricular block (AV block). Primary dysrhythmias and secondary dysrhythmias (i.e., those associated with structural heart disease) are discussed below.

Primary abnormalities in cardiac rhythm: ventricular tachydysrhythmias

LONG QT SYNDROMES

The long QT syndromes (LQTS) are primary disorders of cardiac repolarization in which prolongation of the QT interval corrected for heart rate (QTc) is seen on the surface electrocardiogram (ECG) along with abnormalities of T wave morphology and sinus bradycardia (Schwartz et al., 2000a,b) (Fig. 50.1). Syncope, seizures, and sudden death are the clinical features that are commonly seen, occurring due to ventricular tachycardia (VT), especially polymorphic VT or *torsade de pointes* (Fig. 50.2), which can degenerate into ventricular fibrillation (VF). *Torsade de pointes* is common in all forms of LQTS, and is defined as "turning of the points." which reflects the varying axis of the QRS complex during VT (Schwartz et al., 2000a,b). This dysrhythmia is a subset of polymorphic VT, to be distinguished from monomorphic VT, which has a different morphology and mechanism of development (Viskin et al., 1996; El-Sherif et al., 1997). Monomorphic VT usually results from reentrant mechanisms and typically can be induced by programmed electrical stimulation. On the other hand, polymorphic VT cannot be induced using programmed electrical stimulation, suggesting that the mechanism is unlikely to be primary reentry. *Torsade de pointes*, in fact, is thought to be initiated by abnormal automaticity and then maintained by reentrant mechanisms (Antzelevitch, 1999). Development of early after depolarizations (EADs) appear

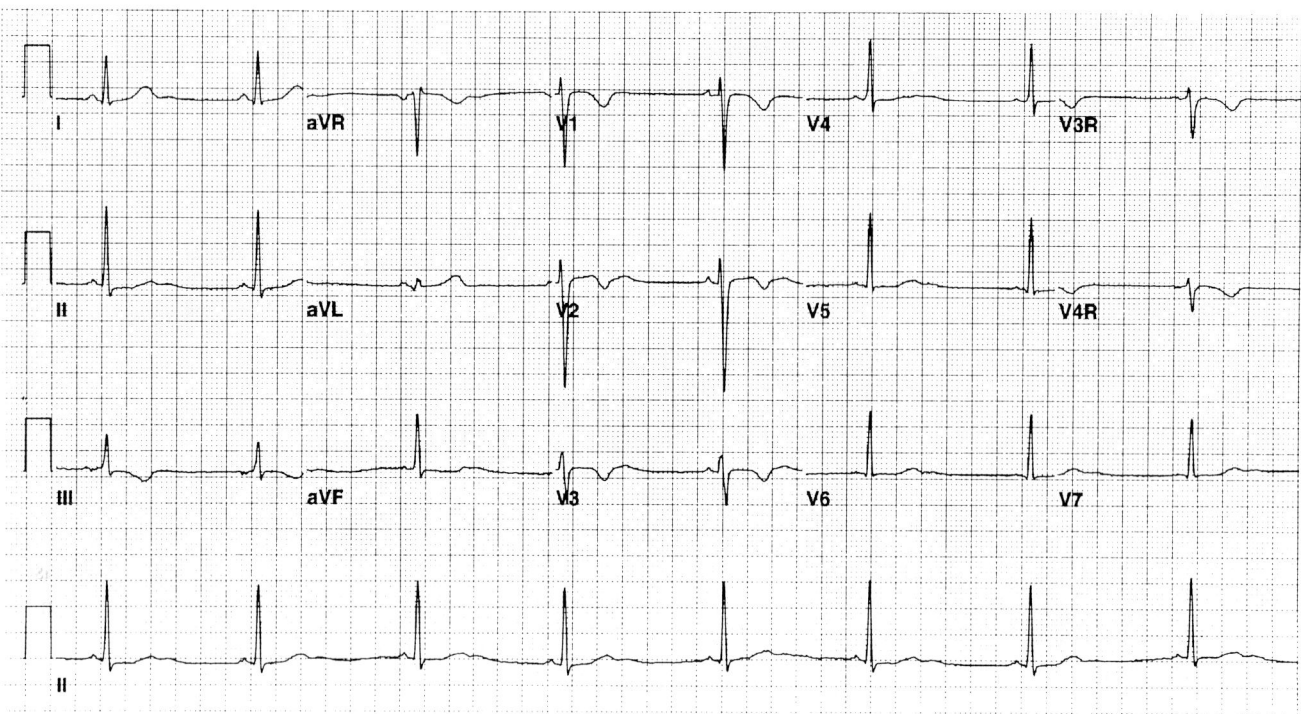

Fig. 50.1. Fourteen year-old female with long QT syndrome. Note the sinus bradycardia (48 bpm), very prolonged QTc of 600 milliseconds, with low amplitude bifid T waves.

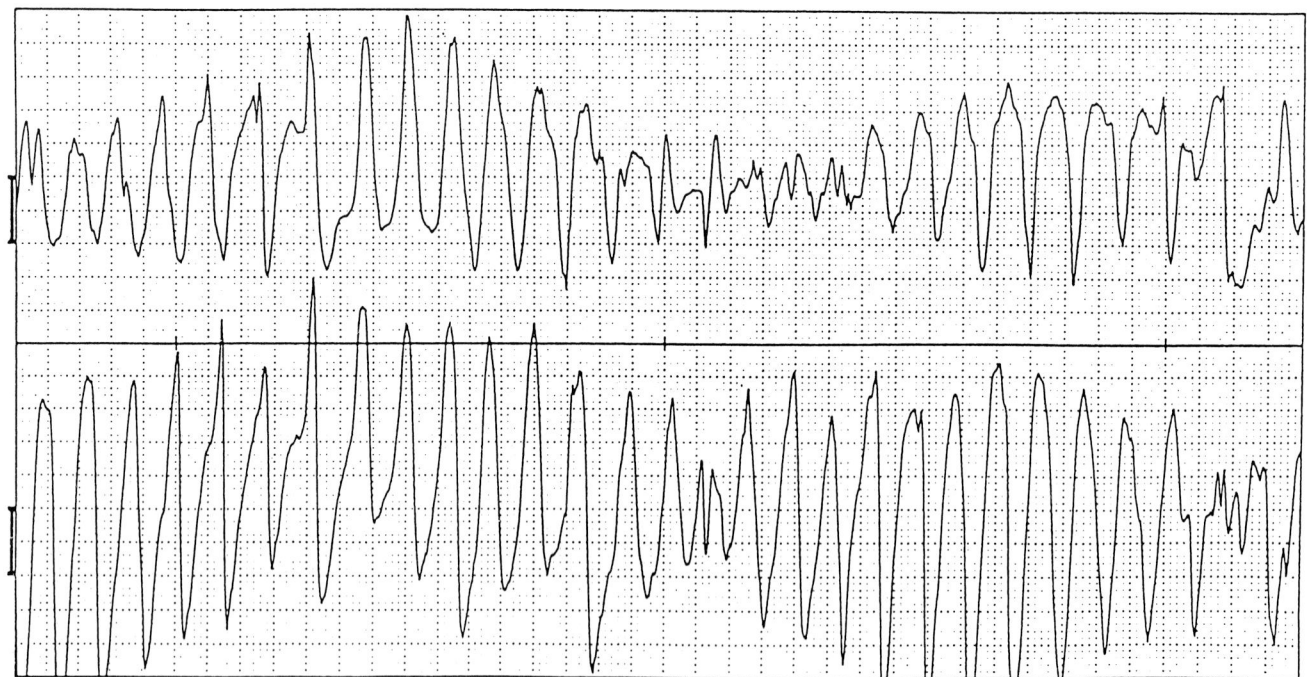

Fig. 50.2. *Torsade de pointes* polymorphic ventricular tachycardia.

to be an important mechanism whereby drug-induced action potential prolongation initiates torsade (January and Riddle, 1989; Verduyn et al., 1997). Under normal conditions, the ventricle is activated from subendocardium to epicardium by impulses arising in the subendocardial Purkinje network. Mapping data in animal models support the idea that the initial beat in torsade arises in the subendocardium, consistent with a triggered beat arising from an

EAD in the Purkinje system (El-Sherif et al., 1996). The conditions that evoke EADs markedly prolong repolarization in the mid-myocardium (M cell region) as well, resulting in a situation where propagation of EAD-related triggered beats from the subendocardium may be blocked in regions where M cell action potentials have become especially long, setting up intramural reentrant excitation with a circuit that varies from beat to beat (Antzelevitch et al., 1995). This perhaps accounts for the distinctive morphology of *torsade de pointes* (Asano et al., 1997; El-Sherif et al., 1997).

Recently, the concept has emerged that defects in currents important for repolarization prolong the action potential but are not directly arrhythmogenic. Rather, action potential duration creates a milieu in which genetically normal, drug-unmodified ion channels or other electrogenic phenomena further prolong repolarization and precipitate arrhythmias.

The long QT syndromes have been classified into acquired and genetically inherited forms. Acquired long QT syndrome is the most common form of LQTS, with drug-induced LQTS particularly common. Drugs implicated in acquired LQTS include antiarrhythmic agents such as quinidine or sotalol, tricyclic antidepressants, antibiotics (especially macrolide antibiotics such as erythromycin), antihistamines such as terfenidate, and inhalational anesthetics. Acquired LQTS has also been seen in association with metabolic derangements including hypokalemia, hypomagnesemia, and hypercalcemia. Additionally, acquired LQTS has been identified in patients with other cardiac diseases such as cardiomyopathies and myocardial ischemia, as well as under circumstances of intracranial disease (i.e., intracranial surgery, subarachnoid hemorrhage, and increased intracranial pressure).

Two forms of inherited LQTS are known: Romano-Ward LQTS (Romano et al., 1963; Ward, 1964) and Jervell and Lange-Nielsen syndrome (Jervell and Lange-Nielsen, 1957). Romano-Ward syndrome is characterized by autosomal dominant inheritance with reduced penetrance and is the most common inherited form of LQTS, estimated to have an incidence of 1 in 10,000 live births worldwide (Priori et al., 1999a,b; Vatta and Towbin, 2000). Jervell and Lange-Nielsen syndrome is a seemingly rare condition, with an estimated incidence of 1 in 1.6 million live births (Priori et al., 1999a,b; Vatta and Towbin, 2000). This latter disorder, which is defined as LQTS associated with sensorineural deafness, has been described as having autosomal recessive inheritance since its initial description in 1957 (Jervell and Lange-Nielsen, 1957). Recent molecular genetic studies, however, have clarified its inheritance, suggesting it to be autosomal dominant LQTS associated with autosomal recessive deafness. Finally, sudden infant death syndrome (SIDS) has been shown to be another presentation of inherited LQTS (Schwartz et al., 2000a,b).

Clinical features

Long QT syndrome is typically identified in individuals presenting with syncope, seizures or sudden cardiac death from episodic ventricular tachydysrhythmias, particularly *torsade de pointes* and ventricular fibrillation (Priori et al., 1999a,b; Schwartz et al., 2000a,b; Vatta and Towbin, 2000). Cardiac dysrhythmias have been reported in up to 24% of cases, but the risk of sudden death has been estimated to be less than 1% per year. These estimates are almost certainly inaccurate, however, since a significant percentage of the 300,000–400,000 sudden deaths occurring in the United States yearly (Myerburg, 1997) are likely to be the result of this disorder (which goes unrecognized); and many living patients are asymptomatic and can have normal QT intervals on screening ECGs due to reduced penetrance. Today, many asymptomatic family members are being identified via screening ECGs and molecular genetic family studies, and, therefore, better estimates are likely in the future.

Since LQTS may be difficult to diagnose, a set of criteria have been developed by Schwartz and colleagues (Schwartz et al., 1991, 2000a,b). These criteria use a point system in the diagnostic scheme, relying heavily on classic features (Table 50.1). This approach is thought to improve diagnostic accuracy by including major criteria (prolonged QTc >440 msec; stress-induced syncope; family history of LQTS) and minor criteria (congenital deafness; T wave alternans; relative bradycardia; abnormal ventricular repolarization) (Fig. 50.3).

The clinical features of LQTS, which occur due to dysrhythmias, are typically associated with triggering events. The most well described triggers include exercise, anxiety or excitement, auditory events (i.e., telephone or alarm clock ringing), swimming or diving into a pool, and postpartum. Some patients have events or die during sleep, which is thought to be associated with bradycardia.

In most cases of LQTS, no other abnormalities occur. However, sensorineural deafness is associated with the Jervell and Lange-Nielsen form of LQTS, distinguishing it from the Romano-Ward syndrome. LQTS has been reported to occur in approximately 1% of children with congenital deafness and this has led to the recommendation for screening ECGs in this group of children. These children also appear to have more severe ECG abnormalities than Romano-Ward syndrome patients and have a worse cardiovascular prognosis. Other abnormalities have been

Table 50.1. Diagnostic Criteria in LQTS

Clinical Finding	Points
*Electrocardiographic Findings	
†QT$_c$	
> 480 ms$^{1/2}$	3
460–470 ms$^{1/2}$	2
450 (male) ms$^{1/2}$	1
‡Torsades de pointes	2
T-wave alterans	1
Notched T wave in three leads	1
§Low heart rate for age	0.5
Clinical History	
‡Syncope	
With stress	2
Without stress	1
Congenital deafness	0.5
#Family History	
¶Family members with definite LQTS	1
Unexplained sudden cardiac death below age 30 among immediate family members	0.5

Scoring: <1 point = low probability of LQTS; 2 to 3 points = intermediate probability of LQTS; > 4 points = high probability of LQTS.
*In the absence of medications or disorders known to affect these ECG features.
†QTc calculated by Bazett's formula, where QTc = QT/√RR
‡Mutually exclusive.
§Resting heart rate below the second percentile for age.
#The same family member cannot be counted twice.
¶Definite lqts is defined by an lqts score > 4.

reported rarely in patients with LQTS. Marks et al. (1995) described LQTS patients with syndactyly; in this patient subset, LQTS appears to be quite severe, with a high percentage dying in infancy. In most of these patients, the initial presentation included 2:1 AV block due to marked QT prolongation. These patients have all been sporadic cases, with both genders being represented. Other patients with LQTS have been described with diabetes mellitus or asthma (Bellavere et al., 1988; Rosero et al., 1999).

Genetics

As previously noted, three forms of inherited LQTS have been described, including autosomal dominant (Romano-Ward syndrome), autosomal recessive (Jervell and Lange-Nielsen syndrome), and sporadic cases. Over the past decade, the genetic aspects of all three forms of LQTS have been unraveled. In 1991, Keating et al identified genetic linkage to the short arm of chromosome 11 (11p15.5) in several families with Romano-Ward syndrome (Keating et al., 1991a,b). Shortly thereafter, we demonstrated genetic heterogeneity and this was confirmed by several laboratories (Benhorin et al., 1993; Curran et al., 1993; Towbin et al., 1992; Towbin et al., 1994). In a collaborative effort (Jiang et al., 1994), linkage was shown for several families

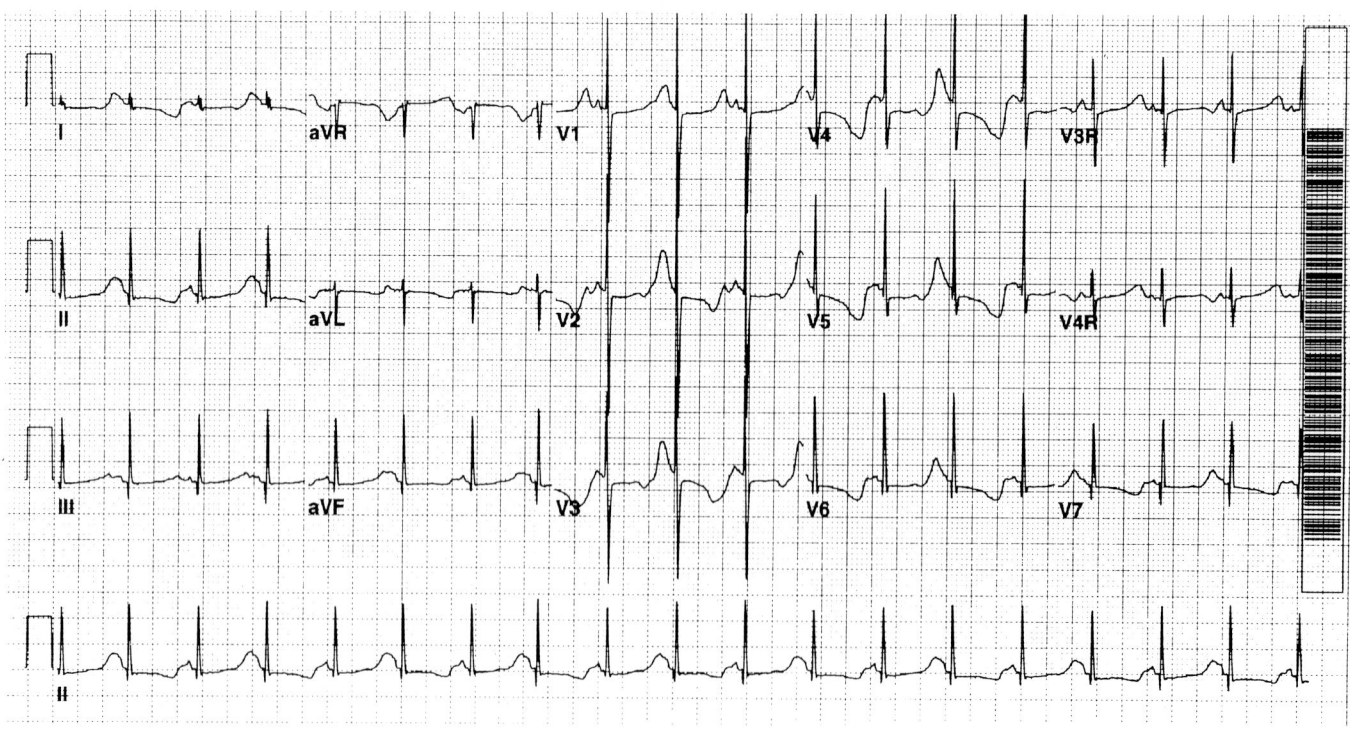

Fig. 50.3. T wave alternans in a child with long QT syndrome.

Genetics of Long QT Syndrome

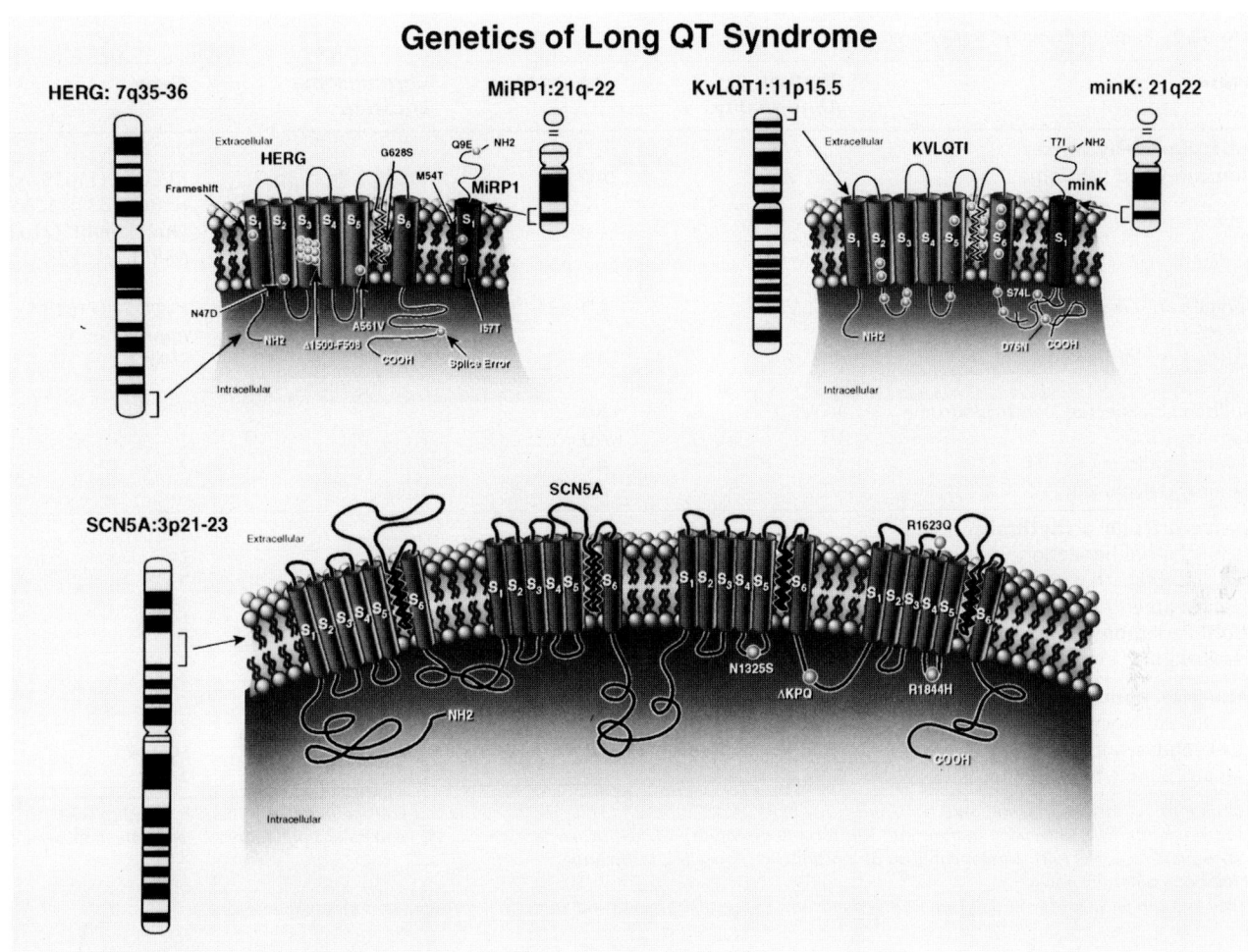

Fig. 50.4. Chromosomal loci and genes responsible for long QT syndrome.

to two new loci, the long arm of chromosome 7 (7q35-36) and the short arm of chromosome 3 (3p21). The three loci were later termed *LQT1* (11p15.5), *LQT2* (7q35-56), and *LQT3* (3p21). A fourth locus (LQT4) on chromosome 4q (4q25-27) was described later (Schott et al., 1995). Most recently, two other genes, both located on chromosome 21q22 (*LQT5, LQT6*), were identified (Barhanin et al., 1996; Sanguinetti et al., 1996a; Abbott et al., 1999) (Fig. 50.4). Penetrance in Romano-Ward syndrome is reduced and in some families, Romano-Ward syndrome appears to occur in a recessively inherited pattern (Priori et al., 1998).

GENE IDENTIFICATION IN ROMANO-WARD SYNDROME

KVLQT1 or *KCNQ1*: the LQT1 gene

The first of the genes mapped for LQTS, termed LQT1, required five years from the time that mapping to chromo-some 11p15.5 was first reported to gene cloning (Table 50.2). This gene, originally named *KVLQT1*, but more recently called *KCNQ1*, is a novel potassium channel gene that consists of 16 exons, spans approximately 400 kb, and is widely expressed in human tissues including heart, inner ear, kidney, lung, placenta, and pancreas, but not in skeletal muscle, liver, or brain. In the original report, 11 different mutations (deletion and missense mutations) were identified in 16 LQTS families, establishing *KVLQT1* as LQT1. To date, more than 100 families with *KVLQT1* mutations have been described. Although most of the mutations are "private" (i.e., only seen in one family), there is at least one frequently mutated region (called a "hot spot") of *KVLQT1* (Chouabe et al., 1997; Li et al., 1998).

Analysis of the predicted amino acid sequence of *KVLQT1* suggests that it encodes a potassium channel α-subunit (Barhanin et al., 1996; Sanguinetti et al., 1996a; Wang et al., 1996) with a conserved potassium-selective pore-signature sequence flanked by six membrane-spanning

Table 50.2. Familial Primary Dysrhythmias

Disease	Rhythm Abnormality	Inheritance	Chromosome Location	Gene
Ventricular arrhythmias				
Romano-Ward syndrome	TdP, VF	AD	11p15.5,7q35,3p21, 4q25,21q22$^\alpha$	KVLQT1 (11p15.5); HERG (7q35); SCN5A (3p21); minK (21q22); MiRP1 (21q22)
Jervell-Lange-Nielsen syndrome	TdP, VF	AD/AR*	11p15.5, 21q22	KVLQT1 (11p15.5); minK (21q22)
Brugada syndrome	VT, VF	AD	3p21	SCN5A
Sudden Unexpected Death Syndrome	VT/VF	AD	?	?
Familial VT	VT	AD	?	?
Familial bidirectional VT	VT	AD	?	?
Familial polymorphic VT	VT	AD	1q42$^\alpha$	?
Supraventricular arrhythmias				
Familial atrial fibrillation	AF	AD	10q22	?
Familial total atrial standstill	SND, AF	AD	?	?
Familial absence of sinus rhythm	SND, AF	AD	?	?
Wolff-Parkinson-White syndrome	AVRT, AF, VF	AD	7q3	?
Familial PJRT	AVRT	AD	?	?
Conduction abnormalities				
Familial AV block	AVB,AF,SND,VT,SD	AD	19q13	?
Lev-Lengre syndrome	AVB,AF,SND,VT,SD	AD	3p21	SCN5A
Familial bundle branch block	RBBB	?	?	?

Abbreviations: AF, atrial fibrillation; AVB, atrioventricular block; AVRT, atrioventricular reciprocating tachycardia; RBBB, right bundle branch block; SD, sudden death; SND, sinus node dysfunction; TdP, torsade de pointes; VT, ventricular tachycardia; VF, ventricular fibrillation; AD, autosomal dominant; AR, autosomal recessive; PJRT, permanent form of junctional reciprocating tachycardia.
$^\alpha$ At least one other unknown.
* Jervell and Lange-Nielsen syndrome: autosomal dominant rhythm abnormality and autosomal recessive sensorineural deafness

segments similar to shaker-type channels (Fig. 50.4). A putative voltage sensor is found in the fourth membrane-spanning domains (S4) and the selective pore loop is between the fifth and sixth membrane-spanning domains (S5, S6). Biophysical characterization of the KVLQT1 protein confirmed that KVLQT1 is a voltage-gated potassium channel protein subunit that requires coassembly (Barhanin et al., 1996; Sanguinetti et al., 1996a) with a β-subunit called minK to function properly (Fig. 50.4). Expression of either KVLQT1 or minK alone results in inefficient (or no) current development. When minK and KVLQT1 are coexpressed in either mammalian cell lines or *Xenopus* oocytes, however, the slowly activating potassium current (I_{ks}) is developed in cardiac myocytes. Combination of normal and mutant KVLQT1 subunits forms abnormal I_{Ks} channels and these mutations are believed to act through a dominant-negative mechanism (the mutant form of KVLQT1 interferes with the function of the normal wild-type form through a "poison pill"-type mechanism) or a loss-of-function mechanism (only the mutant form loses activity) (Shalaby et al., 1997; Wollnick et al., 1997; Demolombe et al., 1998).

Because KVLQT1 and minK form a unit, mutations in *minK* could also be expected to cause LQTS (Sanguinetti et al., 1996a), and this fact was subsequently demonstrated (see "minK: the LQT5 gene"). The vast majority of mutations in *KVLQT1* and *minK* are heterozygous mutations in Romano-Ward syndrome patients (Chouabe et al., 2000; Duggal et al., 1998; Sanguinetti et al., 1996a). *KVLQT1* appears to be the most commonly mutated gene in LQTS.

HERG: the LQT2 gene

After the initial localization of LQT2 to chromosome 7q35-36 by Jiang et al. (1994) (Table 50.2), candidate genes (i.e., genes encoding proteins that could cause repolarization abnormalities if mutated, such as ion channels, modulators of ion channels, members of the sympathetic nervous system) in this chromosomal region were analyzed. *HERG* (*h*uman *e*ther-a-go-go-*r*elated *g*ene), a cardiac potassium channel gene originally cloned from a brain cDNA library (Warmke and Ganetzky, 1994), and which is expressed in neural crest-derived neurons (Arcangeli et al.,

1997), microglia (Pennefather et al., 1998), a wide variety of tumor cell lines (Bianchi et al., 1998), and the heart (Curran et al., 1995), was found to be mutated in patients with clinical evidence of LQTS (Curran et al., 1995). Six LQTS-associated mutations were initially identified in *HERG*, including missense mutations, intragenic deletions, and a splicing mutation. Later, Schulze-Bahr et al. (1995) confirmed *HERG* as the LQT2 gene, identifying mutations in other families. Currently, this gene is thought to be the second most common gene mutated in LQTS (second to KVLQT1). As with *KVLQT1*, "private" mutations that are scattered throughout the entire gene without preferential clustering are seen.

HERG consists of 16 exons and spans 55 kb of genomic sequence (Curran et al., 1995). The predicted topology of *HERG* is shown in Figure 50.4 and is similar to *KVLQT1*. Unlike *KVLQT1*, *HERG* has extensive intracellular amino- and carboxyl-termini, with a region in the carboxyl-terminal domain having sequence similarity to nucleotide binding domains (NBDs).

Electrophysiologic and biophysical characterization of *HERG* expressed in *Xenopus* oocytes established that *HERG* encodes the rapidly activating delayed-rectifier potassium current 1_{Kr} (Sanguinetti et al., 1995; Trudeau et al., 1995) and electrophysiologic studies of LQTS-associated mutations demonstrated a loss-of-function or a dominant-negative mechanism (Sanguinetti et al., 1996b) of action. In addition, protein trafficking abnormalities have been shown to occur (Furutani et al., 1999; Zhou et al., 1998). This channel has been shown to coassemble with β-subunits for normal function, similar to that seen in 1_{Ks}. McDonald et al. (1997) initially suggested that the complexing of HERG with minK is needed to regulate the 1_{Kr} potassium current. Bianchi et al. (1999) provided confirmatory evidence that minK is involved in regulation of both 1_{Ks} and 1_{Kr}. Most recently, Abbott et al. (1999) identified MiRP1 as a β-subunit for HERG (see "MiRP1: the LQT6 gene").

SCN5A: the LQT3 gene

Utilization of the candidate gene approach established that the gene responsible for chromosome 3-linked LQTS (LQT3) (George et al., 1995) is the cardiac sodium channel gene *SCN5A* (Wang et al., 1995b,c) (Table 50.2). *SCN5A* is highly expressed in human myocardium and brain, but not in skeletal muscle, liver, or uterus (Hartmann et al., 1999; Wang et al., 1995b). It consists of 28 exons that span 80 kb and encodes a protein of 2016 amino acids with a putative structure that consists of four homologous domains (DI to DIV), each of which contains six membrane-spanning segments (S1 to S6) similar to the structure of the potassium channel α-subunits (Fig. 50.4) (Gellens et al., 1992). Mutation analysis identified three mutations, one 9-base pair intragenic deletion ($\Delta K_{1505}P_{1506}Q_{1507}$) and two missense mutations ($R_{1644}H$ and $N_{1525}S$) in six LQTS families (Wang et al., 1995b,c); when expressed in *Xenopus* oocytes, all mutations generated a late phase of inactivation-resistant, mexiletine- and tetrodotoxin-sensitive whole-cell current via different mechanisms (Bennett et al., 1995; Dumaine et al., 1996). Two of the three mutations showed dispersed reopening after the initial transient, but the other mutation showed both dispersed reopening and long-lasting bursts. These results suggested that *SCN5A* mutations act through a gain-of-function mechanism (the mutant channel functions normally, but with altered properties such as delayed inactivation) and that the mechanism of chromosome 3-linked LQTS is persistent nonactivated sodium current in the plateau phase of the action potential. An et al. (1998) also showed that not all mutations in *SCN5A* are associated with persistent current and demonstrated that *SCN5A* interacted with β-subunits. Furthermore, mutations in *SCN5A* have been shown to result in widely different clinical phenotypes and different responses to medications (Benhorin et al., 1998; 2000). Novel mutations in *SCN5A* were identified by our laboratory in patients with Brugada syndrome and idiopathic ventricular fibrillation (Chen et al., 1998), disorders with normal QT interval, but ST segment elevation in the right precordial leads (Table 50.2). Electrophysiologically, these mutations result in more rapid recovery from inactivation of the mutant channels or loss of function causing the Brugada syndrome-type phenotype (see section on Brugada syndrome). In addition, mutations in this gene cause conduction system disease (Schott et al., 1999) and sudden infant death syndrome (SIDS) (Schwartz et al., 2000a,b) (Table 50.2).

minK: the LQT5 gene

The *minK* (lsK or KCNE1) gene was initially localized to chromosome 21 (21q22.1) and found to consist of three exons that span approximately 40 kb (Honore et al., 1991). It encodes a short protein consisting of 130 amino acids and has only one transmembrane-spanning segment with small extracellular and intercellular regions (Fig. 50.4). When expressed in *Xenopus* oocytes, it produces potassium current that closely resembles the slowly activating delayed-rectifier potassium current 1_{Ks} in cardiac cells (Barhanin et al., 1996; Sanguinetti et al., 1996a). The fact that the *minK* clone was expressed only in *Xenopus* oocytes and not in mammalian cell lines raised the question whether minK is a human channel protein. With the cloning of *KVLQT1* and coexpression of *KVLQT1* and *minK* in both mammalian cell lines and *Xenopus* oocytes, it became clear that KVLQT1 interacts with minK to form the cardiac slowly activating delayed-rectifier I_{Ks} current (Barhanin et al., 1996; Sanguinetti et al., 1996a); minK alone cannot form a functional channel but induces the I_{Ks} current by interacting with endogenous KVLQT1 protein in *Xenopus* oocytes and mammalian cells. Bianchi et al. (1999) also showed that mutant minK results in abnormalities of I_{Ks} and I_{Kr} and in protein trafficking abnormalities. McDonald et al. (1997) showed that minK also interacts with HERG, regulating I_{Kr}. Splawski et al. (1997b) demonstrated that *minK* mutations cause LQT5 when they identified mutations in two families with LQTS (Table 50.2). In both cases, missense mutations (S74I; D76N) were identified that reduced I_{Ks} by shifting the voltage dependence of activation and accelerating channel deactivation. This was later confirmed by others (Chouabe et al., 2000; Duggal et al., 1998) and further supported by the fact that a mouse model with mutant minK (Vetter et al., 1996) developed a phenotype (which included deafness). The functional consequences of these mutations include delayed cardiac repolarization and hence, an increased risk of dysrhythmias (Chouabe et al., 2000; Duggal et al., 1997; Franqueza et al., 1999).

MiRP1: the LQT6 gene

The *MiRP1* gene (the minK-related peptide 1 or *KCNE2* gene) is a novel potassium channel gene cloned and characterized by Abbott et al. (1999). This small integral membrane subunit protein assembles with HERG (LQT2) to alter its function and enable full development of the I_{Kr} current (Fig. 50.4). MiRP1 is a 123-amino acid channel protein with a single predicted transmembrane segment similar to that described for minK. Chromosomal localization studies mapped *KCNE2* to chromosome 21q22.1, within 79 kb of *KCNE1* (*minK*) and arrayed in opposite orientation. The open reading frames of these two genes share 34% identify and both are contained in a single exon, suggesting that they are related through gene duplication and divergent evolution.

Three missense mutations associated with dysrhythmias were identified in *KCNE2* by Abbott et al., and biophysical analysis demonstrated that these mutants form channels that open slowly and close rapidly, thus diminishing potassium currents. In one case, the missense mutation, a C-to-G transversion at nucleotide 25 that produced a glutamine (Q) to glutamic acid (E) substitution at codon 9 (Q9E) in

the putative extracellular domain of MiRP1, led to the development of *torsade de pointes* and ventricular fibrillation after intravenous clarithromycin infusion (i.e., drug induced). Therefore, like minK, this channel protein acts as a β-subunit but, by itself, leads to risk of ventricular arrhythmia when mutated (Table 50.2). These similar channel proteins (i.e., minK and MiRP1) suggest that a family of channels exist that regulate ion channel α-subunits. The specific role of this subunit and its stoichiometry remain unclear and are currently hotly debated.

JERVELL AND LANGE-NIELSEN SYNDROME

Clinical features

As noted previously, patients with Jervell and Lange-Nielsen syndrome have severe QT interval prolongation, episodic tachydysrhythmias including *torsade de pointes*, syncope and/or sudden death, and congenital sensorineural deafness (Jervell and Lange-Nielsen, 1957; Schwartz et al., 1999). The deafness is autosomal recessive while the LQTS is autosomal dominant but severe (Vatta et al., 2000).

Genetics

Neyroud et al. (1997) reported the first molecular abnormality in patients with JLNS when they reported on two families in which three children were affected by JLNS, finding a novel homozygous deletion-insertion mutation of *KVLQT1* (Table 50.2). A deletion of 7 bp and an insertion of 8 bp at the same location led to premature termination at the C-terminal end of the KVLQT1 channel. At the same time, Splawski et al. (1997a) identified a homozygous insertion of a single nucleotide that caused a frameshift in the coding sequence after the second putative transmembrane domain (S2) of KVLQT1. Together, these data strongly suggested that at least one form of JLNS is caused by homozygous mutations in *KVLQT1*. This has been confirmed by others (Chen et al., 1999; Chouabe et al., 1997; Schulze-Bahr et al., 1997; Tyson et al., 1997; Wollnick et al., 1997).

As a general rule, heterozygous mutations in *KVLQT1* cause Romano-Ward syndrome (LQTS only), whereas homozygous (or compound heterozygous) mutations in *KVLQT1* cause JLNS (LQTS and deafness). The hypothetical explanation suggests that although heterozygous *KVLQT1* mutations act by a dominant-negative mechanism (Mohamad-Pannah et al., 1999), some functional KVLQT1 potassium channels still exist in the stria vascularis of the inner ear. Therefore, congenital deafness is averted in patients with heterozygous *KVLQT1* mutations. For patients with homozygous *KVLQT1* mutations, no functional KVLQT1 potassium channels can be formed. It has been shown by *in situ* hybridization that *KVLQT1* is expressed in the inner ear (Neyroud et al., 1997), suggesting that homozygous *KVLQT1* mutations can cause the dysfunction of potassium secretion in the inner ear and lead to deafness (Vetter et al., 1996). However, it should be noted that incomplete penetrance exists and not all heterozygous or homozygous mutations follow this rule (Priori et al., 1999).

As with Romano-Ward syndrome, if *KVLQT1* mutations can cause the phenotype, it could be expected that *minK* mutations could also be causative of the phenotype (JLNS). Schulze-Bahr et al. (1997), in fact, showed that mutations in *minK* result in JLNS syndrome as well (Table 50.2), and this was confirmed subsequently (Duggal et al., 1998; Tyson et al., 1997). Hence, abnormal I_{Ks} current, whether it occurs due to homozygous or compound heterozygous mutations in *KVLQT1* or *minK*, results in LQTS and deafness.

Genotype-phenotype correlations

Moss et al. (1995) showed that the ECG manifestations of LQTS were in great part determined by the channel mutated. Different T-wave patterns were clearly evident when comparing tracings from patients with mutations in *LQT1*, *LQT2*, and *LQT3*. More recently, Zareba et al. (1998) showed that the mutated gene may result in a specific clinical phenotype with different triggers and may predict outcome. For instance, these authors suggested that mutations in *LQT1* and *LQT2* result in early symptoms (i.e., syncope) but the risk of sudden death was relatively low for any event. In contrast, mutations in *LQT3* resulted in a paucity of symptoms but when symptoms occurred they were associated with a high likelihood of sudden death. Ackerman et al. (1999) and Moss et al. (1999) showed that swimming is a common trigger for symptoms in *LQT1* patients while Wilde and colleagues (1999) have found auditory triggers to be common in *LQT2*. *LQT3*, on the other hand, appears to be associated with sleep-associated symptoms. All of these findings suggest that understanding the underlying cause of LQTS in any individual could be used to improve survival by prevention and gene-specific therapy.

Management

At present, there are three classical modalities for treatment of LQTS that have withstood the test of time: (1) β-adrenergic blocking drugs (β-blockers) (Moss, 1998; Moss et al., 2000), (2) pacemakers (Eldar et al., 1987; Moss et al., 1991, Viskin, 2000), and (3) left cervicothoracic sympathetic ganglionectomy (Moss and MacDonald, 1970; Schwartz et al., 1991). The mortality of untreated symptomatic patients with LQTS exceeds 20% in the year after their first syncopal episode and approaches 50% within ten years of initial presentation (Schwartz, 1985). With institution of the classical therapy, this can be reduced to 2 to 4% in 5 years after initial presentation (Moss et al., 2000; Schwartz, 1985). Despite the lack of a placebo-controlled, randomized clinical trial, strong evidence supports the use of antiadrenergic interventions as the mainstay of therapy for most patients. The trigger for many life-threatening events appears to involve sudden increases in sympathetic activity (i.e., emotional or physical stress), and therefore, antiadrenergic therapy makes physiological sense. Various β-blockers prevent new syncopal episodes in approximately 65 to 75% of patients (Moss et al., 2000). Suppression of complex ventricular arrhythmias, i.e., couplets and VT, seems desirable. The addition of a IB agent (mexiletine) to β-blocker therapy may be helpful, particularly in patients with a mutation in *LQT3* (Schwartz et al., 1995). High-risk patients with drug-resistant, symptomatic ventricular tachycardia are referred for left cardiac sympathetic denervation, which apparently provides additional protection (Moss and MacDonald, 1970; Schwartz et al., 1991). In addition, the use of cardiac pacing as an adjunct to β-blockers appears to be most rational in patients with evidence of pause-dependent or bradycardia-dependent arrhythmias (Eldar et al., 1987; Moss et al., 1991; Viskin, 2000). Symptomatic bradycardia due to LQTS or induced by β-blocker therapy, should also be considered an indication for elective pacing. β-blocker therapy is monitored with treadmill exercise testing with the desired result a blunting of the heart rate response to exercise. Unfortunately, in some patients, this comes at the expense of excessive sinus bradycardia at rest and with minimal levels of exertion. Excessive fatigue, inattentiveness and irritability may result in discontinuance of therapy by the patient. Compliance, especially in the adolescent population, may be enhanced by returning the patient to a relatively normal lifestyle by the elimination of chronotropic incompetence with a pacemaker.

Other less time-tested therapies are also available. In some rare cases, *torsade de pointes* persists despite therapy with the classical modalities. The implantable cardioverter-defibrillator has been used successfully in this setting (Platia et al., 1985; Groh et al., 1996). Up until recently, it had not been considered to be first-line therapy because shocks from the device can precipitate further emotional stress and set off a circuitous response of persistent malignant arrhythmias. However, the Multicenter Automatic Defibrillator Implantation Trial (MADIT), which demonstrated dramatic superiority of therapy with automatic implantable defibrillators over "best conventional therapy" in patients with coronary disease at high risk for ventricular arrhythmias (Moss et al., 1996), has made this therapeutic approach somewhat appealing. It is likely that automatic implantable defibrillators will be used more commonly in LQTS patients due to the results of the MADIT trial. However, whether this is the best approach is not currently clear.

Another new approach to treating patients with LQTS is the so-called "gene-specific" approach. With the identification of the precise molecular defect in some patients with LQTS, specific mechanism-based therapies have been devised and small therapeutic trials performed. Schwartz et al. (1995) were the first to use this approach when they used the sodium channel blocker mexiletine in patients with mutations in the sodium channel gene *SCN5A* (*LQT3*). In these patients the QTc was dramatically shortened in a statistically-significant manner (Fig. 50.5). Patients with

potassium channel mutations (*HERG, LQT2*) treated with mexiletine had no change in the QTc. However, no data currently demonstrate clinical efficacy of this approach in either decreasing the number of syncopal events or improving survival. Other sodium channel blockers have had similar effects (Rosero et al., 1999). Recently, Benhorin et al. (2000) showed that flecainide shortened the QTc in patients with a D1790G *SCN5A* mutation while lidocaine was ineffective, suggesting that allele-specific therapies may be needed. Although the data are intriguing, use of sodium channel blockers alone for patients with *SCN5A* mutations should still be considered experimental. Other gene-specific trials have also been performed with similar results. Compton et al. (1996) used intravenous potassium to elevate the serum potassium to > 4.8 in patients with *LQT2* and found significant shortening of the QTc. Again, no data on survival or symptom improvement exists for this therapy, but this has been confirmed (Choy et al., 1997). Other gene-specific therapeutic approaches are currently being developed (Shimizu et al., 1998).

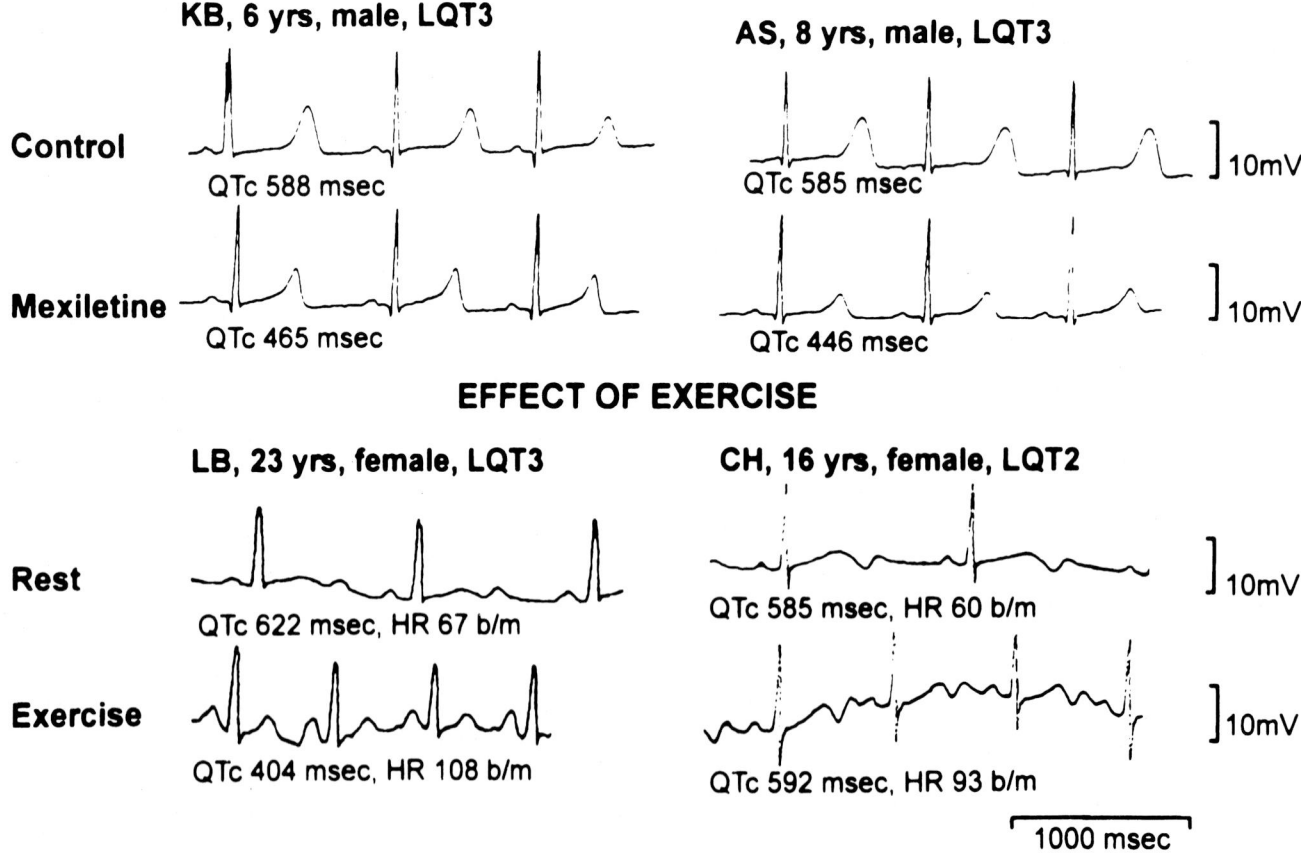

Fig. 50.5. Mexiletine, a sodium channel blocker, shortens the QTc in these two children with extreme QTc prolongation (>580 msec) and an SCN5A mutation.

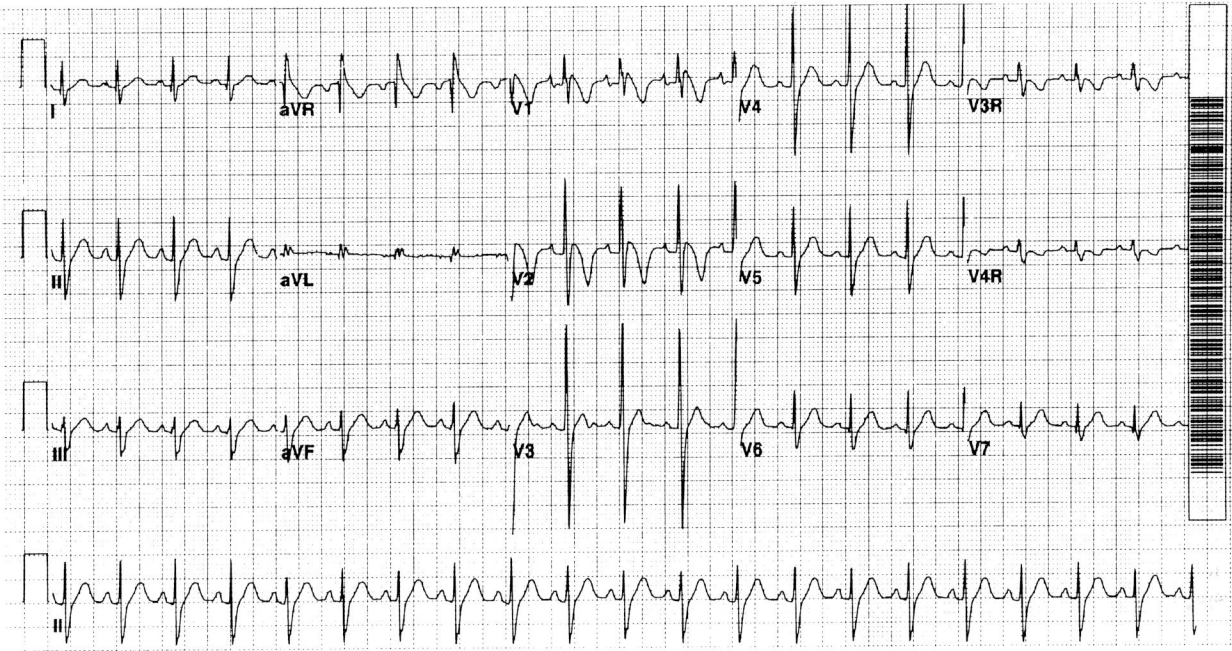

Fig. 50.6. Brugada syndrome in a four-year-old. Note the right ventricular conduction delay and ST segment elevation in leads V1, V2. Procainamide infusion worsened the ST elevation.

BRUGADA SYNDROME

Clinical features

This disorder is characterized by ST-segment elevation in the right precordial leads (V1–V3) with or without right bundle branch block (RBBB) (Fig. 50.6) and episodic ventricular fibrillation (Fig. 50.7). The first identification of the electrocardiographic (ECG) pattern of RBBB with ST-elevation in leads V1–V3 was reported by Osher and Wolff (1953). Shortly thereafter, Edeiken (1954) identified persistent ST-elevation without RBBB in ten asymptomatic males and Levine et al. (1956) described ST-elevation in the right chest leads and conduction block in the right ventricle in patients with severe hyperkalemia. The first association of this ECG pattern with sudden death was described by Martini et al. (1989) and later by Aihara et al. (1990) and further confirmed in 1991 by Pedro and Josep Brugada (1991) who described four patients with sudden death and aborted sudden death with ECGs demonstrating RBBB and persistent ST-elevation in leads V1–V3. In 1992, these authors characterized what they believed to be a distinct clinical and electrocardiographic syndrome. In some patients, even with a positive family history, the surface ECG appears normal. Provocation studies in the catheterization laboratory using ajmaline, flecainide, or procainamide will result in ST-segment elevation in the right precordial leads in affected patients (Brugada et al., 2000).

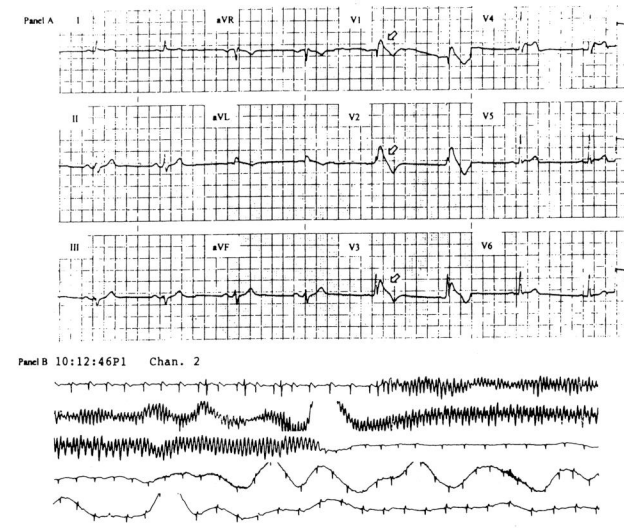

Fig. 50.7. Ventricular fibrillation in a patient with Brugada syndrome.

The finding of ST-elevation in the right chest leads has been observed in a variety of clinical and experimental settings and is not unique or diagnostic of Brugada syndrome by itself. Situations in which these ECG findings occur include electrolyte or metabolic disorders, pulmonary or inflammatory diseases, abnormalities of the central or peripheral nervous system. In the absence of these abnormalities, the term idiopathic ST-elevation is often used and may identify Brugada syndrome patients (Antzelevitch, 1999).

The ECG findings and associated sudden and unexpected death has been reported as a common problem in Southeast Asia where it often affects men during sleep (Nademanee et al., 1997). This disorder, known as Sudden and Unexpected Death Syndrome (SUDS) or Sudden Unexpected Nocturnal Death Syndrome (SUNDS), has many names in Southeast Asia including bangungut (to rise and moan in sleep) in the Philippines; non-laitai (sleep-death) in Laos; lai-tai (died during sleep) in Thailand; and pokkuri (sudden and unexpectedly ceased phenomena) in Japan. General characteristics of SUDS include young, healthy males in whom death occurs suddenly with a groan, usually during sleep late at night. No precipitating factors are identified and autopsy findings are generally negative (Gotoh, 1976). Life-threatening ventricular tachydysrhythmias as a primary cause of SUDS has been demonstrated, with VF occurring in most cases (Hayashi et al., 1985).

BRUGADA SYNDROME AND ARRHYTHMOGENIC RIGHT VENTRICULAR DYSPLASIA

Controversy exists concerning the possible association of Brugada syndrome and arrhythmogenic right ventricular dysplasia (ARVD), with some investigators arguing that these are the same disorder or that at least one is a *forme fruste* of the other (Corrado et al., 1996; Fontaine, 1996; Fontaine et al., 1996; Naccarella, 1993; Ohe, 1996; Scheinman, 1997). However, the classic echocardiographic, angiographic, and magnetic resonance image (MRI) findings of ARVD are not seen in Brugada syndrome patients. In addition, Brugada syndrome patients typically are without the histopathologic findings of ARVD. Further, the morphology of VT/VF differs, as noted in Table 50.2.

Clinical genetics

Most of the families identified to date with Brugada syndrome have autosomal dominant inheritance (Antzelevitch, 1998; Brugada et al., 1997; Gussak et al., 1999; Kobayashi et al., 1996). It appears as if penetrance is reduced, as many patients have a normal ECG and no symptoms until provocation studies are performed. Although the number of families reported has been small, it is likely that this is due to under-recognition as well as premature and unexpected death.

Molecular genetics

In animal studies, blockade of the calcium-independent 4-aminopyridine-sensitive transient outward potassium current (I_{to}) results in surface ECG findings similar to that seen in Brugada syndrome. These include elevated, downsloping ST segments (Antzelevitch, 1999) associated with greater abbreviation in the epicardial action potential compared with the endocardium (which lacks a plateau phase). Loss of the action potential plateau (or dome) in the epicardium but not endocardium would be expected to cause ST segment elevation. Because loss of the dome is caused by an outward shift in the balance of currents active at the end of phase I of the action potential (principally I_{to} and I_{Ca}), autonomic neurotransmitters such as acetylcholine facilitate loss of the action potential dome by suppressing calcium current and augmenting potassium current, whereas β-adrenergic agonists (i.e., isoproterenol, dobutamine) restore the dome by augmenting I_{Ca}. Sodium channel blockers also facilitate loss of the canine right ventricular action potential dome as a result of a negative shift in the voltage at which phase I begins (Antzelevitch, 1999). Based on this information, candidate genes (I_{to}, I_{Ca}, and I_{Na}) were selected for study.

In 1998, our laboratory reported the findings on six families and several sporadic cases of Brugada syndrome (Chen et al., 1998)(Table 50.2). The families were initially studied by linkage analysis using markers to the known ARVD loci and linkage was excluded. Candidate gene screening using the mutation analysis approach of single-strand conformation polymorphism analysis and DNA sequencing was performed and SCN5A was chosen for study, based on physiologic speculation (Antzelevitch, 1999). In three families, mutations in SCN5A were identified (Chen et al., 1998) including a missense mutation (C-to-T base substitution) causing a substitution of a highly conserved threonine by methionine at codon 1620 (T1620M) in the extracellular loop between transmembrane segments S3 and S4 of domain IV (DIVS3 to DIVS4), an area important for coupling of channel activation to fast inactivation; a two-nucleotide insertion (AA) that disrupts the splice-donor sequence of intron 7 of SCN5A; and a one-nucleotide deletion (A) at codon 1397 that results in an inframe stop codon that eliminates DIIIS6, DIVS1 to DIVS6, and the carboxy terminus of SCN5A (Fig. 50.8).

Biophysical analysis of the mutants in *Xenopus* oocytes demonstrated a reduction in the number of functional sodium channels in both the splicing mutation and one-nucleotide deletion mutation, which should promote development of reentrant dysrhythmias. In the missense mutation, sodium channels recovered from inactivation more rapidly than normal, and are temperature-dependent (Dumaine et al., 1999). In this case, the presence of both normal and mutant channels in the same tissue would be expected to promote heterogeneity of the refractory period,

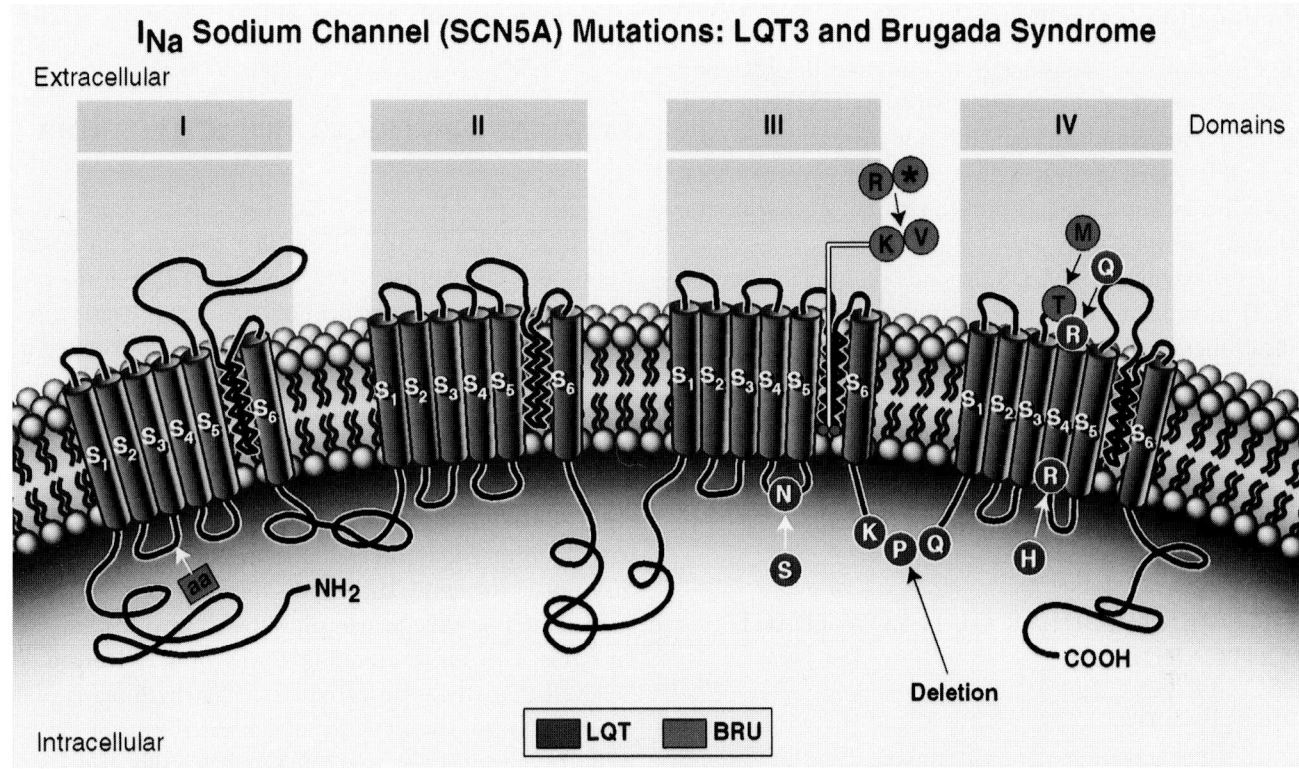

Fig. 50.8. Mutations in SCN5A in patients with Brugada syndrome (green) versus those with long QT syndrome (red).

a well-established mechanism causing dysrhythmias. Inhibition of the sodium channel I_{Na} current causes heterogeneous loss of the action potential dome in the right ventricular epicardium, leading to a marked dispersion of depolarization and refractoriness, an ideal substrate for development of reentrant dysrhythmias. Phase 2 reentry produced by the same substrate is believed to provide the premature beat necessary for initiation of the VT and VF responsible for symptoms in these patients. Interestingly, however, Kambouris et al. (1998) identified a mutation (R1623H) in essentially the same region of *SCN5A* as the T1620M mutation, but the clinical and biophysical features of this mutation were found to be consistent with LQT3 and not Brugada syndrome. More recently, the same authors demonstrated these mutant channels to have a propensity to inactivate without ever opening (i.e., closed state inactivation), suggesting novel physiologic mechanisms can occur in a heterogeneous manner in similar regions of this ion channel (Kambouris et al., 2000).

Therapy

No good medical therapy has been clearly identified for these patients thus far. Belhausen et al. (1999) have argued that quinidine has a role in chronic therapy for these patients but this is based on a small number of clinical vignettes and has not been stringently evaluated. Currently, implantation of an ICD is the therapy of choice but this remains controversial.

SUDDEN UNEXPECTED DEATH SYNDROMES (SUDS)

Clinical features

Sudden unexpected death syndromes (SUDS) is a disorder that occurs in Southeast Asia, particularly Thailand, Cambodia, Japan and the Philippines. The clinical features of this disorder are highlighted by the flamboyant names given this disease in the various Asian countries: SUDS is the most common cause of "natural" death in these countries (Nadamanee et al., 1997). The clinical features include an abnormal surface electrocardiogram with ST-segment elevation in the right precordial leads (V1–V3), with or without right bundle branch block (RBBB). Ventricular fibrillation (VF) leads to the clinical symptoms of syncope, sudden death, and resuscitated sudden death. It has been speculated that SUDS is an allelic form of Brugada syndrome, but this has not been proven, as the gene(s) responsible for SUDS remain unknown (Table 50.2).

Genetics and management

SUDS has not been considered an inherited disorder but we have identified some families in which SUDS is inherited as an autosomal dominant trait. It is not currently clear why SUDS afflicts men almost exclusively but it is certain that this is not transmitted in an X-linked fashion, since male-to-male transmission occurs.

The management of SUDS depends on implantation of an ICD in order to treat rapidly any episodes of VF. No medical therapy has proven effective for this disorder. Another important step necessary for optimal therapy of SUDS is the screening of all family members by surface ECG testing. It is possible that provocation tests, similar to that described in Brugada syndrome, may be useful, but this has not been proven.

RIGHT VENTRICULAR OUTFLOW TRACT TACHYCARDIA

Clinical features

This rare form of VT occurs in the setting of an apparently normal, healthy individual who develops repetitive monomorphic VT arising from the right ventricular outflow tract (RVOT) (Buxton et al., 1983; Palileo et al., 1982; Rahilly et al., 1982). These VTs are characterized by left bundle branch block (LBBB) morphology with an inferior frontal plane axis, which may be either leftward or rightward directed. Unlike ARVD/ARVC which also is associated with LBBB/inferior axis VT, the ECG in normal sinus rhythm is typically normal. VT episodes tend to be characterized by frequent salvos of nonsustained VT or are separated by short periods of normal sinus rhythm and may be entirely asymptomatic. In some cases, however, catecholamines or exercise may provoke sustained episodes of VT.

Genetics

No genetic data exist regarding RVOT VT. It is not known how often genetic inheritance occurs or what type of inheritance pattern occurs. At the molecular level, no gene has been identified.

Management

In some cases, these tachycardias appear to be adenosine-sensitive, terminating with an intravenous bolus of adenosine. In other cases, verapamil has been reported to terminate the VT. Implantation of an ICD may be consid-ered in symptomatic patients with recurrent VT refractory to medical therapies.

FAMILIAL VENTRICULAR TACHYCARDIA

Clinical features

This inherited form of VT was first described in detail by Rubin and colleagues (1992) and is another form of VT that occurs in the absence of structural heart disease. Clinically, these patients present with frequent runs of non-sustained VT at rest (Fig. 50.9), which may decrease or extinguish with exercise (Rubin et al., 1992; Sacks et al., 1978). In some cases, salvos of nonsustained VT may be incessant, causing palpitations, dizziness or syncope. The electrocardiogram is usually normal during sinus rhythm, with a normal QT interval. Electrophysiologic evaluation may not consistently show inducible VT in these patients, suggesting that the mechanism is this dysrhythmia is not re-entry, as with more common forms of VT. Instead, it is believed that this form of inherited dysrhythmia is due to enhanced automaticity (i.e., an increased rate of electrical firing of a ventricular myocyte) or triggering (i.e., results from secondary depolarizations that occur during or immediately after repolarization).

Genetics and management

This inherited tachydysrhythmia is transmitted as an auto-somal dominant trait (Table 50.2) (Wren et al., 1990). It appears to be relatively uncommon but the incidence and prevalence are not known. The therapy of this disorder appears to rely on the use of β-adrenergic blocking agents, which effectively suppresses this rhythm disturbance. In addition, the use of class I and class III antiarrhythmics have reportedly been successful in treating this disorder. The use of ICDs have not been reported in this disorder but this is certainly a likely option in malignant families or difficult cases.

BIDIRECTIONAL VENTRICULAR TACHYCARDIA

Clinical features

Bidirectional ventricular tachycardia occurs as an acquired disorder as well as an inherited abnormality. The acquired form occurs secondary to digitalis intoxication (Schwensen, 1992). The inherited form of VT occurs in the absence of drugs or structural heart disease (Cohen et al., 1989; Gault et al., 1972; Glikson et al., 1991). Clinically, this

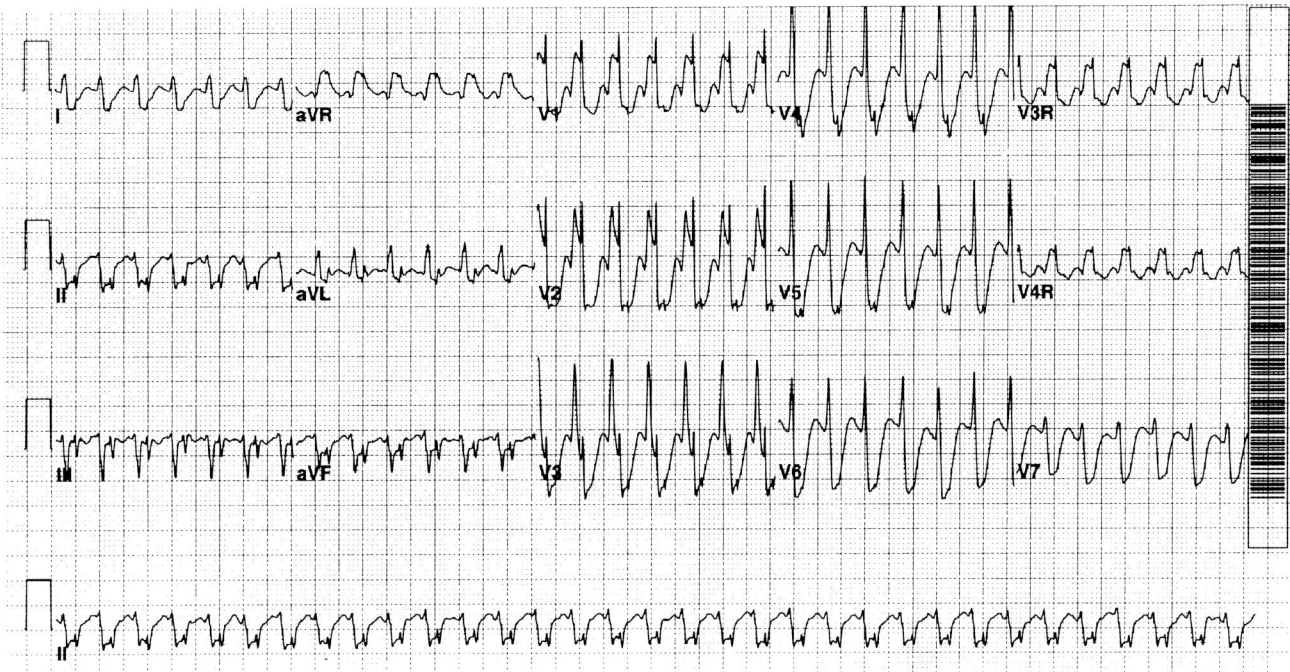

Fig. 50.9. Monomorphic ventricular tachycardia (200 bpm).

disease appears to be catacholamine-sensitive (Coumel et al., 1978; Fisher et al., 1999; Leenhardt et al., 1995; Vlay, 1987), with increased adrenergic stimulation inducing polymorphic ventricular premature complexes followed by directional and polymorphic VT (Coumel et al., 1978). Many patients present during the first decade of life with syncope or sudden cardiac death, although in many cases the individual may be asymptomatic. Bidirectional VT has a characteristic ECG appearance that includes VT with a RBBB morphology, alternation in the frontal plane QRS axis from $-60°$ to $-80°$ to $+120°$, and a rate of 140–200 beats per minute (Rosenbaum et al., 1969). This form of VT may be confused with a supraventricular rhythm arising from above the atrioventricular node, but several differentiating features are known. These include dissociation of the atria from the ventricles during tachycardia and the ability to identify the His bundle during tachycardia (Glikson et al., 1991); both occur with bidirectional VT.

Genetics and management

Although uncommon, this disorder appears to be transmitted as an autosomal dominant trait with variable penetrance (Table 50.2). A family history of syncope or sudden death is reported in 30% of cases. The therapy for this disorder is not completely clarified, but it appears as if exercise or increase in atrial rate by atrial overdrive pacing (Gault et al., 1972; Glikson et al., 1991) suppresses the VT. Recurrence of the

dysrhythmia has been prevented by β-blockers (Cohen et al., 1989). Fisher and colleagues (1999) have reported twenty-five years of follow-up in patients with this form of VT in which medical therapy, predominantly β-blockers, was successfully based on serial exercise-pharmacologic testing. In these patients, early identification of exercise- or catecholamine-induced dysrhythmias, as demonstrated on exercise stress tests predominantly, led to successful therapy.

Recently, Swan et al. (1999) mapped a gene for malignant polymorphic ventricular tachycardia in two families with structurally normal hearts to chromosome 1q42-q43 (Table 50.2). It is likely that this gene is responsible for the catcholamine-sensitive VT. Based on previous genetic studies of ventricular tachydysrhythmias, all of which have been shown to be due to ion channel abnormalities, we could speculate this disorder to be an ion channelopathy; identification of this gene in the future will help to clarify this mystery.

Primary abnormalities in cardiac rhythm: supraventricular dysrhythmias

FAMILIAL ATRIAL FIBRILLATION

Clinical features

Atrial fibrillation (AF) is considered the most common sustained dysrhythmia worldwide (Fig. 50.10) and is believed

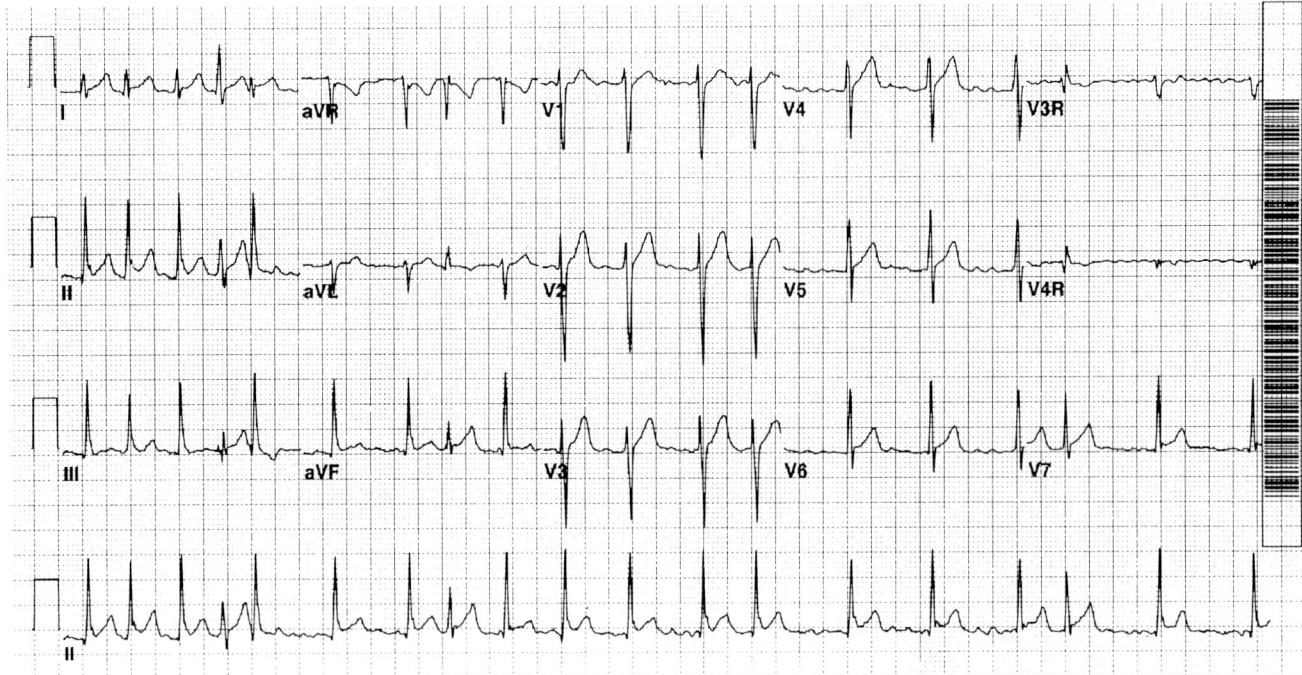

Fig. 50.10. Atrial fibrillation with its irregularly irregular rhythm and fibrillation pattern, which is well seen in the right chest leads (V3R, V4R) and rhythm strip.

to be the most common cause of embolic stroke, accounting for 75,000 strokes per year in the US (Feinberg et al., 1995). Currently, there are more than 3 million cases of AF in the U.S., with an overall prevalence of 0.5–1%, increasing to ~10% in individuals older than age 70 years. Atrial fibrillation accounts for ~1/3 of strokes in people over the age of 65 years and leads to more hospital admissions than any other dysrhythymia (Albers, 1994). AF, however can occur in children and fetal life (Tikanoja et al., 1998).

Genetics

Familial atrial fibrillation is reportedly rare but Brugada and Brugada (1997) identified multiple families with familial AF from Spain and noted the penetrance to be high. Generally, the disease is chronic but some individuals present with paroxysomal AF, some having palpitations. Left atrial dilatation developed in some individuals; syncope and dyspnea also occurs. This disorder appears to be inherited as an autosomal dominant trait and many of these patients develop AF very early in childhood (Beyer et al., 1993; Poret et al., 1996; Tikanoja et al., 1998; Wolff, 1943). Brugada et al. (1997) identified the first locus for familial AF to chromosome 10q22-q24 (Table 50.2) and genetic heterogeneity has also been identified. The genes for familial AF, however, are not yet known.

WOLFF-PARKINSON-WHITE SYNDROME

Clinical features

In the normal heart, the atria and ventricles are electrically connected via a single pathway through the atrioventricular (AV) node. In Wolff-Parkinson-White (WPW) syndrome (1930), an accessory atrioventricular bypass pathway is present, creating the substrate for tachydysrhythmias (Mehdirad et al., 1999). The electrical conduction properties of accessory pathways in WPW syndrome are more like that seen in ventricular myocardium than in AV nodal tissue and may conduct very rapidly with a short refractory period (Chung et al., 1965). During sinus rhythm, ventricular excitation occurs via the accessory pathway prior to excitation through the AV node, a process referred to as pre-excitation. It is this pre-excitation that is responsible for the characteristic ECG findings of a short PR interval and the so-called "delta wave", a slurring of the upstroke of the QRS complex (Fig. 50.11).

The most common dysrhythmia seen in patients with WPW syndrome is orthodromic AV reciprocating tachycardia (AVRT), which uses the AV node as the antegrade limb and the accessory pathway (i.e., bypass tract) as the retrograde limb (Durakovic et al., 1992). This tachydysrhythmia commonly causes palpitations, chest pain, dizziness and lightheadedness, shortness of breath, and in some cases,

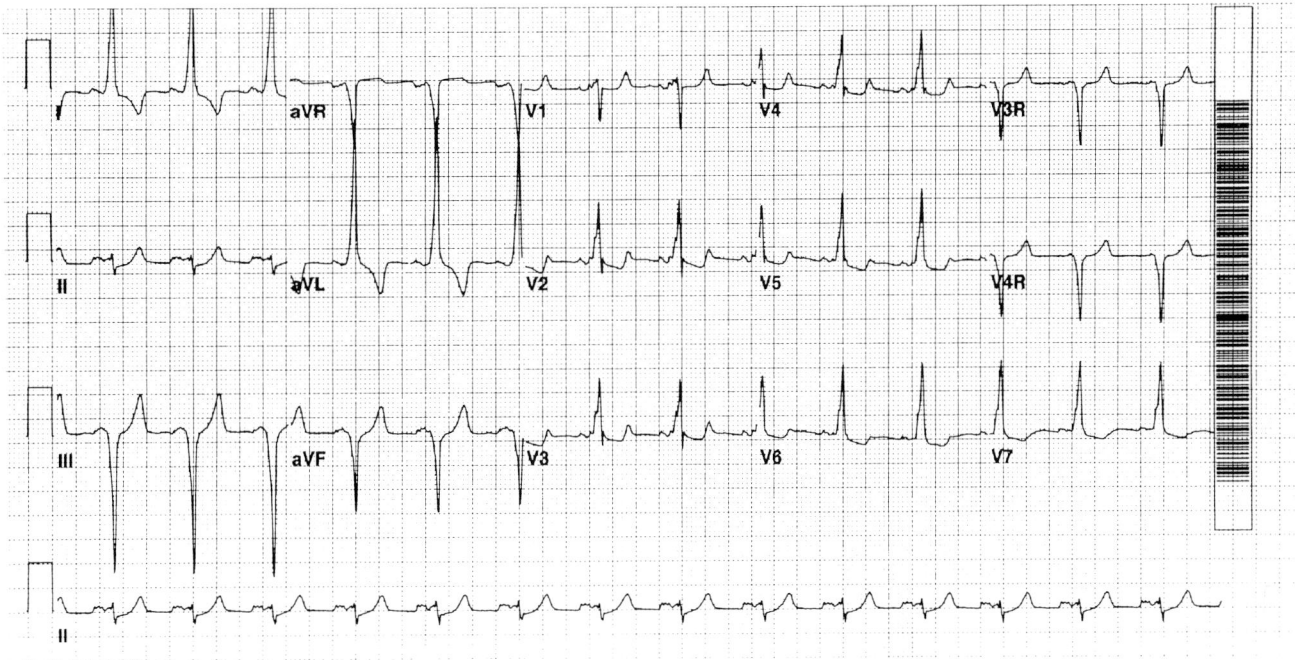

Fig. 50.11. A fifteen-year-old female with Wolff-Parkinson-White syndrome. The electrocardiographic features include a short PR interval and delta wave.

syncope. When sustained, AVRT may precipitate onset of atrial fibrillation, which under certain circumstances may be life-threatening due to its ability to rapidly conduct via the accessory pathway, inducing VF. These patients are therefore at increased risk of sudden death.

Genetics and management

Although most cases of WPW syndrome are believed to be sporadic, autosomal dominant inherited WPW syndrome is well described (Chia et al., 1982; Gillette et al., 1978; Vidaillet et al., 1987). The incidence of pre-excitation in first-degree relatives has been reported to be less than 1%, with a prevalence in the general population of about 0.15% (Chung et al., 1965; Vidaillet et al., 1987). Notably, patients with multiple pathways have an increased prevalence of pre-excitation in first-degree relatives, approximately 1.7%. WPW syndrome may also occur in the setting of congenital heart disease, particularly Ebstein's anomaly, or myocardial disease (i.e., hypertrophic cardiomyopathy). It is not clear whether WPW in this circumstance has increased familial incidence. The permanent form of junctional reciprocating tachycardia (PJRT), in which a septal accessory pathway is present and has similar decremental properties as the AV node, appears to have familial inheritance as well but is probably uncommon. Neither WPW syndrome nor familial PJRT have been deciphered from a genetic standpoint, but linkage has been described for both.

In WPW syndrome, families with primary WPW as well as those with associated autosomal dominant familial hypertrophic cardiomyopathy (FHCM), have been mapped to chromosome 7q3 (MacRae et al., 1995), but the gene remains elusive (Table 50.2). Similarly, the gene(s) for PJRT remains unknown (Table 50.2), although the association with the HLA-Bw41 haplotype (chromosome 6p) has been reported (Perticone and Marisco, 1988).

The current first line therapy for WPW is radiofrequency ablation (RFA) which, in most cases, permanently disrupts the accessory pathway (Jackman et al., 1991). In those small percentage of patients not undergoing RFA, medical therapy may be used.

Primary conduction abnormalities

LEV-LENEGRE PROGRESSIVE CARDIAC CONDUCTION DISEASE

Clinical features

This syndrome, also known as progressive cardiac conduction defect (PCCD), is among the most common cardiac conduction disorders in the world and represents the major cause for pacemaker implantation worldwide at 0.15 pacemaker implantations per 1000 inhabitants per year in developed countries (Schott et al., 1999). PCCD is characterized by progressive worsening of cardiac conduction through the His-Purkinje system, resulting in right or left bundle branch block and widening of the QRS complex (Lenegre and Moreau, 1963; Lev et al., 1970). Patients with this disorder ultimately develop complete AV block (Fig. 50.12) and in many instances present with syncope or sudden death. Etiologically, PCCD has been considered to be a primary degenerative disease or an exaggerated age-related process in which sclerosis of the conduction system occurs.

Genetics

The first gene for PCCD was mapped to chromosome 19q13.3 (Table 50.2) in families with autosomal dominantly transmitted disease (Brink et al., 1995; De Meeus et al., 1995). Genetic heterogeneity was identified when Schott and colleagues demonstrated linkage to chromosome 3p21 and identified mutations in the cardiac sodium channel gene SCN5A (Schott et al., 1999) (Table 50.2). This gene had previously been shown to cause a form of long QT syndrome (LQT3) as well as Brugada syndrome (Chen et al., 1998; Wang et al., 1995b,c).

Management

Patients with PCCD require pacemaker therapy once bradycardia occurs. In cases where syncope precedes diagnosis, immediate implantation is appropriate. Before pacemaker implantation, serial ECGs and Holter monitor studies are necessary for close monitoring.

FAMILIAL COMPLETE ATRIOVENTRICULAR HEART BLOCK

This disorder, when familial, presents with adult onset (age 20–50 years) and has an autosomal dominant inheritance pattern (Connor et al., 1959; Gazes et al., 1965; Waxman et al., 1975). Approximately 50 families have been identified with this disorder and, in all cases, transmission is consistent with autosomal dominant inheritance with full penetrance and variable expression. Whether all of these conditions represent a single disorder is not known. The common presentation of this disease includes one of the following: right bundle branch block (RBBB) alone; left axis deviation (LAD) alone; RBBB plus LAD; or complete heart block (Fig. 50.12). In addition, atrioventricular block has been associated with DCM and skeletal myopathy, and several genetic loci have been identified for those cases (see sections on limb girdle muscular dystrophy and conduction disease with cardiomyopathy, CDDC). As previously noted, another gene has been mapped to chromosome 19q13 in a family with AV block (Table 50.2) but without DCM (Brink et al., 1995), while the gene for Lev-Lenegre progressive cardiac conduction disease (PCCD) has been found to be the cardiac sodium channel gene *SCN5A* (Schott et al., 1999) (Table 50.2).

FAMILIAL TOTAL ATRIAL STANDSTILL

Clinical features

Atrial standstill is characterized by complete absence of spontaneous atrial electrical activity and inability to pace the

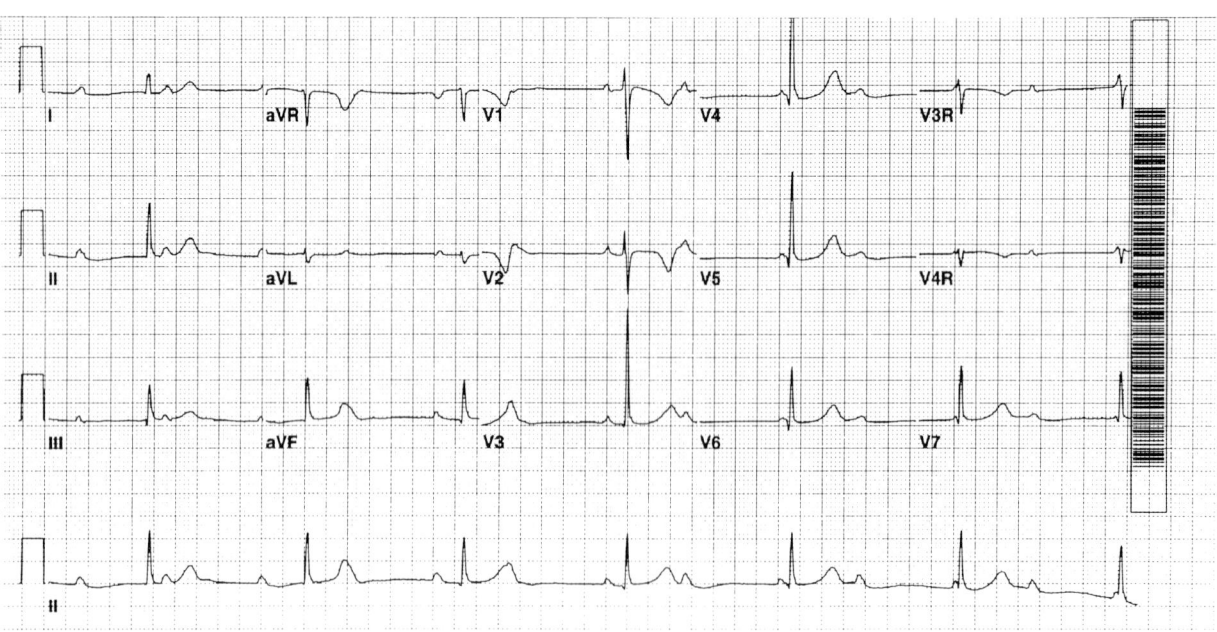

Fig. 50.12. Complete atrioventricular block in this individual with bradycardia.

atria. In addition to loss of electrical activity, there is loss of mechanical function of the atria documented by absence of "a" waves on jugular venous pulse and right atrial pressure tracing, and absence of atrial contraction as detected by echocardiography. Primary atrial standstill can occur as sporadic cases or in families. Familial cases have been reported in an isolated community having a high rate of inbreeding. (Disertori et al., 1983; Shah et al., 1992; Ward et al., 1984). Familial atrial standstill can be associated with other cardiac abnormalities. Ebstein anomaly (ventricular displacement of the tricuspid valve) has been reported in one family with persistent atrial standstill (Pierard et al., 1985). Certain types of muscular dystrophy, Emery-Dreifuss muscular dystrophy, and Kugelberg-Welander syndrome, can present with atrial standstill. These disorders are discussed in further detail below.

Atrial standstill and abnormal sinus node function are common dysrhythmias in familial cases of amyloidosis. Often other systemic effects of amyloidosis, such as peripheral neuropathy, cardiomyopathy, or renal dysfunction, are not seen in these cases. Histologic evidence of amyloid deposits may be identified in atrial or ventricular myocardium (Maeda et al., 1988).

The clinical symptoms of atrial standstill, whether primary or secondary to a systemic disease, may be due to absence of atrial activity or to intermittent atrial tachydysrhythmias. Patients may present with bradycardia due to loss of atrial activity or palpitations, presyncope, dyspnea or chest pain as a result of atrial tachydysrhythmias. A high rate of unexplained sudden death has been reported (Disertori et al., 1983; Ward et al., 1984). Loss of atrial mechanical function may predispose to the development of atrial thrombi, and cerebral and peripheral emboli are reported in up to 30% of cases (Disertori et al., 1983; Pierard et al., 1985).

Genetics and management

The mode of inheritance is not known with certainty, as there are few reports of large affected families, but it is most likely autosomal dominant (Disertori et al., 1983). No gene has been identified thus far (Table 50.2). Treatment consists of permanent ventricular pacing for symptomatic bradycardia and chronic anticoagulation to prevent formation of atrial thrombi.

SINUS NODE DYSFUNCTION

Clinical features

Congenital absence of sinus rhythm (Surawicz and Hariman, 1988) or sinus node dysfunction (Caralis and

Varghese, 1976; Spellberg, 1971) occurs in familial forms. The clinical presentation is generally due to symptomatic bradycardia, but it also may be associated with paroxymal atrial fibrillation and other atrial tachydysrhythmias. Histologic data are limited, but one report of a single member of a family who suffered sudden death showed mononuclear cell infiltration of the sinus node; fibrosis of the sinus, AV nodes, and atrial tissue; and atrophy of the right and left bundle branches (Bharati et al., 1992).

Genetics and management

The inheritance pattern of familial congenital absence of sinus node function is autosomal dominant with a high degree of penetrance (Table 50.2). The gene for this disorder remains unknown. Treatment consists of permanent pacing for symptomatic bradycardia and, unlike persistent atrial standstill, in which the atria are unable to be paced due to inability to produce electrical excitation, atrial or dual-chamber pacing may be used. If atrial fibrillation is a prominent feature, antiarrhythmic medications and/or chronic anticoagulation may be indicated.

Familial dysrhythmias associated with myocardial disease

HYPERTROPHIC CARDIOMYOPATHY (HCM)

Hypertrophic cardiomyopathy (HCM; see Ch. 49) is characterized by myocardial hypertrophy with a wide spectrum of symptoms, including dyspnea, chest pain, and syncope (Maron, 1997). The annual mortality rate was initially reported to be 2 to 4% primarily due to sudden death, often occurring in asymptomatic individuals, but is now believed to be 0.1% per year. This disorder is considered to be the leading cause of sudden death in the young and in athletes (Maron et al., 1996). The annual incidence of sudden death is higher in younger patients with familial HCM than in the elderly. The diagnosis is based on typical clinical features and the demonstration of unexplained left ventricular, right ventricular, or biventricular hypertrophy on two-dimensional echocardiography. The left ventricular hypertrophy is commonly asymmetric, localized to the septum, but may involve the entire ventricle in a concentric pattern (Fig. 50.13). Isolated right ventricular hypertrophy occurs in fewer than 5% of cases. Isolated apical hypertrophy is rare except in Japan where it is claimed to account for 20 to 30% of the cases, or in elderly patients. Dynamic outflow tract obstruction occurs in about 30% of patients.

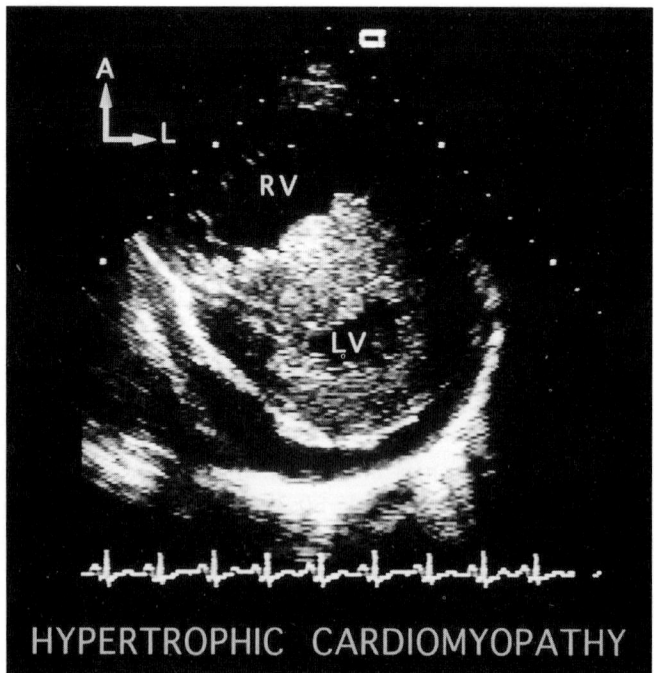

Fig. 50.13. Echocardiogram demonstrating hypertrophic cardiomyopathy with left ventricular posterior wall and interventricular septal hypertrophy.

Histologically, the myocardial hypertrophy consists of myocyte hypertrophy, cellular and myofibrillar disarray, and myocardial fibrosis and one of the hallmarks of familial HCM is myocyte and myofibrillar disarray (Maron et al., 1987).

Mapping of familial hypertrophic cardiomyopathy genes

The first gene for familial hypertrophic cardiomyopathy (FHC) was mapped to chromosome 14q11.2-q12 using genome-wide linkage analysis in a large Canadian family (Jarcho et al., 1989). Soon afterwards, FHC locus heterogeneity was reported (Epstein et al., 1992; Schwartz et al., 1992; Solomon et al., 1990) and subsequently confirmed by Thierfelder et al. (1993) and Watkins et al. (1993) when they mapped the second FHC locus to chromosome 1q3 (Watkins et al., 1993) and of the third locus to chromosome 15q2 (Thierfelder et al., 1993) (Table 50.3). Carrier et al. (1993) mapped the fourth FHC locus to chromosome 11p11.2. Five other loci were subsequently reported, located on chromosomes 7q3 (MacRae et al., 1995), 3p21.2-3p21.3, (Poetter et al., 1996), 12q23-q24.3 (Kimura et al., 1997), 15q14 (Mogensen et al., 1999), and 2q31 (Satoh et al., 1999)(Fig. 50.14). Several other families are not linked to any known FHC loci, indicating the existence of additional FHC-causing genes. These genes have been identified in patients presenting late in childhood or adulthood and not in neonates, infants, and very young children.

Fig. 50.14. Loci, genes and proteins responsible for familial hypertrophic cardiomyopathy. All genes causing HCM encode proteins of the sarcomere.

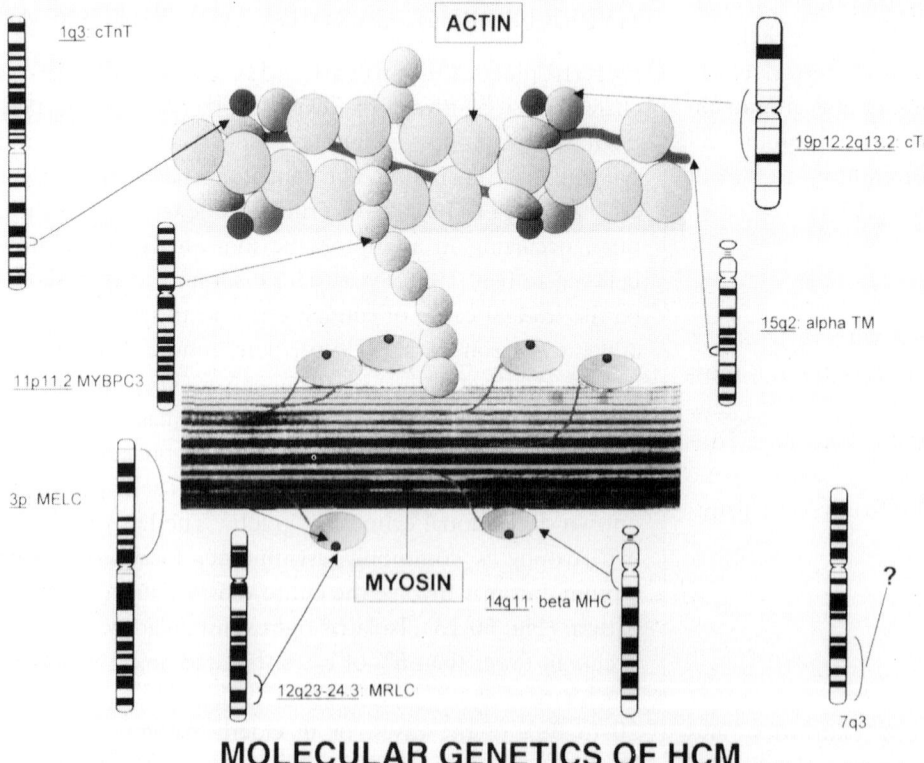

MOLECULAR GENETICS OF HCM

Table 50.3. Familial Disorders of Cardiac Structure Associated with Dysrhythmias

Disease	Rhythm Abnormality	Inheritance	Chromosome Location	Defective Protein
Ventricular arrhythmias				
Hypertrophic cardiomyopathy	VT, VF	AD	1q3; 2q31; 3p21.2; 7q3; 11p11.2; 12q23; 14q11; 15q14; 15q2; 19p12[α]	Cardiac troponin T (1q3); titin (2q31); myosin essential light chain (3p21.2); myosin regulatory light chain (12q23); β-myosin heavy chain (14q11); α-actin (15q14); α-tropomyosin (15q2); cardiac troponin I (19p12.2)
Arrhythmogenic right ventricular dysplasia/cardiomyopathy	VT,VF	AD	1q42-43, 2q32,3p23, 10p12-14, 14q12-22, 14q24.3	?
Arrhythmogenic right ventricular dysplasia/cardiomyopathy with myofibrillar myopathy	VT,VF	AD	10q22.3	?
Familial palmoplantar keratosis (Naxos syndrome)	VT, IVCD	AR	17q21	Plakoglobin
Dilated cardiomyopathy	VT	AD	1q32, 2q31, 5q33, 9q13, 10q21-23, 15q14[α]	Desmin (2q31); δ-sarcoglycan (5q31); α-actin (15q14)
Dilated cardiomyopathy	VT	X-linked	Xp21	Dystrophin
Mitral valve prolapse	AF, ?SD	AD	16p11.2-12.1	?
Barth syndrome	VT	X-linked	Xq28	G4.5 (Tafazzin)
Left ventricular noncompaction	VT	X-linked	Xq28[α]	G4.5 (Tafazzin)
Supraventricular arrhythmias				
Familial amyloidosis	Atrial standstill, AF	AD	TTR locus	Prealbumin (Transthyretin)
Conduction abnormalities				
Idiopathic restrictive cardiomyopathy	AVB,VT	AD,AR	2q31,[α] TTR locus	Desmin (2q31), Prealbumin (Transthyretin)
Familial amyloidosis	AVB	AD	TTR locus	Prealbumin (Transthyretin)
Dilated cardiomyopathy with conduction disease	AVB	AD	1p1-1q1, 3p22, 6q23	Lamin A/C (1p1-1q1)
Holt-Oram syndrome	AVB, AT	AD, X-linked	12q24.1	TBX-5
Familial atrial septal defect	AVB, AF, SD	AD, ?	5q35, 5p	Nkx2–5 (5q35)
LEOPARD syndrome	AVB, BBB, IVCD	AD	17,*	Neurofibromin
Heterotaxy	AVB, SVT, AF	X-linked	Xp26	Zic3
Heterotaxy	AVB, SVT, AF	AD		NODAL, LEFTY A, LEFTY B, Activin type IIB
Neurologic disorders				
Muscular dystrophies				
Duchenne	ST, AT, IVCD, VT	X-linked	Xp21	Dystrophin
Becker	AVB, SVT, AF	X-linked	Xp21	Dystrophin
Limb-girdle	AVB	AR	2p13, 4q12, 5q33-34, 13q12, 15q15, 17q11-12, 17q21[α]	Dysferlin (2p13), β-sarcoglycan (4q12), δ-sarcoglycan (5q33-34), γ-sarcoglycan (13q12), Calpain-3 (15q15), telethonin (17q11-12), α-sarcoglycan (17q21)
Limb-girdle	AVB, VT	AD	1q11-21, 3p25, 5q31, 6q23	Caveolin-3 (3p25)
Facioscapulohumeral	Atrial standstill, AF	AD	4,[α]	?
Emery-Dreifuss	Atrial standstill, AF	X-linked	Xq28	Emerin
Emery-Dreifuss	Atrial standstill, AF	AD	1p1-1q1	Lamin A/C
Myotonic dystrophy	AVB, VT	AD	19q13.3	Myotonin protein kinase
Other neurologic disorders				
Freidreich ataxia	Variable	AR	9q13-31.3	Frataxin
Kearns-Sayre syndrome	AVB	Mitochondrial	mtDNA	tRNA[leu (UUR)]-3243
MELAS syndrome	AVB, VT	Mitochondrial	mtDNA	
MERRF syndrome	AVB, T	Mitochondrial	mtDNA	
McArdle syndrome	SD, AVB	AR, AD	?	?
Kugelberg-Welander syndrome	Atrial standstill, AF, AVB	AR	?	?

Abbreviations: AF, atrial fibrillation; AT, atrial tachycardia; AVB, atrioventricular block; IVCD, intraventricular conduction delay; BBB, bundle branch block; SD, sudden death; SND, sinus node dysfunction; ST, sinus tachycardia; VT, ventricular tachycardia; VF, ventricular fibrillation; AD autosomal dominant; AR, autosomal recessive; mtDNA, mitochondrial genome
[α] *At least one other unknown.*

Gene identification in familial hypertrophic cardiomyopathy

All the disease genes encode proteins that are part of the sarcomere (i.e., a sarcomyopathy), which is a complex structure with an exact stoichiometry and multiple sites of protein-protein interactions (Thierfelder et al., 1994; Towbin, 2000b). The encoded proteins (Fig. 50.15) include three myofilament proteins, the β-myosin heavy chain (β-MyHC) (Geisterfer-Lowrance et al., 1990; Hejtmancik et al., 1991), the ventricular myosin essential light chain 1 (MLC-1s/v) and the ventricular myosin regulatory light chain 2 (MLC-2s/v) (Poetter et al., 1996); four thin filament proteins, cardiac actin (Mogensen et al., 1999), cardiac troponin T (cTnT) (Thierfelder et al., 1994), cardiac troponin I(cTnI) (Kimura et al., 1997) and α-tropomyosin (α-TM) (Thierfelder et al., 1994), and finally one myosin-binding protein, the cardiac-myosin binding protein C (cMyBP-C) (Bonne et al., 1995; Watkins et al., 1995). Titin has recently been described as well (Satoh et al., 1999) (Table 50.3). Each of these proteins is encoded by multigene families that exhibit tissue specific, developmental, and physiologically regulated patterns of expression.

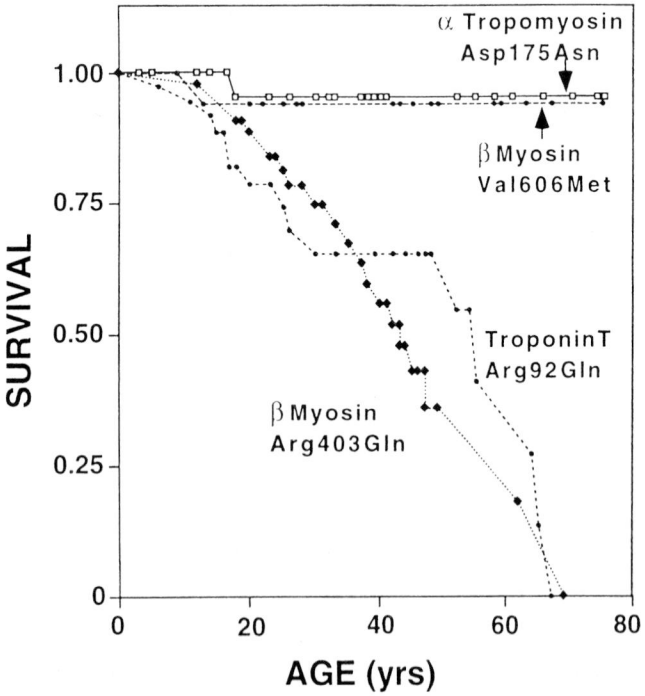

Fig. 50.15. Kaplan-Meier survival curve in hypertrophic cardiomyopathy comparing mutations of β-myosin heavy chain, cardiac troponin T, and α-tropomyosin (with permission).

Thick filament proteins (Fig. 50.14)

1. Myosin subunits Myosin is the molecular motor that transduces energy from the hydrolysis of ATP into directed movement that, drives sarcomere shortening and muscle contraction. Cardiac myosin consists of two heavy chains (MyHC) and two pairs of light chains (MLC), referred to as essential (or alkali) light chains (MLC-1) and regulatory (or phosphorylatable) light chains (MLC-2), respectively (Schiaffino and Reggiani, 1996). The myosin molecule is highly asymmetric, consisting of two globular heads joined to a long rod-like tail. The light chains are arranged in tandem in the head-tail junction. Their function is not fully understood. Neither myosin light chain type is required for the adenosine triphosphatase (ATPase) activity of the myosin head, but they probably modulate it in the presence of actin and contribute to the rigidity of the neck, which is hypothesized to function as a lever arm for generating an effective power stroke. Mutations have been found in the heavy chains and in the two types of ventricular light chains.

Concerning the heavy chains, the β isoform (β-MyHC) is the major isoform of the human ventricle and of slow-twitch skeletal fibers. It is encoded by *MYH7*. At least 50 mutations have been found in unrelated families with FHC, and three hot spots for mutations have been identified, including codons 403, 719 and 741. All but three of these mutations are missense mutations located in the head or in the head-rod junction of the molecule (Bonne et al., 1998). The three exceptions are two 3 bp deletions that do not disrupt the reading frame (codon 10, codon 930) and a 2.4 kb deletion in the 3′ region. In the kindred with the latter mutation, only the proband developed clinical evidence of HCM, which occurred at a very late age of onset (59 years).

Animal models were initially reported by Vikstrom et al. (1996) and Geisterfer-Lowrance et al. (1996). The mice produced by these groups developed HCM-like disease. heterozygotes have been produced with the Arg403Gln mutation and have been shown to have normal survival while homozygotes had premature death, mimicking the human mutations. Fatkin et al. (1999a,b) demonstrated neonatal cardiomyopathy in homozygotes. In addition, Bevilacqua et al. (1999) demonstrated QT dispersion in these animals while Berul et al. (1998) showed gender differences in the electropohysiologic abnormalities seen in these animals

As for the light chains, the isoforms expressed in the ventricular myocardium and in the slow-twitch muscles are the so-called ventricular myosin regulatory light chains (MLC-2s/v) encoded by *MYL2*, and the ventricular myosin essential light chain (MLC-1s/v) encoded by

MYL3. They both belong to the superfamily of EF-hand proteins. Two missense mutations have been reported in *MYL3*, and five in *MYL2*.

2. Myosin binding protein-C (MyBP-C) Myosin binding protein-C (MyBP-C) is part of the thick filaments of the sarcomere, being located at the level of the transverse stripes, 43 nm apart, seen by electron microscopy in the sarcomere A band. Its function is uncertain, but it is believed to play both structural and regulatory roles. Partial extraction of cMyBP-C from rat cardiac myocytes and rabbit skeletal muscle fibers has been shown to alter Ca^{2+}-sensitive tension (Hofmann et al., 1991). In addition, phosphorylation of cMyBP-C was shown to alter myosin cross-bridges in native thick filaments, suggesting that cMyBP-C can modify force production in activated cardiac muscles.

The cardiac isoform of myosin binding protein-C is encoded by *MYBPC3* (Carrier et al., 1997; Watkins et al., 1995), which has three distinct regions that are specific to the cardiac isoform: the NH_2-terminal domain CO lg-l containing 101 residues; the MyBP-C motif (a 105-residue stretch linking the C1 and C2 lg-l domains); and a 28-residue loop inserted in the C5 lg-l domain (Gautel et al., 1995). cMyBP-C is specifically expressed in the heart during human and murine development (Fougerousse et al., 1998; Gautel et al., 1998).

Approximately 30 *MYBPC3* mutations have been identified in unrelated families with FHC. In the majority of cases, the mutations result in aberrant transcripts that are predicted to encode COOH-terminal truncated cardiac MyBP-C polypeptides lacking at least the myosin-binding domain. Of the remaining reported mutations, mutated or deleted proteins occur without disruption of the reading frame; most of these are missense mutations (exons 6, 17, 21, and 23) but a splice donor site mutation (intron 27), and an 18-residue duplication (exon 33) have also been reported (Bonne et al., 1995; Moolman-Smook et al., 1998; Moolman et al., 2000; Rottbauer et al., 1997; Watkins et al., 1995; Yu et al., 1998). In addition, three mutations are predicted to produce either a mutated protein or a truncated one: two are missense mutations in exon 15 and 17 and one is a branch point mutation in intron 23. It has been suggested that most mutations result in a dominant negative action of the mutant protein. Another possibility is defective processing and rapid degradation of partially glycosylated protein. Rapid degradation of a truncated protein may be a critical step preventing myofibrillogenesis, with filament formation (rather than the function of assembled filaments) being disturbed (Fultan and L'Ecuyer, 1993; Gruen and Gautel, 1999; and Moolman et al., 2000).

Recently, a mouse model was reported by McConnell et al. (1999) in which mice expressing altered forms of MYBPC3 were produced. The engineered mutations encoded truncated forms of MyBP-C in which the cardiac myosin heavy chain-binding and titin-binding domain was replaced with novel amino acid residues. Homozygous mice exhibited neonatal onset of a progressive dilated cardiomyopathy with myocyte hypertrophy, myofibrillar disarray, fibrosis, and dystrophic calcification on histopathology. Left-ventricular dilation with reduced contractility was noted on echocardiography in the neonatal period, but myocardial hypertrophy and diastolic dysfunction developed later in the life of these animals. Previously, Yang et al. (1998) reported a mouse model of HCM due to mutant MyBP-C, and this clinical phenotype was more similar to the human disorder. Here, however, the transgenic animals had very high levels of expression of the mutant gene (driven by the α-MHC promoter) and diminished wild-type gene expression.

Thin-filament proteins (Fig. 50.14)

The thin filament contains actin, the troponin complex and tropomyosin. The troponin complex and tropomyosin constitute the Ca^{2+}-sensitive switch that regulates the contraction of cardiac muscle fibers. Mutations were found in α-TM (Thierfelder et al., 1994) and in two of the subunits of the troponin complex: cTnI, the inhibitory subunit, and cTnT, the tropomyosin-binding subunit (Kimura et al., 1997; Thierfelder et al., 1994). Recently, actin mutations have also been reported (Mogensen et al., 1999).

α-Tropomyosin (α-TM) is encoded by *TPM1*. The cardiac isoform is expressed both in the ventricular myocardium and in fast twitch skeletal muscles (Lees-Miller and Helfman, 1991). It shares the overall structure of other tropomyosins—rod-like proteins that possess a simple dimeric α-coiled-coil structure in parallel orientation along their entire length. Four missense mutations were initially described in unrelated FHC families. Two of them, A63V and K70T, are located in exon 2b within the consensus pattern of sequence repeats of α-TM and could alter tropomyosin binding to actin. Mutations D175N and E180G are both located within constitutive exon 5, in a region near the C190 and near the calcium-dependent TnT binding domain. This appears to be a relatively rare cause of HCM. Michelle et al. (1999) recently demonstrated that the known α-TM mutations rely on the calcium-sensitizing effects of these mutations to define the severity of disease.

Cardiac troponin T (cTnT) is encoded by *TNNT2*. In human cardiac muscle, multiple isoforms of cTnT have been described that are expressed in the fetal, adult and diseased heart, and which result from alternative splicing of the single gene *TNNT2*. (Mesnard et al., 1995; Townsend et al., 1995). The precise physiological relevance of these isoforms is currently poorly understood, but the organization of the human gene has been partially established (Forissier et al., 1996; Farza et al., 1998), thus allowing precise identification of the position of the mutations within exons, including those alternatively spliced during development. Eleven mutations (10 missense, 1 deletion) have been found in unrelated FHC families, three of which are located in a hot spot (codon 102).

Cardiac troponin I (cTnI) is encoded by *TNNI3*. The cTnI isoform is expressed only in cardiac muscles (Hunkeler et al., 1991). Cooperative binding of cTnI-actin-tropomyosin is a unique property of the cardiac variant (Solaro and Van Eyk, 1996). To date, six mutations have been identified, all single base substitutions.

α-Cardiac actin (ACTC) was recently identified as a cause of FHC. Mogensen et al. (1999) studied a family with heterogeneous phenotypes, ranging from asymptomatic with mild hypertrophy to pronounced septal hypertrophy and left ventricular outflow tract obstruction. Using linkage analysis and mutation screening, the gene was mapped to chromosome 15q14 with a lod score of 3.6 and a missense mutation (G→T in position 253, exon 5) resulted in an Ala295Ser amino acid substitution. The mutation is localized at the surface of actin in proximity to a putative myosin-binding site. This mutation, which causes FHC, differs from the two mutations reported to cause dilated cardiomyopathy (DCM) that were localized in the immobilized end of actin that cross-binds to the anchor polypeptides in the Z bands (Olson et al., 1998). It appears that mutations near the dystrophin binding region result in DCM while mutations affecting the sarcomeric end result in a HCM phenotype.

Genotype-phenotype relations in familial hypertrophic cardiomyopathy

The pattern and extent of left ventricular hypertrophy in patients with HCM vary greatly even in first-degree relatives, but some families share a high incidence of sudden death. An important issue therefore is to determine whether the genotype heterogeneity observed in FHC accounts for the phenotypic diversity of the disease. However, current results yield preliminary, conclusions because the available data relate to only a few hundred individuals. Several concepts nevertheless begin to emerge, at least for mutations in the *MYH7*, *TNNT2* and *MYBPC3*

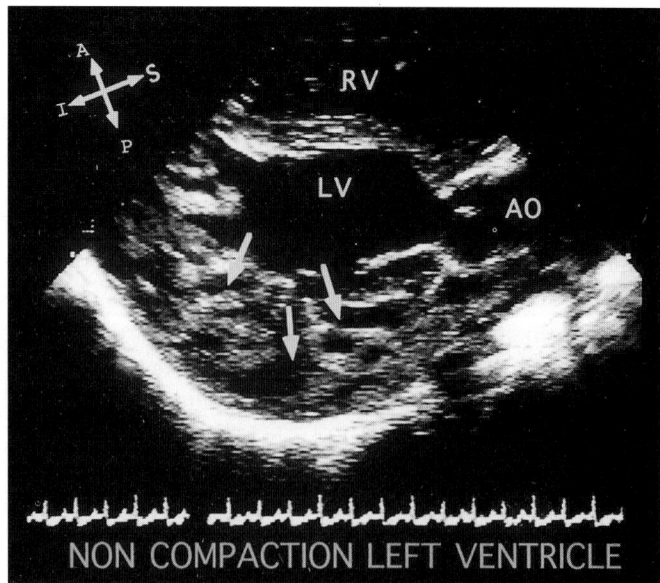

Fig. 50.16. Echocardiogram of left ventricular noncompaction. Note the deep endomyocardial trabeculations in the left ventricle.

genes. For *MYH7*, prognosis for patients with different mutations varies considerably (Watkins et al., 1992). For example, the R403Q mutation appears to be associated with markedly reduced survival, whereas some others, such as V606M, appear more benign (Fig. 50.16). The disease caused by *TNNT2* mutations is usually associated with a 20% incidence of nonpentrance, a relatively mild (and sometimes subclinical) hypertrophy, but a high incidence of sudden death, which can occur even in the absence of significant clinical left ventricular hypertrophy (Moolman et al., 1997; Watkins et al., 1995b). However, one family with a *TNNT2* mutation reportedly had complete penetrance, and echocardiographic data showed a wide range of hypertrophy but no sudden cardiac death (Farza et al., 1998). Thus, more data are needed before final conclusions are drawn. Mutations in MYBPC3 seem to be characterized by specific clinical features with a mild phenotype in young subjects, a delayed age at the onset of symptoms and a favorable prognosis before the age of 40 years (Bonne et al., 1995; Charron et al., 1998; Moolman et al., 2000; Nimura et al., 1998; Watkins et al., 1995a).

Genetic studies have also revealed the presence of clinically healthy individuals carrying a mutant allele (no matter which gene is affected), which is associated in relatives with a typical phenotype of the disease. Several mechanisms could account for the large variability of the phenotypic expression of the mutations: the role of environmental differences and acquired traits (e.g., differences in lifestyle, risk factors, and exercise), and the existence of modifier genes and/or polymorphisms that could modulate the phenotypic expression of the disease. The only significant results obtained so far concern the influence of the angiotensin I converting enzyme insertion/deletion (ACE I/D) polymorphism. Association studies showed that, compared to a control population, the D allele is more common in patients with hypertrophic cardiomyopathy and in patients with a high incidence of sudden cardiac death (Marian et al., 1993; Yoneya et al., 1995). The association between the D allele and hypertrophy is observed in the case of *MYH7* R403 codon mutations, but not with *MYBPC3* mutation carriers (Tesson et al., 1997), raising the concept of multiple genetic modifiers in FHC.

Elucidation of the pathogenesis from genetic models

Based on *in vitro* and *in vivo* studies in genetic animal models of HCM, it now appears that the primary defect is impaired contractility. Analysis of a human heart from a patient with the Arg[403]Gln mutation showed the ratio of myosin to actin was normal (Vybiral et al., 1992), indicating there is no deficiency of the βMHC protein. All of the responsible mutant genes encode for a sarcomeric protein and appear, in some way, to impair systolic contraction or diastolic relaxation. In feline adult cardiac myocytes, in which βMHC is the predominant myosin form, expression of human mutant βMHC gene, Arg[403]Gln, was associated with sarcomere disassembly (Marian et al., 1995). Expression of the human mutant troponin T in this model also induced sarcomere disassembly and was associated with impaired rate of cell shortening as detected by laser (Marian et al., 1997). Furthermore, the expressed mutant protein was incorporated into the sarcomere. In a transgenic mouse, expression of troponin T gene (cTnT-Gln[92]) exhibited sarcomere disarray, increased fibrous tissue, and sudden death, but only minimal hypertrophy (Oberst et al., 1998). In this model increased expression of the mutant protein was associated with a more severe phenotype, confirming the mutant protein has a dominant-negative effect. These results have been confirmed by several investigators (Becker et al., 1997; Geisterfer-Lowrance et al., 1996; Marian et al., 1995; Vikstrom et al., 1996). Expression of the mutant myosin heavy chain gene or the troponin gene in the mouse has, in general, been associated with less hypertrophy than expected (Oberst et al., 1998). Recently, a transgenic rabbit model (rabbit has βMHC as its cardiac myosin) has been developed expressing the βMHC (Arg[403]Gln) mutation that exhibits sarcomere disarray, hypertrophy and increased fibrous tissue virtually identical to that observed in humans (Marian et al., 1999). In addition, α-TM mutations in an animal model

caused cardiac dysfunction as well (Mutuohamy et al., 1999). Thus, the overall postulated pathogenesis of FHCM may be summarized briefly as follows.) The mutant protein is incorporated into the sarcomere and acts as a poison peptide, which impairs contractility of that particular cell, which, in turn, provides the stimulus for the mitogenic response (probably several growth factors) of compensatory hypertrophy. The growth stimulus, as in acquired disorders, appears highly localized and mediated by autocrine or intracrine factors, given that the hypertrophy is localized in many patients, primarily to the interventricular septum. The growth factors also stimulate fibroblast proliferation and increased matrix formation. The relationship between the hypertrophy and increased fibrous tissue response to sudden death and arrhythmias remains to be determined. It is postulated that the fibrous tissue leads to delayed electrical conduction and predisposes to arrhythmias and sudden death. The future elucidation of the molecular basis for the pathogenesis of this disease, however, must provide a rationale for three puzzling, consistent features of the pathology of familial HCM: predominance of hypertrophy in the septum; sarcomere and myocyte disarray; and, the supernormal systolic function. The diastolic stiffness or decreased compliance is expected with hypertrophy whether it is primary or compensatory, but these other features are not seen in compensatory hypertrophy associated with myocardial infarction or pressure overload.

Management

Medical therapy is typically indicated (Spirito et al., 1997). The most commonly used medications include β-adrenergic blockers and calcium channel blockers. Good hydration status is also important. Antiarrhythmic agents are used when necessary; poorly controlled ventricular dysrhythmias or syncope may lead to ICD implantation. In cases where severe obstruction occurs, myomectomy or pacemaker implantation (DDD mode) have been utilized. More recently alcohol ablation has been employed in adults. Cardiac transplantation may be necessary in cases with dilation and systolic dysfunction.

NEONATAL HYPERTROPHIC CARDIOMYOPATHY

Clinically, this appears to be the same disorder as that seen in older children and adults (Towbin and Lipshultz, 1999). Echocardiograms and electrocardiograms tend to mimic the findings described for adults with HCM. However, the underlying causes appear to differ from the sarcomeric gene-related disorders of adults. In the neonate and infant with HCM, abnormalities of mitochondrial function and metabolic disorders tend to predominate. In addition, genetic syndromes are common in this age group as well. Recently, Mott et al. (2000) have demonstrated that Noonan syndrome, mitochondrial myopathies, and metabolic disorders such as glycogen storage diseases predominate along with abnormalities of fatty acid oxidation. Although sarcomeric gene mutations could be involved as well, no patients have been described to date in the literature. Instead, it is likely that the sarcomere is secondarily affected by the mitochondrial and metabolic abnormalities, which probably create an energy production-utilization mismatch.

Finally, neonates with a dilated form of HCM with combined systolic and diastolic dysfunction are well described. In some cases, deep endomyocardial trabeculations are noted, consistent with left ventricular noncompaction (Chin et al., 1990; Ichida et al., 1999) (Fig. 50.15). Males with this abnormality have been shown, in some cases, to carry mutations in G4.5, an X-linked gene (Xq28) that encodes a novel protein called tafazzin (Bione et al., 1996; Bleyl et al., 1997 D'Adamo et al., 1997) (Table 50.3). Although the function of this protein is not known, clinically these children have abnormal mitochondria on electron microscopy and abnormal energy production. Other children with early presentation of dilated HCM have been found to have mitochondrial abnormalities as well and this occurs in both sexes.

Evaluation of these children should include urine for organic acids, serum amino acids, acylcarnitine profile, and skeletal muscle biopsy for microscopy, electron microscopy, and electron transport chain analysis (Towbin and Lipshultz, 1999).

Management

Therapy includes β-adrenergic blockers in patients with HCM and hypercontractile function, with or without obstruction. In metabolic mitochondrial disorders, the metabolic derangement should be treated. Carnitine, coenzyme Q10, riboflavin, thiamine and other vitamins are useful in some cases. When ventricular dysfunction occurs, anticongestive measures are necessary. Dysrhythmias are treated with medical therapy.

DILATED CARDIOMYOPATHY (DCM)

Clinical features

Dilated cardiomyopathy (DCM) (see Ch. 49) is characterized by increased ventricular chamber size, decreased wall thickness, and impaired systolic ventricular function (Towbin, 1999b). Secondary diastolic dysfunction may also occur. Due to the left ventricular dilation, the mitral ring stretches and the development of mitral regurgitation (MR) is common. When MR is significant, left atrial enlargement occurs and the development of pulmonary hypertension may occur. The most common clinical presentation is that of congestive heart failure (CHF), with resting tachycardia (probably due to increased sympathetic tone), dyspnea due to pulmonary edema, hepatomegaly, and poor perfusion due to low cardiac output (Kannel and Belanger, 1991; Senni et al., 1998; Smith, 1985). Syncope and sudden death may occur and in many of these cases VT/VF is the cause (Anderson et al., 1987; Friedman et al., 1991; Hoffman et al., 2000; Sugrue et al., 1992; Tamburro and Wilber, 1992; Wiles et al., 1991). Many patients may have pericardial and/or pleural effusion as well. In addition to the ventricular tachydysrhythmias, SVT can occur. In some patients, conduction abnormalities are prominent.

Genetics

The prevalence of idiopathic DCM has been estimated to be approximately 40 cases per 100,000 (Codd et al., 1989; Manolio et al., 1992; Schocken et al., 1992). Familial DCM is estimated to account for 30% of patients with idiopathic DCM. Inheritance of familial DCM is usually autosomal dominant but X-linked, mitochondrial and autosomal recessive DCM also occurs. Genetic heterogeneity has been found for the autosomal dominant form of DCM. The first autosomal dominant gene was identified by our group on chromosome 1q32 (Durand et al., 1995). Five other chromosomal loci have been identified by us: chromosome 10q21-23, (Bowles et al., 1996) 5q33, (Tsubata et al., 2000) and others including 9q13 (Krajinovic et al., 1995), 15q14 (Olson et al., 1998), 2q31 (Siu et al., 1999) (Table 50.3). Three additional chromosomal loci have been mapped to 1p1-1q1 (Kass et al., 1994), 1q11-1q21 (Van der Kooi, 1997), 3p22-25 (Olson and Keating, 1996), and 6q23 (Messina et al., 1997), in families having DCM in association with conduction defects. One family linked to chromosome 6q23 also has associated limb girdle muscular dystrophy (Messina et al., 1997), while 2 other families had sensorineural deafness (Schonberger et al., 2000). In the families with conduction disease, transient dysrhythmias, which present in the second or third decade, become sustained and commonplace by the third or fourth decade (Graber et al., 1986). The abnormal rhythms included second- or third-degree AV block, atrial fibrillation, or marked bradycardia, commonly requiring a pacemaker. DCM usually developed in the fourth of fifth decade, generally out of proportion to the severity of the rhythm disturbance. Sudden death commonly occurred in the late stages of the disease. On autopsy, marked right and left ventricular dilatation, interstitial fibrosis, myocyte degeneration characterized by cytoplasmic vacuolization, and AV nodal cell replacement by fibrous tissue were noted. The gene for the chromosome 1p–1q-linked disorder was recently shown to be lamin A/C (Fatkin et al., 1999b), the same gene that causes autosomal dominant Emery-Dreifuss muscular dystrophy (Bonne et al., 1999). The other genes have remained elusive (Table 50.3). In the pure forms of familial DCM, three genes have now been identified, α-actin (15q14) (Olson et al., 1998), desmin (2q31) (Li et al., 1999), and δ-sarcoglycan (5q33)(Tsubata et al., 2000) (Table 50.3). In addition to forming portions of the thin filament of the sarcomere, which is essential to the generation of force, α-actin is also an important cytoskeletal protein involved in structural integrity and the transmission of force. Mutations in actin responsible for DCM, are located in the domain that is immobilized and attached to the Z-band or intercalated disc and involved with transmitting force. In contrast, mutations in the actin domain affecting the myosin cross-bridges and the generation of force (sarcomere) give rise to HCM (Mogensen et al., 1999). Desmin is the specific intermediate filament for muscle and an essential cytoskeletal protein for maintaining cardiac structure and for the transmission of force and other signals to the cytoplasm and the nucleus of the cell. Desmin stretches from its attachment to the sarcomere Z-band to the nuclear membrane and other organelles (Fuchs, 1994). Mutations in desmin have been shown to be associated with cardiac and skeletal abnormalities (Milner et al., 1996). A missense mutation (Ile^{451}Met) was recently found to be responsible for DCM in a family without any skeletal or smooth muscle abnormalities. Mutations leading to combined skeletal and cardiac abnormalities have all been in the rod region of desmin. In contrast, the Ile^{451} Met mutation responsible for the restricted cardiac phenotype of DCM encodes for the tail domain of human desmin, located in codon 451 with cytosine substituting for guanine. This would suggest a possible unique cardiac function for the domain in this region. Elimination of the desmin gene in a knockout mouse was associated with a phenotype of DCM exhibiting impaired cardiac function and myocyte necrosis. It is of note that DCM associated with musculoskeletal disorders such as Duchenne muscular dystrophy, are due to dystrophin, muscle Lim protein, metavinculin, α-dystroglycan, α-, β-, and γ-sarcoglycan, all of which are cytoskeletal proteins (Melacini et al., 1999; Maeda et al., 1997; Roberds et al., 1993; Zolk et al., 2000). There is, thus, the strong suggestion that familial DCM may be a disease of the cytoskeletal proteins (Towbin, 1998;

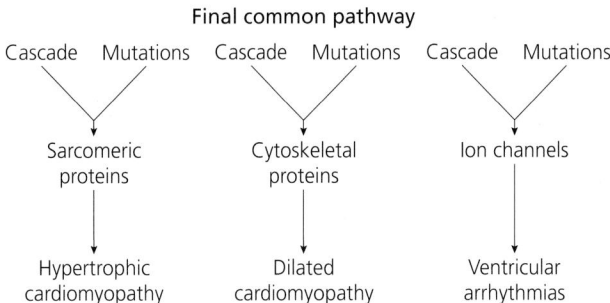

Fig. 50.17. Final common pathway hypothesis. The concept developed here is that phenotypes result from mutations in genes encoding specific subtypes of proteins or cascade pathways which affect the function of these targets. For instance, hypertrophic heart disease results from mutations in sarcomeric proteins or in cascade pathways affecting these target proteins. Similarly, ventricular arrhythmias and dilated, dysfunctional hearts are caused by abnormalities of ion channels and cytoskeletal/sarcolemmal proteins, respectively or cascade pathways involved in the function of these target proteins.

Towbin et al., 1999) analogous to HCM being a disease of the sarcomere (Thierfelder et al., 1994) and long QT syndrome and Brugada syndrome being an ion channelopathy (Towbin, 2000; Vatta et al., 2000). This has been termed by Towbin as the "final common pathway hypothesis" (Towbin, 1998; Towbin et al., 1999) (Fig. 50.17) and the concept has been reiterated recently by Katz (2000a). Our recent identification of defects in δ-sarcoglycan in DCM (Tsubata et al., 2000) further supports this concept.

X-LINKED DILATED CARDIOMYOPATHY (XLCM)

Clinical features

Berko and Swift (1987) reported a five-generation kindred with DCM, X-linked inheritance, and no clinical evidence of skeletal myopathy. Males presented in their teens or early twenties with clinical evidence of mitral regurgitation and an echocardiographic diagnosis of DCM. Episodes of ventricular tachycardia were noted in several patients. The males progressed rapidly (within 1 or 2 years) to death or cardiac transplantation. Manifesting female carriers developed mild cardiomyopathy in the fourth or fifth decade and progressed slowly. Right ventricular endomyocardial biopsy revealed minimal interstitial fibrosis, while postmortem evaluation showed marked dilatation, widespread patchy fibrosis (worst in the posterior wall), and normal mitochondria on electron microscopy. There were no pathognomonic findings differentiating this cardiomyopathy from other dilated forms, except for the apparent X-linked inheritance and elevation of the muscle isoform of creatine kinase (CK-MM) in the serum of affected males and female carriers.

Genetics

Towbin and colleagues (1993) demonstrated linkage of XLCM to the dystrophin (Table 50.4) locus at Xp21 (i.e., the gene responsible for Duchenne and Becker muscular dystrophy) in the family described above, as well as in a second family. Evaluation of the protein defect in XLCM showed absence (or low abundance) of the N-terminal and rod portion of the dystrophin protein while skeletal muscle total protein was normal (Towbin et al., 1993). The 156 kD dystrophin-associated glycoprotein (known as α-dystroglycan) (Towbin et al., 1993; Towbin, 1995), a membrane-bound constituent of the dystrophin-associated glycoprotein (DAG) complex, was decreased in abundance in cardiac tissue as well and it was suggested that the entire DAG complex was involved (Towbin, 1995) (Fig. 50.18). This was later confirmed by others (Bies et al., 1997; Ohlendieck, 1993; Franz et al., 2000; Kaprielian et al.,

Table 50.4. Limb-Girdle Muscular Dystrophies

Designation	Genetic Locus	Defective Protein	Cardiac Disease
Autosomal Dominant			
LGMD 1A	5q31	?	None
B	1q11-21	?	Dysrhythmias, AVB
C	6q23	?	Dysrhythmias, AVB
D	3p25	Caveolin-3	Dysrhythmias, AVB
Autosomal Recessive			
LGMD 2A	15q15	Calpain-3	None
B	2p13	Dysferlin	None
C	13q12	γ-Sarcoglycan	Cardiomyopathy, AVB
D	17q21	α-Sarcoglycan	Cardiomyopathy, AVB
E	4q12	β-Sarcoglycan	Cardiomyopathy, AVB
F	5q33-34	δ-Sarcoglycan	Cardiomyopathy, AVB
G	17q11-12	Telethonin	Cardiomyopathy, AVB

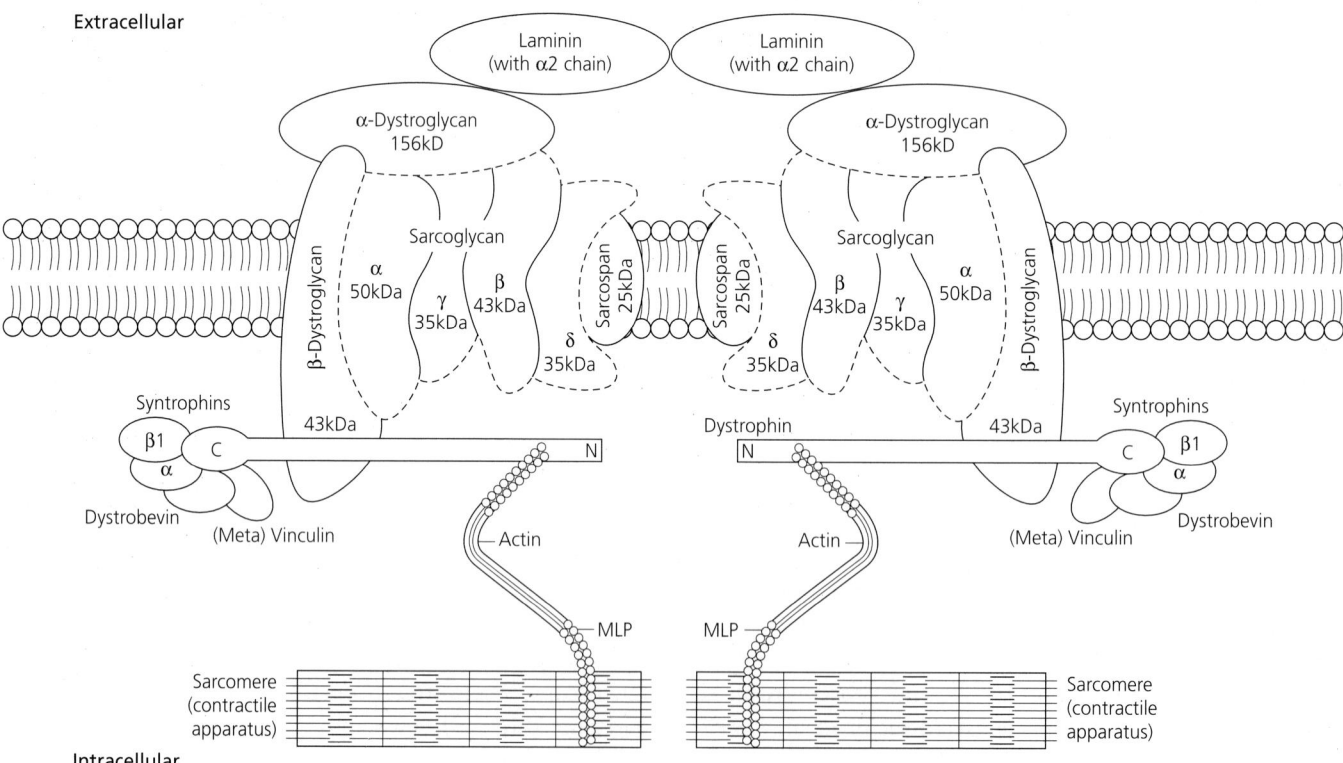

Fig. 50.18. Dystrophin-associated glycoprotein complex (DAG). Abnormalities in proteins comprising this complex result in myocardial disease with or without skeletal muscle disease.

2000). Diverse mutations leading to XLCM have been shown by Towbin and Ortiz-Lopez (1994) Yoshida et al. (1993), Muntoni et al. (1993), Milasin et al. (1996), and Ortiz-Lopez et al. (1997), with most mutations residing in the 5′ portion of the gene. Franz et al. (2000) recently reported on a mutation in exon 29, however. In all cases, it appears that the DCM occurs due to mechanical destablization of the muscle membrane. Recently, novel mutations in the 5′ end of dystrophin, including a transposon (Yoshida et al., 1998) insertion and an *Alu*-rearrangement (Ferlini et al., 1998) were found to result in XLCM.

Management

Treatment of congestive heart failure and ventricular arrhythmias is necessary and transplantation is common. Medical therapy includes an oral anti-congestive regimen of digoxin, diuretic, and an ACE inhibitor such as captopril or enalapril. Recently, the addition of a β-blocker such as metoprolol or carvedilol has become standard practice. Due to the poor systolic function, the potential for the development of thrombi and embolic phenomena has led to the institution of therapy with aspirin or other medications. In some patients inotropic support intravenously is needed; the usual approach includes use of renal-dose dopamine, milrinone and possibly other medications such as dobutamine, epinephrine and norepinephrine. Ventricular assist devices (VADs) or intraaortic balloon pumps may be indicated in severe cases as a bridge to transplantation. VADs have recently been used as a bridge to recovery. Antiarrhythmic agents may be needed in some patients; ICD implantation is reserved for patients with life-threatening dysrhythmias.

CONDUCTION DISEASE WITH DILATED CARDIOMYOPATHY (CDDC)

Clinical features

Families are described with variable conduction disease ranging from first degree atrioventricular block and second degree atrioventricular block which occurs in the second or third decade of life and progresses to complete atrioventricular block over one to two decades (Graber et al., 1986). In these families, dilated cardiomyopathy occurs late in the course of the disease and is out of proportion to the conduction disease severity. Typically, these are autosomal dominant transmitted disorders and in some cases skeletal myopathy is notable. Multiple genes have been identified thus far.

Genetics

Over the past decade several families have been studied using linkage analysis. The first gene for CDDC was identified by Kass et al. (1994) to be a chromosome 1p1-1q1-linked gene (Table 50.3). Subsequently, Olson and Keating mapped a second locus to 3p25-3p22 (1996). In these families, no skeletal myopathy was demonstrated. However, Messina et al. (1997) localized a gene to 6q25 in a family with skeletal myopathy and Van der Kooi et al. (1997) described another family as having limb girdle muscular dystrophy (LGMD1B) with CDDC, which they mapped to chromosome 1q11-1q21. The gene for the 1p1-1q1-linked CDDC was recently identified as lamin A/C (Table 50.3). This gene encodes two proteins that are members of the intermediate filament class of cytoskeletal proteins. The families identified had variable skeletal myopathy as well. The gene also causes autosomal dominant Emery-Dreifuss muscular dystrophy (EDMD), which has a similar phenotype, although skeletal myopathy is central to the diagnosis in these patients (Bonne et al., 1999). In the CDDC patients, tachydysrhythmias including nonsustained VT, supraventricular tachycardia and atrial fibrillation occur in some of the affected patients, including young individuals.

Although the 3p25-p22-linked gene and 6q25-linked gene have not been identified, another group of similar patients have been shown to have mutations in the chromosome 2q-linked gene desmin, a myofibrillar protein that accumulates in the muscle fibers of affected patients (Li et al., 1999). In skeletal and cardiac muscles, normal desmin encircles the Z bands that hold together the actin filaments and help transmit tension along the myofibrils, protecting their structural integrity during repeated muscle contractions over time. Mutant desmin appears to cause fragility of the myofibrils and impair contraction. In mice lacking desmin, the same phenotype occurs but later in life.

Management

The management of conduction system disease requires pacemaker implantation for symptomatic bradycardia signs and symptoms of CHF are treated with standard CHF therapy.

ARRHYTHMOGENIC RIGHT VENTRICULAR DYSPLASIA/CARDIOMYOPATHY (ARVD/ARVC)

Arrhythmogenic right ventricular dysplasia/cardiomyopathy (ARVD/ARVC) is characterized by fatty infiltration

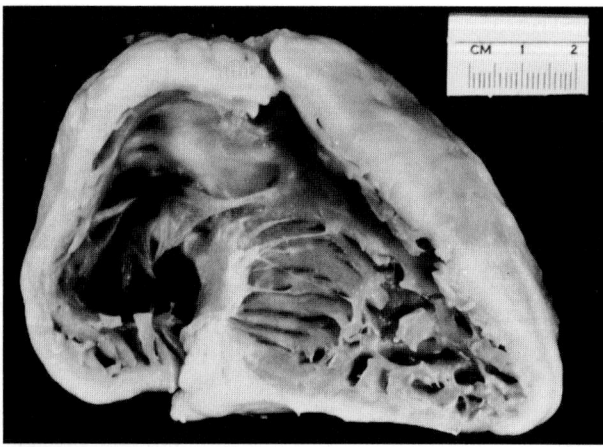

Fig. 50.19. Gross anatomic findings in ARVD. Note the right ventricle free wall thinning with fatty replacement.

of the right ventricle, fibrosis and ultimately thinning of the right ventricular wall (Fig. 50.19) with chamber dilatation (Marcus et al., 1982; Thiene et al., 1988, 2000). The residual myocardial fibers are often embedded in fibrous tissue and this substrate is conducive to right ventricular re-entrant arrhythmias. It is the most common cause of sudden cardiac death in the young in Italy (Thiene et al., 1988) and is said to account for about 17% of sudden death in the young in the United States (Marcus et al., 1980; Shen et al., 1994; Thiene et al., 1988, 2000).

Clinical features

The clinical presentation of ARVD/ARVC is highly variable and includes palpitations, syncope, right heart (or biventricular) failure, or sudden death (Corrado et al., 1997). Some patients may be asymptomatic. Clinical manifestations are rare before puberty, with typical onset between 12–45 years of age, and sudden death is a common first symptom. It has been estimated that 3% to 4% of sudden deaths during sports (and 17% of all sudden deaths in young persons) occur due to this disorder and it is well known that the dysrhythmias in this disease are most likely to occur during exercise.

ARVD/ARVC is extremely difficult to diagnose and since there is no diagnostic standard, consensus criteria were developed (McKenna et al., 1994) on the basis of structural, functional, and electrical manifestations. The structural changes most commonly noted include increased right ventricular chamber size, deep fissuring and trabeculation of the right ventricular outflow tract, localized akinetic or dyskinetic bulges or outpouchings (particularly the infundibulum at the apex and posterior sub-tricuspid areas), and localized thinning of the right ventricular wall (Fontaine et al., 1999).

Morphologically, the most striking feature of ARVD/ARVC is fatty replacement of the epicardium and mid-myocardium of the right ventricular free wall (Thiene et al., 1988; 2000). The endocardium is usually spared, as is the septum. As the disease progresses, the left ventricle may become involved, particularly the epicardial surface. Focal right ventricular thinning, especially in the infundibular region, in the diaphragmatic inferior wall, or at the apex, is typical. Histology demonstrates severe myocardial atrophy with residual myocytes interspersed with fibro-fatty tissue. Evidence of patchy and acute inflammation with myocyte death and focal round cell infiltrate (lymphocytes) are present is approximately 70% of cases (Thiene et al., 1991).

Clinically, the key feature of this disease is its propensity to tachydysrhythmias (Corrado et al., 1997). During sinus rhythm there are abnormalities of the QRS configuration that are due to slow conduction of electrical activity in the Purkinje system of the right ventricular wall, known as parietal block. In addition, there may be abnormalities of repolarization secondary to the underlying abnormal anatomy of the right ventricular free wall and chamber enlargement. These abnormalities include (1) prolongation of the QRS duration in the right precordial leads (V1–V3), representing alterations of conduction delay predominantly affecting the right ventricular free wall, the last portion of the heart to be depolarized; (2) epsilon waves, small electrical potentials occurring immediately after the QRS complex and representing delayed right ventricular depolarization; (3) presence of late potentials by signal averaged ECG, also suggestive of delayed depolarization and typically associated with reduced right ventricular ejection fraction; (4) T wave inversion beyond lead V1 in a patient older than 12 years of age and the extent of T wave inversion correlates with the extent of right ventricular involvement; (5) ventricular dysrhythmias (Fig. 50.20). The ventricular complexes are almost always of left bundle branch block morphology, since they arise from the right ventricular free wall (Fig. 50.21). The propensity for dysrhythmias has been suggested to occur due to abnormalities of cardiac sympathetic innervation, with significant reduction of myocardial β-adrenergic receptor density (Wichter et al., 2000). Due to its high-risk features, it has been suggested that a registry be created (Corrado et al., 2000).

Genetics

ARVD/ARVC is commonly inherited, with a family history of disease being present in 30 to 50% of cases (Corrado et al., 1997). With the exception of a variant of the disease found in Naxos, Greece with a recessive mode of transmis-

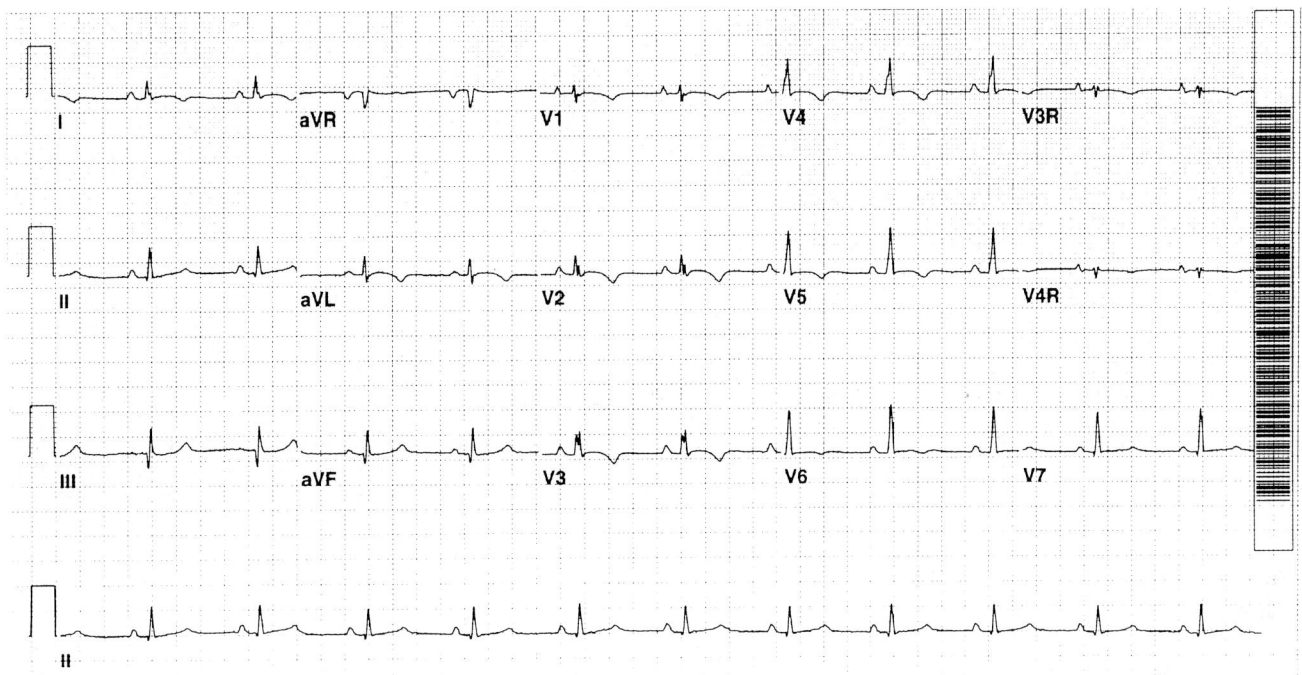

Fig. 50.20. Features of ARVD are seen in this electrocardiogram. Epsilon waves and T wave inversion in the lateral leads are seen.

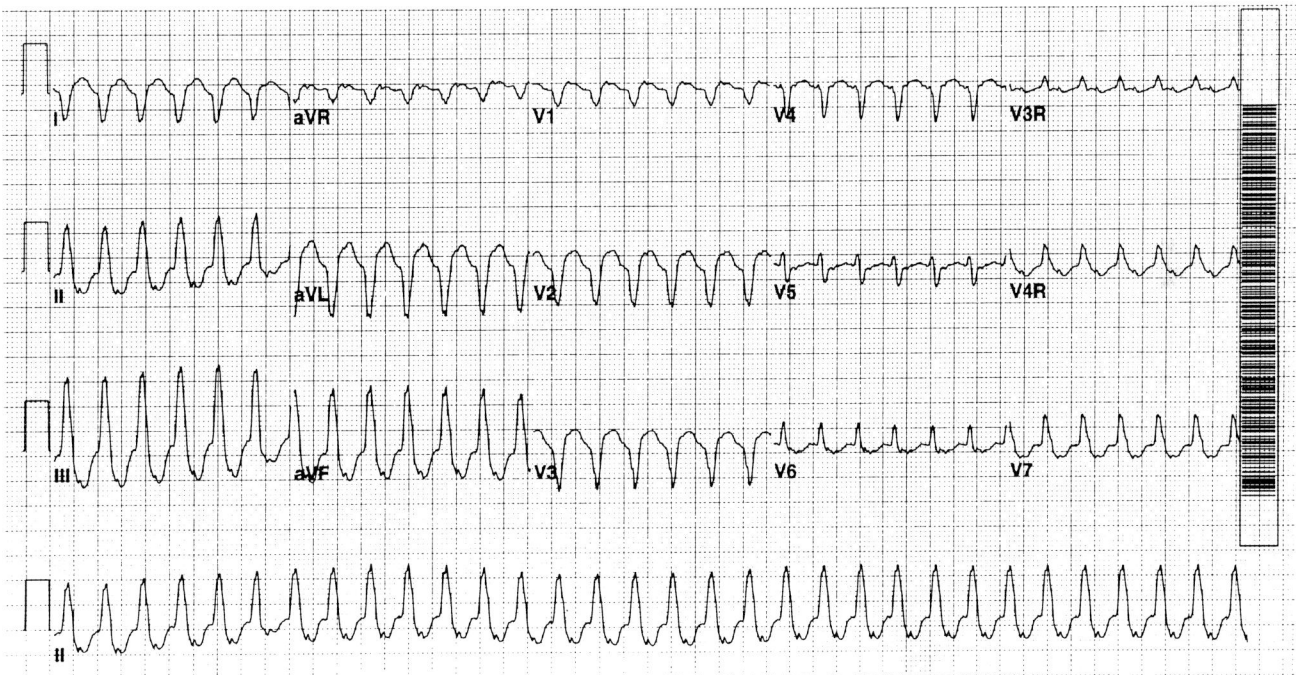

Fig. 50.21. Left bundle branch ventricular tachycardia in ARVD.

sion (Coonar et al., 1998), the disease is transmitted in an autosomal dominant pattern with various degrees of clinical expression. The autosomal dominant form is genetically heterogeneous, with six genes for a pure form of ARVD/ARVC mapped to chromosomes 14q24.3 (ARVD1) (Rampazzo et al., 1994), 1q42-q43 (ARVD2) (Rampazzo et al., 1995), 14q12-q22 (ARVD3) (Severini et al., 1996), 2q32.1-q32.3 (ARVD4) (Rampazzo et al., 1997), 3p23 (ARVD5) (Ahmad et al., 1998), and 10p12-p14 (ARVD6) (Li et al., 2000) (Table 50.3). A locus has also been identified for ARVD/

ARVC associated with myofibrillar myopathy, a skeletal myopathy with axial and distal weakness, myopathic electromyographic findings, and abnormal biopsies with myopathic changes, rimmed vacuoles, accumulation of desmin, dystrophin and sarcoglycan, and myofibril disorganization. This gene was mapped to chromosome 10q22.3 (Table 50.3) and, like the six pure-form loci, the gene has not yet been identified (Melberg et al., 1999).

The lone autosomal recessive form of ARVD/ARVC, Naxos disease, was mapped to chromosome 17q21 (Coonar et al., 1998). This complex disorder consists of ARVD/ARVC associated with diffuse nonepidermolytic palmoplantar keratoderma and wooly hair. Recently, the gene for this disorder was found to be plakoglobin (Table 50.3), a desmosomal protein (McKoy et al., 2000). The autosomal dominant myofibrillar myopathy/ARVC has desmin-like inclusions, suggesting that a similar gene product will be found to cause this disorder, as well as the genes involved in the pure form of ARVD/ARVC.

Management

Medical therapy consists of antiarrhythmic drugs to suppress ventricular arrhythmias, with sotalol (most common), amiodarone, flecainide, and propafenone reportedly used (Wichter et al., 1992; Fontaine et al., 1999). Although sotalol appears to be effective in preventing recurrence of sustained VT, it remains unknown as to whether it is effective in preventing sudden death. In selected patients, catheter ablation of VT has been achieved but recurrences are not uncommon, probably due to the progressive nature of the disease. Implanted cardioverter defibrillators (ICDs) are currently recommended for patients who have had cardiac arrest or are deemed to be at high risk of syncope/ sudden death or who have polymorphic VT (Fontaine et al., 1999). Due to the fatty infiltrate, implantation (and function) of the ICD may be problematic.

RESTRICTIVE CARDIOMYOPATHY

Clinical features

Restrictive cardiomyopathy (RCM) is the least common of the four major categories of cardiomyopathy (Denfield et al., 1997; WHO/ISFC Task Force, 1996). It is a primary abnormality of diastolic function caused by derangement in the dynamics of ventricular filling, resulting in the increase in ventricular end diastolic pressures and dilated atria (Fig. 50.22). Systolic function is usually preserved. Pulmonary hypertension commonly occurs (Ammash et al.,

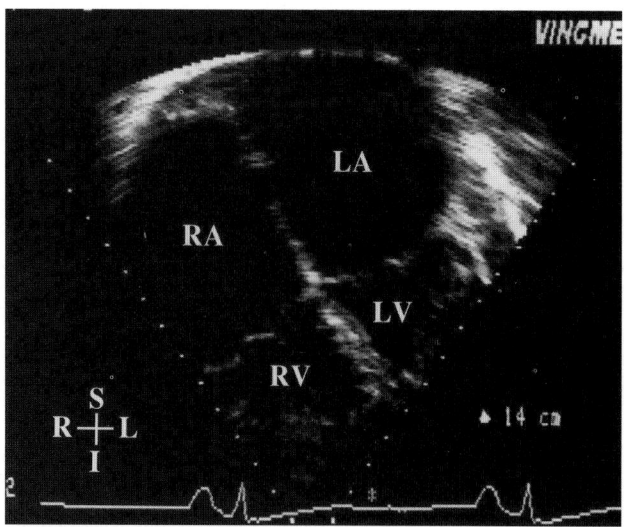

Fig. 50.22. Restrictive cardiomyopathy. This echocardiogram identifies the diagnostic features: dilated atria, normal ventricular size, thickness, and systolic function.

2000). The diagnosis may be made by ECG in which extreme P wave (atrial) voltage and width is notable and an echocardiogram with severe atrial dilation with normal ventricular size and function (Fig. 50.23). Ischemia and ventricular tachydysrhythmias may occur, as does atrial tachydysrhythmias and conduction abnormalities. Sudden death is common (Cetta et al., 1995; Katritsis et al., 1991; Lewis, 1992; Denfield et al., 1997; Rivenes et al., 2000). Secondary RCM can develop in the late stages of HCM (Maki et al., 1990), DCM, valvular, hypertensive and ischemic heart disease or specific heart muscle disease such as amyloidosis (Hirota et al., 1990; Meaney et al., 1976). The most common cause of secondary restrictive cardiomyopathy in adults is due to myocardial amyloid. Patients manifest exercise intolerance due to their inability to increase cardiac output by tachycardia without further compromising ventricular filling. Weakness and dyspnea are often prominent, and chest pain may also occur. At endstage, the findings are those of cardiac failure with anasarca (Ammash et al., 2000; Kushwaha et al., 1997).

Genetics

Mutations in the transthyretin (*TTR*) gene (Jacobson et al., 1997a,b; McCarthy and Kaspar, 1998) which codes for the TTR serum protein, has been found associated with RCM (Table 50.3). This protein contains four subunits each with 127 amino acids, encoded by four exons within a 7 Kb gene. Many *TTR* point mutations cause TTR to form amyloid, which occurs primarily in the heart, leading to heart failure.

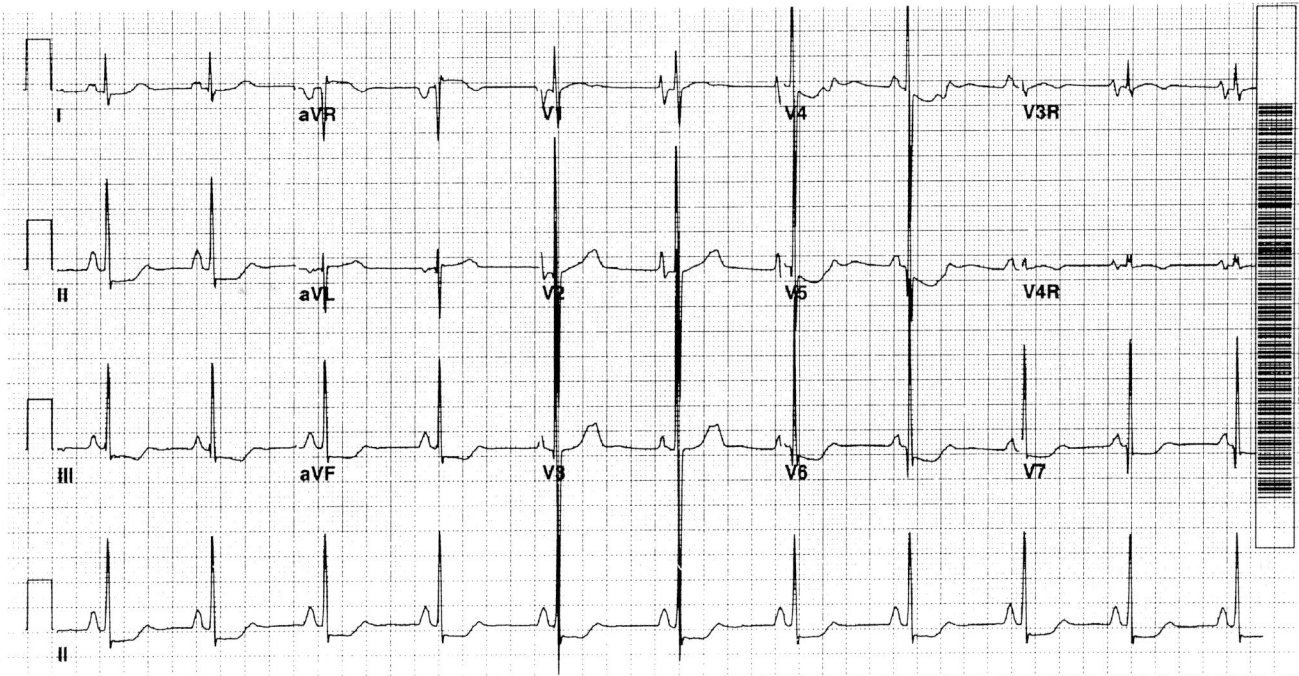

Fig. 50.23. Restrictive cardiomyopathy. Biatrial enlargement (tall, wide P waves) and left ventricular hypertrophy (large voltage QRS in V6) are noted along with ST segment depression in the inferior lateral leads, which is particularly noticeable in the rhythm strip.

Familial forms of restrictive cardiomyopathy have also been seen. In these cases, autosomal dominant and autosomal recessive inheritance has been described. One such family was found to have mutations in the desmin gene (Arbustini et al., 1998) (Table 50.3) and mice have been created with desmin mutations that have a similar phenotype as the clinical condition (Li et al., 1996; Thornell et al., 1997).

Management

In patients with CHF, anticongestive therapy is appropriate (Ammash et al., 2000; Denfield et al., 1997). However, most patients do not improve with any medical therapy and because of the high risk of sudden death, transplantation may be first-line therapy. The use of ICDs is controversial.

Neurologic disorders associated with dysrhythmias and conduction disease

Numerous atrial and ventricular dysrhythmias and myocardial diseases (DCM, HCM, RCM) can be seen in certain familial neurologic diseases. Generally, the most common rhythm disturbances associated with neurologic diseases are due to abnormalities of the cardiac conduction system. The following neurologic disorders will be discussed: Duchenne

muscular dystrophy (DMD), Becker muscular dystrophy (BMD), Emery-Dreifuss muscular dystrophy (EDMD), limb girdle muscular dystrophies (LGMD), congenital muscular dystrophies, myotonic dystrophy (DM), Friedreich ataxia (FA), and mitochondrial myopathies.

DUCHENNE/BECKER MUSCULAR DYSTROPHY (see Ch. 123)

Clinical features

Duchenne muscular dystropohy (DMD) is an X-linked disorder characterized by the early onset of progressive, generalized muscle weakness and "pseudohypertrophy" of certain muscle groups (Cox and Kunkel, 1997; Worton, 1995). The incidence of DMD is estimated to be 1 in 3300 live male births with little ethnic variation, and the calculated mutation rate of 10^4 is an order of magnitude higher than for most other genetic diseases. Approximately 35% of cases arise by spontaneous mutation, with the remaining two-thirds occurring by inheritance of the disease-causing gene from the carrier mother. Female carriers of DMD are usually asymptomatic but occasionally have a slowly progressive myopathy of moderate severity (Hoffman et al., 1992; Politano et al., 1996). This "manifesting female carrier" state occurs in about 8% of carriers and is thought to occur due to the vagaries of random X-inactivation.

Cardiomyopathy may be the first clinical manifestation of female carriers (Mirabella et al., 1993). The disease may also be expressed in females with Turner syndrome having a single X chromosome and in females with X-autosome translocations that disrupt the DMD gene. In the latter case, the translocation not only disrupts the DMD gene but also causes the nonrandom inactivation of the normal allele on the other X chromosome, resulting in the expression of the disease phenotype.

Although evidence of skeletal muscle disease in boys with DMD is evident in the neonatal period, as seen by high serum muscle enzymes (particularly CK-MM), clinical disease is not. There may be mild developmental delay, such as walking later than expected, but weakness is usually not appreciated until at least two to three years of age (Worton, 1995). Early symptoms reported by parents include difficulty in running or climbing stairs, frequent falling, and enlargement of calf muscles. Pelvic girdle weakness is more obvious than shoulder girdle weakness in the early stages. The gait becomes lordotic and waddling, and the child usually walks with the heels raised slightly off the ground (i.e., toe walking). As pelvic girdle weakness increases, the child has increasing difficulty rising from a seated position. In order to rise from the floor to a standing position, the child must brace the arms against the front of the thigh and climb up the legs, the so-called Gowers sign. Muscle pseudohypertrophy usually appears by five to six years of age, with muscle enlargement most commonly occurring in the calf muscles; the quadriceps, infraspinatus, deltoid, and gluteal muscles may also be involved, however. The upper and lower extremities become progressively weaker with age, and joint contractures may appear due to uneven weakness of agonist and antagonist muscles. Contractures of the hip flexors, iliotibial bands, and heel cords develop in 70% of patients between six and 10 years of age. Most patients are wheelchair-bound by the end of the first decade of life. After ambulation is lost, fixed contractures occur and paraspinal muscle weakness leads to progressive kyphoscoliosis. Significant weakness of the respiratory muscles occurs early in the second decade and is a common cause of demise.

While most cases of DMD can be recognized on the basis of the patient's history and clinical signs alone, laboratory evaluation is important to confirm the diagnosis (Cox and Kunkel, 1997). As previously noted, extremely high levels of CK-MM are found in the early stages of disease, as early as birth, and precede evidence of clinical involvement. Other muscle enzymes, including aldolase, SGOT, lactic dehydrogenase (LDH), and pyruvate kinase are also grossly elevated. In the end stages of the disease, enzyme levels fall but do not reach normal values. Electromyographic exam-

ination may also be useful, demonstrating the characteristic features of a myopathy (Engel et al., 1994). Insertional activity is normal or increased initially, but decreases in the advanced stages of the disease, when fibrosis replaces muscle fibers. Fibrillation potentials and positive sharp waves occur in the early stages of the disease due to the splitting of muscle fibers. The motor unit potentials are small and polyphasic, and an early recruitment pattern with minimal effort is present. Mild intellectual impairment is common in patients with DMD. The retardation is present at an early age, is nonprogressive, and does not correlate well with the stage of the disease. Approximately one-third of patients have an IQ < 75, characterized primarily by impaired verbal ability.

The heart is commonly involved in DMD, with electrocardiographic abnormalities and dilated cardiomyopathy being most typical (Perloff et al., 1967; Nigro et al., 1990; Cox and Kunkel, 1997). Cardiac symptoms, however, are unusual before the terminal stages of the disease, probably due to limited physical activity. Congestive heart failure tends to occur (Nigro et al., 1995). A mid-systolic click and late systolic murmur associated with mitral valve prolapse is also common. In addition, an S3 or S4 gallop, sinus tachycardia, and a mitral regurgitation murmur are usually heard along with cardiomegaly and increased pulmonary vascular markings on chest X-ray; at this stage, bilateral diaphragmatic elevations may be seen due to diaphragmatic dystrophy. Unlike the late-onset findings of dilated cardiomyopathy, the electrocardiogram is abnormal early in the course of DMD, with a tall R-wave and an abnormally increased R/S ratio in the right precordial chest leads and a deep, narrow Q-wave in leads I, aVL, V5, and V6 (Perloff et al., 1967). These abnormalities progress over time and are attributed to the finding that the greatest dystrophic myocardial changes are in the posterobasal and contiguous lateral left ventricular myocardium. In addition, P-waves with negative terminal deflections in V1 exceeding 20 ms and 0.1 mV appear in 20–45% of patients and, in the absence of left atrial enlargement on echocardiogram, is attributed to an intrinsic disorder of left atrial or intra-atrial conduction. A short PR interval may be seen in up to 50% of patients but is not thought to be due to a bypass tract as seen in Wolff-Parkinson-White syndrome. Infranodal conduction abnormalities, however, may be seen in patients with DMD and these include complete or incomplete bundle branch block, and left anterior or posterior fascicular block. Atrial and ventricular premature beats and atrial flutter are seen in some patients.

Echocardiography reveals left ventricular dilatation and dysfunction, with significantly reduced shortening fraction or ejection fraction and LV hypokinesis of the posterobasal ventricular wall (Towbin et al., 1993; Nigro et al., 1994; Melacini et al., 1999). Doppler and color Doppler interrogation commonly demonstrate mitral regurgitation, either secondary to the dilated cardiomyopathy or to the associated mitral valve prolapse, which occurs secondary to papillary muscle dysfunction (Sanyal et al., 1980). In some patients systolic function appears normal but diastolic dysfunction is present.

Histopathologic abnormalities of the heart and skeletal muscle are universal in patients with DMD and those of skeletal muscle are widespread even in the early stages of disease (Cox and Kunkel, 1997; Dubowitz, 1985). Typical findings are rounding of the muscle fibers, increased variability in fiber size, increased central nucleation, and fiber splitting. Necrotic and regenerating fibers are present along with large, round hyaline fibers. In the late stages, muscle may be virtually replaced by fat and fibrous tissue. In the heart, degenerative changes in muscle fibers and areas of fibrosis in the ventricles, atria, and conduction system occur, with most pronounced changes in the posterobasal region and adjacent lateral wall of the left ventricle. The underlying cause of cardiac disease is not currently known, but it is speculated that the gene defect in DMD leads to instability of the translated cytoskeletal protein, leading to weakening of the myocyte membrane and subsequent myocyte death due to mechanical stress (Nigro et al., 1994; Towbin et al., 1999).

Genetics

The dystrophin gene (Table 50.3), on the short arm of the X chromosome at Xp21 (Cox and Kunkel, 1997; Sadoulet-Puccio and Kunkel, 1996), may cause either low level production of a nonfunctional protein or complete absence of dystrophin in the heart and skeletal muscle of affected patients when mutated. It is among the largest genes discovered thus far, comprising approximately 2.5 Mb and transcribing a 14 kb mRNA molecule (Hoffman et al., 1987; Koenig et al., 1987; 1988). This cytoskeletal protein-encoding gene is normally expressed in striated and smooth muscle, as well as in brain. In muscle tissue, the dystrophin protein has been localized to the cytoplasmic surface of the sarcolemma and is associated with several integral membrane glycoproteins (Bonnemann et al., 1997). This glycoprotein/dystrophin complex, which involves the sarcoglycans, dystroglycan, syntrophins, and dystrobrevins, connects dystrophin to the sarcolemma and links to the extracellular matrix (Fig. 50.18); it may be involved in the regulation of intracellular calcium which in dystrophin-deficient muscle is

increased along with increased calcium channel transport (Bonnemann et al., 1997; Ervasti and Campbell, 1993; Ozawa et al., 1995; Tinsley et al., 1994).

The diagnostic approaches to DMD have changed dramatically over the past decade. Previously, serum CK-MM level and muscle biopsy were the standard approaches. Today DMD is diagnosed primarily by molecular analysis (Beggs and Kunkel, 1990), which is rapid and accurate and may predict clinical course. Most commonly, dystrophin mutations that cause a frameshift (Koenig et al., 1987; Malhotra et al., 1988; Monaco et al., 1988) of the nucleotide sequence results in the severe form of muscular dystrophy, DMD.

Management

Management of the congestive heart failure associated with the DCM seen in DMD is identical to that used for patients with other causes of heart failure and dysrhythmias. Pacing is not usually necessary.

BECKER MUSCULAR DYSTROPHY

Clinical features

Becker muscular dystrophy (BMD) is an X-linked disorder that differs in both severity and time of onset from DMD (Cox and Kunkel, 1997; Engel et al., 1994), despite being due to allelic mutations in dystrophin, the gene responsible for DMD. BMD appears later and progresses more slowly than DMD, so that survival to middle age is seen. The pattern of muscle weakness, however, is identical to that in DMD, with early involvement of the pelvic girdle and proximal lower extremities (Cox and Kunkel, 1997). The initial signs of weakness usually appear during the second decade, but may occur as late as the third decade. The weakness gradually progresses, with the upper extremities becoming involved after five to ten years. Patients generally remain ambulatory until their mid-thirties. Similar to DMD, muscle hypertrophy is common; intellectual impairment, however, is less common and less severe. As in DMD, life expectancy is also reduced in BMD, with only 50% of patients surviving to 40 years of age.

Cardiac involvement may be seen in adolescence and ultimately affects 80% of patients (Melacini et al., 1996). As in DMD, dilated cardiomyopathy and cardiac failure are the usual abnormalities encountered and are often the ultimate cause of death. Conduction abnormalities manifesting as fascicular block or complete heart block are also seen. As in DMD, muscle enzyme activity is markedly elevated in BMD and preclinical cases may be detected by elevated CK-MM. Electromyographic examination shows a "myopathic" pattern with small, polyphasic motor units and early recruitment of motor units. The histology of BMD is similar to that of other forms of muscular dystrophy. In contrast to DMD, hyaline fibers are rarely seen. Electrocardiographic changes similar to those seen in DMD. Other electrocardiographic abnormalities encountered include left axis deviation, right bundle branch block, left bundle branch block, and complete heart block. The echocardiogram may demonstrate the features of dilated cardiomyopathy.

Genetics and management

BMD is also due to mutations within the dystrophin gene; i.e., it is allelic with DMD (Table 50.3). As is the case with DMD, more than 30% of patients with BMD have no family history of the disease, an indication that they represent spontaneous mutations. The phenotypic difference between DMD and BMD patients has been speculated to be due to frameshift mutations leading to more severe disease (DMD) while out-of-frame mutations cause less severe (BMD) disease (Beggs et al., 1991; Koenig et al., 1989; Malhotra et al., 1988; Monaco et al., 1988). The frameshift hypothesis explains >90% of the cases of DMD versus BMD. The cardiac abnormalities in BMD, as with that described for DMD, require further study (Yoshida et al., 1993). However, cardiomyoypathy is quite common (Melacini et al., 1996; Nigro et al., 1994; 1995; Politano et al., 1996; Quinlivan and Dubowitz, 1992; Saito et al., 1996; Yoshida et al., 1993). The treatment of CHF and arrhythmias is similar to other patients with these signs and symptoms.

Animal models have been created during the past several years that help to characterize the roles of dystrophin and the associated complexes. Loss of function mutations of dystrophin leads to a DMD or BMD phenotype, while utrophin-deficient mice have defects in the post-synaptic membrane folds at the neuromuscular junction. Mice lacking both dystrophin and utrophin display a severe muscular dystrophy with premature death (Deconinck et al., 1997; Grady et al., 1997a,b; Lumeng et al., 1999). Sarcoglycan-deficient mice also demonstrate severe muscular dystrophy but, in addition, severe hypertrophic and/or dilated cardiomyopathy has been seen (Hack et al., 1999; Nigro et al., 1997; Sakamoto et al., 1997). This has recently been supported by the identification of δ-sarcoglycan mutations in humans with FDCM by our laboratory (Tsubata et al., 2000).

Various methods evaluating the possibility of gene therapy for dystrophinopathies have been reported over the past several years in mice with varying degrees of success. Mini-gene and stem-cell transplantation have both been considered promising, using dystrophin and utrophin (Deconinck et al., 1996; Mendell et al., 1995; Phelps et al., 1995; Rafael et al., 1994; Tinsley et al., 1996; Vainzof et al., 1995; Wells et al., 1995).

LIMB-GIRDLE MUSCULAR DYSTROPHY (LGMD) (see Ch. 124)

Clinical features

The LGMDs are a heterogeneous group of muscle disorders first described in 1954 and characterized by predominant weakness and wasting of muscles of the pelvic and shoulder girdle (Walton and Gardner-Medwin, 1988). Facial and extraocular muscles are usually spared. There is broad clinical heterogeneity and this is paralleled by genetic heterogeneity (Bushby and Beckmann, 1995; Bushby, 1995). The heart is affected in several forms of LGMD, including cardiomyopathy (dilated and hypertrophic) and conduction system abnormalities (Bonnemann et al., 1997; Cox and Kunkel, 1997; Melacini et al., 1999). Onset can occur at any age in childhood or adulthood, but usually has its onset after walking has been started. Autosomal dominant and autosomal recessive forms of LGMD have been described, with the age of onset generally earlier in the autosomal recessive forms (Bushby and Beckmann, 1995).

Genetics

A classification scheme for the LGMDs has been devised that depends on the pattern of inheritance (Bushby and Beckmann, 1995). The autosomal dominant forms of LGMD are designated LGMD1 (LGMD1A-1D) while the autosomal recessive forms are designated LGMD2 (LGMD2A-2G). This classification scheme is based on the inheritance and the specific gene causing the disorder (Table 50.4). The majority of recessive LGMDs are due to mutations in the dystrophin-associated protein subcomplex sarcoglycan (Angelini et al., 1999; Bonnemann et al., 1996; Fanin et al., 1997; Jones et al., 1998; Matsumura et al., 1999; Ozawa et al., 1998; Straub and Campbell, 1997; Vainzof et al., 1996; 1999), with LGMD2C-2F being caused by α- (Eymard et al., 1997), β-, γ- and δ- sarcoglycan, respectively (i.e., sarcoglycanopathies) (Table 50.3). Although quite variable in severity, these LGMDs tend to have a course that is often reminiscent of DMD in its severity. In all cases, cardiac disease can occur (Melacini et al., 1999) and includes conduction system disease and cardiomyopathy (HCM and/or

DCM). The other recessive forms of LGMD are caused by mutations in calpain-3 (Richard et al., 1995; 1999), a muscle-specific calcium dependent protease (LGMD2A), resulting in a somewhat milder course than the sarcoglycanopathies. Recently, LGMD2B was characterized as being caused by mutations in dysferlin (Liu et al., 1998; Weiler et al., 1999), a novel muscle protein of uncertain function, and LGMD2G was found to be caused by mutations in the sarcomeric protein telethonin, a protein localized to the Z disc of muscle (Moreira et al., 2000). In this form, cardiomyopathy occurs (Table 50.4).

The autosomal dominant forms of LGMD have been more difficult to identify thus far (DeCoster et al., 1974; Gilchrist et al., 1988). The only gene identified to date is caveolin-3 (McNally et al., 1998), which causes LGMD1D. In LGMC1B, and 1C, and 1D cardiac dysrhythmias can become evident concomitant with the initial stages of muscular weakness (Table 50.3). Cardiomyopathy is found as well (Messina et al., 1997; Van der Kooi et al., 1997) (Table 50.4).

Multiple animal models of the limb girdle muscular dystrophies have been reported, with most having cardiac disease. Cardiomyopathy and premature death consistently occurs. In addition to the murine models, a naturally occurring hamster model with associated cardiomyopathy has been well described and occurs due to δ-sarcoglycan mutation (Allamand and Campbell, 2000; Holt et al., 1998; Nigro et al., 1997; Roberds et al., 1993; Sakamoto et al., 1997; Straub et al., 1998).

EMERY-DREIFUSS MUSCULAR DYSTROPHY

Clinical features

Emery-Dreifuss muscular dystrophy (EDMD) is a relatively rare disorder characterized by weakness in the humero-peroneal distribution, early joint contractures, dilated cardiomyopathy with X-linked inheritance. (Emery, 1989; Emery and Dreifuss, 1966; Toniolo et al., 1998, 1999; Voit et al., 1988). Occasionally, autosomal dominant (Fenichal et al., 1982; Miller et al., 1985) or autosomal recessive (Takamoto et al., 1984; Taylor et al., 1998) inheritance is seen. The onset of disease in these patients occurs between two and ten years of age, with weakness initially noted in the shoulder girdles and upper extremities. Contractures of the elbows and posterior cervical muscles appear early. The disease is slowly progressive, with involvement of the distal leg musculature following that of the upper extremities; contractures of the knees and ankles follow contractures of the elbows. Unlike DMD and BMD, muscle pseudohyper-

trophy does not occur (Emery, 1989). The disease evolves slowly and usually stabilizes in the third decade, with most patients remaining ambulatory. Dilated cardiomyopathy is a common occurrence but the severity of disease varies from family to family (Emery and Dreifuss, 1966; Emery, 1989). Varying degrees of atrioventricular block are common and atrial standstill may occur. These electrical abnormalities may lead to episodes of syncope, transient ischemic attacks, stroke, and sudden death. A pacemaker is commonly required. Atrial fibrillation has also been observed. As in DMD and BMD, muscle enzyme activity is elevated, albeit to a lesser extent. Skeletal muscle biopsy histopathologic findings are similar to those associated with other forms of muscular dystrophy. Type I fiber atrophy has been described in some cases.

Genetics

The gene responsible for X-linked EDMD was localized to Xq28 (Consalez et al., 1991) before being cloned (Bione et al., 1994) (Table 50.3). The gene, called emerin (or STA), was shown to have an open reading frame of 762 nucleotides that encodes a serine-rich 254 amino acid protein with probable mechanical/structural function (Bione et al., 1994). Emerin mRNA shown ubiquitous tissue distribution, with the highest expression in skeletal and cardiac muscles. The cDNA sequence of emerin predicts a tail-anchor membrane protein with amino acid sequence similar to thymopoietins, a group of nuclear lamina-associated proteins (Harris et al., 1995). Nagano et al. (1996) and Manilal et al. (1998) both showed that emerin is a 34kD nuclear membrane protein in skeletal and cardiac muscle, which is absent in EDMD. Emerin belongs to a family of type II integral membrane proteins that are anchored to the inner nuclear membrane via hydrophilic tails, with the remainder of the molecule projecting into the nucleoplasm (Manilal et al., 1998; Morris and Manilal, 1999). This family includes lamins, lamin receptor, and thymopoietin β. Emerin is also found at intercalated disks and are thought to result in conduction defects due to this localization (Cartegni et al., 1997) and its interactions with demosomes and fascial adherans.

The autosomal dominant form of EDMD was initially mapped to chromosome 1 (1q11-q23) and the gene was identified as lamin A/C (Bonne et al., 1999) (Table 50.3). The encoded protein is also a nuclear lamina-associated protein and is expressed in myocytes and adipocytes. In the nuclear inner membrane, this protein has a distribution that mirrors that of emerin (Hegele, 2000). The phenotypic spectrum of this gene appears to be broad when mutated.

In some cases, only a DCM phenotype with conduction disease (Brodsky et al., 2000; Fatkin et al., 1999b) occurs (in the absence of clinical skeletal muscle disease) while in other cases familial Dunnigan-type lipodystrophy occurs (Cao and Hegele, 2000). The nuclear membrane either plays a critical communication role or a structural role through interactions with cytoskeletal proteins (Hegele, 2000; Di Barletta et al., 2000).

Management

The DCM associated with EDMD is treated with the usual anticongestive medical regimen and conduction disease typically requires a pacemaker.

MYOTONIC DYSTROPHY

The most common adult-onset muscular dystrophy in humans, myotonic dystrophy (DM), is a progressive, multisystem disorder that manifests as a highly pathological phenotype of the skeletal muscle, smooth muscle, brain, lens, testicular function, glucose metabolism, and the heart (Forsberg et al., 1990; Harper and Rudel, 1994). The variable phenotype in DM is further expanded by clinical "anticipation", a phenomenon in which the severity of symptoms tends to increase while the age of disease-onset decreases with each successive generation within a family (Howeler et al., 1989). Thus, the spectrum of DM symptoms can vary from mild, where only cataracts develop late

in life, to a severe congenital form associated with skeletal muscle hypotonia, often resulting in respiratory arrest and death. An intermediate adult-onset form also occurs, which manifests with one or more characteristic feature of DM including myotonia (an abnormal muscle membrane depolarization resulting in abnormally delayed muscle relaxation time after strong muscle contraction), skeletal muscle weakness and wasting, cardiac conduction system disease with or without dilated cardiomyopathy, cataracts, endocrine dysfunction, frontal balding, epitheliomas, and mental retardation (Table 50.5).

Clinical features

Although a range of skeletal muscles can be affected in DM, fast twitch muscles are usually more severely affected than slow twitch muscles. During the course of the disease it is common to find early involvement of facial and neck muscles, with later involvement of extensor forearm and anterior tibial muscles, and muscles of hands and feet. The heart is affected in approximately 80% of patients (Melacini et al., 1988; Fragola et al., 1994) and sudden death occurs with a high incidence (15 to 30%). Cardiac abnormalities are primarily conduction disorders, which occur in 45 to 80% of DM patients and the increased incidence of sudden cardiac death occurs from either complete AV block or ventricular dysrhythmias (Fragola et al., 1991; Morgenlander et al., 1993; Olofsson et al., 1988). Disorders of impulse formation in the sinus node also occur and a significant

Table 50.5. Systemic Involvement In Myotonic Dystrophy

Muscle	
Skeletal muscle	Myotonia, weakness and dystrophy predominately of facial, neck and distal limb muscles
Heart	Conduction disorders more prominent than overt cardiomyopathy (dilated)
	Conduction abnormalities include disorders of impulse formation (sinus bradycardia, prolonged SA node recovery time, SA node dysfunction), disorders of impulse conduction (atrioventricular block including 1° through complete AV block; intraventricular conduction defects including fascicular block, bundle branch block), and dysrhythmias including premature atrial beats, atrial fibrillation and flutter, premature ventricular beats and VT
Smooth muscle	Widespread involvement of pharynx, esophagus, colon and uterus
	Delayed relaxation and abnormal peristalsis
CNS	
Brain	Mental retardation, hypersomnolence
Eye	Cataracts, decreased vision independent of cataracts
Endocrine	
Testis	Gonadal atrophy
Metabolism	Abnormal carbohydrate metabolism
Skeletal/Skin	
Skeletal	Cranial and facial abnormalities, talipes
Skin	Premature balding, calcifying epithelioma
Lungs	
Respiration	Hypoventilation

number of patients exhibit sinus bradycardia (Table 50.5). The cardiac conduction abnormalities typically have a gradual but predictable increase in severity, often progressing from intermittent to stable first degree AV block followed by more serious intraventricular block including bundle branch blocks and ultimately progressive AV block to complete heart block (Bulloch et al., 1967; Nguyen et al., 1988; Fragola et al., 1991). Ventricular dysrhythmias, including VT, may also occur.

A rough correlation exists between the severity of the neuromuscular disease and progression of the cardiac features. DM is occasionally associated with overt cardiac failure, with 28% of patients having systolic dysfunction (Badano et al., 1993). Mitral valve prolapse is seen in 17 to 32% of patients as well (Winters et al., 1976; Streib et al., 1995). Like conduction abnormalities, echocardiographic abnormalities usually are more prevalent in older patients with severe neuromuscular symptoms.

Genetics

Myotonic dystrophy, because of its variable presentation, may be under-diagnosed and therefore only conservative estimates of incidence can be made. Currently it is believed that the incidence is 4.5–5.5 per 100,000 live births (Roig et al., 1994). DM is inherited as an autosomal dominant disorder but does demonstrate two unique non-mendelian features. Both the sex and the position of the parent within the pedigree affects the severity of disease in the subsequent generation due to genetic anticipation (Howeler et al., 1989). The adult-onset form is inherited more frequently through the father while congenital DM is almost exclusively maternally inherited.

The gene responsible for DM was initially mapped (Buxton et al., 1992) to the long arm of chromosome 19 (19q13.3); the DM gene was identified as myotonin protein kinase (Brook et al., 1992; Fu et al., 1992; Mahadevan et al., 1992), a serine threonine kinase (DMPK) (Timchenko et al., 1995a) (Table 50.3). The causative mutations are CTG repeat sequence expansions in the 3′ untranslated region of DMPK which causes alterations in the expansion of neighboring genes when large enough (Timchenko et al., 1995b; Thornton et al., 1997). The probability and amplitude of the expansion increases as a function of repeat tract length and the severity of the disease correlates with length of the repeat sequence (Tsilfidis et al., 1992). Two distinct patterns of CTG expansion have been described. Small changes in repeat size appear to predominate at repeat tract lengths less than 150 bps (35 repeats) in length. Such changes in tract size are reflected in the range of repeat tracts observed in the normal population (5–35 repeats). Once a threshold of >50 repeats is reached, however, the pattern of instability appears to change dramatically, causing the frequency of large repeats (>200 repeats) to greatly increase. In congenital DM, enormous expansions occur, reaching expansions of >10kb.

It is currently believed that nuclear retention of mutant DMPK transcripts occur in the nuclei of DM fibroblasts and muscle, causing a decrease in the pool of translatable DMPK mRNA in the cytoplasm (Fu et al., 1993). Titration of CUG-BP (a novel CUG binding protein believed to play a role in processing and/or transport of CUG encoding mRNAs) by the mutant DMPK message could allow DMPK levels to drop below 50% of normal (Klesert et al., 1997; Phillips et al., 1998; Timchenko, 1999). Reddy and colleagues (1996) developed a mouse model in which DMPK is functionally inactivated (DMPK −/−) and showed that loss of DMPK results in late-onset skeletal myopathy characterized by 30 to 50% loss in muscle twitch and tetanic force development by 11 months of age. Ultrastructural changes included Z line loss, mitochondrial and sarcoplasmic reticulum abnormalities, and loss of sarcomere organization suggesting that impaired excitation-contraction coupling or contractile apparatus abnormalities underlie the progressive muscle weakness seen in DM. Although DMPK is clearly an important component of muscle, loss of its expression cannot explain the complete DM phenotype. Timchenko (1999) has suggested that RNA CUG repeats play a significant role in the development of the full phenotype. Wang et al. (1995a) initially demonstrated that DMPK poly A+ RNA is significantly reduced in muscle biopsies from DM patients although total RNA had normal DMPK transcript levels and suggested that the repeat expansion caused abnormalities in RNA processing. Timchenko et al., (2001) further suggested that CUG repeat-containing DMPK RNA could affect processing of other mRNAs, perhaps by sequestering specific RNA-binding proteins and thereby causing tissue-specific abnormalities.

Genetic heterogeneity exists for DM as well. Ranum et al. (1998) identified a second locus for DM, called DM2, on chromosome 3q. Although the gene at this locus is not yet known, it is likely that DM2 could be associated with CTG repeats in a gene different (but similar) from DMPK or with another type of triplet repeat expansion and that RNA processing could modify the clinical features of this gene as well.

Finally, animal models have been created that mimic the clinical findings in humans (Jansen et al., 1996; Reddy et al., 1996; Berul et al., 1999; Saba et al., 1999). These animals continue to be studied in order to further unravel the molecular physiology responsible for this disorder.

Management

The management of DM involves the treatment of the skeletal myopathy with occupational and physical therapy and when needed, use of a wheelchair. Cardiac abnormalities require pacemaker implantation for the conduction disorder and anticongestive therapy for patients with heart failure.

FRIEDREICH ATAXIA (FA)

Clinical features

This is the most common of the hereditary spinal cerebellar degenerations, with an incidence of 1 in 50,000 and carrier frequency of 1 in 110 (Durr et al., 1996). This autosomal recessive form of spinocerebellar degeneration is characterized by progressive limb ataxia, loss of deep tendon reflexes, sensory abnormalities, and musculoskeletal deformities. The symptoms of FA usually appear insidiously during childhood or early adolescence. Progressive weakness of the upper and lower extremities gradually becomes obvious. Gait difficulties are often the first symptom which progress slowly followed by unsteadiness in the arms and hands. Difficulty in writing and handling eating utensils subsequently becomes apparent.

Cardiac involvement (Durr et al., 1996) occurs in 50 to 90% of patients and the most common abnormality is hypertrophic cardiomyopathy; dilated cardiomyopathy occurs rarely. Thus, the most common cardiac symptoms relate to cardiac failure and dysrhythmias (Ackroyd et al., 1984; Alboliras et al., 1986; James et al., 1987). Left ventricular outflow tract obstruction due to asymmetric septal hypertrophy may be evident and approximately 50% of patients die of cardiac disease. Patients are followed for development of dysrhythmias and the signs and symptoms of cardiac failure.

Involvement of the heart is readily detected by electrocardiography and echocardiography (Alboliras et al., 1986). The electrocardiographic abnormalities are found in 90% of patients and include repolarization abnormalities manifesting as inverted or biphasic T-waves in the inferior limb leads and left precordial leads, a short PR interval, left and right ventricular hypertrophy, as well as left and right axis deviation. Premature atrial contractions, atrial flutter/fibrillation, and premature ventricular contractions are common (Ackyroyd et al., 1984; Alboliras et al., 1986). Echocardiography detects cardiac involvement in 60 to 100% of patients with the most common finding being concentric hypertrophy, but asymmetric septal hypertrophy accompanied by systolic anterior motion (SAM) of the mitral valve is also common. Left ventricular chamber diameter may be normal or decreased and fractional shortening or ejection fraction is usually normal although dilated cardiomyopathy (left ventricular dilation and reduced contractility) is seen occasionally. There is no specific treatment for the cardiac manifestations except symptomatic treatment if cardiac failure ensues.

Genetics

Friedreich ataxia is inherited as an autosomal recessive disorder, and parental consanguinity has been noted in some cases. The gene was initially mapped to chromosome 9q13-31.1 (Chamberlain et al., 1988) and in 1996, the gene was identified (Campuzano et al., 1996). This gene encompasses 40 kb, contains five exons, has a 1.3 Kb transcript, and encodes a 210 amino acid protein called frataxin (Table 50.3). The highest level of expression is within the heart, while intermediate levels are seen in liver, skeletal muscle, and pancreas; minimal levels are identified in other tissues, including the brain. Although a few affected patients were found to have a point mutation of frataxin, the majority (~95%) are homozygous for an unstable GAA trinucleotide expansion in the first intron (Campuzano et al., 1996). The remainder of patients are compound heterozygotes for the expansion. In patients homozygous for the expansion, there is a correlation between the number of GAA repeats on the smaller allele, age of onset, disease progression and cardiomyopathy (Durr et al., 1996; Filla et al., 1996; Lamont et al., 1997; Monros et al., 1997; Montermini et al., 1997), confirming that the expansion is the primary cause of disease. The expansion results in severely reduced levels of mature frataxin mRNA (Campuzano et al., 1996). Campuzano et al. (1997) demonstrated that frataxin is localized to the mitochondria, associated with the mitochondrial membranes and crests. They suggested that reduction in frataxin results in oxidative damage. Subsequently, Rotig and colleagues (1997) suggested that frataxin regulates mitochondrial iron transport and that deficiency of iron-sulphur cluster-containing subunits of mitochondrial respiratory complexes I-II and the iron-sulphur protein aconitase occurs. Hence, it appears that Friedreich ataxia is a mitochondrial disorder (Koutnikova et al., 1997; Knight et al., 1998). As these patients have HCM, diabetes, ataxia, and apparent free radical toxicity, the mitochondrial basis of this disorder clarifies the clinical features.

Management

The management of this disorder is symptomatic. The HCM is typically treated with β-blocker or calcium channel blocker while the other symptoms are increasingly treated with mitochondrial-based therapy, such as vitamins and free radical reducing agents (i.e. coenzyme Q10, ibedenone, riboflavin, thiamine, vitamin K).

MITOCHONDRIAL DISORDERS

Mitochondria are intracellular organelles that participate in several metabolic pathways, including ATP synthesis by oxidative phosphorylation (Fig. 50.25) (Towbin, 1999a; Wallace, 1999; Zeviani et al., 1998). Mitochondria are unique organelles because they contain a genome that encodes some of the polypeptides in the oxidative phosphoylation pathway and all the transfer (tRNA) and ribosomal RNA (rRNA). Nuclear genes encode the remaining mitochondrial proteins. Mitochondria self-replicate and are derived from the oocytes. Thus, mutations in the mitochondrial genome are maternally inherited (Wallace, 1999; see Ch. 124)

Clinical features

Cardiac abnormalities are common in mitochondrial disorders and include conduction defects, HCM, DCM, and combined HCM/DCM, which may in part represent progression from the hypertrophic form (Anan et al., 1995; Zeviani et al., 1991). Leber hereditary optic neuropathy (LHON), a disorder in which loss of central vision due to degeneration of the retinal ganglion cells and the optic nerve axons, commonly has associated WPW syndrome (Bower et al., 1992; Federico et al., 1987; Howell and Mackey, 1998; Mashima et al., 1996; Nikoskelainen et al., 1994). Other mitochondrial mutations are also associated with WPW syndrome. These include MELAS syndrome (*m*yopathy, *e*ncephalopathy, *l*actic *a*cidosis, *s*troke-like episodes) (Ciafaloni et al., 1992; Pavalakis et al., 1984) and MERRF syndrome (*m*yoclonic *e*ncephalopathy and *r*agged *r*ed *f*ibers) (Chomyn, 1998; Rowland et al., 1991). Another mitochondrial myopathy associated with cardiac disease is Kearns-Sayre syndrome where DCM and conduction disease are common findings (Tveskov and Angelo-Nielsen, 1990).

Genetics

The human mitochondrial genome (Attardi, 1986) is a small circular DNA molecule (Fig. 50.24) that is maternally inherited. Mitochondrial DNA (mtDNA) encodes 13 of the 69 proteins required for oxidative metabolism, 22 transfer RNAs (tRNAs) and 2 ribosomal RNAs (rRNAs) required

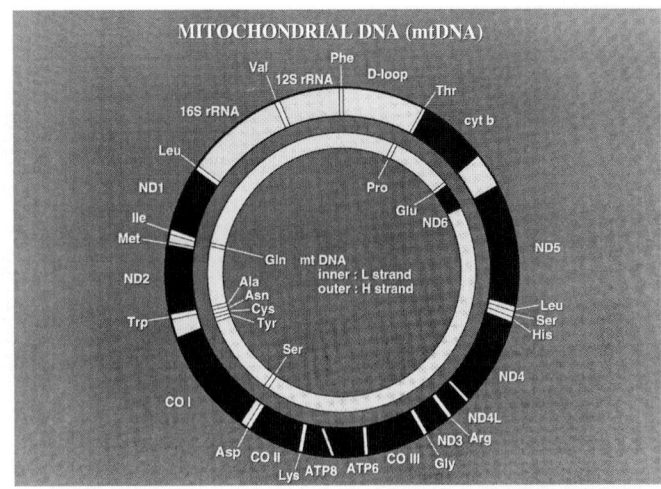

Fig. 50.24. Mitochondrial DNA (mtDNA). A small circular molecule that encodes 13 of the 69 proteins required for oxidative metabolism, 22 tRNAs and 2 rRNAs.

for their translation. Since mtDNA has much less redundancy than the nuclear genome (in which essentially identical information is received from both parents), and tRNAs and rRNAs are present in multiple copies, the mitochondrial genome is an excellent target for mutations giving rise to human disease (Liang and Wong, 1998; Smeitnik and van den Heuvel, 1999). Mitochondria are dependent on nucleocytoplasmic mechanisms for most structural components, but do contribute vital peptides that are central to cellular respiration. The electron transport chain, which generates cellular ATP, is organized into complexes I-IV and the ATP synthase (Complex V) (Fig. 50.25). The 13 mtDNA genes that encode enzymes in the respiratory chain include seven Complex I (Robinson, 1998; Smeitink and van den Heuvel, 1999) subunits, (ND1, 2, 3, 4L, 4, 5, and 6); 1 Complex III subunit (cytochrome b); 3 Complex IV subunits (COI, II, III); and 2 Complex V subunits (ATPase 6 and 8) (Morris et al., 1996; Loeffen et al., 1998; Smeitink et al., 1998). Each cell contains numerous mitochondria and each mitochondrion contains multiple copies of mtDNA. In most mitochondrial disorders, patients carry a mix of mutant and normal mitochondria – a condition known as heteroplasmy, with the proportions varying from tissue-to-tissue and individual-to-individual within a pedigree, in a manner correlating with severity of phenotype.

Mitochondrial diseases often produce disturbances of brain and muscle function, and are usually evident during infancy or early childhood (Zeviani et al., 1998). Cardiac disease is most commonly seen with respiratory chain defects (Anan et al., 1995). Ragged red fibers are present in muscle biopsy specimens (Shoffner et al., 1990) almost invariably when the molecular defect involves mtDNA (Egger et al.,

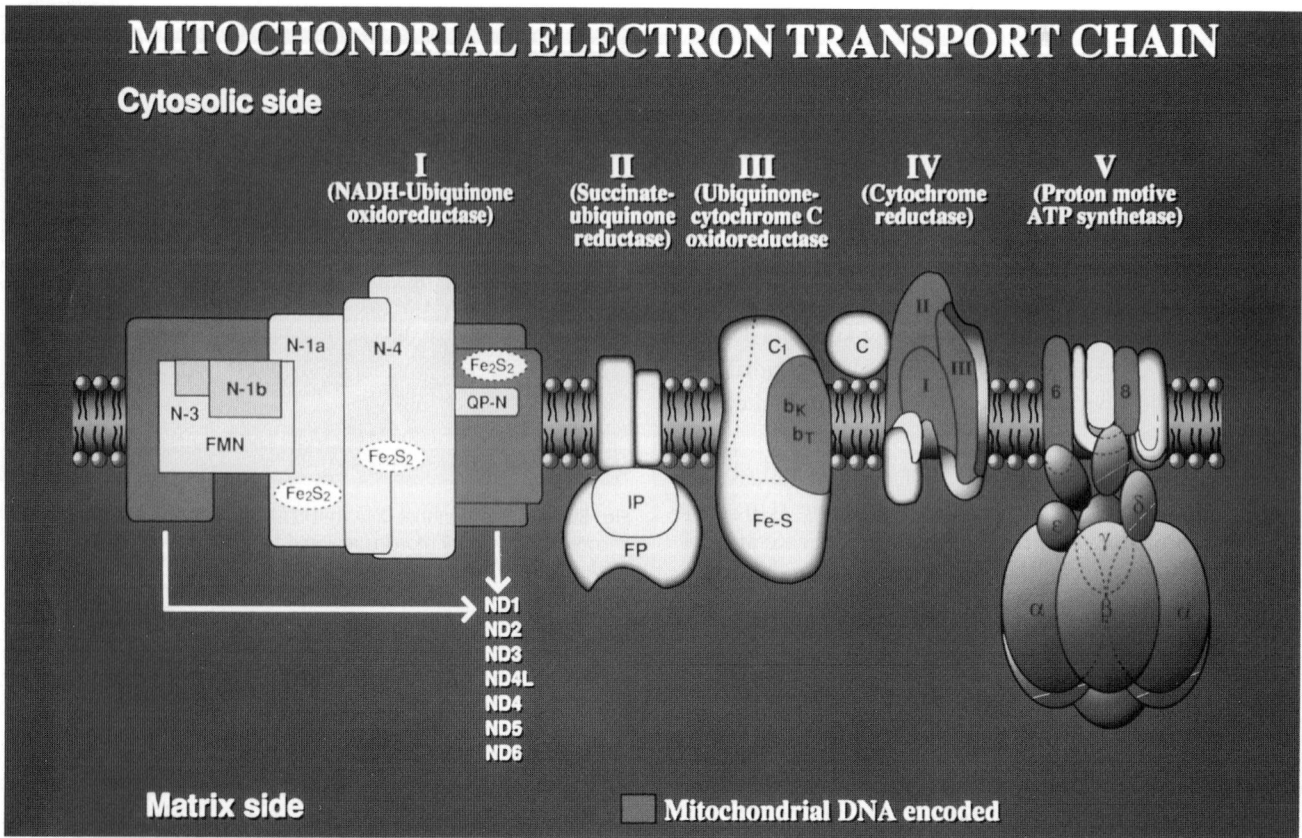

Fig. 50.25. Oxidative phosphorylation pathway.

1981; Chomyn, 1998) (Table 50.3). These defects represent the genetics of ATP production. The diverse clinical syndromes associated with various respiratory chain complexes are thought to result from involvement of tissue-specific isoforms in some cases, involvement of tissue-nonspecific (generalized) subunits in other cases, and the residual enzyme activity in affected tissues (Egger et al., 1981). The cardiac diseases seen associated with mitochondrial defects include both HCM and DCM (Corral-Debrinski et al., 1991; Anan et al., 1995; Smeitink and van den Heuvel, 1999).

Mitochondrial gene mapping, in contrast to the nuclear genome, does not require genetic linkage. One simply has to show that the disease exhibits transmission through all mothers and no fathers in a sufficiently large family. Once this is established, the mitochondrial genome can sequenced to identify the mutation which must be shown to segregate with the disease since there are many apparently harmless polymorphisms.

Management

Therapy for these disorders is generally symptom-based. Conduction disturbance generally requires placement of a permanent pacemaker and heart failure is treated with the usual therapy. In some patients, β-blockers may be useful. Hypertrophic heart disease is usually treated in a fashion similar to that of other forms of HCM. Mitochondrial-based therapy may include coenzyme Q10, carnitine, or vitamins but these therapeutic approaches typically do not alter the clinical course.

KEARNS-SAYRE SYNDROME (KSS)

This mitochondrial myopathy is characterized by ptosis, chronic progressive external ophthalmoplegia, abnormal retinal pigmentation, and cardiac conduction defects, as well as DCM (Tveskov and Angelo-Nielsen, 1990). Hearing loss and limb weakness are frequently associated, as are endocrinopathies such as diabetes mellitus, hypoparathyroidism, and growth hormone deficiency. Approximately 20% of KSS patients have cardiac involvement and, of these, the majority usually have conduction defects causing progressive heart block (Charles et al., 1981; Kenny and Wetherbee, 1990; Roberts et al., 1979). These patients generally have large heterogeneous deletions in the mitochondrial genome, of which tRNA$^{leu(UUR)}$-3243 is most common.

Clinically, conduction abnormalities, bifascicular block or progressive high-grade block may define the requirement for permanent pacemaker implantation. Symptomatic improvement using mitochondrial therapies may occasionally be seen with coenzyme Q10 therapy. The major function of coenzyme Q10 in mitochondria is to shuttle electrons from Complexes I and II to Complex III, while stabilizing the respiratory chain complexes. Vitamins such as phylloquinone (vitamin K1), menadione (vitamin K3), and ascorbic acid (vitamin C) have been used to donate electrons directly to cytochrome c. In addition, the endocrine abnormalities and heart failure should be treated in the usual way.

LEOPARD SYNDROME

LEOPARD syndrome is an inherited disorder involving multiple organ systems. The acronym represents the abnormalities characteristic of this syndrome: multiple *l*entigines, *e*lectrocardiographic conduction abnormalities, *o*cular hypertelorism, *p*ulmonic stenosis, *a*bnormal genitalia, *r*etardation of growth, and sensorineural *d*eafness. The conduction abnormalities include first-degree AV block, intraventricular conduction delay, and bundle branch block (Matthews, 1968; Gorlin et al., 1969). Progression to complete heart block is generally not seen. The gene for LEOPARD syndrome is not known although a report of mapping to chromosome 17 with identification of the neurofibromin gene is documented (Table 50.3). Therapy is supportive.

Congenital heart disease and dysrhythmias or conduction disease (see also Ch. 47)

ATRIAL SEPTAL DEFECTS

Clinical features

Atrial septal defects (ASDs) are common congenital heart malformations that account for more than 10% of isolated congenital heart defects (Hoffman, 1990). Ostium secundum ASDs located in the region of the fossa ovalis is the most prevalent subtype and one thought to arise by malformation of the septum primum. This results in incomplete coverage of the fossa ovalis and shunting across the defect. Blood flow through the ASD depends on a variety of physiologic factors, including the ratio of left-sided (systemic) vs right-sided (pulmonary) resistance, the ratio of left ventricular to right ventricular compliance, and defect size. Uncorrected ASDs can lead to increased pulmonary blood flow with secondary development of pulmonary

artery hypertension, right ventricular hypertrophy, right-sided volume overload, heart failure and death. In addition, ECG abnormalities are common and include variable degrees of atrioventricular block, atrial tachydysrhythmias (such as atrial fibrillation or flutter), and abnormal ECG findings including right bundle branch block, right axis deviation, or right ventricular hypertrophy with strain (Emanuel et al., 1975; Pease et al., 1976).

Genetics and management

Although most cases of ASD are sporadic, autosomal dominant familial transmission has been well reported, particularly ASD associated with conduction system defects (Bizarro et al., 1970; Bjornstad, 1974; Hoffman, 1990; Kahler et al., 1996). Age-related penetrance has also been noted. Linkage analysis initially identified a locus on chromosome 5q35 (Table 50.3) and subsequently mutations in the transcription factor Nkx2–5 were identified (Benson et al., 1998; Schott et al., 1998; Mah et al., 1999). Mutations in this gene were thought to destabilize the protein or disrupt the ability of Nkx2–5 to target DNA binding. Nkx2–5 defects appear to cause haploinsufficiency of a transcription factor meant to play a central role in cardiac morphogenesis, including the atrioventricular node. A second locus (5p) has been identified (Table 50.3) but the gene remains elusive (Benson et al., 1998).

Therapy of ASDs includes diuretic therapy when significant left-to-right shunting occurs. In patients with conduction disease, pacemakers may play a role.

HOLT-ORAM SYNDROME

Da Vinci was the first to recognize that communication between right- and left-sided cardiac chambers resulted from defects in the atrial and ventricular septum. Approximately 100 years later, an association between congenital cardiac malformations, particularly septal defects, and upper limb deformities was first recognized (Pruznanski, 1964), but it was not until 1960 that familial cases of a heart-hand syndrome were described by Holt and Oram (1960). This syndrome, Holt-Oram syndrome (HOS), is characterized by malformed thumbs associated with atrial septal defects (ASDs), normal intelligence and normal (i.e., non-dysmorphic) facial features. Essentially all individuals with HOS exhibit some upper limb skeletal abnormality in the developmental distribution of the pre-axial radial ray (Poznanski et al., 1970; Basson et al., 1994). These skeletal deformities may be bilateral and asymmetric or unilateral and, in either limb, may be mild and subclinical or severe and overt. The most common is malformation of one or more carpal bones. The wrist bones may be absent, misshapen or fused. Another feature, which has been considered to be a typical and expected finding, is a triphalangial or hypoplastic/absent thumb. Some children present with severe foreshortening of the radius that extends proximally in a preaxial distribution to include the humerus and shoulder girdle and may present as phocomelia.

Approximately 75% of individuals with HOS have cardiac manifestations (Basson et al., 1994), which vary in magnitude from severe to clinically insignificant and are not dependent on the severity of skeletal disease. The cardiac abnormalities may manifest as congenital cardiac structural disease or conduction disease. Most commonly, individuals present with ASDs (usually ostium secundum ASD); many individuals, however, have ventricular septal defects (VSDs), typically in the membranous portion of the ventricular septum. Rarely, more complex congenital heart disease occurs (i.e., tetralogy of Fallot, truncus arteriosus, hypoplastic left heart syndrome, heterotaxia, total anomalous pulmonary venous return) (Sletten and Pierpont, 1996; Sahn et al., 1981; Glauser et al., 1989).

Cardiac conduction abnormalities may occur in the presence or absence of structural heart disease, and are commonly progressive. They may manifest initially as sinus tachycardia with mild first-degree atrioventricular block but, over time, the function of the sinus node can deteriorate and, in addition, atrioventricular node block can occur. High-grade heart block and atrial fibrillation may occur in patients with HOS (Sletter and Pierpont, 1996).

Genetics and management

Holt-Oram syndrome has autosomal dominant inheritance with complete penetrance but high variability (Newbury-Ecob et al., 1996). The prevalence is believed to be approximately 1 per 100,000 live births. As 85% of these are due to new mutations, the mutation rate is calculated to be 1 per million (Elek et al., 1991).

No consistent familial cytogenetic abnormalities have been associated with HOS although karyotypic abnormalities have been reported in sporadic cases (Ockey et al., 1967; Turleau et al., 1984). Linkage analysis initially identified a locus on chromosome 12q2 in families with HOS (Table 50.3) and subsequent refining studies localized an HOS gene to chromosome 12q24.1 (Bonnet et al., 1994; Terrett et al., 1994). Cloning of this region identified the human *TBX5* gene (Table 50.3) within this region of the genome and mutation analysis identified disease-causing mutations (Basson et al., 1994, 1995, 1997, 1999; Li et al.,

1997). The gene is expressed in skeletal and cardiac tissue, with TBX5 protein found in the atria and, like the Nkx2–5 mutations in familial ASD, ventricles and haploinsufficiency appears to be the mechanism of disease in many patients (Basson et al., 1999; Bruneau et al., 1999). In others, it is speculated that dominant negative effects occur by stoichiometric inhibition of TBX5 binding to DNA. Genetic heterogeneity exists (Basson et al., 1995) but the remaining genes are currently unknown.

The management of HOS focuses on treatment of the left to right shunt in patients with ASDs or VSDs (potentially requiring diuretics) and ultimately closure of the defect. When more severe congenital heart disease occurs, surgical palliation is required. The conduction disorder must also be monitored closely and in some cases a pacemaker is needed.

LATERALITY DEFECTS

The clinical presentation of children with laterality defects is varied (Gutgesell, 1998; Van Praagh et al., 1992) and include abnormal visceral and atrial situs resulting in situs inversus or heterotaxy, abnormal looping of the cardiac tube resulting in ventricular inversion, and abnormal positioning of the heart in the chest (i.e., dextrocardia) (Sapire et al., 1986; Splitt et al., 1996). In some cases, complex cardiac anomalies occur and may be associated with conduction disease (Dickinson et al., 1979; Wren et al., 1987). Conduction defects occur most often in patients with heterotaxy or with "corrected" transposition of the great arteries (L-TGA).

HETEROTAXY SYNDROME

The fundamental characteristics of heterotaxy syndrome include abnormal symmetry of the viscera and veins (such as lungs, liver, vena cava) and situs discordance between various organ systems, as well as between the various segments of the heart (Freedom, 1972; Gutgesell, 1998; Liberthson et al., 1973; Van Praagh et al., 1992). Patients with heterotaxy have a random orientation of various organs and include asplenia or polysplenia syndrome (Uemura et al., 1995) and loss of pulmonary and cardiac asymmetry (isomersion) at some levels resulting in apparent bilaterally right- or left-sidedness, respectively. Patients with heterotaxy syndromes tend to have significant non-cardiac midline defects as well (Ticho et al., 2000; Rose et al., 1975).

In asplenia syndrome, both lungs are frequently trilobed, both bronchi are eparterial, the spleen is hypoplastic or absent, and the liver commonly overrides the midline. The cardiac abnormalities found in these patients include right atrial appendage isomerism, common atrium, complete atrioventricular canal, double outlet right ventricle, pulmonic stenosis, transposition of the great arteries and anomalous pulmonary venous connections (Gutgesell, 1998; Hashmi et al., 1998; Van Praagh et al., 1992). Atrioventricular block rarely occurs. Several reports of bilateral sinus nodes have been reported and dual AV nodes appear to predispose these patients to SVT, particularly in patients with two ventricles (Wu et al., 1998). The mechanism for SVT has been postulated to be "AV nodal to AV nodal" reentry with the retrograde accessory pathway for SVT mapped to an anterior AV node, left lateral pathway, or tricuspid valve.

Polysplenia or bilateral left-sidedness with mirror image lungs (i.e., both lungs have the appearance of the left lung including two lobes and hyparterial bronchi), anomalous pulmonary venous return, renal to hepatic inferior vena cava segment absence with return of blood from lower body occurring via the azygos or hemiazygos system (Moller et al., 1967). Bilateral left atrial appendages may occur and typical cardiac defects include ASD, VSD, pulmonic stenosis, AV canal, and others. Unlike asplenia, conduction disturbances are common in polysplenia (Momma et al., 1990), including congenital complete atrioventricular block in 20% to 30% of cases (Garcia et al., 1981; Roguin et al., 1984). The mechanism for AV block has been postulated to be due to discontinuity between the AV node and the ventricular conduction pathway, usually at the level of the penetrating bundle (Ho et al., 1992)

VENTRICULAR INVERSION

Isolated ventricular inversion is relatively rare, with the vast majority of patients having associated CHD. In 99% of cases of ventricular inversion, transposition of the great arteries, resulting in physiologically corrected transposition (L-TGA), is associated (Benson et al., 1980; Bharati et al., 1980; Van Praagh et al., 1998). In addition to L-TGA, other lesions include abnormal left-sided systemic tricuspid valves, malformations of the left-sided systemic right ventricle, VSD, pulmonic stenosis, and dextrocardia. Rhythm disturbances are frequently seen including pre-excitation, atrial tachydysrhythmias including atrial fibrillation or flutter or SVT (Benson et al., 1980). In some cases the dysrhythmias occur due to AV valve regurgitation or ventricular dysfunction while other cases are due to accessory pathways. Heart block is also common, even in patients with L-TGA only (i.e., no other associated cardiac lesions)(Daliento et al., 1986; Huhta et al., 1983). The site of block may be above the His bundle, within the His or below. The AV node is usually located anteriorly in the right atrium of patients

with L-TGA that connects right atrium to His bundle which encircles the anterior lateral region of the pulmonary valve. In most cases the posterior AV node is hypoplastic.

GENETICS

Mouse models

Mouse models of aberrant left-right asymmetry have been useful in dissecting the embryological and genetic basis of laterality. The inversus viscerum (iv) mouse, in which heterotaxy occurs in 50% of homozygous progeny (with the remainder developing normal visceral situs) is due to mutations in the left-right dynein (lrd) gene, an axonemal dynein heavy chain gene, which is expressed in the embryonic midline along the node and rostral floorplate (Supp et al., 1997). Another model, the inv mouse, has situs inversus in 85% of cases and heterotaxy in 15% of cases of homozygous offspring and in this mouse the defective gene is an ankyrin-repeat protein called inversin (Morgan et al., 1998).

Other mice thus far developed include a model in which lefty, a ligand in the TGF-β pathway which is important for left-right determination, is selectively disrupted (Meno et al., 1998). In this model, thoracic left isomerism with bilateral left lungs and left atria occurs and appears similar to human polysplenia syndrome. Mice with mutations in the activin receptor type IIB (Act RIIB) gene develop abnormal spleens and other signs of heterotaxia, as well as bilateral right-sidedness of the pulmonary and atrial anatomy consistent with human asplenia syndrome (Yokoyama et al., 1993).

Human genetics

To date a number of genes have been identified for laterality defects. In X-linked heterotaxy, Gebbia and colleagues (1997) identified mutations in Zic3, a zinc-finger transcription factor which functions in the early stages of left-right body axis formation (Table 50.3). In autosomal dominant forms of disease, mutations in the human activin type IIB gene (Kosaki et al., 1999b), NODAL, LEFTY (Kosaki et al., 1999a), and HNF-3β, all transcription factors (Table 50.3) which are members of the TGF-β pathway, have been identified in patients with laterality defects (Kosaki and Casey, 1998; Levin et al., 1995).

FAMILIAL MITRAL VALVE PROLAPSE

Clinical features

Mitral valve prolapse (MVP) is a very common clinical diagnosis, particularly in young, healthy women (Barlow and

Pocock, 1979). The diagnosis is usually made on the basis of auscultatory findings of a midsystolic click with or without a mitral regurgitation murmur heard at the cardiac apex (Bareiss, 1976; Barlow and Pocock, 1979).

Echocardiography may identify the prolapsing valve cusps into the left atrium during systole and the redundant valve leaflets; in cases of mitral regurgitation, Doppler and color Doppler may clearly demonstrate the regurgitant jet. Typical symptoms include chest pain, palpitations, and anxiety. Dysrhythmias are common. The dysrhythmias occurring in the MVP syndrome include atrial premature complexes, nonsustained atrial tachycardia, and nonsustained ventricular ectopy. It has been speculated that MVP has an associated increased risk of sudden death, possibly due to dysrhythmias; severe mitral regurgitation or ruptured mitral chordae tendineae has also been cited as causes of sudden death. In addition, these patients have an increased risk of endocarditis.

Genetics and management

MVP is commonly inherited, with autosomal dominant transmission seen (Devereaux et al., 1982). Expression may be variable, and this depends on age and gender. Full expression is found in young adult women (11 to 50 years of age), affecting approximately 50% of this population in families with MVP. On the other hand, only 10 to 30% of older women, older men and children in affected families demonstrate MVP, consistent with incomplete penetrance.

Recently, linkage to chromosome 16 at 16p 11.2-p12.1 (Table 50.3) was identified in families with MVP (Disse

et al., 1999). Interestingly, males and females were equally affected clinically. This gene has not yet been identified, but we have speculated that a connective tissue protein-encoding gene would be at the root of the abnormality (Towbin, 1999b). MVP commonly accompanies connective tissue disorders, such as Marfan syndrome and Ehlers-Danlos syndrome, which have been shown to occur due to mutations in fibrillin and various collagens. It is likely that MVP syndrome is a form-fruste of a connective tissue disorder (Towbin, 1999b).

The dysrhythmias commonly seen in MVP usually do not require therapy. However, in those cases in which symptoms occur, standard antiarrhythmia therapy (particularly β-blockers) may be necessary. Prophylaxis against endocarditis is also indicated when appropriate.

SUMMARY

The genetics of cardiac disease, including those in which dysrhythmias are primary or secondary findings, has come of age as the 21st century begins. As the Human Genome Project comes to completion, it is expected that further understanding of the genes responsible for the disorders of the heart will also be better understood. In the next decade, the relationships between mutated genes, modifier genes and environmental factors are likely to be important areas of study which will enable better therapies to be developed.

REFERENCES

Abbott GW, Sesti F, Splawski I et al. (1999) *MiRP1* forms l$_{Kr}$ potassium channels with *HERG* and is associated with cardiac arrhythmia. Cell 97:175–187

Ackerman MJ, Tester DJ, Porter CJ, Edwards, WD (1999) Molecular diagnosis of the inherited long-QT syndrome in a woman who died after near-drowning. N Eng J Med 341:1121–1115

Ackroyd RS, Finnegan JA, Green SH (1984) Friedreich's ataxia: A clinical review with neurophysiological and echocardiographic findings. Archives of Diseases of Childhood 59:217–221

Ahmad F, Li D, Karibe A, Gonzalez O et al. (1998) Localization of a gene responsible for arrhythmogenic right ventricular dysplasia to chromosome 3p23. Circulation 98:2791–2795

Aihara N, Ohe T, Kamakura S et al. (1990) Clinical and electrophysiologic characteristics of idiopathic ventricular fibrillation. Shinzo 22 (Suppl. 2):80–86

Albers GW (1994) Atrial fibrillation and stroke: Three new studies, three remaining questions. Arch of Internal Med 154:1443–1448

Alboliras ET, Shub C, Gomez MR et al. (1986) Spectrum of cardiac involvement in Friedreich's ataxia: Clinical, electrocardiographic and echocardiographic observations. Am J Cardiology 58:518–524

Allamand V, Campbell KP (2000) Anual models for muscular dystrophy: valuable tools for the development of therapies. Hum Mol Genet 9:2459–2467

Ammash NM, Seward JB, Bailey KR et al. (2000) Clinical profile and outcome of idiopathic restrictive cardiomyopathy. Circulation 101:2490–2496

An RH, Wang XL, Kerem B et al. (1998) Novel *LQT-3* mutation affects Na+ channel activity through interactions between alpha- and beta 1-subunits. Circulation. Research 83:141–146

Anan R, Nakagawa M, Miayata M et al. (1995) Cardiac involvement in mitochondrial diseases. A study on 17 patients with documented mitochondrial DNA defects. Circulation 91:955–961

Anderson KP, Freedman RA, Maron JW (1987) Sudden death in idiopathic dilated cardiomyopathy. Ann Internal Med 107:104–106

Angelini C, Fanin M, Freda MP et al. (1999) The clinical spectrum of sarcoglycanopathies. Neurology 52:176–179

Antzelevitch C (1998) The Brugada Syndrome. J Cardiovascular Electrophysiology 9:513–516

Antzelevitch C (1999) Ion channels and ventricular arrhythmias: Cellular and ionic mechanisms underlying the Brugada syndrome. Current Opinion in Cardiology 14:274–279

Antzelevitch C, Sicouri S, Luteas A et al. (1995) Regional differences in the electrophysiology of ventricular cells: Physiological and clinical implications. In Zips DP, Jalife J, eds: Cardiac Electrophysiology: From Cell to Bedside. WB Saunders, Philadelphia pp. 228–245

Arbustini E, Morbini P, Grasso M et al. (1998) Restrictive cardiomyopathy, atrioventricular block and mild to subclinical myopathy in patients with desmin-immunoreactive material deposits. J Am College of Cardiology 31:645–653

Arcangeli A, Rosati B, Cherubini A et al. (1997) *HERG*- and IRK-like inward rectifier currents are sequentially expressed during neuronal crest cells and their derivatives. Europ J Neuroscience 9:2596–2604

Asano Y, Davidenko J, Bater WT et al. (1997) Optical mapping of drug-induced polymorphic arrhythmias and torsades de pointes in the isolated rabbit heart. J Am College of Cardiology 29:831–842

Badano L, Autore C, Fragola PV et al. (1993) Left ventricular myocardial function in myotonic dystrophy. Am J Cardiology 71:987–991

Bareiss P (1976) Familial forms of the mid-end systolic click and murmur syndrome with deviations of left ventricular kinetics. Archives of Maladies du Couer et des Vaisseaux 69:71–81

Barhanin J, Lesage F, Guillemare E et al. (1996) KVLQT1 and lsK (*minK*) proteins associate to form the I_{Ks} cardiac potassium current. Nature 384:78–80

Barlow JB, Pocock WA (1979) Mitral valve prolapse, the specific billowing mitral leaflet syndrome, or an insignificant non-ejection systolic click. Am Heart J 97:277–285

Basson CT, Cowley GS, Solomon SD et al. (1994) The clinical and genetic spectrum of the Holt-Oram syndrome (heart-hand syndrome). N Eng J Med 330:885–891

Basson CT, Solomon SD, Welsoman B et al. (1995) Genetic hetero-geneity of heart-hand syndrome. Circulation 91:1326–1329

Basson CT, Bachinsky DR, Lin RC et al. (1997) Mutations in human Tbx5 cause limb and cardiac malformation in Holt-Oram syndrome. Nat Gene 15:30–35

Basson CT, Huang T, Lin RC et al. (1999) Different TBX5 interactions in the heart and limb defined by Holt-Oram syndrome mutations. Proc Nat Acad Sci USA 96:2919–2924

Becker KD, Gottshall KR, Hickey R, Perriard JC, Chien KR (1997) Point mutations in human beta cardiac myosin heavy chain have differential effects on sarcomeric structure and assembly: An ATP binding site change disrupts both thick and thin filaments, whereas hypertrophic cardiomyopathy mutations display normal assembly. J Cell Biol 137:131–140

Beggs AH, Kunkel LM (1990) Improved diagnosis of Duchenne/Becker muscular dystrophy. J Clin Invest 85:613–619

Beggs AH, Hoffman EP, Snyder JR et al. (1991) Exposing the molecular basis for variability among patients with Becker muscular dystrophy: Dystrophin gene and protein studies. Am J Hum Genet 49:54–67

Bellavere F, Ferri M, Guarini L et al. (1988) Prolonged QT period in diabetic autonomic neuropathy: A possible role in sudden cardiac death. British Heart Journal 59:379–383

Belhassen B, Viskin S, Fish R, Glick A, Setbon I, Eldar M (1999) Effects of electrophysiologic-guided therapy with Class IA antiarrhythmic drugs on the long-term outcome of patients with idiopathic ventricular fibrillation with or without the Brugada syndrome. J Cardiovasc Electrophysiol 10:1301–1312

Benhorin J, Kalman YM, Madina A et al. (1993) Evidence of genetic heterogeneity in the long QT syndrome. Science 260:1960–1962

Benhorin J, Taub R, Goldmit M et al. (1998) Effects of flecainide in patients with new SCN5A mutation. Mutation-specific therapy for long-QT syndrome. Circulation 101:1698–1706

Bennett PB, Yazawa K, Makita N George AL Jr (1995) Molecular mechanism for an inherited cardiac arrhythmia. Nature 376:683–685

Benson DW Jr, Gallagher JJ, Oldham HM et al. (1980) Corrected transposition with severe intracardiac deformities with Wolff-Parkinson-White syndrome in a child. Electrophysiologic investigation and surgical correction. Circulation 61:1256–1261

Benson DW, Sharkey A, Fatkin D et al. (1998) Reduced penetrance, variable expressivity, and genetic heterogeneity of familial atrial septal defects. Circulation 97:2043–2048

Berko BA, Swift M (1987) X-linked dilated cardiomyopathy. N Engl J Med 316:1186–1191

Berul CI, Christe ME, Aronovitz MJ et al. (1998) Familial hypertrophic cardiomyopathy mice display gender differences in electrophysiological abnormalities. J Interventional Cardiac Electrophysiology 2:7–14

Berul CI, Maguire CT, Arnovitz MJ et al. (1999) DMPK dosage alterations result in atrioventricular conduction abnormalities in a mouse myotonic dystrophy model. J Clin Invest 103:R1–R7

Bevilacqua LM, Maguire CT, Seidman CE et al. (1999) QT dispersion in α-MHC familial hypertrophic cardiomyopathy in mice. Pediatr Res 45:643–647

Beyer F, Paul T, Luhmer I et al. (1993) Familial idiopathic atrial fibrillation with bradyarrhythmia. Zeitschrift fuer Kardiologie 83:674–677

Bharati S, Rosen K, Stainfeld L et al. (1980) The anatanic substrate for preexcitation in corrected transposition. Circulation 62:831–842

Bharati S, Surawicz B, Vidaillet HJ et al. (1992) Familial congenital sinus rhythm abnormalities: Clinical and pathological correlations. PACE 15:1720–1729

Bianchi L, Wible B, Arcangeli A et al. (1998) *HERG* encodes a K+ current highly conserved in tumors of different histogenesis: a selective advantage for cancer cells? Cancer Res 58:815–822

Bianchi L, Shen Z, Dennis AT et al. (1999) Cellular dysfunction of *LQT5-minK* mutants: abnormalities of I_{ks}, I_{kr} and trafficking in long QT syndrome. Hum Molec Genet 8:1499–1507

Bies RD, Maeda M, Roberds SL, Holder E, Bohlmeyer T, Young JB, Campbell KP (1997) A 5' dystrophin duplication mutation causes membrane deficiency of alpha-dystroglycan in a family with X-linked cardiomyopathy. J Mol Cell Cardiol 29:3175–3188

Bione S, Maestrini E, Rivella S, Mancini M, Regis S, Romeo G, Toniolo D. (1994) Identification of a novel X-linked gene responsible for Emery-Dreifuss muscular dystrophy. Nature Genet 8:323–327

Bione S, D'Adamo P, Maestrini E, Gedeon AK, Bolhuis PA, Toniolo D (1996) A novel X-linked gene, G4.5, is responsible for Barth syndrome. Nature Genet 12:385–389

Bizarro RO Callahan JA, Feldt RH et al. (1970) Familial atrial septal defect with prolonged atrioventricular conduction. Circulation 41:677–683

Bjornstad PG (1974) Secundum-type atrial septal defect with prolonged PR interval and autosomal dominant mode of inheritance. British Heart Journal 36:1149

Bleyl SB, Mumford BR, Thompson V, Carey JC, Pysher TJ, Chin TK, Ward K (1997) Neonatal lethal noncompaction of the left ventricular myocardium is allelic with Barth syndrome. Am J Hum Genet 61:868–872

Bonne G, Carrier L, Bercovici J, Cruaud C, Richard P, Hainque B, Gautel M, Labeit S, James M, Beckmann J et al. (1995) Cardiac myosin binding protein-C gene splice acceptor site mutation is associated with familial hypertrophic cardiomyopathy. Nature Genet 11:438–440

Bonne G, Carrier L, Richard P et al. (1998) Familial hypertrophic cardiomyopathy: From mutations to functional defects. Circ Res 83:580–593

Bonne G, DiBarletta MR, Varnous S et al. (1999) Mutations in the gene encoding lamin A/C cause autosomal dominant Emery-Dreifuss muscular dystrophy. Nat Gene 21:285–288

Bonnemann CG, Passos-Bueno R, McNally EM et al. (1996) Genomic screening for β-sarcoglycan mutations: Missense mutations may cause severe limb-girdle muscular dystrophy type 2E (LGMD2E). Hum Molec Genet 5:1953–1961

Bonnemann CG, McNally EM, Kunkel LM (1997) Beyond dystrophin: Current progress in the muscular dystrophies. Current Opinion in Pediatr 8:569–582

Bonnet D, Pelet A, Legeai-Mallet L et al. (1994) A gene for Holt-Oram syndrome maps to the distal long arm of chromosome 12. Nat Genet 6:405–408

Bower SP, Hawley I, Mackey DA (1992) Cardiac arrhythmia and Leber's hereditary optic neuropathy. Lancet 339:1427–1428

Bowles KR, Gajarski R, Porter P et al. (1996) Gene mapping of familiar autosomal dominant dilated cardiomyopathy to chromosome 10q21-23. J Clin Invest 98:1355–1360

Brink PA, Fereira A, Moolman-Weymar HW et al. (1995) Gene for progressive familial heart block type I maps to chromosome 19q13. Circ 91:1633–1640

Brodsky GL, Muntoni F, Miocic S et al. (2000) Lamin A/C gene mutation associated with dilated cardiomyopathy with variable skeletal muscle involvement. Circ 101:473–476

Brook JD, McCurrach ME, Harley HG et al. (1992) Molecular basis of myotonic dystrophy: Expansion of a trinucleotide (CTG) repeat at the 3′ end of a transcript endcoding a protein kinase family member. Cell 68:799–808

Bushby KMD 1995 Diagnostic criteria for the limb-girdle muscular dystrophic report of the ENC consortium on limb-girdle dystrophies. Neuromuscular Disorders 5:71–74

Buxton AE, Waxman HL, Marchlinski FE et al. (1983) Right ventricular tachycardia: Clinical and electrophysiologic characteristics. Circulation 68:917–927

Buxton J, Shelbourne P, Davies J et al. (1992) Characterization of a YAC and cosmid contig containing markers tightly linked to the myotonic dystrophy locus on chromosome 19. Genomics 13:526–531

Campuzano V, Montermini L, Molto MD et al. (1996) Friedreich's ataxia: Autosomal recessive disease caused by an intronic GAA triplet repeat expansion. Science 271:1423–1427

Campuzano V, Montermini L, Lutz Y et al. (1997) Frataxin is reduced in Friedreich ataxia patients and is associated with mitochondrial membranes. Human and Molecular Genetics 6:1771–1780

Cao H, Hegele RA 2000 Nuclear lamin A/C R482 mutation in Canadian kindreds with Dunnigan-type familial partial lipodystrophy. Human Molecular Genetics 9:109–112

Caralis DG, Varghese PJ 1976 Familial sinoatrial node dysfunction: Increased vagal tone a possible aetiology. British Heart Journal 38:951–956

Carrier L, Hengstenberg C, Beckmann JS et al. (1993) Mapping of a novel gene for familial hypertrophic cardiomyopathy to chromosome 11. Nature Genet 4:311–313

Carrier L, Bonne G, Bahrend E et al. (1997) Organization and sequence of human cardiac myosin binding protein C gene (MYBPC3) and identification of mutations predicted to produce truncated proteins in familial hypertrophic cardiomyopathy. Circ Res 80:427–434

Cartegni L, di Barletta MR, Barresi R et al. (1997) Heart-specific localization of emerin: New insights into Emery-Dreifuss muscular dystrophy. Hum Mol Genet 6:2257–2264

Cetta F, O'Leary PW, Seward JB et al. (1995) Idiopathic restrictive cardiomyopathy in childhood: Diagnostic features and clinical course. Mayo Clin Proc 70:634–640

Chamberlain S, Shaw J, Rowland A et al. (1988) Mapping of mutation causing Friedreich's ataxia to human chromosome 9. Nature 334:248–250

Charles R, Holt S, Kay JM et al. (1981) Myocardial ultrastructure and the development and the development of atrioventricular block in Kearns-Sayre syndrome. Circulation 63:214–219

Charron P, Dubourg O, Desnos M et al. (1998) Clinical features and prognostic implications of familial hypertrophic cardiomyopathy related to the cardiac myosin-binding protein C gene. Circulation 97:2230–2236

Chen Q, Kirsch GE, Zhang D et al. (1998) Genetic basis and molecular mechanism for idiopathic ventricular fibrillation. Nature 392:293–296

Chen Q, Zhang D, Gingell RL et al. (1999) Homozygous deletion in KVLQT1 associated with Jervell and Lange-Nielsen syndrome. Circulation 99:1344–1347

Chia BL, Yew FC, Chay SO, Tan AT (1982) Familial Wolff-Parkinson-White syndrome. J Electrocardiol 15:195–198

Chin TK, Perloff JK, Williams RG, Jue K, Mohrmann R (1990) Isolated noncompaction of left ventricular myocardium. A study of eight cases. Circulation 82:507–513

Chomyn A (1998) The myoclonic epilepsy and ragged-red fiber mutation provides new insights into human mitochondrial function and genetics. Am J Hum Genet 62:745–751

Chouabe C, Neyroud N, Guicheney P, Lazdunski M, Romey G, Barhanin J (1997) Properties of KVLQTIK⁺ channel mutations in Romano-Ward and Jervell and Lange-Nielsen inherited cardiac arrhythmias. EMBO Journal 16:5472–5479

Chouabe C, Neyroud N, Richard PK et al. (2000) Novel mutations in KVLQT1 that affect lKs activation through interactions with IsK. Cardiovasc Res 45:971–980

Choy AM, Lang CC, Chomsky DM et al. (1997) Normalization of acquired QT prolongation in humans by intravenous potassium. Circulation 96:2149–2154

Chung KY, Walsh TJ, Massie E (1965) Wolff-Parkinson-White syndrome. Am Heart J 69:116–133

Ciafaloni E, Ricci E, Shanske S et al. (1992) MELAS: clinical features, biochemistry, and molecular genetics. Ann Neurol 31:391–398

Codd MB, Sugrue DD, Gersh BJ, Melton LJ 3d. (1989) Epidemiology of idiopathic dilated and hypertrophic cardiomyopathy. A population-based study in Olmsted County, Minnesota, 1975–1984. Circulation 80:564–572

Cohen TJ, Liem BL, Hancock W (1989) Association of bidirectional ventricular tachycardia with familial sudden death syndrome. Am J Cardiol 64:1078–1079

Compton SJ, Lux RL, Ramsey MR, Strelich KR, Sanguinetti MC, Green LS, Keating MT, Mason JW (1996) Genetically defined therapy of inherited long-QT syndrome. Correction of abnormal repolarization by potassium. Circulation 94:1018–1022

Connor AC, McFadden JF, Houston BJ et al. (1959) Familial congenital complete heart block: Case report and review of the literature. Am J Obst Gynecol 78:75–79

Consalez GG, Thomas NS, Stayton CL et al. (1991) Assignment of Emery-Dreifuss muscular dystrophy to the distal region of Xq28: The results of a collaborative study. Am J Hum Genet 48:468–480

Coonar AS, Protonotarios N, Tsatsopoulou A et al. (1998) Gene for arrhythmogenic right ventricular cardiomyopathy with diffuse nonepidermolytic palmoplantar keratoderma and wooly hair (Naxos disease) maps to 17q21. Circulation 97:2049–2058

Corrado D, Nava A, Buja G et al. (1996) Familial cardiomyopathy underlies syndrome of right bundle branch block, ST segment elevation and sudden death. J Am Coll Cardiol 27:443–448

Corrado D, Basso C, Thiene G et al. (1997) Spectrum of clinicopathologic manifestations of arrhythmogenic right ventricular cardiomyopathy/dysplasia: A multicenter study. J Am Coll Cardiol 30:1512–1520

Corrado D, Fontaine G, Marcus FI et al. (2000) Arrhythmogenic right ventricular dysplasia/cardiomyopathy: Need for an international registry. Study Group on Arrhythmogenic Right Ventricular Dysplasia/Cardiomyopathy of the Working Groups on Myocardial and Pericardial Disease and Arrhythmias of the European Society of Cardiology and of the Scientific Council on Cardiomyopathies of the World Heart Federation. Circulation 101:E101–106

Corral-Debrinski M. Stepien G, Shoffner JM et al. (1991) Hypoxemia is associated with mitochondrial DNA damage and gene induction. Implications for cardiac disease. J Am Med Assoc 266:1812–1816

Coumel P, Fidelle J, Lucet V, Attuel P, Bouvrain Y (1978) Catecholamine-induced severe ventricular arrhythmias with Adams-Stokes syndrome in children: Report of four cases. Br Heart J 40(Suppl):28–37

Cox GF, Kunkel LM (1997) Dystrophies and heart disease. Curr Opin Cardiol 12:329–343

Curran ME, Atkinson D, Timothy K et al. (1993) Locus heterogeneity of autosomal dominant long QT syndrome. J Clin Invest 92:799–803

Curran ME, Splawski I, Timothy KW et al. (1995) A molecular basis for cardiac arrhythmia: *HERG* mutations cause long QT syndrome. Cell 80:795–803

D'Adamo P, Fassone L. Gedeon A et al. (1997) The X-linked gene G4.5 is responsible for different infantile dilated cardiomyopathies. Am J Hum Genet 6:862–867

Daliento L, Corrado D, Buja G, John N, Nava A, Thiene E (1986) Rhythm and conduction disturbances in isolated, congenitally corrected transposition of the great arteries. Am J Cardiol 58:314–318

De Meeus A, Stephan E, Debrus S et al. (1995) An isolated cardiac conduction disease maps to chromosome 19q. Circ Res 77:735–740

Deconinck N, Ragot T, Marechal G et al. (1996) Functional protection of dystrophic mouse (mdx) muscles after adenovirus-mediated transfer of a dystrophin minigene. Proc Nat Acad Sci USA 93:3570–3574

Deconinck AE, Rafael JA, Skinner JA et al. (1997) Utrophin-dystrophin-deficient mice as a model for Duchenne muscular dystrophy. Cell 90:717–727

DeCoster W, DeReuck J, Thiery E (1974) A late onset autosomal dominant form of limb-girdle muscular dystrophy. Eur Neurol 12:159–172

Demolombe S, Baro I, Pereon Y et al. (1998) A dominant negative isoform of the long QT syndrome 1 gene product. J Biol Chem 273:6837–6843

Denfield SW, Rosenthal G, Gajarski RJ et al. (1997) Restrictive cardiomyopathies in childhood: Etiologies and natural history. Texas Heart Inst J 24:38–44

Devereaux RB, Brown WT, Kramer-Fox R, Sachs I (1982) Inheritance of mitral valve prolapse: Effect of age and sex on gene expression. Ann Int Med 97:826–832

Di Barletta MR, Ricci E, Galluzzi G et al. (2000) Different mutations in the LMNA gene cause autosomal dominant and autosomal recessive Emery-Dreifuss muscular dystrophy. Am J Hum Genet 66:1407–1412

Dickinson DF, Wilkinson JL, Anderson KR, Smith A, Ho SY, Anderson RH (1979) The cardiac conduction system *in situs* ambiguous. Circulation 59:879–885

Disertori M, Guarnerio M, Vergara G et al. (1983) Familial endemic persistent atrial standstill in a small mountain community: Review of eight cases. Eur Heart J 4:354–361

Disse S, Abergel E, Berrebi A et al. (1999) Mapping of the first locus for autosomal dominant myxomatous mitral valve prolapse to chromosome 16p 11.2-p12.1. Am J Hum Genet 65:1242–1251

Dubowitz V 1985 Muscle biopsy: A practical approach. In The muscular dystrophies. London, Bailliere Tindall, 289–404

Duggal P, Vesely MR, Wattanasirichaigoon D, Villafane J, Kaushik V, Beggs AH (1998) Mutation of the gene for IsK associated with Jervell and Lange-Nielsen and Romano-Ward forms of long QT syndrome. Circulation 97:142–146

Dumaine R, Wang Q, Keating MT et al. (1996) Multiple mechanisms of sodium channel-linked long QT syndrome. Circ Res 78:916–920

Dumaine R, Towbin JA, Brugada P (1999) Ionic mechanisms responsible for the electrocardiographic phenotype of the Brugada syndrome are temperature dependent. Circ Res 85:803–809

Durakovic Z, Durakovic A, Kastelan A (1992) The pre-excitation syndrome: Epidemiological and genetic study. Int J Cardiol 35:181–186

Durand JB, Bachinski LL, Bieling LC et al. (1995) Localization of a gene responsible for familial dilated cardiomyopathy to chromosome 1q32. Circulation 92:3387–3389

Durr A, Cossee M, Agid Y et al. (1996) Clinical and genetic abnormalities in patients with Friedreich's ataxia. N Engl J Med 335:1169–1175

Edeiken J (1954) Elevation of RS-T segment, apparent or real in right precordial leads as probable normal variant. Am Heart J 48:331–339

Egger J, Lake BD, Wilson J (1981) Mitochondrial cytopathy. A multisystem disorder with ragged red fibres on muscle biopsy. Arch Dis Child 56:741–752

Eldar M, Griffin JC, Abbott JA et al. (1987) Permanent cardiac pacing in patients with the long QT syndrome. J Am Coll Cardiol 10:600–607

Elek C, Vitez M, Czeizel E (1991) Holt-Oram syndrome. Orv Hetil 132:73–74, 77–78

El-Sherif N, Caref EB, Yin H, Restivo M (1996) The electrophysiological mechanism of ventricular arrhythmias in the long QT syndrome: Tridimensional mapping of activation and recovery patterns. Circ Res 77:474–492

El-Sherif N, Chinushi M, Caref EB et al. (1997) Electrophysiological mechanism of the characteristic electrocardiographic morphology of *torsade de pointes* tachyarrhythmias in the long-QT syndrome: Detailed analysis of ventricular tridimensional activation patterns. Circulation 96:4392–4399

Emanuel R, O'Brien K, Somerville J, Jefferson K, Hegde M (1975) Association of secundum atrial septal defect with atrioventricular conduction abnormalities or left axis deviation. Br Heart J 7:1085–1092

Emery AEH (1989) Emery-Dreifuss syndrome. J Med Genet 26:637–641

Emery AEH, Dreifuss FE (1966) Unusual type of benign X-linked muscular dystrophy. J Neurol Neurosurg Psych 29:338–342

Engel AG, Yamamoto M, Fischbeck KH (1994) Dystrophinopathies. In Engel AG, Franzin-Armstrong C (eds): Myology, 2nd edn. McGraw-Hill, NY, pp. 1133–1187

Epstein ND, Fananapazir L, Lin HJ et al. (1992) Evidence of genetic heterogeneity in five kindreds with familial hypertrophic cardiomyopathy. Circulation 85:635–647

Ervasti JM, Campbell KP (1993) A role for the dystrophin-glycoprotein complex as a transmembrane linker between laminin and actin. J Cell Biol 122:809–823

Eymard B, Romero NB, Leturcq F et al. (1997) Primary adhalinopathy (α-sarcoglycanopathy): Clinical, pathologic and genetic correlation in 20 patients with autosomal recessive muscular dystrophy. Neurology 48:1227–1234

Fanin M, Angelini C (1999) Regeneration in sarcoglycanopathies: Expression studies of sarcoglycans and other muscle proteins. J Neurol Sci 165:170–177

Fanin M, Duggan DJ, Mostacciuolo ML et al. (1997) Genetic epidemiology of muscular dystrophies resulting from sarcoglycan gene mutations. J Med Genet 34:973–977

Farza H, Townsend PJ, Carrier L et al. (1998) Genomic organization, alternative splicing and polymorphisms of the human cardiac troponin T gene. J Mol Cell Cardiol 30:1247–1253

Fatkin D, Christe ME, Aristizabul O et al. (1999a) Neonatal cardiomyopathy in mice homozygous for the Arg403Gln mutation in the alpha cardiac myosin heavy chain gene. J Clin Invest 103:147–153

Fatkin D, MacRae C, Sasaki T et al. (1999b) Missense mutations in the rod domain of the lamin A/C gene as causes of dilated cardiomyopathy and conduction system disease. N Eng J Med 341:1715–1724

Federico A, Aitiani P, Lomonacu B et al. (1987) Electrocardiographic abnormalities in Leber's hereditary optic atrophy. J Inherit Met Dis 10(Suppl 2):256–259

Feinberg WM, Blackshear JL, Laupacis A, Kronmal R, Hart RG (1995) Prevalence, age distribution, and gender of patients with atrial fibrillation. Arch Int Med 155:469–473

Fenichal GM, Sul YC, Kilroy AW, Blouin R (1982) An autosomal-dominant dystrophy with humeroperopelvic distribution and cardiomyopathy. Neurology 32:1399–1401

Ferlini A, Galie N, Merlini L, Sewry C, Branzi A, Muntoni F (1998) A novel Alu-like element rearranged in the dystrophin gene causes a splicing mutation in a family with X-linked dilated cardiomyopathy. Am J Hum Genet 63:436–446

Filla A, De Michele G, Cavalcanti F et al. (1996) The relationship between trinucleotide (GAA) repeat length and clinical features in Friedreich ataxia. Am J Hum Genet 59:554–560

Fisher JD, Krikler D, Hallidie-Smith KA (1999) Familial polymorphic ventricular arrhythmias. A quarter century of successful medical treatment based in serial exercise-pharmocologic testing. J Am Coll Cardiol 34:2015–2022

Fontaine G (1996) Familial cardiomyopathy associated with right bundle branch block, ST segment elevation and sudden death (Letter). J Am Coll Cardiol 28:540

Fontaine G, Piot O, Sohal P et al. (1996) Right precordial leads and sudden death. Relation with arrhythmogenic right ventricular dysplasia. Arch Malaides Coeur Vaisseaux 89:1323–1329

Fontaine G, Fontaliran F, Hebert JL, Chemla D, Zenati O, Lecarpentier Y, Frank R (1999) Arrhythmogenic right ventricular dysplasia. Ann Rev Med 50:17–35

Forissier JF, Carrier L, Farza H (1996) Codon 102 of the cardiac troponin T gene is a putative hot spot for mutations in familial hypertrophic cardiomyopathy. Circulation 94:3069–3073

Forsberg H, Olofsson BO, Eriksson A et al. (1990) Cardiac involvement in congenital myotonic dystrophy. Br Heart J 63:119–121

Fougerousse F, Delezoide AL, Fiszman MY et al. (1998) Cardiac myosin binding protein C gene is specifically expressed in heart during murine and human development. Circ Res 82:130–133

Fragola PV, Autore C, Magni G, Antonini G, Picelli A, Cannata D (1991) The natural course of cardiac conduction disturbances in myotonic dystrophy. Cardiology 79:93–98

Fragola PV, Luzi M, Calo L et al. (1994) Cardiac involvement in myotonic dystrophy. AM J Cardio 74:1070–1072

Franqueza L, Lin M, Splawsky I, Keating MT, Sanguinetti MC (1999) Long QT syndrome-associated mutations in the S4-S5 linker of KVLQT1 pottasium channels modify gating and interaction with minK subunits. J Bio Chem 274:21063–21070

Franz WM, Muller M. Muller OJ et al. (2000) Association of nonsense mutation of dystrophin gene with disruption of sarcoglycan complex in X-linked dilated cardiomyopathy. Lancet 355:1781–1785

Freedom RM (1972) The asplenia syndrome: A review of significant extracardiac structural abnormalities in 29 necropsied patients. J Ped 81:1130–1133

Friedman RA, Moak JP, Garson A Jr (1991) Clinical course of idiopathic dilated cardiomyopathy in children. J Am coll Cardio 18:152–156

Fu Y-H, Pizzuti A, Fenwick RG et al. (1992) An unstable triple repeat in a gene related to myotonic muscular dystrophy. Science 255:1256–1258

Fu Y-H, Friedman DL, Richards S et al. (1993) Decreased expression of myotonin-protein kinase messenger RNA and protein in adult form of myotonic dystrophy. Science 260:235–237

Fuchs E (1994) Intermediate filaments and disease: Mutations that cripple cell strength. J Cell Biol 125:511–516

Fulton AB, L'Ecuyer T (1993) Cotranslational assembly of some cytoskeletal proteins: Implications and prospects. J Cell Sci 105:867–871

Furutani M, Trudeau MC, Hagiwara N et al. (1999) Novel mechanism associated with an inherited cardiac arrhythmia. Defective protein trafficking by the mutant HERG (G601S) potassium channel. Circulation 99:2290–2294

Garcia OL, Metha AV, Pickoff AS et al. (1981) Left isomerism and complete atrioventricular block: A report of six cases. Am J Cardiol 48:1103–1107

Gault JH, Cantwell J, Lev M et al. (1972) Fatal familial cardiac arrhythmias: Histologic observations on the cardiac conduction system. Am J Cardiol 29:548–553

Gautel M, Zuffardi O, Freiburg A, Labeit S (1995) Phosphorylation switches specific for the cardiac isoform of myosin binding protein-C: A modulator of cardiac contraction? EMBO J 14:1952–1960

Gautel M, Furst DO, Cocco A, Schiaffino S (1998) Isoform transitions of the myosin binding protein C family in developing human and mouse muscles: Lack of isoform transcomplementation in cardiac muscle. Circ Res 82:124–129

Gazes PC, Culter RM, Taber E et al. (1965) Congenital familial cardiac conduction defects. Circulation 32:32–34

Gebbia M, Ferrero GB, Pilia G et al. (1997) X-linked situs abnormalities result from mutations in Zic3. Nature Genet 17:305–308

Geisterfer-Lowrance AA, Kass S, Tanigawa G (1990) A molecular basis for familial hypertrophic cardiomyopathy: A beta cardiac myosin heavy chain gene missense mutation. Cell 62:999–1006

Geisterfer-Lowrance AA, Christe M, Conner DA et al. (1996) A mouse model of familial hypertrophic cardiomyopathy. Science 272:731–734

Gellens M, George AL, Chen L et al. (1992) Primary structure and functional expression of the human cardiac tetrodotoxin-insensitive voltage-dependent sodium channel. Proc Nat Acad Sci USA 89:554–558

George AL, Varkony TA, Drakin HA et al. (1995) Assignment of the human heart tetrodotoxin-resistant voltage-gated Na channel α-subunit gene (SCN5A) to band 3p21. Cytogenet Cell Genet 68:67–70

Gilchrist JM, Pericak-Vance M, Silverman L, Roses AD (1988) Clinical and genetic investigation in autosomal dominant limb-girdle muscular dystrophy. Neurology 38:5–9

Gillette PC, Freed D, McNamara DG (1978) A proposed autosomal dominant mode of inheritance of the Wolf-Parkinson-White syndrome and supraventricular tachycardia. J Ped 93:257–258

Glauser TA, Zackai E, Weinberg P, Clancy R (1989) Holt-Oram syndrome associated with the hypoplastic left heart syndrome. Clin Genet 36:69–72

Glikson M, Constantini N, Grafstein Y et al. (1991) Familial bidirectional ventricular tachycardia. Eur Heart J 12:741–745

Gorlin RJ, Anderson RC, Blaw ME (1969) Multiple lentigines syndrome: Complex comprising multiple lentigines, electrocardiographic conduction abnormalities, ocular hypertelorism, pulmonary stenosis, abnormalities of genitalia, retardation of growth, sensorineural deafness, and autosomal dominant hereditary pattern. Am J Dis Child 117:652–662

Gotoh K (1976) A histopathological study on the conduction system of the so-called Pokkuri disease (sudden unexpected cardiac death of unknown origin in Japan). Jpn Circ J 40:753–768

Graber HL, Unverforth DV, Baker PB, Ryan JM, Baba N, Wooley CF (1986) Evolution of a hereditary cardiac conduction and muscle disorder: A study involving a family with six generations affected. Circulation 74:21–35

Grady RM, Merlie JP, Sanes JR (1997a) Subtle neuromuscular defects in utrophin-deficient mice. J Cell Biol 136:871–882

Grady RM, Teng H, Nichol MC et al. (1997b) Skeletal and cardiac myopathies in mice lacking utrophin and dystrophin: A model for Duchenne muscular dystrophy. Cell 90:729–738

Groh WJ, Silka MJ, Oliver RP et al. (1996) Use of implantable cardioverter-defibrillators in the congenital long QT syndromes. Am J Cardiol 78:703–706

Gruen M, Gautel M (1999) Mutations in β-myosin S2 that cause familial hypertrophic cardiomyopathy (FHC) abolish the interaction with the regulatory domain of myosin binding protein-C. J Mol Biol 286:933–949

Gussak l, Antzelevitch C, Bjerregaard P, Towbin JA, Chaitman BR (1999) The Brugada syndrome: clinical, electrophysiological, and genetic considerations. J Am Coll Cardiol 33:5–15

Gutegesell HP (1998) Cardiac malposition and heterotaxy. In The Science and Practice of Pediatric Cardiolgoy. (eds) Garson A, Bricker JT, Fisher DJ, Neish SR Williams & Wilkins, Baltimore, pp. 1539–1562

Hack AA, Cordier L, Shoturma DI et al. (1999) Muscle degeneration without mechanical injury in sarcoglycan deficiency. Proc Natl Acad Sci USA 96:10723–10728

Harper PS, Rudel R (1994) Myotonic dystrophy. In Engel AG, Franzini-Armstrong C (eds) Myology: Basic and Clinical, vol 2; pp 1192–1219

Harris CA, Andryuk PJ, Cline SW et al. (1995) Structure and mapping of the human thymopoietin (TMPO) gene and relationship of human TMPO beta to rat lamin-associated polypeptide 2. Genomics 28:198–205

Hartmann HA, Colom LV, Sutherland ML, Noebels JL (1999) Selective localization of cardiac SCN5A sodium channels in limbic regions of rat brain. Nature Neurosci 2:593–595

Hashmi A, Abu-Sulaiman R, McCrindle BW et al. (1998) Management and outcomes of right atrial isomerism: A 26-year experience. J Am Coll Cardiol 31:1120–1126

Hayashi M, Murata M, Satoh M et al. (1985) Sudden nocturnal death in young males from ventricular flutter. Jpn Heart J 26:585–591

Hegele R (2000) The envelope, please: Nuclear lamins and disease. Nature Med 6:136–137

Heijtmancik JF, Brink PA, Towbin J et al. (1991) Localization of gene for familial hypertrophic cardiomyopathy to chromosome 14q1 in a diverse US population. Circulation 83:1592–1597

Hirota Y, Shimizu G, Kita Y et al. (1990) Spectrum of restrictive cardiomyopathy: Report of the national survey in Japan. Am Heart J 120:188–194

Ho SY, Fagg N, Anderson RH, Cook A, Allan L (1992) Disposition of the atrioventricular conduction tissues in the heart with isomerism of the atrial appendages: Its relation to congenital complete heart block. J Am Coll Cardiol 20:904–910

Hofmann PA, Hartzell HC, Moss RL (1991) Alterations in Ca2+ sensitive tension due to partial extraction of C-protein from rat skinned cardiac myocytes and rabbit skeletal muscle fibers. J Gen Physiol 97:1141–1163

Hoffman EP, Brown RJ, Kunkel LM (1987) Dystrophin: The protein product of the Duchenne muscular dystrophy locus. Cell 51:919–928

Hoffman EP, Arahata K, Minetti C, Bonilla E, Rowland LP (1992) Dystrophinopathy in isolated cases of myopathy in females. Neurology 42:967–975

Hoffman JE (1990) Congenital heart disease: Incidence and inheritance. Ped Clin N Am 37:25–43

Hoffman J, Grimm W, Menz V, Maisch B (2000) Cardiac autonomic tone and its relation to nonsustained ventricular tachyarrhythmias in idiopathic dilated cardiomyopathy. Clin Cardiol 23:103–108

Holt KH, Lim LE, Straub V et al. (1998) Functional rescue of the sarcoglycan complex in the B1014.6 hamster using δ-sarcoglycan gene transfer. Mol Cell 1:841–848

Holt M, Oram S (1960) Familial heart disease with skeletal malformations. Br Heart J 22:236–242

Honore E, Attali B, Heurteaux C et al. (1991) Cloning, expression, pharmacology and regulation of a delayed rectifier K+ channel in mouse heart. EMBO J 10:2805–2811

Howeler CJ, Busch HF, Geraedts JP, Niermeijer MF, Staal A (1989) Anticipation in myotonic dystrophy: Fact or fiction? Brain 112:779–797

Howell N, Mackey DA (1998) Low-penetrance branches in matrilineal pedigrees with Leber hereditary optic neuropathy. Am J Hum Genet 63:1220–1224

Huhta JC, Maloney JD, Ritter DG, Ilstrup DM, Feldt RH (1983) Complete atrio-ventricular block in patients with atrioventricular discordance. Circulation 67:1374–1377

Hunkeler NM, Kullman J, Murphy AM (1991) Troponin I isoform expression in human heart. Circ Res 69:1409–1414

Ichida F, Hamamichi Y, Miyawaki T et al. (1999) Clinical features of isolated noncompaction of the ventricular myocardium. Long-term

clinical course, hemodynamic properties, and genetic background. J Am Coll Cardiol 34:233–240

Jackman WM, Wang X, Friday KJ et al. (1991) Catheter ablation of accessory atrioventricular pathways (Wolff-Parkinson-White syndrome) by radiofrequency current. N Eng J Med 324:1605–1611

Jacobson DR, Ittmann M, Buxbaum JN, Wieczorek R, Gorevic PD (1997a) Transthyretin Ile 122 and cardiac amyloidosis in African-Americans. 2 case reports. Texas Heart Inst J 24:45–52

Jacobson DR, Pan T, Kyle RA, Buxbaum JN (1997b) Transthyretin ILE20, a new variant associated with late-onset cardiac amyloidosis. Hum Mutat 9:83–85

James TN, Cobbs BW, Coghlan HC et al. (1987) Coronary disease, cardioneuropathy, and conduction system abnormalities in the cardiomyopathy of Friedreich's ataxia. Br Heart J 57:446–447

Jansen G, Groenen PJTA, Bachner D et al. (1996) Abnormal myotonic dystrophy protein kinase levels produce only mild myopathy in mice. Nature Genet 13:316–324

January CT, Riddle JM (1989) Early afterdepolarizations: Mechanism of induction and block: A role for L-type Ca²⁺ current. Circ Res 64:977–990

Jarcho JA, McKenna W, Pare JA, Solomon SD, Holcombe RF, Dickie S, Levi T, Donis-Keller H, Seidman JG, Seidman CE (1989) Mapping a gene for familial hypertrophic cardiomyopathy to chromosome 14q1. N Eng J Med 321:1372–1378

Jervell A, Lange-Nielsen F (1957) Congenital deaf-mutism, function heart disease with prolongation of the Q-T interval and sudden death. Am Heart J 54:59–68

Jiang C, Atkinson D, Towbin JA et al. (1994) Two long QT syndrome loci map to chromosome 3 and 7 with evidence for further heterogeneity. Nature Genet 8:141–147

Jones KJ, Kim SS, North KN (1998) Abnormalties of dystrophin, the sarcoglycans and laminin α-2 in the muscular dystrophies. J Med Genet 35:379–386

Kahler RL, Braunwald E, Plauth WH Jr et al. (1966) Familial congenital heart disease: Familial occurrence of atrial septal defect with A-V conduction abnormalities, supravalvular aortic and pulmonic stenosis, and ventricular septal defect. Am J Med 40:384–399

Kambouris NG, Nuss HB, Johns DC, Tomaselli GF, Marban E, Balser JR (1998) Phenotypic characterization of a novel long-qt syndrome mutation (R1623Q) in the cardiac sodium channel. Circulation 97:640–644

Kambouris NG, Nuss HB, Johns DC, Marban E, Tomaselli GF, Balser JR (2000) A revised view of cardiac sodium channel "blockade" in the long-QT syndrome. J Clin Invest 105:1133–1140

Kannel WB, Belanger AJ (1991) Epidemiology of heart failure. Am Heart J 121:951–957

Kaprielian RR, Stevenson S, Rothery SM, Cullen MJ, Severs NJ (2000) Distinct patterns of dystrophin organization in myocyte sarcolemma and transverse tubules of normal and diseased human myocardium. Circulation 101:2586–2594

Kass S, MacRae C, Graber HL et al. (1994) A gene defect that causes conduction system disease and dilated cardiomyopathy maps to chromosome 1p1-1q1. Nature Genet 7:546–551

Katritsis D, Wilmshurst PT, Wendon JA, Davies MJ, Webb-Peploe MM (1991) Primary restrictive cardiomyopathy: Clinical and pathologic characteristics. J Am Col Cardiol 18:1230–1235

Keating MT, Atkinson D, Dunn C, Timothy K, Vincent GM, Leppert M (1991a) Linkage of a cardiac arrhythmia, the long QT syndrome, and the Harvey ras-1 gene. Science 252:704–706

Keating MT, Atkinson D, Dunn C, Timothy K, Vincent GM, Leppert M (1991b) Consistent linkage of the long QT syndrome to the Harvey ras-1 locus on chromosome 11. Am J Hu#aam Genét 49:1335–1339

Kenny D, Wetherbee J (1990) Kearns-Sayre syndrome in the elderly: Mitochondrial myopathy with advanced heart block. Am Heart J 120:440–443

Kimura A, Harada H, Park JE et al. (1997) Mutations in the cardiac troponin I gene associated with hypertrophic cardiomyopathy. Nature Genet 16:379–382

Klesert TR, Otten AD, Bird T, Tapscott SJ (1997) Trinucleotide repeat expansion at the myotonic dystrophy locus reduces expression of DMAHP. Nature Genet 16:402–407

Knight SA, Sepuri NB, Pain D, Dancis A (1998) Mt-Hsp70 homolog, Ssc2p, required for maturation of yeast frataxin and mitochondrial iron homeostasis. J Biol Chem 273:18389–18393

Kobayashi T, Shintani U, Yamamoto T et al. (1996) Familial occurrence of electrocardiographic abnormalities of the Brugada-type. Ann Intern Med 35:637–640

Koenig M, Hoffman EP, Bertelson CJ, Monaco AP, Feener C, Kunkel LM (1987) Complete cloning of the Duchenne muscular dystrophy (DMD) cDNA and preliminary genomic organization of the DMD gene in normal and affected individuals. Cell 50:509–517

Koenig M, Monaco AP, Kunkel LM (1988) The complete sequence of dystrophin predicts a rod-shaped cytoskeletal protein. Cell 53:219–226

Koenig M, Beggs AH, Moyer M et al. (1989) The molecular basis for Duchenne versus Becker muscular dystrophy: Correlation of severity with type of deletion. Am J Hum Genet 45:498–506

Kosaki K, Casey B (1998) Genetics of human left-right axis malformation. Sem Cell Dev Biol 9:89–99

Kosaki K, Bassi MT, Kosaki R, Lewin M, Belmont J, Schauer G, Casey B (1999a) Characterization and mutation analysis of human LEFTY A and LEFTY B, homologues of murine genes implicated in left-right axis development. Am J Hum Genet 64:712–721

Kosaki R, Gebbia M, Kosaki K, Lewin M, Bowers P, Towbin JA, Casey B (1999b) Left-right axis malformations associated with mutations in ACVR2B, the gene for human activin receptor type IIB. Am J Med Genet 82:70–76

Koutnikova H, Campuzano V, Fourty F, Dolle P, Cazzalini O, Koenig M (1997) Studies of human, mouse and yeast homologues indicate a mitochondrial function for frataxin. Nature Genet 16:345–351

Krajinovic M, Pinamonti B, Sinagra G, Vatta M, Severini GM, Milasin J, Falaschi A, Camerini F, Giacca M, Mestroni L (1995) Linkage of familial dilated cardiomyopathy to chromosome 9. Heart Muscle Disease Study Group. Am J Hum Genet 57:846–852

Kushwaha SS, Fallon JT, Fuster V (1997) Restrictive cardiomyopathy N Eng J Med 336:267–276

Lamont PJ, Davis MB, Wood NW (1997) Identification and sizing of the GAA trinucleotide repeat expansion of Friedreich's ataxia in 56 patients. Clinical and Genetic correlates. Brain 120:673–680

Leenhardt A, Lucet V, Denjoy I, Grau F, Ngoc DD, Coumel P (1995) Catecholaminergic polymorphic ventricular tachycardia in children. Circulation 91:1512–1519

Lees-Miller JP, Helfman DM (1991) The molecular basis for tropomyosin isoform diversity. Bioessays 13:429–437

Lenegre J and Moreau PH (1963) Le block auriculo-ventriculaire chronique. Etude anatomique, clinique et histologieque. Arch Mal Coeur 56:867–888

Lev M (1964) Anatomic basis for atrioventricular block. Am J Cardiol 37:742–748

Lev M, Kinare SG, Pick A (1970) The pathogenesis of atrioventricular block in coronary disease. Circulation 42:409–425

Levin M, Johnson RL, Stern CD, Kuehn M, Tabin C (1995) A molecular pathway determining left-right asymmetry in chick embryogenesis. Cell 82:803–814

Levine HD, Wanzer SH, Merrill JP (1956) Dialyzable currents of injury in potassium intoxication resembling acute myocardial infarction or pericarditis. Circulation 13:29–36

Lewis AB (1992) Clinical profile and outcome of restrictive cardiomyopathy in children. Am Heart J 123:1589–1593

Li D, Ahmad F, Gardner MJ et al. (2000) The locus of a novel gene responsible for arrhythmogenic right ventricular dysplasia characterized by early onset and high penetrance maps to chromosome 10p12-p14. Am J Hum Genet 66:148–156

Li D, Tapscott T, Gonzalez O, Burch PE, Quinones MA, Zoghbi WA, Hill R, Bachinski LL, Mann DL, Roberts R (1999) Desmin mutation responsible for idiopathic dilated cardiomyopathy. Circulation 100:461–464

Li H, Chen Q, Moss AJ et al. (1998) New mutations in the *KVLQT1* potassium channel that cause long QT syndrome. Circulation 97:1264–1269

Li QY, Newbury-Ecob RA, Terrett JA et al. (1997) Holt-Oram syndrome is caused by mutations in TBX5, a member of the Brachyury (T) gene family. Nature Genet 15:21–29

Li Z, Colucci-Guyan E, Pincon-Raymond M et al. (1996) Cardiovascular lesions and skeletal myopathy in mice lacking desmin. Dev Biol 175:362–366

Liang MH, Wong LJ (1998) Yield of mtDNA mutation analysis in 2,000 patients. Am J Med Genet 77:395–400

Liberthson RR, Hastreiter AR, Sinha SN et al. (1973) Levocardia with visceral Heterotaxy–isolated levocardia: Pathologic anatomy and its clinical implications. Am Heart J 85:40–54

Liu J, Aoki M, Illa I et al. (1998) Dysferlin, a novel skeletal muscle gene, is mutated in Miyoshi myopathy and limb girdle muscular dystrophy. Nature Genet 20:31–36

Loeffen JL, Triepels RH, van den Heuvel LP et al. (1998) cDNA of eight nuclear encoded subunits of NADH:ubiquinone oxidoreductase: Human complex I cDNA characterization completed. Biochem Biophys Res Commun 253:415–422

Lumeng CN, Phelps SF, Rafael JA et al. (1999) Characterization of dystrophin and utrophin diversity in the mouse. Hum Mol Genet 8:593–599

MacRae CA, Ghaisas N, Kass S et al. (1995) Familial hypertrophic cardiomyopathy with Wolff-Parkinson-White syndrome maps to a locus on chromosome 7q3. J Clin Invest 96:1216–1220

MacRae JR, Wagner GS, Rogers MC, Cament RV (1974) Paroxysmal familial ventricular fibrillation. J Ped 84:515–518

Maeda M, Holder E, Lowes B, Valent S, Bies RD (1997) Dilated cardiomyopathy associated with deficiency of the cytoskeletal protein metavinculin. Circulation 95:17–20

Maeda S, Tanaka T, Hayashi T (1988) Familial atrial standstill caused by amyloidosis. Br Heart J 59:498–500

Mah CS, Vaughan CJ, Basson CT (1999) Advances in the molecular genetics of congenital structural heart disease. Genet Test 3:157–172

Mahadevan M, Tsilfidis C, Sabourin L et al. (1992) Myotonic muscular dystrophy: An unstable CTG repeat in the 3' untranslated region of the gene. Science 255:1253–1255

Maki T, Niimura I, Nishikawa T, Sekiguchi M (1990) An atypical case of cardiomyopathy in a child: Hypertrophic or restrictive cardiomyopathy? Heart Vessels Suppl 5:84–87

Malhotra SB, Hart KA, Klamut HJM et al. (1988) Frame-shift deletions in patients with Duchenne and Becker muscular dystrophy. Science 242:755–759

Manilal S, Recan D, Sewry CA et al. (1998) Mutations in Emery-Dreifuss muscular dystrophy and their effects on emerin protein expression. Hum Mol Genet 7:855–864

Manolio TA, Baughman KL, Rodenheffer R et al. (1992) Prevalence and etiology of idiopathic dilated cardiomyopathy (Summary of a National Heart, Lung and Blood Institute Workshop). Am J Cardiol 69:1458–1466

Marcus FI, Fontaine G (1995) Arrhythmogenic right ventricular dysplasia/cardiomyopathy: A review. PACE 18:1298–1314

Marcus FI, Fontaine GH, Guiraudon G, Frank R, Laurenceau JL, Malergue C, Grosgogeat Y (1982) Right ventricular dysplasia: A report of 24 adult cases. Circulation 65:384–398

Marian AJ, Yu QT, Workman R et al. (1993) Angiotensin-converting enzyme polymorphism in hypertrophic cardiomyopathy and sudden cardiac death. Lancet 342:1085–1086

Marian AJ, Yu QT, Mann DL et al. (1995) Expression of a mutation causing hypertrophic cardiomyopathy disrupts sarcomere assembly in adult feline cardiac myocytes. Circ Res 77:98–106

Marian AJ, Zhao G, Seta Y, Roberts R, Yu QT (1997) Expression of a mutant (Arg92Gln) human cardiac troponin T, known to causes hypertrophic cardiomyopathy, impairs adult cardiac myocyte contractility. Circ Res 81:76–85

Marian AJ, Wu Y, Lim DS (1999) A transgenic rabbit model for human hypertrophic cardiomyopathy. J Clin Invest 104:1683–1692

Marks ML, Trippel DL, Keating MT (1995) Long QT syndrome associated with syndactyly identified in females. Am J Cardiol 10:744–745

Maron BJ (1997) Hypertrophic cardiomyopathy. Lancet 350:127–133

Maron BJ, Bonow RO, Cannon RO III et al. (1987) Hypertrophic cardiomyopathy. Interrelations of clinical manifestations, pathophysiology, and therapy. N Engl J Med 316:780–784

Maron BJ, Shirani J, Poliac LC et al. (1996) Sudden death in young competitive atheletes. J Am Med Ass 276:199–204

Martini B, Nava A, Thiene G et al. (1989) Ventricular fibrillation without apparent heart disease. Description of six cases. Am Heart J 118:1203–1209

Mashima Y, Kigasawa K, Hasegawa H, Tani M, Oguchi Y (1996) High incidence of pre-excitation syndrome in Japanese families with Leber's hereditary optic neuropathy. Clin Genet 50:535–537

Mathews NL (1968) Lentigo and electrocardiographic changes. N Engl J Med 278:780–781

Matsumura K, Saito F, Yamada H, Hase A, Sunada Y, Shimizu T (1999) Sarcoglycan complex: A muscular supporter of dystroglycan-dystrophin interplay? Cell Mol Biol 45:751–762

McCarthy RE 3rd, Kasper EK (1998) A review of the amyloidoses that infiltrate the heart. Clin Cardiol 21:547–552

McConnell BK, Jones KA, Fatkin D et al. (1999) Dilated cardiomyopathy in homozygous myosin-binding protein-C mutant mice. J Clin Invest 104:1771

McDonald TV, Yu Z, Ming Z et al. (1997) A Mink-HERG complex regulates the cardiac potassium current I_{Kr}. Nature 388:289–292

McKenna WJ, Thiene G, Nava A et al. (1994) Diagnosis of arrhythmogenic right ventricular dysplasia/cardiomyopathy. Task Force of the Working Group Myocardial and Pericardial Disease of the European Society of Cardiology and of the Scientific Council on Cardiomyopathies of the International Society and Federation of Cardiology. Br Heart J 71:215–218

McKoy G, Protonotarios N, Crosby A et al. (2000) Identification of a deletion in plakoglobin in arrhymogenic right ventricular cardiomyopathy with palmoplantar keratoderma and wolly hair (Naxos disease). Lancet 355:2119–2124

McNally EM, Moreira ES, Duggan DJ et al. (1998) Caveolin-3 in muscular dystrophy. Hum Mol Genet 7:871–877

Meaney E, Shabetai R, Bhargava V et al. (1976) Cardiac amyloidosis, constrictive pericarditis and restrictive cardiomyopathy. Am J Cardiol 38:547–556

Mehdirad AA, Fatkin D, DiMarco JP et al. (1999) Electrophysiologic characteristics of accessory atrioventricular connections in an inherited form of Wolff-Parkinson-White syndrome. J Cardiovas Electrophysiol 20:629–635

Melacini P, Buja G, Fasoli G et al. (1988) The natual history of cardiac involvement in myotonic dystrophy: An eight year follow-up in 17 patients. Clin Cardiol 11:231–238

Melacini P, Fanin M, Danieli GA et al. (1996) Myocardial involvement is very frequent among patients affected with subclinical Becker's muscular dystrophy. Circulation 94:3168–3175

Melacini P, Fanin M, Duggan DJ et al. (1999) Heart involvement in muscular dystrophies due to sarcoglycan gene mutations. Muscle Nerve 22:473–479

Melberg A, Oldfors A, Bloomstrom-Lundqvist C et al. (1999) Autosomal dominant myofibrillar myopathy with arrhythmogenic right ventricular cardiomyopathy linked to chromosome 10q. Ann Neurol 41:684–692

Mendell JR, Kissell JT, Amato AA, King W, Signore L, Prior TW, Sahenk Z, Benson S, McAndrew PE, Rice R et al. (1995) Myoblast transfer in the treatment of Duchenne's muscular dystrophy. N Engl J Med 333:832–838

Meno C, Shimino A, Saijoh Y et al. (1998) Lefty-1 is required for left-right determination as a regulator of lefty-2 and nodal. Cell 94:287–297

Mesnard L, Logeart D, Taviaux S, Diriong S, Mercadier JJ, Samson F (1995) Human cardiac troponin T: Cloning and expression of new isoforms in the normal and failing heart. Circ Res 76:687–692

Messina DN, Speer MC, Pericak-Vance MA, McNally EM (1997) Linkage of familial dilated cardiomyopathy with conduction defect and muscular dystrophy to chromosome 6q23. Am J Hum Genet 61:909–917

Michelle DE, Albayya FP, Metzger JM (1999) Direct convergent hypersensitivity of calcium-activated force generation produced by hypertrophic cardiomyopathy mutant α-tropomyosins in adult cardiac myocytes. Nature Med 5:1413–1417

Milasin J, Muntoni F, Severini GM et al. (1996) A point mutation in the 5′ splice site of the dystrophin gene first intron responsible for X-linked dilated cardiomyopathy. Hum Mol Genet 5:73–79

Miller RG, Layzer RB, Mellenthin MA et al. (1985) Emery-Dreifuss muscular dystrophy with autosomal dominant transmission. Neurology 35:1230–1233

Milner DJ, Weitzer G, Tran D, Bradley A, Capetanaki Y (1996) Disruption of muscle architecture and myocardial degeneration in mice lacking desmin. J Cell Biol 134:1255–1270

Mirabella M, Servidei S, Manfredi G et al. (1993) Cardiomyopathy may be the only clinical manifestation in female carriers of Duchenne muscular dystrophy. Neurology 43:2342–2345

Mogensen J, Klausen IC, Pedersen AK et al. (1999) Alpha-cardiac actin is a novel disease gene in familial hypertrophic cardiomyopathy. J Clin Invest 103:R39–43

Mohammad-Panah R, Demolombe S, Neyroud N et al. (1999) Mutations in a dominant-negative isoform correlate with phenotype in inherited cardiac arrhythmias. Am J Hum Genet 64:1015–1023

Moller JH, Nakib A, Anderson RC, Edwards JE (1967) Congenital cardiac disease associated with polysplenia, a developmental complex of bilateral "left-sidedness". Circulation 36:789–799

Momma K, Takao A, Shibata T (1990) Characeristics and natural history of abnormal atrial rhythms in left atrial isomerism. Am J Cardiol 65:231–236

Monaco AP, Bertelson CJ, Liechti GS, Moser H, Kunkel LM (1988) An explanation for the phenotypic differences between patients bearing partial deletions of the DMD locus. Genomics 2:90–95

Monros E, Molto MD, Martinez F et al. (1997) Phenotype correlation and intergenerational dynamics of the Friedreich ataxia GAA trinucleotide repeat. Am J Hum Genet 61:101–110

Montermini L, Richeter A, Morgan K et al. (1997) Phenotypic variability in Friedreich ataxia: Role of the associated GAA triplet repeat expansion. Ann Neurol 51:675–682

Moolman JC, Reith S, Uhl K et al. (2000) A newly created splice donor site in exon 25 of the MyBP-C gene is responsible for inherited hypertrophic cardiomyopathy with incomplete disease penetrance. Circulation 101:1396–1402

Moolman-Smook JC, Mayosi B, Brink P, Corfield V (1998) Identification of a new missense mutation in MyBP-C associated with hypertrophic cardiomyopathy. J Med Genet 35:253–254

Moolman JC, Corfield VA, Posen B et al. (1997) Sudden death due to troponin T mutations. J Am Coll Cardiol 29:549–555

Moreira ES, Wiltshire TJ, Faulkner G et al. (2000) Limb-girdle muscular dystrophy type 2G is caused by mutations in the sarcomeric protein telethonin. Nature Genet 2000;24:163–166

Morgan D, Turnpenny L, Goodship J et al. (1998) Inversin, a novel gene in the vertebrate left-right axis pathway, is partially deleted in the inv mouse. Nature Genet 20:149–156

Morgenlander JC, Nohria V, Saba Z (1993) EKG abnormalities in pediatric patients with myotonic dystrophy. Ped Neurol 124–126

Morris AA, Leonard JV, Brown GK et al. (1996) Deficiency of respiratory chain complex I is a common cause of Leigh disease. Ann Neurol 40:25–30

Morris GE, Manilal S (1999) Heart to heart: From nuclear proteins to Emery-Dreifuss muscular dystrophy. Hum Mol Genet 8:1847–1851

Moss AJ (1998) Management of patients with the hereditary long QT syndrome. J Cardiovasc Electrophysiol 9:668–674

Moss AJ, McDonald J (1970) Unilateral cervicothoracic sympathetic ganglionectomy for the treatment of long QT interval syndrome. N Engl J Med 285:903–904

Moss AJ, Liu JE, Gottlieb S, Locati E, Schwartz PJ, Robinson JL (1991) Efficacy of permanent pacing in the management of high-risk patients with long-QT syndrome. Circulation 84:1524–1529

Moss AJ, Zareba W, Benhorin J et al. (1995) ECG T-wave patterns in genetically distinct forms of the hereditary long QT syndrome. Circulation 92:2929–2934

Moss AJ, Hall WJ, Cannom DS et al. (1996) For the MADIT Investigators: Improved survival with an implantable defibrillator in patients with coronary disease at high-risk of ventricular arrhythmias. N Engl J Med 335:1933–1940

Moss AJ, Robinson JL, Gessman L et al. (1999) Comparison of clinical and genetic variables of cardiac events associated with loud noise vs. swimming among subjects with the long QT syndrome. Am J Cardiol 84:876–879

Moss AJ, Zareba W, Hall WJ et al. (2000) Effectiveness and limitations of β-blocker therapy in congenital long-QT syndrome. Circulation 101:616–623

Mott AR, Pac F, Denfield SW et al. (2000) Hypertrophic cardiomyopathy in children. J Am Coll Cardiol, in press.

Muntoni F, Cau M, Ganau A et al. (1993) Deletion of the dystrophin muscle-promoter region associated with X-linked dilated cardiomyopathy. N Engl J Med 329:921–925

Mutuchamy M, Pieples K, Rethinasamy P et al. (1999) Mouse model of a familial hypertrophic cardiomyopathy mutation in alpha-tropomyosin manifests cardiac dysfunction. Circ Res 85:47–56

Myerburg RJ (1997) Sudden cardiac death in persons with normal (or near normal) heart. Am J Cardiol 79:3–9

Naccarella F (1993) Malignant ventricular arrhythmias in patients with a right bundle-branch block and persistent ST segment elevation in V1-V3: a probable arrhythmogenic cardiomyopathy of the right ventricle (Editorial comment). G Italian Cardiol 23:1219–1222

Nademanee K, Veerakul G, Nimmannit S et al. (1997) Arrhythmogenic marker for the sudden unexplained death syndrome in Thai men. Circulation 96:2595–2600

Nagano A, Koga R, Ogawa M et al. (1996) Emerin deficiency at the nuclear membrane in patients with Emery-Dreifuss muscular dystrophy. Nature Genet 12:254–259

Newbury-Ecob R, Leanage R, Raeburn JA, Young ID (1996) The Holt-Oram syndrome: A clinical genetic study. J Med Genet 33:300–307

Neyroud N, Tesson F, Denjoy I et al. (1997) A novel mutation on the potassium channel gene KVLQT1 causes the Jervell and Lange-Nielsen cardioauditory syndrome. Nature Genet 15:186–189

Nguyen HH, Wolfe JT, Holmes DR Jr, Edwards WD (1988) Pathology of the cardiac conduction system in myotonic dystrophy: A study of 12 cases. J Am Coll Cardiol 11:662–671

Nigro G, Comi LI, Politano L, Bain RJI (1990) The incidence and evolution of cardiomyopathy in Duchenne muscular dystrophy. Int J Cardiol 26:271–277

Nigro G, Politano L, Nigro V, Petratta VR, Comi LI (1994) Mutation of the dystrophin gene and cardiomyopathy. Neuromuscular Disorders 4:371–379

Nigro G, Comi LI, Politano L et al. (1995) Evaluation of the cardio-myopathy in Becker muscular dystrophy. Muscle Nerve 18:283–291

Nigro V, Okazaki Y, Belsito A et al. (1997) Identification of the Syrian hamster cardiomyopathy gene. Hum Mol Genet 6:601–607

Niimura H, Bachinski LL, Sangwatanaroj S et al. (1998) Mutations in the gene for cardiac myosin-binding protein C and late-onset familial hypertrophic cardiomyopathy. N Engl J Med 338:1248–1257

Nikoskelainen EK, Sarontaus ML, Huopenen K, Antila K, Hartiala J (1994) Pre-excitation syndrome in Leber hereditary optic neuropathy. Lancet 344:857–858

Oberst L, Zhao G, Park JT et al. (1998) Dominant-negative effect of a mutant cardiac troponin T on cardiac structure and function in transgenic mice. J Clin Invest 102:1498–1505

Ockey CH, Feldman GV, Macaulay ME, Delaney MJ (1967) A large deletion of the long arm of chromosome No. 4 in a child with limb abnormalities. Arch Dis Child 42:428–434

Ohe T (1996) Idiopathic ventricular fibrillation of the Brugada type – an atypical form of arrhythmogenic right ventricular cardiomyopathy. Int Med 35:595

Ohlendieck K, Matsumura K, Ionasescu VV et al. (1993) Duchenne muscular dystrophy: Deficiency of dystrophin-associated proteins in the sarcolemma. Neurology 43:795–800

Olofsson B-O, Forsberg H, Anderson S, Bjerle P, Henriksson A, Wedin I (1988) Electrocardiographic findings in myotonic dystrophy. Br Heart J 59:47–52

Olson TM, Keating MT (1996) Mapping a cardiomyopathy locus to chromosome 3p22-p25. J Clin Invest 97:528–532

Olson TM, Michels VV, Thibodeau SN, Tai Y, Keating MT (1998) Actin mutation in dilated cardiomyopathy: A heritable form of heart failure. Science 280:750–752

Ortiz-Lopez R, Li H, Su J, Goytia V, Towbin JA (1997) Evidence for a dystrophin missense mutation as a cause of X-linked dilated cardiomyopathy. Circulation 95:2434–2440

Osher HL, Wolff L (1953) Electrocardiographic pattern simulating acute myocardial injury. Am J Med Sci 226:541–545

Ozawa E, Yoshida M, Hagiwara Y, Suzuki A, Mizuno Y, Noguchi S (1995) Dystrophin-associated proteins in muscular dystrophy. Hum Mol Genet 4:1711–1716

Ozawa E, Noguchi S, Mizuno Y et al. (1998) From dystrophinopathy to sarcoglycanopathy: Evolution of a concept of muscular dystrophy. Muscle Nerve 21:421–438

Palileo EV, Ashley WW, Swiryn S et al. (1982) Exercise provocable right ventricular outflow tract tachycardia. Am Heart J 104:185–193

Pavlakis SG, Phillips PC, DiMauro S, De Vivo DC, Rowland LP (1984) Mitochondrial myopathy, encephalopathy, lactic acidosis, and strokelike episodes: A distinctive clinical syndrome. Ann Neurol 16:481–488

Pease WE, Nordenberg A, Ladda RL (1976) Familial atrial septal defect with prolonged atrioventricular conduction. Circulation 53:759–762

Pennefather PS, Zhou W, Decoursey TE (1998) Idiosyncratic gating of HERG-like K+ channels in microglia. J Gen Physiol 111:795–805

Perloff JK, Roberts WC, de Leon AC Jr, O'Doherty D (1967) The distinctive electrocardiogram of Duchenne's progressive muscular dystrophy. Am J Med 42:179–188

Perticone F, Marisco SA (1988) Familial case of permanent form of junctional reciprocating tachycardia: Possible role of the HLA system. Clin Cardiol 11:345–348

Phelps SF, Hauser MA, Cole NM et al. (1995) Expression of full-length and truncated dystrophin mini-genes in transgenic mdx mice. Hum Mol Genet 4:1251–1258

Philips AV, Timchenko LT, Cooper TA (1998) Disruption of splicing regulated by a CUG-binding protein in myotonic dystrophy. Science 280:737–741

Pierard LA, Henrard L, Demoulin JC (1985) Persistent atrial standstill in familial Ebstein's anomaly. Br Heart J 53:594–597

Platia EV, Griffith LSC, Watkins L, Mirowski M, Mower MM, Reid PR (1985) Management of the prolonged QT syndrome and recurrent ventricular fibrillation with an implantable defibrillator. Clin Cardiol 8:490–493

Poetter K, Jiang H, Hassanzadeh S et al. (1996) Mutations in either the essential or regulatory light chains of myosin are associated with a rare myopathy in human heart and skeletal muscle. Nature Genet 13:63–69

Politano L, Nigro V, Nigro G et al. (1996) Development of cardiomyopathy in female carriers of Duchenne and Becker muscular dystrophies. J Am Med Ass 275:1335–1338

Poret P, Mabo P, Deplace C et al. (1996) Isolated atrial fibrillation genetically determined? Apropos of a familial history. Arch Mal Coeur Vaiss 89:1197–1203

Poznanski AK, Gall JC Jr, Stern AM (1970) Skeletal manifestations in the Holt-Oram syndrome. Radiology 94:45–53

Priori SG, Schwartz PJ, Napolitano C et al. (1998) A recessive variant of the Romano-Ward long-QT syndrome. Circulation 97:2420–2425

Priori SG, Barhanin J, Hauer RNW et al. (1999a) Genetic and molecular basis of cardiac arrhythmias. Impact on clinical management. Parts I & II. Circulation 99:518–528

Priori SG, Barhanin J, Hauer RN et al. (1999b) Genetic and molecular basis of cardiac arrhythmias: impact on clinical management. Part III. Circulation 99:674–681

Priori SG, Napolitano C, Schwartz PJ (1999c) Low penetrance in the long-QT syndrome. Clinical impact. Circulation 99:529–533

Pruznanski W (1964) Familial congenital malformations of the heart and upper limb. A syndrome of Holt-Oram. Cardiologia 45:21–38

Quinlivan RM, Dubowitz V (1992) Cardiac transplantation in Becker muscular dystrophy. Neuromus Disord 2:165–167

Rafael JA, Sunada Y, Cole NM, Campbell KP, Faulkner JA, Chamberlain JS (1994) Prevention of dystrophic pathology in mdx mice by a truncated dystrophin isoform. Hum Mol Genet 3:1725–1733

Rahilly GT, Prystowsky EN, Zipes DP et al. (1982) Clinical and electrophysiologic findings in patients with repetitive monomorphic ventricular tachycardia and otherwise normal electrocardiogram. Am J Cardiol 50:459–468

Rampazzo A, Nava A, Danieli GA et al. (1994) The gene for arrhythmogenic right ventricular cardiomyopathy maps to chromosome 1q42-q43. Hum Mol Genet 3:959–962

Rampazzo A, Nava A, Erne P et al. (1995) A new locus for arrhythmogenic right ventricular cardiomyopathy (ARVD2) maps to chromosome 1q42-q43. Hum Mol Genet 4:2151–2154

Rampazzo A, Nava A, Miorin M et al. (1997) ARVD4, a new locus for arrhythmogenic right ventricular cardiomyopathy, maps to chromosome 2 long arm. Genomics 45:259–263

Ranum LPW, Rasmussen PF, Benzow KA, Koob MD, Day JW (1998) Genetic mapping of a second myotonic dystrophy locus. Nature Genet 19:196–198

Reddy S, Smith DBJ, Rich MM et al. (1996) Mice lacking the myotonic dystrophy protein kinase develop a late onset progressive myopathy. Nature Genet 13:325–335

Richard I, Bronx O, Allamand V et al. (1995) Mutations in the proteolytic enzyme, calpain 3, cause limb-girdle muscular dystrophy type 2A. Cell 81:27–40

Richard I, Roudant C, Saenz A et al. (1999) Calpainopathy: A survey of mutations and polymorphisms. Am J Hum Genet 64:1524–1540

Rivenes SM, Kearney DL, Smith EO, Towbin JA, Denfield SW (2000) Sudden death and cardiovascular collapse in children with restrictive cardiomyopathy. Circulation 102:876–882

Roberds S, Ervasti JM, Anderson RD et al. (1993) Disruption of the dystrophin-glycoprotein complex in the cardiomyopathic hamster. J Biol Chem 268:11496–11499

Roberts NK, Perloff JK, Kark P (1979) Cardiac conduction in Kearns-Sayre syndrome. Am J Cardiol 44:1396–1400

Robinson BH (1998) Human complex I deficiency: Clinical spectrum and involvement of oxygen free radicals in the pathogenicity of the defect. Biochim Biophys Acta 1364:271–286

Roguin N, Pelled B, Freundlich E, Yaholom M, Riss E (1984) Atrioventricular block in situs ambiguus and left isomerism (polysplenia syndrome). PACE 7:18–22

Roig M, Pere-Ramon B, Navarro C, Brugada R, Losada M (1994) Presentation, Clinical course and outcome of the congenital form of myotonic dystrophy. Ped Neurol 111:208–213

Romano C, Gemme G, Pongiglione R (1963) Antmie cardiache rare in eta pediatrica. Clin Ped 45:656–683

Rose V, Izkawa T, Moes CAF (1975) Syndromes of asplenia and polyspenia: A review of cardiac and non-cardiac malformation in 60 cases with special reference to diagnosis and prognosis. Br Heart J 37:840–852

Rosenbaum MB, Elizari MV, Lazzari JO (1969) The mechanisms of bidirectional tachycardia. Am Heart J 78:4–12

Rosero SZ, Zareba W, Moss AJ et al. (1999) Asthma and the risk of cardiac events in the long QT syndrome. Long QT Syndrome Investigative Group. Am J Cardiol 84:1406–1411

Rotig A, de Lonlay P, Chretien D et al. (1997) Aconitase and mitochondrial iron-sulphur protein deficiency in Friedreich ataxia. Nature Genet 17:215–217

Rottbauer W, Gautel M, Zehelein J et al. (1997) Novel splice donor site mutation in the cardiac myosin-binding protein-C gene in familial hypertrophic cardiomyopathy. Characterization of cardiac transcript and protein. J Clin Invest 100:475–482

Rowland LP, Blake DM, Hirano M et al. (1991) Clinical syndromes associated with ragged red fibers. Rev Neurol 147:467–473

Rubin DA, O'Keefe A, Kay RH, McAllister A, Mendelson DM (1992) Autosomal dominant inherited ventricular tachycardia. Am Heart J 123:1082–1084

Saba S, Vander Brink BA, Luciano B et al. (1999) Localization of the sites of conduction abnormalities in a mouse model of myotonic dystrophy. J Cardiovasc Electrophysiol 10:1214–1220

Sacks HS, Matisonn R, Kennelly BM (1978) Familial paroxysmal ventricular tachycardia of unknown etiology. Proc R Soc Med 68:305–306

Sadoulet-Puccio HM, Kunkel LM (1996) Dystrophin and its isoforms. Brain Pathol 6:25–35

Sahn DJ, Goldberg SJ, Allen HD, Canale JM (1981) Cross-sectional echocardiographic imaging of supracardiac total anomalous pulmonary venous drainage to a vetical vein in a patient with Holt-Oram syndrome. Chest 79:113–115

Saito M, Kawai H, Akaike M, Adachi K, Nishida Y, Saito S (1996) Cardiac dysfunction in Becker muscular dystrophy. Am Heart J 132:642–647

Sakamoto A, Ono K, Abe M et al. (1997) Both hypertrophic and dilated cardiomyopathies are caused by mutation of the same gene, δ-sarcoglycan. Mol Cell 1:841–848

Sanguinetti MC, Jiang C, Curran ME, Keating MT (1995) A mechanistic link between an inherited and an acquired cardiac arrhythmia: *HERG* encodes the I_{Kr} potassium channel. Cell 81:299–307

Sanguinetti MC, Curran ME, Zou A et al. (1996a) Coassembly of *KvLQT1* and *minK* (IsK) proteins to form cardiac I_{Ks} potassium channel. Nature 384:80–83

Sanguinetti MC, Curran ME, Spector PS, Keating MT (1996b) Spectrum of *HERG* K^+-channel dysfunction in an inherited cardiac arrhythmia. Proc Natl Acad Sci USA 93:2208–2212

Sanyal SK, Johnson WW, Dische MR, Pitner SE, Beard C (1980) Dystrophic degeneration of papillary muscle and ventricular myocardium. A basis for mitral valve prolapse in Duchenne's muscular dystrophy. Circulation 62:430–438

Sapire DW, Ho SY, Anderson RH, Rigsby ML (1986) Diagnosis and significance of atrial isomerism. Am J Cardiol 58:342–346

Satoh M, Takahashi M, Sakamoto T, Hiroe M, Marumo F, Kimura A (1999) Structural analysis of the titin gene in hypertrophic cardiomyopathy: Identification of a novel disease gene. Biochem Biophys Res Commun 262:411–417

Schiaffino S, Reggiani C (1996) Molecular diversity of myofibrillar proteins: Gene regulation and functional significance. Physiol Rev 76:371–423

Scheinman MM (1997) Is Brugada syndrome a distinct clinical entity? J Cardiovasc Electrophysiol 8:332–336

Schocken DD, Acrieta MI, Leaverton PE, Ross CA (1992) Prevalence and mortality rate of congestive heart failure in the United States. J Am Coll Card 20:301–306

Schonberger J, Levy H, Grunig E et al. (2000) Dilated cardiomyopathy and sensorineural hearing loss: A heritable syndrome that maps to 6q23-24. Circulation 101:1812–1818

Schott J, Charpentier F, Peltier S et al. (1995) Mapping of a gene for long QT syndrome to chromosome 4q25-27. Am J Hum Genet 57:1114–1122

Schott J-J, Benson DW, Basson CT et al. (1998) Congenital heart disease caused by mutations in the transcription factor Nkx2–5. Science 281:108–111

Schott J-J, Alshinawi C, Kyndt F et al. (1999) Cardiac conduction defects associated with mutations in SCN5A. Nature Genet 23:20–21

Schulze-Bahr E, Haverkamp W, Funke H (1995) The long-QT syndrome. N Engl J Med 333:1783–1784

Schulze-Bahr E, Wang Q, Wedekind H et al. (1997) *KCNE1* mutations cause Jervell and Lange-Nielsen syndrome. Nature Genet 17:267–268

Schwartz PJ (1985) Idiopathic long QT syndrome. Progress and questions. Am Heart J 109:399–411

Schwartz PJ, Locati E, Moss AJ, Crampton RS, Trazzi R, Ruberti U (1991) Left cardiac sympathetic denervation in the therapy of the congenital long-QT syndrome: A worldwide report. Circulation 84:503–511

Schwartz K, Beckmann J, Dufour C et al. (1992) Exclusion of cardiac myosin heavy chain and actin gene involvement in hypertrophic cardiomyopathy of several French families. Circulation Res 71:3–8

Schwartz PJ, Priori SG, Locati EH et al. (1995) Long QT syndrome patients with mutations of the SCN5A and HERG genes have differential responses to Na+ channel blockade and to increases in heart rate. Implications for gene-specific therapy. Circulation 92:3381–3386

Schwartz PJ, Stramba-Badiale M, Segantini A et al. (1998) Prolongation of the QT interval and the sudden infant death syndrome. N Engl J Med 338:1709–1714

Schwartz PJ, Priori SG, Dumaine R et al. (2000a) A molecular link between the sudden infant death syndrome and the long-QT syndrome. N Engl J Med 343:262–267

Schwartz PJ, Priori SG, Napolitano C (2000b) Long QT syndrome. In Zipes DP, Jalife J (eds): Cardiac Electrophysiology: From Cell to Bedside, 3rd edn. Philadelphia, PA, Saunders, pp 597–615

Schwensen C (1992) Ventricular tachycardia as the result of the administration of digitalis. Am Heart J 123:1082–1084

Senni M, Tribouilloy CM, Rodeheffer RJ et al. (1998) Congestive heart failure in the community. Circulation 98:2282–2289

Severini GM, Krajinovic M, Pinamonti B et al. (1996) A new locus for arrhythmogenic right ventricular dysplasia on the long arm of chromosome 14. Genomics 31:193–200

Shalaby FY, Levesque PC, Yang WP et al. (1997) Dominant-negative KvLQT1 mutations underlie the LQT1 form of long QT syndrome. Circulation 96:1733–1736

Shah SK, Subramanyan R, Tharakan J et al. (1992) Familial total atrial standstill. Am Heart J 123:1379–1382

Shimizu W, Kurita T, Matsuo K et al. (1998) Improvement of repolarization abnormalities by a K+ channel opener in the LQT1 form of congenital long-QT syndrome. Circulation 97:1581–1588

Shen WK, Edwards WD, Hammill SC, Gersh BJ. (1994) Right ventricular dysplasia: A need for precise pathological definition for interpretation of sudden death. J Am Coll Cardiol 23:34

Shoffner JM, Lott MT, Lezza AM et al. (1990) Myoclonic epilepsy and ragged-red fiber disease (MERRF) is associated with a mitochondrial DNA tRNA(Lys) mutation. Cell 61:931–937

Siu BL, Nimuira H, Osborne JA et al. (1999) Familial dilated cardiomyopathy locus maps to chromosome 2q31. Circulation 99:1022–1026

Sletten LJ, Pierpont ME. (1996) Variation in severity of cardiac disease in Holt-Oram syndrome. Am J Med Genet 65:128–132

Smeitink J, van den Heuvel L (1999) Human mitochondrial complex I in health and disease. Am J Hum Genet 64:1505–1510

Smeitink JA, Loeffen JL, Triepels RH et al. (1998) Nuclear genes of human complex I of the mitochondrial electron transport chain: State of the art. Hum Mol Genet 7:1573–1579

Smith WM (1985) Epidemiology of congestive heart failure. Am J Cardiol 55:3A–8A

Solaro RJ, Van Eyk J. (1996) Altered interactions among thin filament proteins modulate cardiac function. J Mol Cell Cardiol 28:217–230

Solomon SD, Geisterfer-Lowrance AA, Vosberg HP et al. (1990) A locus for familial hypertrophic cardiomyopathy is closely linked to the cardiac myosin heavy chain genes. CRI-L436, and CRI-L329 on chromosome 14 at q11-q12. Am J Hum Genet 47:389–394

Spellberg RD (1971) Familial sinus node disease. Chest 60:246–251

Spirito P, Seidman CE, McKenna WJ, Maron BJ. (1997) The management of hypertrophic cardiomyopathy. N Engl J Med 336:775–785

Splawski I, Timothy KW, Vincent GM, Atkinson DL, Keating MT (1997a) Brief report: molecular basis of the long-QT syndrome associated with deafness. N Engl J Med 336:1562–1567

Splawski I, Tristani-Firouzi M, Lehmann MH, Sanguinetti MC, Keating MT (1997b) Mutations in the *minK* gene cause long QT syndrome and suppress I_{Ks} function. Nature Genet 17:338–340

Splitt MR, Burn J, Goodship J (1996) Defects in the determination of left-right asymmetry. J Med Genet 33:498–503

Straub V, Campbell KP (1997) Muscular dystrophies and the dystrophin-glycoprotein complex. Curr Opin Neurol 10:168–175

Straub V, Duclos F, Venzke DP et al. (1998) Molecular pathogenesis of muscle degeneration in the δ-sarcoglycan-deficient hamster. Am J Pathol 153:1623–1630

Streib EW, Meyers DG, Sun SF (1985) Mitral valve prolapse in myotonic dystrophy. Muscle Nerve 8:650–653

Sugrue DD, Rodeheffer RJ, Codd MB, Ballard DJ, Fuster V, Gersh BJ. (1992) The clinical course of idiopathic dilated cardiomyopathy. A population-based study. Ann Int Med 117:117–123

Supp DM, Witte DP, Potter SS, Brueckner M (1997) Mutation of an axonemal dynein in the left-right asymmetry mouse mutant inversus viscerum. Nature 389:963–966

Surawicz B, Hariman RJ, (1988) Follow-up of the family with congenital absence of sinus rhythm. Am J Cardiol 61:467–469

Swan H, Piippo K, Viitasalo M et al. (1999) Arrhythmic disorder mapped to chromosome 1q42-q43 causes malignant polymorphic ventricular tachycardia in structurally normal hearts. J Am Coll Cardiol 34:2035–2042

Takamoto K, Hirose K, Uono M, Nokana I (1984) A genetic variant of Emery-Dreifuss disease. Arch Neurol 41:1291–1293

Tamburro P, Wilber D (1992) Sudden death in idiopathic dilated cardiomyopathy. Am Heart J 124:1035–1045

Taylor J, Sewry CA, Dubowitz V, Muntoni F (1998) Early onset autosomal recessive muscular dystrophy with Emery-Dreifuss phenotype and normal emerin expression. Neurology 51:1116–1120

Terrett JA, Newbury-Ecob R, Cross GS et al. (1994) Holt-Oram syndrome is a genetically heterogeneous disease with one locus mapping to human chromosome 12q. Nature Genet 6:401–404

Tesson F, Dufour C, Moolman JC et al. (1997) The influence of the angiotensin I converting enzyme genotype in familial hypertrophic cardiomyopathy varies with the disease gene mutation. J Mol Cell Cardiol 29:831–838

Thiene G, Basso C, Calabrese F, Angelini A, Valente M (2000) Pathology and pathogenesis of arrhythmogenic right ventricular cardiomyopathy. Herz 25:210–215

Thiene G, Nava A, Corrado D, Rossi L, Pennelli N. (1988) Right ventricular cardiomyopathy and sudden death in young people. N Eng J Med 318:129–133

Thiene G, Corrado D, Nava A et al. (1991) Right ventricular cardiomyopathy: Is there evidence of an inflammatory aetiology? Eur Heart J (Suppl D):22–25

Thierfelder L, MacRae C, Watkins H et al. (1993) A familial hypertrophic cardiomyopathy locus maps to chromosome 15q2. Proc Natl Acad Sci USA 90:6270–6274

Thierfelder L, Watkins H, MacRae C et al. (1994) Alpha-tropomyosin and cardiac troponin T mutations cause familial hypertrophic cardiomyopathy: A disease of the sarcomere. Cell 77:701–712

Thornell L-E, Carlsson L, Li Z, Mericskay M, Paulin D (1997) Null mutation in the desmin gene gives rise to a cardiomyopathy. J Mol Cell Cardiol 20:2107–2124

Thornton CA, Wymer JP, Simmons Z, McClain C, Moxley RT (1997) Expansion of the myotonic dystrophy CTG repeat reduces expression of the flanking DMAHP gene. Nature Genet 16:407–409

Ticho BS, Goldstein AM, Van Praagh R (2000) Extracardiac anomalies in the heterotaxy syndromes with focus on anomalies of midline-associated structures. Am J Cardiol 85:729–734

Tikanoja T, Kirkinen P, Nikolajev K, Eresmaa L, Haring P (1998) Familial atrial fibrillation with fetal onset. Heart 79:195–197

Timchenko LT (1999) Myotonic dystrophy: The role of RNA CUG triplet repeats. Am J Hum Genet 64:360–364

Timchenko L, Nastainczyk W, Schneider T, Patel B, Hofmann F, Caskey CT (1995a) Full length myotonin protein kinase (72Kd) displays serine kinase activity. Proc Natl Acad Sci USA 92:5366–5370

Timchenko LT, Monckton DG, Caskey CT (1995b) Myotonic dystrophy: An unstable repeat in a protein kinase gene. Semin Cell Biol 6:13–19

Timchenko NA, Cai ZJ, Welm AL, Reddy S, Ashizawa T, Timchenko LT (2001) RNA CUG repeats sequester CUGBP1 and alter protein levels and activity of CUGBP1. J Biol Chem (in press)

Tinsley JM, Blake DJ, Zuellig RA, Davies KE (1994) Increasing complexity of the dystrophin-associated protein complex. Proc Natl Acad Sci USA 91:8307–8313

Tinsley JM, Potter AC, Phelps SR, Fisher R, Trickett JI, Davies KE (1996) Amelioration of the dystrophic phenotype of mdx mice using a truncated utrophin transgene. Nature 284:349–353

Toniolo D, Bione S, Arahata K (1998) Emery-Dreifuss muscular dystrophy. In: Emery AEH (ED). Neuromuscular disorders. Clinical and molecular genetics Wiley, London; pp 87–103

Toniolo D, Minetti C (1999) Muscular dystrophies: Alterations in a limited number of cellular pathways? Curr Opin Genet Dev 275–282

Towbin JA (1998) The role of cytoskeletal proteins in cardiomyopathies. Curr Opin Cell Biol 10:131–139

Towbin JA (1999a) Pediatric myocardial diseases. Ped Clin N Am 46:289–312

Towbin JA (1999b) Toward an understanding of the cause of mitral valve prolapse. Am J Hum Genet 65:1238–1241

Towbin JA (2000a) Cardiac arrhythmias: The genetic connection. Journal of Cardiovascular Electrophysiology 11:601–602

Towbin JA (2000b) Molecular genetics of hypertrophic cardiomyopathy. Curr Cardiol Rep 2:134–140

Towbin JA, Ortiz-Lopez R. (1994) X-linked dilated cardiomyopathy. N Engl J Med 330:369–370

Towbin JA, Lipshultz SE. (1999) Genetics of neonatal cardiomyopathy. Curr Opin Cardiol 14:250–262

Towbin JA, Pagotto L, Siu B et al. (1992) Romano-Ward long QT syndrome (RWLQTS): Evidence of genetic heterogeneity. Ped Res 31:23A

Towbin JA, Hejtmancik F, Brink P et al. (1993) X-linked cardiomyopathy (XLCM): Molecular genetic evidence of linkage to the Duchenne muscular dystrophy (dystrophin) gene at the Xp21 locus. Circulation 87:1854–1865

Towbin JA, Li H, Taggart T et al. (1994) Evidence of genetic heterogeneity in Romano-Ward long QT syndrome: analysis of 23 families. Circulation 90:2635–2644

Towbin JA (1995) Biochemical and molecular characterization of X-linked dilated cardiomyopathy. In: Clark EB, Markwald RR, Takao A (eds): Developmental Mechanisms of Heart Disease. Futura Publishing, NY, pp. 121–132

Towbin JA, Bowles KR, Bowles NE (1999) Etiologies of cardiomyopathy and heart failure. Nature Med 5:266–267

Townsend PJ, Barton PJ, Yacoub MH, Farza H. (1995) Molecular cloning of human cardiac troponin T isoforms: Expression in developing and failing heart. J Mol Cell Cardiol 27:2223–2236

Trudeau MC, Warmke J, Ganetzky B, Robertson G (1995) HERG, a human inward rectifier in the voltage-gated potassium channel family. Science 269:92–95

Tsilfidis C, MacKenzie AE, Mettler G, Barcelo J, Kroneluk RG (1992) Correlation between CTG trinucleotide repeat length and frequency of severe congenital myotonic dystrophy. Nature Genet 1:192–195

Tsubata S, Bowles KR, Vatta M et al. (2000) Genomic cloning and characterization of mutations in the human δ-sarcoglycan gene in familial and sporadic dilated cardiomyopathy. J Clin Invest 106:655–662

Turleau C, de Grouchy J, Chavin-Colin F et al. (1984) Two patients with interstitial del (14q), one with features of Holt-Oram syndrome. Exclusion mapping of PI (alpha-1-antitrypsin). Ann Genet 27:237–240

Tveskov C, Angelo-Nielsen K. (1990) Kearns-Sayre syndrome and dilated cardiomyopathy. Neurology 40:553–554

Tyson J, Transbjaerg L, Bellman S et al. (1997) IsK and KVLQT1: Mutation in either of the two subunits of the slow component or the delayed rectifier potassium channel can cause Jervell and Lange-Nielsen syndrome. Hum Mol Genet 6:2179–2185

Uemura H, Ho SY, Devine WA, Anderson RH (1995) Analysis of visceral heterotaxy according to splenic status, appendage morphology, or both. Am J Cardiol 76:846–849

Vainzof M, Passos-Bueno MR, Man N, Zatz M (1995) Absence of correlation between utrophin localization and quantity and the clinical severity in Duchenne/Becker dystrophies. Am J Med Genet 58:305–309

Vainzof M, Passos-Bueno MR, Moreira ES et al. (1996) The sarcoglycan complex in the six autosomal recessive limb-girdle muscular dystrophies. Hum Mol Genet 5:1963–1969

Vainzof M, Passos-Bueno MR, Pavanello RC, Marie SK, Oliviera AS, Zatz M (1999) Sarcoglycanopathies are responsible for 68% of severe autosomal recessive limb-girdle muscular dystrophy in the Brazilian population. J Neurol Sci 164:44–49

Van der Kooi AJ, van Meegan M, Leddevhof TM et al. (1997) Genetic localization of a newly recognized autosomal dominant limb girdle muscular dystrophy with cardiac involvement (LGMD1B) to chromosome 1q11-21. Am J Hum Genet 60:891–895

Van Praagh R, Papagiannis J, Gruenfelder J, Bartram U, Mantanovic P (1998) Pathologic anatomy of corrected transposition of the great arteries: Medical and surgical implications. Am Heart J 135:772–785

Vatta M, Li H, Towbin JA (2000) Molecular biology of arrhythmic syndromes. Curr Opin Cardiol 15:12–22

Verduyn SC, Vos MA, Vanderzande J et al. (1997) Further observations to elucidate the role of interventricular dispersion of repolarization and early afterdepolarizations in the genesis of acquired torsade de pointes arrhythmias. A comparison between almokalant and d-sotalol using the dog as its own control. J Am Coll Cardiol 30:1575–1584

Vetter DE, Mann JR, Wangemann P et al. (1996) Inner ear defects induced by null mutation of the IsK gene. Neuron 17:1251–1264

Vidaillet HJJ, Pressley JC, Henke E, Harrell FEJ, German LD (1987) Familial occurrence of accessory atrioventricular pathways (preexcitation syndrome). N Engl J Med 317:65–69

Vikstrom KL, Factor SM, Leinwand LA (1996) Mice expressing mutant myosin heavy chains are a model for familial hypertrophic cardiomyopathy. Mol Med 2:556–567

Viskin S (2000) Cardiac pacing in the long QT syndrome: Review of available data and practical recommendations. J Cardiovasc Electrophysiol 11:593–600

Viskin S, Alla SR, Barron HV et al. (1996) Mode of onset of torsade de pointes in congenital long QT syndrome. J Am Coll Cardiol 28:1262–1268

Vlay SC (1987) Catecholamine-sensitive ventricular tachycardia. Am Heart J 114:455–461

Voit T, Krogman O, Lenard HG et al. (1988) EMD: Disease spectrum and differential diagnosis. Neuropediatrics 19:62–71

Wallace DC (1999) Mitochondrial diseases in man and mouse. Science 283:1482–1488

Walton JN, Gardner-Medwin D (1988) The muscular dystrophies. In Walton J (eds): Disorders of Voluntary Muscle. Churchill-Livingstone, New York, pp 519–568

Wang Q, Curran ME, Splawski I et al. (1996) Positional cloning of a novel potassium channel gene: KVLQT1 mutations cause cardiac arrhythmias. Nature Genet 12:17–23

Wang J, Pegoraro E, Menagazzo E et al. (1995a) Myotonic dystrophy: Evidence for a possible dominant-negative RNA mutation. Hum Mol Genet 4:599–606

Wang Q, Shen J, Splawski I et al. (1995b) SCN5A mutations associated with an inherited cardiac arrhythmia, long QT syndrome. Cell 80:805–811

Wang Q, Shen J, Li Z et al. (1995c) Cardiac sodium channel mutations in patients with long QT syndrome, an inherited cardiac arrhythmia. Hum Mol Genet 4:1603–1607

Ward DE, Ho SY, Shinebourne EA (1984) Familial atrial standstill and inexcitability in childhood. Am J Cardiol 53:965–967

Ward OC (1964) A new familial cardiac syndrome in children. J Irish Med Ass 54:103–106

Warmke JE, Ganetzky B (1994) A family of potassium channel genes related to eag in Drosophila and mammals. Proc Natl Acad Sci USA 91:3438–3442

Watkins H, Rosenzweig A, Hwang DS et al. (1992) Characteristics and prognostic implications of myosin missense mutations in familial hypertrophic cardiomyopathy. N Engl J Med 326:1108–1114

Watkins H, MacRae C, Thierfelder L et al. (1993) A disease locus for familial hypertrophic cardiomyopathy maps to chromosome 1q3. Nature Genet 3:333–337

Watkins H, Conner D, Thierfelder L et al. (1995a) Mutations in the cardiac myosin binding protein-C gene on chromosome 11 cause familial hypertrophic cardiomyopathy. Nature Genet 11:434–437

Watkins H, McKenna WJ, Thierfelder L et al. (1995b) Mutations in the genes for cardiac troponin T and alpha-tropomyosin in hypertrophic cardiomyopathy. N Engl J Med 332:1058–1064

Waxman MB, Catching JD, Felderhof CH et al. (1975) Familial atrioventricular heart block; an autosomal dominant trait. Circulation 51:226–233

Weiler T, Bashir R, Anderson LVB et al. (1999) Identical mutation in patients with limb girdle muscular dystrophy type 2B or Miyoshi myoypathy suggests a role for modifier gene(s). Hum Mol Genet 8:871–877

Wells DJ, Wells KE, Asante EA et al. (1995) Expression of human full-length and minidystrophin in transgenic mdx mice: Implications for gene therapy of Duchenne muscular dystrophy. Hum Mol Genet 4:1245–1250

WHO/ISFC Task Force (1996) Report of the 1995 World Health Organization/International Society of Federation of Cardiology Task Force on the definition and classification of cardiomyopathies. Circulation 93:841–842

Wichter T, Borggrefe M, Haverkamp W, Chen X, Bretihardt G (1992) Efficacy of antiarrhythmic drugs in patients with arrhythmogenic right ventricular disease. Results in patients with inducible and noninducible ventricular tachycardia. Circulation 86:29–37

Wichter T, Schafers M, Rhodes CG (2000) Abnormalities of cardiac sympathetic innervation in arrhythmogenic right ventricular cardiomyopathy: Quantitative assessment of presynaptic norepinephrine reuptake and postsynaptic beta-adrenergic receptor density with positron emission tomography. Circulation 101:1552–1558

Wilde AA, Jongblood RJ, Doevendans PA et al. (1999) Auditory stimuli as a trigger for arrhythmic events differentiate HERG-related (LQTS2) patients from KVLQT1-related patients (LQTS1). J Am Coll Cardiol 33:327–332

Wiles HB, McArthur PD, Taylor AB et al. (1991) Prognostic features of children with idiopathic dilated cardiomyopathy. Am J Cardiol 68:1372–1376

Winters SJ, Schreiner B, Griggs RC, Rowley P, Nanda NC (1976) Familial mitral valve prolapse and myotonic dystrophy. Ann Int Med 85:19–22

Wolff L (1943) Familial auricular fibrillation. N Engl J Med 229:396–397

Wollnick B, Schreeder BC, Kubish C, Esperer HD, Wieacker P, Jensch TJ (1997) Pathophysiological mechanisms of dominant and recessive KVLQTI K+ channel mutations found in inherited cardiac arrhythmias. Hum Mol Genet 6:1943–1949

Worton R (1995) Muscular dystrophies: Diseases of the dystrophin-glycoprotein complex. Science 270:755–756

Wren C, Macartney FJ, Deanfield JE (1987) Cardiac rhythm in atrial isomerism. Am J Cardiol 59:1156–1158

Wren C, Rowland E, Burn J, Campbell RWF (1990) Familial ventricular tachycardia: A report of four families. Br Heart J 1990;63:169–174

Wu MH, Wang JK, Lin JL et al. (1998) Supraventricular tachycardia in patients with right atrial isomerism. J Am Coll Cardiol 32:773–779

Yang Q, Sanbe A, Osinska H et al. (1998) A mouse model of myosin binding protein C human familial hypertrophic cardiomyopathy. J Clin Invest 102:1292–1300

Yokoyama T, Copeland NG, Jenkins NA et al. (1993) Reversal of left-right asymmetry: A situs inversus mutation. Science 260:679–682

Yoneya K, Okamoto H, Machida M (1995) Angiotensin-converting enzyme gene polymorphism in Japanese patients with hypertrophic cardiomyopathy. Am Heart J 130:1089–1093

Yoshida K, Ikeda S, Nakamura A et al. (1993) Molecular analysis of the Duchenne muscular dystrophy gene in patients with Becker muscular dystrophy presenting with dilated cardiomyopathy. Muscle Nerve 16:1161–1166

Yoshida K, Nakamura A, Yazaki M (1998) Insertional mutation by transposable element, L1, in the DMD gene results in X-linked dilated cardiomyopathy. Hum Mol Genet 7:1129–1132

Yu B, French JA, Carrier L et al. (1998) Molecular pathology of familial hypertrophic cardiomyopathy caused by mutations in the cardiac myosin binding protein C gene. J Med Genet 35:205–210

Zareba W, Moss AJ, Schwartz PJ et al. (1998) Influence of the genotype on the clinical course of the long-QT syndrome. N Engl J Med 339:960–965

Zeviani M, Gellera C, Antozzi C et al. (1991) Maternally inherited myopathy and cardiomyopathy with mutation in mitochondrial DNA tRNA (Leu)(UUR). Lancet 338:143–147

Zeviani M, Tiranti V, Piantadosi C (1998) Mitochondrial disorders. Medicine 77:59–72

Zhou Z, Gong Q, Miles L et al. (1998) HERG channel dysfunction in human long QT syndrome. J Biol Chem 263:21061–21066

Zolk O, Caroni P, Bohm M (2000) Decreased expression of the cardiac LIM domain protein MLP in chronic human heart failure. Circulation 101:2674–2677

Molecular basis of human hypertension

Xavier Jeunemaitre
Anne-Paule Gimenez-Roqueplo
Sandra Disse-Nicodeme
Pierre Corvol

The genetic basis of essential hypertension is complex. A number of epidemiologic studies have shown that individual blood pressure levels result from both genetic predisposition and environmental factors. The heritable component of blood pressure has been documented in familial and in twin studies. Evidence suggests that approximately 30% of the variance of blood pressure is attributable to genetic heritability and 50% to environmental influences (Ward, 1990).

Up to now there is no indication on the number of genetic loci involved in hypertension, the frequency of deleterious alleles, their mode of transmission, and the quantitative effect of any single allele on blood pressure. The unimodal distribution of blood pressure within each age group and in each sex strongly suggests that several loci are involved. Several strategies based on the biological tools available at the genetic level and on different approaches for comparing hypertensive and normotensive subjects (case-control studies, family based association studies, sibling pairs studies) have been used to identify major genes or susceptibility genes. Statistical positive results are useful indicators for elucidating the various genetic loci favoring high blood pressure: the discovery of a positive linkage between a given locus and high blood pressure promotes new studies for finding a functional gene variant and for identifying new intermediate phenotypes of the locus. Molecular genetics can unravel an underestimated or even totally unexpected mechanism of blood pressure control and can also eliminate a candidate gene as being an important contributor to familial hypertension.

Over the past few years there has been intensive efforts to identify the genes involved in blood pressure regulation, their respective importance in determining blood pressure level, and sometimes their interaction with other genes and environmental components. Different strategies have been undertaken (Fig. 51.1). A first and successful approach, mainly taken by Lifton and coworkers (1992) has been to identify genes causing some rare mendelian forms of hypertension. This has led to the confirmation of the importance of some enzymes, channels and receptors implicated in sodium handling in the regulation of blood pressure. A second approach has been to study genes that may contribute to the variance of blood pressure due to their well known effect on the cardiovascular system. The genes of the renin-angiotensin-aldosterone system are a good illustration of such a "candidate gene" approach, since this system is involved in the control of blood pressure and in the pathogenesis of several forms of experimental and human hypertension. A third approach has been developed more recently, thanks to progress made on the human genome and on the availability of an ordered human genetic map of several thousand polymorphic markers. This strategy, called

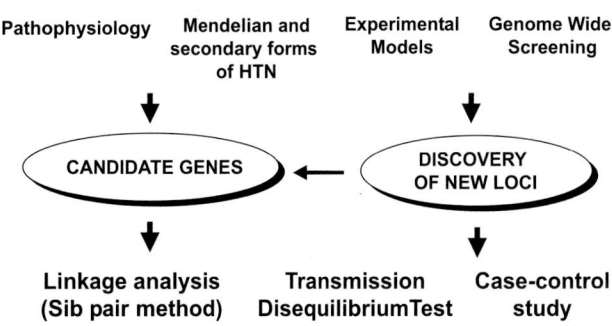

APPLICATIONS OF DIFFERENT STRATEGIES FOR STUDYING THE GENETICS OF HUMAN ESSENTIAL HYPERTENSION

Fig. 51.1 Main strategies used for studying the genetics of arterial hypertension

genome-wide scan (GWS), usually corresponds to the genotyping of a first set of about 400 genetic markers in large familial samples and to the analysis of their cosegregation with either hypertension or blood pressure.

This review will discuss recent results obtained by the molecular analysis of mendelian forms of hypertension, of some candidate genes in human essential hypertension, and by the first GWS reports. No mention will be given to the very fruitful research performed on the genetics of hypertension based on experimental rodent models, for which excellent reviews are available (Dominiczak et al., 1998; Rapp, 2000; Smithies et al., 2000).

Monogenic forms of hypertension

The molecular basis of several rare mendelian forms of hypertension have been recently elucidated. They are usually characterized by an early onset of hypertension, a frequent familial history of stroke, and a strong penetrance. Most of them are also characterized by extracellular volume expansion leading to a suppression of plasma renin activity, confirming the importance of salt and water homeostasis in blood pressure regulation.

GLUCOCORTICOID SUPPRESSIBLE HYPERTENSION

In glucocorticoid suppressible hypertension (GSH) (also called dexamethasone—suppressible aldosteronism or glucocorticoid–remediable aldosteronism), there is a variable degree of hyperaldosteronism and an increased urinary excretion of 18-hydroxylated and 18-oxo-cortisol metabolites, 18-hydroxycortisol and 18-oxocortisol. These abnormalities, including hypertension, can be corrected by the suppression of adrenocorticotropic hormone (ACTH) by dexamethasone. It had been proposed that the disease was due to an abnormality of aldosterone synthase, CYP11B2, in the zona fasciculata the enzyme responsible for the conversion of corticosterone into aldosterone. Lifton et al. (1992) showed that this disorder was linked to an abnormal aldosterone synthase gene. They studied a large kindred and found a gene duplication arising from unequal crossing over, resulting in a fusion of the 11β-hydroxylase (*CYP11B1*) promoter with the coding sequence of aldosterone synthase. The chimeric gene encodes a protein that can hydroxylate cortisol (the steroid substrate present in the zona fasciculata) in the 18-position. This gene is under the control of the 11β-hydroxylase gene regulatory region,

whose expression is under ACTH control and can be down-regulated by exogenous glucocorticoid administration. All the phenotypic abnormalities of GSH could be explained by this mutation.

Since this original description, a few other families affected with this syndrome have been identified. In a case of GSH with an adrenal tumor, we found expression of the chimeric gene in the tumoral tissue and in the zona fasciculata of the surrounding adrenal tissue and observed the sensivity of the corresponding adrenal cells to ACTH (Pascoe et al., 1995). In all families reported so far, the chimeric gene derives from unequal homologous recombination between exons 2 and 4 of the 11β-hydroxylase and aldosterone synthase genes, respectively. It has been shown by site-directed mutagenesis that such hybrid genes expressed in heterologous eucaryotic cells are able to encode chimeric proteins which hydroxylate cortisol in the 18-position (Pascoe et al., 1992). More recently, the transfection into COS-7 cells of a series of *CYP11B1* cDNAs containing various regions of *CYP11B2* sequence showed that two amino acid changes, Ser288Gly and Val320Ala, are sufficient to convert *CYP11B1* into an efficient aldosterone producing enzyme (Curnow et al., 1997). Although these results suggest that a gene conversion involving exons 5 and 6—in which these residues are encoded—could cause a novel form of GSH, no such molecular abnormality has yet been found in a series of patients with essential hypertension and primary aldosteronism (Mulatero et al., 1998).

GSH is probably very rare. The possible locations of the unequal crossover between *CYP11B1* and *CYP11B2* allow its molecular diagnosis by a simple Southern-blot or a long-range PCR assay (11). We could not find any case of GSH through a systematic analysis of more than 200 patients with primary aldosteronism without Conn adenoma (Jeunemaitre et al., unpublished data) and only three French families have been diagnosed up to now. However, one of the major interests of this diagnosis is its therapeutic implication with a clinical and biological improvement with small doses of dexamethasone (Jonsson et al., 1995; Jeunemaitre et al., 1995) which can be associated with an anti-aldosterone treatment and/or a more usual antihypertensive therapy.

Gordon and colleagues described another form of familial primary aldosteronism, called type II (FH-II), that corresponds to few families with about 30% of the affected patients presenting an aldosterone-producing tumor and with probably an autosomal dominant inheritance (Stowasser et al., 1992; Stowasser and Gordon; 2000). The screening of the entire genome in a large family with FH-II recently showed linkage with chromosome 7p22 (Lafferty et al., 2000).

LIDDLE SYNDROME

Liddle et al. (1963) described a family with hypertension and an abnormality of Na+ reabsorption at the level of the renal distal tubule, which simulated primary aldosteronism but had negligible basal and stimulated aldosterone secretion. Blood pressure and hypokalemia were not influenced by spironolactone treatment, but triamterene, a specific inhibitor of the distal renal epithelial sodium channel, corrected these abnormalities. The authors proposed that the primary abnormality was a constitutive activation of the epithelial sodium channel. Some 30 years later, this hypothesis was reinvestigated in the proband and in the originally described pedigree. The index case developed renal failure and renal transplantation corrected the aldosterone and renin responses to salt restriction, showing the involvement of the kidney in the disease (Botero-Velez et al., 1994), making the epithelial amiloride-sensitive sodium channel (ENaC) located in the collecting cortical tubule a logical candidate gene for this disease. This channel consists of at least three homologous subunits, α, β and γ, which act together to confer its low sodium conductance, and its high selectivity for sodium and amiloride (Canessa et al., 1994).

Loss-of-function mutations of either one of the subunits of the ENaC gene result in the recessive form of pseudo-hypoaldosteronism type I, characterized by excessive salt wasting accompanied with hyperkalemic acidosis, increased plasma and urinary aldosterone, and increased plasma renin activity (Chang et al., 1996). Analyzing the original Liddle pedigree, Shimkets et al. (1994) showed complete linkage of the gene encoding the β subunit of this channel, located at chromosome 16p13–12. In this pedigree and in other unrelated kindreds, a premature stop codon, a frameshift mutation and other deleterious mutations were found, all located in the last exon of the gene encoding for the intracellular carboxy-terminal domain of the β subunit (Shimkets et al., 1994). These mutations were showed to be gain-of-function mutations, with an increased amiloride-sensitive Na+ current after transfection of the corresponding mutant subunits together with α and γ wild-type subunits. In a Portugese family affected with this syndrome, we found a 32 base-pair deletion leading to a premature termination of the carboxy-end of the same subunit (Jeunemaitre et al., 1997a,b). A point mutation affecting the same region of the γ subunit has also been found to cause Liddle syndrome (Hansson et al., 1995a), but no mutation of αENaC has been discovered in this syndrome. Comprehensive studies (Snyder et al., 1995; Schild et al., 1996; Staub et al, 1996) have shown that the mechanism by which truncation of the C terminus of the β and γ subunits alter the function of the epithelial sodium

channel was corresponding to a very conserved motif (PPxxY) in the C terminus of all three subunits of the sodium channel. Normally, a specific interaction between the PY motif and cytosolic proteins (Nedd4 and other related WW proteins) leads to degradation of part of the newly synthetized subunits (Rotin et al., 2000) Both truncation or punctual mutation of this PY motif increased surface statement of the mutant proteins and thus increased the number of sodium channels in the apical membrane (Firsov et al., 1996), favoring renal sodium absorption and hypertension.

A GAIN OF FUNCTION MUTATION IN THE MINERALOCORTICOID RECEPTOR

A new monogenic form of hypertension, which could be called pseudoaldosteronism type II, has been recently reported by Geller et al. (2000). It is characterized by an early onset and severe form of hypertension associated with low plasma levels of renin and aldosterone. It is caused by an activating missense mutation (Ser810Leu) of the human mineralocorticoid receptor. This mutation is located within the hormone binding domain and results in constitutive mineralocorticoid receptor activity and in alteration of the receptor specificity. The receptor becomes abnormally activated by progesterone and other steroids lacking 21-hydroxyl groups, which act normally as antagonists. In the family described by Geller and coworkers, all women bearing the mutation had severe pregnancy-induced hypertension with hypoaldosteronism which is likely caused by the massive increased production of progesterone during pregnancy. These original findings open the possibility of such mutations underlying some cases of pregnancy-induced hypertension.

APPARENT MINERALOCORTICOID EXCESS, ULICK SYNDROME

The syndrome of apparent mineralocorticoid excess (AME) is a rare autosomal recessive form of hypertension diagnosed in children and characterized by very early and severe hypertension associated with hyporeninism and hypoaldosteronism (Ulick et al., 1979). It corresponds to a defect of the 11β hydroxysteroid dehydrogenase type 2 (11βHSD2), which is expressed in the kidney and converts cortisol into cortisone and corticosterone into 11-dehydrocorticosterone. Classical deleterious mutations have been found in affected patients being either homozygotes for the mutation, especially in consanguineous families, or composite heterozygtes (More et al., 1995; Stewart et al., 1996; Morineau et al., 1999).

The enzymatic defect leads to increased renal concentrations of cortisol and corticosterone, which are themselves powerful agonists of the human mineralocorticoid receptor contrary to cortisone and 11-dehydrocorticosterone. Thus, affected patients are characterized by high values of the cortisol/cortisone ratio in plasma and urines, and by arterial hypertension, mimicking a primary aldosteronism (Stewart, 1999). The genetic diagnosis can be obtained rapidly by direct sequencing of the five exons of the gene.

PSEUDOHYPOALDOSTERONISM TYPE 2, GORDON SYNDROME

Pseudohypoaldosteronism type 2 (PHA2) also known as Gordon syndrome, is an autosomal dominant form of volume dependent hypertension characterized by hyperkalemia and hyperchloremic acidosis without any glomerular insufficiency (Gordon et al., 1995). The low renin levels are thought to be the consequence of volume repletion whereas plasma aldosterone seems to vary according to the opposite influences of low renin and high potassium levels. At least two arguments suggest a primary renal tubular defect along the distal convoluted tubule: affected patients are highly sensitive to small doses of thiazide diuretics; and the features of PHA-II are the mirror image of the Bartter-Gitelman syndrome in which inactivating mutations in the thiazide-sensitive sodium-chloride cotransporter (SLC12A3) gene have been demonstrated (Simon et al., 1996). However, the pathophysiology of PHA-II is certainly more complex, and other authors have proposed an associated reduced proximal reabsorption, a chloride reabsorption defect, and an altered sensitivity to mineralocorticoids (Schambelan et al., 1981).

Using eight affected but limited families, Mansfield et al. (1997) identified two loci on the long arm of chromosomes 1 and 17, respectively, named PHA2A and PHA2B. Involvement SLCA12A3 was excluded by genetic linkage analysis. The selection and genetic analysis of four French pedigrees led us to exclude these two loci and to identify a third chromosomal region on chromosome 12p, called PHA2C. Exclusion of linkage for these chromosomal regions in two additional affected pedigrees suggests further genetic heterogeneity. Thus, it is expected that molecular genetics of this syndrome will lead to a variety of molecular defects, highlighting the role of either several new components of the same pathway, multiple aldosterone-regulated effectors, or direct or indirect partners of the sodium-chloride cotransporter.

SYNDROME ASSOCIATING ARTERIAL HYPERTENSION AND BRACHYDACTYLY

A rare form of an autosomal dominant syndrome associating arterial hypertension and brachydactyly has been reported in a few families, especially one extended Turkish pedigree (Bilginturan et al., 1973; Luft, 1998). In 100% of the affected patients, hypertension is accompanied by short stature and brachydactyly but with no other special biological or hormonal phenotype (Schuster et al., 1996a). A particular defect of cerebral vascularization—loops in the posterior/inferior cerebellar artery—has been discussed as the possible origin of neurovascular compression and high blood pressure (Naraghi et al., 1997). The gene responsible for the disease has been mapped to chromosome 12p (Schuster et al., 1996b), in a region which is more centromeric than the PHA2C locus, but has not been identified yet.

DISCUSSION

In conclusion, several interesting lessons as well new questions arise from the molecular analysis of these monogenic forms of hypertension:

1. It is clear that single gene mutations can provoke hypertension. Even though blood pressure level results from complex interactions between genes and environment, most of the syndromes identified above are strongly penetrant. Thus, mutations arising at key genes involved in blood pressure regulation are probably sufficient to increase human blood pressure. Whether an ascertainment bias exists for the families collected so far, and whether it explains part of this strong pernetrance will be determined by genetic analysis of extended pedigrees and the detection of other families diagnosed by a systematic, direct molecular investigation.

2. The expression of these mendelian forms of hypertension is probably modulated by the effect of other genes acting on blood pressure. For example, it has been suggested that the impact of the GSH chimeric gene on kalemia and blood pressure varies among families and even differs within a single family (Dluhy and Liftan, 1995). There was also large variability of the disease in the original Liddle pedigree, since some patients had mild hypertension and no hypokaliemia. The same phenotypic variability was also observed in our extended PHA2 family (Disse-Nicodeme et al., 2000).

3. The exact prevalence of the monogenic forms of hypertension might have been underestimated due to the difficulty of establishing the diagnosis by classical biological approaches. In GSH, Liddle and AME syndromes, a genetic test can be performed when the

diagnosis is suspected, which simplifies the diagnosis and may increase the actual number of cases diagnosed.

4. Finally, these findings raise the possibility that similar genetic mechanisms operate in some common forms of essential hypertension with a related phenotype, such as low plasma renin activity, variable hypokalemia, and inappropriately high or low plasma aldosterone. The inheritable salt-dependent form of hypertension (Volpe et al., 1991) might represent the phenotype of more subtle mutations of the genes operating in the caricatural forms of hypertension. This has prompted investigators to study possible association or linkage in patients with essential hypertension. Even though most of the results obtained were negative, interesting polymorphisms were discovered, some of which being detailed in the next section.

Candidate genes in human essential hypertension

Although it is likely that genes interact with each other and with environmental factors (Fig. 51.2), most of the studies performed so far have been conducted in a very simple design, only testing the possible role of each candidate gene, i.e., gene coding for a protein (hormone, enzyme, receptor, channel, etc.) known to be involved in blood pressure regulation.

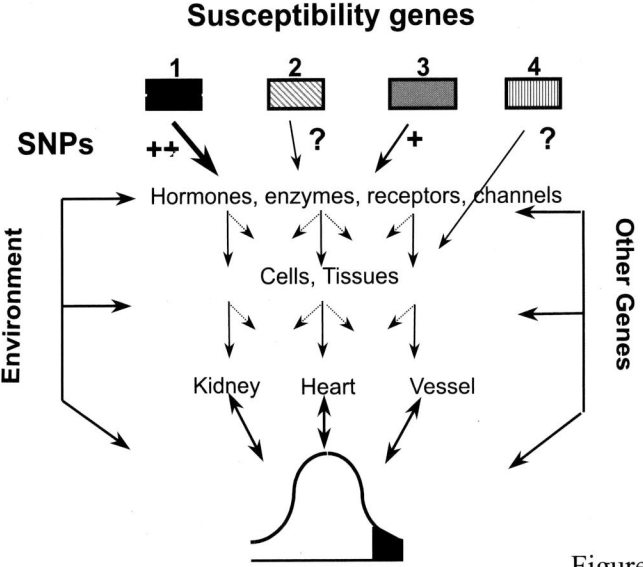

Fig. 51.2. Interaction between genes and environment in the regulation of blood pressure

THE RENIN ANGIOTENSIN SYSTEM

The importance of the renin angiotensin system in salt and water homeostasis and in the regulation of vascular tone, the effectiveness of inhibitors of this system in the treatment of hypertension and of its morbid consequences have justified the genetic analysis of this system for more than ten years. All the genes of the human renin-angiotensin system have been mapped and cloned, and genetic markers identified. Since very complete reviews have already been published on that matter from our group (Corvol et al., 1996; 1997) and others (Rieder and Nickerson, 2000; Danser and Schunkert, 2000; Wang and Staessen, 2000) we will only summarize the main findings obtained that concern essential hypertension, blood pressure regulation or both.

The renin gene

The renin gene is important because the renin angio-tensinogen reaction is the first and rate-limiting step leading to angiotensin II (Ang II) production. Numerous studies have involved renin to some degree in experimental forms of hypertension and in human hypertension. This was especially the case of the fulminant hypertension that develops in transgenic rats harboring the mouse *Ren 2* gene (Mullins et al., 1990) and of the pioneer observation made by Rapp et al (1989) of cosegregation between a renin gene polymorphism and blood pressure level in Dahl rats. In humans, about 30% of subjects with essential hypertension have higher renin levels compared to normotensive subjects of the same age when examined under the same metabolic conditions (Brunner et al., 1972). Interestingly, renin levels seem at least partly heritable, as observed by Grim and colleagues (1980) in twins submitted to very standardized conditions of posture and sodium diet, and more recently confirmed by Rossi et al. (1999). The analysis of 175 sibling pairs and trios who participated to a multicenter trial showed very significant correlations of plasma renin levels either on a high salt ($r=0.36$, $p<10^{-3}$) or on a low salt diet ($r=0.46$, $p<10^{-3}$) (Jeunemaitre et al., unpublished results).

The human renin gene is located on the short arm of chromosome 1 (1q32–1q42) (Cohen-Haguenauer et al., 1983). Association studies – most of them being of limited power – performed with several polymorphisms of the renin gene largely have been negative (Danser and Schunkert, 2000; Morris and Griffiths, 1988; Soubrier et al., 1990; Wang et al., 1999). To explore the potential role of the renin gene as a genetic determinant of hypertension, we analyzed the same renin gene haplotypes in 98 sibling pairs with severe essential hypertension (Jeunemaitre et al., 1992a). Allelic concordance for all sib pairs according to sibship size was not significantly different from that expected under the hypothesis of no linkage reflecting only a small excess of renin alleles shared by the hypertensive sibs (1.44 (+/− 0.6) *versus* 1.36 (+/− 0.6)). These results suggest that the renin gene does not have a frequent and/or important role in the pathogenesis of essential hypertension. However, the definitive exclusion of a contribution of the renin gene in the heritability of essential hypertension will require more powerful linkage studies, such as the use of a reliable renin intermediate phenotype, and a more informative marker of the renin locus. Some of the recent genome scans have found the chromosome 1q32 region as a possible locus for hypertension.

The angiotensin I-converting enzyme

Angiotensin I-converting enzyme (ACE) is a zinc metalloprotease whose main functions are to convert angiotensin I into angiotensin II, and to inactivate bradykinin. It is assumed that this step of the renin angiotensin system is not limiting in plasma, and indeed there is no indication that plasma ACE levels are directly related to blood pressure levels. However, the local generation of angiotensin I and the degradation of a bradykinin might depend on the level of ACE expressed in tissues.

Molecular cloning of the human endothelial ACE cDNA (Soubrier et al., 1988) has revealed that the enzyme consists of two highly homologous and functionally active domains resulting from a gene duplication. The organization of the human *ACE* gene provides further support for the duplication of an ancestral gene (Hubert et al., 1991). There are two *ACE* promoters, a somatic promoter localized on the 5′ side of the first exon of the gene and a germinal, intragenic, promoter located on the 5′ side of the specific testicular *ACE* mRNA (Hubert et al., 1991; Howard et al., 1990; Kumar et al., 1991). The two alternate promoters of *ACE* exhibit highly contrasting cell specificities, as the somatic promoter is active in endothelial, epithelial and neuronal cell types, whereas the germinal promoter is only active in a stage-specific manner in male germinal cells (Howard et al., 1990). It is thought that plasma ACE concentration reflect the level of the synthesis of the enzyme at the somatic level.

For a geneticist, one of the big advantages of plasma ACE concentration as a genetic marker is its large interindividual variation (from 1 to 8 at the extremes of the distribution) and its reproducibility when measured repeatedly in a given subject (Alhenc-Gelas et al., 1991). This important interindividual variability is due, in large part, to a major genetic effect, as shown by Cambien et al., (1988) in a

family population study where there was an intrafamilial resemblance between plasma ACE levels, this effect accounting for approximately 30% and 75% of the ACE variance in parents and in offsprings, respectively.

The role of *ACE* in the genetic control of plasma ACE was assessed using an *ACE* polymorphism. A polymorphism consisting of the presence or the absence of a 287 base-pair DNA fragment was detected (Insertion/Deletion) and used as a marker genotype (Rigat et al., 1990). In this seminal observation of 80 healthy subjects, Rigat and colleagues showed that DD subjects had an immunoreactive ACE level almost twice as high as patients homozygous for the I allele, whereas heterozygous patients had an intermediate ACE level. This I/D polymorphism accounted for 47% of the total variance of serum ACE, showing that the *ACE* locus plays an important role in determining serum ACE levels (Rigat et al., 1990). Like for serum ACE, T-lymphocyte ACE levels are significantly higher in patients homozygous for the D allele than in the other subjects (Costerousse et al., 1993). The *ACE* I/D polymorphism is not directly involved in the genetic regulation of serum and tissue ACE, and the causative variant responsible for the increase in ACE has yet to be found; indeed, another study combining segregation and linkage analysis in 98 healthy nuclear families showed that the *ACE* I/D polymorphism is only a neutral marker in strong linkage disequilibrium with the putative functional variant (Tiret et al., 1992). Soubrier's group performed an extensive study of eight new polymorphisms in 95 healthy nuclear families (Villard et al., 1996). After adjustment for the I/D polymorphism, all polymorphisms of the 5′ group remained significantly associated with ACE levels, which suggested the existence of two quantitative trait loci (QTL) acting additively on ACE levels and which would explain 38% and 49% of the ACE variance in parents and offspring, respectively. More recently, Rieder and colleagues (1999) performed the complete genomic sequence of *ACE* from 11 individuals, representing the longest contiguous scan (24 kb) for sequence variation in human DNA. They identified 78 varying sites in 22 chromosomes that resolved into 13 distinct haplotypes, 17 being in absolute linkage disequilibrium with the *ACE* I/D polymorphism, producing two distinct and distantly related clades and suggesting that the causal variant should be located within the 3′ part of the gene.

The observation that plasma ACE levels are under the direct control of an *ACE* gene variant coupled with the role of the ACE enzyme in two main enzymatic cascades (renin angiotensin system and kallikrein kinin system) in cardiovascular physiology, rapidly made the *ACE* I/D polymorphism one of the most popular markets tested in cardiovascular diseases. The first genome scans performed in a F2 rat population generated from stroke-prone spontaneously hypertensive rats (SHR/SP) and normotensive in genetically hypertensive rats made this hypothesis even more attractive (Hilbert et al., 1991; Jacob et al., 1991). Both groups of investigators found a significant linkage between NaCl loaded hypertension and a gene locus on rat chromosome 10 which contributed as much as 20% of blood pressure variance under high salt intake and that contained the *ACE* locus. Several hundreds of reported and unreported studies have been performed since then (Rieder and Nickerson, 2000; Danser and Schunkert, 2000; Wang and Staessen, 2000). We will only summarize here some of the main findings using *ACE* as a candidate gene for human essential hypertension.

One association study comparing a normotensive and a hypertensive Australian population with two hypertensive parents, showed an association of hypertension with an *ACE* polymorphism (Zee et al., 1992). In fact, the significant difference between the I/D genotype originated only from a subgroup of patients aged 50 years or more, where the D genotype was less frequent than in normotensives. This finding was interpreted as due to an overrisk of cardiovascular events in hypertensive patients carrying the D allele (Morris et al., 1994). Harrap et al. (1993) investigated the distribution of the *ACE* I/D gene polymorphism described above in young adults with contrasting genetic predisposition to high blood pressure (Watt et al., 1992) ("four-corners approach"): young adults with high blood pressure and two parents with high blood pressure did not show any significant difference in the I/D allele frequencies of *ACE* when compared with adults of the same age but with low blood pressure and no genetic predisposition to high blood pressure. Other association studies were also negative (Higashimori et al., 1993; Schmidt et al., 1993). In a large series of hypertensive sib pairs from Utah, we found no evidence of linkage between hypertension and a growth hormone gene polymorphic marker in complete linkage disequilibrium with *ACE* (Jeunemaitre et al., 1992b).

Other positive results suggest however that the *ACE* locus might influence blood pressure variability in a sex-specific manner. This was the case of the analysis of 3095 participants in the Framingham Heart Study (O'Donnell et al, 1998). In a logistic regression analysis, the adjusted odds ratios for hypertension among men for the DD and DI genotypes were 1.59 and 1.18, respectively, *versus* II, whereas no effect was observed in women. Positive results were also observed by Fornage et al., (1998), in the analysis of a large population-based sample of 1488 siblings having a mean age of 15 years and belonging to the youngest generation of 583 randomly ascertained three-generation pedigrees from Rochester, Minnesota. In sex-specific analyses, genetic variation in and around *ACE* explained as much as 35% of the interindividual blood pressure variation in males but not in females. Finally, Julier et al. (1997) conducted an affected sib-pair analysis in French and UK families, based on the fact that one of the principal blood pressure loci in rat hypertensive strains lies on chromosome 10, a region homologous on to human chromosome 17. Significant evidence of linkage was found near two closely linked microsatellite markers, D17S183 and D17S934, that reside 18 cM proximal to *ACE* in the homology region (Julier et al., 1997).

Taken together, these results suggest that *ACE* does not play a major role on blood pressure variance in the overall population, but that it could influence it either in a sex-specific manner or indirectly by its role on different tissues (kidney, heart, vessels) for which several studies indicate a relation with the *ACE* I/D polymorphism (Rieder and Nickerson, 2000; Danser and Schunkert, 2000; Wang and Straessen, 2000).

The angiotensinogen gene

Angiotensinogen (AGT), the renin substrate, is mainly synthesized by the liver and is the unique substrate for renin. Plasma AGT plasma concentration is within a range where variations of its concentration directly affects the angiotensin I production rate. Indeed, angiotensinogen levels are around the K range of renin, and therefore it is logical to suspect that a chronic state of increased plasma angiotensinogen might increase angiotensin I and facilitate hypertension and/or cardiovascular diseases. Its role in human hypertension has been suspected in an epidemiological study where a strong correlation was found between plasma angiotensinogen concentration and blood pressure (Walker et al., 1979), and in another study where offsprings of hypertensive patients had elevated plasma AGT levels (Fasola et al., 1968).

The human angiotensinogen gene belongs to the superfamily of serpins (Gaillard et al., 1989) and is localized to chromosome 1q42.3, in the same region as human renin (Gaillard-Sanchez et al., 1990). With the group of JM Lalouel, we suggested a role of the AGT gene in human essential hypertension (Jeunemaitre et al., 1992c). An extensive study was performed in two large series of hypertensive sibships yielding a total of 379 sib pairs (Salt Lake City, Utah, USA and Paris, France) and using a highly polymorphic microsatellite marker at *AGT*. An excess of *AGT* allele sharing was found mainly in severely hypertensive sibpairs and in men. Other linkage studies have since been reported with controversial results. Caulfield et al. showed a strong linkage and an association of *AGT* to essential hypertension in a set of British families (Caulfield et al., 1994; 1996). To the contrary, no evidence for linkage was found in a large European study involving 630 affected sibling pairs, either in the whole panel or in family subsets selected for severity or early onset of disease (Brand et al., 1998a). Linkage of *AGT* to essential hypertension was also found in 63 affected African Caribbean sibling pairs (Caulfield et al., 1995). Similarly, positive albeit modest significant excess of *AGT* allele sharing was found in 46 extended Mexican American families (Atwood et al., 1997). No linkage was found between *AGT* and hypertension in 310 hypertensive Chinese sibling pairs (Niu et al., 1998; 1999). Altogether, these results probably highlight the modest effect of *AGT* in the overall population and the difficulty of identifying susceptibility genes by linkage analysis in complex diseases.

Among the 15 polymorphisms initially identified (Jeunemaitre et al., 1992a,b,c), two of them leading to aminoacid changes, 174M and M235T, were found to be associated with hypertension and to plasma AGT concentration. This association between plasma angiotensinogen level and the M235T genotype was further confirmed in white children (Bloem et al., 1995). In this study, a strong and independent relationship of serum angiotensinogen with body mass index ($p = 0.0001$) and race ($p = 0.0003$) was also observed. Confirmation of the impact of an increased statement of angiotensinogen on blood pressure was obtained by Smithies and colleagues (2000) who performed genetic manipulations in mice leading to animals having several functional copies of a given gene. Mice bearing one, two, three or four functional angiotensinogen copies displayed a gene-dosage effect on plasma angiotensinogen concentration and blood pressure level, paralleling the M235T variant effect observed in humans (Smithies et al., 1994; Kim et al., 1995). The threonine residue at position 235 is not conserved across species and is in complete linkage disequilibrium with another nucleotide substitution (G->A) at position −6 in the promoter of the gene, both alleles being indistinguishable (Jeunemaitre et al., 1997b). Lalouel and his group were able to show that this variant is associated *in vitro* with increased expression of *AGT* and probably explains the association with increased plasma angiotensinogen (Inoue et al., 1997). However, the true biological effect may be more complex since other polymorphisms, C-532T, C-18T, A-20C, T+31C, also in linkage disequilibrium with G-6A and M235T, might play a role in the variation of transcription of the gene (Corvol and Jeunemaitre, 1997; Sato et al., 1997; Paillard et al., 1999; Ishikawa et al., 2001).

There is a strong effect of race on the allele frequency of most of these polymorphisms. The 235T allele frequency varies from 40% in Caucasians to 80% in the Asian and African-American population and even 93% in Nigerians (Rotimi et al., 1994). This high prevalence of the 235T allele may explain why no relation between 235T or 174M allele frequencies and hypertension was observed in a study of African-Americans (Rotimi et al., 1994). In the Japanese population, a significant association between this allele and high blood pressure was found in several separate case control studies (Hata et al., 1994; Kamitani et al., 1994; Iwai et al., 1994; Morise et al., 1995). These differences in alleles frequencies might also facilitate false positive results in case of admixture in case-control studies (Sharma and Jeunemaitre, 2000).

The association between the M235T polymorphism and essential hypertension has been tested in a large number of case-control studies which have been reviewed recently (Jeunemaitre et al., 1999). A meta-analysis of case-control studies representing on 5493 Caucasian patients showed that the *AGT* 235T allele was significantly but mildly associated with hypertension (odds-ratio: 1.20; 95% [CI]: 1.11 to 1.29; $p < 0.0001$). This association increased in studies with positive family history (OR: 1.42; 95% CI: 1.25 to 1.61, $p < 0.0001$) (Kunz et al., 1997). This polymorphism represents a good example of susceptibility alleles, quite common in the population but that explains only a small part of the blood pressure variance in the overall population.

One possibility is that molecular variants of *AGT* might represent also a susceptible allele for pregnancy-induced hypertension, for which a familial tendency has been documented (Cooper et al., 1988; Liston and Kilpatrick, 1991). Ward et al. (1993) found a significant association between the *AGT* 235T variant and pre-eclampsia in both Caucasian and Japanese samples. Using another strategy, analysis of the allelic inheritance of the GT repeat in 52 sibling pairs of preeclamptic sisters, Arngrimsson et al. (1993) showed a significant linkage between *AGT* and preeclampsia in Icelandic and Scottish families. The association in Japanese women was confirmed in a larger case-control study involving 139 women with pregnancy – induced hypertension and 278 matched controls (Kobashi, 1995). However, other studies limited in their sample size found no indication of association or linkage between pre-eclampsia and *AGT* in Caucasian women (Morgan et al., 1995; Wilton et al., 1995; Guo et al., 1997). More recently, we found a significant increase of the T235 allele frequency in a large series of pre-eclamptic women of African origin ascertained in the Mauritius Island (Poonyth, unpublished data). Interestingly, nulligravid women homozygous T235 have a reduced plasma volume during the follicular phase of the menstrual cycle than those bearing the MT or MM genotype (Bernstein et al., 1998).

The pathogenesis of preeclampsia is probably influenced by a variety of genetic (maternal and paternal) and non-genetic factors. Recent genome-scan studies have reported possible loci on chromosomes 4q (Harrison et al., 1997) and 2p (Arngrimsson et al., 1999; Moses et al., 2000). The gene coding for nitric oxide synthase has also been linked to the pathology (Guo et al., 1999). The possible pathophysiological relationship between *AGT* and pregnancy-induced hypertension may be due to both an increased expression of angiotensinogen in decidual arteries (Morgan et al., 1997) and to a decreased formation of high-molecular mass angiotensinogen (Gimenez-Roquepo et al., 1998) an aggregate form of the protein particularly abundant during pregnancy. We also recently demonstrated that the M235T polymorphism is associated with increased response of plasma AGT to a one-week exposure to ethinyl-estradiol in normovolunteers (Azizi et al., 2000).

From all these studies, *AGT* appears to be involved in the determination of human familial hypertension and some forms of pregnancy-induced hypertension. However, its exact quantitative effect on blood pressure is unknown but might be weak and modulated by a variety of interacting loci and environmental factors accounting for the negative results in some under-powered studies.

The angiotensin II type 1 receptor

Angiotensin II receptors, which mediate all the biological and physiological effects of the renin angiotensin system, are also candidate genes for essential hypertension. The AT_I subtype is a G-coupled receptor inserted into the plasma membrane of angiotensin II target cells, vascular smooth muscle cells, renal vasculature and mesangial cells, adrenal and brain. The human gene (*AT1R*) has been cloned and is located on chromosome 3q21-3q25 (Curnow et al., 1992; Furuta et al., 1992).

In a first series of experiments, we looked for putative molecular variants in the coding region of the gene that would result in an overactivation of the receptor. Such variants have been reported for other G-coupled seven-transmembrane domain receptors, such as the human thyrotropin (Parma et al., 1993) and luteinizing hormone (Shenker et al., 1993) receptors, resulting in a constitutive activation or hyperresponsiveness of the receptor. In the case of hypertension, similar functional variants of angio-

tensin II receptors could theoretically lead to some forms of essential hypertension or to tumoral sporadic primary aldosteronism. However, no evidence of such mutations in the coding region of *AT1R* was found in 60 probands of hypertensive families (Bonnardeaux et al., 1994) and in 20 cases of tumoral primary aldosteronism (Davies et al., 1997). There was no evidence of linkage between a microsatellite marker of *AT1R* and hypertension in a hypertensive sib-pair study. However, an informative diallelic marker A1166C present in the 3′ untranslated region of *AT1R* was found significantly more frequently in 206 hypertensive subjects than in 298 normotensive control population, suggesting that a variant of AT_1 receptor exerts a small effect on blood pressure (Bonnardeaux et al., 1994).

Other polymorphisms have been described, especially at the promoter region of *AT1R*. However, none of these newly characterized polymorphisms has shown evidence for association with hypertension in a large Caucasian population-based sample (Zhang et al., 2000). Recent studies performed in Finland demonstrate suggestion for linkage at the *AT1R* locus and association with the A1166C polymorphism (Kainulainen et al., 1999; Perola et al., 2000). In 218 Caucasian hypertensive patients, we recently found a positive relationship between the acute blood pressure response to Ang II and *AT1R* (Vuagnat et al., 2001). It is interesting to note that the A1166C polymorphism of *AT1R* has also been associated to essential hypertension aortic stiffness (Benetos et al., 1996), left ventricular mass (Osterop et al., 1998) coronary vasoconstriction (Amant et al, 1997), different responses to Ang II in isolated human arteries (van Geel et al., 2000) and myocardial infarction in interaction with the angiotensin I-converting enzyme insertion/deletion polymorphism (Tiret et al., 1994). However, these associations have been disputed in other studies and no relation was found between AT1R density in platelets and the A1166C genotype (Paillard et al, 1999).

OTHER CANDIDATE GENES

α-Adducin

For more than ten years, the group headed by G Bianchi in Milan has extensively studied the possible role of α and β-adducin genes in rat and human hypertension. We will only summarize here some of the main findings obtained with these genes in relation to blood pressure, the more interested reader being invited to read more complete papers on that matter (Bianchi et al., 1985; 1994). Adducin is a cytoskeletal protein that favors the association between spectrin and actin, but it can also directly interact with actin. Thus, it might be involved in cellular signal transduction and interact with membrane cytoskeletal proteins that affect ion transport across the cell membrane. Adducin is an heterodimeric protein that is composed of three subunits α, β and γ. Each subunit is composed of two distinct domains: a N-terminal globular hydrophobic domain and a C-terminal tail responsible of its interaction with actin and spectrin. The α-adducin gene is located at human chromosome 4p16 and has been originally identified due to its proximity with the gene responsible for Huntington disease. The α-adducin gene is widely expressed, but is predominantly expressed in brain and kidney tissue. The β-adducin gene is 50% identical, and is expressed with different tissue-specific isoforms. Thus, there are physiological quantitative and qualitative differences in assembly of these subunits according to the tissue in which they are expressed.

Bianchi and coworkers made the hypothesis that variations in adducin could lead to variations in the activity of ionic transporters or channels, especially the Na-K-Cl cotransporter in the thick ascending limb and the Na-K-ATPase all along the renal tubule, thus leading to increased salt reabsorption and hypertension. The Milan strain of hypertensive rat (MHS) has characteristics that suggest a renal abnormality of sodium handling: increased glomerular filtration rate during the first weeks of life, low renin status, increased sensitivity to furosemide compared to the normotensive strain (MNS) (Bianchi et al., 1985). Differences in the amino acid sequence of the adducin genes between the MHS and the MNS strains could explain a significant part of the blood pressure difference between these 2 strains (Bianchi et al., 1994). Indeed, two amino acid changes were found in the α (F316Y) and β (Q529R) adducin genes (Bianchi et al., 1994). The transfection of wild or mutant subunits in renal epithelial cells showed that these mutations induce an increased activity of the Na-K pump, thus establishing a pathophysiological link with increased renal sodium handling and with high blood pressure.

In humans, several studies are now concordant and establish a relation between the α-adducin gene and salt-sensitivity and blood pressure, even though its effect is probably mild at the population level. In a study involving French and Italian hypertensive sibpairs, significant linkage was found between several markers surrounding the α-adducin locus and essential hypertension (Casari et al., 1995). A positive association was also found when the authors compared the genotype frequencies of the G460W polymorphism of the α subunit of the adducin gene in 190 hypertensive patients and 126 controls. The blood pressure response to the chronic administration of hydrochlothiazide was also significantly more important in subjects bearing the 460W allele, suggesting that this variant could predispose to salt-sensitivity and to hypertension. Since then, other studies have been performed with conflicting results. The association with low-renin status was recently confirmed in a multicenter international study investigating intermediate phenotypes in hypertension (Grant et al., 2001). The exact importance of the adducin locus in human hypertension will probably require large-scale studies as well as search for interaction with other genes and sodium content of the diet.

G-protein beta3 subunit

Several studies have suggested an increased activity of the sodium-proton exchanger in about 50% of subjects with essential hypertension. An increased ion transport activity has also been found in immortalized lymphoblasts and in fibroblasts from hypertensive subjects that might be due to an altered intercellular signal transduction and enhanced activation of pertussis toxin sensitive G-proteins (Siffert et al., 1995). The heterotrimeric G-proteins are formed by the assembly of several subunits α, β, and γ. After having excluded mutations of several of these subunits, Siffert et al (1998) found a very interesting genetic polymorphism (C825T) in the exon 10 of the gene coding for the β3 subunit (GNB3). This polymorphism is not a missense mutation, but favors the use of an alternative splicing of exon 9 of the gene and thus the expression of a protein with a deletion of 41 amino acids. The statement of the deleted protein in insect cells showed that it was functional but that it presents an enhanced reactivity to pharmacologic activators. Finally, in this pionneering study, the 825T allele was more frequent in 426 hypertensives (0.31) than in 427 controls (0.25), suggesting its role as a susceptibility factor for essential hypertension.

However this association with essential hypertension has been since debated. In a population-based study at Augsburg (Germany) selected from the MONICA survey (Schunkert et al., 1998), the C825T polymorphism showed a weak, albeit significant, association with diastolic blood pressure (CC:88.6 mm Hg, CT:90.1 mm Hg, TT:91.8 mm Hg, $p < 0.02$). Interestingly, plasma renin levels were lower in patients in subjects bearing the 825T allele, suggesting that it might be associated with a low renin profile. An association study performed in 110 Australian white hypertensives, each of whom were the offspring of two hypertensive parents, and 189 controls whose parents were both normotensive beyond the age of 50 years, found a significant difference in the 825T allele frequency (0.43 *versus* 0.25, *p* < 0.001) supporting a role for this variant (Benjafield et al., 1998) contrast, Brand et al. (1999a) analyzed the GNB3 variant in two large case-control studies selected for essential hypertension (PEGASE study) and myocardial infarction (ECTIM study). The odds ratios for hypertension and myocardial infarction associated with T-allele carrying were 1.23 (95% confidence interval, 0.94 to 1.62; *p* = 0.13) and 1.11 (95% confidence interval, 0.88 to 1.39; *p* = 0.37), respectively. There was no association of the GNB3 polymorphism with early onset of hypertension, familial history of hypertension, or blood pressure. In a German case-control study involving 479 hypertensives and 1000 gender and age-matched controls, the 825T allele was associated with an odds ratio of 1.5 (95% CI, 1.1 to 2.2) *versus* non-T carriers for the presence of hypertension (Beige et al., 1999). However, in both the whole group and untreated group, blood pressure levels were virtually identical between the genotypic groups. In a study performed in 447 Indians of the Oji-Cree tribe in Canada, the frequency of the 825T allele was 0.50, much greater than those usually observed in Caucasians (Hegele et al., 1998). Surprisingly, the 825T allele was associated with a lower mean systolic blood pressure (CC: 126.7 mm Hg, CT: 123.5 mm Hg, TT: 119.6 mm Hg, *p* < 0.05) and was not associated with significant difference in diastolic blood pressure. A Japanese study seems to confirm these negative results (Kato et al., 1998). The frequency of the 825T allele was very similar (0.49) in 718 subjects with confirmed essential hypertension, 191 with borderline hypertension and 515 controls, all from the Tokyo aera.

In conclusion, the hypothesis of a genetic polymorphism of the GNB3 subunit favoring high blood pressure is attracting by its possible ubiquitous effect, especially on the vascular tone on the renal sodium handling. In this regard, the measurement of this polymorphism in 197 blacks and 190 non Hispanic whites who underwent a monotherapy with hydrochlorothiazide for four weeks, showed that 825TT homozygotes had greater response of both diastolic and systolic blood pressure than the CC homozygotes (Turner et al., 2001).

Subunits of the epithelial sodium channel

The amiloride-sensitive epithelial Na channel (ENaC) is the rate-limiting step of Na^+ reabsorption by the kidney distal tubule. As discussed in the paragraph on Liddle syndrome, the presence of gain of function mutations in the genes coding for the β and γ ENaC subunits suggests the possibility of more subtle polymorphisms at those genes that might modify ENaC activity, especially in salt-sensitive patients or those with a low-renin profile. Several groups have, therefore, extended the screening for mutations in essential hypertension to β and γENaC. In a series of more than 400 hypertensive subjects, we found seven missense mutations at the gene coding for the βENaC subunit, almost all of them in patients of African descent (Persu et al., 1998). Whereas these variants led to no significant increase in Na^+ current after statement in *Xenopus* oocytes, data obtained in human B lymphocytes (Su et al., 1996) suggest that at least one of them (T594M) could have an effect on Na^+ reabsorption. In a case-control study involving black resident of London, Baker et al. (1998) found a significant increase of the 594M frequency in the 206 hypertensive patients (8.3%) compared to the normotensive subjects (2.1%), the statistical significance persisting after adjustment for sex and body-mass index. In the subset of patients in whom plasma renin activity was measured, the T594M polymorphism was also associated with a low renin profile, suggesting that it could raise blood pressure in affected people by increasing renal tubular sodium reabsorption. However, the impact of this polymorphism is still debated.

Several polymorphisms have also been detected in γEnaC. We found four neutral polymorphisms, three in the third exon of the gene (T387C, T474C, C549T) and one in the last exon (C1990G) (Persu et al., 1999). These four variants had similar frequencies in 453 hypertensive and 245 normotensive Caucasian subjects as well as in patients with low-renin profile. We also found two rare mutations in three hypertensive subjects, 594insP and R631H, that produced no significant increase in Na^+ current in *Xenopus* oocytes. Results obtained by other groups (Melander et al., 1998) confirm that this subunit is infrequently involved in essential hypertension.

The analysis of αEnaC showed an interesting missense polymorphism (W493R) located in the extracellular loop of the subunit and in a rather well conserved sequence not far from the amino acids responsible for the sensitivity to amiloride. However, in Caucasians, this polymorphism was found at similar allele frequency in hypertensive and normotensive individuals and did not change the amiloride-sensitive current when expressed in *Xenopus* oocytes (Corvol et al., 1999). Other polymorphisms, G442V at βENaC and T663A at αENaC have been shown to be associated with changes in the aldosterone/potassium ratio in urine and with essential hypertension (Ambrosius et al., 1999). It is also interesting to note that a sibpair linkage study performed on 286 white Australian families showed significant linkage between systolic blood pressure and microsatellites at chromosome 16p12, located in the vincinity of the genes encoding the β and γ subints of ENaC (Wong et al., 1999).

Other candidate genes

Many other genes can be considered as excellent candidates for essential hypertension. A list of more than 100 genes that may act directly or indirectly on blood pressure is easily established (Table 51.1). Among them are genes coding for proteins of the adrenergic systems (dopamine receptors, α and β adrenergic receptors in particular), for proteins involved in the salt-water homeostasis (natriuretic peptides and their receptors, subunits of the epithelial Na channel, renal transporters, kallikrein-kinin system, etc.), for proteins involved in the hormonal regulation of blood pressure (enzymes and receptors of the mineralo and glucocorticoid pathways), for proteins involved in the structure and/or the regulation of vascular tone (endothelins and their receptors in particular).

It is, of course, not possible to summarize here the studies that have been performed for all these candidate genes, except that none of them has been firmly established as bearing polymorphisms strongly favoring changes in blood pressure. For example, the gene coding for the endothelial cell nitric oxide synthase (*NOS*) was very attractive since nitric oxide plays an important role in regulating blood flow and pressure, and since several reports have suggested that hypertensive subjects have a blunted endothelium-dependent vasodilatation that might be secondary to decreased nitric oxide production. However, linkage and case-control studies performed in French hypertensive and normotensive subjects failed to show association or linkage with essential hypertension (Bonnardeaux et al., 1995), suggesting that common variants of this isoform of nitric oxide synthase are not involved in common hypertension. Similar negative results were obtained in humans for the *SA* locus located (Nabika et al., 1995) that was linked to blood pressure levels in several crosses involving different strains of genetically hypertensive rats (Iwai et al., 1992).

The gene coding for aldosterone synthase (*CYP11B2*) is also an attractive candidate. It has been tested for its possible association with essential hypertension (Brand et al., 1998b; Davies et al., 1999; Komiya et al., 2000) and primary aldosteronism (Mulatero et al., 2000). A polymorphism in the promoter region of the gene (C-344T) is located at a steroidogenic transcription factor SF-1 binding site and could play a role in the statement of the gene. Despite the fact that the Ang II, K⁺ and c-AMP-signaling pathways

utilize *in vitro* a CRE-like cis element and another SF-1 binding site that is located closer to the transcription start to regulate human *CYP11B2*, expression (Clyne et al., 1997), the C-344T polymorphism has been associated with variations in plasma aldosterone (Brand et al., 1998b; Hautanen et al., 1999), suggesting that it could favor sodium retention and high blood pressure. Contradictory results have been obtained according to the populations and the biochemical and clinical parameters studied (Kupari et al., 1998; Hautanen et al., 1999; Schunkert et al., 1999; Tamaki et al., 1999).

Genome-wide scan approach in human essential hypertension

Taking into account the major advances accomplished these last years on the genetic and physical map of the human genome, the genomic-wide scan (GWS) approach becomes another major strategy that could allow the identification of major loci implicated in complex traits. Once the regions of interest have been identified, a systematic analysis of their genes is undertaken, firstly based on their possible function, i.e., positional candidate gene approach (Lander and Schork, 1994). Because it does not make any a priori assumption on the genes to identify, this strategy may be promising for discovering new pathways involved in blood pressure regulation. However, there are strong statistical limits to this approach that have been well delineated by several authors (Lander and Kruglyak, 1995; Schork, 1997; Darvasi, 1998; Rao, 2001). Among them, the problem of power to identify loci that have only a small influence on blood pressure level, the requirement of non parametric methods requiring the use of hundreds of sibpairs and/or particular study designs such as discordant sibpairs, the necessity of adjustment of the statistical significance for multiple testing that might prevent the identification of genes with mild effects on the trait, the requirement of replication of any positive result in another sample with the same characteristics using either the same design or a complementary approach such as family-based association studies or case-control studies, the low power of replication for loci with only a small blood pressure effect, the possible heterogeneity of genes causing essential hypertension according to the ethnic background and confounding factors such as obesity or associated diseases like dyslipidemia and diabetes. Finally, one must be aware that GWS, at least in the first stage, does not take into account the interaction between genes and between genes and environment, which are the mechanisms at work at the phenotypic level.

Table 51.1. A list of 100 candidate genes in human essential hypertension

Gene protein

Genes of the renin angiotensin system
AGT angiotensinogen
REN renin
ACE Angiotensin I converting enzyme, DCP1
AT1R Angiotensin II type 1 receptor
ENEP Aminopeptidase A (EC3.4.11.7)
APN Aminopeptidase N (EC3.4.11.2)

Genes of the adrenergic system
ADRA1a Alpha-adrenergic receptor 1a
ADRA1b Alpha-adrenergic receptor 1b
ADRA1d Alpha-adrenergic receptor 1d
ADRA2b Alpha-adrenergic receptor 2b
ADRB1R B1-adrenergic receptor
ADRBK2 B2-adrenergic receptor
BARK1 Beta adrenergic receptor kinase
DRD1 D1a-Dopamine receptor
DRD1B D1b-Dopamine receptor
DRD2 D2-Dopamine receptor
DRD3 D3-Dopamine receptor
DRD4 D4-Dopamine receptor
DRD5 D5-Dopamine receptor
NPY Neuropeptide Y
NPYY1 Neuropeptide Y receptor Y1
PNMT Phenylethanolamine N-methyl transferase

Genes of the kallikrein kinin system
KNG Kininogen
KLK1 Tissue renal/pancreatic kallikrein
BDKRB1 Bradykinin receptor type 1
BDKRB2 Bradykinin receptor type 2

Genes affecting steroids
CYP11B1 11beta hydroxylase
CYP11B2 aldosterone synthase
CYP17 17-alpha-hydroxylase
CYP21 Steroid 21-hydroxylase
CYP27 Steroid 27-hydroxylase
GRL Glucocorticoid receptor
HSD11B1 11-beta-hydroxysteroid dehydrogenase, type 1
HSD11B2 11-beta-hydroxysteroid dehydrogenase, type 2
MLR Mineralocorticoid receptor

Genes directly related to vascular tone
EDN1 Endothelin 1
EDN2 Endothelin 2
EDN3 Endothelin 3
ENDRA Endothelin A receptor
ENDRB Endothelin B receptor
ECE1 Endothelin Converting Enzyme type 1
ECE2 Endothelin Converting Enzyme type 2
NOS1 Nitric oxide synthase 1
NOS2A Nitric oxide synthase 2a
NOS3 Nitric oxide synthase 3
CACNA1C Calcium channel, L-type, a1c subunit
CACNA1H Calcium channel, T-type, a1H subunit
CACNAB1 Calcium channel, L-type, beta1 subunit
CACNAB2 Calcium channel, L-type, beta 2 subunit
CACNAB3 Calcium channel, L-type, beta 3 subunit

Genes directly affecting the salt-water homeostasis
AVP Arginine vasopressin
AVPR1A Arginine vasopressin receptor 1A
AVPR1B Arginine vasopressin receptor 1B; VIBR
AVPR2 Vasopressin V2 receptor; ADHR
NPPA Atrial natriuretic peptide
NPPB Brain natriuretic peptide
NPPC Natriuretic peptide type C
NPR1 Atrial natriuretic peptide receptor; type A
NPR2 Atrial natriuretic peptide receptor; type B
NPR3 Atrial natriuretic peptide receptor; type C
MME Neutral endopeptidase
AQP1 Aquaporin 1
AQP2 Aquaporin 2
AQP3 Aquaporin 3
AQP4 Aquaporin 4
SCNN1A α subunit of the epithelial Na channel
SCNN1B β subunit of the epithelial Na channel
SCNN1C γ subunit of the epithelial Na channel
CLCN1 Chloride channel 1
CLCN2 Chloride channel 2
CLCN3 Chloride channel 3
CLCN4 Chloride channel 4
CLCN5 Chloride channel 5
CLCN6 Chloride channel 6
CLCN7 Chloride channel 7
CLCNKA Chloride channel Kidney A
CLCNKB Chloride channel Kidney B
AE1 CL/HCO3 exchanger
AEBP1 AE1 binding protein
NHE1 Antiporter, sodium-hydrogen ion, amiloride-sensitive
NHE2 Sodium-hydrogen exchanger, type 3, SLC9A2
NHE3 Sodium-hydrogen exchanger, type 3, SLC9A3
NHE4 Sodium-hydrogen exchanger, type 4, SLC9A4
NHE5 Sodium-hydrogen exchanger, type 5, SLC9A5
NHE6 Sodium-hydrogen exchanger, type 6, SLC9A6
NHERF Sodium-hydrogen exchanger regulatory factor, SLC9A3R1
NBC1 Sodium bicarbonate cotransporter, SLC4A4
ROMK1 Inwardly rectifying potassium channel
ROMK2 Inwardly rectifying potassium channel
SLC12A1 Sodium/potassium:chloride transporter-2; NKCC2
SLC12A2 Sodium/potassium:chloride transporter-1; NKCC1
SLC12A3 Thiazide-sensitive Na-Cl transporter; NCCT

Genes affecting metabolism
INSRα Insulin receptor α
INSRβ Insulin receptor β
IRS-1 Insulin Receptor Substrate 1
LEP Leptin
LEPR Leptin receptor
PTHRP Parathyroid hormon-related protein

Genes affecting the vessel structure
ELN Elastin
LAMB1 Laminin B1
COL3A1 Collagen type3 alpha1
CBP2 Collagen binding protein
FBN1 Fibrillin

Table 51.2. Genome wide linkage analysis in human hypertension

Families	Origin	Trait	Location	References
263 nuclear families	UK	Hypertension	11q	Sharma et al. (2000)
55 families with 427 subjects and 69 highly discordant pairs	USA Rochester	BP	2p22, 5q23 6q23, 15q25	Krushkal et al., (1999)
589 families with 975 parents + 1574 offsprings	USA Rochester	BP	5q33	Bray et al., (2000)
694 subjects from 28 families	USA Amish	BP	2q31–34	Hsueh et al., (2000)
1702 subjects from 332 families	USA Framingham	longitudinal BP	17q12–q21	Levy et al., (2000)
679 individuals from 206 families (125 random, 81 obese)	Canada Quebec	BP	2p11–q12.3 5p, 7q32–q36	Rice et al., (2000)
47 affected sibpairs	Finland	Hypertension	3q, 2q, Xp, 22q, 1q	Perola et al., (2000)

Only studies using either hypertension as a qualitative trait or basal blood pressure as a quantitative trait and performed in Caucasian families are reported

Thus, negative results can be obtained for a locus with a true biological and clinical effect that would be detected only if analyzed in combination with other loci or with environment. Despite these limits, several GWS have been reported recently with interesting although contradictory results. A nonexhaustive summary of these studies is presented next and in Table 51.2.

CAUCASIANS

One of the first GWS to be published was that performed by the group of Boerwinkle based on the Family Heart Program in Rochester Minnesota, that included 3974 subjects from 583 families. A first study (Krushkal et al., 1999) was performed based on the selection of 69 sibling pairs highly discordant for their blood pressure level (above the 80th percentile or below the 20th percentile). Four genomic regions (2p22, 5q33, 6q23, 15q25) were suggested to be linked with systolic blood pressure. In a second study (Bray et al., 2000), the authors analyzed the candidate genes contained in the most promising region (5q33), among them the dopaminergic receptor type IA, the α_{1B} adrenergic receptor, and the β_2 adrenergic receptor. For each of those, an extensive search for polymorphisms was performed followed by the genotyping of the population. Most results did not show any consistent association between these polymorphisms and blood pressure. The polymorphism (Arg16Gly) of the β_2 adrenergic receptor appeared as the most interesting because of its association with significant although minor changes (2 to 3 mm Hg) of systolic blood pressure.

Another study was performed in England on 119 Caucasian families selected on the presence of at least three hypertensive subjects in the same sibship (Sharma et al., 2000). The genome scan used 262 markers and identified a suggestive region on chromosome 11q. However, the analysis of 124 additional families did not confirm that location. A statistical simulation confirmed the genetic complexity of essential hypertension with a multipoint exclusion-linkage analysis showing that at least three genetic loci were necessary to explain the familial aggregation of the trait.

The Amish population seems ideal for genetic studies looking at blood pressure because of the size of the families and of the environment which is more standardized than in the other populations, and which prevents alcohol consumption and obesity. The study reported by Hsueh et al. (2000) involved 694 subjects from 28 families, each containing from 3 to 69 individuals. A total of 357 microsatellite markers have been genotyped in 436 parent-siblings couples, 1326 sibling pairs, 1342 relations between first degree-relatives, and 1311 relation between first cousins. In these families, blood pressure heritability was 0.23 for systolic and 0.29 for diastolic, estimations similar to what has been generally observed in the literature. The only region that was linked without ambiguity to the trait was located in 2q31–34 with lod scores of 1.64 for systolic and of 3.36 for diastolic blood pressure.

One of the most recently published GWS is also probably one of the most convincing (Levy et al., 2000). It was performed on 1702 subjects from 332 families selected from the Framingham survey. For each individual, blood pressure was measured at least three times over a period of at least ten years. The trait was corresponding to the blood pressure averaged on this duration and adjusted for age and body-mass-index. A 10-cM genome scan was performed that allowed the analysis of the following relative pairs: 1545 sibling pairs, 933 parent-offsprings pairs, 742 cousin pairs, and 468 pairs of other first-degree relatives. The statistical analysis showed only one region of interest – chromosome 9 – for diastolic blood pressure. For systolic blood pressure, a suggestion for linkage was found for several regions on chromosomes 5, 10 and 17. On chromosome, two regions were suggested, with the one located on 17q12–21 giving the most promising multipoint lodscore (4.7).

This chromosome 17 region corresponds with what was also found by Julier et al., (1997). In this study involving French hypertensive sibpairs, French diabetic pairs with hypertension and UK families, significative linkage and association was found using markers of the same region that contains the ACE locus at its telomeric end. However, no particular gene has been proven as the one responsible for this statistical association, yet. Other arguments make this region of interest. First, it corresponds to the chromosome 10 region in the rat genome, a region that has been shown by two groups as containing a major locus, explaining up to 20% of the blood pressure variance in the stroke-prone SHR rats compared to its normotensive counterpart WKY rats (Hilbert et al., 1991; Jacob et al., 1991). Second, it is also a region containing one of the genes responsible for pseudohypoaldosteronism (*PHA2B*), an autosomal dominant hypertensive condition associated with hyperkalemia despite normal glomerular function (Mansfield et al., 1997). Finally, a missense polymorphism (Gly40Ser) at the glucagon receptor gene located at 17q25 has been associated with hypertension, with an allele frequency of 0.08 in a limited set of Caucasian hypertensives who have two hypertensive parents compared to only 0.01 in normotensive controls (Morris and Chambers, 1996). This polymorphism was not significantly associated with hypertension in the overall sample of 741 French hypertensive subjects compared to 412 controls (Brand et al., 1999b).

The Finnish Twin Cohort Study has also been used for a genome scan analysis of blood pressure (Perola et al., 2000). The strategy was to study a limited number of pairs with a early onset phenotype (mean at discovery 38.3 years) and to diminish the effect of possible confounding factors (at least one sib with body mass index < 27 Kg/m², exclusion of diabetes). Only 47 sibpairs were studied, 36 dizygotic twins, 11 non-twin siblings, in the stage 1 of the analysis. In stage 2, genotyping was focused on the regions of suggestive linkage with the addition of all available family members of the 47 probands (total of 138 subjects). Despite these relatively small numbers, several regions gave a maximum likelihood score > 1.5 (1q, 2q, 22q and Xp). The most

significative result was obtained on chromosome 3q21–25 (MLS=3.38 on the entire sample). This region contains the AT1 receptor gene, and the stronger result was obtained with the intragenic CA repeat at this locus. An analysis of candidate genes in a German population, using blood pressure as a quantitative trait also suggested linkage with the AT1 receptor gene (Nagy et al., 1999).

A GWS was also performed in 125 random and 81 obese families participating in the Québec Family Study (Rice et al., 2000). Multiple linkage regions were suggested for systolic blood pressure, especially on chromosomes 1p, 2p, 5p, 7q, 8q, 19p. One of the main interests of this study was to show the importance of gene-gene or gene-environment interactions, suggested by the fact that most of the regions that were suggested in lean families did not show any linkage when analyzed in families in which one or more members had a body-mass-index > 32 kg/m².

ASIAN

A remarkable effort has been made by Xu and colleagues (1997) to characterize a large population from the Anqing region in China. A GWS using 367 markers was performed in extreme sib pairs (207 discordant, 258 high concordant, and 99 low concordant), selected from a blood-pressure screen of >200,000 Chinese adults, comprises rare but highly efficient extreme sib pairs (207 discordant, 258 high concordant, and 99 low concordant) (Xu et al., 1999). Although no regions achieved a 5% genome wide significance level, maximum LOD-score values were >2.0 (unadjusted $P< 0.001$) for five markers (D3S2387, D11S2019, D15S657, D16S3396, and D17S1303). It was interesting to observe that the suggestive regions were depending on the comparison design and were different for systolic and diastolic blood pressure. By refining the trait definition and genotyping additional markers, the authors highlighted a region on chromosome 15q with a maximum lod score of 3.8 near D15S203 in lower extreme diastolic blood pressure sibling pairs (Xu et al., 1999).

DISCUSSION

These first attempts to identify by a random screening approach genes influencing blood pressure level have the merit to show the difficulty of such strategy. The absence of replication from one sample to another demonstrate the importance of ascertainment methods and possibly the fact that there is no major gene regulating the trait but rather many genes with mild effects that may play a role on basal blood pressure or its evolution with age, reactivity at different stimuli or complications. In this regard, the GWS analysis of pulse pressure in 10 families (440 individuals) in the San Antonio Family Heart Study showed an heritability of 0.21 and suggested four regions, on chromosomes 21, 7, 8 and 18 (Atwood et al., 2001). A suggestive evidence for linkage on chromosome 18q was found with postural systolic blood pressure in 498 white sibling pairs from the Hypertension Genetic Epidemiology Network (Pankow et al, 2000). Using creatinine clearance measurements in a large biracial sample of hypertensive siblings (466 African American subjects and 634 white subjects) from the same network, DeWan et al. (2001) showed that a locus on chromosome 3q may contribute to the degradation of renal function. The careful characterization of intermediate biological and clinical phenotypes and of cardiovascular endpoints in a very large number of hypertensive families will probably highlight the importance of genes not directly to blood pressure level but rather to its regulation and complications.

contributions of several candidate genes to blood pressure variance, the search for major genes contributing to the trait with the temporary (but perhaps definitive) conclusion that there is no major gene explaining high blood pressure in the population. Whereas all these studies need to be confirmed and extended, several main new challenges, among others, will be faced in the first decades of this new millennium that will require using all the tools of modern biological technology: (1) will we be able to subdivide the hypertensive population using genotypes in addition to the classical clinical and biochemical parameters in order to better understand the pathophysiology of hypertension in day-to-day practice, and better predict the risk of cardiovascular events; (2) will we be able to invent new biostatistical tools that will help to identify not only one locus at a time but a combination of interacting genes that are associated in the general population with blood pressure; and (3) will pharmacogenomics predict the risk of side-effects and the efficacy of a particular drug together with the development of new molecular targets.

Conclusion

Molecular genetic studies have revolutionized the physiological approach to arterial hypertension. In the last ten years, they have enabled the identification of most of the mendelian forms of hypertension, the evaluation of the

Acknowledgement

This work was supported by grants from INSERM, Collège de France, Bristol-Myers Squibb, Association Claude Bernard and Association Naturalia and Biologia.

REFERENCES

Alhenc-Gelas F, Richard J, Courbon D, Warnet JM, Corvol P (1991) Distribution of plasma angiotensin I-converting enzyme levels in healthy men: Relationship to environmental and hormonal parameters. J Lab Clin Med 117(1):33–39

Amant C, Hamon M, Bauters C, Richard F, Helbecque N, McFadden EP et al. (1997) The angiotensin II type 1 receptor gene polymorphism is associated with coronary artery vasoconstriction. J Am Coll Cardiol 29:486–490

Ambrosius WT, Bloem LJ, Zhou L, Rebhun JF, Snyder PM, Wagner MA et al. (1999) Genetic variants in the epithelial sodium channel in relation to aldosterone and potassium excretion and risk for hypertension. Hypertension 34(4 Pt 1):631–637

Arngrimsson R, Purandare S, Connor M, Walker JJ, Bjornsson S, Soubrier F et al. (1993) Angiotensinogen: A candidate gene involved in preeclampsia? Nat Genet 4(2):114–115

Arngrimsson R, Sigurard ttir S, Frigge ML, Bjarnad ttir RI, Jonsson T, Stefansson H et al. (1999) A genome-wide scan reveals a maternal susceptibility locus for pre-eclampsia on chromosome 2p13. Hum Mol Genet 8(9):1799–1805

Atwood LD, Kammerer CM, Samollow PB, Hixson JE, Shade RE, MacCluer JW (1997) Linkage of essential hypertension to the angiotensinogen locus in Mexican Americans. Hypertension 30(3 Pt 1):326–330

Atwood LD, Samollow PB, Hixson JE, Stern MP, MacCluer JW (2001) Genome-wide linkage analysis of pulse pressure in Mexican Americans. Hypertension 37 [part 2]:425–428

Azizi M, Hallouin MC, Jeunemaitre X, Guyene T-T, Menard J (2000) Influence of the M235T polymorphism of human angiotensinogen (AGT) on plasma AGT and renin concentrations after ethinylestradiol administration. J Clin Endocrinol Metab 85:4331–4337

Baker EH, Dong YB, Sagnella GA, Rothwell M, Onipinla AK, Markandu ND et al. (1998) Association of hypertension with T594M mutation in beta subunit of epithelial sodium channels in black people resident in London. Lancet 351(9113):1388–1392

Beige J, Hohenbleicher H, Distler A, Sharma AM (1999) G-Protein beta3 subunit C825T variant and ambulatory blood pressure in essential hypertension. Hypertension 33(4):1049–1051

Benjafield AV, Jeyasingam CL, Nyholt DR, Griffiths LR, Morris BJ (1998) G-protein beta3 subunit gene (GNB3) variant in causation of essential hypertension. Hypertension 32(6):1094–1097

Benetos A, Ricard S, Topouchian J, Asmar R, Poirier O, Larosa E et al. (1996) Influence of angiotensin-converting enzyme and angiotensin II type I receptor gene polymorphisms on aortic stiffness in normotensive and hypertensive patients. Circulation 94:698–703

Bernstein IM, Ziegler W, Stirewalt WS et al. (1998) Angiotensinogen genotype and plasma volume in nulligravid women. Obstet Gynecol 92:171–173

Bianchi G, Ferrari P, Trizio D, Ferrandi M, Torielli L, Barber BR et al. (1985) Red blood cell abnormalities and spontaneous hypertension in the rat. A genetically determined link. Hypertension 7(3 Pt 1):319–325

Bianchi G, Tripodi G, Casari G, Salardi S, Barber BR, Garcia R et al. (1994) Two point mutations within the adducin genes are involved in blood pressure variation. Proc Natl Acad Sci USA 91(9):3999–4003

Bilginturan N, Zileli S, Karacadag S, Pirnar T (1973) Hereditary brachydactyly associated with hypertension. J Med Genet 10(3):253–259

Bloem LJ, Manatunga AK, Tewksbury DA, Pratt JH (1995) The serum angiotensinogen concentration and variants of the angiotensinogen gene in white and black children. J Clin Invest 95(3):948–953

Bonnardeaux A, Davies E, Jeunemaitre X, Fery I, Charru A, Clauser E et al. (1994) Angiotensin II type 1 receptor gene polymorphisms in human essential hypertension. Hypertension 24(1):63–69

Bonnardeaux A, Nadaud S, Charru A, Jeunemaitre X, Corvol P, Soubrier F (1995) Lack of evidence for linkage of the endothelial cell nitric oxide synthase gene to essential hypertension. Circulation 91(1):96–102

Botero-Velez M, Curtis JJ, Warnock DG (1994) Brief report: Liddle's syndrome revisited—a disorder of sodium reabsorption in the distal tubule. N Engl J Med 330(3):178–181

Brand E, Chatelain N, Keavney B, Caulfield M, Citterio L, Connell J et al. (1998a) Evaluation of the angiotensinogen locus in human essential hypertension: a European study. Hypertension 31(3):725–729

Brand E, Chatelain N, Mulatero P, Fery I, Curnow K, Jeunemaitre X et al. (1998b) Structural analysis and evaluation of the aldosterone synthase gene in hypertension. Hypertension 32(2):198–204

Brand E, Bankir L, Plouin PF, Soubrier F (1999a) Glucagon receptor gene mutation (Gly40Ser) in human essential hypertension: The PEGASE study. Hypertension 34(1):15–17

Brand E, Herrmann SM, Nicaud V, Ruidavets JB, Evans A, Arveiler D et al. (1999b) The 825C/T polymorphism of the G-protein subunit beta3 is not related to hypertension. Hypertension 33(5):1175–1178

Bray MS, Krushkal J, Li L, Ferrell R, Kardia S, Sing CF et al. (2000) Positional genomic analysis identifies the beta(2)-adrenergic receptor gene as a susceptibility locus for human hypertension. Circulation 101(25):2877–2882

Brunner HR, Laragh JH, Baer L, Newton MA, Goodwin FT, Krakoff LR et al. (1972) Essential hypertension: Renin and aldosterone, heart attack and stroke. N Engl J Med 286(9):441–449

Cambien F, Alhenc-Gelas F, Herbeth B, Andre JL, Rakotovao R, Gonzales MF et al. (1988) Familial resemblance of plasma angiotensin-converting enzyme level: the Nancy Study. Am J Hum Genet 43(5):774–780

Canessa CM, Schild L, Buell G, Thorens B, Gautschi I, Horisberger JD et al. (1994) Amiloride-sensitive epithelial Na+ channel is made of three homologous subunits. Nature 367(6462):463–467

Casari G, Barlassina C, Cusi D, Zagato L, Muirhead R, Righetti M et al. (1995) Association of the alpha-adducin locus with essential hypertension. Hypertension 25(3):320–326

Caulfield M, Lavender P, Farrall M, Munroe P, Lawson M, Turner P et al. (1994) Linkage of the angiotensinogen gene to essential hypertension. N Engl J Med 330(23):1629–1633

Caulfield M, Lavender P, Newell-Price J, Farrall M, Kamdar S, Daniel H et al. (1995) Linkage of the angiotensinogen gene locus to human essential hypertension in African Caribbeans. J Clin Invest 96(2):687–692

Caulfield M, Lavender P, Newell-Price J, Kamdar S, Farrall M, Clark AJ (1996) Angiotensinogen in human essential hypertension. Hypertension 28(6):1123–1125

Chang SS, Grunder S, Hanukoglu A, Rosler A, Mathew PM, Hanukoglu I et al. (1996) Mutations in subunits of the epithelial sodium channel cause salt wasting with hyperkalaemic acidosis, pseudohypoaldosteronism type 1. Nat Genet 12(3):248–253

Clyne CD, Zhang Y, Slutsker L, Mathis JM, White PC, Rainey WE (1997) Angiotensin II and potassium regulate human CYP11B2 transcription through common cis-elements. Mol Endocrinol 11(5):638–649

Cohen-Haguenauer O, Soubrier F, N'Guyene VC, Serero S, Turleau C, Jegou C et al. (1983) Regional mapping of the human renin gene to 1q32 by in situ hybridization. Ann Genet (Paris) 32:16–20

Cooper DW, Hill JA, Chesley LC, Bryans CI (1988) Genetic control of susceptibility to eclampsia and miscarriage. Br J Obstet Gynaecol 95(7):644–653

Corvol P, Jeunemaitre X (1997) Molecular genetics of human hypertension: Role of angiotensinogen. Endocr Rev 18(5):662–677

Corvol P, Soubrier F, Jeunemaitre X (1996) Molecular genetics of hypertension. In Rimoin DL, Connor JM, Pyeritz RE, Emery AEH (eds): Principles and Practice of Medical Genetics, 3E. Churchill Livingstone, NY, pp. 899–908

Corvol P, Soubrier F, Jeunemaitre X (1997) Molecular genetics of the renin-angiotensin-aldosterone system in human hypertension. Pathol Biol (Paris) 45(3):229–239

Corvol P, Persu A, Gimenez-Roqueplo AP, Jeunemaitre X (1999) Seven lessons from two candidate genes in human essential hypertension: Angiotensinogen and epithelial sodium channel. Hypertension 33(6):1324–1331

Costerousse O, Allegrini J, Lopez M, Alhenc-Gelas F (1993) Angiotensin I-converting enzyme in human circulating mononuclear cells: Genetic polymorphism of expression in T-lymphocytes. Biochem J 290(Pt 1):33–40

Curnow KM, Pascoe L, White PC (1992) Genetic analysis of the human type-1 angiotensin II receptor. Mol Endocrinol 6(7):1113–1118

Curnow KM, Mulatero P, Emeric-Blanchouin N, Aupetit-Faisant B, Corvol P, Pascoe L (1997) The amino acid substitutions Ser288Gly and Val320Ala convert the cortisol producing enzyme, CYP11B1, into an aldosterone producing enzyme. Nat Struct Biol 4(1):32–35

Danser AH, Schunkert H (2000) Renin-angiotensin system gene polymorphisms: Potential mechanisms for their association with cardiovascular diseases. Eur J Pharmacol 410(2–3):303–316

Darvasi A (1998) Experimental strategies for the genetic dissection of complex traits in animal models. Nat Genet 18(1):19–24

Davies E, Bonnardeaux A, Plouin PF, Corvol P, Clauser E (1997) Somatic mutations of the angiotensin II (AT1) receptor gene are not present in aldosterone-producing adenoma. J Clin Endocrinol Metab 82(2):611–615

Davies E, Holloway CD, Ingram MC, Inglis GC, Friel EC, Morrison C et al. (1999) Aldosterone excretion rate and blood pressure in essential hypertension are related to polymorphic differences in the aldosterone synthase gene CYP11B2. Hypertension 33(2):703–707

DeWan AT, Arnett DK, Atwood LD, Province MA, Lewis CE, Hunt SC et al. (2001) A genome scan for renal function among hypertensives: The HyperGEN study. Am J Hum Genet 68(1):136–144

Disse-Nicodeme S, Achard JM, Desitter I, Houot AM, Fournier A, Corvol P et al. (2000) A new locus on chromosome 12p13.3 for pseudohypoaldosteronism type II, an autosomal dominant form of hypertension. Am J Hum Genet 67(2):302–310

Dluhy RG, Lifton RP (1995) Glucocorticoid-remediable aldosteronism (GRA): Diagnosis, variability of phenotype and regulation of potassium homeostasis. Steroids 60(1):48–51

Dominiczak AF, Clark JS, Jeffs B, Anderson NH, Negrin CD, Lee WK et al. (1998) Genetics of experimental hypertension. J Hypertens 16(12 Pt 2):1859–1869

Fasola AF, Martz BL, Helmer OM (1968) Plasma renin activity during supine exercice in offsprings of hypertensive parents. J Appl Physiol 25:410–415

Firsov D, Schild L, Gautschi I, Merillat AM, Schneeberger E, Rossier BC (1996) Cell surface expression of the epithelial Na channel and a mutant causing Liddle syndrome: A quantitative approach. Proc Natl Acad Sci USA 93(26):15370–15375

Fornage M, Amos CI, Kardia S, Sing CF, Turner ST, Boerwinkle E (1998) Variation in the region of the angiotensin-converting enzyme gene influences interindividual differences in blood pressure levels in young white males. Circulation 97(18):1773–1779

Furuta H, Guo DF, Inagami T (1992) Molecular cloning and sequencing of the gene encoding human angiotensin II type I receptor. Biochem Biophys Res Commun 183(1):8–13

Gaillard I, Clauser E, Corvol P (1989) Structure of human angiotensinogen gene. DNA 8(2):87–99

Gaillard-Sanchez I, Mattei MG, Clauser E, Corvol P (1990) Assignment by in situ hybridization of the angiotensionogen gene to chromosome band 1q4, the same region as the human renin gene. Hum Genet 84(4):341–343

Geller DS, Farhi A, Pinkerton N, Fradley M, Moritz M, Spitzer A et al. (2000) Activating mineralocorticoid receptor mutation in hypertension exacerbated by pregnancy. Science 289(5476):119–123

Gimenez-Roqueplo AP, Celerier J, Schmid G et al. (1998) Role of cysteine residues in human angiotensinogen. Cys232 is required for angiotensinogen-pro major basic protein complex formation. J Biol Chem 273:3448–3487

Gordon RD, Klemm SA, Tunny TJ, Stowasser M (1995) Gordonis syndrome: A sodium-volume-dependent form of hypertension with a genetic basis. In Laragh JH and Brenner BM (eds): Hypertension: Pathophysiology, Diagnosis and Management. Second Edition. Raven Press, NY, Chapter 125

Grant FD, Romero J, Jeunemaitre X, Hunt SC, Hopkins PN, Hollenberg NH et al. (2001) A homozygous alpha-adducin polymorphism (460Trp) is associated with salt-sensitivity and low renin hypertension in humans. J Hypertens (in press)

Grim CE, Luft FC, Miller JZ, Rose RJ, Christian JC, Weinberger MH (1980) An approach to the evaluation of genetic influences on factors that regulate arterial blood pressure in man. Hypertension 2[suppl2]:1–34–1–42

Guo G, Wilton AN, Fu Y, Qiu H, Brennecke SP, Cooper DW (1997) Angiotensinogen gene variation in a population case-control study of preeclampsia/eclampsia in Australians and Chinese. Electrophoresis 18(9):1646–1649

Guo G, Lade JA, Wilton AN, Moses EK, Grehan M, Fu Y et al. (1999) Genetic susceptibility to preeclampsia and chromosome 7q36. Hum Genet 105(6):641–647

Hansson JH, Nelson-Williams C, Suzuki H, Schild L, Shimkets R, Lu Y et al. (1995) Hypertension caused by a truncated epithelial sodium channel gamma subunit: genetic heterogeneity of Liddle syndrome. Nat Genet 11(1):76–82

Harrap SB, Davidson HR, Connor JM, Soubrier F, Corvol P, Fraser R et al. (1993) The angiotensin I converting enzyme gene and predisposition to high blood pressure. Hypertension 21(4):455–460

Harrison GA, Humphrey KE, Jones N, Badenhop R, Guo G, Elakis G et al. (1997) A genomewide linkage study of preeclampsia/eclampsia reveals evidence for a candidate region on 4q. Am J Hum Genet 60(5):1158–1167

Hata A, Namikawa C, Sasaki M, Sato K, Nakamura T, Tamura K et al. (1994) Angiotensinogen as a risk factor for essential hypertension in Japan. J Clin Invest 93(3):1285–1287

Hautanen A, Toivanen P, Manttari M, Tenkanen L, Kupari M, Manninen V et al. (1999) Joint effects of an aldosterone synthase (CYP11B2) gene polymorphism and classic risk factors on risk of myocardial infarction. Circulation 100(22):2213–2218

Hautanena A, Lankinen L, Kupari M, Janne OA, Adlercreutz H, Nikkila H et al. (1998) Associations between aldosterone synthase gene polymorphism and the adrenocortical function in males. J Intern Med 244(1):11–18

Hegele RA, Harris SB, Hanley AJ, Cao H, Zinman B (1998) G protein beta3 subunit gene variant and blood pressure variation in Canadian Oji-Cree. Hypertension 32(4):688–692

Higashimori K, Zhao Y, Higaki J, Kamitani A, Katsuya T, Nakura J et al. (1993) Association analysis of a polymorphism of the angiotensin converting enzyme gene with essential hypertension in the Japanese population. Biochem Biophys Res Commun 191(2):399–404

Hilbert P, Lindpaintner K, Beckmann JS, Serikawa T, Soubrier F, Dubay C et al. (1991) Chromosomal mapping of two genetic loci associated with blood-pressure regulation in hereditary hypertensive rats. Nature 353(6344):521–529

Howard TE, Shai SY, Langford KG, Martin BM, Bernstein KE. (1990) Transcription of testicular angiotensin-converting enzyme (ACE) is initiated within the 12th intron of the somatic ACE gene. Mol Cell Biol 10(8):4294–4302

Hsueh WC, Mitchell BD, Schneider JL, Wagner MJ, Bell CJ, Nanthakumar E et al. (2000) QTL influencing blood pressure maps to the region of PPH1 on chromosome 2q31–34 in Old Order Amish. Circulation 101(24):2810–2816

Hubert C, Houot AM, Corvol P, Soubrier F (1991) Structure of the angiotensin I-converting enzyme gene. Two alternate promoters correspond to evolutionary steps of a duplicated gene. J Biol Chem 266(23):15377–15383

Inoue I, Nakajima T, Williams CS, Quackenbush J, Puryear R, Powers M et al. (1997) A nucleotide substitution in the promoter of human angiotensinogen is associated with essential hypertension and affects basal transcription in vitro. J Clin Invest 99(7):1786–1797

Ishikawa K, Baba S, Katsuya T, Iwai N, Asai T, Fukuda M et al. (2001) T+31C polymorphism of angiotensinogen gene and essential hypertension. Hypertension 37:281–285

Iwai N, Inagami T (1992) Identification of a candidate gene responsible for the high blood pressure of spontaneously hypertensive rats. J Hypertens 10(10):1155–1157

Iwai N, Ohmichi N, Nakamura Y, Mitsunnami X, Kinoshita M (1994) Molecular variants of the angiotensinogen gene and hypertension in a Japanese population. Hypertens Res 17:117–121

Jacob HJ, Lindpaintner K, Lincoln SE, Kusumi K, Bunker RK, Mao YP et al. (1991) Genetic mapping of a gene causing hypertension in the stroke-prone spontaneously hypertensive rat. Cell 67(1):213–224

Jeunemaitre X, Rigat B, Charru A, Houot AM, Soubrier F, Corvol P (1992a) Sib pair linkage analysis of renin gene haplotypes in human essential hypertension. Hum Genet 88(3):301–306

Jeunemaitre X, Lifton RP, Hunt SC, Williams RR, Lalouel JM (1992b) Absence of linkage between the angiotensin converting enzyme locus and human essential hypertension. Nat Genet 1(1):72–75

Jeunemaitre X, Soubrier F, Kotelevtsev YV, Lifton RP, Williams CS, Charru A et al. (1992c) Molecular basis of human hypertension: Role of angiotensinogen. Cell 71(1):169–180

Jeunemaitre X, Charru A, Pascoe L, Guyene TT, Aupetit-Faisant B, Shackleton CH et al. (1995) [Hyperaldosteronism sensitive to dexamethasone with adrenal adenoma. Clinical, biological and genetic study]. Presse Med 24(27):1243–1248

Jeunemaitre X, Bassilana F, Persu A, Dumont C, Champigny G, Lazdunski M et al. (1997a) Genotype-phenotype analysis of a newly discovered family with Liddle's syndrome. J Hypertens. 15(10):1091–1100

Jeunemaitre X, Inoue I, Williams C, Charru A, Tichet J, Powers M et al. (1997b) Haplotypes of angiotensinogen in essential hypertension. Am J Hum Genet 60(6):1448–1460

Jeunemaitre X, Gimenez-Roqueplo AP, Celerier J, Soubrier F, Corvol P (1999) Angiotensinogen and hypertension. In Dominiczak AF, Connell JMC, Soubrier F, Molecular Genetics of Hypertension. (eds): BIOS Scientific Oxford, pp. 201–230

Jonsson JR, Klemm SA, Tunny TJ, Stowasser M, Gordon RD (1995) A new genetic test for familial hyperaldosteronism type I aids in the detection of curable hypertension. Biochem Biophys Res Commun 207(2):565–571

Julier C, Delepine M, Keavney B, Terwilliger J, Davis S, Weeks DE et al. (1997) Genetic susceptibility for human familial essential hypertension in a region of homology with blood pressure linkage on rat chromosome 10. Hum Mol Genet 6(12):2077–2085

Kainulainen K, Perola M, Terwilliger J, Kaprio J, Koskenvuo M, Syvanen AC et al. (1999) Evidence for involvement of the type I angiotensin II receptor locus in essential hypertension. Hypertension 33(3):844–849

Kamitani A, Rakugi H, Higaki J, Yi Z, Mikami H, Miki T et al. (1994) Association analysis of a polymorphism of the angiotensinogen gene with essential hypertension in Japanese. J Hum Hypertens 8(7):521–524

Kato N, Sugiyama T, Morita H, Kurihara H, Yamori Y, Yazaki Y (1998) G protein beta3 subunit variant and essential hypertension in Japanese. Hypertension 32(5):935–938

Kim HS, Krege JH, Kluckman KD, Hagaman JR, Hodgin JB, Best CF et al. (1995) Genetic control of blood pressure and the angiotensinogen locus. Proc Natl Acad Sci U S A 92(7):2735–2739

Kobashi G (1995) A case-control study of pregnancy-induced hypertension with a genetic predisposition: association of a molecular variant of angiotensinogen in the Japanese women. Hokaido Igaku Zaosshi 70:649–657

Komiya I, Yamada T, Takara M, Asawa T, Shimabukuro M, Nishimori T et al. (2000) Lys(173)Arg and—344T/C variants of CYP11B2 in Japanese patients with low-renin hypertension. Hypertension 35(3):699–703

Krushkal J, Ferrell R, Mockrin SC, Turner ST, Sing CF, Boerwinkle E (1999) Genome-wide linkage analyses of systolic blood pressure using highly discordant siblings. Circulation 99(11):1407–1410

Kumar RS, Thekkumkara TJ, Sen GC (1991) The mRNAs encoding the two angiotensin-converting isozymes are transcribed from the same gene by a tissue-specific choice of alternative transcription initiation sites. J Biol Chem 266(6):3854–3862

Kunz R, Kreutz R, Beige J, Distler A, Sharma AM (1997) Association between the angiotensinogen 235T-variant and essential hypertension in whites: A systematic review and methodological appraisal. Hypertension 30(6):1331–1337

Kupari M, Hautanen A, Lankinen L, Koskinen P, Virolainen J, Nikkila H et al. (1998) Associations between human aldosterone synthase (CYP11B2) gene polymorphisms and left ventricular size, mass, and function. Circulation 97(6):569–575

Lafferty AR, Torpy DJ, Stowasser M, Taymans SE, Lin JP, Huggard P et al. (2000) A novel genetic locus for low renin hypertension: Familial hyperaldosteronism type II maps to chromosome 7 (7p22). J Med Genet 37(11):831–835

Lander ES, Schork NJ (1994) Genetic dissection of complex traits. Science 265(5181):2037–2048

Lander E, Kruglyak L (1995) Genetic dissection of complex traits: Guidelines for interpreting and reporting linkage results. Nat Genet 11(3):241–247

Levy D, DeStefano AL, Larson MG, O'Donnell CJ, Lifton RP, Gavras H et al. (2000) Evidence for a gene influencing blood pressure on chromosome 17: genome scan linkage results for longitudinal blood pressure phenotypes in subjects from the Framingham heart study. Hypertension 36(4):477

Liddle G, Bledsoe T et al. (1963) A familial renal disorder simulating primary aldosteronism byt with negligible aldosterone secretion. Trans Assoc Am Phys 76:199–213

Lifton RP, Dluhy RG, Powers M, Rich GM, Cook S, Ulick S et al. (1992) A chimeric 11 beta-hydroxylase/aldosterone synthase gene causes glucocorticoid-remediable aldosteronism and human hypertension. Nature 355(6357):262–265

Lifton RP (1996) Molecular genetics of human blood pressure variation. Science 272(5262):676–680

Liston WA, Kilpatrick DC (1991) Is genetic susceptibility to pre-eclampsia conferred by homozygosity for the same single recessive gene in mother and fetus? Br J Obstet Gynaecol 98(11):1079–1086

Luft FC (1998) Molecular genetics of human hypertension. J Hypertens 16(12 Pt 2):1871–1878

Mansfield TA, Simon DB, Farfel Z, Bia M, Tucci JR, Lebel M et al. (1997) Multilocus linkage of familial hyperkalaemia and hypertension, pseudohypoaldosteronism type II, to chromosomes 1q31–42 and 17p11–q21. Nat Genet 16(2):202–205

Melander O, Orho M, Fagerudd J, Bengtsson K, Groop PH, Mattiasson I et al. (1998) Mutations and variants of the epithelial sodium channel gene in Liddle's syndrome and primary hypertension. Hypertension 31(5):1118–1124

Morgan L, Baker P, Pipkin FB, Kalsheker N (1995) Pre-eclampsia and the angiotensinogen gene. Br J Obst Gynaecol 102:489–490

Morgan T, Craven C, Nelson L, Lalouel JM, Ward K (1997) Angiotensinogen T235 expression is elevated in decidual spiral arteries. J Clin Invest 100(6):1406–1415

Morineau G, Marc JM, Boudi A, Galons H, Gourmelen M, Corvol P et al. (1999) Genetic, biochemical, and clinical studies of patients with A328V or R213C mutations in 11betaHSD2 causing apparent mineralocorticoid excess. Hypertension 34(3):435–441

Morise T, Takeuchi Y, Takeda R (1995) Rapid detection and prevalence of the variants of the angiotensinogen gene in patients with essential hypertension. J Intern Med 237(2):175–180

Morris BJ, Chambers SM (1996) Hypothesis: glucagon receptor glycine to serine missense mutation contributes to one in 20 cases of essential hypertension. Clin Exp Pharmacol Physiol 23(12):1035–1037

Morris BJ, Griffiths LR (1988) Frequency in hypertensives of alleles for a RFLP associated with the renin gene. Biochem Biophys Res Commun 150:219–224

Morris BJ, Zee RY, Schrader AP (1994) Different frequencies of angiotensin-converting enzyme genotypes in older hypertensive individuals. J Clin Invest 94(3):1085–1089

Moses EK, Lade JA, Guo G, Wilton AN, Grehan M, Freed K et al. (2000) A genome scan in families from Australia and New Zealand confirms the presence of a maternal susceptibility locus for pre-eclampsia, on chromosome 2. Am J Hum Genet 67(6):1581–1585

Mulatero P, Curnow KM, Aupetit-Faisant B, Foekling M, Gomez-Sanchez C, Veglio F et al. (1998) Recombinant CYP11B genes encode enzymes that can catalyze conversion of 11-deoxycortisol to cortisol, 18-hydroxycortisol, and 18-oxocortisol. J Clin Endocrinol Metab 83(11):3996–4001

Mulatero P, Schiavone D, Fallo F, Rabbia F, Pilon C, Chiandussi L et al. (2000) CYP11B2 gene polymorphisms in idiopathic hyperaldosteronism. Hypertension 35(3):694–698

Mullins JJ, Peters J, Ganten D (1990) Fulminant hypertension in transgenic rats harbouring the mouse Ren-2 gene. Nature 344(6266):541–544

Mune T, Rogerson FM, Nikkila H, Agarwal AK, White PC (1995) Human hypertension caused by mutations in the kidney isozyme of 11 beta-hydroxysteroid dehydrogenase. Nat Genet 10(4):394–399

Nabika T, Bonnardeaux A, James M, Julier C, Jeunemaitre X, Corvol P et al. (1995) Evaluation of the SA locus in human hypertension. Hypertension 25(1):6–13

Nagy Z, Busjahn A, Bahring S, Faulhaber HD, Gohlke HR, Knoblauch H et al. (1999) Quantitative trait loci for blood pressure exist near the IGF-1, the Liddle syndrome, the angiotensin II-receptor gene and the renin loci in man. J Am Soc Nephrol 10(8):1709–1716

Naraghi R, Schuster H, Toka HR, Bahring S, Toka O, Oztekin O et al. (1997) Neurovascular compression at the ventrolateral medulla in autosomal dominant hypertension and brachydactyly. Stroke 28(9):1749–1754

Niu T, Xu X, Rogus J, Zhou Y, Chen C, Yang J et al. (1998) Angiotensinogen gene and hypertension in Chinese. J Clin Invest 101(1):188–194

Niu T, Yang J, Wang B, Chen W, Wang Z, Laird N et al. (1999) Angiotensinogen gene polymorphisms M235T/T174M: No excess transmission to hypertensive Chinese. Hypertension 33(2):698–702

O'Donnell CJ, Lindpaintner K, Larson MG, Rao VS, Ordovas JM, Schaefer EJ et al. (1998) Evidence for association and genetic linkage of the angiotensin-converting enzyme locus with hypertension and blood pressure in men but not women in the Framingham Heart Study. Circulation 97(18):1766–1772

Osterop AP, Kofflard MJ, Sandkuijl LA, Ten Cate FJ, Krams R, Schalekamp MA et al. (1998) AT1 receptor A/C1166 polymorphism contributes to cardiac hypertrophy in subjects with hypertrophic cardiomyopathy. Hypertension 32:825–830

Paillard F, Chansel D, Brand E, Benetos A, Thomas F, Czekalski S et al. (1999) Genotype-phenotype relationships for the renin-angiotensin-aldosterone system in a normal population. Hypertension 34(3):423–429

Pankow JS, Rose KM, Oberman A, Hunt SC, Atwood LD, Djousse L et al. (2000) Possible locus on chromosome 18q influencing postural systolic blood pressure changes. Hypertension 36(4):471–476

Parma J, Duprez L, Van Sande J, Cochaux P, Gervy C, Mockel J et al. (1993) Somatic mutations in the thyrotropin receptor gene cause hyperfunctioning thyroid adenomas. Nature 365(6447):649–651

Pascoe L, Curnow KM, Slutsker L, Connell JM, Speiser PW, New MI et al. (1992) Glucocorticoid-suppressible hyperaldosteronism results from hybrid genes created by unequal crossovers between CYP11B1 and CYP11B2. Proc Natl Acad Sci USA 89(17):8327–8531

Pascoe L, Jeunemaitre X, Lebrethon MC, Curnow KM, Gomez-Sanchez CE, Gasc JM et al. (1995) Glucocorticoid-suppressible hyperaldosteronism and adrenal tumors occurring in a single French pedigree. J Clin Invest 96(5):2236–2246

Perola M, Kainulainen K, Pajukanta P, Terwilliger JD, Hiekkalinna T, Ellonen P et al. (2000) Genome-wide scan of predisposing loci for increased diastolic blood pressure in Finnish siblings. J Hypertens 18(11):1579–1585

Persu A, Barbry P, Bassilana F, Houot AM, Mengual R, Lazdunski M et al. (1998) Genetic analysis of the beta subunit of the epithelial Na+ channel in essential hypertension. Hypertension 32(1):129–137

Persu A, Coscoy S, Houot AM, Corvol P, Barbry P, Jeunemaitre X (1999) Polymorphisms of the gamma subunit of the epithelial Na+ channel in essential hypertension. J Hypertens 17(5):639–645

Rao DC (2001) Genetic dissection of complex traits: an overview. Adv Genet 42:13–34

Rapp JP (2000) Genetic analysis of inherited hypertension in the rat. Physiol Rev 80(1):135–172

Rapp JP, Wang SM, Dene H (1989) A genetic polymorphism in the renin gene of Dahl rats cosegregates with blood pressure. Science 243(4890):542–544

Rice T, Rankinen T, Province MA, Chagnon YC, Perusse L, Borecki IB et al. (2000) Genome-wide linkage analysis of systolic and diastolic blood pressure: the Quebec Family Study. Circulation 102(16):1956–1963

Rieder MJ, Nickerson DA (2000) Hypertension and single nucleotide polymorphisms. Curr Hypertens Rep 2(1):44–49

Rieder MJ, Taylor SL, Clark AG, Nickerson DA (1999) Sequence variation in the human angiotensin converting enzyme. Nat Genet 22(1):59–62

Rigat B, Hubert C, Alhenc-Gelas F, Cambien F, Corvol P, Soubrier F (1990) An insertion/deletion polymorphism in the angiotensin I-converting enzyme gene accounting for half the variance of serum enzyme levels. J Clin Invest 86(4):1343–1346

Rossi GP, Narkiewicz K, Cesari M, Winnicki M, Bigda J, Chrostowska M et al. (1999) Genetic determinants of plasma ACE and renin activity in young normotensive twins. J Hypertens 17(5):647–655

Rotimi C, Morrison L, Cooper R, Oyejide C, Effiong E, Ladipo M et al. (1994) Angiotensinogen gene in human hypertension. Lack of an association of the 235T allele among African Americans. Hypertension 24(5):591–594

Rotin D, Staub O, Haguenauer-Tsapis R (2000) Ubiquitination and endocytosis of plasma membrane proteins: Role of Nedd4/Rsp5p family of ubiquitin-protein ligases. J Membr Biol 176(1):1–17

Sato N, Katsuya T, Rakugi H, Takami S, Nakata Y, Miki T et al. (1997) Association of variants in critical core promoter element of angiotensinogen gene with increased risk of essential hypertension in Japanese. Hypertension 30(3 Pt 1):321–325

Schambelan M, Sebastian A, Rector FC (1981) Mineralocorticoid-resistant renal hyperkalemia without salt wasting (type II pseudohypoaldosteronism): Role of increased renal chloride reabsorption. Kidney Int 19(5):716–727

Schild L, Lu Y, Gautschi I, Schneeberger E, Lifton RP, Rossier BC (1996) Identification of a PY motif in the epithelial Na channel subunits as a target sequence for mutations causing channel activation found in Liddle syndrome. EMBO J 15(10):2381–2387

Schmidt S, van Hooft IM, Grobbee DE, Ganten D, Ritz E (1993) Polymorphism of the angiotensin I converting enzyme gene is apparently not related to high blood pressure: Dutch Hypertension and Offspring Study. J Hypertens 11(4):345–348

Schork NJ (1997) Genetically complex cardiovascular traits. Origins, problems, and potential solutions. Hypertension 29(1 Pt 2):145–149

Schunkert H, Hense HW, Doring A, Riegger GA, Siffert W (1998) Association between a polymorphism in the G protein beta3 subunit gene and lower renin and elevated diastolic blood pressure levels. Hypertension 32(3):510–513

Schunkert H, Hengstenberg C, Holmer SR, Broeckel U, Luchner A, Muscholl MW et al. (1999) Lack of association between a polymorphism of the aldosterone synthase gene and left ventricular structure. Circulation 99(17):2255–2260

Schuster H, Wienker TF, Toka HR, Bahring S, Jeschke E, Toka O et al. (1996a) Autosomal dominant hypertension and brachydactyly in a Turkish kindred resembles essential hypertension. Hypertension 28(6):1085–1092

Schuster H, Wienker TE, Bahring S, Bilginturan N, Toka HR, Neitzel H et al. (1996b) Severe autosomal dominant hypertension and brachydactyly in a unique Turkish kindred maps to human chromosome 12. Nat Genet 13(1):98–100

Sharma AM, Jeunemaitre X (2000) The future of genetic association studies in hypertension: Improving the signal to noise ratio. J Hypertens 18:811–814

Sharma P, Fatibene J, Ferraro F, Jia H, Monteith S, Brown C et al. (2000) A genome-wide search for susceptibility loci to human essential hypertension. Hypertension 35(6):1291–1296

Shenker A, Laue L, Kosugi S, Merendino JJ, Minegishi T, Cutler GB (1993) A constitutively activating mutation of the luteinizing hormone receptor in familial male precocious puberty. Nature 365(6447):652–654

Shimkets RA, Warnock DG, Bositis CM, Nelson-Williams C, Hansson JH, Schambelan M et al. (1994) Liddle's syndrome: heritable human hypertension caused by mutations in the beta subunit of the epithelial sodium channel. Cell 79(3):407–414

Siffert W, Rosskopf D, Moritz A, Wieland T, Kaldenberg-Stasch S, Kettler N et al. (1995) Enhanced G protein activation in immortalized lymphoblasts from patients with essential hypertension. J Clin Invest 96(2):759–766

Siffert W, Rosskopf D, Siffert G, Busch S, Moritz A, Erbel R et al. (1998) Association of a human G-protein beta3 subunit variant with hypertension. Nat Genet 18(1):45–48

Simon DB, Nelson-Williams C, Bia MJ, Ellison D, Karet FE, Molina AM et al. (1996) Gitelman's variant of Bartter's syndrome, inherited hypokalaemic alkalosis, is caused by mutations in the thiazide-sensitive Na-Cl cotransporter. Nat Genet 12(1):24–30

Smithies O, Kim HS (1994) Targeted gene duplication and disruption for analyzing quantitative genetic traits in mice. Proc Natl Acad Sci USA 1994;91(9):3612–3615

Smithies O, Kim HS, Takahashi N, Edgell MH (2000) Importance of quantitative genetic variations in the etiology of hypertension. Kidney Int 58(6):2265–2280

Snyder PM, Price MP, McDonald FJ, Adams CM, Volk KA, Zeiher BG et al. (1995) Mechanism by which Liddle's syndrome mutations increase activity of a human epithelial Na+ channel. Cell 83(6):969–978

Soubrier F, Alhenc-Gelas F, Hubert C, Allegrini J, John M, Tregear G et al. (1988) Two putative active centers in human angiotensin I-converting enzyme revealed by molecular cloning. Proc Natl Acad Sci USA 85(24):9386–9390

Soubrier F, Jeunemaitre X, Rigat B, Houot AM, Cambien F, Corvol P (1990) Similar frequencies of renin gene restriction fragment length polymorphisms in hypertensive and normotensive subjects. Hypertension 16(6):712–717

Staub O, Dho S, Henry P, Correa J, Ishikawa T, McGlade J et al. (1996) WW domains of Nedd4 bind to the proline-rich PY motifs in the epithelial Na+ channel deleted in Liddle's syndrome. EMBO J 15(10):2371–2380

Stewart PM (1999) Mineralocorticoid hypertension. Lancet 353(9161):1341–1347

Stewart PM, Krozowski ZS, Gupta A, Milford DV, Howie AJ, Sheppard MC et al. (1996) Hypertension in the syndrome of apparent mineralocorticoid excess due to mutation of the 11 beta-hydroxysteroid dehydrogenase type 2 gene. Lancet 347(8994):88–91

Stowasser M, Gordon RD (2000) Primary aldosteronism: Learning from the study of familial varieties. J Hypertens 18(9):1165–1176

Stowasser M, Gordon RD, Tunny TJ, Klemm SA, Finn WL, Krek AL (1992) Familial hyperaldosteronism type II: Five families with a new variety of primary aldosteronism. Clin Exp Pharmacol Physiol 19(5):319–322

Su YR, Rutkowski MP, Klanke CA, Wu X, Cui Y, Pun RY et al. (1996) A novel variant of the beta-subunit of the amiloride-sensitive sodium channel in African Americans. J Am Soc Nephrol 7(12):2543–2549

Tamaki S, Iwai N, Tsujita Y, Kinoshita M (1999) Genetic polymorphism of CYP11B2 gene and hypertension in Japanese. Hypertension 33(1 Pt 2):266–270

Tiret L, Rigat B, Visvikis S, Breda C, Corvol P, Cambien F et al. (1992) Evidence, from combined segregation and linkage analysis, that a variant of the angiotensin 1-converting enzyme (ACE) gene controls plasma ACE levels. Am J Hum Genet 51(1):197–205

Tiret L, Bonnardeaux A, Poirier O, Ricard S, Marques-Vidal P, Evans A et al. (1994) Synergistic effects of angiotensin-converting enzyme and angiotensin-II type I receptor gene polymorphisms on risk of myocardial infarction. Lancet 344(8927):910–913

Turner ST, Schwartz GL, Chapman AB, Boerwinkle E (2001) C825T polymorphism of the G protein β3-subunit and antihypertensive response to a thiazide diuretic. Hypertension 37 [part 2]:739–743

Ulick S, Levine LS, Gunczler P, Zanconato G, Ramirez LC, Rauh W et al. (1979) A syndrome of apparent mineralocorticoid excess associated with defects in the peripheral metabolism of cortisol. J Clin Endocrinol Metab 19(5):757–764

van Geel PP, Pinto YM, Voors AA, Buikema H, Oosterga M, Crijns HJ et al. (2000) Angiotensin II type I receptor A1166C gene polymorphism is associated with an increased response to angiotensin II in human arteries. Hypertension 35:717–721

Villard E, Tiret L, Visvikis S, Rakotovao R, Cambien F, Soubrier F (1996) Identification of new polymorphisms of the angiotensin I-converting enzyme (ACE) gene, and study of their relationship to plasma ACE levels by two-QTL segregation-linkage analysis. Am J Hum Genet 58(6):1268–1278

Volpe M, Lembo G, De Luca N, Lamenza F, Tritto C, Ricciardelli B et al. (1991) Abnormal hormonal and renal responses to saline load in hypertensive patients with parental history of cardiovascular accidents. Circulation 84(1):92–100

Vuagnat A, Giacche M, Hopkins PN, Hunt SC, Azizi M, Fisher NDL, et al. (2001) Plasma LDL cholesterol is a strong predictor of the blood pressure increase following an acute infusion of angiotensin II. J Mol Med (in press)

Walker WG, Whelton PK, Saito H, Russell RP, Hermann J (1979) Relation between blood pressure and renin, renin substrate, angiotensin II, aldosterone and urinary sodium and potassium in 574 ambulatory subjects. Hypertension 1(3):287–291

Wang WY, Glenn CL, Zhang W, Benjafield AV, Nyholt DR, Morris BJ (1999) Exclusion of angiotensinogen gene in molecular basis of human hypertension: Sibpair linkage and association analyses in Australian anglo-caucasians. Am J Med Genet 87(1):53–60

Wang JG, Staessen JA (2000) Genetic polymorphisms in the renin-angiotensin system: Relevance for susceptibility to cardiovascular disease. Eur J Pharmacol 410(2–3):289–302

Ward R (1990) Familial aggregation and genetic epidemiology of blood pressure. In Laragh JH and Brenner BM (eds): Hypertension: Pathophysiology, Diagnosis and Management. Raven Press, NY, pp. 81–100

Ward K, Hata A, Jeunemaitre X, Helin C, Nelson L, Namikawa C et al. (1993) A molecular variant of angiotensinogen associated with preeclampsia. Nat Genet 4(1):59–61

Watt GC, Harrap SB, Foy CJ, Holton DW, Edwards HV, Davidson HR et al. (1992) Abnormalities of glucocorticoid metabolism and the renin-angiotensin system: A four-corners approach to the identification of genetic determinants of blood pressure. J Hypertens 10(5):473–482

Wilton AN, Kaye JA, Guo G, Brennecke P, Cooper DW (1995) Is angiotensinogen a good candidate gene for preeclampsia? Clin Exp Hypertens 14:251–260

Wong ZY, Stebbing M, Ellis JA, Lamantia A, Harrap SB (1999) Genetic linkage of beta and gamma subunits of epithelial sodium channel to systolic blood pressure. Lancet 1999:353(9160):1222–1225

Xu X, Niu T, Christiani DC, Weiss ST, Zhou Y, Chen C et al. (1997) Environmental and occupational determinants of blood pressure in rural communities in China. Ann Epidemiol 7(2):95–106

Xu X, Rogus JJ, Terwedow HA, Yang J, Wang Z, Chen C et al. (1999) An extreme-sib-pair genome scan for genes regulating blood pressure. Am J Hum Genet 64(6):1694–1701

Zee RY, Lou YK, Griffiths LR, Morris BJ (1992) Association of a polymorphism of the angiotensin I-converting enzyme gene with essential hypertension. Biochem Biophys Res Commun 184(1):9–15

Zhang X, Erdmann J, Regitz-Zagrosek V, Kurzinger S, Hense HW, Schunkert H (2000) Evaluation of three polymorphisms in the promoter region of the angiotensin II type I receptor gene. J Hypertens 18(3):267–272

Preeclampsia

Reynir Arngrímsson

Introduction

Preeclampsia is a common and sometimes dangerous multisystem disorder of pregnancy, especially notable for hypertension and proteinuria. Preeclampsia affects 2% to 6% of pregnant women and progress to eclampsia (convulsions) in about 0.1% of pregnancies. It has remained a leading cause of maternal death not only in developing countries but also in Europe and North America. Women affected in their first pregnancy are at higher risk than those who remain normotensive of developing preeclampsia in subsequent pregnancies (Sibai et al., 1986). Maternal morbidity of moderate preeclampsia ranges from psychological strain to cerebral hemorrhage (Geirsson et al., 1994). In developing countries the mortality among women sustaining eclampsia or severe preeclampsia can be as high as 10% (Duley, 1992).

The fetus is also exposed to the disease, as evident from a higher perinatal mortality rate and more frequent births of small-for-gestational age fetuses, some of whom remain growth-retarded. Failure to recognize the multisystem effects and the varied presentations of the syndrome represents a major source of mortality and morbidity for women.

The central feature related to the cause of preeclampsia is almost certainly to be found in the placental bed where there is failure of maternal adaptation to the invading fetal tissue. Similar pathologic features are observed in placental tissue of preeclamptic women and in pregnancies affected by idiopathic intrauterine growth retardation without hypertensive complications (Khong et al., 1986). Why some patients remain normotensive while others develop preeclampsia is unknown. Family studies show that the susceptibility to develop hypertension and proteinuria in pregnancy may be inherited (Humphries, 1960; Chesley et al., 1968; Cooper and Liston, 1979; Arngrímsson, 1990). Blood relatives of affected women are at significantly higher risk than relatives by marriage. Analysis of various inheritance models in data from several family studies have suggested either dominant inheritance of an autosomal gene with moderate penetrance or multifactorial inheritance as the most likely explanation of this phenomenon (Arngrímsson et al., 1994a). Interestingly both the mother and the fetus seem to contribute to the risk of preeclampsia and that the contribution of the fetus being affected by paternal genes (Lie et al., 1998).

Classification

The classification of hypertensive complications in pregnancy remains confused despite several classification schemes proposed in the last 50 years. This may be because the etiology is not known and the pathologic processes that lead to symptoms in the latter half of pregnancy are incompletely understood. Most classifications depend almost exclusively on the presence of hypertension and proteinuria (Nelson, 1955; Davey and MacGillivray, 1988; Gifford et al., 1990), which are but two manifestations of what likely comprises several disease processes. Preeclampsia, preeclamptic toxemia, pregnancy-induced hypertension, pregnancy-associated hypertension, hypertensive disease of pregnancy, and gestosis are roughly synonymous terms. Here the general term preeclampsia is used to emphasize that there is more to the disease than hypertension.

Hypertension is an imprecise concept based on arbitrary thresholds used to divide normotensive from hypertensive subjects. During pregnancy the most commonly chosen

Table 52.1. Classification of Hypertensive Disorders of Pregnancy

Preeclampsia	Rise in blood pressure in latter half of pregnancy in women who were normotensive before pregnancy; hypertension remits within few months of delivery
Mild	Rise in blood pressure ≥15 mmHg diastolic or ≥30 mmHg systolic from measurement early in pregnancy or bp ≥140/90–170/110 mmHg in late pregnancy if no early reading available; plus proteinuria (≥0.30 g/24 h)
Severe	Blood pressure ≥170/110 mmHg with proteinuria as above
Transient hypertension	Rise in blood pressure as for preeclampsia; no proteinuria
Chronic hypertension	Known essential or secondary hypertension before pregnancy or rise in blood pressure ≥140/90 mmHg before 20 weeks due to coincidental development of new medical cause occurring in pregnancy
Eclampsia	Convulsions in hypertensive pregnancy

threshold is a diastolic blood pressure of 90 mmHg after 20 weeks of pregnancy. This cut-off corresponds to statistical descriptions of the distribution of blood pressure in the population. A diastolic pressure of 90 mmHg is three standard deviations (SD) above the mean for midpregnancy, 2 SD above the mean for 34 weeks gestation, but owing to physiologic rise in blood pressure, only 1.5 SD above the mean at term (MacGillivray et al., 1969). In the latter part of pregnancy, 15% to 20% of pregnant women have at least one blood pressure reading above 140/90, but only 1% of women reach or exceed 170/110 mmHg. Hypertension can therefore be graded as mild to moderate for readings in the range 140–165/90–105 mmHg and severe for readings higher than 170/110 mmHg (Redman, 1989).

Classification schemes for hypertensive complications of pregnancy must also account for increased fetal and maternal mortality and morbidity among women with hypertension accompanied by proteinuria or with eclampsia, compared to those who remain normotensive throughout pregnancy or have only transient hypertension (Page and Christianson, 1976; Gifford et al., 1990). The simplest definition of preeclamptic disorders is therefore a pregnancy-specific syndrome characterized by a group of signs of which at least two must be present (Table 52.1). In preeclampsia, the most common signs are hypertension and proteinuria with onset in the second half of pregnancy. In eclampsia, the most common defining characteristics are hypertension and seizures, since eclampsia can occur without proteinuria (Sibai et al., 1981). This may be an oversimplification because preeclampsia is unpredictable in onset and progress. None of the known features of preeclampsia is specific, and there is no diagnostic test. Clinical judgment must therefore be based on the progression of symptoms and signs and on several biochemical and hematologic parameters. Some patients will present with severe hypertension and little renal involvement; others will have severe proteinuria but mild hypertension. It may even be possible to have preeclampsia

without hypertension (Redman et al., 1977), and some patients have predominantly hepatic involvement (so-called HELLP-syndrome). An abnormal increase in diastolic blood pressure (>15–20 mmHg) must also be considered a warning sign even though it does not reach 90 mmHg (Redman and Jeffries, 1988). Most classification schemes emphasize the importance of diastolic measurements, but high systolic readings should not be disregarded even though the diastolic component is below 90 mmHg.

In other forms of hypertension, high blood pressure is evident from conception, as opposed to preeclampsia where the maternal syndrome only becomes apparent in the latter half of the pregnancy. This is usually due to the presence of essential hypertension or to hypertension secondary to other medical conditions, such as renal disorders or pheochromocytoma evident before pregnancy. Women with preexistent hypertension have high risk of developing superimposed preeclampsia.

Clinical and pathologic findings

The main symptoms and signs of preeclampsia are hypertension, proteinuria, edema, coagulation and platelet disturbances, liver involvement and neurological abnormalities, including cortical blindness and convulsions (Table 52.2). The fetus is also subjected to chronic hypoxia, malnutrition, and growth retardation. These features reflect the pathologic changes that can occur in the brain, liver, kidney, cardiovascular system, and the decidual vessels. A common pathologic factor has not yet been identified, but the disseminated and diverse changes suggest vascular endothelial dysfunction and reduced organ perfusion (Roberts et al., 1989).

Morphologic endothelial cell changes, the so-called glomerular endotheliosis, only have been described best in

Table 52.2. Possible Symptoms and Signs of Preeclampsia Syndrome[a]

System	Pathologic Changes	Symptoms and Signs
Cardiovascular	Increased peripheral resistance Increased arterial sensitivity to angiotensin II Reduced blood volume (hemoconcentration)	Pregnancy-induced hypertension
Renal	Glomerular endotheliosis Reduced glomerular function and renal blood flow Reduced uric acid clearance Acute tubular or cortical necrosis	Proteinuria Hyperuricemia, hypocalcuria Generalized edema Excessive weight gain Ascites, renal failure Respiratory difficulties
Coagulation	Activation of the coagulation system	Reduced platelet count Increased fibrinogen-fibrin turnover Disseminated intravascular coagulation
Hepatic	Infarction and periportal hemorrhages Hepatic rupture	Raised liver enzymes, epigastric pain and vomiting HELLP syndrome, jaundice Hepatic encephalopathy
Nervous system	Reduced perfusion Vasospasm Retinal detachment Cerebral hemorrhage and infarcts	Headaches and hyperreflexia Visual disturbances Convulsions "Hypertensive" encephalopathy
Fetoplacental unit	Failure to adaptation to trophoblast invasion High resistance uterine vasculature Reduced perfusion, hypoxia	Reduced fetal growth Abnormal Doppler waveforms Fetal growth retardation and hypoxia Intrauterine death

[a]Vascular endothelial dysfunction and reduced perfusion are thought to be central to the development of the condition.

the kidneys of pregnant women (Spargo et al., 1959; Sheenan, 1980; Lindheimer et al., 1987) (Fig. 52.1). Changes in endothelial cells within the endomyocardial vessels, with swelling of the cytoplasm and luminal narrowing, occurred in women dying from severe preeclampsia (Barton et al., 1991). This confirms the widespread

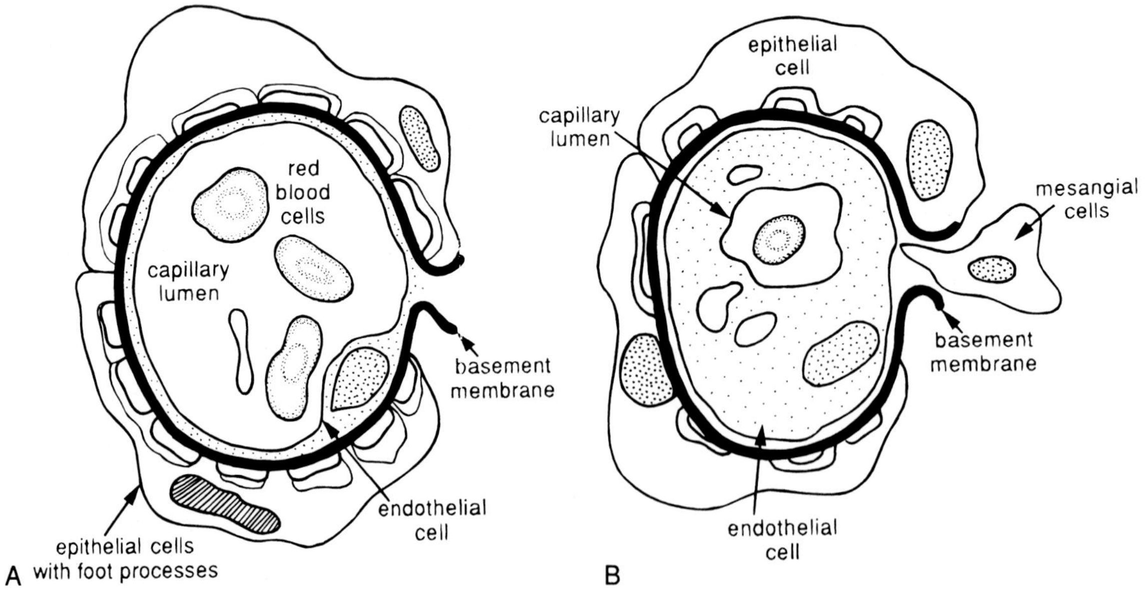

Fig. 52.1. Glomerular endotheliosis has only been described in association with pregnancy and includes capillary ballooning with swollen foamy endothelial cells, which partially obliterate the capillary lumen. The basement membrane and the foot processes of the epithelial cells are intact. A slight increase in mesangial cells may be observed. The severity of changes has been correlated with the degree of hypertension, proteinuria, and hyperuricemia. Capillary loops in normal (A) and preeclamptic glomerulus (B).

endothelial changes throughout the systemic circulation in preeclamsia.

HEMODYNAMIC AND COAGULATION ALTERATIONS

Throughout pregnancy, striking physiologic changes occur to accommodate the growing products of conception. These changes are most profound in the cardiovascular system, kidney, and uterus. During pregnancy blood volume and cardiac output increase 40% to 50% (Walters and Lim, 1975; Clark et al., 1989), while the peripheral resistance falls. The blood pressure declines in early pregnancy (10–15 mmHg) and reaches a nadir in second trimester with some widening of the pulse pressure. It slowly rises again from 16 to 20 weeks onward and returns to the prepregnant state at term (Christianson, 1976). Concomitantly the cardiac output is redistributed in favor of the kidneys and the uteroplacental circulation. The uteroplacental circulation receives 10% to 15% of the maternal cardiac output in the third trimester and the renal blood flow and glomerular filtration increase 50% and 75%, respectively (Davison and Hytten, 1974; Dunlop, 1981). In summary, normal pregnancy is associated with hemodynamic changes of high volume, high flow, and low resistance (Friedman et al., 1991).

In preeclampsia, however, there is failure of the compensatory responses seen in normal pregnancy. The increment in plasma volume is smaller or abolished (Gallery et al., 1979; Hays et al., 1985). Cardiac output has been variably reported as elevated, normal or depressed, while there has been more universal agreement about increased systemic vascular resistance followed by hypertension (Benedetti et al., 1980; Cotton et al., 1988; Wallenburg, 1988). The hemodynamic situation is therefore one of high blood pressure, high resistance and low blood flow, which may result in reduced organ perfusion.

Studies of subcutaneous arteries of women with preeclampsia have shown impaired endothelium-dependent relaxation (McCarthy et al., 1993) and enhanced pressor response to angiotensin II (Aalkjaer et al., 1985). It appears to be an abnormal endothelium-dependent relaxation, rather than smooth muscle dysfunction that contributes to the enhanced peripheral vascular resistance, since endothelium-independent, nitroprusside-mediated relaxation is intact. Local regulation of vasoactive substance, especially in the uterus, may be important in this respect (Gisclard et al., 1988; Broughton-Pipkin, 1988; Bird et al., 1997).

Altered proximal renal tubular function, activation of the coagulation cascade, and increased sensitivity to vasopressors all antedate an overt rise in blood pressure in preeclamptic patients. The cause of increased sensitivity to circulating pressor agents such as angiotensin II (Gant et al., 1973) still needs to be fully elucidated, but may be related to imbalance in production of vascular prostanoids with a higher vasoconstrictor/vasodilator ratio (thromboxane/prostacyclin) than normal (Bussolino et al., 1980; Ylikorkala et al., 1986). Alternatively, there may be altered regulation of angiotensin II receptor concentrations (Baker et al., 1989) or nitric oxide production (Nathan et al., 1995).

The angiotensinogen locus (*AGT*) on the distal long arm of chromosome 1 has been implicated in preeclampsia. In a sample of 32 American primigravid preeclamptic women and 9 women with superimposed preeclampsia, a highly significant association was found with the polymorphism M235T, which lies distal to the coding region for angiotensin II in exon 2 of *AGT*. This was corroborated by findings in a Japanese sample of 13 primigravidae with preeclampsia. When all forms of hypertension in pregnancy were included in the analysis, no association was observed in the American sample, but the Japanese results were highly significant (Ward et al., 1993). Further evidence for possible association with *AGT* (dinucleotide polymorphism in the 3′ flanking region of the gene, *AGT*-CAn) came from a study of Icelandic and Scottish families using the affected pedigree member method (Arngrímsson et al., 1993). The Icelandic families were ascertained through women with severe preeclampsia (160/110 mmHg and proteinuria) or eclampsia with at least two affected relatives alive. The Scottish families were ascertained through patients with severe preeclampsia and at least one affected first-degree relative. When the diagnostic criteria among the relatives was set as transient hypertension and preeclampsia, an association with a highly polymorphic microsatellite marker distal to the angiotensiongen gene (*AGT*-CAn) was observed, but only in families identified through preclamptic probands and not in families with eclamptic probands. More stringent diagnostic criteria revealed higher significance in the preeclamptic families (Arngrímsson et al., 1993). Recently, a study of English families showed transmission distortion at the *AGT*-CAn locus. The allele designated A9 was transmitted more frequently from the mother to the fetus and was associated with low plasma angiotensinogen concentrations and high renin concentrations (Morgan et al., 1999). The same trend was observed with polymorphisms within the angiotensin II type 1 receptor gene, where transmission distortion of alleles associated with low levels of surface receptor expression on platelets was shown (Morgan et al., 1998). Still there is not a universal agreement about the relevance of molecular aberrations within the renin-angiotensinogen system in the development of preeclampsia although this has also been supported by animal studies (Takimoto et al., 1996). For example no evidence of association was found among 76 Scottish primigravid preeclamptic women compared to 99 matched normotensive control subjects (Brock and Hayward, 1994, personal communication). Larger trials are required to estimate the risk associated with molecular variants at *AGT* and the possible physiologic role that these may play during pregnancy. To complicate matters even further, different regulatory mechanisms seem to be involved in the systemic and uterine artery endothelium during pregnancy, e.g., expression of angiotensin II type-1 receptor is different in mental artery endothelium from that seen in uterine arteries (Bird et al., 1997).

Activation of the coagulation system in preeclampsia is evidenced by increased platelet consumption and reduced platelet lifespan (Redman et al., 1978a; Rakoczi et al., 1979; Inglis et al., 1982). One characteristic feature of preeclampsia is maternal hypercoaguable state and intravascular coagulation. About 25% of eclamptic women have thrombocytopenia, and a fall in the platelet count may be an early sign of the start of preeclampsia. Widespread deposition of fibrin, disseminated intravascular coagulation (DIC), and even microangiopathic hemolysis may result. In preeclampsia levels of tissue plasminogen activator (tPA) and plasminogen activator inhibitor-1 (PAI) are increased (Estelles et al., 1987) along with increased levels of plasma von-Willebrand factor and fibronectin (Lockwood and Peters, 1990; Taylor et al., 1991). These factors are also markers for endothelial activation. Reduced expression of endothelial cell-associated anticoagulant proteins has also been shown in preeclampsia including antithrombin III, protein C and protein S. In a series of pregnancies complicated by severe early-onset preeclampsia, 25% of the women had functional protein S deficiency, 18% demonstrated hyperhomocysteinemia and 29% had detectable anticardiolipin antibodies (Dekker et al., 1995). It has also been noted that the prevalence of these abnormalities is 1.5–2.0 times higher in patients who were delivered before 28 weeks of gestation in comparison with patients who were delivered after 28 weeks (van Pampus et al., 1999). The resistance to activated protein C is an inherited mutation of the coagulation factor V gene. The factor V Leiden mutation predisposes to thromboembolic events. The presence of this mutation has been shown to be increased in patients with severe preeclampsia (Dizon-Townson et al., 1996; Lindoff et al., 1997; Grandone et al., 1997). Deletion/insertion polymorhism in the promoter region for PAI gene has also been associated with increased risk of preeclampsia (Yamada et al., 2000). The deletion, 4G, is associated with enhanced gene expression and plasma PAI levels and preeclampsia.

Other symptoms of preeclampsia such as proteinuria and excessive fluid leakage into the interstitial tissue with development of edema may also be related to endothelial dysfunction. Leakage of proteins through the endothelium into the interstitial space causes increased colloid osmotic pressure and leads to reduction in plasma albumin and hemoconcentration (Fadnes and Øian, 1989).

CIRCULATING "TOXINS" THEORIES: TOXEMIA REVISITED

The factors mediating the vascular endothelial dysfunction have not been conclusively identified. A few hypotheses have been advanced. The longest surviving one was postulated before blood pressure measurements became common in clinical practice. Specific toxins produced by the placenta were believed to be released into the bloodstream of the mother (DeLee, 1905), hence the well-known term "toxemia of pregnancy." Modified versions of this theory are still appearing, such as a recent suggestion that poor placental perfusion may result in release of factors from the placenta that stimulate or injure endothelial cells (Rodgers et al., 1988; Smárason et al., 1993). Serum from women with preeclampsia has a greater cytotoxic and mitogenic effect on endothelial cells and fibroblasts, respectively, than serum from healthy pregnant women (Rodgers et al., 1988; Taylor et al., 1990). This effect apparently disappears after delivery, suggesting placental origin of the factor. It has been shown that syncytiotrophoblast micorvillous membranes (STBM) isolated from normal or preeclamptic placentae, specifically inhibit the proliferation of cultured human umbilical vein endothelial cells (HUVEC) (Smárason et al., 1993). The anti-proliferative activity of STBM resides in self-aggregating complex in which eight proteins, namely integrins alpha (5) (CD49e) and alpha (V) (CD51), dipeptidyl peptidase IV (DPP IV, CD26), alpha-actinin, transferring receptor (TfR, CD71), tranferrin, placental alkaline phosphatase (PLAP) and monoamine oxidase A (MAO-A) were identified. Research today suggest that a major part of the antiproliferative activity appears to be related to the adhesion molecules within the complex (Kertesz et al., 2000). Neutrophil activation could also be involved (Lyall and Greer, 1994). Activated neutrophils release substances capable of mediating vascular endothelial damage such as elastase, toxic oxygen radicals and leukotrienes and may thus contribute directly to the vascular lesion in preeclampsia (Greer et al., 1989). Higher concentrations of cytokines and cell adhesion molecules in sera from preeclamptic women (Lyall et al., 1994; Greer et al., 1994) may provide a mechanism by which leukocytes are attracted to the endothelium, thus upsetting the prostaglandin balance and releasing toxic superoxide anions and hydrogen peroxides.

Oxidative stress and toxicity associated with free radicals occurs when excessive production overwhelms defense systems or when protective mechanisms are impaired. Normal equilibrium is maintained by antioxidants such as vitamin E, glutathione peroxidase, superoxide dismutase, and catalase (Halliwell and Gutteridge, 1989). In patients with preeclampsia, high levels of lipid peroxides and oxygen free radicals have been detected before clinical symptoms develop (Ishihara, 1978; Wickens et al., 1981). Low serum concentrations of vitamin E correlate with severity of the disease (Wang et al., 1991). On that basis preeclampsia could be a disease of antioxidant inadequacy and appear when the normal antioxidant equilibrium is upset. Dietary experiments in rats support this notion, as diets low in vitamin E induce fatal eclampsia (Stamler, 1959), and diets rich in peroxidised oils induce preeclamptic-like changes in the kidneys (Kaunitz et al., 1962). Supplementation with vitamins C and E in women at increased risk of preeclampsia has been shown to be beneficial in the prevention of preeclampsia (Chappell et al., 1999), although multicenter trials may be needed to show whether vitamin supplementation affects the occurrence of preeclampsia in low-risk women. Recently, a polymorphism in the glutathion S-transferase P1 gene was associated with increased risk of preeclampsia (Zusterzeel et al., 2000a) and recurrent early pregnancy loss (Zusterzeel et al., 2000b). Glutathione S-transferase is an important biotransformation enzyme involved in detoxification. Genetically determined lower activity of certain isoforms of the enzyme in placenta could be a joint factor in preeclampsia and recurrent miscarriages and explain, in part, some of the observations described in preeclamptic family studies (Cooper et al., 1988; Arngrímsson et al., 1994a).

Hyperlipidemia is a feature of normal pregnancy. Plasma cholesterol and triglycerides rise and there is a further increase in plasma triglyceride and free fatty acids in preeclampsia (Potter and Nestel, 1979). It has therefore been postulated that the disturbances of endothelial function in preeclampsia might be associated with abnormal lipid metabolism and that very-low-density-lipoproteins (VLDL) could be a major contributor in this respect (Arbogast et al., 1994). Alternatively, the endothelial dysfunction may be promted by oxidative stress due to lipid peroxidation.

Preeclampsia is associated with a dyslipidemic pattern similar to that seen in insulin resistance syndrome associated with increased cardiovascular disease risk. This involves hypertriglyceridemia, increased apolipoprotein B concentrations, decreased high density lipoprotein cholesterol and the presence of small dense low density lipoprotein particles (Hubel et al., 1998). Small dense low density lipoprotein (LDL) particles are more prone to oxidative modification than large buoyant low density lipoproteins and these may have adverse effect on the endothelial cell function and contribute to arterial lesions in atherosclerosis (Witztum 1994) and diabetes (Chisolm et al., 1992). Maternal dyslipidemia may have an important role in generation of oxidative stress and development of preeclampsia (Hubel, 1999).

THE PLACENTAL TISSUE

The cause of preeclampsia is connected to the presence of placental tissue because the disorder is specific to pregnancy and it occurs in hydatidiform mole in the absence of a fetus. Pathologic and pathophysiologic changes completely revert within six months postpartum, so the disease is related to the presence of fetal trophoblast tissue or to the maternal adaptation to implantation and placentation (Piering et al., 1993).

At implantation, the fetal trophoblast cells must migrate into the uterine tissues to establish contact with uterine vessels (Fig. 52.2). Simultaneously, trophoblast must be transformed into a well-differentiated tissue capable of extracting nutrients from the mother and transporting those into the fetal circulation. Trophoblast also serves as a barrier between the mother and the fetus and produces substances vital to supporting the pregnancy.

In preeclamptic pregnancies this normal differentiation process is halted. The interstitial cytotrophoblast invasion is abnormally shallow. The cytotrophoblasts are increased in number (Hustin et al., 1984; Arnholdt et al., 1991), but fewer endovascular cytotrophoblast cells are seen. The syncytiotrophoblast mass is smaller (Boyd et al., 1983) with high glycogen content (Arkwright et al., 1993) and greatly distorted microvilli and increased numbers of syncytial sprouts (Alvarez et al., 1972).

The myometrial segments of the arteries maintain their smooth muscle but at diameters of only about 40% of those of the vessels in normal pregnancy (Khong et al., 1986). Fewer vessels are transformed and cytotrophoblast invasion into many of them is patchy and discontinuous (Brosens et al., 1972; Khong et al., 1992).

Some of the spiral arteries in the decidua and myometrium are occluded by a process termed "acute

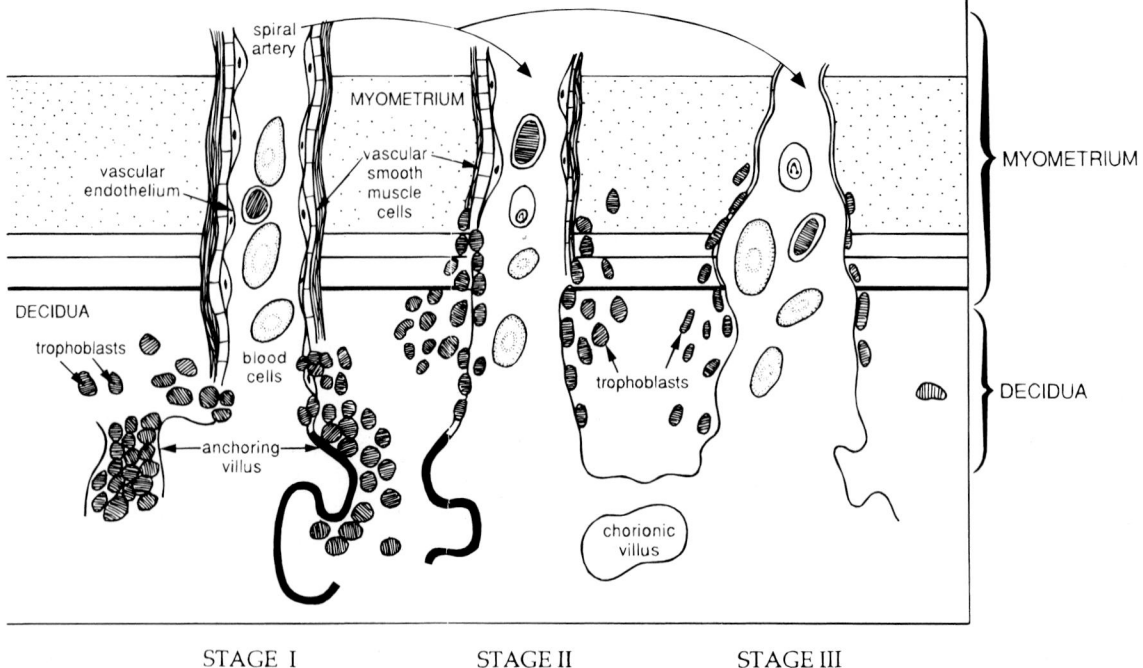

STAGE I   STAGE II   STAGE III

Fig. 52.2. In normal pregnancy, cytotrophoblast cells in the anchoring villi aggregate to form columns that adhere to the uterine epithelium. Early in pregnancy they start to proliferate and migrate in the direction of the maternal spiral arteries through the decidua and into the myometrium. The migration is believed to take place in two waves. The initial wave takes place during the first trimester when the decidua is inhabited (*stage 1*) and the second wave occurs around 15–16 weeks with further invasion into the structures of the myometrium. The cytotrophoblast cells, which form prominent cell layers in early pregnancy, gradually disappear by forming a multinucleate syncytium (the syncytiotrophoblast) with an extensive microvillous brush border. Blood flow to the fetus is established when the cytotrophoblasts invade and modify the uterine arteries. These cells erode the endothelium of the spiral arteries causing extensive changes to the arterial wall (*stage 2*). The internal elastic lamina is replaced by trophoblasts and amorphous extracellular matrix rich in fibrin. As a consequence, the vessels are transformed from being muscular end-arteries into wide sinusoid structures with four to six times the diameter of the same vessel in nonpregnant women (*stage 3*). Curiously, neither the veins nor other branches of the radial arteries (basal arteries) undergoes this process.

atherosis," characterized by aggregates of fibrin, IgM, C_3, apolipoprotein(a), platelets, lipid-loaded macrophages (lipophages or foam cells) and leukocytes, which focally disrupt the endothelium and partially or completely block the spiral arteries (Robertson et al., 1967; Kitzmiller and Beirschke, 1973; Labarrere and Althabe, 1986; MacFadyen et al., 1986). These changes are not confined to the placenta but are also observed in basal arteries in the myometrium and decidua basalis, that is, arteries in which trophoblast invasion is normally absent (Pijnenborg et al., 1991). Placental infarcts are seen in conjunction with acute atherosis of the spiral arteries, but infarction in the placenta is not specific to preeclampsia (Wallenburg et al., 1973; Sheppard and Bonnar, 1980). There is not universal agreement about the pathogenesis of atherosis. Some have compared it to vascular changes in malignant hypertension and suggested that it could be caused by acute hypertension (Robertson et al., 1967), while others argue for the importance of immune mechanisms (Roberts and Redman, 1993).

Over the last few years we have gained more knowledge about trophoblast differentiation and placenta morphogenesis from animal studies. Several specialized trophoblast cell subtypes arise during development. Some cells invade the uterus to promote maternal blood flow to the implantation site and other cells fuse into a syncytium, expand and fold to increase the surface area for efficient transport of nutrients to the fetus. Mutations of many genes in mice lead to defects in placenta development and thus fetal growth restrictions or embryonic mortality. Specific classes of mutant phenotypes observed in the placenta of knockout mice resemble those seen in humans that are associated with preeclampsia and intrauterine growth restriction (Cross, 2000). Although the cause of preeclampsia is unknown, the accumulated evidence strongly implicates the placenta. To understand the development of preeclampsia it is thus important to study the distinct molecular pathways that regulate the differentiation of the various trophoblast cell subtypes. Also it is important to realize that the proliferation, differentiation and morphogenesis of trophoblasts are highly regulated by interactions with adjacent cell types.

Anatomic examination show that the area of the placenta most affected by preeclampsia is the fetal-maternal interface. The cytotrophoblasts in preeclampsia not only have limited capacity for endovascular invasion but also display an altered morphology and tend to remain as individual rounded cells, instead of being invasive with ability to adhere to the vessel wall and replace the vascular endothelium. In healthy pregnancies the molecules expressed on the invasive cytotropoblasts mimic broadly the adhesion phenotype of the endothelial cells they replace, but in preeclampsia the cytotrophoblasts fail to switch their expression profile to that of the endothelial cells (Zhou et al., 1997).

Similar anatomical changes have been described in placenta in the idiopathic intrauterine growth-retardation syndrome (IUGR) where the maternal syndrome of preeclampsia is otherwise absent (Brosens et al., 1977, Gerretsen et al., 1981; McFadyen et al., 1986) and in pregnancies of patients with chronic hypertension and miscarriages (Khong et al., 1986; Pijnenborg et al., 1991). Since a wide spectrum of changes was observed in the placental tissue without clear-cut relation to the clinical signs it was suggested that failure of invasion should be regarded as defective or insufficient physiologic change, rather than as a separate primary pathologic entity of preeclampsia (Pijnenborg et al., 1991). An inherent difference between the various groups of pregnant women may therefore explain the diversity of response to the misbehaving trophoblast tissue.

Epidemiology

PARITY AND AGE

Eclampsia and preeclampsia are more common in primigravidae than parous women, although those once affected have a considerably higher recurrence risk than those who have remained normotensive (Lie et al., 1998). This appears to hold true for the whole spectrum of diseases from eclampsia to mild preeclampsia, and an excess of primigravidae is observed in all age groups (Hauch and Lehman, 1934; Davies et al., 1970). Most studies show a J-shaped curve when relating the incidence of preeclampsia to maternal age (Fig. 52.3). This reflects the high incidence among young women and a high risk among women over the age of 35 years. In addition, a marked rise in maternal mortality affects women over 35 years of age with preeclampsia

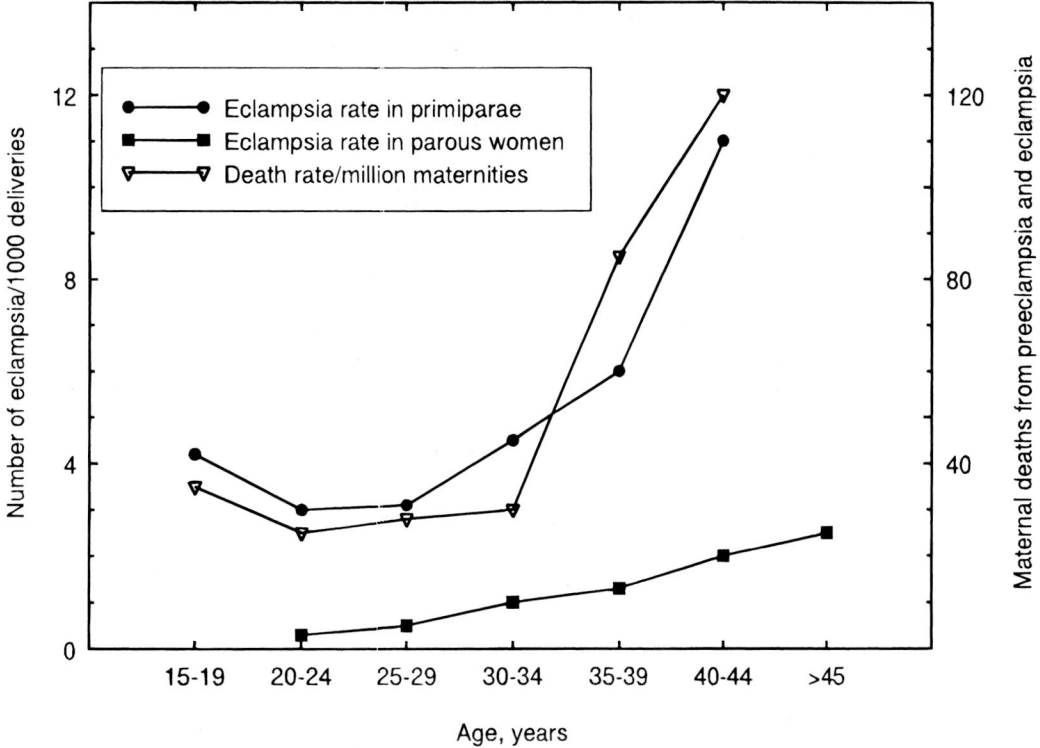

Fig. 52.3. Maternal deaths from preeclampsia and eclampsia by age and effect of age and parity on eclampsia.

(Department of Health, 1979; Augensen and Bergsjö, 1984). The J-shaped incidence curves are truncated at both ends reflecting the reproductive years so the two peaks could reflect two etiologically distinct conditions with a different mean age of onset.

Chesley (1978) demonstrated that parous women with eclampsia are more likely to develop chronic hypertension and thus could retrospectively be diagnosed as having superimposed preeclampsia, but at the time of the pregnancy it can be impossible to distinguish this from "true preeclampsia." This was also the finding of Fisher and colleagues (1973) who described relatively low correlation between clinical diagnosis and renal biopsy findings. Over 75% of the parous women did not have the classical endotheliosis found in the primigravid women, but rather findings consistent with chronic hypertensive or renal disorders. Conversely many of the primigravidae did not have classical renal lesions.

PREECLAMPSIA IN PAROUS WOMEN: RECURRENT PREECLAMPSIA

Preeclampsia may be predominantly a disease of primigravidae, but women with severe preeclampsia in their first pregnancy have a 12 fold higher risk of also being affected in their second pregnancy (Lie et al., 1998) and two to four fold increased chance of hypertensive disease in any subsequent pregnancy over those who are normotensive in their first pregnancy (Sibai et al., 1986). If the first pregnancy is complicated by preeclampsia and intratuterine growth-retardation the risk increases further. It is generally accepted that infants of women with preeclampsia are at higher risk of growth-retardation, but few studies have investigated whether the risk differs by parity. Lin and associates (1982) found that 38% of parous women and 18% of primigravid women with preeclampsia, confirmed by renal biopsy, had small-for-gestational age babies. When adjusted for smoking and race the odds ratio is 29.4 (95% confidence interval: 5.2–167.5) in favor of the parous women (Eskenazi et al., 1993) and the growth retardation is worse in babies of women who develop preeclampsia for the first time in a second pregnancy (Hochner-Celnikier et al., 1993). In general, the course of the disease among the parous women is more severe. The gestational age at first increase in blood pressure and delivery occur earlier than among the primigravid preeclamptic women (Hochner-Celnikier et al., 1993; Eskenazi et al., 1993). The risk of recurrence of preeclampsia is modified by the presence of hypertensive complications, length of gestation at delivery and birthweight during first pregnancy. Normotension indicates low risk of

subsequent hypertension in pregnancy (Campbell and MacGillivray, 1985; Lindeberg et al., 1988). Therefore if the first pregnancy is uncomplicated the risk in a second pregnancy is reduced from 3% to 6% to less than 1%. On the other hand, about a third of affected women in a first pregnancy have hypertension in subsequent pregnancies and about half of these have proteinuria, while 2% are at risk of developing eclampsia (Chesley, 1980; Sibai et al., 1986).

BLOOD PRESSURE IN PREECLAMPTIC WOMEN AND THEIR RELATIVES

Women who develop preeclampsia in their first pregnancy have higher diastolic and mean arterial blood pressures at their first antenatal visit than those who remain normotensive. This difference appears to be sustained throughout pregnancy (Moutquin et al., 1985). Systolic and mean arterial blood pressure are also significantly higher in midtrimester in this group of women, but the predictive value is estimated to be low for both (Fallis and Langford, 1963; Page and Christianson, 1976; Villar and Sibai, 1989; Kyle et al., 1993). These observations suggest that women with preeclampsia are beforehand in the higher centile of the normal distribution for blood pressure. A familial association of blood pressure levels is well known and liability to high blood pressure is inherited as a continuous trait (Ward, 1990). Offspring of women with preeclampsia also appear to have higher systolic blood pressures (Kotchen et al., 1979; Higgins et al., 1980; Seidman et al., 1991) and diastolic blood pressures (Langford and Watson, 1980; Palti and Rothschild, 1989; Seidman et al., 1991) than their peers born of normotensive women (see Ch. 51). They are usually smaller-for-gestational age, but low birthweight has been suggested as a risk factor for hypertension and cardiovascular disease in later life (Barker, 1992). This must be taken into account when later health implications of preeclampsia are considered.

PREEXISTING MEDICAL CONDITIONS AND BODY SIZE

Women with preexisting medical conditions appear to be at substantial increased risk of developing preeclampsia during pregnancy. Best studied are relations with preexisting essential or chronic hypertension, diabetes mellitus and renal dysfunction. Women with known hypertension before pregnancy are 10 times more likely to develop preeclampsia than those who were normotensive (Rey and Couturier, 1994). The longer the hypertension has lasted before the pregnancy the higher is the risk of superimposed hypertension (Sibai et al., 1998). Superimposed preeclampsia was diagnosed in 25% of cases if the women had history of hypertension and in the group that hypertension had been present more than fours years before conception the risk was 35%. Women with chronic hypertension are also more likely to have early onset preeclampsia or recurrence of preeclampsia in more than one pregnancy (Sibai et al., 1991). The women who are at greatest risk of developing preeclampsia are women with long lasting hypertension (more than four years), women with evidence of more severe underlying blood pressure elevation as demonstrated by either left ventricular hypertrophy, a serum creatinin greater than 1.0 mg% or diastolic BP greater than 100 mmHg at less than 20 weeks gestation (Moutquin et al., 1985; Sibai et al., 1998; Sibai et al., 1986; Mabie et al., 1986).

Similarly the risk of preeclampsia is associated with the severity and duration of diabetes mellitus (Chesley, 1978; Dekker et al., 1995). The rate of preeclampsia was in one prospective study found to be from 9% among diet-controled gestational diabetes to 30% among women with White class D, F and R (Garner et al., 1990). Polycystic ovary syndrome (PCOS) has been associated with metabolic changes and insulin resistance. Women with PCOS have been found to be at increase risk of preeclampsia (de Vries et al., 1998).

Other underlying medical problems associated with development of preeclampsia include resistance to activated protein C, functional protein S deficiency and hyperhomocysteinemia (Dekker et al., 1995; Kahn, 1998; Horstkamp et al., 1999). Women with underlying connective tissue disease and inflammatory rheumatic disease (Skomswoll et al., 2000) and women with increase in serum anticardiolipin antibodies (Dekker et al., 1995) are prone to develop preeclampsia and the rate of cesarean section seem to be particular high in this patient group.

Several studies have implied an association between increase in body mass and preeclampsia (Eskenazi et al., 1991; Sibai et al., 1995; Smith, 1947; Stone et al., 1994; Thadhani et al., 1999; Wolfe et al., 1991). Higher rates of preeclampsia seem to follow increasing levels of overweight, ranging from 2.3 to 5.5 fold rise in the risk of developing preeclampsia. Obesity may also contribute to the relation of other risk factors such as hypertension and diabetes with preeclampsia (Barden et al., 1999).

REMOTE PROGNOSIS

Numerous clinical studies have described the remote prognosis after preeclampsia and eclampsia. The estimated incidence of future chronic hypertension has ranged from 0% to 78% with a mean of 23.8% (Chesley, 1978). However, the populations studied, the definitions used, the diagnosis of hypertensive disorders, and duration of follow-up were highly variable.

Although it is still debatable if women with preeclampsia or transient hypertension have an increased risk of future hypertension compared to women at large, there appears to be a contrasting risk between women with preeclampsia and those who remain normotensive (Adams and MacGillivray, 1961; Svenson et al., 1983; Sibai et al., 1986; Selvaggi et al., 1988; Lindeberg et al., 1988). Follow-up studies show that a higher proportion of eclamptic and preeclamptic women have developed chronic hypertension within 10 years of the index pregnancy (4.4%) compared to normotensive women (1.5%) (Sibai et al., 1986). The cumulative risk increased more with age in the eclamptic and preeclamptic group. In women followed for more than 10 years, the proportion was 51% compared to 14% in the normotensive group. Gestational age at first detection of high blood pressure seemed to be an important risk factor. Women with onset of high blood pressure before 31 weeks had a 2.3 times higher risk of developing chronic hypertension than those with later onset. Therefore, women who develop preeclampsia early in pregnancy, apparently have hypertensive complications in more than one pregnancy (recurrent preeclampsia), and those who develop preeclampsia for the first time in their second or later pregnancy are at risk of developing chronic hypertension.

The ultimate way to measure whether the preeclampsia syndrome is a risk factor for future cardiovascular disorders is to determine the proportion of women who develop hypertensive complications or die from such complications. A significant increase in mortality rate has been observed in women (black and white) classified as parous at the time of the index pregnancy (Chesley et al., 1976). The death rate was also significantly higher in black primigravid women but not in primigravid white women. The majority of the deaths (82%) were due to hypertensive cardiovascular complications, which was over three times the rate in women without pregnancy hypertension. Nearly half of this mortality was secondary to cerebral hemorrhage. Women with recurrent preeclampsia syndrome were also at high risk of early death from heart disorders. This has been the case in the Icelandic population as well, where the death rate among women with previous hypertensive complications in pregnancy was significantly higher than expected. About 55% of the excess deaths were attributed to ischemic heart disease. An association with the severity of the pregnancy disease and the risk of developing ischemic heart disease later in life was also noted (Jónsdóttir et al., 1995).

Dyslipoproteinemia and insulin resistance syndrome (dyslipidemia, insulin resistance and compensatory hyperinsulinemia) are features found several years after delivery in women who have experienced eclampsia or preeclampsia during pregnancy (He et al., 1999; Hubel et al., 2000; Laivuori et al., 1996). Other important features are higher apolipoprotein B concentrations, smaller-sized low density lipoproteins, decreased high density lipoprotein (HDL) cholesterol, increased total cholesterol: HDL cholesterol ratio. These metabolic changes could be predisposing factor for cardiovascular disorders. Women who experience recurrent preeclampsia have higher rates of these metabolic abnormalities than those who only experience preeclampsia in first pregnancy or those who remain normotensive throughout all pregnancies (Hubel et al., 2000). Similar changes are found during pregnancy of these women (Hubel et al., 1998; Lorentzen et al., 1998; Sowers et al., 1995).

The clinical symptoms at the time of pregnancy do not allow differentiation between those who are destined to develop chronic hypertension or heart disease in later life and those who will not do so. The same general advice on preventive measures to promote a healthy lifestyle must be targeted to all those at potential risk, at least until it becomes possible to separate subgroups at definite risk in this respect. Blood pressure measurements and follow-up on blood lipids levels may prove to be important preventive steps that should be carried out on a regular basis.

Genetic predisposition in preeclampsia

During the last three decades several studies describe a tendency for preeclampsia and eclampsia to occur more frequently in relatives of affected women compared to population control groups (Table 52.3). This association was first exposed through the work of Humphries (1960) and particularly of Leon Chesley and colleagues (1961, 1968). Since the last part of the 19th century (Elliot, 1873), isolated case reports drew attention to family clustering in both eclampsia and preeclampsia.

Kaku and Nagata (1955) and Browne and Sheumack (1956) suggested that preeclampsia might unmask a familial tendency to essential hypertension. On the other hand, Platt and coworkers (1958) entertained the possibility that incompatibility between mother and fetus was the cause of preeclampsia. This was followed by investigations in the United States and Scotland, which suggested that the disease pattern conformed to inheritance by a single recessive gene, but were unable to distinguish between the roles of the fetal and maternal genotypes. Some evidence pointing to the fetus came from Scottish preeclamptic probands and their relatives (Adams and Finlaysson, 1961; Cooper and Liston, 1979; Liston and Kilpatrick, 1991). Data based on only eclamptic women as index cases mainly supported maternal influences (Chesley and Cooper, 1986); there was no significant difference between the incidence of preeclampsia by whether the daughters were born of an eclamptic pregnancy or another pregnancy. Nor did it matter whether the mother had hypertension on long-term follow-up or if she was normotensive. In order try to distinguish between a maternal, fetal, or maternal-fetal genetic predisposition toward preeclampsia, the incidence of the disease in mothers, mothers-in-law, and matched controls was compared (Sutherland et al., 1981). The results again supported the hypothesis of a single maternal gene, when

Table 52.3. Percentage of Relatives With Hypertension and Proteinuria in Family Studies of Preeclampsia and Eclampsia[a]

Reference	Daughters	Daughters -in-law	Granddaughters	Mothers	Mothers-in-law	Sisters	Control
Humphries (1960)				(28.7)		(14.3)[b]	
Adams & Finlayson (1961)						13.8	4.5[c]
Chesley et al. (1961)	(32)				(37)		
Chesley (1968)	18.2 (25.7)	8	(25)				
Cooper & Liston (1979)				22.8		15.9	
Sutherland et al. (1981)				15.9	4.4		4.2
Chesley & Cooper (1986)	17.5 (26.2)	6.1	16.2				
Cooper et al. (1988)	16 (36)						
Kilpatrick et al. (1989)						11	2
Arngrímsson et al. (1990)	19.2 (25.8)	6.9 (11.2)	16.6 (26.6)				

[a] In many of the studies other criteria were mainly used and diagnosis of hypertension alone or the woman's own affirmation was sufficient for inclusion. The proportion of affected women using these various criteria as published by the authors is presented with parentheses.
[b] Mothers of normotensive women.
[c] Sisters of normotensive women. (Adapted from Arngrímsson, 1990, with permission.)

homozygous, was responsible for severe preeclampsia. The study also convincingly excluded that the inheritance pattern could be wholly ascribed to the fetal genotype. Scottish data, however, cast doubt on the autosomal recessive theory because the prevalence in sisters of affected women was lower than expected. The prevalence among consanguineous couples was also not higher than among offspring of unrelated parents (George et al., 1992). Furthermore, the prevalence among daughters and mothers of preeclamptic women was higher than among sisters. This can in part be explained by the high gene frequency estimated in these studies, but would in most instances indicate that autosomal dominant inheritance is the more plausible explanation. Data from 96 pedigrees selected through probands with eclampsia or severe preeclampsia (defined as blood pressure > 160/110 and proteinuria) showed that autosomal dominant inheritance with reduced penetrance could equally as well explain the familial tendency as the autosomal recessive model previously suggested (Arngrímsson et al., 1990). For the practicing clinician it is important to evaluate predictive factors for any medical conditions. In the case of preeclampsia it has proved difficult to find consistent and simple predictive factors, but among those potentially useful in classifying women into those with high risk and low risk groups is family history (Cincotta & Brenneke 1998; Mogren et al., 1999; Salonen Ros et al., 2000). The increment in rate of preeclampsia in women with positive family history of preeclampsia is reported to be 1.7–4.3 fold. This clinical history identifies women who warrant close clinical surveillance during pregnancy and possibly later in life.

EVIDENCE OF A FETAL INFLUENCE

Several observations support the involvement of the fetus in the development of the disorder. First, in a study of 48 families, Cooper and colleagues (1988) ascertained the pregnancy outcome of 96% of daughters of women with eclampsia and observed that eclampsia was more common in women born of eclamptic pregnancies as compared to their sisters born of a noneclamptic pregnancy. Second, hydatiform molar pregnancies, which possess two sets of paternal chromosomes and have no maternal contribution, are associated with increased risk of preeclampsia (Newman and Eddy, 1988). Oocyte-donation pregnancies are also associated with an increased likelihood of preeclampsia (Serhal and Craft, 1989), as are fetuses with trisomy 13 (Boyd et al., 1987). Association with confined placental mosaicism and uniparental disomy for chromosome 16 has been described (Kalousek et al., 1993). It appears that high populations of trisomic 16 cells in the placenta at term rather than uniparental disomy is linked to preeclampsia (D.K. Kalousek, 1996, personal communication). Careful cytogenetic studies of the term placenta may therefore be appropriate in early-onset, severe preeclampsia.

Data from two reports of monozygotic twins (zygosity determined by questionnaire) has caused considerable confusion for those studying genetic predisposition of preeclampsia. These reports showed lack of concordance for proteinuric preeclampsia and low concordance for transient hypertension among 10 twin pairs (Thompson and Fraser, 1988; Thornton and Onwude, 1991). This would only be explained by involvement of the fetus, a low penetrance of the maternal susceptibility gene(s), or both. By combining the data from these two studies, five or possibly six monozygotic twin pairs were concordant for transient hypertensive disease in pregnancy. The penetrance defined as the percentage of concordant affected cases out of all affected cases was 26%. However, this pooling of the data may not be valid due to different ascertainment, and straight comparison between the sisters may be inappropriate because of different complications experienced by one or the other twin, including stillbirth, previous abortion, or twin pregnancies. In an effort to estimate the liability of developing preeclampsia and gestational hypertension the population-based Swedish Twin Register and the Swedish Medical Birth Register were cross-linked (Salonen Ros et al., 2000). The study included 917 monozygotic and 1199 dizygotic twin pairs. The estimated heritability and non-shared environmental factors were 0.54 and 0.46 respectively for preeclampsia. Corresponding estimates for gestational hypertension alone were 0.24 and 0.76. When considering both diseases as a single entity the heritability estimate was 0.47.

One of the strongest pieces of evidence for fetal involvement has come from population-based data from the Medical Birth Registry of Norway (covering about 1.7 million births) and the Norwegian Central Population Register (Lie et al., 1998). The main outcome showed that both the mother and the fetus contributed to the risk of preeclampsia and that the contribution of the fetus was affected by paternal genes. For women who had experienced preeclampsia in first pregnancy and had a second pregnancy with the same partner, the risk was 11.8 fold compared to those who had been normotensive and not changed partner. In the groups where the women had changed partners between first and second pregnancy the relative risk of preeclampsia was 8.2 fold in second pregnancy for those who had previous preeclamptic pregnancy. If a woman became pregnant by a man who had previously fathered a preeclamptic pregnancy by a different woman, her risk of developing preeclampsia increased about 1.8 fold. If the woman had a half sister who had preeclampsia and with whom she shares the same mother but different fathers the risk is 1.6. If the half-sisters have the same father but different mothers the risk is 1.8. This shows that when women change partners for their second pregnancy their risk of recurrence is reduced but still substantial. Some of the risk of recurrence is however transmitted by the fathers. Men who fathered one preeclamptic pregnancy are nearly as twice as likely to father a preeclamptic pregnancy in a different woman regardless of whether she had already had a preeclamptic pregnancy or not. The fetuses in these pregnancies are paternal half siblings. Given the risk of recurrence carried by related fetuses is as high as the risk of recurrence for related mothers, the contribution of the fetus to the risk may be as large as the mother's own contribution.

HLA AND PREECLAMPSIA

The suggestion that fetal genotype might have a role to play in the development of preeclampsia has triggered some interesting hypotheses of maternal-fetal incompatibility and studies into the role of the major histocompatibility complex. The results have been contradictory and difficult to interpret due to lack of expression of these molecules on the human trophoblast cells that form the barrier between maternal and fetal tissues.

The relatively nonpolymorphic and nonclassic HLA-G antigen is expressed on the placenta. In preeclamptic pregnancies, reduced expression of this antigen correlates with a reduced number of trophoblasts in placental tissue (Colbern et al., 1994). Increased HLA sharing (Jenkins et al., 1978), increased HLA homozygosity (Redman et al., 1978b), and reduced reaction of maternal lymphocytes to paternal lymphocyte stimuli (Sargent et al., 1982) have all been observed. Women of the Zulu tribe with imminent eclampsia are more likely to be heterozygous at the HLA-B locus than normal controls (Johnson et al., 1988). Of the HLA antigens the most frequent association has been with HLA-DR4 type II antigen (Kilpatrick et al., 1987a), but also with DR5 and A30 antigens (Bolis et al., 1987). Some investigators have only observed an association with the exposure of the fetus to HLA-DR antigens (Hoff et al., 1992), while others have stressed that the risk of developing preeclampsia or growth retardation appeared to be higher if both the mother and infants bore HLA-DR antigen (Kilpatrick et al., 1990; Hoff et al., 1993). Not all studies have reported an association with the HLA-DR antigens (Wilton et al., 1990). Most recently, an association

with the rare HLA-A23/29, B44, DR7 haplotype has been described in preeclampsia (RR=3.33) and idiopathic intrauterine growth retardation (RR=4.19) (Peterson et al., 1994). When confounding factors such as gender, gestational age, ethnicity, and mother's stature and body mass were accounted for, the final relative risk was 6.02 for the combined group. This haplotype has previously only been associated with IgA deficiency, common variable immunodeficiency, and gluten-induced enteropathy.

MITOCHONDRIAL ABNORMALITIES

Notwithstanding the evidence for a fetal contribution in the development of preeclampsia, most of the data from familial and segregation studies point to a strong influence from factors within the mother herself. Although it seems clear that maternal susceptibility can not entirely be attributed to mitochondrial genes (Lie et al., 1998), Torbergsen and colleagues (1989) described a family with mitochondrial dysfunction that also had a high prevalence of preeclampsia. Mutations in the tRNA genes were found in these families (Folgero et al., 1996). Further studies have shown that well known mutations of the mitochondrial genome in the placenta tissue are unlikely to play a major part in the development of preeclampsia (Vuorinen et al., 1998). Long-chain 3-hydroxyacyl-CoA dehydrogenase (LCHAD) deficiency is one of recently discovered defects of the mitochondrial fatty acid β-oxidation. Female carriers of LCHAD deficiency are prone to have preeclampsia-like pregnancy complications (Tyni et al., 1998). Diagnosis is suggested by 3-hydroxylated acylcarnitine species in blood and definitive diagnosis can be made by measuring intermediates of fatty acid β-oxidation in fibroblasts or by detecting disease causing mutations (Tyni and Pihko, 1999). Women heterozygous for the mutation are reported to develop acute fatty liver of pregnancy and a high proportion also develop preeclampsia and HELLP syndrome (hemolysis, elevated liver enzymes, and low platelets (Treem et al., 1996, Strauss et al., 1999), but only when they carry an affected fetus (Tyni et al., 1998).

GENETIC MODEL FOR PREECLAMPSIA

In only one family study of preeclampsia have various inheritance models been compared (Arngrímsson et al., 1995). The prevalence among different groups of relatives of eclamptic, proteinuric preeclamptic, and normotensive women in six previous family studies were used to estimate the relative goodness of fit of several genetic models. Of the major gene inheritance mechanisms a model with dominant inheritance of the disease allele and equal penetrance (0.30) of the heterozygous and homozygous genotypes showed best fit. The test statistic for the multifactorial model was slightly higher than for the major gene model, but was still compatible with the data, and the estimate of heritability was 67%. The observed prevalence among sisters of affected probands was 14.3%, which was lower than among daughters/mothers (18.2%). These results differ somewhat from what had previously been concluded when the studies were first published. This may be due to the fact that only the goodness of fit of the autosomal recessive inheritance pattern was tested.

The criteria used in this analysis only allowed inclusion of those individuals who had documented evidence of blood pressure readings and urinary protein levels. The susceptibility to develop preeclampsia could be described as dichotomous expression of an underlying continuous trait that is normally distributed in the population. Individuals above a certain threshold on this liability trait will manifest the illness, and those below it will not do so. The observation of moderately low penetrance indicates that the maternal susceptibility is under strong external influence. The genetic model therefore implies that the woman's susceptibility to develop preeclampsia syndrome depends on both her genotype and an external pathologic factor, such as an abnormal or noncompatible trophoblast tissue. Her mean liability could theoretically be estimated before pregnancy by her genotype. Women in the low mean liability group could tolerate considerable fetal pathology before developing preeclampsia. This might explain why the idiopathic intrauterine growth-retardation syndrome is not always associated with maternal hypertension or proteinuria. Women whose liability falls above a certain threshold level are at risk of developing the syndrome even if only minor abnormalities are detected in the placental tissue (maternal factors predominance). This would explain why severe growth retardation is not a constant feature of the preeclampsia syndrome. Finally women whose liability falls above the threshold and have severe placental tissue changes would be those who develop severe preeclampsia associated with growth retardation, early onset and risk of secondary complications.

Arngrímsson and colleagues (1994a) suggested that the genetic predisposition to preeclampsia in some instances is related to implantation and placentation, a physiologic process that is complex and involves signalling between the developing embryo and the maternal tissue (Fig. 52.4). However, the main question still remains unanswered. Is it failure of the maternal tissue to suppress immune response in the decidua, which is prerequisite for successful invasion

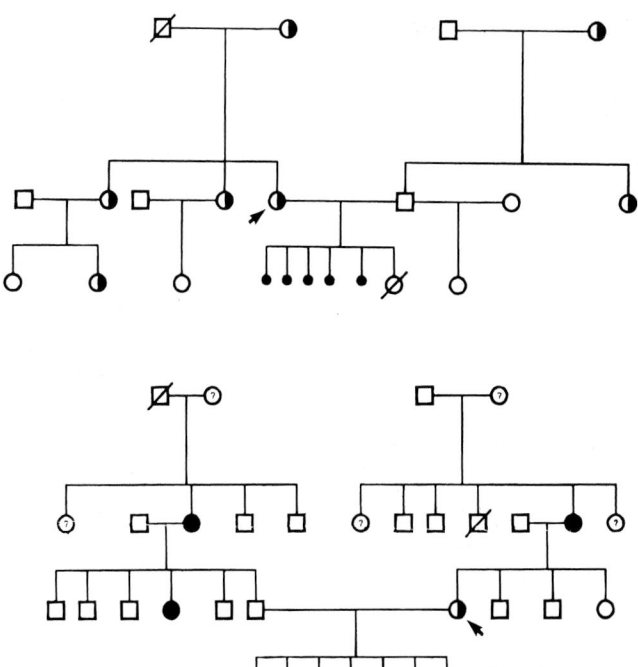

Fig. 52.4. In a study of 44 families, two couples were identified with a definite history of familial preeclampsia and eclampsia. Pregnancies of these couples either ended in early miscarriages (10), severe preeclampsia associated with growth retardation (2), or stillbirth (1). The high rate of miscarriages in these families and a definite link with severe preeclampsia and eclampsia support the notion that aberrant fetomaternal interaction may be a central pathogenic event in some forms of the preeclampsia syndrome, and that the putative genes that favor preeclampsia and eclampsia may be important for successful implantation and maintainance of a healthy pregnancy. ● = Eclampsia, ◑ = preeclampsia, □ = deceased or stillbirth, ○ = miscarriage; ⊘ = unknown pregnancy status. (Adapted from Arngrímsson et al., 1994a, with permission.)

of trophoblast cells, or are there intrinsic abnormalities in the invading trophoblast tissue?

MOLECULAR GENETIC STUDIES IN PREECLAMPSIA

All genetic studies of preeclampsia are hampered by the fact that the phenotype is only expressed in females and only during pregnancy. It is also plausible that the phenotype may be a result of more than one underlying cause. Studies that define the phenotype as either transient hypertension or hypertension and proteinuria will not necessarily identify the gene or genes involved in the development of the underlying condition, that is, the placental pathology, but may rather find association or linkage with genes that make women susceptible to develop these phenotypes under various stimuli. Hence this approach could potentially locate a genetic aberration important in blood pressure regulation. Future studies will aim to identify primary genes (involved in the invasion of the trophoblast cell and the maternal immune suppression function) and susceptibility genes (which make women at risk of developing hypertension, renal complications or both).

Linkage studies of the HLA locus and several random markers have been undertaken using the previously suggested autosomal recessive model without apparent positive findings (Wilton et al., 1990; Hayward et al., 1992; Arngrímsson et al., 1994b). Association' studies have implicated genetic background to some of the biochemical changes seen in preeclampsia. These include the angiotensinogen locus (Arngrímsson et al., 1993; Morgan et al., 1999; Ward et al., 1993), the angiotension II type I receptor (Morgan et al., 1998), nitric oxide synthase (eNOS) (Arngrímsson et al., 1997), which potentially affects the hemodynamic state, and blood pressure regulation. In the coagulation systems factor V Leiden (Kahn, 1998) and plasminogen activator inhibitor-1 (Yamada et al., 2000). In other metabolic systems the metylenetetrahydrofolate reductase (MTHFR) (Dizon-Townson et al., 1996) and the lipoprotein lipase gene (Hubel et al., 1999) have been implicated. Despite these findings, which would in general suggest polygenic mechanism in the development of preeclampsia, it is important to realize that almost as many reports have not confirmed the above associations when repeated in different populations or by different methods. Most of the positive observations carry little increase in risk and can not be used for prediction of preeclampsia. So today little consensus exists among investigators about which polymorphisms, mutations or genes should be called preeclampsia-related genes.

Only one report so far reaches the recommended levels of significance in genome-wide search for a trait locus. Recently, a genome-wide screening of Icelandic families representing 343 affected women, including patients with non-proteinuric preeclampsia (gestational hypertension), proteinuric preeclampsia and eclampsia detected a significant locus on 2p13 with a lod score of 4.70 (Arngrimsson et al., 1999). Interestingly, a fair contribution came from relatively large pedigrees with multiple affected women. At this point it is difficult to assess the contribution of the chromosome 2 locus to preeclampsia cases in general. Under the assumption of dominant model it was estimated that 22% of the families were affected by this mutation. Positive finding has also been reported in data from Australia, in which many families have multiple affected cases (Brennecke, 2000, personal communications). However, given the complexity of the disease phenotype, a reliable assessment of the effect of the chromosome 2 locus will probably have to wait until the gene is identified.

GENE EXPRESSION STUDIES IN PREECLAMPSIA

Successful implantation and placentation rely on complex interactions of cytokines, transcriptional regulators, and growth factors derived from both fetal and maternal tissue. Several growth factors and cytokines have been identified in placental tissue, for example, epidermal growth factor (Hofmann et al., 1988), tumor necrosis factor-α (Austgulen et al., 1992; Li et al., 1992) and transforming growth factors β (Selick et al., 1994). Such factors regulate the proliferation and differentiation of the trophoblast cells at various stages of pregnancy. The actual regulating process is as yet poorly understood. Growth factors may also play an important role in suppressing immunoreaction in the decidua and thus facilitate successful implantation, but one of the fundamental questions in medicine is how human extraembryonic tissues escape rejection by the mother.

Understanding the basic principles of implantation and placentation is essential for interpreting the pathologic process in preeclampsia. Studies into the function and regulation of genes expressed in the placenta are therefore important. Although much has been learned about gene expression in placental cells, few studies have investigated changes in expression patterns in normal and preeclamptic pregnancies.

Expression of plasminogen activator inhibitor type 1 (PAI-1) mRNA and protein is enhanced in syncytiotrophoblasts from women with preeclamptic and growth-retarded pregnancies (Estelles et al., 1994), but elevated levels of PAI-1 have been implicated in mediating the fibrin deposition within occlusive lesions in the spiral arteries.

Changes in the expression pattern of cell membrane molecules on trophoblast and changes in the production of various components of the extracellular matrix as the cells travel deeper into the maternal tissues have been described in preeclampsia (Damsky et al., 1992). Expression of integrins is abnormal in preeclamptic pregnancies and favors those restraining the invasion process.

Among the most potent vasoconstrictor agents are the endothelins, and they are thought to exert their effects locally rather than systemically. (Yanagisawa et al., 1988). Three types are known, but only the ET-1, produced by endothelial cells, is found in the circulation. Production of endothelins appears to be regulated primarily by modulation of mRNA levels. Expression of ET-1 mRNA is significantly higher in the uterine muscle layer during pregnancy than in the nonpregnant state. In preeclampsia, significantly higher ET-1 expression occurs in placental villous tissue (at 32 weeks gestation) than in normotensive pregnancies (38 weeks) (McMahon et al., 1993). Excessive placental secretion of neurokinin B during the third trimester has been reported to be associated with elevation of blood pressure in pregnancy and preeclampsia (Page et al., 2000). The expression of neurokinin B is confined to the outer syncytiotrophoblast of the placenta and significant concentration can be detected as early as week nine of pregnancy.

These studies indicate that local regulation at the cell level may be important for initiation and progress of the pathophysical processes in preeclampsia. Elevated levels of trophoblast PAI-1 may play a role in the initiation of placental damage as well as in associated thrombotic complications. Increased local production of ET-1 can contribute to vasoconstriction and vascular insufficiency and hence fetal growth retardation. Dysregulation of trophoblast cell differentiation, possibly in association with altered growth factor and cytokine activity may explain why cell migration is limited to the decidual portion of the spiral vessels in preeclampsia.

Imprinting is a potentially important mechanism for fetal growth retardation and fetal loss. Severe early-onset growth retardation is known to occur in fetuses with maternal uniparental disomy (Bennet et al., 1992), where growth retardation may be associated with underexpression of imprinted growth-related genes on chromosome 16. This phenomenon is well described in mice (DeChiara et al., 1991). How idiopathic intrauterine grow retardation and possibly preeclampsia may be associated with genetic imprinting awaits future research.

Animal models

There is no spontaneous disease or inducible condition in animals that has general acceptance as a model for preeclampsia. From an evolutionary point of view, preeclampsia is probably a rather recent natural phenomenon, since the disorder has only been detected in humans, and a similar condition has only been seen in closely related species such as the gorilla, the chimpanzee, and the patas monkey, with a possible familial factor beeing detected in the gorillas (Thornton and Onwude, 1992).

The animal models devised to mimic preeclampsia can be divided into the following categories: (1) Uteroplacental ischemia model, with either aortic constriction, placental vascular occlusion or multiple vessel ligation. (2) Dietary manipulation model with either starvation or single or multiple nutrient deficiency. (3) Alterations of vasopressor balance, e.g., with inhibition of nitric oxide synthesis or infusion of thromboxane A_2. (4) Endothelial injury by endotoxin infusion. (5) Gene manipulation of animals. (6) Animals with preexisting disease that predispose to preeclampsia, e.g., renal disease or hypertension.

Experimental preeclampsia-like disease has been induced in various animals by nutritional manipulation and by inducing placental ischemia. Placental ischemia in baboons causes a similar clinical picture as in humans, including typical glomerular changes (Cavanagh et al., 1977; Horvath et al., 1990). A preeclampsia-like syndrome with hypertension and growth retardation has been induced in rats by inhibition of nitric oxide synthesis (Yallampalli and Garfield, 1992; Molnar et al., 1994). Rabbits have also been used for this purpose, and treatment with 17 β-estradiol enhances release of endothelium-derived relaxing factor (nitric oxide) in the uterine vasculature, but not in the systemic circulation (Gisclard et al., 1988). This supports the notion that local regulation of vasoactive substances takes place within the uterus.

Other rat models include vitamin E-deficient rats fed with oxidized lipids, where morphologic and functional abnormalities of the trophoblast have been correlated with clinical and pathologic features resembling eclampsia (Goldstein et al., 1964; Zunker et al., 1965). Transgenic mice model has shown that both renin gene from the father and angiotensinogen gene in the mother contribute to the risk of hypertension during pregnancy (Takimoto et al., 1996).

Management of preeclampsia

Preeclampsia is still among the most common causes of pregnancy-related deaths. Death generally occurs from cerebral hemorrhage, pulmonary edema, anoxic cardiac arrest, or hepatic failure. In order to minimize the morbidity and mortality associated with this condition it is essential that a multidisciplinary approach is established in every referral hospital.

In principle the management of preeclampsia incorporates early diagnosis, well-timed delivery to avoid complications, and postpartum follow-up to define underlying medical problems. Preeclampsia is asymptomatic, and the diagnosis depends on screening pregnant women. It is important to review all pregnant women at the end of the first trimester, divide them into low- and high-risk groups

(Table 52.4), and modify the gap between antenatal visits accordingly. The baseline assessment should include arterial blood pressure measurements and urinary protein analysis. For those in the high-risk category, additional laboratory measurements should include a platelet count, serum creatinine and uric acid, and liver function tests (Redman, 1989). The maternal factors may be easier to identify, but fetal factors only become apparent as pregnancy evolves. At present, several methods are being established to assess fetal health using various biophysical approaches to estimate intrauterine health of the fetoplacental unit. This includes fetal heart rate monitoring and Doppler measurements of flow velocity waveform patterns in the fetal circulation. The latter may be a useful screening test in high-risk pregnancies, allowing identification of fetuses at risk of becoming hypoxic (Bower et al., 1993). Changes in fetal behavior (movements and breathing pattern) and oligohydramnios are all warning signs.

The objective of hospital treatment is to deliver the baby before the disease progresses to the stage of an obstetric emergency (Table 52.5). This stage of the disease is often associated with clinical symptoms such as headache, visual disturbances, hyperreflexia, and epigastrial pain. It is a life-threatening situation and delivery should be immediate after stabilization.

Medical treatment is aimed at controlling the hypertension and avoiding serious complications associated with pressure-induced arterial injury, such as cerebral hemorrhage. Medication must be chosen carefully with regard to its cardiovascular and renal effects. Frequently, it is essential to monitor fluid balance and to treat neurologic problems and coagulation disturbances in patients with severe preeclampsia or imminent eclampsia.

Preeclampsia is associated with an altered intravascular ratio of thromboxane and prostacyclin (Bussolino et al., 1980). This finding and the evidence of activation of the

Table 52.4. Risk Factors for Preeclampsia Divided into Maternal, Fetal, and Environmental Components

Maternal	Fetal	Environmental[a]
First pregnancy	Multiple pregnancies	Infections (viral)?
Previous preeclamptic pregnancy	Oocyte donation pregnancies	Nutritional factors, e.g., low plasma levels of
Family history of preeclampsia or eclampsia	Hydatiform moles	antioxidants
Women under 20 or over 35 years old	Hydrops	
Chronic hypertension or renal disease	Trisomy 13 and triploidy pregnancies	
Collagen vascular disease	Confined placental moscaism (Ch. 16)	
Diabetes mellitus	Uniparental disomy?	
Migraines		
Underweight and short		

[a]Infectious agent has previously been suggested (Kilpatrick et al., 1987b), but definite proof is lacking. Evidence for nutritional factors comes primarily from animal experiments, but dietary supplements of minerals, vitamins, and halibut liver oil have also been shown to cause modest but significant reduction in the incidence of preeclampsia (People's League of Health, 1946).

Table 52.5. Progress and Management of Preeclampsia[a]

Stages of preeclampsia		
Pathologic	Clinical	Management
Primary pathologic changes in the placental bed	Subclinical	Screening and evaluation; baseline assessment Identification of risk factors
Secondary pathologic changes	Hypertension	Frequent monitoring in a day-care unit
Involvement of maternal organs	Preeclampsia	Admission to hospital; short-term medical treatment to prolong the pregnancy to 34–36 weeks
Tertiary pathologic changes	Visual disturbances	Life-threatening situation for mother and baby
Damage to the maternal organs	Eclampsia Renal failure DIC/HELLP syndrome Cerebral hemorrhage	Immediate delivery after stabilization

[a] The diagnosis of suspected preeclampsia should be made early in the hypertensive stage, and follow-up should be at a specialized high-risk clinic. Mild to moderate hypertension alone is in most instances not a reason for hospital admission, but as it is commonly the earliest sign of preeclampsia it demands frequent monitoring in a day-care unit. Women who progress to develop proteinuria should be admitted on the same day to a hospital that can offer continuous monitoring and care by an experienced team.

clotting system with early involvement of platelets (Redman et al., 1978a) have led to the use of low-dose antiplatelet agents (usually low-dose aspirin, 60–150 mg/day) in an attempt to ameliorate or prevent the development of preeclampsia. This treatment inhibits platelet cyclooxygenase and thus the production of the vasoconstrictor and platelet aggregating agent thromboxane A_2. Several small controlled trials have reported a reduction in the incidence of proteinuric preeclampsia when aspirin alone or in combination with other presumed antiplatelet agents (e.g., dipyridamole) has been prescribed. Larger trials have failed to show substantial benefits, and side effects such as hemorrhage remain a concern. (Italian Study of Aspirin in Pregnancy, 1993; Sibai et al., 1993). The largest randomized multicenter trial so far failed to show significant benefit of low-dose aspirin for the prevention and treatment of preeclampsia among almost 10,000 women (CLASP, 1994). Overall the use of aspirin was associated with a 12% reduction in proteinuric preeclampsia (which was not significant), but the treatment did significantly reduce the likelihood of preterm delivery. Low-dose aspirin may be justified in women judged to be especially liable to early-onset preeclampsia severe enough to lead to preterm delivery although definite proof of that may still be lacking (Caritis et al., 1998). Prevention of preeclampsia with vitamin supplementation (E and C vitamins) has been suggested to be beneficial in women falling into the high risk category of preeclampsia (Chappell et al., 1999), although multicenter trials may be needed to confirm this finding.

REFERENCES

Aalkjaer C, Danielsen H, Johannesen P et al. (1985) Abnormal vascular functional morphology in preeclampsia: a study of isolated resistance vessels. Clin Sci 69:477–482

Adams EM, Finlayson A (1961) Familial aspects of preeclampsia and hypertension in pregnancy. Lancet ii:1375–1378

Adams EM, MacGillivray I (1961) Long term effect of preeclampsia and blood pressure. Lancet ii:1373–1375

Alvarez H, Medrano CV, Sala MA, Benedetti WL (1972) Trophoblast development gradient and its relationship to placental haemodynamics II. Study of fetal cotyledons from toxemic placenta. Am J Obstet Gynecol 95:1134–48

Arbogast BW, Leeper SC, Merrick RD et al. (1994) Which plasma factors bring about disturbances of endothelial function in preeclampsia? Lancet 343:340–341

Arkwright PD, Rademacher TW, Dwek RA, Redman CWG (1993) Preeclampsia is associated with an increase in trophoblast glycogen content and glycogen synthase activity, similar to that found in hydatidiform moles. J Clin Invest 91:2744–53

Arngrímsson R (1990) Inheritance and family patterns in pre-eclampsia and eclampsia. Contemp Rev Obstet Gynaecol 2:152–158

Arngrímsson R, Björnsson S, Geirsson RT et al. (1990) Genetic and familial predisposition to eclampsia and pre-eclampsia in a defined island population. Br J Obstet Gynaecol 97:762–770

Arngrímsson R, Purandare S, Connor MJ et al. (1993) Angiotensinogen: a candidate gene in preeclampsia? Nature Genet 4:114–115

Arngrímsson R, Connor JM, Geirsson RT et al. (1994a) Is genetic susceptibility for pre-eclampsia and eclampsia associated with implantation failure and fetal demise? Lancet 343:1643–1644

Arngrímsson R, Geirsson RT, Cooke A et al. (1994b) Renin gene restriction fragment length polymorphisms do not show linkage with preeclampsia and eclampsia. Acta Obstet Gynecol Scand 73:10–13

Arngrímsson R, Björnsson H, Geirsson RT (1995) Analysis of different inheritance patterns in preeclampsia/eclampsia syndrome. Hypertens Preg 14:27–38

Arngrímsson R, Hayward C, Nadaud S et al. (1997) Evidence for a familial pregnancy-induced hypertension locus in the eNOS-gene region. Am J Hum Genet 61:354–362

Arngrímsson R, Sigurdardottir S, Frigge ML et al. (1999) A genome-wide scan reveals a maternal susceptibility locus for preeclampsia on chromosome 2p13. Hum Mol Genet 8:1799–1805

Arnholdt H, Meisel F, Fandrey K, Lohrs U (1991) Proliferation of villous trophoblast of the human placenta in normal and abnormal pregnancies. Virchows Arch B 60:365–372

Augensen K, Bergsjö P (1984) Maternal mortality in the Nordic countries 1970–79. Acta Obstet Gynaecol Scand 63:115–121

Austgulen R, Espevik T, Meesci R, Scott H (1992) Expression of receptors for tumor necrosis factor in human placenta at term. Acta Obstet Gynaecol Scand 71:417–424

Baker PN, Broughton-Pipkin F, Symonds EM (1989) Platelet angiotensin II binding sites in hypertension in pregnancy. Lancet i:1151

Barden AE, Beilin LJ, Ritchie J, Walters BN, Michael C (1999) Does a predisposition to the metabolic syndrome sensitize women to develop preeclampsia? J Hypertens 17:1307–1315

Barker DJP (1992) Fetal and infant origins of adult disease. BMJ

Barton JR, Hiett AK, O'Connor WN et al. (1991) Endomyocardial ultrastructural findings in preeclampsia. Am J Obstet Gynecol 165:389–391

Benedetti TJ, Cotton DB, Read JC et al. (1980) Haemodynamic observations in severe preeclampsia with a flow-directed pulmonary artery catheter. Am J Obstet Gynecol 136:465–470

Bennet P, Vaughan J, Henderson D et al. (1992) Association between confined placental trisomy, fetal uniparental disomy, and early intrauterine growth retardation. Lancet 340:1284–1285

Bird IM, Zheng J, Cale JM, Magness RR (1997) Pregnancy induces an increase in angiotensin II type-1 receptor expression in uterine but not systemic artery endothelium. Endocrinology 138:490–498

Bolis PF, Bianchi MM, La Fianza A et al. (1987) Immunogenetic aspects of preeclampsia. Biol Res Pregn 8:42–45

Bower S, Schuchter K, Campbell S (1993) Doppler ultrasound scanning as part of routine antenatal scanning: prediction of preeclampsia and intrauterine growth retardation. Br J Obstet Gynaecol 100:989–994

Boyd PA, Brown RA, Coghill GR et al. (1983) Measurement of the mass of syncytiotrophoblast in a range of human placentae using an image analysis computer. Placenta 4:255–262

Boyd PA, Lindenbaum RH, Redman C (1987) Pre-eclampsia and trisomy 13: a possible association. Lancet ii:425–427

Brosens IA, Robertson WB, Dixon HG (1972) The role of the spiral arteries in the pathogenesis of preeclampsia. Obstet Gynecol Ann 1:177–191

Brosens I, Dixon HG, Robertson WB (1977) Fetal growth retardation and the arteries of the placental bed. Br J Obstet Gynaecol 84:656–663

Broughton-Pipkin F (1988) The renin-angiotensin system in normal and hypertensive pregnancies. In Rubin PC (ed): Hypertension in Pregnancy. Handbook of Hypertension. Elsevier, Amsterdam, 10:118–151

Browne FJ, Sheumack DR (1956) Chronic hypertension following pre-eclamptic toxaemia: the influence of familial hypertension on its causation. J Obstet Gynaecol Br Commonw 63:677–680

Bussolino F, Benedetto C, Massobrio M, Camussi G (1980) Maternal vascular prostacyclin activity in preeclampsia. Lancet ii:702

Campbell DM, MacGillivray I (1985) Pre-eclampsia in second pregnancy. Br J Obstet Gynaecol 92:131–140

Caritis S, Sibai B, Hauth J et al. (1998) Low-dose aspirin to prevent preeclampsia in women at high risk. National Institute of Child Health and Human Development Network of Maternal-Fetal Medicine. N Engl J Med 338:701–705

Cavanagh D, Rao PS, Tsai CC, O'Connor TC (1977) Experimental toxaemia in the pregnant primate. Am J Obstet Gynecol 128:75–85

Chappell LC, Seed PT, Briley AL et al. (1999) Effect of antioxidants on the occurrence of preeclampsia in women at increased risk: a randomized trial. Lancet 354:810–816

Chesley LC (1978) Hypertensive Disorders in Pregnancy. Appelton & Lange, E. Norwalk, CT

Chesley LC (1980) Hypertension in pregnancy: definitions, familial factor and remote prognosis. Kidney Int 18:234–240

Chesley LC, Cooper DW (1986) Genetics of hypertension in pregnancy: possible single gene control of preeclampsia and eclampsia. Am J Obstet Gynecol 53:851–863

Chesley LC, Cosgrove RA, Annitto JE (1961) Pregnancy in sisters and daughters of eclamptic women. J Pathol Microbiol 24:662–666

Chesley LC, Annitto JE, Cosgrove RA (1968) The familial factor in toxemia of pregnancy. Obstet Gynecol 32:303–311

Chesley LC, Annitto JE, Cosgrove RA (1976) The remote prognosis of eclamptic women: sixth periodic report. Am J Obstet Gynecol 124:446–459

Chisolm GM, Irwin KC, Penn MS (1992) Lipoprotein oxidation and lipoprotein-induced cell injury in diabetes. Diabetes 41:61–66

Christianson RE (1976) Studies on blood pressure during pregnancy I. Influence of parity and age. Am J Obstet Gynecol 125:509–513

Cincotta RB, Brennecke SP (1998) Family history of preeclampsia as a predictor for preeclampsia in primigravidas. Int J Gynaecol Obstet 60:23–27

Clark SL, Cotton DB, DeLee W et al. (1989) Central hemodynamics of normal term pregnancy. Am J Obstet Gynecol 161:1439–1442

CLASP (Collaborative Low-Dose Aspirin Study in Pregnancy) Collaborative Group (1994) Randomised trial of low-dose aspirin for the prevention and treatment of preeclampsia among 9364 pregnant women. Lancet 343:619–629

Colbern GT, Chiang MH, Main EK (1994) Expression of the nonclassic histocompatibility antigen HLA-G by preeclamptic placenta. Am J Obstet Gynecol 170:1244–1250

Cooper DW, Liston WA (1979) Genetic control of severe preeclampsia. J Med Genet 16:409–416

Cooper DW, Hill JA, Chesley LC, Bryans CI (1988) Genetic control of susceptibility to eclampsia and miscarriage. Br J Obstet Gynaecol 95:644–653

Cotton DB, Lee W, Huhta JC et al. (1988) Hemodynamic profile of severe pregnancy-induced hypertension. Am J Obstet Gynecol 158:523–529

Cross JC (2000) Genetic insight into trophoblast differentiation and placental morphogenesis. Semin Cell Dev Biol 11:105–113

Damsky CH, Fitzgerald ML, Fisher SJ (1992) Distribution patterns of extracellular matrix components and adhesion receptors are intricately modulated during first trimester cytotrophoblast differentiation along the invasive pathway in vivo. J Clin Invest 89:210–222

Damsky CH, Sutherland A, Fisher S (1993) Extracellular matrix 5: adhesive interactions in early mammalian embryogenesis, implantation and placentation. FASEB J 7:1320–1329

Davey DA, MacGillivray I (1988) The classification and definition of hypertensive disorders of pregnancy. Am J Obstet Gynecol 158:892–898

Davies AM, Czaczkes KW, Sadosky E et al. (1970) Toxaemia of pregnancy in Jerusalem: epidemiological studies of total community. Isr J Med Sci 6:253–266

Davison JM, Hytten FE (1974) Glomerular filtration during and after pregnancy. J Obstet Gynaecol Br Commonw 81:588–595

DeChiara TM, Robertson EJ, Efstratiadis A (1991) Paternal imprinting of mouse insulinlike growth factor II gene. Cell 64:849–859

Dekker GA, de Vries JI, Doelitzsch PM (1995) Underlying disorders associated with severe early-onset preeclampsia. Am J Obstet Gynecol 173:1042–1048

DeLee JB (1905) Theories of eclampsia. Am J Obstet 51:325–330

Department of Health (1979) Report on confidential enquiries into maternal deaths in England and Wales 1973–75. HM Stationery Office, London

de Vries MJ, Dekker GA, Schoemaker J (1998) Higher risk of preeclampsia in the polycystic ovary syndrome. A case control study. Eur J Obstet Gynecol Reprod Biol 76:91–95

Dizon-Townson DS, Nelson LM, Easton K et al. (1996) The factor V Leiden mutation may predispose women to severe preeclampsia. Am J Obstet Gynecol 175:902–905

Duley L (1992) Maternal mortality associated with hypertensive disorder of pregnancy in Africa, Asia, Latin America and the Caribbean. Br J Obstet Gynaecol 99:547–553

Dunlop W (1981) Serial changes in renal hemodynamics during normal human pregnancy. Br J Obstet Gynaecol 88:1–9

Elliot GT (1873) Case 120: Puerperial Eclampsia in the Eighth Month; Extraordinary Family History. Obstetricial Clinic, Appleton, New York

Eskenazi B, Fenster L, Sidney S (1991) A multivariate analysis of risk factors for preeclampsia. JAMA 266:237–241

Eskenazi B, Fenster L, Sidney S, Elkin EP (1993) Fetal growth retardation in infants of multiparous and nulliparous women with preeclampsia. Am J Obstet Gynecol 169:1112–1118

Estelles A, Gilabert J, Espana F et al. (1987) Fibrinolysis in preeclampsia. Fibrinolysis 1:209–214

Estelles A, Gilabert J, Keeton M et al. (1994) Altered expression of plasminogen activator inhibitor type 1 in placentas from pregnant women with preeclampsia and/or intrauterine growth retardation. Blood 84:143–150

Fadnes HO, Øian P (1989) Transcapillary fluid balance and plasma volume regulation: a review. Obstet Gynecol Surv 44:69–73

Fallis NE, Langford HG (1963) Relation of second trimester blood pressure toxaemia of pregnancy in the primigravid patient. Am J Obstet Gynecology 87:123–125

Fisher KA, Luger A, Spargo BH, Lindheimer MD (1973) Hypertension in pregnancy: clinical-pathological correlation and remote prognosis. Medicine 60:267–276

Folgero T, Storbakk N, Torbergsen T, Oian P (1996) Mutation in mitochondrial transfer ribonucleic acid acid genes in preeclampsia. Am J Obstet Gynecol 174:1626–1630

Friedman SA, Taylor RN, Roberts JM (1991) Pathophysiology of preeclampsia. Clin Perinatol 18:661–682

Gallery EM, Hunyor SN, Györy AZ (1979) Plasma volume contraction: A significant factor in both pregnancy-associated hypertension (preeclampsia) and chronic hypertension in pregnancy. Q J Med 48:593–602

Gant NF, Daley GL, Chand S et al. (1973) A study of angiotensin II pressor response throughout primigravid pregnancy. J Clin Invest 52:2682–2689

Garner PR, D'Alton ME, Dudley DK et al. (1990) Preeclampsia in diabetic pregnancies. Am J Obstet Gynecol 163:505–508

Geirsson RT, Arngrímsson R, Apalset E et al. (1994) Falling population incidence of eclampsia: a case control study of short term outcome. Acta Obstet Gynecol Scand 73:465–467

George K, Vedamony J, Idikulla J, Rao PSS (1992) The effect of consanguinity on pregnancy-induced hypertension. Aust N Z J Obstet Gynaecol 32:231–233

Gerretsen G, Huisjes HJ, Elma JD (1981) Morphological changes of the spiral arteries in the placental bed in relation to preeclampsia and fetal growth retardation. Br J Obstet Gynaecol 88:876–881

Gifford RW, August P, Chesley LC et al. (1990) National high blood pressure education program working group report on high blood pressure in pregnancy. Am J Obstet Gynecol 163:1691–712

Gisclard V, Miller VM, Vanhoutte PM (1988) Effect of 17 β-estradiol on endothelium-dependent responses in the rabbit. J Pharmacol Exp Ther 244:19–22

Goldstein HB, Hochstein P, McKay DG (1964) Tissue metabolism in experimental toxaemia of pregnancy. Am J Obstet Gynecol 88:791–794

Grandone E, Margalione M, Colaizzo D et al. (1997) Factor V Leiden, C > T MTHFR polymorphism and genetic susceptibility to preeclampsia. Thromb Haemost 77:1052–1054

Greer IA, Hadded NG, Dawes J et al. (1989) Neutrophil activation in pregnancy-induced hypertension. Br J Obstet Gynaecol 96:978–982

Greer IA, Lyall F, Perera T et al. (1994) Increased concentration of cytokines II-6 and II-Ira in plasma of women with pre-eclampsia: a mechanism for endothelial dysfunction? Obstet Gynecol 84:937–940

Halliwel B, Gutteridge J (1989) Free Radicals in Biology and Medicine 2nd Ed. p. 236. Clarendon Press, Oxford

Hauch E, Lehman K (1934) Investigation into the occurrence of eclampsia in Denmark during 1918–1927. Acta Obstet Gynecol Scand 14:425

Hays PH, Cruikshank DP, Dunn LJ (1985) Plasma volume determination in normal and preeclamptic pregnancies. Am J Obstet Gynecol 151:958–966

Hayward C, Livingstone J, Holloway S et al. (1992) An exclusion map for pre eclampsia: assuming autosomal recessive inheritance. Am J Hum Genet 50:749–757

He S, Silveira A, Hamsten A et al. (1999) Haemostatic, endothelial and lipoprotein prameters and blood pressure levels in women with a history of preeclampsia. Thromb Haemost 81:538–542

Higgins M, Keller J, Moore F et al. (1980) Studies of blood pressure in young people and its relationship to personal and familial characteristics and complications of pregnancy in mothers. Am J Epidemiol 111:142–155

Hochner-Celnikier D, Shimonovitz S, Bursztyn M et al. (1993) The prognosis of hypertensive disease of pregnancy accompanied by intrauterine growth retardation in relation to parity. Acta Obstet Gynecol Scan 72:531–533

Hoff C, Peevy K, Giattina K et al. (1992) Maternal-fetal HLA-DR relationships and pregnancy-induced hypertension. Obstet Gynecol 80:1007–1011

Hoff C, Peevy K, Spinnato JA et al. (1993) Association between maternal-fetal relationships and fetal growth. Am J Reprod Immunol 30:246–254

Hofmann GE, Rao CV, Carmen FR, Siddiqi TA (1988) [125]I human epidermal growth factor binding to placentas and fetal membranes from various pregnancy states. Acta Endocrinol 117:5239–5334

Horstkamp BS, Kiess H, Kramer J et al. (1999) Activated protein C restistance showns an association with pregnancy-induced hypertension. Hum Reprod 14:3112–3115

Horvath JS, Phippard AF, Gillin AG et al. (1990) A model of preeclampsia including renal histology, in the baboon, abstracted. Proceedings of the Seventh World Congress of Hypertension in Pregnancy, Perugia, 1990

Hubel CA (1999) Oxidative stress in the pathogenesis of preeclampsia. Proc Soc Exp Biol Med 222:222–235

Hubel CA, Lyall F, Weissfeld L et al. (1998) Small low density lipoproteins and vascular cell adhesion molecule (VCAM-1) are increased in association with hyperlipidemia in preeclampsia. Metabolism 47:1281–1288

Hubel CA, Roberts JM, Ferrell RE (1999) Association of pre-eclampsia with common coding sequence variations in the lipoprotein lipase gene. Clin Genet 56:289–296

Hubel CA, Snaedal S, Ness RB et al. (2000) Dyslipoproteinaemia in postmenopausal women with a history of eclampsia. Br J Obstet Gynaecol 107:776–784

Humphries JO (1960) Occurence of hypertensive toxemia of pregnancy in mother-daughter pairs. Bull John Hopkins Hosp 107:271–277

Hustin J, Foidart JM, Lambotte R (1984) Cellular proliferation in villi of normal and pathological pregnancies. Gynecol Obstet Invest 17:1–9

Inglis TC, Stuart J, George AJ, Davies AJ (1982) Haemostatic and rheological changes in normal pregnancy and preeclampsia. Br J Haematol 50:461–65

Ishihara M (1978) Studies on lipoperoxide of normal pregnant women and women with toxaemic pregnancy. Clin Chim Acta 84:1–9

Italian Study of Aspirin in Pregnancy (1993) Low dose aspirin in prevention and treatment of intrauterine growth retardation and pregnancy-induced hypertension. Lancet 341:396–400

Jenkins DM, Need JA, Scott JS et al. (1978) Human leucocyte antigens and mixed lymphocytic reaction in severe pre-eclampsia. B Med J 1:542–545

Johnson N, Moodley J, Hammond MG (1988) Human leucocyte antigen status in African women with eclampsia. B J Obstet Gynaecol 95:877–879

Jónsdóttir LS, Arngrímsson R, Geirsson RT et al. (1995) Increased death rate from ischemic heart disease among women with previous history of preeclampsia syndrome. Acta Obstet Gynecol Scand 74:772–776

Kahn SR (1998) Severe preeclampsia associated with coinheritance of factor V Leiden mutation and protein S deficiency. Obstet Gynecol 91:812–814

Kaku M, Nagata H (1955) Hypertensive lineage and toxemia of pregnancy. Am J Obstet Gynecol 78:399–404

Kalousek DK, Langois S, Barret I et al. (1993) Uniparental disomy for chomosome 16 in humans. Am J Hum Genet 52:8–16

Kaunitz, II, Malins D, McKay DO (1962) Studies of the generalised Shwartzman reaction produced by diet. II. Feeding of oxidised cod liver oil. J Exp Med 115:1127–1136

Kertesz Z, Linton EA, Redman CW (2000) Adhesion molecules of syncytiotrophoblast microvillous membranes inhibit proliferation of human umbilical vein endothelial cells. Placenta 21:150–159

Khong TY, DeWolf F, Robertson WB, Brosens I (1986) Inadequate maternal vascular response to placentation in pregnancies complicated by preeclampsia and small-for-gestational age infants. Br J Obs Gynaecol 93:1049–59

Khong TY, Hilary Sawyer I, Heryer AR (1992) An immunohistologic study of endothelialization of uteroplacental vessels in human pregnancy: evidence that endothelium is focally disrupted by trophoblast in preeclampsia. Am J Obstet Gynecol 167:751–756

Kilpatrick DC, Jazwinska EC, Liston WA, Smart GE (1987a) Severe preeclampsia in multiparous women: indication of an environmental triggering agent? Scott Med J 32:8–10

Kilpatrick DC, Liston WA, Jazwinska EC, Smart GE (1987b) Histocompatibility studies in pre-eclampsia. Tissue Antigens 29:232–236

Kilpatrick DC, Gibson F, Livingstone J, Liston WA (1990) Pre-eclampsia is associated with HLA-Dr4 sharing between mother and fetus. Tissue Antigens 35:178–181

Kitzmiller JL, Beirschke K (1973) Immunofluorescent study of placental bed vessels in preeclampsia. Am J Obstet Gynecol 15:248–251

Kotchen JM, Kotchen TA, Cottrill CM et al. (1979) Blood pressure of young mothers and their children 3–6 years following hypertension during pregnancy. J Chron Dis 36:653–659

Kyle PM, Clark SJ, Buckley D et al. (1993) Second trimester ambulatory blood pressure in nulliparous pregnancy: a useful screening test for pre-eclampsia. B J Obstet Gynecol 100:914–919

Labarrere CA, Althabe OH (1986) Primary chronic abortion, preeclampsia, idiopathic intrauterine growth retardation, hydatidiform mole, and choriocarcinoma: a unifying concept. Am J of Reprod Immunol Microbiol 10:156–157

Laivuori H, Tikkanen MJ, Ylikorkala O (1996) Hyperinsulinemia 17 years after preeclamptic first pregnancy. J Clin Endocrinol Metab 81:2908–2911

Langford HG, Watson RL (1980) Pre-pregnant blood pressure, hypertension during pregnancy, and later blood pressure of mothers and offspring. Hypertension 2: (Suppl I):130–133

Li Y, Matsuzaki N, Masuhiro K et al. (1992) Trophoblast-derived tumor necrosis factor-a induces release of human chorionic gonadotropin using interleukin-6 (IL-6) and IL-6-receptor-dependent system in the normal human trophoblasts. J Clin Endocrinol Metab 74:184–191

Lie RT, Rasmussen S, Brunborg H et al. (1998) Fetal and maternal contributions to risk of pre-eclampsia: population based study. Br Med J 316:1343–1347

Lin CC, Lindheimer MD, River P, Moawad AH (1982) Fetal outcome in hypertensive disorders of pregnancy. Am J Obstet Gynecol 142:255–260

Lindeberg S, Axelson O, Jorner U et al. (1988) A Prospective controlled five-year follow-up study of primiparas with gestational hypertension. Acrta Obstet Gynecol Scand 67:605–609

Lindheimer MD, Chesley LC, Taylor JR et al. (1987) Renal function and morphology in hypertensive disorders of pregnancy. pp. 73–91. In Sharp F, Symonds EM (eds): Hypertension in Pregnancy. Proceedings of the Sixteenth Study Group of the Royal College of Obstetricians and Gynaecologists. Perinatology Press, NY

Lindoff C, Ingemarsson I, Martinsson G et al. (1997) Preeclampsia is associated with a reduced response to activated protein C. Am J Obstet Gynecol 176:457–460

Liston WA, Kilpatrick DC (1991) Is genetic susceptibility to preeclampsia conferred by homozygosity for the same single recessive gene in mother and fetus? B J Obstet Gynecol 98:1079–1086

Lockwood CJ, Peters JH (1990) Increased levels of EDI+ cellular fibronectin precede the clinical signs of preeclampsia. Am J Obstet Gynecol 162:358

Lorentzen B, Birkeland KI, Endresen MJ, Henriksen T (1998) Glucose intolerance in women with preeclampsia. Acta Obstet Gynecol Scand 77:22–27

Lyall F, Greer IA (1994) Pre-eclampsia: a multifacet vascular disorder of pregnancy. J Hypertension

Lyall F, Greer IA, Boswell F et al. (1994) The cell adhesion molecule, VCAM-1 is selectively elevated in serum in pre-eclampsia: does this indicate the mechanism of leucocyte activation? Br J Obstet Gynaecol 101:485–487

Mabie WC, Pernoll ML, Biswas MK (1986) Chronic hypertension in pregnancy. Obstet Gynecol 67:197–205

McCarthy AL, Woolfson RG, Raju SK, Poston L (1993) Abnormal endothelial cell function of resistance arteries from women with preeclampsia. Am J Obstet Gynecol 168:1323–1330

MacFadyen IR, Price AB, Geirsson RT (1986) The relation of birthweight to histological appearances in vessels of the placental bed. Br J Obstet Gynecol 93:476–481

MacGillivray I, Rose GA, Rowe D (1969) Blood pressure survey in pregnancy. Clin Sci 37–395

McMahon LP, Redman CWG, Firth JD (1993) Expression of three endothelin genes and plasma levels of endothelin in preeclamptic and normal gestations. Clin Sci 85:417–424

Mogren I, Hogberg U, Winkvist A, Stenlund H (1999) Family occurrence of preeclampsia. Epidemiology 10:518–522

Molnar M, Suto T, Toth T, Hertelendy F (1994) Prolonged blockade of nitric oxide synthesis in gravid rats produces sustained hypertension, proteinuria, thrombocytopenia and intramurine growth retardation. Am J Obstet Gynecol 170:1458–1466

Morgan L, Crawshaw S, Baker PN, et al. (1999) Maternal and fetal angiotensinogen gene allele sharing in preeclampsia. Br J Obstet Gynaecol 106:244–251

Moutquin JM, Rainville C, Giroux L et al. (1985) A prospective study of blood pressure in pregnancy: prediction of preeclampsia. Am J Obstet Gynecol 15:191–196

Nathan L, Cuevas J, Chandbury G (1995) The role of nitric oxide in altered vascular reactivity of pregnancy in the rat. Br J Pharmacol 114:955–960

Nelson JR (1955) A clinical study of preeclampsia. Part I. J Obstet Gynaecol Br Empire 62:48–57

Newman RB, Eddy EL (1988) Association of eclampsia and hydatidiform mole: case report and review of the literature. Obstet Gynecol Surv 43:185–190

Page EW, Christianson R (1976) The impact of mean arterial blood pressure in the middle trimester upon the outcome of pregnancy. Am J Obstet Gynaecol 125:740

Page NM, Woods RJ, Gardiner SM et al. (2000) Excessive placental secretion of neurokinin B during the third trimester causes pre-eclampsia. Nature 405:797–800

Palti H, Rothschild E (1989) Blood pressure and growth 6 years of age among offspring of mothers with hypertension of pregnancy. Early Hum Dev 19:263–269

People's League of Health (1946) The nutrition of expectant and nursing mothers in relation to maternal and infant mortality and morbidity. J Obstet Gynaecol Br Empire 53:498–509

Peterson RDA, Tuck-Muller CM, Spinnato JA et al. (1994) An HLA-haplotype associated with preeclampsia and intrauterine growth retardation. Am J Reprod Immunol 31:177–179

Piering WF, Garancis JG, Becker CG et al. (1993) Preeclampsia related to a functional extrauterine placenta: report of a case and 25 year follow up. Am J Kidney Dis 21:310–313

Pijnenborg R, Anthony J, Davey DA et al. (1991) Placental bed spiral arteries in the hypertensive disorders of pregnancy. Br J Obstet Gynaecol 98:648–655

Platt R, Stewart AE, Emery EW (1958) The etiology, incidence, and heredity of preeclamptic toxaemia of pregnancy. Lancet 1:552–559

Potter JM, Nestel PJ (1979) The hyperlipidemia of pregnancy in normal and complicated pregnancies. Am J Obstet Gynecol 133:165–170

Rakoczi I, Tallian F, Bagdany S, Gati I (1979) Platelet life-span in normal pregnancy and preeclampsia as determined by non-radioisotope technique. Thromb Res 15:553–556

Redman CWG (1989) Hypertension in pregnancy pp. 515–541. In Turnbull SA, Chamberlain G (eds): Obstetrics. Churchill Livingstone, Edinburgh

Redman CWG, Jeffries M (1988) Revised definition of pre-eclampsia. Lancet i:809–812

Redman CWG, Allington MJ, Bolton FG, Stirrat GM (1977) Plasma beta thromboglobulin in preeclampsia. Lancet ii:248

Redman CWG, Bonnar J, Beilin L (1978a) Early platelet consumption in preeclampsia. BMJ 1:467–469

Redman CWG, Bodmer JG, Bodmer WF, Beilin LJ (1978b) HLA antigens in severe pre-eclampsia. Lancet ii:397–399

Rey E, Couturier A (1994) The prognosis of pregnancy in women with chronic hypertension. Am J Obstet Gynecol 171:410–416

Roberts JM, Redman CWG (1993) Pre-eclampsia: more than pregnancy-induced hypertension. Lancet 341:1447–1451

Roberts JM, Taylor RN, Musci TJ et al. (1989) Preeclampsia: an endothelial cell disorder. Am J Obstet Gynecol 161:1200–1204

Robertson WB, Brosens I, Dixon HG (1967) The pathological reponse of the vessels of the placental bed to hypertensive pregnancy. J Pathol Bacteriol 93:581–592

Rodgers GM, Taylor RN, Roberts JM (1988) Preeclampsia is associated with a serum factor cytotoxic to human endothelial cells. Am J Obstet Gynecol 159:908–914

Salonen Ros H, Lichtenstein P, Lipworth L, Cnattingius S (2000) Genetic effects on the liability of developing preeclampsia and gestational hypertension. Am J Med Genet 91:256–260

Sargent IL, Redman CWG, Stirrat G (1982) Maternal cell mediated immunity in normal and preeclamptic pregnancy. Clin Exp Immunol 50:601

Skomswoll JF, Ostensen M, Irgens LM, Baste V (2000) Pregnancy complications and delivery practice in women with connective tissue disease and inflammatory rheumatic disease in Norway. Acta Obstet Gynecol Scand 79:490–495

Seidman DS, Laor A, Gale R et al. (1991) Pre-eclampsia and offspring's blood pressure, cognitive ability and physical development at 17-year-of age. Br J Obstet Gynaecol 98:1009–1014

Selick CE, Horowitz GM, Gratch M et al. (1994) Immunohistochemical localization of transforming growth factor beta in human implantation sites. J Clin Endocrinol Metab 78:592–596

Selvaggi L, Loverro G, Schena P et al. (1988) Int Gynecol Obstet 27:45–49

Serhal PF, Craft IL (1989) Oocyte donation in 61 patients. Lancet i:1185–1187

Sheenan HL (1980) Renal morphology in preeclampsia. Kidney Int 18:241–252

Sheppard BL, Bonnar J (1980) Ultrastructural abnormalities of placental villi in placentae from pregnancies complicated by fetal growth retardation: their relationship to decidual sprial arterial lesions. Placenta 1:145–156

Sibai BM, McCubbin JH, Anderson GD et al. (1981) Eclampsia. I Observations from 67 recent cases. Obstet Gynecol 58:609–613

Sibai BM, El-Nazer A, Gonzalez-Ruiz A (1986) Severe preeclampsia-eclampsia in young primigravid women: subsequent pregnancy outcome and remote prognosis. Am J Obstet Gynecol 155:1011–1116

Sibai BM, Mercer B, Sinoglu C (1991) Severe preeclampsia in the second trimester: Recurrence risk and long-term prognosis. Am J Obstet Gynecol 165:1408–1412

Sibai BM, Caritis C, Thom E et al. (1993) Prevention of preeclampsia with low-dose aspirin in healthy nulliparous pregnant women. N Engl J Med 329:1213–1218

Sibai BM, Gordon T, Thom E et al. (1995) Risk factors for preeclampsia in healthy nulliparous women: A prospective multicenter study. The National Institute of Child Health and Human Development Network of Maternal-Fetal Medicine Units. Am J Obstet Gynecol 172:642–648

Sibai BM, Lindheimer M, Hauth J et al. (1998) Risk factors for preeclampsia, abruptio placentae, and adverse neonatal outcomes among women with chronic hypertension. N Engl J Med 339:667–671

Smárason AK, Sargent IL, Starkey PM, Redman CWG (1993) The effect of placental syncytiotrophoblast microvillous membranes from normal and preeclamptic women on the growth of endothelial cells in vitro. Br J Obstet Gynecol 100:943–949

Smith CA (1947) The effect of wartime starvation in Holland upon pregnancy and its product. Am J Obstet Gynecol 53:599–606

Spargo B, McCartney CP, Winemiller AB (1959) Glomerular capillary endotheliosis in toxaemia of pregnancy. Arch Pathol 68:593–599

Stamler FW (1959) Fatal eclamptic disease of pregnant rats fed antivitamin E distress diet. Am J Pathol 35:1207–1231

Stone JI, Lockwood CJ, Berkowitz GS et al. (1994) Risk factors for preeclampsia. Obstet Gynecol 83:357–361

Strauss AW, Bennet MJ, Rinaldo MJ et al. (1999) Inherited long-chain 3-hydroxyacyl-CoA dehydrogenase deficiency and a fetal-maternal interaction cause maternal liver disease and other pregnancy complications. Semin Perinatol 23:100–112

Sutherland A, Cooper DW, Howie PW et al. (1981) The incidence of severe pre-eclampsia amongst mothers and mothers in law of preeclamptics and controls. Br J Obstet Gynaecol 88:785–790

Svenson A, Andersch B, Hansson L (1983) A clinical follow-up study of 260 women with hypertension in pregnancy. Clin Exp Hyperten. Hyperten Preg B2:95–102

Sowers JR, Saleh AA, Sokol RJ (1995) Hyperinsulinemia and insulin resistance are associated with preeclampsia in African-Americans. Am J Hypertens 8:1–4

Takimoto E, Ishida J, Sugiyama F et al. (1996) Hypertension induced in pregnant mice by placental renin and maternal angiotensinogen. Science 274:995–998

Taylor RN, Heilbron DC, Roberts JM (1990) Growth factor activity in the blood of women in whom preeclampsia develops is elevated from early pregnancy. Am J Obstet Gynecol 163:1839–1844

Taylor RN, Crombleholme WR, Friedman SA et al. (1991) High plasma cellular fibronectin levels correlate with biochemical and clinical features of preeclampsia but cannot be attributed to hypertension alone. Am J Obstet Gynecol 165:895–901

Thadhani R, Stampfer MJ, Hunter DJ et al. (1999) High body mass index and hypercholesterolemia: risk of hypertensive disorders of pregnancy. Obstet Gynecol 94:543–550

Thompson B, Fraser C (1988) Some aspects of first births and heights of twin sisters of known zygosity. In MacGillivray I, Campbell DM, Thompson B (eds): Twinning and Twins. Wiley, Chichester, UK

Thornton JG, Onwude JL (1991) Preeclampsia: disordance among identical twins. Br Med J 303:1241–1242

Thornton JG, Onwude JL (1992) Convulsions in pregnancy in related gorillas. Am J Obstet Gynaecol 167:240–241

Torbergsen T, Øian P, Mathiesen E, Borud (1989) Pre-eclampsia-a mitochondrial disease. Acta Obstet Gynecol Scand 68:145–148

Treem WR, Shoup ME, Hale DE et al. (1996) Acute fatty liver of pregnancy, hemolysis, elevated liver enzymes, and low platelets syndrome, and long chain 3-hydroxylacy-coenzyme A dehydrogenase deficiency. Am J Gastroenterol 91:2293–3000

Tyni T, Pihko H (1999) Long-chain 3-hydroxyacyl-CoA dehydrogenase deficiency. Acta Paediatr 88:237–245

Tyni T, Ekholm E, Pihko H (1998) Pregnancy complications are frequent in long-chain 3-hydroxyl-coenzyme A dehydrogenase deficiency. Am J Obstet Gynecol 178:603–608

Van Pampus MG, Dekker GA, Wolf H et al. (1999) High prevalence of hemostatic abnormalities in women with a history of severe preeclampsia. Am J Obstet Gynecol 180:1146–1150

Villar MA, Sibai BM (1989) Clinical significance of elevated mean arterial blood pressure in second trimester and threshold increase in systolic or diastolic blood pressure during third trimester. Am J Obstet Gynecol 160:419–423

Vuorinen K, Remes A, Sormunen R et al. (1998) Placental mitochondrial DNA and respiratory chain enzymes in the etiology of preeclampsia. Obstet Gynecol 91:950–955

Wallenburg HC (1988) Hemodynamics in hypertensive pregnancy. In Rubin PC (ed): Hypertension in Pregnancy. Handbook of Hypertension. Elsevier, Amsterdam 10:66–101

Wallenburg HC, Stolte LA, Janssens J (1973) The pathogenesis of placental infarction. I. A morphological study in the human placenta. Am J Obstet Gynecol 116:835–840

Walters WAW, Lim YL (1975) Blood volume and haemodynamics in pregnancy. Clin Obstet Gynecol 2:301–320

Wang Y, Walsh SW, Guo J, Zhang J (1991) The imbalance between tromboxane and prostacyclin in preeclampsia is associated with an imbalance between lipid peroxides and vitamin E in maternal blood. Am J Obstet Gynecol 165:1695–1700

Ward R (1990) Familial aggregation and genetic epidemiology of blood pressure. Laragh JH, Brenner BM (eds): Hypertension:

pathophysiology, diagnosis and managment. Lippincott-Raven, NY, pp. 81–100

Ward K, Hata A, Jeunemaitre X et al. (1993) A molecular variant of angiotensinogen associated with preeclampsia. Nature Genet 4:59–61

Wickens D, Wilkins MH, Luneyc J et al. (1981) Free radical oxidation (peroxidation) products in plasma in normal and abnormal pregnancy. Ann Clin Biochem 18:158

Wilton AN, Cooper DW, Brennecke SP et al. (1990) Absence of close linkage between maternal genes for susceptibility to pre-eclampsia/eclampsia and HLA DRB. Lancet 336:653–657

Witztum JL (1994) The oxidative hypothesis of atherosclerosis. Lancet 344:793–795

Wolfe HM, Zador I, Gross T et al. (1991) The clinical utility of body mass index in pregnancy. Am J Obstet Gynecol 164:1306–1309

Yallampalli C, Garfield RE (1992) Inhibition of nitric oxide synthesis in rats during pregnancy produces signs similar to those of preeclampsia. Am J Obstet Gynecol 169:1316–1320

Yamada N, Arinami T, Yamakawa-Kobayashi K et al. (2000) The 4G/5G polymorphism of the plasminogen activator inhibitor-1 gene is associated with severe preeclampsia. J Hum Genet 45:138–141

Yanagisawa M, Kurihara H, Kimura S et al. (1988) A novel potent vasoconstrictor peptide produced by vascular endothelial cells. Nature 332:411–415

Ylikorkala O, Pekonen F, Viinikka L (1986) Renal prostacyclin and thromboxane in normotensive and preeclamptic pregnant women and their infants. J Clin Endoerinol Metab 63:1307–12

Zhou Y, Damsky CH, Chiu K et al. (1993) Preeclampsia is associated with abnormal expression of adhesion molecules by invasive cytotrophoblasts. J Clin Invest 91:950–960

Zhou Y, Damsky CH, Fisher SJ (1997) Preeclampsia is associated with failure of human cytotrophoblasts to mimic a vascular adhesion phenotype. One cause of defective endovascular invasion in this syndrome? J Clin Invest 99:2152–2164

Zunker HO, Phillips LL, McKay DG (1965) Potassium transport in kidney and placenta in normal pregnancy and in experimental toxaemia. Am J Obstet Gynecol 91:369–376

Zusterzeel PL, Visser W, Peters WH et al. (2000a) Polymorphism in the glutathione S-transferase P1 gene and risk for preeclampsia. Obstet Gynecol 96:50–54

Zusterzeel PL, Nelen WL, Roelfs HM et al. (2000b) Polymorphism in biotransformation enzymes and the risk for recurrent early pregnancy loss. Mol Hum Reprod 6:474–478

Genetic determinants of atherosclerotic heart disease and other occlusive arterial disorders

53

Asad A. Rizvi
Paul D. Thompson
Reed Pyeritz

Introduction

Atherosclerosis is the leading cause of mortality in the USA and other industrialized countries accounting for up to 50% of deaths. In 1997, over 400,000 people died from atherosclerotic heart disease (ASHD) in the USA, over 750,000 were admitted to the hospital with an acute myocardial infarction, and over 600,000 suffered a stroke (Elixhauser et al, 1997). The estimated costs, both direct and indirect (resulting from lost productivity), from cardiovascular diseases in the USA in 2000 are estimated to top 300×10^9 (American Heart Association, 2000). In addition, with the increasingly westernized diets and lifestyles in developing countries and the increasing mean age of many populations, the burden from atherosclerosis will be significantly greater in the twenty-first century (Gaziano, 1998).

However, the last several decades have seen important successes in the treatment and prevention of diseases due to atherosclerosis, important contributors to the 50% decline in age-adjusted mortality rates from all cardiovascular disease. The improvement in death rates from stroke and myocardial infarction are especially impressive (Braunwald, 1997). An explosion in understanding of both the causes and pathogenesis of atherosclerosis has been an important contributor to improved clinical outcomes. Long held to be an inevitable part of the aging process, atherosclerosis is now more clearly understood as a chronic disease, in part inflammatory, that results from the interaction of personal risk factors (most with a strong genetic basis) and environmental factors. A clearer understanding of the genetic basis of atherosclerosis will help elucidate further the etiology and pathogenesis of the disorder, facilitate novel approaches to therapy, and help to prevent overt disease in high-risk individuals. The goals of this chapter are to review the approaches used to identify the genetic risk factors for atherosclerotic heart disease (ASHD) and peripheral vascular disease (PVD), discuss the clinical relevance of these factors, and to highlight the influence that environmental factors play in the expression of these genes.

Difficulties with investigating the genetic bases of atherosclerosis and its associated diseases

The general approaches to investigating the genetic bases of common diseases are reviewed in Ch. 12, and with specific reference to cardiovascular disease elsewhere (Boerwinkle et al., 1996; Kraus, 2000; Pyeritz, 1999, 2001; Roses, 2000; Williams et al., 2000; Winkelmann et al., 2000).

Atherosclerosis is a pathologic process that usually begins in early life (Strong et al., 1999). Thickening of the intimal-medial layers of coronary arteries is present in infants with a statistically higher risk of developing clinical coronary artery disease (Kaprio et al., 1993). However, except for the infrequent opportunities to study human pathologic specimens early in life, the subclinical stages of atherosclerosis remain largely inscrutable in vivo. As a result, most investigations of genetic factors have employed clinical diseases as the phenotypes. These phenotypes nearly always occur as a consequence of advanced atherosclerosis. In this section we discuss the difficulties—best viewed as challenges—posed by this reality. These issues have been recognized for decades (Murphy, 1967), but continue to be overlooked in contemporary investigations.

Table 53.1 lists some of the impediments to studying the genetics of human atherosclerotic diseases. Atherosclerosis

Table 53.1. Impediments to investigating the genetic bases of human atherosclerotic diseases

Both atherosclerosis and atherosclerotic diseases are age-dependent
>   Young people at genetic risk do not manifest disease
>>   Few measures of subclinical phenotypes
>   People at risk may die from other causes before the effects of atherosclerosis are evident

Multiple diseases result from atherosclerosis
>   Are angina/myocardial infarction, stroke and claudication equivalent phenotypes?

Diseases have multiple potential causes
>   Not all myocardial infarctions and strokes are due to atherosclerosis

Most atherosclerotic disease not due to the effect of a single mutant gene
>   Segregation analysis usually not informative

Atherosclerosis is a quantitative trait that is difficult to quantify
>   Occurrence of overt disease may represent a threshold or multiple-hit effect

Genetic risk factors may interact with environmental risk factors

Genetic risk factors act on a background of normal variation, even within families
>   Vessel caliber
>   Circulatory anatomy
>   Activity
>   Nutrition

is a disease of the young that may not become evident until middle age or older. As a result classical family studies, whether rooted in segregation analysis or various other models, are difficult. Relatives in the youngest generations have not lived long enough to express the diseases due to atherosclerosis. Relatives in the oldest generations pose different problems. Some may have died without clear cause or without sufficient documentation to be certain that atherosclerosis was involved. Others may have succumbed for reasons not related to atherosclerosis (such as accidents or cancer) even though they had subclinical arterial disease. Clearly, having some sensitive method for detecting *pathology* at a subclinical stage would be an enormous advantage, especially if the method was noninvasive and relatively inexpensive. This search for reliable surrogate markers is common to investigations of virtually all complex diseases. With respect to atherosclerosis, the detection of calcification of coronary arterial walls by ultrafast computed tomography has been used in some studies (Conti, 2000), although the correlation with clinical outcome remains in question. Magnetic resonance imaging holds some promise for detecting early arterial wall pathology, quantifying the degree of pathology, and analyzing the constituents of atherosclerotic plaques (Skinner et al., 1995, Fayad et al., 2000). Such capabilities would be of value in family and population studies of genetic factors, as well as in investigations of therapies.

Multiple diseases result from atherosclerosis. Are angina, myocardial infarction and sudden cardiac death equivalent phenotypes for genetic studies? Comparing published investigations is hazardous unless the disease phenotypes are the same and defined by equivalent criteria. Are stroke and claudication equivalent phenotypes to whatever measure is employed for coronary artery disease? On the one hand, atherosclerosis is the most common cause of each disease, and many patients with atherosclerosis show two or all three of them. On the other hand, some families show predominantly or exclusively only one of these diseases.

Myocardial infarction and stroke have multiple potential causes besides atherosclerosis, such as vasospasm (potentially drug-induced), emboli and dissection.

Most atherosclerotic disease is not due to the effect of a single mutant gene. We have been spoiled by the remarkable insight gained through study of familial hypercholesterolemia due to mutations in the gene that encodes the receptor for low density lipoprotein (*LDLR*) (see Ch. 91). Over 60 mendelian conditions are associated with coronary artery disease, and 250 are each associated with hypertension and diabetes mellitus, with little overlap (OMIM, 2001). But on a numerical basis, most of the mendelian causes of stroke and coronary artery disease do not involve atherosclerosis (Pyeritz, 2001), and those that do account for a small proportion of the population burden of disease. For example, one in 500 individuals harbors a mutation in *LDLR* that causes familial hypercholesterolemia and elevated LDL cholesterol, which if untreated, carries a very high likelihood of causing ASHD. Familial hypercholesterolemia is one of the most common of the highly penetrant mendelian predispositions to ASHD. However, mutations at this locus account for less than 1% of the disease burden. Thus, the reductionistic approach, while not having reached its limits, will not solve the major questions posed in this chapter.

The search for highly penetrant loci predisposing to common diseases has typically begun with family studies and segregation analysis. However, this approach is usually not informative for detecting defective genes of low penetrance that cause stroke, PVD or ASHD. Newer statistical approaches to this challenge include sib-pair analysis and quantitative trait analyses (see Chs 8 and 12). Unfortunately, atherosclerosis is a quantitative trait that is difficult to quantify. The pathology is often focal rather than uniform within a vessel, so sampling is a major issue. Furthermore, as noted above, noninvasive measures of disease severity are largely lacking. Many studies in the past relied on invasive angiographic methods for quantifying the extent of atherosclerotic disease. While the degree of lumenal occlusion can be measured with reasonable accuracy by contrast radiography, there is poor correlation with the degree of vessel wall involvement, especially at early stages (Glagov et al., 1987; St Goar et al., 1992). Relying on overt disease phenotypes has little role in quantitative trait analysis. The occurrence of overt disease may represent a threshold or multiple-hit effect, with marked variability among individuals, even relatives.

Virtually all genetic risk factors interact with developmental and environmental factors, both those that are (such as age and smoking) and are not epidemiologically identified as independent risk factors for ASHD (Childs, 1999; Ch. 23). Individuals and relatives differ in not only their exposure to environmental risk factors, but how they respond to a given level of exposure. Quantifying such confounders in studies of genetic factors is extraordinarily difficult. A related issue is that genetic risk factors act on a background of normal variation in both physiology and experiences. Examples of the former include arterial caliber, tortuosity, branching patterns and wall characteristics such as reactivity; some and perhaps all of these traits are under genetic control (Herrington and Pearson, 1987). Level of physical activity, intake of vitamins, and diet are examples of confounding variables that, while they might be quantified and analyzed to some degree, complicate interpretation of genetic studies.

Evidence for a genetic basis of ASHD

A variety of formal genetic studies, conducted before much was known about the etiology and pathogenesis of atherosclerosis, suggested increased familial occurrence of ASHD. For example, studies of twins showed concordance rates of ASHD of 20% in monozygotic twins versus 6–8% for dizygotic twins (Cederlof et al., 1967; Hamby, 1981). Other studies found increased risk in offspring of two affected parents compared to when only one parent was affected (Thomas and Cohen, 1955). The marked increased prevalence of ASHD among men compared to women, especially at younger ages, has also been long recognized (Murphy, 1963). Some studies suggested that the offspring of female probands carried an increased risk of developing disease (Slack and Evans, 1966). However, much more refined investigations were necessary to infer a genetic explanation from familial occurrence and sexual predilection.

Risk factors for ASHD have been studied for decades by epidemiologic methods. A set of factors is now well recog-

Table 53.2. Established risk factors for atherosclerotic vascular disease

Male sex
Advanced age
Hypertension
Diabetes mellitus /insulin resistance
Hypercholesterolemia Elevated low-density lipoprotein
Low high-density lipoprotein
Family history of a relative with symptomatic arterial occlusive disease occurring < 55 years of age
Cigarette smoking
Obesity
Inactivity
Elevated serum uric acid

nized (Table 53.2) and widely used in both clinical practice and public health. Familial occurrence of ASHD was one of the first risk factors to be established, and provided the first evidence for a genetic basis for the disorder (Thomas and Cohen, 1955; Hamby, 1981). Clearly, some of the other traditional risk factors, particularly dyslipidemias, obesity, hypertension and diabetes mellitus, occur more commonly in certain families, suggesting a heritable basis for the individual risk factors and at least a partial explanation for the overall importance of family history (Adlersberg et al., 1949; Thomas and Cohen, 1955; Becker et al., 1988). In a study by Blumenthal et al. (1975), children of men with myocardial infarction before age 50 years were three times as likely to have hyperlipidemia than children of controls. Other investigators have confirmed that genetically related risk factors such as hypertension, dyslipidemias, and diabetes mellitus are two to six times as likely in the relatives of cases than controls (Rissanen and Nikkila, 1977; Hamby et al., 1981).

Familial clustering of risk factors that each has its own genetic susceptibilities is one characteristic of a genetic predisposition to a complex disease such as atherosclerosis. Another is earlier than average age of onset in individuals with genetic predisposition. A study in Finland compared the occurrence of ASHD between first-degree relatives of patients with premature fatal or non-fatal myocardial infarction and controls (Rissanen, 1979). The younger the patient at the time of myocardial infarction, the more likely was the occurrence of ASHD in parents and sibs. In patients suffering myocardial infarction before the age 46, the patient's brother was at 7–11-fold higher risk of having ASHD before age 55 than were the brothers of controls (Rissanen, 1979). These findings have been replicated many times. In a study of 421 patients with angiographically proven ASHD and 184 controls, the incidence of ASHD was higher in sibs of cases with a parental history of ASHD compared to both controls and those without a parental history (Hamby et al., 1981). Slack and Evans (1966) found the risk of death from ASHD to be 2.5–7 fold higher in the first-degree relatives of ASHD patients than in relatives of controls. Interestingly, however, the relatives of ASHD patients who lacked other risk factors still appeared to have a higher incidence and earlier onset of ASHD than did patients with ASHD who had traditional risk factors such as dyslipidemia, diabetes mellitus, and hypertension. This suggests that a family history of ASHD is an independent risk factor (Shea et al., 1984, Hopkins et al., 1988; Jorde and Williams, 1988). In a genetic-epidemiologic study looking at 19 independent risk factors for ASHD in 207 patients with myocardial infarction before age 55 compared with 621 controls, the highest risk ratio was for patients with a family history of ASHD (Nora et al., 1980).

Family history is at least as strong an independent risk factor for ASHD in the young patient as some dominantly inherited, highly atherogenic traits. The disease liability among first-degree relatives of the youngest patients approaches 65% in some studies (Nora et al., 1980). For relatives of the oldest cases, the heritable component is only 15–30% (Rissanen et al., 1979). At our current state of knowledge, one-third to one-half of the familial occurrence of ASHD is independent of genetic predisposition to other, established risk factors (Williams et al., 2000).

Changes in classic risk factors over time in individuals and families are likely to be strongly influenced by environmental factors such as diet, smoking, and exercise. However, recent studies suggest that genes affect the intra-individual variation over time in various risk factors including LDL, HDL and systolic blood pressure (Friedlander et al, 1997). There is also evidence suggesting a higher incidence of cardiovascular events in family members of patients with premature PVD compared with controls, suggesting a familial basis for PVD (Valentine et al., 2000).

Finally, linkage analyses in populations with few genetic "founders" have provided evidence for a small number of genes having an important contribution to the risk of coronary artery disease (Pajukanta et al., 2000), although the specific genes have yet to be identified.

Established risk factors for atherosclerosis

The concept of risk factors was first coined by Kannel and co-workers reporting on the findings of the Framingham Heart Study (Kannel et al., 1961). This long-term, multi-generational investigation of a free-living population, which continues today, established much of what we know about the incidence, patterns, associated conditions and natural history of the disease. From this and many other populations, over 300 different factors have been purported to increase the risk of ASHD (Williams et al., 2000). This section deals with those having the strongest support (Table 53.2).

Male gender is a powerful risk factor for atherosclerosis. Between 30–40 years of age, the risk for ASHD is 13-fold higher in men than in women. After the age of 45, the ratio becomes more equitable, but still remains two-fold higher in men. The risk for ASHD associated with hypertension is skewed more in the direction of women. Between the ages of 40–59, the presence of hypertension increases the incidence of ASHD by 2.6-fold for men compared with a 6-fold increase in the risk for women. Hypertension thus appears to be more of a risk factor in women compared with men.

Diabetes mellitus is associated with a 2–3-fold increase of clinical atherosclerotic disease including ASHD, PVD, heart failure and stroke. The effects of diabetes mellitus are more profound in women than in men. In diabetic women, the inherent advantage of gender is lost and diabetic women have a rate of ASHD morbidity and mortality comparable to men (Kannel and McGee, 1979). Diabetes mellitus worsens survival following myocardial infarction particularly in women with a 4-fold higher likelihood of developing heart failure (Abbott et al., 1988). As with hyperlipidemia and hypertension, the risk of ASHD from diabetes mellitus increases with the presence of other risk factors. In addition, impaired glucose tolerance, which does not satisfy the strict definitions for diabetes mellitus, is also associated with increased cardiovascular mortality (Wilson et al., 1991).

Dyslipidemias, consisting of elevated LDL cholesterol or an unusually depressed HDL, are powerful risk factors and may be prerequisite for the development of atherosclerosis in most individuals. Even in the presence of other risk factors, such as diabetes, hypertension and smoking, the incidence of ASHD is low if the serum level of LDL is low. In the Framingham Heart Study, elevation of total cholesterol above 245 mg/dl was associated with a 3-fold increase in the development of ASHD in men compared with a 1.6-fold increase in women. After adjusting for other risk factors, the impact of an elevated cholesterol level remained unchanged for men but was considerably reduced in women (Kannel et al., 1961). The Framingham Study was also the first to establish the continuous, graded relationship between ASHD mortality and serum cholesterol levels over the entire range of normal and elevated levels. The discovery of a 5-fold range of risk within what most laboratories reported as "normal" cholesterol levels caused a major shift in public health efforts. Optimal values appeared to be total cholesterol levels less than 200 mg/dl (Kannel, 1990). Martin and co-workers (1986) showed a doubling in ASHD mortality between total cholesterol concentrations of 153 mg/dl and 226 mg/dl, with an additional doubling between 226 mg/dl and 290 mg/dl. Further confirmation of the role of elevated cholesterol in atherosclerosis has come from therapeutic trials and animal models that have shown regression of disease with lipid lowering therapy (Blankenhorn et al., 1987; 1993; Brown et al., 1990; Kane et al., 1990).

The Framingham Heart Study was also the first to establish the risk associated with a depressed HDL cholesterol. Numerous studies since have confirmed that elevation of either major isoform of HDL (HDL 2 and HDL 3) is associated with a reduced risk of ASHD (Gordon, 1977; 1981; 1989; Miller, 1987; Tall, 1990; 1992). The role of triglycerides as atherogenic molecules is less clear. Although a high fasting triglyceride level is predictive of cardiovascular risk, multivariate adjustment for other risk factors lessens the association (Pasternak et al., 1996; LaRosa et al., 1997). Other studies have suggested elevated triglycerides as an independent risk factor (Stampfer et al., 1996; Gaziano et al., 1997). In a meta-analysis of 17 population-based prospective studies involving 57,000 patients, an increase of 1 mmol/L or 88.6 mg/dl was associated with a 1.32-fold higher risk in men and 1.76-fold in women. After adjusting for other risk factors, the relative risk was 1.14 in men and 1.37 in women (Hokanson and Austin, 1996). In the Copenhagen Male Study, men with the middle and highest triglyceride levels had a relative risk of 1.5 and 2.2 respectively of developing ASHD compared with the lowest third (Jeppesen et al., 1998). High triglyceride levels predict angiographic progression of ASHD disease, especially for lesions less than 50%, and therapy to reduce triglycerides reduces mortality and cardiac events in both primary and secondary prevention trials (Frick et al., 1987; Blankenhorn et al., 1990; Mack et al., 1996; Goldbourt et al., 1998). The association between elevated triglycerides and ASHD may be due to an indirect interaction with the HDL molecule (there is a moderate inverse relationship between the two). However, even after correcting for these effects, elevated triglycerides may still be a risk factor (Austin, 1991).

Smoking increases the risk for ASHD and PVD. The risk for acute myocardial infarction and sudden death is dependent on the number of cigarettes smoked per day rather than the duration of smoking in years. Quitting is associated with a prompt reduction of the risk of sudden death by approximately 50%. In addition, exposure to environmental tobacco appears to be associated with subclinical disease (Howard and Wagenknecht, 1999).

Abnormally high body weight is a risk for ASHD of modest effect (Kaplan, 1992). Obesity also increases the incidence of all major risk factors including dyslipidemias, hypertension and glucose intolerance.

Risk factors for PVD overlap those for ASHD, specifically smoking, dyslipidemia, elevated homocysteine levels, alterations in coagulation factors, diabetes mellitus and elevated Lp(a) (Dobs et al., 1999). In addition to the overlap in risk factors, patients with PVD are 2–3-fold more likely than controls to develop ASHD and cerebrovascular disease (Criqui and Denenberg, 1998).

Emerging risk factors

A number of biological components have been suggested to play a role in increasing or decreasing risk of ASHD (Ridker, 2000) (Table 53.3). Because conclusive epidemiologic, genetic or pathophysiologic data supporting their importance and independence are lacking, we and others term these risk factors "emerging" (Braunwald, 1997). Table 53.4 lists these factors according to their predominant physiologic function and some of the evidence for their etiologic or pathogenetic roles in atherosclerotic disease. Classifying any risk factor within a specific metabolic pathway can be misleading. For example, the peroxisome proliferator-activated receptors (pPAR's) constitute a family of transcription factors that affect adipocyte differentiation, insulin sensitivity and, within the atherosclerotic plaque, foam cell metabolism and smooth muscle cell hyperplasia (Kersten et al., 2000). And this recitation ignores their activities in neoplasia.

Table 53.3. Emerging risk factors of atherosclerotic arterial disease

Hyperhomocysteinemia
Dyslipidemia
Elevated Lp(a)
Atherogenic lipoprotein phenotype
Factors predisposing to thrombosis
Elevated fibrinogen
Elevated factor VII
Elevated factor V
Elevated PAI-1
Markers of inflammation
Elevated C-reactive protein

Table 53.4. Loci with evidence for and against certain genotypes predisposing to atherosclerosis or atherosclerotic arterial disease

Class/Protein	Locus	Genotype	Phenotype	Evidence	References
Blood pressure regulation and complications of hypertension					
Adrenergic recp. α1B	ADRA1B		variation in systolic BP	family and sib pairs, linkage and assoc	Krushkal et al., 1998
Adrenergic recp. β2	ADRB2		variation in systolic BP	locus linked to ADRA1B	Krushkal et al., 1998
Angiotensinogen	AGT	T174M,M235T	↑ extent of CAD	cases	Gardemann et al., 1999
		M235T	↑ [AGT], ↑ CAD, ↑ MI	cases and pop. Controls, Danish	Winkelmann et al., 1999
		M235T	↑ BP	pop., French and Utah	Williams et al., 1994
Angiotensin converting enzyme	ACE	del/del	no ↑ MI	case-referent, Danish	Agerholm-Larsen et al., 1997a
		del/del	no ↑ stroke	case-referent, Danish	Agerholm-Larsen et al., 1997b
		insert/del	no ↑ CAD	females, CAD, Italian	Corbo et al., 1997
		del/del	no ↑ CAD, no ↑ MI	pop, cross-section, German	Winkelmann et al., 1996
		del/del	↑ reduction in [LDL-C]	clinical trial of statin	Marian et al., 1999
Mineralocorticoid recp.	NR3C2	mutations	severe hypertension	families; pregnancy	Geller et al., 2000
NO synthase, endothelial	NOS3	T-786C	↑ coronary spasm	case-control	Yoshimura et al., 2000
Renin	REN	BglI site	essential hypertension	pop. assoc., Arab, US cauc.	Frossard et al., 1999
Glucose regulation					
Glucokinase	GCK	mutations	MODY; gestational DM	pop., Japanese-American men	Stone et al., 1996
		G-30A	glucose tolerance		
Insulin	INS	mutations	DM	cases, families	Vinik and Bell, 1988
Insulin recp.	INSR	V985M	type 2 DM	case-control	't Hart et al., 1999
Calpain-10	CAP10	UCSNP-43	type 2 DM	pop., Mexican-American	Horikawa et al., 2000
Sulfonurea recp.	SUR	SNP	insulin response	cases, French	Reis et al., 2000
Growth factors					
Transforming growth factor-β	TGFB	P10	↓ [TGFβ] in severe CAD	cases with CAD	Grainger et al., 1995
			↑ [TGF], ↑ BP	pop., African-American	Suthanthiran et al., 2000
Hemostasis					
Factor II (prothrombin)	F2	C20210A	↑ MI	young females	Rosendaal et al., 1997
Factor V	F5	Q506 (Leiden)	no ↑ MI or stroke; ↑ VT	Physicians' Health Study	Ridker et al., 1995B
		R485K	↑ CAD	case-control, Chinese	Le et al., 2000
Factor VII	F7	−323 0/10bp	↓ [FVIII] assoc with ↓ MI	case-control, Italian	Di Castelnuovo et al., 2000
		R353Q	↓ [FVII]; no effect CAD	Framingham	Feng et al., 2000
		R353Q, HVR4	↓ [FVII] assoc with ↓ MI	cases with CAD, Italian	Girelli et al., 2000
Fibrinogen	FGA	453G/G	↑ CAD	cases and controls	Yu et al., 1996
		455A	↑ [FGA], no ↑ CAD	pop, Danish	Tybræg-Hansen et al., 1997
Plasminogen activator inhibitor-1	PAI1	4G	↑ MI	case-control, Finnish	Pastinen et al., 1998
Platelet IIIa/IIb glycoprot. recp.		PlA2	↑ MI	case-control, Finnish	Pastinen et al., 1998
		PlA2	↑ MI at early age	case-control	Weiss et al., 1996
Homocysteine metabolism					
Cystathionine β-synthase	CBS	heterozygotes	↑ [Hcy] fast & post-Met	obligate carriers	Franken et al., 1996
					Boers et al., 1985a and b
Methylene tetrahydrofolate reductase	MTHFR	thermolabile variant	↑ CAD	case-control	Kang et al., 1991
		A236V	↑ CAD	case-control	Frosst et al., 1995
		C677T	no ↑ CAD	case-control	Adams et al., 1996

Inflammatory/adhesion molecules

Description	Gene	Variant	Effect	Study	Reference
Adhesion molecule, intracellular	ICAM1	↑ [ICAM]	↑ risk of CVD	pts with renal failure	Stenvinkel et al., 2000
		↑ [ICAM]	↑ risk and severity of CAD	pts. with CAD and controls	Ikata et al., 2000
Adhesion molecule, vascular	VCAM1	↑ [VCAM1]	no predictor of future MI	pop.	de Lemos et al., 2000
C-reactive protein	CRP	↑ [hsCRP]	↑ risk MI and stroke	post-menopausal women	Ridker et al., 2000a
Interleukin 6	IL6	↑ [IL-6]	↑ risk of MI	healthy men	Ridker et al., 2000b
PAF acetylhydrolase (lipoprotein-associated phospholipase)	PLA2G7	↑ levels		coronary event and controls	Packard et al., 2000
Selectin E	SELE	S128R	↑ in young CAD pts.	case-control	Wenzel et al., 1994

Lipid metabolism

Description	Gene	Variant	Effect	Study	Reference
ApoA1	APOA1	↑ [apoAII]	↓ CAD	cases, families	Marshall et al., 1994
ApoAI-ApoCIII-ApoAIV cluster		5 polymorphisms	no ↑ CAD	cases having angiography	Marshall et al., 1994
ApoAII	APOA2	MspI site	no ↑ CAD		Marshall et al., 1994
ApoAIV	APOA4	Glu360His	attenuates ↑ [chol] 2° diet	clinical trial	McCombs et al., 1994
ApoB	APOB	4 polymorphisms	no ↑ CAD		Marshall et al., 1994
		Arg350Gln	↑ [chol], ↑ CAD	pop., Danish	Tybjærg et al., 1998
		inser/del	no ↑ CAD	females, Italian	Corbo et al., 1997
ApoCII	APOC2	TaqI site	no ↑ CAD		Marshall et al., 1994
ApoE	APOE	isoforms	no ↑ CAD		Marshall et al., 1994
		isoforms	no ↑ CAD	elderly Finns	Kuusisto et al., 1995
		3/2	earlier CAD onset	caucasians	Moore et al., 1997
		−219GT	↓ [apoE], ↑ MI	case-control, French men	Lambert et al., 2000
		ε4	↑ severe CAD	CAD cases, caucasian	Wang et al., 1995
Cholesterol ester transfer prot.	CETP	1405 V	↓ CAD	+EtOH, -smoking men, Iceland	Gudnason et al., 1997
Cholesterol-7α hydroxylase	CYP7A1	poly.	linked to [LDL-C]	sib-pairs, linkage and association	Wang et al., 1998
Endothelial lipase	LIPG		↑ expression →↓ [HDL]	mice	Jaye et al., 1999
Hepatic triglyceride lipase	LIPC	−514T	↑ [HDL$_2$-C]	population	Couture et al., 2000
Lecithin cholesterol acetyl transferase 1995	LCAT	heterozygotes	↓ [HDL], ↑ CAD	obligates carriers for LCAT def.	Kuivenhoven et al.,
LDL recp.	LDLR	poly.	linked to atherogenic lipoprotein phenotype	family study	Naggert et al., 1997
		mutations	familial hypercholesterolemia		
Lp(a)	LPA	poly.	↑ CAD	case-control; pop.	see text
Lipoprotein lipase	LPL	mutations	type I hyperlipoproteinemia ↑ [chylomicron], ↑ atherosclerosis		Nevin et al., 1994
			↓ [LPL], ↓ [HDL]		Benlian et al., 1996
		Asn291Ser			Reymer et al., 1995
Microsomal triglyceride transfer prot.	MTP	mutations	abetalipoproteinemia		
Paraoxonase	PON1,2,3	PON1*B+PON2*S	↑ CAD	Asian Indians	Sanghera et al., 1998
		PON1*B	no ↑ CAD	Chinese	Sanghera et al., 1997
		PON1*A/B	no ↑ CAD	Finns	Antikainen et al., 1996

continued

Table 53.4. Loci with evidence for and against certain genotypes predisposing to atherosclerosis or atherosclerotic arterial disease (continued)

Class/Protein	Locus	Genotype	Phenotype	Evidence	References
Muscle metabolism					
Adenosine monophosphate deaminase-1	AMPD1	C34T	$\downarrow$ AMPD1 activity, CAD survival	CAD cases	Anderson et al., 2000
Obesity					
Adrenegic recp.α2b	ADRA2B	poly.	$\uparrow$ obesity	cases	Heinonen et al., 1999
Adrenergic recp.β2	ADRB2	W64A	$\uparrow$ obesity	cases	Large et al., 1997
Adrenergic recp.β3	ADRB3	Trp64R	$\uparrow$ obesity	cases	Nagase et al., 1997 Mitchell et al., 1998
Leptin	LEP	$\uparrow$ [leptin] poly.	$\uparrow$ body mass index no assoc. with obesity	pop.-Mexican-Am and mixed ethnic obese Finns	Weigle et al., 1997 Karvonen et al., 1998
Melanocortin recp.	MC4R	mutations	obesity	cases	Sina et al., 1999
Peroxisome proliferator-activated recp.	PPARA PPARG	poly.	obesity	cases	Valve et al., 1999
Tumor necrosis factor	TNF	poly.	$\uparrow$ BMI, no $\uparrow$ MI	case-control	Herrmann et al., 1998
Uncoupling prot.	UCP2	poly.	variation in metabolic rate	Pima Indians	Walder et al., 1998
Other					
Ataxia telangiectasia locus	AT	heterozygotes	$\uparrow$ risk of death from CVD	obligate carriers	Su and Swift, 2000
Werner syndrome locus	WRN	L1074F	$\uparrow$ CAD	Mexicans, Finns	Castro et al., 2000

Abbreviations: BMI = body-mass index; CAD = coronary artery disease; CVD = cardiovascular disease; del = deletion; insert = insertion; MI = myocardial infarction; poly. = polymorphisms; pop. = population; recp. = receptor; SNP = single nucleotide polymorphism; [] = serum/plasma concentration; $\uparrow$ = elevated; $\downarrow$ = decreased

HYPERHOMOCYSTEINEMIA

Homocysteine (Hcy) is an amino acid and a metabolic intermediate derived from methionine (see Ch. 88). Homocysteine is metabolized to cysteine by a vitamin B_6-dependent transsulfuration reaction, or remethylated to methionine in a reaction dependent on both vitamin B_{12} and folate. Consequently, vitamins B_6 and B_{12} and folate are directly involved in regulating the plasma level of Hcy. Fasting levels greater than 15 mmol/L are generally considered abnormal, but vascular risk is directly associated with plasma Hcy regardless of the absolute levels (Boushey et al., 1995). Among people who have elevated Hcy levels, about one-quarter only demonstrate elevated levels after consuming an oral load of methionine.

The association between atherosclerosis and thrombotic vascular disease was first noted in homocystinuria, a recessive disorder due to cystathionine β-synthase (CBS) deficiency. Individuals with two mutant alleles at the *CBS* locus have remarkably high levels of Hcy, skeletal defects resembling those of the Marfan syndrome, lens dislocation, mental retardation and a tendency to venous thrombosis (Pyeritz, 1993) (see Ch. 88). The most common causes of death are myocardial infarction and stroke, and the arterial pathology is atherosclerotic.

Mild to moderate elevation of Hcy is associated with ASHD, myocardial infarction, PVD, cerebrovascular disease, post-transplant vasculopathy, and mortality form ASHD (Boers et al., 1985a; Clarke et al., 1991; Stampfer et al., 1992; Nygard et al., 1997). The relation between the level of Hcy and vascular disease is graded. For each 5 mmol/L increase in fasting plasma homocysteine level, the incidence of ASHD rises 1.6–1.8 fold (Boushey et al., 1995). In the Physicians Health Study, the adjusted relative risk for myocardial infarction was 3.4 in patients with Hcy levels in the top fifth percentile compared with those with levels in the lowest nintieth percentile (Stampfer et al., 1992). In contrast to cross sectional studies, results from prospective studies have been less consistent. Only two (Stampfer, 1992; Arnesen et al., 1995) of five of the prospective studies have found a significant correlation between Hcy levels and ASHD (Alfthan et al., 1994, Evans et al., 1997, Folsom et al., 1998). More problematic is the fact that when one of these studies (Alfthan et al., 1994) was extended for two years, there was no longer an association between Hcy levels and ASHD (Chasan-Taber et al., 1996). Additional data against the importance of elevated Hcy arose from the Atherosclerosis Risk in Communities Study, in which women but not men with Hcy levels in the top tenth percentile had a higher incidence of ASHD. However, after adjustment for other risk factors, Hcy levels were not signifi-cantly associated with ASHD (Folsom et al., 1998). On the basis of available evidence, screening of baseline homocysteine levels is not indicated in patients with no more than the average population risk of ASHD (Christen and Ridker, 2000).

Homocysteine has a number of biologic effects that could contribute to promoting or accelerating atherosclerois (Table 53.5).

Both genetic and environmental factors influence homocysteine levels (Motulsky, 1996). Low levels of vitamins B_6 and B_{12} and folic acid are more common in patients with elevated Hcy levels. Supplementation with these three cofactors decreases plasma Hcy levels. Folate is the most powerful agent for decreasing plasma levels (Ubbink, 1997). Vitamin B_{12} administration alone is less effective than folate for reducing levels except when associated with overt vitamin B_{12} deficiency (Brattstrom et al., 1988). Vitamin B_6 does not reduce fasting homocysteine levels but because it is a cofactor for CBS, if supplementation reduces Hcy levels after methionine loading, a defect in CBS or vitamin B_6 deficiency is suggested (Brattstrom et al., 1990). Combined supplementation reduces Hcy levels regardless of what the fasting plasma vitamin levels are (Naurath et al., 1995) The use of oral estrogen in men and post-menopausal women is associated with an 11–14% reduction in fasting levels of Hcy (Giri et al., 1998). At the present time no data from large, randomized clinical trials support a benefit from reducing moderately elevated levels of Hcy. Current or future studies in the USA also must recognize that as of 1998, cereal grains are being fortified with folic acid in order to reduce the incidence of neural tube defects (see Ch. 111).

Other factors affecting plasma Hcy include age, gender, renal function, the presence of neoplastic and other proliferative disorders, and certain drugs (Mayer et al., 1996).

Table 53.5. Potentially atherogenic actions of homocysteine

Endothelial dysfunction (Woo et al., 1997)

Endothelial cell injury (Harker et al., 1974; Starkebaum and Harlan, 1986)

Smooth muscle proliferation (Tsai et al., 1994)

Enhanced production of collagen by smooth muscle cells (Majors et al., 1997)

Cysteine deficiency, which impairs fibrillin-1 deposition (Majors and Pyeritz, 2000)

Enhancement of thromboxane A2 formation

Enhancement of platelet aggregation

Inhibition of the effect of endothelium derived relaxing factor

Enhancement of binding of Lp(a) to fibrin

A procoagulant effect (Harpel et al., 1992; Stamler et al., 1993; Mayer et al., 1996; Durand et al., 1997)

Plasma Hcy levels increase with age and although the precise mechanism remains obscure, age-related reductions in CBS activity may play a role (Nordstrom and Kjellstrom, 1992; Ueland et al., 1992). Plasma Hcy levels and serum creatinine are positively correlated, and levels in patients with renal failure may be considerably elevated and may contribute to the associated accelerated vascular disease (Wilcken and Gupta, 1979; Brattstrom et al., 1992; Chaveau et al., 1993). Other conditions associated with elevated plasma Hcy levels include: disease states such as hypothyroidism, systemic lupus, diabetes mellitus, psoriasis, acute lymphoblastic leukemia, breast, ovarian and pancreatic carcinoma; and pharmacologic agents including methotrexate, nitrous oxide, phenytoin, carbamazepine, azaribine, estrogen, cyclosporine, thiazide diuretics and penicillamine (Mayer et al., 1996, Eikelboom et al., 1999).

In the clinic, studying or utilizing Hcy as a risk factor for vascular disease demands attention to several issues. First, the initial blood sample must not only be fasting, but must be processed properly. Because erythrocytes leak Hcy over time, the sample must either be centrifuged promptly to isolate the plasma, or kept on ice for no longer than a couple of hours before processing. Second, the assay must be reliable. High-performance liquid chromatography has been a useful gold-standard, but isotope-dilution GC-MS has much to recommend it (Goodman et al., 1998). The "normal ranges" will vary depending on the assay. Third, little free Hcy circulates. Most Hcy forms a disulfide with itself (creating homocystine) or with cysteine or other compounds with a free sulfhydryl group to form mixed disulfides. Furthermore, all of these moieties are largely bound to plasma proteins. As a result, most epidemiologic studies have focused on the "total" plasma concentration of Hcy. Fourth, the level of Hcy in either fasting or fed states is sensitive to deficiencies of folic acid, vitamin B_6 and vitamin B_{12}. In some clinical settings, the serum levels of these cofactors are measured at the time of assaying Hcy, but this increases the cost. Certainly if the Hcy level is elevated, relative vitamin deficiency must be considered. Finally, people with relative defects in CBS, either due to mutations in *CBS* or deficiency of vitamin B_6, may have plasma Hcy levels in the normal range but hyperhomocysteinemia after a meal. Thus, a thorough evaluation of this risk factor includes assaying the plasma Hcy level two or four hours after a standard dose of oral methionine (0.1g Met/kg body weight).

LP (A)

Lipoprotein (a) (Lp(a)) was first described by Berg (1963) over 35 years ago. Lp (a) has a cholesterol ester-rich core similar to LDL with an additional polypeptide, apo (a), that is covalently linked to the apo B molecule (Scanu et al., 1991). Lp(a) may contribute to vascular disease by a variety of mechanisms: competing with binding for plasminogen thus reducing the amount of plasmin generated and inhibiting fibrinolysis (McLean et al., 1987; Loscalzo, 1990); increasing cholesterol deposition in the arterial wall (Rath et al., 1989); enhancing foam cell formation (Naruszewicz et al., 1992); generating oxygen free radicals in monocytes (Riis-Hansen et al., 1994); promoting smooth muscle proliferation, perhaps by reducing plasma-induced activation of latent TGF-β (Grainger et al. 1993; 1994; Kreuzer et al., 1994); and, inducing chemotactic activity in endothelial cells (Poon et al., 1997). Despite numerous studies showing a positive correlation between Lp(a) levels and ASHD, more recent studies have cast some doubt on the potential role of Lp(a) in ASHD. Prior studies showed that people with Lp(a) levels in the highest quartile have a 2–3 fold higher incidence of myocardial infarction, especially in the young or in those lacking traditional risk factors (Rhoads et al., 1986; Cremer et al., 1994). High levels of Lp(a) have been associated with premature ASHD, family history of myocardial infarction, restenosis following angioplasty, reocclusion following coronary artery bypass surgery, stroke and post-transplant vasculopathy (Durrington et al., 1988; Genest et al., 1992; Berg et al., 1993; Schaefer et al., 1994; Desmarais et al., 1995; Bostom et al., 1996; Chanbless et al., 1996; Van Kooten et al., 1996). Other studies have failed to show an association between Lp(a) and vascular disease. In the Physicians Health Study, 14,916 predominantly white, middle-aged men were examined prospectively and serum Lp(a) did not correlate with future risk of myocardial infarction or stroke (Ridker et al., 1993; 1995a). In the Helsinki Heart Study, baseline Lp(a) levels were similar in patients who developed coronary events and those who did not over a five-year follow-up period (Jauhianen et al., 1991). In a five-year prospective study of French-Canadian men, elevated levels were not an independent risk factor; however, high levels did appear to increase the deleterious effect of high total and LDL cholesterol and detract from the effects of a high HDL (Cantin et al., 1998). In a study of 140 African-American patients, Lp(a) levels were similar in those with and without ASHD (Moliterno et al., 1995). In a recent meta-analysis of 27 studies including both 18 population studies and eight studies of patients with previous disease, involving over 5400 deaths or non-fatal myocardial infarctions, a higher relative risk was reported (1.6–1.7-fold) of mortality from ASHD and or non-fatal MI in patients with the highest third of Lp(a) levels compared with the lowest third (Danesh et al., 2000).

The conflicting data from these studies may result from differences in acquisition of samples during acute illness, inadequate storage of samples, lack of standardized assays, and definitions in endpoints in the studies (Albers and Marcovina, 1994; Kronenberg et al., 1996; Stein and Rosenson, 1997). Based on current evidence, it is debatable whether or not to screen for elevated Lp(a). There is currently a lack of clinical trial data showing a benefit of reducing levels. Dietary intervention, exercise and lipid-lowering therapy appear to have little effect on Lp(a) levels. Estrogen replacement therapy in post-menopausal women, testosterone replacement therapy in men (Zmuda et al., 1996.), and nicotinic acid (Gurakar et al., 1985; Temme et al., 1996; Stein and Rosenson, 1997; Thomas et al., 1997; Espeland et al., 1998;) do reduce serum Lp(a). Also, in men with high LDL and Lp(a) levels, the atherogenic potential of Lp(a) is neutralized by effective reduction in LDL (Maher et al., 1995). In sum, for patients with premature vascular disease but few overt risk factors, screening for elevated Lp(a) may have a role.

FIBRINOGEN

Several large prospective studies from Europe and the United States have shown fibrinogen levels to be an independent predictor of cardiovascular disease, including ASHD (Wilhelmsen et al., 1984; Meade et al., 1986; Kannel et al., 1987; Heinrich et al., 1994). Comparing the highest tertile with the lowest tertile of fibrinogen levels, the odds ratio for ASHD is 2.3 (Ernst and Resch, 1993). In patients with established ASHD, fibrinogen levels are associated with angiographic severity of disease (Lowe et al., 1980; Broadhurst et al., 1990), recurrent ischemic events (Meade et al., 1986), and the risk of restenosis after coronary angioplasty (Montalescot et al., 1995). In non-smoking males, levels of fibrinogen are associated with all-cause and cardiovascular mortality (Rosengren and Wihelmsen, 1996). In patients with non-Q wave myocardial infarction or unstable angina, fibrinogen levels correlate with risk of death or myocardial infarction (Toss et al., 1997). Reducing fibrinogen levels in patients with established ASHD has been shown to reduce the incidence of cardiac death and ischemic stroke (Behar, 1999).

The mechanism by which fibrinogen has a deleterious effect has been extensively studied. In addition to its role in the coagulation cascade, fibrinogen has additional effects including stimulation of smooth muscle proliferation, promotion of platelet aggregation, increased blood viscosity (Meade et al., 1986) and may have mitogenic and angiogenic properties (Smith and Thompson, 1994). Fibrin may also bind to lipoprotein in the intima and may enhance accumulation of extracellular lipid in plaques (Smith and Crosbie, 1991).

Numerous environmental and non-environmental processes influence the level of fibrinogen. Fibrinogen is an acute phase reactant and may only be an inflammatory marker for the atherosclerotic process. Fibrinogen levels are higher in women, increase with age, and are associated with an elevated LDL cholesterol level, depressed HDL cholesterol level, hypertriglyceridemia, obesity, smoking, sedentary lifestyle, family history of premature ASHD, hypertension and diabetes mellitus (Lee et al., 1993; Genest and Cohn, 1995; Tybjaerg-Hansen et al., 1997). Fibrinogen levels are responsive to therapeutic interventions. Smoking cessation, weight loss, exercise, and moderate alcohol consumption have all been associated with a reduction in fibrinogen (Ernst and Resch, 1995). Pharmacotherapy with fibric acid derivatives, including ciprofibrate, bezafibrate, fenofibrate but not gemfibrozil, reduce fibrinogen levels (Niort et al., 1988; Pazzucconi et al., 1992; Otto et al., 1994; De Maat et al., 1994; Koenig et al., 1994). Finally, estrogen replacement in post-menopausal women and estrogen therapy in elderly men reduce fibrinogen levels (Giri et al., 1998; Espeland et al., 1998).

Extensive intra-individual variation in fibrinogen level, disagreement as to the best analytic assay, and a lack of conclusive data that reducing fibrinogen reduces cardiovascular risk limits the widespread use of measuring this risk factor for ASHD.

VARIATION IN OTHER HEMOSTATIC FACTORS

Several lines of evidence suggest that increased coagulability and decreased fibrinolytic activity contribute to the risk of ASHD (Meade et al., 1986; Yarnell et al., 1991; Fowkes et al., 1992; Ernst and Resch, 1993; Folsom et al., 1993; Heinrich et al., 1994; Salomaa et al., 1994; Levenson et al., 1995). Although acute thrombosis of an underlying atherosclerotic vessel is the precipitating event of an acute myocardial infarction, recurrent thrombus formation is an integral part of advanced atherosclerotic lesions (Stary et al., 1989). Various studies suggest that levels of these circulating hemostatic factors are under environmental as well as genetic influences (De Boever et al., 1993; Folsom et al., 1993; Eliasson et al., 1995) (Ch. 70).

FACTOR VII

Girelli and co-investigators (2000) compared 311 patients with angiographically documented ASHD with 133 controls and found no overall difference in frequencies of the various factor VII polymorphisms. This supports data from the Framingham Heart Study (Feng et al., 2000). However, in Girelli's study, patients with ASHD who had not suffered a prior myocardial infarction had a higher frequency of polymorphisms associated with lower levels of factor VII compared with those who had suffered a myocardial infarction (Girelli et al., 2000). This finding suggests that certain factor VII genotypes may protect against the occurrence of myocardial infarction in patients with ASHD.

FACTOR V LEIDEN

The factor V Leiden mutation (Arg506Gln) predisposes to both venous thromboembolism and arterial thrombosis. In the Physicians Health Study, however, the presence of the factor V Leiden allele in healthy men did not appear to increase the risk of myocardial infarction or stroke, although it was associated with venous thromboembolism (Ridker et al., 1995b).

PLASMINOGEN ACTIVATOR INHIBITOR TYPE 1

The plasma levels of plasminogen activator inhibitor type 1 (PAI-1) is the major determinant of plasma fibrinolysis, and elevated PAI-1 levels have been associated with thrombotic disorders (Wiman et al., 1985; Auwerx et al., 1988). PAI-1 levels also influence the risk of reinfarction in patients who have already suffered a myocardial infarction under the age of 45 years (Hamsten et al., 1985). PAI-1 is synthesized in the liver and endothelial cells and is carried by platelets, although it also circulates in the plasma in inactive and active forms bound to vitronectin. Levels of PAI-1 are affected by various cytokines and hormones including insulin and glucocorticoids. Several polymorphisms of the PAI-1 gene have been identified that are associated with increased expression of PAI-1 (Dawson et al., 1993). These will be discussed later in the chapter.

ATHEROGENIC LIPOPROTEIN PHENOTYPE

In addition to quantitative measures of various lipoprotein classes, certain structural variations of lipoproteins are strongly associated with ASHD. The presence of small, dense LDL particles, as measured by increased density on centrifugation, increased mobility on native gel electrophoresis, or an elevated LDL-apo B in the presence of normal cholesterol levels has been associated with a 3-fold increased incidence of ASHD compared to other LDL-cho-

lesterol particles. The occurrence of small, dense LDL, increased triglycerides and low HDL constitutes the atherogenic lipoprotein phenotype. This phenotype has been suggested to have a heritable basis (Sniderman, 1980; Austin et al., 1990; 1998). The genetic determinants for small, dense LDL particles and familial combined hyperlipidemia overlap (Juo et al., 1998).

C-REACTIVE PROTEIN

Various markers of inflammation have been related to the risk of atherosclerotic vascular disease (Table 53.5), and others are reasonable candidates for further investigation (Table 53.6). A major question that needs to be addressed is whether these factors are markers of on-going inflammatory processes, or actually predisposing factors. One such factor is C-reactive protein (CRP), a member of the pentraxin family of evolutionarily ancient proteins. An acute-phase reactant, CRP is synthesized by the liver and lymphocytes (Kilpatrick and Volanakis, 1991). Elevated levels of plasma CRP are strongly associated with the risk of ASHD in both men and postmenopausal women (Rhode et al., 1999; Ridker et al., 2000a). Another example of an indicator of tissue injury and inflammation is interleukin-6. Ridker and colleagues (2000b) examined archived plasma specimens of men who subsequently developed myocardial infarction and found that their baseline IL6 levels were elevated compared to matched controls who did not develop symptomatic ASHD. While this type of investigation has the advantage of examining preclinical phases of diseases, the fundamental issue of whether IL6 is causative or simply a marker of established pathology remains.

The genetic basis of specific risk factors

Most of the molecules that have both a suggested role in the etiology or pathogenesis of atherosclerosis and atherosclerotic diseases and a genetic basis are listed in Table 53.5. Some are reviewed in more detail in this section. Once a locus is identified as significant in etiology, pathogenesis, or both, the analysis needs to be extended to understanding the relevance of specific nucleotide sequence variations. Array and other testing technologies enable the screening of both many sequence variations and many specimens (Cambien et al., 1999; Cheng et al., 1999; Witkowski et al., 2000). This needs to be matched with the ability to store and interpret massive amounts of data, and to look for

Table 53.6. Potential candidate loci that may predispose to atherosclerosis

Protein	Locus(I)
Blood pressure regulation	
Adducin	ADD1, ADD3
Adrenergic recp. α2A	ADRA2
Adrenergic recp. α2C	ADRA2C
Adrenergic recp. β1	ADRB1
Aldosterone synthase	CYP11B2
Angiotensin recp. 1	AGTR1
Angiotensin II receptor type-1B	AGTR1B
Angiotensin II receptor type-2	AGTR2
Anion exchangers	SLC4A3, SLC4A4, SLC4A7
Bradykinin recp. B2	BDKRB2
Endothelins	EDN1, EDN2, EDN3
Endothelin recp.	EDNRA
Glucocorticoid recp.	GCCR
Guanyl cyclase NOS recp.	GUCY1A3, GUCY1B3
Kallikrein 1	KLK1
Kininogen	KNG
NO synthase, neuronal	NOS1
Renin binding protein	RBP
Sodium channel proteins	SCN2A1, etc.
Sodium-hydrogen exchanger	SLC9A3, SLC9A5
Sodium-K-ATPase transporter	
Glucose regulation	
Glucagon receptor	GCGR
Glycogen synthase	GYS1, GYS2
Growth factors	
Platelet-derived growth factor recp.	PDGFR
Platelet activating factor recp.	PTAFR
Platelet-derived growth factors	PDGFA, PDGFB
Thrombospondin-1	THBS1
Transforming growth factor γ	TGFG
Vascular endothelial growth factor	VEGF
Hemostasis	
Antithrombin III	AT3
Platelet activating factor recp.	PTAFR
Platelet activating factor acetylhydrolase	PAFAH1B1
Platelet endothelial cell adhesion molecule 1	PAFAH1B1
Thrombomodulin	THBD
Thromboxane A2 recp.	TBXA2R
Kininogen	KNG
Homocysteine metabolism	
Methionine synthase reductase	MTRR
Inflammatory/adhesion molecules	
NO synthase, inducible	NOS2A
Lipid metabolism	
Fatty acid binding proteins	FABP1–5
HMG CoA reductase	HMGCR
HDL recp.–SRBI	CD36L1
Obesity	
Adrenergic recp. α2B	ADRA2B
Adrenergic recp. β3	ADRB3
Agouti signaling recp.	ASIP
Hormone sensitive lipase	LIPE
Leptin recp.	LEPR
Melanocortin recps.	MC3R, MC5R

patterns that may represent genotype-phenotype correlations (von Kodolitisch et al., 1999).

DYSLIPIDEMIAS (see also Ch. 91)

Twin and family studies reveal that the heritability of most lipoprotein traits is greater than 50%, suggesting that in isolation genetic factors are more important than environmental factors in determining lipoprotein levels in individuals. In addition, about one-quarter to one-third of intra-individual variance in LDL cholesterol and HDL cholesterol over time is attributable to genetic influences (Friedlander et al., 1997). The major portion of this genetic influence is accounted for by multiple genes, each of small effect, combined with rare alleles of some genes that have a large effect. Most dyslipidemias are thus polygenic, complex traits, while a few occur as a result of the profound effects of a specific gene. The number of genetic factors that have been identified as yet is small compared with the number that likely contributes to the heritability of lipid levels in the population (Warden et al., 1993).

One such genetic factor that has been identified is the locus that encodes apolipoprotein E (*APOE*). Apo E alleles cause both variation in cholesterol levels in normolipidemic individuals and type III hyperlipidemia. In western populations, apo E alleles account for 4% of the variation in fasting serum cholesterol levels (Sing and Davignon, 1985; Weintraub et al., 1987; Davignon et al., 1988). In contrast, taken together rare mendelian single gene defects account for 10% or less of the variance of lipoprotein levels in the population. Monogenic disorders of lipid metabolism occur less frequently than 1% of the general population, although they are more frequent in patients with premature ASHD occurring in about 15% of cases (Nora et al., 1980).

Genetic traits are expressed on the background of environmental influences such as diet, exercise, smoking, obesity and alcohol intake. The effects of these and other environmental factors may enhance or reduce the inherent genetic risk of ASHD. For example, The Seven Countries Study revealed a correlation between dietary saturated fat intake, serum cholesterol and ASHD mortality (Keys et al., 1986). Also, the intake of fat, serum cholesterol levels, and the incidence of ASHD and stroke increases progressively among individuals of Japanese ancestry who live in Japan, Hawaii or the US mainland (Kagan et al., 1974; Nichman et al., 1975). Thus, the most common atherogenic alterations in lipoprotein metabolism require the combination of multiple gene effects in addition to environmental factors.

The focus of this section will be to highlight the genetic basis of the more frequently occurring dyslipidemias that contribute to ASHD, as well to highlight the more rare disorders with a genetic basis that also require environmental factors for full expression. These disorders include single gene defects such as the heterozygous form of familial hypercholesterolemia, single gene defects requiring other environmental factors for expression such as type III hyperlipidemia (familial dysbetalipoproteinemia), and polygenic disorders such as atherogenic lipoprotein phenotype and familial combined hyperlipidemia. For a comprehensive discussion of lipoprotein disorders) (see Ch. 91).

TYPE III HYPERLIPIDEMIA (FAMILIAL DYSBETALIPOPROTEINEMIA)

This relatively rare, recessive disorder results in the accumulation of chylomicron remnants and IDL particles. The disorder has a strong association with premature ASHD. Clinically it is manifested by cutaneous xanthomas in 50% of patients, tuberous xanthomas less commonly and rarely with tendon xanthomas. Cholesterol concentrations may be over 300 mg/dl and triglyceride concentrations are usually higher. The frequency in the general caucasian population is about 1 in 5000, however, in survivors of myocardial infarction it is 1 in 100 patients (Uterman, 1985). Over 90% of type III hyperlipidemia patients are homozygous for a common allele of *APOE*, apo ε2. Apo ε2 has only 1–2% of the LDL receptor binding affinity of the more common allele, apo ε3. However, possessing two apo ε2 alleles is necessary but not sufficient for the development of type III hyperlipidemia, since 95% of homozygous individuals do not have the disorder. Additional genetic or environmental factors such as obesity, diabetes, menopause, and physical inactivity probably contribute to the appearance of Type III disease. It has been estimated in population-based studies that apo ε4 alleles determine up to 50% of the variation of serum total cholesterol level in various populations and up to 40% variation in ASHD mortality (Stengard et al., 1998).

FAMILIAL COMBINED HYPERLIPIDEMIA

This is a relatively common disorder that is characterized by varying levels of VLDL, IDL and LDL. The incidence in the general population is about 1 in 200 people (Cabezas et al., 1992). The disorder may present with an elevated cholesterol level, high triglycerides or both, often exceeding 300 mg/dl for both. The disease has an autosomal dominant transmission and is often associated with the small, dense LDL phenotype. Due to the variability in lipoprotein patterns in individuals and families, it is also known as multiple type hyperlipidemia. Due to the lack of a specific marker, it is a difficult disorder to diagnose. Most often the diagnosis is made by family studies documenting an elevation of cholesterol, triglycerides or both. Among survivors of patients with premature myocardial infarction, familial combined hyperlipidemia is the most commonly encountered lipid disorder occurring in up to 11–20% of cases (Nikkila and Aro, 1973).

The defect in familial combined hyperlipidemia appears to be an increased production of apo B and VLDL (Chait et al., 1980; Janus et al., 1980; Grundy et al., 1987). However, this does not appear to be linked to *APOB* (Rauh et al., 1990). A number of genetic loci have been implicated in familial combined hyperlipidemia including a null mutation in the lipoprotein lipase gene and the *APOAI-APOC3-APOA4* gene cluster (Stalenhoef et al., 1984; Babirak et al., 1989; Wojciechowski et al., 1991; Nevin et al., 1994). In addition, *APOE* alleles and environmental factors such as obesity may contribute to the disorder. No one factor explains the mechanism of this disorder (Cabezas et al., 1992), but evidence is mounting for the influence of at least one major gene (Juo et al., 1998).

SMALL, DENSE LDL AND THE ATHEROGENIC LIPOPROTEIN PHENOTYPE

The frequency of this disorder appears to be 20% of the U.S. population. The disorder appears to have an autosomal dominant transmission with variable penetrance. LDL particle size is influenced by various environmental factors such as diet, drugs, exercise and hormonal status. Family studies have suggested a linkage to the LDL receptor locus (*LDLR*) on chromosome 19 (Nishina, 1992). Other studies have suggested a more complex inheritance with contributions from several loci including chromosome 6 linked to the superoxide dismutase gene, chromosome 11 linked to the *APOAI-APOC3-APOA4* gene cluster, and a chromosome 16 link to the cholesterol ester transfer protein gene (*CETP*) (Rotter et al., 1996).

FAMILIAL HYPERCHOLESTEROLEMIA

Familial hypercholesterolemia is due to a defect in the structure or function of the LDL receptor or, less commonly, to a defect in the structure of apo B. The frequency of this disorder is approximately 1 in 500 of the general United States population. However, the disorder has a much higher frequency in French Canadians, Afrikaners and Lebanese in whom the frequency is approximately 1 in 200. The vast majority of patients are heterozygous for a mutation in *LDLR*. In heterozygotes, cholesterol levels classically range between 300–500 mg/dl and elevations are seen from early childhood. At the molecular level, the disorder is heterogeneous with several hundred different mutations of *LDLR* having been discovered. Some *LDLR* mutations produce considerably lower total cholesterol levels. The disorder results primarily in elevated LDL, however, smaller increases occur in VLDL and IDL and there is an inhibition of conversion of cholesterol to bile acids. Clinically patients have tendon xanthomas, preferentially in the achilles tendon, as well as corneal arcus. The probability of tendon xanthomas being present is approximately equal to the age of the patient. The cumulative incidence of ASHD by age 60 is 52% in men and 33% in women heterozygotes. When a patient has inherited a mutation in *LDLR* from each parent, the condition is much more severe, with death from ASHD common before young adulthood.

LOW HDL

High-density lipoproteins are a heterogeneous group of particles consisting of about 50% protein and 50% lipid (Tall, 1990; Karathanasis, 1993). Like the other lipoproteins, HDL consists of a hydrophobic core of cholesterol esters and triglycerides with a surrounding layer of free cholesterol, phospholipids and various proteins. Some of the proteins carried include apo AI, apo A2, apo A4, apo CI, CII, CIII, apo D, E, H, J, lecithin:cholesterol acyl transferase (LCAT), CETP, serum amyloid A, paraoxanase, transferrin and platelet activating factor hydrolase. The mechanism by which HDL particles confer protection against ASHD is postulated to be due to reverse cholesterol transport. Free cholesterol is taken up from cells by free diffusion or a receptor mediated process and then esterified and transported to the HDL core by LCAT. The cholesterol carried by HDL is then brought back to the liver or exchanged for triglycerides from VLDL and IDL particles in the plasma by the action of CETP. HDL is also capable of inhibiting the oxidation of LDL (Parthasarathy et al., 1990). HDL may play additional roles including in host defense.

The several classes of HDL are divided based on size and density and can be separated by gel electrophoresis (Astalos et al., 1993). The major subclasses are HDL 2 and HDL 3 with considerable functional heterogeneity between the various HDL particles, including differences in ability to promote efflux of cholesterol from cells, ability to interact with HTGL and activate LCAT (Karathanasis, 1993; Rader et al., 1993). As a result, all HDL species may not be equally protective (Costel-Burel et al., 1990; Parra et al.,

1992). Genetic factors determine not only the level of HDL but also the amounts of various species. Simple mendelian disorders account for only a small proportion of markedly low or high HDL levels found among individuals.

The majority of disorders resulting in a low HDL level are multifactorial (Breslow, 1996). A number of environmental factors, such as exercise and alcohol consumption, and other disorders, such as diabetes mellitus and excessive BMI (body mass index), contribute to low HDL levels (Williams et al., 1993). However, a number of genes, some known and some inferred, also influence the levels of HDL in plasma as well as the composition of the particles (Almasy et al., 1999). Common variations of the CETP gene influence HDL levels with evidence from both association as well as linkage studies (Kondo et al., 1989; Bu et al.,1994;Agerholm-Larsen et al, 2000). Apo AII gene variations also contribute to apo AI and apo AII levels as well as the composition of HDL (Scott et al., 1985; Warden et al., 1993; Bu et al., 1994). The ratio of apo AII to apo AI affects the ability of HDL to accept cholesterol from cells (Karathanasis, 1993). Mice models have suggested that high apo AII levels can promote atherosclerosis despite high levels of HDL (Warden et al., 1993). Association and linkage studies have shown that variations in the LPL locus also contribute to HDL levels (Heinzmann et al., 1991; Heiba et al., 1993).

APO AI DEFICIENCY

Apo AI is the major protein of HDL and a cofactor for LCAT. Mutations in the apo AI gene result in decreased or completely absent apo AI and as a result virtually absent HDL (Norum et al., 1982; Schaefer, 1984; Karathanasis et al., 1987; Ordovas et al., 1989; Funke, 1991; Matsunaga et al., 1991). Affected individuals have a high incidence of ASHD. On occasion, certain mutations are associated with cerebellar neuropathy, subretinal lipid deposition, tendon xanthomas and planar xanthomas in addition to premature ASHD (Ng et al., 1994).

Hypertension

A full discussion of the genetics of blood pressure regulation can be found in Chapter 51.

The development of hypertension appears to result when patients with specific susceptibility genes are exposed to environmental co-factors resulting in the disease. The range of susceptibility genes varies from rare single gene effects causing secondary hypertension to the much more common polygenic effects. Specific genetic traits related to hypertension (Table 53.5) include abnormalities in sodium-lithium countertransport, urinary kallikrein excretion, high levels of adrenal steroid hormones (glucocorticoid remediable aldosteronism), as well as polymorphisms at the angiotensinogen locus (Williams et al., 1994). Genotype accounts for 18% and 28% of the variation of systolic and diastolic blood pressure, respectively (Mitchell et al., 1996).

DIABETES MELLITUS

A detailed discussion of the genetics of diabetes can be found in Chapter 83.

The familial clustering of small dense LDL, glucose intolerance, hyperinsulinemia, hypertension, elevated VLDL, IDL and depressed HDL in patients with type 2 diabetes mellitus and atherosclerosis has been labelled "syndrome X" (Reaven, 1988).

CIGARETTE SMOKING

Numerous studies have suggested an heritable influence on smoking (Raaschou-Nielsen, 1960; Edwards et al., 1995; Rossing, 1998; Sullivan and Kendler, 1999). In a study of sets of twins raised together and apart, genetic influences accounted for approximately 60% of the liability for smoking (Heath et al., 1993; Kendler et al., 20000. Studies have also shown a heritable influence on the initiation of smoking, number of cigarettes smoked per day, and ability to quit (True et al., 1997; Koopmans et al., 1999). The knowledge of specific genes that account for these effects is still lacking. The habit-forming actions of nicotine occur at nicotinic receptors on cell bodies of dopaminergic neurons in the mesolimbic "reward" system of the brain (also implicated in addiction to cocaine, alcohol and opioids). Genes affecting dopaminergic pathways, nicotinic receptors or both could potentially play a role in the addiction (Comings et al., 1996; Rossing, 1998).

OBESITY (see Ch. 87)

Approximately 40% of variation in body-mass index (BMI) is under genetic control in certain populations (Mitchell et al, 1996), and between 50–80% of changes in BMI over time in an individual is under genetic control (Friedlander et al., 1997). The pattern of obesity is likely to influence the occurrence of ASHD. Fat deposited in the abdomen is more likely to contribute to ASHD than fat in thighs and buttocks. Fat in the abdomen is more metabolically active and there is a higher rate of lipolysis with a resulting increase in

free fatty acids returning to the liver and being incorporated into and secreted as VLDL. The FFA may also inhibit insulin breakdown in the liver (Despres et al., 1990; Kaplan, 1992). Obesity may effect HDL levels through effects on CETP, hepatic triglenoyl lipase (HTGL) and lipoprotein lipase (LPL) (Arai et al., 1994; Dullaart et al., 1994).

HOMOCYSTEINE

Various genetic factors influence homocysteine levels. Cystathionine β-synthase, the enzyme responsible for the metabolism of homocysteine to cystathionine, is markedly reduced in patients with the autosomal recessive condition homocystinuria. About one-half of patients respond clinically to pharmacologic doses of pyridoxine (vitamin B_6). The estimated incidence of *CBS* heterozygotes is 1–2 percent of the general population. While some early studies suggested that up to 80% of patients with hyperhomocysteinemia and vascular disease may be heterozygous for deficiency of CBS (Clarke et al., 1991), other studies have not supported this notion (Tsai et al., 1999; Perry, 1999; de Franchis et al., 2000; Christen et al., 2000).

Methylenetetrahydrofolate reductase (MTHFR) catalyzes the synthesis of 5-methyltetrahydrofolate, important in the remethylation of homocysteine to methionine. A thermolabile variant of MTHFR with reduced enzymatic activity, resulting from a highly prevalent mutation of the MTHFR gene (C677T), has also been associated with higher plasma homocysteine levels especially in the setting of reduced folate levels (Kang et al., 1988a, 1988b; Frosst et al, 1995; Arruda et al., 1997). The result of the point mutation is a substitution of valine for alanine, and a 50% reduction in activity of the enzyme. Approximately 5% of the general population, 17% of patients with ASHD and 28% of patients with premature vascular disease are homozygous for the gene (Kang et al., 1993; Boushey et al., 1995). Thirty-eight percent of French Canadians were found to carry the trait in one study, and 12% were homozygous for the thermolabile variant (Frosst et al., 1995). Overall, the thermolabile variant appears to be 5–14-fold more prevalent amongst the general population in caucasians than the heterozygous state of *CBS* deficiency. A recent meta-analysis, however, failed to show an association between this common genetic trait and the risk of vascular disease (Brattstrom et al., 1998), possibly because an adequate folate intake reduces risk from the mutation.

LP(A)

Lp(a) levels are almost exclusively determined by the apo (a) gene (*LPA*) on chromosome 6 and are very resistant to environment and drug effect. Over 90% of the variance in Lp(a) levels is determined by variation of the apo (a) gene. The apo (a) polypeptide is very similar to plasminogen and contains numerous repetitions of the plasminogen kringle IV domain in slightly differing forms. The number of these sequences determines the length of the apo (a) polypeptide and varies between individuals as a result of differing alleles of the apo (a) gene. Over 30 alleles have been identified, each differing by a single kringle IV domain (Lackner et al., 1991; Boerwinkle et al., 1992).

FIBRINOGEN

Fibrinogen levels appear to be strongly influenced by environmental factors outlined in the previous section. However, two common polymorphisms in the 5′-flanking region of the β-fibrinogen gene also influence levels. The (G455A) and (C148T) substitutions in the 5′ flanking region appear to give rise to the most consistent variation in fibrinogen levels. These polymorphisms account for about 1–3% of the variance in fibrinogen levels (Thomas et al., 1991; Green et al, 1993; Tybjærg-Hansen et al., 1997).

OTHER HEMOSTATIC FACTORS

Several polymorphisms of the factor VII gene have been described. One results from the substitution of G–A in the codon for amino acid 353, which results in the substitution of glutamine for arginine. Individuals who carry this allele display approximately 20% lower factor VII levels compared with those without the polymorphism. Those who are homozygous have even lower factor VII levels (Green et al., 1991). It is estimated that the (Arg/Gln) polymorphism may explain up to 7–8% of the variance of factor VII levels in the population (Feng et al., 2000). Another polymorphism, a 10 base pair insertion/deletion polymorphism in the promoter region of the factor VII gene, may account for up to 40% of the variation in factor VII levels (Marchetti et al., 1993; de Knijff et al., 1994). The presence of this rare insertion allele of 10 base pairs reduces promoter activity. The presence of both of these polymorphisms is associated with reduced levels of factor VII (Green et al., 1991; Silveira et al., 1994; Takamiya, 1995; Bernardi et al., 1996).

A G→A mutation at nucleotide 1691 of the factor V gene produces an amino acid substitution at 506 Arg→Gln, which results in increased levels of activated factor V and an increased resistance to cleavage by activated protein C (Bertina et al., 1994; Voorberg et al., 1994; Zoller and Dahlback, 1994). Recognized in up to 20–65% of patients

with a prior history of deep venous thrombosis and 40–60% of patients with a family history of thrombophilia, factor V Leiden has been associated with an increased risk for myocardial infarction, particularly in young women (Svensson and Dahlback, 1994; Dahlback et al., 1995; Rosendaal et al., 1997). The Physicians Health Study did not find the presence of factor V Leiden to increase the risk of myocardial infarction or stroke in apparently healthy men (Ridker et al., 1995B).

A polymorphism consisting of an additional guanine in a run of 4G nucleotides in the promoter region of the PAI-1 gene appears to influence rates of PAI-1 production (Dawson, 1993). Several studies have shown higher levels of PAI-1 in patients with myocardial infarction and controls who are homozygous for the 4G allele compared with 5G/5G genotype (Dawson et al., 1993; Ye et al., 1995).

Weiss and co-workers (1995; 1996) emphasized the potential importance of platelet membrane glycoproteins in coronary thrombosis. Specifically, the PI^{A2} polymorphism of the platelet glycoprotein IIIa gene was associated with a higher risk of acute coronary thrombosis, especially in patients under age 60. In a case-control study, the odds ratio for acute myocardial infarction or unstable angina was 2.8 compared with controls. In cases under the age of 60, the risk associated with the presence of this particular polymorphism was significantly greater (6.2) compared with controls. The molecular basis for this polymorphism is the substitution of proline for leucine at position 33, which results from a single point mutation (C→T) at position 1565 of exon 2 of the glycoprotein IIIa gene (Weiss et al., 1996).

In a recent report, investigators from the Atherosclerosis Risk in Communities (ARIC) study compared 376 patients, age 45-64, who had suffered an ASHD event with 461 controls for the prevalence of a single nucleotide polymorphism of the thrombomodulin gene (Wu et al, 2001). Thrombomodulin (TM), a transmembrane glycoprotein expressed on the surface of basal endothelial cells, acts by binding and modifying thrombin from a procoagulant moiety to an activator of protein C. A dimorphism consisting of thymidine in place of cytosine at codon 455 results in the substitution of valine for alanine (A455V). Although there was no difference in TM levels between the AA and AV/VV genotypes, the AV/VV genotype was significantly over-represented in cases compared with controls. In addition, the presence of the V allele appeared to impart a 6-fold greater risk of events in blacks although it did not increase the risk in white patients. The study not only highlights a possible new independent risk factor for ASHD but also the importance of taking into consideration the effects of ethnic and racial backgrounds when investigating the genetic bases of atherosclerosis.

Clinical implications

PRIMORDIAL VERSUS PRIMARY PREVENTION

Over the last several decades, there has been a steady decline in the age-adjusted mortality rates from ASHD and stroke. This has been attributed to improvements in treatment as well as a very strong emphasis on primary and secondary prevention through public health campaigns against smoking, early detection and treatment of hypertension, as well as screening and effective treatment of dyslipidemias (Gaziano, 1998). However, with our increasing knowledge and understanding of the genetic basis of atherosclerosis, the door to the next step in prevention, i.e., "primordial prevention", is being opened (Williams et al., 1999; 2000). Primary prevention deals with preventing the first clinical event. Primordial prevention deals with eliminating the risk factors that lead to the primary event, such as eliminating atherosclerosis through earlier modification of individual risk factors, or the prevention of hypertension and diabetes rather than targeting the prevention of end organ damage such as stroke.

Current knowledge of specific genetic disorders underlying atherosclerosis permits identification of individuals at high risk and to target them aggressively with drug therapy and environmental risk factor modification. Two practical, somewhat complementary approaches apply. The first is to screen family members and first degree relatives of individuals presenting with premature ASHD or stroke or PVD for established and, to a certain degree, emerging risk factors. Autosomal dominant disorders such as familial combined hyperlipidemia, familial hypercholesterolemia, and type 2 diabetes mellitus will affect 50% of first degree relatives. Relatives of patients with polygenic disorders would be expected to be affected to an even higher degree (Williams et al., 2000). The other approach to primary prevention would be to seek a family history of premature ASHD more carefully when evaluating individuals for risk factors. We know that a family history of premature ASHD is a strong risk factor, independent of other established risk factors.

The family history can also be a guide as to which emerging risk factors, in addition to the established ones, to examine. Given the long list already available for study (Table 53.5), some prioritization is essential if for no other

than economic reasons. Also, even though a factor can be analyzed at the level of the nucleotide sequence, often a phenotypic assay, such as the serum level, is both more informative and less expensive (Pyeritz, 1999; Wang et al., 1997). However, the allure of DNA analyses is currently strong, and commercial interests are marketing panels of loci, the importance of which may not be established. This puts considerable pressure on the primary care physician and cardiologist to use testing wisely. Furthermore, when adequate clinical validity and utility of a molecular test have or have not been established can be unclear, or at least debatable. And testing for a marker on a research basis carries even higher burdens (Granger et al., 2000).

Gene therapy appears to hold prospects for primordial prevention of a number of disorders that lead to atherosclerosis. In particular, transfer of the LDL receptor gene has been reported through a replication defective adenovirus into the livers of animal models of familial hypercholesterolemia (Ishibashi et al., 1993; Kozarsky et al., 1994). This resulted in expression of LDL receptors in over 50 percent of liver cells and brief normalization of LDL levels; however, the success was short-lived due to an immunologic response against the transfected hepatocytes (Kozarsky et al., 1994). In another study, explanted human liver cells were transfected ex vivo with recombinant murine retroviruses containing the LDL receptor gene. The cells were subsequently reintroduced into the five patients from whom the cells had been taken. LDL receptor expression was observed in hepatocytes obtained by biopsy from three of the five patients at four months (Grossman et al., 1994; 1995; Raper et al., 1996). However, technical challenges such as improving the efficiency of gene delivery and providing a more prolonged expression of delivered genes still remain significant hurdles (Williams et al., 1999).

SECONDARY PREVENTION

With the expansion in knowledge in molecular genetics and the human genome, "functional genomics" will help direct specific therapy towards patients most likely to benefit. At present, genotypic analysis may help confirm specific inherited disorders; however, the clinical applicability is limited apart from the screening of affected relatives.

Conclusion

A family history of premature ASHD is a powerful risk factor for vascular disease and should prompt a more aggressive modification of established risk factors. The genetic basis for this association is now increasingly understood at the molecular level, but considerable additional work is required to understand the interaction of minor genetic variants and environmental factors. In addition, how the multiple genetic variants that predispose to ASHD can be modified to reduce risk is a virtually untapped area of investigation. Ultimately, knowledge of how genetics and environment interact should permit more accurate targeting of hygienic and pharmacological prevention and treatment strategies. In addition, new risk factors under heritable influence are being identified. As a result, earlier recognition of disease and risk factors, more targeted prevention in high risk individuals and families, and novel therapeutic approaches should further reduce morbidity and mortality from these diseases.

REFERENCES

Abbott RD, Donahue RP, Kannel WB, Wilson PWF (1998) The impact of diabetes on survival following myocardial infarction in men vs. women. The Framingham Study. JAMA 260:3456–3460

Adams M, Smith PD, Martin D et al. (1996) Genetic analysis of thermolabile methylenetetrahydrofolate reductase as a risk factor for myocardial infarction. Q J Med 89:437–444

Adlersberg D, Parets AD, Boas EP (1949) Genetics of atherosclerosis. Studies of families with xanthoma and unselected patients with coronary artery disease under the age of fifty years. JAMA 141:246

Agerholm-Larsen B, Nordestgaard BG, Steffensen R et al. (1997a) ACE gene polymorphism: Ischemic heart disease and longevity in 10,150 individuals. Circulation 95:2358–2367

Agerholm-Larsen B, Tybjærg-Hansen A, Frikke-Schmidt R et al. (1997b) ACE gene polymorphism as a risk factor for ischemic cerebrovascular disease. Ann Intern Med 127:346–355

Agerholm-Larsen B, Tybjærg-Hansen A, Schnohr P et al. (2000) Common cholesteryl ester transfer protein mutations, decreased HDL cholesterol, and possible decreased risk of ischemic heart disease. The Copenhagen City Heart Study. Circulation 102:2197–2203

Albers JJ, Marcovina SM (1994) Lipoprotein (a) quantification: Comparison of methods and strategies for standardization. Curr Opin Lipidol 5:417–21

Alfthan G, Pekkanen J, Jauhianen M et al. (1994) Relation of serum homocysteine and lipoprotein (a) concentrations to atherosclerotic disease in a prospective Finnish population based study. Atherosclerosis 106:9–19

Almasy L, Hixson JE, Rainwater DL et al. (1999) Human pedigree-based quantitative-trait—locus mapping: Localization of two genes influencing HDL-cholesterol metabolism. Am J Hum Genet 64:1686–1693

American Heart Association (2000) Heart and Stroke Statistical Update. American Heart Association, Dallas

Anderson JL, Habashi J, Carlquist JF et al. (2000) A common variant of the *AMPD1* gene predicts improved cardiovascular survival in patients with coronary artery disease. JACC 36:1248–1252

Antikainen M, Murtomaki S, Syvanne M et al. (1996) The Gln-Arg 191 Polymorphism of the human paraoxonase gene (HUMPONA) is not associated with the risk of coronary artery disease in Finns. J Clin Invest 98:883–5

Arai T, Yamashita S, Hirano K et al. (1994) Increased plasma cholesteryl ester transfer protein in obese subjects: A possible mechanism for the reduction of serum HDL cholesterol levels in obesity. Arterioscler Thromb 14:1129–36

Arnesen E, Refsum H, Bonaa K et al. (1995) Serum total homocysteine and coronary heart disease. Int J Epidemiol 24:704–709

Arruda VR, von Zuben PM, Chiaparini LC et al. (1997) The mutation Ala677—Val in the methylenetetrahydrofolate reductase gene: A risk factor for arterial disease and venous thrombosis. Thromb Haemost 77:818–21

Astalos BF, Sloop CH, Wong L, Roheim PS (1993) Two dimensional electrophoresis of plasma lipoproteins: Recognition of new apo A-I—combining subpopulations. Biochim Biophys Acta 1169:291–300

Austin MA (1991) Plasma triglycerides and coronary heart disease. Arterioscler Thromb 11:2–14

Austin MA, King MC, Vranizan KM, Krauss RM (1990) Atherogenic lipoprotein phenotype: A proposed genetic marker for coronary heart disease risk. Circulation 82:495–506

Austin MA, Talmud PJ, Luong L-A et al. (1998) Candidate-gene studies of the atherogenic lipoprotein phenotype: aA sib-pair linkage analysis of DZ women twins. Am J Hum Genet 62:406–419

Auwerx J, Bouillon R, Collen D, Gebeors J (1988) Tissue type plasminogen activator antigen and plasminogen activator inhibitor in diabetes mellitus. Arteriosclerosis 8:68–72

Babirak SP, Iverius P-H, Fujimoto WY, Brunzell JD (1989) Detection and characterization of the heterozygote state for lipoprotein lipase deficiency. Arteriosclerosis 9:326–334

Becker DM, Becker LC, Pearson TA et al. (1988) Risk factors in siblings of people with premature coronary heart disease. J Am Coll Cardiol 12:1273–80

Behar S (1999) Lowering fibrinogen levels: Clinical update. BIP Study Group—Bezafibrate Infarction Prevention. Blood Coagul Fibrinolysis 10 Suppl 1:S41–3

Benlian P, De Gennes JL, Foubert L et al. (1996) Premature atherosclerosis in patients with familial chylomicronemia caused by mutations in the lipoprotein lipase gene. N Engl J Med 335:848–854

Berg K (1963) A new serum system in man: The Lp system. Acta Pathol Microbiol Scand 59:369–382

Berg K (1993) Lp(a) lipoprotein: An important genetic risk factor for atherosclerosis. In Lusis AJ, Rotter JI, Sparkes RS (eds): Molecular Genetics of Coronary Artery Disease, Karger, Basel, pp. 189–207

Bernardi F, Marchetti G, Pinotti M et al. (1996) Factor VII gene polymorphisms contribute about one-third of the factor VII level variation in plasma. Arterioscler Thromb Vasc Biol 16:72–6

Bertina RM, Koelman BPC, Koster T et al. (1994) Mutation in blood coagulation factor V associated with resistance to activated protein C. Nature 369:64–7

Blankenhorn DH, Nessim SA, Johnson RL et al. (1987) Beneficial effects of combined colestipol-niacin therapy on coronary atherosclerosis and coronary venous bypass grafts. JAMA 247:3233–3240

Blankenhorn DH, Alaupovic P, Wickham E et al. (1990) Prediction of angiographic change in native human coronary arteries and aorto-coronary bypass grafts. Lipid and non-lipid factors. Circulation 81:470–6

Blankenhorn DH, Azen SP, Kramsch DM et al. (1993) Coronary angiographic changes with lovastatin therapy: The Monitored Atherosclerosis Regression Study (MARS). Ann Intern Med 119:969–976

Blumenthal S, Jesse MJ, Hennekens CH et al. (1975) Risk factors for coronary artery disease in children of affected families. J Pediatr 87:1187–1192

Boers GHJ, Smals AGH, Trijbels FJ et al. (1985a) Heterozygosity for homocystinuria in premature peripheral and cerebral occlusive arterial disease. N Engl J Med 313:709–15

Boers GHJ, Fowler B, Smals AGH et al. (1985b) Improved identification of heterozygotes for homocystinuria due to cystathionine synthase deficiency by the combination of methionine loading and enzyme determination in cultured fibroblasts. Hum Genet 69:164–169

Boerwinkle E, Leffert CC, Lin J et al. (1992) Apolipoprotein (a) gene accounts for greater than 90% of the variation in plasma lipoprotein (a) concentrations. J Clin Invest 90:52–60

Boerwinkle E, Ellsworth DL, Hallman DM, Biddinger A (1996) Genetic analysis of atherosclerosis: A research paradigm for the common chronic diseases. Hum Molec Genet 5:1405–1410

Bostom AG, Cupples LA, Jenner JL et al. (1996) Elevated plasma lipoprotein (a) and coronary heart disease in men aged 55 years and younger. A prospective study. JAMA 276:544–8

Boushey CJ, Beresford SAA, Omenn GS, Motulsky AG (1995) A quantitative assessment of plasma homocysteine as a risk factor for vascular disease: Probable benefits of increasing folic acid intake. JAMA 274:1049–1057

Brattstrom LE, Israelsson B, Jeppesen JO, Hultberg BL (1988) Folic acid—an innocuous means to reduce plasma homocysteine. Scand J Clin Lab Invest 48:215–21

Brattstrom LE, Israelsson B, Norrving B et al. (1990) Impaired homocysteine metabolism in early-onset cerebral and peripheral occlusive arterial disease. Effects of pyridoxine and folic acid treatment. Atherosclerosis 81:51–60

Brattstrom LE, Lindgren A, Israelsson B et al. (1992) Hyperhomocysteinemia in stroke: Prevalence, cause, and relationships to type of stroke and stroke risk factors. Eur J Clin Invest 22:214–21

Brattstrom L, Wilken DE, Ohrvik J, Brudin L (1998) Common methylenetetrahydrofolate reductase gene mutation leads to hyperhomocysteinemia but not to vascular disease: The result of a meta-analysis. Circulation 98:2520–6

Braunwald E (1997) Shattuck Lecture—cardiovascular medicine at the turn of the millennium: Triumphs, concerns, and opportunities. N Engl J Med 337:1360–1369

Breslow JL (1996) Familial disorders of high density lipoprotein metabolism. In Scriver CR, Beaudet AL, Sly WS, Valle D (eds): The Molecular and Metabolic Bases of Inherited Disease. 7th edn. McGraw-Hill, NY

Broadhurst P, Kelleher C, Hughes I et al. (1990) Fibrinogen, factor VII clotting activity and coronary artery disease severity. Atherosclerosis 85:169–73

Brown G, Albers JJ, Fisher LD et al. (1990) Regression of coronary artery disease as a result of intensive lipid lowering therapy in men with high levels of apolipoprotein B. N Engl J Med 323:1289–1298

Bu X, Warden CH, Xia YR et al. (1994) Linkage analysis of the genetic determinants of high density lipoprotein concentrations and composition: Evidence for involvement of the apolipoprotein A-II and cholesteryl ester transfer protein loci. Hum Genet 93:639–48

Cabezas MC, deBruin JWA, Erkelens DW (1992) Familial combined hyperlipidemias: 1973–1991. Netherlands J Med 40:83–95

Cambien F, Poirier O, Nicaud V et al. (1999) Sequence diversity in 36 candidate genes for cardiovascular disorders. Am J Hum Genet 65:183–191

Cantin B, Gagnon F, Moorjani S et al. (1998) Is lipoprotein (a) an independent risk factor for ischemic heart disease in men? The Quebec Cardiovascular Study. J Am Coll Cardiol 31:519–25

Castro E, Edland SD, Lee L et al. (2000) Polymorphisms at the Werner locus: II. 1074Leu/Phe, 1367Cys/Arg, longevity, and atherosclerosis. Am J Med Genet 95:374–380

Cederlof R, Friberg L, Jonsson E (1967) Hereditary factors and "angina pectoris". A study on 5,877 twin-pairs with the aid of Mmailed questionnaires. Arch Environ Health 14:397

Chait A, Albers JJ, Brunzell JD (1980) Very low density lipoprotein overproduction in genetic forms of hypertriglyceridemia. Eur J Clin Invest 10:17–22

Chambless LE, Shahar E, Sharrett AR et al. (1996) Association of transient ischemic attack/stroke symptoms assessed by standardized questionnaire and algorithm with cerebrovascular risk factors and carotid artery wall thickness. The ARIC study, 1987–1989. Am J Epidemiol 144:857–66

Chasen-Taber L, Selhub J, Rosenberg IH et al. (1996) A prospective study of folate and vitamin B_6 and risk of myocardial infarction in US physicians. J Am Coll Nutr 15:136–43

Chauveau P, Bernadette C, Coude M et al. (1993) Hyperhomocysteinemia, a risk factor for atherosclerosis in chronic uremic patients. Kidney Int 43:S72–7

Cheng S, Grow MA, Pallaud C et al. (1999) A multilocus genotyping assay for candidate markers of cardiovascular disease risk. Genome Res 9:936–949

Childs B (1999) Genetic Medicine: A Logic of Disease. Johns Hopkins University Press, Baltimore

Christen WG, Ridker PM (2000) Blood levels of homocysteine and atherosclerotic vascular disease. Curr Atheroscler Rep 2:194–199

Christen WG, Ajani UA, Glynn RT et al. (2000) Blood levels of homocysteine and increased risks of cardiovascular disease: or casual? Arch Intern Med 160:422–434

Clarke R, Daly L, Robinson K et al. (1991) Hyperhomocysteinemia: An independent risk factor for vascular disease. N Engl J Med 324:1149–55

Comings DE, Ferry L, Bradshaw-Robinson S et al. (1996) The dopamine D2 receptor (DRD2) Gene: A genetic risk factor in smoking. Pharmacogenetics 6:73–9

Conti CR (2000) Detecting coronary artery calcification. Clin Cardiol 23:717–718

Corbo RM, Vilardo T, Mantuano E et al. (1997) Apolipoproteins B and E, and angiotensin I-converting enzyme (ACE) genetic polymorphisms in Italian women with coronary artery disease (CAD) and their relationships with plasm lipid and apolipoprotein levels. Clin Genet 57:77–82

Costel-Burel M, Mainard F, Chivot L et al. (1990) Study of lipoprotein particles LpAI and LpAI:AII in patients before coronary bypass surgery. Clin Chem 36:1889–91

Couture P, Otvos JD, Cupples LA et al. (2000) Association of the C-514T polymorphism in the hepatic lipase gene with variations in lipoprotein subclass profiles. Arterioscler Thromb Vasc Biol 20:815–822

Cremer P, Nagel D, Labrot B et al. (1994) Lipoprotein (a) as predictor of myocardial infarction in comparison to fibrinogen, LDL cholesterol and other risk factors: Results from the prospective Gottingen Risk Incidence and Prevalence Study (GRIPS). Eur J Clin Invest 24:444–53

Criqui MH, Denenberg JO (1998) The generalized nature of atherosclerosis: How peripheral arterial disease may predict adverse events from coronary artery disease. Vasc Med 3:241–245

Dahlback B (1995) Inherited thrombophilia: Resistance to activated protein C as a pathogenic factor of venous thrombosis. Blood 85:607–14

Danesh J, Collins R, Peto R (2000) Lipoprotein (a) and coronary heart disease. Meta-analysis of prospective studies. Circulation 102:1082–5

Davignon J, Gregg RE, Sing CF (1988) Apolipoprotein E polymorphism and atherosclerosis. Arteriosclerosis 8:1–21

Dawson SJ, Wiman B, Hamsten A et al. (1993) The two allele sequences of a common polymorphism in the promoter of the plasminogen activator inhibitor-1 (PAI-1) gene respond differently to IL-1 in hepG2 cells. J Biol Chem 268:10739–10745

De Boever E, De Bacquer D, Braeckman L et al. (1995) Relation of fibrinogen to lifestyles and to cardiovascular risk factors in a working population. In J Epidemiol 24:915–21

de Franchis R, Fermo I, Mazzola G, Sebastio G, Di Minno G, Coppola A, Andria G, D'Angelo A (2000) Contribution of the Cystathionine Beta-Synthase gene (844ins68) Polymorphism to the Risk of Early Onset Venous and Arterial Occlusive Disease and of Fasting Hyperhomocysteinemia. Thromb Haemost 84:576-82

de Jong SC, Stehouwer CDA, van den Berg M, Kostense PJ, Alders D, Jakobs C, Palis G, Rawuerda JA (1999) Determinants of Fasting and Post Methionine Homocysteine Levels in Families Predisposed to Hyperhomocysteinemia and Premature Vascular Disease. Arteriosclerosis, Thromb Vasc Biol 19:1316-1324

de Knijff P, Green F, Johansen LG et al. (1994) New alleles in F7 VNTR. Hum Molec Genet 3:384

de Lemos JA, Hennekens CH, Ridker PM (2000) Plasma concentration of soluble vascular cell adhesion molecule-1 and subsequent cardiovascular risk. J Am Coll Cardiol 36:423–426

De Maat MP, Knopscheer HC, Kastelein JJ, Kluft C (1994) Modulation of plasma fibrinogen levels by ciprofibrate and gemfibrozil in primary hyperlipidemia. Blood Coagul Fibrinolysis 5 Suppl 2:17

Desmarais RL, Sarembock IJ, Ayers CR et al. (1995) Elevated serum lipoprotein (a) is a risk factor for recurrence after coronary balloon angioplasty. Circulation 91:1403–9

Despres JP, Moorjani S, Lupien PJ et al. (1990) Regional distribution of body fat, plasma lipoproteins, and cardiovascular disease. Arteriosclerosis 40:497–511

Di Castelnuovo A, D'Orazio A, Amore C et al. (2000) The decanucleotide insertion/deletion polymorphism in the promoter region of the coagulation factor VII gene and the risk of familial myocardial infarction. Thromb Res 98:9–17

Dobs AS, Nieto FJ, Szklo M et al. (1999) Risk factors for popliteal and carotid wall thickness in the Atherosclerosis Risk in Communities (ARIC) Study. Am J Epidemiol 150(10):1055–67

Dullaart PPF, Sluiter WJ, Dikkeschei LD et al. (1994) Effect of adiposity on plasma lipid transfer protein activities: A possible link between insulin resistance and high density lipoprotein metabolism. Eur J Clin Invest 24:188–94

Durand P, Lussier-Cacan S, Blache D (1997) Acute methionine load-induced hyperhomocysteinemia ednhances platelet aggregation, thromboxane biosynthesis, and macrophage-derived tissue factor activity in rats. FASEB J 11:1157–68

Durrington PN, Ishola M, Hunt L et al. (1988) Apolipoprotein (a), AI, and B and parental history in men with early onset ischaemic heart disease. Lancet 1:1070–3

Edwards KL, Austin MA, Jarvik GP (1995) Evidence for genetic influences on smoking in adult women twins. Clinical genetics 47:236–44

Eikelboom JW, Lonn E, Genest J et al. (1999) Homocysteine and cardiovascular disease: A critical review of the epidemiologic evidence. Ann Intern Med 131:363–375

Eliasson M, Asplund K, Evrin PE, Lundblad D (1995) Relationship of cigarette smoking and snuff dipping to pPlasma fibrinogen, fibrinolytic variables and serum insulin: The northern Sweden MONICA study. Atherosclerosis 113:41–53

Elixhauser A, Yu K, Steiner C et al. (1997) Hospitalization in the U.S., Rockville (Md) Agency for Healthcare Research and Quality; 2000HCUP Fact Book No 1, AHRQ Publication no 00–0031

Epstein FH (1964) Hereditary aspects of coronary heart disease. Am Heart J 67:445

Ernst E, Resch KL (1993) Fibrinogen as a cardiovascular risk factor: A meta-analysis and review of the literature. Ann Intern Med 118:956–63

Ernst E, Resch KL (1995) Therapeutic interventions to lower plasma fibrinogen concentration. Eur Heart J 16 Suppl A:47–53

Espeland MA, Marcovina SM, Miller V et al. (1998) Effect of postmenopausal hormone therapy on lipoprotein (a) concentration. Circulation 97:979–86

Evans RW, Shaten J, Hempel JD et al. (1997) Homocysteine and the risk of cardiovascular disease in the Multiple Risk Factor Intervention Trial. Arterioscler Thromb Vasc Biol 17:1947–1953

Fayad ZA, Fuster V, Fallon JT et al. (2000) Noninvasive *in vivo* human coronary artery lumen and wall imaging using magnetic resonance imaging. Circulation 102:506–510

Feng DL, Tofler GH, Larson MG et al. (2000) Factor VII Gene polymorphism, factor VII levels, and prevalent cardiovascular disease. The Framingham Heart Study. Arterioscler Thromb Vasc Biol 20:593–600

Folsom AR, Wu KK, Shahar E, Davis CE (1993) Association of hemostatic variables with prevalent cardiovascular disease and asymptomatic carotid artery atherosclerosis: The Atherosclerosis Risk in Communities (ARIC) study investigators. Arterioscler Thromb 13:1829–36

Folsom AR, Nieto FJ, McGovern PG et al. (1998) Prospective study of coronary heart disease incidence in relation to fasting total homocysteine, related genetic polymorphisms, and B vitamins: The Atherosclerosis Risk in Communities (ARIC) study. Circulation 98:204–10

Fowkes FGR, Connor JM, Smith FB et al. (1992) Fibrinogen genotype and risk of peripheral atherosclerosis. Lancet 339:693–6

Franken DG, Boers GHJ, Blom HJ et al. (1996) Prevalence of familial mild hyperhomocysteinemia. Atherosclerosis 125:71–80

Frick MH, Elo O, Haapa K et al. (1987) Helsinki Heart Study: Primary prevention trial with gemfibrozil in middle-aged men with dyslipidemia. Safety of treatment, changes in risk factors, and incidence of coronary heart disease. N Engl J Med 317:1237–45

Friedlander Y, Austin MA, Newman B et al. (1997) Heritability of longitudinal changes in coronary heart disease risk factors in women twins. Am J Hum Genet 60:1502–1512

Frossard PM, Lestringant GG, Malloy MJ, Kane JP (1999) Human renin gene Bgll dimorphism associated with hypertension in two independent populations. Clin. Genet. 56:428–433

Frosst P, Blom HJ, Milos R et al. (1995) A candidate genetic risk factor for vascular disease: A common mutation in methylenetetrahydrofolate reductase. Nature Genet 10:111–3

Funke H, von Eckardstein A, Pritchard PH et al. (1991) A frameshift mutation in the human apolipoprotein A-I gene causes high density lipoprotein deficiency, partial lecithin:cholesterol-acyl-transferase deficiency, and corneal opacities. J Clin Invest 87:371–76

Gardemann A, Stricker J, Humme J et al. (1999) Angiotensinogen T174M and M235T gene polymorphisms are associated with the extent of coronary atherosclerosis. Atherosclerosis 145:309–314

Gaziano JM (1998) When should heart disease prevention begin? N Engl J Med 338:1690–1692

Gaziano JM, Hennekens CH, O'Donnell CJ et al. (1997) Fasting triglycerides, high-density lipoprotein cholesterol, and risk of myocardial infarction. Circulation 96:2520–5

Geller DS, Farhi A, Pinkerton N et al. (2000) Activating mineralocorticoid receptor mutation in hypertension exacerbated by pregnancy. Science 289:119–123

Genest J Jr, Cohn JS (1995) Clustering of cardiovascular risk factors: Targeting high-risk individuals. Am J Cardiol 76:8A–20A

Genest J Jr, McNamara JR, Ordovas JM et al. (1992) Lipoprotein cholesterol, apolipoprotein AI and B and lipoprotein (a)

abnormalities in men with premature coronary artery disease. J Am Coll Cardiol 19:792–802

Girelli D, Russo C, Ferraresi P et al. (2000) Polymorphisms in the factor VII gene and the risk of myocardial infarction in patients with coronary artery disease. N Engl J Med 343:774–80

Giri S, Thompson PD, Taxel P et al. (1998) Oral estrogen improves serum lipids, homocysteine and fibrinolysis in elderly men. Atherosclerosis 137:359–66

Glagov S, Weisenberg E, Zarins CK et al. (1987) Compensatory enlargement of human altherosclerotic coronary arteries. N Engl J Med 316:1371–1375

Goldbourt U, Brunner D, Behar S, Reicher-Reiss H (1998) Baseline characteristics of patients participating in the Bezafibrate Infarction Prevention Study. Eur Heart J 19 Suppl H:H42–7

Goodman SI, Elsas LJ, Rosenblatt DS (1998) Measurement and use of total plasma homocysteine. 63:1541–1543

Gordon T, Castelli WP, Hjortland MC et al. (1977) High density lipoprotein as a protective factor against coronary heart disease. The Framingham Study. Am J Med 62:707–714

Gordon T, Kannel WB, Castelli WP, Dawber TR (1981) Lipoproteins, cardiovascular disease, and death: The Framingham Study. Arch Intern Med 141:1128–1131

Gordon DJ, Probstfeld JL, Garrison RJ et al. (1989) High density lipoprotein cholesterol and cardiovascular disease: Four prospective American studies. Circulation 79:8–15

Grainger DJ, Kirschenlohr M, Metcalfe JC et al. (1993) Proliferation of human smooth muscle cells promoted by lipoprotein (a) Science 260:1655–8

Grainger DJ, Kemp PR, Liu AC et al. (1994) Activation of transforming growth factor-beta is inhibited in transgenic apolipoprotein(a) mice. Nature 370:460–462

Grainger DJ, Kemp PR, Metcalfe JC et al. (1995) The serum concentration of active transforming growth factor-β is severely depressed in advanced atherosclerosis. Nature Med 1:74–79

Granger CB, Keavney B, Francomano et al. (2000) Recommendations for national and local regulatory authorities concerning research in genetic markers of disease. Am Heart J 140:S3–5

Green F, Kelleher C, Wilkes H et al. (1991) A common genetic polymorphism associated with lower coagulation factor VII levels in healthy individuals. Arterioscler Thromb 11:540–46

Green F, Hamsten A, Blomback M, Humphries S (1993) The role of β-fibrinogen genotype in determining plasma fibrinogen levels in young survivors of myocardial infarction and healthy controls from Sweden. Thromb Haemost 70:915–20

Grossman M, Raper SE, Kozarsky K et al. (1994) Successful ex-vivo gene therapy directed to liver in a patient with familial hypercholesterolemia. Nature Genet 6:335–41

Grossman M, Rader DJ, Muller DW et al. (1995) A pilot study of ex-vivo gene therapy for homozygous familial hypercholesterolemia. Nature Med 1:1148–54

Grundy SM, Chait A, Brunzell JD (1987) Familial combined hyperlipidemia workshop. Arteriosclerosis 7:203–207

Gudnason V, Thromar K, Humphries SE (1997) Interaction of the cholesterol ester transfer protein 1405V polymorphism with alcohol consumption in smoking and non-smoking healthy men, and theefect on plasma HDL cholesterol and apoAI concentration. Clin Genet 51:15–21

Gurakar A, Hoeg JM, Kostner G et al. (1985) Levels of lipoprotein (a) decline with neomycin and niacin treatment. Atherosclerosis 57:293–301

Hamby RI (1981) Hereditary aspects of coronary artery disease. Am Heart J. 101:639–649

Hamsten A, Wiman B, de Faire U, Blomback M (1985) Increased plasma levels of a rapid inhibitor of tissue plasminogen activator inhibitor in young survivors of myocardial infarction. N Engl J Med 313:1557–1563

Harker LA, Slichter SJ, Scott CR, Ross R (1974) Homocysteinemia. Vascular injury and arterial thrombosis. N Engl J Med 291:537–43

Harpel PC, Chang VT, Borth W (1992) Homocysteine and other sulfhydryl compounds enhance the binding of lipoprotein (a) to fibrin: A potential link between thrombosis, atherogenesis and sulfhydryl compound metabolism. Proc Natl Acad Sci USA 89:10193–7

Heath AC, Cates R, Martin NG et al. (1993) Genetic contribution to risk of smoking initiation: Comparisons across birth cohorts and across cultures. J Substance Abuse 5:221–46

Heiba IM, DeMeester CA, Xia YR et al. (1993) Genetic contributions to quantitative lipoprotein traits associated with coronary artery disease: Analysis of a large pedigree from Bogalusa Heart Study. Am J Med Genet 47:875–83

Heinonen P, Koulu M, Pesonen U et al. (1999) Identification of a three-amino acid deletion in the alpha-2B-adrenergic receptor that is associated with reduced basal metabolic rate in obese subjects. J Clin Endocr Metab 84:2429–2433

Heinrich J, Balleisen L, Schulte H et al. (1994) Fibrinogen and factor VII in the prediction of coronary risk. Results from the PROCAM study in healthy men. Arterioscler Thromb 14:54–9

Heinzmann C, Kirchgessner T, Kwiterovich PO et al. (1991) DNA polymorphism haplotypes of the human lipoprotein lipase gene: Possible association with high density lipoprotein levels. Hum genet 86:578–84

Herrington DM, Pearson TA (1987) Clinical and angiographic similarities in twins with coronary artery disease. Am J Cardiol 59:366

Herrmann S-M, Ricard S, Nicaud V et al. (1998) Polymorphisms of the tumour necrosis factor-alpha gene, coronary heart disease and obesity. Eur J Clin Invest 28:59–66

Hokanson JE, Austin MA (1996) Plasma triglyceride level is a risk factor for cardiovascular disease independent of high-density lipoprotein cholesterol level: A meta-analysis of population-based prospective studies. J Cardiovasc Risk 3:213–9

Hopkins PN, Williams RR, Kuida H et al. (1988) Family history as an independent risk factor for incident coronary artery disease in a high risk cohort in Utah. Am J Cardiol 62:703–707

Horikawa Y, Oda N, Cox NJ et al. (2000) Genetic variation in the gene encoding calpain-10 is associated with type 2 diabetes mellitus. Nature Genet 26:163–175

Howard G, Wagenknecht LE (1999) Environmental tobacco smoke and measures of subclinical vascular disease. Environmental Health Perspectives 107 Suppl 6:837–40

Iacoviello L, Di Castelnuovo A, De Knijff P et al. (1998) Polymorphisms in the coagulation factor VII gene and the risk of myocardial infarction. N Engl J Med 338:79–85

Ikata J, Wakatsuki T, Oishi et al. (2000) Leukocyte counts and concentrations of soluble adhesion molecules as predictors of coronary atherosclerosis. Coron Artery Dis 11:445–449

Ishibashi S, Brown MS, Goldstein JL et al. (1993) Hypercholesterolemia in low density lipoprotein knockout mice and its reversal by adenovirus mediated gene delivery. J Clin Invest 92:883–93

Janus ED, Nicoll AM, Turner RR et al. (1980) Kinetic bases of the primary hyperlipidemias: Studies of ApoB turnover in genetically defined subjects. Eur J Clin Invest 10:161–72

Jauhianen M, Koskinen P, Ehnholm C et al. (1991) Lipoprotein (a) and coronary heart disease risk: A nested case-control study of the Helsinki Heart Study participants. Atherosclerosis 89:59–67

Jaye M, Lynch KJ, Krawiec J et al. (1999) A novel endothelial-derived lipase that modulates HDL metabolism. Nature Genet 21:424–428

Jeppesen J, Hein HO, Suadicani P, Gyntelberg F (1998) Triglyceride concentration and ischemic heart disease: An eight year follow-up in the Copenhagen Male Study. Circulation 97:1029–36

Jorde LB, Williams RR (1988) Relation between family history of coronary artery disease and coronary risk variables. Am J Cardiol 62:708–713

Juo S-HH, Bredie SJH, Kiemeney LA et al. (1998) A common genetic mechanism determines plasma apolipoprotein B levels and dense LDL subfraction distribution in familial combined hyperlipidemia. Am J Hum Genet 63:586–594

Kagan A, Harris BR, Winkelstein W Jr et al. (1974) Epidemiologic studies of coronary heart disease and stroke in Japanese men living in Japan, Hawaii and California: Demographic, physical, dietary and biochemical characteristics. J Chronic Dis 27:345–364

Kane JP, Malloy MJ, Ports TA et al. (1990) Regression of coronary atherosclerosis during treatment of familial hypercholesterolemia with combined drug regimens. JAMA 264:3007–3012

Kang SS, Wong PWK, Zhou J et al. (1988a) Thermolabile methylenetetrahydrofolate reductase in patients with coronary artery disease. Metabolism 37:611–13

Kang SS, Zhou J, Wong PWK et al. (1988b) Intermediate homocysteinemia: A thermolabile variant of methylenetetrahydrofolate reductase. Am J Hum Genet 43:414–421

Kang SS, Passen EL, Ruggie N et al. (1993) Thermolabile defect of methylenetetrahydrofolate reductase in coronary artery disease. Circulation 88:1463–69

Kannel WB (1990) Contribution of the Framingham Study to preventive cardiology. J Am Coll Cardiol 15:206–211

Kannel WB, McGee DL (1979) Diabetes and cardiovascular disease. The Framingham Study. JAMA 241:2035–2038

Kannel WB, Dawber TR, Kagan A et al. (1961) Factors of risk in the development of coronary heart disease—Six year follow up experience. Ann Intern Med 55:33–50

Kannel WB, Wolf PA, Castelli WP, D'Agostino RB (1987) Fibrinogen and risk of cardiovascular disease. JAMA 258:1183–6

Kaplan NM (1992) Obesity: Location matters. Heart Dis Stroke 1:148–150

Kaprio J, Norio R, Pesonen E, Sarna S (1993) Intimal thickening of the coronary arteries in infants in relation to family history of coronary artery disease. Circulation 87:1960–1968

Karathanasis S (1993) Lipoprotein metabolism: High density lipoproteins. In Lusis AJ, Rotter JI, Sparkes RS (ed.): Molecular Genetics of Coronary Artery Disease: Candidate Genes and Processes in Atherosclerosis. Karger, Basel, pp. 140–171

Karathanasis SK, Ferris E, Haddad EA (1987) DNA inversion within the apolipoproteins AI/CIII/AIV encoding gene cluster of certain patients with premature atherosclerosis. Proc Natl Acad Sci USA 84:7198–7202

Karvonen MK, Pesonen U, Heinonen P et al. (1998) Identification of new sequence variants in the leptin gene. J Clin Endocrinol Metab 83:3239–3242

Kendler KS, Thornton LM, Pedersen NL (2000) Tobacco consumption in Swedish twins reared apart and reared together. Arch Gen Psychiatry 57:886–92

Kersten S, Desvergne B, Wahli W (2000) Roles of PPARs in health and disease. Nature 405: 421–424

Keys A, Menotti A, Karvonen MJ et al. (1986) The diet and 15-year death rate in the Seven Countries Study. Am J Epidemiol 124:903–915

Kilpatrick JM, Volanakis JE (1991) Molecular genetics, structure, and function of C-reactive protein. Immun Res 10:43–53

Koenig W, Hoffmeister HCA, Nehmer C et al. (1994) How do fibrates lower fibrinogen? The possible role of interleukin-6 suppression (abstr) Blood Coagul Fibrinolysis 5 Suppl 2:16

Kondo I, Berg K, Drayna D, Lawn R (1989) DNA polymorphism at the locus for human cholesterol ester transfer protein (CETP) is associated with high density lipoprotein cholesterol and apolipoprotein levels. Clin Genet 35:49–56

Koopmans JR, Slutske WS, Heath AC et al. (1999) The genetics of smoking initiation and quantity smoked in Dutch adolescent and young adult twins. Behavior Genet 29:383–93

Kozarsky KF, McKinley DR, Austin LL et al. (1994) In vivo correction of low density lipoprotein receptor deficiency in the Watanabe heritable hyperlipidemic rabbit with recombinant adenoviruses. J Biol Chem 269:13695–702

Kraus WE (2000) Genetic approaches for the investigation of genes associated with coronary heart disease. Am Heart J 140:S27–35

Kreuzer J, Lloyd MB, Bok D et al. (1994) Lipoprotein (a) displays increased accumulation compared to low-density lipoprotein in the murine arterial wall. Chem Phys Lipids 67/68:175–90

Kronenberg F, Trenkwalder E, Dieplinger H, Utermann G (1996) Lipoprotein (a) in stored plasma samples and the ravages of time. Why epidemiological studies might fail. Arterioscler Thromb Vasc Biol 16:1568–72

Krushkal J, Xiong M, Ferrell R et al. (1998) Linkage and association of adrenergic and dopamine receptor genes in the distal portion of the long arm of chromosome 5 with systolic blood pressure variation. Hum Molec Genet 7:1379–1383

Kuivenhoven JA, van Voorst tot Voorst EJGM, Wiebusch H et al. (1995) A unique genetic and biochemical presentation of fish-eye disease. J Clin Invest 96:2783–2791

Kuusisto J, Mykkänen L, Kervinen K et al. (1995) Apolipoprotein E4 phenotype is not an important risk factor for coronary heart disease or stroke in elderly subjects. Arterioscler Thromb Vasc Biol 15:1280–1286

Lackner C, Boerwinkle E, Leffert CC et al. (1991) Molecular basis of apolipoprotein (a) isoform size heterogeneity as revealed by pulsed-field gel electrophoresis. J Clin Invest 87:8980–84

Lambert J-C, Brousseau T, Defosse V et al. (2000) Independent association of APOE gene promoter polymorphism with increased risk of myocardial infarction and decreased APOE plasma concentrations—the ECTIM study. Hum Molec Genet 9:57–61

Large V, Hellstrom L, Reynisdottir S et al. (1997) Human beta-2 adrenoceptor gene polymorphisms are highly frequent in obesity and associate with altered adipocyte beta-2 adrenoceptor function. J Clin Invest 100:3005–3013

LaRosa JC (1997) Triglycerides and coronary risk in women and the elderly. Arch Intern Med 157:961–8

Le W, Yu J-D, Lu L et al. (2000) Association of the R485K polymorphism of the factor V gene with poor response to activated protein C and increased risk of coronary artery disease in the Chinese population. Clin Genet 57:296–303

Lee AJ, Lowe GD, Woodward M, Tunstall-Pedoe H (1993) Fibrinogen in relation to personal history of prevalent hypertension, diabetes, stroke, intermittent claudication, coronary heart disease, and family history: The Scottish Heart Study. Br Heart J 69:338–42

Levenson J, Giral P, Razavian M et al. (1995) Fibrinogen and silent atherosclerosis in subjects with cardiovascular risk factors. Arterioscler Thromb Vasc Biol 15:1263–8

Loscalzo J (1990) Lipoprotein (a): A unique risk factor for atherothrombotic disease. Arteriosclerosis 10:671–9

Lowe GD, Drummond MM, Lorimer AR et al. (1980) Relation between extent of coronary artery disease and blood viscosity. BMJ 280:673–4

Mack WJ, Krauss RM, Hodis HN (1996) Lipoprotein subclasses in the Monitored Atherosclerosis Regression Study (MARS): Treatment effects and relation to coronary angiographic progression. Arterioscler Thromb Vasc Biol 16:697–704

Maher VM, Brown BG, Marcovina SM et al. (1995) Effects of lowering elevated LDL cholesterol on the cardiovascular risk of lipoprotein (a). JAMA 274:1771–4

Majors AK, Pyeritz RE (2000) A deficiency of cysteine impairs fibrillin-1 deposition: Implications for the pathogenesis of cystathionine beta-synthase deficiency. Mol Genet Metab 70:252–260

Majors A, Erhart LA, Pezacka EH (1997) Homocysteine as a risk factor for vascular disease. Enhanced collagen production and accumulation by smooth muscle cells. Arterioscler Thromb Vasc Biol 17:2074–2081

Marchetti G, Patracchini P, Papacchini M et al. (1993) A polymorphism in the 5′ coagulation factor VII gene (F7) caused by an inserted decanucleotide. Hum Genet 90:575–6

Marian AJ, Safaci F, Ferlic L et al. (1999) Interactions between angiotensin-l converting enzyme insertion/deletion polymorphism and response of plasma lipids and coronary atherosclerosis to treatment with fluvastatin. J Am Coll Cardiol 35:89–95

Marshall HW, Morrison LC, Wu LL et al. (1994) Apolipoprotein polymorphisms fail to define risk of coronary artery disease. Circulation 89:567–577

Martin MJ, Hulley SB, Browner WS et al. (1986) Serum cholesterol, blood pressure, and mortality implications from a cohort of 361, 662 men. Lancet 2:933–936

Matsunaga T, Hiasa Y, Yanagi H et al. (1991) Apolipoprotein A-I deficiency due to a codon 84 nonsense mutation of the apolipoprotein A-I gene. Proc Natl Acad Sci USA 88:2793–97

Mayer EL, Jacobsen DW, Robinson K (1996) Homocysteine and coronary atherosclerosis. J Am Coll Cardiol 27:517–27

McCombs RJ, Marcadis DE, Ellis J, Weinberg RB (1994) Attenuated hypercholesterolemic response to a high-cholesterol diet in subjects heterozygous for the apolipoprotein A-IV-2 allele. N Engl J Med 331:706–710

McLean JW, Tomlinsosn JE, Kuang WJ et al. (1987) C-DNA sequence of human apolipoprotein (a) is homologous to plasminogen. Nature 330:132–7

Meade TW, Mellows S, Brozovic M et al. (1986) Haemostatic function and ischaemic heart disease: Principal results of the Northwick Park Heart Study. Lancet 2:533–7

Miller NE (1987) Association of high density lipoprotein subclasses and apolipoproteins with ischemic heart disease and coronary atherosclerosis. Am Heart J 113:589–597

Mitchell BD, Kammerer CM, Blangero J et al. (1996) Genetic and environmental contributions to cardiovascular risk factors in Mexican Americans. The San Antonio Family Heart Study. Circulation 94:2159–2170

Mitchell BD, Blangero J, Comuzzie AG et al. (1998) A paired sibling analysis of the beta-3 adrenergic receptor and obesity in Mexican Americans. J Clin Invest 101:584–587

Moliterno DJ, Jokinen EV, Miserez AR et al. (1995) No association between plasma lipoprotein (a) concentrations and the presence or absence of coronary atherosclerosis in African-Americans. Arterioscler Thromb Vasc Biol 15:850–5

Montalescot G, Ankri A, Vicaut E et al. (1995) Fibrinogen after coronary angioplasty as a risk factor for restenosis. Circulation 92:31–8

Moore JH, Reilly SL, Ferrell RE, Sing CF (1997) The role of the apolipoprotein E polymorphism in the prediction of coronary artery disease age of onset. Clin Genet 51:22–25

Motulsky AG (1996) Nutritional ecogenetics: Homocysteine-related arteriosclerotic vascular disease, neural tube defects, and folic acid. Am J Hum Genet 58:17–20

Murphy EA (1963) Genetics and atherosclerosis. In Likoff, Moyer JH (eds): Coronary Heart Disease. NY, Grune & Stratton, pp. 89–94

Murphy EA (1967) Some difficulties in the investigation of genetic factors in coronary artery disease. Canad Med Assoc J 97:1181–1192

Nagase T, Aoki A, Yamamoto M et al. (1997) Lack of association between the trp64arg mutation in the beta-3-adrenergic receptor gene and obesity in Japanese men: a longitudinal analysis. J Clin Endocr Metab 82:1284–1287

Naggert JK, Recinos A III, Lamerdin JE et al. (1997) The atherogenic lipoprotein phenotype is not caused by a mutation in the coding region of the low density lipoprotein receptor gene. Clin Genet 51:236–240

Naruszewicz M, Selinger E, Davignon J (1992) Oxidative modification of lipoprotein (a) and the effect of beta-carotene. Metabolism 41:1215–24

Naurath HJ, Joosten E, Riezler R et al. (1995) Effects of vitamin B12, folate, and vitamin B6 supplements in elderly people with normal serum vitamin concentrations. Lancet 346:85–9

Nevin DN, Brunzell JD, Deeb SS (1994) The LPL gene in individuals with familial combined hyperlipidemia and decreased LPL activity. Arterioscler Thromb 14:869–873

Ng DS, Leiter LA, Vezina C et al. (1994) Apolipoprotein A-I Q(-2) Causing isolated apolipoprotein A-I deficiency in a family with analphalipoproteinemia. J Clin invest 93:223–229

Nichman MZ, Hamilton HB, Kagan A et al. (1975) Epidemiologic studies of coronary heart disease and stroke in Japanese men living in Japan, Hawaii and California: Distribution of biochemical risk factors. Am J Epidemiol 102:491–501

Nikkila EA, Aro A (1973) Family study of serum lipids and lipoproteins in coronary heart disease. Lancet 1:954–59

Niort G, Bulgarelli A, Cassader M, Pagano G (1988) Effect of short-term treatment with bezafibrate on plasma fibrinogen, fibrinopeptide A, platelet activation, and blood filterability in atherosclerotic hyperfibrinogenaemic patients. Atherosclerosis 71:113–9

Nishina PM, Johnson JP, Naggert JK, Krauss RM (1992) Linkage of atherogenic lipoprotein phenotype to the low density lipoprotein receptor on the short arm of chromosome 19. Proc Natl Acad Sci USA 89:708–712

Nora JJ, Lortscher RH, Spangler RD et al. (1980) Genetic-epidemiologic study of early onset ischemic heart disease. Circulation 61:503–508

Nordstrom M, Kjellstrom T (1992) Age dependency of cystathionine beta-synthase activity in human fibroblasts in homocysteinemia and atherosclerotic vascular disease. Atherosclerosis 94:213–21

Norum RA, Lakier JB, Goldstein S et al. (1982) Familial deficiency of apolipoprotein A-I and C-III and precocious coronary artery disease. N Engl J Med 306:1513–19

Nygard O, Nordrehaug JE, Refsum H et al. (1997) Plasma homocysteine levels and mortality in patients with coronary artery disease. N Engl J Med 337:230–6

OMIM. On Line Mendelian Inheritance in Man. McKusick-Nathans Institute for Genetic Medicine, Johns Hopkins University (Baltimore, MD) and National Center for Biotechnology Information, National Library of Medicine (Bethesda, MD), 2000. World Wide Web URL: http://www.ncbi.nlm.nih.gov/omim/

Ordovas JM, Cassidy DK, Civeira F et al. (1989) Familial apolipoprotein A-I, C-III, A-IV deficiency and premature atherosclerosis due to deletion of a gene complex on chromosome 11. J Biol Chem 264:16339–4

Otto C, Pschiere V, Schwandt P, Richter WO (1994) Effect of gemfibrozil treatment on plasma fibrinogen levels in patients with familial hypertriglyceridemia. Blood Coagul Fibrinolysis 5 Suppl 2:11

Packard CJ, O'Reilly DSJ, Caslake MJ et al. (2000) Lipoprotein-associated phospholipase A2 as an independent predictor of coronary heart disease. New Engl J Med 343:1148–1155

Pajukanta P, Cargill M, Viitanen L et al. (2000) Two loci on chromosomes 2 and X for premature coronary heart disease identified in early- and late-settlement populations in Finland. Am J Hum Genet 67:1481–1493

Parra HJ, Arveiler D, Evans AE et al. (1992) A case-control study of lipoprotein particles in two populations at contrasting risk for coronary heart disease: The ECTIM study. Arterioscler Thromb 12:701–07

Pasternak RC, Grundy SM, Levy D, Thompson PD (1996) 27th Bethesda Conference: Matching the intensity of risk factor management with the hazard for coronary disease events. Task Force 3. Spectrum of risk factors for coronary heart disease. J Am Coll Cardiol 27:978–90

Pastinen T, Perola M, Niini P et al. (1998) Array-based multiplex analysis of candidate genes reveals two independent and additive genetic risk factors for myocardial infarction in the Finnish population. Hum Molec Genet 7:1453–1462

Pazzucconi F, Mannucci L, Mussoni L et al. (1992) Bezafibrate lowers plasma lipids, Fibrinogen and platelet aggregability in hypertriglyceridemia. Eur J Clin Pharmacol 43:219–23

Perry DJ (1999) Hyperhomocysteinaemia. Balliere's Best Practice in Clinical Haematology 12:451-77

Poon M, Zhang X, Dunsky KG et al. (1997) Apolipoprotein (a) induces monocyte chemotactic activity in human vascular endothelial cells. Circulation 96:2514–9

Pyeritz RE (1993) Homocystinuria. In Beighton P (ed.): McKusick's Heritable Disorders of Connective Tissue, 5th edn. CV Mosby, St Louis, pp. 137–178

Pyeritz RE (1999) Genetic approaches to cardiovascular disease. In Chien KR (ed.): Molecular Basis of Cardiovascular Disease. Philadelphia: WB Saunders. pp. 19–36

Pyeritz RE (2001) Genetics and cardiovascular disease. In: Braunwald E (ed.). Heart Disease, 6th edn, WB Saunders, Philadelphia, pp. 1977–2018

Raaschou-Nnielsen E (1960) Smoking habits in twins. Dan Med Bull 7:82–88

Rader DJ, Ikewaki K, Duverger N et al. (1993) Very low high density lipoproteins without coronary atherosclerosis. Lancet 342:1455–58

Raper SE, Grossman M, Rader DJ et al. (1996) Safety and feasibility of liver directed ex-vivo gene therapy for homozygous familial hypercholesterolemia. Ann Surg 223:116–26

Rath M, Niendorf A, Reblin T et al. (1989) Detection and quantification of lipoprotein (a) in the arterial wall of 107 coronary bypass patients. Arteriosclerosis 9:579–92

Rauh G, Schuster H, Miller B et al. (1990) Genetic evidence from 7 families that the apolipoprotein B gene is not involved in familial combined hyperlipidemia. Atherosclerosis 83:81–87

Reaven GM (1988) The Banting Lecture: Role of insulin resistance in human disease. Diabetes 37:1595–1607

Reis AF Ye W-Z, Dubois-Laforgue D et al. (2000) Association of a variant in exon 31 of the sulfonylurea receptor 1 (SUR 1) gene with type 2 diabetes mellitus in French Caucasians. Hum Genet 107:138–144

Reymer PWA, Gagné E, Groenemeyer BE et al. (1995) A lipoprotein lipase mutation (Asn291'Ser) is associated with reduced HDL cholesterol levels in premature atherosclerosis. Nature Genet 10:28–34

Rhoads GG, Dahlen G, Berg K et al. (1986) Lp(a) Lipoprotein as a risk factor for myocardial infarction. JAMA 256:2540–4

Rhode LE, Hennekens CH, Ridker PM (1999) Survey of C-reactive protein and cardiovascular risk factors in apparently healthy men. Am J Cardiol 84:1018–1022

Ridker PM (2000) Novel risk factors and markers for coronary disease. Adv Intern Med 45:391–418

Ridker PM, Hennekens CH, Stampfer MJ (1993) A prospective study of lipoprotein (a) and the risk of myocardial infarction. JAMA 270:2195–2199

Ridker PM, Stampfer MJ, Hennekens CH (1995a) Plasma concentration of lipoprotein (a) and the risk of future stroke. JAMA 273:1269–73

Ridker PM, Hennekens CH, Lindpaintner K et al. (1995b) Mutation in the gene coding for coagulation factor V and the risk of myocardial infarction, stroke, and venous thrombosis in apparently healthy men. N Engl J Med 332:912–917

Ridker PM, Hennekens CH, Buring JE, Rifai N (2000a) C-reactive protein and other markers of inflammation in the prediction of cardiovascular disease in women. N Engl J Med 342:836–843

Ridker PM, Rifai N, Stampfer MJ, Hennekens CH (2000b) Plasma concentration of interleukin-6 and the risk of future myocardial infarction among apparently healthy men. Circulation 101:1767–1772

Riis-Hansen P, Kharazmi A, Jauhianen M, Ehnholm C (1994) Induction of oxygen free radical generation in human monocytes by lipoprotein (a) Eur J Clin Invest 24:497–9

Rissanen AM (1979) Familial occurrence of coronary heart disease: Effect of age at diagnosis. Am J Cardiol 44:60–66

Rissanen AM, Nikkila EA (1977) Coronary artery disease and its risk factors in families of young men with angina pectoris and in controls. Br Heart J 39:875–883

Rosendaal FR, Siscovick DS, Schwartz SM et al. (1997) Factor V Leiden (resistance to activated protein C) increases the risk of myocardial infarction in young women. Blood 89:2817–21

Rosengren A, Wilhelmsen L (1996) Fibrinogen, coronary heart disease and mortality from all causes in smokers and nonsmokers. The study of men born in 1933. J Intern Med 230:499–507

Roses A (2000) Genetic susceptibility to cardiovascular disease. Am Heart J 140:S45–47

Rossing MA (1998) Genetic influences on smoking: Candidate genes. Environmental Health Perspect 106:231–8

Rotter JI, Bu X, Camtor R et al. (1996) Multilocus genetic determinants of LDL particle size in coronary artery disease families. Am J Hum Genet 58:585–94

Salomaa V, Rasi V, Pekkanen J et al. (1994) Haemostatic factors and prevalent coronary heart disease: The FINRISK Haemostasis Study. Eur Heart J 15:1293–99

Sanghera DK, Saha N, Aston CE, Kamboh MI (1997) Genetic polymorphism of paraoxonase and the risk of coronary heart disease. Arterioscler Thromb Vasc Biol 17:1067–1073

Sanghera DK, Aston CE, Saha N, Kamboh MI (1998) DNA polymorphisms in two paraoxonase genes (PON1 and PON2) are associated with the risk of coronary heart disease. Am J Hum Genet 62:36–44

Scanu AM, Lawn RM, Berg K (1991) Lipoprotein(a) and atherosclerosis. Ann Intern Med 115:209–18

Schaefer EJ (1984) Clinical, biochemical and genetic features in familial disorders of high density lipoprotein deficiency. Arteriosclerosis 4:303–22

Schaefer EJ, Stefania L-F, Jenner JL et al. (1994) Lipoprotein (a) levels and risk of coronary heart disease in men: The Lipid Research Clinics Coronary Primary Prevention Trial. JAMA 271:999–1003

Scott J, Knott TJ, Priestly LM et al. (1985) High density lipoprotein composition is altered by a common DNA polymorphism adjacent to apolipoprotein A-II gene in man. Lancet 1:770–3

Shea S, Ottman R, Gabrieli C et al. (1984) Family history as an independent risk factor for coronary artery disease. J Am Coll Cardiol 4:793–801

Silveira A, Green FR, Karpe F et al. (1994) Elevated levels of factor VII activity in the postprandial state: Effect of the factor VII Arg—Gln polymorphism. Thromb Haemost 72:734–9

Sina M, Hinney A, Ziegler A et al. (1999) Phenotypes in three pedigrees with autosomal dominant obesity caused by haploinsufficiency mutations in the melanocortin-4 receptor gene. Am J Hum Genet 65:1501–1507

Sing CF, Davignon J (1985) Role of the apolipoprotein E polymorphism and determining normal plasma lipid and lipoprotein variation. Am J Hum Genet 37:268–285

Skinner MP, Yua C, Mitsumori L et al. (1995) Serial magnetic resonance imaging of experimental atherosclerosis detects lesion fine structure, progression and complications *in vivo*. Nature Med 1:69–73

Slack J and Evans KA (1966) The increased risk of death from ischaemic heart disease in first degree relatives of 121 men and 96 women with ischaemic heart disease. J Med Genetics 3:239–257

Smith EB, Crosbie L (1991) Does lipoprotein (a) compete with plasminogen in human atherosclerotic lesions and thrombi? Atherosclerosis 89:127–36

Smith EB, Thompson WD (1994) Fibrin as a factor in atherogenesis. Thromb Res 73:1–19

Sniderman AD, Shapiro S, Marpole DG et al. (1980) Association of coronary atherosclerosis with hyperapobetalipoproteinemia (increased protein but normal cholesterol levels in human plasma low density lipoproteins) Proc Natl Acad Sci USA 77:604–7

Stalenhoef AFH, Malloy MJ, Kane J-P, Havel RJ (1984) Metabolism of apolipoprotein B-48 and B-100 of triglyceride-rich lipoproteins in normal and lipoprotein lipase deficient humans. Proc Natl Acad Sci USA 81:1839–1843

Stamler JS, Osborne JA, Jaraki O et al. (1993) Adverse vascular effects of homocysteine are modified by endothelium-derived relaxing factor and related oxides of nitrogen. J Clin Inv 91:303–18

Stampfer MJ, Malinow MR, Willet WC et al. (1992) A prospective study of plasma homocysteine and risk of myocardial infarction in US physicians. JAMA 268:877–881

Stampfer MJ, Krauss RM, Ma J et al. (1996) A prospective study of triglyceride level, low-density lipoprotein particle diameter, and risk of myocardial infarction. JAMA 276:882–8

Starkebaum G, Harlan JM (1986) Endothelial cell injury due to copper-catalyzed hydrogen peroxide generation from homocysteine. J Clin Invest 77:1370–6

Stary HC (1989) Evolution and progression of atherosclerotic lesions in coronary arteries of children and young adults. Arteriosclerosis 9(suppl I):119–32

Stein JH, Rosenson RS (1997) Lipoprotein (a) excess and coronary heart disease. Arch Intern Med 157:1170–6

Stengard JH, Weiss KM, Sing CF (1998) An ecological study of association between coronary deart disease mortality rates in men and the relative frequencies of common allelic variations in the gene coding for apolipoprotein E. Hum Genet 103:234–41

Stenvinkel P, Lindholm B, Heimburger M, Heimburger O (2000) Elevated serum levels of soluble adhesion molecules predict death in pre-dialysis patients: Association with malnutrition, inflammation, and cardiovascular disease. Nephrol Dial Transplant 15:1624–1630

St Goar FG, Pinto FJ, Alderman EL, Fitzgerald PJ, Stinson EB, Billingham ME, Popp RL (1992) Detection of Coronary Atherosclerosis in Young Adult Hearts Using Intravascular Ultrasound. Circulation 86:756-63

Stone LM, Kahn SE, Fujimoto WY et al. (1996) A variation at position –30 of the beta-cell glucokinase gene promoter is associated with reduced beta-cell function in middle-aged Japanese-American men. Diabetes 45:422–428

Strong JP, Malcom GT, McMahan CA et al. (1999) Prevalence and extent of atherosclerosis in adolescents and young adults. JAMA 281:727–735

Su Y, Swift M (2000) Mortality rates among carriers of ataxia-telangiectasia mutant alleles. Ann Intern Med 133:770–778

Sullivan PF, Kendler KS (1999) The genetic epidemiology of smoking. Nicotine Tobacco Res 1:S51–57

Suthanthiran M, Li B, Song JO et al. (2000) Transforming growth factor-beta-1 hyperexpression in African-American hypertensives: A novel mediator of hypertension and/or target organ damage. Proc Natl Acad Sci USA 97:3479–3484

Svensson PJ, Dahlback B (1994) Resistance to activated protein C as a basis for venous thrombosis. N Engl J Med 330:517–22

Takamiya O (1995) Genetic polymorphism (Arg353Gln) in coagulation factor VII gene and factor VII levels (coagulant activity, antigen and binding ability to tissue factor) in 101 healthy Japanese. Scand J Clin Lab Invest 55:211–15

Tall A (1990) Plasma high density lipoproteins: Metabolism and relationship to atherogenesis. J Clin Invest 86:379–384

Tall A (1992) Metabolic and genetic control of HDL cholesterol levels. J Intern Med 231:661–668

Temme EH, Mensink RP, Hornstra G (1996) Comparison of the effects of diets enriched in lauric, palmitic, or oleic acids on serum lipids and lipoproteins in healthy women and men. Am J Clin Nutr 63:897–903

't Hart LM, Stolk RP, Dekker JM et al. (1999) Prevalence of variants in candidate genes for type 2 diabetes mellitus in the Netherlands: The Rotterdam study and the Hoorn study. J Clin Endocr Metab 84:1002–1006

Thomas A, Kelleher C, Green F et al. (1991) Variation in the promoter region of the β-fibrinogen gene is associated with plasma fibrinogen levels in smokers and non-smokers. Thromb Haemost 65:487–90

Thomas CB, Cohen BH (1955) The familial occurrence of hypertension and coronary artery disease, with observations concerning obesity and diabetes. Ann Intern Med 42:90–127

Thomas TR, Ziogas G, Harris WS (1997) Influence of fitness status on very-low density lipoproteins subfractions and lipoprotein (a) in men and women. Metabolism 46:1178–83

Toss H, Lindahl B, Siegbahn A, Wallentin L (1997) Prognostic influence of increased fibrinogen and C-reactive protein levels in unstable coronary artery disease. Circulation 96:4204–10

True WR, Heath AC, Scherrer JF et al. (1997) Genetic and environmental contributions to smoking. Addiction 92:1277–87

Tsai JC, Perrella MA, Yoshizumi M et al. (1994) Promotion of vascular smooth muscle cell growth by homocysteine: A link to atherosclerosis. Proc Natl Acad Sci USA 91:6369–73

Tsai MY, Welge BG, Hanson NQ, Bignell MK, Vessey J, Schwichtenberg K, Yang F et al (1999) Genetic Causes of Mild Hyperhomocysteinemia in Patients with Premature Occlusive Coronary Artery Disease. Atherosclerosis 143:163-170

Tybjærg-Hansen A, Agerholm-Larsen B, Humphries SE et al. (1997) A common mutation (G-455 A) in the β-fibrinogen promoter is an independent predictor of plasma fibrinogen, but not of ischemic heart disease. A study of 9,127 individuals based on the Copenhagen City Heart Study. J Clin Invest 99:3034–39

Tybjærg A, Steffensen R, Meinertz H et al. (1998) Association of mutations in the apolipoprotein B gene with hypercholesterolemia and the risk of ischemic heart disease. N Engl J Med 338:1577–1584

Ubbink JB (1997) The role of vitamins in the pathogenesis and treatment of hyperhomocysteinemia. J Inherit Metab Dis 20:315–25

Ueland PM, Refsum H, Brattstrom L (1992) Plasma homocysteine and cardiovascular disease. In Francis RB Jr (ed.): Atherosclerotic Cardiovascular Disease, Hemostasis, and Endothelial Function. New York: Marcel Dekker: pp. 183–236

Utermann G (1985) Genetic polymorphism of apolipoprotein E: Impact on plasma lipoprotein metabolism. In: Cripaldi G, Tiengo A, Baggio G (eds.). Diabetes, Obesity and Hyperlipidemias. Vol 3. Elsevier: Amsterdam; 1–11

Valentine RJ, Verstraete R, Clagett GP, Cohen JC (2000) Premature cardiovascular disease is common in relatives of patients with premature peripheral atherosclerosis. Arch Int Med 160:1343–1348

Valve R, Sivenius K, Miettinen R (1999) Two polymorphisms in the peroxisome proliferator-activated receptor-gamma gene are associated with severe overweight among obese women. J Clin Endocrinol Metab 84:3708–3712

van Kooten F, van Krimpen J, Dippel DW et al. (1996) Lipoprotein (a) in patients with acute cerebral ischemia. Stroke 27:1231–5

Vinik A, Bell G (1988) Mutant insulin syndromes. Hormone Metab Res 20:1–10

von Kodolitsch Y, Pyeritz RE, Rogan PK (1999) Splice-site mutations in atherosclerosis candidate genes: relating individual information to phenotype. Circulation 100:693–699

Voorberg J, Roelse J, Koopman R et al. (1994) Association of idiopathic venous thromboembolism with single point mutation at Arg506 of factor V. Lancet 343:1536–6

Walder K, Norman RA, Hanson RL et al. (1998) Association between uncoupling protein polymorphisms (UCP2-UCP3) and energy metabolism/obesity in Pima Indians. Hum Molec Genet 7:1431–1435

Wang SL, McCredie RM, Wilcken DEL (1995) Polymorphisms of the apolipoprotein E gene and severity of coronary artery disease defined by angiography. Arterioscler Thromb Vasc Biol 15:1030–1034

Wang XL, Wang J, McCredie RM, Wilcken DEL (1997) Polymorphisms of factor V, factor VII, and fibrinogen genes: Relevance to severity of coronary artery disease. Arterioscler Thromb Vasc Biol 17:246–251

Wang J, Freeman DJ, Grundy SM et al. (1998) Linkage between cholesterol 7-alpha-hydroxylase and high plasma low-density lipoprotein cholesterol concentrations. J Clin Ivest 101:1283–1291

Warden CH, Fisler JS, Pace MJ et al. (1993) Coincidence of genetic loci for plasma cholesterol levels and obesity in a multifactorial mouse model. J Clin Invest 92:773–779

Weigle DS, Ganter SL, Kuijper JL et al. (1997) Effect of regional fat distribution and Prader-Willi syndrome on plasma leptin levels. J Clin Endocrinol Metab 82:566–570

Weintraub MS, Eisenberg S, Breslow JL (1987) Dietary fat clearance in normal subjects is regulated by genetic variation in apolipoprotein E. J Clin Invest 80:1572–77

Weiss EI, Goldschmidt-Clermont PJ, Grigoryev D et al. (1995) A monoclonal antibody (SZ21) specific for platelet GPIIIa distinguishes PlA1 from PlA2. Tissue Antigens 46:374–81

Weiss EJ, Bray PF, Tayback M et al. (1996) A polymorphism of a platelet glycoprotein receptor as an inherited risk factor for coronary thrombosis. N Engl J Med 334:1090–4

Wenzel K, Felix S, Kleber FX et al. (1994) E-selectin polymorphism and atherosclerosis: An association study. Hum Molec Genet 3:1935–1937

Wilcken DEL, Gupta VJ (1979) Sulfur containing amino acids in chronic renal failure with particular reference to homocysteine and cysteine-homocysteine mixed disulfide. Eur J Clin Invest 9:301–7

Wilhelmsen L, Svardsudd K, Koran-Bengsten K et al. (1984) Fibrinogen as a risk factor for stroke and myocardial infarction. N Engl J Med 311:501–5

Williams PT, Vranizan KM, Austin MA, Krauss RM (1993) Associations of age, adiposity, alcohol intake, menstrual status, and estrogen therapy with high density lipoprotein subclasses. Arterioscler Thromb 13:1654–61

Williams RR, Hunt SC, Hopkins PN et al. (1994) Evidence for single gene contributions to hypertension and lipid disturbances: Definition, genetics, and clinical significance. Clin Genet 46:80–87

Williams RR, Hopkins PN, Stephenson S et al. (1999) Primordial prevention of cardiovascular disease through applied genetics. Prevent Med 29:S41–49

Williams RR, Hopkins PN, Wu LL, Hunt SC (2000) Applying genetic strategies to prevent atherosclerosis. In Khoury MJ, Burke W, Thomson E (eds): Genetics and Public Health Oxford University Press, London in press

Wilson PWF, Cupples LA, Kannel WB (1991) Is hyperglycemia associated with cardiovascular disease? The Framingham Study. Am Heart J 121:586–590

Wiman B, Ljungberg B, Chmielewska J et al. (1985) The role of the fibrinolytic system in deep vein thrombosis. Lab Clin Med 105:265–270

Winkelman BR, Nauck M, Klein B et al. (1996) Deletion polymorphism of the angiotensin I-converting enzyme gene is associated with increased plasma angiotensin-converting enzyme activity but not with increased risk for myocardial infarction. Ann Intern Med 125:19–25

Winkelmann BR, Russ AP, Nauck M et al. (1999) Angiotensinogen M235T polymorphism is associated with plasma angiotensinogen and cardiovascular disease. Am Heart J 137:698–705

Winkelmann BR, Hager J, Kraus WE et al. (2000) Genetics of coronary heart disease: current knowledge and research principles. Am Heart J 140:S11–26

Witkowski NE, Leiendecker-Foster C, Gerry NP et al. (2000) Microarray-based detection of select cardiovascular disease markers. Bio Tech 29:936–8,940,942 passim

Wojciechowski AP, Farrall M, Cullen P et al. (1991) Familial combined hyperlipidemia linked to the apolipoprotein AI-CIII-AIV gene cluster on chromosome 11q23–q24. Nature 349:161–4

Woo KS, Chook P, Lolin YI et al. (1997) Hyperhomocysteinemia is a risk factor for arterial endothelial dysfunction in humans. Circulation 96:2542–4

Wu KK, Aleksic N, Ahn C, Boerwinkle E, Folsom AR, Juneja H (2001) Thrombomodulin Ala455Val Polymorphism and Risk of Coronary Heart Disease. Circulation 103:1386–1389

Yarnell JWG, Baker IA, Sweetman PM et al. (1991) Fibrinogen, viscosity, and white blood cell count are major risk factors for ischaemic heart disease: The Caerphilly and Speedwell Collaborative Heart Disease Studies. Circulation 83:836–44

Ye S, Green F, Henney A et al. (1995) Genetic variation in the promoter of the PAI-1 gene in relation to plasma PAI-1 activity and risk of myocardial infarction: The ECTIM Study. Thromb Haemost 74:837–41

Yoshimura M, Yasue H, Nakayama M et al. (2000) Genetic risk factors for coronary artery spasm: Significance of endothelial nitric oxide synthase gene T-786→C and missense Glu298Asp variants. J Investig Med 48:367–374

Yu Q, Safavi F, Roberts R, Marian AJ (1996) A variant of β fibrinogen is a genetic risk factor for coronary artery disease and myocardial infarction. J Invest Med 44:154–159

Zmuda JM, Thompson PD, Dickenson R, Bausserman LL (1996) Testosterone decreases lipoprotein (a) in men. Am J Cardiol 77:1244–47

Zoller B, Dahlback B (1994) Linkage between inherited resistance to activated protein C and factor V gene mutation in venous thrombosis. Lancet 343:1536–8

Hereditary disorders of the lymphatic and venous systems

54

Robert E. Ferrell
Reed E. Pyeritz

Varicose veins are the result of an improper selection of grandparents.

William Osler, *Aphorism 335*

A large number of mendelian and multifactorial disorders affect, either primarily or secondarily, the development, function and natural history (aging) of veins and lymphatics. This chapter reviews those conditions, likely caused by mutation in a single gene, that include clinically important abnormalities of the systemic veins, lymphatics or both. Specifically excluded are congenital anomalies of veins attached to the heart (see Ch. xx), the large number of conditions that predispose to veno-occlusive disease (see Ch. xx), and conditions associated with external obstruction of venous or lymphatic circulation (e.g., various tumors).

The venous system

The systemic venous system connects capillaries to the right side of the heart, beginning with venules through progressively larger caliber vessels draining into the superior and inferior vena cavae. Veins of all types have the same general structure of arteries of similar caliber in that three layers—intima, media and adventitia—can be distinguished histologically. However, for a given lumenal diameter, the walls of veins are considerably thinner than arteries. Veins lack internal and external elastic laminae, and have considerably fewer and less well organized elastic fibers and smooth muscle bundles in the media compare to arteries.

Veins are distinct from arteries by the presence of valves, which occur in all veins except for the vena cavae and the common iliac veins. Valves are composed of opposing folds of intimal tissue and typically occur just distal (i.e., upstream) from the entry point of a tributary.

DEVELOPMENT OF THE VENOUS SYSTEM

The mature venous system results from a developmental process that is as complex in anatomic terms as anything else occurring in the embryo. Systemic veins arise from the cardinal veins, the principal intraembryonic system, which are present by the end of the fourth week. As development of organs progress, systemic veins disappear and emerge in response to the changing needs of the embryo. Two extraembryonic sets of veins, the vitelline and the umbilical, also participate critically in embryogenesis. The vitelline veins ultimately contribute to the development of the inferior vena cava, the portal veins and the superior mesenteric vein. The umbilical veins regress and are represented postnatally by the ligamenta venosum and teres. Considerable variation in the caliber, location and branching pattern of systemic veins occurs in healthy individuals; the extent to which this variation is genetically controlled is unclear. The extent of this "normal" variation is magnified in many congenital malformation syndromes.

A congenitally narrowed vein, or one represented by a fibrous strand, is often called "atretic". Venous atresia can result from either failure to grow to the requisite size or excessive regression of a once-normal embryologic structure.

DISORDERS OF THE VENOUS SYSTEM

Table 54.1 enumerates the mendelian conditions affecting the venous system. The following sections discuss several of the more important and informative ones.

Table 54.1. Mendelian Disorders with Primary Effects on Veins.

Disorder	Inheritance	OMIM	#Locus	Gene	Features
Cerebral cavernous angiomas-CCM1	AD	116860	7q11-q22	KRIT1	enlarged capillaries in the central nervous system; headache, seizure, hemorrhage; American Hispanic locus
Cerebral cavernous angiomas-CCM2	AD	603284	7p15-p13		same as CCM1
Cerebral cavernous angiomas-CCM3	AD	603285	3q25.2-q27		same as CCM1
Distichiasis and anomalies of the heart and vasculature	AD	126320			
Ehlers-Danlos, classic form	AD	130000	9q34.2-q34.3 q34.3 2q31 17q21.31-q22	COL5A1 COL5A2 COL1A1	thin, fragile skin; bruisability; hyperextensible joints; varicosities
Ehlers-Danlos, vascular form	AD	130050	2q31	COL3A1	bruisability; acrogeria; mild hyperextensibility; arterial and bowel rupture; varicosities
Hereditary neurocutaneous angioma	AD	106070			cutaneous and parenchymal hemangiomatat and AVMs; stroke
Marfan syndrome	AD	154700	15q21.1	FBN1	dolichostenomelia; scoliosis; ectopia lentis; mitral valve prolapse; aortic root dilatation and dissection; varicosities
Multiple cutaneous and mucosal venous malformation (VMCM1)	AD	600195	9p21	TIE2	congenital, progressive varicosities or complex vascular masses; pain, airway obstruction, bleeding
Varicose veins	MF	192200			
Venous malformations with glomus cells (glomangiomas) (VMGLOM)	AD	138000	1p21-p22		congenital cutaneous (not mucosal) lesions; painful; highly variable

Inherited venous malformations

Several autosomal dominant forms consisting primarily of congenital, progressive venous malformation have been described. One form involves both cutaneous and mucosal surfaces (VMCM; OMIM 600195) while another involves only the skin and contains glomus cells (Boon et al., 1999; Irrthum et al., 2001). Both are autosomal dominant and highly variable.

In the former condition, the lesions appear as subcutaneous or submucosal nodules that may or may not appear bluish, depending on their depth. The nodules are easily compressible and, when small, usually not painful. Congenital lesions often enlarge, and new ones emerge, over time; the causes of this evolution are unclear, but trauma, hormones and hemodynamic influences have been suggested (Pasyk et al., 1984; Gallione et al., 1995). Although many people have concerns that are primarily cosmetic, mucosal bleeding can be a problem. The vascular lesions are complex masses of vessels with thin walls, often only composed of an endothelium poorly supported by extracellular matrix. Only the interposition of a capillary bed between the pressures of the arterial side of the circulation prevents more severe hemorrhagic complications.

One form of venous malformations (VMCM1) was initially linked to chromosome 9p by Boon et al. (1994) and confirmed by Gallione et al. (1995). Dumont et al. (1994) had previously mapped the endothelial-specific receptor tyrosine kinase (TEK also called TIE2) to chromosome 9p21. Vikkula et al. (1996) examined TEK in these two families and a C→T transition at nucleotide 2545 which was predicted to lead to an Arg to Trp (R849W) substitution at amino acid 849 of the mature kinase, located in the first intracellular kinase domain. Subsequently, Calvert et al. (1999) examined four additional large VMCM families, of which two were linked to chromosome 9p. One of these segregated for the R849W mutation previously reported in Finnish families while the other had a Y897S mutation, also in first kinase domain. They show that in vitro these two mutations lead to ligand independent hyperphosphorylation of TEK, consistent with a gain of function mutation. Of the remaining two families, one excluded linkage of markers flanking the TEK locus, establishing locus heterogeneity for VMCM. Boon et al. (1999) confirmed this heterogeneity by localizing a second *VMCM* locus to chromosome 1p21-22.

The TIE family of receptor tyrosine kinases, TIE (TIE1) and TEK (TIE2) is expressed almost exclusively in cells of endothelial lineage (Mustonen and Alitalo, 1995). The ligands for TEK are members of the angiopoiten (ANG) family and these ligands appear to have opposing actions on TEK. ANG1 and ANG4 stimulate tyrosine phosphorylation while ANG2 and ANG3 inhibit phosphorylation. Inactivation of TEK results in early embryonic lethality with angiogenic defects throughout the vascular system decreased vessel sprouting and reduced endothelial cell survival (Sato et al., 1995). The mechanism by which activating mutations in TEK lead to the vascular lesions in VMCM is likely to be complex since they lead to focal vascular lesions rather than global disruption of the vascular network.

Cerebral cavernous malformations

Cerebral cavernous angiomas are rare vascular lesions that may involve any part of the central nervous systems (Fig. 54.1). These lesions may cause seizures or focal neurological deficit and predispose to intracranial aneurysms. These outcomes can frequently be avoided by surgical repair. Dubovsky et al., (1995) mapped the first locus for this disorder (CCM1,

OMIM #604214) to 7q11-q22 in a large Hispanic kindred. This localization was confirmed in additional families of Hispanic as well as non-Hispanic ancestry (Gunel et al., 1995; 1996; Marchuk et al., 1995; Johnson et al., 1995). At least two other loci cause this condition (Table 54.2).

Leberge-le Couteulx et al., (1999) reported a physical and transcript map of the *CCM1* locus and identified truncation mutations in the *KRIT1* (Krev Interaction Trapped 1) gene. *KRIT1* encodes a 529 amino acid protein with an amino terminal ankyrin repeat domain and a carboxy-terminal domain which interacts with KREV1, a member of the Ras GTPase family of cell signaling molecules (Serebriiskii et al., 1997). Subsequently, Sahoo et al., (1999) identified seven KRIT1 mutations in 23 distinct CCM1 families. The identical mutation was observed in 16 of 21 Hispanic families supporting the suggestion of a CCM1 founder effect among Mexican Americans (Zhang et al., 2000). At least two other loci, mapped to 7p15-13 and 3q25.2-q27 (Table 54.1) and these three loci appear to account for the majority of CCM families (Craig et al., 1998).

Varicose veins

This term most commonly refers to increased caliber and tortuosity associated with engorgement of the superficial veins of the leg, with the saphenous being the most prominent.

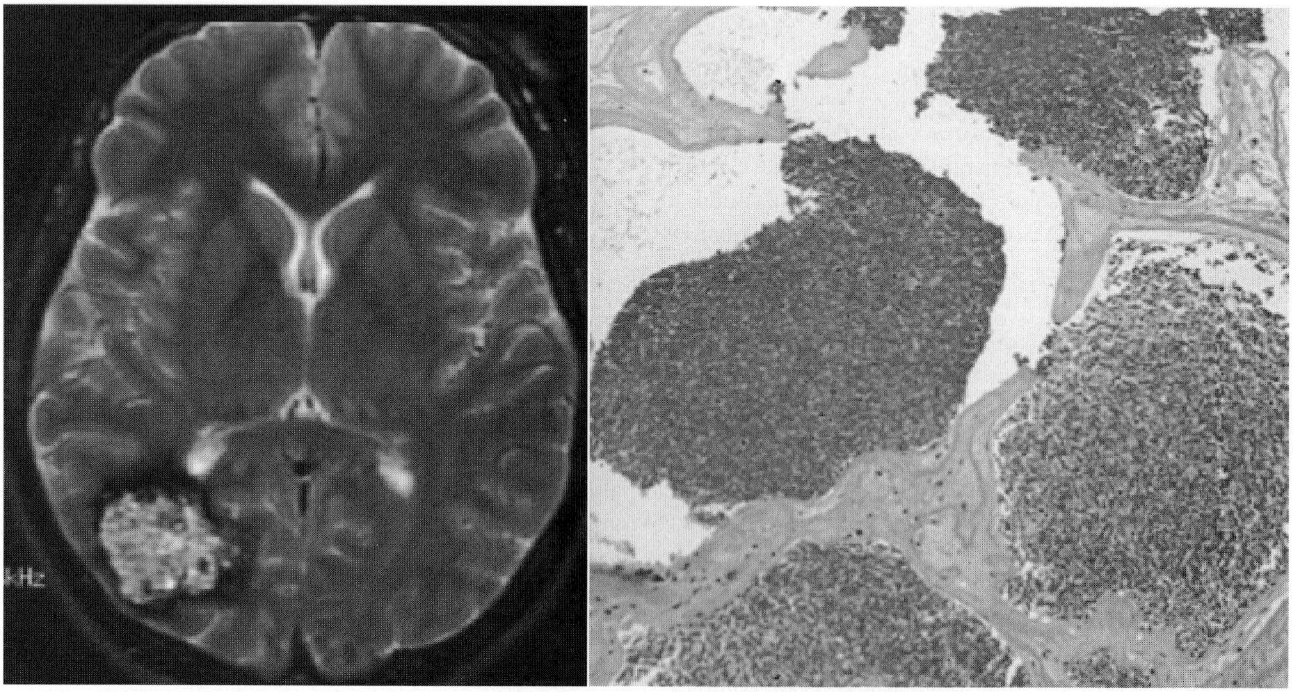

Fig. 54.1. The image on the left, a T2-weighted MRI of the brain, demonstrates a right occipital cavernous malformation in a patient who presented with a left visual field defect. The image on the right is a hematoxylin and eosin stained section through this lesion. Dilated vascular sinusoids lined with endothelium and embedded in a collagenous matrix is the typical histologic appearance of these lesions.

Table 54.2. Mendelian Disorders with Primary Effects on Lymphatics

Disorder	Inheritance	OMIM#	Locus	Gene	Features
Cholestasis-lymphedema syndrome	AR	214900			recurrent cholestasis progressive to jaundice and cirrhosis; leg edema due to lymphatic hypoplasia
Hennekam lymphangiectasia-lymphedema	AR	235510			protein-losing intestinal lyphangiectasia; abnormal facies; digital anomalies; seizures and mental retardation
Hereditary lymphedema I	AD	153100	5q34-q35	FLT4 (VEGFR3)	congenital lymphedema of legs
Hereditary lymphedema II	AD	153200			onset of lymphedema at puberty or later
Hereditary lymphedema, recessive	AR	247440			
Intestinal lymphangiectasia	AD	152800			
Lymphedema and distichasis	AD	153400	16q24.3	FOXC2	bilateral dilated lymphatics and edema; double row of eyelashes with corneal abrasions
Lymphedema and hypothyroidism	AR	247410			
Lymphedema, microcephaly and chorioretinopathy	AD	152950			microcephaly with normal intelligence; congenital or early-onset leg edema; chorioretinopathy with progressive visual impairment
Lymphedema and ptosis	AD	153000			
Lymphedema and yellow nails	AD	153300			
Noonan syndrome	AD	163950			edema; may resolve postnatally; pterygium colli; congenital heart defects

Varicosities may be congenital, but develop in middle-age in the vast majority of affected people. As much as 10% of the population of developed countries have varicosities of the legs, and perhaps 10% of them have symptomatic venous insufficiency. Anything that increases pressure and flow in the superficial veins, such as proximal obstruction (pregnant uterus, tumor) or thrombosis of the deep veins, can increase the lumenal diameter. Little dilatation is necessary before the venous valves become incompetent, which in turn increases pressure upstream and causes further dilatation. Chronic dilatation results in vascular remodeling and persistent valvular failure. The clinical results are discomfort, mild edema, susceptibility to venous rupture with minor trauma, and venous stasis, which increases the susceptibility to thrombosis. About 20% of people with chronic, symptomatic venous varicosities develop skin breakdown (varicose ulcers). Conservative treatment of support stockings and elevation of the legs can provide temporary relief of discomfort, but does not address the fundamental problem. Surgical treatment has involved ligation and stripping of larger vessels and sclerosis of smaller one. In all cases, recurrence rates are high (40%). In 1999, the US Food and Drug Administration approved the use of radio-frequency heat to collapse distended veins. While this procedure is much less invasive than other surgical approaches and produces little short-term disability, the long-term effectiveness is unclear.

The vast majority of venous varicosities are not simply inherited. Multifactorial inheritance has been suggested by several large family studies (Hauge and Gundersen, 1969; Matousek and Prerovsky, 1974). Certain heritable disorders of connective tissue, especially Ehlers-Danlos of the classical and vascular types and the Marfan syndrome, predispose to varicose veins. Whether a specific tendency to defective or absent venous valves is inherited remains uncertain (Leu, 1974). This seems an ideal condition, when examined by some objective measure such as venous diameter or compliance, in which to apply quantitative trait linkage analysis.

Evidence of endothelial cell dysfunction in varicose veins (Barber et al., 1997; Mangiafico et al., 1997) led Sverdlova et al., (1998) to examine the prevalence of a thermolabile variant of methylene-tetrahydrofolate reductase (MTHFR), C677T, in patients with lower limb varicose veins. They observed a two-fold increase in risk of varicose veins among individuals homozygous or heterozygous for the thermolabile allele. The C677T variant of MTHFR is both thermolabile and less active than the normal allele and is associated with elevated levels of plasma homocysteine (Frosst et al., 1995). Hyperhomocysteinemia due to polymorphic variation in

MTHFR, mutations in cystathionine β-synthase, folate and vitamin B_{12} deficiency, and other factors is common, and potentially predisposes to a remarkable range of vascular dysfunction, from occlusive arterial disease to varicose veins (McCully, 1996; Duell and Malinow, 1997).

The lymphatic system

Lymphatics are thin-walled vessels that carry a protein-rich fluid from the periphery back to the central circulation. As in the systemic venous system, unidirectional flow is assisted by valves throughout lymphatics of all calibers. Lymphatics draining the legs, pelvis and abdomen merge into the cisterna chyli, which passes with the aorta through the diaphragm and becomes the thoracic duct. Lymphatics comprising the left jugular, subclavian and mediastinal trunks usually join the thoracic duct as it loops over the left subclavian artery and drains into the left innominate vein. Lymphatic drainage of the right subclavian, jugular and mediastinal trunks usually merge into a right lymphatic duct, which opens into the right innominate vein. However, any of the trunks may open independently into the great veins. Arranged periodically along lymphatic trunks are lymph nodes, comprised of a stroma packed with cells of the immune system, which serve as filters of the lymphatic fluid.

DEVELOPMENT OF THE LYMPHATIC SYSTEM

In both timing and location, the lymphatic and venous systems develop embryologically in close relationship (Van der Putte, 1975). Direct communication occurs around 40 days postconception, whereby the lymphatic drainage of the right and left sides of the upper body, which had collected in bilateral jugular lymph sacs, empty into the ipsilateral jugular veins. Failure or delay in completing these communications leads to widespread distortion of embryonic development termed the "jugular lymphatic obstruction sequence" (Jones, 1997). The clinical consequences of edema distal to the obstruction will vary depending on whether communication is established and when it occurs. Complete absence of communication is lethal. Distention of the jugular sac produces, among other findings, a cystic hygroma, which causes excess skin to grow over the neck, the posterior hairline and hair pattern to be disturbed, and the ears to protrude and rotate. If the jugular sac does not decompress until late in fetal development, the infant will have pterygium colli, or webbing of the neck. Edema of the

hands and feet may not be fully resolved at birth, and permanent effects on digital development will be noted, such as predominance of digital whorls and narrow, hyperconvex nails. If drainage of lymph from the lower quadrants of the fetus is primarily affected, the iliac lymph sacs become distended and excess skin grows over the lower abdomen. Prenatal resolution can result in the prune belly birth defect.

Defective lymphatic development has consequences on the cardiovascular system. Peripheral veins tend to be of large caliber, presumably because of increased venous return from edematous tissues. The frequency of left-side flow defects (e.g., aortic coarctation, bicuspid aortic valve, hypoplastic left heart) is increased, in part due to the space occupied by the distended jugular sacs.

DISORDERS OF THE LYMPHATIC SYSTEM

Diffuse, acquired blockage of lymphatics, such as by fibrosis, tumor or infection (e.g., *Microfilaria bancrofti*), usually results in edema of the body parts distal to the blockage. However, if the thoracic duct is blocked, anastamosing channels develop between the lymphatic system and systemic veins, and edema does not persist.

A prenatal cystic hygroma is often seen in fetal anueploidy. If the fetal karyotype is normal, a cystic hygroma detected in the first trimester carries a good prognosis; if it resolves by the mid-second trimester, little distortion of the infant is likely to be noted (Trauffer et al., 1994).

Both the Turner syndrome (Ch. 45) and the Noonan syndrome (Ch. 47) have prominent, multisystem malformations due to fetal lymphatic obstruction (Witt et al., 1987). Failure of the jugular lymphatic-venous communication to occur may be the major reason that 98% of embryos with a 45,X karyotype do not survive to term.

The National Lymphedema Network, Inc., maintains a list of various support groups; while many pertain to acquired lymphedema, issues pertinent to various congenital and hereditary conditions can be found (www.lymphnet.org).

Hereditary lymphedema I

This condition, often termed Milroy disease after the physician in Omaha, Nebraska who described the phenotype and autosomal dominant inheritance in a family for which he cared (Milroy, 1892), has as its predominant feature congenital edema of the lower half of the body. However, the extent and severity of the edema are highly variable, even within a family (Esterly, 1965). For example, infantile chylous ascites, edema of the hands, and severe scrotal edema occur.

Numerous examples of apparently nonpenetrant individuals have been described. The age of onset of edematous legs ranges from embryonic (as shown by prenatal ultrasound) to middle-age.

The complications of Milroy disease are not solely cosmetic. The medical consequences include hypoproteinemia due to intestinal loss of albumin, increased susceptibility to infection in the affected limb and, in same cases, angiosarcoma.

Management is symptomatic. Elevation of the affected limbs above the level of the heart and form-fitted pressure stockings can afford some relief of discomfort, but only temporary reduction of swelling.

Recently, three groups independently reported linkage between congenital lymphedema and markers at chromosome 5q34-q35 (Ferrell et al., 1998; Witte et al., 1998; Evans et al., 1999). While there was evidence of reduced penetrance in these families, the majority of affected individuals were diagnosed at birth or in early childhood. Lymphangioscintigraphy in affected members of two large, chromosome 5 linked families reveal a variety of lymphangiodysplastic features in both affected and unaffected limbs (Witte et al., 1998), although no clinically normal, obligate mutations carriers were examined. Ferrell et al., (1998) observed non-conservative mutations in the positional candidate gene encoding vascular endothelial growth factor receptor-3 (VEGFR-3, FLT4), and Karkkainen et al. (2000) showed that missense mutations in *VEGFR3* in four independent lymphedema families led to loss of protein kinase activity in the mutant receptor. These four mutations were located in the intracellular kinase domain and appeared to exert a dominant negative effect by interfering with normal signal transduction by the normal allele. In another family of 5 affected relatives, a point mutation causing a histidine-to-arginine substitution segregated with lymphedema (Irrthum et al., 2000). This alteration in the catalytic loop of the protein inhibited autophosphorylation of VEGFR-3, which is consistent with the notion of defective signaling being the fundamental defect in Milroy disease. All families with lymphedema due to VEGFR-3 kinase domain mutations were characterized by congenital onset lymphedema.

VEGFR-3 is expressed in all endothelial cells during early embryogenesis, but in the course of development its expression in vascular endothelial cells declines and in the adult, VEGFR-3 expression is largely restricted to the lymphatic endothelium (Kaipainen et al., 1995; Kukk et al., 1996). In the mouse, ablation of VEGFR-3 expression is lethal at about day eleven of embryonic development due to failure in maturation of the perineural vascular plexus into a dendriform hierarchy of large and small vessels (Dumont et al., 1998). Heterozygous animals (with a single functional *VEGFR3* allele) survive with no obvious vascular or lymphatic phenotype, but these animals have not been carefully characterized. Further evidence of the vascular endothelial growth factors and their receptors in lymphatic development comes from mice which over-express VEGF-C, a primary ligand for VEGFR-3. These mice are characterized by specific lymphatic proliferation and hyperplasia (Jeltsch et al., 1997).

Complex segregation analysis in several large families suggests that more than one locus affects the phenotype (Holberg et al., 2001). Autosomal dominant congenital lymphedema has been reported in the dog (Patterson et al., 1967), the domestic pig (van der Putte 1978) and the cow (Morris et al., 1954).

Hereditary lymphedema II

Lymphedema of onset at puberty or later is phenotypically and undoubtedly genetically heterogeneous. Meige (1898) described eight affected individuals in four generations, and the disorder often bears his eponymous designation. Autosomal dominant inheritance is firmly described in numerous families. However, one or a few cases in a family may represent variable expression of hereditary lymphedema I. The discovery of specific genetic defects, such as *FLT4* in hereditary lymphedema I, should aid categorization in the future.

The extent of edema in families with pubertal or later onset is highly variable. The legs are predominantly affected, but the arms, face and larynx may also be involved (Goodman, 1962; Herbert and Bowen, 1983). Some individuals were first diagnosed with myxedema. Pleural effusions may occur. A few families have shown association with yellow nails (Emerson, 1966); whether this represents a separate condition or not remains unclear (Samman and White, 1964; Wells, 1966).

Angiographic analysis of the lymphatic system suggests primary atresia.

Management of the lower extremity edema is as described for edema of congenital onset.

Lymphedema with distichiasis

A small fraction (~1%) of people with primary lymphedema have a double row of eyelashes (distichiasis) (Dale, 1987), who often come to medical attention first because of corneal abrasions caused by the extra lashes (Fig. 54.2). The edema is not congenital and is bilateral, primarily affecting the legs (Fig. 54.3). The thoracic duct is often absent, while lymphatics in the legs are dilated ("hyperplastic" as opposed to

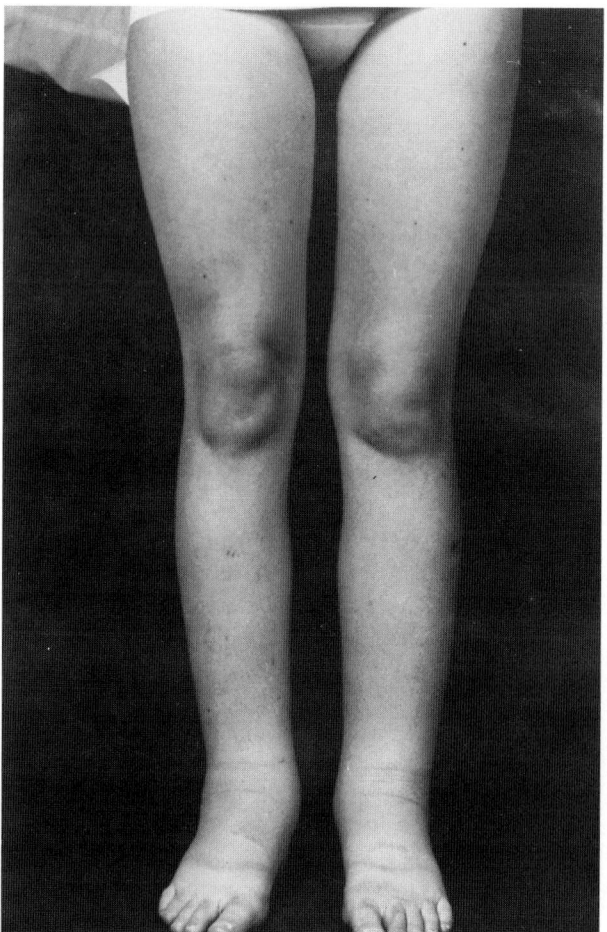

Fig. 54.2. Distichiasis in a young woman with the distichiasis-lymphedema syndrome. The inner row of lashes can irritate the cornea. Courtesy of Drs David Meisler and Elias Traboulsi.

atretic). This condition is associated with congenital heart defects much more so than other forms of hereditary lymphedema (Corbett et al., 1982).

In three families, this phenotype has been linked to 16q24.3 (Mangion et al., 1999) and Fang et al. (2000) showed that the lymphedema-distichiasis syndrome was caused by mutations in the fork head family transcription factor, FOXC2, in two families. Finegold et al. (2001) described extreme phenotypic heterogeneity in 12 lymphedema families with *FOXC2* mutations. Rosbotham et al. (2000) conducted a detailed lymphoscintigraphic study of a large lymphedema/distichiasis family and noted lymphatic abnormalities in a number of clinically normal family members, the absence of lymphatic abnormalities in several clinically affected family members and normal lymphatics in one obligate mutation carrier with only distichiasis as a clinical feature. This study emphasizes the need for detailed characterization of family members in efforts to map genes for lymphedema by linkage analysis.

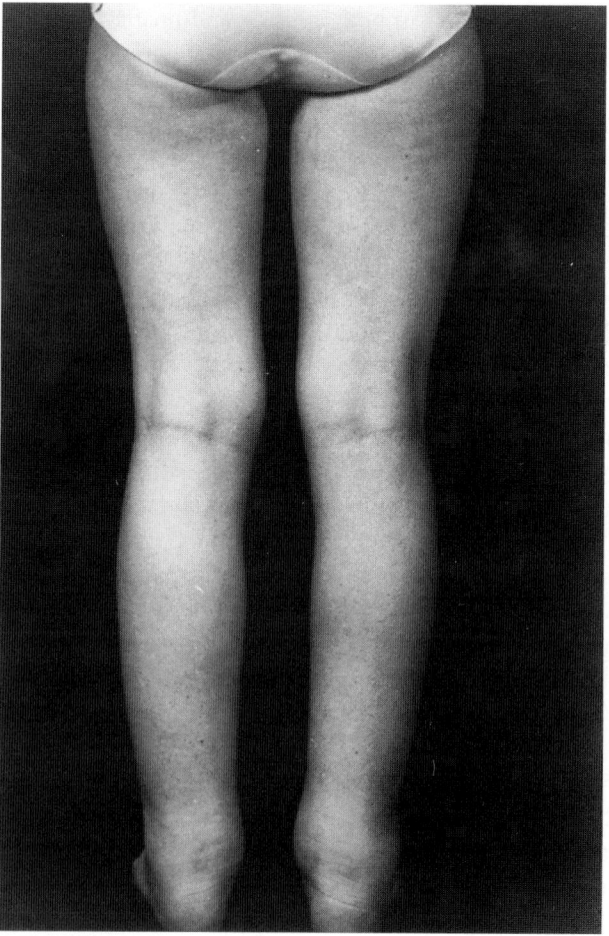

A   B

Fig. 54.3. Lymphedema in a 17-year-old woman with the distichiasis-lymphedema syndrome. She also had a cleft palate. The lymphedema developed around the time of puberty. A lymphangiogram at that time reportedly showed no abnormalities in the legs.

Hennekam lymphangiectasia-lymphedema syndrome

Hennekam syndrome is an autosomal recessive syndrome of intestinal lymphangiectasia, severe lymphedema of the face and genitalia and severe mental retardation (Hennekam et al., 1989). Intestinal biopsies, although quite variable, generally show severe dilatation of the lymphatic channels of the lamina propria with distortion of villi. The characteristic facial features anomalies are attributed to cutaneous over-distention due to jugular lymphatic obstruction during gestation (Jones, 1997).

Lymphedema, microcephaly, chorioretinopathy syndrome

Associations between lymphedema and microcephaly, and microcephaly and chorioretinopathy have long been recognized, but only recently have all three features been described in both sporadic cases and in families (Feingold and Bartoshesky, 1992; Angle et al., 1994). Expression has been quite variable and inheritance consistent with autosomal dominance. The edema is often present at birth, and may regress during childhood, suggesting that the lymphatic system has delayed maturation. The facial features include thick, full cheeks, thick epicanthal folds, ptosis and micrognathia consistent with the "congenital lymphedema facies" (Optiz, 1986). Despite often striking microcephaly, intelligence is average. The eyes show patchy chorioretinal dysplasia that usually progresses; vision can become severely compromised (Limwongse et al., 1999). A kindred with moderately short stature and lacking retinal changes has been reported (Strenge and Froster, 1998).

Cholestasis-lymphedema syndrome

Cholestasis-lymphedema syndrome, also referred to as Aagenaes syndrome, is an autosomal recessive condition of recurrent cholestasis and lymphedema first described by Aagenaes et al., (1968; 1970; 1974) among Norwegian families. Sharp and Krivit (1971) reported a US family of Norwegian ancestry and one British family (Morris et al., 1997) and one Italian family (Vajro et al., 1984) without known Norwegian ancestry have been reported. Aagenaes (1998) reviewed the clinical course of the syndrome from birth to adulthood. During the first months of life, the syndrome is dominated by cholestasis with malabsorption. One of 14 cases died of progressive, intrahepatic cholestasis at two years of age. Nine patients died in childhood of a vitamin K-deficient coagulopathy. Lymphedema may be present at birth or have a childhood onset. Lymphangiography has not been performed in the Norwegian patients. Lymphangiography in the Italian patient revealed no gross abnormalities of the lower limbs, while lymphadenoscintigraphy revealed slow progression of the radiocolloid up to the inguinal lymph nodes and poor liver uptake. The Norwegian families appear ideal for homozygosity mapping to localize the gene causing cholestasis-lymphedema syndrome in this population. Bull et al. (2000) recently mapped a locus causing Aagnaes syndrome to a 6.6 cM interval on chromosome 15q in Norwegian pedigrees.

Disorders affecting veins and lymphatics
(Table 54.3)

KLIPPEL-TRENAUNAY SYNDROME (KTS)

This enigmatic condition may well be heterogeneous, both of cause and actual pathophysiology. In common, but probably incorrect categorization this condition is often termed, "Klippel-Trenaunay-Weber syndrome". The features of KTS are defined by: cutaneous vascular malformations (not, as is frequently assumed, hemangiomata) and other malformations of capillaries, veins and lymphatics; venous varicosities of early onset; and hypertrophy of the underlying bones and soft tissues (Fig. 54.4). Edema and varicosities of affected limbs are common (Fig. 54.5). Lindenauer (1965) suggested that some patients, including several first described by Weber (1907), have arteriovenous malformations accounting for their overgrowth. Cohen (2000) concurs and argues persuasively that the presence of AVMs and limb overgrowth define the Parkes Weber syndrome. Patients with KTS, such as those described first by Klippel and Trenaunay (1900), often have

Table 54.3. Mendelian Disorders Affecting Both Veins and Lymphatics

Disorder	Inheritance	OMIM	# Locus	Gene	Features
Klippel-Trenaunay syndrome	sporadic	149000			cutaneous vascular malformations; segmental, enlargement with bony lesions, esp. of lower limbs; atresia of deep veins and congenital varicosities; atresia of lymphatics

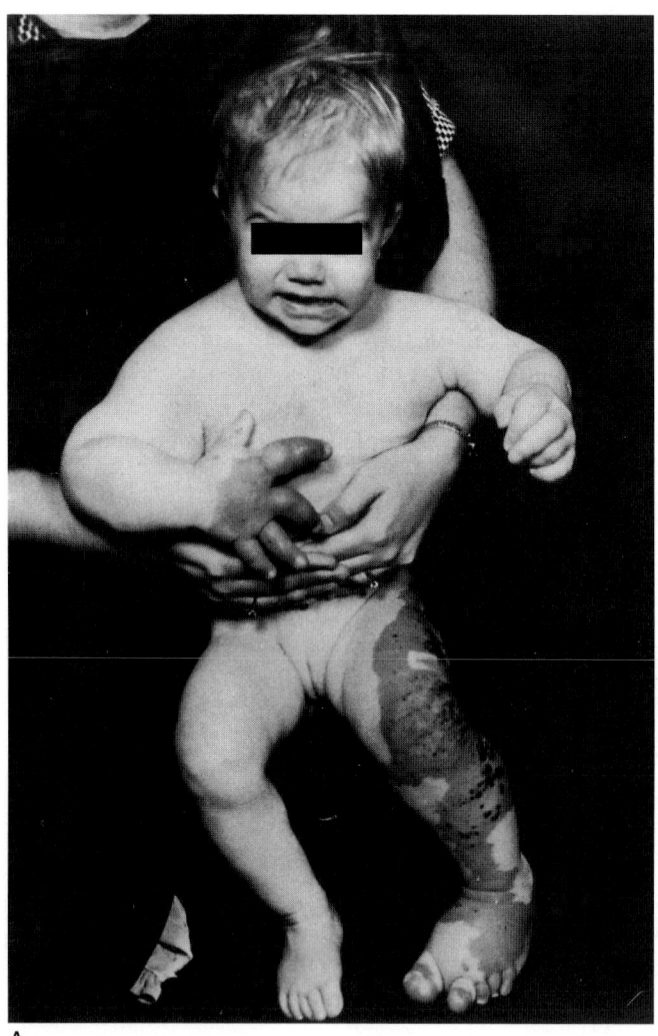

A   B

Fig. 54.4. Klippel-Trenaunay-Weber syndrome in a 14-month-old with marked bony overgrowth.

atresia of deep veins; in this case, superficial varicosities result from increased flow and should not be treated by ligation or "stripping" (Lindenauer, 1965). Indeed, review of clinical results suggests that surgical management of venous varicosities in KTS is unwise (Samuel and Spitz, 1995). In some patients with considerable edema of the affected body part(s), atresia of the lymphatics may be present.

Conservative measures to treat the peripheral edema should be advocated. Amputation of an affected limb may be necessary, either because of debilitating hypertrophy or skin breakdown or thrombophlebitis due to chronic venous stasis (Viljoen, 1988).

Patients with large or multiple arteriovenous malformations (such as are common in Parkes-Weber syndrome) or large hemangiomata are prone to high-output cardiac failure, severe thrombocytopenia due to platelet consumption (Kasabach-Merritt syndrome), and hemorrhage. This combination of complications is uncommon in KTS, in which any consumptive coagulopathy is usually local and associated with mild thrombocytopenia.

Most cases of KTS have been sporadic (Berry et al., 1998), but the increased occurrence of subtle findings of cutaneous vascular malformations or vascular nevi in near relatives suggests the importance of genetic factors (Rigamonti et al., 1988; Aelvoet et al., 1992; Ceballos-Quintal et al., 1996). Alternatively, because minor cutaneous vascular malformations are both common and frequently misinterpreted, their occurrence in relatives of a patient with KTS may be coincidental.

Autosomal dominant inheritance of a susceptibility to vascular maldevelopment, coupled with somatic mutations in the normal allele could result in the segmental findings in this and other disorders, analogous to the "two-hit" mechanism of tumor suppressor genes (Happle, 1993).

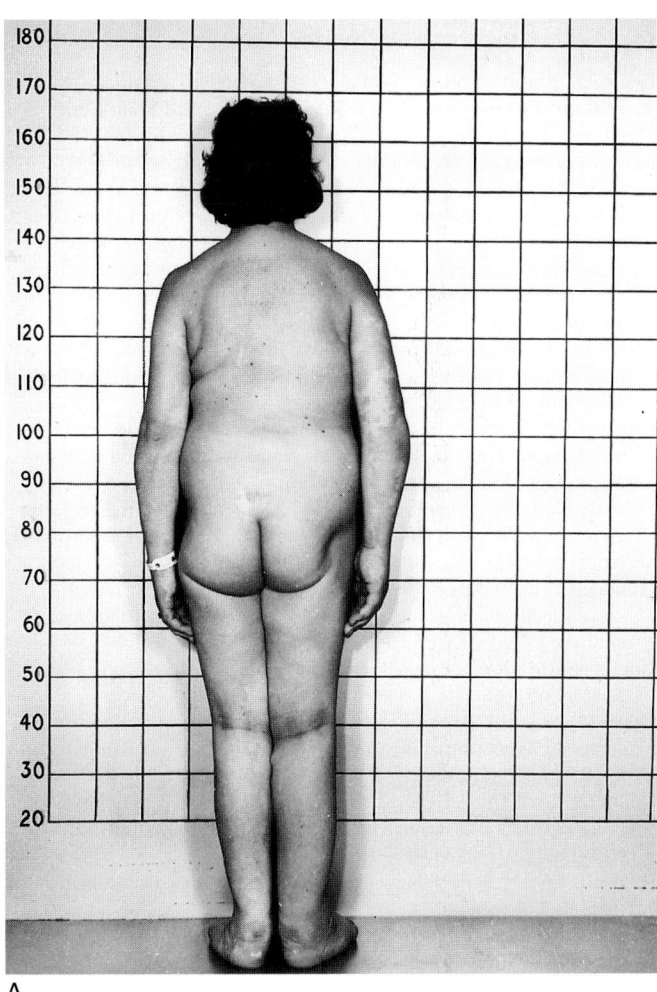

A

B

C

Fig. 54.5. Klippel-Trenaunay-Weber syndrome in a 15-year-old woman with a leg-length discrepancy (and resulting scoliosis), asymmetric lymphedema, and superficial varicosities. This patient was originally published in Harper PS 1971 Klippel-Trenaunay-Weber syndrome. Birth Defects: Orig Art Ser 7(8):315–316

Paternal age was advanced in a series of cases of KTS, a finding consistent with this hypothesis (Lorda-Sanchez et al., 1998). Sperandeo et al. (2000) described a family in which KTS syndrome and Beckwith-Wiedemann syndrome, another syndrome characterized by tissue overgrowth, occurred in first cousins. They noted relaxation of maternal imprinting of the *IGF2* locus in both patients. Interestingly, Whelan et al. (1995) reported a patient with KTS syndrome and a chromosome translocation involving band 11p15, near the location of *IGF2* gene.

REFERENCES

Aagenaes O (1974) Hereditary recurrent-cholestasis with lymphedema-two new families. Acta Paediat Scand 64:465–471 cholestasis from birth. Arch Dis Child 43:646–657

Aagenaes O (1998) Hereditary cholestasis with lymphedema (Aagenaes syndrome, cholestasis-lymphedema syndrome). New cases and follow-up from infancy to adult age. Scand J Gastroenterol 33:335–345

Aagenaes O, Sigstad H, Bjorn-Hansen R (1970) Lymphedema n hereditary recurrent cholestasis from birth. Arch Dis Child 45:690–695

Aagenaes O, Van der Hagen CB, Refsum S (1968) Hereditary recurrent intrahepatic cholestasis from birth. Arch Dis Child 43:646–657

Aelvoet GE, Jorens PG, Roelen LM (1992) Genetic aspects of Klippel-Trenaunay syndrome. Br J Dermatol 126:603–607

Angle B, Holgado S, Burton BK et al. (1994) Microcephaly, lymphoedema, and chorioretinal dysplasia: Report of two additional cases. Am J Med Genet 53:99–101

Barber DA, Wang X, Gloviczki P et al. (1997) Characterization of endothelin receptors in human varicose veins. J Vasc Surg 26:61–69

Berry SA, Peterson C, Mize W et al. (1998) Klippel-Trenaunay syndrome. Am J Med Genet 79:319–326

Boon LM, Mulliken JB, Vikkula M et al. (1994) Assignment of a locus for dominantly inherited venous malformations to chromosome 9p. Hum Mol Genet 3:1583–1587

Boon LM, Brouillard P, Irrthum A et al. (1999) A gene for inherited cutaneous venous anomalies ("glomangiomas") localizes to chromosome 1p21-22. Am J Hum Genet 65:125–133

Bull LN, Roche E, Sang EJ et al. (2000) Mapping of the locus of cholestasis-lympheatoma syndrome (Aagenaes syndrome) to a 6.6 cM interval an chromosome 15q Am J Hum Genet 67:994–999

Calvert JT, Riney TJ, Kontos CD et al. (1999) Allelic and locus heterogeneity in inheritied venous malformations. Hum Mol Genet 8:1279–1289

Ceballos-Quintal JM, Pinto-Escalante D, Castillo-Zapata I (1996) A new case of Klippel-Trenaunay-Weber (KTW) syndrome: Evidence of autosomal dominant inheritance. Am J Med Genet 63:426–427

Cohen MM Jr. (2000) Klippel-Trenaunay syndrome. Am J Med Genet 93:171–175

Corbett CRR, Dale RF, Coltart DJ, Kinmonth JB (1982) Congenital heart disease in patients with primary lymphoedemas. Lymphology 15:85–90

Craig HD, Gunel M, Cepeda O et al. (1998) Multilocus linkage identifies two new loci for a mendelian form of stroke, cerebral cavernous malformation, at 7p15-13 and 3q25.2-27. Hum Mol Genet 7:1851–1858

Dale RF (1987) Primary lymphoedema when found with distichiasis is of the type defined as bilateral hyperplasia by lymphography. J Med Genet 24:170–171

Dobyns WB, Michels VV, Groover RV et al. (1987) Familial cavernous malformations of the central nervous system andretina. Ann Neurol 21:578–83

Dubovsky J, Zabramski JM, Kurth J et al. (1995) A gene responsible for cavernous malformations of the brain maps to chromosome 7q. Hum Mol Genet 4:453–458

Duell PB, Malinow MR (1997) Homocyt(e)ine: an important risk factor for atherosclerotic vascular disease. Curr Opin Lipidol. 8:28–34

Dumont DJ, Anderson L, Breitman ML, Duncan AM (1994) Assigment of the endothelial-specific protein receptor tyrosine kinase gene (TEK) to human chromosome 9p21. Genomics 23:512–513

Dumont DJ, Jussila L, Taipale J et al. (1998) Cardiovascular failure in mouse embryos deficient in VEGF receptor-3. Science 282:946–949

Emerson PA (1966) Yellow nails, lymphoedema, and pleural effusions. Thorax 21:247–253

Esterly JR (1965) Congenital hereditary lymphedema. J Med Genet 2:93–98

Evans AL, Brice G, Sotirova V et al. (1999) Mapping of primary congenital lymphedema to the 5q35.3 region. Am J Hum Genet 64:547–555

Fang J, Dagenais SL, Erickson RP et al. (2000) Mutations in FOXC2 (MFH1), a forkhead family transcription factor, are responsible for the hereditory lymphedema-distichiasis syndrome. Am J Hum Genet 67:1382–1388

Feingold M, Bartoshesky L (1992) Microcephaly, lymphedema, and chorioretinal dysplasia: a distinct syndrome? Am J Med Genet 43:1030–1031

Ferrell RE, Levinson KL, Esman JH et al. (1998) Hereditary lymphedema: evidence for linkage and genetic heterogeneity. Hum Mol Genet 7:2073–2078

Finegold DN, Kimak MA, Lawrence EC et al. (2001) Truncating mutations in FOXC2 cause multiple lymphedema syndromes. Hum Mol Genet 10: in the press

Frosst P, Blom JH, Milos R et al. (1995) A candidate genetic risk factor for vascular disease: a common mutationin methylenetetrahydrofolate reductase. Nat Genet 10:111–113

Gallione CJ, Pasyk KA, Boon LM et al. (1995) A gene for familial venous malformations maps to chromosome 9p in a second large kindred. J Med Genet 32:197–199

Goodman RM (1962) Familial lymphedema of the Meige's type. Am J Med 32:651–656

Gunel M, Awad IA, Anson J, Lifton RP (1995) Mapping a gene causing cerebral cavernous malformation to 7q11.2-q21. Proc Natl Acad Sci USA 92:6620–6624

Gunel M, Awad IA, Finberg K, et al. (1996) A founder mutation as a cause of cerebral cavernous malformation in Hispanic Americans. New Engl J Med 334:946–951

Happle R (1993) Klippel-Trenaunay syndrome: is it a paradominant trait? Br J Dermatol 128:465

Hauge M, Gundersen J (1969) Genetics of varicose veins of the lower extremities. Hum Hered 19:573–80

Hennenkam RCM, Geerdink RA, Hamel BCJ et al. (1989) Autosomal recessive intestinal lymphangiectasia and lymphedema, with facial anomalies and mental retardation. Am J Med Genet 34:593–600

Herbert FA, Bowen PA (1983) Hereditary late-onset lymphedema with pleural effusion and laryngeal edema. Arch Intern Med 143:913–915

Holberg CI, Erickson RP, Bernas MJ et al. (2001) Segregation analyses and a gename-wide linkage search confirm genetic heterogeneity and suggest oligogenetic inheritance in same Milroy congenital primary lymphedema families. Am J Med Genet 98:303–312

Irrthum A, Karkkainen MJ, Devriendt K et al. (2000) congenital hereditary lymphedema caused by a mutation that inactivates VEGFR3 tyrosine kinase. Am J Hum Genet 67:295–301

Irrthum A, Brouillard P, Enjolras O et al. (2001) Lingage disequilibrium narrows locus for venous malformation with glomus cells (VMGLOM) to a single 1.48 Mbp YAC. Eur J Hum Genet 9:34–48

Jeltsch M, Kaipainen A, Joukov V et al. (1997) Hyperplasia of the lymphatic vessels in VEGF-C transgenic mice. Science 276:1423–1425

Johnson EW, Iyer LM, Rich SS, et al. (1995) Refined localization of the cerebral cavernous malformation gene (CCM1) to a 4cM interval of chromosome 7q contained in a well defined YAC contig. Geonome Res 5:368–380

Jones KL (1997) Jugular lymphatic obstruction sequence. pp. 620–621. In Smith's Recognizable Patterns of Human Malformation. 5th edn, Saunders: Philadelphia

Kaipainen A, Karhonen J, Mustonen T, et al. (1995) Expression of the fms-like tyrosine kinase 4 gene becomes restricted to lymphatic endothelium during development. Proc Natl Acad Sci USA 92:3566–3570

Karkkainen MJ, Ferrell RE, Lawrence EC et al. (2000) Missense mutations interfere with VEGFR-3 signalling in primary lymphoedema. Nat Genet 24:25:153–159

Klippel M, Trenaunay P (1900) Du naevus variquex osteo-hypertophique. Arch Gen Med 185:641–672

Kukk E, Lymboussaki A, Taira S et al. (1996) VEGF-C receptor binding and pattern of expression of VEGFR-3 suggests a role in lymphatic vascular development. Development 122:3829–3837

Laberge-le Couteulx S, Jung HH, Labauge P et al. (1999) Trancating mutations in CCM1, encoding KRIT1, cause hereditary cavernous angiomas. Nature Genet 23:189–193

Leu HJ (1974) Familial congenital absence of valves in the deep leg veins. Humangenetik 22:347–349

Limwongse C, Wyszynski RE, Dickerman LH, Robin NH (1999) Microcephaly-lymphedema-chorioretinal Dysplasia: a unique genetic syndrome with variable expression and possible characteristic facial appearance. Am J Med Genet 86:215–218

Lindenauer SM (1965) The Klippel-Trenaunay syndrome: Varicosity, hypertrophy and hemangioma with no arteriovenous fistula. Ann Surg 162:303–314

Lorda-Sanchez I, Prieto L, Rodriquez-Pinilla E, Martinez-Frias ML (1998) Increased parental age and number of pregnancies in Klippel-Trenaunay-Weber syndrome. Ann Hum Genet 62:235–239

Mangiafico RA, Malatino LS, Santonocito M et al. (1997) Plasma endothelin-1 release in normal and varicose saphenous veins. Angiology 9:769–774

Mangion J, Rahman N, Mansour S, et al. (1999) A gene for lymphedema-distichasis maps to 16q24.3. Am J Hum Genet 65:427–432

Marchuk DA, Gallione CJ, Morrison LA et al. (1995) A locus for cerebral cavernous malformations maps to chromosome 7q in two families. Genomics 28:311–314

Matousek V, Prerovsky I (1974) A contribution to the problem of the inheritance of primary varicose veins. Hum Hered 24:225–235

McCully KS (1996) Homocysteine and vascular disease. Nature Med 2:386–389

Meige H (1898) Dystrophie oedemateuse hereditaire. Presse Med 6:341–343

Milroy WF (1892) An undescribed variety of hereditary oedema. NY Med J 56:505–508

Morris AA, Sequeira JSS, Malone M et al. (1997) Parent-child transmission of infantile cholestasis with lymphedema (Aagenaes syndrome). J Med Genet 34:852–853

Morris B, Blood DC, Sidman WR et al. (1954) Congenital lymphatic oedema in Ayrshire calves. Austr J Exp Biol 32:265–274

Mustonen T, Alitalo K (1995) Endothelial cell receptor kinases involved in angiogenesis. J Cell Biol 129:895–898

Opitz JM (1986) On congenital lymphedema. Am J Med Genet 24:127–129

Pasyk KA, Argenta LC, Erickson RP (1984) Familial vascular malformations. Report of 25 members of one family. Clin Genet 26:221–227

Patterson DF, Medway W, Luginbuhl H, Chacks S (1967) Congenital hereditary lymphedema in the dog. J Med Genet 4:145–152

Rigamonti D, Hadley MN, Drayer BP et al. (1988) Cerebral cavernous malformations: incidence and familial occurrence. N Engl J Med 319:343–347

Rosbotham JL, Brice GW, Child AH, et al. (2000) Distichiasis-lymphedema: clinical features, venous function and lymphoscintigraphy. Br J Dermatol 142:148–152

Sahoo T, Johnson EW, Thomas JW, et al. (1999) Mutations in the gene encoding KRIT1, a Krev1/rap1a binding protein, cause cerebral cavernous malformations (CCM1). Hum Mol Genet 8:2325–2333

Samman PD, White WF (1964) The "yellow nail" syndrome. Br J Dermatol 76:153–157

Samuel M, Spitz L (1995) Klippel-Trenaunay syndrome: clinical features, complications and management in children. Br J Surg 82:757–761

Sato TN, Tozawa Y, Deutsch U, et al. (1995) Distinct roles of the receptor tyrosine kinases Tie-1 and Tie-2 in blood vessel formation. Nature 376:70–74

Serebriiskii I, Estojak J, Sonoda G, et al. (1997) Association of Krev1/rap 1a with Krit1, a novel ankyrin repeat-containing protein-encoded by a gene mapping to 7q21-22. Oncogene 15:1043–1049

Sharp HL, Krivit W (1971) Hereditary lymphedema and obstructive jaundice. J Pediat 78:491–496

Sperandeo MP, Ungaro P, Vernucci M et al. (2000) Relaxation of insulin-like growth factor 2 imprinting and discordant methylation at KvMR1 in two first cousins affected with Beckwith-Wiedeman and Klippel-Trenaunay-Weber syndrome. Am J Hum Genet 66:841–847

Strenge S, Froster UG (1998) Microcephaly-lymphedema syndrome: report of a family with short stature as additional manifestation. Am J Med Genet 80:506–509

Sverdlova AM, Bubnova NA, Baranovskaya SS, et al. (1998) Prevalence of the methylenetetrahydrofolate reductase C677T mutations in patients with varicose veins of lower limbs. Mol Genet Metabol 63:35–36

Trauffer PM, Anderson CE, Johnson A, et al. (1994) The natural history of euploid pregnancies with first-trimester cystic hygromas. Am J Obstet Gynecol 170:1279–1284

Vajro P, Romano A, Fontanello A, et al. (1984) Aagenaes syndrome in an Italian child. Acta Paediatr Scand 73:695–696

van der Putte SC (1975) The development of the lymphatic system in man. Adv Anat Embryol Cell Biol 51:3–60

van der Putte SCJ (1978) Congenital hereditary lymphedema in the pig. Lymphol 11:1–9

Vikkula M, Boon LM, Carraway KL, et al. (1996) Vascular dysmorphogenesis caused by an activating mutation in the receptor tyrosine kinase TIE2. Cell 87:1181–1190

Viljoen DL (1988) Klippel-Trenaunay-Weber syndrome (angio-osteohypertrophy syndrome) J Med Genet 25:250–252

Weber FP (1907) Angioma formation in connection with hypertrophy of limbs and hemihypertrophy. Br J Dermatol 19:231–235

Wells GC (1966) Yellow nail syndrome with familial primary hypoplasia of lymphatics, manifest late in life. Proc Roy Soc Med 59:447

Whelan AJ, Watson MS, Porter FD, Steiner RD (1995) Klippel-Trenaunay-Weber syndrome associated with a 5;11 balanced translocation. Am J Med Genet 59:492–494

Witt DR, Hoyme E, Zonana J et al. (1987) Lymphedema in Noonan syndrome: clues to pathogenesis and prenatal diagnosis and review of the literature. Am J Med Genet 27:841–856

Witte MH, Erikson R, Bernas M, et al. (1998) Phenotypic and genetic heterogeneity in familial Milroy lymphedema. Lymphology 31:145–155

Zhang J, Clatterback RE, Rigamonti D, Dietz HC (2001) Mutations in KRIT1 in familial cavernous malformations. Neurosurgery 46:1272–1277

Index

Hepatocardiomuscular carnitine palmitoyl transferase defect, 2560
Hepatocellular carcinoma, 1841–1843
aflatoxins, 1842
mutagenesis, 3616
glucose 6-phosphatase deficiency, 2450
hepatorenal tyrosinemia, 2414
porphyria cutanea tarda, 2607
Hepatocellular differentiation markers, hepatocellular carcinoma, 1843
Hepatocyte nuclear factors. See HNF genes
Hepatocytes
bilirubin uptake, 1797–1798
gene therapy, 888–890, 1807
transplantation, 888–889, 1807
progressive familial intrahepatic cholestasis, 1815
Hepatoerythropoietic porphyria, 2593t, 2603, 2604, 2605, 2607
Hepatorenal tyrosinemia, 2412–2414
Hephaestin, 2639t, 2640
HER2 gene. See NEU gene
Hereditary amyloidoses, 106
Hereditary angioneurotic edema, 105, 2099–2100
systemic lupus erythematosus, 2105
vascular permeability, 2104
Hereditary ataxias, 3109–3123
'with retained tendon reflexes', 3115, 3116
Hereditary benign telangiectasia, 3935
Hereditary bullous dysfunction, 2813t
Hereditary cerebral hemorrhage with amyloidosis
Dutch type, 3214
Iceland type, 3214
Hereditary coproporphyria, 2591, 2608–2610
Hereditary cylindromatosis, 3930t
Hereditary deep corneal dystrophy, 3521
Hereditary elliptocytosis, 1913–1914
Hereditary endotheliopathy with retinopathy, nephropathy and stroke (HERNS), 3212
Hereditary exostoses, 4084–4085, 4147–4149
Hereditary fructose intolerance, 835, 2447–2448, 2473
Hereditary hemochromatosis. See hemochromatosis, hereditary

Hereditary hemorrhagic telangiectasia, 1289t, 1945, 3215, 3934t, 3935–3936
blue rubber bleb nevus syndrome vs, 3935, 3937
Hereditary hyperferritinemia-cataract syndrome, 2657, 3547
Hereditary hypophosphatemic rickets, with hypercalciuria, 2579
Hereditary hypotrichosis. See Marie-Unna syndrome
Hereditary iron-handling disorder, 2657
Hereditary lymphedemas, 1549t, 1550–1551
Hereditary mixed polyposis syndrome, 1838
Hereditary motor and sensory neuropathies. See Charcot-Marie-Tooth disease
Hereditary myasthenias (congenital myasthenias), 3419t, 3421–3426
Hereditary nephropathy, with hyperuricemia, 2468, 2487
Hereditary neurocutaneous angioma, 1547t
Hereditary neuropathy with liability to pressure palsies, 3309, 3311t
allelic heterogeneity and, 641
deletion, 88
Hereditary non-inflammatory arthropathies, 4245–4251
Hereditary non-polyposis colorectal carcinoma, 528t, 537, 1830–1835
available genetic testing, 663t
colorectal carcinoma prevention, 666, 667
frequency, 57
gastric carcinoma, 1840
genes involved, 98
mismatch repair gene mutations, 97, 550–551
MLH1 mutations, 164–165
molecular genetic diagnosis, 741
Muir-Torre syndrome subgroup and, 3948, 3969
ovarian carcinoma, 2367
replication error phenotype, 741, 2364
screening, 656, 657
ureteric carcinoma, 1736
Hereditary orotic aciduria, 1919, 2487–2488
Hereditary panhypopituitary dwarfism, diabetes mellitus, 2234t
Hereditary papillary renal cell carcinoma, 1735

Hereditary persistence of α-fetoprotein, 96–97
Hereditary persistence of fetal hemoglobin, 96–97, 106, 1891t, 1892
mutations of enhancers and promoters, 69
Hereditary polymorphous light eruption, xeroderma pigmentosum vs, 3943
Hereditary progressive autosomal dominant dystonia with marked diurnal fluctuations. See dopa-responsive dystonia
Hereditary pyropoikilocytosis, 1914
Hereditary relapsing pancreatitis, diabetes mellitus, 2234t
Hereditary sensory and motor neuropathies. See Charcot-Marie-Tooth disease
Hereditary sensory radicular neuropathy, 3156–3157, 3159t
Hereditary spherocytosis, 1911–1913
iron overload, 2651
Hereditary urogenital adysplasia, 1663, 1665t, 1671t, 1679t, 1681t
Hereditary vitamin D dependency
type 1, 2572–2574
type 2, 2572t, 2574–2579
Hereditary xanthinuria, 2480–2481
Heregulins, 525
HERG (potassium channel subunit), 613
minK interaction, 1424
HERG gene, 1421f, 1422–1423
Heritability, 457
attention deficit-hyperactivity disorder, 2887
bipolar affective disorder, twin studies, 2939
drug abuse, 2960
interpupillary distance, 3597
lipids, 2504–2506
vs manageability, 52
personality, 2792–2794
strabismus, 3597
Heritability index, drug half-lives, 595
Herlitz junctional epidermolysis bullosa, 3834f–3835f, 3837
mutations, 3839–3843
population genetics, 3883
prenatal diagnosis, 813
Hermanski-Pudlak syndrome, 1945, 3763–3765
diagnosis, 3769

HPS1 gene, 3734, 3740t, 3745–3746, 3765
HPS2 gene, 3746, 3765
inflammatory bowel disease, 1770
lung disease, 1643–1644, 3764
Puerto Rico, 3746, 3763
Hermaphroditism. See also pseudohermaphroditism
true, 2329–2331
Hernia
complete androgen insensitivity, 2325
Marfan syndrome, 3993
HERNS. See hereditary endotheliopathy with retinopathy, nephropathy and stroke
Heroin addiction, 2955
Herpes gestationis, BPAG2, 3847
Herpes simplex virus
gene vectors, 878t, 880–881
transplacental infection, 1020
Herrmann syndrome, diabetes mellitus, 2235t
Hers disease, 2453
HESX1 gene, 950t, 952, 2162t
Heterochromatin, 62, 63–64, 79, 160
C-banding, 695
exchange, uniparental disomy, 118, 120f
Y chromosome, 155–156
Heterochromia
retinoblastoma, 3610
Waardenburg syndrome, 3649
Heterodimers, HLA Class II proteins, 1107
Heteroduplex analysis
hypertrophic cardiomyopathy, 1328–1329, 1352–1353
temperature modulated, 1328
Heterogeneity. See also genetic heterogeneity; locus heterogeneity
clinical, retinopathies, 3556
diabetes mellitus, type 2, 2253–2255
etiologic, 140–141
twin studies, 463–464
high-density lipoproteins, 2521
inflammatory bowel disease, 1762–1764
mitochondrial DNA, 742
multifactorial disorders, 647
phenotypic, PRPN mutations, 2911
phosphoribosylpyrophosphate synthetase locus, 2479
retinopathies, 3556
spinal muscular atrophy, 3359
Heterogeneous mutations, detection, 726–727
Heterokaryons, 2765
Heteromorphisms, 697

Hyperoxaluria type 2, 2775
Hyperparathyroidism
  deafness and renal disease
    syndrome, 3649
  primary, 2203–2212
  surgery criteria, 2214
  vitamin D deficiency, 2571
Hyperparathyroidism-jaw tumor
    syndrome, 2205t,
    2212–2213
Hyperphenylalaninemia 2 mouse,
    Hartnup disease model,
    3941
Hyperphenylalaninemias,
    2405–2410. See also
    phenylketonuria
  neonatal screening, 831–837
Hyperphosphatasemia with
    osteoectasia, 4135–4136
  juvenile Paget's disease, 3570t
Hyperpipecolic acidemia, 2760t,
    2763–2764
L-Hyperpipecolic acidemia, 2764
Hyperplasia, hyperparathyroidism,
    2204
Hyperplastic polyposis, 1838
Hyperprolactinemia, 2170
Hyperprolinemias, 2428
  frequencies, neonatal screening,
    836
Hyperpyrexia. See hyperthermia;
    malignant hyperthermia
Hyperreflexia, hypocalcemia, 2215
Hypersensitivity pneumonitis,
    1650–1651
Hypertelorism (Farag syndrome),
    1284t
Hypertelorism-microtia-clefting
    syndrome, 1290t
Hypertension, 1475–1495,
    1533–1535
  ADPKD genes, 1694
  angiotensin gene mutation, 93
  animal models, 413–414
  atherosclerotic heart disease,
    risk, 1522
  brachydactyly, syndrome
    associating, 1478
  cardiomyopathy diagnosis, 1344
  family history, accuracy, 661
  11β-hydroxylase deficiency, 2293
  mitochondrial DNA, 366–367
  monogenic syndromes, 412
  neurofibromatosis type 1, 3172
  phenotypes, 411, 412
  after pre-eclampsia, 1505
  pregnancy, 1496–1497,
    1504–1505. See also pre-
    eclampsia; pregnancy-
    induced hypertension
  pregnancy loss, 991
  therapy, lipid disorders, 2515t
  transmission/disequilibrium
    test, 418
  Turner syndrome, 1188

Hyperthermia, 1023. See also
    malignant hyperthermia;
    thermochemotherapy
  arthrogryposis, 4216t
  congenital sensory neuropathy
    with anhidrosis,
    3151–3152
  hypohidrotic ectodermal
    dysplasia, 3902
  malformations, 3712
  neural tube defects, 2979
Hyperthyroidism
  activating G protein mutations,
    2192–2193
  activating TSH receptor
    mutations, 2193
  familial, 2141t
  fibrous dysplasia, 4155
Hyperthyroxinemia, 2141t
Hypertransfusion, β-thalassemia,
    1894–1895
Hypertrichosis lanuginosa,
    congenital, 3926t
Hypertrichosis-
    osteochondrodysplasia,
    1290t
Hypertrichosis-osteodysplasia-
    cardiomyopathy, 1290t
Hypertriglyceridemias. See familial
    hypertriglyceridemias
Hypertrophic cardiomyopathy,
    1343–1388, 1403, 1404,
    1435–1441
  central core disease, 3336
  dilated cardiomyopathy vs
    actin mutations, 1393
  mechanisms, 1363
  management, 1383–1388
  mtDNA mutations, 343–347
  Wolff-Parkinson-White
    syndrome, 1346, 1364,
    1433
Hypertrophic pyloric stenosis,
    infantile, 1750–1751
Hyperuricemia, 2469, 2470
  hereditary nephropathy with,
    2468, 2487
Hypervariable regions, HLA
    molecules, 1104, 1106f
Hypervariable repetitive
    minisatellite sequences,
    1866
Hyphema, retinoblastoma,
    3610
Hyplip1 mouse model, 2517
Hyp mouse, X-linked
    hypophosphatemic rickets
    model, 4138
Hypoadrenocorticism, familial,
    2141t
Hypoalphalipoproteinemia,
    2507, 2509t, 2510f,
    2521, 2523
  genetic counseling, 2530
  management, 664t

Hypobetalipoproteinemia, 2509t,
    2519
  lipoprotein levels, 2510f
Hypoblast, 472
Hypocalcemia, 2214–2215
  Albright hereditary
    osteodystrophy, 4139
  tubular stenosis, 4133
Hypocalciuric hypercalcemia. See
    familial hypocalciuric
    hypercalcemia
Hypocatalasemia. See catalase
Hypocholesterolemia, Smith-
    Lemli-Opitz syndrome,
    1256
Hypochondrogenesis, 1068t, 4081
Hypochondroplasia, 4086t
  bibliography, 4107
  fibroblast growth factor receptor
    3 mutations, 4083
Hypocretins. See orexins
Hypodontia, 3718–3719
Hypofibrinogenemia, 1942
Hypogammaglobulinemia, X-
    linked, isolated growth
    hormone deficiency, type
    III, 2164
Hypoglycemia. See also
    hypoketotic hypoglycemia
  Beckwith-Wiedemann
    syndrome, 1730
  FATMO disorders, 2540t,
    2543
  glucose 6-phosphatase
    deficiency, 2450
  glycogen synthetase deficiency,
    2458
  hereditary fructose intolerance,
    2447
  nonketotic, 2543
Hypoglycorrhachia, 2442
Hypogonadism. See also Kallmann
    syndromes
  gonadotropins
    female, 951–952
    male, 964t, 970–971
  hemochromatosis, 2150
  juvenile hemochromatosis, 2654
  X-linked adrenoleukodystrophy,
    2768
  Yq deletions, 1193–1194
Hypogonadotropic
    hypogonadism, 2141t
  deafness, 3654
Hypohidrotic ectodermal
    dysplasia. See anhidrotic
    ectodermal dysplasia
Hypokalemia, 11β-hydroxylase
    deficiency, 2293, 2294
Hypokalemic periodic paralysis,
    3373, 3386–3388, 3389t
  hyperkalemic periodic paralysis
    vs, 3381t
  malignant hyperthermia, 3334
  type 2, 3373, 3388

Hypoketotic hypoglycemia. See
    also nonketotic
    hypoglycemia
  FATMO disorders, 2540t
  management, 2559
Hypoketotic medium-chain
    dicarboxylic aciduria,
    FATMO disorders, 2545,
    2561
Hypokinesia, 3076t
Hypolactasia, 2441–2442
Hypomania, 2937–2938
Hypomelanosis
  of Ito. See pigmentary mosaicism
  phylloid, Patau syndrome, 1160
Hypomelanotic macules, 3179
  tuberous sclerosis, 3180t
Hypoparathyroidism
  biochemical changes, 2219t
  deafness and renal disease
    syndrome, 3649
  nephrogenic diabetes insipidus,
    2175
  primary, 2214–2219
Hypoparathyroidism,
    sensorineural hearing loss
    and renal dysplasia, 1671t
Hypophosphatasia, 4136–4137.
    See also alkaline
    phosphatase, deficiency
Hypophosphatemia,
    hyperparathyroidism, 2204
Hypophosphatemic rickets, 1725,
    4137–4139
  hepatorenal tyrosinemia, 2412
  hereditary, with hypercalciuria,
    2579
  X-linked, 4137–4139
Hypopigmentation. See also
    albinism
  generalized cutaneous,
    3767–3768
  localized, 3770–3771
  tuberous sclerosis, 3179, 3180t
Hypopituitarism, 1074. See also
    anterior pituitary
  18p- syndrome, 2141t
  congenital, 2144
  iatrogenic, 2146
Hypoplasias, 491
Hypoplastic anemia
  congenital. See Diamond-
    Blackfan anemia
  constitutional. See Fanconi
    anemia
Hypospadias, pseudovaginal
    perineoscrotal (5α-
    reductase deficiency),
    963t, 2328–2329
Hyposthenuria, medullary cystic
    disease of kidney, 1699
Hypothalamopituitary-adrenal
    axis, 2279
  feeding and body size,
    2393–2394

Nance syndrome (X-linked recessive mixed deafness with stapes fixation and perilymphatic gusher), 3642, 3646
Naphthoquinone. *See* lawsone
Narcolepsy
    autoantigens, 1998t
    HLA complex, 1997t, 2005
    relative risk, 458
    orexin knockout mice, 2393
Narrative ethics, confidentiality and, 905
Narrow angle glaucoma. *See* closed angle glaucoma
Narrow heritability, 457
Nasal pits, 3711
Nasal polyposis, cystic fibrosis, 1564–1565
Nasal potential differences, cystic fibrosis diagnosis, 1584
Nasal swellings (embryological), 3713
Nasolacrimal groove, 3713
Natal teeth, pachyonychia congenita, 3920
NAT genes, 596–597, 622
Nathalie syndrome, 1297t
National Center for Human Genome Research, 22–23. *See also* National Human Genome Research Institute
National Cholesterol Education Program Expert Panel, 2528
National Coalition for Health Professional Education in Genetics, URL, 744
National Epidermolysis Bullosa Registry, United States, 3882
National Human Genome Research Institute, 23. *See also* National Center for Human Genome Research
National Institutes of Health, Human Genome Project funding, 22
National Marfan Foundation, 4010
National Marrow Donor Program, 1109–1110
Native Americans
    Athabascan type severe combined immunodeficiency disease, 2081
    congenital dislocation of hip, 4239
    mitochondrial DNA haplogroups, 319
    rheumatoid arthritis, 2032
Natural killer cell receptors, T cells, psoriasis, 3917

Natural killer cells, inhibitory receptor systems, 2002
Natural resistance associated microphage protein 1, 1092
    inflammatory bowel disease, 1783
Natural resistance associated microphage protein 2 (divalent metal transporter 1), 2639t, 2640
Natural selection, 44, 47–48, 50, 433–434, 437
    aging and, 576
    inflammatory bowel disease, 1773–1774
    pharmacogenomics, 620–621
Nature, *vs* nurture, 447–448
Naurua, diabetes mellitus, 2253, 2254
Nausea, pregnancy, arthrogryposes, 4183–4185
Navajo Indians, glucose tolerance, 2254
Naxos disease, 1297t, 1401, 1437t, 1446–1447, 1448
NBS-1 gene, 554
NC domains, collagen VII, 3863–3864
Nci I (restriction endonuclease), HPA1 typing, 1966–1967
ND4 mutations, mitochondrial DNA, 649
NDFs (heregulins), 525
NDGR1 gene, complex Charcot-Marie-Tooth diseases, 3311
NDP gene (Norrie syndrome), 3564t, 3611
NDUFS4 mutation, Leigh syndrome, 339–340
NDUFS8 (TYKY) complex I subunit, nuclear DNA mutation, 339
Near haploidy, acute lymphoblastic leukemia, 1986
Necrotizing myopathy-cataract-cardiomyopathy, 1298f
Neel, J.V., 30
NEFH gene, transgenic mice, 3446
NEFL gene, Charcot-Marie-Tooth diseases, 3305, 3310
Negative selection, T cells, 2001
Negro variant, galactosemia, 2445
Neish-Roberts syndrome, 1298f
Neisseria meningitidis. See meningococcal disease
Neisseria spp., complement deficiencies, 2105
Nemaline bodies, 3330
Nemaline myopathy, 4200t
    muscle biopsy, 3323f, 3329–3331

Nematodes, aryl hydrocarbon receptor, 616
NEMO gene. *See IKK-gamma* gene
Neodarwinism, 44
Neonatal adrenoleukodystrophy, 1058–1059, 2760t, 2761–2762, 2763
    biochemistry, 2764, 2778t
    molecular biology, 2764–2765
Neonatal convulsions, benign familial, 3040, 3047, 3051–3052
Neonatal galactosialidosis, 2681
Neonatal hypertrophic cardiomyopathy, 1441–1442
Neonatal MFS, 4002
Neonatal myasthenia gravis, 3426
Neonatal progeria, 1310t
Neonatal purpura fulminans, 1948
Neonatal severe hyperparathyroidism, 2205t, 2206–2209
    phenotypes, 2205t
Neonatal sialidosis, 2680
Neonatal tyrosinemia, 2411–2412
Neonates. *See also* transient bullous dermolysis of the newborn
    abnormal diagnosis, counseling of parents, 863–865
    bilirubin toxicity, 1795–1796
    cardiomyopathy, nDNA mutations, 351–352
    congenital myasthenias, 3421
    congenital recessive ichthyosis, 3791–3792
    death
        genetic counseling, 861–862
        prenatal diagnosis on figures, 909
    Down syndrome, tubular stenosis, 4133
    Ehlers-Danlos syndrome, 4023
    glucose 6-phosphate dehydrogenase deficiency, 1903–1904
    gram-negative septicemia, galactose-1-phosphate uridyltransferase deficiency, 1092
    hemochromatosis, 2642, 2654–2655
    hemolysis, 1959–1966
    hyperbilirubinemia, 1801
    hypopituitarism, 2144
    ichthyosis of, 3795
    oculocutaneous albinism, 3754
    OXPHOS gene mutations, 332t
    phagocytes, 2111
    phenylketonuria, management, 2408
    respiratory adaptation, 1000

rickets, prematurity, 2579
screening, 826–841. *See also* phenylketonuria, neonatal screening
    cystic fibrosis, 828, 836–837, 909, 1561–1562, 1585
    deafness, 3659
    Duchenne muscular dystrophy, 3276
    ethics, 908
    ethics, 908–909
    galactokinase deficiency, 2443
    galactose-1-phosphate uridyltransferase deficiency, 2444–2445
    hepatorenal tyrosinemia, 2413
    homocystinuria, 2421
    legal aspects, 935–936
    molecular genetics, 724
    research ethics, 919
    systemic lupus erythematosus, 2023
    withdrawal syndrome, sodium valproate, 3067
Neoplasms. *See also* malignant change
    ataxia telangiectasia, 3112, 3113
    Beckwith-Wiedemann syndrome, 1730
    screening, 1079
    Bloom syndrome, 3938
    blue rubber bleb nevus syndrome and, 3937
    central nervous system, 3001, 3231–3249
    colorectal carcinomas and, 1830
    chromosomal abnormalities, 690
    chromosome rearrangements, 171
    CYP2D6 gene polymorphisms, 602
    deafness and keratitis with ichthyosis, 3803
    deletion mapping, 13
    Diamond-Blackfan anemia, 1916
    Down syndrome, 1141
    epidermodysplasia verruciformis, 3952, 3963t
    family history, accuracy, 661
    Fanconi anemia, 1917, 4173
    gastrointestinal tract, 1824–1857
    horseshoe kidney, 1685
    hypercalcemia, 2213
    Klinefelter syndrome, 1191
    Maffucci syndrome, 4152
    mitochondria, 381–382

neural tube defects, 763–773, 2981–2982

Preprocollagen type 1 mRNA, 1,25-dihydroxyvitamin D on, 2569

PreproPTH precursor signal sequence, mutation, 2216

Prescription drugs, teratogenesis, 1028–1037

Presenilins, 363
Down syndrome, 1144
genes, 2068. *See also* PS1 gene; PS2 gene

President's Commission for the Study of Ethical Problems, confidentiality and families, 932

Pressure gradients, ventricular outflow tract, hypertrophic cardiomyopathy, 1349

Presymptomatic DNA testing, 725
genetic counseling, 868–869
Huntington disease, 734, 868
myotonic dystrophy, 3413–3414

Presymptomatic genetic testing, 642
multiple sclerosis, 3207

Pre-synaptic congenital myasthenias, 3422t, 3426

Pretibial dystrophic epidermolysis bullosa, 3859, 3879–3880
anchoring fibrils, 3861f–3862f
collagen VII mutation, 3873

Prevalence, incidence vs, retinoblastoma, 3605

Prevalence studies, mental retardation, 1046–1047

Prevention, 46, 50–51, 656, 666
genetic counseling as, 843
neural tube defects, 764, 2981
primary open angle glaucoma, 3499–3500
primordial, 1536

Previous affected child
Down syndrome risk, 1150
genetic counseling, prenatal diagnosis, 854

Previous affected pregnancy, aneuploidy, 772–773
maternal blood fetal cells from, 818

PRH gene (prolactin-releasing hormone gene), 2163t

Prieto syndrome, 2813t

Primary angle-closure glaucoma (primary closed angle glaucoma), 3500–3502

Primary biliary cirrhosis, lipid disorder, 2515t

Primary care physicians
genetic risk assessment and, 669–670
retinoblastoma diagnosis, 3608, 3612–3613

Primary ciliary dyskinesia, 1261
infertility, male, 965t, 972–973

Primary closed angle glaucoma, 3500–3502

Primary congenital glaucoma, 622t, 3506–3509

Primary hyperparathyroidism, 2203–2212

Primary hypoparathyroidism, 2214–2219

Primary lateral sclerosis, 3137–3138
hereditary spastic paraplegias vs, 3131t, 3138t

Primary mutations, Leber hereditary optic neuropathy, 3478

Primary open angle glaucoma, 3492–3500
juvenile, 3504–3506

Primary pigmentary retinopathies, 3572–3573

Primary sclerosing cholangitis, inflammatory bowel disease, 1771–1772

Primates
1,25-dihydroxyvitamin D resistance, 2577
photopigments, 3457–3458

Primers, PCR, Rh genotyping, 1964

Primidone, 1033

Primitive neuroectodermal tumors, 3240–3242

Primitive streak, 473

Primordial germ cells, 967

Primordial prevention, 1536

Principles and practice of medical genetics (Emery and Rimoin), 37, 38

Principles of disease, 38–39

Prion diseases, 2910–2911
ataxia, 3119

Prion protein
Gerstmann-Sträussler-Scheinker disease, 2068
mutations, 2910–2911

Prior probabilities, Bayes theorem, 676
Becker muscular dystrophy carriers, 3279
Duchenne muscular dystrophy, 3274

Pristanic acid
bifunctional protein deficiency, 2773
β-oxidation
fibroblasts, 2778t
lysosomal, 2753
peroxisomal disorders, 2764, 2778

Private mutations, KCNQ1 gene, 1421

PRKCA gene (protein kinase C α gene), 2163t

PRL gene (prolactin gene), 2137, 2163t

PRNP gene, 2910

Probabilities, 675

Probability calculations
linkage analysis, 139
maternal serum alphafetoprotein screening, 773

Probands, 126
pedigrees, 637

Probandwise concordance, twins, 462, 463
bipolar affective disorder, 2939

Probenecid, 2470, 2472

Probes. *See* α-satellites, probes; DNA, probes

Probst bundles, 2998

Probucol, 2530

Procainamide, slow acetylators, 597

Processing, antigens, 1103

PROC gene (protein C), 1948

Procollagens, 4023
type I
arthrochalasis multiplex congenita, 4033–4034
osteogenesis imperfecta type I, 4119–4120
type III, Ehlers-Danlos syndrome type IV, 4028

Product deficit disorders, 449

Prodynorphin gene, 2163t
opioid addiction, 2964

Proficiency testing, molecular genetic diagnosis, 743

Profile pattern analysis, craniofacial disorders, 3693

Profilaggrin, ichthyosis vulgaris, 3789

Progenitor cells. *See* neural stem/progenitor cells

Progeria, 2142t
ataxia telangiectasia, 2088
Cockayne syndrome *vs*, 3945
neonatal (Wiedmann-Rautenstrauch syndrome), 1310t
Tay syndrome, 3800

Progeria syndrome (Hutchinson-Gilford syndrome), 585, 1302t

Progeroid syndromes, 584–585
diabetes mellitus, 2236t

Progesterone
hypospadias and, 2320
recurrent abortion, 985–986

Progestins, on fetus, 1033, 1034

Prognosis, 27

Progressive ataxias from metabolic insufficiency, 3110t, 3111–3112

Progressive bulbar palsy, 3363t, 3365–3366, 3434

Progressive cardiac conduction defect (Lev-Lenegre), 1433–1434

Progressive epilepsy with mental retardation (Northern epilepsy), 3059

Progressive external ophthalmoplegia
chronic, 350, 352–356, 3601
mouse model, 378
psychiatric illness, 367

Progressive familial intrahepatic cholestasis, 622t, 1814–1815

Progressive macrocephaly, 1051

Progressive muscle weakness, mtDNA cytochrome b mutations, 340–342

Progressive myoclonus epilepsies, 3056–3059
dentatorubropallidoluysian atrophy, 3096
type 1, 87t, 88
neuroserpin, 2069–2070

Progressive neurodegenerations, 1058–1059. *See also* specific diseases

Progressive panneuropathy with hypotonia, 3156, 3159t

Progressive pseudorheumatoid disease, 4092t
bibliography, 4110

Progressive spinal muscular atrophy, progressive bulbar palsy *vs*, 3434

Progressive supranuclear palsy, 3081

Progressive synostosis, 3698

Progress zone, limb growth, 479

Prohormone convertase 2 gene, diabetes mellitus, 2259t

Pro-inflammatory cytokines, 1092–1093

Proinsulin, 2390

Prolactin. *See also* hyperprolactinemia
amniocentesis, hypopituitarism, 2145
gene, 2137, 2163t
seizures, 3041

Prolactinoma, familial, 2142t

Prolactin-releasing hormone gene, 2163t

Prolastin (alpha-1-antitrypsin), replacement therapy, 1630

Prolidase deficiency, 2428t, 2429

Proline, inborn errors of metabolism, 2427–2429

Proline oxidase, 2427
deficiency, 2428

Prolyl hydroxylase, 4022

ProMBP, complexing with 3'-phosphoadenosine-5'-phosphosulfate assay specificity, 787